S0-AZQ-870

PATHOLOGIC BASIS *of* DISEASE

Third Edition

STANLEY L. ROBBINS, M.D.

Visiting Professor of Pathology, Harvard Medical School;
Senior Pathologist, Brigham and Women's Hospital, Boston

RAMZI S. COTRAN, M.D.

F. B. Mallory Professor of Pathology, Harvard Medical School;
Chairman, Department of Pathology, Brigham and Women's Hospital, Boston

VINAY KUMAR, M.D.

Professor of Pathology, University of Texas Health Science Center,
Southwestern Medical School, Dallas

1984

W. B. Saunders Company PHILADELPHIA LONDON TORONTO MEXICO CITY RIO DE JANEIRO SYDNEY TOKYO

W. B. Saunders Company: West Washington Square
Philadelphia, PA 19105

1 St. Anne's Road
Eastbourne, East Sussex BN21 3UN, England

1 Goldthorne Avenue
Toronto, Ontario M8Z 5T9, Canada

Apartado 26370—Cedro 512
Mexico 4, D.F., Mexico

Rua Coronel Cabrita, 8
Sao Cristovao Caixa Postal 21176
Rio de Janeiro, Brazil

9 Waltham Street
Artarmon, N.S.W. 2064, Australia

Ichibancho, Central Bldg., 22-1 Ichibancho
Chiyoda-Ku, Tokyo 102, Japan

Library of Congress Cataloging in Publication Data

Robbins, Stanley L.

Pathologic basis of disease.

Includes bibliographical references and index.

1. Pathology. I. Cotran, Ramzi S. II. Kumar, Vinay. III. Title. [DNLM: 1. Pathology. QZ 4 R363p]

RB111.R62 1984 616.07 83-20403

ISBN 0-7216-7597-2

Listed here is the latest translated edition of this book together with the language of the translation and the publisher.

Portuguese (*2nd edition*)—Editoria Interamericana Ltda., Rio de Janeiro, Brazil

Spanish (*1st edition*)—Nueva Editorial Interamericana S.A. de C.V., Mexico 4 D.F., Mexico

Yugoslavian (*1st edition*)—Serbo-Croat, Skolska Knjiga, Zagreb, Yugoslavia

Italian (*2nd edition*)—Piccin Editore, Padova, Italy

Pathologic Basis of Disease ISBN 0-7216-7597-2

Last digit is the print number: 9 8 7 6 5 4 3 2

To
Elly
to
Kerstin
and to
Raminder
with love

PREFACE

The five years since publication of the second edition of this text have witnessed enormous advances in biomedical science, and particularly in the application of basic scientific knowledge to our understanding of the mechanisms of disease. At the same time, the introduction of modern immunologic, radiologic, biochemical, and other diagnostic techniques into clinical disciplines has greatly improved our understanding of the dynamics of diseases and the ability to make meaningful clinicopathologic correlations. Since the study of the dynamics and mechanisms of disease and of clinicopathologic correlations remains the core of Pathology, it has been satisfying and at the same time challenging for the authors to prepare this new edition. The major challenge was to present the new clinical, biomolecular, and morphologic developments, while at the same time not permitting the book to grow larger. In recognition of the constraints on a student's time, a strenuous effort produced about a 10% reduction in size by defining the limits of the subject matter to be included in a teaching text—with emphasis on the word "teaching." We have also strived to maintain the readability, clarity, and organization that have gained previous editions their warm reception by students and faculty. To what extent these challenges have been met, only the readers and time will tell—we can only say that our best efforts were made.

All the chapters have been thoroughly revised and about half the book has been completely rewritten. Rigorous efforts have been made to include those new advances that are pertinent to the pathogenesis of disease, as well as the fundamental morphologic, physiologic, and clinical descriptions that are critical to the understanding of specific disease processes. Throughout the text we have emphasized more common or significant entities, exploring their distribution, origins, and morphologic changes and the resultant clinical manifestations and consequences. Where rare disorders are discussed at some length, it is because they point to critical advances in medical science that may be relevant to other diseases. The book is written primarily for student use throughout the years of medical or dental school, but we believe it should also prove useful to biomedical and basic scientists and to clinicians who wish to learn or review the pathologic basis of disease. Although an encyclopedic reference is not intended, we expect that pathologists and pathology trainees will find the text thorough and well referenced.

The organization of the text retains its compatibility with most teaching programs in pathology. The first one-third is devoted to a discussion of general pathologic processes—cell injury, inflammation, thrombosis, and neoplasia, as well as genetic and immunologic mechanisms of disease. There follow general chapters dealing with diseases caused by the most unwieldly classes of etiologic factors: infectious agents, environmental hazards, and nutritional disturbances. The chapter on Infectious Diseases has been totally rewritten and substantially expanded, dictated by the emergence in the past decade of many types of infections caused by agents that either had been unknown or have been unmasked by modern antibiotic or immunosuppressive therapy. In addition, the great increase in air travel and population movements of the past 20 years now necessitates knowledge of a wide spectrum of infectious diseases, some previously regarded as rare, tropical, or exotic. The later chapters are devoted to a presentation of diseases affecting specific organ systems. In these chapters we have maintained our efforts to organize diseases of each organ system into the most logical categories and to discuss for each, on the one hand, the pathogenetic mechanisms leading to the morphologic changes, and on the other hand, the clinical and physiologic implications of these morphologic changes. In this way, we can only hope that the pathologic lesions and clinical disorders are unfolded as dynamic processes, and that the reader will agree with us that a sound knowledge of pathogenesis and pathology is the solid foundation of clinical medicine.

ACKNOWLEDGMENTS

All authors of texts know how dependent they are on the support of many others in the preparation of a large manuscript. It would take pages to acknowledge everyone who, in one way or another, has provided us with assistance, but certain individuals deserve citation for their invaluable help. To the remainder, wittingly or unwittingly unsung, our apologies and our grateful thanks.

First and foremost it is a pleasure for the two senior authors to welcome aboard Dr. Vinay Kumar as a co-author. No stranger to the world of book-writing, Dr. Kumar has already served as a co-author in *Basic Pathology*, the smaller cousin of this text. His breadth and depth of knowledge, his expertise as a teacher, and the lucidity of his writing have added greatly to this edition.

Preeminent among our staunch supporters are our editorial assistants and secretaries. Dr. Robbins was fortunate to have the extremely able and devoted services of Sandra Jeffries, Marcia Diefendorf, and Laura Duffy. Sandra, in particular, labored through the long and arduous task of researching the literature, editing the manuscript, and endlessly proofreading every page of manuscript and proof, but most of all she was Dr. Robbins' "right hand" and indeed "right brain," providing organization to a perpetually disorganized author. The efforts of Marcia and Laura, while less sustained, were equally critical: typing and retyping manuscript and doing whatever was needed to maintain progress. Playing similar roles for Dr. Cotran were Julie Smith and Leslie White, and for Dr. Kumar, Bernita Shelton. The commitment and standards of excellence of all these "heroes" contributed greatly to such accuracy and style as this text may possess. Also to be acknowledged is the assistance (to Dr. Kumar) of Beverly Shackelford, who willingly helped at critical junctures.

A large number of colleagues have freely offered critiques of segments of the text. Our principal advisors, in alphabetic order, were Drs. Gilbert Brodsky, Michael Gimbrone, John Godleski, James Madara, Fred Schoen, and William Welch, of Boston; and Drs. Maximilian Buja, Jose Hernandez, Patricia Howard-Peebles, Mary Lipscomb, Joseph Rutledge, and Fred Silva, of Dallas. They added much, in their areas of particular expertise, to the authenticity and currency of the writing. Others who offered helpful suggestions included Drs. Abul Abbas, John Farber, Robert Jennings, Morris Karnovsky, Jordan Pober, Nancy Schneider, Wayne Taylor, Manjeri Venkatachalam, Art Weinberg, and Charles White, III. The list of donors of new illustrations to this edition is long and they are acknowledged individually in the figure legends. It is surprisingly difficult to find "photogenic gems" of particular lesions, and without the generosity of numerous colleagues it would not have been possible to add the many new figures to this edition. Dr. Kumar would also like to express gratitude to the library staff at Dallas, in particular to Patricia McKeown, whose expertise in computer-assisted literature search saved countless hours.

We owe a special debt of gratitude to the contributors of special chapters. We were indeed fortunate to have Dr. Franz von Lichtenberg assume responsiblity for the expanded chapter on Infectious Diseases. His expertise and monumental knowledge of this field will be plainly evident in his authoritative contribution. Dr. Gerald Shklar graciously revised his chapter on The Oral Cavity. We are grateful for his continued support. Drs. Martin Mihm and Theodore Kwan were joined by their colleague, Dr. George Murphy, in the extensive and expert revision of the Skin chapter. And Dr. William Schoene was joined by his close associate, Dr. James Morris, in the elegant rewriting of the chapter "The Nervous System." All these contributors have added much authenticity to the coverage of those areas of pathology requiring specialized expertise, and so we consider ourselves fortunate to have and are grateful for their highly valued contributions.

In the last analysis it is the publishers who complete a book. We wish to acknowledge the continued efforts and support of W. B. Saunders, and especially all those directly involved in the preparation of this text. Particularly meritorious is Mr. David Harvey, our copy editor, who patiently and expertly shepherded the original manuscript to its final printed form. Unfailingly he tolerated our numerous changes and graciously acceded to almost all. Like us, his only goal was to achieve the best text of pathology possible, and for sharing this goal with us we are deeply indebted to him.

Not to be forgotten are our patient and supportive wives, Elly Robbins, Kerstin Cotran, and Raminder

Kumar. For their encouragement and willingness to tolerate husbands too busy for other activities, and for their unflagging faith in our efforts, we singly and collectively "doff our hats" and say in all humility "many, many thanks."

Finally, each of us would like to pay tribute to the other members of the author-triumvirate. Working together in the preparation of a text has many similarities to a marital relationship—compromises must be found for honest differences of opinion, suggestions for change carefully weighed and accepted when indicated, and close collaboration maintained throughout the months and years. We are pleased that we began this revision with mutual respect and warm friendship and completed it with an even keener appreciation of each other's efforts, abilities, and dedication to the long and sometimes onerous task.

S.L.R.
R.C.
V.K.

CONTENTS

CELLULAR INJURY AND ADAPTATION

1

INTRODUCTION TO PATHOLOGY

Translated literally, Pathology is the study (*logos*) of suffering (*pathos*) and, indeed, as a science Pathology is intimately concerned with the cause of much of the suffering on this mortal coil, namely why diseases arise and what they do. More specifically it is focused on the structural and functional consequences of injurious stimuli to the cells, tissues, and organs of the body and ultimately the consequences on the entire organism. Just as we live in a constantly changing world, so do the cells and tissues survive in a constantly changing microenvironment. The "normal" or "physiologic" state, then, is achieved by adaptive responses to the ebb and flow of various stimuli permitting the cells and tissues to adapt and to live in harmony within their microenvironment. Thus, homeostasis is preserved. It is only when the stimuli become more severe, or the response of the organism breaks down, that disease results—a generalization as true for the whole organism as it is for the individual cell. There are few new biochemical pathways or new structures that occur in diseased tissues. There is simply modification, loss, or accentuation of existing pathways and structures.[1] In this sense, pathology deals with the study of deviations from normal structure, physiology, biochemistry, and cellular and molecular biology. Not surprisingly, in some instances the study of these deviations has clarified our understanding of the norm.

Traditionally the study of pathology is divided into *General Pathology*, and *Special* or *Systemic Pathology*. The former is the study of the basic reactions of cells and tissues to abnormal stimuli that underlie *all diseases*. The latter examines the specific responses of specialized organs and tissues to more or less well-defined stimuli. In this book we will first cover the principles of general pathology and then proceed to specific disease processes as they affect particular organs or systems.

The four aspects of a disease process that form the core of pathology are: (1) its cause (etiology), (2) the mechanisms of its development (pathogenesis), (3) the structural alterations induced in the cells and organs of the body (morphologic changes), and (4) the functional consequences of the morphologic changes (clinical significance).

1. *Etiology or Cause*. The concept that certain abnormal symptoms or diseases are "caused" is as ancient as recorded history. For the Acadians (2500 BC), if someone became ill, it was either his own fault (for having sinned) or the makings of outside agents, such as bad smells, cold, evil spirits, or gods.[2] In more modern terms, there are the two major classes of etiologic factors: *Genetic* and *Acquired* (infectious, nutritional, chemical, physical, etc.). Knowledge or discovery of the primary etiology remains the backbone on which a diagnosis can be made, a disease understood, or a treatment developed. But the concept of *one cause* leading to *one disease*—developed largely from the discovery of specific infectious agents as the causes of specific diseases—is no longer sufficient. While it is true that there would be no malaria without malarial parasites, no tuberculosis without tubercle bacilli, and no gout without a genetic defect in urate metabolism, not all individuals infected with these organisms or born with the metabolic abnormality develop the disease, or develop it at the same rate and with the same severity. Genetic factors clearly affect environmentally induced maladies, and the environment may have profound influences on genetic diseases. Finally, the humbling fact is that for many of the crippling or killing diseases of modern times, such as arthritis, cancer, and arteriosclerosis, the etiologic agents are largely unknown.

2. *Pathogenesis*. This refers to the sequence of events in the response of the cells or tissues, or the whole organism, to the etiology—from the initial stimulus to the ultimate expression of the manifestations of the disease. The study of these reactions to injury constitutes one of the main domains of the science of pathology. In a great variety of diseases, in which the etiologic agent is still unknown, unclear, or controver-

sial, uncovering the pathogenesis is the only way to devise strategies to treat or to prevent progression of the process. Even when the initial infectious or molecular cause is known, it is many steps removed from the expression of the disease. For example, to understand "Strep throat" as a disease, one has to understand not only how the streptococcus causes red, enlarged, painful tonsils, but also the fever, chills, and headache that ensue; and to know gout is to know not only the molecular pathways of uric acid metabolism, but also the events leading to a painful toe or a kidney stone. Although from the late nineteenth century up to the 1950s pathology was largely limited to the study of the morphologic consequences of disease, chemical and molecular mechanisms clearly underlie the morphologic changes and these, fortunately, have become the business of all basic sciences, including pathology.

3. *Morphologic Changes.* This refers to the structural and associated functional changes in cells or tissues that are either characteristic of the disease or diagnostic of the etiologic process.

4. *Functional Derangements and Clinical Significance.* The nature of the morphologic changes and their distribution in different organs or tissues influence normal function and determine the clinical features (symptoms and signs), course, and prognosis of the disease.

With this preamble, we can turn to the nature, origin, and meanings of cell damage.

CELLULAR INJURY AND ADAPTATION

DEFINITIONS

The normal cell is confined to a fairly narrow range of function and structure by its genetic programs of differentiation and specialization, constraints of neighboring cells, the availability of metabolic substrates, and the finite capacities of its primary and alternative metabolic pathways. The normal cell is said to be in a homeostatic "*steady state,*" able to handle physiologic demands. Somewhat more excessive external stresses or stimuli may bring about a number of *cellular adaptations* in which a new but altered steady state is achieved but in which the cell remains viable. The bulging muscles of the "musclemen" engaged in "pumping iron" are an example of cellular adaptation. The increase in muscle mass reflects the increase in size of the individual muscle fibers, which in turn results from the synthesis of increased numbers of mitochondria and myofilaments. The workload is thus shared by a greater mass of cellular components, and each muscle fiber is spared excess work so that the muscle cell escapes injury. The enlarged muscle cell achieves a new equilibrium, permitting it to survive at a higher level of metabolic activity. This adaptive response is called *hypertrophy.* Other adaptations occur at the level of individual organelles, as will become apparent later.

If the limits of adaptive capability are exceeded, or when no adaptive response is possible, a sequence of events follows, loosely termed *cell injury,* which may range from mild to lethal. Cell injury is *reversible* up to a certain point, but if the stimulus persists or is severe enough from the beginning, the cell reaches the point of no return, and suffers *irreversible cell injury* and cell death. For example, if the blood supply to a segment of the heart is cut off for 10 to 15 minutes, and then restored, the myocardial cells experience injury but can recover and function normally. However, if blood flow is not restored until one hour later, the myocardial fiber dies.[3] *Adaptation, reversible injury,* and *cell death,* then, should be considered states along a continuum of progressive encroachment on the cell's normal function and structure. Whether specific types of stress induce an adaptive response, a reversible injury, or cell death depends on the nature and severity of the stress, and (as we shall see) on many other variables relating to the intrinsic state of the cell itself.

In the following discussion, we will first review the causes, mechanisms, and morphologic patterns of reversible and irreversible cell injury, and then some of the more common forms of adaptive responses involving whole cells or cell organelles. But first a few traditional terms must be introduced, some unfortunately somewhat inaccurate. In older textbooks, reversible or sublethal forms of cell injury were referred to as *degenerations* (hydropic degeneration, waxy degeneration, etc.). This term has a nonspecific connotation implying that "bad things" have happened to the cell—you can understand nobody wants to degenerate! Because of its lack of specificity, the word should be used only as a last resort when a more accurate descriptive term is not available. *Necrosis* refers to the sum of the morphologic changes occurring within dead cells in a *living* tissue. These changes are caused by the cell's own degradative enzymes, and by enzymes and other factors released by infiltrating leukocytes. *Autolysis* is the descriptive term traditionally used for the process of dissolution of dead cells by the cell's own digestive enzymes; after death of the entire organism, when it occurs, it is referred to as *postmortem autolysis.*

GENERAL CONSIDERATIONS

Cell injury is one of the most common cell responses in disease, affecting virtually every cell type in almost all pathologic conditions. It is also seen frequently during normal embryogenesis, as developing structures are replaced by mature tissues, and is also the aim of radiotherapy and chemotherapy for malignant disease. Yet large gaps still exist in our understanding of the process. Some of the most basic questions remain unanswered. For example, how much injury can a cell sustain and, especially, what are the biochemical mechanisms responsible for the transition from reversible to irreversible injury? This is by no means an academic question but has practical importance in medicine. Consider the problem of cell death in the muscle fibers of the heart. Ischemic injury to myocardial cells caused by coronary artery narrowing or occlusion leads to myocardial infarction, one of the most common causes of death in the Western world. Previously it was believed that all muscle cells in areas supplied by an occluded artery were destined for irreversible injury, and a fatalistic view prevailed toward attempting to salvage ischemic myocardium. This is no longer true. It is now possible to protect ischemic myocardium and decrease infarct size in experimental animals by various interventions such as increasing the delivery of metabolic substrates to the ischemic area or administering pharmacologic agents.[4] Although the mechanism of action of these interventions is still unclear, it is likely that they protect the sublethally damaged cells from irreversible injury. Thus, any knowledge we can gather about the events leading to cell death may improve our ability to intervene in the process. Many other examples might be cited, but suffice it to say that a firm understanding of the structural and, more importantly, biochemical events that occur in injured cells is essential to our understanding of all disease processes and their treatment. In the final analysis, if the theologians will permit, we are all a bundle of cells, cast in the form of a biped.

Some general considerations of cell injury will be reviewed first.

1. *There are numerous causes of cell injury,* but the most common are ischemia, chemical injury, and injury produced by infectious agents. In particular, ischemic injury may be a common pathway by which other injurious agents act. For example, some immune reactions, such as the Arthus reaction, cause destruction of vessel walls. The vessel then becomes occluded by a thrombus, resulting in ischemia of the tissue supplied by this vessel. It is important therefore to consider primary causes of cell injury as well as secondary pathways individually.

2. Although it is not always possible to determine the precise biochemical site of action of injurious agents, four intracellular systems are particularly vulnerable: (a) *aerobic respiration* involving oxidative phosphorylation and production of ATP, (b) *maintenance of the integrity of cell membranes* on which the ionic and osmotic homeostasis of the cell and its organelles is dependent, (c) *synthesis of enzymic and structural protein,* and (d) *preservation of the integrity of the genetic apparatus* of the cell.

3. *The structural and biochemical elements of the cell are so closely related that whatever the precise point of initial attack by the damaging agent, injury at one locus leads to wide-ranging secondary effects.* For example, impairment of aerobic respiration and the production of ATP quickly disrupt the energy-dependent sodium pump that maintains the ionic and fluid balance of the cell, resulting in alterations in the intracellular content of ions and water.

4. *The morphologic changes of cell injury become apparent only after some critical biochemical system within the cell has been deranged.* As would be expected, the morphologic manifestations of lethal damage take more time to develop than those of reversible damage. For example, cell swelling is a reversible morphologic change, and this may occur in a matter of minutes; however, unmistakable light microscopic changes characteristic of cell death do not occur in the myocardium until 10 to 12 hours after total ischemia, yet we know that irreversible injury occurs within 20 to 60 minutes.[5] In the kidney deprived of blood supply, tubular cell death occurs within 30 minutes, but cells do not appear histologically dead until 12 hours later.[6] Obviously, ultrastructural alterations occur earlier than light microscopic changes.

Finely drawn is the line between reversible and lethal cell damage. This complexity should come as no surprise. Well known in clinical practice is the vexing question: When did the patient die? Brain function, as determined by the electroencephalogram, may cease hours to days before cardiac or respiratory function stops. Yet, even after all vital signs (e.g., pulse, respiration, and body temperature) indicate the death of the organism, most of the cells within the host continue to survive, as has been amply documented by the use of cadaver organs in transplantation. *The transition from life to death is as difficult to establish for the cell as it is for the whole organism.*

5. *Reactions of the cell to injury depend not only on the type of injury but also on its duration and severity;* thus, small doses of a chemical toxin or ischemia of short duration may induce reversible disturbances in the cell's osmotic and water homeostasis, while large doses of the same toxin or more prolonged ischemia might lead either to instantaneous cell death or to slow, irreversible injury leading in time to cell death.

6. *The result of cell injury depends not only on the type, duration, and severity of the stimulus but also on the type, state, and adaptability of the cell.* The cell's nutritional and hormonal status and its metabolic needs are important in its response to injury. How vulnerable is a cell, for example, to loss of blood supply and hypoxia? The striated muscle cell in the leg can be placed entirely at rest when deprived of its blood supply; not so, the striated muscle of the heart. Exposure of two individuals to identical concentrations of carbon tetrachloride fumes may be without effect in one and may produce cell death in the other. This may be due, as we shall see, to the integrity and amount of the smooth endoplasmic reticulum in the hepatic cells, which converts carbon tetrachloride to toxic free radicals. Differences in the nutritional state or in potentiating factors, such as alcohol consumption, influence the ability of the two individuals and their cells to withstand injury.

CAUSES

The causes of reversible cell injury and cell death range from the external gross physical violence of an automobile accident to internal endogenous causes, such as a subtle genetic lack of a vital enzyme that impairs normal metabolic function. Most adverse influences can be grouped into the following broad categories.

Hypoxia. Hypoxia (lack of oxygen) is probably the most common cause of cell injury and may also be the ultimate mechanism of damage initiated by a variety of physical, biologic, and chemical agents. Hypoxic injury to cells may be caused by the loss of their blood supply, depletion of the oxygen-carrying capacity of the blood, or poisoning of the oxidative enzymes within the cells. Among these, by far the most common is loss of blood supply (*ischemia*). Such impairment of blood flow may be caused by primary arterial disease (atherosclerosis), intravascular clots (thrombi or emboli), or other lesions that narrow or occlude arteries. Thus, heart attacks (myocardial infarction) and strokes (cerebral infarction)—the most frequent and lethal diseases of many industrialized nations—are examples of cell death due to hypoxia related to atherosclerotic narrowing of arteries. Loss of oxygen-carrying capacity is exemplified by many forms of anemia and by carbon monoxide poisoning, in which monoxyhemoglobin replaces oxyhemoglobin and blocks the normal transport of oxygen. Poisoning of the oxidative enzymes within the cells is caused by agents such as cyanide, which inactivates cytochrome oxidase.

Physical Agents. These include mechanical trauma, extremes of temperature (burns and deep cold), sudden changes in atmospheric pressure, radiation, and electric shock (see Chapter 10—Environmental Pathology).

Chemical Agents and Drugs. The list of chemicals that may produce cell injury defies compilation. Simple chemicals such as glucose or salt in hypertonic concentrations may cause cell injury by deranging the fluid and electrolyte homeostasis of cells. Even oxygen, in high concentrations, is severely toxic. The levels of toxicity of certain substances are so high that they are known as *poisons*, and trace amounts of arsenic, cyanide, or mercuric salts may destroy sufficient numbers of cells within minutes to hours to cause death. Other substances, however, are our daily companions: environmental and air pollutants, insecticides, and herbicides; industrial and occupational hazards, such as carbon monoxide, carbon tetrachloride, asbestos, and silica; social stimuli, such as alcohol and narcotic drugs; and the ever-increasing variety of therapeutic drugs. Such drug-induced (iatrogenic) injury has become a truly major cause of illness in modern man; about 5% of hospital admissions are due to illnesses induced by medicines that have been either prescribed or sold "over the counter."

Biologic Agents. These agents range from the submicroscopic viruses to the large tapeworms. In between are the rickettsiae, bacteria, fungi, and higher forms of parasites. The ways by which this heterogeneous group of biologic agents cause injury are diverse and in many cases still mysterious. They will be discussed in greater detail in Chapter 8 (Infectious Diseases).

In general, bacteria cause cell injury by means of secretion of a toxin (exotoxin) or by release of endotoxin from their cell walls when the bacteria are killed, or by induction of immunologic responses to antigens contained within the microbiologic agent. Such mechanisms are also postulated for many of the higher forms of microbiologic agents, such as protozoa, fungi, and worms. Viruses, on the other hand, cause cell injury in different ways. They survive within living cells, where they subvert the metabolism of the host for their own survival. This results in the decreased synthesis of all macromolecules vital to the host. Continued viral replication may therefore interfere with the host's own metabolism; however, this is probably not the explanation for the cell injury and necrosis that follow. It is more likely that viral protein elaborated during viral infection may be directly toxic to the infected cell. There are also nonlethal effects of virus infection. Viral ribonucleic acid (RNA) or deoxyribonucleic acid (DNA) may become incorporated into the genome of the host cell and cause either cell death or cellular transformation, and frequently increased cell proliferation. This last effect may lead to tumor formation, a phenomenon relevant to the viral causation of cancer.

Two other points must be stressed. First, there is a remarkable specificity displayed by many microbiologic agents in terms of the cell type they affect. Thus, the pneumococcus is a common inhabitant of the pharynx, but it rarely causes cell injury in this location. However, when it invades the lung, it finds a suitable environment for growth and produces pneumonia. Second, the effect of any biologic agent depends not only on the virulence of the agent itself but also on the vigor with which the host can mount its defenses. Such defenses include the inflammatory response and a variety of immunologic reactions.

Immunologic Reactions. These may be life-saving or lethal. Although the immune system serves in the defense against biologic agents, immune reactions may, in fact, cause cell injury. The anaphylactic reaction to a foreign protein or a drug is a prime example, and reactions to endogenous self-antigens are thought to be responsible for a number of so-called autoimmune diseases (see Chapter 5).

Genetic Derangements. Genetic defects as causes of cellular injury are of major interest to biologists today (see Chapter 4). The genetic injury may result in as gross a defect as the congenital malformations associated with Down's syndrome (mongolism) or in subtle alterations in the coding of hemoglobin responsible for the production of hemoglobin S in sickle cell anemia. The many inborn errors of metabolism arising from enzymatic abnormalities, usually an enzyme lack, are excellent examples of cell damage due to subtle alterations at the level of the coding in DNA. Some of these errors result in the abnormal accumulation of lipids, carbohydrates, or proteins within the cell.

Nutritional Imbalances. Even today these continue to be major causes of cell injury. Protein-calorie deficiencies cause an appalling number of deaths, chiefly among underprivileged populations. Deficiencies in specific vitamins are found throughout the world. Hypovitaminoses are encountered even in the midst of abundance, but they abound among lower socioeconomic groups in all countries (see Chapter 9).

Ironically, nutritional excesses have become important causes of cell injury among the overprivileged. Excesses of calories, carbohydrates, and lipids are thought to predispose to atherosclerosis. Obesity is an extraordinary manifestation of the overloading of some cells in the body with lipids. But above and beyond such cell changes, obesity has been shown to be associated with the production of hypertension and cardiac disease.

PATHOGENESIS

The problem of unraveling the precise biochemical mechanisms responsible for cell injury has proved to be immensely complex. First, as we have seen, injury to cells may have many causes, and there is as yet no known common final pathway of cell injury. Second, different cell types show differences in their vulnerability to specific stimuli and in their responsive mechanisms. Third, the many macromolecules, enzymes, biochemical systems, and organelles within the cell are so closely interdependent that it is difficult to differentiate the primary target of injury from the secondary ripple effects. Finally, the "point of no return," i.e., the point at which irreversible damage and cell death occur, is still largely undetermined.

With certain injurious agents, the mechanisms and loci of attack are well defined. Cyanide represents an intracellular asphyxiant in that it inactivates cytochrome oxidase. Certain anaerobic bacteria, such as *Clostridium perfringens*, elaborate phospholipases, which attack phospholipids in cell membranes. Other isolated examples exist, but the modes of action of many injurious agents are largely unknown. In the following discussions, we shall concentrate on two of the common causes of cell injury: (1) *hypoxic injury* and (2) some forms of *chemical injury*. These two model systems offer valuable insights into the mode of action of adverse influences on the cell.

Ischemic and Hypoxic Injury

Sequence of Events. The sequence of morphologic changes following acute hypoxic injury has been studied extensively in humans, in experimental animals, and in culture systems,[7, 8] and reasonable schemes concerning the mechanisms underlying these changes have emerged (Fig. 1–1). A useful model for the study of hypoxic injury has been occlusion of one of the main coronary arteries. Besides the relevance of this model to human myocardial infarction, the cellular changes in the heart can also be correlated with biochemical and electrophysiologic alterations.[3]

The first point of attack of hypoxia is the cell's aerobic respiration, i.e., oxidative phosphorylation by mitochondria. As the oxygen tension within the cell decreases, there is loss of oxidative phosphorylation, and the generation of ATP slows down or stops. This loss of ATP—the energy source—has widespread effects on many systems within the cell. Heart muscle, for example, ceases to contract within 60 seconds of coro-

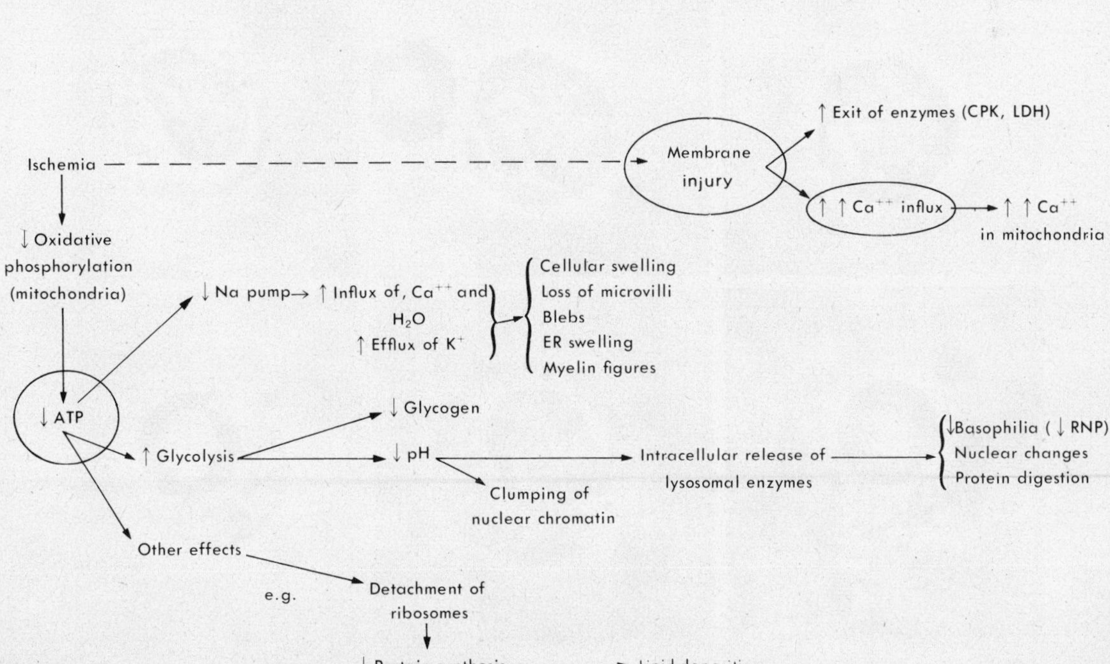

Figure 1–1. Postulated sequence of events in ischemic injury. Note that while the reduced ATP levels have a central role, ischemia may directly cause membrane damage, by currently uncertain mechanisms discussed in the text. The circled events appear to be the three most critical phenomena.

nary occlusion. (Note, however, that noncontractility does not mean cell death.) In particular, maintenance of cell membranes and the activity of their associated enzymes, such as ATPase, are impaired, eventually resulting in cell swelling (see below). The decrease in cellular ATP and associated increase in AMP stimulate the enzyme phosphofructokinase, which results in an increased rate of anaerobic glycolysis to maintain the cell's energy sources by generating ATP from glycogen. Glycogen is thus rapidly depleted, a phenomenon which can be appreciated histologically if tissues are stained for glycogen (such as with the periodic acid–Schiff stain [PAS]). Glycolysis results in the accumulation of lactic acid and inorganic phosphates from the hydrolysis of phosphate esters. *This reduces the intracellular pH.* As we shall see, this reduction in cell pH may have profound effects in later stages of cellular injury. At this early period there is also *early clumping of nuclear chromatin,* which can be seen on electron microscopy.

One of the earliest and most important effects of reduced ATP concentration is *acute cellular swelling* (cellular edema) (Fig. 1–2). You will recall that mammalian cells possess a high intracellular osmotic colloidal pressure, exerted by a greater intracellular than extracellular concentration of protein. On the other hand, sodium and other ions are at a lower intracellular than extracellular concentration. The low intracellular sodium concentration is maintained by an energy-dependent system within the cell membrane (the sodium pump), which also keeps the concentration of potassium significantly higher intracellularly than extracellularly. The ouabain-sensitive enzyme ATPase is involved in this active transport system. *In hypoxia, failure of this active transport, owing to diminished ATP and ATPase, causes sodium to accumulate intracellularly with diffusion of potassium out of the cell.* The net gain of solute is accompanied by an iso-osmotic gain of water and consequent cell swelling. The movement of fluid and ions into the cell is associated with *early dilatation of the endoplasmic reticulum.* The mechanisms of this dilatation are not known, but it occurs before any swelling of mitochondria, Golgi apparatus, or lysosomes.

The next phenomenon to occur is *detachment of ribosomes from the granular endoplasmic reticulum* and *dissociation of polysomes into monosomes,* probably due to disruption of the energy-dependent interactions between the membranes of the endoplasmic reticulum and its ribosomes. If hypoxia continues, other alterations take place and, again, are reflections of increased membrane permeability and diminish mitochondrial function. *Blebs* may form at the cell surface (Figs. 1–3 and 1–4), and cells that possess microvilli (such as proximal tubular epithelial cells) begin to lose their normal microvillous structure.[7, 9] Freeze fracture techniques show aggregation of intramembranous particles of plasma membranes. "Myelin" figures, derived from plasma as well as organellar membranes, may be seen within the cytoplasm or extracellularly. They are thought to result from dissociation of lipoproteins with unmasking of phosphatide groups, promoting the uptake and inter-

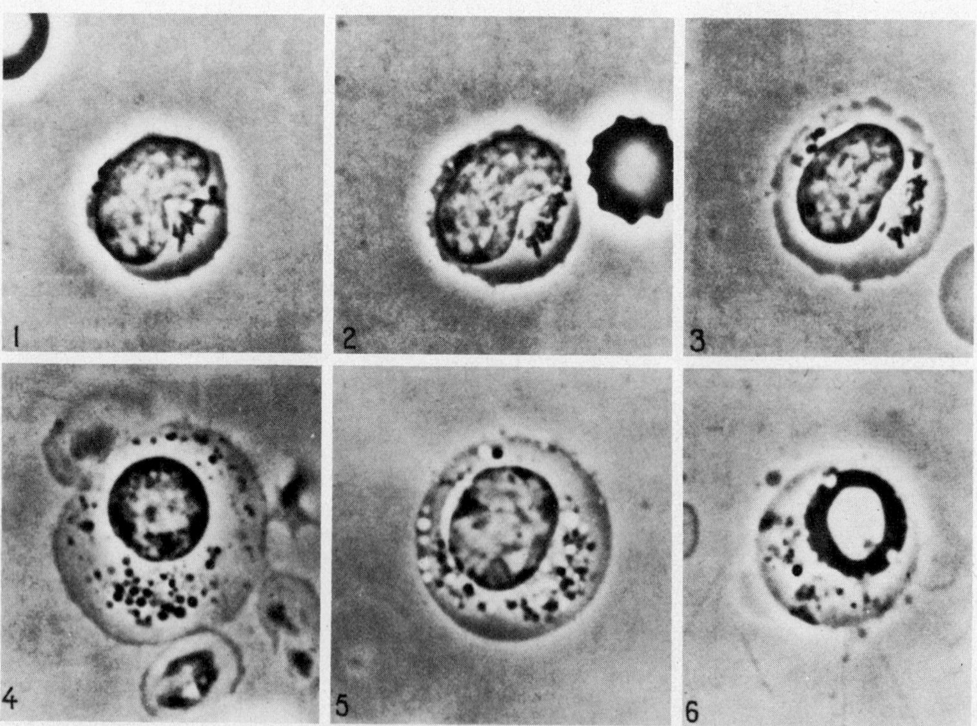

Figure 1–2. Light micrographs depicting stages of cell death in blood lymphocyte. *1,* Normal lymphocyte; *2,* Slight cytoplasmic edema; *3,* Increasing cytoplasmic edema; *4* and *5,* Disappearance of the nuclear depression; *6,* Nuclear pyknosis. (From Bessis, M.: Living Blood Cells and Their Ultrastructure. New York, Springer-Verlag, 1972.)

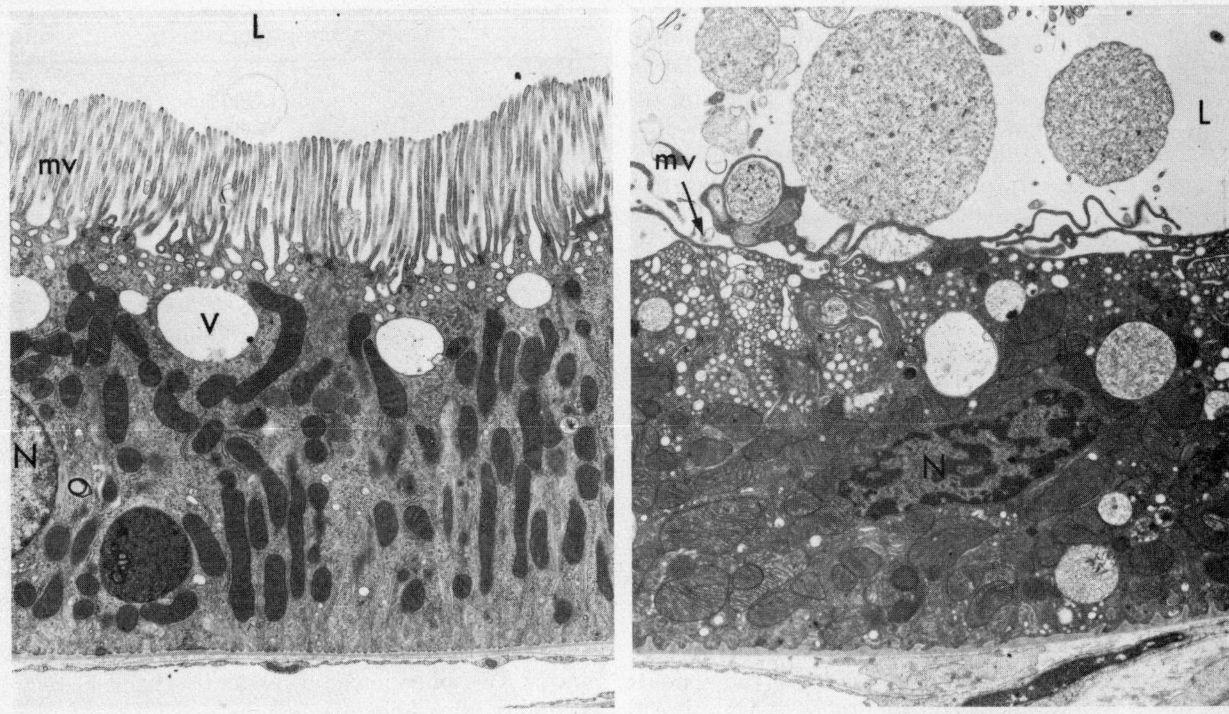

Fig. 1–3

Fig. 1–4

Figure 1–3. Electron micrograph of normal epithelial cell of proximal kidney tubule. Note abundant microvilli (mv) lining the lumen (L). N = nucleus; V = apical vacuoles (which are normal structures in this cell type). (Figs. 1–3 to 1–5 courtesy of Dr. M. A. Venkatachalam, University of Texas at San Antonio.)

Figure 1–4. Epithelial cell of the proximal tubule showing reversible ischemic changes. The microvilli (mv) are lost and have been incorporated in apical cytoplasm; blebs have formed and are extruded in the lumen (L). Mitochondria are slightly dilated. (Compare with Fig. 1–3.)

calation of water between the lamellar stacks of membranes. Changes in the ionic environment and pH of the injured cell probably cause the formation of such myelin figures, since similar alterations can be induced in vitro in model membrane systems. At this time the mitochondria are either normal, or slightly swollen, or actually condensed; the endoplasmic reticulum remains dilated; and the entire cell is markedly swollen, with increased concentrations of water, sodium, and chloride and a decreased concentration of potassium.

All the above disturbances are reversible if oxygenation is restored. However, if ischemia persists, irreversible injury ensues. As will be detailed later, *there is no universally accepted biochemical explanation for the transition from reversible injury to cell death.* However, irreversible injury is associated morphologically with severe vacuolization of the mitochondria (Fig. 1–5), including their cristae (so-called *"high-amplitude swelling"* to differentiate it from the minor degrees of *"low-amplitude swelling"* seen under physiologic conditions); extensive damage to plasma membranes; swelling of lysosomes; and—particularly if the ischemic zone is reperfused—massive calcium influx into the cell. Amorphous densities develop in the mitochondrial matrix (Fig. 1–5). In the myocardium, these are early indications of irreversible injury and can be seen as early as 30 to 40 minutes after ischemia. *Calcium also accumulates in mitochondria after reperfusion.* There

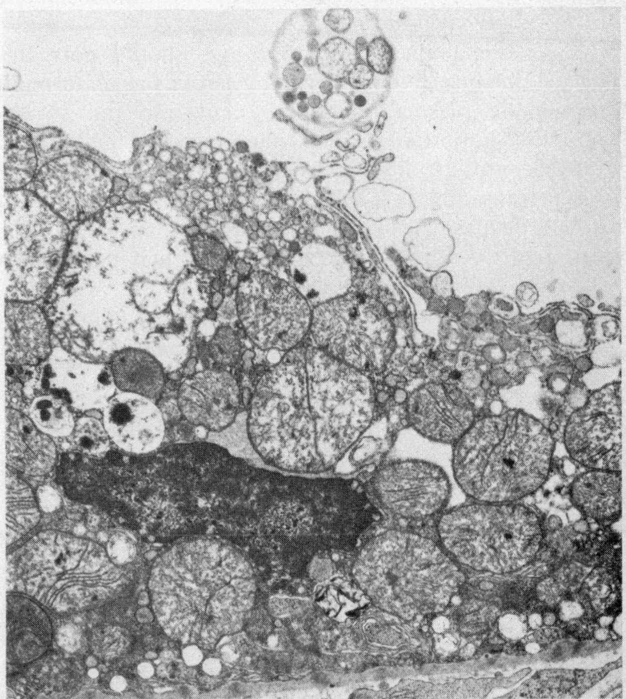

Figure 1–5. Proximal tubular cell showing irreversible ischemic injury. Note the markedly swollen mitochondria containing amorphous densities, disrupted cell membranes, and dense pyknotic nucleus.

is continued loss of proteins, essential coenzymes, and ribonucleic acids from the hyperpermeable membranes. The cells may also leak metabolites, which are vital for the reconstitution of ATP, thus further depleting net intracellular high-energy phosphates.[5, 10]

The falling pH (due to glycolysis, lactate accumulation, and breakdown of phosphate esters) together with changes in the ionic composition of the cell leads to *injury to the lysosomal membranes, followed by leakage of their enzymes into the cytoplasm and activation of their acid hydrolases.* Lysosomes contain RNAases, DNAases, proteases, phosphatases, glucosidases, and cathepsins. Activation of these enzymes leads to enzymatic digestion of cell components evidenced by loss of ribonucleoprotein, deoxyribonucleoprotein, and glycogen. An attractive theory for irreversibility of cell injury was the so-called "suicide-bag hypothesis," which postulated that cell death (suicide) occurred when the lysosomes (bags) ruptured. However, although lysosomal enzymes undoubtedly participate in the digestion and removal of the dead cell, the point of irreversibility has already passed by the time these lysosomes rupture.[11]

At any rate, following cell death, cell components are progressively degraded, and there is widespread leakage of cellular enzymes into the extracellular space and, conversely, entry of extracellular macromolecules from the interstitial space into the dead cells. Finally, the dead cell may become replaced by large masses composed of phospholipids in the form of "myelin figures." These are then either phagocytosed by other cells or degraded further into fatty acids. *Calcification* of such fatty acid residues may occur with the formation of so-called calcium soaps.

At this point in the story, we should note that leakage of intracellular enzymes across the abnormally permeable plasma membrane, and into the serum, provides important clinical parameters of cell death. Cardiac muscle, for example, contains glutamic-oxaloacetic transaminase (GOT), pyruvic transaminases, lactic dehydrogenase (LDH), and creatine kinase (CK). Elevated serum levels of such enzymes, and particularly the isoenzymes specific for heart muscle (e.g., CK-MB), are valuable clinical criteria of myocardial infarction, a locus of cell death in heart muscle discussed in some detail on page 564.

MECHANISMS OF IRREVERSIBLE INJURY. The sequence of events for hypoxia was described as a continuum from its initiation to the ultimate digestion of the lethally injured cell by lysosomal enzymes. But at what point did the cell actually die? How much hypoxia (or, for that matter, any other type of injury) can any cell tolerate without sustaining lethal injury? The duration of hypoxia necessary to induce irreversible cell injury varies tremendously according to the cell type and the nutritional and hormonal status of the animal (Table 1–1). In the liver, between one and two hours of ischemia are required to produce irreversible damage to liver cells. In the brain, neurons suffer irreversible damage after three to five minutes. In the kidney, 20 minutes of ischemia fails to produce cell death, whereas 30 minutes of ischemia induces widespread death among epithelial cells in the proximal tubules. Thus, a difference of 10 minutes of ischemia determines cell life or death. Even within the kidney, different segments of the nephron show varying susceptibility to ischemia. The proximal tubule is by far the most susceptible, and its straight segment is more vulnerable than its convoluted segment.[9] The state of nutrition of the cell is also important. Liver cells of rats fed a normal diet contain abundant glycogen and have a higher potential for survival after ischemia than do the liver cells of starved rats.

Table 1–1. SUSCEPTIBILITY OF CELLS TO ISCHEMIC NECROSIS

High	Neurons (3–5 min)
Intermediate	Myocardium, hepatocytes, renal epithelium (30 min–2 hr)
Low	Fibroblasts, epidermis, skeletal muscle (many hours)

What then are the critical events for lethal hypoxic injury? Two phenomena consistently characterize irreversibility after ischemia and these point the finger to the two most likely events. The first is the *inability to reverse mitochondrial dysfunction* (lack of oxidative phosphorylation and ATP generation) upon reperfusion or reoxygenation, and the second is the development of *profound disturbances in membrane function.*[12]

Mitochondrial Dysfunction. It would be reasonable to consider that progressive depletion of ATP in itself at some critical juncture constitutes a lethal event, but the evidence on this issue is conflicting.[12, 13] In favor of a primary role for ATP depletion are the following observations. High-energy phosphate in the form of ATP is required for many synthetic and degradative processes within the cell.[3] Intravenous infusion or in vivo perfusion of ATP (complexed to $MgCl_2$) improves renal function and histology after renal ischemia and promotes animal survival in shock.[13] In the myocardium, the marked depletion of ATP (90% after 40 minutes of ischemia) is closely related to the development of lethal injury.[5] However, in the ischemic kidney the concentration of ATP falls within a few minutes to a level approximately one-fifth of normal, but no progressive loss occurs over the next 20- or 30-minute period, when the vulnerable epithelial cells pass the "point of no return."[6] Further, if ethionine, an analog of methionine, is administered to experimental animals, ATP levels in the liver decrease to 20% of normal without cell death.[14] Although numerous alterations in mitochondrial structure and function are found in ischemic tissues, it has been possible experimentally to dissociate these changes as well as ATP depletion from the inevitability of cell death.[15, 16] Despite such arguments about the primary role of ATP depletion, there is little doubt that it contributes to the functional and structural consequences of ischemia, as described earlier (Fig. 1–1). In addition, ATP depletion may indirectly participate in the other critical event in ischemia—cell membrane damage (discussed next).[13]

Cell Membrane Alterations. *A great deal of evidence indicates that cell membrane damage is a central factor in the pathogenesis of irreversible cell injury.*[16–18] As should be well-known, the cell membrane consists of a lipid-protein mosaic made up of a bimolecular layer of phospholipids and globular proteins embedded within the lipid bilayer (Fig. 1–6*A*). An intact plasma membrane is essential to the maintenance of normal cell permeability and volume. Loss of volume regulation, increased permeability to extracellular molecules such as inulin, and demonstrable plasma membrane ultrastructural defects occur in the earliest stages of irreversible injury.[19–21]

The biochemical basis of this membrane damage is now under intensive study. Several possibilities exist, but it now appears clear that one important alteration is net loss of phospholipids from cell membranes.[16, 22–24] Normally, the turnover of membrane phospholipids is coupled to their re-synthesis so that the integrity of the cell membrane is maintained. Most membrane phospholipids consist of a 3-carbon glycerol chain in which two fatty acids are esterified to two of the three hydroxyl groups of the glycerol backbone (Fig. 1–6*B*). Degradation of membrane phospholipids involves the action of a *phospholipase A*, which splits off one fatty acid, followed by removal of the second by a lysophospholipase. These enzymes are endogenous to normal cell membranes and their activation is strongly calcium dependent. One postulated explanation for such phospholipid loss is activation of endogenous phospholipases present in the endoplasmic reticulum and plasma membranes, causing increased degradation of phospholipid.[22] This activation of phospholipases may in turn be the result of increased cytosolic calcium concentration induced by ischemia. It should be remembered that the normal intracellular calcium concentration is extremely low ($\pm 10^{-7}$M), and that such calcium is sequestered in

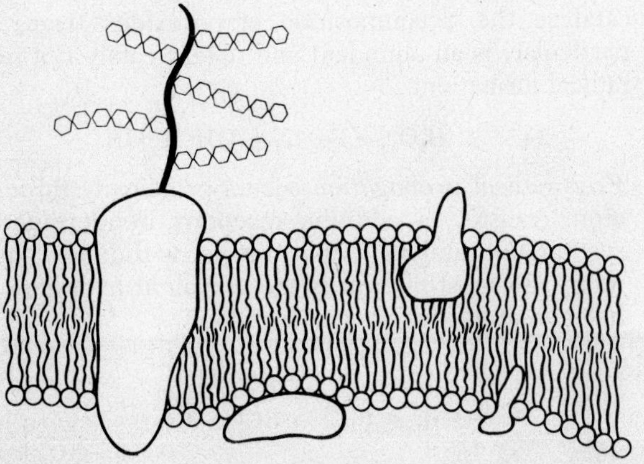

Figure 1–6A. Schematic representation of the plasma membrane. The bilipid layer has its hydrophilic end *(circles)* directed outward and its hydrophobic tails directed inward. Globular proteins are embedded in the lipid, and some span the entire bilayer. The polysaccharide chains of the glycoproteins project above the surface.

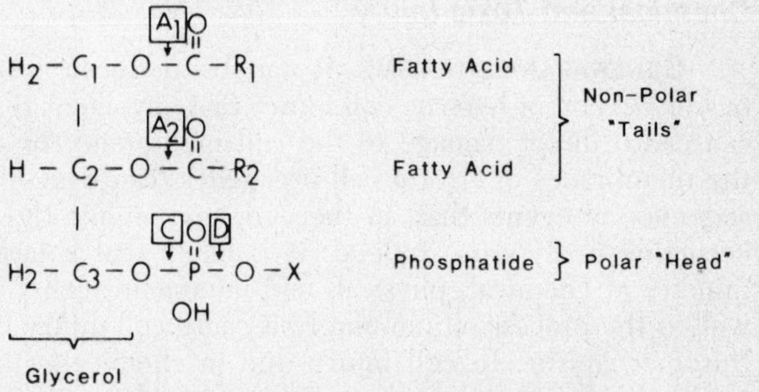

$H_2-C_1-O-\overset{\boxed{A_1}\,O}{\overset{\|}{C}}-R_1$ Fatty Acid

$H-C_2-O-\overset{\boxed{A_2}\,O}{\overset{\|}{C}}-R_2$ Fatty Acid } Non-Polar "Tails"

$H_2-C_3-O-\overset{\boxed{C}\,O\,\boxed{D}}{\overset{\|}{P}}-O-X$ Phosphatide } Polar "Head"

OH

Glycerol

Figure 1–6B. Structure of a phospholipid. Two fatty acids (R_1 and R_2) are esterified to the 1 and 2 carbons of glycerol, and one of a number of polar phosphatides (X) is esterified to the 3 carbon of the glycerol "backbone." The ester bonds linking these functional groups to glycerol can be hydrolyzed by a number of phospholipases as shown on the illustration. (Letters in squares) (From Katz, A.M., and Messineo, F.C.: Lipid-membrane interactions and the pathogenesis of ischemic damage in the myocardium. Circ. Res. *48*:1, 1981. By permission of The American Heart Association, Inc.)

mitochondria (and endoplasmic reticulum). Oxygen deprivation releases sequestered calcium and raises cytosolic calcium.[24] However, there is no clear evidence that increased phospholipid degradation *precedes* plasma membrane damage, at least in myocardial ischemia.[25]

Other mechanisms for membrane damage have been invoked. These include the detergent action of toxic lipid breakdown products, such as unesterified fatty acids (acyl carnitine and lysophospholipids), which accumulate in ischemia;[26, 27] depressed phosphorylation of membrane proteins due to reduction of ATP;[13] decreased synthesis of membrane phospholipids;[16] or release of toxic free radicals by ischemic cells (p. 10). Whatever the mechanism(s), the resultant membrane damage causes further influx of calcium from the extracellular space, where it is present in high concentrations ($>10^{-3}$M), into the cells. When, in addition, the ischemic tissue is reperfused to some extent, as may occur in vivo, the scene is set for a massive influx of calcium. Farber[16] has argued that this calcium influx may be the "coup de grace" that determines irreversible injury, not only after ischemia but also in toxic injury. This author found that agents that block calcium influx (e.g., chlorpromazine, a phenothiazine derivative) prevent irreversible ischemic or toxic injury. Calcium is taken up avidly by mitochondria after reoxygenation and permanently poisons them, inhibits cellular enzymes, denatures proteins, and causes the cytologic alterations characteristic of coagulative necrosis.

It is evident that the precise molecular events that initiate irreversible cell damage are still incompletely understood. Indeed, it may well be that several mechanisms, acting at more than one locus, underlie cell death. *For now it must suffice to say that hypoxia affects oxidative phosphorylation and hence the synthesis of vital ATP supplies, that membrane damage is critical to the development of lethal cell injury, and that calcium ions may under some conditions be important mediators of the biochemical alterations leading to cell death.*

Chemical and Toxic Injury

General Mechanisms. It can be deduced from our discussion of hypoxic cell injury that any agent that can cause direct damage to the cell membrane, or to the membranes of critical cell organelles, can trigger a sequence of events that, in the end, may mimic those occurring in hypoxia. Indeed, it is likely that a large number of chemical, physical, and infectious agents as well as the process of immune lysis cause cell injury by this mechanism. In cell injury due to chemicals, the unanswered question is this—What is the biochemical nature of the interaction between the toxic agent and the particular cell membrane that eventually leads to cell damage and increased permeability? In some cases, the explanations are straightforward. For example, some bacteria, such as *Clostridium perfringens*, secrete phospholipase C (Fig. 1–6*B*), which interacts with the phospholipids of membranes and causes severe and acute permeability changes, with influx of ions and water into the cell. In *mercuric chloride poisoning*, mercury binds to the sulfhydryl groups of the cell membrane and other proteins, causing increased membrane permeability and inhibition of ATPase-dependent transport. Most other toxic chemicals, however, are not biologically active but must be converted to reactive toxic metabolites by specific target cells. Two general mechanisms are postulated to account for membrane damage by such reactive metabolites:[29] (1) *free radical formation* and *lipid peroxidation* (to be discussed in detail presently) and (2) direct *covalent binding* of a metabolite to the macromolecular components (lipid and protein) of the membrane. An example of the latter mechanism is the hepatotoxicity of bromobenzene, although recent evidence questions the extent to which covalent binding can explain lethal damage with this compound.[30]

Free Radicals and Cell Injury. Many forms of toxic injury, as well as a number of important pathologic processes, are caused by the formation of highly reactive free radicals. The processes include chemical and radiation injury, oxygen and other gaseous toxicity, cellular aging, microbial killing by phagocytic cells, inflammatory damage, tumor destruction by macrophages, endothelial injury, and others. Although the role of free radicals in these events will be detailed later, it would be helpful here to review briefly some aspects of free radical pathology that may be shared by these processes. The physicochemical basis for free radical formation and the biochemical reactions leading to cell injury are complex, so a rather oversimplified account will be given. For the hardy, recent reviews and books are available.[31–35]

Free Radical Reactions. The biologically relevant free radicals include metabolic products of exogenous chemicals or drugs (e.g., CCl_3, a product of carbon tetrachloride, CCl_4) or naturally occurring free radicals formed during endogenous, usually oxidative, metabolic reactions (superoxide [O_2^-], hydroxyl [OH ·], singlet oxygen). Free radicals can be most simply defined as atoms or groups of atoms having an odd (unpaired) number of electrons that may enter into chemical-bond formation. They may be positively charged, negatively charged, or neutral.

Free radicals are potentially extremely reactive, are chemically unstable, and usually occur in low concentrations. They generally induce chain reactions that occur slowly under normal conditions but may be rapidly accelerated if chain initiators (e.g., other free radicals) are introduced. Three processes are important in free radical reactions: (1) *initiation*, when free radicals are produced; (2) *propagation*, when new free radicals are formed as a chain reaction; and (3) *termination*, when free radicals are destroyed.

1. The *initiation* of free radicals in biologic materials requires either: (a) a powerful outside energy source (e.g., x-ray or ultraviolet light) or (b) more commonly, interactions of oxygen or other molecules (e.g., CCl_4) with a free electron during oxidation-reduction (redox) reactions.
   a. Free radical formation by *ionizing radiation* is usually mediated through the radiolysis of water: H· and OH· are produced, and the latter in particular is damaging to the cell. If these damages remain unrepaired, mutation ensues (p. 466).
   b. The formation of free radicals during *redox* reactions is crucial because of the ubiquitous nature of these processes in living cells. A free electron can interact with O_2 in the vicinity of electron transfer reactions to produce the highly reactive free radical *superoxide:*

$$O_2 + e^- \rightarrow O_2^-$$

   or in the case of CCl_4:

$$CCl_4 + e^- \rightarrow CCl_3\cdot + Cl^-$$

   In these reactions, transitional metals (e.g., iron, copper) can donate or accept single electrons in their transit from one valency state to another and can catalyze the decomposition of peroxides. Iron, in particular, is an abundant and potent catalyst of free radical formation:

$$Fe^{++} + H_2O_2 \rightarrow Fe^{+++} + OH\cdot + OH^-$$

2. Free radical *propagation* occurs principally through atom transfer or addition reactions, rendering the system autocatalytic. Atom transfer is the most common, and most often it is the univalent hydrogen or halogen atom that is transferred:

$$R\cdot + R_1H \rightarrow RH + R\cdot_1 \text{ or}$$
$$R\cdot + R_1Cl \rightarrow RCl + R\cdot_1$$

   It is thought that the propagation of CCl_4 as a free radical occurs by addition to a preexisting free radical(s):

$$R\cdot + CCl_4 \rightarrow CCl_3\cdot + RCl$$

Addition reactions also contribute to the damage of unsaturated fatty acids in membranes:

$$RCH = CH_2 + CCl_3\cdot \rightarrow RC\cdot = CH_2 + CHCl_3$$

3. *Termination,* or inactivation, of free radicals is obviously of great benefit and indeed is the mechanism by which normal cells protect themselves from free radical injury. In biologic systems, termination is achieved by several means.
   a. Endogenous or exogenous *antioxidants* (e.g., vitamin E; sulfhydryl compounds like cysteine, glutathione, and D-penicillamine; serum proteins, such as ceruloplasmin and transferrin), which either block the initiation of free radical formation or inactivate (e.g., scavenge) free radicals. Sulfhydryls (e.g., reduced glutathione or GSH) allow the hydrogen on —SH to be abstracted by a free radical, and the resultant —S· is combined with another —S to form an oxidized disulfide —S—S:

$$2HO\cdot + 2GSH \rightarrow 2H_2O + G - S - S - G$$

$$H_2O_2 + 2GSH \rightarrow 2H_2O + G - S - S - G$$

   These reactions are catalyzed by GSH peroxidase. Transferrin is thought to act as an antioxidant by binding free iron, which as we have seen can catalyze free radical formation.
   b. Another important reaction is the inactivation of superoxide (O_2^-) catalyzed by the enzyme *superoxide dismutase* (SOD):

$$O_2^- + O_2^- + 2H^+ \rightarrow H_2O_2 + O_2$$

The H_2O_2 is then decomposed by the action of catalase:

$$2H_2O_2 \rightarrow O_2 + 2H_2O$$

Unfortunately, all tissues are not equally endowed with SOD and catalase. Hence, accumulation of both H_2O_2 and/or O_2^- may ensue, and these may undergo the Haber-Weiss reaction to induce another highly toxic free radical (OH·):

$$H_2O_2 + O_2^- \rightarrow OH\cdot + OH^- + O_2$$

The balance of these reactions is unpredictable, but the availability of superoxide dismutase *diminishes* the possibility of production of oxidative free radicals.

Pathologic Consequences of Free Radical Formation

LIPID PEROXIDATION. Free radicals can affect lipids by initiating peroxidation, and can also catalyze amino-acid oxidation, protein-protein cross-linking, and protein strand scission (Fig. 1–7).[35] Here we shall discuss only lipid peroxidation as a mechanism of membrane damage by free radicals. Simply defined, this is deterioration of polyunsaturated lipids[36] and is equivalent to the process by which fats become rancid. Peroxidation involves the direct reaction of oxygen-derived free radicals and lipid to form free radical intermediates and semi-stable peroxides. There results a chain of subsequent autocatalytic reactions of free radicals, propagation reactions that result in membrane damage and the production of terminal aldehydes including malondialdehyde. The latter product is important, since it mediates a variety of cross-linking reactions and can also be quantitated as a measure of the extent of lipid peroxidation.

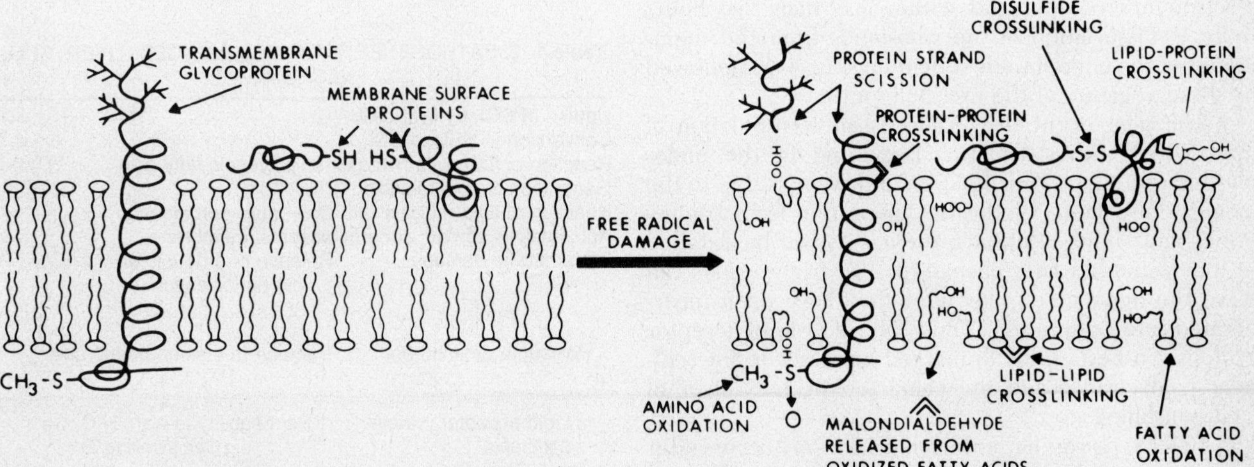

Figure 1–7. Free radical damage to membranes. Free radicals can affect lipids by initiating peroxidation, which leads to short-chain fatty acyl derivatives and the by-product malondialdehyde. Variety of cross-linking reactions can be mediated by malondialdehyde reactions. Free radicals can also catalyze amino acid oxidation, protein-protein cross-linking, and protein strand scission. (From Freeman, B. A., and Crapo, J. D.: Biology of disease: free radicals and tissue injury. Lab. Invest. *47*:412, 1982. © 1982, The Williams & Wilkins Company, Baltimore.)

CCl_4-INDUCED CELL INJURY. One of the best characterized models of lipid peroxidation is the chemical injury produced in the liver by *carbon tetrachloride (CCl_4) poisoning.*[29, 37] This halogenated hydrocarbon is used widely in the dry-cleaning industry and represents a prototype for chemical injury by many similar compounds. The toxic effect of carbon tetrachloride is not due to the CCl_4 molecule but to conversion of the molecule to the *highly reactive toxic free radical* $CCl_3\cdot$ in the smooth endoplasmic reticulum (SER) by the mixed-function (P-450) oxidase system of enzymes involved in the metabolism of lipid-soluble drugs and other compounds.[38] It follows, therefore, that procedures that inhibit the hepatic mixed-function oxidase system reduce the severity of CCl_4 injury. Thus, newborn rats, which do not possess the enzyme, are resistant to the effect of carbon tetrachloride, as are protein-depleted rats whose hepatic drug metabolizing system is markedly diminished. On the other hand, when hepatic mixed-function oxidative activity is increased, as in the adaptive response to administration of phenobarbital (p. 27), the rats become hypersensitive to CCl_4.

At any rate, the free radicals produced locally cause autooxidation of the polyenoic fatty acids present within the membrane phospholipids. There, oxidative decomposition of the lipid is initiated, and organic peroxides are formed after reacting with oxygen (lipid peroxidation). *This reaction is autocatalytic* in that new radicals are formed from the peroxide radicals themselves. Thus, rapid breakdown of the structure and function of the endoplasmic reticulum is due to decomposition of the lipid. *It is no surprise, therefore, that CCl_4-induced liver cell injury is both severe and extremely rapid in onset.* Within less than 30 minutes there is a decline in hepatic protein synthesis of both plasma proteins and endogenous protein enzymes. Swelling of the cisternae of the endoplasmic reticulum can be seen early with the electron microscope, and within less than two hours there is dissociation of the ribosomes from the membranes of the endoplasmic reticulum (Fig. 1–8), followed by disaggregation of the free polysomes.

The next event that occurs is an accumulation of lipid within the cytoplasm, beginning in the endoplasmic reticulum. This lipid accumulation is due to the inability of cells to synthesize lipoprotein from triglycerides and "lipid acceptor protein." As will be detailed in the section on fatty change (p. 19), triglycerides can leave the hepatic cell only after they have been incorporated into lipoprotein. Thus, failure of lipid acceptor protein synthesis leads to marked increases in intracellular triglycerides and the characteristic fatty liver of CCl_4 poisoning.

In CCl_4 poisoning, mitochondrial injury occurs after injury to the endoplasmic reticulum, and this is followed by progressive swelling of the cells due to increased permeability of the plasma membrane. Plasma membrane damage is thought to be caused by relatively stable fatty aldehydes, which are produced by lipid peroxidation in the SER but are able to act at distant sites.[39, 40] Plasma membrane damage also results in a massive influx of calcium, which accumulates in the mitochondria. The progressive damage to the cell after these events is similar to that which occurs in hypoxic injury (Table 1–2).

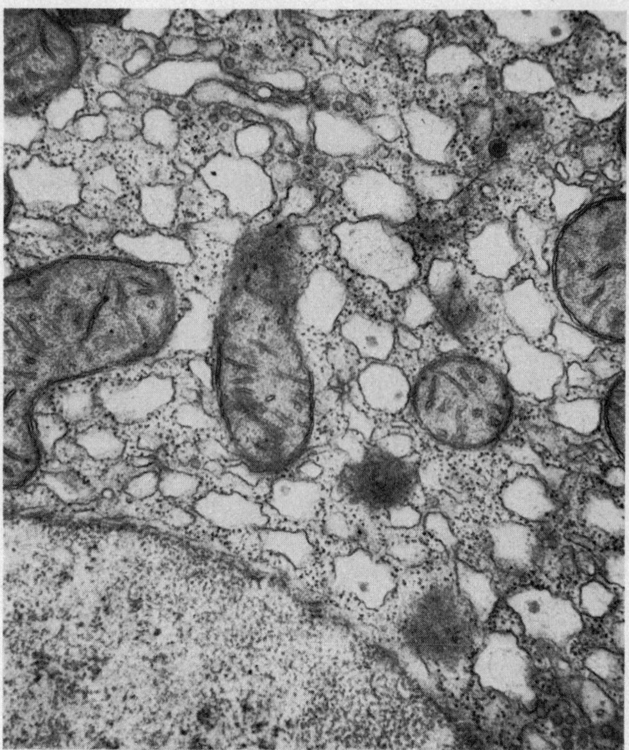

Figure 1–8. Rat liver cell four hours after carbon tetrachloride intoxication with well-developed swelling of endoplasmic reticulum and shedding of ribosomes. Mitochondria at this stage are unaltered. (Courtesy of Dr. O. Iseri.)

Table 1–2. PATHOGENESIS OF CCl_4-INDUCED LIVER CELL NECROSIS

Uptake of CCl_4 by liver cells
Conversion in SER to CCl_3
Reaction of CCl_3 with microsomal polyenoic fatty acid
Generation of lipid radicals
Reaction of lipid radicals with O_2 → *lipid peroxidation*
Autocatalytic spread along microsomal membrane

Membrane damage RER	Release of products of lipid perioxidation
↓	↓
Polysome detachment	Damage to plasma membrane
↓	↓
↓ Lipid acceptor protein synthesis	↑ Permeability to Na^+, H_2O, Ca^{++} Cell swelling
↓	↓
Fatty liver	Massive influx of Ca^{++}
	↓
	Inactivation of mitochondria, cell enzymes, and denaturation of proteins

Other Examples of Free Radical Injury. As stated earlier, free radicals are now thought to be involved in many pathologic and physiologic processes, to be discussed throughout this book. Here we shall introduce only some examples of free radical injury.

Oxygen and Other Gas Toxicity. Exposure to high concentrations of oxygen, ozone, and other gases results in damage to alveolar cells (mainly type I pneumocytes), and this action also appears to be mediated by free radical formation.[41, 42] In addition, the herbicide *paraquat* ingested or injected parenterally causes extensive pulmonary damage, which is enhanced by oxygen and is ascribed to damage by oxygen radicals.[43] Since superoxide dismutase and catalase inactivate some of the toxic radicals of oxygen, administration of these enzymes will diminish the severity of lung damage.

Aging. In its simplest form, the so-called *"free radical" theory of aging* supposes that the formation of free radicals is more frequent in aging organisms, resulting in lipid peroxidation and membrane damage. In fact, the accumulation of the pigment lipofuscin (p. 23) in large amounts in the aging liver and heart is taken as evidence for this theory, since lipofuscin appears chemically to consist of complexes of lipid-protein substances, probably derived through peroxidation of polyunsaturated lipids of subcellular membranes.[44] Theoretically, increased lipid peroxidation with aging might occur as a result of (1) continuous increased formation of free radicals caused by environmental agents; (2) diminished availability of antioxidants for unknown reasons; or (3) a loss or diminution of activity of some of the compounds or enzymes that catalyze the inactivation of toxic free radicals, e.g., superoxide dismutase.

Irradiation Injury. The role of free radicals in tissue damage induced by *irradiation* is well documented. − OH· and H· produced by radiolysis are known to add to the bases of nucleic acids and to abstract hydrogen from pentose to release organic free radicals (p. 464).

Microbial Killing. Bacteria ingested by leukocytes are killed within the phagolysosomes. The lethal damage to bacteria is largely dependent on the oxidative burst that occurs in leukocytes during phagocytosis. The role of generated free radicals in bacterial killing is discussed on page 50.

Inflammation. Oxygen-derived free radicals produced by leukocytes and other cells in the course of inflammation play an important role in inducing tissue damage and in elaborating chemotactic agents (p. 56).[41]

Free radical reactions also account for the therapeutic effects of some drugs, such as antibiotics and anticancer agents,[46] and have also been implicated—often with marginal evidence—in a multitude of other processes including atherosclerosis[47] and cancer.[44]

In concluding this discussion of the pathogenesis of cellular injury induced by hypoxia and chemicals, several points should be made. Cells sustain biochemical injuries long before they undergo alteration in their structure. Alterations in one intracellular locus have ramifications affecting a host of additional systems. The tiny pebble cast into the pool causes only a minute splash, but the ripples propagate and ultimately affect the entire pool. Irreversible injury may well be not the result of damage to a single locus or system, but the summation of many disruptions that eventually overcome the cell's capacity to adapt. Whatever the Achilles' heel(s) of the cell may be, they are undoubtedly biochemical processes that, when dislocated, lead in time to observable morphologic change.

MORPHOLOGY OF CELL INJURY

Ultrastructural Changes

We can now examine the morphologic changes in reversibly and lethally injured cells, and we shall begin with the ultrastructural changes. These have been alluded to in the discussion of the pathogenesis of cell injury; here we shall briefly summarize these changes as they affect various components of the cell.

Changes ascribable to alterations in the plasma membrane are seen early in cell injury, reflecting the disturbances in ion and volume regulation induced by loss of ATP. These include cell swelling, formation of cytoplasmic blebs, blunting and distortion of microvilli, creation of myelin figures, and deterioration and loosening of intercellular attachments. These changes can occur rapidly and are readily reversible. In later stages, breaks are seen in both the membranes enclosing the cell and those of the organelles (Figs. 1–4 and 1–5).

Mitochondrial changes occur extremely rapidly after ischemic injury but are delayed in some forms of chemical injury. Early after ischemia, the mitochondria appear condensed, possibly as a result of condensation of the matrix protein following loss of ATP. However, this is quickly followed by *swelling of mitochondria* due to the ionic shifts that occur in the mitochondrial inner compartment. Characteristic *amorphous densities* appear as early as 30 minutes after ischemia in the myocardium, where they correlate with the onset of irreversibility. These densities consist of lipids or lipid-protein complexes, but with reperfusion, dense granules appear that are very rich in *calcium*. The latter also occur in chemical injury. With irreversible injury also comes increased swelling of mitochondria, which may assume large, bizarre forms. Finally, there is outright rupture of the mitochondrial membranes, followed by progressively increased calcification.

Dilatation of the *endoplasmic reticulum* occurs early after injury, probably owing to changes in ion and water movement. This is followed by detachment of ribosomes and disaggregation of polysomes, with a decrease of protein synthesis (Fig. 1–8). These responses are also reversible, but with further injury (or early on, as in the case of CCl_4, due to lipid peroxidation) there is progressive fragmentation of the endoplasmic reticulum and formation of intracellular aggregates of myelin figures.

Changes in the *lysosomes* generally appear late. In

the stages of irreversible injury, lysosomes may be clear and often swollen, but there is no evidence of leakage of lysosomal enzymes at this stage. However, after the onset of lethal injury, lysosomes rupture and eventually may disappear as recognizable structures from the disfigured carcass of the dead cell. Most of these vanishing lysosomes must have ruptured, but some have fused with the autophagic vacuoles (phagosomes), which now become apparent within the damaged cell.

Light Microscopic Patterns

Before we describe the histologic alterations of reversibly injured and dead cells, let us remember that these are observations made on fixed static cells. Much more dramatic are the dynamic changes that can be seen by phase-contrast microscopy or better still by time-lapse cinemicrography of unfixed cells observed in culture.[48] Here one of the earliest changes is the so-called "irritability" of cells, in which cells move faster, seem to contract, form folds, and throw out pseudopods. These are almost certainly due to alterations in the cytoskeletal system and are reversible. Vacuolization, membrane blebbing, nuclear alterations, and final rupture of the cell can also be directly observed as they occur in the writhing cell if the toxic stimulus is maintained.

In classic pathology, the morphologic changes resulting from nonlethal injury to cells were termed *degenerations,* but today they are more simply designated *reversible injuries.* Two patterns can be recognized under the light microscope: *cellular swelling* and *fatty change.* Cellular swelling appears whenever cells are incapable of maintaining ionic and fluid homeostasis. *Hydropic change* is an older term that merely denotes an extension of cellular swelling, reflecting the intracellular accumulation of greater amounts of water. *Fatty change,* under some circumstances, may be another indicator of reversible cell injury. It is a less universal reaction, principally encountered in cells involved in and dependent on fat metabolism, such as the hepatocyte and myocardial cell. Since it is a form of intracellular accumulation, it is described in detail later in this chapter.

CELLULAR SWELLING. The first manifestation of almost all forms of injury to cells is an increase in their size resulting from a shift of extracellular water into the cell caused by mechanisms described earlier.

Cellular swelling is a difficult morphologic change to appreciate with the light microscope; it may be more discernible at the level of the whole organ. When it affects all cells in an organ, it causes some pallor, increased turgor, and increase in weight of the organ. Microscopically, enlargement of cells is most often discernible by compression of the microvasculature of the organ as, for example, the hepatic sinusoids and the capillary network within the renal cortex. Likewise, the spaces of Disse in the liver may be narrowed. In passing, **loss of glycogen** is another particularly early sign of ischemic injury and can often be appreciated with use of special stains.

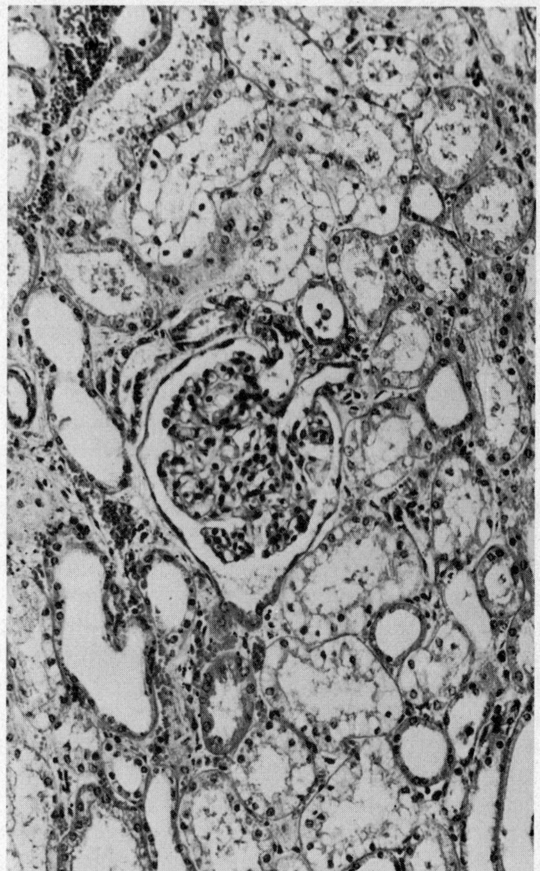

Figure 1–9. Marked cellular swelling (hydropic degeneration) of renal tubular epithelial cells seen in the center field above and below the glomerulus. The cleared, vacuolated cells contain dark displaced nuclei.

If water continues to accumulate within cells, the further swelling is associated with the appearance of small cleared vacuoles within the cytoplasm. These vacuoles presumably represent distended and pinched-off or sequestered segments of the endoplasmic reticulum. This pattern of nonlethal injury is sometimes called "hydropic change" or "vacuolar degeneration" (two terms that are better discarded) and is encountered most often in the epithelial cells of the proximal convoluted tubules of the kidney (Fig. 1–9), liver, or heart following chloroform or CCl_4 poisoning, as well as in certain infections, high fevers, and hypokalemia.

Swelling of cells is a reversible alteration and, indeed, may be without significant functional effect. It is, therefore, an indicator of mild injury and is of principal importance as a possible antecedent to more severe cell injury.

THE NECROTIC CELL. *Necrosis is the sum of the morphologic changes that follow cell death in a living tissue or organ.* Except for "normal" tissues placed immediately in fixatives, necrosis is the major morphologic manifestation of cell death. It has already been made clear that cells die some time before such lethal injury can be identified under the light microscope. In the studies done by Majno and colleagues, it was not possible to make light microscopic diagnoses of ischemic rat liver cell necrosis until seven to eight hours after the cells had died.[49] Ironically, the necrosis was apparent to the naked eye after three to four hours, because the tissue became abnormally opaque and pale at this time. As stated earlier, enzymes are activated and released from the lysosomes of the dead cell, causing *autoloysis.* Moreover, dead cells evoke an inflammatory reaction that brings to the area leukocytes as well as plasma proteins that leak across the small blood vessels. Lysosomal enzymes released by the leukocytes, as well as activated factors from plasma, contribute to further degradation of the dead cells, a process called *heterolysis.*[49]

The dead cell usually shows increased eosinophilia, due in part to the loss of normal cytoplasmic basophilia imparted by the ribonucleoprotein in the cytoplasm (which is scattered and lost during cell death) and in part to increased binding of eosin to denatured intracytoplasmic proteins. The cell may have a more glassy homogeneous appearance than normal cells, due mainly to the loss of glycogen particles, which impart a more granular appearance to the cytoplasm in the normal cell. Eosinophilic globules within the cytoplasm represent swollen mitochondria. When lysosomal enzymes have digested the cytoplasmic organelles, the cytoplasm becomes moth-eaten and vacuolated. Finally, calcification of the dead cells may occur in some instances (p. 35).

Nuclear changes also occur in sublethally and lethally injured cells. The earliest observed ultrastructural change is a reversible clumping of the chromatin to create large aggregates attached to the nuclear membrane and to the nucleolus. As the degradative changes in the cell progress, however, nuclear degeneration may follow along one of two pathways. In some cells, the nucleus progressively shrinks and becomes transformed to a small, dense, wrinkled mass of tightly packed chromatin, an alteration called nuclear **pyknosis.** With time, this chromatin undergoes progressive dissolution **karyolysis,** apparently as a result of the hydrolytic action of the DNAses of lysosomal origin. In other cells, after undergoing **pyknosis,** the nucleus may break up into many clumps, a process called **karyorrhexis.** Eventually the nucleus disappears, and so far as we know, with the exception of the erythrocyte in man, no cell devoid of a nucleus is vital. However, by the time the nucleus has disintegrated, the cell is long dead.

A somewhat distinctive morphologic pattern of cell death has recently been renamed *apoptosis*[50] (derived from Greek for "dropping off"). It usually involves single cells, or clusters of cells, and appears on H and E sections as a round or oval mass of intensely eosinophilic cytoplasm often with pyknotic nuclear fragments. One example is the acidophil or *Councilman body* seen in the liver in toxic or viral hepatitis, but apoptosis also occurs in a variety of other physiologic conditions. It is thought that the alterations initially involve rapid condensation of both nucleus and cytoplasm,[50] but the mechanism of cell injury in apoptosis is unclear, as is its distinctness from the mechanism of necrosis.

TYPES OF NECROSIS. The death of cells is not always followed by immediate dissolution of the cellular carcass. Different pathways may be followed depending on the balance between progressive proteolysis, coagulation of protein, and calcification, resulting in the emergence of distinctive morphologic types of necrosis. Although in all instances these types of necrosis clearly signify previous cell death, the characteristic histologic types sometimes give a clue to the cause of cell injury, and will therefore be described in some detail.

Coagulation Necrosis. Coagulation necrosis is the most common pattern of necrosis and is characterized by conversion of the cell to an acidophilic, opaque "tombstone." This usually occurs with loss of the nucleus but with preservation of the basic cellular shape, permitting recognition of the cell outlines and tissue architecture (Fig. 1–10). For example, an entire renal tubule may undergo coagulation necrosis, but can still be recognized as a tubule owing to preservation of its cylindrical shape and the outlines of the tubular epithelial cells. This pattern of necrosis results most commonly from sudden severe ischemia in such organs as the kidney, heart, and adrenal gland. It can also occur after chemical injury, as in the coagulation necrosis of proximal renal tubules induced by ingestion of mercuric chloride. Presumably, this pattern results from denaturation of proteins soon after the cell has died. The mechanism of such denaturation is poorly understood, but may be similar to the molecular transformations that occur when soluble proteins such as albumin are coagulated by heat or when proteins are fixed by formaldehyde. The proteins are rendered less soluble, thus delaying proteolysis by lysosomal enzymes and preserving, for a few days, the dense eosinophilic coagulate itself. In the course of time, however, these coagulated cells are either liquefied or removed by fragmentation and phagocytosis by invading leukocytes.

Liquefaction Necrosis. Liquefaction necrosis results from the action of powerful hydrolytic enzymes and occurs when autolysis and heterolysis prevail over conditions that favor denaturation of proteins (the latter resulting in coagulation necrosis). This pattern is characteristic of ischemic destruction of brain tissue. It is also commonly encountered in all focal bacterial lesions, presumably because enzymes of bacterial and leukocytic origin contribute to the digestion of dead cells. Such liquefactive necrosis is particularly characteristic of pyogenic microorganisms (staphylococci, streptococci, *E. coli,* and others); the leukocyte-containing proteinaceous fluid composes a large part of what would be called pus (Fig. 1–11). Brain tissue undergoing liquefaction necrosis is eventually converted to a cystic structure filled with debris and fluid. These cysts are the hallmark of areas of past brain infarction.

Enzymatic Fat Necrosis. Enzymatic fat necrosis is the highly specific morphologic pattern of cell death encountered when lipases escape into fatty depots. It is seen in a disease called *acute pancreatic necrosis,* in which there is patchy necrosis of the pancreas and of fatty depots throughout the abdomen caused by pancreatic enzymes released from the injured acinar cells. Powerful lipases and proteases run amuck and enzymatically destroy not only the pancreatic substance itself, but also fat cells in and about the pancreas and throughout the peritoneal cavity. These lipases catalyze the decomposition of triglycerides that leak from adja-

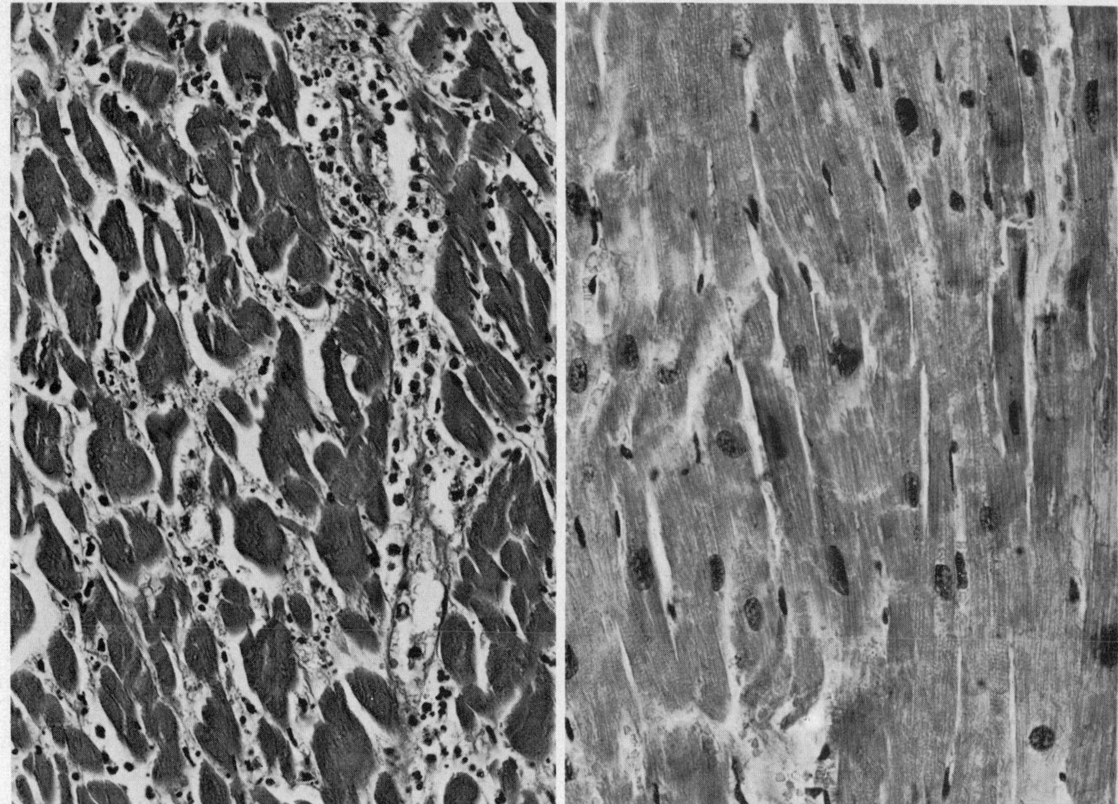

Figure 1–10. Left, necrotic cardiac muscle cells with well preserved outlines. The nuclei have disappeared, and the cytoplasm is coagulated and granular. *Right,* preserved normal muscle for comparison.

cent damaged adipose cells to produce free fatty acids. The necrosis takes the form of foci of shadowy outlines of necrotic fat cells, the lipid content of which has been lipolyzed, surrounded by an inflammatory reaction (Fig. 1–12). The released fatty acids then complex with calcium to create calcium soaps, which appear in tissue sections as amorphous, granular, basophilic deposits. To the naked eye, the necrotic foci appear opaque and

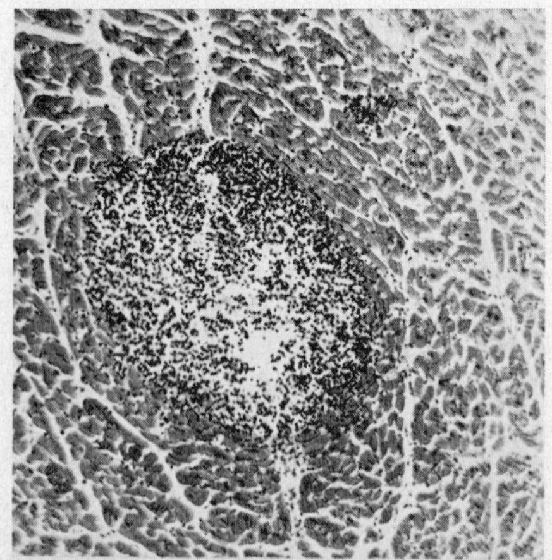

Figure 1–11. A focus of liquefactive digestion in the myocardium. In the involved area, all muscle cells have been destroyed, and the focus is filled with inflammatory white cells.

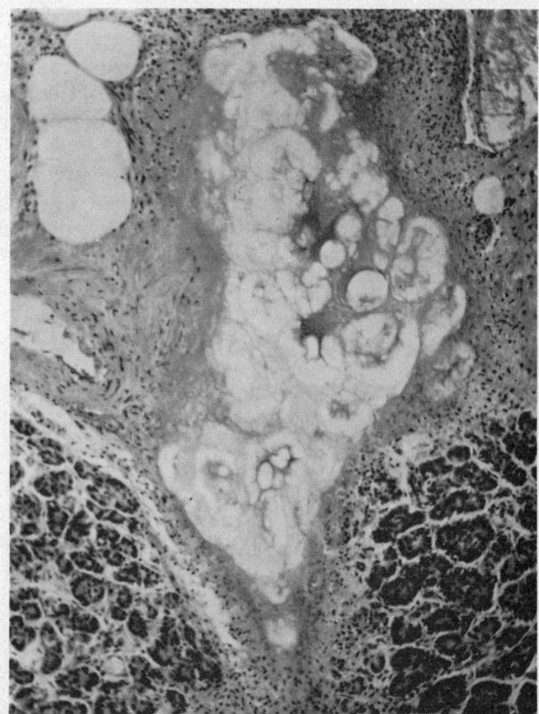

Figure 1–12. A sharply circumscribed focus of enzymatic necrosis of fat. Shadowy outlines of fat cells persist, surrounded by a zone of inflammation. The focus is surrounded by normal pancreatic substance.

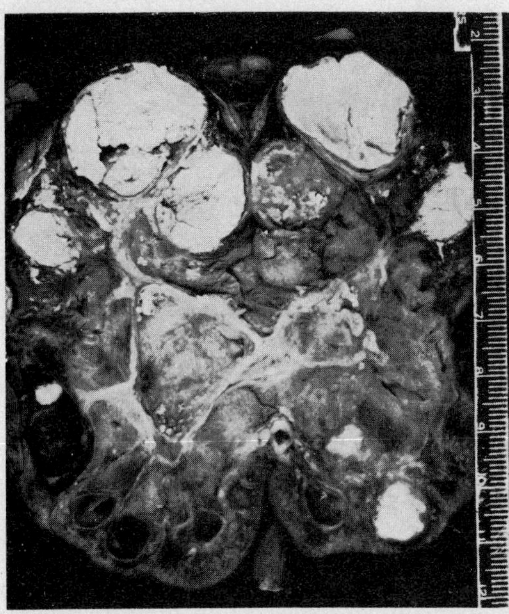

Figure 1–13. A tuberculous kidney with multiple discrete large foci of caseous necrosis. The caseous debris is yellow-white and cheesy.

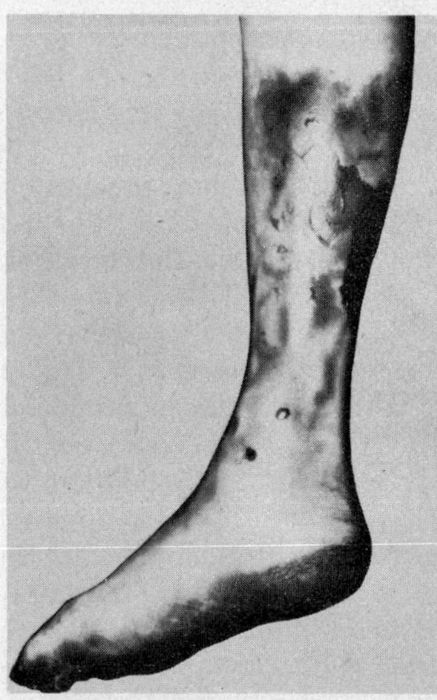

Figure 1–15. Gangrene of the lower leg, sharply delineated from the proximal normal tissues. The affected areas are discolored and the superficial skin and tissues have begun to slough.

chalky-white, and familiarity with the gross and microscopic features of this form of necrosis often enables the surgeon and the pathologist to identify the nature of the acute abdominal emergency.

Caseous Necrosis. This is another distinctive type of necrosis that is a combination of coagulative and liquefactive necrosis encountered principally in the center of tuberculous infections (Fig. 1–13). The characteristic appearance of this type of necrosis is that of soft, friable, whitish-gray debris resembling clumped cheesy material, hence the term caseous necrosis. This appearance has been attributed to the capsule of the tubercle bacillus *Mycobacterium tuberculosis,* which contains lipopolysaccharides, but the exact interaction of this material with dead cells is not well understood. Microscopically the cells are not totally liquefied nor are their outlines preserved, creating a distinctive amorphous granular debris (Fig. 1–14). The caseous necrosis is enclosed within a granulomatous inflammatory wall.

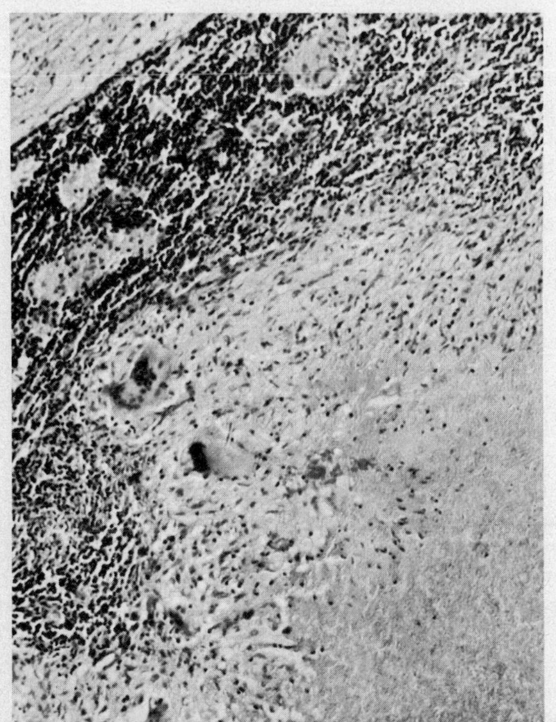

Figure 1–14. A tubercle. A large area of caseous tuberculosis is seen in lower right.

Gangrenous Necrosis. Although gangrenous necrosis in reality does not represent a distinctive pattern of cell death, the term is still commonly used in surgical clinical practice. It is usually applied to a limb, generally the lower leg, which has lost its blood supply and has subsequently been attacked by bacterial agents (Fig. 1–15). The tissues in this case have undergone ischemic cell death and coagulative necrosis modified by the liquefactive action of the bacteria and the attracted leukocytes. When the coagulative pattern is dominant, the process may be termed *dry gangrene.* Alternatively, when the liquefactive action is more pronounced, it may be designated as *wet gangrene.*

INTRACELLULAR ACCUMULATIONS

Under some circumstances, normal cells may accumulate abnormal amounts of various substances. The stockpiled substances fall into three categories: (1) *a normal cellular constituent* accumulated in excess, such as lipid, protein, and carbohydrates; (2) *an abnormal substance,* which may be a product of abnormal metabolism; and (3) *a pigment,* i.e., a colored substance.

These substances may accumulate either transiently or permanently and may be detected by the macroscopic color of the stored material, by its microscopic appearance, by its staining characteristics, by its immunohistochemical specificity, and, most precisely, by biochemical and biophysical determinations. These accumulated substances may be harmless to the cells, but on occasion may also be severely toxic. The location of the substance may be in either the cytoplasm or the nucleus; in the former location *it is most frequently within lysosomes.* In some instances the cell may be producing the abnormal substance, and in others it may be merely storing products of pathologic processes occurring elsewhere in the body.

The processes that result in abnormal intracellular accumulations in non-neoplastic cells are many, but most can be divided into three general types.

1. *A normal endogenous substance is produced at a normal or increased rate, but the rate of metabolism is inadequate to remove it.* An example of this type of process is *fatty change*, one of the most common types of intracellular accumulations occurring in various forms of cell injury.

2. *A normal or abnormal endogenous substance accumulates since it cannot be metabolized.* The most common cause of such failure of metabolism is *lack of an enzyme* that blocks a specific metabolic pathway, so that some particular metabolite cannot be used. Enzyme lack is due to a genetically determined inborn error of metabolism, and resulting diseases are referred to as *storage diseases.* Clinical entities result from the abnormal accumulations and are discussed more fully later (p. 142).

3. *An abnormal exogenous substance is deposited* and accumulates because the cell has neither the enzymatic machinery to degrade the substance nor the ability to transport it to other sites. Accumulations of carbon particles, and such nonmetabolizable chemicals as silica particles are examples of this type of alteration.

Whatever the nature and origin of the intracellular accumulation, it implies the storage of some product by individual cells. If overload is due to a systemic derangement and can be brought under control, the accumulation is reversible. In diabetes mellitus, for example, control of the hyperglycemia may mobilize the abnormal accumulations of glycogen that have collected. On the other hand, in genetic storage diseases, because the metabolic error is not correctable, accumulation is progressive, and the cells may become so overloaded as to cause secondary injury, leading in some instances to death of the tissue and the patient.

INTRACELLULAR ACCUMULATIONS OF LIPIDS

Fatty Change

Fatty change refers to any abnormal accumulation of fat within parenchymal cells. The term embraces the older terms *fatty degeneration* and *fatty infiltration*, which are misleading because neither a degenerative nor an infiltrative process is necessarily involved in the pathogenesis of the lipid accumulation. The more noncommital term *fatty change* embraces the different pathogenetic mechanisms that may lead to accumulation of neutral fat within cells.

Although quite different pathogenetic mechanisms may underlie fatty change, several facts are agreed upon: (1) *The appearance of fat vacuoles within cells, whether small or large, represents an absolute increase in intracellular lipids.* It does not represent so-called unmasking of the normal fat content of cells. (2) The amount of contained fat is not dependent on the pathogenetic mechanism but rather reflects some imbalance in production, utilization, or mobilization of it. The injured cell is incapable of metabolizing or exporting even normal levels of lipids, while the normal cell may synthesize excessive quantities of fat when presented with excess substrate. (3) Fatty change is sometimes preceded by cellular swelling. (4) Although itself an indicator of nonlethal injury, fatty change is sometimes the harbinger of cell death and, in many situations, is encountered in cells adjacent to those that have died and undergone necrosis. Fatty change is often seen in the liver, since it is the major organ involved in fatty metabolism, but it may also occur in heart, muscle, kidney, and other organs.

Pathogenesis of Fatty Liver

An understanding of the mechanisms involved in lipid accumulation in the liver requires familiarity with normal fat metabolism, in which the liver plays a central role.[51, 52] Under normal conditions, lipids are transported to the liver from adipose tissue and from the diet. From adipose tissue, lipids are released and transported in only one form—free fatty acids (FFA). Dietary lipids, on the other hand, are transported either as chylomicra (lipid particles consisting of triglyceride, phospholipid, and protein) or as free fatty acids (the latter being derived mainly from medium-chain triglycerides containing C_8 and C_{10} fatty acids). Free fatty acids enter the liver cell, and most are esterified to triglycerides. Some are converted to cholesterol, incorporated into phospholipids, or oxidized in mitochondria into ketone bodies. Some fatty acids are synthesized from acetate within the liver proper.

In order to be secreted by the liver, intracellular triglyceride must be complexed with specific apoprotein molecules called "lipid acceptor proteins" to form lipoproteins (see also p. 513). The sequence, shown diagrammatically in Figure 1–16, indicates that *excess accumulation of triglycerides within the liver may result from the following six defects,* sometimes acting in combination: (1) *Excessive entry of free fatty acids into the liver.* In starvation, for example, adipose tissue fats are mobilized, and more fatty acids are brought to the liver, where they are synthesized into triglycerides. Corticosteroids also produce lipid mobilization from adipose tissue. (2) *Enhanced fatty acid synthesis.* (3) *Decreased fatty acid oxidation.* Both (2) and (3) result in increased esterification of fatty acids to triglycerides. (4) *Increased esterification of fatty acids to triglycerides,*

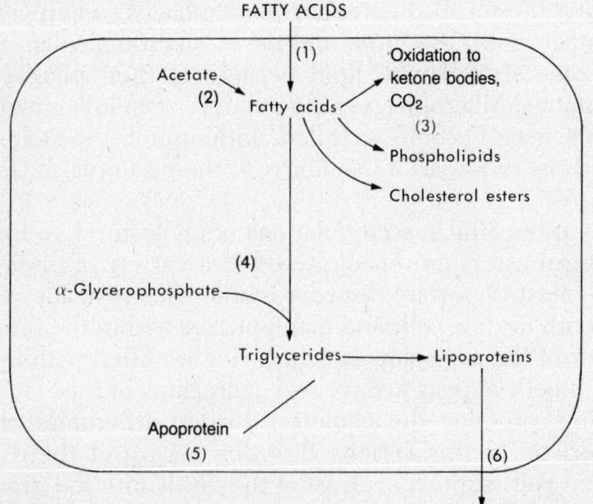

Figure 1–16. Lipid metabolism in the liver cell. The numbers refer to possible sites of abnormalities leading to fatty liver, as indicated in the text. (Modified from Podolsky, D. K., and Isselbacher, K. L.: Derangements of hepatic metabolism. *In* Harrison's Principles of Internal Medicine. New York, McGraw-Hill Book Co., 1983, p. 1778.)

owing to an increase in alpha-glycerophosphate, the carbohydrate backbone involved in such esterification. This is thought to be one effect of alcohol poisoning. (5) *Decreased apoprotein synthesis.* As stressed earlier, this protein is necessary for the conversion of triglycerides to lipoproteins, the only form in which lipid is excreted from the liver. This mechanism has been well established as the cause of fatty accumulation produced by such toxins as carbon tetrachloride and phosphorus, and appears to be the reason for fatty liver in protein malnutrition. (6) *Impaired lipoprotein secretion from the liver.* This seems to be involved in an experimental model of fatty liver induced by the administration of orotic acid.

It should be apparent that different types of disturbances may affect the control of fat transport and metabolism, and that an individual etiologic agent may act at more than one locus within the complex process of fat metabolism. Alcohol, at least in industrialized countries, is perhaps the most common cause of fatty liver. Alcohol is a hepatotoxin that alters mitochondrial and microsomal functions. Increased free fatty acid mobilization, diminished triglyceride utilization, decreased fatty acid oxidation, a block in lipoprotein excretion, as well as direct damage to the endoplasmic reticulum by free radicals produced by ethanol metabolism, have all been implicated, but the major factor remains to be determined.[53, 54]

The significance of fatty change depends on the cause and severity of accumulation. It may have no effect on cellular function when mild. More severe fatty change may impair cellular function, but unless some vital intracellular process is irreversibly impaired (such as in carbon tetrachloride poisoning), fatty change per se is reversible. The liver in the alcoholic, for example, may become enormously enlarged. Such extreme accumulation of fat may indeed be associated with functional deficit and, by a complex process to be described later (Chapter 19), may lead to a progressive form of fibrosis of the liver termed *cirrhosis.* However, in the alcoholic who has not yet developed cirrhosis and who wisely adopts an alcohol-free balanced diet, it is quite remarkable to observe the return of the enlarged fatty liver to normal size, structure, and function. As a severe form of injury, therefore, fatty change may be a harbinger of cell death, *but it should be emphasized that cells may die without undergoing fatty change.*

Fatty change is most often seen in the liver and heart, but it may occur in other organs.

Liver. In the liver, mild fatty change may not affect the gross appearance. With progressive accumulation, the organ enlarges and becomes increasingly yellow until, in extreme instances, the liver may weigh 3 to 6 kg and be transformed into a bright yellow, soft, greasy organ. Such an extreme is most commonly encountered in alcoholics.

Fatty change begins with the development of minute, membrane-bounded inclusions (liposomes) closely applied to the endoplasmic reticulum and probably derived from it.[51] It is first manifested under the light microscope by the appearance of small fat vacuoles in the cytoplasm around the nucleus. As the process progresses, the vacuoles coalesce to create cleared spaces that displace the nucleus to the periphery of the cell (Fig. 1–17). Occasionally, contiguous cells rupture, and the enclosed fat globules coalesce to produce so-called fatty cysts.

Heart. Lipid, as neutral fat, is quite frequently found in heart muscle in the form of small droplets. It occurs in two patterns. In one, prolonged moderate hypoxia, such as that produced by profound anemia, induces a "thrush breast" or "tigered" effect. Here the intracellular deposits of fat create grossly apparent bands of yellowed myocardium, alternating with bands of darker, red-brown, uninvolved myocardium. In the other pattern of fatty change, such as that produced by more profound hypoxia or some forms of myocarditis (e.g., diphtheritic), the myocardial cells are uniformly affected and the entire myocardium becomes flabby. Histologically, the fat in the myocardial cell tends to be distributed in minute cytoplasmic vacuoles that are readily missed on casual inspection of routine tissue stains. It is often necessary to

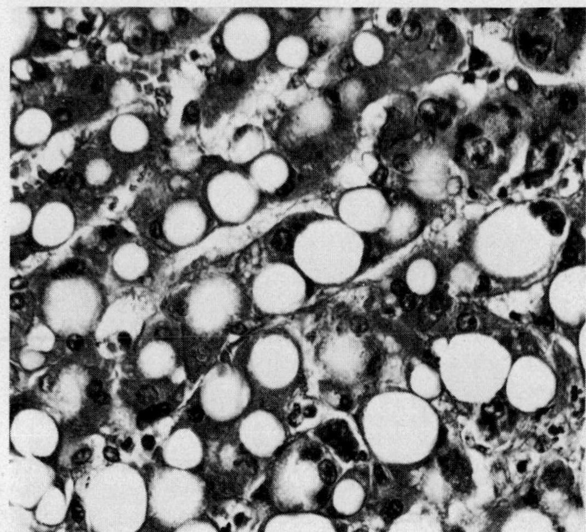

Figure 1–17. High-power detail of marked fatty change of liver. The variability in size of vacuoles is evident. In some cells, the well-preserved nucleus is squeezed into the displaced rim of cytoplasm about the fat vacuole.

apply special fat stains to unmask this change. The mechanism by which the diphtheria bacillus causes a fatty heart is apparently the production of an exotoxin that interferes with the metabolism of carnitine, a cofactor for the oxidation of long-chain fatty acids.

In all organs, fatty change appears as clear vacuoles within parenchymal cells. Intracellular accumulations of water or polysaccharides (such as glycogen) may also produce clear vacuoles, and it becomes necessary to resort to special techniques to distinguish these three types of clear vacuoles. The identification of lipids requires the avoidance of fat solvents commonly employed in paraffin embedding for routine hematoxylin and eosin stains. To identify the fat, it is necessary to prepare frozen tissue sections on either fresh or aqueous formalin-fixed tissues. The sections may then be stained with Sudan IV or Oil Red-O, both of which impart an orange-red color to the contained lipids. The periodic acid–Schiff (PAS) reaction is commonly employed to identify glycogen, although it is by no means specific. When neither fat nor polysaccharide can be demonstrated within a clear vacuole, it is presumed to contain water or fluid with low protein content.

Other Lipid Accumulations

As detailed in the previous section, the overload of parenchymal liver cells by triglycerides is termed "fatty change." By quite different mechanisms, phagocytic cells may become overloaded with lipid (triglycerides and cholesterol). Scavenger macrophages, wherever in contact with the lipid debris of necrotic cells, may become stuffed with lipid because of their phagocytic activities. Macrophages at the margin of an inflammatory focus may become so filled with minute vacuoles of lipids as to impart a foaminess to their cytoplasm *(foam cells)*.

Intracellular accumulations of cholesterol and cholesterol esters are encountered in a variety of diseases. The most important disorder is atherosclerosis, in which smooth muscle cells and macrophages within the intimal layer of the aorta and large arteries are filled with lipid. Such cells appear foamy, and aggregates of them in the intima produce the cholesterol-laden atheromas characteristic of this serious disorder. Many of these fat-laden cells rupture, releasing the lipids into the ground substance of the intima. The mechanisms of lipid accumulation in these cells in atherosclerosis are discussed in Chapter 13. The extracellular cholesterol esters may crystallize in the shape of long needles, producing quite distinctive clefts in tissue sections.

Intracellular accumulations of cholesterol and cholesterol esters within macrophages are also characteristic of acquired and hereditary hyperlipidemic states (p. 515). Usually, these lesions are found in the subepithelial connective tissue of the skin and in tendons, producing tumorous masses known as *xanthomas*.

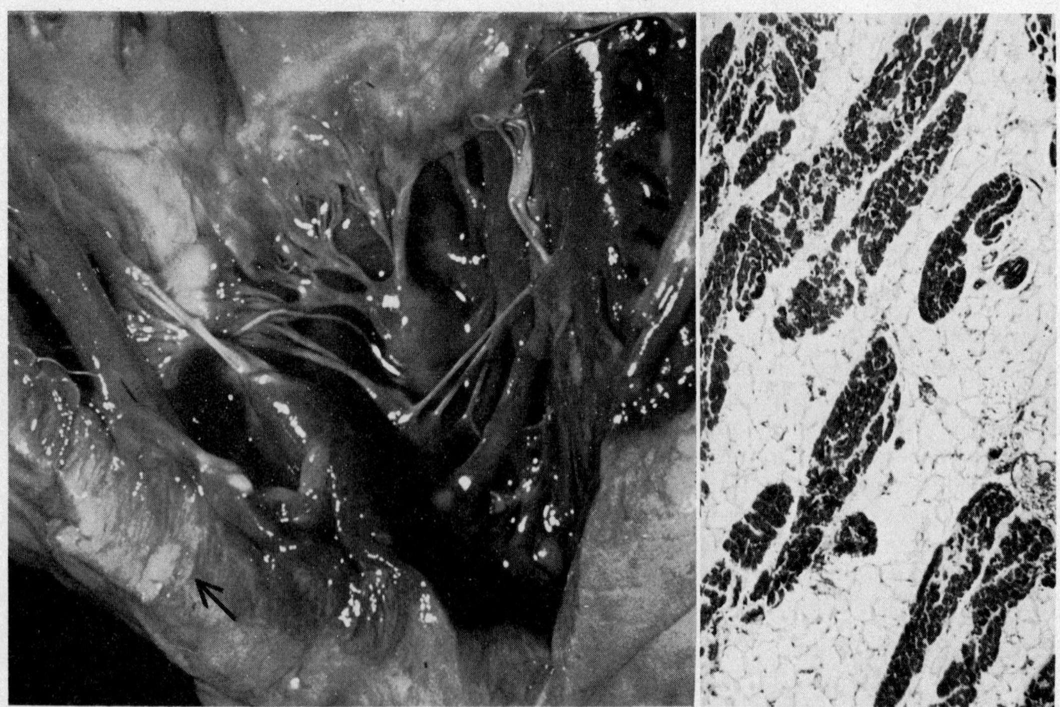

Fig. 1–18

Fig. 1–19

Figure 1–18. Stromal fatty infiltration (fatty ingrowth) of the heart. Streaks of yellow fat extending through the myocardium are visible on cross section of the ventricular wall *(arrow)*. Small, pale yellow deposits are also present subendocardially in the columnae carneae.

Figure 1–19. Stromal fatty infiltration (fatty ingrowth) of the heart. A microscopic detail to demonstrate normal myocardial fibers separated by adult fat tissue.

Stromal Infiltration of Fat or Fatty Ingrowth

This is a form of *accumulation of lipids that has a mechanism and connotation completely different from those of intracellular fatty accumulation.* It is discussed at this time merely to differentiate it from the condition described as fatty change. Fatty ingrowth refers to the accumulation of lipids *within stromal connective tissue cells.*

Fatty ingrowth is most commonly encountered in the heart and pancreas, where adult adipose cells appear within the connective tissue stroma. In the heart, the right ventricle is generally more severely affected than the left. Usually, there is an increase of subepicardial fat that extends in continuity as finger-like projections between the muscle bundles (Fig. 1–18). These insinuations may extend throughout the thickness of the myocardium to appear beneath the endocardium as small yellow deposits. The adult fat cells separate but do not damage the adjacent myocardial cells (Fig. 1–19). In the pancreas, the fat is found in the connective tissue septa of the pancreatic lobules (Fig. 1–20). The glandular tissue may become so dispersed as to be almost invisible on gross inspection. However, if one were to extract the fat from such a pancreas, the normal size, shape, and morphologic characteristics of the organ would be restored.

As far as is known, stromal infiltration of fat rarely affects cardiac or pancreatic function.

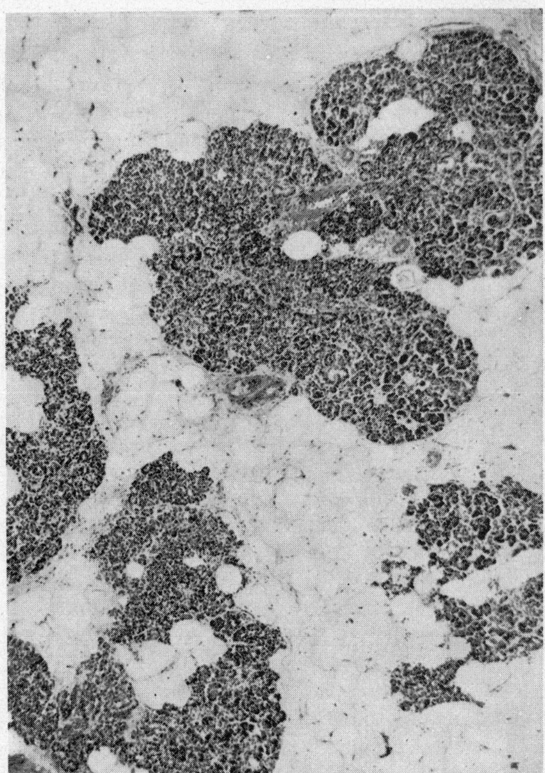

Figure 1–20. Stromal fatty infiltration of pancreas (fatty ingrowth). Large fat cells separating normal acinar glands.

INTRACELLULAR ACCUMULATIONS OF PROTEIN

Excesses of proteins within the cells sufficient to cause morphologically visible droplets occur principally in the renal epithelial cells of the proximal convoluted tubules and in plasma cells. The former example is seen in renal diseases associated with protein loss in the urine (proteinuria). If a protein leaks across the glomerular filter, it passes into the proximal tubule where it is reabsorbed by the epithelial cell through pinocytosis. Pinocytotic vesicles fuse with lysosomes to produce phagolysosomes, which appear as pink hyaline droplets within the cytoplasm of the tubular cell (Fig. 1–21). These aggregations do not impair cellular function. If the underlying cause for the proteinuria can be controlled, the protein excess is metabolized and the droplets disappear.

Plasma cells engaged in active synthesis of immunoglobulins may become overloaded with their synthetic product to produce large, homogeneous eosinophilic inclusions called *Russell bodies.* With an electron microscope, such Russell bodies are localized within hugely distended cisternae of the endoplasmic reticulum, where protein synthesis occurs.[55]

INTRACELLULAR ACCUMULATIONS OF GLYCOGEN

Excessive intracellular deposits of glycogen are seen in patients with an abnormality in either glucose or glycogen metabolism. Whatever the clinical setting, the glycogen masses appear as clear vacuoles within the cytoplasm. Glycogen is best preserved in nonaqueous fixatives; for its localization, tissues are best fixed in absolute alcohol. Staining with Best's carmine or the periodic acid–Schiff (PAS) reaction imparts a rose-to-violet color to the glycogen, and diastase digestion prior to staining will serve as a further control by hydrolyzing the glycogen.

Diabetes mellitus is the prime example of a disorder of glucose metabolism. In this disease, glycogen is found

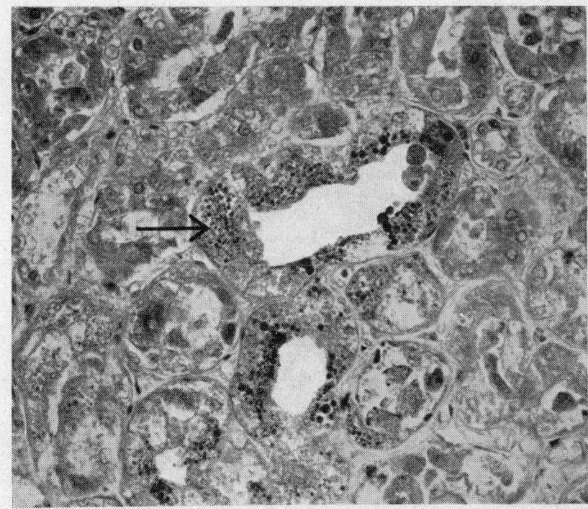

Figure 1–21. Hyaline droplets in the renal tubular epithelium *(arrow).*

in the epithelial cells of the distal portions of the proximal convoluted tubules and sometimes in the descending loop of Henle, as well as within liver cells, beta cells of the islets of Langerhans, and heart muscle cells. The mechanisms involved in the renal change consist of hyperglycemia resulting from impaired insulin function, glycosuria as the blood glucose levels rise above the renal threshold, and tubular reabsorption of the abnormal quantities of glucose in the glomerular filtrate. The glucose is stored in the form of glycogen.

The intracellular glycogen produces marked vacuolization of the cytoplasm to the point at which the cells appear to be entirely cleared (Fig. 1–22). For obscure reasons, glycogen deposition in hepatocytes appears by light microscopy within nuclei, which thus become swollen and clear, giving the nucleus a ground-glass appearance (Fig. 1–23). Such glycogen accumulation is a reasonably common finding at autopsy in diabetic patients as well as in patients receiving intravenous glucose solutions, but it has no clinical or functional significance.

Glycogen also accumulates within the cells in a group of closely related disorders, all genetic, collectively referred to as the *glycogen storage diseases*, or *glycogenoses*. In these disorders, either there is lack of one or several of the enzymes that metabolize normal glycogen, or some abnormal form of glycogen is synthesized and cannot be metabolized. In the various syndromes (discussed in Chapter 4), the intracellular accumulations affect mainly myocardial muscle, skeletal muscle, and hepatic and renal cells. In all instances the glycogen appears as clear, intracytoplasmic vacuoles. These diseases represent instances in which massive stockpiling of substances within cells causes secondary injury and cell death.[56]

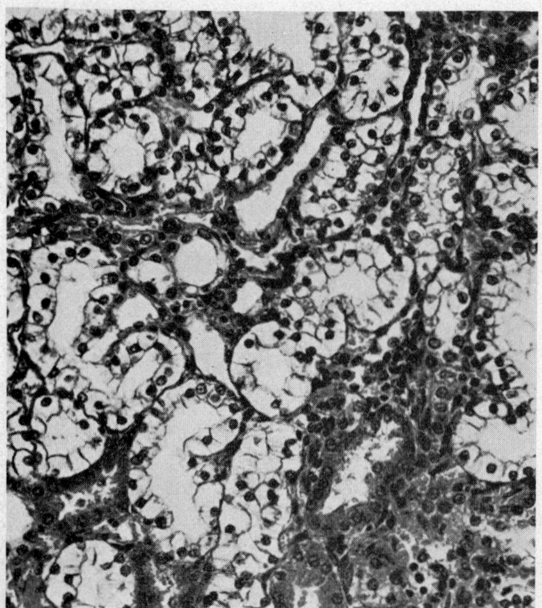

Figure 1–22. Glycogen vacuolation of the kidney. The epithelial cells of the affected tubules have distinct, well-preserved nuclei and sharp cell membranes.

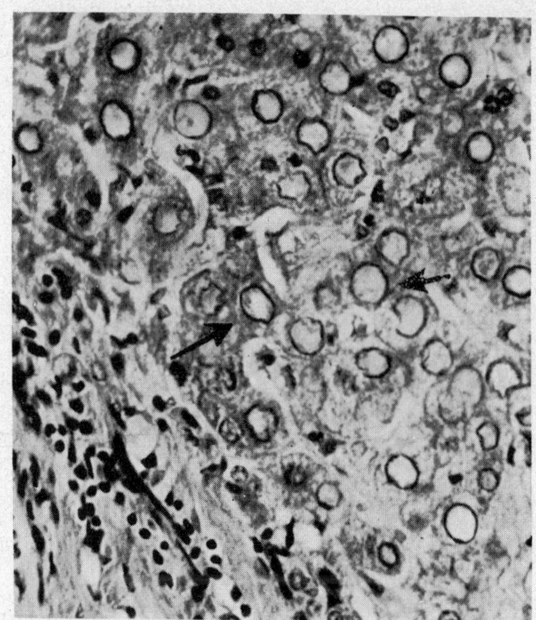

Figure 1–23. Glycogen accumulation in liver cell nuclei. The sharply defined circular nuclei are almost totally "cleared" by the glycogen *(arrows).*

INTRACELLULAR ACCUMULATIONS OF COMPLEX LIPIDS AND CARBOHYDRATES

In certain forms of storage diseases resulting from inborn errors of metabolism, abnormal complexes of carbohydrates and lipids accumulate that cannot be normally metabolized (p. 142). These substances collect within cells throughout the body, principally those in the reticuloendothelial system. In Gaucher's, Tay-Sachs, and Niemann-Pick diseases, the abnormal products are complex lipids, while in the mucopolysaccharidoses they are complex carbohydrates. In the glycolipidoses and mucolipidoses, other more unusual products are accumulated. The abnormal metabolites in all the storage diseases overflow into the blood and are phagocytized by reticuloendothelial cells, which thus become enlarged and develop an apparent foaminess to their cytoplasm, often producing massive splenomegaly and hepatomegaly. The accumulations may also appear in parenchymal cells in the heart, liver, and kidneys, and within ganglion cells of the brain and retina. The precise nature of the stored product rarely can be identified from morphologic examination and requires specific biochemical or enzymic analysis of affected tissues. These intracellular deposits may become extreme and cause death not only of the cell but also of the patient.

INTRACELLULAR ACCUMULATIONS OF PIGMENTS

Pigments are colored substances, some of which are normal constituents of cells (e.g., melanin), while others are abnormal and collect in cells only under special circumstances.[57] The various pigments differ greatly in origin, chemical constitution, and biologic significance. Pigments in pathology are traditionally differentiated into exogenous pigments, coming from outside the body, and endogenous pigments, synthesized within the body itself.

Exogenous Pigments. The most common exogenous pigment is *carbon* or coal dust, which is a virtually ubiquitous air pollutant of urban life. When inhaled, it is picked up by macrophages within the alveoli and is then transported through lymphatic channels to the regional lymph nodes in the tracheobronchial region. Accumulations of this pigment blacken the tissues of the lungs *(anthracosis)* and the involved lymph nodes (Fig. 1–24). In general, anthracosis does not interfere with normal respiratory function nor does it predispose to infection. However, in coal miners and those living in heavily polluted environments, the aggregates of carbon dust may induce a fibroblastic reaction or even emphysema, and thus cause a serious lung disease known as *"coal workers' pneumoconiosis."* The vast amount of carbon in the lungs of city dwellers is a grim reminder of man's devastation of his environment.

Inhabitants living in iron-mining communities may develop a rustlike discoloration of the lungs *(siderosis)*. This pigmentation itself is not associated with tissue damage, but in some areas the iron dust is accompanied by silica dust *(siderosilicosis)*. The silicotic component causes the serious lung disease *silicosis* (p. 435).

As is well known, *tattooing* is a form of localized pigmentation of the skin. The pigments inoculated are phagocytized by dermal macrophages in which they reside for the remainder of the life of the embellished. While the pigments do not evoke any inflammatory response, they have a distressing habit of persisting as a reminder of bygone follies.

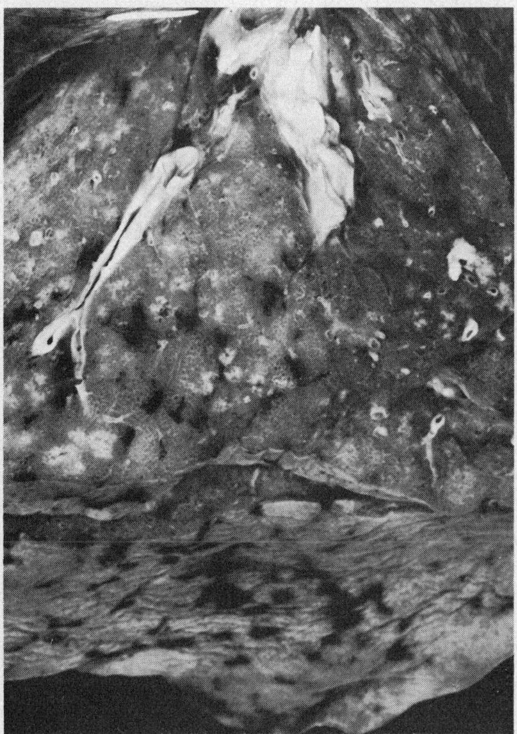

Figure 1–24. Focal black deposits of anthracotic pigmentation in the lung.

Endogenous Pigments. Except for lipofuscin and melanin, all the endogenous pigments are derivatives of hemoglobin.

Lipofuscin. Lipofuscin is an insoluble pigment, also known as lipochrome, ceroid, and "wear-and-tear" or aging pigment. Its importance lies in its being the "telltale" sign of free radical injury and lipid peroxidation. The term is derived from the Latin *(fuscus* = brown), thus brown lipid. In tissue sections it appears as a yellow-brown, finely granular intracytoplasmic pigment. It is seen in cells undergoing slow, regressive changes such as in the atrophy accompanying advanced age and chronic injury, is particularly prominent in the liver and heart of aging patients or patients with severe malnutrition, and is usually accompanied by organ shrinkage *(brown atrophy)*.[58] In the heart there is a linear increase in the amount of pigment with age. This amount may represent as much as 30% of the total solids of the heart muscle fiber by the time a person reaches 90 years of age. In hepatocytes it is not present in children but accumulates in great amounts in the elderly. In the brain the pigment is localized to specific regions, such as the ganglion cells of the hippocampus, and here again the amounts correlate with the age of the individual.

Lipofuscin represents the indigestible residues of autophagic vacuoles (Fig. 1–25) formed during aging or atrophy. Because of the marked insolubility of lipofuscin, chemical analysis has been unsatisfactory, but the pigment appears to be composed of polymers of lipids and phospholipids complexed with protein.[59] *This biochemical composition of lipofuscin suggests that it is derived through lipid peroxidation of polyunsaturated lipids of subcellular membranes* and is consistent with the theory that free radical formation causes the progressive deterioration of cell membranes in aging (see p. 37). The high rate of lipofuscin formation in relatively young people who die of conditions associated with inanition is presumed to result from the lack of dietary antioxidants that help prevent autooxidation.[60] With progressive polymerization, the lipofuscin loses its lipid characteristics, including its solubility in organic solvents and its staining with Sudan dyes.

Lipofuscin itself is not injurious to the cell or to its function. Sometimes, for obscure reasons, pigment that is indistinguishable from lipofuscin undergoes chemical or physical transformation so that it becomes autofluorescent and stains positively with acid-fast stains, the stains used to identify acid-fast tubercle bacilli. To this variant the designation *ceroid* has been given, but it is not believed to be different from lipofuscin. Ceroid can be induced experimentally by deficiency of the antioxidant vitamin E, again suggesting that autooxidation by free radicals is involved in its formation.

Melanin. Melanin (derived from the Greek word *melas*, meaning black) is an endogenous, non–hemoglobin-derived, brown-black pigment formed when the enzyme tyrosinase catalyzes the oxidation of tyrosine to

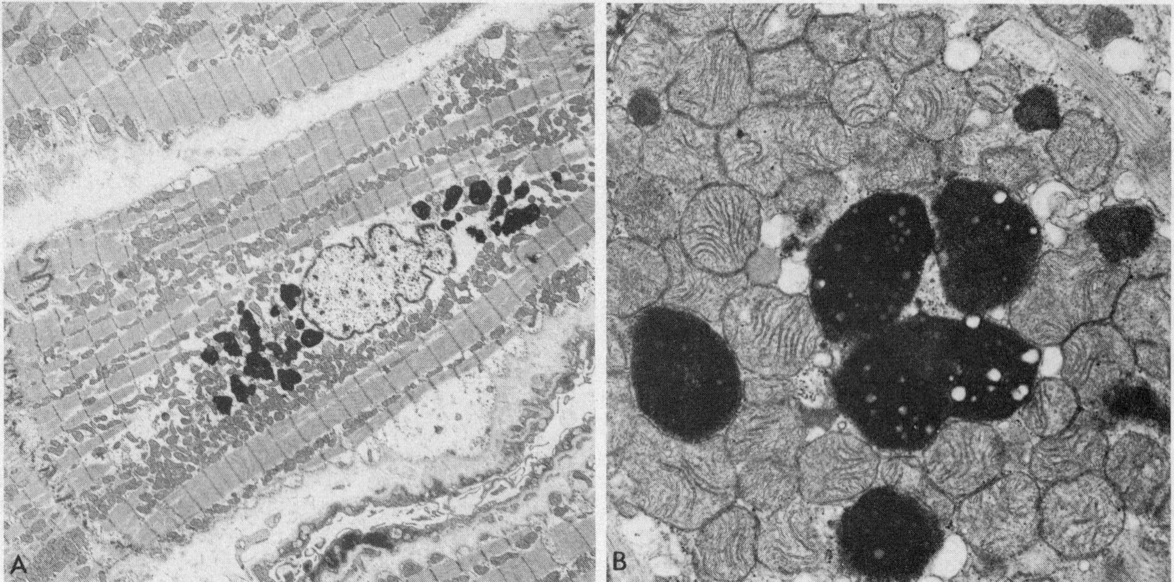

Figure 1–25. Lipofuscin. Lipofuscin granules in myocardial fiber. *A*, Low magnification, showing perinuclear localization. *B*, Electron-dense bodies are composed of lipid-protein complexes. (Courtesy of Dr. Marcel W. Seiler, Boston, MA.)

dihydroxyphenylalanine (DOPA) in melanocytes. It is the skin pigment, and its derivation is discussed in detail on page 1258.

In addition to its function as the skin pigment, melanin is important clinically for several reasons. *First*, both benign and malignant tumors arising from melanocytes are common. The benign mole (pigmented nevus) and its malignant counterpart (the melanoma), an often lethal form of cancer, arise from melanocytes or closely related cells. They are usually pigmented and sometimes the accumulation of melanin imparts an intense black coloration to these lesions (Fig. 1–26). *Second*, disorders of melanin pigmentation are frequent and important clues to disease in other organ systems. For example, hyperpigmentation occurs in Addison's disease, a condition caused by adrenocortical insufficiency secondary to the destruction of adrenal cortex (p. 1235). *Finally*, local disturbances of pigmentation (hyper- or hypomelaninosis) are common features of many skin conditions; for example, hyperpigmentation commonly follows drug eruptions.

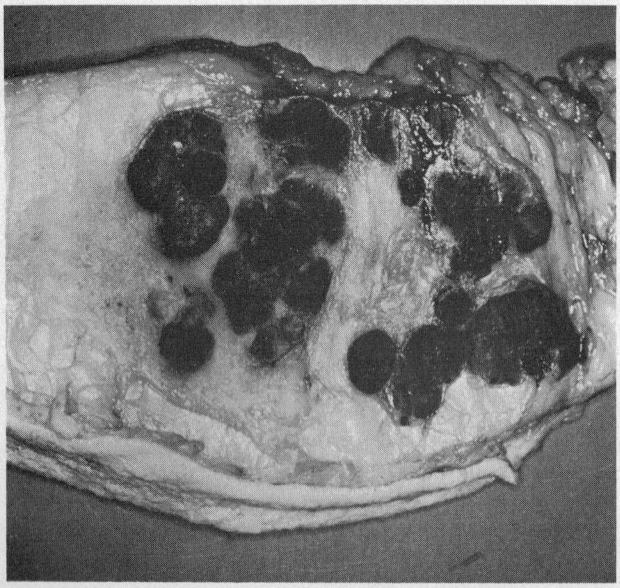

Figure 1–26. Black nodules representing metastatic deposits of malignant melanoma in the breast.

For all practical purposes melanin is the only endogenous *brown-black* pigment. The only other is homogentisic acid, a black pigment that occurs in patients with alkaptonuria, a rare metabolic disease. Here the pigment is deposited in the skin, connective tissue, and cartilage, and the pigmentation is known as "ochronosis" (p. 142).

Hemosiderin. Hemosiderin is a hemoglobin-derived, golden-yellow to brown granular or crystalline pigment in which form iron is stored in cells. Iron metabolism and the synthesis of ferritin and hemosiderin are considered in detail on page 636. Suffice it to say here that iron is normally carried by transport proteins, transferrins. In cells it is normally stored in association with a protein, apoferritin, to form ferritin micelles, which can be identified with the electron microscope as characteristic, closely packed dense particles (61 Å in radius) arranged in tetrads.[61] Ferritin is a constituent of many cell types under normal conditions. *When there is a local or systemic excess of iron, ferritin forms hemosiderin granules*, which are easily seen with the light microscope. Thus, hemosiderin pigment represents aggregates of ferritin micelles (Fig. 1–27). Under normal conditions small amounts of hemosiderin can be seen in the mononuclear phagocytes of the bone mar-

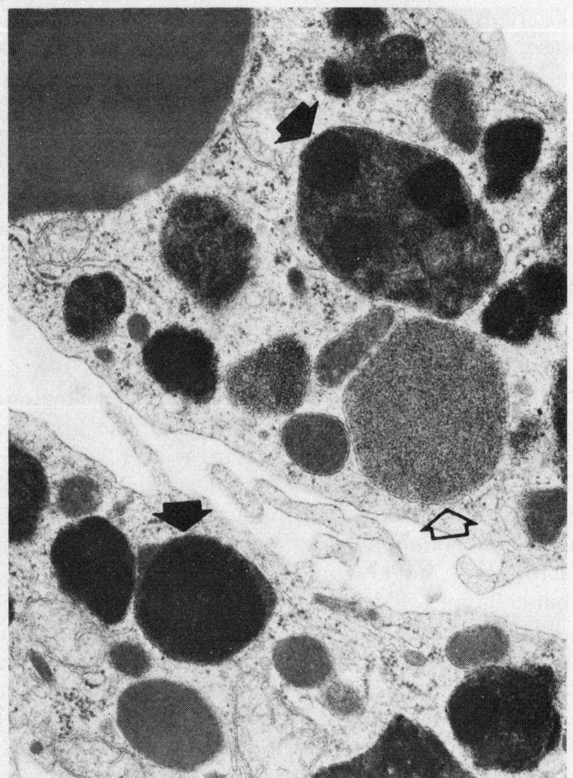

Figure 1–27. Hemosiderin granules in human splenic sinusoidal lining cells. Ferritin micelles *(open arrow)* are concentrated within siderosomes. The osmiophilic (black) material present in some siderosomes *(arrows)* is probably lipid. A recently engulfed (undigested) red blood cell is present in the upper left hand corner. (× 28000.) (Courtesy of Marcel Seiler, M.D., Roxbury Veterans Administration Medical Center.)

row, spleen, and liver, all actively engaged in red cell breakdown.

In many pathologic states, excesses of iron cause hemosiderin to accumulate within cells, either as a localized process or as a systemic derangement. Under all circumstances the hemosiderin (having ferric ions in the ferritin micelles) can be visualized by such histochemical procedures as the Prussian blue reaction. In this reaction, which can be applied to both gross and histologic sections of tissue, colorless potassium ferrocyanide reacts with the ferric ions to create an insoluble blue ferric ferrocyanide. This reaction helps to differentiate the golden pigmentation of hemosiderin from that produced by lipofuscin, and can exclude non–iron-containing melanin.

Local excesses of iron and hemosiderin result from gross hemorrhages or the myriad minute hemorrhages that accompany severe vascular congestion. The best example of localized hemosiderosis is the common bruise. Following local hemorrhage, the area is at first red-blue. With lysis of the erythrocytes, the hemoglobin eventually undergoes transformation to hemosiderin. Macrophages take part in this process by phagocytizing the red cell debris, and then lysosomal enzymes eventually convert the hemoglobin, through a sequence of pigments, into hemosiderin. The play of colors through which the bruise passes reflects these transformations. The original red-blue color of hemoglobin is transformed to varying shades of green-blue, comprising the local formation of biliverdin (green bile), then bilirubin (red bile), and in addition the iron moiety of hemoglobin is deposited as golden-yellow hemosiderin. The chronically congested lung in long-standing heart failure may become pigmented, owing to rupture of capillaries and phagocytosis of erythrocytes by alveolar macrophages.

Whenever there are causes for *systemic overload of iron,* hemosiderin is deposited in many organs and tissues, a condition called *hemosiderosis.* It is seen with (1) increased absorption of dietary iron, (2) impaired utilization of iron, (3) hemolytic anemias, and (4) transfusions, since the transfused red cells constitute an exogenous load of iron. These conditions are discussed on page 924.

The morphologic appearance of the pigment and its staining reactions are identical whatever the mechanism of its accumulation. It appears as a coarse, golden, granular pigment lying within the cell's cytoplasm. When the basic cause is the localized breakdown of red cells, the pigmentation is found at first in the reticuloendothelial cells in the area. In systemic hemosideroses, it is found at first in the mononuclear phagocytes of the liver, bone marrow, spleen, and lymph nodes and in scattered macrophages throughout other organs such as the skin, pancreas, and kidneys. With progressive accumulation, parenchymal cells throughout the body (principally in the liver, pancreas, heart, and endocrine organs) become pigmented.

In most instances of systemic hemosiderosis, the intracellular accumulations of pigment do not damage the parenchymal cells and so do not impair organ function. However, the more extreme accumulations of iron in a disease called *hemochromatosis* (p. 924) are associated with liver and pancreatic damage, resulting in liver fibrosis and diabetes mellitus.

Hematin. Hematin is a hemoglobin-derived pigment whose precise composition is unknown. It is encountered most commonly following a massive hemolytic crisis such as may occur with a transfusion reaction or in malaria, in which the parasite actively destroys red cells. The pigment is also golden-brown and granular and is virtually confined to mononuclear phagocytes. Because the iron is presumably bound into some organic complex with protein, it fails to give a positive reaction with the Prussian blue stain, although the iron is present in the ferric form.

Bilirubin. Bilirubin is the normal major pigment found in bile. It is derived from hemoglobin but contains no iron. Its normal formation and excretion are vital to health, and jaundice is a common clinical disorder due to excesses of this pigment within cells and tissues. Bilirubin metabolism and jaundice are discussed in detail on page 887.

Bilirubin pigment within cells and tissues is only morphologically visible when the patient is rather severely jaundiced for some period of time. Even though this pigment is distributed throughout all tissues and fluids of the body, the *accumulations are most evident in the liver and kidneys.* In the liver, particularly with diseases caused by obstruction of the outflow of bile (such as cancers of the common bile duct or head of the pancreas), bilirubin is encountered within bile sinusoids, Kupffer cells, and hepatocytes. *In all these sites, it appears as a mucoid, green-brown to black, amorphous, globular deposit.* In advanced cases of such obstructive jaundice, the aggregates of pigment may be quite large, creating so-called bile lakes. These may cause necrosis of hepatocytes in the focal area. Bilirubin pigment is encountered in the renal tubular epithelial cells in various forms of jaundice.

ALTERATIONS IN ORGANELLES AND CYTOSKELETON

Certain conditions are associated with rather distinctive alterations in cell organelles or cytoskeleton. Some of these alterations coexist with those described for acute lethal injury; others represent more chronic forms of cell injury, and others still are adaptive responses that involve specific cellular organelles. Here we shall touch on only some of the more common or interesting of these reactions.

LYSOSOMES: HETEROPHAGY AND AUTOPHAGY

As should be well known, lysosomes are membrane-bound cytoplasmic bodies, 0.2 to 0.8 μ in diameter, which contain a variety of hydrolytic enzymes including acid phosphatase, glucuronidase, sulfatase, ribonuclease, collagenase, and so on. These enzymes are synthesized in the rough endoplasmic reticulum and then packaged into vesicles in the Golgi apparatus (Fig. 1–28). At this stage they are called *primary lysosomes.* The latter have different appearances in different cells; for example, in the liver they resemble other Golgi vesicles, while in the neutrophils they have the characteristic appearance of *specific granules.* Primary lysosomes fuse with membrane-bound vacuoles that contain material to be digested (the latter called *phagosomes*), forming *secondary lysosomes* or *phagolysosomes.*

Phagolysosomes originate in one of two ways:

Heterophagocytosis refers to the uptake of materials from the external environment through the process of *endocytosis.* Uptake of particulate matter is known as *phagocytosis,* and that of soluble smaller macromolecules as *pinocytosis.* Heterophagy is most common in the "professional" phagocytes, such as neutrophils and macrophages, but also occurs to a certain extent in many other cell types. Examples of heterophagocytosis include the uptake and digestion of bacteria by neutrophilic leukocytes, the removal of necrotic cells by macrophages, and the reabsorption of protein that may filter across the renal glomerulus by the pinocytotic vesicles of the proximal convoluted tubules (heteropinocytosis).

Autophagocytosis. In many instances, individual cell organelles, such as mitochondria or endoplasmic reticulum, suffer focal injury and must then be digested if the cell's normal function is to be preserved. The lysosomes involved in such autodigestion are called *autolysosomes* and the process is called *autophagy.* Autophagy is particularly pronounced in cells undergoing atrophy.

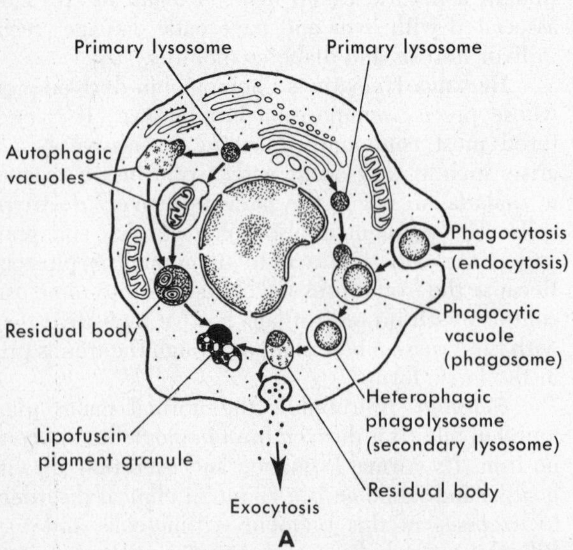

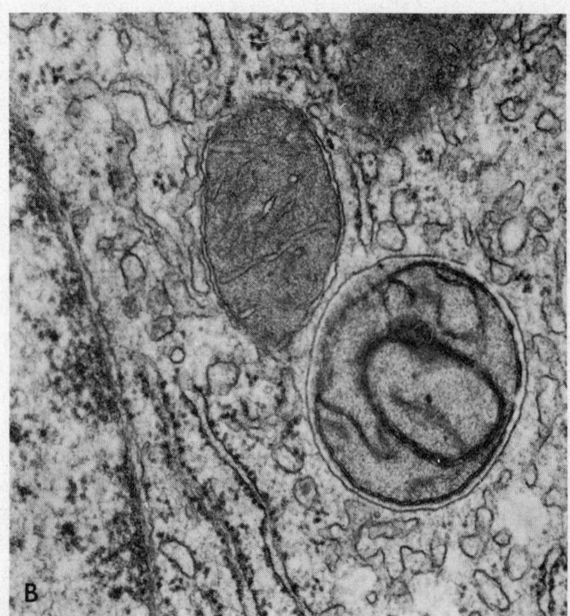

Figure 1–28. *A,* Schematic representation of autophagy *(left)* and heterophagy *(right).* (Redrawn from Bloom, W., and Fawcett, D. W.: A Textbook of Histology. 10th ed. Philadelphia, W. B. Saunders Co., 1975, p. 214.) *B,* Electron micrograph of an autolysosome containing a degenerating mitochondrion and amorphous material. (Courtesy of Dr. Fahimi.)

Both heterophagy and autophagy are very common intracellular processes and will be repeatedly alluded to in subsequent discussions of specific pathologic conditions such as inflammation, atrophy, and others. The enzymes in the lysosomes are capable of breaking down most proteins and carbohydrates, but some lipids remain undigested. Lysosomes with undigested debris may persist within cells as *residual bodies*, or may be extruded. *Lipofuscin pigment* granules, discussed earlier, represent undigested material that results from intracellular lipid peroxidation. Certain indigestible pigments, such as carbon particles inhaled from the atmosphere, or pigment inoculated in tattoos, can persist in phagolysosomes of macrophages for decades.

Lysosomes are also waste baskets in which cells sequester abnormal substances, particularly those of macromolecular nature, when these cannot be adequately metabolized. For example, in some hereditary diseases known as *lysosomal storage* disorders, deficiencies of certain enzymes that degrade mucopolysaccharides cause abnormal amounts of these compounds to be sequestered in the lysosomes. Such diseases are characterized by lysosomal deposits in cells all over the body, particularly in neurons, with often severe neurologic abnormalities.

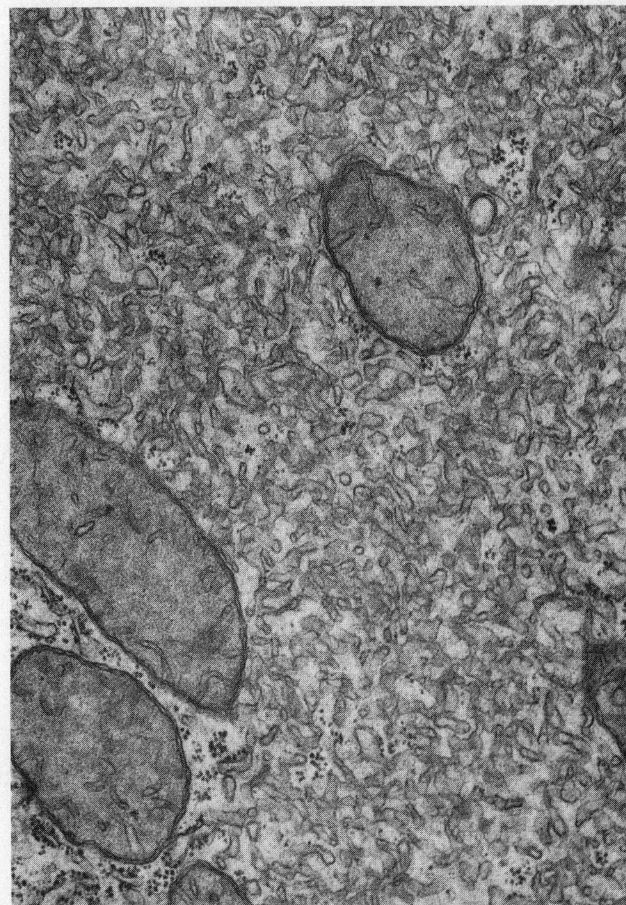

Figure 1–29. Electron micrograph of liver from phenobarbital-treated rat showing marked increase in smooth ER. (From Jones, A. L., and Fawcett, D. W.: Hypertrophy of the agranular endoplasmic reticulum in hamster liver induced by phenobarbital. J. Histochem. Cytochem., *14:215*, 1966. Copyright 1966, The Histochemical Society. Courtesy of Dr. Fawcett.)

HYPERTROPHY (INDUCTION) OF SMOOTH ENDOPLASMIC RETICULUM

This is an interesting adaptive response, first described by Jones and Fawcett[62] in hamster liver cells following administration of phenobarbital to these animals (Fig. 1–29). It is known that protracted human use of this hypnotic agent leads to a state of increased tolerance, so that repeated identical doses lead to progressively shorter time spans of sleep. The patients have thus "adapted" to the medication. The basis of this adaptation has been traced to induction of increased volume (hypertrophy) of the smooth endoplasmic reticulum (SER) of hepatocytes. Phenobarbital and other drugs are detoxified in the SER by the mixed-function oxidase electron transport pathway, the cytochrome P-450–centered drug metabolizing multienzyme complex. P-450 catalyzes the metabolism of a multitude of other exogenous compounds, including potentially carcinogenic hydrocarbons, steroids, and insecticides. It is noteworthy that cells adapted to one drug have increased capacity to detoxify other drugs handled by the system, or endogenous metabolic products, such as bilirubin and bile acids. This cross reactivity among drugs may be either harmful to or protective of the cell. For example, if CCl_4 is administered after phenobarbital, there is increased conversion of CCl_4 to the highly toxic free radical $CCl_3\cdot$, thus allowing very small amounts of CCl_4 to become toxic. On the other hand, the adaptive response may be protective if detoxification of the second agent has a salutary effect. Advantage is taken of such a protective effect in clinical practice. Bilirubin conjugation to bilirubin diglucuronide in the liver is catalyzed by glucuronyl transferase, which is present in the smooth endoplasmic reticulum. In genetic diseases characterized by low transferase activity (e.g., Gilbert's disease), treatment with phenobarbital will induce hyperplasia of the SER, increased enzyme levels, and correction of the defect. Since bilirubin can be excreted only in the diglucuronide form, this will mitigate the increases in blood bilirubin (and the jaundice) characteristic of such diseases.

MITOCHONDRIAL ALTERATIONS

We have seen that mitochondrial dysfunction plays an important role in acute cell injury. In addition, however, various alterations in the number, size, and shape of mitochondria occur in some pathologic conditions. For example, in hypertrophy and atrophy there is an increase and decrease, respectively, in the number of mitochondria in cells. Mitochondria may assume an extremely large and abnormal shape (megamitochondria) (Fig. 1–30). These can be seen in the liver in alcoholic

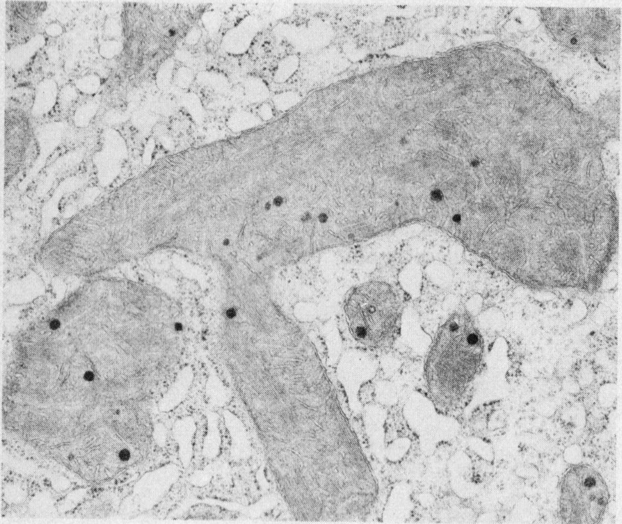

Figure 1–30. Enlarged, abnormally-shaped mitochondria from liver of patient with alcoholic cirrhosis. Note also crystalline formations in mitochondria. (Courtesy of Dr. Marcel W. Seiler, Boston, MA.)

liver disease and in certain nutritional deficiencies, in skeletal muscle fibers in some myopathies, and in other cells in which there is alteration in mitochondrial growth and replication. In addition, large and highly pleomorphic mitochondria are seen commonly in tumor cells.

ABNORMALITIES OF CYTOSKELETON AND MEMBRANE SKELETON

Abnormalities of the cytoskeleton and membrane skeleton are emerging as important determinants of certain disease states, and these will be alluded to repeatedly throughout the book. The *cytoskeleton* consists of microtubules (20–25 nm in diameter), thin actin filaments (6–8 nm), thick myosin filaments (15 nm), and various classes of intermediate filaments (10 nm).[63, 64] Several other nonpolymerized and nonfilamentous forms of contractile proteins also exist. Cytoskeletal abnormalities may be reflected by defects in cell function, such as cell locomotion and intracellular organelle movements, or in some instances by intracellular accumulations of fibrillar material. Only a few examples will be cited.

Functioning myofilaments and microtubules are essential for various stages of leukocyte migration and phagocytosis, and functional deficiencies of the cytoskeleton appear to underlie certain defects in leukocyte movement toward an injurious stimulus (chemotaxis, p. 51), or the ability of such cells to perform phagocytosis adequately. For example, a defect of microtubule polymerization in the *Chédiak-Higashi syndrome*[65] causes delayed or decreased fusion of lysosomes with phagosomes in leukocytes, and thus impairs phagocytosis (p. 52). Cytochalasin B, a drug that inhibits microfilament function, also affects phagocytosis. Other drugs, such as colchicine, cause disruption of microtubules, thus blocking mitosis in the metaphase by inhibiting spindle formation; morphologically, they cause aggregations of crystalline tubulin within the cytoplasm. Defects in the organization of microtubules in sperm inhibit sperm motility and cause male sterility, and a microtubule defect in the cilia of respiratory epithelium interferes with the ability of such epithelium to clear inhaled bacteria and predisposes to lung infections (the immotile cilia syndrome)[66] (p. 729).

As shown in Table 1–3, *intermediate filaments* are constituents of a variety of cell types and can be distinguished biochemically and immunochemically into *keratin* filaments, *neurofilaments*, *glial* filaments, *vimentin*, and *desmin*. Intermediate filaments are thought to mechanically integrate the organelles within the cytoplasm. Two common histologic entities have recently been traced to accumulations of intermediate filaments. One is the *Mallory body*, or "alcoholic hyaline," an eosinophilic intracytoplasmic inclusion in liver cells (Fig. 1–31A), which is highly characteristic of alcoholic liver disease but whose nature until recently has been obscure.[69] Such inclusions are now known to be composed largely of intermediate filaments (Fig. 1–31B) of predominantly *prekeratin* composition,[70] suggesting that a cytoskeletal defect with loss of intracellular organization may be a mechanism of cell injury in alcoholic liver disease.[54] Another is the *neurofibrillary tangle* found in the brains of patients with Alzheimer's disease, an important cause of presenile dementia. These entities are now thought to represent cross-linked neuronal intermediate filaments, and it is believed that such cross-linking may interfere with the dynamics of neuronal cytoskeleton and the maintenance of axons and dendrites.[71]

Finally, mention should be made of defects in the *"membrane skeleton,"* a filamentous meshwork of proteins lining the inner membrane surface of certain cells, particularly erythrocytes.[71] These proteins consist of *spectrin, actin, protein 4.1,* and *ankyrin* (Fig. 1–32), and their interactions determine the structural stability of the cell membrane. It has recently been shown that membrane-skeletal flaws may account for some important red cell disorders (p. 616).[71] For example, in some

Table 1–3. CONTRACTILE AND CYTOSKELETAL FILAMENTS

	Diameter (nm)	Mol. Weight (daltons)	Distribution
Actin	6–8	43	All cells
Myosin	15	450	Most cells
Tubulin (microtubules)	25	110	All cells
Intermediate filaments	8–10		
Keratins		40–65	Epithelial cells
Desmin		50	Muscle cells, fibroblasts
Vimentin		52	All mesenchymal cells ± epithelial cells
Glial filaments		51	Glial cells
Neurofilaments		68, 160, 210	Neurons

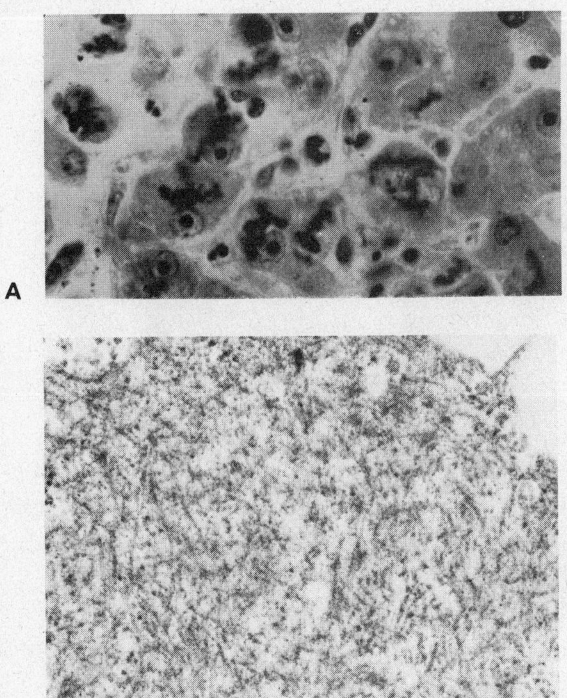

Figure 1–31. *A*, The liver of alcohol abuse (chronic alcoholism). Hyaline inclusions in hepatic parenchymal cells appear as dark, irregular networks disposed about the nuclei. *B*, Electron micrograph of alcoholic hyaline. The material is composed of intermediate (prekeratin) filaments and an amorphous matrix. (Courtesy of Dr. Marcel W. Seiler, Boston, MA.)

patients with *hereditary spherocytosis*, in which the red cells are spheroid rather than discoid (and more prone to fragmentation), the defect in red cell shape is caused by abnormal spectrin molecules that are incapable of binding protein 4.1 and thus unable to maintain the stability of the red cell membrane[72] (Fig. 1–32).

Undoubtedly the burgeoning field of "cytoskeletal pathology" will soon uncover many more instances in which abnormalities of the cytoskeleton or membrane skeleton contribute to the expression of disease.

CELLULAR ADAPTATIONS

Up to this point we have been discussing regressive alterations induced in cells by potentially lethal stimuli. However, cells may escape injury by adaptations to their environment, just as does the individual. Shivering is an adaptive response of the warm-blooded animal to low environmental temperatures. Unpleasant as the sensation may be, the increased muscular activity generates internal heat to compensate for the loss from the surface of the body. The cells do not shiver, but their increased metabolic activity is the ultimate source of the heat. Insofar as the body temperature is supported, no injury results to either the entire organism or its cells. In the same way, insofar as a cell can adapt to an alteration in its environment, it can escape injury. Cellular adaptation, then, is a state that lies intermediate between the normal, unstressed cell and the injured, overstressed cell.

The four most important adaptive changes in cells will be considered here. These include atrophy (decrease in cell size), hypertrophy (increase in cell size), hyperplasia (increase in cell number), and metaplasia (change in cell type).

ATROPHY

Shrinkage in the size of the cell by loss of cell substance is known as atrophy. It represents a form of

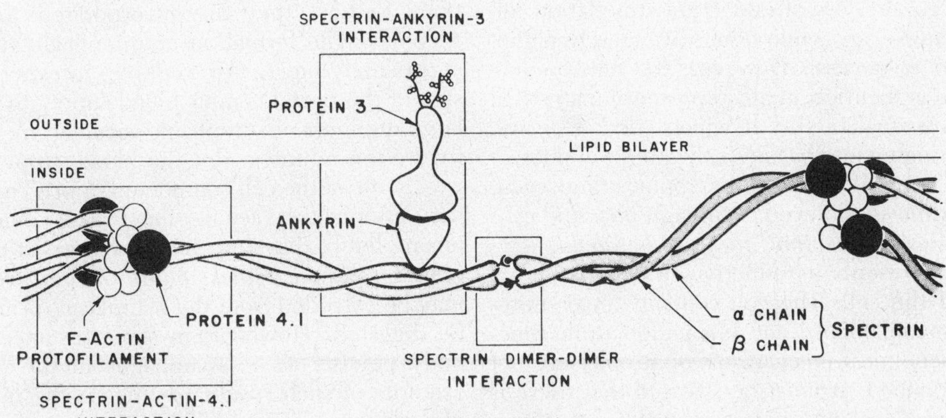

Figure 1–32. One model of the red cell membrane skeleton. Spectrin, a high-molecular-weight, usually flexible molecule, fastens to ankyrin by means of protein 3, an integral membrane protein that spans the lipid bilayer. It establishes lateral connections within the skeleton meshwork, partly by binding to F-actin protofilaments, a binding enhanced by protein 4.1. In hereditary spherocytosis, spectrin lacks the ability to bind protein 4.1. (From Wolfe, L. C., et al.: A genetic defect in the binding of protein 4.1 to spectrin in a kindred with hereditary spherocytosis. N. Engl. J. Med. *307*:1367, 1982. Reprinted by permission from The New England Journal of Medicine.)

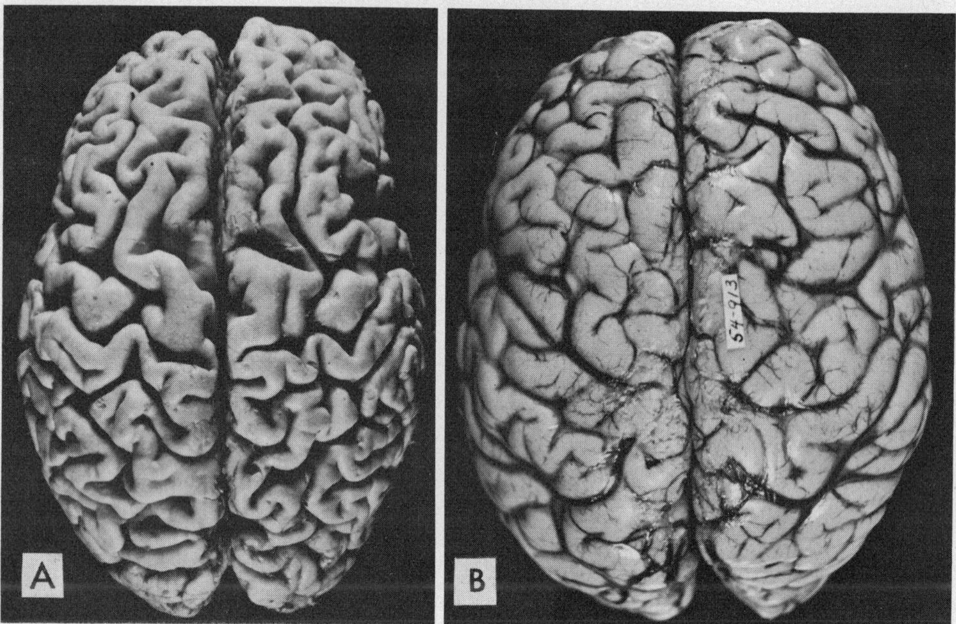

Figure 1–33. *A*, Physiologic atrophy of the brain in an 82-year-old male. The meninges have been stripped. *B*, Normal brain of 36-year-old male.

adaptive response. When a sufficient number of cells are involved, the entire tissue or organ diminishes in size, or becomes atrophic.

The apparent causes of atrophy are (1) decreased workload, (2) loss of innervation, (3) diminished blood supply, (4) inadequate nutrition, and (5) loss of endocrine stimulation. When a limb is immobilized in a plaster cast, or muscles become paralyzed from loss of innervation as in poliomyelitis, atrophy of cells ensues. In late adult life, the brain undergoes progressive atrophy, presumably as arteriosclerosis narrows its blood supply (Fig. 1–33) and the gonads shrink with depletion of endocrine stimulation. Some of these stimuli are physiologic (e.g., the loss of endocrine stimulation following the menopause), while others are clearly pathologic (e.g., loss of nerves). However, the fundamental cellular change is identical in all, representing a retreat by the cell to a smaller size at which survival is still possible. By bringing into balance cell volume and lower levels of blood supply, nutrition, or trophic stimulation, a new equilibrium is achieved. Although *atrophic cells may have diminished function, they are not dead.*

Atrophy represents a reduction in the structural components of the cell. The cell contains fewer mitochondria and myofilaments, and less endoplasmic reticulum. The biochemical mechanisms of atrophy are not very well understood. It must be stressed that there is a finely regulated balance between protein synthesis and degradation in normal cells, and either decreased synthesis, increased catabolism, or both may cause atrophy.[74] Hormones, particularly insulin, thyroid hormones, glucocorticoids, and prostaglandins influence such protein turnover. Thus, only slight increases of degradation over a long period of time may result in atrophy, as seems to occur in some muscle dystrophies.

In many situations atrophy is also accompanied by marked increases in the number of *autophagic vacuoles.* As stated earlier, these are membrane-bound vacuoles within the cell that contain fragments of cell components (e.g., mitochondria, ER), which are destined for destruction, and into which the lysosomes discharge their hydrolytic contents. The cellular components are then digested. *Autophagy* ("self-eating") is a mechanism by which injured organelles are isolated from unharmed organelles. The concentration of hydrolytic proteases within the cell increases in atrophy; however, these enzymes are not simply released into the cytoplasm, since this might lead to uncontrolled cellular destruction. Rather, they are incorporated into autophagic vacuoles. The formation of autophagic vacuoles can be surprisingly rapid. For example, in experimental occlusion of the portal venous blood supply to the liver lobe, large numbers of autophagic vacuoles are formed within five to ten minutes after the blood supply is occluded.

Some of the cell component debris contained within the autophagic vacuole may resist digestion, or be incompletely digested, and may persist as membrane-bound *residual bodies.* Some of these residual bodies may be extruded from the cytoplasm, or may eventually be digested. However, in some instances the residual body persists as a sarcophagus in the cytoplasm. An example of such residual bodies is the *lipofuscin granules,* discussed earlier (p. 23). When present in sufficient amounts, they impart a *brown discoloration* to the tissue (brown atrophy).

Obviously, atrophy may progress to the point at which cells are injured and die. If the blood supply is inadequate even to maintain the life of shrunken cells, injury and cell death may supervene. The atrophic cells are then replaced by connective and adipose tissue. The replacement with adipose tissue gives rise to so-called *stromal fatty infiltration* of tissues (p. 21).

HYPERTROPHY

Hypertrophy refers to an increase in the size of cells and, with such change, an increase in the size of the organ. Thus, the hypertrophied organ has no new cells, just larger cells. The increased size of cells is due not to an increased intake of fluid, called cellular swelling or edema, but to the synthesis of more structural components.

Hypertrophy can be caused by increased functional demand or by specific hormonal stimulation, and may occur under both physiologic and pathologic conditions. The physiologic growth of the uterus during pregnancy involves both hypertrophy and hyperplasia. The cellular hypertrophy is stimulated by estrogenic hormones through smooth muscle estrogen receptors, which allow for interactions of the hormones with nuclear DNA, eventually resulting in increased synthesis of smooth muscle proteins and increase in cell size. This is then physiologic hypertrophy effected by hormonal stimulation. Hypertrophy as an adaptive response was cited earlier in the discussion of muscular enlargement. The striated muscle cells in both the heart and skeletal muscle are most capable of hypertrophy, perhaps because they cannot adapt to increased metabolic demands by mitotic division and the formation of more cells to share the work.

The environmental change that produces hypertrophy of striated muscle appears principally to be increased workload, implying an increase in metabolic activity. There is synthesis of more membranes, more enzymes, more ATP, and more filaments capable of achieving an equilibrium between the demand and the cell's functional capacity. The greater number of myofilaments means an increased workload but with a level of metabolic activity per unit volume of cell not different from that borne by the normal myofilament. Thus, the draft horse readily pulls the load that would break the back of a pony.

Perhaps the best example of adaptive hypertrophy occurs in the heart in a variety of cardiovascular diseases that place increased burdens on the myocardium (Fig. 1–34). In patients with hypertension (high blood pressure), the heart, which must contract against increased pressures in the aorta, hypertrophies and may achieve weights of 700 to 800 gm instead of the normal weight of 350 gm. Similar cardiac hypertrophy occurs secondary to diseased cardiac valves. When valves are damaged, there is incomplete emptying of the cardiac chambers and stretching of the cardiac muscle fibers. The precise signal for hypertrophy under these conditions is unknown. ATP depletion, stretching of muscle fibers, activation by cell degradation products, and hormonal factors (e.g., thyroid hormones) have all been implicated.[75] Whatever the mechanism, there follows increased RNA synthesis, an increased protein synthesis, and the formation of a greater number of all organelles, including mitochondria, sarcoplasmic reticulum, and especially myofibrils.

Although muscular hypertrophy can be most simply seen as the result of increased synthesis of protein, recent studies have suggested that there is in addition a decrease in protein degradation, with a normal or slightly increased amount of protein synthesis. Intracellular enzymes, including proteases, are responsible for such protein degradation, and thus any alterations in these intracellular enzymes may affect cellular protein mass. Whatever the exact mechanism of hypertrophy, however, it eventually reaches a limit beyond which enlargement of muscle mass is no longer able to compensate for the increased burden, and cardiac failure ensues. At this stage, a number of "degenerative" changes occur in the myocardial fibers, of which the most important are lysis and loss of myofibrillar contractile elements. The limiting factors for continued hypertrophy and the causes of regressive changes are

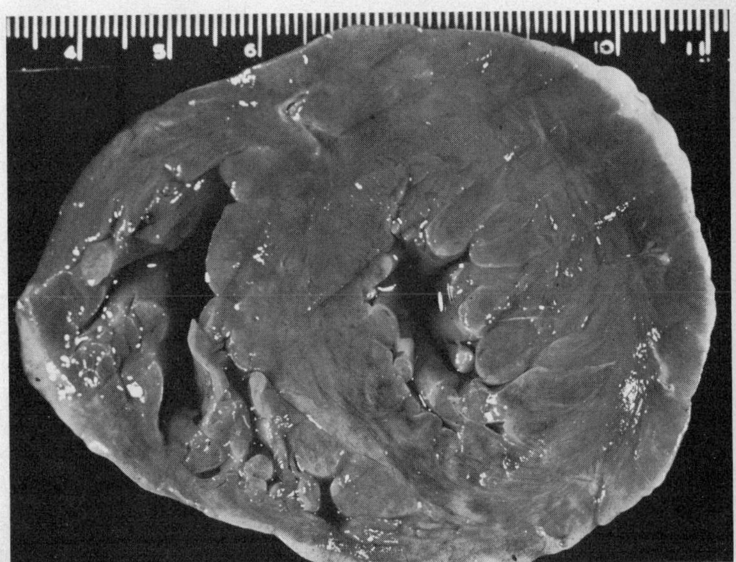

Figure 1–34. Cross section of a heart with marked left ventricular hypertrophy. The left ventricular wall is over 2 cm in thickness (normal = 1–1.5 cm). On the right side of the interventricular septum, the mottled, dark area is a focus of fresh ischemic necrosis (myocardial infarct).

incompletely understood; they may be due to limitation of the vascular supply to the enlarged fibers, diminished oxidative capabilities of mitochondria or to alterations in protein synthesis and degradation.

HYPERPLASIA

Just as enlargement of cells, hypertrophy, represents a response to increased functional demand, cells capable of mitotic division may divide when stressed or stimulated to increased activity. *Hyperplasia therefore constitutes an increase in the number of cells in an organ or tissue, which may then have increased volume.* Hypertrophy and hyperplasia are closely related and often develop concurrently. Both hypertrophy and hyperplasia take place if the cellular population is capable of synthesizing DNA, thus permitting mitotic division.

It should be emphasized initially that not all adult cell types have the same capacity for hyperplastic growth. Although skin epidermis, intestinal epithelium, hepatocytes, fibroblasts, and bone marrow cells can undergo profound hyperplasia, nerve cells and, for all practical purposes, cardiac and skeletal muscle cells have no capacity for hyperplastic growth. Intermediate among these are such tissues as bone, cartilage, and smooth muscle. The determinants of cell growth control are discussed more fully on page 75.

Hyperplasia traditionally has been divided into *physiologic* and *pathologic* hyperplasia.

Physiologic Hyperplasia. The two most common types of physiologic hyperplasia are (1) *hormonal hyperplasia*, best exemplified by the enlargement of the glandular epithelium of the female breast at puberty and during pregnancy, and the physiologic hyperplasia that occurs in the pregnant uterus; and (2) *compensatory hyperplasia*, e.g., the hyperplasia that occurs when a portion of the liver is removed (partial hepatectomy). The ancient Greeks knew of the capacity of the liver to regenerate. According to the myth, Prometheus was chained to a mountain, and his liver was daily devoured by a vulture only to regenerate anew every night.[76] In fact, the mitotic activity of hepatocytes increases after partial hepatectomy, eventually restoring the liver to normal weight. At this time (usually 12 days after partial hepatectomy in the rat), further growth stops. This is therefore a regulated form of hyperplasia that results in *regeneration* of the liver without appreciable increase in size or abnormal function. A similar sequence occurs in the epidermis following skin abrasion. If the superficial skin layers are removed, cells of the basal layer undergo increased mitosis that results in regeneration of the superficial layers and restoration of the original skin.

The model of partial hepatectomy has been especially useful in following the sequence of events in compensatory hyperplasia.[77] In the normal mature liver, only 0.5 to 1.0% of cells are dividing at any one time, as can be proved autoradiographically by injecting tritiated thymidine into the experimental animal. An increase in the number of DNA-synthesizing cells begins

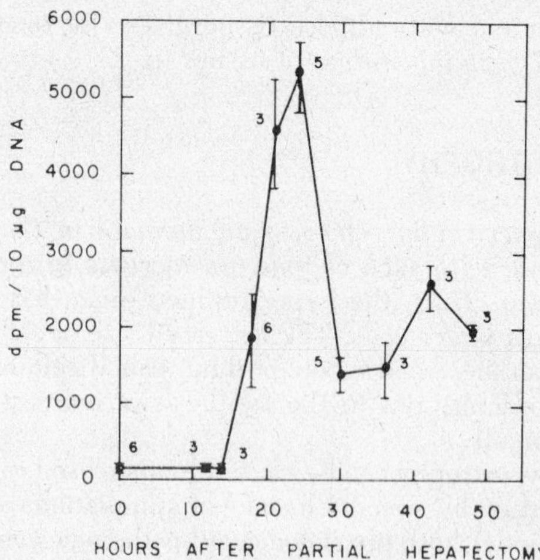

Figure 1–35. One-hour incorporation of ^{3}H-thymidine into hepatic DNA in 200-gm male Sprague Dawley rats at intervals after partial hepatectomy. Vertical lines indicate the standard error of the mean, numbers the number of rats per point. (From Bucher, N. L. R., and McGowan, J. A.: Regulatory mechanisms. *In* Wright, R., Albert, K. G. M. M., Karran, S., and Millward-Sadler, G. H. (eds.): Liver and Bilary Disease. Philadelphia, W. B. Saunders Co., 1979, pp. 210–227.)

as early as 12 hours after hepatectomy and peaks between one and two days, at which time about 10% of all cells may be involved in DNA synthesis (Fig. 1–35). Regeneration is complete by two weeks.

The ultimate mechanism that triggers this form of physiologic hyperplasia is not well understood. Although a number of factors may modify this response (age, sex, nutrition, etc.), there is substantial evidence that circulating humoral regulatory substances *stimulate* or *potentiate* cell growth after partial hepatectomy. The evidence can be summarized as follows:[78] (a) the liver in normal rats can be induced to synthesize DNA after blood transfusions from partially hepatectomized rats, (b) cross-circulation experiments using parabiotic rats (pairs of animals whose circulations are connected surgically) show that DNA synthesis is initiated in the intact liver of the unoperated animal after partial hepatectomy in the other member of the pair, (c) subcutaneous grafts of liver can be induced to synthesize DNA after partial hepatectomy of the host, and (d) primary cultures of differentiated liver cells respond to serum from partially hepatectomized rats by increasing their uptake of tritiated thymidine. The precise growth factors responsible for hepatic regeneration are unclear, but insulin, epidermal growth factor, and possibly glucagon appear to be involved. Alternatively, regeneration may be due to loss of inhibitory substances that in normal liver serve to maintain a low mitotic rate. Such substances, termed "chalones,"[79] have been postulated to control growth of epidermis, bone marrow cells, and other tissues, but thus far a "hepatic" chalone has not been identified (see also p. 76).

Pathologic Hyperplasia. Most forms of *pathologic hyperplasia* present instances of excessive hormonal stimulation of target cells. One of the most common examples is *adenomatous hyperplasia of the* *endometrium.* Following every normal menstrual period, there is a rapid burst of proliferative activity, which might be considered as reparative proliferation or physiologic hyperplasia in the endometrium. As is well known, this proliferation is potentiated by pituitary hormones and ovarian estrogen. It is brought to a halt by the rising levels of progesterone occurring usually about 10 to 14 days before the anticipated menstrual period. In some instances, however, the balance between estrogen and progesterone is disturbed. This results in absolute and/or relative increases in the amount of estrogen, with consequent hyperplasia of the endometrial glands. Although this form of hyperplasia is a common cause of abnormal menstrual bleeding, the hyperplastic process remains controlled nonetheless: if the estrogenic stimulation abates, the hyperplasia disappears. Thus, it responds to regular growth control of cells. As will be discussed in the chapter on neoplasia (p. 230), it is this response to normal regulatory control mechanisms that differentiates benign pathologic hyperplasias from cancer. However, it should be stressed here that *pathologic hyperplasia constitutes a fertile soil in which cancerous proliferation may eventually arise.* Thus, patients with adenomatous hyperplasia of the endometrium are at increased risk of developing endometrial cancer (see p. 1134).

To summarize, hyperplasia (either physiologic or pathologic) is induced by known stimuli. It is a controlled process inasmuch as it stops when the stimulus has ceased. It can, however, repair a defect or reconstitute an organ, and it may serve a useful purpose, such as preparing breast tissue for lactation or compensating for tissue destroyed by disease. Neoplasia obeys none of these rules and serves none of these purposes. It is to be remembered, however, that in a small but real number of instances it appears that the mitotic and metabolic activities that result in hyperplasia provide a subsoil for carcinogenic influences. However, although there are a number of proposed cell cycle models to account for the differences between hyperplasia and neoplasia,[80] none of these is proven.

Although hypertrophy and hyperplasia are, by definition, two distinct processes, it is clear that in many instances both occur together and, further, are triggered by the same mechanism. Estrogen-induced growth in the uterus is the classic example. Uterine epithelium and smooth muscle undergo both increased DNA synthesis and enlargement of cells. In fact, there is probably more hypertrophy than hyperplasia in this condition. Both processes are initiated by binding of estrogen to a receptor complex in the cytoplasm of target cells.[81] Even in nondividing cells that undergo only hypertrophy (such as myocardial fibers), events occur that result in an increase in or derepression of DNA synthesis; the nuclei thus have a much higher DNA content than normal myocardial cells. In fact, a large percentage of cells from severely hypertrophied hearts are polyploid, and large, bizarre nuclei are seen in hypertrophied myocardial fibers. A likely explanation for such polyploidy is that the cells arrest in the G_2 phase of the cell cycle without undergoing mitosis.[76] Baserga suggests that hypertrophy and hyperplasia may to a large extent share common biochemical events, at least until the completion of DNA synthesis.[76] The events that cause a particular cell to block in G_2 and undergo hypertrophy, or go through the full cycle and divide, are under investigation.

METAPLASIA

Metaplasia is a reversible change in which one adult cell type (epithelial or mesenchymal) is replaced by another adult cell type. It, too, may represent an adaptive substitution of cells more sensitive to stress by other cell types better able to withstand the adverse environment. Such adaptive metaplasia is best seen in the squamous metaplasia that occurs in the respiratory tract in response to chronic irritation. In the habitual cigarette smoker, the normal columnar ciliated epithelial cells of the trachea and bronchi are often replaced focally or widely by stratified squamous epithelial cells. Similar changes may be encountered in chronic infections of the bronchi and bronchioles. Stones in the excretory ducts of the salivary glands, pancreas, or bile ducts may cause replacement of the normal secretory columnar epithelium by nonfunctioning stratified squamous epithelium (Fig. 1–36). For less clear reasons, a deficiency of vitamin A induces squamous metaplasia in the respiratory epithelium. In all these instances, the more rugged stratified squamous epithelium is able to survive under circumstances in which the more fragile specialized epithelium most likely would have succumbed.

Metaplastic cells probably arise from abnormal differentiation of undifferentiated stem cells, but there is some evidence of metaplasia also arising from division

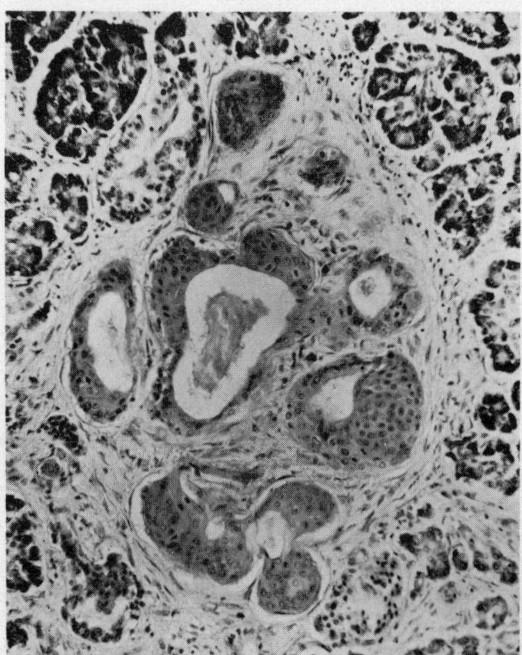

Figure 1–36. Metaplastic transformation of adult columnar epithelial cells to adult stratified squamous cells in pancreatic ducts.

of preexisting differentiated cells.[83] Although the squamous metaplastic cells in the respiratory tract, for example, are capable of surviving, an important protective mechanism—mucus secretion—is lost. Thus, epithelial metaplasia is a two-edged sword and, in most circumstances, represents an undesirable change. *Moreover, the influences that predispose to such metaplasia, if persistent, may induce cancerous transformation in the metaplastic epithelium.* Thus, the common form of cancer in the respiratory tract is composed of squamous cells.

Metaplasia may also occur in mesenchymal cells but less clearly as an adaptive response. Fibroblasts may become transformed to osteoblasts or chondroblasts to produce bone or cartilage where it is normally not encountered. For example, bone is occasionally formed in soft tissues, particularly in foci of injury. This process represents a form of "divergent differentiation." Similar abnormal differentiation is sometimes encountered in tumors in which genetic coding, apparently repressed in the normal cells from which the tumor derived, becomes expressed when the cells lose certain of their controls and become tumorigenic.

DYSPLASIA

Dysplasia is an alteration in adult cells characterized by variation in their size, shape, and organization. It is a controversial term in pathology, used both loosely and commonly. Strictly speaking, *dysplasia means deranged development; however, in common medical usage it is applied to either epithelial or mesenchymal cells, principally the former, that have undergone somewhat irregular, atypical proliferative changes in response to chronic irritation or inflammation.* It is not an adaptive process but is considered here because it is closely related to hyperplasia; indeed, it is sometimes called *atypical hyperplasia.*

Epithelial dysplasia presents as a loss of normal orientation of one epithelial cell to the other, accompanied by alterations in cellular size and shape, nuclear size and shape, and staining characteristics. It is most commonly encountered in the uterine cervix but often affects other epithelia. The dysplastic stratified squamous epithelium is thickened by hyperplasia of basal cells, accompanied by disordered maturation of the cells as they proceed to the surface layers. Mitotic figures are found only in the basal layer in normal cervical mucosa but, in dysplastic cervical epithelium, they may be found in the mid levels or even toward the surface. The increased proliferative activity produces greater amounts of DNA and more intense basophilia of the nuclei (Fig. 1–37). Although mitoses are increased in number, they are not usually abnormal, such as is characteristic of cancer.

Dysplastic changes also are frequently encountered

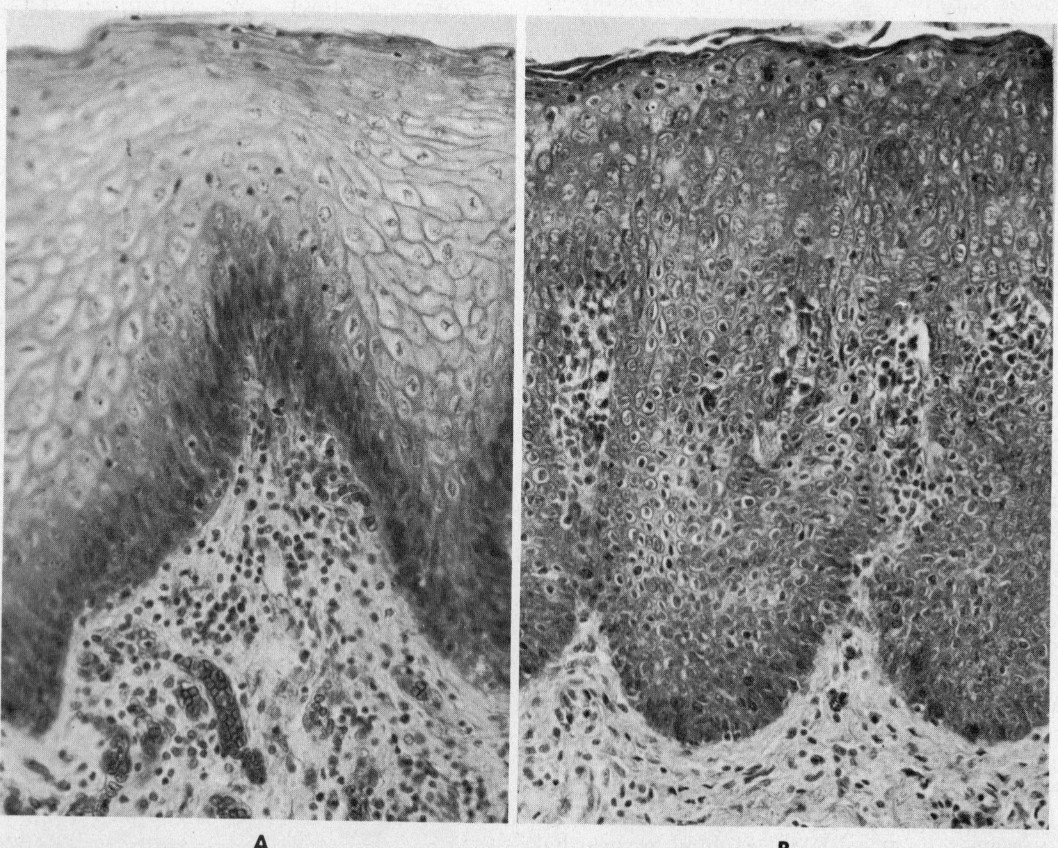

Figure 1–37. *A,* Normal stratified squamous epithelium. *B,* Dysplastic stratified squamous epithelium. The basal cells are hyperplastic and form a zone many cells thick. The dysplastic cells are deeply chromatic and disorganized.

in the metaplastic squamous epithelium of the respiratory tract in habitual cigarette smokers. *In both the cervix and the respiratory tract, such dysplasia is strongly implicated in the causation of cancer.* Dysplastic changes are often found adjacent to foci of cancerous transformation and, in long-term studies of cigarette smokers, epithelial dysplasia almost invariably precedes in time the appearance of cancer. However, from many clinical studies, it is known that dysplasia does not necessarily progress to cancer. The changes may be reversible and, with removal of the inciting causes, the epithelium may revert to normal.

SUNDRY ALTERATIONS

CALCIFICATION

Pathologic calcification implies the abnormal deposition of calcium salts, together with smaller amounts of iron, magnesium, and other mineral salts. It is a common process occurring in a variety of pathologic conditions. When the deposition occurs in dead or dying tissues, it is known as *dystrophic calcification;* it may occur despite normal serum levels of calcium and in the absence of derangements in calcium metabolism. In contrast, the deposition of calcium salts in vital tissues is known as *metastatic calcification,* and it almost always reflects some derangement in calcium metabolism, leading to hypercalcemia.

DYSTROPHIC CALCIFICATION. This alteration is encountered in areas of coagulation, caseous and liquefactive necrosis, and also in foci of enzymic necrosis of fat whenever the necrotic tissue persists for long period of time. Thus, calcification is frequently seen in chronic tuberculosis of the lungs or lymph nodes. It also commonly develops in damaged heart valves, further hampering their function (Fig. 1–38). Calcification is almost inevitable in the atheromas of advanced atherosclerosis, which, as will be seen, are focal intimal injuries in the aorta and larger arteries characterized by the accumulation of lipids (p. 506). Whatever the site of deposition, the calcium salts appear macroscopically as fine, white granules or clumps, often felt as gritty deposits. Sometimes, a tuberculous lymph node is virtually converted to stone.

Histologically, with the usual H and E stain, the calcium salts have a basophilic, amorphous granular, sometimes clumped appearance. They can be *intracellular, extracellular,* or *in both locations.* In the course of time, *heterotopic bone* may be formed in the focus of calcification. On occasion, single necrotic cells may constitute seed crystals that become encrusted by the mineral deposits. The progressive acquisition of outer layers may create lamellated configurations called *psammoma bodies* because of their resemblance to grains of sand. Some types of papillary cancers (e.g., thyroid) are apt to develop psammoma bodies. Strange concretions emerge when calcium iron salts gather about long slender spicules of asbestos in the lung, creating exotic, beaded dumbbell forms.

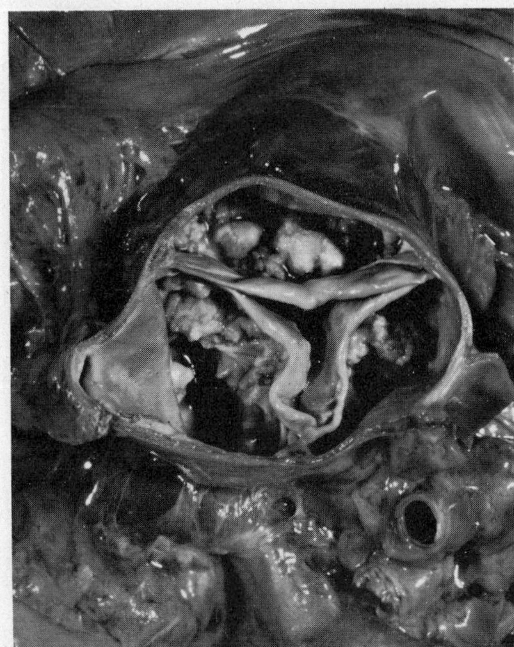

Figure 1–38. Massive calcific nodules in the sinuses of the cusps of the aortic valve—dystrophic calcification of a previously injured tissue. (View is looking down on cusps from aortic side.)

The pathogenesis of dystrophic calcification is beginning to be unraveled.[84, 85] The final common pathway is the formation of crystalline calcium phosphate mineral in the form of hydroxyapatite (a compound with 10 calcium atoms, 6 phosphate, and 2 hydroxyl groups). The process has two major phases: *initiation* and *propagation.* Initiation in *extracellular* sites occurs in membrane-bound *vesicles,* about 200 nm in diameter; in cartilage and bone they are known as *matrix vesicles,* and in pathologic calcification they seem to be derived from degenerating or aging cells. It is thought that calcium is concentrated in these vesicles by its affinity to acidic phospholipids, and phosphates accumulate as a result of the action of membrane-bound phosphatases. Initiation of *intracellular* calcification occurs in the *mitochondria* of dead or dying cells that accumulate calcium, as described earlier. After mineral initiation in either location, propagation of crystal formation occurs, dependent on the concentration of Ca^{++} and PO_4 in the extracellular spaces, the presence of mineral inhibitors, and the presence of collagen. The latter appears to increase the rate of crystal proliferation.

Although dystrophic calcification may be simply a "telltale" sign of previous cell injury, it is often a cause of organ dysfunction. Such is the case in calcific valvular disease and arteriosclerosis, as will become clear in further discussion of these diseases.

METASTATIC CALCIFICATION. This alteration may occur in normal tissues whenever there is hypercalcemia. Hypercalcemia also accentuates dystrophic calcification. The causes of hypercalcemia include hyperparathyroidism, vitamin D intoxication, systemic sarcoidosis, milk-alkali syndrome, hyperthyroidism, idiopathic hypercalcemia of infancy, Addison's disease (adrenocortical in-

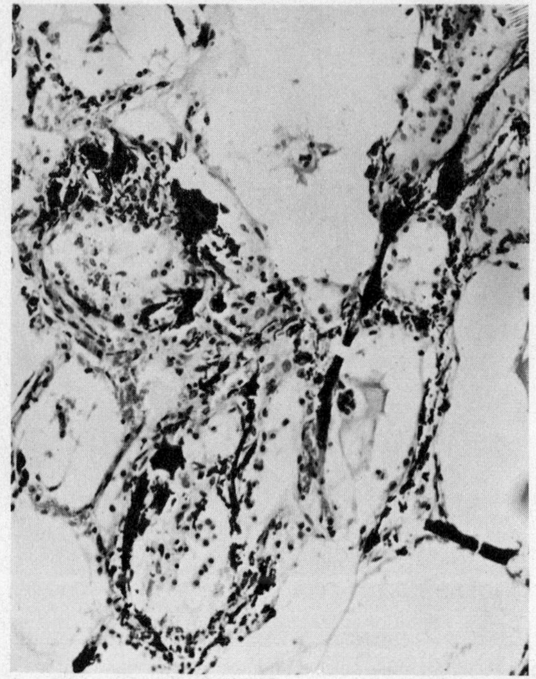

Figure 1–39. Irregular, dark, calcific precipitates within the walls of the pulmonary alveolar septa in a patient with hyperparathyroidism.

sufficiency), increased bone catabolism associated with disseminated bone tumors (such as multiple myeloma and metastatic cancer) and leukemia, and decreased bone formation as occurs in immobilization. Hypercalcemia also arises in some instances of advanced renal failure with phosphate retention, leading to secondary hyperparathyroidism.

Metastatic calcification may occur widely throughout the body but principally affects the interstitial tissues of the blood vessels, kidneys, lungs, and gastric mucosa (Fig. 1–39). In all these sites, the calcium salts morphologically resemble those described in dystrophic calcification. Thus, they may occur as noncrystalline amorphous deposits or, at other times, as hydroxyapatite crystals. Metastatic calcification appears to begin also in mitochondria, except in kidney tubules where it develops in the basement membranes, probably in relation to extracellular vesicles budding from the epithelial cells.

In general, the mineral salts cause no clinical dysfunction but, on occasion, massive involvement of the lungs produces remarkable x-ray films and respiratory deficits. Massive deposits in the kidney (nephrocalcinosis) may in time cause renal damage.

HYALINE CHANGE

The term hyaline is a widely used descriptive histologic term rather than a specific marker for cell injury. *Hyaline refers to any alteration within cells or in the extracellular space, which gives a homogeneous, glassy, pink appearance in routine histologic sections stained with H and E.* It may then represent an intracellular accumulation or be the consequence of extracellular deposits. This tinctorial change is produced by a variety of alterations and does not represent a specific pattern of accumulation. Thus, it is important, when describing hyaline change, to be cognizant of the possible mechanisms of its formation. In some instances the mechanism is clearly known; in others it is obscure.

Some examples of *intracellular hyaline* change are the following: (1) The hyaline droplets seen in the proximal tubular epithelial cells of the kidney have already been referred to (p. 21). In most instances they represent reabsorption of excessive amounts of protein that have leaked across the glomerular filter. (2) In plasma cells, spherical hyaline deposits represent aggregates of immunoglobulin synthesized in the rough endoplasmic reticulum of the cell, so called Russell bodies. (3) Many viral infections are associated with the appearance of hyaline inclusions within either the cytoplasm or the nucleus. In some instances these are accumulations of viral nucleoproteins. (4) As described earlier, the characteristic hyaline inclusions in the liver cells of alcoholics, "alcoholic hyaline," consist of aggregates of prekeratin intermediate filaments.

Extracellular hyaline has been somewhat more difficult to analyze. Collagenous fibrous tissue in old scars may appear hyalinized, but the physicochemical mechanism underlying this change is not clear. In long-standing hypertension and diabetes mellitus the walls of arterioles, especially in the kidney, become hyalinized. As we shall see (p. 518), such *hyaline arteriolosclerosis* in renal vessels has important diagnostic and pathogenetic implications. It appears that much of the hyaline is composed of precipitated plasma proteins that have leaked across injured endothelium into the arteriolar wall. There is also some reduplication of the basement membrane of the arterioles. Another example of extracellular hyaline is the hyalinization of glomeruli of the kidney when these undergo chronic damage. Here the hyaline appears to be a conglomeration of plasma proteins, basement membrane material, and mesangial matrix (p. 993). With H and E stains, the protein *amyloid* (p. 196) also has a hyaline appearance. But this is a very specific fibrillar protein, with a characteristic biochemical composition. Amyloid can be clearly identified by its special staining characteristics with the Congo red stain, with which it appears red and shows bipolar refringence.

Thus, although one continues to use the convenient term hyaline, it is important to recognize the multitude of mechanisms that produce this change and the implications of the alteration when it is seen in different pathologic conditions.

CELLULAR AGING

The process of aging or senescence in the organism involves complex interactions of genetic, metabolic, hormonal, immunologic, and structural influences at the level of organs, tissues, and cells. Here we shall discuss *cellular aging* because it could represent the progressive accumulation, over the years, of alterations in structure and function that may lead to cell death or at least to a diminished capacity of the cell to respond to injury. The pursuit of immortality has preoccupied man since the beginning of time. Yet, although life expectancy has increased in the past century, such achievements as have been made simply allow more people to reach the limit of what appears to be a fixed life span. If the three leading causes of death in the United States—heart disease, stroke, and cancer—were completely eliminated, only 10 to 20 years of additional life could be expected.[85]

The aging of a person can be regarded as the composite effect of aging of cells. But why and how do cells age? We have no answer to these questions, and controversies abound among experts. It is useful, at least as a working concept, to think of two events that lead to cell senescence.[86] The first (and more controversial) *is the existence of a built-in genetic program that limits the replicative life span of various normal somatic cells (clonal senescence).* The second event is the occurrence of alterations in cells no longer capable of mitotic replication, and hence no longer capable of compensating (by increasing the numbers of progeny) for deficiencies in cell numbers, structure, or function. This is called *postreplicative senescence* and could be the consequence of repeated cell injury.

The notion that each cell type has a limited, genetically determined replicative life span has come from tissue culture studies, principally those of Hayflick.[85] He showed that human diploid fibroblast-like cells in culture regularly achieve only 50 ± 10 doublings, after which they undergo senescence and then death of the whole population. (This is in contrast to transformed malignant cells, which replicate indefinitely.) This phenomenon was not related to restrictions imposed by the culture conditions.

Of the mechanisms invoked to explain a limited life span,[87] some postulate changes in the genetic loci that code for proteins involved in correcting the various subtle mutations that occur during the life span of the cell, e.g., DNA repair enzymes (the so-called intrinsic mutagenesis theory of aging). Others invoke changes in expression of the genetic material. Considerable evidence is available suggesting that aging of fibroblasts is accompanied by defects in enzymes, genes, chromosomes, DNA replication, and DNA repair—changes that might be expected if errors in molecules were accumulating.

Some workers consider the limited growth of diploid fibroblasts an artifact of normal culturing procedures.[86] It has been theorized that replicating cells are potentially immortal (i.e., there is no *genetic* limit on the replicative span), but there is always a given probability that mitosis will give rise to cells that divide but *are irreversibly committed to senescence and cell death* (the commitment theory of cell aging).[88] Immortal uncommitted cells are diluted by committed ones and may ultimately be lost in subculturing, thus explaining the eventual cessation of division in culture. Yet the concept of limited replicative ability has great appeal, and a restricted replicative span of fibroblasts has been claimed in some diseases. For example, in diabetes mellitus, decreased growth of fibroblasts in culture has been implicated in the pathogenesis of diabetic microvascular disease.[89]

In contrast to the controversial concept of limited replication, there is agreement that changes that occur in postreplicating cells are important in cellular aging. *Morphologically* postreplicative senescent cells in culture become larger, are occasionally multinucleate, develop vacuoles of various sizes, and are more prone to injury than nonsenescent cells. *In vivo* it is difficult to ascribe any single morphologic or biochemical change to cell aging. In the central nervous system, a well-documented example of age-related cell change is *neuronal cell loss,* which occurs in some of the Purkinje cells in the cerebellum. In neurons, there is also a characteristic "neurofibrillary degeneration" that occurs in aging brains and is more pronounced in patients with senile dementia and Alzheimer's disease, in whom there is premature senility (p. 1414). Structural alterations also occur in the DNA of senescent brain cells. There is also a decrease in the number of varieties of RNA species in senescent whole brain.[90] There are several interpretations of these biochemical derangements in DNA, RNA, and other molecules. A large number of environmental agents, to which aging individuals are increasingly exposed, are capable of causing somatic mutations by their damaging effect on DNA. These include ultraviolet light, x-rays, chemicals, and food products. However, such agents may also affect other cytoplasmic constituents directly (e.g., ER, cell membranes, mitochondria, ribosomes), and it is not possible at present to decide whether molecular injury to DNA or other macromolecules, or both, may contribute to the process.

You will recall that another known morphologic marker for aging is the accumulation of lipofuscin pigment in cells, the yellow-brown wear-and-tear pigment that is the final breakdown product of autophagic vacuoles. The biochemical composition of lipofuscin suggests that it is derived through lipid peroxidation and is consistent with the so-called "free radical theory" of aging, discussed earlier (p. 13).

In the final analysis there is probably no single cause for cellular aging.[85] It is clear that with aging numerous phenotypic alterations appear in both replicating and nonreplicating somatic cells. But which of these is the result of some genotypic programming is unknown.

In closing this consideration of the various forms of cellular derangement, it is apparent that they cover a wide spectrum, ranging from the reversible and irreversible forms of cell injury to the less ominous forms of intracellular accumulations, including pigmentations. Reference will be made to all these alterations throughout this book because all organ injury and, ultimately, all clinical disease arise from derangements in cell structure and function.

1. Hill, R. B.: Pathobiology and disease. *In* Hill, R. B., and LaVia, M. F. (eds.): Principles of Pathobiology. New York, Oxford University Press, 1980, pp. 3–20.
2. Majno, G.: The Healing Hand. Cambridge, MA, Harvard University Press, 1975, p. 43.
3. Jennings, R. B., and Reimer, K. A.: Lethal myocardial ischemic injury. Am. J. Pathol. *102*:241, 1981.
4. Rude, R. E., et al.: Efforts to limit the size of myocardial infarction. Ann. Intern. Med. *95*:736, 1981.
5. Jennings, R. B., et al.: Relationship between high energy phosphate and lethal injury in myocardial ischemia in the dog. Am. J. Pathol. *92*:187, 1978.
6. Vogt, M. T., and Farber, E.: On the molecular pathology of the ischemic renal cell death. Reversible and irreversible cellular and mitochondrial metabolic alterations. Am. J. Pathol. *53*:1, 1968.
7. Trump, B. F., et al.: Cellular reaction to injury. *In* Hill, R., and LaVia, M. (eds.): Principles of Pathobiology. New York, Oxford University Press, 1980, pp. 20–111.
8. Cowley, R. A., and Trump, B. F.: Pathophysiology of Shock, Anoxia and Ischemia. Baltimore, Williams & Wilkins Co., 1981.
9. Venkatachalam, M. A., et al.: Ischemic damage and repair in the rat proximal tubule: Differences among the S_1, S_2, and S_3 segments. Kidney Int. *14*:31, 1978.
10. Welsh, F. A.: Factors limiting regeneration of ATP following temporary ischemia in cat brain. Stroke *13*:234, 1982.
11. Farber, E., et al.: Cell suicide and cell death. *In* Aldridge, W. N. (ed.): Mechanisms of Toxicity. London, Macmillan & Co., 1971, pp. 163–170.
12. Farber, J. L., et al.: The pathogenesis of irreversible cell injury in ischemia. Am. J. Pathol. *102*:271, 1981.
13. Venkatachalam, M. A., et al.: Salvage of ischemic cells by impermeant solute and ATP. Lab. Invest. *49*:1, 1983.
14. Shull, K. H.: Hepatic phosphorylase and adenosine triphosphate levels in ethionine-treated rats. J. Biol. Chem. *237*:1734, 1962.
15. Mittnacht, S., Jr., and Farber, J. L.: Reversal of ischemic mitochondrial dysfunction. J. Biol. Chem. *256*:3199, 1982.
16. Farber, J. L.: Membrane injury and calcium homeostasis in the pathogenesis of coagulative necrosis. Lab. Invest. *47*:114, 1982.
17. Katz, A. M., and Messineo, F. C.: Lipid-membrane interactions and the pathogenesis of ischemic damage in the myocardium. Circ. Res. *48*:1, 1981.
18. Chien, K. R., et al.: Phospholipid alterations in canine ischemic myocardium. Temporal and topographical correlations with Tc-99-m-PPi accumulation and an *in vitro* sarcolemmal calcium permeability defect. Circ. Res. *48*:711, 1981.
19. Burton, K. P., et al.: Lanthanum probe studies of cellular pathophysiology induced by hypoxia in isolated cardiac muscle. J. Clin. Invest. *60*:1289, 1977.
20. Shine, K. I.: Ionic events in ischemia and anoxia. Am. J. Pathol. *102*:256, 1981.
21. Macknight, A., and Leaf, A.: Regulation of cellular volume. Physiol. Res. *57*:510, 1977.
22. Chien, K. R., et al.: Accelerated phospholipid degradation and associated membrane dysfunction in irreversible ischemic injury. J. Biol. Chem., *253*:4809, 1978.
23. Matsumoto, J., et al.: Phospholipid metabolism of dog liver under hypoxic conditions induced by ligation of hepatic artery. Biochim. Biophys. Acta *664*:527, 1981.
24. Nayler, W. G.: The role of calcium in the ischemic myocardium. Am. J. Pathol. *102*:262, 1981.
25. Streenbergen, C., and Jennings, R. B.: Relation between lysophospholipid accumulation and plasma membrane injury during total *in vitro* ischemia in dog heart. J. Mol. Cell. Cardiol., in press.
26. Matthys, E., et al.: Membrane lipid alterations during and after renal ischemia in rats: Lipid hydrolysis, lipid breakdown products and membrane damage. Kidney Int., in press.
27. Neely, J. R., and Fenvray, D.: Metabolic products and myocardial ischemia. Am. J. Pathol. *102*:282, 1981.
28. Higgins, T. J. C., et al.: Interrelationship between cellular metabolic status and susceptibility of heart cells to attack by phospholipase. J. Mol. Cell. Cardiol. *14*:645, 1982.
29. Farber, J. L.: Reactions of the liver to injury: Necrosis. *In* Farber, E., and Fisher, M. M. (eds.): Toxic Liver Injury. New York, Marcel Dekker, 1978.
29. Zimmerman, H. J.: Hepatotoxicity: The adverse effects of drugs and other chemicals on the liver. New York, Appleton-Century-Crofts, 1978.
30. Casini, A., et al.: Mechanisms of cell injury in the killing of cultured hepatocytes by bromobenzene. J. Biol. Chem. *257*:6721, 1982.
31. Pryor, W. A. (ed.): Free Radicals in Biology. New York, Academic Press, Vols. 1–6, 1976–1983.
32. Weiss, S. J., and LoBuglio, A. F.: Phagocyte-generated oxygen metabolites and cellular injury. Lab. Invest. *47*:5, 1982.
33. Mason, R. P., and Chignell, C. F.: Free radicals in pharmacology and toxicology. Pharmacol. Rev. *33*:189, 1982.
34. Autor, A. (ed.): Pathology of Oxygen. New York, Academic Press, 1982.
35. Freeman, B. A., and Crapo, J. D.: Biology of disease: Free radicals and tissue injury. Lab. Invest. *47*:412, 1982.
36. Plaa, G. L., and Witschi, H.: Chemicals, drugs and lipid peroxidation. Am. Rev. Toxicol. Pharmacol. *16*:125, 1976.
37. Recknagel, R. O., and Glende, E. A.: Carbon tetrachloride hepatotoxicity: An example of lethal cleavage. CRC Crit. Rev. Toxicol. *2*:263, 1973.
38. Smuckler, E. A.: Alterations produced in the endoplasmic reticulum by carbon tetrachloride. Panminerva Med. *18*:292, 1976.
39. Roders, M. K., et al.: NADPH-dependent microsomal lipid peroxidation and the problem of pathological action at a distance. New data on induction of red cell damage. Biochem. Pharmacol. *27*:437, 1978.
40. Benedetti, A., et al.: Cytotoxic effects of carbonyl compounds originating from the peroxidation of microsomal lipids. *In* McBrian, D. (ed.): Recent Advances in Lipid Peroxidation. London, Bruenel University Press, 1982.
41. Fantone, J. C., and Ward, P. A.: Role of oxygen derived free radicals and metabolites in leukocyte-dependent inflammatory reactions. Am. J. Pathol. *107*:397, 1982.
42. Suttorp, N., and Simon, L. M.: Lung cell oxidant injury. J. Clin. Invest. *70*:342, 1982.
43. Martin, W. J., et al.: Oxidant injury of lung parenchymal cells. J. Clin. Invest. *68*:1277, 1981.
44. Emanuel, N. M.: Free radicals and the action of inhibitors of radical processes under pathological states and aging in living organisms and man. Q. Rev. Biophys. *9*:283, 1976.
45. Baehner, R. L., et al.: Reduced oxygen byproducts and white blood cells. *In* Pryor, W. (ed.): Free Radicals in Biology. Vol. 5. New York, Academic Press, 1982, p. 91.
46. Doroshow, J., and Hochstein, P.: Redox cycling and the mechanism of action of antibiotics in neoplastic disease. *In* Autor, A. (ed.): Pathology of Oxygen. New York, Academic Press, 1982, p. 245.
47. Peng, S. K., et al.: Effect of auto-oxidation products from cholesterol on aortic smooth muscle cells. Arch. Pathol. Lab. Med. *102*:57, 1978.
48. Bessis, M.: Cell death. Triangle *9*:191, 1970.
49. Majno, G., et al.: Cellular death and necrosis: Chemical, physical, and morphologic changes in rat liver. Virchows Arch., *333*:421, 1960.
50. Searle, J., et al.: Necrosis and apoptosis: Distinct modes of cell death with fundamentally different signficance. Pathol. Annu. *17*(2):229, 1982.
51. Lombardi, B.: Considerations on the pathogenesis of fatty liver. Lab. Invest. *15*:1, 1966.
52. Podolsky, K., and Isselbacher, K. J.: Derangements of hepatic metabolism. *In* Harrison's Principles of Internal Medicine. New York, McGraw-Hill Book Co., 1983, pp. 1773–1779.
53. Lieber, C. S.: Pathogenesis and early diagnosis of alcoholic liver injury. N. Engl. J. Med. *298*:888, 1978.
54. Geokas, M. C., et al.: Ethanol, the liver and the gastrointestinal tract. Ann. Intern. Med. *95*:198, 1981.
55. Gray, A., and Doniach, I.: Ultrastructure of plasma cells containing Russell bodies in human stomach and thyroid. J. Clin. Pathol. *23*:608, 1970.
56. Stanbury, J. B.: The Metabolic Basis of Inherited Disease. 5th ed. New York, McGraw-Hill Book Co., 1983.
57. Wolman, M.: Pigments in Pathology. New York, Academic Press, 1969.
58. Porta, E. A., and Hartcroft, W. S.: Lipid pigments in relation to aging and dietary factors (lipofuscins). *In* Wolman, M. (ed.): Pigments in Pathology. New York, Academic Press, 1969.
59. Toubald, R. D., et al.: Studies on the chemical nature of lipofuscin (age pigment) isolated from normal human brain. Lipids *10*:383, 1975.
60. Koobs, D. H., et al.: The origin of lipofuscin and possible consequences to the myocardium. Arch. Pathol. Lab. Med. *102*:66, 1978.
61. Richter, G. W.: A review. The iron-loaded cell—the cytopathology of iron storage. Am. J. Pathol. *91*:361, 1978.
62. Jones, A. L., and Fawcett, D. W.: Hypertrophy of the agranular endoplasmic reticulum in hamster liver induced by phenobarbital. J. Histochem. Cytochem. *14*:215, 1966.
63. Goldman, R.: Cytoplasmic fibers in mammalian cells: Cytoskeletal and contractile elements. Ann. Rev. Physiol. *41*:703, 1979.
64. Hyams, K., and Roberts, K.: Microtubules. New York, Academic Press, 1979.
65. Nath, J., et al.: Tubulin tyrosinization in normal and Chediak-Higashi syndrome neutrophils. J. Cell Biol. *95*:519, 1982.
66. Eliasson, R., et al.: The immotile cilia syndrome. N. Engl. J. Med. *297*:1, 1977.
67. Lazarides, E.: Intermediate filaments: A chemically heterogeneous, developmentally regulated class of proteins. Annu. Rev. Biochem. *51*:219, 1982.
68. Lazarides, E.: Intermediate filaments—chemical heterogeneity in differentiation. Cell *23*:649, 1981.
69. Phillips, M. J.: Mallory bodies of the liver. Lab. Invest. *47*:311, 1982.
70. French, S. W.: Present understanding of the development of Mallory's body. Arch. Pathol. Lab. Med. *107*:445, 1983.

71. Selkoe, D. J., et al.: Alzheimer's disease: Insolubility of partially purified paired helical filaments in sodium dodecyl sulfate and urea. Science *215*:1243, 1982.
72. Marchesi, V. T.: The red cell membrane skeleton: Recent progress. Blood *61*:1, 1983.
73. Wolfe, L. C., et al.: A genetic defect in the binding of protein 4.1 to spectrin in a kindred with hereditary spherocytosis. N. Engl. J. Med. *307*:1367, 1982.
74. Goldberg, A. L., et al.: Hormonal regulation of protein degradation and synthesis in skeletal muscle. Fed. Proc. *39*:31, 1980.
75. Zak, R.: Cardiac hypertrophy: Biochemical and cellular relationships. Hosp. Pract. *18*:23, 1983.
76. Baserga, R.: Multiplication and Division in Mammalian Cells. New York, Marcel Dekker, 1976.
77. Bucher, N. L. R., and McGowan, J. A.: Liver regeneration. Regulatory mechanisms. *In* Wright, R., et al. (ed.): Liver and Biliary Disease. Philadelphia, W. B. Saunders Co., 1979, pp. 210–227.
78. Bucher, N. L., et al.: Thirty years of liver regeneration: A distillate. Cold Spring Harbor Conferences on Cell Proliferation *9*:15, 1982.
79. Rytömaa, T.: The chalone concept. Int. Exp. Pathol. *16*:135, 1976.
80. Scott, R. E., and Florine, D. L.: Cell cycle models for aberrant coupling of growth arrest and differentiation in hyperplasia, metaplasia and neoplasia. Am. J. Pathol. *107*:342, 1982.
81. Jensen, E. V., et al.: Estrogen interaction with target tissues: Two-step transfer of receptor to the nucleus. *In* O'Malley, B. W. (ed.): Methods in Enzymology. New York, Academic Press, 1975, pp. 156–166.
82. McCarty, K. S., and McCarty, K. S.: Steroid hormone receptors in the regulation of differentiation. Am. J. Pathol. *86*:705, 1977.
83. McDowell, E., et al.: The respiratory epithelium. VII. Epidermoid metaplasia of hamster tracheal epithelium during regeneration following mechanical injury. J. Natl. Cancer Inst. *62*:995, 1979.
84. Anderson, H. C.: Calcific diseases: A concept. Arch. Pathol. Lab. Med. *107*:341, 1983.
85. Kim, K. M.: Pathological calcification. *In* Trump, B., and Arstila, A. (eds.): Pathobiology of Cell Membranes, Vol. 3. New York, Academic Press, 1983.
86. Hayflick, L.: The Biology of Human Aging Adv. Pathobiol. *7*:21, 1980.
87. Martin, G. M.: Cellular aging (Parts I and II). Am. J. Pathol. *89*:484, 1977.
88. Holliday, R., et al.: Cellular aging: Further evidence for the commitment theory. Science *213*:505, 1981.
89. Goldstein, S., et al.: Chronologic and physiologic age affect replicative life span of fibroblasts from diabetic, prediabetic and normal donors. Science *199*:781, 1978.
90. Smith, K. C.: Aging, carcinogenesis, and radiation biology: The role of nucleic acid addition reactions. New York, Plenum Press, 1976.

2 INFLAMMATION AND REPAIR

Inflammation

Inflammation is best defined as *the reaction of vascularized living tissue to local injury.* Invertebrates with no vascular system, single-celled organisms, and multicellular parasites all have their own responses to local injury. These include phagocytosis of the injurious agent; entrapment of the irritant by specialized cells (hemocytes), which then ingest it; and neutralization of noxious stimuli by hypertrophy of the cell or one of its organelles. All these reactions have been retained but what characterizes the inflammatory process in higher forms is *the reaction of blood vessels,* leading to the accumulation of fluid and blood cells. This makes the reaction much more complex but also more fascinating to unravel.

The inflammatory response is closely intertwined with the process of *repair.* Inflammation serves to destroy, dilute, or wall off the injurious agent, but in turn sets into motion a complex series of events that, as far as possible, heal and reconstitute the damaged tissue. Repair begins during the early phases of inflammation but reaches completion usually after the injurious influence has been neutralized. During repair, the injured tissue is replaced by regeneration of native parenchymal cells, by filling of the defect with fibroblastic "scar" tissue, or most commonly by a combination of these two processes.

Humans owe to inflammation and repair their ability to contain injuries and heal defects. Without inflammation, infections would go unchecked, wounds would never heal, and injured organs might remain permanent festering sores. *However, inflammation and repair may be potentially harmful.* Inflammatory reactions underlie the genesis of rheumatoid arthritis, life-threatening hypersensitivity reactions, and some forms of fatal renal disease. Reparative efforts may lead to disfiguring scars or fibrous bands that cause intestinal obstruction or limit the mobility of joints. It is for this reason that our pharmacies abound with so-called "anti-inflammatory drugs," which supposedly limit, control, or modify the normal inflammatory reaction. The ideal drug would be one that enhances the salutary effects of inflammation yet controls its destructive, harmful sequelae. As our understanding of the mechanisms of inflammation increases, so will our ability to control its evolution and to foster its beneficial effects.

HISTORICAL HIGHLIGHTS

The scientific advances of the past 20 years have brought us tantalizingly close to understanding many of the cellular and biochemical events in inflammation, but because inflammation is so often a visible reaction, it has a rich and ancient history, intimately linked to the history of wars, wounds, and infections. Space here does not allow for any but the briefest of historical perspectives. The interested student should read some of *Majno's* historical writings.[1–3]

Cornelius Celsus, a Roman nonmedical writer of the first century AD, described the four cardinal signs of inflammation: *rubor, tumor, calor, and dolor* (redness, swelling, heat, and pain). In 1793, the Scottish surgeon *John Hunter* noted what is now considered an obvious fact: that inflammation is not a disease but a nonspecific response that has a "salutary" effect on its host.[5] Just as *Virchow* (1821–1902) established the concept of "cellular pathology," which was fundamental to the recognition that all disease processes must originate in diseased cells, so it was his pupil *Julius Cohnheim* (1839–1884) who provided one of the first (and still best) microscopic descriptions of inflammation. He observed injured blood vessels in thin, transparent membranes, such as the mesentery and tongue of the frog. Noting the initial vasodilatation and changes in blood flow, the subsequent edema due to increased vascular permeability, and the characteristic leukocyte emigration, he wrote descriptions that can hardly be improved upon.[2–6]

The Russian biologist *Elie Metchnikoff* discovered the process of *phagocytosis* by observing the ingestion of rose thorns by amebocytes of starfish larvae (1882), and of bacteria by mammalian leukocytes (1884). He concluded that the purpose of inflammation was to bring phagocytic cells to the injured area to engulf invading bacteria. At that time, Metchnikoff contradicted the prevailing theory, strengthened by the discovery of antitoxins by Behring and Kitasato (1890), that the purpose of inflammation was to bring in factors from the serum to neutralize the infectious agents. It soon became clear that both cellular (phagocytosis) and serum factors (antibodies) were critical to our defense against organisms, and in recognition of this both Metchnikoff and Paul Ehrlich (who developed the "humoral theory") shared the Nobel Prize in 1908.[7]

To these names must be added that of *Sir Thomas Lewis* who, on the basis of simple experiments involving the triple response in skin (p. 42), established the concept that chemical substances, locally induced by injury, mediate the vascular changes of inflammation. This fundamental concept underlies the important discoveries of *chemical mediators* of inflammation and of potent anti-inflammatory agents.

ACUTE INFLAMMATION

It is common to think of bacteria or other microbes as the cause of inflammation, but almost all the causes of cell injury cited earlier (Chapter 1) may also provoke inflammation. These include physical agents (such as burns, radiation, and trauma), chemical agents (such as caustic substances), and all types of immunologic reactions. The last category, in particular, is integral to various aspects of inflammation. Of necessity, therefore, much of our discussion on the mechanisms of inflammation will require an understanding of some fundamental aspects of immunology, summarized in Chapter 5. (For those not familiar with basic immunologic terms, prereading of Chapter 5 may be useful.)

It is customary to divide inflammation into acute and chronic patterns—useful terms, provided that certain qualifications of their meaning are appreciated.[3] *Acute inflammation* is of relatively short duration, lasting for a few minutes, several hours, or one to two days, and its main characteristics are the exudation of fluid and plasma proteins (edema) and the emigration of leukocytes, predominantly neutrophils. It is more or less stereotypic, regardless of the nature of the injurious agent. *Chronic inflammation*, on the other hand, is less uniform. It is generally of longer duration and is associated histologically with the presence of lymphocytes and macrophages, and the proliferation of blood vessels and connective tissue. But many factors modify the course and histologic appearance of chronic inflammation, and these will become apparent later in this chapter.

Although the basic pattern of acute inflammation is uniform, the intensity and duration of the reaction is determined by both the severity of the injurious agent and the reactive capability of the host. Even slight injury may produce a serious, sustained response in the frail and, conversely, even the most robust may fall prey to a virulent attack, as every victim of a severe burn well knows. Depending on the severity of the injury and the adequacy of the defense, the inflammation may remain localized to its site of origin or may evoke systemic responses.

The arena of the inflammatory response is the vascularized connective tissue, including plasma, circulating cells, blood vessels, and the cellular and extracellular constituents of connective tissue. The student should be familiar with the structure, biology, and biochemistry of these components. The circulating cells that are important in inflammation include *neutrophils*, *monocytes*, *eosinophils*, *lymphocytes*, *basophils*, and *platelets*. The main connective tissue cells are the *mast cells*, which intimately surround *blood vessels*, and the connective tissue *fibroblasts*. The extracellular connective tissue consists of *basement membrane*, the various types of *collagen*, *elastin*, and *proteoglycans* (heparan sulfate, chondroitin sulfate, hyaluronic acid). *Fibronectin* and *laminin* are glycoproteins that, together with some types of collagen (*IV* and *V*), are present in basement membranes (see pp. 78–79).

Certain terms must be defined before we describe the specifics in inflammation. The escape of fluid, proteins, and blood cells from the vascular system into the interstitial tissue or body cavities is known as *exudation*. An *exudate* is an inflammatory extravascular fluid that has a high protein concentration, much cellular debris, and a specific gravity above 1.020. It implies significant alteration in the normal permeability of small blood vessels in the area of injury. In contrast, a *transudate* is a fluid with low protein content (most of which is albumin) and a specific gravity of less than 1.012. It is essentially an ultrafiltrate of blood plasma and results from hydrostatic imbalance across the vascular endothelium (see p. 42). Here, the permeability of the endothelium is normal. *Edema* denotes an excess of fluid in the interstitial tissue or serious cavities; it can be either an exudate or a transudate. *Pus*, a *purulent exudate*, is an inflammatory exudate rich in leukocytes (mostly neutrophils) and parenchymal cell debris. Lysosomal enzymes are present in pus, and the extent of proteolysis that they produce determines the viscosity of the material.

The local clinical signs of acute inflammation are the heat, redness, swelling, and pain immortalized by Celsus. A fifth clinical sign, loss of function (functio laesa), was later added by Virchow.[2] These signs of the inflammatory response are induced by (1) *changes in vascular flow and caliber* (also referred to as hemodynamic changes), (2) *changes in vascular permeability*, and (3) *leukocytic exudation*. These three reactions may overlap, and some share common mediator mechanisms. In general, however, the structural and biochemical basis of each of these responses is sufficiently different to require separate consideration.

CHANGES IN VASCULAR FLOW AND CALIBER

These changes are best observed in thin, transparent injured tissues under the phase microscope, or better still by time-lapse cinematography. They begin very early after injury but develop at varying rates, depending on the severity of the injury. The changes occur in the following order.[8]

1. First, there is *transient vasoconstriction of arterioles*. This is an inconstant finding, and with mild forms of injury it disappears within three to five seconds. With more severe injury, such as a burn, vasoconstriction may last several minutes. The mechanism of constriction is unknown; it may well be neurogenic, but some chemical mediators (to be discussed) induce vasoconstriction when injected in high doses.

2. The next and fundamental event is *vasodilatation*, which first involves the arterioles and then results in opening of new microvascular beds in the area. *Thus comes about the increased blood flow—the hallmark of the early hemodynamic changes in acute inflammation* and the cause of the heat and the redness. At this stage, the increased blood volume in the vasodilated vessels may result in sufficient increases in local hydrostatic pressure to cause fleeting transudation of protein-poor fluid into the extravascular space.

3. *Slowing of the circulation* follows, brought about by *increased permeability of the microvasculature*, with the outpouring of protein-rich fluid into the extravascular tissues. This results in concentration of the red cells in small vessels, and increased viscosity of the blood. In histologic sections, this phenomenon is reflected by the presence of dilated small vessels packed with red cells—termed stagnation or "*stasis*."

4. As stasis develops, one begins to see peripheral orientation of leukocytes, principally neutrophils, along the vascular endothelium, a process termed *leukocytic margination*. Leukocytes stick to the endothelium at first transiently, then more avidly; soon after they migrate through the vascular wall into the interstitial tissue, the latter process being called *emigration*.

The time scale of these events is variable. For example, with mild stimuli the stages of stasis may not become apparent until 15 to 30 minutes have elapsed, whereas with severe injury stasis may occur in but a few minutes. Further, if the injurious agent is diffusible or if there is a gradient of injury, the vessels closest to the stimulus show evidence of severe and rapid hemodynamic changes, whereas those at the periphery have mild alterations. Thus, if a local burn is inflicted on the skin, the area immediately adjacent to the burn may show complete stasis, while more peripheral areas may still be vasodilated.

What brings about the characteristic vasodilatation and acceleration of flow? Here we must go back to 1927 for the classic description by Sir Thomas Lewis of the "*triple response*."[9] Lewis pointed out that when the skin of the forearm of a normal individual is firmly stroked by a blunt instrument, such as the tip of a lead pencil or the edge of a ruler, three separate changes can be observed. First, within seconds, *a dull red line* develops along the line of the stroke. Second, a bright red halo (the *flare*) appears about the stroke mark. Soon thereafter the third feature appears—*swelling* of the stroke mark (the wheal), accompanied by its blanching. Lewis further observed that neither the red stroke mark nor the wheal could be abolished by cutting local sensory nerves to the skin. He thus postulated the release of a humoral *histamine-like substance* (H-substance) by injured tissue as the cause of the dull red line, which he ascribed to vasodilatation, as well as the cause of the wheal, which he attributed to increased vascular permeability. Although more potent chemicals than histamine—the prostaglandins—are now thought to be the mediators of vasodilatation, Lewis' experiments were the first to suggest the action of chemical mediators in inflammation.

CHANGES IN VASCULAR PERMEABILITY

Normal Permeability and Structure of Microcirculation

We have seen that, in the early stages, vasodilatation and increased hydrostatic pressure may result in some degree of *transudation*. However, this is soon dwarfed by *increased vascular permeability and exudation of plasma proteins, the mark of acute inflammatory edema*. Increased permeability in inflammation occurs in the microcirculation, which includes the small arterioles, capillaries, and venules. It is in these segments that exchange of substances between the blood and tissues occurs.

According to Starling's hypothesis, the normal fluid balance is maintained by two opposing sets of forces (Fig. 2–1*A*). Those that cause fluid to move out of circulation are the osmotic pressure of interstitial fluid and the intravascular hydrostatic pressure; those that cause fluid to move in are the osmotic pressure of plasma proteins and the tissue hydrostatic pressure. The balance of these forces is such that there is a net small movement of fluid outward, but this fluid normally drains into the lymphatics, and no edema occurs. Factors that tend either to increase intravascular hydrostatic pressure or to decrease intravascular osmotic pressure will result in increased movement of fluid out of the capillary and the formation of edema. In these instances, however, the edema is a transudate. In inflammatory edema there is loss of high-protein fluid due to a leaky endothelium and therefore *a reduction of the intravascular osmotic pressure*, accompanied by increased osmotic pressure of the interstitial fluid, both leading to impairment of the return of fluid to the blood on the venous end of the capillary (Fig. 2–1*B*). There is thus a marked *outflow* of fluid.

Normal fluid exchange is critically dependent on an intact endothelium. Normal endothelium is a thin, simple, squamous epithelium adapted to permit free, rapid exchange of water and small molecules between

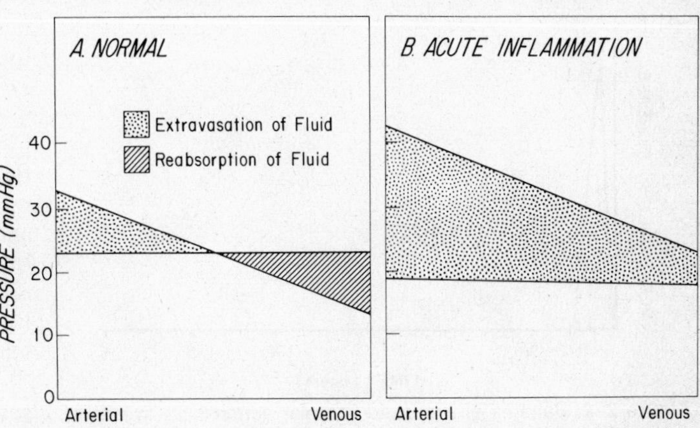

Figure 2–1. Blood pressure and plasma colloid oncotic forces in normal and inflamed tissues. *A*, Normal hydrostatic pressure of about 32 mm Hg at arterial end of capillary and 12 mm Hg at venous end. Mean capillary pressure equals colloid oncotic pressure (horizontal line). *B*, Acute inflammation. Mean capillary pressure is increased because of arteriolar dilatation, while oncotic pressure is reduced because of increased permeability of vascular wall. Result is net excess of extravasated fluid. (Redrawn from Wright, G. P.: An introduction to Pathology. 3rd ed. London, Longmans, Green and Co., 1958.)

plasma and interstitium, but to limit the passage of plasma proteins with increased restriction as the size of the protein increases. The endothelial lining of all arterioles and venules and most capillaries in the body is of the *continuous* type, having an unbroken cytoplasmic layer with closely apposed intercellular junctions. *Fenestrated* endothelium is characteristic of endocrine organs, intestines, and the renal glomerulus, and *discontinuous* or *open* endothelium occurs in the liver, spleen, and bone marrow. Physiologic studies[10,11] explain normal capillary permeability for water and small lipid-insoluble molecules by the existence of water-filled "small pores" 6 nm in radius, or slits about 8 nm wide. There is also a postulated system of large pores (25-nm radius) to account for the small quantities of protein and other large solutes that normally cross the capillary wall.

Although there is agreement among electron microscopists that *micropinocytotic vesicles* represent the large pores, the morphologic equivalent of the small pore system is still uncertain. At present there are two opposing views, based on interpretation of the ultrastructural localization of protein tracers having different molecular weights. One view is that the small-pore system is represented by continuous transendothelial channels formed by fusing pinocytotic vesicles.[12] The other ascribes to the *intercellular junctions* the transfer site of molecules up to 40,000 daltons.[13] Whichever the route in capillaries, it is clear that intercellular junctions are less structurally complex and more permeable in *small venules*.[14] Further, junctions are labile structures and are susceptible to being widened by a variety of physical and chemical factors. As we shall see, most chemical mediators of inflammation cause increased vascular permeability by opening gaps in *intercellular* junctions.

Recent studies suggest that various polyanionic molecules, such as sialoglycoproteins and heparan sulfate, are localized in specific domains on the luminal surface of endothelium (e.g., vesicles, fenestrae, intercellular junctions).[15] These anionic sites may well play a role in normal and increased vascular permeability by repelling anionic molecules and facilitating the transport of cationic proteins. Such a role for anionic sites has been shown in the case of the renal glomerulus (p. 993).

It must be emphasized that, despite its relatively simple structure, the vascular endothelial cell is a functionally and metabolically active cell capable of secretion of a variety of biologically important molecules. These include hormones (prostaglandins), procoagulant (Factor VIII), anticoagulant (plasminogen activator) factors, and connective tissue proteins (e.g., fibronectin).[16–18]

Patterns and Morphologic Basis of Increased Vascular Permeability

Increased vascular permeability is seen clinically as *edema*. It can be demonstrated or quantitated experimentally in several ways, including (1) measurement of the water content of the inflamed tissue; (2) assessment of leakage of intravenously injected dyes (e.g., Evans blue, which binds to serum proteins), causing "blueing" of inflamed sites; (3) measurement of the escape of injected radiolabeled albumin into injured areas; and (4) vascular "labeling" with carbon.[19] With the last technique, colloidal carbon, which contains particles 25 to 30 nm in diameter, is injected intravenously. Normally it is taken up by the reticuloendothelial (mononuclear phagocyte) system, but not by endothelial cells. However, carbon particles leak across injured endothelium but are too large to cross the basement membrane. They are thus trapped between the basement membrane and the endothelium. Leaky vessels are therefore "labeled with carbon" and can be visualized on light and electron microscopy.

With such techniques, varying patterns in the rise and ebb of vascular leakage can be demonstrated in the skin of animals exposed to various types of injury[20] (Fig. 2–2). Three general types of response are recognized: (1) *the immediate-transient response*, (2) *the immediate-sustained* (also called immediate-prolonged) *response*, and (3) *the delayed-prolonged response*.

The immediate-transient response usually begins immediately after injury, reaches a peak by five to ten minutes, and phases out within 15 to 30 minutes. The response is elicited by histamine and most other chemical mediators and by mild injury (such as heating the skin of a guinea pig at 54° C for five seconds) and is also the typical fleeting response of the allergic wheal seen in Type I hypersensitivity (p. 163). Majno and coworkers[19, 21] used the carbon-labeling technique and

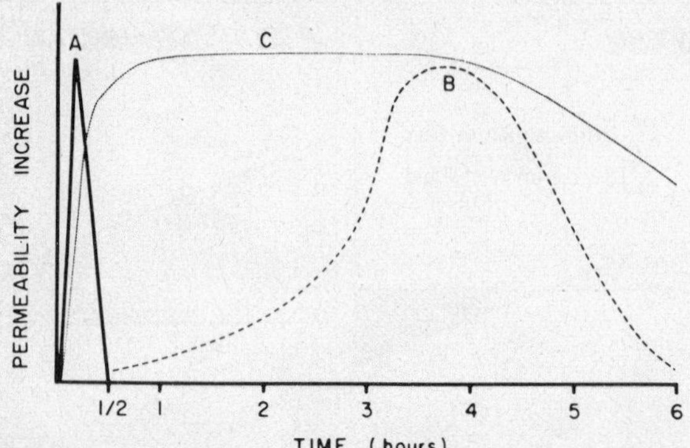

Figure 2–2. Patterns of increased vascular permeability in inflammation. The solid line, A, shows the immediate transient response; the dashed line, B, shows the delayed response; and the thin line, C, shows the immediate sustained response.

found that immediate-transient leakage induced by histamine, serotonin, and bradykinin occurred (1) *exclusively from small- and medium-sized venules* less than 100 μ in diameter, leaving the capillaries unaffected (Fig. 2–3); and (2) through gaps (0.5 to 1.0 μ in width) *between the endothelial cells* (Fig. 2–4). The mechanism by which gaps form turns out to be quite simple: they are caused by actual *contraction* of endothelial cells and widening of the junction.[22, 23] Similar changes are seen in the immediate-transient responses induced by mild thermal injury,[24] and these can be inhibited by antagonists of histamine. Why do histamine-type mediators act exclusively on venules? We do not know for sure, but recent interesting evidence suggests that venular endothelium has a higher concentration of high-affinity binding sites (receptors) for histamine than does arteriolar or capillary endothelium.[25]

Immediate-sustained reactions are encountered in severe injuries, usually associated with necrosis of endothelial cells. Leakage starts immediately after injury, is sustained at a high level for several hours, and continues for one to several days until the damaged vessels are either thrombosed or repaired. *All levels of the microcirculation are affected, including venules, capillaries, and arterioles.* Severe endothelial cell damage, with frequent sloughing of endothelial cells, is present (Fig. 2–5). *Here the mechanism for increased permeability appears to be direct damage by the injurious stimulus.*

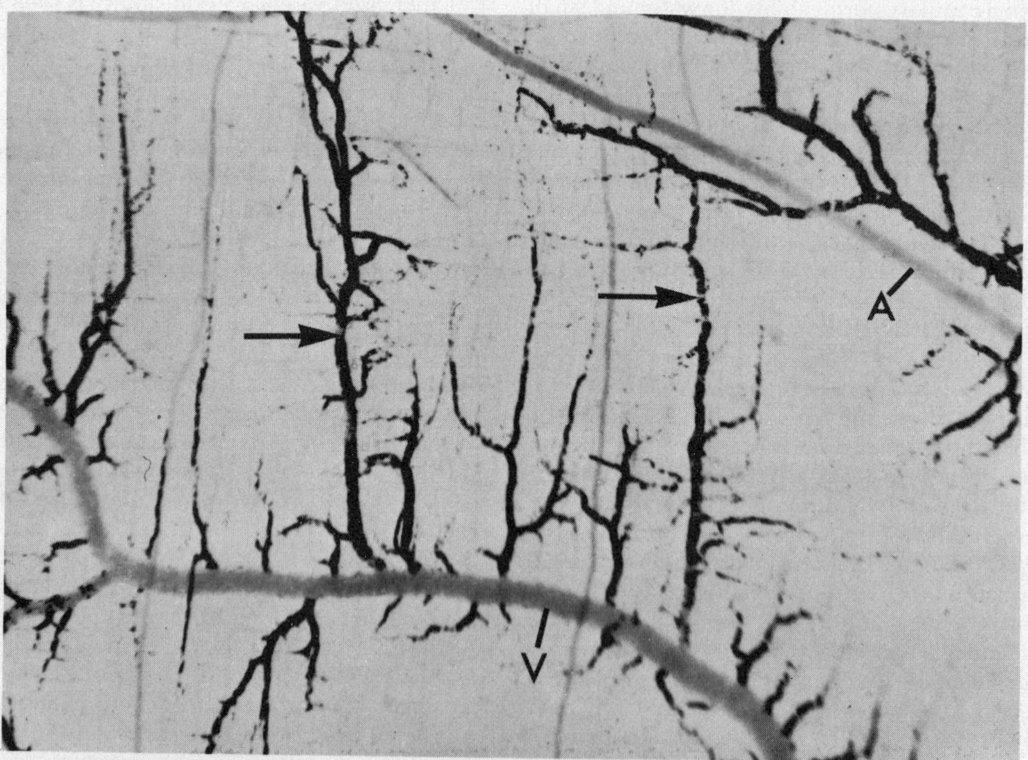

Figure 2–3. Vascular leakage as induced by histamine, serotonin, and bradykinin. This is a laminar muscle of the rat (cremaster), fixed, cleared in glycerin, and examined unstained by transillumination. One hour prior to sacrifice, bradykinin was injected over this muscle, and colloidal carbon was given intravenously; bradykinin caused small gaps to appear between endothelial cells in some vessels (see Fig. 2–4). Plasma, loaded with carbon, escaped, but most of the carbon particles were retained by the basement membrane of the leaking vessels, with the result that these became "labeled" in black. *Note that not all the vessels leak* — only the venules, and then only within a certain caliber range. A = arteriole; V = small vein; arrows point to blackened, leaking venules. The capillary network is very faintly visible in the background. (Courtesy of Dr. Guido Majno, Department of Pathology, University of Massachusetts School of Medicine.)

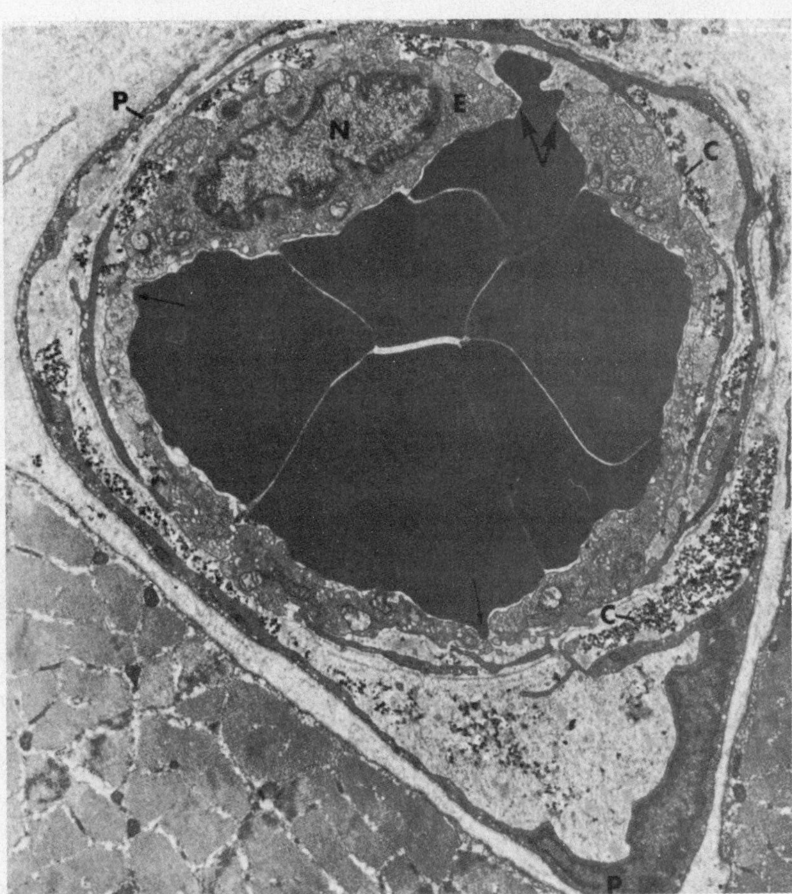

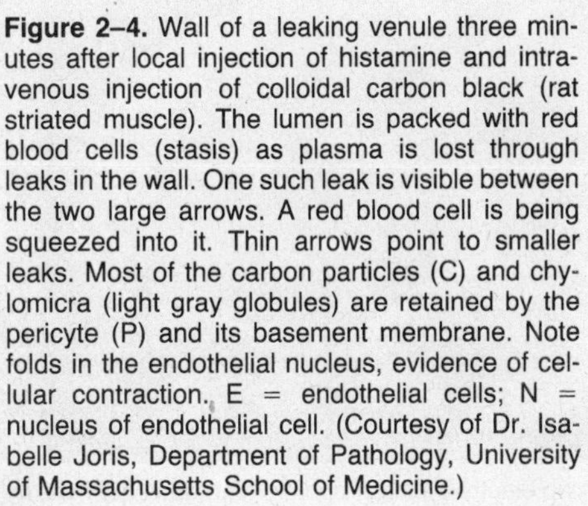
Figure 2–4. Wall of a leaking venule three minutes after local injection of histamine and intravenous injection of colloidal carbon black (rat striated muscle). The lumen is packed with red blood cells (stasis) as plasma is lost through leaks in the wall. One such leak is visible between the two large arrows. A red blood cell is being squeezed into it. Thin arrows point to smaller leaks. Most of the carbon particles (C) and chylomicra (light gray globules) are retained by the pericyte (P) and its basement membrane. Note folds in the endothelial nucleus, evidence of cellular contraction. E = endothelial cells; N = nucleus of endothelial cell. (Courtesy of Dr. Isabelle Joris, Department of Pathology, University of Massachusetts School of Medicine.)

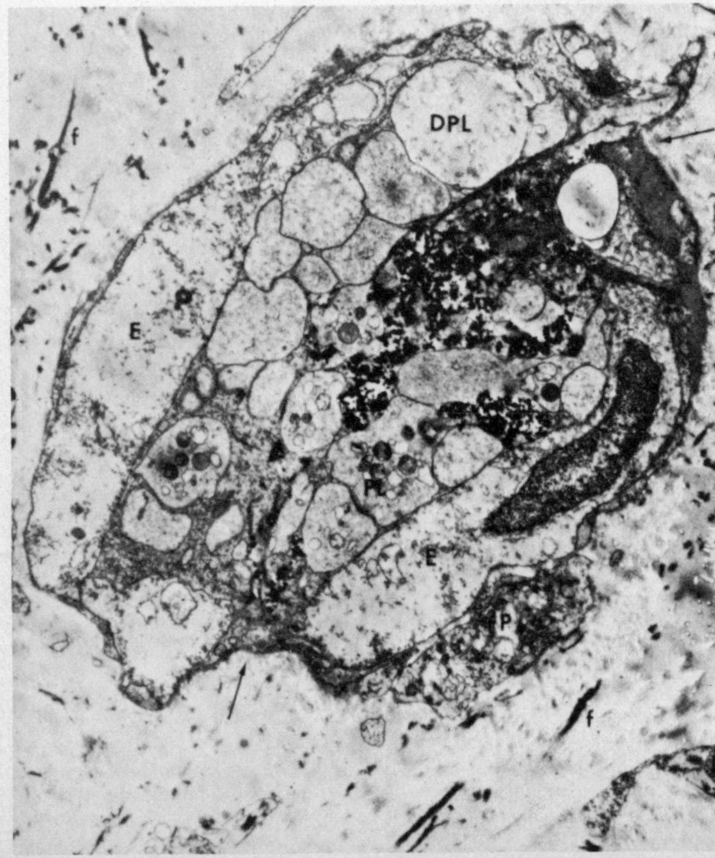

Figure 2–5. Electron micrograph showing effects of direct injury to endothelium by necrotizing thermal stimulus. There is marked swelling of endothelium (E); disruptions (*arrows*) allow leakage of injected carbon particles. Note the platelets (PL) plugging the lumen. DPL = degranulated platelets; P = pericyte; F = fibrin. Compare with Figure 2–4.

The classic example is the increased permeability that occurs after a severe burn.[26]

Delayed-prolonged leakage is a curious type of response that *begins after a delay* and lasts for several hours or even days.[27] This response is rather common, occurring after mild-to-moderate thermal injury, after x-ray or ultraviolet irradiation, with certain bacterial toxins, and in delayed (Type IV) hypersensitivity reactions (p. 169). One common example of a delayed response is seen in sunburn, which is appreciated only several hours after a person has left the beach. In the delayed phase, leakage occurs in both venules and capillaries.[28, 29] Most workers now believe that the delayed leakage is largely due to direct injury to the endothelium by the initial stimulus.[3, 20] Electron microscopy shows the leakage to be predominantly intercellular, but curiously there is no endothelial cell contraction. How gaps form with this type of direct injury and why the leakage is delayed is not known.

Before we leave this discussion, it should be noted that while it is possible to separate the three patterns in the experimental model, the patterns in most inflammatory reactions of man overlap since there is a graded severity of injury from the center to the periphery of injured sites. In addition, different chemical mediators—with histamine-type patterns—may be activated at consecutive phases of the inflammatory response and account for sustained and prolonged responses. However, as mentioned, the allergic wheal is an example of an immediate-transient permeability response, and x-irradiation and ultraviolet rays classically induce delayed-prolonged responses.

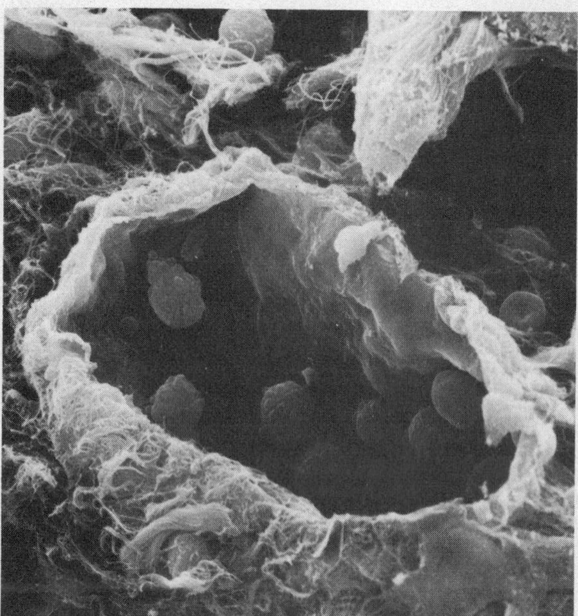

Figure 2–6. Scanning electron micrograph of inflamed venule showing margination and sticking of neutrophils. (Courtesy of Dr. M. J. Karnovsky, Department of Pathology, Harvard Medical School.)

CELLULAR EVENTS: LEUKOCYTIC EXUDATION AND PHAGOCYTOSIS

The accumulation of leukocytes—principally neutrophils and monocytes—is the most important feature of the inflammatory reaction. Leukocytes serve to engulf and degrade bacteria, immune complexes, and the debris of necrotic cells, and their lysosomal enzymes contribute in other ways to the defensive response. But, as we shall see, leukocytes during these defensive reactions also release enzymes, chemical mediators and toxic radicals that may themselves prolong inflammation and increase tissue damage.

The sequence of these "leukocyte events" can be divided into (1) margination, (2) sticking, (3) emigration, (4) phagocytosis and intracellular degradation, and (5) extracellular release of leukocyte products.

Margination

Margination or peripheral orientation of white cells in the moving bloodstream has already been mentioned in the discussion of hemodynamic changes. In normally flowing blood, the red and white cells within microvessels are confined to the axial central column, leaving a relatively cell-free layer of plasma in contact with the vessel wall. As slowing and stagnation of the flow occur, this laminar flow disappears. The white cells appear to fall out of the central column to assume positions in contact with the endothelium (Fig. 2–6). The cells first stumble slowly along the walls of the capillaries and

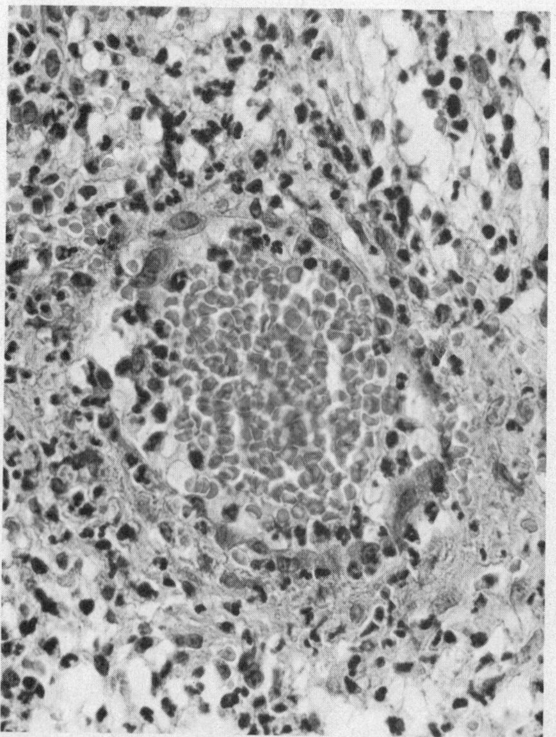

Figure 2–7. A dilated congested venule with peripheral orientation (margination) of neutrophils. Many neutrophils have emigrated into the perivascular edematous tissue.

venules to come to rest finally at some point. In time, the endothelium appears to be virtually lined by such cells, a phenomenon called *pavementing* (Fig. 2–7).

The displacement of white cells to the periphery of the stream may be governed by the laws of physics. In the stagnated blood flow, the red cells tend to stick together and form small clumps or rouleaux, a process that has been referred to as *sludging*. These clumps thus become larger than the white cells and occupy the most rapidly moving central axis of the slowly moving stream, displacing the white cells to the periphery.

Sticking

Following margination, white cells adhere in great numbers to the endothelial surface, resembling "pebbles or marbles over which a stream runs without disturbing them." It must first be said that, under *normal* circumstances, a considerable proportion (as high as 50%) of circulating neutrophils are transiently marginating and sticking (or even emigrating), particularly in the lung, but the numbers adherent are too few to be seen histologically in normal tissues.

Several mechanisms have been postulated in increased adhesiveness of leukocytes in inflammation.[30]

1. *Alterations in cell surface charge*. Both the endothelium and the white cells are covered by negatively charged cell coats and thus are believed to repel each other. It is possible that injury in some way neutralizes these negative charges (either on the endothelium or the neutrophil), causing adhesion. Neuraminidase treatment (which neutralizes sialoproteins) increases neutrophil attachment in endothelial cultures. Neutrophils themselves release cationic proteins that conceivably may serve to neutralize the negative charges. However, this loss of charge may be focal and has been difficult to demonstrate directly.

2. *Divalent ions*, such as Ca^{++}, Mn^{++}, and Mg^{++}, may also play some role in this adherence, serving as bridges between the negative charges on endothelium and white cells or as cofactors in some other enzyme reactions or protein interactions necessary for adhesion. Treatment with EDTA suppresses adhesiveness and addition of these cations increases adhesiveness, both in vivo[31] and in vitro.[30]

3. *Chemical mediators (chemotactic factors)* such as C5a, applied either to neutrophils or to endothelium, increase the adherence of neutrophils to endothelial cells in culture.[30] This suggests that some of the mediators that result in emigration *toward* a focus of injury also cause sticking of leukocytes to the endothelium.

Arachidonic acid metabolites may also be involved. Recent studies show that inhibition of the lipoxygenase pathway of arachidonic acid metabolism *decreases* basal leukocyte adhesion to endothelium in culture,[32] and that lipoxygenase pathway products such as leukotriene B_4 (p. 55) induce increased leukocyte adhesion to endothelium in vivo.

Emigration

Emigration refers to the process by which motile white cells escape from the blood vessels to the perivascular tissues. Neutrophils, eosinophils, basophils, monocytes, and lymphocytes all use the same pathway. Following adhesion, the leukocytes move slightly along the endothelial surface and insert large pseudopods into the junctions between the endothelial cells.[33] They crawl through widened interendothelial junctions, eventually to assume a position between endothelial cell and basement membrane (Fig. 2–8). They may stay at that site for short periods, but they eventually traverse the basement membrane and escape into the extravascular space. Electron microscopy has elegantly shown the incredible plasticity of the white cells as they crawl through the narrow serpentine pathways between endothelial cells.

Red cells may also leave blood vessels, particularly in severe injuries. Unlike the white cell, the red cell seems to be passively and unwillingly shoved out of the leaky, injured vessel by the intraluminal pressure in the wake of emigrating leukocytes.

The cell type present in the inflammatory response varies with the age of the inflammatory lesion and with the type of stimulus. In most types of acute inflammation, *neutrophils predominate in the first six to 24 hours, being replaced by monocytes in 24 to 48 hours*. Although this sequence can be explained in different ways, three factors account for it best: (1) short-lived neutrophils disintegrate and disappear after 24 to 48 hours, while monocytes survive much longer in tissues; (2) monocyte emigration is sustained long after neutrophil emigration ceases;[35] and (3) chemotactic factors for neutrophils and monocytes are activated at different periods of the response. Indeed, *neutrophils release a chemotactic factor for monocytes*, and its activation in the early part of inflammation may call forth the monocytes that predominate later. There are many exceptions to this pattern of cellular exudation: in infection produced by *Pseudomonas* organisms, neutrophils predominate over two to four days; in viral infections, lymphocytes may be the first cells to arrive; in some hypersensitivity reactions, eosinophilic granulocytes may be the main cell type.

Chemotaxis

Chemotaxis may be defined as the unidirectional migration of cells toward an attractant, or more simply locomotion oriented along a chemical gradient. The term should be differentiated from *chemokinesis*, which is the accelerated *random* locomotion of cells. All granulocytes, monocytes, and to a lesser extent lymphocytes respond to such stimuli with various rates of speed.

Many early workers studied chemotaxis, but the development of Boyden's micropore filter technique[36] turned the early expeditions to "fish" for chemoattractants into an international sport![37] With Boyden's technique, leukocytes are placed in one compartment of a

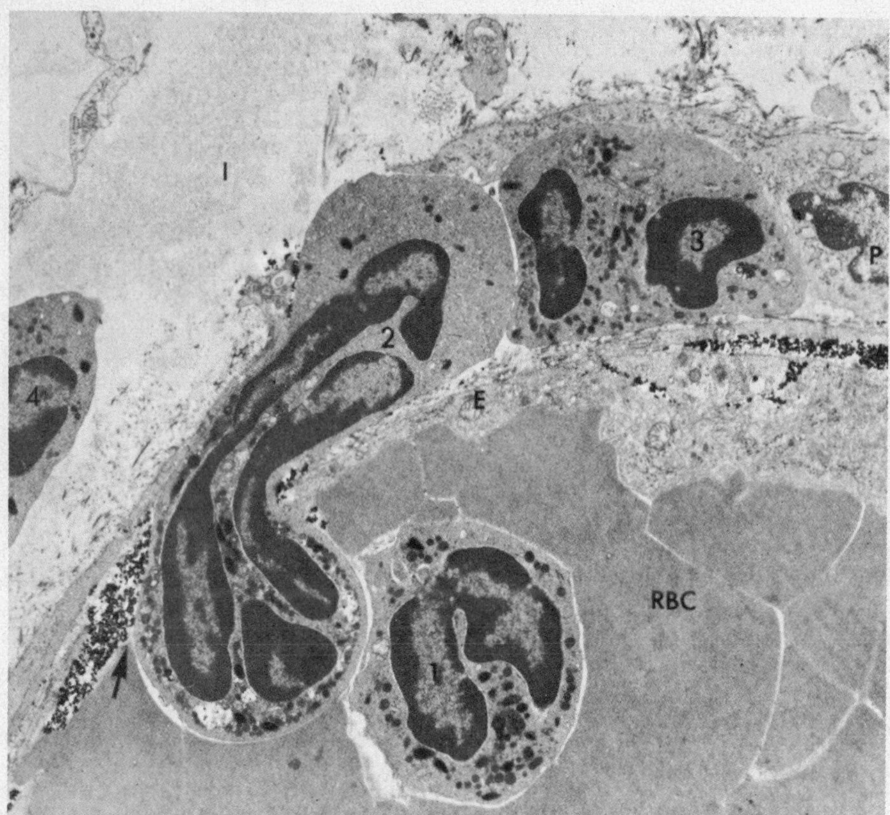

Figure 2–8. Venule ten hours after injection of an inflammation-provoking toxin. Four polymorphonuclear (PMN) leukocytes are seen: 1 is in the lumen; 2 is squeezing through (emigrating from) the lumen into the perivascular space; 3 is trapped between the endothelium (E) and pericyte (P); and 4 is already in the interstitium (I).

chamber, separated by a porous filter membrane from a second compartment in which the chemotactic substance is placed. If a chemotactic influence is present, the leukocytes crawl across the pores of the filter. Quantitation of chemotaxis can be done by counting the cells either on the stained filter membrane or in the second chamber. Direct microscopic observation of leukocytes across a gradient of chemotactic factors is used to check on results obtained by the Boyden technique.[38] Some chemotactic factors operate only on the polymorphonuclear leukocytes, others only on monocytes, and some affect both types of white cells.

Exogenous and endogenous substances can act as attractants. The most significant chemotactic agents for neutrophils are (1) *bacterial products;* (2) *components of the complement system,* particularly C5a; and (3) *products of the lipoxygenase pathway of arachidonic acid metabolism,* particularly leukotriene B_4. The last-named two are discussed in detail in the section on chemical mediators. *Soluble bacterial factors* with chemotactic activity can be isolated from filtrates of a variety of organisms, including *Staphylococcus albus* and *aureus* and *E. coli.* Some of these are peptides that possess an *N*-formyl-methionine terminal amino acid, an observation that led to the synthesis of simple oligopeptides that are highly chemotactic for leukocytes. Others are lipid in nature and resemble the endogenously-produced lipoxygenation products of arachidonic acid metabolism.[39]

But how does the leukocyte "see" (or "smell"?) the chemotactic agents, and how do these diverse substances actually induce directed cell movement? Although not all the answers are known, several important steps are recognized. *First and foremost is the presence of specific receptors for chemotactic agents on the cell membranes of leukocytes.* Schiffman[40] made the interesting observation that synthetic simple formyl methionyl peptides were chemotactic in vitro. The chemotactic activity of such peptides depended not only on their amino acid composition but also on the exact sequence of the amino acids in the peptide chain. This suggested binding of a small portion of the polypeptide chain with a structurally specific receptor on the neutrophil surface. Such receptors have since been identified and quantitated, not only for the synthetic oligopeptides,[41] but also for C5a[42] and for leukotriene B_4.[43] The binding of the ligand to the receptor is rapid, and if about 20% of the receptors are occupied it leads to increased random locomotion as well as chemotaxis. The precise sequence of events from receptor-ligand interaction to actual cell movement is still unclear but appears to involve mobilization of membrane-associated Ca^{++}, Ca^{++} (and Na^{+}) influx into the cell, and increased ionic calcium within the cytosol.[44, 45] The last-named is the key event associated with the assembly of contractile elements responsible for cell movement.

The mechanisms of actual locomotion in leukocytes are beginning to be unraveled.[46] The phagocyte moves by extending a pseudopod that pulls the remainder of the cell in the direction of extension, just as an automobile with front-wheel drive is pulled by the motor in front. The interior of the pseudopod consists of a branching network of filaments composed of *actin,* as well as the contractile protein *myosin.* The phagocyte uses rapid association and dissociation of actin from monomer to fibrillar form to expand and contract the pseudopod when it is required to move. This phenomenon is controlled by calcium ions and a number of regulatory proteins. These include *actin-binding protein,* which organizes actin fibers at right angles to each other, transforming the pseudopod from sol to gel state; *gelsolin,* which binds one end of each actin fragment, preventing reassembly; *acumentin,* a protein that binds to the opposite end of the filament, serving to revert the actin to the sol state; and *calmodulin,* the calcium-binding protein that controls the assembly of myosin molecules. Precisely how myosin interacts with actin in the pseudopod to produce contraction is unknown. However, movement is very dependent on intracytoplasmic calcium gradients that affect both the action of gelsolin on actin and the assembly of myosin filaments.

Chemotactic substances for monocytes include bacterial products, C5a, leukotriene B_4, a factor derived from neutrophils, a factor liberated from activated lymphocytes, and fibronectin fragments.[48]

Eosinophils accumulate in immunologic reactions, particularly at sites of anaphylactic allergy (Type 1 hypersensitivity). In this reaction, IgE-sensitized basophils or mast cells release a variety of factors when they meet specific antigen (p. 164). Some of these factors either are directly chemotactic or enhance other chemotactic agents;[49] these include products of the cyclooxygenase pathway of arachidonic acid metabolism (p. 54), intermediate-molecular-weight peptides, a lipid chemotactic factor (LCF), histamine, prostaglandin D_2, and a small polypeptide called the *eosinophil chemotactic factor of anaphylaxis* (ECF-A). Other eosinophil chemotactic substances include C5a and substances released by activated lymphocytes.

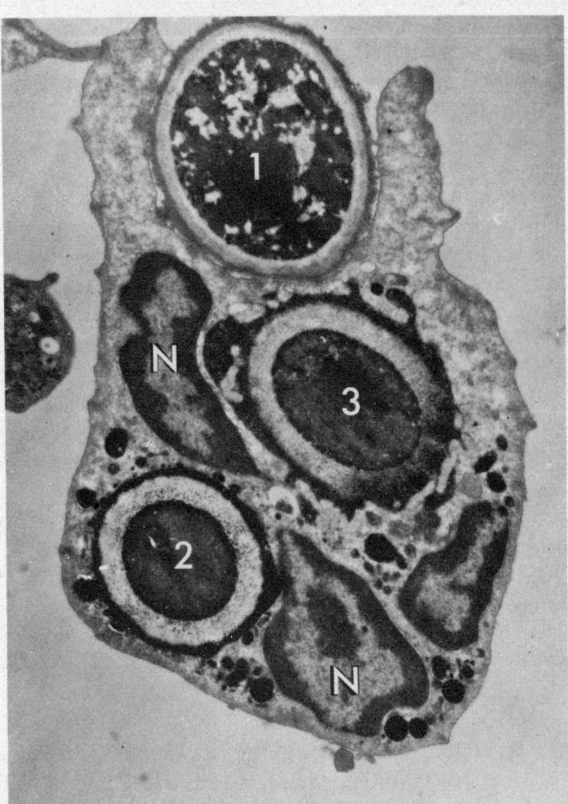

Figure 2–9. Neutrophil, stained for myeloperoxidase (black reaction product), showing phagocytosis of three yeast particles. Particle 1 is being engulfed and particle 2 shows fusion with granules; the granules have emptied their contents around particle 3. N = nucleus. (Courtesy of Dr. M. J. Karnovsky, Department of Pathology, Harvard Medical School.)

Phagocytosis

Phagocytosis and the release of enzymes by neutrophils and macrophages constitute two of the major benefits derived from the accumulation of leukocytes at the inflammatory focus.[50–53] Phagocytosis involves three distinct but interrelated steps (Fig. 2–9). First, the particle to be ingested becomes attached to the surface of the leukocyte, a phenomenon that requires some kind of *recognition* by the leukocyte. The second step is *engulfment,* with subsequent formation of a phagocytic vacuole. The third is *killing and/or degradation* of the ingested material.

1. *Recognition and attachment.* Neutrophils and macrophages on occasion recognize and engulf bacteria or extraneous matter (e.g., latex beads) in the absence of serum, *but most microorganisms are not recognized until they are coated by naturally occurring serum factors called opsonins.* Two opsonins are well characterized: (a) IgG (subtypes 1 and 3), presumably naturally occurring antibody against the ingested particle; and (b) C3b, the so-called "opsonic fragment of C3," generated by activation of complement by immune or nonimmune mechanisms (p. 53). Opsonized particles attach to two corresponding *receptors* on the surface of neutrophils and macrophages: one for the Fc fragment of the IgG molecules (to react with IgG opsonins), and the other a C3b receptor (to react with opsonic C3 fragments). It is no surprise, therefore, that serum of individuals genetically deficient in C3 has impaired opsonic activity.
2. *Engulfment.* This occurs once the phagocyte recognizes a particle's foreignness. Extensions of the cytoplasm (pseudopods) flow around the object to be engulfed, eventually resulting in complete enclosure of the particle by the cytoplasmic membrane of the cell. The limiting membrane of this phagocytic vacuole then fuses with the limiting membrane of the lysosomal granule, resulting in discharge of the granule's contents into the phagolysosome. In the course of this action, the neutrophil and the monocyte become progressively degranulated. *During this process of degranulation there is some leakage of hydrolytic enzymes as well as metabolic products* (e.g., hydrogen peroxide) *from the phagocytizing*

leukocyte into the external medium, probably through unclosed channels from the phagolysosome to the exterior. This process is aptly termed "regurgitation during feeding"; it is important because some of the leaked enzymes have profound proteolytic activity and may cause tissue damage.

An important question concerns how interaction between the leukocyte membrane and the particle to be ingested is translated into the motile and dynamic processes of phagocytosis and degranulation. Several steps in this puzzle are still missing, but many of the events seem to be similar to those occurring during chemotaxis. The process is associated with translocation of calcium ions across the plasma membrane (probably due to activation of membrane phospholipids[54]), which then act as a second messenger and initiate cellular events that involve microfilaments, and possibly microtubules.[47, 55]

3. *Killing and/or degradation.* The ultimate step in phagocytosis of bacteria is killing and degradation. Two categories of bactericidal mechanisms are recognized, oxygen-dependent and oxygen-independent.

   a. *Oxygen-dependent bactericidal mechanisms.* Phagocytosis is an energy-dependent phenomenon that stimulates numerous intracellular events, including a burst in oxygen consumption, glycogenolysis, *increased glucose oxidation via the hexose-monophosphate shunt, and production of active oxygen metabolites.*[56–59] The last is due to the rapid activation of an oxidase (reduced pyridine nucleotide oxidase), which converts NAD(P)H to $NAD(P)^+$ and in the process reduces oxygen to superoxide ion (O_2^-).

$$2\,O_2 + NAD(P)H \xrightarrow{\text{oxidase}} 2\,O_2^- + NAD(P)^+ + H^+$$

Superoxide is then converted into H_2O_2, mostly by spontaneous dismutation. The superoxide is generated on the *outside cell surface* of the leukocyte, but when phagocytosis occurs it ends on the *inside surface* of the phagolysosome.[60] Thus, the hydrogen peroxide is produced within the lysosome. These oxygen metabolites are the principal killers of bacteria, acting in one of two ways:(1) *The H_2O_2-myeloperoxidase-halide system* (myeloperoxidase-dependent killing). The quantities of H_2O_2 produced in the phagolysosome are probably insufficient to induce effective killing of bacteria. However, the azurophilic granules of neutrophils contain the enzyme *myeloperoxidase* (MPO), and *the bactericidal effect of hydrogen peroxide is multiplied several-fold in the presence of myeloperoxidase plus a halide ion such as iodide, bromide, or chloride,*[61] chloride being the physiologically relevant ion. It is now thought that the final reactive radical in this process is HOCl, a powerful oxidant and antimicrobial agent. A similar mechanism is also effective against fungi, viruses, and mycoplasma. Most of the H_2O_2 is eventually broken down by catalase into H_2O and O_2 (p. 11), and some is destroyed by the action of glutathione oxidase.

The most cogent argument for the relevance of the H_2O_2-myeloperoxidase system is the existence of a disease—*chronic granulomatous disease of childhood* (CGD)—characterized by an inherited enzymatic defect that results in the failure of production of H_2O_2 during phagocytosis. Inhibition of the H_2O_2-myeloperoxidase-halide killing system makes these patients unusually susceptible to recurrent infections.

(2) *Myeloperoxidase-Independent Killing.* Studies of myeloperoxidase-deficient leukocytes (a rare disorder) indicate that these cells are capable of effectively killing bacteria (albeit more slowly than control cells). This MPO-independent system also requires oxygen. Superoxide, singlet oxygen, and hydroxyl radicals, extremely reactive radicals also formed during oxidative metabolism, have been implicated in such killing.[62] However, the H_2O_2-myeloperoxidase-halide system is by far the most efficient in neutrophils.[56]

Macrophages under various conditions also produce superoxide and H_2O_2, but do not contain MPO (monocytes do). They may thus kill bacteria by producing sufficient quantities of H_2O_2 or other toxic radicals.

   b. *Oxygen-independent bactericidal mechanisms.*

(1) *Hydrogen ion,* derived from the increased production of lactate or from the action of carbonic anhydrase, results in marked reduction of intravacuolar pH. Few bacteria can continue to grow at a pH of 4.0, and many are actually killed by lactic acid.

(2) The *enzyme lysozyme* attacks bacterial cell walls, especially those of gram-positive cocci, by hydrolyzing the muramic acid-*N*-acetyl glucosamine bond, which is found in the glycopeptide coat of all bacteria.

(3) *Arginine-rich cationic proteins (phagocytin)* of neutrophils can also lyse bacterial membranes.

(4) *Lactoferrin,* an iron-binding protein present in specific granules, is bactericidal.

Following killing, acid hydrolases found in azurophil granules serve to degrade the bacteria within phagolysosomes. The pH of the phagolysosome drops to 4–5 after phagocytosis,[63] this being the optimal pH for the action of such enzymes.

Although most organisms are readily killed by the scavenger cells, some are sufficiently virulent to destroy their captor. Others, such as the tubercle bacillus, appear to survive happily within the phagocyte. Indeed, the persistence of organisms within phagocytes poses a problem in the eradication of such infections as tuberculosis. Thus enclosed, the microorganism is protected against the action of antibacterial drugs as well as other defense mechanisms. When these phagocytic cells migrate through lymphatic pathways, infections such as tuberculosis may be spread.

Extracellular Release of Leukocyte Products

The membrane perturbations that occur in neutrophils and monocytes after receptor-ligand binding during chemotaxis and phagocytosis result in the release of products not only within the phagolysosome, but also potentially into the extracellular space. The most important of these products are (1) lysosomal enzymes; (2) oxygen-derived active metabolites, detailed earlier; and (3) products of arachidonic acid metabolism, including prostaglandins and leukotrienes.

The actual release of lysosomal enzymes during phagocytosis occurs in three ways:

1. As explained earlier, the phagocytic vacuole may remain transiently open to the outside before complete closure of the phagolysosome, permitting escape of lysosomal hydrolases.[64] This is referred to as *regurgitation during feeding.*

2. *Reverse endocytosis* (or frustrated phagocytosis) occurs when white cells are exposed to potentially ingestible materials (such as immune complexes) on flat surfaces, such as capillary endothelium. Attachment of the immune complexes to the leukocyte triggers membrane movements, but because of the flat surface phagocytosis does not occur, and lysosomal enzymes are released into the medium. This interesting phenomenon occurs in certain forms of immune complex–induced glomerular injury (p. 1005).

3. *Cytotoxic release* occurs when the neutrophil dies and is disrupted, its lysosomal enzymes rupturing into the extracellular space. Some particles (urate crystals[66] and silica[67]) are toxic to lysosomal membranes, allowing intracellular release of lysosomal enzymes.

Defects in Leukocyte Function

The significance of emigration, chemotaxis, and phagocytosis in the body's defense against bacterial infections cannot be underestimated. The most telling evidence for an in vivo role for these phenomena is the vulnerability to infection of patients suffering from a deficiency in any of the factors that may affect the white cell—*from the moment it sticks to the endothelium, through its journey across the venular wall, to the ultimate battle within the phagolysosome.* Although the diseases associated with these deficiencies are discussed in later chapters, it is useful here to list the *basic defects* that underlie the specific disorders of leukocytic function:[51, 68, 69]

1. *Defects in numbers of circulating cells* (e.g., neutropenia, toxic depression of bone marrow resulting from radiotherapy or chemotherapy).
2. *Defects in adherence.* These have been reported in diabetics, after acute alcohol intoxication, and after intake of certain drugs such as corticosteroids.
3. *Defects in migration and chemotaxis.* These may be caused by:
   a. *an intrinsic abnormality of leukocytes,* resulting in impaired locomotion or response to chemotactic agents. Examples are the *Chédiak-Higashi syndrome* (a genetic disease in which there are several defects in leukocytes, including impaired chemotaxis), the "lazy leukocyte syndrome," and diabetes.
   b. *a defect in chemotactic factor generation,* such as genetic or acquired C5 deficiency, or immunoglobulin deficiency.
   c. *serum chemotactic inhibitors;* such inhibitors (for example, C5 inactivators) are present in small amounts in normal serum but are markedly increased in patients with cirrhosis, sarcoidosis, and other diseases.
   d. *inhibitors of leukocyte locomotion;* these include some drugs (chloroquine) and poorly defined serum factors present in patients with malignancy, rheumatoid arthritis, and other isolated diseases.
4. *Defects in phagocytosis.* These may also be due to an intrinsic cellular defect (e.g., diabetes, neutrophil "actin dysfunction") or a deficiency of immunoglobulin or complement, resulting in decreased opsonization of particles.
5. *Defect in microbicidal activity.* This may be due to:
   a. *impaired H_2O_2 production,* such as in chronic granulomatous disease (CGD). This is an inherited, most commonly X-linked disease of male children and infants, characterized by recurrent infections and death at an early age. The neutrophils do not develop the typical "respiratory burst" upon phagocytosis. H_2O_2 production is deficient, leading to failure of the important MPO-H_2O_2 halide killing system. Catalase-positive organisms (e.g., *Staphylococcus aureus*), which destroy the little H_2O_2 that is produced, most frequently cause infections, while catalase-negative bacteria or bacteria that form their own H_2O_2 are killed normally by CGD leukocytes.
   b. *myeloperoxidase deficiency;* this is a rare disorder. Because H_2O_2 and O_2^- themselves may be sufficiently bactericidal, most patients are in good health, although some have recurrent infections.
   c. *severe deficiency of leukocyte glucose-6-phosphate dehydrogenase (G6PD);* since this enzyme is required to produce NAD(P)H in the HMP shunt, its absence results in H_2O_2 deficiency and a defect similar to that seen in CGD.
6. *Mixed defects.* In some diseases (e.g., diabetes, Chédiak-Higashi syndrome), more than one defect is involved. In the latter disease, for example, there is

neutropenia, impaired chemotactic response, delayed or decreased fusion of lysosomes with phagosomes, and deficient degranulation. The disease is a rare autosomal recessive disorder, characterized by the presence of giant, lysosome-like granules in the leukocytes and other granule-containing cells. The basic defect may be in microtubule polymerization. Leukocyte defects increase the susceptibility of these patients to infection. As described later (p. 80), corticosteroids also interfere with a variety of leukocyte functions.

CHEMICAL MEDIATORS OF INFLAMMATION

Injury precipitates the inflammatory response, but released chemicals mediate it. Their existence was long suspected for two reasons: (1) Whatever the nature of the injury, the ensuing inflammatory changes constituted a fairly uniform, almost stereotyped reaction. (2) Inflammation developed in tissues deprived of their nervous connections. We have already referred to the classic triple response described by Sir Thomas Lewis and to his suggestion that histamine or histamine-like substances were the cause of the stroke and wheal in this reaction. Some years later it became apparent that histamine could not account for all the features of inflammation. The active search for other mediators has uncovered a perplexing multitude of candidates. The list of possible mediators (almost all discovered from studies in vitro) increases almost daily. We must now determine which are significant in man and what roles each plays.

Mediators can originate from *plasma*, from *cells*, or conceivably from *damaged tissue*. They can be divided into the following groups:

1. Vasoactive amines: histamine and serotonin.
2. Plasma proteases.
   a. the kinin system (bradykinin and kallikrein).
   b. the complement system (C3a; C5a; C5b–C9).
   c. the coagulation-fibrinolytic system (fibrinopeptides, fibrin degradation products).
3. Arachidonic acid (AA) metabolites.
   a. via cyclooxygenase (endoperoxides, prostaglandins, thromboxane).
   b. via lipoxygenase (leukotriene; HPETE; HETE).
   c. nonenzymatically (chemotactic lipids).
4. Lysosomal constituents (neutral proteases).
5. Oxygen-derived free radicals.
6. Acetylated alkyl phosphoglycerides (AGEPC).
7. Lymphokines.
8. Others.

Vasoactive Amines

Histamine and serotonin (5-hydroxytryptamine) are believed to be mediators in the immediate active phase of increased permeability. In humans, histamine is stored and is immediately available largely in the granules of the mast cells and basophils, and in platelets. Serotonin is present in the mast cells of such rodents as rat and mouse, and in platelets.[70] These amines cause vasodilatation and increased vascular permeability, the latter being restricted to venules, as noted earlier. They have vasoconstrictor or dilator effects according to species; the relative activity of serotonin and histamine is also species dependent. For example, the rat is exquisitely more reactive to serotonin than to histamine, whereas the reverse is true in humans. Histamine acts on the microcirculation mainly through H1-type receptors.[70]

Many agents release amines from mast cells.[64] Principal among these are (a) *physical agents*, such as trauma or cold; (b) *immunologic reactions*, through a well-known mechanism involving receptors on the mast cell surface that bind with IgE (p. 164); (c) *C3a and C5a*, fragments of complement that induce release of histamine from mast cells and thus increase permeability (for which reason they are called *anaphylatoxins*); (d) *cationic proteins*, derived from neutrophil lysosomes; and (e) a variety of *low-molecular-weight substances*, such as polymyxin B and compound 48/80, which are potent mast cell degranulators and histamine liberators.

Release of histamine following exposure to the stimulus involves fusion of perigranular membranes to the plasma membrane, and extrusion of the granules, followed by a complex process of regranulation.[72] The mechanism of release[73] involves binding of the ligand with a cell receptor, activation of adenylate cyclase, elaboration of cyclic AMP, and, via phosphorylation of a still undefined intracytoplasmic protein, movement of the granule to the cell surface (see Fig. 5–4, p. 164).

Histamine can be isolated from inflammatory sites in early inflammation, and H1 histamine antagonists suppress the immediate-transient response induced by mild injury. However, the content of histamine dwindles within the first 60 minutes, and antihistaminics have no effect on the delayed permeability responses. *Thus, histamine is important mainly in early inflammatory responses* and in immediate IgE-mediated hypersensitivity reactions.

Release of histamine and serotonin from *platelets* (the platelet release reaction) is stimulated when platelets aggregate after contact with collagen, thrombin, ADP, and antigen-antibody complexes. Platelet release is also activated by a factor produced by basophils and mast cells (platelet-activating factor [PAF]) during IgE-mediated reactions. In this way the platelet release reaction results in increased permeability during immunologic reactions. As will be discussed later, PAF itself has inflammatory properties.

Plasma Proteases

Three interrelated systems—the complement, kinin, and clotting systems—are active within this category. The kinins are highly vasoactive; complement components are both vasoactive and chemotactic.

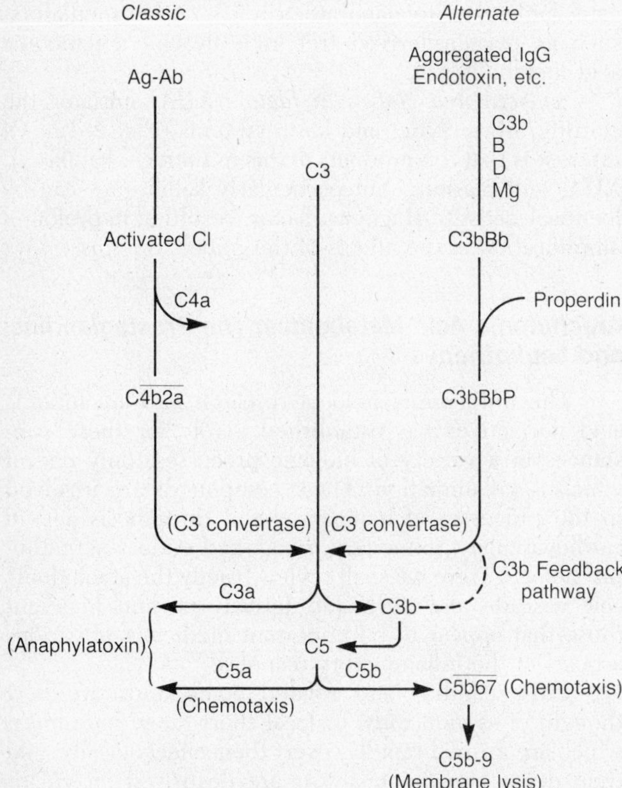

Figure 2–10. The complement system.

The Complement System.[74] This system consists of 18 component proteins (together with their cleavage products), which are found in greatest concentration in plasma. It functions in the immune system by mediating a series of biologic reactions, all of which serve in the defense against microbial agents. These include increased vascular permeability, chemotaxis, opsonization prior to phagocytosis, and lysis of target organisms.

The complement system consists of *activating* and *effector* sequences. Activation occurs either via the *classic* pathway, initiated by antigen-antibody complexes, or by the *alternate* pathway, initiated by a variety of largely nonimmunologic stimuli. As a result of activation, proteolytic cleavage products are produced and it is these that have profound inflammatory effects. The cascade involved in the activation of these various proteins is shown in Figure 2–10.

The *classic pathway* is initiated by binding of an antigen-antibody complex to C1, which self-activates to $\overline{C1}$ and cleaves C4 and C2; the resulting cleavage fragments form a complex C4b2a, also called *C3 convertase*. C3 convertase is an important enzyme, since it splits C3 into two critical fragments, C3a and C3b. C3a is released but C3b forms a trimolecular complex with $\overline{C4b2a}$ (C5 convertase). (C3b is the opsonic C3 fragment alluded to earlier.) C5 convertase interacts with C5 to break off C5a; C5b combines with C6 and C7 into a $\overline{C5b67}$ complex. Further binding of $\overline{C5b67}$ with C8 and C9 produces C5b-9, the final lytic agent of complement.

In the alternative complement pathway (Fig. 2–10), C3 is activated directly (thus bypassing C1, C4, and C2) by such stimuli as bacterial endotoxins, cobra venom, and aggregated globulins. The C3 convertase of this system is formed by interactions of Factors B, D, C3b in the presence of Mg (see also p. 167).

The components of the complement system that have biologic activity in inflammation are as follows:

1. *C3a* increases vascular permeability. In addition to being produced by the classic and alternative pathways, *C3 can be directly cleaved* (at least in vitro) by plasmin, bacterial proteases, and other C3-cleaving enzymes found in various tissues.
2. *C5a* induces increased vascular permeability (being much more potent in this respect than C3a) and is highly chemotactic to neutrophils and monocytes. It is released by complement activation, or direct cleavage by trypsin, bacterial proteases, and enzymes found in neutrophil lysosomes and macrophages.[75].
3. *C3b* is an important opsonin, recognizing receptors on neutrophils, macrophages, and eosinophils.
4. *C5b67* complex produced during activation of the complement system has no permeability effect but is a chemotactic agent. Its role in vivo is unclear.
5. *C5b-9* is the final lytic component of complement and may be involved in injury to parenchymal cells.

The permeability-increasing components of C3a and C5a are called "anaphylatoxins." As mentioned earlier, they act mainly by liberating histamine from mast cells and platelets; their activity can be suppressed by antihistaminics, or by previous depletion of mast cell histamine. It is thus no surprise that they also induce vascular leakage through gaps in the endothelium of venules similar to those induced by histamine. C5a also activates the lipoxygenase pathway of arachidonic acid metabolism in neutrophils and macrophages, leading to the formation of additional mediators of increased permeability and chemotaxis from these cells. Concomitant release of oxygen-derived radicals may also cause endothelial damage and production of other chemotactic lipids, as we shall see (p. 56). Thus, C5a in vivo is a powerful inflammatory agent.

The Kinin System. This system results in the ultimate release of the vasoactive nonapeptide *bradykinin*, a potent agent that increases vascular permeability. *Bradykinin also causes contraction of smooth muscle, dilatation of blood vessels, and pain when injected into the skin. It is not chemotactic.* The cascade that eventually produces kinin is shown in Figure 2–11.[76] It begins with the activation of factor XII of the clotting system (Hageman factor) by contact with surface-active agents, such as glass, collagen, basement membrane material, cartilage, and endotoxin. A fragment of factor XII (prekallikrein activator, or factor XIIA) is produced, and this converts plasma prekallikrein into an active proteolytic form, the enzyme *kallikrein*. The latter cleaves a plasma-glycoprotein precursor, *high-molecular-weight kininogen* (HMWK), to produce *bradykinin* (HMWK also acts as a cofactor or catalyst in the acti-

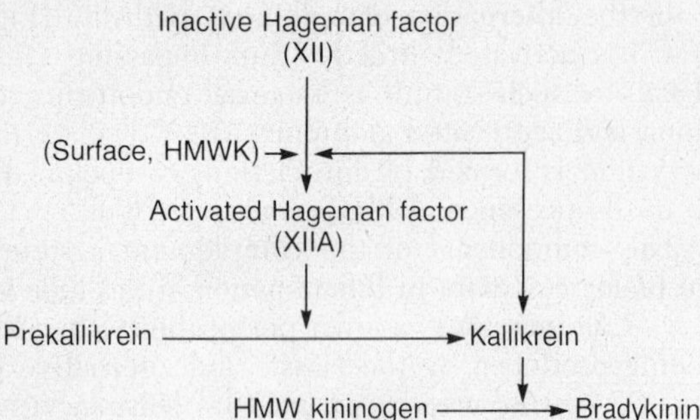

Figure 2–11. The plasma kinin generating system.

vation of Hageman factor). The action of bradykinin is short-lived, since it is quickly inactivated by an enzyme called *kininase. Of importance is that kallikrein itself is a potent activator of Hageman factor,* allowing for autocatalytic amplification of the initial stimulus. Kallikrein itself appears to have chemotactic activity, and causes aggregation of neutrophils in vitro.[77]

THE CLOTTING SYSTEM. This is another group of plasma proteins that can be activated by Hageman factor. The final step of the cascade is the conversion of fibrinogen to fibrin by the action of thrombin. During this conversion *fibrinopeptides* are formed, which induce increased vascular permeability and chemotactic activity for leukocytes.

The *fibrinolytic system* contributes to the vascular phenomena of inflammation in several ways, but mainly by means of the kinin system. Plasminogen activator (released from endothelium, leukocytes, and other tissues) or kallikrein cleaves plasminogen, a plasma protein that binds to the evolving fibrin clot to generate *plasmin,* a multifunctional protease. Plasmin is important in lysing fibrin clots, but in the context of inflammation it has the following actions: (1) it activates Hageman factor (XII), releasing XIIA, which initiates the cascade to generate bradykinin; (2) it cleaves C3, the third component of complement, to produce C3 fragments; and (3) it induces the formation of "fibrin-split products," which may have permeability-inducing properties. Which of these actions is important in vivo is still unknown.

SUMMARY OF PLASMA PROTEASES (Fig. 2–12). From this discussion of the complex mediators generated by the kinin, complement, and clotting systems, a few general conclusions can be drawn:

1. The mediators most likely to be important in vivo are *bradykinin, C3a, and C5a as mediators of increased vascular permeability, and C5a as the mediator of chemotaxis.*

2. *C3 and C5* are central because they can be generated (at least in vitro) by three different groups of influences: (a) classic immunologic reactions; (b) alternate complement pathway activation; and (c) agents with little immunologic specificity, such as bacterial products, plasmin, and some serine proteases found in normal tissue. In addition, C5a, by inducing chemotaxis, activates leukocytes to elaborate or release other mediators, such as oxygen-derived free radicals and arachidonic acid metabolites.

3. *Activated Hageman factor (XIIA)* initiates the clotting, fibrinolytic, and kinin systems (Fig. 2–12). Of interest is that the products of this initiation—kallikrein, XIIA, and plasmin, but particularly kallikrein—can by feedback activate Hageman factor, resulting in profound amplification of the effects of the initial stimulus.

Arachidonic Acid Metabolites: The Prostaglandins and Leukotrienes

The burgeoning field of research into arachidonic acid derivatives has established a role for these substances in a variety of biologic processes, only one of which is inflammation. These compounds are involved in the processes of hemostasis and thrombosis and in cardiovascular, pulmonary, renal, and endocrine pathophysiology. Here we shall review briefly the arachidonic acid cascade and its major derivatives, and highlight those that appear to be important mediators of various aspects of the inflammatory response.[78–82]

Prostaglandins and related compounds are best thought of as *autacoids,* or local short-range hormones, which are formed rapidly, exert their effects locally, and then decay spontaneously or are destroyed enzymatically.[82] Although there are several possible pathways for arachidonic acid metabolism, it appears that specific cells are highly selective in their metabolism of this fatty acid; this selectivity can be linked, on the one hand, with the specific enzyme content of the cell, and on the other, with the function of the biologically active products.

Arachidonic acid (AA) is a 20-carbon polyunsaturated fatty acid (5,8,11,14-eicosatetraenoic acid) that is derived directly from dietary sources or by conversion from the essential fatty acid linoleic acid. It does not occur free in the cell but is normally esterified in

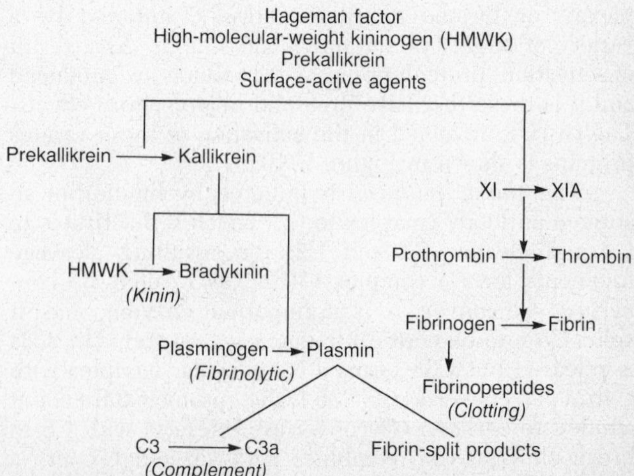

Figure 2–12. Interactions of kinin, clotting, fibrinolytic, and complement systems.

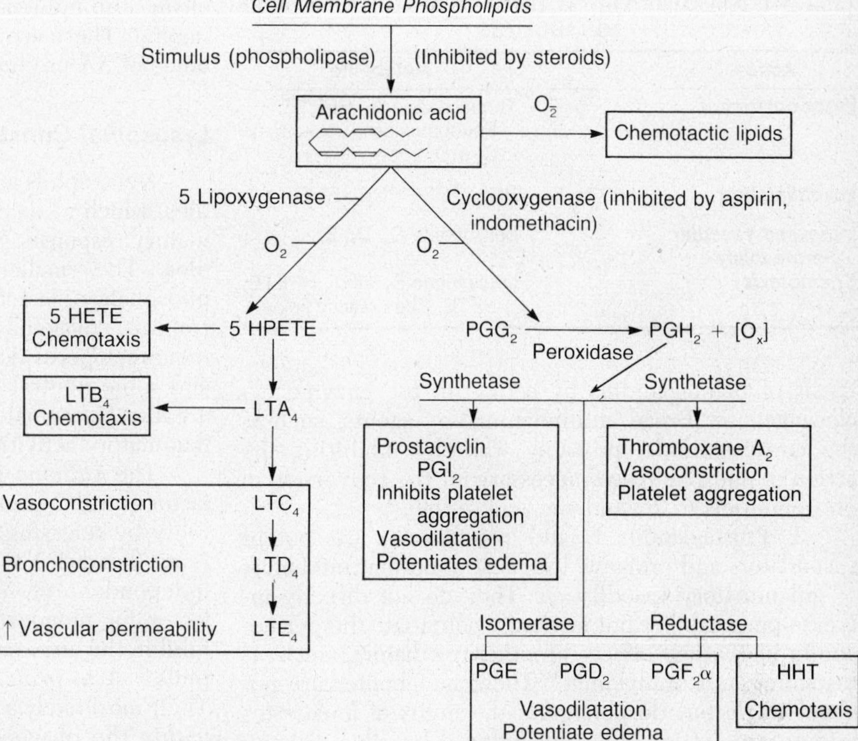

Figure 2–13. Arachidonic acid metabolites in inflammation. The principal mediators and their actions are cited in the text.

membrane phospholipids, particularly in the 2 position of phosphatidylcholine and phosphatidylinositol. In order for arachidonic acid to be utilized by the cell to make prostaglandins, it must first be released from phospholipids. This is accomplished through the activation of cellular phospholipases (phospholipase A2 and, in some cells, phospholipase C) by mechanical, chemical, and physical stimuli or by other mediators (e.g., C5a). Following activation, biosynthesis of the metabolites of arachidonic acid occurs by one of two major pathways (Fig. 2–13).

The Cyclooxygenase Pathway. A fatty acid cyclooxygenase transforms arachidonic acid rapidly into the prostaglandin endoperoxide PGG_2, which in turn is converted by enzymatic peroxidation into PGH_2. In the conversion of PGG_2 to PGH_2, a free radical of oxygen is generated. PGG_2 and PGH_2 stimulate platelet aggregation and release, as well as contraction of vascular smooth muscle. Aspirin, indomethacin, and other nonsteroidal anti-inflammatory drugs inhibit cyclooxygenase. PGH_2 is then converted enzymatically into three products: (1) *thromboxane* A_2 (TXA_2) found in platelets and other cells, a short-lived (half-time of seconds), potent platelet aggregator and blood vessel constrictor; (2) *prostacyclin* (PGI_2) found predominantly in the vessel wall, a potent inhibitor of platelet aggregation and vasodilator; and (3) in many sites the more stable prostaglandins PGE_2, $PGF_{2\alpha}$, *and* PGD_2, which have a variety of actions on vascular tone and permeability. Each of these steps is carried out by specific enzymes (e.g., thromboxane synthetase, prostacyclin synthetase) present within the target cell.

The Lipoxygenase Pathway. This pathway involves the conversion of AA by fatty acid lipoxygenases into hydroperoxy derivatives [hydroperoxy eicosatetraenoic acid (HPETE); 12 HPETE in platelets and 5 and 15 HPETE in leukocytes]. HPETE may undergo peroxidation to HETE, the latter being a potent chemotactic stimulus for neutrophils. 5 HPETE gives rise to the important *leukotrienes,* so designated because of their typical triene chain and their initial isolation from leukocytes. An unstable 5,6 epoxy derivative, *leukotriene* A_4 (LTA_4), is then enzymatically converted to *leukotriene* B_4, or by addition of a glutathione residue to *leukotriene* C_4. The latter is then converted to *leukotriene* D_4 (LTD_4) and subsequently to *leukotriene* E_4. Leukotriene B_4 is a potent chemotactic agent that causes aggregation of leukocytes, and LTC_4, LTD_4, and LTE_4 cause vasoconstriction, bronchospasm, and increased vascular permeability.

A third mechanism of arachidonic acid conversion has been uncovered recently: this involves the nonenzymatic peroxidation of AA by oxygen-derived free radicals, leading to the elaboration of highly chemotactic lipids.[83] The biochemical nature of these products is now under investigation.

The principal actions of arachidonic acid metabolites are summarized in Table 2–1. The evidence for their involvement in inflammation is fast accumulating and can be summarized as follows:

1. Prostaglandins and, more recently, leukotrienes have been detected in the fluids and exudates of inflammatory reactions and in anaphylactic reactions in the lungs.

2. Drugs such as aspirin and indomethacin, which have anti-inflammatory properties, inhibit the biosyn-

Table 2–1. INFLAMMATORY ACTIONS OF ARACHIDONIC ACID METABOLITES

Action	Metabolite
Vasoconstriction	Thromboxane A_2, HPETE, Endoperoxides, Leukotriene C_4 & D_4
Vasodilatation	PGI_2, PGE_1, PGE_2, PGD_2
Increased Vascular Permeability	Leukotriene C_4, D_4, E_4
Chemotaxis	Leukotriene B_4, HHT, HPETE, HETE, Chemotactic lipids

thesis of prostaglandins by acting on the enzyme cyclooxygenase. Broad anti-inflammatory agents, such as the corticosteroids, probably work by inhibiting the action of phospholipases necessary for the conversion of phospholipids to arachidonic acid (p. 80).

3. Prostaglandin E and prostacyclin are potent vasodilators and probably the most important mediators of inflammatory vasodilation. They do not directly increase permeability but markedly potentiate the permeability-increasing effects of other mediators, such as histamine and bradykinin.[86] These metabolites are not chemotactic but do *potentiate* the influx of leukocytes into an area of inflammation induced by other chemotactic mediators.[87] Whether these potentiating effects are due to the vasodilatation or to other mechanisms is uncertain.[88]

4. The cysteinyl-containing leukotrienes C_4, D_4, and E_4 cause intense vasoconstriction and are at least 1000 times as potent as histamine in increasing vascular permeability.[89] The vascular leakage, as with histamine, is restricted to venules. Leukotrienes C_4, D_4 and E_4 are also potent bronchoconstrictors and have now been identified as the previously described slow-reacting substances of anaphylaxis (SRS-A) released from mast cells and basophils.[90–94]

5. Leukotriene B_4 causes conspicuous aggregation and adhesion of leukocytes to venular endothelium and is a powerful chemotactic agent.[95] Some of the other products of lipoxygenase metabolism, such as HETE, are also chemotactic.

6. The prostaglandins are also involved in the pathogenesis of pain and fever in inflammation. PGE_2 causes a marked increase in pain produced by intradermal injection of suboptimal concentrations of histamine and bradykinin, and there is evidence that prostaglandin production may be one of the causes of fever during severe infections.

Admittedly the story of prostaglandins, leukotrienes, and similar products[94, 95] is complex and undoubtedly it will keep changing. Nonetheless for the time being it is clear that inflammatory stimuli induce the synthesis and release of arachidonic acid metabolites; that these metabolites contribute to the genesis of fever, pain, vasodilatation, increased vascular permeability, and leukocytic infiltration in inflammation; and that anti-inflammatory drugs such as aspirin, indomethacin, and corticosteroids, which influence arachidonic acid metabolism, also influence the signs and symptoms of inflammation. These are compelling arguments for the importance of AA products in the inflammatory response.

Lysosomal Constituents

Neutrophils and monocytes contain lysosomal granules, which when released may contribute to the inflammatory response. *Neutrophils* exhibit two types of granules. The smaller *specific* granules contain alkaline phosphatase, lactoferrin, lysozyme, and (in human neutrophils) collagenase. The large *azurophil* granules contain myeloperoxidase, cationic proteins, acid hydrolases, and some neutral proteases (elastase). The latter three are the lysosomal constituents that have potential inflammatory activities.

The *cationic proteins* include (a) an arginine-rich factor (band 2 protein) that increases vascular permeability by releasing histamine from mast cells;[96] (b) proteins (band 1,3,4) that increase vascular permeability independent of histamine release; (c) a chemotactic factor for monocytes; and (d) a factor that appears to inhibit the movement of other neutrophils or eosinophils.[97] *Acid proteases* degrade proteins at an acid pH. Their most likely action is to degrade bacteria and debris *within* the phagolysosomes, but in vitro they also degrade basement membrane–like material. It is doubtful whether they have an extracellular effect in vivo, since optimal low pH values for their action are not reached extracellularly. *Neutral proteases,* on the other hand, are capable of degrading various extracellular components. These enzymes (collagenase, elastase, cathepsin G, etc.) can attack collagen, basement membrane, fibrin, elastin, and cartilage, resulting in the tissue destruction characteristic of purulent and deforming inflammatory processes. Neutral proteases can also release a kinin-like peptide from kininogen.[98]

The *monocytes* and *macrophages* also contain acid hydrolases, collagenase, elastase, and plasminogen activator. These may be particularly active in chronic inflammatory reactions.

Lysosomal constituents thus have numerous and profound effects. It is evident that the intitial leukocytic infiltration, if unchecked, can potentiate further increases in vascular permeability, chemotaxis, and tissue damage. These harmful proteases, however, are held in check by a system of *antiproteases* in the serum and tissue fluids.[99] Foremost among these is *alpha-1-antitrypsin,* which is the major inhibitor of neutrophilic elastase. It follows, therefore, that a deficiency of these inhibitors may lead to unchecked action of leukocyte proteases, as is the case in patients with alpha-1-antitrypsin deficiency (p. 721). *Alpha-2-macroglobulin* is another antiprotease found in serum and various secretions.

Oxygen-Derived Free Radicals

As we have seen, reactive oxygen metabolites elaborated in neutrophils and macrophages after exposure to chemotactic agents, immune complexes, or a phagocytic challenge may be released extracellularly. These metabolites have been implicated in the following responses: (1) *Endothelial cell damage with resultant increased vascular permeability.*[100] For example, activation of C5a in vivo causes neutrophilic aggregation, endothelial cell damage, and increased permeability of lung capillaries; the last-named can be prevented by previous treatment of the animals with H_2O_2 and OH· scavengers, which suggests that these species mediate the endothelial damage.[101] (2) *Generation of chemotactic lipids nonenzymatically from arachidonic acid* (see Fig. 2–13). The superoxide ion and hydroxyl ions seem to be the active radical in this conversion.[83] (3) *Inactivation of antiproteases*, such as alpha-1-antitrypsin, discussed earlier. Potentially this may lead to unopposed protease activity with increased destruction of structural components of tissue, such as elastin. Inactivation appears to result from oxidation by hydroxyl ions (OH·) of methionyl residues on the antiprotease molecule.[99] (4) *Injury to other cell types* (fibroblasts, red cells, parenchymal cells), ascribed to a variety of oxygen metabolites.

It must be emphasized that serum, tissue fluids, and target cells possess antioxidant protective mechanisms that detoxify these potentially harmful oxygen-derived radicals.[101] These have been discussed in Chapter 1, but to repeat, they include: (1) the copper-containing serum protein *ceruloplasmin;* (2) the iron-free fraction of serum *transferrin*; (3) the enzyme *superoxide dismutase*, which is found or can be activated in a variety of cell types; (4) the enzyme *catalase*, which detoxifies H_2O_2; and (5) *glutathione peroxidase*, another powerful H_2O_2 detoxifier. Thus, the influence of oxygen-free radicals in any given inflammatory reaction is the balance between the production and inactivation of these molecules by cells and tissues.

Acetylated Glycerol Ether Phosphocholine (AGEPC; PAF)

AGEPC belongs to the most recently described and novel class of lipid mediators.[82] Its biologic effect has been known for years as *platelet activating factor* (PAF), a factor derived from antigen-stimulated, IgE-sensitized basophils, which causes aggregation of platelets and release of their active constituents (such as histamine and serotonin). The chemical structure of PAF has been documented as AGEPC, and the molecule has been synthesized. In addition to platelet stimulation, AGEPC (in high doses) causes vasoconstriction, and at extremely low concentrations induces vasodilatation and increased vascular permeability with a potency 100 to 10,000 times greater than that of histamine.[102] It also causes increased leukocyte adhesion in vitro[103] and early leukocytic infiltration when injected into the skin.[103A] Thus, AGEPC can elicit at least four of the five cardinal signs of inflammation. A variety of cell types, including basophils, neutrophils, and monocytes, can elaborate AGEPC. It remains to be seen whether AGEPC acts as a mediator in vivo directly, or by releasing other mediators (e.g., leukotrienes)[104] or by both mechanisms.

Lymphocyte Factors

The lymphocyte is involved in the two major types of immunologic reactions: antibody formation and cell-mediated immunity (delayed hypersensitivity). In the latter reaction, sensitized T lymphocytes become activated and release a variety of biologically active compounds, called *lymphokines*. Included are chemoattractants for macrophages, neutrophils, and basophils; inhibitors of macrophage migration, and a factor that increases vascular permeability. Other lymphokines are more relevant to immunologic reactions and will be discussed on page 170. It is important to note, however, that lymphocytes may be abundant in nonimmunologic inflammation and can be activated in vitro by nonimmunologic means, such as exposure to surface-active plant lectins (concanavalin A and phytohemagglutinin).

Other Mediators

Other mediators that have chemotactic activity for leukocytes are fragments derived from the breakdown of collagen[105] or fibronectin,[48] and the platelet-derived growth factor[106] (p. 76). These factors have additional roles in chronic inflammation and wound healing and are discussed further on page 76.

Summary of Chemical Mediators

Table 2–2 summarizes the major actions of the principal mediators. The multiplicity of proposed mediators is eloquent testimony to the current excitement about the biochemical basis of inflammation, but also to the fact that we are still unsure of the precise events involved in mediation of the inflammatory response. When Sir Thomas Lewis suggested histamine, one mediator was clearly not enough. Now we may have too many. Yet from this morass we can tentatively extract a few mediators that may be relevant in vivo (Table 2–3). For increased vascular permeability, histamine, the anaphylatoxins (C3a and C5a), the kinins, and the leukotrienes (C and D) are almost certainly involved, at least early in the course of inflammation. For chemotaxis, complement fragments (particularly C5a), AA lipoxygenase products (leukotriene B_4), and other chemotactic lipids are the most likely protagonists. Also, one cannot deny the important role of prostaglandins in vasodilatation, pain, and fever and in other ways as yet not understood. Lysosomal products, especially neutral proteases, and oxygen-derived radicals are the most likely candidates as causes of the ensuing tissue destruction.

Two points must be reemphasized before the discussion of mediators is closed. The first is that the different mediator systems, although discussed separately, are intimately intertwined. One example, cited earlier, is the role of activated Hageman factor in the kinin, clotting, and fibrinolytic cascades. Another is the

Table 2–2. SUMMARY OF MEDIATORS

Mediator	Source	Action: *Vascular Leakage*	*Chemotaxis*: *Neutrophils*	*Chemotaxis*: *Monocytes*	*Other*
Histamine and Serotonin	Mast cells, basophils, and platelets	+	–	–	
Kinins					
Bradykinin	Plasma substrate	+	–	–	Pain
Kallikrein		–	+	+	
Complement					
C3a	Plasma protein via liver; macrophages	+	–	–	Opsonic fragment (C3b)
C5a		+	+	+	
Prostaglandins	Most cells, from membrane phospholipids	Potentiate other mediators	±	–	Vasodilation, pain, fever
Leukotrienes					
B_4	Leukocytes	–	+	+	
C_4, D_4, E_4	Leukocytes; mast cells	+	–	–	Bronchoconstriction, vasoconstriction
Lysosomal components					
Cationic proteins	Leukocytes	+	–	–	Immobilization of neutrophils
Neutral proteases	Leukocytes	+			Tissue damage
Oxygen Metabolites	Leukocytes	+			Endothelial damage, tissue damage
AGEPC	Mast cells Other cells	+	+	?	Bronchoconstriction

influence of chemotactic agents or phagocytic stimuli themselves on leukocytes; these result in activating the arachidonic acid cascade and releasing proteases and oxygen-derived free radicals from leukocytes. These interactions may explain prolonged inflammatory responses, in which mediators may be activated in sequence. The second point is that with all these mediators there seems to be an intelligent system of checks and balances. If not, we would all be red, bloated, and covered with exudate! But these chemicals either are tightly sequestered within cells or are present in plasma or tissue as precursor forms that must go through many steps before becoming activated. Thus, the biochemical mechanisms responsible for the rate-limiting steps involved are of primary importance in understanding inflammation. Conversely, once activated or released, these mediators are quickly inactivated or destroyed: otherwise, inflammation would never cease! Some of the inactivators are known, such as kininase, which destroys bradykinin; chemotactic factor inactivators, which neutralize C5a; antioxidants, which scavenge oxygen-derived free radicals; and antiproteases, which neutralize elastase and collagenase. Others are more obscure. It is evident, however, that the more we know about these checks and balances, the better we can modify the inflammatory response.

Table 2–3. MOST LIKELY MEDIATORS IN INFLAMMATION

Vasodilation
Prostaglandins
Increased Vascular Permeability
Vasoactive amines
C3a and C5a (through liberating amines)
Bradykinin
Leukotriene C, D, E
Chemotaxis
C5a
Leukotriene B_4
Other chemotactic lipids
Neutrophil cationic proteins
Fever
Endogenous pyrogen
Prostaglandins
Pain
Prostaglandins
Bradykinin
Tissue Damage
Neutrophil and macrophage lysosomal enzymes
Oxygen metabolites

The discussion of mediators completes the basic description of the relatively uniform pattern of the inflammatory reaction encountered in most injuries. Recall that, although hemodynamic, permeability, and white cell changes have been described sequentially and may be initiated in this order, all these phenomena in the fully evolved reaction to injury are concurrent in a seemingly chaotic but remarkably organized multiring circus. As might be expected, many variables may modify this basic process. Particularly important are (1) the nature and intensity of the injury, (2) the site and tissue affected, and (3) the responsiveness of the host—nutrition, adequacy of the cardiovascular system, drug therapy, existence of predisposing disorders such as diabetes mellitus and cancer, and the possible presence of previously acquired immunity to the offender, if it is indeed microbiologic in origin.

Table 2–4. THE MONONUCLEAR PHAGOCYTE SYSTEM (THE RETICULOENDOTHELIAL SYSTEM)

Stem Cells (Committed)	
Monoblasts	BONE MARROW
Promonocytes	
Monocytes	BLOOD
Macrophages	TISSUES Inflammatory macrophages Liver (Kupffer cells) Lung (alveolar macrophages) Connective tissue (histiocytes) Bone marrow (macrophages) Spleen and lymph nodes (fixed and free macrophages) Serous cavities (pleural and peritoneal macrophages) Nervous system (microglial cells) Bone (osteoclasts) Skin (?Langerhans' cells) Lymphoid tissue (?dendritic cells)

THE MONONUCLEAR PHAGOCYTE SYSTEM

The mononuclear phagocyte system (MPS) is the currently favored designation of the reticuloendothelial system (RES). Mononuclear phagocytes have always been known as the scavenger cells of the body. This traditional role, known since Metchnikoff, remains one of their most important functions. In inflammation, they are abundant after the early stages, when they avidly engulf and digest foreign particles, debris from injured cells, red cells, proteins that have leaked out, and even their predecessors, the neutrophils, after the latter have finished their own job of ingestion. Recent research, however, has established that macrophages have much wider functions in biology and pathology.[107–110] They have a fundamental role in specific immunity through a relationship that has developed with the lymphocyte, a role that will be further developed in the chapter on immunity (Chapter 5). Here we shall briefly review the normal physiology of macrophages and their established or postulated roles in inflammation.

Monocytes and macrophages belong to the system of mononuclear phagocytes (Table 2–4). The MPS consists of cells in the bone marrow, peripheral blood, and tissues that are highly specialized for the function of endocytosis (pinocytosis and phagocytosis) and intracellular digestion. In connective tissue they are frequently termed *histiocytes.* They originate from a committed stem cell in the bone marrow through a *monoblast* stage to form the *promonocytes.* Promonocytes are capable of rapid division, giving rise to the peripheral blood *monocyte.* The blood monocyte is a smaller cell, is more functionally active, does not divide, and forms 4 to 8% of the total white count. Its average transit time in the blood is about 32 hours, appreciably longer than that of the neutrophil or eosinophil. The monocyte is characterized by large numbers of pinocytotic vesicles, ruffling of surface membrane, a variable number of lysosomes, and an active Golgi apparatus (Fig. 2–14).

The origin and turnover of all the tissue macrophages in Table 2–4 are not precisely known, but the evidence suggests that they also are derived from blood

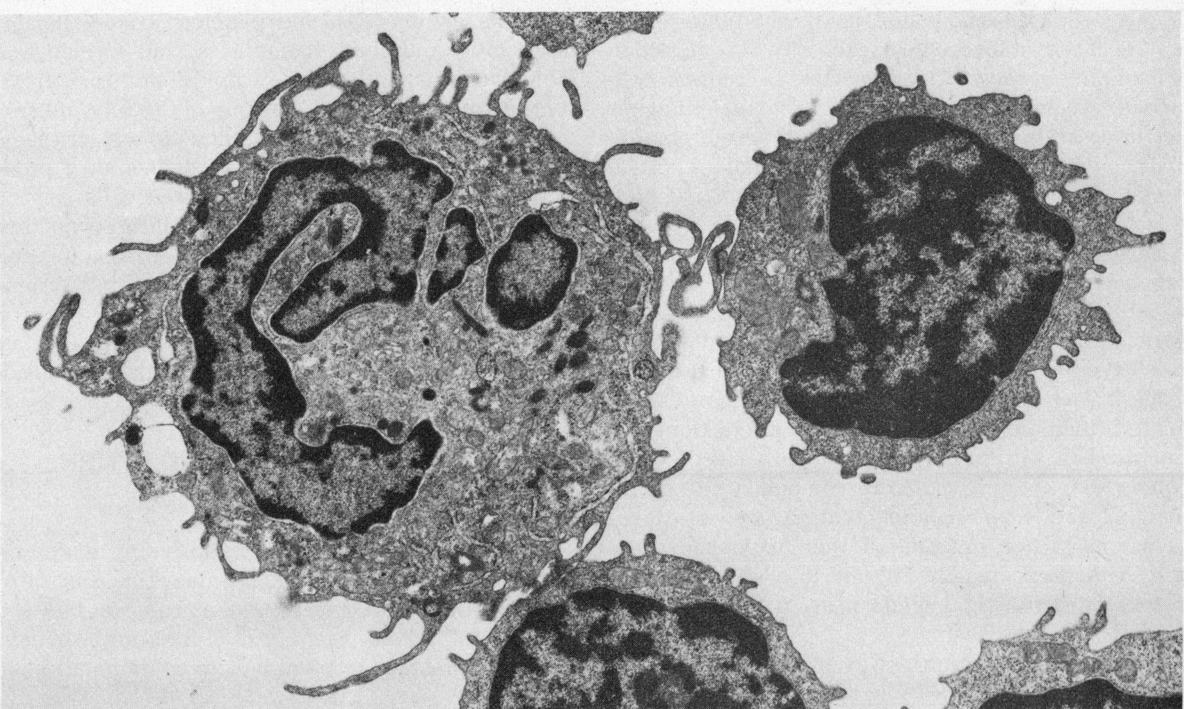

Figure 2–14. Electron micrograph of peripheral blood monocyte (*left*) and lymphocyte. Note the abundant cytoplasm, indented nucleus, ruffled surface membrane, and lysosomes of monocyte.

or marrow precursors by way of blood monocytes. This evidence is most compelling for the alveolar macrophages, peritoneal cells, and Kupffer cells.

There is little question now that the origin of the majority of macrophages in inflammation is the blood monocyte.[111] The conclusive experiments involved "marking" of the monocytes, either by previous injections of ^{3}H-thymidine (which is incorporated only by the precursor monocyte in the bone marrow) or with a cytoplasmic marker in the form of a phagocytized particle such as carbon. Identification of such circulating labeled cells within inflammatory lesions (taken together with the appropriate experimental controls) indicated the source of inflammatory macrophages to be blood monocytes.

Macrophages from various sites share some general properties that make them unique. The morphologic characteristics should be well-known. The cells are highly mobile (although slower than neutrophils). They are capable not only of *phagocytosis* of relatively large particles but also of *pinocytosis* of soluble molecules smaller than 10 nm. The uptake of particles is carried out in part as a result of the presence on the macrophage of cell surface receptors for the Fc fragment of immunoglobulin and the third component of complement (C3b). Macrophages possess a large repertoire of hydrolytic enzymes, which explains their capacity to degrade various materials rapidly. Finally, mononuclear phagocytes have the property of becoming "activated" by external stimuli. The term "activated macrophage" refers to cells that are larger and have a more ruffled cytoplasm, increased numbers of mitochondria, increased levels of hydrolytic enzymes and lysosomes, greater membrane activity with increased endocytosis, more active metabolism, and a greater ability to kill both intracellular bacteria and malignant tumor cells. This state of activation can be triggered by (1) interaction with *immune-sensitized* T lymphocytes, as occurs in cell-mediated reactions (p. 170); or (2) *nonimmunologic direct interactions* that "perturb" the cell membrane, such as contact with fibronectin-coated surfaces, certain bacterial products (such as endotoxin), or other chemicals.

Recently it has emerged that these stimulated macrophages secrete a wide variety of products, many of which are active in inflammation. The spectrum of biologic activities induced is phenomenal—and all from one cell type![107, 112] Further, the versatility of the macrophage is such that secretion of these products can be regulated (increased or decreased) by interactions between the cell and its environment—other cells (e.g., lymphocytes), connective tissue components (e.g., fibronectin), and serum (complement), as well as exogenous agents. Since in addition the macrophages are long-lived and can readily migrate to all tissues, their secretory properties may affect many pathophysiologic responses.

Among the important classes of macrophage products are the following:

1. *Neutral proteases,* such as plasminogen activator, which activates the elaboration of the fibrinolytic agent plasmin; and collagenase and elastase, which degrade connective tissue components.
2. *Complement components* of both the classic and alternate pathways.
3. *Coagulation factors* (e.g., Factor V, thromboplastin), which may be important in converting fibrinogen to fibrin locally.
4. *Chemotactic factors* for neutrophils.
5. *Arachidonic acid metabolites,* both cyclooxygenase and lipoxygenase products, which cause vasodilatation, increased vascular permeability, and chemotaxis.
6. *Reactive oxygen metabolites.*
7. *Growth-promoting factors* for fibroblasts, blood vessels, and myeloid progenitor cells.
8. *Interleukin* I, a polypeptide with far-ranging activities including lymphocyte activation, fever production (endogenous pyrogen), and stimulation of specific protein synthesis by other cells (e.g., acute-phase protein in liver; collagenase in fibroblasts).
9. Other biologically active agents that cause inflammation (AGEPC) or have antiviral activity (interferon).

Although some of these factors seem to be harmful to the individual, the overall effect is beneficial. Macrophages are in a sense allies but, like all powerful allies, they are to be respected and occasionally feared!

Besides its importance in inflammation and immunity, MPS (particularly the Kupffer cells of the liver and splenic macrophages) is the main line of defense against bacteria in the bloodstream and serves to control the hematogenous dissemination of organisms. The system is also involved in the removal and phagocytosis of unwanted materials floating about in the blood or sequestered in organs. Included are obsolescent or injured red cells, white cells, and platelets; coagulation products; antigen-antibody complexes; and foreign macromolecules such as complex lipids and carbohydrates synthesized by the body in some of the inborn errors of metabolism (the basis for so-called storage diseases) (p. 142). The capacity of MPS to recognize such products is remarkable. When dead or injured cells are coated with antibody, they are selectively filtered out by the surveillance system, even though they do not appear to be morphologically abnormal. Thus, the system of phagocytic cells becomes extremely active in a wide variety of hemolytic diseases and anemias and, as we shall see, it is these cells that accumulate hemosiderin in various iron overload states (p. 924).

THE ROLE OF LYMPHATICS AND LYMPH NODES

The system of lymphatics and lymph nodes filters and "polices" the extravascular fluids. Together with the *mononuclear phagocyte system,* it represents a secondary line of defense that is called into play whenever a local inflammatory reaction fails to contain and neutralize injury.

Lymphatics are extremely delicate channels that

are difficult to visualize in ordinary tissue sections because they readily collapse. They are lined by continuous thin endothelium with loose, overlapping cell junctions; scant basement membrane; and no muscular support, except in the larger ducts. Lymph flow in inflammation is increased and helps drain the edema fluid from the extravascular space. Because the junctions of lymphatics are loose, lymphatic fluid eventually equilibrates with extravascular fluid. It has always been a mystery, however, when the lymphatic channels, so thin and without support, do not collapse under the pressure of the edema in the regions of inflammatory reactions. This seems to have been explained by the demonstration of delicate fibrils attached at right angles to the walls of the lymphatic channel and extending into the adjacent tissues. When fluid pressure mounts in the extravascular space, it exerts traction on these fibrils, which then open up the lymphatics and maintain their patency.[114] The traction may further widen the intercellular junctions and provide more ready access for macromolecules themselves. Not only fluid, but leukocytes and cell debris may find their way into lymph.

In severe injuries the drainage may transport the offending agent, be it chemical or bacterial. The lymphatics may become secondarily inflamed *(lymphangitis)*, as may the draining lymph nodes *(lymphadenitis)*. Therefore, it is not uncommon in infections of the hand, for example, to observe red streaks along the entire arm up to the axilla following the lymphatic channels, accompanied by painful enlargement of the axillary lymph nodes. The nodal enlargement is usually caused by hyperplasia of the lymphoid follicles and also by hyperplasia of the phagocytic cells lining the sinuses of the lymph nodes. This constellation of nodal histologic changes is termed *reactive* or *inflammatory lymphadenitis*.

Fortunately, the secondary barriers sometimes contain the spread of the infection, but in some instances they are overwhelmed, and the organisms drain through progressively larger channels and gain access to the vascular circulation, thus inducing a bacteremia. The phagocytic cells of the liver, spleen, and bone marrow contribute the next line of defense, but in massive infections, bacteria seed distant tissues of the body. The heart valves, meninges, kidneys, and joints are favored sites of implantation for blood-borne organisms, and in such a fashion endocarditis, meningitis, renal abscesses, and septic arthritis may develop.

CHRONIC INFLAMMATION

DEFINITION AND CAUSES

Thus far, we have described the inflammatory process in the early reaction to local injury—acute inflammation—usually seen when the stimulus is transient, such as an allergic wheal, a mild burn, or an avirulent infection that is rapidly cleared by the host response. Some of these acute reactions disappear completely, while others are repaired by processes to be discussed in the next section (Repair). In contrast, some inflammatory stimuli may go on for weeks, months, or even years, as in some persistent infections and self-perpetuating immunologic reactions. Persistent inflammatory stimuli lead to *chronic inflammation*. Although the transition from acute to chronic is often difficult to pinpoint, chronic inflammatory responses have some features sufficiently unique to warrant a separate description.

Clinically, chronic inflammation in various organs arises in three ways:

1. It may follow acute inflammation, either because of the persistence of the inciting stimulus, or because of some interference in the normal process of healing. For example, infection of the lung by some species of bacteria may begin as an acute inflammation (pneumonia), but persistence of these organisms or their products leads to tissue destruction, a smoldering inflammation, and a chronic lung abscess.
2. It may be due simply to repeated bouts of acute inflammation, with the patient showing successive attacks of fever, pain, and swelling. Here, histologic examination will show evidence of acute inflammation and healing (between attacks), as seen in recurrent infections of the gallbladder (cholecystitis) and kidney (pyelonephritis).
3. More curiously, chronic inflammation may begin insidiously as a low-grade smoldering response that does not follow classic symptomatic acute inflammation. It is this last form that includes some of the most common and disabling diseases of humans, such as rheumatoid arthritis, tuberculosis, and chronic lung disease. Such diseases occur in one of the following settings:
   a. persistent infection by *intracellular* microorganisms (e.g., tubercle bacilli, viral infection), which are of low toxicity but evoke an immunologic reaction.
   b. prolonged exposure to nondegradable but potentially toxic substances (e.g., silicosis in the lung).
   c. immune reactions perpetuated against the individual's own tissues (autoimmune diseases, such as rheumatoid arthritis).

CELLS AND MEDIATORS

The histologic hallmarks of chronic inflammation are (1) *infiltration by mononuclear cells*, principally macrophages, lymphocytes, and plasma cells; (2) *proliferation of fibroblasts* and, in many instances, *small blood vessels* (Fig. 2–15); and (3) increased connective tissue (fibrosis).

Infiltration by monocytes/macrophages is a particularly important component of chronic inflammation. As discussed previously, monocytes begin to emigrate rather early in acute inflammation, and within 48 hours constitute the predominant cell type. When the monocyte reaches the extravascular tissue it undergoes transformation into a much larger cell, the macrophage,

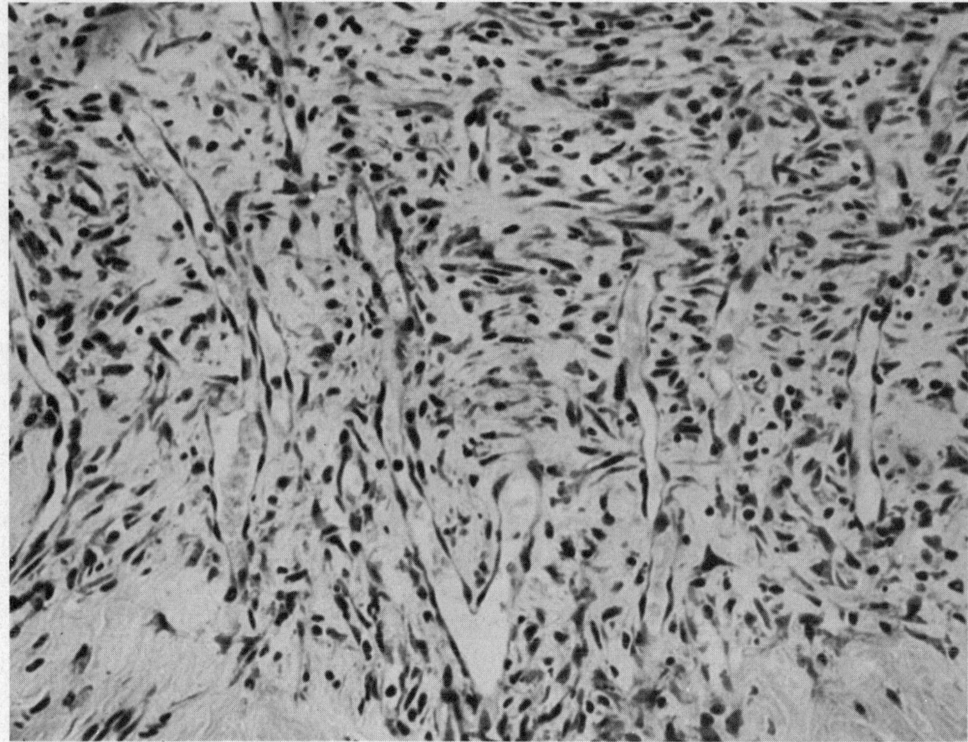

Figure 2–15. Focus of chronic inflammation showing infiltration by mononuclear cells and proliferation of fibroblasts and small vessels. (From Sholley, M. M., et al.: Endothelial proliferation in inflammation. I. Autoradiographic studies following thermal injury to the skin of normal rats. Am. J. Pathol. *89*:277, 1977.)

which may become "activated," as described earlier. In short-lived acute inflammation, if the irritant is eliminated, these macrophages eventually disappear (either dying off or making their way into the lymphatics and lymph nodes). If the injurious agent is not eliminated, as occurs with a tuberculous infection, with some immunologic reactions, or in the presence of a stubborn irritant, macrophages persist for prolonged periods of time.

Accumulation of macrophages occurs in three ways, each predominating in different types of infection:[115]

1. *Continued recruitment of monocytes* from the circulation, which results from the steady release of chemotactic factors. This is numerically the most important source for macrophages. As previously discussed, chemotactic stimuli for monocytes include C5a, fibrinopeptides, neutrophilic cationic proteins, a lymphokine from antigen-stimulated lymphocytes, and fragments from the breakdown of collagen and fibronectin. Each of these may play a role under given circumstances; for example, lymphokines are almost certainly involved during delayed hypersensitivity immune reactions.

2. *Local proliferation* (by mitotic division) *of macrophages* after their emigration from the bloodstream. We have no idea what triggers this division, but no more than two cycles of division occur.

3. *Prolonged survival and immobilization of macrophages* within the site of inflammation. This is especially evident when irritants such as inert lipids and carbon particles are of low virulence.

The mechanisms that lead to the recruitment and proliferation of *fibroblasts* and to collagen accumulation in chronic inflammation are less well understood.[116] A factor derived from platelets (platelet-derived growth factor)[117] as well as proteolytically cleaved fibronectin[118] is chemotactic to fibroblasts in vitro. The platelet-derived growth factor, and factors derived from macrophages and lymphocytes, cause fibroblast proliferation and increased collagen accumulation in vitro (p. 77).[116] It is tempting to speculate that macrophages and lymphocytes, both of which are invariably present in the chronic phases of immune and nonimmune inflammatory reactions, may interact with each other or with other stimuli, leading to the elaboration of factors that induce fibrous tissue proliferation. Whatever the mechanism, continued fibroblast proliferation and collagen deposition are followed by considerable scarring, with resultant deformities, e.g., narrowing of the bowel and adhesions between serosal surfaces.

The mechanisms of vascular proliferation and collagen deposition are discussed on page 76.

Other types of cells present in chronic inflammation are plasma cells, lymphocytes, eosinophils, and mast cells. *Plasma cells* produce antibody, directed either against persistent antigen in the inflammatory site or against altered tissue components (Fig. 2–16). *Lymphocytes* are called for in both antibody and cell-mediated

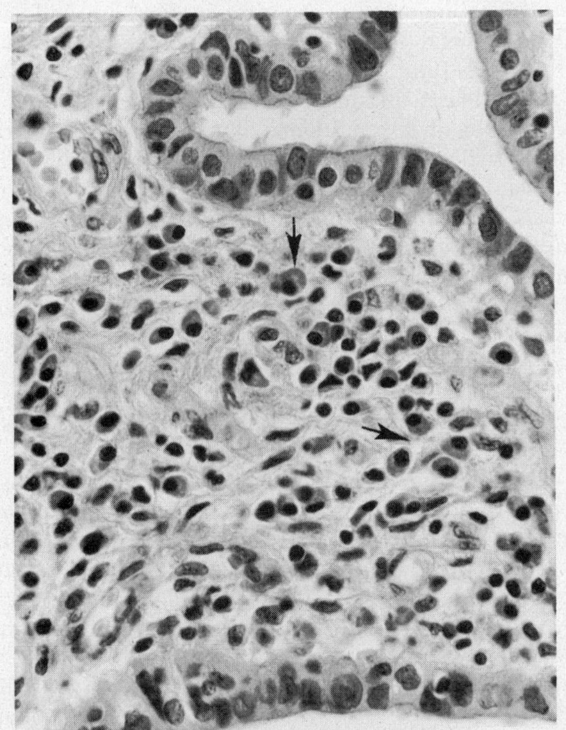

Figure 2–16. Chronic inflammation of the fallopian tube. The subepithelial connective tissue is infiltrated with mononuclear white cells, principally plasma cells marked by eccentric nuclei (*arrows*).

immunologic reactions, but also, for unknown reasons, in nonimmunologic inflammation. *Eosinophils* are characteristic of immunologic reactions mediated by IgE and of parasitic infections, but also are often present for obscure reasons. Eosinophils respond to chemotactic agents derived largely from mast cells (p. 49), and are phagocytic, although to a much lesser degree than are neutrophils. Because they appear late in hypersensitivity reactions, it has been suggested that they serve to terminate such reactions by degrading chemical mediators, and indeed eosinophil granules contain histaminase, which is capable of oxidative deamination of histamine.

It should be pointed out that, although polymorphonuclear leukocytes are usually considered the hallmarks of acute inflammation, many forms of chronic inflammation, lasting for months, continue to show large numbers of neutrophils and to form *pus*. In chronic inflammation of bone (osteomyelitis), a neutrophilic exudate can persist for many months. In actinomycosis, a disease induced by organisms with a particular ability to attract neutrophils, the center of the lesion abounds with neutrophils months or years after the initial infection. Here, then, chronic and acute responses are simply superimposed. Conversely, the presence of lymphocytes does not always mean that inflammation has been present for long periods. This is especially true of viral infections. In acute viral hepatitis or viral myocarditis,

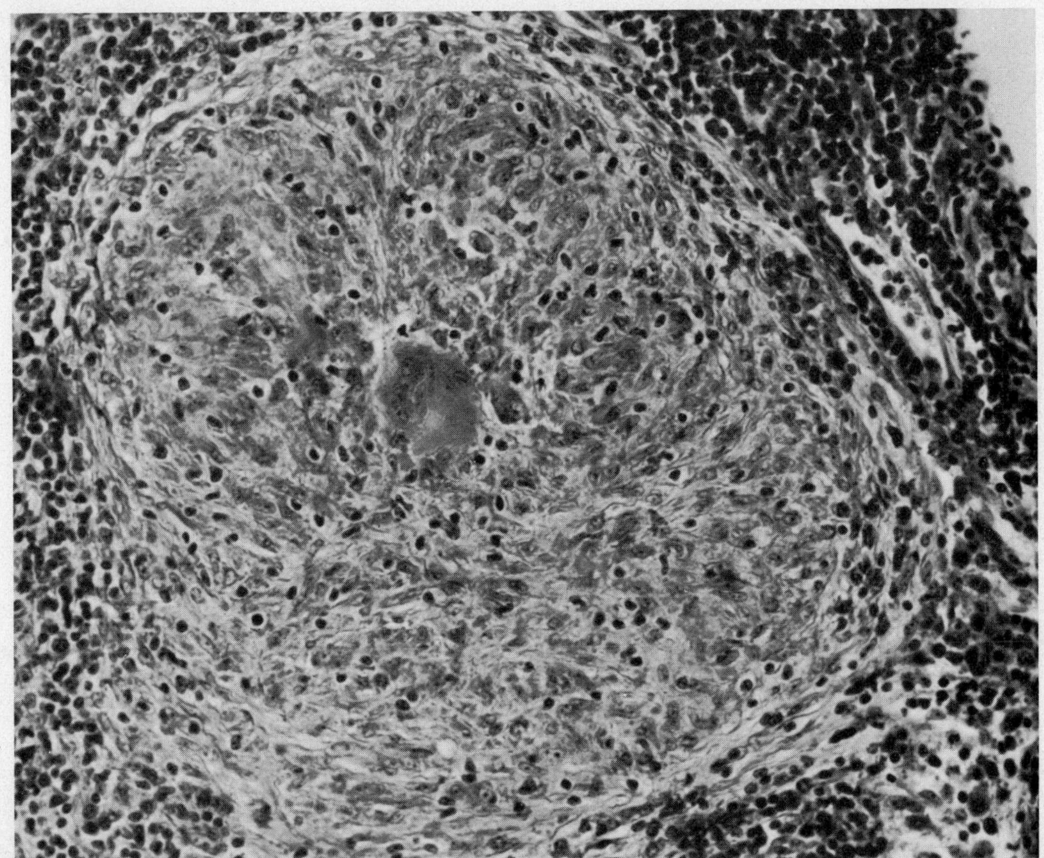

Figure 2–17. A granuloma with a central Langhans'-type giant cell surrounded by chronic inflammatory infiltrate.

for example, lymphocytes predominate even in the first few days of the acute disease.

CHRONIC GRANULOMATOUS INFLAMMATION

Some agents evoke a distinctive pattern of chronic inflammation referred to as granulomatous inflammation. Granulomatous diseases, such as tuberculosis, leprosy, and schistosomiasis, are of major, worldwide, public health importance. *Granulomas are small, 0.5- to 2-mm collections of modified macrophages called "epithelioid cells," usually surrounded by a rim of lymphocytes* (Fig. 2–17). The modified macrophages have abundant, pale-pink, plump cytoplasm, resembling an epithelial cell. Like all macrophages, epithelioid cells are derived from blood monocytes, but the reason for their transformation to this peculiar cell type is poorly understood. They are much less phagocytic than macrophages but are rich in endoplasmic reticulum, Golgi apparatus, vesicles, and vacuoles. Their appearance suggests that the cells may be adapted for extracellular secretion rather than phagocytosis.[120]

Another feature of the granuloma is the presence of *Langhans' or foreign body–type giant cells.* These are formed by the coalescence and fusion of macrophages, with only rare internal nuclear division. They may achieve diameters of 40 to 50 μ and may contain as many as 50 nuclei. The nuclei are sometimes arranged around the periphery (creating a horseshoe pattern), giving rise to the traditional Langhans'-type giant cell (Fig. 2–18). Giant cells also are formed in the presence of large amounts of indigestible material, and indeed they often conglomerate around a foreign body and have scattered nuclei (hence the term foreign body-type giant cell) (Fig. 2–19).

Fibroblasts, plasma cells, and at times neutrophils can be seen in a granuloma, but the presence of the characteristic cell (the epithelioid cell) is required for the diagnosis of granulomatous inflammation. *The diagnosis of granulomatous inflammation based on lymph node biopsy significantly limits the number of possible etiologies.* The classic example of granulomatous disease is tuberculosis, but sarcoidosis, deep fungal infections, reactions to a foreign body, brucellosis, schistosomiasis, cat-scratch fever, syphilis, and leprosy all evoke this pattern. In clinical practice, the most common causes are reaction to a foreign body, tuberculosis, and sarcoidosis.

In tuberculosis, the granuloma is referred to as a *tubercle* and is *classically characterized by the presence of central caseous necrosis.* In contrast, caseating necrosis is rare in other granulomatous diseases. The morphologic patterns in the various granulomatous diseases may be sufficiently different to allow reasonably accurate diagnosis by an experienced pathologist (Table 2–5); however, there are so many atypical presentations that it is always necessary to identify the specific etiologic agent. The agent can be identified histologically (as in the case of a refractile foreign body that can be detected by polarization microscopy), by special stains for organisms (e.g., acid-fast stains for tubercle bacilli), by culture methods (TB, fungus), and by serologic studies (e.g., syphilis). In sarcoidosis, the etiologic agent is unknown and the diagnosis is made by a combination of histologic

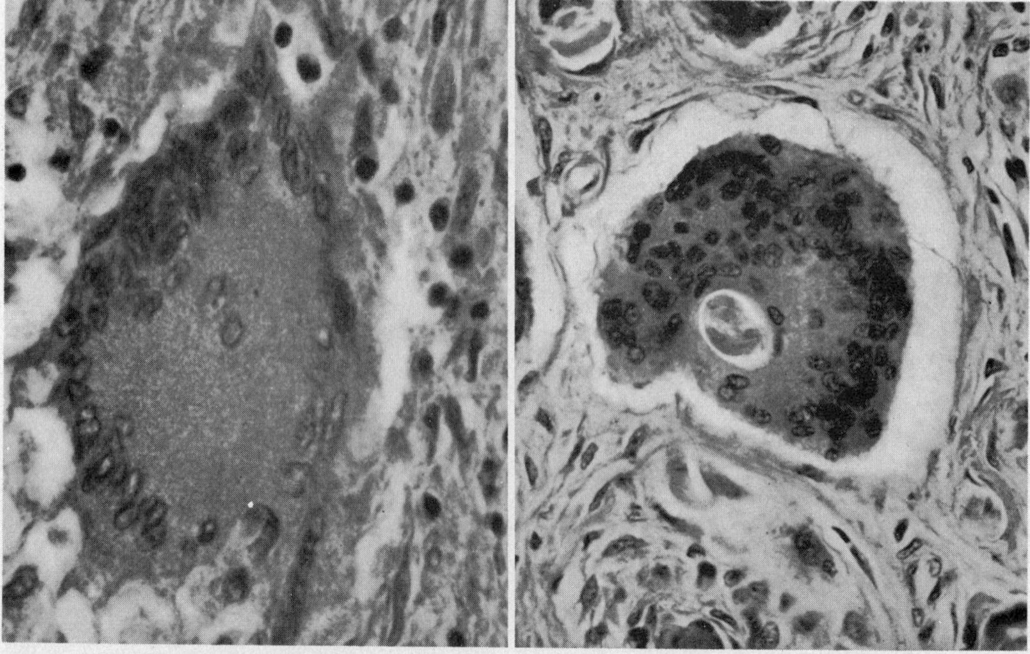

Fig. 2–18 Fig. 2–19

Figure 2–18. Detail of a Langhans'-type giant cell in the margin of a tubercle.

Figure 2–19. Detail of a foreign body–type giant cell containing a foreign body.

Table 2–5. MAJOR GRANULOMATOUS INFLAMMATIONS

Disease	Cause	Tissue Reaction
Tuberculosis	*Mycobacterium tuberculosis*	Noncaseating tubercle (*Granuloma prototype*): A focus of epithelioid cells, rimmed by fibroblasts, lymphocytes, histiocytes, occasional Langhans' giant cell. Caseating tubercle: Central amorphous granular debris, loss of all cellular detail.
Sarcoidosis	Unknown	Noncaseating granuloma: Giant cells (Langhans' and foreign body types); asteroids in giant cells; occasional Schaumann's body (concentric calcific concretion).
Certain fungal infections		Granuloma usually larger than single tubercle with central granular debris; often contains causal organism and recognizable neutrophils.
	Cryptococcus neoformans	Organism is yeast-like, sometimes budding; 5 to 10 μ; large, clear capsule.
	Blastomyces dermatitidis	Organism is yeast-like, budding; 5 to 15 μ; thick, doubly refractile capsule.
	Coccidioides immitis	Organism appears as spherical (30–80 μ) cyst containing endospores of 3 to 5 μ each.
Syphilis	*Treponema pallidum*	Gumma: Microscopic to grossly visible lesion, enclosing wall of histiocytes, fibroblasts and lymphocytes; plasma cell infiltrate; center cells are necrotic without loss of cellular outline.
Cat-scratch fever	Unknown	Rounded or stellate granuloma containing central granular debris and recognizable neutrophils; giant cells uncommon.
Actinomycosis	*Actinomyces bovis*	Granulomatous rim enclosing necrotic and viable polymorphonuclear leukocytes as well as "sulfur granules."

features (absence of caseation necrosis), by clinical findings (p. 390), and by excluding other specific agents.

Two factors appear to determine the formation of granulomas. One factor is evident—the presence of indigestible organisms (such as the tubercle bacillus) or particles (such as mineral oil, complex polysaccharides, and polymers). In addition, experimental studies indicate that *granulomatous inflammation is potentiated by, or sometimes requires, the presence of cell-mediated immunity to the inciting agent.*[120, 123] Indeed, a T-lymphocyte product (lymphokine) enhances the transformation of monocytes to multinucleate giant cells in culture.[123]

To summarize, granulomatous inflammation is a specific type of chronic inflammation characterized by accumulations of modified macrophages (epithelioid cells) and initiated by a variety of infectious and noninfectious agents. The presence of *poorly digestible irritants or cell-mediated immunity to the irritant, or both,* appears to be necessary for granuloma formation.

MORPHOLOGIC PATTERNS IN ACUTE AND CHRONIC INFLAMMATION

The severity of the reaction, its specific causation, and the particular tissue and site involved all introduce morphologic variations in the basic themes of acute and chronic inflammation. For example, the fluid, plasma protein, and cell content of an exudate depend on the specific causative agent and its intensity. Thus, major characteristic patterns of acute and chronic inflammation can be differentiated on the basis of the nature of the exudate and on the morphologic variables introduced by location.

SEROUS INFLAMMATION. This pattern is marked by the outpouring of a thin fluid that, according to the site of injury, is derived from either the blood serum or the secretions of serous mesothelial cells—i.e., the cells lining the peritoneal, pleural, and pericardial cavities and the joint spaces. The skin blister resulting from a burn is a simple example of a serous exudate (Fig. 2–20). The blister represents a large accumulation of fluid, either within or immediately beneath the epidermis of the skin. This type of exudate, seen early in the development of most acute inflammatory reactions, is the dominant pattern in mild injuries and is characteristic of certain causative agents, such as tuberculous pleuritis, often referred to as pleurisy with effusion.

FIBRINOUS INFLAMMATION. The exudation of large amounts of plasma proteins, including fibrinogen, and the precipitation of masses of fibrin are characteristic of certain severe inflammatory responses. They are also

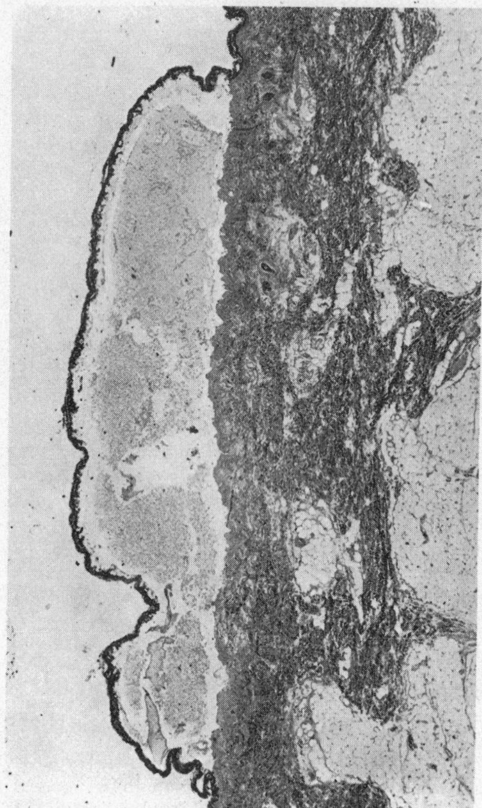

Figure 2–20. A low-power view of a cross section of a skin blister. The epidermis has been lifted off the dermis by the focal collection of fluid.

characteristic of specific types of inflammation, such as rheumatic involvement of the pericardial cavity. Here the pericardial space may become virtually filled with large masses of fibrin. When the epicardium is stripped from the pericardium, the rubbery, adherent fibrin coats both surfaces, simulating the appearance of two slices of buttered bread when pulled apart (*"bread and butter" pericarditis*) (Fig. 2–21). Histologically, fibrin is readily identified by its tangled, threadlike eosinophilic mesh-

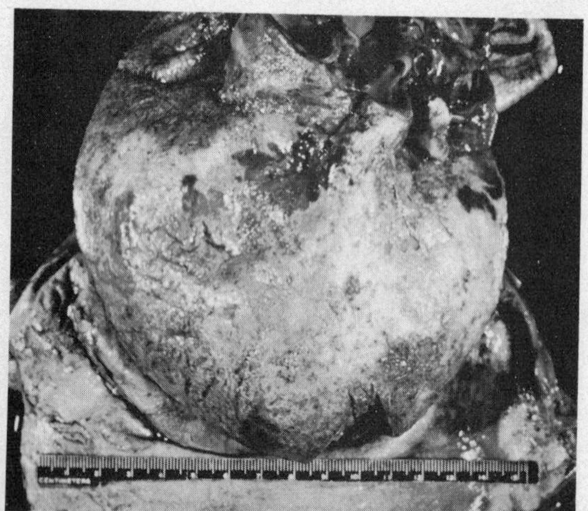

Figure 2–21. A gross view of the heart with a massive, fibrinous, "bread and butter" pericarditis.

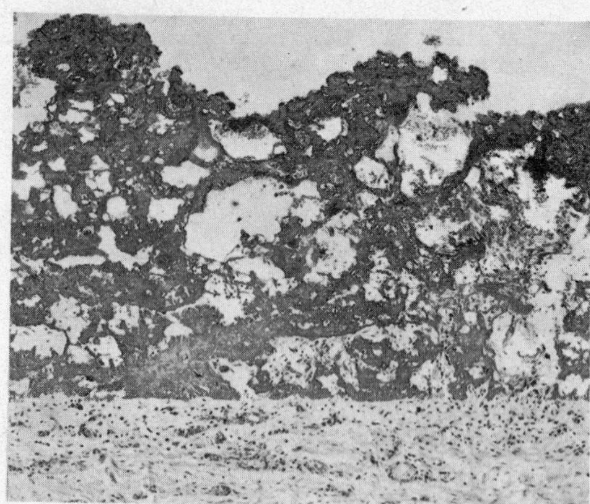

Figure 2–22. The microscopic appearance of the shaggy, amorphous fibrinous exudate.

work, although it occasionally presents as large masses of solid amorphous eosinophilic coagulum (Fig. 2–22).

A fibrinous exudate carries implications not encountered with serous exudates. It invites ingrowth of fibroblasts and capillary buds, which transform the proteinaceous precipitate into a vascularized connective tissue, a process referred to as *organization* of the exudate. Organization of a fibrinous pleuritis or pericarditis may obliterate these serosal cavities and hamper the function of the organs now tied down to surrounding structures. Happily, all fibrinous exudates do not follow such a path, and many are resorbed by fibrinolysis, referred to as *resolution* of the exudate.

SUPPURATIVE OR PURULENT INFLAMMATION. This form of inflammation is characterized by the production of large amounts of pus or purulent exudate. Certain organisms (e.g., staphylococci) produce this localized suppuration and are therefore referred to as pyogenic (pus-producing) bacteria. A common example of an acute suppurative inflammation is acute appendicitis. Here, masses of polymorphonuclear leukocytes are found diffusely or in focal aggregates throughout the mucosa, submucosa, muscularis, and subserosal regions, and coagulated pus may layer the surface as well as fill the lumen (Figs. 2–23 and 2–24). Abscesses (see below) are an example of a localized suppurative inflammation.

Although the various types of exudative reactions have been described separately, mixed patterns develop in many inflammations and are termed serofibrinous or fibrinopurulent. Moreover, the exudation may begin as a serous response in any single inflammatory reaction and, with extension and increasing severity of the reaction, may become predominantly fibrinous and ultimately change into a suppurative exudate.

ABSCESSES. *An abscess is a localized collection of pus* caused by suppuration buried in a tissue, organ, or confined space. It is usually produced by the deep seeding of pyogenic bacteria into a tissue. In its early stages, an abscess is a focal accumulation of neutrophils in a space created either by the separation of preexisting cellular elements or by the liquefactive necrosis of the native cells of the tissue. As it develops, it may expand

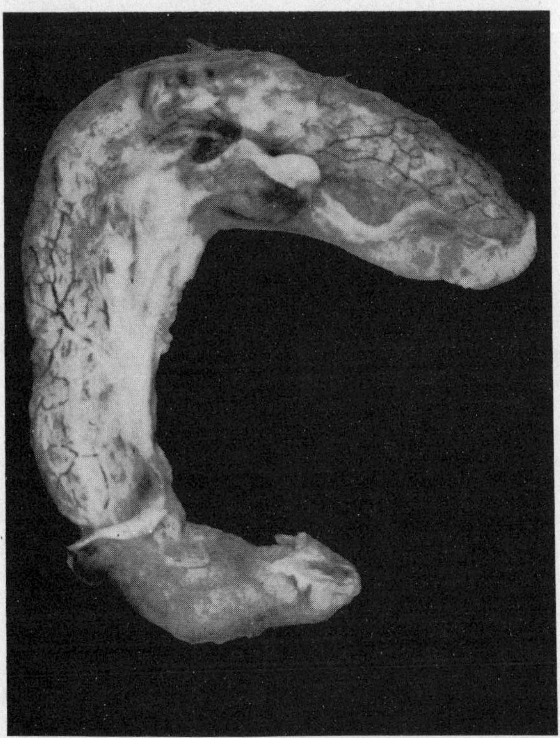

Figure 2–23. A gross view of acute appendicitis. The covering serosa is heavily layered with a pale fibrinosuppurative exudate.

as a result of the progressive necrosis of surrounding cells. The central region at this time appears as a mass of granular, acidophilic, amorphous, semifluid debris composed of the necrotic white cells and tissue cells. There is usually a zone of preserved neutrophils about this necrotic focus, and outside this region vascular dilation and parenchymal and fibroblastic proliferation occur, indicating the beginning of repair. In time, the abscess may become walled off by highly vascularized connective tissue that serves as a limiting barrier to further spread.

Healing of an abscess (to be described under Repair) can occur only after the suppurative exudate and necrotic debris have been removed, since their presence still provokes inflammation. Removal may be accomplished when the abscess burrows to the surface of the organ or tissue (pointing) and discharges its contents by rupture, or by surgical drainage. If evacuation of the abscess does not occur, healing may still take place after total proteolytic digestion of the accumulated tissue and cellular debris. This watery digestate may then be resorbed into the blood.

ULCERS. *An ulcer is a local defect, or excavation, of the surface of an organ or tissue, which is produced by the sloughing (shedding) of inflammatory necrotic tissue.* Ulceration can occur only when an inflammatory necrotic area exists on or near a surface. It is most commonly encountered in three situations: (1) inflammatory necrosis of the mucosa of the mouth, stomach, or intestines; (2) subcutaneous inflammations of the lower extremities in older individuals who have circulatory disturbances that predispose to extensive necrosis; and (3) inflammation of the cervix or the uterus.

Such lesions are best exemplified by the peptic ulcer of the stomach or duodenum. The ulcer craters are usually circular to oval, 0.5 to 4.0 cm in diameter, sharply punched out of the intestinal mucosa. Microscopically, the pattern of the inflammatory reaction depends on the duration of the lesion. In the acute stage, there is intense polymorphonuclear infiltration and vascular dilation in the margins of the defect (Fig. 2–25). With chronicity, the margins and base of the ulcer develop fibroblastic proliferation, scarring, and the accumulation of lymphocytes, macrophages, and plasma cells. Eosinophils may also be very numerous, especially when foreign protein from the cavity of the stomach enters the ulcer and sensitizes the underlying tissues.

MEMBRANOUS (PSEUDOMEMBRANOUS) INFLAMMATION. As the name implies, this form of inflammatory reaction is characterized by the *formation of a membrane usually made up of precipitated fibrin, necrotic epithelium, and inflammatory white cells.* Some prefer to call this reaction "pseudomembranous," since they reserve the term membrane for vital cells and structures. Whatever its designation, the reaction is encountered only on mucosal surfaces, most commonly in the pharynx, larynx, respiratory passages, and intestinal tract (Fig. 2–26). The membrane formation results from an acute inflammatory response to a powerful necrotizing toxin (e.g., the diphtheria exotoxin that causes

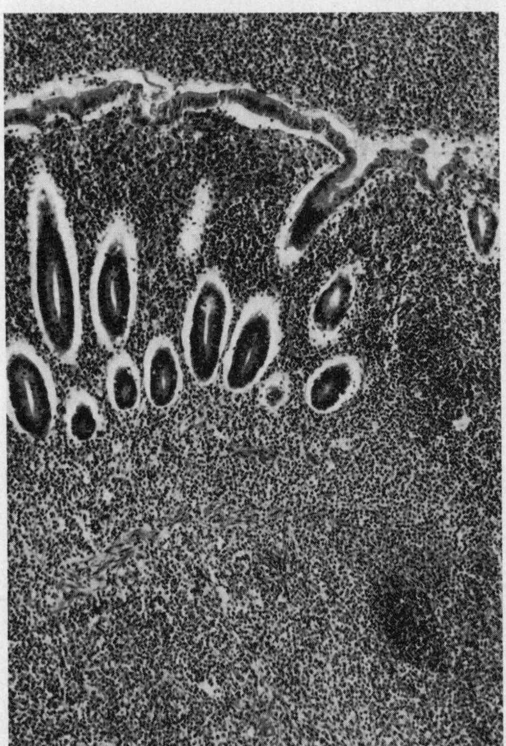

Figure 2–24. A microscopic detail of the wall of an acute suppurative appendicitis. The lumen above the mucosal epithelium is filled with suppurative exudate and the wall is heavily infiltrated with neutrophils, most evident beneath the zone of mucosal glands.

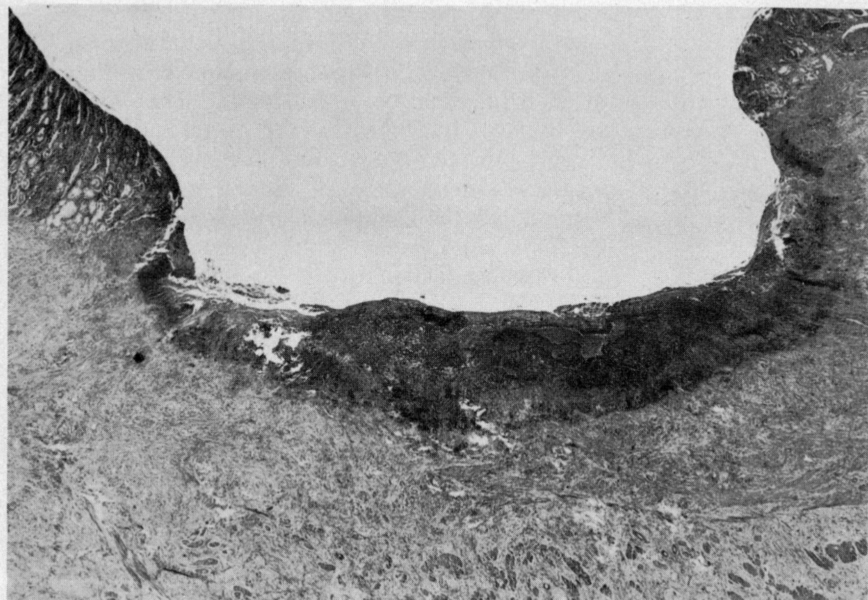

Figure 2–25. A low-power cross section of an ulcer crater with a dark inflammatory exudate in the base.

necrosis of surface epithelial cells and their desquamation or a clostridium toxin that affects the intestinal mucosa). An outpouring of exudate traps the necrotic and cellular debris, producing a dirty gray-white, rubbery membrane on the eroded surface.

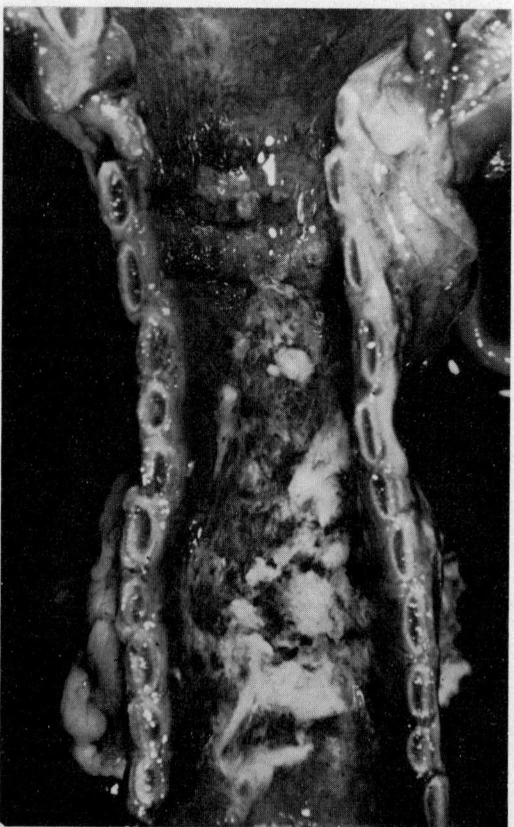

Figure 2–26. Membranous inflammation in the trachea. The membrane appears as large patches of gray-white layered exudate.

SYSTEMIC EFFECTS OF INFLAMMATION

Anyone who has suffered a severe sore throat or a respiratory infection has experienced the systemic manifestations of acute inflammation. Fever is one of the most prominent systemic manifestations, especially when the inflammation is associated with bacteremia. Bacteremia usually induces fever with dramatic swings in temperature, producing so-called spikes on the temperature chart. Violent shaking chills are known to all those who have had the flu.

The elusive cause of *fever* in inflammation is being tracked down, thanks mainly to the work on *endogenous pyrogens* and *prostaglandins*. Endogenous pyrogens are basic proteins of low molecular weight ($\pm$ 15,000) that act on the thermoregulatory centers in the hypothalamus, leading to elevation of the "thermostat" and the development of fever.[124] They can be detected in the blood of experimental animals given endotoxin or antigen-antibody complexes. Endogenous pyrogens are synthesized and released by macrophages (including those of the mononuclear phagocyte system) after activation by phagocytosis, endotoxin, viruses and fungi, immune complexes, and lymphocyte products. Endogenous pyrogen appears to be chemically similar or identical to the macrophage product called *interleukin 1*,[125] which is important in inducing lymphocyte activation during immune reactions (p. 60).

Prostaglandins are also involved in the production of fever. PGE_1 produces fever on injection into the cerebral ventricle of most mammalian species examined.[126] PGE_2 appears in the cerebrospinal fluid during endotoxin fever and disappears when the fever is brought down by inhibitors of prostaglandin synthesis (aspirin). The following sequence of events appears to account for the pathogenesis of fever in man. Endogenous pyrogen is produced by phagocytic leukocytes in response to infections or immunologic or toxic reactions, and is released into the circulation where it interacts with receptors in the thermoregulatory center of the anterior hypothalamus. *Either by the direct action of pyrogen, or through the local production of prostaglandins,* information is transmitted from the anterior through the posterior hypothalamus to the vasomotor center, resulting in sympathetic nerve stimulation, vasoconstriction of skin vessels, decrease in heat dissipation, and fever. Endogenous pyrogen also stimulates the muscle protein degradation characteristic of febrile states.[127]

Leukocytosis is a common feature of inflammatory reactions, especially those induced by bacterial infection. The leukocyte count usually climbs to 15,000 or 20,000 but sometimes may reach extraordinarily high levels of 40,000 to 100,000. These extreme elevations are referred to as *leukemoid reactions,* since they are similar to the white counts obtained in leukemia. The leukocytosis of acute inflammation is usually due to an absolute increase in the number of neutrophils, at the same time increasing the relative proportion in the differential count. The leukocytosis apparently occurs initially because of *accelerated release* of cells from the bone marrow postmitotic reserve pool, and is often associated with a rise in the number of more immature neutrophils in the blood ("shift to the left"). However, prolonged infection also stimulates proliferation of precursors in the bone marrow. Mediators for the accelerated release from the bone marrow have not been well identified, but the increased proliferation may be due to increased production of *colony-stimulating factors* (CSF), factors produced by macrophages and activated T lymphocytes that stimulate mitotic activity in neutrophil precursors in the bone marrow.

Most bacterial infections induce *neutrophilia,* but infectious mononucleosis, whooping cough, mumps, and German measles are exceptions and produce a leukocytosis by virtue of an absolute increase in the number of lymphocytes *(lymphocytosis).* In an additional group of disorders such as bronchial asthma, hay fever, and parasitic infestations, there is an absolute increase in the number of eosinophils, creating an *eosinophilia.* Generally, the magnitude of the eosinophilia is sufficient to raise the relative proportion of these cells in the differential count, but is not sufficient to induce a significant elevation of the total white cell count.

Certain systemic inflammatory states such as typhoid fever, infections caused by viruses, and rickettsiae and certain protozoal infections decrease the number of circulating white cells *(leukopenia).* Leukopenia is also encountered in infections that overwhelm patients debilitated by disseminated cancer or rampant miliary tuberculosis. Under these circumstances, it is theorized that the massive assault upon the body depresses leukopoiesis.

In closing this discussion of inflammation, it is evident that, although the early reaction pattern of the inflammatory response is quite stereotyped, it is soon modified by a number of variables pertaining to both intruder and host that introduce striking departures from the basic theme. Perhaps the most important is the duration of the inflammatory process, but the causative agent, the location of the injury, and the nature of the exudate all contribute heavily to the ultimate character of the reaction. Even these modifiers do not tell the whole story because an important component has, to this point, been omitted—the changes induced by the reparative response. The repair of injury begins almost as soon as the inflammatory changes have begun, and so constitutes a sequence of events as important as that of inflammation.

Healing and Repair

The body's attempts to heal damage induced by local injury begin very early in the process of inflammation and, in the end, result in *repair and the replacement of dead or damaged cells by healthy cells.* Repair usually involves two distinct processes: (1) *regeneration,* which is the replacement of injured tissue by parenchymal cells of the same type, sometimes leaving no residual trace of the previous injury; and (2) *replacement by connective tissue,* which in its permanent stage constitutes a scar. In most instances, both processes contribute to the repair.

The advantages that man may have gained in the evolutionary process have been accompanied by loss of the capacity to regenerate severely damaged organs, and some tissues have no regenerative capacity at all. Because of these limitations, repair usually involves much connective tissue scarring. Such repair may fill defects and more or less restore morphologic continuity, but it replaces specialized cells with nonfunctioning connective tissue and depletes the functional reserve of an organ. In this chapter the healing of *skin wounds* is discussed, as a prototype of the repair process in inflammation, but first some of the general features of regeneration and connective tissue repair are reviewed.

REGENERATION

The cells of the body are divided into three groups on the basis of their regenerative capacity: labile, stable, and permanent cells. Labile cells continue to proliferate throughout life; stable cells retain this capacity, although they do not normally replicate; and permanent cells cannot reproduce themselves after birth.[128]

LABILE CELLS

Under physiologic conditions, these cells continue to proliferate throughout life, replacing cells that are continually being destroyed. Labile cells consist of surface epithelia and blood cells. All epithelial surfaces throughout the body are made up of labile cells. These include the stratified squamous surfaces of the skin, oral cavity, vagina, and cervix; the lining mucosa of all the excretory ducts of the glands of the body, e.g., salivary glands, pancreas, and biliary tract; the columnar epithelium of the gastrointestinal tract, uterus, and tubes; and the transitional epithelium of the urinary tract. In all these sites, the surface cells exfoliate continually throughout life, and the integrity of the epithelium is maintained by a continual proliferation of reserve cells, replacing lost elements. A perfect example is the regrowth of the endometrium following each menstrual period.

When epithelial cells are lost as a result of injury, almost perfect reconstitution may occur by replication of reserve cells. If the defect is small, regeneration is remarkably rapid. The epithelium in the skin of man completely closes over an incised wound within 24 to 48 hours. When injury produces a deep, excavated defect or ulcer, regeneration is completed only after the defect is filled by connective tissue.

The cells of the *splenic, lymphoid, and hematopoietic tissues* are also labile cells. Bone marrow is in a state of active hematopoiesis throughout life. Destruction of hematopoietic cells is rapidly compensated for by proliferation of persisting elements. The embryonic precursors of splenic and lymphoid cells (primitive mesenchymal stem cells) survive postnatally, proliferating and differentiating to replace lost elements. Destruction of large areas of bone marrow, spleen, or lymphoid tissues may radically reduce the local population of stem cells, thus thwarting parenchymal reconstitution and giving rise to focal scarring.

STABLE CELLS

This group normally demonstrates a low normal level of replication. However, these cells can undergo rapid division in response to a variety of stimuli and are thus capable of reconstitution of the tissue of origin.[129] In this category are the parenchymal cells of virtually all the glandular organs of the body, such as liver, kidney, and pancreas; mesenchymal derivatives such as fibroblasts, smooth muscle cells, osteoblasts, and chondroblasts; and vascular endothelial cells. The regenerative capacity of stable cells is best exemplified by the ability of the liver to regenerate after hepatectomy and following toxic, viral, or chemical injury.

Although labile and stable cells are capable of regeneration, it does not necessarily follow that there will be restitution of normal structure. *The underlying framework or supporting stroma of the parenchymal cells must be present to permit orderly replacement. The basement membrane appears to be the main structural component necessary for organized regeneration, forming a "scaffold" for the replicating parenchymal cells.* When basement membranes are disrupted, cells may proliferate in a haphazard fashion and produce disorganized masses of cells bearing no resemblance to the original arrangement. Alternatively, scarring may ensue. To use the liver as an example, hepatitis virus specifically destroys parenchymal cells without injuring the more resistant connective tissue cells or framework of the liver lobule. Thus, after viral hepatitis, regeneration of liver cells may completely reconstitute the liver lobule, and tests for liver function may be entirely normal a few weeks after the illness. By contrast, a large liver abscess that destroys hepatocytes and connective tissue is followed by scarring. In most large injuries, *regeneration proceeds from the margins,* where stable cells remain viable. Central regions where the framework is not preserved are usually replaced by scar tissue.

The *connective tissue cells* (fibroblasts, chondrocytes, and osteocytes) that secrete the connective tissue matrix are quiescent in adult mammals. However, all proliferate in response to injury, and fibroblasts, in particular, proliferate widely, constituting the connective tissue response to inflammation (see below). To this group should be added two significant cell types—vascular endothelium and smooth muscle. Adult *vascular endothelium* has a very slow turnover rate. If, however, a segment of large vessel is denuded of its endothelium by mechanical or chemical means, the cells around the edge of the denuded area quickly migrate into the defect, proliferate, and eventually fill the defect. This proliferation ceases when the defect is reconstituted. A somewhat different type of endothelial response occurs in small vessels (capillaries, venules, and arterioles) of the connective tissue in wound healing. Here, proliferation of endothelium results in the *formation of new capillary beds* that invade the injured inflamed sites. This *neovascularization* is prominent in many chronic inflammatory processes, such as rheumatoid arthritis, and, as we shall see, is also a component of most malignant tumors.[130]

Smooth muscle cells present in the walls of viscera and blood vessels also have a low turnover rate but proliferate under hormonal influences, as seen in the pregnant uterus, and in response to injury, as seen in the walls of large arteries. Indeed, as detailed on page 516, smooth muscle proliferation in the arterial wall is thought to be a major process in the development of atherosclerosis.[131]

PERMANENT CELLS

To this group belong the nerve cells, which cannot undergo mitotic division in postnatal life, and the skeletal and cardiac muscle cells, the regenerative attempts of which (at least in mammals) are of no practical importance. *Neurons* destroyed in the central nervous system (CNS) are permanently lost. They are replaced by the proliferation of the CNS supportive elements, the glial cells. The situation is somewhat more complicated with respect to the neurons of the peripheral nerves, as detailed in Chapter 29. When the cell body is destroyed, the entire structure (i.e., the cell body and extended axon) totally degenerates. If the cell body is spared and only the peripheral axon is injured, regeneration of a new process may proceed from the cell body or from the remaining proximal axonal segment.

With regard to *striated muscle*, evidence for regeneration in man is at best tenuous, most being derived from studies of lower animals. The precise mode of regeneration of *skeletal muscle* is still somewhat uncertain. It may occur (1) from the budding of old fibers, (2) by the fusion of myoblasts, or (3) by transformation of the satellite cells found attached to the sheaths of all multinucleated skeletal cells. If the ends of severed muscle fibers are closely juxtaposed, muscle regeneration in mammals can be excellent, a condition that can rarely be attained under practical conditions.[132] As to *cardiac muscle*, it is fair to state that if cardiac muscle has regenerative capacity, it is limited, and most large injuries to the heart are followed by connective tissue scarring (Fig. 2–27). Certainly, scarring follows the all too common myocardial infarction in man. This point is stressed because of its great clinical importance. Heart attacks are the most common cause of death in industrialized nations, and every myocardial infarction implies some permanent loss of myocardial reserve.

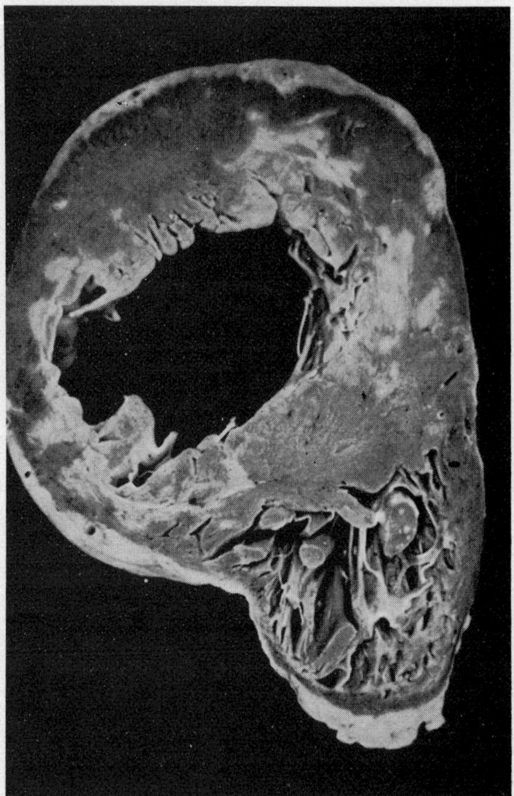

Figure 2–27. Myocardial fibrosis. The cross section of the ventricular myocardium is studded with pale scars of fibrous tissue that have been caused by ischemic necrosis of foci within the myocardium.

REPAIR BY CONNECTIVE TISSUE

GRANULATION TISSUE

As mentioned earlier, healing starts very early in inflammation, when the macrophages begin digesting whatever invading organisms have survived the neutrophilic attack, as well as necrotic debris from dead parenchymal cells and neutrophils. Sometimes as early as 24 hours after injury, fibroblasts and vascular endo-

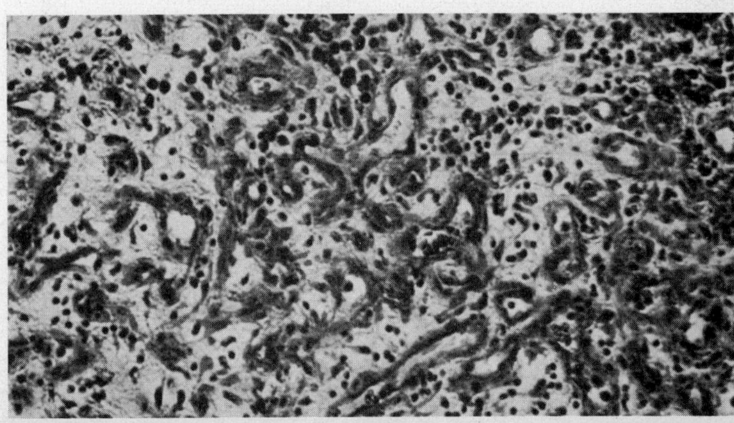

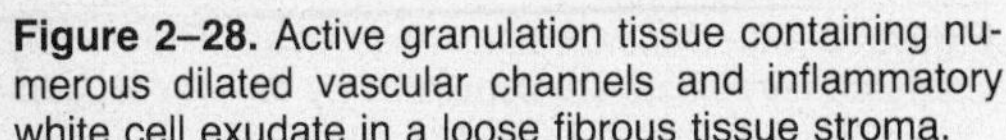

Figure 2–28. Active granulation tissue containing numerous dilated vascular channels and inflammatory white cell exudate in a loose fibrous tissue stroma.

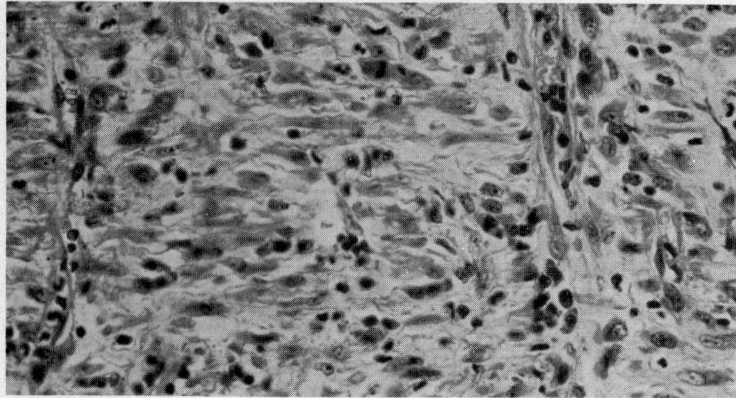

Figure 2–29. Cellular scar composed of packed fibroblasts with only scattered white cells and vascular channels.

thelial cells begin proliferating to form (by three to five days) the specialized type of tissue (granulation tissue) that is the hallmark of healing inflammation. The term "granulation tissue" derives from its pink, soft granular appearance on the surface of wounds, but it is the histologic features that are characteristic: the *proliferation of new small blood vessels and of fibroblasts* (Fig. 2–28).

New vessels originate by budding or sprouting of preexisting vessels, a process (called angiogenesis or neovascularization) that involves migration, proliferation, and maturation of endothelial cells.[130, 133] The buds are solid at first but subsequently become tunneled and permit blood to circulate. These new vessels have leaky interendothelial junctions, allowing the passage of proteins and red cells into the extravascular space.[134] *Thus, new granulation tissue is often edematous.* Indeed, this leakiness accounts for much of the edema that persists in healing wounds, long after the acute inflammatory response has subsided.

In newly developing granulation tissue, fibroblasts hypertrophy, acquire increased amounts of rough endoplasmic reticulum, and appear in histologic sections as large, plump ("juicy") cells.[135] They are active in synthesizing mucopolysaccharides (glycosaminoglycans) and collagen. In early stages, more glycoproteins are formed; later on, collagen predominates. *Many of the large fibroblasts in granulation tissue acquire electron microscopic and biochemical features of smooth muscle cells:* they develop large indented nuclei, prominent bundles of cytoplasmic fibrils with peripheral condensations, and large amounts of actomyosin in their cytoplasm.[136] Further, when strips of granulation tissue are incubated in vitro with smooth muscle–contracting agents (such as bradykinin and serotonin), the strips show significant and reversible contraction.[137] This property almost certainly accounts for the "contraction" of healing wounds seen clinically. The term *"myofibroblast"* has thus been used to refer to these modified granulation tissue fibroblasts.[138]

Macrophages are almost always present in granulation tissue, busily eating up extracellular debris, fibrin, and other foreign matter, and if the appropriate chemotactic stimuli persist, neutrophils, eosinophils, and lymphocytes will also be seen. Mast cells are also present in great numbers. With further healing, there is an increase in extracellular constituents, mostly collagen, with a decrease in the number of active fibroblasts and new vessels (Figs. 2–29, 2–30). Many of the blood vessels characteristic of early stages undergo thrombosis and degeneration, and their various cells are resorbed and digested by macrophages. The end result of granulation tissue is a scar composed of inactive-looking, spindle-shaped fibroblasts; dense collagen; fragments of elastic tissue; extracellular matrix; and relatively few vessels.

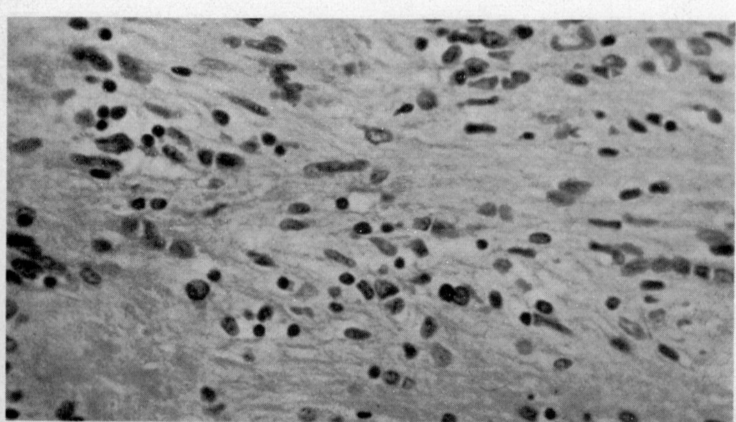

Figure 2–30. Dense collagenous scar. The widely scattered fibroblasts are separated by dense collagen. Only a few inflammatory white cells remain.

INTEGRATION OF PARENCHYMAL REGENERATION WITH CONNECTIVE TISSUE SCARRING

Most bodily injuries are repaired by the regeneration of parenchymal cells, accompanied by more or less connective tissue scarring. Both these processes have been considered separately, but it would be well to discuss their respective contributions to the reparative process of most injuries. An abscess in the cortex of the kidney resulting from a bacterial infection might be used as an example. Regeneration is initiated soon after the inflammatory phase has begun. There is proliferation of the marginal cells beyond the range of the toxic action of the microbial invader. At some point in the margin, there will be a zone where the epithelial cells lining the tubules are destroyed but the more resistant basement membrane is preserved. Here, regeneration of tubular cells may reconstitute the original renal architecture perfectly. At the same time, the central focus of injury may have accumulated a considerable amount of suppurative exudate, filling the central space where all native architecture had undergone liquefactive necrosis. Regeneration cannot create new tubules where the basement membrane has been destroyed. Here, the defect will be filled in by the process of removal of necrotic debris and exudate, followed by the ingrowth of granulation tissue. Glomeruli cannot be regenerated. The anatomic continuity of the tissue is thus restored by a combination of parenchymal regeneration and connective tissue scarring.

The quality and adequacy of the repair of any tissue loss is governed, then, by the regenerative capacity of the affected cells; by the extent of the injury, particularly since it may have destroyed the skeletal framework of the tissue; and by the proliferative activity of the connective tissue stroma, which fills in the defects that remain after parenchymal regeneration has ceased. Although the example of an abscess in the kidney has been used, the essential details do not differ in any tissue composed of parenchymal cells capable of replication.

With this background on parenchymal regeneration and the formation of granulation tissue, we can now turn to a discussion of the healing of skin wounds.

WOUND HEALING

PRIMARY UNION (HEALING BY FIRST INTENTION)

The least complicated example of wound repair is the healing of a clean surgical incision. The tissues are approximated by surgical sutures or tapes, and healing occurs without significant bacterial contamination and with a minimal loss of tissue. Such healing is referred to surgically as "primary union" or "healing by first intention." The incision causes the death of a limited number of epithelial cells as well as of dermal adnexa and connective tissue cells; the incisional space is narrow and immediately fills with clotted blood, containing *fibrin* and blood cells. The fibrin clot is well anchored to the adjacent tissue by the continuity of the fibrin mesh. Dehydration of the surface clot forms the well-known scab that covers the wound and seals it from the environment almost at once. The precise timing of the subsequent events is variable, and the following account merely approximates the times at which they occur.

Within 24 hours, neutrophils appear at the margins of the incision, moving toward the fibrin clot. The epidermis at its cut edges thickens as a result of mitotic activity of basal cells and, within 24 to 48 hours, spurs of epithelial cells from the edges both migrate and grow along the cut margins of the dermis and beneath the surface scab to fuse in the midline, thus producing a continuous but thin epithelial layer. This epithelial response is amazingly fast, and epidermal continuity is reestablished in 24 to 48 hours—long before the subjacent connective tissue reaction has begun to evolve.

By day 3, the neutrophils have largely disappeared and are replaced by macrophages. Granulation tissue progressively invades the incisional space. Collagen fibers are now present in the margins of the incision, but at first these are vertically oriented and do not bridge the incision. Epithelial cell proliferation continues, thickening the epidermal covering layer.

By day 5, the incisional space is filled with granulation tissue. Neovascularization is maximal. Collagen fibrils become more abundant and begin to bridge the incision. The epidermis recovers its normal thickness, and differentiation of surface cells yields a mature epidermal architecture with surface keratinization.

During the second week, there is continued accumulation of collagen and proliferation of fibroblasts. Leukocytic infiltrate, edema, and increased vascularity have largely disappeared. At this time the long process of blanching begins, accomplished by the increased accumulation of collagen within the incisional scar, accompanied by regression of vascular channels. The tensile strength of the wound is still well below that of normal skin, and it will take months or even a year or more for the wound to attain its maximal mechanical strength.

By the end of the first month, the scar comprises a cellular connective tissue devoid of inflammatory infiltrate, covered now by an intact epidermis. It may require almost a year for the scar to be transformed into an acellular, avascular, pale, collagenous scar. The dermal appendages that have been destroyed in the line of the incision are permanently lost; those that have been partially damaged along the lateral margins of the incision may regenerate.

To summarize, in the clean surgical wound, sealing occurs within hours by the formation of a blood clot, the surface of which becomes dehydrated to create the scab. Epithelial continuity is restored within 24 to 48 hours. Fibroblastic bridging does not become evident until three to five days following the incision, and demonstrable collagenization only begins to appear in the latter part of the first week. Thereafter, the process is one of progressive proliferation of fibroblasts, the continued accumulation of collagen, and the slow compression and devascularization of the newly formed connective tissue.

SECONDARY UNION (HEALING BY SECOND INTENTION

When there is more extensive loss of cells and tissue such as occurs in infarction, inflammatory ulceration, abscess formation, or surface wounds that create large defects, the reparative process is more complicated. *The common denominator in all these situations is a large tissue defect that must be filled.* Regeneration of parenchymal cells cannot completely reconstitute the original architecture. Granulation tissue grows in from the margin to complete the repair. This form of healing in skin wounds is referred to as "secondary union" or "healing by second intention."

Secondary healing differs from primary healing in several important respects:

1. Inevitably, large tissue defects initially have more *fibrin* and more necrotic debris and exudate that must be removed. Consequently, the *inflammatory reaction is more intense.* Healing cannot be completed until the inflammatory response has controlled the injurious agent, and the necrotic debris and exudate have been removed at least sufficiently to permit ingrowth of the granulation tissue from the margins.

2. *Much larger amounts of granulation tissue are formed.* When a large defect occurs in deeper tissues, such as in a viscus, granulation tissue bears the full responsibility for its closure, since drainage to the surface cannot occur.

3. Perhaps the feature that most clearly differentiates primary from secondary healing is the phenomenon of *wound contraction*, which occurs in large surface wounds. It has been shown that a defect of about 40 cm^2 in area in the skin of a rabbit is reduced in approximately six weeks to 5 to 10% of its original size, largely by contraction.[139] The mechanism of wound contraction has excited great interest. Shortening of collagen fibers has largely been ruled out. The best evidence implicates contraction of the modified wound fibroblasts or "myofibroblasts" described earlier.[137] Whatever the mechanism, wound contraction contributes heavily to the repair of large surface defects, making it clear that whatever the dimensions of a scar, the initial area of necrosis or tissue loss must have been greater.

As may be expected, events sometimes go awry in wound healing. Many aberrations relate to the management of the wound and the state of health of the wounded person. However, two deviations in particular may occur in the completely normal individual who has received optimal care. The first is the formation of excessive amounts of granulation tissue. The excess, referred to as "*exuberant granulations,*" or more grandiloquently as "*proud flesh,*" may protrude above the margins of the closing defect and block reepithelialization. Happily, the problem is readily managed by either surgical excision or cauterization of the excess. The second abnormality, for mysterious reasons encountered most often in blacks, is *keloid* formation. Here, an abnormal amount of collagen is present in the connective tissue, producing a large, bulging tumorous scar (Fig. 2–31). The tendency to form keloids appears to be an individual genetic characteristic. Keloid formation can be a troublesome problem, particularly on exposed skin areas, since it is disfiguring and exceedingly difficult to manage clinically; excision may be followed only by recurrence.

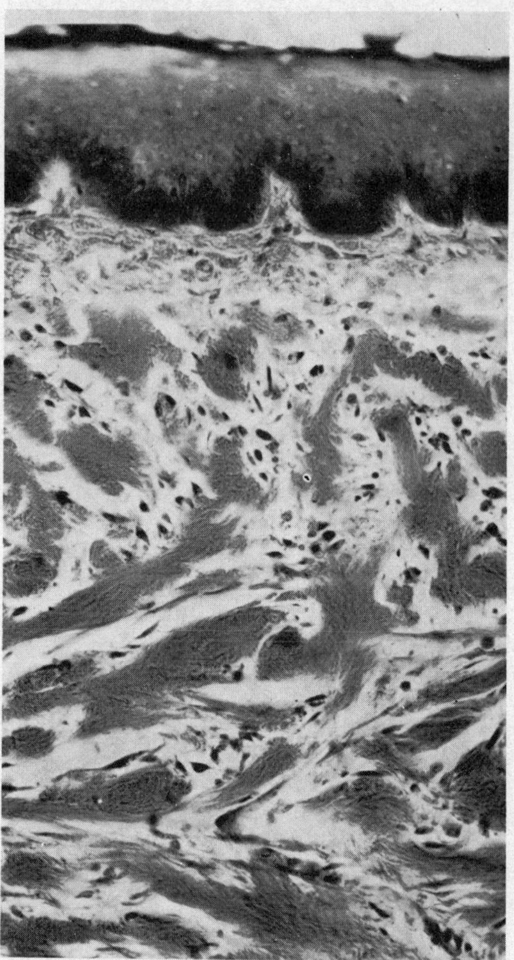

Figure 2–31. Keloid. Deep to the overlying regenerated epithelium there are interlacing broad bands of dense collagen.

MECHANISMS INVOLVED IN REPAIR

Having described the sequence of events in repair, we can now turn to the mechanisms underlying these events. Two features of repair will be addressed: (1)

control of cell proliferation, a process central to the regeneration of parenchymal cells and growth of fibroblasts and blood vessels; and (2) *collagenization* and acquisition of wound strength.

Repeated references have been made in the previous discussion to the proliferation of parenchymal and connective tissue cells in the repair of an injury. What signals do these cells perceive that initiate their proliferation? The answers are not clear. But behind this question lies a central problem in current biomedical research: the manner in which cell proliferation is controlled. The question is of more than theoretical interest, since growth control is fundamental to our understanding of cancer, as we shall see. The literature on this subject is constantly expanding.[141, 142] Here we shall touch only on some aspects of growth control and on the possible stimuli for cell division and multiplication. Short accounts of the subject may be found in Baserga's highly readable book *Multiplication and Division of Mammalian Cells*,[143] and his brief review of the cell cycle.[144]

GROWTH CONTROL AND CELL PROLIFERATION

We have already mentioned the growth characteristics of the three types of cells in mammalian tissues: the labile cells capable of continuous division; the stable cells, quiescent cells that can be stimulated to undergo mitosis; and the permanent nondividing cells. Another way of looking at these cell types is to consider their relationship to the cell growth cycle, which should be familiar to you (Fig. 2–32). *Continuously dividing (labile) cells* follow the cell cycle from one mitosis to the next. *Nondividing (permanent) cells* have left the cell cycle and are destined to senesce and die. *Quiescent (stable) cells* can be considered to be in G_0 but can be stimulated into G_1 by an appropriate stimulus. Arrest at G_2 before entering mitosis results in the appearance of polyploid cells—characteristic of cells that have undergone hypertrophy but cannot undergo division. Except for nondividing tissues, *tissues of adult animals consist of a mixture of cells that includes continuously dividing cells, quiescent cells that occasionally go back to the cell cycle, and nondividing cells*.[142]

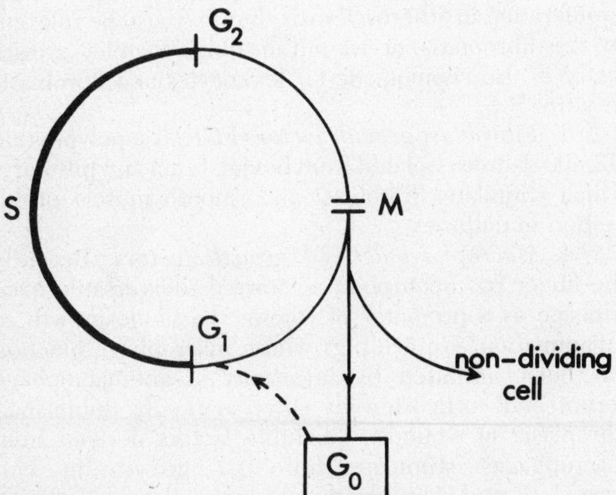

Figure 2–32. Cell populations and the phases of the cell cycle. Continuously dividing cells go around the cell cycle from one mitosis (M) to the next. Nondividing cells have left the cycle and are destined to die without dividing again. Quiescent G_0 cells are neither cycling nor dying and can be induced to reenter the cycle by an appropriate stimulus. (From Baserga, R.: The cell cycle. N. Engl. J. Med. *304*:453, 1981. Reprinted, by permission, from The New England Journal of Medicine.)

Although growth can be accomplished by shortening the cell cycle or decreasing the rate of cell loss (as occurs in tumors), *the most important factors are those that recruit G_0 cells into the cell cycle*. At least three lines of investigation have been pursued to account for the stimulation of cell proliferation. These are: (1) *the action of growth or stimulatory factors;* (2) *the loss of a growth inhibitor normally present in cells (negative feedback);* and (3) *cell-cell or cell-matrix interactions*, which may play a modulatory role in cell proliferation. These are not mutually exclusive phenomena but will be discussed separately for the sake of simplicity.

Stimulatory Hormones and Growth Factors

The existence of stimulatory factors has long been deduced from studies in vivo and from work on cell cultures. First, there is the well-known action of such hormones as estrogens, progesterone, and somatotropin in stimulating growth and function of their target organs. Second, the presence of growth factors in serum was inferred from the finding that serum was necessary for the growth of normal cells in culture. (The serum requirement for epithelial cells is much lower than that for fibroblasts.) Third, studies on regenerating liver after partial hepatectomy,[144] discussed in Chapter 1, indicate the presence of a circulating growth factor as the cause of regeneration.

Although many growth factors (including nutrients) have been uncovered, much remains to be learned about their relevance outside the culture dish. Begging the question of which are the "real" growth factors, current interest is on a number of *polypeptides* present in serum or produced by cells. These stimulate proliferation of a variety of cell types. The list includes insulin, epidermal growth factor, fibroblast growth factor, platelet growth factor, nerve growth factor, the lymphocyte proliferating factors interleukin I and II (p. 171), a macrophage-derived growth factor, and factors produced by cancer cells (sarcoma growth factor).

The most well studied of the factors is *epidermal growth factor* (EGF), a 6045-dalton polypeptide, purified from submaxillary glands of mice or from human urine (urogastrone).[145] EGF enhances epidermal proliferation and keratinization in newborn mice, an activity first discovered by precocious separation of the eyelids of newborn mice (a true eye-opener)! EGF is also mitogenic for fibroblasts in vitro. The mechanism by which EGF stimulates cell division may be a model for other growth factors[146] and involves binding of EGF to specific receptors on the cell membrane, clustering of cell-bound EGF, phosphorylation of EGF receptor protein, internalization and lysosomal degradation of bound EGF, followed eventually by onset of RNA synthesis and a commitment to DNA synthesis. Precisely how the second message—from EGF binding to RNA and DNA synthesis—is transmitted is now under active study.

Inhibitory Factors (Chalones)

An altogether different hypothesis for the control of cell growth proposes that proliferation is controlled by means of *negative feedback*, mediated by *endogenous hormone-like mitotic inhibitors* present in normal mature cells. With injury or upon the proper stimulation, *these substances diffuse out of the injured differentiated cell and permit proliferation of undifferentiated stem cells.*[148, 149] The term *chalone* (from the Greek *chalon*, meaning to slacken a sail in order to slow down the boat) was coined for these inhibitors. The three best studied chalone systems are an epidermal chalone, thought to control cellular proliferation in the skin; a granulocyte chalone, apparently produced by granulocytes to control the total cell population; and a lymphocyte chalone. Chalones are tissue- or cell line–specific (e.g., a skin chalone inhibits only epidermal growth), but not species-specific. The mechanism of inhibition is still highly speculative. It is obvious, however, that for a chalone to be meaningful, one must clearly exclude a direct injurious effect of the presumed chalone on cell structure and function. Although the concept of chalones has not gained wide acceptance, a number of substances have recently been shown to induce true inhibition of cell growth. One example is the inhibition of vascular smooth muscle by heparin-like molecules released from endothelial cells.[150]

Cell-Cell and Cell-Matrix Interactions

When certain normal cell lines are placed in culture, they proliferate, eventually to form a confluent monolayer of cells, *after which proliferation ceases.* Since malignant cells do not display this phenomenon (and continue growing), a clear understanding of the mechanism may shed light on the initiation of neoplastic growth. The cessation of division may in part be ascribed to "contact inhibition," analogous to contact inhibition of cell movement. However, many lines of evidence indicate that it is also dependent on cell density within the culture dish.[151] This *density-dependent regulation of cell growth* may be due to limitation of any one of the various materials in the microenvironment that surrounds the crowded cells, or the number of receptor sites for the growth factors, or accumulation of inhibitors in the culture medium. Whatever the mechanism, *the density-dependent regulation of cell growth is as important in vivo as it is in culture. As stated earlier, most cells capable of regenerating in response to injury usually cease proliferating after the defect caused by the injury has healed.*

Of current interest is the influence of cell-matrix or cell-substrate interactions on cell proliferation.[152] Cells grown in culture on basement membrane–coated dishes have a higher rate of replication when exposed to growth factors than cells grown on plastic. The type of collagen in the matrix, the presence of fibronectin or fibronectin fragments, and the nature of the proteoglycans in the pericellular areas all seem to affect growth in vitro, but the mechanisms involved are unclear. One possible effect is to modify cell shape. It has been shown that highly flattened cells respond to growth factors, while spheroidal cells from the same source no longer respond.[153]

Possible Growth Factors in Healing Wounds

Now that we have discussed some theoretical considerations relating to cell proliferation, the question remains: Are there likely candidates for factors that may influence parenchymal and connective tissue cell proliferation and are required for healing of wounds? From the assortment of possible stimulatory and modulating factors described, the following deserve mention.

1. *Epidermal growth factor (EGF).* As detailed earlier, EGF causes epidermal proliferation and is also mitogenic for fibroblasts. There is substantial evidence that the molecule may have relevance in vivo.

2. *Platelet-derived growth factor (PDGF).* This is a 27,000- to 35,000-dalton polypeptide stored in the platelet alpha granules and released upon platelet activation.[154, 155] It is a powerful mitogen for fibroblasts and smooth muscle cells, and indeed represents the main growth-promoting substance of serum.[154] It is thought to be particularly involved in causing smooth muscle proliferation in atherosclerosis, but may also be relevant to the fibroplasia of wound healing. Platelet growth factor is also chemotactic for leukocytes and fibroblasts in vitro.[106, 117]

3. *Fibroblast growth factor (FGF)* is a polypeptide (13,400 daltons) isolated from bovine brain and pituitary, which stimulates fibroblast and smooth muscle proliferation in culture.

4. *Macrophage-derived growth factors.* Recently the finger has been pointing toward the versatile macrophage as a promoter of connective tissue growth in inflammation. Guinea pigs whose macrophage function has been inhibited by injections of antimacrophage serum and corticosteroids show markedly diminished fibroplasia in wounds.[156] Soluble factors derived from macrophages stimulate fibroblast growth in culture,[116, 157] and new blood vessel growth in vivo.[119] Of interest is that macrophages need to be "activated" by nonimmunologic or immunologic stimuli to express optimal growth-promoting activity.

5. As stated earlier, the presence of *fibrin* is associated with the influx of fibroblasts and new vessels and the formation of granulation tissue in wound healing. Defibrination retards these processes in experimental

wounds.[158] Fibrinogen and fibrin degradation products appear to be chemotactic to leukocytes, including monocytes;[159] fibrin also binds to fibronectin, and fibronectin fragments are chemotactic to fibroblasts.[118] Thus, the effect of fibrin may be indirect. On the other hand, some product of the coagulation system (e.g., thrombin) might be directly mitogenic to fibroblasts and endothelial cells.

An additional component of the connective tissue cellular response in repair is the directional *migration* of both fibroblasts and endothelial cells *into* the wound. What draws these cells? Chemotactic influences for these two cell types are just beginning to be explored; in initial reports, collagen and collagen fragments, proteolytically cleaved fibronectin,[118] platelet growth factor,[117] heparin,[160] and lymphokines[116] have been found to be active in stimulating chemotaxis or chemokinesis of fibroblasts in vitro.

It must be apparent that the nature of the factors that regulate cell growth, and of the stimuli for cell migration and proliferation in inflammatory repair, though of critical importance, is still largely speculative. In the end it may be that growth will depend not on the action of one chemical acting on one cell but on the net effect of many factors that modulate cell growth and migration.

COLLAGENIZATION AND WOUND STRENGTH

The development of wound strength is undoubtedly related to the proliferation of fibroblasts and the laying down of collagen and other extracellular elements in healing wounds.[161, 162] In this section we will briefly review a few details of the biology of connective tissue extracellular matrices and then discuss the development of wound strength.

COLLAGEN

Collagen is the most common protein in the animal world, providing the extracellular framework for all multicellular organisms.[163–165] Without collagen, man would be reduced to a clump of cells, interconnected by a few neurons![166] Collagen consists of a family of molecules, each a genetically distinct type, which are a major component of fibrous tissue, basement membranes, bone, cartilage, and other specialized tissues, such as cornea and heart valves. It is the essential product of the fibroblast that ultimately provides the tensile strength of healing wounds.

The metabolism of collagen in normal tissues involves a balance between biosynthesis and degradation.[167] The fundamental unit of collagen is the collagen molecule (*tropocollagen*)—a long rod, 300 × 1.5 nm, with a molecular weight of 285,000.[168] Each collagen molecule is made up of three separate polypeptide chains (alpha chains) wrapped tightly together into a triple left-handed helix. Based on the biochemical composition of the chains, five major types of collagen are recognized, each characteristic of the tissue from which it is derived (Table 2–6). In types I, II, and III, the interstitial or fibrillar collagens, each native molecule packs with about one-fourth stagger with respect to the adjacent molecules. The overlap produces the characteristic 67-nm banding of the collagen fibril. Types IV and V do not form fibrils, but appear as amorphous materials in interstitial tissue or basement membranes. Synthesis of collagen (Fig. 2–33) is initiated by DNA transcription from specific genes coding for the polypeptide chains, followed by processing of mRNA precursor, and translation (synthesis) of the alpha chains on ribosomes. The alpha chains subsequently come off the ribosomes into the cisternae of the rough endoplasmic reticulum (RER), where they undergo a series of biochemical modifications of the chains, activated by spe-

Table 2–6. GENETICALLY DISTINCT VERTEBRATE COLLAGENS*

Type	Molecular Formula	Native Polymer	Tissue Distribution	Distinctive Features
I	$[\alpha(I)]_2\alpha 2$	Fibril	Skin, tendon, bone, dentin, fascia; widespread	Low content of hydroxylysine; broad fibrils
II	$[\alpha 1(II)]_3$	Fibril	Cartilage, nucleus pulposus, notochord, vitreous body	High content of hydroxylysine: heavily glycosylated
III	$[\alpha 1(III)]_3$	Fibril	Skin, uterus, blood vessels; "reticulin" fibers generally	High content of hydroxyproline; low content of hydroxylysine; few sites of hydroxylysine glycosylation
IV	$[\alpha(IV)_2]\alpha_2(IV)$	Basement lamina	Kidney glomeruli, lens capsule; Descemet's membrane; basement laminae of all epithelial and endothelial cells	Very high content of hydroxylysine; almost fully glycosylated; retains procollagen extension pieces
V	$\alpha A(\alpha B)_2$ or $(\alpha A)_3$ and $(\alpha B)_3$	Unknown	Widespread in small amounts; basement laminae of smooth and striated muscle cells? exoskeleton of fibroblasts and other mesenchymal cells?	High content of hydroxylysine; heavily glycosylated; fails to form native fibrils in vitro

*Modified from Eyre, D. R.: Science *207*:1315, 1980.

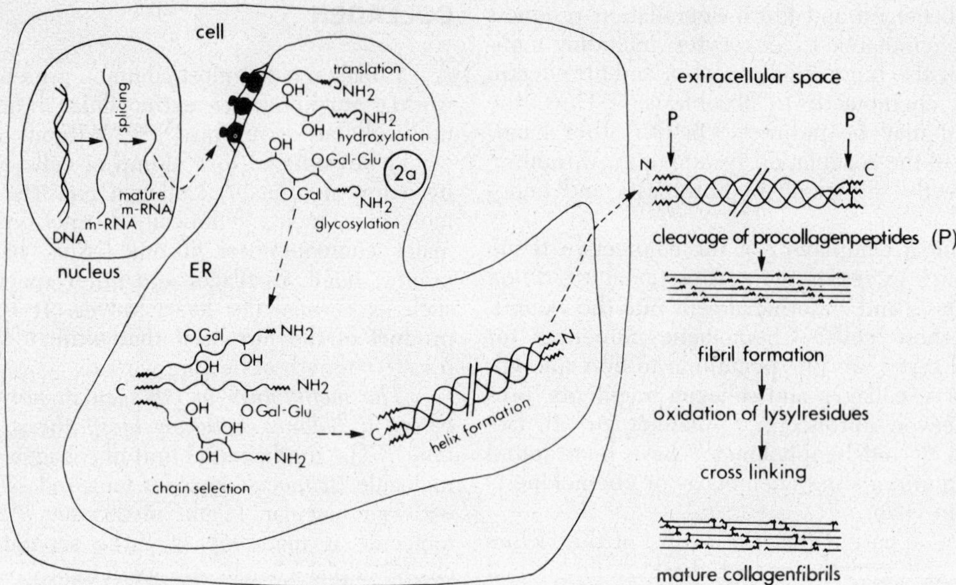

Figure 2–33. Synthesis of collagen. From Krieg, T., et al., Molecular defects of collagen metabolism in the Ehlers-Danlos syndrome. Int. J. Dermatol. *20*:415, 1981. Reproduced with permission.)

cific enzymes. One of these modifications is the hydroxylation of proline in the 4 position, providing collagen with its characteristic high content of hydroxyproline (about 10%). This hydroxylation, which is dependent on the availability of ascorbic acid (vitamin C), is important, since it is necessary to hold the three alpha chains in the cisternae of the RER.[167]

Another critical modification is *lysine oxidation*, since this results in *cross-linkages* between adjacent chains and is *the basis of the structural stability of collagen*. Indeed, inhibition of lysine oxidation results in malformations of the skeleton, skin, and blood vessels, as occurs in some forms of human disorders of collagen (i.e., Marfan's syndrome, p. 137). *Thus, cross-linking is a major contributor to the tensile strength of collagen.*

As mentioned, the triple helix is assembled in the cisternae of the rough endoplasmic reticulum. At this stage the procollagen molecule is still soluble and contains an extra length of polypeptide at the NH_2 terminal end of the chain. It is transported through the Golgi apparatus and larger vacuoles to the cell surface. During or shortly after excretion from the cell, procollagen peptidases clip the terminal peptide chains, promoting formation of fibrils. *It is in the extracellular space that true fibrils form,* and it is these collagen fibrils that give strength to connective tissue.

Collagen fibers are very hardy and in the native state are resistant to digestion. However, *collagenase,* which is present in a variety of cell types (fibroblasts, macrophages, polymorphonuclear leukocytes, synovial cells, and some epithelial cells), can cleave collagen under physiologic conditions, cutting the triple helix into two unequal fragments which are then susceptible to digestion by other proteases. Fortunately, however, collagenase is present in these cells in the inactive form, *procollagenase*. The conditions regulating the activation of the precursor molecule are obviously of great importance but are not well understood. However, it is thought that the collagenase of neutrophils, macrophages, and fibroblasts plays a role in degrading collagen in inflammation and wound healing. This might aid in the "débridement" of injured sites and also in the remodeling of connective tissue necessary for the healing defect. However, it may have a harmful effect, since there is evidence that collagenase contributes to continuing tissue damage in rheumatoid arthritis.[169,170]

Collagen types IV and V, together with laminin, fibronectin, and heparan sulfate proteoglycan, are components of the basement membranes. They exhibit no fibrils, and although readily degraded by selected neutral proteases derived from leukocytes, they are resistant to the collagenases found in skin.[171]

OTHER EXTRACELLULAR CONNECTIVE TISSUE COMPONENTS

Fibroblasts also synthesize *elastic fibers*[172] and secrete the various glycosaminoglycan (GAG) components of ground substances.

Elastic fibers consist of two protein components: the more abundant *elastin,* which is amorphous on electron microscopy, and the *elastic microfibril,* composed of a specialized glycoprotein. Mature elastin fibers are made of individual polypeptide chains, called tropoelastin, about 70,000 daltons, which are covalently connected by cross-linkages (desmosine and isodesmosine).[173] Elastin has an extremely long half-life, exceeding the life of the individual, but a number of elastases produced by certain bacteria, neutrophils, and macrophages may play a role in local degradation of elastic tissue in inflammation.[174] Indeed, as discussed in Chapter 16, unchecked activity of elastase may be a major factor in the pathogenesis of *emphysema*, a common and debilitating disease in which the lung loses its normal elasticity.

Laminin, a large (1,000,000 daltons) glycoprotein, is an integral component of basement membranes and mediates the attachment of epithelial cells to type IV collagen.

Glycosaminoglycans and *proteoglycans* of connective tissue are described in Chapter 28. Some workers believe that a relationship exists between the type of GAG present and the size and orientation of the collagen fibers, which thus influences the tensile strength of the wounds.[162]

Fibronectin is a large (440,000-dalton) glycoprotein consisting of two dimers held together by disulfide bonds. It is associated with cell surfaces, basement membranes, and pericellular matrices, and is produced by fibroblasts, monocytes, endothelial cells, and other cells.[175] An immunologically and structurally similar protein is found in plasma, where it is designated as "cold-insoluble globulin" because of its tendency to coprecipitate with cryofibrinogen. An important characteristic of both cellular and plasma fibronectins is their ability to bind a number of other macromolecules, including collagen, fibrin, heparin, and proteoglycans. For these reasons, it is thought that fibronectin is involved in interactions (e.g., attachment and spreading) of cells upon the matrix substrata.[176] Although the mechanism by which fibronectin regulates such interactions is still unclear, it is concentrated in areas of intense cellular activity during embryogenesis, and in immune reactions, such as delayed hypersensitivity. In healing skin wounds, a large quantity of fibronectin, mostly plasma-derived, appears in the extracellular matrix in the first two days after wounding. Thereafter, fibronectin is actively synthesized by proliferating endothelial cells.[177] There is some evidence that fibronectin in healing wounds may induce cell migration and possibly tissue organization: as alluded to earlier, fibronectin fragments are chemotactic for fibroblasts, and also promote organization of endothelial cells into capillary tubes in vitro.[177A]

Although it is clear that fibroblasts and myofibroblasts are the cells that secrete collagens, elastin, and proteoglycans in healing wounds, the mechanisms that stimulate or terminate such secretion at different phases are poorly understood. Factors derived from macrophages, platelets, and lymphocytes have been shown to stimulate collagen accumulation in cultures; other agents, such as corticosteroids, parathyroid hormone, and a macrophage factor, depress collagen synthesis.[178] Yet another macrophage factor stimulates collagenase formation by fibroblasts.[116] The point to emphasize is that the healing wound is a dynamic and changing environment. It is likely that different mechanisms, occurring at different times and involving interactions between cells and local factors (e.g., oxygen tension, pH, immune reactions), may trigger the release of chemical signals that modulate the synthesis, release, or degradation of extracellular matrix proteins, as well as migration and proliferation of cells. The details of these phenomena are unknown, but it is remarkable that despite the many seemingly disjointed activities, the general pattern of wound healing is so orderly.

WOUND STRENGTH

We now turn to the crucial questions of how long it takes for a skin wound to achieve its maximal strength and which substances contribute to this strength. There are variations that depend on the site of the wound, the species, and the depth of the incision.[162]

From the welter of facts, however, a general impression emerges. Immediately after injury, there is a short lag phase, lasting perhaps a few days and possibly up to 10 to 14 days. There is a rapid increase in wound strength over the next four weeks. This rate of increase then slows and virtually plateaus at approximately the third month after the original incision. This plateau is reached at about 70 to 80% of the tensile strength of unwounded skin, and indeed may persist for life.

Thus, Dunphy reports that "*most wounds involving skin, fascia, or tendon never regain the initial strength of the tissue divided.*"[179] The recovery of tensile strength can therefore be represented by a sigmoid curve terminating in a plateau below the original level of the unwounded skin. The structural or biochemical explanation of this curve still eludes us. It is not merely a function of collagen synthesis, since the curve of tensile strength does not parallel that of collagen increase in the wound. *The later slower rise in tensile strength is not associated with a significant increase in the collagen content of the wound.* It is unlikely that the amount of mucopolysaccharides contribute to tensile strength. It may be related to the type of collagen produced. Thus, while adult skin collagen is type I, collagen deposited early in granulation tissue is type III, that characteristic of embryonic skin. During maturation of the scar, type III is again replaced by adult type I collagen. It seems likely that further quantitative biochemical studies on collagen types and cross-linking may explain many of the mechanical properties of wounds that distinguish them from normal tissue.

In light of these findings, one may properly ask: How can patients be discharged from the hospital within a week of surgery? An interesting study bears on this question. It has been shown that carefully sutured wounds have approximately 70% of the strength of unwounded skin immediately following surgery.[180] Indeed, eight weeks later there was no significant increase in tensile strength despite the presumed proliferation of fibroblasts and synthesis of collagen. The obvious conclusion is that, in the fresh wound, most of its tensile strength depends on surgical skill and the placement of sutures. When the latter are removed at the end of the first week, wound strength is only at approximately the 10% level. However, in addition, it is reasonable to propose that reepithelialization, which occurs within the first days after wounding, provides some strength, and perhaps the early granulation tissue in some way serves as a binding agent or adhesive material.

FACTORS MODIFYING QUALITY OF INFLAMMATORY-REPARATIVE RESPONSE

Many systemic and local host factors influence the adequacy of the inflammatory-reparative response. Only a few of the most important will be discussed here.

SYSTEMIC INFLUENCES

Age is probably not a major influence on the inflammatory-reparative response. There is a prevailing "general wisdom" that the elderly heal more slowly than the young, but very little controlled data in the experimental animal to support this notion.

Nutrition has a profound effect on the healing of wounds.[181] Many workers have confirmed the deleterious effects of prolonged protein starvation on wound healing. Synthesis of collagen appears to be inhibited in protein-deficient animals. A high-protein diet hastens the rate of tensile strength gain. It has not been possible to isolate specific critical amino acids, but it has been said by some and contradicted by others that methionine and cystine supplementations have a beneficial effect on the healing process in the protein-depleted animal. Of the many influences, the best documented is the necessity of adequate levels of vitamin C for the synthesis of normal collagen. As mentioned earlier, vitamin C enhances the conversion of proline to hydroxyproline and lysine to hydroxylysine. Thus, deficiencies of this nutrient (scurvy) result in impaired synthesis of normal collagen. Absence of hydroxyproline will result in failure to achieve fibrillogenesis. Many enzymes, such as the metalloenzymes and DNA and RNA polymerases, are *zinc dependent*. The amount of zinc in tissues and blood may fall to low levels after trauma, and this is particularly noticeable in burn patients. Wound healing is delayed in patients with zinc deficiency and is restored to normal by zinc administration. However, zinc therapy has no effect on wound healing in normal patients.

Hematologic derangements, such as deficiency of neutrophils in the circulating blood (granulocytopenia) or defects in leukocyte chemotaxis and phagocytosis, are well-documented bases for increased susceptibility to bacterial infection. Wound infection greatly slows the entire reparative process. In bleeding disorders there is excessive extravasation of blood into the wounded areas, serving as a substrate for bacterial growth and significantly slowing repair.

Diabetics have an increased susceptibility to serious infections, owing to a variety of factors, including diminished neutrophil chemotaxis and decreased phagocytic capacity. These patients are more vulnerable to bacterial invasion and consequent delays in wound healing.

Corticosteroids have a well-documented anti-inflammatory effect. They inhibit the availability of leukocytes to inflammatory sites and interfere with a variety of their functions, including phagocytosis, intracellular killing, and secretion. One common mechanism for these anti-inflammatory effects may be the ability of glucocorticoids to enhance the production of a specific protein, called *lipomodulin*. Lipomodulin inhibits phospholipase A2, which, as may be recalled (Fig. 2–13), is the enzyme necessary for the release of arachidonic acid from membrane phospholipids. There follows reduced synthesis of active metabolites of arachidonic acid.[182]

The action of steroids on the healing phase is controversial. Inhibition of the synthesis of connective tissues in vitro and in vivo, impairment of granulation tissue formation, decreased production of hydroxyproline, as well as total collagen formation have all been attributed to steroids. However, there is a strong suspicion that these inhibitory effects on the healing process result from suppression of the inflammatory response. If cortisone is administered to animals 2 days after injury, healing does not appear to be impaired, suggesting that it acts early in the response and probably does not primarily affect the healing phase. We may conclude by noting that steroids unquestionably block or retard the inflammatory-reparative response. *Clinically a wound in any patient receiving appreciable amounts of corticosteroids during or following surgery should be watched carefully.*

LOCAL INFLUENCES

Infection is the single most important local cause for delayed healing. Indeed, if one examines the generalized and local factors that adversely influence repair, infection is the final common pathway by which they retard the process of healing.

Adequacy of blood supply in an area of injury is an obvious important influence. From all that has been said before, it must be apparent that vascularization of the focus is a key factor in both inflammation and repair. Arterial disease that limits blood flow and venous abnormalities that retard drainage are well-documented impairments to the healing of wounds.

Foreign bodies and, of course, sutures constitute impediments to healing. The surgeon is faced with the dilemma of an incision that has virtually no intrinsic strength during the immediate postoperative period, save that conferred by sutures, while at the same time the sutures are an obstacle to healing. The puncture wounds in the epidermis invite bacterial contamination, and the suture material excites an inflammatory and foreign body reaction. One old but interesting study contends that a single suture enhances the invasiveness of staphylococci by a factor of 10,000.[183] Fragments of wood, steel, glass, and even bone are equally undesirable. One must walk between Scylla and Charybdis by using sutures judiciously and removing all extraneous foreign bodies.

Tissue in which the injury has occurred. It is apparent that perfect repair can occur only in tissues made up of stable and labile cells, whereas all injuries to tissues composed of permanent cells must inevitably give rise to scarring and, at the most, very slight restoration of specialized elements. The location of the injury, or the character of the tissue in which the injury occurs, is also of considerable importance from yet another standpoint. There are many situations in the body in which inflammations arising within tissue spaces or cavities develop extensive exudates that fill these spaces, but in which there is no associated necrosis of fixed tissue cells. Under these circumstances, repair may occur by digestion of the exudate, initiated by the proteolytic enzymes of leukocytes, and resorption of the dissolved exudate. This mechanism of dealing with an exudative inflammation is called *resolution*. Since no necrosis of fixed tissue cells has occurred, perfect restitution of the preexisting architecture is attained.

An example of resolution may make its meaning more clear. Bacterial infections in the lung cause inflammations that may solidly fill the alveolar spaces with exudate. In many instances the alveolar septa are not damaged, although the lung becomes totally solidified by the inflammatory exudation. Proteolytic digestion of the exudate and resorption or coughing up of the watery digestate permit resolution of the pneumonia and restoration of normal lung structure and function. This same sequence of events is not inevitable in all pneumonias, since infections with more virulent pathogens may cause necrosis of septa and result in fibrous scarring and permanent pulmonary damage. Moreover, for completely obscure reasons, certain pneumonias with or without necrosis sometimes fail to resolve; instead, granulation tissue grows from the septal walls into the exudate and converts it into masses of fibrous tissue, referred to as *organization* of the pneumonia.

These processes of resolution or organization of inflammatory exudates are also observed in inflammations within other tissue spaces of the body—i.e., peritoneal, pericardial, and pleural cavities and joint spaces. Overall, most injuries of the body do not resolve without tissue necrosis, and result in some connective tissue proliferation and therefore some degree of scarring. Finally, even when scarring is complete, there is another hazard consequent upon a lag in the return of tensile strength of the collagen fibers. A rise in tension may bring about undue stretching of the scar, with hernia formation when the abdominal wall is affected.

In concluding this discussion of host factors, it is hardly necessary to point out that many involve issues of considerable clinical importance. The correction of nutritional deficiencies, avoidance of steroid therapy, wise use of sutures, careful débridement and removal of foreign bodies, and, in general, scrupulous attention to all the influences that may hamper the inflammatory response are all responsibilities of the clinician.

PERSPECTIVE ON INFLAMMATORY-REPARATIVE RESPONSE

The full spectrum of events, from the initial reaction to injury to the ultimate tissue repair, has been presented. It must be obvious that an injury may have little consequence and may be dealt with readily, or may culminate in severe destruction and damage. A perspective of the various pathways is offered in Figure 2–34. This overview makes clear that not all injuries result in permanent damage; some are resolved with perfect reconstitution of the native tissue. Most often, however, some residual scarring persists.

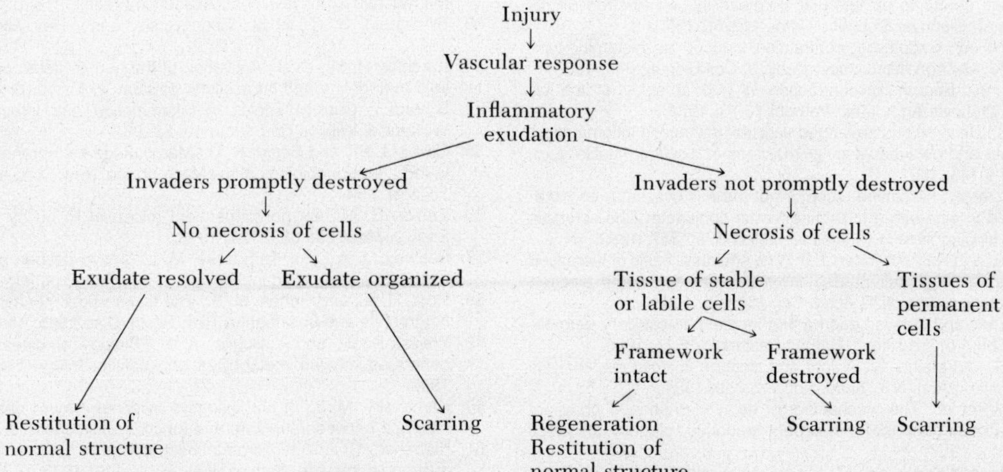

Figure 2–34. Pathways of reparative response.

1. Majno, G.: The Healing Hand: Man and Wound in the Ancient World. Boston, Harvard University Press, 1975.
2. Ryan, G., and Majno, G.: Inflammation. Kalamazoo, Michigan, A Scope Publication, Upjohn Co., 1977.
3. Ryan, G., and Majno, G.: Acute inflammation, a review. Am. J. Pathol. *86*:185, 1977.
4. Majno, G.: Inflammation and infection. Historical highlights. *In* Majno, G., and Cotran, R.S. (eds.): Current Topics in Inflammation and Infection. Baltimore, Williams & Wilkins Co., 1982, p. 1.
5. Hunter, J.: A treatise of the blood, inflammation, and gunshot wounds. Vol. I. London, J. Nicoll, 1794.
6. Cohnheim, J.: Lectures in General Pathology. Translated by McKee, A. D., from the second German edition, Vol. I. London, New Sydenham Society, 1889.
7. Heifets, L.: Centennial of Metchnikoff's discovery. J. Reticuloendothel. Soc. *31*:381, 1982.
8. Zweifach, B. W.: Vascular events in the inflammatory process. *In* Zweifach, B. W., Grant, L., and McCluskey, R. T. (eds.): The Inflammatory Process. 2nd ed. Vol. II. New York, Academic Press, 1973, pp. 3–40.
9. Lewis, T.: The blood vessels of the human skin and their responses. London, Shaw, 1927.
10. Landis, E. M., and Pappenheimer, J. R.: Exchange of substances through the capillary wall. *In* Hamilton, W. F., and Dow, P. (eds.): Handbook of Physiology. Washington, DC, American Physiological Society, Section 2, Vol. II, 1963, pp. 961–1043.
11. Renkin, E. M.: Relation of capillary morphology to transport of fluid and large molecules. A review. Acta Physiol. Scand. (Suppl.) *463*: 81, 1979.
12. Simionescu, N., et al.: Permeability of muscle capillaries to small hemepeptides. Evidence for existence of patent transendothelial channels. J. Cell Biol., *64*:586, 1975.
13. Karnovsky, M. H.: The ultrastructural basis of transcapillary exchange. J. Gen. Phys. *52*:645, 1970.
14. Simionescu, N., et al.: Structural basis of permeability in sequential segments of the microvasculature of the diaphragm. II. Pathways followed by microperoxidase across the endothelium. Microvasc. Res. *15*:17, 1978.
15. Simionescu, M., et al.: Differentiated microdomains on the luminal surface of capillary endothelium. II. Partial characterization of their anionic sites. J. Cell Biol. *90*:614, 1981.
16. Gimbrone, M. A., Jr.: Vascular endothelium and atherosclerosis. *In* Moore, S. (ed.): The Vascular Wall and Atherosclerosis. New York, Marcel Dekker, 1981, pp. 25–51.
17. Cotran, R. S.: The endothelium in inflammation, New insights. *In* Majno, G., and Cotran, R. S. (eds.): Current Topics in Inflammation and Infection. Baltimore, Williams & Wilkins Co., 1982, pp. 18–38.
18. Jaffe, E. (ed.): The Biology of Endothelial Cells. Amsterdam, Martinus Nijhoff, 1983.
19. Majno, G., et al.: Studies on inflammation. II. Effects of histamine and serotonin along the vascular tree: A topographic study. J. Biophys. Biochem. Cytol. *11*:607, 1961.
20. Hurley, J. V.: Acute Inflammation. 2nd ed. Baltimore, Williams & Wilkins Co., 1983.
21. Majno, G., and Palade, G. E.: Studies on inflammation. I. The effect of histamine and serotonin on vascular permeability: An electron microscopic study. J. Biophys. Biochem. Cytol. *11*:571, 1961.
22. Majno, G., et al.: Endothelial contraction induced by histamine-type mediators: An electron microscopic study. J. Cell Biol. *42*:647, 1969.
23. Joris, I., et al.: Endothelial contraction *in vivo*: a study of the rat mesentery. Virchows Arch. (Zell. Pathol.) *12*:73, 1972.
24. Cotran, R. S.: Delayed and prolonged vascular leakage in inflammation. III. Immediate and delayed vascular reactions in skeletal muscle. Exp. Mol. Pathol. *6*:143, 1967.
25. Heltianu, C., et al.: Histamine receptors of the microvascular endothelium revealed *in situ* with a histamine-ferritin conjugate: Characteristic high-affinity binding sites in venules. J. Cell Biol. *93*:357, 1982.
26. Cotran, R. S., and Remensynder, J. P.: The structural basis of increased vascular permeability after graded thermal injury: Light and electron microsopic studies. Ann. N.Y. Acad. Sci. *150*:495, 1968.
27. Sevitt, S.: Early and delayed edema and increase in capillary permeability after a burn of the skin. J. Pathol. Bacteriol. *75*:27, 1958.
28. Cotran, R. S. and Majno, G.: A light and electron microscopic analysis of vascular injury. Ann. N.Y. Acad. Sci. *116*:750, 1964.
29. Hurley, J. V., et al.: The mechanism of delayed-prolonged phase of increased vascular permeability in turpentine-induced pleurisy. J. Pathol. Bacteriol. *94*:1, 1967.
30. Hoover, R. L., and Karnovsky, M. J.: Leucocyte-endothelial interactions. *In* Nossel, H., and Vogel, H. (eds.): Pathobiology of the Endothelial Cell. New York, Academic Press, 1982, pp. 357–367.
31. Atherton, A.: Quantitative investigations of adhesiveness of circulating polymorphonuclear leukocytes to blood vessel walls. J. Physiol. *222*:447, 1972.
32. Gimbrone, M.A., Jr., and Buchanan, M. R.: Interactions of leucocytes with vascular endothelium. Ann. N.Y. Acad. Sci., *77*:171, 1982.
33. Marchesi, V. T.: The site of leucocyte emigration during inflammation. Q. J. Exp. Phys. *46*:115, 1961.
34. Issekutz, A. C., et al.: Enhanced vascular permeability and haemorrhage-inducing activity of rabbit C5ades arg: probable role of polymorphonuclear leukocyte lysosomes. Clin. Exp. Immunol. *41*:512, 1980.
35. Issekutz, T. B., et al.: The *in vivo* quantitation and kinetics of monocyte migration into acute inflammatory tissue. Am. J. Pathol. *103*:47, 1981.
36. Boyden, S.: The chemotactic effect of mixtures of antibody and antigen on polymorphonuclear leukocytes. J. Exp. Med. *115*:453, 1962.
37. Becker, E. L., and Ward, P. A.: Chemotaxis. *In* Parker, C. W. (ed.): Clinical Immunology. Philadelphia, W. B. Saunders, 1980, pp. 272–297.
38. Zigmond, S. M.: Polymorphonuclear leucocyte chemotaxis: Detection of gradient and development of cell polarity. Ciba Found. Symp. *71*:299, 1980.
39. Sahu, S., and Lynn, W. S.: Lipid chemotaxis isolated from culture filtrates of *E. coli* and oxidized lipids. Inflammation *2*:47, 1977.
40. Schiffman, E., et al.: *N*-Formylmethionyl peptides as chemoattractants for leukocytes. Proc. Natl. Acad. Sci. U.S.A. *72*:1059, 1975.
41. Williams, L. T., et al.: Specific receptor sites for chemotactic peptides on human polymorphonuclear leukocytes. Proc. Natl. Acad. Sci. U.S.A. *74*:1204, 1977.
42. Chenoweth, D. E., and Hugli, T. E.: Demonstration of specific C5a receptor on intact human polymorphonuclear leukocytes. Proc. Natl. Acad. Sci. U.S.A. *75*:3943, 1978.
43. Goldman, D. W., and Goetzl, E. J.: Specific binding of leukotriene B_4 to receptors on human polymorphonuclear leukocytes. J. Immunol. *129*:1600, 1982.
44. Ward, P.: The chemotaxis system. *In* Majno, G., and Cotran, R. S. (eds.): Current Topics in Inflammation and Infection. Baltimore, Williams & Wilkins Co., 1982, pp. 54–61.
45. Naccache, P. H., et al.: Mono- and di-hydroxyeicosatetraenoic acids alter calcium homeostasis in rabbit neutrophils. J. Clin. Invest. *67*:1584, 1981.
46. Stossel, T. P.: Actin gelation and the structure of cortical cytoplasm. Cold Spring Harbor Symp. Quant. Biol. *46*:569, 1982.
47. Gallin, J. I.: The cell biology of leucocyte chemotaxis. *In* Weissmann, G. (ed.): Cell Biology of Inflammation. Amsterdam, Elsevier/North-Holland, 1980, p. 340.
48. Norris, D. A., et al.: Fibronectin fragment(s) are chemotactic for human peripheral blood monocytes. J. Immunol. *129*:1612, 1982.
49. Goetzl, G. E., et al.: Biochemical and functional bases of regulatory and protective roles of the human eosinophil. *In* Weissmann, G., et al. (eds.): Advances in Inflammation Research. Vol. 1. New York, Raven Press, 1979, pp. 157–168.
50. Stossel, T. P.: Endocytosis. *In* Cutrecasas, P., and Greaves, M. (eds.): Receptors and Recognition. Vol. 4. London, Chapman and Hall, Ltd., 1978.
51. Johnston, R. B., Jr.: Defects of neutrophil function. N. Engl. J. Med. *307*:426, 1982.
52. Wilkinson, P. C.: Cellular and molecular aspects of chemotaxis of macrophages and monocytes. *In* Nelson, D. S. (ed.): Immunobiology of the Macrophage. New York, Academic Press, 1976, p. 349.
53. Silverstein, S. C., et al.: Endocytosis. Annu. Rev. Biochem. *46*:669, 1977.
54. Korchak, H. M., et al.: Activation of the human neutrophil: The roles of lipid remodeling and intracellular calcium. *In* Majno, G., and Cotran, R. S. (eds.): Current Topics in Inflammation and Infection. Baltimore, Williams & Wilkins Co., 1982, pp. 83–93.
55. Oliver, J. M., and Berlin, R. D.: Macrophage membranes. *In* Nelson, D. L. (ed.): Immunobiology of the Macrophage. New York, Academic Press, 1976, p. 269.
56. Babior, B. M.: Oxygen-dependent microbial killing by phagocytes. N. Engl. J. Med. *298*:659, 721, 1978.
57. Badwey, J. A., and Karnovsky, M. L.: Active oxygen species and the function of phagocytic leukocytes. Annu. Rev. Biochem. *49*:695, 1980.
58. Root, R. K., and Cohen, M. S.: The microbicidal mechanisms of human neutrophils and eosinophils. Rev. Infect. Dis. *3*:565, 1981.
59. Weiss, S. J., and LoBuglio, A. F.: Biology of disease: Phagocyte-generated oxygen metabolites and cellular injury. Lab. Invest. *47*:5, 1982.
60. Karnovsky, M. J., et al.: Oxidative cytochemistry in phagocytosis: The interface between structure and function. Histochem. J. *13*:1, 1981.
61. Klebanoff, S. J.: Antimicrobial mechanisms in neutrophilic polymorphonuclear leukocytes. Semin. Hematol. *12*:117, 1975.
62. Johnston, R. B., and Lehmeyer, J. S.: *In* Michelson, J. (ed.): Superoxide and Superoxide Dismutase. London, Academic Press, 1978.

63. Jacques, Y. V., and Bainton, D. F.: Changes in pH within the phagocytic vacuole of human neutrophils and monocytes. Lab. Invest. *39*:179, 1978.
64. Weissman, G., et al.: Release of inflammatory mediators from stimulated neutrophils. N. Engl. J. Med. *303*:27, 1980.
65. Becker, S. L., and Henson, P. M.: In vitro studies of immunologically induced reaction of mediators from cells. Arch. Immunol. *17*:93, 1973.
66. Weissmann, G., and Pieter, J. A.: Molecular basis of gouty inflammation: Interaction of monosodium urate crystals with lysosomes and liposomes. Nature *240*:167, 1972.
67. Allison, A. C., et al.: An examination of the cytotoxic effects of silica on macrophages. J. Exp. Med. *124*:141, 1966.
68. Babior, B. M., and Crowley, C. A.: Chronic granulomatous disease and other disorders of oxidative killing by phagocytes. *In* Stanbury, J. B., et al. (eds.): The Metabolic Basis of Inherited Disease. New York, McGraw-Hill Book Co., 1983, pp. 1956–1985.
69. Ward, P., et al.: Regulatory dysfunction in leukotaxis. Am. J. Pathol. *88*:701, 1977.
70. Busse, W. W.: Histamine: Mediator and modulator in inflammation. *In* Houck, J. C. (ed.): Chemical Messengers of the Inflammatory Process. Amsterdam, Elsevier/North-Holland, 1979, pp. 1–35.
71. Lagunoff, D.: Membrane fusion during mast cell secretion. J. Cell Biol. *57*:252, 1973.
72. Galli, S. J., et al.: Basophils and mast cells: Morphologic insights into their biology, secretory patterns and function. *In* Ishizaka, K. (ed.): Prog. Allergy *34*:1, 1984.
73. Austen, K. F.: Tissue mast cells in immediate hypersensitivity. Hosp. Pract. *17*:98, 1982.
74. Sandberg, A. L.: Complement. *In* Oppenheim, J., et al. (eds.): Cellular Functions in Immunity and Inflammation. Amsterdam, Elsevier/North-Holland, 1981, pp. 373–395.
75. Ward, P. A., et al.: Complement and chemotaxis. *In* Weissmann, G., et al. (eds.): Chemical Messengers of Inflammation. Vol I of Handbook of Inflammation. Amsterdam, Elsevier/North-Holland, 1979, pp. 153–177.
76. Movat, H. Z.: Kinins and the kinin system as inflammatory mediators. *In* Weissmann, G., et al. (eds.): Chemical Messengers of Inflammation. Vol. I of Handbook of Inflammation. Amsterdam, Elsevier/North-Holland, 1979, pp. 47–112.
77. Wiggins, R. C., and Cochrane, C. G.: Hageman factor and the contact activation system. *In* Weissman, G., et al. (eds.): Chemical Messengers of Inflammation. Vol. I of Handbook of Inflammation. Amsterdam, Elsevier/North-Holland, 1979, pp. 179–196.
78. Weissmann, G.: Prostaglandins in acute inflammation. *In* Current Concepts, Upjohn Co., pp. 5-32, 1981.
78A. Samuelsson, B.: Leukotrienes: Mediators of immediate hypertensitivity reaction and inflammation. Science *220*:568, 1983.
79. Samuelsson, B., and Paoletti, B. R.: Leukotrienes and Other Lipoxygenase Products. New York, Raven Press, 1982.
80. O'Flaherty, J. T.: Lipid mediators of inflammation and allergy. Lab. Invest. *47*:314, 1982.
81. Granström, E., and Hedqvist, P.: Prostaglandins, thromboxanes and leukotrienes. *In* Nossel, H., and Vogel, M. J. (eds.): Pathobiology of the Endothelial Cell. New York, Academic Press, 1982, pp. 287–300.
82. Pinckard, N.: The "new" chemical mediators of inflammation. *In* Majno, G., and Cotran, R. S. (eds.): Current Topics in Inflammation and Infection. Baltimore, Williams & Wilkins Co., 1982, pp. 38–54.
83. Perez, H. D., et al.: Generation of chemotactic lipid from arachidonic acid by exposure to a superoxide generating system. Inflammation *4*:313, 1980.
84. Johnston, M. G., et al.: The distribution of prostaglandins in afferent and efferent lymph from inflammatory sites. Am. J. Pathol. *99*:695, 1980.
85. Rae, S., et al.: Leukotriene B_4, an inflammatory mediator in gout. Lancet *2*:1122, 1982.
86. Williams, T. J., and Peck, M. J.: Role of prostaglandin-mediated vasodilatation in inflammation. Nature *270*:530, 1977.
87. Issekutz, A. C., and Movat, H. Z.: The effect of vasodilator prostaglandins on polymorphonuclear leucocyte infiltration and vascular injury. Am. J. Pathol. *107*:300, 1982.
88. Ameland, E., et al.: Interactions among inflammatory mediators on edema formation in the canine forelimb. Circ. Res. *49*:298, 1981.
89. Dahlen, S. E., et al.: Leukotrienes promote plasma leakage and leukocyte adhesion in postcapillary venules: *In vivo* effects with relevance to the acute inflammatory response. Proc. Natl. Acad. Sci. U.S.A. *78*:3887, 1981.
90. Weiss, W., et al.: Bronchoconstrictor effects of leukotriene C in human subjects. Science *216*:196, 1982.
91. Dahlén, S. E., et al.: Leukotrienes are potent constrictors in human bronchi. Nature *288*:484, 1980.
92. Örning, L., et al.: Leukotriene D. A slow reacting substance from rat basophilic leukemia cells. Proc. Natl. Acad. Sci. U.S.A. *77*:2014, 1980.
93. Lee, C. W., et al.: Generation and metabolism of C6-sulfodipeptide leukotrienes in IgE dependent reactions: Mast cell heterogeneity. *In* Piper, P. (ed.): Proc. Symp. on Leukotrienes and Other Lipooxygenase Products. London, John Wiley & Sons, 1983.
94. Lewis, R. A., et al.: Biology of the C-6 sulfopeptide leukotrienes. *In* Samuelsson, B., and Paoletti, R. (eds.): Advances in Prostaglandin, Thromboxane and Leukotriene Research. Vol. XI. New York, Raven Press, 1983.
95. Palmblad, J., et al.: Leukotriene B_4 is a potent and stereospecific stimulator of neutrophil chemotaxis and adherence. Blood *58*:658, 1981.
96. Weissmann, G. (ed.): Mediators of Inflammation. New York, Plenum Press, 1974.
97. Geotzl, E. J., et al.: A neutrophil-immobilizing factor derived from polymorphonuclear leukocytes. 2. Specificity of action on polymorphonuclear leukocyte mobility. J. Immunol., *111*:938, 1973.
98. Movat, H. Z.: Pathway to allergic inflammation: The sequelae of antigen-antibody complex formation. Fed. Proc. *35*:2439, 1976.
99. Janoff, A., and Carp, H.: Proteases, antiproteases, and oxidants: Pathways of tissue injury during inflammation. *In* Majno, G., and Cotran, R. S. (eds.): Current Topics in Inflammation and Infection. Baltimore, Williams & Wilkins Co., 1982, pp. 62–82.
100. Fantone, J. C., and Ward, P. A.: Role of oxygen-derived free radicals and metabolites in leukocyte-dependent inflammatory reactions. Am. J. Pathol. *107*:397, 1982.
101. Ward, P. A., et al.: Evidence for a role of hydroxyl radical in neutrophil dependent tissue injury. J. Clin. Invest. *72*:789, 1983.
102. Humphrey, D. M., et al.: Vasoactive properties of AGEPC and analogues. Lab. Invest. *46*:422, 1982.
103. Valone, F. H., and Goetzl, E. J.: Enhancement of human leukocyte adherence by the phospholipid mediator AGEPC. Am. J. Pathol. *113*:85, 1983.
103A. Humphrey, D. M., et al.: Induction of leukocytic infiltrates in rabbit skin by acetyl glyceryl ether phosphorylcholine. Lab. Invest. *47*:227, 1982.
104. Lin, A. H., et al.: AGEPC stimulates leukotriene B_4 synthesis in human polymorphonuclear leukocytes. J. Clin. Invest. *70*:1058, 1982.
105. Postlethwaite, E. A., and Kang, A. H.: Collagen- and collagen peptide–induced chemotaxis of human blood monocytes. J. Exp. Med. *143*:1299, 1976.
106. Deuel, T. F., et al.: Chemotaxis of monocytes and neutrophils to platelet-derived growth factor. J. Clin. Invest. *69*:1046, 1982.
107. Nathan, C. F., et al.: The macrophage as an effector cell. N. Engl. J. Med. *303*:622, 1980.
108. Unanue, E., and Rosenthal, A. (eds.): Macrophage Regulation of Immunity. New York, Academic Press, 1980.
109. Van Furth, R.: Mononuclear Phagocytes. Functional Aspects. The Hague, Martinoff Nijhoff Publishers, 1980.
110. Lasser, A.: The mononuclear phagocytosystem: A review. Hum. Pathol. *14*:108, 1983.
111. Volkman, A., and Gowans, J.: The production of macrophages in the rat. Br. J. Exp. Pathol. *46*:50, 1965.
112. Scott, W. A., and Cohn, Z. A.: Secretory products of mononuclear phagocytes. *In* Nossel, L., and Vogel, M. J. (eds.): Pathobiology of the Endothelial Cell. New York, Academic Press, 1982, p. 351.
113. Rosenstreich, D. L.: The macrophage. *In* Oppenheim, J., et al. (eds.): Cellular Functions in Immunity and Inflammation. Amsterdam, Elsevier/North-Holland, 1981, pp. 130–148.
114. Leak, L. V., and Burke, J. F.: Early events of tissue injury and the role of the lymphatic system in early inflammation. *In* Zweifach, B. W., Grant, L., and McCluskey. R. T. (eds.): The Inflammatory Process. Vol. III. New York, Academic Press, 1974, p. 163.
115. Ryan, G. B., and Spector, W. G.,: Macrophage turnover in inflamed connective tissue. Proc. R. Soc. Lond. Biol. *174*:269, 1970.
116. Wahl, S. M., and Wahl, L. M.: Modulation of fibroblast growth and function by monokines and lymphokines. *In* Pick, E. (ed.): Lymphokines. New York, Academic Press, 1981, pp. 179–201.
117. Seppä, H., et al.: Platelet-derived growth factor is chemotactic for fibroblasts. J. Cell Biol. *92*:584, 1982.
118. Tsukamoto, Y., et al.: Macrophage production of fibronectin, a chemoattractant for fibroblasts. J. Immunol. *127*:673, 1981.
119. Polverini, P. J., et al.: Activated macrophages induce vascular proliferation. Nature *269*:804, 1977.
120. Boros, D. L.: Granulomatous inflammation. Prog. Allergy *24*:184, 1978.
121. Unanue, E. R.: The immune granulomas. *In* Samter, M. (ed.): Immunological Diseases. 3rd ed. Boston, Little, Brown & Co., 1978, p. 297.
122. Unanue, E. R., and Benacerraf, B.: Immunological events in experimentally induced granulomas. Am. J. Pathol. *71*:349, 1973.
123. Postlethwaite, A. E., et al.: Formation of multinucleated giant cells from human monocyte precursors. Mediation by a soluble protein from antigen- and mitogen-stimulated lymphocytes. J. Exp. Med. *155*:168, 1982.

124. Atkins, E., and Bodel, P.: Clinical fever: Its history, manifestations and pathogenesis. Fed. Proc. *38*:57, 1979.
125. Dinarello, C. A.: Leukocytic pyrogen. Lymphokines 7:23, 1982.
126. Dinarello, C. A., and Wolff, S. M.: Molecular basis of fever in humans. Am. J. Med. *72*:799, 1982.
127. Barakos, V., et al.: Stimulation of muscle protein degradation and prostaglandin E_2 release by leukocytic pyrogen (interleukin-1). N. Engl. J. Med. *308*:553, 1983.
128. McMinn, R. M. H.: The cellular morphology of tissue repair. Int. Rev. Cytol., *22*:63, 1967.
129. LeBlond, C. P., and Walker, B. E.: Renewal of cell populations. Physiol. Rev. *36*:255, 1956.
130. Folkman, J., and Cotran, R. S.: The relationship of endothelial proliferation to tumor growth. Int. Rev. Pathol. *16*:207, 1976.
131. Ross, R.: Atherosclerosis: A problem of the biology of arterial wall cells and their interactions with blood components. Arteriosclerosis *1*:293, 1981.
132. Hay, E.: Regeneration. New York, Holt, Rinehart & Winston, 1966.
133. Ausprunk, D. H.: Tumor angiogenesis. *In* Houck, J. C. (ed.): Chemical Messengers of the Inflammatory Process. Amsterdam, Elsevier/North-Holland, 1979, pp. 317–351.
134. Schoefl, G. I.: Studies of inflammation. III. Growing capillaries: Their structure and permeability. Virchows Arch. Pathol. Anat. *337*:97, 1963.
135. Ross, R.: Wound healing. Sci. Am. *220*:40, 1969.
136. Ryan, G. B., et al.: Myofibroblasts in human granulation tissue. Hum. Pathol. *5*:55, 1974.
137. Gabbiani, G., et al.: Granulation tissue as a contractile organ. A study of structure and function. J. Exp. Med. *135*:719, 1972.
138. Seemayer, T. A., et al.: The myofibroblast. Pathol. Annu. *15*:443, 1980.
139. Billingham, R. E., and Russell, P. S.: Studies on wound healing, with special reference to the phenomenon of contracture in experimental wounds in rabbit skin. Ann. Surg. *144*:961, 1956.
140. Gabbiani, G., and Rungger-Brändle, E.: The fibroblast. *In* Glynn, L.E. (ed.): Tissue Repair and Regeneration. Vol. 3 of Handbook of Inflammation. Amsterdam, Elsevier/North-Holland, 1981, pp. 1–51.
141. Sato, G. H., and Ross, R. (eds.): Hormones and Cell Culture. Cold Spring Harbor Conf. on Cell Proliferation *6*:1, 1979.
141A. Cold Spring Harbor Conferences on Cell Proliferation. 7–10, 1980–1982.
142. Widdowson, E. M.: First Nobel Conference on the Biology of Human Growth. New York, Raven Press, 1982.
143. Baserga, R.: Multiplication and Division of Mammalian Cells. Biochemistry of Disease. Vol. 6. New York, Marcel Dekker, 1976.
144. Baserga, R.: The cell cycle. N. Engl. J. Med. *304*:453, 1981.
145. Bucher, N. L., et al.: Hormonal factors concerned with liver regeneration. *In* Ciba Foundation Symposium on Hepatotrophic Factors (No. 55, New Series). Amsterdam, Elsevier/North-Holland, 1978, pp. 95–107.
145A. Carpenter, G., and Cohen, S.: Epidermal growth factor. Annu. Rev. Biochem. *48*:193, 1979.
146. Fox, F., et al.: Receptor remodeling and regulation in the action of epidermal growth factor. Fed. Proc. *41*:2989, 1982.
147. Todaro, G. J., et al.: Sarcoma growth factor and other transforming peptides produced by human cells: Interactions with membrane receptors. Fed. Proc. *41*:2296, 1982.
148. Rytömaa, E.: The chalone concept. Int. Rev. Exp. Pathol. *16*:156, 1976.
149. Iversen, O. H.: The chalones. *In* Baserga, R. (ed.): Handbook of Experimental Pharmacology. Vol. 57. Berlin/Heidelberg, Springer-Verlag, 1981, pp. 491–550.
150. Karnovsky, M. J., et al.: Effects of heparin on vascular smooth muscle cell proliferation. Clinical Physiology Series. Am. Phys. Soc. Publ., in press, 1984.
151. Holley, R. W.: Control of growth of mammalian cells in cell culture. Nature *258*:487, 1975.
152. Gospodarowicz, D., et al.: The control of proliferation and differentiation of endothelial cells. *In* Nossel, L., and Vogel, M. J. (eds.): Pathobiology of the Endothelial Cell. New York, Academic Press, 1982, pp. 19–61.
153. Folkman, J., and Moscona, A.: Role of cell shape in growth control. Nature *273*:345, 1978.
154. Ross, R., and Vogel, A.: The platelet derived growth factor. Cell *14*:203, 1978.
155. Deuel, T. F., et al.: Human platelet derived growth factor — purification and resolution into two active protein fractions. J. Biol. Chem. *256*:8896, 1981.
156. Liebovich, S. J., and Ross, R.: The role of the macrophage in wound repair: A study with hydrocortisone and anti-macrophage serum. Am. J. Pathol. *78*:71, 1975.
157. Martin, B., et al.: Stimulation of non-lymphoid mesenchymal proliferation by a macrophage-derived growth factor. J. Immunol. *126*:1510, 1981.
158. Dvorak, H. A., et al.: Fibrin as a component of the tumor stroma: Origins and biological significance. Cancer Metastasis Rev. *1*: , 1983.
159. Richardson, D. L., et al.: Chemotaxis for human monocytes by fibrinogen related peptides. Br. J. Haematol. *32*:507, 1976.
160. Azizkhan, R. G., et al.: Mast cell heparin stimulates migration of capillary endothelial cells *in vitro*. J. Exp. Med. *152*:931, 1980.
161. Ross, R.: The fibroblast and wound repair. Biol. Rev. *43*:51, 1968.
162. Peacock, E. E., and Van Winkle, W.: Wound Repair. 2nd ed. Philadelphia, W. B. Saunders Co., 1976, p. 8l.
163. Eyre, D. R.: Collagen: Molecular diversity in the body's protein scaffold. Science *207*:1315, 1980.
164. Bornstein, P., and Sage, H.: Structurally distinct collagen types. Annu. Rev. Biochem. *49*:957, 1980.
165. Prockop, D. J.: How does a skin fibroblast make type I collagen fibers? J. Invest. Dermatol. *79*:35, 1982.
166. Wuepper, K., et al.: Symposium on the biology of skin. Structural elements of the dermis. J. Invest. Dermatol. *79*:Supp. 1, 1982.
167. Duance, V. C., and Bailey, A. J.: Biosynthesis and degradation of collagen. *In* Glynn, L. E. (ed.): Tissue Repair and Regeneration. Vol. 3 of Handbook of Inflammation. Amsterdam, Elsevier/North-Holland, 1981, pp. 51–111.
168. Prockop, D. J., et al.: The biosynthesis of collagen and its disorders. N. Engl. J. Med. *301*:13, 77, 1979.
169. Harris, E. T., and Crane, S. M.: Collagenases. N. Engl. J. Med. *291*:652, 1974.
170. Krane, S. M.: Collagenases and collagen degradation. J. Invest. Dermatol. *79*:83s, 1982.
171. Sage, H.: Collagens of basement membranes. J. Invest. Dermatol. *79*:51s, 1982.
172. Ross, R., and Bornstein, P.: Elastic fibers in the body. Sci. Am. *224*:44, 1971.
173. Sandberg, L. B., et al.: Elastin structure, biosynthesis, and relation to disease states. N. Engl. J. Med. *304*:566, 1981.
174. Werb, Z., et al.: Elastases and elastic degradation. J. Invest. Dermatol. *79*:154s, 1982.
175. Hynes, R. O., and Yamada, K. M.: Fibronectins: Multifunctional modular glycoproteins. J. Cell Biol. *95*:369, 1982.
176. Virtanen, I., et al.: Fibronectin in adhesion, spreading and cytoskeletal organization of cultured fibroblasts. Nature *298*:660, 1982.
177. Clark, R. A. F., et al.: Fibronectin is produced by blood vessels in response to injury. J. Exp. Med. *156*:646, 1982.
177A. Maciag, T., et al.: Organizational behavior of human umbilical vein endothelial cells. J. Cell Biol. *94*:511, 1982.
178. Castor, C. W.: Autacoid regulation of wound healing. *In* Glynn, L. E. (ed.): Tissue Repair and Regeneration. Vol. 3 of Handbook of Inflammation. Amsterdam, Elsevier/North Holland, 1981, pp. 177–202.
179. Dunphy, J. E. (ed.): Wound Healing. New York, Medcom Press, 1974.
180. Lichtenstein, I. L., et al.: The dynamics of wound healing. Surg. Gynecol. Obstet. *130*:685, 1970.
181. Bourne, G. H.: Nutrition and wound healing. *In* Glynn, L. E. (ed.): Tissue Repair and Regeneration. Vol. 3 of Handbook of Inflammation. Amsterdam, Elsevier/North-Holland, 1981, 1981, pp. 211–234.
182. Claman, H. N.: Glucocorticosteroids. I. Anti-inflammatory mechanisms. Hosp. Pract. *18*:123, 1983.
183. Elek, S. D., and Conen, P. E.: The virulence of *Staphylococcus pyogenes* for man: A study of the problems of wound infection. Br. J. Exp. Pathol. *38*:573, 1957.

FLUID AND HEMODYNAMIC DERANGEMENTS 3

All cells and tissues of the body are critically dependent on a normal fluid environment and on adequate blood supply. Either or both of these supporting systems may be deranged in a wide variety of clinical settings, and therefore fluid imbalances (edema or dehydration) and hemodynamic disturbances (hemorrhage, thrombosis, embolism, and infarction) are not only commonplace, but also life-threatening. Myocardial infarction is the predominant cause of death in industrialized nations (p. 556). Edema of the brain or lungs and pulmonary embolism also are major causes of death. Severe hemorrhage is a frequent cause of morbidity and mortality, especially in this day of automobile and industrial accidents.

EDEMA

Edema is the term generally used for the accumulation of excess fluid in the intercellular (interstitial) tissue spaces or body cavities. Cells, too, may accumulate an abnormal amount of fluid, but this phenomenon is referred to as a "cell swelling" or "cellular edema," described on page 14. Edema may occur as a localized process (for example, the swelling of the leg when the venous outflow is obstructed) or it may be systemic in distribution, as in congestive heart failure or renal failure. When edema is severe and generalized and causes diffuse swelling of all tissues and organs in the body, particularly noticeable in the subcutaneous tissues, it is called *anasarca*. Collection of edema fluid in the peritoneal cavity is known as *ascites;* in the pleural cavity as *hydrothorax;* and in the pericardial sac as *pericardial effusion,* or *hydropericardium.* Noninflammatory edema fluid such as accumulates in heart failure and renal disease is protein poor and is referred to as a *transudate.* In contrast, inflammatory edema related to increased endothelial permeability is protein-rich and is caused by the escape of plasma proteins (principally albumin), and possibly leukocytes, to form an *exudate.* The differentiation of a transudate from an exudate was presented on page 41. Here we are principally concerned with the noninflammatory transudation of fluid related to hemodynamic derangements.

PATHOGENESIS. Water constitutes 60% of the body mass. In a 70-kg man this volume is divided into the various compartments indicated in Table 3–1. Under normal circumstances about 25% of the extracellular fluid is found in the plasma confined to the intravascular compartment. The remainder is interstitial fluid separated from the intravascular fluid by a semipermeable endothelial barrier.

The exchange of fluid between blood plasma and interstitial fluid depends on two sets of forces: the hydrostatic pressure of the blood and osmotic pressure of the tissue fluid, opposed by the oncotic pressure of plasma proteins and hydrostatic pressure within the interstitial fluid (see Starling forces, p. 42).

In health the hydrostatic pressure at the arteriolar end of the capillary bed is about 35 mm Hg. At the venular end it falls to 12 to 15 mm Hg. The oncotic pressure of the plasma is approximately 20 to 25 mm Hg, rising slightly at the venular end as fluid escapes. Thus, with a normal endothelial barrier, fluid escapes from the vascular compartment at the arteriolar end of the capillary bed and is returned at the venular end. There is a small net loss from the vascular compartment into the interstitial tissue spaces, which is drained off through lymphatics, ultimately to be returned to the bloodstream. Despite an active interchange, a steady state is maintained in health with the normal partition of extracellular water between the plasma and interstitial compartments. Edema constitutes in essence an abnormal expansion of the interstitial fluid or the accumulation of fluid in some "third extracellular space" such as the peritoneal or pleural cavity.

The primary causes of edema comprise (1) increased hydrostatic pressure, (2) reduced oncotic pressure, (3) lymphatic obstruction, (4) increased osmotic tension of the interstitial fluid related to sodium retention, and (5) increased endothelial permeability (as discussed on p. 43) (Table 3–2).

Increased hydrostatic pressure may be caused by thrombosis of a vein or any other basis for venous

Table 3–1. DISTRIBUTION OF TOTAL BODY WATER

Compartment	Volume (Liters)	% Lean Body Weight
Total body water	42	60
Extracellular water	14	20
Plasma	3 to 4	4 to 5
Interstitial	11	16
Intracellular water	28	40

obstruction, the edema being localized to the affected part. Congestive heart failure, when it affects right ventricular function, and constrictive pericarditis cause increased hydrostatic pressure throughout the venous system, and thus systemic edema. Left ventricular failure alone produces edema of the lungs.

Reduced oncotic pressure results from either inadequate synthesis or increased loss of albumin. Reduced synthesis is most commonly associated with diffuse liver disease, particularly cirrhosis, but it may also occur with severe protein malnutrition as in kwashiorkor (p. 400). Increased albumin loss is most often encountered with the glomerulopathies that induce the nephrotic syndrome (p. 1011), characterized by: (a) marked proteinuria, (b) hypoproteinemia, and (c) generalized edema. Fundamental to all these disorders is increased glomerular permeability to plasma proteins. Additional causes of albumin loss are protein-losing enteropathies.

Lymphatic obstruction, whether it be due to the spread of cancers, surgical removal of lymph nodes and associated lymphatics, or inflammatory or radiation-induced scarring, is an obvious cause for the development of edema, referred to in this context as *lymphedema* (p. 538). Usually the edema is localized, for

Table 3–2. CAUSES OF EDEMA FORMATION*

I. Increased hydrostatic pressure
   - Congestive heart failure
   - Constrictive pericarditis
   - Venous thrombosis
   - Cirrhosis of liver (ascites)

II. Reduced oncotic pressure of plasma—hypoproteinemia
   - Cirrhosis of liver
   - Malnutrition
   - Protein-losing glomerulopathies—nephrotic syndrome
   - Protein-losing gastroenteropathy

III. Lymphatic obstruction (lymphedema)
   - Cancer
   - Inflammatory scarring
   - Radiation-induced

IV. Sodium retention
   - Excessive salt intake
   - Increased tubular reabsorption of sodium
   - Reduced renal perfusion

V. Increased endothelial permeability
   - Inflammation
   - Burns
   - Trauma
   - Allergic or immunologic reactions

*Modified from Leaf, A., and Cotran, R. S.: Renal Pathophysiology. New York, Oxford University Press, 1980, p. 139.

example, to the lower extremities or a single extremity, upper or lower.

Sodium Retention. An expansion of plasma volume leading to increased transudation occurs. Unlike the other clinical situations already mentioned, the edema here is accompanied by hypervolemia as well as expansion of the interstitial fluid compartment (as detailed below).

The primary causes of generalized noninflammatory edema, with the exception of sodium retention, all produce hypovolemia and a reduction in the circulating blood volume as a secondary consequence. For example, venous and lymphatic obstruction may cause sufficient trapping of fluid in the periphery to reduce the circulating blood volume, but admittedly only rarely. In cardiac failure, blood stagnates in the venous side of the circulation, and so the effective circulating arterial volume falls. Constrictive pericarditis has its greatest effect on the thin-walled venae cavae, and so also impounds blood in the veins. Reduced oncotic pressure with a shift of fluid from the vascular to the interstitial compartment reduces the effective arterial volume. With all these derangements there is lowered renal perfusion, leading to a compensatory increase in the plasma levels of renin, angiotensin, and aldosterone. The increased circulating levels of aldosterone (secondary hyperaldosteronism, see p. 1240) then bring about renal retention of sodium and water, which may restore the deficit in the arterial blood volume; however, the retained sodium and water contribute to the edema. Thus, whatever the primary cause of edema, a high salt diet is likely to worsen the situation, particularly if there is some renal impairment of sodium excretion.

Clinical Derangements Causing Systemic Edema

1. *Congestive heart failure,* whatever the etiology, is the most common cause of edema. The lungs alone may be involved when the failure involves only the left ventricle, but in most cases both sides of the heart are eventually affected, causing systemic edema (p. 548).

2. *Constrictive pericarditis* is an infrequent cause of systemic edema.

3. *Renal diseases,* particularly those forms associated with heavy proteinuria or salt retention, are among the more common clinical causes of generalized edema. In the proteinuric disorders, the edema is likely to appear when the serum albumin concentration falls below 2.5 gm per 100 ml of plasma. As pointed out, the consequent physiologic responses induce renal retention of sodium and water, but the retained water further dilutes the plasma proteins, creating a vicious cycle.

4. *Cirrhosis of the liver* sometimes produces generalized edema, but more often excessive accumulation of fluid within the abdominal cavity—*ascites.* A number of mechanisms are operative. The diffuse hepatocellular damage impairs the capacity of the liver to synthesize albumin, and the extensive fibrous scarring and distortion of the intrahepatic vasculature leads to portal hypertension (discussed on p. 916). Thus, there is trapping of blood within the portal system, thereby reducing the effective arterial blood volume, in turn leading to sec-

ondary hyperaldosteronism. An additional mechanism that causes cirrhotic edema is obstruction of hepatic lymphatics. Thus, a transudate weeps not only from the hepatic capsule, but also from all the peritoneal surfaces. The hypoalbuminemia may also induce peripheral systemic edema.

5. Other clinical states associated with generalized edema include: *protein malabsorption*, *starvation*, and *protein-losing enteropathies*, in which the edema is related to hypoproteinemia; *exogenous estrogens* and *normal pregnancy*, with its increased level of estrogens, which promote sodium retention; *toxemia of pregnancy; hypothyroidism; vitamin B_1 (thiamine chloride) deficiency;* and *"idopathic cyclic edema."* This last-mentioned rare syndrome is seen principally in women. The fact that the edema usually appears in some temporal relation to the menstrual cycle points to a hormonal mechanism possibly related to estrogen levels. In all these varied states, however, the systemic edema is rarely as severe as that encountered in congestive heart failure and renal disease.

Clinical Derangements Causing Localized Edema. *The major causes of localized edema are: (1) impaired venous drainage leading to a local increase in capillary pressure, (2) a local increase in vascular permeability, and (3) lymphatic blockage. Chronic cardiac failure or reduction in the osmotic pressure of the plasma cannot be a primary basis for localized edema.*

1. *Impaired venous drainage*, whatever its basis, can sufficiently elevate the capillary hydrostatic pressure to cause localized edema. Thromboses, such as commonly occur in the deep veins of the leg (p. 97); incompetent venous valves commonly encountered in varicose veins of the lower extremities; and compression of veins by external pressures (tumors, enlarged organs, encircling tight garments, surgical dressings, or plaster casts) may all lead to localized edema. Even in the normal individual, prolonged periods of sitting may induce edema of the feet and ankles as the cessation of the milking action by the leg muscles causes a slight increase in hydrostatic pressure in the major veins that drain the legs.

2. *Increased vascular permeability*, such as occur in inflammatory reactions or in many forms of allergic reactions, is an obvious cause of localized edema, as has been emphasized in Chapter 2.

3. *Obstruction of the lymphatics* by cancers or by traumatic, surgical, inflammatory, or radiation injury may produce edema. The mechanism in all these situations is obvious, since under normal conditions the lymphatics constantly drain small amounts of tissue fluid from the interstitial spaces. Edema is a common sequel to cancer surgery when regional lymph nodes are excised to control the spread of tumor. For example, the dissection of axillary lymph nodes performed in the excision of cancer of the breast quite often results in edema of the arm. The most striking cause of inflammatory obstruction to the lymphatics is encountered in the parasitic infection known as *filariasis*. These parasites penetrate the skin, usually in the feet, and migrate to the inguinal nodes where they cause inflammatory fibrosis and lymphatic obstruction. Massive subcutaneous edema develops in the legs and genitals, with accompanying epidermal thickening (p. 381). The deformed legs come to resemble those of the elephant, hence the clinical designation *elephantiasis*.

Congenital malformation or absence of the lymphatics, such as is encountered in Milroy's disease (p. 538), produces a form of localized lymphedema of the extremities.

MORPHOLOGY. The anatomic changes produced by edema depend on its severity, the rapidity with which it occurs, and the underlying cause. Indeed, the interstitial fluid compartment may expand as much as several liters before edema becomes manifest clinically or morphologically. The two most common systemic causes—cardiac failure and renal disease—produce slightly different patterns of edema. In **cardiac failure,** in which increased capillary pressure is an important contributor, the accumulation of fluid is most severe in the dependent portions of the body, and hence is referred to as **dependent edema.** When the patient is ambulatory, fluid collects first in the lower extremities, particularly over the dorsal aspects of the feet and ankles. If the patient is confined to bed, fluid may accumulate over the sacral region. Changes in position of the recumbent patient may cause the distribution of fluid to shift and most severely affect the lowermost regions of the body.

Edema of renal origin, such as is encountered in the nephrotic syndrome, is generally of greater severity than is cardiac edema. All regions of the body are affected equally, and the edema tends to be generalized. It may, however, be most manifest in those tissues that have a loose connective tissue matrix. **Renal edema is therefore classically identified by edema of the face, particularly of the eyelids.**

In cases in which edema is due to localized disturbances, the distribution depends on the location of the underlying disorder. Whatever the mechanism of origin of edema, whether generalized or localized, finger pressure over edematous subcutaneous tissue will displace the interstitial fluid from the dermal and subcutaneous connective tissues to leave pitted depressions, often referred to clinically as **"pitting edema"** (Fig. 3–1).

Although considerable emphasis has been placed on subcutaneous edema, the visceral tissues likewise participate in generalized edema. Edematous viscera are slightly enlarged, pale, and heavier than normal; show somewhat tense capsules; and, on section, have a glistening appearance.

When well defined, edema is apparent microscopically as a granular, acidophilic, interstitial precipitate that separates the cellular and fibrillar elements of the tissue. This pink, amorphous deposit represents the protein and solutes of the edema fluid. As the parenchymal cells swell, gland lumina and small vessels are compressed.

Edema of the brain and edema of the lungs are the most life-threatening forms of abnormal fluid retention.

Edema of the brain is encountered with brain trauma, infections within the cranial vault (meningitis, brain abscesses, encephalitis), hypertensive crises, and obstruction to the venous outflow of the brain. The edematous brain is heavier than normal; the sulci are narrowed, and the swollen gyri are flattened where they press against the skull. On section, the white matter may appear unusually soft and

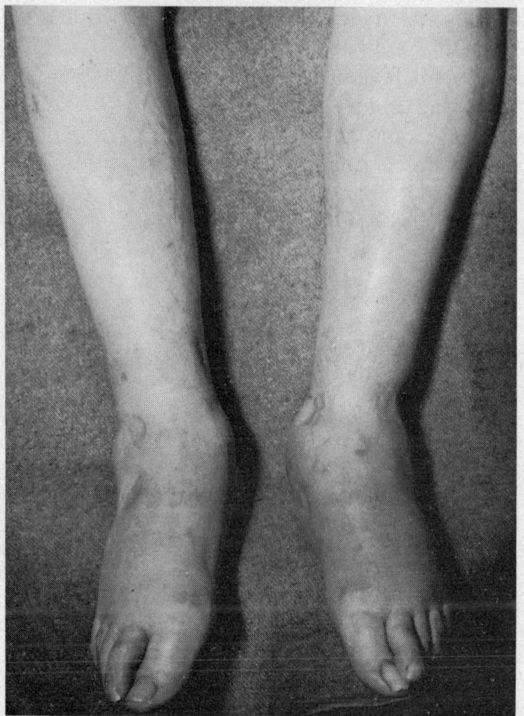

Figure 3–1. Dependent edema of the lower legs, illustrating "pitting" about the ankles.

gelatinous, and the peripheral layer of gray matter is widened. The ventricles are usually compressed. Histologically, there is considerable widening of the interfibrillar spaces of the brain substance; this gives a loose appearance to the white and gray matter. Swelling of the neuronal and glial cells may also be present. The perivascular (Virchow-Robin) spaces become unusually widened and form clear halos about the small vessels.

Pulmonary edema is a very common clinical problem, discussed in some detail on page 710. Here it is necessary to indicate only that it is a major manifestation of left ventricular failure and is also encountered in renal disease, shock, diffuse alveolar damage (p. 714), infections within the lungs, and hypersensitivity states when the lungs are target organs. The edema is usually confined to, or most marked in, the lower lobes. In far-advanced edema, however, all lobes may be involved and assume a rubbery gelatinous consistency. Sectioning of the lobes permits the free escape of frothy, sanguineous fluid representing a mixture of air, blood, and edema. On histologic examination, there is widening of septal walls due to congestion of the capillaries and intraseptal interstitial edema. As the process evolves there is initially the escape of a protein-poor fluid into the alveolar spaces, which is not retained in the histologic section. More severe edema leads to the accumulation of more protein in the edema fluid with the precipitation of a granular, pink coagulate within the alveolar spaces (Fig. 3–2). When present for any period of time, intra-alveolar edema fluid is prone to secondary infection, producing pneumonia, which in this setting is called **hypostatic pneumonia.**

CLINICAL SIGNIFICANCE. In the brain and the lungs, edema may be fatal, but subcutaneous edema and edema of other viscera are usually of little functional significance. Swelling of the brain leads to increased intracranial pressure with resultant headaches, projectile vomiting, and convulsive seizures. Herniation of the brain stem or cerebellar tonsils into the foramen magnum may precipitate death. Cerebral edema may develop within hours of brain injury, requiring immediate corrective steps to save the patient's life. Pulmonary edema is important because it impedes the normal ventilatory function of the lungs. Characteristically, as the respired air bubbles through the proteinaceous fluid within the alveolar spaces, a variety of abnormal breath sounds called rales are produced. In severe pulmonary edema, the collection of fluid in the respiratory passages gives rise to extremely loud rales, popularly and appropriately termed the "death rattle." Edema of the lungs (with the attendant hazards of hypostatic pneumonia) is one of the most serious complications of cardiac and renal insufficiency and frequently triggers the demise of these vulnerable patients.

HYPEREMIA AND CONGESTION

The terms hyperemia and congestion are elegant medical expressions for an increased volume of blood in an affected tissue or part. *Hyperemia, also called active hyperemia to differentiate it from congestion or passive hyperemia,* occurs when arterial and arteriolar dilatation

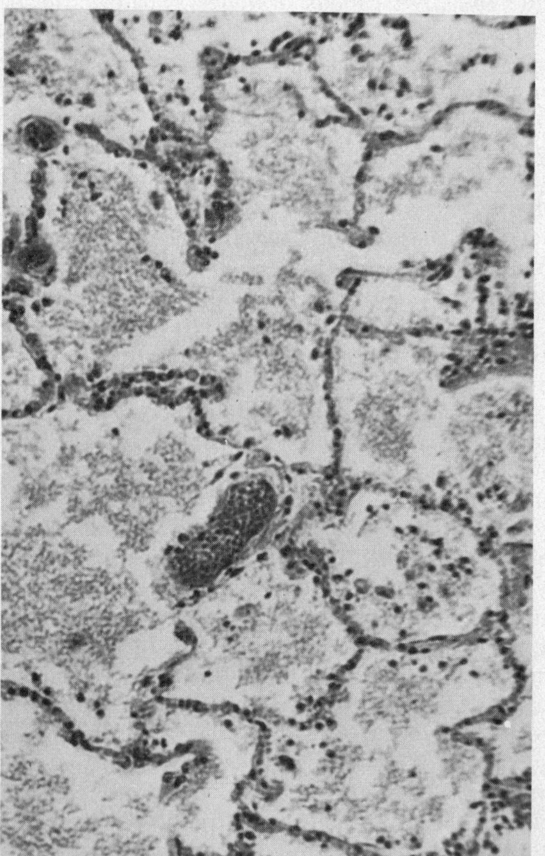

Figure 3–2. Pulmonary edema. The edema fluid in tissue section appears as a granular pink precipitate within the alveoli.

produces an increased flow of blood into capillary beds, with opening of inactive capillaries. Congestion or passive hyperemia, on the other hand, results from impaired venous drainage.

Active hyperemia causes increased redness in the affected part. The arterial and arteriolar dilatation is brought about by sympathetic neurogenic mechanisms or the release of "vasoactive" substances (as discussed in Chapter 2). Active hyperemia of the skin is encountered whenever excess body heat must be dissipated, such as in muscular exercise and febrile states. Hormonal influences such as circulating epinephrine may induce active hyperemia of skeletal muscle, myocardium, and liver at the expense of other circuits in the "fight or flight" response. Blushing is another example of hyperemia induced by neurogenic mechanisms.

Congestion, or *passive hyperemia*, causes an intensified blue-red coloration in affected parts as venous blood is dammed back. The blue tint is accentuated when the congestion leads to an increase of deoxygenated hemoglobin in the blood—*cyanosis*. Congestion may occur as a systemic phenomenon in congestive heart failure when both left and right ventricles are decompensated; may affect only the pulmonary circuit in left ventricular failure; or may affect the entire body, sparing the lungs, in right ventricular decompensation. Congestion can of course occur as a localized process when, for example, the venous return of blood to an extremity is obstructed or involves only the portal circulation when there is portal hypertension secondary to cirrhosis of the liver. *Congestion of capillary beds is closely related to the development of edema, and so congestion and edema commonly occur together.*

MORPHOLOGY. Cut surfaces of acutely hyperemic and/or congested organs are excessively bloody. With long-standing congestion, called chronic passive congestion, the stasis of poorly oxygenated blood causes chronic hypoxia, which may lead to degeneration or even death of parenchymal cells. Minute hemorrhages from capillary rupture may be converted in time to hemosiderin-laden scars. The lungs, liver, and spleen develop the most obvious manifestations of chronic passive congestion.

Chronic passive congestion of the lungs and consequent pulmonary edema are encountered whenever there is elevated left atrial pressure and consequent elevated pulmonary venous pressure. Such changes imply either stenosis of the mitral valve (seen notably in chronic rheumatic heart disease) or any condition leading to reduced left ventricular output. The most extreme form is associated with rheumatic mitral stenosis. Microscopically, the alveolar capillaries become engorged with blood and often become tortuous, with small aneurysmal dilatations (Fig. 3–3). Rupture of distended capillaries may cause minute intraalveolar hemorrhages, and the breakdown and phagocytosis of the red cell debris eventually lead to the appearance of hemosiderin-laden macrophages ("heart failure" cells) in the alveolar spaces. In severe forms of chronic passive congestion, the alveolar septa are widened both by the dilatation of alveolar capillaries and by edema fluid that collects within the interstitium of the alveolar septa (congestion and edema). In time, the edematous septa become fibrotic and, together with the hemosiderin pigmentation, constitute the basis for the designation **"brown induration."** The long-standing congestion and consequent pulmonary hypertension may cause progressive thickening of the walls of the pulmonary arteries and arterioles (p. 713).

Acute and chronic passive congestion of the liver results from right-sided heart failure or, more rarely, from obstruction of the inferior vena cava or hepatic vein. The

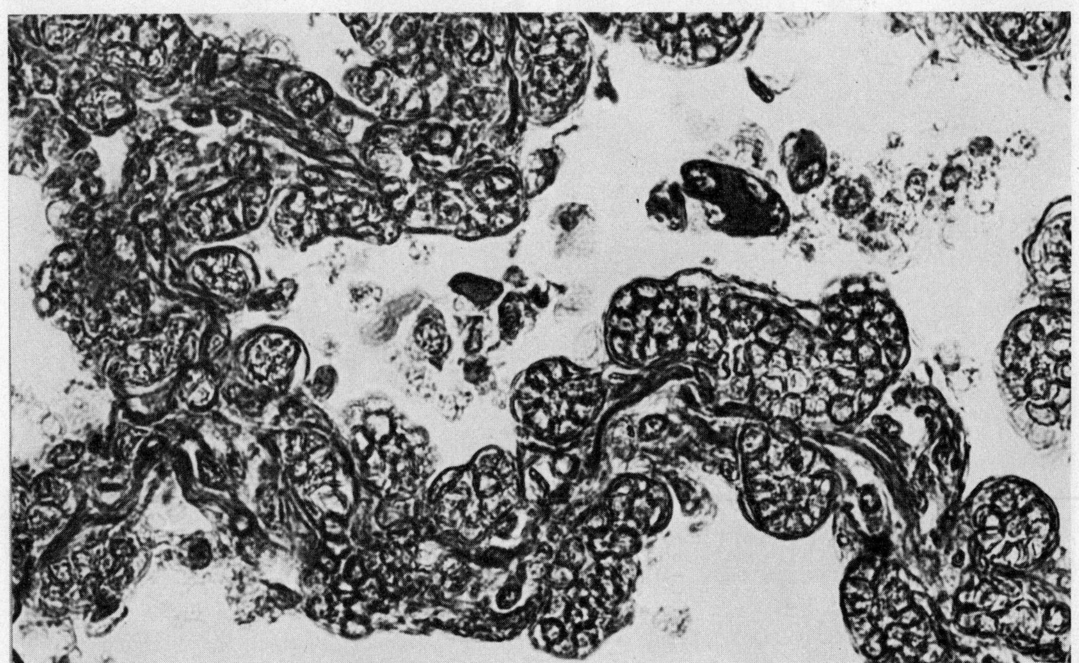

Figure 3–3. Marked congestion of pulmonary alveolar capillaries, a microscopic detail showing the widened and tortuous capillaries. Their lumina now permit the passage of two to three red cells abreast of each other.

first changes include a dusky red cyanosis and increase in liver size and weight. On liver section, there is an excessive ooze of blood, and the central veins may appear prominent. With chronic congestion, the central regions of the lobule become red-blue, surrounded by a yellow-brown zone of uncongested liver substance, descriptively referred to as the **"nutmeg liver"** (Fig. 3–4). Microscopically, the central vein and the vascular sinusoids of the centrilobular regions are distended with blood. The central hepatocytes frequently become atrophic secondary to chronic hypoxia, whereas the peripheral hepatocytes, suffering from less severe hypoxia, develop fatty change.

With severe cardiac failure the central hepatocytes may become necrotic and the centrilobular zone hemorrhagic, producing so-called central **hemorrhagic necrosis** (Fig. 3–5). Arcidi and colleagues suggest that, whereas chronic passive congestion of the liver is related to elevation of the systemic venous pressure, the subsequent development of central hemorrhagic necrosis reflects hypoxia due to reduction in the circulating blood volume and hepatic blood flow.[1] Thus, **centrilobular necrosis** may appear in shock from any cause without preceding chronic passive congestion. With long-standing chronic passive congestion, particularly when associated with death of central hepatocytes, fibrous thickening of the walls of the central veins eventually appears. Extension of this fibrous tissue into the surrounding lobule creates the distinctive anatomic pattern called cardiac sclerosis or sometimes "cardiac cirrhosis" (p. 898).

Chronic passive congestion of the spleen produces at first a slightly enlarged, tense, cyanotic organ that on section freely exudes blood and collapses slightly, so that the capsule becomes wrinkled. With time, the pulp becomes progressively more firm. In the early stages, the spleen usually does not exceed 250 to 300 gm in weight (normal = 150 gm). Microscopically, marked sinusoidal dilatation is present, accompanied by foci of recent hemorrhage and possible hemosiderin deposits. In long-standing chronic congestion, the organ progressively enlarges and may weigh up to 500 to 700 gm. Fibrous thickening and hemosiderin deposits within the edematous, congested, sinusoidal walls produce the characteristic anatomic pattern of **congestive splenomegaly** (p. 700). Sometimes focal hemorrhages, followed by repair, yield **siderofibrotic** nodules of scar tissue laden with hemosiderin.

HEMORRHAGE

Rupture or laceration of a blood vessel is the obvious cause of hemorrhage. If a significant amount of released blood accumulates within a tissue, it may produce a massive clot, referred to as a *hematoma* (Fig. 3–6). For example, with rupture of the aorta, usually due to some underlying aortic disease, large mediastinal or retroperitoneal hematomas may be produced. If the blood escapes into a serous cavity, it is referred to appropriately as *hemothorax*, *hemopericardium*, or *hemoperitoneum*. Smaller hemorrhages, usually encountered in the skin, mucous membranes, and serosal surfaces, are known as *petechiae* (minute), *purpura* (up

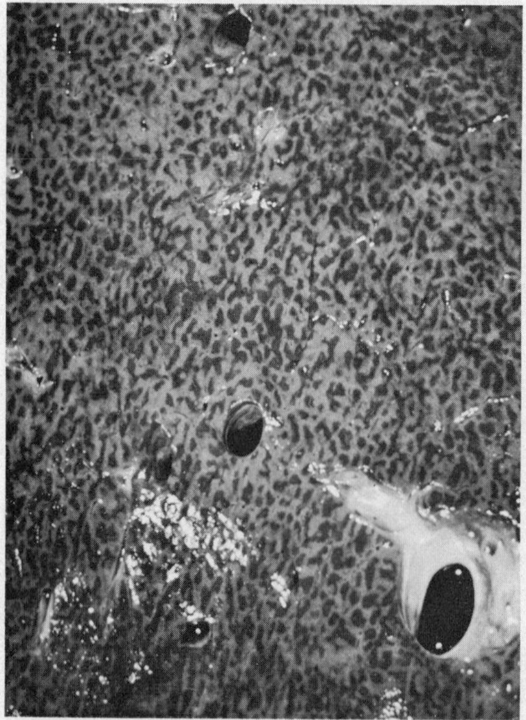

Fig. 3–4

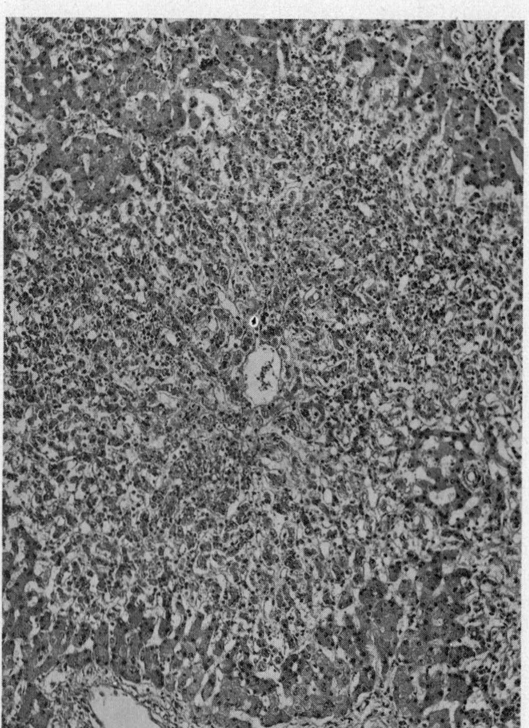

Fig. 3–5

Figure 3–4. Chronic passive congestion of the liver. On the cut surface, the central congested areas appear darker than the pale peripheral portions of the lobules, and thus compose the so-called "nutmeg" pattern.

Figure 3–5. Central hemorrhagic necrosis of the liver. The extravasation of blood into the hepatic parenchyma is accompanied by destruction and disappearance of the centrilobular liver cells.

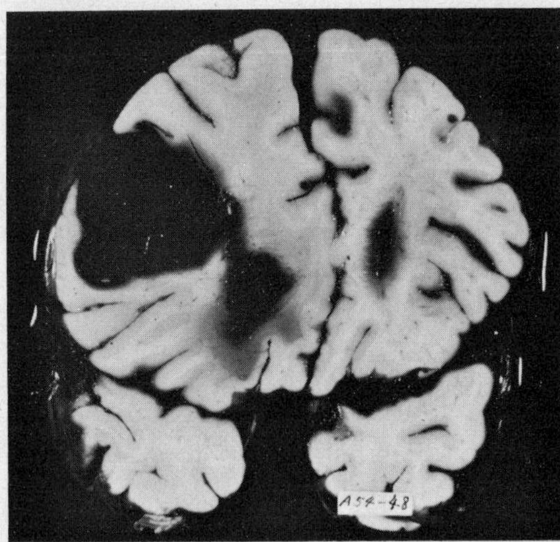

Figure 3–6. Intracerebral hemorrhage. In the transection of the cerebral hemispheres, the large hematoma extends to the cortical surface as well as into the ventricular system, and blood is visible in the lateral ventricle on the opposite side.

to approximately 1 cm), or *ecchymoses* (when large and blotchy). Microscopic hemorrhages may be produced in loose tissues, such as the lung, merely by marked congestion followed by escape of erythrocytes—a phenomenon referred to as *red cell diapedesis*.

The causes of hemorrhage are too numerous to be detailed and include trauma as well as all the diseases that primarily (e.g., atherosclerosis) or secondarily (e.g., an extending erosive cancer) attack vessel walls. Worthy of special mention in this context are hypertension and the hemorrhagic diatheses. Retinal and, more ominously, cerebral hemorrhages are encountered in hypertensive patients. The latter is a frequent cause of death in patients having marked (malignant) hypertension. The hemorrhagic diatheses constitute a group of clinical disorders having in common an increased bleeding tendency. Platelet deficiencies and a lack of any one of the clotting factors are the principal causes of hemorrhagic diatheses (p. 643).

CLINICAL SIGNIFICANCE. The significance of hemorrhage depends on the amount of blood loss, its rate of escape, and the site of the hemorrhage. Acute losses of up to 10 to 20% of blood volume and slow losses of even greater amounts may have no clinical significance. Larger or more rapid losses may cause hemorrhagic (hypovolemic) shock. But even relatively small amounts of hemorrhage in the brain or pericardial sac may produce sufficient increases of pressure to cause death. It is obvious that external bleeding or hemorrhage into the gastrointestinal tract represents a permanent loss of vital iron. However, if bleeding occurs in a body tissue or cavity (peritoneal, pleural), progressive breakdown of the hemoglobin permits resorption of the iron and its reutilization. In the course of this resorption of hemoglobin, increased amounts of bilirubin are formed and may cause transient jaundice. This sequence is associated particularly with massive gastrointestinal bleeding because even though much of the red cell mass is excreted, some is rapidly digested, with rapid resorption of large amounts of the hemoglobin precursor of bilirubin.

THROMBOSIS

Thrombosis is the process of formation of a solid mass from the constituents of the blood within *living* blood vessels or the heart; the resultant mass is termed a *thrombus. A thrombus must be differentiated from a blood clot.* The thrombus is formed by a complex process involving the interaction of blood vessel walls, the formed elements of the blood, notably the platelets, and the plasma coagulants that constitute the blood clotting system. In contrast, a blood clot involves only the coagulation sequence, and thus clotting occurs, as you know, when blood is drawn into a test tube. Clotting also occurs in extravascular accumulations of blood (hematomas), and after death there is postmortem clotting of the blood in the cardiovascular system. The composition of thrombi may also differ from that of blood clots. Thrombi that arise in the rapidly moving arterial or cardiac circulation are composed largely of fibrin and platelets with only a few trapped red and white cells, and thus bear little resemblance to a blood clot. However, with very sluggish venous flow, thrombi may closely resemble blood clots as will shortly be explained.

Clearly the development of a thrombus is life-saving when a large vessel ruptures or is severed. Under these circumstances the thrombus comprises what might better be termed a "hemostatic plug." However, when a thrombus develops in the unruptured cardiovascular system, it may be life threatening. Thrombi may (1) diminish or obstruct vascular flow, causing ischemic injury to tissues and organs, or (2) become dislodged or fragment to create emboli. An *embolus* is an intravascular solid, liquid, or gaseous mass carried in the bloodstream to some site removed from its origin or from its point of entrance into the cardiovascular system. Although there are other forms of emboli, as will soon become clear, most are derived from thrombi. Indeed, thrombosis and embolism are so closely interrelated as to give rise to the term *thromboembolism. Infarcts*, as you recall, are areas of ischemic necrosis of tissues. They are usually caused by thromboembolic occlusion of a vessel. Infarctions of the heart, lungs, and brain collectively account for more deaths than all forms of cancer and infectious disease together. Indeed, ischemic injury of the heart, brain, and lungs, secondary to thromboembolism, and cancer are the dominating clinical problems today in all industralized nations.

PATHOGENESIS. Before turning to the pathogenesis of thrombosis, a brief review of *normal hemostasis* is in order because, to a considerable extent, *thrombosis is the consequence of inappropriate activation of normal hemostasis.*[2]

Normal Hemostasis. Before considering normal hemostasis in some detail, the highlights will be presented first.

1. *With vascular injury there is a brief period of*

vasoconstriction, which in small vessels (principally arterioles) serves to reduce blood loss.

2. *Much more important, the injury to endothelial cells exposes highly thrombogenic subendothelial connective tissue, to which the platelets adhere and undergo so-called contact activation involving shape change, a release reaction, and further aggregation of more platelets.*

3. *Virtually simultaneously, release of tissue factors at the site of injury in combination with platelet factors activates the plasma coagulation sequence.*

4. *Prostaglandins and derivatives are synthesized at the site of injury by endothelial cells and platelets modulating the hemostatic sequence.*

5. *Ultimately a permanent hemostatic plug is produced by the combined activities of endothelial cells, platelets, and the coagulation sequence.*

We can best dissect this complex process by separately considering the three major contributors to it: (1) the vascular wall, (2) platelets, and (3) the plasma coagulant factors of the blood-clotting mechanism.

Table 3–3. ENDOTHELIAL CELL FUNCTIONS

Opposes Blood Clotting/Thrombosis	Predisposes to Blood Clotting/Thrombosis
Intact monolayer is barrier between blood and subendothelial thrombogenic elements	With injury, subendothelial elements exposed, initiates clotting and activates platelets
Glycocalyx contains: anticoagulant heparan sulfate; α-2 macroglobulin—an antiprotease	With injury, tissue factor released, initiates extrinsic pathway clotting
Synthesizes: plasminogen activators; antiaggregating and vasodilating prostacyclin (PGI_2); antithrombin III	Synthesizes factor VIII—von Willebrand protein involved in platelet aggregation.
Converts proaggregating ADP into antiaggregating adenine nucleotides	

Vascular Wall. The major features of the vascular wall for our present interests are (a) the endothelial lining, (b) the subendothelial connective tissue, and (c) the muscular layer.

a. The *endothelial monolayer* serves three important functions: (1) it is a selective permeability barrier; (2) it is a nonthrombogenic surface that insulates circulating blood elements from highly thrombogenic subendothelial connective tissues; and (3) it is an active synthetic-metabolic-secretory tissue that in the normal state inhibits hemostasis and thrombosis but, when injured, promotes these two processes.[3] The selective permeability function assumes greatest importance in atherogenesis, and therefore is discussed on page 513. The thromboresistance of the endothelial lining has been characterized by Gimbrone as "nature's prototype for blood-compatible surfaces."[4] Thus, endothelial injury is a potent thrombogenic influence. So it is that endothelial cells occupy a pivotal role in the initiation and prevention of clotting and thrombosis, as summarized in Table 3–3. The luminal surface of the endothelium is covered by an "endocapillary layer" representing the glycocalyx. Biochemically the glycocalyx is a composite of intrinsic membrane-glycoproteins and glycolipids, as well as membrane-associated polysaccharides and glycosaminoglycans, among which are sialic acid residues and heparan sulfate. This endocapillary layer has a strong net negative charge, which at one time was thought to contribute to thromboresistance by repelling negatively-charged blood elements. However, reduction of the negative charge by removal of sialic acid residues does not alter endothelial-blood compatibility; thus, other explanations have been sought for its thromboresistance. Heparan sulfate in the glycocalyx has certain structural similarities to the anticoagulant heparin. In concert with antithrombin III synthesized by endothelial cells, the heparan sulfate residues could serve to inhibit blood clotting.[5] In addition, an alpha-2 macroglobulin constituting a potent antiprotease is associated with the vascular lining. It serves to inhibit the activation of clotting factors in the coagulation sequence. Endothelial cells also inhibit platelet aggregation by several mechanisms. They have the capacity to convert the strongly proaggregating adenosine diphosphate (ADP) released from platelets to the potent adenine nucleotide platelet inhibitors.[6] *Much more important is their elaboration of one of the prostaglandins (p. 54), namely antiaggregating prostacyclin (PGI_2), also a strong vasodilator.* Indeed, with endothelial cell injury and activation of the coagulation sequence, the formation of thrombin at the site of injury stimulates the surrounding endothelial cells into more active synthesis of PGI_2. The role of PGI_2 is further discussed on page 94. Whatever the mechanism(s), the endothelial surface serves the highly important function of insulating the blood from highly thrombogenic subendothelial elements (described below). In addition, endothelial cells react against blood clots and thrombi by synthesizing plasminogen activators (and inhibitors), which on balance promote fibrinolytic activity in the blood, clear fibrin deposits from the endothelial surface, and also participate in the resolution of intravascular thrombi.

The schizophrenic endothelial cell can promote, on the other hand, hemostasis and thrombosis by virtue of its synthetic-metabolic-secretory activities. Its *prohemostatic functions are mediated by the synthesis and release of substances that act both on the coagulation sequence and on platelets.* The extrinsic clotting pathway can be activated by tissue factor (thromboplastin) present in latent form in endothelium, and released by certain pharmacologic stimuli, endotoxin, and by injury, even if sublethal.[7] Endothelial cells also synthesize and secrete von Willebrand's factor, which is a component of the coagulant factor VIII (factor VIII-VWF). This product is a necessary cofactor for the adherence of platelets to subendothelial components.

b. *The subendothelial connective tissues not only support the endothelial monolayer but are also throm-*

bogenic. Subendothelial cells produce basement membrane collagen, fibrillar collagen, elastin, glycosaminoglycans, and fibronectin. Although other components such as basement membrane and elastin promote platelet adherence, the most potent stimulus is the fibrillar collagen, which provides a substrate for attachment and activation of platelets, and activation of clotting factors in the so-called extrinsic pathway of blood coagulation. Fibronectin serves to stabilize cell-to-cell and cell-to-substrate attachments in the normal endothelial lining. It also becomes cross-linked to fibrin and facilitates anchorage of hemostatic plugs.[8] Thus, damage to the endothelial cell barrier exposes the highly thrombogenic subendothelium to initiate thrombosis and hemostasis.

c. The *muscular layer* of smooth muscle cells in small arteries and arterioles slows blood loss by transient vasoconstriction immediately following an acute vascular injury, thus contributing to hemostasis. Neurogenic mechanisms and vasoactive products released from platelets such as epinephrine mediate the vasoconstriction.

Platelets, it must already be evident, play a central role in normal hemostasis and, therefore, in thrombosis also.[9] Despite their lack of a nucleus, head, and heart, these tiny structures (about 2 μm in diameter) are amazingly versatile. At sites of endothelial cell injury they are capable of (a) adhesion and shape transformation, (b) secretion (release reaction), and (c) aggregation. Collectively the three phenomena are referred to as "platelet activation." In addition, as you remember, platelets are also capable of synthesizing prostaglandin derivatives, notably thromboxane (TxA_2). Even without vascular injury, in some poorly defined manner, perhaps by metabolic support, they maintain the integrity of the normal endothelial layer, since patients who suffer a platelet deficiency (thrombocytopenia) are prone to purpuric bleeding. With vascular and endothelial cell injury, the following sequence of platelet events unfolds.

Adhesion refers to attachment of platelets to sites of endothelial cell injury where subendothelial elements, particularly fibrillar collagen, are exposed (Fig. 3–7). The precise events in collagen-platelet interaction have

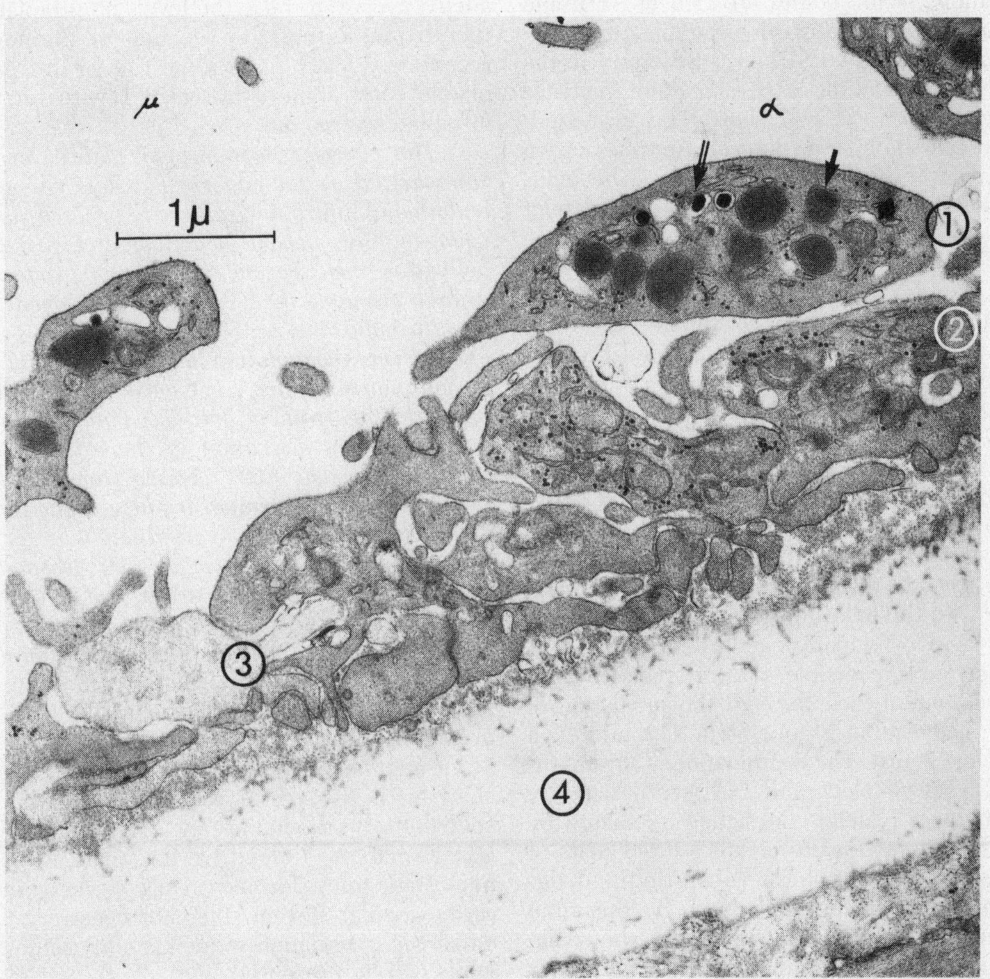

Figure 3–7. Platelet adherence to subendothelial connective tissue at focus of endothelial loss. *1,* Intact platelet with pseudopod (thin arrow is alpha granule, thick arrow is dense body); 2, partially degranulated platelet; *3,* degranulated platelet "ghost"; *4,* internal elastic lamina. (From Haudenschild, C., and Studer, A.: Early interactions between blood cells and severely damaged rabbit aorta. Eur. J. Clin. Invest. 2:1, 1971.)

not yet been fully elucidated. Whether platelets possess specific collagen receptors is uncertain. It may well be that collagen exerts its effect by stimulating TxA_2 synthesis or by initiating a platelet release reaction with the secretion of ADP as the ultimate mediators of adhesion.[10] As already mentioned, von Willebrand factor is necessary for such adhesion. The platelets at first attach themselves by long pseudopods, but then spread broadly to become tightly adherent. The shape transformations are mediated by intraplatelet actomyosin microfilaments and microtubules. In former years the actomyosin was referred to as thrombasthenin—the platelet "muscle."

Secretion—the release reaction—of the contents of platelet granules follows soon after adhesion. Platelets contain two major types of granules—*alpha granules* and *dense bodies*.[11] *Alpha granules* contain fibrinogen, fibronectin, a mitogen known as platelet growth factor, an antiheparin (platelet factor 4), and platelet-specific proteins, i.e., cationic proteins and beta-thromboglobulin. Beta-thromboglobulin has no known function, but when found in the plasma it serves as an indicator of platelet activation. *Dense bodies* are rich in ADP and ionized calcium and also contain histamine, epinephrine, and serotonin (5-HT). Calcium is necessary in the coagulation sequence and the ADP is a potent mediator of platelet aggregation, as will shortly be discussed. With platelet activation and the release reaction, a phospholipid complex called platelet factor 3 becomes activated or in some manner exposed on the platelet surface. This phenomenon is of some importance since it provides a site on the platelet surface where coagulation factors X and V and Ca^{++} bind to activate prothrombin. In this manner, platelet activation contributes to the intrinsic pathway of blood clotting and the formation of thrombin.

Platelet aggregation (implying platelet-platelet interadherence) closely follows platelet adherence and activation. A major contributor to aggregation is the formation of thromboxane A_2 (TxA_2) by activated platelets. TxA_2 is also a vasoconstrictor.[12, 13] In addition, the adherent and activated platelets, which form the initial nidus, release ADP to thus set into motion an autocatalytic reaction with the build-up of an enlarging platelet aggregate known as a "temporary hemostatic plug." This primary aggregation is reversible, but with the activation of the coagulation sequence through the mediation of platelet factor 3, thrombin is generated. Thrombin is a powerful platelet agonist. The combination of thrombin, ADP released from platelets, and TxA_2 synthesized by the platelets induces platelet contraction (mediated by the intraplatelet actomyosin) to create a fused mass of platelets—"viscous metamorphosis"—constituting a definitive or "secondary hemostatic plug." By this time fibrin is formed and deposited within and about the platelet aggregate, comprising in essence a mortar for the "platelet bricks," further stabilizing the plug and anchoring it via fibronectin to its site of origin. Thus a fine mechanism, referred to as a "delicate hemostatic balance," exists at the blood-endothelial cell interface. Under normal conditions the intact endothelial monolayer with its anticlotting features and its synthesis of antiaggregating PGI_2 tends to maintain the fluidity of the blood. However, with the endothelial cell injury and reduction of PGI_2 synthesis, the balance tips in favor of TxA_2 to initiate platelet aggregation and hemostasis.[14]

The precise biochemical events that trigger platelet secretion and aggregation are poorly understood, but this much is known. In vitro a variety of agents—ADP, thrombin, collagen, serotonin, catecholamines, and TxA_2—are platelet activators. Among these, ADP, thrombin, and TxA_2 are probably most important in vivo. These platelet agonists are believed to bind to membrane receptors to inhibit membrane adenyl cyclase. The resultant decreased intraplatelet levels of cyclic adenosine monophosphate (cAMP) then lead to aggregation, involving an interaction between platelet membrane receptors and plasma- or platelet-derived fibrinogen. Increased cAMP levels inhibit aggregation. Prostacyclin, the potent antiaggregating agent, acts by binding to specific platelet receptors and activating adenyl cyclase to raise the levels of intraplatelet cAMP, thereby inhibiting the function of fibrinogen-binding receptors.[15] Ca^{++} plays some role in this process since platelet activation is associated with an increase of intraplatelet calcium.

The complex sequence of platelet events can be summarized as follows: (1) Platelets recognize sites of endothelial injury and adhere to exposed subendothelial collagen, thus becoming activated (Fig. 3–8). (2) With activation they secrete a variety of products stored in granules (among them ADP and fibrinogen) and synthesize thromboxane A_2. (3) Platelet factor 3 is unmasked and activates coagulation factor X to initiate the intrinsic coagulation sequence. (4) Concomitantly, the release of tissue factor from injured cells and endothelial cells participates in activation of the extrinsic coagulation sequence. (5) The ADP released from platelets initiates the formation of a temporary hemostatic plug of aggregated platelets, soon converted into a larger "secondary plug" under the influence of ADP, thrombin, thromboxane—all platelet agonists. (6) The deposition of fibrin (derived from platelets and plasma fibrinogen) into and about the platelet aggregate stabilizes and anchors it.

Thus, a platelet deficiency, either in number or function, will lead to potentially serious bleeding disorders, as discussed on page 643.

Coagulation System. The blood clotting sequence, along with the vessel wall and platelets, is a major contributor to the hemostatic process and also to thrombus formation. Indeed, a thrombus is in a sense a hemostatic plug formed inappropriately in the intact cardiovascular system. It is not necessary to review in detail the coagulation sequence; only some of the highlights will be presented.

The coagulation sequence has been likened to a cascade in which inactive blood zymogens, the clotting factors, are activated into proteolytic enzymes that selectively attack the next zymogen in the sequence,

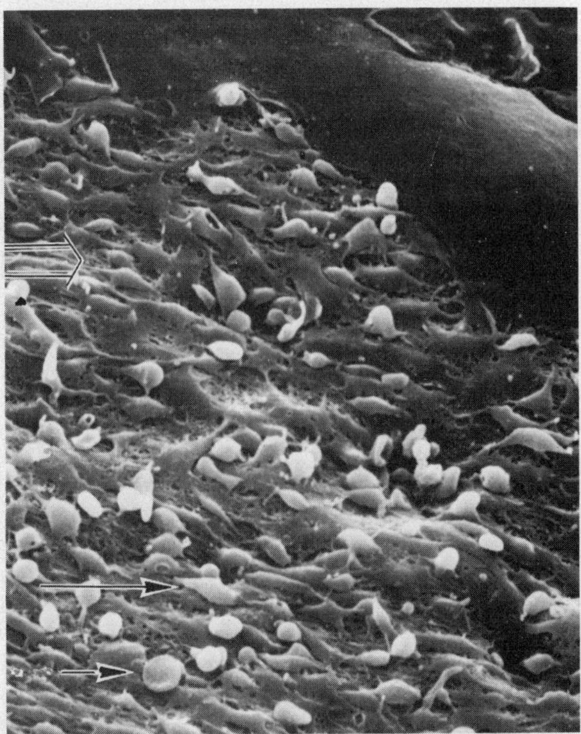

Figure 3–8. Platelet adherence at site of endothelial loss. Margin of endothelial lining with contoured endothelial cell is seen at top right. Short arrow points to a discoid intact platelet with a single pseudopod. Long arrow points to an elongated adherent platelet. Double arrow marks densely adherent platelets appearing as elongated humps fused to the subendothelial layer. (Courtesy of Dr. Christian Haudenschild, Mallory Institute of Pathology.)

converting it into an active enzyme. At each step along the way there is amplification, so that a small initial stimulus ultimately evokes a significant amount of solid fibrin polymer. The cascade begins as two separate pathways that ultimately converge. One is "intrinsic" to the blood and the other is so-called "extrinsic" because it is triggered by the introduction into the blood of tissue factors containing thromboplastin. The intrinsic pathway probably plays the major role in hemostasis following an injury. The "extrinsic" pathway becomes activated in a variety of pathologic situations, e.g., advanced cancer, complications of pregnancy, endotoxemia, and diffuse endothelial damage as in various forms of vasculitis. These conditions may evoke explosive blood clotting throughout the body followed by activation of fibrinolysis (plasmin generation), to produce what will be described as disseminated intravascular coagulation associated with intravascular coagulation and fibrinolysis (p. 649).

Several features of the clotting sequence are germane to thrombosis and merit discussion. A pivotal reaction is the conversion of prothrombin (factor II) to thrombin (factor IIA), which then activates platelets and contributes to the generation of the definitive secondary aggregate of platelets. Simultaneously it converts fibrinogen to fibrin. Both pathways lead to the generation of thrombin, and there is clinical evidence that both may be linked in vivo since a defect in either impinges on the other. In the *intrinsic pathway* there is first activation of factor XII (Hageman factor), converting it into a proteolytic enzyme, factor XIIa. This simple statement belies the complexity and confusion that envelops this phenomenon. Activation of factor XII occurs when fluid blood "contacts" an abnormal surface (glass, various negatively charged surfaces, injured endothelium, collagen). Within a blood vessel, a platelet aggregate overlying a site of endothelial injury behaves in a similar fashion. Additionally, there is an interaction with high-molecular-weight kininogen and conversion of prekallikrein into kallikrein. Kallikrein, once formed, participates in a positive feedback loop, activating more factor XII. Factor XIIa can also activate the complement system by cleaving the C′1,2,4 and C′3 components. The kallikrein likewise converts kininogen precursor into the vasoactive inflammatory mediator bradykinin. Thus, it is evident that three separate but interrelated systems are triggered into action with the conversion of factor XII to its activated form. With the formation of factor XIIa, the cascade proceeds over the span of several minutes to the development of factor Xa.

The *extrinsic pathway* is triggered by a lipoprotein present in "tissue factor" (also known as thromboplastin), normally present on the surface of virtually all cells including endothelial cells. Tissue factor complexes with factor VII to activate it, either by a change in shape or proteolytic cleavage, and the complex then interacts with factor X to form Xa. Thereafter, with the facilitation of calcium ions and phospholipid, prothrombin is converted to thrombin as the two separate pathways of blood clotting converge. For further details on the clotting mechanism, reference may be made to the review by Baugh and Houghie.[16] It should be noted at this time that a lack or defective function of any of the clotting factors or of platelets will induce a bleeding tendency referred to later as a "hemorrhagic diathesis" (p. 643).

ANTICLOTTING MECHANISMS. An intricate system of checks and balances maintains the fluidity of the blood and localizes a clot to the site of injury, thus preventing a chain reaction leading to the coagulation of the entire cardiovascular system. It is noteworthy that sufficient thrombin is generated by the clotting of only 1 ml of blood to coagulate all the fibrinogen in 3 liters of blood. These control mechanisms can be characterized as (a) depletion of clotting factors, (b) clearance of activated factors, (c) plasma inhibition of activated proteases, and (d) fibrinolysis.

Depletion of clotting factors by dilution when there is active blood flow past the local site or by utilization-exhaustion when flow is blocked serves to slow or check the clotting process. *Clearance of activated clotting factors* is accomplished by the liver and reticuloendothelial system.[17] This mechanism is effective only when there is flow of blood from the site of injury. With sufficient stasis the activated factors cannot be washed away to reach the sites of clearance.

Normal human blood contains a variety of *protease*

inhibitors, four of which—antithrombin III, C'1 inactivator, α_2-macroglobulin, and α_1-antitrypsin—act on one or more coagulation factors.[18] Antithrombin III in the presence of heparin is the principal inhibitor of thrombin but it also inactivates clotting factors XIIa, XIa, Xa, and IXa. C'1 inactivator blocks the classic pathway of activation of complement but also neutralizes XIa, XIIa, and plasma kallikrein. It might be noted here that an acquired or hereditary deficiency of or defect in antithrombin III is a major predisposition to thrombosis. The potent antiprotease α_2-macroglobulin also neutralizes thrombin; alone it accounts for about 25% of the total antithrombin activity of normal plasma. Alpha$_1$-antitrypsin inhibits factor XIa and also serves as an antiplasmin. Recently, yet another pathway has been described in vitro for removal of activated coagulation factors. Protein C is a vitamin K–dependent plasma protein. In the presence of an endothelial cell surface cofactor it is converted by thrombin to a protease capable of inactivation of factors Va and VIIIa.[19] Whether this anticoagulation pathway operates *in vivo* is not known.

The *fibrinolytic system* (Fig. 3–9) provides a critically important mechanism for the dissolution of fibrin clots. Involved are the precursor plasminogen, plasminogen activators, antiactivators (which block formation of plasmin), and antiplasmins (which inhibit already formed plasmin). Plasminogen is a β-globulin normally present in the plasma. Plasminogen can be proteolytically converted to plasmin by factor XIIa involving high-molecular-weight kininogen and prekallikrein, or by plasminogen activators within endothelial cells released with cell damage. Plasmin is a powerful proteolytic enzyme capable of cleaving fibrinogen and fibrin to yield split products also called fibrinogen—fibrin degradation products that themselves act as anticoagulants. They delay the polymerization of fibrin, resulting in a poorly formed fibrin clot susceptible to lytic degradation, and also inhibit platelet aggregation. Plasmin also lyses factors V and VIII. In-built systems are present that block the formation and action of plasmin. The major blocker of plasmin formation is α_2-globulin, an antiactivator. Other antiplasmins are α_1-macroglobulins, α_1-antitrypsin, and a fast reacting α_1-globulin—the most potent of the three.[20] Any lack of fibrinolytic function is an important predisposition to thrombosis. In passing, it should be noted that plasmins of exogenous origin such as urokinase or streptokinase are currently employed therapeutically to dissolve thrombi.

Against this background of normal hemostasis we can now consider thrombogenesis.

Thrombogenesis. *Three major influences predispose to thrombosis: (1) injury to endothelium, (2) alterations in normal blood flow, and (3) alterations in the blood (hypercoagulability).*

Endothelial injury is clearly the major and most frequent influence in the induction of thrombosis. This is amply documented in man by the frequency with which thrombi develop on ulcerated plaques in advanced atherosclerosis of the aorta and arteries (p. 506). Diabetics with their predisposition to severe atherosclerosis and hyperlipidemia (rendering platelets prone to aggregation) are extremely vulnerable to arterial thrombi. Thrombi also develop within the cardiac chambers when there has been injury to the endocardium, as may occur with myocardial infarcts, infections of the myocardium, or immunologic myocardial reactions. Inflammatory valve disease (and prosthetic valves) are favored sites for thrombus formation. In addition to such overt causes, microtrauma may be produced by a variety of influences. The hemodynamic stress in hypertension or the turbulent flow in arterial disorders is thought to be injurious to endothelial cells. Other potential bases for damage to endothelial cells are: chemical agents of exogenous origin (derivatives of cigarette smoke, for example) or of endogenous origin (hypercholesterolemia, homocystine); bacterial toxins or endotoxins; and immunologic injuries (in transplant rejection, immune complex deposition). Whatever the cause, damage to endothelial cells has wide ramifications, as has been pointed out.[21] Subendothelial collagen is exposed, tissue thromboplastin is released, and PGI_2 synthesis is locally depleted, as is plasminogen activator. There follows the sequence of adherence of platelets and activation of the clotting sequence.[22] It should be remembered, however, that numerous mechanisms are called into play that serve to prevent or limit thrombus formation; increased synthesis of PGI_2 by endothelial cells and activation of

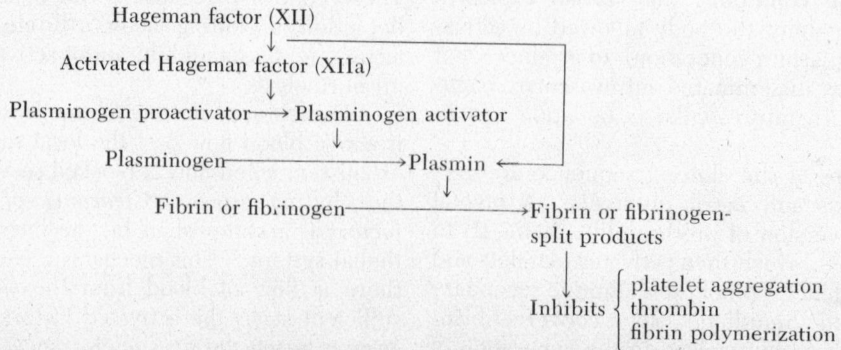

Figure 3–9. The fibrinolytic system.

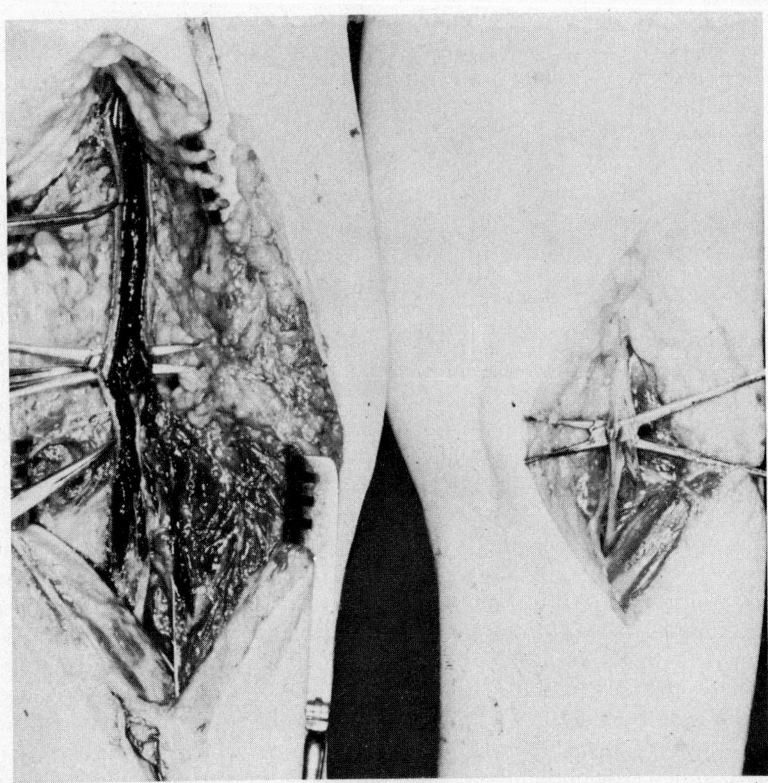

Figure 3–10. The popliteal veins exposed to demonstrate a large thrombus on the left and the normal vein for comparison on the right.

the fibrinolytic sequence are only two examples. Notwithstanding, endothelial injury is a potent thrombogenic influence.

Thrombi are common in the superficial and deep veins of the lower extremities, particularly where there is stasis or sluggish venous drainage of the legs (Fig. 3–10). These circumstances are encountered with varicosities of the superficial veins, which render the venous valves incompetent, and in the deep veins with prolonged bed rest or immobilization of an extremity, which reduces the milking action of muscular activity. Whether some subtle metabolic endothelial injury underlies the thrombus formation in these settings is still a matter of controversy, but if so it is beyond the range of present methods of visualization. It may well be that endothelial injury is not requisite for the formation of thrombi in veins. Stasis alone, as detailed below, may suffice.

Change in laminar flow as encountered with turbulence contributes to the development of arterial and cardiac thrombi, while stasis is probably requisite for venous thrombosis.[23] In normal flow the larger particles, such as white cells and red cells, occupy the central, most rapidly moving axial stream. The smaller platelets are carried in the more slowly moving laminar stream outside the central column. The periphery of the bloodstream adjacent to the endothelial layer moves most slowly and is free of all formed blood elements. Stasis and turbulence (causing countercurrents and local pockets of stasis) provide four important dimensions: (1) they disrupt laminar flow and bring platelets into contact with the endothelium, (2) they prevent the hepatic dilution and clearance of the activated coagulation factors by the fresh flow of blood, (3) turbulence could contribute to endothelial injury and damage to the formed elements of the blood, and (4) the loss of normal blood velocity permits the build-up of thrombi and prevents their being swept away by the moving stream.

The roles of turbulence or stasis are clearly documented in many clinical situations involving both the arterial and venous sides of the circulation. Thrombi often form, as mentioned earlier, overlying ulcerated atherosclerotic plaques. Here the ulceration not only exposes connective tissue elements and lipids in the plaque but also causes local turbulence. Thrombi are also prone to occur in the aorta and arteries within abnormal dilatations referred to as aneurysms. Frequently the thrombus completely fills the abnormal dilatation up to the preexistent normal level of the vessel wall, when laminar flow is presumably reestablished. In the heart, not only do myocardial infarctions provide sites of endothelial injury, but the necrotic muscle does not contract, and so some element of stasis is added. In healed rheumatic heart disease, for example, mitral stenosis causes the left atrium to expand and fail to empty. When arrhythmias such as atrial fibrillation (common in rheumatic heart disease) supervene, the stage is set for atrial and auricular thrombosis.

Stasis is undoubtedly the prime factor in the more slowly moving venous circulation. Most thrombi that develop in abnormally dilated varicose veins arise within the pockets created by venous valves, where presumably there is increased stasis or turbulence.[24] Sevitt examined 50 newly formed thrombi in femoral veins and found no evidence of underlying endothelial damage.[25] However, among 35 macroscopically uninvolved valve pockets, 13 contained a small nidus of one or more of the following elements: red cells, white cells, fibrin strands, or platelet aggregates. While such a small nidus might be washed out with normal flow, stasis might permit its progressive build-up to form a thrombus. The intrinsic clotting system may become activated in sites of marked stasis for reasons that are unclear.[26] The generation of thrombin and fibrin strands might then anchor the nidus to create a setting for superimposed build-up of a thrombus. It is of interest in this connection that in experimental models of atherosclerosis, monocytes-macrophages have been observed to adhere to endothelial surfaces having no overt lesion, but possibly some biochemical or metabolic injury. Conceivably, some analogous endothelial change contributes to the onset of thromboses in veins where there is no obvious endothelial damage. Intriguing as many of these observations are, we must conclude that the mechanism of thrombogenesis within veins that are not the site of obvious endothelial damage is still uncertain.

Stasis may have more subtle origins. Hyperviscosity syndromes such as polycythemia, cryoglobulinemia, and macroglobulinemia increase resistance to flow and induce stasis in small vessels. In sickle cell anemia the deformed red cells tend to log-jam, and the stasis predisposes to thrombosis. Similarly there is a thrombotic diathesis in the rare condition known as giant cavernous hemangioma (Kasabach-Merritt syndrome). Here the neoplastic large vascular spaces result in stasis and turbulence, and also provide poorly endothelialized surfaces that may lead to thromboses both within the tumor and elsewhere. Stasis and turbulence, then, are potent thrombogenic influences, particularly when combined with endothelial injury.

Alterations in the blood (hypercoagulability) have been proposed to explain the increased incidence of thrombosis encountered in certain clinical states referred to as thrombotic diatheses. Hypercoagulability has been defined as "an altered state of circulating blood that requires a smaller quantity of clot-promoting substances to induce intravascular coagulation than is required to produce comparable thrombosis in a normal subject."[21] In many clinical situations, such as extensive burns, severe trauma, shock, disseminated cancer, premature separation of the placenta, and retained dead fetus, explosive thrombosis may occur in small vessels throughout the body to produce so-called disseminated intravascular coagulation (DIC) (p. 649). Moreover, patients with cancer, particularly abdominal cancers such as those of the pancreas, have a well-defined predisposition to phlebothromboses, first noted over a hundred years ago by Trousseau. Since his time, many have confirmed the appearance of venous thrombi, often multiple and sequential at several sites, in patients with various forms of cancer; this condition now is justifiably designated as *Trousseau's syndrome* or *migratory thrombophlebitis* (p. 972).[28, 29] It seems reasonable to assume that both DIC and migratory thrombophlebitis have similar origins, namely the appearance of hypercoagulability of the blood.[30] Although the origin of the hypercoagulable state is still poorly understood, a number of procoagulant factors have been identified in cancer cells that conceivably might be released into the blood to initiate the coagulation sequence.[30A] Among these are tissue factor (analogous to that activating the so-called extrinsic pathway); cancer procoagulant A, which activates clotting factor X; and other procoagulants released from tumor cells along with shed plasma membrane vesicles. Thus, the appearance of hypercoagulability seems entirely plausible in the cancerous state, and it is highly likely that similar mechanisms may be operative in the many other conditions associated with DIC.

In addition to all these situations there are a number of settings in which there is a well-defined increased incidence of thromboses in the absence of identifiable potentiating causes, save possibly for hypercoagulability.[31] Why, for example, should thrombi appear late in pregnancy, and after childbirth, surgery, and various forms of injury? Studies indicate that approximately 70% of elderly patients with hip fractures and 50% of patients undergoing elective hip replacement develop a venous thrombosis.[32] As many as 30% of general surgical patients and 15% of gynecologic patients undergoing a hysterectomy for nonmalignant disease may develop deep vein thrombosis despite the fact that the individuals may be relatively young. If the reason was infusion of tissue factor (thromboplastin) by the antecedent "traumatic" event, one would expect the thrombus to appear virtually at once. The increased incidence of thrombosis during the last trimester of pregnancy, childbirth, and the puerperium is so pronounced as to have received the specific designation "*milk leg*" or "*phlegmasia alba dolens*" (painful white leg) (p. 537). Sometimes the thrombosis appears, as noted, prior to the delivery and therefore before any inciting mechanism can be identified.

The relationship between *oral contraceptives* and thrombosis is discussed in more detail on page 446, but it suffices here to note that when they are used by women between 35 and 45 years of age they increase the risk of pulmonary embolism and myocardial infarction, related to thromboses in the veins of the leg and coronary arteries, respectively. Hypercoagulability is suspected to be the basis of this increased risk.

Despite all the suggestive clinical evidence, there is a paucity of laboratory evidence to support the existence of a hypercoagulable state. The many studies in quest of this "elusive grail" have focused on: (1) increased numbers and/or activation of platelets, (2) raised levels or activation of clotting factors, (3) elevated fibrinogen levels, (4) decreased fibrinolytic activity, and (5) reduced antithrombin III levels. However, so many and such disparate abnormalities have been found as to challenge the significance of all.[33]

The only reasonably well-established hypercoagulable state is a genetic deficiency of antithrombin III. Several kindreds have been identified with blood levels of antithrombin III approximately 50% below the normal range in whom leg vein thromboses were extremely common.[36] It is ironic that the lack of a procoagulant factor may induce a bleeding tendency as occurs in hemophilia (p. 648), but it does not protect against thrombosis. John Hageman, who lacked factor XII (hence the designation "Hageman factor") died of a massive pulmonary embolism from a venous thrombus.[37] We must leave it that the concept of hypercoagulability remains alive, but it is weak and sorely lacks evidence.

MORPHOLOGY. Thrombi may occur anywhere in the cardiovascular system: within the cardiac chambers, arteries, veins, or capillaries. They are of variable size and shape, dictated by their site of origin and the circumstances leading to their development. When formed within a cardiac chamber or the aorta they may have apparent laminations called the "lines of Zahn." These are produced by alternating layers of paler platelets admixed with some fibrin, separated by darker layers containing more red cells. However, the laminations may not be evident in thrombi formed within smaller arteries or veins. Moreover, thrombi formed in the slower-moving flow in veins sometimes closely resemble coagulated blood, but close inspection will reveal traversing or tangled strands of aggregated platelets and fibrin—the lines of Zahn.

In the heart and aorta the thrombi almost always begin at some site of endothelial damage. Thus, the thrombi begin as a layer attached to the underlying wall. Although the mass may expand, the rapid flow of blood usually precludes total occlusion of the chamber or lumen and consequently they are referred to as **mural** thrombi. In small arteries and veins they are more often **occlusive** thrombi. However, contraction of the thrombus often reconstitutes a slitlike lumen, permitting blood flow past the intravascular mass and the build-up of more thrombus, referred to as **propagation of the thrombus.** The head of the thrombus exposed to the flowing stream tends to accumulate platelets and fibrin, creating a white head, while the downstream surface accumulates a dark red stasis tail because of the slowing of the blood flow and turbulence in the lee of the obstructing mass. In this fashion, a large propagating tail may build up, eventually filling the lumen and thus producing an occlusive thrombus. The developing head and long, snakelike tail may not be firmly attached to the underlying endothelium and, since they literally wave in the bloodstream, they sometimes fragment and embolize, as occurs very often with thrombi in the deep veins of the lower extremity.

Occlusive arterial thrombi are encountered, in descending order of frequency, in the coronary, cerebral, iliac, and femoral arteries. Almost always, the arterial thrombus is superimposed upon an atherosclerotic lesion. Uncommonly, other forms of vascular disease such as that produced by the many forms of necrotizing vasculitis (p. 519) and traumatic injury of vessels underlie arterial thrombus formation.

Mural thrombi generally occur in the more capacious lumina of the heart chambers and aorta. Myocardial infarcts or cardiac arrhythmias are common antecedents to the thrombi that form in the heart, while atherosclerosis or aneurysmal dilatations are almost invariable precursors of aortic thrombus formation. The mural thrombi, which are generally formed in these sites, do not fill the entire lumen, since total occlusion would be incompatible with survival except in extraordinarily rare instances (Fig. 3–11).

In addition to arising within the cardiac chambers, thrombotic masses under special circumstances may build up on the heart valves, particularly the mitral and aortic valves. In this setting, the thrombi are referred to as **vegetations.** The most common antecedent is a blood-borne bacterial infection that seeds the heart valves, and thus provides a site of injury on which a thrombotic mass of fibrin and platelets builds up to produce so-called **infective vegetative endocarditis** (p. 580). Less commonly, **nonbacterial bland thrombotic vegetations** (verrucous endocarditis) appear, particularly in patients having systemic lupus erythematosus (p. 187) and in those already debilitated by some fatal illness such as disseminated cancer, advanced tuberculosis, or some lymphomatous-leukemic disorder (although they sometimes appear in young individuals not having a fatal illness). In these settings, hypercoagulability of the blood is predicated but without substantial proof.

Venous thrombi are also known as phlebothromboses. They are almost invariably occlusive and in fact often form quite accurate casts of the vessel in which they arise, even revealing the markings of the venous valves. Thrombi are frequently found in superficial varicose veins, but these rarely embolize and so are more bothersome locally than serious. More ominous, phlebothrombosis is encountered preponderantly in the veins of the lower extremity (90% occur in deep leg veins) in approximately the following descending order of frequency: calf, femoral, popliteal, and iliac veins. Less commonly, venous thrombi may develop in the periprostatic plexus and the ovarian and periuterine veins. This order of frequency varies considerably among the many series of patients reported.[24]

Thrombi must be differentiated from postmortem clots. This may be particularly difficult with venous thrombi formed in a sluggish circulation and therefore having a large component of red cells. The thrombus is generally somewhat friable and firm, whereas the postmortem clot is usually a rubbery, gelatinous coagulum. Thrombi contain lines of Zahn. Thrombi may or may not nicely fit their vascular enclosure, but in all instances they have some attachment to the underlying wall. In contrast, postmortem clots almost always form a perfect cast of the vessel in which they arise, and they can usually be gently lifted out because they are not attached to their site of origin. The postmortem clot may be a cyanotic dark red "currant jelly," or it may have a supernatant portion of coagulated clear plasma "chicken fat"

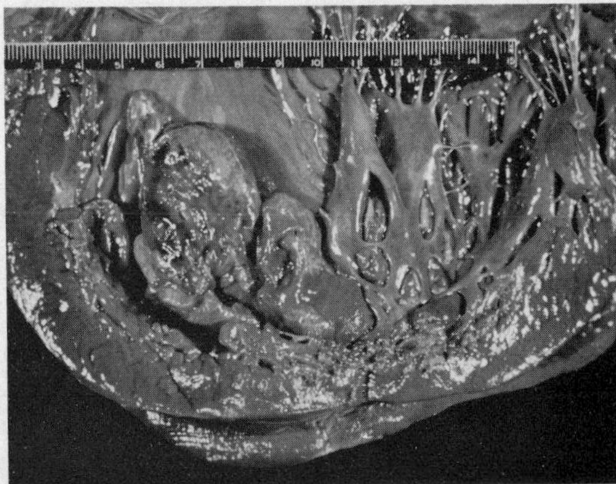

Figure 3–11. Numerous fresh dark mural thrombi attached to the ventricular endocardium.

overlying a portion of darker hue where the red cells have settled. Of great importance is the differentiation of postmortem clotting in, for example, the coronary artery from a valid thrombus that may, indeed, have been the cause of death. The development of postmortem clots is a highly variable phenomenon, since in many patients activation of the fibrinolytic system before or immediately after death prevents postmortem clotting, whereas in others this does not occur, and postmortem clots are abundant.

EVOLUTION OF THE THROMBUS. If a patient survives the immediate ischemic effects of a newly developed thrombus, what happens thereafter? One of a number of pathways may be followed. *The thrombus may (1) propagate and, by its enlargement, eventually cause obstruction of some critical vessel; (2) give rise to an embolus (discussed in the next section); (3) be removed by fibrinolytic action; or (4) become organized.* The last two potentials deserve further consideration. As already indicated, a thrombus provokes prompt activation of the plasminogen-plasmin system. Indeed, in animals it is difficult to create a persistent thrombus because of the prompt and effective fibrinolytic response. Such a happy outcome may also occur in man, and pulmonary thromboemboli have been observed by angiography to shrink rapidly and, indeed, to disappear within days of the appearance of the intravascular obstruction.[38, 39] Resolution occurs mostly within the first few days of development of the coagulum, probably because freshly formed fibrin is more susceptible to lysis than is older fibrin. The efficacy of this response depends on the size of the thrombus, the adequacy of the blood flow in its environs, and the level of the fibrinolytic activity. One study suggests that physical conditioning enhances the fibrinolytic response, giving one rationale for the notion that regular physical exercise lowers the risk of coronary thrombosis and myocardial infarction.[40] Blood flow is crucial, since the occlusive thrombus may induce sufficient stasis to block the delivery of the necessary activated enzymes. Fortunately, fresh clots retract under the action of thrombasthenin of platelet origin. In this manner, even an occlusive thrombus generally leaves a slitlike channel through which some flow continues.

Almost from the beginning of its formation, the trapped white cells and platelets begin to modify the thrombus to initiate the process of *organization.* The neutrophils, and especially the macrophages, phagocytize fragments of fibrin and cell debris; in addition, released lysosomal enzymes, derived both from the white cells and from the platelets, begin to digest the coagulum. When a thrombus is quite large, the central region is protected from the diluting effect of the blood flow about the margins, and here the build-up of lysosomal enzymes may be sufficient to produce *central softening.* Such a sequence is particularly likely to occur in large thrombi within the cardiac chambers or aneurysmal sacs. In passing, bacteremic seeding of such a digestate may convert the softened thrombus to a mass

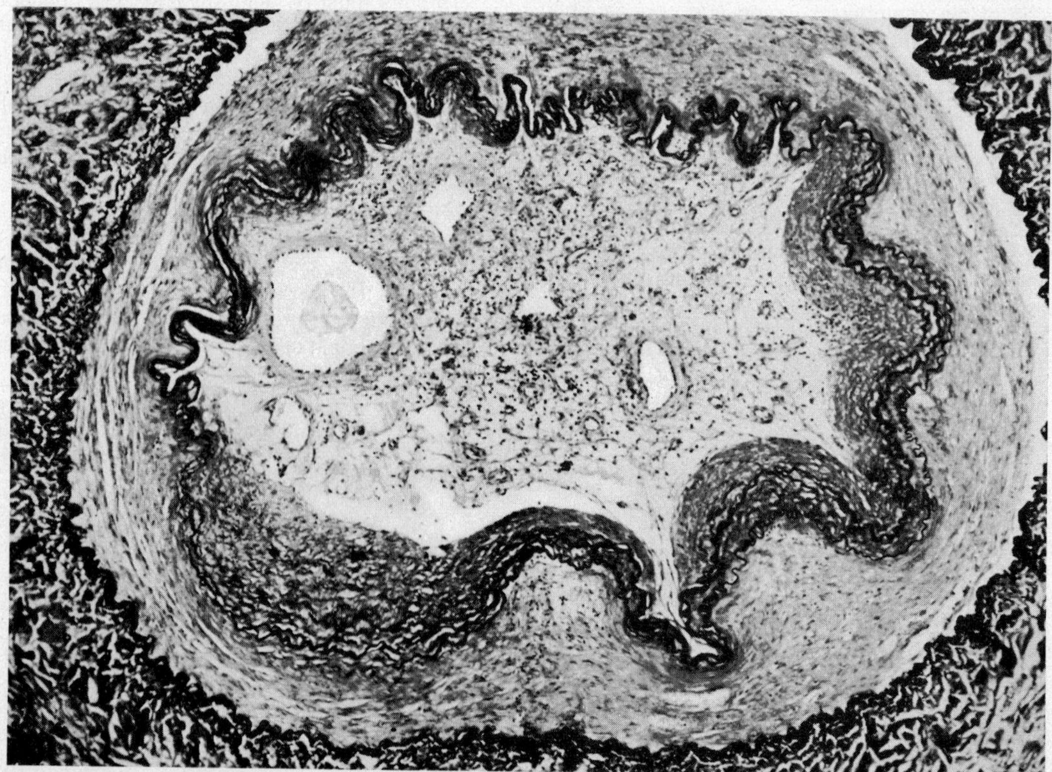

Figure 3–12. A low-power view of a thrombosed artery stained for elastic tissue.The lumen is delineated by the partially degenerated internal elastic membrane and is totally filled with organized clot, now traversed by many newly formed recanalized channels.

of pus. Concurrently fibroblasts and capillaries proliferate and invade the base of the thrombus where it is attached to the underlying vessel wall. Growth factors derived from platelets and monocytes-macrophages probably contribute to this cellular proliferation. In time, the entire intravascular mass is organized and converted essentially into a vascularized connective tissue. The capillary channels may anastomose to produce thoroughfares that traverse the thrombus and, indeed, provide new channels through which blood flow may at least in part be reestablished, a process known as *canalization of the thrombus* (Fig. 3–12). The regrowth of the endothelial cells over the surface of the thrombus covers it, thereby excluding it from the flow of blood. Since fibrous tissue contracts in the course of weeks to months, the thrombus is virtually incorporated within the vessel wall or cardiac chamber as a fibrous lump or thickening (Fig. 3–13).

An overview of the critical steps involved in thrombogenesis and the subsequent events that may follow is given in Figure 3–14.

CLINICAL IMPLICATIONS. The clinical significance of a thrombus depends, as would be expected, on its size and particularly on its site, i.e., arterial or venous.

Arterial thrombi in small vessels are occlusive and usually cause infarction of the dependent tissues (although there are exceptions, as discussed more fully on p. 111). Two of the major killers in affluent societies, myocardial infarction and cerebral infarction (encephalomalacia), are related to thrombi in atherosclerotic vessels. Occlusive arterial thrombi rarely embolize since they are firmly wedged into the vessel at their sites of origin. However, thrombi in the cardiac chambers or

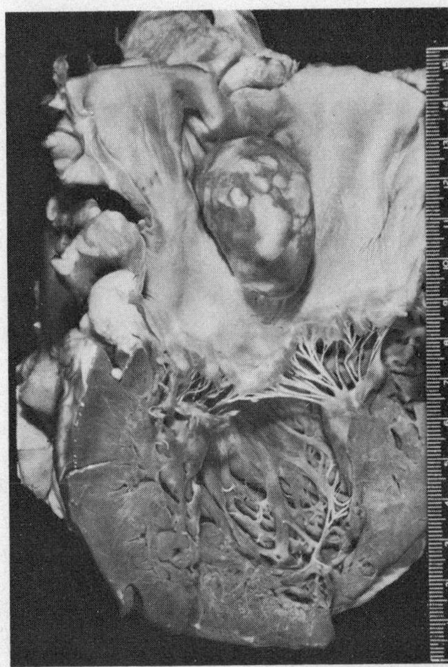

Figure 3–13. An endothelialized mural thrombus within the left atrium of the heart. The surface is smooth and the clot has been converted into a firmly attached globular mass.

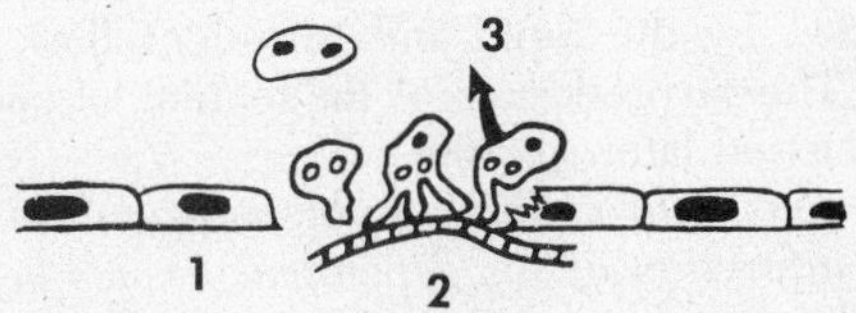

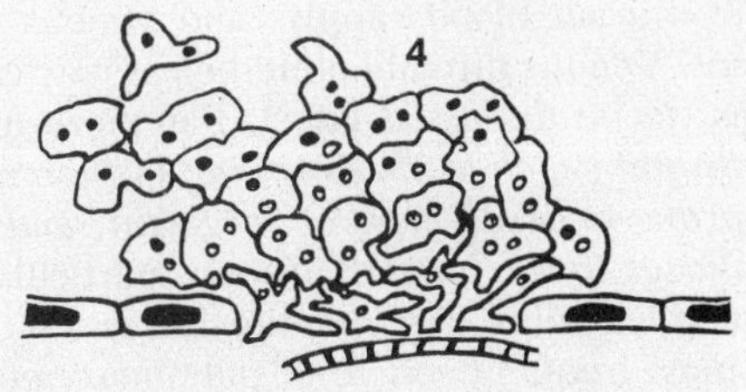

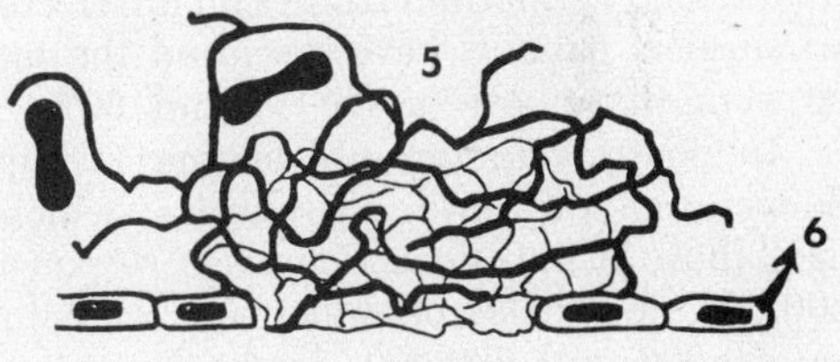

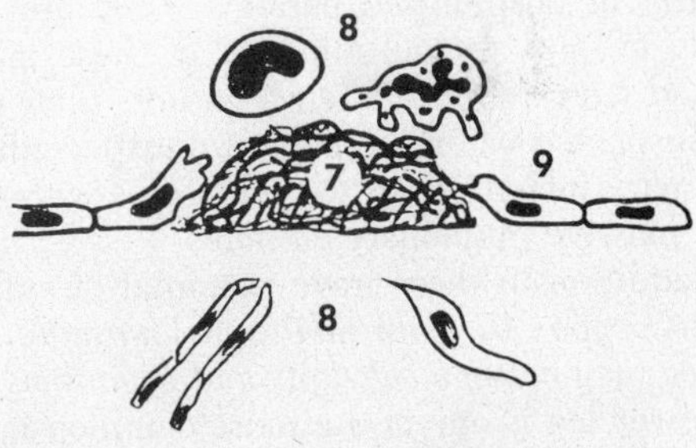

Figure 3–14. Summary of thrombogenesis.

1, *Endothelial injury* releases tissue factor and exposes subendothelial connective tissues. 2, *Platelet adherence* and *plasma clotting system* are triggered. 3, *Granule release* and *prostaglandin generation begin.* 4, *Platelet aggregation* induced by released ADP and *vasoconstriction* (5HT, thromboxanes) result in *primary (temporary) hemostatic plug.* 5, *Thrombin, thromboxanes,* and *endoperoxides* promote *release reaction* and irreversible *aggregation;* amorphous platelet mass and trapped red cells are enmeshed in *fibrin* to form *definitive (permanent) hemostatic plug.* 6, *Endothelial plasminogen activator* and plasma *antithrombin* check rapid clotting. 7, *Clot retraction (platelet contraction) and fibrinolysis* reduce size of plug. 8, *Organization* (ingrowth of capillaries and fibroblasts, infiltration by polymorphonuclear leukocytes, and macrophages). 9, *Endothelial regeneration* gradually repairs the injured area. (Time scale: Steps 1 to 4, seconds to minutes; steps 5 to 7, several minutes to hours; steps 8 and 9, one to several days.) (Courtesy of Dr. Michael Gimbrone, Department of Pathology, Peter Bent Brigham Hospital.)

aorta are prime origins for emboli because they are almost always mural lesions and are vulnerable to fragmentation by the rapid and turbulent flow of passing blood. The favored sites of lodgement of such emboli are discussed later (p. 106).

Venous thrombosis (phlebothrombosis) rarely causes infarction of the dependent tissues because collateral bypass channels soon enlarge sufficiently to maintain the venous drainage of the affected part. There are, however, exceptions where bypasses do not exist as in the ovarian blood supply, and venous infarction may result. Venous thrombi nonetheless may cause local problems (to be discussed later). Far more important, *venous thrombi such as those arising in the veins of the leg are prone to break loose or fragment, and embolize almost always to the lungs.* Thrombi, particularly those in the deep leg veins, e.g., popliteal, femoral, and iliac, are the most frequent source of pulmonary emboli and are major causes of morbidity and mortality, especially in hospitalized individuals. It has been estimated that 20 million deep vein thromboses occur annually in the United States.[41] Postmortem studies on unselected medical and surgical patients have disclosed the incidence of deep vein thrombosis to be 34 and 60%, respectively.[42] In contrast to thrombi arising in superficial varicose veins of the lower extremities, which rarely embolize, those of the deep veins are responsible for over 600,000 new cases of pulmonary embolism and between 50,000 and 200,000 deaths annually in the United States.[43] Potentially lethal deep vein thrombi are all the more important because they are so frequently insidious at their local site of origin. Despite the fact that necropsies reveal deep vein thrombi so frequently in hospitalized patients, they are detected clinically in only a small minority of these individuals (discussed later).[44] More often than not, their presence is first suspected when the patient unexpectedly suffers a pulmonary infarction, or too often dies without warning of a massive pulmonary embolus.

In addition to their grave potential of embolizing, *occlusive venous thrombi in the major outflow vessels of the leg may cause local signs and symptoms.* Edema of the lower leg is one of the more common manifestations. Analogously, thrombosis of the superficial veins of the leg, when varicosities are present, may cause some localized edema and predispose the skin in the affected area to infections following trivial trauma, with the development of indolent varicose ulcers that are most difficult to control. Thrombosed veins may be painful and tender to palpation. Thus, with thrombi in the veins of the calf muscles, dorsiflexion of the foot may elicit pain known as *Homans' sign.* Similarly, simply squeezing the calf muscles will also elicit pain. The painfulness of some thrombosed veins has led clinicians to refer to venous thrombosis as thrombophlebitis. This designation would imply inflammation of the vein wall in association with a thrombus. However, microscopic examination of such veins rarely discloses significant evidence of inflammation, and the origin of the pain remains obscure. The term thrombophlebitis is firmly fixed in clinical parlance, but should be equated with phlebothrombosis.

The many clinical conditions frequently associated with thrombosis have already been mentioned in the discussion of thrombogenesis. However, it should be emphasized that *whatever the clinical setting, advanced age, bed rest, and immobilization increase the risk.* Older patients are more likely to have heart disease with impairment of the circulation, reduced physical activity with less effective venous return from the lower extremities, and more advanced atherosclerosis. Thus, older patients confined to bed for any chronic illness, paraplegics, and even young individuals with an extremity immobilized in a cast are at risk. For these reasons, venous thrombosis and its attendant pulmonary emboli are constant hazards to hospitalized patients.

The clinical diagnosis of *arterial* thrombosis is usually made all too evident by the resultant infarction that it induces. On the other hand, as pointed out, the clinical diagnosis of *venous* thrombosis is extremely difficult. The fallibility of local clinical signs is notorious. Noninvasive techniques, such as ultrasound examination and impedance plethysmography, improve diagnostic accuracy. However, in many instances radiographic venography with a contrast medium is required, or the demonstration of increased radioactivity over the site of an evolving thrombus following the intravenous administration of ^{125}I-labeled fibrinogen.[45] The reliability of these various procedures is beyond our scope and ultimately is very controversial. But most important is a high index of suspicion, greatly aided by a knowledge of the particular clinical settings in which thrombosis is likely to occur.

Current approaches to the prevention and treatment of this condition are relevant to pathogenetic issues. Occupying front stage center today are methods designed to inhibit platelet aggregation.[46] Aspirin, indomethacin, and other aspirin-like drugs have been shown to inhibit cyclooxygenase, which, it will be recalled, is necessary for the synthesis of endoperoxides (p. 54). It was hoped that platelet synthesis of thromboxane A_2 could be lowered to inhibit platelet aggregation and thrombogenesis. However, cyclooxygenase is also requisite for the synthesis of prostacyclin by endothelial cells. In an attempt to resolve this dilemma, very small doses of aspirin have been used because of the evidence that cyclooxygenase in platelets is more susceptible to aspirin inhibition than the enzyme in endothelial cells.[47] More promising are a combination of aspirin and dipyridamole, since the latter is believed to enhance the action of prostacycylin,[48] or the new classes of drugs that serve as prostacyclin receptor agonists, thromboxane receptor antagonists, and thombroxane synthetase inhibitors.[49] All these still experimental approaches have not displaced the use of anticoagulants such as heparin in the patient at risk, but the use of anticoagulation therapy incurs the risk of hemorrhage, particularly in postsurgical patients.

Another form of therapy still under trial involves treating already developed thrombi (particularly arterial thrombi as in the coronaries) with fibrinolytic agents such as streptokinase or urokinase. It is argued that once the thrombus has developed, heparin cannot do more than block its further build-up, whereas fibrinolytics may augment the normal plasminogen system to hasten the removal of the thrombus.[50, 51] The results to-date suggest that streptokinase, when infused within a thrombosed coronary artery within hours of a myocardial infarction, may be beneficial. However, the time limit and difficulty restrict the usefulness of this therapeutic approach.

In closing this discussion of thrombosis, it is important to point out that although many "high-risk" settings are known, thrombogenesis is a puzzling and unpredictable phenomenon. It may occur at any time, under any conditions, and indeed has appeared in young, vigorous individuals without apparent provocation or predisposition.

DISSEMINATED INTRAVASCULAR COAGULATION (DIC)

A variety of disorders ranging from obstetric difficulties to advanced cancer may be complicated by the sudden or insidious development of myriad fibrin thrombi in the microcirculation—DIC—followed soon by active fibrinolysis and a bleeding diathesis. The paradox of a thrombotic disorder leading to a hemorrhagic tendency has been explained as follows. The rapid depletion of fibrinogen and platelets produces what has been called "consumption coagulopathy" or "defibrination syndrome." Simultaneously the fibrinolytic system is activated, leading to proteolytic digestion of clotting factors as well as fibrinogen. In this manner the stimulus to thrombosis leads to a bleeding disorder. It should be noted that DIC is not a primary disorder. Rather, it complicates the course of any disease associated with the introduction or release into the blood of procoagulants or platelet-aggregating factors, e.g., thromboplastin tissue factor, thromboxane A_2, and so forth. It is closely related to several other poorly understood conditions—thrombotic thrombocytopenic purpura, hemolytic-uremic syndrome, amniotic fluid infusion—all characterized by widespread deposition of fibrin and/or aggregation of platelets in the microcirculation. Thus, DIC is discussed on page 649, thrombotic thrombocytopenic purpura on page 646, and the hemolytic-uremic syndrome on page 1048. Only amniotic fluid infusion needs characterization at this point.

AMNIOTIC FLUID INFUSION

As pointed out above, this condition may represent that form of DIC initiated by the entrance of amniotic fluid into the circulation. Whatever its nature it has become one of the principal causes of maternal death, since other major causes of maternal mortality such as pulmonary embolism, toxemia, and hemorrhage have come under control. It is nonetheless rare (approximately one case per 80,000 deliveries), but has a mortality rate approaching 80%.[52] Most fatalities occur during labor and delivery or the immediate postpartum period. Prompt delivery, perhaps by cesarean section, rescues most of the babies.

Most patients with this condition are multiparous and somewhat older than the mean of obstetric patients. Although tumultuous labor, the use of uterine stimulants, traumatic delivery, and large babies have been said to be predisposing influences, these factors are encountered only in a minority of patients. Typically, the condition announces itself by the catastrophic onset of profound cardiovascular shock and respiratory difficulty with deep cyanosis, often accompanied by uterine atony and excessive hemorrhage. Convulsions and coma may appear in some cases just before death. Anatomically, the diagnosis rests on the demonstration in the pulmonary capillaries of components derived from the amniotic fluid: (1) epithelial squames from the fetal skin, (2) lanugo hairs, (3) fat from the vernix caseosa, (4) mucin from the fetal gut, and (5) meconium (Fig. 3–15).[53] Similar debris can sometimes be found in the vessels of other organs. In some cases fibrin thrombi can be shown in the pulmonary microcirculation, but their relative rarity may merely reflect active fibrinolysis.

The pathogenesis of this disorder is still poorly understood. Clearly there is the entrance of amniotic fluid into the maternal circulation made possible by a tear in the placental membranes and rupture of uterine and/or cervical veins. It is further proposed that the fetal head creates a plug in the lower uterine segment permitting uterine contractions to force fluid into the maternal circulation. However, there is some doubt whether obstruction of the pulmonary circulation by the particulate matter of amniotic origin adequately explains all the features of the clinical conditions. Anaphylactic shock, DIC (secondary to the entrance of thromboplastic factors present in the amniotic fluid) with consumption of coagulant factors, platelet aggregation, or the infusion of vasoactive substances derived from the amniotic fluid have all been proposed as alternative mechanisms. Attention has been directed to the possible role of various prostaglandins and thromboxane known to be present in amniotic fluid during labor.[54, 55] Which specific endoperoxide derivative is most important remains unknown, but several prostaglandins (particularly prostacyclin) and thromboxane A_2 have vasoactivity and effects on platelets. Further investigation is required to unravel the cause of, and to determine effective treatment for, this rare but diastrous disorder to spare the infant from being born into a motherless world. To date "this cause of maternal death remains unpredictable and largely unpreventable."[56]

EMBOLISM

An embolus is a detached intravascular solid, liquid, or gaseous mass that is carried by the blood to a site

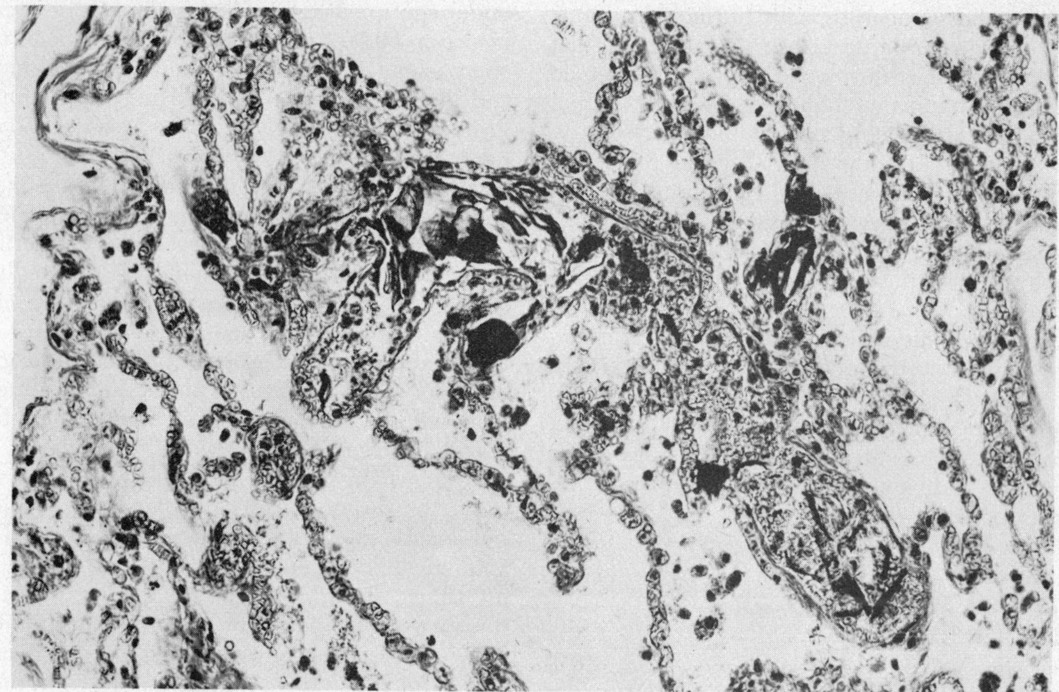

Figure 3–15. Amniotic embolism. Masses of dark mucous debris and desquamated squames are present in the pulmonary vessels and alveolar capillaries.

distant from its point of origin. Virtually 99% of all emboli arise in thrombi (thromboembolism). Rare forms of emboli include fragments of bone or bone marrow, atheromatous debris from ruptured atherosclerotic plaques, droplets of fat, bits of tumor, foreign bodies such as bullets, and bubbles of air or nitrogen. *Unless otherwise qualified, the term embolus implies thromboembolism.* Inevitably, emboli lodge in vessels too small to permit their further passage, resulting in partial or complete occlusion of the vessel. Depending on their site of origin, emboli may come to rest anywhere within the cardiovascular system and are best discussed from the standpoint of whether they lodge in the pulmonary or systemic circulations, thus producing differing clinical effects.

PULMONARY EMBOLISM

This subject is discussed fully on page 711; only an overview is presented here. Occlusion of a large or medium-sized pulmonary artery is embolic in origin until proved otherwise. *Thrombotic occlusion of these vessels is very uncommon* and is virtually encountered only when pulmonary hypertension has led to atherosclerotic or other hypertensive changes in the pulmonary arterial tree. Pulmonary embolism is generally considered to be the third most common acute cause of death in the United States; only heart attacks and strokes have a higher incidence.[43] As pointed out earlier, there are over 600,000 new cases of pulmonary embolism each year in the United States, accounting for approximately 10 to 15% of deaths of hospitalized patients who come to necropsy.[57] It is, then, a clinical disorder of the first magnitude.

Over 95% of all pulmonary emboli arise in thrombi within the large deep veins of the lower legs—popliteal, femoral, and iliac veins (Fig. 3–16). Thrombi within veins of the calf muscles are less likely to cause significant emboli. Similarly, thrombi arising in superficial varicose veins rarely embolize, apart from the extremely small minority that propagate into larger outflow channels. Other sites of venous thrombosis such as the veins in the pelvis—the periprostatic, broad ligament, periovarian, and uterine veins—are also very uncommon sites of origin of emboli.

Dislodgement, in part or whole, of a large venous thrombus produces an embolus that flows with the venous drainage through progressively larger vessels to the right heart. Unless the blood clot is very large, it passes through the capacious chambers and valves of the right side of the heart, and enters the pulmonary arterial circulation. Infrequently, long masses impact astride the bifurcation of the main pulmonary artery to create a *saddle embolus* (Fig. 3–17). More often, they occlude a major pulmonary vessel or pass further out into the periphery of the pulmonary vasculature to occlude smaller vessels. Occasionally, showers of small emboli may have the same effect as a large embolus. Rarely, emboli may enter the right side of the heart and pass through interatrial or interventricular septal defects to gain access to the arterial side of the circulation *(paradoxical embolism).*

The clinical consequences of a pulmonary embolus range from sudden death to the development of a pulmonary infarct, or only a transient pulmonary hem-

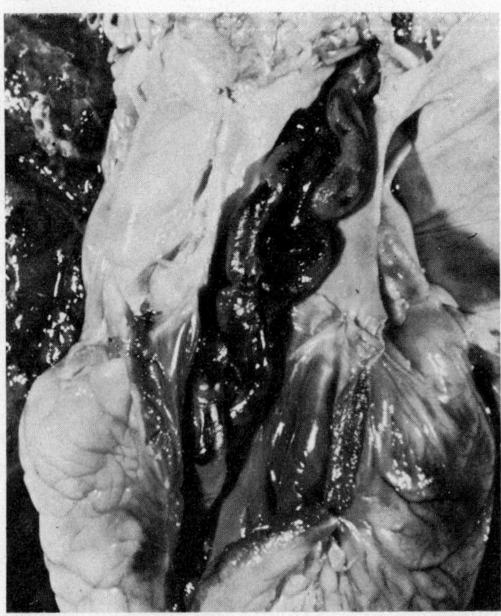

Figure 3–16. A large coiled embolus from the veins of the lower leg lies in the right ventricle and pulmonary artery, almost completely covering the pulmonary valve.

orrhage to mild or no respiratory dysfunction. Many factors, discussed more fully on page 712, govern this variable outcome. Only some cursory comments are offered here. *The size of the embolus (and therefore its site of lodgement within the pulmonary vessels) and the number of emboli are the prime factors in determining the extent of embolic obstruction and the likelihood of survival.*

When more than 50% of the major pulmonary arterial flow is suddenly obstructed, acute right ventricular failure and sudden death are likely. Thus, a large embolus in the main pulmonary artery or in its primary division into right and left branches will probably cause sudden death before the changes of infarction can develop. Reflex or humoral vasoconstriction may worsen the perfusion deficit.[58] *Small emboli are less likely to cause sudden death. They travel out into the more peripheral areas of the lung, where they cause either pulmonary hemorrhages or infarcts.*[59] Obviously, the number of emboli is of importance since all contribute to the extent of embolic obstruction. In this connection, it must be emphasized that the patient with a pulmonary embolus has a 30% chance of developing a second one and, should this happen, a 20% chance that this second episode will be fatal.

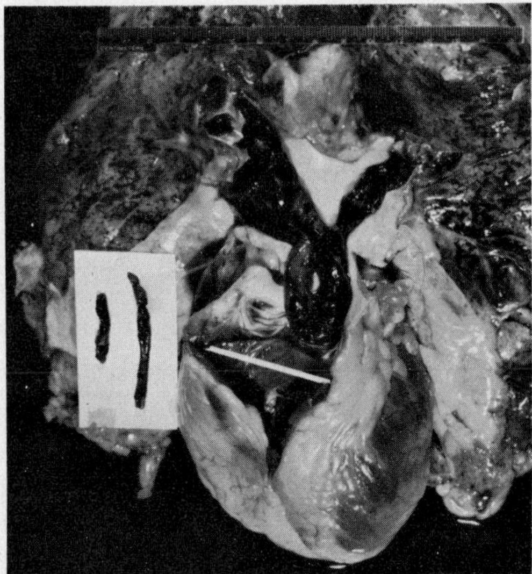

Figure 3–17. A large, Y-shaped saddle embolus from the femoral veins fills the pulmonary artery and its two major divisions.

The cardiopulmonary status of the patient prior to embolism is a key determinant of the outcome. A relatively small embolus may be fatal in an elderly individual with preexisting cardiopulmonary disease, but may have only limited impact on an otherwise healthy young individual. Similarly, the cardiopulmonary status of the patient influences the likelihood of infarction as opposed to hemorrhage. In one study it was shown that the larger the embolus and the more central the site of arterial occlusion, the less likely was there to be infarction. Apparently large emboli tend to permit adequate collateral flow through the bronchial circulation to preserve the vitality of the affected segment of the lung, and thus cause only pulmonary hemorrhage.[59] However, the adequacy of the bronchial circulation is dependent on the cardiac status of the patient; therefore, in an individual with congestive failure, infarction rather than hemorrhage is likely. Smaller emboli that occlude distal branches more surely lead to infarction even in persons without congestive failure.

The persistence of the embolic occlusion bears on the prognosis. It is well recognized that pulmonary emboli, once impacting within the pulmonary circulation, may shatter and travel out into more peripheral areas of the lung. Depending on the size of the fragments, they produce small pulmonary lesions or have no significant effect. At the same time, embolic occlusion activates the fibrinolytic system, as does the original venous thrombus. Sequential angiographic studies indicate that within 24 hours the flow begins to improve, which is attributable to fibrinolytic resolution. In some patients the resolution becomes complete within seven to 30 days.[60] If resolution does not occur, the embolus will undergo organization. The organized clot may partially or totally obstruct the lumen of the vessel. Multiple emboli, whether organized or not, may constitute a significant increased resistance to flow and lead to either acutely developing or chronic pulmonary hypertension.

The promptness of diagnosis and institution of appropriate therapy (general supportive measures, anticoagulation, administration of fibrinolytics, and surgical procedures to prevent recurrent embolization) materially modify the outcome. It is estimated that the mortality rate is 30% in persons whose disease is not diagnosed correctly, dropping to 8% among those for whom treatment is promptly and effectively instituted.[44]

In summary, the major outcomes of a pulmonary embolus can be listed as follows:[61]

1. Resolution by fragmentation or fibrinolysis occurs in 70 to 80%.
2. Pulmonary infarction appears in 10 to 15%.
3. Chronic pulmonary hypertension is a late sequel in about 5%.
4. Death related to the sudden embolic occlusion occurs in about 8 to 12%.

SYSTEMIC EMBOLISM

This term refers to emboli that travel through the arterial circulation. *Most arterial emboli (80 to 85%) arise from thrombi within the heart.*[62] About 60 to 65% arise within the left ventricle secondary to myocardial infarction or some form of cardiomyopathy. An additional 20% stem from mural thrombi in the left atrium secondary to rheumatic heart disease involving atrial fibrillation. Less common sources of arterial emboli include thrombi developing in relation to ulcerated atherosclerotic plaques of the aorta, aortic aneurysms, infective endocarditis, valvular or aortic prostheses, and paradoxical embolism from venous thrombi that gain access to the left side of the circulation through a right-to-left congenital cardiac anomaly. In about 10 to 15% of patients the source of the embolus is unknown.

In contrast to venous emboli, *arterial emboli follow a much more varied pathway, but they almost always cause infarction.* Emboli from infective endocarditis caused by virulent organisms produce septic infarcts that may be rapidly converted to large abscesses. The major sites of lodgement of all systemic emboli are the lower extremities (70 to 75%), the brain (10%), visceral (10%—includes mesenteric, renal, and splenic), and the upper limbs (7 to 8%). The site of lodgement and the size of the embolus within the systemic vessels are obvious critical determinants of its significance. Embolic occlusion of the femoral artery is disastrous inasmuch as it causes infarction (gangrene) of the lower extremity, but it is not necessarily life threatening. In contrast, a much smaller embolus that occludes the middle cerebral artery may lead to death in days, or even hours. On the other hand, impaction in the circle of Willis, depending on the state of the cerebral vessels, may be entirely compensated for by collateral flow. As with pulmonary emboli, prompt diagnosis and effective treatment—general supportive measures, anticoagulation, embolectomy—have greatly improved the prognosis of both life and limb. However, a significant mortality rate persists, largely related to the serious cardiovascular diseases that occasioned the thromboembolism.

AIR OR GAS EMBOLISM (CAISSON DISEASE OR DECOMPRESSION SICKNESS)

Bubbles of air may gain access to the circulation during delivery or abortion when they are forced into ruptured uterine venous sinuses by the powerful contractions of the uterus. Air embolization may also occur during the performance of a pneumothorax when a large artery or vein is ruptured or entered accidentally. It may also be observed when injury to the lung or the chest wall opens a large vein and permits the entrance of air during the negative pressure phase of inspiration. These bubbles of air act as physical masses. Many small bubbles may coalesce to produce frothy, gaseous masses, sufficiently large to occlude a major vessel, usually in the lungs or brain. Aggregates of larger size may become trapped in the chambers of the right heart and block the orifice of the pulmonary artery. Sudden death may result. Large quantities of air, probably somewhere in the neighborhood of 100 cc, are required to produce problems; the small amounts commonly introduced during intravenous therapy are of no significance, since they rapidly dissolve in the plasma.

When air or gas embolism is suspected, it is necessary at autopsy to open the heart and major pulmonary trunks under water to detect the escaping gas. At times the frothy appearance of the blood calls attention to the presence of the gaseous bubbles.

A specialized form of gas embolism, known as *caisson disease* or *decompression sickness*, occurs in persons exposed to sudden changes in atmospheric pressures. When air is breathed under high pressure, increased amounts of the inspired gases dissolve in the blood, tissue fluids, and fat. Nitrogen, in fact, is more soluble in fat than in body fluids, so that obese individuals are at greater risk. If the individual decompresses too rapidly the dissolved oxygen, carbon dioxide, and nitrogen will come out of solution as minute bubbles. The oxygen and carbon dioxide will be rapidly reabsorbed, but the nitrogen, which as mentioned has low *fluid* solubility, may remain as minute bubbles or may coalesce to form large masses of gas within the blood vessels and tissues. The sequence may occur in deep sea and scuba divers who ascend to the surface too rapidly, or during air flight in unpressurized cabins with rapid ascent to high altitudes.

Clinical symptoms arise from several sources. Gaseous bubbles may be formed within the interstitial tissues of the body, particularly within muscles, tendons, and ligaments, as a result of the changing local tissue tensions in these sites. Numerous minute emboli of nitrogen gas may emerge within vessels, causing, in the aggregate, vascular obstructions. Platelets may adhere to these bubbles and release such vasoconstrictive agents as serotonin and epinephrine. Concomitantly, platelet factor 3 may activate the coagulation mechanism. This combination of ischemic influences in and around the joints and skeletal muscles causes the patient to double up in pain, a phenomenon known as *the bends*. The same process may induce ischemic injury to the brain, causing mental disturbances and even coma. A similar mechanism in the lungs evokes edema, hemorrhages, and focal atelectasis or emphysema, leading sometimes to "*the chokes*"—sudden respiratory distress. Gas bubbles may cause infarction of the highly vascularized bones, with destruction of articular surfaces and joints. The heart may also be affected. These symptoms are promptly relieved by placing the individual in a compression chamber where the solution of the bubbles of nitrogen is accomplished by raising the barometric pressure.

FAT EMBOLISM SYNDROME

The fat embolism syndrome is basically characterized by progressive pulmonary insufficiency, mental deterioration, and sometimes renal insufficiency, usually developing 24 to 72 hours after fractures of bones containing fatty marrow, or after severe trauma to adipose tissue. The clinical findings have long been related to the entrance of myriad fat droplets into ruptured vessels, with extensive microembolic occlusions of the pulmonary, renal and cerebral circulations (Fig. 3–18). Currently, however, there is a growing suspicion that the pathogenesis of this condition is more complex, as discussed later.[63] Embolic fat can be identified at necropsy in approximately 90% of patients with multiple traumas and fractures.[64] However, only about 0.5 to 2% of patients with a single fracture or 5 to 10% of those with pelvic or multiple long-bone fractures develop clinical manifestations. Once developed, the syndrome has grave significance and a 10 to 15% overall mortality rate, which, as might be expected, worsens with increasingly severe fractures.

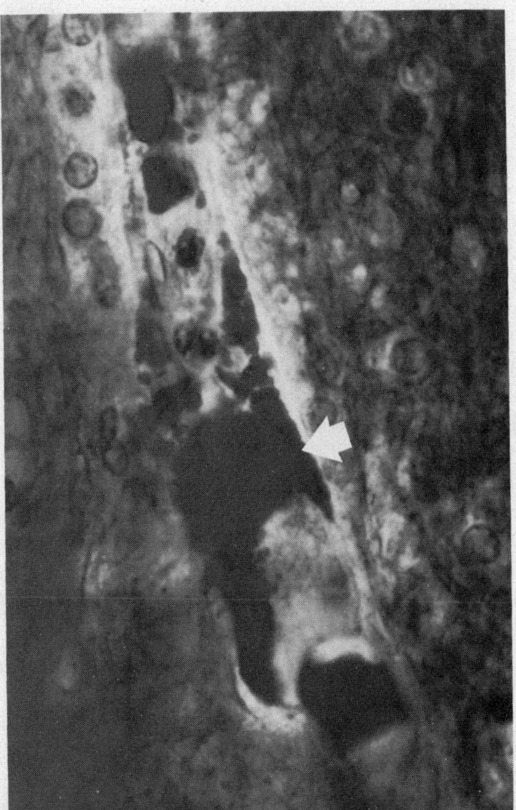

Figure 3–18. Fat embolism in the brain. An aggregate of darkly staining microemboli of fat *(arrow)* blocking a capillary in the brain.

Fat embolism can also be identified at postmortem, usually as a clinically insignificant finding in a variety of nontraumatic conditions such as alcoholism, diabetes mellitus, and chronic pancreatitis. The fact that trauma is not involved in any of these clinical conditions underscores the need to reconsider the pathogenesis of the fat embolism syndrome.

The various causative theories are interrelated and can be characterized as (a) mechanical, (b) emulsion instability-stress, (c) intravascular coagulation, and (d) chemical injury.

The mechanical theory is applicable to cases with severe trauma to adipose tissue or fat-bearing bones. Rupture of small vessels and damage to fat cells set the stage for the entrance of globules. Emboli greater than 20 microns in diameter are filtered out in the lungs to produce respiratory difficulties. Smaller emboli may squeeze through the pulmonary circulation to be dispersed throughout the arterial system, with greatest impact on the brain.

The emulsion instability-stress theory proposes that severe trauma or stress induces physicochemical changes in the blood leading to coalescence of chylomicrons into fat droplets. With any form of stress there is catecholamine release, with mobilization of lipids. The increased blood levels of neutral fats and free fatty acids may then induce the formation of more and larger chylomicrons, which may coalesce to produce the fat emboli. Adhesion and aggregation of platelets would enlarge their physical size.[65]

The coagulopathy theory is basically an extension of the mechanical and emulsion instability hypotheses. It proposes that intravascular coagulation is the major mediator of the obstructive features of the fat embolism syndrome, and that fat emboli potentiate and augment the process. This view of the pathogenesis of the fat embolism syndrome likens it to a specialized form of disseminated intravascular coagulation.

The chemical theory points to free fatty acids in the plasma as a cause of microvascular toxic injury and capillary blockage. Under normal circumstances, free fatty acids in the plasma are bound to albumin and are nontoxic. With stress there is increased mobilization of fatty acids to a level at which all can no longer be bound to albumin. The fatty acids then cause a chemical vascular lesion, principally in the lungs.[66]

All these proposed mechanisms may be valid. The fat embolism syndrome could be initiated by microglobules of fat derived either from injured bone marrow or peripheral fat depots. Stress-emulsion instability might then make a further contribution. Interactions with platelets could initiate intravascular coagulation. Release of fatty acids might then add an element of chemical injury. In this manner, respiratory failure and cerebral injury might occur.[67]

MORPHOLOGY. The diagnosis of this condition when suspected can sometimes be confirmed during the autopsy by gentle pressure on fresh slices of lung tissue immersed in saline, which releases the fat globules and permits them to float to the surface. Microscopic demonstration of the fat emboli within the vessels, principally of the lungs and brain, requires the use of frozen sections and fat stains, thereby avoiding the usual solvents employed in paraffin embedding of tissues. In addition there are a variety of pulmonary changes comprising essentially patchy foci of pulmonary edema, congestive atelectasis, and the escape of protein-rich fluid into the alveolar spaces with the formation of hyaline membranes—findings identical to those in the adult respiratory distress syndrome (p. 714). The central nervous system changes are extremely variable and depend on the severity of brain involvement and the duration of survival. At an early stage the brain may appear entirely normal on gross inspection, but it may contain microemboli of fat, demonstrable by the methods just described. Over the course of a few days, cerebral edema may appear, accompanied by microfoci of hemorrhage, most visible in the white matter.

Well-developed microinfarcts are sometimes present, but are uncommon. Characteristically there are petechiae of the skin (most prominent over the upper body), conjunctivae, and serosal membranes.

The fat embolism syndrome must be suspected when a patient develops sudden respiratory difficulty 24 to 72 hours after severe trauma (usually involving fracture of one or more large bones). However, as mentioned earlier, the syndrome may also occur in a wide variety of other settings, many of which are not associated with trauma. Central nervous system changes are classic but do not always appear. Other frequent features include petechiae on the skin and conjunctivae and fat microglobules in the urine. In some cases there is an abrupt drop in the plasma concentrations of fibrinogen and factors V and VIII as well as a transient fall in the platelet count. The blood levels of lipids, especially free fatty acids, are often elevated, as is the lipase activity. Supportive therapy, directed mainly to improving the respiratory insufficiency, is usually necessary, but as previously noted, 10 to 15% of patients die with the full-blown syndrome.

INFARCTION

An infarct is a localized area of ischemic necrosis in an organ or tissue resulting from sudden reduction of either its arterial supply or venous drainage. The vascular impediment is usually caused by thrombosis and/or embolism. However, vascular occlusion does not necessarily produce an area of ischemic necrosis, as will soon be seen. It may cause only atrophy or focal cell death or may even be without effect.

Interruption of the arterial blood supply to a tissue produces ischemic necrosis more certainly than does venous obstruction. Thrombosis of veins may lead to pulmonary arterial embolism, but if the thrombus remains in situ it may cause only stasis for a brief period until the increased venous pressure distal to the obstruction leads to dilatation of bypasses, which at least partially restores the vascular flow in the affected tissue. However, in organs having a single venous outflow channel devoid of bypass channels, occlusion of this outflow may induce infarction. Examples of this are seen when the venous drainage of the testis or ovary is blocked. Arterial flow must soon come to a standstill, since it has no escape through venous bypasses, and infarction often develops.

Much more rarely, narrowing of a vessel and infarction may be caused by other forms of vascular disease, such as a large atherosclerotic plaque in the wall of a medium- or small-sized artery, or by compression of vessels by expansile tumors or inflammatory fibrous adhesions. Myocardial infarcts may result when marked atherosclerosis severely narrows a coronary artery to a point where the available blood supply is inadequate to meet the myocardial demands (p. 556). Quite recently, spasm of already atherosclerotic and narrowed coronary arteries has aroused interest as another possible mechanism that may contribute to myocardial infarction. Vascular narrowing or occlusion may also result from the twisting of the pedicle of a mobile viscus, such as a loop of bowel or the ovary. The venous drainage or arterial supply of loops of bowel, which become trapped in narrow-mouthed hernial sacs, may also become severely reduced or totally compromised. External pressures and torsions usually lead to embarrassment of venous flow, since the veins are more readily compressed than the arteries.

TYPES OF INFARCTS. Infarcts are classified on the basis of their color and the presence or absence of bacterial contamination. Infarcts are either *anemic (white)* or *hemorrhagic (red)*.

White infarcts are encountered (1) with arterial occlusion and (2) in solid tissues. When a solid tissue is deprived of its arterial circulation, the infarct may be transiently hemorrhagic, but most become pale in a very short time. The reasons for the development of pallor in most organs are as follows. In the area of ischemia, vessels (particularly the capillaries) as well as parenchymal cells are destroyed. At the moment of vascular occlusion, blood from anastomotic peripheral vessels flows into the focus of injury, producing the initial hemorrhagic appearance. If the tissue affected is solid, the seepage of blood is minimal. Soon after the initial extravasation, the red cells are lysed, and the released hemoglobin pigment either diffuses out or is converted to hemosiderin. In solid organs, therefore, the arterial infarct will soon (24 to 48 hours) become pale. The heart, spleen, and kidneys are representative of solid, compact organs that tend to have pale infarcts (Fig. 3–19).

Red infarcts are encountered usually (1) with venous occlusions, (2) in loose tissues, (3) in tissues with a double circulation, and (4) in tissues previously congested. The loose, honeycombed tissue of the lung provides an example of hemorrhagic infarction secondary to arterial obstruction. At the moment of infarction, large amounts of hemorrhage collect in the spongy pulmonary parenchyma, so the arterial infarction re-

Fig. 3–19

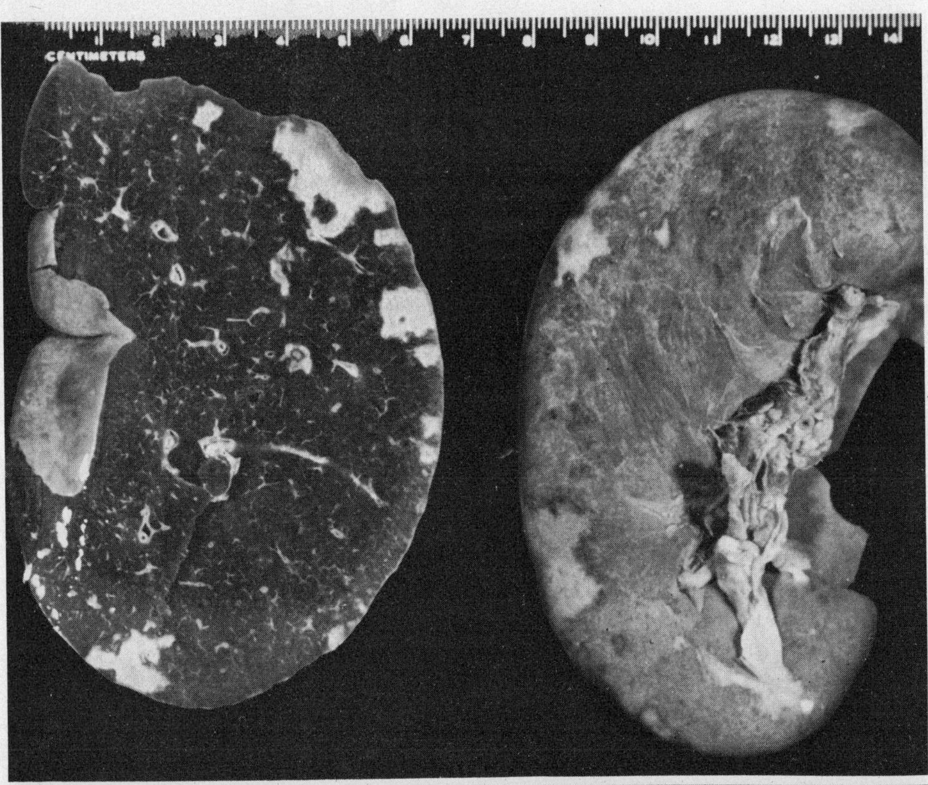

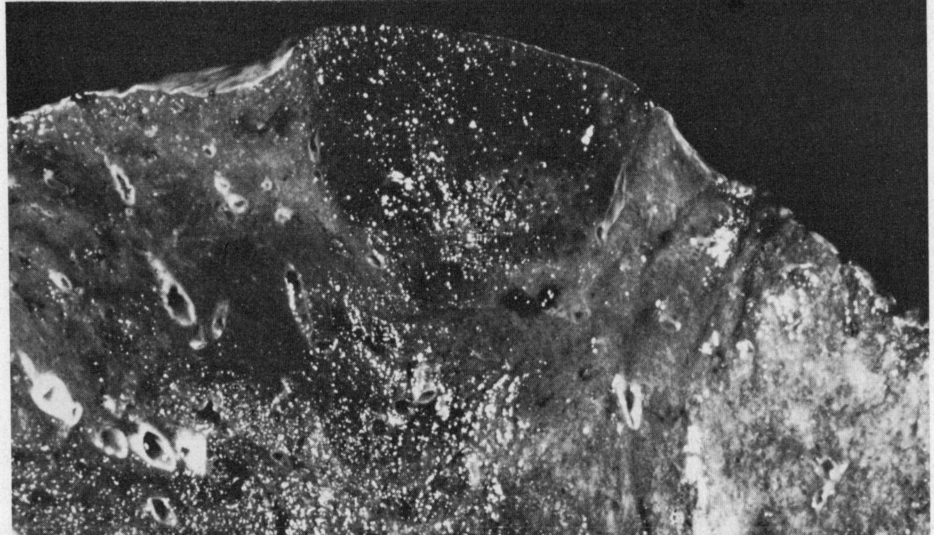

Fig. 3–20

Figure 3–19. Multiple small, peripheral, pale infarcts in a spleen viewed from the capsular surface and in cross section.

Figure 3–20. A sharply circumscribed hemorrhagic infarct in the lung.

mains red (Fig. 3–20). However, pale infarcts may occasionally be encountered in the lung or hemorrhagic infarcts in the compact organs. Prior congestion may lead to hemorrhagic infarction as occurs, for example, with twisting of the pedicle of the ovary. The thin-walled ovarian veins are occluded first, causing intense congestion and infarction with or without occlusion of the artery. The small intestine is another site where red infarcts typically occur. Venous occlusions or even arterial occlusions may cause hemorrhagic infarction of long segments of the intestine. The explanation lies in the rich arterial anastomoses between the many branches of the superior mesenteric artery, which permit arterial flow to the injured segment through anastomosing arcades. Indeed, this type of vascular supply may well protect against ischemic damage (p. 111). Hemorrhagic arterial infarction is sometimes encountered in the brain as well. An embolus to a large artery such as the middle cerebral may produce a nonhemorrhagic area of cerebral infarction. Soon thereafter, the embolus may shatter, and the fragments may move into smaller, more peripheral branches. Reflow through the major trunk may yield extensive hemorrhage into the primary area of ischemic necrosis.

Infarcts are also classified as either *septic* or *bland*, depending on the presence or absence of bacterial infection in the area of necrosis. Bacterial contamination may be due to organisms present in the tissue prior to the development of the ischemic necrosis, as in infarction of a lung already affected by bacterial pneumonia; may be brought to the area by an infected blood clot, as occurs with embolization of a fragment of bacterial vegetation from a heart valve; or may result from bacteremic seeding of the margins of the area of ischemic necrosis.

Morphology. Whether hemorrhagic or pale, all infarcts tend to be wedge-shaped, with the apex of the wedge pointing toward the focus of vascular occlusion. Since all the dependent tissue out to the periphery of the organ is affected, the external aspect of the organ forms the base of the wedge. The exact outline of the infarct may be quite variable, and sometimes maplike patterns result from the preservation of small marginal areas of tissue that have different and unaffected sources of blood supply.

A few hours after onset, all infarcts are somewhat poorly defined, are slightly darker in color than normal, and have a firmer consistency than surrounding normal tissue. During the next 24 hours, the demarcation becomes better defined, and the color change is more intense. In solid organs, the infarct may then appear paler than normal as the small amounts of hemorrhage are lysed, whereas in the spongy tissues the massive hemorrhage makes the lesion red-blue. The firmer consistency of the infarct is due to the suffusion of blood or inflammatory exudation.

In the course of several days, pale infarcts become yellow-white and sharply demarcated, while the appearance of the pulmonary hemorrhagic infarcts remains relatively unchanged. The margins of both types of infarcts tend to become better defined by a narrow rim of hyperemia due to the marginal inflammatory response (Fig. 3–21). The involved surface of the organ is usually covered by an inflammatory exudation, which is commonly fibrinous. In venous thrombosis and infarction as, for example, in the small intestine, the areas of hemorrhagic necrosis may be somewhat poorly delimited.

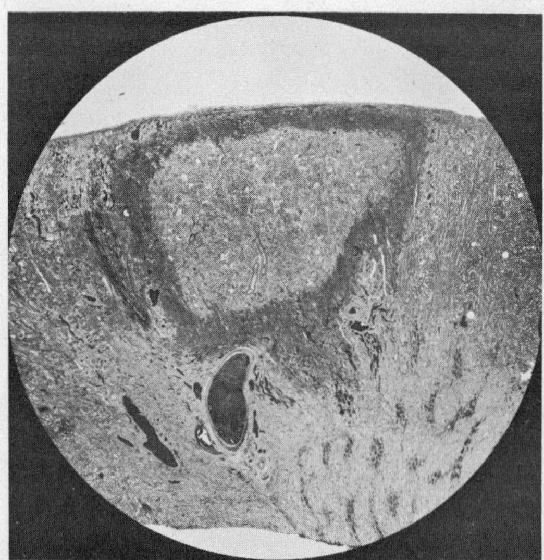

Figure 3–21. A low-power view of a small renal infarct enclosed within a zone of dark hyperemia and hemorrhage.

The characteristic cytologic change of all infarcts, save those in the brain, is ischemic coagulative necrosis of the affected cells (p. 15) (Fig. 3–22). The tissue cells undergo the progressive changes of coagulative necrosis and resorption discussed in Chapter 1. These basic changes

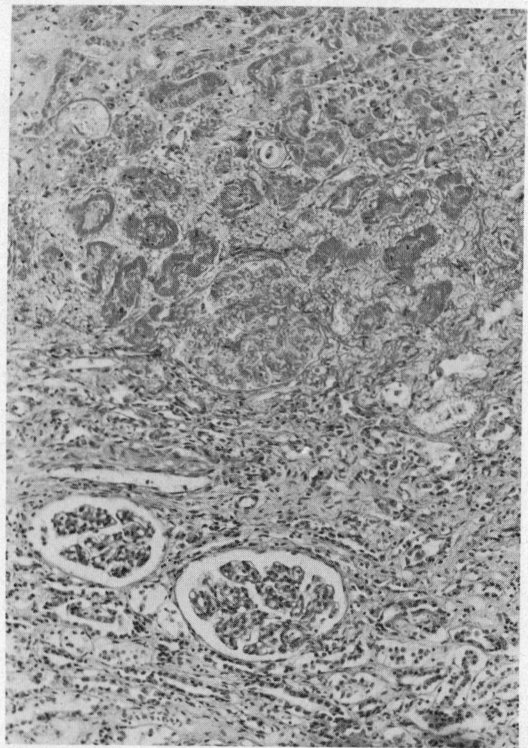

Figure 3–22. The margin of a renal infarct in detail. Outlines of coagulated tubules remain (*above*) and are separated from the normal renal substance by a wide band of fibrosis.

may be considerably masked or modified by the extensive hemorrhage in hemorrhagic infarcts and by the bacterial suppuration in septic infarcts. If the vascular occlusion has occurred only a few hours prior to the death of the patient, there may be no demonstrable cellular change, since there may have been insufficient time for enzymic alteration of the dead cells. If the patient survives for about 12 to 18 hours, only hemorrhagic suffusion may be present.

Inflammatory exudation begins after the first few hours and becomes better defined over the next few days. The inflammatory reaction is followed by a fibroblastic, reparative response beginning in the preserved margins. Some parenchymal regeneration may occur at the periphery where the underlying framework of the organ has been spared. However, in most cases the necrotic focus is eventually replaced by scar tissue. In very large infarcts, replacement of the central necrotic tissue may be long delayed. In some infarcts, months-old, dense, fibrous scar may be found enclosing areas of persistent ischemic necrosis. Ultimately, however, these infarctions end up as fibrous scars, just as do all areas of extensive tissue destruction (Fig. 3–23).

The brain is an exception to these generalizations. When it suffers ischemic necrosis the affected area promptly and rapidly undergoes **liquefaction** (p. 15). The microglia constitute the scavenger cells of the brain, and these phagocytize the cellular debris while the other glial cells in the margins proliferate and invade the area (gliosis) to form the reparative scar.

With septic infarction the lesion is converted to an abscess and, if seen at a very late stage, may be unrecognizable as an infarct. The inflammatory reaction is correspondingly greater, but the eventual sequence of organization follows the pattern already described.

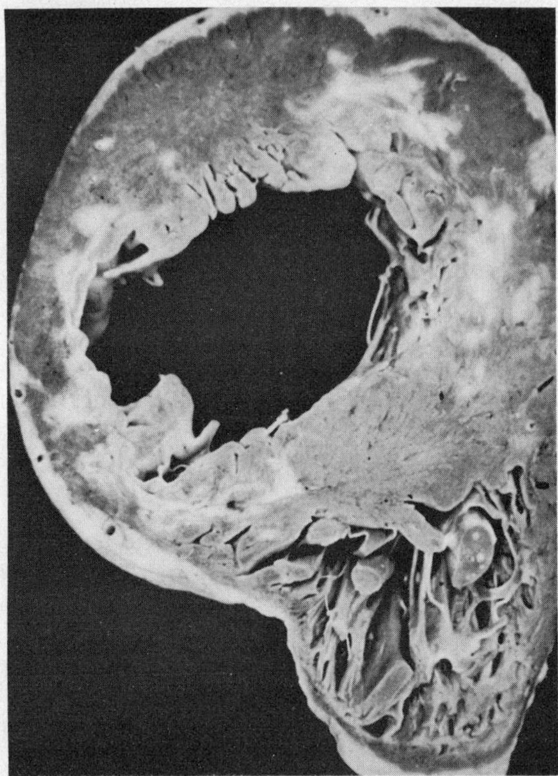

Figure 3–23. Numerous old myocardial infarcts have resulted in scattered pale fibrous scars throughout the myocardium.

FACTORS CONDITIONING SEVERITY OF INJURY RESULTING FROM VASCULAR OCCLUSION. Both arterial and venous vascular obstructions may be without effect or may cause only atrophy or single cell necroses. The extent to which a tissue is disturbed by occlusion of its venous or arterial connections depends on a number of factors: (1) the general status of the blood and the cardiovascular system, (2) the anatomic pattern of the vascular supply, (3) the rate of development of the occlusion, and (4) the vulnerability of the tissue to ischemia.

General Status of Blood and Cardiovascular System. Any systemic alteration that reduces the oxygen-carrying capacity of the blood, or the velocity and volume of blood flow through the tissue, predisposes to infarction. Severe anemia or hypoxemia (as in chronic cardiac or lung disease) also predisposes to infarction. Anemia may exert its effect not only by reduction in the hemoglobin mass but also in other ways. Sickle cell anemia is characterized by logjamming of the misshapen erythrocytes, and the stasis creates tissue hypoxia. Infarctions are common in these patients. In the very aged patient with marked coronary atherosclerosis, myocardial infarction may occur subsequent to the development of severe anemia or sudden drops in blood pressure, even in the absence of total occlusion of a vessel. Cardiac failure, blood loss, and shock impair the oxygenation of all tissues and thereby render tissues vulnerable to further diminution of their vascular supply.

Anatomic Patterns of Arterial Supply. The various tissues and organs of the body receive their arterial supply through one of four patterns: (1) a double blood supply; (2) parallel arterial systems; (3) a "single" arterial supply with rich interarterial anastomoses; and (4) a "single" arterial supply with few anastomoses, insufficient to provide adequate bypass channels, so-called "end arteries." Obviously there are many gradations between the last two patterns. The lungs and the liver are examples of organs fortunately provided with dual blood supplies. In individuals having a normal hematologic and cardiovascular status, the bronchial circulation is often capable of preventing ischemic necrosis when a radicle of the pulmonary artery is obstructed. Similarly, infarction is extremely uncommon in the liver because the portal supply of blood may be adequate even when the hepatic arterial flow is compromised. However, in the presence of cardiac failure, severe anemia, or reduced oxygenation of the blood, occlusion of one system may precipitate ischemic necrosis.

Parallel arterial systems are encountered in the forearm and brain. Either the radial or the ulnar artery is sufficient to sustain the vitality of the tissues of the forearm when the other is occluded. The brain with its circle of Willis is protected from ischemic injury resulting from an occlusion at any point *in* the circle of Willis or in one of the major arteries *supplying* the circle. Such a proposition, of course, implies the absence of preexisting vascular disease within the circle of Willis. These comments should not be construed to apply to the arterial supply to the brain *derived from* the circle of Willis. Occlusion of one of the cerebral or cerebellar arteries will, of course, cause infarction of the dependent region of the brain.

The small intestine is the prototype of a tissue enjoying an arterial supply with rich interarterial anastomoses. The branches of the superior mesenteric artery are interconnected by looping arcades enabling blood to bypass focal occlusion. If, however, one of the primary divisions of the superior mesenteric artery or the main artery itself is obstructed, the arcades cannot provide compensation.

The kidney is the unfortunate victim of an arterial supply composed of "end arteries." The major branches of the renal artery supply well-defined segments of the kidneys, and occlusion of one of the major branches or, of course, the main renal artery is almost invariably followed by ischemic necrosis.

The heart is an example of an organ having an intermediate pattern of fairly rich interarterial anastomoses that may compensate for narrowing or occlusion of one of the three main trunks of the coronary arterial system. Perfusion techniques have confirmed the presence of fine interarterial anastomoses joining each of the major coronary trunks to the others.[68] When one major trunk is compromised, the collateral supply from an unaffected trunk may suffice to prevent ischemic injury.

Thus, the anatomic pattern of the vascular supply of a tissue materially modifies the consequence of a vascular occlusion.

Rate of Development of Occlusion. Slowly developing occlusions are far better tolerated than those occurring suddenly, since they provide an opportunity for alternative pathways and collaterals to become activated.

Vulnerability of Tissue to Ischemia. Tissues of the body vary widely in their susceptibility to ischemic hypoxia. The neurons of the central nervous system are undoubtedly the most sensitive, and complete ischemia for a period of only a few minutes may produce irreversible changes. Indeed, a hierarchy of vulnerability to ischemia has been described for the varying cell types within the brain.[69] Cerebral cortical neurons are most sensitive to ischemia, followed in order by those in the cerebellum and by those in the basal ganglia. The glial cells are more resistant than neurons but also have differing sensitivities. The epithelial cells of the proximal convoluted renal tubules (more so than the other tubular segments) and the myocardial cells are likewise exquisitely sensitive to hypoxia. By contrast, the mesenchymal tissues of the body are in general quite resistant. The robustness of the fibroblast may permit the framework and stroma of a tissue to remain vital despite ischemic necrosis of its more sensitive parenchymal cells.

CLINICAL SIGNIFICANCE OF INFARCTION. In the U.S. over half of all deaths are caused by cardiovascular disease. Most of these cardiovascular deaths result from myocardial and cerebral infarctions. Coronary heart disease alone accounts for about 30% of all the mortality, and myocardial infarction is by far the predominant cause of fatal coronary heart disease. Cerebral infarction (encephalomalacia) is also the most frequent type of central nervous system disease. Pulmonary infarction is an extremely common complication in a variety of clinical settings, as has been indicated, and is reported to be the cause of death in 10 to 15% of hospitalized patients. Renal infarction does not have the paramount importance of these other forms mentioned. It is, nonetheless, an occasional cause of renal failure and death and is a not uncommon cause of clinical signs and symptoms. Ischemic necrosis (gangrene) of the lower extremities is a relatively unusual clinical problem in the population at large but is a major concern in diabetics. Infarction of tissues, therefore, is a common cause of clinical illness.

Thrombosis, embolism, and infarction may strike without notice, but even worse, they are proverbial vultures, stalking every ill, bedridden, and aged patient who regrettably is least able to cope with them.

SHOCK

Shock, often referred to as hemodynamic or vascular collapse, may be caused by any serious assault on the body's homeostasis, such as profuse hemorrhage, severe trauma or burns, extensive myocardial infarction, massive pulmonary embolism, or uncontrolled bacterial sepsis. Although the initiating hemodynamic derangement among such varied clinical conditions may differ, ultimately *all cases of shock are characterized by a disproportion between the circulating blood volume and the volume of the circulatory system that needs to be filled. The disproportion is usually secondary to blood loss, reduced cardiac output, or deranged peripheral vasomotor control. Thus, an effective circulating blood volume cannot be maintained.*[70] *Shock may be defined, then, as a state of inadequate perfusion of all cells and tissues, which at first leads to reversible hypoxic injury, but if sufficiently protracted or grave, to irreversible cell and organ injury and sometimes to the death of the patient.* The cellular hypoxia induces a shift from aerobic to anaerobic metabolism, resulting in increased lactate production and sometimes in lactic acidosis. Thus, the syndrome begins as a hemodynamic problem that eventuates in a cellular oxygen deficit and metabolic derangement.

The clinical signs and symptoms of shock are inconstant and vary with the precipitating insult and the duration of the shock state. The most classic syndrome consists of hypotension, a weak thready pulse, tachycardia, hyperventilation, cool clammy skin, pallor or sometimes cyanosis, oliguria, and variable mental changes (obtundation, restlessness, or apprehension). With shock induced by bacterial sepsis there may at first be peripheral vasodilatation, and the patient may appear warm, dry, and flushed for a time, but with progression the more classic syndrome appears. In addition to the clinical features relating to the shock state, the patient may also manifest the signs and symptoms relating to the precipitating disease, e.g., severe chest pain in myocardial infarction, or the disability and discomfort produced by the trauma or burn.

CLASSIFICATION. The terminology and classification of shock vary. Sometimes the terminology is based on the nature of the precipitating event, e.g., "traumatic shock," "burn shock," and "septic shock." Such terms, however, provide no clue to the pathophysiologic derangement responsible for the shock state. Toward this objective the following classification (Table 3–4) can be offered. Each of the categories represents a distinctive hemodynamic mechanism of reducing the effective circulating blood volume.

Reduced cardiac output, often referred to as *cardiogenic shock*, constitutes in essence "pump failure." Myocardial infarction is overwhelmingly the commonest cause of marked reduction of the cardiac output, but the other conditions cited within this category have the same consequence.

Hypovolemia as a mechanism is frequently called *hemorrhagic shock*. However, hypovolemia may be related to fluid loss, such as vomiting, diarrhea, excessive transudation and exudation of fluid from burn wounds, or sequestration of transudate and exudate in the peritoneal cavity. The basis for the reduction in effective circulating blood volume is obvious.

Pooling of blood in the peripheral circulation is another way in which the effective circulating blood volume may be reduced. Blood may be impounded in the periphery by interference with the neural controls of normal vasomotor function. The arterial pressure is normally maintained by both the cardiac output and the peripheral resistance exerted at the level of peripheral arterioles. With diminution of this peripheral resistance, the capillary and venular beds at first become distended with blood. Venoconstriction may then occur, impounding the blood within the periphery. Bacterial infection, often called *septic* or *bacterial shock*, also produces peripheral pooling. The most common organisms involved are the "gram-negative" endotoxin-producing aerobic rods—*E. coli, Klebsiella pneumoniae, Proteus* species, and *Pseudomonas aeruginosa*—hence the designation *endotoxic shock*.[71] Gram-positive septicemias, particularly pneumococcal or streptococcal, may produce a similar clinical syndrome. Whatever the offending agent, the peripheral circulation is affected. Direct toxic injury possibly induces arteriolar vasodilatation and pooling of blood. The elevated capillary pressure leads to escape of plasma water into the interstitial compartment, further impinging on the circulating blood volume. An inflammatory-immune reaction conceivably leads to the release of vasodilators, such as histamine and complement fractions, further reducing the effective circulating volume.[72] Now it may be apparent why some patients appear warm and flushed. Platelet activation and the formation of thromboxane A_2 may add an element of platelet aggregation, possibly with activation of the clotting sequence and the induction of disseminated intravascular coagulation.[73] There is no dearth of theories.

A number of other mechanisms may induce shock. With *anaphylaxis*, there is production of anaphylatoxins and release of histamine from mast cells, both causing peripheral vasodilatation. Concomitant vascular injury with increased transudation and exudation provides yet another mechanism for disruption of the hemodynamic homeostasis. *Disseminated intravascular coagulation* poses a complex problem. It may in some instances initiate shock. More often, DIC appears as a complication that develops late in shock, initiated by other mechanisms. As pointed out above, it may occur during endotoxic shock, when it appears to be an effect rather than the cause of the shock state. In any event it is clear that in all of the categories, the normal hemodynamics are unhinged and lead to the low-perfusion state characteristic of shock.

Table 3–4. PATHOPHYSIOLOGIC CLASSIFICATION OF SHOCK

Cardiogenic Shock (Pump Failure)—Reduced Cardiac Output
- Myocardial infarction
- Rupture of heart
- Cardiac tamponade
- Pulmonary embolism
- Obstruction to valvular orifice—ball valve thrombus, atrial myxoma
- Arrhythmias—severe bradycardia, ventricular tachycardia, or fibrillation

Hypovolemia
- Hemorrhage
- Fluid loss
  - vomiting
  - diarrhea
  - excessive sweating
  - extensive bone or soft tissue injury
  - burns
  - intraperitoneal sequestration of fluid—ascites, peritonitis, pancreatitis, bowel gangrene

Pooling of Blood in Periphery
- Neuropathic—spinal cord injury, anesthesia, ganglionic and adrenergic blocker drugs
- Bacterial infection—gram-negative endotoxemia, gram-positive septicemia

Other Mechanisms
- Anaphylaxis
- Disseminated intravascular coagulation

PATHOGENESIS. Shock is a progressive disorder that, if unhalted, spirals downward into ever more grave levels of hemodynamic and metabolic deterioration. The pathogenesis is best considered, then, from the standpoint of the evolution of the changes over time. The progression may be tumultuous, and the patient may go into profound shock within minutes of a massive hemorrhage or extensive myocardial infarct involving more than 40% of the left ventricular wall. More often, it evolves over a span of hours. It should be emphasized, however, that *progression is not inevitable and by no means all patients die*. With mild shock, such as may occur in a previously healthy individual with an acute loss of as much as 10% of the normal blood volume, reflex compensatory mechanisms may maintain adequate perfusion of vital organs, and the patient may recover relatively promptly, often without treatment. Even with a more serious insult, therapeutic intervention aimed at restoring the circulating blood volume and arterial pressure can usually interrupt the natural course. Indeed, although death may be caused by the direct effects of hypoxic injury to vital organs, more often the mortality is related to inability to control the initial event that precipitated the shock. Recognizing, then, that the following sequence of events is not inevitable, three somewhat arbitrary stages or phases of shock can be defined.

Stage I. Compensated hypotension—"early shock." Whatever the basis for the reduction in circulating blood volume and hypotension, reflex mechanisms are promptly activated, speeding the heart rate and constricting the peripheral arteriolar bed. As pointed out earlier, in endotoxic shock there may be a transient period of peripheral vasodilatation, but it soon gives way to vasoconstriction. The vasoconstriction is mediated by the discharge of norepinephrine from sympathetic nerve endings, and both norepinephrine and epinephrine from the adrenal. The extent of the constriction differs among the vascular beds. It is most profound in the skin and skeletal muscles, thereby diverting flow elsewhere, particularly to the brain and heart. Cerebral blood vessels lack sympathetic innervation, while the vasculature of the heart, despite its rich sympathetic connections, is largely under the control of local metabolism. At the same time, the renin-angiotensin-aldosterone axis is called into play, which contributes to peripheral vasoconstriction and more gradually restores blood volume by retaining sodium and water. Other humoral factors such as antidiuretic hormone (ADH) and prostaglandins, as well as local autoregulatory mechanisms, also contribute to the response. At this stage in the evolution of the shock state the patient might well manifest tachycardia and some coolness and pallor of the skin, although the function of vital organs is not yet seriously impaired. Therapeutic intervention, if needed, would very likely arrest the progression of the shock state, but in the absence of significant hypotension the gravity of the situation might go unappreciated.

Stage II. Tissue hypoperfusion. If therapy has not been instituted and the compensatory mechanisms, although maximal, are insufficient to correct the deficit in circulating blood volume, the stage of tissue hypoperfusion commences. Even the vital organs—brain, heart, lungs, and kidneys—are affected. The oxygen deficit forces the cells to revert to anaerobic glycolytic metabolism to the extent possible. Pyruvate, formed from the metabolism of glycogen and glucose, is converted to lactic acid. Cellular acidosis may then develop and lactate may spill over into the plasma to produce a lactic acidosis. The reduced hepatic blood flow and impaired clearance of lactate contributes to the *lactic acidosis, which constitutes one of the characteristic metabolic changes in all forms of fully-developed shock.* At the same time, a sequence of microcirculatory changes unfolds to worsen the ever-deepening crisis. In early shock the vasoconstriction that appears under the influence of sympatho-adrenal responses involves both precapillary arterioles and postcapillary venules. Thus, while the flow to the capillary beds is reduced, the capillary pressure is at normal or near-normal levels. However, the vasoconstriction itself contributes to the reduced perfusion of organs. With progressive tissue hypoxia and acidosis the arterioles dilate or, more correctly, can no longer sustain their vasomotor control, but the venules remain constricted. In large measure this differential vasoconstriction reflects the fact that arterioles are more sensitive to oxygen deprivation than are venules. As a consequence there is pooling of blood and stagnant hypoxia in the capillary beds throughout the body. Moreover, the elevated hydrostatic pressure in the capillaries increases the transudation of fluid into the interstitial tissue compartment. Both phenomena thus worsen the deteriorating hemodynamics. Manifestations of organ injury make their appearance, such as mental obtundation and a fall in urinary output, and individuals with preexisting coronary atherosclerosis are at risk of developing a myocardial infarct, or suffer at least depressed cardiac function. It is evident at this point that matters have gone from bad to worse!

Stage III. Cell and organ injury. At some point in the downward spiral, the hypoperfusion and oxygen deficit cause at first reversible, and then irreversible, hypoxic injury to cells. The loss of energy-generating mechanisms impairs membrane transport systems and maintenance of membrane integrity. Increased membrane permeability permits lysosomal enzymes to leak out, contributing to the cell injury and the aggravation of the shock state. The stagnant hypoxia in the capillaries damages endothelial cells, leading to further leakage of fluid and proteins. In animal models, the formation of prostacyclin and TxA_2 has been documented, contributing to the vasodilatation and initiating platelet adhesion and aggregation with the release of vasoactive platelet factors.[73] Activation of the clotting sequence, either by platelet activation or endothelial cell injury, has the potential for inducing DIC—an ominous turn of events.

Cardiac insufficiency is likely to appear in all forms of severe shock; the origin of this failure is not clear. It could be related to global myocardial ischemia, but a circulating cardiotoxic factor—myocardial depressant factor (MDF)—has been identified in both experimental models and in humans during the shock state.[74] MDF is a small polypeptide liberated from the ischemic pancreas that causes direct depression of myocardial function.[75] Ischemic injury to the gastrointestinal mucosa may permit intestinal flora and their products to enter the circulation, a situation that may contribute an element of endotoxic shock to the already grave crisis. Renal damage is likely in advanced shock, producing morphologic changes referred to as *acute tubular necrosis* (ATN); thus, acute renal failure with its electrolyte imbalances makes its unwanted contribution to the already critically ill patient. Is death inevitable at this juncture? Although it may be imminent, there is no evidence that shock in humans ever reaches a stage of irreversibility if the trigger event that initiated the shock can be controlled. Nonetheless, the hypoxic injury to vital organs may be lethal. Shock not only stops the machine, but also wrecks the machinery.

MORPHOLOGY. As expected, the changes induced by shock take the form of ischemic injury. The cellular and subcellular alterations have been meticulously detailed by Trump[76,77] and were described on page 13. While such cellular injury is bodywide, certain organs are more severely affected than others because of shunting of blood to the heart and brain and away from other organs, and because of differing cellular vulnerabilities to hypoxic and metabolic injury.

The principal threats to life stem from injury to the brain, heart, lungs, and kidneys, but morphologic changes are frequent in the gastrointestinal tract, adrenals, and liver.

The **brain** suffers so-called "ischemic encephalopathy," described in detail on page 1389.

The **heart** is affected in all forms of shock, whether cardiogenic in origin or some other form. Obviously in cardiogenic shock there is the primary cardiac or extracardiac disease that initiated the shock syndrome.

Two types of distinctive cardiac change appear in all forms of shock: (1) subepicardial and subendocardial hemorrhages and necroses and (2) zonal lesions, also called banding (Fig. 3–24).[78,79] The necroses range from isolated fiber ischemic lesions to larger areas of involvement comprising micro- or macroinfarcts. The zonal lesions constitute opaque transverse bands (p. 561) within a myocyte usually close to an intercalated disc, accompanied by shortening and scalloping of the sarcomere, fragmentation of the Z bands, distortion of the myofilaments, and displacement of the mitochondria away from the intercalated disc. These lesions are not distinctive of shock and may appear with coronary artery insufficiency.

The **lung** is quite resistant to ischemia and so may not be affected in pure hypovolemic shock. But anatomic alterations are prominent in shock incited by bacterial sepsis and trauma, and are referred to as "shock lung." The pulmonary changes are generically referred to as "adult respiratory distress syndrome" or "diffuse alveolar damage" and are encountered in many other clinical settings (discussed on p. 714). In essence they include severe intraseptal edema, followed later by the collection of edema fluid and exuded plasma proteins within the alveolar spaces.

The **kidneys** are major targets in severe shock, principally affecting the tubules at all levels of the nephron. As stated earlier, the tubular lesions are referred to as acute tubular necrosis (ATN). Once again, ATN is not limited to the shock state and so is described in detail on page 1027.

The **adrenal** lesions encountered in shock constitute the reaction of this gland to all forms of stress, and hence might be designated as the "stress response." These begin as focal depletion of lipids within the cortical cells, transforming them from their usual clear vacuolated state to the nonvacuolated, so-called compact cells (p. 1232). This transformation begins within the zona reticularis and then spreads outward toward the capsule to the adjacent zona fasciculata. Scattered necroses of isolated cortical cells may create apparent lumina or "pseudotubules." The loss of corticolipids has erroneously been interpreted as adrenal exhaustion. Ultrastructural studies, however, show that the compact cells contain increased numbers of organelles, indicating a morphologic response to increased functional activity, with mobilization of the steroids as a response to the stress.

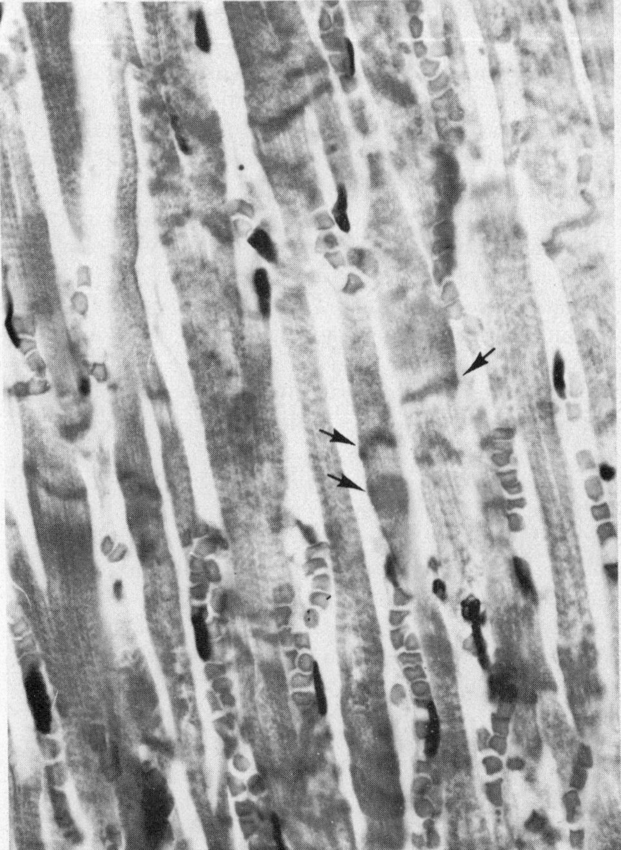

Figure 3–24. Contraction bands *(arrows)* in a heart suffering from hypoperfusion. The heavy bands should not be confused with the more delicate cross striations of cardiac myocytes.

The **gastrointestinal tract** may develop patchy, mucosal hemorrhages and necroses designated as "hemorrhagic gastroenteropathy," described on p. 831.

The **liver** sometimes accumulates fat within the hepatocytes. In severe shock states, central necrosis may appear within the lobule.

With certain exceptions, the cellular and organ changes encountered in shock are reversible if the patient survives. Thus, regeneration of renal tubular cells, adrenocortical cells, hepatocytes, and gastrointestinal mucosa may restore the normal architecture of these organs. Loss of neurons from the brain and of myocytes within the heart and development of pulmonary septal fibrosis may constitute irreversible damage, but cellular injury severe enough to lead to such changes is encountered only in the patient with extreme, usually lethal, forms of shock. In those who survive, therefore, the function of these organs is usually not detectably altered.

CLINICAL CORRELATIONS. The *initial threats* to the life of the patient in shock arise from the medical, surgical, or obstetric catastrophe that initiated the shock state. However, the cerebral and cardiac changes described worsen the early crisis. If these hazards are survived, metabolic acidosis, shifts in electrolyte levels, and respiratory difficulties occur. The pulmonary changes in particular markedly increase the amount of work required for a given level of alveolar ventilation, giving rise to the clinical term "lung stiffness."

The "fortunate" patient survives to enter a *second phase* of clinical problems, dominated by renal dysfunction. This may appear any time from the second to the sixth day and is characterized by a dramatic fall in urine output, reflecting the reduction of renal blood flow and glomerular filtration and the impaired tubular function. The oliguria may persist for days to a few weeks, with urine levels of only a few milliliters a day. The clinical dilemma is now dominated by the signs and symptoms of fluid overload, hyperkalemia, acidosis, and sometimes uremia. Fortunately, ATN is reversible, and with appropriate therapy most patients can be maintained during this period of renal shutdown to recover fully from this phase.

The *third* or *diuretic phase* begins with a steady increase in urine volume, reaching possibly 3 liters per day. This urinary flood heralds a regeneration of the tubular epithelium, but tubular malfunction persists, and various electrolyte imbalances may now occur. For somewhat obscure reasons, in this stage of the course, vulnerability to infections is increased, perhaps because of reduced immunologic competence, and about 20% of deaths from ATN occur during the diuretic phase.

Despite all these therapeutic nightmares, most patients survive when the inciting cause of the shock can be controlled. Thus, patients with hypovolemic and neurogenic shock have the best prognosis. It is those with cardiogenic shock, usually initiated by massive myocardial infarction, and those with "gram-negative" endotoxic shock who have a mortality rate as high as 70 to 80%. It is sad to note that this rate has not been lowered over the last generation, despite all efforts to devise effective therapy.

---

1. Arcidi, J. M., Jr., et al.: Hepatic morphology in cardiac dysfunction: a clinicopathologic study of 1000 subjects at autopsy. Am. J. Pathol. *104*:159, 1981.
2. Schafer, A. I., and Handin, R. I.: The role of platelets in thrombotic and vascular disease. Prog. Cardiovasc. Dis. *22*:31, 1979.
3. Gimbrone, M. A.: Vascular endothelium and atherosclerosis. *In* Moore, S. (ed.): The Biochemistry of Disease. New York, Marcel Dekker, 1981, p. 25.
4. Gimbrone, M. A., Jr.: Endothelial dysfunction and the pathogenesis of atherosclerosis. *In* Gotto, A. M., Jr., Smith, L. C., and Allen, B. (eds.): Atherosclerosis. V. Proceedings of the Fifth International Symposium on Atherosclerosis. New York, Springer-Verlag, 1980, p. 415.
5. Gamse, G., et al.: Metabolism of sulfated glycosaminoglycans in cultured endothelial cells and smooth muscle cells from bovine aorta. Biochim. Biophys. Acta *544*:514, 1978.
6. Pearson, J. D., and Gordon, J. L.: Vascular endothelial and smooth muscle cells in culture selectively release adenine nucleotides. Nature *281*:384, 1979.
7. Colucci, M., et al.: Cultured human endothelial cells generate tissue factor in response to endotoxin. J. Clin. Invest. *71*:1893, 1983.
8. Birdwell, C. R., et al.: Identification, localization and role of fibronectin in cultured bovine endothelial cells. Proc. Natl. Acad. Sci. U.S.A. *75*:3273, 1978.
9. Weiss, H. J.: Platelet physiology and abnormalities of platelet function. N. Engl. J. Med. *293*:580, 1975.
10. Charo, I. F.: Interactions of platelet aggregation and secretion. J. Clin. Invest. *60*:866, 1977.
11. Shattil, S. J., and Bennett, J. S.: Platelets and their membranes in hemostasis: Physiology and pathophysiology. Ann. Intern. Med. *94*:108, 1980.
12. Olley, P. M., and Coceani, F.: The prostaglandins. Am. J. Dis. Child. *134*:688, 1980.
13. Moncada, S., and Vane, J. R.: Arachidonic acid metabolites and the interactions between platelets and blood-vessel walls. N. Engl. J. Med. *300*:1142, 1979.
14. Gerrard, J. M., and White, J. G.: Prostaglandins and thromboxane: "Middlemen" modulating platelet function in hemostasis and thrombosis. Prog. Hemost. Thromb. *4*:87, 1978.
15. Haiviger, J.: Prostacyclin inhibits mobilization of fibrinogen-binding sites on human ADP- and thrombin-treated platelets. Nature *283*:195, 1980.
16. Baugh, R. F., and Houghie, C.: The chemistry of blood coagulation. Clin. Haematol. *8*:3, 1979.
17. Hirsch, J.: Hypercoagulability. Semin. Haematol. *14*:409, 1977.
18. Ogston, D., and Bennett, B.: Naturally occurring inhibitors of coagulation. *In* Ogston, D., and Bennett, B. (eds.): Haemostasis: Biochemistry, Physiology, and Pathology. London, John Wiley and Sons, 1977, p. 202.
19. Esmon, C. T., and Owen, W. G.: Formation and functions of the anticoagulant protein, activated protein C. *In* Bing, D. H., and Rosenbaum, R. A. (eds.): Plasma and Cellular Modulatory Proteins. Boston, Center for Blood Research, 1981, p. 203.
20. Brozovic, M. A.: Mechanisms of deep vein thrombus: A review. J. R. Soc. Med. *72*:602, 1979.
21. Wall, R. T., and Harker, L. A.: The endothelium and thrombosis. Annu. Rev. Med. *31*:361, 1980.
22. Spaet, T. H., and Gaynor, E.: Vascular endothelial damage and thrombosis. Adv. Cardiol. *4*:47, 1970.
23. Wessler, S., and Yiu, E. T.: On the mechanism of thrombosis. Prog. Hematol. *6*:201, 1969.
24. Hume, M., et al.: Venous Thrombosis and Pulmonary Embolism. Cambridge, Harvard University Press, 1970, p. 25.
25. Sevitt, S.: The structure and growth of valve-pocket thrombi in femoral veins. J. Clin. Pathol. *27*:517, 1974.
26. Deykin, D., and Wessler, S.: Activation product, factor IX, serum thrombotic accelerator activity and serum-induced thrombosis. J. Clin. Invest. *43*:160, 1964.
27. Wessler, S., et al.: Estrogen-containing oral contraceptive agents. A basis for their thrombogenicity. JAMA *236*:2179, 1976.
28. Caprini, J. A., and Sener, S. F.: Altered coagulability in cancer patients. CA *32*:162, 1982.
29. Sack, G. H., et al.: Trousseau's syndrome and other manifestations of chronic disseminated coagulopathy in patients with neoplasms. Medicine *56*:2, 1977.
30. Mersky, C.: DIC: identification and management. Hosp. Pract. *17*:83, 1982.
30a. Dvorak, H. F., et al.: Fibrin as a component of the tumor stroma: Origins and biological significance. Cancer Metastasis Rev., *2*:41, 1983.
31. Penner, J. A.: Hypercoagulation and thrombosis. Med. Clin. North Am. *64*:743, 1980.
32. Morris, G. J.: Pre-operative prediction of post-operative deep vein thrombosis. Thromb. Haemost. *41*:27, 1979.
33. Davies, J. A., and McNichol, G. P.: Blood coagulation in pathological thrombus formation and the detection in blood of a thrombotic tendency. Br. Med. Bull. *34*:113, 1978.
34. Poller, L.: Oral contraceptives, blood clotting, and thrombosis. Br. Med. Bull. *34*:151, 1978.
35. Kernoff, B. P. A., and McNichol, G. P.: Normal and abnormal fibrinolysis. Br. Med. Bull. *33*:239, 1977.
36. Marciniak, E., et al.: Familial thrombosis due to antithrombin III deficiency. Blood *43*:209, 1974.
37. Ratnoff, O. D., et al.: The demise of John Hageman. N. Engl. J. Med. *279*:760, 1968.
38. Sabiston, D. C.: Pulmonary embolism. Surg. Gynecol. Obstet. *126*:1075, 1968.
39. Editorial: What happens to blood clots in the lung? Lancet *1*:194, 1978.
40. Williams, R. S., et al.: Physical conditioning augments the fibrinolytic response to venous occlusion in healthy adults. N. Engl. J. Med. *302*:987, 1980.
41. Moser, K. M.: Pulmonary embolism: Where the problem is not. J.A.M.A. *236*:1500, 1976.
42. Le Quesne, L. P.: Diagnosis and prevention of post-operative deep-vein thrombosis. Annu. Rev. Med. *26*:63, 1975.
43. Dalen, J. E., and Alpert, J. S.: Natural history of pulmonary embolism. Prog. Cardiovasc. Dis. *17*:257, 1975.
44. Roberts, J. J.: Controversies and enigmas in thrombo-phlebitis and pulmonary embolism. Perspective on alleged overdiagnosis. Angiology *31*:686, 1980.
45. McNamara, M. F., et al.: Venous disease. Surg. Clin. North Am. *57*:1201, 1977.
46. Hirsh, J.: Platelet inhibitors in the treatment of thrombosis. Clin. Invest. Med. *1*:191, 1978.
47. Hanley, S. P.: Differential inhibition by low-dose aspirin of human venous

prostacyclin synthesis and platelet thromboxane synthesis. Lancet *1*:969, 1981.
48. Salzman, E. W.: Aspirin to prevent arterial thrombosis. N. Engl. J. Med. *307*:113, 1982.
49. Editorial: Prostacyclin in therapeutics. Lancet *1*:643, 1981.
50. Elliot, M. S., et al.: A comparative randomized trial of heparin vs. streptokinase in the treatment of acute proximal venous thrombosis: An interim report of a prospective trial. Br. J. Surg. *66*:838, 1979.
51. NIH Concensus Conference; Thrombolytic therapy in treatment. Br. Med. J. *1*:1585, 1980.
52. Morgan, M.: Amniotic fluid embolism. Anaesthesia *34*:20, 1979.
53. Roche, W. D., and Norris, H. J.: Detection and significance of maternal amniotic fluid embolism. Obstet. Gynecol. *43*:729, 1974.
54. Karim, S. M. M.: Identification of prostaglandins in human amniotic fluid. J. Obstet. Gynaecol. (Br. Commonw.) *73*:903, 1966.
55. Mitchel, M. D, et al.: Thromboxane B_2 in amniotic fluid before and during labour. Br. J. Obstet. Gynaecol. *85*:442, 1978.
56. Editorial: Amniotic fluid embolism. Lancet *2*:398, 1979.
57. McGlynn, T. J., Jr., et al.: Pulmonary embolism. J.A.C.E.P. *8*:532, 1979.
58. Sabiston, D. C.: Pathophysiology, diagnosis, and management of pulmonary embolism. Am. J. Surg. *138*:384, 1979.
59. Dalen, J. E., et al.: Pulmonary embolism, pulmonary hemorrhage, and pulmonary infarction. New Engl. J. Med. *296*:1431, 1977.
60. A National Cooperative Study: The urokinase pulmonary embolism trial. Circulation *47* (Suppl. II):1, 1973.
61. Giudici, J. C., et al.: Pulmonary thromboembolism. I. Current concepts in pathogenesis and diagnosis. Postgrad. Med. *67*:64, 1980.
62. Elliott, J. P., Jr., et al.: Arterial embolization: Problems of source multiplicity, recurrence, and delayed treatment. Surgery *88*:833, 1980.
63. Shier, M. R., and Wilson, R. S.: Fat embolism syndrome: Traumatic coagulopathy with respiratory distress. Surg. Ann. *12*:139, 1980.
64. Palmovic, V., and McCarroll, J. R.: Fat embolism in trauma. Arch. Pathol. *80*:630, 1965.
65. Moylan, J. A., et al.: Fat embolism syndrome. J. Trauma *16*:341, 1976.
66. Riseborough, E. J., and Herndon, J. H.: Alterations in pulmonary function, coagulation and fat metabolism in patients with fractures of the lower limbs. Clin. Orthop. *115*:248, 1976.
67. Gossling, H. R., and Donohue, T. A.: The fat embolism syndrome. J.A.M.A. *241*:2740, 1979.
68. Robbins, S. L., et al.: Demonstration of intercoronary anastomoses in human hearts with a low viscosity perfusion mass. Circulation *33*:733, 1966.
69. Krainer, L.: Pathological effects of cerebral anoxia. Am. J. Med. *25*:258, 1958.
70. Haljamae, H., et al.: Pathophysiology of shock. Pathol. Res. Pract. *165*:200, 1979.
71. Barnett, J. A.: Bacterial shock. J.A.M.A. *209*:1514, 1969.
72. Duff, P.: Pathophysiology and management of septic shock. J. Reprod. Med. *24*:109, 1980.
73. Lefer, A. M.: Role of the prostaglandin-thromboxane system in vascular homeostasis during shock. Circ. Shock *6*:297, 1979.
74. Hess, M. L.: Subcellular function in the acutely failing myocardium. Circ. Shock *6*:119, 1979.
75. Lefer, A. M.: Blood-borne humoral factors in the pathophysiology of circulatory shock. Circ. Res. *32*:129, 1973.
76. Trump, B. F., et al.: The application of electron microscopy and cellular biochemistry to the autopsy. Observations on cellular changes in human shock. Hum. Pathol. *6*:499, 1975.
77. Trump, B. F.: The role of cellular membrane systems in shock. *In* The Cell in Shock. The Proceedings of a Symposium on Recent Research Developments and Current Clinical Practice in Shock. Michigan, Upjohn Symposium, 1974, p. 16.
78. Hackel, D. B., et al.: The heart in shock. Circ. Res. *35*:805, 1974.
79. McGovern, V. J.: Hypovolemic shock with particular reference to the myocardial and pulmonary lesions. Pathology *12*:63, 1980.

4 GENETIC DISORDERS

The study of genetics truly has reached the promised land. The technology is now at hand to manipulate—"engineer"—the genetic code, carrying with it the hope of alleviating or curing mutations but also the awesome potential of unleashing on this already troubled world new, threatening biologic forms. Currently, not a month passes without the description of a new syndrome, a fresh identification of a gene locus, a better appreciation of the interrelationship between genotype and immunologic competence, and a new penetration of the genetic code and its complexities.[1, 2]

In recent years, recombinant DNA technology has truly revolutionized our understanding of both normal and mutated genes. Take, for example, the hemoglobin genes; we can now describe the "microanatomy" of the normal beta-globin gene and define the molecular pathology of the defective beta-globin genes that give rise to hemolytic anemias.[3] The technology to clone human genes, now at hand, has begun to influence our thinking about the diagnosis as well as treatment of genetic disorders. Most genetic disorders are currently detected by identification of abnormal gene products or their clinical effects. Now we can realistically anticipate the detection of abnormal genes before irreversible tissue injury has occurred. For treatment, the exciting possibility of direct gene replacement offers the chances of real "cure" by removing the cause of the disease, instead of attempting to limit the clinical effects produced by defective genes.

Remarkably, most of this progress has been achieved within the past decade. Although it rests on Mendel's brillant observations made over a century ago, his astute deductions were not even related to humans until the early years of the twentieth century. It was only in 1956 that the correct count of man's 46 chromosomes was established by Tjio and Levan.[4] Confronted with myriad genetic diseases, the hapless medical student of today might look back wistfully to not so many years ago when there were relatively few. Today it has become apparent that virtually all diseases arise out of, or are affected by, the genotype.

Traditionally the diseases of humans have been divided into three categories: (1) those environmentally determined, (2) those genetically determined, and (3) those in which both environmental and genetic factors play a role. Microbiologic infections might be representative of the first category; however, even here, with the expansion of knowledge about the role of immune response genes in the control of immunocompetence, it is evident that microbiologic infections are conditioned, as are all disorders to a greater or lesser degree, by the genotype.[5] Perhaps malnutrition is an instance in which the environment totally determines the nature of the disease. But one wonders whether the constitutional ability to sustain such nutritional deficits or to accommodate them is not genetically influenced. Into the third category mentioned above fall many of the important diseases of man such as peptic ulcer, diabetes mellitus, atherosclerosis, schizophrenia, and probably most cancers in which clearly both nature and nurture play significant roles. Gregor,[6] in writing about the life of Charles Darwin, expressed this nature-nurture interrelationship well:

> Between the environment and the genes that determine heredity there exists a highly complex relationship. It seems that genes cannot produce normal individuals unless the environmental factors are also normal. What is inherited is a packet of genes transmitted from the parents with the capacity to respond to environmental conditions in certain ways, some of which are called normal for the species in its normal environment.

Recognizing the complexity of this nature-nurture interplay, our interest here is with those diseases in which nature, i.e., the genetic component, plays a major if not determinant role. Some diseases are associated with genetic abnormalities detectable in the karyotype, many have their origins in mutations of a single gene of large effect (mendelian disorders), and some result from the combined effects of multiple small gene mutations and environmental influences, so-called multifactorial inheritance.

The genetic diseases encountered in medical practice represent only the tip of the iceberg, that is, those with less extreme genotypic errors permitting full embryonic development and live birth. In 1977 it was estimated that 50% of spontaneous abortuses have a demonstrable chromosomal abnormality, and of course this must represent a minimum estimate, since many defects now detectable and many others still beyond our range of identification went unrecognized.[7] About 1% of all newborn infants possess a gross chromosomal abnormality.[8] How many more mutations remain hidden? For years we have marveled at the biologic precision in the processes of mitosis and meiosis, but it is now unmistakably evident that there is far more slippage in these processes than has been appreciated. Fortunately, among the many with mutations, only the "fittest" survive. Nonetheless, in the United States alone these "fittest" add up to 12 million with some genetic disease, imposing in the aggregate an enormous health problem.

It is hardly necessary to emphasize the importance of establishing the nature of the genotypic error in these diseases. It is requisite not only for clinical diagnosis but also for genetic counseling. The *great preponderance of disorders arising out of chromosomal abnormalities can be identified with a high degree of certainty by cytogenetic analysis*, i.e., by examination of the patient's karyotype with methods now available. In appropriate cases, the cytogenetic diagnosis can even be established antenatally. Amniocentesis—the withdrawal of a small sample of amniotic fluid early in pregnancy—provides a means of establishing the karyotype of the fetus from desquamated fetal cells. If a tragic disorder such as trisomy 21 (Down's syndrome) (p. 126), which may be familial in origin, is discovered, the opportunity is provided to terminate the pregnancy. Perhaps even more important, a negative result can alleviate a great deal of harrowing anxiety during pregnancy. In one study dealing with a variety of diseases, approximately 95% of 100 "high-risk" pregnancies were negative for the condition in question. Few medical words are more beautiful than "there is no evidence of the disease."

Mendelian disorders without alteration of the karyotype can frequently be diagnosed by the combined application of biochemistry and genetics, often referred to as biochemical genetics. Included among these diagnosable disorders are the ever-growing list of hemoglobinopathies, serum protein variations, and inborn errors of metabolism. In the live-born patient, biochemical analysis of blood cells or tissue samples discloses most of these abnormalities. The recognition that cultured fibroblasts reveal most of the inborn errors of metabolism, the so-called "missing enzyme" syndromes, permits diagnosis of these entities in the unborn child. For example, Tay-Sachs disease is an inborn error of metabolism that tragically distorts these unfortunate infants and is invariably fatal within months to a few years after birth. Amniocentesis and assay of the fetal cultured cells for the specific enzyme in question makes it possible to diagnose and terminate the unhappy pregnancy. Since the risk of recurrence of this condition in subsequent pregnancies is 25%, it is perhaps even more important to determine that the tragic condition is not present in the next fetus. *Phenylketonuria, histidinemia, and type I glycogen storage disease among the better understood metabolic errors cannot be diagnosed by assay of cultured fibroblasts because fibroblasts do not synthesize phenylalanine hydroxylase, histidase, and hepatic glucose-6-phosphatase.*

The multifactorial disorders can be identified only by analyses of family pedigrees. Although some grotesque malformations result from this mode of inheritance, fortunately many of the multifactorial disorders, such as congenital dislocation of the hip, cleft lip and cleft palate, hypertension, and gout are remediable and compatible with long life. Much can be learned from the use of cytogenetics, biochemical genetics, and amniocentesis to ascertain the orgins of genetic disorders, not only in the patient, but also in the fetus, adding new dimensions to the clinical study of these conditions.

Before we turn to a consideration of specific entities, the normal karyotype will be reviewed, as well as some of the known causes of mutation.

THE NORMAL KARYOTYPE—CYTOGENETICS

For many years, efforts were made to count the chromosomes of man in microscopic sections of testis, leading to the conclusion that each human cell possessed 48 chromosomes. The development of improved tissue culture techniques, the introduction of colchicine into the tissue cultures to stop dividing cells in metaphase, and the use of hypotonic solutions to improve the separation of chromosomes allowed Tjio and Levan in 1956 finally to establish 46 as the correct chromosome count in man.[4] As is well known, these comprise 22 homologous pairs of autosomes and two sex chromosomes, XX in the female and XY in the male. Up until 1970, only limited differentiation of the chromosome pairs was possible, based on their size and the position of the centromere. As is seen in a metaphase spread, the individual chromosomes take the form of two chromatids connected at the centromere to create the familiar "X" or wishbone conformations. *If the centromere connects the chromatids in their center, the chromosome is said to be median or metacentric; if the centromere is eccentrically placed, the chromosome is said to be submedian or submetacentric. In some chromosomes, the centromere is almost, but not quite, at the end of the chromatids. These are acrocentric chromosomes,* all of which can bear small projections on their short arms. The projections are known as *satellites* and are involved in the formation of nucleoli. Probably because of this activity, acrocentric chromosomes are often seen in groups in the metaphase plate, a phenomenon described as satellite association. These details are presented in Table 4–1.

In 1970, Caspersson and colleagues described the identification of each individual chromosome based on a distinctive and reliable pattern of alternating light and dark bands along the length of the chromosome.[9] Their method involved staining with a quinacrine that fluoresces under ultraviolet light. Since then a number of *banding techniques* have been developed that can be categorized briefly as follows:

Table 4–1. KARYOTYPE GROUPINGS OF HUMAN CHROMOSOMES WITHOUT BANDING

Group 1–3 (A)	Two large metacentric chromosomes and one large submetacentric chromosome readily distinguished from each other by size and centromere position
Group 4–5 (B)	Large submetacentric chromosomes that are difficult to distinguish from each other
Group 6–12—X (C)	Medium-sized submetacentric chromosomes. The X chromosome resembles the longer chromosomes in this group. This large group is the one that presents major difficulty in identification of individual chromosomes without the use of banding techniques.
Group 13–15 (D)	Medium-sized acrocentric chromosomes with satellites
Group 16–18 (E)	Relatively short metacentric chromosomes (No. 16) or submetacentric chromosomes (Nos. 17 and 18)
Group 19–20 (F)	Short metacentric chromosomes
Group 21–22—Y (G)	Short acrocentric chromosomes with satellites. The Y chromosome is similar to these chromosomes but bears no satellites.

1. Q bands (from quinacrine) are the fluorescent bands observed after quinacrine mustard staining.

2. G bands (from Giemsa) are stained with Giemsa after various forms of treatment. These have the same locations as the Q bands. A normal male karyotype with G-banding is illustrated in Figure 4–1.

3. R bands (from reverse) are the bands stained after controlled denaturation by heat as well as newer fluorescent techniques. The dark bands in this method correspond to the nonfluorescent bands demonstrated by quinacrine, hence their designation as reverse bands.

4. C bands (from constitutive heterochromatin) are located in the pericentromeric regions except on the Y chromosome.

5. T bands (from terminal) visualize the terminal ends of the arms of the chromosomes. Details of these methods are available in the literature.[10] In recent years, the resolution obtained by banding techniques has been dramatically improved by obtaining the cells in prophase. The individual chromosomes appear markedly elongated and up to 1500 bands per chromosome may be recognized.[11] The use of these banding techniques permits certain identification of each chromosome, as well as chromosomal abnormalities that alter neither chromosome number nor shape.

The banding techniques also distinguish the sex chromosomes, but in addition *the X and Y chromosomes can be identified in interphase nuclei.* In the female, one of the two X chromosomes can be seen in the interphase nucleus as a darkly staining small mass in contact with the nuclear membrane known as the Barr body or X chromatin (Fig. 4–2). In interphase nuclei the other X chromosome is active and is dispersed throughout the nuclear chromatin. With appropriate staining the X chromatin can be readily identified in many cells types, but most often used are smears of squamous cells obtained from scrapings of the buccal mucosa. The generally accepted explanation of the X chromatin is known as the *Lyon hypothesis,* which might also be called the *single active–X hypothesis.* It states that *(a) only one of the X chromosomes is genetically active, (b) the other X of either maternal or paternal origin undergoes heteropyknosis to become the Barr body, (c) inactivation of either the maternal or paternal X occurs at random among all the cells of the blastocyst on or about the 16th day of embryonic life, and (d) inactivation of the same X chromosome persists in all the cells derived from each precursor cell.* Thus, the great preponderance of normal females are in reality mosaics and have two populations of cells, one with an inactivated maternal X and the other with an inactivated paternal X. Herein lies the explanation of why females have the same dosage of X-linked active genes as the male. As will be seen, certain genetic disorders in both the male and the female are characterized by extra X chromosomes. All save one will be inactivated, and thus *the number of Barr bodies in a given nucleus is one less than the number of X chromosomes.* The female with four X chromosomes will present three Barr bodies in her somatic cells, whereas the male with an XXY complement will disclose a single Barr body.

The Y chromosome too can be identified in interphase nuclei. It has one of the most vividly fluorescent segments when stained with quinacrine and examined under ultraviolet light. This fluorescence is vivid enough to be visible in most interphase nuclei, where it is sometimes referred to as the *Y body.* However, since the fluorescent segment of the Y chromosome is genetically inert, it is entirely possible for phenotypically normal males to lack Y bodies.[12]

Before this discussion of the normal karyotype is concluded, reference must be made to the enormous strides achieved in gene mapping (the assignment of gene loci to specific chromosomes). This process has involved the meticulous correlation of phenotypic changes with alterations in the genotype. The whole range of pedigree analysis, cytogenetics, and biochemical genetics has contributed to gene mapping, but the newer methods of *chromosome banding* and *cell hybridization* in particular have immeasurably speeded and facilitated the process.

Cell hybridization or *cell fusion,* sometimes referred to as somatic cell genetics, has provided a powerful tool in gene mapping. It has proved possible to fuse two different cell lines in culture and derive cell hybrids. In such cultures one can observe two different nuclei within a single cytoplasmic mass (a heterokaryon) and, occasionally, fusion of the two nuclei to form a

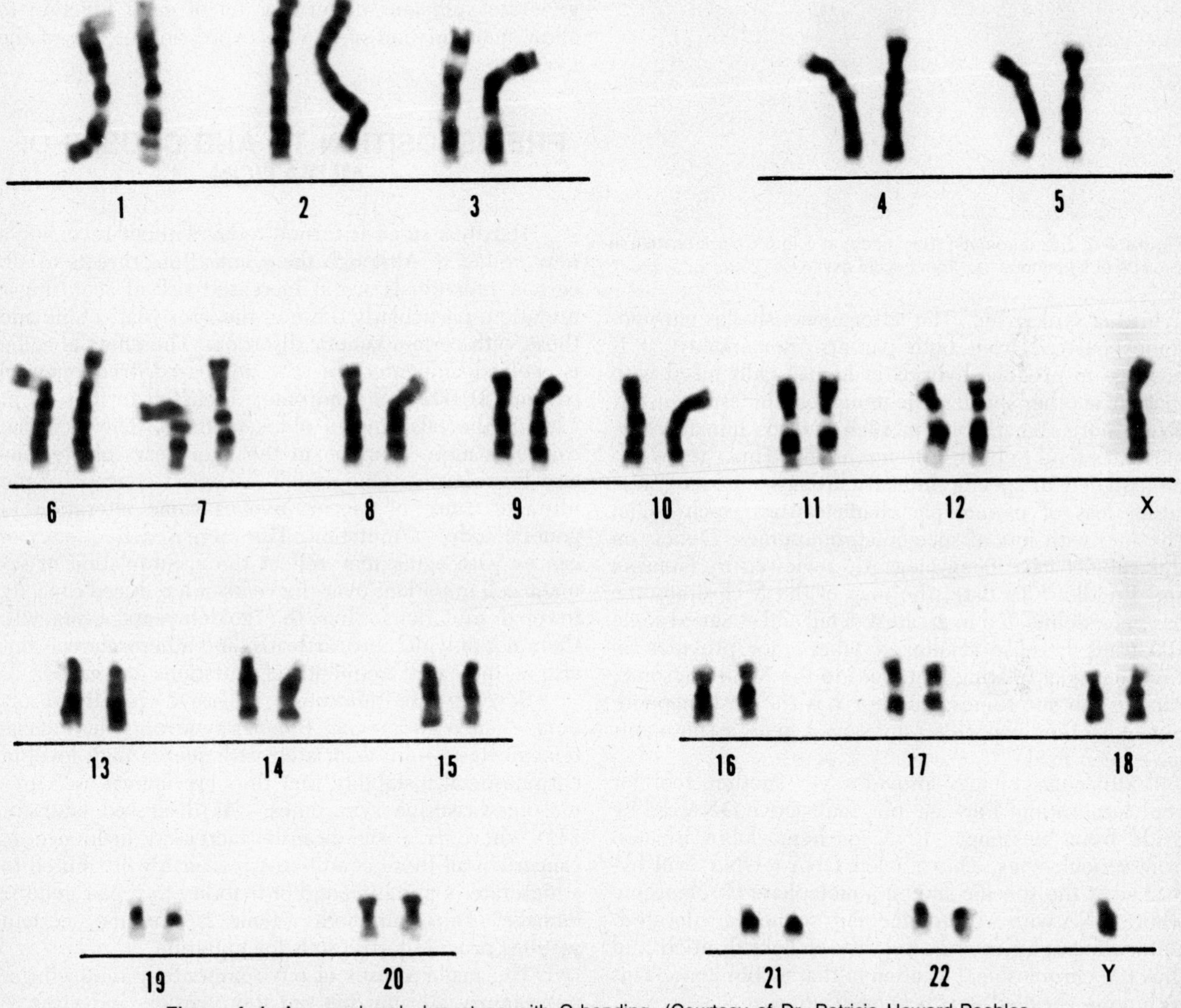

Figure 4–1. A normal male karyotype with G-banding. (Courtesy of Dr. Patricia Howard-Peebles, Southwestern Medical School, Dallas, Texas.)

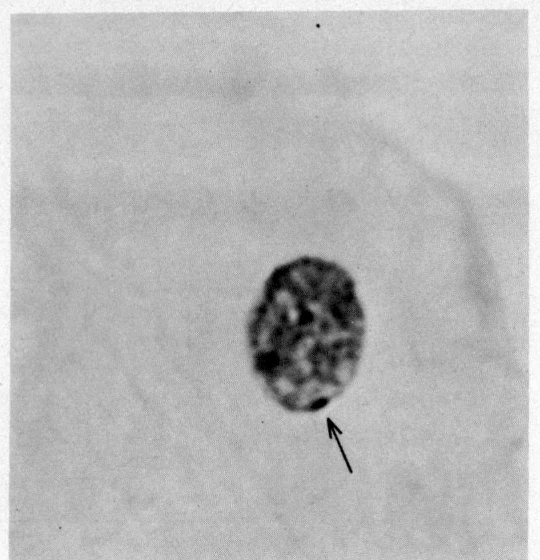

Figure 4–2. Sex chromatin (Barr body) at 5 to 6 o'clock (*arrow*) in nucleus of squamous cell from buccal cavity (×1200).

hybrid (a synkaryon). The latter obviously has chromosomes derived from both parents. Remarkably, it is possible to produce hybrids of human cells fused with those of another species, the mouse or Chinese hamster. Even more remarkably, in such hybrids human chromosomes tend to be lost preferentially. Thus, genes can be assigned to specific human chromosomes by correlating loss of phenotypic characteristics (such as an enzyme) with loss of specific chromosomes. Details on this subject have been elegantly reviewed by Creagan and Ruddle.[13] To date, the map of the X chromosome has been delineated in greatest detail and assigned some 100 traits because sex-linked inheritance provides an easy means of relating mutations to the X chromosome. Among the autosomes, number 1 is the best mapped, but altogether about 350 autosomal gene assignments have been made.[14]

Molecular biology provides yet another tool for gene localization. For example, radioactive DNA can be made from messenger RNA for hemoglobin isolated from reticulocytes. This labeled DNA (cDNA) will hybridize at the specific site on a metaphase chromosome where DNA with a complementary sequence is located. Autoradiography reveals the site of hybridization and thus the chromosomal location of that globin gene. This technique is called *in situ hybridization.*

Even greater precision in the localization and study of genes is made possible by utilizing bacterial enzymes called restriction endonucleases. Each member of this family of enzymes recognizes a specific sequence (i.e., restricted) of nucleotides, and cuts DNA wherever that particular sequence occurs. With these enzymes, therefore, it is possible to generate well-defined fragments of cellular DNA, which are separated electrophoretically and then immobilized on filter paper (the so-called "Southern blot"). A radioactive cDNA probe is then hybridized to the immobilized DNA fragments and its position on the blot is detected by autoradiography; this is similar to the in situ hybridization method. Specific genes are found by cDNA probes to be on DNA fragments of predictable size. If a probe does not hybridize, the gene in question is not present in the DNA segment. If the DNA fragment to which the probe hybridizes is not the normal size, some alteration has occurred in that gene or in its immediately flanking DNA. The clinical utility of this new methodology is already apparent. For example, this method has been used to unravel the molecular lesions of the thalassemias (p. 622),[3] to diagnose sickle anemia antenatally,[15] and to generate sufficient understanding of gene function to allow manipulation of in vivo expression of one of the globin genes.[16]

PREDISPOSITION TO AND CAUSES OF MUTATION

Hardly a stone is turned today without revealing a new mutagen. Although these constitute threats to all, certain individuals are at increased risk of acquiring a mutation, particularly those in the later years of life and those with certain genetic disorders. The effect of aging is well documented by the increased frequency of trisomy 21 (Down's syndrome, discussed further on p. 126) in the offspring of older mothers. The fact that cancer is more common in the later years of life may also be relevant. One widely accepted concept of the ultimate cause of cancer invokes some alteration in genetic code—a mutation. The increased frequency of cancer with aging may reflect the accumulation of somatic cell mutations over the years or a reduced capacity to repair mutations. Thus, the "golden years" bring with them not only debility, arthritis, and atherosclerosis but also an increased frequency of mutations and cancer.

Several rare autosomal recessive genetic disorders—Fanconi's anemia, Bloom's syndrome, and ataxia telangiectasia—are associated with such a high level of chromosomal instability that they are known as "chromosome-breakage syndromes." As discussed later (p. 241), there is a significantly increased incidence of cancers in all these conditions, reasonably attributed to a high rate of mutation and/or inability to repair genetic damage. Thus, although no-one is immune, certain settings provide fertile soils for mutation.

The major causes of environmentally induced genetic injury are ionizing radiation, drugs, and viruses. We must now add to the list, with some alarm, certain components of man's diet as possible mutagens.

The mutagenic potency of ionizing radiation has been clearly established in man, as noted on page 242. Much of this evidence derives from the study of survivors of the atomic blasts. Because of its cumulative effects, *even the repeated smaller doses of radiation energy used in radiotherapy may build up to mutagenic levels.*

The role of drugs and chemical agents in mutagenesis is a complex and controversial issue. Many compounds induce karyotypic aberrations in cell culture or, in animals, malform the fetus when sufficiently large doses are administered during pregnancy. In both settings, it has been impossible to segregate the metabolic and toxic effects of the drugs from their potential to induce direct genetic injury. In cell culture, karyotypic abnormalities can be produced by introducing into the nutrient medium a host of agents, even such seemingly innocent ones as aspirin. In almost all these instances, the evidence suggests that the genetic damage is a consequence of toxic cell injury and reflects irreversible damage to cells destined to die. On the other hand, the nitrogen mustards, azathioprine, and amethopterin are clearly mutagenic both in vivo and in vitro. These agents are capable of binding directly to guanine in DNA, thereby altering the genetic code. These and several other mutagenic agents, including some food additives, have possible implications as carcinogens and are discussed on page 237.

Viruses have been clearly documented as mutagenic in animals, and may well have the same effect in man, as pointed out in the discussion on oncogenic viruses (p. 243). Nononcogenic viruses have also been shown to be mutagenic both in vivo and in vitro. An increased frequency of chromosome breaks has been reported in the leukocytes of patients suffering from measles, chickenpox, mumps, and infectious mononucleosis, but the significance of such leukocytic changes is uncertain. The mere fact that some viruses can induce cellular or developmental abnormalities does not prove alteration of the genome. For example, rubella infections during pregnancy are clearly associated with congenital malformations in the infant (p. 480), but there is no evidence that the teratogenic effect of rubella is associated with genetic injury.

How much mutagenic agents contribute to the production of clinical disease remains uncertain. Unless alterations in the karyotype are induced, one must depend on expressed phenotypic changes, and confirmation of their genetic origin requires detailed analysis of successive generations. The long generation time of man, dispersion of members of families, and problems involved in effecting clinical evaluation of all members of a family have rendered these human studies difficult. Animal models are of only limited usefulness because of the remarkable variation in species susceptibility. For example, cortisone induces congenital malformations in mice and rabbits but not in rats. As far as we know, cortisone has no effect on the genome of man. Despite these complexities, there is little doubt that it is difficult, if not impossible, to escape exposure to environmental mutagens. So-called "spontaneous" mutations may not be entirely accidents of nature. Conceivably, the relationship of aging to mutation merely documents longer exposure to environmental hazards. The term "spontaneous" may merely reflect our ignorance of the importance of the many potentially mutagenic agents to which we are all exposed virtually daily.

Against this background we can now turn our attention to the genetic disorders. *The genetically determined diseases to be considered here can conveniently be divided into four categories: (1) cytogenetic disorders with visible chromosomal abnormalities, (2) mendelian disorders having origin in a mutation of a single gene of large effect, (3) disorders having origin in multifactorial inheritance, and (4) the few entities having variable modes of transmission.* The number of disorders assigned to each of these categories grows apace with each passing year. Undoubtedly we have no more than scratched the surface in investigating these categories. Many of the diseases are rare; a large number confer no serious disadvantage on the host; some will be dealt with in subsequent chapters. Here, we will confine our discussion only to some of those which are more important and common.

CYTOGENETIC DISORDERS

Cytogenetic aberrations underlying these disorders may take the form of an abnormal number of chromosomes or alterations in the structure of one or more chromosomes. The normal 46 count is known as the *(2n) diploid number*. The first meiotic reduction division in the formation of gametes halves the number to the *(n) haploid count of 23*. The normal count would be expressed as 46,XX for the female and 46,XY for the male. Any exact multiple of the haploid number is called *euploid*. However, if an error occurs in meiosis or mitosis, and a cell acquires a chromosome complement that is not an exact multiple of 23, it is referred to as *aneuploidy*. The usual causes for aneuploidy are *nondisjunction* and *anaphase lag*. The former occurs when a homologous pair of chromosomes fails to disjoin at the first meiotic division, or the two chromatids fail to separate either at the second meiotic division or in somatic cell divisions, resulting in two aneuploid cells. The gamete with 24 chromosomes or the somatic cell with 47 chromosomes each has a trisomy for one of the chromosome complements, whereas the other gamete or somatic cell suffers from a monosomy of the same chromosome. In anaphase lag, one homologous chromosome in meiosis or one chromatid in mitosis lags behind and is left out of the cell nucleus. The result is a normal cell and a cell with monosomy. As will be seen, monosomy or trisomy involving the sex chromosomes, or even more bizarre aberrations, yields surprisingly mild phenotypic abnormalities. On the other hand, *monosomy involving an autosome generally represents loss of too much genetic information to permit live birth or even embryogenesis, but a number of autosomal trisomies do permit survival.* With the exception of trisomy 21, almost all yield severely handicapped infants who almost invariably die at an early age.[17]

Here it is necessary to clarify some cytogenetic terminology. Abnormal sex chromosome complements are expressed as 47,XXX or 48,XXXY, for example, indicating the total number of chromosomes present. Both these karyotypes would yield two X-chromatin bodies, but the latter, with a Y chromosome, would be a male. *Irrespective of the number of X chromosomes in the human, the presence of a single Y determines the male sex.* Loss of an X chromosome in the female would lead to a 45,X karyotype, producing the so-called Turner's syndrome. Loss of the X chromosome in the male genotype is lethal. When autosomes are involved, the total chromosome count is given along with the sex chromosome complement, followed by a plus or minus sign, and the specific number of the autosome gained or lost as, for example, 47,XY, +21 (a male with trisomy 21) or 47,XX, +13 (a female with trisomy 13). More than one extra autosome or higher chromosome counts almost always result in abortion.

Occasionally, *mitotic errors in early development give rise to two or more populations of cells in the same individual, a condition referred to as mosaicism.* This can result from mitotic errors during the cleavage of the fertilized ovum or in somatic cells. Mosaicism affecting the sex chromosomes is relatively common. In the division of the fertilized ovum an error may lead to one of the daughter cells receiving three sex chromosomes, while the other receives only one, yielding, for example, a 45,X/47,XXX mosaic. All descendent cells derived from each of these precursors will thus have either a 47,XXX count or a 45,X count. Such a patient would be a mosaic variant of Turner's syndrome, with the extent of phenotypic expression dependent on the number and distribution of the 45,X cells. If the error occurs at a later cleavage, the mosaic will have three populations of cells, with some possessing the normal 46,XX complement, i.e., 45,X/46,XX/47,XXX. Repeated mitotic errors may lead to many populations of cells. Elderly males show a propensity for loss of the Y chromosome in varying proportions of cells.

Autosomal mosaics appear to be much less common than those involving the sex chromosomes. An error in an early mitotic division affecting the autosomes usually leads to a nonviable mosaic with autosomal monosomy. Rarely, the loss of a nonviable cell in embryogenesis is tolerated, yielding a mosaic, e.g., 46,XY/47,XY, +21. Such a patient would be a trisomy 21 mosaic with partial expression of the Down's syndrome depending on the proportion of cells expressing the trisomy.

Any abnormal karyotype may result from a second category of meiotic errors involving structural changes in the chromosome. All these are the consequence of some form of chromosome breakage and loss or rearrangement of material. To designate the location of the structural change, "p" (for petit) denotes the short arm of a chromosome and "q" (the next letter) the long arm. Each arm is then divided into numbered regions (1, 2, 3, etc.) from the centromere outward, and each band within the region is similarly numbered. For example, 1p32 denotes chromosome number 1, short arm, region 3, band 2. However, we can leave such elegant detail to the cytogeneticists and confine further remarks to less detailed nomenclature without indicating the precise locus of breaks and rearrangements.

In *translocation*, a segment of one chromosome is transferred to another (Fig. 4–3). In one form called *balanced reciprocal translocation*, there are single breaks in each of the two chromosomes, with exchange of material. Such a translocation might not be disclosed without banding techniques. A balanced reciprocal translocation between the long arm of chromosome 2, which has been shortened, and the short arm of chromosome 5, which has been lengthened, would be written 46,XX,t(2q−;5p+). This individual has 46 chromosomes with altered morphology of one of the chromosomes 2 and one of the chromosomes 5. Since there has been no loss of genetic material, the individual will be phenotypically normal. However, a balanced translocation carrier is at increased risk of producing abnormal gametes. For example, in the case cited above a gamete containing one normal chromosome 2 and a translocated chromosome 5 may be formed. Such a gamete would be unbalanced since it would not contain the normal complement of genetic material. Subsequent fertilization by a normal gamete would lead to the formation of an abnormal (unbalanced) zygote, resulting in spontaneous abortion or birth of a malformed child. The other important pattern of translocation is called a *Robertsonian translocation* (or centric fusion), a reciprocal translocation between two acrocentric chromosomes. Typically the breaks occur close to the centromeres of each chromosome, affecting the long arm in one and the short arm in the other. Transfer of the segments then leads to one very large chromosome and one extremely small one. Often, the small product is lost (Fig. 4–3); however, it carries so little genetic information that this loss is compatible with a normal phenotype, and Robertsonian translocation between two chromosomes in a group is encountered in apparently normal individuals. The significance of this form of translocation also lies in the production of abnormal progeny, as discussed later with Down's syndrome.

Inversion refers to a rearrangement that involves two breaks within a single chromosome with reincorporation of the inverted segment, thus transforming a sequence along the chromosome from ABCD to ACBD (Fig. 4–3). Such an inversion involving only one arm of the chromosome is known as paracentric. If the breaks are on opposite sides of the centromere, and the inverted segment incorporates the centromere, it is known as pericentric. Inversions are perfectly compatible with normal development.

Deletion occurs when there is a single break in the arm of a chromosome, producing a fragment with no centromere, which is then lost at the next cell division. This might be designated as 46,XY,16p− to indicate loss of some part of the short arm of chromosome 16 (Fig. 4–3). One can specify in which region and at what band the break and deletion has occurred, as, for example, 46,XY,del(16)(p14), meaning a break point in region 1 band 4 of the short arm of chromosome 16.[18]

A *ring chromosome* may be produced when a deletion occurs at both ends of a chromosome with fusion of the damaged ends (Fig. 4–3). If significant genetic material is lost, phenotypic abnormalities result.

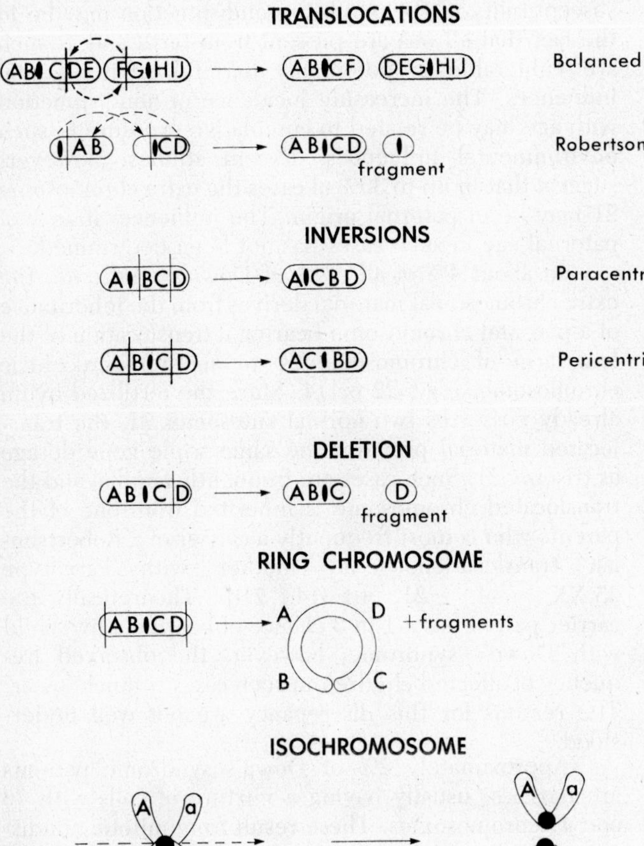

Figure 4–3. Types of chromosomal rearrangements.

This might be expressed as 46,XY,r(14). Ring chromosomes do not behave normally in meiosis or mitosis and usually have serious consequences.

Isochromosome formation results when the centromere divides in a transverse plane rather than in the normal long axis of the chromosome. Thus, the misdivision gives rise to two chromosomes, one consisting of, for example, two short arms only and the other consisting of two long arms (Fig. 4–3). Both these chromosomes now have genetic information that is morphologically identical in both arms.

All these structural anomalies at one time or another have been described for both autosomes and sex chromosomes. The use of banding techniques has begun to disclose an additional great variety of minor structural abnormalities in chromosomes involving differences in the size of certain bands, largely composed of heterochromatin. Since the heterochromatin contains little genetic information that is transcribed into messenger RNA, it would not be expected to have much effect on the phenotype. However, even minor structural changes may have importance. In the process of repair of a break, one or more genes may be lost. It has been observed that even in balanced translocations, which are acquired rather than inherited, mental retardation and other abnormalities may result. Moreover, phenotypically normal parents, who have a balanced structural abnormality such as inversion or a balanced translocation, are more prone to meiotic errors in gametogenesis, and therefore are at increased risk of having miscarriages and/or chromosomally unbalanced and abnormal children.

Many more numerical and structural aberrations can be found in specialized texts, and the number of abnormal karyotypes encountered in genetic diseases increases with each passing month. A number of important abnormal karyotypes are listed in Table 4–2. As pointed out earlier, the clinically important chromosome

Table 4–2. CLINICALLY IMPORTANT AUTOSOMAL CHROMOSOMAL ABNORMALITIES*

Trisomy: 21, 18, 13, 8, 22, 9, mosaicism for trisomic and normal cells
Partial trisomy (duplication†): 21q, 13q, 9p, 4p, 10q, 11q, 7q, 14q, 1q, 3p, 4q, 8q, 10p, 11p, 15q, 20p
Monosomy: 21, 22
Deletion of part of (deficiency†): 5p, 13q, 4p, 18p, 18q, 11q, 7p, 9p, 12p
Duplication-deficiency: 3, 4, 2
Triploidy
Chromosome breakage: Fanconi's anemia, Bloom's syndrome, ataxia telangiectasia, glutathione reductase deficiency

*In each category, abnormalities are listed approximately in order of decreasing frequency.

†Some duplications and deficiencies are really combined duplication deficiencies in which one or the other chromosomal imbalance predominates.

From Miller, O. J., and Breg, W. R.: Autosomal chromosome disorders and variations. N. Engl. J. Med. *294*:596, 1976. Reprinted, by permission, from The New England Journal of Medicine.

disorders represent only the "tip of the iceberg." Chromosome abnormalities are identified in approximately 50% of spontaneous abortuses and in 5% of stillbirths and infants who die in the immediate postnatal period. Even in live-born infants the frequency is approximately 0.5 to 1.0%. Many of the early deaths are attributable to gross structural malformations or severe developmental defects in the brain. However, since some congenital malformations are also associated with mendelian and multifactorial modes of inheritance, these will be described later as disorders with variable modes of transmission.

CYTOGENETIC DISORDERS INVOLVING AUTOSOMES

Several of the major autosomal disorders are presented in Table 4–3.

Trisomy 21 (Down's Syndrome)

Down's syndrome is the most common of the chromosomal disorders and is a leading cause of mental retardation. In the United States the incidence in newborns is about one in 1000. Over 90% of affected individuals have trisomy 21, so their chromosome count is 47 (Fig. 4–4); the others have normal chromosome numbers, but the extra chromosomal material is present as a translocation. As mentioned earlier, the most common cause of trisomy and therefore of Down's syndrome is meiotic nondisjunction. The parents of such children have a normal karyotype and are normal in all respects.

Maternal age has a strong influence on the incidence of Down's syndrome. It occurs once in 1550 live births in women under the age of 20 years, in contrast to one in 25 live births for mothers over 45 years of age.[19] The correlation with maternal age suggests that in most cases the meiotic nondisjunction of chromosome 21 occurs in the ovum. The reason for the increased susceptibility of the ovum to nondisjunction may lie in the fact that all ova are present from birth and as such are vulnerable to potentially harmful environmental influences. The increasing incidence of nondisjunction with age may be related to cumulative exposure to such environmental influences. Recent studies, however, suggest that in up to 30% of cases the extra chromosome 21 may be of paternal origin. The influence, if any, of paternal age in such cases has not been determined.

In about 4% of all cases of Down's syndrome, the extra chromosomal material derives from the inheritance of a parental chromosome bearing a translocation of the long arm of chromosome 21 to another acrocentric chromosome, e.g., 22 or 14. Since the fertilized ovum already possesses two normal autosomes 21, the translocated material provides the same triple gene dosage as trisomy 21. Such cases are frequently familial and the translocated chromosome is inherited from one of the parents who is most frequently a carrier of a Robertsonian translocation, e.g., mother with karyotype 45,XX, −14, −21, +t (14q 21q). Theoretically the carrier parent has a 1 in 3 chance of bearing a live child with Down's syndrome; however, the observed frequency of affected children in such cases is much lower. The reasons for this discrepancy are not well understood.

Approximately 2% of Down's syndrome patients are mosaics, usually having a mixture of cells with 46 and 47 chromosomes. These result from mitotic nondisjunction of chromosome 21 during an early stage of embryogenesis. Symptoms in such cases are variable and milder, depending on the proportion of abnormal cells. Clearly, in cases of translocation or mosaic Down's syndrome, maternal age is of no importance.

The diagnostic clinical features of this condition, listed in Table 4–3, are usually readily evident, even at birth. The flat facial profile, oblique palpebral fissures, and epicanthic folds account for the older, unfortunate designations "mongolism" and "mongolian idiocy." Down's syndrome is a leading cause of mental retardation. The mental retardation is severe; approximately 80% of those afflicted have an I.Q. of 25 to 50. Ironically, these severely disadvantaged children usually have a gentle, shy manner and are far more easily directed than their more fortunate siblings, less adorned with chromosomes. It should be pointed out that some mosaics with Down's syndrome have very mild phenotypic changes and may even have normal or near-normal intelligence.

The prognosis for affected children is uncertain. Even today, about 40% die by age 10, many of infections or cardiac problems in infancy. About 30% have congenital heart disease, most commonly ventricular septal defects. In addition, there is a striking increase in the frequency of acute leukemia in this condition.[20] The acute leukemia is myeloblastic in about one-third of cases and lymphoblastic in two-thirds. In passing, it should be cautioned that these patients also have a predisposition to leukemoid reactions (transient marked elevations in the white cell count) predisposing to

Table 4–3. DISORDERS ASSOCIATED WITH THE AUTOSOMES

Disorder	Examples of Karyotype	Approximate Incidence	Maternal Age	Clinical Features
Down's Syndrome (1 in 1000 births)				
Trisomy 21 type	47,XX, +21 47,XY, +21	Over 90% of cases	Increased	1. Mental retardation 2. Flat facial profile 3. Oblique palpebral fissures
Translocation type	46,XX, −14, +t(14q;21q) 46,XY, −22, +t(21q;22q)	3 to 4% cases	Normal	4. Muscle hypotonia 5. Hyperflexibility 6. Lack of Moro reflex
Mosaic type	46,XX/47,XX, +21	2 to 3% cases	Normal	7. Abundant neck skin 8. Broad and/or short trunk 9. Dysplastic ears 10. Horizontal palmar crease 11. Dysplastic pelvis (by x-ray) 12. Dysplastic middle phalanx (by x-ray) 13. Epicanthic folds 14. Acute leukemia
Trisomy 18 (Edwards' Syndrome) (1 in 5000 births)				
Trisomy 18 type	47,XX, +18 47,XY, +18	90% of cases	Increased	1. Mental retardation and failure to thrive 2. Prominent occiput
Translocation type	46,XX, −D, +t(Dq;18q)	Rare	Normal	3. Micrognathia and low-set ears 4. Hypertonicity
Mosaic type	46,XX/47,XX, +18	10% of cases	Normal	5. Flexion of fingers (second and fifth digits overlapping third and fourth) 6. Cardiac, renal, and intestinal defects 7. Short sternum and small pelvis 8. Abduction deformity of hip
Trisomy 13 (Patau's Syndrome) (1 in 6000 births)				
Trisomy 13 type	47,XX, +13 47,XY, +13	Over 80% of cases	Increased	1. Microcephaly and mental retardation 2. Scalp defect
Translocation type	46,XX, −13, +t(Dq;13q)	10% of cases	Normal	3. Microphthalmia 4. Harelip and cleft palate
Mosaic type	46,XX/47,XX, +13	5% of cases	Normal	5. Polydactyly 6. Rocker-bottom feet 7. Abnormal ears 8. Apneic spells and myoclonic seizures 9. Cardiac dextroposition and interventricular septal defect 10. Extensive visceral defects
Cri du Chat (Cat-cry) Syndrome (1 in 50,000 births)	46,XX,5p– 46,XY,5p–		Normal	1. Mental retardation 2. Microcephaly and round facies 3. Mewing cry 4. Epicanthic folds

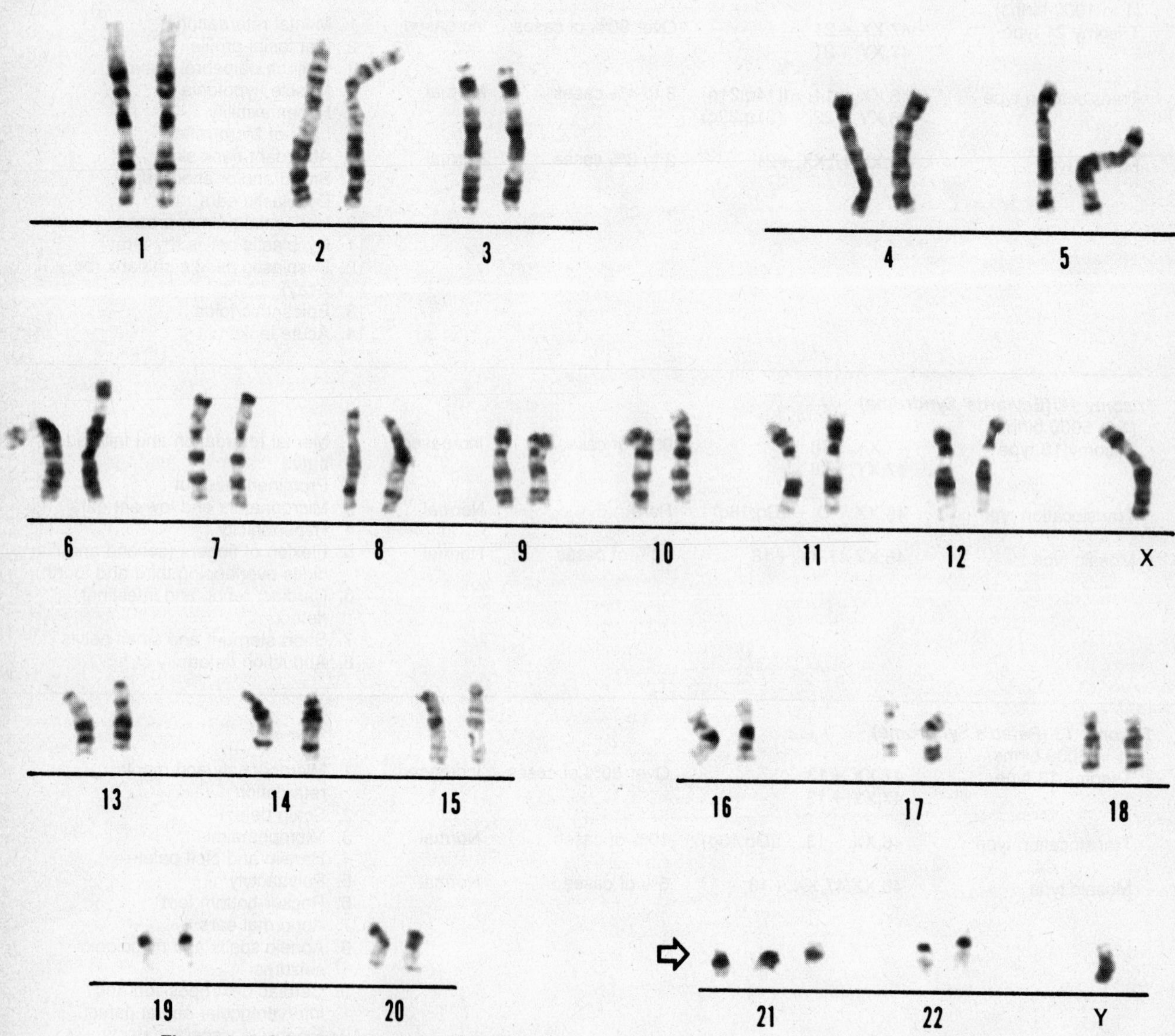

Figure 4–4. G-banded karyotype of a male with trisomy 21. (Courtesy of Dr. Patricia Howard-Peebles, Southwestern Medical School, Dallas, Texas.)

overdiagnosis of leukemia in these already sufficiently troubled unfortunates.[21,22] Despite all these problems, some patients survive into adult life and some into the advanced years. A few of those who survive into middle age have a predisposition to develop premature Alzheimer's disease. Some females with Down's syndrome have had children, but males with this disorder are almost always infertile or lack sexual potency. It should be noted that 50% of the offspring of mothers with Down's syndrome may be normal, since the extra chromosome may not be transmitted to the ovum.

Trisomy 18 (Edwards' Syndrome)

This syndrome, characterized by severe malformations, is fortunately much less common than trisomy 21 (about one in 5,000 to 10,000 live births) but much more severe and wide-ranging. Only 13% of these infants live beyond the age of one year, with an average survival of little more than ten weeks. The major clinical features are presented in Table 4–3. The mental retardation is severe, and cardiac anomalies, most commonly ventricular septal defects, are present in 95% of cases. The great preponderance of infants have an extra chromosome 18 derived from a meiotic error in parental germ cells, most likely those of the mother. About 10% of the patients have mosaicism. Rarely, an unbalanced translocation of the long arm of chromosome 18 to one of the D group underlies this condition. In the case of the trisomies, parents are almost always normal, but the mothers are generally older. In the few instances of trisomy 18 associated with a translocation, one of the parents is a carrier of the abnormal chromosome.

Trisomy 13 (Patau's Syndrome)

Infants with this syndrome have the most severe malformations of all the chromosomal abnormalities (Table 4–3). Microcephaly and mental retardation are marked. Many have arrhinencephaly (congenital absence of those regions of the forebrain derived from the olfactory system) and a variety of abnormalities of the eye ranging from virtual absence of the eyes to cyclopia (single eye with the nose absent or located as a tubular appendage above the eye). Most of these patients have a complete trisomy 13, but a few have an unbalanced translocation of the long arm of 13, usually to one of the other D group, or mosaicism with a trisomy 13 cell line. The congenital malformations are so extreme that only a few infants live longer than one year, and in fact most die soon after birth.

Other Trisomies

A variety of other trisomies have now been described, particularly those involving chromosome 8, 9, or 22. In addition, partial trisomies have been identified for virtually every chromosome in the complement. These are all too rare to merit description here but can be found in specialized texts.[23]

Cri du Chat Syndrome (5p −)

Deletion of the short arm of chromosome 5 (5p −) (Fig. 4–5) was so named because affected infants up to the age of one year have the characteristic cry of a cat. The major clinical features are given in Table 4–3. The mental retardation is quite severe, and congenital heart anomalies (usually ventricular septal defects) are present in about 25%. In general, these children thrive better than those with the trisomies, and some survive into adult life. As the infant grows older, the kitten cry and high vocal register improve, rendering diagnosis more difficult.

Other deletion syndromes involving virtually every chromosome have been identified with the new banding techniques. A variety of congenital malformations are encountered in association with the deletions, including abnormalities of the brain, mental retardation, microcephaly, hypertelorism, congenital heart disease, and malformations of the face, hands, and ears.

CYTOGENETIC DISORDERS INVOLVING SEX CHROMOSOMES

The genetic diseases associated with karyotypic changes involving the sex chromosomes are far more common than those related to autosomal aberrations. The syndromes associated with an extra X or Y chromosome are generally benign because, as you recall, all but one X chromosome are inactivated to appear as X chromatin or Barr bodies, and the Y chromosome seems to be genetically inert except for its role in sex determination (p. 133). However, the absence of one sex chromosome can have serious consequences. As mentioned earlier, there is a very high prenatal mortality with the 45,X karyotype, and even live-born infants have an increased risk of early death. The 45,Y karyotype is lethal.

A few features are common to all sex chromosome disorders. *In general they induce subtle, chronic complaints relating to sexual development and fertility.* They are often difficult to diagnose at birth, and many are first recognized in adult life. In general, the higher the number of X chromosomes, in both male and female, the greater the likelihood of mental retardation. Although the condition can often be detected by visualization of X chromatin or Y chromatin in interphase nuclei, such methods are not as reliable as cytogenetic analysis of the karyotype. The most important disorders arising in aberrations of sex chromosomes are cited in Table 4–4 and will be described briefly.

Klinefelter's Syndrome

Also called *testicular dysgenesis,* Klinefelter's syndrome is one of the most frequent forms of genetic disease involving the sex chromosomes, as well as one of the most common causes of hypogonadism in the male. The incidence of this condition is approximately

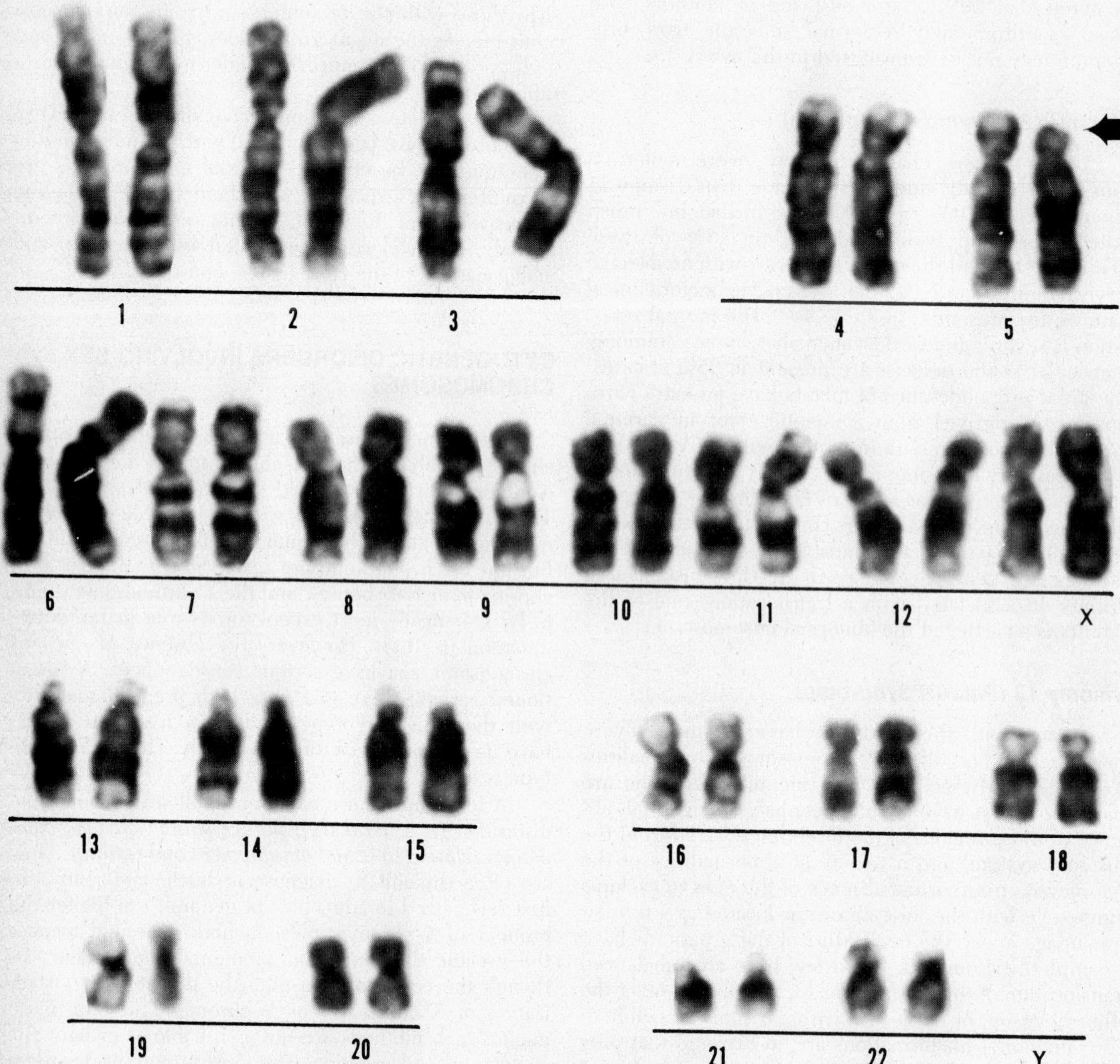

Figure 4–5. Karyotype of a female with the cri du chat syndrome (5p –). (Courtesy of Dr. Patricia Howard-Peebles, Southwestern Medical School, Dallas, Texas.)

Table 4–4. DISORDERS ASSOCIATED WITH THE SEX CHROMOSOMES

Disorder	Examples of Karyotype	X-Chromatin Pattern	Approximate Incidence	Maternal Age	Clinical Features
Klinefelter's Syndrome	47,XXY 46,XY/47,XXY	+ +	1 in 850 male births	Slightly increased	1. Testicular atrophy and azoospermia 2. Eunuchoid bodily habitus 3. Increase in sole to os pubis length 4. Gynecomastia 5. Female distribution of hair 6. Mental retardation
Variants of Klinefelter's Syndrome	48,XXXY 49,XXXXY 48,XXYY	+ + + + + +	Rare	Increased	1. More severe mental retardation 2. Cryptorchidism 3. Hypospadias 4. Radioulnar synostosis
Double Y Males	47,XYY	Negative	1 in 1000 male births	Normal	1. Phenotypically normal 2. Most over 6 feet tall 3. (?) Increased aggressive behavior
Turner's Syndrome (Gonadal Dysgenesis)	45,X	Negative	1 in 3000 female births	Normal	1. Short stature 2. Primary amenorrhea 3. Infertility 4. Webbing of neck 5. Cubitus valgus 6. Peripheral lymphedema 7. Broad chest and wide-spaced nipples 8. Low posterior hairline 9. Pigmented nevi 10. Coarctation of aorta
Defective second X chromosome	46,XXp – 46,XXq – 46,X,r(X) 46,X,i(Xq)	+ (small) + (small) + + (large)		Normal Normal Normal Normal	
Mosaicism	45,X/46,XX	Usually +		Normal	
Multiple X Females	47,XXX 48,XXXX	+ + + + +	1 in 1200 female births	Increased	1. Mental retardation 2. Menstrual irregularities 3. Many normal and fertile
True Hermaphrodites			Rare	Normal	1. Testicular and ovarian tissue 2. Varying genital abnormalities
Most cases	46,XX	+			
Some mosaics	46,XX/47,XXY	+			
Rare case of double fertilization	46,XX/46,XY	+			

1 in 850 live male births. It can rarely be diagnosed before puberty, particularly since the testicular abnormality does not develop before early puberty. The major clinical features are presented in Table 4–4. Particularly characteristic are the eunuchoid bodily habitus with abnormally long legs, the small atrophic testes often associated with a small penis and the lack of such secondary male characteristics as deep voice, beard, and male distribution of pubic hair. Confirmatory laboratory findings are (1) positive X chromatin, (2) absence or striking reduction of sperm in the seminal fluid, (3) increased urinary excretion of follicle-stimulating hormone, and (4) lower than normal serum testosterone levels.

Klinefelter's syndrome has two important clinical significances: (1) it is an important cause of sterility in the male; and (2) it is often associated with a slight decrease in intelligence, but some patients have an I. Q. in the normal range. The reduced spermatogenesis is related to several patterns of morphologic change in the testis. In some patients, the testicular tubules are totally atrophied and are replaced by pink, hyaline, collagenous ghosts. In others, the dysgenesis is manifested by apparently normal tubules interspersed with atrophic tubules. In some patients, all tubules are primitive and appear embryonic, consisting of cords of cells that never developed a lumen or mature spermatogenesis. Hyperplasia of the Leydig cells has been reported in all these variants. According to some authors, however, there is no true Leydig cell hyperplasia but the Leydig cells appear prominent owing to atrophy and crowding of the tubules.[24]

The classic pattern of Klinefelter's syndrome has a 47,XXY karyotype, accounting for the positive sex chromatin test (82% of cases). This complement has been explained by nondisjunction during the meiotic divisions in one of the parents. The extra X chromosome might therefore be of either maternal or paternal origin.[25] Advanced maternal age and irradiation of either parent have been suggested as relevant in the etiology of this condition. In addition to this classic karyotype, some patients with Klinefelter's syndrome have been found to have a variety of mosaic patterns, most of them being 46,XY/47,XXY. Others are 47,XXY/48,XXXY and variations of this theme. Rare individuals have also been found to possess 48,XXXY or 49,XXXXY karyotypes.

With increasing numbers of X chromosomes, patients exhibit a progressively greater reduction in intelligence. Concomitantly, such polysomic X individuals have further physical abnormalities including cryptorchidism, hypospadias, more severe hypoplasia of the testes, and skeletal changes such as prognathism and radioulnar synostosis. Such severely affected individuals are likely to have had considerably older mothers.

XYY Syndrome

Supernumerary Y's may be found in the male, giving rise to 47,XYY, or even greater Y polysomy. The diagnosis usually rests on identification of more than one Y chromatin body in interphase nuclei, but false-positive errors may result because of fluorescent segments on non-Y chromosomes, and false-negative errors may result because of possible mosaicism or technical deficiencies. Chromosome analysis is far more accurate. Approximately one in 1000 live-born males has one of these karyotypes. Nearly all are phenotypically normal, but the individuals frequently are excessively tall and may be susceptible to severe acne. From present data it appears that the intelligence of these individuals is in the normal range.

Most controversial is the impact of extra Y chromosomes upon behavior. These karyotypes have been identified with increased frequency among inmates of penal institutions. The behavioral difficulties take the form of antisocial (not violent), delinquent, impulsive acting-out disorders.[26] From recent studies it appears that only about 1 to 2% of individuals with XYY phenotypes exhibit such deviant behavior; the overwhelming preponderance are no more antisocial than their peers who are less richly endowed with Y chromosomes. At present, the situation is far from clear and long-term prospective study of infants with these karyotypes is required.

Turner's Syndrome

Although Turner's syndrome is generally equated with a 45,X karyotype, about one-half of the patients are in fact mosaics with two or three cell lines, one of which is 45,X. Because the mosaics do not completely express the classic phenotype, a wide range of clinical severities is found. Moreover, the clinical manifestations vary with age. Other karyotypic findings include structural deletions or rearrangements of one of the X chromosomes. At the outset, it should be emphasized that only about 3% of fetuses with the 45,X karyotype survive to birth. There is an increased postnatal mortality as well. Surviving infants generally present edema (due to lymph stasis) of the dorsum of the hand and foot, and sometimes swelling of the nape of the neck. The latter is related to markedly distended lymphatic channels, producing a so-called cystic hygroma (p. 544). As these infants develop, the swellings subside but often leave persistent looseness of skin on the back of the neck and bilateral neck webbing. Congenital heart disease is also common, particularly preductal coarctation of the aorta and aortic stenosis with endocardial fibroelastosis, anomalies that may account for some of the early deaths.

The principal clinical features in the adolescent and adult are cited in Table 4–4. At puberty there is failure to develop normal secondary sex characteristics. The genitalia remain infantile, breast development is inadequate, and there is little pubic hair. The mental status of these patients is usually normal, but a few may exhibit some retardation. Of particular importance in establishing the diagnosis in the adult is the shortness of stature (rarely exceeding 150 cm in height) and the amenorrhea. In this regard, approximately one-third of women who present with primary amenorrhea have a chromosome anomaly and about half of these have the 45,X karyotype.[27] Typically the ovaries are reduced to atrophic fibrous strands, devoid of ova and follicles, and are termed *"streak ovaries."* There appears to be loss of germ cells at or before birth.[28] The reduced estrogen output by the ovaries leads to elevated pituitary gonadotropin secretion. However, it should be noted that a few women with this condition have been reported to be fertile.

Because of the frequency of mosaicism, the clinical signs and symptoms may be exceedingly subtle. Mosaicism also introduces difficulties in confirming the diagnosis by study of somatic cells for X chromatin or cytogenetic analysis, since a significant proportion of cells may have the normal XX karyotype. Structural abnormalities of the X chromosome are found in 28% of patients with Turner's syndrome,[29] the most common being isochromosome of the long arm of X [46,X,i(Xq)]. Deletion of the short arm, i.e., 46,XXp− is also seen in some cases. These abnormalities may be present in all the cells or in association with a 45,X line (mosaics).

Multi-X Females

Karyotypes with one to three extra X chromosomes have been described and are not uncommon, being found in about one in 1200 newborn females. The diagnosis should be readily made by the demonstration of two or more X chromatin bodies, but this technique may well miss a significant number of cases identifiable by karyotype. Most of these women, according to current thought, are entirely normal. However, a variety of random findings may be present. As mentioned, there is an increased tendency to mental retardation in proportion to the number of extra X chromosomes. Thus, mental retardation is seen in all with the 49,XXXXX karyotype, whereas most with 47,XXX are unaffected. Some women have amenorrhea or occasionally other menstrual irregularities.

Hermaphroditism and Pseudohermaphroditism

The problem of sexual ambiguity is exceedingly complex, and only limited observations are possible here. For more details, reference should be made to specialized texts.[30, 31] It may be no surprise to medical students that the sex of an individual can be defined on several levels. Genetic sex is determined by the presence or absence of a Y chromosome. No matter how many X chromosomes are present, a single Y chromosome dictates testicular development and the genetic male gender. The initially indifferent gonads of both the male and female embryos have an inherent tendency to feminize, unless influenced by Y chromosome–dependent masculinizing factors. The testis organizing genes, (H-Y genes) have been located on the short arm of Y. The H-Y gene product (H-Y antigen) can be detected serologically on male cells. *Gonadal sex* is based on the histologic characteristics of the gonads. *Ductal sex* depends on the presence of derivatives of the müllerian or wolffian ducts. *Phenotypic* or *genital sex* is based on the appearance of the external genitalia. Sexual ambiguity is present whenever there is disagreement among these various criteria for determining sex.

The term true hermaphrodite *implies the presence of both ovarian and testicular tissue. In contrast, a* pseudohermaphrodite *represents a disagreement between the phenotypic and gonadal sex,* i.e., a female pseudohermaphrodite has ovarian gonads but male external genitalia; a male pseudohermaphrodite has testicular tissue but female-type genitalia. Disappointingly, karyotypic analyses have not shed much light on these difficult problems of intersex. Indeed, as will be seen, hormonal influences may induce sexual ambiguity completely apart from the genotype of the individual.

True hermaphroditism, implying the presence of both ovarian and testicular tissue, is an extremely rare condition. In some cases there is a testis on one side and an ovary on the other, while in other cases there may be combined ovarian and testicular tissue, referred to as ovotestes. Such abnormal gonads most often are found in the abdomen but can lie anywhere along the tract of testicular descent into the scrotum. Most of these individuals have a uterus and other ductal structures reminiscent of those found in both male and female. The external genitalia are usually ambiguous, and could be interpreted as a bifid scrotum or enlarged labia with a small penis or enlarged clitoris. A large majority of such individuals yield a positive test for X chromatin but all are also positive for the H-Y antigen, suggesting the presence of at least a part of the Y chromosome. Included among the sex chromatin–positive true hermaphrodites are XX/XXY mosaics and chimeras (XX/XY), the latter resulting from the fertilization of a binucleate ovum by two sperms, one bearing an X and the other a Y chromosome. Many XX true hermaphrodites, however, do not seem to have a Y-bearing cell line, and in such cases translocation of the H-Y gene–bearing segment of the Y chromosome to either an X chromosome or an autosome has been suggested. Thus, true hermaphrodites are a heterogeneous group, having in common the presence of two X chromosomes as well as a complete or partial Y chromosome, at least in some of the cells.

Female pseudohermaphroditism is much less complex. The genetic sex in all cases is XX and the development of the gonads (ovaries) and internal genitalia is normal. Only the external genitalia are ambiguous or virilized. The basis of female pseudohermaphroditism is excessive and inappropriate exposure to androgenic steroids during the early part of gestation. Such steroids are most commonly derived from the fetal adrenal affected by congenital adrenal hyperplasia, which is transmitted as an autosomal recessive trait. Biosynthetic defects in the pathway of cortisol synthesis are present in these cases that lead secondarily to excessive synthesis of androgenic steroids by the fetal adrenal cortex (p. 1241). Less commonly, the virilizing steroids are maternal in origin. Androgen-secreting maternal tumors (e.g., the Sertoli-Leydig cell tumor), or more commonly administration of androgens or progestins to the mother during pregnancy, underlie such cases.

Male pseudohermaphroditism represents the most complex of all disorders of sexual differentiation since the development of "maleness" requires not only the differentiation of male gonads and genitalia, but also active suppression of the inherent tendency of the fetus to feminize. A brief review of normal male differentiation will help our understanding of the patterns of male pseudohermaphroditism. Under the influence of the Y chromosome (H-Y antigen), the primordial gonad differentiates into the testis. Further steps involve on the one hand, inhibition of müllerian ducts by the Sertoli cell–derived müllerian duct inhibitory factor and on the other hand, secretion of testosterone by the Leydig cells, which in turn regulates the male differentiation of the wolffian ducts, urogenital sinus, and external genitalia. The secretion of testosterone by the Leydig cells is regulated by human chorionic gonadotropins (HCG) as well as luteinizing hormone (LH). The action of testosterone and the gonadotropins requires specific interaction with the appropriate receptors on the target tissues.

With this overview, we can discuss the definition and classification of male pseudohermaphroditism. Male pseudohermaphrodites are individuals who possess a Y chromosome, and thus their gonads are exclusively testes but the genital ducts or the external genitalia are incompletely differentiated along the male phenotype. Their external genitalia are either ambiguous or completely female. On the basis of the etiology, male pseudohermaphroditism has been divided into six categories (Table 4–5).[31] However, it is beyond our scope to discuss these disorders individually, and therefore only a few general comments will be offered. The karyotype in all cases, except in some variants with dysgenetic testes, is XY. The presence of Y chromosome dictates testicular differentiation, and therefore testes can be identified, either readily or with some difficulty, in most cases. In the gonadal dysgenesis pattern the aberrations in testicular organogenesis may be so severe that the gonad is represented only by a fibrous streak. Except for variants with dysgenetic testes, all other forms are familial, although there is no single pattern of transmission. Of considerable clinical significance is the fact that about one-third of male pseudohermaphrodites, especially those whose condition is associated with testicular dysgenesis, develop testicular tumors of germ cell origin. The risk is so great that prophylactic gonadectomy is recommended.

Table 4–5. MALE PSEUDOHERMAPHRODITISM

A. Testicular unresponsiveness to HCG and LH
B. Inborn errors of testosterone biosynthesis
   1. Enzyme defects affecting synthesis of both corticosteroids and testosterone (variants of congenital adrenal hyperplasias)
   2. Enzyme defects primarily affecting testosterone biosynthesis by the testes
C. Defects in androgen-dependent target tissues
   1. End-organ insensitivity to androgenic hormones, e.g., complete syndrome of androgen insensitivity (testicular feminization) and variant forms
   2. Defects in testosterone metabolism by peripheral tissues, e.g., 5 α-reductase deficiency
D. Dysgenetic male pseudohermaphroditism
E. Defects in synthesis, secretion, or response to müllerian duct inhibitory factor
F. Maternal ingestion of estrogen and progestins

Modified from Grumbach, M. M., and Conte, F. A.: Disorders of sex differentiation. *In* Williams, R. H. (ed.): Textbook of Endocrinology. Philadelphia, W. B. Saunders Co., 1981, p. 423.

MENDELIAN DISORDERS

All mendelian disorders are the result of expressed mutations in single genes of large effect transmitted by autosomal dominant, autosomal recessive, or X-linked modes of inheritance. It is not necessary to detail Mendel's laws here, since every student in biology, and possibly every garden pea, has learned about them at an early age. Only some comments of medical relevance will be made.

The number of mendelian disorders has grown to monumental proportions. In the recent edition of his book, McKusick has listed 2786 disorders.[32] It is estimated that every individual is a carrier of five to eight deleterious genes.[33] Fortunately, most of these are recessive and therefore do not cause serious phenotypic effects. About 80 to 85% of these mutations are familial. The remainder represent new mutations.

When dealing with mendelian disorders, a number of considerations must be kept in mind, some of which apply equally to autosomal dominant, autosomal recessive, and X-linked mutant genes. Most obvious, the mutation may be acquired de novo by an affected individual. Obviously, such a proband (index patient) will have a normal family pedigree but, on the other hand, will be the forebear of affected generations to come. The extent to which mutations are expressed varies widely. Two variants associated with autosomal dominant inheritance are recognized: (1) When individuals who have a mutant gene fail to express it, the trait is said to demonstrate reduced penetrance. *Penetrance* is expressed in mathematical terms: thus, 50% penetrance indicates that 50% of those who carry the gene express the trait. The factors that affect penetrance are not clearly understood, but this possibility is of obvious importance in genetic counseling. (2) In contrast to penetrance, if a trait is seen in all the individuals carrying the mutant gene but is expressed differently among individuals, the phenomenon is called *variable expressivity*. For example, polydactyly may be expressed in the toes or in the fingers as one or more extra digits.

Some autosomal mutations produce partial expression in the heterozygote and full expression in the homozygote. Sickle cell anemia is caused by substitution of normal hemoglobin (HbA) by hemoglobin S (HbS). The molecular basis for the formation of hemoglobin S is presented on p. 618, but here it is sufficient to note that when an individual is homozygous for the mutant gene, all of the hemoglobin is of the abnormal HbS type, and even under normal atmospheric pressures of oxygen the disorder is fully expressed, i.e., sickling deformity of all red cells and hemolytic anemia. In the heterozygote only a proportion of the hemoglobin is HbS (the remainder being HbA), and therefore red cell sickling and possibly hemolysis occur only when there is exposure to lowered oxygen tension. This is referred to as the sickle cell trait to differentiate it from full-blown sickle cell anemia.

Although gene expression is usually described as dominant or recessive, it should be remembered that in some cases both alleles of a gene pair may be fully expressed in the heterozygote—a condition called *codominance*. Histocompatibility and blood group antigens are good examples of codominant inheritance as well as *polymorphism*. The latter implies the existence of multiple allelic forms of a single gene.

A single mutant gene may lead to many end effects, termed *pleiotropism*, and conversely mutations at several genetic loci may produce the same trait *(genetic heterogeneity)*. Sickle cell anemia may serve as an example of pleiotropism. In this hereditary disorder, not only does the point mutation in the gene give rise to HbS, which predisposes the red cells to hemolysis, but the abnormal sickled red cells tend to cause a logjam in small vessels; the vascular embarrassment in turn induces a variety of end-organ effects, including splenic fibrosis, organ infarcts, and bone changes. The numerous differing end-organ derangements are all related to the primary defect in hemoglobin synthesis. On the other hand, profound childhood deafness, an apparently homogeneous clinical entity, results from 16 different types of autosomal recessive mutations. Recognition of genetic heterogeneity is not only important in genetic counseling, but is also relevant in the understanding of the pathogenesis of some common disorders, such as diabetes mellitus (p. 975).

BIOCHEMICAL BASIS OF MENDELIAN DISORDERS

Mendelian disorders result from alterations involving single genes, implying that these diseases result from a primary abnormality in a *single protein molecule*. Broadly speaking, three kinds of proteins may be affected by mutation—enzymes, structural proteins, and regulatory proteins. To some extent the pattern of inheritance of the disease is related to the kind of protein affected by the mutation. In general, *diseases resulting from mutations involving enzyme proteins are inherited as autosomal recessives*. In such cases, equal amounts of the normal as well as the defective enzyme are synthesized in the heterozygotes, and usually the natural "margin of safety" ensures that cells with half their usual complement of the enzyme will function normally. On the other hand, *mutations involving key structural proteins, such as collagen, or those involving regulatory proteins, such as membrane receptors, are usually dominant*. The biochemical derangements underlying autosomal dominant diseases are generally much more complex and difficult to characterize.

To aid our understanding of the pathogenesis of mendelian disorders, we can classify the mechanisms of single gene disorders into five categories: *(1) enzyme defects and their consequences; (2) defects in membrane receptors and transport systems; (3) alterations in the structure, function, or quantity of nonenzyme proteins; (4) mutations resulting in unusual reactions to drugs; and (5) unknown mechanisms*. It should be understood that this is a provisional classification subject to modification as the biochemical basis of the large number of diseases in the unknown category begins to unfold.

ENZYME DEFECTS AND THEIR CONSEQUENCES. Mutations may result in the synthesis of a defective enzyme or in a reduced amount of a normal enzyme. In either case, the consequence is a metabolic block. Figure 4–6 provides an example of an enzyme reaction in which the substrate S is converted by intracellular enzymes E_1, E_2, and E_3 into an end product P through intermediates I_1 and I_2. In this model the final product P exerts feedback control on enzyme E_1. A minor pathway producing small quantities of M_1 and M_2 also exists. The biochemical consequences of an enzyme defect in such a reaction may lead to two major consequences: (1) *Accumulation of the substrate*, which, depending on the site of block, may be accompanied by accumulation of one or both intermediates. Moreover, an increased concentration of I_2 may stimulate the minor pathway and thus lead to an excess of M_1 and M_2. Under these conditions tissue injury may result if the precursor, the intermediates, or the products of alternate minor pathways are toxic in high concentrations. For example, in galactosemia, the deficiency of galactose-1-phosphate uridyltransferase (p. 491) leads to the accumulation of galactose and consequent tissue damage. A deficiency of phenylalanine hydroxylase (p. 490) results in the accumulation of phenylalanine. Excessive accumulation of complex substrates within the lysosomes due to deficiency of degradative enzymes is responsible for a group of diseases generally referred to as *lysosomal* storage diseases (p. 142). (2) *An enzyme defect can lead to a metabolic block and a decreased amount of end product* that may be necessary for normal function. For example, a deficiency of melanin may result from lack of tyrosinase, which is necessary for the biosynthesis of melanin from its precursor tyrosine. This results in the

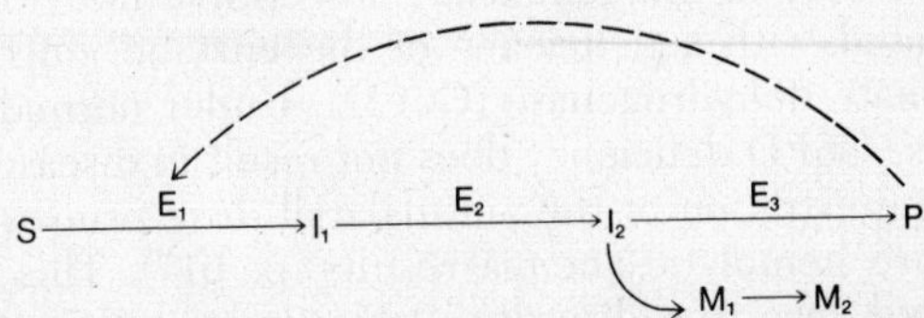

Figure 4–6. A schema illustrating the conversion of a substrate (S) to the end product (P), through several intermediates (I), brought about by enzymes (E). P exerts feedback inhibition of E_1. M denotes products of minor pathways.

clinical condition called albinism, to be discussed later (p. 141). If the end product is a feedback inhibitor of the enzymes involved in the early reactions (in Fig. 4–6 it is shown that P inhibits E_1), the deficiency of the end product may permit overproduction of intermediates and their catabolic products, some of which may be injurious at high concentrations. A prime example of a disease with such an underlying mechanism is the Lesch-Nyhan syndrome (p. 1358).

DEFECTS IN RECEPTORS AND TRANSPORT SYSTEMS. Many biologically active substances have to be actively transported across the cell membrane. This is generally achieved by one of two mechanisms—through initial binding to a specific receptor site followed by internalization, or via a "carrier" protein. A genetic defect in a receptor-mediated transport system is exemplified by familial hypercholesterolemia, in which inadequate synthesis of receptors leads to defective transport of low-density lipoproteins (LDL) into the cells and secondarily to excessive cholesterol synthesis by complex intermediary mechanisms (p. 139). In Hartnup's disease, on the other hand, the transport system for tryptophan (and certain other amino acids) across the intestinal cells is defective. Since tryptophan is a precursor of the vitamin nicotinamide, symptoms of pellagra (p. 415) develop. More than 20 inherited disorders of membrane transport have been described in humans. Most affect the gut, the kidney, or both.

ALTERATIONS IN STRUCTURE, FUNCTION, OR QUANTITY OF NONENZYME PROTEINS. Genetic defects resulting in alterations of structural proteins often have widespread secondary effects, as exemplified by sickle cell disease (p. 618). Indeed, the hemoglobinopathies, sickle cell disease being one, all of which are characterized by defects in the structure of the globin molecule, best exemplify this category. In contrast to the hemoglobinopathies, the group of thalassemias results from mutations in genes that *regulate the rate of globin chain synthesis*. They are associated with reduced amounts of structurally normal alpha- or beta-globin chains (p. 622). Other examples of genetically defective structural proteins that we shall discuss in this chapter involve collagen and are exemplified by Marfan's and Ehlers-Danlos syndromes.

GENETICALLY DETERMINED ADVERSE REACTIONS TO DRUGS. Certain genetically determined enzyme deficiencies are unmasked only after exposure of the affected individual to certain drugs. This special area of genetics, called pharmacogenetics, is of considerable clinical importance.[34] The classic example of drug-induced injury in the genetically susceptible individual is associated with a deficiency of the enzyme glucose-6-phosphate dehydrogenase (G6PD). Under normal conditions, G6PD deficiency does not result in disease, but on administration of the antimalarial drug primaquine, a severe hemolytic anemia results (p. 617). This is an X-linked recessive disorder. An estimated 100 million people throughout the world have some degree of G6PD deficiency. It has been suggested that the deficiency confers some protection against the parasitization of red cells by the malarial parasite, which may explain in evolutionary terms why such a gene mutation appears with such frequency.

UNKNOWN MECHANISMS. Despite our extensive knowledge of the biochemical basis of many genetic disorders, the list of "unknowns" remains large. Included in this category, regrettably, is one of the commonest genetic diseases, cystic fibrosis. Other important unknowns include neoplasms such as retinoblastoma, familial colonic polyposis, neurofibromatosis, and neuromuscular disorders, including Huntington's disease and myotonic dystrophy.

Despite the usefulness of a pathogenetic classification, based on the nature of the underlying biochemical defect, mendelian disorders are generally classified according to their mode of inheritance, a tradition followed in the succeeding sections.

AUTOSOMAL DOMINANT DISORDERS

Autosomal dominant inheritance has the following characteristics:

1. *Affected patients have an affected parent and forebears back to the point in the ancestry at which the mutant gene arose through an acquired mutation.*
2. *Unaffected relatives do not transmit the condition.*
3. *Offspring of an affected person and a normal mate have a 50–50 chance of being affected.*
4. *In the rare case in which two affected heterozygotes mate, there is a 3 out of 4 chance of offspring being affected (1 chance in 4 of homozygous normal, 2 chances in 4 of heterozygous affected; and 1 chance in 4 of homozygous affected).*

We can do no more than scratch the surface in discussing the impressive array of autosomal dominant mendelian diseases. Some of these conditions are more logically discussed in other chapters. Listed alphabetically, they are:

- achondroplasia—a form of dwarfism (p. 1321)
- Huntington's chorea—a neurologic disorder (p. 1416)
- lymphedema, hereditary (Milroy's disease) (p. 538)
- nephropathy with deafness (Alport's syndrome) (p. 1026)
- polycystic kidney disease (p. 1000)
- polyposis of the colon, certain forms of—multiple benign colonic tumors (p. 867)
- sickle cell anemia—a hemoglobinopathy (p. 618)
- spherocytosis—a form of hemolytic anemia (p. 616)
- telangiectasia, Osler's—widespread vascular malformations (p. 542)
- thalassemia—a red cell disorder (p. 622)
- tuberous sclerosis—a multisystem disease affecting principally the brain (p. 1428)
- von Willebrand's disease—a bleeding diathesis (p. 648)

A few autosomal dominant conditions not considered

elsewhere follow, either because of their frequency or because they illustrate significant genetic principles.

Marfan's Syndrome

Marfan's syndrome is an uncommon but interesting *disorder of the connective tissues of the body, manifested principally by changes in the skeleton, eyes, and cardiovascular system.*[35] Because affected individuals have unusually long, slender extremities, particularly elongation of the fingers, this entity has also been termed *"arachnodactyly"* (spider fingers). Approximately 85% of the cases are familial and transmitted by autosomal dominant inheritance. The remainder are sporadic and arise from new mutations.[36] In contrast to Down's syndrome in which the risk for the offspring rises with maternal age, it is the paternal age that is important in the sporadic cases of Marfan's syndrome; fathers of affected children are about seven years older than the average.

There is considerable range in the severity of clinical manifestations among affected individuals. This range has been attributed to variable expressivity of the mutant gene as well as possible genetic heterogeneity (p. 134). For unknown reasons, males transmit the familial disease far less often than females, perhaps because they have reduced fertility as compared with affected females.

Skeletal abnormalities are the most striking feature of Marfan's syndrome. Typically, the patient is unusually tall with exceptionally long extremities and long, tapering fingers and toes. Interestingly, it is the forearms (distal) and thighs (proximal) that contribute most to this extremity elongation. The joint ligaments in the hands and feet are lax, suggesting that the patient is double-jointed; typically, the thumb can be hyperextended back to the wrist. The head is commonly dolichocephalic (long-headed) with bossing of the frontal eminences and prominent supraorbital ridges. President Lincoln is suspected to have had Marfan's syndrome and represents a classic example of the condition. A variety of spinal deformities may appear, including kyphosis, scoliosis, or rotation or slipping of the dorsal or lumbar vertebrae. The chest is classically deformed, presenting either pectus excavatum (deeply depressed sternum) or a pigeon-breast deformity. Subcutaneous fat is usually scant, and muscular development is poor; thus, these patients have a long. gaunt appearance, sometimes marked by the many distortions of the bodily habitus mentioned.

The **ocular changes** take many forms. Most characteristic is bilateral subluxation or dislocation (usually outward and upward) of the lens, referred to as ectopia lentis. This abnormality is so uncommon in those who do not have this genetic disease that the finding of bilateral ectopia lentis should raise the suspicion of Marfan's syndrome. Cataracts, retinal detachment, secondary glaucoma, and a wavy, tremulous iris on rapid eye motion may also be present. All these ocular changes relate to a basic defect in connective tissue and impaired support of the ocular structures.

Cardiovascular lesions are the most life-threatening features of this disorder. Of greatest importance is the development of cystic medionecrosis (p. 522) of the aorta, which predisposes to aneurysmal dilatation and sometimes rupture. The medial weakening and dilatation principally affect the ascending aorta, but in a few cases have involved the aortic arch and the descending and abdominal aorta. Sometimes the pulmonary artery is concomitantly affected. Histologically, the changes in the aorta are virtually identical to those found in cystic medionecrosis not related to Marfan's syndrome, and constitute depletion and fragmentation of elastic laminae of the media associated with increased vascularity of the media and adventitia. Along with disruption of the elastic fibers there is deposition of a metachromatic amorphous intercellular substance, which can be histochemically identified as acid mucopolysaccharides. In very severe cases, large clefts or cystic areas may be seen within the increased ground substance (Fig. 4–7). There is some associated increase in collagen fibers and smooth muscle cells. The latter become disoriented and enlarged and may

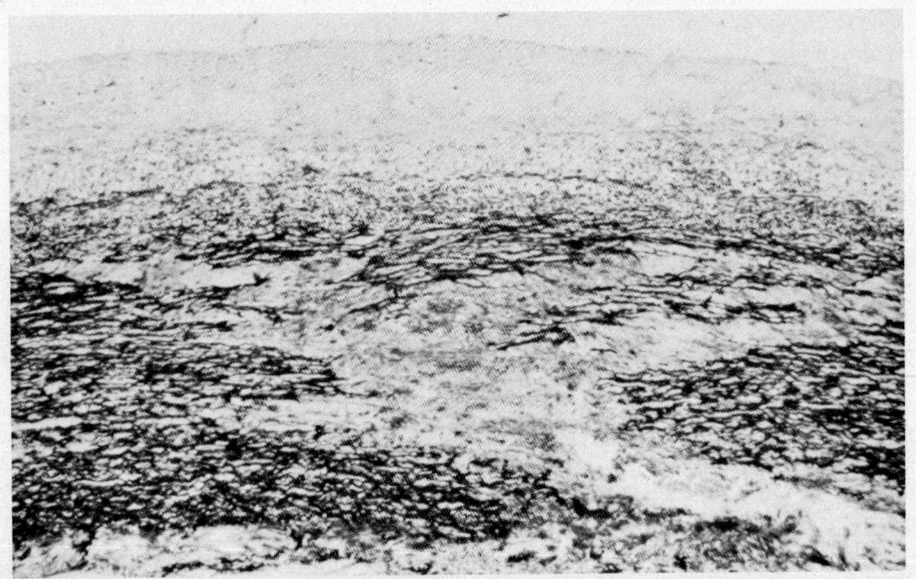

Figure 4–7. Idiopathic medial necrosis. The large defect in the laminar pattern of the aortic wall is highlighted by the elastic tissue stain.

even come to lie at abnormal, oblique, or right angles to the layers of elastic tissue. Loss of medial support results in progressive dilatation of the aortic valve ring and the root of the aorta, giving rise to severe aortic incompetence. Weakening of the media also predisposes to an intimal tear, which may initiate an intramural hematoma that cleaves the layers of the media to produce a so-called dissecting aneurysm (p. 522). After cleaving the aortic layers for considerable distances, sometimes back to the root of the aorta or down to the iliac arteries, the hemorrhage often ruptures through the aortic wall. Such a calamity is the cause of death in 30 to 45% of these individuals and may occur at any age; it has been reported in a 4-year-old child. Even when dissection does not occur, the dilatation of the aorta may involve the aortic valve ring, leading to aortic regurgitation.

A variety of other cardiac lesions are often found in these patients. Loss of connective tissue support in the mitral valve leaflets may make them soft and billowy, creating the so-called "floppy valve." Valvular lesions, along with shortening of the chordae tendineae, frequently give rise to mitral regurgitation. Similar changes may affect the tricuspid, and rarely the aortic, valves. Although mitral valve lesions are more frequent, they are clinically less important than aortic valve lesions. Hemodynamic dysfunction secondary to the valvular changes often leads to cardiomegaly.

As mentioned at the outset, there is great variation in the clinical expression of this genetic disorder. Patients with prominent eye or cardiovascular changes may have few skeletal abnormalities, while others with striking changes in bodily habitus have no eye changes. All combinations and permutations may be encountered, and in some affected individuals the signs and symptoms are exceedingly subtle. Failure to identify these formes frustes in family pedigrees may account for the misinterpretation that the patient represents a fresh mutation.

It is disappointing to report that, despite all the striking clinical findings, the basic nature of the underlying connective tissue defect is still obscure. Indeed, there is still uncertainty whether the hereditary defect primarily involves elastic fibers or collagen fibers. Conceivably, both are affected concomitantly. Most of the evidence supports the concept that some subtle biochemical or metabolic defect in collagen accounts for its premature degeneration or "aging."[37]

Much interest has centered around the concept that the basic defect in Marfan's syndrome is decreased formation of cross-linkages in collagen and elastic fibers, which impairs their tensile strength. Indeed, in certain animal models, defects in collagen cross-linkages do lead to marfanoid manifestations. For example, rats fed sweet pea meal derived from the seeds of *Lathyrus odoratus* develop remarkably similar skeletal changes and dissecting aneurysms of the aorta. The active ingredient responsible for the production of *lathyrism* is beta-aminopropionitrile, which blocks cross-linkages in collagen and elastin fibers by inhibiting the enzyme lysyl-oxidase (p. 78). Since lysyl-oxidase is a copper-dependent enzyme, the search for possible genetic metabolic derangements lead to *Menke's syndrome*, an X-linked recessive disorder of man marked by a block in the intestinal absorption of copper. In this rare metabolic disorder, changes in aortic collagen and elastin are present that may well be attributable to the deficiency of the cross-linking enzyme lysyl-oxidase. *However, there is no evidence of any impairment of copper metabolism or lysyl-oxidase activity in Marfan's syndrome.* Defective cross-link formation could also be brought about by a number of other mechanisms. These include structural abnormalities involving critical lysine or histidine residues in the collagen chains, presence of cross-link inhibitors analogous to β-aminopropionitrile, or altered fibril stability resulting from defects in the synthesis of proteoglycans. Some preliminary evidence for defective biosynthesis of type I collagen in aortic explants has been obtained,[38] and abnormalities of cross-links in collagen obtained from several patients with Marfan's syndrome have also been noted.[39] Although deranged synthesis of ground substance by Marfan's fibroblasts has also been reported,[40] the bulk of the evidence now favors a primary defect in the collagen.

As an autosomal dominant syndrome to be anticipated in 50% of the offspring of an affected parent, Marfan's syndrome is of tragic significance. The average age at death is between 30 and 40 years.[41] The great majority of these deaths are caused by rupture of dissecting aneurysms, followed in importance by cardiac failure. Unhappily, there are no satisfactory means of consistently preventing these calamitous consequences, even when the diagnosis is established at an early age. Therapy to lower the blood pressure, sometimes followed by replacement of the aortic arch with a prosthesis, has yielded encouraging results in some patients.

Neurofibromatosis (von Recklinghausen's Disease)

Neurofibromatosis is a relatively common disorder with a frequency of almost one in 3000.[42] Although approximately 50% of the patients have a definite family history consistent with autosomal dominant transmission, the remainder appear to represent new mutations, perhaps affecting the same gene or genes. In familial cases, the expressivity of the disorder is variable but the penetrance is 100%. There is more than one form of neurofibromatosis, pointing to genetic heterogeneity. Most common is the classical neurofibromatosis, which has three major features: (1) multiple neural tumors dispersed anywhere on or in the body; (2) numerous pigmented skin lesions, some of which are "café au lait" spots; and (3) pigmented iris hamartomas, also called Lisch nodules. A bewildering assortment of other abnormalities may accompany these cardinal manifestations.

The neurofibromas arise within or are attached to nerve trunks anywhere in the skin, including the palms and soles, as well as in every conceivable internal site, including the cranial nerves (particularly the acoustic nerve). Acoustic neuromas when they occur in classical neurofibromatosis are unilateral in contrast with the presence of bilateral tumors in the **central or acoustic form of neurofibromatosis.** On the surface of the body they generally occur in profusion and range from discrete, soft, yielding, subcutaneous nodules less than 1 cm in diameter to moderate-sized pedunculated lesions, to huge, multilobar pendulous masses, 20 cm or more in greatest diameter. Similar tumors may occur internally, and in general the deeply situated lesions tend to be large. On gross examination, the neurofibromas vary from spherical to cylindrical to beaded, sometimes tortuous (plexiform) masses. They may or may not be encapsulated. Microscopically they are composed of a proliferation of all the elements in the peripheral nerve including neurites, Schwann cells, and fibroblasts. Typically, these components are dispersed in a loose, disorderly pattern, often in a loose, myxoid stroma. Elongated, serpentine Schwann cells predominate, with their slender, spindle-shaped nuclei. The loose disorderliness of the microscopic architecture helps to differentiate these neural tumors from related neurilemmomas (schwannomas). Neurilemmomas composed entirely of Schwann cells virtually never undergo malignant transformation, whereas the neurofibromas of von Recklinghausen's disease become malignant in about 10 to 15% of patients. Malignant transformation is most common in the very large tumors attached to large nerve trunks of the neck or extremities. The superficial lesions, despite their size, rarely become malignant.

The cutaneous pigmentations, the second major component of this syndrome, are present in over 90% of patients. Most commonly they appear as light brown **"café au lait"** macules, with generally smooth borders, often located over nerve trunks. They are usually round to ovoid, with their long axes parallel to the underlying cutaneous nerve. Although normal individuals may have a few café au lait spots, it is a clinical maxim that when six or more spots over 1.5 cm in diameter are present, the patient is likely to have neurofibromatosis.

Lisch nodules are present in over 94% of patients who are 6 years or older. They do not produce any symptoms but are helpful in establishing the diagnosis.

A wide range of associated abnormalities has been reported in these patients. Perhaps most common (30 to 50% of patients) are skeletal lesions, which take a variety of forms, including (1) erosive defects due to contiguity of neurofibromas to bone, (2) scoliosis, (3) intraosseous cystic lesions, (4) subperiosteal bone cysts, and (5) pseudarthrosis of the tibia. Other types of tumors are encountered more frequently in neurofibromatosis than in the general population, including meningiomas, gliomas, Wilms' tumors, rhabdomyosarcomas, pheochromocytomas, medullary thyroid cancers, among others. Pheochromocytomas are found in about 1% of patients with this genetic disease, and conversely 5 to 20% of patients with pheochromocytomas have neurofibromatosis. Stricture of the aqueduct of Sylvius, leading to hydrocephalus, may occur as a consequence of some peculiar overgrowth of the neuroglial cells.

Although some patients with this condition have normal mentality, there is an unmistakable tendency for reduced intelligence. When neurofibromas arise within the gastrointestinal tract, intestinal obstruction or gastrointestinal bleeding may occur. Narrowing of a renal artery by a tumor may induce hypertension. The range of clinical presentations is almost limitless, but ultimately the diagnosis rests on the concurrence of multiple café au lait spots and multiple skin tumors. However, these cardinal features may not be well developed at birth, and in many patients the disease is not discovered until adult life. The skin pigmentations become more evident with age as giant melanosomes in epidermal cells accumulate melanin, and the neural tumors, though small at first, slowly enlarge.

There are three other genetic variants of neurofibromatosis,[42] of which only the central or acoustic form is common enough to merit discussion. In these patients, bilateral acoustic nerve tumors are invariably present with or without skin tumors. Café au lait spots are present but Lisch nodules in the iris are not found. Patients with central or the acoustic form breed true, but it is not yet clear whether this trait is allelic with classical neurofibromatosis.

von Hippel-Lindau Disease

Von Hippel-Lindau disease is a rare autosomal dominant disorder characterized by *a variety of benign and malignant neoplasms widely dispersed throughout the body.* The most common and characteristic neoplasms are retinal hemangioblastoma (retinal angiomatosis), sometimes referred to as von Hippel's tumor, and hemangioblastoma of the cerebellum, sometimes called Lindau's tumor. The next most common tumors are hemangioblastoma of the medulla oblongata or spinal cord; angiomas of the liver and kidney; adenomas of the kidney and epididymis, renal cell carcinoma; adrenal pheochromocytoma; and cysts of the pancreas, kidney, and epididymis. Less frequently present are angiomas and cysts in a number of other organs, including lungs, spleen, omentum, adrenal gland, and ovary. In this roster the most important are the hemangioblastomas of the central nervous system, since these are the immediate cause of death in over half of all patients. The retinal angiomatosis is also of significance because it causes visual disturbances that are the presenting symptoms in many patients. Attention should also be directed to the renal cell carcinoma, since this is found in about one-fourth of the patients and is a major cause of death when present. All these neoplasms are rarely detectable at birth, and in most patients diagnosis is not made until the fourth decade of life.[43]

Phenotypic expression of this disease is wide-ranging, and no individual has all the tumors mentioned. Those unfortunate enough to have an intracranial hemangioblastoma or renal cell carcinoma usually follow a progressive downhill course to death at an early age.

Familial Hypercholesterolemia

This "receptor disease" is the consequence of a mutation in the gene encoding specific cell membrane receptors involved in the transport and metabolism of cholesterol. The loss of feedback control leads to elevated levels of cholesterol that induce premature atherosclerosis and greatly increase the risk of myocardial infarction.[44]

Familial hypercholesterolemia is possibly the most frequent mendelian disorder. Heterozygotes with one mutant gene representing about one in 500 individuals have from birth a two- to threefold elevation of plasma cholesterol, leading to tendinous xanthomas and premature atherosclerosis in adult life (p. 507). Homozygotes having a double dose of the mutant gene are much more severely affected and may have five- to sixfold elevations in plasma cholesterol levels. These individuals develop skin xanthomas and coronary, cerebral, and peripheral vascular atherosclerosis at an early age. Myocardial infarction may develop before the age of 20 years (p. 556). Large-scale studies have found that familial hypercholesterolemia is present in 3 to 6% of survivors of myocardial infarction.

An understanding of this disorder requires that we briefly review the normal process of cholesterol metabolism and transport. Cholesterol performs vital structural and metabolic functions in the body. About 93% of the body's total cholesterol is located within cells, whereas 7% circulates in the plasma. Low-density lipoproteins (LDL) constitute the major transport form of cholesterol in the plasma. There appear to be two mechanisms for removal of LDL from plasma, one mediated by a receptor-dependent process and the other by a receptor-independent pathway. Many cell types, including fibroblasts, smooth muscle cells, hepatocytes, and adrenocortical cells, possess high-affinity LDL-receptors and acquire cholesterol from LDL by a sophisticated transport process (Fig. 4–8). The first step involves binding of LDL to cell surface receptors, which are located in specialized regions of the plasma membrane called coated pits. Following binding, the coated pits containing the receptor-bound LDL are internalized by invagination to form coated vesicles, after which they migrate within the cell to fuse with the lysosomes. Here the LDL molecule is enzymatically degraded, the apoprotein part being hydrolyzed to amino acids, whereas the cholesteryl esters are broken down to free cholesterol. This in turn crosses the lysosomal membrane to enter the cytoplasm, where it is utilized for membrane

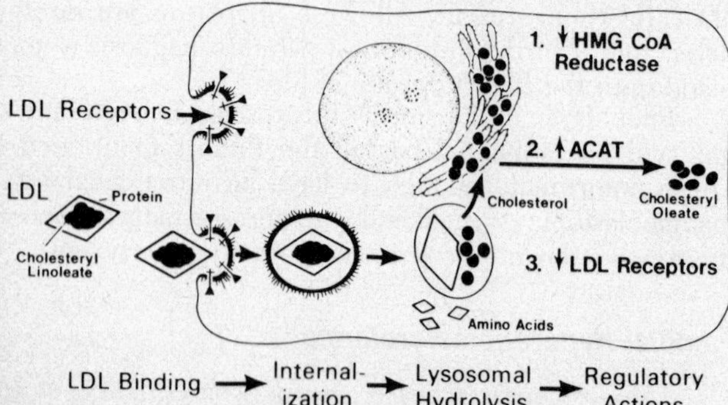

Figure 4–8. Sequential steps in LDL receptor pathway in cultured mammalian cells. LDL = low-density lipoprotein; HMG CoA reductase = 3-hydroxy-3-methyl-glutaryl CoA reductase; ACAT = acyl-coenzyme A:cholesterol acyltransferase. (From Goldstein, J. L., and Brown, M. S.: The LDL receptor defect in familial hypercholesterolemia. Implications for pathogenesis and therapy. Med. Clin. North Am. *66*:335, 1982.)

synthesis and as a regulator of cholesterol homeostasis. Three separate processes are affected by the released intracellular cholesterol. First, it *suppresses* cholesterol synthesis within the cell by inhibiting the activity of the enzyme 3-hydroxy-3-methylglutaryl (3HMG) CoA reductase, which is the rate-limiting enzyme in the synthetic pathway. Second, the cholesterol *activates* the enzyme cholesterol acyltransferase, which favors esterification and storage of excess cholesterol. Third, cholesterol *suppresses* the synthesis of cell surface LDL receptors, thus protecting the cells from excessive accumulation of cholesterol.

The transport of LDL not involving LDL receptors alluded to earlier appears to take place in the cells of the mononuclear phagocytic system, but may also occur in other cells (p. 514). The amount catabolized by this pathway is directly related to the plasma cholesterol level.

As mentioned earlier, familial hypercholesterolemia results from mutation in the gene specifying the receptor for LDL. Heterozygotes with familial hypercholesterolemia possess only 50% of the normal number of high-affinity LDL receptors, since they have only one normal gene. As a result of this defect in transport, the catabolism of LDL by the receptor-dependent pathway is impaired and the plasma level of LDL increases approximately twofold. With an increase in the plasma LDL, a new steady state is achieved in which the absolute amount of LDL catabolized by the receptor-dependent pathway is near normal since the elevation of the plasma LDL "compensates" for the defective transport. The price the body pays for such compensation is increased susceptibility to atherosclerosis. Homozygotes have virtually no normal LDL receptors in their cells and have much higher levels of circulating LDL. In addition to defective LDL transport, both the homozygotes and heterozygotes have increased synthesis of LDL. In homozygotes production of LDL is estimated to be two- to threefold above normal, whereas in heterozygotes there is a 30% increase. The mechanism of increased synthesis that contributes to hypercholesterolemia has been clarified recently by the study of a rabbit model of familial hypercholesterolemia.[44A] It appears that the lack of LDL receptors on the liver cells increases the conversion of very-low-density lipoproteins into LDL via the formation of intermediate-density lipoprotein (see Fig. 12–12).

We mentioned earlier the receptor-independent transport of LDL into the phagocytic cells. Normally, the amount of LDL transported along this pathway is less than that mediated by the receptor-dependent mechanisms. However, in the face of hypercholesterolemia there is a marked increase in the LDL receptor-independent traffic of LDL-cholesterol into the cells of the mononuclear phagocyte system and possibly the vascular walls. This is responsible for the appearance of xanthomas and may also contribute to the pathogenesis of premature atherosclerosis.

Although familial hypercholesterolemia results from mutation in a single gene, three distinct types of mutations affecting the LDL gene have been recognized (genetic heterogeneity). These are: (1) *Receptor-negative disease*, characterized by the absence of functional receptors. The LDL binding by cells from homozygotes with receptor-negative disease is less than 2% of normal. (2) *Receptor-defective disease*, in which the mutant allele specifies a receptor protein with reduced binding activity. Cells from homozygotes bind from 2 to 20% of normal LDL particles. (3) *Internalization defect*, which is extremely rare and is characterized by the presence of a receptor protein that can bind LDL normally but cannot internalize the bound LDL.

These recent discoveries of the crucial role of LDL receptors in cholesterol homeostasis have stimulated several studies designed to lower plasma cholesterol by increasing the number of LDL receptors.[45] For example, certain compounds that inhibit intracellular cholesterol synthesis are capable secondarily of increasing cellular LDL receptors. Although intracellular cholesterol synthesis is suppressed, the body stores of cholesterol are not depleted since adequate delivery of cholesterol into the cells continues by the improved receptor-mediated transport at lower levels of plasma LDL. Such approaches may be beneficial not only in familial hypercholesterolemia, but also in cases in which plasma LDL levels are elevated owing to nongenetic factors (see p. 515 for other forms of hypercholesterolemia).

AUTOSOMAL RECESSIVE DISORDERS

Autosomal recessive inheritance is the single largest category of mendelian disorders. Nonetheless, the mutant genes are relatively rare in the population, and so the following features obtain:

1. *In most instances the phenotypic change is not present in the parents, forebears, or relatives of the affected individual, but both parents carry the unexpressed recessive gene, i.e., they are carriers.*
2. *Siblings of an affected child have a 1 in 4 chance of being affected.*
3. *Consanguinity is more common among parents of affected children than among parents of normal children; moreover, the rarer the disease, the greater the likelihood of parental consanguinity.*

The category of autosomal recessive disease includes almost all the inborn errors of metabolism. As mentioned previously, these are syndromes in which the gene mutation leads to deficient functional activity of a specific enzyme. The various consequences of enzyme deficiencies were discussed on page 135. Mechanisms other than enzyme deficiency may also be involved. Increasingly we have become aware that there is another category of genetic metabolic diseases characterized by inborn errors of transport. These are essentially "membrane disorders." The Fanconi syndrome, characterized by glycosuria, aminoaciduria, chronic acidosis, vitamin D–resistant rickets, and osteomalacia, represents such a transport disorder. In some cases, the transport defects have been traced to defects in membrane receptors.[46] Thus, autosomal recessive errors in metabolism involve a wide range of mechanisms. Some of these conditions are presented elsewhere in this text, as follows:

- adrenogenital syndrome—an endocrinopathy (p. 1241)
- alpha-1-antitrypsin deficiency—associated with pulmonary disease (p. 721)
- cystic fibrosis of the pancreas—a childhood disorder (p. 493)
- galactosemia—a childhood disorder (p. 491)
- muscular dystrophy—one form (p. 1308)
- osteopetrosis—a skeletal disorder (p. 1321)
- phenylketonuria—a childhood disease (p. 490)
- severe combined immunodeficiency—a primary immunodeficiency (p. 207)
- Wilson's disease (p. 932)

A few additional autosomal recessive disorders that involve multiple organs will be described here.

Albinism

Among the genetic metabolic disorders, albinism is, happily, one of the less serious. It constitutes the hereditary inability to synthesize melanin. There are two clinical variants: ocular albinism and oculocutaneous albinism. In the former, which in the vast majority of cases is inherited as an X-linked recessive, the lack of pigmentation is limited to the eye; in the latter, hair, skin, and eye pigmentation is affected.[47]

Six genetic variants of oculocutaneous albinism have been identified, all transmitted as autosomal recessive traits. In four of the six genetic forms, there are associated defects in other organ systems, notably the hematopoietic cells. In two, the lack of skin and eye pigmentation is the dominant clinical feature. In one of these two, called "tyrosinase negative," the melanocytes lack tyrosinase; in the other, called "tyrosinase positive," there is no deficiency of tyrosinase and the precise biochemical defect is unknown. As you recall, tyrosine is the substrate from which melanin is produced. Tyrosinase catalyzes the formation of dihydroxyphenylalanine (dopa) from tyrosine. Dopa is one of the intermediaries in the formation of the dark brown-black pigment melanin. Whether due to a defect in the handling of the basic substrate or to a defect in its metabolic conversion, the end result is an albino individual. In both types of metabolic defect, individuals have a dermatosensitivity to solar exposure, greater in the tyrosinase–negative type. When exposed to sunlight, the skin is prone to develop wrinkles, but more important, there is an increased frequency of solar keratosis and basal cell and squamous cell carcinomas.

In the eye, the lack of pigment in the iris and retina leads to exquisite sensitivity to bright light and impaired visual acuity. Astigmatism, myopia, and other visual disturbances may also be present. The lack of the "sun shield" in the skin and eye predisposes to actinic-induced melanocarcinomas at these sites.

Alkaptonuria (Ochronosis)

In this autosomal recessive disorder, *the lack of homogentisic oxidase blocks the metabolism of phenylalanine-tyrosine at the level of homogentisic acid.* Thus, homogentisic acid accumulates in the body. Some is excreted and imparts a black color to the urine, if allowed to stand and undergo oxidation.

The retained homogentisic acid selectively binds to collagen in connective tissues, tendons, and cartilage, imparting to these tissues a blue-black pigmentation **(ochronosis)** most evident in the ears, nose, and cheeks. **The most serious consequences of ochronosis, however, stem from deposits of the pigment in the articular cartilages of the joints.** In some obscure manner, the pigmentation causes the cartilage to lose its normal resiliency and become brittle and fibrillated.[48] Wear-and-tear erosion of this abnormal cartilage leads to denudation of the subchondral bone, and often tiny fragments of the fibrillated cartilage are driven into the underlying bone, worsening the damage. The vertebral column, particularly the intervertebral disc, is the prime site of attack, but later the knees, shoulders, and hips may be affected. The small joints of the hands and feet are usually spared.

Although the metabolic defect is present from birth, the degenerative arthropathy develops slowly and usually does not become clinically evident until the fourth decade of life. While it is not life threatening, it may be severely crippling. The disability may be as extreme as that encountered in the severe forms of osteoarthritis (p. 1349) of the elderly, but unfortunately in alkaptonuria the arthropathy occurs at a much earlier age.

Lysosomal Storage Diseases

A group of relatively rare genetic metabolic diseases are characterized by a lysosomal enzyme deficiency that results in the accumulation in secondary lysosomes of some material that would ordinarily be metabolized, hence the designation *"lysosomal storage diseases."* They are considered here as a group because almost all are transmitted as autosomal recessives. Despite the fact that they are uncommon, they are of importance for many reasons: (1) the specific enzyme deficiency has been identified in most; (2) some of these conditions are the most devastating of childhood; (3) amniocentesis permits identification of most conditions in fetal cultured fibroblasts, providing the opportunity to terminate the pregnancy; (4) heterozygotes can be detected, permitting genetic counseling; and (5) most important of all, attempts to treat some of these diseases by administration of exogenous enzymes are now being actively investigated.

Several distinctive and separable conditions are included among the lysosomal storage diseases (Table 4–6). They can be divided into rational categories based on the biochemical nature of the accumulated metabolite, thus creating such subgroups as *the glycogenoses, sphingolipidoses (lipidoses), mucopolysaccharidoses, and mucolipidoses.* Within a category the individual entities may closely resemble one another, not only clinically but also biochemically. The chemical interrelationships among the sphingolipidoses, for example, are emphasized in Figure 4–9, where it is evident that the individual conditions result from a variety of enzyme blockages affecting different levels in the pathways of complex lipid degradation. It therefore is often necessary, and always desirable, to confirm clinical impressions by biochemical identification of the accumulated metabolite and/or the enzyme deficiency. Only one among the many glycogenoses results from a lysosomal enzyme deficiency, and so this family of storage diseases will be considered later (p. 150). Only the most common disorders among the remaining groups will be considered here; the others must be relegated to specialized texts.[49]

TAY-SACHS DISEASE (G_{M2}-GANGLIOSIDOSIS TYPE 1). The autosomal recessive Tay-Sachs disease is the prototype and the most important of the gangliosidoses. As can be seen from Table 4–6, there are other gangliosidoses separated into G_{M1} and G_{M2} categories, each further subdivided into distinctive entities. Tay-Sachs disease, a G_{M2}-gangliosidosis, is particularly prevalent among Jews, in particular among those of Eastern European (Ashkenazic) origin in whom a carrier rate of one in 30 has been reported.[50] The specific enzyme dysfunction in Tay-Sachs disease is a deficiency of hexosaminidase A, while the activity of the other isoenzyme, hexosaminidase B, is increased. Hexosaminidase A catalyzes the degradation of G_{M2}-ganglioside, and so in this condition it accumulates.

The hexosaminidase A is absent from virtually all the tissues that have been examined, including leukocytes and plasma, and so G_{M2}-ganglioside accumulates in many tissues (e.g., heart, liver, spleen), but it is the involvement of neurons in the central and autonomic nervous systems and retina that dominates the clinical picture. Depending on the duration of survival, the weight of the brain may be normal or decreased, but in patients surviving one or more years it is usually increased, sometimes more than 50%, owing to the accumulation of ganglioside in cells. The increase in weight is accompanied by enlargement of the cerebral gyri and narrowing of the sulci. Paradoxically, the cerebellum and brain stem may concomitantly undergo atrophy. On histologic examination, the neurons are ballooned with cytoplasmic vacuoles, each of which comprises a markedly distended lysosome filled with gangliosides (Fig. 4–10). Stains for fat such as oil red O and Sudan black are positive. Under the electron microscope, several types of cytoplasmic inclusions can be visualized, the most prominent being whorled configurations within lysosomes composed of onionskin layers of membranes (Fig. 4–10).[51] In time there is progressive destruction of neurons, proliferation of microglia, and accumulation of complex lipids in phagocytes within the brain substance. A similar process occurs in the cerebellum as well as in neurons throughout the basal ganglia, brain stem, spinal cord, and dorsal root ganglia, and the neurons of the autonomic nervous system.[52] The ganglion cells in the retina are similarly swollen with G_{M2}-ganglioside, particularly at the margins of the macula. A **cherry-red spot** thus appears in the macula, representing

Table 4–6. LYSOSOMAL STORAGE DISEASES

Disease	Enzyme Deficiency	Major Accumulating Metabolites
Glycogenosis		
Type 2—Pompe's disease	α-1,4-glucosidase (lysosomal glucosidase)	Glycogen
Sphingolipidoses		
G_{M1}-gangliosidosis:	G_{M1} ganglioside β-galactosidase	G_{M1}-ganglioside, galactose-containing oligosaccharides
Type 1—infantile, generalized		
Type 2—juvenile		
G_{M2}-gangliosidosis:		
Tay-Sachs disease	Hexosaminidase A	G_{M2}-ganglioside
Sandhoff-Jatzkewitz disease	Hexosaminidases A and B	G_{M2}-ganglioside, globoside
Sulfatidoses:		
Metachromatic leukodystrophy	Aryl sulfatase A	Sulfatide
Multiple sulfatase deficiency	Aryl sulfatases A, B, C; steroid sulfatase; iduronate sulfatase, heparan *N*-sulfatase.	Sulfatide, steroid sulfate, heparan sulfate, dermatan sulfate
Krabbe's disease	Galactosylceramidase	Galactocerebroside
Fabry's disease	α-Galactosidase A	Ceramide trihexoside
Gaucher's disease	Glucocerebrosidase	Glucocerebroside
Niemann-Pick disease	Sphingomyelinase	Sphingomyelin
Mucopolysaccharidoses		
Several types (see Table 4–7)	Several types (see Table 4–7)	Dermatan sulfate, heparan sulfate, keratan sulfate, chondroitin sulfate
Mucolipidoses (ML)		
I-cell disease (MLII) and pseudo-Hurler polydystrophy (MLIII)	Intralysosomal deficiency of acid hydrolases that fail to localize in the lysosomes owing to poor phosphorylation; the enzyme levels increase in extracellular fluids	Mucopolysaccharide, glycolipid
Other Diseases of Complex Carbohydrates		
Fucosidosis	α-Fucosidase	Fucose-containing sphingolipids and glycoprotein fragments
Mannosidosis	α-Mannosidase	Mannose-containing oligosaccharides
Aspartylglycosaminuria	Aspartylglycosamine amide hydrolase	Aspartyl-2-deoxy-2-acetamidoglycosylamine
Other Lysosomal Storage Diseases		
Wolman's disease	Acid lipase	Cholesterol esters, triglycerides
Acid phosphate deficiency	Lysosomal acid phosphatase	Phosphate esters

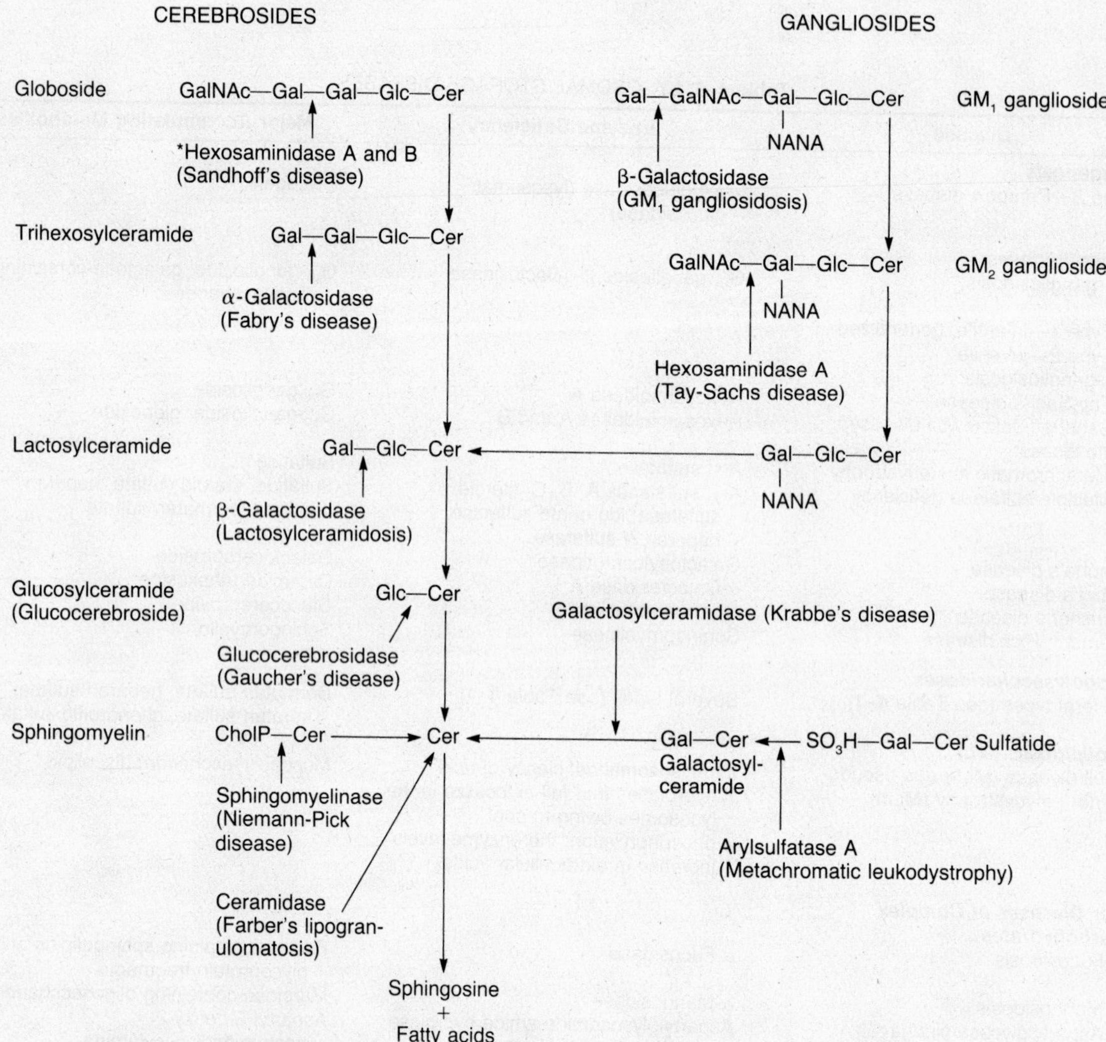

Figure 4–9. Site of enzymatic defects in sphingolipidoses and diseases produced by the lack of enzymes. *Both hexosaminidase A and B can cleave the terminal *N*-acetylgalactosaminyl residue of globoside; therefore, globoside does not accumulate in Tay-Sachs disease, in which only hexosaminidase A is deficient. GalNAc = *N*-acetylgalactosamine; Gal = galactose; Glc = glucose; Cer = ceramide; CholP = phosphorylcholine. (Modified from Jackson, L. G., and Schimke, R. N. (eds.): Clinical Genetics. New York, John Wiley & Sons, 1979, p. 159.)

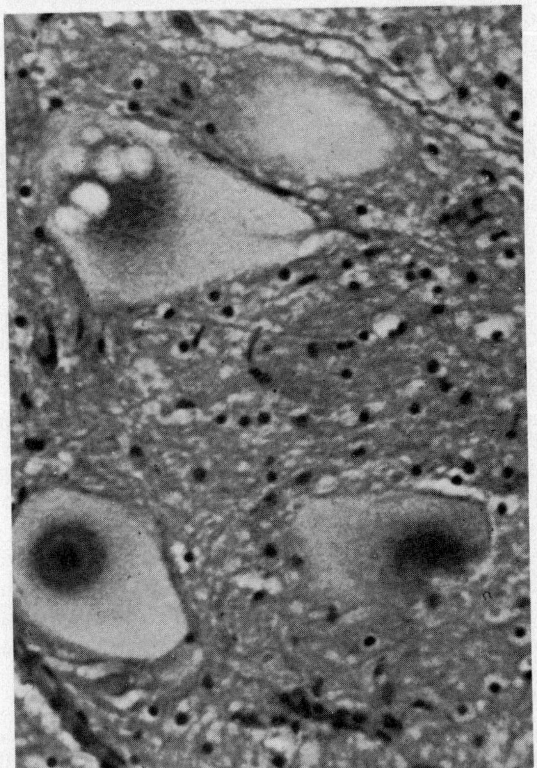

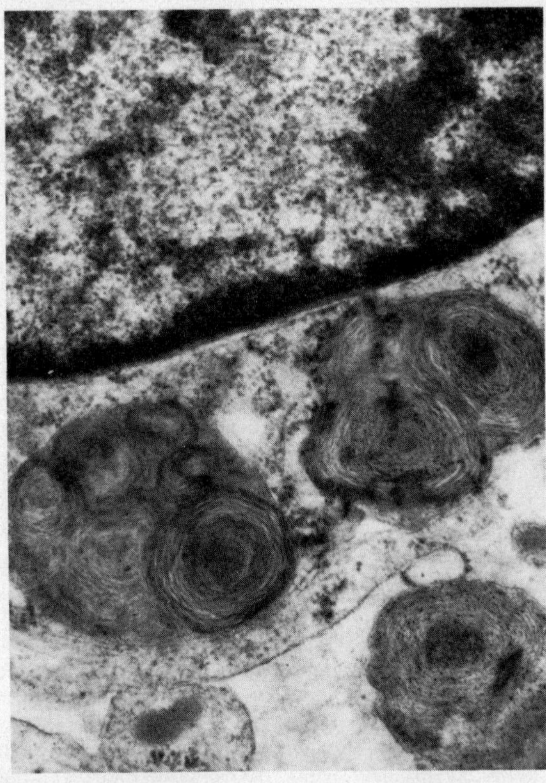

Figure 4–10. Ganglion cells in Tay-Sachs disease. *A,* Under the light microscope, a large neuron at the top has obvious lipid vacuolation with karyolysis and granularity of nucleus. *B,* Portion of a neuron under the electron microscope shows prominent lysosomes with whorled configurations. Part of the nucleus is shown above. (Electron micrograph courtesy of Dr. Joe Rutledge, Southwestern Medical School, Dallas, Texas.)

accentuation of the normal color of the macular choroid contrasted with the pallor produced by the swollen ganglion cells in the remainder of the retina. As the retinal ganglion cells die from the accumulation of lipid, the cherry-red spot may disappear in patients with protracted disease.

Affected infants appear quite normal at birth but begin to manifest signs and symptoms at about 6 months of age. There is relentless motor and mental deterioration, beginning with motor incoordination, mental obtundation leading to muscular flaccidity, blindness, and increasing dementia. The blindness and progressive mental deterioration account for the older designation of this condition as *amaurotic (having blindness) familial idiocy.* Sometime during the early course of the disease the characteristic, but not pathognomonic, "cherry-red" spot appears in the macula of the eye grounds in almost all patients. Over the span of one or two years a complete, pathetic vegetative state is reached, followed, usually too late, by death at 2 to 3 years of age.

Antenatal diagnosis is possible by identification of the deficiency of hexosaminidase A in cultured fibroblasts derived from amniotic fluid. It is important to note, however, that perfectly normal individuals have been identified who lack detectable hexosaminidase A activity but can nonetheless catabolize G_{M2}-ganglioside.[53] It is also possible to identify heterozygote carriers who have enzyme levels intermediate between controls and homozygous affected infants. Although the intravenous administration of purified hexosaminidase A is being explored as a therapeutic modality, early results have not been encouraging; however, it is too soon to draw conclusions.

NIEMANN-PICK DISEASE. This autosomal recessive disorder is characterized by a deficiency of the sphingomyelin-cleaving enzyme sphingomyelinase, resulting in the accumulation of sphingomyelin as well as cholesterol in reticuloendothelial and parenchymal cells in many organs throughout the body. On the basis of the distribution of the involved organs and the nature of sphingomyelinase deficiency, five clinically distinguishable phenotypes (types A to E) have been delineated. Remarks here will be largely confined to type A, representing 75 to 80% of all cases. *It is the severe infantile form with extensive neurologic involvement, marked visceral accumulations of sphingomyelin, and progressive wasting and early death within the first three years of life.* To provide a perspective on the differences between the variants of Niemann-Pick disease we need only point out that in type B, for example, patients have organomegaly but generally no central nervous system involvement. Type C resembles type A but the disease appears later in life, generally in the teens. Recent evidence points to genetic heterogeneity within this group of disorders. For example, it is now established that clinical phenotypes A and C result from mutations involving two separate genes.[54] More details on the other clinical phenotypes can be found in specialized texts.[49]

In the classic infantile type A variant, the deficiency of sphingomyelinase is almost complete. Sphingomyelin is a ubiquitous component of cellular (including organellar) membranes, and so the enzyme deficiency blocks degradation of the normal turnover of the lipid, resulting in its progressive accumulation within secondary lysosomes, particularly within reticuloendothelial cells (Fig. 4–11). Affected cells become enlarged sometimes to 90 μ in diameter, secondary to the distention of lysosomes with sphingomyelin and cholesterol. Innumerable small vacuoles of relatively uniform size are created, imparting a foaminess to the cytoplasm. In frozen sections of fresh tissue, the vacuoles stain for fat with Sudan black B and oil red O. The PAS reaction is variable but may be positive. Electron microscopy confirms that the vacuoles are engorged secondary lysosomes that often contain membranous cytoplasmic bodies (MCB) resembling concentric lamellated myelin figures. Sometimes the lysosomal configurations take the form of parallel palisaded lamellae, creating so-called "zebra bodies."[54A] Isolation and analysis of these cellular inclusions confirm that they principally contain sphingomyelin.

The lipid-laden phagocytic foam cells are widely distributed in the spleen, liver, lymph nodes, bone marrow, tonsils, gastrointestinal tract, and lungs. In addition, the hepatoparenchymal cells are sometimes vacuolated, as well as Schwann cells in the peripheral nerves. The involvement of the spleen generally produces massive enlargement, sometimes to ten times its normal weight, but the hepatomegaly is usually not quite so striking. The lymph nodes are generally moderately to markedly enlarged throughout the body. Often the color of these organs is paler than usual owing to the massive accumulations of sphingomyelin.

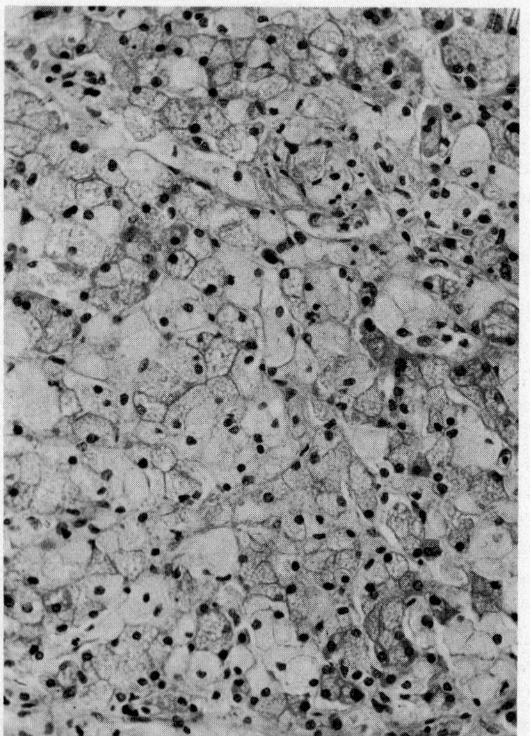

Figure 4–11. Niemann-Pick disease in bone marrow. The marrow space is virtually filled with fairly regular lipophages.

Involvement of the brain and eye deserve special mention. The brain in advanced cases is generally decreased in weight and unusually firm. The gyri are shrunken and the sulci widened. Paradoxically, the cortex is somewhat softer than usual, while the underlying white matter is abnormally firm. Vacuolation and ballooning of neurons is the dominant histologic change, which in time leads to cell death and loss of brain substance.[52] This neuronal involvement is diffuse throughout the cerebrum, cerebellum, brain stem, and spinal cord and extends to the ganglion cells in the peripheral plexuses as well. A retinal cherry-red spot similar to that seen in Tay-Sachs disease (p. 142) is present in about one-third to one-half of affected individuals. Its origin is similar to that described in Tay-Sachs disease, except that the accumulated metabolite is sphingomyelin.

It is evident from the morphologic changes that these tragic infants are devastated by the accumulations of sphingomyelin and cholesterol. Clinical manifestations may even be present at birth but almost certainly become evident by six months of life. The infants typically have a protuberant abdomen because of the hepatosplenomegaly. Accumulation of sphingomyelin and cholesterol in subcutaneous phagocytic cells may produce small skin xanthomas. Once the manifestations appear, they are followed by progressive failure to thrive, vomiting, fever, and generalized lymphadenopathy as well as progressive deterioration of psychomotor function. Death comes as a release, usually within the first or second year of life.

Although Niemann-Pick disease may be suspected in an infant with hepatosplenomegaly, mental retardation, and foam cells in the bone marrow, biochemical analysis of affected cells to identify the specific accumulated metabolite and/or enzyme deficiency is necessary to establish the precise diagnosis. This is readily accomplished in biopsies of liver, spleen, or bone marrow and in cultured fibroblasts. Affected individuals as well as heterozygous carriers can be recognized antenatally by enzyme assays in cultured fibroblasts obtained by amniocentesis.

GAUCHER'S DISEASE. This autosomal recessive disorder is characterized by a deficiency of glucocerebrosidase. As a result, glucocerebroside accumulates, principally in the reticuloendothelial cells of the body but sometime also in central nervous system neurons. In the normal individual, glucocerebrosides are continually formed from the catabolism of glycolipids derived mainly from the cell membranes of senescent leukocytes and erythrocytes. This pathway is the predominant source of glucocerebrosides that accumulate within the reticuloendothelial cells; the accumulations in the neurons may in part be derived from the turnover of gangliosides in the nervous system, which is quite rapid in the neonatal period. Three clinical subtypes of Gaucher's disease have been distinguished. *The classic form, called type I, is the adult type of Gaucher's disease, sometimes called the noncerebral form, in which the storage of* *glucocerebrosides is limited to the reticuloendothelial system throughout the body without involving the brain. Splenic, hepatic, and skeletal involvements dominate this pattern of the disease.* It is found principally in Jews of European stock and accounts for at least 80% of all cases of Gaucher's disease. Patients with this disorder have reduced but detectable levels of glucocerebrosidase activity. Longevity is shortened but not markedly. *The type II form of Gaucher's disease is the infantile acute cerebral pattern. This infantile disease has no predilection for Jews. In these patients there is virtually no detectable glucocerebrosidase activity in the tissues.* Hepatosplenomegaly is also seen in this form of Gaucher's disease, but the clinical picture is dominated by progressive central nervous system involvement, leading to death at an early age. A third pattern, type III, is sometimes distinguished, intermediate between types I and II. These patients are usually juveniles, have the systemic involvement characteristic of type I, but have progressive central nervous system disease that usually begins in the second or third decade of life. The levels of glucocerebrosidase activity in this variant are intermediate between those found in types I and II. These specific patterns run within families, and so appear to be distinct entities, possibly resulting from different mutations of the affected gene.

The glucocerebrosides accumulate in massive amounts within phagocytic cells throughout the body and sometimes in neurons. These distended reticuloendothelial cells, known as **Gaucher cells**, are found in the spleen, liver, bone marrow, lymph nodes, tonsils, thymus, and Peyer's patches. Similar cells may be present, both in the alveolar septa and air spaces in the lung. In contrast to the lipid storage diseases already discussed, Gaucher cells rarely appear vacuolated but instead have a fibrillary type of cytoplasm likened to crumpled tissue paper (Fig. 4–12). Gaucher cells are often enlarged, sometimes up to 100 μm in diameter, and have one or more dark, eccentrically placed nuclei.[52] PAS staining is usually intensely positive. Under the EM, the fibrillary cytoplasm can be resolved as elongated, distended lysosomes, containing the stored lipid in stacks of bilayers.[55]

The accumulation of Gaucher cells produces a variety of gross anatomic changes. The spleen is enlarged in the adult form of the disease, sometimes up to 10 kilos. It too may appear uniformly pale or have a mottled surface owing to focal accumulations of Gaucher cells. The lymphadenopathy is mild to moderate and is bodywide. The accumulations of Gaucher cells in the bone marrow may produce small focal areas of bony erosion or large, soft, gray tumorous masses that cause skeletal deformities or destroy sufficient bone to give rise to fractures. Occasionally, aggregates of distended phagocytes are found in the lungs and other organs, particularly the endocrine glands. In patients with cerebral involvement, Gaucher cells are seen in the Virchow-Robin spaces, and arterioles are surrounded by swollen adventitial cells. Neurons appear shriveled and are progressively destroyed.

The clinical course of Gaucher's disease depends on the clinical subtype. In the type I pattern, symptoms and signs first appear in adult life secondary to splenomegaly or hepatomegaly. Bone marrow involvement may produce skeletal pain or disturbed motor function. Anemia, leukopenia, and thrombocytopenia (often with a hemorrhagic diathesis) reflect either marrow involvement or are the consequence of a hypersplenic syn-

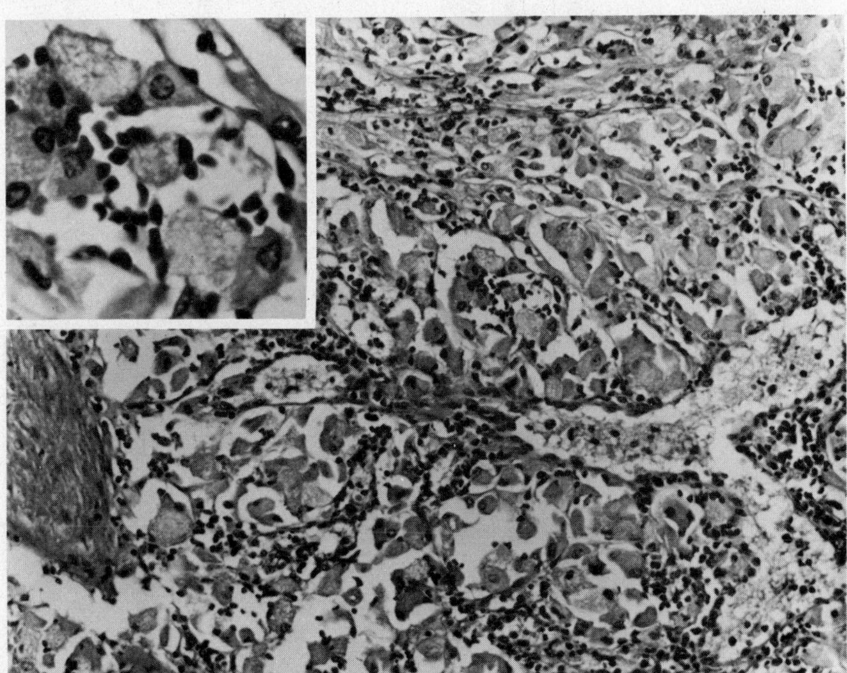

Figure 4–12. Gaucher's disease involving the spleen. The entire field is made up of lipid-laden cells of varying size with sharp cell boundaries, abundant granular cytoplasm, and small eccentric nuclei. Inset shows Gaucher cells at higher magnification. (Courtesy of Dr. Joe Rutledge, Southwestern Medical School, Dallas, Texas.)

Table 4–7. MUCOPOLYSACCHARIDOSES (MPS)

Name*	Genetics	Accumulated Product	Enzyme Deficiency	Life Expectancy	Intelligence	Clinical Features
MPS I H (Hurler)	AR	Heparan sulfate Dermatan sulfate	α-L-iduronidase	6 to 10 years	Retarded	1. Onset 6 to 8 months 2. Dwarfism 3. Large, long head 4. Flat, broad nose with upturned nostrils 5. Corneal clouding 6. Hepatosplenomegaly 7. Valvular lesions 8. Coronary artery lesions 9. Skeletal deformities 10. Joint stiffness
MPS I S (Scheie)	AR	Heparan sulfate Dermatan sulfate	α-L-iduronidase	Normal	Normal	1. Onset after 5 years 2. Near-normal height 3. Corneal clouding 4. Aortic valvular lesions 5. Finger stiffness
MPS I H-S (Hurler-Scheie)	AR Genetic Compound of MPS I H and I S genes	Heparan sulfate Dermatan sulfate	α-L-iduronidase	Third decade	Mild retardation (may be normal)	1. Onset infancy 2. Dwarfism 3. Facial and bony lesions of Hurler's syndrome 4. Cardiac lesions
MPS II (Hunter) (Wide range of severity)	X-R	Heparan sulfate Dermatan sulfate	L-iduronosulfate sulfatase	Second decade to normal	Mild retardation to normal	1. Similar to Hurler's syndrome, but a. No corneal clouding b. Retinal degeneration c. Deafness d. Nodular skin infiltrates

MPS III (Sanfilippo A)	AR	Heparan sulfate	Heparan sulfate sulfamidase	Second to third decade	Retarded	1. Onset after 3 years 2. Normal growth 3. Hurler facies 4. No corneal clouding 5. Mild somatic features with severe mental retardation
(Sanfilippo B)		Heparan sulfate	*N*-acetyl-α-D-glucosaminidase			
(Sanfilippo C)		Heparan sulfate	Acetyl CoA:α-glucosaminide-*N*-acetyltransferase			
(Sanfilippo D)		Heparan sulfate	*N*-acetyl-α-D-glucosaminide-6-sulfatase			
MPS IV (Morquio) (Wide range of severity, possibly several forms with different enzyme deficiencies)	AR	Keratan sulfate Chondroitin sulfate	*N*-acetylgalactosamine-6-sulfatase	Third to sixth decade	Normal	1. Dwarfism 2. Thoracolumbar gibbus 3. Kyphoscoliosis 4. Facies similar to Hurler's syndrome 5. Corneal clouding 6. Aortic valvular lesions 7. Joint hypermobility 8. Genu valgum
MPS VI (Maroteaux-Lamy) (Wide range of severity)	AR	Dermatan sulfate	*N*-acetylgalactosamine-4-sulfatase	Second decade	Normal	1. Similar to Hurler's syndrome, but a. Preservation of intelligence b. Longer survival c. Striking white cell inclusions
MPS VII (Glucuronidase deficiency disease)	AR	Dermatan sulfate Heparan sulfate Chondroitin sulfate	β-Glucuronidase	(?) Some restriction	Retarded	Variable

*MPS V is no longer used.
AR = Autosomal recessive; X-R = X-linked recessive.

drome. Although the disease is progressive in the adult, it is compatible with long life. In types II and III, central nervous system dysfunction, convulsions, and progressive mental deterioration dominate, although organs such as the liver, spleen, and lymph nodes are also affected.

The diagnosis of homozygotes and the detection of heterozygous carriers can be made through measurement of glucocerebrosidase activity in peripheral blood leukocytes or in extracts of cultured skin fibroblasts. Biochemical analysis of the stored glycolipid may also be used as a diagnostic test. Prenatal diagnosis is also possible using cultured fetal fibroblasts.

Great excitement has attended the discovery that infusion of human placental glucocerebrosidase into some patients with type I Gaucher's disease resulted in definite mobilization of stored metabolite from the liver, with some improvement in the clinical condition of the patient.[56] Although these therapeutic efforts are too recent for full evaluation, they offer the first ray of hope in what heretofore has been a bleak outlook.

MUCOPOLYSACCHARIDOSES (MPS). The mucopolysaccharidoses are another form of lysosomal storage disease. They make up a group of closely related syndromes that result from genetically determined deficiencies of specific lysosomal enzymes involved in the degradation of mucopolysaccharides (glycosaminoglycans). The mucopolysaccharides that accumulate in the MPS are dermatan sulfate, heparan sulfate, keratan sulfate, and chondroitin sulfate.[57] The enzymes involved in each of the MPS cleave terminal sugars from the polysaccharide chains disposed along a polypeptide or "core protein." When there is a block in the removal of a terminal sugar, the remainder of the polysaccharide chain is not further degraded, and thus these chains accumulate within lysosomes in various tissues and organs of the body. Severe somatic and neurologic changes result.

Several clinical variants of MPS, classified numerically from MPS I to MPS VII, have been described, each resulting from the deficiency of one specific enzyme. All the MPS except one are inherited as autosomal recessives; one variant, called Hunter syndrome, is an X-linked recessive (Table 4–7). Within a given group (e.g., MPS I, characterized by a deficiency of α-L-iduronidase) subgroups exist that result from different mutant alleles at the same genetic locus. Thus, the severity of enzyme deficiency and the clinical picture even within subgroups is often different.

In general, the MPS are progressive disorders, characterized by involvement of multiple organs, including liver, spleen, heart, and blood vessels. Most are associated with coarse facial features, clouding of the cornea, joint stiffness, and mental retardation. Urinary excretion of the accumulated mucopolysaccharides is often increased.

The accumulated mucopolysaccharides are generally found in reticuloendothelial cells, endothelial cells, intimal smooth muscle cells, and fibroblasts throughout the body. Common sites of involvement are thus the spleen, liver, bone marrow, lymph nodes, and blood vessels and also the heart.

Microscopically, affected cells are distended and have apparent clearing of the cytoplasm to create so-called "balloon cells." The cleared cytoplasm can be resolved as numerous minute vacuoles which, under the electron microscope, can be visualized as swollen lysosomes filled with a finely granular PAS-positive material that can be identified biochemically as mucopolysaccharide.[58] Similar lysosomal changes are found in the neurons of those syndromes characterized by central nervous system involvement. In addition, however, some of the lysosomes in neurons are replaced by lamellated zebra bodies like those seen in Niemann-Pick disease. These peculiar intracellular inclusions are seen most often in Hurler's syndrome and the more severe forms of the Sanfilippo syndrome.[59] Hepatosplenomegaly, skeletal deformities, valvular lesions, and subendothelial arterial deposits, particularly in the coronary arteries and lesions in the brain, are common threads that run through all the MPS. In many of the more protracted syndromes, coronary subendothelial lesions lead to myocardial ischemia. Thus, myocardial infarction and cardiac decompensation are common causes of death.

Some data relating to clinical manifestations and life expectancy are provided in Table 4–7. Further details can be found in a recent review.[60] With these syndromes, biochemical identification of the accumulated metabolite and/or specific enzyme deficiency is necessary to differentiate one syndrome unmistakably from the others. Prenatal diagnosis is now possible. Hope runs high that replacement enzyme therapy may be of benefit in these disorders.

Glycogen Storage Diseases

A number of genetic syndromes have been identified that result from some metabolic defect in the synthesis or catabolism of glycogen. The best understood and most important category includes the *glycogen storage diseases* resulting from a hereditary deficiency of one of the enzymes involved in the synthesis or sequential degradation of glycogen. Depending on the tissue or organ distribution of the specific enzyme in the normal state, *glycogen storage in these disorders may be limited to a few tissues, be more widespread while not affecting all tissues, or be systemic in distribution.*

On the basis of the specific enzyme deficiency and resultant pattern of glycogen accumulation, eight syndromes have been differentiated, some of which are being further subdivided (Table 4–8). Most are inherited as autosomal recessive conditions. One of the variants, the liver phosphorylase deficiency syndrome, is also X-linked. The individual entities differ in their clinical severity. Type II associated with lysosomal glucosidase deficiency is devastating; most infants die at an early age. The same is true of the branching enzyme deficiency. On the other hand, the variants characterized by a deficiency of liver or muscle phosphorylase and the debranching enzyme variant are relatively mild conditions compatible with long survival.

The significance of a specific enzyme deficiency is

best understood from the perspective of the normal metabolism of glycogen (Fig. 4–13). As is well known, glycogen is a storage form of glucose. Glycogen synthesis begins with the conversion of glucose to glucose-6-phosphate by the action of a hexokinase (glucokinase). A phosphoglucomutase then transforms the glucose-6-phosphate to glucose-1-phosphate, which in turn is converted to uridine disphosphoglucose. A highly branched, very large polymer is then built up (molecular weight up to 100,000,000), containing up to 10,000 glucose molecules linked together by alpha-1,4-glucoside bonds. The central spine gives off many branches joined by alpha-1,6-glucoside linkages requiring brancher enzymes. The glycogen chain and branches continue to be elongated by the addition of glucose molecules mediated by glycogen synthetases. During degradation the phosphorylases split glucose-1-phosphate from the glycogen until about four glucose residues remain on each branch, leaving a branched oligosaccharide called limit dextrin. This can be further

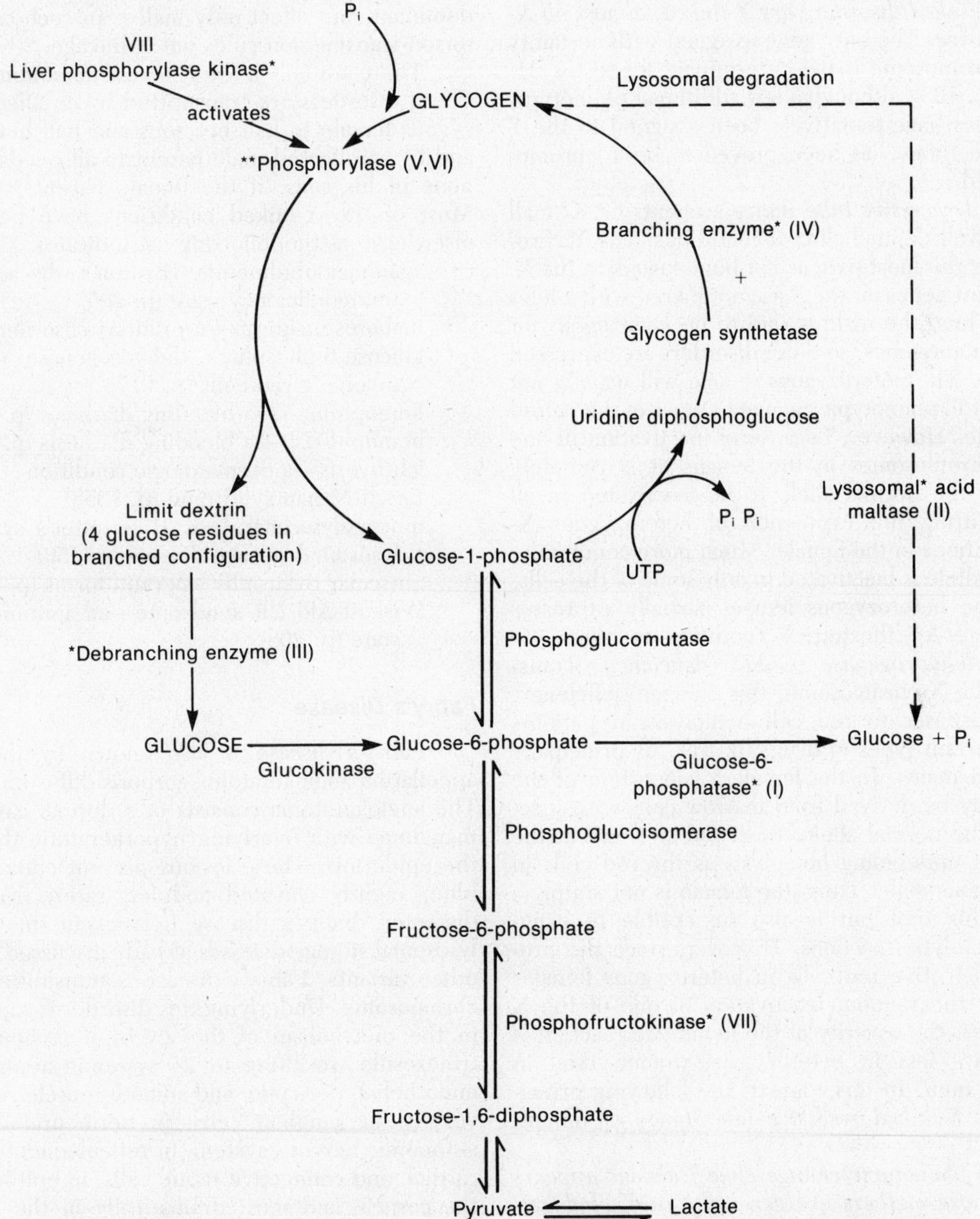

Figure 4–13. Pathways of glycogen metabolism. Asterisks mark the enzyme deficiencies associated with glycogen storage diseases. Roman numerals indicate the type of glycogen storage disease associated with the given enzyme deficiency. Types V and VI result from deficiencies of muscle and liver phosphorylases, respectively. (After Howell, R. R., and Williams, J. C.: The glycogen storage disease. *In* Stanbury, J. B., et al. [eds.]: Metabolic Basis of Inherited Diseases. 5th Ed. New York, McGraw-Hill Book Co., 1982, p. 144.)

degraded only by the debranching enzyme. In addition to these major pathways, glycogen is also degraded in the lysosomes by acid maltase. If the lysosomes are deficient in this enzyme, the glycogen contained within them is not accessible to degradation by cytoplasmic enzymes such as phosphorylases. The principal features of the glycogenoses are summarized in Table 4–8.

SEX-LINKED (X-LINKED) DISORDERS

All sex-linked disorders are X-linked, almost all X-linked recessive. The only gene assigned with certainty to the Y chromosome is the determinant for testes (H-Y antigen, p. 133); although a few additional phenotypic characteristics have tentatively been assigned to the Y chromosome, none has been proved to be Y chromosome–related.

X-linked recessive inheritance accounts for a small number of well-defined clinical conditions. The Y chromosome, for the most part, is not homologous to the X, and so mutant genes on the X are not paired with alleles on the Y. Thus, the male is said to be *hemizygous* for X-linked mutant genes, so these disorders are expressed in the male. The heterozygous female will usually not express the full phenotypic change because of the paired normal allele. However, because of inactivation of one of the X chromosomes in the female, it is remotely possible for the normal allele to be inactivated in all cells, permitting full expression of heterozygous X-linked conditions in the female. Much more commonly, the normal allele is inactivated in only some of the cells, and thus the heterozygous female partially expresses the disorder. An illustrative condition is *glucose-6-phosphate dehydrogenase (G6PD) deficiency.* Transmitted on the X chromosome, this enzyme deficiency, which predisposes to red cell hemolysis in patients receiving certain types of drugs (p. 617), is principally expressed in males. In the female a proportion of the red cells may be derived from marrow cells with inactivation of the normal allele. Such red cells are at the same risk of undergoing hemolysis as the red cells in the hemizygous male. Thus, the female is not simply a carrier of this trait but is also susceptible to drug-induced hemolytic reactions. However, since the proportion of defective red cells in heterozygous females depends on the random inactivation of one of the X chromosomes, the severity of the hemolytic reaction is almost always less in heterozygous women than in hemizygous men. In this context, the following principles govern *X-linked recessive* inheritance of mutant genes:

1. *The phenotypic change almost always appears in males whose mothers are generally unaffected heterozygous carriers.*
2. *Each son of a carrier female has a 1 in 2 chance of being affected.*
3. *Affected males cannot transmit the mutant genes to their sons but do transmit it to all their daughters, who will almost always be unaffected heterozygous carriers.*
4. *Unaffected males never transmit the gene.*
5. *Full phenotypic expression of the condition is possible in the rare homozygous female who has a carrier or homozygous affected mother and affected father.*

A distinction should be made between *sex-linked* disorders and *sex-limited* diseases. The latter are autosomally transmitted but expressed in one sex for physiologic, rather than genetic, reasons. For example, certain patterns of baldness are inherited as autosomal dominant, but affect only males. In such cases, father-to-son transmission rules out X-linkage.

There are only a few *X-linked dominant* conditions. These disorders are transmitted by an affected heterozygous female to half her sons and half her daughters, and by an affected male parent to all his daughters but none of his sons, if the female parent is unaffected. Most of the X-linked conditions have been covered elsewhere, as the following list indicates.

- agammaglobulinemia (Bruton's disease)—an immunodeficiency state (p. 205)
- diabetes insipidus—a pituitary disorder (p. 1200)
- glucose-6-phosphate dehydrogenase deficiency—involving red cells (p. 617)
- hemophilia A—a bleeding diathesis (p. 648)
- hemophilia B—a bleeding diathesis (p. 649)
- ichthyosis—a dermatologic condition
- Lesch-Nyhan syndrome (p. 1358)
- mucopolysaccharidosis II (Hunter's syndrome)—a lysosomal storage disease (p. 150)
- muscular dystrophy—certain forms (p. 1308)
- Wiskott-Aldrich syndrome—an immunodeficiency state (p. 208)

Fabry's Disease

Fabry's disease is also known by the imposing appellation angiokeratoma corporis diffusum universale. The angiokeratoma consists of a dermal cavernous hemangioma with overlying hyperkeratotic thickening of the epidermis. These lesions present clinically as red-blue, slightly elevated nodules, rarely over 1 cm in diameter. Fabry's disease belongs to the category of lysosomal storage diseases already discussed. Unlike the other variants, Fabry's disease is transmitted on the X chromosome. Underlying this disorder is a genetic error in the metabolism of the glycosphingolipid ceramide trihexoside, resulting in its systemic accumulation in endothelial, pericytic, and smooth muscle cells of blood vessels; in ganglion cells; in perineural cells of the autonomic nervous system; in reticuloendothelial, myocardial, and connective tissue cells; in epithelial cells of the cornea; and most dramatically in the kidney glomeruli and tubules. The deficient lysosomal enzyme has been identified as trihexosylceramide α-galactosidase (Fig. 4–9). The storage product imparts a foaminess to the affected cells which, on higher resolution, can be resolved as lamellated whorls reminiscent of myelin

Table 4–8. PRINCIPAL FEATURES OF GLYCOGENOSES

	Type and Frequency	Enzyme Deficiency	Morphologic Changes	Clinical Features
I	Hepatorenal— von Gierke's disease ~ 1 per 100,000	Glucose-6-phosphatase	Hepatomegaly—intracytoplasmic accumulations of glycogen and small amounts of lipid; intranuclear glycogen. Renomegaly— intracytoplasmic accumulations of glycogen in cortical tubular epithelial cells.	Failure to thrive, stunted growth, hepatomegaly and renomegaly. Hypoglycemia due to failure of glucose mobilization, often leading to convulsions. Hyperlipidemia and hyperuricemia resulting from deranged glucose metabolism; many patients develop gout and skin xanthomas. Bleeding tendency due to platelet dysfunction. Mortality approximately 50%.
II	Generalized glycogenosis—Pompe's disease ~ 1 per 100,000	Lysosomal glucosidase (acid maltase)	Mild hepatomegaly—ballooning of lysosomes with glycogen creating lacy cytoplasmic pattern. Cardiomegaly—glycogen within sarcoplasm as well as membrane bound. Skeletal muscle—similar to heart.	Massive cardiomegaly, muscle hypotonia, and cardiorespiratory failure within 2 years. A milder adult form with only skeletal muscle involvement presenting with chronic myopathy.
III	Cori's disease ~ 1 per 100,000	Amylo-1,6-glucosidase (debrancher enzyme)	Mild-to-marked hepatomegaly—cells similar to type I. Mild-to-moderate cardiomegaly—cells similar to type II. Skeletal muscle—similar to type II.	Similar to type I but usually milder. Compatible with normal longevity.
IV	Brancher glycogenosis 1 per 500,000	Amylo-1,4:1,6-transglucosidase (brancher enzyme)	Accumulation of abnormal glycogen (amylopectin) in liver cells, cardiac and skeletal muscle, and brain; intracytoplasmic accumulations of a hyaline, fibrillar, PAS-positive material that is diastase resistant. In time, development of cirrhosis of liver.	Hepatomegaly, splenomegaly, ascites, and liver failure. Lethal within 2 years.
V	McArdle's syndrome 1 per 500,000	Muscle phosphorylase	Skeletal muscle only—accumulations of glycogen predominantly in subsarcolemmal location	Painful cramps associated with strenuous exercise. Myoglobinuria occurs in 50% of cases. Onset in adulthood (>20 years). Muscular exercise fails to raise lactate level in venous blood. Compatible with normal longevity.
VI	Hers' disease 1 per 200,000	Liver phosphorylase	Only hepatomegaly—scattered cytoplasmic vacuoles, occasionally lipid vacuoles; no intranuclear glycogen.	Hepatomegaly. Mild clinical course.
VII	Tarui's disease 1 per 500,000	Muscle phosphofructokinase	Only skeletal muscle and erythrocytes studied—subsarcoplasmic glycogen similar to that in type V.	Similar to type V.
VIII	1 per 100,000	Deficient activity of phosphorylase kinase	Hepatomegaly—similar to type VI.	X-linked recessive. Hepatomegaly and mild clinical course.

figures.[61] In adolescence and young adult life, skin lesions (angiokeratomas) and central nervous system symptoms dominate the presentation of this disease, but most patients die in middle life of progressive renal failure due to the kidney involvement.

Fragile X–Syndrome

An X-linked pattern of mental retardation has been seen in many kindreds with familial mental retardation. As in the case of other X-linked disorders, males are affected and the carrier females are unaffected or minimally affected. In recent years, a subdivision of this disorder became diagnosable cytogenetically by the identification of a fragile site on the long arm of X chromosome.[62] This is now thought to be a frequent cause of retardation in males. The fragile site is usually seen as discontinuity of staining (Fig. 4–14) in an unbanded karyotype. It should be pointed out that such fragile sites have also been found on several autosomes without any obvious associated clinical disorder. Demonstration of the fragile sites requires culture of cells in folic acid deficient media and is not yet a routine diagnostic tool.

DISORDERS WITH MULTIFACTORIAL INHERITANCE

As pointed out earlier, the multifactorial disorders are believed to result from the combined actions of environmental influences and two or more mutant genes having additive effects. The genetic component, then, exerts a dosage effect—the greater the number of inherited deleterious genes, the more severe the expression of the disease. Because environmental factors significantly influence the expression of these genetic disorders, the term *polygenic inheritance* is misleading.

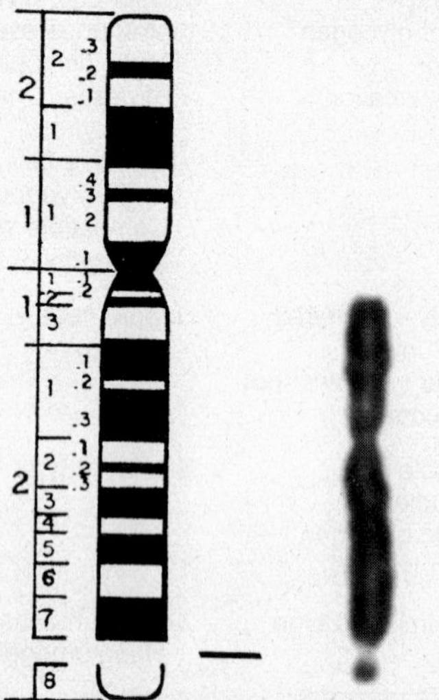

Figure 4–14. Fragile X, seen as discontinuity of staining. (Courtesy of Dr. Patricia Howard-Peebles, Southwestern Medical School, Dallas, Texas.)

A number of normal phenotypic characteristics are governed by multifactorial inheritance, such as hair color, eye color, skin color, height, and intelligence. These characteristics exhibit a continuous variation in population groups, producing the standard bell-shaped curve of distribution. However, environmental influences significantly modify the phenotypic expression of multifactorial traits. For example, certain subsets of diabetes mellitus have many of the features of a multifactorial disorder. It is well recognized clinically that individuals often first manifest this disease following weight gain. Thus, obesity as well as other environmental influences unmasks the diabetic genetic trait. Nutritional influences may cause even monozygous twins to achieve different heights. The culturally deprived child cannot achieve his or her full intellectual capacity.

The following features characterize multifactorial inheritance. These have been established for the multifactorial inheritance of congenital malformations and, in all likelihood, obtain for other multifactorial diseases.[63]

1. *The risk of expressing a multifactorial disorder is conditioned by the number of mutant genes inherited. Thus, the risk is greater in sibs of patients having severe expressions of the disorder.*
2. *Environmental influences significantly modify the risk of expressing the disease.*
3. *The rate of recurrence of the disorder (in the range of 2 to 7%) is the same for all first-degree relatives, i.e., parents, sibs, and offspring, of the affected individual. Thus, if parents have had one affected child, the risk that the next child will be affected is between 2 and 7%. Similarly, there is the same chance that one of the parents will be affected.*
4. *The likelihood that both identical twins will be affected is significantly less than 100%, but is much greater than the chance that both nonidentical twins will be affected. Experience has proved, for example, that the frequency of concordance for identical twins is in the range of 20 to 40%.*
5. *The risk of recurrence of the phenotypic abnormality in subsequent pregnancies depends on the outcome in previous pregnancies. When one child is affected there is a 2 to 7% chance that the next child will be affected, but after two affected sibs the risk rises to about 9%.*
6. *Severity of expression of the disease may range along a bell-shaped curve or may be discontinuous. Despite the polygenic mode of inheritance, a threshold may exist beyond which individuals are at risk. Thus, for some multifactorial disorders it appears that inheritance of a certain number of mutant genes is required before the disorder is expressed. As stated before, however, environmental influences still play a role.*

Assigning a disease to this mode of inheritance must be done with caution. It depends on many factors, but first of all on familial clustering and the exclusion of mendelian and chromosomal modes of transmission. A range of levels of severity of a disease is suggestive of multifactorial inheritance but, as pointed out earlier, variable expressivity and reduced penetrance of mendelian mutant genes may also account for this phenomenon. Because of these difficulties there is often disagreement as to whether the pedigree conforms to a mendelian or multifactorial pattern, as is the case, for example, with diabetes mellitus and epilepsy. The problem is well put in the statement: "multifactorial inheritance is a geneticist's nightmare."

In contrast to the mendelian disorders, which must be considered uncommon, the multifactorial group includes some of the most common ailments to which humans are heirs. Among newborns and infants, the following multifactorial disorders are considered elsewhere:

- anencephaly—a neurologic malformation (p. 1425)
- cleft lip with or without cleft palate (p. 785)
- congenital heart disease, several forms of (p. 585)
- pyloric stenosis (p. 808)
- spina bifida, many types of (p. 1427)

In adults the following conditions are believed to have multifactorial origins:

- diabetes mellitus (possibly certain subsets) (p. 975)
- epilepsy
- gout, in some cases (p. 1356)
- Hirschsprung's disease (possibly) (p. 855)
- hypertension (p. 1041)

As our awareness of the subtle, and sometimes not so subtle, impact of the genotype on the expression of many diseases increases, the future roster of multifactorial disorders will undoubtedly be larger.

DISORDERS WITH VARIABLE GENETIC BACKGROUNDS

To this category belong those conditions associated with a variety of genotypic aberrations.

CONGENITAL MALFORMATIONS

Congenital malformations are structural abnormalities that are extremely common causes of spontaneous abortion, stillbirth, and pediatric disease. About 2% of newborns have such malformations.[63] Since they have greatest clinical impact in postnatal life and infancy, they are considered in greater detail on page 479. You should note that the term congenital means "born with." *Only some of the congenital anomalies are genetic in origin and have variable modes of transmission*, including (1) cytogenetic aberrations, (2) mendelian inheritance, and (3) multifactorial inheritance. *Some are due to environmental influences* such as fetal exposure to teratogenic drugs or viral infections during pregnancy. The well-known case of thalidomide toxicity is an example of a gestational teratogen. Infants born of mothers who had taken this drug during pregnancy have congenital malformations (seal limbs) that are *not* of genetic origin. Similarly, several viral infections, rubella being the best known, induce fetal malformations. Moreover, many congenital malformations are of completely obscure origin.

It is important to identify the genotypic aberrations underlying those malformations of genetic origin. Those involving cytogenetic aberrations are often sporadic, owing to errors in gametogenesis. For example, Klinefelter's syndrome (47,XXY) and Turner's syndrome (45,X) are both characterized by structural anomalies, but neither of these conditions is familial, so that the risk of recurrence in subsequent pregnancies is considerably less than in the case with the mendelian and multifactorial modes of inheritance. It is also important to point out that multiple malformations often occur in consistent patterns to create syndromes. Some syndromes having different modes of transmission resemble each other closely. Thus, it is possible to confuse one related to a sporadic chromosomal anomaly with another having mendelian origins. The significance of such a misinterpretation in genetic counseling is obvious, since the mendelian disorder might well be autosomal dominant and carry a 50% risk for subsequent offspring.

EHLERS-DANLOS SYNDROMES (EDS)

Contortionists must have or should have one of the EDS. *Basic to all the variants is some defect in connective tissue*, more specifically collagen, leading to hyperelasticity and fragility of the skin accompanied by striking loose-jointedness. The hyperelasticity of the skin and loose-jointedness permit grotesque contortions, such as bending the thumb backward to touch the forearm and bending the knee forward to create almost a right angle. However, a predisposition to joint dislocation is one of the prices paid for this virtuosity. The skin is extraordinarily stretchable, but in younger individuals it appears to have normal elasticity, returning to its normal position promptly on release. Later the elasticity is lost, and the skin becomes saggy and hangs in folds and wrinkles. It is extremely fragile and vulnerable to trauma. Minor injuries produce gaping defects, and surgical repair or any surgical intervention is accomplished with great difficulty because of the lack of normal tensile strength. The basic defect in connective tissue may lead to internal complications, such as diaphragmatic hernia; spontaneous rupture of the intestine; and rupture of arteries, including dissecting aneurysms of the aorta.

Eight distinctive variants of the EDS have been identified. All are characterized by some abnormality in collagen synthesis or fibrogenesis. The distinctive clinical and genetic features of these are summarized in Table 4-9. Further details can be found in recent reviews.[65, 66]

NEOPLASIA

Cancer and genotype are intimately related on a variety of levels. There is a strong possibility that some

Table 4–9. THE EHLERS-DANLOS SYNDROME*

Type and Inheritance	Basic Defect	Clinical Features: *Joints*	Clinical Features: *Skin*	*Other Features*
Autosomal Dominant Forms				
EDS I	Unknown. Collagen fibers of increased diameter and irregular shape identified in some cases	Hypermobility, dislocations, and early onset osteoarthritis	Hyperextensible, fragile, bruisable with thin "cigarette paper" scars	Premature rupture of fetal membranes; tearing out of sutures and poor wound healing
EDS II	Unknown	Extensibility only slightly increased and may be localized to hands and feet	Minimal involvement, slight tendency to bruising but no scarring	All features much milder than type I
EDS III	Unknown	Severe generalized hyperextensibility	Insignificant involvement	—
EDS VIII	Unknown	Mild hypermobility	Moderate fragility with scarring, mild hyperextensibility, and bruising	Severe periodontitis with alveolar bone resorption
Autosomal Recessive Forms				
EDS IV (Autosomal dominant also reported)	Defective synthesis of type III collagen, especially in tissues containing smooth muscles, e.g., blood vessels	Mild involvement or normal.	Pale, thin skin; no hyperextensibility but easy bruisability, with ecchymoses after minor trauma; no delay in wound healing	Rupture of bowels and great vessels due to weakness of wall
EDS VI	Deficiency of enzyme lysyl hydroxylase leading to reduced formation of hydroxylysine, which in turn leads to deficiency in hydroxylysine-derived cross-links	Moderate hyperextensibility, severe kyphoscoliosis	Thin, pale, hyperextensible, and fragile	Ocular fragility with rupture of cornea, and sclerae and retinal detachment
EDS VII	Deficiency of enzyme procollagen-*N*-peptidase; persistence of *N*-terminal peptides in procollagen impairs aggregation of collagen fibers	Severe hyperextensibility; short stature, dislocation of joints common	Moderately hyperextensible and bruisable	—
X-linked Recessive Form				
EDS V	Possible deficiency of the cross-linking enzyme lysyl oxidase	Minimal hypermobility	Markedly hyperextensible; moderate increase in bruisability and fragility	Floppy mitral valve

*Modified from Krieg, T., et al.: Molecular defects in collagen metabolism in the Ehlers-Danlos syndrome. Int. J. Dermatol. *20*:415, 1981; and Minor, R. R.: Collagen metabolism: A comparison of diseases of collagen and diseases affecting collagen. Am. J. Pathol. *98*:225, 1980.

alteration of the genetic code—namely, one or more mutations—initiates the formation of malignant neoplasms, as discussed on page 248. Well documented is the fact that certain inherited genotypes predispose to the development of cancers (p. 263). For example, inheritance of a specific autosomal dominant mutation clearly predisposes to the development of retinoblastomas. At yet another level are the cytogenetic abnormalities observed in cancer cells. Both numerical and structural alterations in chromosomes have been observed in cancer cells in vitro as well as in the cells of malignant neoplasms of both animals and man. These and the questions raised about their pathogenetic significance are discussed on pages 231 and 677. There is still another level where the genome and cancer interrelate, namely, the chromosomal breakage syndromes predisposing to both mutations and cancers. Four autosomal recessive diseases—Fanconi's anemia, Bloom's syndrome, ataxia telangiectasia, and xeroderma pigmentosum—are characterized by an increased susceptibility to various forms of neoplasia. The fundamental defect in all four of these conditions may be an inability to repair DNA mutations acquired during life, thus increasing the risk of developing cancer (p. 241).

So we come to the end of this chapter, but by no means the end of the role of genetics in the diseases of man. Additional instances appear throughout this book.

1. Kronenberg, H. M.: Looking at genes. N. Engl. J. Med. *307*:50, 1982.
2. McKusick, V. A.: The anatomy of the human genome. Am. J. Med. *69*:267, 1980.
3. Benz, E. H., and Forget, B. G.: The thalassemia syndromes: Models for molecular analysis of human disease. Annu. Rev. Med. *33*:363, 1982.
4. Tjio, J. H., and Levan, A.: The chromosome number of man. Hereditas *42*:1, 1956.
5. Childs, B.: Persistent echoes of the nature-nurture argument. Am. J. Hum. Genet. *29*:1, 1977.
6. Gregor, A. S.: Charles Darwin. London, Angus & Robertson, 1967.
7. Carr, D. H., and Gideon, M.: Population cytogenetics of human abortuses. *In* Hook, E. B., and Porter, I. H. (eds.): Population Cytogenetics. Studies in Humans. New York, Academic Press, 1977, p.1.
8. Hook, E. B., and Hamerton, J. L.: The frequency of chromosomal abnormalities detected in consecutive newborn studies—differences between studies—result by sex and severity of phenotypic involvement. *In* Hook, E. B., and Porter, I. H. (eds.): Population Cytogenetics. Studies in Humans. New York, Academic Press, 1977, p. 63.
9. Caspersson, T., et al.: Analysis of human metaphase chromosome set by aid of DNA-binding fluorescent agents. Exp. Cell Res. *62*:490, 1970.
10. Priest, J. H.: Medical Cytogenetics and Cell Culture. Philadelphia, Lea & Febiger, 1977.
11. Francke, U., and Oliver, N.: Quantitative analysis of high-resolution trypsin-Giemsa bands of human prometaphase chromosomes. Hum. Genet. *45*:137, 1978.
12. Gerald, P. S.: Sex chromosome disorders. N. Engl. J. Med. *294*:706, 1976.
13. Creagan, R. P., and Ruddle, F. H.: New approaches to human gene mapping by somatic cell genetics. *In* Yunis, J. J. (ed.): Molecular Structure of Human Chromosomes. New York, Academic Press, 1977, p. 90.
14. Shows, T. B., and McAlpine, P. J.: The 1979 catalog of human genes and chromosome assignments. Cytogenet. Cell Genet. *25*:117, 1979.
15. Chang, Y. C., and Kan, Y. W.: A sensitive new prenatal test for sickle-cell anemia. N. Engl. J. Med. *307*:30, 1982.
16. Ley, T. J., et al.: 5-Azacytidine selectively increases beta-globin synthesis in a patient with β^+ thalassemia. N. Engl. J. Med. *307*:1469, 1982.
17. Martin, G M., and Hoehn, H.: Genetics and human disease. Hum. Pathol. *5*:387, 1974.
18. An international system for human cytogenetic nomenclature (1978). Birth defects: Orig. Art Ser. XIV (8), New York. The National Foundation, 1978.
19. Thompson, J. S., and Thompson, M. W.: Genetics in Medicine. Philadelphia, W. B. Saunders Co., 1980, p. 152.
20. Fabia, J., and Drolette, M.: Malformations and leukemia in children with Down's syndrome. Pediatrics *45*:60, 1970.
21. Rosner, F., and Lee, S. L.: Down's syndrome and acute leukemia: Myeloblastic or lymphoblastic. Am. J. Med. *53*:203, 1972.
22. Breg, W. R.: Down syndrome: A review of recent progress in research. Pathobiol. Annu. *7*:257, 1977.
23. deGrouchy, J., and Turleau, C.: Clinical Atlas of Human Chromosomes. New York, John Wiley & Sons, 1977.
24. Ahmad, K. N., et al.: Leydig cell volume in chromatin-positive Klinefelter's syndrome. J. Clin. Endocrinol. Metab. *33*:517, 1971.
25. Race, R. R., and Sanger, R.: Xg and sex-chromosome abnormalities. Br. Med. Bull. *25*:99, 1969.
26. Money, J., et al.: Cytogenetics, hormones and behavior disability: Comparison of XXY and XYY syndromes. Clin. Genet. *6*:370, 1974.
27. Sarto, G. E.: Cytogenetics of 50 patients with primary amenorrhea. Am. J. Obstet. Gynecol. *119*:114, 1974.
28. Weiss, L.: Additional evidence of gradual loss of germ cells in the pathogenesis of streak ovaries in Turner's syndrome. J. Med. Genet. *8*:540, 1971.
29. Summit, R. L.: Abnormalities of sex-chromosomes. *In* Kaback, M. M. (ed.): Genetic Issues in Pediatric and Obstetric Practice. Chicago, Year Book Medical Publishers, 1981, p. 70.
30. Simpson, J. L.: Disorders of sexual differentiation: Etiology and clinical delineation. New York, Academic Press, 1976.
31. Grumbach, M. M., and Conte, F. A.: Disorders of sex differentiation. *In* Williams, R. H. (ed.): Textbook of Endocrinology. Philadelphia, W. B. Saunders Co., 1981, pp. 423–506.
32. McKusick, V. A.: Mendelian Inheritance in Man. 5th ed. Baltimore, John Hopkins Press, 1978.
33. Erbe, R. W.: Principles of medical genetics. N. Engl. J. Med. *294*:381, 480; 1976.
34. Vessell, E. S.: Pharmacogenetics: Multiple interactions between genes and environment as determinants of drug response. Am. J. Med. *66*:183, 1979.
35. Payvandi, M. N., et al.: Cardiac, skeletal and ophthalmologic abnormalities in relatives of patients with Marfan's syndrome. Circulation *55*:797, 1977.
36. McKusick, V. A.: The Marfan syndrome. *In* McKusick, V. A. (ed.): Heritable Disorders of Connective Tissue. St. Louis, C. V. Mosby Co., 1972, p. 61.
37. Hirst, A. E., Jr., and Gore, I.: Marfan's syndrome: A review. Prog. Cardiovasc. Dis. *16*:187, 1973.
38. Scheck, M., et al.: Aortic aneurysm in Marfan's syndrome: Change in the ultra-structure and composition of collagen. J. Anat. *129*:645, 1979.
39. Boucek, R. J., et al.: The Marfan syndrome: A deficiency in chemically stable collagen cross-links. N. Engl. J. Med. *305*:988, 1981.
40. Lamberg, S. I., and Dorfman, A.: Synthesis and degradation of hyaluronic acid in cultured fibroblasts of Marfan's disease. J. Clin. Invest. *52*:2428, 1973.
41. Murdoch, J. L., et al.: Life expectancy and causes of death in the Marfan syndrome. N. Engl. J. Med. *286*:804, 1972.
42. Riccardi, V. M.: Von Recklinghausen neurofibromatosis. N. Engl. J. Med. *305*:1617, 1981.
43. Horton, W. A.: Von Hippel-Lindau disease: Clinical and pathological manifestations in nine families with 50 affected members. Arch. Intern. Med. *136*:769, 1976.
44. Goldstein, J. L., and Brown, M. S.: The LDL receptor defect in familial hypercholesterolemia. Implications for pathogenesis and therapy. Med. Clin. North Am. *66*:335, 1982.

44A. Goldstein, J. L., et al.: Defective lipoprotein receptors and atherosclerosis. Lessons from an animal counterpart of familial hypercholesterolemia. N. Engl. J. Med. *309*:288, 1983.

45. Brown, M. S., and Goldstein, J. L.: Lowering plasma cholesterol by raising LDL-receptors. N. Engl. J. Med. *305*:515, 1981.
46. Jacobs, S., and Cuatrecasas, P.: Cell receptors in disease. N. Engl. J. Med. *197*:1383, 1977.
47. Witkop, C. J.: Depigmentations of the general and oral tissues and their genetic foundations. Ala. J. Med. Sci. *16*:327, 1979.
48. O'Brien, W. M., et al.: Biochemical, pathologic and clinical aspects of alcaptonuria, ochronosis and ochronotic arthropathy. Review of world literature (1584–1962). Am. J. Med. *34*:813, 1963.
49. Stanbury, J. B., et al.: The Metabolic Basis of Inherited Disease. 5th ed. New York, McGraw-Hill Book Co., 1982, p. 751.
50. Schneck, L., et al.: The gangliosidoses. Am. J. Med. *46*:245, 1969.
51. Volk, B. W., et al.: The gangliosidoses. Hum. Pathol. *6*:555, 1975.
52. Arey, J. B.: The lipidoses: Morphologic changes in the nervous system in Gaucher's disease, G_{M2} gangliosidoses and Niemann-Pick disease. J. Clin. Lab. Sci. *5*:475, 1975.
53. Tallman, J. F., et al.: Ganglioside catabolism in hexosaminidase A–deficient adults. Nature *252*:254, 1974.
54. Besley, G. T. N., et al.: Somatic cell hybridization studies showing different gene mutations in Niemann-Pick variants. Hum. Genet. *54*:409, 1980.

54A. da Silva, V., et al.: Niemann-Pick's disease. Clinical, biochemical and ultrastructural findings in a case of infantile form. J. Neurol. *211*:61, 1975.

55. Lee, R. E., et al.: Gaucher's disease: Clinical, morphologic and pathogenetic considerations. Pathol. Annu. *12*:309, 1977.
56. Desnick, R. J.: Treatment of inherited metabolic diseases: An overview. *In* Kaback, M. M. (ed.): Genetic Issues in Pediatric and Obstetric practice. Chicago, Year Book Medical Publishers, 1981, p. 525.
57. Dorfman, A., and Matalon, R.: The mucopolysaccharidoses (a review). Proc. Natl. Acad. Sci. U. S. A. *73*:630, 1976.
58. Loeb, H., et al.: Biochemical and ultrastructural studies in Hurler's syndrome. J. Pediatr. *73*:860, 1968.
59. Legum, C. P., and Schor, R. S.: The genetic mucopolysaccharidoses and mucolipidoses: Review and comment. Adv. Pediatr. *22*:305, 1976.
60. McKusick, V. A., and Neufeld, E.: The mucopolysaccharide storage diseases. *In* Stanbury, J. B., et al. (eds.): Metabolic Basis of Inherited Disease. 5th ed. New York, McGraw Hill Book Co., 1982, p. 751.
61. Bagdade, J. D., et al.: Fabry's disease: A correlative clinical, morphological and biochemical study. Lab. Invest. *18*:681, 1968.
62. Sutherland, G. R.: Heritable fragile sites on human chromosomes. I. Effect of composition of culture medium on expression. Am. J. Hum. Genet. *31*:125, 1979.
63. Holmes, L. B.: Congenital malformations. N. Engl. J. Med. *295*:204, 1976.
64. Carter, C. O.: Genetics of common disorders. Br. Med. Bull. *25*:52, 1969.
65. Krieg, T., et al.: Molecular defects in collagen metabolism in the Ehlers-Danlos syndrome. Int. J. Dermatol. *20*:415, 1981.
66. Minor, R. R.: Collagen metabolism: A comparison of diseases of collagen and diseases affecting collagen. Am. J. Pathol. *98*:225, 1980.

5 DISEASES OF IMMUNITY

The immune response is an exquisitely specific yet highly versatile two-edged sword. Although it is vital for survival in the often hostile microbiologic environment, an immune reaction may cause fatal disease, as in the case of an overwhelming hypersensitivity reaction to the sting of a bee. Indeed, a host of disorders affecting all organ systems are clearly attributable to immunologic reactions to exogenous agents or to the abnormal emergence of immunity against one's own tissues and cells. This chapter will review some fundamentals of the immune system and consider the role of this system in the production of disease.

BASIC IMMUNOLOGY

GENERAL FEATURES OF THE IMMUNE SYSTEM

The immune response comprises all the phenomena that result from the specific interaction of cells of the immune system with antigens. Entrance of an antigen into the body can have two possible outcomes: (1) a *humoral immune response*, involving the synthesis and release of antibody molecules within the blood and extracellular fluids; or (2) *cell-mediated immunity*, manifested by production of "sensitized" lymphocytes capable of interacting with the antigen by means of special structures on the cell surface (receptors). In the first type of reaction, the humoral antibodies can combine with antigens such as bacterial toxins and cause neutralization of the toxin, or they can coat the antigenic surfaces of microorganisms and render them susceptible to lysis by complement or to phagocytosis by macrophages. In the second type of reaction, the sensitized cells are responsible for such actions as rejection of foreign tissue grafts and resistance against many intracellular microbes, e.g., viruses, fungi, and some bacteria.

The principal cellular component in both types of reactions is the lymphocyte. Thus, lymphoid tissues of the body, including the thymus, lymph nodes, spleen, bone marrow, and circulating lymphocytes, are the essential structural components of the immune response. The two major types of lymphocytes involved in the immune response are bursa-dependent lymphocytes (B cells) and thymus-dependent lymphocytes (T cells). These two lymphocyte classes differ in their ontogeny and in the functions that they perform. B lymphocytes are the progenitors of plasma cells that secrete antibodies, while T lymphocytes are the mediators of cell-mediated immunity. Macrophages also constitute an essential part of the immune apparatus. Although they do not produce antibodies or give rise to sensitized cells themselves, they play an important role in the induction of most immune responses and in the expression of the cell-mediated immune response. These and other cellular components of the immune response are briefly described below, to be followed by a brief description of the HLA complex, since it is relevant to several immunologically mediated diseases and to rejection of transplants.

T Lymphocytes

Like B lymphocytes, T lymphocytes are present in the peripheral lymphoid tissues as well as in circulating blood. *In contrast to B cells, they are found mainly in the area between the follicles and in the deep cortex of the lymph nodes, and mainly in the periarteriolar sheaths of the spleen.* In the peripheral blood they constitute 70 to 80% of all lymphocytes. T lymphocytes are long-lived, and they form a large, recirculating pool of cells. Their functions can be divided into two broad categories:

1. *Cellular immune reactions.* These include several phenomena in which T cells play a pivotal role. Examples are delayed hypersensitivity reactions, resistance against infection by certain bacteria and viruses,

rejection of solid organ transplants, and possibly resistance against tumors.

2. *Regulatory functions.* T cells perform important functions in modulating the immune response mediated by other T cells and B cells. This regulatory function can be expressed as facilitation or suppression of an immune response. Accordingly, *T-helper cells* provide "help" to B cells and other T cells to respond optimally in response to certain antigens, while *T-suppressor cells* can suppress the immune response. More recently, *inducer T cells* that serve to induce the helper or suppressor cells have also been described.

In view of these multiple T-cell functions, one might ask whether they are all carried out by a single set of T cells, or whether there are several subpopulations among T cells, each capable of mediating only certain functions. The answers to these questions have been provided by studies of the Lyt antigen system in mice and by the development of monoclonal anti-T cell antibodies in humans. Monoclonal antibodies are secreted by clones of hybridoma cells derived by the fusion of a B cell producing the desired antibody and a mouse myeloma cell. Because one of the fusion partners (myeloma cell) is cancerous, the hybrid is virtually immortal and its progeny continue to secrete antibodies identical in specificity to that produced by the sensitized parent B cell.

The two most widely used groups of anti-T monoclonal antibodies are referred to as OKT and Leu.[1, 2] By utilizing these it has been possible to delineate several functionally distinct subpopulations of human T cells, and to identify distinct stages in T cell differentiation. Antibodies, designated OKT1 (Leu-1), OKT3 (Leu-4), and OKT11 (Leu-5) react with virtually all the T cells in the peripheral blood; therefore, the antigens corresponding to these antibodies (designated similarly OKT1, OKT3, and OKT11) can be considered common markers of all mature T cells. Among these mature T cells, OKT4 (Leu-3) is expressed in 60% (i.e., 60% are OKT1$^+$, 3$^+$, 11$^+$, and T4$^+$), whereas 30% of the peripheral T cells express OKT8. Most of the latter also express OKT5 antigen. The OKT4$^+$ and OKT8$^+$/5$^+$ cells are non-overlapping; more important, they express distinct functional properties. The OKT4$^+$ cells have been defined as the helper/inducer subset, since they serve as helpers in antibody synthesis and generation of cytotoxic T cells. On the other hand, OKT8$^+$/5$^+$ cells include cytotoxic T cells and suppressor T cells. The ratio of OKT4/OKT8 cells in the peripheral blood is approximately 2;[1] this may be altered in various disease states, as discussed later in this chapter. Within the human thymus, several stages of T cell differentiation have been recognized by the use of monoclonal anti-T cell antibodies. Over 90% of the thymocytes express OKT10, whereas this antigen is not expressed on mature post-thymic T cells.[3] In severe combined immunodeficiency, a disorder characterized by defective maturation of T cells (p. 207), OKT10 cells immunologically not competent may be found in the peripheral blood.

In summary, monoclonal anti-T cell antibodies have not only been of help in a better understanding of T-cell physiology but also aided considerably in defining the aberrations associated with various disorders of the immune system. Many such applications of these hybridoma antibodies will be cited in this chapter and in the consideration of hemopoietic malignancies. Mature T cells in the peripheral blood, in addition to reacting with OKT3 antibodies, also form spontaneous rosettes with sheep erythrocytes (E). This property (E rosetting) is utilized clinically for enumeration of T cells.

B Lymphocytes

B lymphocytes are present in the blood and lymphoid tissue, including bone marrow. In human blood they constitute 10 to 20% of the lymphocyte population. *In lymph nodes they are found in the superficial cortex, forming lymphoid follicles. In the spleen they are found in the white pulp organized as lymphoid follicles, usually having pale staining central areas called germinal centers.* As is well known, B cells express surface immunoglobulin (Ig), which is thought to be identical in specificity to the immunoglobulins secreted when the B cell becomes a plasma cell. Ig on the B-cell surface can be identified by fluorescence microscopy after the cells have been incubated with anti-Ig antibodies labeled with fluorescein isothiocyanate. This procedure is utilized clinically to identify and quantitate B cells. In addition to Ig, B cells express two other receptors on their surface: a receptor for the Fc portion of IgG (Fc receptor) and a receptor for the third component of complement (C3b receptor). The function of these receptors in the immune response is not entirely clear, but they can be used as markers of B cells. The cell membrane of B cells bearing C3b receptors binds sheep erythrocytes (E) coated with IgM antibody (A) and complement (C′) to form so-called EAC′ rosettes. This technique is sometimes used to enumerate B cells in human peripheral blood.

In recent years a variety of monoclonal antibodies, produced by the hybridoma technique, that recognize B-cell antigens have been described.[4] At present they are not as widely used as the monoclonal antibodies reactive with T lymphocytes.

Macrophages

The origin and differentiation of macrophages have been discussed earlier in Chapter 2. Macrophages are widely distributed in the lymphoid tissue as well as in the circulating blood (as monocytes). In the lymph nodes they are present in the walls of sinuses as well as among the cells of the deep cortex. Macrophages play several roles in the immune response. First, they are required to "process" and present the antigen to immunocompetent cells. The presence of HLA-D/DR antigens (p. 161) on the macrophages is considered critical for the antigen-presenting functions. Second, macrophages act as powerful effector cells in certain cell-mediated immune reactions, appearing in response to products of

T-lymphocyte activation (lymphokines). Third, macrophages produce a number of soluble factors that profoundly influence the growth and function of lymphocytes as well as nonlymphoid cells such as fibroblasts, smooth muscle, and endothelial cells (p. 61).

The macrophage cell membrane has two important receptors: one for the Fc portion of IgG and the other for activated C3 (complement). Both these receptors help in phagocytosis of particulate matter. For example, antibody-coated ("opsonized") bacteria are readily ingested, because the Fc portion of the IgG coating the bacterium can bind to the macrophage Fc receptor. These receptors are also convenient markers for the study of macrophages in blood and lymphoid cell suspensions. Sheep erythrocytes (E) coated with IgG anti–sheep red cell antibodies (A) form rosettes (EA rosettes) with macrophages via the Fc portion of IgG.

Other Cell Types

K CELLS. *These cells are characterized by the presence of an Fc receptor, but they lack surface Ig and surface markers of T cells and are nonphagocytic.* Thus, they lack typical markers for B cells, T cells, or macrophages. Morphologically, they resemble small or medium-sized lymphocytes and are sometimes included in the group called "null cells." (Null cells constitute a heterogeneous group of cells, all of which lack well-defined cell-surface markers for T cells, B cells, and macrophages.) K cells, by virtue of their Fc receptor for IgG, can lyse antibody-coated target cells by means of a nonphagocytic mechanism. This process, called *antibody-dependent cellular cytotoxicity (ADCC)*, is discussed later under Type II hypersensitivity (p. 166), and its possible role in destruction of tumor cells will be described later (p. 258).

NK CELLS. In recent years much interest has focused on a novel cell type, called the natural killer (NK) cells. These cells are capable of lysing a variety of tumor cells, virus-infected cells, and some normal cells, *without previous sensitization.* NK cells are found in the peripheral blood and the lymphoid tissues of man as well as a variety of animal species.[5] Although NK cells share some cell surface antigens with T cells and macrophages, and possess Fc receptors, they are believed to be distinct from mature T cells, B cells, or macrophages. Morphologically they are somewhat larger than small lymphocytes and possess granules in their cytoplasm; they have therefore been described as *large granular lymphocytes.* Because of their ability to lyse tumor cells and virus-infected cells in vitro, without previous immunization, they are considered to be important as the first line of defense against tumors and virus infections.

DENDRITIC AND LANGERHANS' CELLS. These include a population of cells, all characterized by dendritic cytoplasmic processes and the presence of large amounts of cell surface HLA-D/DR antigens.[6] Dendritic cells are found in the lymphoid tissues, and somewhat similar cells within the epidermis have been called Langerhans' cells. By virtue of cell surface HLA-D/DR antigens, dendritic cells and Langerhans' cells are extremely efficient in antigen presentation, and some investigators believe that they are the most important antigen-presenting cells in the body. It should be noted that, unlike macrophages, they are either weakly phagocytic (Langerhans' cells) or not phagocytic (dendritic cells). Nevertheless, they are believed to be a part of the mononuclear phagocytic system.

HISTOCOMPATIBILITY ANTIGENS

Although originally identified as antigens that evoke rejection of transplanted organs, histocompatibility antigens are now considered important in the regulation of the immune response as well as in resistance/susceptibility to a growing list of diseases. The structure and organization of histocompatibility antigens and the corresponding histocompatibility genes are complex and still incompletely understood. Here we will summarize only the salient features of human histocompatibility antigens, primarily to facilitate an understanding of their role in rejection of organ transplants and disease susceptibility. A detailed description may be found in specialized texts.[7]

It is well known that when an individual receives an organ transplant obtained from a genetically dissimilar donor, the transplanted organ is rejected by immunologic mechanisms. In this process of rejection, the recipient's immune system recognizes the histocompatibility antigens displayed on the cell surfaces of the donor organ. Several genes code for histocompatibility antigens, but those that code for the most important transplantation antigens are clustered on a small segment of chromosome 6. This cluster of genes constitutes the human major histocompatibility complex (MHC) and is also known as the HLA complex (Fig. 5–1). It is equivalent to the murine H-2 complex.

The term HLA refers to human leukocyte antigens, since MHC-encoded antigens were initially detected on the white cells. Four closely linked loci, designated HLA-A, -B, -C, and -D/DR, form the human HLA complex. A feature common to all the HLA loci is the high degree of polymorphism, i.e., the existence of multiple allelic forms in a population. Each of the several allelic determinants at these loci is identified by a number, e.g., HLA-A1, HLA-B5, and so forth. Already over 40 antigens have been recognized at the HLA-B

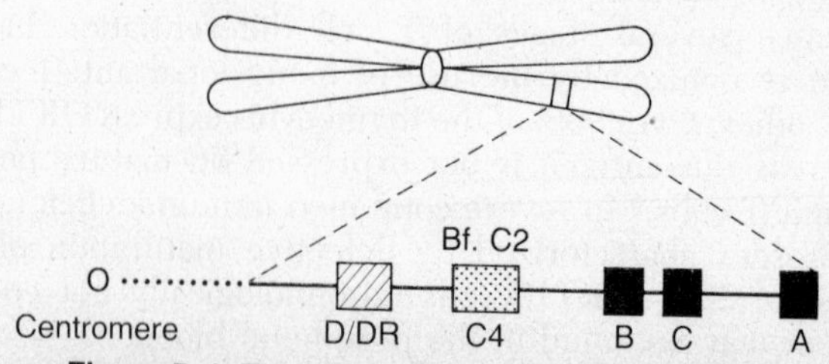

Figure 5–1. The HLA complex on chromosome 6.

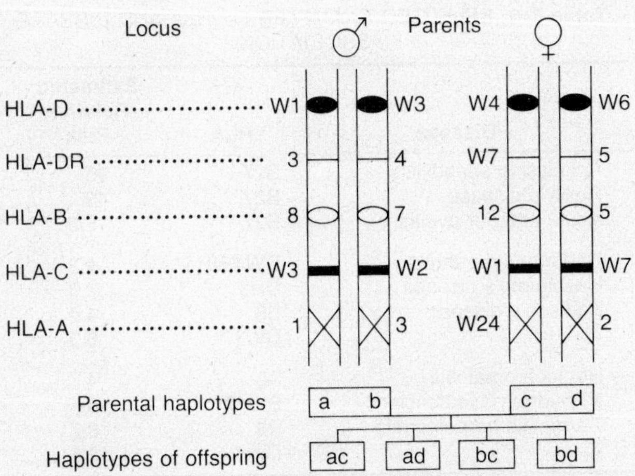

Figure 5–2. Inheritance of HLA haplotypes. The paternal haplotypes are indicated by *a* and *b* and the maternal haplotypes by *c* and *d*. The possible haplotype combinations of offspring are indicated, assuming no crossing over; e.g., ac = HLA-DW1, 4; -DR 3, W7; -B 8, 12; -CW 3, W1; -A1, W24.

locus. Those antigens that have been defined only provisionally are designated by a W (for international workshop), e.g., HLA-BW21. Every individual inherits only one determinant from each parent and can express no more than two different antigens for every locus (Fig. 5–2). Antigens coded by HLA-A, -B, and -C loci (also called class I antigens) are similar in many respects. They are 44,000 molecular weight glycoproteins, which are represented on virtually all the nucleated cells. Since class I antigens evoke the formation of humoral antibody in genetically nonidentical recipients, it is possible to obtain antibodies reactive against them. This makes it possible to type class I antigens by conventional serologic techniques such as antibody- and complement-mediated cytotoxicity.

HLA-D antigens differ in several respects from class I antigens. They were initially defined by a functional test called the *mixed lymphocyte reaction*. This reaction occurs when lymphocytes from two individuals who differ at the HLA-D locus are cultured together in vitro. T lymphocytes from one individual can recognize ("see") foreign HLA-D antigens on the cells of the other individual and respond by proliferation, which can be measured. If the individuals share the same HLA-D antigens, proliferation does not occur. By using the mixed lymphocyte reaction, it has been possible to provisionally identify 12 HLA-D antigens designated HLA-DW1 through HLA-DW12. In recent years, efforts to define the HLA-D antigens by serologic techniques have led to the identification of closely related (if not identical) -DR (D-related) antigens. Collectively, the HLA-D/DR antigens are called class II antigens and they are coded by a segment of HLA that corresponds to the I region of the murine H-2 complex. The bulk of the available data indicates that most or all of these antigens are products of Ir (immune response) genes, which determine individual patterns of responses to foreign antigens. Unlike class I antigens, D/DR antigens have a restricted tissue distribution, being found mainly on B lymphocytes, monocytes/macrophages, dendritic/Langerhans' cells, and some endothelial cells. Chemically, HLA-DR antigens are quite distinct from class I antigens in that they are found on a 2-chain molecule, with molecular weights of 34,000 (α-chain) and 29,000 (β-chain). Several other less well-defined class II antigens have also been found recently; these include -MB, -MT, and -SB antigens.

In addition to histocompatibility antigens, structural genes for complement components (C4, C2, and Bf of the alternate pathway) are also closely linked to the HLA complex (Fig. 5–1).

Inheritance of HLA Haplotypes

A set of closely linked genes on one chromosome constitutes a haplotype, and these tend to be inherited en bloc. In the case of the human major histocompatibility complex it includes one gene each from HLA-A, -B, -C, -D, and -DR loci. Haplotype analysis is of importance in family studies and in organ transplantation. An illustration of inheritance of HLA is provided in Figure 5–2. There are two paternal and two maternal haplotypes. Each parent is depicted as being heterozygous at all loci, and the two parents do not share any common HLA-specificities. The offspring can have only four possible combinations of haplotypes. There is a 25% chance that two siblings will be HLA-identical (i.e., share both haplotypes). An additional 50% will share one haplotype, and 25% will not share any haplotype. Parents share one haplotype with all children and differ in the other. However, if both parents had shared one haplotype, there would be a 1 in 2 chance of parents and offspring being identical. The degree of haplotype-sharing is of fundamental importance in predicting graft survival. In the above example, crossing-over was not considered, although it is possible and can lead to formation of a new haplotype.

Significance of HLA Complex

In Organ Transplantation. As mentioned earlier, HLA antigens were discovered in the course of transplantation studies, and continue to present formidable barriers to the success of clinical organ transplantation. HLA antigens of the graft evoke both humoral and cell-mediated responses, which lead eventually to graft destruction, as discussed on page 171. Since the severity of the rejection reaction is related to the degree of HLA disparity between the donor and recipient, HLA typing is of immense clinical significance in the selection of the donor-recipient combinations.

Regulation of Immune Response. In mice, a set of genes that control the magnitude of both cellular and humoral immune responses has been mapped within the I region of the murine major histocompatibility complex (H-2 complex). In humans, there is accumulating evidence that immune response (Ir) genes map in the -D/DR region of the HLA complex and that -D/DR antigens may be the products of Ir genes. For example, the magnitude of IgE antibody response to a ragweed allergen (Ra 5) has been found to be highly associated with HLA-DR2, suggesting Ir-gene control. The mechanisms by which Ir genes regulate the immune response are not entirely clear and are beyond the scope of this discussion.

Cell-to-cell Interactions in Immune Response. The ultimate expression of the immune response, both humoral and cellular, depends on an intricate and finely orchestrated interaction among several cell types. It is well-known, for example, that in the process of antigen presentation macrophages must interact with T cells and B cells, and in many cases T-helper cells have to interact with B cells or other effector T cells. T-suppressor cells can signal other immune cells to dampen or limit the immune reactivity. These interactions are critically dependent on cell surface HLA antigens. Many such interactions involve the recognition of class II HLA antigens, which you may recall are distributed almost exclusively on cells of the immune system.

Role in Host Defense. As we shall discuss later, cytotoxic T lymphocytes are believed to be important in resistance against virus infections and tumor cells (p. 258). The protective effects of cytotoxic T cells lie in their ability to lyse virus-infected or neoplastic cells. In this process of T cell–mediated lysis, class I antigens have been found to be of paramount importance. It has been discovered, for example, that cytotoxic T cells, specifically sensitized against a virus, can lyse the virus-infected cells only in association with class I HLA molecules. In other words, cytotoxic T cells cannot recognize the viral antigens independent of the HLA molecules. One explanation of this phenomenon (called *HLA restriction*) is that HLA antigens provide specific sites that are modified by virus infection and that the virus-modified self-HLA antigens provide the target antigen for cytotoxic T cells (Fig. 5–3). In this context, the presence of class I HLA antigens on virtually every somatic cell may be viewed as an evolutionary step designed to help in the elimination of abnormal or altered cells.

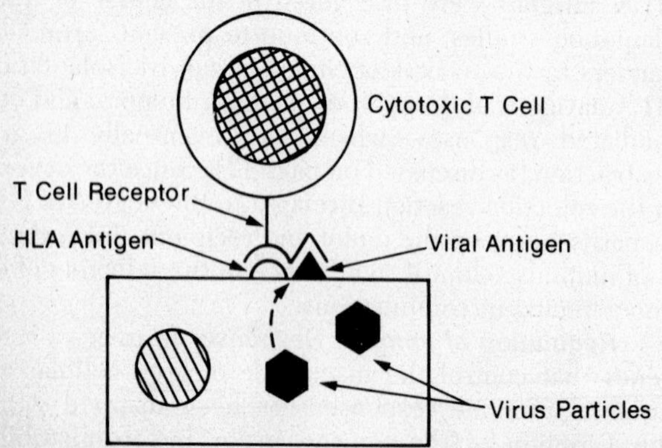

Figure 5–3. Schematic illustration of the role of HLA antigens in the lysis of virus-infected cell by cytotoxic T lymphocytes.

Table 5–1. SELECTED EXAMPLES OF HLA AND DISEASE ASSOCIATION

Disease	HLA	Estimated Relative Risk
Ankylosing spondylitis	B27	90
Reiter's disease	B27	48
Acute anterior uveitis	B27	16.9
Rheumatoid arthritis	DW4/DR4	4.2
Hashimoto's disease	DR3	2.6
Addison's disease	B8	4.0
	DW3	6.3
Hemochromatosis	A3	4
21-hydroxylase deficiency	BW47	15
Dermatitis herpetiformis	B8	8.7
	DW3	13.5

HLA and Disease Association. A variety of diseases have been found in association with certain HLA types (Table 5–1). The best known is the association between ankylosing spondylitis and HLA-B27; individuals who possess HLA-B27 antigen have a 90-fold greater chance (relative risk) of developing this disease than those who are negative for HLA-B27. The diseases that show association with HLA can be broadly grouped into the following categories: (1) *inflammatory diseases* including ankylosing spondylitis and several postinfectious arthropathies, all associated with HLA-B27; (2) *inherited errors of metabolism*, e.g., hemochromatosis (HLA-A3) and 21-hydroxylase deficiency (HLA-BW47); (3) *autoimmune diseases* including autoimmune endocrinopathies, associated with alleles at the DR locus; and (4) *complement deficiency* syndromes. The mechanisms underlying these associations are not understood at present. Clearly, with diseases as diverse as enzyme deficiency syndromes and autoimmune disorders, no single mechanism of association is likely. In view of the physiologic role of the HLA complex in regulation of the immune response, it is somewhat easier to speculate on the possible mechanisms that may underlie the associations with immunologically mediated diseases. The following two mechanisms have been proposed.[8]

1. *Involvement of immune response genes.* It was mentioned previously that immune response (Ir) genes appear to exist within the HLA complex of humans. If so, an association between certain autoimmune diseases and HLA antigens (see Table 5–1) may be explained on the basis of closely linked Ir genes that regulate the levels of auto-antibody responses. (See p. 179 for further discussion.)

2. *Direct participation of HLA macromolecules in disease.* There are two possible mechanisms by which HLA molecules may participate directly in disease. First, pathogens may share a cross-reacting antigen with HLA and be protected from an immune response by the host's tolerance for self-HLA antigens ("molecular mimicry"). Second, certain HLA molecules may provide receptors for viruses, and this may either facilitate virus-cell interaction or provide a target for host immune cells to destroy virus-infected cells. In the former case, the

presence of a given HLA type would favor virus-induced disease, whereas in the latter case it would favor removal of virus-infected cells.

DISORDERS OF THE IMMUNE SYSTEM

Having reviewed some fundamental aspects of immunology, we can now turn to general disorders of the immune system and some specific immunologic diseases. These will be discussed under four broad headings: (1) *hypersensitivity reactions*, which form the mechanisms of immunologic injury in a variety of diseases discussed throughout this book; (2) *autoimmune diseases*, which are caused by immune reactions against "self"; (3) *amyloidosis*, a poorly understood disorder having immunologic associations; and (4) *immunologic deficiency syndromes*, which result from rather distinct, often genetically determined defects in some components of the normal immune response.

MECHANISMS OF IMMUNOLOGIC TISSUE INJURY (HYPERSENSITIVITY REACTIONS)

Humans live in an environment teeming with substances capable of producing immunologic responses. Contact with antigen leads not only to induction of a protective immune response, but also to reactions that can be damaging to tissues. Exogenous antigens occur in dust, pollens, foods, drugs, microbiologic agents, and chemicals, and in many blood products used in clinical practice. The immune response that may result from such exogenous antigens take a variety of forms, ranging from annoying but trivial discomforts such as itching of the skin to potentially fatal disease such as bronchial asthma. The various reactions produced are called *hypersensitivity reactions*, and these can be initiated either by the interaction of antigen with humoral antibody or by cell-mediated immune mechanisms.

Disorders resulting from tissue-damaging immune reactions have been categorized in a variety of ways, but only two classifications will be reviewed here. The first (Table 5–2) divides the immunologically mediated disorders into three categories on the basis of the source of the offending antigen—exogenous, homologous, or autologous.[9] This classification is of value because it indicates that some disorders—those due to exogenous antigens—are essentially environmental and as such are theoretically preventable. Poison ivy contact dermatitis could be eradicated as a disease by mere avoidance of contact with the plant, as could hay fever resulting from inhalation of plant pollens. On the other hand, many of the most important immune diseases are caused by homologous and autologous antigens intrinsic to humans. The disorders triggered by homologous antigens result from the genetic and antigenic dissimilarities between individuals. Transfusion reactions and graft rejection are examples of immunologic disorders evoked by homologous antigens. Appropriate cross-matching of donor and recipient could preclude such reactions. Unfortunately, as discussed later, we do not yet have enough knowledge to match the donor and recipient accurately enough to prevent rejection of organs, nor are we likely to control erythroblastosis fetalis in the newborn (p. 486) by imposing the requisite of blood group compatibility on individuals who intend to marry. The third category of disorders, those incited by autologous antigens, comprises the important group of autoimmune diseases, to be discussed later in this chapter. These diseases appear to arise because of the emergence of immune responses against "self" antigens.

Table 5–2. IMMUNE DISORDERS CLASSIFIED BY SOURCE OF ANTIGEN

Exogenous	Atopic disease (e.g., poison ivy contact dermatitis; reactions to plant pollens, sera, and drugs)
Homologous	Reactions to isoantigens (e.g., transfusion reactions, erythroblastosis fetalis, transplant rejection)
Autologous	Autoimmune diseases (e.g., systemic lupus erythematosus, rheumatoid arthritis, Sjögren's syndrome)

The second classification (Table 5–3) is based on the immunologic mechanism that mediates the disease. This approach is of value in clarifying the manner in which the immune response ultimately causes tissue injury and disease. In Type I disease, the immune response releases vasoactive substances that act on smooth muscle and vessels, thus altering their function. In Type II disorders, humoral antibodies participate directly in injuring cells by predisposing them to phagocytosis or lysis. Type III disorders are best remembered as "immune complex diseases," in which humoral antibodies bind antigens and activate complement. The fractions of complement then attract neutrophils which, partly through the release of neutrophilic lysosomal enzymes, produce tissue damage. Type IV disorders involve tissue injury in which cell-mediated immune responses with sensitized lymphocytes are the cause of the cellular and tissue injury. Prototypes of each of these immune mechanisms are presented in the following sections.

TYPE I HYPERSENSITIVITY (ANAPHYLACTIC TYPE)

Anaphylaxis may be defined as a rapidly developing immunologic reaction occurring within minutes after the combination of an antigen with antibody bound to mast cells or basophils in individuals or animals previously sensitized to the antigen. It may occur as a systemic disorder or a local reaction. The systemic reaction

Table 5–3. MECHANISMS OF IMMUNOLOGICALLY MEDIATED DISORDERS

Type	Prototype Disorder	Immune Mechanism
Type I, Anaphylactic type	Anaphylaxis, some forms of bronchial asthma, atopy	Formation of IgE (cytotropic antibody) → release of vasoactive amines from basophils and mast cells
Type II, Cytotoxic type	Autoimmune hemolytic anemia, erythroblastosis fetalis, Goodpasture's disease	Formation of IgG, IgM → binds to antigen on target cell surface → phagocytosis of target cell or lysis of target cell
Type III, Immune complex disease	Arthus reaction, serum sickness, systemic lupus erythematosus, certain forms of acute glomerulonephritis	Antigen-antibody complexes → activated complement → attracted neutrophils → release of lysosomal enzymes
Type IV, Cell-mediated (delayed) hypersensitivity	Tuberculosis, contact dermatitis, transplant rejection	Sensitized T lymphocytes → release of lymphokines and other effector mechanisms

usually follows an intravenous injection of an antigen to which the host has already become sensitized. Often within minutes a state of shock is produced, which is sometimes fatal. Local reactions depend on the portal of entry of the allergen, and take the form of localized cutaneous swellings (skin allergy, hives), nasal and conjunctival discharge (allergic rhinitis and conjunctivitis), hay fever, bronchial asthma, or allergic gastroenteritis (food allergy).

In humans, Type I reactions are mediated by IgE antibodies.[10] In guinea pigs and mice (but apparently not in humans), 7S IgG immunoglobulins can also mediate anaphylactic reactions, albeit less efficiently than IgE. IgE is present in serum in very low concentrations and is also encountered bound to mast cells and basophils. An allergen stimulates IgE production by lymphocytes and plasma cells, principally in tonsillar tissue, Peyer's patches, and the lamina propria of gastrointestinal and other mucosal surfaces. The synthesis of IgE antibodies requires T-helper cells. Normally, however, this process is actively suppressed by T-suppressor cells. Once IgE antibodies are formed in response to an allergen, they have a strong tendency to attach to mast cells and basophils through cell surface receptors for the Fc portion of IgE heavy chain (Fig. 5–4). When a mast cell or basophil, armed with cytophilic IgE antibodies, is reexposed to the specific allergen, a series of reactions takes place, leading eventually to the release of a variety of powerful vasoactive mediators. This first step in this sequence is the binding of antigen (allergen) to the IgE antibodies previously attached to the mast cells. In this process, multivalent antigens bind to more than one IgE molecule and cause cross-linkage of adjacent IgE antibodies. The bridging of IgE molecules leads to perturbations of the IgE-Fc receptors and initiates two parallel and interdependent processes—one leading to mast cell degranulation with discharge of preformed (primary) mediators and the other involving de novo synthesis and release of secondary mediators such as leukotrienes.

Degranulation of mast cells is an active process that requires influx of calcium and depends on an intact glycolytic pathway. Involved in the complex sequence is a rapid and transient increase in cAMP, which activates cAMP-dependent protein kinases. These in turn are responsible for phosphorylation of the membrane around mast-cell granules. Phosphorylation and other alterations of the perigranular membranes render them permeable to water and calcium, resulting in marked swelling of the granules (visible under the electron microscope). Simultaneously, calcium-activated enzymes release energy required for the assembly of microtubules and microfilaments. These contractile elements of the cytoskeleton cause the movement of swollen granules toward the cell surface, where they fuse

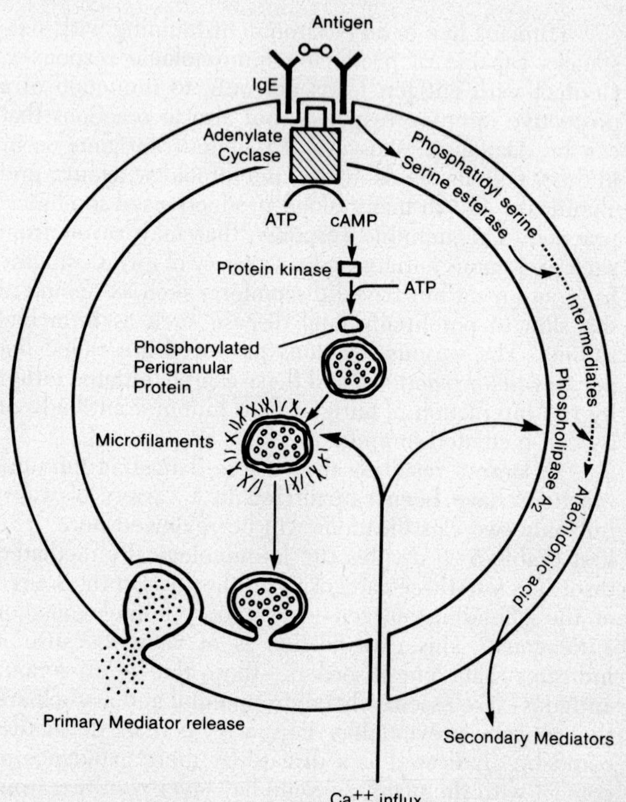

Figure 5–4. Schematic view of mast cell activation, degranulation, and secretion. (Adapted from Austen, K. F.: Tissue mast cells in immediate hypersensitivity. Hosp. Pract. *17*(No. 11):98, 1982. Reprinted with permission. Original drawing by Bunji Tagawa.)

with the cell membrane and spill their contents. As indicated earlier, the biologically active compounds contained within the mast cell granules are called the primary mediators; they include: (1) *histamine*, which causes intense bronchial smooth muscle contraction, increased vascular permeability, and increased secretion by nasal, bronchial, and gastric glands; (2) *eosinophil chemotactic factor of anaphylaxis* (ECF-A), which accounts for the presence of these cells in allergic reactions; and (3) a distinct, *neutrophil chemotactic factor*, which has also been identified more recently. In addition to these mediators, human mast cell granules contain impressive amounts of neutral proteases, whose normal function or role in disease is not yet clear.

The events resulting in the de novo synthesis of mast cell–derived secondary mediators take place within the cell membrane. The first step in this process is activation of a serine esterase, which through several intermediate steps leads to the formation of phosphatidylcholine. This compound somehow causes increased membrane permeability to calcium, which in turn activates phospholipase A_2. Next, phosphatidylcholine is metabolized by the phospholipase to yield arachidonic acid. This, you may recall, is the starting material for the synthesis of prostaglandins and leukotrienes (p. 55). It should be pointed out that the *secondary mediators*, including arachidonic acid metabolites, are formed not only by activated mast cells, but also by other leukocytes.[11] They can be divided into two groups:

Arachidonic Acid Metabolites. The metabolism and derivatives of arachidonic acid were discussed earlier in relation to inflammation. In the past, before they were chemically identified, many of the arachidonic acid derivatives involved in anaphylaxis were designated as slow-reacting substance of anaphylaxis (SRS-A) since their release was much slower as compared with histamine and they caused a much more prolonged contraction of bronchial smooth muscle. SRS-A has now been shown to be composed of leukotrienes C_4, D_4, and E_4.[12] It should be pointed out that these lipoxygenase derivatives of arachidonic acid are produced not only by mast cells but also by neutrophils and macrophages. Leukotrienes C_4 and D_4 are believed to be the major mediators of bronchospasm in systemic anaphylaxis, and on a molar basis they are 4000 times more potent than histamine. Leukotriene B_4 (not a component of SRS-A) is the most powerful natural chemotactic substance known. It acts on eosinophils, neutrophils, and macrophages. In addition to the leukotrienes, prostaglandins derived by the activation of the cyclooxygenase pathway are also produced during anaphylaxis. Mast cells form PGD_2, a potent vasodilator, and PGI_2, which causes disaggregation of platelets.

Platelet Activating Factors (PAF). These constitute the other group of secondary mediators. These low-molecular-weight lipids (acetylated glycerol ether phosphocholine, p. 57) released from basophils, as well as macrophages, cause platelet aggregation and noncytotoxic release of histamine from the platelets.

Eosinophils, which are attracted to the site of mast cell degranulation, apparently function to neutralize the effects of the mediators by releasing enzymes such as histaminase.[13] Thus, they may serve to *end* the reaction initiated by contact with allergen. It is thus apparent that in this type of reaction the mast cell—present in the connective tissue around blood vessels and bearing specific IgE recognition units—responds to a foreign material by inducing increased vascular permeability and recruiting both cells and serum factors, without necessarily inducing the extensive tissue damage characteristic of complement-mediated antigen-antibody reactions. Although this may serve to limit most reactions, an uncontrolled response may lead to profound consequences, as we shall see.

Systemic Anaphylaxis

In man, systemic anaphylaxis may occur after administration of heterologous proteins in the form of antisera, hormones, enzymes, polysaccharides, and drugs (such as the antibiotic penicillin). The severity of the disorder varies with the level of sensitization. However, the shock dose of antigen may be exceedingly small, as, for example, the tiny amounts used in ordinary skin testing for various forms of allergies. Within minutes after exposure, itching, hives, and skin erythema appear, followed shortly thereafter by a striking contraction of respiratory bronchioles and the appearance of respiratory distress. Laryngeal edema will result in hoarseness. Vomiting, abdominal cramps, diarrhea, and laryngeal obstruction follow, and the patient may go into shock and even die within the hour. At autopsy, some patients may be found to have pulmonary edema and hemorrhage, while others show hyperdistention of the lungs along with right-sided cardiac dilatation, a reflection of the constricted pulmonary vasculature. It is obvious that the effect of anaphylaxis must always be borne in mind when a therapeutic agent is administered. Although patients at risk can generally be identified by a previous history of some form of allergy, the absence of such a history does not preclude the possibility of an anaphylactic reaction. It is somewhat frightening to know that perhaps as many as one in five patients receiving penicillin develop some sensitivity to this drug and that 100 to 500 individuals die each year from penicillin anaphylaxis in the United States.

Local Anaphylaxis

These reactions are exemplified by so-called atopic allergy, *atopy* being the term introduced in 1923 to imply a propensity to develop such allergic reactions. In more modern terms, atopy is defined as a genetically controlled predisposition to the production of specific IgE antibodies upon inhalation or ingestion of minute amounts of antigen. About 10% of the population suffers from allergies involving localized anaphylactic reactions to extrinsic allergens such as pollen, animal dander, house dust, fish, and the like. Specific diseases include urticaria, angioedema, allergic rhinitis (hay fever), and asthma—all to be discussed elsewhere in this book. Of interest is the familial predisposition to the development of this type of allergy. A positive family history of allergy is found in 50% of atopic individuals. The mode of inheritance is unclear, but it is most likely multifactorial. Several genes seem to be involved and it has been suggested that genetic regulation of atopy is exerted at two levels. The total ability to produce IgE antibodies regardless of the allergen appears to be regulated by genes not linked to HLA, whereas the ability to respond specifically to a given allergen seems to be controlled by immune response genes within or linked to HLA.[14, 15] Although there are no significant associations between HLA antigens and atopic diseases as a group, significant association between some HLA loci and immune responses against certain allergens has been noted (e.g. DW 2 and ragweed allergen 5). Furthermore, IgE antibody production to some pollen extracts has been correlated with specific HLA haplotypes in certain families.[15]

TYPE II HYPERSENSITIVITY

This type of hypersensitivity is mediated by antibodies directed toward antigens present on the surface of cells or other tissue components. The antigenic determinants may be intrinsic to the cell membrane, or an exogenous antigen adsorbed on the cell surface. In either case the hypersensitivity reaction results from the binding of antibodies to normal or altered cell surface antigens. Two or possibly three different antibody-dependent mechanisms are involved in this type of reaction (Fig. 5–5).

Complement-Mediated Cytotoxicity. In this reaction, antibody (IgM or IgG) reacts with an antigen present on the surface of the cell, causing activation of the complement system and resulting in direct membrane damage and lysis. In addition, the antibody-coated cells become susceptible to phagocytosis. This type of reaction most commonly involves blood cells—red blood cells, white blood cells, and platelets—but the antibodies can also be directed against extracellular tissue (e.g., glomerular basement membrane in anti-GBM nephritis, p. 1004). Clinically, cytotoxic reactions occur in the following situations: (1) *transfusion reactions,* in which cells from an incompatible donor react with autochthonous antibody of the host; (2) *erythroblastosis fetalis,* in which there is an antigenic difference between the mother and the fetus, and antibodies from the mother (of the IgG class) cross the placenta and cause destruction of fetal red cells; (3) *autoimmune hemolytic anemia, agranulocytosis,* or *thrombocytopenia,* in which, for obscure reasons, individuals produce antibodies to their own blood cells, which are then destroyed; (4) *certain drug reactions,* in which antibodies are produced that react with the drug, which may be complexed to red cell antigen (p. 629).

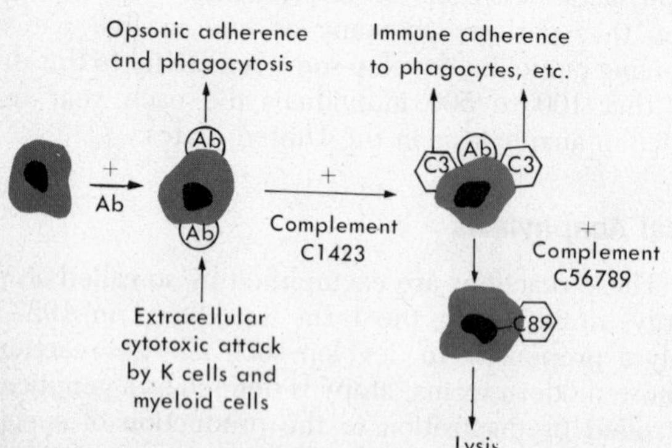

Figure 5–5. Type II antibody-dependent cytotoxic hypersensitivity. Antibodies directed against cell surface antigens cause cell death not only by C-dependent lysis but also by adherence reactions leading to phagocytosis or through nonphagocytic extracellular killing by certain lymphoreticular cells (antibody-dependent cell-mediated cytotoxicity). (Redrawn from Roitt, I.: Essential Immunology. 3rd ed. Oxford, Blackwell Scientific Publications, 1977.)

Antibody-Dependent Cell-Mediated Cytotoxicity (ADCC). Although complement-mediated lysis and phagocytosis are the best known mechanisms of cytotoxicity in vivo, the operation of a quite distinct cytotoxic mechanism is suggested by experiments in which target cells coated with low concentrations of IgG antibody can be killed by a variety of *nonsensitized* cells that have Fc receptors. The latter bind to the target by their receptors for Fc fragment of IgG, and cell lysis proceeds without phagocytosis. ADCC may be mediated by monocytes, neutrophils, eosinophils, and K cells (p. 160). So far, ADCC has been studied only in vitro, and whether it plays a positive role in antibody-mediated cytotoxicity in vivo remains an open question. Conceivably it could be relevant to the destruction of targets too large to be phagocytosed, such as parasites or tumor cells (p. 258), and it may also play some role in graft rejection.

Although cytotoxicity is the most common consequence of the interaction between antibody and cell-bound antigen, this may not always be the case. In recent years, a variety of diseases resulting from non-cytotoxic interactions between cell surface receptors and antireceptor antibodies have been described. For example, in myasthenia gravis, muscle weakness results from impaired neuromuscular transmission brought about by anti–acetylcholine receptor antibodies (p. 1311). Whether such antibody-mediated diseases should be classified as Type II or segregated into a new category (Type V) is a matter of semantics we can leave for the experts.

TYPE III HYPERSENSITIVITY (IMMUNE COMPLEX–MEDIATED)

This type of hypersensitivity reaction is induced by antigen-antibody complexes that produce tissue damage as a result of their capacity to activate a variety of serum mediators, principally the complement system. The toxic reaction is initiated when antigen combines with antibody, either within the circulation (circulating immune complexes) or at extravascular sites where antigen may have been deposited (in situ immune complexes). Some forms of glomerulonephritides in which immune complexes are formed in situ on the glomerular basement membrane are discussed later on page 1004. Complexes formed in the circulation produce damage, particularly as they localize within blood vessel walls or when they are trapped in filtering structures such as the renal glomerulus. It should be pointed out at the outset that the mere formation of antigen-antibody complexes in the circulation does not imply the presence of disease; indeed, immune complexes are formed during many immune responses, and may perhaps represent a normal mechanism of antigen removal. The factors that determine whether the immune complexes formed in circulation will be pathogenic are not fully understood, but some possible influences will be discussed later.

Two general types of antigens cause complex-mediated injury: the antigen may be *exogenous*, such as a foreign protein, a bacterium, or a virus, but under some circumstances the individual can produce antibody against self-components—*endogenous antigens*. The latter can be trace components present in the blood or, more commonly, antigenic components in cells and tissues. Immune complex–mediated diseases can be generalized, involving vessels in many organs (acute serum sickness), or may be localized to particular organs such as the kidney (glomerulonephritis), joints (arthritis), or only the small blood vessels of the skin (the local Arthus reaction).

Wherever complexes deposit, the mediation of tissue damage is similar (Fig. 5–6). *Central to this mechanism is activation of the complement cascade (p. 53) and the elaboration of biologically active fragments.* As will be recalled, complement activation (1) releases C3b, the opsonin that promotes phagocytosis of particles and organisms; (2) yields chemotactic factors, which direct the migration of polymorphonuclear leukocytes and monocytes (C5 fragments, and $\overline{C5b67}$); (3) releases anaphylatoxins (C3a and C5a), which increase vascular permeability and cause contraction of smooth muscle; and (4) causes cell membrane damage and even cytolysis (C5–9).

Phagocytosis of antigen-antibody complexes by leukocytes drawn in by the chemotactic factors results in the release or generation of a variety of proinflammatory substances including prostaglandins, vasodilator peptides, and more chemotactic substances, as well as several lysosomal enzymes including proteases capable of digesting basement membrane, collagen, elastin, and cartilage. Tissue damage may also be mediated by free oxygen radicals produced by activated neutrophils.[16] Immune complexes have several other effects: they cause aggregation of platelets and activate Hageman factor; both of these reactions augment the inflammatory process and initiate the formation of microthrombi (Fig. 5–6). The resultant pathologic lesion is termed vasculitis if it occurs in blood vessels, glomerulonephritis if it occurs in renal glomeruli, arthritis if it occurs in the joints, and so on.

It is clear from the above that only complement-

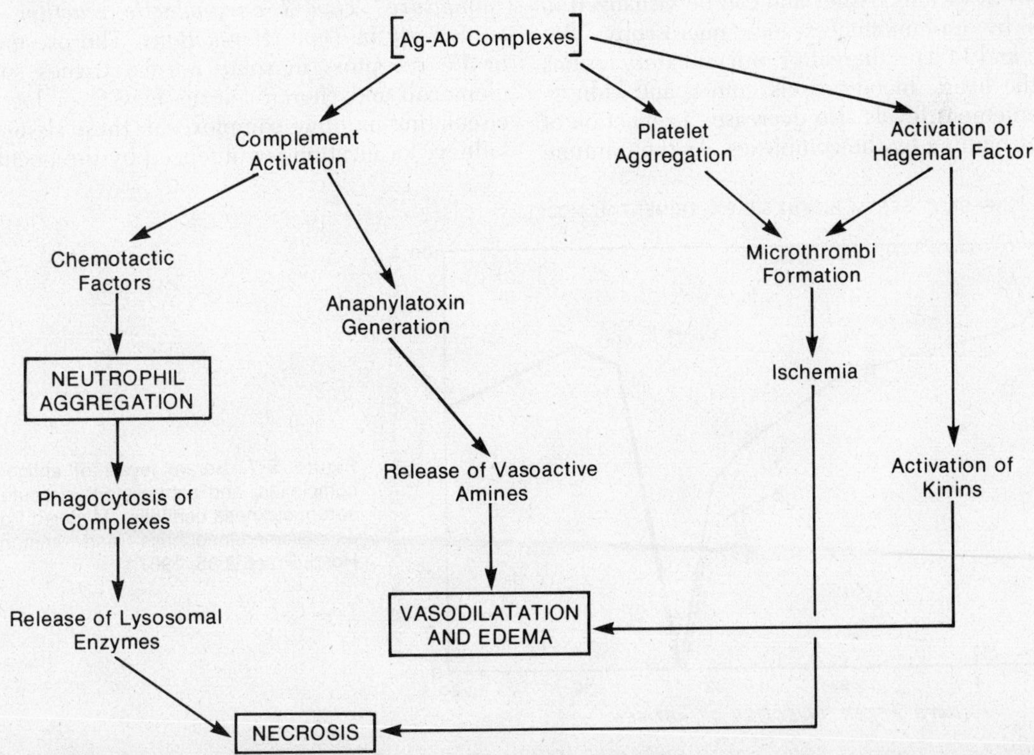

Figure 5–6. Schematic representation of the pathogenesis of immune complex–mediated tissue injury. The morphologic consequences are depicted as boxed areas.

fixing antibodies will induce these lesions, i.e., IgG and IgM but not IgA, IgD, or IgE. Furthermore, experimental manipulations that eliminate serum complement, such as injections of cobra venom or anticomplement antisera, inhibit these reactions. Also, if the animal's neutrophils are depleted, there might be some slight increase in permeability to proteins, but severe injury will not develop because there is a lack of the tissue-damaging effects of these cells.[17]

Systemic Immune Complex Disease

Serum sickness, acute or chronic, is a systemic disorder caused by the formation of small, soluble antigen-antibody aggregates within the circulation. In man, serum sickness is manifested by the appearance of urticaria, fever, edema, generalized lymphadenopathy, and occasionally arthritis, glomerulonephritis, and vasculitis. It occurs about eight to 12 days following the use of some therapeutic antiserum (e.g., horse tetanus antitoxin) or a drug.

The experimental model of acute serum sickness has clarified the mechanism of injury in a variety of human glomerular and connective tissue diseases.[18] To produce acute serum sickness, a rabbit is injected with a large dose of foreign protein, e.g., bovine serum albumin (Fig. 5–7). In the first week of illness the animal is asymptomatic despite the presence of free antigen in the circulation. Antibody first appears in the serum after about one week, but it quickly complexes to antigen, forming small antigen-antibody complexes in the presence of antigen excess. These deposit in the blood vessels of various tissues and can be visualized in the lesions by immunofluorescence microscopy. Between eight and 14 days thereafter, inflammatory lesions appear in the heart, blood vessels, joints, and kidney. Serum complement levels also decrease, a reflection of complement binding by the complexes. As the immune response continues, antibody excess develops, forming large immune complexes that are taken up by the mononuclear phagocyte system (MPS). At this time the lesions begin to resolve and symptoms disappear. From Figure 5–7 it is clear that the development of lesions in acute serum sickness corresponds with the appearance of small antigen-antibody complexes and is not related to free antigen or free antibody.

There are no completely satisfactory explanations for the peculiar localization of immune complexes in certain tissues in the body. Some facts, however, are pertinent.[19] The most pathogenic *complexes are those of small or intermediate size formed in antigen excess,* presumably because they circulate longer, bind less avidly to phagocytic cells, and therefore have the opportunity to localize in blood vessels, whereas larger complexes formed in antibody excess are taken up by the mononuclear phagocyte system. Since the MPS normally serves to sequester circulating immune complexes, it follows that *overload or intrinsic dysfunction of the MPS will increase the probability of tissue deposition* and immune complex–mediated injury. In order for the complexes to penetrate across the endothelium into the blood vessel wall, an increase in vascular permeability must occur. It is thought that IgE antibody induced by the antigen shortly after injection binds to circulating basophils and releases platelet activating factor (PAF). The latter induces platelets to aggregate and release their amines (serotonin and histamine) through the platelet-release reaction (p. 94). These amines then separate the endothelial cells and allow the complexes to enter the vessel wall.[20] *This is then a "miniature" Type I anaphylactic reaction, occurring transiently in Type III reactions.* The presence of C3b or Fc receptors in some normal tissues such as the glomeruli and choroid plexus may favor localization of circulating immune complexes in these tissues.[21] In the kidney, localization is influenced by the peculiar hemo-

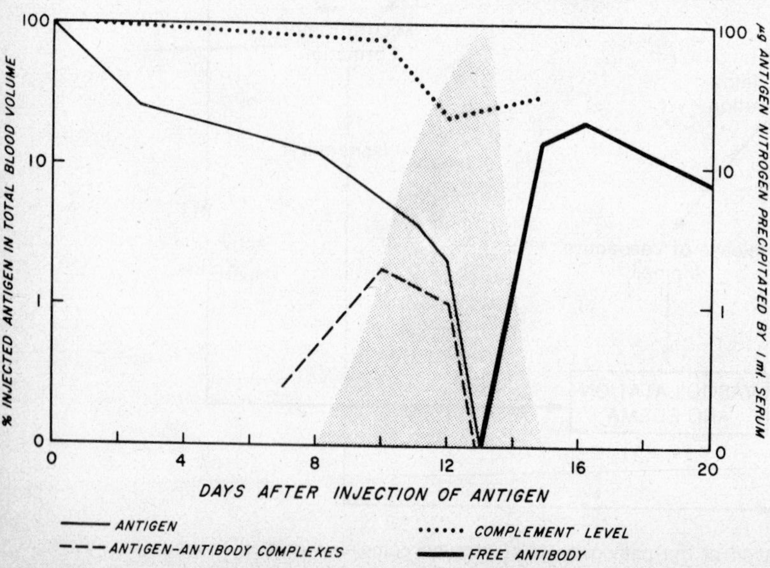

Figure 5–7. Serum levels of antigen, antibody, complexes, and complement in acute "one-shot" serum sickness nephritis. (Modified from Dixon, F. J.: Glomerulonephritis and immunopathology. Hosp. Pract. 2:35, 1967.)

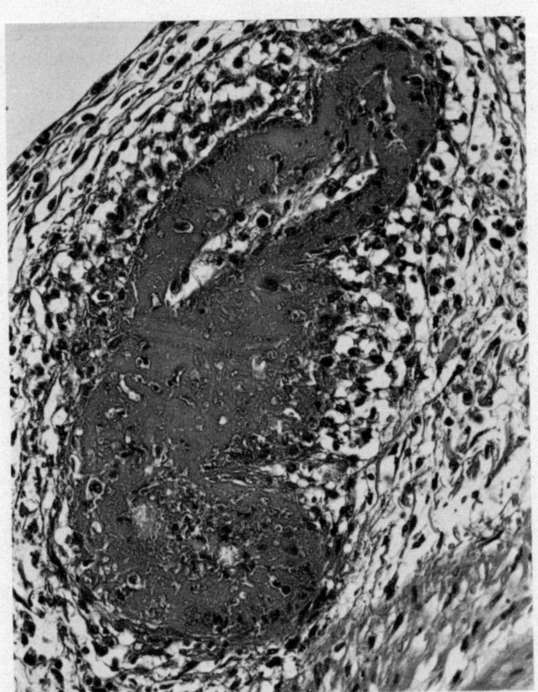

Figure 5–8. Immune complex vasculitis. Acute fibrinoid necrosis of walls of small vessels.

dynamic factors that obtain within the glomerular capillary wall, the nature of the antigen, the avidity of the antibody, and the charge of the immune reactants[21–23] as discussed on page 1003.

The vascular lesions resulting from immune complex deposition take the form of acute necrotizing vasculitis, with deposits of fibrinoid and intense neutrophilic exudation permeating the entire arterial wall, much like the changes that we shall describe in polyarteritis nodosa (Fig. 5–8). Affected glomeruli are hypercellular because of swelling and proliferation of endothelial and mesangial cells, accompanied by neutrophilic and monocytic infiltration. *The complexes can be seen on immunofluorescence microscopy as granular lumpy deposits of immunoglobulin and complement,* and on electron microscopy as electron-dense deposits along the glomerular basement membrane (Figs. 21–9 and 21–12 on pp. 1004 and 1009). The endocarditis takes the form of edema and increased vascularity of the heart valves, and the vegetations that develop over the inflamed valves have more than a passing resemblance to acute rheumatic lesions.

A chronic form of serum sickness results from repeated or prolonged exposure to an antigen. Continuous antigenemia is necessary for the development of chronic immune complex disease, since, as stated earlier, complexes in antigen excess are the ones most likely to deposit in vascular beds. Chronic immune complex disease is observed most commonly in the kidney, and the resultant lesion is called *membranous glomerulonephritis* because the complexes deposit along the glomerular basement membrane, thus resulting in thickening of this structure (p. 1012).

Local Immune Complex Disease (Arthus Reaction)

The Arthus reaction may be defined as a localized area of tissue necrosis resulting from acute immune complex vasculitis and usually elicited in the skin. The reaction can be produced experimentally by intracutaneous injection of antigen in *an immune animal having circulating antibodies against the antigen.* Because of the excess of antibodies, as the antigen diffuses into the vascular wall, large immune complexes are formed, which precipitate locally and trigger the inflammatory reaction already discussed. Unlike IgE-mediated Type I reactions, which appear immediately, the Arthus lesion develops over a few hours and reaches a peak four to ten hours after injection, when it can be seen as an area of visible edema with severe hemorrhage followed occasionally by ulceration. Immunofluorescent stains will disclose complement and immunoglobulins and fibrinogen precipitated within the vessel walls, usually the venules. On light microscopy, these produce a smudgy eosinophilic deposit that obscures the underlying cellular detail, an appearance termed *"fibrinoid" necrosis* of the vessels (Fig. 5–8). Rupture of these vessels may produce local hemorrhages, but more often the vascular lumina undergo thrombosis, adding an element of local ischemic injury.

TYPE IV HYPERSENSITIVITY (CELL-MEDIATED)

This type of hypersensitivity is initiated by specifically sensitized T lymphocytes. It includes the classic *delayed-type hypersensitivity reactions* and *cell-mediated cytotoxic reactions.* It is the principal pattern of immunologic response to a variety of intracellular microbiologic agents, particularly *M. tuberculosis,* but also to many viruses, fungi, protozoa, and parasites. So-called "contact skin sensitivity" to chemical agents and graft rejection are other instances of cell-mediated reactions.

Delayed-Type Hypersensitivity

The best known example of delayed hypersensitivity is the *tuberculin reaction,* which is performed by the intracutaneous injection of tuberculin, a protein-lipopolysaccharide component of the tubercle bacillus. In a previously sensitized individual, reddening and induration of the sites appear in eight to 12 hours, reach a peak in 24 to 72 hours, and thereafter slowly subside. An extremely sensitive patient may indeed develop necrosis at the site of injection. Morphologically the lesion is characterized by the accumulation of mononuclear cells in the subcutaneous tissue and deep and superficial dermis[24] (Fig. 5–9). There is predominant accumulation around small veins and venules, producing a characteristic perivascular "cuffing." Varying numbers of polymorphonuclear leukocytes may also be present, depending on the intensity of the reaction and the amount of necrosis. A small number of basophils are

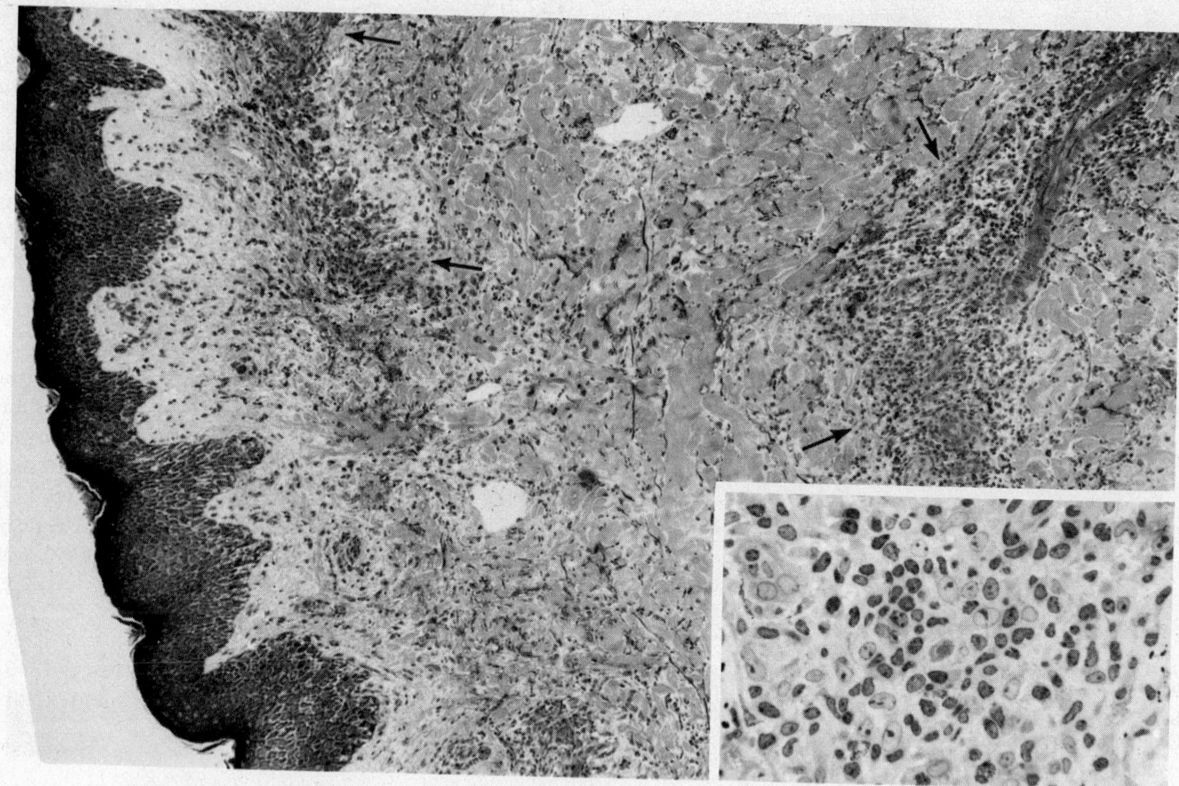

Figure 5–9. A 48-hour delayed hypersensitivity skin reaction in man elicited with tuberculin. There are superficial and deep perivascular infiltrates of mononuclear cells *(arrows)*. Note edema *(pale areas)* of superficial dermis. *Inset*: Higher-power view of mononuclear perivascular infiltrate. (From Dvorak, H.: Delayed hypersensitivity. *In* Zweifach, B. W., et al. (eds.): The Inflammatory Process. Vol. III. New York, Academic Press, 1974.)

usually present at the site of cutaneous delayed hypersensitivity reaction in man, but in certain species they may form a prominent part of the cellular reaction.[25] Increased vascular permeability is a constant feature beginning four to six hours after injection of antigen and reaching a peak by 12 to 24 hours. Fibrin deposition in the interstitium appears to be the main cause of the *induration*, which is characteristic of delayed hypersensitivity skin lesions. Such induration can be prevented by anticoagulants in experimental animals and in man.

Delayed hypersensitivity reactions are initiated by specifically sensitized T lymphocytes, generated during the initial contact with the antigen; some of the memory cells remain in the circulation for a long time, often several years. When the individual is reexposed to the specific antigen (e.g., tuberculin), memory T lymphocytes are stimulated to divide and release a variety of biologically active molecules called *lymphokines*. The function of lymphokines is to amplify the inflammatory response by recruiting inflammatory cells, activating them, and keeping them at the site. In a fully developed delayed hypersensitivity reaction, therefore, only a very small percentage of the mononuclear cell infiltrate is made up of antigen-sensitive T cells that initiated the reaction. Among the lymphokines *the most important appear to be the ones that result in the accumulation and activation of macrophages within the lesion*. Macrophages are required for the development of the prominent inflammatory reaction and tissue damage in delayed hypersensitivity reactions. The various ways by which activated macrophages induce tissue injury and continued inflammation were discussed in detail in the chapter on the inflammatory response (Chapter 2).

Lymphokines. A variety of lymphokines, detected usually by diverse functional assays, has been described.[26] However, it is not yet clear how many chemically distinct molecules are involved, nor how many of the lymphokine activities detected in vitro are relevant in vivo. Some of the important lymphokines are listed below:

1. *Macrophage migration inhibition factor (MIF)*. As its name implies, this substance inhibits the normal active migration of macrophages. MIF, like most other lymphokines that have been characterized, is of relatively low molecular weight and lacks immunologic specificity. Thus, it is not antibody-like. MIF is a glycoprotein, of about 20,000 to 40,000 molecular weight, which can be generated in vitro by interaction of immune T cells with antigen and with nonspecific polyclonal mitogens such as concanavalin A.

2. *Interferons*. Interferons were originally described for their antiviral activity, but it is now known that they represent a family of molecules that can also exert immunomodulatory effects. The interferon produced by sensitized T cells is called gamma-interferon, and it is chemically distinct from the alpha- and beta-

interferons induced by viruses. Gamma-interferon (in addition to its antiviral effect) can also activate macrophages to increased levels of metabolic activity accompanied by greater ability to kill tumor cells and ingested microbes. Until recently, this effect was ascribed to an independent lymphokine termed macrophage activating factor (MAF).[26A] Whether MAF activity also resides in molecules other than gamma-interferon is presently unknown.

3. *Chemotactic factors.* These are for neutrophils, eosinophils, basophils, monocytes, and other lymphocytes.

4. *Interleukin 2.* This substance, also called T-cell growth factor, is produced by antigen- or mitogen-activated T cells. In turn it causes proliferation of the T cells involved in mediating cellular immunity.

5. *Transfer factor.* This is an ill-defined substance (present only in humans), which has been found to transfer tuberculin sensitivity to previously unsensitized individuals.

6. *Others.* Several other lymphokines, including lymphotoxins that kill tumor cells in vitro and permeability increasing factors, have been described.

T Cell–Mediated Cytotoxicity

Cytotoxicity signifies a lethal effect on a cell, and in its most severe form leads to cell lysis, or *cytolysis.* We have seen that in Type II antibody-mediated cytotoxic reactions, circulating antibody can coat cell-surface antigens and result in either phagocytosis of the cells by macrophages or their lysis by way of the complement system. It has also been noted that antibody-dependent cytotoxicity (ADCC) can be effected by monocytes, neutrophils, eosinophils, and K cells. NK cells are known to be cytotoxic to tumor cells without previous immunization. Here we will consider yet another form of cytotoxicity in which sensitized T cells kill antigen-bearing target cells.

In response to certain antigens including virus-infected cells, tumor cells, and incompatible (allogeneic) tissue cells, the immune system responds by the generation of cytotoxic T cells (CTLs). The process of CTL generation is complex and still incompletely understood. Some aspects of this process are considered later in relation to rejection of organ transplants. We do know, however, that cytotoxic T cells and their precursors belong to a distinct subset of T cells characterized by the presence of OK T5/T8 antigens on their surface. The process of T cell–mediated lysis is initiated by the recognition of a cell-surface antigen by the corresponding receptor on the CTL. In this process, the CTL binds avidly and specifically to its target cell and then delivers a somewhat mysterious lytic signal, which leads eventually to permeability changes in the target cell membrane. Progressive damage to the target cell membrane finally leads to its rupture. The CTL itself survives the encounter and is then recycled to kill other target cells. It should be remembered that CTL-mediated cytolysis is highly specific and that adjacent ("innocent bystander") cells are not damaged. Critical to such specificity is the ability of CTLs to recognize the cells bearing the appropriate target antigens. It is now abundantly clear that cell-surface HLA antigens play an extremely important role in the process by which CTLs recognize their target cells. For example, CTL generated during a virus infection can recognize the virus-infected cell only in association with self cell-surface HLA antigens.[27] To explain this phenomenon of HLA-restricted killing it has been suggested that infection of a cell with virus leads to alterations in the cell-surface HLA antigens; the modified HLA antigens differ from normal self-HLA antigens ("altered self") and so evoke cytotoxic T cells capable of recognizing "altered self" and thereby killing the virus-infected target cells (Fig. 5–3). The lysis of virus-infected cells by CTL prior to the synthesis of new virions can lead in due course to elimination of the viral infection. Tumor antigens expressed on the cancer cells may also be viewed as modified self-antigens, thus evoking a CTL response that may contribute to immunosurveillance (p. 258).

TRANSPLANT REJECTION

Transplant rejection is discussed here because it appears to involve several of the hypersensitivity reactions discussed above. One of the goals of present-day immunologic research is successful transplantation of tissues in humans without immunologic rejection. Although the surgical expertise for the transplantation of skin, kidneys, heart, lungs, liver, spleen, bone marrow, and endocrine organs is now well in hand, it regrettably outpaces thus far our ability to confer on the recipient permanent acceptance of foreign grafts. Although advances in transplantation biology have increased our ability to achieve better matches between the tissue antigens in donors and recipients, much remains to be done. Histocompatibility, a concept necessary for an understanding of transplant rejection, was reviewed earlier (p. 160). Here we shall cover the mechanisms involved in rejection and the anatomic changes and patterns of rejection injury.

MECHANISMS INVOLVED IN REJECTION. Graft rejection depends on recognition by the host of the grafted tissue as foreign. The antigens responsible for such rejection in humans are those of the major histocompatibility antigen system (HLA). *Rejection is a very complex process in which both cell-mediated immunity and circulating antibodies play a role;* moreover, the relative contribution of these two mechanisms to rejection varies among grafts and is often reflected in the histology of the rejected organs.

T Cell–Mediated Reactions. The critical role of T cells in transplant rejection has been documented both in humans and in experimental animals. But how do T lymphocytes cause graft destruction? Both generation of CTL and delayed hypersensitivity reactions (discussed earlier) seem to be involved (p. 169). The generation of CTL and antibodies in response to allogeneic HLA

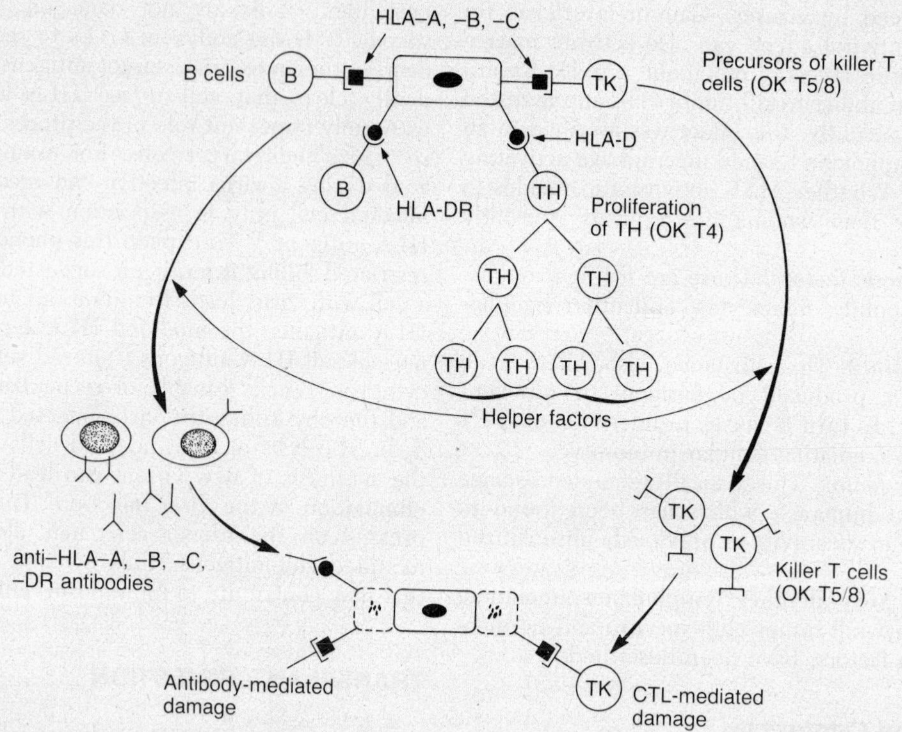

Figure 5–10. Schematic representation of the possible mechanisms and interactions involved in the immunologic destruction of a histoincompatible tissue graft. Both class I and class II antigens are represented on parenchymal cells for simplicity. TH = T-helper cells; TK = T-killer cells and their precursors.

antigens is depicted schematically in Figure 5–10. The T cell–mediated reaction is initiated when the recipient's lymphocytes encounter the donor's HLA antigens. The presentation of the foreign HLA antigens may take place within the grafted organ (as depicted) or after the shed donor antigens are carried to the regional lymph nodes. It is believed that the donor lymphoid cells ("passenger lymphocytes") and dendritic cells contained within the graft are the most important immunogens, since they are rich in both class I and class II antigens. Two distinct subsets of T cells are involved in the generation of CTL. The OK T4–positive T-helper cells (TH) are triggered into proliferation by recognition of the HLA-D specificities, in a manner similar to the mixed lymphocyte reaction in vitro (p. 161). At the same time, OK T5/8–positive precursors of CTL ("pre-killer T cells"), which bear receptors for class I antigens, differentiate into mature CTLs. The differentiation of CTLs from their precursors is greatly augmented and facilitated by soluble "helper factors" secreted by the proliferating T-helper cells. The mature CTLs so generated are specifically directed against the donor's class I HLA antigens and can therefore lyse virtually any nucleated cell within the graft. In addition to the specific cytotoxic T cells, sensitization also leads to the generation of OK T4–positive, lymphokine-secreting T cells, which in turn recruit macrophages as well as other lymphocytes (not shown in Fig. 5–10). This scheme of events has been pieced together mostly from experimental studies in vitro and is supported by recent observations in humans. In one study, T4- and T5/T8-positive T lymphocytes could be identified in rejected skin transplants by the use of monoclonal antibodies and immunoperoxidase techniques.[28] However, it is still not clear which of the two mechanisms, cytotoxicity by OK T5/8 CTL or the inflammatory response (delayed hypersensitivity) induced by OK T4–positive cells, is more important in vivo. Furthermore, whether the primary targets of CTL in vivo are parenchymal cells or blood vessels is also debatable. Although it is generally assumed that direct parenchymal cell destruction by CTLs is the major cause of organ failure, some studies suggest that, at least in the case of skin grafts, ischemia resulting from vascular damage may precede direct lysis of the parenchymal cells.[29]

Antibody-Mediated Reactions. Earlier studies suggested no role for humoral antibody, since transplantation immunity could not be transferred by serum. It is now thought, however, that humoral responses are important in at least two types of rejection in human kidney transplant recipients:

(1) *Preformed circulating antibodies* occur in transplant recipients who have encountered the foreign antigen *before transplantation.* This may occur as a result of presensitization of a recipient by blood transfusions, previous pregnancies, or infections with HLA cross-reacting bacterial or virus-surface antigens. In this circumstance, rejection occurs almost immediately after transplantation owing to the fixation of circulating anti-donor antibody to the vascular bed of the graft. The

antigenic components of endothelial cells are the initial point of contact of the host immune recognition and effector mechanisms. The resulting reaction is termed "hyperacute rejection." The antidonor antibodies responsible for hyperacute rejection may be directed against HLA or blood-group antigens. Recent evidence suggests that certain non-HLA antigens present only on endothelial cells, and monocytes may also be relevant.

(2) In recipients not previously sensitized to transplantation antigens, exposure to the class I and class II HLA antigens of the donor may evoke antibodies, as depicted in Figure 5–10. The antibodies formed by the recipient may cause injury by several mechanisms including complement-dependent cytotoxicity, antibody-dependent cell-mediated cytolysis, and the deposition of antigen-antibody complexes. *The initial target of these antibodies in rejection appears to be the graft vasculature.* Thus, antibody-dependent rejection phenomena in the kidney are reflected histologically by a vasculitis, sometimes referred to as "rejection vasculitis." The interaction of specific antibody with antigen initiates complement-dependent tissue injury and triggers other mediators of inflammation, namely, platelet aggregation and release and neutrophil lysosomal leakage as well as coagulation, fibrinolysis, and activation of the kinin cascade (p. 53).[30, 31]

MORPHOLOGY OF REJECTION REACTIONS. In the past, two morphologic patterns of rejection were recognized, based on the intensity of the reaction. First-set rejection applied to the initial rejection of a skin allograft, while second-set rejection designated a rejection of a second skin allograft from the same donor to the same recipient. Since it is now appreciated that a potential recipient can become sensitized by other pathways, such as pregnancy, this older terminology has been replaced by the terms "hyperacute, acute, and chronic rejection."[31] *The morphologic changes in these patterns will be described as they relate to renal transplants.* Similar changes are encountered in any other vascularized organ transplant.

Hyperacute Rejection. This form of rejection is due to the presence in the recipient of **preformed** circulating antibodies directed against donor-specific antigens. It usually occurs within minutes after transplantation and can be recognized by the surgeon just after the graft vasculature is anastomosed to the recipient's. In contrast to the nonrejecting kidney graft, which rapidly regains a normal pink coloration and normal tissue turgor and promptly excretes urine, a hyperacutely rejecting kidney rapidly becomes cyanotic, mottled, and flaccid and may excrete a mere few drops of bloody urine. In some cases, the process occurs more slowly over a period of hours or one to two days. This variation in onset appears to relate directly to the recipient's titer of circulating cytotoxic complement-dependent antibody. The histologic lesions are characteristic of the classic Arthus reaction. In the first hour, increased numbers of neutrophils are present on the arteriolar endothelium and within the glomerular and peritubular capillaries. Immunoglobulin and complement deposit in the vessel wall, and electron microscopy will disclose early endothelial injury together with fibrin-platelet thrombi. **These early lesions point to an antigen-antibody reaction at the level of vascular endothelium.** Subsequently these changes become diffuse and intense, the glomeruli undergo thrombotic occlusion of the capillaries, and fibrinoid necrosis occurs in arterial walls (Fig. 5–11). The kidney cortex then undergoes outright infarction necrosis, and such nonfunctioning kidneys are eventually removed. Fortunately, cross-matching of the donor's lymphocytes with the recipients' serum prior to transplantation has diminished the incidence of this dramatic complication.

Acute Rejection. This may occur within days of transplantation in the untreated recipient or may appear suddenly months or even years later, when immunosuppression has been employed and terminated. As suggested earlier, acute graft rejection is a combined process in which both cellular and humoral tissue injury play parts. In any one patient, one or the other mechanism may predominate. Histologically, humoral rejection is associated with vasculitis, whereas cellular rejection is marked by an interstitial mononuclear cell infiltrate.

Acute cellular rejection is most commonly seen within the initial months after transplantation and is often accompanied by the abrupt onset of clinical signs of renal failure. Histologically, there may be extensive interstitial mononu-

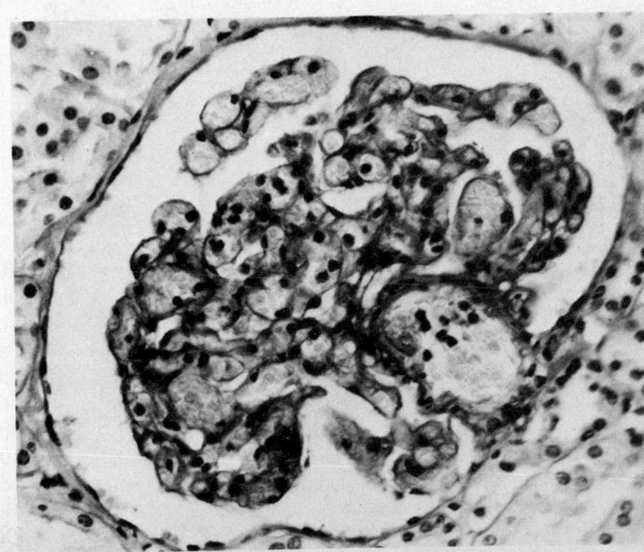

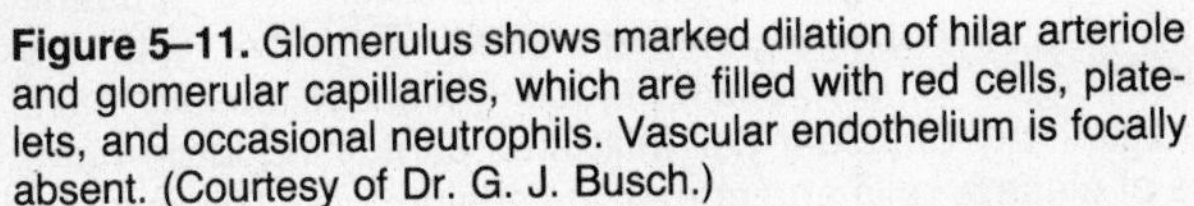

Figure 5–11. Glomerulus shows marked dilation of hilar arteriole and glomerular capillaries, which are filled with red cells, platelets, and occasional neutrophils. Vascular endothelium is focally absent. (Courtesy of Dr. G. J. Busch.)

clear cell infiltration and edema, as well as mild interstitial hemorrhage (Fig. 5–12). In man, the mononuclear cell infiltrate consists primarily of medium-sized and small lymphocytes along with some large "transformed" lymphocytes, which have abundant basophilic cytoplasm and a vesicular nucleus. Some plasma cells can also be identified, especially in long-standing cases. Glomerular and peritubular capillaries contain large numbers of mononuclear cells that may also invade the tubules, causing focal tubular necrosis. The recognition of cellular rejection is important since, in the absence of an accompanying arteritis, patients respond promptly to immunosuppressive therapy.

Acute rejection vasculitis (humoral rejection) is seen most commonly in the first few months after transplantation or when immunosuppressive therapy is discontinued. Such patients show immediate and persistent poor function of the graft and do not respond to high-dose immunosuppressive therapy. The histologic lesions consist of necrotizing vasculitis with endothelial necrosis; neutrophilic infiltration; deposition of immunoglobulins, complement, and fibrin; and thrombosis. The process may evolve to extensive glomerular necrosis and cortical arteriolar thrombosis, with resulting cortical infarction. Almost all these patients will also have evidence of acute cellular rejection. More common than this acute type of vasculitis is so-called **subacute vasculitis**, which is also seen in greatest intensity during the first months after transplantation. Clinically, patients with subacute vasculitis have a course punctuated by repeated episodes of clinical rejection with altered renal function. The arterial lesions are rather characteristic. **The major alterations are in the intima,** which is markedly thickened by a cushion of proliferating fibroblasts, myocytes, and foamy macrophages, often leading to luminal narrowing or obliteration. The thickened intima may be infiltrated by scattered neutrophils and mononuclear cells, and the walls of most of these arteries show deposits of immunoglobulin and complement.

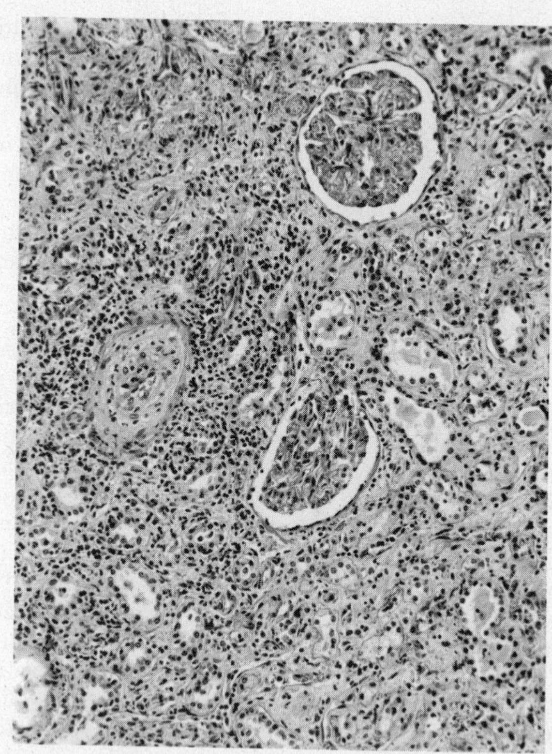

Figure 5–13. Chronic transplant rejection of kidney. There is marked tubular atrophy, increased interstitial fibrosis, and mononuclear cell infiltration. The vessel at left center has a markedly thickened wall with virtual obliteration of the lumen. The glomeruli show some ischemic axial thickening.

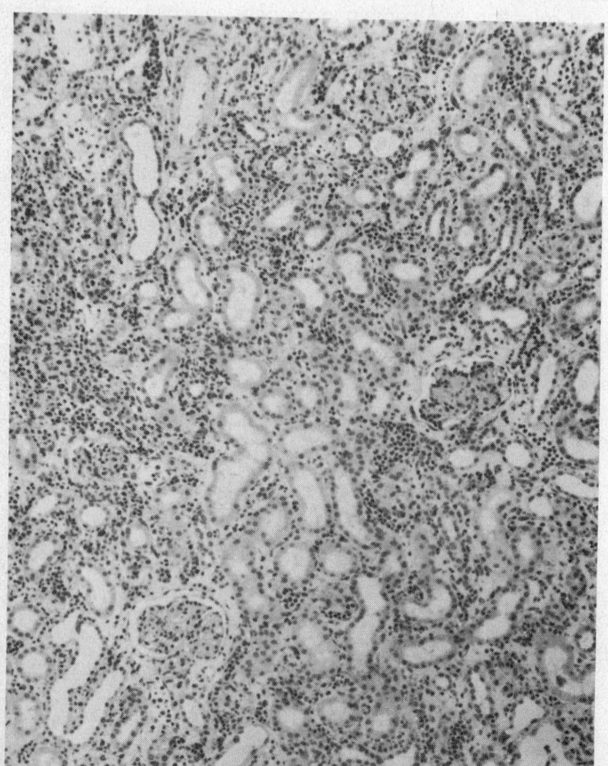

Figure 5–12. Acute cellular rejection of a renal allograft manifested by a diffuse interstitial mononuclear cell infiltrate and interstitial edema with separation of tubules. (Courtesy of Dr. G. J. Busch.)

Chronic Rejection. Since most instances of acute graft rejection are more or less controlled by immunosuppressive therapy, chronic changes are commonly seen in the renal allograft (Fig. 5–13). Patients with chronic rejection present clinically with a progressive rise in serum creatinine (an index of renal dysfunction) over a period of four to six months. **The vascular changes** consist of dense intimal fibrosis, principally in the cortical arteries, the lesion probably being the end stage of the proliferative arteritis described in acute and subacute stages. These vascular lesions result in renal ischemia manifested by glomerular ischemic simplification and obsolescence, interstitial fibrosis and tubular atrophy, and shrinkage of the renal parenchyma. The decline in renal function is proportional to the degree of interstitial fibrosis and tubular atrophy. An acute arteritis may sometimes be superimposed on the chronic lesions, and in these instances immunoglobulin and complement are present, suggesting a humoral rejection crisis. Together with the vascular lesions, chronically rejecting kidneys usually have interstitial mononuclear cell infiltrates containing large numbers of plasma cells and numerous eosinophils. This is taken as an indication of chronic cell-mediated rejection, but in truth it must be said that differentiation of the pathogenetic mechanisms in chronic graft rejection is much more difficult than it is in the acute forms and is further complicated by the contribution of ischemic damage to progressive renal dysfunction.

The glomeruli in chronic graft rejection show no consistent pattern of injury. They may be entirely normal in appearance, or may show ischemic changes, while some may show extensive widening of the subendothelial spaces by deposits of amorphous, relatively electron-lucent material, believed to represent, in part, degradation products of fibrin.[32–34] In some patients these late glomerular changes may be difficult to distinguish from recurrent glomerular disease.

METHODS OF INCREASING GRAFT SURVIVAL

1. Since HLA antigens are the major targets in transplant rejection, minimization of the HLA disparity between the donor and recipient would be expected to influence graft survival. Historically, attempts at reducing donor-host histoincompatibility have involved matching for class I antigens, since serologic typing for class II antigens has not been widely available. Indeed, in the case of intrafamilial (related donor) kidney transplants, a markedly beneficial effect of matching for class I antigens has been observed. For example, HLA-identical sibling transplants have survival rates of about 90% at three years, whereas the graft survival is reduced to 75% if the donor and recipient share only one haplotype. These strikingly beneficial effects of matching are not seen in the case of cadaver renal transplants. Thus, there is only 10 to 15% better graft survival when donor and recipient are matched fully for class I antigens (HLA-A and -B) as compared with totally unmatched combinations. The reasons for this disparity between matched intrafamilial and cadaveric renal grafts can best be explained in terms of the role of HLA-D/DR (class II) antigens in graft rejection. Within families, matching at the HLA-A and -B loci usually ensures matching at the closely linked HLA-D/DR locus, whereas this is much less likely when the donor and recipient are unrelated. This implies, then, that *matching at the -D/DR locus may be crucial to graft survival.* Preliminary data obtained from several centers support this view.[35] With a combination of D/DR matching and compatibility for class I antigens, an 80 to 85% two-year survival of cadaver renal transplants is being obtained.

2. Except in the case of identical twins, who are obviously matched for all possible histocompatibility antigens, *immunosuppressive therapy* is a practical necessity in all other donor-recipient combinations. Even HLA-identical siblings may differ at several minor histocompatibility loci, which can evoke slow rejection. At present, drugs such as azathioprine, steroids, and Cyclosporin are commonly employed. Antilymphocyte globulin (ALG) is also utilized in some cases. Trials with monoclonal antibodies to defined T-cell subsets are also under way. Although immunosuppression has produced significant gains in terms of graft survival, it should be remembered that immunosuppressive therapy is like the proverbial double-edged sword. The price paid in the form of increased susceptibility to opportunistic fungal, viral, and other infections is not small.

3. Paradoxical as it may seem, *previous blood transfusions* have been definitely proved to be of benefit in allowing greater survival of the transplanted kidneys, especially in cadaver renal transplants.[36] Although blood transfusions do carry the definite risk of presensitization, such risk is small, contrary to earlier expectations. The exact mechanisms underlying this peculiar observation are unknown, but several possibilities have been suggested; these include a nonspecific decrease in cell-mediated immunity, activation of suppressor cells, impairment of the mononuclear phagocyte system, and formation of "blocking" antibodies.[37] This continues to be an area of active research.

Finally, the goal of transplantation immunologists is to create a donor-specific transplantation tolerance, so as to avoid graft rejection even in the absence of perfect HLA-matching and without the dreadful effects of nonspecific immunosuppression. Although several experimental models are currently being tested, the goal remains elusive.

TRANSPLANTATION OF HEMATOPOIETIC CELLS. Mention should be made of the special features of transplantation of bone marrow. Use of this form of therapy for hematologic malignancies, aplastic anemias, and certain immune deficiency states is increasing. In most of the conditions in which bone marrow transplantation is indicated, the recipient is lethally irradiated either to destroy the malignant cells (e.g., leukemias) or to create a graft bed (aplastic anemias). Two major problems arise in bone marrow transplantation: graft-versus-host disease (GVH) and rejection of the transplant. *Graft-versus-host disease* occurs in any situation in which immunologically competent cells or their precursors are transplanted into immunologically crippled recipients. Recipients of bone marrow transplants are immunodeficient because of either primary disease or prior treatment of the disease with drugs or irradiation. When such recipients receive normal bone marrow cells from allogeneic donors, the immunocompetent T cells derived from the donor marrow recognize the recipient's tissue as "foreign" and react against them. The relevant antigens, as might be expected, belong to the HLA complex. Antirecipient CTL as well as lymphokine-producing T cells are generated. Although any organ may be affected, the predominant clinical manifestations of GVH relate to the involvement of skin, liver, and intestinal mucosa. GVH disease and its attending complications, mainly infections, are often lethal; better matching of the donor and recipients at the HLA locus reduces the possibility of a GVH reaction. Another approach, which has been quite successful in mice, is to remove all the mature T cells from the donor bone marrow prior to transplantation. This can be achieved by pretreating the bone marrow cells with anti–T cell antibodies and complement. A similar procedure is now being tested in humans.[38]

Even in those cases in which GVH disease is mild, there remains the problem of rejection of the grafted marrow. What effector system can reject the donor marrow cells in the recipients whose immune responses have been suppressed by lethal irradiation? The answer comes from experiments in mice in which it has been demonstrated that the cells that reject bone marrow transplants are resistant to acute lethal irradiation, and are distinct from T or B cells or macrophages. In mice, these cells resemble natural killer cells.[39] In humans, however, the mechanism of bone marrow graft rejection is still poorly understood, and the participation of NK cells is unproven.

AUTOIMMUNE DISEASES

The evidence is now compelling that an immune reaction against "self-antigens"—autoimmunity—is the cause of certain diseases in humans.[40] This concept is not new and dates back to at least 1904, when Donath and Landsteiner[41] described a complement-dependent autohemolytic serum antibody. Since then, a growing number of diseases have been attributed to autoimmunity (Table 5–4),[42] but it must be confessed that in many the evidence is not firm. This is because autoantibodies can be found in the serum or tissues of a remarkably large number of apparently normal individuals, particularly in older age groups.[43] Apparently innocuous autoantibodies are also formed following damage to tissue and, according to some, these serve a physiologic role as carriers of tissue breakdown products.[44] Furthermore, recent investigations of cellular interactions involved in the normal immune response indicate that recognition of self-histocompatibility antigens is required for normal cell-to-cell interactions (p. 162). These observations indicate that some forms of autorecognition are normal and physiologic. How then does one define "pathologic" autoimmunity?

Ideally, at least three requirements should be met before a disorder can be categorized as truly due to autoimmunity: (1) the presence of an autoimmune reaction, (2) clinical or experimental evidence that such a reaction is *not secondary* to tissue damage but is of primary pathogenetic significance, and (3) the absence of another well-defined cause of the disease. Unfortunately, these requirements are met in only a few diseases such as systemic lupus erythematosus (SLE) and autoimmune blood dyscrasias. Most others remain in the category of probable autoimmune disorders until definitive evidence is obtained (Table 5–4).

The autoimmune disorders form a spectrum on one end of which are conditions in which autoantibodies are directed against a single organ or tissue, therefore resulting in localized tissue damage. A classic example is Hashimoto's thyroiditis, in which the antibodies have absolute specificity for thyroid constituents. At the other end of the spectrum is SLE in which a diversity of antibodies result in widespread lesions throughout the body. In SLE, autoantibodies react with nuclear constituents of virtually every cell within the organism. In the middle of the spectrum falls Goodpasture's syndrome, in which antibodies to basement membranes of lung and kidney induce lesions and symptoms in these organs. It is obvious that autoimmunity implies loss of self-tolerance, and the question arises as to how this happens. Before we look for answers to this question, we should review the mechanisms of immunologic tolerance and self-tolerance.[45]

IMMUNOLOGIC TOLERANCE

Immunologic tolerance is a state in which the individual is incapable of developing an immune response to a specific antigen. Self-tolerance refers to lack

Table 5–4. PROBABLE AUTOIMMUNE DISEASES

Disorder	Probable Antigen(s)
Systemic	
Systemic lupus erythematosus	Numerous nuclear and cellular components
Rheumatoid arthritis	IgG
Dermatomyositis	Nuclear antigens; myosin (?)
Scleroderma	Nuclear antigens; IgG
Sjögren's syndrome	Salivary gland; thyroid; nuclear antigens; IgG
Mixed connective tissue disease	Ribonucleoprotein
Blood	
Autoimmune hemolytic anemia	Erythrocyte antigens
Idiopathic thrombocytopenic purpura	Platelet surface antigens
Neutropenia and lymphopenia	Leukocyte surface antigens
Other Organs	
Hashimoto's thyroiditis	Thyroglobulin and microsomal antigens
Thyrotoxicosis	Cell-surface TSH receptors
Goodpasture's syndrome	Kidney and lung basement membranes
Pernicious anemia	Parietal cell antigens; intrinsic factor
Myasthenia gravis	Acetylcholine receptors
Primary biliary cirrhosis	Mitochondria; bile duct cells
Chronic active hepatitis	Liver cells, virally infected
Ulcerative colitis	Colonic mucosal cells
Autoimmune adrenalitis	Adrenal cells
Insulin-dependent diabetes (type I)	Islet cell antigens
Pemphigus vulgaris	Intercellular substance of mucosa and skin
Sympathetic ophthalmia	Uvea
Temporal arteritis	Blood vessel antigens
Acute idiopathic polyneuritis	Peripheral nerve myelin
Insulin-resistant diabetes	Insulin receptors

of responsiveness to an individual's antigens, and obviously underlies our ability to live in harmony with our own cells and tissues. It is important to note that tolerance obeys the same laws of antigen specificity that characterize other immune responses, and thus is restricted to the antigens used to induce tolerance. The initial observation on tolerance underlined the importance of *maturity* of the immune system in acquisition of self-tolerance. Owen found in 1945 that if dizygotic calf twins shared the same placental circulation, they also shared red cells and were tolerant later in life of each other's red cells and tissue cells.[46] If, however, they did not share the same circulation, red cells from one twin injected into the other during adult life induced a strong immunologic reaction. Owen correctly concluded that foreign antigens introduced into a host during neonatal life before maturation of the immune apparatus would induce life-long tolerance of these antigens. Thus, if the lymphoid tissues are exposed to foreign cells around the perinatal period, they will treat these as "self-components" later in life.

Later studies showed that adult animals can be rendered tolerant when the antigen is administered in certain forms or doses. A molecular configuration not conducive to easy phagocytosis favors tolerance over immunity; for example, monomeric (nonaggregated) bovine gamma globulin (BGG) is tolerogenic in mice, whereas aggregated BGG is strongly immunogenic. *Antigen dose* is also important in tolerance induction. Mice pretreated with repeated small doses of bovine serum albumin (BSA) (1 μg) or very large doses (1000 μg) and then challenged with a highly antigenic form of BSA fail to produce anti-BSA antibody. Those pretreated with intermediate doses produce a good secondary response.[47] Thus, tolerance is produced both at very low antigen dosage (*low-zone tolerance*) and at very high antigen dosage (*high-zone tolerance*).

Several mechanisms, albeit not well understood, have been postulated to explain the tolerant state. Two of these are worth consideration:

CLONAL DELETION. According to this concept initially developed by Burnet, immature clones of lymphocytes that bear receptors for self-antigens are eliminated (deleted) from the lymphoid system during development. This seemed to be a reasonable explanation for the observations made by Owen on dizygotic calf twins (see above) and was also supported by the Nobel prize–winning experiments of Medawar in which mice exposed to foreign histocompatibility antigens in utero became tolerant to them in adult life. According to this hypothesis autoimmune diseases are thought to result from the emergence of "forbidden clones" of lymphocytes reactive against self-antigens, probably owing to somatic mutations. Although this theory has gone a long way to increase our understanding of immunology, it cannot account for all the known facts regarding tolerance. *The strongest evidence against the clonal deletion hypothesis is the presence of lymphocytes in normal human beings and animals that bear surface receptors for autoantigens.* This finding is not compatible with the deletion of autoreactive clones during development. To resolve this dilemma, some investigators have presented a modified version of the clonal deletion hypothesis. It is suggested that during development the immature B cells go through a phase during which contact with an antigen leads to functional paralysis without physical deletion.[48] According to this concept, described as "clonal anergy," autoreactive lymphoid cells continue to exist and express receptors for self-antigens but cannot be triggered to form antibody. Whether or not clonal anergy operates in vivo to maintain self-tolerance, there is little doubt that in vitro immature B cells are far more sensitive to tolerogenic signals than adult B cells.

SUPPRESSION OF AUTOREACTIVE LYMPHOCYTES. Although some form of clonal deletion or anergy may indeed contribute to maintenance of self-tolerance, several lines of evidence suggest that additional "fail-safe" mechanisms must also be involved. A most compelling argument derives from the ease with which autoantibodies can be formed in humans during a number of infectious processes in vivo and by stimulation of B cells in vitro. In several experimental models, autoimmune disorders can be readily induced by immunization with autoantigens. It seems highly unlikely that infectious agents and immunization protocols can readily trigger immunocompetent autoreactive cells if they do not already exist in vivo. These observations can most readily be explained if one assumes that functionally competent autoreactive cells are normally present and that self-tolerance is maintained by mechanisms that actively suppress immune responses against self. Notice that this concept differs from clonal anergy in that the autoreactive cells are believed to be intrinsically capable of responding *unless* restrained by suppressor mechanisms. Several such suppressor mechanisms have been proposed:

Suppressor Cells. T cells capable of suppressing the response of T-helper cells and B cells are generated during the course of immune response to a variety of heterologous antigens. It is believed that T-suppressor cells are part of the normal regulatory circuits, which control the magnitude and the duration of an immune response.[49] It has also been suggested that one of the physiologic functions of T-suppressor cells may be to prevent autoimmune reactions.[50] Loss of suppressor cells might then lead to immune reactions against "self." The association between loss of T-suppressor cells and the emergence of autoimmunity in some human autoimmune diseases (p. 183) and in experimental models supports this concept of self-tolerance.

Suppressive Factors in Serum. In many experimental models, immune complexes formed in antibody excess can suppress an ongoing immune response.[45] Several mechanisms have been suggested including: (1) masking of the antigen by excess antibody, thus preventing further interaction with antigen receptor–bearing lymphocytes; (2) binding of the immune complexes to T-suppressor cells that bear an IgG Fc receptor, thus activating the suppressor T-cell circuit; and (3) blocking the activity of cytolytic T cells by binding of the circulating antigen-antibody complex to the antigen receptor on the T-cell surface. In addition to immune complexes, humoral antibodies directed against the antigen-combining site of the T-cell receptor (*anti-idiotypic antibodies*), could combine with, and thereby block, the antigen receptor of autoreactive lymphocytes. Some or all of these mechanisms not only could be involved in restraining immune response against self, but also might contribute to the failure of immune surveillance against tumor cells.

In closing this discussion it should be pointed out that the concepts of clonal deletion and peripheral suppression should not be viewed as mutually exclusive. Prevention of autoreactivity is such an important "goal" for the body that it is likely to involve a series of mechanisms. According to one view, clonal anergy may be the major mechanism of self-tolerance in the neonatal state. However, since approximately 10^{11} new lymphocytes (some potentially autoreactive) are generated every day during adult life, it is conceivable that at least some of the autoreactive lymphocytes may "leak" through the barrier exerted by clonal anergy. These would then have to be restrained by the suppressor influences. Self-tolerance is so vital that it would not be surprising if there were several lines of defense to maintain it.[51]

Cellular Basis of Tolerance. To understand the cellular basis of tolerance, one must recall that the antibody response against several antigens requires the cooperation of T-helper cells with antibody-secreting B cells. In this process the T-helper cells recognize the carrier determinants, whereas the B cells recognize the haptenic determinants and form antihapten antibodies (Fig. 5–14). It follows then that, regardless of the mechanism (i.e., clonal anergy or suppressor influences), tolerance can be maintained if either the T-helper cells or B cells (or both) are rendered inactive. Indeed, experiments performed by Weigle indicate that both T-helper cells and B cells can be rendered tolerant under appropriate conditions.[52] T and B cells differ with respect to the dosage of antigen required to induce tolerance and the escape from the tolerant state. In general, T-helper cells are easily rendered tolerant with small doses of the antigen (low-zone tolerance) and the tolerance is long-lasting. On the other hand, B-cell tolerance requires exposure to larger amounts of antigen and is relatively short-lived. In the case of self-tolerance it is proposed that the inability to respond results from T-cell tolerance, whereas B cells are fully competent. It follows, therefore, that if the nontolerant B cells could be activated, autoimmunity might result. This and other mechanisms of autoimmune diseases will be discussed next.

MECHANISMS OF AUTOIMMUNE DISEASES

Although it would be attractive to explain all autoimmune diseases by a single mechanism, it is now clear that there are a number of ways by which tolerance can be bypassed, thus terminating a previously unresponsive state to autoantigens. More than one defect

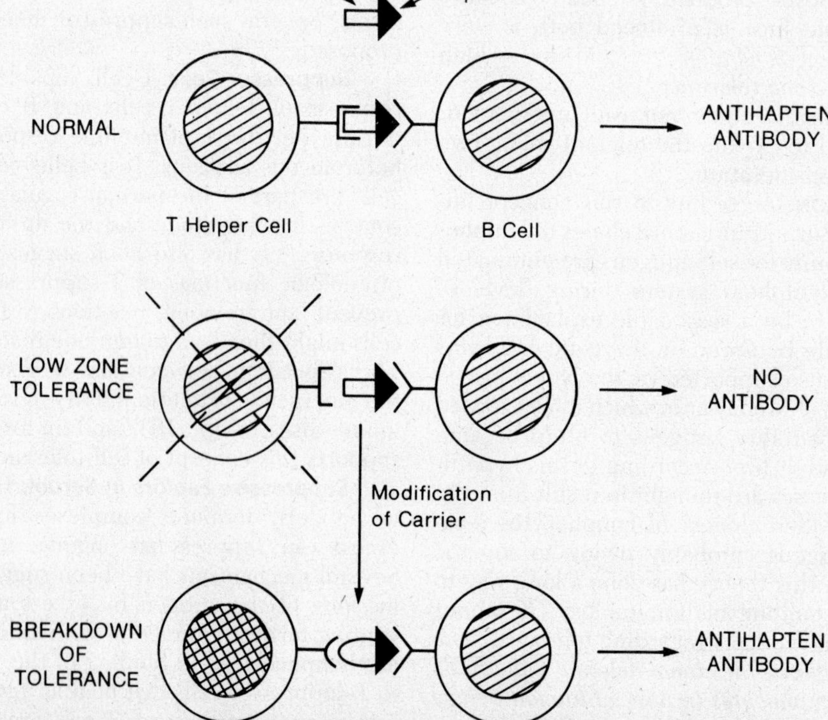

Figure 5–14. Low-zone tolerance and its breakdown by modification of the native carrier determinant. The altered carrier is recognized by nontolerant T-helper cells.

might be present in each disease, and the defects will vary from one disorder to the other. Further, *the pathogenesis of autoimmunity appears to involve immunologic, genetic, and viral factors* interacting through complicated mechanisms that are poorly understood. Here we can only scratch the surface of the rapidly evolving area of investigation into the mechanisms of autoimmunity. We will first discuss the initiating immunologic mechanisms and then briefly review the role of genetic and viral factors.

The *initiating mechanisms* in autoimmunity can best be understood in terms of those discussed for tolerance. Three general mechanisms for loss of self-tolerance have been postulated:

Bypass of T-helper Cell (Low-Zone) Tolerance. It can be deduced from our discussion of low-zone tolerance that it may be broken if T-cell tolerance for the carrier is lost or bypassed (Fig. 5–14). Bypass can be accomplished experimentally in several ways, some of which may have relevance to human autoimmunity.

1. *Modification of the molecule.* If a potentially autoantigenic determinant (hapten) is complexed to a new carrier, the carrier part of the complex may be recognized by nontolerant T cells as foreign. The latter would then cooperate with hapten-specific B cells, leading to the production of autoantibodies. This modification of the molecule could arise in several ways:
   a. *Complexing of Self-Antigens With Drugs or Microorganisms.* Autoimmune hemolytic anemia associated with drugs (e.g., antihypertensive agent alpha-methyldopa) may be due to an alteration of the red cell surface, thus providing a new carrier for an Rh antigen-hapten that stimulates B cells.
   b. *Partial Degradation of Autoantigen.* This could expose new antigenic determinants. Thus, partially degraded collagen and enzymatically altered thyroglobulin or gamma globulin are more immunogenic than the native species. The autoantibodies to gamma globulin (rheumatoid factor) induced during some bacterial, viral, and parasitic infections may well be due to alterations of gamma globulin by either the microorganisms or lysosomal hydrolases.
2. *Cross reactions.* Several infectious agents cross-react with human tissues through their haptenic determinants. The infecting microorganisms may trigger an antibody response by presenting the cross-reacting haptenic determinant in association with their own carrier to which the T-helper cells are not tolerant. The antibody so formed may then damage the tissue that shares the cross-reacting determinants. There is evidence that rheumatic heart disease sometimes follows streptococcal infection because an antibody to streptococcal M protein cross-reacts with the M protein in the sarcolemma of cardiac muscle.
3. *Polyclonal B-cell activation.* Another mechanism by which the T-cell tolerance may be bypassed is through the direct activation of autoreactive B cells. Several microorganisms and their products are capable of causing polyclonal (i.e., antigen nonspecific) activation of B cells.[53] The best investigated among these is bacterial lipopolysaccharide (endotoxin), which can induce mouse lymphocytes to form anti-DNA, antithymocyte, and anti–red cell antibodies in vitro. Epstein-Barr virus (EBV) is another potent stimulator of B cells and is suspected to be associated with rheumatoid arthritis, as we shall discuss elsewhere (p. 1351). It should be pointed out that the B-cell activation observed in human and animal models of autoimmune diseases could also result from genetically determined, intrinsic B-cell abnormalities or loss of T-suppressor cell influence. These are discussed below.

Loss of T-suppressor Function. It may be expected from our discussion of T-suppressor cells that any loss of suppressor T-cell function will contribute to autoimmunity. Experimental evidence, indeed, suggests that this is true. For example, following early thymectomy, which depletes T cells, leghorn chickens develop a more severe form of autoimmune thyroiditis than would occur spontaneously. There is also evidence for an age-associated loss of T-suppressor cells in the NZB/NZW (F1) mice, which develop an autoimmune disease similar to SLE as they age. Defects in T-suppressor cell function and/or numbers have also been reported in human SLE and several organ-specific autoimmune disorders.[54, 55] However, as we shall discuss later (p. 183), it is not yet resolved whether the abnormalities of T-suppressor cells are critical in the initiation or maintenance of autoimmunity.

Emergence of a Sequestered Antigen. Regardless of the exact mechanism by which self-tolerance is achieved (clonal deletion or suppressive influences), it is clear that induction of tolerance requires interaction between the antigen and the immune system. It follows, then, that any self-antigen that is completely sequestered is likely to be viewed as foreign if introduced into the circulation, and an immune response will follow. Spermatozoa, myelin basic protein, and lens crystallin may fall into this category of sequestered antigens. Indeed, trauma to the testes involving the release of sperm into the tissues is followed by the appearance of antibodies to spermatozoa.[56] Injection of the basic protein of myelin into rats results in so-called allergic encephalomyelitis. Seductive as this theory may be, it is probably not a major mechanism of autoimmune reactions in humans and is applicable only to the special situations cited above.

Several other immunologic abnormalities, including thymic defects and defects in macrophages, have also been implicated in loss of self-tolerance. For a discussion of these, the reader is referred to a recent review.[45]

GENETIC FACTORS IN AUTOIMMUNITY. There is compelling evidence, both in laboratory animals and in humans, that genetic factors determine the incidence and the nature of autoimmune diseases.[57] A familial increased incidence of several autoimmune diseases, such as SLE, Hashimoto's thyroiditis, and pernicious anemia, has been noted, and it is strongly suspected that at least some of the genes conferring susceptibility (or resistance) to autoimmune diseases are located within the HLA complex. Many autoimmune disorders show associations with HLA antigens, in particular those coded by the -D/DR locus (p. 162). You may recall that this locus is homologous to the murine I region where several immune response (Ir) genes have been mapped. Indeed, one mechanism of the association may be that certain HLA-linked Ir genes regulate the magnitude of the autoantibody response. In mice, immune responses to a variety of autoantigens such as thyroglobulin, insulin, collagen, and myelin basic protein are regulated by Ir genes. Since the HLA genes are involved in the regulation of lymphocyte interactions (p. 162), it is also conceivable that their effects are manifested through aberrant immunoregulation (e.g., T-suppressor cell function).

Viruses in Autoimmunity. Evidence for viral involvement in autoimmune diseases comes principally from study of the spontaneous autoimmune disease of NZB mice. Additional evidence, however, derives from studies on virally induced experimental demyelinating diseases of the nervous system (e.g., Marek's disease of chickens), which bear a strong resemblance to human neurologic disorders such as postinfectious encephalomyelitis.[58]

Viruses theoretically may trigger autoimmune reactions in several ways. First, viral antigens and autoantigens may become associated to form immunogenic units and bypass T-cell tolerance, as described earlier (p. 179). Second, some viruses (such as EBV) are nonspecific, polyclonal B-cell mitogens and may thus induce formation of autoantibodies. Third, viral infection may result in loss of suppressor T-cell function by mechanisms that at present are not entirely clear. To present the other side of the coin, there are those who believe that the presence of viruses in autoimmune diseases is merely another *consequence* of the genetic defects in immune regulation rather than the cause of autoimmunity.[59] (See also p. 182.)

It must be obvious that there is no dearth of speculation about the origins of autoimmunity and that all theories are built on fragmentary observations held together by gossamer threads. However, it is likely that the tremendous advances now being made in basic immunology will soon separate fact from fancy.

Mechanisms of Tissue Damage in Autoimmune Diseases. Theoretically, autoimmune tissue injury could be mediated by antibodies or by T cell–mediated reactions. However, at present there is much better evidence for the participation of antibodies in autoimmune tissue injury. This may relate in part to the relative ease with which antibodies can be detected. Both Types II and III hypersensitivity mechanisms have been implicated. For example, opsonization and phagocytosis of red blood cells seems to be the principal mechanism of red cell destruction in autoimmune hemolytic anemia (p. 628). On the other hand, fixation of anti–basement membrane antibody and complement to the glomerular basement membrane seems to be the trigger for glomerular injury in Goodpasture's syndrome (p. 1010). Both of these are examples of Type II hypersensitivity. Type III reactions, initiated by deposition of circulating immune complexes, are the major mechanisms of tissue injury in SLE. In addition to their cytotoxic effects, antibodies may also induce diseases by a variety of other mechanisms. In one group of autoimmune disorders, formation of antireceptor antibodies leads to a variety of disease manifestations. Included in this group are: (1) myasthenia gravis, in which anti-acetylcholine-receptor antibodies lead to impairment of myoneural transmission by accelerating the degradation or blocking of muscle acetylcholine receptors (p. 1311); (2) Graves' disease, in which antibodies to the TSH receptor on thyroid cells mimic the action of normally activated TSH receptor, leading to hyperthyroidism (p. 1210); and (3) certain forms of diabetes mellitus, in which anti-insulin receptor antibodies render the cells resistant to the action of insulin (p. 980). In pernicious anemia, on the other hand, the autoantibodies are formed against a biologically active molecule, the intrinsic factor, which is blocked or neutralized, leading to impaired absorption of vitamin B_{12}.

As stated earlier, the autoimmune diseases of man range from those in which the target is a single tissue, such as the autoimmune hemolytic anemias and thyroiditis, to those in which a host of self-antigens evoke a constellation of reactions against many organs and systems. In this chapter we will deal principally with those presumed autoimmune diseases that are primarily of a systemic nature, and we will leave most single-tissue diseases to specific chapters throughout the book. For reference, however, Table 5–4 lists both systemic and organ-specific autoimmune disorders.

In some of the systemic autoimmune diseases the lesions tend to occur in and about blood vessels, causing deposits of fibrinoid material, followed in time by deposition of collagen; thus, at one time they were considered to be "collagen diseases." However, ultrastructural and biochemical studies have shown that collagen is not deranged in these disorders save perhaps secondarily, and this group of entities is now referred to by the more noncommittal term "*connective tissue diseases.*" Under this general term are included SLE, scleroderma, polymyositis-dermatomyositis, Sjögren's syndrome, mixed connective tissue disease, rheumatoid arthritis, and polyarteritis nodosa and its variants. Polyarteritis, however, is probably not of autoimmune origin and is discussed later with other diseases of blood vessels. Rheumatoid arthritis will be discussed in Chapter 28.

SYSTEMIC LUPUS ERYTHEMATOSUS (SLE)

Systemic lupus erythematosus is the classic prototype of the multisystem disease of autoimmune origin, characterized by a bewildering array of autoantibodies, particularly antinuclear antibodies. *Acute or insidious in its onset, it is a chronic, remitting and relapsing, often febrile illness characterized principally by injury to the skin, joints, kidney, and serosal membranes.* Virtually every other organ in the body, however, may also be affected. At one time SLE was thought to be a fairly rare disease, but improved methods for detecting antinuclear antibodies have shown it to be as prevalent as one in 2000.[60] SLE is predominantly a disease of women (female:male ratio of 9:1) and usually arises in the second and third decades, but may become manifest at any age, even in early childhood.[61]

ETIOLOGY AND PATHOGENESIS. Although the etiology of SLE remains unknown, the appearance of the limitless number of antibodies in these patients against self-constituents indicates that the *fundamental defect in SLE is a failure of the regulatory mechanisms that sustain self-tolerance.* Antibodies have been identified against an array of nuclear and cytoplasmic components of cells that are neither organ- nor species-specific. Apart from their value in the diagnosis and management of patients with SLE, these antibodies are of major pathogenetic significance, as, for example, in the immune complex–mediated glomerulonephritis so typical of this disease.

Antinuclear antibodies (ANA) are directed against deoxyribonucleoprotein, double- and single-stranded DNA, RNA and RNA-associated proteins, histone, nucleoli, and a soluble non-nucleic acid glycoprotein (Sm antigen). Some of these antibodies are found in other connective tissue disorders, but the *the presence of antibody to native (double-stranded) DNA is virtually diagnostic of SLE.* Several techniques are utilized to detect ANAs. The most commonly employed clinically is the immunofluorescence test for ANA (FANA). Three other techniques are also used: (1) the detection of antibodies to extractable nuclear antigens (ENA); (2) measurement of anti–native DNA antibody; and (3) the LE cell test. The first two are becoming increasingly available as well as important in the diagnosis of SLE and other connective tissue disorders.[62, 63]

The indirect immunofluorescence test for ANA is positive in 99% of patients with SLE. Although this test is quite sensitive, it is not specific. Ten per cent of normal individuals have low titers of these antibodies. It is also positive in a number of other collagen diseases including Sjögren's syndrome (68%), scleroderma (60 to 70%), and rheumatoid arthritis (20 to 40%). A lower incidence is also encountered in a miscellaneous group of other diseases. Antibodies to many nuclear components may produce a positive FANA result. The pattern of nuclear fluorescence suggests the type of antibody present in the patient's serum. For instance, anti-DNA antibodies may ring the internal circumference of the nucleus and produce a "shaggy" or "peripheral" pattern. A "nucleolar" pattern refers to the presence of a few discrete spots of fluorescence within the nucleus, and represents antibodies to nucleolar RNA. This pattern has been reported most often in patients with scleroderma (progressive systemic sclerosis), and when seen the nucleolar pattern should make one entertain this diagnosis. A homogeneous nuclear pattern may reflect antibodies to deoxyribonucleoprotein, and speckled nuclear fluorescence, to extractable nuclear antigen (ENA). It must be emphasized, however, that the patterns are not absolutely specific for the type of antibody.

Extractable nuclear antigens consist of several antigenic components including an RNA-associated protein (RNP), the Sm antigen, and the SS-A and SS-B antigens.[63] Antibodies to these antigens are determined either by immunoprecipitation techniques or by hemagglutination, when red blood cells are coated with ENA. Anti-RNP antibodies in high titer are always present in the mixed connective tissue disease (p. 195), and in addition are present in 40% of patients with SLE. Antibodies to the Sm antigen are present almost exclusively in SLE (in up to 30% of cases) and often appear in the absence of RNP antibodies. SS-B and SS-A antibodies are present in some cases of SLE and in Sjögren's syndrome (p. 189).

Despite the impressive array of *antinuclear autoantibodies,* there is no evidence that any of them are directly cytotoxic; indeed, their intracellular nuclear targets are probably inaccessible to the blood-borne immunoglobulins. ANA, however, are clearly responsible for the production of the characteristic *LE bodies and LE cells.* Although the autoantibodies cannot penetrate healthy cells, they can attack the nuclei of damaged cells. Within 15 seconds of contact with ANA serum, nuclei in injured cells lose their chromatin pattern and become homogeneous. The nucleus concomitantly swells and is extruded to create an LE body. *This LE body is extremely chemotactic for phagocytes, and in the presence of complement it is engulfed by a neutrophil or macrophage to create the typical LE cell* (Fig. 5–15). *The LE cell is thus composed of an LE body engulfed by a phagocyte.* It is rarely seen in blood smears, presumably because damaged nucleated cells are exceedingly rare in the circulating blood. In the LE cell test, however, the agitation of withdrawn blood injures a sufficient number of leukocytes to expose nuclei to the ANA. The LE cell test is positive in up to 70% of patients. In tissue sections, LE bodies can be seen principally in the renal glomerulus and interstitium as round basophilic structures, also called *hematoxylin bodies* (Fig. 5–16). Although these are found in only 20% of cases, they are pathognomonic of SLE.

Granted all these antibodies, what initiates their emergence, usually in the second and third decades of life? The general theories of autoimmunity were described earlier; here we shall refer only to those relevant to SLE.

Genetic Factors. As already discussed, considerable evidence supports a genetic prediposition to a variety of autoimmune diseases. The evidence for SLE is equally impressive. According to one study, in 66% of monozygotic twin pairs both members had clinical SLE, whereas the rate of concordance in dizygotic twins is about 3%.[64] Other evidence supporting a genetic basis for SLE comes from the association with HLA antigens. In data compiled from North American Caucasian populations, a significant positive correlation with DR2 and

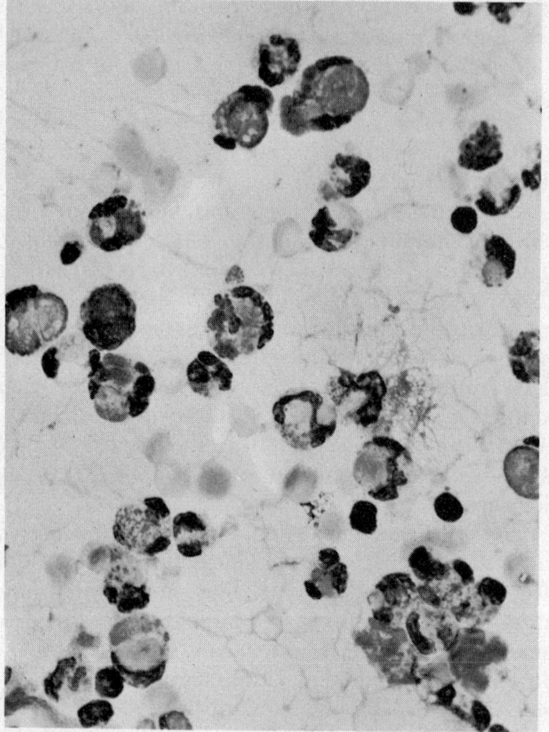

Figure 5–15. A cluster of LE cells (in vitro reaction) demonstrating homogeneous inclusions that have distorted the enclosing polymorphonuclear leukocytes.

DR3 has been noted.[65] In other populations, association with A1 and B8 has been observed. However, since A1, B8, and DR3 are in linkage disequilibrium (i.e., tend to occur together more frequently than expected by chance), this association may not be entirely unforeseen. The role of the HLA genes in the pathogenesis of SLE can be only a matter for speculation at present. On the basis of our knowledge of the role of the HLA-D/DR region in the regulation of immune response (p. 161), it has been suggested that immune response genes linked to HLA-DR3 may allow for a generalized hyperresponsiveness, whereas excessive immune response to specific antigens such as nucleic acids may be related to the genes linked to HLA-DR2. *Another intriguing association is noted between SLE and inherited deficiencies of complement components* (especially C2 and C4). The fact that individuals heterozygous for C2 deficiency who have *adequate* serum complement levels also have increased incidence of SLE indicates that the level of complement per se is not involved in the susceptibility to SLE.[66] It may be recalled that the C2 and C4 genes are located within the HLA region, and therefore genetically determined deficiencies of these complement components may merely reflect association with certain immune response genes. In addition to the well-known associations between HLA and SLE, it should be pointed out that two or three genes outside the HLA also determine susceptibility to SLE. How these multiple genetic influences interact is unknown, although several interesting speculations have been made.[67]

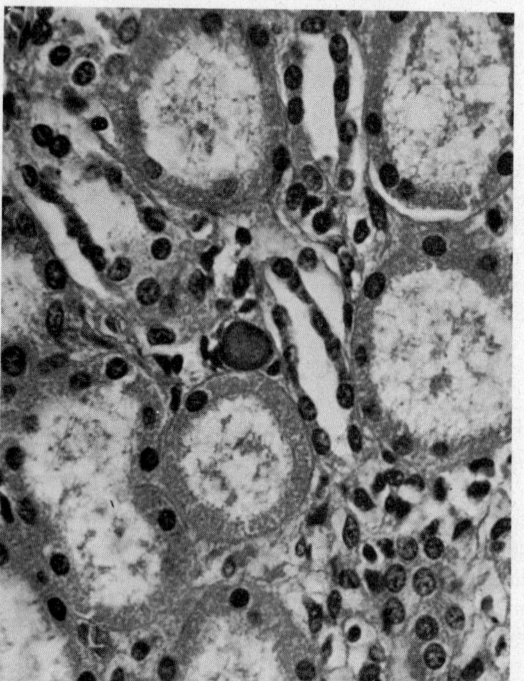

Figure 5–16. A hematoxylin body within the interstitium of the kidney, presumably a residual of a former focus of inflammatory activity.

Nongenetic Factors. There are many indications that, in addition to genetic factors, several *environmental* or nongenetic factors must be involved in the pathogenesis of SLE. The most clear example of the impact of nongenetic factors comes from the observation that drugs such as hydralazine, procainamide, and D-penicillamine can induce an SLE-like response in humans.[68] *Viruses* have also been suspected to be the cause of SLE.[45] Most evidence stems from the study of spontaneous SLE-like disease in NZB and (NZB × NZW)F1 hybrid mice. These mice express high levels of C-type viruses throughout their life, and viral antigen-antiviral immune complexes can be recovered from the glomeruli of (NZB × NZW)F1 mice. However, careful genetic analyses have revealed that the presence of C-type viruses or virus proteins is not essential for development of autoimmunity in NZB mice. Viruses or viral antigens when present do, however, play a role in the pathogenesis of tissue damage by inducing the formation of viral-antiviral immune complexes.[69] The evidence for a role of viruses in human SLE is even more tenuous. Several reports have suggested the presence of C-type virus particles or antigens on a variety of tissues of SLE patients, but most such observations have not been reproduced widely. Although the search continues, the consensus appears to be that viruses are not the primary cause of SLE. *Sex hormones* seem to exert an important influence on the occurrence and manifestations of SLE. During the reproductive years the incidence of SLE is ten times greater in women, and exacerbation of the disease has been noted during normal menses and pregnancy. Some recent data suggest that lupus patients have an alteration in estrogen metabolism that results in hyperestrogenic effects.[70]

Immunologic Factors. With all the immunologic findings in SLE patients, there can be little doubt that some *fundamental derangement of the immune system* is involved in the pathogenesis of SLE. A variety of immunologic abnormalities affecting both T cells and B cells have been detected in patients with SLE.[71, 72] Until recently, derangements in T-suppressor cells (TSC) have received the most attention, since a primary defect in TSC could initiate autoantibody formation as discussed previously (p. 179). Although defective or deficient TSC functions in vitro have been reported in patients with SLE,[73] the significance of these findings is not entirely clear. Several recent observations suggest that the defects in TSC are not seen consistently and that their presence does not necessarily imply the existence of autoimmunity.[74] For example, in one study 20% of the clinically normal family members demonstrated defective TSC function, although statistically no more than 5% of the unaffected family members would be expected to develop SLE.[75, 76]

Abnormalities in B cells are much more consistent and less controversial.[71, 77] B cells from the peripheral blood of lupus patients show eight to ten times higher spontaneous proliferative activity in vitro, and secrete excessive quantities of immunoglobulin directed against self- and non–self-antigens. The basis for the sustained polyclonal B-cell hyperactivity appears to be an inherent (genetically determined) defect in B cells and not a consequence of T-suppressor cell abnormalities.[78] Finally, although macrophages have not received much attention in SLE, defects in their functions could also contribute to the pathogenesis of autoimmunity. In patients with SLE, the Fc receptor–mediated uptake of circulating immune complexes by mononuclear phagocyte system is markedly impaired,[79] thereby facilitating their tissue deposition and the consequent inflammatory response.

Recent studies on the immunologic profiles of several strains of autoimmune mice, other than the classical NZB and (NZB × NZW)F1, have provided a new perspective on the immunopathogenesis of human SLE.[77] The lessons learned from these studies are best summarized in the words of R.S. Schwartz:[67]

> "Each of these inbred lines of mice has distinct immunologic, genetic and hormonal features. Yet each develops one or more characteristic lesions of SLE. These various models add to the evidence that SLE is a syndrome that can result from several different pathways. Each inbred strain presents a genetic window through which one of the pathways to lupus can be perceived. It would thus be surprising if a single mechanism could explain SLE in a genetically heterogenous human population. There is, therefore, no place for dogmatism in formulating notions about the etiology of SLE."

The mechanisms of tissue damage in SLE are for the most part those discussed under hypersensitivity reactions. Formation of immune complexes made up of DNA–anti-DNA is of prime pathogenetic importance in the development of vascular and glomerular lesions in SLE. The evidence can be summarized as follows:[79] (1) immunoglobulins and complement can be identified by fluorescence microscopy in glomeruli in a granular pattern (p. 1005); (2) when immunoglobulins are eluted from kidneys, they react with double-stranded DNA, single-stranded DNA, and RNA-protein; and (3) immune complexes can be readily detected in the serum of patients with active lupus nephritis.

A second type of tissue damage is that induced by specific antibodies directed against particular cell types. Antibodies against erythrocytes, platelets, and neutrophils may be the cause of the hemolytic anemia, thrombocytopenia, and neutropenia, respectively. In addition, antibodies against neurons may be responsible for the central nervous system manifestations.[80]

To summarize, the evidence to date suggests that SLE results from a state in which there is a heightened immune response to "self-antigens," determined by defects in regulatory genes and potentiated or modulated by hormonal or environmental factors. The lesions in SLE are caused largely by the deposition of DNA–anti-DNA complexes and in part by direct damage to cells by autoantibodies.

MORPHOLOGY. The morphologic changes in SLE are extremely variable, reflecting the variability of the clinical manifestations and the course of the disease in individual patients. It can also be said that none of these morphologic changes is pathognomonic. It is the constellation of clinical, serologic (particularly the presence of ANA), and morphologic changes that characterize the disease. Table 5–5 lists the percentage of patients showing involvement of individual organs. The most characteristic lesions are found in the blood vessels, kidneys, connective tissue, and skin.

An acute necrotizing **vasculitis involving small arteries and arterioles** is present in most affected tissues. The arteritis is characterized by fibrinoid deposits in the vessel walls. In chronic stages, vessels undergo fibrous thickening with luminal narrowing. Frequently a perivascular lymphocytic infiltrate is present, sometimes accompanied by significant edema and an increase in ground substance. In the spleen these vascular lesions involve the central penicilliary arteries and are characterized by marked perivascular fibrosis, producing so-called **"onionskin" lesions** (Fig. 5–17). Immunoglobulins, DNA, and C3 have been found in these

Table 5–5. DISTRIBUTION OF ORGAN INVOLVEMENT IN SYSTEMIC LUPUS ERYTHEMATOSUS

	Approximate Percentage of Cases
Skin	80
Joints*	80–90
Kidneys*	70
Heart*	50
Serous membranes*	40
Lungs	10–20
Liver	25–30
Spleen	20
Lymph node enlargement	60
Gastrointestinal tract	30
Central nervous system	30
Peripheral nervous system	11
Eyes	20

*Lesions cause major clinical symptoms.

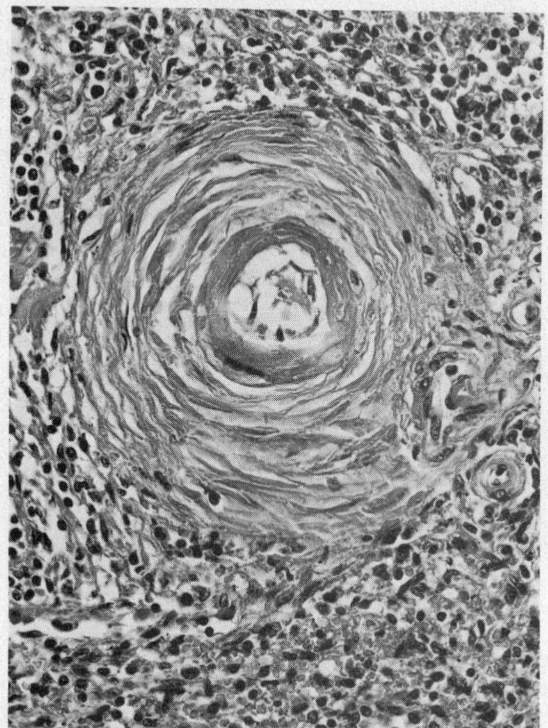

Figure 5–17. Lupus erythematosus—concentric periarterial fibrosis in the spleen.

vessel walls, supporting the theory that they may be immune DNA–anti-DNA complexes.

Kidney. On light microscopic examination, the kidney appears to be involved in 60 to 70% of cases, but **if immunofluorescence and electron microscopy are included in the examination of biopsy material, almost all cases of SLE will show some renal abnormality.**[81, 82] According to the W.H.O. morphologic classification of lupus nephritis, five patterns are recognized: (1) normal by light, electron and immunofluorescent microscopy (class I), which is quite rare; (2) mesangial lupus glomerulonephritis (class II); (3) focal proliferative glomerulonephritis (class III); (4) diffuse proliferative glomerulonephritis (class IV); and (5) membranous glomerulonephritis (class V). These lesions are discussed further in the chapter on renal diseases (p. 1021).

Mesangial lupus nephritis is the mildest of the lesions and is seen in those patients who have minimal clinical manifestations such as mild hematuria or proteinuria. It occurs in approximately 10% of the patients. There is slight-to-moderate increase in the intercapillary mesangial matrix as well as in the number of mesangial cells. Despite the very mild histologic changes, granular mesangial deposits of immunoglobulin and complement are frequently present. The WHO classification subdivides mesangial lupus nephritis into a group characterized by mesangial deposits but no changes in mesangial cellularity (class IIA), and another subgroup in which increase in mesangial cellularity can be observed by light microscopy (class IIB).[81]

Focal proliferative glomerular lesions are seen in about one-third of initial biopsies of these patients. As the name implies, this is a focal lesion, affecting usually less than 50% of the glomeruli and only portions of each glomerulus. Typically, one or two tufts in an otherwise normal glomerulus exhibit swelling and proliferation of endothelial and mesangial cells, infiltration with neutrophils, and sometimes fibrinoid deposits and intracapillary thrombi (Fig. 5–18). Hematoxylin bodies may be present, and fragmentation and breakdown of nuclei produces an appearance described as "nuclear dust." Focal lesions may be associated with rather mild clinical manifestations: recurrent hematuria and moderate proteinuria with only occasional mild renal insufficiency. However, some patients with focal lesions may have more severe clinical disease progressing to renal failure.[82, 83]

Diffuse proliferative glomerulonephritis is the most serious of the renal lesions in SLE, occurring in 45 to 50% of patients. Anatomic changes are dominated by proliferation of endothelial, mesangial, and sometimes epithelial cells (Fig. 5–19). Most or all glomeruli are involved in both kidneys, and the entire glomerulus is almost always affected. Patients with diffuse lesions are usually overtly symptomatic, showing microscopic or gross hematuria, proteinuria including the nephrotic syndrome, hypertension, and frequently a diminution of glomerular filtration rate.

Membranous glomerulonephritis occurs in 10% of patients and is a designation given to glomerular disease in which the principal histologic change consists of widespread thickening of the capillary walls. The lesions are very similar to those encountered in idiopathic membranous glomerulonephritis, described more fully on page 1013. Patients with this histologic change almost always have severe proteinuria or the overt nephrotic syndrome.

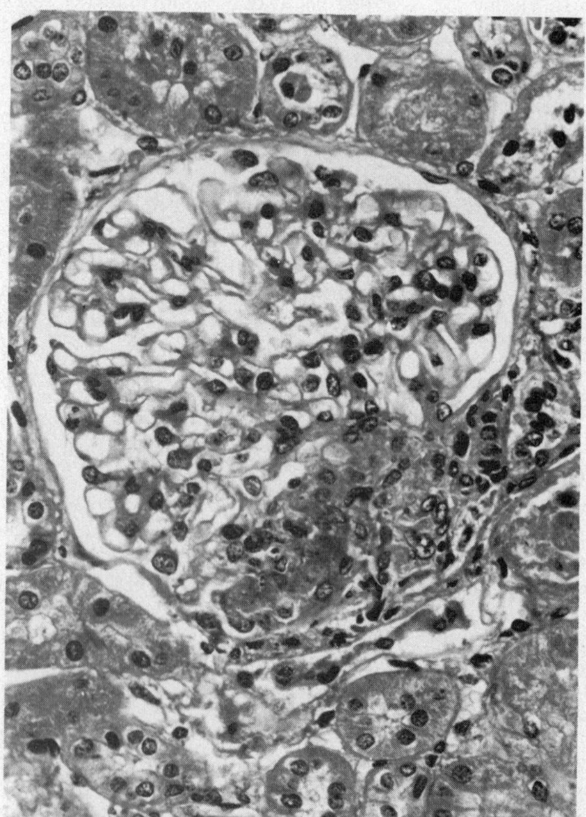

Figure 5–18. Segmental proliferation and necrosis of a glomerular lobule from a case of focal proliferative lupus nephritis. (Courtesy of Dr. Fred Silva, Department of Pathology, Southwestern Medical School, Dallas, Texas.)

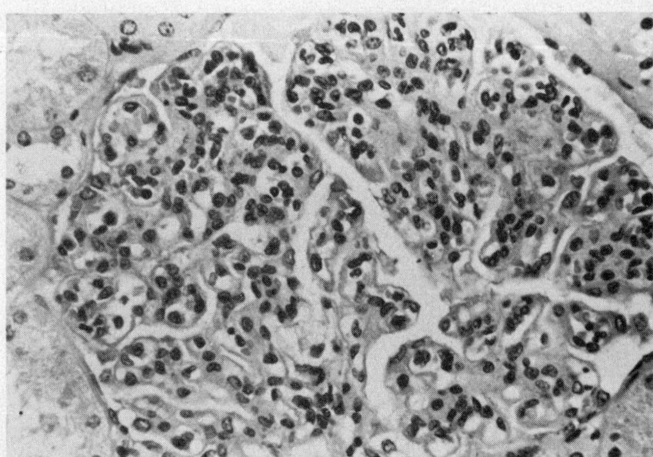

Figure 5–19. Diffuse proliferative lupus nephritis. Note hypercellularity throughout glomerular tuft.

All four types are thought to have the same general pathogenetic mechanism, that is, the deposition of DNA–anti-DNA complexes within the glomeruli. Thus, deposits of immunoglobulin and complement—sometimes localized to the mesangium only, sometimes along the entire basement membrane, and sometimes massively throughout the entire glomerulus—are characteristic features (Fig. 5–20). Why this same pathogenetic mechanism produces such different histologic lesions (and clinical manifestations) in different patients is not entirely clear. It is likely, as we shall see (p. 1003), that the physical and chemical characteristics of the complexes as well as the state of the glomerular capillary wall both play a role in the pattern of deposition of complexes and also in the histologic change.

Electron microscopy demonstrates electron-dense deposits (presumably immune complexes) in three locations within the glomerulus. (1) In the membranous type the deposits are predominantly between the basement membrane and the visceral epithelial cell (subepithelial), a location similar to that of deposits in other types of membranous nephropathy. (2) All histologic types show large amounts of deposits in the mesangium. (3) Subendothelial deposits (between the endothelium and the basement membrane) are particularly characteristic of SLE, since they are present in few other types of glomerulonephritis (Fig. 5–21). When extensive, subendothelial deposits create a peculiar thickening of the capillary wall, which can be seen by means of light microscopy as a "wire loop" lesion (Fig. 5–21 *A*). Such "wire loops" are often found in the proliferative type of glomerulonephritis but can also be present in the focal and membranous types. They usually reflect active disease and are generally a poor prognostic sign.

Although the specific types of lesions may persist in individual patients throughout the course of the disease, cases of mesangial or focal glomerulonephritis can progress to diffuse proliferative glomerulonephritis, with a more serious clinical course.[83]

In addition to these glomerular lesions, vasculitis similar to that seen in all affected tissues and organs is generally found in cortical arterioles. Accompanied by edema and a perivascular infiltrate, it is often responsible for ischemic necrosis of affected glomeruli or dependent tubules. Hematoxylin or LE bodies may be found in such areas of injury.

There is also increasing interest in **the interstitial and tubular lesions frequently present in patients with SLE,** especially in association with diffuse proliferative glomerulonephritis. In a few cases, tubulointerstitial lesions may be the dominant abnormality. As we shall see in the chapter on kidney diseases (p. 991), granular deposits composed of immunoglobulin and complement similar to those seen in glomeruli are present around the tubules in about 50% of patients with SLE, a pattern indicative of so-called tubular immune complex disease. Antibody eluted from these deposits, like that in the glomeruli, reacts with DNA.

Skin. The skin is often involved. Characteristic erythema affects the facial "butterfly" area (bridge of the nose and cheeks) but also the extremities and trunk. Urticaria, bullae, maculopapular lesions, and ulcerations also occur. Exposure to sunlight incites or accentuates the erythema. Histologically, the involved areas show liquefactive degeneration of the basal layer of dermis together with edema at the dermal junction. In the dermis there are variable degrees of fibrosis, marked perivascular mononuclear infiltrate, and

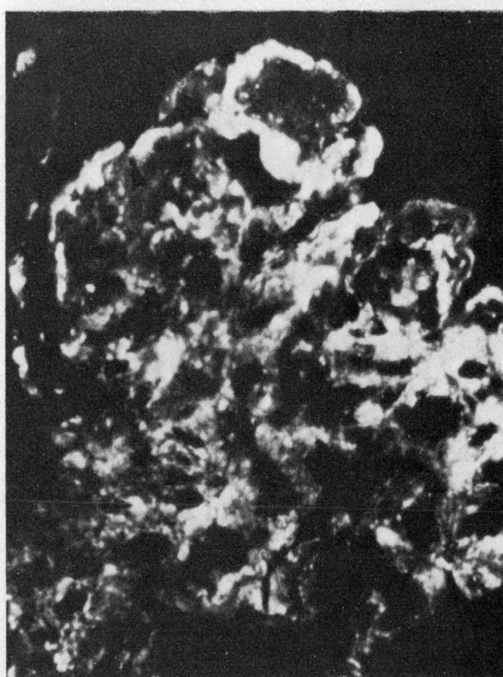

Figure 5–20. Immunofluorescence micrograph stained for IgG from glomerulus with diffuse proliferative lupus nephritis showing abundant deposition of immunoglobulin.

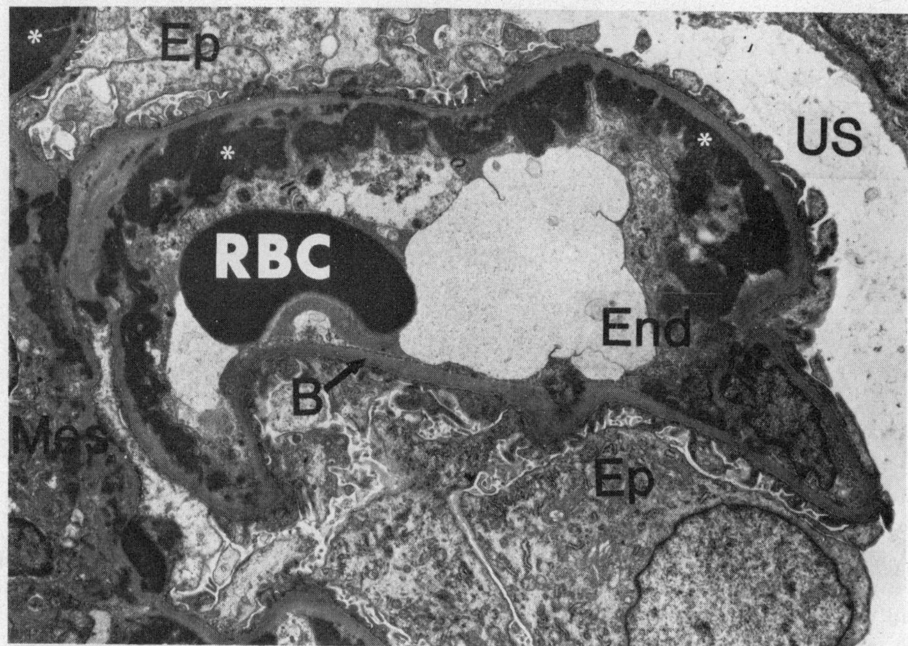

Figure 5–21. Electron micrograph of renal glomerular capillary loop from patient with systemic lupus erythematosus nephritis. Subendothelial dense deposits correspond to "wire loops" seen by light microscopy. End-endothelium; Mes-mesangium; Ep-epithelial cell with foot processes; RBC-red blood cell in capillary lumen; B-basement membrane; US-urinary space; *-electron-dense deposits in subendothelial location. (Courtesy of Dr. Edwin Eigenbrodt, Department of Pathology, Southwestern Medical School, Dallas, Texas.)

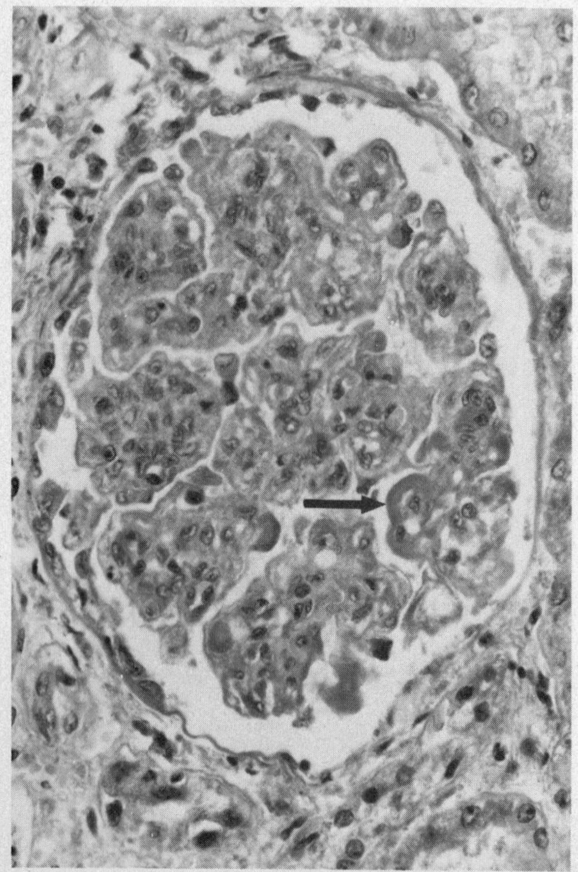

Figure 5–21A. Lupus nephritis. A glomerulus with "wire loop" thickening of the basement membrane.. (Courtesy of Dr. Fred Silva, Department of Pathology, Southwestern Medical School, Dallas, Texas.)

occasionally fibrinoid change in the vessel wall. **Immunofluorescence microscopy shows deposition of immunoglobulin and complement along the dermoepidermal junction.** The presence of immunoglobulin in both involved and noninvolved skin in SLE distinguishes the skin lesions from those seen in other connective tissue disorders such as dermatomyositis and scleroderma, as well as chronic discoid lupus erythematosus. In the latter disorders, only involved areas of the skin are positive. The origin of the immune deposits is not certain; it is unlikely that they represent circulating immune complexes, but more probable that they could be nuclear antigens released from necrotic epidermal cells reacting with antinuclear antibodies present in the circulation.[84]

Joints. Joint involvement is frequent, the typical lesion being a nonerosive synovitis with little deformity. The latter fact distinguishes this arthritis from that seen in rheumatoid disease. In the acute phases of arthritis in SLE there is exudation of neutrophils and fibrin into the synovium, and a perivascular mononuclear cell infilrate in the subsynovial tissue, but the severe mononuclear infiltration of the subsynovium and the intense synovial hyperplasia characteristic of rheumatoid arthritis are unusual.[85]

Central Nervous System. The pathologic basis of CNS symptoms is ascribed principally to acute vasculitis, with occlusion of small arteries causing infarcts or hemorrhages. Of interest is the deposition of immune complexes in the choroid plexus,[86] which is very similar to the renal glomerulus in some of its anatomic and filtration characteristics. Some of the neurologic manifestations may also be due to the occurrence of antineuronal cytoplasmic antibodies.[80]

Pericarditis and Other Serosal Cavity Involvement. Inflammation of the serosal lining membranes may be acute, subacute, or chronic. During the acute phases, the mesothelial surfaces are sometimes covered with fibrinous exudate. Later they become thickened, opaque, and coated with a shaggy fibrous tissue that may lead to partial or total obliteration of the serosal cavity. In areas of acute involvement, even when the pericardial sac appears normal on gross inspection, there is microscopic evidence of edema; focal vasculitis with a perivascular, mononuclear, inflammatory infiltrate; and fibrinoid necrosis, sometimes containing hematoxylin bodies. These acute changes are replaced in time by fibroblastic proliferation, together with diffuse or focal lymphocytic and plasma cell infiltration.

Heart. In addition to pericarditis, cardiac valves or myocardium is affected in about half of the cases. The endocardial alterations **(nonbacterial verrucous endocarditis or Libman-Sacks endocarditis)**, when present, constitute one of the most striking anatomic findings of lupus erythematosus. Vegetations occurs on the mitral and tricuspid valves. These may be small, warty excrescences or in some cases, friable, berry-like masses of amorphous material that vary in size from less than 1 mm to 3 or 4 mm in diameter (Fig. 5–22). They may occur singly, but more often occur multiply in random fashion anywhere on the valvular leaflets, usually on the surfaces exposed to the forward flow of blood but sometimes behind the cusps. Infrequently, the vegetations extend onto the mural endocardium of the cardiac chambers or onto the chordae tendineae.

The vegetations in SLE must be differentiated principally from those formed in bacterial endocarditis and acute rheumatic endocarditis. In infective endocarditis, the vegetations tend to be considerably larger (0.5 to 2.0 cm) than those in lupus, and only rarely are they as widely dispersed. More often, infective vegetations occur singly or in two or three discrete foci, and only very infrequently are they positioned behind the cusps. In rheumatic endocarditis, the vegetations are small, are confined to the lines of closure of the leaflets on the surface exposed to the forward flow of blood, and almost never extend behind the cusps.

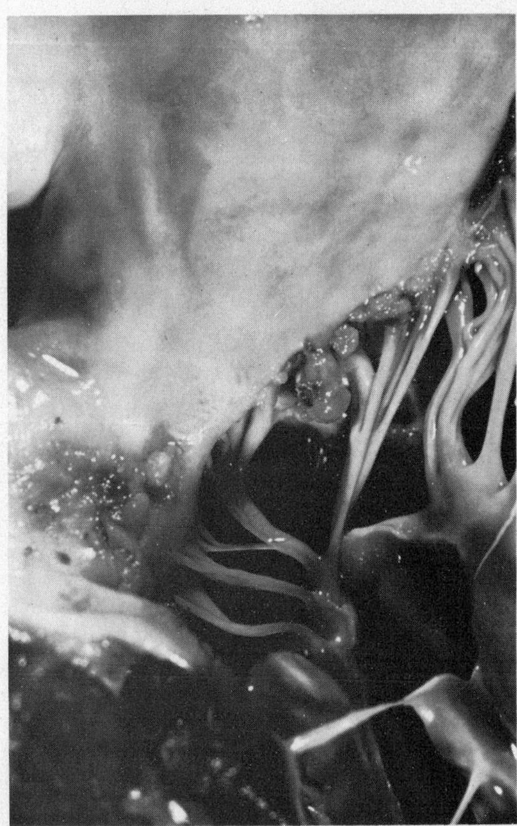

Figure 5–22. Libman-Sacks endocarditis of the mitral valve in lupus erythematosus. The small vegetations attached to the margin of the valve leaflet are easily seen.

Characteristic histologic alterations in Libman-Sacks endocarditis are found underlying the vegetations. Increased ground substance, "fibrinoid necrosis," and, in the later stages, increased vascularization, fibroblastic proliferation, and neutrophilic and mononuclear cell infiltration constitute the inflammatory changes. The vegetation itself may be composed in part of fibrin, but more characteristically is made up of necrotic debris, fibrinoid material, and trapped disintegrating fibroblasts and inflammatory cells. Hematoxylin bodies are sometimes found within the fibrinoid. Organization may, in time, convert the vegetation into a nodule of organized connective tissue. Focal areas of acute-to-chronic inflammation containing fibrinoid may be found throughout the heart in the connective tissue of the endocardium and myocardium, about blood vessels, and in the interfascicular connective tissue planes. Myocardial arterioles and small arteries may suffer acute necrotizing injury with mural deposition of fibrinoid, but myocardial fibers are injured by resultant ischemia only in the florid, acute cases when the vascular damage is severe and causes thromboses of luminia.

Spleen. The spleen may be moderately enlarged. Capsular thickening is common, as is follicular hyperplasia. Plasma cells are usually numerous in the pulp and can be shown to contain immunoglobulins of the IgG and IgM variety by fluorescence microscopy. As mentioned above, the central penicilliary arteries show thickening and perivascular fibrosis, producing the so-called "onionskin" lesions.

Lungs. In addition to pleuritis and pleural effusions, interstitial pneumonitis and diffuse fibrosing alveolitis can occur in SLE. As its name indicates, fibrosing alveolitis consists of filling of the alveolar spaces with fibrous tissue, often containing many inflammatory cells. There is evidence that DNA–anti-DNA complexes may contribute to the pathogenesis of this alveolitis.

Other Organs and Tissues. Acute vasculitis may be seen in the portal tracts of the liver accompanied by lymphocytic infiltrates, creating nonspecific portal triaditis. LE cells in the bone marrow may be strongly indicative of lupus erythematosus. Lymph nodes may be enlarged and contain hyperactive follicles as well as plasma cells, changes that are of interest in view of the etiology of this disease. Focal fibrinoid necrosis in lymph nodes may suggest the possibility of a connective tissue disorder.

CLINICAL COURSE. The most common clinical manifestations of systemic lupus erythematosus are articular pain, usually involving the hands or feet but also the larger joints (92%); fever (84%); skin eruptions, including butterfly rash (72%); renal manifestations, including hematuria, proteinuria, hypertension, and the nephrotic syndrome (60%); pleuritis and pleural effusions (50%); cardiopulmonary abnormalities, including symptoms and signs of pericarditis (50%); and neurologic manifestations (25%), including convulsive disorders, peripheral neuropathies, and mental dysfunction. Lymph node enlargement indicative of hyperactivity of the immune system occurs in about 50% of patients, and splenomegaly in 10%. Hematologic abnormalities include leukopenia, thrombocytopenia with bleeding tendency, and hemolytic anemia.

The course of the disease is variable and almost unpredictable. Rare acute cases result in death within weeks to months. More often, with appropriate therapy, the disease is characterized by flareups and remissions spanning a period of years or even decades. During acute flareups, increased formation of immune complexes and the accompanying complement activation often result in hypocomplementemia. Disease exacerbations are usually treated by corticosteroids or immunosuppressant drugs, which often control acute manifestations. Even without therapy, some patients may run a benign course with skin manifestations and mild hematuria for years. The outcome has improved significantly in the recent past. In one recent large multicenter study the survival was 90% at one year, 77% at five years, and 71% at ten years.[87] This apparent improvement derives in part from earlier diagnosis and recognition of the milder forms of the disease. The most common cause of death is renal failure, followed by intercurrent infections.[87] Cardiac failure, hemorrhages, and central nervous system disease may also contribute.

As mentioned earlier, involvement of skin along with multisystem disease is fairly common in SLE. In addition, two syndromes have been recognized in which the cutaneous involvement is the most prominent or exclusive feature.

Chronic Discoid Lupus Erythematosus. Chronic discoid lupus erythematosus is a disease in which the skin manifestations mimic systemic lupus erythematosus but systemic manifestations are rare. It is characterized by the presence of skin plaques showing varying degrees of edema, erythema, scaliness, follicular plugging, and skin atrophy surrounded by an elevated erythematous border. The face and scalp are usually affected, but widely disseminated lesions occasionally occur. The disease is usually confined to the skin, but 50% of patients with discoid lupus develop multisystem manifestations after many years.[88] The LE cell test is rarely positive, but about 35% of patients show a positive ANA test. Antibodies to double-stranded DNA are rarely present, and immunofluorescence studies of skin biopsies show the same deposition of Ig and C3 at the dermal-epidermal junction that is seen in SLE. *However, in contrast to SLE, normal uninvolved skin does not show such fluorescence.*

Subacute Cutaneous Lupus Erythematosus. This condition also presents with predominant skin involvement and can be distinguished from chronic discoid LE by several criteria.[89] It is characterized by widespread but superficial and nonscarring lesions. There usually is clinical evidence of mild systemic disease, and patients often have clearly abnormal levels of antinuclear antibodies, particularly antibodies to the SS-A antigen (p. 181). Furthermore, unlike discoid LE, a distinct association with HLA-B8 and -DR3 antigens has also been noted. Thus, the term subacute LE seems to define a group intermediate between SLE and lupus localized only to skin.

Drug-Induced Lupus Erythematosus. An interesting syndrome develops in patients receiving a variety of drugs, including hydralazine (given for hypertension), procainamide, isoniazid, and D-penicillamine, to name only a few. These patients develop antinuclear antibodies and anti–single-stranded DNA antibodies, but anti–double-stranded DNA antibodies are found only rarely. Patients receiving hydralazine may develop a multisystem lupus syndrome with skin and joint manifestations, but without renal involvement and hypocomplementemia. As a rule, drug-induced lupus improves spontaneously following withdrawal of the drug. Recent theories emphasize genetic defects in the origin of the autoimmunity in drug-induced SLE ("lupus diathesis"). Persons having the HLA-DR4 antigen are at increased risk of developing drug-induced SLE, and these patients seem to have a genetically determined inability to acetylate the amine or hydralazine moiety of these compounds adequately through the hepatic *N*-acetyltransferase system. Presumably these "slow acetylators" develop accumulations of nonacetylated metabolites of these drugs, which covalently bind to a nucleoprotein or to cellular macromolecules, producing antigenic complexes. Antinuclear antibodies and eventually lupus disease are thus induced.[90] If these observations are correct, this would be an interesting example of how a genetic *metabolic* defect may lead to autoimmunity.

SJÖGREN'S SYNDROME

Sjögren's syndrome is a clinicopathologic entity characterized by dry eyes (keratoconjunctivitis sicca) and dry mouth (xerostomia) resulting from immunologically mediated destruction of the lacrimal and salivary glands. It occurs as an isolated disorder (primary form) also known as the *sicca syndrome,* or more often in association with another autoimmune disease (secondary form). Among the associated disorders, rheumatoid arthritis is the most common, but some patients have SLE, polymyositis, scleroderma, vasculitis, mixed connective tissue disease, or thyroiditis.[91]

ETIOLOGY AND PATHOGENESIS. As we shall see in the description of morphology, the decrease in tears and saliva (sicca syndrome) is the result of *lymphocytic infiltration* and fibrosis of the lacrimal and salivary glands. The infiltrate contains predominantly T cells (both OK T4 and OK T8) and some B cells, including plasma cells that secrete antibody locally.[92] Most of the infiltrating T cells are OK T4–positive and may serve as helper cells for antibody synthesis. It is not clear, however, whether the tissue damage is mediated by the few cytotoxic T cells that infiltrate the gland or by autoantibodies, several of which can be found in the serum. About 75% of patients have rheumatoid factor (p. 181) irrespective of whether coexisting rheumatoid arthritis is present or not. ANA are detected in 60 to 70% of patients and a positive LE test in 25%. A whole host of additional antibodies have been identified, including autoantibodies to salivary duct cells, smooth muscle mitochondria, gastric parietal cells, and thyroid antigens. Recently, antibodies directed against two extractable nuclear antigens (p. 181) have been detected in the sera of patients with Sjögren's syndrome. These antigens have been called by various names, but at present most authors designate them as SS-A and SS-B (SS = sicca syndrome).[63] Antibodies to SS-B are considered highly specific for Sjögren's syndrome. They are found in 60 to 70% of patients with primary Sjögren's syndrome and in 70 to 80% of patients with Sjögren's syndrome and associated SLE. Anti–SS-A antibodies are found in a smaller percentage (14%) of patients with Sjögren's syndrome, and are also detected in other collagen vascular diseases. Therefore, SS-A antibodies without the concomitant presence of anti–SS-B are not considered specific for Sjögren's syndrome. In Sjögren's syndrome associated with rheumatoid arthritis, there is a high frequency of antibodies to yet another nuclear antigen called rheumatoid associated nuclear antigen (RANA). Both serologic and immunogenetic studies suggest that patients with secondary Sjögren's syndrome (associated most often with rheumatoid arthritis) make up a subset that is distinct from those with primary Sjögren's syndrome. The latter seem to show higher frequency of HLA-DR-3, whereas patients with associated rheumatoid arthritis show a positive correlation with HLA-DR4.

As might be expected from the presence of autoantibodies, a variety of functional abnormalities have been detected in the T cells, B cells, and macrophages, many of which are similar to those described in SLE and need not be repeated (p. 183).[93] Although it seems logical to assume that autoimmunity is involved in the pathogenesis of Sjögren's syndrome, the triggering mechanisms are not clear. As in SLE, genetic predisposition, viruses, and deranged immunoregulation are suspected, but the evidence is even more nebulous.

MORPHOLOGY. As mentioned earlier, lacrimal and salivary glands are the major targets of the disease, although other exocrine glands including those lining the respiratory and gastrointestinal tract may also be involved.

The earliest histologic finding in both the major and minor salivary glands is **periductal lymphocytic infiltration.** The cells are predominantly small lymphocytes, but large lymphocytes and plasma cells may also be present as well as lymphoid follicles with germinal centers (Fig. 5–23). The ductal lining epithelial cells may show hyperplasia, thus obstructing the ducts. Later there is atrophy of the acini, fibrosis, and hyalinization, and still later in the course, atrophy and fatty replacement of parenchyma. In some cases the lymphoid infiltrate may be so intense as to give the appearance of a lymphoma; however, the benign appearance of lymphocytes, the heterogeneous population of cells, and the preservation of lobular architecture of the gland differentiate the lesions from those of lymphoma.

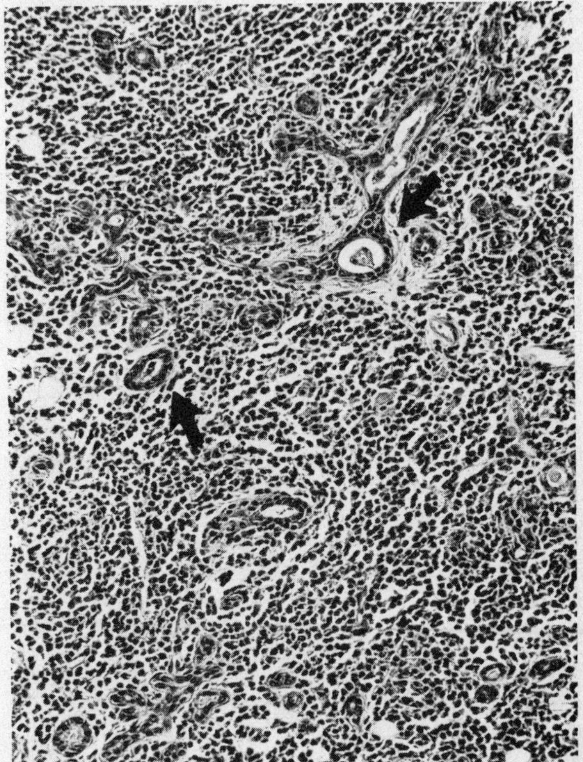

Figure 5–23. Sjögren's syndrome—submandibular gland. The intense lymphocytic and plasma cell infiltration virtually obscures the native architecture. Only a few residual ducts *(arrows)* can be identified.

The lack of tears leads to drying of the corneal epithelium, which becomes inflamed, eroded, and ulcerated; the oral mucosa may atrophy with inflammatory fissuring and ulceration; and dryness and crusting of the nose may lead to ulcerations and even perforation of the nasal septum. When the respiratory passages are involved, secondary laryngitis, bronchitis, and pneumonitis may appear. Atrophic gastritis may also occur. In approximately 25% of cases, extraglandular tissues such as kidneys, lungs, and muscles are also involved. In contrast with SLE, glomerular lesions are extremely rare in Sjögren's syndrome. However, defects of tubular function, including renal tubular acidosis, uricosuria, and phosphaturia, are often seen and are associated histologically with a **tubulointerstitial nephritis** (p. 1040). There is infiltration of the renal interstitium by monocytes, plasma cells, and macrophages and often a pronounced degree of fibrosis. Tubules are atrophied and may be invaded by lymphoid and plasma cells.

CLINICAL MANIFESTATIONS. The keratoconjunctivitis produces symptoms of blurring of vision, burning and itching, and accumulated thick secretions in the conjunctival sac. The xerostomia results in difficulty in swallowing solid foods, a decrease in the ability to taste, cracks and fissures in the mouth, and dryness of the buccal mucosa. Parotid gland enlargement is present in half the patients; dryness of the nasal mucosa, epistaxis, recurrent bronchitis, and pneumonitis are other symptoms. The 60% of patients who have an accompanying connective tissue disorder such as rheumatoid arthritis also have the symptoms and signs of that disorder.

The combination of lacrimal and salivary gland inflammatory involvement was once called *Mikulicz's disease*. However, the entity has now been replaced by the noncommittal *Mikulicz's syndrome*, broadened to include lacrimal and salivary gland enlargement, whatever the cause. In addition to Sjögren's syndrome, sarcoidosis, leukemia, lymphoma, and other tumors produce Mikulicz's syndrome. Thus, biopsy of the lip (to examine minor salivary glands) is frequently required to aid in the diagnosis.

The lymph nodes of patients with Sjögren's syndrome show not only enlargement but also a pleomorphic infiltrate of cells with frequent mitoses. The appearance has been described as "pseudolymphoma," since all the criteria of malignant lymphoma are not satisfied. However, clear-cut malignant lymphomas mostly of the B-cell type have developed in the salivary glands and lymph nodes in some patients and it is believed that patients with Sjögren's syndrome have an approximately 40-fold higher risk of developing lymphoid malignancies.[91] This has led to the statement that the disorder lies "somewhere between hyperplasia and neoplasia."

SCLERODERMA (PROGRESSIVE SYSTEMIC SCLEROSIS)

Although the term "scleroderma" is ingrained in the literature through common usage, this disease is better named progressive systemic sclerosis (PSS), since it is characterized by excessive fibrosis *throughout the body*. The skin is most commonly affected, but the gastrointestinal tract, kidneys, heart, muscles, and lungs also are frequently involved. In some patients the disease appears to remain confined to the skin for many years, but in the majority it progresses to visceral involvement and death from renal failure, cardiac failure, pulmonary insufficiency, or intestinal malabsorption. Women are affected two to fives times as often as men. Although it usually appears in the third to fifth decade, no age is immune—the disease has been identified in infants 6 months old and in patients of advanced years.

ETIOLOGY AND PATHOGENESIS. Progressive systemic sclerosis is a disease of unknown etiology. Three main lines of investigation have been pursued to explain the excessive deposition of collagen. One is concerned with the factors leading to altered collagen synthesis, another with possible immunologic derangements, and still another with microvascular abnormalities.

In spite of the widespead and striking overgrowth of connective tissue, there is no clear-cut evidence for an abnormality in collagen metabolism as the primary defect in this disease. Cultured fibroblasts from skin of patients with PSS have an increased capacity to synthesize collagen,[95] without any decrease in the ability to degrade it.[96] Although augmented collagen synthesis is established, the nature of the forces that "charge" these cells remains elusive. Is there an intrinsic defect in fibroblasts or are they responding to external stimuli? We cannot answer this question with certainty, but a hypothesis has been proposed that links abnormal cell-mediated immunity to excessive fibroblast activity.[97] According to this, the initial event is T-cell sensitization to collagen, resulting in a delayed-type hypersensitivity reaction and elaboration of lymphokines. The lymphokines then attract fibroblasts and stimulate them to produce collagen, which in turn triggers further lymphokine production by the sensitized T cells. In support of this hypothesis can be cited the demonstration of cell-mediated immunity to collagen in some patients, and the ability of lymphokines to attract and stimulate fibroblasts in vitro.[97]

A variety of serologic abnormalities have also been reported in PSS. Approximately 50% of cases have mild hypergammaglobulinemia; also detected are a variety of autoantibodies including rheumatoid factor (20 to 30% of cases), anti–smooth muscle antibodies (40 to 60% of cases), and antinucleolar antibodies (40 to 50% of cases). The last-named produce a characteristic "nucleolar pattern" of fluorescence in the indirect immunofluorescence assay (p. 181). Recently two antinuclear antibodies more or less unique to scleroderma have been described.[98] One of these reacts with a nonhistone nuclear protein called Scl-70 while the other is an anticentromere antibody. Although these two antibodies are not believed to be involved in the pathogenesis of scleroderma, they may prove to be useful diagnostic tools.[99] The anticentromere antibody is found in a much higher frequency in individuals with CREST syndrome, a variant of PSS that tends to remain localized to the skin for long periods (see p. 193).

The third hypothesis lays the primary blame on small blood vessels—the so-called microvascular hypothesis.[100] According to this, widespread damage to the small blood vessels and their subsequent narrowing leads to ischemic injury followed by scarring. In support of this hypothesis can be cited the narrowing of small arteries (150 to 500 μ in diameter) together with mononuclear infiltrates in the connective tissue seen early in the course of lesion development. Of interest is the demonstration that the vascular lesions in the kidney, to be described later, contain IgG and complement as well as antibody to nuclear antigens, thus suggesting that these are caused by immune complexes, as postulated for SLE.[101] Although these findings suggest immunologic injury of the vasculature, other investigators have described a poorly defined endothelial cell toxic factor in the serum of patients with PSS.[102] The microvascular hypothesis appears attractive because of its simplicity, but the evidence supporting its role in the pathogenesis of PSS is not particularly impressive.

MORPHOLOGY. Virtually all organs may be involved in PSS. The prominent changes occur in the skin, alimentary tract, musculoskeletal system, and kidneys; but lesions also are often present in the blood vessels, heart, lungs, and peripheral nerves. A great majority of patients have diffuse, sclerotic atrophy of the skin, which usually begins in the fingers and distal regions of the upper extremities and extends proximally to involve the upper arms, shoulders, neck, and face. In the early stages, affected skin areas are somewhat edematous and have a doughy consistency. Histologically there is edema and perivascular lymphocytic infiltrates, together with swelling and degeneration of collagen fibers, which become eosinophilic. Capillaries may show thickening of the basal lamina, endothelial cell damage, and partial occlusion.[103] With progression, the edematous phase is replaced by progressive fibrosis of the dermis, which becomes tightly bound to the subcutaneous structures. There is marked increase of compact collagen in the dermis along with thinning of the epidermis, loss of rete pegs, atrophy of the dermal appendages, and hyaline thickening of the walls of dermal arterioles and capillaries (Fig. 5–24). Often, pigmentation resulting from increased melanin in the basal layer of the epidermis darkens the areas. In advanced stages, the fingers take on a tapered, claw-like appearance with limitation of motion in the joints (Fig. 5–25), and the face becomes a drawn mask. Loss of blood supply may lead to cutaneous ulcerations and to atrophic changes in the terminal phalanges. Sometimes the tips of the fingers undergo autoamputation.

Alimentary Tract. The alimentary tract is affected in over half the patients. Progressive atrophy and collagenous fibrous replacement of the muscularis may develop at any level of the gut but is most severe in the esophagus (Fig. 5–26). The lower two-thirds of the esophagus often develops a rubber hose inflexibility and usually has the most marked narrowing. The mucosa may be thinned and ulcerated, and there is excessive collagenization of the lamina propria and submucosa. Similar changes occur in the walls of the small intestine and colon. Loss of villi and microvilli is the anatomic basis for the malabsorption syndrome sometimes encoun-

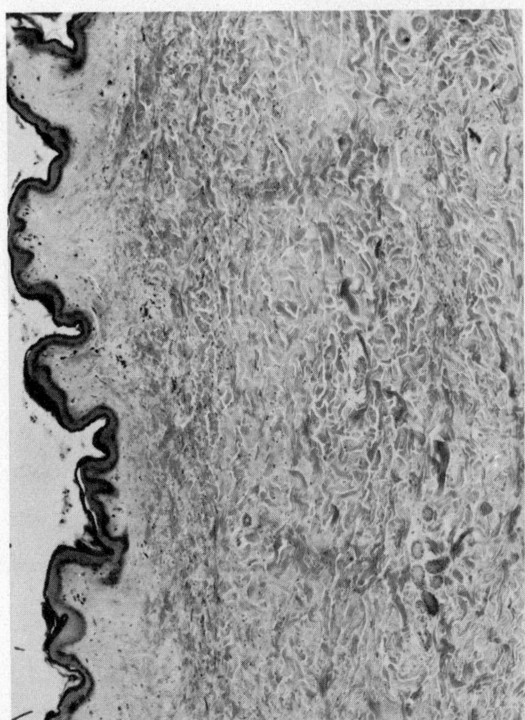

Figure 5–24. Scleroderma. Atrophy of skin with dense sclerosis of dermal tissue and atrophy of skin adnexa.

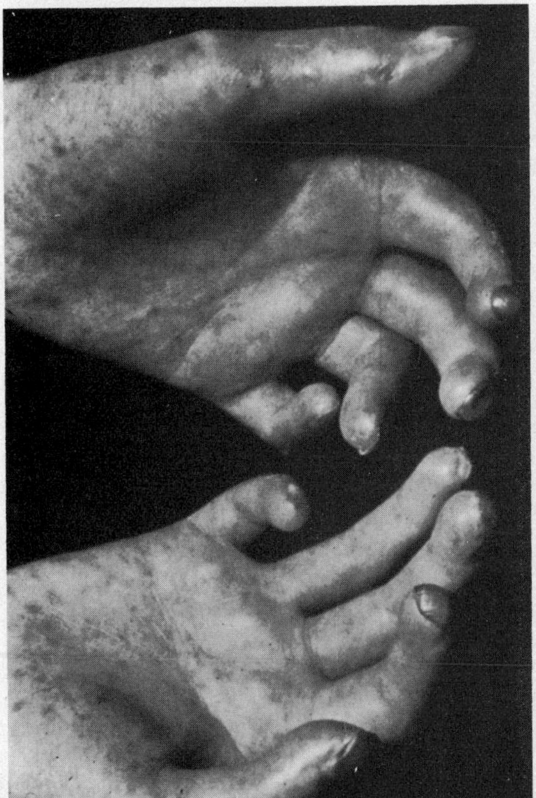

Figure 5–25. Advanced scleroderma. The extensive subcutaneous fibrosis has virtually immobilized the fingers, creating a clawlike flexion deformity.

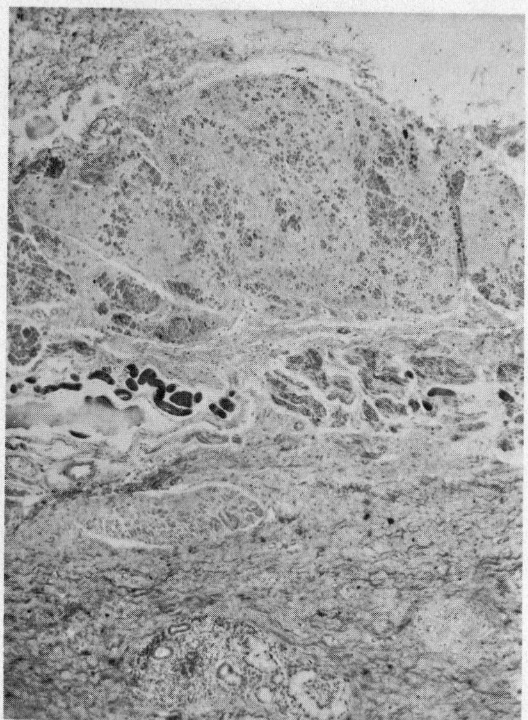

Figure 5–26. Extensive fibrous replacement of the musculature of the esophagus. Isolated striated muscle fibers of the pharyngeal constrictor muscles are present.

tered. Vessel walls contain perivascular mononuclear cell infiltrates and show hyaline collagenous thickening.

Musculoskeletal System. Inflammatory synovitis is common in PSS. The changes consist of infiltrates of lymphocytes and plasma cells, sometimes gathered into focal aggregates, associated with hypertrophy and hyperplasia of the synovial soft tissues. Fibrosis later ensues. It is evident that these changes are closely reminiscent of rheumatoid arthritis, but joint destruction is not common in PSS. As in polymyositis (p. 193), the muscles may be affected, beginning usually with the proximal groups. Interfiber edema and perivascular infiltrates of lymphocytes and plasma cells make up the early changes, followed by progressive interstitial fibrosis and sometimes regressive alterations in the fibers themselves. However, in systemic sclerosis, the primary change involves the interstitium, while in polymyositis, fiber damage is a prominent early lesion. Thickening of the basement membrane of the microcirculation and microvascular sclerosis accompany the interstitial fibrosis.

Kidneys. Renal abnormalities occur in two-thirds of patients with PSS.[104] The most prominent are those in the vessel walls. Interlobular arteries (150 to 500 μ in diameter) show intimal thickening as a result of deposition of mucinous or finely collagenous material, which stains histochemically for glycoprotein and acid mucopolysaccharides (Fig. 5–27). There is also concentric proliferation of intimal cells. These changes may resemble those seen in malignant hypertension, but it has been stressed that in scleroderma the alterations are restricted to vessels 150 to 500 μ in diameter and are not always associated with hypertension. Hypertension, however, occurs in 30% of patients with scleroderma, and in 7 to 10% takes an ominously malignant course (malignant hypertension). In hypertensive patients, vascular alterations are more pronounced and are often associated with fibrinoid necrosis involving the arterioles together with thrombosis and infarction. When this occurs it becomes difficult to differentiate the lesions of scleroderma from those of other types of malignant hypertension (p. 1046). Such patients often die of renal failure, which accounts for about 50% of deaths in patients with PSS. Glomerular changes are nonspecific and mainly consist of slightly increased cellularity of the mesangium and localized irregular thickening of the basement membrane. Some of these changes may be related to the hypertension.

Lungs. A diffuse interstitial and alveolar fibrosis may appear in the lungs, with variable fibrous thickening of small pulmonary vessels. In some instances the alveolar walls thicken, and in others there is an apparent distention of alveolar spaces and rupture of septa, leading to cystlike cavities. In other stages, honeycomb changes and severe interstitial fibrosis may ensue. Thus, patients with PSS have a pulmonary picture very much like that of idiopathic pulmonary fibrosis (p. 747), and indeed PSS must be considered in the differential diagnosis of diffuse pulmonary interstitial disease.

Other Organs. Small arterial lesions similar to those seen in the kidneys are present in many organs including the skin, muscle, gastrointestinal tract, pancreas, synovium, vasa vasorum, and central nervous system. In the heart, interstitial fibrosis with perivascular infiltrates can occur; the fibrosis may involve the conduction system, leading to AV conduction defects and arrhythmias, or may result in progressive cardiac failure. Sometimes a peripheral neuropathy occurs owing to loss of blood supply to the axis cyclinders, resulting from perineurial and vascular sclerosis.

CLINICAL COURSE. In most cases, the disease presents with symmetric edema and thickening of the hands

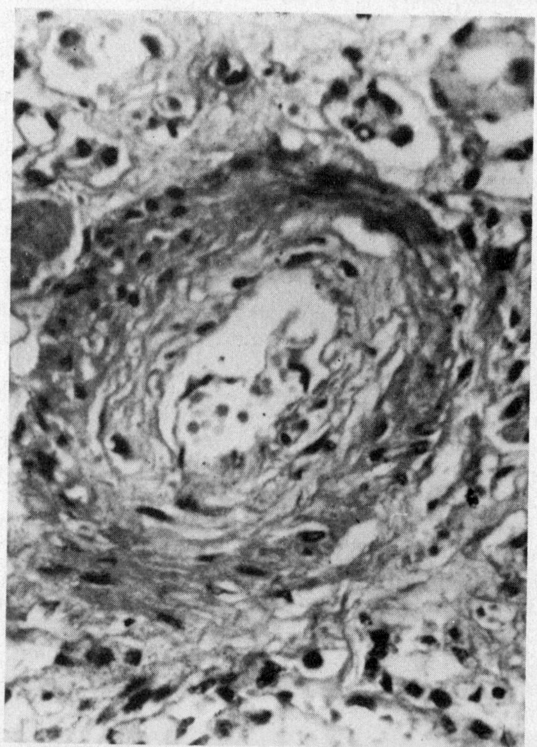

Figure 5–27. Scleroderma. Small renal artery showing intimal thickening.

and fingers or with Raynaud's phenomenon (p. 529). Articular manifestations in the form of pain and stiffness of the finger and knee joints may mimic rheumatoid arthritis. Dysphagia attributable to esophageal fibrosis is present in more than 50% of patients. Abdominal pain, intestinal obstruction, or malabsorption syndrome with weight loss and anemia reflect involvement of the small intestine. Respiratory difficulties due to the pulmonary fibrosis may result in right-sided cardiac dysfunction, and myocardial fibrosis may cause either arrhythmias or cardiac failure. Mild proteinuria occurs in up to 70% of patients, but rarely is the proteinuria so severe as to cause a nephrotic syndrome. The most ominous manifestation is malignant hypertension, with the subsequent development of fatal renal failure, but in its absence progression of the disease may be slow. The disease tends to be more severe in blacks, especially black females.

In recent years a somewhat benign variant of PSS has been recognized, the so-called CREST syndrome, characterized by calcinosis (C), Raynaud's phenomenon (R), esophageal dysfunction (E), sclerodactyly (S), telangiectasia (T), and the presence of anticentromere antibodies.[105] Patients with the CREST syndrome have relatively limited involvement of skin, often confined to fingers and face, and calcification of the subcutaneous tissues. Raynaud's phenomenon and involvement of skin are the initial manifestations and often the only manifestation for several years. Involvement of the viscera, including esophageal lesions, pulmonary hypertension, and biliary cirrhosis, occur late, and in general these patients live longer than those with PSS and diffuse visceral involvement at the outset.

Localized scleroderma, to be distinguished from PSS, is characterized by skin manifestations only. *Morphea* (one of the localized forms) refers to the presence of localized patches of violaceous or lilac, sometimes itchy skin lesions that may appear on any part of the body. Morphea may be widespread and chronic and may involve the fingers with contractures. Since the localized forms do not involve the internal organs, it is unlikely that they have any relationship to PSS.

POLYMYOSITIS-DERMATOMYOSITIS

Polymyositis refers to a chronic inflammatory myopathy of uncertain etiology. It is commonly discussed with the other connective tissue diseases because some patients have manifestations that mimic SLE, scleroderma, or rheumatoid arthritis, and by implication an immunologic origin is suspected. Although a rare disease, it is one of the more common myopathies. Muscular weakness is present in all cases, but in some it is accompanied by a prominent skin rash, termed "dermatomyositis."

The feature that distinguishes this disorder from other myopathies is the nature of the pathologic lesions in the muscles, i.e., degeneration of individual groups of muscle fibers accompanied by a prominent interstitial infiltrate of chronic inflammatory cells. The disease is most common in the 40- to 60-year-old age group, but a variant affecting children between the ages of 5 and 15 years is also recognized. Overall, females are affected about twice as often as males. The clinical expressions of polymyositis are extremely varied and so have been subclassified as follows:[106]

1. *Typical adult myositis*. This is a disease of insidious onset with symmetric weakness of proximal limb and trunk muscles, without dermatitis or with an atypical skin rash.

2. *Typical adult dermatomyositis*. This disorder is of acute or subacute onset, occurs in women, and is associated with a classic rash on the face and progressive muscular weakness.

3. *Dermatomyositis or polymyositis with malignancy*. The association of malignancy with polymyositis or dermatomyositis has long been apparent. The reported incidence of underlying malignancy varies from 9 to 14% depending on the design of the study.[106, 107] Higher incidence seems to be associated with dermatomyositis than with polymyositis. Children seem to be at less risk. The most common associated cancers are carcinoma of the lung and breast, but carcinomas of the stomach, kidney, uterus, and ovary and (rarely) lymphomas have been described. It is a curious fact that removal of cancer may result in clinical remission of the associated dermatomyositis.

4. *Childhood dermatomyositis*. This is an acute or chronic disease, usually with both myositis and rash. Widespread vasculitis of the skin leads to ulcerations and sometimes to calcifications; vasculitis within the gastrointestinal tract adds a prominent element of intestinal manifestations.

5. *Polymyositis or dermatomyositis with other connective tissue disorders*. In some patients the myositis is either preceded or followed by manifestations characteristic of scleroderma, arthritis, SLE, or Sjögren's syndrome.

ETIOLOGY AND PATHOGENESIS. Although the cause of the disease is unknown, its close association with other connective tissue diseases of presumed autoimmune etiology points to an immunologic origin. Some patients have antinuclear antibodies and rheumatoid factor, but the specificities of the antinuclear antibodies detected in this disease have not been fully defined. Most of the autoantibodies seem to react with extractable nuclear antigens, and preliminary data suggests that some of the antibodies (PM-1 and Jo-1) are found primarily in polymyositis-dermatomyositis.[63] Antibodies to purified human myoglobin have also been identified in the serum of some patients with polymyositis.[108] In childhood dermatomyositis, immune complexes, which may be responsible for vasculitis, have been detected within the circulation and blood vessels.[109]

There is also evidence suggesting cell-mediated immune reactions. Experimentally, polymyositis can be induced in guinea pigs or rats by injection of muscle homogenate in Freund's adjuvant, and the disease can be transferred by lymphocytes.[110] When incubated in skeletal muscle homogenates, lymphocytes from patients with polymyositis produce a lymphokine that is capable of lysing human fetal muscle in culture.[111] Whatever mechanism stimulates cell-mediated immunity to endogenous antigens (muscle) is as obscure as it is in other autoimmune diseases. Of interest, however, is the report of multiple cases within the same family, and the association of polymyositis with C2 deficiency[112] and with HLA-DR 3, suggesting that genetic factors may be involved in the pathogenesis.[113]

MORPHOLOGY

Striated Muscle. Involvement of striated muscles is present in all cases of polymyositis and dermatomyositis. The first groups to be affected are almost always the proximal muscles of the lower and upper extremities. Thereafter, the muscles of the pelvic and shoulder girdles, neck, posterior pharynx, intercostals, and diaphragm may be affected. In severe cases, the involvement may be more generalized.

At the onset, the muscles are normal in gross appearance, possibly slightly enlarged owing to diffuse edema. With advance of the disease, they become atrophic and yellowish-gray as the muscle fibers are replaced by fibrous tissue and fat. Histologically, the early changes comprise a slight interfiber edema, perhaps accompanied by a scant interstitial infiltrate of lymphocytes and histiocytes. In the full-blown stage of the disease, focal or extensive muscle fiber death becomes apparent in the form of vacuolation and fragmentation of the sarcoplasm. Usually readily evident is invasion of necrotic fibers by scavenger phagocytic cells engulfing the cellular debris. At this stage, a prominent mononuclear interstitial inflammatory infiltrate is apparent, sometimes focal, sometimes widespread. Regeneration of injured but surviving muscle cells may become apparent in the later stages, producing large vesicular sarcolemmal nuclei accompanied by sarcoplasmic basophilia (Fig. 5–28).[114] In advanced cases, fatty ingrowth and dense fibrosis (containing irregular amorphous deposits of calcium) replace large areas of muscle substance. Electron microscopy has yielded the findings that we would expect in cells undergoing severe injury and death. Focal degeneration of myofibrils, shredding of myofilaments, the formation of so-called "cytoplasmic" and "targetoid" bodies, and increased numbers of autophagic vacuoles and residual bodies have all been noted.

Skin. The typical skin rash of dermatomyositis occurs in about 40% of all patients with polymyositis. It takes the form of a dusky erythematous eruption on the malar eminences and bridge of the nose in a butterfly distribution, quite similar to that seen in SLE. However, the facial rash is frequently accompanied by a similar eruption on the V of the neck, forehead, and shoulders, and front and back of the upper chest. In some cases, a dusky lilac suffusion occurs on the upper eyelids, called the heliotrope rash, which is considered by some to be pathognomonic of dermatomyositis. Histologically, the early changes consist of slight edema in the dermis and a perivascular lymphocytic and histiocytic infiltrate, sometimes associated with overlying hyperkeratosis, parakeratosis, and liquefactive degeneration at the epidermal-dermal junction. Dermal atrophy, fibrosis, and calcification may ensue in the late stages.

Other Systems. In common with the other connective tissue diseases, many organs and systems may be affected. Articular reactions are not usually prominent but may closely resemble rheumatoid arthritis. Involvement of the viscera, including kidneys, lungs, and gastrointestinal tract, has been described in polymyositis.[115] In childhood forms of the disease, an acute necrotizing vasculitis resembling polyarteritis nodosa may be seen.

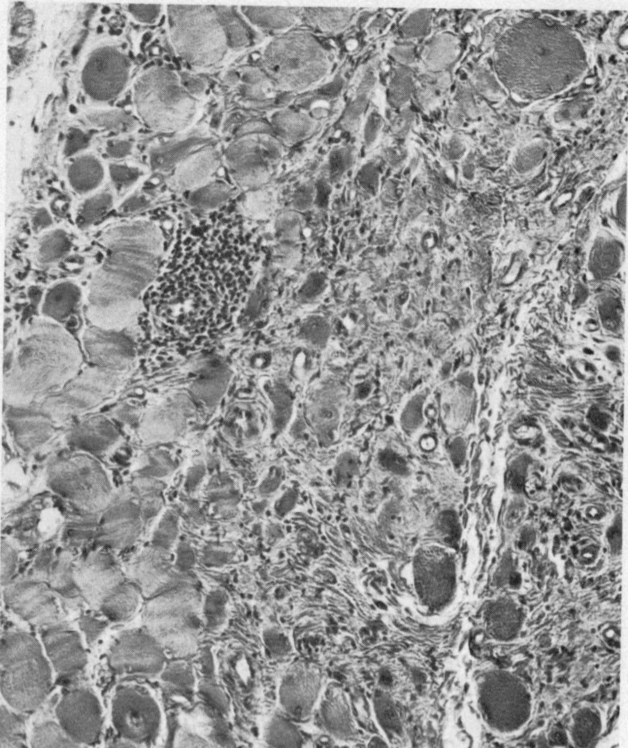

Figure 5–28. A section of striated muscle with interstitial fibrosis, leukocytic infiltration, muscle cell atrophy, and variability in muscle fiber size due to regenerative activity.

It is apparent that there are many morphologic similarities among the so-called connective tissue diseases. Myopathy may be found in SLE, rheumatoid arthritis, systemic sclerosis, and rheumatic fever as well as polymyositis. In all, an interstitial inflammatory reaction is present but not the extensive muscle fiber injury and necrosis seen in dermatomyositis. Similarly, acute arteritis is common to many but, of course, is most characteristic of polyarteritis nodosa. Although ischemic muscle damage may occur in polyarteritis, the myopathy is far more destructive in polymyositis and is disproportionate to the arterial involvement.

CLINICAL FEATURES. Muscle weakness, tenderness on palpation, muscular pain, and eventual motor disability are the most important clinical findings. The proximal nature of the muscular involvement helps to differentiate this disease from some of the dystrophies (p. 1308). In chronic cases, the patient may be confined to a wheelchair or bed. The skin rash may be followed by sufficient dermal fibrosis and skin atrophy to cause stiffness of the fingers. Raynaud's phenomenon occurs in about one-third of the patients. The involvement of joints is usually mild and rarely causes joint destruction. Dysphagia, due to involvement of the pharyngeal muscles, can be a disabling and serious clinical problem. When visceral involvement occurs, colicky abdominal pain and constipation complicate the musculoskeletal disability. The diagnosis depends on (1) demonstration of elevated serum enzymes derived from muscle (glutamic-oxaloacetic transaminase and aldolase), (2) detection of excessive creatinuria, (3) electromyographic evidence of muscle disease, and (4) morphologic confirmation of the nature of the muscle involvement. With regard to the biopsy, it must be recalled that the disease may be focal, and careful search must be made for appropriate biopsy sites in order to avoid a false-negative diagnosis.

MIXED CONNECTIVE TISSUE DISEASE (MCTD)

This term was coined in 1972 to describe a group of patients who were identified clinically by the coexistence of features suggestive of SLE, polymyositis, and scleroderma and serologically by high titers of antibodies to ribonucleoprotein (RNP), an extractable nuclear antigen.[116] Two other factors were initially considered important in lending distinctiveness to MCTD—the paucity of renal disease and an extremely good response to corticosteroids, both of which could be considered as indicative of a good long-term prognosis.

These patients may present with arthritis, swelling of the hands, Raynaud's phenomenon, abnormal esophageal motility, myositis, leukopenia, and anemia, fever, lymphadenopathy, and hypergammaglobulinemia. These manifestations suggest SLE, polymyositis, and scleroderma. The incidence ratio of females to males is 12:1, most patients presenting between the ages of 30 and 60. Although serologic overlap with SLE occurs, the unifying feature of MCTD is the speckled pattern of nuclei on immunofluorescence (p. 181) and the presence of antibodies against ribonucleoproteins in extremely high titers. Over the last ten years, as more patients with clinical and serologic features consistent with the diagnosis of MCTD have been identified, a controversy has developed over whether MCTD constitutes a distinct collagen disease or is a heterogeneous mixture of subsets of SLE, scleroderma, and polymyositis.[117] Several additional facts, some of which have emerged in long-term follow-up of patients with MCTD, are relevant to this issue: (1) The "overlap" of symptoms is not necessarily concurrent; often the appearance of symptoms more or less characteristic of SLE, scleroderma, polymyositis, or even rheumatoid arthritis is sequential.[118] (2) A small but definite proportion (5 to 10%) of the patients develop renal disease.[119] (3) Long-term prognosis with steroid or other therapy does not appear to be distinctly superior to that of other related diseases. (4) In the follow-up of the original patients there appeared to be a tendency for evolution into progressive systemic sclerosis. (5) Not everyone with high titer anti-RNP antibodies has clinical features of MCTD. "Typical" cases of SLE as well as scleroderma also have a high frequency of anti-RNP antibodies. Conversely, all patients with "overlap" symptoms do not have high anti-RNP titers.

Those who continue to support the notion of MCTD as a distinct disorder argue that whereas the presence of anti-RNP antibody by itself is not diagnostic, the associated absence of antibodies to native DNA and Sm antigen, which characterize SLE, is important in defining MCTD. Although the precise incidence of nephritis in patients with MCTD is not known, the incidence of severe nephritis, destructive arthritis, or severe CNS involvement is distinctly less than that in classical SLE. On balance it seems that the status of MCTD as a distinct entity will remain unresolved until careful long-term prospective studies with clearly defined clinical, serologic, and genetic criteria are performed.

POLYARTERITIS NODOSA (PN) AND OTHER VASCULITIDES

Polyarteritis nodosa belongs to a group of diseases characterized by necrotizing inflammation of the walls of blood vessels and showing strong evidence of an immunologic pathogenetic mechanism. The general term *noninfectious necrotizing vasculitis* differentiates these conditions from those due to direct infection of the blood vessel wall (such as occurs in the wall of an abscess) and serves to emphasize that any type of vessel may be involved—arteries, veins, or capillaries.

Noninfectious necrotizing vasculitis is encountered in many clinical settings. Many classifications are available, and these depend on the size of the involved blood vessels, the anatomic site, the histologic character of the lesion, or the clinical manifestations.[120] A detailed classification and description of vasculitides is presented in the chapter on the diseases of blood vessels, where the immunologic mechanisms are also discussed (p. 520).

POSSIBLE IMMUNE DISORDERS

Immunologic mechanisms are suspected of contributing to a large number of diseases in addition to those already described in this chapter. Some of these entities will be discussed in the chapters dealing with individual organs and systems. One disease—amyloidosis—requires description at this point. New observations provide strong evidence that some derangement in the immune apparatus underlies this disease, and as a systemic disease it cannot be assigned to any single organ or system.

AMYLOIDOSIS

Amyloid is a pathologic proteinaceous substance, deposited between cells in various tissues and organs of the body in a wide variety of clinical settings. Because amyloid deposition appears so insidiously, and sometimes mysteriously, its clinical recognition ultimately depends on morphologic identification of this distinctive substance in appropriate biopsies. Macroscopically, painting the cut surface of affected organs with an iodine solution imparts to sufficiently large deposits of amyloid a yellow-red color that is transformed into blue or violet after the application of dilute sulfuric acid. This technique was first employed over a century ago by Virchow, who interpreted the results to be starchlike, hence the designation "amyloid." *With the light microscope and standard tissue stains, amyloid appears as an amorphous, eosinophilic, hyaline, extracellular substance that, with progressive accumulation, encroaches on and produces pressure atrophy of adjacent cells.* To differentiate amyloid from other hyalin deposits (e.g., collagen, fibrin) a variety of histochemical techniques (p. 201) are employed. Perhaps most widely used is the Congo red stain, which under ordinary light imparts to tissue deposits a pink or red color, but far more dramatic and specific is the green birefringence of the stained amyloid when observed by polarizing microscopy (Fig. 5–29).

The clinical circumstances under which amyloidosis appears as well as the distribution of the deposits throughout the body are extremely varied. Numerous attempts have been made to discern clinical and anatomic categories within the wide range of presentations, but with only limited success. In the past, classifications depended principally on presumed patterns of distribution of deposits among the organs of the body. One putative pattern involved mainly the heart, gastrointestinal tract, skin, nerves, and tongue and was encountered largely in patients free of any concomitant or underlying disease, hence its designation as *primary amyloidosis*. Another variant encountered in patients with some chronic inflammatory disease was referred to as *secondary amyloidosis*, with major involvement of the liver, spleen, kidneys, and adrenals. There are, however, innumerable discrepancies and overlaps in these categories, although (as will be seen) they possess a germ of truth. More recently, attention has been directed to the chemical composition and origins of amyloid as possible bases for classification. Despite the fact that all deposits have uniform appearance and tinctorial characteristics, *it is quite clear that amyloid is not a chemically distinct entity*. There are two major and several minor biochemical forms. These are deposited by several different pathogenetic mechanisms, and therefore amyloidosis should not be considered a single disease; rather, it is a group of diseases sharing in common the deposition of similar-appearing proteins. At the heart of the morphologic uniformity is the remarkably uniform physical organization of amyloid protein, which we will consider first. This will be followed by a discussion of the chemical nature of amyloid.

PHYSICAL NATURE OF AMYLOID. Although amyloid has a remarkably bland, uninteresting appearance under the light microscope, high resolution has disclosed a remarkably complex substructure.[121] *The amorphous deposits are in fact largely made up of nonbranching fibrils of indefinite length and a width of approximately 7.5 to 10 nm* (Fig. 5–30). This electron microscopic structure is identical in all types of amyloidosis. The fibrils may appear singly, in laterally aggregated bundles, or in an interlocking meshwork. In addition to these nonbranching slender fibrils, a minor second

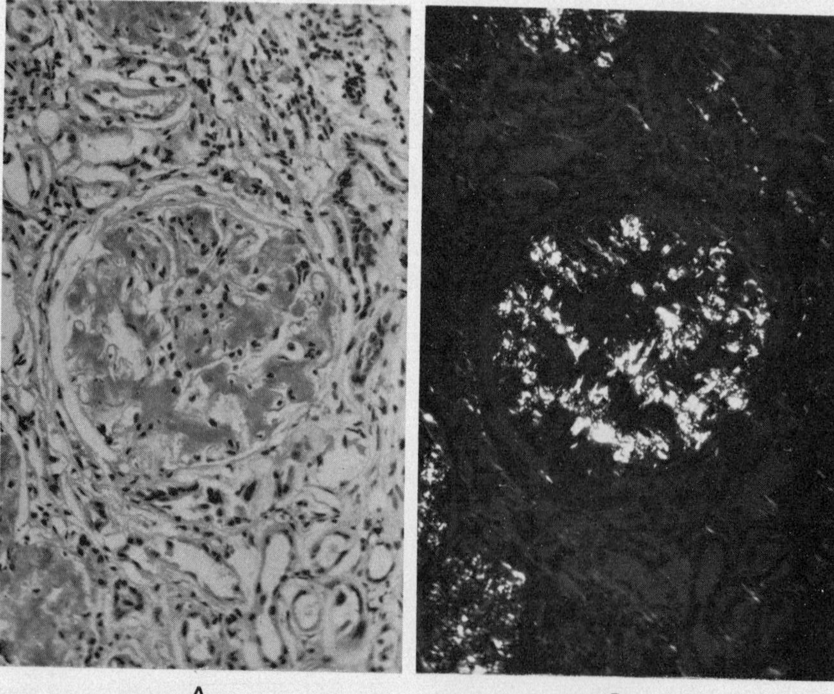

Figure 5–29. *A*, Amyloidosis of the glomerulus. *B*, Note birefringence of the deposits after Congo red staining. (From Cohen, A. S.: The constitution and genesis of amyloid. Int. Rev. Exp. Pathol. *4*:172, 1965.)

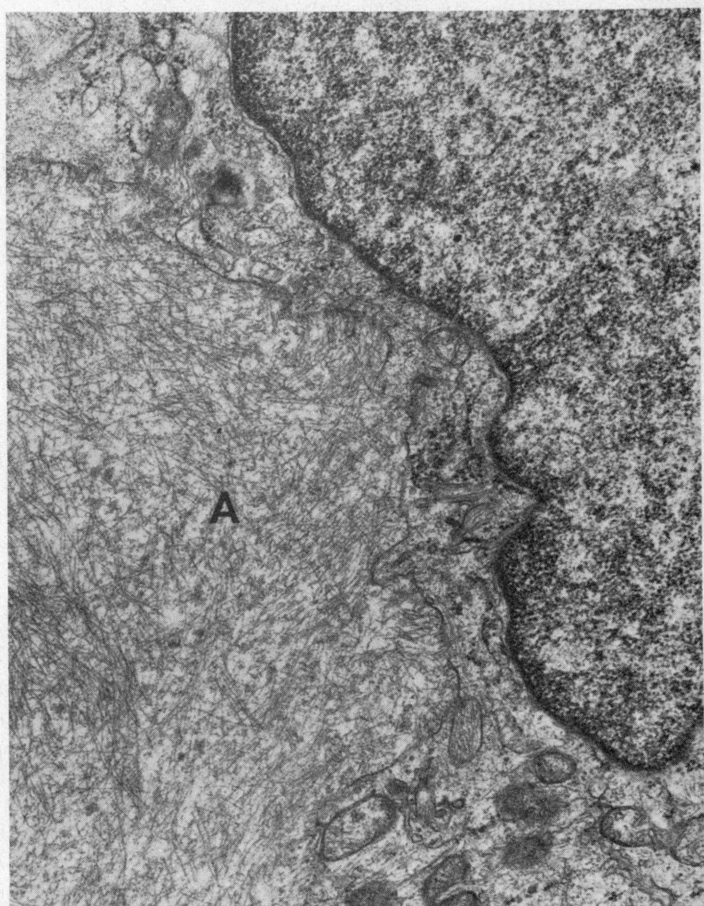

Figure 5–30. Amyloidosis of the spleen under the electron microscope. The amyloid deposit *(A)* adjacent to a reticular cell contains a feltwork of delicate fibrils (×22,500). (From Cohen, A. S.: The constitution and genesis of amyloid. Int. Rev. Exp. Pathol. *4*:178, 1965.)

component is always present in amyloid, known as the P component. Under the electron microscope it appears as a pentagonal, doughnut-shaped structure having an external diameter of approximately 9 nm and an internal diameter of 4 nm. Each pentagon is composed in turn of five globular subunits. Stacking of these "doughnuts" may create short rods.

It now appears to be reasonably well established that *the major factor responsible for the optical features by which amyloid deposits are classically identified in histologic section is the physicochemical aggregation of amyloid fibrils, yielding a "cross-β" pleated sheet on x-ray crystallographic analysis.*[122] Stated in another way, any fibrillar protein deposition that yields a β-pleated sheet will give rise to what is recognized as amyloid. This physicochemical aggregation gives to amyloid its polariscopic characteristics. The increased intensity of the birefringence of Congo red–stained amyloid is related to the high order of regularity and parallelism of the dye molecules bound to the aggregated fibrils.

Chemical Nature of Amyloid. Major advances in our understanding of amyloidosis have emerged from the clarification of the chemical structure of amyloid fibril proteins that constitute approximately 90% of the amyloid material, the remaining 10% being the P component, which is a glycoprotein.[122, 123] *Two chemically and antigenically distinct major classes of amyloid fibril proteins have been identified; one called AL (amyloid light chain) is derived from plasma cells (immunocytes) and contains immunoglobulin light chains; the other, designated AA (amyloid associated), is a unique non-immunoglobulin protein of uncertain origin.*

These two amyloid proteins are deposited in distinct clinicopathologic settings. The AL protein is made up of complete immunoglobulin light chains, the *N*-terminus of light chains, or both. Most of the AL proteins analyzed are composed of λ light chains or their fragments, but in some cases κ chains have been identified. As might be expected, the amyloid fibril protein of the AL type is produced by immunoglobulin-secreting cells, and their deposition is associated with some form of B-cell dyscrasia. The archetype is multiple myeloma, a tumor of plasma cells that may be associated with the deposition of amyloid of the AL type. In multiple myeloma it can be demonstrated that the amyloid fibril protein is derived from the circulating light chains (i.e., Bence Jones protein, p. 689). In fact, Glenner has been able to create a fibrillar precipitate that has the typical ultrastructure of amyloid fibrils by proteolytic digestion of λ Bence-Jones proteins in vitro.[122]

The second major class of amyloid fibril protein (AA) does not have structural homology to any known protein. It has a molecular weight of 8500 and consists of 76 amino acid residues. The AA protein is found in those clinical settings alluded to earlier as "secondary amyloidosis." AA fibrils are believed to be derived from a larger precursor in the serum called SAA (serum amyloid associated) protein. SAA is an α_1-globulin that is antigenically related to the AA protein, and has a molecular weight of 160,000–180,000. In the serum it is associated with a high-density lipoprotein from which a smaller 12,000–14,000 dalton subunit can be obtained.[124] Amino acid sequencing of this subunit has revealed that SAA is identical to AA for at least the first 55 amino acid residues, suggesting strongly that AA is derived from SAA by proteolytic cleavage.[123]

Two other biochemically distinct proteins have been found in amyloid deposits.[122] The normal plasma protein prealbumin seems to be the major protein constituent of amyloid in fairly diverse clinical settings. These include the Portugese and Swedish polyneuropathic forms of familial amyloidosis,[125, 126] senile cardiac amyloidosis,[127] and senile cerebral amyloid.[128] The other uncommon form of amyloid protein deposited within the medullary carcinoma of thyroid shares chemical structure with the hormone calcitonin and is believed to be derived from the prohormone form of thyrocalcitonin.

The P component is distinct from the amyloid fibrils but is closely associated with them in all forms of amyloidosis. It constitutes approximately 10% of the amyloid substance and has been found to be identical to a normal α_1 serum glycoprotein. It has a molecular weight of 180,000–220,000 daltons and a striking structural homology with C-reactive protein, which is an acute-phase reactant.

Classification of Amyloidosis. Amyloidosis has been classified in a variety of ways. On the basis of tissue distribution of amyloid deposits, one could classify amyloid into *generalized*, involving several organ systems, or *localized*, when the deposits are limited to a single organ or tissue such as the heart. Traditionally, a generalized pattern of amyloid deposition has been subclassified into *primary amyloidosis* when no obvious predisposing cause could be discerned, or *secondary amyloidosis* when it was found in association with chronic inflammatory conditions. Amyloidosis associated with multiple myeloma has usually been granted a separate category since the pattern of tissue involvement more closely resembles primary amyloidosis, although it is secondary to a known predisposing condition. The *hereditary forms* of amyloidosis constitute a separate, albeit heterogeneous, group since the individual inherited forms have their own distinctive patterns of organ involvement. Some of the difficulties encountered in finding appropriate "pigeon holes" for the diverse settings in which amyloid is deposited in the tissues are understandable. Amyloidosis, we now know, is not a single disease except by morphologic criteria, and therefore it seems logical to take into account the chemical nature of the amyloid fibril proteins in arriving at a scientifically accurate and clinically useful classification. The so-called primary amyloidosis and myeloma-associated amyloidosis may be grouped into a single category of *immunocyte-derived amyloidosis*, since an overt or covert disorder of B cells underlies the deposition of AL proteins in all these cases. The term secondary amyloidosis, used to designate amyloidosis associated with chronic inflammatory disorders, may best be replaced by the term *reactive systemic amyloidosis* as suggested by Glenner, since even the so-called primary amyloidosis is secondary to B-cell dyscrasias.[122] A schema based on our current knowledge of amyloidosis is presented in Table 5–6.

Immunocyte Dyscrasias with Amyloidosis. Amyloidosis in this category is usually systemic in distribution and is of the AL type. In many of these cases, the patients have some form of plasma cell dyscrasia. Best defined is the occurrence of systemic amyloidosis in 5 to 15% of patients with multiple myeloma, a form of plasma cell neoplasia characterized by multiple osteolytic lesions throughout the skeletal system (p. 689). The cancerous plasma cells in multiple myeloma characteristically synthesize abnormal amounts of a single specific immunoglobulin (monoclonal gammopathy), producing an M (myeloma) protein spike on serum electrophoresis. In addition to the synthesis of whole immunoglobulin molecules, only the light chains (referred to as Bence Jones protein) of either the kappa or the lambda variety may be elaborated and found in the serum. By virtue of the small molecular size of the Bence Jones protein, it is frequently excreted in the urine. Almost all the patients with myeloma who develop amyloidosis have Bence Jones proteins in the serum or urine or both, but it should be remembered that a great majority of myeloma patients who have free light chains do not develop amyloidosis. Clearly, therefore, the presence of Bence Jones proteins, although necessary, is by itself not enough to produce amyloidosis. We shall discuss later the other factors relating to the pathogenesis of amyloidosis (p. 200). Amyloidosis may also be encountered in a variety of other B-cell neoplasms that are much less common. These include Waldenström's macroglobulinemia, heavy-chain disease, solitary plasmacytomas, and nodular malignant lymphoma.[122] All these conditions are examples of a monoclonal gammopathy.

The great majority of patients with AL amyloid do not have classic multiple myeloma or any other overt B-cell neoplasm; such cases have been traditionally classified as "primary amyloidosis" since their clinical features derive from the effects of amyloid deposition without any other associated disease. However, in a vast majority of such cases, monoclonal immunoglobulins and/or free light chains can be found in the serum or urine.[128A] Most of these patients also have a modest increase in the number of plasma cells in the bone marrow, which presumably secrete the precursors of AL protein. Clearly, these patients have an underlying B-cell dyscrasia ("covert myeloma") in which production of an abnormal protein, rather than production of tumor masses, is the predominant manifestation. Whether the condition of most of these patients would evolve into

Table 5–6. CLASSIFICATION OF AMYLOIDOSIS

Clinicopathologic Category	Associated Diseases	Major Fibril Protein	Chemically Related Protein
Immunocyte dyscrasias with amyloidosis	Multiple myeloma, monoclonal gammopathy, and other B-cell neoplasms	AL	Immunoglobulin light chains
Reactive systemic amyloidosis	Chronic inflammatory conditions, Hodgkins disease, and other nonlymphoid solid tumors	AA	SAA
Hereditary amyloidosis (several subtypes)			
1. Familial Mediterranean fever		AA	SAA
2. Neuropathic forms (several),			
e.g., Portuguese		AF_p	Prealbumin
Swedish		AF_s	Prealbumin
Localized			
1. Endocrine,			
e.g., Medullary carcinoma		AE_t	Thyrocalcitonin
2. Senile,			
e.g., Cardiac		AS_c	Prealbumin
Cerebral		AS*	Prealbumin

*Nomenclature of fibril protein not established.

Based on Glenner, G. G.: Amyloid deposits and amyloidosis. The β-fibrilloses. N. Eng. J. Med. *302*:1283, 1980; and Husby, G.: A chemical classification of amyloid. Correlation with different types of amyloidosis. Scand. J. Rheumatol. *9*:60, 1980.

AL = amyloid light chain; AA = amyloid associated (protein); AF = amyloid familial; AF_p = AF Portuguese; AF_s = AF Swedish; AE_t = amyloid endocrine, thyroid; AS = amyloid senile; AS_c = AS cardiac.

multiple myeloma if they lived long enough can only be a matter for speculation.

Reactive Systemic Amyloidosis. The amyloid deposits in this pattern are systemic in distribution and are composed of AA protein. This category is commonly referred to as "secondary amyloidosis" since it is believed to be secondary to the associated inflammatory condition. The feature common to most of the conditions associated with reactive systemic amyloidosis is protracted breakdown of cells resulting from a wide variety of infectious and noninfectious chronic inflammatory conditions. At one time tuberculosis, bronchiectasis, and chronic osteomyelitis were the most important underlying conditions, but with the advent of effective antimicrobial chemotherapy the importance of these conditions has diminished. More commonly now, reactive systemic amyloidosis complicates rheumatoid arthritis, other connective tissue disorders such as dermatomyositis and scleroderma, and inflammatory bowel disease, particularly regional enteritis and ulcerative colitis. Among these, the most frequent associated condition is rheumatoid arthritis. Amyloidosis is reported to occur in 14 to 26% of patients with rheumatoid arthritis.[129] These figures obtained from autopsy studies may be somewhat higher than the true frequency of amyloidosis in an unselected group of rheumatoid arthritis patients. Reactive systemic amyloidosis may occur in association with non–immunocyte-derived tumors, the two most common being renal cell carcinoma and Hodgkin's disease.

Heredofamilial Amyloidosis. A variety of familial forms of amyloidosis have been described. Most of them are rare and occur in limited geographic areas. The most common and best studied is an autosomal recessive condition called *familial Mediterranean fever*. This is a febrile disorder of unknown cause characterized by attacks of fever accompanied by inflammation of serosal surfaces, including peritoneum, pleura, and synovial membrane. This disorder is encountered largely in individuals of Armenian, Sephardic Jewish, and Arabic origins. It is associated with widespread tissue involvement indistinguishable from reactive systemic amyloidosis. Quite interestingly, the amyloid fibril proteins are identical to AA proteins, suggesting that they may be related to the recurrent bouts of inflammation that characterize this disease.

In addition to familial Mediterranean fever, which as stated is autosomal recessive, a large number of obscure hereditary disorders having autosomal dominant modes of transmission are associated with fairly specific patterns of organ involvement. They are so rare that none merits specific description. Suffice it that they can be broken down into the following categories based on the principal sites of amyloid deposition: (1) neuropathies, (2) nephropathies, (3) cardiopathies, and (4) miscellaneous. Familial clusters within each of these categories have been described in different parts of the world. For example, neuropathic amyloidosis has been identified in individuals in Portugal, Japan, Sweden, and the United States. As mentioned previously, in two of the neuropathic forms (Portuguese and Swedish) the amyloid fibril has been characterized as being related to serum prealbumin.

Localized Amyloidosis. Sometimes amyloid deposits are limited to a single organ or tissue without involvement of any other site in the body. The deposits may produce grossly detectable nodular masses or be evident only on microscopic examination. Nodular (tumor-forming) deposits of amyloid are most often encountered in the lung, larynx, skin, urinary bladder, tongue, and region of the eye.[128A] Frequently there are infiltrates of lymphocytes and plasma cells in the periphery of these amyloid masses, raising the question of whether the mononuclear infiltrate is a response to the deposition of amyloid or instead is responsible for it. At least in some cases the amyloid consists of AL protein[122] and may therefore represent a localized form of immunocyte-derived amyloid. However, not enough information is available to enable generalizations to be made about the nature of localized amyloid.

Microscopic deposits of localized amyloid may be found in tissues and tumors of the APUD system: medullary carcinoma of the thyroid gland, islet tumors of the pancreas, pheochromocytomas, and undifferentiated carcinomas of the stomach and in the islets of Langerhans in patients with diabetes mellitus. In all these settings it is suspected that the amyloidogenic proteins are derived by enzymic conversion of the polypeptide hormones or prohormones. This is confirmed in at least one case: medullary carcinoma of the thyroid, in which the amyloid material seems to be related to the hormone thyrocalcitonin.

Amyloid of Aging. There is a well-documented correlation between amyloid deposition and aging. In elderly patients (usually in the eighth and ninth decades of life) amyloid deposits can often be found in the heart, brain, pancreas, and spleen.[130] Although in many instances the amyloidosis does not produce clinical disease, cardiac amyloidosis, as will be pointed out, can become sufficiently advanced to be grossly evident and cause serious cardiac dysfunction. Chemically, both senile cardiac and cerebral amyloid have been found to be related to prealbumin.

PATHOGENESIS OF AMYLOID FORMATION. It is now generally accepted that the two major forms of amyloid proteins, AL and AA, are derived from proteolytic cleavage of their precusor proteins, immunoglobulin light chains and SAA, respectively.[122, 131] But several questions remain unanswered. What triggers the production of amyloidogenic precursors? What are the cells and sites involved in the degradation of the precursor proteins? Why do only a small fraction of those at risk develop amyloidosis? At present we can only make "intelligent guesses."

Taking first the case of reactive systemic amyloidosis, we know that patients with chronic inflammatory diseases have elevated serum levels of SAA. Thus, it may be presumed that an excess of the precursor is related to the formation of amyloid. Unfortunately, the situation is much more complex. SAA behaves as an acute-phase reactant, and although its serum concentration in healthy individuals is very low, the levels rise several hundred–fold within 24 hours of acute inflammatory stimuli. The major site of synthesis of SAA, at least during the acute-phase reaction, is the liver.[124] Experimentally, it is possible to stimulate the production of hepatic SAA by a soluble factor released by activated macrophages. In chronic inflammation, therefore, it could be conjectured that increased production of SAA is in response to sustained activation of macrophages. However, it is not yet clear whether liver is the only site of SAA production. Granulocytes, fibroblasts, and spleen have also been implicated. Increased production of SAA may be an important risk factor in the pathogenesis of amyloidosis, but its breakdown also appears to be involved. Although the exact mechanism by which SAA is metabolized is not clear, it has been reported that membrane-bound serine esterases of blood monocytes can degrade SAA.[132] It is conceivable, then, that some acquired or genetic defect in the monocyte-mediated degradation of SAA may result in its incomplete cleavage into insoluble AA intermediates. In addition to the monocyte-related proteolysis, a poorly defined serum factor capable of degrading AA proteins in vitro has also been demonstrated. Preliminary reports suggest that the serum amyloid degrading activity is reduced in patients with amyloidosis associated with rheumatoid arthritis and familial Mediterranean fever.[133, 134] Another factor relevant to the handling of SAA may be the type of SAA formed. On the basis of physicochemical characteristics, at least six species of SAA proteins have been discovered.[124] Whether some are more prone to abnormal degradation, and thus more amyloidogenic, remains to be investigated.

The case of immunocyte-derived amyloid (AL) is somewhat less complex. We know with certainty both the source and the identity of the precursor proteins (i.e., immunoglobulin light chains). As already discussed, the derivation of amyloid-like fibrils from Bence Jones proteins in vitro has also been demonstrated. Unknown, however, is why only a small fraction of individuals with circulating free light chains develop amyloidosis. Conceivably some light chains are more amyloidogenic than others. In addition to their amyloidogenic potential, the subsequent cleavage of light chains may also be important, as discussed above.

In summary, both the overproduction of precursor proteins, and their defective degradation, seem to be involved in the pathogenesis of amyloid fibril formation.[131] Since the amyloid fibrils are insoluble in physiologic fluids, it must be that the process of fibrillogenesis takes place in proximity to the sites of deposition. The cells involved in the conversion of the precursor proteins into the fibrils are not fully characterized, but macrophages seem to be the most likely candidates. Whether the conversion of the soluble precursors into amyloid occurs intracellularly within phagocytes or close to the plasma membrane in the ground substance is not yet resolved.

MORPHOLOGY. There are no consistent or distinctive patterns of organ or tissue distribution of amyloid deposits in any of the categories cited. Nonetheless, a few generalizations can be made. Amyloidosis secondary to chronic inflammatory disorders tends to yield the most severe systemic involvements. Kidneys, liver, spleen, lymph nodes, adrenals, and thyroid, as well as many other tissues, are classically involved. Although immunocyte-associated amyloidosis cannot reliably be distinguished from the secondary form by its organ distribution, more often it involves the heart, gastrointestinal tract, peripheral nerves, skin, and tongue. In addition, bizarre distributions, such as amyloidosis of the eye and respiratory tract, are encountered more often in patients with immunocyte-associated amyloidosis. However, the same organs affected by reactive systemic amyloidosis (secondary amyloidosis), including kidneys, liver, and spleen, may also contain deposits in the immunocyte-associated form of the disease. Certain common features characterize amyloidosis wherever it is deposited. When present in only small amounts, it produces no apparent gross abnormalities. Often the presence of small amounts of amyloid is not suspected macroscopically until after the surface of the cut organ is painted with iodine and sulfuric acid. With larger amounts the involved organ often assumes a rubbery, firm consistency and a waxy, gray appearance.

Histologically, the depositions always begin between cells, often closely adjacent to basement membranes. With progression, and as the amount of amyloid accumulates, nodular masses fuse and encroach on neighboring cells. In the advanced stages of this process, large masses of amyloid completely entrap and, in time, destroy the cellular constituents of the involved organ.

The histologic diagnosis of amyloid is based almost entirely on its staining characteristics. The most commonly used staining technique utilizes the dye Congo red, which under ordinary light imparts a pink or red color to amyloid deposits. Under polarized light the Congo red–stained amyloid shows a green birefringence (Fig. 5–29). This reaction is shared by all forms of amyloid and is due to the cross-β-pleated configuration of amyloid fibrils. A recent report suggests that AA and AL amyloid can be distinguished in histologic sections. AA protein loses affinity for Congo red after incubation of tissue sections with potassium permanganate, whereas AL proteins and other chemical forms of amyloid do not.[135] Other methods of differentiating amyloid from hyaline deposits include somewhat less specific histochemical techniques. For example, amyloid is metachromatic (violet to pink) with crystal or methyl violet. It yields secondary fluorescence in ultraviolet light with the dyes thioflavine T and S. For routine diagnosis, birefringence after Congo red staining is the most widely practiced and reliable tool. Confirmation can be obtained by electron microscopy. AA protein (unlike AL protein) is not denatured by formalin fixation, and hence it is possible to identify this specific form of amyloidosis in paraffin-embed-

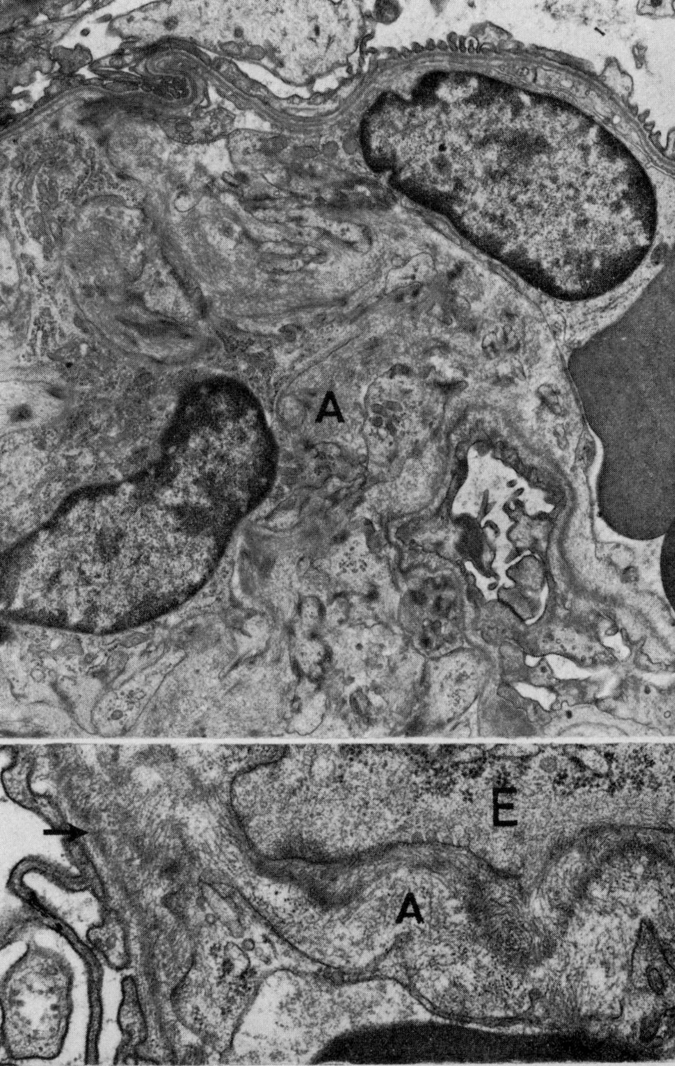

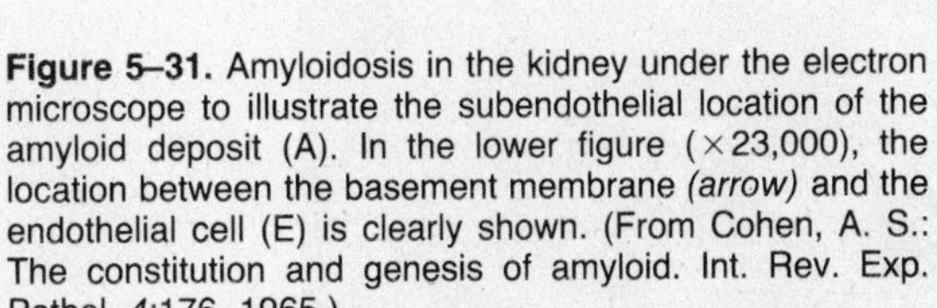
Figure 5–31. Amyloidosis in the kidney under the electron microscope to illustrate the subendothelial location of the amyloid deposit (A). In the lower figure (×23,000), the location between the basement membrane *(arrow)* and the endothelial cell (E) is clearly shown. (From Cohen, A. S.: The constitution and genesis of amyloid. Int. Rev. Exp. Pathol. *4*:176, 1965.)

ded tissue sections by the immunoperoxidase method, or by extraction and subsequent chemical analyses.[136]

Since the pattern of organ involvement in different clinical forms of amyloidosis is variable, each of the major organ involvements will be described separately.

Kidney. Amyloidosis of the kidney is the most common and potentially the most serious form of organ involvement. In most reported series of patients with amyloidosis, renal amyloidosis is the major cause of death. On gross inspection, the kidney may appear normal in size and color or it may be enlarged, pale gray, and firm. Often the cortical surface shows a slight undulation due to subcapsular masses of amyloid. It is not unusual, however, for the kidney to be shrunken and contracted even in the absence of other intercurrent nephropathies. This contraction is attributable to vascular narrowing induced by the deposition of amyloid within arterial and arteriolar walls.

Histologically, the selective sites of amyloid involvement are primarily the glomeruli, but the interstitial peritubular tissue, arteries, and arterioles are also affected. The glomerular deposits first appear as subtle thickenings of the mesangial matrix, accompanied usually by barely discernible, uneven widening of the basement membranes of the glomerular capillaries. In time, the mesangial depositions and the depositions along the basement membranes cause capillary narrowing and distort the glomerular vascular tuft. With the electron microscope, the fibrillar accumulations begin on the endothelial side of the basement membrane and then appear to flood over the basement membrane to abut the contiguous podocytes (Fig. 5–31). In many instances, the epithelial cells lose their foot processes. With progression of the glomerular amyloidosis, the endothelial cells are enveloped, the capillary lumina are obliterated, and the obsolescent glomerulus is flooded by confluent masses or interlacing broad ribbons of amyloid (Fig. 5–32). Often the enlarged damaged vascular tufts obliterate the urinary space, and with time all normal architecture is wiped out.

The peritubular deposits also begin in apposition to the tubular basement membranes, and progressively extend into the intertubular connective tissue as well as encroach on the tubular lumina. The overlying tubular epithelium may be unaffected or may undergo regressive changes. Often, proteinaceous casts fill these tubular lumina. In cases of myeloma-associated amyloidosis, the casts sometimes exhibit birefringence with Congo red stain, suggesting that they are composed of amyloid proteins. The vascular involvement takes the form of pink, hyaline thickening of arterial and arteriolar walls, often with narrowing of the lumina. With such ischemia, widespread tubular atrophy and interstitial fibrosis superimpose themselves upon the basic deformity produced by the amyloidosis.

Spleen. Amyloidosis of the spleen may be inapparent grossly or may cause moderate-to-marked splenomegaly (up to 800 gm). It is believed that the amyloid deposits begin in the perifollicular regions, but almost always, by the time they are observed in postmortem studies, the deposits are far more widespread. For completely mysterious reasons, one of two patterns emerges. In one the deposit is largely limited to the splenic follicles, producing tapioca-like granules on gross inspection, designated "sago" spleen. Microscopy indicates that the amyloid is laid down in a lacy pattern surrounding individual or nests of follicular cells, but eventually in more marked cases it fuses into a conglomerate mass, replacing the follicle. In the other pattern, the amyloid

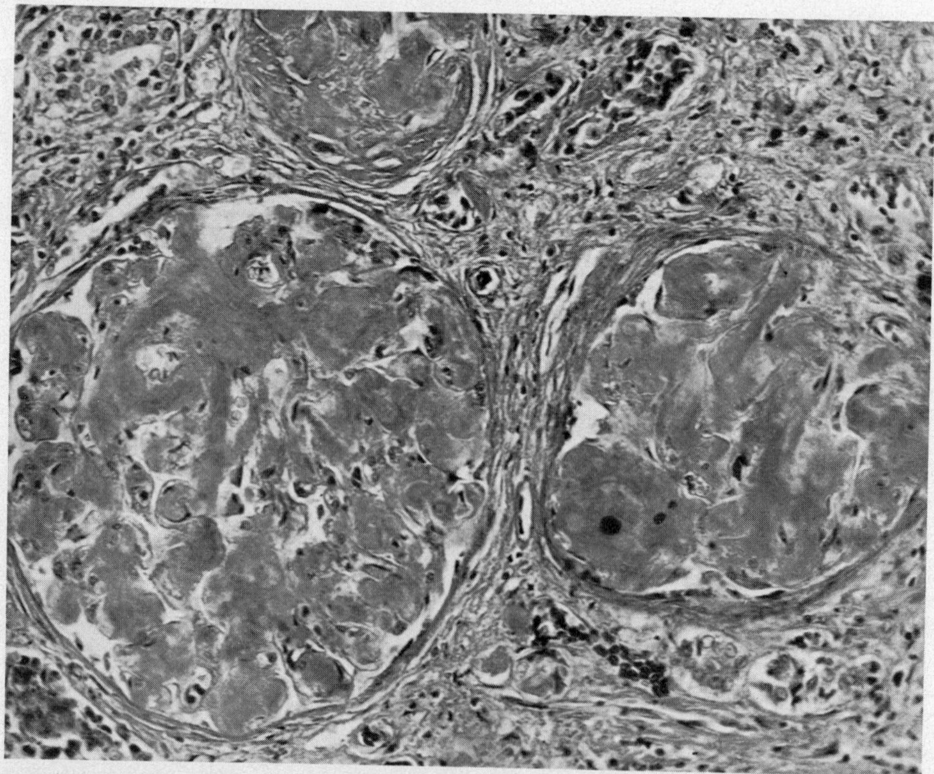

Figure 5–32. Amyloidosis of the kidney. The glomerular architecture is almost totally obliterated by the massive accumulation of amyloid.

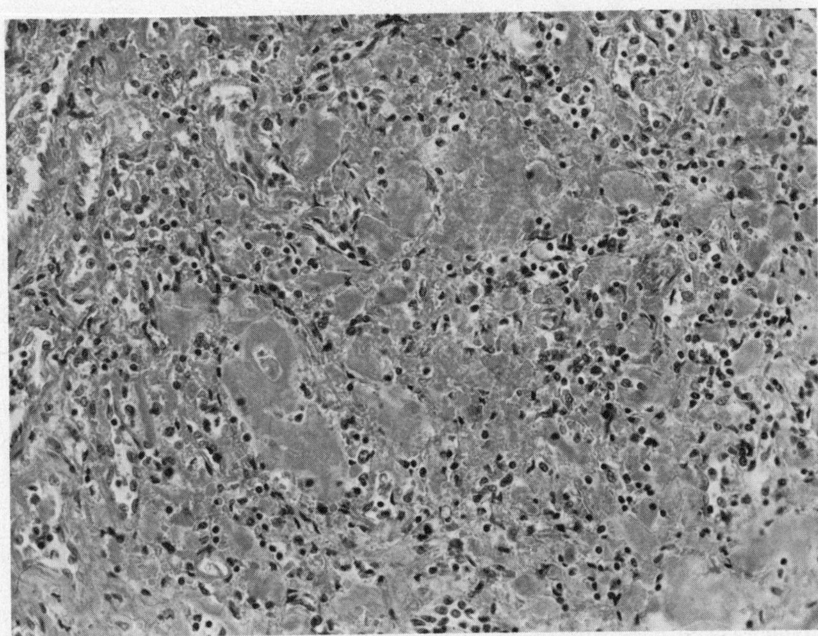

Figure 5–33. Amyloidosis of the spleen. The coalescent masses of amyloid surround the spleen cells.

appears to spare the follicles and instead involves the walls of the splenic sinuses and connective tissue framework. The pulp is therefore affected rather than the follicles (Fig. 5–33). Here again, fusion of the early deposits gives rise to large, maplike areas of amyloidosis, creating what has been designated the "lardaceous" spleen (Fig. 5–34). Ultrastructural studies indicate that the early deposits always occur between cells or in immediate apposition to the basement membranes of the mononuclear phagocytic (reticuloendothelial) cells of the splenic sinuses, as well as within the walls of small blood vessels.

Liver. Amyloidosis of the liver was found in 52 of 53 patients with reactive systemic and in 17 of 20 patients with immunocyte associated disease in one large series.[137] Here again, the deposits may be grossly inapparent or may cause moderate-to-marked hepatomegaly. With enlargement, the liver assumes a pale, waxy-gray, firm appearance. The amyloid appears first in the space of Disse and then progressively encroaches on adjacent hepatic parenchymal cells and sinusoids. In time, deformity, pressure atrophy, and eventual disappearance of hepatocytes occur, causing total replacement of large areas of liver parenchyma (Fig. 5–35). Vascular involvement and Kupffer cell depositions are frequent. Normal liver function is usually preserved despite sometimes quite severe involvement of the liver.

Heart. Amyloidosis of the heart may occur in any form of systemic amyloidosis, much more commonly in persons with immunocyte-derived disease. In some patients it represents an isolated organ involvement, and almost invariably the patient is over 70 years of age **(amyloid of aging)**. The heart may be enlarged and firm but more often shows no significant changes on cross section of the myocardium. Somewhat distinctive findings, when present, are pink-to-gray pinpoint or nodular elevations of the endocardium, having a dewdrop appearance. Histologically, the deposits begin in focal subendocardial accumulations and within the myocardium between the muscle fibers. Expansion of these myocardial deposits eventually causes pressure atrophy of myocardial fibers (Fig. 5–36). Vascular and subepicardial accumulations may also occur. In most cases the deposits are separated and widely distributed, but when subendocardial the conduction system may be damaged, accounting for the electrocardiographic abnormalities noted in some patients.[138]

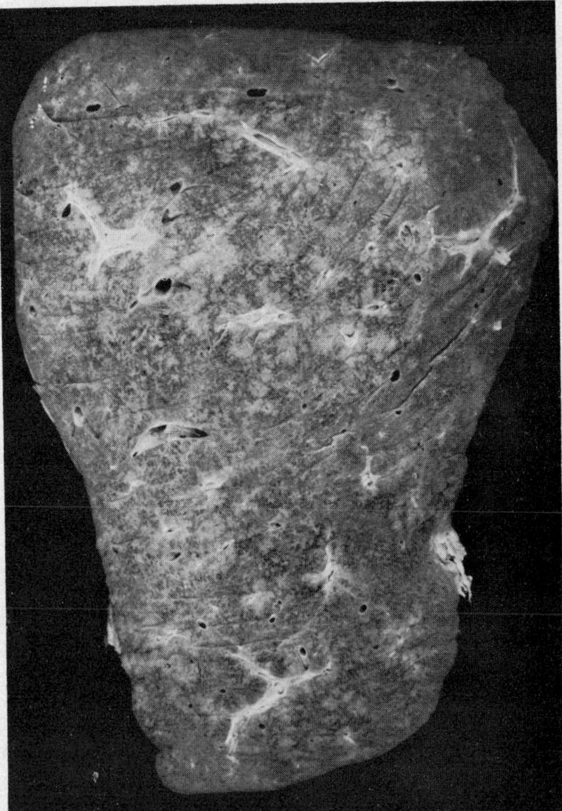

Figure 5–34. Amyloidosis of spleen. The focal deposits appear paler than the surrounding substance and in some areas are confluent. The pattern is that known as "lardaceous."

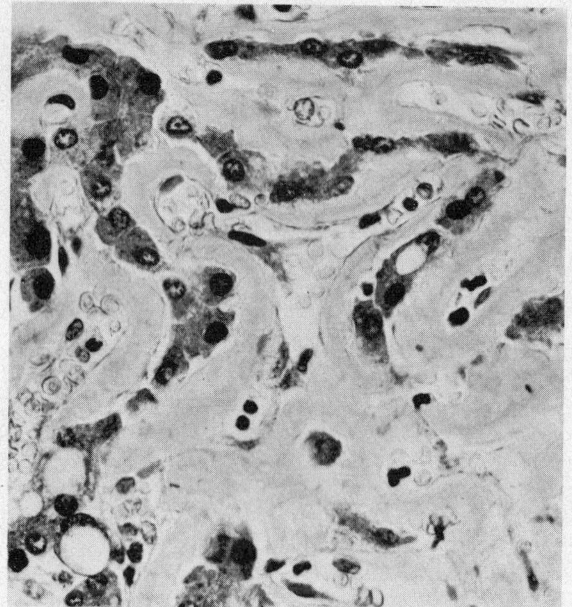

Figure 5–35. Amyloidosis of the liver. Pressure atrophy of hepatic cords by amyloid. Some cells are compressed and distorted, while others have been replaced by the amyloid deposit.

Other Organs. Amyloidosis of other organs is generally encountered in systemic disease. The adrenals, thyroid, and pituitary are common sites of involvement. In the adrenals, the intercellular deposits begin adjacent to the basement membranes of the cortical cells, usually first in the zona glomerulosa. With progression, the deposits encroach on cortical cells and advance into the deeper layers of the cortex. Large sheets of amyloid may replace considerable amounts of the cortical parenchyma. Similar patterns are seen in the thyroid and pituitary. The gastrointestinal tract may be involved at any level, from the oral cavity (gingiva, tongue) to the anus. The early lesions are largely perivascular in origin but eventually extend to involve the adjacent areas of the submucosa, muscularis, and subserosa. Coalescence of these small deposits may produce plaques or bands of firm gray substance. Nodular depositions in the tongue may cause macroglossia, giving rise to the designation **"tumor-forming amyloid of the tongue."** The respiratory tract may be involved focally or diffusely from the larynx down to the smallest bronchioles. Once again, the deposits are often perivascular in location, found in the submucosa, but enlargement may yield plaques, nodules, or polyps that protrude directly beneath the covering epithelium. Amyloidosis of the central nervous system has been reported within so-called plaques in the brain in elderly patients having Alzheimer's disease, and has been found in peripheral neuropathies, particularly in certain heredofamilial syndromes. Curiously, amyloid infiltrations of the carpal ligaments may give rise to the carpal tunnel syndrome.

CLINICAL CORRELATION. Amyloidosis may be found as an unsuspected anatomic change, having produced no clinical manifestations, or it may cause death. The symptomatology depends, as you might expect, on the magnitude of the deposits and on the particular sites or organs affected. Clinical manifestations at first are often entirely nonspecific, such as weakness, weight loss, lightheadedness, or syncope. Somewhat more specific findings appear later and most often relate to renal, cardiac, and gastrointestinal involvement, but hepatomegaly and splenomegaly and alterations in serum proteins may also be present.

Renal involvement is the dominating and most life-threatening feature of most cases of reactive systemic (secondary) amyloidosis, including those patients with familial Mediterranean fever. It may also be present (although less consistently) in patients with amyloidosis associated with immunocyte dyscrasias. Proteinuria and protein and occasionally cellular casts are the principal urinary findings in renal amyloidosis. The proteinuria of renal amyloidosis is an important cause of the nephrotic syndrome (p. 1011), since it may be sufficiently severe to induce hypoalbuminemia. Progressive obliteration of glomeruli in advanced cases ultimately leads to renal failure and uremia. It is worth noting that, unlike most causes of renal failure, amyloidosis is not usually associated with hypertension.

Cardiac amyloidosis is extremely common in patients with immunocyte-derived amyloidosis, but is less frequently present in those with reactive systemic amyloidosis. It is also encountered in familial Mediterranean fever and other familial forms of amyloidosis, and as an "isolated" involvement in patients of advanced age, when it is sometimes called senile cardiac amyloidosis. Whether clinical manifestations will appear depends on the severity and extent of the amyloid deposits. When symptomatic, the typical presentation is the insidious

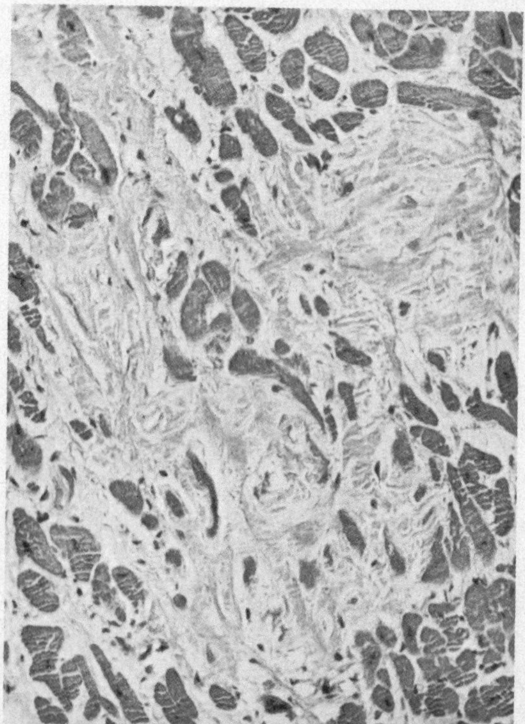

Figure 5–36. Amyloidosis of aging in the heart. The amyloid surrounds isolated myocardial fibers and has caused atrophy of others.

onset of congestive heart failure. Heart sounds are often faint, and the electrocardiogram frequently shows low voltage. The most serious aspects of cardiac amyloidosis are the conduction disturbances and arrhythmias. Indeed, in patients with significant cardiac amyloidosis, as many as half die suddenly of an arrhythmia. This form of heart disease responds poorly to digitalis therapy; in fact, fatal arrhythmias may be precipitated by digitalis administration. Occasionally, cardiac amyloidosis produces a restrictive pattern of cardiomyopathy and masquerades as chronic constrictive pericarditis (p. 599).

Gastrointestinal amyloidosis may be entirely asymptomatic or present in a variety of ways. Nodular (tumor-forming) amyloidosis of the tongue may cause sufficient enlargement and inelasticity to hamper speech and swallowing. Depositions in the stomach and intestine may lead to disturbances in digestion, malabsorption, and diarrhea. There is a current belief that many of these symptoms result from the involvement of the autonomic nerves and ganglia within the gastrointestinal tract.[139] Many more clinical signs and symptoms may appear, and these are available in an excellent recent review.[128A]

Even when amyloidosis is suspected on the basis of the clinical findings, resort must be made to biopsy and morphologic demonstration of the depositions to confirm the clinical impression. The most common sites biopsied are the kidney, when renal manifestations are present, or rectal or gingival tissue in patients suspected of having systemic amyloidosis. Gingival and/or rectal biopsies are positive in the majority of advanced cases with systemic disease. Sometimes the amyloid in these biopsy sites is restricted to perivascular locations and is not readily evident on usual tissue sections so that Congo red staining and polariscopic examination are requisite. Obviously a negative biopsy does not rule out amyloidosis, since the particular site selected may have been spared.

In suspected cases of immunocyte-associated amyloidosis, serum and urine protein electrophoresis and immunoelectrophoresis should be performed. Bone marrow aspirates in such cases often show plasmacytosis even in the absence of overt multiple myeloma. Estimation of SAA protein level is not commonly available, and in any case of no particular help, since elevation of SAA proteins often occurs in several acute and chronic inflammations without amyloidosis.

The prognosis for patients with generalized amyloidosis is poor. Those with immunocyte-derived amyloidosis (not including multiple myeloma) have a median survival of 14 months after diagnosis. Patients with myeloma-associated amyloidosis have a worse prognosis. The outlook for patients with reactive systemic amyloidosis is somewhat better and depends to some extent on the control of the underlying condition. Resorption of amyloid after treatment of the associated condition has been reported,[140] but the exact frequency of such a fortunate outcome is difficult to ascertain since there is no quantitative method for estimating the amyloid mass in the body.

IMMUNOLOGIC DEFICIENCY SYNDROMES

The immunologic deficiency syndromes are experiments of nature that beautifully document the complexities inherent in man's immune system. Nowhere has relevance of the individual components of immunologic function been more distinctly shown than when deficiencies of single components have given rise to distinctive disorders. Indeed, many of the important concepts of immunology either arose from or were confirmed by the study of clinical examples of specific immunodeficiencies. Traditionally, immunodeficiency disorders are considered according to the primary component or components involved, i.e., the B cell, the T cell, the undifferentiated stem cell, or complement; however, in view of the major cell interactions between T and B lymphocytes and macrophages, these distinctions are not clear-cut. Indeed, dissection of the underlying bases of various immunodeficiency states with monoclonal antibodies is beginning to reveal that several states of antibody deficiency are related to abnormal regulation by T-helper or -suppressor cells.[141]

Immunodeficiencies can also be divided into the primary immunodeficiency disorders, which are almost always genetically determined, and secondary immunodeficiency states, arising as complications of infections, malnutrition, aging, or side effects of immunosuppression, irradiation, or chemotherapy for cancer and other autoimmune diseases. Both primary and secondary immunodeficiency disorders are being discovered with increasing frequency because of new laboratory methods that can detect various cellular and humoral components of the immunologic reaction.[142] Here we shall briefly discuss some of the more important primary immunodeficiencies, and a mysterious and often lethal condition called acquired immunodeficiency syndrome.

PRIMARY IMMUNODEFICIENCIES

The primary immunodeficiency diseases are genetically determined and may affect specific immunity (i.e., humoral and cellular) or nonspecific host defense mechanisms mediated by complement proteins, and cells such as phagocytes or NK cells. Most primary immunodeficiencies manifest themselves in infancy, between 6 months and 2 years of life, and are noted because of the susceptibility of infants to recurrent infections. Detailed classification of the primary immunodeficiencies according to the suggested cellular defect may be found in the WHO report on immunodeficiency and other specialized sources.[143] Only a few examples will be presented here.

X-linked Agammaglobulinemia of Bruton

This is one of the most common forms of primary immunodeficiency and is characterized by the virtual absence from the serum of immunoglobulins, although small amounts of IgG may sometimes be present. It is an X-linked disease restricted to males, but there is no linkage with other markers on the X chromosome. Severe recurrent infections may begin as early as 8 months of age, when maternal immunoglobulins are depleted, but sometimes three years elapse before repeated infections call attention to the disorder. The most common offending organisms are pyogenic (e.g., staphylococcus, *Hemophilus influenzae*), and patients have recurrent conjunctivitis, pharyngitis, otitis media, bronchitis, pneumonia, and skin infections.

The classic characteristics, first described by Bruton, are those that would be expected from a primary B-cell deficiency. B cells are virtually absent in the blood except in very rare cases. Pre-B cells, which are large lymphoid cells with intracytoplasmic IgM but no surface immunoglobulins, have recently been found in normal numbers in some of these patients. Thus, the basic defect seems to be failure of pre-B cells to mature into B cells.[144] The lymph nodes and spleen lack germinal centers, and plasma cells are absent from the lymph nodes, spleen, bone marrow, and connective tissue. Tonsils in particular are poorly developed or rudimentary. In those rare cases in which B cells are present, they usually fail to respond to mitogenic or antigenic stimuli in vitro and are incapable of secreting immunoglobulin.[145] There are, however, normal numbers of circulating and tissue T cells, and T-cell function as measured by delayed hypersensitivity tests and allograft rejection is normal. As mentioned, patients are agammaglobulinemic or severely hypogammaglobulinemic, and they fail to produce antibodies to bacteria or viruses and in response to many vaccines. There is a remarkably high incidence of various autoimmune connective tissue diseases in these patients, and about one-third of them may develop an indolent form of rheumatoid-like arthritis, which responds to gamma-globulin therapy. Dermatomyositis, lupus erythematosus, and diffuse vasculitis are also rather common in these patients. Children can resist many virus infections without difficulty (e.g., measles, varicella, and mumps) and also resist infections by mycobacteria and low-grade pathogens reasonably well. This is a reflection of their normal phagocytic cell-mediated immunologic functions or abilities. Curiously, however, they are unable to resist infection by hepatitis virus, which may cause either severe liver destruction or chronic active hepatitis, and may be predisposed to cerebrospinal fluid infections caused by polioviruses and different types of ECHO viruses.

Common Variable Immunodeficiency

This rather poorly defined category is *by far the most common form of immunodeficiency with serious clinical impact.* It represents a group of syndromes that occur in both males and females, can be congenital or acquired, and appear at any time between the ages of 2 and 80 years. Some of the cases are familial, but there is no clear-cut mode of transmission. The group has in common (1) clinical manifestations of antibody deficiency, such as recurrent pneumococcal pneumonia or infections; and (2) a persistent hypogammaglobulinemia, which may affect all the immunoglobulins. However, agammaglobulinemia of the degree seen in Bruton's disease is unusual.

There are other differences also. Patients with common variable immunodeficiency are often affected with a sprue-like malabsorption syndrome that seems to be related to gluten sensitivity. Infestation by the protozoon *Giardia lamblia* is also quite common. Another feature is the frequent occurrence of noncaseating granulomas in the liver, lungs, spleen, and skin without any consistent microbial cause. Most of the patients have normal levels of circulating B cells. Histologically, the B-cell areas, i.e., the lymphoid follicles in the nodes, spleen, and gut, may look markedly hyperplastic, suggesting that B cells can proliferate in response to antigens, but they fail to mature into immunoglobulin-secreting plasma cells. In some patients the basis of the defect in immunoglobulin secretion seems to be an inability to glycosylate the heavy chain.[145] In other patients, the B cells appear to be intrinsically normal but there are abnormalities in immunoregulatory T cells. Both lack of T-helper function[146] and excessive suppressor-cell function have been described.[147] Also included in this obviously heterogeneous group are some patients with associated defects in cell-mediated immunity and macrophage functions.[148]

These patients also have a high frequency of autoimmune diseases including rheumatoid arthritis, pernicious anemia, and hemolytic anemia. Lymphoid malignancy also sometimes develops several years after immunologic deficiency is diagnosed.

Isolated IgA Deficiency

This is a very common immunodeficiency that occurs in about one in 600 individuals and consists of the virtual absence of *both serum and secretory IgA.* It may be familial or acquired in association with toxoplasmosis, measles, or some virus infection. Most of these individuals are completely asymptomatic, but some have repeated sinopulmonary infections caused by both bacteria and viruses. In addition, these patients have a high incidence of respiratory tract allergy and a variety of autoimmune diseases, particularly SLE and rheumatoid arthritis. The basis of the increased frequency of autoimmune and allergic diseases is not known. Since secretory IgA normally acts as a mucosal barrier against foreign proteins and antigens, it could be speculated that unregulated absorption of foreign protein antigens triggers abnormal immune responses in vivo.

The basic defect is in the differentiation of IgA B lymphocytes. Normally, the first IgA B cells are detected in the 12-week-old fetus. These immature cells have surface IgM and IgD in addition to IgA. Transition to mature IgA B cells starts at birth, and in adults only 10% of the IgA B cells express surface IgM and IgD;

the majority express only IgA. In most patients with selective IgA deficiency, the number of IgA-positive B cells is normal, but most of them express the immature phenotype and very few of these cells can be induced to transform into IgA plasma cells in vitro.[149] Other mechanisms such as IgA-specific T-suppressor cells and inadequate T-helper cells have also been implicated. However, whether these abnormalities are primary or arise as a consequence of the IgA deficiency is not entirely established.[149]

DiGeorge's Syndrome (Thymic Hypoplasia)

This is an example of selective T-cell deficiency and derives from failure of development of the third and fourth pharyngeal pouches. The latter give rise to the thymus, the parathyroids, some of the clear cells of the thyroid, and the ultimobranchial body. Thus, these patients have total absence of cell-mediated immune responses (due to lack of thymus), tetany (due to lack of parathyroids), and congenital defects of the heart and great vessels. In addition, the appearance of the mouth, ears, and facies may be abnormal. Absence of cell-mediated immunity is reflected in low levels of circulating lymphocytes and a poor defense against certain fungal and viral infections. Sometimes the lymphocyte counts may be normal, in which case virtually all the lymphocytes are B cells. Plasma cells are present in normal numbers in lymphoid tissues, but the thymic-dependent paracortical areas of the lymph nodes and the periarteriolar sheaths of the spleen are depleted. Immunoglobulin levels tend to be normal.

Support for the idea that this syndrome is directly attributable to maldevelopment of the thymus also comes from the successful treatment of some patients with this disease with thymic hormones (thymosin), by transplantation of fetal thymus or thymic epithelium. The syndrome is not genetically determined but appears to be the result of an intrauterine accident before the eighth week of gestation. Patients with "partial" DiGeorge's syndrome who have an extremely small but histologically normal thymus have also been recorded. T-cell function improves with age in these children, so that by 5 years of age many have no T-cell deficit.

Severe Combined Immunodeficiency (SCID)

This is an extremely serious form of inherited immunodeficiency syndrome characterized by defects in both T cell–mediated and humoral immunity. This disorder is heterogeneous with respect to both pattern of inheritance and underlying defects in T and B cells. Two modes of transmission are recognized—autosomal recessive and X-linked recessive. Many patients with the autosomal recessive form of SCID lack the enzyme adenosine deaminase (ADA) in their cells. The implications of enzyme deficiency in the pathogenesis of the immunologic abnormalities is discussed later.

Although all patients show impairment of both T- and B-cell functions, in general there is greater loss of T-cell immunity. Most patients are severely lymphopenic and lack mature T lymphocytes in the blood. The few T cells found in the circulation bear the OK T9 and OK T10 antigens characteristic of very immature intrathymic T cells.[150] When bone marrow cells from some SCID patients are incubated with normal thymic epithelial cells or thymic hormones, they fail to differentiate normally suggesting a defect in the stem cells.[151] However, other patients have shown improvement in T-cell functions after transplantation of thymus, which suggests that the defect may lie in the ability of the thymus to provide signals for differentiation of stem cells.[152] It seems, therefore, that there are two mechanisms of impaired T-cell immunity in SCID: a defect in stem cells, or abnormal differentiation of normal stem cells due to thymic abnormalities.

Investigations into the basis of impaired humoral immunity also indicate heterogeneity. Some patients have a stem cell defect, leading to an extreme paucity of mature B cells in the peripheral blood, whereas others have normal or even increased B cells that are unable to function.[153] In the latter group of patients, lack of adequate T-helper cells and/or excessive T-suppressor cell function have been implicated.[153]

In summary, SCID in most cases results from defects of lymphoid stem cells involving both T-cell and B-cell precursors. As might be expected, lymph nodes, spleen, tonsils, and appendix show virtual absence of any lymphoid tissue, but the pathognomonic histologic finding is in the thymus gland, which fails to descend from the neck into the anterior mediastinum and is devoid of lymphoid cells or Hassell's corpuscles. The blood vessels are very small, indicating that the thymus is fetal rather than involuted. The gland seems to be arrested at the stage at which it resembles the thymus of a 6- to 8-week-old fetus. Infants are incapable of any of the immunologic functions—they do not produce antibodies, exhibit very small amounts of IgG and no IgM or IgA in the serum, fail to reject allografts, or develop delayed hypersensitivity reactions. They succumb during the first year of life, usually to such opportunistic organisms as *Pseudomonas* or *Candida* or fatal viral infections. Since SCID is usually caused by defects in stem cells, grafting of normal bone marrow stem cells is the treatment of choice. In some patients, full immunologic reconstitution can be achieved by transplantation of sibling bone marrow. However, graft-versus-host disease mediated by the T cells within the donor bone marrow poses a serious problem that limits the effectiveness of this form of treatment (p. 175).

Approximately 50% of patients with the autosomal recessive form of SCID lack the enzyme adenosine deaminase (ADA) in their red cells and leukocytes. This enzyme is involved in the metabolism of nucleic acids by converting adenosine to inosine. Deficiency of ADA leads to the accumulation of adenosine and its derivatives such as deoxy-ATP, which may be lymphocytotoxic or may interfere with pyrimidine biosynthesis. *Because ADA is also absent in amniotic cells, this finding is of practical importance, since it enables the prenatal diagnosis of this immunodeficiency by culture of amniotic cells.* Of the thousands of Caucasians who have been screened for ADA, all but one of the ADA-deficient infants had severe combined immunodeficiency.[154] In addition to bone marrow transplantation, treatment of this variant of SCID has been attempted by infusion of normal ADA-containing erythrocytes. This has resulted in immunologic improvement in some, but not all, patients.[155]

Immunodeficiency with Thrombocytopenia and Eczema (Wiskott-Aldrich Syndrome)

This remarkable syndrome has been called "curious," "enigmatic," or "confusing," because its immunologic defects are so difficult to explain. It is an X-linked recessive disease characterized by thrombocytopenia, eczema, and a marked vulnerability to recurrent infection, ending in early death. The thymus is morphologically normal, at least early in the course of the disease, but there is progressive secondary depletion of lymphocytes in the peripheral blood and in the paracortical (thymus-dependent) areas of the lymph nodes, with variable loss of cellular immunity. Patients may show normal responses to such protein antigens as tetanus and diphtheria toxoid, but classically show a poor antibody response to polysaccharide antigens. IgM levels in the serum are low, but levels of IgA and IgE may be normal or elevated. Patients are also prone to the development of malignant lymphomas. Whether the failure to respond to polysaccharides results from a defect in antigen recognition and processing, or a qualitative deficiency of lymphocyte B-cell function, is unclear. Transfer factor has been reported to be beneficial in some patients with this disease, and results of bone marrow transplantation appear to be particularly encouraging.[156]

ACQUIRED IMMUNE DEFICIENCY SYNDROME (AIDS)

The first indication of this mysterious disease appeared in June, 1981, when the Center for Disease Control (CDC) of the United States reported five cases of *Pneumocystis carinii* pneumonia in homosexual men in the Los Angeles area.[157] Within a month it was reported that a rare malignant tumor called Kaposi's sarcoma (p. 543) had been found in 26 young homosexual males, four of whom also had *Pneumocystis carinii* pneumonia.[158] By mid-1983 the CDC had received reports of approximately 1350 cases of AIDS with multiple opportunistic infections with or without Kaposi's sarcoma in previously healthy individuals, with an alarming overall mortality of 41%.[159, 159A]

As might be expected, there is a rapidly growing body of literature devoted to various aspects of AIDS. Here we will summarize only the salient epidemiologic, clinical, morphologic, and immunologic features, and follow with a brief discussion of the possible etiologic factors.

For *epidemiologic* studies, CDC defines a case of AIDS as a "disease, at least moderately predictive of a defect in cell-mediated immunity, occurring in a person with no known cause for diminished resistance to that disease." Such diseases include Kaposi's sarcoma, *Pneumocystis carinii* pneumonia, or other serious opportunistic infections.[159] It should be borne in mind that this is a working definition that may not necessarily delineate a specific disease in terms of etiology and pathogenesis. Approximately 90% of the reported cases have occurred in the United States, most of them concentrated in six large metropolitan areas including New York, Newark, San Francisco, Los Angeles, Miami, and Houston. However, AIDS has also been reported from several countries around the world. In the U.S. approximately 75% of the patients are homosexual or bisexual males, but an increasing number of heterosexual (male and female) patients are being reported. This varied population of AIDS victims includes intravenous drug users, female partners of intravenous drug users, hemophiliacs,[160] infants of possibly affected mothers, individuals receiving blood transfusions from donors who subsequently developed AIDS, and Haitian refugees in the United States. The Haitian patients are unique in that they do not share the known risk factors common to most other AIDS victims, such as homosexual life style, intravenous drug abuse, or intimate contact with affected individuals.[160A]

Clinically, the typical patient is a young homosexual male presenting with fever, weight loss, and persistent generalized lymphadenopathy. Pneumonia caused by the opportunistic protozoon, *Pneumocytis carinii,* which very rarely affects healthy individuals, is seen in approximately 50% of cases.[159, 161] A variety of other (often multiple) opportunistic pathogens including aspergillus, candida, cryptococcus, cytomegalovirus, toxoplasma, atypical mycobacteria, and herpes viruses have also been found in these patients.[162] In addition to opportunistic infections, over one-third of the patients also present with Kaposi's sarcoma, a multicentric neoplasm,[159, 163] which is extremely rare in the United States (p. 1270). Unlike the sporadic cases, Kaposi's sarcoma in patients with AIDS follows an aggressive clinical course characterized by widespread involvement of the skin and early involvement of the lymph nodes and viscera. This pattern resembles that seen in immunosuppressed renal transplant recipients.[164] In addition to Kaposi's sarcoma, diffuse undifferentiated non-Hodgkin's lymphoma (Burkitt-like) has been reported and is considered to be a part of the AIDS syndrome.[165, 166] This full-blown picture may be preceded by a prodrome (lasting for several months) characterized by recurrent fever, weight loss, and lymphadenopathy.

As might be expected from the clinical picture, there is a profound suppression of cell-mediated immunity in every patient, but, somewhat surprisingly, humoral immunity remains intact.[167] These patients have a lymphopenia with a selective impairment of T cell–mediated reactions, such as cutaneous delayed hypersensitivity, and several other parameters of in vitro T-cell functions. A particularly consistent finding is an inversion of the ratio of T-helper/inducer cells (OK T4) to cytotoxic/suppressor (OK T8) T cells. Normally this ratio is approximately 2, whereas in the AIDS patients a ratio of 0.5 is not uncommon. This inversion results primarily from a severe deficiency of OK T4–positive cells, which act as helper/inducer cells in both cell-mediated and humoral immunity. It should be noted, however, that inversion of the OK T4/T8 ratio is not a specific test for AIDS, since a similar change commonly occurs during the course of several acute viral infections such as hepatitis and infectious mononucleosis. Total serum immunoglobulin levels are either normal or elevated owing to a polyclonal hypergammaglobulinemia. High antibody titers (often rising during the course of observation) are seen against Epstein-Barr (EBV), cytomegalovirus (CMV), and herpes simplex virus.[163]

The anatomic changes in the tissues are neither specific nor diagnostic. They reflect morphologic manifestations of immunodeficiency, infections with multiple opportunistic pathogens, and unusual neoplasms.[167A] At autopsy, **lymph nodes** usually show marked lymphoid cell depletion affecting both the cortical and paracortical areas. There is, in some cases, an associated proliferation of blood vessels and the presence of a plasma cell infiltrate. In the empty-looking lymph nodes, the presence of infectious agents and/or neoplasms may not be readily apparent, yet careful examination often reveals the presence of viral inclusions (CMV), atypical acid-fast bacilli or fungi, sometimes within the few remaining histiocytes. Tumors found in association with AIDS, such as Kaposi's sarcoma (p. 543) and a variety of non-Hodgkin's lymphomas (p. 658), may also involve lymph nodes in addition to extranodal tissues. In contrast with the picture of lymphoid cell depletion noted in fatal cases, antemortem specimens may reveal marked hyperplasia of the lymphoid follicles, paracortex, or sinusoidal histiocytes. These reactions presumably represent reactions to infectious agents prior to the onset of severe immunologic failure. In addition to lymph nodes, other lymphoid tissues such as spleen, thymus, Peyer's patches, appendix, and bone marrow also reveal marked hypocellularity in fatal cases. Changes related to **opportunistic infections** are widespread and may be present in virtually every organ, but the central nervous system, lungs, and gastrointestinal tract are prominently involved. In the context of profound immunodeficiency, the inflammatory reactions in response to infections may be sparse or atypical. For example, in the lungs mycobacteria do not evoke the formation of well-defined granulomas, because T-cell immunity is suppressed. As mentioned earlier, Kaposi's sarcoma is the neoplasm most commonly associated with AIDS. Although histologically similar to the "classical" Kaposi's tumor, it is distinguished by multifocal presentation and aggressive clinical course. The next most common types of neoplasm seen in AIDS victims are the non-Hodgkin's lymphomas. These are usually of the aggressive histologic varieties such as undifferentiated non-Burkitt's type and immunoblastic sarcomas.

Although it is quite clear that the common denominator in these patients is a severe and selective immunodeficiency, the cause of this state remains unknown. The clustering of cases in large metropolitan centers among male homosexuals raises the possibility that an infectious agent, possibly a virus, transmitted by close contact may be involved. Homosexual males are known to be at greater risk for acquisition of sexually transmitted diseases as well as common viral infections such as hepatitis B, CMV, and EBV.[168] The occurrence of AIDS in female sex partners of intravenous drug abusers (a high-risk group themselves) indicates that the mysterious "AIDS agent" could be sexually transmitted even among heterosexuals. The possibility of a parenteral route of transmission is strongly suggested by the spread of AIDS in hemophiliacs, in habitual users of intravenous drugs, and in some recipients of blood transfusion. It should be noted that among hemophiliacs those who receive lyophilized factor VIII concentrates are at greatest risk. These preparations of factor VIII are derived by pooling material obtained from several thousand blood donors.[169] Although the transmissible agent hypothesis seems plausible, the identity of the causative organism is a matter for speculation. CMV has been considered a candidate virus since it is known to be immunosuppressive, can be transmitted sexually, and most of the male homosexuals have serologic evidence of previous CMV infection. Even before the current epidemic of AIDS, CMV was linked to the causation of Kaposi's sarcoma based on seroepidemiologic studies and on the finding of CMV-DNA in the genome of Kaposi's sarcoma cells.[170, 171] More recently, some investigators have focused on the human T-cell leukemia virus (HTLV) as a possible etiologic agent.[159A] This retrovirus is horizontally transmitted and is associated with certain T-cell malignancies (pp. 243 and 678). HTLV is capable of infecting human T cells and could possibly cause suppression of cell-mediated immunity. In preliminary studies, 25 to 40% of AIDS patients have been found to have anti-HTLV antibodies, and in a few cases HTLV DNA has been found in the patients' T cells. It should be pointed out, however, that none of this evidence is conclusive and that all the suggested agents could merely be opportunistic infections occurring in the setting of severe immunosuppression.

Although an infectious etiology of AIDS seems plausible, this hypothesis leaves certain nagging questions unanswered. Why have only certain segments of the male homosexual population been affected? Why the sudden outbreak of a new epidemic? To explain these and similar questions, the synergistic action of several other factors has been postulated. Genetic predisposition, for one, may be an important influence. Noteworthy in this connection is the significantly increased frequency of HLA-DR5 antigen in homosexual as well as nonhomosexual males with Kaposi's sarcoma.[163] Changing sexual practices, particularly repeated contacts with multiple anonymous partners (which characterize many of the patients), may have increased the risk of recurrent and eventually persistent viral infections. The recent increase in the use of recreational drugs such as amyl nitrite (which could be immunosuppressive) may be a cofactor. The immunosuppressive effects of intravenously administered sperm in mice may also be relevant, since repeated exposure to spermatozoa (through abrasions) could very well occur in homosexual males with multiple partners.[172] Emergence of a new mutant strain of virus has also been the subject of speculation. A host of other possible contributing factors could be cited, but suffice it to say that the syndrome of AIDS is likely to be multifactorial in origin, resulting from the exposure of genetically susceptible individuals to a variety of known and as yet undiscovered environmental agents, creating in the final analysis a severely immunocompromised individual who falls easy prey to opportunistic infections and perhaps "opportunistic" Kaposi's sarcoma and lymphoma.

GENETIC DEFICIENCIES OF THE COMPLEMENT SYSTEM

Inherited deficiencies of complement proteins represent primary immunodeficiency states but, unlike the other forms described previously, do not involve primary defects in the lymphocytes. However, the various components of the complement system play a critical role in inflammatory and immunologic responses (p. 53). Advances in laboratory methods to quantitate complement components have revealed that deficiency of specific complement components may predispose to certain diseases, much like the predisposition that occurs with selective deficiencies of the immune system, discussed earlier. The end result of defects in complement, particularly C3, is an increased susceptibility to bacterial infection and with C2 deficiency, a greater risk of connective tissue diseases similar to those that occur in the primary immunodeficiencies. The deficiencies of the later acting components of the classic pathway (C5–8) result in recurrent neisserial infections. Thus far, hereditary deficiencies have been described for almost all the classic components of the complement system and two of the inhibitors.[173] Some of these deficiencies occur rather often: for example, the C2 deficiency gene occurs with a frequency of about 1% in the general population.

The most important of these conditions are: deficiency of C1 inhibitor, causing *hereditary angioedema;* C2 deficiency, because it is such a common defect and is associated with connective tissue diseases; and C3 deficiency, because of its association with life-threatening bacterial infections. Each of these will be described here only briefly.

HEREDITARY ANGIOEDEMA ($C\bar{1}$ INHIBITOR DEFICIENCY). Genetic deficiency of $C\bar{1}$ inhibitor is associated with a syndrome that consists of recurrent attacks of swelling, involving the subcutaneous tissue, gastrointestinal tract, bronchi, and lungs. Laryngeal edema and intestinal obstruction are serious complications. Although these attacks are often spontaneous, they can be triggered by trauma, menstruation, and possibly mental stress.[174] The disease is most crippling during adolescence and tends to subside in the fifth decade of life. Inheritance is autosomal dominant, most affected members being heterozygous.

$C\bar{1}$ inhibitor is a serum glycoprotein that inactivates $C\bar{1}s$, the activated first component of complement. In addition, it inhibits plasmin, kallikrein, and activated Hageman factor (factor XIIa), all of which are involved in increased vascular permeability. *Deficiency of the inhibitor, therefore, will leave unchecked the complement cascade* and possibly other proinflammatory factors, and thus result in increased permeability. But what triggers the initial activation of C1 responsible for the attacks of hereditary angioedema? One pathway that has been postulated is as follows: trauma or tissue damage results in activation of Hageman factor, which in turn triggers clotting, kinin generation, and fibrinolysis, resulting in the generation of plasmin, which is known to activate C1. Indeed, during the attacks, patients exhibit levels of free $C\bar{1}s$ that cannot be found in the circulation of normal individuals. Recently, two forms of therapy have been introduced that take into account these considerations of pathogenesis: tranexamic acid, which inhibits plasminogen, and danazol, which causes increased synthesis of $C\bar{1}$ esterase inhibitor.

C2 DEFICIENCY. This is the most commonly occurring complement deficiency. In one survey there were five heterozygotes in 250 normal blood donors, and one homozygote among 10,000 normal blood donors.[66] It is transmitted as an autosomal codominant trait. Heterozygotes have half the normal C2 concentration. *About half the affected homozygotes develop either an SLE-like disease, discoid lupus, or some other connective tissue disorder.* This association can be explained in several ways. One possibility is that deficiency of the early components of complement predisposes the individual to viral infections that may be involved in the induction of SLE (p. 182). However, since heterozygotes who have adequate complement levels to resist infections also have a greater-than-normal incidence of SLE, it is likely that the association of the C2 deficiency gene with lupus disease is not causal but is rather a result of linkage to some other gene, which determines the predisposition to SLE; genes determining C2 levels are linked to histocompatibility genes and may be in linkage disequilibrium with certain immune response genes. It must be stated, however, that the SLE-type disease associated with C2 deficiency is atypical in that there is a low incidence of antibodies to DNA, low incidence of renal disease, and infrequent finding of immunoglobulin and complement in the skin and kidney.[66]

C3 DEFICIENCY. In the heterozygous form of congenital C3 deficiency, C3 serum levels are 50% of normal values, but affected individuals have no clinical abnormalities. The homozygous form is extremely rare, but most affected children show increased susceptibility to infection with encapsulated bacteria. Although these children's clinical history is remarkably similar to that of agammaglobulinemic patients, they have normal immunoglobulin levels and can respond to infection with antibody formation. Acquired C3 deficiencies are much more common, and some are associated with a peculiar form of chronic renal disease, to be discussed later (see p. 1016).

EPILOGUE

It is evident from this chapter that the versatile immune system, designed to protect the individual from exogenous agents and from potentially antigenic self-components, may fail in a multitude of ways. The resulting disorders range from too little (immunologic deficiency) to too much (the autoimmune diseases), and include every shade of hyperactivity and abnormal reactivity in between. Not covered in this chapter are the sundry neoplasms of the lymphoid system (p. 658), which represent abnormal proliferations of the immune system, or the numerous immunologic disorders affecting specific organ systems. It will become apparent that the latter contribute to a host of acute and chronic crippling diseases, discussed in other chapters. The immune system is still the darling of basic scientists and physicians alike, and so we can anticipate much more information about basic immunology and many more immunologic disorders to fill more pages of future textbooks!

---

1. Reinherz, E.L., and Schlossman, S.F.: The characterization and function of human immunoregulatory T lymphocyte subsets. Immunol. Today *2*:69, 1981.
2. Haynes, B.F.: Human T cell antigens as defined by monoclonal antibodies. Immunol. Rev. *57*:1, 1981.
3. Reinherz, E.L., and Schlossman, S.F.: Regulation of the immune response—inducer and suppressor T-lymphocyte subsets in human beings. N. Engl. J. Med. *303*:370, 1980.
4. Foon, K.A., et al.: Surface markers on leukemia and lymphoma cells: Recent advances. Blood *60*:1, 1982.
5. Herberman, R.B. (ed.): NK cells and other natural effector cells. New York, Academic Press, 1982.
6. Steinman, R.M.: Dendritic cells. Transplantation *31*:151, 1981.
7. Kostyu, D., and Amos, D.B.: The major histocompatibility complex: Genetic polymorphism and disease susceptibility. *In* Stanbury, J.B., et al. (eds.): Metabolic Basis of Inherited Disease. 5th ed. New York, McGraw-Hill Book Co., 1982, p. 77.
8. DeWolf, W.C., et al.: HLA and disease—current concepts. Hum. Pathol. *11*:332, 1980.
9. Bellanti, J.A.: Immunology. 2nd ed. Philadelphia, W.B. Saunders Co., 1978, pp. 471–621.
10. Ishizaka, K.: Cellular response in the IgE antibody response. Adv. Immunol. *23*:1, 1976.
11. Schwartz, L.B., and Austen, K.F.: Mast cells and mediators. *In* Lachmann, P.J., and Peters, D.K. (eds.): Clinical Aspects of Immunology. 4th ed. Oxford, Blackwell Scientific Publications, 1982, p. 130.
12. O'Flaherty, J.T.: Lipid mediators of inflammation and allergy. Lab Invest., *47*:314, 1982.
13. Butterworth, A.E., and David, J.R.: Eosinophil function. N. Engl. J. Med. *304*:154, 1981.
14. Marsh, D.G., et al.: The epidemiology and genetics of atopic allergy. N. Engl. J. Med. *305*:1551, 1981.
15. deWeck, A.A., et al.: HLA and allergy. *In* Dausset, J., and Svejgaard, A. (eds.): HLA and Disease. Copenhagen, Munksgaard, 1976.
16. McCormick, J.R., et al.: Suppression by superoxide dismutase of immune complex–induced pulmonary alveolitis and dermal inflammation. Am. J. Pathol. *102*:55, 1981.
17. Sell, S.: Immunopathology. Am. J. Pathol. *90*:215, 1978.
18. Germuth, F.G., Jr.; Comparative histologic and immunologic study in rabbits of induced hypersensitivity of the serum sickness type. J. Exp. Med. *97*:257, 1953.
19. Mannik, M.: Pathophysiology of circulating immune complexes. Arthritis Rheum. *25*:783, 1982.
20. Henson, P.M.: Mechanisms of tissue injury produced by immunologic reactions. *In* Bellanti, J.A. (ed.): Immunology. 2nd ed. Philadelphia, W.B. Saunders Co., 1978, pp. 292–354.
21. Williams, R.C.: Immune complexes: A clinical perspective. Am. J. Med. *71*:743, 1981.
22. Gallo, G.R., et al.: Nephritogenicity and differential distribution of glomerular immune complexes related to immunogen charge. Lab. Invest. *48*:241, 1983.
23. McCluskey, R.T.: Modification of glomerular immune complex deposits. Lab. Invest. *48*:241, 1983.
24. Adelman, N.E., et al.: Lymphokines as inflammatory mediators. *In* Cohen, S., et al. (eds.): Biology of the Lymphokines. New York, Academic Press, 1979, p. 15.
25. Dvorak, H.F., et al.: Expression of cell-mediated hypersensitivity *in vivo*—recent advances. Int. Rev. Exp. Pathol. *21*:120, 1980.
26. Rocklin, R.E., et al.: Mediators of immunity: Lymphokines and monokines. Adv. Immunol. *29*:56, 1980.

26A. Nathan, C.F., et al.: Identification of interferon-γ as the lymphokine that activates human macrophage oxidative metabolism and antimicrobial activity. J. Exp. Med. *158*:670, 1983.

27. Zinkernagel, R.M.: Major transplantation antigens in host response to infection. Hosp. Pract. *13*:83, 1978.
28. Bhan, A.K., et al.: T cell subsets in allograft rejection. In situ characterization of T cell subsets in human skin allografts by the use of monoclonal antibodies. J. Immunol. *129*:1578, 1982.
29. Dvorak, H.F., et al.: Rejection of first set skin allografts in man. The microvasculature is the critical target of the immune response. J. Exp. Med. *150*:322, 1979.
30. Busch, G., et al.: Hyperacute renal allograft rejection in the primate. Am. J. Pathol. *80*:1, 1975.
31. Russell, P.S., and Winn, H.J.: Transplantation. N. Engl. J. Med. *282*:786, 1970.
32. Busch, G., et al.: Human renal allografts: Analysis of lesions in long-term survivals. Hum. Pathol. *2*:253, 1971.
33. Porter, K.A.: Renal transplantation. *In* Heptinstall, R.H.: Pathology of the Kidney. Boston, Little, Brown & Co., 1983, p. 1455.
34. McPhaul, J.J., et al.: Renal transplantation: Some comtemporary problems. *In* Wilson, C.B., et al. (eds.): Immunologic Mechanisms of Renal Disease. New York, Churchill Livingstone, 1979, p. 323.
35. Berg, B., and Ringden, O.: Correlation between relative response in mixed lymphocyte culture, HLA-D and -DR typing, and graft survival in renal transplantation. Transplantation *33*:291, 1982.
36. Opelz, G., and Terasaki, P.I.: International study histocompatibility in renal transplantation. Transplantation *33*:87, 1982.
37. Moore, S.B.: The enigma of blood transfusion and kidney transplantation. Mayo Clin. Proc. *57*:431, 1982.
38. Filopovich, A.H., et al.: Pretreatment of donor bone marrow with monoclonal antibody OKT3 for prevention of acute graft-versus-host disease in allogeneic histocompatible bone marrow transplantation. Lancet *1*:1266, 1982.
39. Kiessling, R., et al.: Evidence for a similar or a common mechanism for natural killer cell activity and resistance to hemopoietic grafts. Eur. J. Immunol. *7*:655, 1977.
40. Talal, N.: Autoimmunity: Genetic, Immunologic, Virologic and Clinical Aspects. New York, Academic Press, 1977.
41. Donath, J., and Landsteiner, K.: Uber paroxysmal Hamoglobinurie. Munch. Med. Wochenschr. *51*:1509, 1904.
42. Dameshek, W., and Schwartz, S.O.: The presence of hemolysins in acute hemolytic anemia. N. Engl. J. Med. *218*:75, 1938.
43. Weksler, M.E.: The senescence of the immune system. Hosp. Pract. *16*:53, 1981.
44. Graber, P.: Hypothesis. Autoantibodies and immunologic theories. An analytic review. Clin. Immunol. Immunopathol. *4*:453, 1975.
45. Theofilopoulos, A.N., and Dixon, F.J.: Autoimmune diseases. Immunopathology and etiopathogenesis. Am. J. Pathol. *108*:321, 1982.
46. Owen, R.D.: Immunogenetic consequences of vascular anastomoses between bovine twins. Science *102*:400, 1945.
47. Mitchison, N.A.: Induction of immunologic paralysis in two zones of dosage. Proc. R. Soc. Med. (Series B) *161*:275, 1964.
48. Nossal, G.J.V., and Pike, B.L.: Clonal anergy: Persistence in tolerant mice of antigen-binding B lymphocytes incapable of responding to antigen or mitogen. Proc. Natl. Acad. U.S.A. *77*:1602, 1980.
49. Gershon, R.K.: Suppressor T cells: A miniposition paper celebrating a new decade. *In* Forugereau, M., and Daussett, J. (eds.): Immunology 80—Progress in Immunology. London, Academic Press, 1980, p. 373.
50. Golub, E.S.: Suppressor T cells and their possible role in the regulation of autoreactivity. Cell *24*:595, 1981.
51. Teale, J.M., and Mackay, I.R.: Autoimmune diseases and the theory of clonal abortion. Is it still relevant? Lancet *2*:284, 1979.
52. Weigle, W.O.: Analysis of autoimmunity through experimental models of thyroiditis and allergic encephalomyelitis. Adv. Immunol. *30*:159, 1980.
53. Goodman, M.G., and Weigle, W.O.: Role of polyclonal B cell activation in self/non-self discrimination. Immunol. Today *2*:54, 1981.
54. Raveche, E.S., et al.: Lymphocytes and lymphocyte functions in systemic lupus erythematosus. Semin. Hematol. *16*:344, 1979.
55. Berrih, S., et al.: Evaluation of T-cell subsets in myasthenia gravis, using anti-T cell monoclonal antibodies. Clin. Exp. Immunol. *45*:1, 1981.
56. Hekman, A., and Rumke, P.: Autoimmunity and isoimmunity against spermatozoa. *In* Miescher, P.A., and Muller-Eberhard, H.J. (eds.): Textbook of Immunopathology. Vol. II, 2nd ed. New York, Grune & Stratton, 1976, pp. 947–962.

57. Rose, N.R., et al.: Genetic control of autoimmune disease. *In* Rose, N.R., et al. (eds.): Developments in immunology. Vol. 1. New York, Elsevier/North Holland, 1978.
58. Lampert, P.W.: Autoimmune and virus-induced demyelinating diseases. Am. J. Pathol. *91*:176, 1978.
59. Winchester, R.J. (ed.): New directions for research in SLE. Arthritis Rheum. *21*(Suppl.):1, 1978.
60. Christian, C.L.: Systemic lupus erythematosus. Clinical manifestations and prognosis. Arthritis Rheum. *25*:887, 1982.
61. Platt, J.L., et al.: Systemic lupus erythematosus in the first two decades of life. Am. J. Kid. Dis. *2*(Suppl. 1):212, 1982.
62. Lorincz, L.L., et al.: Anti-nuclear antibodies. Int. J. Dermatol. *20*:401, 1981.
63. Tan, E.M.: Antinuclear antibodies in diagnosis and management. Hosp. Pract. *18*:79, 1983.
64. Walport, M.J., et al.: The immunogenetics of SLE. Clin. Rheum. Dis. *8*:3, 1982.
65. Winchester, R.J., and Nunez-Roldan, A.: Some genetic aspects of systemic lupus erythematosus. Arthritis Rheum. *25*:833, 1982.
66. Schur, P.H.: Complement and lupus erythematosus. Arthritis Rheum. *25*:793, 1982.
67. Schwartz, R.S.: Immunologic and genetic aspects of systemic lupus erythematosus. N. Engl. J. Med. *30*:803, 1979.
68. Harmon, C.E., and Portanova, J.P.: Drug-induced lupus: Clinical and serologic studies. Clin. Rheum. Dis. *8*:121, 1982.
69. Datta, S.K., et al.: Genetic studies of autoimmunity and retrovirus expression in crosses of New Zealand black mice. I. Xenotropic virus. J. Exp. Med. *147*:854, 1978.
70. Lahita, R.G., et al.: Abnormal estrogen and androgen metabolism in the human with systemic lupus erythematosus. Am. J. Kid. Dis. *2*(Suppl. 1):206, 1982.
71. Steinberg, A.D., et al.: Studies of immune abnormalities in systemic lupus erythematosus. Am. J. Kid. Dis. *2*(Suppl. 1):101, 1982.
72. Decker, J.L., et al.: Systemic lupus erythematosus: Evolving concepts. Ann. Intern. Med. *91*:587, 1979.
73. Morimoto, C., et al.: Alterations in immunoregulatory T cell subsets in active systemic lupus erythematosus. J. Clin. Invest. *66*:1171, 1980.
74. Nakamura, Z.I., et al.: Reevaluation of suppressor cell function in systemic lupus erythematosus. Clin. Immunol. Immunopathol. *24*:72, 1982.
75. Miller, K.B., and Schwartz, R.S.: Familial abnormalities of suppressor cell function in systemic lupus erythematosus. N. Engl. J. Med. *30*:803, 1979.
76. Smolen, J.S., et al.: Heterogeneity of immunoregulatory T-cell subsets in systemic lupus erythematosus. Correlation with clinical features. Am. J. Med. *72*:783, 1982.
77. Dixon, F.J.: Murine lupus: An overview. Arthritis Rheum. *25*:721, 1982.
78. Manny, N., et al.: Synthesis of IgM by cells of NZB and SWR mice and their crosses. J. Immunol. *122*:1220, 1979.
79. McCluskey, R.T.: Evidence for an immune complex disorder in systemic lupus erythematosus. Am. J. Kid. Dis. *2*(Suppl. 1):199, 1982.
80. Williams, G.N., et al.: Brain reactive lymphocytotoxic antibody in the cerebrospinal fluid of patients with systemic lupus erythematosus: Correlation with central nervous system involvement. Clin. Immunol. Immunopathol. *18*:126, 1981.
81. Silva, F.G.: The nephropathies of systemic lupus erythematosus. *In* Rosen, S. (ed.): Contemporary Issues in Surgical Pathology. Vol. I. Pathology of Glomerular Diseases. New York, Churchill Livingstone, 1983, p. 79.
82. Appel, G.B., et al.: Renal involvement in systemic lupus erythematosus (SLE): A study of 56 patients emphasizing histologic classification. Medicine *57*:371, 1978.
83. Baldwin, D.S.: Clinical usefulness of the morphologic classification of lupus nephritis. Am. J. Kid. Dis. *2*(Suppl. 1):142, 1982.
84. Gilliam, J.N., et al.: Immunoglobulin in clinically uninvolved skin in systemic lupus erythematosus. J. Clin. Invest. *53*:1434, 1974.
85. Goldberg, D., and Cohen, A.S.: Synovial membrane histology in the differential diagnosis of rheumatic diseases. Medicine *57*:239, 1978.
86. Atkins, C.J., et al.: The choroid plexus in systemic lupus erythematosus. Ann. Intern. Med. *76*:65, 1972.
87. Ginzler, E.M., et al.: A multicenter study of the outcome in systemic lupus erythematosus. Arthritis Rheum. *25*:601, 1982.
88. Gilliam, J.N., and Sontheimer, R.D.: Skin manifestations of SLE. Clin. Rheum. Dis. *8*:207, 1982.
89. Sontheimer, R.D., et al.: Serologic and HLA associations in subacute lupus erythematosus, a clinical subset of lupus erythematosus. Ann. Intern. Med. *97*:664, 1982.
90. Woosley, R.L., et al.: Effect of acetylator phenotype on the rate at which procainamide induces antinuclear antibodies and the lupus syndrome. N. Engl. J. Med. *298*:1157, 1978.
91. Moutsopoulos, H.M. (Moderator) NIH Conference: Sjögren's syndrome (sicca syndrome): Current issues. Ann. Intern. Med. *92*(Part 1):212, 1980.
92. Adamson, T.C., et al.: Immunohistologic analysis of lymphoid infiltrates in primary Sjögren's syndrome using monoclonal antibodies. J. Immunol. *130*:203, 1983.
93. Fauci, A.S., and Moutsopoulos, H.M.: Polyclonally triggered B cells in the peripheral blood and bone marrow of normal individuals and in patients with systemic lupus erythematosus and primary Sjögren's syndrome. Arthritis Rheum. *24*:577, 1981.
94. Symposium on the fibrotic processes. Ann. Rheum. Dis. *36*(Suppl. 2), 1977.
95. Gay, R.E., et al.: Collagen types synthesized in dermal fibroblast cultures from patients with early progressive systemic sclerosis. Arthritis Rheum. *23*:190, 1980.
96. Uitto, J., et al.: Scleroderma: Increased biosynthesis of triple helical type I and type III procollagens associated with unaltered expression of collagenase by skin fibroblasts in culture. J. Clin. Invest. *64*:921, 1979.
97. Haynes, D.C., and Gershwin, M.E.: The immunopathology of progressive systemic sclerosis (PSS). Semin. Arthritis Rheum. *11*:331, 1982.
98. Tan, E.M., et al.: Diversity of antinuclear antibodies in progressive systemic sclerosis: Anti-centromere antibody and its relation to CREST syndrome. Arthritis Rheum. *23*:617, 1980.
99. Gershwin, M.E.: Editorial: Slow progress in scleroderma. Ann. Intern. Med. *97*:776, 1982.
100. Fries, J.F.: The microvascular pathogenesis of scleroderma: An hypothesis. Ann. Intern. Med. *91*:788, 1979.
101. McCoy, R., et al.: The kidney in progressive systemic sclerosis: Antibody elution studies. Lab. Invest. *35*:124, 1976.
102. Kahaleh, M.B., et al.: Endothelial injury in scleroderma. J. Exp. Med. *149*:1326, 1979.
103. Fleischmajer, R., et al.: Skin capillary changes in early systemic scleroderma. Arch. Dermatol. *112*:1553, 1976.
104. Oliver, J.A., and Cannon, P.J.: The kidney in scleroderma. Nephron *18*:141, 1977.
105. Rodnan, G.P.: Classification and nomenclature of progressive systemic sclerosis. Clin. Rheum. Dis. *5*:5, 1979.
106. Bohan, A., et al.: An analysis of 153 patients with polymyositis and dermatomyositis. Medicine *56*:255, 1977.
107. Callen, J.P., et al.: The relationship of dermatomyositis and polymyositis to internal malignancy. Arch. Dermatol. *116*:295, 1980.
108. Nishikai, M., and Homma, M.: Anti-myoglobin antibody in polymyositis. Lancet *2*:1205, 1972.
109. Packhan, L.M., and Cooke, N.: Juvenile dermatomyositis: A clinical and immunologic study. J. Pediatr. *96*:226, 1980.
110. Currie, S., et al.: Immunological aspects of polymyositis: The in vitro activity of lymphocytes on incubation with muscle antigen and with muscle cultures. Q. J. Med. *157*:63, 1971.
111. Dawkins, R.L., and Zilko, P.J.: Polymyositis and myasthenia gravis: Immunodeficiency disorders involving skeletal muscle. Lancet *1*:200, 1975.
112. Agnello, V.: Complement deficiency states. Medicine (Baltimore) *57*:1, 1978.
113. Hirsch, T.J., et al.: HLA-DR antigens in polymyositis: Evidence for clinical immunogenetic heterogeneity. Arthritis Rheum. *23*:689, 1980.
114. Schwarz, H.A., et al.: Muscle biopsy in polymyositis and dermatomyositis: A clinicopathologic study. Ann. Rheum. Dis. *39*:500, 1980.
115. Callen, J.P.: Dermatomyositis. Int. J. Dermatol. *18*:423, 1979.
116. Sharp, J.C., et al.: Mixed connective tissue disease—an apparently distinct rheumatic disease syndrome associated with specific antibody to a ribonucleoprotein antigen. Am. J. Med. *52*:148, 1972.
117. Black, C.: Comment—Mixed connective tissue diseases. Br. J. Dermatol. *104*:713, 1981.
118. Bennett, R.M., and O'Connell, D.J.: Mixed connective tissue disease: A clinicopathologic study of 20 cases. Semin. Arthritis Rheum. *10*:25, 1980.
119. Nimel-Stein, S.H., et al.: Mixed connective tissue disease: A subsequent evaluation of the original 25 patients. Medicine *59*:239, 1980.
120. Fauci, A.S., et al.: The spectrum of vasculitis. Clinical, pathologic, immunologic and therapeutic considerations. Ann. Intern. Med. *89*:660, 1978.
121. Cohen, A.S., and Shirohama, T.: Electron microscopic analysis of isolated amyloid fibrils from patients with primary, secondary and myeloma associated disease. A study utilizing shadowing and negative staining techniques. Isr. J. Med. Sci. *9*:849, 1973.
122. Glenner, G.G.: Amyloid deposits and amyloidosis. The β-fibrilloses. N. Engl. J. Med. *302*:1283 and *302*:1333, 1980.
123. Franklin, E.C.: The amyloid disease. *In* Lachmann, P.J., and Peters, D.K. (eds.): Clinical Aspects of Immunology. 4th ed. Oxford, Blackwell Scientific Publications, 1982, p. 1231.
124. McAdam, K.P.W.J., et al.: The biology of SAA: Identification of the inducer, in vitro synthesis, and heterogeneity demonstrated with monoclonal antibodies. Ann. N.Y. Acad. Sci. *389*:126, 1982.
125. Costa, P.P., et al.: Amyloid fibril protein related to prealbumin in familial amyloidotic polyneuropathy. Proc. Natl. Acad. Sci. U.S.A. *75*:4499, 1978.

126. Benson, M.D.: Partial amino acid sequence homology between an heredofamilial amyloid protein and human plasma prealbumin. J. Clin. Invest. *67*:1035, 1981.
127. Sletten, K., et al.: Senile cardiac amyloid is related to prealbumin. Scand. J. Immunol. *12*:503, 1980.
128. Shirahama, T., et al.: Senile cerebral amyloid. Prealbumin as a common constituent in the neuritic plaque in the neurofibrillary tangle and in the microangiopathic lesion. Am. J. Pathol. *107*:41, 1982.
128A. Kyle, R.A.: Amyloidosis. Clin. Haematol. *11*:151, 1982.
129. Husby, G.: Amyloidosis in rheumatoid arthritis. Ann. Clin. Res. *7*:154, 1975.
130. Wright, J.R., et al.: Relationship of amyloid to aging, review of the literature and systematic study of 83 patients derived from a general hospital population. Medicine *48*:39, 1969.
131. Cohen, A.S., et al.: Editorial—Amyloid proteins, precursors, mediator, and enhancer. Lab Invest. *48*:1, 1983.
132. Lavie, G., et al.: Degradation of amyloid precursor SAA by blood monocytes—roles in pathogenesis. J. Exp. Med. *148*:1020, 1978.
133. Kedar, I., et al.: Degradation of amyloid by a serum component and inhibition of degradation. J. Lab. Clin. Med. *99*:693, 1982.
134. Maury, P.J., and Teppo, A.: Mechanism of reduced amyloid—a degrading activity in serum from patients with secondary amyloidosis. Lancet *2*:234, 1982.
135. Van Rijswijk, M.H., and Van Heusden, C.W.G.J.: The potassium permanganate method: A reliable method for differentiating amyloid AA from other forms of amyloid in routine laboratory practice. Am. J. Pathol. *97*:43, 1979.
136. Shtrasburg, S., et al.: Demonstration of AA-protein in formalin-fixed, paraffin-embedded tissues. Am. J. Pathol. *106*:141, 1982.
137. Briggs, G.W.: Amyloidosis. Ann. Intern. Med. *55*:943, 1961.
138. Wright, J.R., and Calkins, E.: Amyloid in the aged heart: Frequency and clinical significance. J. Am. Geriatr. Soc. *23*:97, 1975.
139. Montiero, J.G.: The digestive system in familial amyloidotic polyneuropathy. Am. J. Gastroenterol. *60*:47, 1973.
140. Dickman, S.H., et al.: Resolution of renal amyloidosis. Am. J. Med. *63*:430, 1977.
141. Reinherz, E.L., and Rosen, F.S.: New concepts of immunodeficiency. Am. J. Med. *71*:511, 1981.
142. Ammann, A.J., and Fudenberg, H.H.: Immunodeficiency diseases. *In* Stites, D.P., et al. (eds.): Basic and Clinical Immunology. 4th ed. Los Altos, Lange Medical Publications, 1982, p. 395.
143. WHO Report: Immunodeficiency. Clin. Immunol. Immunopathol. *13*:296, 1979.
144. Pearl, E.R., et al.: B lymphocyte precursors in human marrow: An analysis of normal individuals and patients with antibody deficiency states. J. Immunol. *120*:1169, 1978.
145. Rosen, F.: Genetic defects in gamma globulin synthesis. *In* Stanbury, J.B., et al. (eds.): Metabolic Basis of Inherited Disease. 5th ed. New York, McGraw-Hill Book Co., 1982, p. 1921.
146. Reinherz, E.L., et al.: Immunodeficiency associated with loss of T4+ T-cell function. N. Engl. J. Med. *304*:811, 1981.
147. Waldman, T.A., et al.: Role of T-suppressor cells in the pathogenesis of common variable hypogammaglobulinaemia. Lancet *2*:609, 1974.
148. Eibl, M.M., et al.: Defective macrophage function in a patient with a common variable immunodeficiency. N. Engl. J. Med. *307*:803, 1982.
149. Conley, M.E., and Cooper, M.D.: Immature IgA B-cells in IgA deficient patients. N. Engl. J. Med. *305*:495, 1981.
150. Reinherz, E.L., et al.: Abnormalities of T-cell maturation and regulation in human beings with immunodeficiency disorders. J. Clin. Invest. *68*:699, 1981.
151. Incefy, G.S., et al.: In vitro differentiation of human marrow T-cell precursors by thymic factors in severe combined immunodeficiency. Transplantation *32*:299, 1981.
152. Hong, R.M., et al.: Reconstitution of B- and T-lymphocyte function in severe combined immunodeficiency disease after transplantation with thymic epithelium. Lancet *2*:1270, 1976.
153. Pahwa, S.G., et al.: Heterogeneity of B-lymphocyte differentiation in severe combined immunodeficiency disease. J. Clin. Invest. *66*:543, 1980.
154. Rosen, F.S.: Immunodeficiency. *In* Benacerraf, B. (ed.): Immunogenetics and Immunodeficiency. Lancaster, England, Medical Technical Publishing Co., 1975.
155. Mitchell, B.S., et al.: Purinogenic immunodeficiency disease: Clinical features and molecular mechanism. Ann. Intern. Med. *92*:826, 1980.
156. Parkman, R., et al.: Correction of Wiskott-Aldrich syndrome by bone marrow transplantation. N. Engl. J. Med. *298*:921, 1978.
157. CDC: *Pneumocystis* pneumonia—Los Angeles. M.M.W.R. *30*:250, 1981.
158. CDC: Kaposi's sarcoma and *Pneumocystis* pneumonia among homosexual men—New York City and California. M.M.W.R. *30*:305, 1981.
159. CDC: Update on acquired immune deficiency syndrome (AIDS)—United States. M.M.W.R. *31*:507, 1982.
159A. Research News: Human T-cell leukemia virus linked to AIDS. Science *220*:806, 1983.
160. Desforges, J.F.: AIDS and preventive treatment in hemophilia. N. Engl. J. Med. *308*:94, 1983.
160A. Pitchenik, A.E., et al.: Opportunistic infections and Kaposi's sarcoma among Haitians: Evidence of a new acquired immunodeficiency state. Ann. Intern. Med. *98*:277, 1983.
161. Follansbee, S.E., et al.: An outbreak of *Pneumocystis carinii* pneumonia in homosexual men. Ann. Intern. Med. *96*:705, 1982.
162. Special Report: Epidemiologic aspects of the current outbreak of Kaposi's sarcoma and opportunistic infections. N. Engl. J. Med. *306*:248, 1982.
163. Friedman-Klein, A.E., et al.: Disseminated Kaposi's sarcoma in homosexual men. Ann. Intern. Med. *96*:693, 1982.
164. Hardy, M.A., et al.: De novo Kaposi's sarcoma in renal transplantation. Case report and a brief review. Cancer *38*:144, 1976.
165. Editorial: Acquired immunodeficiency syndrome. Lancet *1*:22, 1983.
166. CDC: Diffuse, undifferentiated non-Hodgkins lymphoma among homosexual males-U.S. M.M.W.R. *31*:277, 1982.
167. Fauci, A.S.: The syndrome of Kaposi's sarcoma and opportunistic infections: An epidemiclogically restricted disorder of immunoregulation. Ann. Intern. Med. *96*:777, 1982.
167A. Reichert, C.M., et al.: Autopsy pathology in the acquired immune deficiency syndrome. Am. J. Pathol. *112*:357, 1983.
168. Durock, D.T.: Opportunistic infections and Kaposi's sarcoma in homosexual men. N. Engl. J. Med. *305*:1465, 1981.
169. Editorial: Acquired immune deficiency syndrome: The past as prologue. Ann. Intern. Med. *98*:401, 1983.
170. Giraldo, G., et al.: Antibody patterns to herpes virus in Kaposi's sarcoma. II. Serologic association of American Kaposi's sarcoma with cytomegalovirus. Int. J. Cancer *22*:126, 1978.
171. Giraldo, G., et al.: Kaposi's sarcoma and its relationship to cytomegalovirus (CMV). III. CMV, DNA and CMV antigens in Kaposi's sarcoma. Int. J. Cancer *26*:23, 1980.
172. Hurtenbach, V., and Shearer, G.M.: Germ cell induced immune suppression in mice. Effect of inoculation of syngeneic spermatozoa on cell mediated immune responses. J. Exp. Med. *155*:1719, 1982.
173. Glass, D.N., et al.: Inherited abnormalities of the complement system. *In* Stanbury, J.B., et al. (eds.): Metabolic Basis of Inherited Disease. 5th ed. New York, McGraw-Hill Book Co., 1982, p. 1934.
174. Frank, M., et al.: Hereditary angioedema. The clinical syndrome and its management. Ann. Intern. Med. *84*:580, 1976.

6 NEOPLASIA

In the United States each year well over 1,000,000 individuals learn for the first time that they have some type of cancer, but fortunately many of these tumors can be cured. Nonetheless, according to American Cancer Society estimates, cancer will cause about 450,000 deaths in 1984, accounting for about 23% of all deaths—the largest proportion to date.[1] Only cardiovascular diseases cause more deaths. The discussion that follows deals with both benign tumors and cancers; understandably, the latter receive more attention. The focus is on the basic morphologic and behavioral characteristics and our present understanding of their origins. There follows in Chapter 7 the clinical aspects and implications. Although the discussion of therapy is beyond our scope, with many forms of malignancy, notably the leukemias and lymphomas, there are now dramatic improvements in the five-year survival rates. A greater proportion of cancers are being cured or arrested today than ever before.

DEFINITIONS

Neoplasia literally means "new growth" and the new growth is a "neoplasm." The term "tumor" was originally applied to the swelling caused by inflammation. Neoplasms also may induce swellings, and by long precedent the non-neoplastic usage of "tumor" has passed into limbo; thus, the term is now equated with neoplasm. Oncology (Greek "oncos" = tumor) is the study of tumors or neoplasms. *Cancer is the common term for all malignant tumors.* Although the ancient origins of this term are somewhat uncertain, it probably derives from the Latin for crab, "cancer"—presumably because a cancer "adheres to any part that it seizes upon in an obstinate manner like the crab." A major focus of pathology is the anatomic differentiation of benign and malignant tumors, carrying with it the implication of their probable clinical behavior. It will become evident, however, that all benign tumors are not completely innocent, just as all malignant tumors are not completely evil. Moreover, some neoplasms fall in the gray area both clinically and anatomically between benign and malignant.

Although all physicians know what they mean when they use the term "neoplasm," it has been surprisingly difficult to develop an accurate definition. The eminent British oncologist Sir Rupert Willis has come closest—"A neoplasm is an abnormal mass of tissue, the growth of which exceeds and is uncoordinated with that of the normal tissues and persists in the same excessive manner after cessation of the stimuli which evoked the change."[2] To this characterization we might add that the abnormal mass is purposeless, preys on the host, and is virtually autonomous. It preys on the host insofar as the growth of the neoplastic tissue competes with normal cells and tissues for energy supplies and nutritional substrate. Inasmuch as these masses may flourish in a patient who is wasting away, they are to a degree autonomous. Later it will become evident that such autonomy is not complete. All neoplasms ultimately depend on the host for their nutrition and vascular supply; many forms of neoplasia require endocrine support.

NOMENCLATURE

All tumors, benign and malignant, have two basic components: (1) proliferating neoplastic cells that constitute their *parenchyma* and (2) *supportive stroma* made up of connective tissue, blood vessels, and possibly lymphatics. Although parenchymal cells represent the proliferating "cutting edge" of neoplasms and so determine their nature, the growth and evolution of neoplasms are critically dependent on their stroma. An adequate stromal blood supply is requisite and the stromal connective tissue provides the framework for the parenchyma. In some tumors the stromal support is scant, and so the neoplasm is soft and fleshy. Sometimes the parenchymal cells stimulate the formation of an abundant collagenous stroma—referred to as *desmoplasia.* Such tumors as, for example, some cancers of the female breast are stony hard or scirrhous. The nomenclature of tumors is, however, based on the parenchymal component. *The suffix "oma" denotes a benign neoplasm.* Benign mesenchymal tumors (those arising in muscle, bones, tendon, cartilage, fat, vessels, and lymphoid and fibrous tissue) are classified histogenetically according to parenchymal cell type, e.g., lipoma, fibroma, angioma. Benign epithelial neoplasms are variously classified, some on the basis of their cells of origin, others on microscopic architecture, and still others on their macroscopic patterns.

Adenoma is the term applied to the benign epithelial neoplasm that forms glandular patterns, as well as to the tumors derived from glands but not necessarily reproducing glandular patterns. On this basis a benign epithelial neoplasm that arises from renal tubular cells growing in the form of numerous tightly clustered small glands would be termed an adenoma, as would a heterogeneous mass of adrenal cortical cells growing in no distinctive pattern. Benign epithelial neoplasms producing microscopically or macroscopically visible fingerlike or warty projections from epithelial surfaces are referred to as *papillomas*. Those that form large cystic masses as in the ovary are referred to as *cystadenomas*. Some tumors produce papillary patterns that protrude into cystic spaces and are called *papillary cystadenomas* (Fig. 6–1). When a neoplasm, benign or malignant, produces a macroscopically visible projection above a *mucosal* surface and projects, for example, into the gastric or colonic lumen, it is termed a *polyp*. The term polyp preferably is restricted to benign tumors. Malignant polyps are better designated polypoid cancers.

Malignant tumor nomenclature essentially follows the same schema used for benign neoplasms with certain additions. *Cancers arising in mesenchymal tissue are called sarcomas* (Greek "sarc-" = fleshy) because they usually have very little connective tissue stroma and so are fleshy: e.g., fibrosarcoma, liposarcoma, and leiomyosarcoma for smooth muscle cancer, and rhabdomyosarcoma for a cancer arising in striated muscle. *Malignant neoplasms of epithelial cell origin, derived from any of the three germ layers, are called carcinomas.* Thus, cancer arising in the epidermis of ectodermal origin is a carcinoma, as is a cancer arising in the mesodermally derived cells of the renal tubules and the endodermally derived cells of the lining of the gastrointestinal tract. Carcinomas may be further qualified. One with a glandular growth pattern microscopically is termed an *adenocarcinoma,* and one producing recognizable squamous cells arising in any of the stratified squamous epithelia of the body would be termed a *squamous cell carcinoma*. It is further common practice to specify, when possible, the organ of origin, e.g., a renal cell adenocarcinoma or bronchogenic squamous cell carcinoma. Not infrequently, however, a cancer is composed of very primitive, undifferentiated cells and must be designated merely as a poorly differentiated or undifferentiated malignant tumor or, when possible, undifferentiated carcinoma or undifferentiated sarcoma.

In most neoplasms, benign and malignant, the parenchymal cells bear a close resemblance to each other, as though all were derived from a single cell, as indeed we know to be the case with many cancers. Infrequently, divergent differentiation of a single line of parenchymal cells creates what are called *mixed tumors*. The best example is the *mixed tumor of salivary gland origin*. These tumors contain epithelial components scattered within a myxoid stroma that sometimes contains islands of apparent cartilage or even bone (Fig. 6–2). All of these elements, it is believed, arise from epithelial and myoepithelial cells of salivary gland origin; thus, the preferred designation of these neoplasms is *pleomorphic adenoma*. This schizophrenic morphology presumably reflects variable expression of several programs of differentiation that are repressed and hidden in the genome of all cells in a multicellular organism. The great majority of neoplasms, even mixed tumors, are composed of cells representative of a single germ layer. The *teratoma*, in contrast, is made up of a variety of parenchymal cell types representative of more than one germ layer, usually all three. They arise from totipotential cells and so are principally encountered in the gonads, but rarely in sequestered primitive cell rests elsewhere. These totipotential cells differentiate along various germ lines, producing, for example, tissues that can be identified as skin, muscle, fat, gut epithelium, tooth structures, and, indeed, any tissue of the body (Fig. 6–3). A particularly common pattern is the ovarian *cystic dermoid teratoma* that differentiates principally along ectodermal lines to create a cystic tumor lined by skin replete with hair, sebaceous glands, and tooth structures. Its true teratomatous origin is often disclosed by accompanying foci of muscle, bone, and cartilage. The cystic dermoid teratoma usually behaves

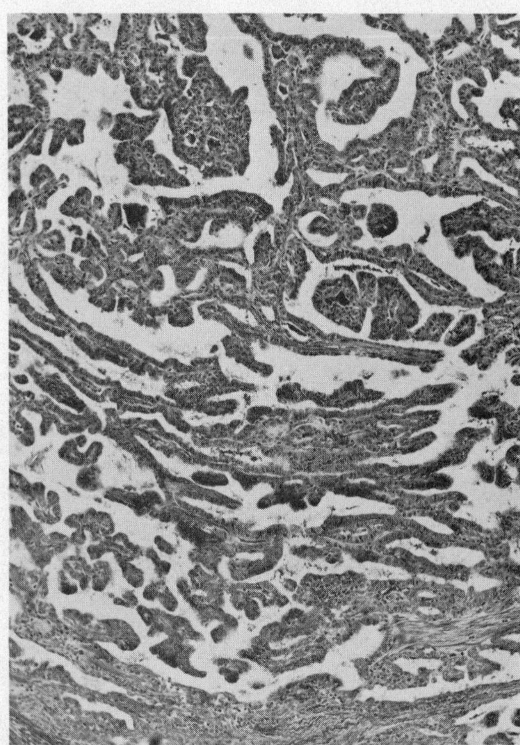

Figure 6–1. Papillary cystadenoma. The papillary tumor fills a small cystic space.

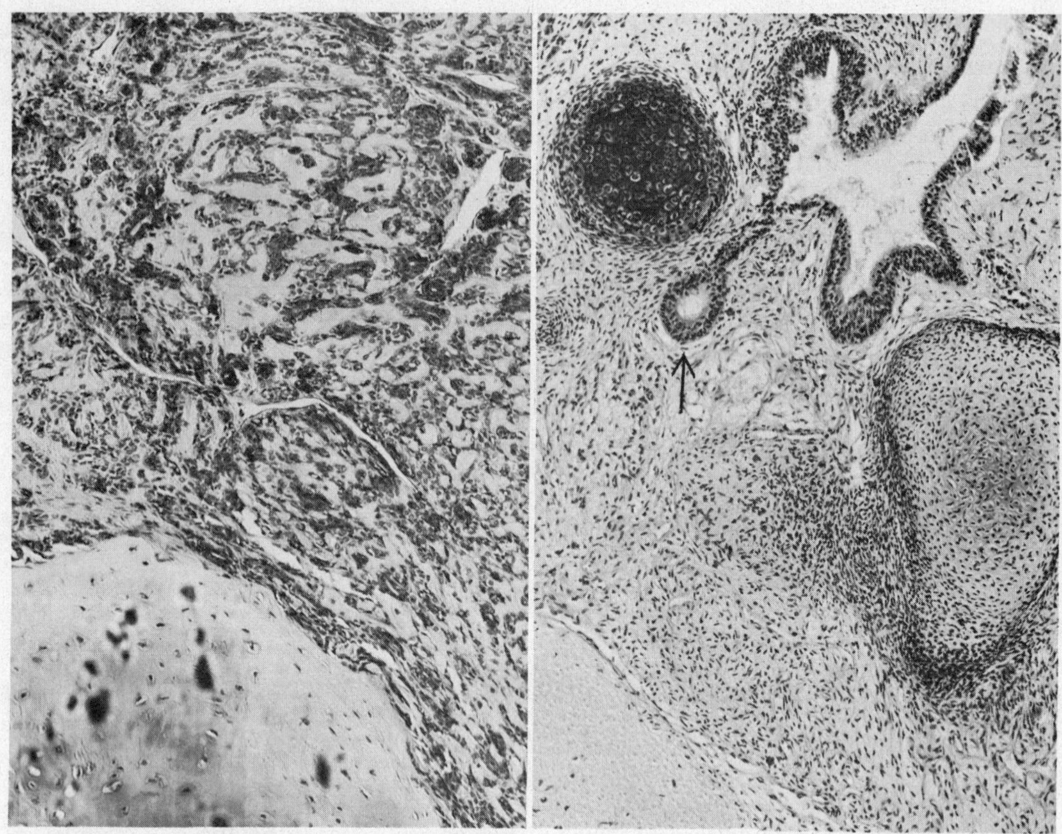

Fig. 6–2

Fig. 6–3

Figure 6–2. A mixed tumor of salivary gland origin (pleomorphic adenoma). There is a large plate of pseudocartilage in the lower field. The remainder of the tumor is composed of small cords and nests of epithelial cells separated by pale areas of loose connective tissue.

Figure 6–3. A teratoma. Three distinct types of adult tissues are seen: a circular island of darkly stained cartilage (mesodermal) in the upper left, a large nest of stratified squamous epithelial cells (ectodermal) on the right, and in the center a gland space lined by columnar cells resembling intestinal tract mucosa (endodermal) *(arrow).*

as a benign neoplasm, but the noncystic, solid, more variegated teratoma is frequently malignant (p. 1095).

The nomenclature of the more common forms of neoplasia is presented in Table 6–1. It is evident from this compilation that there are some inappropriate but deeply entrenched usages. For generations, carcinomas of hepatocytic origin have been called "hepatomas," although correctly they should be referred to as hepatocellular carcinomas, or liver cell carcinomas. Analogously, carcinomas of melanocytes, e.g., melanocarcinomas, are stubbornly called "melanomas," just as certain carcinomas of testicular origin are referred to as seminomas. Other instances will be encountered in which innocent designations belie ugly behavior. Irrational as such usage may be, it is probably more irrational to expect man to be rational. The converse is also true when ominous terms are applied to usually trivial lesions. An ectopic rest of normal tissue is sometimes called a *choristoma*—as, for example, a rest of adrenal cells under the kidney capsule (p. 497). Occasionally a pancreatic nodular rest in the mucosa of the small intestine may mimic a neoplasm, providing some partial justification for the use of a term that implies a tumor. Analogously, aberrant differentiation may produce a mass of disorganized but mature specialized cells or tissue indigenous to the particular site, referred to as a *hamartoma* (p. 497). Thus, a hamartoma in the lung may contain islands of cartilage, blood vessels, bronchial-like structures, and lymphoid tissue. Indeed, sometimes the lesion is purely cartilaginous, or purely angiomatous. Although these might be construed as benign neoplasms, the complete resemblance of the tissue to normal cartilage or blood vessels and the occasional admixture of other elements favors a hamartomatous origin. In any event, the hamartoma is totally benign.

The nomenclature of tumors is important, since specific designations have specific clinical implications. The historically sanctified term "seminoma" connotes a form of carcinoma that tends to spread to lymph nodes along the iliac arteries and aorta. These cancers in their sites of origin in the testes tend to be resectable in almost all cases. Further, the spread into the abdominal lymph nodes, should it be present, can usually be eradicated by radiotherapy; thus, very few patients with seminomas die of their neoplasm. By contrast, the embryonal carcinoma of the testis is not radiosensitive, tending to invade locally beyond the confines of the

Table 6–1. NOMENCLATURE OF TUMORS

Tissue of Origin	Benign	Malignant
I. Composed of one parenchymal cell type		
A. Tumors of mesenchymal origin		*Sarcomas*
(1) Connective tissue and derivatives		
fibrous tissue	fibroma	fibrosarcoma
myxomatous tissue	myxoma	myxosarcoma
fatty tissue	lipoma	liposarcoma
cartilage	chondroma	chondrosarcoma
bone	osteoma	osteogenic sarcoma
(2) Endothelial and related tissues		
blood vessels	hemangioma capillary cavernous sclerosing	angiosarcoma
	hemangioendothelioma	endotheliosarcoma, Kaposi's sarcoma
lymph vessels	lymphangioma	lymphangiosarcoma
synovia		synovioma (synoviosarcoma)
mesothelium (lining cells of body cavities)		mesothelioma (mesotheliosarcoma)
brain coverings	meningioma	
glomus	glomus tumor	
? endothelial or mesenchymal cells		Ewing's tumor
(3) Blood cells and related cells		
hematopoietic cells		myelogenous leukemia monocytic leukemia
lymphoid tissue		malignant lymphomas lymphocytic leukemia plasmacytoma (multiple myeloma)
monocyte-macrophage; Langerhans' cells		histiocytosis X, ? histiocytic lymphoma ? Hodgkin's disease
(4) Muscle		
smooth muscle	leiomyoma	leiomyosarcoma
striated muscle	rhabdomyoma	rhabdomyosarcoma
B. Tumors of epithelial origin		*Carcinomas*
stratified squamous	squamous cell papilloma	squamous cell or epidermoid carcinoma
basal cells of skin or adnexia		basal cell carcinoma
skin adnexal glands:		
sweat glands	sweat gland adenoma	sweat gland carcinoma
sebaceous glands	sebaceous gland adenoma	sebaceous gland carcinoma
epithelium lining		
glands or ducts—well-differentiated group	adenoma papilloma papillary adenoma cystadenoma	adenocarcinoma papillary carcinoma papillary adenocarcinoma cystadenocarcinoma
poorly differentiated group		medullary carcinoma undifferentiated carcinoma (simplex)
respiratory tract		bronchogenic carcinoma bronchial "adenoma"
neuroectoderm	nevus	melanoma (melanocarcinoma)
renal epithelium	renal tubular adenoma	renal cell carcinoma (hypernephroma)
liver cells	liver cell adenoma	hepatocellular carcinoma
bile duct	bile duct adenoma	bile duct carcinoma (cholangiocarcinoma)
urinary tract epithelium (transitional)	transitional cell papilloma	papillary carcinoma transitional cell carcinoma squamous cell carcinoma
placental epithelium	hydatidiform mole	choriocarcinoma
testicular epithelium (germ cells)		seminoma embryonal carcinoma
II. More than one neoplastic cell type—mixed tumors—usually derived from one germ layer		
salivary glands	mixed tumor of salivary gland origin (pleomorphic adenoma)	malignant mixed tumor of salivary gland origin
renal anlage		Wilms' tumor
III. More than one neoplastic cell type derived from more than one germ layer—teratogenous		
totipotential cells in gonads or in embryonic rests	teratoma, dermoid cyst	Malignant teratoma and teratocarcinoma

testis and to spread throughout the body. By the time most of these neoplasms are discovered, the overall two-year survival is about 50%, despite all therapeutic efforts. There also are other varieties of testicular neoplasms, and so the designation "cancer of the testis" tells little of its clinical significance.

CHARACTERISTICS OF BENIGN AND MALIGNANT NEOPLASMS

In the great majority of instances, the differentiation of a benign from a malignant tumor can be made morphologically with considerable certainty; sometimes, however, a neoplasm defies categorization. It has been said, "All tumors need not of necessity be either benign or malignant." Certain anatomic features may suggest innocence while others point toward cancerous potential. Ultimately, all morphologic diagnosis is subjective and constitutes prediction of the future course of a neoplasm. Occasionally this prediction is confounded by a marked discrepancy between the morphologic appearance of a tumor and its biologic behavior: an innocent face may mask an ugly nature. However, such deception or ambiguity is not the rule; in general, there are criteria by which benign and malignant tumors can be differentiated, and they behave accordingly. These differences can conveniently be discussed under the following headings:

(1) Differentiation and anaplasia
(2) Rate of growth
(3) Encapsulation—invasion
(4) Metastasis

A concluding chart on page 229 summarizes the differential points.

DIFFERENTIATION AND ANAPLASIA

The terms *differentiation* and *anaplasia* apply to the parenchymal cells of neoplasms. *Differentiation refers to the extent to which parenchymal cells resemble comparable normal cells, both morphologically and functionally.* Well-differentiated tumors are thus composed of cells resembling the mature normal cells of the tissue of origin of the neoplasm. Poorly differentiated or undifferentiated cancers have primitive-appearing, unspecialized cells (Figs. 6–4 and 6–5). *In general, all benign tumors are well differentiated.* The neoplastic cell in a benign smooth muscle tumor—a leiomyoma—so closely resembles the normal cell as to make it impossible to recognize it as a tumor cell on high-power examination. Only the massing of these cells into a nodule discloses the tumorous nature of the lesion. One may get so close to the tree that one loses sight of the forest. In such benign tumors, mitoses are extremely scant in number, and the few present are normal in appearance. Not infrequently, mitoses seem to be ab-

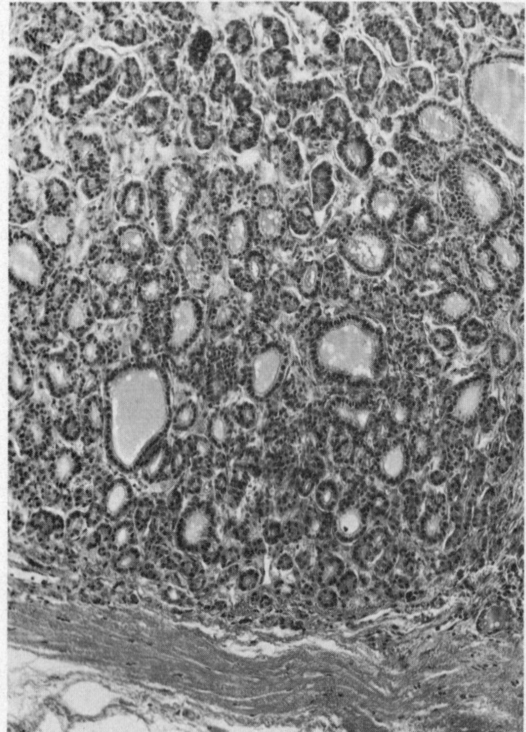

Fig. 6–4

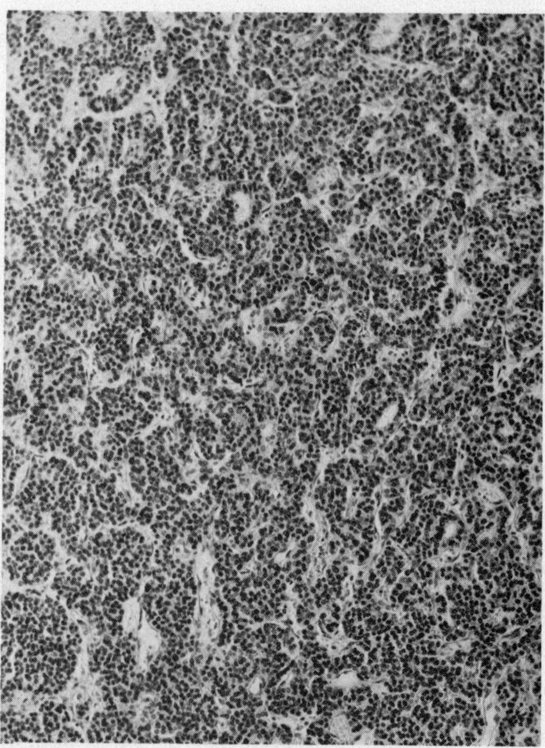

Fig. 6–5

Figure 6–4. A well-differentiated benign thyroid adenoma. The fibrous capsule is in the lower field. The tumor faithfully reproduces thyroid follicles filled with colloid.

Figure 6–5. A moderately poorly differentiated thyroid carcinoma. The tumor cells comprise disorganized cords of cells, and only occasional follicular spaces suggest a thyroid origin.

sent, raising the interesting question of how the tumor achieved its bulk. *Malignant neoplasms, in contrast, range from well differentiated to undifferentiated.*

Anaplasia is a characteristic of cancerous cells and so constitutes one of the features that marks a tumor as malignant. It implies some lack of differentiation of tumor cells. Literally, anaplasia means "to form backward," implying a reversion from a high level of differentiation to a lower level. However, there is substantial evidence that cancers arise from reserve or stem cells present in all specialized tissues. The well-differentiated cancer evolves from maturation or specialization of undifferentiated cells as they proliferate, whereas the undifferentiated malignant tumor derives from proliferation without maturation of reserve cells. Lack of differentiation, then, is not the consequence of dedifferentiation. The conceptual issue is more than academic. Many cells lose their capacity to replicate as they become specialized, but in neoplasia replicative capability may be retained along with specialization.

Lack of differentiation or anaplasia is marked by a number of morphologic and functional changes. Both the cells and their nuclei characteristically display pleomorphism—variation in size and shape. Cells may be found that are many times larger than their neighbors, and other cells may be extremely small and primitive-appearing. Characteristically, the nuclei contain an abundance of DNA and are extremely dark staining (hyperchromatic). The nuclei are disproportionately large for the cell, and the nuclear-cytoplasmic ratio may approach 1:1 instead of the normal 1:4 or 1:6. The nuclear shape usually is extremely variable, and the chromatin often is coarsely clumped and distributed along the nuclear membrane. Large nucleoli are usually present in these nuclei, reflecting the synthetic activity of these cells. Undifferentiated tumors usually possess large numbers of mitoses, reflecting the proliferative activity of the parenchymal cells. Often, the number of mitoses is used as a parameter of the level of aggressiveness of a cancer. In borderline neoplasms when it is difficult to judge whether they are benign or malignant, the decision is sometimes made on the basis of the number of mitoses present. However, as will be seen, tumor growth is not solely dependent on replicative activity. Moreover, the presence of mitoses does not necessarily indicate that a tumor is malignant.

More important as a diagnostic feature of malignant neoplasia are atypical and bizarre mitotic figures sometimes producing tripolar, quadripolar, or multipolar spindles (Fig. 6–6). Often, the mitotic jumble possesses abnormally large spindles in one area and shrunken, puny spindles in other regions. Another important feature of anaplasia is the formation of *tumor giant cells,* some possessing only a single huge polymorphic nucleus, while others have two or more nuclei. These giant cells are not to be confused with inflammatory Langhans' or foreign body giant cells, which possess many small, normal-appearing nuclei. In the cancer giant cell, the nucleus is hyperchromatic and is too large in relation to the cell (Fig. 6–7).

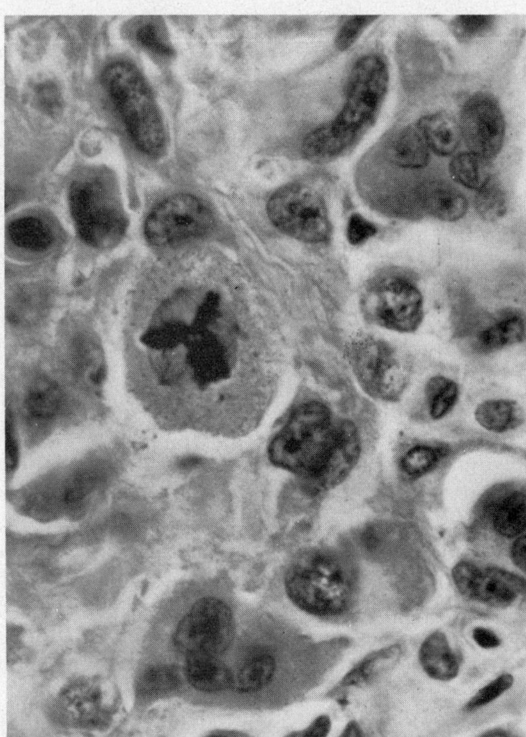

Figure 6–6. High-power detail of anaplastic tumor cells to show cell and nuclear variation in size and shape. The prominent cell in the center field has an abnormal tripolar spindle.

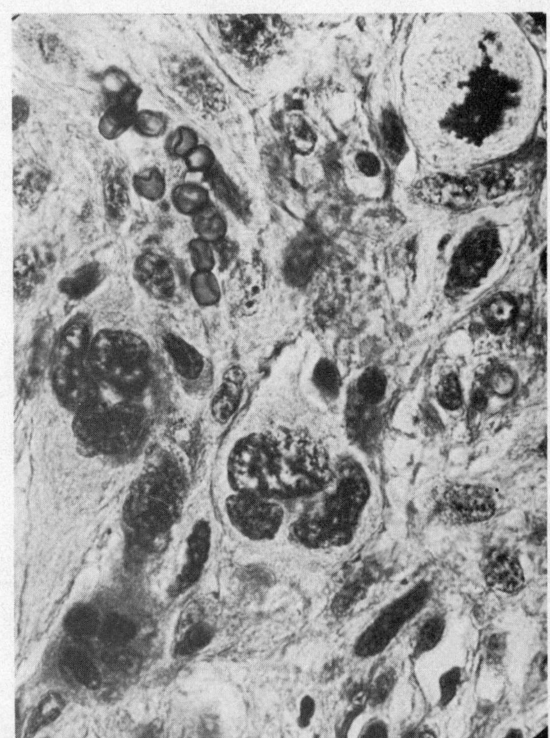

Figure 6–7. Anaplastic tumor cells with prominent multinucleate tumor giant cells and an abnormal mitotic figure in the upper right field.

The orientation of anaplastic cells to each other varies among cancers. In some better differentiated lesions, the cells reproduce a well-defined architecture resembling, to some extent, the tissue of origin. Thus, the gland patterns in adenocarcinomas of the thyroid sometimes resemble normal follicles. At the other end of the spectrum is the very anaplastic cancer, made up of cells that not only are very deviant but whose orientation to each other is helter-skelter. Sheets or large masses of tumor cells grow in an anarchic, disorganized fashion. Although these growing cells obviously require a blood supply, often the connective tissue–vascular stroma is scant, and indeed in many anaplastic tumors large central areas undergo ischemic necrosis.

Electron microscopic, histochemical, and immunocytochemical studies have extended the characterization of neoplastic cells.[3] The cells of benign neoplasms have virtually all the usual ultrastructural features of their normal forebears. Similarly, the well-differentiated cancer cell deviates little from the normal. In undifferentiated cancer cells, having progressively more marked anaplasia, the internal structures have unusual appearances such as accentuation of the nuclear chromatin in clumps along the nuclear membrane, simplification of the rough endoplasmic reticulum, an increase of free ribosomes, and greater pleomorphism of the mitochondria. Various elements may be missing, reduced in size or number, or disturbed throughout the cell in abnormal patterns. However, the cytoskeleton may be markedly retained even in undifferentiated tumor cells. Most normal cells in the body contain three classes of filamentous structures: (1) microfilaments containing actin, (2) microtubules containing tubulin, and (3) intermediate-sized filaments (about 10 nm in diameter.)[4] Presently, at least five types of intermediate filaments have been identified: neurofilaments, glial filaments, cytokeratin, vimentin, and desmin,[5] as pointed out on p. 28. Each of these filaments is restricted to certain cell types (Fig. 6–8). Identification of a particular type by electron microscopy, and the use of specific antibodies with immunofluorescence or immunoperoxidase methods, is proving to be a valuable aid in the diagnosis and identification of the histogenetic origin of many tumors. For example, cytokeratin is present exclusively in cells of epithelial and mesothelial origin, and therefore is a marker for carcinoma or mesothelioma, ruling out the possibility that an undifferentiated cancer is a sarcoma.[6, 6A] In some instances, large amounts of cytokeratin are produced by a neoplasm. The cells in well-differentiated carcinomas taking origin from the keratinocytes of the epidermis (squamous cell or epidermoid carcinomas) elaborate sufficient cytokeratin to produce

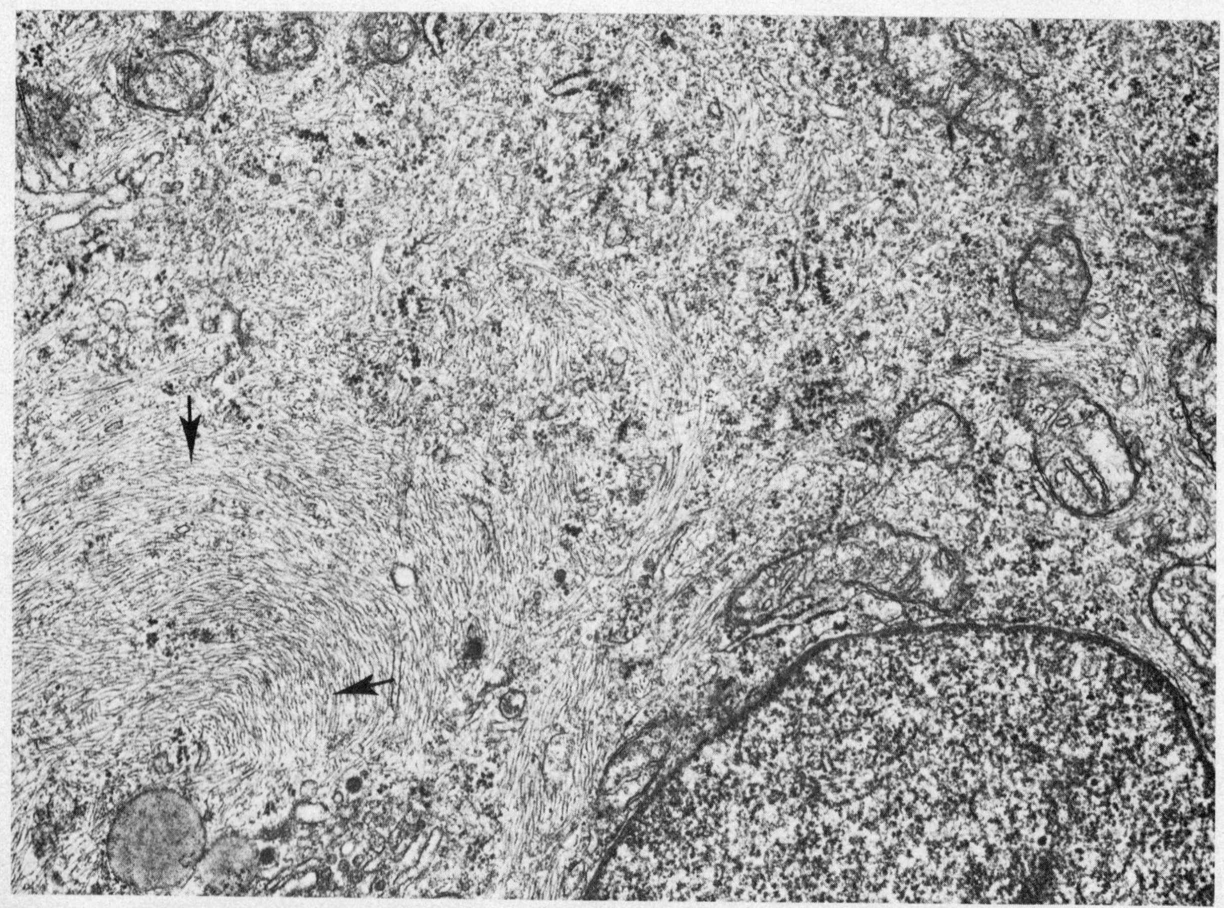

Figure 6–8. Transmission micrograph of an osteoblast to demonstrate the abundant parallel arrays of intermediate filaments compatible with vimentin *(arrows)* (× 8000). (Courtesy of Dr. M. Warhol, Brigham and Women's Hospital.)

intracellular globular masses of hyaline-appearing keratin, readily visible in routine H and E stains under the light microscope. Desmin has so far been described only in muscle cells and neurofilaments in the neuronal line. Thus, intermediate filaments and immunocytochemical methods have provided a new dimension in the characterization of cancers.[7]

The tumor cell's functional sophistication correlates with its level of morphologic differentiation. Well-differentiated cancer cells may elaborate the characteristic products of their normal counterparts, e.g., mucin by carcinomas of the colon, steroids by adrenocortical carcinomas, and bile by hepatocellular carcinomas. The enzyme profiles of differentiated neoplasms also differ little from those of their normal forebears; thus, prostatic carcinomas often elaborate acid phosphatase, while osteogenic sarcomas produce alkaline phosphatase. Undifferentiated cancers, however, may lose these specialized functional characteristics. Thus, poorly differentiated hepatocellular carcinomas may be incapable of synthesizing bile and, similarly, undifferentiated prostatic carcinomas may not elaborate acid phosphatase.

The functional capacity of some cancer cells may exceed, in a sense, that of their normal forebears. For example, in the process of neoplastic transformation, some cancer cells express genetic programs normally expressed only in embryonic cells. Thus, a variety of carcinomas produce fetal antigens as well as tumor neoantigens (p. 268). Identification of fetal antigens in the blood (as discussed later) is used to detect and follow the course of many forms of cancer. In addition, malignant tumors may elaborate hormones and other bioactive products not found in the normal cells from which the tumors arose; this is referred to as *ectopic hormone production*. Thus, certain bronchogenic carcinomas elaborate parathormone, adrenocorticotropic hormone, prostaglandins, and others; renal cell carcinomas may produce erythropoietin. Many other examples might be cited. The systemic consequences of these secreted tumor products induce what are referred to as "paraneoplastic syndromes," described on page 255.

Despite all the ordinary and extraordinary functional capabilities of cancer cells, *the differentiation of benign from malignant tumors rests on their morphology*—more specifically, parenchymal differentiation. The fact that cancers have some degree of anaplasia has been usefully exploited in the cytologic diagnosis of cancer, described later (p. 265). *Anaplasia and evidence of invasion of surrounding structures constitute the two major criteria for the diagnosis of cancer in its primary site of origin.* Later, we shall see that cancers may disseminate (metastasize), and when this has occurred the nature of the primary lesion is no longer in doubt, since *benign tumors never metastasize*.

RATE OF GROWTH

The generalization can be made that *most benign tumors grow slowly over a period of years, whereas most cancers grow rapidly, sometimes at an erratic pace*, and eventually spread and kill their hosts. However, such an oversimplification must be extensively qualified. In truth, little is known about the cell kinetics of benign tumors. The impression that most benign tumors grow slowly derives largely from clinical observation of animals and humans having such neoplasms. Indeed, some may seem to be dormant for years with no increase in size. However, some benign tumors have a higher growth rate than malignant tumors.[8] Moreover, the rate of growth of benign neoplasms may not be constant over time. Factors such as hormone dependence, adequacy of blood supply, and very likely unknown influences may affect their growth. For example, leiomyomas (benign smooth muscle tumors) of the uterus are very common. Not infrequently, repeated clinical examination of women bearing such neoplasms over the span of decades discloses no significant increase in size. After the menopause, the neoplasms may atrophy and later be found to be replaced largely by collagenous, sometimes calcified, tissue. On the other hand, leiomyomas frequently enter a growth spurt during pregnancy. Presumably these neoplasms are to some extent dependent on the circulating levels of steroid hormones, particularly estrogens.

In general, *the growth rate of tumors correlates with their level of differentiation, and thus most malignant tumors grow more rapidly than benign lesions.* There is, however, a very wide range in behavior. At one extreme are the highly aggressive cancers that seem to appear suddenly, increase in size virtually under observation, and explosively disseminate to cause death within a few months of discovery. At the other extreme are some that grow more slowly than benign tumors and may even enter periods of dormancy lasting for years. Indeed, on occasion, cancers have been observed to decrease in size and even spontaneously disappear, but the handful of "miracles" fills only a small volume.[9] To examine this variable behavior more closely, we must consider what is known about: (1) the life history of cancer, involving the cell kinetics of cancer growth; and (2) the influences that modify the growth of malignant tumors.

Both clinical and experimental observations indicate that it takes years for a cancer to produce a clinically overt mass. Most cancers are monoclonal in origin, resulting from the clonal expansion of a single cell that has undergone neoplastic transformation.[10] Evidence for this concept derives from the studies of neoplasms in black women, who often express two isoenzymes of glucose-6-phosphate dehydrogenase (G6PD), each coded by a gene locus on one of the X chromosomes. As explained on page 120, there is random inactivation of one X chromosome in all cells of the female embryo at about 16 days of development. Thus, females are a complex of two populations of cells, each having only one active X chromosome of maternal or paternal origin. Most neoplasms in these women express only a single G6PD variant.[11] If the neoplasms were polyclonal, chance would dictate the two variant forms of G6PD. Additional evidence for the monoclonality of some tumors comes from plasma cell neoplasms. These synthesize a single specific immunoglobulin or fragment of this immunoglobulin, indicating identical genetic programming in all the neoplastic cells, and documenting that all were derived from a single precursor. Nonetheless, in a minority of instances, cancers appear to be polyclonal and sometimes multifocal in origin as, for example, the more-than-chance occurrence in women of lobular cell carcinomas in both breasts simultaneously. In any event, if a cancer is monoclonal and the original transformed cell is about 10 μ in diameter, it will take 30 doublings to produce a mass 1 cm in diameter. Studies of many cancers and leukemias reveal that the doubling time of the neoplastic cells varies enormously, even among histogenetically similar tumors.[12] It may be as long as 260 hours, and indeed may be longer than that of comparable normal cells. Thirty doublings might then require about a year to produce a 1-cm mass if all the cells continue to proliferate and none die or are lost. However, cancer cells are less cohesive than normal cells (for reasons discussed later) and so there is continuous shedding of cells, as well as cell maturation and death.[13] The rate of cell loss per unit of time has been calculated to reach 80 to 90% of the rate of cell birth.[14] Moreover, in most cancers only 30 to 80% of cells are in the replicating pool. Growth rate is determined, then, by the excess of cells produced over those lost per unit of time. Thus, to reach a size of 1 cm might require many years and a computer to calculate precisely, given the three variables. Now it should be evident why the frequency of mitoses in a neoplasm is at best an inaccurate criterion of rate of growth. A cancer could rapidly increase in size, with relatively slow division of cells, if all remained in the replicating pool and none were lost by shedding or maturation and death. These cell kinetics also make evident that *the evolution of a cancer involves more than loss of growth controls and rapid proliferation; it may also represent a disorder of differentiation, maturation, and death of cells.*

Longitudinal studies of patients with carcinoma of the cervix corroborate these theoretical calculations. The Papanicolaou cytologic test (described on p. 265) permits the discovery of extremely small cervical carcinomas when they are only *foci of intramucosal anaplasia without evidence of penetration of the basement membrane, so-called carcinoma in situ (ca-in-situ)* (Fig. 6–9). Such lesions produce no grossly visible change in the cervix, although many can be detected by colpomicroscopy. The peak incidence of in situ cervical carcinoma occurs between 25 and 35 years of age. The average age of patients with clinically overt cancer is 40 to 45 years. It must follow, therefore, that it requires about 10 to 15 years for these neoplasms to evolve from the in situ stage to clinically overt neoplasms.[15] Whether there is continuous growth during this time period, or instead a long interval of dormancy followed by activity, is not known. In either case, it is apparent that a clinically evident neoplasm is only the tip of the iceberg.

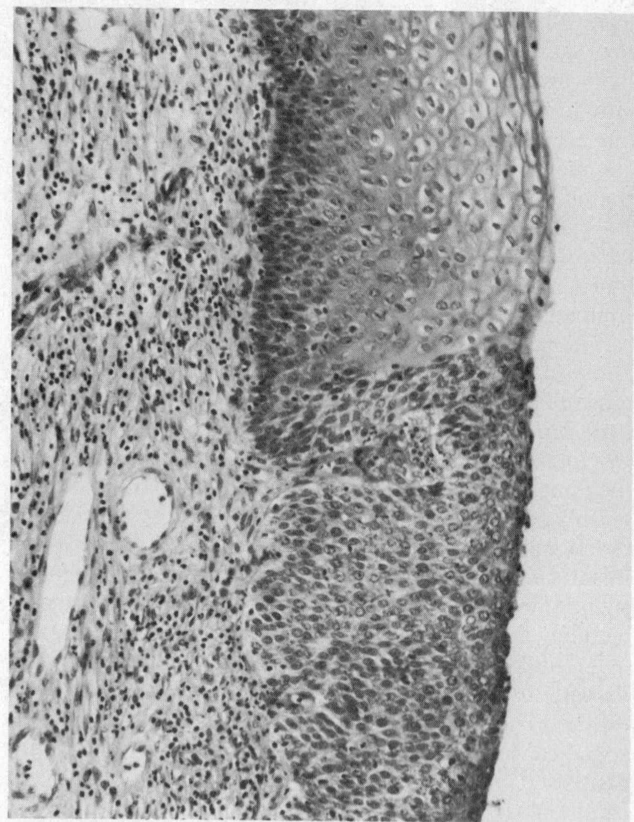

Figure 6–9. Carcinoma in situ of cervix. The normal cervical mucosa is above. There is a sharp transition to the hyperchromatic disorderly cancer cells below, showing no evidence of normal maturation from basal layer to surface. There is no extension of cancer beyond the confines of the mucosa.

Many influences involving the neoplasm and host modify the growth rate of cancers and, possibly, benign tumors as well. Blood supply, nutrition, the defensive immune response of the host, and, in some tumors, endocrine support are the most important influences. Folkman and collaborators have demonstrated that the development of an adequate vascular supply is critical to the growth and development of a cancer as well as its metastases.[16] When they injected cancer cells into the nonvascularized anterior chamber of a rabbit eye, nodules greater than 1 to 2 mm in diameter did not develop. However, the same cells introduced into a vascularized area of the eye developed a stromal blood supply and rapidly overgrew the eye.[17] It was possible to show that the neoplastic cells elaborate a soluble *tumor angiogenesis factor (TAF)* that promotes vascularization of the stroma and permits the progressive growth of solid tumors.[18] The identification of TAF raised the interesting possibility that cancer growth could be blocked by inhibiting the angiogenesis factor. Indeed, an "anti-angiogenesis" factor has been extracted from cartilage, a tissue that normally lacks vascularization. Infusion of an extract of cartilage reduces the growth rate of experimental neoplasms in animals.[19] More recently it was shown that heparin also promotes angiogenesis, and protamine (a heparin antagonist) not only inhibits angiogenesis but also suppresses tumor growth.[20]

Thus, it is clear that tumor growth is dependent on blood supply. Often, primary tumors and their metastases outgrow their blood supply and undergo central ischemic necrosis, where the tumor cells are most remote from the vascular supply of the surrounding normal tissue. Thus, with cancers, the primary lesions and their secondary implants may enlarge progressively while the central regions of necrosis expand. Cancer cells in their growth are also dependent on an adequate supply of nutrients and indeed, when deprived, continue to replicate for a few days and then rapidly die.[21] Many cancers, particularly those arising in hormonally responsive tissues, e.g., breast, uterus, endometrium, ovary, and prostate, are dependent on endocrine support. Steroid sex-hormone receptors have been identified in the epithelial cells of these tissues and their cancers that play roles in the modulation of cell growth in response to varying hormone levels.[22, 23] Exploitation of this endocrine dependence in the treatment of cancers arising in these sites is discussed in some detail on pages 1104 and 1188. It is clear that more is involved in the growth of neoplasms than meets the eye clinically.

ENCAPSULATION—INVASION

Nearly all benign tumors grow as localized expansile masses enclosed within a fibrous capsule. They remain localized to their site of origin and cannot disseminate throughout the body. The capsule comprises an enclosing fibrous membrane, in part derived from the fibrous stroma of the surrounding normal tissues and in part elaborated by the tumor. Such encapsulation tends to contain the benign neoplasm as a discrete, readily palpable, and easily movable mass that can be surgically enucleated (Figs. 6–10 and 6–11). However, the centrifugal growth does cause compression atrophy of contiguous structures. The benign adenoma of the anterior pituitary may destroy all residual normal pituitary parenchyma trapped between the expanding lesion and the sella turcica.

Although encapsulation is a characteristic of benign neoplasms, lack of a capsule does not make a neoplasm malignant. Some benign tumors, such as the leiomyoma in the uterus, remain discrete but are not encapsulated; however, since it is surrounded by compressed myometrium, it can be enucleated. Similarly, hemangiomas (neoplasms composed of tangled blood vessels) are often unencapsulated, and indeed may appear to permeate the site in which they arise (commonly the dermis of the skin). Similarly, certain other benign neoplasms, particularly in the dermis, are unencapsulated. Despite their infiltrative growth and lack of capsule, these new growths never metastasize and so are considered benign.

Cancers are almost never encapsulated and are characterized by infiltrative, erosive growth that extends crablike feet into adjacent tissues (Fig. 6–12). Slowly expanding malignant tumors may develop an apparently

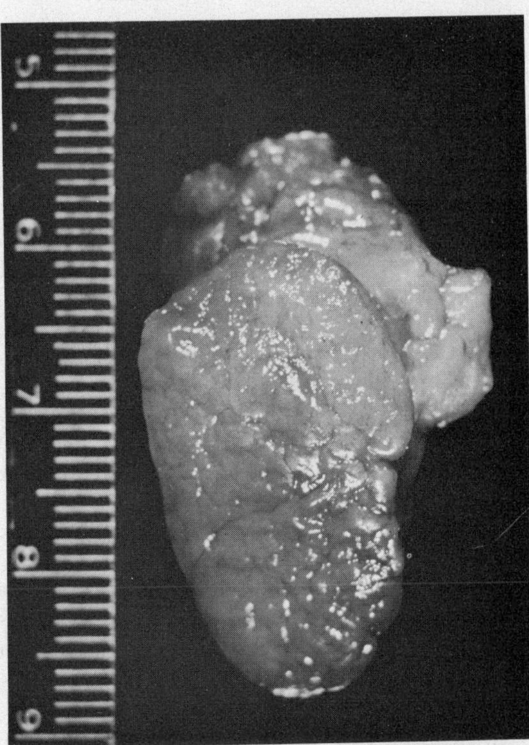

Fig. 6–10

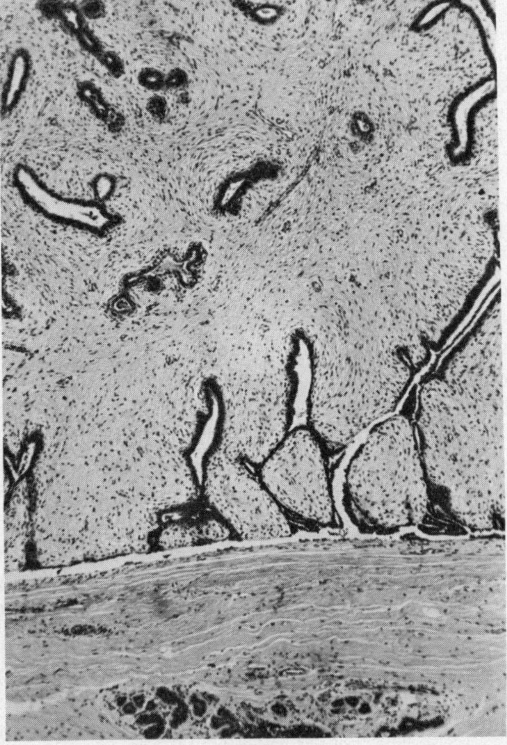

Fig. 6–11

Figure 6–10. Gross view of fibroadenoma of breast. The discrete tumor bulges above the level of the surrounding breast substance as it extrudes from its tight encapsulation.

Figure 6–11. Microscopic view of fibroadenoma of breast seen in Figure 6–10. The fibrous capsule *(below)* separates the sharply delimited tumor mass from the surrounding breast substance.

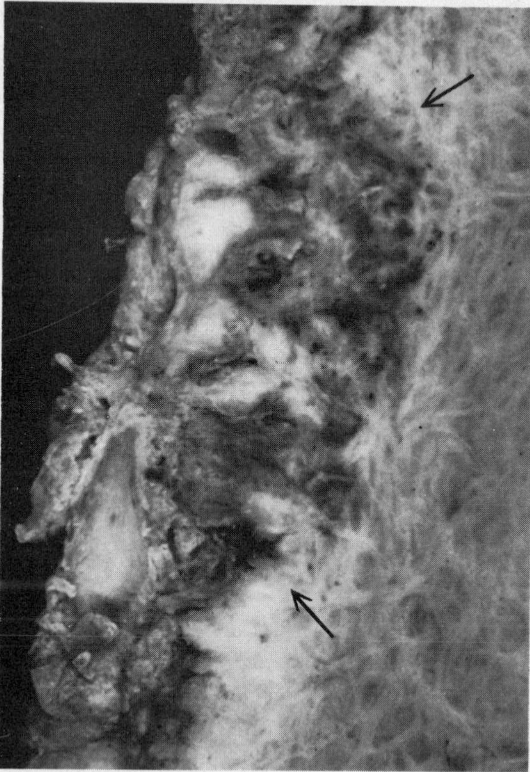

Fig. 6–12

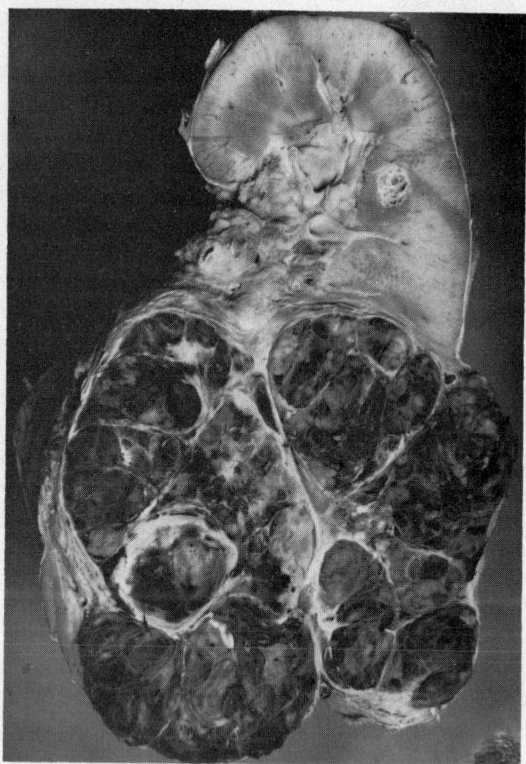

Fig. 6–13

Figure 6–12. Close-up view of adenocarcinoma of endometrium. The malignant tumor *(arrows)* extends into the underlying muscular wall of the uterus. There is no sharp line of delimitation from the surrounding normal tissue.

Figure 6–13. Renal cell carcinoma. The malignancy deceptively appears to be well encapsulated.

enclosing fibrous membrane and may push along a broad front into adjacent normal structures (Fig. 6–13). However, histologic examination will almost always disclose tiny pseudopods indicative of penetrating spread.

Most cancers are obviously invasive and can be expected to penetrate the wall of the colon or uterus, for example, or fungate through the surface of the skin. They recognize no normal anatomic boundaries and often permeate lymphatics, blood vessels, and perineural spaces. Such invasiveness makes their surgical resection exceedingly difficult and generally requires removal of a considerable margin of apparently normal tissues about the infiltrative neoplasm; this is referred to as "radical surgery." *Next to the development of metastases, invasiveness is the most reliable feature that differentiates malignant from benign tumors.*

Although all tissues in the body can be invaded by cancers, there are differences in their vulnerability. The connective tissue stroma of organized tissues is the favored invasive path of most malignant tumors. Within the connective tissue, elastin fibers are much more resistant to the destructive effects of cancers than the collagen fibers. This difference may relate to a high ratio of collagenase relative to elastase in malignant invading tumors. In addition, elastin is extremely inert metabolically and has little or no turnover; it may therefore resist enzymic digestion. Collagen, on the other hand, is more vulnerable to degradation, having a half-life of about 60 days. Nonetheless, densely compacted collagen such as is encountered in membranes, tendons, joint capsules, and so forth, resists invasion for long periods of time. Cartilage is probably the most resistant of all tissues to invasion, but it is not absolute. Several factors have been invoked: (1) the physicochemical characteristics of the matrix, (2) the biologic stability and slow turnover of cartilage, and (3) the elaboration of inhibitory substances such as anti-angiogenesis factor or inhibitors of enzymes involved in the growth and invasiveness of cancer cells.[24, 25] Arteries are much more resistant to invasion than veins and lymphatic channels. The resistance to invasion is conventionally ascribed to the thickness of the arterial walls, but it may also be attributable to the elastin content of arterial walls and their elaboration of protease inhibitors.[26]

Despite extensive study, the mechanisms that make cancer invasive are still poorly understood.[27] There are observations in support of and against each of the following possible processes: (1) physical pressure, (2) reduced adhesiveness and cohesiveness of tumor cells, (3) increased motility of tumor cells, (4) loss of "contact inhibition," and (5) the release of destructive enzymes. Expansile physical pressure may account for compression atrophy and destruction of abutting normal cells in solid organs such as the liver and kidney, and may contribute to penetration of loosely organized connective tissue. However, mechanical factors cannot explain why certain malignant tumors, e.g., some in the gut, permeate the bowel wall without bulging into the lumen.

Cancer cells are less adhesive to structures or substrate and less cohesive than normal cells, but it is highly doubtful whether these attributes contribute significantly to invasiveness.[28] The bases of this altered behavior are still poorly understood, but presumably involve the many surface changes (to be described) associated with neoplastic transformation. The role of locomotion or cell motility in invasiveness is equally controversial.[29] Most malignant cells are capable of locomotion, and during invasion cytoplasmic processes can often be seen protruding between, and indeed into, contiguous normal cells. Such behavior could contribute to invasiveness. Another attribute is that cancer cells will pile up into multilayered, disorganized masses when grown in a culture flask. In contrast, normal cells, when grown in culture, will only form a monolayer covering the surface of the medium, described as "confluence" (Fig. 6–14). When they come into contact with each other in the course of achieving confluence, further cell division and mobility cease in the direction of the cell's contact; this is referred to as "contact inhibition." Unfortunately, poor correlation has been found in cancer cells between "contact inhibition" in culture and invasiveness in vivo.[30]

Malignant tumor cells elaborate a number of enzymes, some released from their surfaces, capable of destroying host tissues in their immediate environment.[31] Among the many tissue-destructive factors are collagenases, lysosomal hydrolases, and plasminogen activator. Many human cancers possess higher levels of lytic enzymes than corresponding normal tissues or benign tumors, and so importance has been ascribed to these destructive enzymes in the invasiveness of cancers, although this has not been established. Conceivably, destruction or disruption of normal tissues by enzymatic action might prepare potential pathways for expansile growth and locomotion, while reducing inhibitory contacts.[27] Other factors might be mentioned. There is considerable evidence in lower animals and some evidence in man that cancers possess tumor-specific antigens, and evoke both a humoral and local cell-mediated immune response. The local immune response induces an inflammatory reaction, and the edematous disruption and possible destruction of abutting tissues might open pathways favorable for tumor permeation.

Attractive as each of these possibilities may appear, the contribution of each is still uncertain. It must be remembered that some normal cells, e.g., leukocytes and trophoblasts, are also capable of invasion. There are no indications that the cellular activities of malignant and nonmalignant cells are different qualitatively, except for the speculation that they are unregulated, and therefore more aggressive in the cancerous phenotype.

METASTASIS

Metastases are tumor implants discontinuous with the primary tumor. The metastases themselves may secondarily give rise to other metastases. *Metastasis*

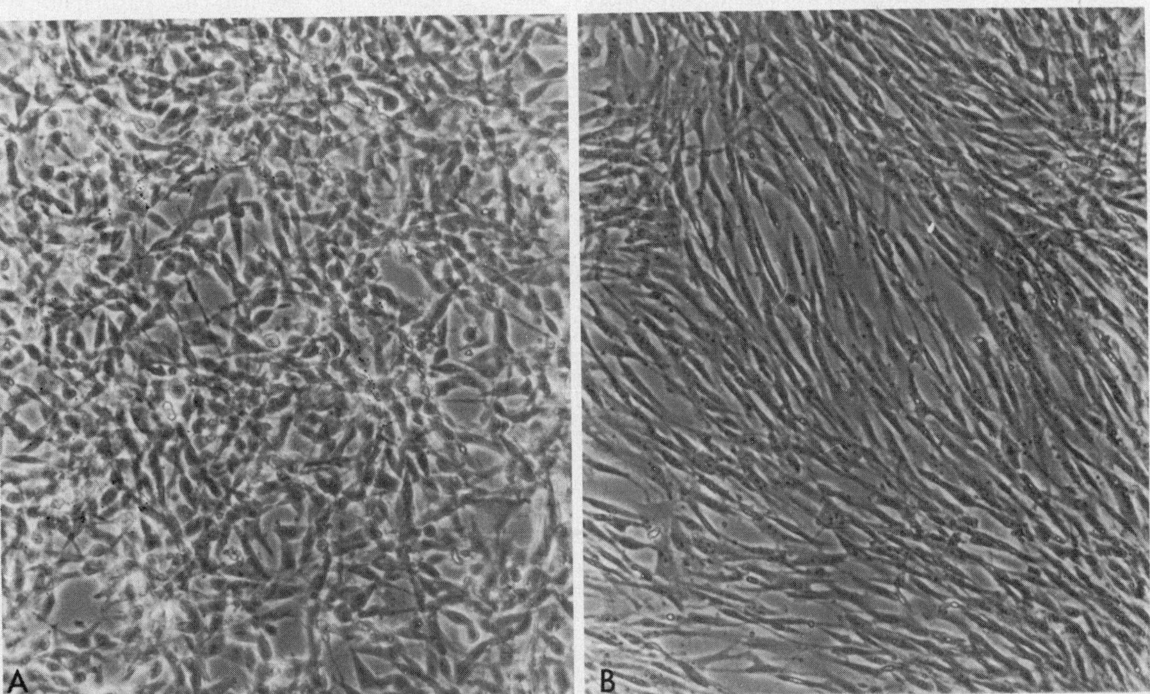

Figure 6–14. Phase-contrast photography of living cell cultures. *A*, The helter-skelter piled-up disarray of virally transformed hamster fibroblasts. *B*, For contrast, the orderly oriented monolayer of normal hamster fibroblasts. (Courtesy of Dr. Thomas Wright, Department of Pathology, Harvard Medical School.)

unequivocally marks a tumor as malignant because benign neoplasms do not metastasize. The invasiveness of cancers permits them to penetrate into blood vessels, lymphatics, and body cavities, providing the opportunity for spread. *With few exceptions, all cancers can metastasize.* The major exceptions are most malignant neoplasms of the glial cells in the central nervous system, called gliomas, and basal cell carcinomas of the skin. Both are highly invasive forms of neoplasia (the latter being known in the older literature as rodent ulcers because of their invasive destructiveness), but they rarely metastasize.

In general, the more aggressive, the more rapidly growing, and the larger the primary neoplasm, the greater the likelihood that it will metastasize or already has metastasized. However, there are innumerable exceptions. Small, well-differentiated, slowly growing lesions sometimes metastasize widely, and conversely, some rapidly growing lesions remain localized for years. No judgment can be made, then, about the probability of metastasis from pathologic examination of the primary tumor. Many factors relating to both invader and host are involved, as will be pointed out later.

Pathways of Spread

Dissemination of cancers may occur through one of four pathways: (1) direct seeding of body cavities or surfaces, (2) transplantation, (3) lymphatic permeation, and (4) embolization through blood vessels. Each of these pathways will be described separately.

SEEDING OF BODY CAVITIES AND SURFACES. This may occur whenever a malignant neoplasm penetrates into a natural "open field." Most often involved is the peritoneal cavity, but any other cavity—pleural, pericardial, subarachnoid, and joint spaces—may be affected. Such seeding is particularly characteristic of carcinomas arising in the ovaries, when not infrequently all peritoneal surfaces become coated with a heavy layer of cancerous glaze. Remarkably, the tumor cells may remain confined to the surface of the coated abdominal viscera without penetrating into their substance. Superficial seedings have as much impact on the host as deep seedings. Sometimes, mucus-secreting ovarian and appendiceal carcinomas fill the peritoneal cavity with a gelatinous neoplastic mass referred to as *"pseudomyxoma peritonei."*

TRANSPLANTATION. This term refers to the mechanical transport of tumor fragments by instruments or gloved hands. That this can occur is amply documented by the ease of tumor transplantation in animals. Transplantation of cancers has also taken place along needle tracks following aspiration biopsy. Fortunately, however, mechanical transport is a rare pathway of tumor dissemination in man, a tribute to either judicious surgical care or the inability of tumor cells to survive when artificially displaced.

LYMPHATIC SPREAD. Transport through lymphatics is the most common pathway for the initial dissemination of carcinomas, but it should be emphasized that sarcomas may also use this route. Past emphasis on lymphatic spread for carcinomas and hematogenous spread for sarcomas is misleading, since ultimately there are numerous interconnections between the vascular and lymphatic systems.[32] The precise steps are still somewhat uncertain, but most of the evidence suggests that invasive cancer cells, when they reach a lymphatic channel, actively migrate through interendothelial cell junctions by a process resembling reverse diapedesis to gain access to the lumen and then embolize to regional nodes (Fig. 6–15). *The pattern of lymph node involvement follows the natural routes of drainage.* Since carcinomas of the breast usually arise in the upper outer quadrants, they generally disseminate first to the axillary lymph nodes. Cancers of the inner quadrant may drain through lymphatics to the nodes within the chest along the internal mammary arteries. Thereafter, the infraclavicular and supraclavicular nodes may become involved. Bronchogenic carcinomas arising in the major respiratory passages metastasize first to the perihilar tracheobronchial and mediastinal nodes. However, local lymph nodes may be bypassed—"skip metastasis"—because of venous-lymphatic anastomoses, or when there has been inflammatory or radiation-induced obliteration of channels.

In many cases the regional nodes serve as effective barriers to further dissemination of the tumor, at least for a time. Conceivably the cells, after arrest within the node, may be destroyed. A tumor-specific immune response initiated by the tumor-specific antigens (described later) may participate in this cell destruction. In addition, non–immunologically sensitized "natural killer" (NK) cells (p. 160) may also participate in tumor cell destruction.[33] Drainage of tumor cell debris and/or tumor antigens will also induce reactive changes within nodes. Thus, enlargement of nodes may occur either from the spread and growth of cancer cells or from follicular hyperplasia, proliferation of paracortical T cells, and sinus histiocytosis (proliferation of sinus endothelial cells and histiocytes) initiated by the products released from the primary lesion or from tumor cells

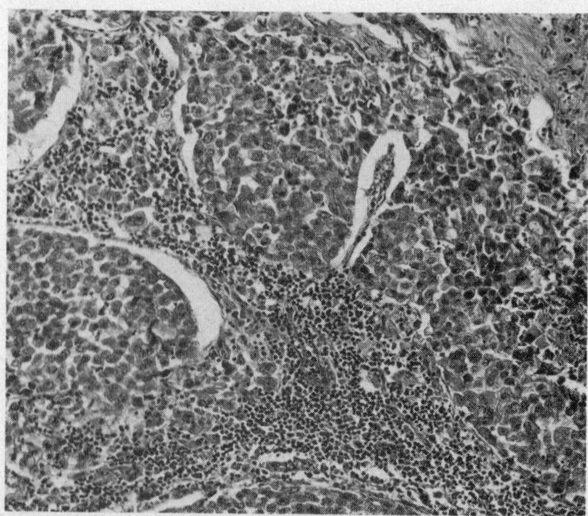

Figure 6–15. Portion of a lymph node with sinuses distended by metastatic tumor.

destroyed within the nodes. It should be noted therefore that *nodal enlargement in proximity to a cancer does not necessarily mean dissemination of the primary.*

HEMATOGENOUS SPREAD. This pathway is typical of sarcomas but also is not uncharacteristic of carcinomas. Arteries, as mentioned, are less readily penetrated than veins. However, arterial spread may occur when tumor cells pass through the pulmonary capillary beds or pulmonary arteriovenous shunts, or when pulmonary metastases themselves give rise to additional tumor emboli. In such arterial spread, a number of factors (to be discussed) condition the patterns of distribution of the metastases. With venous invasion, the blood-borne cells follow the venous flow, draining the site of the neoplasm. Understandably, the liver and lungs are most frequently secondarily involved in such hematogenous dissemination (Fig. 6–16). All portal area drainage flows to the liver, and all caval blood flows to the lungs. Cancers arising in close proximity to the vertebral column often embolize through the paravertebral plexus, and this pathway is probably involved in the frequent metastases to the skull of neuroblastomas of the adrenal gland, in pelvic metastases of pancreatic carcinoma, and in vertebral metastases of carcinomas of the thyroid and prostate.

Certain cancers have a propensity for invasion of veins. The renal cell carcinoma often invades the branches of the renal vein and then the renal vein itself to grow in a snakelike fashion up the inferior vena cava, sometimes reaching the right side of the heart. Hepatocarcinomas often penetrate portal and hepatic radicles to grow within them into the main venous channels. Remarkably, such intravenous growth may not be accompanied by widespread dissemination. Histologic evidence of penetration of small vessels at the site of the primary neoplasm is obviously an ominous feature. However, such changes must be viewed guardedly because, for reasons discussed below, they do not indicate the inevitable development of metastases.

Events Involved in Metastasis

The development of a metastasis involves a complex sequence of interdependent events best conceptualized as a stairway (Fig. 6–17) where each sequential step must be successfully surmounted to eventually produce a secondary implant.[31, 34] The initial steps in this sequence have been discussed elsewhere, and so we may pick up the sequence where tumor cells have invaded the vascular or lymphatic channels. They may either grow at the site of penetration or, because of their loss of cohesiveness, be swept away as individual cells or small embolic clumps. In this exposed situation they are vulnerable to humoral or cell-mediated immune responses and to nonimmune defenses such as destruction by activated macrophages or natural killer cells. Conversely, they may become coated with polymerized fibrin[35, 36] or platelet aggregates, both of which could enhance survival of intravascular cancer cells, and therefore the formation of metastases. The cells that survive must then arrest in the capillary beds of distant organs either by adherence to endothelial cells or attachment

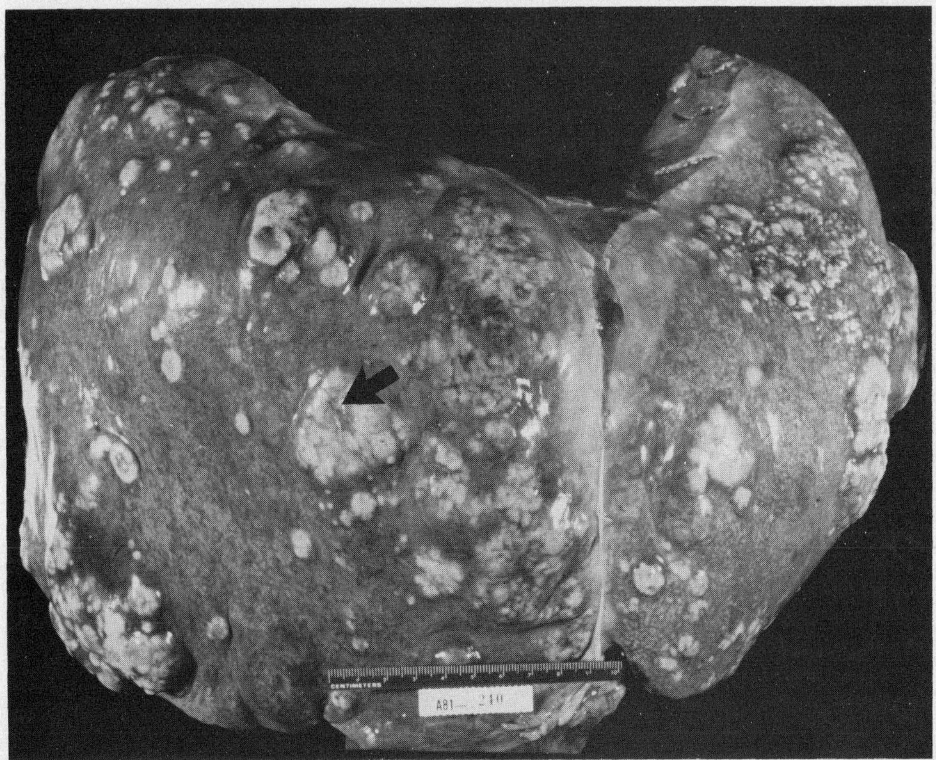

Figure 6–16. Metastatic carcinoma to liver. Note umbilication *(arrow)* of large implant caused by central necrosis of tumor. (Courtesy of Dr. Lawrence Weiss, Brigham and Women's Hospital.)

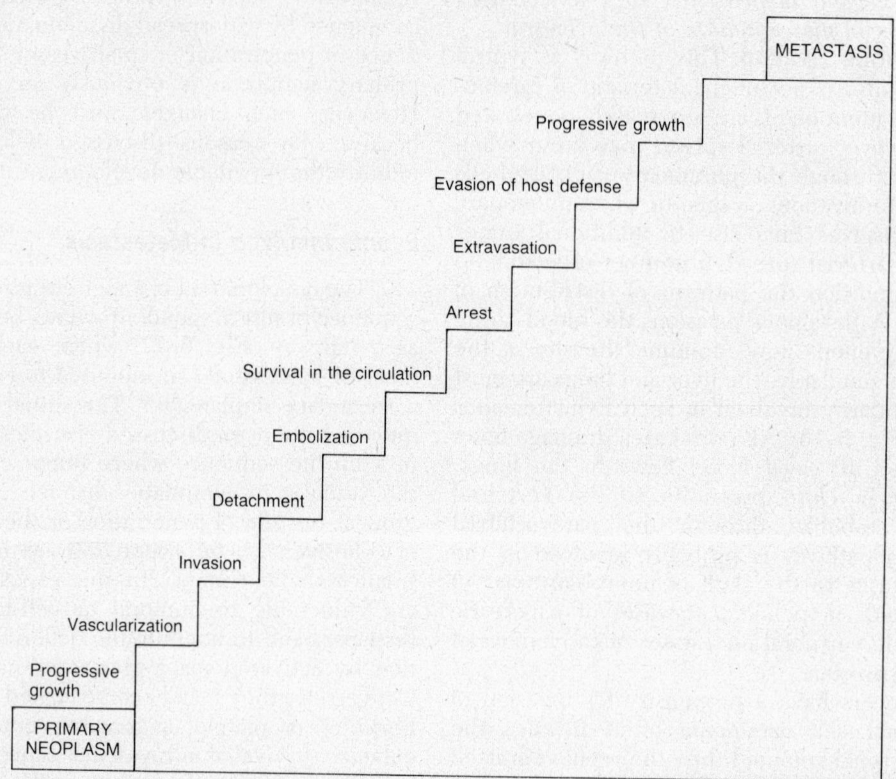

Figure 6–17. Essential steps in the formation of a metastatic lesion. Failure to complete any of the steps will lead to no secondary growth. (Drawn from Hart, I. R., and Fidler, I. J.: The implications of tumor heterogeneity for studies on the biology and therapy of cancer metastasis. Biochim. Biophys. Acta *651*:37, 1981. Reproduced with permission.)

to vascular basement membrane exposed by endothelial cell retraction.[37] As discussed below, the arrest of circulating tumor cells is not merely haphazard. Extravasation of cells at sites of arrest presumably involves the same ill-defined influences that determine the invasiveness of primary neoplasms. Thereafter the metastasis must avoid the host immune response, develop its own vascularization, and in this way, unfortunately, produce a secondary implant that often presages the beginning of the end for the patient.

Several other phenomena bear on the metastatic process. There is good documentation that all cancers in humans are made up of diverse subpopulations of cells having differing biologic characteristics. Cells obtained from individual tumors have been shown to differ with respect to their antigenic properties, karyotypes, growth rate, hormone receptors, ability to invade, and, of particular interest here, metastatic capabilities.[38] This *tumor heterogeneity* could, of course, reflect a polyclonal origin of a single neoplasm but it most likely results from acquired mutations in the genetically unstable replicating cells of monoclonal origin. This heterogeneity is closely linked to what has been called *"tumor progression," i.e., the progressive acquisition by a neoplasm of such individual and separable characteristics as invasiveness, metastatic potential, hormonal responsiveness, and others.* Progression implies that over the course of its evolution a cancer, or particular subpopulations or clones, acquire, for example, an increased growth rate or the capacity to invade or to metastasize. In keeping with this concept, specific sublines can be isolated from a heterogeneous tumor having considerably higher metastatic potential than others.[39] Growth of such a clone would yield a neoplasm capable of metastasis. Thus, the basal cell carcinoma has the capacity to invade but not to metastasize. Conversely, some ovarian carcinomas may seed (metastasize) throughout the peritoneal cavity but not invade the intra-abdominal organs. Metastatic potential is an attribute that may or may not be acquired by one or more sublines within a malignant tumor during its evolution. Thus, some cancers acquire this regrettable capability early, perhaps during its *in situ* stage, while others may develop this ugly attribute only late or possibly never. It is evident that heterogeneity and tumor progression introduce elements of uncertainty into clinical judgments about the best approach to its therapeutic management.

Because of the many interdependent events involved, most blood-borne cancer cells fail to complete successfully all the steps involved in the establishment of metastases. Indeed, in experimental models it can be shown that only between 0.1 and 1% of intravenously injected cells survive for more than 24 hours.[40] Death of the cells occurs in such experiments before an immune response is mounted, and so they must fall prey to other defenses such as activated macrophages or natural killer cells.[33] *For these reasons the finding of tumor cells within vascular channels in a microscopic slide of a cancer, although ominous, cannot be equated with metastasis.*

For some long time the distribution of metastases in the body was thought to be largely haphazard, dependent only on the natural lymphatic and vascular connections of the primary neoplasm. The concept of "favorable" and "unfavorable" soil was invoked to explain the relative rarity of metastases in certain organs or tissues, e.g., in the spleen and skeletal muscles. However, in experimental systems the location of metastases has been shown to be nonrandom, and so influences must condition the trapping of tumor cells in specific locations, as discussed below. During transport through the blood a variety of interactions occur such as homotypic adhesion of tumor cells to form multicell emboli, and adhesion of tumor cells to platelets, lymphocytes, and noncirculating host cells, that undoubtedly affect the location of cancer cell arrest and survival.[41, 42] In addition, poorly understood surface properties of circulating cancer cells and host normal cells, possibly receptors, have been shown to lead to specific localization of metastases. Ingeniously, it has been possible to select sublines from a variety of tumors—notably the B16 mouse melanoma—that will selectively "home" to specific organs, e.g., the lung, liver, brain, or ovary.[43] Pursuing this strange phenomenon further, it has been shown that cancer cells that preferentially "home" to the lung will also localize selectively within lung tissue implanted in the thigh. Indeed, it is possible to confer on sublines a preference for the lung by fusing onto them vesicles of plasma membrane derived from pulmonary homing sublines.[44] It appears, therefore, that at least certain experimental neoplasms possess surface properties or receptors specific for certain normal tissues. Whether these phenomena have applicability to man is not known, but it is a curious fact that bronchogenic carcinomas have a high propensity for metastasizing to the adrenal glands, and renal cell and breast carcinomas have a preference for the lungs, bones, and brain. Thus, factors still unidentified may influence the localization of all metastases. There is more to the metastatic process than the mere casting free of cells into the languid or rushing streams of lymph and blood.

With this overview of the specific characteristics of benign and malignant tumors, the differential features are summarized in Table 6–2.

GRADING AND STAGING OF CANCER

Comparison of end results of various forms of cancer treatment, particularly between clinics, requires some degree of comparability of the neoplasms being assayed. To this end, systems have been devised to express, at least in semiquantitative terms, the level of differentiation—*grade*, and extent of spread of a cancer within the patient—*stage*, as parameters of the clinical gravity of the disease.

Grading of a cancer is based on the cytologic differentiation of the tumor cells and the number of mitoses within the tumor as presumed correlates of the neoplasms' aggressiveness and level of malignancy. Thus, cancers are classified as Grades I to IV with increasing anaplasia. Criteria for the individual grades vary with each form of neoplasia and so will not be detailed here, but all attempt, in essence, to judge the extent to which the tumor cells resemble or fail to resemble their normal counterparts. One of the most widely used systems is Broder's grading, usually applied to squamous cell carcinomas of the skin. Unfortunately, the grading of cancers is replete with shortcomings. The level of differentiation may differ somewhat from one area to the next in large tumors, creating sampling errors. As has been indicated, with tumor progression the level of differentiation may change. Most often, cancers become progressively more undifferentiated as more vigorous, less specialized clones outgrow the better differentiated ones. Infrequently, cancers may become better differentiated, documented by the transformation of highly aggressive neuroblastomas into benign ganglioneuromas. Moreover, the correlation between histologic appearance and biologic behavior is less than perfect. In recognition of these problems and in order to avoid spurious quantification, it is more common practice to characterize a particular neoplasm in descriptive terms, e.g., well-differentiated, mucin-secreting adenocarcinoma of the stomach, or highly undifferentiated, rapidly growing (more than ten mitoses

Table 6–2. COMPARISONS BETWEEN BENIGN AND MALIGNANT TUMORS

Characteristics	Benign	Malignant
Differentiation—anaplasia	Well-differentiated; structure may be typical of tissue of origin	Some lack of differentiation with anaplasia; structure is often atypical
Rate of growth	Usually progressive and slow; may come to a standstill or regress; mitotic figures are rare and normal	Erratic and may be slow to rapid; mitotic figures usually numerous and abnormal
Encapsulation—invasion	Usually encapsulated, but rarely capsule is lacking; generally cohesive and expansile	Invasive without encapsulation; usually infiltrative, but may be seemingly cohesive and expansile
Metastasis	Absent	Frequently present; the larger and more undifferentiated the primary, the more likely are metastases

per ten high-power fields) retroperitoneal malignant tumor—probably sarcoma.

The staging of cancers is based on the size of the primary lesion, its extent of spread to regional lymph nodes, and the presence or absence of blood-borne metastases. Two major staging systems are currently in use, one developed by the Union Internationale Contre Cancer (UICC) and the other by the American Joint Committee (AJC) on Cancer Staging. The UICC employs a so-called *TNM system*—T for primary tumor, N for regional lymph node involvement, and M for metastases. The TNM staging varies slightly for each specific form of cancer, but there are general principles. With increasing size the primary lesion is characterized as T1 to T4. Occasionally a T0 is added to indicate an in situ lesion. N0 would mean no nodal involvement, while N1–N3 would denote involvement of an increasing number and range of nodes. M0 signifies no distant metastases, while M1 or sometimes M2 indicates the presence of blood-borne metastases and some judgment as to their number.

The AJC employs a somewhat different nomenclature and divides all cancers into Stages 0 to IV, incorporating within each of these stages the size of the primary lesion as well as the presence of nodal spread and distant metastases. The use of these systems of staging and more details will emerge later in the consideration of specific tumors. However, it merits emphasis here that staging of neoplastic disease has assumed great importance in the selection of the best form of therapy for the patient, as is most clearly exemplified in the treatment of Hodgkin's disease (p. 674).

ATTRIBUTES OF TRANSFORMED (CANCER) CELLS

When normal cells are exposed in vitro to carcinogenic influences (chemical carcinogens, oncogenic viruses, radiant energy), they acquire many altered characteristics involving growth behavior and morphology, as well as others, and are said to have undergone transformation. Parenthetically, normal cells when maintained in vitro for some time may "spontaneously" undergo transformation. However, transformation is not a sudden change that occurs all at once. Instead, it appears to be a gradual process in which successive generations of cells exposed to a carcinogen or repeatedly subcultured become ever more deviant until finally irreversible transformation is achieved. Such fully transformed cells upon transplantation into syngeneic hosts, are capable of producing tumors. Earlier, some or many of the cells cultured in vitro, when removed from the carcinogenic environment, may be capable of reversion to normal, and may or may not in vivo be capable of forming tumors on transplantation.[45] Thus, the evidence suggests that *transformation followed by cancerous potential is a dynamic process involving more than one generation of cells, each exhibiting greater deviation from the norm.* Moreover, cell proliferation is required to "fix" the transformed state permanently. This concept of the sequential development of cancerous transformation is of some clinical importance. Cells from certain human brain tumors and animal neoplasms, when grown in culture and treated with cAMP, have been induced to differentiate into specialized normal cells, suggesting the turning off of the cancerous transformation process. This so-called "reverse transformation" has been achieved with other agents that apparently induce mature differentiation of cells.[45A] The highly malignant neuroblastoma in children has been known to change into the more differentiated benign ganglioneuroma. In these instances, the neoplastic transformation had apparently not passed the "point of no return." Regrettably, however, most cancers in man are made up of irreversibly transformed cells that do not revert to "tame little pussycats."

The intracellular, presumably molecular event or events that bring about the conversion of normal cells to cancer cells is of course a critical issue that is still under investigation. But whatever is involved, the phenotype of the cancer cell differs in many ways from the normal.[46] These differences can be arbitrarily divided into: (1) altered growth properties in vitro and in vivo; (2) morphologic changes; (3) karyotypic changes; (4) antigenic changes; (5) metabolic deviations; and (6) altered surface characteristics. It must be emphasized, however, that none of these deviations from the norm is invariably present in all transformed cells, and so none can be considered as a marker of the cancerous phenotype. *The only certain proof of cancerous conversion is the ability of the cells to grow when implanted into an appropriate host and eventually to cause the death of the host.* It is still not clear whether such destructive behavior results from some genetic change, i.e., a mutation, or is caused by some modification of gene expression, i.e., is epigenetic. But in either event the cancerous phenotype, once firmly imprinted, is almost always persistent and transmitted from one generation to the next. What then are the salient features of cancer cells?

ALTERED GROWTH PROPERTIES

Cancer cells can be characterized as antisocial, fairly autonomous units that appear to be indifferent to the constraints and regulatory signals imposed on normal cells.

Unregulated proliferation is a fundamental feature of all neoplastic cells, benign as well as malignant. They appear to have acquired the inbuilt capacity for continued replication in the absence of mitogenic stimuli.[47] Loss of response to regulatory controls is a favored theory.[48]

Failure to maturate may play as important a role in the altered growth of cancers cells as unregulated proliferation. When cells fail to maturate, they live much longer than normal cells because there is no

As is evident from Table
deletions or translocations ha
lymphomas and solid tumors
the translocation 8;14 in the c
a monoclonal B-cell malignan
particularly frequent in certa
662). There is a great deal c
that the Epstein-Barr virus
causation. Conceivably, eithe
a single B cell renders it
transformation by the EBV,
act in concert to induce th
later.[57] The meningioma is an
ally benign) of particular inter
specific chromosomal abnorm
neoplasms arising, as the na
inges, have either a partial
chromosome 22. Recent stud
approximately half of the long
associated with benign behav
by complete loss of the chro
behavior ensues with local in

In addition to the specifi
certain tumors, a wide range
and structural chromosomal ab
present in solid neoplasms. Th
secondary changes acquired
progression. Whether such ac
are associated with altered b
intense study.[58]

ANTIGENIC CHANGES

Cancer cells, when trans
by carcinogenic agents (chem
ergy), express a range of ant
also found in normal cells, e.
or organ specific, and ABO
they express a great many *t*
that may or may not be prese
any event are more abundant
it might be noted that these
provide so-called "markers" o
they can be used sometimes
nocytochemical procedures to
tologically. Some are produce
released into the blood in
detectable by sensitive imm
provide clinical evidence of th
The questions arise: (1) are
found only in the tumor cel
antigens? and (2) do the sp
humans express tumor-specifi
requires separate consideratio

The neoantigens of experi
are membrane-associated, are
from histocompatibility antige
plantation immunity. A syng
nized against viable tumor cel

terminal differentiation. In the normal epidermis, when a basal cell divides, one daughter cell remains undifferentiated to replace its forebear, but one undergoes differentiation into an anucleate squame and is desquamated. In this way the normal thickness is maintained. Failure of terminal differentiation would produce a tumor. Thus, at least some cancers may arise as the result of disordered differentiation of normal cells.

Transplantability. Individual malignant cells can be readily explanted into appropriate culture media or living syngeneic hosts. In contrast, it is difficult and sometimes impossible to establish primary in vitro cultures of many forms of mature, specialized normal cells.

Cancer cells are "immortal." They can be indefinitely subcultured in vitro or be transplanted from one to another appropriate host. Indeed, many tumor cell lines, such as the Ehrlich ascites tumor, have been maintained in vitro for decades.

Loss of contact inhibition. As pointed out earlier, normal cells in vitro cease locomotion and division when confluence of a monolayer has been achieved. Cancer cells, in contrast, pile up on each other to create multilayered, disorderly masses. Although it would appear that malignant cells have escaped from cell-to-cell control signals, in the process referred to as "contact inhibition," the excessive cellular proliferation may relate to decreased susceptibility to "density-dependent inhibition of growth."

Cancer cells require lower serum concentrations for optimal growth, do not require anchorage, and so will grow in semisolid or fluid media.[47, 49] It appears that they are less dependent than normal cells on serum factors and solid substrate, e.g., basement membrane, for their growth.

Malignant cells achieve higher densities in the culture than normal cells, and do not arrest at the G_0 stage in the cell cycle at high density or in low serum media.[50] They are, therefore, less subject to *"density-dependent inhibition of growth,"* probably because they are less dependent on growth factors such as those in serum and are also capable of bypassing cell cycle restriction points that would normally arrest a cell from entering the S phase of DNA synthesis.

MORPHOLOGIC CHANGES

As already indicated in the discussion of differentiation and anaplasia, the malignant phenotype is usually associated with morphologic changes that, indeed, underlie the anatomic diagnosis of cancer. However, the changes may be subtle and, in some instances, deceptively absent. Repeatedly one reads in the literature of a "benign metastasizing whateveroma." Since benign tumors do not metastasize, such lesions are testaments to the fact that some malignant tumors have none of the morphologic attributes expected in the transformed phenotype (Fig. 6–18).

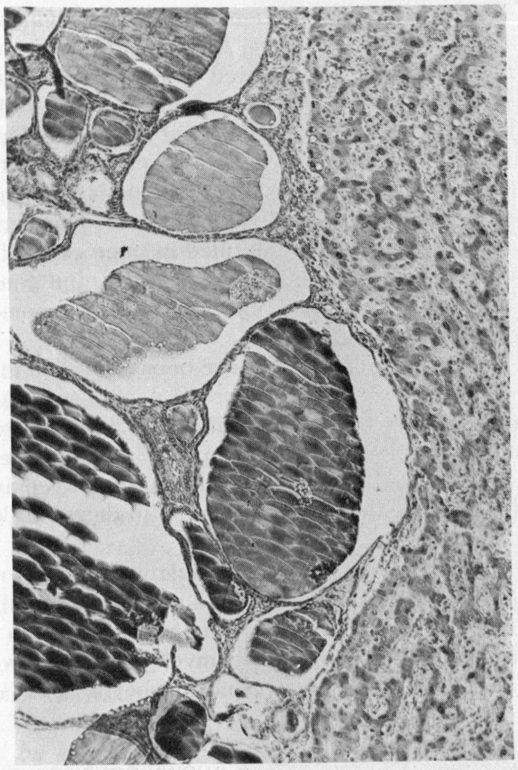

Figure 6–18. Metastatic thyroid carcinoma in liver. The tumor is formed of well-developed follicles filled with colloid and lined by flattened, innocent-appearing cells. Only the intrahepatic location discloses the true malignant character of the neoplasm.

KARYOTYPIC CHANGES

With each passing year it becomes more certain that the malignant cells of most types of human cancer have chromosomal abnormalities, and in many types of cancer the defects are consistent.[51] Most of the chromosomal alterations only became evident with the advent of the newer high-resolution banding techniques that now reveal 1200 (sometimes more) specific bands within the karyotype. The most common findings are either a band deletion usually involving autosomes 1, 3, 11, or 13 in solid tissue cancers (e.g., carcinomas of the lung, ovary, and pancreas and neuroblastomas) or a translocation most often between 8 and 14 or between 22 and 9 among the lymphomas and leukemias.[52] More rarely a trisomy of autosome 8 or 12 is present in certain forms of lymphoma/leukemia. The fact that in many forms of cancer the chromosomal abnormality is nonrandom has led some investigators to propose that the secrets of cancer are locked within certain genes—"oncogenes"—and that alteration of these "oncogenes" or rearrangements of the DNA code permit these genes to be expressed (discussed later).[53] It should be noted, however, that not all cells with karyotypic abnormalities are necessarily malignant: witness the many mutations not necessarily associated with neoplasia as in such genetic disorders as Down's syndrome, Turner's syn-

drome, and other conditio
Moreover, certain benign
gioma, are regularly associa
as pointed out below. Th
appear to be important, and
to the cancerous phenotype
remain instances of maligr
accompanied by genomic a
changes have not been iden
myelogenous or lymphoblas
bly further penetrations in
disclose them.

Specific abnormalities h
than 20 tumors, with the
come. Some of the better e
sented in Table 6–3.[54] It is
tations of space to discuss
will document their potenti
fication, and prognosis.[55]

Chronic myelogenous le
nant disease associated wit
change, described in some d
90% of affected adults have
erythroid, megakaryocytic, a

Table 6–3. NEOPLASMS WITH A

Leukemias
Chronic myelogenous leukemi
Acute nonlymphocytic leukemi
M1
M2
M3
M4*
M4*, M5*
M1, M2, M4, M5, M6
Chronic lymphocytic leukemia
Acute lymphocytic leukemia
L1-L2
L2§
L3
Lymphomas
Burkitt's, small noncleaved cell
Follicular small cleaved,* follicu
Small cell lymphocytic*
Small cell lymphocytic, transfor
Carcinomas
Neuroblastoma, disseminated
Small cell lung carcinoma
Papillary cystadenocarcinoma c
Constitutional retinoblastoma*
Retinoblastoma†
Aniridia-Wilms' tumor*
Wilms' tumor†
Benign solid tumors
Mixed parotid gland tumor
Meningioma

*Consistent chromosomal defects r
†Few cases described.
‡Chromosomes 6, 10, 17, and 19 r
§Drawn and slightly modified from

leading to the malignant phenotype. The nuclear T antigens of DNA viruses, on the other hand, are intrinsic to the transforming process.

Only a very few human cancers express "private" tumor-specific antigens comparable with those in chemically induced neoplasms, and an additional few have common tumor antigens shared with similar and sometimes dissimilar neoplasms. *Most human cancers totally lack tumor-specific antigens or, at most, are very weakly immunogenic.* The cells of human cancers, however, do have many of the previously mentioned tumor-associated antigens also present in smaller amounts in normal cells. Some of these tumor-associated antigens are fetal antigens found normally in embryonic cells. These fetal antigens are discussed in greater detail later (pp. 268 and 873), but will be briefly characterized here. One, alpha-fetoprotein (AFP) is mainly associated with hepatocarcinomas, yolk-sac tumors, a few other neoplasms, and some non-neoplastic conditions discussed on page 938.[64] Another, carcinoembryonic antigen (CEA), is principally associated with carcinomas of the colon, but is also encountered with those of the respiratory tract, pancreas, mammary gland, and others.[65] It suffices here to note that they are not tumor-specific antigens since they are also found in non-neoplastic conditions.

The tumor neoantigens most closely approximating the TSTAs of experimentally-induced neoplasms have been best studied in malignant melanomas, the form of clinical cancer most clearly associated with an immune response. In an analysis of about 50 patients with this neoplasm, only a few were found to have IgG antibodies specific for their own neoplasm. The large majority of patients had nonspecific antibodies reactive with a wide variety of other tumor types as well as normal cells. In the past, such widely reacting antibodies have been mistakenly taken to indicate tumor-specific immunity.

Recently, a new so-called "Ca antigen" has been described in a wide variety of malignant tumors, but not all—putatively a marker for human cancer cells.[66, 67] This widely shared tumor-associated antigen was not identified in benign tumors nor in any normal tissue, save for the epithelium of the normal fallopian tube and urinary tract. Whether these normal cells actually possess the Ca antigen, or instead have a cross-reacting normal antigen, is at present unclear. The validity of this "tumor" antigen for human cancer remains to be established, but it must be cautioned that similar claims in the past have often fallen by the wayside.

Despite the lack of immunologic evidence of tumor-specific antigens in the cancers of humans, there is histologic evidence suggesting cell-mediated reactions to tumor-associated antigens in some malignant neoplasms. Certain carcinomas of the lung, testis, and breast, malignant melanomas, and Hodgkin's disease are heavily infiltrated by lymphocytes and macrophages. In a few instances the immunocompetent cells have been shown to be sensitized to the tumor antigens. Whether the presence of such a cellular response indicates an improved prognosis, as some contend, is still controversial.[68] The presumed defensive role of these sensitized cells is best exemplified in Hodgkin's disease, as discussed on page 670. Other indirect evidence of an apparent immune response to human cancers is the increased frequency of malignant neoplasms in immunocompromised individuals, a topic to be explored more fully in the consideration of host-neoplasm interactions (p. 258). It is possible, therefore, that human cancers do express neoantigens, but it is too soon to say whether clinical neoplasms elaborate in the strictest sense tumor-specific antigens. Whether specific or not, the question may be asked: if the antigens evoke immune responses, how do the tumors escape destruction? This brings up the controversial subject of *immunologic surveillance*, discussed later (p. 258).

METABOLIC CHANGES

So many metabolic deviations from the normal have been described in experimentally transformed and human cancer cells that it is only possible to skim the surface of this vast subject. However, certain generalizations can be made. (1) *The better the differentiation and the slower the rate of division of the cancer cell, the closer its metabolism approximates that of its normal forebear, and vice versa.* (2) *All highly anaplastic cancer cells tend toward a common simplified metabolic and enzyme pattern, sometimes referred to as "the biochemical convergence of tumors."* Weinhouse has put it well: "The highly neoplastic cell which has been transplanted many generations is like a stripped-down racing car in which other metabolic activities have been subordinated to the overwhelming compulsion to divide."[69] (3) *None of the metabolic deviations constitutes a hallmark of the malignant phenotype.* Instead, they appear to reflect the activated state of proliferating cells and so may also be present in rapidly dividing non-neoplastic cells. (4) *None of the metabolic deviations is thought to be the fundamental event responsible for the emergence of the cancer phenotype.* Rather, they appear to be secondary to cancerous transformation. With this overview, a few of the more outstanding alterations will be cited.

Long ago Warburg called attention to what he construed to be a fundamental metabolic alteration in cancer cells, namely, an unusually high rate of anerobic metabolism even in the presence of oxygen—so-called "aerobic glycolysis." It is now well recognized that this metabolic change merely reflects rapid growth of cells, whether neoplastic or non-neoplastic. There is increased synthesis of cellular constituents required for cell division and increased shedding of surface components. Considerable importance has been ascribed by some to impaired control of cholesterol synthesis in cancer cells.[70] As a result, it is contended that all membranes within cancer cells have an enriched cholesterol content with alteration of the cholesterol/phospholipid ratio. It is further proposed that the membrane changes comprise early events in tumorigenesis accounting for the described deviations in social behavior, shape, and membrane transport of cancer cells. However, there is not universal agreement on such a proposal. Identifiable in many cancer cells are increased glutamate and glutamine oxidation, increased polyamine synthesis and accumulation, alterations in mitochondrial bioenergetics, synthesis of aberrant proteins and glycoproteins (such as tumor-associated antigens), and sometimes synthesis of "ectopic" hormones as well as other bioactive abnormal products producing paraneoplastic syndromes (p. 255). Alterations in enzymes are frequently present, but are too diverse and numerous to be detailed. In general, there is a tendency to revert to fetal-type isoenzymes as the level of differentiation falls. For example, an alkaline phosphatase called the Regan isozyme is produced by about 10% of cancers. It is of interest because it is normally produced by placental tissue, suggesting derepression of an embryonic program. In several experimental tumor cell lines, abnormal function of membrane $Na^{+}K^{+}$-ATPase has been identified that renders the sodium pump inefficient. Sometimes particular enzyme changes have unusual clinical significance. Terminal deoxynucleotidyl transferase (TdT) is typical of T- and null-cell lymphocytes (rarely of pre–B cells and early myeloid forms). Thus, when present in acute leukemia, it suggests a lymphoid origin. Conversely, the cells of acute lymphocytic leukemia often lack an enzyme required for the synthesis of the amino acid asparagine. The survival of these leukemic cells is therefore dependent on asparagine produced in the liver. The enzyme lack has been exploited by administering L-asparaginase to these patients in the hope of depriving the leukemic cells of required asparagine. Thus, although the biochemical and metabolic analyses of cancer cells have yielded no profound insights into the nature of the cancerous transformation, a few findings have proved clinically useful.

CELL SURFACE AND MEMBRANE CHANGES

Changes in the plasma membrane and at the interface between transformed cells and normal cells would seem a priori to be critical to the aggressive behavior of the malignant phenotype. Indeed, a large number of alterations have been identified, but it is not clear whether they are primary or secondary. Proteolytic treatment of normal cells confers on them many of the properties of transformed cells. Moreover, the literature abounds with conflicts over the validity and significance of each of the alterations. Nonetheless, certain changes are reasonably well established, and attention will be directed to these.[71]

Neoplastic cells, whether derived from transformed cultures or from neoplasms in vivo, generally, but not invariably, reveal:

–A loss, diminution, or in some cases acquisition of such surface specializations as microvilli, pseudopodia, and filopodia.

–Alterations in cell junctions.

–Inconstant cytoskeletal alterations.

–Changes in surface-associated glycoproteins and proteins, particularly enzymes affecting membrane transport and, possibly, invasiveness.

–Changes in glycolipids and lipids affecting permeability, surface receptors, and surface antigens.

–Enhanced lectin agglutinability.

–Changes in responsiveness to inhibitory and stimulatory putative growth factors.

–Alterations of surface-associated and intracellular ions.

The above represents a very incomplete listing, but it indicates the scope of the changes. Rather than commenting on each, some synthesis will be attempted.

In the perspective of the many morphologic changes in tumor cells previously described, it is no surprise that surface morphologic changes are also present. In general, they take the form of simplification and disorganization of specialized features. Thus, *tumor cells often exhibit diminution or loss of microvilli, pseudopodia, and filopodia and a tendency toward "rounding-up."* Such cytopodia as persist are often distorted or elongated, and occasionally replaced by blebs.[72] However, such findings are not universal, and certain types of tumor cells often acquire extraordinary microvilli or cytopodia not present in their normal counterparts (Fig. 6–19). Closely related to the changes in cell shape are alterations in the cytoskeleton. These were mentioned on page 28, but in general there is disorganization of microtubules and microfilaments in tumor cells. Intermediate filaments may be diminished in number, but more often they are abundant and provide a means of identifying the histogenetic origin of the tumor cell.

A number of cell surface and membrane alterations may have importance in the abnormal social behavior of cancer cells. A fundamental feature is enhanced transmembrane transport of nutrients, for example, into the cell and metabolites out of the cell, potentiating increased metabolic activity and replication. Typically, *there also is increased synthesis, incorporation, and, in particular, shedding of surface and membrane components.*[73] Of major current interest is the cell surface glycoprotein fibronectin, formerly known as LETS (large external transformation-sensitive) protein. There is a general, although imperfect, correlation between the level of tumorigenicity and the extent of loss by shedding of fibronectin from cell surfaces.[74] Loss of fibronectin may contribute to the reduced adhesiveness and cohesiveness of cancer cells. Other glycoproteins, both integral to the plasma membrane and extrinsic (within the glycocalyx), are altered.[75] While some are lost, new glycoproteins appear that probably reflect tumor neoantigens. Shed fibronectin is found in the plasma as cold-insoluble globulin; the increased plasma levels in patients with cancer may contribute to the coagulopathy occasionally observed in these patients (p. 98). Other procoagulant factors are also released by certain cancer cells, contributing possibly to the coagulopathy.[76]

Surface glycolipids, some of which constitute receptors, are reduced in many cancer cells. These recep-

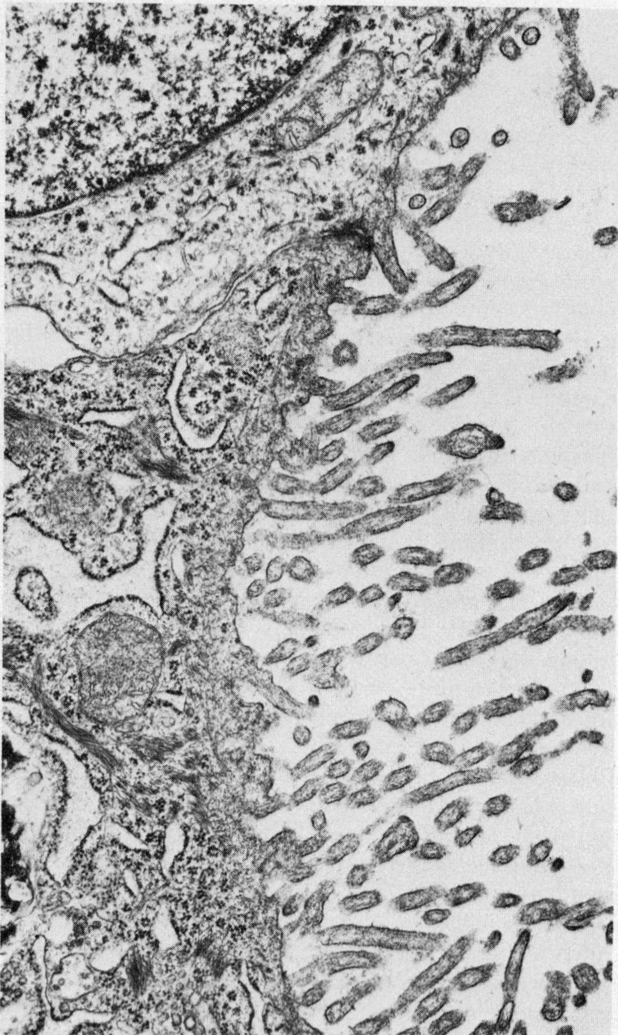

Figure 6–19. A malignant mesothelial cell displaying numerous slender, wavy cytopodia projecting from the cell surface. The normal mesothelial cell lacks cytopodia but they are acquired in inflammatory and neoplastic states (× 8000). (Courtesy of Dr. M. Warhol, Brigham and Women's Hospital.)

tors play roles in the localization of metastases, and the actions of hormones and possibly growth-stimulatory and -inhibitory substances, e.g., chalones.[77] Deletion of these molecules may be important to the loss of growth regulation. Cancer cells have an increased ability to take up solutes from their environment, which function may play a role in the diminished density-dependent inhibition of growth by conferring an advantage in the competition for nutrients.

Cell junctions are another feature affecting social behavior. Desmosomes involved in cell-to-cell attachment would be expected to be reduced in number in tumor cells with their lowered adhesiveness and cohesiveness, as indeed they are in some cancer cells. However, recent studies point out that a normal complement may be present in the primary lesion and within the hepatic metastases.[78] It is significant, then, that cells may detach and spread to distant sites despite retention of desmosomes. On the other hand, gap or communicating junctions are frequently diminished or absent.[79] Such junctions have been attributed importance in the transmission of chemical signals between cells, and so any reduction in the number of these junctions might play a role in the diminished contact inhibition characteristic of cancer cells.

Several other surface features are worthy of note. Most tumor or transformed cells agglutinate at a much lower concentration of lectins than their normal counterparts. Lectins comprise plant and invertebrate divalent molecules that cross-link sugars on adjacent cells. Increased lectin agglutinability is poorly understood; it has been attributed to their redistribution related to increased mobility within the cell membrane. Lectin agglutinability and receptor shifts correlate well with loss of growth regulation. A host of membrane enzyme changes have been described. The production and release of the serine protease, plasminogen activator, is thought to be important to cancer transformation. Other proteases are also released. Such enhanced fibrinolytic and proteolytic activity could contribute to the invasiveness of cancer cells.[80] Increased amounts of galactosyltransferase are released by many types of tumor cells. Detection of this enzyme in the blood is now used clinically as an indicator of the presence of a cancer, as discussed on page 1107. Another surface-related enzyme of great current interest is a protein phosphorylating kinase. It is a major feature of the transforming activity of certain oncogenic viruses (p. 247). Adenyl cyclase is another surface-associated enzyme that mediates the synthesis of cAMP from ATP. As you know, cAMP is thought to be an intracellular messenger. For example, hormones that bind to membrane receptors assert their intracellular actions by modifying cAMP levels. It is, therefore, of great interest that reduced cAMP levels are commonly found in transformed cells, suggesting lack of regulatory signals involved in control of cell growth and division. Underlying the lower levels of cAMP are reductions in membrane adenyl cyclase and increases in cyclic nucleotide phosphodiesterase involved in its breakdown.[81]

Enough has been said about cell surface and membrane changes to make evident the many deviations from normal that are sometimes, or usually, found in cancer cells. Collectively these alterations provide reasonable explanations for many of the attributes of the malignant phenotype, e.g., altered social behavior, surface antigens, invasion, and others. Thus, there is a widely held view that, in the last analysis, "cancer is a membrane disease."

With this survey of the salient features of the malignant phenotype, we can turn to the search for the cause or causes of cancer.

CARCINOGENIC AGENTS AND THEIR CELLULAR INTERACTIONS

A large number of agents induce neoplastic transformation of cells in vitro and cancers in experimental animals. They can be divided into the following categories: (1) chemical carcinogens; (2) radiant energy; (3) oncogenic viruses; and (4) others. Radiant energy and certain chemical carcinogens are documented causes of cancer in humans, and the evidence linking viruses to certain types of clinical neoplasia grows ever stronger. Indeed, epidemiologic studies hint strongly that 80 or even 90% of human cancers are the result of life style and other environmental influences.[82] The following discussion will deal largely with observations of particular pertinence to humans and relevant experimental data. Agents will be considered separately, but it is important to note that several may act in concert or synergize the effects of others. *There is strong experimental evidence that neoplastic transformation is a progressive process involving multiple steps and "multiple hits."* Thus, chemical carcinogens may initiate the process that is completed by oncogenic viruses.[83] It is possible, therefore, that at least some cancers in humans are the consequences of the unfortunate confluence of several of the carcinogenic influences discussed here.

Table 6–4. MAJOR CHEMICAL CARCINOGENS

Direct-Acting Carcinogens
- *Alkylating agents*
  - beta-propiolactone
  - dimethylsulfate
  - diepoxybutane
  - anticancer mustards (cyclophosphamide, chlorambucil, busulfan, melphalan, and others)
- *Acylating agents*
  - 1-acetyl-imidazole
  - dimethylcarbamyl chloride

Procarcinogens that Require Metabolic Activation
- *Polycyclic and heterocyclic aromatic hydrocarbons*
  - benz(a)anthracene
  - benzo(a)pyrene
  - dibenz(a,h)anthracene
  - 3-methylcholanthrene
  - 7,12-dimethylbenz(a)anthracene
- *Aromatic amines, amides, azo dyes*
  - 2-naphthylamine (beta-naphthylamine)
  - benzidine
  - 2-acetylaminofluorene
  - dimethylaminoazobenzene (butter yellow)
- *Natural plant and microbial products*
  - aflatoxin B_1
  - mitomycin C
  - griseofulvin
  - cycasin
  - safrole
  - betel nuts
- *Others*
  - nitrosamine and amides
  - carbon tetrachloride
  - ethionine

CHEMICAL CARCINOGENS

Although John Hill earlier called attention to the association of "immoderate use of snuff" and the development of "polypusses" (polyps), we owe largely to Sir Percival Pott our awareness of the potential carcinogenicity of chemical agents. Pott astutely related the increased incidence of scrotal skin cancer in chimney sweeps to chronic exposure to soot. A few years later, on the basis of this observation, the Danish Chimney Sweeps Guild ruled that its members must bathe daily. No public health measure since that time has so successfully controlled a form of cancer! Over the succeeding two centuries, hundreds of chemicals have been shown to transform cells in vitro and to be carcinogenic in animals.[84, 85] Some of the most potent (e.g., the polycyclic aromatic hydrocarbons) have been extracted from fossil fuels or are products of incomplete combustions. Some are synthetic products created by industry or for the study of chemical carcinogenesis. Some are naturally occurring components of plants and microbial organisms. Most important, a significant number (including, ironically, some medical drugs) have been strongly implicated in the causation of cancers in humans.

All the chemical carcinogens fall into one of two categories: (1) direct-acting (also known as activation-independent) compounds; or (2) procarcinogens that require metabolic conversion in vivo or enzymatic conversion in vitro to produce metabolites capable of transforming cells, referred to as "ultimate carcinogens." Intermediate products in this metabolic conversion are sometimes referred to as "proximate carcinogens." The major agents in these two categories are listed in Table 6–4. A few comments follow about some of these agents.

Types of Chemical Carcinogens

Direct-Acting Alkylating Agents. Although these agents are activation-independent, they may be chemically or enzymatically inactivated. In general, they are weak carcinogens. Nonetheless, they have importance because many therapeutic agents (e.g., cyclophosphamide, chlorambucil, busulfan, melphalan, and others) fall into this category. These are used as anticancer drugs, but regrettably have been documented to induce lymphoid neoplasms, leukemia, and other forms of cancer.[86] In one survey of patients receiving alkylating agents in the treatment of disseminated ovarian cancer, the risk of leukemia was increased 17-fold in those who survived for at least two years.[87] Alkylating agents appear to exert their therapeutic effects by interacting with and damaging DNA, but it is precisely these actions that render them also carcinogenic.[88, 89]

Polycyclic Aromatic Hydrocarbons. These agents represent some of the most potent carcinogens known. They require metabolic activation but can also be metabolized to noncarcinogenic products. These strong carcinogens can induce tumors in a wide variety of tissues and species. Painted on the skin they cause skin cancers, injected subcutaneously they evoke sarcomas, or introduced into a specific organ they cause cancers locally. Such pluripotency denotes potent carcinogenicity, which depends on the balance between conversion to active and inactive metabolites. The formation of the final reactive products—the "ultimate carcinogens"—has been elegantly detailed for many of the aromatic hydrocarbons.[90] Involved are microsomal endoplasmic reticulum–associated monooxygenases belonging to a family of cytochromes, principally P-450 and P-448.[91] These enzyme systems require NADPH as a cofactor, and utilize molecular oxygen for their oxidative activity. A comparable system may be located in the nucleus. The "ultimate carcinogens" for many of the polycyclic hydrocarbons are now known to be dihydrodiol epoxides.[92] *These epoxides are strong electrophilic reactants and combine with nucleophilic sites in the target cells, including DNA, RNA, and proteins.*[92] Electrophilic reactants are positively charged molecules that form covalent bonds with electron-deficient nucleophilic atoms. Since some of the polycyclic procarcinogens may be metabolized to several electrophilic products and since there are very likely multiple reactive sites in the macromolecules of cells, covalent bonding must occur at many sites within the cell. The polycyclic hydrocarbons are of particular interest as carcinogens because they are produced in the combustion of tobacco, particularly with cigarette smoking or possibly in the process of cooking, especially broiling or smoking of meats and fats.[93]

AROMATIC AMINES AND AZO DYES. Agents in this category were the first to reveal the requirement for metabolic activation of most carcinogens. They do not usually cause cancer at the point of application; instead, they exert their effects at sites of release of the ultimate electrophilic reactant. The carcinogenicity of most aromatic amines and azo dyes is exerted mainly in the liver, where the "ultimate carcinogen" is formed by the intermediation of the cytochrome P-450 oxygenase systems. Thus, fed to rats, acetylaminofluorene and the azo dyes induce hepatocellular carcinomas, but not cancers of the gastrointestinal tract. An agent implicated in human cancers, beta-naphthylamine, is an exception. It has in the past been responsible for a 50-fold increased incidence of bladder cancer in heavily exposed workers in aniline dye and rubber industries.[94] After absorption it is hydroxylated into an N-OH derivative and then detoxified by conjugating with glucuronic acid. Other products are also formed but are less strong electrophiles. When excreted in the urine, the nontoxic conjugate is split by the urinary enzyme glucuronidase to again release the electrophilic reactant, thus inducing bladder cancer. Regrettably, humans are one of the few species to possess the urinary glucuronidase. Some of the azo dyes were developed to color food, e.g., butter yellow to give margarine the appearance of butter, and scarlet red to impart the seductive coloration of certain foods such as maraschino cherries. These dyes are now federally regulated in the United States because of the fear that they may be dangerous to humans.

NATURALLY OCCURRING CARCINOGENS. Among the approximately 30 known chemical carcinogens produced by plants and microorganisms, the potent hepatic carcinogen aflatoxin B_1 is most important. It is produced by some strains of *Aspergillus flavus* that thrive on improperly stored grains and peanuts. A strong correlation has been found between the dietary level of this hepatocarcinogen and the incidence of hepatocellular carcinoma in some parts of Africa and the Far East.[95, 96] The aflatoxin, along with other procarcinogens, requires metabolic activation by hepatic microsomal oxygenases to yield a dihydrodiol epoxide as the "ultimate carcinogen." It may be noted that infection with hepatitis B virus has also been strongly correlated with these cancers, raising the possibility that the aflatoxin and the virus collaborate in the production of this form of neoplasia, as discussed on page 936.[97]

NITROSAMINES AND AMIDES. These carcinogens are of interest because of the possibility that they may be formed in the gastrointestinal tract of humans (p. 426) and so may contribute to the induction of some forms of cancer, particularly gastric carcinoma. Like most other carcinogens, the nitroso- compounds require activation, which again involves the microsomal P-450 system. The ultimate carcinogenic derivatives are alkyl diazonium ions that are strongly electrophilic.

MISCELLANEOUS AGENTS. *Scores of other chemicals* have been indicted as carcinogens. Only a few that represent important industrial hazards will be mentioned. Occupational exposure to *asbestos* has been associated with an increased incidence of bronchogenic carcinomas, mesotheliomas, and gastrointestinal cancers, as discussed in detail on p. 440. It is somewhat sobering to realize that a number of cases of mesothelioma have been reported among individuals whose only exposure to asbestos was household contact with asbestos workers. Concomitant cigarette smoking heightens the risk of bronchogenic carcinoma manyfold.[98] Vinyl chloride is the monomer from which the polymer polyvinyl chloride is fabricated. It was first identified as a carcinogen in animals, but investigations soon disclosed a scattered incidence of the extremely rare hemangiosarcoma of the liver among workers exposed to this chemical. There are some tentative data among those heavily exposed, suggesting in addition an excess mortality from tumors of the brain, lung, and lymphatic and hematopoietic systems.[99] The oncogenicity of vinyl chloride is dose related, raising the issue of whether individuals living in proximity to factories that release fumes into the ambient air may not also be at risk. Chromium, nickel, and other metals, when volatilized and inhaled in industrial environments, have caused cancer of the lung. Skin cancer associated with arsenic is also well established. Similarly, there is reasonable evidence that many insecticides, such as aldrin, dieldrin, and chlordane and the polychlorinated biphenyls are carcinogenic in animals, and the unpleasant citations could be continued.

In summary, save for a few direct-acting carcinogens, most of the strong chemical agents are procarcinogens requiring metabolic transformation into "ultimate carcinogens." The liver is by far the major site of both metabolic activation and detoxification. Its ability to perform these conflicting functions is materially enhanced by previous or simultaneous exposure to drugs and chemicals, e.g., phenobarbital, insecticides, and herbicides that are also detoxified by the same microsomal ("mixed function oxidases") system and so induce higher levels of the enzymes. Nutrition, age, and hormones also modify the enzyme levels. All these influences, then, modify the rate of activation of procarcinogens, but at the same time the rate of detoxification.[100] The carcinogenicity of a chemical hangs on this balance and, regrettably, ways have not been found to alter it favorably. *There is strong evidence that both direct and activation-dependent carcinogens exert their effects by interaction with DNA or, more simply, that they are mutagenic,* as discussed below. However, many also bind to RNA and proteins and, through epigenetic pathways, could modify gene expression.

Steps Involved in Chemical Carcinogenesis

Neoplastic transformation of cells in culture and the induction of cancers in vivo by chemical carcinogens is a dynamic process. It involves sequential generations of cells over a variable span of time—depending mainly on cell type, species, reactivity of the carcinogen or its metabolites, and especially on dosage. During the process, at least two stages can be identified in experimental systems: *initiation* and *promotion*. In all probability these stages are also involved in the "spontaneous" emergence of cancers in humans. *Initiation results from the exposure of cells or tissues to an appropriate dose of a carcinogenic agent; an initiated cell is in some manner permanently altered, rendering it likely to give rise to a tumor.* However, initiation alone is not sufficient for tumor formation. Cell replication, at least one cycle, must follow to complete the "biochemical lesion."[101] Initiation, therefore, is at least a two-step phenomenon. In the classic model system, the exposure of mouse skin to an initiating agent evokes few or no tumors. Moreover, the treated skin appears histologically normal. Subsequent painting of the skin by repetitive, sufficiently large doses of a promoting agent over the span of months evokes at first a large number of papillomas, which in about one year are transformed into carcinomas. *Promoters can therefore be defined as agents that increase the tumorigenic response when applied after the initiator in amounts above a threshold level.* By themselves, most promoters produce no tumors. However, with sufficiently strenuous application some promoters, notably phorbol esters, will evoke tumors, although not on a scale comparable in time or number with the combination of initiator and promoter.[102] Several points are noteworthy in the initiation-promotion sequence. Some chemicals are "complete carcinogens" that with sufficiently large doses act as both initiators and promoters. Indeed, a single "hit" may suffice. However, most chemicals are "incomplete carcinogens" that require promoters to induce tumors. *Tumors do not result when the promoting agent is applied before, rather than after, the initiating agent.* However, since initiation is irreversible, withholding the promoting agent for months or even up to a year has been shown still to result in the production of skin tumors.[103] Because of the irreversibility of the effects of initiators, multiple divided doses will achieve the same result as a comparable total dose administered at one time. In contrast, there is a threshold level for promoters and their effects are reversible; thus, subthreshold or widely spaced doses are without effect.

Promoters, since they enhance tumorigenesis, are in a sense carcinogens. They constitute a diverse group of chemicals. Best studied is the phorbol ester 12-O-tetradecanoylphorbol-13-acetate derived from croton seed oil. A few other promoters of relevance to humans are phenols (found in tobacco tars), phenobarbital, saccharin, cyclamates, and various hormones, notably estrogens. Phorbol ester, about which most is known, does not require metabolic conversion, is not an electrophilic reactant, and so does not bind covalently to cellular macromolecules. It has a variety of effects in mouse epidermis, the most significant being increased cell replication, induction of enzymes, retardation of terminal differentiation, and modification of the membranes of cells grown in vitro.[104] How it exerts these effects, and which are critical to its enhancement of tumor induction, is unclear. One theory proposes that promoters derepress synthetic programs and thus activate cell replication.[105] Alternatively, membrane actions may mediate the changes. Other mechanisms may be involved with some of the promoters. Phenobarbital may act by increasing the levels of the cytochrome-P-450 microsomal oxydase system involved in metabolic conversion and detoxification (p. 27).[106]

Certain promoters may contribute to cancers in humans. Saccharin and cyclamates have been shown to promote the induction of bladder cancer in rats previously given marginal doses of carcinogens.[107] Whether these artificial sweeteners are also initiators or promoters in humans is a hotly debated issue, addressed on page 426. Suffice it here to note that epidemiologic studies, while yielding conflicting results, disclose no solid evidence of carcinogenicity in the dosages customarily used by humans. Hormones such as the estrogens serve in animals as promoters of liver tumors. The prolonged use of diethylstilbestrol is implicated in the production of postmenopausal endometrial carcinoma and in the causation of vaginal cancer in offspring exposed in utero, as discussed on page 1120. The action of many promoters is limited to specific cells and tissues. With such specificity, surface receptors or target cells are postulated.[108] However, some promoting agents act in a nonspecific manner to exert their effects widely. We must accept that the role of promoters is still far from clear, but a number of agents to which humans are exposed are known to be promoters and may play a role in the production of clinical cancer.

The study of chemical carcinogens has yielded important insights into the nature of oncogenic transformation of cells.[101, 109] Because DNA is a primary target of all carcinogenic chemicals (or their ultimate metabolites), it seems most likely that *some alteration of the genetic code, generically referred to as a somatic mu-*

tation, is a critical feature of the transforming process. However, nonmutational epigenetic mechanisms cannot be excluded as alternative or collaborative pathways, as discussed later in more detail. The carcinogens—DNA adducts—have been shown to impair template activities during replication and transcription, thus in effect inducing miscoding errors and expanding mutations.[110] Each carcinogen interacts with DNA in specific ways that differ in their effects. For example, alkylating agents have been shown to alkylate the N-7 position of guanine, which is nonmutagenic, but also the O-6 position, which is strongly mutagenic and concomitantly carcinogenic. Thus, *it is not the extent of total binding but rather the specific sites of binding that is important.* Corroborating DNA as the primary target, normal cells can be converted to cancer cells by transfection (transfer of genes by recombinant DNA techniques) with DNA from chemically transformed cells.[111] Intriguing as this observation may be, transformation has also been accomplished by transfection with genes from normal cells, as further elaborated on page 248, but in either event alteration of the genome appears to be central to the transforming process.

Significant Features of Chemical Carcinogenesis

Most known chemical carcinogens are mutagenic in at least one test system.[112, 113] The Ames test is the most widely employed. *Salmonella typhimurium* mutants incapable of synthesizing histidine are grown on histidine-deficient medium and exposed to potential carcinogens along with liver homogenate, to provide the necessary enzymes for metabolic conversion. If the metabolites are mutagenic, some of the organisms back-mutate from a defective to a functional histidine gene, thus permitting bacterial growth. The number of colonies is a rough measure of the level of mutagenicity. Chemical carcinogens have also been shown to be mutagenic in mammalian cell cultures. *The initiation-induced mutation, however, can be repaired;* conversely, when there is a defect in DNA repair as occurs with certain hereditary disorders, xeroderma pigmentosum for example, there is increased vulnerability to cancers. However, not all carcinogens are mutagens, and conversely some mutagens are noncarcinogenic.[114] There is nonetheless a high correlation between carcinogenicity and mutagenicity, but the fact that it is not absolute underscores the possibility that nonmutational pathways may also lead to the malignant phenotype.

Cell replication is required for "fixation" of the transformed state. During the preneoplastic phase, perhaps before fixation of the initiation occurs, reversal is possible with return of the cells to normal differentiation.[115] What precisely occurs with "fixation" is still not clear, but it is speculated that in the process of cell division the initiation "lesion" in DNA leads to ever greater errors in the genetic code. Indeed, the contribution of promoters to the formation of tumors may be the induction of cell replication. Thus, regenerative activity following cell death, whatever the cause, favors the development of cancers in humans and experimental animals.[115] Indeed, "complete carcinogens" may depend for their potency not only on their electrophilic reactivity, but also on their toxicity, causing cell death followed by regenerative activity. Hyperplastic states in humans are also fertile soils for tumor formation. During the latent period between the application of an initiator and the appearance of tumors, "preneoplastic" enzyme-altered foci have been described in chemical model systems, and cell proliferation is thought to be obligatory to their induction.[116]

Since malignant transformation can be the result of the additive effects of multiple small exposures to initiators, there is no "safe" threshold level for carcinogens. However, during the intervals between subcarcinogenic exposures, repair of the initiation lesion or terminal differentiation of affected cells may interrupt the transforming process.

Diverse oncogenic influences may act in concert to induce cell transformation. Cells previously exposed to radiant energy are more vulnerable to chemical carcinogens, and the latter synergize the transforming action of oncogenic viruses.[83] Thus has arisen the concept of cocarcinogenesis. Tobacco smoke residue, with its polycyclic aromatic hydrocarbons, also contains nitrosamines, and other chemicals that may serve as cocarcinogens. In addition it contains phenolic promoters, making it a dangerous witches' brew. The increasing frequency of cancer with advancing age in humans might well be due to cumulative exposure over the years to a variety of carcinogenic influences, although other explanations may exist.

Finally, *neoplastic transformation by chemical agents is a multistage and possibly "multihit" process involving successive generations of cells, each approaching more closely the malignant phenotype.* Not only is initiation and promotion involved, but also tumor progression with the evolution of successive clones of cells, one or more of which ultimately escapes regulatory controls.

With the rapidly lengthening list of indicted compounds, mention should be made here of the growing uneasiness about the criteria for labeling substances carcinogenic. Phenobarbital is a known promoter in animals and, to this extent, is carcinogenic. Massive pharmacologic doses of phenobarbital have produced nodules in the livers of certain mice, but the drug is without effect in rats. There have been no reports of an increased incidence of cancer in patients with epilepsy receiving this drug over prolonged periods of years. Should phenobarbital be labeled a carcinogen? We find ourselves in the dilemma in which tests employing large, nontherapeutic dosages in laboratory animals suggest or establish the carcinogenicity of a chemical, and negative epidemiologic surveys in humans do not provide total reassurance. Will cancers appear much later? How much of the usual incidence of cancer is related to these suspected, and still other unsuspected, chemical agents? On the one hand, withdrawal of falsely accused substances might impair the quality of life: on the other hand, inadequate surveillance could impair the quantity of life. It is a thorny issue that cannot be dismissed. Chemicals are known causes of cancer in humans and it is indeed possible, as others have said, that "we swim in a sea of carcinogens."

RADIATION CARCINOGENESIS

Radiant energy, whether in the form of the ultraviolet (UV) rays of sunlight or ionizing electromagnetic and particulate radiation, can transform virtually all cell types in vitro and induce neoplasms in vivo in both humans and experimental animals.[117, 118] UV light is clearly implicated in the causation of skin cancers, and ionizing radiations of medical, occupational, and, lamentably, atomic bomb origins have produced a variety of forms of malignant neoplasia. Although the contribution of radiation to the total human burden of cancer is probably small, the well-known latency of radiant energy and its cumulative effect require extremely long periods of observation and make it difficult to ascertain its total significance. Only now, almost four decades later, is an increased incidence of breast cancer becoming apparent among females exposed during childhood to the A-bomb.[119] Moreover, its possible additive or synergistic effects on other potential carcinogenic influences add yet another dimension. Although the mode of action of radiant energy on target cells is still imperfectly understood, the weight of evidence implicates the production of damage to DNA. The effects of UV light on DNA differ somewhat from that of ionizing radiations, requiring separate consideration of these two forms of radiant energy.

Ultraviolet Rays

There is ample evidence from epidemiologic studies that **UV rays** derived from the sun induce an increased incidence of squamous cell carcinoma, basal cell carcinoma, and melanocarcinoma of the skin.[120] The degree of risk depends on the intensity of exposure and the quantity of light-absorbing "protective mantle" of melanin in the skin. Thus, persons of European origin who have fair skin that repeatedly gets sunburned but stalwartly refuses to tan, and who live in locales receiving a great deal of sunlight (e.g., Queensland, Australia, closest to the equator), have the highest incidence of melanocarcinoma.[121] UV rays have a number of effects on cells including inhibition of cell division, inactivation of enzymes, induction of mutations, and, in sufficient dosage, killing of cells. These biologic effects are discussed in greater detail in the general consideration of radiant energy (p. 464). Although other mechanisms such as chain breakage, formation of abnormal cross-links, and base destruction are not precluded, the carcinogenicity of UV light is attributed to its formation of pyrimidine dimers in DNA. When unrepaired, these dimers lead to larger transcriptional errors and, in some instances, cancer. Recent studies in mice suggest that more is involved than UV-induced mutations alone.[122] The UV light simultaneously activates T-suppressor cells and so inhibits cell-mediated immunity, which permits the emergence of highly antigenic skin tumors.[123] Whether these findings apply to humans is still under study, but in any event the UV-induced mutations apparently serve as the initiating mechanism and the immune changes as either potentiators or promoters.

Supportive evidence for the mutagenic effects of UV radiant energy comes from a small group of autosomal recessive hereditary diseases, all characterized by some anomaly in DNA metabolism, particularly repair mechanisms. Several methods of DNA repair have been identified: (1) in situ restoration of the damage by enzymatic mechanisms; (2) reversal of UV-induced dimers by visible light, or its spontaneous "decay" to some innocuous form; (3) removal and replacement ("cut and patch") of the abnormal DNA segment; and (4) the development of alternative pathways despite persistence of the DNA lesion. In mammalian cells, removal and replacement appears to be most important. Essentially, a defect in a single strand is excised by endonucleases and replaced using the intact strand of DNA as a template.

Much of our present awareness of the probable role of mutations in the induction of cancer comes from investigations of the increased vulnerability of individuals with xeroderma pigmentosum (XP) to cancer.[124] Those with this condition can be divided into several distinct groups, each having some defect in excision-repair of DNA, the major subset lacking endonucleases for excision of the dimer.[125] With such impairments these individuals have a markedly increased predisposition to skin cancers, predominantly in the sun-exposed areas of the body. In vitro skin fibroblasts from these patients are also abnormally sensitive to UV light as well as to some chemical carcinogens. However, it is of interest that there is *no* increased incidence of the common forms of lethal cancer, e.g., carcinomas of the lung, breast, and colon in XP.[126] Possibly, different tissues have differing mechanisms of DNA repair, or there are other pathways to cancer than damage to DNA. Three other hereditary "chromosome instability syndromes"—ataxia telangiectasia, Fanconi's anemia, and Bloom's syndrome—are also characterized by predisposition to cancer.[127] In ataxia telangiectasia there is a predisposition to leukemia, thought to relate to the lack of a full complement of endonucleases and thus an inability to excise and repair gamma ray-induced DNA damage. However, other factors such as an immune deficiency, characteristic of this condition, may also be involved. The molecular defect in DNA repair in Fanconi's anemia and Bloom's syndrome has not been clearly defined, but there are observations suggesting defects in DNA repair and/or DNA replication.[128, 129] Individuals with Bloom's syndrome have a markedly increased incidence of all forms of cancer, including the most common types. *These syndromes offer strong evidence that defective DNA metabolism and, more specifically, repair mechanisms predispose to cancer, and therefore that alterations in DNA represent at least one pathway to neoplastic transformation.*

Ionizing Radiation

Electromagnetic (x-rays, gamma rays) or particulate (alpha particles, beta particles, protons, neutrons) radiations are all carcinogenic. Therapeutic irradiation has unmistakably been responsible for an increased incidence of cancer.[130] At one time, radiation treatments were used for many benign conditions, such as ankylosing spondylitis (a form of arthritis of the spine). Follow-up of these patients has revealed a 10- to 12-fold increase in incidence of leukemia, which peaked three to five years after the therapeutic irradiation. All types of leukemia were seen, except for chronic lymphocytic leukemia. Slightly more than a twofold increased incidence of other forms of cancer occurred somewhat later, peaking at about 10 to 14 years.[131] Similarly, female patients who had received radiotherapy to the pelvic region for benign and malignant disorders experienced a three- to fourfold increased incidence of leukemia.[132] Both thyroid cancer patients treated with ^{131}I and polycythemia vera patients who received ^{32}P later suffered from an excess of leukemia. Head and neck irradiation, particularly in infants and children, is followed—sometimes as much as 35 years later—by thyroid cancers in 9% of those exposed.[133] Even diagnostic irradiation has been implicated; x-ray examination of pregnant women has been substantiated as a cause of an increased frequency of leukemia in the exposed children.

Occupational exposure to irradiation has long been a well-known source of cancer in humans.. Early radiologists, unaware of the danger, often exposed their hands to test the effectiveness of their machines, and thereby incurred skin cancers. They also suffered a large excess of leukemia deaths as compared with other physicians. Happily, more scrupulous avoidance of exposure has eradicated this occupational hazard. Approximately 10% of watch-dial painters, who pointed their fine brushes with their lips and thus absorbed considerable amounts of ^{226}Ra, later developed bone sarcomas and antral carcinomas.[134] A major form of occupational exposure is the mining of ores containing radioactive elements. As high as a tenfold increased frequency of lung cancers has been observed among these miners both in central Europe and in the Rocky Mountain regions of the United States.

Were all this evidence not enough, further documentation of the carcinogenicity of radiation comes from the long-term follow-up of approximately 100,000 atomic bomb blast survivors and controls in Hiroshima and Nagasaki. At Hiroshima, the radiation consisted principally of a mixture of gamma rays and neutrons, and in Nagasaki, predominantly gamma rays. In individuals most heavily exposed at Hiroshima, the annual leukemia incidence rate reached the astounding level of approximately 140 per 100,000 about six years after exposure. All types of leukemia increased, except chronic lymphocytic leukemia. It is significant that even 20 to 25 years after the exposure, the leukemia risk was still higher for the heavily exposed than for the controls. An excess mortality from thyroid, breast, and pulmonary carcinoma has also become apparent in the survivors about 20 years following the exposure.

To conclude this doleful litany, mention should be made of the residents of the Marshall Islands who were exposed on one occasion to accidental fallout from a hydrogen bomb test that contained thyroid-seeking radioactive iodines. As many as 90% of the children under the age of 10 years on Rongelap Island developed thyroid nodules within 15 years, and it is significant that about 5% of these nodules proved to be thyroid carcinomas.[135] It is evident that radiant energy—whether absorbed in the pleasant form of sunlight, through the best intentions of a physician, or by the tragic victim of an atomic bomb blast—has awesome carcinogenic potential.[136]

Mechanisms of Radiation Carcinogenesis

Although radiant energy is clearly oncogenic, the precise event responsible for neoplastic transformation is obscure. Radiant energy damages DNA, alters proteins, and inactivates enzymes, perhaps by disruption of specific cysteine residues and hydrogen bonds. It also injures membranes. How it exerts all these effects is still debated (see the general discussion of radiant energy on p. 464). Two theories dominate current thinking: (1) the radiation directly ionizes critical cellular macromolecules; or (2) according to the "indirect theory," it first interacts with water or molecular oxygen to produce free radicals that mediate the damage. Through either pathway the DNA sustains injury, thus in effect inducing a somatic mutation. Other theories of the carcinogenicity of ionizing radiation persist. One holds that latent oncogenic viruses are activated; this is most convincing with relation to certain forms of murine neoplasia. Another proposal is that radiation-induced neoplastic transformation is the result of cell-killing followed by regenerative replication. Possibly the combination of radiation-induced DNA errors and heightened cell replication might lead to cancer formation. However, in the last analysis *the carcinogenicity of ionizing radiation appears to correlate best with its mutagenicity.* In turn, the mutagenicity depends on a number of factors including (1) radiation quality, (2) dose, (3) dose rate, (4) DNA repair, and (5) host factors. On a dose-for-dose basis, particulate radiations having high LET (linear energy transfer) values (p. 465), such as neutrons and alpha particles, are more dangerous than low LET radiations, such as x-ray and gamma rays.

Ill-defined host factors also play a role. Clearly, fetuses, infants, and children are more vulnerable than adults. Thyroid cancer following radiation to the head and neck in adults is rare compared with its frequency in persons irradiated in childhood. Immune competence, hormonal influences, and cell type influence the carcinogenicity of radiation. Indeed, in humans there is a hierarchy of vulnerability of radiation-induced cancers.

Most frequent are the leukemias, save for chronic lymphocytic leukemia, which, for unknown reasons, almost never follows radiation injury. Cancer of the thyroid follows closely but only in the young. In the intermediate category are cancers of the breast, lungs, and salivary glands. In contrast, skin, bone, the gastrointestinal tract, and other organs and tissues (including lymphoid tissue) are relatively resistant to radiation-induced neoplasia, even though the gastrointestinal mucosal cells are vulnerable to the cell-killing effects of radiation and the skin is in the pathway of all external radiation. Nonetheless, the physician dare not forget—any cell can be transformed into a cancer cell by sufficient exposure to radiant energy.

ONCOGENIC VIRUSES

Oncogenic viruses can induce cancers in a wide range of species from amphibia to man's closest relatives, the primates, so it seems illogical to believe that humans alone in the animal kingdom are immune. However, decades of search have yielded no conclusive evidence of the viral causation of any type of human cancer; only the unglamorous benign wart and some closely related lesions have been documented to be viral induced. Nonetheless, there is much smoke, as will become evident, and one day the fire may be discovered.

A large number of RNA- and DNA-containing viruses are oncogenic to certain cells in vitro and to particular species in vivo. The RNA oncogenic viruses are better known as oncornaviruses (*onco*genic-*RNA* virus) or retroviruses, since they all code for a reverse transcriptase critical to their transforming function. The major implicated agents are presented in Table 6–5. Taken as a whole, they make up a diverse collection with no evident correlations between vulnerable host or type of tumor, and taxonomic status or size (complexity) of agent. Nononcogenic viruses are infectious agents; however, oncogenic viruses, with rare exceptions (e.g., the lymphomasarcoma/leukemia retrovirus in cats), do not spread horizontally. In addition, the DNA papilloma viruses causing warts and related lesions in humans may spread by contact with infected animals or contaminated environment. The reasons for the noncontagiousness in general of oncogenic viruses vary somewhat with the particular agent, and will emerge in later discussions. A brief overview of the clinically important categories of oncogenic viruses follows.

RNA Oncogenic Viruses

RNA tumor viruses (retroviruses) can induce lymphomas, leukemias, sarcomas, and mammary carcinomas in a wide variety of animals—chickens, rodents, cats, cattle, and primates—and are the apparent cause of many naturally occurring leukemias and lymphomas in several animal species. The viruses have in common the following features: (1) They have a single-stranded RNA genome enclosed within a virus-specified glycoprotein envelope. Specific cell surface receptors for the viral glycoproteins account for the particular cytotropism of the various agents. (2) Some are competent viruses (possess all the genes necessary for viral replication), and are able to replicate within permissive cells and simultaneously transform them. In this circumstance, virions can be visualized in the transformed cells. Others are defective viruses but can be "rescued" by cocultivation with helper viruses. In nonpermissive cells, transformation may occur but the virus cannot replicate. (3) The viral nucleoid is centrally placed in most retroviruses—so-called "type C" viruses. The MMTV (mouse mammary tumor virus) has an eccentric core and is a type B virus. (4) All have a reverse transcriptase coded by the viral genome, which mediates the synthesis of a complementary copy of DNA, using the viral RNA as a template. The DNA may then be integrated into the genome of the host cell as a "provirus." (5) They either carry a specific transforming gene (oncogene) or become associated with an indigenous cellular "protooncogene" critical to their transforming capacity.

The methods of transmission of retroviruses in their natural hosts vary with the particular agent. For example, with the avian leukosis virus causing leukemia in chickens, the provirus is integrated into the genome of the host's cells and so is transmitted as a congenital infection through the ovum. In contrast, the feline leukemia virus is infectious because it is transmitted horizontally in the saliva of affected cats. Other RNA viruses are transmitted congenitally (perhaps transplacental). The MMTV follows yet another route, being transmitted through the milk of infected animals. Bittner showed that newborn mice of high-incidence strains developed few mammary tumors if nursed by low-incidence foster mothers.[137] Contrarily, mammary carcinomas developed regularly in low-incidence nurslings if they were suckled by high-incidence foster mothers. Thus, the vectors of spread of the retroviruses are totally dissimilar to those of nontumor viruses.

Recently, exciting new findings have raised the possibility that a retrovirus may be implicated in the causation of a form of human neoplasia. A unique type-C retrovirus designated HTLV has been associated with an uncommon form of human T-cell lymphoma/leukemia.[138] The same or virtually identical viral agents have been implicated in endemic pockets of this disease in southwestern Japan and in West Indian blacks, suggesting horizontal transmission of the agent. However, the disease may also occur sporadically and is now being described around the world.[139, 140] Only a sample of the rapidly accumulating circumstantial evidence incriminating this particular agent will be offered. HTLV, like all retroviruses, codes for a reverse transcriptase. In animals, T-cell leukemias of retroviral origin are well documented. Nucleic acid hybridization reveals nucleotide sequences in leukemic cells of humans homologous to HTLV. Cultured neoplastic T cells from leukemic patients release type-C virus (HTLV). The virus will induce continuous proliferation in vitro of normal cord-blood T cells, strongly reminiscent of neoplastic trans-

Table 6–5.

Some Oncogenic RNA-Containing Viruses (Retrovirus Family)

Genus	*Virus*	*Host of Origin*	*Oncogenic Potential*
Type B oncovirus	Mammary tumor virus	Mouse	Mammary adenocarcinoma
Type C oncovirus	Rous sarcoma virus	Fowl	Fibrosarcoma, spindle cell sarcoma
	Fujinami virus	Fowl	Myxosarcoma
	Lymphoid leukosis viruses	Fowl	Lymphoid leukemia, erythroblastosis, osteopetrosis, nephroblastoma, sarcoma(?)
	Myeloblastosis viruses	Fowl	Myeloblastosis, erythroblastosis(?)
	Myelocytomatosis viruses (MC29, CMII)	Fowl	Myelocytomas, liver and kidney carcinomas
	MH2	Fowl	Endotheliomas, liver and kidney carcinomas
	OK10	Fowl	Endotheliomas and/or carcinomas
	Erythroblastosis viruses	Fowl	Erythroblastosis, sarcomas
	Gross leukemia viruses	Mouse	Thymic lymphosarcomas, lymphoid and myeloid leukemias
	Graffi leukemia virus	Mouse	Myeloid leukemia
	Rauscher, Kirsten, Friend } erythroleukemia viruses	Mouse	Erythroblastosis, polycythemia, lymphoid leukemia
	Moloney leukemia virus	Mouse	Lymphoid leukemia (T cells)
	Abelson leukemia virus	Mouse	pre–B-cell lymphosarcoma
	Harvey, Kirsten } sarcoma viruses	Mouse/Rat	Pleomorphic sarcomas
	Moloney sarcoma virus	Mouse	Rhabdomyosarcoma
	Myeloproliferative virus	Mouse	Erythroleukemia, myeloid leukemia
	FBJ sarcoma virus	Mouse	Osteosarcoma
	Feline leukemia virus	Cat	Lymphosarcoma
	Feline sarcoma virus	Cat	Fibrosarcoma
	Bovine lymphosarcoma virus	Cattle	Lymphosarcoma, leukemia
	Simian sarcoma virus	Woolly monkey	Fibrosarcoma
	Gibbon ape leukemia viruses	Gibbons	Myeloid (granulocytic) leukemia, lymphosarcoma

formation. The pursuit of further evidence substantiating the retroviral origin of this clinical disease is now in full cry. As pointed out on page 209, the HTLV is also under study as a possible cause of the various forms of neoplasia seen in patients with the acquired immune deficiency syndrome (AIDS).

DNA Oncogenic Viruses

Four families of DNA viruses are capable of causing tumors in animals, one of which is also strongly implicated in human cancers. In addition, the hepatitis B virus, for which there is no known counterpart in other species, is strongly linked to hepatocellular carcinoma in humans.

The *papovavirus* family contains three members: (1) *pa*pilloma virus, (2) *po*lyoma virus, and (3) *va*cuolating virus (the original name for SV-40). Many types of papilloma virus have now been identified; they cause papillomas in rabbits (Shope papilloma) that often progress to cancers, and these agents also cause warts, condyloma acuminatum, and laryngeal papilloma (all benign lesions) in humans.[141] It is of significance that on occasion the condyloma acuminatum gives rise to a squamous cell carcinoma, and in the rare clinical disease epidermodysplasia verruciformis (caused by several subtypes of papilloma virus) the warts often progress to squamous cell carcinomas when one particular subtype is involved. The papilloma viruses may be spread horizontally by infected animals or contaminated environment. There is some evidence that viral-induced warts may also be spread from human to human, but the contagiousness, at best, is very low. Recently the question has been raised as to whether certain papilloma viruses are involved in the production of cervical cancer in humans (p. 1124). Polyoma virus is so named because it produces a variety of neoplasms in several species of animals, but it has not been implicated in any form of human tumor. The SV-40 virus, whose natural hosts are a variety of monkeys, is of interest because it was found to be present in the monkey cells used in the large-scale production of poliomyelitis vaccine. Thus, thousands of individuals inadvertently received the agent and, while it is capable of transforming human cells in culture, there is no substantial evidence of tumorigenesis in immunized individuals.[142] Recently, two viruses designated BK and JC, both closely related to SV-40, have been isolated from humans, and transform animal cells in culture and induce neoplasms in newborn hamsters.[143] There is no evidence that either agent is carcinogenic in humans, but the JC virus is strongly implicated in the causation of the neurologic disorder progressive multifocal leukoencephalopathy (p. 1386).

Table 6–5 (cont'd)

Some Oncogenic DNA-Containing Viruses

Family	*Virus*	*Host of Origin*	*Oncogenic Potential*
Papovavirus	Papilloma virus	Various mammals, including man	Papillomas, may progress to carcinoma
	SV40	Rhesus, cynomolgus, and cercopithecus monkeys	Fibrosarcomas, ependymomas (in hamsters)
	Polyoma	Mouse	Adenomas, adenocarcinomas, hemangiomas, fibromas, fibrosarcomas
Adenovirus	Various strains of human, simian, bovine, and avian origin		Sarcomas (in hamsters)
Herpesvirus	Frog herpesvirus	Leopard frog	Adenomas, adenocarcinomas, osteochondroma(?)
	Marek's disease	Fowl	Neurolymphomatosis; not strictly neoplastic
	Guinea pig herpesvirus	Guinea pig	Lymphocytic leukemia
	Herpesvirus ateles	Spider monkey	Lymphoma, lymphoblastic leukemia
	Herpesvirus saimiri	Squirrel monkey	Lymphoma, lymphoblastic leukemia
	Herpes simplex 1	Man	Squamous cell carcinoma (??)
	Herpes simplex 2	Man	Cervical carcinoma (?)
	Epstein-Barr virus	Man	Burkitt's lymphoma, nasopharyngeal carcinoma
Hepatitis virus	Hepatitis B	Man	Hepatocarcinoma (?)
Poxvirus	Shope fibroma	Rabbit	Fibroma
	Yaba virus	Rhesus monkey	Fibroma-like nodular hyperplasia; not neoplastic
	Molluscum contagiosum	Man	Nodular epidermal hyperplasia; not neoplastic

The evidence that these viruses are causally associated with the tumors listed is, in most cases, strong if not definite. However, (?) indicates reasonable doubt and (??) considerable doubt that the virus plays an etiologic role in tumor production.

From Wyke, J. A.: Oncogenic viruses. J Pathol. *135*:39, 1981. Reproduced with permission.

Adenoviruses are common causes of minor respiratory tract and conjunctival infections in humans. Three human adenoviruses—types 12, 18, and 31—are strongly oncogenic in newborn hamsters and transform rodent cells in culture, but they have no similar effect in humans or their cells.

The *herpesviruses* are responsible for a variety of forms of cancer and proliferative diseases in several vertebrate animal species. There is also much evidence, all circumstantial, implicating these agents in the cause of certain forms of cancer in humans. The findings fall short of fulfilling Koch's postulates but they point strongly to a role for the Epstein-Barr virus (EBV) in the causation of African Burkitt's lymphoma, and somewhat less strongly to a similar role with undifferentiated nasopharyngeal carcinoma.[144, 145] Both these neoplasms are reviewed in detail on pages 662 and 764, respectively. Burkitt's lymphoma is a neoplasm of B lymphocytes that is the commonest childhood tumor in Central Africa and New Guinea, where EBV is endemic. A morphologically identical lymphoma also occurs sporadically throughout the world, but there is little evidence that EBV plays any role in its induction. As you may know, EBV is known to be the cause of infectious mononucleosis. What, then, underlies the change in its behavior leading to the induction of African Burkitt's lymphoma? Additional influences appear to be involved.[146] In normal individuals, effective humoral and cell-mediated immune responses control the viral invasion, accounting for the self-limited nature of infectious mononucleosis. In Africa, on the other hand, concomitant malaria or some other disorder impairs the immune competence of individuals, and thus EBV is able to replicate freely within B cells and so activate them into clonal expansion and proliferation, favoring the appearance of mutational errors. Particularly critical appear to be translocations from chromosome 8 mainly to 14 and, less often, to 2 or 22. Preliminary observations suggest that the breakpoint in chromosome 8 is close to a possible "oncogene." Transposition of this gene into the immediate vicinity of an immunoglobulin gene on chromosomes 14, 2, or 22, already actively functioning because of the viral infection, might favor enhanced expression of the oncogene.[148] In this connection, similar translocations are encountered in sporadic cases of non-African Burkitt's lymphoma not associated with the EBV, and so other exogenous stimuli may assume the role of the EBV. It thus appears that under appropriate circumstances, particularly immunologic incompetence, EBV may initiate oncogenesis.

There is substantial evidence supporting the role of immunoincompetence in viral tumorigenesis, some presented later (p. 259). AIDS, mentioned earlier in connection with the HTLV (p. 209), provides an example. Infections, presumably opportunistic (only arising in predisposed persons), are extremely frequent in these individuals, such as with *Pneumocystis carinii* and, of particular interest to our discussion, also with EBV and cytomegalovirus (CMV). Many other opportunists also find "snug harbors" in these immunocompromised individuals, as pointed out on page 208.[148A] The strikingly high attack rate of malignant neoplasia is relevant in these circumstances, taking the forms of either Kaposi's sarcoma or Burkitt's lymphoma.[149, 150] Traces of the CMV have been identified in the sarcoma cells, and of EBV in the lymphoma cells.[151] Enough has been said to justify present concern about the potential oncogenicity of the herpesviruses.

There is substantial but not totally convincing evidence associating another member of the herpes group with human cancer. Seroepidemiologic data link herpes simplex type 2 (HSV-2) to carcinoma of the cervix. Moreover, viral DNA has been identified in tumor cells.[152] More is detailed about the HSV-2 and cervical carcinoma on page 1124, but for now we can leave it that the possibility that the viral infection is merely coincidental has not been ruled out.

The *poxviruses*, to date, have not been associated with human neoplasms.

Mechanisms of Action of Viruses

Great strides have been made in dissecting the molecular mechanisms involved in experimental, viral-induced malignant transformation. Only an overview can be offered here, but excellent reports are available.[138, 153] Since the RNA and DNA viruses act in different manners they require separate consideration.

Concepts about the mechanism(s) of action of the oncogenic RNA retroviruses are not only changing rapidly, but are exploding. Much that might be said, then, will undoubtedly require modification in the near future, and it seems best to limit remarks to "the state of the art." Oncogenic retroviruses achieve a stable association with the host cell by integration of the provirus into the genome of infected cells. However, cell replication only leads to viral replication when the DNA provirus contains a linear sequence of three genes necessary for viral replication. One gene (called "gag") codes for a polyprotein that can be cleaved into four virion core proteins. Next to it is a gene ("pol") coding for the reverse transcriptase. The third gene ("env") specifies the envelope glycoproteins. At both the 3′ and 5′ ends of this proviral gene sequence there are nucleotide segments, referred to as long terminal repeat (LTR) units (Fig. 6–20). The LTR unit appears to be a control-promoter sequence that probably has importance in regulating replication of the contiguous proviral genome. Loss of one of the three genes yields a defective, incompetent virus incapable of replication, which can, however, be rescued by coinfection with nondefective helper viruses. It is significant that retroviruses appear to be capable of integration into multiple sites within the host DNA, which may have relevance in their oncogenicity, as will be seen. Nonetheless, the tumors they evoke are monoclonal and so the cells of the tumor all have identical sites of integration, a point of some importance in proposed mechanisms of action of certain retroviruses.

In addition to their basic replicative structure, retroviruses can be divided into two categories: those that also contain the genetic information for transforming cells—a so-called "oncogene," and those without transforming oncogenes. How the retroviruses without transforming genes cause tumors will be discussed presently. There is now substantial evidence that retroviruses having *onc* genes acquired them through genetic recombinations very likely with cellular genes.[154] Genetic loci homologous to viral *onc* genes have been detected in the normal genome of virtually all vertebrates examined from chickens to humans.[155] It thus appears that (1) *retroviruses having oncogenes are likely to have acquired them as captives during infections of evolutionary antecedents, and* (2) *normal cells in both animals and humans possess apparent protooncogenes—"the enemy within."* What "turns on" these genes is not clear but, as indicated below, it may depend on genetic or epigenetic control mechanisms or some mutation in the protooncogene itself.

In the context of present proposals about the derivation of viral *onc* genes from cellular *onc* genes, a construct can be offered as to how retroviruses not possessing their own transforming *onc* genes act. Since proviral integration occurs at multiple sites, *chance insertion of a provirus with its promoter LTR next to a cellular* onc *gene would result in tumorigenesis.* In fact, the complete viral sequence is not needed; defective (or incomplete) viruses are no less able to transform cells than replicative viruses. Indeed, it has been shown that integration of the LTR unit alone may suffice, suggesting

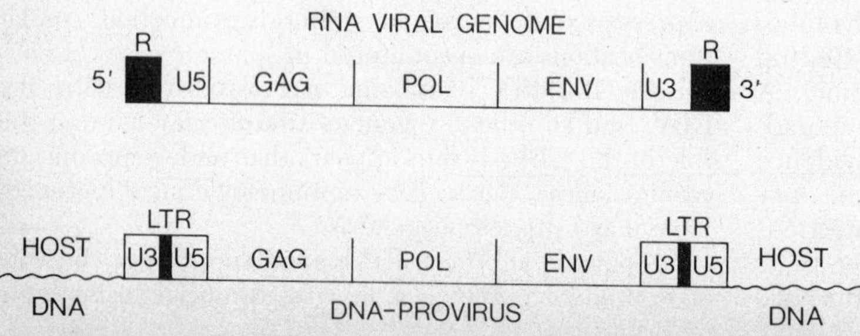

Figure 6–20. R = repeat sequence of nucleotides; U = unique sequence of nucleotides; LTR = long terminal repeat sequences.

once again that tumor formation hinges on regulation or mutation of cellular-potential *onc* genes.[156] Could chemical- and radiation-induced mutations directly involve protooncogenes or affect control sequences adjacent to indigenous oncogenes? Dosage of the *onc* gene product might be critical to viral transformation[147] but these speculations remain to be proved.

Granting the presence of *onc* genes, whether viral or cellular in origin, how do they effect cell transformation? One potential pathway has been identified with some of the retroviruses—namely, the synthesis of oncogene-coded transforming protein. Best defined is a phosphoprotein produced by the avian sarcoma virus oncogene having a molecular weight of 21,000, called p21. It is a protein kinase catalyzing the preferential phosphorylation of acceptor proteins and, in particular, of tyrosine.[157] Phosphorylation is known to regulate enzyme activity. Moreover, the protein kinase has been shown to be largely associated with the membranes of tumor cells, and so presumably may alter membrane function and the social behavior of transformed cells.[158] A further point of interest: some transforming proteins are structurally related to growth factors, such as platelet-derived growth factor, known to be mitogenic to normal cells. Transforming proteins have also been associated with several other retroviruses, but not all, and so it may not be the only pathway of tumorigenesis with these agents. It is evident that, despite significant gaps in our knowledge, deep penetrations have been made into the oncogenicity of retroviruses, and it is further evident that a fundamental feature is their interaction with cellular genes indigenous to the host cells.

The mechanism(s) of action of the DNA oncogenic viruses appears to differ from that of the RNA viruses. With the former, virus cannot be isolated from transformed cells since transformation is incompatible with replication of the virus. Infectious virus can, however, be rescued with SV-40 and some of the other DNA agents by co-cultivation with permissive cells. However, polyoma- and adenovirus-induced neoplasms are completely virus-free. This observation gave rise to the "hit-and-run" concept, implying that a virus might be able to induce heritable uncontrolled proliferation and then be eliminated. *However, tumor cells transformed by all DNA oncogenic viruses are, in fact, synthesizing virus-coded proteins termed T antigens.*[159] Further analysis reveals that the polyoma and SV-40 viruses in fact induce three T antigens referred to as large-T, middle-T, and small-T.[160] With SV-40, large-T is found in the nucleus complexed to a protein of 53,000 daltons (53K) of cellular origin. The complex is bound to the integrated viral DNA, suggesting that it is intimately involved in both viral replication and neoplastic transformation. *An apparently identical 53K transforming protein has also been identified in a variety of neoplastic cells transformed by other DNA viruses. Significantly, a similar transforming protein has been identified in cells transformed by EBV, chemical carcinogens, and spontaneous teratocarcinomas, raising the possibility that it is a fundamental mediator of transformation.*[161, 162] However, with some oncogenic DNA viruses, e.g., polyoma virus, large-T is not necessary, nor sufficient for transformation; there are, however, small amounts of 53K protein but it is not bound to polyoma T antigen. Instead, with this virus, middle-T complexes to the cell membrane and is associated with kinase activity,[163] producing some similarity to certain of the retroviruses.

It is apparent that there are differences in mode of action among the DNA viruses and between the DNA and RNA agents, but a few similarities as well. Like the retroviruses, only small pieces of the oncogenic DNA viral genome are required for transformation of cells in vivo or in vitro.[164] The critical segment appears to be located in the "early" region (where transcription begins) of the viral genome. Whether this segment of the viral DNA contains an oncogene or a control region analogous to that in retrovirus is not clear. There is no evidence as yet that the viral DNA must integrate in a particular chromosome or at a specific site.[165] Neither is there any evidence that transforming DNA segments or genes are derived from normal host genes, as is the case with the retroviruses. All that can be said is that integration of complete oncogenic DNA viral genomes into permissive host cells provides a mechanism for viral survival and replication. In contrast, tumorigenesis is the consequence of integration of noninfectious incomplete genomes or fragments into nonpermissive cells that, in some way, perturbs the homeostasis of the cells and leads to the formation of transforming proteins. So we must conclude that with all oncogenic viruses, despite penetrations into their mechanisms of action, complete understanding still eludes us.

OTHER CARCINOGENS

In addition to the three well-defined categories of agents, many other carcinogenic influences have been identified both in experimental systems and in humans.[166] First, the major implicated agents will be cited briefly followed by some speculations about their mechanisms of action. Asbestos fibers are widely recognized carcinogens (p. 439), which readily induce mesothelial tumors in rats and mice following intrapleural or intraperitoneal injection. This agent also causes a markedly increased incidence of bronchogenic carcinomas and mesotheliomas (both pleural and peritoneal) as well as gastrointestinal cancers in chronically exposed humans. Although chemical interactions cannot be ruled out, it is currently believed that asbestos serves largely as a promoter.[166A] In the induction of bronchogenic carcinoma, the asbestos fibers may also serve as "carriers" of other carcinogens such as cigarette smoke residues. Other types of inhaled fibers, including glass, wool, and cotton, have been associated with cancers of the lungs, pleura, mouth, nose, and air sinuses in humans, but only very rarely. Macromolecules such as saturated iron oxide have been implicated, as well as implanted sheets of plastics and metal. Parenthetically, there is no substantial evidence to date that the use of synthetic prostheses such as heart valves or vascular grafts has led to tumors. The scattered reports of cancer induction associated with prostheses are anecdotal and difficult to interpret. *Particularly important in endemic regions is the significantly increased frequency of bladder cancer with* Schistosoma haematobium *infections of the urinary bladder*. In Egypt, where *Schistosoma* is endemic, carcinoma of the bladder is the most common type of cancer in males.[167] *Clonorchis sinensis* infection of the biliary tract represents a well-defined predisposition to cancer at its sites of localization. Many reports call attention to the association of cancers with chronic inflammation and scarring—"*scar cancers,*" although this is a somewhat controversial issue. For example, cancers have appeared within scarred areas caused by nondegradable foreign bodies. More relevant is the increased incidence of lung carcinomas attributed to the chronic scarring induced by a variety of infections, particularly chronic tuberculosis.[168] Analogously, ill-fitting dentures and chronic irritation resulting from jagged fragments of teeth have induced an increased incidence of carcinoma in the chronically injured mucosa of the oral cavity. There is no clear understanding of the carcinogenicity of these diverse influences, and one must assume that widely differing mechanisms are involved.

In concluding this presentation of oncogenic agents, several points should be noted. Although a large number of chemical agents (Table 6–6) have almost certainly caused cancer in humans, many others cannot at this time be exonerated freely; indeed, some are strongly suspected, such as oncogenic viruses, artificial sweeteners, and nitroso compounds. Neither can any agent be dismissed on grounds of level of exposure; many agents, even at low levels of exposure, could act in concert or sequentially to "do their dirty deed." Thus, the notion of "tolerable levels of exposure" is fraught with risk. And finally, the great diversity of the oncogenic influences invites the speculation that all must ultimately exert their effects by common intracellular pathways.

Table 6–6. CHEMICALS STRONGLY IMPLICATED AS CARCINOGENS IN HUMANS*

	Site of Tumor Formation
Industrial	
2-Naphthylamine	Urinary bladder
Benzidine	Urinary bladder
4-Aminobiphenyl	Urinary bladder
Bis(chloromethyl) ether	Respiratory tract
Bis(2-chloroethyl) sulfide (mustard gas)	Respiratory tract
Vinyl chloride	Liver
Tars, soots, and oils	Skin, lungs
Chromium compounds	Lungs
Nickel compounds	Lungs, nasal sinuses
Asbestos	Pleura, peritoneum, respiratory and GI tracts
Benzene	Bone marrow
Medical	
Inorganic arsenic	Skin
Alkylating agents (melphalan, cyclophosphamide, chlorambucil, dihydroxybusulfan, and others)	Acute nonlymphocytic leukemia, bladder (cyclophosphamide), other sites
Methoxypsoralen	Skin cancer
Phenacetin-containing drugs	Renal pelvis, ?bladder
Diethylstilbestrol	Vagina (prenatal exposure) Endometrium (postnatal exposure)
Androgenic anabolic steroids	Liver
Cultural	
Cigarette smoke	Lungs, urinary tract, esophagus, others
Chewing tobacco and betel nuts	Buccal mucosa
Aflatoxins	Liver

*A conservative list for which there is substantial documentation. Many other chemicals are suspect. Modified from Miller, E. C., and Miller, J. A.: Mechanisms of chemical carcinogenesis. Cancer *47*:1055, 1981; and Hoover, R., and Fraumeni, J. F.: Drug-induced cancer. Cancer *47*:1071, 1981.

PATHOGENESIS OF CANCER

Although the precise molecular events responsible for oncogenesis in humans is still unknown, evidence is beginning to converge about fundamental features of the process. Many observations suggest that *malignant transformation is the result either of abnormal expression of genes normally present in the genome of the host cell or of some modification of an endogenous gene or genes. In either event, gene products such as transforming proteins are produced that alter cell differentiation, replicative activity, and social behavior.* Still unresolved is the issue of whether somatic mutations or epigenetic mechanisms permit expression of the modified gene function or, as seems most likely, genetic changes interact with epigenetic phenomena.

Only some of the observations relating indigenous genes to oncogenesis will be reiterated. You recall that retroviral *onc* genes are homologous to sequences in the normal DNA of host cells, and so are thought to constitute "captured" host genes. In addition, with the retroviruses not possessing transforming genes, only a very small fragment of the viral genome (about 7%) is necessary for neoplastic transformation.[170] This non–protein-coding fragment is thought to represent the terminal control unit associated with the viral genome. It exerts its effect, then, by altering the expression of indigenous genes, particularly protooncogenes identified in the cells of all vertebrates, including humans. Another piece of evidence is the transformation of cells by transfection with small fragments of DNA (about the size of a gene) derived from normal cells.[171, 172] Whether the transforming fragment is a protooncogene or a regulatory gene is irrelevant—"indigenous" genes from normal cells transformed other cells. The work of Mintz and Fleischman provides further support to the tumorigenicity of the "normal" genome,[173] demonstrating that it is possible to produce teratocarcinomas by merely implanting normal germ cells or early embryonic cells of mice into ectopic sites in adult syngeneic recipients. Moreover, under particular in vitro conditions, teratocarcinoma cells were induced to differentiate into apparently normal specialized cells, indicating retention of normal genetic programs of the cancerous cells.[174] Even more impressive, the microinjection of teratocarcinoma cells into embryos at the blastocyst stage led to the development of a normal mosaic mouse whose tissues were derived from both the tumor cells and the normal recipient embryo.[175] In this remarkable experiment, the tumor genome retained the capacity to program differentiation into the various specialized cells of a multicellular organism. Thus, *normal cells can be transformed into cancer cells, at least into teratocarcinoma cells, by only an abnormal environment, and abnormal cancer cells can be made to revert to normal programs. The mechanism for the induction of the teratocarcinoma was inherent in the "normal" genome.* It is possible, therefore, that abnormal expression of indigenous *onc* genes, whether related to altered genetic or to epigenetic controls, may underlie tumor formation in humans. By dosage effect, sufficient amounts of transforming proteins could be produced to convert normal cells to cancer cells.

Recent findings, however, suggest an alternative "pathway" to the production of human oncogenes, namely the subtlest of alterations in an indigenous gene converting it into a transforming gene. A small segment of DNA containing about 6600 nucleotide base pairs has been isolated from two human bladder carcinomas that transforms normal fibroblasts in vitro, and that is identical to a normal homologous human gene save for swapping (transversion) of a base pair from guanosine-cytosine to adenine-thymine at a specific position in the gene.[176, 177] The oncogene has been sequenced and has remarkable homology to an RNA tumor virus oncogene. Further, it codes for a 21,000-dalton transforming phosphoprotein differing from the protein product of the protooncogene only in the 12th amino acid where a glycine is replaced by a valine. An almost identical mutated protooncogene has been isolated from many other solid tissue cancers of humans also encoding a p21,000 protein. In one instance the cellular oncogene has been shown to have considerable homology with the gene coding for platelet-derived growth factor, and the transforming protein to have a close structural relationship to the growth factor. The circle grows ever tighter! The question must then be raised: "Does oncogenesis in humans begin when such a point-mutation arises because of some carcinogenic influence or, instead, may protooncogenes be lurking within, which remain latent, only to surface in tumorigenesis when other conditions, genetic or epigenetic, favor their expression?"

That protooncogenes are hidden in the normal genome of vertebrates is entirely compatible with our present concepts of ontogeny. All cell types in a multicellular organism have identical genetic information. Differentiation results from the selective and temporally sequenced activation and suppression of genes according to the Jacob-Monod operon model. Recall the synthesis of hemoglobin F in the fetus that is permanently "turned off" early in life. Model systems document the suppressibility of the neoplastic genotype. With temperature-sensitive mutants of the Rous sarcoma virus, for example, a few degrees' difference in the temperature of the culture determines whether the normal or the tumor phenotype will be expressed.[178] At the nonpermissive temperature the cells harbor the provirus but are not transformed, presumably because transcriptase or translation of the *onc* gene is blocked. Cell hybrids (described on p. 120) provide another model of suppression of the transforming genotype.[179] When a malignant cell line capable of inducing tumors in appropriate hosts is hybridized with a nonmalignant cell line, malignancy is suppressed in the hybrids. These hybrids on replication tend to lose chromosomes, with resumption of the malignant phenotype. In this system, "malignancy" behaves as a genetic recessive or is dependent on gene dosage effect.

Many hypothetical mechanisms involving genetic or epigenetic pathways have been proposed for inappropriate activation or suppression of genes in the "normal" genome. Most invoke some genetic rearrangement such as trisomy, transpositions, and translocations (karyotypically visible transpositions), any one of which might alter control segments and/or have dosage effects.[147] An example of gene dosage is the trisomy, usually of chromosome 15, seen in some B-cell lymphomas and leukemias.[180] The fact that trisomy 15 is a primary event and not an epiphenomenon is supported by its being present in leukemias induced by oncogenic viruses, radiation, and various chemical carcinogens as well as in spontaneously arising murine leukemias.[181, 182] Transpositions are now thought to commonly occur "spontaneously" in normal organisms and produce phenotypic modifications that can be tested for survival advantage in the evolutionary process. Programmed transpositions may be involved in normal cell differentiation. They are made possible by the presence of certain short sequences in the DNA ("transposons") that constitute substrates for various recombinational enzymes ("transposases").[126] Such shuffling of genes profoundly alters the expression of entire segments of the genetic code. The Philadelphia chromosome of chronic myelogenous leukemia is a form of transposition. In ataxia telangiectasia a translocation affecting chromosome 14 is often present, as it is in the lymphoid cells of the leukemia that tends to arise in these individuals. Burkitt's lymphoma and some other lymphoproliferative disorders are characterized by an 8:14 translocation (p. 669).[183, 184] Significantly, in a number of instances the breakpoints in the two chromosomes involved in the translocation occurred at loci of a putative "oncogene" in one and at an immunoglobulin gene in the other. At completion of the translocation, the oncogene was positioned immediately adjacent to the immunoglobulin gene. Activation of the immunoglobulin gene by some antigenic challenge may then lead to active expression of the oncogene. It suffices that there are many examples in humans and animals in which gene dosage and shuffling of the normal genome (as with a translocation) apparently have led to the malignant phenotype, lending some credibility to the concept that neoplastic transformation could be the consequence of mutation of a protooncogene into an oncogene or altered expression of genes indigenous in the host. Indeed, it may well be that two or more mutations are necessary, one conferring enhanced replicative capability, and another affecting control regions and permitting escape from normal regulatory signals.

Despite all the evidence pointing to genetic mechanisms in the induction of cancer, abnormal gene expression could be caused by *epigenetic mechanisms*, i.e., cytoplasmic regulatory products affecting transcription or translation.[185] According to this view, *neoplasia emerges as a result of some derangement of cellular differentiation and maturation imposed by abnormalities in epigenetic regulatory mechanisms.* Fetal characteristics are retained in tumor cells, e.g., the elaboration of "fetal antigens," the reversion to fetal isoenzyme profiles, and the capacity for sustained replication. Failure of differentiation and maturation confers longer cell survival, and so tumor growth may be related to accumulation of cells, as noted earlier (p. 221). Protooncogenes in vertebrate cells have been so highly conserved in phylogeny that they must be important, perhaps in regulation of growth and differentiation. Some epigenetic alteration in their expression might then underlie cancer. The possibility that epigenetic mechanisms may account for heritable cellular changes is no more surprising than the fact that liver cells produce liver cells and endometrial cells produce endometrial cells, all derived from a single ovum. Many other findings support the epigenetic model of carcinogenesis. All carcinogens are not mutagens.[186] Reversion of malignant cells to noncancer cells has been observed in both clinical and experimental settings. Mention has already been made of the highly malignant neuroblastoma that sometimes matures and differentiates into a benign ganglioneuroma.[187] Neuroblastoma cells in culture can be induced chemically to revert to stable, nondividing, apparently normal nerve cells.[188] Perhaps most convincing was the development of a normal mosaic mouse when teratocarcinoma cells were introduced into a mouse blastocyst; the genome in the tumor cells was evidently intact. It is not profitable to pursue further this now historic controversy over the "genetic" (somatic mutation) versus "epigenetic" initiation of cancer since at present the final answer is not known. It is not necessary that one or the other pathway be correct. It seems reasonable from present observations that an oncogene may become expressed because of mutagenic events alone or because of a mutagenic event coupled with epigenetic alterations.

Finally, it should be pointed out that *host factors may well play a role in the emergence of cancers.* The mere presence of a potentially transforming mutation does not necessitate its expression. In addition to the intracellular or local controls already discussed, systemic controls may exist such as the immune system. Many clinical observations, some cited earlier with respect to the acquired immune deficiency syndrome (p. 208), indicate that individuals suffering from an immunodeficiency are at greater risk of developing a cancer.[189] You recall that individuals who develop ultraviolet-induced skin cancers often have skin anergy. The cancer-prone chromosomal breakage syndrome ataxia telangiectasia is characterized by a selective deficiency of serum IgA and other deficits in cellular immunity. An X-linked immunodeficient syndrome was described in 1981 in which individuals infected with EBV are prone to develop malignant lymphoproliferative disorders.[190] Other examples might be cited, but it is sufficient that there are many suggestions of host-controlling influences. Regrettably, it is all too plain from the prevalence of cancer that they are less than perfect.

EPILOGUE

In concluding this consideration of neoplasia (and the reader may well say—and not a moment too soon!), it is evident that the ultimate changes that confer the malignant phenotype remain a mystery. Whatever these changes may be, the suspicion grows ever stronger that some alteration in the DNA code (a mutation) underlies them. Not clear as yet is whether acquisition of such a mutation spells the onset of a cancer. Perhaps some secondary event, genetic or epigenetic, must follow to permit enhanced expression of the acquired oncogene. It now appears that protooncogenes lurk within many or all of us awaiting (as we all do) the opportunity for self-expression. The accumulating data also make evident that the line separating "cancer" from "the normal" is exquisitely fine, contributing no doubt to the difficulty in defining it. But subtle as it may be, it cannot for long remain hidden with the monumental search now being devoted to its discovery.

1. American Cancer Society: Cancer Statistics, 1984. CA *34*:7, 1984.
2. Willis, R.A.: The Spread of Tumors in the Human Body. London, Butterworth & Co., 1952.
3. Allred, L.E., and Porter, K.R.: Morphology of normal and transformed cells. In Hynes, R.O. (ed.): Surfaces of Normal and Malignant Cells. New York, John Wiley & Sons, 1979, p. 21.
4. Lazarides, E.: Intermediate filaments as mechanical integrators of cellular space. Nature *283*:249, 1980.
5. Gabbiani, G., et al.: Immunochemical identification of intermediate-sized filaments in human neoplastic cells. A diagnostic aid for the surgical pathologist. Am. J. Pathol. *104*:206, 1981.
6. Schlegel, R., et al.: Immunoperoxidase localization of keratin in human neoplasms. A preliminary survey. Am. J. Pathol. *101*:41, 1980.

6A. Nagle, R.B., et al.: The use of antikeratin antibodies in the diagnosis of human neoplasms. Am. J. Clin. Pathol. *79*:458, 1983.

7. Trojanowski, J.Q., et al.: Neuronal origin of human esthesioneuroblastoma demonstrated with antineurofilament monoclonal antibodies. N. Engl. J. Med. *307*:159, 1982.
8. Hill, B.T.: The management of human solid tumours: some observations on the irrelevance of traditional cell cycle kinetics and the value of certain recent concepts. Cell Biol. Int. Rep. *2*:216, 1978.
9. Everson, T.C., and Cole, W.H.: Spontaneous Regression of Cancer. Philadelphia, W. B. Saunders Co., 1966.
10. Nowell, P.C.: The clonal evolution of tumor cell populations. Science *194*:23, 1976.
11. Fialkow, P.J.: Clonal origin of human tumors. Biochim. Biophys. Acta *458*:283, 1976.
12. Baserga, R.: Multiplication and Division in Mammalian Cells. New York, Marcel Dekker, 1976.
13. Black, P.H.: Shedding from normal and cancer-cell surfaces. N. Engl. J. Med. *303*:415, 1980.

14. Baserga, R.: The cell cycle. N. Engl. J. Med. *304*:453, 1981.
15. Johnson, L.D., et al.: Epidemiologic evidence for the spectrum of change from dysplasia to carcinoma-in-situ to invasive cancer. Cancer *22*:901, 1968.
16. Folkman, J., et al.: Growth and metastasis of tumor in organ culture. Cancer *16*:453, 1963.
17. Gimbrone, M.A., Jr., et al.: Tumor dormancy *in vivo* by prevention of neovascularization J. Exp. Med. *136*:261, 1972.
18. Folkman, J., and Cotran, R.S.: Relation of vascular proliferation to tumor growth. Int. Rev. Exp. Pathol. *16*:207, 1976.
19. Langer, R., et al.: Control of tumor growth in animals by infusion of an angiogenesis inhibitor. Proc. Natl. Acad. Sci. U.S.A *77*:4331, 1980.
20. Taylor, S., and Folkman, J.: Protamine is an inhibitor of angiogenesis. Nature *297*:307, 1982.
21. Schiaffonati, L., and Baserja, R.: Different survival of normal and transformed cells exposed to nutritional conditions non-permissive for growth. Cancer Res. *37*:541, 1977.
22. Baster, J.D., and Funder, J.W.: Hormone receptor. N. Engl. J. Med. *301*:1149, 1972.
23. Hoffman, P.G., and Siiteri, P.K.: Sex steroid receptors in gynecologic cancer. Obstet. Gynecol. *55*:648, 1980.
24. Keuttner, K.E., et al.: Morphological studies on the resistance of cartilage to invasion by osteosarcoma cells *in vitro* and *in vivo*. Cancer Res. *38*:277, 1978.
25. Brem, H., and Folkman, J.: Inhibition of tumor angiogenesis mediated by cartilage. J. Exp. Med. *141*:427, 1975.
26. Rifkin, D.B., and Crowe, R.M.: Isolation of a protease inhibitor from tissues resistant to tumor invasion. Hoppe Seylers Z. Physiol. Chem. *358*:1525, 1977.
27. Mareel, M.M.: Recent aspects of tumor invasiveness. Int. Rev. Exp. Pathol.. *22*:65, 1980.
28. Weinstein, R.S., et al.: The structure and function of intercellular junctions in cancer. Adv. Cancer Res. *23*:23, 1976.
29. Strauli, P., and Weiss, L.: Cell locomotion and tumor penetration. Eur. J. Cancer *13*:1, 1977.
30. Tickle, A.A., et al.: Cell movement and the mechanism of invasiveness: A survey of the behavior of some normal and malignant cells implanted into the developing chick wing bud. J. Cell Science *31*:293, 1978.
31. Hart, I.R., and Fidler, I.J.: Cancer invasion and metastasis. Q. Rev. Biol. *55*:121, 1980.
32. delRegato, J.A.: Pathways of metastatic spread of malignant tumors. Semin. Oncol. *4*:33, 1977.
33. Herberman, R.B., and Ortaldo, J.R.: Natural killer cells: Their role in defenses against disease. Science *214*:24, 1981.
34. Poste, G., and Fidler, I.J.: The pathogenesis of cancer metastasis. Nature *283*:139, 1980.
35. Dvorak, H.F., et al.: Induction of a fibrin-gel investment: An early event in line 10 hepatocarcinoma growth mediated by tumor-secreted products. J. Immunol. *122*:166, 1979.
36. Chew, E.C., and Wallace, A.C.: Demonstration of fibrin in early stages of experimental metastases. Cancer Res. *36*:1904, 1976.
37. Kramer, R.H., and Nicolson, G.L.: Interactions of tumor cells with vascular endothelial cell monolayers: A model for metastatic invasion. Proc. Natl. Acad. Sci. U.S.A. *76*:5704, 1979.
38. Hart, I.R.: The selection of characterization of an invasive variant of the B16 melanoma. Am. J. Pathol. *97*:587, 1979.
39. Fidler, I.J., and Kripke, M.L.: Metastasis results from preexisting variant cells within a malignant tumor. Science *197*:893, 1977.
40. Fisher, B., and Fisher, E.R.: Experimental studies of factors influencing hepatic metastases. I. The effect of number of tumor cells injected and time of growth. Cancer *12*:926, 1959.
41. Karpatkin, S., and Pearlstein, E.: Role of platelets in tumor cell metastases. Ann. Intern. Med. *95*:636, 1981.
42. Nicolson, G.L., et al.: The role of fibronectin in adhesion of metastatic melanoma cells to endothelial cells and their basal laminae. Exp. Cell. Res. *135*:461, 1981.
43. Brunson, K.W., et al.: Selection and altered tumor cell properties of brain-colonizing metastatic melanoma cells selected from B16 melanoma. Int. J. Cancer *23*:854, 1979.
44. Poste, G.: The influence of cell surface properties on the arrest of circulating melanoma cells. *In* Hynes, R.O., and Fox, C.F. (eds.): Tumor Cell Surfaces and Malignancy. New York, Alan R. Liss, 1980, p. 737.
45. Editorial: Is cancer irreversible? Br. Med. J. *2*:585, 1978.
45A. Editorial: Reversal of cancer. Lancet *1*:799, 1983.
46. Iype, P.T., et al.: Markers for transformation in rat liver epithelial cells in culture. Ann. N.Y. Acad. Sci. *349*:312, 1980.
47. Hull, L.A.: Progress towards a unified theory of the mechanisms of carcinogenesis: Role of cell cycle restriction points. Med. Hypotheses *7*:187, 1981.
48. Vaheri, A., and Mosher, D.F.: High molecular weight, cell surface–associated glycoprotein (fibronectin) lost in malignant transformation. Biochim. Biophys. Acta *516*:1, 1978.
49. Riddle, V.G.H., et al.: Growth control of normal and transformed cells. J. Supramol. Struct. *11*:529, 1979.
50. Allen, T.D., and Iype, P.T.: Ultrastructural morphology of three-dimensional colonies of cells derived from a hepatocellular carcinoma. J. Cancer Res. Clin. Oncol. *95*:225, 1979.
51. Mitelman, F., and Levan, G.: Clustering of aberrations to specific chromosomes in human neoplasms. IV. A survey of 1871 cases. Hereditas *95*:79, 1981.
52. Yunis, J.J.: The chromosomal basis of neoplasia. Science *221*:227, 1983.
53. Rowley, J.: Identification of the constant chromosome regions involved in human hematologic malignant disease. Science *216*:749, 1982.
54. Yunis, J.J.: Chromosomes and cancer: New nomenclature and future directions. Hum. Pathol. *12*:494, 1981.
55. Rowley, J.D.: Chromosome abnormalities in human leukemia. Annu. Rev. Genet. *14*:17, 1980.
56. Rowley, J.D.: Ph[1]-positive leukaemia including chronic myelogenous leukaemia. Clin. Haematol. *9*:54, 1980.
57. Klein, G.: The relative role of vital transformation and specific cytogenic changes in the development of murine and human lymphomas. Haematol. Blood Transfus. *26*:3, 1981.
58. Sandberg, A.A., et al.: Chromosomes and causation of human cancer and leukemia. XLII. Ph[1]-positive ALL: An entity within myeloproliferative disorders? Cancer Genet. Cytogenet. *2*:145, 1980.
59. Damjanov, I., and Knowles, B.B.: Biology of disease: Monoclonal antibodies and tumor-associated antigens. Lab. Invest. *48*:510, 1983.
60. Old, L.J., and Stockert, E.: Immunogenetics of cell surface antigens of mouse leukemia. Annu. Rev. Genet. *11*:127, 1977.
61. Embleton, M.J., and Baldwin, R.W.: Antigenic changes in chemical carcinogenesis. Br. Med. Bull. *36*:83, 1980.
62. Law, L.W., et al.: Tumor antigens on neoplasms induced by chemical carcinogens and by DNA- and RNA-containing viruses: Properties of the solubilized antigens. Adv. Cancer Res. *32*:201, 1980.
63. Old, L.J.: Cancer immunology: The search for specificity. GHA Clowes Memorial Lecture. Cancer Res. *41*:361, 1981.
64. Abelev, G.I.: Alpha-fetoprotein in ontogenesis and its association with malignant tumors. Adv. Cancer Res. *14*:295, 1971.
65. Gold, P., and Freedman, S.O.: Demonstration of tumor-specific antigens in human colonic carcinomata by immunological tolerance and absorption techniques. J. Exp. Med. *121*:439, 1965.
66. Ashall, F., et al.: A new marker for human cancer cells. I. The CA antigen and the Ca_1 antibody. Lancet *2*:1, 1982.
67. McGee, J.O'D., et al.: A new marker for human cancer cells. II. Immunohistochemical detection of the Ca antigen in human tissues with the Ca_1 antibody. Lancet *2*:7, 1982.
68. Ioachim, H.L.: The stromal reaction of tumors: An expression of immune surveillance. J. Natl. Cancer Inst. *57*:465, 1976.
69. Weinhouse, S.: Enzyme activities in tumor progression. In Edsall, J.T. (ed.): Amino Acids, Proteins and Cancer Biochemistry. New York, Academic Press, 1960, p. 109.
70. Coleman, P.S., and Lavietes, B.B.: Membrane cholesterol, tumorigenesis, and the biochemical phenotype of neoplasia. CRC Crit. Rev. Biochem. *11*:341, 1981.
71. Nicolson, G.L.: Transmembrane control of the receptors on normal and tumor cells. II. Surface changes associated with transformation and malignancy. Biochim. Biophys. Acta *458*:1, 1976.
72. Trump, B.F., et al.: Cell surface changes in preneoplastic and neoplastic epithelium. Scan. Electron Microsc. *3*:43, 1980.
73. Black, P.H.: Shedding from normal and cancer-cell surfaces. N. Engl. J. Med. *303*:1415, 1980.
74. Chen, L.B., et al.: Possible role of fibronectin in malignancy. J. Supramol. Struct. *12*:139, 1979.
75. Warren, L., and Buck, C.A.: The membrane glycoproteins of the malignant cell. Clin. Biochem. *13*:191, 1980.
76. Dvorak, H.F., et al.: Induction of a fibrin-gel investment: An early event in line 10 hepatocarcinoma growth mediated by tumor-secreted products. J. Immunol. *122*:166, 1979.
77. Critchley, D.R.: Glycolipids as membrane receptors important in growth regulation. *In* Hynes, R.O. (ed.): Surfaces of Normal and Malignant Cells. New York, John Wiley & Sons, 1979, p. 63.
78. Jesudason, M.L., and Iseri, O.A.: Host-tumor cellular junctions: An ultrastructural study of hepatic metastasis of bronchogenic oat cell carcinoma. Hum. Pathol. *11*:66, 1980.
79. Lowenstein, W.R.: Junctional intercellular communication and the control of growth. Biochim. Biophys. Acta *560*:1, 1979.
80. Roblin, R.: Plasminogen activator production as a possible biological marker for human neoplasia: Some fundamental questions. In Ruddon, R. (ed.): Biological Markers for Neoplasia: Basic and Applied Aspects. New York, Elsevier Press, 1978, p. 421.
81. Graham, J.M.: Surface membrane enzymes in neoplasia. *In* Hynes, R.O. (ed.): Surfaces of Normal and Malignant Cells. New York, John Wiley & Sons, 1979, p. 199.

82. Doll, R., and Peto, R.: The causes of cancer: Quantitative estimates of avoidable risks of cancer in the United States today. J. Natl. Cancer Inst. *66*:1191, 1981.
83. Fisher, P.B., et al.: Interactions between initiating chemical carcinogens, tumor promoters, and adenovirus in cell transformation. Teratogen. Carcinogen. Mutagen. *1*:245, 1980.
84. Weisburger, J.H., and Williams, G.M.: Metabolism of chemical carcinogens. *In* Becker, F.F. (ed.): Cancer, A Comprehensive Treatise. Vol. 1. New York, Plenum Press, 1982, p. 241.
85. Miller, E.C.: Some current perspectives on chemicals in humans and experimental animals: Presidential address. Cancer Res. *38*:1479, 1978.
86. Harris, C.C.: A delayed complication of cancer therapy—cancer. J. Natl. Cancer Inst. *63*:275, 1979.
87. Reimer, R.R., et al.: Acute leukemia after alkylating-agent therapy of ovarian cancer. N. Engl. J. Med. *297*:177, 1977.
88. Rosner, F.: Acute leukemia as a delayed consequence of cancer chemotherapy. Cancer *37*:1033, 1976.
89. Bergsagel, D.E., et al.: The chemotherapy of plasma cell myeloma and the incidence of acute leukemia. N. Engl. J. Med. *301*:743, 1979.
90. Sims, P.: The metabolic activation of chemical carcinogens. Br. Med. Bull. *36*:11, 1980.
91. White, R.E., and Coon, M.J.: Oxygen activation by cytochrome P-450. Annu. Rev. Biochem. *4*:315, 1980.
92. Miller, E.C., and Miller, J.A.: Mechanisms of chemical carcinogenesis. Cancer *47*:1055, 1981.
93. Sugimura, T., et al.: Activation of chemicals to proximal carcinogens. Dev. Toxicol. Environ. Sci. *8*:205, 1980.
94. Kleinfeld, M., et al.: Bladder tumors in a coal tar dye plant. Ind. Med. Surg. *35*:570, 1966.
95. Miller, J.A., and Miller, E.C.: Carcinogens occurring naturally in foods. Fed. Proc. *35*:1360, 1976.
96. Peers, F.G., et al.: Dietary aflatoxins and human liver cancer. A study in Swaziland. Int. J. Cancer *17*:167, 1976.
97. Sumithran, E., and MacSween, R.N.M.: An appraisal of the relationship between primary hepatocellular carcinoma and hepatitis B virus. Histol. Pathol.. *3*:447, 1979.
98. Selikoff, I.J., et al.: Asbestos exposure, smoking and neoplasia. J.A.M.A. *204*:106, 1968.
99. Waxweiler, R.J., et al.: Neoplastic risk among workers exposed to vinyl chloride. Ann. N.Y. Acad. Sci. *271*:40, 1976.
100. Wattenburg, L.W.: Inhibitors of chemical carcinogenesis. Adv. Cancer Res. *26*:197, 1978.
101. Farber, E.: Chemical carcinogens. N. Engl. J. Med. *305*:1379, 1981.
102. Iversen, U.M., and Iversen, O.H.: The carcinogenic effect of TPA (12-O-tetradecanoylphorbol-13-acetate) when applied to the skin of hairless mice. Virchows Arch. B *30*:33, 1979.
103. Van Duuren, B.L., et al.: Effect of aging in two-stage carcinogenesis on mouse skin with phorbol myristate acetate as promoting agent. Cancer Res. *38*:865, 1978.
104. Blumberg, P.M.: In vitro studies on the mode of action of phorbol esters, potent tumor promoters. CRC Crit. Rev. Toxicol. *8*:153, 1980.
105. Pitot, H.C., et al.: The natural history of carcinogenesis: Implications of experimental carcinogenesis in the genesis of human cancer. J. Supramol. Struct. Cell Biochem. *16*:133, 1981.
106. Pitot, H.C.: Drugs as promoters of carcinogenesis. *In* Estabrook, R.W., and Lindenlaub, E. (eds.): The Induction of Drug Metabolism. Stuttgart-New York, Schattauer Verlag, 1979, p. 471.
107. Cohen, S.M., et al.: Promoting effect of saccharin and DL-tryptophan in urinary bladder carcinogenesis. Cancer Res. *39*:1207, 1979.
108. Pitot, H.C., et al.: Quantitative evaluation of the promoting by 2,3,7,8-tetrachlorodibenzo-p-dioxin of hepatocarcinogenesis from diethylnitrosamine. Cancer Res. *40*:3616, 1980.
109. Chan, G.L.: On the nature of oncogenic transformation of cells. Int. Rev. Cytol. *70*:101, 1981.
110. Weinstein, I.D.: Current concepts and controversies in chemical carcinogenesis. J. Supramol. Struct. Cell Biochem. *17*:99, 1981.
111. Shih, L., et al.: Passage of phenotypes of chemically transformed cells via transfection of DNA and chromatin. Proc. Natl. Acad. Sci. U.S.A. *76*:5714, 1979.
112. Straus, D.S.: Somatic mutation, cellular differentiation, and cancer causation. J. Natl. Cancer Inst. *67*:233, 1981.
113. Ames, D.N.: Identifying environmental chemicals causing mutations in cancer. Science *204*:587, 1979.
114. Rinkus, S.J., and Lagator, M.S.: Chemical characterization of 465 known or suspected carcinogens and their correlation with mutagenic activity in the *Salmonella typhimurium* system. Cancer Res. *39*:3289, 1979.
115. Columbano, A., et al.: Requirement of cell proliferation for the initiation of liver carcinogenesis as assayed by three different procedures. Cancer Res. *41*:2079, 1981.
116. Farber, E., and Cameron, R.: The sequential analysis of cancer development. Adv. Cancer Res. *31*:125, 1980.
117. Storer, J.B.: Radiation carcinogenesis. *In* Becker, F.F. (ed.): Cancer: A Comprehensive Treatise. New York, Plenum Press, 1982, p. 629.
118. Upton, A.C.: Physical carcinogenesis: Radiation-history and sources. In Becker, F.F. (ed.): Cancer: A Comprehensive Treatise. New York, Plenum Press, 1982, p. 551.
119. Takanaga, M., et al.: Breast cancer in Japanese A-bomb survivors. Lancet *2*:924, 1982.
120. Urbach, F.: Ultraviolet radiation: Interaction with biological molecules. *In* Becker, F.F. (ed.): Cancer: A Comprehensive Treatise. New York, Plenum Press, 1982, p. 617.
121. Viola, M.V., and Houghton, A.N.: Solar radiation and cutaneous melanoma. Hosp. Pract. *17*:97, 1982.
122. Kripke, M.L.: Immunological mechanisms in UV radiation carcinogenesis. Adv. Cancer Res. *34*:69, 1981.
123. Fisher, M.S., and Kripke, M.L.: Suppressor T lympho-control. The development of primary skin cancers in ultraviolet irradiated mice. Science *216*:1133, 1982.
124. Cleaver, J.E., and Bootsma, D.: Xeroderma pigmentosum. Biochemical and genetic characteristics. Annu. Rev. Genet. *9*:19, 1975.
125. Bootsma, D.: Xeroderma pigmentosum. *In* Hanawalt, P.C., Friedberg, E. C., and Fox, C.F. (eds.): DNA Repair Mechanisms. New York, Academic Press, 1978, p. 589.
126. Cairns, J.: The origins of cancer. Nature *289*:353, 1981.
127. Setlow, R.B.: Repair deficient human disorders and cancer. Nature *271*:713, 1978.
128. Remsen, J.F., and Cerutti, P.A.: Deficiency of gamma-ray excision repair in skin fibroblasts from patients with Fanconi's anemia. Proc. Natl. Acad. Sci. U.S.A. *73*:2419, 1976.
129. German, J., et al.: Bloom's syndrome. V. Surveillance for cancer in affected families. Clin. Genet. *12*:162, 1977.
130. Boice, J.D.: Cancer following medical irradiation. Cancer (Suppl.) *47*:1081, 1981.
131. Court-Brown, W.M., and Doll, R.: Mortality from cancer and other causes after radiotherapy for ankylosing spondylitis. Br. Med. J. *2*:1327, 1965.
132. Hutchison, G.B.: Leukemia in patients with cancer of the cervix uteri treated with radiation. A report covering the first five years of an international study. J. Natl. Cancer Inst. *40*:951, 1968.
133. Favus, M.J., et al.: Thyroid cancer occurring as a late consequence of head and neck irradiation: Evaluation of 1056 patients. N. Engl. J. Med. *294*:1019, 1976.
134. Evans, R.D., et al.: Radiogenic tumors in the radium and mesothorium cases studied at M.I.T. *In* Mays, C.W., et al. (eds.): Delayed Effects of Bone-Seeking Radionuclides. Salt Lake City, University of Utah Press, 1969, p. 157.
135. Report of the United Nations Scientific Committee on the Effect of Atomic Radiation: Official Records of the General Assembly, 20-7 Session, Ionizing Radiation Levels and Effects, Vol. II. Suppl. 25. (A.8725). New York, United Nations, 1972.
136. Hirohata, T.: Radiation carcinogenesis. Semin. Oncol. *3*:25, 1976.
137. Bittner, J.J.: Some possible effects of nursing on the mammary gland tumor incidence in mice. Science *84*:162, 1936.
138. Gallo, R.C., and Wong-Staal, F.: Retroviruses as etiologic agents of some animal and human leukemias and lymphomas and as tools for elucidating the molecular mechanisms of leukemogenesis. Blood *60*:545, 1982.
139. Kadin, M.E., and Kamoun, M.: Nonendemic adult T-cell leukemia/lymphoma. Hum. Pathol. *13*:691, 1982.
140. Catovsky, D., et al.: Adult T-cell lymphoma-leukaemia in blacks from the West Indies. Lancet *1*:639, 1982.
141. Editorial: Human papillomaviruses and neoplasia. Lancet *2*:435, 1983.
142. Mortimer, E.A., Jr., et al.: Long-term follow-up of persons inadvertently inoculated with SV40 as neonates. N. Engl. J. Med. *305*:1517, 1918.
143. Howley, P.M.: DNA sequences of human papovavirus BK. Nature *284*:124, 1980.
144. Epstein, M.A., and Achong, B.G.: The relationship of the virus to Burkitt's lymphoma. *In* Epstein, M.A., and Achong, B.G. (eds.): The Epstein-Barr Virus. Berlin, Springer-Verlag, 1979, p. 331.
145. Klein, G.: The relationship of the virus to nasopharyngeal carcinoma. *In* Epstein, M.A., and Achong, B.G. (eds.): The Epstein-Barr Virus. Berlin, Springer-Verlag, 1979, p. 339.
146. Editorial: New clinical manifestations of Epstein-Barr virus infection. Lancet *2*:1253, 1982.
147. Klein, G.: The role of gene dosage and genetic transpositions in carcinogenesis. Nature *294*:313, 1981.
148. Lenoir, G.M., et al.: Correlation between immunoglobulin light chain expression and variant translocation in Burkitt's lymphoma. Nature *293*:474, 1982.
148A. Editorial: Acquired immunodeficiency syndrome. Lancet *1*:161, 1983.
149. Ziegler, J.L., et al.: Outbreak of Burkitt's-like lymphoma in homosexual men. Lancet *2*:631, 1982.
150. Koziner, B., et al.: Opportunistic infections and Kaposi's sarcoma in homosexual men. N. Engl. J. Med. *306*:933, 1982.
151. Drew, W.L.: Cytomegalovirus and Kaposi's sarcoma. Lancet *2*:125, 1982.
152. McDougall, J.K., et al.: Cervical carcinoma: Detection of herpes simplex

virus RVA in cells undergoing neoplastic change. Int. J. Cancer *25*:1, 1980.

153. Wyke, J.A.: Oncogenic viruses. J. Pathol. *135*:39, 1981.
154. Wong-Staal, F., et al.: Three distinct genes in human DNA related to the transforming genes of mammalian sarcoma retroviruses. Science *213*:226, 1981.
155. Bishop, J.M.: Enemies within: The genesis of retrovirus oncogenes. Cell *23*:5, 1981.
156. Weinberg, R.A.: Alteration of the genomes of tumor cells. Cancer *52*:1971, 1983.
157. Hamlyn, P., and Sikora, K.: Oncogenes. Lancet *2*:326, 1983.
158. Hunter, T.: Protein phosphorylated by the RSV transforming function. Cell *22*:647, 1980.
159. Huebner, R.J., et al.: Specific adenovirus complement-fixing antigens in virus-free hamster and rat tumors, with preliminary observations on similar antigen in other virus-induced tumors. Proc. Natl. Acad. Sci. U.S.A. *50*:379, 1963.
160. Crawford, L.V.: Transforming genes of DNA tumor viruses. Cold Spring Harbor Symp. Quant. Biol. *44*:9, 1980.
161. Dippold, W.G., et al.: p53 transformation-related protein: Detection by monoclonal antibody in mouse and human cells. Proc. Natl. Acad. Sci. U.S.A. *78*:1695, 1981.
162. Rotter, V., et al.: Abelson murine leukemia virus-induced tumors elicit antibodies against a host cell protein, p50. J. Virol. *36*:547, 1980.
163. Schaffhausen, B.S., et al.: Phosphorylation of polyoma T antigens. Cell *18*:935, 1979.
164. Israel, M.A., et al.: Interrupting the early region of polyoma virus DNA enhances tumorigenicity. Proc. Natl. Acad. Sci. U.S.A. *76*:3713, 1979.
165. Croce, C.M.: Integration of oncogenic viruses in mammalian cells. Int. Rev. Cytol. *71*:1, 1981.
166. Brand, K.G.: Cancer associated with asbestosis, schistosomiasis, foreign bodies and scars. *In* Becker, F.F. (ed.): Cancer: A Comprehensive Treatise. New York, Plenum Press, 1982, p. 661.
166A. Mossman, B.T., and Craighead, J.E.: Mechanisms of asbestos carcinogenicity. Environ. Res. *25*:269, 1981.
167. Eisebai, I.: Parasites in the etiology of cancer-bilharziasis and bladder cancer. CA *27*:100, 1977.
168. Auerbach, O., et al.: Scar cancer of the lung. Increase over a 21-year period. Cancer *43*:636, 1979.
169. Karp, R.D., et al.: Tumorigenesis by Millipore filters in mice: Histology and ultrastructure of tissue reactions as related to pore size. J. Natl. Cancer Inst. *51*:1275, 1973.
170. Neel, B.G., et al.: Avian leukosis virus-induced tumors have common proviral integration sites and synthesize discrete new RNAs: Oncogenesis by promoter insertion. Cell *23*:323, 1981.
171. Cooper, G.M., et al.: Transforming activity of DNA of chemically-transformed and normal cells. Nature (Lond.) *284*:418, 1980.
172. Rigby, P.W.: The detection of cellular transforming genes (news). Nature *290*:186, 1981.
173. Mintz, B., and Fleischman, R.A.: Teratocarcinomas and other neoplasms as developmental defects in gene expression. Adv. Cancer Res. *34*:211, 1981.
174. Rheinwald, J.G., and Green, H.: Formation of a keratinizing epithelium in culture by a cloned cell line derived from a teratoma. Cell *6*:317, 1975.
175. Illmensee, K., and Mintz, B.: Totipotency and normal differentiation of single teratocarcinoma cells cloned by injection into blastocysts. Proc. Natl. Acad. Sci. U.S.A. *73*:549, 1976.
176. Tobin, C.T., et al.: Mechanism of activation of a human oncogene. Nature *300*:143, 1982.
177. Reddy, E.P., et al.: A point mutation is responsible for the acquisition of transforming properties by the T24 human bladder carcinoma oncogenes. Nature *300*:149, 1982.
178. Pacifici, M., et al.: Transformation of chondroblasts by Rous sarcoma virus and synthesis of the sulphated proteoglycan. Cell *11*:891, 1977.
179. Stanbridge, E.J., et al.: Human cell hybrids: Analysis of transformation and tumorigenicity. Science *215*:252, 1982.
180. Wiener, F., et al.: Chromosome 15 trisomy in spontaneous and carcinogen-induced murine lymphomas of B-cell origin. Int. J. Cancer *27*:51, 1981.
181. Spira, J., et al.: Chromosomal, histopathological and cell surface marker studies on Moloney virus induced lymphomas. Leuk. Res. *5*:113, 1981.
182. Wiener, F., et al.: Non-random duplication of chromosome 15 in murine T-cell leukemias: Further studies on translocation heterozygotes. Int. J. Cancer *26*:661, 1980.
183. Manolova, Y., et al.: The same marker chromosome, mar17p+, in four consecutive cases of multiple myeloma. Hereditas *90*:307, 1979.
184. Mitelman, F.: Marker chromosome 14q+ in human cancer and leukemia. Adv. Cancer Res. *34*:141, 1981.
185. Braun, A.C.: An epigenetic model for the origin of cancer. Q. Rev. Biol. *56*:33, 1981.
186. Segaloff, A.: Steroids and carcinogenesis. J. Steroid Biochem. *6*:171, 1975.
187. Dyke, P.C., and Mulkey, D.A.: Maturation of ganglioneuroblastoma to ganglioneuroma. Cancer *20*:1343, 1967.
188. Kimhi, Y.C., et al.: Maturation of neuroblastoma cells in the presence of dimethyl sulfoxide. Proc. Natl. Acad. Sci. U.S.A. *73*:462, 1976.
189. Purtilo, D.T.: Malignant lymphoproliferative diseases induced by Epstein-Barr virus in immunodeficient patients, including X-linked cytogenetic and familial syndromes. Cancer Genet. Cytogenet. *4*:251, 1981.
190. Purtilo, D.T.: Immune deficiency predisposing to Epstein-Barr virus-induced lymphoproliferative diseases: The X-linked lymphoproliferative syndrome as a model. Adv. Cancer Res *34*:279, 1981.

CLINICAL ASPECTS OF NEOPLASIA 7

The ultimate importance of neoplasms is their effect on their hosts. This chapter is concerned with certain general clinical aspects of neoplasia in humans and some of the specific neoplasms that arise in supporting tissues (e.g., connective tissue, fat, and muscle) common to all organs. The three general areas of clinical importance are (1) the interactions between tumor and host, (2) the factors involved in predisposition to neoplasia, and (3) the diagnosis of neoplasia in the clinical and laboratory setting.

TUMOR-HOST INTERACTIONS

Neoplasms are essentially parasites. Some cause only trivial mischief but others are catastrophic. Tumor-host interactions are, however, a two-way street, and the host impinges on the tumor as well. First we shall consider the effects of the tumor on the host, and then the converse.

EFFECTS OF TUMOR ON HOST

All neoplasms, even those that are benign, may induce morbidity and mortality. Obviously, cancers are far more threatening but benign tumors are not necessarily trivial. Save for the in situ stage of cancers, all neoplasms, benign as well as malignant, constitute masses, and every abnormal mass requires investigation to determine its nature. This issue comes into sharpest focus with masses in the female breast. Carcinoma of the breast is the most frequent form of cancer in females, but even more common are a variety of non-neoplastic lesions, collectively referred to as fibrocystic disease, that often present as a mass or more often as multiple, even bilateral, masses. Although clinical examination (palpation, mammography, aspiration of a cyst) permits an educated guess as to the nature of the disease, and although cancer is usually a single mass, only morphologic examination of a biopsy or of the excised lesion reliably differentiates the benign from the cancer. Innumerable other difficult differentials could be cited, e.g., polypoid lesions of the colon and papillary lesions of the bladder, but it is sufficient to note that any growth may be a cancer until proved otherwise. Clinical experience teaches that some lesions are less worrisome than others. Soft, discrete, subcutaneous lipomas and small, discrete, hemangiomas of the skin, for example, are commonplace and almost never transform to cancers; they do not signal immediate surgery. Leiomyomas of the uterus are the most common form of benign neoplasia in females, typically presenting as spherical masses readily palpable on pelvic examination that enlarge very slowly over the span of many years, and sometimes plateau in growth after achieving a certain size. In contrast, the leiomyosarcoma is rare and generally increases in size within a relatively short period of observation (months). On these grounds, static or virtually static uterine masses are sometimes managed by "watchful waiting" if they cause no other clinical problems such as pelvic discomfort or vaginal bleeding. However, leiomyosarcomas make up about 3% of uterine cancers (dominated by cervical and endometrial carcinomas), and many leiomyosarcomas arise in leiomyomas. The patient is not a statistic; the most benign neoplasm, wherever it occurs, is the excised one.

LOCAL AND HORMONAL EFFECTS. Neoplasms, both benign and malignant, may have adverse effects on the host because they (1) obstruct or destroy critical structures by virtue of their location, (2) have functional activity such as hormone production, (3) cause bleeding, (4) ulcerate through natural surfaces leading to secondary infections, and (5) become infarcted. Any one of these consequences may prove fatal even when induced by benign tumors. Understandably, the potential for such adverse effects is much greater with malignant neoplasms, and indeed may be caused by any one or more of their metastases. In addition, *cancers often induce cachexia and sometimes so-called "paraneoplastic syndromes,"* both discussed later. An example of disease related to critical location is the pituitary adenoma. Although this is benign and possibly not productive of hormone, its expansile growth can destroy the remaining pituitary and thus lead to serious endocrinopathy. Analogously, cancers arising within or metastatic to an endocrine gland may cause an endocrine insufficiency by destroying the gland. Neoplasms in the gut, both benign and malignant, may cause obstruction as they enlarge. Infrequently, the peristaltic pull telescopes the neoplasm and its affected segment into the downstream segment, producing an obstructing intussusception (p.

852). Neoplasms arising in endocrine glands may produce manifestations by elaboration of hormones. Such functional activity is more typical of benign tumors than cancers, which may be sufficiently undifferentiated to have lost such capability. A benign beta-cell adenoma of the pancreatic islets less than 1 cm in diameter may produce sufficient insulin to cause fatal hypoglycemia. In addition, nonendocrine tumors may elaborate hormones or hormone-like products. The erosive destructive growth of cancers and the expansile pressure of a benign tumor on any natural surface, such as the skin or mucosa of the gut, may cause ulcerations, secondary infections, and bleeding. Indeed, melena (blood in the stool) and hematuria, for example, are characteristic of neoplasms of the gut and urinary tract, respectively. Neoplasms may cause disease in unusual ways. A mobile organ bearing a large tumor may, in some unknown manner, undergo torsion, thereby cutting off the venous drainage and sometimes also the arterial supply (Fig. 7–1). This complication most often occurs with benign ovarian neoplasms that become infarcted, and so cause acute lower abdominal pain and sometimes bleeding into the peritoneal cavity. Neoplasms, benign as well as malignant, may then cause problems in varied ways, but all are far less common than the cachexia of malignancy.

CACHEXIA. *Cachexia refers to the constellation of progressive weakness, malaise, loss of appetite, and wasting, which is so very common in the terminal stages of cancer.* Usually, but not always, there is a direct correlation between the size and extent of spread of the malignant tumor and the severity of the cachexia, and so it becomes more profound as the disease advances. On occasion, however, it becomes manifest with remarkably small primary lesions. Commonplace as it is, cachexia is still poorly understood.[1] It probably is not caused by the nutritional demands of the tumor. Cancers never grow as rapidly as the fetus, yet many a postpartal mother when getting on the scale laments that she did not suffer just a little bit of "cachexia." One theory proposes that cancers release peptides or other factors into the serum that derange the nutritional homeostasis of the host,[2] but if such products are present they have not been well documented. A peripheral resistance to insulin not related to a reduction in membrane receptors has also been described.[3] Thus, the cachexia of cancer is likened to the catabolic state of uncontrolled diabetes mellitus. Alternatively, it may well be secondary to a decrease in nutritional intake related to anxiety, grief, and depression only too natural in the mortally ill patient. In some instances it could be related to the anatomic location of the neoplasm and its metastases, or to the systemic and gastrointestinal effects of anticancer therapy.[4] In addition, infections are common in persons with advanced cancer because of impaired immune responses, which may contribute to the general catabolic state. Thus, it is likely that cancerous cachexia, although poorly understood, has many origins, one or more of which may be dominant in the individual patient.

PARANEOPLASTIC SYNDROMES. Symptom complexes in cancer-bearing patients that cannot readily be explained, either by the local or distant spread of the tumor or by the elaboration of hormones indigenous to the tissue from which the tumor arose, are known as *paraneoplastic syndromes.*[5] These occur in about 15% of patients with advanced malignant disease. However, paraneoplastic syndromes occasionally appear as the first

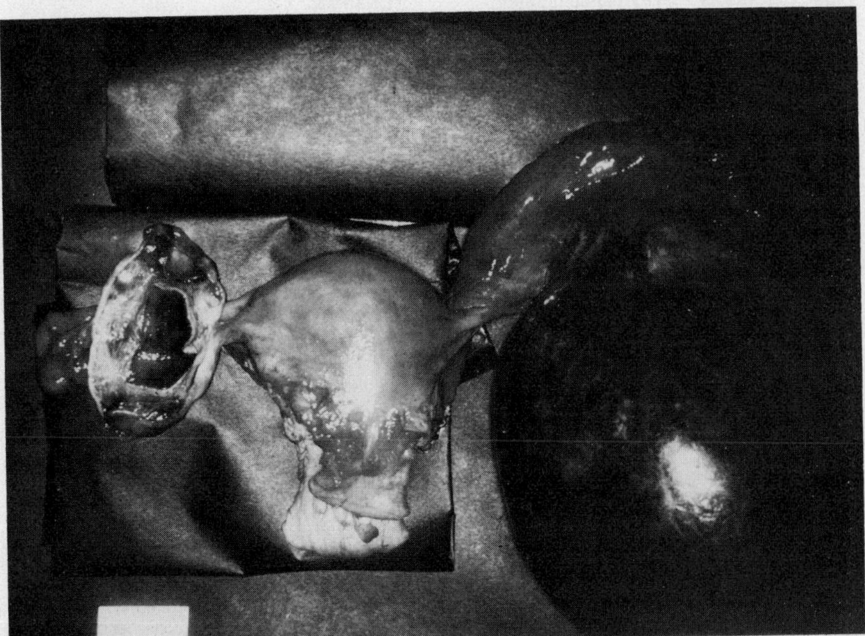

Figure 7–1. Torsion of a large, benign ovarian tumor *(right)* that has induced hemorrhagic infarction of the neoplasm. Compare the size of this tumor with the normal uterus and essentially normal hemisected ovary on the left. (Courtesy of Dr. Robert L. Ehrmann, Brigham and Women's Hospital.)

manifestation of an occult, extremely small neoplasm.[6] A classification of paraneoplastic syndromes and their presumed origins is presented in Table 7–1. A few comments on some of the more common and interesting syndromes follow.

The *endocrinopathies* are frequently encountered paraneoplastic syndromes. Since the native cells giving rise to the cancer are not of endocrine origin, the functional activity is referred to as *ectopic hormone production*. In some instances the elaboration of the hormone or hormone-like substance is attributed to derepression of hidden genetic programs, as, for example, the formation of insulin by fibrosarcomas (usually retroperitoneal) or erythropoietin by renal cell carcinomas. In many instances the neoplasms giving rise to the paraneoplastic endocrinopathies take their origin from specialized neurosecretory cells widely distributed in the tissues and organs of the body during embryogenesis. These cells have the capacity for *a*mine *p*recursor *u*ptake and *d*ecarboxylation, and so are called APUD cells. They are thus able to synthesize a variety of amine and polypeptide hormones, discussed in some detail on page 842. Morphologic and histochemical studies indicate that oat cell carcinomas of the lung, bronchial adenomas, undifferentiated carcinomas of the gastrointestinal tract and pancreas, thyroid medullary carcinomas, pancreatic islet tumors, and carcinoids of the gastrointestinal tract are derived from APUD cells, and

Table 7–1. PARANEOPLASTIC SYNDROMES

Clinical Syndrome	Major Forms of Underlying Cancer	Causal Mechanism
Endocrinopathies		
Cushing's syndrome	Bronchogenic carcinoma Malignant thymoma Pancreatic carcinoma	Adrenocorticotropin or ACTH-like substance
Hyponatremia	Bronchogenic carcinoma Intracranial neoplasms	Antidiuretic hormone or ADH-like substance
Hypercalcemia	Bronchogenic oat cell carcinoma Bronchogenic squamous carcinoma Renal carcinoma Endometrial carcinoma Others	Parathormone or PTH-like substance, prostaglandins
Hyperthyroidism	Blood dyscrasias Bronchogenic carcinoma Prostatic carcinoma	Thyroid-stimulating hormone or TSH-like substance
Hypoglycemia	Fibrosarcoma Other mesenchymal sarcomas Hepatocellular carcinoma	Insulin or insulin-like substance
Carcinoid syndrome	Argentaffinomas Bronchial adenoma (carcinoid) Pancreatic carcinoma Gastric carcinoma	Serotonin, bradykinin, ?histamine ?prostaglandins
Polycythemia	Renal carcinoma Cerebellar hemangioma Hepatocellular carcinoma	Erythropoietin
Nerve and Muscle Syndromes		
Myasthenia Disorders of central and peripheral nervous systems	Bronchogenic carcinoma Breast carcinoma Ovarian carcinoma	?Immunologic, ?toxic
Dermatologic Disorders		
Acanthosis nigricans	Gastric carcinoma Lung carcinoma Uterine carcinoma	?Immunologic, ?toxic
Dermatomyositis	Bronchogenic, breast carcinoma	?Immunologic, ?toxic
Osseous, Articular, and Soft Tissue Changes		
Hypertrophic osteoarthropathy and clubbing of fingers	Bronchogenic carcinoma	Unknown
Vascular and Hematologic Changes		
Venous thrombosis (Trousseau's phenomenon)	Pancreatic carcinoma Bronchogenic carcinoma Other cancers	?Hypercoagulability—procoagulant factors
Disseminated intravascular coagulation	Advanced cancers	?Hypercoagulability
Marantic endocarditis (nonbacterial thrombotic vegetations)	Advanced cancers	?Hypercoagulability
Anemia	Thymic neoplasms	Unknown
Leukemoid reaction	Thymic neoplasms Bronchogenic carcinoma Gastric carcinoma	Unknown
Renal Dysfunction		
Insufficiency	Leukemia/lymphoma Multiple myeloma	Various
Nephrotic syndrome	Lung carcinoma Stomach carcinoma Colon carcinoma	?Tumor antigens—immune complexes

so the neoplasms are *APUDomas.* Herein may lie the explanation for the elaboration of amine and polypeptide hormones or closely related substances by many of the tumors commonly associated with paraneoplastic syndromes.[7]

Hypercalcemia is probably the most common paraneoplastic syndrome, and conversely overtly symptomatic hypercalcemia is most often related to some form of cancer rather than hyperparathyroidism. Two general processes are involved in cancer-associated hypercalcemia: (1) osteolysis induced by cancer whether primary in bone, such as multiple myeloma, or metastatic to bone from any primary; and (2) the production of a calcemic humoral substance by extraosseous neoplasms.[8] The nature of the calcium-mobilizing tumor product is still uncertain. At one time it was thought to be usually parathyroid hormone or a functionally active fragment of the hormone.[9] However, measurable levels of these products in the serum are often lacking or extremely low in patients with cancer-related hypercalcemia.[10] More recently prostaglandin E (PGE) has become the favored candidate.[11] The commonest neoplasm associated with hypercalcemia and PG synthesis is the squamous cell bronchogenic carcinoma, rather than undifferentiated (oat cell) cancers of the lung (more often associated with well-defined endocrinopathies).

The *neuromyopathic paraneoplastic syndromes* take diverse forms, such as peripheral neuropathies, cortical cerebellar degeneration, a polymyopathy resembling to some extent polymyositis (p. 193), and a myasthenic syndrome similar to *myasthenia gravis* (p. 1310). The etiology of these syndromes is poorly understood, and both immunologic reactions to necrotic tumor cells that cross-react with target tissues and toxic products released by the neoplasm have been vaguely proposed.[12]

Acanthosis nigricans is characterized by gray-black patches of verrucous hyperkeratosis on the skin (p. 1274). This disorder occurs very rarely as a genetically determined disease in juveniles or adults. In addition, particularly in those over the age of 35, the appearance of such lesions is associated in about 50% of cases with some form of cancer. Sometimes the skin changes appear before discovery of the cancer. It is important to remember, however, that in the remaining nongenetic cases there is no underlying cancer, but some endocrinopathy or in fact no associated disease.

Clubbing of fingers and hypertrophic osteoarthropathy, described more fully on page 1333, are encountered in 1 to 10% of patients with bronchogenic carcinomas. Rarely, other forms of cancer are involved. Although the osteoarthropathy is seldom seen in noncancer patients, clubbing of the fingertips may be encountered in liver diseases, diffuse lung disease, congenital cyanotic heart disease, ulcerative colitis, and other disorders.

Several *vascular and hematologic manifestations* may appear in association with a variety of forms of cancer. As mentioned in the earlier discussion of thrombosis (p. 98), *migratory thrombophlebitis* (Trousseau's syndrome) may be encountered in association with deep-seated cancers, most often with carcinomas of the pancreas or lung. Disseminated intravascular coagulation (DIC) may complicate a diversity of clinical disorders, as pointed out on page 649. Among these is advanced cancer. In this setting, hypercoagulability is postulated, attributed to the synthesis and/or release of platelet-aggregating factors and procoagulants (p. 98) from the tumor or its necrotic products. Bland, small, nonbacterial fibrinous vegetations sometimes form on the cardiac valve leaflets (more often on left-sided valves than on right), particularly in patients with advanced cancer (Fig. 7–2). These lesions are called *nonbacterial thrombotic endocarditis (NBTE) or marantic (derived from marasmus) endocarditis.* As the term marantic endocarditis indicates, these valvular vegetations are most often associated with the terminal phase of wasting disease. However, NBTE sometimes occurs in nonwasted, occasionally young individuals who do not have cancer; this is discussed in more detail on page 584. Whatever the setting, the vegetations are potential sources of emboli that assume increased importance in the young nonterminal patient.

Renal dysfunction is occasionally encountered in patients with advanced cancer. Often it takes the form of nonspecific renal insufficiency caused by direct infiltration of the kidneys by such neoplasms as lymphoma and leukemia or by cancerous obstruction of the ureters, or it occurs as a secondary consequence of hypercalcemia, DIC, or systemic amyloidosis. More intriguing is the appearance of the nephrotic syndrome in association with membranous glomerulopathy (p. 1012). Distinctive in the glomerular membranous involvement is the deposition of immune complexes, and in the cancer setting the inciting antigens appear to be the fetal antigens and other tumor-associated antigens described in Chapter 6.[13] The nephrotic syndrome has occurred with a wide variety of forms of cancer, but is particularly associated with those of the lung, stomach, and colon.

The paraneoplastic syndromes sometimes provide important diagnostic clues to as yet undiscovered cancers, and at other times cause serious, even lethal, disease.

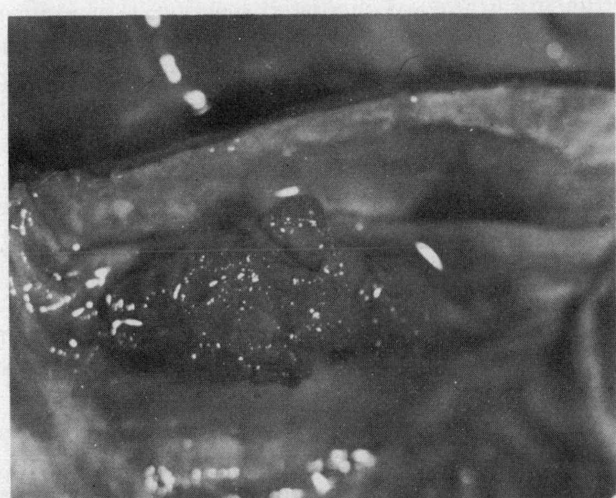

Figure 7–2. A small, protruding marantic vegetation on the aortic valve.

EFFECTS OF HOST ON TUMOR

Host influences impact on the tumor, but unfortunately are usually outweighed by the effects of the tumor on the host. It has been suggested that the nutrition of the host modifies tumor growth. Dietary restriction, at least in the animal, impedes tumor growth[14] and it has been speculated that the cachexia of malignancy represents a "last-ditch defense." However, there is no evidence that tumors can be deprived of critical substrates by any diet that will not simultaneously kill the host. On the contrary, there is some evidence, albeit still controversial, that a deficiency of vitamin A and its analogs (retinoids) may promote tumor formation in both animals and humans and conversely that the administration of retinoids may control some cancers (p. 405).[15] Certain malignant neoplasms, notably some carcinomas of the female breast and the prostate, have steroid hormone dependence, and so can sometimes be controlled for variable periods of time by measures that reduce or oppose the circulating levels of steroid hormones. Hence, tamoxifen, an antiestrogenic agent, is sometimes used in conjunction with surgery or radiation in the treatment of breast carcinoma, and estrogens in prostatic carcinoma to oppose endogenous androgens. Thus, neoplasms are not totally autonomous. Even more important, however, is the question whether the immune system of the host exerts a controlling or a protective influence.

THE IMMUNE RESPONSE AND IMMUNOSURVEILLANCE. Consideration of the role of host immunity in the possible prevention or control of neoplasms requires an examination of some of the experimental data as well as the evidence in humans. Most, but not all, experimentally induced tumors express tumor-specific transplantation antigens (TSTAs), and all tumors have nonspecific, tumor-associated antigens. These antigens evoke immune reactions effected largely by cell-mediated immunity, but humoral mechanisms also participate. Immune reactions and their mediators in general are extensively discussed on page 158; it is necessary here only to briefly characterize the mediators of antitumor reactions. Four basic categories of effector cells participate in the cell-mediated reaction: (1) *specifically sensitized cytolytic T (thymus-dependent) lymphocytes* that recognize on contact membrane-associated tumor antigens; (2) *killer (K) cells* possessing F_c receptors that recognize antibody-coated tumor cells and destroy them by antibody-dependent cellular cytotoxicity (ADCC); (3) *macrophages* specifically armed to destroy tumor cells by a lymphokine "macrophage arming factor" elaborated by sensitized T cells. In addition to this specific macrophage reactivity, nonspecific activation of macrophages can be effected by a variety of immunostimulants including BCG (bacille Calmette Guérin), *Corynebacterium parvum*, levamisole, and endotoxin; and (4) *natural killer (NK)* cells capable of destroying tumor cells without specific sensitization.

In passing, it might be noted that interferons contribute to these cell-mediated reactions. Although the details are unclear, stimulation of ADCC and enhanced macrophage and NK-cell activity are produced by interferon. Humoral antibodies also participate in the immune response to experimentally evoked neoplasms. By activation of complement, they may lyse target tumor cells or, by coating target cells, potentiate ADCC. Thus, it is possible in tumor-bearing animals to document the development of antibodies and sensitized immunocompetent cells targeted on the tumor cells and their antigens. Indeed, an animal can be immunized against a tumor by passive transfer of sensitized cells from a tumor-bearing donor. However, Prehn pointed out that the immune response may not always be protective.[16] Co-cultivation of tumor cells in vitro with a small number of specifically sensitized T cells *increases* the rate of growth of the tumor cells. A higher ratio of T cells to tumor cells exerts an inhibitory effect.[17] Moreover, "blocking factors" are sometimes produced in the immune response that prevent killing of tumor cells by sensitized T cells. These factors may be free tumor-associated antigens, antibodies, or antigen-antibody complexes; most likely the last.[18] Antibody presumably masks tumor cell antigens. Antigen might occupy recognition sites on T cells while the immune complexes could function through either of these pathways. To complicate matters further, "unblocking factors" have also been identified. In any event, it is clear that the mere appearance of an immune reaction cannot be equated with a beneficial effect on tumors. There is, therefore, a strong suspicion that NK cells and macrophages, rather than specifically-sensitized T cells, are the most effective antitumor mediators.[19, 20]

In view of all the evidence from animals, it was natural to assume an immune response to cancers in humans and that possibly this response maintained "*immunosurveillance*" against the emergence of cancers, at least reducing their number. As long ago as the turn of the twentieth century, Ehrlich, with amazing foresight, first suggested the existence of "positive mechanisms" against the innumerable "aberrant cells" that must appear throughout the life of an individual. Decades later, this concept was formalized and translated into immunologic terms by Thomas and Burnet.[21, 22] It has been argued that the occurrence of cancers in humans does not invalidate immunosurveillance, since there are many mechanisms by which they might escape, as follows.[19]

Sneaking through. Spontaneous cancers in humans either may lack sufficiently strong neoantigens to evoke an immune response, or may induce low-zone tolerance (p. 179). Alternatively, the weak immunologic challenge may be inadequate to control the emerging tumor, so that later the mass becomes too large for immunologic destruction.

Antigen modulation. Cancer cells continually shed surface-associated antigens, or they may permit stearic shifts in antigens, modifying their recognition by immune effectors. In addition, with tumor progression, new clones and new antigens appear.

Immunosuppression. Cancer-bearing hosts often

demonstrate increased numbers or increased function of suppressor T cells, and "immunoregulatory globulins" have also been described that suppress cell-mediated responses. It is well documented that patients with advanced cancer are usually immunocompromised.

Serum blocking factors. As mentioned earlier, these serum factors may inhibit cell-mediated reactions.

Tumor enhancement. At the outset, the low ratio of sensitized immunocompetent cells to tumor cells may stimulate rather than control tumor growth.

Genetic inability to respond. Individuals who develop a tumor may lack particular immune-response genes to the tumor antigens, or the antigens may be sufficiently similar to normal histocompatibility antigens to escape recognition as "nonself."

It is necessary to emphasize at this point that, although most cancers in humans do not have tumor-specific antigens comparable with the TSTAs of experimentally-induced cancers, they nonetheless apparently express a variety of tumor-associated antigens (p. 233). Sometimes there is a prominent lymphocyte-macrophage infiltration within and about the neoplasm, particularly with seminomas and Hodgkin's disease, taken to imply a defensive immune response (Fig. 7–3). Tumor-associated antigens can be demonstrated by immunofluorescent and immunoperoxidase techniques. These antigens are referred to as "tumor markers" of aid in the histologic diagnosis of neoplasms. Further, the antigens provide an opportunity to localize the cancer and its possible metastases by the intravenous administration of appropriate exogenous radiolabeled antibodies. Moreover, identification in the blood of tumor-associated antigens such as "fetal antigens" and many others is widely used clinically to detect the possible presence of a neoplasm and its posttherapy recurrence. Thus, there is evidence of tumor-associated antigens that may evoke immune responses. Correlations have been drawn between the level of these responses, the presence or absence of "blocking factors," and the clinical course of the lesion, particularly with melanocarcinomas, Burkitt's lymphoma, leukemia, and osteogenic sarcoma.[23, 24] However, more rigorous study of this issue casts doubts on the beneficial effects of immune responses because the important role of NK cells was not taken into account in most studies claiming favorable effects. It is highly significant that, at the present time, *no well-documented, clear-cut benefits have been achieved with any form of immunotherapy for the many types of cancer investigated, with the possible exception of osteogenic sarcoma.*[25]

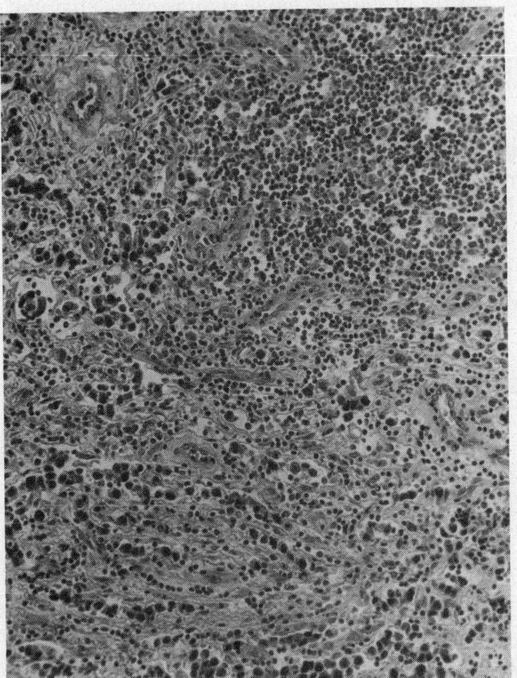

Figure 7–3. A seminoma of the testis with cords of anaplastic tumor cells *(below)* and an abundant infiltrate of lymphocytes, most evident at above right.

Just as the effectiveness of the indigenous immune response in controlling overt cancers in humans, and immunotherapy, have not to the present time proved very effective, so the concept of immunologic surveillance has been challenged. First, let us consider some of the observations that support it. It is argued that, despite the widespread prevalence in vertebrate species of protooncogenes, as noted in Chapter 6, their failure to evoke tumors may, at least in part, be a testament to effective immunosurveillance.[26] Such spontaneous neoplasms as do appear in animals and humans either lack tumor neoantigens or are very weakly immunogenic.[27] The strongest argument in favor of immunosurveillance is the increased frequency of cancers in immunosuppressed hosts.[28] Experimental induction of neoplasms with oncogenic viruses is clearly enhanced by previous immunosuppression, but the enhancement is less definitive with chemical carcinogens. In humans, about 5% of individuals with a congenital immunodeficiency develop cancers, 200 times the expected rate. Analogously, 5 to 7% of transplant recipients maintained on immunosuppressive therapy for long periods develop neoplasms.[29] However, it should be noted that most of these so-called cancers are lymphomas, often immunoblastic sarcomas (p. 664), although in addition there is a slightly increased incidence of carcinomas of the skin and lip and in situ carcinoma of the cervix.

Nevertheless, some have questioned the pertinence of these findings to the validation of immunologic surveillance.[30] It is noted that among immunologic cripples there is no excess risk of the commonest cancers in humans, i.e., bronchogenic carcinoma in males and breast carcinoma in females. The fact that most of the so-called neoplasms are lymphomas and immunoblastic sarcomas raises the issue of whether these lesions are truly neoplastic. Could they represent abnormal immunoproliferative responses to microbial infections, reflect deficiencies in normal immunologic regulatory controls, or, conceivably, be reactions triggered by the grafts and the many therapeutic agents used in transplant patients?[31, 32] Moreover, it is pointed out that "nude" mice lacking both hair and a thymus gland, and thus suffering from grossly impaired cell-mediated immunity, have no increased incidence of spontaneous tumors, nor are they more susceptible to the carcinogenic effects of oncogenic chemicals and viruses.[33] It should be pointed out, however, that these animals have a markedly shortened life span with a consequently reduced risk; further, they possess very effective non–T cell–mediated surveillance mechanisms such as an abundance of NK cells.[34] Other contrary evidence might be cited, but it suffices that *at present the existence of immunologic surveillance in humans has not been clearly established.*

Despite the generally negative evidence about the effectiveness of immune responses, the potential role of NK cells should not be overlooked.[35] The various functions of these cells are discussed on page 160, but it is relevant here to note that they exert nonspecific cytotoxicity for malignant cells, are capable of producing interferon, and in turn are stimulated to increased functional activity by interferon. Increased resistance to tumor growth has been observed in animals with high NK activity[36] and can be transferred by infusions of NK cell–enriched populations. Unfortunately, patients with advanced cancers have been shown to have deficient immune competence, NK activity, and interferon production; although these changes may have antedated and predisposed to the cancers, the best evidence indicates that they are tumor induced.[37, 38] In an effort to stimulate both specific and nonspecific reactivity against tumors, interferon is being employed in cancer patients.[39] It is too soon to draw any conclusions about the effectiveness of this form of therapy, save that results to date (admittedly from studies of patients with advanced neoplasms) offer no evidence that it is superior to any of the more established modalities of treatment.[40] Its effectiveness in early cancer is still under investigation. Thus, while the many attempts to exploit the immune response and NK-cell and macrophage activity in the treatment of cancers have not yet achieved the hoped-for results, refinements in methods such as antigen enhancement, more potent monoclonal antibodies, and linkage of antitumor toxic agents to antibodies may one day bear fruit.

PREDISPOSITION TO CANCER

Everyone would like to know that there is very little likelihood that he or she will ever develop a cancer. It is unfortunate that such reassurance cannot be offered, because for better or for worse it is impossible to predict who is destined to develop a malignant neoplasm. Nonetheless, a number of factors relating to both patient and environment have been identified that influence the individual's predisposition.

GEOGRAPHIC AND RACIAL FACTORS

In some measure, an individual's likelihood of developing a cancer is expressed by national incidence and mortality rates. For example, it is sobering to realize that residents of the United States have about a one in five chance of dying of cancer. There were, it is estimated, about 450,000 deaths from cancer in 1984 representing 23% of all mortality and 870,000 new cases of life-threatening cancer diagnoses.[41] These data do not include an additional 400,000 for the most part readily curable, nonmelanoma cancers of the skin and 40,000 to 50,000 cases of carcinoma in situ, largely of the uterine cervix. The major organ sites affected and their overall frequency are cited in Table 7–2. The rank order of these forms of malignant neoplasia has not materially changed over the past few decades save for a progressive decline in death rates from carcinoma of the stomach in both males and females. Lung cancer has led the grim parade in males since the mid-1950s, as has carcinoma of the breast in females. However, the death rates for many forms of cancer have significantly changed over the past years (Table 7–3).[41A] Many of the temporal comparisons are noteworthy. In males the overall cancer death rate has significantly increased, whereas in females it has fallen slightly. The increase in males can be laid largely at the doorstep of lung cancer. The improvement in females is mainly attributable to a significant decline in death rates from cancers of the uterus, stomach, and liver, notably carcinoma of the cervix, one of the most frequent forms of malignant neoplasia in females. Striking is the alarming increase

Table 7–2. ESTIMATED CANCER INCIDENCE FOR 1983 BY SITE AND SEX

Male (422,500)			Female (432,500)		
Rank	Site	No. cases (%)	Rank	Site	No. cases (%)
1	Lung	94,000 (22)	1	Breast (invasive)	114,000 (26)
2	Prostate	75,000 (18)	2	Colorectum	65,000 (15)
3	Colorectum	61,000 (14)	3	Lung	41,000 (9)
4	Bladder	28,000 (7)	4	Endometrium	39,000 (9)
5	Hodgkin's disease and lymphomas	21,000 (5)	5	Hodgkin's disease and lymphomas	19,300 (4)
6	Stomach	14,800 (4)	6	Cervix (invasive)	16,000 (4)
7	Leukemia	13,200 (3)	7	Pancreas	12,100 (3)
8	Pancreas	12,900 (3)	8	Leukemia	10,700 (2)

Drawn from the American Cancer Society: Cancer Facts and Figures, 1983.

Table 7–3. 25-YEAR TRENDS IN AGE-ADJUSTED CANCER DEATH RATES PER 100,000 POPULATION 1951–53 TO 1976–78

Sex	Sites	1951-53	1976-78	Percent Changes	Comments
Male	All Sites	171.9	215.7	+ 25	Steady increase mainly due to lung cancer.
Female	All Sites	146.4	136.1	− 7	Slight decrease.
Male	Bladder	7.2	7.2	*	Slight fluctuations; overall no change.
Female	Bladder	3.1	2.1	− 32	Some fluctuations; noticeable decrease.
Male	Breast	0.3	0.3	*	Constant rate.
Female	Breast	26.0	27.1	+ 4	Slight fluctuations; overall no change.
Male	Colon & Rectum	25.8	26.4	*	Slight fluctuations; overall no change.
Female	Colon & Rectum	24.8	20.0	− 19	Slight fluctuations; noticeable decrease.
Male	Esophagus	4.7	5.4	+ 15	Some fluctuations; slight increase.
Female	Esophagus	1.2	1.5	*	Slight fluctuations; overall no change in females.
Male	Kidney	3.4	4.7	+ 38	Steady slight increase.
Female	Kidney	2.1	2.2	*	Slight fluctuations; overall no change.
Male	Leukemia	7.9	8.8	+ 11	Early increase, later leveling off.
Female	Leukemia	5.4	5.2	*	Slight early increase, later leveling off.
Male	Liver	6.7	4.8	− 28	Some fluctuations. Steady decrease in both
Female	Liver	7.6	3.6	− 53	sexes.
Male	Lung	25.5	69.3	+ 172	Steady increase in both sexes due to cigarette
Female	Lung	5.0	17.8	+ 256	smoking.
Male	Oral	5.9	5.8	*	Slight fluctuations; overall no change in both
Female	Oral	1.5	2.0	*	sexes.
Female	Ovary	8.1	8.6	+ 8	Steady increase, later leveling off.
Male	Pancreas	8.6	11.2	+ 30	Steady increase in both sexes, then leveling off.
Female	Pancreas	5.5	7.1	+ 29	Reasons unknown.
Male	Prostate	21.0	22.6	+ 8	Fluctuations all through period; overall no change.
Male	Skin	3.1	3.4	*	Slight fluctuations; overall no change in both
Female	Skin	1.9	1.9	*	sexes.
Male	Stomach	22.8	9.3	− 59	Steady decrease in both sexes; reasons unknown.
Female	Stomach	12.3	4.3	− 65	
Female	Uterus	20.0	8.7	− 57	Steady decrease.

*Percent changes not listed because they are not meaningful.
From American Cancer Society: Cancer Facts and Figures, 1983, p. 11.

in deaths from carcinoma of the lung in both sexes. Although the percentage change is greater for females than males, this is merely the spurious consequence of the relative rarity of cancer of the lung in females years ago. The rising slope of the curve is about the same in both sexes, and neither current-day efforts to control smoking nor "low tar" cigarettes have yet shown signs of reducing the awesome mortality rate. Although in females carcinomas of the breast are about three times more frequent than those of the lung, the striking difference in cure rates makes it highly likely that lung cancer will become the number one killer cancer if the increase in frequency does not slow or, better, fall. The decline in the number of deaths caused by uterine cancer probably relates largely to the earlier diagnosis and better cure rate made possible by the Papanicolaou smear. Much more mysterious is the downward trend in deaths from stomach and liver carcinomas. Could this be due to a decrease in some dietary carcinogens?

Remarkable differences can be found in the incidence and death rates of specific forms of cancer around the world. For example, the death rate for stomach carcinoma in both males and females is seven times higher in Japan than in the United States. In contrast, the death rate from carcinoma of the lung is slightly more than twice as great in the United States as in Japan and, indeed, in Scotland is almost twice as high as in the United States. Skin cancer deaths, largely caused by melanocarcinomas, are six times more frequent in New Zealand than in Iceland, which is probably attributable to differences in sun exposure. While racial predispositions cannot be ruled out, it is generally believed that most of these geographic differences are the consequence of environmental influences. This is best brought out by comparing mortality rates for Japanese born in the United States of immigrant parents (Nisei) with those of long-term residents of both countries. Table 7–4 indicates that Nisei have intermediate standardized mortality ratios, pointing strongly to environmental rather than racial (genetic) predisposition. However, what are the environmental influences that account for a death rate from breast carcinoma in females of 33.8 in Denmark in 1976–77 and only 23.5 in Sweden? Equally enigmatic are the prostatic mortality rates of 3.6 in Japan as compared with approximately 23 in both France and the United States. Many hypotheses have been offered. For example, with breast carcinoma, differences in number of pregnancies, age of the mother

Table 7–4. STANDARDIZED MORTALITY RATIOS FOR CANCER IN VARIOUS SITES

	Japanese	Nisei	U.S. White
Stomach	100	38	17
Intestines	100	290	490
Pancreas	100	170	270
Lung, bronchus	100	170	320
Leukemia	100	150	270

Adapted from Haenszel, W., and Kurihara, M.: Studies of Japanese migrants. I. Mortality from cancer and other diseases among Japanese in the United States. J. Natl. Cancer Inst. *40*:43, 1968.

at first birth, and breast-feeding practices may be involved since they tend to reduce the uninterrupted cyclic estrogenic stimulation of the breast, particularly in the early decades. Analogously, coital frequency, number of sexual partners, history of venereal disease, dietary fat, and other environmental influences have been invoked for prostatic carcinoma.[42] These and other cultural and environmental hypotheses are more fully discussed in later chapters, but none offer entirely satisfactory explanations. Thus, it is impossible to rule out racial genetic predisposition. In this connection, the age-standardized mortality rate for prostate cancer in United States blacks is more than twice the rate of whites. But proof of genetic predisposition requires rigorous comparisons controlled for the infinite number of environmental and cultural variables found in free-living populations. Until such time as these are available, which may be never, the remarkable geographic variations in frequency of specific forms of cancer warrant a search for their possible exogenous origins.

AGE AND CHILDHOOD CANCER

Age is an important influence on the likelihood of being afflicted with cancer. As everyone knows, most carcinomas occur in the later years of life (55 years and over). Each age group has its own predilection to certain forms of cancer, as is evident in Table 7–5. Here the striking increase in mortality from cancer in the age group 55 to 74 years should be noted. The decline in deaths in the 75-years-and-over group merely reflects the dwindling population reaching this venerable age.

Table 7–5.

MORTALITY FOR THE FIVE LEADING CANCER SITES FOR MALES BY AGE GROUP, UNITED STATES-1978

All Ages	Under 15	15–34	35–54	55–74	75+
Lung 71,006	Leukemia 550	Leukemia 827	Lung 10,124	Lung 46,049	Lung 14,646
Colon & Rectum 25,696	Brain & Central Nervous System 344	Brain & Central Nervous System 467	Colon & Rectum 2,462	Colon & Rectum 13,717	Prostate 12,298
Prostate 21,674	Bone 47	Hodgkin's Disease 335	Pancreas 1,262	Prostate 9,047	Colon & Rectum 9.325
Pancreas 11,010	Connective Tissues 43	Testis 329	Brain & Central Nervous System 1,282	Pancreas 6,490	Pancreas 3,208
Stomach 8,529	Kidney 39	Melanoma of Skin 261	Leukemia 1,065	Stomach 4,558	Bladder 3.172

Source: Vital Statistics of the United States, 1978.

MORTALITY FOR THE FIVE LEADING CANCER SITES FOR FEMALES BY AGE GROUP, UNITED STATES-1978

All Ages	Under 15	15–34	35–54	55–74	75+
Breast 34,329	Leukemia 411	Breast 585	Breast 8,205	Breast 17,403	Colon & Rectum 12,626
Colon & Rectum 27,573	Brain & Central Nervous System 275	Leukemia 493	Lung 4,679	Lung 14,463	Breast 8,129
Lung 24,080	Bone 45	Brain & Central Nervous System 347	Colon & Rectum 2,210	Colon & Rectum 12,551	Lung 4,819
Uterus 10,842	Kidney 44	Uterus 295	Uterus 2,111	Ovary 5,992	Pancreas 3,939
Ovary 10,651	Connective Tissues 43	Hodgkin's Disease 223	Ovary 2,029	Uterus 5,480	Uterus 2,954

Source: Vital Statistics of the United States, 1978.
From: CA-A Cancer Journal for Clinicians *33*:11, 1983. Reproduced with permission.

Also to be noted is that children under the age of 15 are not spared. Indeed, cancer accounts for slightly more than 10% of all deaths in this group in the United States, and is second only to accidents. Acute leukemia and neoplasms of the central nervous system are responsible for approximately 60 to 75% of these deaths.[43] The most common form of neoplasia (p. 1247) in infants under 1 year of age is neuroblastoma, followed in descending order by Wilms' tumor; rhabdomyosarcoma of the head, neck, and genitourinary tract; and retinoblastoma. Acute leukemias, particularly acute lymphoblastic leukemia, are also prone to occur in children under 5 years in the United States, western Europe, and Japan; it is more common in whites than blacks in the U.S. A predisposition to leukemia is encountered in such inherited disorders as Down's syndrome and in Fanconi's anemia and Bloom's syndrome, characterized by chromosomal instability.[44] Ionizing radiation and alkylating agents are also potent leukemogenic influences in children. Fortunately, dramatic therapeutic results are now being achieved with many of these forms of childhood neoplasia. For example, with acute lymphoblastic leukemia a better than 50% five-year survival can now be effected. Over 90% of children with Wilms' tumor confined to the kidney are alive at 5 years, and most are likely to be cured.[45] Comparably encouraging results could be cited for rhabdomyosarcomas. The occurrence of cancer is always disturbing at any age and particularly lamentable in the young, but there is now solid basis for optimism about the control and possible cure of many forms of childhood malignancies.

ENVIRONMENTAL AND CULTURAL INFLUENCES

Cancer risks lurk behind virtually every door. They can be found in the environment and particularly within certain occupations. Mention has already been made of the carcinogenicity of ultraviolet rays and many drugs. Asbestos, vinyl chloride, and 2-naphthylamine can serve as examples of occupational hazards, and many others are discussed on page 459. The risks may be incurred in life style and personal exposures, for example, the role of nutrition, considered on page 426. Overall, mortality data indicate that persons more than 25% overweight have a higher death rate from cancer than their "trim" neighbors. Alcohol abuse alone increases the risk of carcinomas of the oropharynx (excluding lip), larynx, and esophagus, and through the intermediation of alcoholic cirrhosis, carcinoma of the liver.[46] Smoking, particularly of cigarettes, has been implicated in cancer of the mouth, pharynx, larynx, esophagus, pancreas, and bladder, but most significantly is responsible for about 83% of lung cancer among males and 43% among females (p. 442). Indeed, cigarette smoking has been called the single most important environmental factor contributing to premature death in the United States. Alcohol and tobacco together multiply the danger of incurring cancers in the upper aerodigestive tract.[47] The risk of cervical cancer is linked to age at first intercourse and the number of sex partners. These associations point to a possible causal role for venereal transmission of cervical viral infections. It begins to appear that everything one does to gain a livelihood or for pleasure is either fattening, immoral, illegal, or, most distressing, oncogenic.

HEREDITY

One frequently asked question is: "My mother and father both died of cancer. Does that mean I am doomed to get it?" On the basis of current knowledge, the answer must be carefully qualified.[48, 49] The evidence now indicates that for a large number of types of cancer, including the most common forms, there exist not only environmental influences but also hereditary predispositions. For example, lung cancer is in most instances clearly related to cigarette smoking, yet mortality from lung cancer has been shown to be four times greater among nonsmoking relatives (parents and siblings) of lung cancer patients than among nonsmoking relatives of controls. Similar data (a twofold increase) obtain with smoking relatives. So it appears that genetic influences may contribute to the development of cancer even when there are clearly defined environmental factors. A genetic predisposition to breast cancer in females can also be shown. What role heredity plays in the predisposition to particular breast cancers cannot be quantified. Clearly, women who have no family history of this cancer may develop the disease, but presumably those from breast-cancer families are at some increased risk. A two-mutation theory has been proposed for the inherited predisposition to cancer. Inheritance of a mutant gene through the germ cells slightly increases the risk of a specific form of cancer, but a second somatic mutation is necessary to raise the risk substantially. In the absence of the inherited germinal mutation, two somatic mutations would be required to potentiate tumorigenesis. Thus, inheritance of a predisposition to cancer or, in fact, a subsequent somatic mutation does not imply inevitability; still other influences, possibly environmental, may be necessary for the development of a tumor. Autosomal dominant patterns of transmission can be identified in many instances of hereditary predisposition, but often the predisposition does not follow strict mendelian patterns.

In general, the risk of the same neoplasm developing in close relatives of a cancer patient is about three times greater than in control populations. There is an even greater familial risk with particular forms of cancer, notably embryonal tumors of childhood and carcinomas of the breast and colon. In families in which tumors develop earlier than the usual age or at multiple foci, the risk may be increased many-fold. Childhood retinoblastoma offers the most striking example of the role of heredity. About 60% of these neoplasms are nonhereditary and usually unilateral; the remainder are hereditary and more often bilateral. The risk of tumor in a carrier of the autosomal dominant mutation is about

95%, i.e., 100,000 times greater than it is in the child who does not carry the mutant gene.[51] Bilateral cases are almost always genetic, but unilaterality does not exclude heredity. Because the mutation does not have 100% penetrance, unaffected carriers may pass the mutation to their offspring. It is of interest in terms of the origins of cancer that children have been cured of their ocular retinoblastomas only to develop, in a higher-than-chance frequency, osteogenic sarcoma of the long bones. Multiple polyposis coli is another hereditary disorder marked by an extraordinarily high risk of cancer. Individuals who inherit the autosomal dominant mutation have at birth, or soon thereafter, innumerable polypoid adenomas of the colon, and in virtually 100% of cases are fated to develop a carcinoma of the colon by age 50. A list of some of the more common cancerous and precancerous disorders in which heredity plays a major role is presented in Table 7–6.

It is impossible to estimate the contribution of heredity to the total human burden of cancer. However, the best "guesstimates" suggest that about 5% of all cancers are genetic.[52] The remainder, then, must be largely environmental in origin or so-called "spontaneous," but it is highly likely that genetic predisposition contributes to some proportion of so-called "environmental" and "spontaneous" cancers. For example, individuals with the autosomal recessive "chromosome breakage syndromes" such as xeroderma pigmentosum only develop their cancers of the skin with exposure to the mutational effects of radiant energy. Heterozygotes who do not manifest these recessive "breakage syndromes" are also at increased risk.[53] The converse is equally true: environmental factors must contribute to the initiation of many hereditary neoplasms. *It is best then to consider heredity and environment as the two ends of a spectrum of predisposing influences.* At the extremes are those neoplasms fated to appear because of heredity or because of environment, but in between are the great majority of cancers that have varying proportions of both influences, depending on where they fall within the spectrum.

Table 7–6. HEREDITARY CANCEROUS AND PRECANCEROUS DISORDERS

Disorder	Predominant Tumors
Autosomal Dominant Inheritance	
Retinoblastoma	Retinoblastoma, sarcomas—orbital (following radiation) and at remote sites
Neurofibromatosis	Neurogenic sarcoma, acoustic neuroma, pheochromocytoma
Familial polyposis coli	Colonic cancer, adenomatous polyps
Gardner's syndrome	Colonic cancer, adenomatous polyps, osteomas
Peutz-Jeghers syndrome	Controversial whether predisposes to colonic cancer
Hereditary multiple endocrine neoplasia syndrome— type I (MEN I)	Tumors of pituitary gland, parathyroid gland, and pancreatic islet cells
Multiple endocrine neoplasia syndrome—type II (MEN II)	Medullary carcinoma of thyroid, pheochromocytoma, and parathyroid disease
Cutaneous malignant melanoma	Cutaneous malignant melanoma, other cancers
Von Hippel-Lindau disease	Hemangioblastoma of cerebellum, hypernephroma, and pheochromocytoma
Cancer-family syndrome	Adenocarcinomas (primarily of colon and endometrium)
Breast cancer in association with other malignant neoplasms	Breast cancer, sarcoma, leukemia, and brain tumor
Autosomal Recessive Inheritance	
Xeroderma pigmentosum	Basal and squamous cell carcinoma of skin, malignant melanoma
Fanconi's anemia	Leukemia and lymphoma
Bloom's syndrome	Acute leukemia, various carcinomas
Ataxia telangiectasia	Acute leukemia, lymphoma, and possibly gastric cancer
Turcot's syndrome	Colonic polyps, cancer, and brain tumors

PREDISPOSING DISORDERS

The only certain way to avoid cancer is not to be born: to live is to incur the risk. However, the risk is greater than average under many circumstances, as is evident from the predisposing influences discussed earlier. Certain clinical conditions are also of importance. It has already been sufficiently emphasized that cell replication is involved in cancerous transformation, and thus regenerative, hyperplastic, and dyplastic proliferations are fertile soils for the origin of a malignant neoplasm. There is a well-defined association between certain forms of endometrial hyperplasia and endometrial carcinoma (p. 1134), and between cervical dysplasia and cervical carcinoma. The bronchial mucosal metaplasia and dysplasia of habitual cigarette smokers are ominous antecedents of bronchogenic carcinoma. About 80% of heptocellular carcinomas arise in cirrhotic livers, which are characterized by active parenchymal regeneration. Other examples could be offered, but although these settings constitute important predispositions it must be appreciated that in the great majority of instances they are not complicated by neoplasia.

Certain non-neoplastic disorders—*the chronic atrophic gastritis of pernicious anemia; solar keratosis of the skin; the chromosomal breakage syndromes; chronic ulcerative colitis; and leukoplakia of the oral cavity, vulva, and penis*—have such a well-defined association with cancer that they have been termed "*precancerous conditions.*" This designation is somewhat unfortunate since in the great majority of instances no malignant neoplasm emerges. Nonetheless, the term persists because it calls attention to the increased risk. Analogously, certain forms of benign neoplasia constitute "precancerous conditions." The villous adenoma of the colon, as it increases in size, develops cancerous change in up to 50% of cases. The myriad adenomatous colonic polyps characteristic of familial multiple polyposis coli are almost always followed eventually by carcinoma of the colon. The multiple neurofibromas of the hereditary neurofibromatosis often give rise to neurogenic sarcomas. It might be asked: Is there not a risk with all benign neoplasms? Although some risk may be inherent, a large cumulative experience indicates that *most benign neoplasms do not become cancerous*. Nonetheless, numerous examples could be offered of cancers arising, albeit rarely, in benign tumors: for example, a leiomyosarcoma beginning in a leiomyoma, and carcinoma appearing in long-standing pleomorphic adenomas. Generalization is impossible because each type of benign neoplasm is associated with a particular level of risk ranging from virtually never to frequently. Only follow-up studies of large series of each neoplasm can establish the level of risk, and always the questions remain: Was the tumor an indolent form of cancer or was there a malignant focus in the benign tumor?

LABORATORY DIAGNOSIS OF CANCER

Every year the approach to laboratory diagnosis of cancer becomes more complex, more sophisticated, and more specialized. It may come as a rude surprise that, for virtually every neoplasm mentioned in this text, a number of subcategories have been characterized by the experts; but we must walk before we can run. Each of the following sections attempts to present the "state of the art," avoiding details of method.

HISTOLOGIC DIAGNOSIS

Despite man's ingenuity in inventing amazingly sophisticated instrumentation, the anatomic diagnosis of neoplasms is largely accomplished by "eyeballing." In some part a science, and in larger part an art, it is heavily dependent on the brain behind the eyes behind the microscope. However, a great deal of objectivity has been added to the subjective interpretation by numerous modalities such as transmission electron microscopy, scanning electron microscopy, histochemistry, immunofluorescent and immunocytochemical techniques, and others. Thus, previously hidden cellular details such as organellar structure, intracellular filaments, antigenic markers (to be described), and particular enzymes are now identifiable and permit more certain identifications. For example, desmosomes together with microvilli almost always signify an epithelial origin of a cancer. Endocrine cells bear membrane-bound, dense-core granules. Myoglobin or myosin antibodies permit the immunocytochemical identification of mesenchymal tumor cells. In particular, tumor markers (cited below) have come to the fore. The clinician, too, makes a very important contribution to accurate histologic diagnosis. The tissues submitted for anatomic diagnosis must be representative of the lesion. Obvious as this may sound, large neoplasms often have areas of necrosis; a relatively small breast carcinoma may be enveloped by non-neoplastic fibrocystic disease, and a bronchoscopic biopsy of the margins of a focus of bronchial mucosal change may disclose only cellular atypia and fail to contain the central more definitive cancerous changes. There is much to recommend in the needle biopsy approach, which is highly satisfactory in particular situations, but the risk of sampling error is a serious consideration. The clinician makes a further contribution to the accuracy of diagnosis by circumspect handling of the specimen, avoiding crushing, tearing, and electrodesiccation distortions, and by prompt preservation or fixation of specimens. Often underappreciated is the importance of adequate clinical information; maximal anatomic diagnostic accuracy cannot be achieved in a clinical vacuum. The cellular changes introduced by previous radiotherapy are easily misinterpreted as cancer. The reparative changes of a previous bone injury may, at times, mimic an osteogenic sarcoma.

When general anesthesia is required for biopsy of, say, a deeply situated large breast mass, a "frozen section" anatomic diagnosis can be rendered within minutes, permitting the required definitive surgery. Although "frozen sections" do not provide the fine cytologic detail of the more time-consuming paraffin sections, they are nonetheless entirely satisfactory and accurate in experienced hands. Occasionally the lesion may be difficult to evaluate, and so a definite diagnosis is not rendered. Better to impose on the patient the discomfort and expense inherent in a second surgical procedure than to embark on surgery based on a wrong diagnosis. Except for the rare instances of rapidly growing sarcomas, usually in children, there is no evidence that a few days' delay between biopsy and definitive surgery imposes any danger of dissemination of the cancer.

CYTOLOGIC DIAGNOSIS

Next best to histologic diagnosis of cancer is the cytologic method first described by Papanicolaou in 1928[54] and confirmed in 1943[55] This method has been most widely applied in the detection of carcinoma of the cervix and carcinoma of the endometrium. The secretions obtained on an endocervical swab or aspiration, or those derived from a cervical scraping, are smeared onto a slide, quickly fixed, and stained.

As pointed out earlier, cancer cells have lowered cohesiveness and have a range of morphologic changes encompassed by the term anaplasia. Thus, shed cells can be evaluated for the features of anaplasia indicative of their origin in a cancer (Figs. 7–4 and 7–5). In contrast to the histologist's task, judgment here must be rendered on the basis of individual cell cytology or (at most perhaps) on that of a clump of a few cells without the supporting evidence of architectural disarray, loss of orientation of one cell to another, and (perhaps most important) evidence of invasion. This method permits differentiation among normal, dysplas-

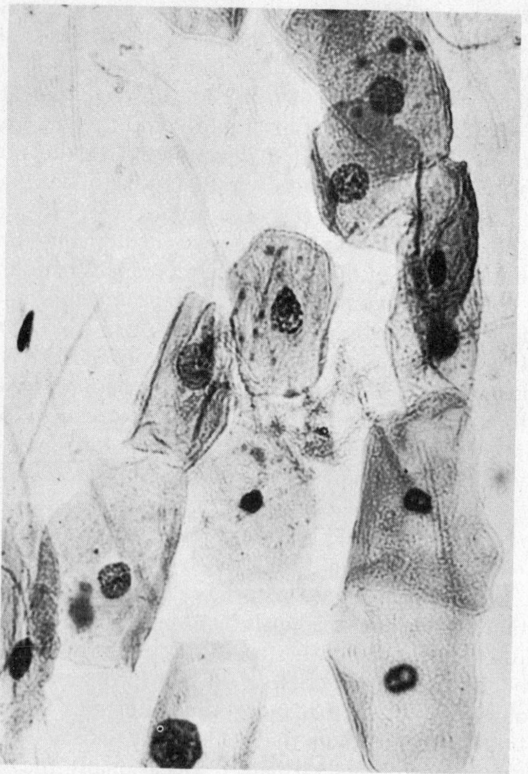

Figure 7–4. Exfoliative cell smear showing normal cytologic flora of the genital tract. Cells are largely flattened surface squamous epithelial cells.

tic, and cancerous cells, and in addition permits the recognition of cellular changes characteristic of carcinoma in situ. The following terminology is frequently used:

Class I: Normal
Class II: Few atypical cells—repeat
Class III: Dysplasia—sometimes subdivided into mild, moderate, and severe
Class IV: Carcinoma in situ
Class V: Cancer

Many other classifications are in use but, whatever the terminology, an accuracy approaching 100% can be achieved in laboratory interpretation of the cytologic smear. There are, however, false-negative errors introduced by misdirected or inadequate sampling. These are greatest when cytologic diagnosis is applied to nongynecologic disease: e.g., sputum; bronchial brushings; abdominal, pleural, joint, and cerebrospinal fluids; urinary sediment; gastric brushings; biliary and pancreatic duct aspirations; and needle aspirations of breast, prostatic, thyroid, and other lesions. Despite the possibility of false-negative errors, a positive finding indicates the existence of a cancer that is best substantiated by biopsy and histologic examination before surgery is embarked upon. Cytologic examination has contributed greatly to the striking reduction in the mortality rate of uterine cancer in the United States and other countries over the past few decades. Women at risk, and indeed entire populations, can be screened for lesions that might well escape detection otherwise.

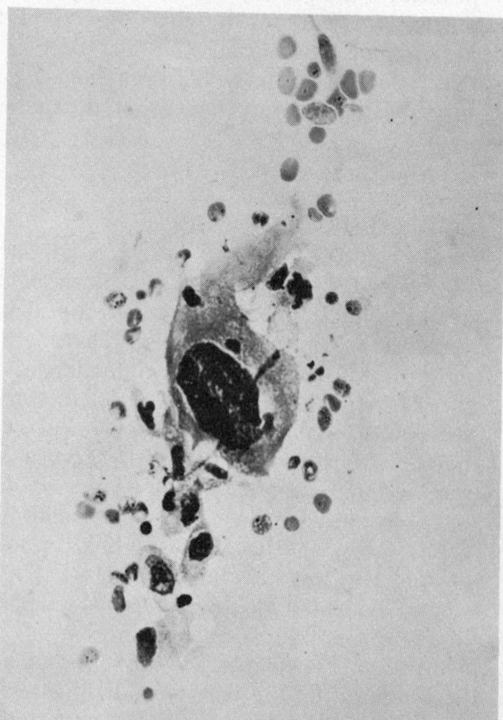

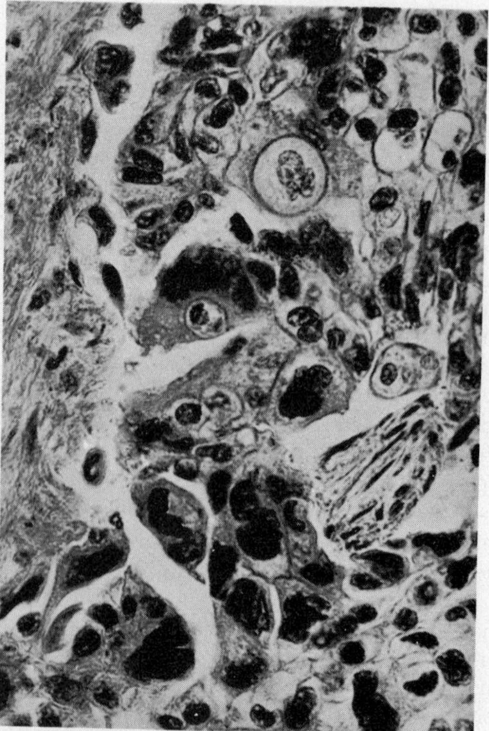

Figure 7–5. On the left is an exfoliative cell smear of vaginal secretions from a patient with a cervical cancer. Contrast the large, malignant anaplastic cell with the normal cells in Figure 7–4 (same magnification). On the right is a tissue section of the resected tumor showing the anaplastic cells in situ.

TUMOR MARKERS

With advances in the development of specific radiotherapeutic and chemotherapeutic protocols for particular cancers, accurate and precise morphologic diagnosis has assumed increased importance. Although in many instances cancers are sufficiently well differentiated to permit ready identification on routine microscopic sections, diagnostic difficulities not infrequently arise, particularly with undifferentiated neoplasms and in establishing the origin of a metastasis. Thus, efforts have been made to characterize "markers" of specific forms of neoplasia that would at least narrow the range of possibilities. Mention was made on page 265 of the use of immunocytochemical methods to identify markers (e.g., enzymes, antigens, intermediate filaments) in the anatomic differential diagnosis of tumors (Fig. 7–6). The markers have also been shown to have clinical importance: (1) By their release into the circulation, they provide a means of screening individuals or populations for the possible presence of a particular form of cancer, thus permitting appropriate clinical verification. (2) Since the plasma level of the marker is a function of the total body burden of cancer, some estimate or prognosis is possible; more important, however, the level reflects the effectiveness of therapy and subsequent possible recurrences. (3) Still highly experimental is the use of radiolabeled antibodies (optimally monoclonal) to the markers, which might be administered to appropriate patients in an effort to localize, by radioscanning techniques, not only the primary lesion but also metastases.[56] (4) If antibodies of sufficient affinity and specificity could be developed, it might be possible to couple them with antitumor agents and thus bring the therapeutic agent to bear directly on the cancer cells wherever they are dispersed. The last two clinical applications are still in the exploratory stage, but the use of markers to facilitate anatomic and clinical diagnosis and follow-up are now well established.

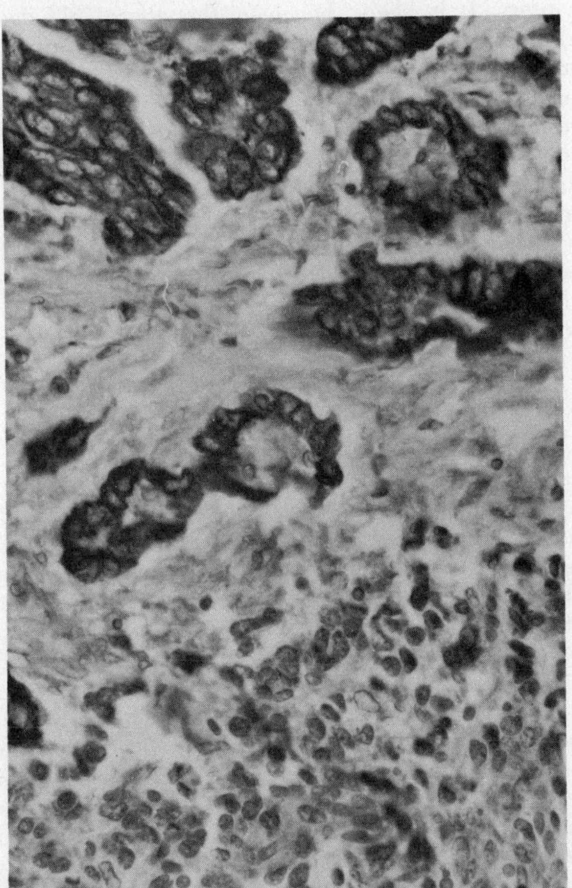

Figure 7–6. An antikeratin immunoperoxidase strain of a mixed adenocarcinoma and undifferentiated carcinoma of the lung. The atypical gland patterns above are stained dark, indicating a positive antikeratin reaction. The undifferentiated cancer cells below are keratin negative.

Table 7–7. APPLIED TUMOR MARKERS

Markers	Principal Application
Immunologic	
E rosettes	Leukemia/lymphoma T cells
Monoclonal antibodies	Leukemia/lymphoma T and B cells
Specific heavy-chain immunoglobulins	Leukemia/lymphoma B cells
Kappa, lambda light chains	Leukemia/lymphoma B cells
Intermediate Filaments	Identification of histogenesis of tumor cells (see p. 220)
Tumor-Associated Antigens	
Carcinoembryonic antigen	Colonic, pancreatic, bronchogenic, gastric, and breast carcinomas and other forms of cancer
Alpha-fetoprotein	Hepatocellular carcinoma, germ cell tumors (principally yolk-sac and endodermal sinus derivatives)
Pancreatic oncofetal antigen	Pancreatic, bronchogenic, and gastric carcinomas and others
Hormones	
Human chorionic gonadotropin	Choriocarcinoma, hydatidiform mole, seminoma, embryonal and teratocarcinoma of the testis, ovarian carcinoma, and others
Human placental lactogen	Trophoblastic neoplasms
Calcitonin	Thyroid medullary carcinoma
Ectopic hormones	See paraneoplastic syndromes (p. 255)
Serum Enzymes	
Acid phosphatase, tartrate-inhibitable	Prostatic carcinoma
Galactosyltransferase II	Pancreatic, gastric, and breast carcinomas

The roster of tumor markers grows longer every month. Some are of principal use in morphologic diagnosis, a few only clinically, but most contribute to both. Those that have been available sufficiently long to be adequately tested are listed in Table 7–7 along with the malignancies for which they have the greatest value.[57, 58] A few comments on some of the more important markers follow.

Immunologic markers have become important adjuncts to the specific chracterization of lymphoid leukemias and lymphomas.[59] It is now possible to subdivide these disorders into T (thymic-dependent) and B (bone marrow–derived) subsets by several techniques, most specifically by monoclonal antibodies (p. 666), and to further differentiate monoclonal neoplastic proliferations from polyclonal lesions that are more likely to be non-neoplastic. For example, the finding that all lymphocytes within a marrow infiltrate are synthesizing kappa light chains argues strongly for their leukemic or lymphomatous origin rather than their being a nonspecific inflammatory reaction. It is not necessary to delve into the technical details involved in these immunologic assays, save to mention that specific antisera, some monoclonal, are now available for the various immunoglobulin chains. These can be coupled with fluorescent dyes and so localized in tissue sections by ultraviolet microscopy. Alternatively, the antibodies can be complexed with horseradish peroxidase, which will react with a chromogen to yield a distinctive precipitate wherever the peroxidase-antibody complex is bound (the immunoperoxidase method). Still in development are a variety of monoclonal antisera capable of reacting with subtypes of T and B cells to provide more accurate subclassification, and the establishment of more precise prognoses and treatment protocols for each particular form of leukemia and lymphoma of lymphoid origin.

The *fetal tumor–associated antigens*, sometimes called *oncofetal antigens*, were the first tumor markers to be described. Initially, carcinoembryonic antigen (CEA), a normal glycoprotein in the embryonic tissue of the gut, pancreas, and liver during the first two trimesters, was believed to be specific for adenocarcinomas of the colon when detected in the plasma in postnatal life.[60] However, with the subsequent development of more sensitive radioimmunoassays, it became apparent that CEA could be demonstrated in the plasma with many endodermally derived cancers (particularly pancreatic, gastric, and bronchogenic) as well as in many other forms of malignancy. Moreover, small quantities are present in the plasma in habitual cigarette smokers, and minimal-to-moderate amounts in alcoholic cirrhosis, pancreatitis, inflammatory bowel disease, peptic ulcer, and other non-neoplastic disorders. Moreover, the level of CEA elevation in the plasma is a function of the body burden of cancer. Thus, large or disseminated cancers produce high plasma levels, but the early potentially curable lesions reveal only modest or marginal levels. It has thus become apparent that CEA assays lack both specificity and the sensitivity required for the detection of early cancers. Nonetheless, quantitative CEA determinations are still very useful in providing presumptive evidence of the presence of colonic cancers, since they yield the highest plasma levels and have proved of great worth in helping to establish a prognosis and in post-therapeutic monitoring of possible recurrences.[61, 62] Further details on this tumor marker may be found on page 873.

Alpha-fetoprotein (AFP) is another well-established tumor marker, discussed in some detail on page 000. This glycoprotein is synthesized normally early in fetal life by the yolk sac and fetal liver. Abnormal plasma elevations are encountered in adults with cancers arising principally in the liver and from yolk sac remnants. Elevated plasma AFP is also found less regularly in teratocarcinomas and embryonal cell carcinomas of the testis, ovary, and extragonadal sites, which presumably contain yolk sac remnants, and occasionally in carcinomas of the stomach and pancreas. Like CEA, non-neoplastic conditions including cirrhosis, toxic liver injury, hepatitis, and pregnancy (especially with fetal distress or death) also may cause minimal-to-moderate plasma elevations of AFP. While there is, then, some problem with specificity, marked elevations of the plasma AFP level have proved a highly useful indicator of carcinomas arising in the liver and from yolk sac or endodermal sinus derivatives (pp. 938 and 1094).[63] Parenthetically, fetal neural tube defects such as anencephaly and spina bifida produce elevations of the amniotic fluid AFP, thus providing an opportunity for prenatal diagnosis.

More details on the established tumor markers will appear in discussions of various forms of cancer in later chapters. It is likely, however, that these "old dogs" will be augmented or replaced in the near future by some of the new markers currently being tested. Attention was called early to a "ca antigen" reported to be present in a wide variety of cancers (p. 234). Another promising candidate is tissue polypeptide antigen (TPA), found in the plasma in patients with a wide variety of cancers, and in the urine in bladder cancer.[64, 65] It is further likely that, as appropriate monoclonal antibodies become available, more tissue and tumor-specific antigens will be characterized (some are already available), providing the long-sought-after specific markers for all forms of cancer.[66]

TUMORS COMMON TO ALL ORGANS

Mesenchymal derivatives (such as connective tissue, fat, blood vessels with their endothelial cells and smooth muscle cells, histiocytes, and Schwann cells) are found in all organs and tissues of the body. Thus, mesenchymal tumors are common to all organs. As you know, mesenchymal cells retain their multipotentiality; thus, fibroblasts may differentiate into osteoblasts, and smooth muscle cells can elaborate collagen and become phagocytic. Thus, while neoplasms derived from mesenchymal cells may be differentiated along a single line such as the lipoma, fibrosarcoma, or leiomyoma, mesenchymally derived tumors not infrequently display the multipotentiality of mesenchymal cells and so produce mixed patterns such as angiolipomas, fibromyxochondromas, or other combinations. It is not possible to describe the range of neoplasms resulting from such versatility. Only the more common patterns, mostly differentiated along a single line, are presented in the following sections, excluding those of blood vessels, cartilage, and bone, which are described elsewhere.

FIBROMA AND FIBROSARCOMA

Many types of mesenchymal cells—macrophages, endothelial cells, mesothelial cells, Schwann cells, and others—may differentiate into fibroblasts. In the context of the abundance of these cells and, of course, fibroblasts throughout the body, it is surprising that fibromas and fibrosarcomas are relatively uncommon neoplasms. Much more common are a loosely defined group of localized overgrowths of fibroblastic cells, collectively referred to as *fibromatoses*. These range from the post-inflammatory keloid to non-neoplastic fibroses, such as palmar or plantar fibromatoses, to lesions intermediate between the fibroma and fibrosarcoma, which, for lack of a better designation, are called desmoid tumors. Since the fibromatoses, including the desmoid tumor, are principally related to the musculoskeletal system, they are considered in Chapter 28. Remarks here are confined to the rare fibroma and the slightly more common fibrosarcoma.

True fibromas (or lesions referred to as fibromas) are, for unknown reasons, found in only a relatively few sites in the body. Ovarian fibromas may arise from stromal cells. Circumscribed nodules referred to as fibromas occur in relation to the teeth. Neurofibromas derived from Schwann cells are found along nerve trunks. Whatever their origin, these benign neoplasms are composed of typical spindled fibroblasts, either closely packed with scant intervening collagen or separated by abundant collagen (Fig. 7–7). The consistency of these usually firm masses depends on the amount of collagen. All are pearly gray and rarely have areas of hemorrhage, cystic softening, or necrosis. The cells may be laid down in random array or sometimes are aligned parallel to each other to make up broad ribbons. In well-differentiated tumors, mitoses are rare, but in so-called "cellular fibromas," scattered mitoses can be found; thus, the differentiation between "cellular fibromas" and fibrosarcomas becomes difficult. Although criteria vary, up to three mitoses per ten high-power fields is often used as the dividing line.[67] The differentiation of fibromas from such neoplasms as the leiomyoma, also composed of spindle cells, may sometimes be difficult. Useful methods include the trichrome stain to highlight the amount and distribution of the collagen; the phosphotungstic acid-hematoxylin stain to reveal slender, wavy fibroglial fibers; and silver impregnations to disclose the delicate, lattice-like fibrillar reticulin enclosing individual cells.

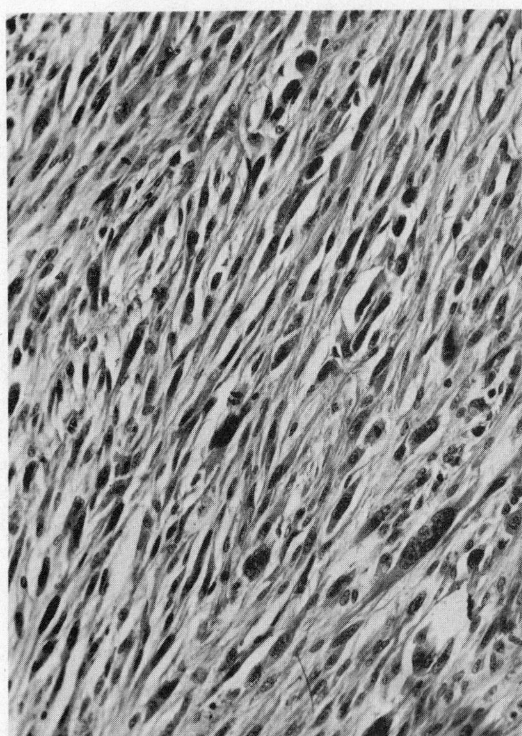

Figure 7–8. Fibrosarcoma. There is considerable anaplasia of cells with marked variation in size and shape. Scattered giant cells are readily evident.

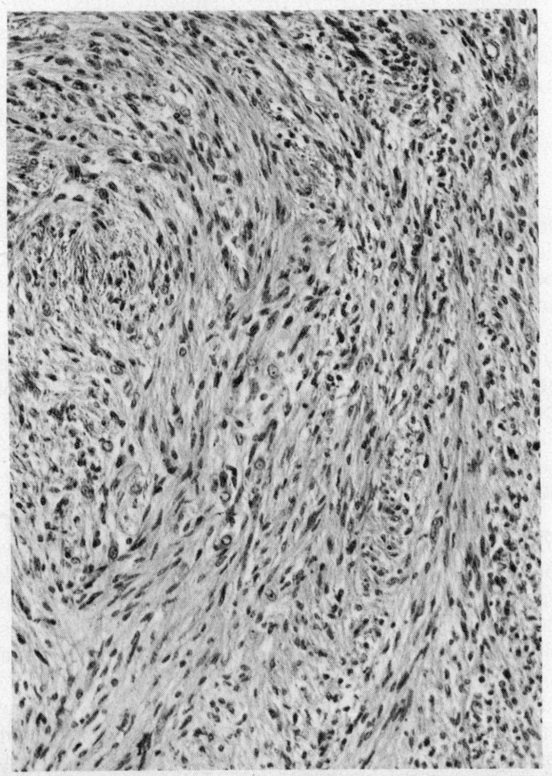

Figure 7–7. Fibroma. The tumor is made up of regular, well-formed fibrocytes and fibroblasts laid down in parallel bands.

Fibrosarcomas may be located anywhere but are most frequent in the retroperitoneum, followed by the superficial or deep tissues of the extremities. Typically, they are unencapsulated, infiltrative, soft, pearly gray to white masses, often having areas of hemorrhage and necrosis. Better differentiated neoplasms may appear deceptively encapsulated. Histologic examination discloses all degrees of differentiation, from slowly growing tumors that closely resemble "cellular fibromas" except for their having more than three mitoses per ten high-power fields, to wildly anaplastic neoplasms dominated by bizarre giant cells and frequent mitoses (Fig. 7–8). Identifying the fibroblastic origin of these undifferentiated lesions is often difficult and sometimes impossible. The special stains previously mentioned may be helpful. As alluded to earlier, all manner of mixed cell patterns may be encountered with areas of myxomatous, lipomatous, chondromatous, and osteomatous tissue within a basically fibromatous neoplasm. Whether to encumber such lesions with such compound designations as fibromyxosarcoma depends on the prominence of the additional elements and, in the last analysis, is highly subjective.

The clinical significance of ovarian, dental, and neural fibromas is considered elsewhere. The outlook for fibrosarcomas depends, of course, on their size, extent of spread, and level of differentiation and mostly on their location and, therefore, resectability. Overall, in adults, about one-quarter will have metastasized by the time of diagnosis. For the remaining nondisseminated lesions, only very radical resection when possible will prevent local recurrence, usually within months. The prognosis for children is somewhat better than that for adults.

MYXOMA

Myxomas are extremely rare neoplasms encountered virtually in adults only, and principally within skeletal muscle, in retroperitoneal tissue, subcutaneously, and rarely in bone (jaws). They seldom occur in children. Much more common are myxoid areas in other forms of mesenchymal neoplasia. However, such areas often are merely loose edematous connective tissue, which invites the overuse of such diagnoses as fibromyxoma, myxolipoma, and the like.

True myxomas range in size from small subcutaneous masses to large neoplasms in skeletal muscle or in the retroperitoneal region, which sometimes weigh over 1000 gm. They often infiltrate into contiguous structures and therefore may be difficult to excise. Grossly, they are pale gray, gelatinous, sometimes slimy masses that are almost never encapsulated. Histologically, large stellate or spindle-shaped cells are seen floating, as it were, in an abundant acid mucopolysaccharide ground substance. Often the ground substance is traversed by thin strands of collagen fibrils. Mitotic activity usually is not evident. When changes suggestive of malignant transformation are present, it is highly likely that the lesion represents an area of myxoid change in some other form of mesenchymal sarcoma, most commonly **liposarcoma.** Pure myxosarcomas are exceedingly rare, if indeed they occur. Polypoid, sometimes papillary, neoplasms termed "myxomas" also arise in the cardiac chambers, usually within the atria (p. 605). Although they resemble histologically the other myxomas already described, they often have a greater variability in structure since they arise from multipotential mesenchymal cells.

LIPOMA AND LIPOSARCOMA

Lipomas are extremely common benign tumors, found principally in the subcutaneous tissues (on the neck and trunk and less often on the face, hands, and feet), but they also occur in deeper structures such as in the retroperitoneum, skeletal muscle, mediastinum, gastrointestinal tract, and indeed in any location where fat is normally found. Children are rarely affected; most patients are in the fifth or sixth decade of life. There appears to be a correlation between the development of these neoplasms and obesity. Most often they occur singly or in limited numbers, but occasionally multiple lipomatous masses affect an entire extremity, for example, or other region, sometimes in association with other endocrine and neurologic disturbances. Whether such lipomatosis is neoplastic or instead an exaggerated differentiation of connective tissue into fatty tissue is not clear.

In a subcutaneous location the true lipoma is small (1 to 4 cm in diameter), poorly delimited, and thinly encapsulated and has the appearance of typical adult adipose tissue. Demarcation of the tumor may be difficult because of its poor encapsulation and the tendency for lobules to project into surrounding fatty tissue. Hemorrhage and necrosis are uncommon. On microscopic section, most of these lesions are indistinguishable from adult fat; however, admixtures of fibrous tissue may occasionally be present. Other mesenchymal elements are sometimes present, for example, in the angiolipoma, fibrolipoma, or myelolipoma (containing hematopoietic tissue).

Benign lipomas are of little clinical significance, save for their cosmetic effects. More deeply situated lesions may cause pressure symptoms on contiguous structures, but as with all masses they require differentiation from more ominous lesions. It is doubtful that liposarcomas ever arise in preexisting lipomas.

Liposarcomas are not only the most common soft tissue sarcoma in adults, but are also among the most pleomorphic of all neoplasms. Relative to lipomas, they are extremely uncommon. Occurrence in childhood is exceptional.

In contrast to lipomas, most liposarcomas arise in deep structures such as the retroperitoneum, mesentery, and axilla and very rarely in subcutaneous locations. On gross inspection these tumors tend to have a somewhat more opaque gray-white to yellow appearance than lipomas, and are usually poorly delimited and not encapsulated. They may achieve massive size (many kilograms) and invade surrounding structures, and so they commonly grow about blood vessels and enclose neighboring organs. Areas of cystic softening, hemorrhage, and necrosis are frequently present. Many times they assume a myxoid gelatinous appearance.

The range of histologic variability of these forms of cancer has led to their being divided into four types: (1) well differentiated, (2) myxoid, (3) round cell, and (4) pleomorphic.[68, 69] The **well-differentiated liposarcoma** is easily misinterpreted as a lipoma. It is composed almost always of adult-appearing fat cells, which, however, generally retain a rim of discernible cytoplasm about the large central fatty vacuole and in addition have prominent nuclei, displaying the anaplasia of malignancy. Variable amounts of myxomatous tissue may be present, as well as occasional stellate and spindle cells having only scant, small, cytoplasmic fatty vacuoles. The **myxoid liposarcoma** is the most common variant. It contains rather primitive mesenchymal-appearing cells, dispersed throughout an abundant ground substance. The neoplastic cells range from adult-appearing fat cells to stellate, pleomorphic, more primitive-appearing cells with cytoplasmic processes containing minute vacuoles (Fig. 7–9). Tumor giant cells may appear but are not common, and mitoses are few in number. Typically, there is a prominent vascularization in the form of branching capillary channels that produce a "chicken-wire" pattern. The **round cell liposarcoma** is composed of masses of small round cells having distinct acidophilic cytoplasm and prominent anaplastic nuclei. Occasional cells bearing fatty vacuoles, referred to as lipoblasts, are requisite for the diagnosis. Mitoses are much more common in this pattern, and sometimes the cells are segregated into small clusters or pseudoglandular arrangements by traversing strands of connective tissue. The **pleomorphic pattern** is a highly undifferentiated, wildly anaplastic lesion, readily confused with a variety of other poorly differentiated mesenchymal sarcomas. Paradoxically, the cells in the pleomorphic variant may contain little or no fatty vacuolation, and thus some pleomorphic liposarcomas may represent, in final analysis, malignant neoplasms arising from relatively primitive mesenchymal cells.

The clinical behavior of liposarcomas is as varied as their histology. The well-differentiated and myxoid liposarcomas are usually locally invasive and may stubbornly recur following incomplete excision, but they rarely metastasize. Occasionally the recurrences are delayed for as long as years or even decades. In contrast, round cell and pleomorphic patterns may be highly aggressive lesions, with widespread metastases as well as local recurrence, with a five-year survival rate of less than 20%.

LEIOMYOMA AND LEIOMYOSARCOMA

Tumors composed of smooth muscle cells range from the clearly benign leiomyoma to anaplastic leiomyosarcomas. Intermediate variants have been segregated into a group called "smooth muscle tumors of uncertain malignant potential." In addition, one distinctive variant that arises most often in the gastrointestinal tract is called an "epithelioid smooth muscle tumor" or "leiomyoblastoma." Leiomyomas and leiomyosarcomas are found most often in the uterus, and indeed the leiomyoma is the most frequent tumor in women. Rarely these smooth muscle tumors take origin from the muscularis of the gut or the media of blood vessels, and thus may occur in any organ or tissue of the body. Because of the locations in which they are preponderant, the leiomyoma and cellular leiomyomas are described on page 1136, the leiomyoblastoma on page 827, and the leiomyosarcoma on page 1140. It suffices to note here that the benign and intermediate lesions are generally discrete, albeit not encapsulated tumors that sometimes achieve extremely large size (15 to 20 cm in diameter). Even leiomyosarcomas may appear deceptively encapsulated, but occasionally they display their true nature by obvious aggressive, infiltrative growth. The leiomyomas and leiomyoblastomas are firm and pearly gray to white on transection, and so must be differentiated on both gross and microscopic levels from fibromas and neurofibromas. The leiomyosarcoma has the typical soft, fish-flesh appearance, often punctuated by areas of hemorrhage, necrosis, and cystic degeneration, requiring differentiation from the fibrosarcoma.

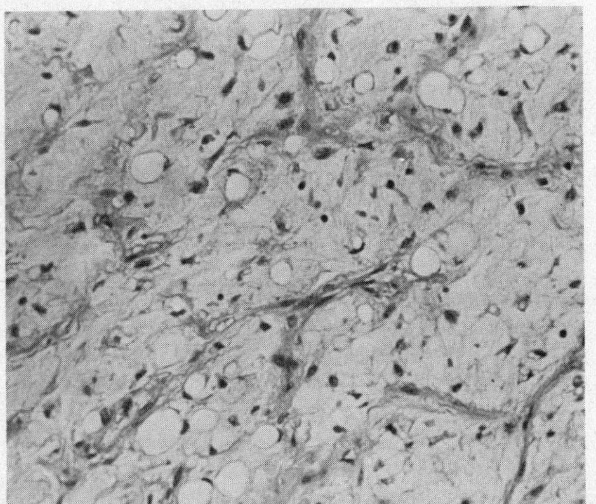

Figure 7–9. Myxoid liposarcoma with abundant ground substance in which are scattered adult-appearing fat cells and more primitive cells, some containing small lipid vacuoles.

BENIGN AND MALIGNANT MESENCHYMOMA

These very rare lesions, composed of two or more mesenchymal elements in addition to fibrous tissue, are perhaps better characterized by the term *"mixed mesenchymal tumors."* The benign variant is most often located in or about the kidney and is composed of a haphazard mixture of adult fat, fibrous tissues, and tangled blood vessels through which are scattered nests or masses of smooth muscle cells. Occasionally there are islands of cartilage, bone, and lymphoid tissue as well as other mesenchymal elements. Because all are extremely mature, these lesions have been interpreted by some as hamartomas (p. 497) rather than neoplasms.

Requisite for the diagnosis of malignant mesenchymoma are at least two or, more rigorously, three cancerous mesenchymal elements within the neoplasm. Since fibroblastic cells are universally present in all neoplasms, particularly those of mesenchymal origin, areas of fibrosarcoma are not accepted by most experts as evidence of variable differentiation. Thus, a liposarcoma or a leiomyosarcoma containing areas of fibrosarcoma would not justify the designation "malignant mesenchymoma," which is best restricted to neoplasms having at least three of the following elements—leiomyosarcoma, myxosarcoma, liposarcoma, chondrosarcoma, osteogenic sarcoma, and hemangioendotheliosarcoma. These cancers may arise anywhere in the body, but are most often found in the extremities and retroperitoneum. Both adults and children may be affected. Aggressive infiltrative neoplasms, they occasionally metastasize and are directly responsible for death in over 50% of adults and about 40% of children.

1. Theologides, A.: Pathogenesis of cachexia in cancer. A review and a hypothesis. Cancer *29*:484, 1972.
2. Theologides, A.: Cancer cachexia. Cancer *43*:2004, 1979.
3. Schein, P.S., et al.: Cachexia of malignancy: Potential role of insulin in nutritional management. Cancer *43*:2070, 1979.
4. Copeland, E.M., III, et al.: Nutrition and cancer. Int. Adv. Surg. Oncol. *4*:1, 1981.
5. Stolinsky, D.C.: Paraneoplastic syndromes. West. J. Med. *132*:189, 1980.
6. Nathanson, L., and Hall, T.C.: Lung tumors: How they produce their syndromes. Ann. N.Y. Acad. Sci. *230*:367, 1974.
7. Gould, V.E., et al.: The APUD cell system and its neoplasms. Observations on the significance and limitations of the concept. Surg. Clin. North Am. *59*:93, 1979.
8. Stewart, A.F., et al.: Biochemical evaluation of patients with cancer-associated hypercalcemia. Evidence for humoral and nonhumoral groups. N. Engl. J. Med. *303*:1377, 1980.
9. Benson, R.C., Jr., et al.: Immunoreactive forms of circulating parathyroid hormone in primary and ectopic hyperparathyroidism. J. Clin. Invest. *54*:175, 1974.
10. Raisz, I.G., et al.: Comparison of commercially available parathyroid hormone immunoassays in the differential diagnosis of hypercalcemia due to primary hyperparathyroidism or malignancy. Ann. Intern. Med. *91*:739, 1979.
11. Metz, S.A., et al.: Prostaglandins as mediators of paraneoplastic syndromes: Review and update. Metabolism *30*:299, 1981.
12. Croft, P.B., and Wilkinson, M.: The incidence of carcinomatous neuropathy with special reference to carcinoma of the lung and breast. In Brain, R., and Norris, F.H. (eds.): The Remote Effects of Carcinoma on the Nervous System. New York, Grune & Stratton, 1965.
13. Eagen, J.W., and Lewis, E.J.: Glomerulopathies of neoplasia. Kidney Int. *11*:297, 1977.
14. Clayson, D.B.: Nutrition and experimental carcinogenesis. Cancer Res. *35*:3292, 1975.
15. Editorial: Vitamin A and cancer. Lancet *1*:575, 1980.
16. Prehn, R.T.: The immune reaction as a stimulator of tumor growth. Science *176*:170, 1972.
17. Prehn, R.T.: Do tumors grow because of the immune response of the host? Transplant. Rev. *28*:34, 1976.
18. Sjögren, H.O., et al.: Suggestive evidence that the "blocking antibodies" of tumor-bearing individuals may be antigen-antibody complexes. Proc. Nat. Acad. Sci. U.S.A. *68*:1372, 1971.
19. Siegel, B.V.: Tumor immunity. An overview. Am. J. Pathol. *93*:515, 1978.
20. Henney, C.S., et al.: Natural killer cells, in vitro and in vivo. Am. J. Pathol. *93*:459, 1978.
21. Thomas, L.: Reactions to homologous tissue antigens in relation to hypersensitivity. *In* Lawrence, H.S. (ed.): Cellular and Humoral Aspects of Hypersensitive States. New York, Hober-Harper, 1959, p. 259.
22. Burnet, F.M.: The concept of immunological surveillance. Prog. Exp. Tumor Res. *13*:1, 1970.
23. Canevari, S., et al.: Humoral cytotoxicity in melanoma patients and its correlation with the extent and course of the disease. Int. J. Cancer *16*:722, 1975.
24. Carpentier, N.A., et al.: Circulating immune complexes and the prognosis of acute myeloid leukemia. N. Engl. J. Med. *307*:1174, 1982.
25. Terry, W.D.: Immunotherapy of malignant melanoma. N. Engl. J. Med. *303*:1174, 1980.
26. Klein, G.: Immune and non-immune control of neoplastic development: Contrasting effects of host and tumor evolution. Cancer *45*:2486, 1980.
27. Hewitt, H.B., et al.: A critique of the evidence of active host defence against cancer based on personal studies of 27 murine tumours of spontaneous origin. Br. J. Cancer *33*:241, 1976.
28. Good, R.A.: Relations between immunity and malignancy. Proc. Natl. Acad. Sci. U.S.A. *69*:1026, 1972.
29. Penn, I., and Starzl, T.E.: Malignant tumors arising *de novo* in immunosuppressed organ transplant recipients. Transplantation *14*:407, 1972.
30. Drew, S.I.: Immunological surveillance against neoplasia: An immunological quandary. Hum. Pathol. *10*:5, 1979.
31. Schwartz, R.S.: Immunoregulation. Oncogenic viruses and malignant lymphomas. Lancet *1*:1266, 1972.
32. Melief, C.J.M., and Schwartz, R.S.: Immunocompetence and malignancy. *In* Becker, F.F. (ed.): Cancer: A Comprehensive Treatise. Vol. 1. New York, Plenum Press, 1982, p. 161.
33. Rygaard, J., and Povlsen, C.O.: The nude mouse versus the hypothesis of immunological surveillance. Transplant. Rev. *28*:43, 1976.
34. Kiessling, R., et al.: Killer cells: A functional comparison between natural, immune T-cell and antibody-dependent in vitro systems. J. Exp. Med. *143*:772, 1976.
35. Herberman, R.B., and Ortaldo, J.R.: Natural killer cells: Their role in defenses against disease. Science *214*:24, 1981.
36. Riccardi, C., et al.: Transfer to cyclophosphamide-treated mice of natural killer (NK) cells and in vivo natural reactivity against tumors. J. Immunol. *126*:1284, 1981.
37. Friedman, H., et al.: Tumor-induced immunosuppression. Am. J. Pathol. *93*:499, 1978.
38. Kadish, A.S., et al.: Natural cytotoxicity and interferon production in human cancer: Deficient natural killer activity and normal interferon production in patients with advanced disease. J. Immunol. *127*:1817, 1981.
39. Priestman, T.J.: Interferons and cancer: The end of the beginning or the beginning of the end? Clin. Oncol. *7*:271, 1981.
40. Sikora, K.: Does interferon cure cancer? Br. Med. J. *281*:855, 1980.
41. American Cancer Society: Cancer Statistics, 1984. CA *34*:7, 1984.
41A. American Cancer Society: Cancer Facts and Figures, 1982, p. 11.
42. Schottenfeld, D.: The epidemiology of cancer. An overview. Cancer *47*(Suppl.):1095, 1981.
43. Jones, P.M.: Cancer in children. Practitioner *222*:221, 1979.
44. Fraumeni, J.F., Jr.: Constitutional disorders of man prediposing to leukemia and lymphoma. Natl. Cancer. Inst. Monogr. *32*:221, 1969.
45. Sinks, T., and Sumer, L.F.: Advances in childhood solid tumors. Adv. Pediatr. *25*:415, 1978.
46. Keller, M. (ed.): Some consequences of alcohol use. I. Alcohol and cancer. *In* Alcohol and Health. Second Special Report to the United States Congress. United States Department of Health, Education, and Welfare. Rockville, MD, National Institute on Alcohol Abuse and Alcoholism, 1974, p. 69.
47. Schottenfeld, D.: Alcohol as a cofactor in the etiology of cancer. Cancer *43*:1962, 1979.
48. Harris, C.C., et al.: Individual differences in cancer susceptibility. Ann. Intern. Med. *92*:809, 1980.
49. Lynch, H.T.: Genetics, etiology, and human cancer. Prev. Med. *9*:231, 1980.
50. Knudson, A.G., et al.: Heredity and cancer in man. Prog. Med. Genet. *9*:113, 1973.
51. Knudson, A.G.: Genetics and etiology of human cancer. Adv. Hum. Genet. *8*:1, 1977.
52. Knudson, A.G.: Genetics and cancer. *In* Burchenal, J.H., and Oettgen, H.F. (eds.): Cancer. Achievements, Challenges and Prospects for the 1980s. Vol. 1. New York, Grune & Stratton, 1981, p. 381.
53. Swift, M., et al.: Malignant neoplasms in the families of patients with ataxia telangiectasia. Cancer Res. *36*:209, 1976.
54. Papanicolaou, G.N.: New cancer diagnosis. *In* Proceedings of the Race Betterment Conference. Battle Creek, Michigan, Race Betterment Foundation, 1928, p. 528.
55. Papanicolaou, G.N., and Traut, H.: Diagnosis of Uterine Cancer by the Vaginal Smear. New York, The Commonwealth Fund, 1943.
56. McIntire, K.R.: Tumor markers for radioimmunodetection of cancer. Cancer Res. *40*:3083, 1980.
57. Ewing, H.P., et al.: Tumor markers. Curr. Probl. Surg. *19*:53, 1982.
58. Holyoke, E.D., et al.: Biologic markers in cancer diagnosis and treatment. Curr. Probl. Cancer *6*:1, 1981.
59. Jaffe, E.S., et al.: Functional markers: A new perspective on malignant lymphomas. Cancer Treat. Rev. *61*:953, 1977.
60. Gold, P., and Freedman, S.O.: Demonstration of tumor-specific antigens in human colonic carcinomata by immunological tolerance and absorption techniques. J. Exp. Med. *121*:439, 1965.
61. Szymendera, J.J., et al.: Predictive value of plasma CEA levels: Preoperative prognosis and postoperative monitoring of patients with colorectal carcinoma. Dis. Colon Rectum *25*:46, 1982.
62. Green, J.B., III, and Trowbridge, A.A.: The use of carcinoembryonic antigen in the clinical management of colorectal cancer. Surg. Clin. North Am. *59*:831, 1979.
63. Rouslahti, E., and Seppala, M.: Alpha-fetoprotein in cancer and fetal development. Adv. Cancer Res. *29*:275, 1979.
64. Menendez-Botet, C.J., et al.: A preliminary evaluation of tissue polypeptide antigen in serum or urine (or both) of patients with cancer or benign neoplasms. Clin. Chem. *24*:868, 1978.
65. Kumar, S., et al.: The clinical significance of tissue polypeptide antigen (TPA) in the urine of bladder cancer patients. Br. J. Urol. *53*:578, 1981.
66. Neville, A.M., et al.: Monoclonal antibodies and human tumor pathology. Hum. Pathol. *13*:1067, 1982.
67. Prat, J., and Scully, R.E.: Cellular fibromas and fibrosarcomas of the ovary: A comparative clinicopathologic analysis of 17 cases. Cancer *47*:2663, 1981.
68. Enzinger, F.M., and Winslow, D.J.: Liposarcoma: A study of 103 cases. Virchows Arch. (Pathol. Anat.) *335*:367, 1962.
69. Enterline, H.T.: Liposarcoma—a clinical and pathological study of 53 cases. Cancer *13*:932, 1960.

INFECTIOUS DISEASES

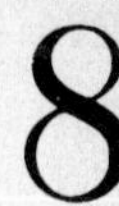

FRANZ VON LICHTENBERG, M.D.

Viral, Chlamydial, Rickettsial, and Bacterial Diseases

*Infectious diseases of limited geographic distribution are marked by an asterisk.

INTRODUCTION

Ever since Pandora opened her mythical box, infectious diseases have plagued humanity, evolving with changing life conditions and population expansion. Indigenous cultures in equilibrium with their endemic infectious diseases have been devastated by contact with infections of modern civilization; indeed, more American Indians may have died of measles than of the white man's bullets.[1] As urban populations expanded, insanitary crowding invited the great medieval pandemics of plague and cholera, which now persist only in localized pockets. Even today, societies in densely populated developing countries are prey to tuberculosis, leprosy, malaria, filariasis, and schistosomiasis. Smallpox alone is back in Pandora's box, thanks to the only wholehearted international preventive campaign ever undertaken.

Medical practices too have altered the panorama of infectious diseases. Since Jenner's time, vaccines have curbed many infections including diphtheria, whooping cough, paralytic poliomyelitis, and measles. Since the discovery of penicillin by Fleming, generations of new antibiotics and microbicidal drugs have radically changed the prevalence and course of most infectious diseases so that they now rarely appear in their classical forms. Yet for some, especially many viral infections, we still lack adequate prevention and treatment. Even preventable infectious disorders keep festering amid urban and rural squalor and during war and famine. Neither affluence nor improved medical technology have curbed the spread of venereal infections. In fact, medical technology itself is responsible for a new category of microbial diseases called "opportunistic infections." "Altered hosts" who receive cytotoxic and immunosuppressive therapy for tumors and tissue transplants become vulnerable to infections that are usually innocuous or dormant in normal adults. Invasive hospital procedures such as intubation, catheterization, or prosthetic implantation have provided new opportunities for such infections to gain entry.[2]

Bacteria are masters of genetic engineering, which they use to ensure their diversity and selective survival. Antibiotics have magnified selection pressures and, when given in subcurative doses, favor the emergence of resistant clones that can ignite dangerous hospital epidemics.[3] "New diseases" appear from time to time. Venereal syphilis was unknown before the siege of Naples in 1494. Legionnaires' disease made its debut in Philadelphia in 1976; its causative agent has now been recognized as a member of an entirely new class of bacterial pathogens. At the time of this writing, an epidemic of "acquired immune deficiency syndrome" (AIDS) is being reported.[4]

In this age of international travel and vast population displacements, diseases are "exotic" only to the eye of the beholder, and the global view of infectious diseases is amply justified. For convenience, *geographically restricted diseases*, including those in the U.S., are marked by an asterisk in this chapter. Some, however, will increasingly appear outside their known perimeters as global distances keep shrinking; others illustrate important pathogenic mechanisms and have therefore been referred to briefly, as necessary.

Infectious diseases are the consequence of host-parasite interactions, and we shall first review the principles involved, together with the contributions of microbiology and immunology.

FACTORS RELATING TO PARASITE

Cooperation between microorganisms and higher phyla is the rule; disease is the exception.[5] No animal is free of smaller life except when reared as a germ-free laboratory artifact. Normal humans would be at risk of a vitamin K deficiency without their gut flora, which synthesize this essential nutrient. We are blissfully unaware of the Dermatonyssus mites that scavenge our hair follicles. Relationships that benefit both host and fellow passenger are termed *symbiotic*. *Commensals* share the host's food intake. *Saprophytes* harmlessly thrive on human excreta. *True parasites are those that interfere with the host's integrity and function, and the degree of such interference is a measure of their virulence or pathogenicity and of the adaptation of the host.* Long-standing human parasites tend to cause milder disease than those newly introduced, perhaps because sustained coexistence within a single host best subserves the perpetuation of the parasite—"selfish genes."

Human parasites belong to many plant and animal phyla, and range in size from the 20-nm poliovirus to the 10-m tapeworm *Taenia saginata*. Most are "microbes," i.e., are microscopic in size. Biochemically, the smallest viruses code for only three polypeptides, while the molecular complexity of helminths almost equals that of man. Speed of genetic variation depends on reproductive rate rather than size, and therefore fast-multiplying agents are better able to stay ahead of their host's defensive maneuvers. Some infectious organisms are *invariably pathogenic* for humans and their recovery in culture always signifies disease. Others must be regarded as *facultative pathogens* capable of either *colonization*, *invasion*, or both in succession; positive cultures of such organisms must therefore be interpreted cautiously, especially if the lesions in the host are incompatible with the particular agent found. The fungus *Candida albicans* offers a prime example. This organism is found in the oral cavity, gastrointestinal tract, and vagina of many normal individuals. Only in the predisposed host is it capable of producing opportunistic infections. With present-day methods of perpetuating life, the list and diversity of facultative human pathogens keeps expanding, and few organisms colonizing humans can any longer be regarded as categorically innocuous.

Parasites vary with regard to the tissue and cellular microenvironment best suited to their survival and reproduction. For some, the skin provides the optimal habitat; for others, a mucosal surface; and for still others, the internal environment of the host. Some organisms are *extracellular parasites* and reproduce only outside of cells, but in this environment are vulnerable to phagocytosis. Other *obligate intracellular parasites* require an intracellular microenvironment or must replicate in the nucleus of the host cell, as is the case with some viruses. Some parasites can reproduce only within specific cell types or cellular organelles, which they seek out within the host. Still other organisms are *facultative intracellular parasites* that can survive and reproduce either outside of or within cells (Table 8–1). The ability of microorganisms to convert from one state or habitat to another must always be kept in mind. Indeed, the higher parasite phyla have complex *life cycles* and must pass through alternate forms and hosts or environmental niches, in order to infect man.

Many biomechanisms underlie the tendency of organisms to seek and colonize specific host tissues or cells; this is referred to as *tropism*, and is most highly developed among the obligate intracellular parasites. It seems likely that receptor-ligand interactions, thus far demonstrated in only a few cases, eventually will clarify the exquisite specificities of certain viruses such as rabies or poliomyelitis for the central nervous system (neurotropism), as well as certain bacterial specificities like that of gonococcal pili for mucosal cells (Fig. 8–1).[6] Parasite entry into host cells can be *passive* (i.e., by phagocytosis, pinocytosis, or membrane fusion (as with

Table 8–1. CLASSES OF HUMAN ENDOPARASITES AND THEIR HABITATS

Taxonomic Class	Size	Site of Propagation	Sample Species and Its Disease	
Viruses	20–30 nm	Obl. intracellular	Poliovirus	Poliomyelitis
Chlamydiae	200–1000 nm	Obl. intracellular	*C. trachomatis*	Trachoma
Rickettsiae	300–1200 nm	Obl. intracellular	*R. prowazekii*	Typhus fever
Mycoplasmas	125–350 nm	Extracellular*	*M. pneumoniae*	Atypical pneumonia
Bacteria, spirochetes, mycobacteria	0.8–15 μm	Cutaneous	*Staphylococcus epidermidis**	Wound infection
		Mucosal	*Vibrio cholerae*	Cholera
		Extracellular	*Streptococcus pneumoniae*	Pneumonia
		Fac. intracellular	*Mycobacterium tuberculosis*	Tuberculosis
Fungi Imperfecti	2–200 μm	Cutaneous	Tinea pedis	Athlete's foot
		Mucosal	*Candida albicans**	Oral thrush
		Extracellular	*Sporothrix schenkii*	Sporotrichosis
		Fac. Intracellular	*Histoplasma capsulatum*	Histoplasmosis
Protozoa	1–50 mm	Mucosal	*Giardia lamblia*	Giardiasis
		Extracellular	*Trypanosoma gambiense*	Sleeping sickness
		Fac. intracellular	*Trypanosoma cruzi**	Chagas' disease
		Obl. intracellular	*Leishmania donovani*	Kala-azar
Helminths	3 mm–10 m	Mucosal	*Enterobius vermicularis*	Oxyuriasis
		Extracellular	*Wuchereria bancrofti*	Filariasis
		Intracellular	*Trichinella spiralis**	Trichinosis

* = Has alternate life stage, habitat, or disease form, described in text; Obl. = obligate; Fac. = facultative.

coated viruses)) or *active* and energy-requiring (as with rickettsiae or protozoa).

TRANSMISSION OF INFECTIOUS AGENTS

Organisms causing infectious disease may be transmitted to vulnerable hosts through a variety of pathways:

1. *Direct spread* by contact or airborne particles from sick individuals to healthy hosts is characteristic of *contagious* infection such as childhood measles or chickenpox. Such spread may result in epidemics. In some instances, short- or long-term asymptomatic carriers or shedders act as human reservoirs.

2. Spread may also occur by way of *contaminated water, food, or soil* from human or environmental reservoirs. The proverbial "Typhoid Mary," carrying *typhoid bacilli* in her gallbladder and stool, constituted such a human reservoir. *Legionella* may be disseminated from water tanks or cooling devices in which conditions for the proliferation of this bacterium are favorable. *Naegleria fowleri,* an ameboflagellate living in overgrown summer ponds, is an example of a free-living organism that can produce lethal meningoencephalitis in young healthy divers by penetrating the cribriform plate of the nasal roof.[7]

3. Infections can be acquired *prenatally,* passed from mother to fetus via the placenta, or *perinatally,* transmitted during or shortly after delivery.

4. Infections transmitted to humans from an animal host or reservoir are termed *zoonotic.* This occurs with all classes of parasites from viruses (e.g., equine encephalitis) to helminths (e.g., the pig roundworm, Trichinella). Zoonotic infections can be more or less pathogenic for humans than for their normal animal hosts. Some bat species harbor the lethal rabies virus with relative impunity, while the cowpox virus, causing disease in its natural host, is innocuous enough for man to serve as a vaccine against smallpox.

In sum, transmission of infection involves a number of factors including parasite biology, vector competence, human behavior, and environmental conditions. Epidemiologic science analyzes all these factors in the hope

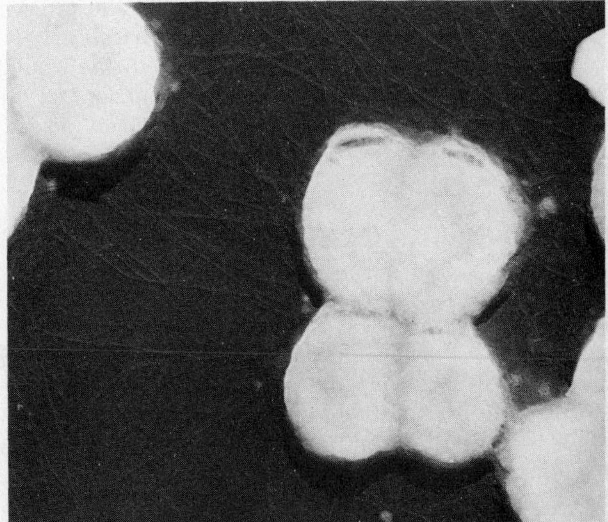

Figure 8–1. Gonococci with pili (as seen by scanning electron microscopy). (Courtesy of Dr. Nicholas Guerina, Department of Pathology, Brigham and Women's Hospital.)

of devising methods of preventing disease transmission, still by far the best way of controlling human infections.[8]

FACTORS RELATING TO HOST

Fortunately there are many *host barriers to infection* that prevent access of parasites to their required environment or, failing that, can suppress infection or curtail its spread. These barriers and defenses take many forms, including (1) the intact integument and mucosal surfaces and secretions; (2) phagocytic white cells that are promptly marshaled to sites of entry; (3) the resident mononuclear-phagocyte (reticuloendothelial) system that effectively polices the internal environment for errant organisms; and (4) the all-important immune system. Phagocytosis (p. 49) and immunity (p. 158) have already been discussed. Overall, normal human barriers to infection are quite effective considering the ample opportunity that microbes have to consort with man. Only four of each ten exposures to gonococci actually result in gonorrhea, and it takes 10^8 vibrios, when ingested by human volunteers with normal gastric juices, to produce cholera.[9] However, normal barriers do occasionally fail, as is evident by the frequency of infectious disease.

The route by which infection enters may be (1) respiratory; (2) oral-fecal; (3) transmucosal; or (4) transcutaneous, usually aided by trauma, arthropod vectors, needles, or other contaminated devices. Most human pathogens follow a preferential route, but this does not preclude other possible entry sites. For instance, the bulk of tuberculous infections arise by droplet aspiration, but some may begin through the swallowing of infected milk or contaminated skin puncture. Moreover, the site of entry does not necessarily conform to the site of disease. The best example is the tropism of many viruses. The polioviruses first insensibly replicate in permissive host cells along the GI tract, but then exert their destructive effects on neuronal targets, the anterior horn cells of the spinal cord. The tetanus bacilli may be confined to an inconspicuous contaminated skin wound while their toxin disrupts axonal transmission in the spinal cord. Usually, however, infection and disease localize and spread together.

HOST-PARASITE RELATIONSHIPS

Whether exposure to an infectious organism will result in disease is determined by the *virulence (or pathogenicity) of the invader* and by the *resistance of the host*. Although *infection* and *infectious disease* are words often used interchangeably, they are not synonymous. Thus, the ability of an organism to establish itself in a given host is termed its *infectivity*, and its disease-producing potential is referred to as *virulence*. The terms *resistance* and *virulence* are broad generalizations based on the complex host-parasite interplay that takes place at the molecular level. *High virulence implies the capability of causing disease in normally resistant people, i.e., in the majority of an exposed population. Low virulence denotes an agent effective only in hosts with low resistance, such as an opportunistic agent causing disease in hosts with impaired defense mechanisms, particularly impaired immune responses.*

The multiple parasite properties and products that, in their composite, determine virulence are only partly known; because of their variety and complexity they will be discussed as each microbial class is introduced below. Host resistance, too, is clearly multifactorial, based on genetics, anatomy, and physiology as well as on the functions of the immune system. Thus, poor circulatory or ventilatory status, debilitating systemic disease, or localized organ impairments can be equally predisposing to infectious disease as the better-known defects of phagocyte or immune function; several resistance factors can be simultaneously impaired in malnutrition, alcoholism, diabetes, and chronic hepatic or renal failure.

The concept of *pathogenicity* involves all the following:

1. *The ability to establish infection and reproduce inside a host* by overcoming normal defenses or by taking advantage of defective host barriers.
2. *The generation of products* such as endotoxins, exotoxins, lytic enzymes, and other substances that *directly damage host tissue* beyond its normal repair capacity.
3. The *induction of host-cellular responses* that, although directed against the invader, may cause additional host damage. Thus, the immune response to the hepatitis viruses mediates the destruction of liver cells harboring viral or viral-directed antigens. Closely related is the phenomenon of cross reaction between microorganisms (nonself antigens) and self antigens, which constitutes a possible mechanism of the induction of autoimmune diseases (p. 179).

In the microbiologists' view, pathogenicity is linked to specific virulence factors such as the phage-induced exotoxin of *Corynebacterium diphtheriae* without which this organism acts as a commensal. To the cell biologist and immunologist, host resistance is paramount. For example, during an epidemic of meningococcal infection, some contacts develop meningitis, but others carry the meningococcus in their nasal secretions for weeks without ill effect. Similarly, infections with *herpes simplex* virus I are common and may remain indefinitely dormant, detectable only by antibody titer. However, such infections may episodically generate fever blisters or, in predisposed individuals such as the immunosuppressed, may cause lethal pneumonia or encephalitis (p. 285).

Once introduced, pathogens may stay confined to their entry site or, if motile or reproducing beyond the capacity of host defenses to contain them, will spread, sometimes throughout the body. The routes of spread initially follow tissue planes of least resistance and the regional lymphatic and vascular anatomy. Thus, the virulent nonselective staphylococci may first induce a locally expanding skin abscess (furuncle). Depending on virulence and host resistance, this local infection may then lead to regional *lymphangitis* and *lymphadenitis*, followed by *bacteremia* (blood-borne infection) and colonization of distant organs. In the case of other, more fastidious pathogens, *tropism* determines the primary sites of tissue damage. Once a portal of entry has been gained, there is always the potential for spread to other sites. Transient viremia, bacteremia, or parasitemia is common during the early stages of apparently localized infections, but it is usually curtailed as host leukocytic and immune responses come into play. When these are defective in an altered host or when the invader is highly virulent, spread will ensue. Major, sustained bloodstream invasion is obviously a feared consequence of any infection and is often fatal.

HOST TISSUE RESPONSES TO INFECTION

In contrast to the almost unlimited molecular diversity of parasites, human cell types and their patterns of response are limited, as are the mediator mechanisms directing these responses. At the microscopic level, therefore, many pathogens evoke identical reaction patterns, and few of the features are unique to or pathognomonic of each agent.

Broadly speaking, there are five microscopic patterns of reaction:

1. *Exudative inflammation*. This is the familiar reaction to acute tissue damage described in Chapter 2, with increased vascular permeability and leukotaxis, predominantly of neutrophils. Massing of neutrophils results in the formation of pus. The rapidly dividing organisms that evoke this response, many of them bacteria of extracellular habit, are called "pyogenic." The chronic or healing phase of this pattern is often termed "nonspecific chronic inflammation."

2. *Necrotizing inflammation*. When tissue damage is initially severe, as in the case of highly virulent or toxic microorganisms, cell death can become the dominant feature, with relatively few reactive exudative components. These lesions may come to resemble ischemic necrosis. This reaction is also prone to appear when opportunistic pathogens acutely infect a host lacking cellular defenses.

3. *Granulomatous inflammation*. This pattern, dominated by aggregates of mononuclear phagocytes, is usually evoked by relatively slow-dividing infectious agents and by those of relatively large size, unmanageable by neutrophils alone; it is also common among the facultative intracellular organisms. Granulomas are among the more distinctive microscopic lesions and therefore suggest certain specific agents as their likely cause (p. 343).

4. *Interstitial inflammation*. Diffuse, predominantly mononuclear interstitial infiltration is a common feature of all chronic inflammatory processes, but when it occurs acutely and in pure form, it is often a response to a viral agent. It also may arise in other infections that stimulate intense lymphocytic reactions, as in early treponemal diseases. This histologic pattern is often quite difficult to interpret in terms of its possible cause.

5. *Cytopathic-cytoproliferative inflammation*. When cell damage of a distinctive type precedes cell destruction, it may initiate cell replication and the formation of inclusion bodies or polykaryons. Such a reaction suggests an obligate intracellular parasite, usually a virus, even when the stromal inflammatory activity is relatively minor.

The above patterns of tissue reaction are useful as working tools in analyzing microscopic features of infective processes, but they rarely appear in pure form because they frequently overlap. More important, they are not exclusively due to infectious processes, but can also be seen in tissue responses to physicochemical agents or in inflammatory diseases of unknown etiology. Their most useful role is that of complementing a patient's clinical and microbiologic findings. If all three sets of observations are mutually compatible, diagnosis is assured; if not, the evidence must be reviewed for possible error or artefact. Histopathologic diagnosis, therefore, plays an important role in deciphering the nature of an infectious disease.

VIRAL DISEASES

Viruses are obligate intracellular parasites whose effects on host cells range from lytic destruction, with fast viral replication, to mutual integration, with long-term persistence of the infection. Induction of neoplastic cell transformation (p. 243) is yet another consequence of viral infection in animals, but yet to be proved in humans. Specific cell membrane proteins or lipids are the attachment sites or receptors for viruses that determine their host range and tropisms. Viral cell entry is usually analogous to that of hormones or other ligands. Once firmly bound, they enter coated pits to be transferred into cytoplasmic vacuoles (pH 5.0) named endosomes. Some viruses fuse with endosome membranes and release their nucleocapsid into the cytosol (influenza virus); others delay this process until their carrier endosome fuses with the nuclear membrane (polyoma virus) or with other organelles. Some, like the Sendai virus, enter host cells directly by fusing their coat with the plasma membrane.[10]

Infection of target cells commonly results in "lytic viral infection" followed by viremia. The dissemination of viral particles through the blood is generally brief and abates as neutralizing host antibody rises. Direct cell-to-cell spread is also important and can be promoted by viral gene products that induce host cell fusions, observable as multinucleate cells or "polykaryons." New antigens or viral "neoantigens" may appear in the host cell plasma membrane. In *lytic viral infection* the cellular host is directed to produce large numbers of progeny virus. Some viral gene products inhibit the host cell's own metabolic pathways, such as the sigma-3 protein of the reovirus, an ADP-ribosyl transferase that blocks polypeptide assembly on host cell ribosomes.[11] Others utilize the substrates and enzymes of host cells for their own reproduction, and direct host ribosomes and Golgi systems to manufacture viral proteins and glycoproteins while host DNA polymerases are spurred to replicate viral genome. In addition, viruses may alter cytoskeletal components such as vimentin.[12] These subversive viral activities result in changes in cell shape and staining, visible as "cytopathic effects." When seen in tissue or culture, these abnormalities (such as *viral inclusions*) are often distinctive of specific viruses. Inclusions can be intranuclear, intracytoplasmic, or both; they represent either collections of virions (adenovirus) or altered cell products and dead virions (herpesvirus). Some inclusions are diagnostically useful, as in smallpox or herpesvirus infection, but it should be noted that *similar inclusions can have nonviral causes. Conversely, in many important viral infections inclusion bodies do not occur and their absence, therefore, does not preclude a viral etiology.* Immunofluorescent methods for viral antigens, tissue culture, and serology must often be used to establish the specific viral etiology.

Instead of inducing cell lysis, viruses can persist in cells to establish long-term *latency.* The basis for this relationship is poorly understood. One mechanism appears to be the ability to lyse the primary phagosome membrane of macrophages and thus escape into the cytosol (vaccinia virus). Other viruses develop a close integrative association with the host cell nucleus or cellular organelles. Thus, herpes zoster–varicella virus can be cultured from spinal and trigeminal ganglia in many symptomless carriers.[13] In other latent viral infections and with the so-called *"slow viruses"* (causing lethal neurologic disease, see p. 1385), the site and form of their long-term latency is not known. However, dormant infections can be reactivated, particularly when host defenses are modified, as exemplified by herpes relapse following even trivial events such as ultraviolet light exposure, emotional stress, or menstruation.

Neutralizing antibodies are important for host defense during viremia, especially by arboviruses and enteroviruses, but are not effective against cell-to-cell or axonal virus propagation. *Cell-mediated immunity is the main host defense.* Involved are: (1) natural killer cells that detect and destroy virus-infected host cells; (2) activated macrophages that serve as both virus killers and cell scavengers; and (3) cytotoxic T cells activated by helper T cells, which must recognize both viral neoantigens and HLA gene products for specific cell lysis.[14] Contributing greatly to the immune response are *interferons,* which either directly inhibit viral intracellular multiplication or enhance cell-mediated responses. Indeed, interferons are the fastest acting antiviral defense mechanism known, but are more effective in early than in established disease.[15] The critical importance of the immune response in defense against viral disease is clearly documented by the effects of immunoincompetence, particularly of T-cell function. Children with the Wiskott-Aldrich syndrome (p. 208), having a deficiency of cell-mediated immunity, fail to develop a typical measles rash and instead may die of giant cell pneumonia. Drug-immunosuppressed patients infected with measles may develop subacute sclerosing panencephalitis (p. 000) even while generating high specific antibody titers. Thus, an intact T-cell system is the major defense against viral disease. However, it is sometimes a two-edged sword. Mice prenatally infected with lymphocytic choriomeningitis are tolerant to this virus and, despite life-long infection, do not develop disease. When sensitized T lymphocytes from postnatally infected mice are adoptively transferred to these recipients, tolerance is broken and lethal meningoencephalitis ensues. By analogy, it is thought that the severity of acute viral hepatitis relates to the adequacy of the immune response. In most normal individuals with an adequate immune reaction, hepatocytes containing viral antigens are destroyed, accounting for the acute hepatic disease. By contrast, in the absence of an adequate immune response, there is no acute disease but instead the development of an asymptomatic carrier state.[16]

Our current understanding of the pathogenesis of viral lesions is insufficient to relate the genetic and biochemical characteristics of each species to the human disease it causes. Both the measles paramyxovirus and a togavirus causing German measles produce similar erythematous skin rashes; conversely, a single herpes virus—the cytomegalovirus—causes divergent clinical syndromes in newborns, in adults, and in immunosuppressed patients. Table 8–2 attempts to list currently known significant human pathogens by predominant disease presentation, rather than by microbiologic criteria. It should be kept in mind that viral diseases are, by definition, systemic infections, and if severe can result in multiorgan and multisystem lesions. *In all sites of involvement, virus infections evoke inflammatory infiltrates composed principally of lymphocytes and macrophages.* Frequently this reaction is found within the interstitium; however, with severe disease parenchymatous cells may also be destroyed, calling forth a neutrophilic infiltration. In active viral infections, the sheer bulk and dispersion of these leukocytic infiltrates may affect vital functions of the neural or cardiac conduction systems.

VIRAL RESPIRATORY DISORDERS

Viral respiratory disorders are caused by many species and serotypes (Table 8–2). They are the most frequent and least preventable of all human infectious diseases, and range in severity from the discomforting but self-limited common cold to life-threatening pneumonia, seen most often in debilitated, hospitalized, or immunosuppressed individuals. Moreover, viral infections of the lung predispose to bacterial superinfection; the rare cases of lethal bacterial pneumonia that originate outside hospitals are usually preceded by a respiratory viral prodrome. The basis of this viral-induced predisposition is not well understood but may involve breakdown of local host barriers, bronchial obstruction, and impairment of phagocyte competence.

Many agents are capable of causing respiratory disease, ranging from *upper respiratory tract infections (URIs)* such as rhinitis, sinusitis, otitis media, pharyngitis, or tonsillitis to *lower respiratory infections (LRIs)* named, as one descends the respiratory tree, laryngotracheobronchitis, bronchiolitis, interstitial pneumonia, and pleuritis. Each viral species may produce one or more of these patterns of disease. Coxsackie viruses are especially versatile: besides nonspecific URIs, certain A strains cause herpangina, a blistering inflammation of the pharynx that must be differentiated from herpes or measles, and the mysterious hand-foot-and-mouth disease. Coxsackie B viruses can cause pleuritis (pleurodynia), myocarditis, or the Guillain-Barré syndrome, and have been implicated in the possible causation of insulin-dependent diabetes mellitus.[17] Echoviruses characteristically produce a pharyngitis with a macular or petechial skin rash, and can also induce myocarditis. Types A, B, and C influenza viruses are the dominating causes of lower respiratory infection marked by fever, myalgias, and headaches (the flu syndromes), but extrapulmonary complications may appear or even be lethal, as, for example, interstitial myocarditis or Reye's syndrome (p. 941) following aspirin therapy.[18] Rhinoviruses

Table 8–2. VIRAL DISEASES AND THEIR PATHOGENS

Predominant Clinical Presentation	Viral Species	Family of Viruses	Genomic Type†	Disease Expression
Respiratory	Adeno	Adeno	DS DNA	Upper, lower respiratory infection, conjunctivitis.
	Echo	Entero*	SS RNA	Pharyngitis, skin rash, URIs
	Rhino	Rhino*	SS RNA	Upper respiratory infection
	Coxsackie	Entero*	SS RNA	Pleurodynia, herpangina, hand-foot-and mouth disease
	Influenza	Orthomyxo	SS RNA‡	Influenza
	Parainfluenza	Paramyxo	SS RNA‡	Lower respiratory infection
	Respiratory syncytial	Paramyxo	SS RNA‡	Bronchiolitis
Digestive				
Salivary gland	Mumps	Paramyxo	SS RNA‡	Mumps, pancreatitis, orchitis
Intestine	Rota	REO	DS RNA‡	Childhood diarrhea
	Parvo	Parvo	SS DNA	Traveler's diarrhea
Liver	Dane particle	Hepato	SS DNA	Hepatitis B
	Hepatitis A	Picorna	DS, SS, DNA	Hepatitis A
	Uncharacterized agents	—	—	Non-A, non-B hepatitis
Epidermal-Epithelial				
Warty growths	Verruca	Papova	DS DNA	Common wart
	Papilloma	Papova	DS DNA	Venereal wart
	Molluscum	Pox	DS DNA‡	Molluscum contagiosum
Exanthemas	Rubeola	Paramyxo	SS DNA‡	Measles
	Rubella	Toga	SS DNA	German measles
Vesicular eruptions	Small pox	Pox	DS DNA‡	Smallpox
	Cowpox	Pox	DS DNA‡	Vaccinia
	Varicella-zoster (HZV)	Herpes	DS DNA	Chickenpox, shingles
	Simplex I (HSV I)	Herpes	DS DNA	Fever blisters
	Simplex II (HSV II)	Herpes	DS DNA	Genital herpes
Hemolymphopoietic	Cytomegalo (CMV)	Herpes	DS DNA	Cytomegalic inclusion disease
	Epstein-Barr (EBV)	Herpes	DS DNA	Infectious mononucleosis
CNS (excluding systemic and arbovirus infections)	Polio	Entero*	SS RNA	Poliomyelitis
	Rabies	Rhabdo	SS RNA‡	Rabies (hydrophobia)
	JC-	Papova	DS DNA	Progressive multifocal leukoencephalopathy
Arthropod-borne				
Hemorrhagic fevers (partial listing)	Dengue	Toga	SS RNA	Dengue, dengue hemorrhagic fever
	Yellow fever	Toga	SS RNA	Yellow fever
	Regional hemorrhagic fevers	Arena	SS RNA	Bolivian, Argentinian, Lassa fever
		Bunya	SS RNA‡	Crimean hemorrhagic fever
		Unknown	—	Korean, Marburg disease
Encephalitides		Toga	SS RNA	Eastern, Western, Venezuelan equine, St. Louis, California, Japanese B encephalitis
Uncertain Pathogenicity		Reo	DS RNA‡	
		Corona	SS RNA‡	
		Retro	SS RNA‡	Human T-cell leukemia

* = Subclass of Picornaviridae (SS RNA); †SS = single-stranded, DS = double-stranded; ‡ = has transcriptase.

are the major causes of the all-too-common cold. Respiratory syncytial viruses and parainfluenza viruses are especially important in infants and children, and can produce lethal bronchiolitis (croup) or pneumonia. Adenoviruses (31 known serotypes) can cause severe sporadic pneumonia, but are more frequently responsible for milder URI outbreaks. Some adenovirus serotypes cause pharyngoconjunctival fever (febrile pharyngitis with unilateral conjunctivitis); serotype B causes alarming epidemics of bilateral hemorrhagic keratoconjunctivitis without respiratory symptoms. Still other adenoviruses have been isolated during a whooping cough–like syndrome.

All these respiratory agents are contagious and are acquired largely by the respiratory route from a sick, incubating, or convalescing individual. An asymptomatic adenovirus carrier state is known among children. For all the agents the incubation time is generally brief, sometimes less than 24 hours.

MORPHOLOGY. The morphologic changes vary for each level of the respiratory tract affected. **URIs** are marked by mucosal hyperemia and swelling, with a nonspecific but predominantly lymphomonocytic and plasmocytic infiltration of the submucosa accompanied by overproduction of mucous secretions. The swollen mucosa and viscid exudate may plug the nasal channels, sinuses, or eustachian tubes and lead to suppurative secondary bacterial infection. Viral-induced tonsillitis with enlargement of the lymphoid tissue within Waldeyer's ring is more characteristic of the young. Histologically, there is lymphoid hyperplasia, usually unassociated with suppuration or abscess formation such as is encountered with streptococci or staphylococci, but bacterial superinfection may transform the picture.

Laryngotracheobronchitis and bronchiolitis often accompanying the common "chest cold" are characterized by vocal cord swelling, abundant mucous exudation, and mucosal changes analogous to those encountered in the URI. Impairment of bronchociliary function invites bacterial superinfection with more marked suppuration. Plugging of small airways may give rise to focal lung atelectasis. In the more severe bronchiolar involvements, widespread plugging of secondary and terminal airways by cell debris, fibrin, and inflammatory exudate may, when prolonged, invite organization and fibrosis giving rise to so-called **viral obliterative bronchiolitis** and to permanent lung damage.

Viral pneumonias, like bacterial pneumonias, take a variety of anatomic forms. They may be patchy or disseminated, interstitial or consolidated, compatible with restoration of normal structure or responsible for permanent damage. In early and milder expressions of viral pneumonia, the involvement is patchy and restricted to an interstitial inflammatory reaction, with edema and mononuclear infiltration of the alveolar septa. The air spaces remain clear save for scattered alveolar macrophages—**"interstitial pneumonia."** The radiographic or clinical findings are not characteristic and may also be produced by **Mycoplasma pneumoniae.** With progression or in more severe involvements, the septal thickening and inflammatory infiltrate become more marked, and type II pneumonocytes round up and desquamate into the alveolar spaces. Leakage of fibrinogen may disrupt the lining epithelial cells with the formation of hyaline membranes layering the septal walls (Fig. 8–2). These changes resemble those of the adult respiratory distress syndrome (diffuse alveolar damage, p. 714). In severe, fulminating, influenzal viral pneumonia, widespread fibrinohemorrhagic alveolar consolidation is superimposed on the changes described. In many instances, however, the consolidative changes reflect bacterial superinfection. Those viruses that have the power to cause necrosis (e.g., the adenovirus and herpesvirus families) can evoke neutrophilic responses indistinguishable from bacterial superinfection. In the usual case, in the absence of parenchymal necrosis, the changes are entirely reversible, with restoration of the normal architecture. However, with protracted involvement or when there have been areas of necrosis, the inflammatory changes give way to interstitial fibrosis and organization of alveolar plugs that fuse with the septa. These changes give rise to the fine reticular or "ground-glass" pattern sometimes seen on chest radiography.

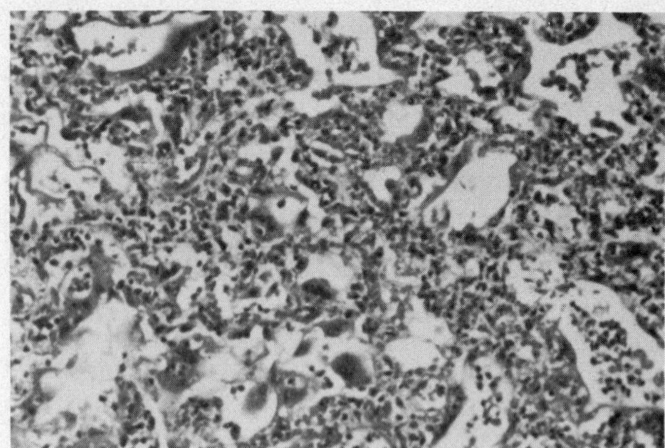

Figure 8–2. Interstitial type of viral pneumonia: thickened, infiltrated septa; hyaline membranes; pneumonocyte desquamation; and syncytium formation.

CLINICAL COURSE. Most URIs are transient or self-limited infections that produce manifestations too well-known to merit repetition. The proverbial "take a couple of aspirins and give me a call tomorrow" is statistically sound advice. Nonetheless, these involvements require prompt attention in infants, the elderly, diabetics, and persons with preexisting chronic respiratory disease, since they impair ventilation and resistance to superimposed bacterial infection.

The LRIs such as bronchiolitis, atypical pneumonia, and the flu syndrome are far more serious. They may be associated with marked hypoxia even when there is only minimal clinical evidence of alveolar consolidation; often there are dramatic changes on the chest film without altered physical signs; hence, the designation "*atypical pneumonia.*" Regression of radiographic changes may lag behind improvement of the clinical status. Confusing clinical pictures may also arise from bacterial or multiple opportunistic superinfections. Although recovery from influenza without sequelae is the rule, thousands died daily during the winter of 1918 (the year of the "swine flu") frequently of bacterial pneumonia or sepsis. Outside the context of a known epidemic, etiologic diagnosis is difficult and is usually confirmed only during convalescence by rising serum antibody titers. In extreme cases, resort may be made to lung biopsy, but only the herpes and measles viruses and CMV produce diagnostic inclusion bodies (pp. 282, 284, 287) by light microscopy. Other viruses may be detectable by immunocytochemical methods. Vaccines and antiviral drugs have been only partially successful against respiratory viral infections, especially against established disease.

VIRAL DISORDERS OF DIGESTIVE TRACT

Mumps

Mumps is an acute, contagious childhood disease characterized by inflammation and swelling of the parotid glands and, less often, the other salivary glands. It may also involve the pancreas, testes, ovaries, and (rarely) the central nervous system or other systemic organs. Although usually mild, mumps occasionally causes acutely incapacitating, painful illness, especially in adult patients, or may leave permanent tissue destruction in its wake. With the advent of an attenuated live vaccine, its frequency has sharply declined.

Mumps is caused by a paramyxovirus, usually acquired by respiratory droplet infection. Its peak incidence is in 5- to 15-year-olds. Asymptomatic or very mild infection is common; most, but not all, adults are now largely immune. Incubation takes two to four weeks, and parotid swelling is preceded by fever, malaise, and headache. The usual duration of the acute illness is one or two weeks with gradual clinical improvement. Atypical presentations lacking parotid enlargement include abdominal pain, painful testicular swelling, or generalized lymphadenopathy and splenomegaly.

The parotitis is bilateral in about 70% of cases or unilateral in 20%, but in about 10% there is only sublingual involvement. Affected glands are enlarged, have a doughy consistency, and are moist, glistening, and reddish-brown on cross section. Testicular swelling may be spectacular, with parenchymal hemorrhage. **Microscopically,** at the peak of mumps parotitis, the gland interstitium is diffusely infiltrated by inflammatory edema and histiocytes, lymphocytes, and plasma cells, which compress acini and ducts. Sometimes there is focal necrosis and spillage of exudate into the epithelial structures. In the enzyme-rich pancreas, mumps lesions become more destructive, causing parenchymal and fat necrosis and polymorphonuclear cell infiltration. Similarly, in the testis, tightly contained by the albuginea, tissue swelling may result in necrosis of seminiferous tubules with neutrophilic infiltration and focal hemorrhages and microinfarctions, thus accounting for the permanent fibrous scars sometimes left by mumps orchitis.[19] Encephalitis or encephalomyelitis, when they occur, are usually mild and lack distinctive pathologic features. The mumps virus does not produce characteristic cell inclusions.

The gland regions are tender and swollen, with pain on mastication, and the overlying skin is tense but not red. Involvement of other organs may precede, accompany, or follow the parotitis. Orchitis, the most frequent (20%), is usually unilateral and is therefore rarely a cause of male sterility. Pancreatitis, when severe, is detectable by elevation of serum lipase and by the other signs and symptoms of pancreatic necrosis (p. 963). The diagnosis of mumps is usually clinical, can be confirmed by convalescent serum titers, and, in the context of an outbreak, offers little difficulty. The parotitis is usually transient and leaves no sequelae. Even mumps pancreatitis tends to be relatively mild and does not relapse. Sporadic deaths due to complicating myocarditis have been recorded. Mumps and measles live vaccines are now customarily administered together in childhood and should eventually make these infections vanish.

Viral Enteritis and Diarrhea

Viruses are major causes of acute diarrheal diseases previously attributed to other or uncertain causes. Two types of enteropathogenic viruses—rotaviruses and parvoviruses—have now been characterized by immunoelectron microscopy, and more may yet be discovered.

Rotaviruses are best visualized in negatively stained electron micrographs of stool ultrafiltrates, and thus far have not been adapted to tissue culture; however, specific Enzyme-Linked Immuno-Sorbent Assays (ELISA) are now available.[20] Transmission is oral-fecal; children of weaning or older ages are most susceptible. Antibodies to rotavirus build up rapidly in normal humans, rendering most adults immune. The peak prevalence of disease is during the winter months in temperate climes, the dry season in the tropics. In the United States rotaviruses account for well over 50% of all childhood diarrheas; in developing countries, plagued by many diarrheal pathogens, they are responsible for between 12 and 38%. Fortunately, rotavirus diarrhea tends to be mild. Indeed, after its 48-hour incubation the diarrhea rarely lasts more than a few days (maximum eight), but fever, vomiting, and loss of appetite are frequent and induce dehydration and electrolyte imbalance, which can be lethal. Animal studies and small bowel biopsies have shown mixed inflammatory infiltration of the lamina propria, shortening of villi, and cellular hyperplasia of mucosal crypts.[21]

Parvoviruses are also detectable by stool electron microscopy. No suitable culture medium has yet been devised. The entry route is digestive. Adults, as well as children, are susceptible. Epidemics, usually local in scope, occur year-round, and in earlier reports the virus was named after each affected locality (e.g., "Norwalk agent"). Parvovirus infection is one of the known causes of "traveler's diarrhea." The incubation period can be as brief as 18 hours; the diarrhea is watery, without tenesmus, and usually abates in one or two days, although some patients may experience more prolonged and severe symptoms. Immunity follows infection but seems to vary individually in degree and duration. Histologic findings in small bowel biopsies of human volunteers largely parallel those reported in rotavirus infection.[22] These changes last longer than do the clinical symptoms. Among the numerous causes of the adult diarrheal syndrome, parvovirus infections rank as relatively benign, and require little more than bed rest and compensatory oral fluid intake.

Viral Hepatitis

Infections caused by the human hepatitis viruses and their role in cirrhosis and liver cancer are discussed on page 936. Impairment of liver function may also occur in many other systemic viral infections, most commonly those of the herpesvirus family. Both the CMV and the EB virus (Table 8–2) produce focal hepatocellular necrosis with some regularity, especially after transfusions or organ transplants. The herpes zoster–varicella and herpes simplex viruses can produce severe liver cell necrosis in immunosuppressed individuals (p. 284). In addition, the yellow fever and hemorrhagic fever viruses (p. 290) can cause liver failure in previously normal persons.

EPIDERMAL-EPITHELIAL VIRAL DISORDERS

Epithelial Warty Growths

These are listed in Table 8–2 and discussed in Chapter 27. Common features of these benign growths are: (1) exuberant, but self-limited epithelial proliferation; (2) cytopathic changes in maturing epithelial cells (inclusion bodies or koilocytosis); and (3) predominantly mononuclear stromal and basal inflammatory infiltration.

Measles (Rubeola)

Thanks to a 95% effective live attenuated vaccine, measles is now well on its way toward extinction in the United States and Europe, and worldwide eradication is under serious contemplation.[23] For many centuries, rubeola was near universal among children 3 to 7 years old. It is an acute, febrile, systemic viral infection usually beginning with coryza and conjunctivitis, followed by typical spotty lesions inside the mouth, lymphoreticular hyperplasia, and a blotchy, generalized, erythematous (morbilliform) rash.

The measles virus, an RNA paramyxovirus, is highly contagious by droplet aspiration and is transmissible via the placenta. Incubation averages ten days; fever and rash peak promptly within a few days and then gradually resolve during one or two weeks, barring complications. Photophobia and eye-burning are the first symptoms; a spotty enanthem that blisters and ulcerates deep in the cheek mucosa near the opening of Stensen's ducts ("Koplik's spots") is diagnostic even before the rash begins. Swollen lymph nodes or splenic enlargement also occur early, and respiratory symptoms, especially dry cough, may be prominent; about one-fifth of patients have lung opacities on chest radiograph. The rash is blotchy, reddish-brown, and barely elevated; begins behind the ears; travels down the neck, trunk, and extremities; and rarely becomes confluent. Except in severe, hemorrhagic "black measles," it blanches on pressure. Earache, bellyache, and other miscellaneous symptoms may confuse the picture, especially when the rash is subtle or does not appear. The fever and symptoms usually abate as the rash blanches with mild epidermal scaling, and recovery is followed by immunity. Although generally benign in normal children, measles can be serious, especially in the very young, very old, and immunosuppressed, either by causing neural or visceral viral damage or, more commonly, because of bacterial superinfections. In children and adults of tropical countries, the illness can cause mortality rates of up to 12%. Measles encephalomyelitis or interstitial, sometimes "giant cell," pneumonia can be a life-threatening acute complication. Moreover, measles has also been incriminated on varying evidence in long-term sequelae, especially in subacute sclerosing panencephalitis (p. 1385), minimal disease nephrotic syndrome (p. 1014), juvenile diabetes mellitus (p. 972), and thrombocytopenic purpura (p. 644). Unlike German measles (see below), rubeola during pregnancy does not cause fetal congenital anomalies.

Histologically, the rash is produced by dilated skin vessels, edema, and a moderate, nonspecific, mononuclear perivascular infiltrate. Ulcerated mucosal lesions in the oral cavity are marked by necrosis, neutrophils, and neovascularization. The lymphoid organs typically have marked follicular hyperplasia, large germinal centers, and randomly distributed multinucleate giant cells, called Warthin-Finkeldey cells, with eosinophilic nuclear and cytoplasmic inclusion bodies (Fig. 8–3). These are pathognomonic of measles, and on occasion permit its diagnosis from histologic examination of the lymphoid structures of an excised appendix.

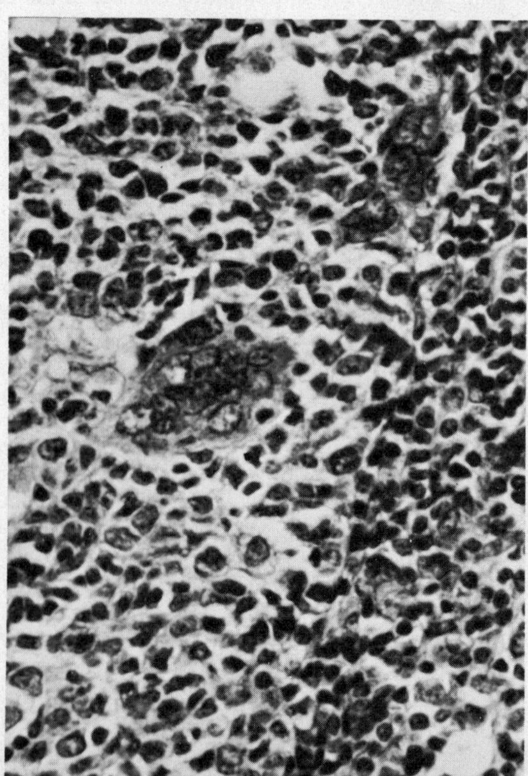

Figure 8–3. Measles giant cells in appendix.

The milder forms of measles pneumonia show the same peribronchial and interstitial mononuclear infiltration seen in other nonlethal viral infections. In severe or neglected cases, bacterial superinfection may be a cause of death. Sometimes, diagnostic giant cells can be detected in the sputum. In debilitated children, especially those with mucoviscidosis, Wiskott-Aldrich syndrome, or lymphoreticular malignancies, measles pneumonia can be protracted and lead to respiratory failure. In such instances the virus may persist in respiratory secretions for months, long after the rash has disappeared. Uncommonly, postmeasles encephalomyelitis develops, caused, it is suspected, by an autoimmune reaction.

German Measles (Rubella)

Rubella, sometimes called "three-day measles," is a highly contagious but mild childhood systemic febrile viral infection characterized by a morbilliform (measles-like) rash and swelling of the posterior cervical lymph nodes. It is caused by a *togavirus* unrelated to the measles virus, and has a longer incubation period and a briefer, more benign course. In passing, it might be noted that *erythema infectiosum* and *roseola infantum* are two additional mild exanthematous eruptions of childhood presumed to be caused by less common, not yet identified, viruses. Rubella tends to be more discomforting in adults, and is sometimes accompanied by joint pain and swelling reminiscent of rheumatic fever. The principal public health importance of rubella derives from its power to cause severe congenital malformations, mostly cardiac, when transmitted from mother to fetus (p. 480). The disease is virtually always nonfatal.

Smallpox (Variola)

The causative agent of smallpox, a 160-nm particle containing double-stranded DNA and terminal transcriptase, has finally been confined to cold storage in a few high-security reference centers. The last documented case of human smallpox occurred during a 1978 laboratory outbreak. All suspected cases since then have proved to be deceptive "look-alikes," some due to the distantly related monkeypox virus or to hemorrhagic varicella (p. 285). Thus culminates the long and stormy history of cowpox vaccination, which began with Jenner's alertness to the well-known fact that milkmaids, unlike others of their time, rarely had their faces disfigured by pockmarks.[24]

MORPHOLOGY. Smallpox began with a viremic phase 12 days after passage by inhalation. Its well-synchronized rash turned from macules to vesicles and pustules over two to six days, covering the skin and mucous membranes. As intraepidermal vesicles formed by cell disruption, the basal epidermal layer was destroyed, followed by inflammatory infiltration beginning in the dermis and spilling into the vesicle to form a pustule (Fig. 8–4) In severe cases there was bleeding into the vesicles and pustules, producing black, "hemorrhagic smallpox." Characteristic of active skin lesions were altered epidermal cells containing eosinophilic intracytoplasmic bodies **(Guarneri bodies).** Lymphoreticular hyperplasia, scattered foci of inflammation in internal organs or the CNS, and changes incident to bacterial superinfection, dehydration, and shock were often present in lethal cases. Usually, in the course of days, the vesicles ruptured and exfoliated, gradually turning to depressed pockmarks as the patient convalesced.

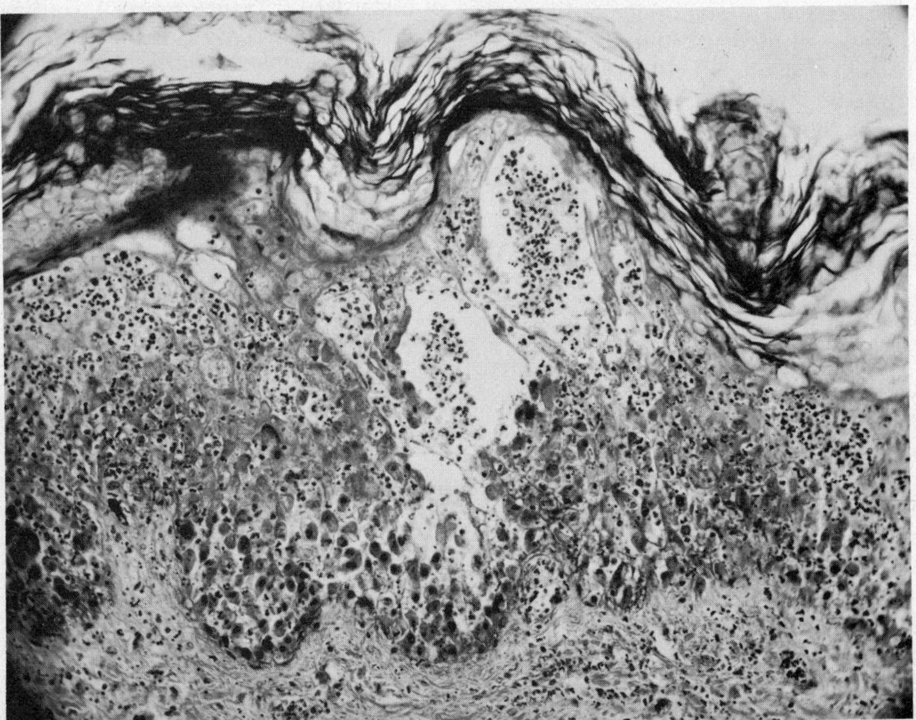

Figure 8–4. Smallpox—a view of a characteristic vesicle with separation of the epidermal cells and a leukocytic exudate within the vesicle.

Should one be faced with a suspect case of smallpox today, the patient should be isolated and contacts limited to vaccinated health personnel. Expert examination of vesicle fluid by electron microscopy is a critical step in confirming the diagnosis. To maintain past gains, surveillance may be necessary for the next decade.

HERPESVIRUS DISEASES

The herpesviruses listed in Table 8–2 are responsible for a wide range of infections from the trivial "cold sore" to lethal disseminated disease. Most frequently seen in medical practice are their acute systemic manifestations such as chickenpox or infectious mononucleosis. Herpetic infections are widely prevalent throughout the world and their frequency increases with age from womb to grave; by maturity most adults carry one or another of these viruses or sometimes several, but the vast bulk of these infections are latent. Overt diseases then represent only "the tip of the iceberg." Both newly acquired and activated latent infections can cause clinical disease. Whatever their clinical presentation, cutaneous or hemolymphopoietic, all herpetic infections must be considered as systemic, and this is particularly true in immunodeficient and otherwise predisposed hosts. The protean and grave, systemic nature of these infections is most striking in a hospital setting, compared to the largely benign forms of disease seen in the community which still make up the bulk of cases.

All the virions of the herpes family look similar by electron microscopy, just as their viral inclusions are indistinguishable by light microscopy, with the exception of those induced by the cytomegalovirus (p. 287). Yet each herpesvirus species is genetically and antigenetically distinct, and each differs in the disease spectrum it causes. Herpes viruses have marked host species specificity although, rarely, zoonotic infection by simian herpesviruses have induced severe illness in primate workers or fanciers.

Herpes Simplex (HSV I) and Herpes Genitalis (HSV II) Infections

Herpes simplex is transmitted by physical contact such as kissing, and is thus spread among family members and friends. About half of all babies in the United States are born with IgG antibodies to this agent transmitted across the placenta. As this immunity dissipates, new infections are acquired until, by age 45, close to 70% of people have become serologically positive—most without ever experiencing signs of disease, others after one or several episodes of "fever blisters" or "cold sores." Only very few suffer major illnesses. By contrast, HSV II is transmitted by sexual contact or during birth; it is less prevalent overall, but is likewise cumulative with age. Its incidence rises with the number of sexual partners, and has therefore greatly increased in today's permissive society. Genital herpes has engendered considerable anxiety because of its possible role in the causation of cervical cancer, discussed in more detail on page 1125. Both infections are difficult to prevent; there is as yet no vaccine.

The spectrum of both herpesvirus infections includes:

1. *latency*—the virus slowly reproduces in trigeminal or other ganglia; diagnosis is made only by antibody titer.
2. *skin or mucosal vesicles* (fever blisters, cold sores, aphthous stomatitis, genital herpes).
3. *severe vesicular eruption of the eye or skin* (herpes keratoconjunctivitis, eczema herpeticum, Kaposi's varicelliform eruption).
4. *severe CNS lesions* (herpes simplex encephalitis, transverse myelitis).
5. *opportunistic localized lesions of internal organs* (herpes esophagitis, herpes simplex pneumonitis).
6. *overwhelming disseminated opportunistic infection* with focal necrosis of many organs in neonates and compromised adults.

Herpesvirus lesions, wherever located, are marked by cytopathic changes, principally the formation of Cowdry type A intranuclear inclusions. As the virions multiply within nuclei, the chromatin first fades to a lavender tinge on H and E staining and loses definition. Darkly stained chromatin clumps then cluster against the nuclear membrane and may herniate through it imparting a spiked contour, while **the nuclear center, now containing live and dead virions and debris, is transformed into a large acidophilic inclusion separated from the nuclear rim by an artifactual cleft.** Cell and nuclear size increase only slightly, in contrast to the striking enlargements induced by the CMV (p. 287). However, cell fusions may produce inclusion-bearing **"polykaryons" or giant cells,** which can also be found in smears of blister fluid **("Tzanck preps"),** confirming the diagnosis of a herpetic infection (Fig. 8–5). More definitive identification of the herpesvirus within cells can be achieved by immunofluorescent methods.

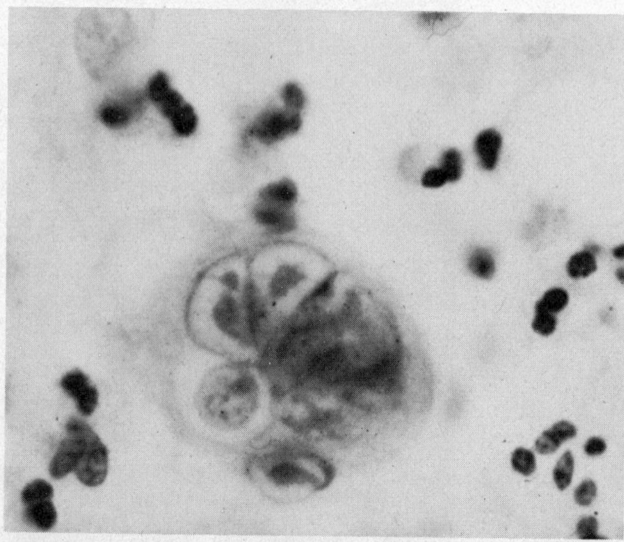

Figure 8–5. Herpes simplex. Typical polykaryon with Cowdry type A intranuclear inclusions as seen in a Tzanck prep of a skin vesicle.

Fever blisters or **cold sores** favor the facial skin around mucosal orifices (lips, nares) but may occur in other regions. Their distribution does not follow skin dermatomes, and bilateral lesions are common. Intraepithelial vesicles are created by intracellular edema and the ballooning degeneration of epidermal cells. The vesicles tend to burst, collapse, and crust promptly, but some may result in superficial ulcerations. Predisposing factors include old age, sunlight, respiratory infections, menstruation, and occasionally some underlying serious illness or hidden malignancy.

Genital herpes is characterized by vesicles on the genital mucous membranes as well as external genitalia. On moist mucosal surfaces the vesicles are transient and rapidly converted into superficial ulcerations, rimmed by an inflammatory infiltrate. The cellular changes are those already described. Large, solitary herpetic ulcers on the genitalia or lips, with swelling of satellite lymph nodes, may simulate a primary syphilitic chancre (p. 336).

Aphthous stomatitis refers to a vesicular eruption that may extend from tongue to retropharynx, usually encountered in children and caused by HSV I. It must be differentiated from other vesicular eruptions in childhood, particularly that caused by Coxsackie virus, which tends to be milder and limited to the pharynx and tonsils. The herpetic infection may induce cervical lymphadenopathy and fever, but is self-limited.

Herpes keratoconjunctivitis of one or both eyes is similar to skin herpes but tends to ulcerate the delicate and gliding epithelia. It is frequently recurrent and is prone to bacterial superinfection; it may therefore cause corneal clouding, deep inflammation, and eventual blindness. Several antiviral drugs, including acyclovir, can ameliorate this disorder.[25]

Kaposi's varicelliform eruption is a generalized vesiculating involvement of the skin occurring mainly in immunodeficient persons and those with previous dermatitis.

Eczema herpeticum is even more severe and is characterized by confluent, pustular, or hemorrhagic blisters. Bacterial superinfection is common, as is dissemination of the viral infection to internal viscera. Both these patterns of herpetic dermatitis can prove fatal.

Herpes simplex encephalitis is described on page 1383. This highly lethal involvement of the brain, usually by HSV I, appears in the absence of a skin rash. With state-of-the-art therapy, the salvage rate has increased modestly.

Visceral and disseminated herpes infections are usually encountered in particular clinical settings. Esophagitis almost always represents activation of a latent infection in hospitalized patients with some form of underlying cancer or under immunosuppressive treatment. The mucosal vesicles and ulcerations are no different from those already described, but are readily superinfected by bacteria or fungi. Similarly, herpes bronchopneumonia, often necrotizing, is seen in predisposed individuals, particularly when an airway must be inserted through oral herpes territory.[26] Disseminated infection most often occurs in neonates, particularly premature babies, or those with abnormal immune systems. Usually, HSV II is transmitted during passage through the birth canal of infected mothers; this can be prevented by cesarean delivery when the risk is known. The disseminated disease in the neonate may be mild, but is more often fulminating with generalized lymphadenopathy, splenomegaly, and necrotic foci throughout the lungs, liver, adrenals, and CNS. Brain damage may persist in the few infants who recover. Disseminated infections may also arise in adults, most often during cancer chemotherapy or immunosuppression following marrow and organ transplants. Necrotic foci may be present throughout the body, particularly in the liver and lungs, leading to hepatic failure or death from respiratory complications. In all these visceral and disseminated involvements, typical intranuclear inclusions often provide the etiologic diagnosis but may not be present in all of the lesions.

Chickenpox (Varicella) and Herpes Zoster

These two seemingly disparate disorders are both caused by the herpes zoster virus (HZV) and are therefore closely related.

Chickenpox is an acute, highly contagious, but mild systemic viral infection with a vesicular, generalized skin eruption. It is usually of little consequence in normal children, but in those with immunodeficiencies may cause pneumonitis, encephalitis, and disseminated visceral lesions, including purpuric skin lesions. Severe neonatal disease may occur when the mother becomes infected shortly before delivery, but, unlike german measles, infection during gestation does not induce congenital malformations in the offspring. In the usual childhood form of chickenpox the infection is acquired through the respiratory route, and after two to three weeks of silent incubation is followed by a viremia. A generalized rash appears, progressing rapidly from a macular to a vesicular stage without forming pustules. Each individual lesion resembles *"a dew drop on a rose petal."* Usually, several crops of lesions succeed each other, traveling from the trunk centrifugally to the face and extremities. *The lack of synchrony best differentiates this eruption from that caused by smallpox.* However, the rare, severe form may resemble hemorrhagic smallpox. Blistering may also occur on the buccal mucosa. Wherever they appear, the vesicles rupture, the rash crusts and scales, and the condition resolves within about a week. However, lymph node swelling may persist for some time. The rare adult patient with varicella tends to be sicker than the child, with a greater tendency to develop pneumonitis or encephalitis. More often, infection with HZV remains latent in adults or else appears as herpes zoster.

Herpes zoster, also known as "shingles," represents a reactivation of a latent HZV infection as shown by its greater frequency with advancing age. Adults with "shingles" can transmit varicella to children, but not vice versa. The pathogenesis of herpes zoster involves a previous attack of chickenpox followed by years of latency of the HZV virus in the sensory dorsal root ganglia. During an attack of "shingles," reactivated virus travels centrifugally from the ganglia to the skin of the corresponding dermatomes, resulting in a localized vesicular eruption; this is similar to that of chickenpox but differentiated by the often intense itching, burning, or sharp pain in the affected skin segment because of a simultaneous radiculoneuritis. Indeed, the pain may be disproportionate to the rash, especially when the trigeminal branches are involved; such involvement may induce a facial paralysis (Ramsay Hunt syndrome). In more than 50% of cases, only a single unilateral thoracic dermatome is involved, but several crops of lesions may arise or recur after long intervals. Sometimes the eruptions are bilateral. Herpes zoster lesions are prone to appear in persons with advanced neoplastic disease, such as Hodgkin's or other lymphomas, or following immunosuppressive drugs; in these circumstances it may become disseminated and hemorrhagic, with widespread mucosal and visceral necrosis but only a feeble inflammatory response. In contrast, in the absence of a predisposing factor, "shingles" tends to follow a protracted but benign course.

The varicella-zoster skin vesicles are identical morphologically to those caused by HSV I and are replete with intranuclear inclusions. In chickenpox vesicles tend to remain intraepithelial, and healing therefore occurs by regeneration, leaving no scars. Traumatic rupture of the vesicles and bacterial superinfection lead to destruction of the basal epidermal layer, with a commensurate greater inflammatory response and a greater tendency to residual scarring. Hence, the sound basis for the admonition "Don't scratch it"! In severe varicella, focal hemorrhages may occur into and around the blisters.

Herpes zoster is marked by a dense, predominantly mononuclear infiltrate into the sensory ganglia. Neurons and their supporting cells develop typical herpetic intranuclear inclusions, and occasional neurons may undergo necrosis with permanent loss. Interstitial pneumonia resembling that of other viral infections, encephalitis, and transverse myelitis are other potential sequelae of herpes zoster. Moreover, immunosuppressed patients may develop severe, necrotizing visceral lesions similar to those of disseminated herpes, often together with other opportunistic infections.

Cytomegalic Inclusion Disease (CID)

Cytomegalic inclusion disease is an exceedingly protean viral disease caused by CMV, a member of the herpesvirus group. Several serotypes of CMV have been isolated in man that differ in antigenicity and possibly in their pathogenetic properties. Congenital infection contracted in utero bears little resemblance to the postnatally acquired disease in infants, which in turn differs from the infection in adults.

The infectious agent is spread through (1) intrauterine transmission to the fetus following a newly acquired infection or reactivation of a latent infection in the mother, (2) perinatal transmission to the fetus as it passes through the birth canal of a mother with a cervicovaginal infection, (3) respiratory droplet transmission among children and possibly between adults, (4) blood transfusions (in about 5% of blood donors the circulating leukocytes show latent CMV infections), (5) transplantation of virus-infected grafts from a donor with latent infection, (6) venereal transmission (virus has been isolated from both semen and vaginal fluid), and (7) transmission through mother's milk.[27]

By isolation of virus from secretions of the oral cavity or urine or by rising antibody titers, it has been shown that there are three peak periods of contraction of the virus. The first is in utero. Such infections may remain latent and have little effect on the fetus, or they may have a devastating impact on the brain and kill in utero or within the first weeks of life. The second peak occurs after birth and after the loss of maternal antibodies; thus, about 10% of all infants develop complement-fixing antibodies during the first year of life. Some of these infections may be acquired in the birth canal or during breast-feeding. Most of these children, whatever the severity of the infection, continue to excrete virus for many months to years. There follows a period up to age 15 years during which the frequency of identifiable antibody increases more slowly, from approximately 10 to 20%. The third peak occurs after age 15, when the frequency of infection again rises. In the aggregate, between 50 and 80% of adults show evidence of exposure to CMV in the form of complement-fixing antibodies. Primary infection in adults is usually followed by only transient excretion of virus in the throat or urine for a few days to weeks. However, a pregnant female acquiring a new infection will excrete virus from the throat, urine, and cervix and even in the breast milk throughout pregnancy and for months afterward. *Despite the high frequency of infection in adults, it is almost always latent and asymptomatic unless the patient is immunocompromised (e.g., AIDS, p. 208) or debilitated.*[28] However, healthy adults who receive transfusions of large volumes of blood from multiple donors may acquire CID. Whether symptomatic infections in adults, or even in children, represent reactivation of endogenous latent virus or acquisition of a fresh infection often remains uncertain.

In neonates, full-blown, congenital, "classic" CID closely resembles erythroblastosis fetalis. Affected infants are often premature or below average birth weight, and at birth or soon after manifest a hemolytic form of anemia, jaundice, thrombocytopenia, purpura, hepatosplenomegaly (due to extramedullary hematopoiesis), pneumonitis, deafness, chorioretinitis, and, most important, neurologic manifestations associated with extensive brain damage. At least half the infants with such severe disease die; some survive but are mentally retarded, while others with perhaps less overwhelming infection completely recover. However, it is now clear that *most congenital infections, perhaps as many as 90% evoke no clinical manifestations at birth.* Despite this benign presentation, in rare cases, brain damage becomes evident over the span of the next few years. Between the extremes of classic CID and asymptomatic infections are those infants who suffer relatively minor illnesses, taking the form of hematologic derangements (often with purpura), mild respiratory disease, transient forms of hepatitis, or simply failure to thrive. Hepatosplenomegaly is often present in those with mild manifestations, and some have clinical evidence of neurologic involvement.

Congenital CID is therefore an unpredictable disease, and even those with mild or asymptomatic infections may suffer serious consequences years later, as shown in Figure 8–6.

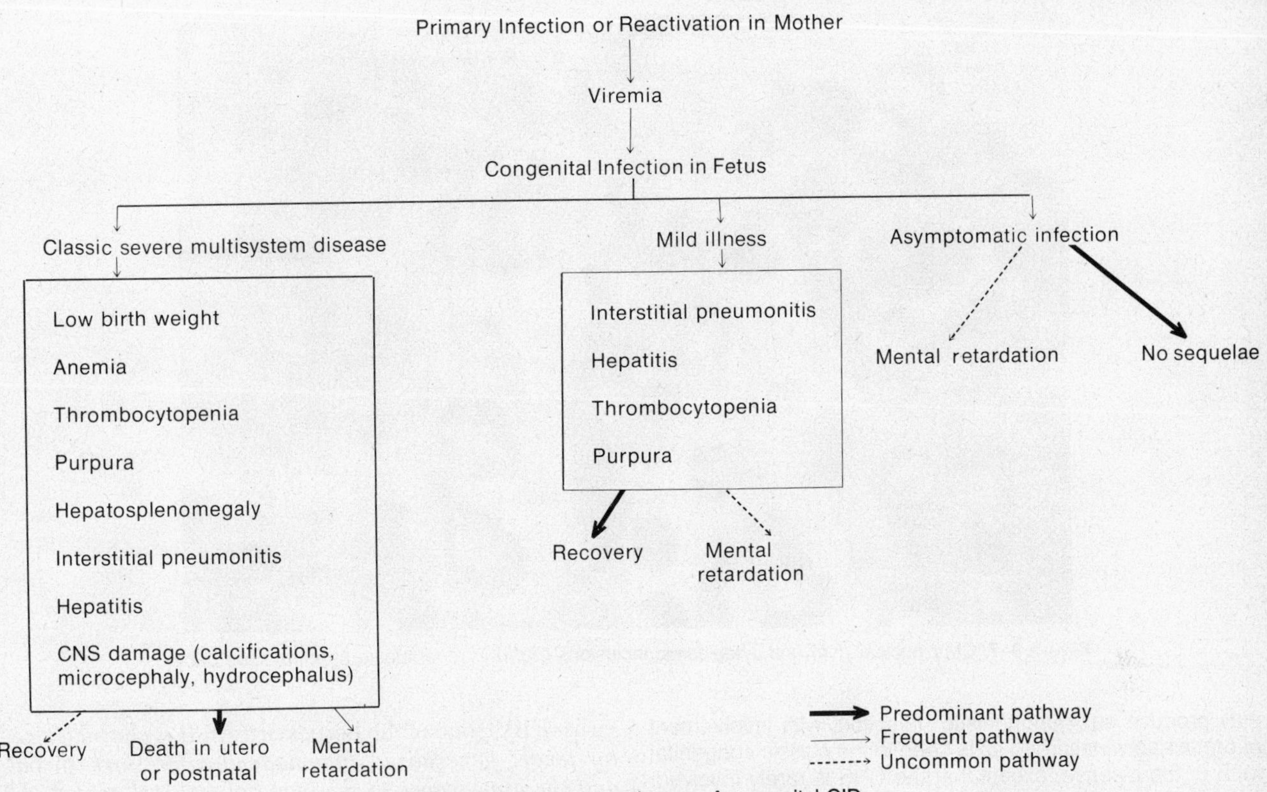

Figure 8–6. Potential pathways of congenital CID.

In classic CID the most prominent and characteristic findings are markedly enlarged cells, with large pleomorphic nuclei harboring basophilic intranuclear inclusions. **The inclusion may have a diameter of half that of the nucleus and, like those of HSV, is surrounded by a clear halo, sharply demarcating it from the nuclear membrane.** Basophilic smaller cytoplasmic inclusions are also present that probably represent viral coat protein or complete viral units (Fig. 8–7). Cells so affected may remain vital and evoke no inflammatory reactions, but others die, and the necrotic debris evokes a leukocytic response. Inclusions and focal necroses may be identified in virtually any organ but are found most often, in descending order of frequency, in the salivary glands, kidneys, liver, lungs, gut, pancreas, thyroid, adrenals, and brain. Cytomegalic inclusions are often abundant in the renal tubular epithelium and occasionally within endothelial cells of glomeruli. Desquamation of tubular cells sometimes permits diagnosis of this disease by examination of the urinary sediment. Similar cellular changes are often present in hepatocytes, and almost always in the lining cells of portal bile ducts. Extramedullary hematopoiesis may induce marked hepatic as well as splenic enlargement. In some infants there are focal hepatic necroses. Lung changes take the form of an interstitial pneumonitis, accompanied by the characteristic intracellular inclusions in the alveolar lining cells and in endothelial cells of septal capillaries as well as in alveolar macrophages. Depending on the severity of the infection, intra-alveolar edema, proteinaceous exudate, and focal hyaline membranes may appear. Cytomegalic changes, focal necroses, or even sharply punched-out ulcerations may occur in the small and large intestines.

Damage to the brain is the most lethal aspect of classic CID. **Two types of lesions** are seen—focal acute inflammatory changes, with inclusion-bearing giant cells distributed principally in a narrow band in the subependymal and subpial tissue, and necrotic lesions irregularly scattered in the cerebrum. Most characteristic of CID is the tendency for these lesions to be located about the lateral ventricles and the aqueduct, down to the fourth ventricle. Frequently the foci of injury become calcified, and the location of these calcifications about the ventricles provides one of the most important clinical diagnostic clues to this infection. The ganglion cells within and about the areas of focal damage show all ranges of injury from chromatolysis to frank necrosis, and microcephaly or hydrocephalus sometimes develops.

In less severe expressions of congenital CID, cytomegaly and inclusions are generally less frequent and less widely distributed. Sometimes, multinucleated giant cells appear in the liver, particularly in those children in whom the principal clinical manifestations are related to hepatitis. Here again, as in the classic disease, the distribution and severity of the changes are variable.

Infections acquired postnatally tend, on the whole, to be asymptomatic but sometimes induce mild, transient illness. Symptoms and signs, when they appear, are extremely varied and include hepatosplenomegaly with or without evidence of hepatitis, interstitial pneumonitis, or enterocolitis secondary to ulcerative lesions in the intestines. Only rarely is the central nervous system obviously infected.

As unpredictable as CID is in childhood, it is even more so in adulthood. Much depends on the immunologic competence of the adult. In severely compromised hosts, CID

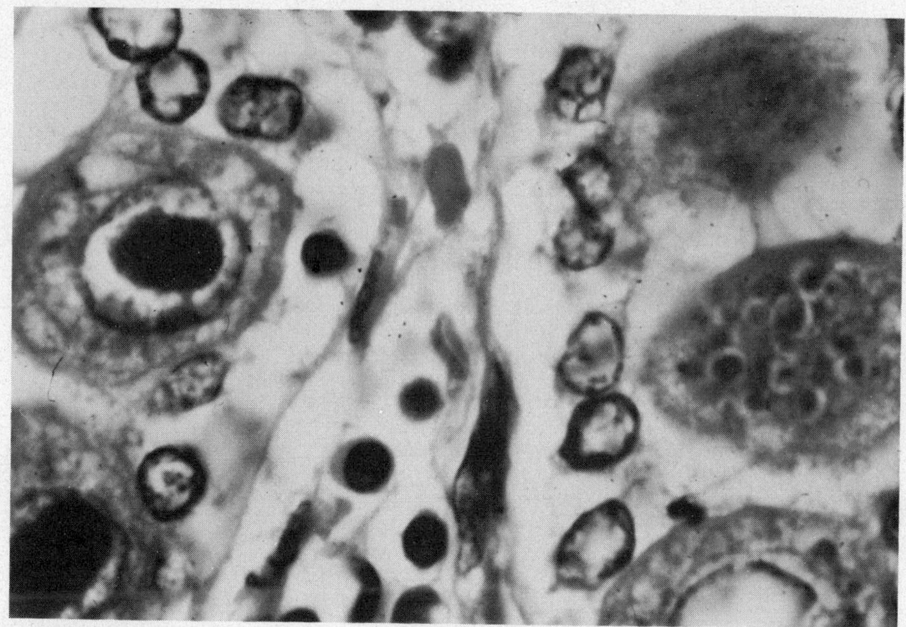

Figure 8–7. CMV nuclear *(left)* and cytoplasmic inclusions *(right)* in renal tubule of an infected baby.

may produce an "opportunistic" infection, with involvement of organs as widespread as is seen in the classic congenital form of the disease, except that the CNS is rarely involved. Indeed, in such cases it is quite common to find concomitant invasion by other "opportunists" such as fungi and *Pneumocystis carinii* (p. 365). More often in adults, CID affects only the lungs and intestinal tract. The pulmonary changes are similar to those described in the congenital form of the disease.[30] In the small and large intestine, ulceroinflammatory lesions develop, often accompanied by the characteristic cytomegaly and inclusions within local endothelial and mucosal cells. Rarely, intestinal perforations may ensue.

The significance of viral infection in adults is variable. Patients may recover following a brief or, more often, prolonged episode of respiratory illness. However, in others it represents "the last straw" superimposed upon an underlying fatal disease.

Otherwise healthy children or adults may develop an infectious mononucleosis–like syndrome especially following transfusion of large volumes of blood from donors with latent CMV infections.[31] These patients manifest fever with lymphocytosis and atypical lymphocytes in the circulating blood, closely resembling infectious mononucleosis and distinguished from it only by the persistently negative heterophil tests. Almost always this syndrome is self-limited and followed by complete recovery. It should thus be evident that CMV is an agent of relatively low virulence, the pathogenicity of which is inversely proportional to the resistance of the host. It presents its most ferocious face to those least equipped to confront it—the fetus and the immunologically incompetent and debilitated.

Infectious Mononucleosis (IM)

Infectious mononucleosis is a benign, self-limited lymphoproliferative disease caused by the Epstein-Barr virus (EBV), one of the herpesviruses. *It is characterized by fever, generalized lymphadenopathy, sore throat, and the appearance in the blood of atypical activated T lymphocytes (mononucleosis cells).* IM also affects the spleen, liver, and less often the heart, lungs, kidneys, hematopoietic system, and CNS. Thus, it may mimic other disorders, particularly viral hepatitis. Conversely, other viral agents, notably CMV, may produce clinical syndromes that can only be differentiated from the EBV disease serologically. EBV is also strongly suspected of contributing to the causation of African (endemic) Burkitt's lymphoma and nasopharyngeal carcinoma, but is not regularly found in patients with Burkitt's lymphoma outside of Africa (p. 662).

IM occurs principally in late adolescence or young adulthood, but may occasionally arise in children and the aged. It is more frequent in upper socioeconomic classes in developed nations. The reasons for this distribution are as follows: In most of the world, natural primary infection with EBV generally occurs in childhood and is usually asymptomatic. These inapparent infections confer immunity to the virus. However, many persons without disease, perhaps as many as 20% of the population in western countries, continue harboring infected lymphocytes and shedding infectious virus from their oropharynx.[33] In privileged societies, contact with such reservoir hosts may be delayed until late adolescence or young adulthood; in these delayed primary infections, symptomatic IM appears.

The EBV virus is transmitted from person to person, often by kissing, with transfer of virally contaminated saliva. In a susceptible seronegative host (lacking antibodies), the virions invade and replicate within salivary gland epithelial cells and then enter B cells in the lymphoid tissues, which possess receptors for the virus.[34] A replicative virus cycle ensues, with dissemination of the agent either through the bloodstream or by the spread of the infected B cells themselves. In either event, death of the infected B cells with viremia produces an acute febrile reaction and specific immunologic responses. As antibodies appear, infectious virus disappears from the blood. IgM and later IgG antibodies to viral capsid antigen can be demonstrated. Virus neutralizing antibodies and antibodies to virus-directed B-cell membrane antigens also appear. These peak about two weeks after the infection and persist throughout life. Other virus-determined antibodies arise, and also transient heterophil (Paul-Bunnell) antibodies, whose association with EBV is still not well understood.

Although infectious B cells and free virions disappear from the blood following the humoral-antibody response, *EBV-transformed B lymphocytes carrying the virus genome integrated into their own DNA continue to be present in the circulation.*[34] Such cells, if explanted in culture, are capable of indefinite reproduction ("in vitro immortality"), whereas cultures of normal B lymphocytes can be grown only for brief periods. In this latent form, the virus does not cause a full cytocidal replicative viral cycle. However, expression of at least some of the virus-determined antigens continues, within these B cells, particularly a lymphocyte-detected membrane antigen. This membrane antigen is recognized by T-killer cells, and stimulates their multiplication. *These T-killer cells are the atypical cells seen in the blood in mononucleosis,* and it is the stimulation of T cells throughout the body that is responsible for the lymphadenopathy and hepatosplenomegaly. The sore throat so typical of this disease in its early stage may be due to necrosis of B cells and possibly epithelial cells in the early virus replicative cycle in the oropharynx. The progressive increase in virus-specific antibodies and T-killer cells eventually brings the disease under control and eliminates the latently infected B cells.

Thus, in summary, the B cells in IM are infected and develop virus-directed membrane antigens that evoke a killer-cell (T-cell) response as the ultimate cause of the lymphoidal and visceral reaction throughout the body.[34]

MORPHOLOGY. Anatomic studies have been confined largely to excised lymph nodes and liver biopsies, and to the rare patients who have died of rupture of the spleen or other complications.[35, 36]

The **peripheral blood** usually shows an absolute lymphocytosis with a total white cell count between 12,000 and 18,000, 95% of which are lymphocytes. Many of these are atypical T lymphocytes approximately 12 to 16 microns in diameter, with an abundant, finely granular, basophilic cytoplasm. The nucleus is variable in shape and may be round, ovoid, folded, or bean shaped. The nuclear chromatin usually is finely divided but may be clumped. Nucleoli are generally absent. The most distinguishing features are small fenestrations or vacuolations in the cytoplasm. These abnormal cells are usually sufficiently distinctive to permit the diagnosis of IM on peripheral blood smear.

The **lymph nodes** are moderately enlarged throughout the body, principally in the posterior cervical, axillary, and groin regions. They show striking immunoproliferation of T cells in their paracortical zones, which become flooded by lymphocytes of varying size. There is, in addition, some B-cell reaction within the follicles. These become enlarged with prominent germinal centers, exhibiting many mitoses, or may become blurred as the follicular center cells intermingle with the perifollicular and paracortical cells. This lymphoproliferative reaction distorts but does not totally efface the normal architecture.[36] **Occasionally, large binucleate cells, "Reed-Sternberg–like" cells (p. 670), are found in these nodes**, and so the changes of IM must be differentiated from those of Hodgkin's disease (p. 670). Leukemia, too, must be ruled out by observing the normal but immunostimulated patterns of lymph node architecture characteristic of IM.

The **spleen** is usually enlarged to two to three times its normal size and is soft and fleshy with a hyperemic cut surface. The trabecular markings and follicular structure may become indistinct. Histologically, there may be prominence of the splenic follicles, or the architecture may be blurred by the heavy accumulation of immunostimulated lymphocytes. These cells sometimes infiltrate the trabeculae and the capsule, and may contribute in this way to easy rupture, an important clinical complication of this condition. Increased numbers of plasma cells are often present.

The **liver** is sufficiently affected in most cases to cause elevated serum levels of glutamic pyruvic transaminase (SGPT) and other enzymes, but it is usually only mildly or moderately enlarged and is otherwise not unusual in its gross appearance. Histologically, there are three principal alterations: portal infiltrations, consisting almost entirely of abnormal mononuclear cells; invasion of the sinusoids by the same cells; and areas of scattered parenchymal necrosis filled with mononuclear cells. These changes may be difficult to differentiate from viral hepatitis.[37]

The **central nervous system** may be affected with congestion, edema, and perivascular mononuclear infiltrates in the leptomeninges. Focal aggregates of mononuclear cells may occur in the perivascular areas of the brain substance. Myelin degeneration and destruction of axis cylinders in the peripheral nerves are on the whole infrequent.

An interstitial "viral-type" pneumonitis has been observed in the lungs, and atypical lymphocytes have been described in the heart and bone marrow.

CLINICAL COURSE. Diagnosis of IM can sometimes be difficult because of its varied presentations and must be based on the sum of clinical, hematologic, and serologic findings. The disease often starts with chills, fever, malaise, sore throat, and painful enlargement of the cervical nodes. Pharyngitis and tonsillitis may be associated with a creamy exudate over these structures. Fine pinpoint petechiae in the palate are present at the height of the illness in somewhat fewer than half of the cases. Differential diagnosis must include streptococcal sore throat, but microbiologic study will fail to incriminate any bacterial agent. A macular skin rash resembling rubella develops in 10 to 15% of cases. Splenomegaly may give rise to left upper quadrant pain or discomfort, and there may be tender hepatic enlargement, indigestion, and inappetence. The differential diagnosis in such cases is often infectious (viral) hepatitis. In other instances, the striking lymphocytosis associated with the lymphadenopathy raises the specter of leukemia. The clinical course is usually one of progressive improvement after two to four weeks of febrile illness, but the intercurrence of hepatic involvement or myocarditis with its associated T-wave abnormalities may prolong the malady. Fatalities are rare in normal immunologic reactors and are attributable to rupture of the spleen or to such intercurrent infections as pneumonia and meningitis.

The hematologic findings, i.e., the elevated white count with a relative lymphocytosis and recognition of the atypical lymphocytes, are crucial to the diagnosis. Abnormal levels of sheep red cell agglutinins are usually present in titers greater than 1 to 64 (the Paul-Bunnell heterophil test). These antibodies are not significantly absorbed by guinea pig kidneys, but are absorbed by beef erythrocytes. Far more specific are the serodiagnostic procedures relating to the EBV antibodies discussed earlier.

Several kindreds of the X-linked recessive lymphoproliferative syndrome marked by an immunodeficiency state (described on p. 669) have been studied whose anomalous responses to the EBV included acutely lethal mononucleosis, development of autoimmune disease, and the delayed appearance of lymphomatous malignancies and leukemia.[38] These observations and those on African Burkitt's lymphoma, both involving herpesviruses, constitute a link between defective T-cell function, viral oncogenesis, and chromosomal translocations in the induction of neoplasia (p. 248).

ARBOVIRUS DISEASES*

There are over 60 known diseases, some widespread, others strictly local, caused by arthropod-borne arboviruses. Table 8–2 lists those causing encephalitis in the U.S. and the best-known hemorrhagic fevers, including yellow fever and dengue. *Arbovirus diseases are confined to the distribution of their specific insect vectors and animal reservoirs, but can become epidemic when there is man-to-man transmission by a ubiquitous insect vector*, as has happened in the past with *Aedes aegypti*–borne yellow fever. Since viral encephalitis is described on page 1383, we shall limit this discussion to the hemorrhagic fevers.

Hemorrhagic Fevers, Dengue, Yellow Fever*

Korean and dengue hemorrhagic fevers have caused fatalities among the military in Southeast Asia. These disorders start suddenly with chills, headache, and muscle and joint pains, followed by widespread skin and scleral bleeding, thrombocytopenia, proteinuria, and renal failure, usually within three to five days. Shock and hypothermia are ominous, preterminal signs. Those who survive the first seven to ten days of illness gradually recover, but proteinuria and oliguria may persist for weeks. Each arbovirus species differs in its clinical expression: jaundice, melena, cardiac arrhythmia, pneumonitis, or CNS symptoms are characteristic of some variants and absent in others.

Dengue is ordinarily a benign, flulike tropical disease well characterized by its popular name, "breakbone fever." However, a potentially lethal hemorrhagic variant occurs, principally among children in countries of the Eastern Pacific perimeter, e.g., Thailand and Pakistan. Recently a large epidemic broke out in Cuba. The DIC-like syndrome is predominantly elicited by dengue virus of serotype II and may possibly be related to partial host immunity.[39] Pulmonary and cerebral hemorrhages are frequent lethal complications.

Yellow fever in monkeys has migrated as far north as the Yucatan peninsula, causing small human epidemics in rural Latin America, but none comparable to those that forced the abandonment of the first attempt to build the Panama Canal. It differs from other arbovirus infections in its profound effect on the liver and marked jaundice. However, the latter may complicate many viral and bacterial infections, and, perhaps for these reasons, yellow fever outbreaks sometimes remain undiagnosed until several deaths have occurred.

Gross autopsy findings in hemorrhagic dengue may be limited to multiple bleeding points and hematomas, or may include shock-related abdominal congestion and centrilobular liver necrosis. In yellow fever, the liver is soft, heavy, yellow in color, and spotted by numerous hemorrhages. Histologically, it is characterized by (1) midzonal liver cell necrosis, which may spread to the entire lobe in severe cases; (2) **acidophilic degeneration of individual liver cells with cell and nuclear shrinkage, followed by hyaline condensation of the cytoplasm and extrusion of the rounded "Councilman" body into the sinusoidal lumen;** (3) fatty degeneration of liver cells and sometimes of the renal tubular and myocardial cells as well; and (4) amorphous intranuclear eosinophilic debris, which can be seen sometimes in degenerating hepatocytes (Torres bodies) (although not considered true viral inclusions, they may serve as a diagnostic clue).[40] Although Councilman bodies are distinctive in yellow fever, they can also be seen in other liver diseases, notably viral hepatitis.

In all cases of hemorrhagic fevers of longer duration, lymph node swelling and splenic enlargement are found related to proliferation and activation of reticuloendothelial cells and macrophages with marked erythrophagocytosis. Other organs may show focal parenchymal necroses, but inflammatory infiltration is usually not pronounced, unless due to bacterial superinfection. Diagnostic viral cell inclusions are not seen in sites of damage. The kidneys frequently show glomerular fibrin thrombi, and these may be found in other small vessels as an expression of DIC. In addition, there may be tubular necrosis with individual cell desquamation in convoluted tubules, mixed protein, heme, and red cell casts, and cortical edema. For a detailed description of regional hemorrhagic fevers, specialized texts should be consulted.[41]

Prudent symptomatic management of fluids, electrolytes, and clotting parameters has reduced the mortality rate of the hemorrhagic fevers. Nonetheless, it remains high in the most fulminant cases, even among the vigorous and young, and specific antiviral treatment is not available.[42] Arbovirus infections (e.g., Lassa virus) may also strike suddenly among health workers and in laboratories.

VIRAL DISEASES OF CENTRAL NERVOUS SYSTEM

These diseases are described in detail in Chapter 29. Here we shall only outline their principal varieties: (1) *The CNS is the direct target for the so-called neurotropic viruses (e.g., the polio-, rabies, and encephalitis viruses) that cause acute injury; it can also be acutely damaged by other systemic viral infections,* including those with prominent skin or visceral manifestations (Table 8–2). (2) Severe, progressive chronic CNS injury may occur long after subclinical or acute infection by the measles virus (subacute sclerosing panencephalitis) or by a papovavirus (JC virus) (progressive multifocal leukoencephalopathy). (3) Relentless CNS destruction due to a new class of infectious agent, the slow viruses, occurs many years after infection (Jakob-Creutzfeldt disease) (p. 1387). (4) Inflammatory damage to the CNS may also arise days or weeks after the clinical cure of an otherwise benign viral infection or following apparently uneventful antiviral vaccination (postviral and postvaccinal encephalitis; the Guillain-Barré syndrome). Presumptive evidence of a viral cause has also been presented for certain insidious CNS disorders of unknown etiology (e.g., multiple sclerosis).

In all the viral involvements of the CNS, *manifestations of the morphologic changes and therefore clinical expression depend largely on the localization of the damaged neurons and axons.* Viruses with highly selective target neurons, as in rabies or poliomyelitis, produce the most distinctive findings. Rabies alone among the neurotropic viruses induces diagnostic cell inclusions (Negri bodies). Those agents that widely involve the brain often provide no histopathologic clue to their etiology. Therefore, virologic and serologic studies and, in some cases, electron microscopy or immunoperoxidase methods are essential diagnostic tools.

VIRAL HEART DISEASE

These diseases are discussed in Chapter 13. *It is unusual for viral infections to present clinically with isolated cardiac symptoms such as pericarditis, heart failure, or arrhythmias related to myocardial involvement in the absence of other systemic manifestations.* More commonly, myocarditis or pericarditis occur as complications of systemic viral disorders. Significantly, the cardiac lesions are not necessarily proportional to the overall severity of a viral infection, and so mild, sometimes forgotten, past illnesses may underlie a clinical cardiomyopathy or an interstitial myocardial fibrosis of unknown cause.

SUSPECTED VIRAL DISEASES

There is a strong suspicion, based largely on epidemiologic evidence, that cat-scratch disease, Kawasaki's disease (mucocutaneous lymph node syndrome), and the acquired immune deficiency syndrome (AIDS) are of viral origin.

Cat-Scratch Disease

This self-limited condition, usually manifested by localized lymphadenopathy, is seen oftener in children (80%) than in adults. Usually it takes the form of enlargement of lymph nodes, most frequently in the axilla and neck, one or more weeks usually following a feline scratch but occasionally a splinter or thorn. A raised, inflammatory nodule, vesicle, or eschar may or may not appear at the site of skin injury. Systemic manifestations are usually minimal, such as fever, mild neutrophilia or eosinophilia, and accelerated sedimentation rate. Very uncommonly, splenomegaly, mild encephalitis, thrombocytopenia, pneumonia, or focal demineralizing bone lesions have been reported, suggesting systemic spread.

The major anatomic changes involve the nodes of drainage, which may become significantly enlarged and sometimes fluctuant. Early in the condition there is a nonspecific reactive lymphadenitis. (p. 656). Thereafter, sarcoid-like granulomas (p. 391) may develop throughout the lymph node, around its capsule, and in the walls of draining veins. Coalescence of these granulomas produces the most distinctive phase of the disease with the formation of "stellate abscesses," i.e., irregular, central accumulations of vital and disintegrating neutrophils surrounded by a prominent rim of palisaded epithelioid macrophages. Although such abscesses are distinctive, they are not pathognomonic and are similar to the lesions of lymphogranuloma venereum. Special stains for bacterial and fungal agents are negative.

Although viral or chlamydial isolates have been reported from cat-scratch lesions, the evidence is not convincing. The diagnosis can often be made on clinical grounds and strongly suspected from the morphologic findings. A skin test, using sterilized exudate from known cases, is positive in over 90% of clinical cases (but it is also positive in 5% of normal individuals and over 10% of veterinarians having no history of disease).

*Kawasaki's Disease (Mucocutaneous Lymph Node Syndrome, MLNS)**

Several outbreaks of this unusual syndrome, first recognized in Japan,[43] have appeared among infants and young children in the continental U.S. and Hawaii since 1979. The disease may be preceded by a viral upper respiratory infection. It begins with fever (unresponsive to antibiotics); dramatic reddening of the conjunctivae, lips, oral mucosa, and tongue; and reddening and edematous swelling of the palms and soles. These changes are eventually followed by skin desquamation around the tips of the fingers and toes. In addition there may be an exanthematous rash or cervical lymphadenopathy not unlike those seen in several childhood viral infections. Mild elevations of liver enzymes are common and sometimes there is diarrhea or mild aseptic meningitis. Joint pain and swelling may suggest a rheumatoid or collagen-vascular disease.

The feature that distinguishes Kawasaki's disease from the usual childhood viral syndromes is inflammatory involvement of the small and medium-sized coronary artery branches, and sometimes of the peripheral arteries as well. Arteriography may reveal that these changes often reverse during convalescence. In the rare, fatal case, they take the form of segmental necrotizing arteritis with focal aneurysms and dense perivascular inflammatory infiltration.[44] The vascular alterations are indistinguishable from so-called "infantile periarteritis nodosa," regarded as an aberrant form of the adult disease (p. 520).[45]

All efforts to isolate viruses or rickettsiae from Kawasaki patients have been unsuccessful thus far, and so the possibility has been raised of a delayed immune response to an unknown preceding viral agent.[46] Occasionally, sudden death from coronary occlusion occurs in these patients after uneventful convalescence from MLNS.

Acquired Immune Deficiency Syndrome (AIDS)

This still mysterious epidemic disease has only recently come to attention, principally among: (1) male homosexuals; (2) hemophiliacs receiving multiple transfusions or factor VIII concentrate; (3) Haitians, both immigrants and nonimmigrants; and (4) drug addicts.[47] Currently, the disease is also being described in prostitutes and individuals without any known predisposing factors. Transmission from addict husbands to their wives (all heterosexual) has also been reported.[48] To date, no spread to medical, hospital, and laboratory personnel has been detected.

Although the cause of this disorder is unknown, viruses are strongly suspected. A favored candidate at the time of writing is the human T-cell leukemia/lymphoma virus (p. 678). Whatever the cause, there is a progressive, nonselective loss of cellular immunity due to depletion of T-helper/inducer cells while the T-suppressor cell population remains normal or increases in number.[49, 50] Thus, AIDS patients become vulnerable to a wide spectrum of opportunistic infectious agents as their disease progresses, including CMV, herpes simplex II and Epstein-Barr viruses, atypical mycobacteria, *Pneumocystis carinii*, fungi, and intestinal cryptosporidia. Typically, multiple invaders are present, either concurrently or sequentially, and as one is brought under control by therapy it is replaced by another. The unique feature that made this condition recognizable as a new disease is the occurrence in many of these relatively young patients of a rapidly progressive form of Kaposi's sarcoma (p. 1270), diffusely involving both skin and internal organs.[51] Because of the prominent role immunodeficiency plays in this condition, it is described in more detail on page 543.

CHLAMYDIAL DISEASES

Chlamydiae are obligate intracellular organisms, larger than viruses, which possess both DNA and RNA and form their own cell walls, much like bacteria. They also respond to wide-spectrum antibiotics. Chlamydiae are passively taken up into phagocytic vacuoles of host cells in which they multiply, alternating between large (1000 nm) and small (200 to 300 nm) forms (*"initial"* vs. *"elementary" bodies*). Cytoplasmic chlamydial inclusions, important in microscopic diagnosis, consist of aggregates of these bodies in their vacuoles; they are best visualized by immunofluorescence or in Giemsa-stained cell smears. By an unknown mechanism, chlamydiae inhibit the fusion of lysosomes with primary phagosomes, and are thus protected from attack by proteases and oxygen-derived free radicals.

Chlamydiae synthesize their own nucleic acids but not their own ATP, and unlike viruses they cannot dictate host cell synthesis of new products. They have therefore served as unique models for analyzing parasite-host cell metabolic interactions.[52] Some human chlamydial infections such as inclusion body conjunctivitis and ornithosis are acute; others such as trachoma or venereal disease tend to be protracted, causing chronic inflammatory reactions, including granulomas. Both antibodies and cellular immunity are induced, but neither seems to cope effectively with established chronic infections. The subclassification of chlamydiae is still in a state of flux. Table 8–3 lists the known serotypes and corresponding human diseases.

Table 8–3. HUMAN CHLAMYDIAL DISEASES AND SPECIES

Species and Serotype	Diseases	Transmission
Chlamydia psittaci	Ornithosis (psittacosis)	Aspiration of bird-contaminated particles
Chlamydia trachomatis		
A, B, Ba, C	Trachoma	Repeated contact, fomites, insects
D, E, F, G, H, I, J, K	Inclusion conjunctivitis	Birth canal infection (infants) Sexual contact, swimming (adults)
"	Nongonorrheal urethritis	Sexual contact
"	Postgonorrheal urethritis	Sexual contact
"	Proctitis, pharyngitis, cervicitis, arthritis, etc.	Sexual contact
L_1, L_2, L_3	Lymphogranuloma venereum	Sexual contact

Ornithosis (Psittacosis)

Ornithosis is caused by *C. psittaci,* transmitted to man by inhalation of dust-borne contaminated excreta from infected birds. Not just parrots, but many species of birds from canaries to seagulls, sick or ostensibly well, may harbor and transmit this infection.[53] Rarely, the disease is acquired through the bite of a bird or by direct contact with a patient. Household and larger epidemics have been reported. In man, *inhalation of the agent may lead to an asymptomatic infection, a transient flulike illness, or to a serious, even fatal, pneumonia.*

The incubation period varies from one to three weeks and is followed by the relatively sudden onset of fever and chills, malaise, headache, sore throat, and a nonproductive cough of variable severity. As in viral pneumonitis, dyspnea and hyperpnea may be pronounced at a time when cough, sputum, and chest physical signs are scarce or absent. X-ray findings do not always convey the extent of interstitial lung involvement. However, in the severest cases, there is pulmonary edema, alveolar damage, and consolidation; bacterial superinfection may further complicate the picture.

The lung has focal, dusky areas of increased consistency and hyperemia and is increased in weight. The pleural surfaces are usually not affected. The bronchi and bronchioles show little change but in some cases considerable hyperemia, edema, and mucopurulent exudation are present, probably owing to secondary bacterial contamination. Histologically, there is edema and mononuclear leukocytic infiltration within the alveolar septa. Seroproteinaceous fluid or fibrin may accumulate in the air spaces, accompanied by mononuclear leukocytes. The alveolar septal cells are often hypertrophic and cuboidal. Occasionally, **intracytoplasmic bodies can be identified in these alveolar cells with the Giemsa or immunofluorescent technique.** They appear as coccoid bodies, 0.25 to 4.0 μ, dark blue on Giemsa stain of smears or sections. Necrosis of alveolar septa may lead to the formation of abscesses accompanied by neutrophilic infiltration or hemorrhages. There is focal variation in the severity of lung involvement. The hilar nodes are usually enlarged and edematous, and show reticuloendothelial hyperplasia and acute lymphadenitis. **Lethal generalized disease**, seen mainly in epidemics, is marked by focal necroses in the liver and spleen, and diffuse mononuclear infiltrative changes in the kidneys, heart, and (sometimes) brain. The reticuloendothelial cells of the liver may contain intracytoplasmic elementary bodies. Similar foci may be present in the spleen accompanied by diffuse reticuloendothelial hyperactivity. Swelling of cardiac muscle fibers and interstitial edema can occur in the heart. The CNS changes consist of nonspecific edema, congestion, and occasional foci of hemorrhage, both in the brain substance and in the meningeal coverings.

In the usual case, after two to three weeks of illness, the condition improves spontaneously or with therapy, and most patients recover. A fourfold rise in specific antibody to *C. psittaci* is considered diagnostic and can be confirmed by yolk sac or tissue culture inoculation. The prognosis is dependent on the virulence of the infective agent, and fatality rates ranging from 5 to 40% have been reported. It is important to note that immunity to this infection is incomplete, and the carrier state may persist for years following recovery from active disease.

Chlamydial Urethritis and Cervicitis

These venereal infections are now the most frequent forms of chlamydial disease in the U.S., where more than half a million new cases of "nongonorrheal urethritis" are being reported annually, largely in males. Close to 50% are due to one of eight serotypes of *C. trachomatis* (Table 8–3). Chlamydiae can also be cultured from 30 to 50% of the asymptomatic female partners of these infected males, and from women with chronic cervicitis. The range and location of lesions caused by the chlamydiae parallel those of the gonococcus (p. 310). In the male, the urethritis may extend to produce acute epididymitis; in the female, extension results in salpingitis and pelvic inflammatory disease. Indeed, *C. trachomatis* may eventually replace the gonococcus as the foremost venereal pathogen in the U.S. and Europe. Infants born of infected mothers may acquire inclusion conjunctivitis and sometimes neonatal pneumonia, infections that may also be acquired by adults.[54] In addition, the role of chlamydiae in triggering Reiter's syndrome (p. 1362) is currently under study.

The symptoms, signs, and pathologic lesions of chlamydial urethritis and cervicitis are also remarkably similar to those related to *Neisseria gonorrhoeae*, but the incubation time for chlamydial infection is longer and the duration of symptoms more prolonged. The infection is often recognized by its persistence following treatment for gonorrhea ("postgonococcal urethritis"). Microscopically, both organisms cause suppurative exudation, but in chlamydial infection one sees inclusions in epithelial cells rather than cocci in the leukocytes of the exudate. Former dependence on the demonstration of typical inclusions in cell smears has been alleviated by the use of culture on McCoy cells, and of fluorescent antibodies that reveal both inclusions and elementary bodies and provide greater diagnostic accuracy. A microcomplement fixation test for type-specific chlamydial antibody is also available in specialized venereal disease centers and is applicable to cervical secretions as well as to serum.

Inclusion Conjunctivitis

This is a benign, self-limited, suppurative conjunctivitis that occurs in newborns of mothers having *C. trachomatis* birth canal infections. Adults acquire this disease by contamination with genital secretions or by bathing in unchlorinated swimming pools ("swimming pool conjunctivitis"). *The chlamydial inclusions seen in the exudate are identical with those of trachoma,* but this more benign conjunctivitis is due to a different group of *C. trachomatis* serotypes (Table 8–3).

The incubation time, as assessed in newborns, varies from five to 12 days and the disease can last for several months if untreated. It is characterized by conjunctival hyperemia, edema, and a monocyte rich purulent exudate, which diminishes after the first two weeks. In adult patients, lymphocytic infiltration is prominent, but lymph follicle formation is rare and the pannus (inflammatory membrane) and corneal scarring seen in trachoma do not occur. Certain differentiation from trachoma depends on type-specific antisera and on the immunoperoxidase and serologic methods employed for the diagnosis of urethral and cervical infections.

*Trachoma**

Trachoma is a chronic suppurative eye disease with follicular keratoconjunctivitis caused by subtypes of *C. trachomatis* (Table 8–3). It is one of the leading global causes of blindness. Although the agent is widespread in many countries, *progressive trachoma is seen mostly in dry and sandy regions and among poor people and nomads.* In these endemic areas, the infection is acquired during childhood by repetitive exposures over months or years. The responsible chlamydial strains have been shown to enter cultured human cells only with difficulty.[55]

Trachoma is transmitted by direct human contact, by contaminated particles (fomites) and, very likely, by flies also. Infections can be either self-limiting or progressive; the latter type passes from a suppurative stage resembling inclusion conjunctivitis to deeper tissue involvement, with lymphoplasmocytic infiltration and formation of lymphoid cell follicles. The upper limbus of the cornea and the upper tarsal plate tend to be most severely involved by epithelial hyperplasia and follicular hypertrophy. Soon, the conjunctiva ulcerates, and penetration into the cornea leads to pannus formation, fibroblast ingrowth, scarring, and eventual blindness. The scarring also hampers closure of the eyelids, in turn promoting bacterial superinfection. Furrowing of the mucosa overlying the tarsal plate and pitting of the upper rim of the limbus are characteristic late deformities of trachoma. *Tragically, despite the good response of this infection to sulfonamides and antibiotics, many young people in developing countries have lost their eyesight to trachoma for lack of access to medical care.*[56]

Lymphogranuloma Venereum (LGV)

Lymphogranuloma venereum (or inguinale) is a venereally transmitted disease caused by the L–1, 2, or 3 serotypes of *C. trachomatis*. It is not to be confused with granuloma inguinale, a bacterial venereal infection (p. 339). In contrast to other relatively superficial chlamydial infections, following the initial involvement of the genitalia, it promptly involves the lymph nodes, and in its rare generalized form can even cause distant lesions in many organs of the body. Largely a disease of tropical climes, its prevalence is low in the U.S., although it continues to be imported and is often spread to multiple sexual partners together with other venereal infections.

LGV infections resulting from heterosexual intercourse localize on the external genitals of either sex, but in males they tend to spread to inguinal nodes, in females to deep and perirectal lymph nodes.[57] Since the external lesions on the genitalia are painless, late stages of the infection are sometimes discovered, especially in females. Labial, buccopharyngeal, digital, or anorectal infections spreading to the corresponding lymphatic draining sites may result from variant sexual behavior or from incidental or laboratory contact, posing difficult diagnostic problems. *A history of rapidly developing tender, matted, fluctuant lymph node swellings (buboes) should arouse suspicion of LGV* but can be mimicked by other infections.

The clinical disease is best considered by stages. Chlamydial entry and tissue invasion are asymptomatic. The *first disease stage* is heralded by the appearance of genital or anorectal lesions at the site of introduction of the agent; however, in more than one-half of reported cases, these either are inapparent or never develop. About one to two weeks later, the *second stage* is initiated by the progressive swelling and enlargement of the regional nodes of drainage, either unilateral or bilateral. This stage may last from days to many weeks. Much later, *a third stage is encountered in a small percentage of the patients, consisting of either elephantiasis of the genitals due to lymphatic obstruction or, in females, of fibrous strictures of the rectum due to inflammatory scarring.* Patients in these late stages may have hyperglobulinemia, presumably related to the plasmocytosis found in the lesions.

The earliest lesion is a small intraepidermal or subepidermal vesicle that soon ruptures to create a shallow inflammatory ulcer, either genital or extragenital. The surface of the ulcer is bathed in a neutrophilic exudate. The ulcer base shows a fairly nondescript mononuclear leukocytic infiltration accompanied by edema, fibroblastic proliferation, some vascular engorgement, and endothelial cell hyperplasia. Occasionally, granulomas similar to those that occur in the lymph nodes occur in the base of these ulcerations. Chlamydial inclusions may be seen in the phagocytes within these lesions.

The regional lymphadenitis is characterized by the progressive swelling of the nodes, creating large, painful buboes. The nodes first are discrete, but as the inflammatory reaction extends into the perinodal tissue, they become matted together. Early in the disease, they have a pink, hyperemic, succulent appearance, but as the inflammatory reaction matures, suppurative necrosis transforms them into fluctuant sacs. These buboes may rupture through the overlying hyperemic skin to produce draining sinuses.

Histologically, the nodes first show nonspecific, diffuse reticuloendothelial hyperplasia and permeation by mononuclear leukocytes. However, aggregates of macrophages soon develop into small granulomas. The centers then become necrotic to create minute abscesses. **As these lesions coalesce, they form irregular linear or branching "stellate abscesses,"** consisting of focal areas of suppuration enclosed within a granulomatous wall, a lesion distinctive but not pathognomonic of LGV (recall cat-scratch fever and certain fungal infections).[58] The centers of the abscesses contain neutrophils in varying stages of preservation, about which there is a radially arranged palisade of epithelioid cells, sometimes replete with Langhans' or foreign body giant cells (Fig. 8–8). Elementary or inclusion bodies can sometimes be visualized in these cells with Giemsa stain or immunofluorescent methods. About the enclosing wall there is an intense infiltrate of plasma cells and lymphocytes. Blood vessels in this inflammatory wall are dilated and often show endothelial proliferation.

With chronicity the infection may last for many weeks or months, leading to considerable fibroblastic proliferation and scarring of the nodes. **Thus, the late sequelae of LGV stem from fibrosis and lymphatic blockage;** chlamydial inclusions become scarce and may not be found, and granulomas may be absent, although plasma cell infiltrates tend to persist. Marked edema and **elephantiasis of the female external genitalia** is known as **"esthiomene." Elephantiasis of the penis may develop.** Because of the drainage of the infection to the perirectal and deeper pelvic nodes in the female, chronic fibrosis about the rectum produces strictures that are sometimes difficult to differentiate from rectal carcinoma.[57]

The diagnosis of LGV can usually be suspected by the clinical finding of large, fluctuant buboes or draining sinuses, especially if they bulge both above and below the inguinal fold, divided by a "groove." Similarly, the combination of rectal stricture and perineal deformity in a young female is highly suggestive. *Characteristic histologic lesions with inclusion bodies confirm the diagnosis.* The *Frei test,* formerly the mainstay of diagnosis, is a delayed-hypersensitivity skin reaction using antigen from yolk sac cultures of *C. trachomatis.* Because this antigen crossreacts with other more common chlamydiae, it is no longer widely used. The LGV complement fixation antigen shows similar cross reactivity, although high titers of this test are of some diagnostic help. A serotype-specific microimmunofluorescent test for L-type chlamydiae has recently been developed but is as yet available only in specialized centers. Definitive diagnosis can also be made from aspirates of buboes by growth of the agent in tissue culture. Early stages of the infection respond slowly to antibiotics, but the fibrosing late lesions may require surgical intervention. It should not be overlooked that *LGV patients frequently harbor other venereal diseases, including latent syphilis.*

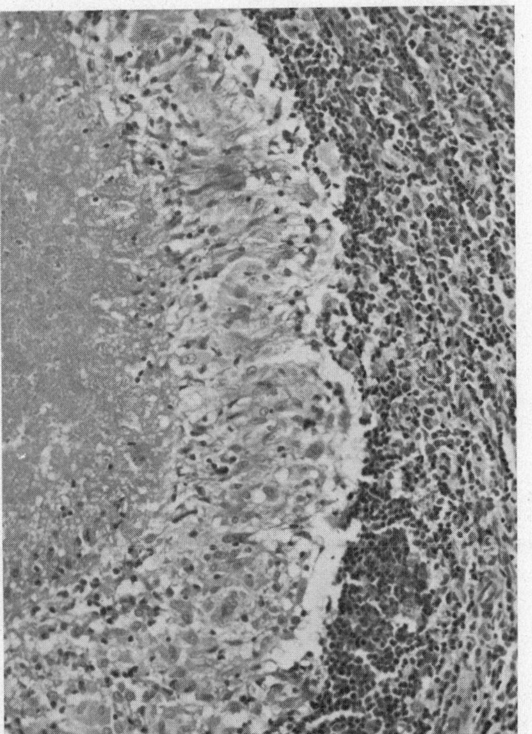

Figure 8–8. Lymphogranuloma venereum. The margin of a characteristic "stellate" abscess rimmed by a granulomatous reaction.

RICKETTSIAL DISEASES

Rickettsiae are small, bacteria-like, *obligate intracellular parasites* with leaky cell walls that can peacefully perpetuate themselves in arthropod vectors by transovarial transmission,[59] but promptly change to a pathogenic mode when deposited in mammalian tissue. Here, they actively penetrate host cells and, *after briefly lodging in phagosomes, escape into the cytosol where they multiply, free of lysosomal attack.* Rickettsiae do not produce toxins and the manner by which they damage tissues is uncertain; activation of endogenous phospholipase A^2 could explain the necrosis, hemolysis, and disseminated intravascular coagulation (DIC) that complicate severe rickettsial infections.[60] A listing of rickettsial species and diseases is given in Table 8–4.

Rickettsiae begin multiplying at the inoculation site where *a dark, swollen, crusted skin lesion (eschar) may or may not be formed.* Hence, they disseminate via the bloodstream, causing an acute febrile reaction. *All but one rickettsial species (that of Q fever) share an affinity for the endothelium of small blood vessels. Swelling and spotty destruction of these cells results in bleeding, sometimes thrombosis, and in purpuric skin rashes.* These are especially severe in Rocky Mountain spotted fever (RMSF), whose agent also invades arteriolar smooth muscle cells. Perivascular inflammatory cells, especially mononuclear phagocytes, take up, disseminate, and ultimately dispose of the rickettsiae, but the effector mechanism by which the rickettsiae are killed in their intracytoplasmic sanctuaries is unclear. Cell-mediated immunity has been linked with host recovery and, following vaccination or cure, protective antibodies against reinfection are generated, resulting in lasting immunity. However, late recurrences may ensue, especially in typhus fever caused by *R. prowazekii,* indicating that the immune responses are not always totally effective and that this agent can assume a latent form. *Inflammatory responses to rickettsiae are typically mononuclear aggregates or "nodules" composed of activated macrophages and lymphocytes,* and are best appreciated in CNS lesions. Neutrophils appear mainly at sites of necrosis. The antibodies to rickettsiae that

Table 8–4. SUMMARY OF CERTAIN IMPORTANT EPIDEMIOLOGIC AND CLINICAL CHARACTERISTICS OF RICKETTSIAL DISEASES

Disease	Epidemiologic Features *Geographic Occurrence*	*Vector*	Reservoir	Usual Incubation Period (days)	Eschar	Rash *Distribution*	Rash *Type*
Typhus Group							
Primary louse-borne typhus	Worldwide	Louse	Man	12 (8–15)	None	Trunk to extremities	Macular, maculopapular
Brill-Zinsser disease	Worldwide	Recrudescence of primary attack	—	—	None	Trunk to extremities	Macular, maculopapular
Murine typhus	Scattered pockets, worldwide	Flea	Rodents	12 (6–14)	None	Trunk to extremities	Macular, maculopapular
Spotted Fever Group							
Rocky Mountain spotted fever	Western hemisphere	Tick	Ticks, rodents	6 (2–12)	None	Extremities to trunk, palms, soles	Macular, maculopapular, petechial
Tick typhus	Mediterranean littoral, Africa, Asia	Tick	Ticks, rodents	12 (7–18)	Frequent	Trunk, extremities, face, palms, soles	Macular, maculopapular, petechial
Rickettsialpox	USA, USSR, Korea	Mites	House mouse	12 (9–24)	Usually present	Trunk, face, extremities	Papular, vesicular
Scrub typhus	Japan, SW Asia and SW Pacific	Mite	Mites, rodents	11 (6–21)	Frequent	Trunk to extremities	Macular, maculopapular, evanescent
Q fever	Worldwide	Inhalation	Ticks, mammals	14 (9–20)	None	None	None

Modified from Murray, E. S.: Introduction to rickettsial disease. *In* Beeson, P. B., and McDermott, W. (eds.): Cecil-Loeb Textbook of Medicine. 14th ed. Philadelphia, W. B. Saunders Co., 1975, p. 249.

appear during the second week of infection cross-react with the stable laboratory OX strains of the common gram-negative bacillus *Proteus vulgaris*, providing the widely available Weil-Felix test used to identify current or past rickettsial infections *by group but not by species*. It is being replaced by more specific rickettsial complement fixation and agglutination tests. Given the urgency of early treatment for such life-threatening infections as RMSF and typhus, direct demonstration of rickettsiae by immunofluorescence is increasingly replacing the temperamental special stains formerly used in tissue biopsies.

Typhus Fever

There are three forms of typhus fever: (1) epidemic (or primary) louse-borne typhus, (2) Brill-Zinsser disease (a recrudescence of an earlier louse-borne infection), and (3) murine or flea-borne typhus fever. All three diseases are clinically and pathologically similar. They differ principally in their epidemiology, severity, and causative agents. Epidemic typhus has always been one of the horrors of war. Hans Zinsser's book, *Rats, Lice and History*[61] vividly describes its role in past campaigns, including the defeat of Napoleon. This disease again became epidemic during World War II, and in 1975 in strife-torn Uganda, and now awaits its next opportunity (if there are any survivors of nuclear bombs).

The typhus agent, *Rickettsia prowazekii*, approximately 300 nm in diameter, bears three known antigens, one associated with the cell wall; another with the cytoplasm; and a third, soluble erythrocyte-sensitizing antigen. It is transmitted from man to man by human head and body lice (*Pediculus humanus capitis* or *corporis*), which are themselves infected by biting a typhus patient during the febrile period of the disease. In the few sporadic human infections reported, the flying squirrel may act as a reservoir host.[62] The organisms multiply within the cells lining the gut of the louse and pass out with the feces. When the louse feeds, its human victim scratches the irritated site, thereby introducing the infective feces into the skin puncture. A local area of hemorrhage may mark the site of the bite, but an eschar is not common. *It is also possible to contract the disease without being infested by lice;* thus, transfer has occurred merely by contact of a skin abrasion with contaminated clothing.

After an eight- to 15-day incubation period, headache, weakness, chills, and fever appear, followed in a few days by a generalized skin rash. During the period of chills and fever, blood-borne dissemination is taking place. At first the rash is maculopapular and pink to bright red, and pressure will blanch it, but during the second week lesions become darker and fixed. Characteristically, the rash begins on the trunk and extends centrifugally. In very severe cases, the individual macules and papules coalesce to produce irregular mottling and maplike blotches. During the second week, there is usually CNS involvement in the form of apathy, progressing to dullness, stupor, and even coma; sometimes this progression is punctuated by episodes of wild delirium. If the patient recovers, the rash begins to fade and the temperature begins to subside toward the end of the third week. Most fatalities occur during the second and third weeks of the illness. During some epidemics, the mortality from typhus has risen to 50%, but today, with effective antibiotics, the death rate is below 10%.

In milder cases, the macroscopic changes are limited to the skin rash and small hemorrhages incident to the vascular lesions. In more severe cases with DIC there may be areas of necrosis of the skin with gangrene of the tips of the fingers, nose, ear lobes, scrotum, penis, and vulva. In such cases, irregular ecchymotic hemorrhages may be found internally, principally in the brain, heart muscle, testes, serosal membrane, lungs, and kidneys.

The microscopic findings in all cases tend to be far more widespread than the gross alterations would suggest. Most prominent are the small vessel lesions that underlie the rash, and the focal areas of hemorrhage and inflammation in the various organs and tissues affected[63] Endothelial proliferation and swelling in the capillaries, arterioles, and venules may narrow the lumina of these vessels. Rickettsiae can usually be demonstrated by immunofluorescent methods in these cells. Surrounding the involved vessels, a cuff of inflammatory mixed leukocytes is usually present (Fig. 8–9). The vascular lumina are sometimes thrombosed but necrosis of the vessel wall is unusual

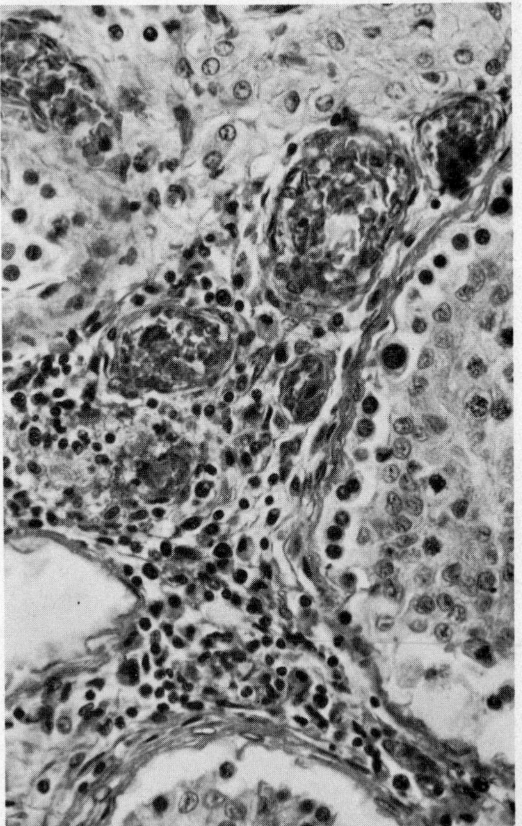

Figure 8–9. Testis in typhus fever with a focus of interstitial leukocytic infiltrate and acute vascular lesions.

in typhus, as compared with RMSF. It is the vascular thromboses that lead to the gangrenous necroses of the skin and other structures.

In the brain of untreated cases, the small vessel lesions tend to be limited to the gray matter and are often associated with focal microglial proliferations mixed with other leukocytes to produce the characteristic "typhus nodule" (Fig. 8–10). Microglial cells are also diffusely increased in numbers throughout the brain. Mononuclear cell meningitis, ring hemorrhages about the small vessels, and, occasionally, degenerative changes in ganglion cells may occur (presumably on an ischemic basis). In addition, an interstitial pneumonitis may be present, sometimes accompanied by exudative consolidation of alveoli, most likely due to secondary bacterial invaders. Typically, there is also nonspecific lymphadenitis and splenitis.[63] Diffuse perivascular mononuclear cell infiltrations as well as foci resembling the typhus nodules of the brain may appear in the heart, kidney, testes, and liver.

Because all the rickettsial infections resemble one another, the differential diagnosis of typhus fever can be difficult. Moreover, infections such as typhoid fever, meningococcemia, measles, and those caused by arboviruses produce similar febrile reactions with a rash. A high titer in the Weil-Felix reaction, although not specific, is strongly suggestive. Specific serologic tests (complement fixation and agglutination) are very important in establishing the precise diagnosis, but these become unequivocally positive only during the second week.

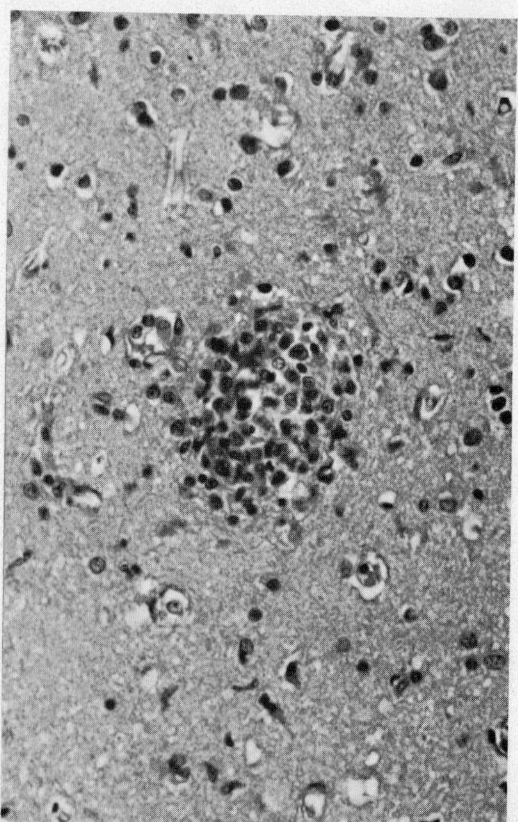

Figure 8–10. A typhus nodule in the brain.

Brill-Zinsser disease is a recrudescent form of epidemic typhus, appearing as a relatively mild febrile illness years after the initial attack of typhus. In the U.S., this condition occurs mostly in Eastern European immigrants. The causative agent is, of course, that of epidemic typhus, but the factors that precipitate such recrudescence are unknown. In the few lethal cases studied, the histopathologic changes are essentially the same as in epidemic typhus, but the disease tends to be milder, and only rarely are focal necroses and gangrene encountered.[64]

Murine typhus is an endemic form of rickettsial infection, somewhat milder than epidemic typhus. It is transmitted to man by rat fleas, and has a natural animal reservoir in rats and mice. Domestic cats and the cat flea have also been incriminated. The causative agent is *R. mooseri (typhi).*[65] Mortality from this infection is low in the U.S., but both the frequency and the mortality continue to be significant in Mexico. The anatomic changes are similar to those of epidemic typhus. Specific serologic tests are required to differentiate this disease from epidemic typhus.

Rocky Mountain Spotted Fever (RMSF)*

Spotted fevers are a group of rickettsial infections characterized by a prominent hemorrhagic rash. All are transmitted from animal reservoirs to man by ticks or mites, each disease linked to particular wild or domestic reservoir hosts, insect vectors, and ecologic settings (Table 8–4). Because there is no easy way of controlling the hosts and vectors or human contact with the latter, small outbreaks of spotted fevers are likely to continue throughout the world.

The prototype disease is RMSF caused by *R. rickettsi* and transmitted by several species of hard ticks. The disease is limited to North and South America and is reported during every tick season in the Carolinas, in Virginia, up the Eastern seaboard, and (less frequently) elsewhere in the U.S. Ironically, it is uncommon in the Bitterroot Valley of Montana where it was originally discovered by H. T. Ricketts, the single-minded microbe hunter who died of the infection he had described so well. In the last decade the annual number of cases in the U.S. has more than doubled. Although no age group is spared, many infections occur in children.

Patients with RMSF may or may not recall the infective tick bite. A primary lesion that becomes hemorrhagic and necrotic and may lead to an eschar is rarely observed at the site of the bite. About two to 12 days later, a full-blown rash ensues. This is at first maculopapular, pink, and predominantly peripheral in distribution, in contrast to the centrally distributed rash of typhus fever. Characteristically, the palms of the hands and soles of the feet are involved. Patients at this time are markedly febrile with chills, mental apathy, and sometimes stupor. In the course of the next few days, the rash extends centripetally and becomes hemorrhagic. In more severe cases, coalescence of lesions produces large, mottled ecchymoses or geographic maplike patterns. Because the organisms penetrate deeply into the vessel walls, the vascular lesions that underlie the rash often lead to acute necrosis, fibrin extravasation, and thrombosis of the small blood vessels, including arterioles (Fig. 8–11). Foci of necrotic skin are thus induced, particularly on the fingers, toes, elbows, ears, and scrotum. Vascular necrosis and thrombosis are far more frequent with RMSF than with typhus and may mimic the necrotizing vasculitis of the collagen-vascular diseases. DIC is the harbinger of death in severe cases. The perivascular inflammatory response is otherwise similar to that of typhus, particularly in the brain, skeletal muscle, lungs, kidneys, testes, and heart muscle. The vascular necroses in the brain may involve larger vessels and produce focal areas of ischemic demyelinization or microinfarcts. A pneumonitis of primary rickettsial origin is present in severely affected patients and often predisposes to a secondary bacterial infection.

Antibiotic and supportive therapy has reduced the mortality rate to 3 to 10%. Deaths are due to shock, DIC, renal failure, and CNS damage. RMSF is especially severe in black patients with G6PD deficiency or other hemoglobinopathies. The anatomic changes of RMSF resemble, to a considerable extent, those of typhus, meningococcemia, and other bacterial and viral diseases responsible for hemorrhagic rashes, and these conditions must be ruled out by appropriate laboratory tests. Diagnosis is urgent, since the prognosis depends on the duration of illness before therapy is instituted. Immunofluorescent staining of rickettsiae in skin biopsies can be of help.[66] A gas-liquid chromatographic method for early detection of rickettsial antigen in serum has recently been described.[66A] Specific antibody tests become positive only later in the course.

*Scrub Typhus (Tsutsugamushi Fever)**

Scrub typhus caused by *R. tsutsugamushi* is a mite-borne rickettsial disease endemic largely in Southeast Asia, the U.S.S.R., Australia, and the Pacific regions. It bears many resemblances, both clinically and pathologically, to both typhus and spotted fever. *It is characterized by fever, headache, lymphadenopathy, and sometimes a maculopapular rash.* In most cases, but not all, an eschar develops "right at the site of the bite of a mite"—to be more accurate, the bite of the larval form of the mite. There is a wide reservoir of infection in wild rodents. The mites themselves provide another reservoir.

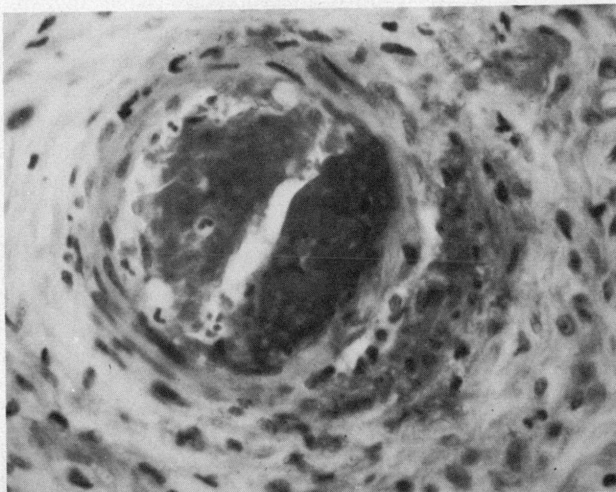

Figure 8–11. RMSF arteritis with mural thrombus and red cell extravasation.

The disease begins in most patients *with the appearance of an eschar,* which may be large, indurated, and black, at the cutaneous site of attachment of the larval mite. The organisms multiply, drain to regional nodes to produce lymphadenopathy, and then disseminate through the blood system. Once again, the skin, brain, lung, serosal surfaces, kidney, heart, and other organs are affected in a distribution similar to that of typhus and spotted fevers. Vascular necrosis and thrombosis is much less frequent in this condition, and so the rash is rarely hemorrhagic. Also, the perivascular inflammatory response is far less prominent. In the brain, the lesions usually consist of a few minor vascular and perivascular reactions, with the occasional formation of glial nodules. A scant meningitis may be present, characterized principally by an accumulation of mononuclear cells in the subarachnoid space. Interstitial pneumonitis of rickettsial origin, sometimes with a superimposed bacterial pneumonia, is encountered in more severe cases. Somewhat distinctive of this condition is the tendency for involvement of serous surfaces, i.e., peritonitis, pleuritis, and pericarditis.[67]

The mortality rate has in the past been reported to be high, but since laboratory diagnosis has made it possible to recognize mild infections and since antibiotic therapy became effective, fatalities have become rare (about 2%). The diagnosis rests with identification of the causative agent and with specific serologic tests.[68]

Q Fever

Human Q fever, caused by *Coxiella burnetii,* is usually transmitted to man by the respiratory route from infected animals, especially sheep and cattle. *Unlike other rickettsial infections, Q fever causes no eschar or skin rash* and can therefore mimic other infections that induce headache, cough, myalgia, swollen lymph nodes, or hepatosplenomegaly.[69]

In nature, this zoonosis is spread by ticks among many wild animal species, sheep, and cattle. Since the rickettsia is exceptionally resistant to drying, it can also be transmitted by inhalation of airborne particles—human infection is most frequently airborne; those handling pregnant or lactating cows or sheep, drinking unpasteurized milk, or working in slaughter-houses are at highest risk. Individuals even a mile distant from an infected herd are known to have become infected. *A negative occupational history, therefore, does not exclude this infection, although a positive one suggests it.*

The usual incubation period is three weeks; the onset of the disease with fever is sudden but in about ten days is followed by slow convalescence. Bradycardia, hepatosplenomegaly, and myalgias are among the more frequent findings. The mortality rate is less than 1% even without treatment. Respiratory involvement ranges from only a dry cough to severe interstitial pneumonitis resembling viral pneumonia, ornithosis, or "primary atypical pneumonia." Pulmonary bacterial superinfection or, rarely, infection of the heart valves or progressive liver failure (which may be indistinguishable from viral hepatitis) account for the few deaths.

In fatal cases **there is an interstitial pneumonia virtually indistinguishable from viral pneumonia or "primary atypical pneumonia."** Nearly confluent involvement of both lower lobes is characteristic. The alveolar walls are thickened by edema and a predominantly mononuclear infiltrate with focal exudation of fibrin and mononuclear, sometimes foamy, phagocytes. Necrosis of alveolar walls or extensive consolidation may develop, probably from bacterial superinfection. In severe prolonged disease, small granulomas may appear in the spleen, liver, or bone marrow, some with epithelioid cells radially arranged around a fat-containing vacuole ringed by fibrinoid material (ring granulomas).[70,71] These changes are suggestive but not diagnostic of Q fever. Focal perivascular inflammatory infiltrates may be seen in many other organs, and very rarely (in patients with immunodeficiencies) rickettsial endocarditis.

On Australian sheep farms and California cattle-raising areas, Q fever is well-known, but in areas of lower endemicity it is often not suspected until more common fevers have been ruled out. Sometimes it may be diagnosed only retrospectively. The Weil-Felix test is of no help, but a complement fixation test using a *C. burnetii* antigen obtained from chick embryo cultures ("phase 2 antigen") is available. A fourfold rise in titer or a single high titer should confirm the diagnosis after the second week. Although *C. burnetii* can be visualized in biopsies by immunofluorescent staining, this is rarely necessary except in prolonged and atypical cases.

MYCOPLASMA DISEASES

Mycoplasmas are also called pleuropneumonia-like organisms (PPLOs) or Eaton agents. They are almost ubiquitous in nature both as saprophytes and as parasites, yet their biology and pathogenicity are perhaps the least well understood of any infectious agent.[72] They resemble the so-called L-forms of bacteria and are tiny organisms (125 to 350 nm) of polymorphous shape that form slow-growing, small, sometimes fried-egg–shaped colonies on special cell-free media. They can also be grown in yolk sac or tissue cultures. Not only are they the tiniest free-living organisms known, but they are also the cause of many important diseases of fowl and cattle; indeed, mycoplasmas have been isolated from a vast number of animals and plants, far down the evolutionary scale.

M. pneumoniae, a proved human pathogen causing primary atypical pneumonia, behaves as an extracellular human parasite and incites epithelial damage in the airways, eliciting predominantly mononuclear inflammatory reactions resembling those in viral infections. Host responses to other mycoplasmas in man and in animals differ widely in course and character; some resemble gram-negative infections, resulting in neutrophil-rich purulent exudate. Small wonder, then, that from time to time mycoplasmas are cultured from diseases of obscure cause, such as infections of the lower urinary tract (p. 1030).

Mycoplasma Pneumonia

It is estimated that *M. pneumoniae* causes about 10 to 30% of primary interstitial pneumonias, mostly in adolescents and young adults. These infections are sometimes epidemic among military recruits and in closed institutions. The pulmonary involvement is very similar to that of viral pneumonia, described on page 280. In the few fatal cases studied,[73] the pulmonary changes induced by the mycoplasma were complicated by bacterial superinfection. *M. pneumoniae* elicits both 19S and 7S complement-fixing antibody. *It also elicits, in about 40% of infections, immunoglobulins that agglutinate human Group-O red cells at 4°C—"cold agglutinins," a test frequently used to confirm the diagnosis. It is also sometimes the cause of false-positive serologic tests for syphilis or streptococcal infections.* Although the mycoplasma pneumonia may last for weeks, even after the fever abates, mild infections detectable only by the cold agglutinin test are most common. Death is rare, and treatment with wide-spectrum antibiotics is effective.

BACTERIAL, SPIROCHETAL, AND MYCOBACTERIAL DISEASES

The extracellular bacterial pathogens of man must resist early engulfment by neutrophils in order to gain a foothold in host tissue, and many have remarkably effective mechanisms to favor their survival. Some generate toxins lethal for leukocytes and other host cells, e.g., the gas-forming anaerobes, and anthrax bacilli. Others, such as the pneumococci, solve their survival problems by forming slippery hydrophilic capsules that resist attachment to wandering neutrophils. Pneumococcal capsules also weakly activate the alternate complement pathway, but high-affinity binding via Fc receptors is delayed until macrophages have ingested sufficient numbers for effective antigen presentation and opsonizing antibody can be formed by specific B-cell clones. In addition, the pneumococci are capable of more than 80 permutations of their capsular polysaccharides, so that in repeated infection the host is unlikely to recognize the new serotype. *Borrelia recurrentis*, a spirochete, is programmed to switch on new sets of antigenic surface determinants repeatedly before each successive clone is exterminated. This results in several clinical bouts of relapsing fever. Programmed antigenic variation or plasmid-induced antigenic variation is common among bacteria, but the full significance of either in the pathogenesis of human infection is still to be clarified.[74]

Facultative intracellular bacteria such as the tubercle bacillus, *Brucella*, and other chronic infectious agents lack mucoid capsules and quick-acting toxins. *They counteract phagocyte aggression* ***after*** *being interiorized, either by inhibiting fusion of phagocytic vac-*

uoles with lysosomes or by somehow shielding themselves from the free radicals and enzymes generated around them. Unlike viruses and rickettsiae, they cannot leave the phagosomes. Nonetheless, they have the potential of establishing latent foci of infection capable of long-term reactivation, often resulting in granulomatous lesions. Bacterial survival in the face of effective phagolysosome fusion is attributed to specific surface components, the best-known examples being the long-chain lipids and waxes of mycobacterial cell walls, such as "cording factor" (p. 342). Experimental analysis of phagosome function in intracellular infections is continuing[75] and should promote an understanding of the initiation and chronicity of several important human diseases, especially those in which foamy macrophages containing many large phagosomes are features, e.g., leprosy, leishmaniasis, rhinoscleroma, malakoplakia (p. 1069), and the so-called xanthogranulomatous infections (p. 1035).

Having established themselves, bacteria can damage host tissues directly in a number of ways.

1. Species capable of fast geometric multiplication soon reach sufficient numbers to compete with the nutritional requirements of host tissues; at the same time, their waste products may alter the local pH or oxygen tension or otherwise interfere with eukaryotic cell metabolism.

2. The list of potentially harmful compounds synthesized by bacteria is virtually endless, yet *relatively few bacterial products have been proved to have defined deleterious effects in vivo.* Many bacterial leukocidins, hemolysins, hyaluronidases, coagulases, fibrinolysins, and others extracted from bacterial cultures act on their respective substrates in vitro, but their role in human disease remains presumptive. By contrast, in a few specific instances *the so-called bacterial "exotoxins" directly determine disease manifestations by known molecular mechanisms.* Diphtheria toxin is a prime example; the structural gene coding for its production resides in a lysogenic bacteriophage that infects *Corynebacterium diphtheriae.* The toxin is a proenzyme protein composed of a C-terminal fragment essential for attachment and entry into cells and an enzymatically active N-terminal fragment that catalyzes the transfer of ADP-ribose from NAD into covalent linkage with elongation factor 2, thus halting the assembly of polypeptides on host cell ribosomes.[76] The toxic proenzyme of certain strains of *Pseudomonas aeruginosa,* named exotoxin-A, acts in an identical manner.[77] The heat-labile enterotoxins of *Vibrio cholerae* and of *Escherichia coli* are likewise ADP-ribosyl transferases, but these enzymes catalyze transfer from NAD to the guanyl-nucleotide–dependent regulatory component of adenylate cyclase, thereby generating excess cAMP. *Although the molecular mechanisms of all these enzymes are related, they differ in their final pathogenic results:* release of enterotoxin in the gut lumen activates the secretion of its mucosa, resulting in voluminous diarrhea and in loss of water and electrolytes; by contrast, wide dissemination of diphtheria toxin is first manifested by neural and myocardial dysfunction.

The gram-positive anaerobic clostridia are virtuosos of bacterial enzyme synthesis. *C. perfringens,* the agent of gas gangrene, literally digests host tissues, including the relatively resistant collagens. Its alphatoxin is a lecithinase that disrupts plasma membranes, including those of red and white blood cells. More selective and subtle are the toxins of *C. tetani,* a wound contaminant, and of *C. botulinum,* which grows in poorly preserved food rather than in human tissue. Tetanospasmin finds its way to the presynaptic terminals of the spinal interneurons, where it interferes with the release of inhibitory transmitter substance, thus inducing the violent muscular contractions that characterize tetanic spasm. Botulinus toxins block the release of cholinergic neurotransmitters by intracellular Ca^{++}, particularly at the neuromuscular junctions, resulting in progressive paralysis of the limbs, breathing muscles, and cranial motor nerves. *Tetanus and botulinus toxins are so selective that the changes by which they kill can scarcely be visualized even by electron microscopy,* and their potency is such that a pinch of either would theoretically suffice to depopulate an entire megalopolis.

Toxin production by bacteria can be encoded by their own chromosomes as a stable species marker, but it can also be phage transmitted (as in diphtheria) or can be conveyed between bacterial strains or species by plasmids via the long sexual pili of these organisms. Thus, the enterotoxic ADP-ribosyl transferase of *E. coli* has proved to be plasmid transmissible. DNA hybridization methods are being developed to determine the presence or absence of toxin-encoding plasmids in isolates of enteric bacteria, having rich promise of future clinical applications.[78] The *bacterial cytogenetics of toxin production are analogous to those of antibiotic resistance;* here, too, resistance sometimes depends on a specific inactivating enzyme, such as a beta-lactamase (penicillinase) encoded within plasmids transmitted from one bacterial strain or species to another.[79]

3. *Bacterial cell walls, especially those of gram-negative organisms, contain lipopolysaccharide-protein complexes, the so-called "endotoxins,"* released mainly by disintegrating pathogens. The protein moiety of these molecules varies by species and can be discriminated by serotyping, but their lipopolysaccharide "business end" is shared between species and accounts for the striking systemic effects (such as high fever, increased capillary permeability, shock, and DIC) seen in many severe infections. Some of the effects of endotoxins are attributable to their disruption of polymorphonuclear leukocytes with the release of their endogenous enzymes and pyrogens. Foci of necrosis in internal organs, including bilateral renal cortical necrosis (p. 1050), such as occur in endotoxemia, can be experimentally reproduced by repeated endotoxin injections (the "Shwartzman reaction"), or by blockade of the reticuloendothelial system prior to endotoxin challenge. Patients with gram-negative infections who undergo urinary catheterization or bowel surgery are candidates for endotoxemia, but thanks to better understanding and use of antibiotics, this complication has occurred less often lately.

4. Bacteria contain many particulate and soluble

antigens that evoke strong, often lasting host immune responses, both humoral and cellular. Antibodies cross-reacting with other parasite species are not unusual and, in some chronic infections such as syphilis, antibodies to common cell antigens, called reagins, are formed, and are indeed used for serologic diagnosis. *Host defense against bacterial infections depends on phagocyte competence and on intact complement and immune systems* (Chapters 2 and 5). Acting in concert, they must overcome the evasive parasite maneuvers outlined. In some instances, phagocyte competence bears the brunt of the defense; in others, the immune system. Many extracellular bacteria are vulnerable to circulating antibodies and are readily opsonized, while intracellular organisms succumb mainly to macrophages activated by cellular immunity. Some infections can be efficiently prevented by vaccination: e.g., immunization with modified bacterial toxins (toxoids) will provide a safeguard against the ill effects of tetanus or diphtheria. By contrast, previous exposure to staphylococci provides little protection against repeat challenge, and here resistance to infections depends largely on the host phagocytes.

In the altered host, any of the links in the chain of host defense can be weakened and, by analyzing these defects, critical effector systems for different pathogens can be defined. For example, patients with defective leukocyte granules, as in the Chédiak-Higashi syndrome (p. 51), suffer from recurrent acute bacterial infections, especially by staphylococci. Individuals deficient in the 5th and later components of complement are especially vulnerable to Neisseria bacteremia.[80] T-cell immunosuppressed patients frequently reactivate dormant infections by tubercle bacilli or other intracellular parasites.

Part of the abnormalities seen in acute infectious diseases can be host mediated. In acute infections, neutrophil pyrogens cause fever and neutrophil proteases contribute to liquefaction necrosis and abscess formation. In chronic granulomatous infection due to facultative intracellular parasites such as the tubercle bacillus, the hypersensitivity mechanisms causing cell damage have been difficult to dissociate from those responsible for host resistance (p. 343). Thus, the defensive response of the host can be regarded as a two-edged sword. On the one hand, it is critical to overcoming an infection; on the other hand, it may itself contribute to the production of damage. Perhaps for that reason, in chronic infections *immunomodulatory T-cell circuits*[81] *come into play that spontaneously dampen host inflammatory responses and render them more tolerable.* In more practical terms, suppression of cell-mediated immunity by drugs is usually countervailing in chronic infection, although corticoid anti-inflammatory drugs have limited uses in reducing tissue responses when given concomitantly with specific antibiotics (e.g., in tuberculous meningitis).

When chronic infection becomes overwhelming, antigen-specific immunomodulation is sometimes replaced by a state of profound, nonselective host anergy in which there is unresponsiveness of T cells to common skin antigens (e.g., those of fungi or streptococci), loss of a previous reaction to tuberculin, and depressed lymphocyte response to mitogens. This can be accompanied by marked B-cell stimulation and hypergammaglobulinemia of a polyclonal type, a state best exemplified in late, lepromatous leprosy. The progressive downhill course that results from this anergy is seemingly irreversible, but has been reported to be reversed by vaccination with mycobacterial antigens.[82]

Table 8–5 provides a working classification of bacterial diseases that takes into account shared clinical and pathologic features likely to be considered in their differential diagnosis.

PYOGENIC COCCI

Organisms of this group evoke neutrophilic exudations and together account for most suppurative lesions seen in medical practice, either as a pus-filled, walled-off abscess or as a spreading "cellulitis" or "phlegmon." In the lung, suppuration may focally involve the terminal airways and alveoli (bronchopneumonia) or extend diffusely throughout the lobe (lobar pneumonia). Exudative and purulent lesions in other anatomic sites have been given specific names, to be cited below. In hospital practice other bacterial groups, especially the common gram-negative "rods" (Table 8–5), have become increasingly important causes of suppurative lesions that are seldom sufficiently distinctive grossly or microscopically to suggest a particular causation. Microbiologic culture is therefore essential in all pyogenic infections.

Staphylococcal Infections

Micrococcus pyogenes var. aureus and *var. dermatitidis (albus)*, i.e., the coagulase-positive and -negative "staph.," *can infect any body site. S. aureus* is the foremost cause of skin abscesses (furuncles, carbuncles) and of deep-seated suppuration in bones (osteomyelitis), and often contaminates traumatic and surgical wounds. Frequently it infects the lung, inducing severe, suppurative, often abscess-forming bronchopneumonia. *S. aureus* is also a rare cause of severe, invasive enterocolitis. It may disseminate from any site to produce septicemia, endocarditis, or pyemia (metastatic abscesses). Strains infecting only the keratinized skin layer cause a honey-colored crusting dermatitis named "impetigo." Staphylococcal toxins are involved in the "scalded skin syndrome" of babies, in food poisoning, and in the "toxic shock syndrome" of young women. *S. albus* is a less virulent pathogen; it often infects surgical wounds or lodges on prosthetic implants, necessitating their removal.

Diverse strains pervade our homes and hospitals and inhabit the nasopharynx and skin of most people. Few are virulent *S. aureus*, but otherwise healthy people may carry them or be periodically afflicted by mild skin or upper respiratory infections, spreading them to others by contact or droplet infection. Carriers and their infected ambience can be monitored by culture

Table 8–5. BACTERIAL, SPIROCHETAL, AND MYCOBACTERIAL DISEASES

Clinical/Microbiologic Category	Species	Frequent Disease Presentations
Infections by Pyogenic Cocci	*Staph. aureus, epidermidis*	Abscess, cellulitis, pneumonia, septicemia
	Streptococcus hemolyticus, viridans	URI, erysipelas, scarlet fever, septicemia
	Streptococcus pneumoniae (Pneumococcus)	Lobar pneumonia, meningitis
	Neisseria meningitidis (Meningococcus)	Cerebrospinal meningitis
	Neisseria gonorrheae (Gonococcus)	Gonorrhea
Septic Gram-Negative Infections, Common	**Escherichia coli* **Klebsiella pneumoniae* **Enterobacter (Aerobacter) aerogenes* **Proteus* sp. *(mirabilis, morgagni,* etc.*)* **Serratia marcescens* **Pseudomonas* sp. *(aeruginosa,* etc.*)*	Urinary tract infection, wound infection, abscess, pneumonia, septicemia, endotoxemia, endocarditis, etc.
Septic Gram-Negative Infections, Rare	**Legionella* sp. *(pneumophilia,* etc.*)*	Legionnaire's disease
	Klebsiella rhinoscleromatis, ozenae	Rhinoscleroma, ozena
	Hemophilus ducreyi	Chancroid (soft chancre)
	Calymmatobacterium donovani	Granuloma inguinale
	Bartonella bacilliformis	Carrión's disease (Oroya fever)
Contagious Childhood Bacterial Diseases	*Hemophilus influenzae* ("H. flu")	Meningitis, URI, LRI
	Hemophilus pertussis	Whooping cough
	Corynebacterium diphtheriae	Diphtheria
Enteropathic Infections	Enteropathogenic *E. coli* *Shigella* sp. *Vibrio cholerae*, etc. *Campylobacter fetus, jejuni* Salmonella sp. (1000 strains)	Invasive or noninvasive gastroenterocolitis, some with septicemia
	Salmonella typhi	Typhoid fever
Clostridial Infections	*Clostridium tetani*	Tetanus (lockjaw)
	Clostridium botulinum	Botulism (paralytic food poisoning)
	Clostridium perfringens, septicum, etc.	Gas gangrene, necrotizing cellulitis
	**Clostridium difficile*	Pseudomembranous colitis
Zoonotic Bacterial Infections	*Bacillus anthracis*	Anthrax (malignant pustule)
	**Listeria monocytogenes*	Listeria meningitis, listeriosis
	Yersinia pestis	Bubonic plague
	Francisella tularensis	Tularemia
	Brucella melitensis, suis, abortus	Brucellosis (undulant fever)
	Pseudomonas mallei, pseudomallei	Glanders, melioidosis
	Leptospira sp. (many groups)	Leptospirosis, Weil's disease
	Borrelia recurrentis	Relapsing fever
	Spirillum minus, Streptobacillus moniliformis	Rat-bite fever
	Uncharacterized treponema-like agent	Lyme disease
Human Treponemal Infections	*Treponema pallidum*	Venereal, endemic syphilis (lues)
	Treponema pertenue	Yaws (frambesia)
	Treponema carateum (herrejoni)	Pinta (carate, mal del pinto)
Mycobacterial Infections	**Mycobacterium tuberculosis hominis, bovis* (Koch's bacillus)	Tuberculosis (phthisis)
	M. leprae (Hansen's bacillus)	Leprosy
	**M. kansasii, avium, intracellulare, fortuitum*, etc.	"Atypical mycobacterial infections"
	M. ulcerans	Buruli ulcer
Actinomycetaceae	**Nocardia asteroides*	Nocardiosis
	Actinomyces israelii	Actinomycosis

*Important opportunistic infections.

and phage typing; by these methods hospital strains, often antibiotic resistant, can be distinguished from community imports and traced back to individual infected cases. Beta-lactamase producers were the first penicillin-resistant hospital strains to achieve notoriety. Recently, methicillin-resistant strains have emerged unresponsive to most antibiotics and have become a cause of wide concern.

Staphylococci are infective only in large numbers. *S. albus* usually requires a breach of host barriers to enter. *S. aureus*, on the other hand, can infect the skin or respiratory tract without any overt preceding lesion, but is more likely to do so when there is lowered local resistance or an antecedent viral infection. *Once established, untreated infections frequently become invasive and progressive.* Even small skin lesions strategically located cannot be ignored (e.g., those of the upper lip or around the eye where the veins connect with dural sinuses). Walled off abscesses near a body surface may heal uneventfully by spontaneous rupture or after surgical drainage. On the other hand, deep rupture into a serosal cavity induces a severe empyema, suppurative peritonitis, or pericarditis. Rather than causing abscess formation, highly virulent strains may produce poorly demarcated, spreading cellulitis or interstitial pneumonia, or may enter the bloodstream early, skipping lymphatic spread. *A sudden rise in body temperature in any person having a staphylococcal infection should therefore receive prompt medical attention because of the implicit danger of endocarditis and of metastatic abscesses.*

Regional lymphadenitis secondary to an *S. aureus* infection is seldom as severe as the primary suppurative lesion it drains, but involvement of local veins may induce infected thrombi that can release pyemic bacterial clumps or septic emboli, more likely than transient bacteremias to implant on heart valves or in distant organs such as the lung, brain, meninges, or kidneys. *S. aureus endocarditis can be right- or left-sided and still ranks as the most frequent, destructive, and lethal form of vegetative endocarditis (p. 580). S. aureus* also may implant in large arteries, giving rise to mycotic aneurysms (p. 529). Staphylococcal septicemia originates, in order of frequency, from lesions of the skin, lungs, kidneys, intestinal tract, or bones. In its fulminant form (so-called gram-positive shock), it kills before subsidiary lesions develop, but when less fulminant it may permit the formation of metastatic abscesses. *S. aureus sepsis constitutes a medical emergency with a continuing high mortality rate despite antibiotics. S. dermatitidis sepsis tends to be more chronic and less dramatic.*

Culture is seldom falsely negative with staphylococcal infections and is the mandatory first diagnostic step in any suspected case, including antibiotic sensitivities to guide therapy. *Coagulase and hemolysin production are markers of virulence although their role in the pathogenesis of lesions is unclear.* Equally unclear is the role of the numerous putative toxins, enzymes, and antigens other than the enterotoxin. Possibly in vivo, *S. aureus* protein A might inactivate immunoglobulins by binding to the Fc fragment; *in any case, protective immunity against these infections is, for clinical purposes, nonexistent.* Staphylococci are catalase producers and are therefore particularly dangerous for patients with impaired phagocyte numbers or functions (p. 654), who often suffer from repeated furuncles and other infections. They are also frequent invaders of patients with granulomatous disease of childhood (p. 51).

Staphylococcal infections occur in any body site, but only the most common forms will be described here.

FURUNCLE AND CARBUNCLE

The furuncle, or boil, is a focal suppurative inflammation of the skin and subcutaneous tissue, either solitary or multiple, or recurrent in successive crops. Beginning in a single hair follicle (folliculitis), a boil develops into a growing and deepening abscess that eventually "comes to a head" by thinning and rupturing the overlying skin. *A carbuncle involves a deeper suppuration that spreads laterally beneath the deep subcutaneous fascia and then burrows superficially to erupt in multiple adjacent skin sinuses* (Fig. 8–12). Furuncles occur anywhere in the skin, but are most common in moist, hairy areas such as the face, neck, axillae, groin, legs, and submammary folds. Carbuncles typically appear beneath the skin of the upper back and posterior neck, where fascial planes favor their spread. Persistent abscess formation of apocrine gland regions, most fre-

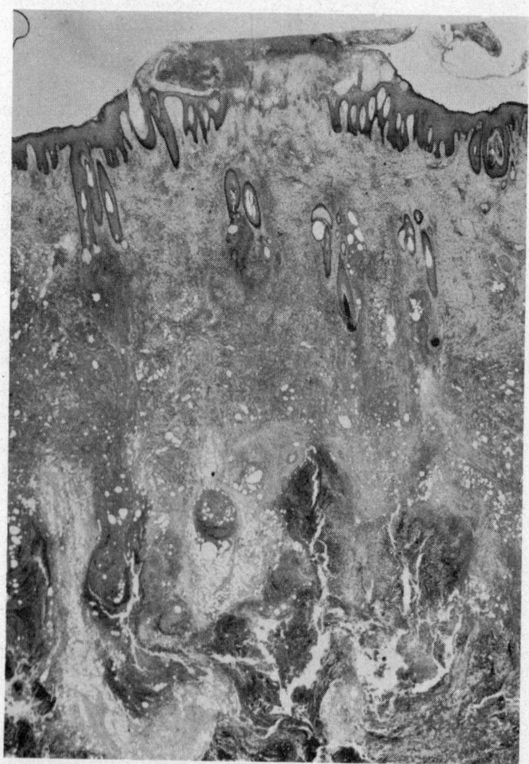

Figure 8–12. Staphylococcal carbuncle at low power showing deep-seated suppuration.

quently of the axilla, is known as *hydradenitis suppurativa*. Those of the nailbed *(paronychia)* or on the palmar side of the fingertips *(felons)* are exquisitely painful. They may follow trauma or embedded splinters, and if deep enough may destroy the bone of the terminal phalanx or detach the fingernail. The anatomic features of abscesses related to localized infections are detailed in Chapter 2. Although painful and disfiguring, most heal by themselves or after drainage, possibly leaving a small scar. However, spread and septic complications may occur, more often in diabetics or otherwise predisposed persons. Not all localized skin suppurations are caused by staphylococci; many other pyogenic organisms can cause similar lesions.

IMPETIGO

In contrast to the burrowing staphylococcal infections, those causing impetigo are strictly localized to the horny layer of the skin. Staphylococcal and streptococcal impetigo are described on page 1299.

INFECTIONS OF SURGICAL WOUNDS

Postoperative wound infections are often but not always caused by staphylococci, including their antibiotic-resistant strains, sometimes traceable to carriers on the surgical team. Sutures and foreign bodies favor the persistence of such infections; inhalation anesthesia carries the risk of spread to the lungs. *Most surgical wound infections remain superficial, but only adequate drainage of all purulent pockets can stem their progress; antibiotics alone are not effective as long as sequestered pus remains.*

UPPER RESPIRATORY INFECTIONS

Staphylococci are more likely to colonize than to infect the upper airways, which must be kept in mind when interpreting throat cultures, but patients with agranulocytosis or who are severely debilitated can suffer severe, even necrotizing staph. pharyngitis, tonsillitis, sinusitis, otitis, or retropharyngeal phlegmons. Trauma or impacted foreign bodies in these regions increase the risk. Unless treated, these infections may become life threatening. *Suppurative sialoadenitis* occurs in dehydrated patients, and in those with ductal obstruction by a sialolith as bacteria invade via the ducts and spread throughout the gland. None of these head and neck lesions is exclusively caused by staphylococci.

STAPHYLOCOCCAL BRONCHOPNEUMONIA

Although the anatomic changes conform to the general pattern described on page 733, *this bronchopneumonia is noted for its marked destructiveness.*[83] The mucosa of the secondary and tertiary bronchi is promptly ulcerated as purulent inflammation erodes their walls, branching out into multiple alveolar abscesses. Escape of air into the lung interstitium may occur in children and add to the ventilatory encroachment by forming air cysts that compress the surrounding lung. *Fulminant infections may spread through the lung septa as well as the airways to induce an interstitial pattern of inflammation.* More commonly, in adults, abscesses break into the pleura, resulting in empyema (p. 758); or bronchopleural fistulas if untreated, septic spread and complications are likely. Staphylococcal pneumonia is a particular risk in patients with pulmonary viral infections. Other predisposing conditions include chronic pulmonary congestion and edema, chronic bronchiectasis, obstructive lung disease, bronchial asthma, and cystic fibrosis.

STAPHYLOCOCCAL FOOD POISONING

This disorder results from the ingestion of preformed enterotoxin and must not be confused with invasive staphylococcal enterocolitis or the food poisoning caused by *Clostridium botulinum* (p. 325). *It usually manifests itself as an acute, self-limited GI upset with nausea, vomiting, abdominal cramps, diarrhea, and prostration occurring within one to six hours of ingestion of the offending food*, usually custards, milk products, or unrefrigerated meat. Recovery is equally prompt and a fatal outcome is rare. As in other noninvasive enteritides, mucosal lesions are not demonstrable. The toxigenic staphylococcus must be recovered by culturing the food rather than the patient's excreta. Frequently, the correct diagnosis can be presumed on the simple basis of the brief incubation and duration of this disorder, compared with other food poisonings.

TOXIC SHOCK SYNDROME

This sporadic, unexpected, and sometimes fatal febrile illness of young women is characterized by volume-resistant shock, a diffuse macular rash, conjunctivitis, sore throat, and a pronounced GI upset. It can rapidly progress to renal and pulmonary failure and death.[84, 85] It is usually associated with the use of vaginal tampons during menstruation from which staphylococci with unique toxins have been cultured; highly absorbent tampons, left in longer than usual, seem to increase the risk. A similar syndrome has been described in children with staphylococcal skin infection, but the responsible toxin has not yet been characterized. *The toxic shock syndrome is easily confused with gram-negative endotoxemia and with acute infections of other causes*, such as leptospirosis (p. 332). Culture of the cervical secretions or the skin supports the diagnosis and permits selection of the appropriate antibiotic. During convalescence, scaling of the skin of the extremities is commonly seen.

Streptococcal Infections

Although the morbidity related to these infections has decreased since the introduction of penicillin, streptococci still rank among the major human pathogens even where medical care is readily available and much more so among the underprivileged. Broadly speaking, *they cause two patterns of disease: (1) suppurative spreading infections, and (2) poststreptococcal hypersensitivity disease.* Suppurative inflammations may arise in any site; they are characterized by a thin, nonviscid exudate and a tendency to spread widely. The poststreptococcal syndromes comprise *rheumatic fever* (p. 571), *immune complex glomerulonephritis* (p. 1007), and *erythema nodosum* (p. 1288). Only the disorders resulting directly from streptococcal invasion will be discussed here. However, the potential for poststreptococcal complications, sometimes following seemingly unimportant upper respiratory tract infections, makes prophylaxis and control a special concern.

A great many groups and subtypes of these organisms have been identified by cultural, biochemical, and immunologic criteria. For our purposes, it suffices that the most common causes of disease in humans are the Lancefield group A beta-hemolytic streptococci, particularly *S. pyogenes*. Group B organisms are found in perinatal sepsis and infections of the newborn; rarely, groups C and G or others cause respiratory infections. "Untypable" alpha (green) hemolytic organisms found in mouth flora, such as *S. viridans*, may cause endocarditis, usually in persons suffering from previous cardiac abnormalities (p. 580). More frequent today is bacterial endocarditis due to the D-group anaerobic *S. faecalis* (better known as the *enterococcus*), which is also an important cause of other miscellaneous infections, especially of the urinary tract. Septicemia and endocarditis by another D-group anaerobe, *S. bovis*, is commonly and mysteriously associated with a carcinoma of the colon, and this has led to the discovery of occult cancers on several occasions. Greater precision in the typing of these organisms has been achieved with monoclonal antibodies, revealing that strains causing throat infections differ somewhat from those causing cutaneous infections.

Streptococci are covered by slippery hyaluronate capsules. Their underlying cell wall contains an M protein closely linked to virulence, and antibodies against any of its 70 subtypes confer immunity against organisms bearing the particular subtype. Lipoteichoic acid, also contained in the cell wall, is required for recognition of and adhesion to host cell membranes. A peptidoglycan forming the structural backbone of the cell wall has pyrogenic and weak endotoxic properties. Several diffusible products are believed to have a role in pathogenicity, but the only one for which there is conclusive proof is *erythrogenic toxin*. It is responsible for the rash of *scarlet fever*, which blanches upon injection of specific antibody. The relative resistance of streptococci to killing by leukocytes is thought to be related to their NAD-ase, which interrupts leukocytic metabolism by diffusing out of the phagosome. *Streptokinase*, an activator of plasminogen, and streptodornase, a desoxyribonuclease that depolymerizes nuclei of dead leukocytes, could account for the characteristically thin, fluid exudate of streptococcal infections, favoring spread. The main importance of *streptolysin O*, a hemolysin found in the beta group, is the persistently high antibody (ASLO) titer it induces, providing a useful marker for the diagnosis and epidemiologic study of streptococcal and poststreptococcal diseases.

Host factors are also important in shaping the fate of streptococcal infections. Many normal persons carry upper respiratory strains only potentially dangerous to others. Indirect spread of streptococci rarely occurs since desiccation makes them nonvirulent. Clinical infection is usually acquired from close contact with carriers or those with active disease, and only with inocula of millions of organisms. Therefore, outbreaks of *streptococcal pharyngitis* are most common in schools and among family members, peaking in wintertime. However, relatively few among the many who are colonized develop disease. *Nevertheless, both persons with inapparent and those with overt streptococcal infections can develop ASLO titers and are at risk of subsequent poststreptococcal sequelae.* Skin infections such as *pyoderma, impetigo, and erysipelas* correlate with crowding, poor hygiene, and warm, moist tropical climates and sometimes follow minor trauma, cuts, and insect bites.

Natural and acquired, strain-specific resistance explains part of the epidemiologic patterns of streptococcal disease. The peak incidence of respiratory disease is in the 5- to 20-year-old age group. Younger children characteristically have milder infections; older people have fewer instances of both colonization and disease. However, no age group is completely immune.

Streptococcal Upper Respiratory Tract Infections

The intensity of nasopharyngeal lesions varies among individuals. Mild lesions, especially in toddlers, may resemble the common cold. Even older children and young adults often show only a reddened throat and mild pain on swallowing, indistinguishable from an adenovirus infection. The more severe, typical case is marked by edema, pain, involvement of the epiglottis, and punctate abscesses of the tonsillar crypts, sometimes accompanied by cervical lymphadenopathy but usually in the absence of rhinitis. Because streptococcal infections have much greater potential for local and systemic complications than viral throat infections, throat culture is requisite in all such instances. With extension of the pharyngeal infection there may be encroachment upon the airways, especially if there is peritonsillar or retropharyngeal abscess formation ("quinsy sore throat"). These lesions are characterized by vasodilation, spreading edema, and intense diffuse neutrophilic exudation, often with a liberal admixture of mononuclear phagocytes, a pattern analogous to that of streptococcal cellulitis. Only rarely are there drainable collections of pus. Fever, chills, and malaise are common systemic manifestations, hinting at bacteremia and possible spread to the heart, lung, or other viscera. Other complications, now rare in the penicillin era, are otitis media, mastoiditis, and spread to the meninges, dural sinuses, or brain. Always in the background is the threat of poststreptococcal complications.

SCARLET FEVER

This febrile exanthematous disorder is *an acute streptococcal pharyngitis or tonsillitis accompanied by a rash due to the production of an erythrogenic toxin.* Scarlet fever is rare before the age of 3 years or over the age of 15. This upper age limit reflects previous exposure to, and the development of immunity to, the erythrogenic toxins of which three variants are known.

The disease begins as a pharyngitis and tonsillitis, with a fiery red color to the pharyngeal mucosa and frequently small crypt abscesses with punctate exudate in the enlarged tonsils. The tongue is bright red and the papillae are edematous—"raspberry tongue"—or, when the mucosa is coated and the papillae protrude, "strawberry tongue." The punctate erythematous rash appears one to three days later and is diffuse, bright violaceous red, and most abundant over the trunk and inner aspects of the arms and legs. The face is also involved, but usually a small area about the mouth remains relatively unaffected, to produce the so-called circumoral pallor. Toward the end of the first week, the pharyngitis and rash begins to subside and the skin begins to scale and desquamate.

Microscopically, there is a characteristic acute, edematous, neutrophilic inflammatory reaction within the affected tissues, i.e., the oropharynx, skin, and lymph nodes. The inflammatory involvement of the epidermis is usually followed by hyperkeratosis of the skin, which accounts for the scaling during defervescence.

Scarlet fever has an incubation period of two to five days. Headache, nausea, vomiting, chills, and fever may appear early, ushering in the sore throat and diagnostic exanthem. Antibiotics have shortened the traditional one-week duration of the illness and prevented its invasive complications elsewhere in the head and neck; however, *scarlet fever is notorious for poststreptococcal sequelae and timely treatment is therefore of the essence.* Rarely used today is the Dick test to determine susceptibility to infection; the appearance of local erythema following a skin injection of erythrogenic toxin indicates a lack of immunity.

STREPTOCOCCAL SKIN INFECTIONS

Impetigo (p.1299) can be caused by streptococci as well as by staphylococci; indeed, poststreptococcal diseases are increasingly being reported in children with this apparently benign infection. *Streptococcal folliculitis, pyoderma, wound infections, lymphatic spread, and sepsis* may be indistinguishable from analogous lesions of staphylococcal origin. However, *streptococcal infections more often induce lymphangitic "red streaks" along the course of draining lymphatics, and less frequently cause focal tissue necrosis or abscess formation.* The exceptions are wound infections by microaerophilic (largely group D) streptococci, which may be complicated by gram-negative organisms. Such lesions are suppurative or gangrenous and undermining, and may burrow deeply into subcutaneous tissues and muscles, forming multiple small pockets of pus to create a *"phlegmon."*

Erysipelas is the most classical cutaneous streptococcal infection. It is commonly seen in warm climates and is caused chiefly by the beta-hemolytic group A and occasionally by group C organisms. *Erysipelas presents as a rapidly spreading, erythematous cutaneous swelling,* which may begin on the face or, less frequently, on the body or an extremity. The disease is uncommon before the age of 20 years and occurs chiefly in middle adult life. Certain individuals appear to be predisposed and suffer repeated attacks.

Anatomically, the disease is characterized by an irregular, spreading, maplike area of brawny erythema that has a sharp, well-demarcated, serpiginous border. A "butterfly" distribution is common in the face (Fig. 8–13). The skin of the affected part is thickened and has a consistency described as **tallow-like.** Gross areas of suppuration are uncommon. Red streaks of lymphangitis occasionally extend from the margins to the local nodes of drainage, and these nodes are often enlarged by acute lymphadenitis (p. 656). Histologically, there is a diffuse, acute edematous, neutrophilic, interstitial reaction in the dermis and epidermis extending into the subcutaneous tissues. The leukocytic infiltration is more intense about vessels and the skin adnexa. Microabscesses may be formed but tissue necrosis is usually minor.

Since the inflammation rarely causes significant tissue destruction, resolution usually permits complete restitution of normal architecture. In addition to the local symptoms, regional lymphadenopathy, constitutional reactions, skin rash, bacteremia, and metastatic foci of infection may all follow, unless the disorder is treated promptly.

OTHER STREPTOCOCCAL INFECTIONS

Spread of the beta-hemolytic group A streptococci to the *lungs, heart valves, or meninges is rare,* but can quickly become life threatening. These organisms pose a particular hazard to splenectomized or splenic-dys-

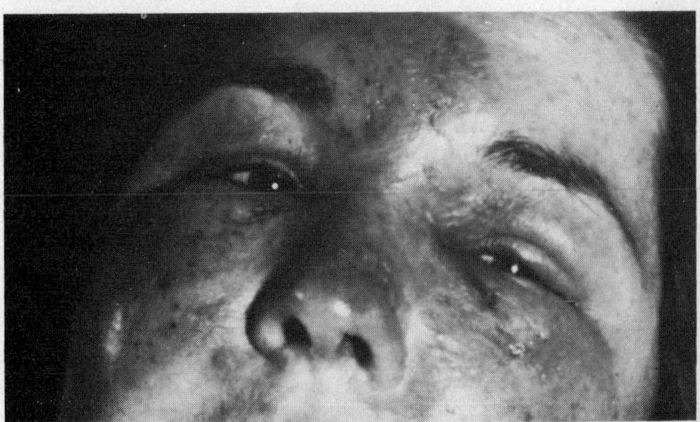

Figure 8–13. Streptococcal erysipelas.

functional patients in whom they tend to cause fulminant septicemia. *Puerperal sepsis* and perinatal *streptococcal disease*, caused by group A organisms, were formerly common on obstetric wards. Long ago, Semmelweiss discovered that these infections were transmitted by the doctors' own contaminated hands. Now these complications of childbirth have become rare, along with the classical "phlegmasia alba dolens," a spreading pelvic lymphangitis with edema, and the bluish "phlegmasia cerulea," which resulted from major vein thrombosis. Nonetheless, group B streptococci are still the most prominent cause of perinatal sepsis. Infections caused by the D-group of streptococci, including the *enterococci*, differ quite sharply from those related to the other strains discussed. Analogous to the gram-negative rods (p. 310), the D-group is sometimes responsible for cholecystitis; urinary, GI, and postsurgical infections; endocarditis; and septicemia.

Pneumococcal Infections

The pneumococcus has now been reclassified as *Streptococcus pneumoniae.* Pneumococci are responsible for most cases of lobar pneumonia (p. 734), but can also cause bronchopneumonia, empyema, URIs (especially of the middle ear, sinuses, and mastoids), and severe meningitis or brain abscess. Less commonly they produce suppurative arthritis, endocarditis, or peritonitis. Severe infections may lead to pneumococcal bacteremia.

Like the streptococci, pneumococci are found in the nasal secretions of up to 60% of normal adults during the winter months. Despite their almost undiminished sensitivity to penicillin, this endemicity makes them the leading cause of death from pneumonia even today, but now *most deaths occur among the aged, debilitated, and immunosuppressed.*[86]

The polysaccharides of pneumococcal capsules, already discussed as virulence factors (p. 300), elicit strain-specific protective antibodies. Over 80 antigenic serotypes are known; a combination of the 14 most frequent has proved satisfactory, but not uniformly effective, as a prophylactic vaccine.[87] The peptidoglycans of the pneumococcal cell wall have pyrogenic and weak endotoxic effects. Pneumococci are usually alpha-hemolytic and produce the enzyme L-alanine muramyl-amidase, but there is no certain evidence that they produce any diffusible toxins, and so there is as yet no satisfactory explanation for the "toxemic symptoms" and the DIC syndrome seen in bacteremic patients. In contrast to streptococcal exudate, pneumococcal pus tends to be thick and viscid because fibrin and nuclear DNA are not lysed. Drainage of pneumococcal empyema is notoriously difficult.

Pneumococcal Pneumonia

Pneumococci are responsible for 90% of lobar pneumonias and also account for a considerable number of bronchopneumonias, especially in debilitated patients in whom one often sees a partly confluent pattern of alveolar consolidation (for detail, see p. 733). Since similar disease patterns can be caused by strains of *Klebsiella pneumoniae, Hemophilus influenzae,* and *S. pyogenes*, radiographic and clinical findings cannot reliably differentiate among these causes. *Smears of sputum or bronchial washings showing profuse gram-positive diplococci followed by culture are necessary to prove a pneumococcal origin.*

The precise steps involved in the development of pneumococcal lobar pneumonia are still uncertain. Person-to-person droplet transmission may occur but is probably not the most important method of spread. More likely the disease springs from endogenous sources: the normal lung defenses such as mucus trapping, ciliary action, cough reflex, and intra-alveolar macrophage-clearing may restrict pneumococci to their harmless existence in the pharynx. Presumably, derangements in one or more of these defenses permit downward spread of diplococci into the lungs. Predisposing influences include anesthesia, alcoholism, cigarette smoking, previous viral infection (especially influenza), or some derangement in the epiglottal reflex. Once within alveoli, rapidly explosive spread occurs through the bronchioles and pores of Kohn, facilitated by edematous exudation, until entire lobes or large areas of a lobe are affected.

Other Pneumococcal Lesions

Pneumococcemia is in many ways similar to meningococcemia (p. 1236) and its outlook is of similar gravity; it is especially fulminant in asplenic patients. *Pneumococci are major causes of bacterial meningitis in the adult* (p. 1378) and still one of the most lethal of meningeal infections *unless diagnosed and treated in the early stages. Pneumococcal peritonitis* is uncommon, except in patients with chronic ascites. It has repeatedly been described in association with the nephrotic syndrome.

Meningococcal Infections

These gram-positive diplococci colonize the upper respiratory mucosae and often quietly reside there, but in susceptible individuals they may invade to cause purulent meningitis or bacteremia. A fulminant form of meningococcemia is the Waterhouse-Friderichsen syndrome (p. 1236), and there is also a chronic recurrent form. Involvement of the lung parenchyma, joints, endocardium, and pericardium and even of the conjunctivae and genitalia have all been sporadically observed, but *meningitis is the predominant manifestation in at least two-thirds of all invasive meningococcal infections.*

Nine serogroups of *Neisseria meningitidis* classified by antigens in their polysaccharide capsules are known. They possess proteases that cleave the heavy chain of IgA immunoglobulins and these may permit them to colonize the mucosa of the upper respiratory tract.

Substrates poor in iron seem to enhance the virulence of strains of meningococci,[88] a possible factor in fulminant meningococcemia. Another virulence factor is the lipopolysaccharide of meningococcal cell walls, which has the properties of an endotoxin and can induce shock and DIC. Carrier rates and case rates of these organisms rank higher than those of pneumococci in persons between 1 month and 15 years of age, but the reverse is true in older individuals. Both rates rise precipitously during epidemics of cerebrospinal meningitis as a particular meningococcal strain gains dominance. Characteristically, clustered infections or small epidemics occur in families or institutions when one member develops meningitis. Once in a decade, major epidemics occur, most notably in the "meningitis belt" of subsaharan Africa, or in U. S. military recruits among whom strain-specific vaccination has had preventive success. Both infection and colonization leave behind protective antibodies but not against a new strain.

Inflammation at the usual portal of entry, the nasopharynx, is often trivial and may be confused with a common cold. Invasion, possibly with bacteremia, may follow and result in (1) purulent meningitis; (2) meningococcal septicemia of moderate, fulminant, or chronic form; (3) both meningeal and septic involvement; or (4) any of the other, rarer localizations already enumerated.

The acute suppurative meningitis caused by meningococci is described on p. 1378 and the meningococcemia on p. 1236. About one-quarter of all infections with these agents present as septicemia with only a mild, rather nondescript febrile syndrome. One must therefore be aware of meningococcal bacteremia as a cause of fever, looking for skin lesions and petechiae (Fig. 8–14) and taking appropriate cultures. The proportion of meningococcal strains resistant to sulfonamides has now increased worldwide, but these and other antibiotics have improved mortality rates substantially. Even more important have been early diagnosis, contact tracing, and general hygiene, including isolation procedures.

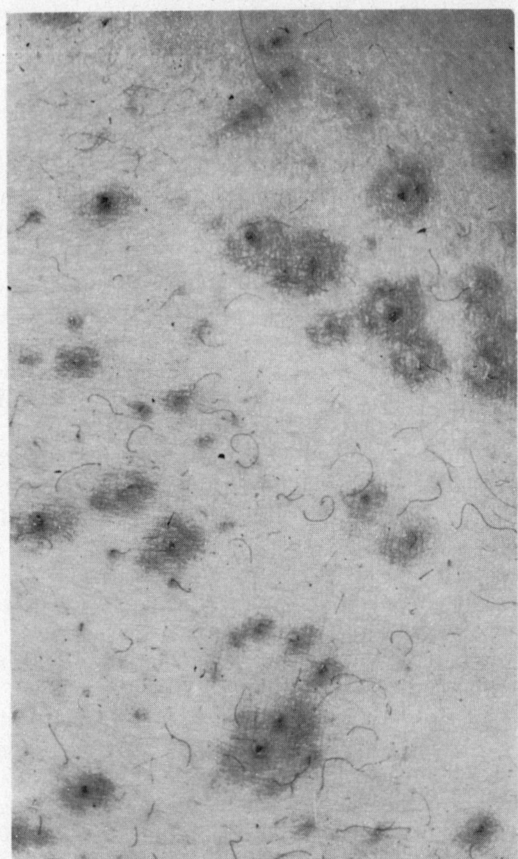

Figure 8–14. Close-up view of skin with the characteristic petechial rash of meningococcemia.

Gonococcal Infections

Gonococci, pyogenic gram-negative diplococci, are well known as the cause of the common gonorrheal urethritis—popularly named "clap." Less commonly, the infection begins with gonococcal pharyngitis or proctitis, depending on sexual practices. Silent infection is widespread and favors easy transmission. Conjunctivitis may appear in adults from autoinoculation, but is more common in neonates of mothers having an acute infection. Young girls cared for by infected adults or sharing their linen and towels may contract gonococcal vaginitis. Rarely, a skin wound may be the portal of entry. Gonococci spread from the anterior urethra retrograde to the male or female internal genitalia, where they produce chronic purulent inflammations or pelvic inflammatory disease. In the female, painful gonococcal perihepatitis may ensue; further spread in either sex can result in bacteremia-septicemia with prominent skin rash or arthritis, or in endocarditis or meningitis.

In smears of exudate, *Neisseria gonorrhoeae* is often seen inside host phagocytes. It lacks a true polysaccharide capsule, but possesses pili that are important in mediating its attachment to columnar and transitional epithelial cells (Fig. 8–1). It does not attach to squamous epithelia. "Smooth" strains poor in pili are less virulent and are prone to cause asymptomatic urethritis or cervicitis. Gonococcal cell walls contain lipopolysaccharides with endotoxic properties. An IgA protease produced by these organisms may be of help in establishing the microbe in its mucosal habitat. Mucus and menstrual flow favor bacterial colonization and invasion; by contrast, normal human serum containing IgM and complement is bacteriostatic for some gonococcal strains. Convalescing patients generate specific opsonizing antibody, but it is not always protective, and reinfection by either the same or another strain of gonococci is now so frequent that six-week follow-up cultures have become routine regardless of clinical course. Whether an effective vaccine can ever be devised is uncertain.[89] High-grade penicillin resistance in gonococci is usually due to one of two known beta-lactamase plasmids, and there also are now mutant strains with *relative* penicillin resistance, but 90% of all U.S. infections have remained penicillin sensitive. Given the frequency of low-grade and asymptomatic infections (50% in females),[90] culture on sensitive media (Thayer agar) is superior to other diagnostic procedures such as examination of stained smears of exudate. The presence of gonorrhea does not preclude syphilis or other venereal infections.

GONORRHEA

Gonorrhea may not be the most frequent infectious disease—that distinction belongs to the common cold—but it is today the most frequent reportable communicable disease in the U.S. In 1977 there were over one million reported cases (up from a low of approximately 200,000 in 1957). There was a significant increase in incidence during the Vietnam war followed by a slow downward trend. Many cases are never diagnosed or reported, thwarting efforts to trace contacts. Individuals with inapparent gonococcal infection and multiple sexual partners play a large role in transmission. Statistics on sexual contact numbers and on repeat infections sometimes strain human credulity. One individual is said to have experienced 45 consecutive acute attacks of gonorrhea.

Gonococci prosper best in warm, mucus-secreting epithelia such as the anterior urethra, accessory urethral glands, Bartholin's and Skene's glands, and cervix. The infantile vagina is also susceptible but not the squamous epithelium of the adult vagina. From its initial sites, infection extends to the prostate, seminal vesicles, and epididymis in the male. In the female, it commonly nests in the fallopian tubes, thence extending to adjacent structures, but only rarely to the endometrium. *These deeper localizations tend to become chronic and much more difficult to eradicate (p. 1114).*

The initial infection becomes manifest approximately two to seven days after an exposure by the appearance of suppurative exudation. In the male there is first discharge of a mucopurulent exudate from the anterior urethra and meatus. The infection is limited largely to the superficial mucous membranes and accessory glands. The meatus becomes hyperemic, edematous, and obviously inflamed. Early gonorrhea is of little consequence if the disease is effectively treated at this stage and does not spread upward in the genital tract. However, **in untreated disease, it extends into the posterior urethra and to the major glands of the male genital tract.** Gonococcal epididymitis is characteristic of the neglected case, but the testis is remarkably resistant and orchitis rarely develops, save for a superficial reaction to the adjacent epididymal lesion. Secondary infections in the prostate, seminal vesicles, and epididymides are chronic, persistent, and suppurative, with abscess formation and destruction of the local structures. Urethral strictures and permanent sterility may result, a sequence rare in the penicillin era. **It is the asymptomatic male carrier who represents the greatest hazard to his female partners and is most likely to develop arthritis or gonococcemia.**

In the female, reddening and edema of the urethral meatus is often much less conspicuous, but abscess formation with bulging of Bartholin's and Skene's glands is common. **Cervicitis is the rule, but gives rise to few specific symptoms. Gonococcal salpingitis may seal the tubes, resulting in pyosalpinx—pus-filled tubes, which may become hugely distended.** Bilateral, tubal involvement obviously interferes with fertility. Tubo-ovarian abscesses and pelvic peritonitis result from further extension and may create multiple adhesions or points of blockage of the oviducts, later giving rise to sterility. **Gonococci are the most common cause of "pelvic inflammatory disease" (PID) in young women vs. gram-negative bacteria in older ones** (p. 1114). All the gonococcal lesions mentioned are characterized at the outset by nonspecific exudative and purulent reactions followed by granulation tissue and scarring as chronicity increases; plasma cells are often prominent but gonococci may be difficult to find microscopically, even on special staining.

Clinically, with upward spread of the infection, persistent discharge, painful urination, impotence in the male, and chronic leukorrhea in the female appear. Salpingitis often causes severe lower abdominal pain, menstrual cramps, pain on defecation, intestinal disturbances, and signs and symptoms of pelvic peritonitis or adhesions. Spread into the peritoneum in females can result in perihepatitis, manifested by stabbing right upper quadrant pain (the Fitz-Hugh-Curtis syndrome). *More important, gonococcal bacteremia is demonstrable by culture in up to 3% of infected persons,* many without symptoms, and can occur in patients with only pharyngitis or proctitis. Symptomatic gonococcemia is rarely as fulminant as meningococcemia, which it otherwise resembles, and generally skin lesions are less prominent (p. 1236). The hemorrhagic rash, when present, is found mostly on the extremities and is related to vasculitis of the dermal vessels. Two forms of gonococcal arthritis are known: (1) an acute polyarticular type free of culturable gonococci, clinically resembling active rheumatoid arthritis or Reiter's syndrome (p. 1362), which may coincide with bacteremic skin lesions; and (2) a more chronic form involving only one or a few joints, with purulent exudate and positive cultures. The frequency of gonococcemia and arthritis has lately been increasing in women, while that of gonococcal endocarditis and meningitis has become vanishingly low.

In sum, the clinical presentations of gonococcal infection range from the obvious (acute anterior urethritis following a sexual exposure) to the arcane (gonococcemia or arthritis, sometimes without a venereal history).

GRAM-NEGATIVE "RODS"

Here we deal with a miscellany of organisms (Table 8–5), formerly known mainly as causes of urinary and intra-abdominal infections and of rare pneumonias. All members of this group have lipid-rich cell walls, are nonsporulating, and, except for Enterobacter sp., are only facultative anaerobes. Drug resistance is frequent among these "rods" and difficult to predict owing to their liberal exchange of plasmids and resistance (R) factors acquired by conjugation and transduction. Since the therapeutic revolution of the 1950s and 1960s, these organisms have increasingly replaced the antibiotic-sensitive pyogenic cocci as causes of various septic and suppurative disorders. Together with the group D streptococci, they now account for the bulk of hospital-acquired and opportunistic bacterial infections, as well as for many terminal complications in advanced chronic diseases.[91] At the same time, these gram-negative "rods" continue infecting normal hosts in the community, usually in more tractable forms than in the hospital setting. As in the case of the pyogenic cocci, their clinical and pathologic features overlap, and species identification by culture remains the cornerstone of diagnosis and management.

Escherichia coli *Infections*

This multitalented enteric gram-negative bacillus is best known as a noninvasive commensal that grows in mass culture in the human and animal gut lumen, perhaps keeping other more harmful bacteria from proliferating. However, *E. coli* is also genetically the most versatile of bacteria and is both the recipient and source of many plasmid- and phage-mediated gene exchanges. Of the hundreds of *E. coli* serotypes arising from this genetic potpourri, only a few are virulent for normal humans and possess invasiveness or one of the other three mechanisms of enteropathogenicity discussed later (p. 318). Each of these disease roles is related to different *E. coli* plasmids and serotypes, and each can thus be acquired by an otherwise harmless *E. coli* strain. Here we are concerned only with *E. coli* as a urinary and septic pathogen.

Urinary tract infections with *E. coli* begin in the bladder (cystitis), with or without extension to the kidneys (pyelonephritis). *Indeed,* E. coli *accounts for the preponderance of primary uncomplicated urinary tract infections,* i.e., when there is no obvious cause for urinary stasis such as an obstructing ureteral stone or enlarged prostate. Other gram-negative "rods" (Proteus, Enterobacter, Pseudomonas, etc.) become prevalent with complicated, obstructive pyelonephritis. In most cases the organisms gain access to the bladder urine through the urethra, sometimes aided by catheterization or instrumentation (urethral dilation, cystoscopy, etc.). Here, they induce an acute inflammatory mucosal reaction. Retrograde spread up the ureters is the usual pathway of development of acute pyelonephritis, marked by focal suppuration within the renal parenchyma (p. 1032).

E. coli is also a common cause (along with Enterobacter and Proteus organisms) of suppurative infections within the abdominal cavity. Thus, enteric organisms are found in acute appendicitis, acute cholecystitis, cholangitis, diverticulitis, and perforated gallbladder or peptic ulcer. In addition, *E. coli* is a common member of mixed wound infections and suppuration in and about the anus (ischiorectal abscess, pilonidal sinus). In a hospital setting, it is also found among the gram-negatives that invade the respiratory tract of debilitated patients, and may cause severe hemorrhagic bronchopneumonias. But the most feared consequence of infections with these organisms is the development of *gram-negative bacteremia.* Once a rare clinical problem, its incidence has increased 20-fold over the past two decades. Fatality rates in gram-negative bacteremias approach 50%, and cause over 100,000 deaths annually in the U.S. Death may be due to uncontrolled endotoxemic febrile reactions, metastatic dissemination of organisms, or endotoxic induction of DIC and shock.

Many factors contribute to this growing clinical problem. The infections are difficult to eradicate because of microbial drug resistance. In the effort to control the local disease, administration of antimicrobial agents suppresses other drug-sensitive organisms, leaving the resistant gram-negatives to proliferate and spread into the blood. This unfortunate sequence is particularly liable to occur in predisposed hospitalized patients, such as the very young and very old, and those having diabetes mellitus, hematologic or neoplastic disorders, or some basis for depressed immunity. *Not all patients with gram-negative bacteremias have obvious local suppurative disease.* In fact, transient contamination of the blood is commonplace in daily life. In the normal individual this is of no consequence, but those with lowered resistance are at risk of developing gram-negative sepsis.

Pathologic lesions caused by invasive ***E. coli*** are usually of the suppurative type and lack specific distinguishing features other than the occasional production of gas, which may mimic that of clostridial infection (p. 326) but differs in odor. ***E. coli*** infections or mixed infections can indeed become gangrenous, especially those arising in abdominal viscera.

Rigors and spiking temperatures are seldom absent when *E. coli* sepsis ensues, and are particularly frequent when there is gram-negative cholangitis or liver abscess formation.

Klebsiella and Enterobacter Infections

K. pneumoniae (also known as Friedländer's bacillus) and *Enterobacter aerogenes* are common enterobacteria, so closely related that they are, for practical purposes, indistinguishable. Their disease spectrum includes severe pneumonia, lobular or lobar; urinary tract infection; and miscellaneous septic lesions, but no enterotoxicity. *K. pneumoniae* is an aerobic lactose-fermenter with a thick mucoid capsule. It is rarely a commensal of the mouth and throat in normal individuals, but is found there in about 20% of hospital patients. Lung infections probably come about by inhalation or aspiration, especially in patients who have difficulty swallowing, who are intubated, who have tracheostomies, or who have poor ciliary function due to alcoholism or chronic obstructive lung disease. *K. pneumoniae* is also a cause of urinary tract infections, particularly when there is urinary tract obstruction, and is frequently present in mixed infections of the biliary tract. Uncommonly, suppuration in the sinuses, middle ears, mastoids, and meninges is attributable to this organism. It is important to identify this pathogen in all these settings because it is more resistant to antibiotics than *E. coli* and is therefore of graver significance.

K. pneumoniae usually produces a bronchopneumonia similar to that caused by other gram-negative bacilli, but distinguished by its tendency to abscess formation and pleural involvement, especially in the settings of aspiration or preexisting chronic lung disease. In some individuals, usually alcoholics acquiring their infection outside the hospital, Friedländer's bacillus causes a primary, lobar pneumonia quickly involving one or more lobes of the lung, indistinguishable clinically from pneumococcal lobar pneumonia. Although this organism is responsible for only 1 to 2% of all lobar pneumonias, it is important to identify it not only because *K. pneumoniae* responds to different antibiotics, but also because it tends to destroy the lung parenchyma, thus causing a much higher mortality than pneumococcal infections.

Friedländer's pneumonia is marked by widespread consolidation of the lung parenchyma, which ensues within the first few days, and may be limited to a portion of a lobe but more often affects a whole lobe or multiple lobes. The lung has the solidified "plaster cast" appearance similar to that seen in pneumococcal pneumonia. Each lung may weigh up to 1500 gm. The pleural surfaces are covered by a fibrinosuppurative exudate. On transection, the parenchyma is usually uniformly gray to gray-red. Copious, mucoid, slimy pus exudes from the cut surface and clings to the sectioning knife and hands.

Histologically, the pneumonic consolidation is characterized by filling of the alveoli with a mucoid suppurative exudate heavily laden with large numbers of encapsulated bacilli. Neutrophils and macrophages make up the dominant leukocytic response (Fig. 8–15). **One of the characteristic features of Klebsiella pneumonia is the development of numerous small focal abscesses.** Fibrin is generally not as copious as in the pneumococcal pneumonias.

Clinically the disease begins suddenly with the onset of chills, fever, pleuritic pain, cough, and the expectoration at first of sanguineous, then frankly sanguinopurulent, mucoid sputum. Shortness of breath, dyspnea, and cyanosis may become evident within the first 48 hours. Patients have difficulty in raising the thick, tenacious sputum. When examined, it is usually loaded with the encapsulated bacilli. If the infection is aborted by antibiotic therapy, considerable resolution may follow, but residual scarring frequently follows abscess formation, and widespread organization of the exudate may leave dense, fibrous pleural adhesions and permanently solidified parenchyma. Before the advent of antibiotics, the mortality rate was over 50%; it is now much lower. Occasionally an acute pneumonia is followed by persistent chronic pulmonary infection, and Klebsiella sp. have been repeatedly cultured in chronic bronchitis, bronchiectasis, and lung abscesses.

K. pneumoniae septicemia, evidenced by chills, fever, malaise, and prostration, may occur in the course of the pneumonia or other localizations of this pathogen. Sometimes it appears without obvious focal infection. These gram-negative bacteremias can be extremely fulminating, and patients usually succumb without the development of metastatic tissue lesions.

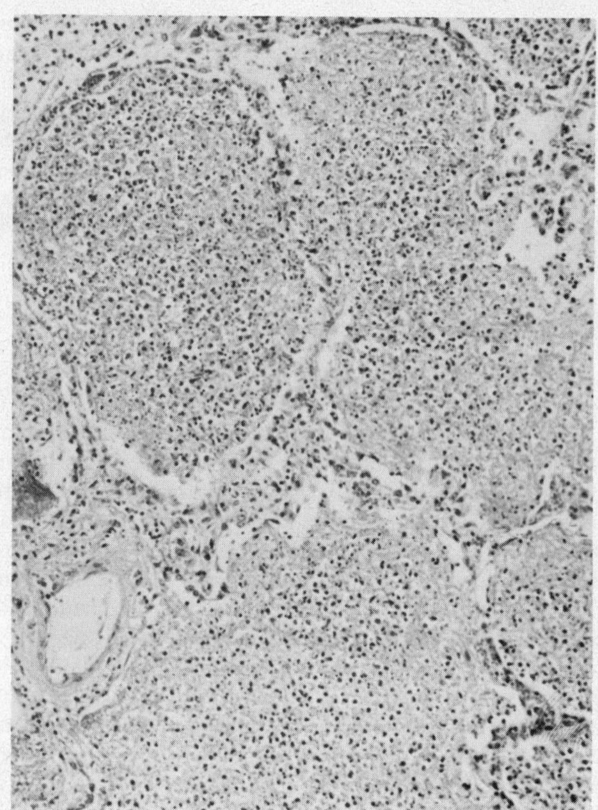

Figure 8–15. Klebsiella pneumonia. Note intra-alveolar exudate and destruction of alveolar septa.

Proteus and Serratia Infections

The spectrum of diseases caused by *Proteus mirabilis,* a motile gram-negative bacillus, is similar to that of *E. coli* and *K. pneumoniae.* It is most frequently a chronic urinary pathogen and is sometimes associated with xanthogranulomatous pyelonephritis, described on page 1035. Proteus pneumonia is uncommon and is usually found in debilitated hospitalized patients. The involvement tends to be lobular and most often in the posterior segment of an upper lobe, especially the right one, as in aspiration pneumonia. Abscess formation is frequent.

Serratia marcescens infection, likewise, is often manifest as a pneumonia, but can involve many other organ systems, including the upper respiratory tract, normally a rare habitat of this organism. Infections are mostly limited to debilitated or immunosuppressed individuals, generally within hospitals. One claim to fame of this red-pigmented nosocomial pathogen is its former use as an "innocuous germ." It was commonly used for teaching medical students how to culture bacteria; on one occasion, it was even aerosolized throughout the New York subway system in a study of the logistics of germ warfare. Fortunately, no epidemic followed among the normal individuals placed at risk—an instructive, if involuntary, demonstration of the importance of host factors in the pathogenesis of gram-negative bacterial infections.[92]

Pseudomonas Infections

P. aeruginosa is of low virulence for normal individuals owing to its poor resistance to natural host barriers, especially to neutrophilic phagocytosis. However, it commonly causes acute nosocomial and opportunistic gram-negative infections in the predisposed. *P. maltophilia* and *P. cepacia* are similar in pathogenicity but are less commonly seen. Once established, Pseudomonas pathogenicity is high. Several toxins have been isolated from its various strains, including the ADP-ribosyl transferase named exotoxin A, a "lethal toxin" that shocks and kills rabbits in microgram amounts, and a "leukocidin," but their in vivo significance has not yet been clearly established. Some strains of *P. aeruginosa* cause chronic infections of the urinary tract, external ear, and respiratory tree, especially in patients with mucoviscidosis and recurrent bronchopneumonias. Formerly known as *Bacillus pyocyaneus*, this microbe has become one of the most common and severe secondary invaders. It is widely distributed throughout hospitals and has been cultured from wash basins, respiratory tubing, nursery cribs, and even antiseptic-containing bottles. It also subsists on the moist skin or in the gut of some normal people, and colonizes the pharynx of patients receiving antibiotics. From these multiple sources, it gives rise to miniepidemics in nurseries, intensive care units, and *particularly burn units where it ranks first as a cause of skin infections and generalized sepsis*. Indeed, the current practice of early coating of burn surfaces with antibacterial agents or grafting was devised primarily to guard against surface contamination of the wound by Pseudomonas and other ambient organisms.[93] Premature infants, patients with neutropenia or any form of extensive wound, and immunosuppressed individuals are also at high risk.

In addition to causing infections on the surface of the body, Pseudomonas may primarily involve the urinary tract or initially present as a pneumonia, in each case incurring the risk of bacteremia and disseminated gram-negative sepsis. Regardless of the source, the lung is frequently seeded and the resultant pneumonia then becomes a prominent part of the sepsis. Early lung involvement, whether by air or bloodstream, is thus an ominous sign; urinary Pseudomonas infections tend to be less rampant and may follow a chronic recurrent course. Successful therapy of these infections depends as much on host defenses (particularly, on a normal neutrophilic response) as on the appropriateness of the antibiotic. This gram-negative "rod" has the pernicious habit of replacing other pathogens as they are suppressed, so that persisting infections often turn out to be superinfections by Pseudomonas for which the initial treatment is no longer appropriate—hence, the importance of follow-up cultures in hospitalized patients.

Microscopically, ***P. aeruginosa*** infection in the altered host is the prototype of a necrotizing inflammation. Masses of proliferating organisms cloud the host tissue with a bluish haze, concentrating in the wall of blood vessels, where host cells undergo coagulation necrosis and nuclei fade away. This picture of "gram-negative vasculitis" accompanied by thrombosis and hemorrhage, while not pathognomonic, is highly suggestive of ***P. aeruginosa.*** The surprising scarcity of neutrophils in these sites is partly a function of previous systemic neutropenia, partly of violent necrosis. Grossly, Pseudomonas pneumonia distributes through the terminal airways in a "fleur-de-lis" pattern, with a striking alternation of whitish necrotic and dark red hemorrhagic areas. In skin burns, these organisms proliferate wildly, penetrating deeply into the veins to induce massive bacteremias. Well-demarcated necrotic and hemorrhagic skin lesions of oval shape often arise during these bacteremias and are named ecthyma gangrenosum. At their bases these lesions show the same Pseudomonas vasculitis seen in the lung. DIC is frequent with bacteremia. The heart valves may also become infected,[94] and when the brain is seeded cortical foci of necrosis may appear with inflammation of the leptomeninges.

Pseudomonas infections of persons with normal white cell defenses usually take the form of suppurative lesions, such as abscesses and streaky infiltrates in pyelonephritic kidneys (Chapter 21). Occasionally, pigment-producing strains of *P. aeruginosa* impart a bluish tinge to the accumulating pus (hence the term pyocyaneus). Suppurative meningitis may follow long-neglected otitis, particularly when other organisms have been suppressed by antibiotics.

With the more effective antibiotics now available, Pseudomonas mortality is abating but still quite high; antibiotic choice is especially critical for hospital strains that exchange resistance plasmids with other bacteria.

Legionella Infections

When lethal pneumonia struck a group of participants at the 1976 convention of the American Legion in Philadelphia, the microbe hunt that ensued led to the unexpected finding of a hitherto unknown gram-negative bacterial pathogen, *Legionella pneumophila*. It was first visualized by silver staining and immunofluorescence in infected human tissue, then cultured on special media. Further study revealed that Legionella had been described as a "rickettsia-like organism" as early as 1947[95] and had been the unrecognized cause of sporadic cases of pneumonia for many years. The new Legionella became identified as the type species of a family of gram-negative bacterial pathogens that includes *L. micdadei* (the "Pittsburgh pneumonia agent"), *L. bozemanii*, *L. dumoffii*, and *L. gormanii*, previously known only as scattered isolates. Finally, Legionella's transmission was found to be respiratory, and a major environmental source was located in water reservoirs and cooling units of air-conditioning systems containing blue/green algae and free-living amebae, among which Legionella sp. can apparently survive for years.[96]

Legionella sp. are small, gram-negative flagellated rods of somewhat polymorphous shape with typical cell walls. They are best visualized by immunofluorescence, which permits identification of the various species. They can also be visualized (more easily on smears than in tissue) with the Dieterle silver stain, or by other special methods.[97] *L. micdadei* is weakly acid-fast in tissue but not in culture. Legionella sp. release catalase and other enzymes, and their cell walls have endotoxic properties; none are encapsulated. Thus far, six serotypes of *L. pneumophila* have been identified; however, although some are more frequent pathogens than others, serotype bears no relation to disease severity. Indeed, the basis of Legionella pathogenicity is still uncertain. It is readily engulfed by neutrophils and mononuclear phagocytes, and is efficiently killed by activated monocytes, but not by macrophages,[97] in whose phagosomes it may actually multiply early in the disease.[98] The role of host resistance is important, since most isolated cases have been in immunosuppressed or compromised hospital patients. Community outbreaks traceable to a common water source have been characterized by two sharply different patterns of disease: (1) Pontiac fever, a mild, nonfatal, self-limited systemic febrile disease; and (2) legionnaires' disease, a severe pneumonia with a fatality rate of 15 to 20% among patients not receiving appropriate antibiotic therapy. As with other gram-negatives, the severest infections have occurred in predisposed, hospitalized human hosts.[99]

After an incubation period of five days, legionnaires' disease is marked by the gradual onset of fever, dry cough, malaise, chest and abdominal pain, confusion, and sometimes diarrhea. As in typhoid fever, the pulse rate may be surprisingly slow relative to the fever and the leukocyte counts may not be impressive. Severe cases typically manifest scanty blood-streaked sputum, increasing respiration rate, high fever, and disproportionate systemic symptoms. Death may follow from respiratory failure or, in some cases, from a shocklike syndrome with DIC and renal failure. Erythromycin and other broad-spectrum antibiotics abbreviate the illness when given in a timely manner. *L. bozemanii* infections are the severest, and no survivors have yet been reported.

All Legionella species produce a lobular pneumonia of fibrinopurulent type that tends to be confluent, sometimes to the point of appearing lobar. Even early, a relatively high ratio of mononuclear phagocytes to neutrophils is characteristic. In the center of the lung lesions, phagocytes are destroyed and their nuclei broken up ("leukocytoclasis"), but intact macrophages congregate about the necrotic zone. Still more peripherally pneumonocyte proliferation, hyaline fibrin membranes lining alveolar spaces, and edema are present; in immunosuppressed or respirator-assisted patients, these changes may closely resemble diffuse alveolar damage and signal the development of DIC. Bacteria are copious in the leukocytoclastic areas and are seen inside large, intact, bubbly-appearing macrophages as well as in neutrophils. Secondary inflammation of the walls of small pulmonary arteries and veins is often intense and accompanied by thrombosis. Abscesses are frequent, but tend to be small and rarely confluent. These destructive lesions explain the tendency to organization and scarring and account for the patient's prolonged convalescence. Fibrinous pleuritis is often relatively modest and the fluid in the pleural spaces is more often serous than purulent. The larger airways are only moderately affected compared with the bronchioles, which are largely plugged with exudate, perhaps explaining the scarcity of sputum. Even when the involvement is lobar, the lesions tend not to be all of the same stage as is characteristic of pneumococal pneumonia. In sum, the picture is one of a confluent bronchopneumonia of bacterial type, and differs sharply from the interstitial pattern seen in viral and in some rickettsial infections.

Bacteremia has been repeatedly demonstrated in patients with pulmonary involvement. Organisms, and sometimes small foci of cell necrosis, can also be found in hilar nodes and in various parenchymal organs, but significant involvements outside the lung have thus far been seen only in the kidneys (microscopic hematuria and unexplained renal failure are not uncommon in legionnaires' disease).

The sporadic appearance of Legionella pneumonia in vulnerable patients, its confluent lobular distribution, and its "toxic" symptoms all parallel the presentation of other gram-negative pneumonias, but the sputum may be scanty and poor in leukocytes, and may fail to yield a convincing, rich growth of organisms on routine media. Even on special media, growth is slow, and thus early diagnosis often requires invasive procedures such as lung aspiration or biopsy to identify the organisms. The radiographic changes parallel the distribution and diversity of the lung lesions, and recede only slowly.

Anaerobic Gram-Negative Bacterial Infections

Of approximately 400 gram-negative anaerobic species found as commensals in the human bowel, vagina, and mouth, only a few become invasive. However, the frequency of this event is underestimated because, in lung abscesses formed by aspiration or in infections initiated by trauma or fecal leakage, these organisms are often present along with other bacteria and are revealed only by rigorously anaerobic methods of culture. The possible presence of anaerobes must therefore be remembered in abdominal sepsis, pelvic inflammatory disease, and lung abscesses, and in septicemias arising from these and other conditions.

The genera Bacteroides, Fusobacterium, Peptococcus, and Peptostreptococcus are the most frequent anaerobic isolates other than Clostridia (p. 324). The two dominant groups are *Bacteroides fragilis*, a gut-dwelling organism, and *Bacteroides melaninogenicus*, a mouth commensal, also incriminated in periodontal disease (p. 773). Both groups are composed of several species or subspecies and several hundred strains are known, but all seem to behave similarly. These organisms gain a foothold through a break in normal defense barriers; colonization along with another, more virulent bacterial invader; and proliferation in devitalized tissue. The virulence factors of Bacteroides are still only partly known. The cell-wall lipopolysaccharide endotoxin differs chemically from that of other gram-negatives and fails to gel limulus lysate except at high doses; it also does not provoke the Shwartzman phenomenon, and only rarely does *B. fragilis* bacteremia result in DIC or bleeding. On the other hand, pathogenic *B. fragilis* has a polysaccharide capsule that appears to facilitate its adhesion to peritoneal mesothelium.[100] It also elaborates a collagenase and a superoxide dismutase.

B. melaninogenicus, alone or in association with aerobic organisms, is found in abscesses and phlegmons mostly above the diaphragm, e.g., in the floor of the mouth, the retropharynx, and even the lung and brain. *B. fragilis* is typically a cause of or participant in intra-abdominal and retroperitoneal sepsis, and in pelvic peritonitis of women beyond their twenties; sometimes it infects surgical abdominal wounds. It may also be present in lung abscesses. In all these lesions, the pus is often discolored and foul smelling, especially in lung abscesses, and the suppuration is often poorly walled off. Otherwise, these lesions pathologically resemble those of the common pyogenic infections.

The outcome of Bacteroides infections depends on the patient's resistance; young women with pelvic infections do relatively well. Debilitated hosts have a high incidence of septicemia and a high mortality rate. *B. fragilis* is a collector of R factors and shows multiple and variable resistance to standard antibiotics. Surgical drainage is as essential as the use of combinations of antibiotics. Patients so treated have greatly reduced mortality rates in the range of 10%,[101] but it is likely that others in whom the anaerobes were not recognized have been recorded as therapy failures under miscellaneous diagnoses.

CHILDHOOD BACTERIA

Three bacterial species, *Hemophilus influenzae*, *Bordetella pertussis*, and *Corynebacterium diphtheriae*, preferentially infect children after maternal antibody protection has been lost and before contact with these and other bacteria has generated some level of self-protection. Adults only occasionally suffer infection, largely those predisposed by viral illness, alcoholism, or chronic disease. At the turn of the century, 80% of all U.S. children contracted whooping cough; diphtheria was also quite common, with a 35% mortality rate. Routine administration of vaccine at 1 year of age has ended these pandemics but has not completely eradicated either disease. *Hemophilus influenzae* ("H. flu") is currently the biggest problem, especially in children under 1 year of age not protected completely by vaccine; it is also a true tissue invader, whereas *B. pertussis* and *C. diphtheriae* infect only luminal surfaces, causing disease mainly by their toxin production.

Hemophilus influenzae *Infections*

This encapsulated coccobacillary or pleomorphic gram-negative organism causes principally meningitis and upper respiratory infections, but sometimes also pneumonia and miscellaneous suppurative infections. Many *H. influenzae* infections are of only moderate severity and are antibiotic-responsive, but *H. influenzae* meningitis, bronchiolitis, or obstructive epiglottitis in children can rapidly become life threatening and currently impose about an 8% mortality rate.

More than 90% of human *H. influenzae* disease is accounted for by encapsulated type B strains, but other strains, even nonencapsulated ones, are occasionally pathogenic, as are two related species, *H. parainfluenzae* and *H. aphrophilus*. The organism's mucoid capsule, as with pneumococci, has an antiphagocytic role with specific antisera it yields a quellung (swelling) reaction, useful for diagnosis. A limulus lysate assay for endotoxin is sometimes positive in cerebrospinal fluid during meningitis. A capsular polyribophosphate, the B antigen is the bacterium's principal seroreactant and is also the antigen used for vaccination. Unfortunately, the youngest children who need protection most are those who show weak antibody responses to B antigen. There is cross reactivity between antigens of Hemophilus and certain strains of *E. coli*, which may explain age-related immunity and also may make possible the development of a more effective vaccine through genetic engineering.

No more than 6% of healthy children carry type B *H. influenzae* organisms in their mouths, but many children carry other strains. Infection enters by the respiratory route and cases appear in small clusters or sporadically among members of day-care centers or families, rather than in meningococcus-like epidemics. The peak incidence of meningitis is at 1 year of age, ranging from 2 months to 7 years. The meningitis may appear suddenly or after a seemingly trivial prodrome mistaken for earache or for infant diarrhea. Neck stiffness or clear-cut neurologic signs of meningitis may not be evident. Because of endotoxin release by the bacteria, systemic manifestations are pronounced and, especially in young children, progression of the disease can be surprisingly fast. All too often, delayed treatment results in death or permanent neural damage. Patients with "flu" epiglottitis or respiratory or systemic infections tend to be somewhat older.

The diagnosis of an *H. influenzae* infection is often suggested by finding gram-negative coccobacillary forms in exudate or in the spinal fluid. Culture on special enrichment medium is effective, and rapid tests for B-antigen by counterimmunoelectrophoresis, latex agglutination, or ELISA are available and are highly specific. Currently, most *H. influenzae* strains respond to antibiotics, but resistant beta-lactamase–bearing organisms are increasing in number.

***H. influenzae* lesions, like those of pneumococci, are exudative and rich in neutrophils and in fibrin, which gives the exudate a plastic quality and makes for slow resolution or sometimes organization and fibrous scarring. Respiratory infections** range from trivial involvements of the pharynx, middle ear, sinuses, or tonsils resembling viral URIs to severe febrile bacteremic illnesses sometimes resistant to routine antibiotics. **Acute epiglottitis** and related involvements are more frequently caused by *H. influenzae* than by any other pathogen. The uvula, epiglottic folds, and/or vocal cords rapidly become red and swollen, virtually suffocating the patient, sometimes within less than 24 hours, unless an airway is promptly established. **Descending laryngotracheobronchitis** may also result in airway obstruction as the smaller bronchi are plugged by dense, fibrin-rich exudate. These airway disorders are pediatric emergencies and have high mortality rates. ***H. influenzae* pneumonia** occurs in both children and adults; it either may follow an upper respiratory infection or bacteremia, i.e., may present as worsening of a previous respiratory disease, or may be a new complication of some other locus of infection.[102] When it follows viral or other bacterial lung infection, it acquires special severity. Pulmonary consolidation is usually lobular and patchy, but when confluent and involving entire lung lobes it may be indistinguishable from pneumococcal pneumonia, except by microbiologic study.

H. influenzae is the most common single cause of **suppurative meningitis** in children up to 5 years of age, after which the meningococcus takes over temporary primacy. Its pathology is described in detail on page 1378 but resembles that of other pyogenic infections. However, the meningeal exudate is usually tenacious because of its rich fibrin content.

Other infections may be caused by this agent. An **acute purulent conjunctivitis** in children, "pink eye," long attributed to the Koch-Weeks bacillus, has now been proved to be due to *H. influenzae*. Like other gram-negatives, this organism can also cause septicemia, endocarditis, pyelonephritis, cholecystitis, and suppurative arthritis, usually in predisposed older individuals. All these lesions show the common anatomic characteristics of pyogenic infections, whose cause can be established only by cultural or serologic methods.

Whooping Cough (Bordetella pertussis)

B. pertussis, formerly misclassified as a *Hemophilus*, causes an acute, highly communicable childhood disease characterized by violent, near-asphyxiative paroxysms of coughing followed by a loud inspiratory "whoop." In mild cases, the classical paroxysms are attenuated or absent, and the infection may pass for a nondescript "bronchitis." Whether adenoviruses can produce a syndrome mimicking whooping cough remains controversial.[103] *B. pertussis* is a pleomorphic gram-negative coccobacillus, as are its rarer relatives, *B. parapertussis* and *B. bronchiseptica*. It produces endotoxin and agglutinogens, but only one of its 49 demonstrable antigens has histamine-sensitizing and lymphocytosis-promoting properties and is thought to represent its exotoxin. The organism has a strong tropism for the brush border of the bronchial epithelium, where it proliferates and whence its toxin diffuses to neural and other remote tissues. *As the bacilli multiply entangled with the tracheobronchial cilia, diffusion of exotoxin is thought to account for the subsequent epithelial damage, enhanced cough reflex, neurotoxicity, and characteristic lymphocytosis of the disease.* The toxin also stimulates insulin production and there is often weight loss during whooping cough despite adequate nutrition and only moderate fever. The Bordetella itself remains superficially located and the disease symptoms outlast these bacteria, perhaps because the toxin, once intracellular, is inactivated rather slowly.[104] Long-lasting immunity follows vaccination, as it does the disease. Whooping cough is therefore no longer inevitable, but currently about 12,000 cases occur annually in the U.S., sometimes in local epidemics. Diseased, incubating, and convalescent patients all transmit pertussis to nearby nonimmune persons by droplet aspiration (dried Bordetella dies promptly). Immune persons generate mucosal antibody, mostly of the IgA class, which prevents epithelial attachment and thus establishment of the bacteria. The disease, although sometimes uncomfortably prolonged, is self-terminating, and death from complications is rare.

Following the incubation period of seven to ten days (rarely longer), the **catarrhal period** of coughing, sneezing, and signs of a URI develop. These symptoms are caused by a neutrophilic exudation limited largely to the mucosal epithelium of the upper airways. Large numbers of organisms are now demonstrable on the surface of the epithelium and entangled within the cilia of the columnar lining cells (Fig. 8–16). As the disease enters the stage of paroxysmal coughing, necrosis of the midzonal and basal portions of the pseudostratified columnar epithelium becomes evident, accompanied by an outpouring of a mucopurulent exudate and a mild leukocytic infiltrate in the submucosal tissues. With further progression the inflammatory reaction permeates the walls of the trachea and bronchi, and there is striking enlargement of the bronchial mucosal lymph follicles and peribronchial lymph nodes. A copious exudate accumulates in the air passages at this time. In the blood, lymphocytosis (up to 90% mature lymphocytes) occurs, together with a rise in the total white cell count, indicating a vigorous immune response; this finding is also helpful in diagnosis.

In severe cases, the necrotic epithelium may desquamate, but genuine ulceration is uncommon. Mild interstitial pneumonitis may sometimes ensue, but alveolar consolida-

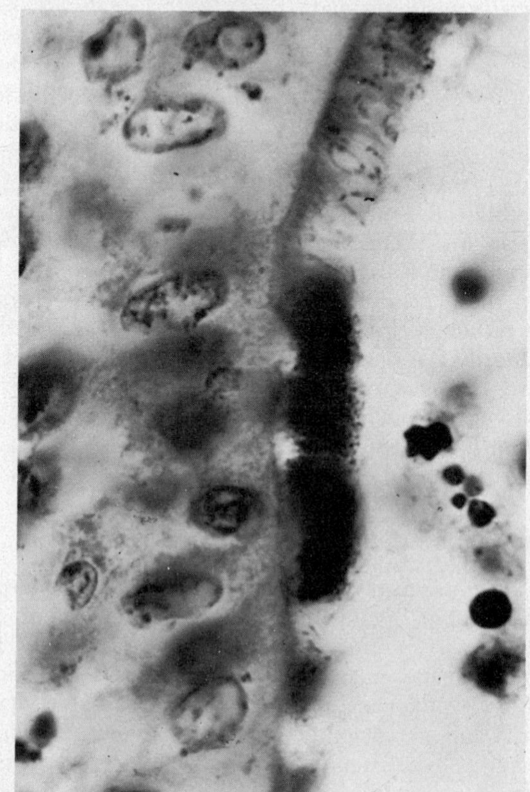

Figure 8–16. Whooping cough. High-power detail of columnar epithelium of a bronchus with bacilli entangled within the cilia.

tion is rare and is usually due to secondary bacterial invaders. Rarely, the violent coughing may rupture alveoli and result in interstitial lung emphysema interspersed with areas of atelectasis. Even subcutaneous emphysema (p. 724) may develop.

Nosebleeds, rupture of superficial vessels in the mucosa of the alimentary tract, hemorrhages into the sclera or conjunctiva, petechial hemorrhages into the serosal linings of the body cavities, petechiae in the skin of the face and neck, and punctate hemorrhages in the brain sometimes appear as a consequence of the explosive coughing and hypoxia. Convulsions appear in about 10% of full-blown cases, probably related to the hypoxia and intracerebral hemorrhages. Posttussis encephalitis is an infrequent and obscure complication.

Convalescence usually follows the paroxysmal stage. Infrequently, bacterial pneumonia or otitis media may complicate the clinical course.

Diphtheria

Diphtheria is an acute communicable disease caused by phage-bearing, exotoxin-producing *Corynebacterium diphtheriae*. In classic *pharyngeal* diphtheria a localized inflammatory membrane of the upper respiratory tract contains the bacteria, while systemic spread of the exotoxin evokes lesions in other organs including the heart and nerves (for discussion of the toxin, see p. 301). In unvaccinated populations, children between 2 and 15 years of age are at highest risk. *Cutaneous* diphtheria originating from neglected skin wounds occurs in adults, especially in combat troops in the tropics or skid-row derelicts in cities.

Although vaccination has made diphtheria a rare childhood disease, many adults vaccinated more than ten years previously are not fully protected, nor are illegal immigrants or their children, and it is among such persons that small epidemics still occur in the U.S. The current incidence is only a few hundred cases per year, but it is slowly rising and the infections are still too often fatal among the totally unprotected. Moreover, the slackening state of prophylaxis in the U.S. raises the specter of larger epidemics. Sporadic respiratory diphtheria, cutaneous diphtheria, and the rare umbilical and conjunctival infections have become difficult diagnostic challenges. Wound infections manifested by nondescript, membrane-covered chronic ulcers are prone to go unrecognized until toxemic manifestations have appeared. Early diagnosis is vital since the systemic effects respond only to prompt administration of antitoxin.

During its one- to seven-day incubation period, *C. diphtheriae* proliferates at its site of implantation, usually the mucosa of the nasopharynx, oropharynx, larynx, or trachea. Reimplantation and satellite lesions in other sites, e.g., the esophagus or lower airways, are common. Edema and hyperemia of the affected epithelial surface appear first. In the next few days, the elaboration of exotoxin causes necrosis of the epithelium, accompanied by an outpouring of large amounts of a dense fibrinosuppurative exudate. **The coagulation of this exudate on the ulcerated necrotic surface creates a tough, dirty gray–to-black, superficial membrane** (Fig. 8–17), **sometimes called a "pseudomembrane."** This harbors sloughed necrotic epithelial cells as well as a profusion of the organisms. Neutrophilic infiltration in the underlying tissues becomes progressively more intense and is accompanied by marked vascular congestion, interstitial edema, and fibrin exudation. When the membrane is torn off its highly vascularized bed, oozing of blood occurs. Occasionally, inflammation and necrosis of the subjacent tissues permit spontaneous dislodgement and aspiration of the membrane, resulting in acute respiratory obstruction. Similar membrane formation and inflammatory reactions occur in many other localizations of the organisms. With control of the infection, the membrane either sloughs or is removed by enzymatic digestion, the inflammatory reaction subsides, and the local mucosal defect is closed by regeneration. The regional nodes of drainage respond with a nonspecific acute lymphadenitis, most dramatically expressed during the severe "bull's neck" type of diphtheria.

Although the bacterial invasion remains localized, generalized reticuloendothelial hyperplasia of the spleen and lymph nodes ensues, owing to the absorption of soluble exotoxin into the blood. **The exotoxin may cause fatty myocardial change, polyneuritis with degeneration of the myelin sheaths and axis cylinders, and (less com-**

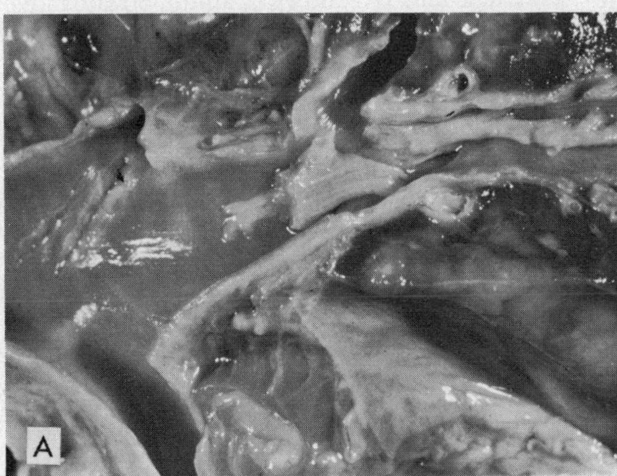

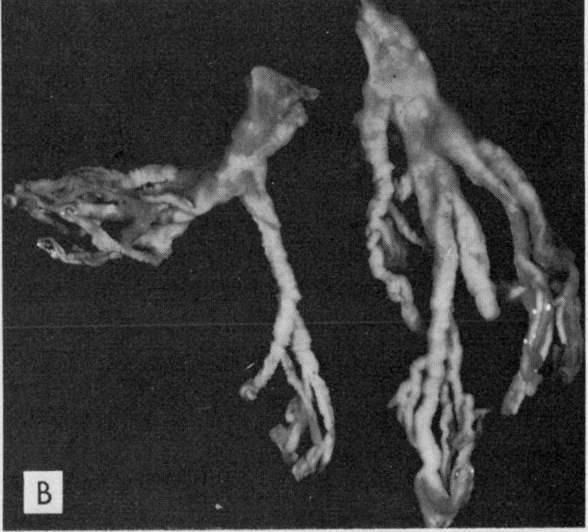

Figure 8–17. Membrane of diphtheria lying within transverse bronchus *(A)* and forming a perfect cast (removed from lung) of the branching respiratory tree *(B)*.

monly) fatty change or even focal necroses of parenchymal cells in the liver, kidneys, and adrenals. Occasionally, in more severe cases, the scattered cardiac muscle fibers undergo degeneration or necrosis.[105] These organ alterations are largely reversible and are rarely followed by permanent scarring, but both motor and sensory nerve fibers may fail to regenerate adequately, and minimal interstitial myocardial fibrosis may persist. Some long-lasting cardiac conduction defects may thus have originated during childhood diphtheria.[106]

Clinically, pharyngeal diphtheria begins with insidiously developing sore throat accompanied by fever, malaise, chills, and weakness. *During full-blown membrane formation, laryngeal and tracheal involvement may cause severe respiratory distress, crowing respiration, cyanosis, and even sudden asphyxiation from the dislodgement and aspiration of the necrotic membrane.* Involvement of the heart (seen in those with severe infections) usually does not become manifest until five to seven days after the local changes have developed. When sufficiently severe, it may cause cardiac arrhythmias or decompensation and death. Neurologic manifestations can start as early as two to three days into the illness, but usually develop considerably later, frequently not becoming evident until the acute infection has subsided (referred to as postdiphtheritic neuritis). Weakness and paralyses of the soft palate, extraocular muscles of the eye, and even of the extremities, occur in less than one-quarter of the cases. Many of these neurologic disturbances slowly subside, but some may persist.

The clinical diagnosis is usually apparent from the characteristic membrane. However, specific identification of pathogenic organisms by culture is required since other (e.g., fungal or fusospirochetal) infections can mimic diphtheria. Special fibrin-containing media must be used for culture because streptococci are often simultaneously present in diphtheria-infected throats, and positive cultures should always be tested by gel diffusion for toxigenicity to avoid confusion with commensal mouth diphtheroids. Susceptibility to diphtheria can be determined by the *Schick test,* the intradermal injection of purified toxin. Within 24 hours, nonimmune individuals develop reddening at the site of injection, which enlarges and becomes edematous over the succeeding five to seven days.

The mortality rate for persons receiving antitoxin promptly is now extremely low. In the untreated, death may be due to respiratory obstruction, myocardial failure, or overwhelming toxemia and shock. The key to diphtheria control is vaccination and revaccination of all those at risk.

ENTEROPATHOGENIC BACTERIA

Besides the bacterial species listed as common enteropathogens in Table 8–5, other organisms can cause intestinal disorders, most notably *Clostridium difficile* and the enterotoxin-producing or invasive staphylococci. Conversely, some enteropathogens can infect organs other than the gut. The diarrheal syndrome, a common denominator of enteric infections, also has many noninfectious causes and can vary greatly in severity. Thus far, *three mechanisms are known by which bacteria cause diarrhea:* (1) direct invasion of the gut wall, (2) release of enterotoxins, and (3) the recently discovered hypersecretory state elicited by bacterial adhesion to mucosal epithelial cells.[107] Only invasive enteropathogens cause substantial leukocytic infiltration and exudation into the stool; adhesive or toxin-producing serotypes induce large diarrheal fluid losses in the absence of exudate or definable anatomic mucosal lesions. This distinction is fundamental to the diagnosis and management of bacterial enteritis, and makes direct microscopic stool examination for leukocytes an important aid in diagnosis.

In some bacterial species, enteropathogenicity is stably transmitted by chromosomal DNA; in others, like *E. coli,* it is acquired via plasmids. It is often desirable, therefore, in enteric infection to go beyond cultural identification of the bacterial species. Serotyping, or the newer methods of DNA blotting or DNA-RNA hybridization, far more specifically characterize the responsible organism.[78, 79] With new methods and culture media, there can be few cases of infectious enteritis without a known etiologic agent today. Enteric infection in the predisposed host should be of as much concern as respiratory infection. Corticosteroids and immunosuppressive drugs sometimes used to treat idiopathic ulcerative colitis increase the pathogenicity of many enteric organisms; moreover, slowing of intestinal transit by antispasmodic drugs favors intraluminal bacterial proliferation, and can thus aggravate and prolong enteric infection. The differential diagnosis between bacterial and idiopathic ulcerative colitis is thus especially crucial (see p. 859).

E. coli *Enteric Infections*

Although *E. coli* is a normal commensal of the human GI tract, it has long been known as a cause of diarrhea and dysentery (painful bowel movements) in infants, children, and adults. Through plasmids, certain serotypes have acquired invasiveness, enteroadhesiveness, or enterotoxicity. *Invasiveness* has been associated mainly with the O-group of *E. coli* (O28, O112, O115, O136), but is not limited to these strains. Most enteroinvasive epidemics in the U.S. occur in the Southwestern states among agricultural migrants or among children on Indian reservations. In developing countries these strains are frequent causes of dysentery. They produce inflammation and partial destruction of the colonic mucosa, similar to that of shigellosis, but milder as a rule (p. 321). After one to two days of incubation, enteroinvasive *E. coli* abruptly give rise to diarrhea, cramping pain, tenesmus, fever, and malaise of about one week's duration. Stools are watery and often contain flecks of mucus and neutrophilic exudate.

The *toxigenic E. coli* strains, also principally of the

O-group (O6, O15, O26, O55, and O111, among others), release a plasmid-acquired enterotoxin whose mode of action parallels that of *Vibrio cholerae* (p. 323). In this more common version of diarrheal disease, the mucosa, though severely deranged in its function, remains morphologically intact; stools have the rice-water quality seen in cholera. The disease in adults is usually mild, limited to three to seven days; in children, the diarrhea may be more severe and prolonged and dehydration can lead to death without careful fluid management. The enterotoxin found in pediatric infections is heat stable, whereas that in adult traveler's diarrhea seems to be heat labile. Enterotoxic *E. coli* are widely disseminated in third-world countries, most of whose adult inhabitants become immune to the native flora. Nonimmune travelers are therefore vulnerable; perhaps one-third of all cases of "Montezuma's revenge" are due to enterotoxic *E. coli*, thus emphasizing the benefits of prophylactic antibiotic use (others are due to parvovirus or to protozoal infections that fail to respond).

A new type of *E. coli enteroadhesive enteritis*, first recognized in piglets (K88 strain), is being seen in humans.[107] Activated by plasmids, the bacterial pili (normally initiating conjugation and DNA exchange) adhere instead to a receptor on the enteric epithelial cell membrane. On electron microscopy, bacteria are solidly anchored on the luminal surface of mucosal cells, which undergo cytoplasmic cupping and vacuolization. The mechanisms by which these organisms induce diarrhea are still poorly understood, but appear to be distinct from those involved in the production of enterotoxin.

Salmonella Infections

These members of the gram-negative coliform group are among the foremost causes of food- and water-borne enteric infections in the world, although only about 25,000 cases are reported annually in the U.S. A biochemical classification recognizes only three human species: (1) *S. typhi* (the cause of classical typhoid fever), (2) *S. choleraesuis*, and (3) *S. enteritidis* (variably causing acute enteritis, or septicemia). However, well over 1000 serotypes of the *S. enteritidis* group have been identified, the most prevalent in the U.S. being *S. typhimurium, S. enteritidis, S. newport*, and *S. heidelberg*.

Salmonellae are versatile in antigenicity and disease manifestations, and may cause (1) typhoid fever; (2) enteric fevers, which basically resemble typhoid fever but are milder; (3) "Salmonella food poisoning," a form of acute gastroenteritis; (4) gram-negative septicemia; (5) localized abscesses and inflammatory foci in almost any organ of the body, including the bones and arteries; and (6) a chronic carrier state. They are acquired by ingestion of contaminated food or water. Small numbers will not produce disease, except in persons lacking gastric acidity. *S. typhi* is shed by infected humans, including convalescents, and by chronic carriers without overt disease who harbor the organisms in their gallbladders. The main reservoir is humans. Personal hygiene, water and insect control, and food inspection have done more than vaccines to prevent typhoid fever, but it remains widespread in developing countries, migrants from which are potential sources of infection. Other salmonellae come principally from animals and their food products, which they widely contaminate; poultry are particular hazards. So many turtles carry salmonellae that they are banned as children's pets in the U.S.

Salmonellae have flagellar, somatic, and outer coat antigens (named H, O, and Vi antigens, respectively), but their pathogenicity remains poorly understood. They lack enterotoxins, but are capable of invading intestinal mucosal cells to cause degenerative changes in the brush border and apical cytoplasm.[108] They also induce luminal fluid accumulation in the isolated ileal loop prior to mucosal ulceration.[109] The manner in which salmonellae traverse the gut epithelium has not yet been adequately explained. After invasion they are taken up by neutrophils and macrophages within the lamina propria, and can multiply for a time inside the phagosomes of these cells. Their ultimate destruction by phagocytes coincides with the onset of clinical convalescence.

TYPHOID FEVER

Luminal proliferation of *S. typhi*, mucosal penetration, uptake by macrophages, and dissemination to the lymphatic structures of the gut and mesentery are the earliest events in typhoid fever and are completed within the incubation period of one to two weeks. Bacteremia then ensues during the first week of clinical disease.

The organisms cause enlargement of reticuloendothelial and lymphoid tissue throughout the body. Proliferation of phagocytes swells the lymphatic submucosal nodules of the entire gut, mainly Peyer's patches of the terminal ileum. These become sharply delineated, plateau-like elevations up to 8 cm in diameter, bulging into the intestinal lumen (Fig. 8–18). Concomitantly, the mesenteric lymph nodes, the spleen, and often the liver increase in size. In untreated cases, during the second week, the mucosa over the swollen ileal lymphoid tissue is shed, resulting in oval ulcers with their long axes in the direction of bowel flow (Fig. 8–19), a pattern seen only in typhoid fever and Yersinia infections (p. 323). Intestinal tuberculosis, by contrast, produces circular or transverse ulcers. Bleeding from typhoidal ulcers is usually scant, but can sometimes become uncontrollable. Perforation, although rare, has been the cause of many fatalities. Once past the peak of the disease, the ulcers slowly heal and the lymphatic structures amazingly regenerate without permanent scarring.

Histologically, there is both local and systemic mobilization and accumulation of mononuclear phagocytes throughout the lymphoreticular system. The macrophages are large, plump, and rounded rather than epithelioid, and form small nodular aggregates rather than full-fledged tuberculoid granulomas. Quite distinctly, they are filled **with red cells (erythrophagocytosis), nuclear debris, and bacilli during the height of the disease.** The bacteria are

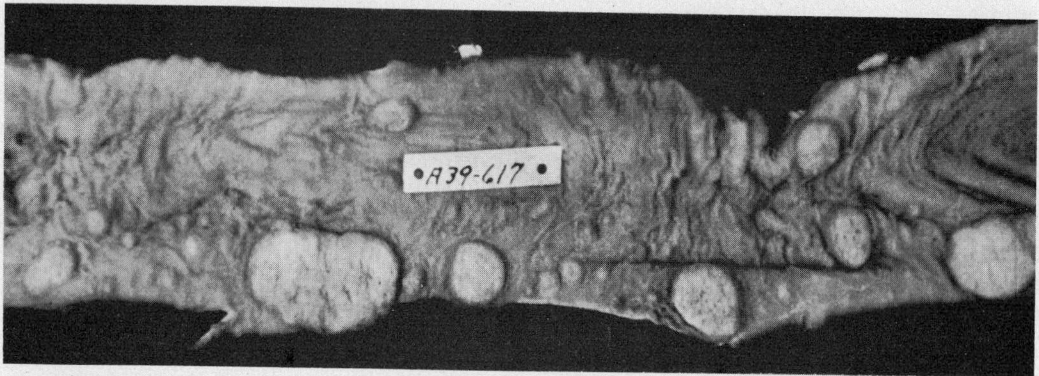

Figure 8–18. Typhoid fever. Gross view of markedly hyperplastic lymphoid follicles in opened ileum.

usually scarce and are better seen after polychrome methylene blue staining than with Gram stains. Intermingled with the phagocytes are lymphocytes and plasma cells in liberal numbers, but granulocytes are typically quite scarce and congregate mainly near the ulcerated surface of Peyer's patches (Fig. 8–20). Not surprisingly, there is neutropenia in the peripheral blood. Despite the distinctiveness of these enteric findings, the pathologic diagnosis must still be confirmed by culture on appropriate enteric media.

The spleen is usually markedly enlarged, soft, and bulging, with uniformly pale red pulp and obliterated follicular markings. Microscopically, it has marked sinus histiocytosis and reticuloendothelial proliferation, replicating the changes seen in the lymphoid tissues of the gut and elsewhere; splenic rupture is uncommon, compared with that in infectious mononucleosis (p. 288). The liver shows small, randomly scattered foci of trabecular necrosis in which the parenchyma is replaced by phagocytic mononuclear cell aggregates, called **"typhoid nodules"**; these nodules also occur in the bone marrow. Treatment can, of course, arrest or modify all these classical lesions. Fatty change may appear in the liver of patients erroneously kept on liquid diets. Tetracycline treatment may result in microvesicular fatty liver change and in hepatic failure with jaundice (similar to the acute jaundice syndrome seen in pregnancy) (p. 890). A more frequent complication is pneumonia, generally due to intercurrent bacterial superinfection. ***S. typhi,*** like other salmonellae, can localize in many sites including the conjunctivae, meninges, joints, kidney, and gallbladder, but despite the early bacteremia of typhoid fever, only gallbladder infections attain a frequency of 3%, that of the carrier state. This may or may not be associated with gallstones and often requires cholecystectomy to terminate the carrier state.

Classical typhoid fever is ushered in by malaise, headache, and fever with afternoon spikes that progressively mount each day. The fever stabilizes during the second week (the fastigium) and then gradually declines during the third and fourth weeks. Recurrent chills may appear, reflecting the bacteremia. A variety of abdominal symptoms (distention, colicky pain, or constipation alternating with diarrhea) point to the intestinal involvement.

During the second week, a characteristic skin rash, described as "rose spots" (1- to 5-mm red macules that blanch upon pressure), may appear, often on the lower anterior chest and upper abdomen. This eruption is rarely conspicuous and fades quickly. Characteristically, there is splenohepatomegaly, bradycardia, and leuko-

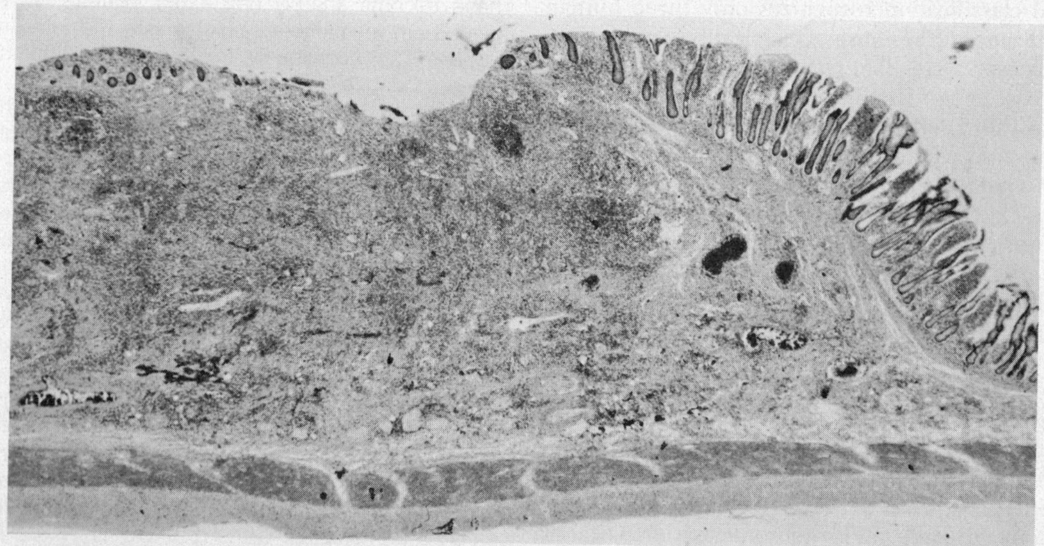

Figure 8–19. Typhoid fever. Low-power view of cross section of a markedly enlarged and disrupted lymphoid follicle in ileum, with necrosis of overlying mucosa.

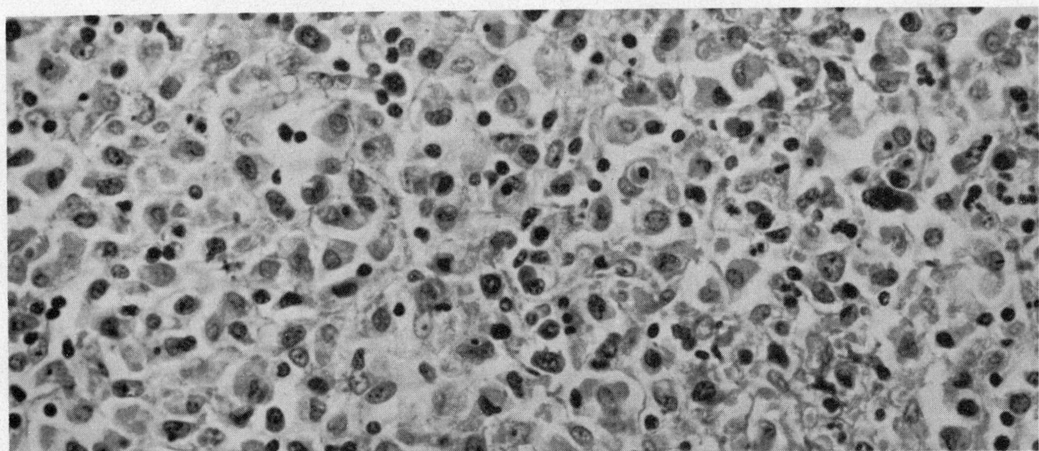

Figure 8–20. Typhoid fever. High-power detail of massed phagocytic cells in center of a reactive lymphoid follicle. Scattered cells contain phagocytized red and white cells.

penia. It will be recalled that neutrophils participate but little in the defensive response; the brunt of the attack is borne by reticuloendothelial cells and macrophages.

The combination of bradycardia and leukopenia in a patient who has an apparently severe septic, febrile illness is sufficiently unusual to suggest the diagnosis of typhoid fever. It can be confirmed by *isolation of the organism from the blood* during the first week in about 90% of cases, falling to 50% by the third week. *Bacilli may appear in the stools early, but are regularly recoverable only during the third to fifth weeks.* Urine cultures become positive during the third to fourth weeks in about one-quarter of patients. Antibodies, as identified by the Widal reaction, are demonstrable during the second week of illness, with progressively rising titers during the subsequent two weeks.

Since typhoid fever became sporadic in the U.S., its diagnosis has often been delayed, but appropriate antibiotics still abort its course and anatomic progression. Resistance (R) factors have now appeared in several countries, so that sensitivity testing and careful antibiotic selection have become mandatory. Infants, children, and the elderly are at highest risk, but death from classical typhoid fever, usually from intestinal perforation or hemorrhages or intercurrent pneumonic infections, still occurs in all age groups among the medically underserved.

Other Salmonella Infections

Food poisoning with vomiting and diarrhea represents the mildest expression of the Salmonella disease spectrum. Its incubation and duration are brief; its systemic effects slight; complications are rare and fatalities unknown. It often presents as a local epidemic traceable to a single food source. Little is known of its pathology except that lesions appear to be limited to the colon, are superficial, and heal promptly. Biopsies have shown mixed inflammatory cell infiltration of the lamina propria of the gut mucosa with superficial epithelial erosions; in a few cases, however, the lesions were severe enough to resemble those of idiopathic ulcerative colitis.[110]

Enteric fevers caused by *S. typhimurium, S. enteritidis, S. choleraesuis,* and other miscellaneous *salmonellae* have features and severity intermediate between those of salmonella food poisoning and typhoid fever. Occasionally, however, *S. typhimurium* infection has proved fatal. *Salmonella bacteremia* can also occur in the absence of intestinal lesions or symptoms, as a febrile septic disease with or without any localizing signs. Occasionally, *S. typhi* bacteremia recurs in an adult carrier who may only dimly recall having had enteric fever during childhood. Localized infections—pyelonephritis, cholecystitis, meningitis, pericarditis, mycotic aneurysm, endocarditis, and salpingitis—due to various Salmonella species may occur. Patients with hemoglobinopathies, especially with hemoglobin S disease (p. 618) are prone to prolonged Salmonella bacteremias and osteomyelitis. Patients, mostly in Egypt and Brazil, with Schistosoma infections may secondarily acquire chronic salmonellosis, arising from either urinary tract[111] or enteric lesions.[112] Treatment of both the helminthic and the Salmonella infection is necessary in such instances because the bacteria adhere to and symbiotically thrive on the parasite's tegument.[113]

Bacillary Dysentery (Shigellae)

Dysentery means diarrhea with abdominal cramps and tenesmus, symptoms that may have many diverse causes, including heavy metal poisoning. Only the full term *bacillary dysentery* is used synonymously with *shigellosis.* The shigellae are a group of slender, gram-negative, coliform facultative anaerobes; they produce an acute colitis clinically manifest as dysentery or, in milder infections, as diarrhea. They resemble the salmonellae in causing disease by invasion of the gut, but differ from them in three respects: (1) shigellae as a group are transmitted between humans, and unlike some salmonellae lack important animal reservoirs; (2)

lesions are largely confined to the colonic mucosa and, rarely, the terminal ileum; and (3) organisms tend to remain localized to the gut wall, sometimes spreading as far as the draining lymph nodes but without significant bacteremia or invasion of distant organs.

Shigellae are pathogenic when as few as 10 to 100 bacteria are ingested. They persist in stools for only several weeks after convalescence, and chronic asymptomatic carriers are very rare. Shigellae do not survive well outside the feces, and fecal contamination of food, water, or eating utensils is probably the most important mode of spread, whether through handling or insect-borne. Today, shigellosis in developed countries occurs mostly as sporadic cases or in small clusters among travelers to locales where effective sanitation is lacking. However, the infection may sometimes appear without any known source, and its recognition is always important because of its potential severity and public health implications. Small epidemics have started within closed institutions or communities that share food supplies. Some of the severest outbreaks have been in nurseries, but occasionally major epidemics spread like wildfire, as during the 1968 invasion of the U.S. by the classical Shiga bacillus (*S. dysenteriae* 1) from Central America.

There are four species: *S. dysenteriae*, *S. flexneri*, *S. boydii*, and *S. sonnei*; each is further subdivided into numerous serologic subtypes. At one time *S. dysenteriae* was the dominant cause of disease in the U.S. as well as in Central and South America, but now *S. flexneri* and *S. sonnei* are the causes of most sporadic disease in industrialized nations. All strains elaborate an endotoxin but, in addition, *S. dysenteriae produces a powerful exotoxin known as Shiga neurotoxin.* In animals the neurotoxin causes diarrhea and hindquarter paralysis. What role it plays in adult human disease is uncertain. The pathogenesis of shigellosis has been studied in animal models, most recently in nonhuman primates[114]; three steps appear to be involved: (1) replication of organisms in the terminal small intestine and colon, (2) penetration of the bowel mucosa directly across epithelial cells, and (3) replication and bacterial colonization within the lamina propria. This same sequence is thought to apply to man.[115] The subsequent appearance of intestinal ulcers is attributable to the activity of liberated endotoxin. Lately, shigellae have been acquiring a miscellany of R factors for antibiotics compounding the therapeutic problem. Sensitivity testing of the isolate thus becomes critical to shorten Shigella excretion and protect the patient from clinical relapse.

In severe bacillary dysentery the colonic mucosa becomes hyperemic and edematous; enlargement of the lymphoid follicles creates small, projecting nodules. **Within the course of 24 hours a fibrinosuppurative exudate diffusely covers the mucosa and produces a dirty gray–to-yellow pseudomembrane.** The inflammatory reaction within the intestinal mucosa builds up, the mucosa becomes soft and friable, and irregular superficial ulcerations appear. If the infection is severe, large tracts may be denuded, leaving only islands of preserved mucosa (Fig. 8–21). Usually, all the ulcerations are superficial and rarely extend below the mucosal level. Macroscopically, they are not distinctive from the lesions of active idiopathic ulcerative colitis. Perforation is an uncommon complication.

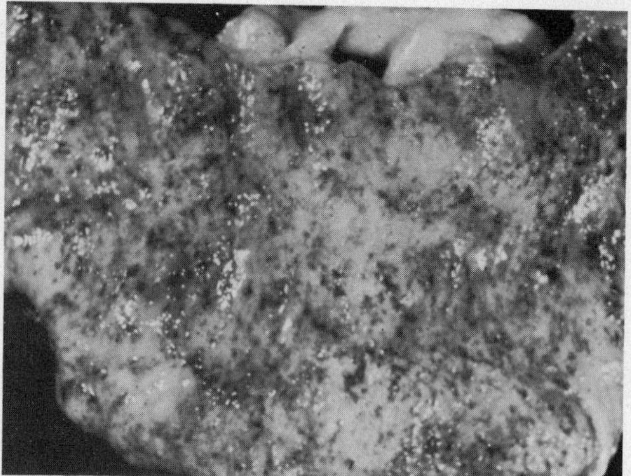

Figure 8–21. Shigella colitis with edema, ulceration, and pseudomembrane formation.

Histologically, there is a predominantly mononuclear leukocytic infiltrate within the lamina propria, but the surfaces of the ulcers are covered with an acute, suppurative, neutrophilic reaction accompanied by congestion, marked edema, fibrin deposition, and thromboses of small vessels. As the disease progresses, the ulcer margins are transformed into active granulation tissue. When the disease remits, this granulation tissue fills the defect, and the ulcers heal by regeneration of the mucosal epithelium.

The incubation period of bacillary dysentery is less than 48 hours. Disease due to *S. dysenteriae* may be fulminating and in epidemics there have been death rates of up to 20 to 50%. Such severity is unusual in infections by the other Shigella species. The classic severe case begins abruptly with watery diarrhea, nausea, and vomiting, often with crampy abdominal pain partly alleviated by bowel movements. Bowel movements may exceed 50 per day. The stools are scanty, mucoid, stained with blood, and flecked with pus. Numerous neutrophils can be seen microscopically. Headache and fever follow the onset of diarrhea. If fluids and electrolytes are not adequately maintained, dehydration, prostration, and impaired mental status may ensue; occasionally in such "toxic" patients, neck stiffness is noted. Unmitigated, severe acute Shigella dysentery is among the most miserable of human diseases, worse than cholera. Fortunately, milder diarrheal cases that spontaneously remit at home are more common. However, all infections, severe or mild, must be traced and treated in order to prevent further spread. Stool culture on enteric media is still the cornerstone of diagnosis.

Cholera (Vibrio cholerae)*

Vibrios are comma-shaped, gram-negative organisms, readily cultured on selective media and sometimes directly visible in stools by microscopy or immunofluorescence. *V. cholerae* has been the cause of seven great pandemics of diarrheal disease, the latest one during the years 1961 to 1974. In addition to its three classical serotypes, the somewhat less pathogenic *V. cholerae El Tor* has recently been spreading. The so-called *non-cholera vibrios* such as *V. parahaemolyticus*, acquired from raw or poorly cooked seafood, cause milder diarrheal illness as a rule. *V. alginolyticus* and the recently isolated *V. vulnificus* are sea-water adapted and, unlike the enteropathogenic vibrios, cause skin infections and systemic sepsis.[116] The Campylobacters are closely related to the Vibrios.

Cholera has been endemic as a childhood and adult disease in the watershed of the Ganges River for as long as can be remembered, and its pandemics have always traveled westward into Europe and Africa. In rural Bangladesh, India, and Indonesia, cholera, especially when inadequately treated, still takes a gigantic toll, particularly among children. The deaths are all the more tragic because the infection is more readily controlled than those caused by shigellae and other enteroinvasive pathogens. A minor outbreak was reported in the southwest of the U.S. in 1978, not traceable to any imported source.[117]

V. cholerae is transmitted by the fecal-oral route, and its long-term excretion by convalescents and asymptomatic carriers contributes greatly to its spread. *Its pathogenicity is entirely attributable to an enterotoxin (p. 301), which activates the adenylate cyclase of the plasma membranes of the crypt epithelium of the small bowel.* Massive secretion of isotonic fluid ensues, overwhelming the reabsorptive capacity of the colon and resulting in the typical, dilute, rice-water or straw-colored diarrhea of cholera containing flecks of mucus, but few if any leukocytes.[118] Fortunately, the absorptive function of the gut remains intact so that the massive Na, K, HCO_2, and fluid losses can be replaced by oral formulas. The untreated adult patient presents a pitiful picture of dry mouth, sunken eyes, weak pulse, lethargy, and anuria. There may be bouts of vomiting and normal or even low body temperature. With fluid replacement and other supportive therapy, complete recovery is the rule, the mortality rate being now less than 1%; without adequate therapy, it ranges up to 50%. Deaths are mostly caused by dehydration, hypovolemic shock, and metabolic acidosis.

V. cholerae does not invade or damage the gut mucosa. The vibrios, if stained by immunofluorescence, do not pass beyond the epithelial brush border. The mucosal lamina propria usually shows congestion and a moderate infiltration of mononuclear inflammatory cells. Where cholera is endemic, such changes in the crypt-to-villus ratio (normally 1:3) as may appear in the jejunal mucosa are usually related to diet and chronic exposure to various enteric pathogens rather than to the vibrios. Interestingly, there is often hyperplasia of the lymphoid cells of Peyer's patches, and sometimes also of the mesenteric lymph nodes and spleen.[119] In sum, the few histologic alterations seen in biopsies of cholera patients in no way reflect the dramatic functional effects of cholera toxin. Fatal cases may reveal the consequences of hypovolemic shock and electrolyte imbalance, e.g., lung edema with hyaline membranes and thickened alveolar septa, or focal myocardial necrosis; terminal bronchopneumonia may complicate the picture.

Immunity to cholera does not seem to be lasting, since reinfection is common and the currently available vaccine composed of killed vibrios protects only partially for three to six months, motivating a search for more effective immunogens.[120]

Campylobacter Enteritis

Until recently, this comma-shaped, flagellated, gram-negative organism was classified with the vibrios. Only when special cultural conditions permitted its isolation did it become apparent that it was an important cause of invasive enterocolitis and septicemia in man that had frequently been missed by routine cultures for the coliforms and enterobacteria. Currently, *Campylobacter (fetus) jejuni* is responsible for 5 to 11% of all cases of diarrhea and dysentery in U.S. hospitals, equaling or surpassing the salmonellae as an enteric pathogen.[121] Another species, *C. (fetus) intestinalis,* is an infrequent but important opportunistic pathogen that is similar to other nonenteric gram-negatives already discussed in causing localized and generalized sepsis.

Much less is known about the epidemiology of *C. jejuni* than of the salmonellae, but there appear to be parallels: both these infections can be zoonotic, poultry is a known source for both, and epidemics are usually modest in size, affecting both adults and children. Sporadic infections may be derived from dogs, many of which are carriers.

Like salmonellae, C. jejuni is enteroinvasive and causes disorders ranging from subclinical infection to incapacitating dysentery. Abdominal pain is a frequent complaint and may precede the diarrhea. Nausea, headache, myalgia, and fever are the most common symptoms; stools are foul-smelling, containing exudate and streaks or microscopic amounts of blood. Pain may persist after diarrhea ceases and the average duration of illness is about five days.

Inflammation involves the entire gut from the jejunum to the anus. The colonic mucosa appears friable or superficially eroded on proctoscopy. Comma-shaped organisms can be seen in the mucosa and lamina propria by electron microscopy. Under the light microscope, **there may be colonic crypt abscesses and ulcerations resembling those of chronic ulcerative colitis.** Small bowel biopsies show hyperemia, edema, and inflammatory infiltrates of neutrophils, lymphocytes, and plasma cells in the lamina propria, with some decrease of the crypt-villus ratio.[122] Septicemia is uncommon and the infection has rarely been fatal, but correct identification of this agent and appropriate antibiotic regimens are obviously important since they can shorten the clinical course and prevent further transmission.

Yersinia Enteritis

One relative of the plague bacillus, *Y. enterocolitica,* has now entered the constellation of enteropathogens and is being reported with increasing frequency, though not equaling that of *Campylobacter*. It too requires special media for identification. Both zoonotic and case-to-case transmission occur. A passive hemagglutination test is now available for diagnosis.

The organism may involve the upper as well as the lower digestive tract and sometimes causes pharyngitis or tonsillitis, along with cervical lymph node enlargement. Most frequently involved are the distal ileum and colon. The ulcerative intestinal lesions are not unlike those of typhoid fever, but histologically, microabscesses of the lymphoid tissues rimmed by mononuclear phagocytes can be identified that resemble the "stellate abscesses" of lymphogranuloma venereum and the lesions of cat-scratch disease. Thus, in its granulomatous characteristics, **Yersinia enterocolitis** is distinctive from other enteric infections. Mesenteric lymphadenitis is prominent, attributable to the necrotizing and suppurative lesions of the gut.

Because of its deeply invasive propensity, *Y. enterocolitica* belongs to the more severe and potentially lethal causes of dysentery. Its diarrheal syndrome resembles that of other enteroinvasive infections and abdominal pain is usually present, sometimes sufficiently severe to lead to surgical exploration.[123] Its destructive potential explains both the relatively prolonged disease caused by the agent and the urgency of appropriate antibiotic therapy.[124] An arthritic syndrome of obscure pathogenesis may complicate the clinical course. A hemagglutination test is available for diagnosis.

CLOSTRIDIA

The clostridia are a large family of gram-positive, sporulating anaerobes, sometimes shaped like a tennis racket. They are inhabitants of the animal gut and their spores widely pervade pastures and garden soil. Only a few species are important causes of human disease (Table 8–5). Clostridia are better adapted to their gut-and-soil cycle than to mammalian tissue, which they invade only under favorable conditions for their growth: low oxygen tension, previous tissue damage, or poor phagocytic defense. Each human pathogenic species produces powerful specific toxins that can give rise to life-threatening illnesses, sometimes even in the absence of tissue invasion (p. 301). Toxin release by clostridia requires germination of spores and proliferation without interference by competing flora. These conditions explain the relative rarity and severity of clostridial disease. Conversely, clostridial spores can be incidentally present in normal skin, clean wounds, and infections due to other pathogens; therefore, isolation of these organisms in anaerobic culture is not necessarily diagnostic of clostridial disease.

Tetanus (C. tetani)

Tetanus is a severe, acute disease characterized by convulsive contractions of voluntary muscles, induced by the powerful neurotoxin elaborated by *C. tetani*, one of the most violent poisons known to man (p. 301). Tetanus resembles diphtheria insofar as the bacterial infection remains localized, but absorption of the exotoxin produces major systemic effects.

The spores of the organisms, derived from the excreta of horses and other animals, are widely distributed and are often ingested with plants and vegetables, but are incapable of germinating or generating toxin in the gut. Tetanus, therefore, usually results from spore contamination of penetrating wounds that permit the development of deep-seated mixed infections providing both low oxygen tension and devitalized tissue necessary for germination of the spores; hence, the need for careful débridement of tissue injuries and for the "laying open" of deep wounds suspected of harboring spores. Clean wounds devoid of tissue necrosis such as needle or nail punctures provide less opportunity for spore germination, but do not preclude tetanus. "Skin popping" or "mainlining" drug addicts are occasional victims. Newborn infants may be infected by fecal soiling of the umbilical cord stump, particularly when the squatting position or birthing chairs are used without proper attention to possible contamination. The incidence of neonatal tetanus has been greatly reduced by maternal vaccination during pregnancy, since maternal antibodies are passed to the infant.[125] In the U.S. the use of tetanus booster doses has lowered the annual incidence of tetanus to about 70 cases.

Tetanus bacilli elaborate a hemolysin (tetanolysin) and a neurotoxin (tetanospasmin), but only the latter accounts for the manifestations of disease. When released into the bloodstream, tetanospasmin attaches to the peripheral endings, mainly of motor neurons, then travels along nerves to enter and concentrate in the cell bodies situated in the CNS, but without affecting their function. *Only when it passes across the synapse into the presynaptic terminals of inhibitory spinal interneurons do the symptoms of tetanus appear.* How the toxin interferes with release of inhibitory impulses is not known, but an increase in muscle tone results, giving rise to the spastic contractions characteristic of the disease.[126] Loss of sympathetic inhibition induces an accelerated heart rate, hypertension, or other symptoms of cardiovascular instability. The toxin can be neutralized by antitoxin only before it combines with receptor nerve fibers; thereafter, its progressive effects are inexorable. Toxin cannot cross the blood-brain barrier and the patient's alertness and mentation remain tragically intact.

The usual incubation period is one to two weeks but may be shorter or even months long, depending on suitability of local conditions for spore germination and the distance the toxin must travel along peripheral nerves from the wound to the CNS. The disease is ushered in by stiffness of voluntary muscles, usually first in the muscles of the jaw, followed by rigidity and tonic spasms of the facial muscles and then of the muscles of the trunk. As a consequence, there may be difficulty in opening the jaw (trismus), giving rise to the lay term "lockjaw." Facial involvement sometimes causes a sardonic smile (risus sardonicus), and contractions of the back muscles produce backward arching, or opisthotonos. Minimal stimuli, such as a noise or if the patient is gently moved, may set these affected muscles into violent, painful contractions. Dysphagia and respiratory difficulty develop with progression of the disease, and maintenance of an airway is routinely necessary to avoid asphyxiation.[127]

The morphologic changes are usually quite minimal. Examination of the local injury discloses only a nonspecific inflammatory reaction and tissue necrosis, due usually to a mixed bacterial flora that may include gram-positive bacilli suggestive of ***Clostridium tetani.*** The neurologic changes are equally nonspecific and inconstant; they consist of swelling of the motor ganglion cells of the spinal cord and medulla associated with nuclear swelling and chromatolysis.

Diagnosis depends largely on the clinical findings. The administration of wound exudate to guinea pigs is helpful, as this induces muscle spasms when the exotoxin is present. Active immunization with tetanus toxoid protects against this disease but the immunity fades within five to ten years. Prompt administration of antitoxin may block the development of clinical disease by effective neutralization of exotoxin before it becomes bound to nerve cells. At experienced intensive care centers the mortality rate from clinical tetanus has been lowered from about 60% to about 20% today. Once the attack passes, it leaves no permanent sequelae.

Botulism

The most common form of this severe paralyzing illness is *food poisoning caused by the ingestion of preformed* C. botulinum *neurotoxin.* Rarely, botulism may be caused by *wound infection* or even more rarely by overgrowth of *C. botulinum* in the relatively germ-free intestines of infants. The usual source of *C. botulinum* spores in infants is contaminated honey.[128] Sporadic adult patients in whom no source of food poisoning could be found may have contracted the disease in a similar manner. Six specific subtypes of *C. botulinum* exotoxin have been identified but all evoke identical clinical manifestations, although type A is the most lethal. The spores of the organisms are widely distributed in soil and on plants and vegetables. They are extremely resistant to drying and can withstand boiling for many hours. Appropriate anaerobic conditions for germination and toxin production are provided in processed or canned food kept without refrigeration, particularly when home-prepared and inadequately sterilized.[129] A pH of 4.6 or lower is required for spore germination. The contaminated food may not appear to be spoiled since pure cultures of this organism fail to produce gas bubbles or gross alterations in the color or taste of the food. The preformed toxin is heat labile and is destroyed by boiling for ten minutes. However, the toxin is resistant to gastric digestion and is readily absorbed into the blood.

Botulinus toxins (p. 301) are composed of two polypeptides, neither of which is separately neurotoxic. The intact toxin attaches to the synaptic vesicles of cholinergic nerves, where it blocks the release of acetylcholine. This blockage is potentiated by nerve activity at the neuromuscular junction. The result is a descending form of paralysis from the cranial nerves down to the extremities.[130] Although the severest poisonings begin within a few hours, onset can be treacherously delayed for up to eight days and is preceded by vomiting, diarrhea, and abdominal bloating. Cranial nerve palsies, ptosis, diplopia, dysphagia, and voice changes develop together with marked dryness of the mouth and, frequently, paralytic ileus. Paralysis of the respiratory muscles may precede that of the extremities. The patient remains mentally alert and afebrile and cerebrospinal fluid is normal. Once the toxin has entered the synapses, it can no longer be inactivated by antitoxin, and only intensive supportive care is possible; this salvages close to 85% of victims. Recovery of motor function is slow but permanent. Most deaths are caused by respiratory infections. Infant botulism occurs below 9 months of age; it may manifest itself as sudden infant death (SIDS) (p. 495) or as constipation, generalized weakness, respiratory difficulty, and lack of spontaneous movement. Appropriately treated babies have a lower mortality rate than adults.

Although depletion of acetylcholine in nerve endings is biochemically demonstrable, the anatomic findings are poorly defined and nonspecific. They consist of visceral and CNS hyperemia, accompanied by minute thromboses of small vessels, chiefly in the brain and brain stem. Similar thrombi may be found occasionally in other organs. The combination of respiratory difficulty and vascular stasis induces hypoxic injury to ganglion cells in the CNS. Variable degrees of hypoxic damage may be found in the kidneys and heart muscle.

The diagnosis is supported by electromyographic studies and confirmed by demonstration of the toxin in the food, blood, or feces by inoculation into mice or rats. Botulism is as rare as it is difficult to eradicate. About ten outbreaks per year each involving one to seven people occur in the U.S., most originating from home-made food products, and a few from improperly prepared commercial canned foods. Awareness of the danger is the only practical preventive measure available.

Septic Clostridial Infections

The clostridia considered here differ from the above-mentioned organisms by their invasive potential. In addition, *C. perfringens (welchii),* the prototype organism of this group, can cause food poisoning with sudden vomiting and diarrhea, induced by its enterotoxin. This disorder develops within a few hours of contaminated food ingestion and is over within less than two days; it lacks the neurologic involvement of botulism but shares its noninvasive pathogenesis. A severe, necrotizing (i.e., invasive) form of enteritis can be caused by *C. perfringens,* but has been reported only in the malnourished (e.g., in World War II–impoverished children) and in vegetarian New Guinea natives after they have feasted on pigs. This disease probably occurs in the U.S. but there are few well-documented reports.

C. perfringens and its relatives *C. septicum, C. novyi, C. sordellii, C. bifermentans,* and other rare or untypable clostridia most frequently cause disease by invasion of traumatic or surgical wounds such as the amputation stumps of patients with gangrene of the leg. Clostridial sepsis is an ever-present threat when abortions are performed under unhygienic conditions. Rarely, peritoneal or generalized sepsis originating in ischemic or perforated bowel initiates infections. *C. perfringens* is both the most frequent and the most virulent invader in these settings and is the richest in its production of enzymes and toxins (p. 301). Regardless of site, *C. perfringens* tissue invasion results either in *necrotizing cellulitis* in which gas is not formed and muscle necrosis is not extensive, or in outright *gas gangrene (clostridial myonecrosis)*, the most severe form of anaerobic infection.[131]

Clostridial cellulitis, which originates in wounds, differs from infections caused by the pyogenic cocci by its foul odor, its thin and discolored exudate, and by the relatively prompt and wide tissue destruction that results in undermining edema and sloughing of the skin. Histologically, the amount of tissue necrosis is disproportional to the modest number of intact neutrophils which increase only after these lesions begin to demarcate and build up granulation tissue along their edges. Very similar lesions can be caused by other organisms such as ***Enterobacter*** (p. 311), the anaerobic streptococci (p. 306), or enteric bacteria, including ***E. coli*** (p. 311). Direct smears and cultures are helpful in making these distinctions and in instituting the correct therapy.

Gas gangrene is the most extreme form of necrotizing clostridial infection. It usually begins in a previous tissue injury and rapidly spreads to contiguous connective tissue and muscle. Large traumatic wounds, "pyogenic" infections, and foreign bodies containing calcium or silicates frequently provide the appropriate lowering of the wound oxygen tension for germination of spores. Gas gangrene is particularly prone to occur in compound fractures, where the bone splinters provide foreign bodies. In the same way, embedded debris or dirt provides both particulate matter and small amounts of calcium. Uterine gas gangrene usually follows "back-room" abortion. The clostridial collagenases aid in the spread of infections by destruction of the connective tissue framework (p. 301), and the clostridial lecithinases attack cell membranes. The destroyed tissue provides additional anaerobiosis for further microbial growth, with subsequent augmentation of the infection in a vicious cycle.

Gas gangrene usually becomes manifest within one to three days of injury and is characterized by marked edema and enzymic necrosis of involved muscle cells (Fig. 8–22). The extensive fluid exudation causes swelling of the affected region; the overlying skin becomes tense and pale from pressure. Necrosis or rupture of the skin may follow the formation of large bullous vesicles. The wound at this time

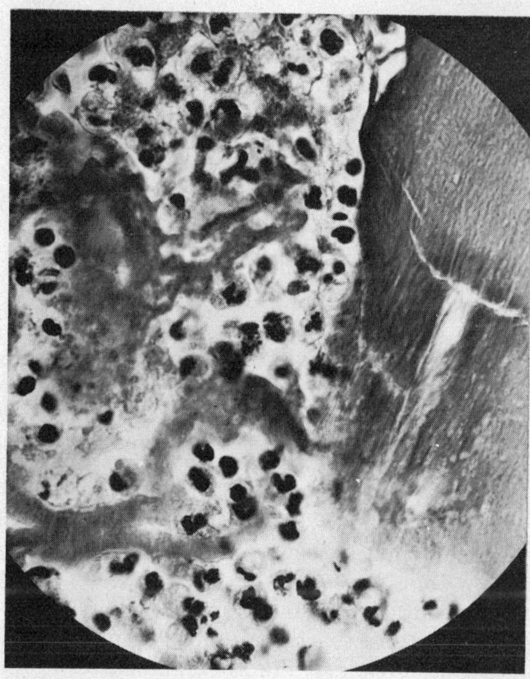

Figure 8–22. Gas gangrene. Histologic detail of enzymatic lysis of muscle cells with accompanying leukocytic exudation.

contains large amounts of a serosanguineous exudate, but there is surprisingly little suppurative reaction.

Gas bubbles caused by fermentative reactions appear early in the gangrenous tissues, accompanied by the release of heme pigment into the exudate and affected tissues. The endothelial linings of the local blood vessels are stained by this hemolytic reaction, and injury to vascular walls may cause local thromboses. Numerous vegetative bacilli are present within the exudate. As the infection progresses, the inflamed muscles become soft, blue-black, friable, and sometimes almost semifluid as the result of the massive proteolytic action of the released bacterial enzymes. Absorption of the elaborated enzymes and invasion of the blood by the bacteria terminally induces hemolytic discoloration of the endothelial lining of the entire cardiovascular system and the formation of gas bubbles throughout the body, particularly in the liver, which create a "Swiss cheese" pattern. The bubbles are sometimes visible by x-ray inside major veins or in the liver (p. 942). Systemic changes are especially common and quick to develop in postabortion clostridial sepsis.

The initial clinical symptoms are pain and distention of tissues. Serosanguineous, slightly foul-smelling fluid exudes from the area of tissue injury, and very soon gas bubbles cause *crepitus* in the regions of bacterial growth. The absorbed toxins cause a rise in pulse rate often markedly out of proportion to the rise in temperature. Active hemolysis may cause *rapid drops in the red cell count and hematocrit,* accompanied by jaundice. At the time of death, no intact red cells may be left in circulation. Death is usually preceded by a period of prostration and shock. Treatment with polyvalent antitoxin and hyperbaric oxygen prevent the terminal complications and have reduced the mortality rate to about 5 to 15%, but adequate débridement and cleansing of extensive tissue injuries is the proverbial "ounce of prevention worth a pound of cure."

Pseudomembranous Colitis (Clostridium difficile)

Severe colitis with pseudomembrane formation accompanied by diarrhea and clinical toxemia is caused by the enterotoxin of *C. difficile,* when this organism is able to proliferate in the gut. Normally it is a minor commensal. Infection usually appears in severely ill patients, especially those receiving wide-spectrum antibiotics. Particularly implicated are clindamycin, lincomycin, and more recently the cephalosporins, but the organism can be controlled by vancomycin, another potentially life-saving antibiotic. In some instances, pseudomembranous colitis has complicated Crohn's disease, ulcerative colitis, or ischemic bowel disease (Chapter 18) and hence must be suspected when a patient with these diseases takes a turn for the worse or fails to respond to ostensibly adequate treatment.[132] Infrequently, pseudomembranous colitis appears in otherwise healthy, sometimes quite young individuals. The pathogenesis of the colonic lesions, though clearly linked to *C. difficile* enterotoxin, is not yet fully understood.

Macroscopically, patchy flecks of grayish-brown–to-black pseudomembrane cover part of the diffusely hyperemic colonic mucosa, confluent in some areas, small and punctate in others. These membranes are soft and rich in mucus and necrotic debris. They are more easily wiped off than Shigella membranes, but on removal expose mucosal erosions. Microscopically, the earliest change is necrosis of mucosal cells accompanied by an intense infiltration of neutrophils and hypersecretion of mucus. This gives rise to so-called "explosive lesions," consisting of abscesses in one or several adjacent crypts from which a mucus- and leukocyte-rich exudate erupts like a minivolcano to cover the surrounding mucosal pits. With progression, there is total necrosis and denudation of the epithelium and a dense mixed inflammatory infiltration of the lamina propria, but the inflammation remains relatively superficial and spreads laterally rather than in depth. The clostridia remain intraluminal. Thrombosis of submucosal venules is a characteristic feature.

C. difficile colitis must be distinguished clinically from invasive Shigella, staphylococcal, or *C. perfringens* enteritis, each of which can be pseudomembranous. Early identification of this condition permits gratifyingly prompt control by appropriate antibiotic therapy. Several approaches are in use for diagnosis. The fecal extracts of suspected patients can be screened for *C. difficile* toxin, using antibodies cross-reactive against a similar toxin of *C. sordellii;* better quantitative data are obtained by titering stool filtrates for cytopathic effects on HeLa cell monolayers.[133] Quantitative stool culture of *C. difficile* is the best diagnostic procedure currently available but its results are necessarily delayed. Diagnostic clues may be a finely bosselated mucosal pattern on postevacuation x-ray contrast enema, or the typical early "explosive" colonic mucosal lesions on endoscopy.[134] However, the clinical diagnosis of pseudomembranous colitis still remains relatively inaccurate, especially in the early stages when treatment would be most effective.

ZOONOTIC BACTERIA

The zoonotic bacteria are a heterogeneous group (Table 8–5) having as a common denominator one or more animal reservoirs.[135] These are transmitted to humans from their animal hosts by direct contact, environmental contamination, insect vectors, or consumption of the animal products. The various resultant diseases, while very dissimilar, merit consideration together because their animal sources are traceable and their transmission can be and has been lowered by public health measures.[136] Other bacteria not included here as zoonotic may also be harbored by animals (e.g., salmonellae, clostridia) but these organisms are widely disseminated in water, soil, or food, which constitute major sources of infection, and have therefore proved more difficult to control. Awareness of the rarer zoonoses can sometimes be life saving.

Anthrax (Bacillus anthracis)

Bacillus anthracis is a highly pathogenic, encapsulated, gram-positive, large, spore-bearing organism found in many species of animals, particularly cattle, sheep, horses, swine, and goats. The spores are extremely resistant to adverse influences, persist in soil and in other sites for years, resist boiling for at least ten minutes, and withstand many of the common chemical disinfectants. When these bacilli grow in vivo they elaborate toxic fractions. These have been identified as: (1) a protective antigen having antiphagocytic activity, (2) an edema factor, and (3) a "lethal factor" having cytotoxicity. Human anthrax is uncommon but can be of great severity. In approximately 95% of cases it is contracted as a skin infection by contact with spore-bearing soil, contaminated hides, animal carcasses, or animal products (such as bone meal fertilizer).[137] The local lesion is graphically described as a *malignant pustule.* However, the organism or its spores may also be airborne, resulting in a diffuse pneumonic consolidation; this clinical variant is designated *woolsorters' disease.* In both forms, bacteremia may ensue if the body defenses are overwhelmed.

In the usual *cutaneous* form of the disease, the organism apparently gains entry through a skin injury. Textile workers, farmers, stevedores, and those in leather industries are at greatest risk. Spores can also be transmitted by contaminated instruments, e.g., in barber shops. *Man-to-man* transmission occurs infrequently, if at all. *Pulmonary* anthrax is particularly apt to occur in industries dealing with raw wool products.

In **cutaneous anthrax** following an incubation period of several days, a small, red, macular lesion appears, resembling a flea bite. The macule enlarges and becomes edematous to create a papule, and then a pustule that is filled with thin, bloody, purulent exudate, imparting a dark purple–

black color to the skin. The surrounding tissues become edematous. **This combination of a relatively small hemorrhagic pustule with extensive brawny edema is the "malignant pustule"** described above and should arouse suspicion of *B. anthracis* infection. In the course of the first week of the disease, the pustule ruptures and a tough black eschar forms, but the circumferential edema continues to expand. Satellite vesicles commonly appear about the primary lesion and the regional nodes become moderately enlarged owing to a nonspecific lymphadenitis. In contrast to the relatively painless malignant pustule, the nodes are very tender. Reddened lymphatics can often be found along the course of drainage. In mild infections, there may be only a blackish skin ulcer with little edema, and without microscopy or culture the diagnosis may be missed.

Histologically, the inflammatory reaction consists principally of intense edema, vascular congestion with hemorrhages, and necrosis of tissues resembling infarction. The leukocytic response is relatively deficient in contrast to the amount of tissue necrosis, and consists of a mixture of neutrophils and mononuclear white cells. In the usual case, the inflammatory process slowly subsides following this stage, and the disease remains localized to the initial site of entry and the regional nodes of drainage. However, if the invasion is more extensive, bacteremia may follow and give rise to meningitis or to localizations in the lungs, gut, or other tissues.

A diffuse pneumonia (woolsorters' disease) develops from the inhalation of spores, characterized by an extensive serofibrinous exudation throughout large areas of the lung that may produce total lobar consolidations. The striking characteristics of this pneumonia are the relative paucity of neutrophils, the tendency to develop hemorrhagic necrosis of alveolar septa, and the overwhelming abundance of bacteria within the inflammatory exudate. Thrombosis of small veins and arteries and profuse endothelial vascular damage by proliferating bacteria are found in severe pulmonary anthrax.[138] Frequently, septicemia develops and causes death within a short time.

Systemic manifestations may be relatively mild in the cutaneous form, but the bacteremic and pneumonic forms are marked by high fever with signs of respiratory distress and often severe prostration. There usually is only moderate elevation of the white cell count, and leukopenia sometimes develops. Electrolyte imbalances, hemoconcentration, and DIC may lead to death. Diagnosis rests on the identification of bacteria in the lesions or in the blood. With penicillin therapy, the fatality rate in cutaneous anthrax is now quite low (2 to 3%), but woolsorters' disease still has a high mortality, even if treated.

The discovery and culture of the anthrax bacillus and its spores, independently accomplished by Koch[139] and Pasteur,[140] was a true milestone in biology. These studies finally disposed of the theory of spontaneous generation and inspired Koch's postulates on which modern bacteriology is founded.

Listeriosis (Listeria monocytogenes)

Listeria monocytogenes is a gram-positive, microaerophilic, motile rod that grows well on ordinary media and, in tissue, often forms aggregates resembling Chinese letters. It is found in many mammals and fowl, and in silage, sewage, milk products, and human stools. An opportunistic agent, its chief victims are pregnant women and their fetuses, and elderly, sick, or immunosuppressed patients.[141] Some infections have been traced to unpasteurized milk or to domestic pets; others appear to have been acquired from human carriers or those with a latent infection, sometimes in such odd locations as the male urethra and semen. Best documented is transplacental transmission; significantly, the maternal infection may be mild or inapparent, whereas that of the fetus is severe, causing abortion, stillbirth, or neonatal sepsis (granulomatosis infantiseptia). Meningeal involvement is predominant in both neonatal infections and in opportunistic adult disease.[142] Rare manifestations of listeriosis include septicemia with hepatosplenomegaly, mimicking infectious mononucleosis; subacute endocarditis; and localized infections of the skin, conjunctiva, pharynx, and cervical lymph nodes. The conjunctival, so-called oculoglandular form of listeriosis is the human equivalent of the keratoconjunctivitis seen three to five days after conjunctival inoculation of the guinea pig—the Anton test—used to document infection by virulent strains of *L. monocytogenes*.

In acute human infections, ***L. monocytogenes*** evokes an exudative pattern of inflammation with numerous neutrophils. The **meningitis** it causes is macro- and microscopically indistinguishable from that caused by other pyogens (p. 1378); the finding of gram-positive, mostly intracellular bacillary rods in the CSF is virtually diagnostic. More varied lesions may be encountered in neonates and predisposed adults. Focal abscesses alternate with grayish or yellow nodules representing necrotic amorphous basophilic tissue debris. These can occur in any organ, including the lung, liver, spleen, and lymph nodes. In infections of longer duration, macrophages appear in large numbers, eventually to dispose of the necrotic remnants, but true epithelioid cell granulomas are rare.[143] In infants born live with Listeria sepsis, there is often a papular red rash over the extremities, and listerial abscesses can be seen in the placenta. A smear of the meconium will disclose the gram-positive organisms.

Mortality from listeriosis, despite its sensitivity to antibiotics, has remained high and seems to depend in part on the promptness with which therapy is instituted.

Plague (Yersinia pestis)*

Yersinia pestis (formerly *Pasteurella pestis*), the cause of plague, is a polymorphous gram-negative bacillus that appears safety pin–shaped or bipolar when stained with methylene blue. It perpetuates itself in nature by infecting many species of wild animals, including 200 rodent species. In the U.S., plague is fortunately rare (less than 20 cases per year) and is largely limited to the western states from Colorado to California; squirrels are the principal reservoir. Infection is usually transmitted to adult males and children of both sexes by fleas, less frequently by other insects or by direct contact. Variations of this endemic pattern prevail in all continents, except in plague-free Australia. Manchuria and Vietnam are major endemic sites.

Periodically, the plague bacilli erupt from their wild animal reservoirs to infect large populations of flea-bearing urban house rats. First rats, then people begin dying and an epidemic spreads in waves of successively increasing virulence. Individual cases range from "minor plague" to septicemic plague with DIC (the modern name of the "black death"), which kills within 24 hours. As rats and susceptible people are decimated, the epidemic slowly becomes milder and recedes. Today focal outbreaks are likely to be controlled more promptly and no global pandemics of plague have occurred since 1894 to 1900.

The extraordinary lethal power of *Y. pestis* derives from its apparently unrestricted proliferation in human tissue; clouds of bacteria obliterate all normal architecture.[145] In addition, the fraction I glycoprotein of the bacterial capsule has antiphagocytic properties, and a potent gram-negative endotoxin is probably responsible for the septic shock, delirium, and DIC in severe infections. *The disease in man presents in four forms: (1) bubonic plague, the most frequent form; (2) pneumonic plague, either primary or following the bubonic pattern; (3) septicemic plague without localizing symptoms, the severest form; and (4) "plague minor," an abortive infection with only mild constitutional symptoms and lymphadenopathy.* The importance of pneumonic plague is that it greatly facilitates person-to-person air droplet transmission. A striking leucocytosis is present in all forms. Patients with plague must by law be quarantined, and those with pneumonia require the most stringent isolation precautions.

The distinctive histologic characteristics of plague are: (1) the dramatic proliferation of the organisms; (2) the early appearance of a protein- and polysaccharide-rich effusion, with few inflammatory cells but with marked tissue swelling, followed by (3) necrosis of tissues and blood vessels with hemorrhage and thrombosis (Fig. 8–23); **and (4) neutrophilic infiltrates that progressively accumulate in the demarcation zone around the necrotic areas as healing begins.**[145] This sequence is prototypic of necrotizing inflammation caused by the most virulent bacterial pathogens.

The **bubonic pattern** begins abruptly with high temperature, chills, tachycardia, and headache, soon followed by mental confusion, delirium, and prostration. The site of entry of the organisms is usually on the legs and may be undetectable, but at times is marked by a vesicle, pustule, or small necrotizing ulceration. The regional nodes of drainage characteristically become enlarged, sometimes to 5 cm in diameter. In the course of a few days, the individual nodes become matted together to form the characteristic "bubo," hence the name of this condition. Macroscopically, the nodes are soft, pulpy, frequently hemorrhagic, and plum-colored. A fibrinous hemorrhagic exudate surrounds them. At later stages the nodes and perinodal tissue may undergo total infarction. As the process extends into the subcutaneous tissues, the lesion may rupture through the skin and produce draining sinuses.

In **septicemic cases,** the nodes throughout the body develop localized areas of necrosis; the spleen and liver become enlarged owing to a diffuse reticuloendothelial hyperplasia. In fulminating cases a bacteremia induces DIC with widespread hemorrhages, thromboses, and necroses,

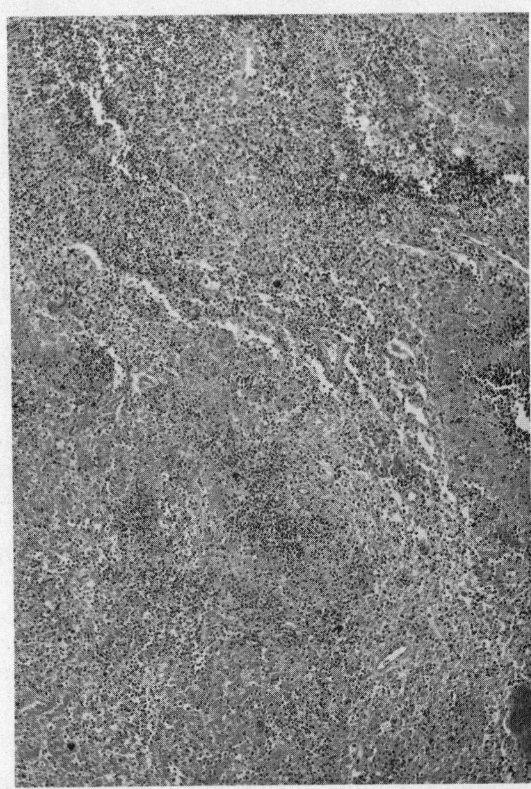

Figure 8–23. Plague. Low-power view of total hemorrhagic necrosis in a lymph node.

creating large, maplike ecchymotic areas of discoloration and necrosis of the skin, serosal linings of cavities, endocardium, epicardium, and sometimes other internal organs.

About 5% of bubonic patients develop the **pneumonic form,** which also occurs as a primary pattern after airborne infection. The lungs are heavy, red, and edematous and show patchy-to-confluent areas of hemorrhagic, gray consolidation. Fibrinous pleuritis is present in most cases. The characteristic necrotizing, hemorrhagic inflammation of plague is evident. The alveolar spaces are filled with bloody serous fluid. The white cell response is chiefly neutrophilic. Organisms abound in the lesions, causing an almost unrestricted destruction and necrosis of underlying architecture. The sputum is abundant and blood-stained and teems with ***Y. pestis.***

Before the advent of antibiotics, mortality from the bubonic form varied between 50 and 90%, and the pneumonic or septicemic forms were almost invariably fatal. Today, with appropriate antibiotic therapy, mortality is about 5 to 20%. Although *Y. pestis* has not developed resistance to antibiotics, their efficacy depends greatly on timing. When given later than 24 hours after onset of the pneumonic or septicemic forms of the disease, little benefit is noted. A vaccine offering six months' protection is available for workers likely to be exposed to *Y. pestis.*

Tularemia (Francisella tularensis)

Tularemia shares several key features with endemic plague: a wild animal source, transmissibility by arthropods, prominent lymph node swellings, and the occurrence of pneumonia.[144] However, its agent, a small pleomorphic gram-negative coccobacillus, though equally infective, belongs to a different genus, is less virulent, has only a relatively feeble endotoxin, and is a facultative intracellular parasite. In contrast to plague, *F. tularensis* causes protracted, granulomatous lesions as the infection runs its long, debilitating, but rarely fatal course.

The causative agent is carried by a wide spectrum of wild and domestic animals and their ticks. Rabbits are the source of 90% of infections in the U.S., where only about 200 cases are reported yearly. Tularemia is, however, endemic throughout the world, causing close to half a million infections per year. The U.S.S.R. has one of the highest rates. Hunters, farmers, butchers, cooks, and housewives handling infected animals are at risk, but the agent can be transmitted by carcass-contaminated water or by insect bite, and *F. tularensis* is a well-known cause of laboratory infections. Although it is said that the organism can enter the unbroken skin, its likeliest portals are skin abrasions and the conjunctival, digestive, and respiratory mucosae.[146] Yet, despite its high transmissibility from outside sources, man-to-man transmission is unrecorded, even from pneumonic patients shedding numerous bacteria.

Four clinical presentations are traditionally distinguished: the "ulceroglandular," "oculoglandular," "glandular," and "typhoidal," but these categories overlap, and pneumonia may arise in any to become the dominant clinical problem.[147] The incubation period ranges from one to 21 days with a mean of three to four days. Duration of the disease ranges from three weeks to three months, but is abbreviated by prompt treatment. In the most common pattern, *ulceroglandular tularemia*, a local skin lesion first develops, usually on the hands, arms, or face (bubonic plague favors the legs). It changes from a rapidly growing papule to a pustule that ulcerates. Next, the draining lymph nodes enlarge and sometimes become fluctuant or ulcerate through the skin via sinus tracts. Within a week of onset, a bacteremic phase is ushered in by fever, chills, headache, digestive symptoms, and muscle and joint pains. Generalized lymphadenopathy and splenomegaly soon develop. However, in contrast to plague, there is seldom a brisk leukocytosis. In some patients, an erythematous maculopapular rash appears, thought to represent a hypersensitivity reaction. Bacteremia is usually curtailed within two to three weeks but the infection may continue festering in local sites for months. Focal or confluent pulmonary opacities with hilar lymphadenopathy may appear on x-ray examination. Some patients develop involvements of the meninges, pericardium, heart valves, or bones. Patients with severe pneumonia and those with endotoxemic shock represent the gravest forms of disease. The convalescence is protracted.

In *oculoglandular tularemia*, the first papular lesions appear in the conjunctiva, then become pustular and ulcerate, accompanied by a lymphadenopathy involving mostly the preauricular, submaxillary, and superior cervical nodes. Severe ulcerations involving the bulbar conjunctiva may penetrate the sclera to enter the eye chambers and even propagate into the optic nerve, destroying vision. Rarely, there is no initial ulceration or it may occur in the *oropharynx*.

In *glandular tularemia*, localized or systemic lymphadenopathy appears as the first manifestation. If fever, hepatosplenomegaly, and toxemia are the presenting features, resembling Salmonella sepsis, the *typhoidal* form is diagnosed. In the absence of a history of infective contact, both these last two patterns are likely to be mistaken for other more frequent systemic illnesses, yet the pathologic processes are the same as those in ulceroglandular disease.

The initial skin lesions resemble pyogenic ulcerations and are neutrophil rich. Later, disseminated lesions undergo complete central necrosis, rimmed by epithelioid macrophages interspersed with giant cells to thus greatly resemble tubercles. As local lymph nodes begin to swell, they are at first firm and discrete owing to nonspecific lymphadenitis, but with the formation of abscesses they become soft, fluctuant, matted, and sometimes bubo-like. Grossly, they contain foci of purulent necrosis corresponding to the suppurative necrotic and granulomatous changes seen histologically. Similar, smaller lesions may also appear in more distant lymph nodes and organs including the liver, lung, serosa, heart, or bones. By contrast, the enlarged spleen shows only nonspecific inflammatory infiltration and lymphoreticular hyperplasia. The focal necrotic lesions in the lung are often surrounded by alveolar consolidation and accompanied by serous or purulent pleuritis and hilar lymphadenopathy, mimicking primary tuberculosis. Healing of large tularemic lung foci or draining buboes often leaves deforming scars because of their destructive character, but the smaller lesions heal without residuals.

The diagnosis can be established by several methods. Pleomorphic coccobacilli are readily visualized with methylene blue on smears of bubo aspirates. Isolation of the organism on special media should be attempted only by vaccine-protected personnel. Agglutinins take about two weeks to reach diagnostic levels. A skin test (Foshay's) is available but seldom used. Early antibiotic treatment is beneficial but less so during the chronic granulomatous phase, and it must be sustained in order to prevent relapse. Death from tularemia still occurs, especially in developing countries, but less frequently than the 1 to 6% of cases formerly reported. It should be noted here that an acute febrile disease resembling tularemia can be caused by *Pasteurella multocida*, usually following a dog or cat bite.

Brucellosis

Brucellosis is a systemic febrile disease with exasperatingly varied clinical presentations that can be acute, intermittent, or chronic. The infection is seldom acutely life threatening and sometimes vague enough to suggest neurosis or malingering.

Brucellae are gram-negative, facultative, intracellular coccobacilli that produce an endotoxin. They originate from livestock (cows for *B. abortus*, goats for *B. melitensis*, and swine for *B. suis*); rarely, dogs also transmit the infection (*B. canis*). All brucellae possess cell wall components enabling them to multiply in human macrophages until these cells become immunologically activated.[148] Skin tests have proven unreliable although they induce strong delayed hypersensitivity, and high serum agglutinin titers are therefore the mainstay of diagnosis. Culture requires special media and precise oxygen pressure; the organisms are hard to stain or find in tissue samples and can only intermittently be recovered from the blood.

Thanks to pasteurization of milk, pruning of diseased herds, and vaccination of animals, the annual incidence of brucellosis in the U.S. (caused mainly by *B. suis* and *B. abortus*) is down to less than 200 cases.[149] Most of these infections are derived from animal contact rather than from ingestion of milk or meat, but imported, unpasteurized goat cheese has also been a source of *B. melitensis*. Meat-packers and veterinarians are at greatest risk and occasional infections have arisen in laboratory workers. Brucellosis is, however, prevalent throughout the developing world, where *B. melitensis* predominates. The incubation period varies widely from one week to several months. First described as "undulant fever" with periodic exacerbations and partial remissions, this course applies to only a fraction of all cases. Brucella infection can be entirely *subclinical;* it can also be *acute, relapsing*, or *chronic* with only *systemic manifestations* and few localizing clinical signs; or it can be dominated by *localized lesions* of the bones, joints, lung, kidney, and other sites, even the heart valves. Skin lesions are rare, and leukopenia with lymphocytosis is more frequent than an elevated white cell count.

Acute brucellosis of less than one month's duration is the usual form among the occupationally infected.[150] It may resemble a systemic viral disease with chills, fever, headache, bone and joint pains, mild lymph node enlargement, and sometimes hepatosplenomegaly. Pronounced lassitude and mental depression are frequent complaints. It resolves spontaneously without treatment. Relapses are common and localized complications may ensue, prolonging the illness. *Chronic brucellosis* may be marked by transient fever (seldom rising above 40°C), episodes of sweating, obscure abdominal and musculoskeletal pains, neuralgias, weakness, weight loss, and sometimes anemia. Personality changes sometimes appear, bordering on psychosis, often misinterpreted because of the lack of physical findings. Splenic enlargement is seen in 10 to 20% of patients, and liver enlargement in 5%. The differential diagnosis includes occult neoplasm or lymphoma. Among the *localized lesions* most frequently due to *B. suis*, lumbar spondylitis or paravertebral abscess, monoarticular arthritis or multiple joint swellings are the most common, but destructive osteomyelitis is rare. Uncommonly, epididymo-orchitis appears, or kidney infections with chronic pyuria that resembles renal tuberculosis clinically. Likewise, chronic granulomatous Brucella pneumonia can mimic mycobacterial infection (p. 340).

Following a brief bacteremic phase, ***Brucella*** diffusely colonizes the lymphoreticular system, with consequent proliferation of macrophages and lymphocytes. Soon, granulomas form; some of them are centrally necrotic, containing numerous neutrophils, especially in ***B. suis*** infection; others may lack necrosis and resemble sarcoid lesions[151] (p. 391). Granulomas and diffuse mononuclear infiltrates result in hepatosplenomegaly. Large, destructive localized lesions, at the sites mentioned earlier, resemble abscesses or focal infarcts. Sometimes they give a spotted appearance to the spleen. In some cases the lesions are all microscopic, but generally they are grossly visible as yellow foci, which riddle organs throughout the body. They may eventually calcify and become detectable by x-rays. Extensive ***Brucella*** pneumonia, like that of tularemia, is focally destructive, granulomatous, and accompanied by hilar lymph node enlargement. It can be difficult to differentiate from tuberculosis. Most patients, however, have few or no focal pulmonary lesions.

When liver biopsy is resorted to for diagnosis, small granulomas may be found and must be differentiated from those of sarcoidosis, miliary tuberculosis, or other chronic infections. Brucellae can seldom be visualized in such lesions, and culture of the biopsy material is therefore necessary. No human vaccine is available in the U.S., but the infection responds to sustained treatment with antibacterial agents. U.S. mortality is now lower than the 2% formerly reported.

Glanders and Melioidosis*

Glanders, caused by *Pseudomonas mallei*, a small, gram-negative, nonmotile, nonsporing bacillus, occurs either as a severe acute disease or takes the form of a protracted infection resembling tuberculosis.[152] The organism is harbored by horses, mules, and donkeys and spreads on contact with broken skin or rarely is airborne. Uncommon but still endemic in South America, Asia, and Africa, the disease is very rare in the U.S. and the few cases seen are imported.

Acute glanders consists essentially of a rapidly developing, overwhelming pyemia. The incubation period of only one to five days is followed by the rather sudden onset of severe, prostrating infection with constitutional signs, i.e., fever, malaise, chills, nausea, vomiting, and generalized aches and pains.

A local papular abscess develops at the sites of inoculation, and the organism spreads from this site along the lymphatics to the regional nodes. Multiple satellite abscesses may occur along the pathways of drainage. The organism rapidly invades the blood to cause generalized pyemic abscesses in many organs and tissues, particularly in the lungs, liver, spleen, and muscles. Meningitis, osteomyelitis, and polyarthritis may all develop in the course of a few days. Diagnosis is frequently made by the demonstration of complement-fixing antibodies. Culture is hazardous and best left to reference laboratories.

Chronic glanders takes the form of a low-grade, febrile, infectious disease characterized by draining abscesses of the skin, lymphadenopathy, splenomegaly, and hepatomegaly. In time, the suppurative reaction becomes granulomatous, often simulating tuberculosis. The lesions are not pathognomonic, and diagnosis rests on the serologic or cultural identification of the organism. Over half of these patients eventually die of their infection.

Melioidosis bears a marked similarity to glanders; its agent, *P. pseudomallei*, causes disease in rodents, dogs, felines, and equines, among others, and widely contaminates soil and water in the Southeast Asian countries of Kampuchea, Laos, Thailand, Malaysia, and Burma. Infection is acquired principally from soil or water. In the endemic foci, mild-to-inapparent as well as severe human melioidosis occurs. Moreover, although the incubation period can be as short as two days, latencies of several years' duration have been observed.[153] Among the U.S. military, melioidosis has been named the "Vietnamese time bomb." As in glanders, the acute lesions tend to be necrotic abscesses, and the chronic ones, granulomas.

Clinically, any organ or tissue can be involved, but in acute infections the lung is usually most prominently affected and shows a necrotizing, sometimes cavitating bronchopneumonia that tends to become confluent. Such infections, even with broad-spectrum antibiotic treatment, still carry a mortality rate approaching 50%; in the more chronic forms, combinations of antibiotics and surgical drainage have been reasonably effective.

Leptospirosis and Weil's Disease

Leptospirae are tightly wound spirochetes about the size of treponemes (p. 335), often shaped like a shepherd's crook. They are widespread saprophytes and animal pathogens, only accidentally infecting man. All pathogenic leptospirae belong to the species-complex *L. interrogans* composed of many serogroups, including *icterohaemorrhagiae*, *canicola*, *autumnalis*, *grippotyphosa*, and *hebdomadis*, in descending order of frequency of disease in the U.S. All these agents can cause either mild or severe disease. *Anicteric or mild leptospirosis (which makes up 90% of all cases) is an acute, self-limited, febrile illness with protean symptoms. Severe infection with jaundice, bleeding, and renal failure is called Weil's disease or icterohemorrhagic fever*, the form of leptospirosis originally described, and the one responsible for most deaths.

Leptospirae indiscriminately infect wild and domestic animals, including the ubiquitous rodents; dogs and other reservoir hosts develop interstitial nephritis and chronically shed leptospirae in their urine. The organisms survive well in warm alkaline waters or moist soils. Human carriers do not seem to exist. Leptospirosis is both urban and rural; rodent-infested slums in developing countries abound with the disease. Contact with animals or soil and water or aerosol exposure may transmit the infection to man. In the U.S. less than 120 cases are reported yearly, mostly from southern locations; less than one-third of these occur among high-risk occupations, e.g., farming, abattoir work, trapping, and veterinary medicine.

Anicteric (mild) leptospirosis is typically a biphasic febrile disease.[154] During the initial *septicemic phase*, leptospirae can be cultured from the blood and CSF; during the second, *immune phase*, they are found only in the urine. The incubation period ranges from five to 14 days and the disease from one to three weeks, but relapses are common. The temperature often rises abruptly with chills, headache, and severe muscle pain, or with nausea and vomiting. Within three to seven days the fever defervesces, only to recur one to three days later, this time at a lower level, but often accompanied by signs of meningeal irritation; it is at this stage that the true diagnosis may first be suspected. Cases with less typical courses are easily mistaken for viral meningitis. In the more severe *Weil's disease*, the biphasic course is obscured by the early advent of jaundice, renal failure, purpura, or hypotension, sometimes within two to three days of onset, peaking during the second week. Conjunctival irritation and hyperemia appears early in both mild and severe leptospirosis. In the army outbreak of "Fort Bragg fever," there was also a sentinel pretibial skin rash.

During the early septicemic phase of **benign infection** leptospirae quickly disseminate and can be visualized by silver stain or immunofluorescence scattered through the liver, spleen, kidney, CNS, muscles, and other sites without apparent cellular reaction. Only later do mononuclear cell infiltrates become prominent, mostly in sites of focal cell necrosis such as striated muscle or kidney. Similarly, in early disease, inflammatory cells are lacking in the CSF although leptospirae are present (sometimes in profusion); lymphocytes appear only during the immune phase, thus mimicking the picture of viral "aseptic meningitis."

Detailed morphologic information is available only on **Weil's disease**. Basically, it is characterized by hemolysis, jaundice, focal hemorrhages, hepatic cholestasis with mild focal hepatocyte degeneration, interstitial nephritis with tubular necrosis, focal necroses of voluntary muscle fibers, and generalized reticuloendothelial activation. Petechial and ecchymotic hemorrhages are impressive and widespread, involving any organ, notably the liver and including the conjunctivae. The liver is slightly enlarged and discolored by bile and capsular hemorrhages. The kidneys are swollen and bile-stained and, with continuing renal failure, uremic pericarditis and related findings may appear (p. 996). Histologically, the lobular and trabecular liver architecture is preserved, but cholestasis and scattered dead hepatocytes and regenerative mitotic figures are found. A few acidophilic, Councilman-like bodies may be present or there may be focal ballooning of hepatocytes in the midzonal or centrolobular region.[155] Kupffer cells are increased in number and show erythrophagocytosis. Autolytic changes of the liver occur quickly in Weil's disease and may thus blur the relevant histologic findings. The renal glomeruli are normal but there is focal interstitial infiltration of lymphoplasmocytic cells of variable intensity. Acute tubular necrosis (p. 1027) is regularly present. The muscles of the extremities may show hemorrhages and necrosis of individual muscle fibers or, more frequently, loss of striations and hyaline change with bunching of the nuclei, thus accounting for the marked muscle pain and tenderness experienced by many patients. With prolonged survival, there is sarcolemmal and fibroblastic proliferation. The spleen and lymph nodes are only moderately enlarged by nonspecific reticuloendothelial hyperplasia. Interstitial myocarditis, anterior uveitis, and nerve palsies are known to occur, but are uncommon.

Tropical and military physicians are familiar with leptospirosis, but sporadic mild cases in the U.S. often remain undiagnosed and unreported. A clue to the diagnosis of Weil's disease is the relatively severe jaundice in a febrile, hemorrhagic illness in the face of only mild abnormalities in liver functions, a constellation of findings that should exclude the more common viral hepatitis (p. 900).[156] The jaundice is attributable largely to the combination of hemolysis and cholestasis. As with the other sporadic zoonoses, clinical awareness is paramount. Early in the infection, the diagnosis can be confirmed by blood or CSF culture; later, by urine culture. More frequently it is confirmed by species-specific microagglutination tests. Complete recovery is the rule in mild leptospirosis. In Weil's disease the mortality rate has ranged from 15 to 40%, largely owing to renal failure, but dialysis, improved supportive care, and possibly early antibiotics should now substantially reduce this rate.

Relapsing Fever (Borrelia recurrentis)*

There are two pathogenetic forms of relapsing fever. (1) *Tick-borne* disease is caused by several regional species of Borrelia and is transmitted to man from small animal reservoirs by soft ticks of the Ornithodoros genus. It occurs throughout the world wherever these ticks reside, including the wilderness areas of the sunbelt states in the U.S.; it is relatively benign, with a 2 to 4% mortality. (2) *Louse-borne* relapsing fever is due solely to *B. recurrentis;* it is transmitted from man to man by body lice and has no known animal source. It is most prevalent in the countries of the eastern horn of Africa and in the Andean highlands, and occurs in many other countries, particularly among the poor, but not in the U.S. In times of war and upheaval, louse-borne relapsing fever has become epidemic, most recently in the U.S.S.R. and North Africa. The louse-borne form is severe (4 to 40% lethal).

Tick-borne borreliae are carried by chipmunks, rats, lizards, and owls. Infected ticks expand the reservoir by transovarian propagation. They can survive 12 years between meals. Lice, during their briefer and meaner existence, carry borreliae only transiently but transmit them to man by biting or by being crushed or defecating at a skin defect. Prevention of the disease by control of wilderness ticks is almost impossible, but ridding people of lice seems attainable.

Borreliae are spirochetes (20 μ long) that can be visualized with the Wright-Giemsa method used on blood smears. They possess a surface coat whose antigens undergo a genetically programmed series of changes during infection, thought to result from mutations.[157] Borreliae also produce endotoxins,[158] which contribute to their pathogenicity. They are sensitive to immobilizing and directly bactericidal host antibodies. The recurrent attacks of fever so characteristic of this condition can be explained as follows: After introduction into a vulnerable host the spirochetes reach the bloodstream, where they proliferate and produce a spirochetemia. In several days the organisms are cleared from the blood as antibodies appear and the fever falls. However, among the spirochetes sequestered in the body a new antigenic variant emerges and invades the blood, with recurrence of the fever. In louse-borne disease only a few relapses are usual, but the tick-borne infection typically is associated with three or more, perhaps extending over a span of months. Although the pattern of the clinical relapses is basically similar, they tend to become gradually milder and eventually disappear. There is no satisfactory understanding of the ultimate spontaneous resolution of the infection, but possibly cross reactivity of the accumulating antibody specificities could account for it.

The acute febrile attack of relapsing fever appears after an incubation period of four to 18 days (mean, one week). It begins abruptly with fever, chills, headaches, myalgias, nausea and vomiting, photophobia, and abdominal tenderness. The fever rises each afternoon to around 40°C for two to seven days, accompanied by flushing of the face, dizziness, confusion, or delirium. Neurologic symptoms, such as neck stiffness, seizures, cranial nerve palsies, or coma occur in almost one-third of louse-borne cases, more rarely in the tick-borne; conversely, an erythematous rash reminiscent of typhus fever (a possible source of confusion) is more likely in the tick-borne version. Typically, the fever drops sharply by crisis after three to six days to end the first bout, and the patient recovers only to relapse after a seven- to nine-day interval. Hepatosplenomegaly may appear in both forms of the disease. Any one of the febrile attacks may be complicated by hypotension or shock, hepatic failure with jaundice, or cardiac symptoms. Such ominous features are seen mainly in the severest infections, usually in the fatal cases of louse-borne fever.

During each attack, large numbers of spirochetes flood the bloodstream and can be found in lesser numbers in the CSF, urine, or sputum. Direct microscopy of these sources is the preferred and promptest diagnostic method. Rickettsial infections (suggested by the clinical picture and by the frequent false-positive reactions to anti-OX antibodies in relapsing fever) must be ruled out. Culture of borreliae is feasible, but not generally available.

In fatal louse-borne disease, the spleen is moderately enlarged (300 to 400 gm) and histologically reveals focal necrosis and miliary collections of mixed leukocytes, including neutrophils. Numerous borreliae are seen about these foci. There is also congestion and hypercellularity of the red pulp with erythrophagocytosis. The liver shows congestion and Kupffer cell prominence as well as scattered septic foci similar to those in the spleen, and these may also be present in other organs including the heart, kidney, and meninges. Scattered hemorrhages resulting from DIC are frequently found in serosal and mucosal surfaces, skin, and viscera. Pulmonary bacterial superinfection is a frequent complication. Biopsy of the skin rash discloses vasodilation with a dense perivascular inflammatory infiltrate of mononuclear leukocytes, but the intense endothelial reaction and necrotizing vasculitis of rickettsial lesions are missing. Exceptionally, both Borrelia and ***R. rickettsii*** can be transmitted simultaneously by the same vector.

Several broad-spectrum antibiotics effectively suppress Borrelia infection and lower mortality. However, they can also induce so-called Jarisch-Herxheimer reactions—abrupt temperature rise, rigors, leukopenia, and fall in blood pressure that accompanies clearing of borreliae from the bloodstream. Accelerated destruction of spirochetes with release of endotoxin is postulated. This crisis is usually over within two hours and is followed by remission; however, it can occasionally lead to cardiac arrhythmias and asystole.[159]

Rat-Bite Fever

Two infections of similar presentation are associated with rat bites: that caused by *Spirillum minus* (sodoku) and that by *Streptobacillus moniliformis* (also named Haverhill fever). Both are obviously related to urban slum conditions and to lapses of pest control, and both present with swelling of the puncture site and local lymphadenopathy, followed by an acute febrile illness with a rash over the extremities resembling a viral infection. The incubation period of the spirillar form of rat-bite fever is longer (one to four weeks) than the streptobacillary form (one to two days). The former has a tendency to remit and exacerbate over a period of up to eight weeks. It is best diagnosed by animal inoculation of blood or by examination of blood under dark field or in Giemsa-stained smears. Streptobacillary infections average a briefer duration of one to two weeks, but often are accompanied by arthralgia or by symmetric swelling, heat, and redness of the large joints of the extremities, which may prolong the course of this infection. Diagnosis of streptobacillary infection is achieved by blood culture or agglutinin titers. No pathologic findings have been reported for either entity, except for one lethal case of *Streptobacillus* endocarditis.

*Lyme Disease**

Lyme disease, first described in 1972, is an inflammatory disorder transmitted by the newly recognized species of hard ticks, *Ixodes dammini.* It begins with a characteristic skin rash, *erythema chronicum migrans,* which is followed by either a migratory polyarthritis or by a more persistent arthritis of large joints. Variable neurologic or cardiac abnormalities may appear weeks or months after the initial skin lesions have subsided. In Europe only the skin erythema is found, but in the U.S. the biphasic Lyme disease is more usual and has now been reported from many locales, particularly from the summer resorts of the North Atlantic coast where *I. dammini* abounds. In the West, *I. pacificus* has been the vector.

Three to 20 days after a tick bite, one or several slowly enlarging erythematous skin lesions appear, which continue expanding as their central portion blanches. The margins are red, hot, and prominent but fade after two to three weeks (occasionally longer, after briefly relapsing). Sometimes between two weeks and six months later, half of the patients with skin lesions develop arthritis, usually in one or both knees or in other large joints in a recurrent or migratory fashion. The joints become painful, swollen, and hot and a few patients go on to develop chronic arthritis. Biopsies of these joints have shown intense neutrophilic infiltrates and synoviocytic proliferation. Uncommonly, meningoencephalitis or facial palsy appears, or a stiff neck, with white cells in the CSF. Some patients show manifestations of myocardial involvement, e.g., atrioventricular block, pericarditis, and (rarely) left ventricular dysfunction. No valvular lesions have been reported. Typically, the erythrocyte sedimentation rate is elevated, and there is cryoglobulinemia with elevated IgM and circulating immune complexes. The clinical disease may resemble rheumatoid arthritis, but lacks the characteristic rheumatoid factor or antinuclear antibody.[160]

Recently, a treponema-like spirochete was isolated from *I. dammini* that induces erythematous skin lesions in New Zealand rabbits after they have been bitten by infected ticks. Moreover, the serum of patients with Lyme disease was shown to have high antibody titers to this agent, and in a few cases the treponeme itself has now been cultured. The evidence for the spirochetal cause of this heretofore mysterious condition seems strong and is a testament to intensive investigations over a decade.[161]

TREPONEMES

Three pathogenic treponemes infect man—*T. pallidum, T. pertenue,* and *T. carateum* (Table 8–5). *T. pallidum* is the cause of syphilis and is by far the most important and best studied of the treponemes. *T. pertenue,* the cause of yaws, after nearing extinction as the result of an international eradication campaign, has since rebounded in several tropical countries. *T. carateum* continues flourishing in the remote corners of Latin America where pinta has always been a part of life. The treponemes are superbly adapted human parasites matching high infectivity, including transmission to the unborn fetus, with low virulence, long periods of latency, and lifelong persistence in the untreated host. Despite their antigenicity they produce no known toxins or tissue-destructive enzymes. Many of their lesions are linked to the hosts' immune responses, such as mononuclear cell infiltrates, proliferative vascular changes, and (sometimes) granuloma formation. Notwithstanding their slow progression the lesions may eventually become destructive, maiming, or lethal.

Human treponemes also pose peculiar diagnostic problems: they cannot be cultured in ordinary media, or passed on to animal hosts other than primates; and they are often difficult to stain and detect in diseased tissues, requiring special procedures—silver stains, immunofluorescence, or dark-field examination. Chief reliance for diagnosis is placed on serological tests that must be interpreted with caution.

Syphilis (Treponema pallidum)

Syphilis, also called lues, is a venereal disease of insidious and furtive habit. Neither the *primary chancre* nor the *secondary stage*, which takes the form of a rash, is accompanied by disturbing symptoms. The disease then enters a period of latency for years or decades, sometimes to be followed by the *tertiary stage* with its seriously disabling or fatal lesions. The late manifestations are localized principally to the cardiovascular and central nervous systems; other organs or structures are affected less frequently.

Immediately after World War II, there was an alarming increase in the incidence of new cases of syphilis in the U.S., reaching a rate of 70 per 100,000 population. A dramatic postwar decline to a rate of 3.8 followed in the mid-1950s, attributable largely to mass blood testing and the effectiveness of penicillin in the treatment of this disease. But the rate has resurged since and infection has increasingly shifted to younger individuals. The incidence is also increasing in male homosexuals. Socioeconomic factors and changing sexual mores have been significant influences in this trend. However, there has been a decline in the incidence of late sequelae and of congenital syphilis.

The *causative agent* is a 10- to 13-μm slender, corkscrew-shaped spirochete, invisible by usual stains and detectable only by silver impregnation, dark-field examination, or immunofluorescent techniques. Treponemas are readily killed by soap and antiseptics, cold, or drying. *Sexual intercourse is the usual mode of transmission* although bacteria-laden secretions can also transfer the disease by other intimate contact. *Transplacental transmission occurs readily* and active disease during pregnancy results in congenital syphilis in the fetus.

T. pallidum produces no demonstrable endo- or exotoxins. It has a double cell wall, and the outer one contains ligands for a wide variety of host cell membranes to which it is found to adhere, and from which it is capable of acquiring host proteins during infection.[162] Syphilis is one of the infections in which downward modulation of host lymphocyte responsiveness by a serum factor occurs,[163] and this early weakening of host immune reactivity may contribute to the latency and chronicity of ongoing infection. Yet even while treponemal infection actively proceeds, patients with syphilis develop immunity to challenge. About two weeks after the initial chancre, they become resistant to reinfection and, despite reexposure, do not develop a second chancre. Treatment very early in the disease may block this development, called "chancre immunity."

Spirochetal antigens evoke host antibodies of two types: (1) *nonspecific antibodies, which react with a lipoidal antigen derived from beef heart (cardiolipin); and (2) specific antibodies to spirochetal antigens.* The nontreponemal antibodies (formerly called "reagins") can be detected by readily performed, inexpensive complement-fixation or flocculation serologic tests for syphilis (STS), such as Wassermann, Kahn, Kline, Hinton, and VDRL. A rapid plasma reagin card test (RPR), which is simple to perform, is also available. However, *since these serologic tests for syphilis do not detect specific treponemal antigens, they can also be positive in a great variety of nonluetic illnesses,* yielding what are known as *biologic false-positives* (BFP). BFP may be encountered in smallpox vaccination, infectious mononucleosis, leprosy, autoimmune diseases, viral hepatitis, and heroin addiction as well as in many acute febrile illnesses.

More specific than the STS are tests based on the detection of treponemal antigens. The *Treponema pallidum* immobilization test (TPI) determines the ability of the patient's serum to abolish the mobility of a strain of live *T. pallidum.* A fluorescent treponemal antibody (FTA) test has been further refined by absorption of nonspecific spirochetal group antibodies from the patient's serum in the so-called fluorescent treponemal antibody absorption test (FTA-ABS), and is now the standard method used. The specific tests may be less practical for population screening but have far greater sensitivity and specificity than the STS. Thus, it is advisable to follow up positive STS results with one of the more specific methods.

The natural course of acquired syphilis evolves in three stages. The *primary stage* follows an incubation period of 10 to 90 days (average, three weeks) and is marked by the development of the chancre at the site of treponemal invasion. Regional nontender adenopathy soon follows. Even before the chancre appears, a spirochetemia seeds tissues throughout the body, thus providing the basis for the later disseminated lesions of secondary and tertiary syphilis. The chancre usually heals in three to 12 weeks with or without therapy, and the patient then appears entirely well.

The *secondary stage* follows in approximately two weeks to six months (average, six to eight weeks). It is characterized by a generalized or, less often, a localized skin eruption. These manifestations too disappear spontaneously in about four to 12 weeks. The two early stages may be extremely subtle or occult. A chancre on the cervix or in the oropharynx would not be noted. The rash might be trivial and fleeting. *Many patients with unmistakable evidence of late syphilis recall no earlier manifestations.*

Following the secondary stage the patient again enters a period of apparent well-being referred to as *latent syphilis*, lasting years or decades. Only then may the lesions of *tertiary syphilis* appear. *These generally take one of three forms: (1) localized destructive lesions (gummas) of virtually any tissue, e.g., liver, bones, testis, or skin; (2) cardiovascular lesions; or (3) CNS involvement.* However, many patients never develop tertiary lesions. Studies of untreated syphilitics indicate that about one-third achieve spontaneous cure with reversion of all serologic abnormalities. Another one-third continue to have positive serologic tests but die of unrelated causes. Only the remaining one-third develop the grave lesions of tertiary disease.[164, 165]

Whatever the stage of the disease and location of the lesions, *histologic hallmarks of the inflammatory reaction are obliterative endarteritis and plasma cell infiltrates.* Small arteries and arterioles in the inflammatory reaction exhibit swelling and proliferation of endothelial cells to produce concentric "onionskin" layers that markedly narrow the lumen. About these vessels there is prominent perivascular cuffing by plasma cells.

Acquired Primary Syphilis

In the **primary stage the chancre usually occurs on the glans penis in males and on the vulva or cervix in females.** In approximately 10% of cases the chancre may be extragenital: lips, fingers, oropharynx, anorectum, or some other site. In about 50% of females and 30% of males, primary lesions either never develop or are not detected.

The chancre usually begins as a solitary, slightly elevated, firm, reddened papule that varies in size up to several centimeters in diameter. It then superficially erodes to create a clean-based, shallow ulceration on the surface of the slightly elevated papule. The contiguous induration characteristically creates a button-like mass directly subjacent to the eroded skin or mucosa, providing the basis of the designation **hard chancre.** Superimposed secondary bacterial infection may impart a suppurative exudation.

Histologically, the chancre is characterized by an intense mononuclear leukocytic infiltration, chiefly of plasma cells with scattered macrophages and lymphocytes (Fig. 8–24). This inflammatory infiltrate is embedded in increased ground substance, rich in glycosoaminoglycans, and bordered by a proliferative vasofibroblastic response that makes up the margins of the ulcer. Obliterative endarteritis, as described, is present within this inflammatory reaction.

Treponemes are not evident without special staining, but with silver impregnations or immunofluorescent techniques they can often be visualized in the surface layer of the ulceration or in the scant overlying exudate. The regional nodes are usually enlarged and may show nonspecific acute or chronic lymphadenitis (p. 656) or a plasma cell–rich infiltrate, or may contain focal epithelioid cell granulomas.

The primary stage of syphilis and its accompanying early spirochetemia are remarkable for the absence of systemic signs and symptoms. Not all syphilitic chancres are typical in appearance or location, and therefore dark-field identification of treponenes provides the most definitive and earliest means of diagnosis. Treponenes can sometimes be aspirated from the enlarged regional nodes after they have disappeared from the chancre. *During the earliest weeks of syphilis the STS and specific tests for antitreponemal antibodies are usually negative.* Adequate treatment with penicillin during the primary stage prevents the development of secondary syphilis and, in most patients, maintains seronegativity or converts serodiagnostic tests to negative. In a few patients, despite adequate therapy, serologic tests remain positive, a phenomenon described as *sero-fastness.*

Secondary Syphilis

The secondary stage is characterized by widespread mucocutaneous lesions that are often generalized over the entire body, including the mucous membranes of the oral cavity, palms of the hands, and soles of the feet. Most often the rash is macular, with discrete red-brown lesions, rarely over 5 mm in diameter. In other cases, follicular, pustular, annular, and scaling lesions may predominate.[166] Vesicular bullous and ulcerative lesions are uncommon. Reddened mucous patches may appear in the mouth or vagina. All the mucocutaneous lesions harbor organisms, but the most contagious are the wet types of mucous patches and skin

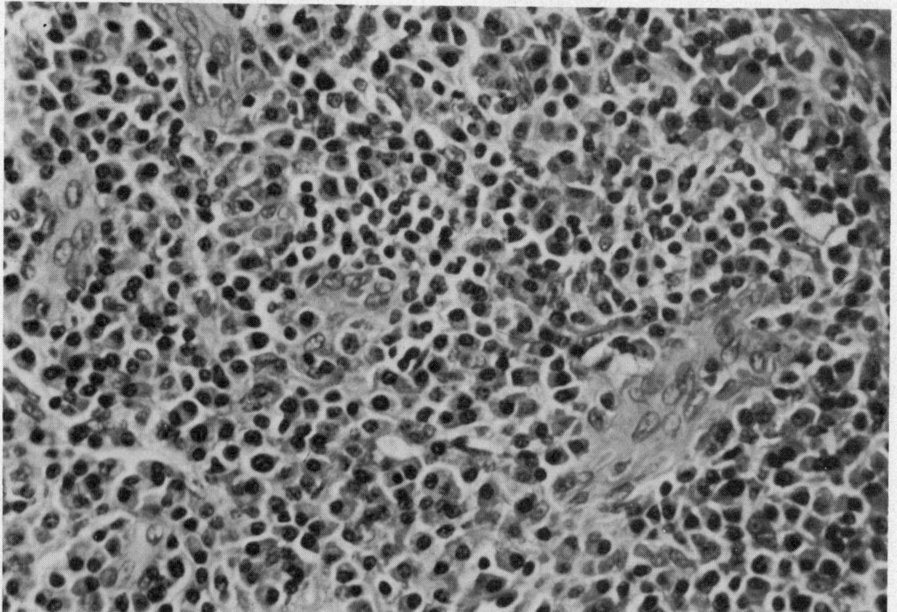

Figure 8–24. Syphilitic chancre: diffuse plasmocytic infiltration and endothelial proliferation.

lesions. Histologically, the inflammatory reaction in the foci of mucocutaneous involvement resembles that found in the chancre. However, there is less intensity to the plasma cell infiltrate and it is ordinarily confined to perivascular cuffing. When the rash is distinctly papular it is usually accompanied by thickening of the epithelium and elongation of the rete pegs. Ulceration modifies the macroscopic and microscopic appearance by the development of suppurative exudation. Occasionally, secondary syphilitic lesions are better localized. Thus, papular lesions in the region of the penis or vulva may become large, elevated, broad plaques. They sometimes also occur on the lips and perianal region. **These flat, red-brown elevations (up to 2 to 3 cm in diameter) are designated condylomata lata and are distinct from condylomata acuminata or venereal warts** (p. 1082). The overlying epithelium is intact and hyperplastic unless secondarily traumatized or infected. Histologically, there is a characteristic plasma cell infiltrate, as well as the characteristic vascular obliterative endarteritis. Many spirochetes may be found in these condylomata. The generalized lymphadenopathy of secondary syphilis is often nonspecific, rarely of a granulomatous type.

The lesions of secondary syphilis are not of themselves pathognomonic since there is such variability in their form. However, the diagnosis of syphilis must be suspected when a disseminated rash develops in a patient who appears to be relatively well except for generalized adenopathy, sore throat, or bone pain. In other bacteremic states associated with rashes, marked constitutional signs of fever, chills, malaise, and prostration usually accompany the skin lesions. A history of primary chancre cannot be relied on to confirm the diagnosis of secondary syphilis since in many patients the primary stage may have passed completely unnoticed. Thus, syphilis may be confused with other noninfectious skin diseases.

A minority of patients with secondary syphilis develop a subacute meningitis, iritis, hepatitis, periostitis, or an immune complex glomerulopathy leading to the nephrotic syndrome (p. 1011). *At this stage of the disease the STS and treponemal tests are almost always positive.* Once again the opportunity is provided to treat these patients and prevent the development of tertiary syphilis.

Tertiary Syphilis

Late syphilitic disease, which develops in only one-third of the untreated patients, is becoming increasingly rare. The cardiovascular system is most commonly affected (80 to 85%). CNS involvement accounts for about 5 to 10%. Gummas in the liver and other sites make up the remainder. These localizations are not mutually exclusive.

Cardiovascular syphilis, principally involving the aorta, may become manifest years to decades after the initial infection. It is an extremely serious disorder that causes considerable inflammatory scarring of the media of the aorta (mesaortitis) with weakening and dilation (aneurysm formation), widening and incompetence of the aortic valve ring, and narrowing of the mouths of the coronary ostia (p. 531).

Central nervous system syphilis, or neurosyphilis (p. 1381), is another late manifestation and takes one of several forms, designated as meningovascular syphilis, tabes dorsalis, and general paresis of the insane. Focal gummas in the brain or cord occur very infrequently. In addition, patients with ataxia and sensory loss from spinal cord syphilis may undergo a rapidly destructive degenerative arthritis of the knee joint (Charcot's joint).

The **syphilitic gumma** is a late-appearing focal area of nonsuppurative inflammatory destruction. It is characterized by a peculiar, rubbery, "gummatous" necrosis, most commonly found in the liver, bones, and testes. Gummas may occur singly or multiply, and vary in size from microscopic defects to large tumorous masses of necrotic material. Erosion of a superficial cutaneous or submucosal gumma may yield a ragged ulcer that is extremely persistent and resistant to local therapeutic measures.

In the liver, scarring due to gummas may cause a distinctive hepatic lesion known as **hepar lobatum** (p. 933). Gummas in bones cause focal areas of destruction, may erode the cortical surfaces and lead to fractures, and sometimes extend into joints to destroy the articular surfaces. A testicular gumma may cause enlargement and simulate a tumor, but later produce fibrous scarring.

Histologically, active gummas consist of a center of a coagulated, necrotic material with faint persistence of the shadowy outlines of dead tissue cells and vessels (Fig. 8–25). The margins of the gumma are composed of plump or palisaded macrophages and fibroblasts that may resemble the epitheliod cells of the tubercle surrounded by large numbers of mononuclear leukocytes, chiefly plasma cells. The small vessels in the wall are narrowed by the obliterative endarteritis found in other syphilitic lesions. Treponemes are scant in these gummas and are extremely difficult to demonstrate.

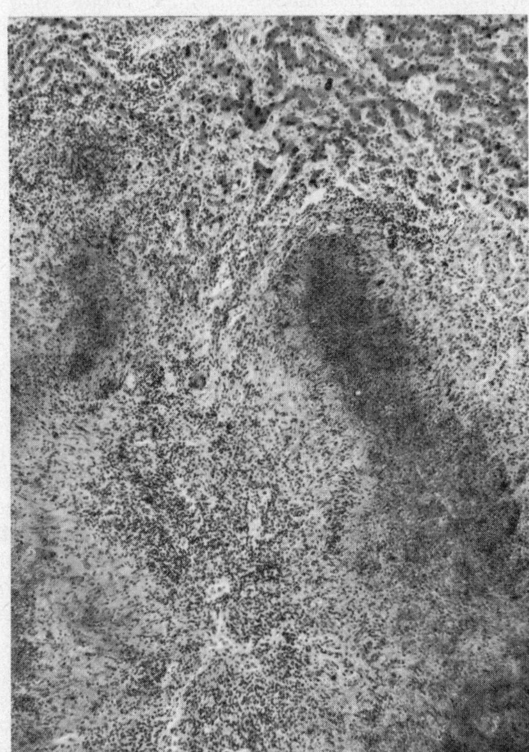

Figure 8–25. Syphilitic gumma of liver with central necrosis.

Gummas at times may be microscopic in size, producing a lesion virtually indistinguishable from the granulomas of tuberculosis or Boeck's sarcoid, without additional evidence of the causative agent.

Congenital Syphilis

Congenital syphilis may be contracted by a fetus born up to five years after the mother first becomes infected, but exceptions have been noted. The more recent the infection, the more certain the involvement of the fetus and the more florid the congenital disease; yet, adequate therapy early in pregnancy will completely protect the child. The treponemes do not invade the placental tissue or the fetus until the fifth month of gestation, and therefore syphilis is an uncommon cause of early abortion. Instead, it causes late abortion, stillbirth, or death soon after delivery, or it may persist in latent form to become apparent only during childhood or adult life.[167]

In the **perinatal** and **infantile** forms of congenital syphilis, the most striking lesions affect the mucocutaneous tissues and bones. A diffuse rash develops, which differs from that of the acquired secondary stage in that there can be extensive sloughing of the epithelium, particularly on the palms and soles and about the mouth and anus. These lesions teem with spirochetes. There is also a generalized luetic osteochondritis and periostitis that affects all bones, most prominently the nose and lower legs. Destruction of the vomer causes collapse of the bridge of the nose and later on the characteristic saddle deformity. Periostitis of the tibia leads to excessive new bone growth on the anterior surfaces and produces anterior bowing, or saber shin. There is also widespread disturbance in endochondral bone formation. The epiphyses become widened as the cartilage overgrows. Cartilage is found as displaced islands within the metaphysis. Throughout this area, there is an overall increase in fibrous tissue accompanied by the characteristic mononuclear leukocytic and vascular changes of syphilitic infections.

The **liver** usually is severely affected in congenital syphilis. Diffuse fibrosis permeates lobules to isolate hepatic cells into small nests, accompanied by the characteristic white cell infiltrate and vascular changes. Gummas are occasionally found in the liver, even in very early cases.

The **lungs** may be affected by a diffuse interstitial fibrosis that produces a marked increase in their consistency. In the syphilitic stillborn they appear as pale, virtually airless organs **(pneumonia alba).**

The generalized spirochetemia may lead to diffuse interstitial inflammatory reactions in virtually any other organ of the body, e.g., the pancreas, kidneys, heart, spleen, thymus, and endocrine organs. In the CNS meningovascular syphilis may develop. Eye changes consist of an interstitial keratitis or a choroiditis with focal or diffuse inflammatory scarring of the choroid. Abnormal pigment production in focal areas may produce the spotted retina of congenital syphilis.

The late-occurring form of congenital syphilis is distinctive in that *interstitial keratitis* is often accompanied by *periostitis, saber shins, and saddle deformity of the nose. In addition, there are characteristic alterations in tooth formation owing to spirochetal infection during the stages of development (Hutchinson's teeth). The incisor teeth are somewhat smaller than normal and have a screwdriver shape, or are sometimes even more pointed, to produce a peg-shaped or pumpkin-seed deformity. The defective formation of enamel results in notching of the biting margins of the incisors. Dental x-ray examinations show characteristic changes even before the teeth erupt. Other lesions resembling tertiary syphilis may develop but, for unknown reasons, cardiovascular syphilis is quite uncommon. On the basis of the meningovascular involvement, eighth nerve deafness and optic nerve atrophy may develop as these cranial nerves are damaged by the surrounding inflammatory reaction. Among these many possible findings, most characteristic of delayed or "tardive" congenital syphilis is the triad: interstitial keratitis, Hutchinson's teeth, and eighth nerve deafness.*

In contrast to many other bacteria, *T. pallidum* for many decades has remained sensitive to penicillin and to other antibiotics, and its prescribed treatment schedules have remained virtually unchanged.

*Yaws, Bejel, and Pinta**

These three treponematoses caused by spirochetes morphologically identical to *T. pallidum* are much less common. Although they share some similarities with syphilis, there are important differences in epidemiology as well as organ involvement. Yaws is a disease of the moist tropics, bejel one of desert zones, and pinta is limited to rural foci in Latin America. *All are transmitted by person-to-person contact but they are not venereal diseases.* Like syphilis, *bejel* is a chronic disorder with onset most often in childhood. The initial lesion involves the mucocutaneous surfaces. *Yaws* begins with a large, raised skin ulcer, the "mother yaw." Late in the course, bones may also be involved by gummatous lesions. However, CNS and cardiovascular lesions, which are the hallmark of tertiary syphilis, are rarely if ever seen. *Pinta,* unlike yaws and bejel, is purely a skin disease causing unsightly pigment changes, and is therefore less serious. All the nonvenereal treponematoses evoke humoral antibodies that give positive serologic tests for syphilis and seem to protect the bearer from venereal lues.

UNCOMMON BACTERIA

The five diseases to be briefly discussed here are rare in the U.S., but each presents a distinctive pattern of pathology. Since only modest research efforts have been expended, their pathogenesis has remained obscure. (See also Whipple's disease, p. 848.)

*Rhinoscleroma**

This is a destructive chronic infection of the nose and upper airways caused by an encapsulated, gram-negative bacillus related to *Klebsiella pneumoniae* (p. 311). In its endemic regions—parts of the U.S.S.R.,

Europe, Latin America, and the Near East—rhinoscleroma is a well-known cause of facial deformity and of dangerous upper airway obstruction.[168] The agent, *K. rhinoscleromatis*, is absent from the normal human microflora, but is readily cultured from rhinoscleroma lesions. Its transmission is not understood and its response to treatment is slow. The disease progresses insensibly from an initial stage resembling an ordinary cold to an atrophic stage in which the respiratory mucosa appears dry and granular, and finally to a nodular stage characterized by the growth of tumor-like submucosal masses caused by granulomatous inflammation. These swellings obliterate the nares, deform the face by distending the nasal structures, and creep downward into the pharynx and larynx with consequent anosmia, dysphonia, and airway obstruction. Isolated laryngeal involvement is rare but more dangerous, since it may lead to early death by suffocation. Microscopically, the lesions are replete with foamy macrophages, some quite large or multinucleate (Mikulicz cells). Aggregates of these foam cells are interspersed within well-vascularized fibrous stroma, which also contains lymphocytes and plasma cells. Contained within the cytoplasmic vacuoles of macrophages are encapsulated diplobacilli, best evidenced by silver staining. The overlying epithelium shows proliferation, sometimes squamous metaplasia, or even pseudoepitheliomatous change.

Ozena

This disease is also a rare, severe, chronic rhinitis. However, instead of swelling it causes atrophy of the turbinates accompanied by a foul-smelling greenish exudate, nasal obstruction, and eventual anosmia. *Klebsiella ozaenae* is thought to be the responsible agent, but mixed cultures with other gram-negative bacilli have sometimes been cultured from these lesions. The histologic picture is one of nonspecific exudative and necrotizing inflammation.

Granuloma Inguinale (Calymmatobacterium donovani)

Granuloma inguinale—not to be confused with lymphogranuloma venereum (p. 294)—is a chronic, venereally transmitted disease with ulcerating and granulating lesions of the genital skin and mucosae that become quite disabling and deforming. The agent, *C. donovani*, is a tiny, encapsulated, facultative, intracellular bacillus, sometimes referred to as a Donovan body. Granuloma inguinale is encountered world-wide, with the highest incidence in New Guinea and India. It is uncommon in Europe and the U.S. The usual mode of transmission is by sexual contact, but for unknown reasons males are predominantly affected. Under highly endemic conditions nonvenereal transmission can also occur.[169]

After an incubation period of three days to several months, the initial lesion appears as a papule on genital, perineal, or more rarely extragenital sites (e.g., the lips). This enlarges, ulcerates, and begins spreading and festering as an elevated, creeping sore with a necrotic center and an indurated, raised border. Satellite papules and ulcers may appear along the lymphatic drainage. In the long chronicity of this infection, the ensuing fibrosis may cause dense scarring, and sometimes keloid formation (Fig. 8–26). Unlike lymphogranuloma venereum, however, the lymph nodes remain uninvolved and rectal strictures are not formed.

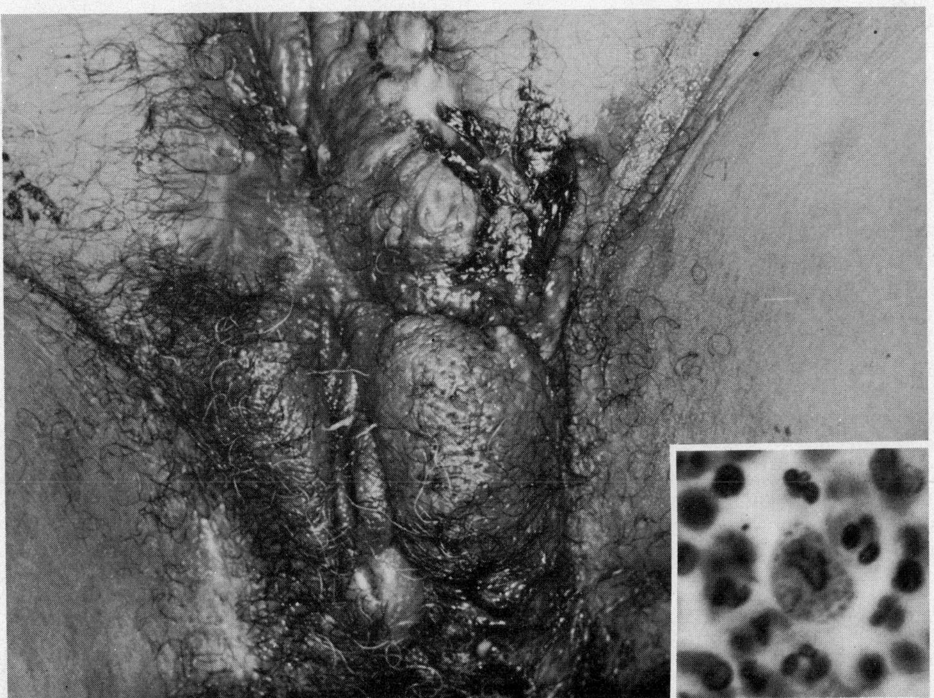

Figure 8–26. Granuloma inguinale of vulva. Inset shows a macrophage in high-power detail filled with faintly visible Donovan bodies.

At the base of the ulcer and in the papillary dermis of the bordering skin or mucosa, microabscesses are formed, merging with the underlying, richly vascularized granulation tissue that constitutes the bulk of the lesion. In the most active, superficial sites, Donovan bodies can be seen in vacuolated macrophages. In H and E–stained sections, they appear as faintly bluish dots sticking to the contour of a vacuole. With Giemsa or silver stains, many more organisms are usually apparent, some in neutrophils but mostly in macrophages. Deep to the granulation tissue, there is fibrosis and mononuclear cell infiltration. Along the expanding borders of the ulcer, the epidermis shows marked acanthosis and sometimes pseudoepitheliomatous hyperplasia. Granuloma inguinale usually remains localized wherever the lesion first appears but rarely, in pregnant women with involvement of the uterine cervix, metastatic dissemination to bones, joints, and other skin sites has been observed.[169] Diagnosis is usually made by the demonstration of Donovan bodies in silver or Giemsa-stained smears or in biopsy tissue. Timely chemotherapy prevents the disfiguring lesions seen in neglected cases.

Chancroid, Soft Chancre (Hemophilus ducreyi)

Chancroid is an acute venereal disease characterized by the development of a necrotic ulcer, the *soft chancre,* at the site of inoculation of *H. ducreyi* on the genitals. This organism is highly infectious, and autoinoculation can lead to multiple chancres. The disease is transmitted by sexual intercourse and infection occurs through skin or mucous membrane abrasions. The organism has been isolated from the penile smegma and vaginal secretions of patients without manifestations of the disease. In the U.S. approximately 800 cases of chancroid are reported every year.[170] It is more widely prevalent in the Orient, West Indies, and North Africa.

The soft chancre usually occurs on the penis and about the labia minora and majora, approximately three to five days after infection. A small macule that becomes papular and then forms an intradermal abscess develops at the site of invasion. The overlying skin sloughs to produce a draining ulcer, which is at first shallow but may enlarge to 2 to 3 cm in diameter. The well-developed ulcer is covered with a necrotic, purulent slough and bears a resemblance to the chancre of syphilis, but is less indurated as a rule. In about 50% of cases, the regional nodes undergo painful inflammatory hyperplasia over the course of one to two weeks. Suppuration may occur in these sites to produce fluctant masses (buboes) that drain to the skin surface.

Histologically, the soft chancre presents three zones. The surface of the ulcer is composed of disintegrating leukocytes and red cells. Deep to this level, there is a zone of granulation tissue with hyperplasia of the endothelial cells in the small vessels, as well as a marked inflammatory reaction within and about the vessel wall. This vasculitis often leads to intravascular thrombosis or necrosis of the vessel wall. Deep to the granulation tissue, there is a third zone of more chronic inflammatory reaction with fibroblastic proliferation infiltrated with mononuclear leukocytes. The regional nodes of drainage present the same alterations of the involved vessels. Abscesses may form in the centers of these inflamed nodes and, by coalescence, may create large areas of suppurative necrosis.

Clinically, the chancre is not particularly painful; however, the regional nodes of drainage are extremely tender, presumably owing to tension. The constitutional symptoms that accompany this disease are mild.

The diagnosis of chancroid can be established by the isolation of *H. ducreyi.* A skin test for chancroid is available, but remains positive for several years after an acute infection.

*Carrión's Disease (Bartonellosis)**

The endemic zone of *Bartonella bacilliformis* infection is limited to that of its sandfly vector, *Phlebotomus verrucarum,* which thrives in the Northern Andes at altitudes between 700 and 2500 m, largely within Peru. *B. bacilliformis* initially infects erythrocytes, causing an acute, febrile illness *(Oroya fever)* associated with hemolytic anemia and hepatosplenomegaly. This is followed by an eruptive phase in which the bartonellae localize in the skin, giving rise to numerous highly vascularized, nodular collections of inflammatory cells. The mortality rate is high in the initial hemolytic phase. The skin lesions usually develop after immunity is acquired and can be treated with chloramphenicol. Rarely, human infections with animal hemobartonellae have been reported in U.S. laboratory workers.[171]

MYCOBACTERIA

Mycobacteria share the basic structure of all bacterial organisms but have distinctive phosphoglycolipids, phospholipids, and waxes in their cell walls. Their family includes pathogens for many animals from mammals to mollusks, as well as free-living mycobacteria that sometimes contaminate laboratory samples and give rise to confusion with human pathogens. Besides the tubercle and leprosy bacilli, there are about 30 other human pathogenic species, called the atypical mycobacteria, which have been classified by their rate of growth, reaction to light, and production of pigment on artificial media. The most important human mycobacteria tend to be slow dividers and are facultative intracellular invaders, and some thrive best at low body temperatures. Their relatively modest infectivity contrasts with their marked ability to persist in tissues either in dormant form or as chronic, destructive pathogens. *Owing to their waxy cell components, many mycobacteria are acid fast,* i.e., they retain the red dye carbolfuchsin after rinsing with acid solvents. One of the pathogenic mycobacteria, the lepra bacillus, has never been successfully cultured. Others have special growth requirements, and even under optimal aerobic conditions they take several weeks to form colonies, so that cultures must be maintained and periodically monitored accordingly. Animal inoculation, formerly the mainstay of diagnosis, is today used mainly for experimental purposes.

Tuberculosis

Tuberculosis is a worldwide, chronic, communicable disease caused by the "Koch bacillus," *Mycobacterium tuberculosis*, which usually affects the lungs but may cause lesions in any organ or tissue of the human body. It evokes focal granulomatous inflammatory reactions that typically undergo central caseous necrosis. *These "caseating granulomas" are the histologic hallmarks of tuberculosis, but since similar lesions can have other infectious and noninfectious causes, tubercle bacilli should always be demonstrated in order to confirm the histologic diagnosis of tuberculosis.*

Two species of tubercle bacilli infect humans: *M. tuberculosis hominis* and *M. tuberculosis bovis*. Human tubercle bacilli are ordinarily transmitted by inhalation of infective droplets coughed or sneezed into the air by a patient with open lesions, i.e., with tuberculous foci in the lungs that are in communication with the airways. Bacilli remain viable in wet sputum for months and even in dried sputum particles for weeks. Most infections are acquired by sustained exposure rather than casual contact, perhaps because respiratory defense mechanisms are able to screen out or kill small numbers of mycobacteria. Rarely, the conjunctivae or the abraded or punctured skin serve as portals of entry. Bovine tubercle bacilli are transmitted by milk from diseased cows and first produce intestinal or tonsillar lesions. In developed countries, disease control in dairy herds and pasteurization of milk have virtually eradicated this mode of transmission, and in the U.S., tuberculosis is now considered to be due to human bacilli unless proved otherwise. Elsewhere, extrapulmonary tuberculosis is sometimes due to bovine bacilli or to distinctive local human strains.[172]

INCIDENCE. Although tuberculosis is now both treatable and to some degree preventable, it is still the single most important bacterial infection worldwide. Its true incidence cannot be precisely determined because (1) only a fraction of persons with *M. tuberculosis* manifest clinical disease at any one time; (2) all infected persons remain indefinitely at risk of developing active disease; and (3) case reporting, even in developed countries, is always incomplete. In 1974, a W.H.O. committee estimated the worldwide prevalence of active disease at 7 million. It is important at this point to distinguish infection from disease. *Most exposed individuals do not develop clinical disease—only an asymptomatic infection—and are converted to tuberculin reactors without necessarily developing disease.* In 1980, of a total U.S. population of 216 million, an estimated 15 million were *tuberculin reactors*, but only 30,000 *active* clinical cases were reported that year. In 1982, this number declined to 27,500.[173] Thus, in terms of active disease, tuberculosis ranks behind the avalanche of 1 million plus venereal infections recorded yearly in the U.S., but in terms of the total number of people infected, it retains its traditional primacy among bacterial infections. Worldwide there is much variation in the incidence and mortality associated with clinical tuberculosis. The current U.S. case rate is 12.4 per 100,000, but there are pockets around the globe with a staggering rate of 350 per 100,000. Likewise, in the U.S. mortality rates have fallen slowly to about 2 per 100,000, whereas they are many times higher in the developing countries. Many factors contribute to this marked variation. *Tuberculosis flourishes wherever there is poverty, malnourishment, and lack of adequate medical care.* Much of the decline of tuberculosis in the U.S. occurred before the advent of effective antibiotic therapy, owing to better living conditions. Unfortunately, those segments of the U.S. population who have benefited least from the improved quality of life, e.g., inner city blacks and Hispanics, continue to succumb to tuberculosis in unacceptably high numbers. These patients constitute a human reservoir of infection. In addition to socioeconomic factors, there seem also to be *racial or ethnic differences*. Africans, American Indians and blacks, and Eskimos are especially vulnerable, possibly because they have been unexposed until the recent past. Blacks in the U.S. Army have significantly higher morbidity rates from tuberculosis than whites. The possibility that these racial differences have genetic origins cannot be ruled out; however, they seem not to be related to the HLA antigens. Moreover, no racial or economic *group* has proved resistant to sustained exposure, although susceptibility clearly differs among *individuals*. Thus, in the past, there has been a higher incidence of the disease in males than in females, perhaps because of greater exposure. Diabetes mellitus, alcoholism, malnutrition, congenital heart disease, chronic lung disease (particularly silicosis), and in fact any debilitating or immunosuppressive condition (e.g., Hodgkin's disease) predispose to active disease. Occupational hazards exist for physicians and hospital personnel.

A significant change in the age distribution of tuberculosis has occurred in the U.S. Outside the inner city reservoirs of infection, where young adults are still at high risk, tuberculin reactivity and peak morbidity and mortality have all shifted from the 20-year-olds to the 50- and 60-year olds. Childhood tuberculosis has declined most sharply—less than 5% of teenagers now react to tuberculin; conversely, peak mortality from tuberculosis in white males now occurs around age 54, and in white females after age 65. Thus, tuberculosis in the U.S. is today mainly a disease of the elderly who became infected earlier in life before transmission declined.[174]

CAUSATIVE ORGANISM. *M. tuberculosis hominis* is a slender, delicately beaded rod averaging 4 microns in length when stained by the Ziehl-Neelsen or fluorescent dye methods. It is undetectable by Gram stain or routine histologic techniques. Its dividing time is of the order of 48 hours and growth in culture is slow; therefore, direct microscopic diagnosis in sputum, sediments, exudates, or biopsy specimens is time saving, although culture is still needed to rule out artifacts and verify the species. It should be remembered, however, that it takes 10^4 bacteria per ml of tissue for them to be visually detected. A recently devised gas chromatographic method for traces of tuberculostearic acids may prove helpful when microscopic examination fails to yield mycobacteria after painstaking search.[175]

Tubercle bacilli are strict aerobes; they thrive at a Po_2 of 140 mm Hg and this may explain their tendency to cause disease in the subapical portions of the lung (Po_2 = 130 mm Hg), and to become scarcer in necrotic tissue lacking blood-borne oxygen. Their growth is also inhibited by a pH lower than 6.5 and by long-chain fatty acids. On the other hand, *M. tuberculosis* can persist in dormant form in old necrotic and calcified lesions capable of reinitiating growth, even when virtually undetectable by microscopy.

PATHOGENESIS. The *pathogenesis* of tuberculosis involves four considerations: (1) the virulence of *M. tuberculosis*, (2) the role of induced hypersensitivity, (3) the role of immunity or resistance, and (4) the genesis of the granulomatous pattern of reaction so characteristic (but not necessarily diagnostic) of tuberculosis.

M. tuberculosis has no known exotoxins, endotoxins, or histolytic enzymes. A variety of antigens (approximately 30) can be identified, but these seem to play no role in virulence. More important appears to be the microbial content of extractable *mycosides* (covalently linked complex lipids and carbohydrates), *which appear to be directly related to bacterial virulence.* One derivative, called "cord factor" (trehalose 6–6 dimycolate), is essential for the in vitro growth of *M. tuberculosis* in a pattern of "serpentine cords." Organisms growing in this fashion are virulent in animals. If "cord factor" is extracted from tubercle bacilli they are rendered avirulent. Cord-forming strains also possess a sulfated glycolipid (sulfatide), which prevents the fusion of phagosomes with the lysosomes and favors the intracellular survival of mycobacteria within macrophages.[176] Several of the mycobacterial cell wall constituents, including wax D (a glycolypid) and muramyl dipeptide (a small water soluble component), when injected with tuberculoprotein (itself weakly immunogenic) induce strong hypersensitivity to tuberculin and so act as adjuvants. Thus, *lipid fractions contribute both to virulence and to the sensitivity state associated with tuberculosis.*

The emergence of *hypersensitivity* to the tubercle bacillus plays a dominant role in the tissue destruction encountered in this disease. About two to four weeks after infection by the tubercle bacillus, sensitization appears as measured by the tuberculin test. The test antigen is purified protein derivative (PPD), derived from the culture medium in which tubercle bacilli have grown. In the widely employed Mantoux or Tine tests, an intradermal injection of PPD will evoke in the sensitized individual an area of induration (not simply erythema) at least 5 mm in diameter in 48 hours. Indeed, in the very sensitive, the site may become necrotic. *A tuberculosensitivity reaction signals infection in the host (but not necessarily disease).* It results from acquisition of delayed (cell-mediated) hypersensitivity (Type IV) (p. 169).

Once an individual becomes tuberculin positive, he usually remains so for the rest of his life. The basis of such long-lasting sensitivity is uncertain but is thought to be the persistence of bacilli, either latent or actively multiplying. In support of this view, some sensitized individuals after an intensive course of chemotherapy become tuberculin negative, taken to mean eradication of all viable bacilli. Repeated PPD skin testing can itself be temporarily sensitizing, but permanent sensitivity is conferred only by intact bacilli, virulent or attenuated. *False-negative* reactions (about 5%), if not due to technical failure, may be caused by viral infection or vaccination, drugs, steroid hormones, malnutrition, neoplasms, sarcoidosis, immunosuppression, or other poorly understood interfering factors including the waning of cellular immune responses during advanced age. Rarely, but most important, *true tuberculin anergy* can be due to overwhelming disseminated tuberculosis itself and may be accompanied by a nonselective suppression of skin responses to other antigens. *False-positive* tuberculin tests have resulted from previous host experience with atypical mycobacteria.[177]

The appearance of tuberculin sensitivity heralds a change in the host's response to the bacilli. On first exposure, tubercle bacilli act as inert particulate matter, and evoke a nonspecific neutrophilic inflammatory response. During this period, bacilli enter phagocytes (Fig. 8–27), but multiply unchecked and can drain via lymphatics and blood stream to distant sites, where they may die, remain dormant, or later induce foci of disease. *Once sensitization appears the inflammatory reaction becomes granulomatous and, as cited earlier, the centers*

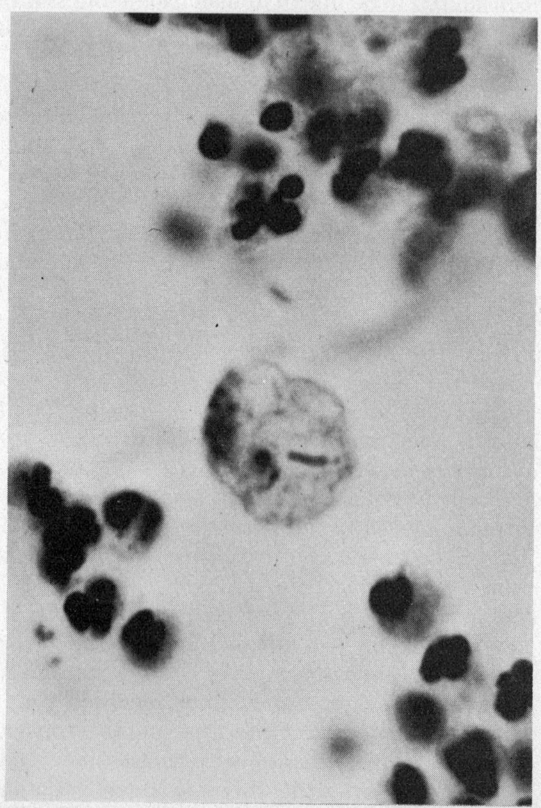

Figure 8–27. A mononuclear phagocyte with an engulfed tubercle bacillus.

of the granulomas often undergo caseation necrosis, to form typical tubercles. Thus, hypersensitization underlies the caseating destruction of tissue encountered in tuberculous lesions, but these damaging effects are counterbalanced by a concomitant increase in resistance to the infecting organisms. As already discussed (p. 170), the sensitized T cells generated during delayed hypersensitivity reactions release lymphokines on exposure to the specific antigen. *These lymphokines include several soluble mediators that are chemotactic to macrophages, induce aggregation of macrophages at sites of infection, and, most important, activate macrophages, i.e., enhance their phagocytic and microbicidal potentials.*[178] *Thus, hypersensitivity is associated with an increased capacity to phagocytose and inhibit the intracellular replication of tubercle bacilli, and yields an increased resistance to the disease.*

Numerous efforts have been made to determine whether hypersensitivity and immunity (resistance) are two concurrent phenomena or two expressions of a single process. In human and experimental disease, anergy (loss of delayed hypersensitivity to tuberculoprotein) is associated with severe, uncontrolled infection (loss of resistance). Thus, the two processes seem closely intertwined. However, recent experimental evidence suggests that delayed hypersensitivity and increased resistance may be mediated by different T-cell subsets.[179] If in natural infection with tubercle bacilli both the T-cell subsets are sensitized simultaneously, hypersensitivity and resistance develop together. When normal individuals are vaccinated with a preparation of avirulent tubercle bacilli—bacille Calmette Guérin (BCG)—the vaccinated individuals become tuberculin positive, but there is no agreement as to whether they also acquire resistance to a virulent infection. Estimates of the protective efficacy of BCG range from nil to 80%.[180] Although this issue is clouded by several technical and epidemiologic complexities, most experts believe that BCG vaccination is inadvisable in areas with a low incidence of tuberculosis, where most young adults are tuberculin negative, because the opportunity is lost to detect the onset of infection and potential disease by monitoring the tuberculin reaction.[181] Opinions are divided on whether BCG should be used in highly endemic populations.

Tuberculosis is the prototype granulomatous disease of man. *Other granulomatous conditions include sarcoidosis, brucellosis, tularemia, syphilis, leprosy, glanders, lymphogranuloma inguinale, cat-scratch fever, berylliosis, and some of the mycoses. Uncommonly, granulomas are found within neoplasms and as reactions to lipids or in diseases of obscure nature such as Wegener's granulomatosis* (p. 523). The basic characteristics of granulomatous inflammation were discussed on page 64. Here it suffices to recall that *the tubercle comprises an organized microscopic aggregation of plump, rounded histiocytes (macrophages) that vaguely resemble epithelial cells and are therefore called epithelioid cells.* Epithelioid cells are closely aggregated together; have an abundant, eosinophilic, faintly granular cytoplasm and vesicular nuclei; and rarely contain stainable bacteria. There may also be Langhans' multinucleate giant cells, formed by the fusion of macrophages or internal nuclear division without cytoplasmic division (p. 64). About the granuloma, a peripheral collar of plump fibroblasts interspersed with lymphocytes is found. The description just given represents the *"hard" tubercle,* so designated because of the absence of central necrosis and softening. More often, the central region of the tubercle undergoes a characteristic form of granular, caseous necrosis (p. 17). This *"soft" tubercle* is the most characteristic hallmark of tuberculosis (Fig. 8–28). Although a variety of other less typical inflammatory changes may be caused by tubercle bacilli, such as purulent and fibrotic lesions, tubercles can always be found if properly sought.

The basis for the granulomatous reaction in tuberculosis has been intensively studied and it is clear that T-cell sensitivity is involved. Sensitized T cells yield the chemotactants and migration inhibiting factor (MIF), and so contribute to the aggregation of macrophages, which then transform to epithelioid cells. The mechanism of epithelioid cell formation is uncertain. Under the electron microscope, epithelioid cells show highly ruffled, interdigitating cell membranes; well-developed endoplasmic reticulum; abundant mitochondria; and large Golgi complexes. Their cytoplasm contains numerous vesicles, but dense, lysosome-like bodies are not typically seen. Thus, their ultrastructure suggests they are better equipped for secretory functions than for phagocytosis,[182] and may represent a form of macrophage specialized for the extracellular secretion of digestive enzymes. The mechanism of caseous necrosis, the other hallmark of a tuberculous granuloma, is also poorly understood. Its appearance coincides with the acquisition of delayed hypersensitivity. Although there is little doubt that the formation of epithelioid cell granulomas in tuberculosis and several other infectious disorders is immunologically mediated, it should be pointed out that epithelioid cell transformation of macrophages can also be brought about by nonimmunologic mechanisms. Thus, in one study it was demonstrated that muramyl dipeptide could produce epithelioid cell granulomas in T cell–deficient animals, presumably by a direct activation of macrophages.[183]

In conclusion, although much remains unknown about the pathogenesis of tissue response in tuberculosis, it is abundantly clear that the fundamental reaction is granulomatous, frequently with central caseation necrosis, and that immunity and hypersensitivity both play major roles in the evolution of the disease.

Primary Tuberculosis

Primary tuberculosis is defined as infection of an individual lacking previous contact with or immune responsiveness to tubercle bacilli. In primary lung infection, a single lesion (known as Ghon focus) is usually found immediately subjacent to the pleura in the lower part of the upper lobes or upper part of the lower lobes of one lung, rarely elsewhere. These localizations reflect the areas receiving the greatest volume flow of inspired air. Bilateral or multiple foci are very

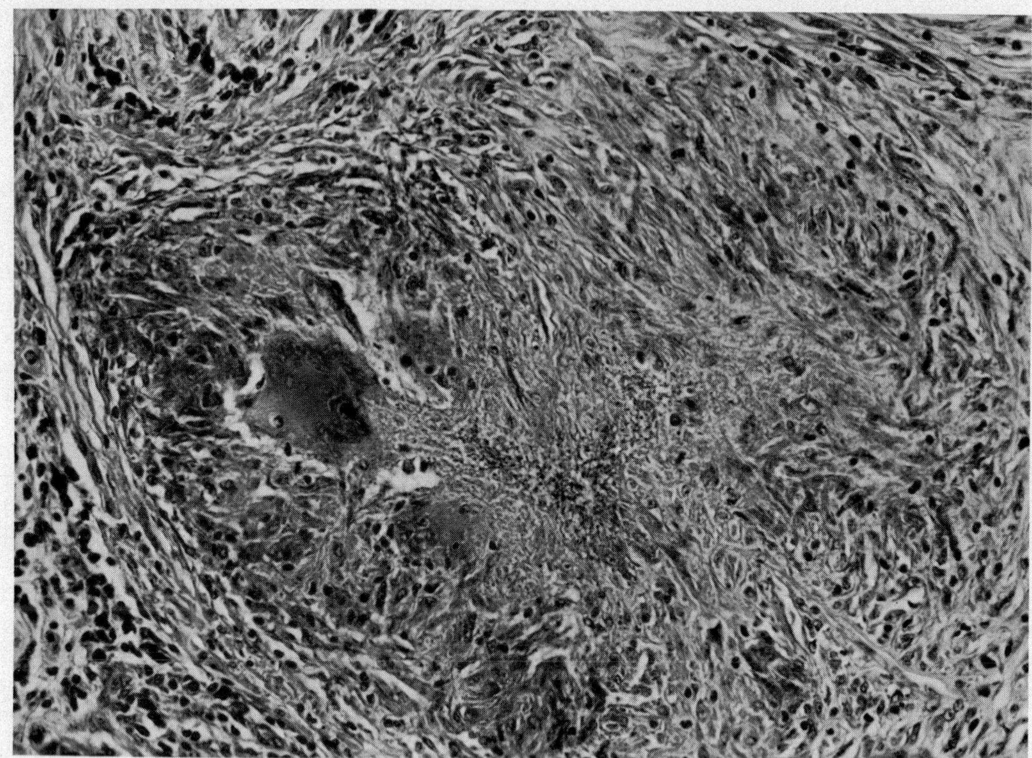

Figure 8–28. A tubercle with giant cell and central caseous necrosis.

infrequent. An active Ghon focus is a 1.0- to 1.5-cm area of gray-white inflammatory consolidation circumscribed from the surrounding lung parenchyma. The consolidated focus becomes granulomatous and then develops a soft, caseous, necrotic center by the second week. Tubercle bacilli, either free or within phagocytes, drain along the regional peribronchial lymphatic channels to the tracheobronchial **lymph nodes** and there evoke caseating granulomas. As a rule, the nodal involvement happens only on one side, that of the lung focus. The combination of the primary lung lesion and lymph node involvement is referred to as the **Ghon complex.**

In most cases, primary tuberculosis does not progress and undergoes shrinkage with fibrosis, calcification, and sometimes ossification, with fibrous scarring and puckering of the pleural surface. Occasionally, the pleural reaction may also become calcified. At the same time, fibrocalcific scarring replaces most of the tuberculous foci in the regional tracheobronchial nodes. Healed primary complexes are frequently quite small and may be hard to detect by either pathologic or x-ray studies. However, the infecting organisms are not totally eradicated, and viable bacilli may persist for years and perhaps for life.

Primary tuberculosis does not always follow a self-terminating course. *Progressive primary tuberculosis* is relatively rare and is more likely to affect children, although adult onset has become more frequent in those countries in which tuberculin conversion has shifted to the older age groups. In the so-called "childhood form," the primary lung focus rapidly enlarges, erodes into the bronchial tree, and gives rise to new satellite lung lesions. This is accompanied and sometimes overshadowed by caseous enlargement of the hilar lymph nodes to the point of forming mediastinal masses that can encroach upon major bronchi and hamper air flow. At the same time, these highly active lesions may seed the bloodstream with tubercle bacilli, resulting in life-threatening *miliary dissemination (or tuberculous meningitis* (p. 1379) (Fig. 8–29). In adults, primary tuberculosis tends to pursue a less rampant course and therefore it is less readily distinguished from the secondary disease. It can be suspected in an adult when radiographs show the subapical lung portions to be spared of lesions in the presence of mediastinal lymph node enlargement, a rare distribution in the usual, secondary form of tuberculosis.

When primary tuberculous infection occurs at the less common portals of entry (GI tract, oropharyngeal lymphoid tissue, skin), primary complexes, similar to the pulmonary form, evolve at these sites and in the corresponding draining nodes.

SECONDARY TUBERCULOSIS

Secondary or postprimary tuberculosis is that phase of tuberculous infection that arises in a previously sensitized individual, whether the tubercle bacilli are derived from endogenous or exogenous sources. Most cases of secondary tuberculosis represent reactivation of asymptomatic primary disease, and may occur at any time following a primary infection, sometimes many decades later, presumably whenever defenses are lowered. Much less commonly, significant exposure to exogenous organisms may trigger the onset of secondary

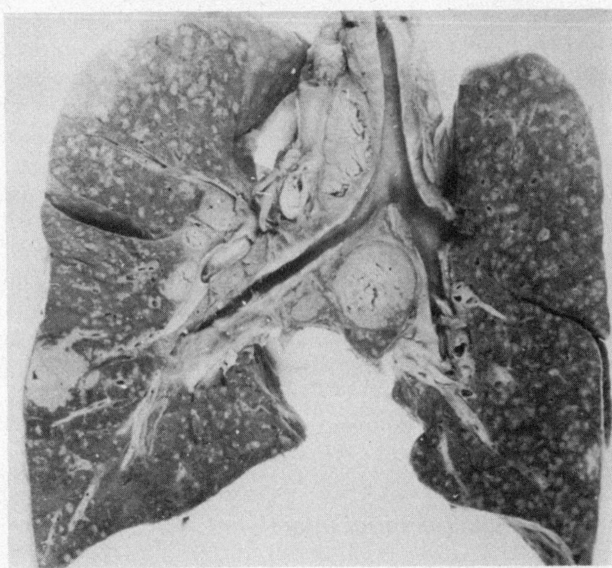

Figure 8–29. Progressive (childhood) primary tuberculosis: pneumonic focus (*left,* near pleura), massive caseous hilar lymphadenitis, and miliary tubercles throughout lung. Note tracheal displacement.

disease. This phase of the disease is sometimes inappropriately called "adult" or "reinfection" tuberculosis. (Secondary tuberculosis can arise in children, and primary tuberculosis in adults.)

Secondary tuberculosis begins in the apical or posterior segments of one or both upper lobes, appearing close to the clavicle in chest films. Such lesions are referred to as Simon's foci and are believed to be seeded during the early period of tuberculosis bacteremia, favored by the high Po_2 of the region. The minimal pulmonary lesion in the apex consists of a 1- to 3-cm focal area of caseous consolidation, usually within 1 to 2 cm of the pleural surfaces. Far less commonly, reactivation occurs in other parts of the lung. Perhaps because of the prompter phagocytosis and destruction of bacilli by activated macrophages in the partly resistant individual, satellite lesions in the regional nodes are distinctly rare and lung lesions are more apt to remain localized or progress slowly; however, at the same time, caseation occurs more rapidly, as does fibrotic walling off of the lesions.

Histologically, the reaction consists of tubercle formation with formation of epithelioid cells, Langhans' giant cells, caseation, fibrosis, and lymphocytic infiltration. When tuberculosis strikes immunosuppressed patients, there may be virtual absence of any reactive cells and the lesions may therefore be represented by cell-poor nondescript foci rich in mycobacteria. Conversely, the lesions may be rich in neutrophils, especially where cavities are formed from large coalescent caseous lesions, and have eroded into the airways.

The course of apical infection is extremely varied. (1) The pathologic process may undergo healing, scarring, and calcification to yield apical, **fibrocalcific "arrested" tuberculosis.** (2) The initial parenchymal infection may spread to the other areas of the lung through one of several pathways to create **progressive pulmonary tuberculosis** (p. 740). (3) It may extend to the pleura to produce pleural fibrosis, pleural adhesions, inflammatory pleural effusions, or, by direct extension of the bacilli into the pleural cavity, lead to a **tuberculous empyema.** (4) When the pulmonary lesions erode into bronchi, the material may be coughed up and seed the mucosal lining of the bronchioles, bronchi, and trachea **(tracheobronchial tuberculosis),** or organisms may become implanted in the larynx to produce laryngeal tuberculosis. (5) Swallowed bacilli can become trapped by the lymphoid patches of the small and large bowel to cause **intestinal tuberculosis.**

(6) **Miliary tuberculosis** may result when the organisms gain access to the lymphatics and blood to seed distant organs. The term miliary is descriptive of the small, yellow-white, barely visible lesions, which resemble canary bird seeds, or millet seeds. When the organisms erode into a **pulmonary artery,** the miliary dissemination may be limited to the lungs as the organisms are trapped in the alveolar capillary circulation. When the seeding of the pulmonary arteries is heavy and organisms get through the alveolar capillaries, or when a caseous focus erodes into a **pulmonary vein,** systemic dissemination follows and miliary lesions may develop in virtually any organ of the body. It is, however, well known that certain tissues are remarkably resistant to tuberculous infection, and therefore it is rare to find tubercles in the heart, striated muscle, thyroid, and pancreas. Favored sites of miliary localization are the bone marrow, eye grounds, lymph nodes, liver, spleen, kidneys, adrenals, prostate, seminal vesicles, fallopian tubes, endometrium, and meninges. Involvement of the eye grounds, bone marrow, and liver offers valuable clinical opportunities to diagnose miliary tuberculosis. The tubercles can be visualized in many instances in the eye grounds by simple fundoscopic examination, and can often be identified in marrow and liver biopsies, even when there is no functional impairment of these organs. (7) **Progressive, isolated-organ tuberculosis** may occur in any one of the organs or tissues commonly affected by miliary dissemination. Most likely, in the course of lymphatic or hematogenous dissemination of bacilli, organisms are rapidly destroyed in all other sites save for the particular tissue involved in the isolated tuberculous process. The most common sites of such isolated-organ tuberculosis are the cervical lymph nodes (scrofula), meninges (tuberculous meningitis), kidneys (renal tuberculosis), adrenals (formerly an important cause of Addison's disease—p. 1235), bones (tuberculous osteomyelitis), and the fallopian tubes and epididymides (genital tuberculosis). From such focal lesions, further dissemination or seeding may occur and thus, in renal tuberculosis, it is common for infective material to drain through the urine and cause tuberculous cystitis. In the same way, tuberculous salpingitis is often followed by tuberculous endometritis and tuberculous pelvic peritonitis. Tuberculous epididymitis may be followed by extension of the tuberculous infection into the testes, and spread from the prostate and seminal vesicles may affect other organs in the genitourinary tract. In vertebral tuberculosis (Pott's disease), long fistulas may form along the psoas muscle to open and drain in the groin region. Long-lasting tuberculous lesions of all types may stimulate the reticuloendothelial system sufficiently to result in systemic secondary **amyloidosis,** (p. 195), but this is rare in treated individuals.

Before this discussion is concluded, attention should be drawn to the need for positive identification of acid-fast tubercle bacilli in the anatomic lesions. Granulomatous lesions are not confined to tuberculosis, as pointed out earlier. Acid fastness is shared by other mycobacteria and by nocardia (p. 349). A diagnosis of tuberculosis should never be made definitive unless typical mycobacteria are seen in typical lesions or tubercle bacilli have been unmistakably identified by culture.

Unfortunately, in all but the most rampant forms of tuberculosis, acid-fast bacilli in the diseased tissues are relatively scarce and therefore quite difficult to find. The most likely sites of their localization are recent necrotic foci still containing nuclear fragments; epithelioid cells rarely contain the bacilli. Even when they are not visible under the microscope, enough bacilli may be present in the tissues or in secretion such as sputum or gastric washings to be cultured successfully.

CLINICAL COURSE. The clinical signs and symptoms of pulmonary tuberculosis are as *varied* as the anatomic lesions. A minute focus of tuberculosis may be totally occult, while extensive tuberculosis is almost invariably accompanied by systemic reactions. Except in progressive primary disease, *primary tuberculosis is usually an entirely silent process.* In most cases, primary infection, past or present, is detected only by tuberculin testing of the individual or by routine roentgenography with visualization of a focus of scarring or calcification in the appropriate location in the lung parenchyma or tracheobronchial nodes. Occasionally the individual may have low-grade fever and lack of appetite.

Secondary tuberculosis may also be asymptomatic when the condition is confined to minimal lesions within the lung apices. *More often, however, these patients have insidious onset of temperature elevations (usually most marked in the midafternoon), night sweats, weakness, fatigability, and loss of appetite and weight.* As lung tissue is destroyed and bronchi are invaded, there is often productive cough, blood-streaked sputum, or hemoptysis. In other instances, pleural effusion may dominate the clinical picture. In advanced lesions, dyspnea and orthopnea may be present. When the process affects other organs the clinical manifestations are referable to these localizations: for example, meningitis or renal disease. When the disease is miliary in its dissemination and does not produce focalizing signs or detectable lesions, the symptom complex may be that of a fever of unknown origin (FUO). Because of their small size, miliary tubercles are often undiscovered by chest radiography.

The diagnosis of all forms of tuberculosis depends on identification or isolation of the causative organism. Tuberculin testing can be helpful, especially in children, or when recent conversion in an adult can be documented. Otherwise, skin reaction is of little diagnostic value, for reasons given earlier. Neither does the failure to demonstrate tubercle bacilli in sputum or other secreta rule out the diagnosis of tuberculosis, since occasionally the lesions are not in contact with natural channels of drainage in the so-called "closed" case. Biopsy may have to be resorted to in such instances.

In recent years, the diagnosis of tuberculosis in North America has become more difficult since the number of "classical" cases has declined and more patients now present with "occult" or atypical disease.[184] Most common among the *atypical presentations* are late generalized infections in older people, some of which present as puzzling hematologic syndromes, leukemoid reactions, or myelophthisic anemias. Reactivation of tuberculosis in the course of a preexisting major illness, e.g., malignancies or chronic renal failure and dialysis, also poses diagnostic problems.[185] In all these clinical settings, many of which are associated with acquired immunosuppression, one should remain alert to the possibility of tuberculosis, especially if the patient develops unexplained pyrexia. Fortunately, in all but those with advanced neglected disease, present methods of treatment with rifampicin, isoniazid, paraminosalicylates, and/or streptomycin can be expected to arrest progression and effect cure.

Atypical Mycobacterial Infections

The so-called atypical mycobacteria are related to *Mycobacterium tuberculosis*, but differ significantly in their distribution and pathogenicity. Formerly uncommon, the prevalence of atypical mycobacteriosis is on the rise in Europe and in parts of the U.S.[186]

Atypical mycobacteria are widespread in the environment, in soil, water, plants, and animal excreta. Many are saprophytic or have very low pathogenicity. Skin test data in the southern U.S. suggest that many false-positive tuberculin reactors have been *exposed* to such organisms, but *progressive disease* caused by "atypicals" is less frequent and is predominantly opportunistic, affecting mainly those with reduced immunity (e.g., AIDS, p. 208) or a preexisting lung disease. Human infections are derived directly from the environment and, unlike tuberculosis, there is no evidence for person-to-person transmission. The lesions associated with mycobacterioses vary considerably and range from granulomas to nodular foam cell lesions and to purulent and necrotizing inflammation. Five patterns of diseases may be seen: (1) *Pulmonary disease*, produced by *M. kansasii* or *M. avium-intracellulare*, mainly affects white males over the age of 45 years with preexisting chronic bronchitis and emphysema; this is the most common form of mycobacteriosis. (2) *Lymphadenitis*, mainly affecting children, is produced by *M. avium-intracellulare* and/or *M. scrofulaceum*. (3) *Ulcerative skin lesions* caused by *M. ulcerans*[187] or *M. marinum* are endemic in Australia, parts of Africa and Latin America. (4) *Injection abscesses* caused by *M. fortuitum* and *M. chelonei* occur sporadically all over the world. (5) In severely immunosuppressed patients, life-threatening *bacteremias* may occur, based on widespread lymphoreticular involvement, principally by *M. avium-intracellulare*. The diagnosis of mycobacterioses rests on culture in specialized media and differential biochemical tests. Since many of these organisms are free living or saprophytic, it is sometimes difficult to distinguish contamination or colonization from true infection. This difficulty arises mainly in patients with pulmonary fibrosis or cavitation resulting from previous tuberculosis or chronic obstructive airway disease. There is at present no satisfactory laboratory method of making this distinction, and therefore in some cases therapeutic trial may be the only recourse. Unfortunately, some species respond only poorly or not at all to antituberculous drugs or antibiotics.

Leprosy (Mycobacterium leprae)*

Leprosy, or Hansen's disease, is an indolent, chronic mycobacterial infection of very low communicability involving mainly the skin and peripheral nerves. It is caused by the acid-fast bacillus *M. leprae*. Endemic foci of the disease are encountered throughout the world, principally in tropical climes. Once endemic in the U.S., especially in Hawaii, it is no longer common in this country and most of the approximately 2700 known cases are concentrated in a single facility in Carville, Louisiana. Obviously, intercontinental travel may deliver an affected individual to any physician.

M. leprae is less strongly acid fast than *M. tuberculosis*, requiring modified staining methods. It divides every 13 days, the slowest known rate of any bacterial pathogen, and fails to thrive at temperatures exceeding 36°C. It is an intracellular parasite with a strong tropism for macrophages and Schwann cells. Since all attempts at culture in vitro have thus far failed, not much is known of its intrinsic virulence factors, except that it lacks exotoxins and lytic enzymes. The nine-banded armadillo with its body temperature of 32° to 35°C offers an animal model in which the disease can be studied. Indeed, a disease closely resembling human leprosy has been identified in wild armadillos killed in Louisiana.[188] Like *M. tuberculosis*, *M. leprae* evokes delayed hypersensitivity detectable by skin testing with lepromin—a killed extract made from *M. leprae* lesions. Sensitized individuals develop a tuberculin-like reaction in 48 hours and a papular reaction at the local site three to four weeks later. Humoral antibodies can be demonstrated in these patients, but they are not in any way protective.

Based on host resistance, leprosy takes one of several clinical forms. Its two polar forms, *tuberculoid leprosy (TT)* and *lepromatous leprosy (LL)*, are associated with intact as opposed to severely impaired cell-mediated immunity. In between these two extremes there is a spectrum of so-called *borderline cases*, representing variable degrees of host resistance. The borderline forms are less stable clinically and may change slowly to one of the more stable polar categories, often after an episode of clinical activity named a "reactional state" which punctuates the slow progression of the disease.

Patients with TT respond to *M. leprae* by mounting a vigorous T cell–mediated immunity, and as in the case of tuberculosis, the sensitized T cells cause local aggregation and activation of macrophages, resulting in the formation of typical *tuberculoid granulomas with few surviving bacilli in the lesions*. The 48-hour lepromin skin test, an indication of delayed hypersensitivity to lepra bacilli, is strongly positive in TT. In sharp contrast to the tuberculoid form, LL is associated with lack of T cell–mediated immunity, and therefore with poor host resistance. Enormous numbers of *M. leprae* can be seen within macrophages, which seem unable to destroy them or limit bacterial growth, perhaps because of lack of activating signals derived from sensitized T cells (Fig. 8–30). Lepromatous lesions show nodular or diffuse aggregates of foamy macrophages rather than epithelioid cell granulomas, and their lepromin skin test is negative. As might be expected, in LL the disease is much more extensive and progressive, and more difficult to cure. The tissue reactions, bacillary load and lepromin test are variable in the intermediate forms and depend on their position within the spectrum of leprosy.

Patients with LL often have a polyclonal hypergammaglobulinemia, which is due perhaps to the lack of T-suppressor cells and massive exposure to lepra antigens. Obviously these antibodies offer little protection against the bacilli. On the contrary, the formation of antigen-antibody complexes may lead to erythema nodosum leprosum (ENL), a potentially life-threatening reaction. This may occur when lepromatous patients are treated with drugs, thereby releasing large amounts of antigenic material from the lysed bacteria. As in the case of other immune complex–mediated disorders, ENL is associated with vasculitis (responsible for erythematous skin nodules), arthralgias, fever, and sometimes, glomerulonephritis. By contrast, tuberculoid patients may experience "borderline reactions," i.e. erythematous swellings of skin lesions, followed by clinical improvement and increased reactivity to lepromin.

Although the profound depression of T cell–mediated immunity in lepromatous leprosy is well established, the basis of immunologic failure is still a mystery. At onset it appears that the defect is selective for the lepra bacilli, since reactions to other T-cell antigens remain intact.[189] In some fully developed cases, however, patients are anergic to several commonly used skin-test antigens. Presumably this is secondary to the destruction of T-cell areas of the lymph nodes by the disease. An inherited basis for the initial specific T-cell deficiency is strongly suspected but no clear genetic markers have been identified. In some families with tuberculoid leprosy, association with HLA-DR2 has been noted. In the vast majority, however, despite a vigorous search, associations with the HLA region have not been detected.

Transmission of leprosy is direct from active cases, mostly LL. The mode of entry is unknown, but probably involves droplet aspiration or skin contact. Tuberculoid patients are not contagious. Infection requires prolonged close contact (years), such as occurs within a family, and once acquired the disease usually pursues an extremely slow course, spanning decades. Indeed, most lepers die with their disease rather than of it. The vital organs and CNS are rarely affected.

In **LL**, once the organism invades, a bacteremia follows that often persists during the course of active disease. From the blood, organisms preferentially localize in the skin,

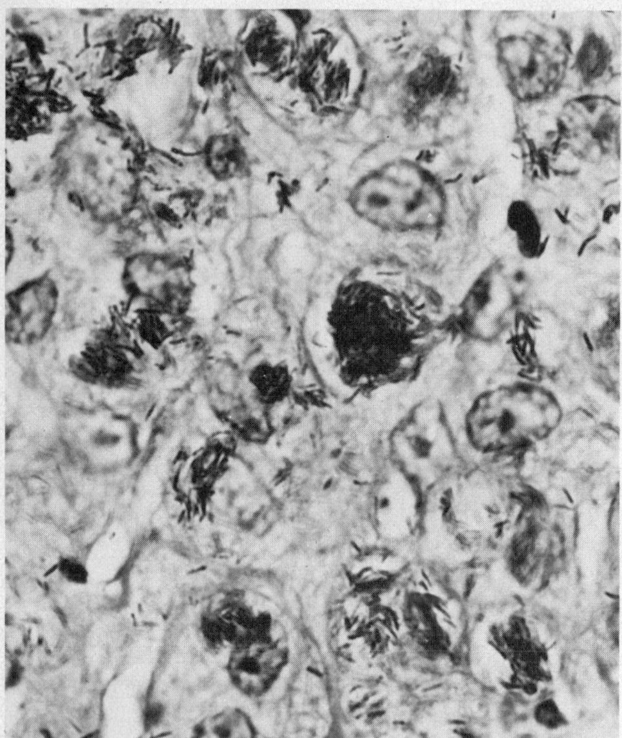

Figure 8–30. Leprosy. High-power view of acid-fast bacilli proliferating in foamy macrophages.

peripheral nerves, anterior eye, upper airways (down to the larynx), testes, and hands and feet. This distribution appears to reflect the fact that the organisms are able to proliferate only in cooler tissues. Wherever they localize they evoke an aggregation of lipid-laden macrophages (lepra cells), often filled with masses of acid-fast bacilli (globi) (Fig. 8–31). These reactions induce macular, papular, or nodular lesions in the skin, with a predilection for the face, ears, wrists, elbows, knees, and buttocks. The distribution of these skin lesions can be symmetric or even diffuse and thus difficult to notice. With progression the nodular lesions predominate, and they may sometimes coalesce to yield a distinctive face deformity known as **leonine facies**. Most skin lesions are hypoesthetic or anesthetic. Lesions in the nose may cause persistent inflammation and bacilli-laden exudate, and may cause airway obstruction, or sometimes collapse of the bridge of the nose or perforation of the septum. The peripheral nerves may be affected (usually symmetrically), especially the ulnar and peroneal nerves where they come near the skin surface. Loss of sensation and trophic changes in the hands and feet may follow the nerve lesions. Although the nerves are laden with bacilli, clinically evident neurologic involvement is not as prominent in LL as in the TT form since there is less intraneuronal inflammation. Lymph nodes show aggregation of foamy histiocytes in the paracortical (T-cell) areas, with enlargement of geminal centers. In advanced disease, similar aggregates of macrophages are also present in the splenic red pulp and in the liver. Testes are usually extensively involved, with destruction of the seminiferous tubules and consequent sterility. Gynecomastia is also a frequent finding.

TT begins with much more localized macular skin lesions. The macules, at first erythematous, enlarge and develop irregular shapes with indurated, elevated, hyperpigmented margins and depressed pale centers (central healing). The skin lesions are usually neither numerous nor bilaterally symmetric. Nerve involvement dominates this form of the disease, typically of the ulnar and peroneal nerves. The nerves are enclosed within granulomatous inflammatory reactions, and if small enough (e.g., the peripheral twigs) may be totally destroyed. The neural involvement thus often induces skin anesthesias and skin and muscle atrophy. The trophic changes render the patient liable to trauma of the affected parts with the development of indolent skin ulcers. When the neurologic and trophic involvements are advanced, contractures, paralyses, and autoamputation of fingers or toes may ensue. Facial nerve involvement can lead to paralysis of the lids, with keratitis and corneal ulcerations. Microscopically, all sites of involvement disclose granulomatous lesions closely resembling hard tubercles. As mentioned, bacilli are almost never identified in these lesions.

The diagnosis of leprosy can be made by skin biopsy, scrapings of lesions, or nasal smears. Evaluation of the biopsy findings and lepromin test are essential steps in classifying the disease form and in planning treatment. Both forms are characterized by great chronicity, with periods of quiescence punctuated by reactional states. Therapy with sulfones must be long-term, taking years, not months, and resistance to these drugs has recently become an increasing problem. The tuberculoid form has the better prognosis and response and in most cases does not materially shorten the patient's life span. Long-standing LL may lead to death from

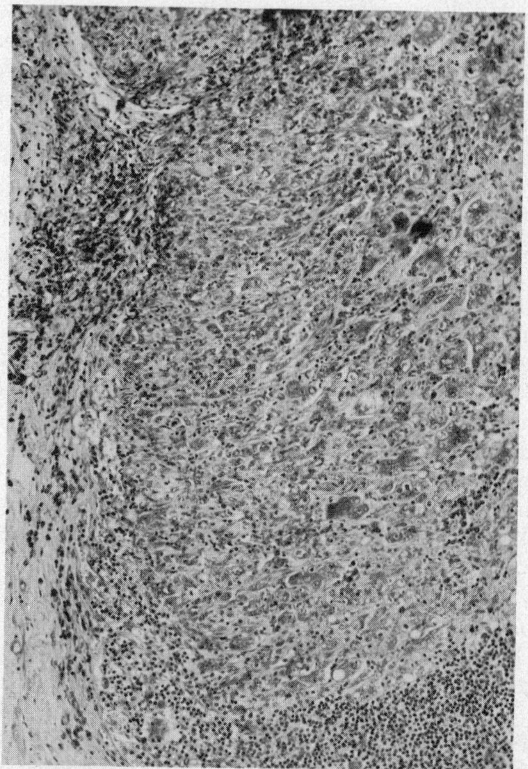

Figure 8–31. Leprosy. Portion of a lepromatous mass composed of typical lepra cells.

intercurrent disease, usually bacterial infection or secondary amyloidosis. The historical ostracism of patients with Hansen's disease has at last been overcome, and with proper care their most disfiguring and disabling lesions can be prevented or rehabilitated. An experimental vaccine is soon to undergo clinical trial.

ACTINOMYCETALES

Although traditionally discussed along with fungi, actinomycetales are closely related to mycobacteria. They show some similarities to fungi, such as branching and the formation of a mycelial network, but the presence of muramic acid in their cell walls and the absence of a membrane-bound nucleus clearly aligns them with the bacteria. Of the several genera included in this group, Actinomyces and Nocardia are the most important human pathogens.

Nocardiosis

The nocardiae are long, filamentous, gram-positive, aerobic bacteria that often aggregate in branching chains. They are weakly acid fast and can be stained by the methods used for *M. leprae* but not by the Ziehl-Neelsen stain for *M. tuberculosis*. They also differ from tubercle bacilli in their culture requirements, which are less fastidious, and by their extracellular habitat during infection. Approximately 1000 cases of nocardiosis are reported every year in the U.S., but there are probably many more. Ninety per cent are caused by *N. asteroides* and the rest by *N. brasiliensis* and *N. caviae*. Most patients who develop nocardiosis are chronically ill or immunosuppressed; transplant rejection, corticosteroid therapy, and alveolar proteinosis (p. 746) are frequent antecedents. In cases without known predisposing condition (mostly skin infections), *N. brasiliensis* is the predominant pathogen.

Little is known of the transmission of nocardiae and it is unclear whether the nosocomial form of nocardiosis represents *new* infection or activation from a commensal state. There is no evidence of person-to-person spread. The lung and skin are the usual primary sites. In the U.S., localized pulmonary disease is the most common form; second is severe, disseminated nocardiosis, including spread to the CNS. Localized skin infection, or mycetoma (p. 359), is uncommon in the U.S., but is endemic in Mexico and elsewhere in Latin America.

In the lung, nocardiae typically cause single or multiple, chronic, necrotizing, walled-off abscesses. Similarly, primary skin lesions are necrotizing or purulent, or both. Grossly nocardial lung abscesses are irregular in shape, with a soft purulent center surrounded by a broad rim of organizing pneumonia, much like the lesions caused by pyogenic bacteria. Fibrosis is seen only in long-standing lesions or during the healing stage, which is characteristically protracted. Pleural involvement is frequent, giving rise to fibrinous pleuritis or sometimes empyema. Microscopically there is widespread necrosis, with a fibrinous exudate rich in neutrophils. In contrast to tuberculosis, granulomas are not formed. The organisms do not stain with H and E and are therefore easily missed in routine sections. Gram staining and a modified acid-fast stain have to be utilized in suspected cases. Fragmentation of the filamentous nocardiae could cause confusion with tubercle bacilli, but staining and culture of the organisms differentiate the two. Nocardia grows out slowly on fungal and mycobacterial media, as well as on other media. In lung lesions, nocardiae appear as discrete filaments, but in mycetomas of the skin they form mycelial colonies not unlike those of ***Actinomyces*** except for their acid-fastness.

The clinical presentation of pulmonary nocardiosis can be confusing and the disease is often unsuspected until late in its course, after the common bacteria have been excluded and response to antibiotics has been disappointing. Dissemination can give rise to meningitis or symptoms of space-occupying lesions in the brain that are due to the formation of cerebral abscesses. In immunosuppressed patients, aggressive diagnostic evaluation for nocardiosis is warranted. If examination of sputum, pleural fluids, and bronchial washings is not helpful, open lung biopsy may be required. Most patients respond to sulfonamide therapy.

Actinomycosis

Actinomycosis is a chronic suppurative infection localized chiefly to the neck, lung, or abdomen. The lesions, which spread by contiguity, are markedly indurated and contain multiple abscesses that drain to the surface by sinuses. The discharge from the sinuses typically contains grossly visible yellowish colonies called sulfur granules. Most human infections are caused by *Actinomyces israelii*; other species including *A. viscosus*, *A. odontolyticus*, and *A. naeslundii* rarely produce disease. The actinomycetes are gram-positive, non–acid-fast, strictly anaerobic bacteria that are easily overgrown by other organisms and difficult to culture. They are commensals within the oral cavity (tonsillar crypts, tartar of teeth), alimentary tract, and vagina, invading only when the tissue is devitalized by trauma (e.g., dental surgery) or bacterial infections. Actinomycotic lesions often contain other bacteria including fusiform bacilli, gram-negative bacilli, and various streptococci. However, Actinomyces is capable of producing lesions in man and experimental animals without any synergistic bacterial flora. Unlike nocardiae, actinomycetes are not opportunists. They infect apparently healthy individuals, when local conditions favorable for their growth are created by trauma or tissue devitalization. All infections are derived endogenously and there is no person-to-person spread. Three classical forms of actinomycosis are recognized: cervicofacial, abdominal, and thoracic, but the disease frequently presents in atypical fashion and can be confused with other infections or even neoplasms.[190]

Cervicofacial actinomycosis is the most frequent pattern. At first the gingiva and adjacent soft tissues become swollen and indurated, but the lesion is not extremely painful.

In the course of time, a large, woody swelling develops, characteristically over the angle of the jaw, reminiscent of the actinomycotic infection in cattle—"lumpy jaw." These infections are characterized by great chronicity, burrowing, and invasive spread: thus, in the cervicofacial disease the **inflammation often extends to the skin to perforate and form multiple sinuses**. Periostitis and osteomyelitis with extensive destruction of bone (jaw or vertebral) are common accompaniments. The histology can be briefly characterized as central suppurative necrosis surrounded by granulation tissue and intense fibrosis. Often included in the granulation tissue are many foamy histiocytes and plasma cells. The center of each abscess usually contains a bacterial colony consisting of intertwined radiating filaments (the "rays"), capped by eosinophilic hyaline material (the "clubs"), creating a sunburst pattern. These are the sulfur granules seen macroscopically (Fig. 8–32). Otherwise, the tissue response in actinomycosis is entirely nonspecific and the diagnosis must be made by identification of the causative agent. Sometimes an astute clinical observer will note diagnostic "sulfur granules" in the draining pus. For more certain identification, cultures may be required.

Abdominal actinomycosis arises from invasion of the intestinal mucosa, most commonly of the appendix or colon. There ensues an acute and chronic inflammatory reaction that penetrates the wall of the bowel to produce a localized peritoneal abscess, which then may extend into adjacent loops of bowel, the retroperitoneal tissues, and anterior abdominal wall and may sometimes dissect to the skin surface with the formation of draining external sinuses. Organisms may reach the liver either by the hematogenous route or by direct continuity, causing extensive liver abscesses. Further spread may then lead to subdiaphragmatic infections, and eventual penetration of the diaphragm and intrathoracic infections. The increasing use of intrauterine contraceptive devices has led to the emergence of a pelvic form of the disease affecting the uterine cervix, fallopian tubes, ovary, and adjacent pelvic viscera.

Thoracic actinomycosis, either primary or following penetration of a subdiaphragmatic infection, causes lung abscesses that sometimes result in pulmonopleural fistulas, or empyema. Further spread may erode the ribs and anterior chest wall or extend into the vertebral column and pericardial cavity. Even in the presence of destructive local lesions, actinomycosis evokes few systemic symptoms, and the relative well-being of a patient bearing a large fistula-forming inflammatory mass is a valuable clinical clue. Actinomyces respond well to sustained antibiotic treatment.

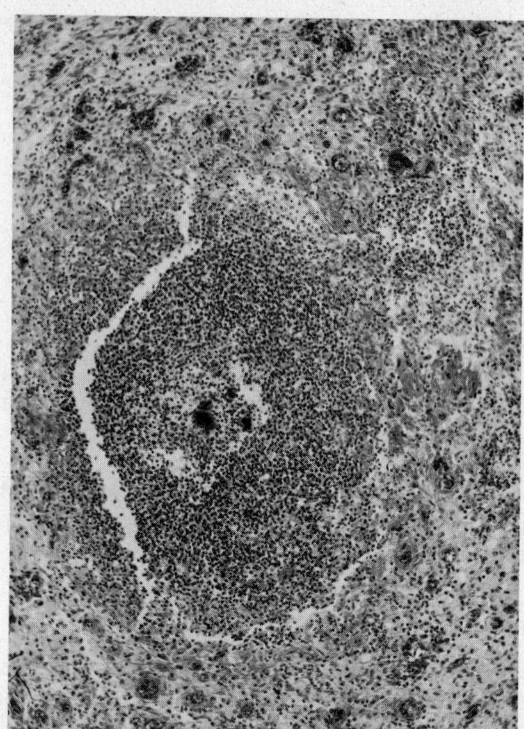

Figure 8–32. Actinomycotic abscess containing colonies of fungi (sulfur granules) appearing as black masses within center of abscess.

Fungal, Protozoal, and Helminthic Diseases and Sarcoidosis

Fungal Diseases
- Deep fungi
  - Candidiasis (moniliasis)
  - Mucormycosis (zygomycosis)
  - Aspergillosis
  - Cryptococcosis *(Cryptococcus neoformans)*
  - Blastomycosis *(Blastomyces dermatitidis)**
  - Paracoccidioidomycosis (South American Blastomycosis)*
  - Coccidioidomycosis *(Coccidioides immitis)**
  - Histoplasmosis *(Histoplasma capsulatum)*
  - Unusual deep fungal infections*
- Superficial fungi (dermatophytes)

Protozoal Diseases
- Luminal protozoa
  - Amebiasis *(Entamoeba histolytica)*
  - Amebic meningoencephalitis
  - Giardiasis *(Giardia lamblia)*
  - Infections by Cryptosporidium and Isospora spp.
  - Trichomoniasis *(Trichomonas vaginalis)*
  - Pneumocystosis *(Pneumocystis carinii)*
- Blood and tissue protozoa
  - Malaria (Plasmodium sp.)*
  - Babesiosis (Babesia sp.)*
  - African trypanosomiasis *(Trypanosoma brucei, rhodesiense, gambiense)**
- Intracellular protozoa
  - Chagas' disease *(Trypanosoma cruzi)**
  - Leishmaniasis (Leishmania sp.)*
  - Toxoplasmosis *(Toxoplasma gondii)*

Helminthic Diseases
- Intestinal roundworms
  - Ascariasis *(Ascaris lumbricoides)*
  - Trichuriasis (Trichuris sp.)
  - Enterobiasis (oxyuriasis)
  - Hookworm disease (Necator, Ancylostoma spp.)
  - Strongyloidiasis *(Strongyloides stercoralis)*
  - Capillariasis *(Capillaria philippinensis)**
- Tissue roundworms
  - Visceral larva migrans *(Toxocara canis, cati)*
  - Other occult zoonotic tissue helminths*
  - Guinea worm infection *(Dracunculus medinensis)**
  - Trichinosis *(Trichinella spiralis)*
  - Filariasis*
    - Lymphatic filariasis *(Wuchereria bancrofti, Brugia malayi)**
    - Onchocerciasis*
    - Minor tropical filariae (Loa, Mansonella, Dipetalonema spp.)*
    - Zoonotic filariasis *(Dirofilaria immitis, D. tenuis, Brugia beaveri)*
- Cestodes, tapeworms
  - Intestinal tapeworm infections
  - Cysticercosis
  - Echinococcosis (hydatid disease)
- Trematodes (flukes)
  - Fascioliasis (liver fluke, *Fasciola hepatica)*
  - Clonorchiasis and opisthorchiasis*
  - Fasciolopsiasis*
  - Paragonimiasis (lung fluke, pulmonary distomiasis)*
  - Schistosomiasis (bilharziasis)*

Sarcoidosis (Boeck's Sarcoid)

*Infectious diseases of limited geographic distribution are marked by an asterisk.

FUNGAL DISEASES

Only a few fungal species commonly infect humans (Table 8–6), yet taken together they rank closely behind viruses and bacteria as causes of disease and are neither rare nor exotic. In tissues, fungi reproduce by simple division of round, yeastlike forms or of slender, tubular hyphae whose aggregation forms a mycelium. Rarely, fruiting bodies named conidia or sporangia are also formed, but the rich diversity of free-living and sexual reproductive stages is missing; in fact, some species form infective spores only in nature or in culture and these differ sharply from their tissue forms, which are noninfective (dimorphic fungi).

Fungal cells are relatively large (Table 8–1) and their walls contain ergosterol and beta-linked polysaccharides rather than the bacterial peptidoglycans. Some species have slimy, antiphagocytic capsules; others have wall components resistant to phagolysosomal attack. *Fungi therefore can imitate the whole gamut of bacterial pathology from acute pyogenic to chronic granulomatous infection, and may not reveal their presence until identified by laboratory methods.* Fortunately, their sturdy cell walls make fungi detectable microscopically even in the midst of necrosis; however, some are so adherent and tightly bound that they are rarely detectable in body fluids or exudates and tissue samples are required to find them. Often, fungal morphology is distinctive enough for tentative microscopic species identification, but only culture is definitive. Fungal pathogens grow well, if slowly, on appropiate media, but so do contaminating spores of free-living or commensal fungi. Therefore, *culture and tissue diagnosis combined provide the most useful information.*

Pathogenic fungi elaborate mycotoxins and enzymes but, with few exceptions, their role in human disease is still unclear. Their antigens, rich in polysaccharides, are sometimes diagnostically detectable; some can induce strong hypersensitivity responses of Types III and IV (p. 166). Phagocytic competence plays a large role in antifungal defense,[191] and patients with fewer than 1000 leukocytes are as vulnerable to fungi as to bacteria. *Steroids and immunosuppressive drugs favor fungal infections of all varieties and species.* In altered hosts, fungal growth is often florid and widespread, with sparse cellular response. It extends into vessel walls to generate thrombosis and infarction. Thus, the combination of necrotic abscesses and infarcts should arouse suspicion of a fungal cause.

Fungal pathogens are subdivided into those that remain *superficial* (i.e., restricted to the epidermal surface) and those that invade deep organs and tissues *(deep fungi)*. More important, some species are considered *opportunistic*, others truly *pathogenic* (i.e., capable of infecting normal persons) (see Table 8–6). Some pathogenic fungi are restricted geographically, and the diseases they cause are called *endemic mycoses*. Opportunistic fungi are cosmopolitan and owe their present high frequency largely to medical progress—maintenance of critically ill patients, immunosuppressive drugs, steroids and antibiotics (themselves initially discovered in the Penicillium mold); all these factors facilitate opportunistic fungal growth, as do modern invasive hospital procedures and prostheses. Although the pathogenic fungi do not require such help, they can be roused from a dormant state or aggravated by similar factors.

Several fungal species do not conform neatly to the

Table 8–6. COMMON DEEP FUNGAL INFECTIONS

Species	Forms	Best Staining Methods*	Portal of Entry	Distribution of Lesions
World-wide Fungi				
Candida† (*albicans, krusei, tropicalis*, etc.)	Nonbranching pseudohyphae; yeasts	Gram, PAS, MSS	GI, skin, intravenous	Superficial, deep, or systemic
Cryptococcus neoformans†	Encapsulated yeasts, single budding	Mucicarmine, PAS	Respiratory	Meninges, lung, systemic
Aspergillus (*fumigatus, niger*, etc.)	Branching hyphae; occ. conidia	PAS, MSS	Respiratory	(1) Endobronchial, noninvasive (2) Invasive: lung, upper respiratory, systemic
Genus Mucorales (Mucor, Absidia, Rhizophus)	Branching hyphae; rare sporangia	PAS, MSS	Respiratory	Upper respiratory, lung, systemic
Torulopsis glabrata	Small yeasts	PAS, MSS	Oral?	Systemic
Sporothrix schenkii†	Small yeasts	PAS	Skin	Skin; lymph nodes
Endemic Fungi‡				
Blastomyces dermatitidis†	Yeasts with single broad-based budding	PAS, H&E	Respiratory	Lung, systemic with typical skin lesions
Paracoccidioides brasiliensis†	Yeast with multiple budding	PAS, H&E	Respiratory	Lung, systemic
Coccidioides immitis†	Spherule with endosporulation	PAS, H&E	Respiratory	Lung, systemic, meninges
Histoplasma capsulatum†	Small yeast with single budding	MSS	Respiratory	Lung, systemic, can involve any organ

*PAS = Periodic acid–Schiff; MSS = methenamine silver; H&E = hematoxylin-eosin.
† = Fungi that can infect hosts without known predisposing factors.
‡ = Limited in their geographic distribution, except *H. capsulatum*.

definitions just outlined. Thus, *Candida albicans*, considered an opportunist, can cause mild disease in ostensibly normal individuals. It can also progress from innocuous colonization to superficial and deep invasion, depending largely on diminishing host resistance (p. 274). In the case of the endemic mycoses, the number of infected persons detectable by skin testing with fungal antigens may be in the millions, but progressive disease is limited to only a fraction, namely, those lacking a vigorous specific immune response (see coccidioidomycosis, p. 357). Thus, the dividing lines between fungal categories cannot be considered hard and fast. When host resistance is at its lowest ebb, specific chemotherapy can sometimes do no better than to induce a succession of opportunistic infections, each harder to eradicate than its predecessor. In such patients, even superficial dermatophytic fungi have become invasive (*Trichophyton beigeli*)[192] and even tissue invasion by primitive algae (Prototheca sp.) has been observed.[193]

DEEP FUNGI

Candidiasis (Moniliasis)

Candidae are the most frequent causes of human fungal disease. *C. albicans* is the most common species and can infect normal as well as altered hosts. In the latter, it is joined by other less pathogenic Candida species. All appear in tissues as nonbranching, boxcar-like chains of tubular cells, called pseudohyphae, from which small 2- to 4-μ yeast forms bud off, named blastospores. Either form or both may be seen in diseased tissues. Candida stains well with Gram, PAS, and silver stains (Fig. 8–33).

Candida albicans is found in the oral cavity, GI tract, and vagina of a great many normal individuals. The normal bacterial microflora at these mucocutaneous surfaces has an inhibitory influence on the growth of Candida, and therefore its suppression (e.g., by antibiotics) or changes in pH may permit the fungus to proliferate. Three disease patterns are seen. (1) *Superficial proliferation* occurs at sites normally colonized by the fungus. (2) *Deep invasion* occurs from destructive surface lesions when there is a systemic impairment of host defenses; widespread dissemination of the fungus may follow. (3) *Direct inoculation into the bloodstream* can give rise to severe disseminated candidiasis in immunocompromised patients; the sources may be iatrogenic (e.g., intravenous lines, catheters, peritoneal dialysis, cardiac surgery) or may be related to intravenous drug abuse with contaminated needles. Thus, the disease spectrum of candidiasis ranges from the domain of office dermatology to that of the intensive care unit.

The most common forms of candidiasis involve the mucosae of the oral cavity and vagina. Here the fungus covers the mucosae in curdy white patches or large, almost fluffy membranes, easily detached, leaving a reddened, irritated underlying surface. The histologic

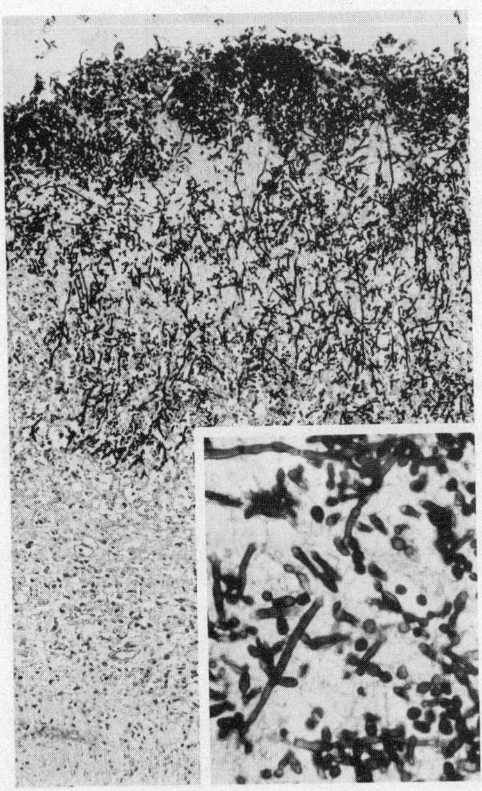

Figure 8–33. Monilial ulcer of esophagus with slender filamentous and yeast forms (silver stain).

changes are nonspecific, save for the identification of the fungus.

Candidiasis of the oral cavity is known as **oral thrush.** It is most commonly encountered in newborns who are bottle-fed; as the normal microflora develops only after birth, oral candidiasis may resolve without any treatment. In adults, it is often seen during therapy with broad-spectrum antibiotics. In immunodeficient and immunosuppressed individuals, particularly those with depressed T-cell function, oral thrush is often the first indication of impending dissemination. Vaginal candidiasis in adults may also arise in any of the above circumstances, but also **is commonly encountered in otherwise healthy young women taking oral contraceptives or during pregnancy.** The common forms of **oral** and **vaginal** candidiasis usually respond to topical therapy, but **cutaneous** eczematoid lesions may arise in moist wet areas of the skin, i.e., between the fingers and toes and in inguinal creases, inframammary folds, and the anogenital region. Microscopically, these lesions show nonspecific, acute, and chronic inflammation, with microabscesses, but in their chronic states granulomatous reactions may develop. Sometimes, hypersensitivity dermal reactions develop in sites remote from the infections, and are known as candidids or id reactions. The fingernails may develop chronic onychia.

Candidiasis of the skin is often associated with diabetes mellitus or with exposure of the skin to excessive moisture. Burn victims are also predisposed to cutaneous colonization and infection. In most of these instances the cutaneous disease responds readily to treatment of the underlying condition and local therapy. On the other hand, *chronic mucocutaneous candidiasis,* lacking obvious antecedents, is quite persistent and difficult to treat. The bases of this clinical pattern are quite heterogeneous. Some patients are found to have inherited or acquired defects in T cell–mediated immunity manifested by cutaneous anergy, impaired production of lymphokines, or ill-defined serum factors that inhibit lymphocyte activation; others have defects in neutrophil and monocyte functions as well. In yet another group, there are inherited polyendocrine deficiencies (hypoparathyroidism, hypoadrenalism, and hypothyroidism). Persistent mucocutaneous candidiasis therefore requires careful investigation of its predisposing conditions.[193A]

Severe, *invasive candidiasis* with visceral dissemination is indicative of a serious underlying disorder associated with immunosuppression or with phagocyte depletion. The portal of entry into the blood may be a destructive superficial lesion such as esophagitis (Fig. 8–33) or direct inoculation as previously discussed. Candidal sepsis may be less rampant than bacterial, but it eventually causes similar systemic manifestations, including shock and DIC. Although no organ is immune, the kidney, heart valves, lung, and liver are the most frequent targets of candidal sepsis.

Renal involvement, seen in over 90% of invasive cases, is characterized by the presence of innumerable microabscesses in both the cortex and medulla. Microscopically, the yeast or pseudohyphal forms of the fungus can be seen to occupy the center of the lesion with a surrounding area of necrosis and polymorphonuclear infiltrate. Some may be found inside glomerular capillary loops. **Candida endocarditis** resulting from direct inoculation of the fungi into the bloodstream gives rise to large, friable vegetations that frequently break off and occlude large arterial branches, sometimes those of an extremity. In the **lungs,** Candida lesions are often extensive and polymorphous; they may be cannonball-shaped or irregular, and are often hemorrhagic and partly infarct-like owing to invasion of vascular walls. Meningitis, intracerebral abscesses, enteritis, endophthalmitis, multiple subcutaneous abscesses, arthritis, and osteomyelitis are some of the other presentations of disseminated candidiasis. In any of these locations, the fungus may evoke little or no inflammatory reaction or may cause the usual suppurative response. In older or treated lesions, a granulomatous reaction is sometimes seen. Lesions indistinguishable from those of disseminated candidiasis are occasionally caused by ***Torulopsis glabrata,*** normally a mouth commensal. This fungus does not produce thrush or dermatitis. It can be distinguished by the tiny size of its blastospores (2 to 3 μ), the only form in which it appears in tissues, or in culture.

The diagnosis of Candida infection requires reasoned judgment. It should be remembered that candidae are normal inhabitants of the sputum and moreover are often secondary invaders in other infections. Therefore, the mere culture of *Candida albicans* from oral or pulmonary lesions does not necessarily indicate a primary candidal infection. The skin test with fungal antigens is of little diagnostic value since the organisms are so prevalent in the general population. Even candidemia and candiduria can be either transient or indicative of systemic infection. Therefore, positive cultures must be interpreted in the light of patient status and the character of the lesions found, as discussed earlier. Similarly, the presence of humoral antibodies to candidal antigens is of little diagnostic value unless rising titers can be demonstrated. A diagnostic approach with some promise is the quantitative detection of fungal antigens in the circulation, but this is still in an experimental stage. Tissue diagnosis, of course, is definitive.

Mucormycosis (Zygomycosis)

Mucormycosis is an uncommon opportunistic fungal infection. The causative agents belong to the family of phycomycetes, or "bread mold fungi," of which three genera are the most important human pathogens—Rhizopus, Mucor, and Absidia. The resultant diseases are entirely similar and are collectively referred to as mucormycosis or zygomycosis. Their incidence has lately been increasing because this disease tends to occur in chronically, often fatally debilitated patients who are kept alive by current improved forms of therapy. Thus, mucormycosis is most often encountered in patients with diabetic acidosis, advanced malignancy, leukemia, lymphoma, or some immunodeficiency (including transplantation cases), and in those receiving broad-spectrum antibiotic, steroid, or cytotoxic therapy. Many of these infections are hospital acquired (nosocomial).

The three primary sites of invasion are the nasal sinuses, lungs, and GI tract, depending on whether the spores (widespread in dust and air) are inhaled or ingested. When spores implant in the nasal cavities, the fungus may spread into the sinuses, orbit, and brain, giving rise to **rhinocerebral mucormycosis.** This form of the disease is most commonly but not exclusively seen in association with diabetic ketoacidosis. The phycomycetes, more than any other fungus, have a predilection for invading arterial walls and may thus permeate arteries to reach the periorbital tissues and cranial vault. A meningoencephalitis may follow or, in some cases, cerebral infarctions appear when the arterial invasions induce thrombosis. At other times the cerebral hemispheres are directly invaded by the fungi. Any of these localizations may lead to local infarctions or to hematogenous dissemination. The nonseptate, wide (6 to 50 μ) fungal hyphae with marked right-angle branching are readily demonstrated in the necrotic tissues, stained with H and E or special fungal stains (Fig. 8–34).

Lung involvement may be secondary to rhinocerebral disease, or it may be primary in patients with hematologic neoplasms. **Gastrointestinal mucormycosis** can occur, usually in association with malnutrition, particularly in children. In the lungs and GI tract the organisms show the same propensity for invading arterial walls. The tissue lesions consist of foci of suppurative necrosis in which hyphae can readily be identified. Occasionally, the fungi can be seen growing in tissues as if in culture medium without evoking an inflammatory reaction.

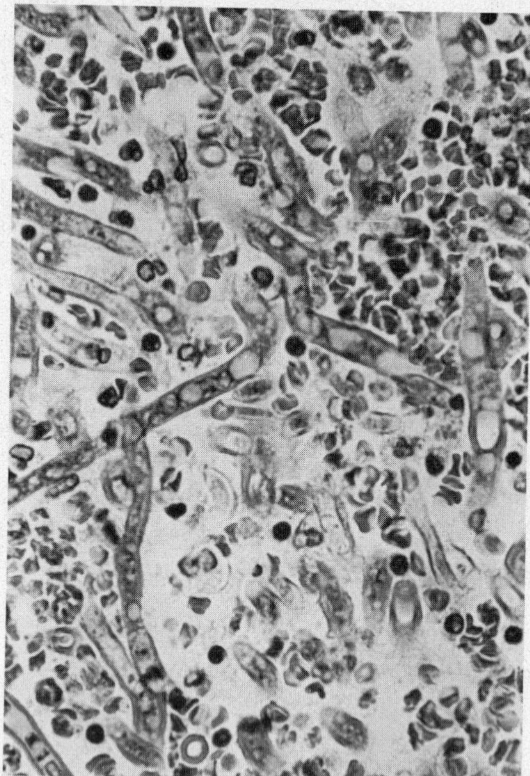

Figure 8–34. Mucormycosis. Note broad hyphae with irregular bulges, some segments showing the empty appearance characteristic of fixed specimens. Branching of hyphae is typically at 90 degrees. The fungi sit amid crenated red cells and leukocytes in the lumen of a thrombosed vessel.

Mucormycosis is a grave disorder because it is largely an opportunistic disease in an already mortally ill patient. Occasional patients, especially those with nasal infections, have recovered following antibiotic therapy combined with surgery.

Aspergillosis

Several different diseases are caused by members of the genus Aspergillus, most commonly *A. fumigatus* and *A. niger*. These can be divided into three categories: (1) *allergic*, (2) *colonizing*, and (3) *invasive*. In addition, aflatoxin elaborated by *A. flavus*, a species not infectious for man, is an important liver poison and potential hepatic carcinogen (p. 936).

Allergic aspergillosis may manifest itself as *bronchial asthma*, similar clinically to other forms of extrinsic asthma. In nonatopic individuals, sensitization to the Aspergillus spores may produce an *allergic alveolitis* by inducing type III and type IV hypersensitivity reactions (p. 166). Both these forms of allergic aspergillosis result from inhalation of spores, without actual colonization of the respiratory mucosa. A third pattern, called *allergic bronchopulmonary aspergillosis*, is associated with hypersensitivity arising from superficial colonization of the bronchial mucosa. Often this occurs in previously asthmatic patients, whose symptoms become more severe and chronic.

Colonizing aspergillosis (aspergilloma) implies growth of the fungus in pulmonary cavities with minimal or no invasion of the tissues. The cavities usually result from preexisting tuberculosis, bronchiectasis, or old infarcts or abscesses. Proliferating masses of fungal hyphae called "fungus balls" can be seen as brownish masses lying free within the cavities. The surrounding reaction may be sparse or there may be chronic inflammation and fibrosis. Patients with aspergillomas usually have recurrent hemoptysis.

Invasive aspergillosis is an opportunistic infection confined to immunosuppressed and debilitated hosts. The primary lesions are usually in the lung, but widespread hematogenous dissemination with involvement of the heart valves, brain, and kidneys is now increasingly common. The **pulmonary lesions** take the form of necrotizing pneumonia with sharply delineated, rounded gray foci with hemorrhagic borders, often referred to as target lesions. Since invasive aspergillosis is rapidly progressive, chronic granulomatous reactions are rarely seen. In the tissues, Aspergillus appears as septate filaments 5 to 10 μ thick, branching at more acute angles than Mucor. Its fruiting body resembles a holy water sprinkler (aspergillum), hence its name. Like the Phycomycetes, Aspergillus has a tendency to invade blood vessels, and thus areas of hemorrhage and infarction may be superimposed on the suppurative tissue reactions.

In addition to life-threatening deep invasion of the lungs, Aspergillus can produce primary lesions localized to the eyes, paranasal sinuses, and/or external ear in apparently healthy individuals.

Invasive aspergillosis is now a common and serious hospital problem. It is difficult to diagnose because aspergilli are rarely demonstrable in the patient's sputum or blood. It should be suspected in any severely debilitated person who suddenly takes a turn for the worse. The diagnosis usually depends on demonstration of the fungus in the tissues. Serology is of limited value but recent attempts to demonstrate *Aspergillus* antigens appear promising. Aspergillus spores are widely distributed in the environment and the fungus is frequently cultured by simply exposing media to hospital air. Contaminated rooms are difficult to rehabilitate and are an obvious hazard for immunosuppressed patients.

Cryptococcosis (Cryptococcus neoformans)

Cryptococcosis may arise in healthy individuals, but more commonly it occurs as an opportunistic infection, particularly in patients with leukemia, lymphoma, or Hodgkin's disease. It is caused by *Cryptococcus neoformans,* a round-to-oval yeast about 5 to 10 μ in diameter that reproduces by unequal budding. It has a distinctive, very prominent, heavy, gelatinous capsule that creates an apparent clear halo about the agent in tissue sections or exudate (Fig. 8–35). A useful laboratory aid in the identification of this organism is the introduction of India ink into exudate suspected of harboring these fungi. The ink provides a contrast medium that clearly outlines the heavy, translucent coat. The capsular polysaccharides also have a strong affinity for the mucicarmine stain, a helpful feature in tissue diagnosis.

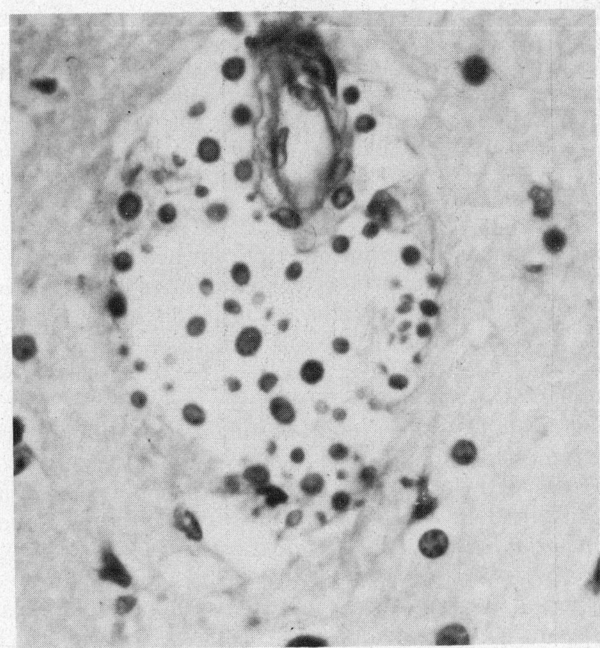

Figure 8–35. Cryptococcal proliferation in Virchow-Robin perivascular space of brain—a "soap-bubble lesion" (PAS stain).

Birds, especially pigeons, excrete infective cryptococci without themselves suffering disease. Inhalation of the infective forms is the usual mode of infection, and therefore the lung is the primary site of localization. However, pulmonary infection may remain mild and asymptomatic even while the fungus is spreading to other organs, most notably the CNS, for which it seems to have a special predilection. Clinically, therefore, *the most frequent manifestation of cryptococcal infection is meningitis.* Other forms, in order of severity, affect only the lung, or both lung and brain, or multiple disseminated organs.

The tissue response to cryptococcus is extremely variable.[194] In immunosuppressed patients they may evoke virtually no inflammatory reaction, and gelatinous masses of fungi may develop as though in a culture medium. In normal reactors or protracted disease, the fungi often induce a chronic granulomatous reaction composed of macrophages, lymphocytes, and foreign body–type giant cells. Neutrophils and suppuration may also occasionally be seen. Thus, cryptococcal meningitis may disclose a pure culture of gelatinous organisms without accompanying white cells. In about half the cases the infection extends into the brain substance about the perivascular spaces, and sometimes enters the gray matter to produce small cysts filled with organisms and their mucinous secretions, the characteristic "soap-bubble" lesions (Fig. 8–35). Rarely, there is granulomatous arteritis of the circle of Willis.

The lung involvement is equally variable. There may be one or more circumscribed foci or a diffuse pattern of infiltration. The lung nodules may be composed of "naked" masses of organisms or, more likely in chronic cases, granulomatous infiltrate. Similar involvement of hilar lymph nodes may be evident. Chronic infection, especially in patients without underlying immunodeficiency, may produce solid lesions that remain stationary and may be mistaken for tumors (cryptococcomas). From their primary sites cryptococci may disseminate widely by the bloodstream to the skin, liver, spleen, adrenals, bones or other tissues, usually in debilitated or severely immunosuppressed patients. Rarely, isolated lesions of the skin or of a joint are found without clear evidence of systemic invasion.

Pulmonary cryptococcosis can be differentiated from other lung infections by identification of the fungus in sputum (using the India ink technique) or at biopsy. CNS cryptococcosis has an insidious onset, characterized by headache, dizziness, or cranial nerve impairments. Usually the patient has little fever and sometimes the picture is misinterpreted as tuberculous meningitis. Diagnosis is aided by the demonstration of cryptococci in the CSF. Since the capsular antigens are shed in body fluids, *their detection by the latex cryptococcal agglutinin test (LCAT) is an extremely valuable diagnostic tool.* This test is positive in the CSF of over 90% of cases of cryptococcal meningitis and therefore has improved early diagnosis and treatment, without which the mortality rate of cryptococcal meningitis is high. Even with the latest antifungal drugs, immunosuppressed patients fare poorly, but the outlook is better for normal reactors.

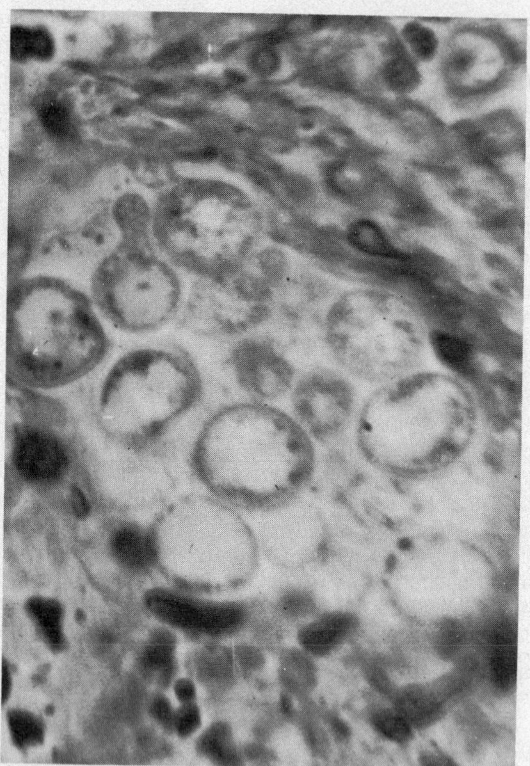

Figure 8–36. Blastomycosis with a cluster of organisms, one of which is in the process of reproduction by budding.

Blastomycosis (Blastomyces dermatitidis)*

Blastomycosis is a chronic infection characterized by focal suppurative and granulomatous lesions, principally in the lungs and skin. The disease is virtually limited to North America, particularly in the Mississippi–Ohio River basins and the Middle Atlantic states, but sporadic cases have been reported in Central and South America, as well as in Africa. Males are affected nine times more often than females. The causative organism assumes a yeast form in tissue lesions and is round-to-oval, 5 to 25 μ in diameter with a thick refractile (double-contoured) wall. Symmetrically budding forms generating *daughter cells with a broad base (4 to 5 μ) are quite characteristic* (Fig. 8–36). The source of infection and route of transmission to humans are still somewhat uncertain. There are only a few reports of recovery of this agent in soil samples from farms or woods. Small epidemics have occurred among hunters. The disease is acquired by spore inhalation and therefore its primary localization is in the lung. From here, hematogenous fungal dissemination may occur, most commonly to the skin and sometimes to the bones, but virtually any organ may be involved. Cutaneous, osseous, or genital lesions are sometimes present without apparent pulmonary involvement, but in all cases the portal of entry is believed to be the lung.

Pulmonary blastomycosis may take one of several forms, most often that of a **solitary focus** of consolidation or of transient bilateral foci sometimes with involvement of regional nodes, simulating the Ghon complex of tuberculosis. These lesions usually heal, leaving behind a small fibrotic scar. Primary infection may be accompanied by erythema nodosum of the skin. Calcification of healed lesions, unlike those of tuberculosis or histoplasmosis, is uncommon. More rarely, **progressive lung disease** ensues, leading to miliary abscesses throughout the lung or to extensive focal consolidation with formation of cavities. Histologically, some of these lesions are rich in neutrophils and abscess-like; others show tubercle-like granulomas; most have a suppurative center surrounded by epithelioid macrophages and giant cells. Grumous caseation necrosis occurs less commonly than in tuberculosis or histoplasmosis, with which the lesions may otherwise be confused. Histologic diagnosis depends on demonstration of characteristic double-contoured fungi, sometimes within giant cells.

Skin involvement, with or without lesions in other organs, is frequent in the progressive form of blastomycosis. The cutaneous lesions tend to appear on the hands, face, feet, wrists, and ankles but eventually involve unexposed regions as well. They begin as indolent, chancre-like papules, but over the course of weeks or months become large, fleshy, fungating ulcers with raised, red, verrucous advancing margins. With healing the central regions may become scarred and depressed, while the disease activity continues at the periphery dotted by numerous microabscesses. Grossly, these skin ulcers have sometimes been confused with carcinomas. Histologically too, the cutaneous lesion may be mistaken for malignancy owing to the striking **pseudoepitheliomatous hyperplasia**, which can mimic squamous cell carcinoma. The epithelium is extensively thickened, showing irregular cellular proliferation. The rete pegs are broadened, extend down into the underlying subepidermal connective tissue, and appear to anastomose deeply. However, there is no anaplasia or invasive growth, as in true neoplasia. Microabscesses, granulomas, and hybrids of both lesions are seen chiefly in the dermis, but extend up into the epidermis. They are surrounded by exuberant granulation tissue. Fungi are usually plentiful in the microabscess-studded ulcer base, but may become sparse in healing skin lesions.

The symptoms of pulmonary blastomycosis are nonspecific and can resemble those of tuberculosis, other mycoses (especially histoplasmosis, which is endemic in the same regions), or lung tumors. The skin lesions may be confused with malignant ulcers. Diagnosis requires identification of the causative agent in exudates or tissue sections. When open lesions are present, diagnosis is best made by examination of KOH-treated sputum or bronchial aspirate.[195] Skin tests and serologic procedures, although available, are of doubtful reliability. Self-limited forms of blastomycosis do not require antifungal drugs. Late progressive stages respond poorly to available drugs and have a high mortality rate.

*Paracoccidioidomycosis (South American Blastomycosis)**

This fungal infection is focally endemic in the area extending between Mexico to the north and Argentina to the south, with most cases occurring in Brazil, Venezuela, and Colombia. It predominantly affects male agricultural workers. The yeast form of *Paracoccidioides brasiliensis,* the causative fungus, is large (10 to 60 μ) and shows characteristic *multiple budding* around a mother cell, resulting in the formation of a fungal rosette or *"ship's wheel image."* The infection is acquired by inhalation, but pulmonary lesions are neither distinctive nor usually dominate the clinical picture. Much more commonly, extrapulmonary spread produces *a mucocutaneous lesion (often in the mouth, nose, or larynx), a spreading lymph node infection, or (sometimes) systemic dissemination.* Infection of mucous membranes may take the form of an inflammatory papilloma that resembles the early stages of blastomycosis. Drainage from this lesion may give rise to a striking involvement of the regional nodes. Lymphadenopathy is sometimes encountered in patients who do not have a well-defined mucocutaneous lesion. When *P. brasiliensis* disseminates, the skin, GI tract, lungs, liver, and other organs may be affected. In all these sites, microabscesses or granulomatous inflammatory reactions develop, resembling those of blastomycosis. The chief differential diagnostic point is the demonstration of the much larger, double-contoured organisms that produce multiple buds.

Coccidioidomycosis (Coccidioides immitis)*

Coccidioidomycosis, caused by inhalation of the spores of *Coccidioides immitis,* is an acute or chronic infection that bears many similarities to tuberculosis. It commonly occurs as an acute, primary, self-limited pulmonary involvement with or without systemic manifestations, but in some cases progresses to disseminated disease. The primary pulmonary involvement is usually asymptomatic or mild, but induces delayed hypersensitivity to the fungal antigens. In a few cases, progression or reactivation of the primary involvement leads to destructive lesions in the lungs or, more important, to disseminated disease throughout the body in a fashion reminiscent of progressive tuberculosis.

Coccidioidomycosis is most prevalent in the Southwest and Far West of the United States and is particularly common in the San Joaquin Valley of California; in this locale, it is sometimes known as "valley fever." It also occurs in Mexico and parts of South America. Risk of infection is highest where carrier bats and birds have their nests. In tissue sections the fungus appears as a thick-walled, nonbudding spherule 20 to 60 μ in diameter, often filled with small endospores (Fig. 8–37). Rupture of the spherule with release of endospores is the method of reproduction, but this tissue form is noninfectious. In nature or artificial culture, reproduction is by boxcar-like arthrospores, easily detached and disseminated by air. Extreme caution is needed in handling this dimorphic fungus in the laboratory. Animals as well as man can be infected.

Approximately 60% of patients with primary coccidioidomycosis are unaware of the infection. Only skin sensitization to coccidioidin or spherulin (fungal antigens) discloses the existence of a past or present infection. Almost 80% of the population of the San Joaquin Valley are coccidioidin positive. In about 10% of patients the lung lesions evoke fever, cough, and pleuritic pains, accompanied by erythema nodosum or erythema multiforme (i.e., the "valley fever" complex).

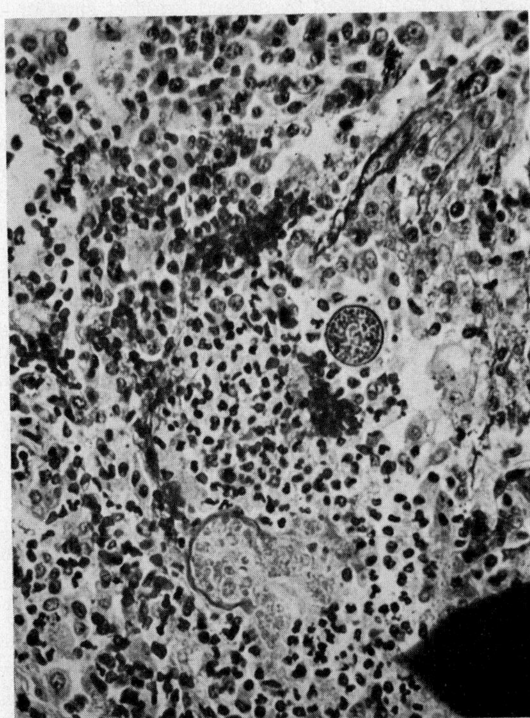

Figure 8–37. Coccidioidomycosis with several microorganisms filled with endospores. One has been caught at the moment of rupture with release of daughter spores.

The presentation of **primary pulmonary coccidioidomycosis** most commonly takes the form of a solitary gray-white focus of consolidation, 2 to 3 cm in diameter, in the middle or lower lung fields. Occasionally a more diffuse pneumonic consolidation or multiple scattered foci of consolidation appear. Hilar lymphadenopathy may be present to mimic, with the parenchymal lesion, the Ghon complex of tuberculosis. More often, however, lymphadenopathy is absent.

Histologically, two reaction patterns are seen. In cases in which there is florid proliferation of fungi, the response tends to be suppurative. More often, in instances with slower rates of fungal reproduction, granuloma production occurs, closely resembling tubercles. Fungal spherules usually are readily evident in the macrophages or giant cells within the granulomas. When the spherules rupture to release the endospores, a pyogenic reaction is superimposed (Fig. 8–37). Similar granulomas may appear in the draining lymph nodes. With time these active lesions fibrose and calcify. Thus, in many patients, only the telltale radiographic calcifications and positive skin reactions reveal the past existence of the infection.

In the great majority of patients, even those who are symptomatic, the primary pulmonary form of the disease is self-limited, like primary tuberculosis. However, about 0.2% of infected white males and twice as many black or Asian males develop progressive coccidioidomycosis, possibly because they fail to mount an adequate cell-mediated immune response to the primary disease. Such individuals do not have dermal hypersensitivity at the time of the spread of the disease.

Anatomically, the progressive disease usually takes the form of more extensive focal involvement of the lungs, frequently accompanied by spread to other sites of localization, principally the meninges, bones, adrenals, lymph nodes, spleen, and liver. In some patients, meningeal involvement may appear to be the sole localization. Progressive pulmonary coccidioidomycosis produces areas of gray-white consolidation, cavitation, scarring, and calcification, simulating progressive tuberculosis. A particularly "malignant" complication of this fungal infection is widespread miliary dissemination throughout the body. Coccidioidomycosis may involve the skin, possibly as a primary site, but more often as a manifestation of progressive disease in which the cutaneous involvement is only one site of hematogenous dissemination. At all these sites the inflammatory response may be purely granulomatous, pyogenic, or mixed. Purulent lesions dominate in patients with the least resistance and with widespread dissemination.

Most individuals with progressive disease have chills, fever, night sweats, weakness, and weight loss, accompanied by a cough productive of mucopurulent sputum. This sputum may harbor the pathognomonic microorganisms and thus permit a direct diagnosis. Unlike several of the previously discussed fungal diseases, *serologic tests are extremely valuable in establishing the diagnosis. With the reactive antibodies, precipitin, latex particle agglutination, or immunodiffusion tests are positive in virtually every symptomatic case.* Complement-fixing antibodies in the CSF are diagnostic of coccidioidal meningitis. The skin tests with coccidioidin or spherulin are of value only in epidemiologic studies. The prognosis in coccidioidomycosis is generally favorable, but becomes increasingly grave with the systemic dissemination of the organisms and the development of infections in the bones or CNS, which require long-term antifungal treatment, itself a cause of many complications.[196]

Histoplasmosis (Histoplasma capsulatum)

Infection by the dimorphic fungus *H. capsulatum* is a world-wide endemic condition almost rivaling the frequency of tuberculosis in the United States today, especially in the Ohio–Mississippi River region. It is acquired by dust inhalation from bird or bat droppings or from contaminated soil, and has been spread widely by birds such as pigeons or nesting starlings. The organism grows in mycelial form in soil or on special media at room temperature, producing sprouting conidia of two sizes. The smaller ones (microconodia) are easily detached, windborne, and infectious; the larger, tuberculate ones (macroconodia) are virtually diagnostic of *H. capsulatum* by their shape. At 37° C on agar or in mammalian tissues there is conversion to a primitive 2- to 5-μ yeast form with a thin cell wall, but lacking a true capsule (despite the organism's misleading name). These yeast forms are best visualized with the methenamine silver stain but are practically invisible in routine H and E sections. Neither they nor the patient bearing these forms can transmit the infection.

The clinical presentations and morphologic lesions of histoplasmosis strikingly parallel those of tuberculosis and coccidioidomycosis. Depending on host resistance and immunocompetence, the fungus may induce: (1) latent asymptomatic infection; (2) self-limited primary pulmonary involvement; (3) chronic, progressive, even cavitary pulmonary disease; (4) rapid, widely disseminated systemic involvement, and (5) localized lesions in one or more organs.

Latent or asymptomatic histoplasmosis can be discovered only by the finding of fibrocalcific residues at sites of past localization of the organisms, most often the lungs or hilar lymph nodes, accompanied by a positive histoplasmin skin test (analogous to the tuberculin test). In contrast to the Ghon complex of tuberculosis (p. 344), latent histoplasma foci are often multiple.

Primary pulmonary histoplasmosis is the most common clinical presentation. It occurs in otherwise healthy individuals (usually adults) as a mild, self-limited, febrile respiratory infection. Chest x-rays reveal hilar adenopathy with or without one or more focal pulmonary parenchymal shadows. Erythema nodosum or erythema multiforme sometimes appear, more commonly in females than in males. Rarely, this pattern is complicated by pericarditis arising by spread of the infection from adjacent involved nodes.

Chronic pulmonary histoplasmosis is the counterpart of secondary tuberculosis. It is characterized by uni- or bilateral apical infiltrates that may progressively enlarge and cavitate as the disease spreads throughout the lung fields. Preexisting chronic lung disease favors the spread of infection. The most common clinical manifestations are cough, fever, night sweats, and weight loss. Death may occur from progression of the pulmonary lesions, dissemination of the infection, cor pulmonale, or bacterial superinfection. However, about one-third of cases spontaneously improve, usually those with limited apical involvement.

Disseminated histoplasmosis may follow either primary or chronic pulmonary disease, but more often appears as an acute, relentlessly progressive infection in the very old, the very young, or those with impaired cell-mediated immunity. Characteristically, these patients have fever, generalized lymphadenopathy, abdominal symptoms, hepatosplenomegaly, wasting, anemia, leukopenia, and thrombocytopenia and may become jaundiced owing to extensive hepatic involvement. Often, meningitis becomes the dominant feature of the disease. This overwhelming dissemination of the fungi is often associated with anergy to histoplasmin.

In addition to these three classical clinical patterns, histoplasmosis sometimes presents in other ways. Rarely, extension of infection from mediastinal nodes gives rise to progressive scarring and contraction of the mediastinal structures—*sclerosing mediastinitis*—even as fungi become quite scarce. Compression of nerves, pulmonary veins, pulmonary arteries, superior vena cava, and esophagus may occur. More commonly, healing or healed, calcified or noncalcified, sometimes laminated pulmonary coin lesions or hilar lesions come to clinical attention on chest radiographs in the absence of other signs or symptoms. When solitary, these are called *histoplasmomas* and must be differentiated from other pulmonary granulomas and tumors (Fig. 8–38). Rarely, calcified histoplasmomas lacking viable fungi erode into a bronchus, and patients cough up the calcified debris (broncholithiasis). Diagnosis of such lesions is usually made after surgical excision by demonstration of the residual fungal cell walls on silver staining. Another uncommon presentation of histoplasmosis is the development of active localized disease in scattered organs. Thus, bilateral adrenal destruction may coexist with or follow only minor respiratory involvement and can lead to adrenal insufficiency (Addison's disease) (p. 1235). Endocarditis, chronic meningitis, granulomatous hepatitis, or gastrointestinal ulcerative involvement have all been reported.

In otherwise healthy adults, histoplasmosis is characterized by the formation of epithelioid cell granulomas at the sites of localization of the fungus. These granulomas usually undergo coagulative necrosis and coalesce to produce larger areas of consolidation, but they may also liquefy to form cavities.[197] With spontaneous or drug control of the infection, the lesions undergo fibrosis and often calcification. Histologic differentiation from tuberculosis, sarcoidosis, and coccidioidomycosis requires identification of the yeast forms that persist in the lesions for many years even into the calcific stage. The macroscopic lesions of active **granulomatous histoplasmosis** in the lung and hilar lymph nodes appear as gray-white foci of consolidation and scarring. In the **chronic pattern of disease** these lesions are usually apical, with retraction and thickening of the apical pleura. Further progression involves more and more of the lung parenchyma, focally, sometimes with cavity formation, albeit somewhat less often than in tuberculosis. In **fulminant disseminated histoplasmosis,** epithelioid cell granulomas are not well formed but instead there are focal accumulations of activated mononuclear phagocytes stuffed with fungal yeasts throughout the tissues and organs of the body. The cells of the reticuloendothelial system in particular become overloaded with yeast forms, reminiscent of kala-azar (Fig. 8–39) (p. 372).

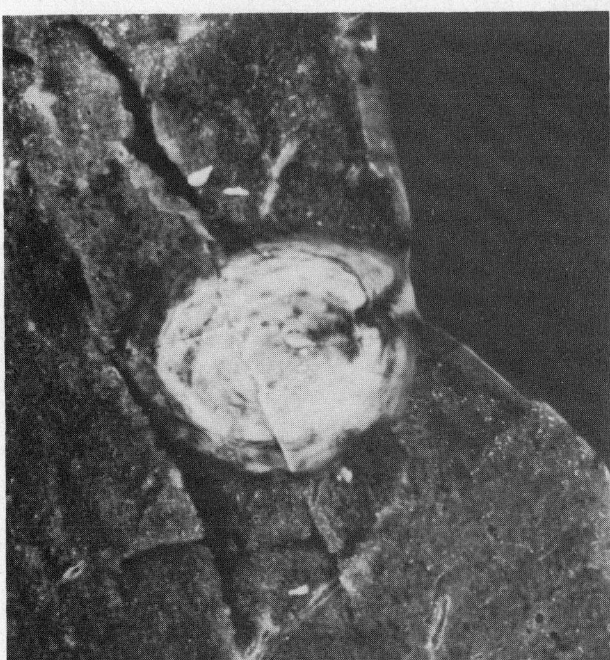

Figure 8–38. Histoplasmosis. Laminated granuloma of lung—a stationary disease form.

The clinical diagnosis of histoplasmosis depends largely on awareness of its protean presentations. The histoplasmin skin test is helpful but may be falsely negative in those with overwhelming infection. Tests for Histoplasma antibodies, although available, suffer from a large proportion of false-positive and false-negative results. Definitive diagnosis is best made by culture (which may, however, require up to four weeks) or by direct demonstration of the characteristic small yeast forms in tissues or smears that must be differentiated from the yeast forms of Candida and torulopsis.[198] Too often in the past, Histoplasmosis has been mislabeled as tuberculosis.

*Unusual Deep Fungal Infections**

Among the many rare and tropical deep fungal infections,[199] only two will receive brief mention here. *Mycetomas* are localized deforming tumefactions with multiple draining sinuses, most commonly of the foot (Madura foot).[199] Many fungal species can cause these

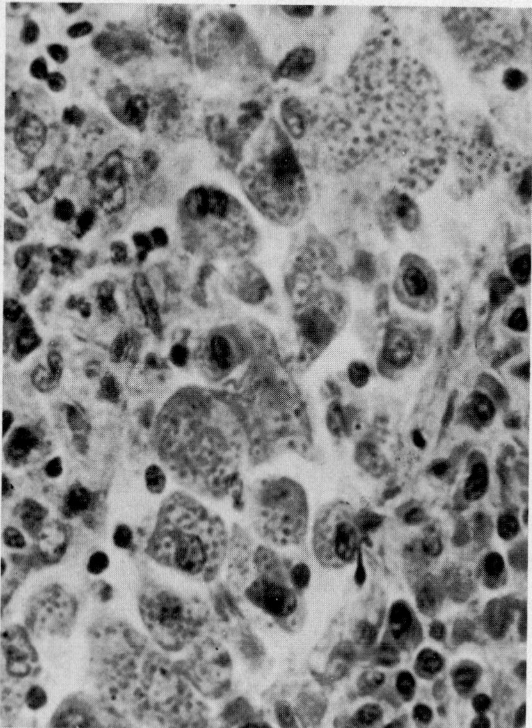

Figure 8–39. Disseminated histoplasmosis in a lymph node. The central phagocytes are stuffed with minute fungal yeasts.

lesions, as well as some of the Actinomycetes, and their etiologic diagnosis is in the realm of specialized mycology. The commonest cause in Central and North America is *Nocardia brasiliensis* (p. 349). *Characteristic of mycetomas is the aggregation of fungi in masses or "grains" analogous to the sulfur granules of Actinomyces* (p. 349). By the time mycetomas are seen, the deep tissues and underlying bones and joints are usually involved and surgical therapy is necessary.

Chromomycosis causes large, warty, ulcerative skin lesions of the extremities with pseudoepitheliomatous epidermal hyperplasia. It occurs in the rural areas of the Caribbean, including Puerto Rico, and is due to a group of fungi forming pigmented spores and hyphae, most often *Fonsecaea pedrosoi.* This condition may be confused with a skin tumor.

SUPERFICIAL FUNGI (DERMATOPHYTES)

These infections of the epidermis, hair, or nails by fungi that generally spare the deeper tissues are described in Chapter 27. They rarely are life threatening but the unsightly skin lesions, hair loss, and itching can cause great distress to those affected. *In most cases, the causal fungus can be visualized if not identified by microscopic examination of skin scrapings and hair shafts.*

Dermatophytes are classified largely on the basis of their preference for the hairy or glabrous skin, and whether they localize in moist or dry skin areas. *Tinea* is caused by fungi of the Trichophyton and Microsporum groups and named according to its location, e.g., *tinea capitis* (of the head) or *barbae* (of the bearded area). Especially well known is *tinea pedis* (athlete's foot), an itching infection spreading from the interdigital folds to the soles of the feet, which can give rise to distant hypersensitivity reactions that can become incapacitating. Several forms of superficial mycosis are grossly distinctive, such as *piedra,* manifested by dark, hard nodules of the hair shafts, but identification by culture is necessary since treatment of these conditions varies according to species.

Onychomycosis, (fungal infections of nails) can be caused by Candida sp. as well as by Trichophyton and other dermatophytes. Likewise, *otomycosis* can be caused by the potentially invasive species—Candida or Aspergillus.

PROTOZOAL DISEASES

Parasitic protozoa (Table 8–7) are among the foremost causes of disease and death in developing countries. They are also widely prevalent in U.S. and other industrial nations, but are less often lethal. Unlike lower forms, pathogenic protozoa are motile, favoring both invasion and evasion. They do not, however, secrete exotoxins, as can certain bacteria. Their reproductive life cycles and host adaptations are more complex than those of bacteria and fungi, and have just begun to be understood at the biochemical and molecular level, raising hopes of eventual control.[200] We shall divide them here into: (1) mucosal (or luminal), (2) bloodstream, and (3) intracellular pathogens, although some life cycles may bridge these categories.

Luminal protozoa, like human mucosal bacteria, include both commensals and parasites; some are opportunistic invaders. Several harmless amebic species inhabit the human gut (e.g., *Entamoeba coli*) and must be differentiated from the pathogenic *E. histolytica.* Within the latter species, strain differences clearly influence amebic virulence.[201] *The harmful effects of entamoebae on cells, both in vivo and in vitro, appear to be exerted only over a short range or by direct contact.*[202, 203] Lectin-like ligands have been concentrated from pathogenic amebic cultures that could facilitate target cell binding. The protozoa appear to open tiny channels in the plasma membrane of the host cell, leading to electrolyte imbalance and lysis.[204] The host cell remnants can then be ingested by the amebae. This lytic process helps to explain the relatively mild inflammatory responses characteristic of destructive amebic lesions (hence, the name *E. histolytica*). Similar short-range effects have been postulated for the cell damage caused by *Giardia lamblia* and *Pneumocystis,*[205, 206] but these interactions are still quite poorly understood.

Host defenses are equally important in determining the outcome of luminal parasite-host interactions. Cortisone therapy sometimes transforms amebiasis from a

Table 8–7. PROTOZOA PATHOGENIC FOR HUMANS

Species	Order	Form, Size*	Disease
Luminal			
Entamoeba histolytica	Amebae	Trophozoite 15–50 μ (cyst slightly smaller)	Amebic dysentery Liver abscess
Balantidium coli	Ciliates	Trophozoite 50–100 μ	Colitis
Naegleria fowleri	Ameboflagellates	Trophozoite 10–20 μ	Meningoencephalitis
Acanthamoeba sp.	Ameboflagellates	Trophozoite 15–30 μ	Same or Ophthalmitis
Giardia lamblia	Mastigophora	Trophozoite 11–18 μ (cyst slightly smaller)	Diarrheal disease Malabsorption
Isospora belli	Coccidia	Oocyst 10–20 μ	Chronic enterocolitis and/or malabsorption
Cryptosporidium sp.	"	Oocyst 5–6 μ	
Trichomonas vaginalis	Mastigophora	Trophozoite 10–30 μ	Urethritis, vaginitis
Pneumocystis carinii	?	Trophozoite 6–8 μ, cyst 4–6 μ	Opportunistic lung infection
Bloodstream			
Plasmodium vivax	Hemosporidia	Trophozoites, schizonts, gametes (all small and inside red cells)	Benign, tertian malaria
P. ovale	"		" " "
P. malariae	"	"	Quartan malaria
P. falciparum	"	"	Malignant tertian malaria
Babesia microti, bovis	Hemosporidia	Trophozoites inside red cells	Babesiasis
Trypanosoma brucei, rhodesiense, gambiense	Hemoflagellates	Trypomastigote 14–33 μ	African sleeping sickness
Intracellular			
Trypanosoma cruzi	Hemoflagellates	Trypomastigote 20 μ (amastigote smaller)	Chagas' disease
Leishmania donovani	Hemoflagellates	Amastigote 2 μ	Kala-azar
Leishmania tropica, mexicana, brasiliensis	Hemoflagellates	Amastigote 2 μ	Cutaneous and mucocutaneous leishmaniasis
Toxoplasma gondii	Coccidia (Eimeriae)	Tachyzoite 4–6 μ (cyst larger)	Toxoplasmosis

*Found in human host.

moderate to a severe infection.[207] Pneumocystis pneumonia in adult patients is virtually unheard of in the absence of immunosuppression.[208] *Mild or subclinical luminal infections constitute the vast endemic background upon which severe protozoal disease occurs only episodically.* As a rule, host immune responses are not greatly challenged by luminal parasitic infections; thus, antibodies to *E. histolytica* are regularly found only when invasive disease is present and amebic reinfections are quite frequent. Loss of normal host immune defense greatly facilitates progressive or lethal mucosal protozoal disease.

Bloodstream protozoa as a group are extraordinarily infective. Thus, a single Rhodesian trypanosome, when inoculated into a susceptible mouse, can kill the animal within a few days. Humans, too, sometimes succumb to this parasite acutely within a few weeks.[209] However, propagation of the parasite species is better served by a more lasting equilibrium between host immune responses and the evasive maneuvers of the parasite. Thus, infections by African trypanosomes soon evoke strong host immune responses, but the trypanosomes evade these by programmed antigenic variation and survive, ultimately to penetrate the blood-brain barrier and cause chronic sleeping sickness. Certain malarial sporozoites early during infection take refuge in hepatocytes, where these "hypnozoites" remain dormant until they reemerge to cause relapses.[210] During active infection, malarial trophozoites are partly protected from lethal host antibody within red cells. While thus temporarily sheltered, they somehow dampen the host's specific immune responses, meanwhile generating variant antigenic clones.[211] Binding of plasmodia to red cells is ensured by specific receptor molecules, and their entry by induction of a vacuole in red cells.[212]

The mechanisms by which blood and tissue parasites cause damage and destroy cells are quite diverse. Malarial trophozoites damage red cells by actively metabolizing their heme, thereby generating waste pigments that are found in many of the characteristic lesions of malaria. In malignant tertian malaria, parasitized red cells develop tiny surface knobs, rendering them adhesive to vascular endothelium. Small vessels within viscera and the CNS thus become plugged with parasitized red cells, inducing severe microvascular disturbances.[213] During their acute, uncontrolled proliferation, both malarial and trypanosomal organisms can elicit severe systemic effects such as shock, pulmonary edema, and DIC. Activation of host mediators such as the kinins and lipoxygenase products has been shown to occur,[214] but the responsible parasite products have not yet been identified with certainty.

Intracellular protozoa behave much like intracellular rickettsiae or chlamydiae. Leishmanias propagate exclusively in macrophages, which phagocytize them. The survival of the parasite within the phagolysosomes of these cells is attributed to their surface glycoprotein products and enzymes known as "excreted factors.[215] Little is yet known about the tropisms of intracellular protozoa, but temperature sensitivity is important in determining leishmanial localizations.[216] *Trypanosoma cruzi* and *Toxoplasma gondii* actively invade parenchymal cells, including those of the myocardium. Intracellular survival of parasites is accomplished either by their escaping from phagolysosomes into the host cell cytosol or by their altering primary phagosomal membranes to thus block fusion with lysosomes.[217] Each parasite appears to have a unique mechanism for intracellular survival. The virulence of intracellular protozoa is closely linked to their ability to proliferate within cells, sometimes literally causing cells to burst and die. Alternatively, they may reduce a host cell to a membranous cyst-envelope.[218] When host immunity is normal such cell destruction is usually focal and piecemeal, but when response is inadequate (as in infants, the elderly, and the immunosuppressed) parasitic proliferation can be virtually unrestrained and the severity of the disease thereby heightened.[218]

Host defense against intracellular parasites is largely dependent on cell-mediated mechanisms. Activated macrophages are the major or, in the case of leishmaniasis, the sole immune effectors known. With *Trypanosoma cruzi* and *Toxoplasma gondii*,[219] humoral antibodies may play capacitating or auxiliary roles. Even when not protective, parasite-specific antibodies are diagnostically helpful in intracellular protozoal infections. Moreover, long-sustained stimulation of the host immune system by intracellular parasitism may induce antibodies reactive with host endothelia or with the ground substance component laminin, such as appear in chronic Chagas' disease.[220] Advanced stages of visceral leishmaniasis result in an even more profound derangement characterized by suppressed cell-mediated immunity, together with polyclonal B-cell stimulation and marked hyperglobulinemia.[221] Thus, the pathogenesis of intracellular protozoal disease is partly controlled and modulated by the immune system of the host.

Much more has recently been learned about protozoan-host interactions and is well reviewed in a monograph.[222]

LUMINAL PROTOZOA

Amebiasis (Entamoeba histolytica)

Amebiasis is primarily an infection of the colon, followed in some cases by spread to the liver, lungs, and brain. The disease is limited to human and nonhuman primates and ranges from mild chronic diarrhea in cases with minimal colonic involvement to severe purging dysentery in those with extensive ulcerations of the colonic mucosa. Far more common than symptomatic amebiasis is the entirely asymptomatic carrier state, the reservoir responsible for transmission of the disease.

The responsible organism, *E. histolytica*, is a deceptively simple trophozoite (15 to 40 μm in diameter) with a relatively small nucleus, distinctive by its tiny central karyosome and aggregated RNA-DNA at the nuclear membrane and by its bubbly cytoplasm containing many glycogen rosettes (Fig. 8–40). The outer cytoplasmic zone ("ectoplasm") is clear and forms pseudopods. The parasite derives its energy largely from

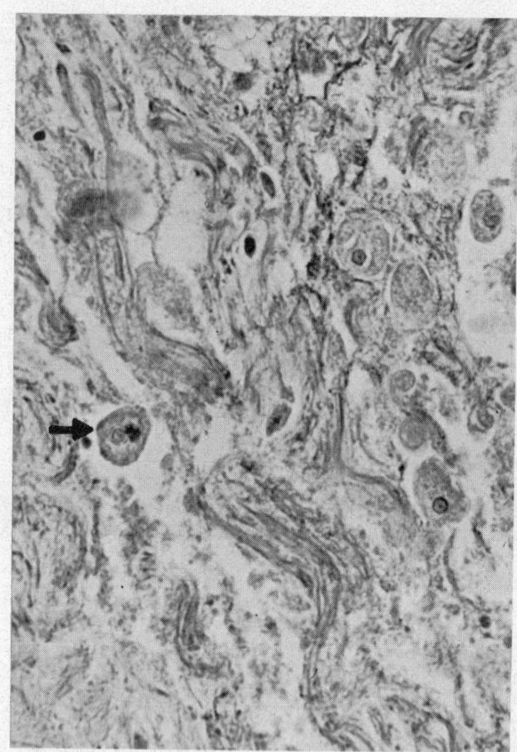

Figure 8–40. Amebiasis of colon. Histologic detail of vegetative parasites is shown. Arrow points to an ameba with a phagocytized red cell.

anaerobic glycolysis. Mitochondria, typical lysosomes, Golgi bodies, and rough endoplasmic reticulum are lacking. Because *E. histolytica* is actively phagocytic and may contain red-cell or other cell debris, *it can be confused with host macrophages, but in its fresh state its motility is much more explosive; it also differs from the nonpathogenic intestinal amebae (E. coli, E. nana, and others) by its nuclear characteristics and its red cell ingestion.* Under unfavorable conditions, *E. histolytica* forms a quadrinucleate cyst that survives in the outer environment. This is the infective form that reverts in the gut to the motile trophozoite after digestion of the cyst wall by gastric juice, thus completing the parasite's simple life cycle. Asymptomatic infected persons are called cyst-passers.

Entamoeba strains differ greatly in virulence; those with small, temperature-insensitive trophozoites are considered nonpathogenic. It therefore is not known what proportion of the population of cyst-passers is capable of transmitting amebic disease. In the U.S. and Europe, cyst-passers do not exceed 3 to 5% of adults and children. In 1980 only about 5000 cases of clinical intestinal amebiasis were reported in the U.S. (if, indeed, reliably identified),[223] but the trend over the last decade has been upward and there is now a resurgence among travelers, refugees, immigrants, and urban homosexuals.[224] High endemicity persists in many developing, though not necessarily tropical, communities. Mortality rates continue especially high in Mexico, Colombia, and India. Fecal contamination of food and water is the mode of transmission.

The cecum and ascending colon are affected most often, followed in order by the sigmoid, rectum, and appendix. However, in severe, full-blown cases the entire colon is involved. The amebae invade the crypts of the colonic glands and then burrow through the tunica propria, but are usually halted in their progress by the muscularis mucosae. At this level, they fan out laterally to create a minute undermined ulceration having a flask shape, i.e., a narrow neck and broad base. As the undermining progresses, the overlying surface mucosa is deprived of its blood supply, and sloughs. In this fashion, progressively larger ulcerations are produced that maintain their typical undermined shape and fairly clean bases.

The earliest amebic lesions seen in man and experimental animals are accompanied by neutrophilic responses, but **later ulcers are often notoriously poor in host inflammatory cells because the tissue destruction is due largely to liquefactive necrosis.** Yet, occasionally, advanced amebic gut lesions have vigorous inflammatory reactions, perhaps initiated by bacterial superinfection.[225] Only rarely do the ulcerations coalesce to denude entire segments of the bowel mucosa. The mucosa between ulcers is often normal or mildly inflamed, in contrast to chronic ulcerative colitis (p. 859). Penetration of the bowel wall is rare but may occur, especially in children or immunosuppressed patients. An amebic peritonitis ensues. Another less common lesion is the ameboma, a napkin-like constrictive lesion that represents a profuse granulation tissue response sometimes confused grossly and radiologically with a tumor of the colon.[226]

In about 40% of autopsy cases, amebae penetrate vessels and are drained to the liver to produce solitary, less often multiple, discrete abscesses, some exceeding 10 cm in diameter. They have a very scant inflammatory reaction in their margins and only a shaggy fibrin lining. Because of hemorrhage into the partially digested liver debris, the abscess cavities are sometimes filled with a chocolate-colored, relatively odorless, pasty material often likened to anchovy paste, but the abscess contents can be of any color and secondary bacterial infection may convert these lytic lesions into frank suppurative abscesses. Solitary abscesses are most frequent in the right lobe. Following the development of hepatic lesions the lung may become involved, either by drainage of parasites through the blood vessels or by their direct penetration through the liver capsule, diaphragm, and pleural cavities to enter the lung parenchyma, again usually on the right side. Extension into the pericardial sac from a left-sided liver abscess or the formation of bronchopleural fistulas occurs in similar fashion. In other cases, infection may spread into the kidney, stomach, and duodenum or reenter the colon. One or several abscesses may develop in the brain by embolic dissemination of the amebae. **In all sites of localization the reaction is that of local lysis of tissues accompanied by a scant inflammatory infiltrate, principally of mononuclear cells.** Rarely, amebic cutaneous ulcers arise in the margins of a surgical wound of a patient who has had intestinal surgery during an active infection, or these may spontaneously arise in the perineum of a patient with neglected ulcerative rectal lesions. Rarely, they occur on the penis as the result of anal intercourse.

Important clinical features are as follows: (1) The intestinal manifestations of amebiasis range from acute to chronic, and from mild or no discomfort to classic dysentery with tenesmus and bloody stools. Invasive colonic amebiasis is rarely painless; usually there is cramping pain. (2) There may be long intervals between the travel that led to infection and the appearance of acute symptoms, during which the patient may either be symptom free or complain of only mild episodes of alternating constipation and diarrhea. (3) Liver, lung, or brain abscesses may present as solitary lesions in the absence of intestinal symptoms. (4) One of the clinical signs of an amebic liver abscess is exquisite tenderness at its point nearest the liver capsule. (5) Lung abscesses tend to evacuate via the bronchi, leading to massive coughing-up of chocolate-colored material lacking the repulsive malodorousness of anaerobic bacterial lung abscesses. (6) A high unilateral paralyzed diaphragm with basilar pleural effusion is a valuable radiographic sign of a liver abscess on that side. (7) Punctate ulcers of the lower colon in the face of intervening areas of normal mucosa may be a good proctoscopic clue suggesting amebic colitis *but, in the final analysis, only the reliable identification of entamoebae in the lesions by an expert observer lends security to diagnosis.* A number of serologic tests, including immunofluorescence and complement fixation, have shown good sensitivity and specificity and can be of great help, but only in the invasive and extraintestinal forms of amebiasis.[227]

Severe complications of amebiasis have followed surgical intervention for presumptive appendicitis or diverticulitis.[228] Cutting through the infected tissues will disseminate the parasite unless this is prevented by vigorous concurrent antiamebic drug treatment. Drug-resistant strains, however, have recently been spreading. *Similarly, amebic gut perforation or systemic infection can follow if a patient with active colitis is given corticosteroids for presumed idiopathic ulcerative colitis.*

Balantidium coli (Table 8–7) is a large, ciliate intestinal parasite prevalent in pigs, rats, and primates. It occasionally infects man, causing lesions very similar in type to those of acute *E. histolytica* infections.[228A] Balantidiasis occurs mostly in the tropics, among malnourished individuals; in the U.S., cases have been reported from prisons and institutions for the mentally retarded.

Amebic Meningoencephalitis

Only in 1965 did it become known that the free-living ameboflagellate *Naegleria fowleri* could cause an acute meningitis by entering the arachnoid space through the perforated cribriform plate of the nose.[6] Acanthamoeba, another free-living species able to induce cytopathic effects in tissue culture,[229] also has caused sporadic cases of human meningoencephalitis, mainly in immunosuppressed patients.[230] The aggregate yearly number of such cases in the U.S. is fortunately quite small, but Naegleria can kill a healthy youngster within a few days despite all medical efforts. In amebic meningoencephalitis there is usually a history of prolonged diving into stagnant waters. In the U.S., lakes and impoundments from Virginia southward have been the main sources of infection, but in Europe chlorinated swimming pool infections have also been reported. Currently it is not clear what factors induce virulence in naegleriae, which are ordinarily innocuous and widely distributed in nature. Thermal pollution is suspected to be a factor, and if this is true the number of cases is likely to increase.

Incubation takes about five to six days. Neurologic deficit and coma progress rapidly, accompanied by fever, severe bifrontal headache, nausea, vomiting, and stiff neck. The CSF shows elevated protein, normal or low sugar, and pleocytosis as in bacterial meningitis, but red cells are copious and *part of the cell count is often contributed by the proliferating amebae, which may not be recognized by the examiner or Coulter counter.*[6]

In CSF smears or tissue sections, these amoebae microscopically resemble human cells even more than do entamoebae. They have a relatively large nucleus, small cytoplasmic mass, and may easily be mistaken for round cell infiltrates or tumor cells. However, in fresh preparations or cultures their motility is characteristic. Pathologic lesions are limited to the olfactory nerves and brain. There is clouding of the meninges with focal hemorrhages, often accompanied by extensive fibrinoid necrosis and thrombosis of blood vessels. There may also be necrosis of nerve tissue.

Several cases of chronic keratitis of the eye due to Acanthamoeba-induced ulceration have been reported in adult patients in the absence of CNS involvement and have proved difficult to cure.[231]

Giardiasis (Giardia lamblia)

Intestinal flagellates of the Giardia group infect both animals and humans; infections of cats and beavers may possibly be transmitted to humans. The human parasite, *G. lamblia,* is the world's most prevalent pathogenic gut protozoan, especially if both asymptomatic and symptomatic infections are counted. *Giardia trophozoites live in the duodenum and give rise to the only other life form, infective cysts that are intermittently shed into the stools.* Estimates of prevalence by stool examination therefore err on the low side. Recently, 15% of random sera from residents of one city in the U.S. had antibodies specific for *G. lamblia,*[232] but even in Bolivia, where more than 50% of stools contain Giardia or its cysts, only a fraction of infected people concurrently experience diarrhea, and only a small segment of the latter develop prolonged or recurrent digestive troubles or the intestinal malabsorption syndrome. *Contaminated drinking water is the usual source of cysts.* In many cities such as Leningrad and Moscow, the tourist returns home with diarrhea, while the natives seem unaffected, whether shedding Giardia cysts or not. By contrast, when a previously safe water system is contaminated, epidemics can be community wide. Such observations strongly suggest *that predisposing host factors are important in Giardia pathogenesis.*[233] Severe giardiasis is sometimes seen in patients with low serum IgA or with low overall immunoglobulin levels, but is not limited to these groups. Young children in day care centers or living in institutions have high Giardia infection rates, but again only 17% of the infected 1- to 3-year-olds have significant disease.[234] Indeed, there is evidence that the youngest children derive protection from maternal breast-feeding, but not from cow's milk. In parts of Latin America where Giardia prevalence reaches 50% or more, diarrhea and malabsorption are in fact more common in older children and adults, but other intestinal parasites and pathogens may cloud the issue. Even normal persons in these areas show blunting of intestinal villi and hypercellularity of the lamina propria that would be interpreted as malabsorptive changes in the U.S. In sum, our understanding of giardiasis remains quite limited, and even the basic issue of how the parasite damages the host gut is still unresolved.

Giardia lamblia trophozoites are pear shaped and binucleate, and in smears, when looked at en face, have a surrealistic, siren-like appearance. On cross section, however, they are sickle shaped and their concavity holds the brushlike sucker plate best seen by electron microscopy. These plates are the parasite's means of epithelial attachment. Trophozoites appear in the stools only during diarrheal episodes. At other times they are replaced by smaller, quadrinucleate ovoid cysts, sometimes mistaken for parasite eggs. Diagnostic *duodenal aspiration is much more reliable than stool examination.* An ELISA test for Giardia antigens in stools has recently become available.

Duodenal biopsies are often teeming with Giardia organisms lining the surface of the epithelial brush border, but the intestinal morphology may range from virtually normal to markedly abnormal. Most commonly there is clubbing of villi and a decreased villus-crypt ratio, with a mixed inflammatory infiltrate of the lamina propria. The brush borders of the absorptive cells appear damaged on electron microscopy.[235] Sometimes there is virtual absence of villi, resembling the atrophic stage of gluten-induced enteropathy (p. 847). In giardiasis with immunoglobulin deficiencies, follicular hypertrophy of the mucosal lymphoid tissue has been a frequent finding, but the same syndrome can occur without such changes.[136] In some cases a scarcity or absence of plasma cells in the lamina propria has been noted.

Mild indigestion or diarrhea may be the only symptoms of pathogenic Giardia infection; more suggestive is copious, watery diarrhea lasting days or weeks with flatulence and cramps followed by bulky, semisolid, malodorous stools, sometimes recurrent. Chronic giardiasis can cause malabsorption and weight loss or growth retardation as well as lactose intolerance and disaccharidase deficiency. Protein and fat loss can be considerable and vitamin B_{12} deficiency may occur,[205] but the disease is virtually never fatal. All too often the diagnosis is delayed until empirical treatment for other presumed agents has proved ineffective. *G. lamblia* responds well to several antiparasitic drugs.

Infections by Cryptosporidium and Isospora spp.

These two rare parasites can cause diarrheal and malabsorption syndromes resembling those caused by Giardia, but they belong to entirely different species. Cryptosporidium is a tiny parasite whose micro- and macrogametes, arrayed along the brush border of the gut epithelium, resemble globs of basophilic mucus (Fig. 8–41), and it therefore seems likely that this infection is often unrecognized. Most well-studied cases have occurred in immunosuppressed patients, particularly in the AIDS syndrome (p. 208).[237] Diarrhea in these cases has been chronic and debilitating, and has responded poorly to all kinds of therapy. The disease has usually been diagnosed by biopsy or electron microscopy, although the parasites can be visualized quite readily in stool filtrates by a sucrose flotation method.

Isospora belli, I. hominis and *I. natalensis* are intracellular parasites of the phylum Coccidia, widespread parasites of mammals and birds that sporadically infect the human intestine. Oocysts, the infective forms, are released into the stool, where they have occasionally been identified; in other cases, intestinal biopsy has shown the trophozoites or gametes of Isospora in the epithelial cells. Diarrheal disease ranges from acute to chronic and in a few cases has caused death by malnutrition and superinfection. Tissue eosinophilia may accompany the diarrheal picture, but eosinophilia in the blood is not a specific feature. Therapy is similar to that for Toxoplasma (p. 373).

Trichomoniasis (Trichomonas vaginalis)

The most frequent venereal parasitic infection is caused by *T. vaginalis,* a flagellate 15 to 18 μ in length, shaped like a turnip, with a single nucleus and three to four anterior flagellae. Its single posterior flagellum is provided with an axostyle and an undulating membrane, visible only on high magnification. This powerful motor system permits the organism to flit about actively when a fresh preparation from an inflamed urethra or vagina is examined microscopically. There is no cyst form; transmission is generally direct via sexual intercourse. Indirect transmission by contaminated articles is possible, but unlikely because the parasite cannot survive for long in the environment. *Optimal conditions for its long-term colonization exist in the vaginas of postpubertal women; in selected groups consulting the gynecologist, estimates have ranged up to 40%.*[238] *Immature female genitalia are refractory, probably by virtue of their fermentative bacterial flora. Infection of the male urethra, the second most common site, is less persistent but may be followed by involvement of the seminal vesicles and prostate.*

T. vaginalis is a near-commensal, producing symptoms only in a fraction of infected persons, mainly in those bearing recent infections. When genital inflammatory lesions are severe, interaction of *T. vaginalis* with bacterial pathogens must be suspected, even if many trichomonads are found. Burning, itching, and discharge are the most frequent symptoms in both males and females, especially before or during micturition. The discharge is typically described as scanty and frothy, most often noticed in the morning. Sometimes there is increased frequency of voiding. Rarely, with involvement of the posterior male urethra, seminal vesicles, or prostate, there is perineal tenderness and these organs may feel boggy on rectal examination.

Typically, there is spotty reddening and edema of the affected mucosa, sometimes with small blisters or granules, referred to as "strawberry mucosa." Histologically, the mucosa and superficial submucosa may be infiltrated by lymphocytes and plasma cells and polymorphonuclears when lesions are intense. The discharge is rarely frankly purulent as in gonorrheal or chlamydial infection. Aside from the presence of parasites, there are no specific pathologic features. The trichomonads are best seen in fresh preparations diluted with warm saline, but some authorities recommend smears stained by the Giemsa method. **When organisms are scarce, they are rarely the cause of disease.** Culture methods are available in specialized laboratories should visual inspection fail.[239]

Trichomonads are only faintly stained on Pap smears and therefore are sometimes missed. Although they have been said to contribute to the induction of cervical dysplasia or neoplasia, this correlation has not held up under rigorous study. *T. vaginalis* is curable with nitroimidazole compounds but rare resistant strains have been reported.

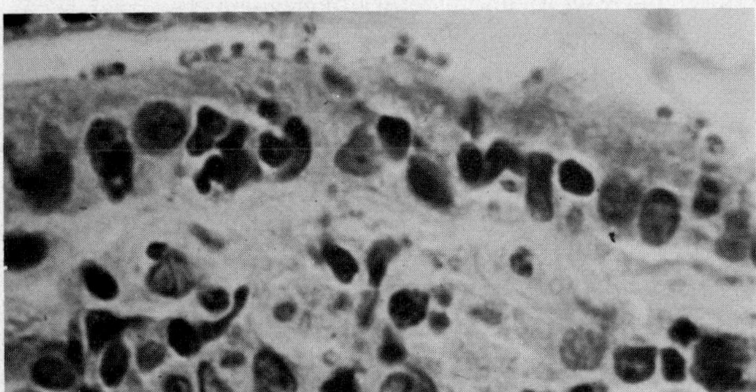

Figure 8–41. Cryptosporidium macro- and microgametes sitting on brush border of gut epithelium. Note inflammatory cells.

Pneumocystosis (Pneumocystis carinii)

This normally latent parasite causes pneumonia almost exclusively in adult immunosuppressed patients and in protein- and calorie-deficient children. In animals, latent infection by species-adapted Pneumocystis can be activated by long-term corticosteroids as may also be encountered in hospital patients. However, the infection may not always be endogenous since case clustering has been observed in the wards of children's hospitals, and since infection rates vary from hospital to hospital. Indeed, pneumocystosis was first described as an epidemic among malnourished and premature children in Europe and in Iran when it was misleadingly named "interstitial plasma cell pneumonia."[240] In the more feebly responding immunosuppressed adult, the interstitial plasma cell and macrophage component is often missing or minor.

The **trophozoites** of ***P. carinii*** are best seen by scanning electron microscopy; they graze on alveolar lining cells by means of long cytoplasmic extensions or "phylopodia,"[206] resulting in pneumocyte death, desquamation, and compensatory proliferation. The alternate **cyst form** has a cell wall stainable by silver impregnation, is cup or boat shaped, and is approximately 4 to 6 μ in size (about the size of Histoplasma fungi). Cysts are mostly extracellular but can be taken up and killed by macrophages. They are diagnostic by their central dark dots or lateral crescent profiles (Fig. 8–42). **Neither parasite form can be clearly seen in the routine H and E stain; rather, the alveolar spaces are filled by an amphophilic, foamy, amorphous material resembling proteinaceous edema fluid, composed of proliferating parasites and cell debris.** Usually there is an accompanying mild interstitial inflammatory reaction with widening of the septa, protein and fibrin exudation, escape of red cells, and sometimes the formation of hyaline membranes. These changes are reminiscent of diffuse alveolar damage (p. 714). Affected lung appears airless, red, and beefy, heightening that similarity, and occasionally there is even granuloma formation. Not infrequently there is concurrent infection by opportunistic bacteria, fungi, or viruses, especially CMV. Since pneumocystosis often supervenes as the terminal complication of other pulmonary infections or systemic diseases, its lesions vary and **it can only be diagnosed with certainty by the direct demonstration of the parasite** in bronchoscopic or open lung biopsies, with use of special stains.[241] **Parasites rarely escape from the consolidated terminal air spaces they inhabit and can only exceptionally be spotted in the sputum.**

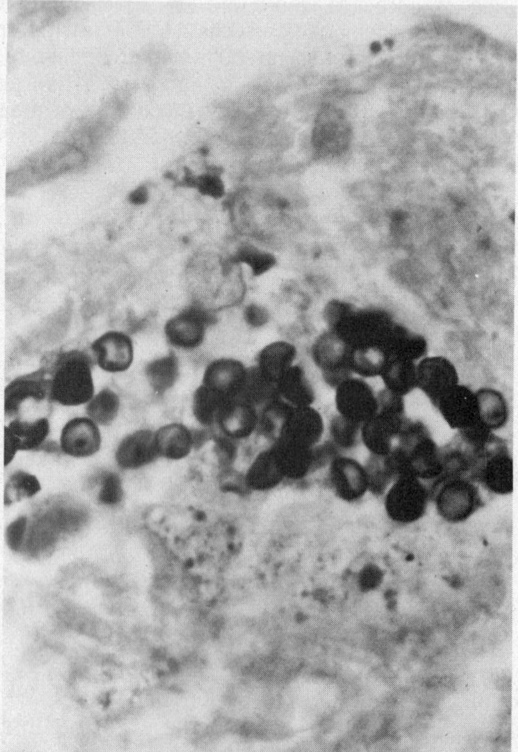

Figure 8–42. *Pneumocystis carinii* stained by methenamine silver technique. Only the cyst forms take up the stain, showing the typical cup shape and central dot. Note also typical foamy amorphous exudate filling alveolus.

Typically, this disease presents as the sudden onset of fever, dyspnea, hypoxia, and a new lung shadow on x-ray films, leading to deterioration of a previously stable and controlled patient under treatment for Hodgkin's lymphoma or another malignancy, or receiving high doses of steroids. Individuals afflicted with AIDS (p. 208) are also at risk. Less often there is also a cough. These nondescript features could herald a large variety of opportunistic lung infections besides *P. carinii.* Unfortunately, a reliable serodiagnostic test for parasite *antigen* is not yet available and the host is often too immunosuppressed to mount an appropriate *antibody* response. Pneumocystosis, therefore, sometimes goes unrecognized, resulting in a very high mortality. Early treatment can significantly improve the outlook for recovery. Nowadays, therefore, patients at risk frequently receive prophylactic drug combination therapy in an attempt to avert open lung biopsy.[242] For these reasons, classical widespread pneumocystosis is becoming an increasingly rare picture at autopsy.

BLOOD AND TISSUE PROTOZOA

*Malaria (Plasmodium sp.)**

Four species of plasmodia—*P. vivax, P. ovale, P. malariae,* and *P. falciparum*—are responsible for malaria, one of the most common ailments of mankind. Distributed throughout the tropics and subtropics, malaria is particularly prevalent in Africa and Asia where millions are infected and the heaviest toll of mortality falls on children under 4 years of age. The prevalence of the disease is directly related to that of its insect vectors, more than a dozen species of Anopheles mosquitos. Attempts to eradicate the infection have foundered, partly owing to socioeconomic factors and partly because of the unexpected proliferation of insecticide-resistant mosquitos and drug-resistant parasites. Nonetheless, the hyperendemic insect breeding grounds have been narrowed, and vectorially transmitted malaria is now extremely rare in developed countries. Malarial spread by worldwide jet travel continues, however, each case representing a potential new endemic focus. Since the parasites invade the blood they can be transmitted by transfusion or among drug addicts. In such nonendemic settings, the lack of familiarity with malaria and its many clinical facets contributes to the danger of a missed diagnosis.

All four species of Plasmodia have complex sexual cycles in their insect vectors, ending with the production of sporozoites, which are inoculated into the mammalian host by mosquito bite. Only female anophelines take blood meals and so "only the female is dangerous."

Sporozoites are antigenically distinct from all subsequent developmental parasite forms, and during their brief journey from the skin to liver cells they are vulnerable to specific antisporozoite antibodies. In an immune or vaccinated host, these antibodies may abort infection by coating the plasma membrane of the sporozoite before it can invade the host liver cell.[243] Within the hepatocyte the parasite transforms and divides (exoerythrocytic cycle), eventually to reenter the bloodstream in the form of merozoites capable of invading and multiplying in red cells. *Merozoites* are also antigenically distinct, and outside of red cells they are vulnerable to specific antibody.[244] *They initiate the intraerythrocytic asexual cycle responsible for most of the anatomic and clinical features of malaria; merozoites grow to become trophozoites, which upon division form numerous schizonts. Released by rupture of the erythrocytes, these reenter other red cells to begin a new cycle.* After a few cycles, intraerythrocytic gametocytes, i.e., male and female offspring, are added to the cyclically generated asexual forms. Although *gametocytes* are not numerous, they are relatively long-lived and are the only forms capable of initiating the insect cycle when taken up by mosquitos.

Each species of Plasmodium produces a somewhat distinctive disease pattern related in part to the timing of its asexual intraerythrocytic cycle. *P. vivax* and *P. ovale* infections are rarely fatal and are marked by fever spikes roughly 48 hours apart: *benign tertian malaria.* With *P. malariae* the spikes occur at 72-hour intervals; this infection is prone to long periods of latency: *benign quartan malaria. P. falciparum* is responsible for the highest parasitemias and for the bulk of mortality due to malaria. The fever in this pattern of infection is often irregular but may show periodicity at 48-hour intervals: *malignant tertian malaria.* In all forms the red cell destruction causes anemia and, at the same time, malarial pigment produced by the parasite's digestion of heme is released. The damaged red cells and malarial pigment are removed from the blood by the monocyte-phagocyte reticuloendothelial system, inducing splenomegaly and hepatomegaly as well as the pigmentation seen in these enlarged organs and in the bone marrow. The "malignant" nature of *P. falciparum* may relate to several factors: unlike other Plasmodia that prefer either young or older red cells, it indiscriminately parasitizes all red cells with glycophorin receptors[212] of any age, resulting in high and steeply rising parasitemias; it also induces sticky knobs in the erythrocyte membranes, which results in plugging of small vessels and tissue hypoxemia or ischemic necrosis (p. 361). This process is particularly dangerous in the small vessels of the brain.

Host factors also condition the occurrence and severity of malarial disease and even its geographic distribution. Protein-calorie malnutrition in African and Asian children compounds the systemic effects of malaria, and favors chronicity and other lethal complications. However, cerebral malaria is less common among these partly immune children than it is among nonimmune visitors.[245] Blackwater fever, a form of hemoglobinuric renal failure seen in *P. falciparum* infection, is infrequent today and may have represented the concurrence of drug or alcohol toxicity or possibly other factors with severe malaria. Sickle cell hemoglobin (S) tends to limit parasitemia, forcing the parasite to leave the red cell as its heme starts sickling. Endemic malaria is therefore less lethal in the hemoglobin (S) heterozygote (p. 618) and its geographic distribution mirrors that of the sickle cell genes. There is suggestive, but no conclusive, evidence that G6PD deficiency may also offer some protection although it also induces hemolysis when antimalarial drugs are given.[246] The Duffy blood group factor appears to be necessary for *P. vivax* red cell penetration, and black persons without that red cell receptor are therefore refractory to benign tertian malaria.[247]

Few observations are available on the morphologic changes in the nonfatal forms of malaria caused by ***P. vivax, P. malariae,*** and ***P. ovale.*** In ***P. falciparum*** infection, depending on its duration, **the spleen is markedly enlarged** and may exceed 1000 gm. During the acute stage of the disease, the splenic enlargement is moderate and the substance congested or hemorrhagic. The capsule is thin and rupture of the spleen may occur, but is rare. As the disease becomes more chronic there is increased cellularity and fibrosis, creating a solid enlargement. The capsule is thickened and on cross section the splenic substance is gray or black and brittle, traditionally described as "ague cake."

Histologically, in the acute stages there is marked splenic congestion along with hypertrophy and phagocytic activity of the reticuloendothelial cells and macrophages. Parasites may be seen within the trapped red cells. With chronicity, the congestion increases and the phagocytic cells become more prominent, sometimes forming solid masses. They are laden with a finely divided brown-black malarial pigment called hemozoin. The pigment has a granular appearance, does not react with stains for ferrous iron, and is faintly birefringent. It resembles hematin, a product of red cell autolysis sometimes seen in congested organs. Accompanying the phagocytosis of pigment there is engulfment of parasites, leukocytic debris, and red cell debris. In the late stages of malaria, as the spleen continues to enlarge, the fibrous trabeculae thicken as the organ hardens and blackens.[245]

The liver is likewise enlarged in malaria. In acute malaria, this enlargement is only moderate and is accompanied by considerable hyperemia. As the infection becomes chronic or reinfections occur, the increase in size progresses and the organ becomes more firm and pigmented. The principal changes are found in the **Kupffer cells,** which are enlarged and hyperplastic; these become heavily laden with malarial pigment, parasites, and cellular debris (Fig. 8–43); some pigment may also be found in the parenchymal cells. The changes in the bone marrow and lymph nodes are of similar nature. Pigmented phagocytic cells may be found dispersed throughout the body in the subcutaneous tissues, lungs, and other sites, particularly when infection has saturated the principal reticuloendothelial organs.

The kidneys are often enlarged and congested. A dusting of pigment is often present in the glomeruli, and the tubules may contain hemoglobin casts, particularly in falciparum malaria.

In malignant falciparum malaria, there may be ex-

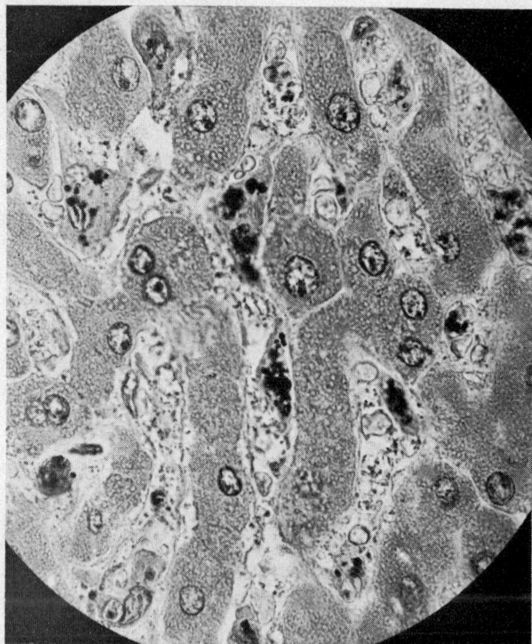

Figure 8–43. Malaria in liver with pigment-laden Kupffer cells.

treme congestion of the brain vessels so that they become plugged with parasitized red cells, each cell containing a single dot of hemozoin pigment (Fig. 8–44). About these vessels, there are ring hemorrhages that are probably related to local hypoxia incident to the vascular stasis. Small focal inflammatory reactions (called malarial or "Dürck's granulomas") may occur about these vessels. These granulomas consist of a small focus of ischemic necrosis surrounded by a microglial reaction. With more severe hypoxia, there is degeneration of ganglion cells, focal ischemic softening, and occasionally a scant inflammatory infiltrate in the meninges. Nonspecific focal hypoxic lesions in the heart may be induced by the progressive anemia and circulatory stasis in chronically infected patients. In some, the myocardium also shows focal interstitial inflammatory infiltration.[248] Usually the pathophysiologic disturbances in malignant tertian malaria far outweigh the anatomic abnormalities found. Thus, in the nonimmune patient, pulmonary edema or shock with DIC are frequent causes of death, sometimes in the absence of other characteristic lesions.

The popular image of malaria is limited to its classical, febrile paroxysm as might be present in a nonimmune adult visitor to the tropics. After an incubation period of one to two weeks and three or four days of a nondescript malaise or fever, the disease declares itself by mounting fever to 40°C or higher, accompanied by chills and rigors. There is dry flushing of the skin, restlessness, intractable headache and body aches, and sometimes delirium. A few hours later, sweating begins, the fever declines, and lassitude follows. After a day or two of respite another paroxysm begins. In developed countries this classical pattern is largely seen in returned travelers or in foreign visitors with severe acute *P. falciparum* infections (sometimes modified by ineffective previous drug prophylaxis). It may also occur with transfusion or addict malaria or during a late relapse of a previously treated chronic latent benign tertian or quartan malaria, especially after splenectomy or immunosuppression.

Ironically, the classical clinical picture accounts for only a fraction of the spectrum of malarial disease. Latent endemic infection is far more frequent, particularly in the wet tropics where malaria transmission is constant, such as in West Africa.[245] Here, the survivors of early childhood infection have developed partial immunity and have low parasitemias, with or without hepatosplenomegaly or mild febrile episodes. In countries with alternating dry and rainy seasons, such as western Latin America, the disease attack rate increases along with the breeding mosquitos (the estivoautumnal pattern) even though few attacks are of the classical type. Overt disease in endemic areas may present in many ways. In young children it can easily be mistaken for pneumonia, diarrheal disease, or typhoid fever. Older children are the chief victims of the relatively rare nephrotic syndrome (p. 1011) associated principally with *P. malariae* infection.[249] Alternatively, endemic malaria may present as a chronic anemia with hepatosplenomegaly; as a protracted, febrile disorder of unknown cause; as renal shutdown; or as the insidious onset of jaundice and hepatic failure.

Catastrophic *P. falciparum* infection is most likely to develop in nonimmune teenagers or adults and in splenectomized individuals. This often lethal form of the disease is characterized by any or all of the following features: cerebral involvement with delirium progressing to coma; hypothermic shock (algid malaria); pulmonary edema; DIC; renal shutdown with hemoglobinuria; and liver failure.

Whatever the clinical pattern, the mainstay of diagnosis is identification of parasites in the blood smear. Indeed, there is a clear correlation between

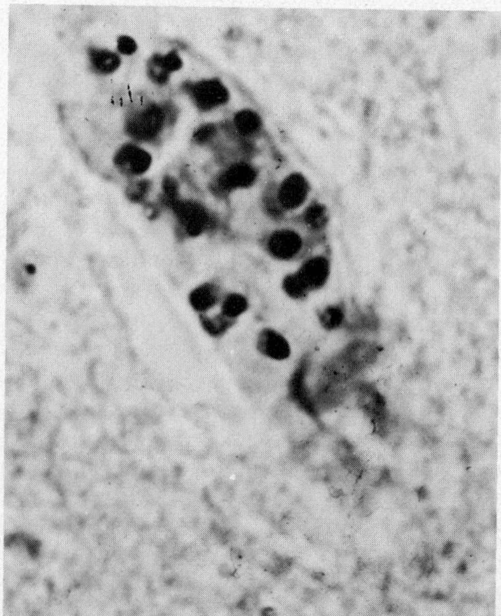

Figure 8–44. Cerebral malaria. High-power view of *P. falciparum* trophozoites, each with a pigment dot, occupying all red cells of a distended brain capillary.

severity of illness and level of blood parasite count. Differentiation among the four species of Plasmodia is today a specialized skill that depends on subtle morphologic features of the parasites. Many drugs have been developed for the prevention and treatment of malaria, but the Plasmodia have been equally adept at developing drug resistance.[250] Recently a culture method for the blood forms of the plasmodia has been devised and is being used for the production of purified and cloned parasites and their antigens. This Trager culture method also permits sensitivity testing analogous to that employed with bacteria but, with appropriate geographic information, effective therapy can often be started before drug sensitivities have been measured. Treatment of malaria is no longer the simple matter it was in the days before the development of drug-resistant strains. Malaria vaccine research has progressed, but its ultimate success still remains uncertain.[251]

*Babesiosis (Babesia sp.)**

B. microti, *a distant relative of the Plasmodia, causes an acute, sometimes prolonged illness that may be incapacitating but is rarely fatal.* It is seen mostly along the Eastern seaboard and on the islands of Nantucket and Martha's Vineyard. The cattle parasites *B. bovis* and *B. bigemina* can also sporadically infect asplenic humans to produce a rapidly fatal febrile infection with hemolysis and renal failure; these are rare infections, but they occur worldwide.

The first human *B. microti* infection was recognized in 1969 and less than 100 symptomatic cases have been reported to date, all but a few in persons older than 40 years.[252] Serologic surveys indicate, however, that asymptomatic infection may be widespread among residents and visitors of all ages in the Northeastern summer resort areas. *B. microti* is transmitted by the bite of the tiny nymphal stage of the hard tick *Ixodes dammini,* whose adult stage feeds on deer and field mice. Ticks can transmit the parasite transovarially. Nymphs are active between May and September; human disease trails this timetable by about one month. Man is thus an accidental and often unaware victim of a natural infection cycle. *B. microti,* once introduced, invades the red blood cells and can be mistaken for *P. falciparum,* but does not produce any pigment. Infections have been acquired by blood or platelet transfusion from asymptomatic donors. Since donors are currently not serologically screened for Babesia, the scope of babesiasis as a cause of posttransfusion fever is unclear.

Headache, fever, chills, myalgia, and fatigue suggesting a "summer flu" may be the only symptoms of babesiasis. The fever usually lasts no longer than one week and recovery is spontaneous but slow. Severe disease, mostly in splenectomized patients or in those debilitated by chronic diseases, can be prolonged or recurrent and can be accompanied by vomiting, hemolysis, jaundice, hemoglobinuria, renal failure, even coma and death. *The level of the* B. microti *parasitemia is a good indication of the severity of infection;* only 1% of erythrocytes are infected in mild cases, but rapidly rising parasitemia above 30% of red cells is seen in infections that become life threatening. *B. bovis,* with its 60% or higher lethality, resembles severe *B. microti* infection.

In fatal cases the anatomic findings are mainly those related to shock and hypoxia, and include jaundice, hepatic necrosis, acute renal tubular necrosis, hemolysis, hemoglobinuria, anemia, and, sometimes, hemorrhagic manifestations.[253] There is no rash or primary eschar that might suggest a tick connection. Diagnosis must be made microscopically by Giemsa-stained blood smears. The intraerythrocytic organisms are tiny and difficult to see on routinely stained tissue sections.

African Trypanosomiasis (Trypanosoma rhodesiense, gambiense)*

The name sleeping sickness by which human infections with the African trypanosomes *T. brucei rhodesiense* and *T. brucei gambiense* are known more aptly describes the condition of medical students during a postprandial lecture. In truth, *African trypanosomal disease covers several clinical stages: (1) an acute febrile attack with purpura and DIC; (2) chronic, episodic fever with lymph node swelling and splenomegaly; and eventually (3) progressive brain dysfunction leading to cachexia and death.* All three disease stages may appear sequentially, or only the chronic stages may be apparent. *T. rhodesiense* infection is often acute and virulent and its tsetse fly *(Glossina)* vector prefers the Savannah plains of East Africa; *T. gambiense* infection tends to be chronic and its vector thrives best in the West African bush. Although Gambian and Rhodesian sleeping sickness have been described as different diseases, there is some overlap as well as regional variation in their disease manifestations. Not surprisingly, both infections have turned up on occasion on the "tropical island" of Manhattan, one of the world's crossroads. All the rare U.S. cases are imported. The vector species Glossina exists only in Africa where its bite also transmits *T. brucei brucei,* which is prevalent among wild animals and cattle and is the ancestor species to which humans have become refractory. *T. brucei* ravages cattle and sheep over millions of square miles of Africa. Wild animals can also serve as reservoirs for *T. rhodesiense,* whereas *T. gambiense* is largely a vector carried from person to person. Tsetse flies seem to be angered by noisy Land Rovers, and safari hunters are known to be at risk.[254]

Bloodstream trypanosomes (trypomastigotes) are fusiform, flagellate, motile protozoa marked by an undulating membrane along the length of the organism. After inoculation of salivary forms by the tsetse, the parasites metamorphose and proliferate at the local site and gain entry to the lymphatics and bloodstream to induce a parasitemia. Within the blood they become vulnerable to opsonizing antibodies specific for their glycoprotein surface antigens. However, these parasites are able to generate a seemingly endless sequence of surface variant antigens, each composed of a single glycoprotein, so that a successor clone begins proliferating before antibody has eradicated its predecessors. This genetically programmed sequence[255] explains the persistent bouts of fever. The chronic assault on the host immune system, especially on the B cells, results in lymphoreticular hyperplasia with lymphadenopathy and splenomegaly. Concomitantly there is a striking IgM hypergammaglobulinemia. Only part of this immunoglobulin is directed specifically against trypanosomal antigens. Much of it may be an expression of polyclonal B-cell activation. Cellular immunity is also weakened.[256] Nonetheless, trypanosomes are vulnerable to neutrophil and macrophage destruction because they lack catalases and other scavengers of oxygen radicals produced by the phagocytes. The precise mechanism of trypanosomal-induced tissue injury is unknown. Antigen-antibody complexes may release kinins and other mediators of inflammation, which may contribute.[257] The release of lysosomal enzymes from degenerating phagocytes could also be a factor.

A large, red, rubbery chancre may form at the site of the insect bite; it is more frequently seen in Rhodesian trypanosomiasis. It teems with parasites and shows intense inflammatory infiltration, largely mononuclear, as well as vasodilatation and interstitial edema. With advancing chronicity of the disease, the lymph nodes and spleen enlarge owing to hyperplasia, accompanied by an infiltrate of lymphocytes, plasma cells, and macrophages that must ultimately dispose of the killed parasites. Trypanosomes are small, difficult to visualize except in "overstained" Giemsa sections. They tend to concentrate in capillary loops such as the choroid plexus and glomeruli. In time, and more often in prolonged Gambian disease, the parasites breach the blood-brain barrier and invade the CNS, to induce initially a leptomeningitis extending into the perivascular Virchow-Robin spaces and eventually a demyelinating panencephalitis. Particularly prominent in all sites of leukocytic infiltration are plasma cells containing glycoprotein globules, often referred to as flame cells or Mott cells (named after the first author to describe these brain changes). Severe acute trypanosomiasis may be followed by DIC, by an interstitial myocarditis, or by lethal bacterial superinfection. Chronic disease leads to progressive cachexia, and these patients, devoid of energy and normal mentation, literally waste away.

The onset of clinical manifestations is more frequently acute in the Rhodesian illness than in the Gambian variety, in which successive bouts of fever are spaced by latent periods of variable length, sometimes months to years. Until CNS manifestations appear the disease is often confused with other chronic infections, but can be diagnosed by visualizing the parasites. During early parasitemia these are easily seen on blood smears. In more chronic stages they may be detectable in the bone marrow, lymph nodes, and spleen, though usually not in great numbers. When parasites cannot be found, the characteristic IgM hyperglobulinemia is of some diagnostic value. Usually there is also anemia, granulocytopenia, and an elevated sedimentation rate. In most cases, if the patient with Gambian disease survives long enough, the meningoencephalitic phase makes its appearance. There is headache and lethargy that over the course of time progresses to a pathetic, vegetative state: drooping eyelids; open, mute mouth; total lack of response to external stimuli; and finally, death in coma. The devastating cerebral manifestations have been attributed to generation of phenylpyruvate and indol-3 ethanol by the trypanosomes in the brain.[257A] Early African trypanosomiasis is treatable but there is no satisfactory cure for advanced sleeping sickness, although organic arsenicals are sometimes employed to halt further progression.

INTRACELLULAR PROTOZOA

Chagas' Disease (Trypanosoma cruzi)*

Also called American trypanosomiasis, Chagas' disease ranges from Texas to Argentina. Its acute stage may be asymptomatic or marked by fever and acute myocarditis. Its chronic phase results in progressive cardiac failure and is the most important cause of death from heart disease in several Latin American countries. In Brazil, but not elsewhere, chronic Chagas' disease is also a cause of megaesophagus (p. 798) and megacolon (p. 855). An autochthonous case of Chagas' disease has been reported from California.

Dogs and wild animals, especially the opossum and armadillo, are hosts of *T. cruzi* strains, but humans are the principal source of human disease. The parasite is transmitted by "kissing bugs" (triatomidae) that hide in the cracks of rickety houses and feed on their sleeping inhabitants at night while contaminating their bites by defecation. Infection can also be acquired by transplacental passage, transfusion, or laboratory accident.

T. cruzi, a fusiform hemoflagellate with an undulating membrane, circulates but does not multiply within the bloodstream. Rather, it invades tissue cells and assumes a leishmanial form, which then divides, eventually to reinvade the blood. Progressive multiplication within the parasitized cells produces intracellular pseudocysts packed with organisms (Fig. 8–45). As the disease progresses, parasitemia decreases but the tissue forms persist, causing either progressive acute infection, latent infection of indefinite duration, or latency followed by chronic infection.

In *acute disease*, damage results from direct invasion of cells by the parasites and from the consequent inflammatory changes. An erythematous swelling—the chagoma—may appear at the site of the bite, only to regress spontaneously. Rarely, the portal of entry may be the conjunctiva, producing unilateral edema, preauricular lymphadenopathy, and sometimes exophthalmos (Romaña's sign). Transient parasitemia undoubtedly follows all infections, including those with seemingly localized reactions, yet many individuals never show any further manifestations other than detectable antitrypanosomal antibodies. If acute Chagas disease does develop it is marked by high parasitemia and fever, principally with cardiac involvement, but sometimes with generalized lymphadenopathy or splenomegaly also. Acute cha-

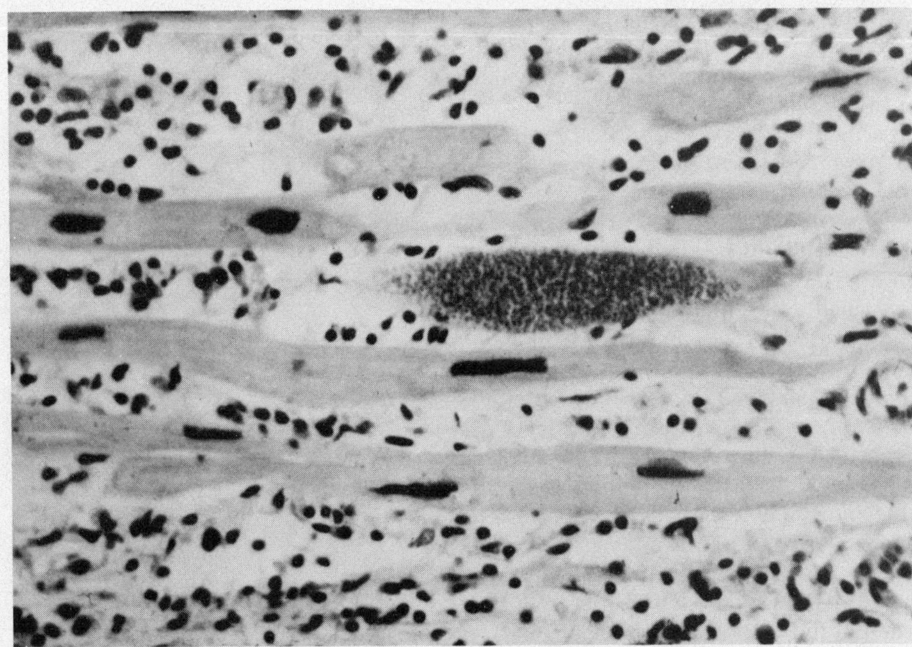

Figure 8–45. Chagasic myocarditis showing *T. cruzi*–filled pseudocyst, interstitial edema, and mononuclear infiltration.

gasic myocarditis may be mild, detectable only by transient ECG changes, but in severe disease rapidly progressive cardiac dilatation and failure may ensue. Meningitis rarely occurs, mainly in newborns and young children. Death follows in about 5 to 10% of acute cases, generally from involvement of the heart. More often the febrile reaction and cardiac changes slowly regress as parasites virtually disappear from both the blood and tissues, and a latent period of variable duration follows.

Chronic disease usually arises in young and mature adults and presents mainly as the progressive onset of cardiac failure. At this late stage the parasitemia remains scanty, and the organisms within the tissues are likewise often vanishing in number and difficult to find in histologic sections. Nonetheless, there is striking inflammatory infiltration of the myocardium and sometimes of the skeletal muscles, completely out of proportion to the demonstrable parasites. The pathogenesis of chronic Chagas' disease is unknown. An autoimmune reaction mediated by cytotoxic T cells and by antibodies, reactive with human endocardial, myocardial, and striated muscle cells and endothelium (EV1 antibodies) has been postulated.[258] However, it is not clear whether these immune reactions are the cause or the result of the tissue damage.

In **lethal acute chagasic myocarditis** the anatomic changes are diffusely distributed throughout the heart. Clusters of leishmanial forms swell individual myocardial fibers to create intracellular pseudocysts. There is focal myocardial cell necrosis accompanied by extensive, dense, acute interstitial inflammatory infiltration throughout the myocardium (Fig. 8–45), and there is often four-chamber cardiac dilatation.

In **chronic Chagas' disease** the heart is typically dilated, rounded in shape, and increased in size and weight. Often there are mural thrombi that, in about one-half of autopsy cases, have given rise to pulmonary or systemic emboli or infarctions. Histologically, there is interstitial and perivascular inflammatory infiltration composed mainly of lymphocytes, plasma cells, and monocytes. It is heaviest in the right bundle branch of the cardiac conduction system.[259] Scattered foci of myocardial cell necrosis can sometimes be seen. There is also interstitial fibrosis, especially toward the apex of the left ventricle, which may undergo aneurysmal dilatation and thinning (a suggestive, but not pathognomonic, feature of chronic chagasic myocarditis). In the Brazilian endemic foci, as many as one-half of the patients with lethal carditis also have dilatation of the esophagus or colon, apparently related to damage to the intrinsic innervation of these organs. However, at the late stages when such changes appear, parasites cannot be found within these ganglia.

As many as 10% of the rural population in endemic foci suffer from chronic chagasic heart disease. Symptoms and signs range from right bundle branch block to progressive cardiac decompensation or thromboembolic manifestations, and to sudden death without previous warning. At this late stage organisms can rarely be identified in the blood, but complement-fixing antibodies can usually be demonstrated. A more laborious, but sometimes necessary, diagnostic measure is xenodiagnosis, i.e., identification of parasites in laboratory-bred triatomids two weeks after they have been allowed to feed on the patient's skin. New drugs have improved the outlook for patients with acute infection, but none have proved of value in chronic disease.[260]

*Leishmaniasis (Leishmania sp.)**

All clinical forms of leishmaniasis are caused by a single parasite stage, the tiny ($< 3\ \mu$), nonflagellated intracellular amastigote, recognizable in tissue sections or smears by its two basophilic dots, its nucleus, and the kinetoplast, the latter sometimes bar shaped. All are transmitted by the bite of sandflies, i.e., by diverse Phlebotomus sp. in the old world, or by Lutzomyia sp. in the new. Nevertheless, *the disease manifestations caused by these organisms vary greatly by parasite species, continent, and endemic region of origin.* Until the taxonomy of the leishmaniae can be further defined through monoclonal antibodies or kinetoplast DNA hybridization studies,[261] the traditional classification will be followed here, which differentiates visceral *leishmaniasis or kala-azar* (caused by *L. donovani)* from *mucocutaneous leishmaniasis or espundia* (due to *L. brasiliensis*) and *cutaneous leishmaniasis or tropical sore* (due to *L. tropica* and *L. mexicana*). All these infections occur largely in poor people in remote locations, and so prevention and treatment have fallen behind those of other parasitic infections. The relatively rare imported cases seen in the U.S. occur in anthropologists, Peace Corps workers, and occasionally the overseas military.

Kala-azar (Hindi for "black fever") results from the widespread invasion of the mononuclear-phagocyte system by *L. donovani.* It is an insidiously developing but severe systemic disease marked by hepatosplenomegaly, lymphadenopathy, pancytopenia, fever, and weight loss. The reticuloendothelial blockade produced by overloading the phagocytic cells with leishmaniae, coupled with pancytopenia, predispose patients to intercurrent bacterial infections, the usual cause of death. Hemorrhages related to thrombocytopenia may also be fatal.

At autopsy the spleen, liver, and lymph nodes are all enlarged. Often the spleen reaches gigantic size (up to 3 kg); lymph nodes may achieve a diameter of 4 to 5 cm; the hepatomegaly is generally less extreme. In all these organs the phagocytic cells are markedly swollen and stuffed with leishmaniae (Fig. 8–46). The flooding of the spleen with infected macrophages, accompanied by marked plasmocytosis, obscures the organ's normal architecture. In the late stages of the disease the liver becomes increasingly and irreversibly fibrotic. Phagocytic cells crowd the bone marrow and may also be found in the lungs, GI tract, kidneys, pancreas, testes, and other organs. Often there is hyperpigmentation of the skin in the extremities, accounting for the Indian designation of this condition. In the kidneys, immune complex deposition as well as mesangial proliferation are sometimes observed,[262] and in advanced cases amyloid deposition is frequent.

Usually no local lesions occur at the site of the sandfly bite, but in African disease there may be a "primary chancre," which generally regresses before systemic manifestations insidiously develop, sometimes a year later. Periods of spiking fever ensue, followed by remissions and relapses. Most patients come to medical attention at an advanced stage of disease showing hepatosplenomegaly, lymphadenopathy, and pancytopenia. Serum albumin is usually low, *globulin is markedly elevated, predominantly the IgG fraction* (as opposed to IgM elevation in African trypanosomiasis). Clotting abnormalities are frequent. Patients who recover from systemic *kala-azar,* usually by treatment, may develop extensive skin involvement (post–Kala-azar dermal leishmanoids) manifested as disfiguring papular or nodular lesions reminiscent of severe lepromatous leprosy. Histologically, these nodules contain numerous histiocytes stuffed with *L. donovani.* Unfortunately, such cases are among the worst responders to chemotherapy.

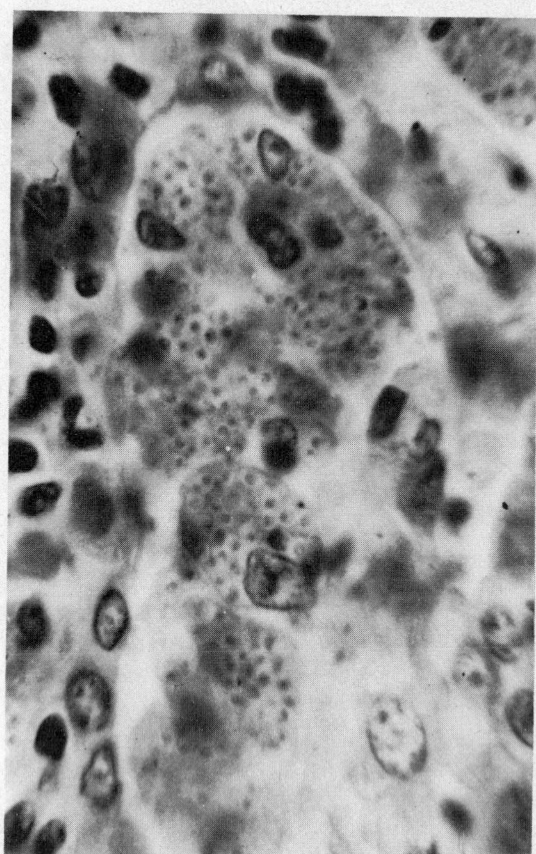

Figure 8–46. Visceral leishmaniasis (kala-azar). Phagocytes within a lymph node are laden with Leishmania.

Diagnosis is best achieved by the demonstration of *L. donovani* in smears, tissue sections, or cultures in special biphasic media; skin testing with leishmanin is used to evaluate host reactivity, but may be negative in patients with advanced disease.

Parasite strain is important in determining the clinical manifestations of kala-azar and its patterns of transmission. Thus, in the Near East, the Mediterranean basin, and North China, visceral leishmaniasis affects mainly rural children, and dogs are the main reservoir host *(L. infantum).* Brazilian infection is also dog related, but the parasite differs biologically from that of the old world. In India, much of kala-azar is urban, young adults are mainly affected, and man himself is the principal reservoir.

Mucocutaneous leishmaniasis is endemic in the hinterlands of several South American countries, including Brazil,[263] and is caused by several species or strains of New World leishmaniae. It begins as a chronic skin ulcer (tropical sore) of the leg, forearm, trunk, or face. Before or after the ulcer regresses, sometimes even years later, *secondary moist, ulcerating, or nonulcer-*

ating lesions develop around or close to the mucocutaneous junctions; these may localize in the larynx, nasal septum, anal zone, or vulva, and can be destructive and disfiguring. These lesions undergo spontaneous exacerbations or remissions and usually last for a long time. Their histopathology varies with their activity and duration. Initially, a mixed inflammatory infiltrate with numerous parasite-containing histiocytes is seen together with many lymphocytes and plasma cells. Later the tissue reaction becomes granulomatous and the number of parasites declines; it is therefore important to sample for parasites at or near the raised growing border of ulcerated lesions where they are likeliest to persist.[264] Giemsa-stained impression smears prepared from biopsy specimens are likeliest to show leishmaniae. Eventually, the lesions remit and scar. A disturbing feature of mucocutaneous leishmaniasis is that even while a treated or untreated lesion seems to be healing, leishmaniae may remain present and reactivation may occur after long intervals. Although the granulomatous host response is associated with containment of the infection, it also aggravates the tissue destruction. The role of host immunoregulation in leishmaniasis is less well understood than in leprosy, with which it otherwise shares many analogies.[265]

Cutaneous leishmaniasis exists in both the Old and New Worlds. Oriental tropical ulcer is caused by *Leishmania tropica* and *is a relatively mild and localized disease compared with the mucocutaneous variant.* It is seen in much of Southern Asia and parts of Africa. An analogous chronic, self-healing cutaneous ulcer occurs in parts of Latin America, and typically affects the ear, i.e., the preferred biting site of the local sandflies. American cutaneous leishmaniasis is caused by *L. mexicana,* whose southernmost territory overlaps with that of *L. brasiliensis.* These two parasite species can now be distinguished by an ingenious new test involving hybridization of kinetoplast DNA.[261]

Tropical ulcers are single and are usually located on exposed parts of the body; after a long incubation period, they begin as an itching papule surrounded by induration; this turns into a shallow, slowly expanding ulcer with irregular borders; healing is even slower than onset, but *most lesions involute within six months without requiring treatment.* Microscopically, the tissue reaction is granulomatous. Parasites are scarce in fully-developed lesions, though detectable by culture, and cutaneous Leishmania hypersensitivity is strong. Problems arise in endemic foci where the local strains of *L. tropica* or *L. mexicana* are quite virulent and may cause expanding or recurrent lesions that require treatment. Several such foci exist in Africa, Southern Russia and in Brazil.

Diffuse cutaneous leishmaniasis is the rarest form of dermal infection, thus far found only in Ethiopia and adjacent East Africa and in Venezuela, Brazil, and Mexico. *It too begins as a single skin nodule, but continues spreading until the entire body may be covered by bizarre nodular lesions, some resembling keloids or large verrucae, some imitating the nodules of lepromatous leprosy.* These lesions do not ulcerate. Microscopically, they show vast aggregates of foamy macrophages containing myriads of leishmanial organisms. Characteristically, the patients are anergic not only to leishmanin, but also to other skin antigens; because of their similarity to lepromatous patients, they are often erroneously sent to leprosaria. These infections have been notoriously difficult to cure by drug treatment. This form of leishmaniasis seems to be closely associated with impaired T-cell immunity, but whether it is causal or secondary is not clear. There is also some evidence that diffuse cutaneous leishmaniasis may be caused by specific strains of *L. mexicana* or perhaps by a separate species of Leishmania.[263]

Toxoplasmosis (Toxoplasma gondii)

T. gondii is a coccidian parasite that infects many animal species. Its definitive hosts are domestic cats and some wild felines, in whose intestines sexual reproduction results in the formation of fertile oocysts. When shed in the feces these are highly infective for most animals, including humans. The tissue forms of *T. gondii* are $3 \times 6\ \mu$, bow-shaped *tachyzoites* and larger *cysts* containing many *bradyzoites.* These can also transmit the infection to humans or animals, chiefly by ingestion of uncooked meat.[266] The versatile life cycle of this parasite has made it prevalent throughout the animal world. Human infection is also worldwide and tends to be nearly universal in the humid tropics, but somewhat rarer in dry or cold climates. *In the U.S., between 15 and 50% of the population have antibodies to T. gondii, with regional variations.*

T. gondii is delicately adapted to intracellular survival in its many hosts and therefore rarely causes disease. In immunocompetent adult persons, toxoplasmosis is usually mild and self-terminating and the bulk of infections remain subclinical. *Most of the toll is borne by fetuses, babies, and immunosuppressed individuals of any age.*[218, 266] In these predisposed groups toxoplasmosis can be devastating, causing severe CNS damage or blindness. For these reasons, pregnant women should avoid contact with infected or potentially infected cats and abstain from uncooked meat. Entering through the gut, *T. gondii* spreads systemically, to penetrate into virtually any type of host cell, phagocytic or not. The parasite initially spreads from cell to cell as a tachyzoite; later it multiplies inside single cells to form microscopic cysts that can remain dormant for long periods. Small numbers of these cysts are formed in subclinical infections, detectable only by subinoculation into toxoplasma-free mice. *In infections of normal adults, it is therefore futile to look for parasites in tissue sections.* By contrast, in newborns and the immunosuppressed, as the infection mounts, myriad tachyzoites can usually be found in the lesions. Examined under oil, they reveal their characteristic sickle-shaped contour and tiny single nucleus, distinct from the double basophilic dots of the Trypanosoma-Leishmania family. Even more distinctive, but few in number, are the cysts that represent dead "nurse" cells filled with hundreds of bradyzoites. Toxoplasma is undetectable in blood or body fluids, but *high or rising antibody titers can be demonstrated by immunofluorescence or the Sabin-Feldman dye test.* In newborn infections, specific IgM antibodies are especially significant since they are less likely to have been passively transferred from the mother.

Several clinical forms of toxoplasmosis are recognized. (1) Acute infection in the normal adult commonly manifests itself as lymphadenopathy with or without fever, mimicking the onset of a lymphoma or a viral infection. The diagnosis is usually suggested by examination of an excised lymph node. (2) Found in infants and children, but rarely in normal adults, is the severe acute febrile form with evidence of pneumonia, liver dysfunction, or even myocarditis. (3) Maternal infection during early pregnancy may be entirely asymptomatic but placental involvement can result in stillbirth, or neonatal jaundice, pneumonia, myocarditis, or encephalitis, often with lethal results. Nonfatal infection of the fetus leads to brain damage, hydrocephalus, mental retardation, seizures, deafness, or other permanent neurologic deficits. (4) Activation of a dormant Toxoplasma infection in an immunosuppressed individual most frequently expresses itself as an acute, progressive encephalitis that, because of the rapidity of onset of coma, may remain clinically unrecognized. (5) Toxoplasma retinochoroiditis that can lead to blindness and glaucoma is a rare complication of chronic toxoplasmosis, sometimes seen in corticosteroid-treated individuals.

The morphologic pattern most often seen in otherwise normal adults is toxoplasma lymphadenitis. It is suggested by the triad of follicular hyperplasia, sinus histiocytosis, and scattered focal accumulations of small numbers of epithelioid-type macrophages not forming well-defined granulomas. The disorder is more frequent in young women than in males, and cervical lymph nodes, especially those in the posterior neck, are most often affected.[267] Once suggested, the diagnosis can be confirmed by serologic titer. The disease is self-terminating. If the infection reverts to a chronic phase, the hazard to a fetus born later is minor compared with that of maternal infection acquired during pregnancy.

Neonatal toxoplasmosis is characterized by destructive lesions in multiple organs, notably the brain. Similar, but usually less destructive, lesions occur in the **severe form of acute toxoplasmosis,** rarely seen in the normal adult. In the CNS, microglial nodules with many tachyzoites appear, particularly about the ventricles and aqueduct, followed by extensive necrosis, vascular thrombosis, and intense inflammation. Obstruction of the foramina is frequent, resulting in hydrocephalus. If the infant survives long enough, these lesions eventually calcify. As the disease persists, Toxoplasma cysts frequently develop in the nervous tissue. In the infant, brain changes are often accompanied by liver cell necrosis and sometimes by adrenal necrosis. The lung and heart may also be focally necrotic and inflamed. There is extramedullary hematopoiesis.

Cysts in the brain are also a frequent feature in the ***Toxoplasma* encephalitis of immunosuppressed patients.** These cysts may rupture and release swarms of bradyzoites to excite a microglial nodular reaction. Other organs, including the myocardium, may also show scattered parasites and focal inflammatory mononuclear infiltrates.[216]

In ***Toxoplasma* chorioretinitis,** destruction of the retina by tachyzoites is accompanied by a granulomatous reaction in the choroid and sclera, perhaps because the chronicity of the lesion permits the cellular hypersensitivity response to express itself.

Because of the huge disparity between the number of persons infected by Toxoplasma and the sporadic overt illnesses it causes, this parasite is rarely identified as the cause of its various protean manifestations. Direct demonstration of *T. gondii* in tissue, the definitive diagnostic confirmation, is rarely achieved during the life of the patient when it is most needed. It is therefore prudent to obtain and compare the specific antibody titers at time of admission to the hospital, at the acute stage, and after some time interval for specific antibody titers whenever this infection is suspected.[218, 266] Adult toxoplasmosis is treatable by a combination of drugs, but the damage to the fetus is irreversible.

HELMINTHIC DISEASES

Helminths are the largest and most highly evolved and accomplished endoparasites of man because they rely on the longevity of individual worms rather than on their multiplication inside the host. Procreation is by eggs or larvae, which must be cycled through the environment or through intermediate hosts before humans can be infected again. Helminths have strict host specificities either for a definitive species in whom sexual reproduction takes place, or for their intermediate hosts or vector in whom reproduction is asexual. They achieve only stunted development in unsuitable hosts, e.g., when humans are infected with animal filariae.[268] Each species of parasitic helminth has its own intricately designed life cycle, seemingly fragile in its dependence on human or animal behavior, yet effective enough in some cases to maintain infections in millions of people.[269] Individual worm burdens in humans tend to be stable and long-lasting. Even reinfection does not often result in linear increases because the helminth-infected host builds up an immunity or because establishment of a single worm interferes with the development of others (e.g., the solitary pig tapeworm, *Taenia solium*). Under endemic conditions, most persons harbor a few worms and are free of disease; only a minority becomes heavily infected and ill. The enormous global prevalence figures reported—400 million infections with Ascaris, and 250 million with schistosomes—must therefore be viewed as representing helminthic frequency and not necessarily helminthic disease.

Many helminthic disease manifestations depend on the worms' habitat or migration routes. On the basis of the habitat of the adult form, we can divide these parasites in an oversimplified manner into *intestinal* and *blood-tissue helminths.* However, several gut-dwelling worms have tissue-migrating larvae and the tapeworms can be human gut or tissue dwellers, depending on whether man serves as their definitive or their intermediate hosts. The only intracellular form among the human parasitic helminths is the muscle larva of *Trich-*

inella spiralis, whose longevity compensates for the fleeting existence of its adult parent.

The pathogenesis of helminthic diseases has been slow to unravel. *Intestinal helminths* can behave as commensals (i.e., as "accidental pathogens"), as opportunists, or even, if sufficiently numerous, as virulent pathogens. *Adult worms can cause disease by (1) competing for essential host nutrients (e.g., vitamin B_{12} depletion by* Diphyllobothrium latum); *(2) mechanically obstructing or perforating the GI tract* (Ascaris lumbricoides); *(3) blood-sucking [hematophagy] (the hookworms,* Ancylostoma *and* Necator); *(4) inducing inflammatory and malabsorptive changes in the gut* (Strongyloides stercoralis); *or (5) inducing host hypersensitivity reactions (many helminths).* Hypersensitivity reactions are often caused by the migratory larval stages of those helminths that must invade tissues and undergo several molts in order to reach maturity in the gut. During that process, there is attrition of the less vigorous invasive larvae and shedding of surface antigens and somatic components. Although there is little evidence that these are toxic to the host, there is no doubt of their antigenicity and capacity to stimulate host antibodies and cellular immune responses. Nevertheless, the migratory schedules and antigenic variations of the developing forms permit a significant proportion to evade host defenses and reach the privileged gut environment. During reinfection, with host antibodies and memory cells poised to react to early helminth antigens, the number of developing forms able to reach their ultimate habitat is drastically reduced. Immunosuppression can dramatically abolish this protection. Even *eosinophilia*, a hallmark of normal host immune responses to the richly glycosylated helminth antigens, can be abolished in an altered host.

Intestinal roundworms require only resistance to the host digestive juices as their condition of survival, but tissue-dwelling worms have developed elaborate mechanisms to evade host cellular defenses and antibodies. (1) In developing flatworms and flukes, antigenic variations analogous to those of molting helminth larvae occur in their cytoplasmic tegument.[270] (2) There is surface acquisition of host-derived molecules such as red cell and histocompatibility antigens, which serve to partially disguise the parasite's identity.[271] (3) A general reduction in helminth surface antigenicity occurs, whose nature is still not fully understood.[272] (4) Enzymes of larval and adult blood flukes can cleave host immunoglobulins, leading to complement consumption[273] and inactivation of clotting factors.[274] (5) Cystic tapeworm larvae release sulfated polysaccharides, which inhibit mediators of inflammation and can generate their own lipoxygenase products, thus inhibiting platelet aggregation.[275] (6) Leukocytes contacting the worm surfaces and phagocytosing their tegumental products soon detach themselves owing to the very high turnover of tegumental parasite glycoproteins and phospholipids.[276] (7) Some helminths generate products that directly suppress the host immunocompetent cells[277] or elicit specific T-suppressor cells, dampening immune responses.[278] As research continues, other ingenious evasive maneuvers of tissue helminths will probably be added to this compilation.

Helminth challenge of an already infected host is always less likely to result in disease than primary infection, for the reasons already given, yet acquired resistance to a naturally occurring helminth infection is rarely complete. What generally ensues is the undisturbed survival of the established adult worms in the face of increased and accelerated attrition of the challenge-larvae, so that only a reduced number of new worms is added to the existing load. This "concomitant immunity"[279] is known to be T lymphocyte–dependent but its effector mechanisms are multiple and complex. In the schistosome experimental model, both antibodies and host effector cells are required for parasite killing, i.e., the process is antibody-dependent, cell-mediated (ADCC). *Eosinophils are concentrated at the parasite-killing sites in vivo; in vitro,* they can kill early parasite forms in the presence of specific antibody by discharging reactive oxygen products, phospholipase A_2, and basic proteins against the invader's tegument.[280] Similar evidence exists for other leukocytes, including macrophages.[281] It is thus still unclear whether eosinophils have a unique, protective role against helminth parasites or whether they simply act in concert with other leukocytes.[282]

Adult tissue-dwelling helminths generate eggs or larvae in volumes many times their own. Both parents and offspring are rich sources of excretory-secretory products, some functioning as proteolytic enzymes,[283] others as powerful, soluble, or particulate antigens capable of evoking strong host immune responses. Thus far, evidence is scant that these products are cytotoxic,[284] but circulating helminth antigens and antigen-antibody complexes can readily be detected and may play an important role in producing some of the lesions encountered, e.g., nephritis complicating schistosomiasis or filariasis.[285] More important, helminth antigens can evoke various forms of local or systemic hypersensitivity reactions or, quite frequently, combinations of reactions,[286] and it is generally agreed that the *disease potential of tissue helminths is largely due to their capacity to induce a spectrum of host hypersensitivities.* Tests for helminth-specific antibodies have been quite useful in epidemiologic studies and for clinical diagnosis, particularly when the parasites themselves are difficult to detect. The identification and use of antigens highly purified by monoclonal antibodies should further enhance their clinical value.[287] By contrast, vaccination against helminths has thus far reached practical application only in the veterinary field.

INTESTINAL ROUNDWORMS

Ascariasis (Ascaris lumbricoides)

The largest (up to 35 cm long) and most common of the intestinal roundworms, *A. lumbricoides* is distributed worldwide and is indistinguishable from *A. suis*, the pig roundworm. It is spread between humans by fecal-oral transmission. In most infected persons, *A. lumbricoides* acts as a commensal, stays in the gut lumen, produces no disease, and eventually dies spontaneously and is shed. Infection is most common in children, becoming rarer from the second decade on. Eggs are excreted with the feces; larvae are liberated when Ascaris eggs are swallowed and reach the stomach. Following systemic tissue migration, they reenter the gut from the lung via the trachea and larynx, and mature into adults.

Disease ensues under three circumstances. (1) Repeated seasonal entry of Ascaris larvae may result in allergic respiratory symptoms. (Ascaris polysaccharide antigen strongly stimulates IgE antibody formation and has become a standard tool in basic immunology research.) (2) Heavy infection may obstruct a gut segment or sphincter. (3) Agitated worms may enter the appendix or common bile duct and cause perforation or bacterial infection with peritonitis, cholangitis, or sepsis. Allergic ascariasis with hypereosinophilia, asthma, or urticaria is a seasonal phenomenon in parts of the Near East, especially the Arabian peninsula.[288] A more serious form has resulted from a massive oral load of pig ascaris eggs eaten during a college fraternity prank, inducing a spectacular allergic pneumonitis.[289] Pyloric obstruction by worms, best demonstrated by barium swallow, sometimes becomes an emergency in children, especially in the tropics, and can usually be alleviated without surgery. By contrast, appendiceal perforation requires emergency operation to avoid life-threatening bacterial and helminthic peritonitis. Near the perforated organ, Ascaris worms or eggs are found in the acute, fibrinopurulent exudate. Ascariasis of the common duct causes jaundice and gram-negative sepsis, and can simulate severe hepatitis of other causes; fortunately, it is extremely rare. Although Ascaris infections have been linked to seizure disorders in children and to anemia or failure to gain weight, none of these charges have stood up to rigorous examination. It is interesting but still insufficiently documented that Ascaris-infected populations tend to have fewer allergies of the atopic type.

Trichuriasis (Trichuris sp.)

T. trichiura, the whipworm, is a small intestinal roundworm up to 5.0 cm long with an attenuated anterior end (its "whip"). It is a very common, worldwide parasite whose life cycle lacks a tissue phase and it is simply transmitted by fecal contamination. It causes disease so rarely that the presence of its eggs in the stools serves largely as an indication to be alert for other parasites. However, poor children in the tropics or mentally retarded individuals sometimes acquire enough of these worms to make their cecum and colon appear villous. This comes about because the worms bury their anterior ends in the crypts of the mucosa, with their thicker half floating in the lumen. Massively infected persons may suffer from persistent diarrhea and tenesmus, and sometimes the load of worms combined with the edematous state of the mucosa produces sufficient obstruction and straining at stool to cause intussusception or rectal prolapse.[290] Eosinophilia is common in heavy infections, the only ones meriting treatment with a vermifuge.

Enterobiasis (Oxyuriasis)

The pinworm, *Enterobius vermicularis,* is a tiny roundworm up to 13 mm long with prominent lateral ridges (alae), whose habitat is the gut. It causes the well-known night itch of children, and can be passed to siblings and sometimes to adults. Female worms migrate nightly to the anal skin for egg-laying, causing intense pruritus, insomnia, and irritability. Diagnosis can sometimes be made simply by inspection of the anus for worms. Enterobius eggs also stick to a piece of Scotch tape placed over the anus, which can then be directly examined under the microscope. The response of night itch to modern vermifuges is near miraculous, but reinfection is very common.

Intense, neglected enterobiasis can be complicated by spreading eczematous skin eruptions, and infection can be transferred to the nares. Enterobius has been suspect as a cause of symptoms simulating appendicitis and is regularly discovered in appendectomy specimens; however, its size is too small to obstruct the lumen and trigger bacterial superinfection (Fig. 8–47). Rarely, female worms migrate from the anus into the vagina to reach the fallopian tube and pelvic peritoneum. Egg-laying in these sites results in chronic granulomatous inflammation plus scarring, which may simulate bacterial or tuberculous pelvic inflammatory disease, thus producing a diagnostic conundrum when the pelvic lesions are discovered years after active enterobiasis has ceased.[291]

Hookworm Disease (Necator, Ancylostoma spp.)

Unlike other intestinal roundworms, *Necator americanus* and *Ancylostoma duodenale,* with their sharp mouthplates, penetrate into the duodenal and jejunal mucosa and feed on blood. A considerable proportion of the blood is wastefully excreted into the intestinal lumen. Nevertheless, iron deficiency anemia due to hookworm alone is seen only in heavy infections, such as may still be found in some tropical countries and in the Appalachian region of the U.S. In many instances of tropical anemia, hookworm disease potentiates the effects of malnutrition, malaria, or mixed parasitic infections of various kinds.

The parasite's life cycle requires hatching of infective larvae following fecal deposition in the soil. Penetrating the unshod skin of human feet, the larvae then undergo systemic migration and reach the lungs, from which they reenter the gut by being coughed up and swallowed. Adult worms are up to 10 mm long and each can waste up to 43 μl of host blood per day.[292] Hookworm anemia is most common where human fecal contamination of the soil is heavy, e.g., in children of village communities in the tropics, especially those

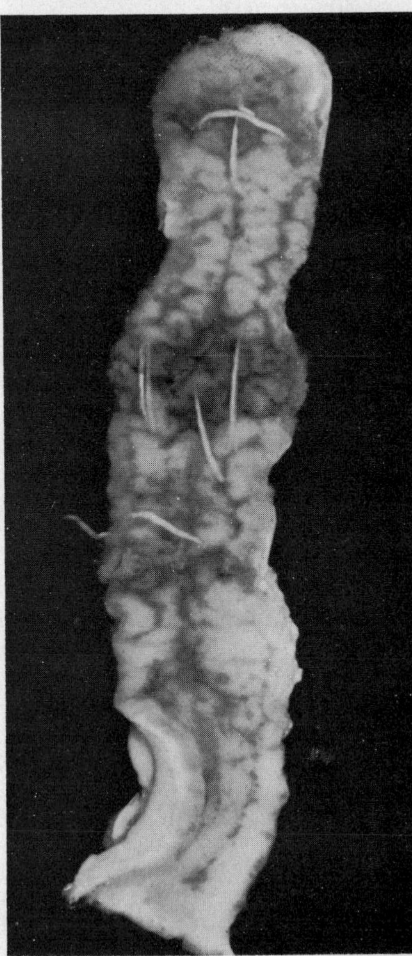

Figure 8–47. Pinworms in appendix.

whose diet contains little iron. In such populations, one also sees hypoalbuminemia and/or intestinal malabsorption, but this may be a combined effect of the parasites and poor nutrition. Treatment of the hookworms and iron supplementation may sometimes unmask an underlying macrocytic anemia due to folate deficiency. The declining frequency of hookworm infection in older persons in endemic areas suggests acquired immunity; complete protection has been achieved in the dog by a radiated live hookworm larval vaccine. The most effective measure against human hookworm anemia has been construction of rural latrines, as documented in Puerto Rico and the southern U.S.[293]

The lesions in the gut are relatively minor; punctate hemorrhages may be seen, but villous atrophy, when present, probably has other causes, and the biting defects caused by the worms are promptly regenerated after vermifuge treatment. Larval migration through the lung is generally silent.

Strongyloidiasis (Strongyloides stercoralis)

The mature parthenogenetic *S. stercoralis* female is small enough (up to 1 mm) to be almost entirely buried in a single intestinal crypt of the duodenum or upper jejunum where these worms reside. Thus, like other intestinal roundworms, *S. stercoralis* is a luminal dweller, but it more readily damages the absorptive surface of the gut, giving rise to chronic enteritis and the malabsorptive syndrome. Moreover, its life cycle permits larvae to become infective both in contaminated soil and in the host intestine itself, especially in malnourished and immunosuppressed individuals. This internal recycling of worms may result in Strongyloides hyperinfection, i.e., in a progressive, potentially lethal accumulation of worms and migratory larvae.[294] Strongyloides eggs mature high in the intestine and the resulting larvae are easily missed on stool examination; duodenal aspiration or biopsy may sometimes be required for diagnosis. Transmission resembles that of hookworms and is more frequent in the rural tropics, but is not limited to these locales. Strongyloidiasis occurs throughout the U.S. and is especially frequent in the Appalachian region. Severe cases occur in institutions for the retarded or insane where fecal contamination is a fact of life. Elsewhere in the Americas, Brazil has been a major focus for many years.

In hypersensitive persons, larval skin penetration may give rise to an urticarial eruption that fades in a few days, but this is rarely recorded or remembered in the endemic setting. Similarly, larval lung migration at about seven days usually passes with a slight coughing episode, unless infection has been massive. The chronic, intestinal phase of infection may also remain asymptomatic but more often results in intermittent bouts of diarrhea, with or without evidence of malabsorption. Some patients, such as West Indian immigrants to Britain or the U.S., manifest a spruelike syndrome with weight loss, fatty stools, and a protein-losing enteropathy, which gradually disappears after therapy.[295] Endogenous hyperinfection, as seen in protein-deprived children or immunosuppressed patients, is a grave illness, marked by nausea, fever, diarrhea, and (sometimes), paralytic ileus (an especially ominous sign). Concomitantly, there may be gram-negative sepsis, pneumonia, or meningitis, complications that tend to recur even after antibiotic treatment unless the underlying strongyloidiasis is also cured. Persistent eosinophilia is the rule in moderate infection, but this decreases in the hyperinfected, altered host.

The lesions of strongyloidiasis mirror the clinical events. In mild, subclinical infection there may only be focal erythema and eosinophilia of the duodenal mucosa; females, eggs, and larvae, are found burrowed in mucosal crypts (Fig. 8–48). In malabsorptive cases, the lamina propria is heavily infiltrated, the mucosal villi are blunted, the lacteals are dilated, and there is widespread mucosal edema. With hyperinfection, there is often ulceration of the small bowel; the invasive, filariform larvae of the worm, larger in size than the rhabdoid larvae of the lumen, are found in submucosal lymphatics and blood vessels of the small bowel, surrounded by florid inflammation. Lower down, in the colon, they are seen mostly in the submucosa and muscularis, provoking focal accumulations of macrophages and lymphoid cells, but rarely well-defined epithelioid cell granulomas; the absence

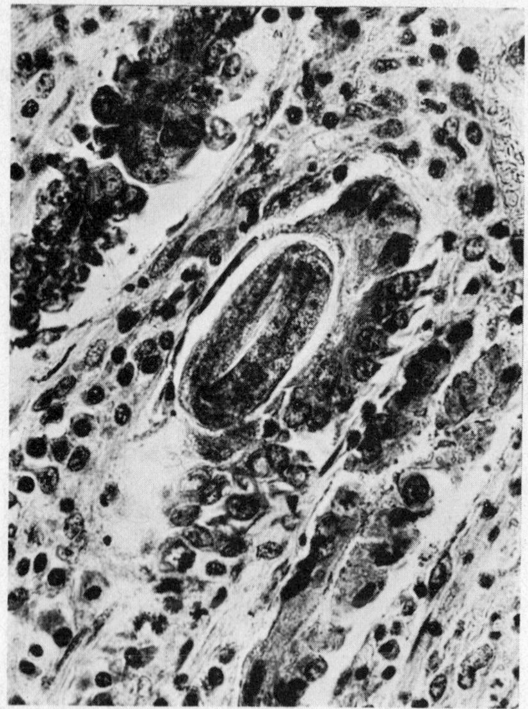

Figure 8–48. Strongyloidiasis in duodenal mucosa with a central, coiled rhabditoid larva.

of a vigorous tissue response may be an indication of the depressed T-cell function found in such patients. In fatal infections the body is literally "riddled with worms."[296] Migrating filariform larvae are most frequently seen in the lung, often associated with hemorrhage but with little focal inflammation. They may also appear in any other organ, including the liver and the CNS. Septic bacterial foci facilitated by the hyperinfection and depressed immunity are commonly seen at this stage, and hemorrhagic pneumonia is often the final insult.

Strongyloidiasis persists as a public health problem because of the same fecal contamination that permits other intestinal roundworms to prosper. It is, however, a more serious disease requiring as careful an evaluation and treatment as any life-threatening bacterial or viral illness.

Capillariasis (Capillaria philippinensis)*

These slender roundworms, up to 4.3 mm long, cause an endemic protein-losing enteropathy in communities of the Philippines and Northeast Thailand. They are capable of an endogenous cycle not involving tissue migration that can give rise to massive intestinal worm loads, sometimes producing malnutrition and cachexia. The infection is acquired from uncooked fish that contains the larvae of this helminth. The eggs of *C. philippinensis* resemble those of *Trichuris trichiuria*, but can be differentiated by careful examination, especially when larvae are also present in the stools.[297]

TISSUE ROUNDWORMS

Visceral Larva Migrans (Toxocara canis, cati)

Toxocariasis is a *zoonotic* infection, acquired by children from puppies or kittens—the normal hosts—in whom the parasite undergoes full development. In man, the accidental host, worm development is stunted at the larval stage, but before these larvae die in the various organs they have reached, they can cause significant tissue destruction and hypersensitivity reactions. A hypereosinophilic syndrome with fever and hepatosplenomegaly is the usual clinical presentation, at times with prominent GI or respiratory symptoms or, rarely, visual impairment.[298] Unlike the intestinal roundworms, which are diagnosable by stool examination or duodenal aspirate, Toxocara larvae can be seen only in tissue samples. In the absence of such direct identification, serologic tests are helpful in dealing with this *occult parasitic infection.*[299]

Toxocara, a large roundworm of the Ascaris family, is exquisitely adapted to canines or felines, which transmit the larvae transplacentally to their progeny; unless wormed early, these pets will shed many eggs into the environment in which children live and play. Ingested eggs liberate the larvae, which then enter the circulatory system and thus can reach any organ in the body.

The larvae are about 400 × 20 μ in size and provoke large, eosinophil-rich inflammatory foci with central necrosis, often containing numerous Charcot-Leyden crystals. Larvae, particularly disintegrating ones, may be difficult to locate in such foci and may required step-sectioning of the entire biopsy sample. During active infection the liver is generally enlarged and may appear studded with grayish-tan nodules up to 1 cm in diameter containing eosinophils, plasma cells, and scattered giant cells; there is also diffuse portal inflammatory infiltration with eosinophils and plasma cells. The lung may similarly show diffuse interstitial eosinophilia, resembling that seen in the acute allergic phase of human ascariasis or in Loeffler's syndrome (p. 748). Focal lung granulomas may appear around disintegrating Toxocara larvae.[300] Many other organs, including the heart, CNS, and rarely the eye, may show similar foci, and the consequent endophthalmitis may lead to retinal detachment and blindness, usually unilateral.

The active stage of toxocariasis begins suddenly or insidiously and lasts for several weeks or months, subsiding after two weeks in most cases. Manifestations are protean and include fever, cough, nausea, anorexia, bodyaches, weight loss, drenching sweats, asthma or urticaria, enlarged tender liver, lymphadenopathy, strabismus, and a host of other confusing complaints. However, the affected child rarely loses all energy or appears very sick. Persistent eosinophilia of up to 40% of the differential count is an important clue and there may be pronounced hyperglobulinemia. Eventually, if contact with infected pets is removed, the infection is self-terminating, but its course can be shortened and complications perhaps prevented by treatment.

Toxocariasis should be suspected in children living in crowded households with pets, in those with pica (compulsive dirt-eating), and in the presence of unexplained hepatomegaly, eosinophilia, or hyperglobulinemia. It is likely that subclinical infections are much more frequent than the overt.

*Other Occult Zoonotic Tissue Helminths**

Other helminths give rise to hypereosinophilic syndromes resembling that of visceral larva migrans, but are sufficiently uncommon to merit only brief mention. *Angiostrongylus cantonensis*, a parasite of the rat, causes eosinophilic meningitis in a wide area of the South Pacific, including Hawaii, and in Thailand, Vietnam, and Taiwan.[301] *Gnathostoma spinigerum*, a roundworm of cats and dogs, causes a striking eosinophilia and a CNS syndrome similar to that seen with *A. cantonensis*.[302] India, Thailand, and Japan are the main endemic foci. Lesions and symptoms tend to be more severe than in angiostrongyliasis. *Angiostrongylus costaricensis* is a parasite of the wild rat transmitted to humans, mostly children, by garden slugs.[303] Its territory ranges from Venezuela to Texas. Pain in the right iliac fossa, fever, and anorexia are the presenting symptoms, with marked leukocytosis and eosinophilia. An appendiceal or paracecal mass is sometimes discovered by palpation or x-ray examination and is due to egg-laying in the feeding arterioles of that region, resulting in a granulomatous, coalescent inflammatory swelling containing numerous ova. *Anisakis marina* is a large roundworm transmitted to humans when raw or smoked fish products are consumed. Released into the human stomach, the infectious Anisakis larva actively burrows into the gastric or cecal wall where it eventually disintegrates, giving rise to large inflammatory masses of eosinophil-rich granulation and fibrous tissue with focal granulomas.[304] *Ancylostoma braziliense* and *A. caninum* are hookworms adapted to dogs and cats, which confine their migration to the human skin and subcutaneous tissue, thereby causing a "creeping eruption" of inflamed worm tunnels that heal after the zoonotic larvae succumb.[305] Similar lesions can be caused by Gnathostoma and certain arthropods. Creeping eruption is common in the southeastern U.S. and in Puerto Rico and is most frequently contracted on sandy beaches where bathers frolic with dogs and cats.

The entities mentioned do not by any means exhaust the known varieties of zoonotic human helminth infections. The list grows longer yearly and may never be completed!

Guinea Worm Infection (Dracunculus medinensis)*

The guinea worm, a long, thin tissue helminth up to 120 cm in length, belongs to a species distinct from the filariae of similar shape (p. 381). It causes disabling and painful inflammatory swellings of the skin. The ancient practice of removing the worm from its superficial location by winding it up on a stick is the probable origin of the caduceus, the emblem of medicine. *Guinea worm disease* is most common in parts of India and of West Africa, but occurs throughout the tropics. Buried in the human subcutaneous tissue, the adult worm discharges larvae into water via skin blisters. The freshwater cyclops serves as the intermediary host and new patients become infested by drinking from infested water. Provision of protected water breaks the cycle. Migration and maturation of worms may take as long as a year. Once in its final skin habitat, the worm causes swelling and blisters that often are located on the outer malleolus of the foot, but also may appear in any other part of the skin. The lesions enlarge, becoming hard and edematous with the formation of multiple blisters and tracks that are prone to bacterial superinfection. The worm rears its ugly head where a blister has recently burst and thus becomes amenable to extraction. Death and degeneration of the worm lead to subcutaneous abscess formation and eventual calcification. Eosinophilia is found both in the blood and in the edematous granulation tissue that borders the local reaction to the worm. Some patients additionally manifest urticaria, and others become disabled by pain or inability to walk. Therapy consists of extraction of the worm by the traditional winding technique, or the administration of nitroimidazole drugs that simultaneously kill the worm[306] and reduce inflammation.

Trichinosis (Trichinella spiralis)

Trichinosis is a common disease throughout the world contracted by eating meat containing viable cysts of *Trichinella spiralis*. In man the parasite larva localizes principally within the striated muscles and therefore evokes generalized muscular aches and pains. However, during the early stage of infection the lungs, brain, heart, and other structures are also invaded.[307] The disease is transmitted by the ingestion of inadequately cooked meat. Smoked meats are also dangerous since they are not cooked.

The larvae of the parasite encyst within the muscles of a wide variety of carnivores and omnivores. The chief reservoir for man is the infected pig (sometimes bear meat or other wild game). More stringent regulations—a decrease in garbage feeding of pigs, sterilization of garbage, and deep-freezing of pork—have markedly reduced the incidence of this disease in many countries. A 1950 U.S. study disclosed trichinosis in 16% of postmortems, but in 1968 the rate had fallen to 4.2%. During this same time span, the incidence of the disease in slaughtered pigs fell from 11 to 0.5%. No regulation is 100% fail-safe, and therefore trichinosis may prove difficult to eradicate completely.

After ingestion of contaminated meat, the larvae are released in the stomach by proteolytic digestion of the cyst wall and attach themselves to the mucosa of the duodenum. As they mature into adult worms, they induce a mild transitory enteritis and malabsorption. About one week after copulation, a host of larvae are produced that penetrate the lacteals and eventually are drained into the blood. In this manner, the migrating larvae are disseminated and produce cell damage throughout the body, e.g., in the lung, heart, and brain. Meanwhile the adult worms die and are expelled. The larvae next invade striated skeletal muscle cells and modulate them to create an intracellular environment suitable for their own growth and maturation. This remarkable biologic coexistence of skeletal muscle cell and larvae has led to the muscle cell being called a "nurse cell."[308]

After the first week of its intracellular existence, the larvae become enclosed within a membrane produced by the host muscle cells (Fig. 8–49), which persists for the life of the larvae, possibly for years. Death of the larva and its "nurse" incites an inflammatory reaction characterized principally by lymphocytes and eosinophils. In time the dead larva calcifies. Therefore, infections in both animals and man can be recognized by microscopic identification of the viable or calcified larvae within striated skeletal muscle fibers. The most intense parasitization is encountered in the most active muscles of the body having the richest blood supply, i.e., the diaphragm, extraocular eye muscles, laryngeal muscles, and deltoid, gastrocnemius, and intercostal muscles. During active trichinosis there is often focal basophilic degeneration of muscle fibers, a lesion that should motivate a careful search for Trichinella larvae. The calcified foci left by dead larvae are characteristic enough to permit retrospective diagnosis even decades later.

During the invasive phase of trichinosis, cell destruction can be widespread and sometimes even lethal. Thus, in the heart, acute inflammatory changes are found during the early stages of the infection in the form of a patchy but widely scattered interstitial myocarditis, **but the larvae do not become encysted.** Instead they undergo necrosis and therefore cannot be identified. The inflammatory pattern in the myocardium is fairly nonspecific save for the prominence of eosinophils and some giant cells. Ultimately, fibrous scarring ensues. In the **lungs,** the reaction to the trapped larvae may consist only of edema and focal hemorrhages, but in some cases a marked leukocytic reaction with large numbers of eosinophils may appear, attributed to an allergic response. **Invasion of the CNS** is reflected by a diffuse lymphocytic and mononuclear infiltration in the leptomeninges, and by the development of focal gliosis in and about the small capillaries of the brain substance, infiltrated with lymphocytes and eosinophils. Sometimes, necrotic larvae can be identified within these inflammatory nodules.

In most clinical cases, a history of the ingestion of improperly cooked pork products can be obtained. Trichinae are killed by cooking at a minimum temperature of 60°C for at least 30 minutes per pound of meat. Freezing the meat for 20 days at a temperature of −15°C (5°F) will also effectively destroy the trichinae. In U.S. locations, therefore, outbreaks of trichinosis occur mostly among ethnic groups processing their own traditional pork dishes for festive occasions or among fanciers of wild game and exotic meats. However, the disease may appear anywhere and may mimic a variety of other infections, as well as the collagen-vascular diseases and hematologic disorders. The period of invasion of the intestinal mucosa may be marked by

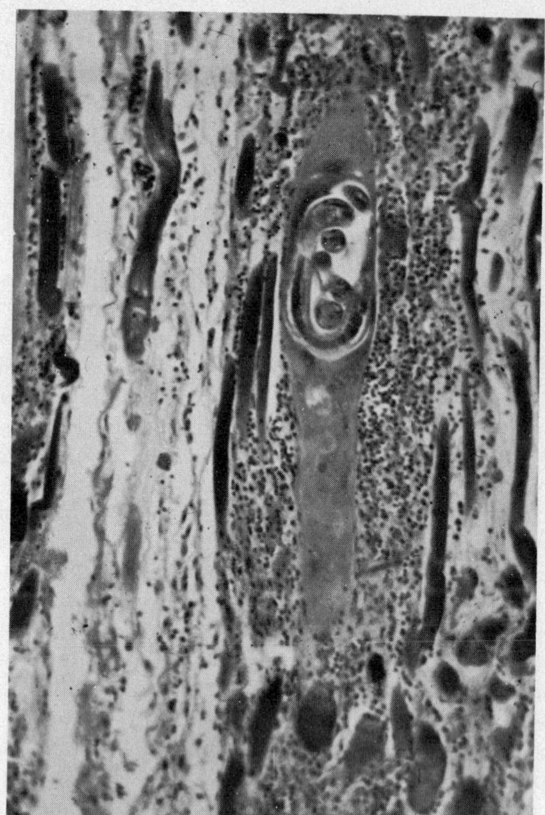

Figure 8–49. Trichinosis with a coiled encysted parasite larva within skeletal muscle.

vomiting and diarrhea, symptoms that suggest "food intoxication." During the hematogenous dissemination and the muscular invasion, widespread aches and pains and fever appear. Particularly characteristic are periorbital and facial edema. Eye movement and breathing and swallowing may be painful; patients often complain of backache and aching pain in the legs or joints. Often the invasion of the lung evokes cough and dyspnea, the latter materially contributed to by the involvement of the respiratory muscles. The CNS invasion may lead to headaches, disorientation, delirium, and a variety of other signs and symptoms strongly suggestive of a diffuse encephalitis. Cardiac failure may appear when the myocardial injury is severe. But the combination of fever, muscle tenderness, eosinophilia, and swelling of the eyelids is most typical.[309] The eosinophilia can account for 70% of the total white count. After the third week of the disease, serologic tests are positive except in overwhelming disease. A skin test is also available. Muscle biopsy, best taken near the tendinous insertion of the deltoids or gastrocnemius muscles, is definitive even earlier.[310]

The mortality rate for trichinosis is low, but overwhelming infection may cause death when patients with severe involvement of the respiratory muscles develop intercurrent pulmonary bacterial infections or cardiac failure. Anti-inflammatory and symptomatic treatment will greatly reduce the severity of patient discomfort, but whether antihelminthic treatment is useful after larval invasion has occurred is debatable. Fortunately, mild and subclinical Trichinella infections are the rule, and severe ones the exception. Experimentally, even a minimal primary infection confers strong immunity to subsequent challenge, which may also be true of mild clinical infections. Several defensive mechanisms have been identified. At the time of adult worm development in the gut, a rapid rejection phenomenon is seen by which most female parasites are shed from the host mucosa before being able to deposit their larval progeny.[311] Newborn larvae, but not their later stages, are also susceptible to attack by eosinophilic and neutrophilic granulocytes in the presence of specific antibody.[312] Once ensconced in their "nurse cells," however, Trichinella larvae are protected from both immune and phagocytic destruction.

*Filariasis**

Human filarial infections are widely endemic in the insect-ridden lowlands and coastal plains of the tropics; animal filariae occasionally infect man in temperate as well as in tropical zones. *Tropical filariasis* can be subdivided into (1) lymphatic filariasis, (2) onchocerciasis or "river blindness," and (3) the lesser tropical filarial infections. The best-known *zoonotic filariae* are those of dogs and raccoons.

Tropical filariasis is one of the great forgotten diseases of mankind. Progress in preventing and treating filariasis has been agonizingly slow. It is estimated that 240 million people are infected by lymphatic filariae. Onchocerca infects about 40 million Africans. Much smaller numbers suffer disabling filarial disease, but the reduction of the working force increases the devastating impact of recurrent drought and famine on poor agricultural communities, such as those of India or of the Sahel region of Africa. Filariasis still exists in Puerto Rico, but in the continental U.S. only scattered cases are seen among immigrants and returnees from endemic regions; a large epidemic arose in U.S. Marines during the WW II Pacific campaign.[313]

Filariae are long, stringlike nematodes whose fertilized females release tiny microfilariae into the lymph, blood, or skin. When taken up by biting insects, these microfilariae molt and metamorphose into infective third-stage larvae, ready to infect a new host via the vector's proboscis. Migration from the biting site to their definitive habitat in the human body and maturation to the mating stage may take several months. Untreated human filariae survive for many years while maintaining steady microfilarial production. In lymphatic filariasis only part of the infected human population shows parasitemia at any one time; those with early infections and those with acquired immunity to microfilariae have "occult filariasis," i.e., infection undetectable by blood concentration methods.[314] Infective larvae, adult worms, and microfilariae each have separate as well as shared antigens, and human immune responses vary individually and over the long duration of the disease. They range from virtual unresponsiveness to vigorous hypersensitivity, and these variations account in part for the protean manifestations of filariasis, making its diagnosis and management difficult. Epidemiologic data suggest that acquired immunity to human filariae exists, but its mechanism is uncertain, as is the mode by which filariae evade the host defenses.[315]

Lymphatic Filariasis *(Wuchereria bancrofti, Brugia malayi)**

Wuchereria bancrofti measures up to 100 mm in length and is distributed worldwide in all tropical countries. *B. malayi,* somewhat smaller (25 mm long), is limited to Southeast Asia from Ceylon to the Philippines and is found as far north as central China. *W. bancrofti* has no known animal reservoir and can be transmitted to monkeys only with difficulty. *B. malayi* has strains that can infect monkeys and cats (potential reservoir hosts). Mosquito vectors vary by species; urban bancroftian filariasis found in the slums of many large tropical cities is transmitted mainly by *Culex fatigans.* As a rule, these infections are milder than those of rural filariasis, which is transmitted by any one of 80 mosquito species, depending on locality. Malayan filariasis also has multiple mosquito vectors.

Expatriates develop acute symptoms several months after contracting infection, but most residents in endemic areas remain indefinitely asymptomatic. The acute phase manifests itself as bouts of fever, lymphangitic streaking of an extremity, transient intrascrotal pain and swelling, urticarial rashes, or tender lymphadenopathy, together with restlessness and apprehension. Eosinophilia is regularly seen, but microfilaremia may or may not be detectable. Acute symptoms often subside spontaneously but may recur or gradually shade into the chronic phase.

Chronic filariasis is characterized by persistent lymphedema of the scrotum, penis, or vulva; the leg; or even the breast or arm (the latter particularly in the Pacific focus). Frequently there is hydrocele, sometimes grotesque, and lymph node enlargement. Rupture of a lymphatic varix may occur, leading to chyluria. Nodular inflammatory lesions or bacteriologically sterile abscesses may appear in the epididymis, along the spermatic cord, in an extremity, or around the external genital organs. In severe and long-lasting infections, chylous weeping of the enlarged scrotum may ensue (lymph scrotum) or a chronically swollen leg may develop tough subcutaneous fibrosis and epithelial hyperkeratosis, named "elephantiasis" (Fig. 8–50). Elephantoid skin shows dilatation of the dermal lymphatics with widespread lymphocytic infiltrates and focal cholesterol deposits; the epidermis is thickened and hyperkeratotic.

Histologically, when adequately sought, adult filarial worms are found in lymphatics or nodes in all infections. They are usually few in number, either live, or dead and calcified. Some have mild or no inflammatory reaction, although the lymphatics may be dilated and tortuous (lymphangiectasis). Lymphatic dilatation and perilymphatic and nodal nonspecific inflammation are more common in symptomatic filariasis. An intense eosinophil inflammation is seen in patients with recurrent filarial funiculoepididymitis, proba-

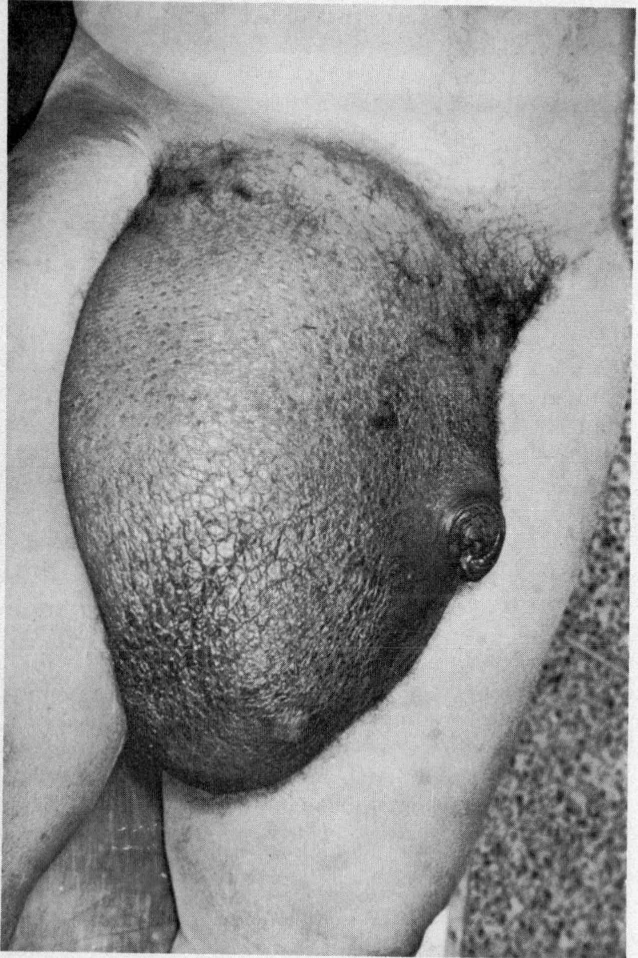

Figure 8–50. Elephantiasis of scrotum due to filariasis.

bly immunologically determined. In these lesions, lymphangitis extends far beyond the nesting points of the parasites themselves and may be hemorrhagic or fibrinous. The severest inflammatory lesions occur around disintegrating worms. Acute inflammation is followed by granulomatous foci that can be mistaken for mycobacterial lesions unless the parasite's cuticular remnants are recognized. Organization of the endolymphatic exudate results in polypoid infoldings of the vessel with persisting eosinophil and lymphocytic infiltration, a picture highly suggestive of lymphatic filariasis even if worms cannot be demonstrated. In endemic areas, filarial skin lesions often become superinfected by bacteria, with resulting cellulitis or abscess formation. In time the hydrocele fluid, which often contains cholesterol crystals, red cells, or hemosiderin, induces thickening and calcification of the tunica vaginalis. Microfilariae are difficult to find in histologic sections. Thus, the diagnosis frequently rests on combined clinical and pathologic criteria unless an adult parasite is found.

In Southeast India, Singapore, and sporadically elsewhere, occult filariasis may not be associated with microfilaremia or lymphatic obstruction. Instead there is a marked eosinophilia with asthma-like respiratory complaints or generalized lymphadenopathy ("tropical eosinophilia" or "eosinophilic lung"), related to high titers of antimicrofilarial antibody capable of triggering mast cell degranulation.[316] In tropical eosinophilia, besides eosinophil infiltration of the lung or lymphoreticular organs, dead microfilariae are found surrounded by stellate, hyaline eosinophilic precipitates embedded in small epithelioid cell granulomas (Meyers-Kouvenaar bodies).

Epidemiologic data suggest that filarial infection is cumulative over time and that chronic disease requires regular exposure. Prevention of mosquito-borne infection is clearly the best hope for controlling filariasis. Diethylcarbamazine, now the standard treatment, effectively clears microfilariae from the circulation, but has adverse side effects and only limited activity against adult worms. A number of promising alternative drugs are under study, but no antifilarial drug can reverse established chronic lymphedema or hydrocele, and even surgery is only partially successful in these conditions. About half of the chyluria patients submitted to diagnostic lymphangiograms sclerose their varix and are cured without operation.[317]

ONCHOCERCIASIS*

Onchocerca volvulus, the largest of the human filariae, reaches up to 50 cm in length; it is transmitted by blackflies (Simulium sp.) rather than by mosquitos. The adult worm preferentially nests in the subcutaneous tissue and discharges its microfilariae into the interstitium of the skin rather than into the blood. The adult worms may eventually elicit unsightly subcutaneous nodules, but the most significant lesions of onchocerciasis are blindness and dermatitis caused by millions of microfilariae accumulated in the skin and in the eye chambers. The disease is often manifested only by pruritus. Onchocerciasis occurs in Africa and parts of Yemen and in an area ranging from Southern Mexico to Northern Brazil.

Severe infection results in chronic dermatitis with focal darkening or loss of pigment in the skin and scaling; later there is epidermal atrophy, or subcutaneous edema with redundancy and thickening of the dermis. These stages of dermatitis have been graphically named "leopard skin," "lizard skin," and "elephant skin."[318] Lymph nodes, especially those of the groin, may show lymphocyte depletion and fibrosis and this may be followed by elephantiasis ("hanging groin"), seen mainly in Africa; in Yemen, onchocerciasis is associated with a marked papular dermatitis and with greatly enlarged lymph nodes, usually involving only one extremity.[319] Severe dermatitis is much less common in Latin America, and the nodules more frequently localize in the upper part of the body, often overlying bony prominences.

Histologic reactions to the adult worms are initially exudative, but later become granulomatous and fibrotic and eventually may calcify (Fig. 8–51). Reactions to live microfilariae are scanty and predominantly mononuclear and eosinophilic. At the later stages of dermatitis, there is subcutaneous edema, epidermal thickening, and hyperkeratosis with patchy pigment incontinence or hyperpigmentation, and finally fibrosis and dermal atrophy. The progressive eye lesions begin with punctate keratitis along with small, fluffy opacities of the cornea caused by degenerating microfilariae, which evoke an eosinophilic infiltration. This is followed by sclerosing keratitis, which opacifies the cornea, beginning at

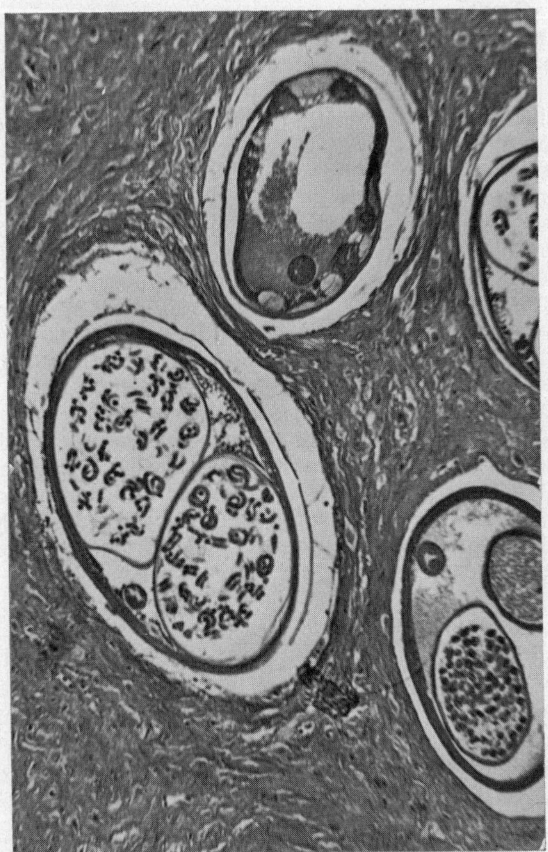

Figure 8–51. Onchocerciasis *(Onchocerca volvulus)* with gravid filaria enclosed in a subcutaneous fibrous nodule.

the scleral limbus. In addition, microfilariae in the anterior eye chamber give rise to iridocyclitis, sometimes ending in glaucoma; involvement of the choroid and retina, although less frequent, eventually results in atrophy and irreversible loss of vision, sometimes affecting the optic nerve itself.[318] Unfortunately, antimicrofilarial drugs can cause an allergic flareup of the skin and eye lesions ("Mazzotti reaction").

Microfilariae reach the inner organs as well and can sometimes be detected in the urinary sediment,[320] but diagnosis is usually made by skin biopsy and direct microscopy.

Minor Tropical Filariae (Loa, Mansonella, Dipetalonema spp.)*

These species rarely cause incapacitating illness. *Loa loa* elicits transitory skin swellings caused by migrating adult worms, preferentially beneath the conjunctiva (it is sometimes called the "eye worm"). *D. streptocerca* may cause itchy skin nodules or lesions that can be confused with leprosy or onchocerciasis.[321] All the species give rise to eosinophilia, and sometimes fever. Diagnosis and treatment are the domain of experienced consultants.

Zoonotic Filariasis *(Dirofilaria immitis, D. tenuis, Brugia beaveri)*

Few physicians recall that biting arthropods can inoculate man with filariae adapted to other mammalian species. The dog heartworm, *D. immitis*, when transmitted to humans, develops only to its larval stage. Usually, a single larva is embolized from the right heart chambers into a pulmonary artery branch where it succumbs, giving rise to a small pulmonary infarct or coin lesion readily mistaken on x-ray examination for a tumor or other infection. Microscopically, such a lesion shows infarcted lung tissue in its center and granulomatous inflammation in its periphery; eosinophils may or may not abound in the specimen, and are rarely elevated in the blood. The causal worm in a feeding artery can easily be missed. The internal cuticular ridges of Dirofilaria, seen in cross section, are pathognomonic.[322]

D. tenuis, a parasite of the raccoon, also causes abortive infections in man, in the form of either inflammatory subcutaneous nodules that come to surgery as presumed granulomas or dermatofibromas, or with other miscellaneous diagnoses. The conjunctiva has been a preferred site for *D. tenuis* larvae.[268] The larval worm occupies the center of the lesion, which is granulomatous and eosinophilic with marked peripheral fibrosis. *D. immitis* is endemic throughout the U.S., but *D. tenuis* infection prevails mostly in the South, especially in Florida.

Brugia beaveri, a parasite of the raccoon and the lynx, is a relative of the tropical Brugia sp. and, similarly, homes to lymph vessels and nodes. This infection has been reported along the Eastern seaboard from New York State to Quebec. The usual history is one of a single swollen lymph node, often in the neck or thoracic region, without any systemic manifestations. The differential diagnosis of lymphoma is often raised and the lymph node is then excised, resulting in cure. The correct diagnosis can be missed unless sufficient histologic sections are taken to discover a single, immature filaria, either intact or damaged, usually present at or near the lymph node hilus. The lymph node itself shows variable follicular hyperplasia, eosinophilia, or reticulosis. Peripheral eosinophilia is absent, and specific serologic tests are not yet available.[323]

None of the three animal filariae reviewed here are common causes of disease nor do they cause serious human illnesses, but they can give rise to puzzling diagnostic problems.

CESTODES, TAPEWORMS

Tapeworms are intestinal parasitic flatworms (Platyhelminthes); some species may achieve lengths of 3 to 6 m. They possess a small head or scolex generating thousands of rectangular proglottids that articulate with each other and make up the bulk of the worm. *Human tapeworm infections take one of two forms:* (1) that in which the mature tapeworm is attached to the intestinal wall, and (2) that in which the larval forms invade the organs of the body to produce so-called larval cestodiasis (cysticercosis).

Intestinal Tapeworm Infections

Among the many tapeworm species, four in particular may cause intestinal disease in man: *Taenia saginata* (beef), *T. solium* (pork), *Hymenolepis nana* (dwarf), and *Diphyllobothrium latum* (fish). Infection caused by these parasites is worldwide in distribution and is usually contracted by the ingestion of undercooked meat or fish. The meat of the intermediate host animals contains encysted larvae that excyst in the human intestinal tract and then mature into adults. These worms attach themselves to the bowel wall by their scolex bearing hooks and sucker plates. The mature worm then progressively develops to the extraordinary lengths mentioned above. Adult tapeworms are well-adapted hermaphroditic parasites that seem to regulate their own numbers; thus, *T. solium* occurs singly as an example of "concomitant immunity." In many patients, tapeworms evoke no clinical signs or symptoms.

Clinical manifestations may arise, however, from (1) the physical mass of worms causing intestinal obstruction or (2) the competitive uptake of vitamin B_{12} to induce a megaloblastic anemia (p. 630). Systemic manifestations, including dizziness, restlessness, inability to concentrate on schoolwork, and others, have also been described.

The diagnosis of intestinal tapeworm infection is usually made by the finding of proglottids in the stools, more rarely by finding eggs, or by radiography (with contrast media) outlining the large tapeworms. Since all Taenia sp. eggs are similar, identification of the worm species depends on detailed examination of the proglottid. Careful stool examination is required after a vermifuge to make sure that the worm's scolex has been expelled, since otherwise the worm will regenerate. Removal of the scolex by colonoscopy is one of the crowning achievements of modern medical technology,[323A] but a good vermifuge can do the same job with less effort.

Cysticercosis

Man becomes the *definitive host* of the adult tapeworm, *T. solium,* by acquiring its *larvae* from pork meat. By contrast, unwitting ingestion of Taenia *eggs* deposited on fecally contaminated vegetables or self-contamination with such eggs converts man into the *intermediate host.* This is a more serious condition since each ingested egg spawns a hexacanth embryo, which penetrates the gut and is disseminated through the blood to develop into a cystic larva (cysticercus) in any body site, including the CNS or heart. Depending on the number and location of *cysticerci,* infections vary from inconsequential to life threatening.

Cysticerci may be found in any organ but preferred localizations are the brain, muscles, skin, and heart. They are ovoid, white-to-opalescent parasite cysts, rarely exceeding 1.5 cm in size, which contain an invaginated scolex bathed in clear cyst fluid (Fig. 8–52). The cyst wall is over 100 μ thick, is rich in glycoproteins, and evokes remarkably little host reaction as long as it remains intact. Once implanted, cysticerci endure in their dormant condition for many years, but eventually degenerate or break open and induce granuloma formation, focal scarring, and calcification, sometimes visible on radiographs as round, opaque densities. Rarely, a cysticercus may proliferate to larger size or to a branching, racemose stage.

Subcutaneous cysticerci form palpable nodules and are often removed by excision biopsy after which the larvae can be visualized. Even degenerate cysticerci are recognizable by their many tiny, sharktooth-shaped birefringent hooklets, which are nearly indestructible. The finding of cutaneous cysts virtually guarantees CNS involvement, but the converse is not true. Cysts may involve the meninges, gray or white matter, sometimes even the sylvian aqueduct or ventricular foramina so as to block spinal fluid circulation.

Neurologic symptoms are protean, seizures being the most common. Occasionally, a cysticercus floating in a ventricle causes a rise of intracranial pressure and headache each time the patient lies down. Cysticerci of the psychomotor cortex may cause tumor-like localizing signs, but these are often absent even in heavy infections. Whether personality or psychiatric abnormalities can ensue from cysticercosis is controversial.[324] Bizarre symptoms also occasionally arise from myocardial cysticercosis. CT scans have greatly increased diagnostic accuracy and, in combination with x-ray studies, can detect both mild and severe CNS cysticercosis. An improved serologic test (ELISA) is also available. Thus, for the first time, large numbers of infected patients are now being found in the American Southwest and urban Northeast, many among Hispanics or Koreans. The problem is vastly greater in countries where there is

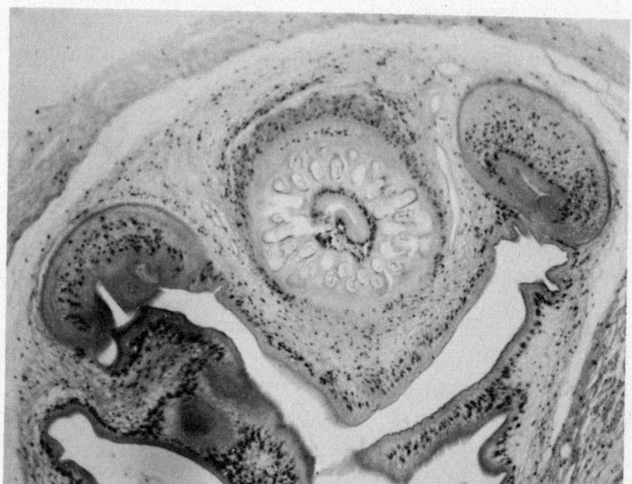

Figure 8–52. Cysticercus in subcutaneous tissue showing inverted scolex with sectioned hooklets *(center)* and suction cups *(both sides).*

fecal contamination of agricultural soil and where pork is a prized item in the diet. (The larvae of *T. saginata*, the cattle tapeworm, do not thrive in man.) Appropriate drug therapy effectively suppresses this parasite but has no effect on old or calcified foci.[325] Although infected persons show dermal hypersensitivity to cyst fluid, allergic or hypereosinophilic episodes are uncommon in cysticercosis.

Echinococcosis (Hydatid Disease)

Adult tapeworms of the genus Echinococcus are small and give their canine hosts little trouble. The intermediary hosts, including man, bear the brunt of the disease. Man becomes the accidental host by ingesting canine tapeworm eggs; these hatch in the duodenum, releasing invasive embryos that traverse the mucosa, enter portal branches, and are swept first into the liver, then to any other organ of the body. After long periods of silent growth, large parasitic cysts—*hydatids*—are formed in the liver and elsewhere; these can cause disease by compressing vital structures, by spilling allergenic cyst fluid, or by spawning proliferative "daughter cysts" that engage in tumor-like parasite growth. Bacterial superinfection converts the cyst into a large abscess. The disease, therefore, presents in many diverse clinical forms.

Echinococcus granulosus, causing unilocular hydatid cysts, is the most prevalent species. Its European strain cycles between dogs and sheep. Human infection is cosmopolitan, but is most common in the sheep-raising areas of the Western U.S., Australia, New Zealand, Argentina, the Eastern Mediterranean, and the Near East. A Northern strain of this parasite has a wild-animal cycle involving wolves and deer; human cases are seen mainly in subarctic regions, including Alaska, Canada, and Siberia, and are usually quite severe. Two other echinococci are transmitted only by feral cycles. *E. multilocularis* is transmitted to moles and rodents by wild canines and sled dogs. In man, it causes *multilocular* (or alveolar) *hydatid cysts with unrestricted budding and without scolices*, which invade the liver much like a malignant tumor. This species shares the Arctic distribution of *E. granulosus*, but also exists in Central and Eastern Europe. *E. vogeli*, cycled between wild dogs and pacas, is responsible for multilocular hydatids in Northern Latin America and Panama.[326]

About two-thirds of human *E. granulosus* cysts are found in the liver, 5 to 15% in the lung, and the rest in bones, brain, or other organs. In the various organs, the larvae lodge within the capillaries and first incite an inflammatory reaction composed principally of mononuclear leukocytes and eosinophils. Many such larvae are destroyed but others encyst. The cysts begin at microscopic levels and progressively increase in size, so that in five years or more they may have achieved dimensions over 10 cm in diameter. Enclosing an opalescent fluid is an inner, nucleated, germinative layer and an outer, opaque, non-nucleated layer. **The outer non-nucleated layer is quite distinctive and has innumerable delicate laminations** as though made up of many layers of gelatin. Outside this opaque layer, there is a host inflammatory reaction that produces a zone of fibroblasts, giant cells, and mononuclear and eosinophilic cells. In time, a dense fibrous capsule forms. When these cysts have been present for about six months, "daughter cysts" develop within them. These appear first as minute projections of the germinative layer, which develop central vesicles and thus form tiny "brood capsules." Scolices of the worm develop on the inner aspects of these brood capsules and separate from the germinative layer to produce a fine, sandlike sediment within the hydatid fluid (Fig. 8–53).

This is the sequence followed in the soft tissues, such as the liver, that permit the progressive enlargement of the cyst. When the original implantation occurs in bone, the hydatid vesicle usually develops near the epiphyseal end or in vertebrae and flat bones. Fibrous adventitial encapsulation of the larva does not occur, and as it grows and develops it permeates the spongy trabeculation of the bone to produce multiple microcystic diverticula. The intervening fragments of bone undergo pressure atrophy and frequently the bone cortex is eroded, so that spontaneous fractures are not uncommon.[327] Cysts that locate in the lung eventually erode into bronchi and are dramatically coughed up, fluid, membrane, and all; this sometimes results in spontaneous cure but, rarely, freak penetration of a cyst into pulmonary vessels or heart chambers may cause lethal embolism. Liver and other abdominal cysts eventually become leaky, resulting in sterile inflammation or bacterial superinfection. This causes shrinkage, fibrosis, and eventual calcification of the cyst and destruction of the parasite structure, with only the patho-

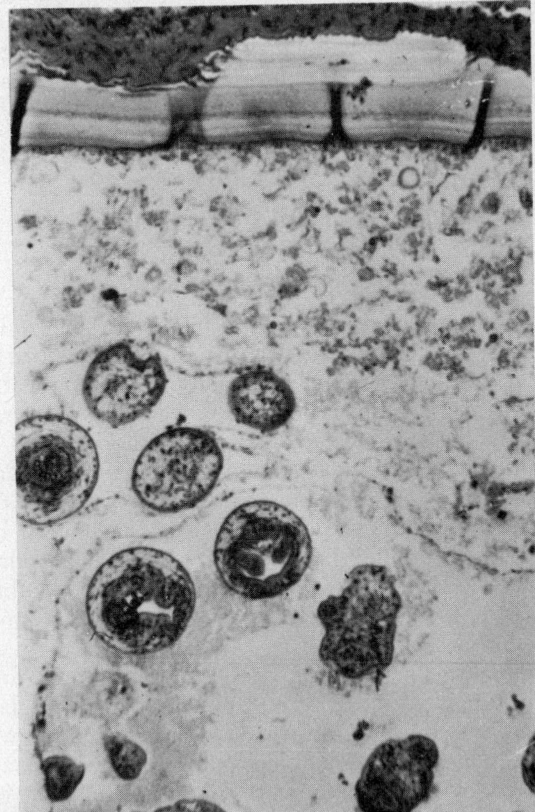

Figure 8–53. Echinococcosis. Wall of a cyst with laminated outer layer and inner germinative layer *(above)*. The cystic lumen contains many daughter "brood" capsules.

gnomonic, hooklet-bearing, degenerate scolices remaining intact amid the pastelike, yellow, cholesterol-rich debris.[328] Cyst rupture into a large bile duct can result in acute cholangitis or cholecystitis.

As is evident from its many localizations, disease due to the dog tapeworm may present in various mystifying guises. The clinical symptoms of unilocular hydatid disease derive mainly from its complications, e.g., from compression of or rupture into vital structures. Except in the brain or heart, the parenchymal atrophy caused by the gradual expansion of the cyst can be remarkably silent. However, external leakage of cyst fluid caused by trauma or surgical spillage can spark an acute anaphylactic attack with severe allergic symptoms accompanied by hypereosinophilia.[327] Surgical removal of these cysts is hazardous because spillage can also result in multiple cysts throughout the abdomen, unless they are sterilized by injection before excision.

Eosinophilia may or may not be present. Serologic tests for *E. granulosus* antigen and antibodies have been much improved and CT scans have greatly increased the accuracy of diagnosis. Drug therapy is moderately successful in sterilizing the cysts, but some have to be surgically removed.

E. multilocularis larvae, which generate *alveolar cysts* with budding and invasive growth in the human liver, cause manifestations virtually indistinguishable from those of a primary liver cell tumor; the cysts can, in fact, invade the caval or portal veins or metastasize to the lung. Various combinations of drugs and surgery have been tried in this unusual infection with only moderate success. The untreated disease has been 100% lethal.

TREMATODES (FLUKES)

Fascioliasis (Liver Fluke, Fasciola hepatica*)*

Human fascioliasis is caused by the hermaphroditic flatworm *F. hepatica* (in Hawaii also *F. gigantica*), a trematode (fluke) normally adapted to sheep and cattle. The disease is acquired by eating watercress contaminated with the metacercarial form of the parasite. Its acute stage, marked by fever and abdominal pain, results from tissue migration and maturation of worms that eventually settle in the lumen of the gallbladder/or bile ducts; the chronic stage is characterized by biliary obstructive symptoms. The disease is worldwide in both temperate and tropical zones; in the U.S. it is most frequent in Puerto Rico.[329]

The leaf-shaped adult parasites are up to 4 cm long; in the lumen of the biliary tree, they produce inflammation, intermittent obstruction, and dilatation with considerable thickening of the wall. *F. hepatica* releases large amounts of proline, presumed to stimulate bile duct or gallbladder hyperplasia and fibrosis.[330] The operculated Fasciola eggs, excreted via the feces, are diagnostic, although rarely present in large numbers.

In the U.S., most cases are sporadic, but in European countries where family farms are more prevalent, larger community outbreaks have occurred, usually three months after consumption of contaminated watercress (the time needed for maturation of the flukes). The early symptoms of the acute disease are malaise, intermittent fever, night sweats, weight loss, and right upper quadrant pain and are not distinctive; not all patients show eosinophilia or urticarial rashes or elevated sedimentation rates. The acute phase is self-terminating, but treatment with drugs will shorten its course and prevent later biliary obstructive complications that include colicky pain, jaundice, and bacterial superinfection. Occasionally, ectopic migration of worms produces painful subcutaneous nodules.

During the early migratory phase of fascioliasis, there is hepatomegaly with hemorrhagic-necrotic worm tracts, best seen in the subcapsular portion of the liver and sometimes resulting in peritoneal hemorrhage also. These lesions are replete with eosinophils and other inflammatory cells, but they ultimately heal, leaving only minor scars. Chronic Fasciola cholecystitis and cholangitis resemble the lesions caused by biliary calculi, but often show marked local eosinophilic infiltration, and there is hyperplasia of the bile duct epithelium, which is thrown into redundant infoldings. In the human liver, pericholangitis and periportal fibrosis are usually minimal.

With replacement of family farming by agribusiness in the U.S., fascioliasis is destined to vanish. Meanwhile, it continues sporadically to pose a diagnostic and epidemiologic challenge.

*Clonorchiasis and Opisthorchiasis**

These two smaller liver flukes (up to 1.5 cm long) differ from *F. hepatica* in many respects: (1) they are acquired by the eating of raw freshwater fish or crayfish that harbor metacercariae; (2) they commonly infect man, and dogs and cats in large numbers; (3) they colonize the small and large intrahepatic bile ducts, and therefore produce chronic cholangitis with extensive liver damage and intrahepatic gallstones; and (4) they are associated with a high frequency of cholangiocarcinoma.

Clonorchis sinensis is widespread in the Far East, ranging from Korea and Japan to Indochina, and is especially common in Hong Kong. *Opisthorchis viverrini* is hyperendemic in parts of Thailand and Laos. *O. felineus* is reported mainly from Poland and the Soviet Union. Oriental liver fluke disease lacks an early tissue-invasive phase but instead develops in a chronic and insidious fashion. Persons infected by few worms may remain asymptomatic indefinitely. In heavier infections, anorexia, diarrhea, slight jaundice, and right upper quadrant discomfort are the most common complaints. Liver enlargement and eosinophilia may be present. Only by cholangiography or arteriography can the marked anatomic changes be appreciated: the hepatic vessels are stretched and narrowed, while the ducts show multiple irregularities and narrowings, often with berry-like dilatations. Sometimes the shadows caused by the leaf-shaped worms are also visible. Diagnosis is made by finding the tiny (30-μ), thick-walled, operculated eggs of these parasites in the stools.

At autopsy, the liver is often enlarged; on section, it shows irregularly-dilated bile ducts lined by fibrous tissue. The parasites can sometimes be flushed out and examined by compressing the organ, but more often are found only microscopically. In complicated cases, there is often cholestasis, bacterial superinfection, or multiple stone formation. In the earliest lesions, microscopic evidence of inflammation of the bile ducts is usually modest and eosinophilia is uncommon. Unlike schistosome eggs (p. 388), the tightly-sealed eggs of the liver flukes cause little or no granulomatous inflammation. However, metaplasia and proliferation of the bile duct epithelium are marked and there is periductal fibrosis.[331] The gallbladder may also be parasitized and inflamed, especially in *O. viverrini* infection. In some cases the pancreatic ducts show epithelial metaplasia and partial obstruction, but the large, extrahepatic bile ducts are seldom abnormal. Cholangiocarcinoma, a rare tumor in the West, is a common form of cancer where Oriental liver flukes are endemic.

Therapeutic agents are available that are likely to diminish morbidity in the future; prevention of fecal contamination of fish ponds by humans and domestic animals is the long-term solution.

*Fasciolopsiasis**

The large intestinal fluke *Fasciolopsis buski* (up to 7 cm long) localizes principally within the small bowel, where it usually causes rather mild inflammatory changes. For the most part these infections are found in India and China and other countries around the Indian Ocean. The pig is a major reservoir. When humans or animals deposit eggs in fresh water, a larval form, the miracidium, hatches and invades an appropriate snail. Within this host, the larvae are transformed to cercariae, which upon leaving the snail become encysted on water plants.

Man contracts the infection by the ingestion of the contaminated plants or water. The cysts are dissolved in the upper intestinal tract, and the larval forms emerge, mature into adult worms, and become attached to the mucosa of the small bowel by means of their suckers. At the local sites of involvement, a hemorrhagic inflammation ensues which is at first fairly nonspecific, although principally characterized by eosinophils. As these focal injuries progress, actual abscesses may develop in the mucosa, with considerable destruction of the intestinal mucosa.

As a consequence of these anatomic lesions in the small bowel, patients often have abdominal pain and diarrhea. When the infection is very severe, a generalized, constitutional febrile reaction sometimes appears, accompanied by facial and periorbital edema. Very infrequently, tangled masses of worms may produce acute intestinal obstruction. Diagnosis is made by identification of the characteristic eggs in the feces.

*Paragonimiasis (Lung Fluke, Pulmonary Distomiasis)**

Flukes of the genus *Paragonimus* are small flatworms, 1.2 cm long, which cause cystic and inflammatory lesions mainly in the lung, more rarely in the brain and abdominal and other organs. Uncooked crabs and crayfish containing the metacercarial form are the main sources of human infection, and the parasite's life cycle is maintained by many hosts including dogs, cats, and humans. Chronic cough, bronchiectasis, and hemoptysis are the most common manifestations. Formerly believed to be due to a single species *(P. westermani)* and limited to the Far East and Philippines, paragonimiasis caused by five other species has now been found in many parts of the tropics including Central and South America and West Africa. In the U.S., clinical cases in Asian immigrants have recently increased in number.

Paragonimus eggs are coughed up, swallowed, and excreted with the feces. They hatch in water and release their miracidia, which then enter several susceptible snail species and develop into cercariae. When liberated, these attack various second intermediate crustacean hosts in which they encyst, to be eaten by man or other definitive hosts.

The ingested young flukes excyst and traverse the gut wall, peritoneum, and diaphragm on their way to the lung, usually without causing significant lesions or symptoms; however, parasites that die in ectopic locations can give rise to focal abscesses, e.g., in the gut wall, pancreas, or brain. Such ectopic lesions are most common in heavily infected individuals; cerebral paragonimiasis, simulating brain tumors, epilepsy, or meningitis, is therefore most common in highly endemic areas such as Korea, Japan, and parts of China, where local brain calcifications are frequent x-ray findings. Once arrived in their definitive habitat, the lung, the parasites incite an encapsulating inflammatory host reaction rich in eosinophils, and end up forming multiple cysts, each a few centimeters in size. Here they lay large numbers of thick-shelled, operculated eggs, which add to the inflammatory process by inciting a granulomatous reaction. Sooner or later, Paragonimus cysts rupture into bronchioles, and their eggs, together with exudate and blood, begin to be expectorated or swallowed.[332] Chronic bronchial irritation by the long-lived worms and their eggs and by occasional dead parasites then leads to focal organizing pneumonitis and bronchiectasis. There frequently is bacterial superinfection. At this stage, the clinical picture often simulates tuberculosis, and in the Orient these two infections frequently coexist. Pure paragonimiasis less frequently involves the lung apices and subpleural parenchyma than does tuberculous infection. Abdominal symptoms are rarely present without significant pulmonary pathology.

Histopathologically, the lesions of paragonimiasis are varied. The cysts in the lungs form abscess-like collections of eosinophils mixed with Charcot-Leyden crystals. In the cyst wall and around eggs extruded from cysts, granulomas arise. Similar changes are seen in cerebral and ectopic Paragonimus lesions. Fibrous scarring then ensues, extending outward in radial fashion to further complicate the picture. Peripheral blood eosinophilia is inconstant, and diagnosis depends almost exclusively on identification of the parasite eggs in the sputum or feces.

The severity of the disease depends on the intensity of infection and ranges from mild to lethal. Clinical diagnosis is difficult, sometimes only recognizable when the characteristic lung cysts containing brownish material are visualized in a surgical or autopsy specimen, or when eggs are demonstrated on a smear.

*Schistosomiasis (Bilharziasis)**

Man is the host of several species of schistosomes that reproduce sexually in the venous bloodstream. The adult parasites are well adapted to their human habitat and cause few changes, but the numerous eggs they lay elicit hypersensitivity granulomas in many organs; these ultimately result in fibrosis of the liver or in obstructive uropathy, and less frequently in lesions of other organs including the CNS. The disease occurs throughout the tropics wherever the parasite's specific snail intermediate hosts are found. Of the 250 million people estimated to bear these infections, about 5% may suffer severe disease. Schistosomiasis therefore ranks high among the chronic endemic infections of mankind.[333]

Six schistosome species are known to infect man. The major ones are *S. mansoni* (Africa, Latin America, the Caribbean, parts of the Near East); *S. japonicum* (China, the Philippines, other parts of the Far East); and *S. haematobium* (Africa and parts of the Near East). Most species seek the portal vein branches as their habitat, but *S. haematobium* prefers the pelvic vena caval tributaries. Several species, but not *S. mansoni*, can also naturally infect animal reservoir hosts other than nonhuman primates,[334] and several animal schistosomes can cause abortive human infections in which the parasites die largely in the skin, giving rise to a hypersensitivity dermatitis named "swimmer's itch" or cercarial dermatitis. This self-terminating disorder occurs in both temperate and tropical settings, including the U.S.

Endemic human schistosomiasis is transmitted by water contact. The free-swimming, fork-tailed *cercariae* released by infected snails quickly burrow through the human epidermis, converting to young worms or *schistosomula*. These enter the bloodstream, pausing in the lung at four to 14 days, and continue recycling until they reach the intrahepatic portal radicles where they mature, finally descending into the mesenteric or pelvic venules where they begin their mating and egg-laying. Schistosome eggs measure up to 150 μ in length, too large to traverse capillaries; they are faintly yellow and translucent with a terminal *(S. haematobium)* or lateral *(S. mansoni)* spine, and contain a miracidial embryo. When mature eggs are deposited in water with human feces or urine, the miracidium hatches and seeks the specific intermediate snail host in which the asexual part of the life cycle is completed, culminating in the reemergence of *cercariae*. The early stages of infection are usually silent, but a fleeting rash may sometimes mark the penetration sites, and sometimes cough, fever, eosinophilia, and asthma-like symptoms appear. Each fertilized female in perpetual copulation with a male can lay up to 500 eggs per day. The 1.5-cm long adult worm pair, wedged into a venule near the gut or urinary lumen, expels its eggs, and these are either extruded into the feces or urine or caught in the wall of the conduit, or swept back by the bloodstream into the liver or lung. Although this early stage of the infection is usually asymptomatic, some individuals, often visitors from outside the endemic area, become febrile during this period, with high eosinophilia, hepatosplenomegaly, diarrhea, or allergic manifestations: this symptom complex is named acute schistosomiasis, toxemic schistosomiasis, or Katayama fever (in Japan). It, too, reverses spontaneously over several weeks and, as oviposition and egg excretion continue, the disease then enters a period of clinical latency. In most light infections, latency continues indefinitely; in severe ones, chronic disease makes its appearance years later.[335]

PATHOGENESIS. Adult schistosomes do not incite significant host/tissue reactions until they die or are killed by drugs. The dead parasites give rise to scattered, large, necrotic granulomas; these are too few in number to explain the manifestations of the disease. By contrast, the eggs, often numbered in millions, are known to release soluble antigens through their porous egg shells during their two- to three-week life span, thus inciting host cellular immunity and hypersensitivity. Those eggs that impact in small vessels are soon surrounded by granulomas containing macrophages and lymphoid and granulocytic elements, and rich in eosinophils. Schistosome granulomas (Fig. 8–54) attain diameters of 500 μ or more, and thus encroach on vessels and parenchymal tissues. However, as the infection turns chronic, granuloma sizes decrease through a complex regulatory process of immune modulation.[336] After several weeks, schistosome eggs die and are destroyed. Each individual granuloma then heals with or without fibrous scarring, but new crops of granulomas continue appearing until the adult worms are killed or rendered infertile. Schistosome granulomas are immunologic and biochemical "factories" processing parasite egg antigens and somatic components and generating a host of enzymes, lymphokines, and other mediators.[337–340] They have served as useful experimental models of cell-mediated hypersensitivity; however, the manner in which the severe fibrotic lesions of chronic schistosomiasis derive from these focal lesions is still uncertain except for a clear relationship to the magnitude of worm and egg burdens.[335]

MORPHOLOGY. The lesions of schistosomiasis vary by species, intensity of infection, and stage. Asymptomatic subjects with light *S. mansoni* or *S. japonicum* infections

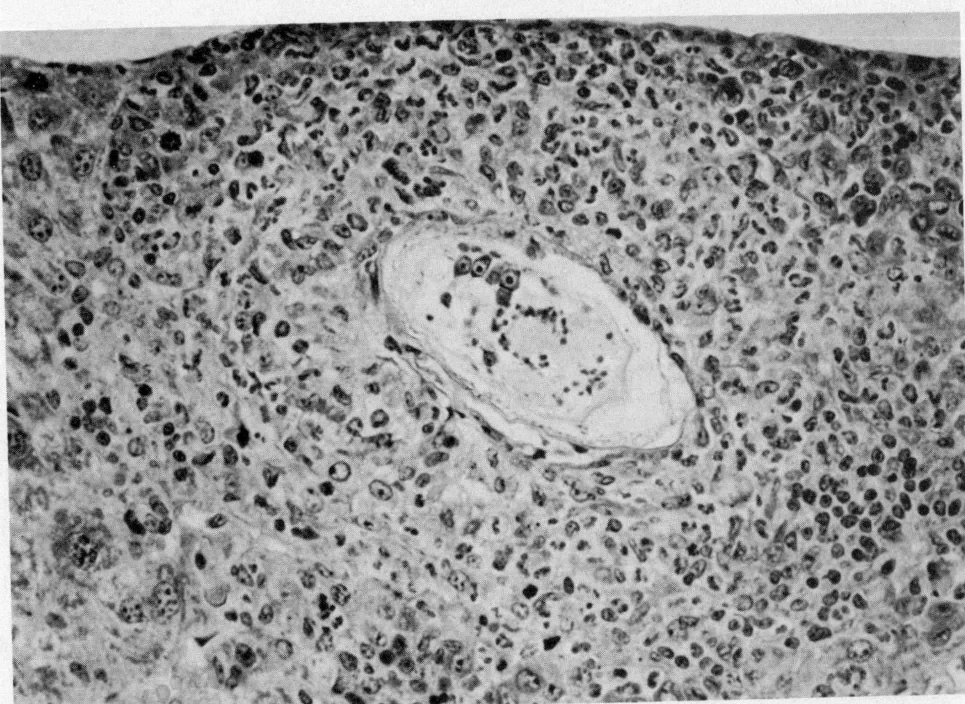

Figure 8–54. *Schistosoma mansoni* granuloma with miracidium-containing egg *(center)* and numerous scattered eosinophils.

may have only scattered eggs and granulomas in the gut, liver, and lung, with sporadic eggs elsewhere in the body. Pinhead-sized, white granuloma nodules are best seen beneath the liver capsule; often, the liver is darkened by regurgitated heme-derived pigment from the hematophagous schistosome gut. Like malaria pigment, schistosome pigment is Prussian blue–negative, and accumulates in Kupffer cells and splenic macrophages without any known adverse consequences.

In severe *schistosomiasis mansoni* or *japonica* the liver is dark in color, showing a bumpy but not a nodular surface, distinct from that of ordinary cirrhosis. In addition to granulomas, the cut surface of the organ shows widespread fibrous portal enlargement without distortion of the intervening parenchyma by regenerative nodules. The cut surfaces of the fibrous triads simulate the cross section of a clay pipe stem, giving rise to the term "pipe-stem fibrosis."[341] Some portal triads may lack a perceptible vein lumen, and corrosion casts show widespread distortion and blockage of the portal vascular bed (Fig. 8–55). This accounts for pre-sinusoidal portal hypertension along with severe congestive splenomegaly, esophageal varices, superficial venous collaterals, and ascites. Jaundice, hepatocellular necrosis, and dysfunction tend to follow only after variceal hemorrhage has taken place.

Schistosome eggs diverted to the lung via portal collaterals, when large in number, may produce granulomatous pulmonary arteritis as they impact, leading to intimal hyperplasia, progressive arterial obstruction, and ultimately heart failure (cor pulmonale). Histologically, arteries in the lungs show disruption of the elastica layer by granulomas and scars, luminal organizing thrombi, and angiomatoid lesions similar to those of idiopathic pulmonary hypertension (p. 713). In addition, patients with hepatosplenic Mansoni's schistosomiasis have an increased frequency of mesangioproliferative or membranous glomerulopathy and some glomeruli show deposits of immunoglobulin or complement, but rarely of schistosome antigen.[342]

In *S. haematobium* infection, the pathologic conditions differ sharply from those of oriental and Mansoni's schistosomiasis. Bladder inflammatory patches due to massed egg deposition may appear early, and later become rough sandy or fibrous patches. When these lesions become confluent, the entire bladder mucosa may become surrounded by a calcified egg layer, visible radiographically as a dense concentric rim (calcified bladder). Inflammation and fibrosis similarly invade the ureteral wall, leading to multiple ureteral stenoses or to irregular dilatation and hydronephrosis. Owing to their patchy distribution, *S. haematobium* eggs, even

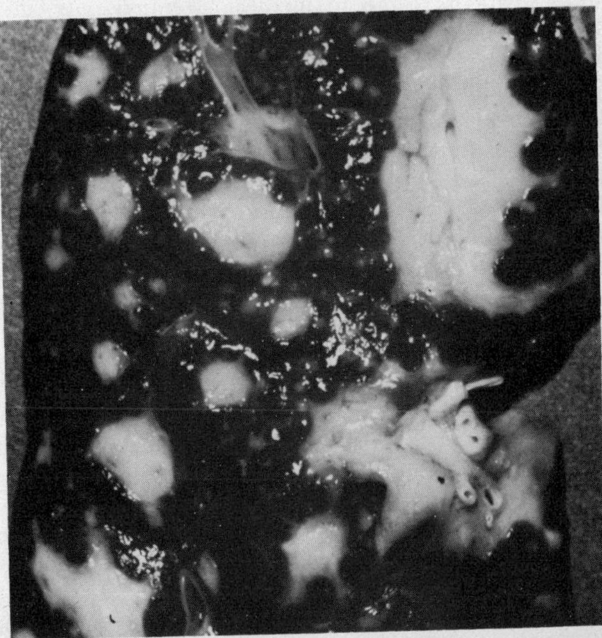

Figure 8–55. Liver pipe-stem fibrosis due to chronic *Schistosoma japonicum* infection.

when small in number, can obstruct the lower ureters. During the early inflammatory stage, these lesions are reversible, but eventually reflux nephropathy (p. 1034) with interstitial inflammation, cortical atrophy, or bacterial superinfection may result in renal failure and death. This is common in hyperendemic Egypt but seen less often in subsaharan Africa. There is also a demonstrable association between urinary schistosomiasis and bladder cancer; the tumor occurs in younger persons, and is predominantly squamous rather than the transitional cell type (p. 1072).[343] By contrast, the severe liver and lung lesions of *S. mansoni* and *S. japonicum* are rare in urinary schistosomiasis.

Ectopic egg deposition has been reported in many organs, usually without major consequences, but *S. japonicum* infection of the brain or meninges can give rise to scattered or massed egg lesions and to miscellaneous neurologic symptoms. *S. mansoni* and, more rarely, *S. haematobium* eggs can mass in the spinal cord or cauda equina, with consequences ranging from transverse spinal cord necrosis to transient paralysis. These latter lesions are unrelated to the intensity or duration of schistosome infection, and constitute a cogent argument for treating even lightly infected patients.

CLINICAL COURSE. *Schistosomiasis mansoni* is an insidious, chronic disease. In its endemic areas infected children may appear reasonably well, although they often have significant hepatomegaly. Albuminuria is somewhat more frequent in asymptomatic infected than in uninfected individuals. Hematuria is the first indication of *S. haematobium* infection, and is so common in parts of Africa that it is regarded as a normal sign of puberty. The peak incidence of severe hepatosplenic schistosomiasis with portal hypertension and the obstructive uropathy of urinary schistosomiasis is during the early twenties at a time when egg excretion may already have begun to decline. Superinfection with hepatitis B virus, frequent in the tropics, is known to aggravate and modify schistosomal liver disease. All too often, patients come to medical attention only after experiencing a life-threatening esophageal hemorrhage or when already showing a rising BUN. Others may present with anemia, hypersplenism, and retarded somatic development. Some are diagnosed and treated in their teens for protein-losing enteropathy due to schistosomal colonic polyposis, a disease form seen mainly in Near Eastern countries. The infection can also masquerade in other confusing ways.

Diagnosis is best made by finding the characteristic eggs in the feces or urine. Concentration methods are useful when eggs are scarce. Rectal biopsy, compressed between slide and coverglass and examined unstained, is sometimes necessary. Liver biopsy can be useful, but needle biopsy should not be used to determine whether pipe-stem fibrosis is present; that evaluation is best made by ultrasound study. A profusion of serologic tests for schistosomiasis exists; those employing egg antigens are the most reliable,[344] but parasitologic diagnosis is to be preferred since quantitative stool or urine egg counts render a useful estimate of the infection load. Treatment with newer drugs has been highly effective and often curative, but must always be followed up with repeated egg counts over several months, since the worms sometimes recover or reinfection may supervene, and there have been indications of relative drug resistance by some schistosome strains.[345] Although the cycle of transmission can be effectively broken by stopping fecal contamination of water sources, schistosomiasis is likely to continue as a threat to health for the foreseeable future. *S. mansoni* infection continues to be endemic in Puerto Rico, and imported clinical cases are no longer rare in the continental U.S.

SARCOIDOSIS (BOECK'S SARCOID)

Sarcoidosis is a disease of unknown cause characterized by noncaseating granulomas in many tissues and organs.[346, 347] Since a number of other diseases may produce noncaseating granulomas, including tuberculosis, tertiary syphilis, fungal infections, and berylliosis, the histologic diagnosis is largely made by exclusion. Because it is a multisystem disorder, sarcoidosis may present in many clinical guises, but bilateral hilar lymphadenopathy or lung involvement occur and are visible on a chest x-ray in 90% of cases. Eye and skin lesions are next in frequency. The Kveim reaction (skin test) is frequently positive.

Sarcoidosis is an uncommon but not rare disorder, most frequent between the ages of 20 and 35. It is more common in women than in men. Overall it is ten times more common in blacks than in whites in the U.S. There are striking geographic differences in the frequency of this disease. A much higher prevalence has been found among both blacks and whites in the southeastern part of the U.S. than elsewhere in this country. There are also puzzling national and ethnic differences. In New York City, a prevalence of approximately 30 cases per 100,000 has been reported, and in Stockholm, Sweden, a prevalence as high as 64 was found. The disease is almost unknown among Chinese and Southeast Asians. Among residents of North London, the prevalence per 100,000 was 27 for those born in the United Kingdom, 97 among Irishmen, and approximately 200 among West Indian men. The basis for these differences remains obscure.

ETIOLOGY AND PATHOGENESIS. Central to all investigations into the causation of this disease is the distinctive granulomatous nature of the tissue response. This in itself strongly suggests an immunologically mediated disease, of the delayed hypersensitivity type, with an as yet unidentified cause. Numerous agents, some common (atypical mycobacteria, beryllium) and some exotic (pine pollen, resin, even clay!) have been considered, but have never been proved to be causative. Some undetected virus is the current favorite candidate.[346]

Despite the etiologic desert, the field of pathogenesis is fertile with enticing leads. *A host of abnormal and sometimes paradoxical immunologic findings have been identified in these patients.* Although the granulomas suggest delayed hypersensitivity, *individuals with this disease have apparently deficient T-cell responses,* as evidenced by cutaneous anergy to a variety of antigens (such as tuberculin) as well as to chemical cutaneous allergens (such as 2,3-dinitrochlorobenzene, DNCB). Peripheral blood T lymphocytes are reduced sufficiently to cause an absolute lymphopenia. The number of circulating B cells, however, is normal. *These patients have hyperreactive B cells and enhanced humoral immunity,* as evidenced by hypergammaglobulinemia with abnormally high levels of antibodies to commonly encountered antigens.

Despite the deficient T-cell responses and the lymphopenia, the number of T cells in the affected *lungs* is markedly increased, and such T cells are clearly *activated.*[348, 349] Recent studies show that, in patients with active pulmonary sarcoidosis, the increase in lung T cells is made up primarily of helper lymphocytes, in a ratio of ten T-helper cells to one T suppressor. In contrast, the proportion of T helpers to T suppressors in the blood is reduced from 2:1 to 0.8:1. Thus, the granulomatous formation in the lung can be ascribed to a marked increase in T-helper cell effect without control by suppressors. Conversely, in peripheral blood there is sufficient suppressor activity to explain the cutaneous anergy. The activated T cells in the lung and the lymphokine-induced influx of monocytes are responsible for the granuloma formation, as well as for the resultant alveolitis and progressive pulmonary fibrosis.

Although the etiologic agent or agents remain unknown, there is a strong suggestion that patients destined to develop sarcoidosis respond in an abnormal manner because of some inherent immunologic derangement.

MORPHOLOGY. Pathologic involvement of virtually every organ in the body has been cited at one time or another.[350]

Lymph nodes are involved in almost all cases. The most typical groups affected are the hilar and mediastinal nodes, but any other node in the body may be involved, particularly the cervical, epitrochlear, preauricular, and postauricular nodes. The tonsils are affected in about one-quarter to one-third of cases. The nodes are characteristically enlarged, discrete and sometimes lobulated. When viewed in chest films, the bilateral hilar lymphadenopathy is referred to as "potato nodes." Typically, the affected nodes in the acute stages of the disease are soft and succulent, but in the more advanced, chronic stages they may become somewhat fibrotic. Histologically, all involved nodes show the classic **noncaseating granulomas** (Fig. 8–56). These make up an aggregate of tightly, clustered epithelioid cells, often with Langhans' or foreign body–type giant cells.

In the long chronicity of the disease, the granulomas may become enclosed within fibrous rims or eventually be replaced by hyaline fibrous scars. Two other microscopic features are often present in the granulomas: (1) laminated concretions composed of calcium and proteins known as Schaumann bodies, and (2) stellate-shaped inclusions known as asteroid bodies enclosed within giant cells (Fig. 8–57). The latter are found in approximately 60% of the granulomas. It is hardly necessary to point out that none of these microscopic features are pathognomonic of sarcoidosis, because noncaseating granulomas may be found in other conditions, as previously mentioned, and asteroid and Schaumann bodies may be encountered in other granulomatous diseases, e.g., berylliosis.

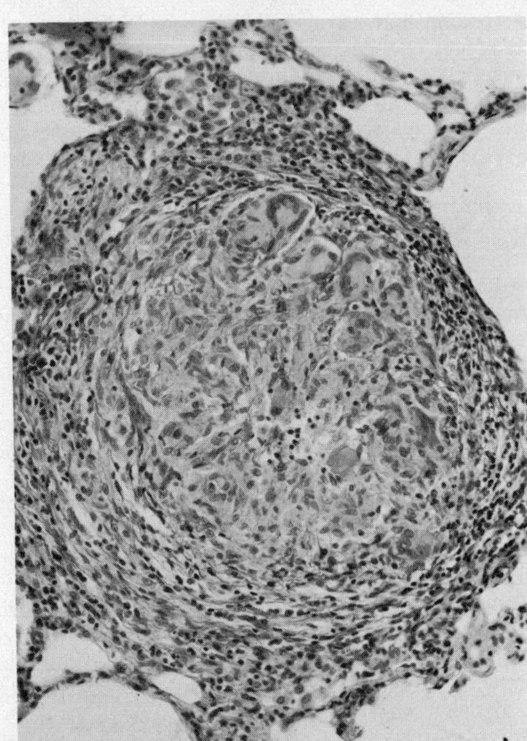

Figure 8–56. A characteristic sarcoid "noncaseating" granuloma in lung with many giant cells.

The **lungs** are common sites of involvement. Macroscopically, there is usually no demonstrable alteration, although at times the coalescence of granulomas may produce

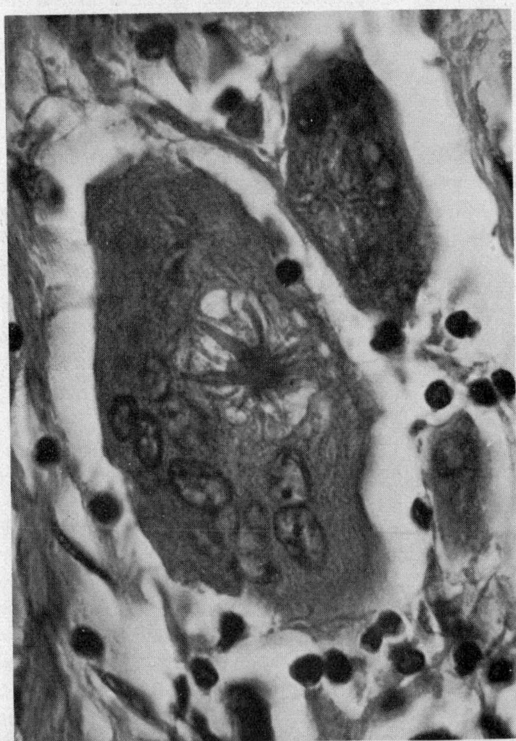

Figure 8–57. Characteristic asteroid body within a giant cell.

small nodules that are palpable or visible as 1- to 2-cm, noncaseating, noncavitated consolidations. Histologically, the lesions are distributed throughout the parenchyma, usually bilaterally, with some tendency to localize about blood vessels, bronchi, and lymphatics. The wide distribution in these organs suggests a hematogenous dissemination of some etiologic agent. In occasional cases cellular proliferative granulomas are present, but there appears to be a strong tendency for lesions to heal in the lungs, so that more often varying stages of fibrosis and hyalinization are found, causing diffuse pulmonary fibrosis (p. 747). There is, in fact, a strong suspicion that, in many cases of systemic sarcoidosis in which the lungs are not apparently involved at postmortem examination, previous lesions may have been present but have since disappeared.

The **spleen** is affected microscopically in about three-quarters of the cases, but enlarged in only 18%. On occasion, granulomas may coalesce to form small nodules that are barely visible macroscopically. The capsule is not involved. Histologically, the cellular proliferative granulomas or fibrosing or totally hyalinized lesions are dispersed throughout the splenic pulp.

The **liver** is affected slightly less often than the spleen. It may also be moderately enlarged and may contain scattered granulomas, more in portal triads than in the lobular parenchyma. Needle biopsy may permit the identification of these focal lesions.

Bone marrow is an additional favored site of localization. Roentgenographic changes can be identified in about one-fifth of cases of systemic involvement. The radiologically visible bone lesions have a particular tendency to involve phalangeal bones of the hands and feet, creating small circumscribed areas of bone resorption within the marrow cavity or a diffuse reticulated pattern throughout the cavity, with widening of the bony shafts and often new bone formations on the outer surfaces. Histologically, numerous characteristic sarcoid nodules are present in the marrow cavity.

Skin lesions are encountered in one-third to one-half of the cases. These are, in fact, the best-known lesions of sarcoidosis and were the ones first described by Boeck. Sarcoidosis of the skin assumes a variety of macroscopic appearances, e.g., discrete subcutaneous nodules; focal, slightly elevated, erythematous plaques; or flat lesions that are slightly reddened and scaling, and resemble those of lupus. Lesions may also appear on the mucous membranes of the oral cavity, larynx, and upper respiratory tract. In all instances, noncaseating granulomas are found histologically in the sites of involvement. Occasionally, deeply situated nodules, characteristic of erythema nodosum (p. 1288), have been described as sensitivity reactions.

Involvement of the **eye, its associated glands, and the salivary glands** occurs in about one-fifth to one-half of the cases. The ocular involvement takes the form of iritis or iridocyclitis, either bilaterally or unilaterally. As a consequence of these inflammatory involvements, corneal opacities, glaucoma, and total loss of vision may occur. The posterior uveal tract is also affected, but less commonly, with resultant choroiditis, retinitis, and optic nerve involvement. These ocular lesions are frequently accompanied by inflammations in the lacrimal glands with suppression of lacrimation. Bilateral sarcoidosis of the parotid, submaxillary, and sublingual glands completes **the combined uveoparotid involvement designated as Mikulicz's syndrome.**

Sarcoid granulomas occasionally occur in the heart, kidneys, CNS, and endocrine glands, particularly in the pituitary, as well as in other body tissues.

CLINICAL COURSE. Because of its varying severity and the inconstant distribution of the lesions, sarcoidosis is a protean clinical disease. In many patients, it is entirely asymptomatic and is discovered incidentally at autopsy. In still other instances, the disease is discovered unexpectedly on routine chest films as bilateral hilar adenopathy. Peripheral lymphadenopathy, cutaneous lesions, eye involvement, splenomegaly, or hepatomegaly may each be a presenting manifestation. In the great majority of cases, however, patients seek medical attention because of the insidious onset of respiratory abnormalities (shortness of breath, cough, chest pains, hemoptysis) or of constitutional signs and symptoms (fever, fatigue, weight loss, anorexia, night sweats). Occasionally a systemic hypersensitivity reaction appears with the fairly acute onset of fever, erythema nodosum, and polyarthritis, associated with bilateral hilar adenopathy. Hyperglobulinemia, hypercalcemia, hypercalcinuria, and resorptive or "punched-out" cystic lesions in the phalangeal bones are strongly supportive of the diagnosis, but any one or all of these features may be absent.

Because of these variable and nondiagnostic clinical symptom complexes, resort is frequently made to lymph node or liver biopsy and to the Kveim test. The latter is performed by intracutaneous injection of a standardized preparation of antigen (a saline suspension of sarcoidal tissue, usually from the spleen or lymph nodes). Positive reactions occur in 60 to 85% of patients and are indicated by a papule four to six weeks later. For confirmation, skin biopsy of the test site should reveal noncaseating granulomas. Although false-positive results have plagued earlier uses of the tests, the use of current carefully controlled antigens reduces the incidence of false-positive reactions to 2%.[351]

Sarcoidosis follows a fairly unpredictable course characterized by either progressive chronicity or periods of activity interspersed by remissions, sometimes permanent, that may be spontaneous or initiated by steroid therapy. Overall, 65 to 70% of affected patients recover with minimal or no residual manifestations. Twenty per cent have permanent loss of pulmonary function or some permanent visual impairment. Of the remaining 10%, some die of cardiac or CNS damage, but most succumb to progressive pulmonary fibrosis and cor pulmonale (p. 747). Patients presenting with hilar lymphadenopathy alone (stage I) have the best prognosis, followed by those with adenopathy and pulmonary infiltrates (stage II). Those presenting with pulmonary disease and no adenopathy (stage III) have few spontaneous remissions and are most likely to develop chronic pulmonary fibrosis.[352]

1. McNeill, W. H.: Plagues and Peoples. Garden City, New York, Anchor Press, Doubleday, 1976.
2. Meyerowitz, R. L.: The Pathology of Opportunistic Infections. With Pathogenetic, Diagnostic and Clinical Correlations. New York, Raven Press, 1983.
3. Murray, B. E., and Moellering, R. C., Jr.: Patterns and mechanisms of antibiotic resistance. Med. Clin. North Am. *62*:899, 1978.

4. Centers for Disease Control Task Force on Kaposi's Sarcoma and Opportunistic Infections: Epidemiological aspects of the current outbreak of Kaposi's sarcoma and opportunistic infections. N. Engl. J. Med. *306*:248, 1982.
5. Thomas, L.: Thoughts for a countdown. *In* The Lives of a Cell; Notes of a Biology Watcher. New York, Viking Press, 1974, pp. 6–10.
6. Smith, H., et al. (eds.): The Molecular Basis of Microbial Pathogenicity. Berlin, Dahlem Conference, 1980, pp. 41–54.
7. Duma, R. L.: Primary amebic meningoencephalitis. CRC Crit. Rev. Clin. Lab. Sci. *2*:163, 1972.
8. Benenson, A. S. (ed.): Control of Communicable Diseases in Man. 12th ed. Washington, D.C., American Public Health Association, 1975.
9. Hornick, R. B., et al.: The Broad Street pump revisited; response of volunteers to ingested cholera vibrios. Bull. N.Y. Acad. Med. *47*:1192, 1971.
10. Bukrinskaya, A. G.: Penetration of viral genetic material into host cell. *In* Lauffer, M. A., et al. (eds.): Advances in Virus Research. Vol. 72. New York–London, Academic Press, 1982, pp. 141–204.
11. Sharpe, A. H., and Fields, B. N.: Reovirus inhibition of cellular DNA synthesis: Role of the S1 gene. J. Virol. *38*:389, 1981.
12. Sharpe, A. H., et al.: The interaction of mammalian reoviruses with the cytoskeleton of monkey kidney, CV-1 cells. Virology *120*:399, 1982.
13. Warren, K. G., et al.: Isolation of latent herpes simplex virus from the superior cervical and vagus ganglions of human beings. N. Engl. J. Med. *298*:1068, 1978.
14. Doherty, P. C.: Cell-mediated immunity in viruses and intracellular bacteria. Clin. Rheum. Dis. *4*:549, 1978.
15. Hirsch, M. S., and Hammer, S. M.: Nucleoside derivatives and interferons as antiviral agents. *In* Remington, J. S., and Swartz, M. N. (eds.): Current Clinical Topics in Infectious Diseases. New York, McGraw-Hill Book Co., 1982, pp. 30–55.
16. Chisari, F. V., et al.: Cellular reactivity in hepatitis B virus-induced liver disease. *In* Vyas, G. N., et al. (eds.): Viral Hepatitis: A Contemporary Assessment of Etiology, Epidemiology, Pathogenesis and Prevention. Philadelphia, Franklin Institute Press, 1978, p. 245.
17. Craighead, J. E.: Viral diabetes mellitus in man and experimental animals. Am. J. Med. *70*:127, 1981.
18. National Surveillance for Reye's Syndrome: Update: Reye's syndrome and salicylate usage. M.M.W.R. *31*:55, 1981.
19. Gall, E.: Mumps orchitis histopathology. Am. J. Pathol. *23*:637, 1947.
20. Yolken, R. H., and Kapikian, A. Z.: Rotavirus. *In* Mandell, G. L., et al. (eds.): Principles and Practice of Infectious Diseases. New York, John Wiley & Sons, 1979, pp. 1268–1281.
21. Holmes, I. H., et al.: Infantile enteritis viruses: Morphogenesis and morphology. J. Virol. *16*:937, 1975.
22. Schreiber, D. S., et al.: The small intestinal lesion induced by Hawaii agent acute infectious non-bacterial gastroenteritis. J. Infect. Dis. *129*:705, 1974.
23. Hinman, A. R.: World eradication of measles. Rev. Infect. Dis. *4*:933, 1982.
24. Fenner, F.: Global eradication of smallpox. Rev. Infect. Dis. *4*:916, 1982.
25. Numerous authors (8 reports): Acyclovir in the normal host. *In* Acyclovir Symposium. Am. J. Med. *23*:281–290, 1982.
26. Nash, G.: Necrotizing tracheobronchitis and bronchopneumonia consistent with herpetic infection. Hum. Pathol. *12*:283, 1972.
27. Weller, T. H.: The cytomegalovirus: Ubiquitous agents with protean clinical manifestations. N. Engl. J. Med. *285*:203, 267, 1971.
28. Betts, R. F.: Syndromes of cytomegalovirus infection. Adv. Intern. Med. *26*:447, 1980.
29. Stern, H.: Cytomegalovirus infection. Br. J. Clin. Pract. *29*:245, 1975.
30. Craighead, J. E.: Cytomegalovirus pulmonary disease. Pathobiol. Annu. *5*:197, 1975.
31. Sterner, G., et al.: Acquired cytomegalovirus infection in older children and adults. Scand. J. Infect. Dis. *2*:95, 1970.
32. Epstein, M. A., and Achong, B. G.: Pathogenesis of infectious mononucleosis. Lancet *2*:1270, 1977.
33. Henle, W., et al.: Epidemiologic aspects of Epstein-Barr virus and Epstein-Barr virus–associated disease. Ann. N.Y. Acad. Sci. *354*:326, 1980.
34. Ho, M. J.: The lymphocyte in infections with Epstein-Barr virus and cytomegalovirus. J. Infect. Dis. *143*:857, 1981.
35. Kass, E. H., and Robbins, S. L.: Severe hepatitis in infectious mononucleosis: Report of a case with minimal clinical manifestations and death due to rupture of the spleen. Arch. Pathol. *50*:644, 1950.
36. Custer, R. P., and Smith, E. B.: The pathology of infectious mononucleosis. Blood *3*:830, 1948.
37. Sullivan, B. H., et al.: The liver in infectious mononucleosis. Am. J. Dig. Dis. *2*:210, 1957.
38. Purtilo, D. T.: Immune deficiency predisposing to Epstein-Barr virus–induced lymphoproliferative disease: The X-linked lymphoproliferative syndrome as a model. Adv. Cancer Res. *34*:279, 1981.
39. Halstead, S. B., et al.: Original antigenic sin in dengue. Am. J. Trop. Med. Hyg. *32*:154, 1983.
40. Strano, A. J.: Yellow fever. *In* Binford, C. H., and Connor, D. H. (eds.): Pathology of Tropical and Extraordinary Diseases. Washington, D.C., Armed Forces Institute of Pathology, 1976, pp. 1–4.
41. Child, P. L.: Viral hemorrhagic fevers. *In* Binford, C. H., and Connor, D. H. (eds.): Pathology of Tropical and Extraordinary Diseases. Washington, D.C., Armed Forces Institute of Pathology, 1976, pp. 5–10.
42. Clayton, A. J., and Best, H. R.: Controlling the exotic diseases. Can. Med. Assoc. J. *123*:863, 867, 1980.
43. Kawasaki, T., et al: A new infantile acute febrile mucocutaneous lymph node syndrome (MLNS) prevailing in Japan. Pediatrics *54*:271, 1974.
44. Fujiwara, H., and Hamashima, Y.: Pathology of the heart in Kawasaki's disease. Pediatrics *61*:100, 1978.
45. Crocker, D. W., et al.: Aneurysms of the coronary arteries. Report of 3 cases in infants and review of the literature. Am. J. Pathol. *33*:819, 1957.
46. Melish, M. E.: Kawasaki syndrome: A new infectious disease. J. Infect. Dis. *143*:317, 1981.
47. Editorial: Acquired immunodeficiency syndrome. Lancet *1*:161, 1983.
48. Harris, C., et al.: Immunodeficiency in female sexual partners of men with the acquired immunodeficiency syndrome. N. Engl. J. Med. *308*:1181, 1983.
49. Guarda, L. A., et al.: Lymphadenopathy in homosexual men. Morbid anatomy with clinical and immunologic correlations. Am. J. Clin. Pathol. *79*:559, 1983.
50. Reichert, C. M., et al.: Autopsy pathology in the acquired immune deficiency syndrome. Am. J. Pathol. *112*:357, 1983.
51. Urmacher, C., et al.: Outbreak of Kaposi's sarcoma with cytomegalovirus infection in young homosexual men. Am. J. Med. *72*:569, 1982.
52. Moulder, J. W.: The cell as an extreme environment. Proc. R. Soc. Lond. *204*:199, 1979.
53. Schachter, J.: Chlamydial infections. N. Engl. J. Med. *298*:428, 490, 540, 1978.
54. Beem, M., and Saxon, E.: Respiratory tract colonization and a distinctive pneumonia syndrome in infants infected with Chlamydial trachomatis. N. Engl. J. Med. *296*:306, 1977.
55. Gordon, F. B., and Quan, A. L.: Isolation of the trachoma agent in cell culture. Proc. Soc. Exp. Biol. Med. *118*:354, 1965.
56. Nichols, R. I. (ed.): Trachoma and related disorders caused by chlamydial agents. Proceedings of a Symposium held in Boston, MA, 1970. International Congress Series No. 223. Amsterdam, Excerpta Medica, 1971.
57. Stewart, D. B.: The gynecological lesions of lymphogranuloma venereum and granuloma inguinale. Med. Clin. North Am. *48*:773, 1964.
58. Jorgensen, L.: Lymphogranuloma venereum. A study of the pathology and the pathogenetic problem based on observation of eight cases examined post-mortem. Acta Pathol. Microbiol. Scand. *47*:113, 1959.
59. Burgdorfer, W., and Brinton, L. P.: Mechanisms of transovarial infection of spotted fever rickettsiae in ticks. Ann. N.Y. Acad. Sci. *266*:61, 1975.
60. Winkler, H. H., and Miller, E. T.: Phospholipase A activity in the hemolysis of sheep and human erythrocytes by *Rickettsia prowazeki*. Infect. Immun. *29*:316, 1980.
61. Zinsser, H.: Rats, Lice and History. Boston, Atlantic Monthly Press, Little Brown & Co., 1935.
62. Duma, R. J., et al.: Epidemic typhus in the United States associated with flying squirrels. J.A.M.A. *245*:2318, 1981.
63. Wolbach, S. B.: The Pathology of the Rickettsial Diseases of Man. Boston, Harvard University Press, American Association for the Advancement of Science Monograph, 1948.
64. Murray, E. S., and Snyder, J. C.: Brill-Zinsser disease. The interepidemic reservoir of epidemic louse-borne typhus fever. Rome, Proc. 6th International Congress on Microbiology *11*:31, 1953.
65. Mooser, H., et al.: Rats as carriers of Mexican typhus fever. J.A.M.A. *47*:4, 1931.
66. Walker, D. H., et al.: Laboratory diagnosis of Rocky Mountain spotted fever by immunofluorescent demonstration of *Rickettsia rickettsii* in cutaneous lesions. Am. J. Clin. Pathol. *69*:619, 1978.
66A. Brooks, J. B., et al.: Rapid differentiation of Rocky Mountain spotted fever from chickenpox, measles, enterovirus infections and bacterial meningitis by frequency-pulsed electron capture gas-liquid chromatographic analysis of sera. J. Clin. Microbiol. *14*:165, 1981.
67. Allen, A. C., and Spitz, S. A.: A comparative study of the pathology of scrub typhus and other rickettsial diseases. Am. J. Pathol. *21*:603, 1945.
68. Berman, S. J., and Kundin, W. P.: Scrub typhus in South Vietnam. A study of 87 cases. Ann. Intern. Med. *79*:26, 1973.
69. Grove, D. I.: Q fever. Aust. Fam. Physician *9*:680, 1980.
70. Dupont, H. C., et al.: Q fever hepatitis. Ann. Intern. Med. *74*:198, 1971.
71. Pellegrin, M., et al.: Granulomatous hepatitis in Q fever. Hum. Pathol. *77*:51, 1980.
72. Chanock, R. M.: Mycoplasma infections of man. N. Engl. J. Med. *273*:1199, 1257, 1965.
73. Maisel, J. C., et al.: Fatal *Mycoplasma pneumoniae* infection with isolation of organisms from the lung. J.A.M.A. *202*:287, 1967.
74. Mäkelä, P. F., et al.: Evasion of host defenses (Group Report). *In* Smith,

J. J., et al.: (eds.): The Molecular Basis of Microbial Pathogenicity. Berlin, Dahlem Konferenzen, 1980, pp. 175–198.
75. Cohn, A. Z.: The activation of mononuclear phagocytes. Fact, fancy and future. J. Immunol. *121*:813, 1978.
76. Pappenheimer, A. M., and Gill, D. M.: Diphtheria. Science *182*:353, 1973.
77. Iglewski, B. H., and Kabat, D.: NAD-dependent inhibition of protein synthesis by *Pseudomonas aeruginosa* toxin. Proc. Natl. Acad. Sci. U.S.A. *72*:2284, 1975.
78. Moseley, S. L., et al.: Detection of enterotoxigenic *Escherichia coli* by DNA colony hybridization. J. Infect. Dis. *142*:892, 1980.
79. O'Brien, T. F., et al.: Molecular epidemiology of antibiotic resistance in Salmonella from animals and human beings in the United States. N. Engl. J. Med. *307*:1, 1982.
80. Peter, G., et al.: Meningococcal meningitis in familial deficiency of the 5th component of complement. Pediatrics *67*:882, 1981.
81. Gershon, R. K.: Introduction, Symposium on Immunoregulation (5 papers). Fed. Proc. *38*:2051, 1979.
82. Mehra, V., et al.: Activated suppressor cells in leprosy. J. Immunol. *129*:1946, 1982.
83. Wolleman, O. J., and Finland, M.: Pathology of staphylococcal pneumonia complicating clinical influenza. Am. J. Pathol. *19*:23, 1943.
84. Chesney, T. J., et al.: Clinical manifestations of toxic shock syndrome. J.A.M.A. *246*:741, 1981.
85. Abdul-Karim, S. W., et al.: Toxic shock syndrome: Clinicopathologic findings in a fatal case. Hum. Pathol. *12*:16, 1981.
86. Austrian, R.: Pneumococcus; the first one hundred years. Rev. Infect. Dis. *3*:183, 1981.
87. Finland, M.: Conference on the pneumococcus. Summary and comments. Rev. Infect. Dis. *3*:358, 1981.
88. Brener, D., et al.: Increased virulence of *Neisseria meningitidis* after in vitro iron limited growth at low pH. Infect. Immun. *33*:59, 1981.
89. Tramont, E. C., et al.: Gonococcal pilus vaccine. Studies of antigenicity and inhibition of attachment. J. Clin. Invest. *68*:881, 1981.
90. Barlow, D., and Phillips, I.: Gonorrhoea in women. Diagnostic, clinical and laboratory aspects. Lancet *1*:761, 1978.
91. Bennett, J. V.: Incidence and nature of endemic and epidemic nosocomial infections. *In* Bennett, J. V., and Brachman, P. S. (eds.): Hospital Infections. Boston, Little, Brown & Co., 1979, Chap. 13.
92. Yu, V. L.: *Serratia marcescens*. Historical perspective and clinical review. N. Engl. J. Med. *300*:887, 1979.
93. Order, S. A., and Moncrief, J. A.: The Burn Wound. Springfield, IL, Charles C Thomas, 1965.
94. Cohen, P. S., et al.: Infective endocarditis caused by gram-negative bacteria. A review of the literature, 1945–1977. Prog. Cardiovasc. Dis. *22*:205, 1980.
95. Blackmon, J. A., et al.: Legionnaires' disease. Pathological and historical aspects of a "new" disease. Arch. Pathol. Lab. Med. *102*:337, 1978.
96. Rowbotham, T. J.: Preliminary report on the pathogenicity of *Legionella pneumophila* for fresh water amoebae. J. Clin. Pathol. *33*:1170, 1980.
97. Horwitz, M. A., and Silverstein, S. C.: Activated human monocytes inhibit the intracellular multiplication of legionnaires' disease bacteria. J. Exp. Med. *154*:1618, 1981.
98. Winn, W. C., and Meyerowitz, R. L.: The pathology of the Legionella pneumonias. Hum. Pathol. *12*:401, 1981.
99. England, A. C., and Fraser, D. W.: Sporadic and epidemic nosocomial legionellosis in the United States. Epidemiologic features. Am. J. Med. *70*:707, 1981.
100. Zaleznik, D. F., and Kasper, D. L.: The role of anaerobic bacteria in abscess formation. Annu. Rev. Med. *33*:217, 1982.
101. Gorbach, S. L., and Bartlett, J. G.: Anerobic infections. N. Engl. J. Med. *290*:1177, 1237, 1289, 1974.
102. Lerner, A. M.: Gram-negative pneumonias. D. M. *27*:1, 1981.
103. Olson, L. C.: Pertussis. Medicine *54*:427, 1975.
104. Pittman, M.: Pertussis toxin: The cause of the harmful effects and prolonged immunity of whooping cough. A hypothesis. Rev. Infect. Dis. *1*:401, 1979.
105. Boyer, N. H., and Weinstein, L.: Diphtheritic myocarditis. N. Engl. J. Med. *239*:913, 1948.
106. Butler, S., and Levine, S. A.: Diphtheria as a cause of late heart block. Am. Heart J. *5*:592, 1930.
107. Rothbaum, R., et al.: A clinicopathologic study of entero-adherent *Escherichia coli:* A cause of protracted diarrhea in infants. Gastroenterology *83*:441, 1982.
108. Sprinz, H., et al.: Histopathology of the upper small intestine in typhoid fever. Am. J. Dig. Dis. *11*:615, 1966.
109. Rout, W. R., et al.: Pathophysiology of salmonella diarrhea in the rhesus monkey: Intestinal transport, morphological and bacteriological studies. Gastroenterology *67*:59, 1974.
110. Mandal, B. K., and Mani, V.: Colonic involvement in salmonellosis. Lancet *1*:887, 1976.
111. Farid, Z., et al.: Chronic salmonellosis, urinary schistosomiasis and massive proteinuria. Am. J. Trop. Med. Hyg. *21*:578, 1972.
112. Rocha, H., et al.: Prolonged Salmonella bacteremia in patients with *Schistosoma mansoni* infection. Arch. Intern. Med. *128*:254, 1971.
113. Young, S. W., et al.: Interactions of salmonellae and schistosomes in host-parasite relations. Trans. R. Soc. Trop. Med. Hyg. *67*:797, 1973.
114. Rout, W. R., et al.: Pathophysiology of shigella diarrhea in the rhesus monkey: Intestinal transport, morphological and bacteriological studies. Gastroenterology *68*:270, 1975.
115. Levine, M. M., et al.: Pathogenesis of *Shigella dysenteriae* 1 (Shiga) dysentery. J. Infect. Dis. *127*:261, 1973.
116. Kelly, M. T., and McCormick, W. F.: Acute bacterial myositis caused by *Vibrio vulnificus*. J.A.M.A. *246*:72, 1981.
117. Blake, P. A., et al.: Cholera—a possible endemic focus in the United States. N. Engl. J. Med. *302*:305, 1980.
118. Carpenter, C. C. J.: Mechanism of bacterial diarrheas. Am. J. Med. *68*:313, 1980.
119. Dammin, G. J.: Vibrio-caused diseases: Cholera. *In* Binford, C. H., and Connor, D. H. (eds.): Pathology of Tropical and Extraordinary Diseases. Washington, D.C., Armed Forces Institute of Pathology, 1976, pp. 137–144.
120. Rappaport, R. S., et al.: Development of a vaccine against experimental cholera and *Escherichia coli* diarrheal disease. Infect. Immun. *32*:534, 1981.
121. Blaser, M. J., and Reller, L. B.: Campylobacter enteritis. N. Engl. J. Med. *305*:1444, 1983.
122. Colgan, T., et al.: *Campylobacter jejuni* enterocolitis. A clinicopathologic study. Arch. Pathol. Lab. Med. *104*:571, 1980.
123. Vantrappen, G., et al.: Yersinia enteritis and enterocolitis: Gastroenterologic aspects. Gastroenterology *72*:220, 1977.
124. Dammin, G. J.: Acute diarrhea and dysentery caused by *Yersinia enterocolitica*. *In* Binford, C. H., and Connor, D. H. (eds.): Pathology of Tropical and Extraordinary Diseases. Washington, D.C., Armed Forces Institute of Pathology, 1976, pp. 162–164.
125. Berggren, G. G., et al.: Traditional midwives, tetanus immunization and infant mortality in rural Haiti. Trop. Doct. *13*:79, 1983.
126. Furste, W. J.: Proceedings, 5th International Conference on Tetanus, Sweden. J. Trauma *20*:101, 1980.
127. Weinstein, L.: Tetanus. N. Engl. J. Med. *289*:1129, 1973.
128. Feldman, R. A. (ed.): A seminar on infant botulism. Rev. Infect. Dis. *1*:612, 1979.
129. Merson, M. H.: Current trends in botulism in the U.S. J.A.M.A. *229*:1305, 1974.
130. Simpson, L. L.: The action of botulinal toxin. Rev. Infect. Dis. *1*:656, 1979.
131. Darke, S. G., et al.: Gas gangrene and related infections: Classification, clinical features and aetiology, management and mortality. A report of 88 cases. Br. J. Surg. *64*:104, 1977.
132. Trnka, Y. M., and Lamont, J. T.: Association of *Clostridium difficile* toxin with symptomatic relapse of chronic inflammatory bowel disease. Gastroenterology *80*:693, 1981.
133. Thelestam, M., and Bronnegard, M.: Interaction of cytopathogenic toxin from *Clostridium difficile* with cells and tissue culture. Scand. J. Infect. Dis. *22*(Suppl.):16, 1980.
134. Seppala, K., et al.: Colonoscopy in the diagnosis of antibiotic-associated colitis: A prospective study. Scand. J. Gastroenterol. *16*:465, 1981.
135. Schultz, M. G.: Emerging zoonoses. N. Engl. J. Med. *308*:1285, 1983.
136. Stoenner, H. (eds.): Bacterial diseases. *In* Steele, J. H. (chief ed.): Zoonoses. CRC Handbook Series, 1981, Vols. 1,2.
137. Lamb, R.: Anthrax. Br. Med. J. *1*:157, 1973.
138. Dutz, W., and Kohout, E.: Anthrax. Pathol. Annu. *6*:209. 1971.
139. Koch, R.: Untersuchungen über Bakterien. Die Aetiologie der Milzbrand Krankheit begründet auf die Entwicklungsgeschichte des *Bacillus anthracis*. Beitr. z. Biol. d. Pflanzen (Breslau) *2*:277, 1877.
140. Pasteur, L.: Charbon et virulence. Bull. Acad. Med. (Paris) *7*:253, 1878.
141. Robertson, M. H.: Listeriosis. Postgrad. Med. J. *53*:618, 1977.
142. Gantz, N. M., et al.: Listeriosis in immunosuppressed patients. Am. J. Med. *58*:637, 1975.
143. Ishak, K. G.: Listeriosis. *In* Binford, C. H., and Connor, D. H. (eds.): Pathology of Tropical and Extraordinary Diseases. Washington, D.C., Armed Forces Institute of Pathology, 1976, pp. 178–186.
144. Butler, T.: Plague and tularemia. Pediat. Clin. North Am. *26*:355, 1979.
145. Smith, J. H.: Plague. *In* Binford, C. H., and Connor, D. H. (eds.): Pathology of Tropical and Extraordinary Diseases. Washington, D.C., Armed Forces Institute of Pathology, 1976, pp. 130–134.
146. Teutsch, S. M., et al.: Pneumonic tularemia on Martha's Vineyard. N. Engl. J. Med. *301*:826, 1979.
147. Miller, R. P., and Bates, J. H.: Pleuropulmonary tularemia. A review of 29 patients. Am. Rev. Respir. Dis. *99*:31, 1969.
148. Smith, H.: Survival of vegetative bacteria in animals. Symp. Soc. Gen. Microbiol. *28*:299, 1976.
149. Wise, R. I.: Brucellosis in the United States. Past, present and future. J.A.M.A. *244*:2318, 1980.
150. Harris, H. J.: Brucellosis (Undulant Fever): Clinical and Subclinical. New York, Paul B. Hoeber, 1950.

151. Spink, W. W.: The Nature of Brucellosis. Minneapolis, University of Minnesota Press, 1956.
152. Sanford, J.: Pseudomonas species (including melioidosis and glanders). *In* Mandell, G. L., et al. (eds.): Principles and Practice of Infectious Disease. New York, John Wiley & Sons, 1979, pp. 1720–1726.
153. Piggott, J. A.: Melioidosis. *In* Binford, C. H., and Connor, D. H. (eds.): Pathology of Tropical and Extraordinary Diseases. Washington, D.C., Armed Forces Institute of Pathology, 1976, pp. 169–174.
154. Jacobs, R.: Leptospirosis. Medical staff conference, University of California, San Francisco. West. J. Med. *132*:440, 1980.
155. Dooley, J. R., and Ishak, K. G.: Leptospirosis. *In* Binford, C. H., and Connor, D. H. (eds.): Pathology of Tropical and Extraordinary Diseases. Washington, D.C., Armed Forces Institute of Pathology, 1976, pp. 101–106.
156. Arean, V. M.: The pathologic anatomy and pathogenesis of fatal human leptospirosis (Weil's disease). Am. J. Pathol. *40*:393, 1962.
157. Felsenfeld, O.: Borreliae, human relapsing fever, and parasite-vector-host relationships. Bact. Rev. *29*:46, 1965.
158. Galloway, R. E., et al.: Activation of protein mediators of inflammation and evidence for endotoxemia in *Borrelia recurrentis* infection. Am. J. Med. *63*:933, 1977.
159. Judge, D. M., et al.: Louse-borne relapsing fever in man. Arch. Pathol. *97*:136, 1974.
160. Dammin, G. J.: Two new diseases and a new tick. Infect. Dis. Pract. *4*:1, 1980.
161. Steere, A. C., et al.: The spirochetal etiology of Lyme disease. N. Engl. J. Med. *308*:733, 1983.
162. Alderete, J. F., and Baseman, J. B.: Surface-associated host protein on virulent *Treponema pallidum*. Infect. Immun. *26*:1048, 1979.
163. Friedman, P. S., and Turk, J. L.: A spectrum of lymphocyte responsiveness in human syphilis. Clin. Exp. Immunol. *21*:59, 1975.
164. Gjestland, T.: The Oslo study of untreated syphilis; an epidemiological investigation of the natural course of the syphilitic infection, based upon a restudy of the Boeck-Bruusgaard material. Acta Derm. Venereol. (Oslo) *35*, Suppl. 34, 1955.
165. Rockwell, D. H., et al.: The Tuskegee study of untreated syphilis. Arch. Intern. Med. *114*:792, 1964.
166. National Centers for Disease Control (U.S. Public Health Service), Venereal Disease Program: Syphilis, a Synopsis. Washington, D.C., U.S. Government Printing Office, 1967.
167. Tavs, L. E.: Syphilis. Major Probl. Clin. Pediatr. *19*:222, 1978.
168. Kerdel-Vegas, F., et al.: Rhinoscleroma. Springfield, IL, Charles C Thomas, 1963.
169. Kuberski, T.: Granuloma inguinale (donovanosis). Sex. Transm. Dis. *7*:129, 1980.
170. Hammond, G. W., et al.: Epidemiologic, clinical, laboratory and therapeutic features of an urban outbreak of chancroid. Rev. Infect. Dis. *2*:867, 1980.
171. Dooley, J. R.: Haemotropic bacteria in man. Lancet *2*:1237, 1980.
172. Grange, J. M.: Tuberculosis. The changing tubercle. Br. J. Hosp. Med. *22*:540, 1979.
173. Center for Disease Control. M.M.W.R. *30*:640, 1982.
174. Stead, W. W., and Dutt, A. K.: What's new in tuberculosis (editorial). Am. J. Med. *71*:1, 1981.
175. Odham, G., et al.: Demonstration of tuberculostearic acid in sputum from patients with pulmonary tuberculosis by selected ion monitoring. J. Clin. Invest. *63*:813, 1979.
176. Goren, M. B.: Immunoreactive substances of mycobacteria. Am. Rev. Respir. Dis. *125* (Suppl.):50, 1982.
177. Chaparas, D., et al.: Antigenic relationships of various mycobacterial species with *Mycobacterium tuberculosis*. Am. Rev. Respir. Dis. *117*:1091, 1978.
178. Patterson, R. J., and Goumans, G. P.: Demonstration in tissue culture of lymphocytic mediated immunity to tuberculosis. Infect. Immun. *1*:600, 1970.
179. Orme, I. M., and Collins, F. M.: T cell subsets in acquired immunity to *M. tuberculosis*. Am. Rev. Respir. Dis. *127* (Part 2):195, 1983.
180. Luelmo, F.: BCG vaccination. Am. Rev. Respir. Dis. *125* (Part 2):70, 1982.
181. Centers for Disease Control: Recommendations of the Public Health Service Advisory Committee on Immunization Practices: BCG vaccine. M.M.W.R. *28*:241, 1979.
182. Turk, J. L.: Delayed hypersensitivity. New York, Elsevier/North Holland, 1980, p. 275.
183. Tanaka, A., et al.: Epithelioid cell granuloma formation requiring no T-cell function. Am. J. Pathol. *106*:165, 1982.
184. Enarson, D. A., et al.: Failure of diagnosis as a factor in tuberculosis mortality. Can. Med. Assoc. J. *118*:1520, 1978.
185. Andrew, O. T., et al.: Tuberculosis in patients with end-stage renal disease. Am. J. Med. *68*:59, 1980.
186. Girard, W. M., et al.: Epidemiology of atypical mycobacterial disease in Texas and Louisiana. Bull. Int. Union Tuberc. *51*:262, 1976.
187. Connor, D. H., et al.: Infections by *Mycobacterium ulcerans*. *In* Binford, C. H., and Connor, D. H. (eds.): Pathology of Tropical and Extraordinary Diseases. Washington, D.C., Armed Forces Institute of Pathology, 1976, pp. 226–235.
188. Marchiondo, A. A., et al.: Naturally occurring leprosy-like disease of wild armadillos. Ultrastructure of lepromatous lesions. J. Reticuloendothel. Soc. *27*:311, 1980.
189. Van Voorhis, W. C., et al.: The cutaneous infiltrates of leprosy. Cellular characteristics and the predominant T-cell phenotypes. N. Engl. J. Med. *307*:1593, 1982.
190. Brown, J. R.: Human actinomycosis: A study of 181 subjects. Hum. Pathol. *4*:319, 1973.
191. Diamond, R. D., et al.: Damage to pseudohyphal forms of *Candida albicans* by neutrophils in the absence of serum *in vitro*. J. Clin. Invest. *61*:349, 1978.
192. Yung, C. W., et al.: Disseminated *Trichosporon beigelii* (cutaneum). Cancer *48*:2107, 1981.
193. Sudman, M. S.: Protothecosis. A critical review. Am. J. Clin. Pathol. *61*:10, 1974.
193A. Edwards, J. E., Jr. (Moderator): UCLA Conference. Severe Candida infections: Clinical perspective, immune defense mechanisms and current concepts of therapy. Ann. Intern. Med. *89*:91, 1978.
194. Baker, R. D., and Haugen, R. R.: Tissue changes and tissue diagnosis in cryptococcosis. Am. J. Clin. Pathol. *24*:14, 1955.
195. Sarosi, G. A., and Davies, S. F.: Blastomycosis. Am. Rev. Respir. Dis. *120*:911, 1979.
196. Drutz, D. J., and Catanzano, A.: Coccidioidomycosis. Am. Rev. Respir. Dis. *117*:559, 1978.
197. Straub, M., and Schwarz, J.: Histoplasmosis, coccidioidomycosis and tuberculosis: A comparative pathological study. Pathol. Microbiol. *25*:421, 1962.
198. Macher, A.: Histoplasmosis and blastomycosis. Med. Clin. North Am. *64*:447, 1980.
199. Binford, C. H., and Dooley, J. R.: Diseases caused by fungi and actinomycetes. *In* Binford, C. H., and Connor, D. H. (eds.): Pathology of Tropical and Extraordinary Diseases. Washington, D. C., Armed Forces Institute of Pathology, 1976, pp. 551–609.
200. UNDP/WORLD BANK/WHO Special Programme for Research and Training in Tropical Disease: Proceedings of a Symposium, Geneva, 1980, Schwabe and Co. Tropical Disease Research Series, 1981.
201. Diamond, L. S.: Techniques of axenic cultivation of *Entamoeba histolytica* Schaudinn, 1903 and E. histolytica-like amebae. J. Parasitol. *54*:1047, 1968.
202. Takeuchi, A., and Phillips, B. P.: Electron microscopic studies of experimental *Entamoeba histolytica* infection in the guinea pig. I. Penetration of the intestinal epithelium by trophozoites. Am. J. Trop. Med. Hyg. *24*:34, 1975.
203. Ravdin, J. I., et al.: Cytopathogenic mechanisms of *Entamoeba histolytica*. J. Exp. Med. *152*:377, 1980.
204. John, D. E., et al.: Characterization of a membrane pore forming protein from *Entamoeba histolytica*. J. Exp. Med. *156*:1677, 1982.
205. Meyer, E. A., and Radulescu, S.: Giardia and giardiasis. Adv. Parasitol. *17*:1, 1979.
206. Murphy, M. J., et al.: *Pneumocystis carinii:* A study by scanning electron microscopy. Am. J. Pathol. *86*:387, 1977.
207. Stuiver, P. C., and Goud, T. J. L.: Corticosteroids and liver amoebiasis. Br. Med. J. *2*:394, 1978.
208. Hughes, W. T., et al.: Intensity of immunosuppressive therapy and the incidence of *Pneumocystis carinii* pneumonitis. Cancer *36*:2004, 1975.
209. Ormerod, W. E.: Human and animal trypanosomes as world public health problems. Pharmacol. Ther. *6*:1, 1979.
210. Krotoski, W. A., et al.: Observations on early and late post-sporozoite tissue stages in primate malaria. 1. Discovery of a new latent form of *Plasmodium cynomologi* (the hypnozoite) and failure to detect hepatic forms within the first 24 hours after infection. Am. J. Trop. Med. Hyg. *31*:24, 1982.
211. Barnwell, J. W., et al.: Altered expression of *Plasmodium knowlesi* variant antigen on the erythrocyte membrane in splenectomized Rhesus monkeys. J. Immunol. *128*:224, 1982.
212. Howard, R. J. et al.: Studies on the role of red blood cell glycoproteins as receptors for invasion by *Plasmodium falciparum* merozoites. Mol. Biochem. Parasitol. *6*:303, 1982.
213. Udeinga, I. J., et al.: Falciparum malaria-infected erythrocytes specifically bind to cultured human endothelial cells. Science *213*:555, 1981.
214. Tizard, I., et al.: Biologically active products from African trypanosomes. Microbiol. Rev. *42*:661, 1978.
215. Mauel, J.: The biology of the macrophage-leishmania interaction. *In* Van den Bossche, H. (ed.): The Host-Invader Interplay. Amsterdam, Elsevier/North Holland Biomedical Press, 1980, pp. 165–178.
216. Sacks, D. L., et al.: Thermosensitivity patterns of old vs. new world cutaneous strains of Leishmania growing within mouse peritoneal macrophages in vitro. Am. J. Trop. Med. Hyg., *32*:300, 1983.
217. Jones, T. C.: Interactions between murine macrophages and obligate intracellular protozoa. Am. J. Pathol. *102*:127, 1981.

218. Krick, J. A., and Remington, J. S.: Toxoplasmosis in the adult. An overview. N. Engl. J. Med. *298*:550, 1980.
219. Brener, Z.: Immunity to *Trypanosoma cruzi*. Adv. Parasitol. *18*:247, 1980.
220. Szarfman, A., et al.: Antibodies to laminin in Chagas' disease. J. Exp. Med. *155*:1161, 1982.
221. Ghose, A. C., et al.: Serological investigations on Indian kala-azar. Clin. Exp. Immunol. *40*:318, 1980.
222. Mettrick, D. F., and Desser, S. S.: Parasites—Their World and Ours. Amsterdam, Elsevier Biomedical Press, 1982, 465 pp.
223. Krogstad, D. J., et al.: Amebiasis. Epidemiological studies in the United States, 1971–1974. Ann. Intern. Med. *88*:89, 1978.
224. Phillips, S. C. et al.: Sexual transmission of enteric protozoa and helminths in a venereal disease clinic population. N. Engl. J. Med. *305*:603, 1981.
225. Brandt, H., and Pérez-Tamayo, R.: The pathology of human amebiasis. Hum. Pathol. *1*:351, 1970.
226. Radke, R. A.: Ameboma of the intestine; an analysis of the disease as presented in 78 collected and 41 previously unreported cases. Ann. Intern. Med. *43*:1048, 1965.
227. Yang, J., and Kennedy, M. T.: Evaluation of an enzyme-linked immunosorbent assay for the serology of amebiasis. J. Clin. Microbiol. *10*:778, 1979.
228. McCoy, G. W., et al.: Epidemic amebic dysentery; the Chicago outbreak of 1933. N. I. H. Bulletin No. 166. Washington, D. C., U. S. Government Printing Office, 1963.
228A. Arean, V. M., and Koppisch, E.: Balantidiasis. A review and report of cases. Am. J. Pathol. *32*:1089, 1056.
229. Culbertson, C. G., et al.: Experimental infection of mice and monkeys by Acanthamoeba. Am. J. Pathol. *35*:191, 1959.
230. Martinez, A. J.: Is Acanthamoeba encephalitis an opportunistic infection? Neurology *30*:567, 1980.
231. Brown, W. J., and Voge, M.: Neuropathology of Parasitic Infections. Oxford, Oxford University Press, 1982, pp. 1–21.
232. Smith, P. D., et al.: IgG antibody to *Giardia lamblia* detected by enzyme-linked immunosorbent assay. Gastroenterology *80*:1476, 1981.
233. Moore, G. T., et al.: Epidemic giardiasis at a ski resort. N. Engl. J. Med. *281*:402, 1969.
234. Black, R. E., et al.: Giardiasis in day care centers: Evidence of person-to-person transmission. Pediatrics *60*:486, 1977.
235. Yardley, J. H., and Bayliss, T. M.: Giardiasis. Gastroenterology *52*:301, 1967.
236. Smith, P. D., et al.: Chronic giardiasis: Studies on drug sensitivity, toxin production and host immune response. Gastroenterology *83*:797, 1982.
237. Weinstein, L., et al.: Intestinal cryptosporidiosis complicated by disseminated CMV infection. Gastroenterology *81*:584, 1981.
238. Honigberg, B. M.: Trichomonads of importance in human medicine. *In* Kreier, J. P. (ed.): Parasitic Protozoa. Vol. 2. New York, Academic Press, 1978, pp. 469–550.
239. McCann, S. J.: Comparison of direct microscopy and culture in the diagnosis of trichomoniasis. Br. J. Vener. Dis. *50*:450, 1974.
240. Vanek, J., and Jirovec, O.: Parasitäre Pneumonie. "Interstitielle" Plasmazellen-Pneumonie der Frühgeborenen, verursacht durch *Pneumocystis carinii*. Zentralbl. Bakteriol. *158*:210, 1952.
241. Pintozzi, R. L., et al.: The morphological identification of *Pneumocystis carinii*. Acta Cytol. *23*:35, 1979.
242. Wilber, R. B., et al.: Chemoprophylaxis for *Pneumocystis carinii* pneumonitis. Am. J. Dis. Child. *134*:643, 1980.
243. Yoshida, N., et al.: Hybridoma produces protective antibodies against the sporozoite stage of malaria parasites. Science *207*:71, 1980.
244. McGregor, I. A.: Immunology of malarial infection and its possible consequences. Br. Med. Bull. *28*:22, 1972.
245. Edington, G. M.: Pathology of malaria in West Africa. Br. Med. J. *1*:715, 1967.
246. Marin, S. K., et al.: Severe malaria and glucose-6-phosphate dehydrogenase deficiency: A reappraisal of the malaria/G-6-P.D. hypothesis. Lancet *1*:524, 1979.
247. Miller, L. H., et al.: The Duffy blood group phenotype in American blacks infected with *Plasmodium falciparum* in Vietnam. Am. J. Trop. Med. Hyg. *27*:1261, 1977.
248. Spitz, S.: The pathology of malaria. Milit. Surg. *99*:555, 1946.
249. Hendrickse, R. G., et al.: Quartan malaria nephrotic syndrome. Collaborative clinicopathologic study in Nigerian children. Lancet 1:1143, 1972.
250. Wernsforder, W. H., and Kouznetsov, R. L.: Drug-resistant malaria—occurrence, control and surveillance. Bull. W.H.O. *58*:341, 1980.
251. Cohen, S.: Progress in malaria vaccine development. *In* Mettrick, D. F., and Desser, S. S. (eds.): Parasites, Their World and Ours. Amsterdam, Elsevier Biochemical Press, 1982, pp. 408–411.
252. Dammin, G. J., et al.: The rising incidence of clinical Babesia microti infection. Hum. Pathol. *12*:398, 1981.
253. Dammin, G. J.: Babesiosis. *In* Weinstein, L., and Fields, B. (eds.): Seminars in Infectious Disease. New York, Stratton Intercontinental Medical Book Corp., 1978, pp. 169–199.
254. Ashworth, T. G., and Goldsmid, J.: A re-assessment of the epidemiology and clinico-pathological features of human trypanosomiasis in Rhodesia. Centr. Afr. J. Med. *21* (Suppl.):1, 1975.
255. Borst, J. P., et al.: DNA rearrangements involving the genes for variant antigens in *Trypanosoma brucei*. Cold Spring Harbor Symp. Quant. Biol. *45*:935, 1980.
256. Mansfield, J. M.: Immunobiology of African trypanosomiasis. Cell. Immunol. *39*:204, 1978.
257. Morrison, W. I., et al.: The pathogenesis of experimentally induced *Trypanosoma brucei* infection in the dog. I. Tissue and organ damage. Am. J. Pathol. *102*:168, 1981.
257A. Seed, J. R., et al.: Pathophysiological changes during African trypanosomiasis. *In* Mettrick, D. F., and Desser, S. S. (eds.): Parasites, Their World and Ours. Amsterdam, Elsevier Biomedical Press, 1982, pp. 255–257.
258. Teixeira, A. R.: Chagas' disease: Trends in immunologic research and prospects for immunoprophylaxis. Bull. W.H.O. *57*:697, 1979.
259. Andrade, Z. A., et al.: Histopathology of the conducting tissue of the heart in Chagas' myocarditis. Am. Heart J. *95*:316, 1978.
260. Gutteridge, W. E.: Prospects for chemotherapy in Chagas' disease. *In* Van den Bossche, H. (ed.): The Host-Invader Interplay. Amsterdam, Elsevier/North Holland Biomedical Press, 1980, pp. 583–594.
261. Wirth, D.: Rapid identification of Leishmania species by specific hybridization of kinetoplast DNA in cutaneous lesions. Proc. Natl. Acad. Sci. U.S.A. *79*:6999, 1983.
262. deBrito, T., et al.: Glomerular involvement in kala-azar. Am. J. Trop. Med. Hyg. *24*:8, 1975.
263. Neva, F. A.: Diagnosis and treatment of cutaneous leishmaniasis. *In* Remington, J. S., and Schwartz, M. N. (eds.): Current Clinical Topics in Infectious Diseases. New York, McGraw-Hill Book Co., 1980, pp. 364–380.
264. Connor, D. F., and Neafie, R. C.: Cutaneous leishmaniasis. *In* Binford, C. H., and Connor, D. H. (eds.): Pathology of Tropical and Extraordinary Diseases. Washington, D. C., Armed Forces Institute of Pathology, 1976, pp. 258–264.
265. Ridley, D. S.: A histologic classification of cutaneous leishmaniasis and its geographical expression. Trans. R. Soc. Trop. Med. Hyg. *74*:1069, 1977.
266. Frenkel, J. K.: Toxoplasmosis in and around us. Bioscience *23*:343, 1973.
267. Dorfman, R. F., and Remington, J. S.: Value of lymph-node biopsy in the diagnosis of acute acquired toxoplasmosis. N. Engl. J. Med. *289*:878, 1973.
268. Beaver, P. C., and Orihel, T. C.: Human infection with filariae of animals in the United States. Am. J. Trop. Med. Hyg. *14*:1010, 1965.
269. Love, M.: The alien strategy. Not all parasites trust to luck. Nat. Hist. *89*:30, 1980.
270. Dean, D. A.: Decreased binding of cytotoxic antibody by developing *Schistosoma mansoni:* Evidence for a surface change independent of host antigen adsorption and membrane turnover. J. Parasitol. *63*:418, 1977.
271. Sher, A., et al.: Acquisition of murine major histocompatibility complex gene products by schistosomula of *Schistosoma mansoni*. J. Exp. Med. *148*:46, 1978.
272. Sher, A., and Moser, G.: Immunologic properties of developing schistosomula. Am. J. Pathol. *102*:121, 1981.
273. Ouaissi, M. A., et al.: Interaction between *Schistosoma mansoni* and the complement system: Role of immunoglobulin G, Fc peptides in the activation of the classical pathway by schistosomula. J. Immunol. *127*:1556, 1981.
274. Tsang, V. C., and Damian, R. T.: Demonstration and mode of action of an inhibitor for activated Hageman factor (factor XIIa) of the intrinsic blood coagulation pathway from *Schistosoma mansoni*. Blood *49*:619, 1977.
275. Leid, W. D., et al.: A parasite trypsin inhibitor with specificity for classical and alternative pathway activation of complement. Fed. Proc. *42*:1246, 1983.
276. Samuelson, J. C., et al.: Schistosomula of *Schistosoma mansoni* clear concanavalin A from their surface by sloughing. J. Cell. Biol. *94*:355, 1982.
277. Hofstetter, M., et al.: Modulation of the host response in human schistosomiasis. IV. Parasite antigen induces release of histamine that inhibits lymphocyte responsiveness in vitro. J. Immunol. *130*:1376, 1983.

278. Piessens, W. F., et al.: Antigen specific suppressor cells and suppressor factors in human filariasis with *Brugia malayi*. N. Engl. J. Med. *302*:833, 1980.
279. Smithers, S. R., et al.: Host antigens in schistosomiasis. Proc. R. Soc. Series B *171*:483, 1969.
280. Butterworth, A. E., et al.: Damage to schistosomula of *Schistosoma mansoni* induced directly by eosinophil major basic protein. J. Immunol. *122*:221, 1979.
281. James, S. L., et al.: Macrophages as effector cells of protective immunity in murine schistosomiasis. II. Killing of newly transformed schistosomula by macrophages activated as a consequence of *Schistosoma mansoni* infection. J. Immunol. *128*:1535, 1982.
282. Capron, A., et al.: Effector mechanisms of immunity to schistosomes and their regulation. Immunol. Rev. *61*:41, 1982.
283. Senft, A. W., et al.: Hemoglobinolytical activity of serum in mice infected with *Schistosoma mansoni*. Am. J. Trop. Med. Hyg. *30*:96, 1981.
284. Phillips, S. M., et al.: The immunologic modulation of morbidity in schistosomiasis. Studies in athymic mice and in vitro granuloma formation. Am. J. Trop. Med. Hyg. *29*:820, 1980.
285. Da Silva, L. C., et al.: Kidney biopsy in the hepatosplenic form of infection with *Schistosoma mansoni* in man. Bull. W.H.O. *42*:907, 1970.
286. Askenase, P. W.: Immune inflammatory responses to parasites: The role of basophils, mast cells and vasoactive amines. Am. J. Trop. Med. Hyg. *26*:96, 1977.
287. Cross, G. A. M.: New technologies for parasitology. *In* Mettrick, D. F., and Desser, S. S. (eds.): Parasites, Their World and Ours. Amsterdam, Elsevier Biomedical Press, 1982, pp. 3–12.
288. Gelpi, A. P., and Mustafa, A.: Ascaris pneumonia. Am. J. Med. *44*:377, 1968.
289. Phills, J. A.: Pulmonary abnormalities and eosinophilia due to *Ascaris suum*. N. Engl. J. Med. *286*:965, 1972.
290. Chanco, P. P., Jr., and Vidad, J. Y.: A review of trichuriasis, its incidence, pathogenicity and treatment. Drugs *15* (Suppl.):87, 1978.
291. Symmers, W. St. C.: Pathology of oxyuriasis. Arch. Pathol. *50*:475, 1950.
292. Rep, B. H.: Pathogenicity of hookworms. The significance of population regression for the pathogenicity of hookworms. Trop. Geogr. Med. *32*:251, 1980.
293. Ashford, B. K.: Ankylostomiasis in Puerto Rico, 1900. *In* Kean, B. H., et al. (eds.): Tropical Medicine and Parasitology; Classic Investigations. Vol. 2. Ithaca, Cornell University Press, 1978, pp. 314–317.
294. Scowden, E. B., et al.: Overwhelming strongyloidiasis. An unappreciated opportunistic infection. Medicine *57*:527, 1978.
295. Milner, P. F., et al.: Intestinal malabsorption in *Strongyloides stercoralis* infection. Gut *6*:574, 1965.
296. De Paola, D, et al.: Enteritis due to *Strongyloides stercoralis*. A report of five fatal cases. Am. J. Dig. Dis. *7*:1086, 1962.
297. Fresh, J. W., et al.: Necropsy findings in intestinal capillariasis. Am. J. Trop. Med. Hyg. *21*:169, 1972.
298. Snyder, C. H.: Visceral larva migrans: Ten years' experience. Pediatrics *28*:85, 1961.
299. Glickman, L., et al.: Toxocara-specific antibodies in the serum and aqueous humor of a patient with presumed ocular and visceral toxocariasis. Am. J. Trop. Med. Hyg. *28*:29, 1979.
300. Kayes, S. G., and Oaks, J. A.: Development of the granulomatous response in murine toxocariasis. Am. J. Pathol. *93*:277, 1978.
301. Nye, S. W., et al.: Lesions of the brain in eosinophilic meningitis. Arch. Pathol. *89*:9, 1970.
302. Chitanondh, H., and Rosen, L.: Fatal eosinophilic encephalomyelitis caused by the nematode *Gnathostoma spinigerum*. Am. J. Trop. Med. Hyg. *16*:638, 1967.
303. Morera, P.: Life history and redescription of *Angiostrongylus costaricensis* Morera and Céspedes, 1971. Am. J. Trop. Med. Hyg. *22*:613, 1973.
304. Pincus, G., et al.: Intestinal anisakiasis. First case reported from the United States. Am. J. Med. *59*:114, 1975.
305. Meyers, W. M., and Neafie, R. C.: Creeping Eruption. *In*: Binford, C. H., and Connor, D. H. (eds.): Pathology of Tropical and Extraordinary Diseases, Washington, D.C., Armed Forces Institute of Pathology, 1976, pp. 437–439.
306. Lucas, A. O., et al.: Niridazole in guinea worm infection. Ann. N. Y. Acad. Sci. *160*:729, 1969.
307. Gould, S. E.: Trichinosis in Man and Animals. Springfield, IL, Charles C Thomas, 1970.
308. Despommier, D.: Adaptive changes in muscle fibers infected with *Trichinella spiralis*. Am. J. Pathol. *78*:477, 1975.
309. Most, H.: Trichinosis—preventable yet still with us. N. Engl. J. Med. *298*:1178, 1978.
310. Kagan, I. G.: Serodiagnosis of trichinosis. *In* Cohen, S., and Sadun, E. (eds.): Immunology of Parasitic Infections. Oxford, Blackwell Scientific Publications, 1976, pp. 143–151.
311. Castro, G. A.: Regulation of pathogenesis in disease caused by gastrointestinal parasites. *In* Johnson, R. (ed.): Physiology of the Gastrointestinal Tract. New York, Raven Press, 1982, pp. 1381–1406.
312. Kazura, J. W., and Grove, D. J.: Stage-specific antibody-dependent eosinophil-mediated destruction of *Trichinella spiralis*. Nature *274*:588, 1978.
313. Wartman, W. B.: Filariasis in American armed forces in World War II. Medicine *26*:333, 1947.
314. Lie Kian, J.: Occult filariasis: Its relationship with tropical pulmonary eosinophilia. Am. J. Trop. Med. Hyg. *11*:646, 1962.
315. Piessens, W. F.: Immunology of lymphatic filariasis and onchocerciasis. *In* Cohen, S., and Warren, K. S. (eds.): Immunology of Parasitic Diseases. 2nd ed. Oxford, Blackwell Scientific Publications, 1982, pp. 622–653.
316. Ottesen, E. A., et al.: Specific allergic sensitization to filarial antigens in tropical eosinophilia syndrome. Lancet *1*:1158, 1979.
317. Gandhi, G. M.: Role of lymphangiography in management of filarial chyluria. Lymphology *9*:11, 1976.
318. Connor, D. H., and Neafie, R. C.: Onchocerciasis. *In* Binford, C. H., and Connor, D. H. (eds.): Pathology of Tropical and Extraordinary Diseases. Washington, D. C., Armed Forces Institute of Pathology, 1976, pp. 360–381.
319. Bartlett, A., et al.: Variation in delayed hypersensitivity in onchocerciasis. Trans. R. Soc. Trop. Med. Hyg. *72*:372, 1978.
320. Buck, A. A., et al.: Serum immunoglobulin levels in five villages of the Republic of Chad and in onchocerciasis patients with and without microfilariae. Z. Tropenmed. Parasitol. *24*:21, 1973.
321. Meyers, W. M., et al.: Human streptocerciasis. A clinico-pathologic study of 40 Africans (Zairians) including identification of the adult filaria. Am. J. Trop. Med. Hyg. *21*:528, 1972.
322. Dayal, Y., and Neafie, R. C.: Human pulmonary dirofilariasis. A case report and review of the literature. Am. Rev. Respir. Dis. *112*:437, 1975.
323. Coolidge, C., et al.: Zoonotic Brugia filariasis in New England. Ann. Intern. Med. *90*:341, 1979.
323A. Descombes, P., et al.: Endoscopic discovery and capture of *Taenia saginata*. Endoscopy *13*:44, 1981.
324. Brown, W. J., and Voge, M.: Neuropathology of Parasitic Infections. Oxford, Oxford University Press, 1982, pp. 108–136.
325. Botero, D.: Treatment of cysticercosis with praziquantel in Colombia. Am. J. Trop. Med. Hyg. *31*:811, 1982.
326. D'Allessandro, R. L., et al.: *Echinococcus vogeli* in man with a review of polycystic disease in Colombia and neighboring countries. Am. J. Trop. Med. Hyg. *28*:303, 1979.
327. Katz, A. M., and Pan, C. T.: Echinococcus disease in the United States. Am. J. Med. *25*:759, 1958.
328. Wilson, J. F., et al.: Cystic hydatid disease in Alaska. A review of 101 autochthonous cases of *Echinococcus granulosus* infection. Am. Rev. Respir. Dis. *98*:1, 1968.
329. Bendezu, P., et al.: Human fascioliasis in Corozal, Puerto Rico. J. Parasitol. *68*:297, 1982.
330. Isseroff, H., et al.: Fascioliasis: Role of proline in bile duct hyperplasia. Science *198*:1157, 1977.
331. Tansurat, P.: Opisthorchiasis. *In* Marcial-Rojas, R. A. (ed.): Pathology of Protozoal and Helminthic Diseases. Baltimore, Williams & Wilkins Co., 1971, pp. 536–545.
332. Meyers, W. M., and Neafie, R. C.: Paragonimiasis. *In* Binford, C. H. and Connor, D. H. (eds.): Pathology of Tropical and Extraordinary Diseases. Washington, D. C., Armed Forces Institute of Pathology, 1976, pp. 517–523.
333. Warren, K. S.: The relevance of schistosomiasis. N. Engl. J. Med. *303*:203, 1980.
334. Hillyer, G. V.: Schistosomiasis. *In* Steele, J. H. (ed.): CRC Handbook Series in Zoonoses; Section C: Parasitic Zoonoses. Vol. III. Boca Raton, FL, CRC Press, 1982, pp. 177–209.
335. Nash, T. E. (Moderator): Schistosome infections in humans. Perspectives and recent findings. Ann. Intern. Med. *97*:740, 1982.
336. Domingo, E. O., and Warren, K. S.: Endogenous desensitization: Changing host granulomatous response to schistosome eggs at different stages of infection with *Schistosoma mansoni*. Am. J. Pathol. *52*:369, 1968.
337. Boros, D. L.: Granulomatous inflammations. Prog. Allergy *24*:183, 1978.
338. Colley, D. G.: The immunopathology of schistosomiasis. Recent Adv. Clin. Immunol. *1*:101, 1977.
339. Weinstock, J. V., and Boros, D. L.: Alteration of the granulomatous

response in murine schistosomiasis by the chronic administration of captopril, an inhibitor of angiotensin-converting enzyme. Gastroenterology *81*:48, 1981.

340. Wyler, D. J., et al.: Hepatic fibrosis in schistosomiasis: Egg granulomas secrete fibroblast-stimulating factor in vitro. Science *202*:438, 1978.
341. Symmers, W. St. C.: Note on a new form of liver cirrhosis due to the presence of the ova of Bilharzia haematobia. J. Pathol. Bacteriol. *9*:237, 1903.
342. Andrade, Z. A., and Rocha, H.: Schistosomal nephropathy. Kidney Int. *16*:23, 1979.
343. Cheever, A. W.: Schistosomiasis and neoplasia (Editorial). J. Natl. Cancer Instit. *61*:13, 1978.
344. Mott, K. E., and Dixon, H.: Collaborative study on antigens for immunodiagnosis of schistosomiasis. Bull. W.H.O. *60*:729, 1982.
345. Jansma, W. B., et al.: Experimentally produced resistance of *Schistosoma mansoni* to hycanthone. Am. J. Trop. Med. Hyg. *26*:926, 1977.
346. Daniele, R. P.: Sarcoidosis. Diagnosis and management. Hosp. Pract. *18*:113, 1983.
347. Fanburg, B. C. (ed.): Sarcoidosis and Other Granulomatous Diseases. Marcel Dekker, New York, 1983.
348. Crystal, R. G., et al.: Pulmonary sarcoidosis: A disease characterized and perpetrated by T lymphocytes. Ann. Intern. Med. *94*:73, 1981.
349. Hunninghake, G. W., and Crystal, R. G.: Pulmonary sarcoidosis. A disorder mediated by excess helper T-lymphocyte activity at sites of disease. N. Engl. J. Med. *305*:429, 1981.
350. Thrasher, D. R., and Briggs, D. D.: *In* Pulmonary sarcoidosis. Clin. Chest. Med. *3*:537, 1982.
351. Siltzbach, L. E.: Sarcoidosis. *In* Fishman, A. P. (ed.): Pulmonary Diseases and Disorders. New York, McGraw-Hill Book Co. 1980, pp. 889–908.
352. Romer, F. K.: Presentation of sarcoidosis and outcome of pulmonary changes. Dan. Med. Bull. *29*: 27, 1982.

NUTRITIONAL DISEASE 9

It is a sad commentary on our world when the effort to avoid or reduce caloric consumption preoccupies vast segments of some societies while less fortunate populations, mainly in developing countries, are dying for want of food. Indeed, over half the entire population of the world struggles to survive on diets grossly inadequate in calories or proteins.[1] This deprivation exacts its heaviest toll from infants and children. Half of all deaths in these starving populations occur in children under 5 years of age, yielding infant mortality rates many times higher than those encountered in affluent countries. In addition to such gross malnutrition, specific deficiency states, such as the avitaminoses, often accompany protein-energy malnutrition, but may also occur despite a sufficient caloric intake.

For optimal health, about 45 to 48 dietary nutrients are currently thought to be essential. These include, in addition to the well-known vitamins, nine amino acids (lysine, threonine, leucine, isoleucine, methionine, tryptophan, valine, phenylalanine, and histidine); two polyunsaturated fatty acids (linoleic and arachidonic—although it is possible that the latter can be synthesized in the body from the former); and a large number of elements. Some of these elements are major constituents of the body such as Na, K, Ca, Mg, P, Cl, S, C, H, O, Fe, and N, whereas others are required only in small amounts and so are referred to as trace elements, e.g., zinc, copper, manganese, iodine, cobalt, molybdenum, chromium, selenium, vanadium, nickel, and possibly silicon, fluorine, tin, and arsenic. The essentiality of all these trace elements has not been well established and only three or four (copper, zinc, iodine, and possibly selenium) are associated with well-documented deficiency syndromes.[2]

Nutritional disease in humans may be of primary dietary origin or may result from secondary (conditioned) malnutrition, as indicated in Table 9–1.

Primary malnutrition is caused by lack of a reasonably balanced diet and is largely a socioeconomic problem that tends to be endemic in the underprivileged and war-torn societies of the earth. The malnutrition found in Africa, Asia, and Central and South America, for example, is largely of primary origin. In these regions of the world the precarious and marginal food supply, caused by drought and poverty, and the disruptions of war render starvation a daily threat to survival. Sometimes, despite an adequate caloric intake, the diet is so restricted that one or more essential nutrients are lacking. For instance, a deficiency of thiamine chloride sometimes accompanied by other avitaminoses may appear in individuals subsisting largely or solely on polished rice. However, primary malnutrition may be unexpectedly encountered among populations living under far more halcyon conditions. In a ten-state nutrition survey in the United States, a surprisingly high incidence of nutritional deficiencies of iron, vitamin A, vitamin C, riboflavin, and folic acid was found.[3] Principally affected were poverty-stricken families, and particularly young women who had had numerous closely spaced pregnancies. Primary malnutrition may well be encountered, therefore, in countries where nutritional inadequacies are little suspected.

Secondary or conditioned malnutrition is usually a sporadic condition that arises in the midst of dietary plenty. This is the pattern of malnutrition often found among hospitalized patients. For some reason the body is unable to utilize the ingested nutrients, and a deficiency state results, despite the intake of adequate amounts and kinds of food. Secondary malnutrition may be *self-induced* and related to drugs, alcohol, or food faddism. The prime example of self-induced conditioned malnutrition related to an *aberrant diet* is chronic alcoholism; the "empty" calories of ethanol too often replace a balanced diet. Psychogenic dysphagia (formerly called anorexia nervosa), bizarre eating habits, food faddism such as "strict vegetarianism" with no use of any animal products, or adolescent diets of soft drinks and fried potatoes are additional examples of dietary aberrations that may lead to malnutrition. *Increased metabolic requirements* are important causes of conditioned malnutrition. Such may be encountered with rapid adolescent or catch-up growth; during pregnancy and lactation; with illness and prolonged fevers; and with excessive physical activity of long duration. *Inability to ingest or absorb foodstuffs* may be seen in those

Table 9–1. ORIGINS OF MALNUTRITION

Primary malnutrition
a. poverty
b. inadequate food supply
c. nutritionally restricted diet
Secondary or conditioned malnutrition
a. aberrant diet
b. increased metabolic requirements
c. inability to ingest or absorb diet
d. impaired utilization
e. abnormal losses
f. drug induced

with inadequate dentition, diseases of the oropharynx and esophagus, obstructive jaundice, pancreatic disorders, and gastrointestinal disease, for reasons that are obvious. *Impaired utilization* is exemplified by diabetes mellitus (p. 972) in which the lack of effective insulin action leads to all manner of secondary metabolic derangements involving not only carbohydrates, but fats and proteins also. *Excessive losses* of requisite nutrients may be seen in severe renal disease or enteropathies that induce excessive excretion of proteins and electrolytes, or in profuse sweating or protracted lactation. *Drugs* may also induce nutritional deficiences. For example, phenytoin, used in the treatment of epilepsy, may lead to a conditioned deficiency of folic acid, and oral contraceptives increase the requirement for vitamin B_6 and impair the metabolism of folic acid. It should be evident that secondary or conditioned malnutrition has little relationship to the availability of food, and so may be encountered whenever there is some basis for disturbance or derangement of the nutritional homeostasis. Depending on its cause, the conditioned malnutrition may involve one nutrient (e.g., inability to absorb vitamin B_{12} in pernicious anemia due to a lack of gastric intrinsic factor), several nutrients (e.g., malabsorption of lipids and lipid-soluble vitamins in obstructive jaundice), or all (e.g., psychogenic dysphagia).

Overt morphologic lesions are relatively late manifestations of deficiency states. Long before anatomic changes become evident, the nutritional deficiency slowly depletes the body stores and can be discovered at this stage only by biochemical measurements. During this period of depletion, relatively nonspecific clinical signs and symptoms may occur, even in the absence of well-developed tissue lesions. For example, vitamin C deficiency eventually causes scurvy, principally marked by a bleeding tendency and, in growing children, derangement of epiphyseal bone formation. However, such changes may appear only after many months of a grossly scorbutigenic diet. Antedating these morphologic manifestations, the patient may have evidence of generalized weakness, apathy, or conceivably a subtle impairment of wound healing relating to deranged collagen synthesis. Even earlier, perhaps many months earlier depending on the body's reserve of vitamin C, low levels of ascorbic acid may be detected in the plasma, whole blood, or white blood cells by assays. Thus, deficiency states may exist, even in the absence of morphologic and sometimes clinical changes.

PROTEIN-ENERGY MALNUTRITION

Marasmus-Kwashiorkor

Protein-energy malnutrition (or, as it is sometimes called, protein-calorie malnutrition) is a global problem of staggering dimensions. Although all ages may be affected, infants and children are usually most severely affected. It is estimated that approximately 400 million preschool children in developing nations suffer protein-energy malnutrition to a greater or lesser degree. It takes one of two somewhat distinctive clinicopathologic forms—(1) marasmus or (2) kwashiorkor—but frequently the distinction between these two syndromes is blurred with intermediate expressions. *Marasmus is the consequence of a deficiency in total calories* as is encountered in mild-to-severe starvation. Adipose tissue and muscle are lost in a graduated fashion. *Kwashiorkor, on the other hand, is the consequence of a relative or absolute deficiency of protein despite sometimes adequate total calories.* The term "kwashiorkor" is derived from the Ghanian language and means "the sickness that the older one gets when the next baby is born," i.e., when the older child is deprived of breast-feeding and weaned largely on a diet of carbohydrates. In many instances, features of both disorders appear. The child with marasmus who develops a protein-losing intestinal infection may develop many of the characteristics of kwashiorkor and, alternatively, diets deficient in both total calories, and particularly in protein calories, may induce hybrid kwashiorkor-marasmus syndromes.

Poverty and a lack of food are the all-too-frequent bases of protein-energy malnutrition, but the problem in developing countries is far more complex. Intercurrent infectious diarrhea, childhood exanthems, intestinal parasitism, and ignorance about dietary requirements all contribute to the appearance of these childhood scourges. In eighteen "Western" countries with gross national product (GNP) above $2000 per capita, the infant mortality rate in 1970–75 ranged from 11 to 30 per 1000 live births. Contrast this with 42 countries with GNP below $300 per capita, where the infant mortality rate in 1970–75 ranged from 45 to 208 per 1000 live births.[4] For obscure reasons, marasmus and kwashiorkor have differing incidences in varying parts of the world. In Lebanon and Iraq, for example, over 90% of children with protein-energy malnutrition are marasmic; in Gambia, marasmus predominates, but in nearby Uganda, kwashiorkor is more frequent.[5]

The reason why some infants with protein-energy malnutrition become marasmic while others develop kwashiorkor is not understood, but the relative lack of proteins in the diet is thought to be the differential feature. Other experts contend, however, that the difference between the two conditions resides in the metabolic adaptations to the dietary inadequacies, with or without such secondary conditioning influences as infection or diseases. It is postulated that in marasmic children the deficient diet is compensated for by mobilization of body stores and tissues, thereby maintaining the serum protein levels, albeit at the cost of progressive wasting away of fat and muscle. In kwashiorkor the metabolic adaptation does not seem to be capable of maintaining serum protein levels, but induces widespread protein deprivation throughout the viscera of the body along with hypoalbuminemia and edema.[5]

The clinical manifestations of *kwashiorkor* vary but include growth failure, edema, enlargement of the liver due to the accumulation of fat, anemia, hair changes, and dermatoses. The child is often apathetic and anorexic, cries a great deal, and is withdrawn and irritable. The edema may be generalized or localized to the upper or lower extremities. There is always hypoalbuminemia and a decrease in total serum protein. The severity of the edema may not correlate with the level of protein deficiency and hypoalbuminemia.[5A] It has been proposed that along with the loss of serum albumin there is a concomitant loss of trace elements, one of which—vanadium—may be involved in the regulation of sodium and water metabolism.[6]

The skin lesions are pathognomonic when present but are not requisite for the diagnosis. Areas of depigmentation or hyperpigmentation or, in white infants, patches of dusky erythema lead to the characteristic "crazy pavement" appearance (Fig. 9–1). There is extensive desquamation in severe cases. The hair changes consist of pallor, straightening (if the normal hair is curly), fineness of texture, and loose attachment of the roots, as evidenced by the ease with which the hair is pulled out. A "flag sign" may appear as alternating bands of light (depigmented) and dark areas in the hair, which in essence record alternating periods of good and bad nutrition. (Fig. 9–2) The liver is usually enlarged and fatty, but never cirrhotic. The anemia may be normocytic, normochromic, or of a mixed type, with concomitant iron and folic acid deficiencies. *These presenting signs are not seen in marasmus.* Other signs may be present, depending on previous nutrition and adequacy of the diet. For example, the extent to which manifestations of a deficiency of vitamin A or thiamine appear is a function of previous nutrition, dietary intake of these essential nutrients, infection, and a host of other factors.

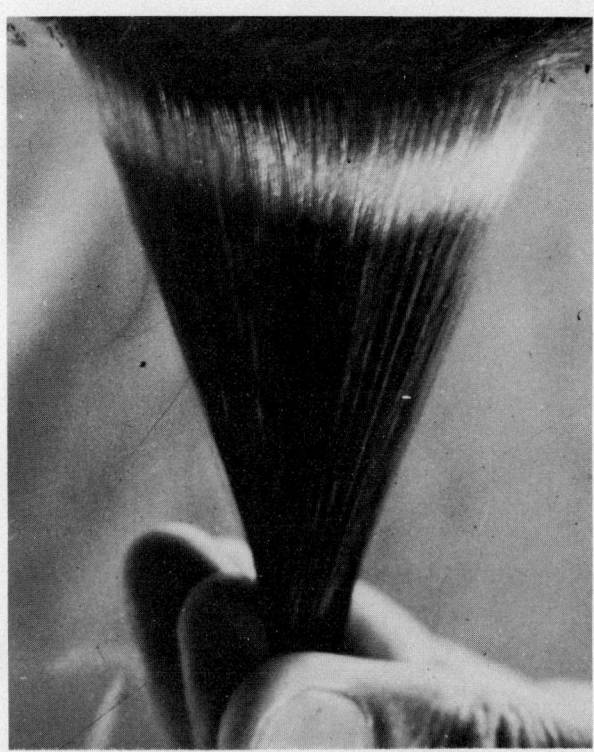

Figure 9–2. Kwashiorkor "flag sign." A tuft of hair in an infant showing a striking band of depigmentation, marking a period of severe malnutrition. (Courtesy of Dr. N. Scrimshaw, Massachusetts Institute of Technology; and the Institute of Nutrition of Central America and Panama.)

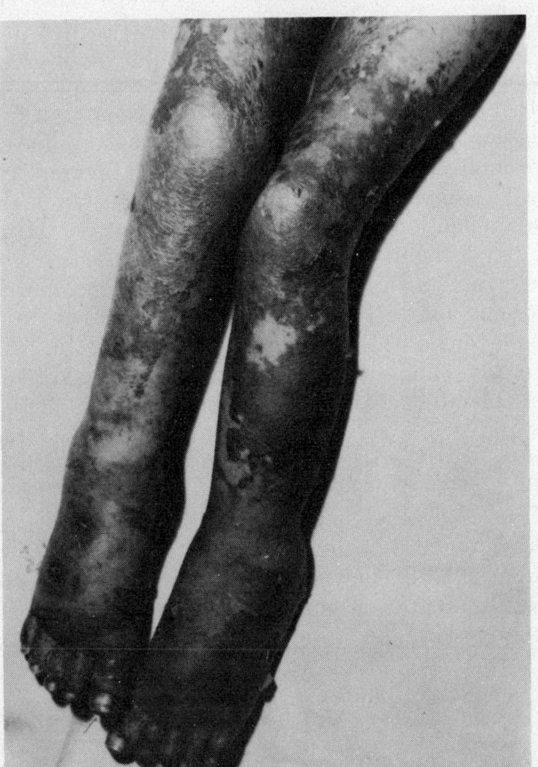

Figure 9–1. Kwashiorkor. Lower extremities of child showing the distinctive skin lesions and edema. (Courtesy of Dr. N. Scrimshaw, Massachusetts Institute of Technology; the Institute of Nutrition of Central America and Panama; and Science *133*:2039, 1961. Copyright 1961 by the American Association for the Advancement of Science.)

The *marasmic* child is obviously wasted, with broomstick arms and legs from which the skin hangs pathetically loose (Fig. 9–3). The face becomes pinched and wizened, imparting a prematurely aged appearance. There is more of a defect in weight than in height, and these children, in contrast to those with kwashiorkor, are alert and hungry and will eat ravenously if given food. The total serum proteins are usually normal. The marasmic child may develop signs of superimposed kwashiorkor following the protein catabolic response to a chronic infection, and conversely treatment of acute kwashiorkor may reveal a marasmic child beneath the edema.

The term protein-calorie malnutrition has been used to explain a kwashiorkor-like syndrome in medical and surgical adult patients in large urban hospitals.[7, 8] These patients present with lethargy, weight loss, anemia, hypoalbuminemia, fatty liver, and gastrointestinal changes. Edema may or may not be present. Usually there are no hair "flag signs" or dermatologic changes. Some chronic debilitating or wasting disease accounts for the inanition and malnourishment. With superimposed infection there is further catabolism and nitrogen loss, as well as increased utilization of nutrients in an already depleted individual. In this manner, a kwashiorkor-like state may develop in adults, even in affluent societies.

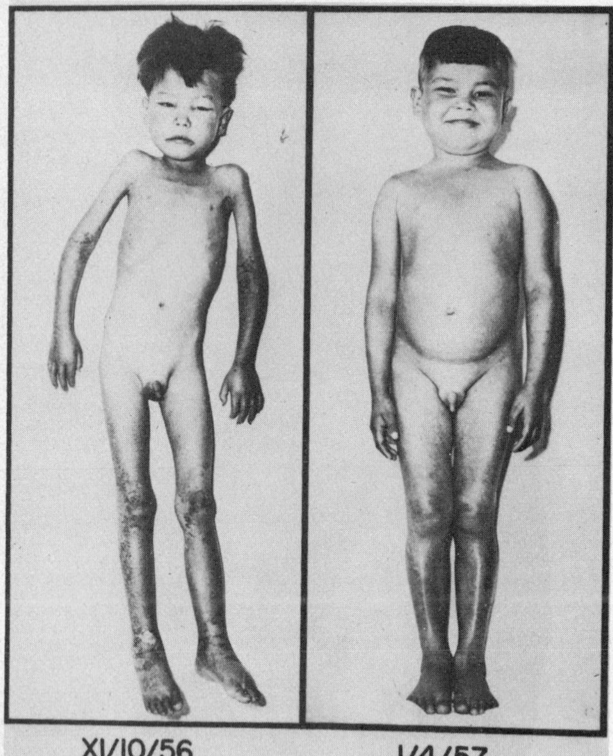

Figure 9–3. Within every marasmic child *(left)* is a sturdy, smiling youngster; seen *(right)* after two months of adequate nutrition. (Courtesy of Dr. N. Scrimshaw, Massachusetts Institute of Technology; and the Institute of Nutrition of Central America and Panama.)

MORPHOLOGY. The anatomic changes in protein-energy deficiency can be generalized as hypoplasia and atrophy of tissues. The anatomic changes are quite similar in both marasmus and kwashiorkor, but extreme examples of these two syndromes show certain differences, principally involving the small bowel mucosa and the liver.

The small bowel in fully expressed kwashiorkor often shows marked atrophy of the mucosa. Such changes are rarely encountered in marasmus. The mucosal atrophy may be patchy or widespread and involve virtually the entire jejunum. It may also vary from mild to severe. The basic anatomic changes consist of diminution or loss of **villi and microvilli with atrophy of the absorptive covering cells.**[9] There is a concomitant infiltrate of lymphocytes and plasma cells into the lamina propria; in some cases there is an increased number of fat vacuoles within the absorptive cells, apparently reflecting some delay in fat transport.[10] Histochemical studies also disclose a decrease in the carbohydrate-splitting enzymes in the brush border of the absorbing cells, such as lactase, sucrase, and maltase. All these changes are reversible in time with restoration of an adequate diet.

The **liver** in kwashiorkor, but not marasmus, is extremely fatty (Fig. 9–4). These changes are thought to be caused by decreased synthesis of the protein carriers necessary to the formation of lipoproteins, the form in which fat is mobilized from the liver. Some observers have described material resembling alcoholic hyalin in such livers.[11] For obscure reasons, cirrhosis almost never develops.

In marasmus, **anemia** may be present but is usually mild. Typically it is normochromic-normocytic and attributed to reduced erythropoietin levels secondary to the lowered metabolic oxygen demand of the wasted body. Concomitant deficiencies of iron or folate may complicate the anemia, adding elements of the microcytic-hypochromic anemia of iron lack (p. 635) to the macrocytic-hyperchromic anemia of folate deficiency (p. 634).

In kwashiorkor the anemia may also be normochromic-normocytic, resulting in part from marrow erythrohypoplasia or atrophy related to the severe protein deficiency, and in part from decreased synthesis of erythropoietin. Infections and marginal iron and folate intake may lead to the marrow changes associated with these deficiencies and a polymorphic anemia in the peripheral blood.

The **immune system** is adversely affected in both kwashiorkor and marasmus, particularly in the former. The thymus becomes atrophic in severe instances of both conditions, with reduction in the number and function of circulating T cells. B-cell function (antibody responses) is likewise depressed. Thus, these children are unusually vulnerable to infections. A vicious circle then ensues in which the infection adversely affects the nutritional status, and the malnourishment worsens the infection.[12]

Controversy persists as to whether clinical and anatomic changes induced by protein-energy malnutrition are totally reversible with restoration of a normal diet. Although most of the manifestations may clear, there is still uncertainty about the long-term effects of protein-calorie malnutrition on physical growth and development or intellectual development. It has been exceedingly difficult to establish objective measurements and clear-cut controls for comparisons. With respect to physical growth and development, some published findings point to retardation in height and weight at age 6 to 12 years in those who had survived protein-energy malnutrition during infancy, but others disagree.[13] These height-weight differences, however, were limited to boys only. Even more important is the growing conviction that food deprivation has a detrimental effect on intellectual development. In the past, this impairment has been ascribed to the social and intellectual environment in which the malnourished child was raised. However, the evidence grows stronger that the single variable of dietary deprivation in infancy and early childhood significantly impairs subsequent levels of intellectual performance and attainment.[13, 14] The first two years of life is a critical period. Studies indicate that the adult number of neurons is achieved perhaps as early as 20 weeks after conception. Throughout the first two years of life, however, there is glial proliferation and further development of neuronal connections as well as myelination of fibers. Thus, protein-energy malnutrition during this growing period has many long-lasting consequences.

VITAMINS

The following discussion of each of the various vitamins deals largely with the clinicoanatomic changes encountered in humans, the basis and prevalence of the deficiency state, and such aspects of the metabolism of the nutrient as are relevant to the pathogenesis of the changes.

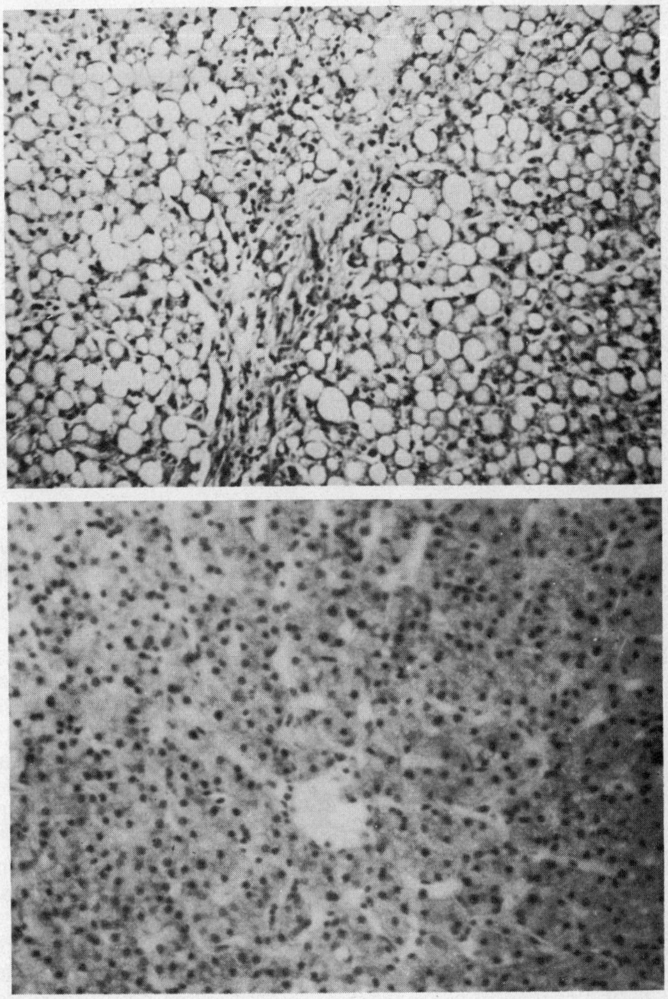

Figure 9–4. Kwashiorkor. The fatty liver is shown above. Contrast with normal liver *(below)* after adequate nutrition for a period of weeks. (Courtesy of Dr. N. Scrimshaw, Massachusetts Institute of Technology; and the Institute of Nutrition of Central America and Panama.)

FAT-SOLUBLE VITAMINS

Avitaminoses of the fat-soluble vitamins—A, D, E, and K—may occur as primary deficiency states in economically deprived populations or as secondary conditioned deficiencies throughout the world, for reasons discussed earlier. Principal among these secondary conditioning influences are such disorders as biliary tract and pancreatic dysfunction and the large category of malabsorption syndromes that affect fat absorption in general and, concomitantly, absorption of the fat-soluble vitamins. Since fat-soluble vitamins are generously stored chiefly in the liver, diffuse advanced liver disease may lead to a conditioned deficiency. However, the normal reserves of fat-soluble vitamins are substantial, and so deficiency states develop only after protracted negative balances.

Vitamin A

[Well-established deficiency states: Blindness; xerophthalmia (conjunctival keratinization); keratomalacia (corneal conjunctival opacity with alteration of the cornea); follicular (papular) hyperkeratosis of the skin; squamous metaplasia of the mucosal linings of the respiratory, gastrointestinal, and genitourinary tracts and of the ducts of glands.]

[Possible consequences: Predisposition to epithelial cancers of the skin, lungs, bladder, and colorectum; retarded skeletal growth in infancy and childhood anemia.]

Vitamin A exists in the body in a variety of chemical forms, and it is best to clarify the terminology at the outset. Vitamin A alcohol is referred to as retinol. There are at least two forms of vitamin A alcohol—A_1 (retinol) and A_2 (3-dehydroretinol). *Retinyl ester* refers to vitamin A ester. The aldehyde form of vitamin A is known as *retinal* and the acid as *retinoic acid.* Provitamin A, found largely in leafy green and yellow vegetables such as carrots and sweet potatoes, is referred to as carotene, of which the most important is beta-carotene, consisting essentially of two linked vitamin A molecules. In addition, there is now a large variety of synthetic products comprising analogs of vitamin A, known collectively as *retinoids.* As will be seen, excesses of vitamin A may induce an important clinical syndrome known as hypervitaminosis A. With the recent interest in the possible use of vitamin A in the treatment of various proliferative and neoplastic epithelial lesions, great effort has been made to synthesize retinoids having antiproliferative activity that can be administered in large amounts without the toxic effects of the naturally occurring vitamin A compounds.

Basis and Prevalence of Deficiency State. The preponderance of vitamin A in the normal Western diet is in the form of retinol or esters derived from liver, dairy products, or vitamin pills. Some from natural vegetable sources is in the form of carotenes, which are split in the intestinal mucosal cell into retinol. Bile and normal pancreatic function is critical to the absorption of these fat-soluble products. Normal blood levels of vitamin A are maintained by the daily intake and by hydrolysis of the stored hepatic retinyl esters, releasing retinol into the blood, which is then bound to retinol-binding protein (RBP), an alpha-1-globulin, in turn complexed to prealbumin.

Primary deficiency of vitamin A is endemic in certain areas of the world—Central America, the Middle East, and in and about India. In these regions, it is the principal cause of blindness, which usually develops during childhood but may not appear until adult life. Poverty and its attendant malnutrition is likely to be the root cause of the deficiency state in these endemic areas; in addition, a woeful lack of knowledge about nutrition undoubtedly contributes since food sources of vitamin A are generally plentiful in these locales. A primary vitamin A deficiency may also occur sporadically in any part of the world because of a grossly inadequate diet. More often the sporadic disorder is a secondary conditioned state related to the impaired fat absorption of biliary tract and pancreatic disease, or some other malabsorptive disorder. Occasionally, diffuse liver disease or protein malnutrition result in inadequate synthesis of plasma transport proteins, depriving the tissues of vitamin A. Under these circumstances, serum vitamin A levels may be spuriously depressed and may not accurately reflect body stores. Moreover, diffuse liver disease may impair the ability to store retinyl esters, thereby potentiating a deficiency state whenever there is a prolonged negative balance.

The pathogenesis of the tissue changes in vitamin A deficiency is best understood in the context of the morphology of the lesions.

Morphology

Epithelial Metaplasia. For reasons yet unknown, vitamin A is necessary for the maturation and differentiation of the specialized epithelial surfaces of the body, e.g., the mucous membranes of the eyes; the mucosa of the respiratory, gastrointestinal, and genitourinary tracts; the lining epithelia of gland ducts; and the ducts of skin appendages. Wolbach and Bessey characterized the general nature of these epithelial changes as "atrophy of the epithelium concerned, reparative proliferation of the basal cells, and growth and differentiation of the new products into a stratified keratinizing epithelium."[15] From this description, it is apparent that in the sites mentioned the normal epithelium, whatever its type, is replaced by inappropriate keratinized, stratified squamous epithelium (Fig. 9–5). If the epithelium is normally stratified and keratinized as is the skin, it becomes excessively keratinized. The nonkeratinized, stratified squamous mucosa, such as is found in the conjunctiva, cornea, and vagina, becomes keratinized. When the epithelium is more specialized, e.g., the columnar epithelium of the respiratory tract, cuboidal epithelium that lines ducts, or transitional epithelium of the urinary tract, the changes take the form of atrophy of the normal mucosa and replacement by squamous differentiation of basal stem cells.

In the eye, the scleral and corneal conjunctivae become keratinized. The mucous cells in these surfaces disappear and, along with this change, the lining of the ducts of the tear gland is replaced by keratinized, stratified squamous epithelium. The keratin debris plugs the ducts and so the normal moist, mucosal surfaces become dry, granular, and roughened, resembling skin **(xerophthalmia).** The keratin debris accumulates in whitish, meringue-like plaques (Bitot's spots). These modifications lead to significant irritation in the orbit. Visual acuity is impaired by the keratinization and thickening of the corneal mucosa. This surface may ulcerate and lead to softening and opacity of the cornea with secondary infection. As the corneal involvement progresses, vascularization and infiltration by inflammatory cells hasten the softening and sometimes lead to frank perforation. These corneal changes are referred to as **keratomalacia.**

In the respiratory tract, including the nose, nasopharynx, and sinuses, replacement of the normal columnar **ciliated epithelium by nonciliated, stratified squamous epithelium** seriously impairs the normal defensive function of the mucosa. Ciliary action is thus lost, and the normal secretions are suppressed. The desquamated keratin debris acts as foreign bodies that predispose to superimposed infections. The epithelial changes in the nose provide a source of diagnostic scrapings, which may reveal keratinized scales in place of the usual cells, an aid in the diagnosis of this avitaminosis.

In the urinary tract, particularly in the renal pelvis and bladder, **the keratin debris may serve as a nidus for the formation of urinary tract stones,** which further predispose to inflammatory changes and infections.

Changes in the skin take the form of hyperplasia and hyperkeratinization of the epidermis, and plugging of the hair shafts and sebaceous gland ducts by piled-up masses of keratin, which produce numerous minute papules and give a rough, sandpaper-like texture to the skin. The condition is known as **follicular or papular hyperkeratosis or dermatosis.** Similarly, plugging of the ducts of the salivary glands and pancreas may give rise to significant digestive disturbances.

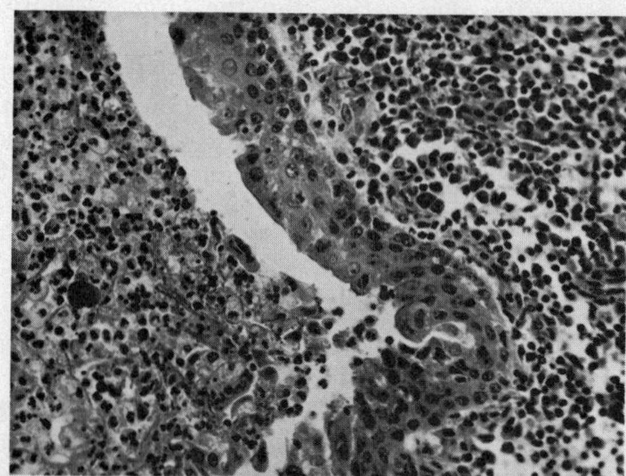

Figure 9–5. Squamous metaplasia of the epithelial lining of a duct in the pancreas.

There is great current interest in the possibility that **vitamin A, carotene, and the synthetic retinoids may protect humans against the development of skin, bladder, lung, stomach, and colorectal cancer.** More specifically, the evidence, albeit not strong, points to a possible lower than normal dietary intake of vitamin A and carotene-containing foods among victims of these forms of neoplasia, particularly squamous cell carcinoma of the lung.[16, 17] Similarly, vitamin A and its analogs inhibit the carcinogenicity of chemical carcinogens, oncogenic viruses, and irradiation in experimental animals and in cell culture.[18, 19] There are the additional findings of regression of basal cell carcinomas with topical application of retinoids, and regression of papillomas of the urinary bladder with oral administration. In passing, it might be mentioned that there are numerous reports of the efficacy of retinoids in treatment of a number of non-neoplastic but proliferative skin conditions, including psoriasis, lichen planus, ichthyosis, plantar warts, and others.[20] Heartening as these data may be, other studies indicate that vitamin A and its synthetic analogs have in certain experimental protocols demonstrated cell-activating properties and induced tumor formation.[21] Dosage, route of administration, and the particular experimental model employed may be involved in these contradictory findings. The issue remains moot, but most of the evidence suggests that retinoids in some way reduce the predisposition to cancer, perhaps by maintenance of normal cell differentiation.

Even more uncertain is the role of this nutrient in skeletal growth and in red cell formation. Infants suffering from a severe lack of vitamin A have been reported to have retarded growth, but concomitant nutritional deficiencies have not been rigorously ruled out. Equally controversial is the role of a lack of vitamin A in the induction of anemia.[22] It is suggested that in some way the nutrient contributes to the mobilization of iron stores, and so a deficiency may impair hemoglobin synthesis.

PATHOGENESIS. *Blindness, in subdued or even bright light, depending on the severity of the deficiency state, is the best elucidated consequence of a lack of this vitamin.* For providing an understanding of this phenomenon, Wald received the Nobel Prize for Medicine in 1967.[23] Critical to vision are the photosensitive pigments—rhodopsin in rods and iodopsin in cones (they differ only in the protein bound to the vitamin A moiety). In both pigments, 11-*cis*-retinal constitutes the crucial prosthetic group. On exposure to light, there is dissociation of the pigment into its protein and retinal, which then isomerizes to the all-*trans* form with the release of a quantum of energy. Reisomerization to the *cis* form occurs in the dark, but only after conversion of retinal to retinol. Thus the 11-*cis*-retinol must be oxidized to the retinal form with reformation of the photosensitive pigment. However, some of the retinal becomes an inactive isomer and so is permanently lost. Thus, a constantly available source of additional vitamin A is necessary to maintain adequate levels. With moderate lack of vitamin A, the pigment is depleted principally in the rods, producing night blindness. With more extreme deficiencies, both rods and cones are affected, producing blindness even in bright light.

In sharp contrast to the understanding of the role of vitamin A in vision, very little is known about how vitamin A maintains the integrity of epithelial cells and prevents keratinizing metaplasia and, possibly, tumor induction. A number of disparate observations have been made. It has been observed that epithelial cells possess specific vitamin A binding proteins, but their role in the homeostasis of the cell is not established.[24] Conceivably, the protein-vitamin complex is transported into the nucleus where it modifies gene translation (like the steroid hormones), thereby playing a role in the proliferation and differentiation of the cell.[25] Oral retinoids have been reported to enhance regression of the atypical metaplasia of the bronchial mucosa seen in heavy cigarette smokers.[26] The vitamin may also be involved in intracellular glycosylation reactions, which could help to maintain the integrity of mucus-secreting cells. Other findings point to maintenance of both plasmalemmal and organellar membranes and to regulation of prostaglandin synthesis. With respect to the putative antitumor effect of vitamin A, it is proposed that, in addition to its role in the differentiation of cells, it enhances the immune reactivity of the host by stimulation of T-killer cells and T-cell cytotoxicity, possibly contributing to so-called tumor surveillance (itself a controversial issue).[27, 28] Alternatively, there are reports suggesting that retinoids inhibit neoplastic transformation of cells (at least in vitro) by restoration of contact inhibition and density-dependent growth inhibition.[29] It is clear that many observations have been made, but their implications need to be clarified. One can only conclude that, in some way, vitamin A and its analogs play some role in normal cell growth and differentiation.

CLINICAL MANIFESTATIONS. Visual abnormalities and changes in the eyes and conjunctivae are major clinical features of a lack of vitamin A. Impaired vision in subdued light (nyctalopia) or even blindness in bright light (hemeralopia) are highly suggestive of the deficiency state in the absence of other abnormalities in the visual apparatus. However, as is evident from the above morphologic discussion, xerophthalmia and keratomalacia in the course of time may lead to extensive erosions, ulcerations, and even destruction of the eyeball. Keratinizing metaplasia of the respiratory tract predisposes to infections, and similar changes in the urinary tract may predispose to urinary tract infections or urolithiasis. Sometimes the hyperkeratotic papular dermatitis suggests the presence of the deficiency state. However, to confirm the diagnosis it is necessary to demonstrate reduced serum values for vitamin A and/or carotene; when they fall below 10 and 20 μg per 100 ml, respectively (normal, 20 and 40 or over), the deficient state is probably present. You recall that such values are reliable only when plasma protein levels are normal.

TOXICITY. Although normal levels of vitamin A are requisite for health, excessive amounts (hypervitaminosis A) are dangerous. In infants, ingestion of excessive dosages has led to increased intracranial pressure with drowsiness, vomiting, bulging of the fontanelles, peeling of skin, loss of hair, hepatomegaly, and bone pain with radiologic evidence of periosteal neo-osteogenesis. In adults, headache, dizziness, blurred vision, diplopia, nausea, vomiting, drowsiness, peeling of the skin, and hepatic enlargement (sometimes with liver injury, portal hypertension, and ascites) may appear. Indeed, with more chronic toxicity, a variety of mental disturbances have developed that closely mimic schizophrenia or depression. Less disturbing is the appearance of yellowing of the skin, particularly of the palms, related to the carotenemia produced by the consumption of monster amounts of carrots (rabbits and carrot freaks, take note). Although the skin pigmentation of carotenemia is easily confused with jaundice, it does not produce yellowing of the sclerae.

Vitamin D

[Deficiency state: Rickets and osteomalacia]

A deficiency of vitamin D, if sufficiently severe and protracted, leads to the classic skeletal disorders—rickets (in growing infants and children whose epiphyses have not yet closed) and osteomalacia (in adults). *Both conditions are basically characterized by inadequate or delayed mineralization of newly laid-down osteoid, and therefore an excess of osteoid. In the case of rickets, there is also defective mineralization of epiphyseal cartilage. Since vitamin D plays a critical role in the maintenance of normocalcemia, the inadequate mineralization associated with vitamin D deficiency is often attributed solely to hypocalcemia.* The basis of the skeletal disorders, however, is more complex. Abnormally low levels of serum calcium alone inevitably induce hyperfunction of the parathyroid glands, and the excess *parathormone* causes a skeletal disorder known as osteitis fibrosa (p. 1329), seen with all forms of hyperparathyroidism. *Thus, a deficiency of vitamin D induces not only abnormal serum levels of calcium and phosphate, but also secondary hyperparathyroidism and consequently skeletal morphologic changes that constitute a combination of rickets (or osteomalacia) and osteitis fibrosa.* Our consideration of hypovitaminosis D, rickets, and osteomalacia, then, must concern itself not only with the metabolism of vitamin D, but also with that of calcium and phosphate, as well as the interplay of the altered parathyroid and thyroid (calcitonin) function that ensues. For clarity, these pathogenetic metabolic considerations will be presented first.

PATHOGENESIS. *There are two generic causes of rickets and osteomalacia: (1) vitamin D deficiency or abnormal metabolism of the vitamin and (2) a deficiency or deranged utilization of inorganic phosphorus.*[30] Both etiologies derange calcification of the skeleton, but with respect to the first it is now clear that vitamin D itself is not active in calcium metabolism. *It must first undergo conversion to its active metabolite, 1-alpha, 25-dihydroxyvitamin D_3 [1,25-$(OH)_2D_3$], which in essence constitutes a hormone since it is formed in the kidney and acts on distant target organs.*

There are two native forms of the vitamin: vitamin D_3 (cholecalciferol) and vitamin D_2 (ergocalciferol), both of which are essentially steroids. Since vitamin D_2 is metabolized in a manner similar to vitamin D_3, it will not be discussed further. Vitamin D_3 may be endogenously derived from 7-dehydrocholesterol, an intermediate in cholesterol biosynthesis. Upon exposure to ultraviolet light, 7-dehydrocholesterol (provitamin D_3) in the skin is transformed first into previtamin D_3, which, without further exposure to light, slowly equilibrates into vitamin D_3.[31] Vitamin D_3 may also be derived from a variety of animal products, particularly liver. With sufficient exposure to sunlight, no dietary source of vitamin D is required. Persons living in the northern hemisphere almost always require exogenous vitamin D.

Dietary D_3 is absorbed in the small intestine, requiring, as do other fats, normal biliary function. After absorption or endogenous synthesis, it is transported in the blood to the liver bound to an alpha-1-globulin. Here it is either stored (other storage sites are fat depots and muscle) or undergoes metabolic conversion to 25-hydroxy-vitamin D_3 (25 OHD_3) by a 25-hydroxylase located primarily in the endoplasmic reticulum of hepatocytes. The 25-hydroxyvitamin D_3 formed in the liver is then transported to the kidney, bound to the alpha-l-globulin transport protein in the blood. *In the kidney it undergoes the final step in its evolution into 1,25-$(OH)_2D_3$—referred to as the vitamin D hormone or calciferol* (Fig. 9–6). Involved in this conversion is the 1-alpha-hydroxylase found in the mitochondria of the renal proximal convoluted tubule cells.[32] It has always been said that the 1-alpha-hydroxylase is found only in the kidney since nephrectomy in animals totally blocks the conversion of 25 OHD_3 into 1,25-$(OH)_2D_3$. However, high plasma levels of the hormone have been identified in a patient maintained on dialysis whose kidneys had been surgically removed.[33] Thus, extrarenal sites may also possess the requisite hydroxylase, or alternative explanations must exist.

The 25-hydroxyvitamin D_3 may undergo other metabolic conversions. The kidney, intestine, and cartilage have a 24R,25-OHD_3 hydroxylase that produces 24,25-$(OH)_2D_3$, a metabolite much less active than the hormone. What initiates conversion of 25-OHD_3 into 24,25-$(OH)_2D_3$ is still somewhat unclear but will be discussed later. Possibly it has a special metabolic role.[34] There are still other metabolites such as 25R,26-$(OH)_2D_3$ into which 25-hydroxyvitamin D may be converted, but these need not be detailed.

As with all steroid hormones, cellular receptors appear to mediate the intracellular function of 1,25-$(OH)_2D_3$.[35] High-affinity receptors have been located in the nuclei of the villus cells of the small intestine; the crypt cells of the small and large intestines; osteoblasts, osteocytes and chondrocytes of bone; parathyroid glands; distal tubules of the kidney; podocytes of the glomerulus; basal cells of the skin; endocrine cells of the stomach; and the TSH-producing cells of the pituitary.[36] It has been shown that in certain hereditary forms of rickets (described later as vitamin D–dependent rickets) skin fibroblasts also possess receptors, providing a ready source of cells for study.[37] Whether all of these cells possessing receptors play a role in calcium and phosphorus metabolism is not certain, but clearly the intestines, bone, parathyroids, and kidneys are involved.

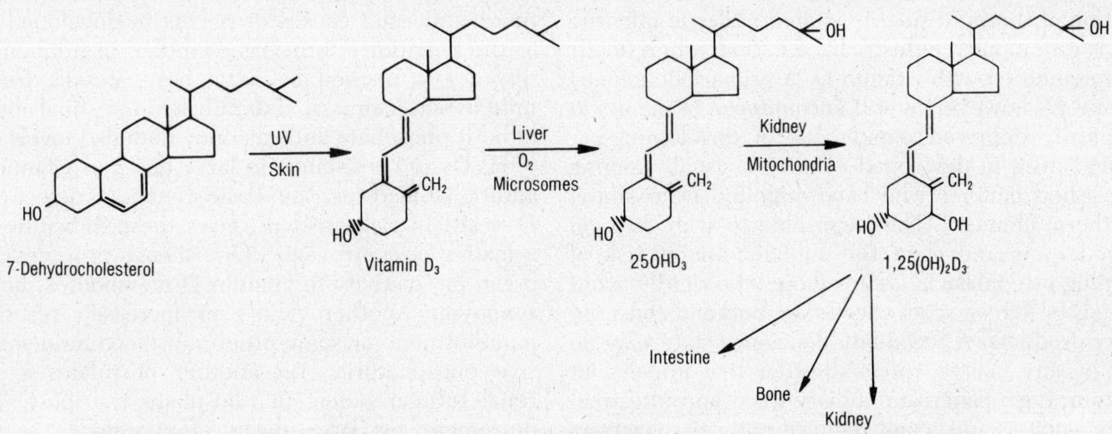

Figure 9–6. Functional metabolism of vitamin D including its biosynthesis by a photolysis reaction in the skin. Note that the final active form, 1,25$(OH)_2D_3$, is made exclusively in the kidney and functions in intestine, bone, and kidney. UV = ultraviolet light. (From DeLuca, H. F.: Vitamin D metabolism and function. Arch. Intern. Med. *138*:838, 1978. Copyright 1978, American Medical Association.)

Despite the remarkable increase in our understanding of the metabolites of vitamin D, there are still gaps in our knowledge about their precise roles in the economy of calcium and phosphorus. *1,25-$(OH)_2D_3$ elevates the plasma calcium level principally by increasing the active transport of calcium from the lumen of the small intestine into the blood.*[38] In intestinal mucosal cells, the hormone stimulates the synthesis of a calcium-binding protein presumably active at the brush border of the cells. A question remains as to whether the carrier protein initiates absorption or merely facilitates calcium transport across the cell membrane. Whichever the case, once within the mucosal cells, the calcium is transferred across the cell to the blood. The hormone participates in the active transport of phosphate by a process quite independent of calcium transport. *In this manner the hormone serves to elevate the plasma calcium and phosphorus concentrations to supersaturated levels. Such levels are requisite for mineralization of newly formed bone.* Whether the hormone is also directly involved in the mineralization of osteoid surprisingly is still uncertain. As you know, normocalcemia is also necessary for normal function of nerve and muscle (including myocardium) and normal membrane permeability and blood clotting. *The active hormone has additional functions: it increases, minimally, renal absorption of calcium in the distal tubules and, together with parathormone, mobilizes calcium and phosphate from the bone-fluid interface,* both serving to further support the serum levels of calcium and phosphorus. The mobilization of minerals in bone probably also involves the synthesis of transport proteins similar to those described in the intestine, since this function can be blocked by previous administration of actinomycin D, which inhibits protein synthesis.

Vitamin D is regulated by the serum levels of both 1,25-$(OH)_2D_3$ and calcium. Although high blood levels of the hormone exert some control of the hepatic 25-hydroxylase, the control is crude since increased dietary intake of the vitamin induces increased formation of 25-OHD_3 despite high blood levels of the hormone. The fine tuning is performed by 1,25-$(OH)_2D_3$. High levels of the hormone suppress the renal 1-alpha-hydroxylase and turn on the 24R-hydroxylase, producing the less active 24,25-$(OH)_2D_3$, while the converse occurs with low levels. *Thus, regulation of the circulating level of 1,25-$(OH)_2D_3$ constitutes a typical endocrine feedback loop.* As mentioned, the serum levels of calcium also constitute a regulatory mechanism, but only through the intermediation of parathormone. In animals, low calcium diets induce secretion of parathormone, the parathyroid hormone, in the presence of vitamin D, increasing the activity of the 1-alpha-hydroxylase and suppressing the 24R-hydroxylase, while high calcium diets do the converse. So it is that, *with hypocalcemia, there is increased activity of the 1-alpha-hydroxylase, and the resultant 1,25-$(OH)_2D_3$ stimulates the absorption of calcium in the distal renal tubules, and mobilization of calcium from bone, but the primary response is increased intestinal absorption.* If for any reason the diet is severely lacking in calcium, or the intestine fails to respond, there is mobilization of calcium from bone. *1,25-$(OH)_2D_3$ does not require parathyroid hormone for its intestinal function, but the mobilization of calcium from bone is dominantly a parathyroid hormone function, with 1,25-$(OH)_2D_3$ playing only a permissive role.*[34]

Finally, it should be pointed out that the serum level of phosphate also plays some as yet poorly understood role in the regulation of 1,25-$(OH)_2D_3$. As with calcium, hypophosphatemia induces synthesis of 1,25-$(OH)_2D_3$, while elevated levels of phosphate lead to the metabolically less active 24,25-$(OH)_2D_3$.

BASIS AND PREVALENCE OF DEFICIENCY STATE. It should be clear from the preceding discussion that many disturbances in vitamin D, calcium, or phosphorus metabolism may lead to defective mineralization of the skeleton.[39, 40] There are many possible causes, but the major ones can be briefly characterized as follows.

Vitamin D Lack. A lack of vitamin D may arise because of: (1) insufficient endogenous synthesis; (2) a primary deficiency state due to a dietary lack of the nutrient; or (3) a secondary deficiency caused by malabsorption of the lipid-soluble vitamin. Classic infantile rickets is rare in most industrialized nations where foods are supplemented with vitamin D. A primary deficiency of vitamin D, however, is still encountered in infants in economically deprived populations of developing nations, and even in developed countries, usually among impoverished families who have migrated from sunny to northern climes.[41] The very elderly who live on restricted diets and shun the sunlight are at risk of developing osteomalacia, as are those who rigidly avoid fatty foods or live on strict vegetarian diets and consume no dairy products. A secondary deficiency state may be caused by any malabsorptive disorder that impairs fat absorption, e.g., pancreatic, biliary tract, and intestinal diseases, such as sprue and regional enteritis. Gastrectomy, for poorly understood reasons, may also induce a secondary deficiency state.

Chronic Renal Failure. The development of rickets or osteomalacia with chronic renal failure is not solely due to loss of renal parenchyma, and with it the ability to convert 25-OHD_3 into 1,25-$(OH)_2D_3$. In renal failure, the development of systemic acidosis may also contribute by altering the metabolism of vitamin D and the renal and intestinal handling of calcium and phosphorus.

Hypophosphatemia. A dietary lack of phosphorus sufficient to produce a primary deficiency state is highly unlikely except in extreme instances of protein malnutrition. A secondary deficiency, however, may develop in peptic ulcer patients on long-term antacids containing aluminum hydroxide, which forms insoluble complexes with phosphorus, blocking its absorption. Several forms of renal tubular disorders may also cause hypophosphatemia. One disorder known as *renal tubular acidosis* is characterized by hypophosphatemia, hyperphosphaturia, systemic acidosis, and impaired intestinal absorption of calcium. The increased renal excretion of phosphate may at least in part be attributable to the acidosis. The metabolic acidosis may also contribute to the development of rickets and osteomalacia by impairment of vitamin D metabolism. Another renal tubular disorder associated with hypophosphatemia is the *Fanconi syndrome,* which basically consists of a general proximal tubular dysfunction with impaired reabsorption of phosphate, glucose, amino acids, and bicarbonate. Thus, hyperphosphaturia, hypophosphatemia, aminoaciduria, glycosuria, and often systemic acidosis appear, as well as other metabolic defects. Analogous dysfunctions may also develop in the course of a variety of diseases, e.g., hereditary disorders of cystine metabolism, Wilson's disease, multiple myeloma, and lead poisoning. In these conditions, the hypophosphatemia is also caused by increased renal loss and the accompanying acidosis. Hypophosphatemia is a prominent feature of certain familial disorders to be discussed next.

Hereditary Diseases. Two genetic disorders are significant causes of rickets or osteomalacia: (1) *X-linked hypophosphatemia,* also known as *vitamin D–resistant rickets* (autosomal dominant) and (2) *vitamin D–dependent rickets* (autosomal recessive). X-linked hypophosphatemia, with a gene frequency in the general population of about one in 25,000, has become one of the more important causes of rickets in developed nations as the nutritional form has dwindled in frequency. The disorder is marked by hypophosphatemia, frequently mild hypocalcemia, and diminished intestinal absorption of both phosphate and calcium. Reduced levels of 1,25-$(OH)_2D_3$ and resistance to large doses of vitamin D are additional features. The basic metabolic defect (vitamin D–resistant rickets) that causes these difficulties is still a matter of controversy. One theory proposes an end-organ insensitivity to vitamin D metabolites, hence the synonym. Another points to increased reactivity to parathormone or some other substance inducing excessive phosphaturia. Yet another postulates a primary renal tubular defect in phosphate transport. The requirement for large doses of vitamin D as well as phosphate is notable with this disorder.

Vitamin D–dependent rickets is also characterized by hypophosphatemia and often by severe skeletal disease, which usually becomes manifest only in adult life as osteomalacia. Two forms of this usually autosomal recessive disease have been identified. In type I the defect is thought to be a "missing enzyme," namely the 1-alpha-hydroxylase required for conversion of 25-OHD_3 to 1,25-$(OH)_2D_3$.[42] In the type II form of the disease there is a defect in cellular uptake of the vitamin D active hormone.[37]

Drug-Induced Rickets and Osteomalacia. Many drugs, including virtually all the anticonvulsants such as phenytoin and phenobarbital, may lead to the skeletal disorders. It is proposed that the use of such drugs increases the hepatic degradation of steroid hormones, including vitamin D. Simultaneously, the drugs may directly impinge on major target sites of calcium metabolism, i.e., inhibition of calcium transport in the intestines and of the bone-resorptive response to parathyroid hormone and 1,25-$(OH)_2D_3$.[43]

It is sufficient to note that, although the skeletal disorders may be produced by a deficiency of vitamin D, in reality they represent common anatomic end points of a wide range of clinical derangements that impinge on vitamin D, calcium, and phosphorus metabolism.

NORMAL BONE DEVELOPMENT AND MAINTENANCE. An understanding of the morphologic changes in rickets and osteomalacia would be greatly facilitated by a review of normal bone development and maintenance (p. 1319). Here the following cursory comments must suffice.

The skeleton is formed by two totally distinct processes—*intramembranous ossification,* involving primarily the development of the flat bones, and endochondral ossification, which accounts primarily for the formation of the long tubular bones. With intramembranous bone formation, mesenchymal cells differentiate directly into osteoblasts, which synthesize the largely (90 to 95%) collagenous matrix. After fetal life, this matrix is laid down in the form of lamellar bone with the collagen fibrils aligned in parallel arrays. During fetal development, or whenever there is excessively rapid bone formation as in certain diseases, the matrix collagen is haphazardly laid down, producing what is called "woven" bone. *Bone matrix prior to its mineral-*

ization is called osteoid. The factors that initiate mineralization of osteoid are still poorly understood.[44] The plasma levels of calcium or phosphorus are critical, but osteoblasts also play some little understood role. Other influences include the fibrillation and maturation of collagen involving the development of intra- and intermolecular cross-links; the ground substance (glycosaminoglycans) of the matrix; and vitamin K–dependent, calcium-binding proteins. The mineral salts laid down are largely composed of calcium phosphate admixed with other trace elements. At first the calcium phosphate is deposited as amorphous granules, but in the course of days these deposits mature into crystalline formations of hydroxyapatite.

Endochondral ossification refers to the process of epiphyseal cartilaginous growth of the long tubular bones. The cartilage is progressively replaced by osteoid, which is then mineralized. The rate of synthesis of cartilaginous matrix by chondroblasts is precisely matched by resorption and replacement by osteoid at the metaphyseal interface. At this interface, the spicules of cartilage must first undergo provisional mineralization before being resorbed and replaced by osteoid, which then undergoes mineralization to create bone. Even in bones formed by endochondral ossification, expansion in diameter occurs by direct synthesis of osteoid by periosteal osteoblasts, while endosteal osteoclasts resorb the inner surface of the cortex to maintain its appropriate thickness.

By the time of epiphyseal closure, the development of the skeleton in terms of its basic size is virtually complete. However, bone maintenance involves continued osteoclastic bone resorption and concurrent osteoblastic activity throughout life, along the cortex, as well as the bony trabeculae. Indeed, in young adults the turnover rate of total skeletal calcium may reach 15 to 18% per year. A relatively steady state is maintained during early adult life by remarkable matching of the rate of bone formation and bone resorption. In middle to later adult life, bone resorption dominates, and with it skeletal mass is progressively lost. The loss may achieve pathologic dimensions to produce the condition known as osteoporosis (p. 1327). In any event, for our purposes, attention is called to the constant deposition of osteoid during adult life to replace bone lost by resorptive processes.

At sites of osteoblastic activity, about 1 micron of osteoid is produced daily. Since total mineralization lags by about 12 to 15 days behind such osteoid synthesis, *bone at virtually all ages contains osteoid seams about 12 to 15 microns in thickness. If mineralization is delayed or inadequate, as occurs in both rickets and osteomalacia, the osteoid seams thicken, a development that is referred to as hyperosteoidogenesis.* It is now possible, with the use of tetracycline, to quantitate quite precisely the rate of mineralization of osteoid. This antibiotic, when administered orally or parenterally to an animal or human, chelates within two hours with the amorphous bone minerals freshly deposited in osteoid. The tetracycline can be visualized in undecalcified bone sections by its fluorescence under ultraviolet light. Normally with a single administration of tetracycline the labeled osteoid is about 4 to 5 microns in width. By the use of time-spaced doses of the drug, it is possible to evaluate the rate of bone formation by the mean distance between the two fluorescent lines.[45] Thus, tetracycline labeling greatly facilitates the histologic visualization of the inadequate or delayed mineralization of rickets and osteomalacia.

MORPHOLOGY. The basic derangement is the same in osteomalacia and rickets, namely, delayed and/or inadequate mineralization, and hence an excess of osteoid. The anatomic changes in rickets, however, are complicated by inadequate provisional mineralization of epiphyseal cartilage leading to deranged endochondral ossification. It is desirable, then, to consider the simpler case of osteomalacia first.

Basically, osteomalacia consists of a subtle loss of skeleton and is one of a group of metabolic bone diseases, inducing so-called osteopenia. Hyperosteoidosis is requisite for the histologic diagnosis. However, excess osteoid is also seen in other skeletal disorders such as Paget's disease and osteitis fibrosa, but in these conditions there is no defect in mineralization, and in fact an increased rate. In contrast, the excess osteoid in osteomalacia is the result of a delay in mineralization. In some areas the newly laid down osteoid shows no mineralization.[46] Unmineralized osteoid in usual hematoxylin and eosin stains appears as pink-staining matrix complete with osteocytes within lacunae and osteoblasts aligned along the surface. Mineralized osteoid tends to stain more violet to blue, reflecting the basophilia of the bone salts. Such tinctorial features are better appreciated in undecalcified bone sections. Even better discrimination can be achieved by tetracycline labeling if the patient has received the antibiotic prior to bone biopsy. Since tetracycline binds only to newly deposited amorphous calcium phosphate, in osteomalacia the tetracycline band may be absent, narrowed, or sometimes widened—the last reflecting delay in maturation of the bone salts. The osteoblasts, arrayed along the surface of the bone matrix, are generally flattened and inactive. There is no fibrosis of the marrow in areas of cancellous bone.

Subtle differences exist between the histologic features of the bony changes associated with hypovitaminosis D and those occurring with phosphate deprivation.[30] In the former, the changes already described are complicated by an element of osteitis fibrosa, resulting from secondary hyperparathyroidism, for reasons given earlier (p. 406). With osteitis fibrosa, there is hyperosteoidosis, often of woven (irregularly laid down) bundles of collagen, but no significant lack of mineralization. In addition, there are increased numbers of osteoclasts and osteoblasts, and marrow fibrosis. All these alterations may complicate the microscopic findings in the osteomalacia of vitamin D lack. In contrast, phosphate deficiency is not associated with hypocalcemia, and thus there is no secondary hyperparathyroidism. The osteomalacia then is not obscured by features of osteitis fibrosa.

Gross morphologic changes of osteomalacia are notable for their absence in most cases. There is indeed an overall loss of mineralized bone, but in the absence of bending deformities, which are infrequent, or fractures, which may occur in this weakened skeleton, the bony contours are not affected. Radiologically, it may be possible to appreciate some loss of calcium, but the interpretation of skeletal x-ray films is difficult because of variation in film exposure and development. Although techniques such as photonbeam absorptiometry and neutron activation of calcium provide methods of quantitating the amount of calcium in the skeleton, these research tools are not often available for clinical diagnostic purposes.

Rickets in the growing infant or child presents histologic changes that are identical to those already described in osteomalacia in the adult. In addition, however, there are striking alterations in endochondral ossification at the epiphyses. These will be listed first and then described in somewhat greater detail.

1. Failure of deposition of minerals into the mature cartilaginous spicules at the metaphyseal interface.
2. Failure of the cartilage cells to mature and disintegrate, with resultant overgrowth of cartilage.
3. Persistence of distorted irregular masses of unmineralized cartilage, many of which project into the marrow cavity.
4. Deposition of unmineralized osteoid matrix on cartilaginous remnants with formation of a disorderly, totally disrupted osteochondral junction.
5. Abnormal overgrowth of capillaries and fibroblasts into the disorganized zone.
6. Bending, compression, and microfracture of soft, weakly supported osteoid and cartilaginous tissue, with resultant skeletal deformities.

Failure of mineralization of the palisade of cartilaginous spicules is the fundamental defect. The cartilage cells that have aligned themselves between the finger-like projections of matrix fail to degenerate or are not invaded properly by capillary fibroblasts. As a result, the continued growth leads to an excess of cartilage. The epiphysis becomes widened, and large, irregular, tonguelike processes of cartilage extend toward the shaft of the bone. In the plane of section, many of these cartilaginous projections may appear as large plates or islands of cartilage totally detached from the adjacent epiphysis. The osteochondral junction, which is normally quite regularly arrayed, becomes completely jagged and disorderly. About and between the cartilaginous masses and spicules, osteoid matrix is produced by the normally functioning osteoblasts, but the matrix does not become mineralized and therefore accumulates in excess (Fig. 9–7). Accompanying increased vascularization and fibrosis are present in the affected area, undoubtedly contributed by an element of osteitis fibrosa. Some calcification may be present in the scattered osteoid spicules in a spotty fashion, possibly related to varying levels of vitamin D deficiency, but in the florid advanced cases mineralization is notably deficient or absent. This zone of disorderly osteoid matrix and cartilage in the metaphysis is soft, and may become distorted under the stress of weight-bearing. The entire metaphyseal areas supported only by soft osteoid tissue and cartilage may become compressed, contributing to widening of the external diameter of the bone. The bone may bend, or the epiphysis may be displaced out of line, so that it is no longer at right angles to the long axis of the bone. These displacements and microscopic fractures cause further disarray of the rachitic zone and lead to hemorrhages, hemosiderosis, and fibrosis.

In the areas of membranous bone, there is a failure of mineralization of newly formed osteoid tissue with accompanying increased fibrosis and vascularization.

Gross skeletal lesions are usually readily evident in rickets. The degree of deformity depends on the severity of the rachitic process, its duration, the rate of growth of the individual, and the stresses and tensions to which the bones are subject. Age is a particularly important factor, not only with respect to the growth rate, but also insofar as it conditions the type of stress. Obviously, the very young infant lying in bed is subject to different pressures and stresses from those of the child of 2 or 3 years who is already walking. During infancy, the nonambulatory child places greatest stress upon the head and chest. The softened occipital bones may become flattened and the cranium can be buckled inward by pressure but, with release of the pressure, elastic recoil snaps the bones back into their original positions. This clinical sign is known as **craniotabes.** It is best elicited in the frontal regions where there is greatest curvature of the skull. An excess of osteoid tissue produces **frontal bossing** and a **squared appearance to the head.** The chest becomes markedly deformed because of the overgrowth of cartilage and osteoid tissue at the costochondral junction, giving rise to the **"rachitic rosary."** The weakened metaphyseal area here is subject to the stress of gravity and the pull of the respiratory muscles, and thus becomes progressively depressed. Along with this depression, the sternum and anterior portion of the rib cage tend to protrude and create the **pigeon-breast deformity.** The diaphragm causes a sharp depression that girdles the thoracic cavity at the lower margin of the rib cage **(Harrison's groove).** In the young infant, the pelvis may become deformed by the stress of gravity.

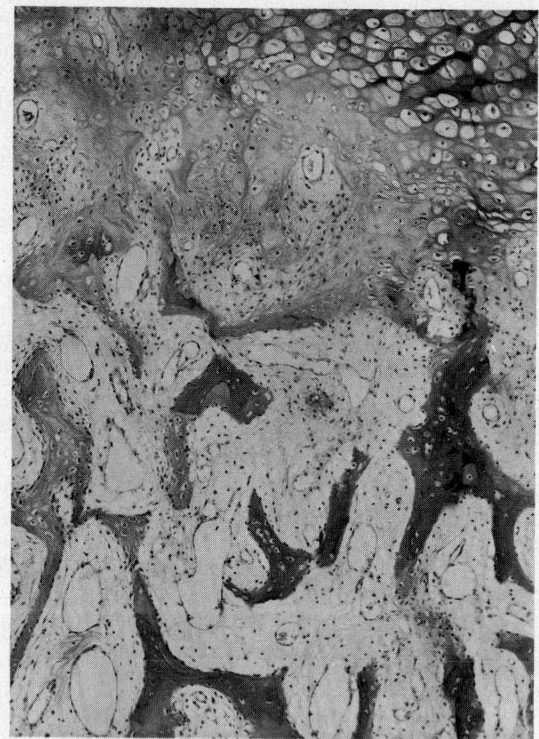

Figure 9–7. A detail of a rachitic costochondral junction. The palisade of cartilage is lost. Some of the trabeculae are old, well-formed bone, but the paler ones consist of unmineralized osteoid tissue.

When the child begins to ambulate, in addition to these deformities, changes occur in the vertebral column, pelvis, and long bones. Commonly, a sharp forward curvature of the lumbar spine develops (lumbar lordosis), which may further accentuate the pelvic deformity. Support of the body weight leads to deformities in the long leg bones, and since these children frequently tend to sit and support themselves with their hands rather than stand, deformities occur in the long bones of the upper extremities also. It should be emphasized here that the skeletal alterations described represent a florid, far advanced case and that suboptimal or varying levels of vitamin D intake may modify the derangements to the point at which alterations are so subtle that they escape detection.

TOXICITY. Large excesses of vitamin D are well tolerated. Extreme overdosage (in the range of 1000 times the normal intake) is extremely uncommon, but may cause hypercalcemia and consequent hypercalciuria. The high calcium levels are probably attributable to increased absorption of calcium from the intestinal tract as well as to mobilization of skeletal calcium.[47] As a consequence of the increased levels of blood calcium, metastatic calcifications may occur and the hypercalciuria predisposes to the formation of renal stones (p. 1052). Sufficient renal damage may occur to cause renal failure. In addition, many nonspecific complaints such as nausea, vomiting, diarrhea, and signs of general toxicity may appear.

Vitamin E

Although vitamin E has been known as an essential nutrient for years, only recently have well-defined deficiency states been identified. *Clearly it plays an important role as an antioxidant.* It protects labile vitamin A against oxidation, DNA from denaturation by free radicals, and the phospholipids within cellular and organellar membranes against peroxidative attack by free radicals; it thus may control the amounts of lipofuscin and ceroid (both peroxidation products of membrane lipids), which accumulate within cells with aging, injury, and atrophy.[48] You recall that free radicals are continuously generated within the body and that there are numerous mechanisms by which the body rids itself of them (detailed on p. 11). Among these defenses are normal levels of vitamin E.

The requirement for the antioxidant activity of vitamin E depends to an extent on the level of easily peroxidized polyunsaturated fatty acids (PUFA) in the diet. The greater the intake of PUFA, the greater the need for vitamin E. Similarly, the selenium intake is important, since it also serves an antioxidant role as an integral part of the enzyme glutathione synthetase, capable of destroying peroxides by converting them into harmless alcohols.[49]

Absorption of vitamin E is essentially dependent on normal biliary, pancreatic, and intestinal function. A deficiency state virtually only develops with maldigestion and malabsorption of fats such as is most prone to appear with sprue and cystic fibrosis of the pancreas. In the absence of such underlying disorders there has been a conspicuous failure to identify a well-defined deficiency syndrome in otherwise normal humans. This is all the more surprising in light of the many well-recognized and diverse disorders that a deficiency of this nutrient produces in experimental animals, including fetal resorption; male sterility; encephalomalacia; muscular dystrophy; an exudative diathesis; and hemolytic anemia, to mention only the best defined. Notwithstanding, no analogous or related disorders have been clearly identified in human volunteers despite extraordinarily prolonged experimental restriction of vitamin E intake. Adult males were placed on a diet containing less than 2 mg vitamin E per day for approximately seven years (recommended daily allowance 8 to 10 mg daily). Although the plasma concentration fell to about 20% of the normal level, the only observable change in the subjects was an increased susceptibility of erythrocytes to hemolysis by hydrogen peroxide, and there was no evidence of a significant anemia.[50] The only naturally occurring clinical condition that is comparable is increased red cell hemolysis and edema in low-birth-weight infants maintained on formulas of cow's milk with added vegetable oils and iron, attributed to a low ratio of vitamin E to polyunsaturated fatty acids.[51] Significantly, a diet deficient only in vitamin E for over six months failed to reproduce this syndrome in premature infants.[52] It must be concluded that although vitamin E may protect red cells against oxidative hemolysis by hydrogen peroxide, there is no evidence that it is a necessary erythropoietic factor in humans.[53]

In part, the failure to identify a vitamin E deficiency syndrome in otherwise normal humans may relate to the fact that the nutrient is ordinarily plentiful in an average diet since it is abundantly available in cooking oils, whole grains, and a wide variety of leafy green vegetables in the form of four tocopherols and four tocotrienols, all of which have vitamin E activity. The major form of vitamin E in the normal diet is the alpha tocopherol. Nonetheless, low levels of vitamin E have been identified in the plasma of patients with fat malabsorption. Such individuals have been observed to be at risk of developing myopathic and neuropathic abnormalities.[53a] The spinocerebellar degeneration closely mimics that encountered in abetalipoproteinemia.

On the basis of its well-defined antioxidant activity, vitamin E is now being employed in the treatment of a variety of diseases in which oxidative injuries are implicated. Only a few examples will be cited, but for more details reference may be made to Horwitt.[54] Vitamin E has been effective in preventing or reducing the severity of retrolental fibroplasia in premature infants exposed to prolonged high-oxygen tensions in incubators.[55] Presumably the vitamin inhibits the formation of oxygen-derived free radicals. Analogously, it has been used in conjunction with the administration of oxygen to infants with bronchopulmonary dysplasia or the respiratory distress syndrome. Other conditions for which pharmacologic doses of vitamin E are employed include the hemolytic anemia of low-birth-weight infants, the shortened red cell survival of patients with cystic fibrosis, and the myopathies and cerebellar dysfunction in patients with hereditary abetalipoproteinemia. In addition, hereditary disorders associated with a deficiency of glutathione synthetase and glucose-6-phosphate dehydrogenase have been said to benefit from large doses of vitamin E. Many other disorders might be mentioned, but it should be emphasized that although encouraging results have been reported in some of these situations, it is not clear that the therapy merely corrects a deficiency state. Despite exhortations in advertisements, there is almost certainly no evidence that vitamin E supplementation in reasonably nourished individuals has any beneficial effect on resistance to infections, muscular strength, or cardiac function, or, unfortunately, on potency or fertility.

Vitamin K

[Deficiency state: Hypoprothrombinemia]

The fat-soluble vitamin K is necessary for the synthesis of the functionally active clotting factors II (prothrombin), VII, X, and XI. A deficiency of vitamin K and the consequent hypoprothrombinemia is recognized in the laboratory by prolongation of the prothrombin time (indicating delayed clotting) and in the patient by a predisposition to hemorrhage, referred to as a "hemorrhagic diathesis." The four clotting factors are all "K-dependent proteins" since the vitamin is a required cofactor for a hepatic microsomal carboxylase that converts glutamyl residues in the already synthesized proteins into gamma-carboxyglutamyl residues. *It is the carboxylated proteins that have clotting activity, whereas the precursor proteins are inactive.* Carboxylation of prothrombin permits it to bind calcium and then interact with phospholipid and factor Xa in the clotting sequence. Calcium binding by the other clotting factors also depends on carboxylation. A number of other K-dependent proteins requiring carboxylation for calcium binding have now been identified in the kidney, placenta, lungs, and spleen, and within renal calculi. An additional calcium-binding protein, known as osteocalcin, may play a role in the mineralization of bone.[56]

The precise molecular events involved in the carboxylation reactions are still somewhat uncertain. The vitamin must be present in a reduced form and in the course of the carboxylation reactions is oxidized to an epoxide by either enzymatic or superoxide activity.[57] The oxidized form is ineffective as a cofactor for the hepatic carboxylase. However, the vitamin epoxide can be reversibly reduced by a hepatic vitamin K epoxide reductase that restores its activity. These details help to explain the mode of action of some of the commonly used clinical anticoagulants. Warfarin, a derivative of coumarin, antagonizes vitamin K activity by inhibiting the epoxide reductase necessary for establishing the physiologic function of the vitamin.[58]

Three closely related compounds all possess vitamin K activity: K_1 (phylloquinone), widely distributed in leafy green vegetables; K_2 (menaquinone), synthesized by microorganisms including the intestinal flora; and K_3 (menadione), a synthetic product. *Although the normal intestinal flora synthesize relatively large amounts of vitamin K, this supply is not sufficient to obviate the need for dietary sources.* A primary deficiency of vitamin K rarely occurs since the normal diet contains an abundance of this nutrient. A conditioned deficiency is far more likely. Impaired absorption of this fat-soluble vitamin may result from conditions inducing fat malabsorption, such as a lack of bile salts (as in obstructive jaundice), pancreatic disease, or diffuse intestinal disorders. Since the body stores of vitamin K, principally in the liver, are relatively small, only a few weeks of negative balance may induce hypovitaminosis K. *Prolonged oral administration of antibiotics, which may destroy the intestinal flora, in association with a marginal dietary intake or impaired absorption, is a well-recognized pathway to the development of a deficiency state.*[59] The neonate is at particular risk of developing *hemorrhagic disease of the newborn,* since the hepatic reserves are very small, and intestinal colonization has not yet fully developed. Moreover, human milk contains less vitamin K than does cow's milk, so that breast-fed infants are particularly at risk. Administration of vitamin K to the mother before delivery is now being reassessed in favor of direct administration to the newborn because recent studies suggest either that this vitamin does not cross the placental barrier or that the uptake by fetal plasma is poor.[59A]

The hemorrhagic diathesis associated with hypoprothrombinemia is identical to that occurring with a deficiency of other clotting factors. It is manifested by a predisposition to ecchymoses, nosebleeds, hematuria, melena, and, in particular, hemorrhages related to surgery, as in the relief of biliary tract obstructions. An additional potentially grave complication is intracranial hemorrhage. Obviously many of these manifestations are more bothersome than serious, but some may be fatal. The bleeding tendency responds promptly with a rise in prothrombin levels within 12 hours after intravenous administration of one of the forms of vitamin K.

WATER-SOLUBLE VITAMINS

Included in this category are a constellation of B vitamins (B complex) and vitamin C (ascorbic acid.) In addition, there are several water-soluble nutrients variously referred to as vitamins—pantothenic acid, biotin, lipoic acid—known to be essential in lower animals, but not well correlated with deficiency states in man. It is worth noting only that excessive consumption of raw egg-white and prolonged parenteral alimentation have been reported to induce a scaly dermatitis and alopecia that responded to the administration of biotin.[60]

As a group, water-soluble vitamins differ in several important respects from fat-soluble vitamins. Since most are rapidly and readily absorbed from the alimentary tract, conditioned deficiencies due to malabsorption are extremely infrequent. On the other hand, since most are not endogenously synthesized by man and some are only scantily stored, a continued dietary intake of many of these vitamins is essential as deficiency states may appear with relatively brief periods of negative balance. Most of the water-soluble vitamins are widely available: the B complex in a variety of foods, principally cereal grains, leafy green vegetables, yeast, liver, and milk; and vitamin C in citrus fruits, vegetables, and some meats.

Ascorbic acid does not require metabolic transformation, but the various members of the B complex all must undergo metabolic transformations that convert them into coenzymes or cofactors essential for a variety of metabolic processes. *The B complex can be roughly divided into two groups: those involved in the intracellular metabolism of carbohydrates, fats, and proteins and those related to red cell production.* The former group includes thiamine, niacin (nicotinic acid), riboflavin, and pyridoxine. These members of the B complex are often referred to as the "energy-releasing vitamins." Despite the widespread metabolic reactions in which these nutrients participate, deficiencies of the individual vitamins tend to affect only specific organ systems, e.g., the heart and nervous system in thiamine deficiency or the skin and mucous membranes in riboflavin deficiency. The reasons for such specific target action are uncertain. The hematopoietic B vitamins comprise vitamin B_{12} (cobalamin) and folic acid. A deficiency of either leads to a megaloblastic anemia and, notably, pernicious anemia in the case of vitamin B_{12}.

Thiamine

[Deficiency state: Beriberi]

Thiamine deficiency principally damages the nervous system (dry beriberi) and the cardiovascular system (wet beriberi). The vitamin is a highly water-soluble nutrient, made up of a substituted pyrimidine linked to a substituted thiazole by a methylene bridge. It is widely distributed in the cells of man where it undergoes phosphorylation into the coenzyme *thiamine pyrophosphate,* also known as *cocarboxylase.* In this form, it participates in the oxidative decarboxylation of alphaketoacids, such as the conversion of pyruvate to acetyl CoA by pyruvate dehydrogenase and the conversion of alpha-ketoglutarate to succinyl CoA by alpha-ketoglutarate dehydrogenase. The pyrophosphate is also a cofactor for the enzyme transketolase, which is a key component of the pentose pathway of carbohydrate metabolism. A decrease in red cell transketolase activity, reversed by in vitro addition of thiamine pyrophosphate, serves as a widely applied clinical diagnostic test for thiamine deficiency. In addition, some recent evidence suggests that thiamine or its derivatives may participate in neural conduction by mechanisms independent of its enzymatic functions. The vitamin or its esters can be found in axonal membranes of nerves. After neural stimulation, the vitamin is broken down into its constituent components.

Basis and Prevalence of Thiamine Deficiency State. Thiamine, widely available in a variety of foodstuffs, is readily and rapidly absorbed through the upper intestinal tract. Absorption is unaffected by most intestinal disorders except those that produce severe anorexia and vomiting or marked gastrointestinal hypermotility. Significant amounts are stored in various organs, principally in striated muscle. A primary deficiency state of thiamine is largely encountered in Southeast Asia and India, where populations subsist largely on polished rice or milled grains from which the vitamin has been depleted by removal of the outer husks. Similarly, in South America and Africa, diets made up largely of cassava, which totally lacks thiamine, may lead to beriberi. Thiamine deficiency is encountered globally, principally among alcoholics having both a poor nutritional intake and frequent bouts of vomiting. Other pathways that may induce a deficiency state are the increased losses caused by diuretic therapy, hemodialysis, and peritoneal dialysis. In addition, certain raw foods such as fish, shrimp, clams, mussels, and raw meats contain a thiaminase and so may contribute to a deficiency. An uncommon inborn error of metabolism involving the enzyme transketolase may greatly potentiate the development of morphologic changes incident to thiamine deficiency.

Pathogenesis. The reasons why the nervous system and heart are the two major targets of thiamine deficiency are still poorly understood. Mention has already been made of a possible role for the vitamin in neural conduction, but this still does not explain the apparent toxic changes seen in the central nervous system in some cases of beriberi. It is known that pyruvic acid tends to accumulate in severe thiamine deficiency. One theory postulates that pyruvate is itself toxic and may damage neurons and nerve trunks. Alternatively, nervous tissue is heavily dependent on carbohydrate for its energy requirements and so may suffer because of the important role of thiamine pyrophosphate in carbohydrate metabolism. These and other speculations are still highly tentative. Even more obscure is the basis for myocardial injury.

Morphology.

Heart. The changes may be slight or absent, even in cases that are otherwise consistent with the diagnosis of cardiac beriberi. A particular problem has been that most well-studied cases have been alcoholics possibly suffering from the cardiac effects of alcohol (p. 597). In better defined examples of thiamine deficiency, particularly those of acute onset, the heart is characteristically dilated and flabby and may be somewhat paler than normal. The dilatation may affect all chambers or, at times, one side more than the other. No endocardial or valvular alterations are produced. Interstitial edema is the most consistent finding. Although microscopic changes such as fatty change and marked swelling of myocardial fibers have been described quite consistently in animal experiments, similar lesions in man are rare. The acute myocardial necrosis encountered in animals is rarely present in clinical cases.

In man, gross and microscopic cardiac lesions in beriberi are not pathognomonic and are useful only in supporting the clinical diagnosis. The genesis of these cardiac changes is unclear.

Nervous Tissues. Here again, there is a paucity of critical information. For the most part, the changes affect the motor and sensory peripheral nerves, the spinal cord, and the brain stem. In the peripheral nerves, there is fatty degeneration of the myelin sheaths. This usually begins in the sciatic nerve and its branches but may ascend to involve the spinal cord and, in time, other peripheral nerves. In severe cases, the polyneuropathy frequently takes the form of an ascending symmetric peripheral neuropathy. In far-advanced deficiency states, degenerative changes involve not only the myelin sheath but also the axon process, which may become fragmented. Histologically, however, these peripheral cord and nerve lesions are not different from those found in other conditions such as diabetes, pernicious anemia, and pellagra. Moreover, it has been pointed out that many of the so-called cases of beriberi in which these lesions are present probably represent multivitamin deficiencies.

Brain. Congestion and edema have been described as the result of a lack of thiamine. In the medulla and pons, cerebellum, and dorsal root ganglia, neuronal degenerative changes have been observed, such as chromatolysis and alterations in the size and staining characteristics of the nuclei. These changes may account for the **Wernicke-Korsakoff syndrome** (described later) encountered in alcoholics. **In Wernicke's syndrome the changes are found principally in the mamillary bodies, the related walls of the third ventricle, and the aqueduct and tegmentum of the medulla.** In these areas, the ganglion cells have the degenerative changes already described and the vessels may show dilatation or rupture with focal and ring petechial hemorrhages. It has been observed that many patients with Wernicke's syndrome have an abnormality in a thiamine-requiring transketolase, since the enzyme binds thiamine phyrophosphate less avidly than the normal transketolase.[61]

CLINICAL MANIFESTATIONS. Beriberi may occur in a chronic or subacute form, usually dominated by involvement of the nervous system, or in an acute, virtually fulminating form, dominated by cardiovascular manifestations. But there is sometimes overlap, and one pattern may be superimposed on the other. Why only one or the other of these syndromes should appear in the individual patient is not understood, but the reason may relate to the severity and acuteness of onset of the deficiency state.

The neurologic manifestations without cardiac decompensation and peripheral edema constitute dry beriberi. This syndrome is manifested by numbness and tingling of the legs, sensory disturbances of the affected parts, tenderness of the calf muscles, and atrophy and weakness of muscles of the extremities, with depression and loss of reflexes. All these findings relate to the previously described peripheral neuropathy of thiamine deficiency. Typically the changes are symmetric and affect the distal regions of limbs more severely than the proximal. Such neuropathy is most often encountered in malnourished chronic alcoholics, but it should be cautioned that identical clinical and anatomic changes may be caused by alcoholism alone. In a small minority of patients with a deficiency of this vitamin, usually but not exclusively chronic alcoholics, the central nervous system is affected, producing the Wernicke-Korsakoff syndrome.[63] The *Wernicke component* is clinically characterized by paralysis or weakness of eye movements (ophthalmoplegia), ataxia of gait, and progressive mental deterioration; the *Korsakoff component* by amnesia, confabulation, and learning difficulties. The two conditions, however, are now thought to be only variable presentations of one disorder. Thus, symptoms usually begin with those relating to Wernicke's encephalopathy, but in time may progress to the Korsakoff psychosis. Indeed, with thiamine administration, many or all of the features of Wernicke's syndrome may improve only to be replaced by manifestations of Korsakoff's psychosis, which are refractory to therapy in most instances.[64]

The cardiovascular involvement of thiamine deficiency may lead to a so-called high cardiac output state related to peripheral vasodilatation, which in some cases is followed by myocardial failure and peripheral edema (wet beriberi).[65] The high-output state may precede the development of cardiac failure, and generally implies a less severe deficiency of the vitamin than is associated with frank myocardial decompensation. It is characterized by peripheral vasodilatation with increased arteriovenous shunting of blood. As a consequence, the patient has ruddy, warm, dry skin, a decreased circulation time; and a normal to slightly increased venous pressure. The decrease in circulation time in association with a failing circulatory system is an uncommon clinical combination that should raise the suspicion of this deficiency state. With acute fulminant beriberi, biventricular failure ensues, with all the findings anticipated in congestive heart failure (p. 548). The peripheral edema is usually striking, particularly in the lower extremities, but it may also affect the trunk, face, and body cavities.

Anorexia, weight loss, and debility are often present in patients with vitamin B_1 deficiency. The clinical diagnosis can be confirmed by the erythrocyte transketolase assay mentioned earlier, by measurement of blood thiamine, and, most definitively, by the clinical response to thiamine administration.

TOXICITY. Although transient mild symptoms such as dizziness and flushing may be produced in certain individuals upon administration of thiamine hydrochloride, massive doses have been given without untoward effects.

Riboflavin

[Deficiency state: Ariboflavinosis]

Riboflavin is an essential cofactor in the oxidation-reduction reactions of the flavoprotein coenzymes flavin mononucleotide and flavin adenine dinucleotide. Thus, it is critical to the function of such enzymes as cytochrome-C reductase, succinate dehydrogenase, and monamine oxidase, to mention only a few. Riboflavin is widely distributed in both plant and animal foods, as riboflavin, riboflavin phosphate, or as a constituent of the flavoproteins. It is rapidly absorbed in the gastrointestinal tract. As a constituent of all cells, it is stored throughout the body; in contrast to most members of the B complex, the stores of riboflavin are sufficient to prevent a deficiency state despite a negative balance for many months. Nonetheless, ariboflavinosis still occurs as a primary deficiency state among persons in economically deprived and developing countries. Under such circumstances, it is frequently accompanied by deficiencies of other vitamins and proteins. In industrialized nations, a deficiency is most likely to be encountered in alcoholics and in individuals with chronic infections, advanced cancer, or other debilitating diseases. Transient mild deficiency states may occur during pregnancy and lactation, and during the rapid growth of adolescence, when there is increased requirement for the vitamin.

MORPHOLOGY. Ariboflavinosis is associated with changes at the angles of the mouth (known as cheilosis or cheilitis), glossitis, and ocular and skin changes. In addition, some patients develop a normochromic, normocytic anemia caused by hypoplasia of the red cell precursors in the bone marrow.

Cheilosis. Cheilosis or, as it is sometimes called, cheilitis is usually the first and most characteristic sign of this deficiency state. However, identical lesions are found in aged individuals with poor dentition who are not vitamin deficient. It begins as areas of pallor at the angles of the mouth, with first a hyperkeratosis of the epidermis and a dermal inflammatory infiltrate. Cracks or fissures may appear, radiating from the corners of the mouth, and tending to become secondarily infected and macerated. In far-advanced cases, the oral mucous membrane at the angles of the mouth and the vermilion border of the lips are similarly affected.

Glossitis. The tongue may take on a magenta hue, strongly resembling the red-blue coloration of cyanosis. Presumably this alteration reflects atrophy of the mucosa of the tongue (Fig. 9–8).

Ocular Lesions. The eye changes may be classified as superficial interstitial keratitis. In the earlier stages, the superficial layers of the cornea are invaded by capillaries. Interstitial inflammatory infiltration and exudation follow to produce opacities and even ulcerations of the corneal surface. The lesion usually affects both eyes, but in certain instances it may be unilateral. Conjunctivitis is a common accompaniment.

Dermatitis. A greasy, scaling dermatitis occurs over the nasolabial folds and may extend into a butterfly distribution to involve the cheeks and skin about the ears. Scrotal and vulvar lesions are common. In well-defined cases, atrophy of the skin may develop. It should be emphasized that the histologic changes are not in themselves distinctive or pathognomonic of ariboflavinosis; it is their distribution that suggests the diagnosis.

Bone Marrow. Erythroid hypoplasia is typically present, but is usually not marked.

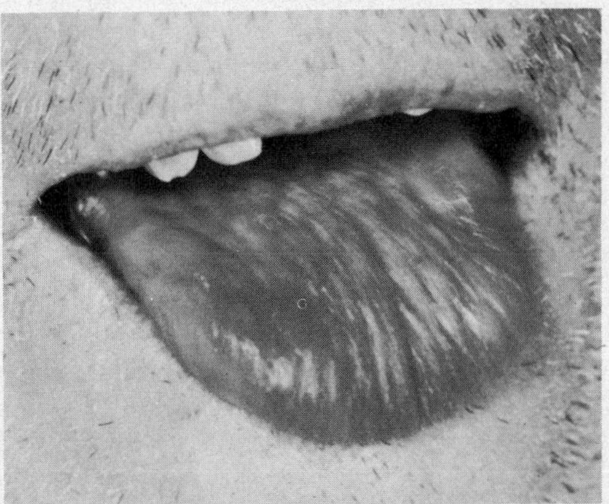

Figure 9–8. The glazed, shiny, atrophic tongue of riboflavin deficiency.

None of the findings just described is specific for riboflavin deficiency, since similar lesions are encountered with pyridoxine deficiency, for example, but in the aggregate they are highly suggestive. There is no clear understanding of why these specific target tissues are affected with the lack of a nutrient that has bodywide functions. Several reports indicate an important role for riboflavin in protein synthesis but it is not clear that a derangement in this process accounts for the lesions described, save possibly for the erythroid hypoplasia and anemia.[66]

Niacin

[Deficiency state: Pellagra]

Niacin is the generic term for nicotinic acid and its derivatives (e.g., nicotinamide) having the functional activity of nicotinic acid. Unlike the other B vitamins, niacin can be endogenously synthesized from dietary tryptophan. For this reason, the required dietary intake depends on the tryptophan content of the diet. Thus, pellagra is in most instances the result of a deficiency of both tryptophan and niacin in the diet.

Niacin is a component of the two important coenzymes nicotinamide adenine dinucleotide (NAD) and nicotinamide adenine dinucleotide phosphate (NADP), which are involved in a great variety of oxidation-reduction reactions, particularly in the electron transport of cellular respiratory reactions. It is widely distributed in most foods and is particularly abundant in whole grain cereals, liver, beef, pork, fruit, and most vegetables. For a long time, it was somewhat of a mystery that pellagra was an endemic disease in corn-eating populations of Central and Southern America, the Mideast, and Africa. The niacin content of the maize, which is the dietary staple in these areas, is no lower than in some grains unassociated with endemic pellagra. Recent studies have shown that maize has a high leucine content that antagonizes the synthesis of NAD and NADP. *Thus, pellagra is revealed as not only a deficiency disease, but also a disorder dependent on the specific amino acid content of the diet.* Awareness of this problem, more adequate diets, and food supplementation have greatly reduced the incidence of endemic pellagra. The disease is still encountered sporadically, however, principally among alcoholics (usually in combination with other vitamin deficiencies) and those suffering from chronic debilitating illnesses such as tuberculosis, cirrhosis of the liver, and cancer. It may also occur with protracted diarrheal states and diets grossly deficient in protein. *Two uncommon disorders affecting tryptophan metabolism may be complicated by pellagra: (a) the carcinoid syndrome, in which most of the tryptophan is usurped by the neoplasm for the formation of serotonin; and (2) Hartnup disease, in which several amino acids, including tryptophan, are poorly absorbed from the diet.*

MORPHOLOGY. The term pellagra, strictly speaking, refers to rough skin. The clinical syndrome, however, is classically identified by most clinicians as the three D's—dermatitis, diarrhea, and dementia.

The **dermatitis** occurs on the body symmetrically and, while it may affect any region, tends to be most severe in areas of exposure to chronic irritation or sunlight, such as the face, dorsa of the hands, wrists, elbows, and knees, and in the inframammary and perineal folds. The margins of these areas of involvement are usually sharply demarcated from normal skin, and this provides one of the more important features differentiating it from other types of dermatitis. The changes consist at first of redness and thickening of the skin with hyperkeratosis and scaling (Fig. 9–9). These early alterations are followed by increased vascularization and chronic inflammation with edema of the subepithelial dermal connective tissue, followed eventually by desquamation of the epidermis. Areas of depigmentation and increased pigmentation may develop. At this stage a variegated dermatitis is present, with brown scaly areas alternating with areas of depigmented, shiny, atrophic skin. With chronicity, the skin may become markedly thickened by subcutaneous fibrosis and scarring. Lesions similar to these may occur in mucous membranes, particularly the oral cavity and vagina. In the mouth, the early stages are marked by vascular congestion and edema of the tongue, and later by atrophy of the mucous membrane and ulceration, so that the tongue becomes red, swollen, and beefy, a form of glossitis reminiscent of the black tongue found in animals.

The **diarrhea** exhibited by patients with pellagra is presumed to be due largely to mucous membrane lesions that have anatomic changes similar to those in the skin. In experimental animals, the first histologic alterations represent vascularization, edema, and inflammation of the submucosal connective tissue of the intestinal lining, which lead to atrophic mucosal glandular changes and eventual atrophy and ulceration of the overlying mucous membrane. These lesions may be found throughout all levels of the intestine but are most prominent in the esophagus, stomach, and colon.

The **dementia** is based on degeneration of the ganglion cells of the brain, accompanied by degeneration of the tracts of the spinal cord. These spinal cord lesions bear a close resemblance to alterations in the posterior columns observed in pernicious anemia, and raise the question of whether a deficiency of another factor in the B complex, such as B_{12}, may also be implicated. Macrocytic anemia may appear in some cases.

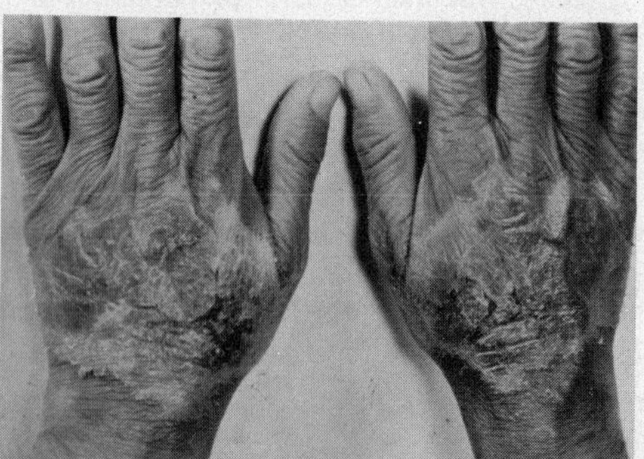

Figure 9–9. The sharply demarcated, characteristic scaling dermatitis of pellagra.

Two of the most dominant complaints of these patients are persistent fatigability and weakness, which have been misinterpreted as malingering or neurosis. Although the skin manifestations eventually appear, they may at times be delayed until significant involvement of the intestinal tract or central nervous system has already developed. Other less prominent clinical features include abdominal pain, dysphagia, proctitis, and vaginitis. It is difficult to explain the precise constellation of clinicoanatomic findings in pellagra on the basis of the known widespread functions of niacin.

TOXICITY. The parenteral administration of niacin quite commonly produces transient peripheral vasodilation, burning sensations in the mouth, nausea, and abdominal cramps. Oral niacin does not produce these symptoms. No persistent ill effects have been described from the administration of doses well in excess of the therapeutic range.

Vitamin B_6 (Pyridoxine)

A primary, clinically overt deficiency of vitamin B_6 is rare in humans, but subclinical conditioned deficiency states, paradoxically, are thought to be quite common. Three naturally occurring substances (pyridoxine, pyridoxal, and pyridoxamine) possess vitamin B_6 activity and are generically referred to as pyridoxine. All are equally active metabolically and all are converted in the tissues to the coenzyme form, pyridoxal 5-phosphate. The coenzyme participates as cofactor for a large number of enzymes involved in transaminations, carboxylations, and deaminations involving lipids, amino acids, nucleic acid, and glycogen in the brain.[67] It is of particular importance in the metabolism of tryptophan, the transmethylation of methionine, and the synthesis of delta-aminolevulinic acid (the heme precursor). Pyridoxal phosphate is also involved in stabilizing muscle phosphorylase and, in some poorly understood fashion, in the transmission of neural impulses.

The vitamin is abundantly available in the usual diet since it is widely present in virtually all foods, principally meats, liver, vegetables, and whole grains. It appears to be readily absorbed from dietary sources through pathways that are still unclear. However, food processing may destroy the pyridoxine, accounting for episodes of severe vitamin B_6 deficiency and convulsions in infants fed badly controlled dried milk preparations, which responded promptly to the administration of B_6.[68] The neurologic manifestations probably stem from complex interrelationships between pyridoxal-5-phosphate and the major brain neurotransmitters such as gamma-aminobutyric acid, which serves an inhibitory function. Normally there are substantial reserves of this vitamin in the body in association with muscle phosphorylase. In addition, the bacterial flora of the gut is able to synthesize vitamin B_6, providing another, but limited, source of the nutrient.

Primary deficiency states are very rare in adults, even in third-world countries; the requirement for this nutrient decreases with general malnutrition and with the lower levels of metabolic activity of aging. However, secondary hypovitaminosis B_6 may be precipitated by the increased requirement for the nutrient during pregnancy and lactation, by hyperthyroidism, and with high-protein diets. During pregnancy there is a marked gradient in the distribution of pyridoxine in favor of the fetus, thus depleting the mother. Breast-feeding by such mothers may lead to a deficiency state in the infants. Alternatively, interference with pyridoxine metabolism in a variety of clinical circumstances may induce a conditioned deficiency. Acetaldehyde, a metabolite of ethanol, displaces pyridoxal phosphate from proteins and thus increases the degradation of the coenzyme. Estrogens, including those contained in oral contraceptives, block the function of the coenzyme in tryptophan metabolism. Isoniazid, employed in the treatment of tuberculosis, combines with pyridoxal or pyridoxal phosphate to metabolically inactivate the vitamin. Penicillamine also forms an inactive product with pyridoxal phosphate.

The clinical manifestations of pyridoxine deficiency have been most clearly delineated in experimental subjects given the antagonist desoxypyridoxine, and include seborrheic dermatitis, cheilosis, glossitis, angular stomatitis, peripheral neuropathy, and sometimes convulsions. The anatomic changes underlying these findings are identical to those described with other members of the B complex. Infants born of vitamin-deficient mothers have suffered mental retardation. Rare cases of so-called hypochromic pyridoxine-responsive anemia have also been reported.

It is not possible to clearly relate all the signs and symptoms cited above to the known metabolic functions of vitamin B_6. However, the anemia probably relates to the role of this nutrient in the synthesis of the heme precursor delta-aminolevulinic acid. The neurologic sequelae may relate to the role of pyridoxal phosphate in brain metabolism and in the synthesis of neurotransmitters, as mentioned earlier. However, there is no clear explanation for the skin and mucosal changes or their particular localizations.

In closing, mention should be made of certain genetic disorders referred to as *vitamin B_6 dependency syndromes.*[69] In one, a familial form of infantile convulsions and fatal brain damage, an apoenzyme for glutamic acid decarboxylase is defective in binding pyridoxal phosphate. Thus, there is decreased synthesis of the neurotransmitter gamma-aminobutyric acid. The pyridoxine-responsive anemia mentioned earlier may represent another genetic defect that requires increased levels of vitamin B_6 for heme synthesis. Patients with homocystinuria, which is due to a deficiency of cystathione synthetase, are improved by the administration of large doses of vitamin B_6. The same can be said of patients with xanthurenic aciduria related to a deficiency of the pyridoxal phosphate-dependent enzyme kynureninase. Thus, it is clear that an inadequacy of B_6 involves more than merely a deficient diet.

Folic Acid

[Deficiency state: Megaloblastic anemia]

A deficiency of this nutrient induces a megaloblastic anemia, but it is important to note that a lack of vitamin B_{12} produces an identical hematologic picture. However, a deficiency of the latter also leads to neurologic damage, thus giving rise to the term "combined systems disease" (anemia and nervous system involvement). The distinction, then, between the anemia of folate deficiency and that related to a lack of vitamin B_{12} assumes great clinical importance: failure to recognize a B_{12} deficiency anemia and consequent treatment of the patient with folates will result in hematologic improvement, but will not stem the progressive neurologic damage.

Folic acid is the common name for pteroylmonoglutamic acid. The terms "folic acid" and "folates" are used generically for all derivatives of folic acid. *Folates of exogenous origin are essential in humans for the transfer of 1-carbon units, such as methyl and formyl groups, to various organic compounds.* Thus, folates serve as coenzymes in a wide variety of intracellular metabolic processes, discussed in the later consideration of the anemia of folate deficiency (p. 634). Largely in the form of polyglutamate conjugates, folates are abundant in virtually all raw foods, particularly vegetables and fruits. Intestinal conjugases are able to split the polyglutamates, yielding mono- and diglutamates that are readily absorbed in the proximal jejunum. Once absorbed, the folates are transported in the blood complexed to specific binding proteins. Some of the folate is excreted in the bile, but is reabsorbed in the gut, thus constituting an enterohepatic circulation. The reserves of folate in the body, principally in the liver, are relatively modest, and a deficiency state in the form of a megaloblastic anemia may arise within months of the onset of a marked negative balance.

A deficiency state may arise because of an inadequate dietary intake or, less commonly, from inadequate absorption or an increased requirement.[70] *Despite the abundance of folates in raw foods, cooking may deplete the content.* Dietary polyglutamates (depending on the specific form) are very sensitive to heat, and steaming or frying of foods for five to ten minutes may cause loss of up to 95% of the folate content. When coupled with a marginal diet, such as is encountered in many chronic alcoholics or in the very elderly living essentially on tea and toast, a deficiency state may well arise.

Inadequate absorption may occur for a number of other reasons.[71] Intestinal conjugases required for splitting polyglutamates into absorbable mono- or diglutamates may be rendered inactive either by inhibitors found in beans and other legumes or by simple lowering of the intestinal pH by acidic foods, such as orange juice. Moreover, there are suggestions that even the monoglutamates found in various foodstuffs vary in their absorbability. In addition, impaired folate absorption is encountered in gluten-sensitive enteropathy (celiac disease), tropical sprue, and Crohn's disease, and after partial gastrectomy or gut resection.[72] An *increased requirement* may also produce a relative deficiency state. This is particularly important during pregnancy and lactation, when the requirement may rise twofold.[73] An increased requirement is also encountered in any disorder associated with a high rate of cell division, such as occurs in the bone marrow in hemolytic anemias and in myeloproliferative disorders, or indeed during the very active growth phases of infancy and adolescence. Recently, folate deficiency has been implicated in so-called hyperalimentation-associated megaloblastic anemia in which the alcohol in the infusate is thought to increase the loss of folate in the bile. It should also be pointed out that, although they do not strictly speaking represent a deficiency state, *many drugs are folate antagonists* and thus may induce a megaloblastic anemia similar to that encountered in a primary deficiency. Indeed, one of these agents—methotrexate—is an effective antineoplastic precisely because it interferes with folate metabolism in the synthesis of DNA.[74] In addition, some anticonvulsants (e.g., phenytoin, phenobarbital) and estrogens (including oral contraceptives) have also been implicated.

Folate deficiency impairs purine, and thus DNA synthesis. *As a consequence, rapidly dividing cells, such as red cell precursors in the bone marrow, suffer from retarded synthesis of DNA relative to the cytoplasm (asynchrony). Thus, the cells become large but cannot divide, and so become megaloblastic.* The megaloblasts in turn produce abnormally large red cells (macrocytes). Moreover, the megaloblastic precursors in the bone marrow are extremely vulnerable to destruction, and so are ineffective in erythropoiesis. In addition, cellular asynchrony may be encountered in the rapidly dividing mucosal epithelium of the gastrointestinal tract, producing large atypical cells, another feature of megaloblastic anemia. More is said about these changes and diagnostic tests in the later discussion (p. 635).

Vitamin B_{12} (Cobalamin)

[Deficiency state: Megaloblastic anemia and neurologic damage]

At the outset, some terminology should be clarified. A lack of vitamin B_{12}, which may arise for many reasons (discussed later), results in megaloblastic anemia. Among the reasons is a lack of gastric intrinsic factor (IF) required for absorption of the nutrient. The most common condition associated with a lack of IF is the megaloblastic anemia termed pernicious anemia, related to an autoimmune reaction against IF or its parietal cell sources. Thus, pernicious anemia is marked by a deficiency of vitamin B_{12}, but it is not correct to term all B_{12} deficiency megaloblastic states pernicious anemia.

Vitamin B_{12}, or cobalamin, is a complex metallo-organic compound synthesized only by a variety of microorganisms, including some found in the intestinal flora of humans. Animals in the food chain acquire this nutrient from the microorganisms growing in soil, water, the intestines, and rumen. Thus, the chief dietary sources of vitamin B_{12} are animal meats and dairy products. Vegetables and fruits are totally lacking in this nutrient, save for their possible contamination by microorganisms or their products. Cyanocobalamin is the therapeutic, stable, synthetic form of the vitamin stabilized by linkage to cyanide. *A deficiency of cobalamin, whether primary or conditioned, leads to megaloblastic anemia characterized not only by hematologic abnormalities and changes in the rapidly dividing mucosal cells of the gut, but also by damage to the nervous system.* The combination is sometimes referred to as "combined systems disease." The intestinal flora of humans does not provide sufficient vitamin B_{12} to satisfy the minimal daily requirement. The *absorption and metabolism* of vitamin B_{12} is included in the discussion of pernicious anemia (p. 631). It will suffice here to note that a lack of B_{12} inhibits DNA synthesis and concomitantly deranges lipid metabolism with the formation of abnormal fatty acids. Incorporation of these fatty acids into myelin may underlie the neurologic abnormalities of a vitamin B_{12} lack.

BASIS OF DEFICIENCY STATE. A primary deficiency state of vitamin B_{12} due to a dietary lack is very uncommon save among strict vegetarians who eat no animal products of any kind. *In industrialized nations, a lack of vitamin B_{12} is for all practical purposes a conditioned deficiency state resulting from malabsorption of cobalamin.*[75] There are a great many causes of malabsorption, but the four most common are: (1) lack of intrinsic factor (IF), (2) chronic pancreatitis, (3) small intestine bacterial overgrowth, and (4) ileal disease.

A lack of IF is the most common cause of cobalamin malabsorption. This is the fundamental defect responsible for pernicious anemia, but surgical removal of the parietal cell–containing region of the stomach is another possible mechanism. Rarely it is due to a genetic abnormality manifested as a defect in secretion of IF.

Cobalamin malabsorption occurs in about 40% of adults with chronic pancreatitis, and in virtually all patients with pancreatic cystic fibrosis. Various hypotheses have been offered, such as failure of the pancreas to neutralize by its alkaline secretions the gastric acidity, thus hampering absorption. Alternatively, failure of pancreatic proteases to release IF from gastric binding proteins may block the formation of IF-B_{12} complexes in the duodenum, necessary to prevent degradation of the vitamin in the jejunum. Other speculations have also been offered.

Bacterial overgrowth in the small intestine leads to a deficient absorption because the bacterial flora successfully competes for the uptake of the nutrient, or bacterial toxins interfere with absorption. Thus, vitamin B_{12} deficiency may occur in patients who undergo intestinal surgery with the formation of blind loops permitting bacterial overgrowth, or who have numerous diverticula of the small intestine.

Ileal disorders, such as Crohn's disease, or ileal resections cause malabsorption by removal of the critical segment of bowel where IF-B_{12} complexes are absorbed. Celiac disease and tropical sprue cause B_{12} deficiency by altering the absorptive surface of the ileum.

Other less common causes of malabsorption include achlorhydria, perhaps because the lack of acid-peptic function may inhibit the initial cleavage of animal proteins with the release of cobalamin, as well as marked gastric hyperacidity such as occurs in the Zollinger-Ellison syndrome (p. 987), since a low pH within the ileum is not favorable for mucosal cell uptake of B_{12}. Several drugs (including neomycin, colchicine, and para-aminosalicylic acid), ethanol, and vitamin C in megadoses interfere with absorption. Indeed, it has been shown that when large doses of vitamin C are added to food, the amount of vitamin B_{12} that can be assayed in it drops significantly. Thus, the current fad for ingestion of large doses of vitamin C for control of respiratory infections may have highly undesirable side effects.

MORPHOLOGY. Whatever its basis, the lack of B_{12} is manifested by a megaloblastic anemia, by alteration in the gastric mucosal cells (identical to those produced by folate deficiency), and notably by demyelination followed by axonal degeneration, and possibly neuronal death. Peripheral neuropathy and degeneration of the posterior and lateral spinal cord columns are the typical sites of involvement. Rarely, the cerebrum itself is involved.[76] More details about these morphologic changes are presented in the consideration of pernicious anemia (p. 631).

Vitamin C

[Deficiency state: Scurvy]

Humans, and their even more long-suffering friends, guinea pigs, as well as other primates and some exotic flying mammals, have lost the capacity to synthesize ascorbic acid (vitamin C). All other mammals, and even such lowly forms as amphibians and reptiles, have the talent to synthesize ascorbic acid from carbohydrate precursors.[77] Man lacks a single critical enzyme—L-gluconolactone oxidase—necessary for its biosynthesis. The enzyme may well have been lost through an evolutionary mutation, and so we are all "walking inborn errors of metabolism."

BASIS OF DEFICIENCY STATE. Fortunately, vitamin C is richly abundant in many foodstuffs (fruits, vegetables, liver, fish, and milk) and is quite resistant to most methods of food processing, so scurvy is uncommon in countries having adequate food supplies. A deficiency state does, however, appear sporadically even in well-nourished populations, particularly among infants in the first year of life whose artificial milk formulas are not fortified with vitamins, and in the very elderly, especially those living alone on restricted diets. Scurvy is encountered endemically among the grossly malnourished poor of developing countries. Vitamin C is rapidly and readily absorbed in the small intestine, and only extensive mucosal disease hinders this process. Thus, conditioned deficiency states are uncommon. Even prolonged periods of negative balance fail to produce scurvy since the vitamin is stored in many tissues and organs throughout the body, principally in the adrenal and pituitary glands. Other sites also have substantial reserves, including the brain, liver, spleen, pancreas, kidney, and heart muscle. For many reasons, then, vitamin C deficiency and scurvy are uncommon.

PATHOGENESIS. The function of ascorbic acid and ascorbates in the body, which is most clearly established, involves the synthesis of collagen.[78] Specifically, *ascorbate is required for: (1) activation of prolyl and lysyl hydroxylase from inactive precursors; (2) hydroxylation of proline and lysine residues in already synthesized collagen polypeptides; and (3) aggregation of hydroxylated polypeptide chains into the triple helix of collagen, prior to its secretion from the cell.* With a deficiency of ascorbate and failure of hydroxylation, there is incomplete intra- and intermolecular cross-linkage, yielding collagen fibrils that lack tensile strength, have increased solubility, and are more vulnerable to enzymatic degradation.[79] Among the various types of collagen, that which has the highest content of hydroxyproline is most affected, namely the collagen in blood vessel adventitia and media and in basal laminae.

Many other functions have been ascribed to ascorbate, some without solid substantiating evidence. Among the better established are the following. Ascorbic acid is readily oxidized and reversibly reduced. It is first reduced to the free radical 3-monodehydroascorbate, then converted to dehydroascorbate. The free radical is, however, a relatively nonreactive species. In its redox function, ascorbic acid may play a role in electron transfer in the cell.[80] It may also act to prevent oxidation of tetrahydrofolate to conserve an active folate pool. Ascorbic acid detoxifies histamine in guinea pigs, and may play a similar role in man; thus, a deficiency may possibly potentiate the development of capillary leakage and hemorrhage in scurvy.[81] There is some evidence that, with depressed ascorbate levels, normal leukocyte function is deranged.[82] Neutrophil and macrophage mobility and phagocytic activity have been reported to be depressed with hypovitaminosis C.[83] Ascorbic acid also appears to play a role in the metabolism of iron, possibly by facilitating absorption or by maintaining the reduced state of stored iron. In any event, scorbutics sometimes develop an iron deficiency anemia.

Almost all the clinical and anatomic features of scurvy can be derived from the above-described functions of ascorbic acid. The clinical features will be described first, followed by the major anatomic changes.

CLINICAL MANIFESTATIONS. Scorbutic adults typically manifest, for poorly understood reasons, hyperkeratotic papular perifollicular skin lesions. They also have a hemorrhagic diathesis and often develop a skin purpura, or sometimes ecchymoses (Fig. 9–10). Typically, these hemorrhagic lesions are located on the backs of the lower extremities. Hemorrhages may also occur into the muscles of the extremities, the joints, and sometimes the nailbeds (splinter hemorrhages). There is poor wound healing and dehiscence of recently healed wounds. The teeth may become loosened, accompanied by gingivitis and bleeding into the gingiva.

Because the tissues and bones of children are in a state of active growth, infantile scurvy is more florid

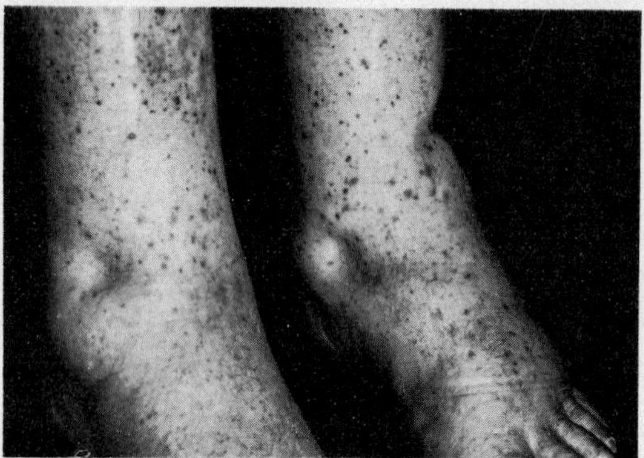

Figure 9–10. The lower extremities of a patient with marked malnutrition, nutritional edema, and petechial hemorrhages related to low levels of vitamin C.

than the adult form. As pointed out, the deficiency state is usually encountered in bottle-fed babies and first becomes manifest by a variety of vague changes, such as loss of appetite, listlessness, weight loss, irritability, and pallor. Soon more specific changes appear, similar to those described in adults. In addition, both endochondral and membranous bone formation are affected because of the collagen defect and its impact on the formation of osteoid. *Subperiosteal hemorrhages and joint hemorrhages are particularly characteristic in infancy.* Such skeletal hemorrhages tend to make the children lie quietly to spare unnecessary motion, with legs characteristically flexed onto the abdomen or in the frog position, relieving tension on the muscles, tendons, and fasciae. Children sometimes suffer subarachnoid or intracerebral hemorrhages, but these are fortunately infrequent. Both infants and adults are classically anemic. The cause of this anemia is still controversial. It may in part be related to numerous hemorrhages, but the alterations in iron metabolism mentioned earlier may contribute.

The disturbances in wound healing and bone development are reasonably attributed to the impact of scurvy on collagen synthesis. Analogously, the predisposition to hemorrhage may stem from the lack of collagenous support of small vessels, but it may also reflect the loss of the detoxifying effect of ascorbate on histamine. As you recall, histamine is a powerful vasodilator, and with increased levels of this vasoactive substance, marked capillary dilatation with opening of interendothelial junctions may all predispose to rupture of small vessels, which are inevitably subject to the minor trauma of usual daily life. The loosening of the teeth would also reflect a loss of collagenous support.

MORPHOLOGY.

Wound Healing. The failure of formation of collagen is most evident in the repair of wounds. Histologically and ultrastructurally, fibroblasts are unaltered,[79] as is fibroblastic proliferation in the reparative phase of wound healing. However, the granulation tissue differs from normal in that it contains an abundant amorphous, granular ground substance deficient in collagen. Hemorrhages are prone to occur in such loosely supported fibrovascular tissue. In the same way, walling-off of infections is inadequate and abscesses are poorly delimited for long periods.

Bone Formation. The formation of the protein-collagen osteoid matrix of bone is vital for normal bone development and growth. In scurvy, **the primary deficiency is in the formation of osteoid matrix, not in the mineralization or calcification such as occurs in rickets.** As a consequence, membranous bone growth and endochondral bone formation are severely disrupted. The total disorganization of the epiphyseal line of growth parallels that found in rickets. The palisade of cartilage cells is formed as usual and is provisionally calcified but, in the scorbutic state, the osteoblasts are incapable of forming bone matrix. Resorption of the cartilaginous matrix then fails or slows and, as a consequence, there is an overgrowth or persistence of cartilage with downgrowth of long spicules and projection of cartilaginous masses and plates into the marrow shaft, producing a change quite similar to that seen in rickets (Fig. 9–11). The usual formation of new osteoid matrix on the degenerating spicules is absent, and the persistent cartilage becomes patchily or completely calcified.

On microscopic inspection it becomes evident that the basic defect is in osteoid formation, not mineralization (Fig. 9–12). Fibroblasts proliferate in this scorbutic zone and form a loose, disorganized connective tissue, but no collagen is formed. Thus, structural strength is markedly decreased, and the stress of weight-bearing or muscle tension may produce actual dislocation of the epiphysis. The soft, poorly formed bone is subject to compression and distortion, because virtually all the stability of this area rests upon calcified, cartilaginous matrix, which is totally inadequate as a substitute for normal bone. The weakened capillaries in the area rupture easily, particularly when stress on the bone causes

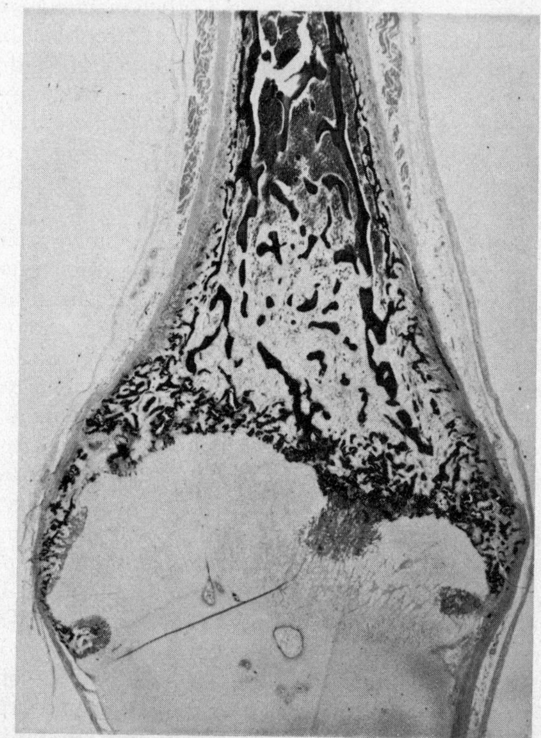

Figure 9–11. A longitudinal section of a scorbutic costochondral junction with widening of the epiphyseal cartilage and projection of masses of cartilage into the adjacent bone.

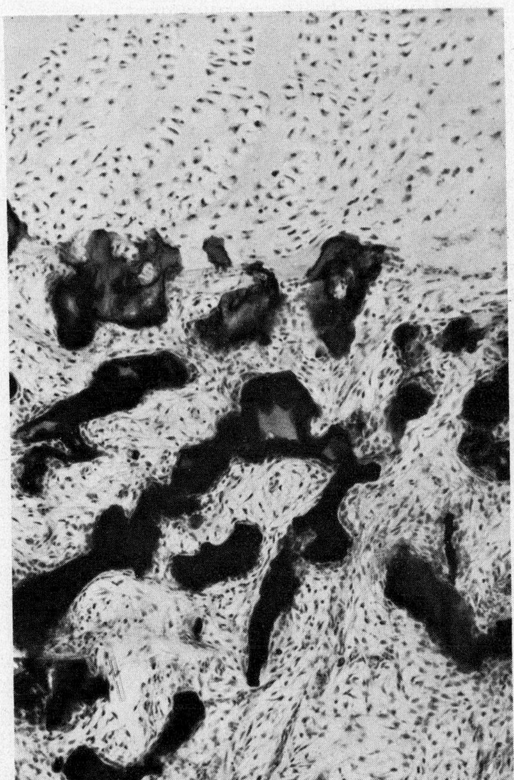

Figure 9–12. A detail of a scorbutic costochondral junction. The orderly palisade is totally destroyed. There is dense mineralization of the spicules present but no evidence of newly formed osteoid.

unusual tensions or fractures. Massive red blood cell extravasation may therefore occur in the epiphyseal area. **The periosteum is loosely attached and extensive subperiosteal hematomas are common, as is bleeding into the joints.** At a later stage, blood pigment derived from such hemorrhage is deposited within macrophages and fibroblasts in these areas.

In the classic clinical case of infantile or childhood scurvy, many of the skeletal deformities and alterations are due to the superimposed hemorrhages and fractures. In experimental animals, far less disorganization is observed.

Formation of Teeth. In experimental animals, striking changes occur in teeth. The clinical counterpart of these changes in infants and adults is less clearly defined and is described in Chapter 17 (p. 770). Resorption of the alveolar bone causes the teeth to loosen, fall out, or become displaced out of line.

Gingivitis. Swelling, hemorrhages, and secondary bacterial infections of the gingival margins are common in severely scorbutic patients. The deficiency of vitamin C does not of itself cause the inflammation, but rather impairs the normal defensive responses of the mucous membranes. Thus, the massive gingival enlargement so characteristic of scurvy results from the combined effects of lack of vitamin C and nonspecific inflammation.

Hemorrhagic Diathesis. Hemorrhages constitute one of the most striking clinical and anatomic manifestations of scurvy. The basis for, and usual localizations of, these hemorrhages have already been detailed. Hemorrhages into the gingivae may occur, but carefully controlled studies indicate that this extravasation is largely due to poor oral hygiene and areas of localized infection rather than solely to vascular disease (Fig. 9–13). Histologically, the vessels may appear to be entirely normal, for the alterations are beyond the range of microscopic visualization.

THE MEGADOSE CONTROVERSY. In the past, the claim was made by the Nobel Laureate Linus Pauling that megadoses of ascorbic acid (up to 10 gm/day—recommended daily allowance 46 mg) taken prophylactically would prevent the common cold or abort it after the onset of infection.[84] A flurry of excitement followed with copious consumption of the vitamin. However, carefully controlled clinical studies have failed to demonstrate any significant benefit, save possibly for modest alleviation of the severity of the symptoms.[85, 86]

More recently, Pauling and co-workers proposed that "increasing ascorbate intake could produce measurable benefits in both the prevention and the treatment of cancer."[87] They proposed that ascorbic acid counters the invasiveness of cancers by favoring collagenous encapsulation, and might control or prevent tumors by enhancing immunocompetence, or possibly by antagonizing known environmental carcinogens such as nitrosamines. Here again, the theory was put to test by controlled clinical studies, which failed to demonstrate any benefit to patients with advanced cancer.[88] Another more recent study proposes that vitamin C has a particular toxicity for malignant melanoma cells in culture.[89] Such cells contain elevated copper concentrations and, in theory, ascorbate could interact with the copper ions to generate toxic free radicals. Although it is possible that large doses of vitamin C may be helpful with certain forms of malignant neoplasia, few believe that the vitamin is of benefit in the prevention or treatment of most if not all cancers.

The doubtful benefits of megadoses of vitamin C must be placed in the perspective of possible untoward effects. Ascorbic acid does not have high toxicity even when taken in large doses, but a variety of harmful effects have been reported: predisposition to calcium oxalate and urate calculi, decreased availability of vitamin B_{12}, enhancement of metal toxicity, decreasing tolerance to a rapid rise to high altitude, potentiation of aspirin-induced mucosal ulcerations, interactions with drug metabolism, and the possibility of mutagenesis

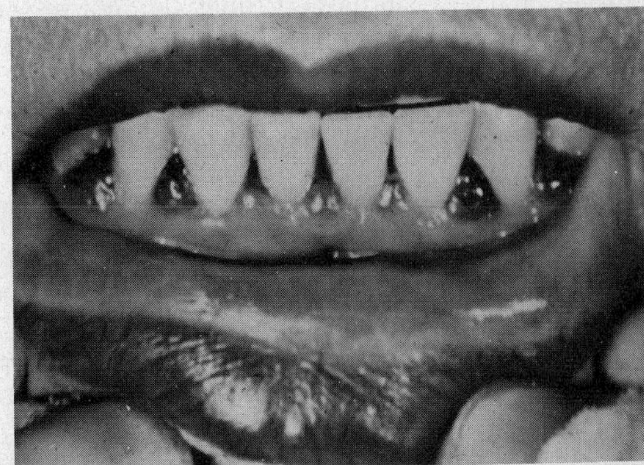

Figure 9–13. Scorbutic hemorrhagic sponginess of the interdental gingival papillae.

from ascorbate metabolites.[82] These untoward effects may not be life-threatening, but the question arises: Do the benefits outweigh the risks?

MINERALS

A number of minerals are no less essential for health than are the vitamins. Some, such as iron, calcium, and phosphorus, are required in large amounts. Others fall into the category of trace elements. Since calcium and phosphorus have already been considered in the discussion of vitamin D (p. 406), only iron and certain of the trace elements require further comment.

Iron

[Deficiency state: Microcytic, hypochromic anemia]

As a global cause of deficiency disease, iron is probably no less important a nutrient than protein. In the U.S., *iron deficiency anemia* related principally to inadequate intake is said to be present in 25% of infants, 15 to 20% of menstruating women, and 30 to 40% of pregnant women. *Less severe levels of iron lack, insufficient to produce anemia,* may be present in as many as 50% of all infants, menstruating women, and pregnant women. In contrast, only about 3% of adult males are similarly affected.[75] A lack of iron is virtually endemic in economically deprived populations and among those who, for religious or economic reasons, seldom eat meat. Hookworm infection (causing intestinal bleeding) continues to be a major cause of iron deficiency where the parasite is prevalent. Iron deficiency anemia is considered on page 635. Here we are concerned only with iron as a nutrient and the basis of a deficiency state.

The total iron content of the body, ranging from 2 gm in small women to 6 gm in large men, is an extremely closely guarded constant, regulated by restricting the amount absorbed to the relatively small fixed daily losses. About two-thirds of this total pool is found in hemoglobin, and somewhat less than one-third in storage iron as ferritin and hemosiderin (representing a mobilizable reserve), in various cells and tissues of the body. The remainder is present in myoglobin and iron-containing enzymes, and a very small amount in transport in the blood as transferrin. In the normal adult approximately 24 mg of iron is required daily for the production of red cells, 95% of which is derived from senescent erythrocytes and the remainder from the dietary intake or the reserve.

The regular daily loss of iron in the normal adult is extremely small, averaging about 1 mg per day. Most of this loss occurs as a result of desquamation of cells from the skin, the mucosal lining of the gut, and the genitourinary systems. During the rapid growth periods of childhood and adolescence, the daily need for iron is about 1.5 mg per day. Women, during reproductive life, may lose as much as 20 mg during a single menstrual period and up to 700 to 800 mg during a normal pregnancy (creating an average daily loss of 2.5 mg). Thus, the normal daily iron requirement in normal adult males is of the order of 1 mg per day; for menstruating women, about 1.5 to 2 mg per day; and during pregnancy, about 2.5 mg per day. During the reproductive years, therefore, young women run a far greater risk of iron deficiency than do males. These losses must be compensated for by the daily absorption of iron from the diet.

The normal Western diet contains approximately 10 to 20 mg of iron per day, only about 5 to 10% of which can be absorbed if iron balance is to be maintained. The mechanism regulating iron absorption is discussed on page 636. Iron occurs in the diet in two basic forms. That contained in meat, fowl, and fish is heme iron; in this form the iron is readily absorbed by intestinal mucosal cells, mainly in the duodenum and upper jejunum, and is not affected by other components of the diet. Inorganic iron found in fruits, vegetables, cereals, and eggs is largely trivalent iron, sometimes in the form of hydroxides complexed to proteins, amino acids, and organic acids. Such iron must be released from its complexes and reduced to the divalent state in the stomach and upper small intestine. The iron so released is chemically reactive and is bound to factors in the gastric juice, as well as amino acids liberated by proteolytic digestion of polypeptides, to form soluble, absorbable complexes. Ascorbic acid is yet another ligand that facilitates iron absorption by the formation of small complexes at the low pH levels of the stomach. Conversely, however, phosphate and phytates in the diet may form insoluble complexes with the iron derived from nonheme sources. An atrophic gastritis with secondary achlorhydria or hypochlorhydria is frequently associated with iron deficiency, but for reasons that still are not clear (Fig. 9–14). On the one hand, the acid peptic environment of the stomach favors release and reduction of nonheme iron and the formation of absorbable complexes. On the other hand, achlorhydria has been observed in individuals for years without the appearance of iron deficiency. Yet total or partial gastrectomy may induce an iron deficiency state. There is much still to be learned.

Basis of Deficiency State. The possible origins of an iron deficiency state can be categorized as: (1) inadequate diet, (2) impaired absorption, (3) increased requirements, or (4) excessive losses of blood.

An *inadequate diet* is a very rare cause of iron deficiency in industrialized countries having abundant food supplies, but it is by no means infrequent in deprived populations of the third world. It is, however, still encountered in privileged societies as a sporadic problem among infants, since milk is a relatively poor source of iron, and among adults, particularly the very elderly, when food faddism or poor dentition leads to very restricted diets. Strict vegetarians who consume no meat, fowl, fish, or eggs are at risk, although the minimal daily requirements can be met by cereals (especially if fortified), fruits, and vegetables.

Impaired absorption as encountered in sprue, other forms of intestinal steatorrhea, and chronic small bowel diarrhea may lead to a deficiency state even in the

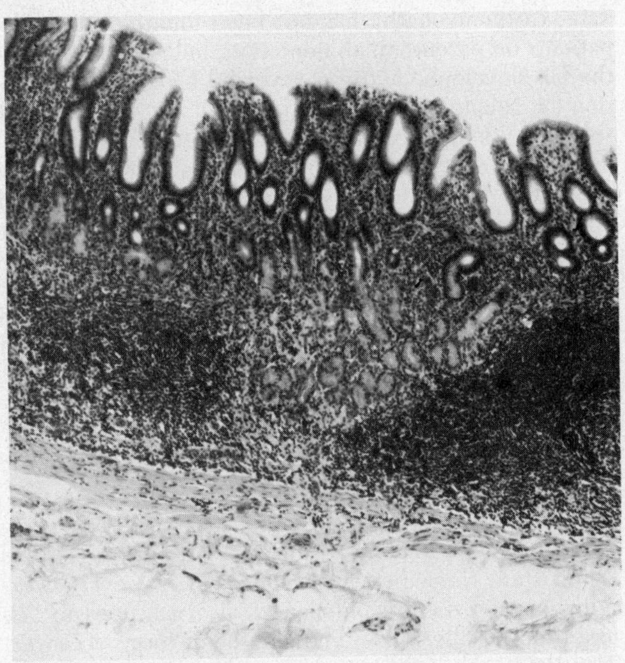

Figure 9–14. Chronic atrophic gastritis with thinning of the gastric mucosa, atrophy of the glands, and an intense lymphocytic infiltration of the lamina propria.

absence of blood loss. The content of the diet, as is evident from the preceding discussion, may also affect absorption.

Increased requirement is an important potential cause of iron deficiency. It has already been emphasized that growing infants and children, adolescents, and premenopausal (and particularly pregnant) women have a much greater requirement for iron than do adult men, which accounts for the prevalence data on iron deficiency cited earlier.

Loss of blood from the body is the most important cause of iron deficiency. Bleeding within the tissues or cavities of the body may be followed by total recovery and recycling of the iron. External hemorrhage or blood loss, as may occur from the gastrointestinal, genitourinary, or respiratory tracts, is the major cause of iron loss. Particularly important are occult bleeding from the gastrointestinal tract (e.g., neoplasms, peptic ulcers, gastritis, and hookworm infections) and menorrhagia (excessive menstrual bleeding) or metrorrhagia (abnormal vaginal bleeding).

In practical terms, an iron deficiency in adult males and postmenopausal women in the Western world should be considered to be caused by gastrointestinal blood loss until it is proved otherwise. To prematurely ascribe an iron lack in such individuals to any of the other possible origins is to run the risk of missing an occult gastrointestinal cancer or other bleeding lesion.

Trace Elements

Trace elements play critical roles in many vital homeostatic functions. Zinc, copper, manganese, and selenium, for example, are crucial components of a wide variety of enzymes ranging from oxidases and dehydrogenases to DNA and RNA polymerases. Other trace elements, such as iodine, are essential for the synthesis of thyroid hormone. Although 14 trace elements (previously listed on page 399) are thought to be essential for humans, only within the relatively recent past have deficiency states of four—zinc, copper, selenium, and iodine—been clearly characterized. Undoubtedly deficiencies of other elements have occurred, but their delineation has proved difficult.

A deficiency of a trace element may have the same origins as, say, a lack of a vitamin; however, three influences are particularly relevant. Total parenteral nutrition of patients, for whatever the reason, may well lead to a critical deficiency. Factors in the diet may interfere with absorption of trace elements, as was first noted among inhabitants of Egypt and Iran subsisting largely on unrefined cereals. Sufficient phytic acid and fiber were present in the diet to bind zinc and block absorption. Similarly, calcium or other divalent cations may interfere with absorption, presumably by competing for receptor sites. Finally, an inborn error of metabolism may lead to a deficiency syndrome of both zinc and copper.

With these few general comments, the clinical effects of a lack of zinc, copper, and selenium will be described briefly. Iodine lack is discussed with the thyroid disorders (p. 1212).

Zinc deficiency was first recognized among inhabitants of Iran and Egypt because of their cereal grain diets, mentioned above.[90] With less restricted diets, a deficiency of zinc would be very unusual since the metal is reasonably abundant in meats, shellfish, fish, whole grain cereals, and legumes. Zinc is an essential component of more than 20 metalloenzymes including DNA and RNA polymerases, carbonic anhydrase, alcohol dehydrogenase, and alkaline phosphatase. It has not been possible to neatly relate a particular clinical finding with impaired function of a specific enzyme or enzymes. With children and adults, the consequences of a chronic zinc deficiency are anemia and retarded growth and sexual maturation. In adults, retarded growth, poor wound healing, testicular atrophy with hypogonadism, anemia, and skin lesions have been attributed to zinc deficiency. Other changes, less certainly related, include diarrhea, mental lethargy, and depression. The older beliefs that a zinc deficiency impaired wound healing and hepatic capacity to oxidize alcohol may well prove to be correct. *Zinc deficiency must at least be suspected in any case of obscure retarded growth and sexual maturation.* The diagnosis is relatively easily established by determining the zinc levels in plasma, serum, hair, urine, or red cells. Depressed levels of zinc-dependent enzymes are further suggestive of the diagnosis. Brief mention should also be made of a rare autosomal recessive disorder characterized by faulty intestinal zinc absorption, leading to a profound deficiency of the metal along with skin lesions (acrodermatitis enteropathica), alopecia, and diarrhea.[91] Oral zinc supplementation is promptly curative.

Copper in appropriate amounts is critical to health, but

but an excess of copper in the body accounts for the genetic disorder known as Wilson's disease (p. 932). Copper deficiency produces well-defined clinical changes, principally involving hematopoiesis, the central nervous system, and the maintenance of vascular and skeletal integrity. The element is an essential component of several metalloenzymes, most of which are oxidases. As noted in the discussion of Wilson's disease, after absorption copper is transported to the liver where it is bound to an alpha-2-globulin to form ceruloplasmin. This nontoxic complex is released into the plasma, and in this form copper is circulated throughout the body. Ceruloplasmin is a ferroxidase and catalyzes the oxidation of ferrous to ferric iron to regulate heme synthesis. Thus, anemia and sometimes neutropenia are features of copper deficiency. The metal and its enzymes are also involved in myelin synthesis or maintenance; hence, impaired myelination is encountered in animals with a lack of copper. Copper is critical to the function of several enzymes within the central nervous system, including dopamine-beta-hydroxylase, involved in the synthesis of neurotransmitters. The copper metalloenzyme—lysyl oxidase—is requisite for the formation of cross-linkages of elastin, hence the impairment of vascular integrity in deficient states. Analogously, the cross-linkages in collagen are deficient, impairing bone formation and maintenance. A number of other critical metalloenzymes such as cytochrome oxidase, lysine oxidase, and cupro-zinc proteins function as superoxide dismutases, quenching highly reactive singlet oxygen radicals. To a considerable extent, the syndrome of human copper deficiency can be deduced from these metabolic functions; it comprises principally anemia, neutropenia and osteoporosis. In infants and children, depigmentation of hair, skin lesions, and various central nervous system abnormalities such as hypotonia and psychomotor retardation may also be present.[92] Such changes are most often encountered in five specific clinical settings: (1) prematurity; (2) generalized malnutrition and prolonged diarrhea in infancy; (3) persistent intestinal malabsorption; (4) infants or adults on long-term use of chelating agents; and (5) the rare X-linked recessive condition known as *Menke's kinky hair disease*. The outstanding clinical feature of the last entity, as the name implies, is a strange steel-wool consistence to the hair, often accompanied by bone changes, abnormalities of the blood vessels, and progressive neurologic deterioration, ending in death in infancy. The basis for this hereditary disorder appears to be some defect in the intestinal absorption of copper.[93]

Selenium deficiency has been incriminated over the past decade as a cause of a congestive cardiomyopathy (p. 596), mainly in children and young women living in selenium-deficient rural areas of China.[94] This cardiac disorder has been designated *Keshan disease*. In 1981 an apparently identical cardiomyopathy was described in an occidental patient who had received nutritional support through intravenous feeding for two years, and also had malabsorption and gastrointestinal disease.[95] To date, cardiomyopathy has not been identified in other patients on parenteral alimentation, but skeletal myopathy has developed and was reversed by the administration of selenomethionine. It is still not certain that selenium deficiency alone accounts for these clinical findings, since other deficiency states may have been present.[96] Nonetheless, selenium is a component of glutathione peroxidase, an enzyme that plays a major role in the scavenging of free oxygen radicals. Why the cardiac muscle or skeletal muscles should bear the brunt of a lack of this enzyme is not clear, and the existence and importance of a specific deficiency of selenium awaits further clarification.

NUTRITIONAL EXCESSES AND IMBALANCES

The well-defined nutritional diseases discussed thus far all stem from dietary deficiencies. However, overnutrition and dietary imbalances also may lead to diseases such as obesity, and possibly some forms of cancer. The latter relationship is currently a matter of great concern. Both subjects are discussed in the following sections.

Obesity

Few subjects are more talked about, are less often corrected, and have supported more authors (of diet books) than obesity. Indeed, obesity has assumed near-epidemic proportions in many Western countries, particularly in the United States. It is the result of the intake of calories in excess of utilization, in essence the storage of unneeded energy in fat cells. Viewed in this way, obesity could have had evolutionary benefits permitting survival over periods of food deprivation. Regrettably the world is now divided into "haves," constantly surrounded by an excess of food and often obese, and the "have nots," largely in third-world countries, who die by the thousands from starvation.

The definition of obesity and how it is best determined are both very controversial. For our purposes, obesity is generally gauged by body weight relative to height when compared with norm standards (categorized by sex, age, and approximate body frame). On this basis, *obesity is defined as a body weight 20% or more above the norm.* By these standards, it is estimated that about 20% of middle-aged males and 40% of middle-aged females in the United States are obese. Dissatisfactions with the norm standards (e.g., they have recently been revised upward) have led to an alternative definition—*the ideal weight for an individual represents his or her weight at the age of 25 years.* Here again, loss in muscle and skeletal mass that occurs with aging could well mask the accumulation of a good deal of adipose tissue. Thus, some prefer to compare the amount of subcutaneous fat as measured by the thickness of skin folds (conventionally in the triceps and subscapular areas) with norm standards. There are, then, difficulties with the clinical determination of obesity, particularly when it is not marked. It would be much easier and far more satisfying to define it as "any individual who is as fat as you are whom you do not like."

We come now to another vexed issue—does obesity predispose to excess morbidity and mortality? On the one hand, obesity has been referred to as "adiposity in excess of that consistent with good health."[97] Indeed, life insurance studies propose that being overweight imposes a significant excess mortality as follows:

	Excess Mortality*	
	Men	**Women**
10% overweight	13%	9%
20% overweight	25%	21%
30% overweight	42%	30%

On the other hand, it is pointed out that weight reduction is only rarely of benefit in the treatment of most diseases.[98] Another analysis also contends that there is no strong evidence that obesity shortens survival.[99] As is so frequently the case, the truth probably lies somewhere in the middle. Although mild obesity may not be harmful (except to the ego), marked obesity must be considered a health hazard and a predisposition to a number of clinical disorders, some of great importance.

Hypertension is unmistakably correlated with obesity.[100] In the long-term Framingham study, the risk of developing hypertension among previously normotensive individuals was proportional to the degree of overweight. In those 20% overweight, the risk was eight times greater than among those 10% underweight, and the likelihood of developing subsequent hypertensive cardiovascular disease was ten times greater.[102] Numerous hypotheses have been offered in explanation of the development of high blood pressure with obesity, but all are highly speculative.

Adult onset (non–insulin-dependent) diabetes is strongly associated with obesity. Over 80% of patients with this disorder are more than 20% overweight. Indeed, the diabetes is often unmasked by the accumulation of excess fat and often reverts to a subclinical state with weight loss. Obesity appears to produce *insulin resistance* in the peripheral tissues by: (1) reducing the number of cell membrane insulin receptors and (2) inducing some intracellular abnormality in glucose metabolism distal to the receptor mechanism. More details can be found on page 979.

Adiposity clearly predisposes to *hyperlipoproteinemia.* The association is relatively weak with the low-density lipoproteins (LDL) carrying most of the cholesterol in the blood, but strong with the very-low-density lipoproteins (VLDL) containing most of the circulating triglycerides. Thus, obesity predisposes to types IIB and IV hyperlipoproteinemia, the former often referred to as "overindulgence hyperlipoproteinemia." With increasing stores of adipose tissue there is increased hepatic synthesis of VLDL, and in addition increased mobilization of fatty acids, providing the substrate for increased hepatic triglyceride synthesis. However, as discussed on page 513, LDL is ultimately derived from both VLDL and high-density lipoproteins (HDL). Through this indirect pathway, obesity has some effect on blood LDL levels, which are thought to play a major role in atherogenesis.

Cholelithiasis (gallstones) is six times more frequent in obese than in lean subjects. The mechanism is mainly an increase in total body cholesterol, increased cholesterol turnover, and augmented biliary excretion of cholesterol in the bile, leading to supersaturation and the formation of gallstones.

Hypoventilation syndrome refers to a constellation of respiratory abnormalities encountered in the very obese. It has been called *pickwickian syndrome* after the fat lad who was constantly falling asleep in Dickens' "Pickwick Papers." Hypersomnolence both at night and during the day is characteristic and is often associated with apneic pauses during sleep, polycythemia, and eventual right-sided heart failure. The complete explanation of the hypoventilation syndrome is complex, but is, at least in part, attributable to the increased burden on chest wall movement imposed by the subcutaneous fat.[102]

The literature is replete with contradictions about the association of all levels of adiposity with *ischemic heart disease,* with particular reference to angina pectoris, myocardial infarction, and sudden coronary death. Clearly, obesity is associated with hypertension, diabetes mellitus, and certain forms of hyperlipoproteinemia that predispose to atherosclerosis and coronary artery disease. However, these associations are strongest with marked obesity. Thus, Keys states: ". . . the idea has been greatly oversold that the risk of dying prematurely or having a heart attack is directly related to the relative body weight. For middle-aged men, the best prospect for avoiding death in 10 or 15 years is to be about average or a bit over in relative weight. The risk rises somewhat with departure in either direction from the happy middle ground, but risk increases substantially only at the extremes of under- and overweight."[103] A subsequent analysis supported this view. In a series of women there was only a weak association between myocardial infarction or angina pectoris and moderate obesity, but a well-defined increased frequency of these forms of ischemic heart disease with marked obesity.[104] However, other studies implicate even less extreme obesity and propose that weighing more or less than the average carries with it an increased mortality.[105] We must leave it that even when other potentially confounding variables have been rigorously excluded, *marked obesity and possibly lesser degrees constitute a definite predisposition to ischemic heart disease, especially to angina pectoris and sudden coronary death, and indirectly to myocardial infarction.*

Stroke and obesity is another area in which the literature is filled with opposing viewpoints. One study

*Drawn from Build and Blood Pressure Study: Overweight: Its Significance and Prevention. 1959 Society of Actuaries, data from Metropolitan Life Insurance Company.

contended that men who were overweight at 20 years of age and then gained 30 or more pounds thereafter had a twofold increase in the incidence of stroke.[106] Others deny any relationship and maintain that it is not the obesity per se, but the related hypertension.

Equally contentious is the relationship between adiposity and *cancer*, particularly cancers arising in the endometrium and breast. Here the problem is complicated by the role of particular foods, such as animal fats, which may have been consumed in excess in the production of obesity. This subject is explored in the following section on diet and cancer.

More clear-cut is the predisposing influence of marked adiposity on the development of *degenerative joint disease (osteoarthritis)*. This form of arthritis, which typically appears in older individuals, is attributed in large part to the cumulative effects of wear and tear. It is reasonable to assert that the greater the body burden of fat, the greater is the trauma to joints with decades of use. We may conclude by saying that obesity clearly contributes to some conditions, notably hypertension, diabetes mellitus, hyperlipoproteinemia, gallstone formation, hypoventilation syndrome, and osteoarthritis, but the magnitude of its influence as an independent variable on such important conditions as ischemic heart disease and stroke still requires clarification.

Diet and Cancer

There is great concern today in governmental, scientific, and lay circles about the possibility that what we eat or fail to eat contributes to the causation of cancer. The fears are that overnutrition and obesity may in some way predispose to cancers,[107] or more specifically that the diet may contain carcinogens, cocarcinogens, or tumor promoters, or may possibly lack some protective ingredient.[108] The grounds for this concern are as follows. It is frequently contended that 80 to 90% of cancers in the United States and other industrialized nations can be attributed to life style (including diet) and environmental influences.[109] This estimate is based on the theory that the lowest rate of occurrence of any form of cancer in any country around the world represents the "natural" or baseline rate. Any increased frequency of the specific form of neoplasia in any other locale must, then, be the result of personal and environmental influences. While there are many potentially carcinogenic influences prevalent in the environment, epidemiologic studies, attempting to control for the many variables, point to diet as a major factor. Support for this view comes from various sources. Actuarial records show an excess mortality from cancer of 16% for men and 13% for women, respectively, who are 20% or more above ideal weight. Cancer of the stomach is about five times more frequent in Japan than in the United States, whereas the reverse holds true for cancer of the colon. Japanese families that migrate to the United States begin to acquire an incidence rate for both forms of cancer approximating that of their new home. Over the span of generations, the incidence rates come ever closer to those prevailing in the native-born population of the United States.[110] Although there are obvious environmental differences between the two countries, both are highly industrialized and have comparable air pollution and cigarette smoking practices; thus, the diet is suspected. Even more convincing is the laboratory evidence from animals. Restriction of dietary intake lowers the spontaneous incidence of cancers in a variety of animals, and also reduces the incidence and progression of experimentally induced neoplasms.[111]

Three aspects of diet have evoked concern: (1) its possible content of exogenous carcinogens; (2) the potential that carcinogens might be endogenously synthesized from dietary components; and (3) a possible lack of protective factors.[112, 113] *Relative to exogenous carcinogens,* it was pointed out in Chapter 6 (p. 248) that some naturally occurring carcinogens may be present in the diet, e.g., aflatoxins. The high incidence of hepatocarcinoma in Africa may be attributable to contamination of grains and ground nuts by aflatoxin B, resulting from the growth of *Aspergillus flavus*. Aromatic polycyclic hydrogens could be produced in the broiling and smoking of meats and fish (p. 238). Of great current interest is the controversy about the dangers of the artificial sweeteners saccharin and cyclamates, mentioned on page 239. It is sufficient to say that, despite earlier alarm, more recent rigorously controlled analyses have failed to reveal any significant increase in the frequency of bladder cancer among users of artificial sweeteners.[115-117] However, a very weak oncogenic effect, which might be potentiated by concurrent exposure to more clearly established carcinogens, has not been ruled out. In experimental animals the long-term administration of saccharin or cyclamate following a small dose of a well-defined carcinogen evokes bladder cancer. In this setting the artificial sweeteners appear to act as promoters, since alone they are without effect.[118] Thus, although saccharin and cyclamates are probably not significant initiators of cancer, the possibility that they might enhance the action of concurrent carcinogenic influences dictates the need for caution in their use, particularly during pregnancy and in the young with long years of potential exposure ahead of them.

Concern about the *endogenous synthesis of carcinogens or promoters* from components of the diet relates principally to gastric, mammary, and endometrial carcinomas. With gastric carcinoma, nitrosamines and nitrosamides are in the spotlight. These compounds could be formed in the body from nitrites and amines or amides derived from digested proteins.[119] Sodium nitrite is added as a flavor and color preservative to foods such as processed meats, which cannot be heated sufficiently to destroy botulinal spores. Sodium nitrite is also present in some common vegetables. Nitrates are abundant in the soil and water and can be reduced to nitrites by bacterial action in the gut. There is, then, the potential for the endogenous production of carcinogenic agents from dietary components, which might well have an effect on the stomach exposed to the highest concentrations.

With carcinoma of the breast in postmenopausal women, and endometrial carcinoma, epidemiologic studies implicate diets high in animal meats and fats, and overnutrition (obesity).[120, 121] There is no shortage of theories to explain these associations. Dietary fat might serve as a vehicle for liposoluble carcinogens, cocarcinogens, or promoters. Alternatively, increased synthesis of estrogens might be involved. As detailed on page 446, estrogens are strongly implicated (probably as promoters) in the development of endometrial carcinoma (p. 1138) and are suspect with regard to breast cancer (p. 1179). A high fat intake might increase the plasma cholesterol level, which serves as a substrate for estrogen and, to a lesser extent, androgen synthesis. Estrogen metabolism might be altered in obese individuals with increased synthesis of the potentially more dangerous estrone (estradiol) and decreased synthesis of "antiestrogenic" 2-hydroxyestrone. Concomitantly, there might be increased conversion of androstenedione (of adrenal origin) to estrone in the mammary and peripheral fat depots. Indeed, the normal fat stores in the breast would increase local tissue levels. These hypothecations have been buttressed by animal studies showing an increased incidence of carcinogen-induced breast cancers when the fat level in the diet is raised.[122] Seductive as all these observations may be, uncertainties persist. There are reports denying any effect of obesity on the incidence of breast cancer.[123] Other studies contend that the amount of vegetable fats or dairy products in the diet correlate better with the incidence of breast carcinoma than do animal fats.[124, 125] More claims and counterclaims might be cited, but suffice to say that the role of nutritional influences in the induction of postmenopausal breast cancer and endometrial cancer is still uncertain but "suspicioid."[126]

Low fiber and a high animal fat intake have been implicated in the causation of colonic cancer.[127] The most convincing attempt to explain these associations is the following. A high animal fat diet might have two effects. The high fat intake would increase the level of bile acids in the gut, which in turn would modify the intestinal flora, favoring the growth of microaerophilic bacteroides. It is then proposed that either the bile acids themselves, or metabolites of the bile acids produced by the bacteroides, might serve as carcinogens or promoters.[128] Furthermore, a low fiber content in the diet would decrease stool bulk and slow transit time, thereby exposing the mucosa to the putative offenders longer. Alternatively, certain types of fiber might bind carcinogens and thereby protect the mucosa. Reduction in stool bulk would also lessen the dilution of offending products. Unfortunately, attempts to document these theories in patients and experimental animals have on the whole led to contradictory results.[129, 130] A recent prospective study in men further confounds the issue. Although it could not provide statistically significant data on colorectal cancer, it indicated a significant reduction in *total* cancer mortality among individuals on high fiber intake, related largely to apparent protection against lung carcinoma.[131] This surprising finding, if confirmed, casts serious doubts about the notion that high fiber intake protects against colorectal cancer by local actions within the gut. Confusion reigns supreme.

It is obvious that the nutrition–cancer story is still unfolding. Many additional pieces of it might be mentioned, e.g., the possible protective roles of vitamins A and C, and the tenuous evidence linking other forms of cancer such as those of the esophagus, prostate, and ovary to nutritional influences. For the present, however, we must leave it that, while there are reasons for suspecting nutritional influences in the development of at least certain forms of cancer, definitive proof is still lacking.

---

1. Brown, C.B.: The incidence of protein-energy (calorie) malnutrition of early childhood. Guy's Hosp. Rept. *120*:129, 1971.
2. Casey, C.E., and Hambidge, K.M.: Trace element deficiencies in man. *In* Draper, H.E. (ed.): Advances in Nutritional Research. Vol. III. New York and London, Plenum Press, 1980, p. 23.
3. Ten-State Nutritional Survey, 1968–1970. Center for Disease Control. Nutrition Program. Department of Health, Education and Welfare Publication No. (HSM) 72–8131. Atlanta, 1972.
4. Editorial: Infant mortality, economics, and arms. Lancet *2*:193, 1982.
5. Thanangkul, O., et al.: Clinical aspects of protein deficiency with special reference to protein-calorie malnutrition (PCM) in children. J. Nutr. Sci. Vitaminol. (Tokyo) *26*:189, 1980.

5A. Golden, M.H.N.: Protein deficiency, energy deficiency and the oedema of malnutrition. Lancet *1*:126, 1982.

6. Editorial: Nutritional oedema, albumin and vanadate. Lancet *1*: 646, 1981.
7. Bistrian, B. R., et al.: Protein status of general surgical patients. J.A.M.A. *230*:858, 1974.
8. Bistrian, B.R., et al.: Prevalence of malnutrition in general medical patients. J.A.M.A. *235*:1567, 1976.
9. Shiner, M., et al.: The jejunal mucosa in protein-energy malnutrition. A clinical, histological and ultrastructural study. Exp. Mol. Pathol. *19*:61, 1973.
10. Nassar, A. M.: Ultrastructural changes in the mucosa of the small intestine due to protein-calorie malnutrition. J. Trop. Pediatr. *26*:62, 1980.
11. Webber, B. L., and Freiman, I.: The liver in kwashiorkor. Arch. Pathol. *98*:400, 1974.
12. Beisel, W. R.: Symposium on the impact of infection on nutritional status of the host. Am. J. Clin. Nutr. *30*:1203 and 1439, 1977.
13. Pereira, S. M., et al.: Physical growth and neurointegrative performance of survivors of protein-energy malnutrition. Br. J. Nutr. *42*:1979.
14. Evans, D., et al.: Intellectual development and nutrition. J. Pediatr. *97*:358, 1980.
15. Wolbach, S. B., and Bessey, O. A.: Tissue changes in vitamin deficiencies. Physiol. Rev. *22*:233, 1942.
16. Editorial: Vitamin A, retinol, carotene and cancer prevention. Br. Med. J. *281*:957, 1980.
17. Editorial: Vitamin A and cancer. Lancet *1*:575, 1980.
18. Verma, A.K., et al.: Correlation of the inhibition by retinoids of tumor promoter–induced mouse epidermal ornithene decarboxylase activity and of skin tumor promotion. Cancer Res. *39*:419, 1979.
19. Harisiadis, L., et al.: A vitamin A analogue inhibits radiation-induced oncogenic transformation. Nature *274*:486, 1978.
20. Orfano, S.: Oral retinoids—present status. Br. J. Dermatol. *103*:473, 1980.
21. Schroder, E. W., and Black, P. H.: Retinoids: Tumor preventors or tumor enhancers? J. Natl. Cancer Inst. *65*:671, 1980.
22. Editorial: Vitamin A deficiency and anemia. Clin. Nutr. *37*:38, 1979.
23. Wald, G.: The molecular basis of visual excitation. Nature *219*:800, 1968.
24. Chytil, F., and Ong, D. E.: Cellular retinol and retinoic acid-binding proteins in vitamin A action. Fed Proc. *38*:2510, 1979.
25. Ong, D.E., et al.: Cellular binding proteins for vitamin A in colorectal adenocarcinoma of rat. Cancer Res. *38*:4422, 1978.
26. Gouvera, J.: Degree of bronchial metaplasia in heavy smokers and its regression after treatment with a retinoid. Lancet *1*:710, 1982.
27. Denner, E. G., and Lotan, R.: Effects of retinoic acid on the immune system: Stimulation of T killer induction. Eur. J. Immunol. *8*:23, 1978.
28. Micksche, M., et al.: Stimulation of immune response in lung cancer patients by vitamin A therapy. Oncology *34*:234, 1977.
29. Adamo, S., et al.: Retinoic acid–induced changes in saturation density and adhesion of transformed mouse fibroblasts. Proc. Am. Assoc. Cancer Res. *19*:27, 1978.

30. Teitelbaum, S. L.: Pathological manifestations of osteomalacia and rickets. Clin. Endocrinol. Metab. *9*:43, 1980.
31. Holick, M.G., and Clark, M.G.: The photobiogenesis and metabolism of vitamin D. Fed. Proc. *37*:2567, 1978.
32. Brunette, M.G., et al.: Site of 1,25-dihydroxy-vitamin D_3 synthesis in the kidney. Nature *276*:287, 1978.
33. Barbour, G.L., et al.: Hypercalcemia in an anephric patient with sarcoidosis: Evidence for extrarenal generation of 1,25-dihydroxy vitamin D. N. Engl. J. Med. *305*:440, 1981.
34. DeLuca, H.F.: Vitamin D: Revisited 1980. Clin. Endocrinol. Metab. *9*:3, 1980.
35. Roth, S.P., and Henry, H.L.: Recent advances in the understanding of the metabolism and functions of vitamin D. Clin. Orthop. *149*:249, 1980.
36. Stumpf, W.E., et al.: Target cells for 1,25-dihydroxyvitamin D_3 in the intestinal tract, stomach, kidney, skin, pituitary, and parathyroid. Science *206*:1188, 1979.
37. Eil, C., et al.: A cellular defect in hereditary vitamin D–dependent rickets, type II. Defective nuclear uptake of 1,25-dihydroxyvitamin D in cultured skin fibroblasts. N. Engl. J. Med. *304*:1588, 1981.
38. Goldsmith, R.S.: Calcium, phosphate and vitamin D. Orthop. Clin. North Am. *10*:319, 1979.
39. Dent, C.E.: Rickets in osteomalacia of various origins. Birth Defects *6*:79, 1971.
40. Marie, P.J., et al.: Histological osteomalacia due to dietary calcium deficiency in children. N. Engl. J. Med. *307*:584, 1982.
41. Stamp, T.C.B., et al.: Nutritional osteomalacia and late rickets in greater London, 1974–1979: Clinical and metabolic studies in 45 patients. Clin. Endocrinol. Metab. *9*:81, 1980.
42. Scriver, C.R., et al.: Serum 1,25-dihydroxyvitamin D levels in normal subjects and in patients with hereditary rickets or bone disease. N. Engl. J. Med. *299*:976, 1980.
43. Hahn, T.J.: Drug-induced disorders of vitamin D and mineral metabolism. Clin. Endocrinol. Metab. *9*:107, 1980.
44. Raisz, L.G.: Direct effects of vitamin D and its metabolites on skeletal tissue. Clin. Endocrinol. Metab. *9*:27, 1980.
45. Frost, H.M.: Tetracycline-based histological analysis of bone remodelling. Calcif. Tissue Res. *3*:211, 1969.
46. Bordier, P., et al.: Vitamin D metabolites and bone mineralization in man. J. Clin. Endocrinol. Metab. *46*:284, 1978.
47. Follis, E.H.: Hypervitaminosis D. Am. J. Clin. Pathol. *26*:400, 1956.
48. Oski, F.A.: Vitamin E: A radical defense. N. Engl. J. Med. *303*:454, 1980.
49. Scott, M.L.: Advances in our understanding of vitamin E. Fed. Proc. *39*:2736, 1980.
50. Horwitt, M.K., et al.: Erythrocyte survival and reticulocyte levels after tocopherol depletion in man. Am. J. Clin. Nutr. *12*:99, 1963.
51. Ritchie, J.H., et al.: Edema and hemolytic anemia in premature infants: A vitamin E deficiency syndrome. N. Engl. J. Med. *279*:1185, 1968.
52. Panos, T.C., et al.: Vitamin E and linoleic acid in the feeding of premature infants. Am. J. Clin. Nutr. *21*:15, 1968.
53. Drake, J.R., and Fitch, C.D.: Status of vitamin E as an erythropoietic factor. Am. J. Clin. Nutr. *33*:2386, 1980.
53a. Bieri, J. J., et al.: Medical uses of vitamin E. N. Engl. J. Med. *308*:1063, 1983.
54. Horwitt, M.K.: Therapeutic uses of vitamin E in medicine. Nutr. Rev. *38*:105, 1980.
55. Hittner, H.M., et al.: Retrolental fibroplasia: Efficacy of vitamin E in a double blind clinical study of preterm infants. N. Engl. J. Med. *305*:1365, 1981.
56. Lian, J.B., et al.: Properties and biosynthesis of a vitamin K–dependent calcium-binding protein in bone. Fed. Proc. *37*:2615, 1978.
57. Bell, R.G.: Metabolism of vitamin K and prothrombin synthesis: Anticoagulants and the vitamin K–epoxide cycle. Fed. Proc. *37*:2599, 1978.
58. Suttie, J.W.: The metabolic role of vitamin K. Fed. Proc. *39*:2730, 1980.
59. Ansell, J.E., et al.: The spectrum of vitamin K deficiency. J.A.M.A. *238*:40, 1979.
59A. Shearer, M.J., et al.: Plasma vitamin K in mothers and their new-born babies. Lancet *2*:460, 1982.
60. Mock, C.M., et al.: Biotin deficiency: An unusual complication of parenteral alimentation. N. Engl. J. Med. *304*:820, 1981.
61. Blass, J.P., and Gibson, G.E.: Abnormality of a thiamine-requiring enzyme in patients with Wernicke-Korsakoff syndrome. N. Engl. J. Med. *297*:1367, 1977.
62. Editorial: Cardiovascular beriberi. Lancet *1*:1287, 1982.
63. Feinberg, J.F.: The Wernicke-Korsakoff syndrome. Am. Fam. Physician *22*:129, 1980.
64. Bonjour, J.P.: Vitamins and alcoholism. IV. Thiamine. Int. J. Vitamin Nutr. Res. *50*:321, 1980.
65. Wakabayashi, A., et al.: A clinical study on thiamine deficiency. Jap. Circ. J. *43*:995, 1979.
66. Perry, G.M., et al.: The effect of riboflavin on red-cell vitamin B_6 metabolism and globin synthesis. Biomedicine *33*:36, 1980.
67. Minns, R.: Vitamin B_6 deficiency and dependency. Dev. Med. Child Neurol. *22*:795, 1980.
68. Molony, C.J., and Parmalee, A.H.: Convulsions in young infants as a result of pyridoxine deficiency. J.A.M.A. *154*:405, 1954.
69. Mudd, S.H.: Pyridoxine-responsive genetic disease. Fed. Proc. *30*:970, 1971.
70. Bernstein, L.H., et al.: The absorption and malabsorption of folic acid and its polyglutamates. Am. J. Med. *48*:570, 1970.
71. Colman, N., et al.: Prevention of folate deficiency by food fortification. IV. Identification of target groups in addition to pregnant women in an adult rural population. Am. J. Clin. Nutr. *28*:471, 1975.
72. Chanarin, I., and Bennett, M.C.: Absorption of folic acid and D-xylose as tests of small-intestinal function. Br. Med. J. *5283*:985, 1962.
73. Colman, N., et al.: Prevention of folate deficiency in pregnancy by food fortification. Am. J. Clin. Nutr. *27*:339, 1974.
74. Steffins, R., et al.: Drug-induced megaloblastic anemias. Semin. Hematol. *10*:235, 1973.
75. Herbert, V.: The nutritional anemias. Hosp. Pract. *15*:65, 1980.
76. Shorvon, F.D.: The neuropsychiatry of megaloblastic anaemia. Br. Med. J. *281*:1036, 1980.
77. Chatterjee, I.B.: Ascorbic acid metabolism. World Rev. Nutr. Diet. *30*:69, 1978.
78. Editorial: The function of ascorbic acid in collagen formation. Nutr. Rev. *36*:118, 1978.
79. Levene, C.I., et al.: Scurvy: A comparison between ultrastructural and biochemical changes observed in cultured fibroblasts and the collagen they synthesize. Virchows Arch. (B) Cell Pathol. *23*:825, 1977.
80. Weis, W.: Ascorbic acid and electron transport. Ann. N.Y. Acad. Sci. *258*:190, 1975.
81. Chatterjee, I.B., et al.: Effect of ascorbic acid on histamine metabolism in scorbutic guinea pigs. J. Physiol. (Lond.) *251*:271, 1975.
82. Editorial: Ascorbic acid: Immunological effects and hazards. Lancet *1*:308, 1979.
83. Thomas, W.R., and Holt, P.G.: Vitamin C and immunity: An assessment of the evidence. Clin. Exp. Immunol. *32*:370, 1978.
84. Pauling, L.: Vitamin C and the Common Cold. San Francisco, W. H. Freeman & Co., 1971, p. 26.
85. Coulehan, J.L.: Ascorbic acid and the common cold. Reviewing the evidence. Postgrad. Med. *66*:153, 1979.
86. Anderson, T.W., et al.: Winter illness and vitamin C: The effect of relatively low doses. Can. Med. Assoc. J. *112*:823, 1975.
87. Cameron, E., Pauling, L., and Leibovitz, B.: Ascorbic acid and cancer: A review. Cancer Res. *39*:663, 1979.
88. Creagan, E.T., et al.: Failure of high dose vitamin C (ascorbic acid) therapy to benefit patients with advanced cancer: A controlled trial. N. Engl. J. Med. *1*:687, 1979.
89. Bram, S., et al.: Vitamin C preferential toxicity for malignant melanoma cells. Nature *284*:629, 1980.
90. Halsted, J.A., et al.: A conspectus of research on zinc requirements of man. J. Nutr. *104*:345, 1974.
91. Hambidge, K.M., et al.: Zinc and acrodermatitis enteropathica. *In* Hambidge, K.M., and Nichols, B.L. (eds.): Zinc and Copper in Clinical Medicine. New York, Spectrum, 1978, p. 81.
92. Graham, G.C.E., and Cordano, A.: Copper deficiency in human subjects. *In* Prasad, A.S. (ed.): Trace Elements in Human Health and Diseases. Vol. 1. New York, Academic Press, 1976, p. 363.
93. Danks, D.M., et al.: Menke's kinky hair disease. Further definition of the defect in copper transport. Science *179*:1140, 1973.
94. Keshan Disease Research Group of the Chinese Academy of Medical Sciences: Epidemiologic studies on the etiologic relationship of selenium and keshan disease. Chin. Med. J. (Eng.) *92*:477, 1979.
95. Johnson, R.A., et al.: An occidental case of cardiomyopathy and selenium deficiency. N. Engl. J. Med. *304*:1210, 1981.
96. Young, V.R.: Selenium: A case for its essentiality in man. N. Engl. J. Med. *304*:1228, 1981.
97. Albrink, M.J.: Overnutrition and the fat cell. *In* Bondy, P.K., and Rosenberg, L.E. (eds.): Duncan's Diseases of Metabolism, 7th ed. Philadelphia, W. B. Saunders Co., 1974, p. 426.
98. Mann, G.V.: The influence of obesity on health. N. Engl. J. Med. *291*:178, 1974.
99. Andres, R.: Effect of obesity on total mortality. Int. J. Obes. *4*:381, 1980.
100. Dustan, H.P.: Obesity and hypertension. Compr. Ther. *6*:29, 1980.
101. Alexander, J., et al.: Report of the Hypertension Task Force—Current Research and Recommendations from the Task Force on Therapy. Preg. Obesity, Vol. 9, Bethesda, U.S. Dept. HEW Publication #NIH 79-1631.
102. Luce, J.M.: Respiratory complications of obesity. Chest *78*:626, 1980.
103. Keys, A.: Overweight, obesity, coronary heart disease and mortality. Nutr. Rev. *38*:297, 1980.
104. Noppa, H., et al.: Obesity in relation to morbidity and mortality from cardiovascular disease. Am. J. Epidemiol. *3*:682, 1980.
105. Sorlie, P., et al.: Body build and mortality. The Framingham Study. J.A.M.A. *243*:1828, 1980.

106. Heyden, S., et al.: Weight and weight history in relationship to cerebrovascular and ischemic heart disease. Arch. Intern. Med. *128*:956, 1971.
107. Editorial: Obesity: The cancer connection. Lancet *1*:1223, 1982.
108. Gori, G.B.: Dietary and nutritional implications in the multifactorial etiology of certain prevalent human cancers. Cancer *43*:2151, 1979.
109. Doll, R., and Peto, R.: The causes of cancer: Quantitative estimates of avoidable risks of cancer in the U.S. today. J. Natl. Cancer Inst. *66*:1191, 1981.
110. Haenszel, W., and Kurihara, M.: Studies of Japanese migrants. I. Mortality from cancer and other diseases among Japanese in the United States. J. Natl. Cancer Inst. *40*:43, 1968.
111. Clayson, D.B.: Nutrition and experimental carcinogenesis. A review. Cancer Res. *35*:3292, 1975.
112. Miller, A.B.: Nutrition and cancer. Prev. Med. *9*:189, 1980.
113. Habs, M., and Schmahl, D.: Diet and cancer. J. Cancer Res. Clin. Oncol. *96*:1, 1980.
114. United States Department of Health, Education & Welfare: Histopathologic evaluation of tissues from rats following continuous dietary intake of sodium saccharin and calcium cyclamate for a maximum period of two years. Final Report (Project P-169-170). Washington, D.C., U.S. Dept. of H.E.W., Public Health Service, F.D.A., 1973.
115. Hoover, R.N., and Strasser, P.H.: Artificial sweeteners and human bladder cancer. Preliminary results. Lancet *1*:837, 1980.
116. Morrison, A.S., and Buring, J.E.: Artificial sweeteners and cancer of the lower urinary tract. N. Engl. J. Med. *302*:537, 1980.
117. Editorial: Saccharin and bladder cancer. Lancet *1*:855, 1980.
118. Cohen, S.M., et al.: Promoting effect of saccharin and DL tryptophan in urinary bladder carcinogenesis. Cancer Res. *39*:1207, 1979.
119. Tannenbaum, S.R.: Ins and outs of nitrites. Sciences *20*:7, 1980.
120. Vorherr, H.: Breast cancer in relation to overnutrition. Klin. Wochenschr. *58*:167, 1980.
121. Armstrong, B., and Doll, R.: Environmental factors and cancer incidence and mortality in different countries with special reference to dietary practices. Intl. J. Cancer *16*:617, 1975.
122. Carrol, K.K., et al.: Dietary fat and mammary cancer. Can. Med. Assoc. J. *98*:590, 1968.
123. Adami, H.O., et al.: Influence of height, weight, and obesity on risk of breast cancer in an unselected Swedish population. Br. J. Cancer *36*:787, 1977.
124. Enig, M.G., et al.: Dietary fat and cancer trends—a critique. Fed. Proc. *37*:2215, 1978.
125. Gaskill, S.P., et al.: Breast cancer mortality and diet in the United States. Cancer Res. *39*:3628, 1979.
126. Lipsett, M.B.: Interaction of drugs, hormones and nutrition in the causes of cancer. Cancer *43*:1967, 1979.
127. Reddy, B.S.: Dietary fiber and colon cancer: Epidemiologic and experimental evidence. Can. Med. Assoc. J. *123*:850, 1980.
128. Weisburger, J.H., et al.: Nutrition and cancer—on the mechanisms bearing on causes of cancer of the colon, breast, prostate and stomach. Bull. N.Y. Acad. Med. *56*:673, 1980.
129. Graham, S.: Diet and cancer. Am. J. Epidemiol. *112*:247, 1980.
130. Burkitt, D.P.: Colonic-rectal cancer: Fiber and other dietary factors. Am. J. Clin. Nutr. *31*:S58, 1978.
131. Kromhaut, D., et al.: Dietary fibre and 10-year mortality from coronary heart disease, cancer and all causes. Lancet 2:518, 1982.

10 ENVIRONMENTAL PATHOLOGY

The statement that man has misused and abused his environment is by now a weary cliché. However, the gravity of the deterioration is not widely appreciated. A few of the opening remarks of The Global 2000 Report to the President of the United States provide a perspective: "If present trends continue, the world in 2000 will be more crowded, more polluted, less stable ecologically, and more vulnerable to disruption than the world we live in now. Serious stresses involving population, resources, and environment are clearly visible ahead."[1] The number, complexity, and magnitude of the looming problems boggle the mind. For example, if present trends continue, the world's population will grow from 4 billion in 1975 to 10 billion by 2030 and will approach 30 billion by the end of the 21st century, closely approximating estimates of the maximal carrying capacity of our planet. We are fast running out of forests, arable land, and potable water. Although the resources of such fuels as coal, oil, gas, and uranium may be sufficient, theoretically, for centuries, they will inevitably be monopolized by industrialized countries—at a price—leaving over half of humanity in desperate need. The concentrations of carbon dioxide and ozone-depleting chemicals in the atmosphere are clearly on the rise and will have momentous impact. Solar radiation is readily transmitted through the atmosphere, but the heat radiated by the earth is at least partially trapped by the mantle of CO_2. Thus, atmospheric CO_2 exerts a "greenhouse" effect. Doubling the level of atmospheric CO_2, which could occur in the next century with the present rate of fossil fuel combustion, would raise the global temperature 2° to 3°C. The temperature shift would not only profoundly affect the ecology of all living things, but also might melt the polar ice caps enough to raise the worldwide sea level as much as 5 meters and possibly force abandonment of coastal cities. The normal ozone layer of the atmosphere serves as an ultraviolet filter. Depletion of the ozone shield would expose all living matter to potentially lethal or mutagenic levels of solar radiation and increase the frequency of skin cancers in humans. The doleful litany could be extended, but it will suffice to say that no longer can we complacently assume "there will always be a tomorrow" without taking measures to ensure it.

Environmental factors also contribute to most of the afflictions of mankind. The term "environmental disease" applies ultimately to every disease not strictly inherent in the genes. The disorders included within this designation range from global problems, such as starvation, to self-imposed disorders, such as bronchogenic carcinoma related to smoking. In this chapter we can deal only with the disorders caused by air pollution and chemical (including drugs) and physical agents. Such diseases collectively account for only a small fraction of environment-connected morbidity and mortality, but have a disproportionate importance because they could be prevented.

AIR POLLUTION: PNEUMOCONIOSES

One of the dubious by-products of "civilization" is air pollution. The atmospheric levels of ozone, NO_2, CO, SO_2, and total suspended particulates are currently monitored in the United States. As judged by these criteria, the overall air quality in the United States is said to be improving.[2] Nonetheless, "unhealthful" levels of pollutants are recorded on occasional days in many urban areas. New York and Los Angeles, representing 8% of the total population of the United States, were found "not to enjoy" excessive levels of pollutants, principally carbon monoxide, more than two-thirds of the year. Urban air has also been found to contain 100- to 10,000-fold the rural levels of lead, zinc, arsenic, cadmium, cobalt, chromium, carbon, silicon, and benzo [*a*]pyrene, to mention only a few of the airborne "embellishments."[3] Aerosolized lead is of particular interest. Less than two decades ago, more than 200,000 tons of lead per year were discharged in motor exhaust in the United States.[4] The increasing use of lead-free gasoline has reduced this contamination. Now there is serious doubt about the catalytic devices employed to reduce the emission of oxides of nitrogen. Particulates generated by these catalysts contain copper, chrome, nickel, platinum, aluminum oxide, barium, and other metals. Are we jumping out of the frying pan into the fire? However, the dangers imposed by these contaminants are dwarfed by the hazards inherent in smoking, particularly cigarette smoking. Each of these forms of air pollution compounds the effects of the others.

Air pollution in general, and cigarette smoking in particular, contribute to the causation and aggravation of lung diseases such as chronic bronchitis and emphysema (collectively referred to as chronic obstructive pulmonary disease, p. 717). They also play a role in worsening upper respiratory infections and asthma. Collectively, such pulmonary diseases now cause more morbidity and mortality than cancer of the lungs, despite the rising incidence of this form of neoplasia. It has been difficult, however, to identify the specific untoward pulmonary effects of each of the pollutants found in the atmosphere. Many are inspired at the same time; the level of each continuously varies and the combined or sequential effects of several agents may be quite different from those of one agent alone.[5, 6] Adding to the problem are pulmonary hypersensitivity reactions. The hazards of cigarette smoking go well beyond the lungs and so will be considered separately. First, the pulmonary disorders associated with certain general airborne chemical and physical agents will be detailed. A more complete listing is presented in Table 10–1.

The *pneumoconioses* are directly related to air pollution. The term "pneumoconiosis" refers to the presence of dust in the lung and the lung's reaction to it. Currently it applies to any aerosol, whether particulate or in the form of fumes or vapors. The most important pneumoconioses, all having the potential of progressing to irreversible nodular or diffuse collagenization of the lungs, are: (1) coal workers' pneumoconiosis, (2) silicosis, (3) asbestosis, and (4) berylliosis. There are, in addition, many other less common and less important noncollagenous pneumoconioses produced by the inhalation of less irritating dusts: siderosis (iron dust), stannosis (tin dust), and baritosis (barium dust). The specific lesions caused by the more widespread dusts are presented in succeeding sections; however, certain pathogenetic generalizations apply to all.

The development of a pneumoconiosis is critically dependent on: (1) the amount of dust retained in the lung and airways, (2) the size and shape of the particles, and (3) their solubility and cytotoxicity.

The amount of dust retained depends on three variables—its concentration in the ambient air, the duration of the exposure, and the effectiveness of clearance mechanisms. Over 80% of larger particles (6 μ in diameter or greater) are either filtered out in the vibrissae of the nares or, after impaction on the linings of nasal passageways or larger airways, are removed within hours by mucociliary clearance mechanisms. Extremely small particles under 0.5 μ in diameter may remain suspended in the air and be exhaled. The most dangerous particles range from 1 to 5 μ in diameter; these penetrate to the respiratory bronchioles and air spaces, where they impact or settle. There are exceptions to these generalizations. Asbestos fibers, sometimes up to 100 μ in length, may remain suspended in the moving air columns to penetrate into the respiratory bronchioles and alveoli. Their low density relative to their size produces buoyancy, or what is referred to as a slow falling rate. However, even particles that reach the distal components of the lung may be removed by phagocytic macrophages. It is important to note in this connection that cigarette smoking, alcoholism, and hypersensitivity reactions significantly impair the clearance effectiveness of macrophages and so may contribute to the development of a dust-caused pneumoconiosis.[7] The epithelial cells that line large and small airways, and those in the alveoli, have also been shown to engulf particles, but the role that these cells play in the clearance of the lung is still under investigation.[8] *Thus, exposure-load is important only insofar as it exceeds clearance mechanisms.*

The size and shape of particles determine to a considerable extent the location and nature of the primary damage. Larger particles tend to be deposited within the airways, principally the respiratory bronchioles. These narrow passages offer the greatest impedance to air flow and, by slowing the air stream, permit larger, heavier particles to settle and impact before they reach the alveoli. Thus, the larger the particle, the more proximal the deposition. Smaller particles in the range of 2 μ or less in size are likely to cause damage primarily within the alveoli.[8A] Much of this understanding of the localization of lesions is owed to the present use of whole-lung thin (Gough) sections. These allow an overall view of the precise distribution of lesions and their relationship to the structural components of the lung.

The solubility and cytotoxicity of particles, influenced to a considerable extent by their size, modifies the nature of the pulmonary response. In general, the smaller the particle, the more likely and the more rapidly toxic levels will appear in the pulmonary fluids, depending of course on the solubility of the agent. Thus, finely divided dust may induce acute exudative reactions. In contrast, larger particles resist dissolution and so may persist within the lung parenchyma for years. They tend to evoke fibrosing collagenous pneumoconioses such as is characteristic of silicosis. The interplay of these variables is an important factor in determining whether or not a pneumoconiosis develops, and its nature. There is a relatively narrow margin between safety and danger. Against this background we turn to a consideration of the more common pneumoconioses.

COAL WORKERS' PNEUMOCONIOSIS (CWP)—PROGRESSIVE MASSIVE FIBROSIS (PMF)

Coal workers' pneumoconiosis (CWP) is a relatively benign form of pulmonary involvement caused by the accumulation of coal dust in those who have worked in heavily polluted underground mines for years (usually more than ten). Although a slight cough and some blackish sputum may be present, most of these miners have no dyspnea and mild, if any, disturbances in ventilatory function.[9] However, a small number of those with CWP become symptomatic, sometimes years after exposure to coal-mine dust has ceased, as progressive pulmonary scarring develops. This pattern of disease is referred to as progressive pulmonary fibrosis (PMF), or

Table 10–1. PHYSICAL AND CHEMICAL IRRITANTS: WORKING CLASSIFICATION OF THEIR PULMONARY EFFECTS

Category of Agents	Effect on Lung	Agent	Circumstances of Exposure, Including Occupation(s) or Industry at Risk
Inorganic dusts	1. Pneumoconiosis (noncollagenous)	Carbon, tin, iron, coal, graphite	Mining, welding
	2. Acute silicolipoproteinosis	Free silica (uncombined SiO_2)	Tunnelling, sandblasting: exposure to high doses of fine particles
	3. Pneumoconiosis (collagenous)		
	a. Nodular	Free silica	Hardrock mining of any sort; quarrying, stonecutting and dressing; foundry, pottery, and enamel workers
	b. Diffuse	Asbestos (all fiber types)	Asbestos mining, milling and manufacturing; insulating
		Fume and other fine silica	Sandblasting
		Beryllium	Fluorescent light and space industry
	c. Complicated	An altered response to usually nonfibrogenic dust	Coal miners (progressive massive fibrosis)
	4. Neoplasia (lung)	Asbestos (all fiber types)	Mining and industrial exposures
		Radioactive dusts	Mining operations
		Metal mining	Hematite, chrome
		Metal refining	Nickel, chrome
	5. Neoplasia (pleura)	Asbestos (excluding anthophyllite)	Industrial exposure more at risk than mining exposures
	6. Chronic bronchitis	All dusts, given a high enough dose	Probably all types of exposure
Organic dusts	1. Asthma-like reactions	Enzymes of *B. subtilis*	Manufacture of detergents
		Western red cedar dust	Wood workers
	2. Late onset airflow obstruction (eventually irreversible)	Cotton, hemp, flax, and jute	Processing of vegetable fiber, especially carding of cotton
	3. Hypersensitivity pneumonitis	Fungal spores, especially *M. faeni*	Haymaking, grain handling, mushroom cultivating, sugar cane picking or processing the residue
	4. Chronic bronchitis	Organic material (nonspecific)	Grain handling
	5. Chronic interstitial pneumonia	Vaporized mineral oil	Smoking blackfat tobacco (Guyana); certain industrial exposures
Chemicals, including fumes and vapors	1. Acute pulmonary edema	Oxides of nitrogen	Silo filling, fire fighting
		Phosgene	Fire fighting
		Certain insecticides, e.g., paraquat	Accidental ingestion
	2. Asthma-like reactions	Complex platinum salts	Platinum refining
		Aluminum solder flux	
		Toluene di-isocyanate (TDI)	Manufacture of polyurethane plastic
	3. Acute bronchitis	TDI (in heavier doses)	Manufacture of polyurethane plastic
		SO_2	Pulp and paper mills
		NH_3	Refrigeration industry
		Vanadium	
	4. Chronic bronchitis	All the aforementioned agents in lower dose	As above
	5. Pneumonitis	Cadmium, Hg, Mn	
Radiation	1. Pneumonitis	X-radiation	Medical treatment
	2. Neoplasia	Radioactive dusts	Uranium and other mining

From Beeson, P. B., McDermott, W., and Wyngaarden, J. B. (eds.): Cecil Textbook of Medicine 15th ed. Philadelphia, W. B. Saunders Co., 1979, p. 984.

sometimes as complicated CWP. It is important to note that *PMF is a generic term referring to progressive, disabling, sometimes fatal pulmonary scarring that may complicate any form of severe primary pneumoconiosis.*

To distinguish advanced CWP from mild PMF and mild CWP from so-called pulmonary anthracosis is difficult, both clinically and anatomically.[10] Over the span of decades of living in the dust-polluted atmosphere of cities, virtually everyone accumulates dust-laden macrophages in the lungs, particularly cigarette smokers. Some of the particulate matter is carbonaceous. When the accumulation is heavy the macrophages aggregate into small accumulations, especially about respiratory bronchioles, to produce what is known as *pulmonary anthracosis*. By and of themselves these changes are banal and cause no respiratory difficulties or radiographic changes, nor do they predispose to other forms of pulmonary disease. In coal miners, similar accumulations of coal dust–laden macrophages appear in the early stages of CWP. However, the much heavier exposure to coal dust among miners soon leads to larger, more intensely pigmented aggregations of macrophages classically referred to as *"coal dust macules."* With the accumulation of more and more coal dust, the macules eventually become fibrotic. There is no problem in differentiating pulmonary anthracosis from fibrosing CWP, but at an earlier, milder stage there are no well-defined criteria to determine where anthracosis ends and CWP begins. So it is that the reported incidence of CWP based on anatomic criteria among coal workers ranges from 25% to greater than 90%.[10, 11] Small wonder that clinicians and radiologists have resorted to nonanatomic criteria such as abnormal ventilatory studies or focal densities on chest x-ray.[12] Whatever the precise incidence, the increased dependence on coal as a source of energy promises a rise in the incidence of this condition.

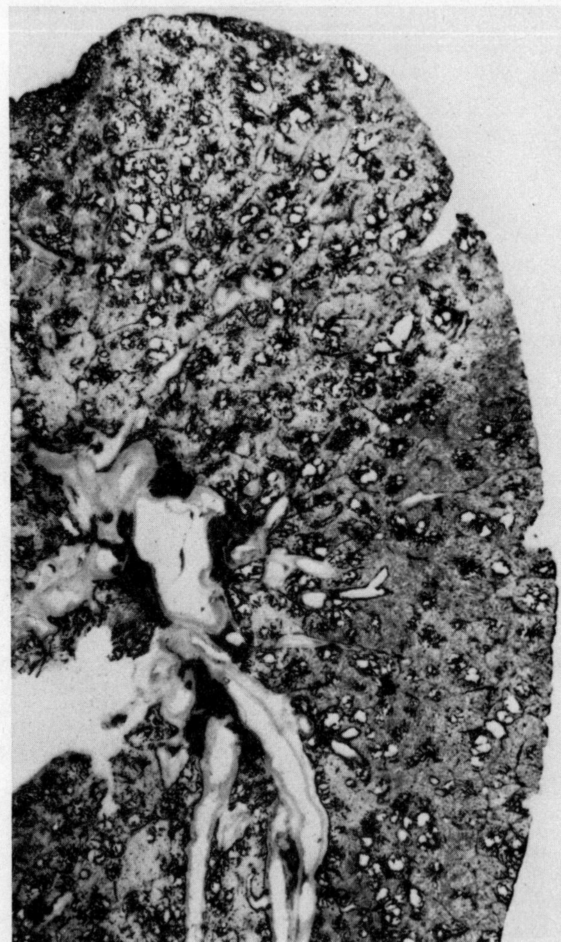

Figure 10–1. Coal workers' pneumoconiosis. Focal accumulations of black coal dust about small airways are readily evident throughout the lung. There is some tendency for more heavy involvement of the upper lobe. (Courtesy of Dr. Werner Laquer, Dr. Jerome Kleinerman, and the National Institute of Occupational Safety and Health.)

MORPHOLOGY. In uncomplicated CWP, the pleura and the cut surfaces of the lung are mottled by focal blue-black pigmentations. The pigmented foci, representing macules, are generally distributed throughout the lungs but tend to be more numerous in the upper lobes (Fig. 10–1). They range from a few millimeters to 1 cm in diameter, depending on the severity of the coal dust accumulation. Generally, there is no pleural thickening or adhesions. As the process advances, the focal pigmentations become somewhat fibrotic and firm to palpation, and are eventually converted into discrete black fibrotic nodules. Close inspection may disclose distended air spaces in and about these nodules. The lymph nodes in the peribronchial hilar and para-aortic regions are usually somewhat enlarged and densely pigmented. By definition, in uncomplicated CWP there are no large confluent areas of pigmentation or fibrosis.

Microscopically, the macule comprises at first an aggregation of intact, dust-laden macrophages disposed principally about respiratory bronchioles, extending into and filling adjacent alveoli. Aggregates of macrophages may also be located about small pulmonary arteries as well as within involved lymph nodes. As the size of the macule increases with the accumulation of coal mine dust, first a fine network of reticulin is deposited and then progressively increasing amounts of collagen. At this stage of the disease, many of the macrophages may have died with release of the pigment into the reactive fibrosis. Eventually the scarring may create relatively circumscribed gray-black nodules of collagen up to 2 cm in diameter surrounded by masses of free carbon particles, as well as dust-laden macrophages. The scarring may obliterate adjacent alveoli and cause distention of those in the periphery of the foci of fibrosis to produce focal emphysema (p. 718). When this process occurs about the ramifications of pulmonary arteries, the arterial walls undergo fibrosis and thicken, with markedly narrowed lumens constituting "obliterative vasculitis." Often, chronic bronchitis and bronchiolitis, as well as centrilobular emphysema, supervene (p. 718). However, controversy continues as to whether these secondary diseases are sequelae of CWP or merely associations.[13]

PMF may occur on a background of nodular CWP. It is characterized by large, sometimes massive, intensely blackened scars that exceed 2 cm in diameter and sometimes achieve dimensions of 5 to 10 cm.[14] The scarred areas are usually bilateral and may occur anywhere in the lungs, but are most common in the upper regions of the upper and lower lobes. When attached to the pleura they may cause retraction and thickening of the pleura (Fig. 10–2). Typically,

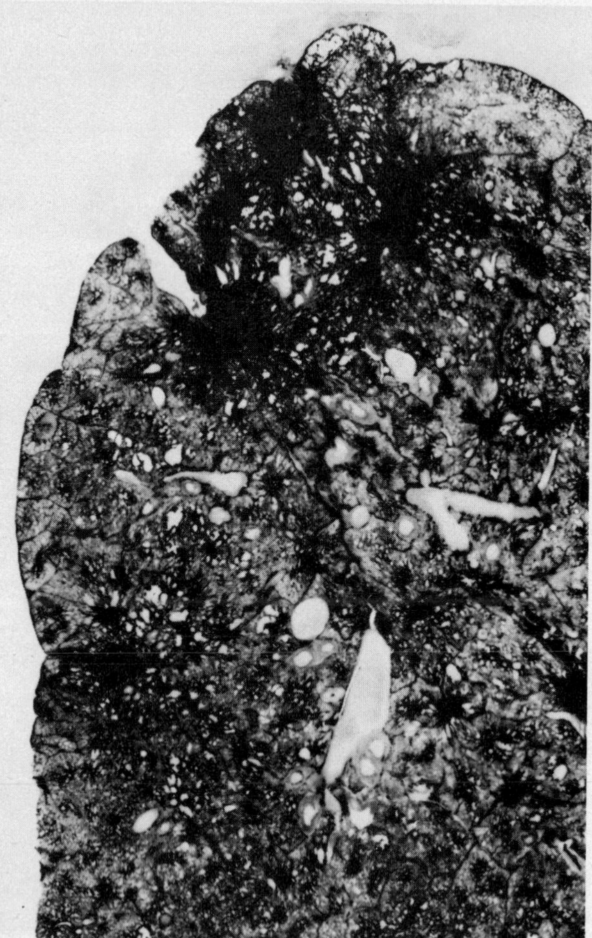

Figure 10–2. Progressive massive fibrosis superimposed on coal workers' pneumoconiosis. The large blackened scars are principally located in the upper lobe. Note extensions of scars into surrounding parenchyma and retraction of adjacent pleura. (Courtesy of Dr. Werner Laquer, Dr. Jerome Kleinerman, and the National Institute of Occupational Safety and Health.)

the scars have irregular borders with long, streaming extensions into the surrounding lung substance. Coalescence of such lesions may replace large areas of lung substance, justifying the sometimes used designation "black lung disease." Occasionally the centers of scars are converted into cavities filled with a fluid to semifluid "India ink." The surrounding air spaces are usually markedly distended or may even appear honeycombed.

Microscopically, the massive scars comprise varying proportions of dense collagen and carbon pigment. The walls of respiratory bronchioles and pulmonary vessels trapped within the scar are thickened or their lumens are obliterated. The vascular changes may account for the central necrosis and cavitation of some scars. Surprisingly, there is only a scant infiltrate of lymphocytes and plasma cells about the areas of fibrosis.

Depending on the extent of the scarring and involvement of the pulmonary vasculature, right ventricular hypertrophy (cor pulmonale) may be present. In addition, miners who have rheumatoid arthritis and simultaneously either CWP or PMF sometimes develop apparent rheumatoid lesions in the lungs. They consist of rubbery-to-firm nodules, 0.5 to 5.0 cm in diameter, usually having foci of opaque necrosis and sometimes central liquefaction, cavitation, and calcification. On microscopic examination they strongly resemble subcutaneous rheumatoid nodules (p. 1352) with central fibrinoid necrosis, and a characteristic enclosing inflammatory reaction. Caplan correctly related these lesions in miners to the concomitant rheumatoid arthritis, and hence **the combination of pneumoconiosis, rheumatoid arthritis, and the distinctive pulmonary lesions is known as Caplan's syndrome.**[15] This syndrome is also associated with silicosis, asbestosis, and other dust-caused pneumoconioses, raising the question of its genesis.[16]

PATHOGENESIS. Three mechanisms have been proposed to explain the fibrosing reaction that supervenes on the coal macule. Silica, a known potent stimulus to pulmonary fibrosis, may be admixed with the coal dust even in "soft" coal mines. There may be release of "fibroblast growth factor" (p. 61) from the activated macrophages.[17] But it might well be that coal mine dust, however inert, when phagocytized in sufficient amounts can injure and destroy macrophages and thus initiate a chronic inflammatory response.

More vexing is the question of what accounts for the transformation of CWP into PMF. Five influences either singly, in sequence, or in concert may be involved: (1) the total burden of lung dust, (2) obliterative vascular lesions, (3) concomitant silica, (4) intercurrent tuberculosis, and (5) immunologic mechanisms. A number of autopsy studies show a fairly strong correlation between the dust content of the lung and the severity of the pulmonary reaction, supporting the dose-duration theory. Obliteration of pulmonary arterial branches and ischemia provides another reasonable basis for extension of pulmonary damage.[18] Silica may contribute to the development of PMF since surveys have correlated the level of quartz in the dust with the tendency of CWP to progress into PMF.[19] For many years there was a suspicion that intercurrent infection with mycobacteria, whether virulent or relatively avirulent, might underlie the development of PMF. This view was based on the past high incidence of tuberculosis in coal miners (40% of cases with PMF). However, the two conditions are now known to be coincidental and only related insofar as poor living and working conditions underlie both. The association of Caplan's syndrome, which has well-defined immunologic origins, with dust-caused pneumoconioses raises the possibility that immunologic factors may be involved in the transition of CWP into PMF. However, the rarity of Caplan's syndrome in coal workers, and the failure to document regularly immunoglobulins or sensitized T cells in the fibrosing reactions of PMF, argue against an important role for immunity in the progression of the pulmonary lesions. The weight of evidence suggests that, as coal dust accumulates, CWP converts into PMF. The other cited influences may augment or hasten the process but are not central.

CLINICAL COURSE. As already mentioned, CWP is usually asymptomatic. It can only be suspected by the occupational history and confirmed clinically by the finding of diffuse radiologic nodularities ("tattooing") on chest film. In the unusual instance a chronic dry cough and exertional dyspnea may appear, but these symptoms may be related more to the concomitant airway disease and emphysema than to the CWP itself.

PMF, by contrast, is a serious, disabling disease. At the outset it is manifested by dyspnea on effort, but as the pulmonary lesions advance the dyspnea worsens until it becomes evident at rest. The chronic cough is productive of coal dust–laden sputum, and sometimes rupture of a lung cavity may lead to an alarming release of jet-black sputum. Poorly localized chest pain is common, as is a purulent bronchitis related to intercurrent bacterial infection. In advanced cases, manifestations of pulmonary hypertension and right heart hypertrophy may appear (p. 569). Fever is uncommon, but if it appears, superimposed tuberculosis must be suspected. Although the incidence of this infection in coal miners has been rapidly decreasing, it is still more prevalent than in nonmining populations. The large areas of scarring are readily visualized on chest x-ray. As pointed out, patients with concurrent rheumatoid arthritis may develop Caplan's syndrome, and with it progression of their symptoms. Still under study is the frequency of lung cancer in coal miners. While there is some disagreement among reports, the majority claim no increase in prevalence when confounding influences, such as cigarette smoking, are carefully excluded.[20] There is, however, a predisposition to carcinoma of the stomach, but for no other form of cancer.[21] Suspected causes include swallowed carcinogens such as polycyclic hydrocarbons, or beryllium present in coal dust, or perhaps the common practice among coal miners of chewing tobacco (since smoking is forbidden within mines), but in truth the explanation is elusive.

SILICOSIS

Silica dust is a potent pulmonary irritant that may cause an acute or chronic pulmonary reaction, depending on intensity of exposure and particle size. The term "acute" as used here refers to the development of an exudative pneumonitis closely resembling pulmonary alveolar proteinosis (p. 746) months or a very few years after intense exposure to finely divided silica dust. Respiratory failure rapidly ensues (which often cannot be reversed by therapy) and death usually occurs within a year or two. In contrast, chronic silicosis is insidious in onset and is compatible with long survival. However, it may slowly progress to respiratory failure and death. This pattern is seen following the slow accumulation over the span of years to decades of larger, more persistent particles of silica in the lungs, with the formation of collagenous nodules wherever they are implanted. Because of the persistence of the silica within the lungs, the disease may first appear and the pulmonary lesions progress long after exposure has ended. Chronic fibrosing nodular silicosis may be complicated by Caplan's syndrome and is also associated with a ten- to 30-fold increased incidence of tuberculosis.[22]

Next to oxygen, silicon is the most common element in man's environment. It occurs in the earth's crust mainly in the form of silicon dioxide, comprising a tetrahedron with a central silicon atom surrounded by four symmetrically situated oxygen atoms. The tetrahedral structure is in some way linked to the fibrosing reaction and is characteristic of the three principal crystalline pathogenic forms of silica—quartz, cristobalite, and tridymite (in ascending order of fibrogenicity). Amorphous forms of silica such as diatomaceous earth have little pathogenicity. Silica dusts are encountered in many industries, particularly in the mining of gold, tin, and copper; stone cutting and polishing; glass manufacture; foundry work; sand blasting; and the fabrication of pottery and porcelain. Particle size is of importance. Those larger than 5 to 10 μ, such as beach sand, are screened or cleared out by normal defense mechanisms. Extremely small particles, less than 0.5 μ in diameter, may remain airborne and be exhaled. The most dangerous are those in the range of 1 to 2 μ. Obviously, intensity and duration of exposure are also important.

PATHOGENESIS. The events that transpire in the induction of the fibrous nodular scarring of chronic silicosis are still somewhat controversial.[23] On this much there is general agreement: (1) deposition of silica particles within respiratory bronchioles and associated alveoli; (2) phagocytosis by macrophages; (3) fusion of the particle-containing phagosome with lysosomes; (4) lysis of phagolysosomes and cells with release of particles; (5) reingestion of particles by other macrophages with continuation of the cycle.[24] Two issues, however, remain unresolved: the basis for the cytotoxicity and the closely related fibrogenicity of silica.[25] A favored theory of toxicity proposes the production of silicic acid by the partial dissolving of the silica particle. The acid's exposed hydroxyl radicals act as donors of hydrogen, with bonding to the phosphate groups of membrane phospholipids leading to damage to lysosomal and plasma membranes.[26] Thereafter, cell death is caused by an influx of calcium ions.[27] In support of this membrane-damaging effect of silica is the correlation between its cytotoxicity and hemolytic activity. There is no dearth of proposals about the ultimate stimulus for collagen synthesis. A favored view is that macrophages activated by phagocytosis of particles release a "fibroblast growth factor" (p. 61).[28] However, immunologic mechanisms have also been suggested. It is known that patients with silicosis usually have increased serum immunoglobulins and often have high serum titers of rheumatoid factor and antinuclear antibody.[29] There is also a greater than chance association between silicosis and autoimmune diseases, particularly progressive systemic sclerosis. Most convincing is the evidence that silica-activated T cells release a factor (? lymphokine) capable of stimulating collagen synthesis in fibroblast cultures. Seductive as these findings may be, the ultimate cause of cell death and stimulus for collagen synthesis in silicosis are still under study.

The pathogenesis of acute silicosis is even less well

understood, but acute toxicity, related to release of silicic acid from finely divided particles, is assumed.

MORPHOLOGY. The anatomic changes of **acute silicosis** closely resemble pulmonary alveolar proteinosis (p. 746) and will not be detailed here. Basically, they consist of large areas of pale gray consolidation produced by filling of the alveoli by amorphous lipoproteinous debris accompanied by an alveolar septal infiltration of mononuclear inflammatory cells. This interstitial reaction differentiates acute silicosis from alveolar proteinosis. A fibrinous pleuritis is often present in acute silicosis.

Chronic nodular silicosis is characterized at the onset by tiny collagenous nodules, more palpable as a fine, sand-like texture than visible. The parenchymal involvement initially tends to be located in the upper lobes and about the hilar regions, but may extend throughout the lungs in severe cases or with progression of the disease. The tiny nodules slowly enlarge, and some coalesce to produce minute areas of readily visible scarring. In time the discrete nodules coalesce with the formation of stony-hard, large fibrous scars, usually in the upper lobes. Pleural involvement creates dense fibrous plaques as well as adhesions that bridge and may even obliterate the pleural cavities. Sometimes the centers of the scars undergo central cavitation, because of either ischemia or superimposed tuberculosis. As the scarring progresses typically the upper lobes are contracted and the lower lobes expand to accommodate (Fig. 10–3). Often the collagenous nodules or scars are blackened by concomitant accumulations of coal dust. The lung parenchyma between the scars may be compressed or emphysematous. Thus, honeycombing develops and is sometimes accompanied by subpleural bullae. Calcification may appear within the scarred areas. Similar collagenous nodules appear within the lymph nodes and classically undergo calcification, producing so-called "eggshell" shadows on chest x-rays. These standard alterations may be complicated by tuberculous lesions with their foci of caseation and cavitation, or by the appearance of the gray-white necrotic lesions of Caplan's syndrome (p. 434).

In late cases that come to autopsy, discrete hyalinized collagenous nodules are seen about the respiratory bronchioles, associated alveoli, pulmonary arteries, and paraseptal and subpleural tissues. The collagen is laid down in concentric laminations, often separated by narrow, cleftlike spaces that may contain crystalline spicules presumably of silica. There is surprisingly scant lymphocytic and occasionally plasma cell infiltrate about such foci. With enlargement, contiguous nodules are enclosed within encircling collagenous layers and, in this fashion, the scarring extends and encroaches on respiratory bronchioles, contributing to bronchiolar obstruction and hyperinflation of alveoli (Fig. 10–4). Similar involvement of the pulmonary arteries adds an element of ischemia to the progression of the disease. The intervening lung parenchyma is hyperinflated or emphysematous. **Of importance in the differentiation of chronic silicosis from other forms of collagenous pneumoconiosis is the polariscopic demonstration of birefringent particles of silica within the fine, cleftlike spaces between the collagenous lamellae of the silicotic nodules. Cavitation may occur in uncomplicated silicosis, but when present should raise the suspicion of intercurrent tuberculosis or Caplan's syndrome.**

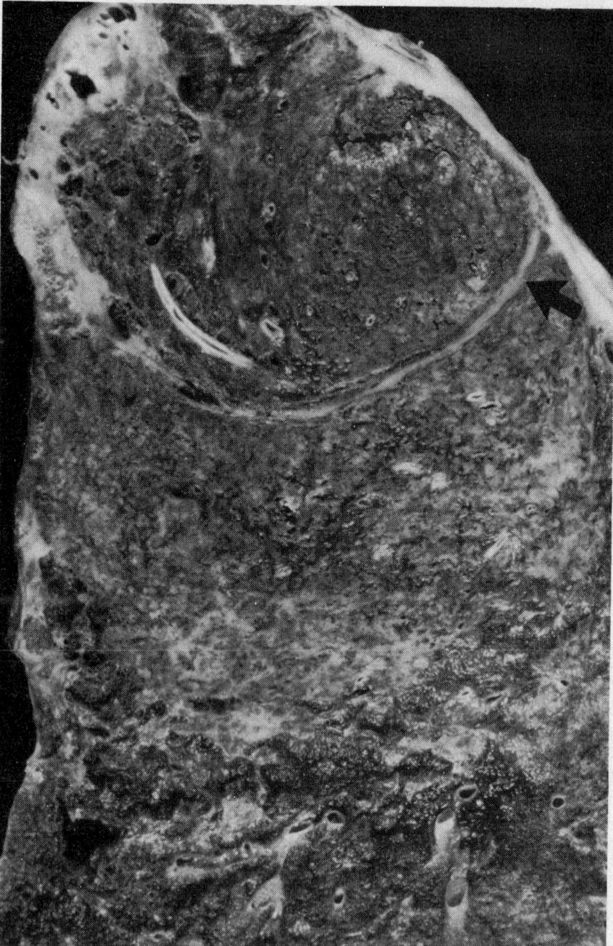

Figure 10–3. Advanced silicosis seen on transection of lung. Scarring is almost confluent, occupying most of upper lobe and contiguous region of lower lobe. Arrow indicates interlobar fissure. Several tuberculous cavities are present in apex. Note dense pleural thickening. (Courtesy of Dr. John Godleski, Brigham and Women's Hospital.)

CLINICAL COURSE. The clinical manifestations of acute silicosis were presented at the outset. Chronic silicosis is extremely insidious, and radiographic findings may appear years before there is any clinical evidence of respiratory dysfunction. Typically, the early phase of fine nodularity imparts a "snowstorm" appearance on chest radiograph. However, with progression there is a tendency for the disease to become more severe in the mid-lung fields (Fig. 10–5). At this stage there is marked decrease in lung compliance and in gas diffusion, and so dyspnea on exertion becomes evident. The breathlessness may at first be mild, but typical of silicosis is its relentless, slow progression, long after all further exposure has ceased. This clinical picture may be complicated by the development of rheumatoid arthritis (Caplan's syndrome), chronic bronchitis, emphysema, cor pulmonale, or pulmonary tuberculosis. Although the disease by and of itself is slow to kill, it may make respiratory cripples of its victims. Obviously, an occupational history is of critical importance in establishing the diagnosis. The only bright note is that there appears to be no increased prevalence of bronchogenic carcinoma or other forms of cancer, including mesotheliomas, in this form of pneumoconiosis.

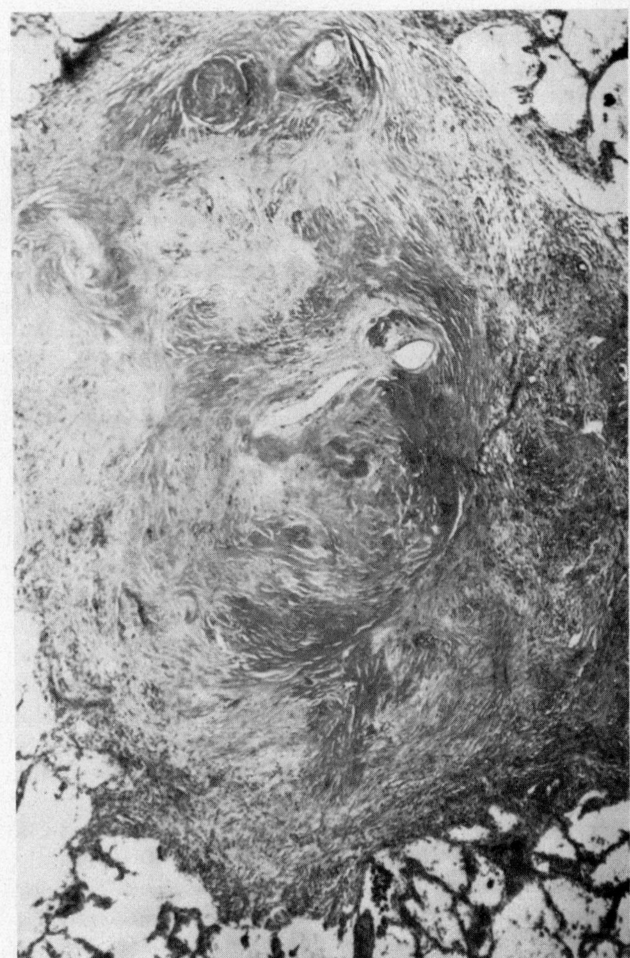

Figure 10–4. Several coalescent collagenous silicotic nodules. (Courtesy of Dr. John Godleski, Brigham and Women's Hospital.)

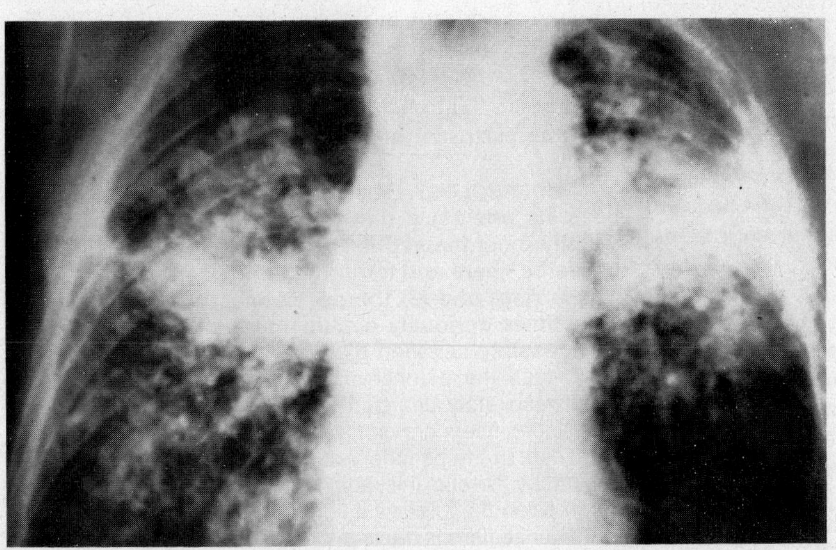

Figure 10–5. Striking bilateral radiodensities in mid-lung fields produced by silicosis.

ASBESTOSIS AND ASBESTOS-RELATED LESIONS

Overexposure to asbestos dust has been called "one of the worst industrial health tragedies in history."[30] It is estimated that 8000 to 10,000 deaths will be caused annually from now to the end of the century by asbestos-related diseases. Inhalation of asbestos may cause not only a pneumoconiosis—asbestosis—but also an increased incidence of mesothelioma, bronchogenic carcinoma, and other forms of cancer.[31] These consequences may not appear until decades later, often long after exposure has ceased. Virtually every urban dweller is exposed to small amounts of asbestos dust in the air because it is so widely used in innumerable products, e.g., sewage and water conduits, flooring and roofing products, insulation, brake linings, clutch casings, and coating compounds. Even water supplies and foods become contaminated by the airborne pollution. Obviously, workers involved in the mining, fabrication, and installation of asbestos and its products are at greatest risk. Almost 40% of a group of shipyard pipe coverers were found to have asbestosis.[32] However, the exposure may be indirect: secretaries in mills, those living in the immediate area of a mill, and families of asbestos workers have suffered an increased incidence of mesotheliomas.[33] While there is a general relationship between intensity of exposure and the development of asbestos and related lesions (neoplasms), no specific threshold level has been established.

Asbestos is a family of fibrous silicates divided into curled serpentines and straight amphiboles. Chrysotile, a serpentine, is the predominant form used commercially (over 90%); two amphiboles—crocidolite and amosite—account for most of the rest. All fibers, whether curled or straight, vary from 0.1 to 1.5 μm in diameter and usually range up to 50 μm in length, although they may be considerably longer. All types of fibers are pathogenic; chrysotile is probably the major air pollutant, but these fibers tend to fragment in the respiratory tract and so are more readily cleared. The long amphiboles, particularly crocidolite, are more strongly implicated in the induction of cancers, and there is great concern over their increased use during the building boom that followed World War II.[34]

Once deposited in the lungs, some fibers are phagocytized by macrophages and within these cells acquire a coating of complexes of hemosiderin and glycoproteins to produce highly distinctive long, beaded *ferruginous bodies,* often with clubbed ends (Fig. 10–6). The axial core of the ferruginous body is the optically transparent asbestos fiber, and the iron-protein accretion appears golden yellow. Particularly long fibers may be enclosed within foreign body giant cells. Several points should be noted: (1) Most fibers remain uncoated, for unknown reasons. (2) There is no strict correlation between the burden of asbestos in the lung and the development of pulmonary disease. Thus, ferruginous bodies can often be found in the absence of disease. (Parenthetically, these observations point to the importance of host factors in the equation.) (3) Other types of fibers, e.g., glass, cotton, may also acquire a coating to become ferruginous bodies.[35] However, for all practical purposes the great majority have an asbestos core, and so ferruginous bodies are sometimes loosely termed *asbestos bodies.* (4) The longer the fiber, the more likely is the formation of a ferruginous body. As noted, chrysotile tends to fragment and so most ferruginous bodies contain amphiboles. (5) Uncoated fibers and fragmented fibers may not be visible by light microscopy, and so special techniques such as electron or phase microscopy of digested lung tissue are required to quantitate the amount of asbestos in the lung.

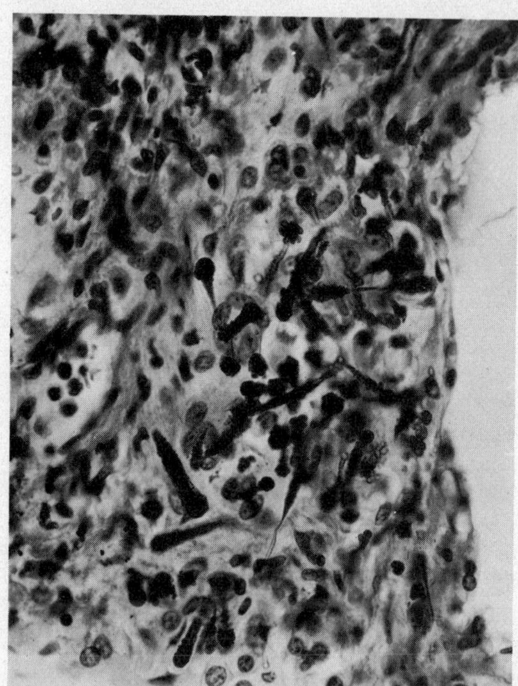

Figure 10–6. Asbestosis of lung in high-power detail to demonstrate pathognomonic "ferruginous bodies."

The morphology of asbestosis will be presented before the pathogenesis of asbestos-related lesions is considered. The neoplasms are discussed elsewhere with the particular organ affected.

MORPHOLOGY. The characteristic changes of asbestosis are: (1) a diffuse interstitial fibrosis (p. 747) initially most marked in the lower lobes (Fig. 10–7); (2) asbestos fibers and ferruginous bodies within the areas of scarring; and (3) the development of small-to-large, sometimes curiously circumscribed, dense, hyalinized, and possibly calcified plaques of the parietal pleura. At the outset, the parenchymal fibrosis is located principally about respiratory bronchioles and alveolar ducts where relatively long fibers are deposited. The fibrosis is usually most prominent in the periphery of the lobes and may be accompanied by fibrotic thickening of the visceral pleura. With progression the interstitial fibrosis extends centrally and the more dense fibrous tracts interconnect, while the intervening unaffected air spaces undergo dilatation to yield a coarse honeycomb pattern. With marked involvement, the middle

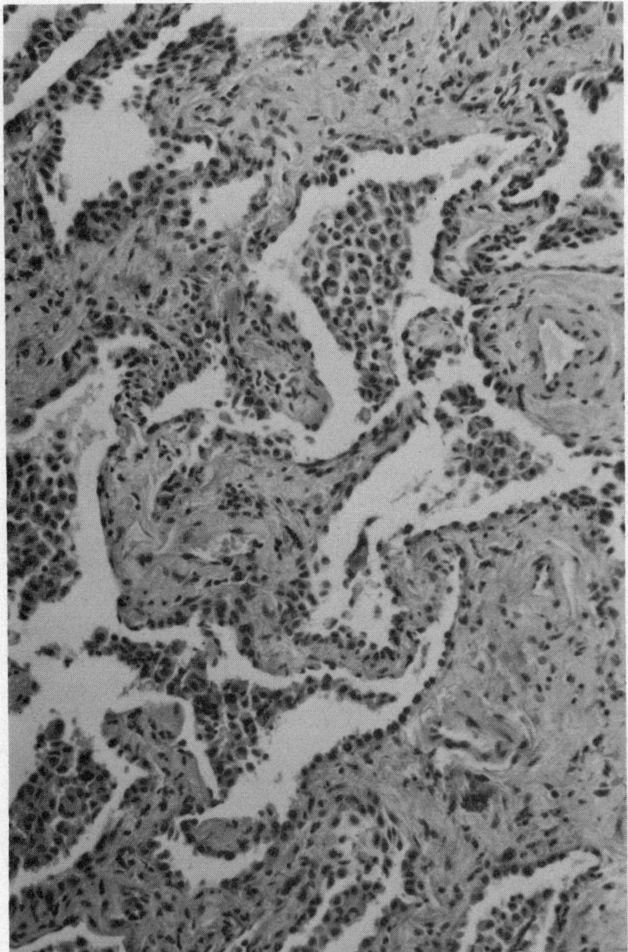

Figure 10–7. Asbestosis. Striking interstitial fibrosis with marked thickening of septal walls. Clusters of macrophages are present within air spaces. (Courtesy of Dr. John Godleski, Brigham and Women's Hospital.)

and upper lobes of the lungs are affected and the scarring becomes heavier. Ferruginous bodies and asbestos fibers are usually detectable under the light microscope within the fibrous scars, lying free within air spaces or enclosed within macrophages or giant cells in the air spaces. Calcification of the parenchymal scars is not common.

The dense fibrocalcific **parietal** pleural plaques are distinctive but not pathognomonic of asbestosis. They tend to occur on the anterior and posterolateral aspects of the parietal pleura and over the dome of the diaphragm; the apices are rarely affected (Fig. 10–8). There is no relationship between the localization of the fibrotic thickening of the visceral pleura and the plaques, nor with adhesions if any between the pleural surfaces.

A number of complications may supervene. Marked emphysema may appear between areas of interstitial fibrosis. Secondary bronchiectasis or Caplan's syndrome (p. 434) may complicate the picture. The scarring may narrow or obliterate pulmonary arteries and arterioles, leading to pulmonary hypertension and cor pulmonale.

There is a markedly increased incidence of pleural and peritoneal malignant mesotheliomas, and bronchogenic carcinomas, and a less striking increase in cancers of the upper and lower gastrointestinal tract and kidney, and lymphomas of the oral cavity and gastrointestinal tract.[35A] These neoplasms may appear in association with asbestosis of the lungs, but sometimes in the absence of significant pulmonary interstitial fibrosis. The incidence of mesotheliomas is increased over 100-fold but they are still less common than bronchogenic carcinoma. The incidence of bronchogenic carcinomas is increased four- to fivefold over that in the non–asbestos exposed. Concurrent cigarette smoking greatly magnifies the risk of bronchogenic carcinoma to 50 to 90 times that of nonsmokers who have had no exposure to asbestos (correlated with the pack-years of smoking). Curiously, concurrent cigarette smoking does not increase the risk of malignant mesothelioma.

PATHOGENESIS. The precise basis for the fibrous reaction to inhaled asbestos fibers is poorly understood, as are the mechanisms involved in the induction of cancers. Size and conformation of fibers and clearance mechanisms may explain the tendency for the parenchymal lesions of asbestosis to begin in the lower lobes and peripherally. Chrysotile, because of its curled conformation, is relatively resistant to air flow and so is deposited in the upper respiratory tract where most is cleared by mucociliary action. The straight amphiboles create less air resistance and so are carried into the periphery. Short fibers may be removed by phagocytosis and transported through the lymphatics to regional lymph nodes. The long amphiboles tend to be re-

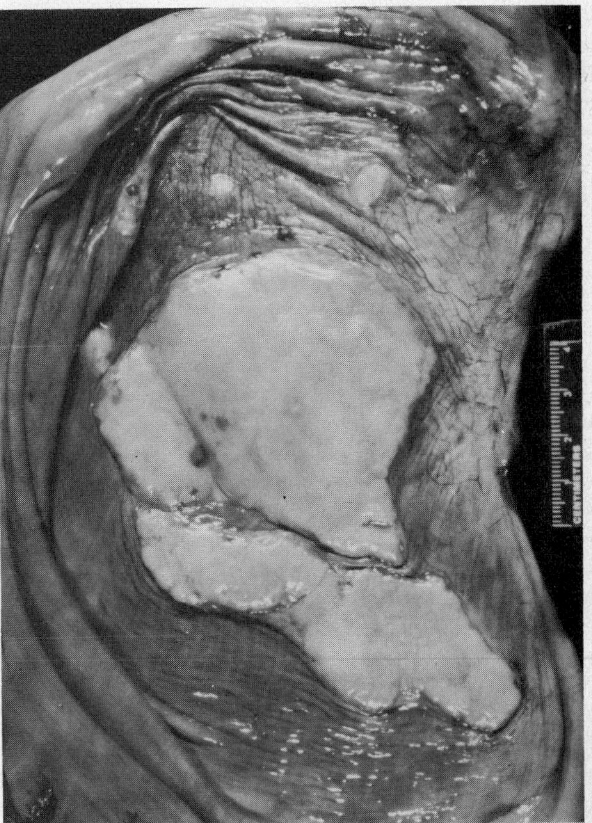

Figure 10–8. Asbestosis. Several discrete, characteristic fibrocalcific plaques on pleural surface of diaphragm. (Courtesy of Dr. John Godleski, Brigham and Women's Hospital.)

tained.[36] Most are carried by macrophages across the wall of the bronchioles and alveolar ducts into the interstitium where the fibrosis is most marked. Fibers may also be taken up by the epithelial cells lining the airways and, through uncertain pathways, move into the submucosal interstitium.[37] The basis for the fibrogenesis is unclear and a number of possibilities have been suggested. Chrysotile, because of its magnesium content, damages lysosomal and plasma membranes of cells in vitro.[38] As with silica, membrane damage could lead to calcium influx and death of macrophages and epithelial cells, thereby setting up a chronic inflammatory fibrotic reaction. Significantly, chrysotile, when added to fibroblast cultures, stimulates the production of reticulin and collagen. There are in addition many hints of asbestos-induced alterations in the immune system, e.g., reduced numbers of circulating T cells, elevated immunoglobulins, and defective cell-mediated immunity.[38A] How these changes relate to the fibrosing reaction is not clear, but it has been proposed that activated macrophages may release growth factors stimulating fibroblasts.[39] Another possibility is that oxygen-derived free radicals liberated by macrophages active in phagocytosis might trigger the injury. There is no dearth of speculation.

Many other puzzles remain. Although there is an imperfect correlation between the pulmonary burden of asbestos fibers and the development of parenchymal fibrosis (implicating host factors), there is in general a good correlation between body burden and the predisposition to asbestos-related neoplasms. However, mesotheliomas occasionally develop with seemingly minimal exposure, or indeed rarely in the apparent absence of exposure. Possibly, unknown exposure to very fine asbestos dust had occurred, leaving no detectable fibers in the lungs. The evidence is strong that crocidolite followed by amosite is more tumorigenic than chrysotile. The mechanism of carcinogenicity is not known. It is speculated that asbestos may act as a promotor enhancing the carcinogenicity of initiating influences, being an irritant rendering cells more vulnerable to carcinogenic influences. In this connection, it has been shown that in organ cultures of hamster tracheal explants, asbestos induces squamous metaplasia of the respiratory lining epithelium.[39A] Conceivably the fibers also act as "carriers" of the carcinogens contained in cigarette smoke, accounting for the striking increased frequency of bronchogenic carcinoma in persons doubly exposed to asbestos and smoking. How then to account for the increased frequency of gastrointestinal neoplasms and mesotheliomas of the parietal pleura and peritoneum with asbestos exposure? The former could be related to inhaled fibers coughed up and swallowed, or to the small amounts of asbestos in drinking water, beverages, and foods. However, the feeding of asbestos to rodents has not induced tumors in the gut. Alternatively, inhaled fibers have been reported to be translocated through lymphatics and blood vessels.[40] For want of a better explanation, this pathway is invoked in the origin of the parietal fibrocalcific plaques and mesotheliomas in the pleura and peritoneum.[41]

CLINICAL COURSE. The manifestations of asbestosis are entirely nondistinctive and include dyspnea; chronic dry cough; predisposition to recurrent respiratory infections, particularly viral; and sometimes weight loss. Respiratory failure may eventually appear. Caplan's syndrome or pulmonary hypertension with the development of cor pulmonale may complicate the clinical course. The pneumoconiosis is slowly progressive even after further exposure has ceased, and death usually occurs within 12 to 20 years of the onset of symptoms. Not infrequently the fatality relates to the late-appearing cancers. Mesotheliomas (discussed in detail on p. 760) are only rarely encountered in the absence of significant exposure to asbestos, but have been reported to occur in up to 10% of heavily exposed workers, sometimes 40 to 50 years after all exposure has ceased.[42] The death rate from bronchogenic carcinoma is increased severalfold among nonsmokers, rising as cited to 90-fold among heavy cigarette smokers.[43] There is also almost a twofold increased incidence of carcinomas of the oropharynx, esophagus, and colon. Thus, although asbestos is an air pollutant, it has wide-ranging neoplastic consequences, most evident in those whose tissues are doubly insulted by smoking.

BERYLLIOSIS

Heavy exposure to airborne, finely divided beryllium or its salts induces an acute chemical pneumonitis, while more protracted exposure to lower levels of these pollutants may cause pulmonary and systemic granulomatous lesions. Minor epidemics of pulmonary berylliosis occurred in the United States in the mid-1940s among workers involved in the manufacture of fluorescent lamps that incorporated powdered beryllium compounds.[44] This use of beryllium has been discontinued, but because of its high tensile strength and resistance to fatigue and heat, beryllium is now increasingly used in electronic, ceramic, aerospace, nuclear energy, and other industries.[45] Those involved in the mining and extraction of the metal from ore are also at risk. Occasional instances of berylliosis have been encountered in individuals who live close to industries using this metal. For reasons that are not clear, there is a striking individual susceptibility to berylliosis since even in high-risk occupations less than 2% of those exposed develop untoward reactions. Several observations suggest that delayed (Type IV) hypersensitivity is involved in the pathogenesis of the lesions. The pneumoconiosis tends to be more frequent in individuals who have returned to their hazardous occupation after some period of absence. Patients with berylliosis often have a positive skin test to this metal and can also be shown to have sensitized T cells. Moreover, the characteristic lesion in chronic berylliosis is granuloma formation (classically a delayed hypersensitivity response).

MORPHOLOGY. Acute berylliosis is basically a toxic or allergic pneumonitis sometimes accompanied by an acute rhinitis, pharyngitis, and tracheobronchitis. The mucosal surfaces are red and edematous and on microscopic examination disclose a nonspecific acute inflammation. The lungs are congested, edematous, and heavy. The histologic reaction is essentially that of an acute inflammatory exudation filling the alveoli with edema fluid, fibrin, red cells, and neutrophils, creating a bronchopneumonic pattern. Lymphocytes, plasma cells, and occasional neutrophils infiltrate the septal walls. In the course of days, the alveolar exudate is largely replaced by macrophages and lymphocytes, sometimes enmeshed in fibrin. As the disease evolves, the alveolar exudate may be resorbed, accompanied by marked clinical improvement, or it may become organized along with the development of septal fibrosis. When organization occurs it produces a gas-diffusion block, which may be fatal. **In acute berylliosis, granulomas are not formed.**

Chronic berylliosis, better known as **beryllium granulomatosis,** is characterized by granuloma formation and a diffuse interstitial inflammatory reaction. Grossly, the lungs may reveal very few changes save possibly for some increase in weight and slight reduction in crepitation. More severe involvement may be accompanied by ill-defined areas of increased consistence and sometimes focal honeycombing. Palpable nodules up to 3 cm in diameter are occasionally found.[46] Enlargement of the hilar lymph nodes is infrequent, but pleural thickening may appear late in the course of severe disease. Cor pulmonale (p. 569) is sometimes encountered.

Microscopically, well-developed epithelioid granulomas strongly resembling those of sarcoidosis are diffusely scattered in the interstitial tissue and are particularly frequent in subpleural septal, peribronchial, and perivascular locations (Fig. 10–9). With electron microscopy the epithelioid cells can be seen to have very prominent Golgi complexes, suggesting secretory activity.[47] Prominent in the granulomas are Langhans'-type giant cells and an enclosing mantle of lymphocytes, presumably T cells. **Three types of inclusions may also be present in these granulomas, sometimes within the giant cells:** (1) a spiculated crystal, 3–10 μ in length, which is birefringent and is composed of calcium carbonate; (2) a concentrically laminated Schaumann body, up to 50 μ in diameter, formed by successive layers of protein, calcium, and iron; and (3) the most unusual—stellate acidophilic asteroids—composed of lipoprotein membrane aggregates and almost always found within giant cells. Although striking, these inclusions are not limited to berylliosis and are found in sarcoidosis and other pulmonary diseases.[48] As mentioned, a diffuse and often extensive interstitial inflammatory reaction accompanies the granulomatous response. Initially it takes the form of septal edema with an infiltrate of lymphocytes, macrophages, and plasma cells, but as the disease progresses, fibrosis ensues. It is this aspect of chronic berylliosis that most significantly deranges pulmonary function.

Accompanying the chronic pulmonary lesions may be granulomatous involvement of the liver, kidney, spleen, lymph nodes, and skin. Chronic persistent ulcerations of the skin replete with a granulomatous reaction may develop at sites of scratches or injuries where beryllium has been absorbed.

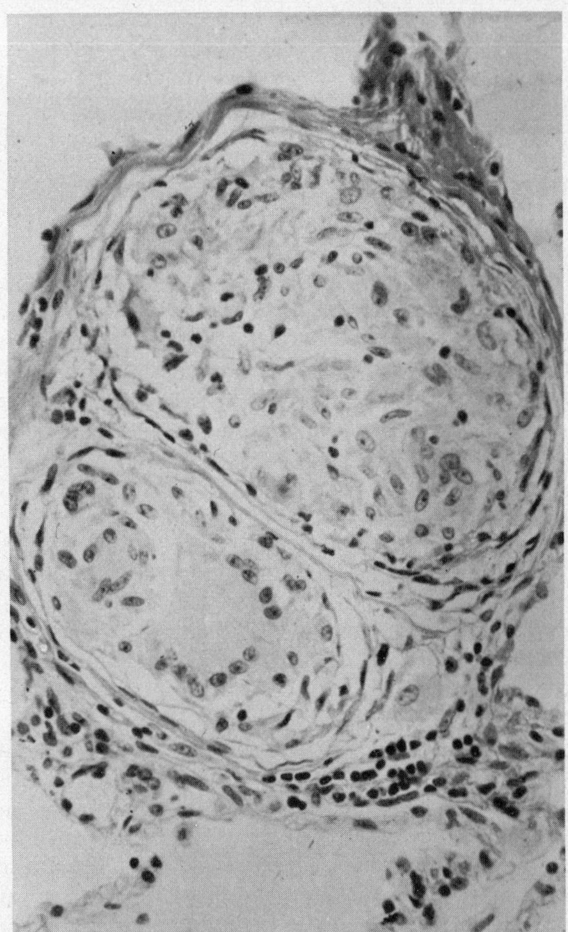

Figure 10–9. The well-developed granulomas of pulmonary berylliosis.

CLINICAL COURSE. *Acute berylliosis* may erupt as a fulminating illness within days of a massive exposure, or may be more insidious in onset. In either case, the major clinical features are rapidly progressive dyspnea, cough, and findings suggestive of pulmonary edema on physical examination and chest film. The ventilation-perfusion derangement induces hypoxemia and sometimes cyanosis. Most cases resolve within weeks to a few months with no residuals, but some are fatal. Approximately 5 to 10% progress to chronic disease.

The *chronic granulomatosis* is far more insidious in onset and usually becomes manifest months to years after initial exposure to beryllium. Sometimes the disease first appears long after all exposure has ended. Exertional dyspnea is usually the presenting symptom, but as the disease progresses, dyspnea may appear even at rest. These manifestations are indistinguishable from those produced by other chronic lung disease, including the other forms of severe pneumoconiosis. Chest radiographs usually disclose scattered nodular opacities accompanied by a diffuse linear and reticular pattern, but hilar adenopathy is uncommon.[49] Diffuse chronic disease of the lungs may lead to cor pulmonale. The diagnosis depends on a history of exposure supported by the demonstration of sensitized T cells, using the macrophage migration inhibition or lymphocyte transformation tests. Chemical assays of urine or lung samples are not generally useful because of the frequency of false-negative results. In most cases the course spans years or decades, sometimes terminating in death from cardiac or respiratory failure. There is now substantial evidence that significant occupational exposure to beryllium induces a twofold increased incidence of bronchogenic carcinoma,[50] which is no surprise in the light of the carcinogenicity of beryllium in animals.[51]

OTHER DUST DISEASES

There are many other forms of pulmonary dust disease in addition to those already discussed; however, most are less life-threatening than the collagenous pneumoconioses. They can be roughly segregated into three categories: (1) noncollagenous inorganic dust pneumoconiosis; (2) asthma; and (3) extrinsic allergic alveolitis.

The *noncollagenous inorganic dust pneumoconioses* include, in addition to uncomplicated coal workers' pneumoconiosis, such entities as siderosis, stannosis, baritosis, and other less common conditions. All of these noncollagenous pneumoconioses are characterized by focal accumulations of the particular dust in the lung to create macules resembling the coal-dust macule. Only very rarely are the pulmonary changes productive of respiratory difficulty, but in the exceptional instance with severe exposure any one of these disorders may prove fatal.

Asthma has many origins, as is evident in the full discussion on page 727. Whatever its origin, the disease is characterized by paroxysms of bronchospasm and bronchial changes that induce obstructive narrowing of the airways. One clinical pattern is known as occupational or industrial asthma because the attacks are triggered by a large variety of dusts—grain, wood, animal hair and dander, and others encountered in the workplace.

Extrinsic allergic alveolitis is a distinctive hypersensitivity pulmonary reaction to inhalation of one of a large number of organic dusts. It differs from asthma inasmuch as it takes the form of an interstitial inflammatory reaction, sometimes granulomatous, at the level of respiratory bronchioles and alveoli. Such inflammation is generally reversible, but may progress to diffuse interstitial pulmonary fibrosis and permanent respiratory insufficiency. Various inhaled allergens are involved, such as spores of molds, pollens, animal and industrial particulates, and chemical fumes. The most important of these sensitivity disorders is *farmers' lung*, which typically appears within hours of the inhalation of spores derived from a thermophilic actinomycete that grows on improperly dried and stored hay. More details on these dust-related hypersensitivity diseases are available on page 744 and in a recent report.[52]

Byssinosis is an uncommon pulmonary disorder caused by organic dusts derived from cotton, flax, and hemp. It may first appear within weeks to months of onset of the occupational exposure, and takes more the form of an asthmatic bronchitis than involvement of the distal lung structures, such as occurs with the other organic dusts causing extrinsic allergic alveolitis. The basis for the lesions is not clear, but the evidence that they are hypersensitivity induced is not strong.

TOBACCO SMOKING

No discussion of disease related to air pollution would be complete without mention of the most common and dangerous pollutant—tobacco smoke. This subject has been so widely heralded in lay and scientific reports and is so frequently cited throughout the book that only a brief summary is necessary here. Cigarette smoking, as is well known, is the principal offender, with a direct correlation between the level of exposure (number of cigarettes daily and years of use) and morbidity and mortality. In one report the overall current mortality rate for male cigarette smokers, irrespective of quantity, was 1.7-fold (70% excess mortality) greater than that of nonsmokers.[53] In different terms, the life expectancy of a 30- to 35-year-old, two-pack-a-day male is about ten years shorter than a comparable nonsmoker. Low "tar" and nicotine cigarettes (less than 1.2 mg nicotine and less than 17.6 mg "tar") lower the mortality ratio about 15 to 20%. Cigar and pipe smoking are not without risk but are significantly less hazardous than cigarette smoking. The "passive smoker" in the immediate vicinity of the smoker is the proverbial "innocent bystander," but fortunately appears to be at only slightly increased risk of developing chronic bronchitis and some reduction in maximal exercise capacity.

Although great emphasis has been placed (and with justification) on the role of cigarette smoking in the causation of bronchogenic carcinoma, there is a long roster of other diseases caused or contributed to by smoking. Presently it includes coronary heart disease; atherosclerosis; cancers of the larynx, oral cavity, esophagus, urinary bladder, pancreas, and kidney (in males); emphysema and chronic bronchitis (together producing chronic obstructive lung disease); peptic ulcer; and, with smoking during pregnancy, reduced birth weight and increased perinatal mortality. Coronary heart disease is the chief contributor to the excess mortality among cigarette smokers. Habitual heavy use of cigarettes is a major risk factor for systemic atherosclerosis, including arteriosclerotic aneurysm of the aorta and ischemic peripheral arterial disease. Disorders of the lung (notably bronchogenic carcinoma, followed by chronic obstructive lung disease) and systemic atherosclerosis are the second and third most important contributors to the excess mortality. Cigarette smoking has been rated as the major single cause of cancer mortality in the United States.[54] It is said to be responsible for about 83% of lung cancers among males and 43% among women (Fig. 10–10). As you recall from an earlier discussion (p. 240), tobacco smoke is a veritable "witches' brew" containing polycyclic aromatic hydrocarbons, aromatic amines, phenols, nickel and other metals, carbon monoxide, hydrocyanic acid, and other "delicacies." Chronic obstructive lung disease related to pulmonary emphysema and chronic bronchitis not only exacts an increased death toll but is second only to coronary artery disease as a cause of smoking-related morbidity. No small wonder that cigarette smoking has been declared "the single most important environmental

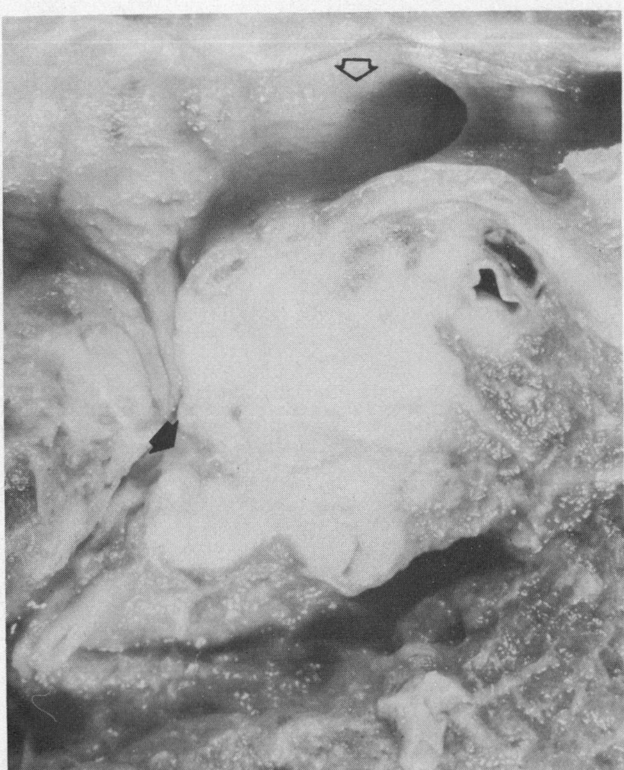

Figure 10–10. Bronchogenic carcinoma seen on transection of main stem bronchus *(upper left)* with marked narrowing of one branch *(closed arrow)* without involving the other *(open arrow).* (Courtesy of Dr. John Godleski, Brigham and Women's Hospital.)

factor contributing to premature mortality in the United States."[53]

CHEMICAL AND DRUG INJURY

All chemicals or drugs in sufficient quantity are capable of causing injury or even death. About 10,000 fatalities in the United States annually result from a self-inflicted overdose of these agents. One half are the deliberate action of those driven to take leave of this mortal coil ere their time. The other half are accidental deaths, and some (on the order of 100 to 200) are the consequence of busy, exploratory little hands. For every fatal accidental poisoning in children under the age of 5 years, it is estimated that there are possibly 3000 nonfatal accidental poisonings, adding up to the astounding number of about 300,000 annually. These mainly result from inhalation or ingestion of common agents or drugs found in most homes, such as cleaning fluids, polishing compounds, and aspirin. Some drug injuries fall into the category of iatrogenic disease from physician-prescribed drugs. There are no reliable data on the annual number of fatal adverse drug reactions in the United States, but in all probability there are thousands. Only a sampling of these chemical and drug-induced injuries can be covered here.

THERAPEUTIC AGENTS: ADVERSE DRUG REACTIONS

The search for better control of illnesses has led to ever more potent therapeutic agents, which regrettably at the same time often have greater potential for inducing iatrogenic disease. Some general comments on adverse drug reactions (ADRs) are offered first, followed by a consideration of a few frequently involved drugs. More details are available in specialized texts.[55]

Few medical subjects have been more exploited for "scare" headlines in the lay press than ADRs. It has been asserted that "bad prescriptions" kill tens of thousands a year.[56] More sober analyses indicate that ADRs are responsible for about 2000 to 3000 deaths annually. Although each death is tragic, many are the result of a calculated risk knowingly assumed by the patient and doctor. A patient with leukemia may suddenly develop an acute blast crisis that threatens immediate death from leukostasis (plugging of blood vessels with leukemic cells). In a desperate effort to prolong life, large doses of cytotoxic or immunosuppressive drugs may be administered with full recognition of the potential of fatal opportunistic infections or a fatal bleed from suppression of thrombopoiesis. Should a drug-related fatality here be labeled an "adverse drug reaction?" On the other hand, a fatal anaphylactic reaction in an individual taking prescribed penicillin for a respiratory viral infection, where penicillin is most unlikely to be effective, constitutes a deplorable adverse reaction. Clear distinction must be made, then, between unwarranted adverse reactions and those that follow the use of a potentially harmful drug for justified clinical reasons. The former have been referred to by Ingelfinger as "adverse drug reactions that count."[58] There is in fact no undisputed definition of an ADR, but the following is most acceptable: *An adverse drug reaction constitutes any response to a medically employed drug which is noxious and unintended and which occurs at doses used in man for prophylaxis, diagnosis, or therapy, excluding failure to accomplish the intended purpose.* In these terms, ADRs probably occur in 3 or 4% of general hospital patients and are fatal in about one-tenth of these instances.[59, 60]

Adverse reactions may arise for one of many reasons.

1. *Overdosage.* This may occur by error, of course, but more often it represents a deliberate gamble impelled by the medical situation, e.g., the use of larger amounts of digitalis in a patient dying of cardiac failure and unresponsive to usual doses of the agent.

2. *Side effects.* Streptomycin, for example, has a well-known toxicity for the inner ear. A particularly distressing side effect seen with increasing frequency is the development of a second neoplasm subsequent to the use of antineoplastics for a primary form of cancer. The risk with alkylating agents is well-known, but the alternative is less than optimal therapy of the primary tumor.[61, 62] Analogously, doxorubicin (Adriamycin) and daunorubicin are extremely effective antineoplastics,

but both may induce myocardial injury (p. 602) (Fig. 10–11).

3. *Extension effects.* A marked hypoglycemic reaction may follow the use of a small dose of insulin in a patient who has marked reactivity to insulin.

4. *Drug interaction.* The desired anticoagulation effect of coumarin may be dissipated by repeated simultaneous use of phenobarbital. Barbiturates, you may remember (p. 27), induce the synthesis of more mixed-function oxidases in the liver that also metabolize coumarin. Thus, the patient may develop a thrombotic episode despite adequate therapeutic levels of coumarin.

5. *Idiosyncrasy.* Such adverse reactions are totally unpredictable: for example, anemia following one application of chloramphenicol ophthalmic solution.

6. *A hypersensitivity reaction* to an agent. These may range from a relatively trivial fever or mild skin rash to life-threatening anaphylaxis.[63] It is worth noting that drug-induced anaphylactic death is most often related to penicillin.

The limitations of space do not permit even a

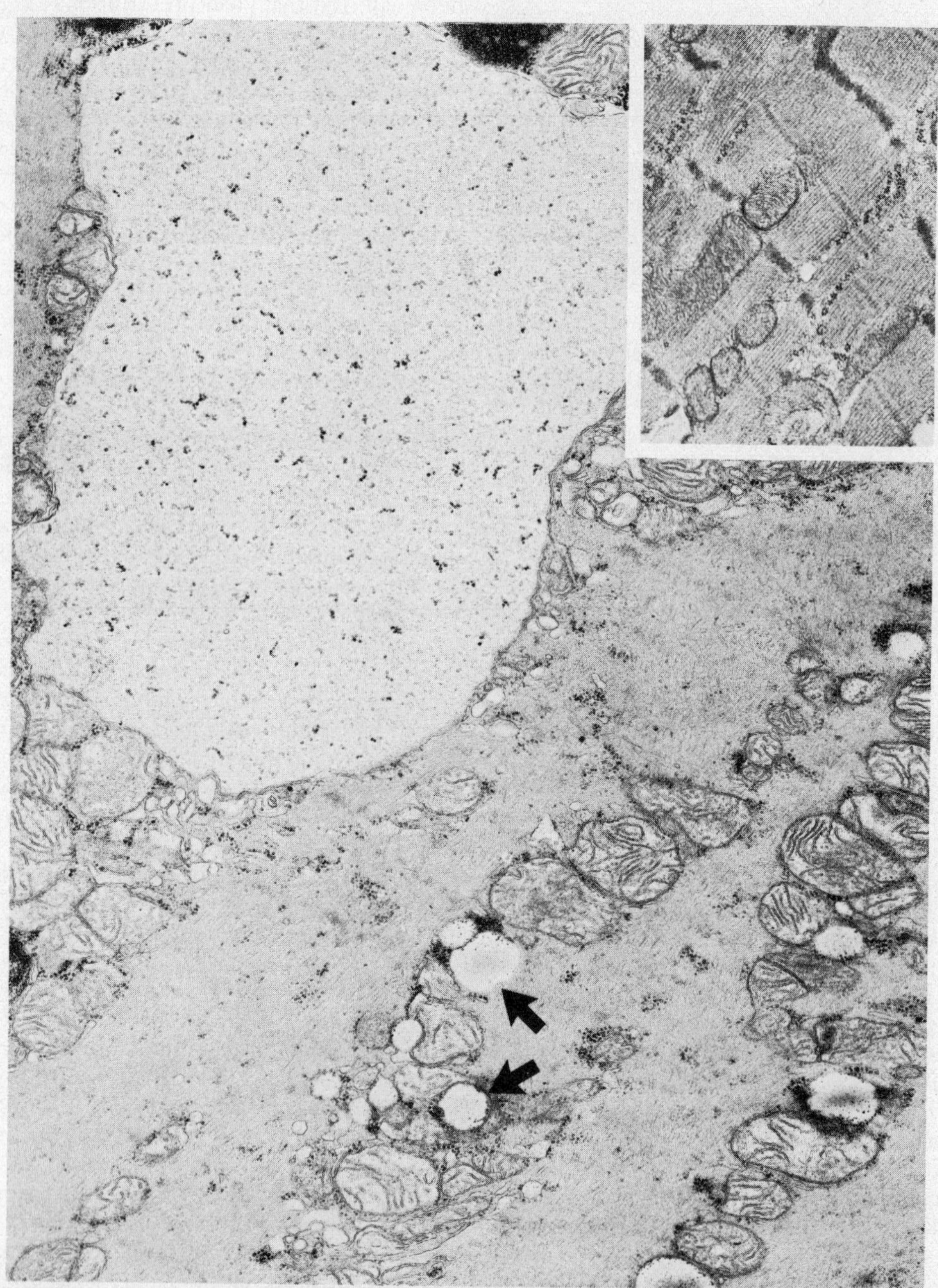

Figure 10–11. Doxorubicin (Adriamycin) cardiotoxicity. Electron micrograph reveals swelling of myofibers with loss of myofibrils (compare with normal in inset). There is also swelling of endoplasmic reticulum, producing small vacuoles *(arrows)* as well as large vacuole *(upper left)* (×17,000). (Courtesy of Dr. Frederick Schoen, Brigham and Women's Hospital.)

cursory account of the particular agents involved in ADRs. In most analyses they fall into the following categories, in descending order of frequency: antibiotics, digitalis glycosides, antineoplastics, hypnotics and sedatives, tranquilizers and antidepressants, insulin, antihypertensives, analgesics, and diuretics. The resultant reactions range widely, but five major patterns may be identified.

1. *Blood dyscrasias* are common and serious adverse reactions. They may take the form of pancytopenia, agranulocytosis, thrombocytopenia, hemolytic anemia, or megaloblastic anemia. Some of these reactions are known side effects of drugs such as anticancer agents; in other instances they represent immunologic hypersensitivity responses such as may occur with penicillin; but most distressing are the totally unexpected idiosyncratic reactions.

2. *Skin eruptions*—macular, papular, vesicular, bullous, exfoliative, or urticarial—are frequent but fortunately are generally not life-threatening. In addition, hypersensitivity responses such as may follow the use of barbiturates or sulfonamides may cause erythema multiforme or erythema nodosum.

3. *Hepatic reactions* range from the more or less benign to the catastrophic. Fatty change (as may occur with tetracycline) or cholestasis (induced by androgens or chlorpromazine) is generally transient and reversible when the drug is withdrawn (Fig. 10–12). More serious are the varying severities of acute to chronic drug-induced hepatitis. Massive hepatic necrosis, as may be produced by halothane, is often fatal.

4. *Renal reactions* may be trivial with transient proteinuria or hematuria, or fatal. In some instances these reactions are predictable because of the known nephrotoxicity of such drugs as amphotericin, but often the renal toxicity is the consequence of a hypersensitivity reaction such as sometimes follows the use of sulfonamides.

5. *Lung reactions* are a well-known threat with the use of certain agents such as bleomycin, ranging from pulmonary congestion, edema, and hemorrhage to the more ominous interstitial fibrosing pneumonitides.

Some of the more common offenders and their possible consequences are presented in Table 10–2.

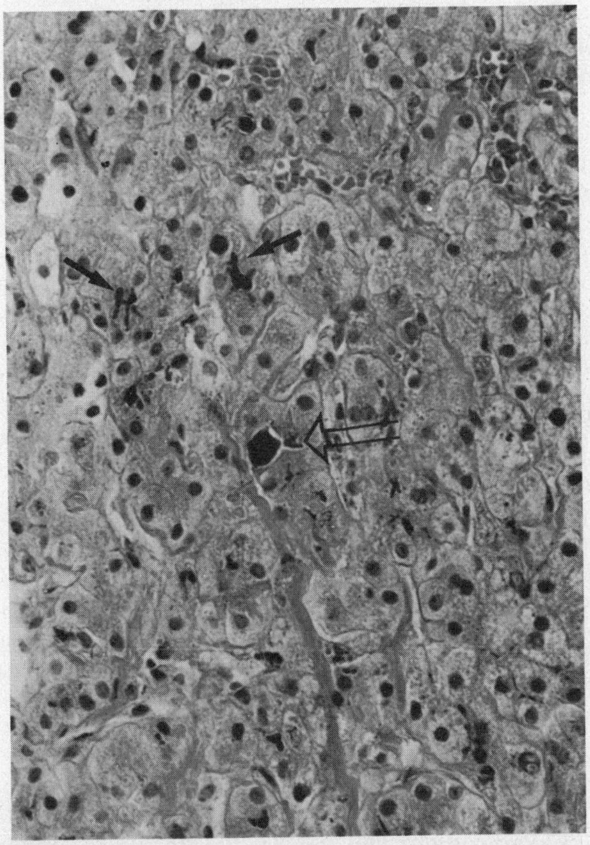

Figure 10–12. Cholestasis induced by chlorpromazine. Inspissated bile plugs can be seen in canaliculi between liver cells *(single arrows)* and in single ductule *(double arrow)*.

Analgesics

Analgesics have the potential for mischief largely because they are popped into mouths as often and as freely as candy. Particularly implicated in adverse reactions are aspirin (acetylsalicyclic acid) and proprietary mixtures of aspirin, phenacetin, caffeine, and acetaminophen. About 30 million pounds of aspirin are produced each year in the United States! Adverse reactions to this drug may result from direct toxicity or a hypersensitivity reaction. Before safety packaging was introduced, accidental deaths in infants and children were all too frequent from the ingestion of 2 to 4 gm (6 to 12

Table 10–2. COMMON DRUGS RESPONSIBLE FOR ADVERSE REACTIONS

Blood Dyscrasias	**Hepatic Reactions**
Pancytopenia	***Hepatitis to massive necrosis***
Chloramphenicol	Halothane
Phenytoin	Methoxyflurane
Trimethadone	Methyldopa
Cytotoxics	Isoniazid
Agranulocytosis	Phenytoin
Chloramphenicol	Tetracyclines
Sulfonamides	***Cholestatic Jaundice***
Phenylbutazone	Phenothiazines
Indomethacin	Chlorpromazine
Cytotoxics	Androgens
Thrombocytopenia	Oral contraceptives
Quinidine	Erythromycin
Quinine	**Renal Reactions**
Furosemide	Penicillamine
Aspirin	Sulfonamides
Indomethacin	Penicillin
Hemolytic Anemia	Phenindione
Methyldopa	Phenacetin
Levodopa	Amphotericin
Isoniazid	**Lung Reactions**
Sulfonamides	Bleomycin
Penicillin	Busulfan
Dermatologic Reactions	Methotrexate
Penicillin	Nitrofurantoin
Sulfonamides	Azathioprine
Barbiturates	
Phenytoin	
Phenylbutazone	

adult-size tablets) at one time. One dose of 15 gm is fatal in adults. The toxic reaction is marked by severe metabolic derangements. High blood levels of aspirin stimulate the respiratory centers, producing at first a respiratory alkalosis as excessive amounts of CO_2 are blown off. Compensatory mechanisms then lead to a metabolic acidosis with excessive excretion of sodium, potassium, and water. A serious, even fatal, hypokalemia may result. The syndrome is further complicated by the almost invariable concurrence of severe vomiting (related to the aspirin-induced gastritis) with its additional losses of fluid, acid salts, and other electrolytes. You recall that aspirin also blocks cyclooxygenase, which is the key enzyme in the synthesis of prostacyclin (PGI_2) and thromboxane A_2 (p. 54). The net effect is a bleeding diathesis related either to the antiaggregating action of prostacyclin, or to thrombocytopenia secondary to the widespread platelet aggregation induced by the thromboxane. Thus, petechial hemorrhages may appear in the skin as well as in the internal viscera and serosal membranes. In children, high levels of toxicity sometimes produce microvesicular fatty change in the liver, resembling that seen in Reye's syndrome (p. 941). At the same time aspirin has a potent effect on the gastric mucosal barrier, leading to erosive hemorrhagic gastritis (p. 809). This gastric reaction, however, may be beneficial because it sometimes initiates prompt and copious vomiting that expels the unabsorbed drug. Most often, death is preceded by a period of coma. When seen early, most victims can be saved by gastric lavage, hemodialysis, and effective control of the blood pH and serum electrolytes.

Hypersensitivity reactions to aspirin take many forms, such as an asthmatic attack, a multiform skin rash—erythema, angioedema, urticaria, eczema, even extensive desquamation—or, worst of all, an anaphylactic attack.[64]

Chronic analgesic abuse with the consumption of large amounts of proprietary mixtures for long periods of time may cause a potentially fatal renal disease referred to as *chronic interstitial nephritis* or *analgesic nephropathy,* discussed in detail on page 1037. It is only necessary here to point out that the particular agent implicated is still uncertain, but greatest suspicion is directed at phenacetin or a combination of phenacetin and aspirin. Almost always, affected individuals have consumed more than 3 kg of analgesics (and sometimes up to 30 kg) over the span of years. Anemia and gastritis may accompany the renal involvement.

Barbiturates

An overdose of barbiturates has long been in vogue as a method of suicide. Accidental poisoning is also encountered, particularly in children and in adults who unknowingly take excessive amounts of these drugs. There is a wide range of individual susceptibility to barbiturates, and relatively small amounts may induce dangerous blood levels in some. Furthermore, alcohol and the barbiturates produce additive depressant effects on the central nervous system. Both agents are metabolized in the liver by the mixed-function microsomal oxidase system and, while the body will adapt to the continued exposure to barbiturates and to some extent to alcohol, the latter, in sufficient amounts, may damage the liver cell and render it unable to metabolize barbiturates. Similarly, any liver disease impairs the metabolism of barbiturate and permits it to reach toxic levels in the blood even after relatively moderate doses.

It is difficult to set a specific lethal threshold for the barbiturates because of the many factors that influence their pharmacodynamics. The short-acting barbiturates, such as secobarbital, are in general more toxic than the long-acting, such as phenobarbital. Even in the absence of the predisposing influences mentioned above, as little as 3 gm of the short-acting barbiturates or 5 gm of the long-acting agents may be potentially fatal in the normal adult. Contrariwise, recovery of an attempted suicide has been reported after an overdose as large as 30 gm of phenobarbital.

The anatomic changes found after a fatal overdose depend on the rapidity of death, and may be remarkably few. When first ingested, and with relatively small doses, barbiturates depress brain function only at the higher centers; with time and increasing dosage, the vital lower centers are depressed as well, including those in the medulla. Depression of the respiratory centers may slow the breathing rate sufficiently to produce respiratory acidosis and systemic hypoxia. The combined effects of the hypoxia and the direct action of the drug on the medullary vasomotor centers may induce vascular collapse and shock (p. 112).

With survival for a few days the respiratory depression predisposes to the development of bronchopneumonia, worsening the hypoxia. Sometimes the hypoxia is sufficiently marked to damage the renal tubules. In addition, skin and blood vessel lesions may also develop in these patients, perhaps from hypersensitization to the drug or its metabolites (which presumably act as haptens). Large bullous vesicles are the most common form of skin reaction. These lesions are so typical as to be referred to as "barbiturate blisters." In some patients, generalization of the bullous lesions produces exfoliative dermatitis. In others, the skin changes take the form of an itching maculopapular rash—so-called eczematous dermatitis (p. 1282). Occasionally, widespread hypersensitivity angiitis develops, closely resembling polyarteritis nodosa (p. 520). Despite its depressant action on the brain, in many cases the neuronal changes are exceedingly scanty or take the form of nonspecific hypoxic injury; thus, even in fatal cases, the diagnosis of this form of poisoning rests largely on chemical identification of the drug in body fluids and tissues.

Estrogens and Oral Contraceptives (OCs)

The potential dangers involved in the use of estrogenic preparations and oral contraceptives (as formulated in the past) have long been issues of contention, and to some extent still are. However, the accumulating evidence now permits some reasonably firm conclusions. Turning first to estrogens, there is now fairly general agreement that *elevated endogenous levels of estrogens* and *prolonged use of exogenous estrogens induce an increased incidence of endometrial cancer (p. 1138).*[65] The relative risk of exogenous agents increases with duration of use and dosage, and in various surveys ranges from four- to 15-fold with more than five years of use.[66, 67] In addition, *clear cell adenocarcinoma of the vagina* has occurred in the teen-aged offspring of mothers who had taken diethylstilbestrol during the pregnancy.[68] Fortunately, the risk appears to be quite small since the vaginal neoplasm has appeared in only 0.14% of these young women. More often, only the benign precursor lesion—*adenosis of the vagina*—develops. Most of the evidence indicates that estrogens act as tumor promoters, as discussed on page 239.

The relationship of exogenous estrogens to the induction of breast carcinoma is still being argued. Basically similar studies have come to remarkably dissimilar conclusions. Most analyses report no increased risk even after long-term use of diethylstilbestrol,[69, 70] but a few find a small increase in risk—usually less than twofold.[71] One retrospective survey disclosed an even stronger association (tenfold increased risk) between exogenous estrogens and breast cancer among naturally menopausal women 45 to 54 years of age, but this discrepant finding requires confirmation.[72]

In addition to their potential oncogenicity, estrogens may have other adverse effects. The long-term use of estrogens (and oral contraceptives) has more than doubled the risk of the development of gallstones in women.[73] In addition, estrogen therapy for prostatic cancer has been reported to increase the mortality rate from coronary heart disease, presumably by predisposing to coronary thrombosis, but another report suggests that menopausal estrogen therapy protects women from this form of heart disease.[74] It is obvious that the relationship of estrogens to heart disease is far from settled.[75]

Oral contraceptives (OCs) as formulated in the past two decades have undoubtedly had adverse effects, both in terms of morbidity and mortality. Thus, the formulations have been significantly changed within the past few years with withdrawal of sequential OCs and reduction in the estrogenic and progestogenic dosages in the combined pills. Adequate data are not yet available on the risks, if any, incurred in the use of these "minipills." The data presented here relate to past use of combined preparations, but they have pertinence because they point to possible future dangers and their long-term effects are still being expressed. Precise morbidity and mortality rates vary among the many analyses available and so only the following generalizations are warranted.[76-79]

1. *Overall, OC users experienced a fivefold higher death rate from circulatory disease than "never-users."* Included in this designation are: myocardial infarction, venous thromboses with pulmonary embolism (Fig. 10–13), subarachnoid hemorrhage, cerebral hemorrhage, malignant hypertension, cardiomyopathy, and mesenteric artery thrombosis.

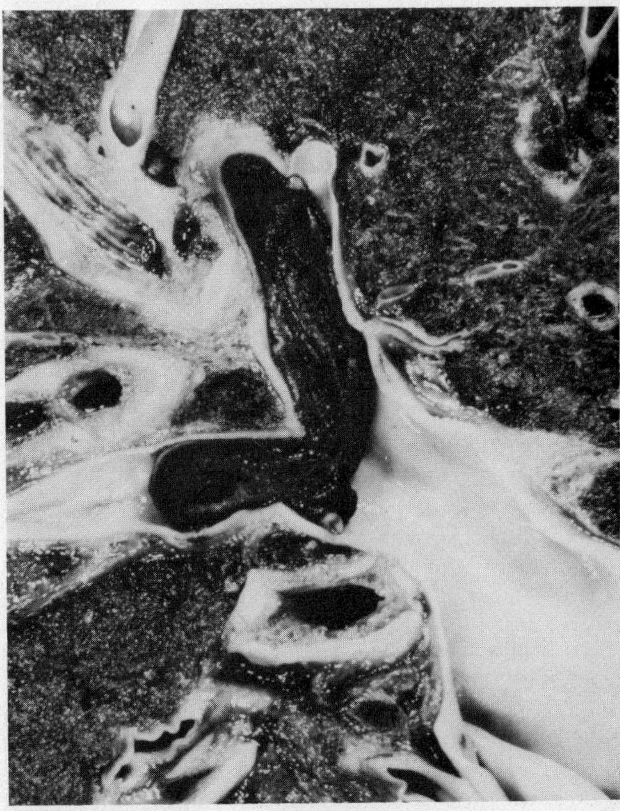

Figure 10–13. Pulmonary saddle embolus at bifurcation of pulmonary artery to right lung in a 34-year-old woman with six years of use of oral contraceptives. (Courtesy of Dr. John Godleski, Brigham and Women's Hospital.)

2. With use for five years or more there is an even greater risk of death from circulatory disease, but a few studies do not correlate risk with duration of use.[80]

3. *These risks do not apply to all women equally; women over 35 face the greatest hazards.*

4. Cigarette smoking (by itself a well-known predisposition to many circulatory diseases) multiplies the danger of many forms of circulatory disease two- to fivefold.

5. Among nonsmoking women under 35 years of age, there is an increased risk but it is very small. In contrast, smoking women over 35 years of age have the highest risk of death from circulatory disease.

6. After fewer than five years of use of OCs, discontinuance restores control levels of risk within a month. With more than five years of past use, the risk remains slightly above control levels, especially that of subarachnoid hemorrhage.

The use of OCs then significantly increases the risk of potentially fatal circulatory diseases, particularly in women over the age of 35 and with concurrent heavy use of cigarettes. However, risk estimates must be placed in the context of the frequency of the disease. Myocardial infarction, for example, is extremely uncommon in premenopausal women in the absence of such well-defined risk factors as hypertension, cigarette smoking, and hyperlipoproteinemia. Thus it has been pointed out that a fivefold increased risk of death from circulatory disease among OC users means a reduction in the chances of survival during a year from 99,995 to 99,975 per 100,000 women, representing two-hundredths of 1%.[81] Moreover, the risks must also be placed in the context of those involved in unwanted pregnancies where other methods of contraception are not readily available or are unacceptable.

Understandably, a great deal of attention has been directed to the possible effects of long-term use of OCs on the incidence of cancers of the breast and reproductive system. Indeed, sequential preparations were withdrawn from the marketplace because one (Oracon) was implicated in the induction of endometrial carcinoma. There is no evidence that combination OCs have increased the frequency of endometrial neoplasia. The issue is less clear with respect to cervical cancer because of so many confounding variables, discussed on page 1124. However, a recent report points to an increased risk of this form of cancer with combined OCs, particularly after more than five years of use.[81A] On the contrary, they may exert a protective effect against endometrial cancer[82] and also possibly a protective effect against ovarian cancer in women who have reached 40 to 60 years of age, but not in younger women.[77, 82A] When we turn to OCs and breast cancer, the issue is confused and confusing. There are reports of "no-risk,"[83] others pointing to "a slightly increased risk,"[84] and still others indicating "a substantially increased risk" but only among premenopausal women and particularly after more than five years of OC use by women under 25 who have had no pregnancies.[85] It is fruitless to attempt to resolve these differences; for the present it is prudent to consider the weight of evidence as favoring "some risk, but how much is unclear." It is of interest in this connection that OC use exerts a clear-cut protective effect against benign cystic hyperplasia and fibroadenoma of the breast.[84] The extent of protection appears to correlate with the duration of use; with four or more years of use the risk of developing benign breast disease is about halved. A similar level of protection against rheumatoid arthritis has been reported.[85A] Finally, a predisposition to the rare liver cell adenoma and a much less substantial predisposition to hepatocellular carcinoma have been associated with long-term use.[86] Although the relative risk with the liver cell adenoma is very high, the great rarity of this form of benign neoplasia keeps the incidence very low. The data are less well-defined with hepatocellular carcinomas but, once again, in the absence of well-defined predisposing factors (discussed on p. 936) this form of cancer is most uncommon in premenopausal women. It is evident that OCs pose the proverbial problem—do the risks outweigh the benefits?

NONTHERAPEUTIC AGENTS

The particular agents discussed in the following section were selected because of the following considerations: (1) the frequency of adverse reactions to the agent, (2) the potential clinical gravity of the reaction, or (3) the current interest in the agent(s) as a societal and environmental problem.

Ethyl Alcohol

Excessive consumption of ethanol has assumed epidemic proportions in both developed and developing countries. It is estimated that 8 to 12% of the adult American population (as well as those of other industrialized nations) are heavy drinkers. Of even greater concern is the growing problem of teenage alcohol abuse. It is fruitless to enter into the controversy on the definition of "heavy drinking" or "alcohol abuse"; defining it is as difficult as characterizing pornography, about which one sage Justice of the Supreme Court of the United States said, "I can't define pornography but I know it when I see it." Operationally, drinking can be considered excessive when it adversely affects health, work performance, or psychologic and societal relationships.

Bypassing the psychologic and sociologic aspects of alcohol abuse, from the medical standpoint it can be crudely divided into acute and chronic alcoholism. The functional effects of acute alcoholism are well known to any college student. Less well-known is the growing evidence that chronic ethanol consumption has wide-ranging deleterious effects on the cells and organs of the body quite apart from associated nutritional deficits.

Acute alcoholic intoxication is directly related to blood alcohol levels. Following ingestion ethanol is absorbed unaltered, largely in the small intestine but some in the stomach. Concomitant consumption of food slows the rate of absorption by delaying the emptying time of the stomach. After absorption, the alcohol is distributed to all the tissues and fluids of the body in direct proportion to the blood level. Less than 10% of the absorbed alcohol is excreted unchanged in the urine, sweat, and breath. The remainder is metabolized in the liver, largely by the cytoplasmic enzyme alcohol dehydrogenase, requiring NAD (nicotinamide adenine dinucleotide) as a cofactor.[87] Two additional pathways may participate in ethanol oxidation, a catalase—H_2O_2—and a microsomal ethanol oxidizing system, but the quantitative contribution these pathways make in the absence of alcoholic liver damage is small.[88] The major dehydrogenase pathway catabolizes alcohol first into acetaldehyde, which is then converted by a hepatic acetaldehyde dehydrogenase to acetyl CoA and acetate, and ultimately into CO_2 and water.

The rate of metabolism of alcohol is relatively constant—about 150 mg per kg of body weight per hour (about 1 oz 90-proof whiskey or 10 oz beer per hour). There is some evidence that chronic alcoholics develop some tolerance by virtue of an increased rate of metabolism. Indeed, modest elevations in blood alcohol levels in chronic alcoholics may improve their performance. Chronic exposure leads to some poorly defined adaptive capacity to perform motor and cognitive tasks at blood alcohol levels that would affect the uninitiated.[89] To date, no inborn errors of alcohol metabolism have been identified to corroborate the "Honest, honey, all I had was one beer."

Acute alcoholism exerts its effects mainly on the central nervous system, but as is evident on page 920, it may induce changes in hepatic structure remarkably quickly. Alcohol is a depressant of the central nervous system, affecting first subcortical structures (probably the high brain stem reticular formation) that modulate cerebral cortical activity. It should be sobering that acute alcoholism contributes significantly to over 50% of motor vehicle fatalities. At progressively higher blood levels lower medullary centers may be affected, including those regulating respiration, and respiratory arrest may follow. These neurologic effects may relate to impaired mitochrondrial function, but neuronal structural changes are usually not evident in acute alcoholism. Occasionally, in fatal cases, there is cerebral edema, possibly secondary to hypoxia.

There is a reasonable correlation between blood alcohol levels and the depth of impairment of CNS function in nonhabituated drinkers. In individuals of average size, consumption of 180 ml of distilled spirits on an empty stomach in a relatively short time will result in a blood alcohol level of approximately 100 mg per 100 ml. This level will induce obvious ataxia and is considered by most jurisdictions as the legal upper limit of sobriety. Drowsiness occurs at about 200 mg per 100 ml, stupor at 300 mg, and 400–500 mg will produce profound anesthesia, if not death. Fortunately, fatal levels are rarely encountered because "blessed stupor" intervenes. Even when large quantities are gulped rapidly with more bravado than brains, life-saving vomiting often occurs because of gastric irritation.

Chronic alcoholism is associated with a variety of morphologic alterations elegantly detailed by Edmondson.[89A] However, nutritional deficiencies, drug addiction, and infections often accompany the chronic alcoholism, and so it has been difficult to segregate the toxic effects of alcohol from these other confounding influences. In addition, some of the adverse effects may relate to the resulting blood levels of acetaldehyde rather than to the alcohol per se.[90] Thus, some prefer to designate the following changes "alcohol-related conditions." Notwithstanding, experimental studies indicate that administration of alcohol to laboratory animals induces a variety of adverse effects on cells and organs. Mitochondrial changes have been noted in hepatocytes and other cells.[90] Indeed, there is convincing evidence that alcohol is a direct hepatotoxin in humans that induces fatty liver (p. 920) and subsequently, in many instances, alcoholic cirrhosis (p. 917). Chronic alcohol abuse is the major cause of cirrhosis in most industrialized countries.[91] In addition, alcoholics are prone to a variety of forms of cancer—oropharynx (excluding lip), larynx, esophagus, and, through the intermediation of cirrhosis, hepatocellular carcinoma. Cigarette smoking multiplies the cancer risk many times.[92] They also are prone to gastrointestinal derangements including esophageal lacerations (p. 800), gastritis (p. 809), peptic ulcer (p. 814), and chronic relapsing pancreatitis (p. 966). In all of these conditions it is likely that alcohol is only one contributing influence. Striated muscle damage is also more frequent in alcoholics than in casual drinkers, inducing what has been referred to as alcoholic cardiomyopathy and alcoholic myopathy.[93] The changes range from regressive alterations in the mitochondria and endoplasmic reticulum to more overt cell necroses.[94] The nervous system, as might be expected, is affected in chronic alcohol abuse. Peripheral neuritis with degeneration of myelin sheaths is a well-known complication in these individuals, but it might largely be attributable to concomitant vitamin deficiencies, particularly of thiamine. Cerebral atrophy with intellectual impairment and cerebellar atrophy have been directly related to chronic alcohol toxicity.[95] Similarly and most unhappily the heavy use of ethanol during pregnancy has resulted in growth retardation and irreversible mental deficiency in the child.[96] With regard to these neurologic changes, other contributing influences have not been rigidly excluded. For example, the Wernicke-Korsakoff syndrome (p. 1421), virtually restricted to chronic alcoholics, responds in most instances to thiamine therapy. Thus, chronic alcoholism is associated with a variety of adverse effects, but with some individuals it may only be one of the contributing influences.

Methyl Alcohol

Methyl alcohol is more widely available than is generally appreciated. It may be used to denature ethanol and is found in solvents, Sterno, paint removers, and antifreezes. The toxic dose may be as small as 20 ml. Poisoning may also result from the inhalation of fumes in industry. When ingested, methyl alcohol causes patchy edema and hemorrhages in the stomach. On inhalation, edema and hemorrhage occur into the lung tissues, chiefly in the subpleural regions. However, methyl alcohol exerts it prime toxic effect after absorption by its oxidation to formaldehyde and formic acid, which in sufficient amounts inhibit hexokinase activity. A metabolic acidosis follows, related in part to the formation of formic acid and in part to depressed hexokinase function. At the same time, both metabolites, principally the formaldehyde and the deranged glucose metabolism, cause degeneration of the receptor cells of the retina with associated degeneration of the optic disc and nerve.

Although methanol and its derivatives, once absorbed, are widely distributed in the body, proportional to the water content of the various tissues, it is hypothesized that it exerts its principal effect on the retina, owing to the high water content of the eye.[97] Swelling of the brain and brain stem may also occur, accompanied by marked congestion of the cerebral vessels. Degenerative changes may develop in 12 to 24 hours in the cortical nerve cells with exposure to large doses. The central nervous system and retinal damage accounts for the major clinical features of the poisoning—variable degrees of central nervous system depression to frank coma and visual impairment—which sometimes results in total blindness. Both the eye and brain changes are reversible if the injury is mild, and recovery is possible with effective treatment and cessation of exposure.

Carbon Monoxide

Carbon monoxide (CO) is a nonirritating, inert gas, without color, taste, or odor, produced by the imperfect oxidation of combustible, carbon-containing material. It is released by internal combustion engines, improperly vented furnaces, and industrial processes that burn fossil fuels. Natural gas, in contrast to the illuminating gas produced in the past, contains no CO. Inhalation of a 1% concentration of CO may prove fatal within 10 to 20 minutes, depending on the degree of physical activity and the respiratory rate of the individual. Some concept of the apparent insignificance of this fatal level can be gained from the fact that the exhaust from automobile motors contains approximately 7%. Indeed, it has been estimated that the average car in a small closed garage would create lethal levels within five minutes. Since the absorption of this agent may be cumulative, toxic effects depend on the total exposure, i.e., the concentration in the inspired air and the duration of exposure. Levels lower than 1% in the inspired air may cause slowly developing, delayed damage and result in death even after removal from further exposure.

Carbon monoxide acts as a systemic asphyxiant. Its affinity for hemoglobin is 200 times greater than that of oxygen. The formation of a relatively stable carboxyhemoglobin destroys the oxygen-carrying capacity of hemoglobin. Symptoms related to a systemic hypoxia begin to appear when the hemoglobin is 20 to 30% saturated with carbon monoxide. When the hemoglobin is 60 to 70% saturated, unconsciousness and death are likely. Lower levels may produce mental confusion that renders the victim incapable of self-help.[98] Once carboxyhemoglobin is formed, the body rids itself of it slowly over the span of days, as the carbon monoxide is displaced by the pressure and mass action of inspired oxygen. The hypoxia most profoundly affects the central nervous system.

ACUTE POISONING. In acute, fatal cases the blood appears a bright cherry-red and produces marked hyperemia of all the tissues. Striking hyperemia, edema, and diffuse punctate hemorrhages throughout the cerebral hemispheres are frequent, but more obvious hypoxic neuronal changes are infrequent. Rarely, in the acute case, the muscle cells of the myocardium, the hepatic cells, and the epithelial cells of the proximal convoluted tubules of the kidneys suffer from hypoxic fatty damage. Death usually ensues too rapidly in acute monoxide poisoning to permit the full development of these visceral lesions.

In fatal exposure, the brain hypoxia leads to the insidious onset of loss of consciousness, progressing into deep coma and death. When the exposure has not been too great and the tissue hypoxia not too profound, complete recovery is possible without residual defects. However, central nervous system residuals, such as impairment of memory, vision, hearing, and speech, may remain in some patients after recovery.[99]

CHRONIC POISONING. Chronic poisoning may result from prolonged inhalation of relatively low levels of monoxide gas. This low-grade hypoxia insidiously gives rise to changes in the central nervous system. Degeneration of the cortical and nuclear ganglion cells may be widespread or may take the form of patchy, asymmetric lesions. The most common finding is symmetric degeneration of the basal ganglia, particularly the lenticular nuclei.[100] Hypoxic degenerative fatty changes in the kidney, liver, and heart are much more common in chronic intoxication than in acute. Clinically, in addition to the insidious onset of disturbances in brain function, these chronically exposed patients may suffer from renal, hepatic, or cardiac failure, which results in death days or weeks after the last exposure. However, chronic poisoning is usually nonfatal, and complete recovery is the rule. It should be emphasized that the tissue lesions of monoxide poisoning are not pathognomonic but merely reflect nonspecific severe hypoxemia.

Kerosene

Kerosene is one of the most frequent forms of accidental poisoning in children living in rural areas and among lower income groups where homes are heated by kerosene stoves. The victims generally range in age from one to six years. Presumably they mistake the colorless liquid for water or they are enticed into tasting the pink or blue fluid created by the introduction of dyes into the kerosene. Although kerosene may be ingested, the major clinical manifestations of this poisoning result from inhalation of the agent with the induction of a fulminant bronchopneumonic process having the characteristics of a lipid pneumonia (p. 749). Kerosene is also a narcotic and produces drowsiness and somnolence so that the onward progression of the respiratory symptoms in the sleeping unobserved child may pass unnoticed until too late.

Chloroform and Carbon Tetrachloride

Chloroform and carbon tetrachloride are infrequent causes of accidental and occupational poisoning. Both products are used in the home and in industry as components of cleaning fluids and degreasing agents. There is marked individual susceptibility to both so that similar levels of exposure may produce widely differing severities of injury. Chloroform and carbon tetrachloride toxicity induce central fatty change and, when more severe, necrosis of the liver (Fig. 10–14). Chronic alcoholism appears to potentiate this toxicity. When inhaled in sufficiently large amounts, these agents may cause profound central nervous system depression and death. Lower levels of exposure may lead to extensive necrosis of the renal tubular epithelium. The pathogenesis of these cell injuries was discussed earlier on page 12. If the hepatic and renal damage is sufficiently limited to permit survival, regeneration of preserved cells may restore both structure and function. Large amounts of both carbon tetrachloride and chloroform are retained in fat tissues throughout the body. The slow release of

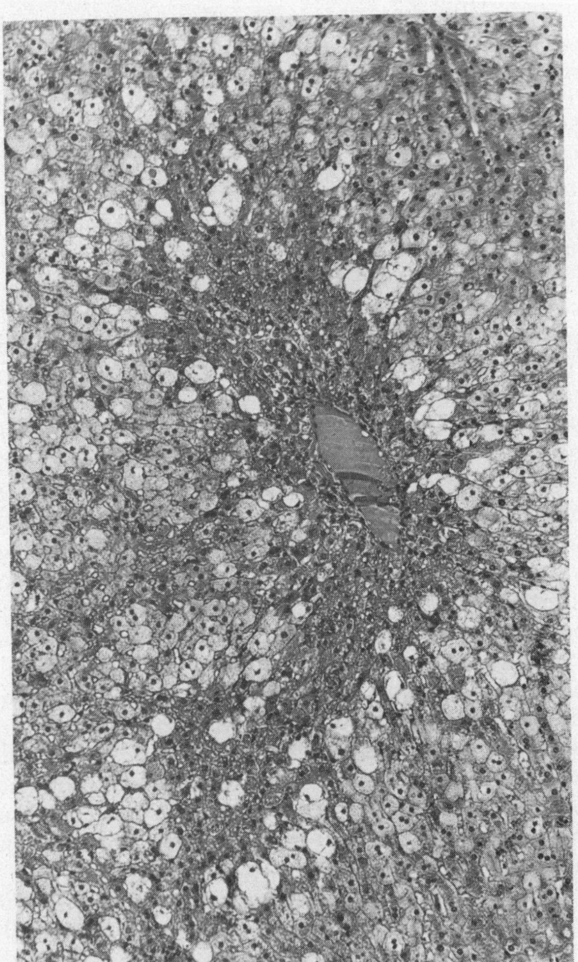

Figure 10–14. CCl_4 hepatotoxicity with necrosis of cells about central vein and fatty change in surrounding cells.

these stores into the blood, and then the breath, permits the clinical diagnosis of these intoxications long after exposure.[101]

Insecticides

The widespread use of these agents in the past and their well-established toxicity for animal life have justifiably evoked a great deal of concern. Indeed, fatal poisonings by pesticides have been reported. However, controls on the use of these agents in the United States have led to a decreasing number of annual fatalities.[102] Many more nonfatal poisonings must have occurred.

Insecticides fall into two broad classes: (1) *chlorinated hydrocarbons* (e.g., aldrin, chlordane, DDT, dieldrin, heptachlor, and lindane) and (2) *organophosphorous compounds* (e.g., malathion and parathion). Human exposure is, of course, greatest among those involved in the manufacture of these agents, and farmers or commercial sprayers who use them frequently. Absorption may occur through the respiratory, skin, or gastrointestinal routes. Since these agents are very resistant to degradation, they persist in soil and water and so contaminate all levels of the human food chain. Analyses have revealed traces of DDT in many animal products, vegetables, and fruits, including infant foods and milk.[103] Both categories of pesticides are lipophilic and accumulate in fat stores through the body. Because of their persistence, toxicity may result from chronic exposure to small daily increments.

The *chlorinated hydrocarbons* principally affect the central nervous system and at first induce hyperexcitability, which may be followed by delirium and convulsions. This phase may be followed by progressive central nervous system depression with paralysis, coma, and death. In experimental animals, similar neurologic effects (accounting for their effectiveness as insecticides) are associated with pyknosis and shrinkage of the ganglion cells of the cerebral cortex and spinal cord. Chronic exposure in humans has induced fatty change in the liver, which may progress to liver necrosis. Adrenal necroses have been observed in dogs, but not in humans. However, it is of interest that analogs of DDT have been used clinically in the treatment of some adrenal hyperfunctional states.

The *organophosphorous insecticides* are basically inhibitors of acetylcholinesterase. Thus, acetylcholine accumulates at synaptic junctions and induces a range of neurologic manifestations, the most serious of which are muscle twitching that progresses to flaccid paralysis and cardiac arrhythmias. Ultimately, respiratory depression and coma may lead to death.

It is well that the potential hazards of these insecticides have been recognized and their use controlled, but at the same time their potential usefulness cannot be ignored.

Polychlorinated Biphenyls (PCBs)

The PCBs are closely related chemically to DDT. Indeed, there is a fear that DDT vapor may be transformed by the ultraviolet rays in sunlight into PCBs. Once widely used in paper coatings, printing inks, adhesives, and hydraulic fluids, the industrial use of PCBs has been restricted to "closed" systems in transformers and capacitors because of their toxicity.[104] However, humans are still exposed to these toxic agents from the open burning and incineration of industrial and municipal wastes, by vaporization from coatings, and from their disposal into municipal sewers and industrial waste dumps. In Japan, toxicity from PCBs was traced to contaminated cooking oils.[105] The extreme persistence of PCBs in the environment is of major concern, since they are resistant to all natural processes of decay. It is estimated that 25,000 tons of PCBs are added each year to the expanding environmental burden, creating an impressive reservoir of toxicity.

In humans, PCBs induce such disorders as chloracne, impaired vision, impotence, and possibly infertility. These changes may not appear for many months after exposure. Toxicologic studies in animals have revealed immunosuppression; hepatic, renal, and intestinal lesions; and reproductive defects. One is driven to ask: Is there no satisfactory substitute for these chemicals?

Mushroom Poisoning

Many species of mushrooms are toxic and cause usually nonfatal gastrointestinal or cardiac disturbances but a few, *Amanita muscaria* and particularly *A. phalloides*, may be lethal.

Amanita muscaria contains a parasympathomimetic alkaloid-muscarine, as well as other substances, which act on the central nervous system. These induce symptoms principally of parasympathetic stimulation: pupillary constriction, sweating, salivation, nausea, vomiting, diarrhea, abdominal pain, bradycardia, dyspnea, and hypotension. In severe poisoning, confusion, hyperexcitability, and delirium may appear. Although death may occur following ingestion of *A. muscaria*, recovery is the rule with supportive therapy. *A. phalloides*, in contrast, induces a 30 to 50% fatality rate. Two toxins have been identified in this "angel of death." One, known as phallin, is a thermolabile hemolysin that is destroyed by cooking and digestion and so plays little role in the potentially fatal outcome. The other toxin, called amanitin, combines with and inhibits RNA polymerase and so blocks the synthesis of messenger RNA. For six to 24 hours following ingestion there are no symptoms, but then marked nausea, violent abdominal cramps, vomiting, diarrhea, and cardiovascular collapse become manifest. In severe intoxications, headache, confusion, convulsions, and coma follow and often lead to death. The major morphologic changes are found in the liver and kidneys, but skeletal muscle, heart, and the neurons in the brain may also suffer damage. The hepatic damage takes the form of centrilobular and sometimes massive necrosis. The kidney usually reveals fatty changes and necrosis of the proximal convoluted tubules. If the victim survives, hepatic fibrosis, resembling that seen in postnecrotic cirrhosis (p. 923), may remain as a permanent residual.

Cyanide

No substance lends itself better to "evil doings" than cyanide. Less than 0.1 gm of a highly absorbable inorganic salt may be lethal. It acts as a cellular asphyxiant by combining with the trivalent iron of cytochrome oxidase, disrupting oxidative respiration. The most pleasant comment that can be made about this poison is that nitrite constitutes a highly effective antidote if administered soon enough. Nitrite converts hemoglobin into methemoglobin, which successfully competes for the cyanide complexed to cytochrome oxidase. With dissociation of the oxidase-cyanide complex, enzymatic function and cell respiration are restored.

Poisoning may result from the inhalation of *hydrocyanic acid gas* with such rapid absorption that death may occur within minutes. The ingestion of *inorganic salts* or *cyanide-containing organic compounds* kills more slowly, possibly within a few hours (depending on dosage).[106] It is worthy of note that the seeds and pits of certain fruits and plants (peach, apricot, bitter almond, wild black cherry) harbor cyanide-containing substances such as amygdalin that may release the poison on digestion. Indeed, cyanide poisoning has been reported from the use of laetrile, which contains an extract of apricot pits.[107] Parents of young children should be alerted to the fact that elderberry and hydrangea plants also contain trace amounts of cyanide. However, the poison is not cumulative and is detoxified in the body to thiocyanate. Toxic levels depend, therefore, on rates of absorption and detoxification.

The clinical course of *acute cyanide poisonings* is, as mentioned, extremely brief. The first symptom to appear is rapidly progressive dyspnea related to literal strangulation of every cell in the body. At autopsy, there may be petechiae in the skin, mucous membranes, and serosal membranes.[108] It is not clear whether these lesions result from generalized vascular injury or from the combination of profound hypoxia and the severe convulsive seizures. Particularly characteristic is the cherry-red color of the fully oxygenated blood (reminiscent of carbon monoxide poisoning, see p. 450) since, with the loss of cytochrome oxidase, the poisoned cells cannot use oxygen. All the tissues have a pungent, bitter-almond odor that is, in fact, detectable clinically and so may permit a prompt diagnosis with immediate initiation of life-saving therapy. When the poison is taken orally, edema, hemorrhage, and necrosis of the gastric mucosa may result. The brain may show minimal-to-slight edema with petechial hemorrhages, but insufficient time elapses for the development of more obvious anoxic lesions.

Chronic cyanide poisoning may occur from repeated absorption of small amounts of poison over the course of days to weeks if the increments exceed the rate of detoxification. The tissue hypoxia under these circumstances is progressive but not immediately fatal. Slowly developing changes affect the brain, liver, and kidneys. Grossly, the brain may appear entirely normal, but on microscopic section, degeneration of ganglion cells is usually evident, sometimes to the point at which these cells become totally necrotic and disappear and are said to have "dropped out." Hypoxic fatty change of the renal convoluted tubular epithelial cells and centrilobular fatty change of the liver may also be present.

Clinically, progressive disturbance of cerebral function in the chronic form leads to the development of unconsciousness and frank coma. When the patient survives for a sufficient time, symptoms of impaired liver and renal function may become manifest. Clinical recognition of this form of poisoning before irreversible brain damage has occurred should permit curative intervention.

Mercury

This metal was once used in the silvering of mirrors and the production of felt hats, and workers often developed toxic mental changes, called madness, hence the phrase "mad as a hatter," hallowed by Lewis Carroll. Mercuric chloride was also once a favored agent among suicides. It is still used in industry in photoengraving and tool hardening. Certain insecticides and fungicides contain mercury compounds. Toxicity due to mercury is rare today, but occasional outbreaks of poisoning still occur, e.g., the one involving the inhabitants of Minimata, Japan. The poisonings were traced back to contaminated fish derived from a coastal body of water polluted by mercury-bearing industrial wastes. Another tragic outbreak occurred in Iraq when grain intended for planting and pretreated with a mercurial fungicide was used in the making of bread.[109] The Japanese experience called attention to a global problem. Mercury was once used in antifouling paints on ships, and trace amounts of this element are still present in waters throughout the world. However, the minute quantities encountered in fish found in open waters are of no clinical significance because in small doses mercury does not accumulate in the body, being excreted through the kidneys, colon, bile, sweat, and saliva.

Mercury causes cellular damage principally by combining with sulfhydryl groups of membranes and enzymes, and has its greatest effect on mitochondrial oxidative processes. Mercuric compounds are more toxic than mercurous. There was once a belief that poisoning from inorganic compounds differed from that caused by organic compounds, but current evidence is against such a notion save that inorganic salts are more rapidly absorbed.[110] Toxicity may result from inhalation of vaporized metallic mercury, by absorption of mercuric compounds through the skin, or through the gastrointestinal route. The principal organs affected are the gastrointestinal tract, kidneys, and central nervous system.[111] The anatomic changes in acute poisonings differ somewhat from those in chronic toxicity.

Acute poisoning is usually caused by the intentional or accidental ingestion of a soluble mercuric salt, e.g., mercuric chloride. Acute erosive lesions may develop within a day in the oral cavity and also in the gastric mucosa. Later, focal necroses and ulcerations may appear in the colonic mucosa. The kidney is a major target, since mercury is excreted through the urine. With high toxic levels an acute tubular necrosis (ATN) results with, at first, vacuolization of epithelial lining cells in the proximal tubules, followed by the death and often calcification of these cells. Ultrastructural studies reveal abnormalities in the endoplasmic reticulum, ribosomes, and mitochondria, which may develop irregular calcium matrix densities.[112] With very high levels of this poison, other tubular segments of the nephron may also be affected. These alterations are very similar to those encountered in other forms of nephrotoxic nephritis, except that the calcification tends to be more prominent in mercury poisoning. Although manifestations of central nervous system dysfunction may appear in acute poisonings, characteristic morphologic lesions have not been identified in the brain apart from cerebral edema.

Chronic poisoning has been reported from the ingestion of food contaminated by fungicide and canned fish derived from polluted coastal waters, and from the use of dermatologic ointments to induce skin lightening. The incremental accumulation of mercury is in part eliminated through the salivary glands, causing excessive salivation. The metal deposits on the gingival margins, especially when a gingivitis is present, to produce a discoloration closely resembling the "lead line" (p. 455), and also causes loosening of the teeth. Chronic gastritis often appears, sometimes accompanied by mucosal ulcerations. A nephrotoxic nephritis with renal insufficiency may develop, but more often a nephrotic syndrome (p. 1011) appears along with its characteristic heavy proteinuria. Both membranous (p. 1012) and proliferative (p. 1007) glomerulonephritis have been observed on light and electron microscopy.[113] The glomerular changes suggest an immune complex disease, caused possibly by a mercury-protein complex as the antigenic stimulus. The heavy proteinuria in these glomerulopathies may lead to tubular reabsorption of protein, with the formation of eosinophilic droplets within the tubular epithelial cells (Fig. 10–15).[114] Scattered foci of atrophy throughout the cerebral cortex; atrophy of the occipital lobes, which produces enlargement of the occipital horns of the lateral ventricles; and atrophy of the cerebellar folia have been described in the brain. It is these changes in the central nervous system that account for all of the neurologic abnormalities in chronic mercury poisoning such as headache, loss of memory, emotional instability, tremors, muscular incoordination, and deafness, progressing in some cases to coma and death.

Lead

Lead poisoning has been aptly called "the silent epidemic." The metal accumulates in the body and thus small, daily increments may reach toxic levels that wreak silent havoc, principally in the brain. Lead poisoning is a widespread hazard, but it occurs particularly as an occupational disease of adults and in slum children heavily exposed to peeling lead paint in dilapidated houses. Occupational exposure is principally encountered in industries extracting and processing lead and its products, in recycling of lead by burning storage batteries, and also with paint spraying and intense exposure to gasoline-burning engines in garage or highway work. Mass screening programs confirm that underprivileged children are indeed at increased risk, but also reveal that the problem is widespread in the United States.[115] Blood lead levels that exceed the accepted limit of 30 μg per deciliter were found in 1.9% of the population from 6 months to 74 years of age, but significantly in 4% of children aged 6 months to 5 years. Most frequently affected and having the highest blood lead levels were black, inner-city children from low-income families. In this group, 18.6% had blood lead levels above the accepted limit, in contrast to 4.5% of comparable white children. This racial difference remains unexplained since location, style of living, and type of housing were the same for whites and blacks. Children are exposed to lead in the dust, dirt, soil, paint, air, and sometimes water. Despite current restrictions on the use of lead in paint, a 1978 survey indicates that in the United States about one-third of dwellings were built before 1940, when lead paint was in common use. The exposure may in fact begin in utero

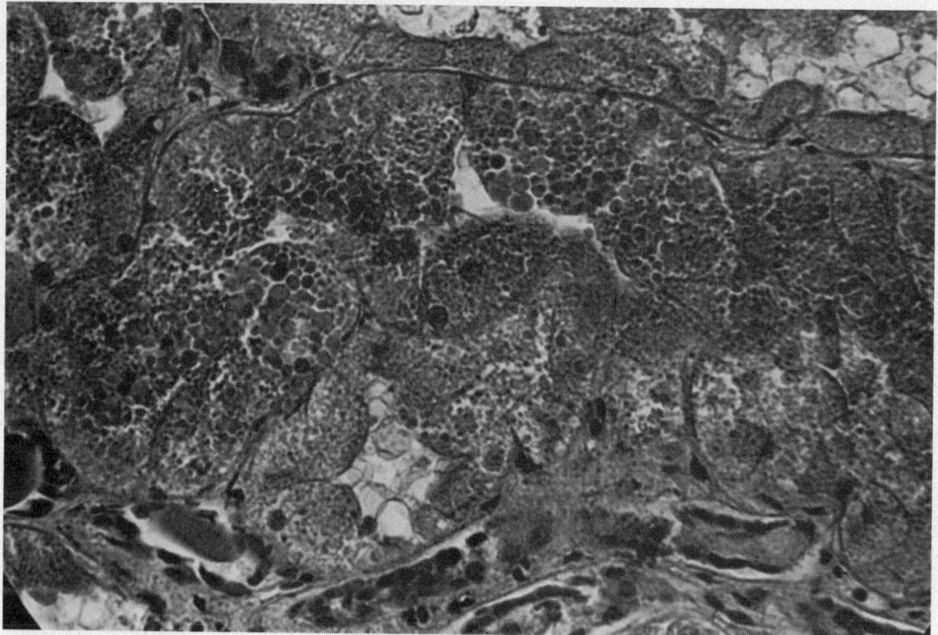

Figure 10–15. Large eosinophilic droplets of resorbed protein are evident in cells of renal tubules in mercury poisoning.

because lead crosses the placental barrier, and mental retardation has been observed in infants whose mothers drank lead-contaminated water during pregnancy. Air pollution has been reduced by a decrease in the use of leaded gasoline and a reduction of lead in gasoline and in automobile-emissions, and with it has come a lowering of the mean blood lead level in the United States population.[116] Although the contribution of this air pollution is now said to be not significantly contributory,[117] even small amounts add to the total body burden of this cumulative poison. Additional sources of lead, principally for children, are ceramics, decorative decals on glassware, and newsprint.

Lead may be absorbed from the gastrointestinal tract or through the respiratory tract. Much of the lead in circulation is deposited in bones; thus, large amounts may accumulate in the skeletal reservoir and, on release, contribute to the blood levels. Although 30 μg of blood lead is considered to be a "safe" upper limit, there are concerns with this standard. Most children with moderate elevations above this level are not obviously poisoned. Much more important, in some instances, levels well below the accepted limit have induced electroencephalographic alterations in central nervous system function.[118] Thus, "low" blood levels of lead may sometimes be neurotoxic. At levels within or near the accepted limit, lead inhibits enzymes (such as aminolevulinic acid dehydratase, ferrochelatase, and pyrimidine 5′-nucleotidase), increases erythrocyte protoporphyrin, and disturbs the metabolism of vitamin B and cortisol. These toxic effects may appear quite suddenly with intense exposure (such as may occur with inhalation of aerosolized lead during battery burning) or they may arise insidiously from the slow build-up of the body burden. There is, however, no clear clinical delineation between the acute and chronic forms of toxicity. The major targets affected are the hematopoietic, nervous, and gastrointestinal systems, but the kidneys may also suffer damage.

Mild anemia is typically present, as is basophilic stippling of large numbers of red cells. Inhibition of levulinic acid dehydratase and ferrochelatase, involved in heme synthesis, impair the incorporation of iron into the porphyrin ring and heme synthesis and simultaneously increase protoporphyrin in erythrocytes. Thus, there is reduction in red cell formation.[119] At the same time, lead appears to inhibit Na-K-ATPase in erythrocyte membranes, and so membrane maintenance is impaired. Thus, increased fragility of erythrocytes adds a hemolytic component to the anemia. The origin of the basophilic stippling is not clear, but may relate to inhibition of the nucleotidase.

Encephalopathy occurs principally in children. The brain is markedly edematous, with flattening of the gyri and narrowing of the sulci (Fig. 10–16). Microscopically, there may be demyelination of the cerebral and cerebellar white matter, and death of ganglion cells with diffuse astrocytic proliferation. Often there is proliferation of the endothelium of small capillaries in the areas of damage. The neuronal loss is attributed to lead-induced inhibition of mitochondrial oxidative phosphorylation. In adults, the central nervous system is less often affected, but frequently a peripheral neuritis with myelin degeneration appears, typically involving the motor innervation of the most commonly used muscles. Thus, the extensor muscles of the wrist and fingers are often the first to be affected, followed by paralysis of the peroneal muscles.

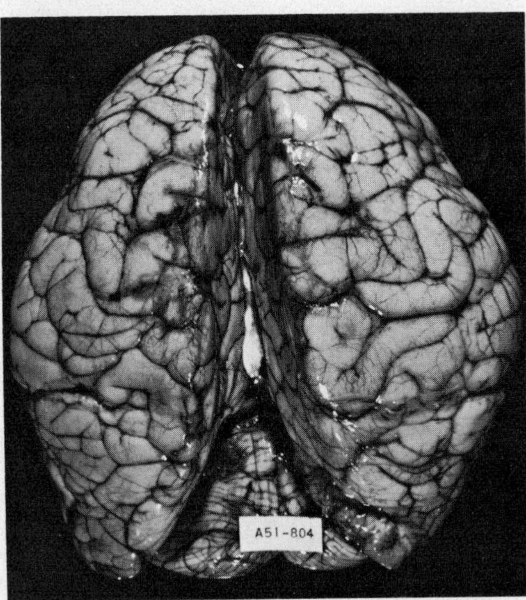

Figure 10–16. Cerebral edema in lead poisoning. The gyri are flattened and widened, and the sulci are narrowed and relatively inapparent.

The gastrointestinal tract is a major source of clinical manifestations. Lead "colic" characterized by extremely severe, poorly localized abdominal pain is often associated with sufficient spasm and rigidity of the abdominal wall to create the impression of an acute "surgical abdomen." Notwithstanding, the only morphologic finding in the gastrointestinal tract is a "lead line" of precipitated lead sulfide along the gingival margins. This discoloration is rare in children and not seen in edentulous individuals. Moreover, although typical of lead poisoning, it may be encountered in other circumstances such as mercury poisoning.

Renal proximal tubular acidosis (the Fanconi syndrome) (p. 408) may possibly become evident because of transport defects secondary to altered function of membrane enzymes. Morphologically, the only changes to be seen are acid-fast intranuclear inclusions, principally in the epithelial cells of the proximal tubules. These inclusions are at least in part composed of lead-protein complexes.

The diagnosis of lead poisoning in adults can often be suspected by the findings of anemia and red cell stippling associated with an elevated blood lead level. A gingival lead line, abdominal colic, and finger, wrist, or foot drop, when present, add weight to the suspicion. In children, the toxicity may be much more insidious, and sometimes only lethargy, stupor, and motor ataxia call attention to the possibility of lead intoxication. These nonspecific findings, however, may be suddenly followed by the rapid development of convulsions and coma. In this age group, sufficient lead may have accumulated in the skeleton to produce striking radiodensities along the epiphyseal lines (Fig. 10–17). The diagnosis can be confirmed in all age groups by the demonstration of increased urinary excretion of aminolevulinic acid and coproporphyrin, increased red cell protoporphyrin, and reduced red cell aminolevulinic acid dehydratase. The lead level in the blood is only confirmatory if it exceeds 60 mg per dl but, as pointed out, lower levels may be toxic. More reliable as a measure of the body burden is the amount of lead excreted in the urine following the administration of a chelating agent. The gravity of lead poisoning in children should not be underestimated. Lead encephalopathy, once it appears, may cause, at the least, behavioral disturbances or mental retardation, and at the most, sudden death.

Arsenic

Arsenic poisoning, once a favorite pastime of the Borgias, is today happily uncommon. The various arsenical salts, oxides, and arsene gas are all highly dangerous. Arsenicals are used in fruit sprays, weed killers, insecticides, rat poisons, and a number of industrial processes. Acute poisonings, usually suicidal or homicidal, are rarely encountered, but chronic poisonings by long exposure to arsenical dusts, arsene gas in industry, or foods bearing a coating of arsenic-containing plant sprays still account for occasional deaths. Arsenic binds with sulfhydryl groups. Thus, in chronic poisoning, the hair, nails, and surface squames of the skin accumulate detectable amounts. By binding to sulfhydryl groups in proteins, arsenic interferes with many enzyme functions essential to cellular metabolism.

The manifestations of arsenic poisoning depend on the dose ingested. At little as 30 mg of arsenic trioxide may be fatal. Large doses of this potent poison kill within an hour or two, usually by the induction of peripheral vasodilation, reduction in effective circulating

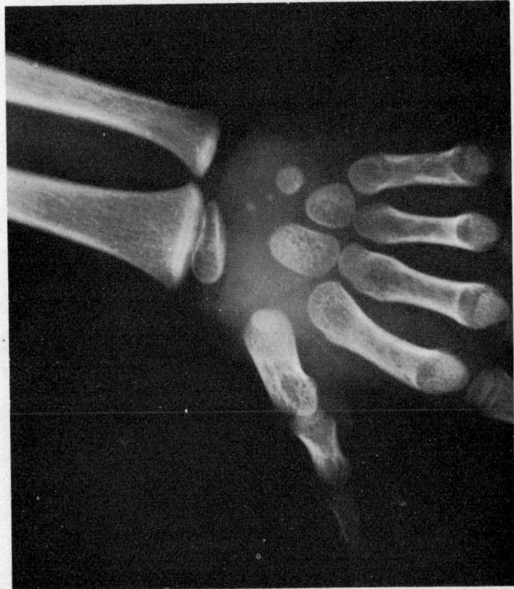

Figure 10–17. Lead deposits in epiphyses of wrist have caused a marked increase in their radiodensity so that they are as radiopaque as the cortical bone.

blood volume, and shock. It is believed that arsenic acts as a depressant on the central nervous system and induces paralysis of vasomotor control. When it is taken orally, the vascular collapse is often preceded by nausea, vomiting, and severe abdominal pain. With large doses, death may occur so rapidly that sufficient time does not elapse for the development of significant morphologic lesions in either the brain or gastrointestinal tract.

With less extreme levels of poisoning, *the major anatomic changes are found after the first day in the vascular system, brain, gastrointestinal tract, and skin.* Generalized visceral hyperemia develops with petechial hemorrhages in the serous membranes and skin; the latter changes are caused by necrotizing damage to capillary walls. With survival for two or three days, intestinal lesions are encountered chiefly in the stomach in the form of congestion and edema, replaced soon with petechial hemorrhages and foci of dark red-black coagulation necrosis. Sloughing of these necrotic areas produces ulcerations that may be dispersed or may coalesce to form large, denuded, raw surfaces. Similar lesions may become evident in the remainder of the intestinal tract. Lesions may also appear in the brain in the course of two to three days. These take the form of widespread petechial hemorrhages, apparently due to necrosis of the capillary walls, together with marked diffuse cerebral edema. Thromboses may occur in these injured vessels and give rise to focal areas of infarction within the brain substance. When patients with high toxic doses survive for four to five days, fatty changes in the parenchymal cells of the kidneys and liver may occur, accompanied sometimes by fatty change of the myocardium. In these patients, there is rapid onset of vascular collapse and central nervous system depression, followed by coma and death within hours. In less acute forms, the presenting signs and symptoms may be marked vomiting followed by severe, persistent, watery diarrhea. Central nervous system depression and vascular collapse may follow.

With low-level chronic poisoning, the major changes involve the gastrointestinal tract, nervous system, and skin. Vascular lesions and petechial hemorrhages are not prominent. In the intestinal tract, congestion, edema, and small superficial ulcerations may develop in the stomach and small intestine. The changes in the nervous system appear to be most prominent in the peripheral nerves, with myelin degeneration and destruction of axis cylinders. Brain lesions are uncommon. Focal or large confluent areas of dark brown–black pigmentation occur in skin areas that are normally most deeply pigmented. The palms of the hands and soles of the feet develop thickening of the keratin layer of the skin. These skin lesions have progressed occasionally to the formation of epithelial carcinomas. The kidneys and liver may also suffer damage similar to that encountered in acute intoxication. In addition, there may be an increased incidence of lung cancer and hepatic angiosarcomas in vineyard workers chronically exposed to arsenical pesticides.

The clinical characteristics of chronic poisoning differ from those in the acute form. At the onset, generalized weakness and malaise appear insidiously, followed by muscular weakness of the hands and feet. Some cases develop frank paralysis and anesthesia in the areas of neural involvement. Frequently, the diagnosis is first suspected by the characteristic pigmentary changes in the skin.

Drug Addiction

Drug addiction continues to be a major societal and medical problem in the United States and many other countries. Precise data are not available, but the Drug Enforcement Administration estimates that there are more than 600,000 opioid addicts in the United States. Drug abuse is the leading cause of death in New York City for those between the ages of 15 and 35 years.[120] It is particularly tragic that one-third of these fatalities occur in teenagers.

There appears to be no end to the variety of agents that have been injected, ingested, or sniffed in the search for "a new experience" or to dodge "the slings and arrows" of everyday life. The federally regulated agents that are too freely available on the street can be divided into (1) psychodepressants (principally the barbiturates, (2) opioids (principally heroin), and (3) psychostimulants and hallucinogens (principally amphetamines, cocaine, mescaline, lysergic acid diethylamide [LSD] and marijuana). It has been difficult to segregate the adverse consequences of various agents. Almost invariably, more than one has been used either simultaneously or sequentially. Many of the narcotics, particularly heroin, are diluted ("cut") by a variety of substances such as quinine, talc, or lactose that themselves may induce pharmacologic, allergic, or foreign body reactions. Further, the methods commonly employed in the preparation of a "shot" are less than fastidious. One report notes that about one-third of a series of heroin addicts had, on occasion, dissolved the drug in water from the toilet.[121] The weird litany could be continued, but it is clear that only some adverse effects may be directly related to the drug itself.

The following remarks will largely pertain to narcotic (principally heroin) addiction, but first some brief observations on marijuana and LSD.

Marijuana (cannabis) has come under intense scrutiny as evidence has waxed and waned that its use may entail unwanted side effects. Studies in animals and humans indicate that habitual smoking of cannabis, like cigarette smoking, may cause chronic bronchitis, obstructive disease of the airways, and (most significantly) metaplastic and dysplastic changes in the bronchial epithelium.[122] Moreover, one cannabis cigarette yields 70 to 500% more carcinogenic hydrocarbons than one tobacco cigarette.[123] Other less well-documented adverse effects have been reported. Changes in reproductive function have been observed, such as a decrease in the sperm count in humans and animals, alterations in the ovulatory cycle in rhesus monkeys, and increased pregnancy loss rate in monkeys.[124] Most controversial are possible deleterious effects on the central nervous system. Changes in memory and learning ability, emotional instability, and microscopic evidence of abnormalities in synaptic junctions have all been reported.[124A] However, a recent report concluded after a year's study of all the evidence that, despite possible short-term adverse psychologic and intellectual effects, there is no convincing evidence of long-term neurologic deficits.[124B] At present, the only reasonable verdict that can be rendered is that, with the evidence at hand, "pot" cannot be convicted of being unequivocally dangerous but neither has it been proved harmless. Until more is known, therefore, it might be prudent to heed the title of a recent book: "*Keep Off The Grass.*"[125]

LSD has been accused of a variety of adverse effects, but for every claim to be found in the literature there is a counterclaim. Earlier reports of an increased frequency of chromosomal abnormalities in the lymphocytes of habitual users have not been confirmed by controlled studies.[126] Equally questionable is an increased frequency of congenital defects in infants born to heavy users of this agent. Less easily dismissed is the question: Does chronic use of LSD predispose to psychiatric illness? There is good neuropharmacologic evidence that LSD depresses the activity of serotonin-containing neurons and, by altering normal pathways of neurotransmission, could exert a direct effect on brain function.[127] There is, in addition, a clinical study suggesting that users of various psychostimulants have an increased incidence of mental disorders.[128] Here the issue arises—which agent, combination of agents, or sequence of agents is implicated? Moreover, it must be questioned whether individuals with preexisting personality disorders tend to indulge in psychostimulants. The jury is still out on LSD and so, at present, the drug is neither "guilty" nor "not guilty."

Heroin is the most commonly used narcotic and the major source of the morbidity and mortality associated with drug addiction. Untoward complications may stem from: (1) the pharmacologic action of the agent, (2) reactions to possible contaminants, (3) hypersensitivity reactions to the drug or its contaminants, and (4) diseases contracted in the course of its use. A consideration of sudden death in drug addicts illustrates some of these pathways. About 20% of narcotic-related fatalities are intentional suicides or homicides, the remaining 80% being caused by "acute reactions" or overdoses. Three overdose syndromes can be distinguished: (a) profound respiratory depression, (b) arrhythmias and cardiac arrest, and (c) severe pulmonary edema.

The respiratory depression may be a direct pharmacologic effect resulting from the use of an amount of heroin in excess of that to which the body is accustomed. There is no way of gauging the precise amount of heroin in preparations bought "on the street." "Pushers" have been known to sell virtually pure heroin to rid themselves of unwanted customers. Moreover, tolerance to drugs falls during periods of withdrawal, such as occurs with incarceration or hospitalization, and so previously used dosages become excessive. The precise basis for arrhythmias and cardiac arrest is somewhat uncertain, but it could be due to quinine, frequently used as a "cutting agent" to dilute the heroin. Severe pulmonary edema (the third of the overdose syndromes) has been referred to as "narcotic lung."[129] Whatever their basis, overdose reactions that fall precariously short of fatal are not unusual in the life of an addict–until . . .

A variety of less dramatic adverse consequences are also associated with the narcotic habit. Most appear to be secondary to contaminants introduced with the drug. Significantly, physician addicts have been known to have no adverse physical effects even after long-term use of addictive drugs. The various morphologic lesions are best considered according to the tissue or organ involved.[130]

Cutaneous lesions are probably the most frequent telltale sign of heroin addiction. They take a variety of forms including scarring at injection sites ("tracks"), hyperpigmentations over commonly used veins, thrombosed veins, skin abscesses, cellulitis, ulcerations, urticaria (presumably secondary to the release of histamine by heroin), and sometimes, for inexplicable reasons, massive swelling of the extremity.[131]

Cardiovascular lesions are being reported with increasing frequency.[132] Bacteremia is seen in about 10% of cases. It is most commonly caused by *Staphylococcus aureus*, but virtually every other microbial agent in the book has been implicated at one time or another, including nonpathogen forms. Infective endocarditis is probably the most costly price for the heroin habit. The exact incidence of this complication is not known, but it is not uncommon. The disease differs somewhat from that encountered in the general population. The patients are usually younger and male; preexistent heart disease is uncommon; the valves of the right side of the heart, particularly the tricuspid, are often involved; and the most common infecting organisms (accounting for almost two-thirds of all cases) are first *S. aureus* and second *Candida albicans*, in that order.[133] The endocarditis usually conforms to the "acute" pattern. Addicts are particularly prone to blood-borne infections; there is repeated introduction of organisms, malnutrition is frequently present, and many, for poorly understood reasons, suffer from immunologic incompetence.

Disseminated necrotizing angiitis resembling polyarteritis nodosa may be encountered. It may relate to hypersensitivity to the narcotic or its diluting agent, but alternatively, hepatitis B antigenemia may underlie the vascular disease. Affected arteries tend to be located in the kidney, liver, and small bowel and may induce renal failure.[134] A variety of other pulmonary vascular lesions have been observed and are described later.

Pulmonary lesions are frequent in narcotic addicts and have been attributed to respiratory depression, shock, and hypersensitivity.[129] The most common form, referred to as "narcotic lung," is pulmonary edema, sometimes hemorrhagic, resembling that seen in the "adult respiratory distress syndrome" (p. 714) (Fig. 10–18). Often these changes are accompanied by broncho-

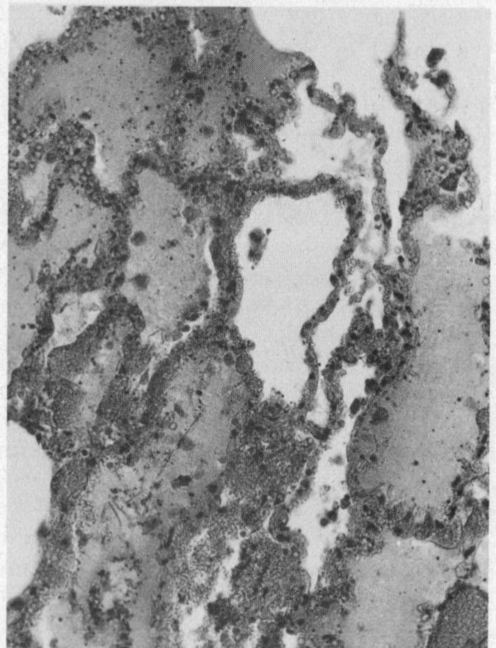

Figure 10–18. Lung of a heroin addict with patchy edema and atelectasis. Many of the alveolar spaces are filled iwth a proteinaceous fluid.

pneumonia, focal atelectasis, emphysema, aspiration of gastric contents, and mononuclear cell accumulations within the alveoli and alveolar walls. Less common and more distinctive is a constellation of pulmonary vascular changes all of which induce, to a greater or lesser extent, obstruction to the pulmonary blood flow, sometimes accompanied by cor pulmonale. They comprise thromboses, plexiform and angiomatoid lesions (presumably representing residuals of organized thrombi), and arterial wall thickenings.[135] Even more distinctive are foreign body granulomas, sometimes within the walls of pulmonary arteries but at other times located about the vessels or within adjacent alveolar septa. These lesions are essentially reactions to particulate matter introduced with the injection, possibly to the "cutting agent" such as talc (a silicate) or to other contaminants. The talc crystals are readily visualized by polarized light (Fig. 10–19).

The *liver* and *biliary tract* are abnormal in 75 to 80% of addicts. The most frequent change is periportal infiltrations of mononuclear cells. This "triaditis" is most consistent with chronic persistent hepatitis and, in most instances, is attributable to infection with the hepatitis B virus acquired by a sharing of needles.[136] Other common findings are fatty change and cirrhosis in about 30% of all long-term addicts (probably related to alcohol abuse).[137] Foreign body granulomas and marked congestion may be present. For poorly understood reasons, the gallbladder is frequently distended with thick bile, and the porta hepatic lymph nodes are often strikingly enlarged, sometimes tenfold.

Renal structural changes are almost invariably present.[138] In most instances they consist of only minimal increases in mesangial matrix deposits in the glomeruli. More significant forms of glomerulopathy may also occur, such as the focal glomerulitis or diffuse proliferative glomerulonephritis associated with infective endocarditis. In addition, focal glomerulosclerosis (p. 1015) or membranoproliferative glomerulonephritis (p. 1016) are

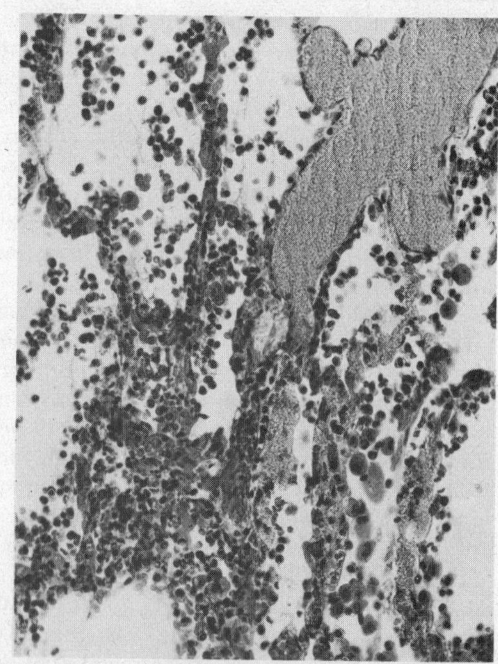

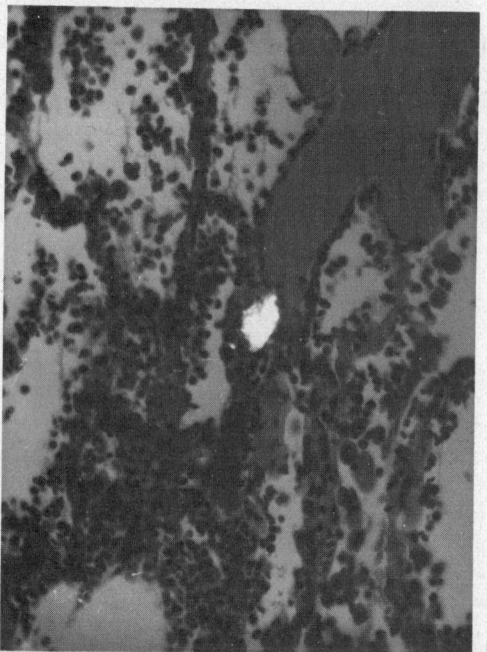

Figure 10–19. Lung of a heroin addict. The alveoli contain many desquamated mononuclear cells. A large congested vessel is seen at upper right, and immediately below it is a small collection of crystalline material seen better under polarizing light (B) as doubly refractile deposits of talc.

sometimes present and induce the nephrotic syndrome.[139]

A miscellany of additional problems complicate the lives of addicts. They are at risk of developing tetanus secondary to deep-seated skin infections resulting from "skin-popping" (subcutaneous inoculations). Peripheral neuropathy, spinal cord transverse myelopathy of an acute necrotizing nature, acute-to-chronic myopathy sometimes mysteriously involving muscles remote from injection sites, and osteomyelitis are relatively infrequent sequelae of addiction. Other problems could be cited, but it is evident that the price of addiction is more than the cost of the drug.

Industrial Carcinogens

It is widely held that life style and environmental influences play some role in the initiation of 80 to 90% of human cancers.[140] These influences range from personal practices (e.g., diet, smoking, alcohol consumption, exposure to therapeutic drugs or sunlight) to more generalized hazards such as air and water pollution and industrial carcinogens. Most of these influences have been considered elsewhere; here, our concern is with the carcinogenic hazards encountered in the workplace.

Human ingenuity in synthesizing new chemical agents outruns the ability to establish their safety. The number of organic chemicals synthesized since 1940 has doubled approximately every eight years.[141] At present, about 45,000 substances are listed in the Environmental Protection Agency's inventory of chemicals in commercial use. Among the 7000 tested, one-fifth have been labeled carcinogenic, but with some there is still disagreement. The problems involved in determining the carcinogenicity of an agent were discussed on page 240. For example, large doses are administered to experimental animals in an attempt to reduce the latent period involved in the induction of tumors. If the dosages far exceed those that might apply to human experience, do they fairly evaluate clinical carcinogenicity? Notwithstanding these difficulties, there is substantial evidence that occupational exposure has induced cancers in workers, and indeed it is estimated that 1 to 5% of all human cancers are job related.[142] A few of the most hazardous industrial agents are cited in Table 10–3. Further information on this important issue can be found in the Report of the Subcommittee on Environmental Carcinogenesis, National Cancer Advisory Board[143] and in the scholarly study of Schottenfeld and Haas.[144]

PHYSICAL INJURIES

The many forms of physical energy that may give rise to injury can be classified into four groups: mechanical violence, changes in temperature, changes in atmospheric pressure, and electromagnetic energy. Of the physical agents, mechanical violence exemplified by the everyday occurrence of auto accidents is the most frequent cause of injury encountered in clinical practice. Much detail on mechanical injuries is unnecessary in general pathology, since only rarely do such cases necessitate pathologic study save for legal purposes. Changes in atmospheric pressure and hypothermia are relatively uncommon causes of injury but hyperthermia (burns) are all too common. Radiation injuries, too, have assumed frightening importance as potential causes of widespread destruction.

MECHANICAL VIOLENCE

Injury from mechanical violence may occur whenever a mass hits the body, the body collides with a stationary mass, or, as sometimes occurs, both body and mass are in movement at the moment of impact. Several categories of tissue injury or wounds may result, which can be grouped broadly into: (1) soft tissue injuries, (2) bone injuries, and (3) head injuries. Injuries of the bones (p. 1325) and of the head (p. 1398) involve specialized problems best considered in the chapters dealing with these structures. Soft tissue injury falls principally into the realms of surgery, inflammation, and repair and involves no special problems in anatomic pathology. However, a few brief definitions are in order. An *abrasion* represents the mechanical tearing away of superficial layers or the entire thickness of the epidermis. A *laceration* is a split or tear in tissues that results from stretching beyond the tensile strength of the structure. Although commonly used interchangeably with the term "cut," strictly speaking, the latter is better referred to as an *incised wound.* A *contusion* is an injury caused by a blunt force that injures small blood vessels and causes interstitial bleeding, usually without disruption of the continuity of the tissue. A bruise of the skin is an example of a contusion. Sometimes deep-seated contusions of skeletal muscle, for example, may occur without evident injury to the skin or subcutaneous tissues. Analogously, laceration of the liver and spleen may be encountered in victims of an automobile accident without demonstrable damage to the abdominal wall. The possible systemic reactions to mechanical trauma are presented in the consideration of shock (p. 112).

CHANGES IN TEMPERATURE

As a homeothermic animal, man must maintain his internal temperature within the narrow range of 31° to 41°C, and even this upper limit can be tolerated only very briefly. However, it is by no means certain that the lower temperature cited represents an absolute limit, since at the present time our knowledge of the reactions of the body tissues to cold is being rapidly expanded by the use of hypothermia as a potential clinical tool in surgery.

Since abnormally high and low temperatures produce different patterns of tissue damage and have different pathogenetic mechanisms, they will be discussed separately.

Table 10–3. CERTAIN INDUSTRIAL AGENTS ASSOCIATED WITH CANCER-FEDERALLY REGULATED CARCINOGENS*

	Animal Studies		
Agent	***Species***	***Route of Administration***	***Target Organs and Lesions***
Asbestos fibers	Rat Rat Rat, hamster, rabbit	p.o. Inhalation Intrapleural	Multiple Lung, mesothelioma Mesothelioma
Occupation: Asbestos miners; Asbestos textile makers; auto brake repairers; cement mixers; construction workers; cutters and layers of water pipes; insulation cord makers; insulators; shipyard workers			
Coke oven emissions (aromatic hydrocarbons including benzo[a]-pyrene)	Multiple	Skin Intratracheal	Lung Local sarcomas, lung
Occupation: Coke oven workers			
α-Naphthylamine	Dog Mouse Hamster	p.o. p.o., s.c. p.o.	Negative Inconclusive Negative
Occupation: Chemical synthesizers; dye makers; rubber workers			
β-Naphthylamine	Dog Monkey	s.c., p.o. p.o.	Bladder Bladder
Occupation: Research workers			
4-Aminodiphenyl	Mouse Dog	p.o. p.o.	Bladder, liver Bladder
Occupation: Diphenylamine workers; research workers			
Benzidine and its salts	Mouse Dog	s.c.	Liver, ear duct, intestine Bladder
Occupation: Biochemists; dye workers; medical laboratory workers; organic chemical synthesizers; plastic workers; rubber workers; wood chemists			
Vinyl chloride	Rat	Inhalation	Skin, lung, osteochondroma
Occupation: Organic chemical synthesizers; polyvinyl resin makers; rubber workers			
Chloromethyl methyl ether (CMME)	Mouse	Skin, s.c.	Carcinoma, sarcoma
Occuption: Organic chemical synthesizers			
Bis (chloromethyl) ether (BCME)	Mouse Rat	Skin, s.c. s.c.	Olfactory esthesioneuroepithelioma, lung adenoma, papilloma, carcinoma Fibrosarcoma
Occupation: Ion exchange resin makers; laboratory workers; organic chemical synthesizers; polymer makers			

*From Schottenfeld, D. M., and Haas, J. F.: Carcinogens in the workplace. Ca *29*:144, 1979.

Abnormally Low Temperatures

The effects of hypothermia depend on whether there is whole body exposure or exposure only of parts. The frostbitten toe may be irreparably damaged, but death may result when the whole body is exposed, without inducing apparent necrosis of cells or tissues. The systemic homeostatic mechanisms are more vulnerable to hypothermia than are individual cells.

LOCAL REACTIONS. Chilling or freezing of cells and tissues causes injury in two ways:

1. Direct effects are probably mediated by physical dislocations within cells and the high salt concentrations incident to the crystallization of the intracellular water. In vitro, this mechanism of cellular injury can be largely prevented by glycerol (used as a preservative in sperm "banks").

2. Indirect effects are exerted by microcirculatory changes. Depending on the rate at which the temperature drops and its duration, slowly developing chilling may induce vasoconstriction and some cellular injury, followed by paralysis of vasomotor control and consequent vasodilation and increased permeability, leading to edematous changes. Alternatively, with sudden sharp

Table 10–3. CERTAIN INDUSTRIAL AGENTS ASSOCIATED WITH CANCER-FEDERALLY REGULATED CARCINOGENS* *(Continued)*

Clinical and Epidemiologic Studies				
Route of Absorption	***Latency (years)***	***Relative Risk***	***Target Organs and Lesions***	**Comments**
Lung Oral	15–50	1.5–12 100+ 1.5–3	Lung Mesothelioma Gastrointestinal tract (esophagus, stomach and large intestine)	Lung cancer synergism between asbestos and cigarette smoking. Because of rarity of mesothelioma in absence of asbestos exposure, relative risk estimate has limited meaning. The number of potentially exposed workers is some 1.6 million. Current estimates of proportionate mortality in heavily exposed workers are lung cancer (20–25%), mesothelioma (7–10%) and gastrointestinal cancers (8–9%).
		2.7	Lung Kidney	Animal studies refer to benzo[a]pyrene, though other aromatic hydrocarbons found in emissions are also carcinogenic in various animal systems. Risk of lung cancer in humans increases with duration and intensity of exposure.
Lung Skin	22	8.4	Bladder	Some questions remain as to whether or not observed human carcinogenicity is due to contamination with β-naphthylamine.
Lung Skin	16	87	Bladder	Previously widely used in dyestuffs, as an antioxidant for rubber and in rubber-coated cables. Little commercial production since 1972.
Lung Skin	15–35		Bladder	Formerly used as a rubber antioxidant and as a dye intermediate. No longer commercially produced. Fifty-three bladder tumors in 315 exposed workers; 1 case occurred with only 133 days of exposure.
Lung Skin Oral	16	14	Bladder	Medical personnel using benzidine to test for occult blood.
Lung ?Skin	12–29	Marked increase 1.6 (?)	Angiosarcoma of the liver Lung Brain	Full potential risk of cancer and hepatobiliary tract disease in humans is not yet established.
Lung Skin	10–15	8	Lung	Small cell carcinomas. Human exposures generally involve both CMME and BCME.
	10–15	100	Lung	Small cell carcinoma.

drops in temperature that are persistent, the vasoconstriction and increased viscosity of the blood in the local area may essentially cause ischemic injury. In this situation, only after the temperature begins to return toward normal do the vascular injury and increased permeability with exudation become evident. However, during the period of ischemia, hypoxic changes and infarction necrosis of the affected tissues may develop.

The anatomic changes can be anticipated from the preceding remarks. Exposure to long-continued nonfreezing temperature, such as occurs in *immersion or trench foot,* induces first a waxy-gray pallor to the extremity, sometimes marked by blotchy, mottled cyanosis. The vasodilatation in vessels that later develops leads to exudation of large amounts of proteinaceous fluid, producing swelling and large epidermal vesicles or bullae. With more severe cold injury, as seen in *frostbite,* degenerative myelin changes often occur in the peripheral nerves, giving rise to sensory and motor disturbances. In some cases, thrombosis may occur and may lead to gangrenous necrosis of the affected part. When the chilling reaches freezing temperatures, gangrene is more certain. If gangrene does not occur, the hypoxia may cause sufficient cellular damage to lead to residual atrophy and fibrosis of the skin and its adnexal structures.

SYSTEMIC REACTIONS. When the entire body is exposed to low temperatures, there is at first marked vasoconstriction of the skin vessels, and as a result the skin becomes extremely pale. As the hypothermia continues, marked peripheral vasodilatation and hyperemia develop. Cooling of the peripheral blood soon causes depression of the temperature in the vital organs, particularly the brain, though the usual mechanism of death appears to be circulatory failure. Sudden acute chilling may cause death within a relatively short time without apparent alteration of the bodily tissues. Under these circumstances, there may be no pathognomonic anatomic changes demonstrable at the time of postmortem examination. Sometimes, widespread thromboses appear with infarctions of internal organs. Acute necrotizing pancreatitis has also been observed.[145] With more slowly developing, protracted hypothermia, the anatomic changes are usually limited to the superficial tissues and extremities, and resemble those described in the local reactions.

Thermal Burns

Thermal burn injury causes approximately 10,000 deaths annually in the United States, so is obviously a problem of considerable clinical magnitude. A large proportion of the fatalities occur among children and young adults. The clinical significance of a burn is determined by the following variables: (1) the percentage of the total body surface involved, (2) the depth of injury of the surface burn, and (3) the possible development of internal injuries from inhalation of hot gases and fumes. These variables require that surface burns be segregated from internal heat injury.

SURFACE BURNS. The amount of surface area involved and the intensity and duration of hyperthermia determine the clinical significance of a burn. Obviously the larger the area, the more grave the prognosis. At one time, involvement of 50% of the body surface was almost always fatal. With the great improvements in therapy, there is no upper limit that can be said to be uniformly fatal, but much depends on the depth of injury. The older terminology of first-, second-, and third-degree burns has now been replaced by the division into "partial-" or "full-thickness" burns. This distinction has clinicopathologic significance, since a full-thickness burn implies an open wound from which large amounts of fluid and plasma proteins may be lost. Moreover, a full-thickness burn may not be capable of self-repair and often requires grafting, since there has been destruction of the dermal appendages from which reepithelialization occurs. Partial-thickness burns, which imply a low intensity of heat (43° to 46°C), induce injury in part by accelerated metabolism of cells, in part by inactivation of temperature-critical enzymes, and in part by inducing vascular injury. As is well-known, the area becomes reddened as small blood vessels dilate, followed soon by increased capillary permeability with exudation of serous or protein-rich fluid, creating the typical "burn blister." The surface epithelial cells in the partial-thickness burn likewise give evidence of deranged membrane permeability with nuclear and cellular swelling. Depending on the variables of temperature and time, transepidermal necrosis may occur. If the skin has not been totally incinerated, the epithelial cells may disclose nuclear pyknosis and granular coagulation of the cytoplasm.[146] The dermal collagen takes on the appearance of a homogeneous gel. The cytologic changes just described may affect ever deeper cells, including fibroblasts and endothelial and skeletal muscle cells. With intense heat there may be coagulation of the blood vessels and little evidence of exudation, but at the peripheral and deep borders between the nonviable and viable tissue, the described cellular and vascular changes will be evident as well as the inflammatory response.[147]

With burns of more than 20% of the body surface, systemic reactions become more important than the local injury. *Shock is the most important postburn concern* (p. 112). It may be partly neurogenic in origin but soon thereafter is related to the massive outpouring of an exudate. *Progressive loss of plasma water induces hypovolemia and hemoconcentration.* Plasma proteins are simultaneously lost and over the span of hours, with hemodilution, the plasma oncotic pressure falls to aggravate the fluid loss. In addition, *burns are frequently accompanied by acute gastroduodenal ulcerations* (Curling's ulcers) (p. 813). *Intravascular hemolysis* may occur at temperatures over 38°C and lead to hemoglobinuria as one of the features of the renal changes in shock.

Sepsis resulting from burn-wound infection is probably the single most important cause of death in the seriously burned patient. In a large study by Teplitz, 74% of fatalities died with a significant degree of burn-wound infection.[148] The burn wound is generally sterile for a period of approximately 24 hours after injury. Bacteria then contaminate the surface and rapidly proliferate to staggering numbers in the range of 100,000 to hundreds of millions of bacteria per sq cm of the burn-wound injury. These bacteria progressively invade the deeper layers, eventually to reach the subjacent viable tissue. Although staphylococci and streptococci have been chief offenders in the past, the gram-negative bacilli, predominantly *Pseudomonas aeruginosa*, but sometimes other gram-negative rods, have now become the major clinical problem. These organisms liberate products that of themselves are capable of producing endotoxic shock, but in addition there is direct invasion of the viable subjacent tissue that leads to massive infection of the subcutaneous fat as well as deeper tissues. *P. aeruginosa* has a predilection for penetration of the blood vessel walls to produce bacteremias. The vulnerability to bacterial infection is not attributable solely to devitalization of tissues. Thermal injury has been reported to induce immunosuppression either because of the appearance in the serum of an immunosuppressive factor or because of activation of T-suppressor cells.[149, 150] Impaired phagocytic function of macrophages has also been described and attributed to loss of their capacity to elaborate fibronectin, which facilitates attachment of bacteria to the cell membrane prior to engulfment.

Not only is the burn area itself colonized by bacteria, but the entire skin surface of the patient harbors organisms that have the distressing potential of producing infections at venipuncture sites, septic phlebitis in veins used for fluid replacement therapy, and infections in and around tracheostomies.

INTERNAL THERMAL INJURY. Individuals trapped in a burning building who inhale noxious fumes and heat may develop thermal injuries at any level of the respiratory tract from nose and mouth to the peripheral pulmonary parenchyma. Oral cavity burns may appear analogous to surface burn—partial- to full-thickness. The epiglottis is often charred. The laryngeal and tracheobronchial mucosa may be severely injured, with secondary intense hyperemic edema that threatens the airway. Most distressing is the development, hours to one or two days later, of the *acute respiratory distress syndrome* (p. 714) with severe pulmonary transudation and exudation. These pulmonary complications are present in 30% of patients dying within either the immediate resuscitative or postresuscitative periods. In addition to pulmonary edema, secondary infections with the development of bronchopneumonia, intra-alveolar hemorrhages, and atelectasis are frequently found.

Thus, the severely burned patient confronts not only the effects of the direct injury but, even more important, its serious systemic consequences.

HEAT STROKE. Heat stroke may result from either inability to dissipate the heat generated by the endogenous metabolic processes in febrile patients or exposure of the whole body to elevated ambient temperatures. When the body temperature reaches 40°C or higher, generalized peripheral vasodilatation occurs with sequestration of large volumes of blood, leading to a reduction in the effective circulating volume. If the compensatory mechanisms are not adequate, volume flow to the brain and heart is reduced, manifested principally by stimulation of the medullary centers and tachypnea and tachycardia. These physiologic adjustments are soon followed by irregular breathing and heart rate. Persistence of the hyperthermia and peripheral pooling of blood will soon lead to hypoxic injury of cells and with it derangement of the intracellular sodium pump, leading to excessive shifts of potassium into the extracellular fluid and blood. Hyperkalemia thus develops. When death occurs it is related to respiratory, circulatory, or electrolyte imbalances. If the body temperature reaches the excessive levels of 41° to 44°C for even a relatively brief period of time, some of the cellular changes described in the discussion of local reactions to extreme heat may appear before death occurs.[151, 152]

CHANGES IN ATMOSPHERIC PRESSURE

The direction of the pressure change (since in general the body withstands increases of pressure better than decreases), the magnitude of the change, and the rate of change all modify the extent, nature, and severity of the tissue damage. For example, sudden violent increases in pressure cause trauma by compression of the thorax and abdomen, while the subsequent negative wave of pressure results in explosive rupture of the respiratory tree or hollow viscera. The same pressure changes, applied slowly, might be without effect.

Changes in atmospheric pressure cause injuries in one of three ways: (1) sudden increases or decreases of pressure may produce mechanical damage—blast injury; (2) with sudden decrease in pressure, free gaseous bubbles may be released in the blood and act as emboli, described earlier as caisson disease (p. 106); and (3) in low atmospheric pressures, lowered oxygen tension in the inspired air causes systemic hypoxia as is seen in high-altitude reactions. Only the first of these three forms of injury requires description here.

Blast Injury

Blast injury is incurred from sudden violent changes in pressure as in an explosion. The forces may be transmitted by air (air blast) or water (immersion blast). These two forms of injury differ in several respects. In air blast, compressive waves impinge against the body, usually from one direction, followed by a sudden wave of decreased pressure exerting a negative force effect. Pressure on the exposed side of the body may collapse the thorax, rupture solid viscera, and cause widespread hemorrhages. The compressive wave may also enter the body orifices, particularly the respiratory passages, and produce multiple pulmonary hemorrhages associated with rupture of alveolar walls or massive laceration. Visceral infarctions due to mysteriously developing gaseous emboli have been noted in animals experimentally exposed to blast injury.

In immersion blast, the pressure is applied to the body from all sides, tending to force the body up out of water. Persons floating in an erect position are lifted slightly, if at all, and thus sustain severe injuries to the lower half of the body, while individuals floating horizontally on the surface may simply be tossed out of the water virtually unharmed. The positive pressure in immersion blast compresses the abdomen and causes lacerations of the diaphragm and compressive rupture of the hollow viscera of the intestines as well as solid organs, i.e., spleen, kidneys, and liver. The wave of compression may enter the anal orifice and produce an explosive effect on the large bowel. Rupture of the intestines may also occur from sudden expansion of the abdominal contents during the ensuing negative phase of pressure.

ELECTRICAL INJURIES

The passage of an electrical current through the body may be without effect or may cause tissue injury or sudden death. Many variables are involved: (1) the nature of the current (direct or alternating), (2) its amperage, (3) its voltage, (4) the path of the current through the body, (5) the resistance of the intervening tissues, and (6) the duration of exposure. Each of these variables modifies the nature and extent of the injury. Alternating current is more dangerous than direct current because it induces strong, sometimes violent muscular contractions—witness the unfortunate individual who cannot let go of a high-tension wire. The intensity of electrical flow through the tissues is a function of its amperage and voltage and the resistance of the tissues. Depending on the duration of the exposure, the passage of the current may create significant amounts of heat to produce electrothermal burns. The pathway that the current takes is of critical importance, since electrical energy disrupts normal neural impulses. Thus, the flow of current through the brain may interrupt the normal cardiac and respiratory impulses from the medulla (the mechanism of death in electrocution). A similar flow of current through the lower part of the body might induce injury but not death.

The tissues of the body in general are good conductors of electricity and transmit this current to some point of exit in contact with the ground. Local injuries are usually produced at the skin sites of entry and exit, since the skin has the highest resistance to the flow of electrical energy. Once having entered the body, the current tends to flow in all directions and passes in a broad front through the cross-sectional areas that intervene between its entrance and exit points. The high potentials thus dispersed may cause little damage except possibly for their action upon neuroregulatory mechanisms.

Much of the damage caused by electrical energy is due to the production of heat. The greater the resistance to conductance, the greater the heat. Skin has the highest resistance to conductance, with dry and thick skins being more resistant than moist or thin skins; dry and thick skins thus generate more heat. The surface area making up the contact with the electrical current also modifies the total amount of heat developed within cells. It has already been indicated that, when the contact surfaces are large, dispersion of the energy load lowers the heat generation to which individual cells are exposed. A similar potential applied in a concentrated focus might produce serious damage. It is this principle that permits the passage of high electrical potentials through broad cross-sectional areas of the body without causing morphologic alterations.

The morphologic effects of the passage of an electrical current vary from superficial skin burns to deep visceral lesions. With high-intensity current, linear arborizing burns known as "lightning marks" appear on the skin. Usually, burn marks are found at the points of entry and exit of the current. Low-intensity currents, transmitted through water or when there is a good contact surface as with moist skin, may cause no skin reaction and yet be of sufficient intensity to produce death by disturbing the cardiac or pulmonary rhythmic impulses. The internal morphologic effects are varied and depend on the voltage and amperage of the current. Lightning may cause sufficient heat and production of steam to explode solid organs and even fracture bones. Focal hemorrhages from rupture of small vessels may be seen in the brain. Sometimes death is preceded by violent convulsions related to the passage of the current through the nervous system.

RADIATION INJURY

Radiant energy provides an invaluable modality of clinical diagnosis and cancer treatment, but at the same time it is both a potent mutagen and a carcinogen and can be terrifyingly destructive, as was all too graphically documented at Hiroshima and Nagasaki.[153] Here we are concerned with its potential for injuring cells, tissues, and indeed the entire organism. We will not delve into the details of the physics of radiation, which is better left to specialized texts.[154, 155] It suffices for our purposes that radiation may occur in two forms: (1) electromagnetic waves (x-rays and gamma rays), (2) energetic charged particles (alpha, beta—also known as electrons, protons, pi-mesons, and heavy ions) as well as neutral high-energy particles, e.g., neutrons. All these forms of radiation exert their effects on cells by the transfer of energy to the molecules and atoms within the cell. With sufficient energy transfer orbiting, electron(s) may be separated from the atomic nucleus, producing *ionization* of the atom or molecule. Transfer of less energy may only move the electron into an orbit more distant from the nucleus—*excitation*. Both the ionized and excited states are unstable and have great potential for chemical reactions, but the biologic effect of radiation on cells is induced largely by ionization.

MECHANISMS OF ACTION. It is somewhat anticlimactic to admit that, although we know that radiation largely causes ionization of matter, we still do not understand precisely how radiant energy exerts its biologic effect on the cell. Two proposals have been made: (1) the *"target theory,"* also known as the "direct hit," "quantum hit," or "direct action" theory; and (2) the *"indirect action"* theory.[156]

The *target theory"* proposes that radiant energy acts by direct hits on target molecules within the cell. It is possible that a single hit might ionize and inactivate a single vital compound or a substance, thus damaging or even killing the cell. Equally possible is the requirement that multiple targets must be hit or a single target must be hit more than once. These three possibilities are sometimes referred to as (1) single-hit, (2) multitarget, and (3) multihit models.[157] The cumulative evidence suggests that DNA is the most vulnerable target of radiation and, more specifically, the linkage and bonds within the DNA molecule.[158] However, the macromolecules within membranes, enzymes, and other constituents are also damaged by radiation.

The *"indirect action theory"* proposes that radiant energy exerts its effect by producing free "hot" radicals within cells, according to the following sequence: Absorbed radiant energy leads to the radiolysis of cell water and the formation of the ionized water molecules H_2O^+ and H_2O^-. These dissociate to form the free radicals H· and OH·, which in turn initiate a chain of reactions with themselves, their own reaction products, and tissue water to form other reactive radicals, such as $H_2O_2^{\cdot}$ and $HO_2^{\cdot}$. Ultimately, these free radicals interact with critical components, among which membranes, nucleic acids and enzymes are the most important. In this sequential manner, a crucial biochemical change takes place, causing cell damage or death (p. 10).

The transfer of energy to a target atom or molecule from the incident source of radiant energy occurs within microfractions of a second, yet its biologic effect may not become apparent for minutes or even decades. *Radiation therefore has a latency.*[159] During this latent period, it must be assumed (although it is poorly understood) that sequential reactions are occurring that ultimately exert a detectable functional or morphologic effect. Both "direct" and "indirect" actions of radiation could start such a chain reaction, but the "indirect theory" would relate better to its latent effect.

QUANTITATION OF RADIATION. *The biologic effect of radiation is largely dependent on the total dosages and the rate of its delivery and absorption.* Later we shall discuss the variable sensitivity of the differing cells and tissues in the body to radiation, but here it should be emphasized that all living matter can be destroyed by radiant energy. Critical, then, to the biologic effects of radiation is dosage.

The *quantitation of radiation* is expressed in several kinds of units for the various forms of radiant energy. X-rays or gamma rays are measured in *roentgens (R)*. A roentgen unit is a measure of the ionization produced by electromagnetic radiation in air, defined as the quantity of radiation required to induce in 1 cc of air an emission equivalent to 1 electrostatic unit of charge. Roentgens deal with air exposure, but it is obvious that more important is the quantity absorbed. The *rad (r)* is the quantity of radiation based on the absorption of 100 ergs of energy per gm of target tissue. For example, one roentgen will lead to the absorption of about 87 ergs per gm of tissue.

A recently introduced unit of radiation measurement is the gray (gy), which equals 100 rads. Thus, one centigray equals one rad. Radionuclides are quantitated in terms of their instantaneous rate of disintegration measured in curies (ci) and their half-life. One curie of radioactive isotope undergoes 3.7 times 10^{10} disintegrations per second. The half-life of the isotope defines the time during which one half of the unstable atoms of the isotope will have disintegrated.

BIOLOGIC EFFECTS OF RADIATION. The discussion of the impact of radiation on cells and tissues will be divided into the following: (1) general considerations, (2) effects on cells and tissues, (3) changes induced in certain specific organ systems, and (4) effects of total body irradiation.

General Considerations. The amount of biologic damage induced by radiant energy is determined by the character of the radiation, i.e., the type of electromagnetic wave or particle, the total amount of radiation administered and absorbed (namely, total dose), and the time frame within which this amount is delivered. Although all forms of radiation ultimately induce ionization of atoms and molecules within cells, two characteristics referred to as *"relative biologic effectiveness" (RBE)* and *"linear energy transfer" (LET)* materially modify the extent and distribution of the damage in tissues. The LET defines the amount of energy transferred per unit path length and involves such considerations as mass, charge, and velocity. *The LET value of a form of radiation indicates the likelihood of its having an effect within a target area.* Alpha particles, for example, because of their relatively low velocity, large mass, and high charge, have a much higher LET potential than high-velocity, smaller beta particles of the same energy, which penetrate more deeply but deliver less energy per unit path length. Gamma rays have a relatively low LET because of their penetrability, thus dissipating their energy over a long distance. Because incident "collisions" along the path of charged particles slows their velocity, the LET gradually increases along the track even though some of the energy may have been leached out by transfer to target atoms and molecules. As the particle comes to rest there is a dramatic increase in the LET, referred to as the "Bragg peak." *The RBE relates to the amount of cellular damage caused by a specific amount of radiant energy.* For example, 1 rad of absorbed energy delivered by x-rays is deposited in a fairly uniform distribution within a field of cells. Thus, although many cells may be affected, none may absorb sufficient energy to be seriously damaged. On the other hand, if the same dose were absorbed from alpha particles the energy distribution would be spotty and random, but it might be lethal to every cellular target that was hit. The RBE, then, relates the absorbed dose of radiant energy to its biologic effect.

It may already be evident that the different forms of radiant energy vary in their ability to penetrate tissues. But penetrance is equally dependent on the nature of the target matter that constitutes the collision course of the radiation. Slow-moving, highly charged particles of large mass may have a high LET but they penetrate less deeply through the skin than fast-moving, lighter, lower-charged beta particles of the same energy that have a lower LET. Thus, alpha radiation has more effect on superficial tissues such as the skin and subcutaneous structures than beta radiation, which reaches much deeper levels. The penetrability of electromagnetic radiation depends largely on its energy. Much deeper penetration is achieved by 100-kV generated roentgen rays than by that produced by 10-kV machines.[160] As mentioned, the various cells and tissues of the body differ in their resistance to penetration by radiant energy. The outer keratinous shell of man is an excellent, albeit not impermeable, radiation shield. Once penetrated, however, the subcutaneous tissues offer far less resistance. With respect to living matter, penetration is a function of the number of interactions between the radiant energy and target matter that eventually absorbs all the energy in the radiation. Penetration ceases once all energy has been dissipated.

The rate of delivery significantly modifies the biologic effect. Although the effect of radiant energy is cumulative, when delivered in divided doses or fractions, as is the practice in radiotherapy, cells may be able to repair some of the damage sustained during the intervals. Evidence of such repair is provided by a few genetic disorders such as *xeroderma pigmentosum*, discussed on page 241. Individuals with this condition have a greatly increased vulnerability to skin cancers related to an inability to repair sunlight-induced dimers in the DNA of epidermal cells. *Thus, fractional dosages of radiant energy have a cumulative effect only to the extent that repair during the intervals is incomplete.* Radiotherapy of tumors exploits the fact that, in general, normal cells are capable of more rapid recovery, and so do not sustain as much cumulative radiation injury as tumor cells.

The oxygenation of cells and tissues modifies the effect of radiation—"the oxygen effect." Radiant energy may interact with molecular oxygen to induce free radicals such as superoxide. According to the indirect action theory, these free radicals may then interact with atoms and molecules to amplify the impact of radiation on cells. "The oxygen effect" assumes particular importance in the radiotherapy of neoplasms. When the centers of rapidly growing tumors are poorly vascularized, and therefore somewhat hypoxic, radiotherapy is rendered somewhat less effective.

Effects on Cells and Tissues. Radiant energy may (1) immediately kill cells; (2) block their replicative capacity; or (3) induce a number of nonlethal alterations of specific macromolecules, including enzymes and cell membranes, or induce a variety of mutations that may or may not be lethal, but some of which may be carcinogenic, as detailed on page 242. The first two are most easily documented in cell culture by quantitating the number of postradiation cells capable of replicating. The loss from this replicating pool can be expressed as "reproductive death."

The vulnerability or radiosensitivity of the many specialized forms of cells and tissues in the body varies widely. In general, *cells are sensitive to radiant energy in direct proportion to their reproductive or mitotic activity and in inverse proportion to their level of specialization.*[161] The same generalization applies to cancers. The more rapidly growing and undifferentiated the neoplasm, the more likely it will be radiosensitive. In general, tumors arising from radiosensitive tissues are themselves radiosensitive. The relative radiosensitivities of cells and associated cancers are given in Table 10–4, modified from Rubin and Casarett.[162]

Although some useful generalizations regarding the relative radiosensitivity of cells and their cancers are possible, there are many strange exceptions. For example, lymphocytes are exquisitely radiosensitive. While some are rapidly dividing, others are long-lived, perhaps for the lifetime of man; but as far as we now know, most are vulnerable to relatively low levels of radiation. The seminoma, which arises from germ cells, is radiosensitive as Table 10–4 indicates, but the embryonal carcinoma that is believed to arise from germ cells is radioresistant. Other factors may play a role here, and perhaps the immune response (more evident

Table 10–4. RADIOSENSITIVITY OF SPECIALIZED CELLS AND THEIR TUMORS

Radiosensitivity	Normal Cells	Tumors
High	Lymphoid, hematopoietic (marrow), germ cells, intestinal epithelium, ovarian follicular cells	Leukemia-lymphoma, seminoma, dysgerminoma, granulosa cell carcinoma
Fairly high	Epidermal epithelium, adnexal structures (hair follicles, sebaceous glands), oropharyngeal stratified epithelium, urinary bladder epithelium, esophageal epithelium, gastric gland epithelium, ureteral epithelium	Squamous cell carcinoma of skin, oropharyngeal, esophageal, cervical and bladder epithelium, adenocarcinoma of gastric epithelium
Medium	Connective tissue, glia, endothelium, growing cartilage or bone	Endothelio- and angiosarcomas, astrocytomas, the vasculature and connective tissue elements of all tumors
Fairly low	Mature cartilage or bone cells, mucous or serous gland epithelium, pulmonary epithelium, renal epithelium, hepatic epithelium, pancreatic epithelium, pituitary epithelium, thyroid epithelium, adrenal epithelium, nasopharyngeal nonstratified epithelium	Liposarcoma, chondrosarcoma, osteogenic sarcoma, adenocarcinoma of: breast epithelium, hepatic epithelium, renal epithelium, pancreatic epithelium, thyroid epithelium, adrenal gland epithelium, colon epithelium, squamous cell cancer of the lung
Low	Muscle cells, ganglion cells	Rhabdomyosarcoma, leiomyosarcoma, ganglioneuroma

Adapted from Rubin, R., and Casarett, G. W.: Clinical Radiation Pathology. Philadelphia, W. B. Saunders Co., 1968, p. 903.

in the case of the seminoma) cooperates to enhance the lethal effect of radiation. Such exceptions underscore the necessity for conservatism in prognosticating the possible effectiveness of radiotherapy in the treatment of a specific tumor in the individual patient.

All cells can be affected by radiant energy and, indeed, all living matter can be killed by radiation. The changes involve both the cytoplasm and the nucleus, but the latter appears to be more radiovulnerable. During the initial response to radiant injury, there is cellular swelling, cytoplasmic vacuolization, and alterations in plasma membranes. Mitochondria enlarge and assume distorted shapes, and some are disrupted. These mitochondrial changes may be secondary to other metabolic dislocations, since many observations suggest that mitochondria themselves are relatively radioresistant.[163] The endoplasmic reticulum is also affected, but lysosomes appear to be more resistant and are often increased in number.[164]

Nuclear changes are marked and include nuclear swelling, vacuolation, focal disappearance of the nuclear membrane, and, in severely affected cells, nuclear pyknosis or lysis. Following radiation injury, cells often assume bizarre sizes and shapes, sometimes with the formation of giant cells containing an extremely pleomorphic nucleus or more than one nucleus. Such nuclear pleomorphism and cellular distortion may persist for years after the radiation exposure.

Although, as pointed out, radiant energy may alter proteins and thus inactivate enzymes and injure membranes, the most vulnerable target within the cell is thought to be DNA. All manner of structural defects can be induced including the formation of pyrimidine dimers, cross-links, single-strand or double-strand breaks, and various rearrangements. If they are not immediately lethal they introduce errors in transcription that may lead to uncontrolled proliferation and the induction of cancer, as discussed in detail on page 248, or alternatively they block cell replication by interference with and/or delay of the mitotic process. It is proposed that genetic programs for the synthesis of mRNA and such vital enzymes as thymidine kinase and DNA polymerase are inhibited or blocked and so synthesis of DNA comes to a halt. For this reason, replicating cells requiring synthesis of DNA are more susceptible to radiation injury. All phases of the cell generation cycle can be affected by radiation, but the G_2 phase (just prior to mitosis) and the M (mitotic) phase are more vulnerable than the S (synthetic) and G_1 phases. It follows, therefore, that slowly dividing cells are less radiosensitive, probably because they have a longer time to recover from the radiation injury before they go into mitosis. Again, any and all of these effects are dose rate–dependent.

A wide range of chromosomal and chromatid mutations is induced by radiation, including deletions, breaks, translocations, interadherence of chromosomes, fragmentation, and indeed all forms of abnormal chromosome morphology.[155] The mitotic spindle often becomes disorderly or even chaotic. Polyploidy and aneuploidy may be encountered. As is well-known, radiation injury has the potential of inducing neoplasia with all its attendant karyotypic abnormalities (p. 231). *The constellation of cellular pleomorphism, giant cell formation, conformation changes in nuclei, and mitotic figures creates a more than passing similarity between radiation-injured cells and cancer cells, a problem that plagues the pathologist when evaluating postirradiation tissues for the possible persistence of tumor cells.* None of these mitotic and chromosomal mutations are diagnostic of radiation, since they can be produced also by certain chemicals.

Vascular changes are prominent in all irradiated tissues (dose rate–dependent), be they normal or neoplastic. Endothelial cells are only moderately radioresponsive but, with the intensive therapy administered to tumors, radiational changes are almost always seen in the vasculature of the neoplasm itself and in the normal tissues interposed between the source of the radiation and the neoplasm. During the immediate postirradiation period, vessels may show only dilatation, accounting for the erythema of the skin seen so often in radiotherapy. Later or with higher dosages, a variety of regressive changes appear, including endothelial cell swelling and vacuolation or even dissolution with total necrosis of the walls of small vessels (such as capillaries and venules). Affected vessels may rupture, yielding hemorrhages, or they may thrombose. For reasons unknown, these vascular changes are peculiarly spotty in their distribution along the course of a vessel and so, in the same tissue section, some channels are affected and others spared. In some part, the cancericidal effectiveness of radiation is attributable to such vascular damage. At a later stage, endothelial cell proliferation and collagenous hyalinization with thickening of the media are seen in irradiated vessels, resulting in marked narrowing or even obliteration of the vascular lumina (Fig. 10–20).[165]

Organ System Changes. The effects of radiation on certain specific organs and systems are worthy of special citation because of either the particular vulnerability of the organ or its frequent involvement.[166]

The *skin* is in the pathway of all intentionally or accidentally delivered external radiation. The changes encountered range from mild postirradiation (two to three days) erythema to late-appearing cancers. Depending on the dose rate and penetrability of the radiant energy, one may observe postirradiation (two to three weeks) edema and epithelial desquamation (four to six weeks). Chronic radiodermatitis takes many forms including blotchy, increased pigmentation or depigmentation, hyperkeratosis, epilation (one to two months), skin atrophy, dermal and subcutaneous fibrosis, and, in some instances, telangiectases and ulcerations (six months to five years) (Fig. 10–21). The epidermal cells may show any of the general cytologic alterations described previously, while the underlying dermis exhibits the characteristic radiation-induced vascular changes accompanied by hyaline collagenization of connective tissue and basophilic degeneration of elastic fibers. The atrophy, depigmentation, and telangiectasia commonly persist for decades.[167] Squamous cell skin cancers may

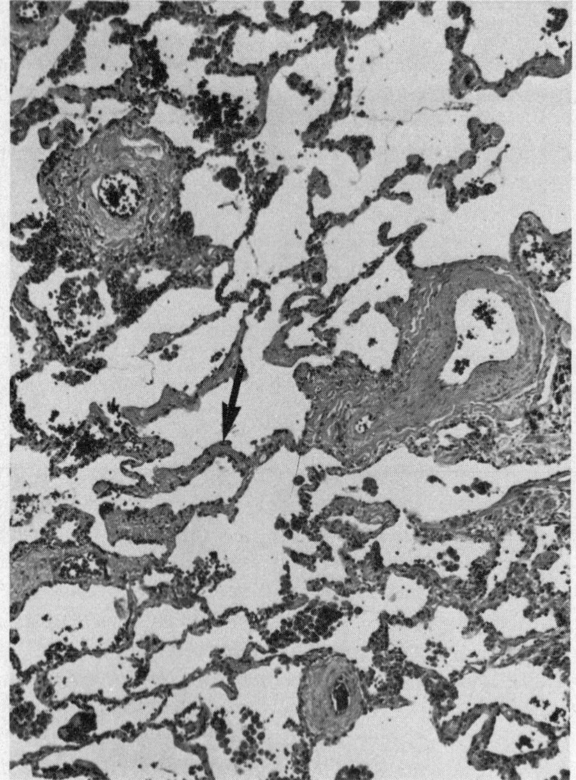

Figure 10–20. Chronic radiation damage to lungs. Note collagenous hyaline thickening of blood vessel walls and fibrosis of septal walls *(arrow)*.

appear years later (average eight to ten), sometimes as long as 56 years later.

The *hematopoietic and lymphoid systems* are extremely susceptible to radiant injury. With high dose levels and large exposure fields, severe lymphopenia may appear within hours of radiation, along with shrinkage of the lymph nodes and spleen. Radiation directly destroys lymphocytes, both in the circulating blood and in tissues (nodes, spleen, thymus, gut) and causes all the cytologic disorganizations already described. With sublethal doses of irradiation, regeneration is prompt, however, from viable precursors, leading to restoration of the normal lymphocyte complement of the blood within weeks to months. The circulating granulocyte count may at first rise but begins to fall toward the end of the first week. Levels near zero may be reached during the second week. If the patient survives, recovery of the normal granulocyte counts may require two to three months. Platelets are similarly affected, with the nadir of the count occurring somewhat later than that of the granulocytes, while recovery is similarly delayed. The hematopoietic cells in the bone marrow are also quite sensitive to radiant energy, including the red cell precursors. The marrow may become virtually acellular weeks after heavy exposure and may contain only varying numbers of disintegrated cells. Erythrocytes are radioresistant, but anemia may appear after two to three weeks and be persistent for months because of marrow damage. Obviously, the severity of the blood and marrow depletion and its clinical significance depend on the dosage of radiation and the extent of marrow damage. Whole body irradiation may be lethal. Localized exposure may have no effect on the circulating blood counts. The neutropenia and thrombocytopenia are responsible for increased susceptibility to infections and bleeding diatheses in the postirradiation period. If the patient survives these hazards and the hypoxic injury resulting from the anemia, regeneration from primitive precursors may yield complete recovery.

Studies of the survivors of the atomic bomb blasts have unmistakably demonstrated the leukemogenic effect of radiation (p. 470).

The *gonads* in both the male and female, particularly the germ cells, are highly vulnerable to radiation injury, and sterility is a frequent residual of such damage. In the testis, spermatogonia, then spermatocytes, spermatids, and spermatozoa are radiosensitive in the order given. The cytologic changes to be observed are those already described (p. 467) but, as late residuals, there may be total atrophy and fibrosis with hyalinization of the testicular tubules. Sertoli cells and interstitial cells are radioresistant. Within the ovary, the germ cells and even more so the follicular granulosal cells are vulnerable. Indeed, for given dosages of the same form of radiation, sterility is more frequent in the female than in the male, principally because of radiation destruction of the ovarian follicles. Cessation of menses and menopausal changes may be temporary or permanent, depending on the dosage of radiation. In passing, it should

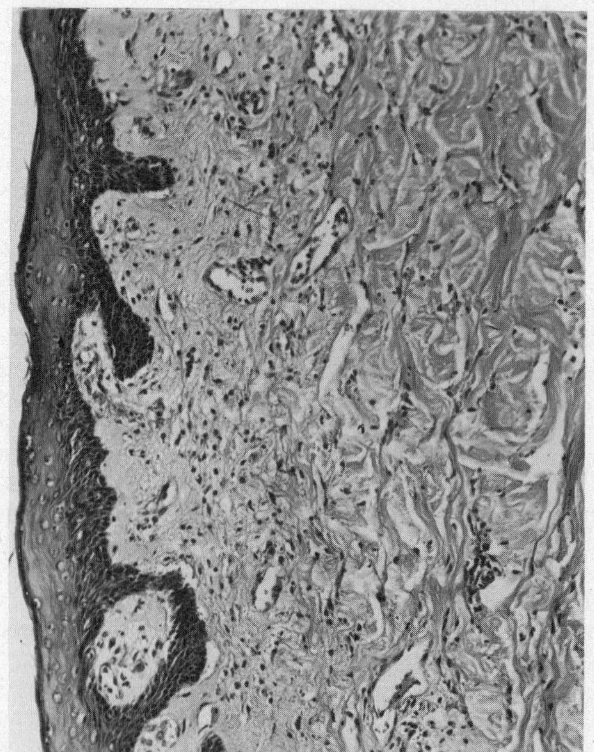

Figure 10–21. Chronic radiodermatitis. There is collagenous hyalinization of dermis, atrophy of skin appendages, and numerous dilated vascular telangiectases.

be noted that the uterus and cervix are quite radioresistant and hence permit the installation of radioactive elements into the uterine cavity for the treatment of endometrial carcinomas.

The *lungs*, because of their rich vascularization, are vulnerable to radiation injury, and shortness of breath, coughing, and even acute fatal respiratory insufficiency may appear within weeks to months following sufficient exposure of large segments of the lung fields. During the acute phase, the endothelial cell changes described in the blood vessels are seen in the alveolar capillaries. The increased vascular permeability may lead to marked pulmonary congestion, edema, fibrin exudation, the formation of hyaline membranes, and even total filling of the air spaces by a rich proteinaceous and cellular debris, creating changes very similar to those of bacterial pneumonia. Later changes include fibrosis of the alveolar walls and the described vascular wall thickening and luminal obliteration (Fig. 10–20). The respiratory dysfunction may be crippling or fatal since the "radiation pneumonitis" creates a profound alveolocapillary block. Bronchogenic carcinomas have occurred after prolonged inhalation of radioactive dusts by persons working in uranium mines.

The *gastrointestinal tract* is quite radiosensitive and is frequently affected in all forms of deep radiation. Soon after exposure, patients often have loss of appetite, nausea, and vomiting, and many develop severe diarrhea for a period of days. As might be expected, the intestinal epithelium is vulnerable because of its high turnover rate, and all forms of nuclear and cellular pleomorphism along with mitotic abnormalities are seen in mucosal cells in the postirradiation period. Mucosal edema, hyperemia, and ulcerations may appear, accompanied by vascular and connective tissue changes in the submucosa at all levels from the mouth to the anus. Later effects comprise mucosal and submucosal atrophy and fibrosis, accompanied sometimes by similar atrophy and fibrosis of the muscularis. These changes may indeed cause intestinal and esophageal strictures or even complete obstruction.

Nervous tissue is quite radiosensitive during embryonic development when nerve cells and glial cells are especially affected; relatively small doses of radiation in animals have caused severe damage to the developing central nervous system. Adult nervous tissue, on the other hand, is relatively radioresistant. Sufficiently high doses even in the adult may damage astrocytes and cause late-appearing injury to neurons.[168] However, functional changes may appear during the immediate postirradiation period even though no morphologic changes are visible in the neurons. Necrosis of the brain and spinal cord has been reported following high dosages of radiation, presumably owing to involvement of the small blood vessels.

Ultimately, all organs and cells are vulnerable to sufficiently high levels of radiant energy, but those not already mentioned are relatively radioresistant: e.g., the thyroid, parathyroid, pituitary, and adrenal glands; the liver; mature bone; and cartilage. Growing bone and cartilage are, however, relatively radiosensitive and development has been stunted in survivors of atomic bomb blasts who were exposed during childhood.[168] Even though the kidneys are not very radiosensitive, they sometimes develop so-called radiation nephritis, following sufficient exposure.

Total Body Radiation. Exposure of large areas of the body to even very small doses of radiation may have devastating effects.[169] As little as 100 to 300 rads of radiant energy in total body exposure delivered in one dose may induce an "acute radiation syndrome." To place this radiation level in context, it must be appreciated that 4000 rads or more are often used in carefully shielded patients in the radiotherapy of tumors. Warren has provided an excellent summary of the significance of various levels of whole body exposure (Table 10–5).[170] The lethal range for man begins at about 300 rads of total body radiation, but is quite certain at 1000 rads.

Table 10–5. EXPECTED SHORT-TERM EFFECTS FROM ACUTE WHOLE BODY RADIATION

Dose in Rads	Probable Effect
10 to 50	No obvious effect except, probably, minor blood changes
50 to 100	Vomiting and nausea for about one day in 5 to 10% of exposed personnel. Fatigue, but no serious disability. Transient reduction in lymphocytes and neutrophils.
100 to 200	Vomiting and nausea for about one day, followed by other symptoms of radiation sickness in about 25 to 50% of personnel. No deaths anticipated. A reduction of approximately 50% in lymphocytes and neutrophils will occur.
200 to 350	Vomiting and nausea in nearly all personnel on first day, followed by other symptoms of radiation sickness, e.g., loss of appetite, diarrhea, minor hemorrhage. About 20% die within 2 to 6 weeks after exposure; survivors convalesce for about 3 months, although many have a second wave of symptoms at about 3 weeks. Up to 75% reduction in all circulating blood elements.
350 to 550	Vomiting and nausea in most personnel on first day, followed by other symptoms of radiation sickness, e.g., fever, hemorrhage, diarrhea, emaciation. About 50% die within one month; survivors convalesce for about 6 months.
550 to 750	Vomiting and nausea (or at least nausea) in all personnel within 4 hours after exposure, followed by severe symptoms of radiation sickness, as above. Up to 100% die, few survivors convalesce for about 6 months.
1000	Vomiting and nausea in all personnel within 1 to 2 hours. All die within days.
5000	Incapacitation almost immediately (minutes to hours). All personnel will die within one week.

From Warren, S.: The pathology of ionizing radiation. *In* Bioastronautics Data Book. 2nd ed. Washington, D.C., NASA, 1973.

Depending on time-dose relationships, three acute radiation syndromes may develop: (1) hematopoietic, (2) gastrointestinal, and (3) cerebral.

The *hematopoietic syndrome* is encountered with the absorption of between 100 and 300 rads. It usually begins with mild gastrointestinal symptoms related to injury to the radiosensitive mucosal lining of the gut; these subside and are followed by changes in the peripheral blood in turn associated with progressive atrophy of lymph nodes, spleen, and bone marrow. The first alteration in the circulating blood is marked depression of lymphocytes, which may become maximal in 24 to 36 hours. This is followed in two to three days by the progressive development of thrombocytopenia, neutropenia, and eventually anemia. As a consequence of these changes, bleeding problems or infections may make their appearance.

The *gastrointestinal syndrome* occurs with a larger dose of absorbed radiation, on the order of 300 to 1000 rads. It makes its appearance with nausea, vomiting, and severe diarrhea. The loss of fluids may lead to dehydration, contraction of the effective circulating blood volume, vascular collapse, and death, usually within three to four days. These clinical signs and symptoms are related to widely scattered cell death throughout the body, particularly prominent in the actively replicating mucosal cells of the gastrointestinal tract. If the acute vascular collapse is effectively treated by massive plasma replacement, the hematopoietic syndrome almost always makes its appearance one to two days later.

The *cerebral syndrome* appears when the absorbed dose is greater than 1500 to 2000 rads. It is always fatal and is characterized by listlessness and drowsiness, soon followed by convulsions, coma, and death within one to two hours.

Absorption of 100 to 200 rads may or may not be lethal, but in any event it usually induces transient nausea and vomiting, sometimes followed by alterations in the peripheral blood similar to those described above. This is the mildest form of "acute radiation syndrome" associated with total body exposure.

In addition to these more or less "acute syndromes," total body irradiation may result in a number of late-appearing sequelae. These have been graphically documented in the survivors at Hiroshima and Nagasaki; the tragic consequences of the atomic blasts will be briefly reviewed "lest we forget." Morgan has movingly detailed the events.[153] The great preponderance of the more than 100,000 immediate or relatively early fatalities at these cities were the result of blast injuries and the following fire storms that engulfed these cities. Thousands more died from "acute radiation syndromes" and their sequelae. Months to years later a variety of forms of neoplasia began to appear. A 20-fold increased incidence of acute leukemia has occurred in those who were less than 10 years or over 50 years of age at the time of the blasts. The latent period for the appearance of these leukemias in children was approximately five to ten years, whereas in adults it was 10 to 20 years. These disorders took the forms of acute lymphocytic, acute myelogenous, and chronic myelogenous leukemia but, for unknown reasons, chronic lymphocytic leukemia was rarely induced. In children under 10 years of age at the time there has been an increased incidence of breast cancer (in females) and thyroid cancer as well as possibly lymphoma, multiple myeloma, and cancers of the stomach, esophagus, urinary tract and salivary glands.[171, 172] Individuals 50 years of age or older at the time of exposure have suffered a notable increase in the incidence of lung cancer. These postirradiation oncogenic changes are discussed in greater detail on page 242. In addition, atomic bomb survivors have developed lenticular opacities and persistent chromosomal aberrations in lymphocytes. Even those exposed in utero were not spared and have manifested an increased frequency of microcephaly and mental retardation.[173]

The atomic blasts make all too evident the injury-producing potential of radiant energy, albeit of enormous doses delivered within an instant in time. Because of its cumulative effects there is understandably great concern about low-level radiation, as may be emitted from nuclear reactors and improper disposal of nuclear wastes. To date, clear documentation of carcinogenicity has not appeared, but the long latency is not comforting. There is ample evidence that low-level radiation may be carcinogenic. Solar radiation and the diagnostic and therapeutic uses of this form of energy have caused cancers, as pointed out (p. 241). In few areas of medicine is the old dictum more applicable—be sure that the treatment is not worse than the disease.

NONIONIZING RADIATION

It would be imprudent to conclude a chapter on environmental pathology without calling attention to the possible dangers of ultrasound, microwave, and laser energy. Although all of them find increasingly wide usage for medical, domestic, and industrial purposes, few data are available regarding their impact on man.[174] The cell destructiveness of laser beams is currently under exploration in many forms of therapy. Experiments in lower animals have shown that microwaves may cause cellular changes in the lens, bone marrow, and endocrine glands and may possibly have DNA-damaging potential. Unquestionably, some of this injury is due to the thermal effect, which is of course the virtue of this form of radiation in microwave ovens. Ultrasound, too, has been shown to alter nerve transmission in lower animal forms, but once again it may relate to thermal effects. With the growing use of sonography in obstetrics and the widespread domestic and industrial use of ultrasonic cleaning devices and microwave ovens, we can only hope that these forms of energy will prove to have no late-appearing adverse effects.

1. Barney, G. O.: The Global 2000 Report to the President of the United States: Entering the 21st Century. Pergamon Press, New York, 1980, p. 1.
2. Environmental Quality—1980. The 11th Annual Report of the Council on Environmental Quality. Washington, D.C., U.S. Government Printing Office, 1980, p. 146.
3. Natusch, D.F.S., and Wallace, J.R.: Urban aerosol toxicity: The influence of particle size. Science *186*:695, 1974.
4. United States Public Health Service: Symposium on Environmental Lead Contamination. Publication No. 1440, March, 1966.
5. Selikoff, I. J.: Widening perspectives of occupational lung disease. Prev. Med. *2*:412, 1973.
6. Boren, H.G.: Pathobiology of air pollutants. Environ. Res. *1*:178, 1967.
7. Green, G.M., and Carolin, D.: The depressant effect of cigarette smoke on the in vitro antibacterial activity of alveolar macrophages. N. Engl. J. Med. *276*:422, 1967.
8. Mossman, B.T., et al.: Interaction of crocidolite asbestos with hamster respiratory mucosa in organ culture. Lab. Invest. *36*:131, 1977.
8A. Abraham, J.I.: Recent advances in pneumoconioses: The pathologist's role in etiologic diagnosis. Monographs in Pathology *19*:96, 1978.
9. Lamb, D.: Physiological/pathological correlations in coal workers' pneumoconiosis. Bull. Physiopathol. Resp. *11*:471, 1975.
10. Fisher, E.R., et al.: Objective pathological diagnosis of coal workers' pneumoconiosis. J.A.M.A. *245*:1829, 1981.
11. Cassidy, E.P.: The national coal workers autopsy study. The development and implementation of an occupational necropsy study. Arch. Pathol. *94*:133, 1972.
12. Morgan, W.K.C., et al.: Respiratory disability in coal miners. J.A.M.A. *243*:2401, 1980.
13. Cockroft, A., et al.: Postmortem study of emphysema in coalworkers and non-coalworkers. Lancet *2*:600, 1982.
14. Kleinerman, J., et al.: Pathology standards for coal workers' pneumoconiosis. Arch. Pathol. Lab. Med. *103*:375, 1979.
15. Caplan, A.: Certain radiological appearances in the chests of coal miners suffering from rheumatoid arthritis. Thorax *8*:29, 1953.
16. Benedek, T.G.: Rheumatoid pneumoconiosis. Documentation on onset and pathogenetic considerations. Am. J. Med. *55*:5151, 1973.
17. Guidotti, T.S.: Coal workers' pneumoconiosis and medical aspects of coal mining. South. Med. J. *72*:456, 1979.
18. Sweet, D.V., et al.: The relationship of total dust, free silica, and trace metal concentrations to the occupational respiratory disease of bituminous coal miners. Am. Ind. Hyg. Assoc. J. *35*:479, 1974.
19. Seaton, A., et al.: Quartz and pneumoconiosis in coal miners. Lancet *2*:1272, 1981.
20. Rooke, G.B., et al.: Carcinoma of the lung in Lancashire coal miners. Thorax *34*:229, 1979.
21. National Institute of Occupational Safety and Health: Mortality among coal miners covered by the UMWA Health and Retirement Funds. Research Report No. 77–155. Rockville, MD, NIOSH, 1977.
22. Snider, D.E.: The relationship between silicosis and tuberculosis. Am. Rev. Respir. Dis. *118*:455, 1978.
23. Reiser, K.M., and Last, J.A.: Silicosis and fibrogenesis: Fact and artifact. Toxicology *13*:51, 1979.
24. Heppleston, A.G.: The fibrogenic action of silica. Br. Med. Bull. *25*:282, 1969.
25. Harington, J.S.: Fibrogenesis. Environ. Health Perspec. *9*:271, 1974.
26. Davies, T.E., and Allison, A.C.: Secretion of macrophage enzymes in relation to the pathogenesis of chronic inflammation. *In* Nelson, D.S. (ed.): Immunobiology of the Macrophage. New York, Academic Press, 1976, p. 427.
27. Kane, A.B., et al.: Dissociation of intracellular lysosomal rupture from cell death caused by silica. J. Cell Biol. *87*:643, 1980.
28. Kilroe-Smith, T.A., et al.: An insoluble fibrogenic factor in macrophages from guinea pigs exposed to silica. Environ. Res. *6*:298, 1973.
29. Jones, R.M., et al.: High prevalence of antinuclear antibodies in sand blasters' silicosis. Am. Rev. Respir. Dis. *113*:393, 1976.
30. Editorial: New York Times, Sept. 7, 1982.
31. Craighead, J.E., and Mossman, B.T.: The pathogenesis of asbestos-associated diseases. N. Engl. J. Med. *306*:1446, 1982.
32. Murphy, R.L., Jr., et al.: Effects of low concentrations of asbestos: Clinical, environmental, radiologic and epidemiologic observations in shipyard pipe coverers and controls. N. Engl. J. Med. *285*:1970, 1971.
33. Vianna, N.J., and Polan, A.K.: Non-occupational exposure to asbestos and malignant mesothelioma in females. Lancet *1*:1061, 1978.
34. Becklake, M.R.: Exposure to asbestos and human disease. N. Engl. J. Med. *306*:1480, 1982.
35. Churg, A.M., and Warnock, M.L.: Asbestos and other ferruginous bodies: Their formation and clinical significance. Am. J. Pathol. *102*:447, 1981.
35A. Ross, R., et al.: Asbestos exposure and lymphomas of the gastrointestinal tract and oral cavity. Lancet *2*:1118, 1982.
36. Brain, J.D., et al.: Pulmonary distribution of particles given by intratracheal instillation or by aerosol inhalation. Environ. Res. *11*:13, 1976.
37. Lee, K.P., et al.: Pulmonary response and transmigration of inorganic fibers by inhalation exposure. Am. J. Pathol. *102*:314, 1981.
38. Craighead, J.E., et al.: Comparative studies on the cytotoxicity of amphibole and serpentine asbestos. Env. Health Perspect. *34*:37, 1980.
38A. Kagan, E., et al.: Immunological studies of patients with asbestosis. I. Studies of circulating lymphoid numbers and of humoral immunity. Clin. Exp. Immunol. *28*:268, 1977.
39. Heppleston, A.G.: Silica and asbestos: Contrast in tissue response. Ann. N.Y. Acad. Sci. *330*:725, 1979.
39A. Woodworth, C.D., et al.: Squamous metaplasia of the respiratory tract. Possible pathogenic role in asbestos-associated bronchogenic carcinoma. Lab. Invest. *48*:578, 1983.
40. Bignon, J., et al.: Human and experimental data on translocation of asbestos fibers through the respiratory tract. Ann. N.Y. Acad. Sci. *330*:745, 1979.
41. Auerbach, O., et al.: Presence of asbestos bodies in organs other than the lung. Chest *77*:133, 1980.
42. Selikoff, I.J., et al.: Asbestos disease in United States shipyards. *In* Selikoff, I.J., and Hammond, E.C. (eds.): Health Hazards of Asbestos Exposure. Ann. N.Y. Acad. Sci. *330*:295, 1979.
43. Selikoff, I.J., et al.: Mortality effects of cigarette smoking among non-smokers rising to 80- to 90-fold among amosite asbestos factory workers. J. Cancer Inst. *65*:507, 1980.
44. Hardy, H.L., and Tabershaw, I.R.: Delayed chemical pneumonitis occurring in workers exposed to beryllium compounds. J. Industr. Hyg. Toxicol. *28*:197, 1946.
45. Hasan, F.M., and Kazemi, H.: Chronic beryllium disease: A continuing epidemiologic hazard. Chest *65*:3, 1974.
46. Iaumi, T., et al.: The first seven cases of chronic beryllium disease in ceramic factory workers in Japan. Ann. N.Y. Acad. Sci. *278*:636, 1976.
47. Jones Williams, W.: Beryllium disease—pathology and diagnosis. J. Soc. Occup. Med. *27*:93, 1977.
48. Freiman, D.G., and Hardy, H.L.: Beryllium disease. The relation of pulmonary pathology to clinical course and prognosis based on a study of 130 cases from the U.S. Beryllium Case Registry. Hum. Pathol. *1*:25, 1970.
49. Constantinidis, K.: Acute and chronic beryllium disease. Br. J. Clin. Pract. *32*:127, 1978.
50. Wagoner, J.K., et al.: Beryllium: An etiologic agent in the induction of lung cancer, non-neoplastic respiratory disease, and heart disease among industrialized exposed workers. Environ. Res. *21*:15, 1980.
51. Groth, D.H.: Carcinogenicity of beryllium: Review of the literature. Environ. Res. *21*:56, 1980.
52. Reynolds, H.Y.: Hypersensitivity pneumonitis. Clin. Chest Med. *3*:503, 1982.
53. United States Department of Health, Education and Welfare: Smoking and Health 1979: A report to the Surgeon General. Public Health Service No. 79-50066. Rockville, MD, 1979.
54. United States Department of Health and Human Services: The health consequences of smoking: Cancer. A report of the Surgeon General, 1982. Washington, D.C., Public Health Service, Office of Smoking and Health, U.S. Government Printing Office, 20402.
55. Martin, E.W.: Hazards of Medication. Philadelphia, J.B. Lippincott Co., 1978.
56. Rensberger, B.: Bad prescriptions kill thousands a year. New York Times, Jan. 28, 1976.
57. Silverman, M., and Lee, P.E.: Pills, Profits, and Politics. Berkeley, University of California Press, 1974.
58. Ingelfinger, F.J.: Adverse drug reactions that count. N. Engl. J. Med. *294*:1003, 1976.
59. Smidt, N.A., and McQueen, E.G.: Adverse reactions to drugs: A comprehensive hospital inpatient survey. N.Z. Med. J. *76*:397, 1972.
60. Levy, M.: Hospital admissions due to adverse drug reactions. Am. J. Med. Sci. *277*:49, 1979.
61. Bergsagel, D.E., et al.: The chemotherapy of plasma cell myeloma and the incidence of acute leukemia. N. Engl. J. Med. *301*:743, 1979.
62. Baccarani, M., et al.: Second malignancy in patients treated for Hodgkin's disease. Cancer *46*:1735, 1980.
63. Greenberger, P.A.: Adverse drug reactions. Compr. Ther. *6*:22, 1980.
64. Chasee, F.H., and Settipane, G.A.: Aspirin intolerance. I. Frequency in an allergic population. J. Allergy Clin. Immunol. *53*:193, 1974.
65. Jick, H., et al.: Replacement estrogens and endometrial cancer. N. Engl. J. Med. *300*:218, 1978.
66. Antunes, C.M.F., et al.: Endometrial cancer and estrogen use: Report of a large case-controlled study. N. Engl. J. Med. *300*:9, 1979.
67. Gusberg, S.B.: The changing nature of endometrial cancer. N. Engl. J. Med. *302*:729, 1980.
68. Welch, W.R., et al.: Pathology of prenatal diethylstilbestrol exposure. Pathol. Annu. *13*:201, 1978.

69. Bibbo, M.: A twenty-five year follow-up study of women exposed to diethylstilbestrol during pregnancy. N. Engl. J. Med. *298*:763, 1978.
70. Ryan, K.J.: Diethylstilbestrol: Twenty-five years later. N. Engl. J. Med. *298*:794, 1978.
71. Hoover, R., et al.: Menopausal estrogens and breast cancer. N. Engl. J. Med. *295*:401, 1976.
72. Jick, H., et al.: Replacement estrogens and breast cancer. Am. J. Epidemiol. *112*:586, 1980.
73. Small, D.: Hormone use to change normal physiology—is the risk worth it? N. Engl. J. Med. *294*:219, 1976.
74. Ross, R., et al.: Menopausal oestrogen therapy and protection from death from ischaemic heart disease. Lancet *1*:858, 1981.
75. Editorial: Oestrogens and atheroma. Lancet *2*:508, 1978.
76. Stadel, B.V.: Oral contraceptives and cardiovascular disease. N. Engl. J. Med. *305*:612, 672, 1981.
77. Royal College of General Practitioners Oral Contraceptive Study: Oral contraceptives, venous thromboses, and varicose veins. J. R. Coll. Gen. Pract. *28*:393, 1978.
78. Royal College of General Practitioners Oral Contraceptive Study: Further analyses of mortality in oral contraceptive uses. Lancet *1*:541, 1981.
79. Population Reports: OCs—update of usage safety and side effects. Population Information Program. Johns Hopkins University. Series A. No. 5, 1979.
80. Slone, D., et al.: Risk of myocardial infarction in relation to current and discontinued use of oral contraceptives. N. Engl. J. Med. *305*:420, 1981.
81. May, D.: Mortality associated with the pill (letter). Lancet *2*:921, 1977.
81A. Vessey, M.P., et al.: Neoplasia of the cervix uteri and contraception. A possible adverse effect of the pill. Lancet *2*:930, 1983.
82. Weiss, N.S., and Sayvetz, T.A.: Incidence of endometrial cancer in relation to the use of oral contraceptives. N. Engl. J. Med. *302*:551, 1980.
82A. Cramer, D.W., et al.: Factors affecting the association of oral contraceptives and ovarian cancer. N. Engl. J. Med. *307*:1047, 1982.
83. Gambrell, R.D., Jr., et al.: Breast cancer and oral contraceptive therapy in premenopausal women. J. Reprod. Med. *23*:265, 1979.
84. Kelsey, J.L., et al.: Oral contraceptives and breast disease. Am. J. Epidemiol. *112*:577, 1980.
85. Pike, M.C., et al.: Breast cancer in young women and use of oral contraceptives. Possible modifying effect of formulation and age at use. Lancet *2*:926, 1983.
85A. Vandenbrouche, J.P., et al.: Oral contraceptives and rheumatoid arthritis: Further evidence for a preventive effect. Lancet *2*:838, 1982.
86. Neuberger, J., et al.: Oral contraceptive–associated liver tumours: Occurrence of malignancy and difficulties in diagnosis. Lancet *1*:273, 1980.
87. Isselbacher, K., Jr.: Metabolic and hepatic effects of alcohol. N. Engl. J. Med. *296*:612, 1977.
88. Thurman, R.G.: Hepatic alcohol oxidation and its metabolic liability. Fed. Proc. *36*:1640, 1977.
89. Mendelson, J.H., and Mello, N.K.: Biologic concomitants of alcoholism. N. Engl. J. Med. *301*:912, 1979.
89A. Edmondson, H.A.: Pathology of alcoholism. Am. J. Clin. Pathol. *74*:725, 1980.
90. Cedarbaum, A.I., and Rubin, E.: Molecular injury to mitochondria produced by ethanol and acetaldehyde. Fed. Proc. *34*:20, 1975.
91. Editorial: Toward prevention of alcoholic liver disease. Lancet *2*:353, 1978.
92. Schottenfeld, D.: Alcohol as a co-factor in the etiology of cancer. Cancer *43*:1962, 1979.
93. Editorial: Alcoholic cardiomyopathy. S. Afr. Med. J. *53*:917, 1978.
94. Rubin, E., et al.: Muscle damage produced by chronic alcohol consumption. Am. J. Pathol. *83*:499, 1976.
95. Lee, K., et al.: Alcohol-induced brain damage and liver damage in young males. Lancet *2*:759, 1979.
96. Editorial: Alcoholic disease. Lancet *1*:1105, 1982.
97. Keeney, A.H., and Mellinkoff, S.M.: Methyl alcohol poisoning. Ann. Intern. Med. *34*:331, 1951.
98. Polson, C.J., and Tattersall, R.N.: Clinical Toxicology. Philadelphia, J. B. Lippincott Co., 1969, p. 578.
99. Dalgaard, J.B.: Post-mortem findings in carbon monoxide deaths. Acta Pathol. Microbiol. Scand. *154* (Suppl.): 186, 1962.
100. Dutra, F.R.: Cerebral residua of acute carbon monoxide poisoning. Am. J. Clin. Pathol. *22*:925, 1952.
101. Stewart, R.D., et al.: Diagnosis of solvent poisoning. J.A.M.A. *193*:115, 1965.
102. Hayes, W.J., Jr., and Vaughn, W.K.: Mortality from pesticides in the United States in 1973 and 1974. Toxicol. Appl. Pharmacol. *42*:235, 1977.
103. Matsumura, F., and Madhukar, B.V.: Exposure to insecticides. Pharmacol. Ther. *9*:27, 1980.
104. Calabrese, E.J., and Sorensen, A.J.: The health effects of PCB's with particular emphasis on human high risk groups. Rev. Environ. Health *2*:285, 1977.
105. Kuratsune, M., et al.: Epidemiologic study on Yusho. A poisoning caused by ingestion of rice oil contaminated with a commercial brand of polychlorinated biphenyls. Environ. Health Perspect. *1*:119, 1972.
106. Humbert, J.R., et al.: Fatal cyanide poisoning. Accidental ingestion of amygdalin. J.A.M.A. *238*:482, 1977.
107. Braico, K.T., et al.: Laetrile intoxication. Report of a fatal case. N. Engl. J. Med. *300*:238, 1979.
108. Gettler, A.O., and St. George, A.V.: Cyanide poisoning. Am. J. Clin. Pathol. *4*:429, 1934.
109. Amin-Zaki, L., et al.: Methyl mercury poisoning in Iraqi children: Clinical observations over two years. Br. Med. J. *1*:613, 1978.
110. Kark, R.A.P., et al.: Mercury poisoning and its treatment with *N*-acetyl-D,L-penicillamine. N. Engl. J. Med. *285*:10, 1971.
111. Troen, P., et al.: Mercuric chloride poisoning. N. Engl. J. Med. *244*:459, 1951.
112. Ganote, C.E., et al.: Acute mercuric chloride nephrotoxicity. Lab. Invest. *31*:633, 1974.
113. Kibukamusoke, J.W., et al.: Membranous nephropathy due to skin-lightening cream. Br. Med. J. *2*:646, 1974.
114. Oliver, J., et al.: Cellular mechanism of protein metabolism in the newborn. I. The structural aspects of proteinuria, tubular absorption, droplet formation and the disposal of proteins. J. Exp. Med. *99*:589, 1954.
115. Mahaffey, K.R., et al.: National estimates of blood lead levels: United States, 1976–1980: Association with selected demographic and socioeconomic factors. N. Engl. J. Med. *307*:573, 1982.
116. Centers for Disease Control: Blood lead levels in United States population. M.M.W.R. *31*:132, 1982.
117. Bryce-Smith, D., and Stephens, R.: Exposure to lead. Lancet *1*:877, 1981.
118. Otto, D.A., et al.: Effects of age and body lead burden on CNS function in young children. I. Slow cortical potentials. Electroencephalogr. Clin. Neurophysiol. *52*:229, 1981.
119. White, J.M.: Lead and haemoglobin synthesis: A review. Postgrad. Med. J. *51*:755, 1975.
120. Johnson, R.B., and Lukash, W.M. (eds.): Summary of Proceedings of the Washington Conference on Medical Complications and Drug Abuse. Washington, D.C., Am. Med. Assoc. Comm. Alcohol and Drug Dependence, Dec. 7, 1972.
121. Bewley, T.H., et al.: Morbidity and mortality from heroin dependence. Part II. Br. Med. J. *1*:730, 1968.
122. Patrick, G.B.: Marijuana and the lung. Postgrad. Med. *67*:110, 1980.
123. Korcok, M.: Marijuana warnings: New evidence against the "soft" drug. Can. Med. Assoc. J. *123*:575, 1980.
124. Cordova, T., et al.: The ovulation blocking effect of cannabinoids: Structure-activity relationships. Psychoneuroendocrinology *5*:53, 1980.
124A. Ellitt, J.: Many questions, fewer answers, about pot. J.A.M.A. *243*:15, 1980.
124B. Committee to study the health-related effects of cannabis and its derivatives, National Academy of Sciences, Institute of Medicine: Marijuana and health. Washington, D.C., National Academy Press, 1982.
125. Nahas, G.G.: Keep Off The Grass: A Scientific Inquiry Into The Biological Effects of Marijuana. New York, Pergamon Press, 1979.
126. Robinson, J.P., et al.: Chromosomal aberrations and LSD: A controlled study of 50 psychiatric patients. Br. J. Psychiatr. *125*:238, 1974.
127. Jacobs, B.L., and Trulson, M.E.: Mechanisms of action of LSD. Am. Sci. *67*:396, 1979.
128. McLellan, A.T., et al.: Development of psychiatric illness in drug abusers: Possible role of drug preference. N. Engl. J. Med. *301*:1310, 1979.
129. Siegel, H.: Human pulmonary pathology associated with narcotic and other addictive drugs. Hum. Pathol. *3*:55, 1972.
130. Ostor, A.G.: The medical complications of narcotic addiction. Med. J. Aust. *1*:410, 448, 497, 1977.
131. Vollum, D.: Skin lesions in drug addicts. Br. Med. J. *2*:647, 1970.
132. Lewis, R.J.: Infections in heroin addicts. J.A.M.A. *223*:1036, 1973.
133. Kaplan, E.L., et al.: A collaborative study of infective endocarditis in the 1970's. Emphasis on infections in patients who have undergone cardiovascular surgery. Circulation *59*:327, 1979.
134. Citron, D.P., et al.: Necrotizing angiitis associated with drug abuse. N. Engl. J. Med. *283*:1003, 1970.
135. Tomashefski, J.F., and Hirsch, C.S.: The pulmonary vascular lesions of intravenous drug abuse. Hum. Pathol. *11*:133, 1980.
136. Miller, D.J., et al.: Chronic hepatitis associated with drug abuse: Significance of hepatitis B virus. Yale J. Biol. Med. *52*:135, 1979.
137. Belb, A.M., et al.: The spectrum and causes of liver disease in narcotic addicts. Am. J. Gastroenterol. *67*:314, 1977.
138. Cunningham, E.E., et al.: Heroin nephropathy: A clinical, pathologic and epidemiologic study. Am. J. Med. *68*:47, 1980.
139. Treser, G., et al.: Renal lesions in narcotic addicts. Am. J. Med. *57*:687, 1974.
140. Doll, R., and Peto, R.: The causes of cancer: Quantitative estimates of avoidable risks of cancer in the United States today. J. Natl. Cancer Inst. *66*:1191, 1981.

141. Reif, A.E.: The causes of cancer. Am. Sci. *69*:437, 1981.
142. Wynder, E.L., and Gori, G.B.: Contribution of the environment to cancer incidence. An epidemiologic exercise. J. Natl. Cancer Inst. *58*:825, 1977.
143. Subcommittee on Environmental Carcinogenesis, National Cancer Advisory Board: General criteria for assessing the evidence for carcinogenicity of chemical substances. J. Natl. Cancer Inst. *58*:461, 1977.
144. Schottenfeld, D., and Haas, J.F.: The workplace as a cause of cancer. Clin. Bull. *8*:54, 1979.
145. Savides, E.P., and Hoffbrand, B.I.: Hypothermia, thrombosis and acute pancreatitis. Br. Med. J. *1*:614, 1974.
146. Cuppage, F.E., et al.: Morphologic changes in rhesus monkey skin after acute burn. Arch. Pathol. *195*:402, 1975.
147. Cotran, R.S., and Remensnyder, J.P.: The structural basis of increased vascular permeability after graded thermal injury—light and electron microscopic studies. Ann. N.Y. Acad. Sci. *150*:495, 1968.
148. Teplitz, C.: Pathology of burns. *In* Artz, C.P., and Moncrief, J.A. (eds.): The Treatment of Burns. 2nd ed. Philadelphia, W. B. Saunders Co., 1969.
149. Constantian, M.: Association of sepsis with immunosuppressive polypeptide in the serum of burned patients. Ann. Surg. *188*:209, 1978.
150. Ninnemann, J., et al.: Thermal injury–associated immunosuppression. Occurrence and in vitro blocking effect of post-recovery serum. J. Immunol. *122*:1736, 1979.
151. Malamud, N., et al.: Heat stroke. A clinico-pathologic study of 125 fatal cases. Milit. Surg. *99*:397, 1946.
152. Clowes, G. H., Jr., and O'Donnell, T.F., Jr.: Heat stroke. N. Engl. J. Med. *291*:564, 1974.
153. Morgan, C.: Hiroshima, Nagasaki and the RERF (Radiation Effects Research Foundation). Am. J. Pathol. *98*:843, 1980.
154. Johns, H.E., and Cunningham, J.R: The Physics of Radiology. 3rd ed. Springfield, IL, Charles C Thomas, 1969.
155. Pizzarello, D.J., and Witcofski, R.L.: Basic Radiation Biology. 2nd ed. Philadelphia, Lea & Febiger, 1975.
156. Dalrymple, G.V., et al. (eds.): Medical Radiation Biology. Philadelphia, W. B. Saunders Co., 1973.
157. Prasad, K.N.: Human Radiation Biology. Hagerstown, MD, Harper & Row, 1974, p. 58.
158. Hutchinson, F.: The molecular basis for radiation effects on cells. Cancer Res. *26*:2045, 1966.
159. Rugh, R.: Damage to cells by ionizing radiation. Atompraxis *14*:13, 1968.
160. Tessmer, C.F.: Radiation effects in skin. *In* Berdjis, C.C. (ed.): Pathology of Irradiation. Baltimore, Williams & Wilkins Co., 1971, p. 146.
161. Anderson Hospital and Tumor Institute: Cellular Radiation Biology. Eighteenth Symposium on Fundamental Cancer Research, Houston, 1964. Baltimore, Williams & Wilkins Co., 1965.
162. Rubin, P., and Casarett, G.W.: Clinical Radiation Pathology. Philadelphia, W. B. Saunders Co., 1968, pp. 850, 894, and 903.
163. Tsinga, E., and Casarett, G.W.: Mitochondria and radiation sensitivity of cells. U.S. Atomic Energy Commission Report UR-666, 1965.
164. Ghidoni, J.J.: Light and electron microscopic study of primate liver 36 to 48 hours after high doses of 32 million electronvolt protons. Lab. Invest. *16*:268, 1967.
165. Benson, E.P.: Radiation injury to large arteries. 3. Further examples with prolonged asymptomatic intervals. Radiology *106*:195, 1973.
166. Fajardo, L.P., and Berthrong, M.: Radiation injury in surgical pathology. Am. J. Surg. Pathol. *2*:159, 1978.
167. Cade, S.: Radiation-induced cancer in man. Br. J. Radiol. *30*:393, 1957.
168. Zeman, W.: Introduction to neuropathology related to physical forces. *In* Minckler, J. (ed.): Pathology of the Nervous System. Vol. 1. New York, McGraw-Hill Book Co., 1968, p. 862.
169. Conard, R.A., and Hicking, A.: Medical findings in Marshallese people exposed to fallout radiation. J.A.M.A. *192*:457, 1965.
170. Warren, S.: The Pathology of Ionizing Radiation. Springfield, IL, Charles C Thomas, 1961.
171. Finch, S.E.: The study of atomic bomb survivors in Japan 1979/80. Ind. Med. *66*:899, 1979.
172. Okita, T.: Review of 30 years of study of Hiroshima and Nagasaki atomic bomb survivors. II. Biological effects. J. Rad. Res. (Suppl.) *16*:49, 1975.
173. Troup, G.M.: Symposium: The delayed consequences of exposure to ionizing radiation. Pathology studies at the Atomic Bomb Casualty Commission. Hiroshima and Nagasaki, 1945–1970. II. Growth and development. Hum. Pathol. 2:493, 1971.
174. Michaelson, S.M., et al.: Fundamental and Applied Aspects of Nonionizing Radiation. New York, Plenum Press, 1975.

11 DISEASES OF INFANCY AND CHILDHOOD

Children are not merely "little people" nor are their disorders merely variants of the diseases of adult life. Most of these conditions are unique to or at least take distinctive forms in this stage of life, and so merit the designation pediatric diseases. Collectively they exact a heavy toll. Considering all ages from birth to senility, "certain diseases of early infancy" constituted the tenth leading cause of death in the United States in 1977. As would be expected, the chances for survival of live-born infants improve with each passing week. The mortality rate in the first week of life is over ten times greater than in the second week. Ironically, this striking differential represents, at least in part, a triumph of improved medical care. Better prenatal care, more effective methods of monitoring the condition of the fetus, and more frequent resort to cesarean section before term when there is evidence of fetal distress all contribute to bringing onto this "mortal coil" live-born infants who in past years might have been stillborn. These represent, then, an increased number of "high-risk" infants. Nonetheless, the infant mortality rate in the United States has shown a gratifying decline from a level of 20.0 deaths per 1000 population in 1970 to 12.8 in 1980. However, before we derive comfort from these data, we must also note that the infant mortality rate in the U.S. is still well above that of many other developed nations, particularly Scandinavia and the Netherlands.

Each stage of development of the infant and child is prey to a somewhat different group of disorders. The data available permit a survey of four time spans: (1) the neonatal period (the first four weeks of life), (2) infancy (the first year of life), (3) 1 to 4 years of age, and (4) 5 to 14 years of age. The single most hazardous period in life is unquestionably the neonatal period. Never again is the individual confronted with more dramatic challenges than in the transition from dependent intrauterine existence to independent postnatal life. From the moment the umbilical cord is severed, the circulation to the heart is radically rerouted. Respiratory function must take over the role of oxygenation of the blood. Maintenance of body temperature and other homeostatic constants must now be borne alone by the fledgling organism. All these adaptations render the neonate particularly vulnerable.

The major causes of death in infancy (the first year of life) are cited in Table 11–1. The 1980 rate from all causes, 1288 deaths per 100,000 population, has decreased significantly as compared with 1606, the rate that prevailed in 1975. It is evident that congenital anomalies, respiratory distress syndrome, immaturity, birth trauma, birth asphyxia, complications of pregnancy, pneumonia, meningitis, diseases of the nervous system, and accidents represents the leading causes of death in the first year of life.

Once the infant survives the first year of life, the outlook brightens measurably. However, it is sobering to realize that in the next two age groups—1 to 4 and 5 to 14—accidents have become the leading cause of death (Table 11–1). Among the natural diseases, in order of importance, congenital anomalies, malignant neoplasms, and pneumonia assume major significance. It would appear then that, in a sense, life is an obstacle course. Fortunately for the great majority of us, the obstacles are surmounted, or even better, bypassed. We can now take a closer look at the specific conditions encountered during the various stages of infant and child development.

BIRTH WEIGHT AND GESTATIONAL AGE

It has been known for many years that infants born before completion of the normal gestation period have higher morbidity and mortality rates than full-term infants. Understandably, the vital organs of preterm infants are immature and therefore unable to adapt readily to early extrauterine existence. As might be expected, infants who have failed to complete normal intrauterine growth weigh less than full-term infants. In view of this association between low birth weight and immaturity in preterm infants, birth weight has traditionally been used as a guidepost for fetal maturity. Thus, in the past premature infants have been defined as those having birth weight less than 2500 gm, regardless of the age of gestation. Although birth weight is indeed an important predictor of neonatal mortality (Table 11–2), it is somewhat inaccurate to define prematurity by birth weight alone, since weight is but one of the several parameters of intrauterine growth. *Not in every case do fetal maturity and birth weight go hand in hand.* For example, an infant weighing 2300 gm but born at 34 weeks of gestation is likely to be more immature and therefore at greater risk of suffering the consequences of organ system immaturity (e.g., respiratory distress syndrome, RDS p. 482) than the 2300-gm full-term infant with functional maturity of the lungs

Table 11–1. SELECTED CAUSES OF DEATH IN INFANCY AND CHILDHOOD*

Causes	Under 1 yr	1–4 Yr	5–14 Yr
All causes	1288.3	63.9	30.6
Certain conditions originating in perinatal period	643.7	0.7	0.0
Disorders relating to short gestation and unspecified low birth weight	103.2		
Newborns affected by complications of placenta, cord, and membranes	27.9		
Birth trauma	29.9		
Birth asphyxia	34.4		
Respiratory distress syndrome	141.2		
Hemolytic disease of newborn due to isoimmunization, and other perinatal jaundice	2.6		
All other conditions originating in perinatal period	304.5		
Congenital anomalies	260.9	8.0	1.6
Pneumonia	28.3	2.0	0.5
Diseases of respiratory system (excluding pneumonia)	20.5	2.0	0.6
Septicemia	6.8	0.6	0.1
Intestinal infectious diseases	3.6	0.2	0.0
Meningitis	12.5	1.7	0.1
Diseases of nervous system and sense organs (excluding meningitis)	15.2	3.7	1.8
Malignant neoplasms, including neoplasms of lymphatic and hematopoietic tissues	3.2	4.5	4.3
Cystic fibrosis	1.1	0.3	0.6
Accidents and adverse effects (including motor vehicle)	33.0	25.9	15.0
All other causes	259.4	14.4	5.9

*Death rates per 100,000 population in a specified group. Data for the year 1980 provided by Statistical Resource Branch, Division of Vital Statistics, National Center for Health Statistics, Hyatsville, MD.

and little risk of developing RDS. As discussed below, these "small-for-dates" infants, who constitute a full one-third of low-birth-weight infants, are also a high-risk group, but the underlying basis for their problems is quite distinct. In recent years, therefore, a system of classification that takes into account both gestational age and birth weight has gained acceptance. Infants are classified as being appropriate for gestational age (AGA), small for gestational age (SGA), and large for gestational age (LGA). Those whose birth weight falls between the 10th and the 90th percentile for a given gestational age are considered AGA, whereas those who fall above or below these norms are classified as LGA or SGA respectively. With respect to gestational age, infants born before 37 or 38 weeks are considered *preterm*, while those delivered after the 42nd week are considered *postterm*. Figure 11–1 presents several possible categories of infants when both gestational age and birth weight are taken into account. It also demonstrates that the risk of neonatal mortality as well as morbidity are strongly influenced by both birth weight and gestational age. For example, infants born before the 34th week with birth weights between 1000 and 1500 gm have a 50% mortality and 90% morbidity; however, within the same weight category, birth after the 34th week reduces the risk of mortality to 13% but the chances of morbidity remain high at 86%. These figures reflect the somewhat distinctive distribution of diseases within each of the birth weight–gestational age groups, which are discussed in specialized texts.[1] Here we will discuss briefly SGA infants to highlight the utility of this classification, since such infants make up a significant fraction of those of low birth weight.

SMALL-FOR-GESTATIONAL-AGE (SGA) INFANTS

Most experts agree that *at least one-third of infants who weigh less than 2500 gm are born at term and that they are therefore undergrown rather than immature.* Impaired intrauterine growth underlies SGA. It may result from a variety of factors, which can be grouped

Table 11–2. NEONATAL MORTALITY RATE BY BIRTH WEIGHT AT UNIVERSITY OF COLORADO MEDICAL CENTER, 1958 TO 1968

Birth Weight (gm)	No. Admitted	No. Died	Mortality Rate (%)
4001 +	531	4	0.8
3501–4000	2528	7	0.3
3001–3500	6040	22	0.4
2501–3000	4977	29	0.6
2001–2500	1429	40	3.0
1501–2000	449	63	14.0
1001–1500	190	83	44.0
501–1000	108	97	90.0
500 or less	35	35	100.0

Reproduced with permission from Lubchenko, L. O.: Survival of the newborn infant. *In* Paxon, C. L., Jr. (ed.): Van Leeuwen's Newborn Medicine. 2nd ed. Copyright © 1979 by Year Book Medical Publishers, Inc., Chicago.

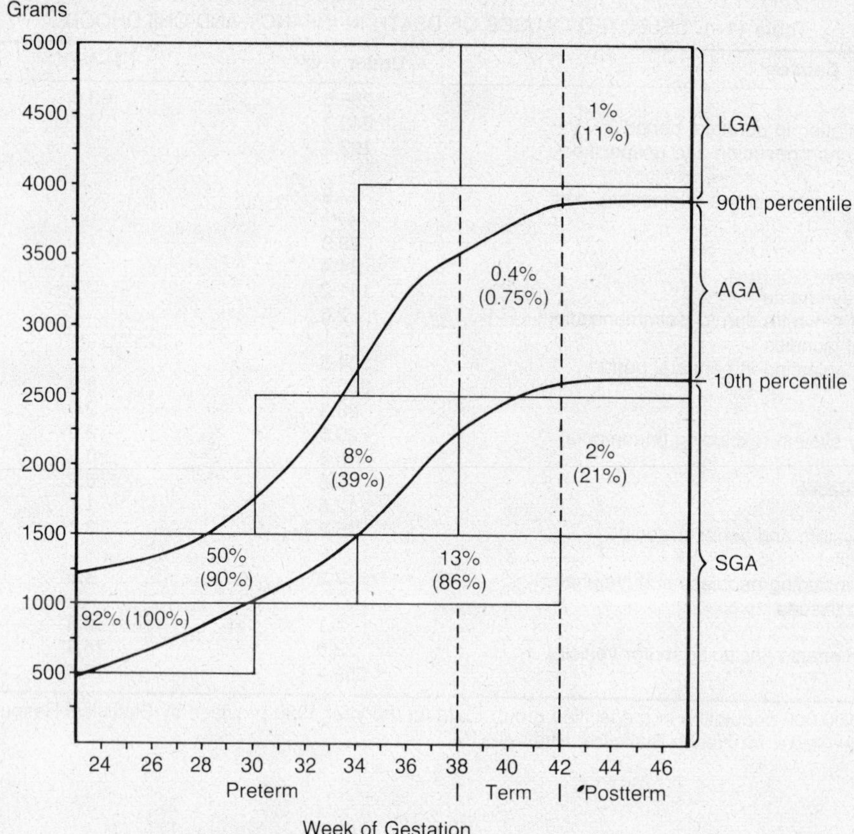

Figure 11–1. Neonatal mortality and morbidity according to birth weight and gestational age. Within each of the three gestational age groups (preterm, term, and postterm), infants are further divided into three categories on the basis of birth weight: large for gestational age (LGA), appropriate for gestational age (AGA), and small for gestational age (SGA). Thus, a total of nine major groups can be defined by the use of these criteria. Several subgroups, represented as boxes enclosed within continuous lines, are also shown. In each such subgroup, the risk of mortality and morbidity (in parentheses) is expressed as percentages. For example, infants born between the 30th and 38th week, weighing 1500 to 2500 gm, have an 8% risk of mortality and 39% risk of morbidity. (Modified from Lubchenco, L. O.: The High Risk Infant. Philadelphia, W. B. Saunders Co., 1976, pp. 104 and 112.)

broadly into three categories—fetal, placental, and maternal. (1) The factors associated with the fetus are those that reduce its growth potential despite an adequate supply of nutrients from the mother. Prominent among such fetal conditions are chromosomal disorders, congenital anomalies, and congenital infections. Although the higher incidence of congenital malformations in small-for-dates infants is well established, the basis of this association is not clearly understood. (2) In the third trimester of pregnancy, vigorous fetal growth places heavy demands on the uteroplacental supply line. *Placental insufficiency*, therefore, is an important cause of growth retardation. This may result from infections, tumors, or vascular lesions such as infarctions. In some cases the placenta may be small without any detectable underlying cause. (3) By far the most common factors associated with SGA infants are *maternal*. Vascular diseases such as toxemia and chronic hypertension are often the underlying cause. Although maternal undernutrition may well be expected to affect fetal growth, the association between SGA and the nutritional status of the mother is controversial. The list of other maternal conditions associated with SGA is long,[1] but some of the avoidable factors worth mentioning are maternal narcotic abuse, alcohol intake, and heavy cigarette smoking. The specific anatomic findings in SGA infants vary with the causes discussed above. In general, however, several organs such as brain, heart, and spleen tend to be heavier than expected for the body weight, and as might be anticipated the histologic maturation of organs such as kidney and lungs is more appropriate for the gestational age than the body weights.

IMMATURITY OF ORGAN SYSTEMS

A major problem confronting the preterm infant regardless of birth weight is the functional and sometimes structural immaturity of various organs. Those who are also SGA are understandably the most seriously handicapped. Since immaturity may be the direct cause of death in very early preterm infants and significantly biases the probable outcome of others, it is appropriate to consider the features of immaturity of the more vital organs.

LUNGS. During the first half of fetal life, the development of the lungs consists essentially of the formation of a system of branching tubes from the foregut that eventually give rise to the trachea, bronchi, and bronchioles. The alveoli only begin to differentiate at approximately the seventh month of gestation. They are at first imperfectly formed, with thick walls and large amounts of inter- and intralobular connective tissue. The vascularization is buried within this connective tissue and is not in immediate contact with the alveolar spaces (Fig. 11–2). The epithelium lining the air spaces at this time is cuboidal and not anatomically suited to effecting the rapid transfer of oxygen to the blood. Between the 26th and 32nd weeks of gestation, the cuboidal epithelium shows transition to the flat, type I alveolar epithelial cells as well as type II cells that contain lamellar bodies (see also p. 706). Further maturation of lungs leads to reduction in the interstitial tissues and increasing numbers of capillaries. However, even at full term the alveoli are small and the septa are considerably thicker than in the adult. Most of the cells lining the alveoli are type I cells. The type II cells appear in small clusters, mainly at the branching points of alveolar ducts.

The immature lungs, then, are grossly unexpanded, red, and meaty. The alveolar spaces are incompletely expanded and usually contain pink proteinaceous precipitate and occasional squamous epithelial cells. The presence of large amounts of amniotic debris, such as squames, lanugo hair, and mucus, usually indicates prenatal respiratory distress. Although lungs of stillborn infants usually sink when immersed in water, the "floating test" is not a critical index of postnatal respiration. Despite the fact that infants may have breathed prior to death, the very weak respiratory muscles and shallow respiration, with little exchange of air or resorption of the contained air, may both cause the lungs to sink when placed in water. Contrariwise, bacterial growth may produce gas that will create buoyancy in the lungs.

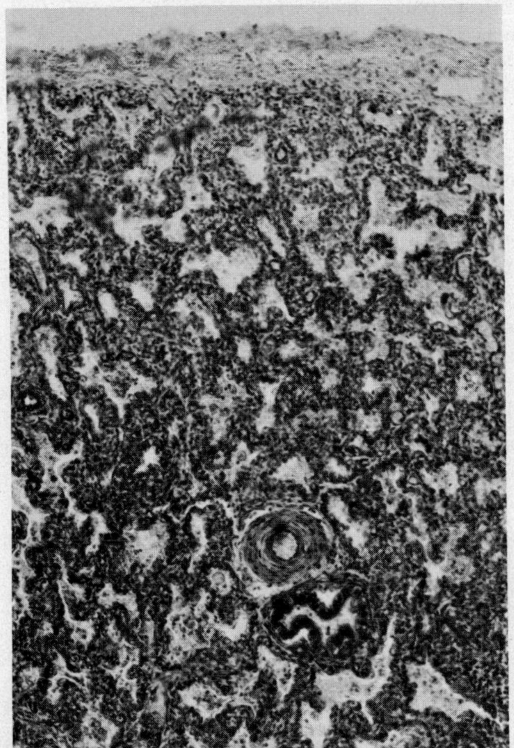

Figure 11–2. Immaturity of lung from a 6-month fetus. The septa are thick and cellular, and the alveolar spaces are small.

KIDNEYS. In the preterm infant the formation of glomeruli is incomplete. Primitive glomeruli can be seen in the subcapsular zone. These structures have an organoid, glandular appearance imparted by the presence of cuboidal cells in the parietal and visceral layers of Bowman's capsule. However, the deeper glomeruli are well formed and renal function is adequate to permit survival.

BRAIN. The brain is also incompletely developed in the preterm infant. The surface is relatively smooth and devoid of the typical convolutions found in the cerebral hemispheres of the adult. The brain substance is soft, gelatinous, and easily torn, and the definition between white and gray matter is somewhat ill defined. This lack of separation is in large part attributable to poorly developed myelination of the nerve fibers. Notwithstanding this underdevelopment, to the best of our present knowledge the vital brain centers are sufficiently developed even in the very immature infant to sustain normal central nervous system function. However, homeostasis is not perfect, and the preterm infant has difficulty in maintaining a constant normal level of temperature and has poor vasomotor control, irregular respirations, muscular inertia, and feeble sweating. None of these difficulties is incompatible with survival.

LIVER. The liver, although large relative to the size of the preterm infant, suffers from lack of physiologic maturity. Some of this increase in size is due to persistence of extramedullary hematopoiesis in this organ. Many or most of the functions of the liver are marginally adequate to carry out the demands placed upon them. Almost all newborns and particularly those of low birth weight have a transient period of physiologic jaundice within the first postnatal week. This jaundice stems from both breakdown of fetal red cells and inadequacy of the biliary excretory function of liver cells. Deficiencies of bilirubin glucuronyl transferase, hydroxylating enzymes, and protein synthetic capacity, to name only a few hepatic systems, all characterize the immature liver.

APGAR SCORE

The Apgar score devised by Dr. Virginia Apgar represents a clinically useful method of evaluating the physiologic condition and responsiveness of the newborn infant, and hence its chances of survival.[2] Table 11–3 indicates the five parameters to be scored and how they are quantitated. The newborn infant may be evaluated at one minute or at five minutes. A total score of 10 indicates an infant in the best possible condition. The correlation between the Apgar score and the mortality

Table 11–3. EVALUATION OF THE NEWBORN INFANT

Sign	0	1	2
Heart rate	Absent	Below 100	Over 100
Respiratory effort	Absent	Slow, irregular	Good, crying
Muscle tone	Limp	Some flexion of extremities	Active motion
Response to catheter in nostril (tested after oropharynx is clear)	No response	Grimace	Cough or sneeze
Color	Blue, pale	Body pink, extremities blue	Completely pink

Sixty seconds after the complete birth of the infant (disregarding removal of the cord and placenta) the five objective signs above are evaluated and each is given a score of 0, 1, or 2. A total score of 10 indicates an infant in the best possible condition.

Modified from Apgar, V.: A proposal for a new method of evaluation of the newborn infant. Anesth. Analg. *32*:260, 1953.

during the first 28 days of life is very impressive. Infants with a five-minute Apgar score of 0 to 1 have a 50% mortality within the first month of life. This drops to 20% with a score of 4, and to almost 0% when the score is 7 or better.[3]

BIRTH INJURIES

Birth injuries constitute an important cause of illness or death in infants as well as in children during the first years of life. Understandably, LGA infants are at a greater risk of sustaining birth injuries, but no group is immune. Preterm AGA or SGA infants, although smaller, have higher associated morbidity since they are the least equipped to adapt. Anatomic immaturity may also increase the risk of some forms of birth injuries (e.g., intraventricular hemorrhage). These injuries may affect any part or any region of the body but most commonly involve the head, skeletal system, liver, adrenals, and peripheral nerves. Considering the violent expulsive forces to which the fragile fetus is exposed, it is quite surprising that birth injuries are so relatively uncommon. It is important to stress that although some birth injuries are avoidable, some are unavoidable even with optimal obstetric care. If the process of birth were not laborious to mother and infant, why would it have been termed "labor?"

Morbidity associated with birth injury may be acute (such as that due to fractures) or the result of later appearing sequelae, such as following damage to nerves or the brain. The distribution of injuries (other than cephalhematoma, which is hardly to be considered an injury) in a large municipal hospital is as follows, in descending order of frequency: clavicular fracture, facial nerve injury, brachial plexus injury, intracranial injury, humeral fracture, and lacerations.[4] Among these, intracranial injuries are the most ominous. Discussion of the other birth injuries may be found in a 1981 review.[5]

Caput succedaneum and *cephalhematoma* are so common even in normal uncomplicated births that they hardly merit the designation birth injury. When the head is the presenting part, some portion of the scalp is exposed in the progressively dilating cervical os. As the fetus is subjected to the compressive forces of labor, fluid tends to accumulate in the small area of the scalp that presents in the cervical os and is not exposed to the increased uterine pressure. *The progressive accumulation of interstitial fluid in the soft tissues of the scalp gives rise to a usually circular area of edema, congestion, and swelling called a caput succedaneum.* When the presenting part of the fetus is not the head, similar edema may involve whatever region presents in the cervical os. *Hemorrhage may occur into these areas of edema and, when it involves the scalp, produces a cephalhematoma.* Usually the blood accumulates between the outer table of the calvarial bone and the pericranial or periosteal membrane. The swelling does not cross the cranial sutures and is therefore distinct from a caput succedaneum, which occurs more superficially in the soft tissues of the scalp. Both forms of injury are of little clinical significance and are of importance only insofar as they must be differentiated from skull fractures with attendant hemorrhage and edema. In approximately 25% of cephalhematomas there is an underlying skull fracture.

The skull bones may be fractured or may override each other, particularly when there is some disturbance in the ordinary mechanism of labor. Precipitate or sudden delivery with incomplete molding of the head, overenthusiastic use of forceps, and prolonged intense labor with disproportion between the size of the fetal head and birth canal are some of the common circumstances that surround the occurrence of these skull injuries.

Intracranial hemorrhage is probably the most common important birth injury. These hemorrhages are generally thought to be related to excessive molding of the head or sudden pressure changes in its shape as it is subjected to the pressure of forceps or sudden precipitate expulsion. Prolonged labor, anoxia, hemorrhagic disorders, or intracranial vascular anomalies are important predispositions. The hemorrhage may arise in tears in the dura, particularly in the falx cerebri and tentorium cerebelli; the dural sinuses may be stretched beyond their elastic limit and may rupture; the substance of the brain may be torn or bruised, leading to intraventricular hemorrhages or bleeding into the brain substance; or vessels that traverse the subdural space may be ruptured. Whatever their origin, intracranial hemorrhages are of great importance, since they cause sudden increases in intracranial pressure; damage to the brain substance; herniation of the medulla or base of the brain into the foramen magnum; and serious, frequently fatal depression of function of the vital medullary centers.

CONGENITAL MALFORMATIONS

Congenital malformations can be defined as structural defects that are present at birth, but some, such as cardiac defects and renal anomalies, may not become clinically apparent until years later. It is estimated that about 2% of newborns have a major malformation, defined as a malformation having either cosmetic or functional significance.[6] As indicated in Table 11–1, they are the leading cause of infant mortality. Moreover, they continue to be a significant cause of illness, disability, and death throughout the early years of life. In a real sense, malformations found in live-born infants represent the less serious developmental failures in embryogenesis that are compatible with live birth. Perhaps 20% of fertilized ova are so anomalous that they are blighted from the outset. Less severe anomalies may be compatible with early fetal survival, only to lead to spontaneous abortion. As one descends the scale of severity, a level is reached that permits more prolonged intrauterine survival, with some disorders terminating in stillbirth, and those still less significant permitting live birth despite the handicaps imposed.

Here we should distinguish between malformations and deformations. *Malformations represent primary errors in morphogenesis; deformations arise later in fetal life and represent alterations in form or structure resulting from mechanical factors.* We shall consider deformations at the end of this section. Malformations may present in several patterns. Some such as congenital heart defects involve single body systems, whereas in other cases multiple malformations involving many organs and tissues may coexist. Multiple congenital anomalies may have their origin in a single localized aberration in organogenesis leading to secondary ripple effects in other organs. For example, early urethral obstruction may secondarily affect renal morphogenesis as well as lead to defects in the lower limbs due to compression of blood vessels. Such a pattern of cascade effects is called a *malformation sequence*. On the other hand, a patient may have several defects that cannot be explained on the basis of a single localized initiating malformation. These are called *malformation syndromes*. Most often they are caused by a single etiologic agent, e.g., viral infections that simultaneously affect several tissues.

ETIOLOGY. Known causes of human malformations can be grouped into two major categories—genetic and environmental (Table 11–4). Almost two-thirds, however, have no recognized cause.

Malformations that are genetic in origin can be divided into three groups: (1) those associated with chromosomal aberrations, (2) those arising in gene mutations, and (3) those resulting from multifactorial inheritance. Since the precise environmental and genetic factors responsible for the malformations in the third group are largely unidentified, they are often included in the unknown category (Table 11–4). You may recall from the chapter on genetic disorders (Chap. 4) that virtually all the chromosomal syndromes are characterized by congenital anomalies. Chromosomal abnormalities are present in approximately 4 to 5% of live-born infants with congenital malformations (p. 123). Only one reaches the birth frequency of one in 1000 total births, namely, trisomy 21 (Down's syndrome) (p. 126). Next in order of frequency are Klinefelters, Turner's, and trisomy 13 (Patau's syndrome). The remaining chromosomal syndromes associated with malformations are far more rare. The great preponderance of these cytogenetic aberrations arise as defects in gametogenesis and so are not familial. There are, however, transmissible chromosomal abnormalities, as for example the translocation form of Down's syndrome passed from one generation to the next, thus constituting a familial pattern of structural abnormalities.

Table 11–4. CAUSES OF CONGENITAL MALFORMATIONS IN HUMANS

Cause	Incidence (%)
Genetic	
Known genetic transmission	20
Chromosomal aberration	4–5
Multifactorial	? (Included in unknown)
Environmental	
Infections	2–3
Rubella	
Cytomegalovirus	
Herpesvirus hominis	
Toxoplasma gondii	
Syphilis	
Drugs and Chemicals	4–6
Androgenic hormones	
Folic acid antagonists	
Thalidomide	
Organic mercury	
Alcohol	
Warfarin	
Irradiation	1
Unknown	65–70

Modified from Bolande, R. P.: Developmental pathology. Am. J. Pathol. *94*:642, 1979.

Major malformations may be determined by single genes of large effect, thus representing mendelian disorders. On the whole these are relatively uncommon and do not have a birth frequency of one in 1000 births. Among these rare entities are the relatively less serious limb malformations: polydactyly, syndactyly, and brachydactyly. However, as pointed out below, there is still some question about the mode of transmission of some of these, and multifactorial inheritance cannot be totally excluded. In addition, there are a number of malformation syndromes in which multiple anomalies occur in disorders having mendelian modes of transmission, as for example Marfan's syndrome and the mucopolysaccharidoses.

Multifactorial inheritance is believed to underlie the most common major malformations, particularly when the malformation is single, i.e., not associated with other malformations. You may recall from the earlier discussion in Chapter 4 that multifactorial inheritance is involved in many of the physiologic characteristics such as height, weight, and blood pressure. Such phenotypic characteristics fall on a continuous or gaussian distribution curve. Similarly, in the case of malformations, the liability to a disorder (determined by genetic and environmental factors) is a continuous variable, but there is in addition a "threshold" that divides individuals with and without the disorder. Thus, it would appear that the inheritance of a certain number of mutant genes and their interaction with the environment is required before the disorder is expressed. In the case of congenital dislocation of the hip, for example, depth of the acetabular socket and laxity of the ligaments are believed to be genetically determined, whereas a significant environmental factor is believed to be frank breech position in utero with hips flexed and knees extended. In most instances, however, the nature of genetic and environment factors and their interplay are unknown. The approximate frequency and sex ratio of the common single malformations in Great Britain are presented in Table 11–5, and there is no reason to doubt the applicability of these data to other countries having relatively advanced medical services. These malformations have been described in the appropriate chapters of this book.

Environmental influences such as viral infections, drugs, and irradiation to which the mother was exposed during pregnancy may induce malformations in the fetus and infant. Many viruses have been implicated, including the agents responsible for rubella, cytomegalic inclusion disease, herpes simplex, varicella-zoster infection, influenza, mumps, and enterovirus infections. Among these, the rubella virus and the cytomegalovirus of cytomegalic inclusion disease are the most important. With all viruses, the gestational age at which the infection occurs in the mother is critically important. *The at-risk period for rubella infection extends from shortly before conception to the 16th to 20th week of gestation,* the hazard being greater in the first eight weeks than the second eight weeks. Various studies indicate that with infection in the first four-week period, approximately 50% of live-born infants will have malformations, a risk so great that abortion is often advised. The incidence of malformations is reduced to 20% and 7% if infection occurs in the second or third month of gestation, respectively. The fetal defects are extremely varied, but the major triad comprises cataracts, heart disease, and deafness, referred to as the "rubella syndrome." The cardiac lesions take many forms, particularly persistent ductus arteriosus, pulmonary artery hypoplasia, pulmonary valve stenosis, aortic stenosis, ventricular septal defect, and tetralogy of Fallot. Other possible concomitant defects are microphthalmia, microcephaly, mental retardation, hepatomegaly, splenomegaly, and retardation of both intrauterine and postnatal growth.

Intrauterine infection with the cytomegalovirus is the most common fetal viral infection, the incidence being estimated to be four to ten infected infants per 1000 births. This viral disease is considered in detail elsewhere (p. 286), and it suffices here to indicate that the highest at-risk period appears to be the second trimester of pregnancy. Since organogenesis is largely completed by the end of the first trimester, congenital malformations occur less frequently than in rubella; nevertheless, the effects of virus-induced injury on the formed organs are often severe. Involvement of the central nervous system is a major feature, and the most prominent clinical changes are mental retardation, microcephaly, deafness, and hepatosplenomegaly. Several other abnormalities are detailed in the discussion of this condition on page 286. The other viral agents previously mentioned have at one time or another been implicated as infective causes of congenital malformations, but the number of reported cases is far fewer and the evidence less substantial.

A variety of drugs and chemicals have been suspected to be teratogenic. However, in view of the complex interactions between genetic and environmental factors in the pathogenesis of most common malformations, it is difficult to establish a definite role of a suspected teratogen. Furthermore, the more widely used is a potential teratogen and the more common a suspected malformation, the more often will they be associated by chance. Perhaps only 4 to 6% of congenital malformations are caused by drugs and chemicals. The list of chemicals and drugs definitely known to cause malformations includes thalidomide, folate antagonists, androgenic hormones, alcohol, anticonvulsants, warfarin (oral anticoagulant), and organic mercury. Here we will review the teratogenic action of two agents: thalidomide, which caused an epidemic of malformations in the early 1960s, and alcohol, which is widely used but poorly appreciated as a teratogenic agent. Thalidomide, once popular as a tranquilizer in Europe, is one of the few drugs that causes an extremely high frequency (50 to

Table 11–5. APPROXIMATE FREQUENCY AND SEX RATIO OF THE MORE COMMON MAJOR CONGENITAL MALFORMATIONS IN GREAT BRITAIN

Malformation	Frequency/1000 Total Births	Approximate Sex Ratio (Male:Female)
Congenital heart defects	6.0	1.0
Pyloric stenosis	3.0	4.0
Spina bifida cystica	2.5	0.6
Anencephaly	2.0	0.3
Cleft lip (± cleft palate)	1.0	1.8
Congenital dislocation of the hip (late diagnosis)	1.0	0.14

From Carter, C. O.: Genetics of common single malformations. Br. Med. Bull. *32*:21, 1976.

80%) of malformations in those exposed to the drug during a vulnerable period. Although the characteristic anomalies of the thalidomide syndrome affect the limbs, several other organs may be affected, depending on the period of exposure during embryogenesis. The limb abnormalities range from severe, such as amelia (absence of limbs) and phocomelia ("seal limbs," absence of limb with hands or feet attached directly to the trunk), to minor, such as hypoplasia of the thumb. *Alcohol*, perhaps the most widely used agent today, has only recently been recognized as a teratogen. Although the exact frequency of alcohol-induced malformations is difficult to ascertain, current estimates range from one to five live births per 1000.[7] Affected infants show growth retardation, microcephaly, atrial septal defect, short palpebral fissures, maxillary hypoplasia, and several other minor anomalies. These together are labeled the *fetal alcohol syndrome*. The level of alcohol consumption necessary to produce this has not been established with certainty. Suffice it to say that in most cases the mothers are chronic alcoholics who have consumed alcohol throughout gestation.

Irradiation, in addition to being mutagenic and carcinogenic, is teratogenic. Exposure to heavy doses of irradiation during the period of organogenesis leads to malformations such as microcephaly, blindness, skull defects, spina bifida, and other deformities. Such exposure occurred in the past when irradiation was used to treat cervical cancer. Similarly, exposure to radioactivity from atomic bomb explosions in Japan led to an increased incidence of malformations. Whether lower doses of irradiation such as those used in diagnostic x-rays are also teratogenic is not known.

PATHOGENESIS. The pathogenesis of congenital malformations is complex and still poorly understood. Certain general principles of developmental pathology that are relevant regardless of the etiologic agent will be discussed first. *The timing of the prenatal insult has an important impact on both the occurrence and the type of malformation produced.* The intrauterine development of humans can be divided into two phases: the embryonic period occupying the first nine weeks of pregnancy, and the fetal period terminating at birth. In the *early embryonic period* (first three weeks after fertilization), an injurious agent damages either enough cells to cause death and abortion, or only a few cells, presumably allowing the embryo to recover without developing defects. Between the third and ninth weeks the embryo is extremely susceptible to teratogenesis, and the peak sensitivity during this period is between the fourth and fifth weeks. It is during this period that organs are being created out of the germ cell layers. The process of organogenesis including the intricate morphogenetic movements is extremely susceptible to injury, regardless of its nature. The *fetal period* that follows organogenesis is marked chiefly by the further growth and maturation of the organs, with greatly reduced susceptibility to teratogenic agents. Instead the fetus is susceptible to growth retardation or injury to already formed organs. For example, in the first trimester, viral infections such as rubella produce malformations by disrupting the developmental program, but later during pregnancy the result of virus infections is usually tissue injury accompanied by inflammation such as congenital encephalitis. Timing of the teratogenic insult is also important with respect to the specific malformation produced. During the period of morphogenesis, different organs are being formed both simultaneously and sequentially, but each organ has a critical period during which it is most susceptible to induction of malformation. It is therefore possible for a given agent to produce different malformations if exposure occurs at different times of gestation. In general, malformations resulting from incomplete morphogenesis usually have their origin when the development of the organ in question is not yet completed. For example, a ventricular septal defect may occur from exposure to a teratogen before six weeks of gestation, since the ventricular septum closes at this time. Similarly, cleft lip must occur before closure of the lip at 36 days. It must be remembered, however, that knowledge of embryologic timetables does not allow an estimate of the particular time when the malformation was produced; one can only say that the teratogen acted prior to a given time.

In producing malformations, *teratogens may act at several levels. These include cell proliferation, cell migration, differentiation, and in some instances damage to formed and differentiated organs.* Inhibition of cell proliferation or cell death occurring at critical points in development can lead to serious malformations. Failure of planned cell death may also produce malformations such as syndactyly. As indicated earlier, cell migrations play an important role in morphogenesis. Orderly migrations take place in matrices, which may be disrupted by teratogenic agents. For example, in experimental animals, disturbance in collagen-matrix formation by cadmium produces major craniofacial anomalies since the migration of neural crest cells is inhibited. Anticonvulsant drugs, on the other hand, impair the appropriate differentiation of the mesenchyme and give rise to cleft palate in rodents. It must be remembered in this context that although a given teratogen may initiate its action primarily by affecting proliferation, migration, or differentiation, interference in any one of these mechanisms may lead to a cascade of effects in all three processes. Although the risk of malformations is reduced after morphogenesis is complete, differentiated tissues may also be affected by teratogens. For example, focal cell death in differentiated tissues caused by anoxia, chemicals, or virus infections can lead to formation of fluid- or blood-filled blebs that can result in significant local malformations.

Another important principle of teratology relates to the *role of heredity in the susceptibility to malformations.* Here we are not concerned with genetic factors in the etiology of malformations, but with the role of heredity in predisposition to the effects of known teratogens. The best example to illustrate this principle is cleft palate induced by cortisone in mice. A given dose of cortisol administered to the mother produces 100% incidence of cleft palate in the progeny of A strain mice but only 20% in C57BL/6 mice. This has been related to the frequency of receptors for corticosteroids in the two strains of mice. Although no such clear example has been found in human teratogenesis, it is considered very likely that the effect of environmental teratogens is modified by the genotype. At yet another level is the *role of heredity in predisposition to certain specific malformations*. Taking again an example from inbred mice, C57BL/6 mice have a low incidence of "spontaneous" ventricular septal defect, but they do not have atrial septal defects. Exposure to the drug dextroamphetamine produces ventricular septal defects in approximately 10% of the offspring. Conversely, the A/J strain of mice have a low incidence of "spontaneous" atrial septal defect, but no ventricular septal defect. Exposure to dextroamphetamine increases the incidence of atrial septal defects to 13%. Thus, the same teratogen produces different septal defects in two strains of mice. Human studies tend to support this notion of genetic predisposition to certain types of malformations. Affected members of a family tend to have the same anomaly, e.g., ventricular septal defect.

With this overview of some general mechanisms whereby congenital malformations may arise, we can now discuss deformations that represent the effects of abnormal mechanical forces on the developing fetus.

DEFORMATIONS

Deformations are common problems, affecting approximately 2% of newborn infants to varying degrees. Fundamental to the pathogenesis of deformations is localized or generalized compression of the growing fetus by abnormal biomechanical forces, leading eventually to a variety of structural abnormalities. In contrast with malformations, there is no intrinsic defect in morphogenesis, although fetal malformations may initiate a sequence of changes that ultimately lead to deformations. The most common underlying factor responsible for deformations is *uterine constraint*. Between the 35th and 38th week of gestation, rapid increase in the size of the fetus outpaces the growth of the uterus, and the relative amount of amniotic fluid (which normally acts as a cushion) also decreases. Thus, even the normal fetus is subjected to some form of uterine constraint. However, several factors increase the likelihood of excessive compression of the fetus, including maternal conditions such as first pregnancy, small uterus, malformed (bicornuate) uterus, and leiomyomas. Factors relating to the fetus, such as multiple fetuses, oligohydramnios, and abnormal fetal presentation, may also be involved. These and other details of deformations are discussed in specialized texts.[8]

Here we will present only one example of deformations resulting from relative lack of amniotic fluid, called the *oligohydramnios sequence*. A deficiency of amniotic fluid, with consequent increase in uterine constraint, may have a variety of causes, including chronic leakage of amniotic fluid due to rupture of the amnion, or uteroplacental insufficiency resulting from maternal hypertension or severe toxemia. Occasionally the oligohydramnios sequence may be initiated by a fetal malformation such as renal agenesis, leading to lack of urine, which is a major constituent of amniotic fluid during pregnancy. The affected newborn presents with facial abnormalities including flattened nose and accordion ears. More serious are abnormalities of the limb joints, which are in aberrant positions and often stiff owing to poor mobility in utero. Hips may be dislocated. Growth of the chest wall and the contained lungs is compromised so that the lungs often achieve only a four- to five-month level of maturation. Several other less striking abnormalities are also apparent. Fortunately, deformations in general carry a much better prognosis than malformations and a much lesser risk of recurrence in subsequent infants.

RESPIRATORY DISTRESS SYNDROME IN NEWBORN

Respiratory distress is one of the most common and life-threatening complications to confront the newborn infant. It can have many origins, including (1) excessive sedation of the mother, with consequent depression of respiration in the infant; (2) brain injury, with failure of the central respiratory centers; (3) feeble respiratory efforts secondary to immaturity of the lungs and skeletal muscles (primary atelectasis); (4) aspiration during birth of blood clot and amniotic fluid when the amniotic debris (i.e., desquamated keratotic squames, mucus, lanugo hairs, proteinaceous precipitate, and blood) blocks ventilatory function; and (5) asphyxiating coils of umbilical cord about the neck of the infant. *But more important than all these by an order of magnitude is the idiopathic respiratory distress syndrome (RDS).* Despite the striking improvement in neonatal intensive care in the last two decades, RDS still takes the lives of about 7000 infants every year in the United States.

RDS is also known as hyaline membrane disease (HMD), highlighting one of the major pulmonary anatomic findings in this disease. In most cases this disorder presents in stereotyped fashion, which is best characterized by the following typical clinical setting. The infant is almost always preterm and appropriate for gestational age (p. 475), and there are strong, but not invariable, associations with diabetes in the mother and with delivery by cesarean section. Resuscitation may be necessary at birth, but usually within a few minutes rhythmic breathing and normal color are reestablished. However, soon afterward, often within 30 minutes, breathing becomes more difficult, there is retraction of the lower ribs and sternum on inspiration, and an expiratory grunt becomes audible. Over the span of the next few hours the respiratory distress becomes worse, the rate of breathing increases to over 100 breaths per minute, and cyanosis becomes evident. Despite the labored breathing, little actual ventilation occurs, and fine rales can now be heard over both lung fields. Chest x-ray at this time usually reveals uniform minute reticulogranular densities, producing a so-called "ground-glass" picture. At first the administration of 40 to 50% oxygen to the infant lessens the cyanosis; indeed, during the next 12 to 24 hours recovery may ensue, but in the full-blown condition the respiratory distress persists, cyanosis increases, and even the administration of 80% oxygen by a variety of ventilatory methods fails to improve the situation. Flaccidity, unresponsiveness, and periods of apnea may now appear and may presage death. However, if therapy staves off death for the first three or four days, the baby has an excellent chance of recovery.[9]

Etiology and Pathogenesis. The pathogenesis of RDS is still incompletely understood, but a number of significant observations have been made. Immaturity of the lungs is the most important subsoil on which this condition develops. It may be encountered in full-term infants, but is much less frequent than in those "born before their time into this breathing world."[10] The incidence of RDS is inversely proportional to gestational age. It is estimated to occur in about 60% of infants born at less than 28 weeks of gestation, 15 to 20% of those born between 32 and 36 weeks, and less than 5% of those born after 37 weeks of gestation.[11] Although the point is still somewhat controversial, a good deal of evidence indicates that cesarean section, when performed before the 38th week of gestation, increases the risk of RDS—with a virtual exponential increase with each week of prematurity.[12] Infants of diabetic mothers, as contrasted with those of nondiabetic mothers, have almost a sixfold increased risk, even when all other confounding variables are taken into account.[13, 14] The sex of the infant is also a factor, males being affected 1.5 to 2 times more often than females.

All the above-mentioned clinical observations bear on what is now considered to be the *fundamental defect in RDS—a deficiency of pulmonary surfactant.* Surfactant is a generic name for surface active compounds synthesized by the lung. It consists predominantly of phosphatidylcholine and smaller amounts of phosphatidylglycerol. Surfactant reduces surface tension within the alveoli so that less pressure is required to hold alveoli open, and maintains alveolar expansion by varying surface tension with alveolar size. It is synthesized by type II alveolar cells and can be visualized under the electron microscope as lamellar osmiophilic bodies. At birth, the first breath of life requires high inspiratory pressures to expand the lungs. With normal levels of surfactant the lungs retain up to 40% of the residual air volume after the first breath; thus, subsequent breaths require far lower inspiratory pressures. With a deficiency of surfactant the lungs collapse with each successive breath, and so the infant must work as hard with each successive breath as it did with the first. Progressive atelectasis and reduced lung compliance then lead to a train of events as depicted in Figure 11–3, resulting in a protein-rich, fibrin-rich exudation into the alveolar spaces with the formation of hyaline membranes. Built into the sequence of events are feedback loops, which constitute vicious cycles that progressively increase the severity of the disease once it has begun. The fibrin-hyaline membranes constitute barriers to gas exchange, leading to CO_2 retention and hypoxemia, worsening the acidosis and subsequent events. The hypoxemia itself further impairs surfactant synthesis. Only effective supportive therapy permitting regeneration of the type II pneumocytes and increased surfactant synthesis can lead to recovery from this condition.

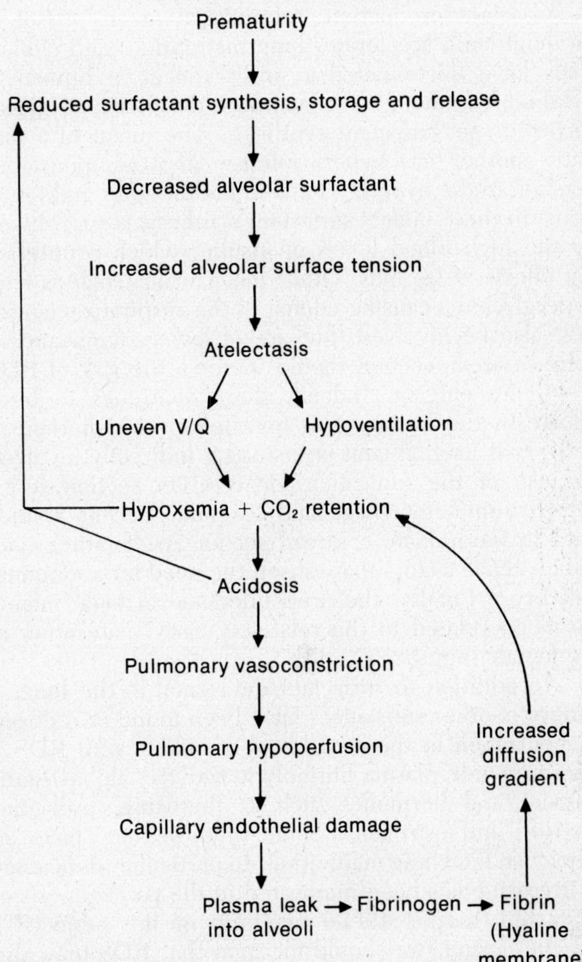

Figure 11–3. Schematic outline of pathophysiology of respiratory distress syndrome. V/Q = ventilation-perfusion ratio. (From Boyle, R. J., and Oh. W.: Respiratory distress syndrome. Clin. Perinatol. 5:283, 1978 Reproduced with permission.)

Immaturity of the fetal lung in preterm infants is the basis of surfactant deficiency. The production of surfactant increases gradually after the appearance of type II alveolar cells, but the largest increase occurs after 35 weeks of gestation. Thus, preterm infants have a deficiency of surfactant relative to their needs.

The effect of maternal diabetes in the pathogenesis of RDS is somewhat complex and involves a consideration of the action of adrenal steroids on surfactant production. The evidence is now convincing that glucocorticoids induce the formation of enzymes involved in surfactant production. Administration of cortisol to the fetal lamb accelerates lung maturation, and clinical trials have documented a similar effect in humans.[15] Insulin, it is thought, antagonizes the action of glucocorticoids on surfactant synthesis. The infant of a diabetic mother has hyperinsulinism as a compensatory reaction to the hyperglycemia in both mother and fetus. Thus, in these infants surfactant synthesis is suppressed by the high blood levels of insulin, which counteract the effects of steroids. Other mechanisms such as fetal hyperglycemia causing edema of the respiratory center may also be involved, but are of lesser significance.[16] Why cesarean section should increase the risk of RDS is still an enigma. Indeed, there continues to be a debate in the literature as to whether this method of delivery is itself at fault or instead is indirectly involved because of the indication for cesarian section, e.g., antepartum hemorrhage and toxemia. Recent studies tend to incriminate cesarean section itself rather than the obstetric factors that caused the need for abdominal delivery.[17] Finally, the preponderance in male infants has been related to the relatively early maturation of the female lung.[18]

In addition to surfactant deficiency in the lung, a variety of other substances have been found in reduced concentration in the cord blood of infants with RDS.[19] These include plasma fibrinolytic activity, alpha-1-antitrypsin, and hormones such as thyroxine, prolactin, cortisol, and estrogens. Some of these may have an impact on fetal lung maturation. In particular, deficiency of thyroxine has been implicated in the pathogenesis of RDS, but there is still no unanimity on this subject.[20]

In closing, we should mention that RDS may also occur in adults (p. 714). Surfactant deficiency is the most common cause of RDS in newborns, but any agent capable of causing diffuse alveolar damage can result in similar respiratory problems in both infants and adults.

MORPHOLOGY. The lungs are extremely distinctive on gross examination. Although of normal size, they are solid, airless, and reddish purple like the liver, and usually sink in water.[21] On low-power microscopic examination, they give the appearance of a solid tissue. The alveoli are small and crumpled, but the proximal alveolar ducts and bronchi are overdistended. When the infant dies early in the course of the disease, necrotic cellular debris is present in the terminal bronchioles and alveolar ducts. Later, the necrotic material becomes incorporated within pink hyaline membranes that line the alveolar ducts and random alveoli, mostly the proximal alveoli (Fig. 11–4). The membranes stain for lipid, are Feulgen positive (indicative of nuclear debris), and give strong immunofluorescent reactions for fibrin. At one time the membranes were thought to be composed solely of inspissated amniotic secretions, but it has been clearly shown that they are largely made up of fibrinogen and fibrin admixed with cell debris derived chiefly from necrotic alveolar-lining pneumocytes.[22] The sequence of events that lead to the formation of hyaline membranes was depicted in Figure 11–3. To this sequence can be added necrosis of alveolar lining cells due to anoxia. There is a remarkable paucity of inflammatory reaction associated with these membranes. An additional prominent feature is intense vascular congestion accompanied by distention of the lymphatics, which are often engorged with a protein-rich fluid. The lesions of hyaline membrane disease are never seen in stillborn infants and those live-born babies who die within a few hours after birth.

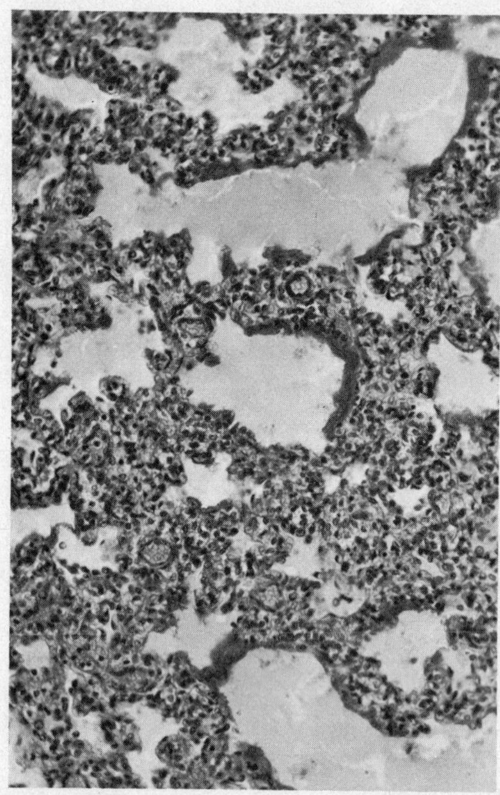

Figure 11–4. Hyaline membrane disease. There is alternating atelectasis and emphysema of the alveoli, and many air spaces are filled with fluid and lined by thick hyaline membranes.

In infants who survive more than 48 hours reparative changes are seen in the lungs. The alveolar epithelium proliferates over the surface of the membrane, essentially to incorporate it within the alveolar septum. At other places the membrane may be desquamated into the air space, where it may undergo partial digestion or phagocytosis by macrophages. Concentric lamellar bodies within type II pneumocytes (morphologic markers of surfactant synthesis) can be found, but are decreased in number.

CLINICAL COURSE. It is difficult to express a clinical course and prognosis for this disease, since so much depends on the maturity and birth weight of the infant, the therapy employed, and the promptness of institution of the therapy. Overall, the mortality rate is approximately 20 to 30%, reaching levels exceeding 50% in infants in the range of 1000 gm body weight. The major threat to life is inadequate pulmonary exchange of oxygen and carbon dioxide, and with it a metabolic acidosis. The keystone of treatment is the delivery of oxygen to these severely hypoxic infants, usually accomplished by a variety of ventilatory assist methods. Such therapy carries with it the now well-recognized hazard of oxygen toxicity. High concentrations of oxygen administered for prolonged periods have been proved to

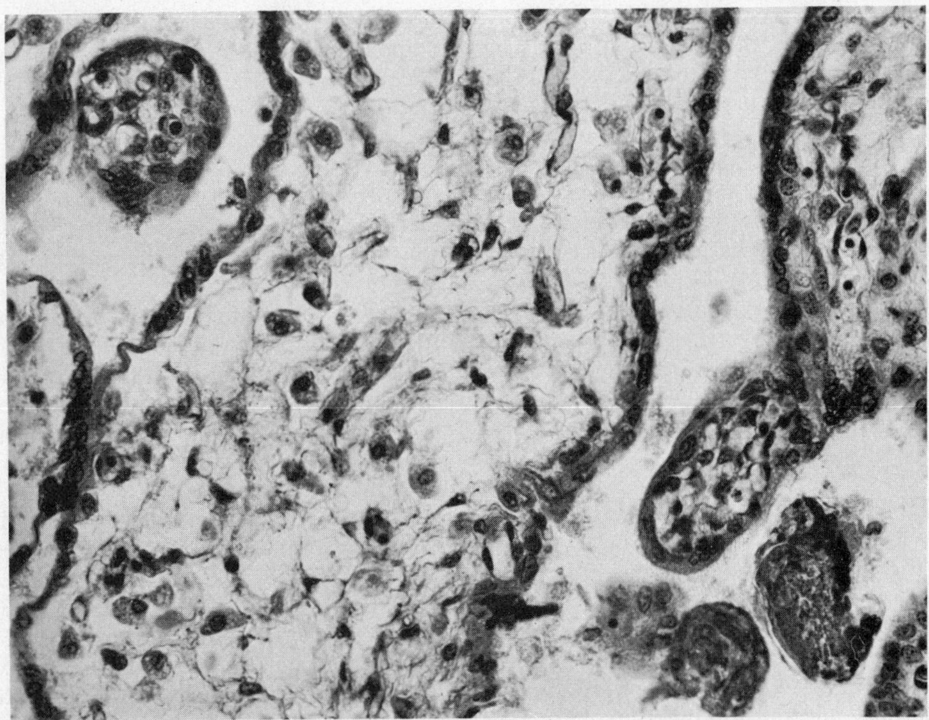

Figure 11–7. High-power detail of a plancental villus to demonstrate edema and round-to-oval Hofbauer cells.

Clinical Features. The clinical manifestations of the three patterns of erythroblastosis should be readily evident from the preceding discussion. They range from pallor, possibly accompanied by hepatosplenomegaly in the infant with congenital anemia (to which may be added jaundice with more severe hemolytic reactions) to the most gravely ill child with intense jaundice, widespread edema, and signs of neurologic involvement in the pattern referred to as hydrops fetalis. The anemia may be so profound as to induce respiratory distress and signs of cardiac decompensation. The combination of hepatic hypoxia, massive extramedullary hematopoiesis, and accumulated bilirubin may add an element of hepatic failure to the symptom complex.

In the last 15 years, remarkable success has been achieved in the prophylaxis of Rh hemolytic disease. As mentioned earlier, administration of anti-D immunoglobulin to Rh-negative (previously nonsensitized) women within 72 hours of delivery of an Rh-positive child prevents Rh immunization in the vast majority of cases. Obviously such treatment has to be employed not only after the first but also following each subsequent childbirth. Although experience has indicated that the use of immunoprophylaxis is highly successful in preventing Rh sensitization, it is not perfect. Approximately 2% of women at risk develop anti-D antibodies in the last trimester or within 72 hours after labor, and thus fail to benefit from Rh immunoprophylaxis.[32] Some of these cases may result from unrecognized previous Rh-positive abortions, but most are believed to be due to significant transplacental bleeds during the early part of the third trimester. In principle, it should be possible to prevent sensitization in such women and thereby increase the success of Rh immunoprophylaxis if anti-D immunoglobulin is administered antepartum at 28 or 34 weeks of gestation as well as postpartum. Although the success of such an approach has been documented in some studies, antepartum administration of anti-D immunoglobulins is still not a widely accepted practice. Doubts have been expressed about its cost effectiveness, especially in view of the fact that Rh immunoglobulin at present can be prepared only in humans by deliberate immunization of Rh-negative persons.[32]

Despite all efforts to prevent incompatibility reactions, it is still necessary to monitor the infant at birth for indications of impending disease. The most important clue to potential disease is a positive direct Coombs' test on fetal cord blood, which detects the presence of antibody globulin coating the fetal red cells. In the *direct* Coombs' test, antiserum (Coombs' serum) against human gamma globulin induces agglutination of red cells coated with specific antibodies. An *indirect* Coombs' test employs normal red cells exposed first to the suspected serum and then treated with Coombs' serum, which then induces agglutination of the red cells if anti–red cell antibodies are present in the suspected serum. Postnatally, the severity of the hemolytic reaction can be monitored by the rapidity of the rise and the ultimate levels of the unconjugated bilirubin in the serum of the infant. The levels may be normal at birth because of placental clearance of the bilirubin, but in severe hemolytic disease they rise rapidly within the first day of life to reach extremely high levels (over 20 mg/dl). Premature or low-birth-weight infants are at greatest risk because their conjugating and excretory systems are less able to cope with the bilirubin overload.

The availability of tests to monitor the severity of the hemolytic reaction has opened a variety of avenues for the treatment of hemolytic disease of the newborn. When analysis of amniotic fluid discloses critical levels of bilirubin, premature delivery may be induced if the fetus is judged to be viable with regard to size. Earlier, the complex and still somewhat hazardous procedure of intrauterine fetal transfusion may be attempted. Postnatally, a variety of supportive measures may be employed, including phototherapy (visual light oxidizes toxic indirect bilirubin to harmless, readily excreted, water-soluble dipyrroles) and, in severe cases, total exchange transfusion of the infant.

INBORN ERRORS OF METABOLISM

The number of now well-characterized inborn errors of metabolism has become astronomic and far beyond our scope. Most of these conditions are exceedingly rare. Some were discussed earlier, in the chapter on genetic disorders (p. 141). Only two, phenylketonuria and galactosemia, are selected for inclusion here because, in both, prompt recognition in the first days of life permits the institution of an appropriate dietary regimen that can prevent early death, or, even worse, survival with mental retardation.

PHENYLKETONURIA (PKU)

Phenylketonuria is an autosomal recessive disorder expressed in the homozygote, characterized by a lack of phenylalanine hydroxylase, which if untreated leads to hyperphenylalaninemia and usually mental retardation. This description applies to the great majority of patients with *classic PKU*, but several significant exceptions have been noted in recent years.[33, 34] For example, it is quite clear that hyperphenylalaninemia is not necessarily associated with the stigmata of PKU. Those with so-called "benign hyperphenylalaninemia" do not develop mental retardation except in the few cases with marked elevation of blood phenylalanine levels (p. 491). On the other end of the spectrum are some patients in whom neurologic impairment occurs despite dietary control of phenylalanine intake. These complexities are clearly significant since it can no longer be assumed that an infant with elevated phenylalanine level requires the rigors of dietary restrictions, nor can the mere restriction of phenylalanine intake be considered adequate for every infant with hyperphenylalaninemia. A detailed discussion of phenylalanine metabolism is beyond our scope, but a brief overview is warranted to obtain some insight into the varieties of hyperphenylalaninemia.

In a normal child, less than 50% of the dietary phenylalanine is utilized for polypeptide and protein synthesis; most of that remaining is converted to tyrosine by means of hydroxylation. This reaction requires the phenylalanine hydroxylating system, which has several components in addition to the hepatic enzyme phenylalanine hydroxylase (PH) (Fig. 11–8).[35] Two of the components, tetrahydrobiopterin (BH_4) and dihydropteridine reductase (DHPR), are relevant for our discussion. During the hydroxylation of phenylalanine to tyrosine, BH_4, which is the coenzyme for PH, is converted to dihydrobiopterin (BH_2). The latter is then reduced back to BH_4 by the enzyme DHPR. As indicated in Figure 11–8, the regeneration of BH_4 is tightly coupled to the hydroxylation of phenylalanine. In addition to their role in phenylalanine metabolism, DHPR and BH_4 are involved in the hydroxylations of tyrosine and tryptophan, a fact that is relevant to the pathogenesis of the variant forms of PKU. With this background we can discuss the genetic and phenotypic variants of hyperphenylalaninemia.[33-35]

The classic form of PKU is believed to result from an almost complete lack (<0.27% of normal) of hepatic PH (PH° phenotype), whereas a less severe deficiency of PH (PH^-) may lead to benign hyperphenylalaninemia. In the latter condition hepatic PH activity varies between 1.5 and 34.5% of normal, presumably owing to the presence of several distinct mutations at the PH locus. The levels of hydroxylase activity in turn determine the plasma phenylalanine levels. Those with the PH° phenotype usually have sustained and marked hyperphenylalaninemia (>1 mM/liter; normal <0.12) when ingesting a normal diet, whereas phenylalanine levels range from 0.12 to 1.0 mM in patients with the PH^- phenotype. The frequencies of the PH° and PH^- phenotypes vary widely in different populations, but in general PH° is more common (three- to fourfold) than PH^- in most population groups. Among whites in the United States the frequency of the PH° phenotype is estimated to be one in 11,000; it is higher in Celtic-derived people and Central Europeans. *Approximately 3 to 10% of patients with PKU have an underlying deficiency of enzymes other than PH.*[36] In one variant form the enzyme dihydropteridine reductase (DHPR) is lacking, whereas in another there is defective synthesis of dihydrobiopterin (BH_2) leading secondarily to a lack of tetrahydrobiopterin (BH_4) (see Fig. 11–8). As mentioned earlier, DHPR and BH_4 are required not only for phenylalanine metabolism but also for the hydroxylation of tyrosine and tryptophan, an essential step in the synthesis of their neurotransmitter metabolites. In such cases, the successful control of hyperphenylalaninemia by dietary measures fails to arrest the progressive neurologic damage since the synthesis of neurotrans-

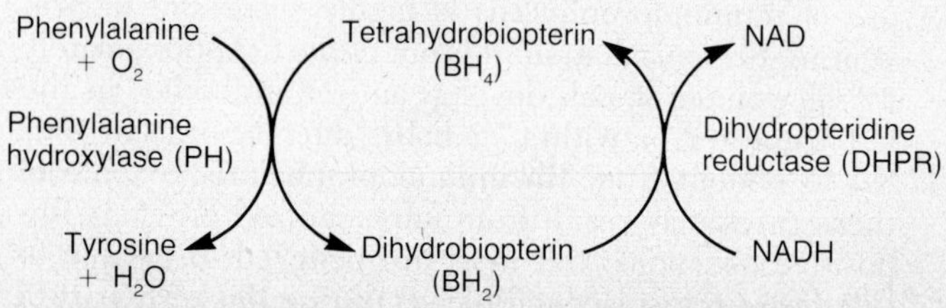

Figure 11–8. The phenylalanine hydroxylase system.

mitters remains impaired. At present the variant forms of PKU can be distinguished from classic PKU only in specialized laboratories.[36]

With a block in the conversion of phenylalanine to tyrosine, several minor metabolites of phenylalanine are synthesized in excessive amounts. These include phenylpyruvic acid, phenyllactic acid, phenylacetic acid, and O-hydroxyphenylacetic acid, all of which are excreted in the urine. The peculiar musty or mouselike odor of untreated patients has been attributed to the presence of phenylacetic acid in the sweat. The basis of mental retardation in PKU is not entirely clear; excessive amounts of phenylalanine or its metabolites are probably involved. Although there is no straightforward or consistent relationship between plasma phenylalanine levels and brain development, it is generally considered that persons with plasma levels above 1 mM per liter (>16.5 mg/dl) are at a high risk of developing mental retardation. This includes all patients with the PH^{o} phenotype and a few of those with the PH^{-} phenotype. In variant forms of PKU, the additional lack of neurotransmitters (derived normally from tyrosine and tryptophan) contribute to the neurologic deterioration.

The only significant morphologic changes found in classic PKU are limited to the brain, and these are variable and nonspecific and cannot be related biochemically to the metabolic changes in these patients. Usually the brain decreases in weight. Defective development of myelin or the formation of an abnormal myelin produces spongy, focal lesions of the white matter.[37] With progression of the disorder, these defects become more evident, the demyelination becomes widespread, and the spongy foci are replaced by areas of gliosis.[38] The precise basis for these neurologic changes is still uncertain, but present indications point to some impairment in synthesis of cerebral lipids caused by the deranged metabolism in these infants.

Infants with classic PKU are apparently normal at birth with no elevation of serum phenylalanine levels. Usually, however, by day 3 or 4 the serum phenylalanine levels begin to rise and in most cases exceed 1 mM per liter (>16.5 mg/dl). Manifestations of brain involvement in the form of abnormal electroencephalographic findings, seizures, and bizarre behavior become evident within three or four months in the untreated infant. Without dietary intervention, the cerebral damage progresses to reach its maximum at age 2 to 3 years. Most untreated patients have IQ values below 20, and less than 4% achieve scores greater than 50 to 60. Characteristically these infants develop the musty or mouselike odor previously mentioned and often eczema of the skin. Because of the deranged tyrosine metabolism, little or no melanin is synthesized, and therefore these patients frequently have unusually fair skin, blonde hair, and blue eyes even when the parents have very dark complexions.

With an appropriate special diet, free of phenylalanine and supplemented with tyrosine, blood levels of phenylalanine can be maintained near normal levels in the classic form and the mental retardation can be prevented. The IQ scores of treated children are near normal and the greatest benefit occurs if treatment is instituted within the first month of life. A controversial issue not yet resolved is the question of when to discontinue treatment. Although earlier it was thought that dietary restrictions of phenylalanine could be terminated after 4 to 5 years of age, some later studies indicate a fall in IQ several years after the cessation of treatment. Until this issue is resolved, most authorities recommend continued treatment into adulthood.[33]

In view of the disastrous but preventable effects of PKU in untreated individuals, great emphasis has been placed on early detection of affected infants. Neonatal screening for elevated blood phenylalanine levels is now widely practiced in the United States and several European countries. However, the screening procedures employed, the Guthrie bacterial inhibition assay and the fluorometric methods, cannot distinguish between various forms of hyperphenylalaninemias, and the diagnosis of PKU requires further metabolic testing.

GALACTOSEMIA

Two forms of galactosemia have been identified, each resulting from a hereditary deficiency of an enzyme involved in the metabolism of galactose. The more common form involves *a lack of galactose-1-phosphate uridyl transferase* blocking the metabolism of galactose in Reaction 2, as is shown in the accompanying diagram. The other form of galactosemia involves a deficiency of galactokinase, also transmitted as an autosomal recessive trait. In contrast to the transferase deficiency, this form is relatively benign and does not cause mental retardation but only the development of cataracts (opacification of the ocular lens); it will not be considered further here.

Estimates of the prevalence of the transferase deficiency range from one in 40,000 to one in 60,000. With a total lack of transferase activity, infants cannot

Reaction 1 $\quad \text{Galactose + ATP} \xrightarrow{\text{Galactokinase}} \text{Galactose-1-phosphate + ADP}$

Reaction 2 $\quad \text{Galactose-1-phosphate + UDP-glucose} \xrightleftharpoons{\text{Galactose-1-phosphate uridyl transferase}} \text{UDP-galactose + glucose-1-phosphate}$

Reaction 3 $\quad \text{UDP-galactose} \xrightleftharpoons{\text{UDP-galactose-4-epimerase}} \text{UDP-glucose}$

metabolize galactose-1-phosphate; when untreated, they develop progressive mental retardation and die early in infancy. Heterozygotes have half the normal level of transferase and are spared the consequences suffered by the homozygote. The lack of transferase activity results from a mutation that leads to the production of an enzymatically inactive protein, which shows antigenic cross reaction with the normal enzyme, suggesting some minor change in the amino acid sequence. Another mutation at the transferase locus results in the synthesis of a protein that possesses only 50% of the normal enzyme activity; this is referred to as the Duarte variant. These individuals are phenotypically normal and can be detected only by assay of enzyme activity.

With the rise in blood galactose levels, galactosuria appears, accompanied by generalized aminoaciduria resulting from impaired renal tubular reabsorption. The diagnosis is suspected by the finding of reducing substances in urine that are not positive for glucose. It can be readily established by a variety of tests. The transferase is normally found in liver cells, leukocytes, and erythrocytes, and sensitive enzyme assays permit identification of the enzyme lack in these cells. Similarly, antenatal diagnosis of this metabolic disorder is possible in cultured fibroblasts derived from amniotic fluid. Heterozygotes having a less severe deficiency in the transferase can also be detected. The elevated galactose levels in the blood and urine are less specific but are valuable clues to the existence of this condition.

In the untreated homozygous disease, infants appear normal at birth, but soon after milk feeding has been instituted develop listlessness, vomiting, diarrhea, and failure to thrive. Jaundice appears early and may seem to be a continuation of the neonatal physiologic jaundice. Soon thereafter, hepatomegaly, splenomegaly, and cataracts develop along with signs of hepatic failure. The liver damage may induce a prothrombin deficiency and a hemorrhagic tendency together with lowered glucose levels and attendant hypoglycemic symptoms. Mental retardation may now become evident. The downward course of the disease may be quite rapid with progressive motor and mental deterioration, leading to death from inanition, secondary infections, or hepatic failure. In particular these infants may develop fulminant *Escherichia coli* septicemia, due possibly to the entry of bacteria from the gut mucosal cells damaged by galactose-1-phosphate.

The involvement of the brain is surprisingly subtle. Nonspecific but definite alterations appear in the central nervous system. Loss of nerve cells, gliosis, and edema are particularly prevalent in the dentate nuclei of the cerebellum and the olivary nuclei of the medulla. There is similar gliosis in the cerebral cortex and white matter, but only occasional damage in the basal ganglia.[39]

Although other organs such as the kidney and eyes are affected, the liver changes are most striking. The early hepatomegaly is due largely to fatty change, but in time cirrhosis supervenes (Fig. 11–9). Microscopically, there is extensive fat throughout the liver lobule as well as bile stasis, both within ductules at the periphery of the lobule and within biliary canaliculi. Often, liver cells are arranged in a rosette-like fashion about the bile plugs. With progression of the disease, a delicate fibrosis appears first in the periportal regions and eventually extends to produce scars bridging adjacent portal tracts. These liver changes have a remarkable resemblance to those found in patients with the cirrhosis of alcohol abuse. Occasionally, in addition to fat the liver cells contain an excess of glycogen.

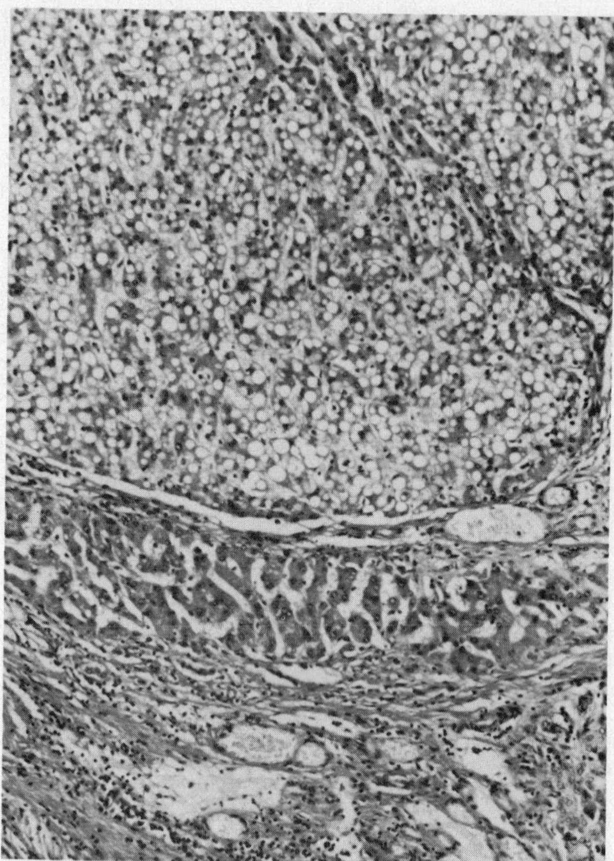

Figure 11–9. Galactosemia. Liver shows extensive fatty change and a delicate fibrosis. (Courtesy of Dr. Joe Rutledge, Southwestern Medical School, Dallas Texas.)

The correlation of the morphologic changes in classic galactosemia with the metabolic derangement in galactose metabolism is not entirely clear. Currently it is proposed that, with the build-up of galactose-1-phosphate behind the transferase block, alternate metabolic pathways are activated with the formation of galactitol. It is postulated that the accumulation of galactitol within the lens leads to hyperosmolarity and excessive imbibition of water to induce the cataracts. The reason for the hepatotoxicity remains obscure. It is of interest that persons with a galactokinase deficiency and high levels of both blood galactose and galactitol do not develop liver damage. Whether galactitol or galactose is directly responsible for the changes in the central nervous system is also unclear.

Early recognition of the homozygous form of the disease, withdrawal of milk from the diet, and substitution of a galactose-free diet spare the infant the clinical and morphologic consequences, and normal development into adulthood may be expected. If treatment is delayed until the onset of symptoms, the neurologic damage seems to be irreversible, although improvements in cataracts and in liver functions may be noted. Delay in the institution of dietary treatment may produce other effects that may not be recognized for many years. In a 1981 study of 18 galactosemic women, 12 were found to have ovarian atrophy. As compared with the six patients who did not have hypogonadism, the affected women were diagnosed and treated at a later age after birth.[40]

CYSTIC FIBROSIS (CF, MUCOVISCIDOSIS)

Among the genetic pediatric disorders, CF is probably the most important. It is very common and frequently fatal in childhood and young adult life. The cause is unknown, *but it is basically a disorder of exocrine glands affecting both mucus-secreting and eccrine sweat glands throughout the body.* The abnormally viscid mucous secretions in the excretory pancreatic ducts leading to their cystic dilatation and fibrous atrophy of the dependent exocrine glands first drew attention to this condition, and gave rise to the designation *cystic fibrosis.* Later it became evident that the mucoid secretions throughout the body were abnormal, and thus this condition became known as *mucoviscidosis.* However, it was then recognized that elevation of sweat sodium chloride and, to a lesser extent, potassium is characteristically present from birth and throughout life, making it evident that more than mucous glands are involved in this disorder, and so the less restrictive term cystic fibrosis is again favored. Nonetheless, the obstruction of organ passages by the abnormally behaving mucus leads to most of the clinical features of this disorder, i.e., chronic pulmonary disease, pancreatic insufficiency, steatorrhea, malnutrition, hepatic cirrhosis, intestinal obstruction, and other complications. These manifestations may appear at any point in life from before birth to much later in childhood or even in adolescence.

INCIDENCE. Most of the evidence favors the view that cystic fibrosis follows simple autosomal recessive transmission. Homozygotes fully express this syndrome. Heterozygotes have no recognizable clinical symptoms. The frequency of cystic fibrosis in whites is approximately one in 2000. Orientals and blacks are seldom affected, but racial intermarriages have disseminated the disease. On the basis of the frequency of affected homozygotes in the white population, it is estimated that one in 20 individuals must be heterozygous carriers. Because of the high frequency of this condition, there is speculation that heterozygotes may have a slight survival advantage, but this hypothesis remains to be proved.

ETIOLOGY AND PATHOGENESIS. No pediatric disease has received more intensive study nor aroused more controversy than CF. Despite all the studies, no unifying concept has yet emerged that satisfactorily explains the abnormalities involving both mucous and sweat glands or unravels the basic metabolic defect. Since CF is a mendelian disorder, one would expect it to be the result of mutation in a single gene, giving rise to a single protein defect (p. 135). However, it has not been possible to identify the abnormal gene product, and therefore detection of heterozygotes is still not feasible. Only a brief survey of the various lines of investigation can be offered here; for more details reference should be made to appropriate reviews.[41, 42]

Before we discuss the various hypotheses, it is worth emphasizing that tissues other than the exocrine secretory glands appear to be normal; that, despite the abnormal behavior of the mucous secretions in CF, the mucous glands themselves are morphologically normal before they are damaged by the disease; and finally that the only consistent biochemical abnormality is the elevation in sweat sodium and chloride levels. Any credible hypothesis must then take into account and explain all these features of cystic fibrosis. The current research into the pathogenesis of CF can be grouped into three major lines of investigation, discussed below.

Physicochemical Properties of Exocrine Secretions. Since the major anatomic changes in CF result from the obstruction of exocrine gland ducts by abnormally behaving mucus, much effort has been spent in the analysis of mucus. Although it is often considered that the mucus secreted by CF patients is more viscid, objective studies to support this notion are scant. Increased viscosity has been documented in pancreatic secretions but not in sputum or other secretions.[41, 43] Turning next to the biochemical composition of the mucus, some authors have reported that mucus obtained from intestinal goblet cells of CF patients is more highly glycosylated,[44] but the generality or significance of this observation remains to be established. It has also been proposed that hypersecretion of calcium by mucous glands is a primary abnormality. Since the solubility of glycoproteins can be decreased by excessive calcium, this would seem to be a plausible hypothesis. However, increased calcium has only been demonstrated in submaxillary saliva obtained from CF patients, and other secretions including tracheobronchial mucus and sweat have a normal calcium content.

Regulation of Exocrine Gland Secretions. Since no consistent abnormality has been found in the composition of the secretions, other investigators have focused on the regulation of exocrine gland functions. *Factors known to regulate secretory processes include intracellular calcium and the activity of the autonomic nervous system.*[45] Increased levels of intracellular calcium have been reported in cells obtained from CF patients, and on the basis of this observation a hypothesis has been proposed that relates the abnormalities in sweat and other exocrine glands to a central disorder of calcium homeostasis.[46] However, whether increased intracellular calcium is a cause of the exocrine gland abnormalities or results from a primary disorder of sodium transport is not clear, so that this hypothesis, like most others, remains in the realm of speculation.[47] Evaluation of the autonomic nervous system in patients with CF has revealed abnormalities. Heightened alpha-adrenergic and cholinergic function and impaired beta-adrenergic responses have been reported.[48] Hyporesponsiveness to beta-adrenergic stimuli has also been confirmed in vitro in the form of reduced cAMP response of leukocytes to beta-adrenergic stimulation. This is explained in part by the reduction of cell membrane beta-adrenergic receptors in leukocytes of CF patients.[49] Whether these observations reflect the presence of a membrane defect in the secretory epithelium as well remains unknown.

Abnormalities in Serum. For over two decades various investigators have reported finding serum factors that inhibit ciliary activity in vitro in such disparate animal models as rabbit tracheal epithelium and gills of oyster. Depending on the investigator and the assay system employed, such factors have been called "mucociliary inhibitors"[50] or "ciliary dyskinesia substances."[51] More recently, such factors have also been obtained from saliva, urine, and supernatants of fibroblasts and leukocytes cultured in vitro. Since measurements in the assay systems employed for the detection of these factors are subjective, much disagreement has been generated regarding the validity and reproducibility of such data.[41] Nevertheless, interest continues, since the reported in vitro effects of these factors (i.e., inhibition of ciliary activity and excessive mucus production in the rabbit tracheal epithelium) mimic some of the expressions of CF in vivo. Attempts are under way to biochemically characterize the mucociliary inhibitors, and preliminary data suggest they are low-molecular-weight glycoproteins.[52, 53] If upon further characterization the mucociliary inhibitor is found to be the product of the CF gene, it could be extremely useful in heterozygote screening. As mentioned earlier, 5% of the population is believed to carry the deleterious gene, and at present there is no reliable method for heterozygote detection.

MORPHOLOGY. The anatomic changes are highly variable and depend on which glands are affected and on the severity of this involvement.[54] In some infants, the disease is quite mild and does not seriously disturb their growth and development, and they readily survive into adolescence or adult life. In others, the pancreatic involvement is severe and impairs intestinal absorption because of the pancreatic achylia, and so malabsorption, inanition, and stunted development not only seriously hamper life but shorten survival. In others, the mucous secretion defect leads to obstruction of bronchi and bronchioles and crippling fatal pulmonary infections. Thus, cystic fibrosis may be compatible with long life or may cause death in infancy.

Pancreatic abnormalities are present in approximately 80% of patients. In the milder cases, there may be only accumulations of mucus in the small ducts with some dilatation of the exocrine glands. In more advanced cases, usually seen in older children or adolescents, the ducts are totally plugged, causing atrophy of the exocrine glands and progressive fibrosis (Fig. 11–10). Because many of these children are being kept alive by appropriate therapy, the advance of the disease sometimes leads to total atrophy of the exocrine portion of the pancreas, leaving only the islets within a fibrofatty stroma. The total loss of pancreatic exocrine secretion impairs fat absorption, and so avitaminosis A may contribute to squamous metaplasia of the lining epithelium of the ducts in the pancreas, which are already injured by the inspissated mucous secretions. In part because of the absence of the pancreatic amylases and in part owing to the deranged gastrointestinal mucous secretions, thick tenacious plugs of viscid mucous may be found in the small intestine of infants. Sometimes these cause small bowel obstruction known as **meconium ileus.**

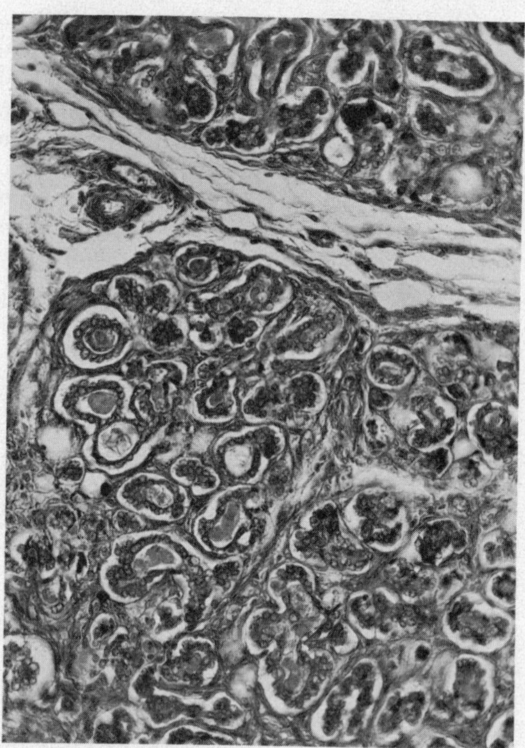

Figure 11–10. Cystic fibrosis of pancreas. Ducts are dilated and plugged with mucin, and parenchymal glands are totally atrophic and replaced by fibrous tissue.

The **liver involvement** follows the same basic pattern. Bile canaliculi are plugged by mucinous material. When this is of long duration, progressive bile duct proliferation and portal fibrosis appear along with a periportal mononuclear cell infiltration. Thus, biliary cirrhosis (p. 928) with its diffuse hepatic nodularity may develop in the longer surviving cases. Such severe hepatic involvement is encountered in only approximately 5% of patients, although minor hepatic changes such as diffuse fatty change are fairly common.

The **salivary glands** are frequently involved with histologic changes similar to those described in the pancreas: progressive dilatation of ducts, squamous metaplasia of the lining epithelium, and glandular atrophy followed by fibrosis.

The **pulmonary changes** are seen in almost every case and are the most serious complications of this disease. These stem from the viscous mucous secretions of the submucosal glands of the respiratory tree with secondary obstruction and infection of the air passages. Grossly, the lungs may be emphysematous or atelectatic, depending on whether the mucus plugs cause subtotal or total obstruction of the respiratory passages. The bronchioles are often distended with thick mucus associated with marked hyperplasia and hypertrophy of the mucus-secreting cells. Superimposed infections give rise to severe chronic bronchitis and bronchiectasis (p. 729). In many instances, lung abscesses develop. *Staphylococcus aureus* and *Pseudomonas aeruginosa* are the two most common organisms responsible for lung infections. For reasons not entirely clear, a mucoid form of *P. aeruginosa* seems to be emerging as the most frequent respiratory pathogen in CF. Its prevalence does not seem to be related to long-term antibiotic therapy.[55] Once this organism is acquired, it seems to persist for long periods, presumably owing to its ability to escape phagocytosis and its impermeability to antibiotics.

A variety of other morphologic changes may be present; important among these are the obstruction of wolffian duct derivatives, i.e., the epididymis and vas deferens, which are responsible for azoospermia and infertility in 95% of the males who survive to adulthood.

CLINICAL COURSE. Few childhood diseases are as protean as cystic fibrosis in clinical manifestations. The symptomatology may range from mild to severe, from onset at birth to first becoming evident years later, and from syndromes that present essentially as cardiopulmonary disease to those that present as intestinal obstruction or as prolapse of the rectum due to chronic constipation. In the classic case, the disorder is discovered in a child between the second and twelfth month of life who comes to attention because of malodorous steatorrhea and recurrent chronic pulmonary infections. Severely affected newborns may fail to regain their birth weight. In others (approximately 5 to 10%), the meconium ileus produces intestinal obstruction and, indeed, such may occur in utero and lead to perforation of the gut. The pancreatic insufficiency induces a malabsorption syndrome manifested principally as inanition, fat intolerance, steatorrhea, and deficient absorption of the fat-soluble vitamins A, D, and K (p. 403). Avitaminosis K may in turn lead to bleeding tendencies. In almost all instances, if the infant or child survives long enough, chronic cough, obstructive pulmonary disease, and persistent pulmonary infections develop and are responsible for approximately 80 to 90% of deaths.

Early diagnosis of this condition continues to be a problem; considerable numbers of patients are not identified until after death. Attention to the nutritional status of the patient and antibiotic control of pulmonary infections significantly prolong survival, if the disease can be identified early. Most reliable is the sweat test as formulated by the Cystic Fibrosis Foundation: "The diagnosis of cystic fibrosis must include a carefully performed quantitative pilocarpine iontophoretic sweat test which is interpreted by an experienced physician. Generally the test should be carried out in duplicate or repeated at least one time." A positive sweat test in the presence of one or more of the major clinical features provides reasonable evidence of the disease.

Better medical care of these patients has produced heartening improvement in the outlook for this disease. Not more than two decades ago, most patients died in infancy; today the mean survival is in the range of 20 years. Despite survival into adult life, most affected males are aspermic because of regressive changes in the epididymis, raising once again the puzzling problem of how the frequency of this serious deleterious gene or genes is maintained in the white population.

SUDDEN INFANT DEATH SYNDROME (SIDS)

The Second International Conference on Causes of Sudden Death in Infants formulated the most widely accepted definition of SIDS as follows: "the sudden and unexpected death of an infant who was either well or almost well prior to death, and whose death remains unexplained after the performance of an adequate autopsy."[56] Clearly, this definition reflects our ignorance of the very basis of this tragic disorder. Not surprisingly, therefore, the literature has been flooded with hypotheses, speculations, and conjectures, many of which have not stood the test of time. Favored today is the view that these infants have a defect in the autonomic regulation of respiratory or cardiac functions. Here we will review the salient epidemiologic, anatomic, and pathophysiologic studies that have contributed to the formulation of some working hypotheses. A detailed discussion of these may be found in several reviews.[57-59]

Also called "crib death" or "cot death," this stunning family tragedy is by no means uncommon, since it is estimated to account for about 10,000 deaths annually in the United States. As infantile deaths due to nutritional problems and microbiologic infections have come under control in countries enjoying higher standards of living, SIDS has assumed greater importance and is now one of the major causes of mortality in 2- to 4-month-old infants. Around the world it causes from one to five deaths per 1000 live births.

Most of these infants are between the ages of 2 and 4 months. Most die at home, usually during the night after a period of sleep. Only rarely is the catastrophic event observed, but even when seen it is reported that the apparently healthy infant mysteriously and suddenly turns blue, stops breathing, and becomes limp without emitting a cry or struggle. Most have had minor manifestations of an upper respiratory infection preceding the fatal event.

In recent years the term "near-SIDS" has been applied to those infants who could be resuscitated after such an episode. There is little doubt that this term is diagnostically imprecise and that many such infants have definable underlying diseases. However, since some of the apparently normal "near-misses" have been reported to succumb later to SIDS, considerable interest is centered around the definition of potentially significant but subtle cardiovascular or pulmonary abnormalities in these infants.[58]

Circumstances surrounding these deaths have been explored in great detail and have yielded some significant observations, but the basic mystery has not been resolved. *There is considerable evidence that as a group these infants are different from normal infants in a great many respects.*[60] At autopsy, their crown-to-heel length, head circumference, and weight gain are significantly lower than in controls. The growth retardation involves not only the skeletal system but also the brain and other organs. In general they are less active during life than their sibling controls, nurse less effectively, and in many respects are less robust than normal infants of comparable birth weight and age. However, none of these characteristics—singly or in combination—is sufficiently clear-cut to identify infants at particular risk.

Attempts to develop a profile of the family setting have yielded the following correlates: premature birth, with resultant lower birth weight; families from lower socioeconomic groups, particularly minority groups; large families; overcrowded homes; and young mothers. The risk is increased if the mother smoked cigarettes or abused narcotics (particularly methadone). The latter is associated with a markedly increased risk, independent of socioeconomic status. However, it should be emphasized that no infant is immune, and SIDS has occurred despite optimal home conditions. Although there is no evidence for any genetic predisposition, there is an unmistakable tendency for this tragedy to recur within families. Among siblings of affected infants, crib death is four to seven times more common than in the population at large.

At autopsy a variety of findings have been recorded. An increase in the thickness of small pulmonary arteries due to medial smooth muscle hypertrophy and hyperplasia has been noted. This, along with gliosis in the brain stem, has been taken to indicate the presence of chronic hypoxia. Some investigators have reported that many of these infants have right ventricular hypertrophy, but whether this is primary or a consequence of pulmonary arterial changes is unresolved. Histologic abnormalities in the conduction system—the bundle of His and the sinoatrial node—have also been reported by some, but not confirmed by others. These infants also frequently exhibit retention of hepatic extramedullary hematopoiesis and periadrenal "brown" fat, and an increased volume of adrenal chromaffin cells. It is tempting to speculate that all these changes relate to chronic hypoxemia, retardation of normal development, and chronic stress.[61] Petechiae in the pleura and epicardium as well as pulmonary congestion and edema compatible with hypoxic death are often found, but these could be agonal changes. There may also be some histologic evidence of recent respiratory infection, but these changes are generally considered to be of no lethal significance. Although autopsy fails to provide a clear cause of death, it is clear that as a group most of these infants do reveal subtle morphologic abnormalities, albeit of uncertain significance.

Understandably, a large number of etiologic and pathogenic postulations have been offered. Infection, particularly viral infection, is thought by some to be important. In support is cited the frequent history of antecedent viral infection and the increased frequency of both SIDS and viral infections in winter months. Virus can often be recovered from a variety of tissues post mortem, but in a significant proportion of infants no virus is isolated. Moreover, the isolation rate for virus in these circumstances does not differ significantly from that in infants dying of other causes. Viral infections are now believed merely to unmask or exaggerate other regulatory abnormalities of respiration.

Currently favored is the possibility of an *instantaneous interruption of some basic physiologic function involving either the heart or respiration. There is a belief, disputed by some, that even normal infants have electrical instability of the heart as a consequence of the normal remodeling process of the cardiac conduction system.* As the heart grows larger, there is resorption of some conduction fibers and growth of others, yielding an unstable condition. In support of the cardiac theory, electrocardiographic abnormalities (prolonged Q-T interval) have been cited in some "near-SIDS" and normal infants between the ages of 2 and 4 months, a period corresponding to the peak incidence of SIDS. These have been attributed to some imbalance in the function of the sympathetic nervous system.[57] Other indications of autonomic dysfunction, such as alterations in the heart rate and rhythm, have also been suspected. Conceivably, these less robust and more fragile infants might be more vulnerable to cardiac irregularities. However, there is no unanimity as to whether the morphologic evidence supports such a notion.

Interruption of respiratory function that may arise centrally or peripherally[62] continues to be a seductive hypothesis. In favor of a central dysfunction is the observation that, in some infants with episodes of "near-SIDS" that eventually culminated in sudden death, there is a history of repeated spells of apnea, some of which are prolonged (>15 sec). Sleep could well be a predisposing factor, since it depresses central respiratory activity. Similarly, apneic episodes are more common with infection and in infants of low birth weight. Central hypoventilation is also associated with use of methadone by the mother, which as mentioned earlier greatly increases the risk of SIDS. Alternatively, the respiratory defect may be peripheral. It has been shown that in the young infant the airway is particularly vulnerable to narrowing at the oropharyngeal level when there is marked muscle relaxation during deep sleep, a large tongue, and a hypermobile mandible. Inapparent infections may compound the problem by triggering laryngeal spasm or pathways involving recently described postlaryngeal receptors, leading to reflex apnea. The repeated episodes of hypoxia could be responsible for the changes in pulmonary vasculature and astrogliosis of the brain stem already mentioned, although at present it is not possible to establish a clear cause-and-effect relationship between the anatomic and functional changes. In conclusion, although mystery still surrounds these deaths, most investigators now believe that infants at risk have subtle physiologic handicaps, some of which may have been acquired before birth.

TUMORS AND TUMOR-LIKE LESIONS OF INFANCY AND CHILDHOOD

Only 2% of all malignant tumors occur in infancy and childhood; nonetheless, cancer (including leukemia) is the leading cause of death from disease in the United States in children beyond infancy and up to 14 years of age. According to the Vital Statistics of the United States in 1980, neoplastic disease accounted for approximately 9.2% of all deaths in this cohort; only accidents caused more. Benign tumors are even more common than cancers. Most benign tumors are of little concern, but rarely they cause serious disease or even death by virtue of their location or rapid increase in size.

It is surprisingly difficult to segregate on morphologic grounds true tumors or neoplasms from tumor-like lesions in the infant and child. Displaced cells and masses of tissue may be present from birth that are normal in appearance histologically but nonetheless grow at approximately the same rate as the growth of the fetus and infant. Indeed, few neoplasms grow as rapidly as the normal embryo. Should such displaced cells and masses be construed as new growths or simply as malformations that enlarge along with the child? In recognition of these intergrades between normal tissue growth and true neoplasia, several special categories of tumor-like lesions have been created.

CHORISTOMAS

The term choristoma has been applied to microscopically normal cells or tissues that are present in abnormal locations. Generally a choristoma is a cohesive mass of aberrant or heterotopic tissue, e.g., a rest of pancreatic tissue found in the wall of the stomach or small intestine, or a small mass of adrenal cells found in the kidney, lungs, ovary, or elsewhere. Rarely, choristomas take the form of scattered, normal-appearing cells found in inappropriate locations. The heterotopic rests are usually of only academic interest, but they can be confused clinically with neoplasms. Rarely, they are sites of origin of true neoplasms, producing the paradox of an adrenal carcinoma arising in the ovary. Even more rarely, an aberrant rest of splenic tissue may perpetuate abnormal hypersplenic function following removal of the definitive spleen (p. 699).

HAMARTOMAS

The term hamartoma designates an excessive focal overgrowth of mature normal cells and tissues in an organ, composed of identical cellular elements. Although the cellular elements are mature and identical to those found in the remainder of the organ, they do not reproduce the normal architecture of the surrounding tissue. The line of demarcation between a hamartoma and a benign neoplasm is at best tenuous and is variously interpreted. Hemangiomas, lymphangiomas, rhabdomyomas of the heart, adenomas of the liver, and developmental cysts within the kidneys, lungs, or pancreas are construed by some as hamartomas and by others as true neoplasms. The frequency of these lesions in infancy and childhood gives credence to the belief that they are developmental aberrations, meriting the designation hamartoma. In support of this view, some of these tumors, principally hemangiomas, spontaneously regress and completely disappear. Whatever the interpretation, they are often present at birth, and for a time may rapidly enlarge along with the growth of the infant and child. In the course of such growth they can become bothersome clinical problems, as discussed below.

BENIGN TUMORS AND TUMOR-LIKE LESIONS

Reference has already been made to the difficulty in distinguishing benign tumors from hamartomas. The benign neoplasms are far more common in infancy and childhood than are cancers. Virtually any histologic pattern may be encountered, but within this wide array hemangiomas, lymphangiomas, and teratomas deserve special mention. They are described in greater detail in appropriate chapters, but here a few comments will be made about their special features in childhood.

Hemangiomas (p. 539) are the most common tumors of infancy. Architecturally they do not differ from those encountered in adults. In children most are located in the skin, particularly on the face and scalp, where they produce flat-to-elevated, irregular, red-blue masses; sometimes large lesions are referred to as "port-wine stains." They may enlarge along with the growth of the child, but in many instances, as mentioned, they spontaneously regress. In addition to their cosmetic significance, they can represent one facet of some hereditary disorder, such as von Hippel-Lindau disease. On very rare occasions, vascular tumors, particularly those in the liver and soft tissues, demonstrate malignant changes.

A wide variety of lesions are of lymphatic origin. Some of them—*lymphangiomas*—are hamartomatous or neoplastic in origin, whereas others appear to represent abnormal dilations of preexisting lymph channels known as *lymphangiectasis.* The lymphangiomas (p. 544) are usually characterized by cystic and cavernous spaces. Lesions of this nature may occur on the skin but more importantly are encountered in the deeper regions of the neck, axilla, mediastinum, retroperitoneal tissue, and elsewhere (Fig. 11–11). Although histologically benign, they tend to increase in size after birth, both by the collection of fluid and by the budding of preexisting spaces. In this manner they encroach on vital structures such as those in the mediastinum or nerve trunks in the axilla to constitute serious clinical problems. Lymphangiectasis, in contrast, usually presents as a diffuse swelling of a part of or all of an extremity; considerable distortion and deformation may result as a consequence of the spongy, dilated subcutaneous and deeper lymphatics. However, the lesion is not progressive and does

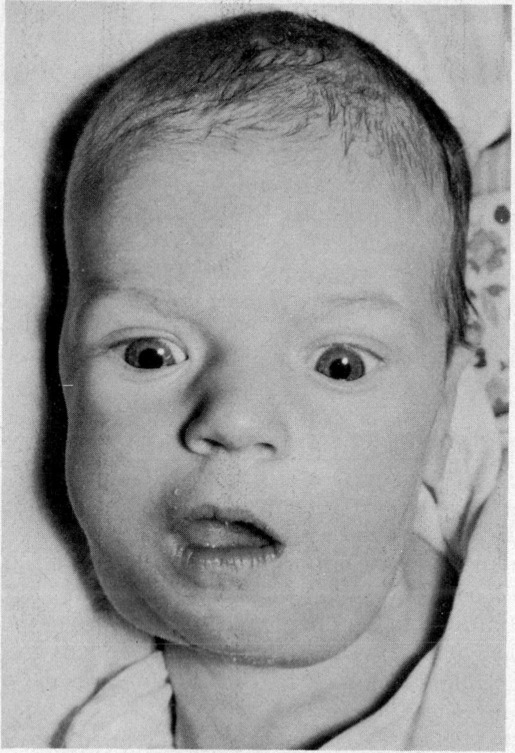

Figure 11–11. Infant with a submandibular lymphangioma causing irregular swelling beneath chin and in right buccal region.

not extend beyond its original location. Nonetheless, it gives rise to difficult corrective cosmetic problems.

Teratomas (p. 231) may occur as well-differentiated cystic lesions—dermoid cysts that are usually benign—or as solid malignant teratomas. They exhibit two peaks in incidence; the first at approximately 2 years of age and the second in late adolescence or early adult life. The first peak probably represents congenital neoplasms; the later-occurring lesions may merely be more slowly growing lesions of prenatal origin. Most teratomas of infancy and childhood arise in the sacrococcygeal region. Other sites include the gonads, mediastinum, base of the skull, roof of the pharynx, hard or soft palate, and base of the tongue. Sacrococcygeal teratomas occur in one out of 20,000 to 40,000 live births and are noted four times more frequently in females than in males. Approximately 75% of these are histologically mature (p. 155) with a benign course, and of the remainder about 12% are unmistakably malignant and lethal. Most of the benign teratomas are encountered in younger infants (below the age of 4 months), whereas children with malignant lesions tend to be somewhat older.[63]

MALIGNANT TUMORS

Cancers of infancy and childhood differ in many respects from those of later life. Our purpose here is to point out these differential features rather than describe individual neoplasms, which are considered in later chapters dealing with the appropriate organs.

TYPES. Although any type of cancer may arise in the early years of life and indeed in utero, the distribution of common cancers of infancy and childhood differs sharply from that of adults. Carcinomas of the skin, lung, breast, prostate, and colon (to mention only some of the more common tumors) constitute the burden of neoplasia in adults, but these lesions are distinctly uncommon in childhood. Instead, the usual origins of childhood cancers are the hematopoietic system, nervous tissue (including the central and sympathetic nervous system, adrenal medulla, and retina), soft tissues, bone, and kidney. *Eight neoplasms exhibit sharp peaks in incidence in children under 5 years of age:* (1) leukemia (principally acute lymphocytic leukemia), (2) neuroblastoma (Fig. 11–12), (3) Wilms' tumor, (4) liver cancer, (5) retinoblastoma, (6) rhabdomyosarcoma, (7) teratoma, and (8) ependymoma. Other forms of cancer are also common in childhood but do not have the same striking early peak. The distribution of these cancers is roughly indicated in Table 11–6. Within this large array, leukemia alone accounts for more deaths in children under 15 years of age than all the other tumors collectively. In order of importance it is followed by neuroblastoma, Wilms' tumor, lymphoma, and osteogenic sarcoma. Collectively, these five forms of neoplasia account for almost three-fourths of all neoplastic deaths in this age group.

GENETICS AND ORIGINS. As earlier discussions have noted (pp. 155 and 248), *genetic mutations underlie certain tumors, many of which occur in childhood.* In some instances the mutation produces both an increased predisposition to cancer and concomitant congenital malformations. These associations provide, in some instances, easily detected clinical syndromes having a strong potential for the later appearance of a neoplasm. For example, the child with congenital aniridia is vulnerable to Wilms' tumor. Usually the *a*niridia is also associated with *g*enitourinary malformations and mental *r*etardation (AGR complex). Hemihypertrophy (gross asymmetry of the body) carries with it an increased risk

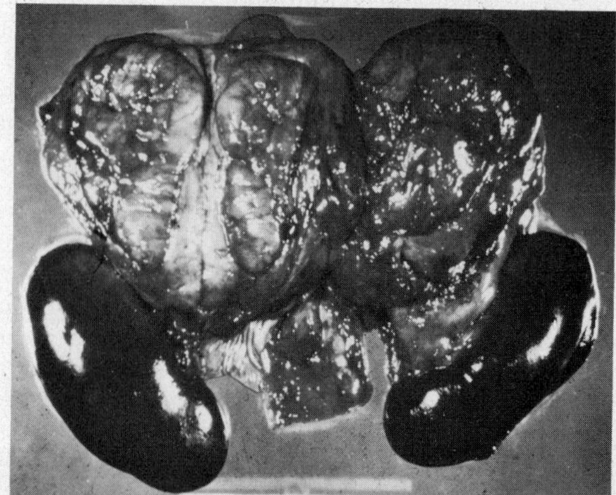

Figure 11–12. Bilateral adrenal neuroblastomas that dwarf the kidneys.

Table 11–6. COMMON MALIGNANT NEOPLASMS OF INFANCY AND CHILDHOOD

0 to 4 Years	5 to 9 Years	10 to 14 Years
Leukemia	Leukemia	
Retinoblastoma	Retinoblastoma	
Neuroblastoma	Neuroblastoma	
Wilms' tumor		
Hepatoblastoma	Hepatocarcinoma	Hepatocarcinoma
Soft tissue sarcoma (especially rhabdomyosarcoma)	Soft tissue sarcoma	Soft tissue sarcoma
Teratomas		
CNS tumors	CNS tumors	
	Ewing's tumor	
	Lymphoma	Osteogenic sarcoma
		Thyroid carcinoma
		Hodgkin's disease
		Carcinoma of colon

of Wilms' tumor, hepatoblastoma, and adrenocortical carcinoma. These and other associations have been reviewed.[64]

Cancer-predisposing mutations may take the form of cytogenetic aberrations. A child with trisomy 21 (Down's syndrome) has about a one in 200 chance of developing leukemia, representing a ten- to 15-fold increased attack rate. A small number of cases of neuroblastoma and Wilms' tumor show associations with specific deletions of chromosomes 13 and 11 respectively, often accompanied by several other congenital malformations.[65] Those with the chromosomal breakage syndromes have a high frequency of leukemias (p. 264).

Gene mutations with autosomal dominant modes of transmission underlie certain forms of neoplasia (p. 264). Principal among these autosomal dominant tumors is the retinoblastoma (derived from neuroblasts in the retina), but the evidence grows stronger with each passing year that Wilms' tumor and neuroblastoma also have similar modes of transmission. Knudson proposes a two-mutation theory for these childhood cancers in which the first mutation is prezygotic in germinal cells, providing a subsoil for the second mutation early in life, which initiates the cancer.[66] In sporadic cases, both mutations might occur as postzygotic events, more likely initiating tumor development at a later age. However, it must be emphasized that even with the retinoblastoma and all other tumors with mendelian transmission, only a proportion of all patients with such neoplasms have well-defined, familial hereditary backgrounds. It has been estimated that only 40% of all cases of retinoblastoma are hereditary; the remainder are sporadic. With the prezygotic familial tumors there is a much greater likelihood of bilateral lesions, and the mean age of appearance is significantly lowered. Moreover, those with "cancer genes" are more susceptible to other forms of cancer, sometimes expressed as a risk of the order of 10 to 15%.[67]

Several cautions must be noted. Gene carriers do not inevitably develop neoplasms, and in the case of the retinoblastoma there is a 10% chance that the carrier will not develop a tumor (90% penetrance). With Wilms' tumor the penetrance is estimated to be 60%. Moreover, bilateral neoplasms, as for example Wilms' tumors, may be encountered in children with unaffected parents. According to Knudson's two-hit hypothesis, reduced penetrance may be explained by the absence of the second or somatic event in the carriers of the first mutation. This may also account for the less than 100% concordance in monozygotic twins.

Environmental influences also contribute significantly to the origin of childhood cancers. Best documented is the carcinogenic potential of radiant energy. The nuclear fallout of the atomic bombs has yielded a 1.5- to 1.8-fold increased incidence of cancer deaths (excluding leukemia) in survivors who received 200 rads or more of ionizing radiation. Decades later, an increased incidence of carcinoma of the thyroid has been found in children who received therapeutic irradiation of the head or neck in early life.[68] Ironically, other types of malignant neoplasms have followed the radiotherapy of retinoblastomas, Wilms' tumors, and neuroblastomas. Chemical agents (including drugs) also contribute to the origin of malignant neoplasms. Vaginal adenosis—glandular inclusions thought to be precancerous—and vaginal adenocarcinoma have developed in children whose mothers received stilbestrol between the eighth and 18th week of pregnancy.[69] Most of these cancers occur late in the second decade or early in the third decade of life. Viruses likewise may contribute to the origin of childhood neoplasms. Although the implication is far from established, Burkitt's lymphoma (p. 662), suspected of being caused by the Epstein-Barr virus, is the most common form of lymphoma in childhood. Thus, it is evident that all the environmental influences thought to have carcinogenic potential in adults may induce cancers in early life.

CLINICAL BEHAVIOR. Cancers of infancy and childhood behave quite differently from those of later life. They tend to be more rapidly growing and as a result often produce disproportionately large masses in the young. Bilateral neuroblastomas of the adrenals may induce a protuberant abdomen, as may other intra-abdominal masses. Often they are readily evident on visual inspection when the child is lying down. For unknown reasons, even large masses are not associated with early anemia, loss of weight, or cachexia in this age group. Instead, the clinical manifestations often resemble those of an infectious process, with fever and malaise. Many are responsive to irradiation and chemotherapy, and remarkable results have been achieved with these modalities in certain forms of cancer. For example, two-year survival rates of almost 95% have been reported after the combined use of surgery and chemotherapy in the treatment of Wilms' tumor in children in whom the tumor is limited to the kidney.[70]

Spontaneous differentiation of some childhood tumors, for example, the embryonic neuroblastoma, into the relatively benign ganglioneuroma has been unmistakably documented in some patients. Remarkably, spontaneous regression of neuroblastomas occurs most commonly in patients with small primary tumors and extensive metastases involving liver, skin, and bone marrow (but not bone). Most of these patients are infants with a median age of 3 months, and according to some authors they should be classified into a special category called stage IV-S (special).[71] In contrast, those who have metastases to the bone (stage IV) are usually older (median age 1 year) and usually have aggressive tumors. The cumulative mortality for all ages is about 50%.[72] The recognition of stage IV-S neuroblastomas has generated much interest since clarification of the mechanisms underlying spontaneous regression could advance our understanding of tumor biology. In one study it was found that children with stage IV disease, but not stage IV-S, had high serum levels of ferritin associated with inhibition of T-cell E-rosette formation in vitro.[73] This suggests that immunologic factors may underlie the sharp difference in the biologic behavior of this tumor. According to Knudson, however, the stage IV-S neuroblastoma may be viewed not as a malignant disseminated tumor but as multiple foci of hyperplastic neural crest cells that bear only one of the two mutations required for development of malignancy (p. 499). This interesting hypothesis is testable since hyperplastic foci would have a polyclonal origin, whereas truly malignant tumors are monoclonal.[74]

Depressing as the development of a cancer is in a child, the outlook is not entirely bleak. Moreover, clinical experience has shown that when metastases or recurrences have not taken place after a period of time represented by the patient's age at the time of removal of the lesion plus nine months, the probability is strong that a complete cure has been effected. In other words, cancers of infancy and childhood declare themselves early, and so both parents and patients can be reassured after an appropriate time interval that they no longer live under the sword of Damocles.

In this chapter, it must be apparent that we have only skimmed the surface of the large catalog of pediatric diseases. The disorders presented, however, are among the most common and important and rightfully belong within the scope of general medical knowledge. As stated at the outset, the major disorders of infancy and childhood are peculiar to the age group. Only a few, such as neoplasms, and infections, also affect adults, and then they usually present different morphologic and clinical features. The disorders of children and of adults differ more than the child from the adult.

1. Avery, G.B. (ed.): Neonatal Pathophysiology and Management of the Newborn. 2nd ed. Philadelphia, J.B. Lippincott Co., 1981, p. 205.
2. Apgar, V.: A proposal for a new method of evaluation of the newborn infant. Curr. Res. Anesth. Analg. *32*:260, 1953.
3. Drage, J.S., and Berendes, H.: Apgar scores and outcome of the newborn. Pediatr. Clin. North Am. *13*:635, 1966.
4. Gresham, E.L.: Birth trauma. Pediatr. Clin. North Am. *22*:317, 1975.
5. Curran, J.S.: Birth-associated injury. Clin. Perinatol. *8*:111, 1981.
6. Holmes, L.B.: Congenital malformations. N.Engl. J. Med. *295*:204, 1976.
7. Golbus, M.D.: Teratology for the obstetrician: Current status. Obstet. Gynecol. *55*:269, 1980.
8. Smith, D.W.: Recognizable patterns of human deformation. Identification and management of mechanical effects on morphogenesis. Major Probl. Clin. Pediatr. *21*:1, 1981.
9. Wung, J.T., et al.: CDP: A major breakthrough. Pediatrics *58*:783, 1976.
10. Editorial: Born before their time into this breathing world. Br. Med. J. *2*:1403, 1976.
11. Boyd, R.J., and Oh, W.: Respiratory distress syndrome. Clin. Perinatol. *5*:283, 1978.
12. Usher, R., et al.: Respiratory distress syndrome in infants delivered by cesarean section. Am. J. Obstet. Gynecol. *88*:806, 1964.
13. Robert, M.F.: Association between maternal diabetes and the respiratory distress syndrome of the newborn. N. Engl. J. Med. *294*:357, 1976.
14. Cuestas, R.A.: Low thyroid hormones and respiratory distress syndrome of the newborn. N. Engl. J. Med. *295*:297, 1976.
15. Liggins, G.C., and Howie, R.N.: A controlled trial of antepartum glucocorticoid treatment for prevention of respiratory distress syndrome in premature infants. Pediatrics *50*:515, 1972.
16. Morrison, J.C., et al.: Lecithin-sphingomyelin ratio and RDS in patients with diabetes mellitus: Possible mechanisms. South. Med. J. *73*:912, 1980.
17. Goldberg, J.D., et al.: Cesarian section indication and the risk of respiratory distress syndrome. Obstet Gynecol. *57*:30, 1981.
18. Nielsen, H.C., et al.: Sex differences in human fetal lung maturation. Pediatr. Res. *13*:261, 1979.
19. Avery, M.E., et al.: The Lung and its Disorders in the Newborn Infant. 4th ed. Philadelphia, W. B. Saunders Co., 1981, p. 247.
20. Klein, A.H., et al.: Thyroid function studies in cord blood from premature infants with and without RDS. J. Pediatr., *98*:818, 1981.
21. Lauweryns, J.M.: Hyaline membrane diseases: A pathological study of 55 infants. Pediatrics *50*:515, 1972.
22. Gitliln, D., and Craig, J.M.: Nature of the hyaline membrane in asphyxia of the newborn. Pediatrics *17*:64, 1956.
23. Volpe, J.J.: Neonatal intraventricular hemorrhage. N. Engl. J. Med. *304*:886, 1981.
24. Harvey, D., et al.: Risk of respiratory distress syndrome. Lancet *1*:42, 1975.
25. Young, B., et al.: Intravenous dexamethasone for prevention of neonatal respiratory distress: A prospective controlled study. Am. J. Obstet. Gynecol. *138*:203, 1980.
26. Fujiwara, T., et al.: Artificial surfactant therapy in hyaline-membrane disease. Lancet *1*:55, 1980.
27. Bownan, J.M.: Rh erythroblastosis. Semin. Hematol. *12*:189, 1975.
28. Cherry, S.H.: Current concepts in hemolytic disease and blood group incompatibility. Mt. Sinai J. Med. *47*:454, 1980.
29. Grundbacher, J.F.: The etiology of ABO hemolytic disease of newborn. Transfusion *20*:563, 1980.
30. Editorial: Haemolytic disease of the newborn due to antibodies other than rhesus anti-D. Br. Med. J. *283*:514, 1981.
31. Harper, R.G., et al.: Kernicterus. Clin. Perinatol. *7*:75, 1980.
32. Nusbacher, J., and Bove, J.R.: Rh immunoprophylaxis: is antepartum therapy desirable? N. Engl. J. Med. *303*:935, 1980.
33. Scriver, C.R., and Clow, C.L.: Phenylketonuria: Epitome of human biochemical genetics. N. Engl. J. Med. *303*:1336 and 1394, 1980.
34. Guttler, F.: Hyperphenylalaninemia. Acta Pediatr. Scand. (Suppl.) *280*:9, 1980.
35. Scirver, C.R., and Clow, C.L.: Phenylketonuria and other phenylalanine hydroxylation mutants in man. Annu. Rev. Genet. *14*:179, 1980.
36. Kaufman, S.: Differential diagnosis of variant forms of hyperphenylalaninemia. Pediatrics *65*:840, 1980.
37. Malamud, N.: Neuropathology of phenylketonuria. J. Neuropathol. Exp. Neurol. *25*:254, 1966.
38. Salguero, I.F., et al.: Neuropathologic observations in phenylketonuria. Trans. Am. Neurol. Assoc. *93*:274, 1968.
39. Smetana, H.F., and Olen, E.: Hereditary galactose disease. Am. J. Clin. Pathol. *38*:3, 1962.
40. Kaufman, J.R., et al.: Hypergonadotropic hypogonadism in female patients with galactosemia. N. Engl. J. Med. *304*:994, 1981.
41. Davis, P.B., and Di Sant'Agnese, P.A.: A review: Cystic fibrosis at forty—Quo vadis. Pediatr. Res. *14*:83, 1980.
42. Littlefield, J.W.: Research on cystic fibrosis (editorial). N. Engl. J. Med. *304*:44, 1981.

43. King, M.: Is cystic fibrosis mucus abnormal? Pediat. Res. *15*:120, 1981.
44. Wesley, A.W., et al.: Differences in mucus glycoproteins of small intestines from subjects with and without cystic fibrosis. Adv. Exp. Med. Biol. *144*:145, 1982.
45. Schultz, I., and Stolze, H.H.: The exocrine pancreas: The role of secretagogues, cyclic nucleotides, and calcium in enzyme secretion. Annu. Rev. Physiol. *42*:127, 1980.
46. Shapiro, B.L., and Lam, L.F.-H.: Calcium and age in fibroblasts from control subjects and patients with cystic fibrosis. Science *216*:417, 1982.
47. Sorcher, E.J., and Breslow, J.L.: Cystic fibrosis: A disorder of calcium stimulated secretion and transepithelial sodium transport. Lancet *1*:368, 1982.
48. Davis, P.B., et al.: Abnormal adrenergic and cholinergic sensitivity in cystic fibrosis. N. Engl. J. Med. *302*:1453, 1980.
49. Galant, S.P., et al.: Impaired beta adrenergic receptor binding and function in cystic fibrosis neutrophils. J. Clin. Invest. *68*:253, 1981.
50. Bowman, B.H., et al.: Studies of cystic fibrosis utilizing mucociliary activity in oyster gills. Fed. Proc. *39*:3195, 1980.
51. Wilson, G.B., and Bahm, V.J.: Synthesis and secretion of cystic fibrosis ciliary dyskinesia substances by purified subpopulation of leukocytes. J. Clin. Invest. *66*:1010, 1980.
52. Carson, S.D., and Bowman, B.H.: Cystic fibrosis. I. Fractionation of the mucociliary inhibitor from plasma. Pediatr. Res. *16*:13, 1982.
53. Blitzer, M.G., and Shapira, E.: A purified serum glycopeptide from control and cystic fibrosis patients. I. Comparison of their mucociliary activity on rabbit tracheal explants. Pediatr. Res. *16*:203, 1982.
54. Oppenheimer, E.H., and Easterly, J.R.: Pathology of cystic fibrosis. Review of literature and comparison with 146 autopsied cases. Perspect. Pediatr. Pathol., *2*:241, 1975.
55. Case records of the Massachusetts General Hospital. N. Engl. J. Med. *304*:831, 1981.
56. Bergman, A., et al.: Sudden infant death syndrome. Proceedings of the Second International Conference on Causes of Sudden Death in Infants. Seattle, University of Washington Press, 1970.
57. Schwartz, P.J.: The sudden infant death syndrome. Rev. Perinatol. Med. *4*:475, 1981.
58. Shannon, D.C., and Kelly, D.H.: SIDS and near-SIDS. N. Engl. J. Med. *306*:959 and 1023, 1982.
59. Valdes-Dapena, M.A.: Sudden infant death syndrome, a review of medical literature, 1974–1979. Pediatrics *60*:597, 1980.
60. Valdes-Dapena, M.A.: Sudden unexplained infant death 1970–1975: An evolution in understanding. Pathol. Annu. *12*:117, 1977.
61. Naeye, R.L.: Hypoxemia and the sudden infant death syndrome. Science *186*:837, 1974.
62. Avery, M. E., and Frantz, I. D.: To breathe or not to breathe. What have we learned about apneic spells and sudden infant death? N. Engl. J. Med. *309*:107, 1983.
63. Valdiserri, R.O., and Yunis, E.J.: Sacrococcygeal teratomas. A review of 68 cases. Cancer *48*:217, 1981.
64. Bolande, R.P.: Neoplasia of early life and its relationships to teratogenesis. Perspect. Pediatr. Pathol. *3*:145, 1976.
65. Schimke, R.M.: Genetics and cancer in children. Current Concepts. *In* Kaback, M.M. (ed.): Genetic Issues in Pediatric and Obstetric Practice. Chicago, Year Book Medical Publishers, 1981, p. 413.
66. Knudson, A.G.: Genetics and cancer. Am. J. Med. *67*:1, 1980.
67. Abramson, D.H., et al.: Second tumors in non-irradiated bilateral retinoblastoma. Am. J. Ophthalmol. *87*:624, 1979.
68. Favus, M.J.: Thyroid cancer occurring as a late consequence of head and neck irradiation; evaluation of 1056 patients. N. Engl. J. Med. *294*:1019, 1976.
69. Herbst, A.L., et al.: Clear cell adenocarcinoma of the genital tract in young females: Registry report. N. Engl. J. Med. *287*:1259, 1972.
70. D'Angio, G.J., et al.: The treatment of Wilms' tumor: Results of the second national Wilms' tumor study. Cancer *47*:2302, 1981.
71. Evans, A.E., et al.: A review of 17 IV-S neuroblastoma patients at the Childrens Hospital of Philadelphia. Cancer *45*:833, 1980.
72. Evans, A.E.: Staging and treatment of neuroblastoma. Cancer *45*:1799, 1980.
73. Hann, H.L., et al.: Biologic differences between neuroblastoma stages IV-S and IV. Measurement of serum ferritin and E-rosette inhibition in 30 children. N. Engl. J. Med. *305*:425, 1981.
74. Knudson, A.G., and Meadows, A.T.: Regression of neuroblastoma IV-S: A genetic hypothesis. N. Engl. J. Med. *302*:1254, 1980.

12 BLOOD VESSELS

NORMAL

In order to understand the diseases that affect the vessels, we should consider some of the distinctive anatomic and functional characteristics of these structures.[1] *Arteries* are divided into three categories based on their size and certain histologic features: (1) large or elastic arteries, including the aorta; (2) medium-sized or muscular arteries, also referred to as distributing arteries; and (3) small arteries (usually less than 2 mm in diameter) that course, for the most part, within the substance of tissues and organs. All arteries characteristically possess three coats—*a tunica intima, a tunica media, and a tunica adventitia*—most clearly distinguished in the larger vessels. As the vessels diminish in caliber, the three separable coats become progressively indistinct and eventually are no longer identifiable at the level of the arterioles.

The **large elastic arteries** of the body include the aorta and its major branches: the innominate, the subclavian, the beginning of the common carotid, and the origins of the pulmonary arteries. The *tunica intima* of these vessels is composed of a smooth layer of thin endothelial cells based on a delicate basement membrane that penetrates between the subendothelial connective tissue and the underlying smooth muscle cells. At birth, the tunica intima is quite thin. Throughout life, the intima thickens by the progressive accumulation of connective tissue matrix as well as myointimal cells. The outer limit of the tunica intima is demarcated by a poorly defined zone of longitudinally dispersed elastic fibers that create a thick felting of elastic tissue. These fibers are not compacted into a discrete internal elastic lamina in vessels of this caliber, as is the case in the muscular arteries (see below), and are poorly separated from the elastic fibers contained within the media.

The *tunica media*, or muscular layer, is rich in elastic tissue in the large arteries, hence their designation as elastic arteries. The elastic fibers of the media are disposed in fairly compact fenestrated layers separated by alternating layers of smooth muscle. Condensation of the elastic tissue at the outer limit of the media produces a poorly defined external elastic membrane. Since the elastic fibers are sensitive to injury, elastic tissue stains may reveal the first indications of abnormality.

The *tunica adventitia* is a poorly defined layer of investing connective tissue in which elastic and nerve fibers and small, thin-walled nutrient vessels, the vasa vasorum, are dispersed. These nutrient vessels are derived from exiting arterial branches at points where they pass through the adventitia of the main vessel. In the aorta, vasa course back into the wall and can usually be identified in the outer third of the media. They ramify into minute, poorly defined channels but fail to enter the inner one-third of the media or the intima. Arterial walls in general are poorly vascularized. The inner layers depend largely on direct imbibition from the vessel lumen for their nutritional needs.

Aging is accompanied by a continuous slow increase in the thickness of the intima. This *diffuse intimal thickening* is caused by the accumulation of smooth muscle–like cells (myointimal cells), surrounded by extracellular matrix.

The elastic content of the media of these large vessels provides great resilience, and their rebound following systole aids in the forward propulsion of the blood. In the aging process, the elastic fibers deteriorate and are replaced by fibrous tissue. With this loss of elasticity, these vessels expand less readily, particularly when blood pressure is increased. The loss of elasticity further predisposes to stretching and elongation and accounts for the progressive development of tortuosity in these arteries in the older age groups.

In the **muscular arteries of medium size,** the three coats are well defined and are derived by gradual transition from the layers in the larger elastic arteries. The outer limit of the *tunica intima* is clearly defined by a compact, wavy internal elastic membrane. Normally this membrane is a single discrete layer; occasionally, two layers may be present, but reduplication or fibrillation generally denotes an increased formation of elastic tissue incident to such abnormal stress as hypertension. *The internal elastic lamina is not a continuous structure but is interrupted by fenestrae, through which medial smooth muscle cells may migrate into the intima.*

The *tunica media* is largely made up of circular or spiral smooth muscle cells arranged in concentric layers. Fine elastic fibers can be visualized only with elastic tissue stains or on electron microscopy. The outer limit of this coat is marked by a well-defined external elastic membrane that is usually somewhat less well developed and delineated than is the internal membrane (Fig. 12–1). The *tunica adventitia* resembles that in the large vessels but contains more abundant nerves, reflecting the role these vessels play in the autonomic regulation of blood flow.

In **small arteries** there is progressive loss first of the external elastic membrane and then of the internal elastic membrane so that, at the prearteriole level, the definition between the three coats is virtually lost. The tunica adventitia is of relatively greater thickness in these small vessels and approximately equals that of the tunica media. As the vessels approach the order of arterioles, the wall comprises an endothelial lining based on a scant subendothelial connective tissue, a layer of muscular media, and an investment of collagenous adventitia. The thickness of the wall is usually about equal to the diameter of the lumen of the vessel. The arterioles are richly supplied by nervous connections with the autonomic nervous system, and these vessels constitute the major site of autonomic control of vascular flow. In this role, the small arteries and the arterioles bear the brunt of elevations of blood pressure and respond to these abnormal stresses by marked alterations in their structure (to be detailed later).

The differentiation of these three types of arteries is of considerable importance in pathology, since each class of vessel tends to have its own pattern of pathologic lesions. Thus, it will be shown that in the various types of arteriosclerosis, atheromatosis is most typical of the elastic and muscular arteries, medial calcific sclerosis occurs in the muscular arteries, and in the small arteries and arterioles arteriosclerosis takes the form of diffuse thickening of the vascular wall by proliferation of fibromuscular tissue and hyalinization.

Veins in general are thin-walled vessels with relatively large lumina. The three separable coats seen in the arteries are not well defined in the veins. The tunica intima is composed largely of an endothelial lining based on a scant connective tissue layer. Internal elastic membranes delimiting the outer extent of the tunica intima can be well identified only in the largest veins. The media is poorly developed, is prominent only in the largest veins, and at best is unevenly distributed and provides very inadequate support in the thinned-out areas. Veins are thus predisposed to abnormal irregular dilatation, compression, and easy penetration by tumors and inflammatory processes. Valves, essentially endothelial folds, are found in many veins, particularly those in the extremities. These valves break the column of blood and reduce the hydrodynamic load in the propulsion of blood back toward the heart.

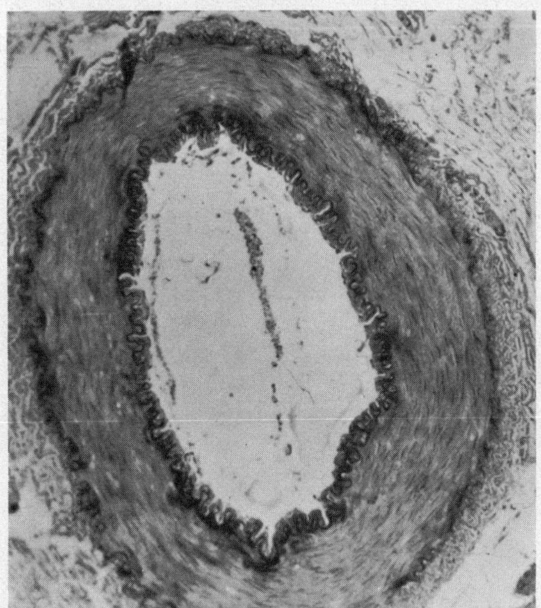

Figure 12–1. A normal muscular artery with clearly defined internal and external elastic membranes.

The **lymphatics** are extremely thin-walled structures, difficult to identify in tissue sections because of their tendency to collapse under ordinary tissue pressures. Clear identification depends on the recognition of thin-walled, endothelium-lined channels devoid of blood cells. The major lymphatics, however, possess a thin supporting muscular wall as well as valves. Histologically, therefore, it is sometimes difficult to distinguish these major trunks from blood vessels.

Although the major function of the lymphatics is as a protective drainage system, they also constitute an important pathway for the dissemination of disease by the conduction of bacteria and tumor cells to distant sites. The role that the lymphatics also play in the normal return of interstitial tissue fluid to the blood must not be overlooked and has been referred to previously (p. 61). Obstruction of these channels causes lymphedema.

Vascular endothelium and smooth muscle, the main components of the vascular wall (Fig. 12–2), play important roles in all types of vascular pathology. Much has been learned about the properties of the cells in these tissues, and a few points will be highlighted here.

The single layer of continuous *endothelium* lining arteries and veins forms the unique thromboresistant layer between blood and potentially thrombogenic subendothelial tissues. The integrity of endothelium is a fundamental requirement for maintenance of normal structure and function of the entire vessel wall. Besides inducing the obvious thrombotic phenomena, endothelial injury may be responsible, at least in part, for the initiation of atherosclerosis and the vascular lesions

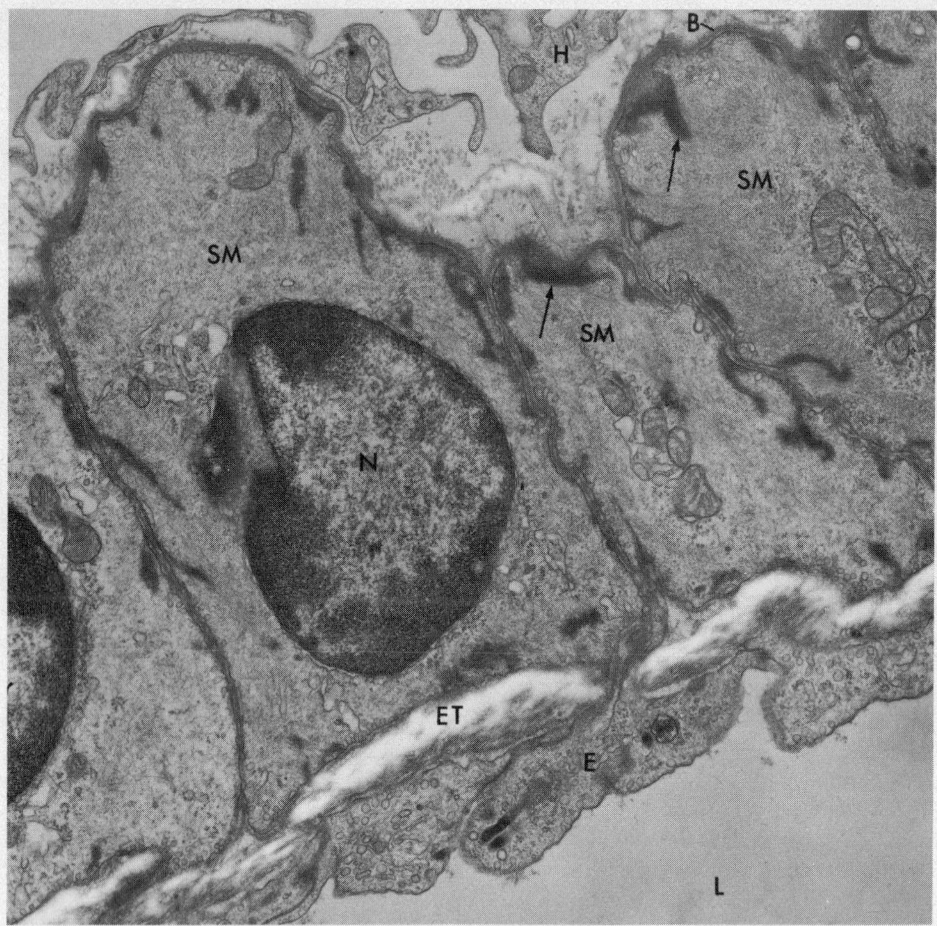

Figure 12–2. Wall of small artery in myocardium of a mouse. Continuous endothelium (E) is separated from smooth muscle layer (SM) by a thin elastica (ET)—unstained. Note peripheral bands in smooth muscle cells *(arrows)* and prominent external basement membrane (B). L = lumen; H = perivascular fibroblast.

of hypertension. Ultrastructurally, arterial endothelium resembles other continuous endothelia in its content of organelles and its rich supply of pinocytotic vesicles (Fig. 12–2). In addition, it contains unique, rod-shaped cytoplasmic organelles of unknown function (the *Weibel-Palade bodies*), which serve as specific markers for endothelium.[2] Like other endothelia, normal arterial endothelium is a semipermeable membrane, controlling the transfer of small and large molecules into the arterial wall.[3] It transports relatively slight amounts of proteins (e.g., horseradish peroxidase, ferritin, and low-density lipoprotein [LDL]) through pinocytotic vesicles. In most arterial regions, the intercellular junctions are normally impermeable to such molecules, but intercellular junctions are relatively labile structures that may widen under the influence of hemodynamic factors (such as high blood pressure) and possibly of vasoactive agents.[4]

Vascular endothelium is a biochemically versatile tissue capable of many synthetic and metabolic functions (Table 12–1). For example, endothelial cells produce prostaglandins (particularly PGI_2), the procoagulant factor VIII (antihemophilic factor), specific types of collagen (III, IV), plasminogen activator, and heparin-like surface proteoglycans. Further, endothelial cells appear to possess receptors for such powerful vasoactive agents as angiotensin II and for hormones such as insulin. As mentioned earlier, endothelial cells can also actively contract. Thus, this thin cell, hardly visible in routine histologic sections, is not a simple passive membrane, as previously thought, but an active participant in the interaction between blood and tissues.[3-7]

With regard to *vascular smooth muscle cells*, recent work has shown these to be capable of a great many

Table 12–1. PROPERTIES OF VASCULAR ENDOTHELIUM

Permeability barrier
Antiplatelet and anticoagulant
Prostacyclin (PGI_2)
Plasminogen activator
Heparin/heparan sulfate
Procoagulant
Von Willebrand factor (factor VIII—antigen)
Metabolism of vasoactive mediators
Bradykinin degradation
Angiotensin converting enzyme
Arachidonic acid metabolism (PGI_2)
Extracellular matrix production
Collagen, elastin, proteoglycans, fibronectin, laminin
Immunologically relevant antigens
ABO; HLA-ABC; HLA-DR

functions.[8] In addition to their already established role in vasoconstriction and dilatation, smooth muscle cells are capable of synthesizing various types of collagen, elastin, and the proteoglycans of the extracellular space. As we shall see, these cells rather than fibroblasts are responsible for the intimal collagenization in atherosclerosis. They can also migrate and proliferate, and both these processes appear to be fundamental to the reaction of the vessel wall to injury. Like fibroblasts, smooth muscle cells also have receptors for low-density lipoprotein as well as the complement of enzymes that regulate intracellular cholesterol metabolism (p. 514). Finally, although not normally phagocytic, these cells can be stimulated to perform pinocytosis and phagocytosis and to develop a variety of hydrolytic enzymes, processes that may be important in lipid accumulation in the vessel wall during atherosclerosis.

PATHOLOGY

Although vessels are secondarily affected by lesions in adjacent structures, primary vascular disease is the major concern of this chapter. In general, all types of vascular diseases are significant because they may (1) weaken the walls of vessels and lead to dilatation or rupture, (2) narrow the lumina of vessels and produce ischemia, or (3) damage the endothelial lining and provoke intravascular thrombosis.

The most important primary vascular diseases affect the arteries and, of these, the most prevalent and clinically significant is atherosclerosis. In the course of time, this disorder affects virtually every individual to some degree. The other arterial diseases are very much less common but, in the individual instance, may be responsible for considerable disability and even death. Certain of the venous disorders, such as varicose veins, are also very commonly encountered in clinical practice, in a frequency that almost approaches that of atherosclerosis. In general, however, these diseases of veins are more noteworthy for the disability they produce than for their importance as causes of death, but this should not imply that venous diseases are unimportant. Many are disabling to the point of crippling, and certain disorders, such as phlebothrombosis, may lead to death by embolism. Diseases of arteries, veins, and lymphatics will be discussed separately. Tumors of these vessels, however, will be considered as a group, since these neoplasms are for the most part quite similar clinically and anatomically, irrespective of their origin in an artery, vein, or lymphatic.

ARTERIES

CONGENITAL ANOMALIES

It is surprising that the development of the far-flung complicated branching and anastomosing system of blood vessels and lymphatics results so consistently in a fairly standard or normal anatomic pattern. It is, therefore, not surprising that many aberrations from the classic pattern may be found. Most of the anomalies in the course and distribution of arteries are of importance only in surgical operative technique, in which recognition of the deviation is important to the surgical dissection. Occasionally, however, these minor anomalies have a greater significance in potentiating or even preventing disease. For example, a double renal arterial supply may prevent infarction of a kidney when one of the vessels is occluded by a thrombus or embolus. On the other hand, by crossing anterior to the ureter, the aberrant renal vessel may compress the ureter, obstruct the outflow of urine, and eventually cause serious renal disease (hydronephrosis). In a somewhat analogous fashion, maldevelopment of a major coronary branch may predispose the myocardium to infarction. Among these diverse vascular anomalies, two merit consideration, the developmental or berry aneurysm, and arteriovenous fistulas or aneurysms. Berry aneurysms involve cerebral vessels only and are discussed in Chapter 29.

ARTERIOVENOUS FISTULA OR ANEURYSM

Abnormal communications between arteries and veins may arise as developmental defects, from rupture of an arterial aneurysm into the adjacent vein, from penetrating injuries that pierce the wall of artery and vein and produce an artificial communication, and from inflammatory necrosis of adjacent vessels. The communication, therefore, is in only certain instances developmental in origin. The connection between artery and vein may consist of a well-formed vessel or a vascular channel formed by the canalization of a thrombus, or may be mediated through an aneurysmal sac. Such lesions are extremely rare and are usually small. They are of some clinical significance, since they short-circuit blood from the arterial to the venous side and throw an increased burden upon the right side of the heart, predisposing to cardiac failure. Sometimes the very tortuous mass of vessels that presumably represents an arteriovenous aneurysm is designated as a *cirsoid aneurysm.*

ARTERIOSCLEROSIS

Arteriosclerosis literally means "hardening of the arteries," but more accurately it refers to a group of disorders that have in common thickening and loss of elasticity of arterial walls. Three distinctive morphologic variants are included within the term arteriosclerosis: *atherosclerosis,* characterized by the formation of atheromas (fibrofatty intimal plaques); *Mönckeberg's medial calcific sclerosis,* characterized by calcification of the media of muscular arteries; and *arteriolosclerosis,* marked by proliferative or hyaline thickening of the walls of small arteries and arterioles. These three forms are relatively easily distinguished by their morphologic appearance. More than one pattern can be identified in the same individual in different vessels or even in the same vessel. In particular, atherosclerosis and Mönckeberg's medial sclerosis often occur together, in the arteries of the legs of aged individuals. Because atherosclerosis is by far the most common and important form of arteriosclerosis, the terms are generally used interchangeably unless otherwise specified.

ATHEROSCLEROSIS (AS)

Among the diseases in the Western world, atherosclerosis is overwhelmingly in first place. Global in distribution, it has reached alarming epidemic proportions in economically developed societies. Although any artery may be affected, the aorta and the coronary and cerebral systems are the prime targets, and *so myocardial infarcts* (heart attacks) and *cerebral infarcts* (strokes) are the two major consequences of this disease. Myocardial infarcts (MIs) alone account for 20 to 25% of all deaths in the United States, almost entirely attributable to AS. This vascular disorder also causes a variety of other less calamitous events that add to its toll, including chronic ischemic heart disease, gangrene of the legs, mesenteric occlusion, and ischemic encephalopathy. At present, about 50% of all deaths in the U.S. are attributed to arteriosclerosis-related diseases. Its variable severity among nations, individuals, and social and ethnic groups is evidence that AS is not an inevitable consequence of life. An understanding of why some individuals have only mild disease while others are severely affected and discovery of the cause of this rampant disorder are two of the most urgently sought goals of medical research today.

DEFINITION. Atherosclerosis is a disease of large and medium-sized muscular arteries (e.g., coronary, carotid, arteries of the lower extremities) and the large elastic arteries, such as the aorta and iliac vessels. *The basic lesion—the atheroma or fibrofatty plaque—consists of a raised focal plaque within the intima, having a core of lipid (mainly cholesterol, usually complexed to proteins, and cholesterol esters) and a covering fibrous cap.* These atheromas are sparsely distributed at first, but as the disease advances they become more and more numerous and sometimes literally cover the entire intimal surface of severely affected arteries. As the plaques increase in size, they progressively encroach on the lumen of the artery as well as on the subjacent media. Consequently, atheromas compromise arterial blood flow and weaken affected arteries, sometimes resulting in aneurysms. Many eventually undergo a variety of complications, e.g., calcification, ulceration, thrombus formation, and aneurysmal dilatation (p. 511). In the progression of this vascular disease, no symptoms may be produced for 20 to 40 years or longer and, unless the lesions precipitate clinical manifestations by virtue of organ injury, they may remain undiscovered until postmortem examination. In the absence of such organ injury, AS can be recognized during life only by angiography or, in some cases, by radiologic visualization of the deposits of calcium in the advanced atheromas.

EPIDEMIOLOGY AND INCIDENCE. Much attention has been paid to the epidemiology and incidence of AS because the variable occurrence and severity of this disease among individuals and groups may provide important clues to its pathogenesis. Epidemiologic data are largely expressed in terms of ischemic heart disease (IHD), also called coronary heart disease (CHD), since the arterial lesions of AS remain silent until they provoke morbidity or mortality from symptomatic "atherosclerotic events." Indeed, most statistical data on AS compare the number of deaths caused by coronary heart disease. It must be stressed that this is not an entirely accurate reflection of AS, since other complex factors contribute to death (especially sudden death) after myocardial infarction (p. 565).

Death rates from cardiovascular disease (heart, brain, kidneys) in the United States rose from 14% of all deaths in 1937 to 54% in 1968, almost all cases being related to AS. The enormous increase over the span of 30 years amply justifies the term epidemic, but happily the rates appeared to plateau in the late 1960s, and in 1975, for the first time, showed a statistically significant decline. From 1968 to 1978, the reduction in IHD mortality averaged about 27% overall for persons 36 to 74 years of age (Fig. 12–3).[9] As we shall see, some believe that this downward trend in IHD mortality may be related to the average decrease in serum cholesterol levels in the general population, probably related to changing diets.

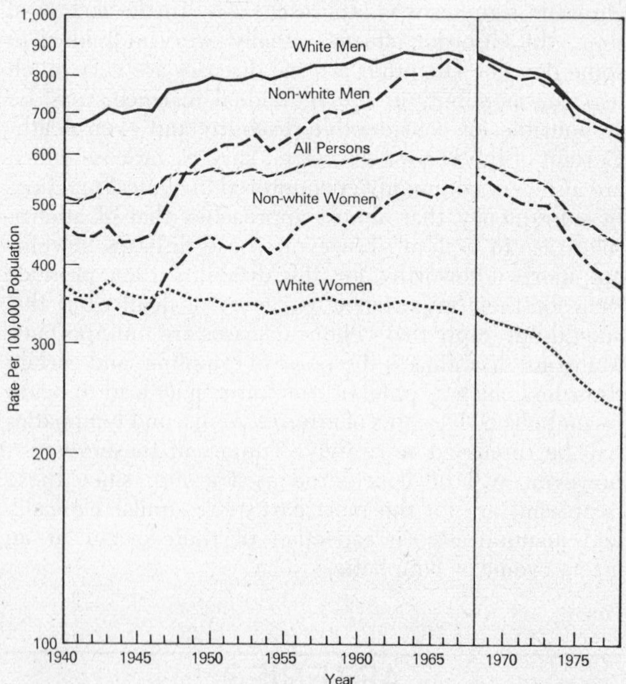

Figure 12–3. Declining mortality rates. Mortality rates for coronary heart disease, age-adjusted, persons aged 35 to 74, by sex–color; United States, 1940–78. From Arteriosclerosis, 1981. Report of the Working Group on Arteriosclerosis of the National Heart, Lung, and Blood Institute. Vol. 2. Reproduced with permission.

Nevertheless, the death rate from IHD in the United States is still among the highest in the world, lower than Finland and Scotland, but above that of other well-developed affluent countries such as Canada, France, Germany, and the Scandinavian countries. Conversely, the rates are remarkably lower in Asia (including Japan, China, India, and much of Southeast Asia), the Near and Middle East, Africa, and South and Central America. For men between the ages of 35 and 64, for example, the death rate in Japan is about one-sixth that in the U.S. Japanese who migrate to the U.S. and adopt the life style and diet of their new home acquire the predisposition to AS evident in the resident American population. There is thus a strong impression that differences in diet, life style, and personal habits may be important in the pathogenesis and progression of this disease. Nevertheless, epidemiologic studies have not shown the reasons for differences between cultures that appear to be at least superficially similar. For example, why is the mortality rate from IHD for North American men under age 55 higher than that of Swedes of the same age group? Genetic factors may explain such differences, but no clear-cut patterns have emerged.

Risk Factors. Epidemiologic studies indicate that certain genetic or acquired factors increase the risk of AS. Some of these, such as age, sex, and familial predisposition, are alas the irreversible companions of our lives, but others are clearly or potentially reversible.

Age has a dominant influence on the development of clinically significant AS. Clinically overt AS, as evidenced by death rates from ischemic heart disease, rises with each decade even up to age 85, although death due to acute myocardial infarction seems to decline slightly after age 75. There is of course a close relationship between age and the severity of AS.[11] Interestingly, despite the fact that clinically overt AS is a disease of aging, fatty deposits—termed *fatty streaks*—are present in the aorta in all infants by the age of 1 year and begin to appear in the coronary arteries at age 10. However, as will be discussed, there is doubt whether the fatty streak is the universal precursor of the atheromatous plaque.

There are striking *sex differences* in the incidence and severity of AS.[12] Death rates from IHD are significantly higher in males until age 75 to 85 when the incidences approach equality. Significantly, myocardial infarction is uncommon in premenopausal women, and in the age group of 35 to 55 the mortality rate of white males is over five times that of white females. Naturally, other risk factors influence the relative risk of IHD in females; the rate is increased in women with a history of heavy smoking, prolonged oral contraceptive intake, or diabetes.

Some families suffer an increased frequency of heart attacks at an early age (so-called premature), presumably indicating *familial predisposition*. This may represent the clustering of other risk factors within families rather than a unique genetic predisposition. In particular, hyperlipidemia (genetic or diet-induced), hypertension, and diabetes all tend to be familial. Nevertheless, there are families with high attack rates of IHD in which none of the known risk factors appears to operate but the determinants of such susceptibility are unclear.[12A]

Granted that residency in certain affluent areas of the world, increasing age, and sex define the population at risk, not all members of this population develop clinically apparent AS. Other significant "risk factors" that predispose to AS and IHD have been identified by means of a number of prospective studies in well-defined population groups, such as the famed Framingham (Massachusetts) Study.[13] *Of the various risk factors, four are considered of prime importance: (1) hyperlipidemia, (2) hypertension, (3) cigarette smoking, and (4) diabetes. Of these, the first three are the principal culprits.*

HYPERLIPIDEMIA AND DIET. The evidence is overwhelming that hyperlipidemia is associated with an increased incidence of premature IHD. Here we shall review some of the epidemiologic evidence. The relationship between lipid metabolism and AS is discussed later (p. 513).

With few exceptions, populations having relatively high levels of cholesterol have higher mortality from IHD. The Framingham study showed that in men and women 35 to 44 years of age, serum cholesterol levels of 265 mg/100 ml or over are associated with a five times higher risk of developing coronary artery disease than are levels below 220 mg/100 ml. *The most striking association is with elevated levels of low-density lipoprotein (LDL)*, the lipoprotein moiety richest in cholesterol, but *hypertriglyceridemia* with increased concentrations of very-low-density lipoprotein (VLDL) also appears to increase risk. In contrast, serum levels of high-density lipoprotein (HDL) are inversely related to risk: the higher the level, the lower the risk.[14-16]

Hyperlipidemia may be secondary to some well-known causes such as nephrotic syndrome (p. 1011) or hypothyroidism (p. 1204), or may be the direct consequence of a single gene defect, as in the familial hypercholesterolemias discussed earlier (p. 140). Complex inheritance factors may also predispose to hypercholesterolemia in some patients. Nevertheless the level of plasma cholesterol is measurably influenced by the dietary intake of total calories of cholesterol, saturated fat, and polyunsaturated fat, i.e., by dietary habits. Further, although there are skeptics,[17] it is thought that there is a direct relationship between diet, hyperlipidemia, and the development of coronary heart disease. The evidence linking these three events can be summarized as follows:[18]

1. Dietary cholesterol intake from 0 to 600 mg per day is closely related to plasma cholesterol levels, and dietary saturated fatty acids elevate plasma cholesterol levels, whereas polyunsaturated fatty acids reduce them.
2. Low-cholesterol, low-saturated-fat, polyunsaturate-rich therapeutic diets reproducibly lower plasma cholesterol levels up to 10 to 20%.
3. Populations with sharply lowered dietary cholesterol and saturated fatty intake have lower plasma cholesterol levels and reduced IHD.

4. Immigrants from populations having low plasma cholesterol to ones in which it is high develop cholesterol levels comparable with their host populations. As mentioned above, in Japanese emigrés the gradient for the crucial three variables (saturated fat, blood lipids, and IHD) increases from indigenous Japanese to emigrant Japanese to native Caucasians.

5. Animal studies, particularly in subhuman primates, reveal an unequivocal relationship between dietary cholesterol or saturated fat, plasma cholesterol levels, and AS.[19]

6. Partly as a result of campaigns by many organizations, principally the American Heart Association, cholesterol intake in the American population has declined since 1970, and the polyunsaturated/saturated ratio in dietary fat has increased. Concurrently, there was a definite lowering trend in serum cholesterol levels of adult Americans, and a significant downward trend (27%) in IHD mortality occurred among persons 36 to 74 years of age.[9]

There are always, of course, two sides to the coin.[17] The opposing view is that the data summarized above are at most only circumstantial evidence; that recent *prospective* intervention studies have failed to demonstrate statistically significant associations between diet and IHD risk; that the reduced mortality from IHD may be due to reduced cigarette smoking or other risk factors; that dietary modification (polyunsaturate-rich diets) may not be safe; and that the preoccupation with diet has hampered the study of genetic factors and the effects of exercise, life habits, and so on.

HYPERTENSION. Elevated blood pressure unequivocally accelerates atherogenesis and increases the incidence of IHD and cerebral vascular disease.[20] The higher the blood pressure, the greater the risk. In the Framingham study, the incidence of IHD in men aged 45 to 62 with blood pressures exceeding 160/95 was more than five times that in normotensive men (BP 140/90 or less). Diastolic hypertension is the more important correlate. The risk of IHD in individuals with diastolic pressures greater than 105 mm Hg is four times that of individuals with pressures 84 mm Hg or less.[21] After age 45, the scales tip toward hypertension as a greater risk factor than hypercholesterolemia. Antihypertensive therapy reduces the incidence of strokes, and possibly also of IHD.

CIGARETTE SMOKING. There is a clear-cut association between *cigarette smoking* and susceptibility to IHD. In men who smoke one or more packs of cigarettes per day, the death rate from IHD is 70 to 200% higher than that for nonsmokers, and the risk is particularly significant in younger men. At autopsy, the degree of aortic and coronary AS is greater in smokers than in nonsmokers. The main influence of smoking appears to be on the incidence of sudden death. Cessation of cigarette smoking in high-risk men is followed by a reduction in the risk of dying from IHD,[22] although it may require 10 to 20 years for the risk to equal that of nonsmokers. The declining death rate from IHD in the recent past may be related, at least in part, to the 25% decrease in cigarette smoking among men. A major unresolved problem is smoking among teen-agers, especially the increase among teen-age girls.

DIABETES. Diabetes is associated with an increase in AS observed at autopsy, a twofold increase in incidence of myocardial infarction in diabetics as compared with nondiabetics, an increased tendency toward cerebral thrombosis and infarction, and an eight- to 150-fold increased frequency of gangrene of the lower extremities. Although the problem of assessing the contribution of AS per se to risk is complicated by the widespread presence of *microvascular changes* in the diabetic state, the main factor appears to be AS.

OTHER RISK FACTORS. A host of other influences, sometimes called *"soft risk factors,"* have been identified that increase the severity of AS,[20] but the data are less definitive than for the major risk factors cited above. Evidence for a role of *physical activity* in protecting against fatal ischemic heart disease and possibly coronary atherosclerosis is increasing.[9, 20] In the Framingham study, the most sedentary men (about 15% of the participating males) had about three times the risk of the 15% most active physically.[13] Some studies have shown that vigorous activity (e.g., in longshoremen and transport workers) is associated with a lower risk of IHD. Physically active groups have elevated levels of serum HDL, which may protect from the development of AS. Physical activity also causes increases in heart volume and mass, increased cardiac capillary vascularity, and a decrease in heart rate—all of which may protect from the effects of ischemic damage.

Obesity is correlated with an increased risk of dying from the clinical complications of AS, since obese individuals tend to have more severe hyperlipidemia, hypertension, and diabetes mellitus. The Framingham study, however, suggests that obesity is a risk factor independent of such associations.

The role of *stress* and *behavior patterns* is now receiving considerable attention. Although it is common belief that stressful life events are related to the risk of coronary disease, the statistical evidence has only recently become available.[24] Several epidemiologic studies suggest that men with Type A behavior patterns (characterized by competitiveness, impatience, and hostility) have a higher rate of CHD than men judged to be of the less competitive behavior pattern, Type B.[25] However, the specific coronary-prone behavior profiles and the physiologic mechanisms linking behavior to CHD are unclear.

Each of the major risk factors noted earlier contributes individually to the possible development of clinically significant AS, but multiple factors exert more than an additive effect. In the Framingham study, for example, when three risk factors were present (hyperlipidemia, hypertension, and smoking), the rate of heart attacks was seven times greater than when there were none; when two risk factors were present, the risk was increased fourfold; and with one risk factor, the increase was twofold. These relationships are shown in Figure 12–4. However, none of these factors is either necessary

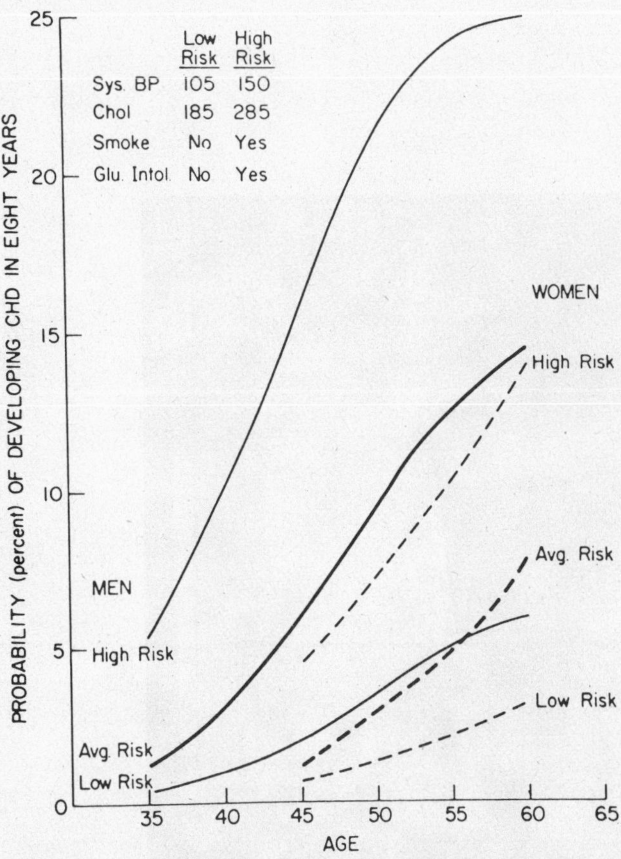

Figure 12–4. Graph of added risks. Probability of developing coronary heart disease in eight years according to age, sex, and risk category (The Framingham Heart Study). (From Braunwald, E. (ed.): Heart Disease. A Textbook of Cardiovascular Medicine. Philadelphia, W. B. Saunders Co., 1984, p. 1209.)

or sufficient for the development of AS, and some cardiac patients have no obvious risk factor. Thus, the etiology and pathogenesis of AS remain subjects of lively speculation and controversy. Before we delve into pathogenesis it is desirable to understand the morphology of the lesions.

MORPHOLOGY. Descriptions of the morphology of atherosclerosis have been confounded by the heterogeneity of the histologic lesions present, and the difficulty in assessing the relationship of one lesion to the other. Despite this, two well-accepted lesions can be described[19, 26, 27]: (1) the **atheromatous plaque,** which is by far the most important lesion, being the principal cause of arterial narrowing in adults, and (2) the **fatty streak,** which is present universally in children, even in the first year of life, and is important mainly as a possible precursor of the atheromatous plaque.

The Atheromatous Plaque. **This is the fundamental lesion of AS,** also called the fibrous, fibrofatty, lipid, or fibrolipid plaque. Plaques are white to whitish-yellow in appearance, protrude into the lumen of the artery, and vary in size from 0.3 to 1.5 cm in diameter, but they sometimes coalesce to form larger masses (Figs. 12–5 and 12–6). On section, the luminal surface tends to be firm and white and the deep portions yellow, whitish-yellow, and soft. The center of larger plaques may exude a yellow, grumous fluid, from which the name *atheroma*—the Greek word for gruel—is derived. **The distribution of atherosclerotic plaques in humans tends to be quite constant and differs from the distribution of fatty streaks.** The abdominal aorta is much more involved than the thoracic aorta, and aortic lesions tend to be much more prominent around the ostia of its major branches. In descending order (after the lower abdominal aorta), the most heavily involved vessels are the coronary arteries (usually within the first 6 cm), the popliteal arteries, the descending thoracic aorta, the internal carotids, and the vessels of the circle of Willis. Vessels of the upper extremities are usually spared, as are mesenteric arteries and renal arteries, except at their ostia.

Histologically, the plaques are localized to the intima and consist of (1) increased numbers of lipid-laden intimal smooth muscle cells and macrophages; (2) an accumulation of connective tissue including collagen, elastic fibers, and proteoglycans; and (3) intracellular and extracellular lipid deposits (Fig. 12–7). These occur in varying proportions in different plaques, giving rise to a spectrum of lesions. Typically, the plaques are composed of a superficial part (the fibrous cap), made up of collagen in which there are variable numbers of smooth muscle cells, and a deeper or central part in which there is a disorganized mass of lipid material, cholesterol clefts, and cellular debris, and variable amounts of fibrin and other plasma proteins (Fig. 12–8). The lipid is primarily cholesterol and cholesteryl ester. The lipid-laden cells assume the appearance of "foam cells." Current studies indicate that such foam cells consist of lipid-filled smooth muscle cells as well as blood-derived macrophages.[27-30] Cells within the plaque and in the deeper

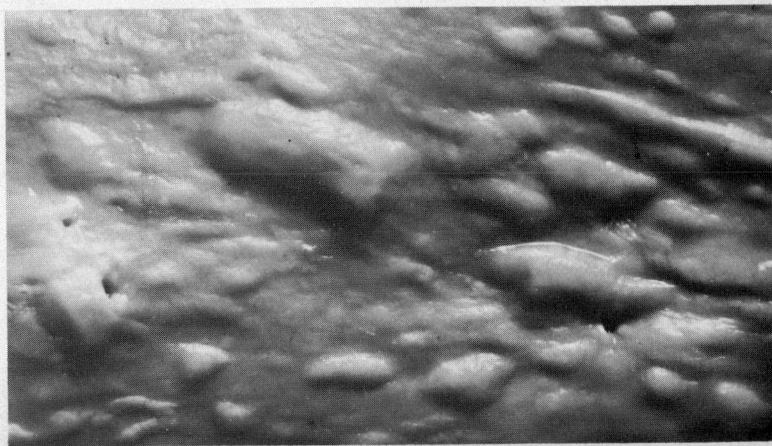

Figure 12–5. Close-up of atheromatous plaques as seen from luminal surface of aorta (× 2.5). (From Benditt, E. P.: The origin of atherosclerosis. Sci. Am. *236*:74, 1977. Copyright © 1977 by Scientific American, Inc. All rights reserved.)

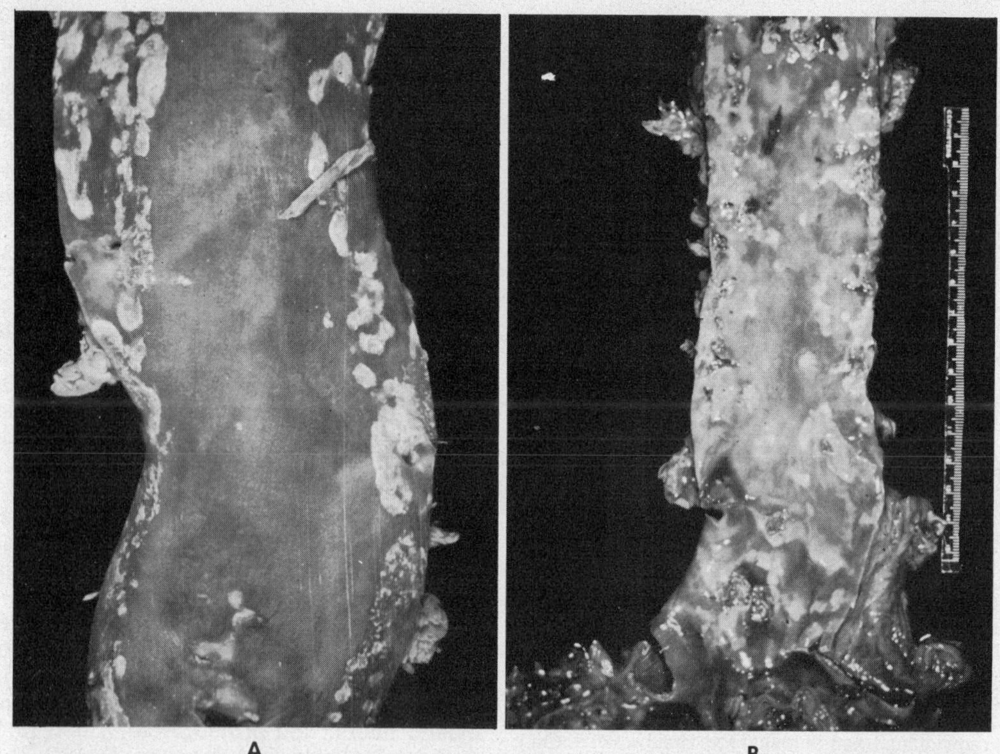

Figure 12–6. *A,* Atherosclerosis. Early stage with widely scattered, barely elevated intimal plaques. *B,* More extensive lesions.

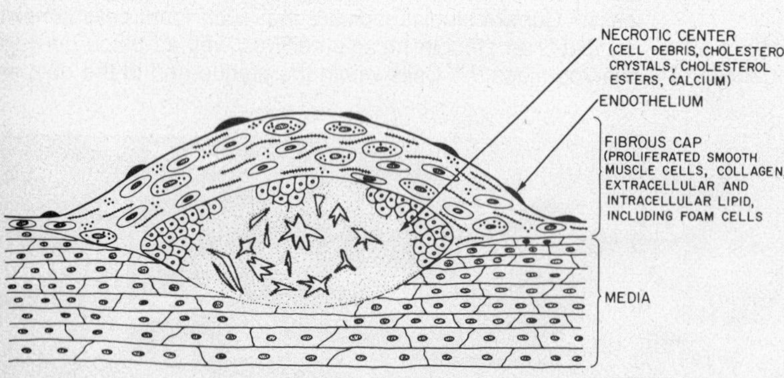

Figure 12–7. Major components of advanced (clinically important) atherosclerotic plaque. (Modified from Wissler, R. W., and Vesselinovitch, D.: Animal models of regression. *In* Schettler, G., et al. (eds.): Atherosclerosis IV. Berlin, Springer-Verlag, 1977, p. 377.)

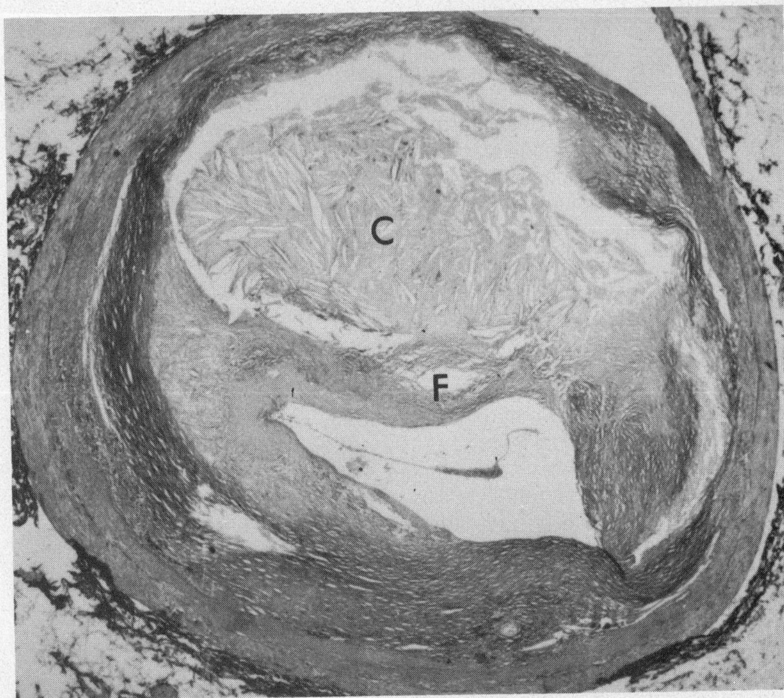

Figure 12–8. Atheromatous plaque. F = fibrous cap; C = central lipid core with typical cholesterol clefts. (Courtesy of Dr. C. Haudenschild, Boston University Medical Center.)

deposits are also surrounded by extracellular material consisting of proteoglycans, elastic fibers, collagen, and cell debris. Variations in the histology of plaques involve the relative numbers of smooth muscle cells, the amount of collagen and extracellular matrix, and especially the lipid content. The most typical atheromas contain rather abundant lipid. Nevertheless, **many plaques are composed mostly of smooth muscle cells and fibrous tissue** (Fig. 12–9), and coronary artery lesions are often largely fibrous.[31] Inflammatory cells, including neutrophils and lymphocytes, are sometimes present. Vascularization of margins of the lesions may develop. In advanced AS, progressive fibrosis may convert the fatty atheroma to a fibrous scar.

Fully developed atheromatous plaques may undergo a series of changes that result in so-called **"complicated plaques"**:

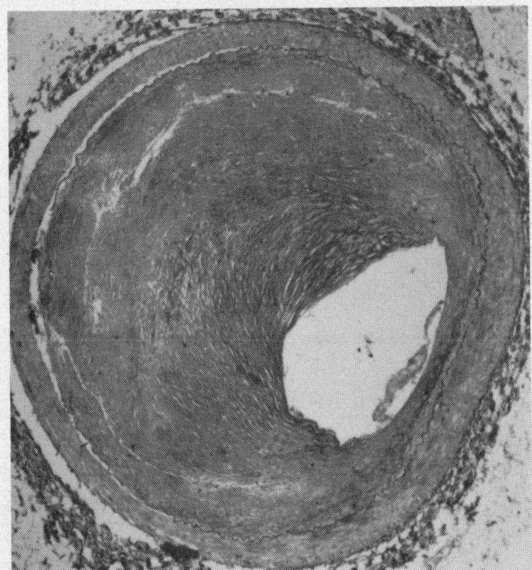

Figure 12–9. Largely fibrous atheromatous plaque narrowing the coronary artery. Compare with plaque in Figure 12–8, which has a lipid core.

1. Almost always, atheromas in advanced disease undergo patchy or massive **calcification.** In severe atherosclerotic disease, arteries may be converted to virtual pipe stems, and the aorta may assume an eggshell brittleness.

2. **Ulceration** of the luminal surface and rupture of the atheromatous plaques may result in discharge of the debris into the bloodstream, producing microemboli **(cholesterol emboli).**

3. Superimposed **thrombosis**, the most feared complication, may occur on fissured or more often ulcerated lesions. Thrombi may either occlude the lumen or become incorporated within the intimal plaque (Fig. 12–10).

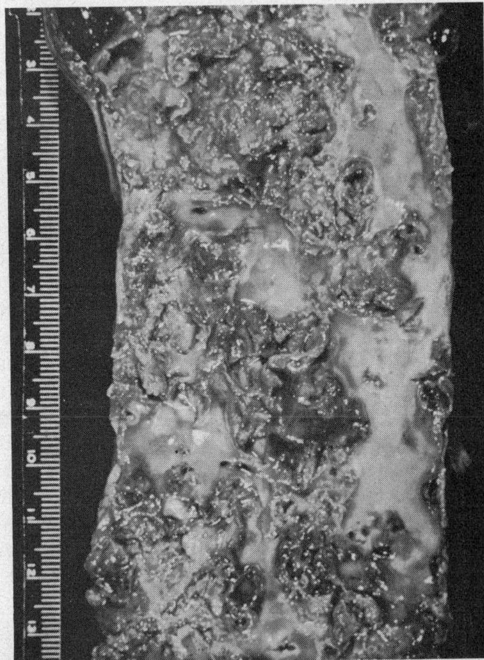

Figure 12–10. Mural thrombosis on underlying atherosclerosis.

4. **Hemorrhage** into the plaque may occur, especially in the coronary arteries, from rupture of either the overlying endothelium or the thin-walled capillaries that vascularize the plaque. The resulting hematoma may remain localized within the intima or rupture into the lumen. Phagocytosis of this extravasated blood leads to the hemosiderin-laden macrophages frequently observed in plaques.

5. Although atherosclerosis is basically an intimal disease, in severe cases the underlying media undergoes considerable pressure atrophy and loss of elastic tissue, causing sufficient weakness to permit **aneurysmal dilatation.** This process is discussed more fully on page 530.

Although AS is a universal disease, "complicated lesions" are seen only in individuals with extremely advanced disease. In predisposed individuals and populations, the entire abdominal aorta may become virtually "one continuous, complicated lesion." The thoracic aorta, including the arch, is usually less severely affected and, remarkably, in the absence of intercurrent syphilitic aortitis, the root of the aorta (the first 4 to 6 cm) is almost always totally spared, even in those with advanced abdominal aortic disease. **Although any form of atheromatosis is serious, it is the "complicated lesion," in particular superimposed thrombosis, that gives this disease its grave clinical significance.**

The Fatty Streak. Fatty streaks are important not because of any disturbance in blood flow that they may cause, but because they may—only **may**—be the precursors of the more ominous atheromatous plaques. The lesions begin as multiple yellow spots less than 1 mm in diameter and grow into elongated streaks, still no more than 1 to 2 mm wide but up to 1 cm long or even longer. They are usually flat or, if elevated, no more than 1 mm above the intimal surface. They may be very hard to see macroscopically but can be stained with Sudan IV, which colors the lesion bright orange. The fatty streak has a rather characteristic histologic appearance, and its hallmark is **lipid deposition in the intima** (Fig. 12–11). It is made up of a variable number of cells, some of which are elongated smooth muscle cells filled with intracytoplasmic lipid droplets while others are large and ovoid, and almost certainly blood-derived macrophages. Lipid is also present extracellularly, and proteoglycans, collagen, and elastic fibers are present in variable amounts.

Fatty streaks appear in the aortas of all children older than one year, regardless of geography, race, sex, or environment. They may be present at birth. At this early age, the lesions are localized to the thoracic aorta and, in particular, in the aortic valve ring region and the area of the ductus arteriosus scar—**locations that are rarely involved by atheromas in adults.** Fatty streaks also occur around the ostia of the costal, lumbar, and abdominal branches. The extent of aortic intimal surface covered by fatty streaks increases with age from about 10% in the first decade to 30 to 50% in the third decade. They subsequently decrease in number as atheromatous plaques begin to predominate. Coronary artery fatty streaking is first observed at about 10 years of age in all populations. **Of interest is that streaks in the coronary artery are most abundant in the proximal segment of the left coronary artery, about 2 cm distal to the left coronary ostium, a location that does correspond to the sites of the atheromatous plaques that develop later.**[32]

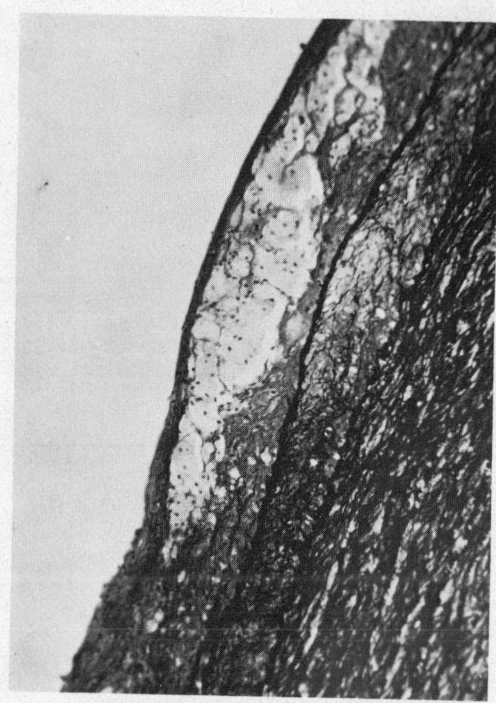

Figure 12–11. Fatty streak—a subintimal collection of foam cells or lipophages.

Now we can return to the unresolved question of whether the fatty streak is the early or precursor form of the important fibrous plaque. In support of this theory, one can cite first the basic resemblance between the histologic features of both conditions, at least at a superficial level: both involve the intima, are characterized by lipid deposition, and exhibit smooth muscle cells within the lesion. Second, in the coronary arteries (in contrast to the aorta), fatty streaks and atheromatous plaques occur in the same locations in the proximal segments. Third, experimental data suggest that lesions similar to human fatty streaks may progress to become fibrolipid plaques.[33] Opposing evidence includes the fact that fatty streaks occur first in the thoracic aorta, while atheromatous plaques develop in the abdominal aorta. More important, aortic fatty streaks are as prevalent and extensive in those geographic areas where the extent of advanced atherosclerosis is relatively low[34] as in those where there is a strong predisposition to AS, suggesting that human aortic fatty streaks are reversible and may be unrelated to atheromas. Although evidence for regression in humans is equivocal, regression has been accomplished in primates by converting from a high- to a low-cholesterol diet.[35] Finally, there are some differences in the chemical composition of the two lesions, particularly with regard to fatty acids, lipoprotein, residual cholesterol, and fibrinogen.[36]

It appears, then, that *fatty streaks are of universal occurrence and distribution, and most, especially those in the aorta, either disappear or remain harmless. In certain locations (e.g., in coronary arteries) and especially in the predisposed individual, these streaks may conceivably evolve into fibrous plaques, but the issue is still unsettled.*[9]

There are other lesions described under different names that should be briefly mentioned. A structure referred to as the **"intimal cushion,"** intimal pad, musculoelastic plaque, or mucoid fibromuscular plaque represents small areas of white thickening at the site of arterial forks or ostia of branch vessels. Microscopically, the thickening is due to accumulation of smooth muscle cells and extracellular matrix in the intima, small but variable amounts of collagen, and **virtually no lipid.** When diffuse, some authors refer to this lesion as **diffuse intimal thickening.**[37] There are some who believe that intimal thickening is a normal response to hemodynamic stress, and others who consider it a stage in the evolution of AS. Similarly, so-called **gelatinous lesions**[27] are characterized by loosely packed, thick, linear collagen bundles that sometimes lie between sparse smooth muscle cells, within abundant pools of plasma insudate. They contain large amounts of LDL and fibrinogen, with little residual cholesterol, in contrast to the fatty streaks and plaques. They have been implicated in plaque growth but have not yet been studied sufficiently.[36]

Having discussed the range of atheromatous lesions, *we should stress again that the most important lesion in terms of its pathologic consequence is the atheromatous plaque, in particular the complicated plaque.* In the capacious aorta, the important complications of these plaques are large mural thrombi that may dislodge and yield peripheral embolism, aneurysmal dilatation due to impingement of the atheromatous plaques on the media, or rupture of cholesterol emboli into the bloodstream. Occlusion of the lumen of the aorta is unusual, since a rapidly moving bloodstream in the center usually prevents massive thrombi. However, in smaller arteries, particularly those in the brain and heart, the narrowing by atheromatous plaques, especially if accompanied by thrombosis or hemorrhage, will lead to occlusion and may be the ultimate event causing strokes and myocardial infarction.

PATHOGENESIS. The search for the etiology and pathogenesis of AS, as for those of cancer, has become an insistent "golden grail." The subject has tantalized investigators from the days of Virchow. Here we shall present only an overview of the various proposals concerning the pathogenesis of AS. For more detailed information, reference should be made to various subject reviews or books.[9, 19, 39-45]

Any concept of the pathogenesis of AS should account for (1) the role of the important risk factors, particularly hyperlipidemia; (2) the focal nature of the lesions and their localization in the intima; (3) the presence of lipid in most lesions; and (4) the mechanisms of smooth muscle proliferation, which appears to be a fundamental and early event in the development of AS.

No single theory copes adequately with all these observations. Historically, two hypotheses were dominant until recently. The first, originally termed "*the imbibition hypothesis*" by Virchow in 1856, held that cellular proliferation in the intima was a form of "low-grade inflammation" as a reaction to increased filtration of plasma proteins and lipids from the blood. Over the years, this concept has undergone modification to become the so-called "lipid," "insudation," or "infiltration" hypothesis. As we shall see later, this proposal has been incorporated in the more modern "reaction to injury" hypothesis dominant today. The second or "*encrustation theory*," often ascribed to Rokitansky, postulated that small thrombi composed of platelets, fibrin, and leukocytes collected over foci of endothelial injury and that the organization of such thrombi and their gradual growth resulted in plaque formation.[46] Few now believe that thrombus encrustation is the sole determinant of AS, but parts of this theory still prevail, i.e., it is thought that endothelial injury, with associated platelet deposition, plays a role in the genesis of the atheromatous plaque. We will first review some aspects of lipid metabolism that are particularly relevant to AS and then present some current theories of pathogenesis.

Role of Lipids in Atherosclerosis. Evidence that lipids play an important role in AS has been reviewed previously and can be summarized as follows:

1. Full-blown AS can be produced in almost all species of experimental animals by feeding them diets that raise the plasma cholesterol level.
2. Symptomatic AS develops infrequently in man, even in the face of other predisposing factors, unless the mean plasma cholesterol exceeds about 160 mg/dl.
3. The probability of the development of myocardial infarction increases in proportion to the plasma cholesterol level.
4. Genetic disorders that cause elevated plasma cholesterol levels, such as familial hypercholesterolemia (p. 140) or cholesteryl ester storage disease, produce fatal AS in childhood despite the lack of any other contributing factors such as hypertension, smoking, or diabetes mellitus.[47]
5. Although trauma to the intima (such as denudation of the endothelial lining) causes proliferative thickening of the arterial wall in experimental animals, the resultant lesion either regresses or resembles a benign scar unless the animal's blood cholesterol level is elevated, at which time lipid is deposited in the lesion and life-threatening AS results.
6. The lipid in atheromatous plaques is largely derived from the lipoproteins in the bloodstream.

As is well-known, all lipids in plasma circulate in combination with protein.[48, 49] The plasma lipoproteins are a family of globular particles, each consisting of a core of neutral lipid (primarily triglyceride or cholesteryl ester) surrounded by a coat composed of polar lipids (phospholipid and free cholesterol) and apoprotein. Plasma lipoproteins can be divided into four types, dependent on their electrophoretic mobility and sedimentation properties: (1) *chylomicrons*, which have the lowest density, are composed primarily of triglyceride, and are found in plasma only after a meal; (2) *very-low-density lipoprotein* (VLDL), which mainly transports triglycerides that have been synthesized in the liver; (3) *low-density lipoprotein* (LDL), and (4) *high-density lipoprotein* (HDL). LDL and HDL function primarily in the transport of endogenous cholesterol to body cells. *About 70% of the total plasma cholesterol level in normal Americans is contained in LDL, the lipoprotein most strongly correlated with AS.* Lipids form 75% of the mass of LDL, and of this 50 to 60% is cholesterol, mostly in the form of cholesteryl esters present in the core of the particle.

Endogenous and exogenous cholesterol are transported by various lipoproteins via two separate pathways (Fig. 12–12).[48] In the *endogenous pathway*, VLDL, containing triglycerides and three apoproteins (E,C, and B100), is transported from the liver to adipose tissue and muscle, where a sequence of events occurs that transforms VLDL, via the formation of intermediate-density lipoprotein (IDL), to LDL. This sequence includes the hydrolysis of triglycerides by the capillary endothelial enzyme lipoprotein lipase, removal of apoproteins E and C, and increase in the cholesteryl ester content of the particles. Thus, the core of LDL is composed almost exclusively of cholesteryl ester and the coat of only one protein, apoprotein B100. Two-thirds of the resultant LDL is metabolized by liver cells and other cells in extrahepatic tissues (adrenal cells, fibroblasts, smooth muscle cells, lymphoid cells, endothelial cells) by the *LDL receptor pathway* detailed on page 140. It will be recalled from the discussion of the genetic disturbances of cholesterol metabolism that this pathway is the means by which nonhepatic cells control the cholesterol needed for membrane synthesis; in the presence of low concentrations of extracellular LDL, more receptors are elaborated, and vice versa. The remaining one-third of LDL is degraded by LDL receptor–independent mechanisms (Fig. 12–12). These include the scavenger cells of the mononuclear phagocyte system, which, as discussed later, have receptors for *modified LDL*. In addition, non–receptor-mediated fluid and adsorptive endocytosis also occur in various cells, particularly in the presence of high LDL concentrations.

As the membranes of cells from extrahepatic tissues undergo turnover and death, they release unesterified cholesterol into the plasma, and this is transported by HDL (Fig. 12–12). Through the action of the plasma enzyme lecithin:cholesterol acyl transferase (LCAT) the cholesterol from HDL is delivered to IDL and eventually to LDL. Epidemiologic and experimental studies have shown an inverse relationship between the level of HDL and the development of AS. Although several mechanisms have been proposed for this protective action of HDL, none is proved. Probably the HDL fraction, usually low in cholesterol and rich in phospholipids, facilitates clearance of cholesterol from the arterial smooth muscle cells and its transport to the liver, where it may be excreted rather than reutilized in further synthesis of LDL.

In the *exogenous pathway* (Fig. 12–12), dietary cholesterol is incorporated into chylomicrons, hydrolyzed by endothelial lipoprotein lipase into cholesteryl ester-rich chylomicron remnants, which are then taken up by the liver through a receptor-mediated mechanism. Some of the cholesterol in the liver is excreted as free cholesterol or bile acids into the intestines.

A number of genetic and acquired derangements influence both exogenous and endogenous pathways of cholesterol metabolism, result in hyperlipoproteinemia,

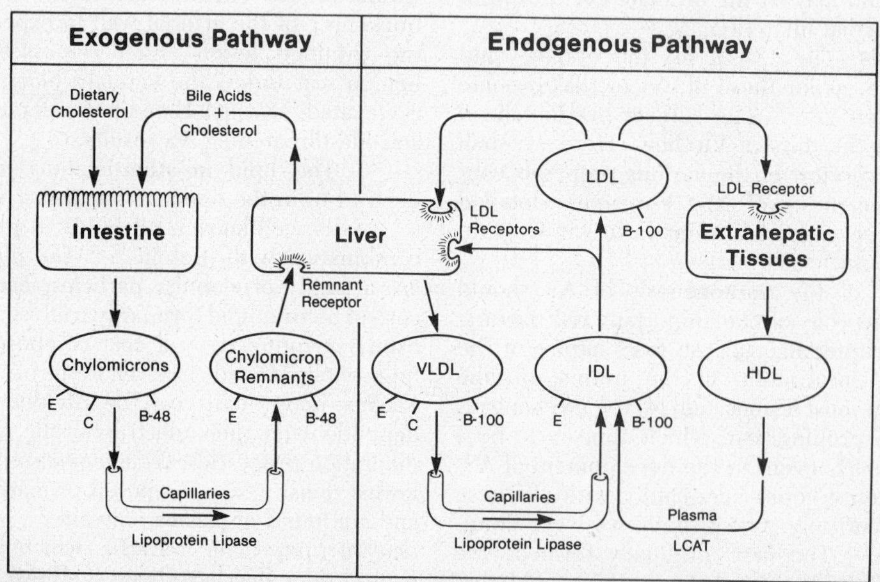

Figure 12–12. Pathways for receptor-mediated metabolism of lipoproteins carrying endogenous and exogenous cholesterol. HDL = high-density lipoprotein; LCAT = lecithin:cholesterol acyltransferase; LDL = low-density lipoprotein; IDL = intermediate-density lipoprotein; VLDL = very-low-density lipoprotein. The distinction between exogenous and endogenous cholesterol applies to the immediate source of the cholesterol in plasma lipoproteins. After the exogenous cholesterol has been delivered to the liver and has been secreted in VLDL, it is considered endogenous cholesterol. Note that HDL is the lipoprotein that removes cholesterol from extrahepatic cells. (From Goldstein, J. L., et al.: Defective lipoprotein receptors and atherosclerosis. N. Engl. J. Med. *309*:288, 1983. Reprinted, by permission, from The New England Journal of Medicine.)

and predispose to the development of AS. The hyperlipoproteinemias are classified as either primary genetic defects in lipid metabolism, or secondary to some other underlying disorder such as nephrotic syndrome or diabetes mellitus (Table 12–2). Some genetic disorders, such as familial hypercholesterolemia (p. 139), are single-gene dominant-recessive disorders, but many have a polygenic complex mode of inheritance and are markedly influenced by environmental factors, including diet (e.g., polygenic hypercholesterolemia). As stated earlier, elevated LDL levels are most closely linked to the development of AS, but both increased VLDL and decreased HDL serum concentrations are also correlated with increased risk.

The mechanisms by which these lipid alterations promote AS are still poorly understood but are currently under intensive study. Clearly, the cholesterol in atheromatous plaques is derived from plasma lipoproteins, as both apoprotein B and LDL have been localized in atherosclerotic lesions. Lipids, mostly cholesteryl esters, accumulate in the plaque extracellularly and within *foam cells*, which, as noted earlier, appear to consist of both smooth muscle cells and macrophages. However, neither smooth muscle cells nor macrophages exposed to naturally occurring LDL in vitro accumulate substantial amounts of cholesterol.

How, then, do these cells become loaded with lipids? In the smooth muscle cell of the lesions, it is conceivable that a defect in any of the steps in the LDL receptor pathway may lead to a positive cholesterol balance and lipid accumulation. Particularly appealing are in vitro studies showing that modifications of LDL (such as by altering its charge) may bypass the receptor-dependent uptake of LDL in smooth muscle cells, in favor of receptor-independent bulk adsorptive endocytosis. In the case of macrophages, modification of LDL by acetylation,[43, 50] or by treatment with malondialdehyde[51] (a product of the platelet release reaction), or by exposure of LDL to endothelial cells,[52] leads to binding of such *modified LDL* to receptors on the surface of the macrophage. Unlike the case in the regular LDL pathway, uptake by the modified LDL receptors is not followed by feedback inhibition of such receptors; thus, lipid progressively accumulates within the macrophages, transforming then to foam cells. In addition, β-VLDL, a cholesterol-rich lipoprotein, which appears in the plasma only after high-cholesterol feeding, is also taken up by macrophages and results in the formation of foam cells.[53] The accumulation of cholesteryl esters in macrophages under these conditions is markedly reduced in the presence of high concentrations of HDL, a finding consistent with the cholesterol-clearing property of the latter class of lipoproteins.[43] The latter experiments emphasize the importance of *egress* of cholesterol from the vessel wall—in addition to influx into the vessel wall—in the overall lipid deposition. Although the relevance of these in vitro studies on lipid accumulation in man is unproved, it is probable that interactions of lipoproteins with platelets, endothelial cells, macrophages, and smooth muscle cells are involved in the net lipid accumulation occurring in atheromatous plaques.[48]

Theories of Atherosclerosis. We can now turn to some of the current theories concerning AS (Fig. 12–13).

REACTION TO INJURY (OR RESPONSE TO INJURY) HYPOTHESIS. This theory, largely based on Virchow's insudation theory, states that *the lesions of atherosclerosis are initiated as a response to some form of injury to arterial endothelium* (Fig. 12–13, *left*).[41, 42] The injury may be subtle or may be outright desquamation of endothelial cells. Focal sites of injury lead to increased permeability to plasma constituents, and permit platelets and/or monocytes to adhere to endothelium or subendothelial connective tissue. Factors released from platelets or monocytes or some plasma constituent then lead to migration of smooth muscle from the media into the intima, followed by proliferation. Concomitantly, large amounts of connective tissue matrix are formed and lipid accumulates. Single or short-lived injurious events are followed by regeneration of endothelium, restoration of the endothelial barrier, and regression of the lesion. However, repeated or chronic injury will finally result in the development of an atheromatous plaque.

Table 12–2. THE HYPERLIPOPROTEINEMIAS*

Name and Increased Lipoprotein Class	Type	Prevalence	Primary Disorders	Secondary Disorders
Hypertriglyceridemia, exogenous (chylomicrons)	I	Rare	Familial lipoprotein lipase deficiency	SLE
Hypercholesterolemia (LDL)	IIa	Moderately common	Familial hypercholesterolemia (LDL receptor defects)	Nephrotic syndrome; hypothyroidism
Combined hyperlipidemia (LDL and VLDL)	IIb	Common	Familial, unclassified (dietary excess)	Nephrotic syndrome; stress-induced.
Remnant hyperlipidemia (β-VLDL)	III	Rare	Familial dysbetalipoproteinemia (broad-beta disease)	Hypothyroidism; monoclonal gammopathies
Endogenous hypertriglyceridemia (VLDL)	IV	Common	Familial (mild) Tangier disease	Diabetes mellitus; alcohol; uremia; stress; oral contraceptives
Mixed hypertriglyceridemia (VLDL & chylomicrons)	V	Fairly common	Familial combined hyperlipidemia	Alcohol; oral contraceptives; diabetes

*Modified from Havel, R. J., et al.: Lipoproteins and lipid transport. *In* Bondy, P.K., and Rosenberg, L.E. (eds.): Metabolic Control and Disease. 8th ed. Philadelphia, W.B. Saunders Co., 1980, pp. 393–494.

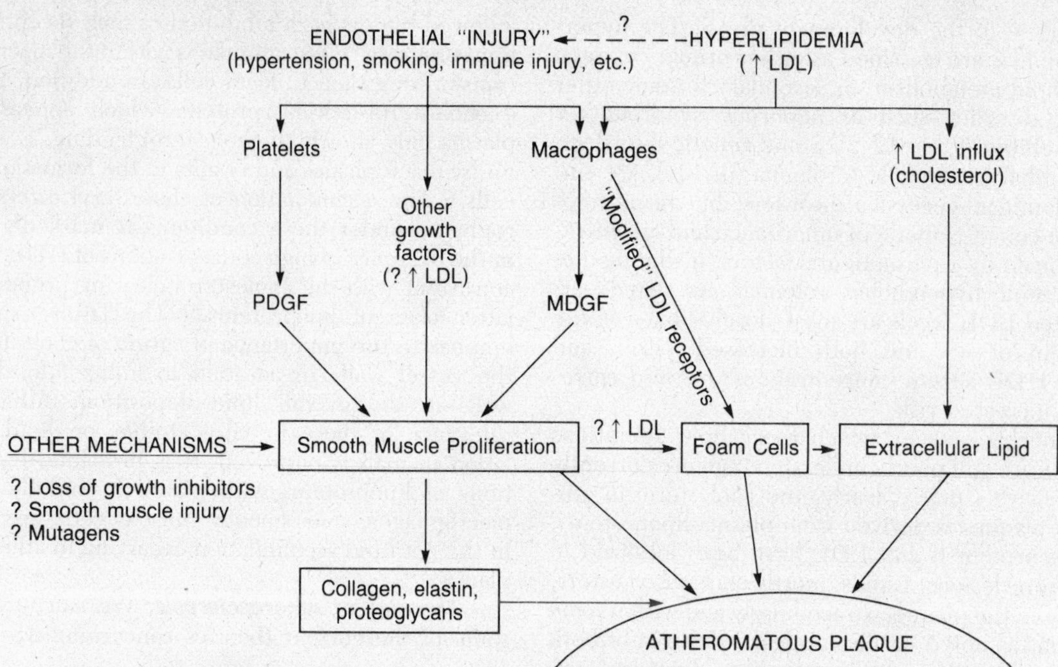

Figure 12–13. Proposed sequences involving endothelial injury, hyperlipidemia, and other mechanisms in the pathogenesis of the atheromatous plaque. Many of the mechanisms are based on in vitro studies. ? Refers to unproved or controversial sequences. Denuding or nondenuding endothelial injury causes platelet and monocyte macrophage adhesion to injured sites; factors derived from these cell types (PDGF, MDGF) or factors derived from the blood (e.g., hyperlipidemic LDL) cause smooth muscle migration and proliferation in the intima. Foam cells are derived from smooth muscle cells by as yet poorly understood mechanisms, and from macrophages in part by uptake via "modified" LDL receptors. The extracellular lipid is derived partly from direct migration from the serum and partly from breakdown of foam cells. The atheromatous plaque is composed of proliferating smooth muscle cells, their secreted extracellular matrix, foam cells, extracellular lipid, and necrotic debris. Hyperlipidemia *may* contribute to atherogenesis by: (1) increasing the influx of LDL, (2) causing endothelial injury, (3) directly inducing smooth muscle proliferation, and (4) influencing the formation of foam cells. Note that smooth muscle proliferation may also be induced directly by several postulated mechanisms *(left)*.

Let us examine the various components of this hypothesis. The fact that endothelial injury may cause proliferation of vascular smooth muscle has been shown experimentally after many forms of injury,[55] including balloon denudation, hemodynamic (arteriovenous fistulas), immunologic (immune complex deposition),[57] physical (irradiation), and chemical (homocystine)[58] endothelial injury. Of importance is the possibility that chronic hyperlipidemia in itself may initiate endothelial injury by some still unknown mechanisms.[59] Risk factors such as hypertension and cigarette smoking may also cause endothelial damage or increased endothelial permeability.[60] The list of other potential endothelium-damaging agents includes drugs, endotoxemia,[61] and viruses.[62] Of interest is the presence of foci of *spontaneous* increased endothelial permeability in apparently normal experimental animals (e.g., pigs) that eventually develop AS at these sites.[63] It is conceivable that such "spontaneous" foci are caused by normal hemodynamic forces ("shear stress"), possibly explaining the distribution of plaques at branch and fork points of arteries and in portions of the abdominal aorta.[38]

It should be stressed that frank endothelial denudation is not a necessary requirement for this theory. Some evidence suggests that foci of heightened endothelial permeability,[64] increased leukocyte adhesion,[28] decreased endothelial surface anionic sites,[65] and increased endothelial cell replication[66] occur early in the course of experimental hypercholesterolemia, *without* overt endothelial desquamation. Such alterations, referred to as endothelial "dysfunction,"[5] broaden the original concept of overt endothelial injury as the initiator of atherosclerosis.

The second component of the hypothesis is *smooth muscle proliferation in the intima.* The proliferating cells originate from cells migrating from the media and possibly also from preexisting myointimal cells. Several smooth muscle mitogens have been implicated in such proliferation. Principal among these is the *platelet-derived growth factor* (PDGF) (p. 76),[67] present in the alpha granules, and released after platelet adhesion to foci of injury. That the platelet mitogen may be active in vivo is suggested by the protective effect afforded by experimentally induced thrombocytopenia or by administration of inhibitors of platelet aggregation in some models of experimental AS.[67] Macrophage-derived growth factor[69] (MDGF, p. 76), LDL from hypercholesterolemic serum,[19] or other circulating hormones may also supply the growth-stimulating effect. Whatever the stimulus, it is the smooth muscle cells that elaborate the extracellular components of the atheromatous plaque: collagen, elastic tissue, and proteoglycans. Further, the smooth muscle cells accumulate large amounts of cholesterol and cholesteryl esters and, together with infiltrating macrophages, give rise to the foam cells in the plaque (p. 515). The *extracellular* lipid in the plaque results from plasma insudation directly into the intima and from necrosis of foam cells and release of their contents. It is of importance that in most experimental models, and also by analogy in man, smooth muscle proliferation ceases when the endothelial damage has been repaired. Endothelial repair occurs by migration and proliferation of endothelial cells from the periphery of the injured site.[71]

The third aspect of the response to injury hypothesis is its *relationship to hyperlipidemia.* As shown in Figure 12–13 (*right*), hyperlipidemia may interact with the vascular response to injury in several ways:[19, 45] (1) endothelial damage increases the insudation of plasma lipids into the vessel wall; (2) chronic hyperlipidemia may in itself cause endothelial injury; (3) certain components of hyperlipidemic serum may directly stimulate smooth muscle proliferation; and (4) hyperlipidemia favors platelet aggregation and release of PDGF—PDGF in turn increases LDL receptors on smooth muscle cells and thus increases their rate of uptake of lipid in addition to triggering smooth muscle growth.

Although the concept of endothelial injury, coupled with the effects of hyperlipidemia, is an attractive mechanism of atherogenesis, *the development of the atheromatous plaque could also be explained if smooth muscle proliferation was in fact the initial event.* Endothelial injury may then be a secondary phenomenon, or may indeed accentuate the lesion, but would be neither the first nor a necessary event. It is possible, for example, that amounts of lipid (or some lipid component) that would normally reach the smooth muscle layer in hypercholesterolemic individuals may somehow alter smooth muscle cells and trigger their proliferation. Or it may be that genetic or acquired defects of the smooth muscle themselves may induce the initial proliferative response. Two theories to account for such a primary effect on smooth muscle have been proposed and will be briefly discussed next.

MONOCLONAL HYPOTHESIS. Benditt and Benditt studied the distribution of A- or B-isoenzyme of X-linked glucose-6-phosphate dehydrogenase (G6PD) in atheromatous plaques of black women heterozygous for this enzyme.[72] As expected, it was found that segments of uninvolved aortic intima and media contained both A- and B-isoenzymes. *However, fibrous plaques contained either A or B, and only seldom contained both.* This monotypic nature of the smooth muscle cells in the plaque was interpreted as evidence that plaques may therefore be equivalent to benign monoclonal neoplastic growths (such as leiomyomas) and are initiated by a mutation. The mutagenic effect may be from an exogenous chemical (e.g., hydrocarbons), endogenous metabolite (e.g., cholesterol or some of its oxidants), or a virus. The monoclonality of a majority of plaques has since been both confirmed and denied;[73] it appears that most are oligoclonal (composed of a few clones) rather than monoclonal. The significance of this appealing hypothesis is still unclear, but it has served to direct attention to possible smooth muscle mutagens as initiators of smooth muscle proliferation.

DISTURBANCES IN GROWTH CONTROL. Other hypotheses accounting for smooth muscle proliferation in AS implicate loss of "growth control" in the cells of the media.[74] Although these concepts are still largely speculative, there is evidence supporting a role for inhibitors in growth regulation of the arterial wall; indeed, factors that inhibit cell growth in culture have been isolated from aortic walls. One of these is a heparin-like molecule elaborated by endothelial[75] and smooth muscle cells. Presumably, focal loss of these inhibitors (possibly initiated by injury) may lead to smooth muscle proliferation. The importance of identifying such inhibitors is that they may be of potential therapeutic value. Indeed, administration of heparin inhibits smooth muscle proliferation induced experimentally by endothelial injury.[76]

Figure 12–13 illustrates some of the proposed mechanisms of atherogenesis, emphasizing the reaction to injury sequences and the role of hyperlipidemia. The most currently plausible theory is the reaction to injury hypothesis, if the term "injury" is broadened to encompass subtle, nondenuding, functional endothelial damage or injury primarily to smooth muscle cells. It is very likely that there is no one cause of AS, no single initiating event, and no exclusive pathogenetic mechanism. *Clinically significant AS appears to be a disease of multiple origins.* In some individuals, severe or repeated endothelial injury may induce AS with relatively normal LDL levels. In others, such as those with extreme hyperlipidemia, endothelial injury may not be necessary to trigger the same events. Perhaps the cumulative effect of many factors is involved, as seems evident from epidemiologic studies. In short, despite all that has been learned, the cause of AS is still unknown. At this stage, it is perfectly reasonable to attempt to halt AS during its progression rather than at its inception. The investigation of serum lipids, the study of risk factors and their manipulation, and the emphasis on prevention and treatment of thrombotic complications constitute attempts to approach the problem in this manner.

CLINICAL SIGNIFICANCE. The clinical manifestations of AS are as varied as the vessels affected and the extent of the atheromatous change. The lesions themselves do not cause symptoms or signs. They cause clinical disease only by (1) narrowing the vascular lumina to cause ischemic atrophy; (2) sudden occlusion of the lumen by superimposed thrombosis or hemorrhage into an atheroma, producing frank infarction; (3) providing a site for thrombosis and then embolism; or (4) weakening the wall of a vessel, followed possibly by aneurysm formation or rupture. Although theoretically any organ or tissue in the body may be so involved, symptomatic atherosclerotic disease is most often localized to the heart, brain, kidneys, lower extremities, and small intestine.

The importance of such vascular disease was amply documented by some of the epidemiologic data cited earlier in this discussion. It will be further documented throughout the remaining chapters of the book, since vascular disease constitutes a significant part of all organ and system pathology.

Given the fact that AS and CHD are virtually epidemic in affluent populations, methods of possible control are understandably major concerns of these groups. A number of clinical trials of prevention of AS and CHD have been instituted. All make the assumption that five factors capable of alteration are of cardinal importance: diets high in cholesterol and saturated fat, hypercholesterolemia, hypertension, cigarette smoking, and diabetes. A review of clinical trials is beyond our scope. Suffice it to say here that the evidence is good that control of hypertension and cigarette smoking diminishes the risk of CHD. With regard to diabetes, there are two opposing camps, one defending and the other denying a role for control of blood sugar in the progression of AS. Finally, controversy still exists concerning the possibility of influencing hyperlipidemia and CHD through dietary alterations. This issue was discussed earlier in the chapter. Many, but not really all, investigators believe that dietary reduction of plasma cholesterol and cholesterol LDL levels would retard the progression of AS, but opinions on the strength of the probability vary widely, since CHD risk is multifactorial. However, experts on all sides of the controversy advocate a reduction in fat intake, avoidance of obesity, moderation of salt intake, cessation of smoking, and the pursuit of physical activity as ways of life that are likely to reduce overall risk. This consensus should not be overlooked in the continuing debate about the issues involved in the relationship between diet and coronary heart disease.[17]

MÖNCKEBERG'S ARTERIOSCLEROSIS (MEDIAL CALCIFIC SCLEROSIS)

Medial sclerosis is characterized by ringlike calcifications within the media of medium-sized to small arteries of the muscular type. Although Mönckeberg's medial calcific sclerosis may occur together with atherosclerosis in the same individual or even in the same vessel, *the two disorders are totally distinct anatomically, clinically, and presumably etiologically.* The vessels most severely affected are the femoral, tibial, radial, and ulnar arteries and the arterial supply of the genital tract in both sexes. The coronary arteries are likewise subject to medial calcinosis. Both sexes are affected indiscriminately. This disorder is rare in individuals under 50 years of age. Its genesis is still obscure, but according to prevailing concepts, medial calcification is related to prolonged vasotonic influences. In animals, analogous medial calcifications can be produced by the prolonged intravascular infusion of such vasoconstrictors as epinephrine and nicotine.

The disorder is characterized by ringlike or plate calcifications within the wall of a vessel that create a "gooseneck lamp" nodularity on palpation. The calcification is not associated with any inflammatory reaction, and the intima and adventitia are largely unaffected. Commonly, bone and even marrow may form within the calcific plaques. Frequently, coexistent atheromas complicate the histologic changes (Fig. 12–14).

This disorder is of relatively little clinical significance. It accounts for roentgenographic densities in the vessels of the extremities in aged individuals, but it is to be remembered that the lesions do *not* produce narrowing or occlusion of vascular lumina.

ARTERIOLOSCLEROSIS

Included under this heading are two entities: hyaline arteriolosclerosis and hyperplastic arteriolosclerosis. Although both lesions are clearly related to elevations of blood pressure, other etiologies may also be involved.

Hyaline Arteriolosclerosis

This condition is encountered frequently in elderly patients, whether normotensive or hypertensive, but is more generalized and more severe in patients with hypertension. The condition is also seen commonly in diabetes, and forms part of the microangiography characteristic of diabetic disease (p. 982). Whatever the clinical setting, the vascular lesion consists of a homogeneous, pink, hyaline thickening of the walls of arterioles with loss of underlying structural detail and with narrowing of the lumen (Fig. 21–54, p. 1045). Under the electron microscope, irregular thickening of the basement membrane can be visualized, and there is deposition of amorphous extracellular substance within the vessel wall. Often, smooth muscle cells are trapped within these deposits. Intimal and medial collagenization adds to the hyaline changes of the arteriolar walls.

It is believed that the lesions reflect leakage of plasma components across vascular endothelium. Presumably, the chronic hydrodynamic stress of hypertension or a metabolic stress in diabetes accentuates endothelial injury, thus resulting in leakage and hyaline deposition. Whatever the pathogenesis, the narrowing of the arteriolar lumina causes impairment of the blood supply to affected organs, particularly well exemplified in the kidneys. Thus, *hyaline arteriolosclerosis is a major morphologic characteristic of benign nephrosclerosis* in which the arteriolar narrowing causes diffuse renal ischemia and symmetric contraction of the kidneys (p. 1045).

Hyperplastic Arteriolosclerosis

The hyperplastic type of arteriolosclerosis is generally related to more acute or severe elevations of blood pressure and is therefore characteristic of malignant hypertension (diastolic pressures usually over 110

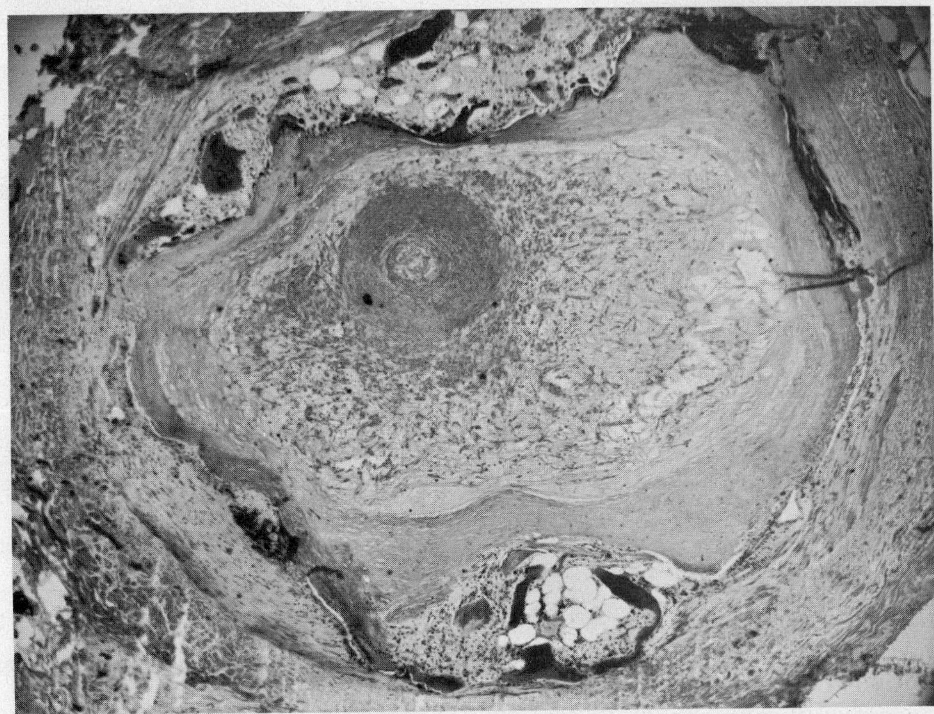

Figure 12–14. Mönckeberg's medial calcific sclerosis and atherosclerosis. Vessel lumen is markedly narrowed by intimal atherosclerosis. Dark, medial, calcific deposits with bone and bone marrow formation (at 6 o'clock) indicate the presence of Mönckeberg's sclerosis.

mm Hg) (p. 1041). This form of arteriolar disease can be identified under the light microscope by virtue of its onionskin, concentric, laminated thickening of the walls of arterioles with progressive narrowing of the lumina (Fig. 12–15). Under the electron microscope, these reduplicated cells have the appearance of smooth muscle. The basement membrane is likewise thickened and reduplicated. Frequently, but not invariably, these hyperplastic changes are accompanied by deposits of fibrinoid and acute necrosis of the vessel walls, referred to as *necrotizing arteriolitis*. The arterioles in all tissues throughout the body may be affected, favored sites being the kidney, periadrenal fat, gallbladder, peripancreatic, and intestinal arterioles. Why these vessels should show more pronounced change than others is not clear. Not infrequently, the two forms of arteriolosclerosis coexist in the same vessel.

INFLAMMATION—THE VASCULITIDES

Arteritis is encountered in a diversity of diseases and clinical settings.[77-79] The terms arteritis, vasculitis, and angiitis are used interchangeably because veins and capillaries may be involved in some of the conditions. In some instances, arteritis is produced when an artery is injured directly by a specific agent, such as by direct bacterial invasion, irradiation, mechanical trauma, and toxins. The most important entities, however, are the so-called "noninfectious necrotizing vasculitides." Although all are characterized by inflammation and necrosis of blood vessels, they are segregated into a number of distinctive clinicopathologic syndromes affecting multiple organ systems. Many of these entities appear to have an immunologic basis. Vasculitis, also of immune origin, is a component of systemic lupus erythematosus

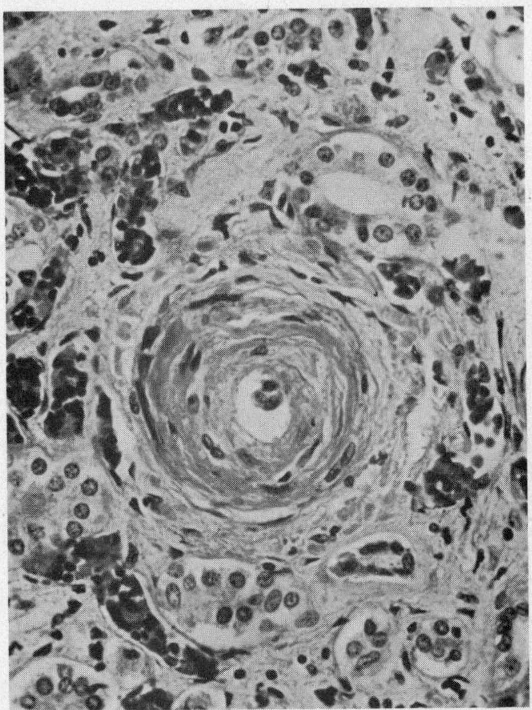

Figure 12–15. Hyperplastic arteriolosclerosis of small vessel in kidney. Patient was a young man who died with blood pressure 310/160.

(SLE) and sometimes complicates the other connective tissue disorders, such as scleroderma, polymyositis, rheumatoid arthritis, and rheumatic fever.

Before discussing some of the syndromes, we shall briefly review pathogenetic mechanisms that may be common to many vasculitides.

Etiology and Pathogenesis of Vasculitis. Although little is known about etiologic agents, many types of vasculitis are thought to be induced by immunologic mechanisms, and the evidence for this can be summarized as follows:[77–79]

1. The vascular lesions resemble those found in experimental immune complex–mediated conditions, such as the local Arthus phenomenon and serum sickness.

2. Vasculitis is found in association with SLE, scleroderma, dermatomyositis, and Sjögren's syndrome. DNA–anti-DNA immune complexes and complement are present in the vascular lesions in these conditions.

3. In patients with mixed cryoglobulinemia, IgG, IgM (antibody to IgG), and complement components have been seen in involved vessels.

4. Drugs such as sulfonamides, penicillin, thiouracil, iodides, and arsenicals have often been associated with the development of vasculitis. In most of these, the lesion described has been that of microscopic polyarteritis (hypersensitivity angiitis).

5. The most impressive evidence is the demonstration of a high incidence of hepatitis B antigenemia (HBsAg) and circulating HBsAg–anti-HBs immune complexes in the sera of some patients with vasculitis.[80] Moreover, HBs antigen, immunoglobulins, and complement occur in the vascular lesions. Indeed, it has been estimated that hepatitis B antigen may be the inciting agent in between 25 and 40% of patients with necrotizing vasculitis. The occurrence of vasculitis in drug addicts may be due to the high incidence of hepatitis B antigenemia in these individuals, but other infectious agents may also be possible causes.

Other pathogenetic mechanisms should be considered. The presence of mononuclear cells and granulomas in some vasculitides suggests cell-mediated immunity, which may be directed against foreign antigens or endogenous components of the vessel wall. In fact, cell-mediated immunity to arterial wall antigens has been described in one form of vasculitis, temporal arteritis. Alternatively, autoantibodies against vessel wall antigens may play a role, as they do in some glomerular diseases. Defects in immunoregulation, well described in SLE (p. 181), may predispose to the development of vasculitis. All these mechanisms, however, are less well established than those of immune complex–mediated damage in vasculitis.

Classification. Many classifications of vasculitis are available and depend on the size of the involved blood vessels, the anatomic site, the histologic characteristic of the lesion, or the clinical manifestations. However, there is considerable clinical and pathologic overlap among these disorders, and some have thus been considered as "groups." Table 12–3 lists the most important groups of vasculitis as currently classified.

Table 12–3. CLASSIFICATION OF VASCULITIS

I. Polyarteritis nodosa group of systemic necrotizing vasculitis
   - A. Classic polyarteritis nodosa
   - B. Allergic angiitis and granulomatosis (Churg-Strauss variant)
   - C. Systemic necrotizing vasculitis "overlap syndrome"

II. Hypersensitivity angiitis
   - A. Serum sickness and serum sickness–like reactions
   - B. Henoch-Schönlein purpura
   - C. Vasculitis associated with connective tissue disorders
   - D. Essential mixed cryoglobulinemia with vasculitis
   - E. Malignancy

III. Wegener's granulomatosis

IV. Lymphomatoid granulomatosis

V. Giant cell arteritides
   - A. Temporal arteritis
   - B. Takayasu's arteritis

VI. Mucocutaneous lymph node syndrome (Kawasaki's disease)

VII. Thromboangiitis obliterans (Buerger's disease)

VIII. Miscellaneous (Others)

POLYARTERITIS NODOSA (PAN) GROUP

This group is characterized by systemic involvement with the vasculitic process and includes the first recognized *classic* type of vasculitis, also called the *macroscopic* form of PAN. *Classic PAN* is a disease of small or medium-sized muscular arteries, characteristically involving renal and visceral vessels and sparing the pulmonary circulation.[81]

Morphology. Classic PAN may affect any artery of medium or small size in any organ or system of the body. The more usual sites of involvement in autopsy series are the kidneys (85%), heart (75%), liver (65%), and gastrointestinal tract (50%), followed by the pancreas, testes, skeletal muscle, nervous system, and skin. Grossly, the individual lesions involve sharply localized segments of vessel with a predilection for branching points and bifurcations. The lesions may be inapparent on macroscopic inspection, but the affected vessels may have nodular gray or red swellings. Rarely, small aneurysmal dilatations or perivascular hematomas may result from weakening or rupture of the wall. Intravascular thrombosis is a frequent sequel to the acute vasculitis. Ulcerations, infarctions, ischemic atrophy, or hemorrhages in the areas supplied by these vessels may provide the first clue to the existence of the underlying disorder.

Microscopically, the changes in the vessels may be divided into acute, healing, and healed stages; within the same case of the classic type of polyarteritis one frequently sees all three lesions, although in other cases one stage may predominate. The **acute lesions** are characterized by fibrinoid necrosis, which may affect only the intima, but often extends to involve the full thickness of the arterial wall, particularly in small arteries (Fig. 12–16). Numerous leukocytes, including neutrophils, may be present in the inflammatory lesions and in perivascular tissue, and there may be a perivascular cuff of cells. The necrosis may involve the entire circumference of the wall but is often localized to a segment. The affected portion may bulge in an aneurysmal fashion, and these aneurysms can frequently be demonstrated by arteriography. It is during this acute stage that the lumen becomes thrombosed (Fig. 12–17) and destruc-

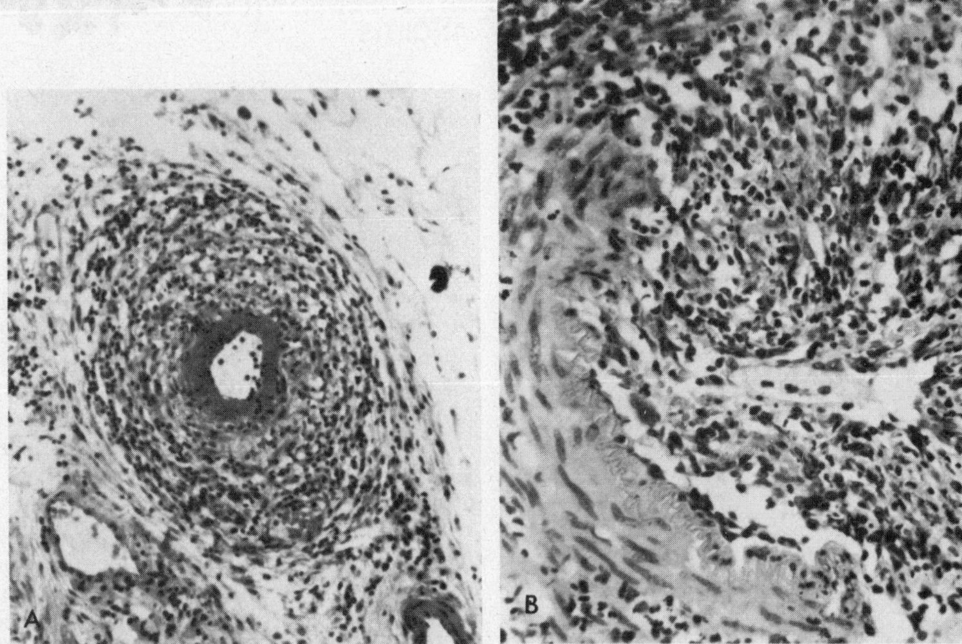

Figure 12–16. *A,* Polyarteritis nodosa. There is fibrinoid necrosis of intima and a severe inflammatory infiltrate throughout the arterial wall. *B,* Higher-power view showing infiltrate of neutrophils and mononuclear cells in vessel wall.

tion of the elastica, particularly the internal elastic membrane, can be demonstrated. Eosinophils and mononuclear cells may be numerous and may represent over half of all white cells present.

Healing lesions are characterized by fibroblastic proliferation in addition to the continuing necrotizing process. Fibroblasts are often found arranged concentrically in the intima, and usually cause thickening of the wall and narrowing of the lumen. The leukocytic infiltrate will now exhibit large numbers of macrophages and plasma cells. The fibroblastic proliferation may extend into the surrounding adventitia, producing the firm nodularity that is sometimes grossly apparent. Thrombosis, if present, becomes organized, and the entire vessel wall then becomes transformed into a fibrous cord.

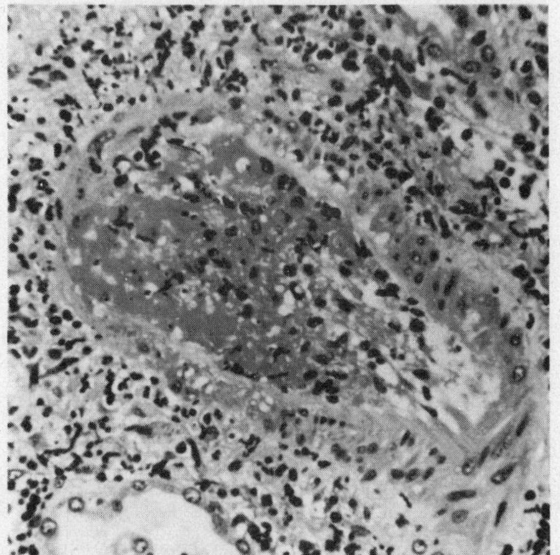

Figure 12–17. Polyarteritis nodosa. Small renal artery showing segmental fibrinoid necrosis of vessel wall and thrombotic occlusion of lumen. Note that part of vessel wall *(bottom right)* is uninvolved.

The **healed lesions** consist merely of marked fibrotic thickening of the affected arterial wall. Scattered lymphocytes, plasma cells, and occasional deposits of calcium may mark for long periods the site of the previous acute damage. Elastic tissue stains are valuable in detecting healed polyarteritis, since they can disclose loss or fragmentation of the internal elastic lamina and its replacement by fibrous tissue (Fig. 12–18).

Although these stages have been described separately, all three may coexist in different loci, either within the same vessel or in different vessels. Only rarely are all lesions at one stage of inflammatory activity. When all signs of activity have regressed, it is sometimes difficult to establish the diagnosis of PAN morphologically, since all that remains is fibrous scarring of nonspecific character.

Clinical Course. Classic PAN is a disease of young adults, although it may occur in children and older individuals. It affects men more frequently than women, in the ratio of 2 to 3:1. Since the vascular involvement is haphazard and widely scattered and induces infarctions of varying ages in affected organs, it is obvious that the clinical signs and symptoms of these disorders may be varied and puzzling. Indeed, the dominant clinical characteristics of PAN are such nonspecific systemic reactions as low-grade fever, malaise, weakness, leukocytosis, and symptoms referable to many systems. The course may be acute, subacute, or chronic and is frequently remittent, with long intervals of freedom from symptoms. The most common manifestations are fever of unknown etiology and weight loss; hematuria, albuminuria, and renal failure attributable to the renal involvement; hypertension, usually developing rapidly;

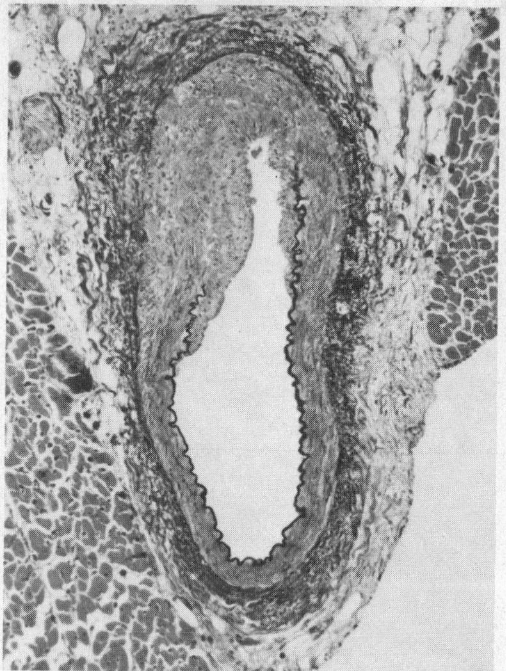

Figure 12–18. Elastic tissue stain of artery showing healed polyarteritis at lower left corner. The internal elastic lamina is destroyed and there is thickening of intima and media.

abdominal pain, cramps, and melena due to vascular lesions in the alimentary tract; diffuse muscular aches and pains; and peripheral neuritis, which is predominantly motor. About 30% of patients with PAN have the hepatitis B antigen in their serum.[82]

The clinical diagnosis can usually be definitely established only by the identification of the vascular lesions. Clinically involved tissue is best for histologic examination, such as kidney, tender muscles, subcutaneous nodules, and skin lesions. Angiography shows vascular aneurysms in 50% of cases. Death may occur during an acute fulminant attack but it may follow a protracted course. Previous data have indicated that up to two-thirds of untreated patients die of renal failure, cerebral hemorrhage, or intestinal infarction within one year. More recent studies, however, showed a five-year survival of 57% for those given corticosteroid therapy, and of 80% for those given corticosteroids and cyclophosphamide,[79] which supports an immunologic origin for this disorder. Effective treatment of the hypertension is a prerequisite for a favorable prognosis.

Allergic granulomatosis and angiitis (the Churg-Strauss syndrome) has been distinguished from classic PAN because of a strong association with bronchial asthma and eosinophilia, the frequent involvement of pulmonary and splenic vessels, and the presence of intra- and extravascular granulomas. The vascular lesions, however, may be histologically identical to those of classic PAN. Vasculitis and granulomas occur in lungs, peripheral nerves, and skin, with a striking infiltration of vessels and perivascular tissues by eosinophils.

HYPERSENSITIVITY (LEUKOCYTOCLASTIC) ANGIITIS

This group, also called microscopic polyarteritis, is differentiated from PAN because smaller vessels are affected (arterioles, venules, and capillaries). Further, in a single patient, all lesions tend to be of the same age. It is a rather frequently encountered type of vasculitis that typically involves the skin, mucous membranes, lungs, brain, heart, gastrointestinal tract, kidneys, and muscle. In many cases a possible antigen can be traced as the precipitating cause. Drugs (penicillin), microorganisms (beta-hemolytic streptococci), heterologous protein, and tumor antigens have been implicated as triggers of the disorder.[83]

In general, muscular and large arteries are spared; thus, macroscopic infarcts similar to those seen in PAN are uncommon. Histologically, fibrinoid necrosis may be present, but in some lesions the change is limited to infiltration with neutrophils, which become fragmented as they flood the vessel wall. The term "leukocytoclastic angiitis" is given to such lesions. *The disease may be confined to the skin (cutaneous vasculitis),* in which it is manifested by palpable purpura (Fig. 12–19), but, as mentioned earlier, almost all organs can be affected and lung involvement is common. The renal lesions tend to be limited to the glomerular tufts. In some patients they are focal and segmental, but in some they may progress to affect all glomeruli, resulting in a lesion identical to that seen in so-called *crescentic glomerulonephritis* (p. 1009). Patients with such glomerular lesions develop rapidly progressive renal failure. Immunoglobulins and

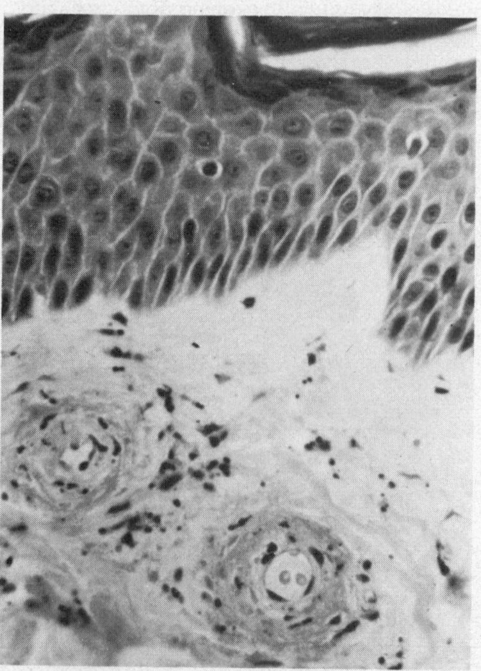

Figure 12–19. Hypersensitivity angiitis affecting skin. Note fragmented nuclei of neutrophils in vessel walls and perivascular spaces.

complement components are present in the vascular lesions of the skin, especially if these are examined within 24 hours of development. With the exception of those who develop crescentic glomerulonephritis, most patients respond well simply to removal of the offending agent.

Disseminated vascular lesions of hypersensitivity angiitis may appear in a number of rather distinct syndromes. These include Henoch-Schönlein purpura, essential mixed cryoglobulinemia, vasculitis associated with some of the connective tissue disorders, and vasculitis associated with malignancy. These are discussed under the specific entities elsewhere in this book.

WEGENER'S GRANULOMATOSIS

This rare form of necrotizing vasculitis is characterized by (1) *acute necrotizing granulomas* of the upper and lower respiratory tract (nose, sinuses, and lung); (2) *focal necrotizing vasculitis*, most prominent in the lungs and upper airways but affecting other sites as well; and (3) renal disease in the form of focal or diffuse necrotizing glomerulitis.

As with polyarteritis, males are more frequently affected than females, and the peak incidence is in the fifth decade. The typical clinical features include a persistent pneumonitis with bilateral nodular and cavitary infiltrates (95%), chronic sinusitis (90%), mucosal ulcerations of the nasopharynx (75%), and evidence of renal disease (80%).[85]

Skin rashes, muscle pains, articular involvement, and mono- or polyneuritis occur in 25 to 60% of patients, and about 50% have fever. Untreated, the course of the disease is malignant, 82% of patients dying within one year, with a mean survival of five months. *During recent years, however, this grim prognosis has been improved dramatically by the use of immunosuppressive drugs such as cyclophosphamide; up to 90% of patients respond to such therapy, and in the majority the remission appears complete.*

MORPHOLOGY. Involvement of the respiratory tract takes the form of focal acute necrosis in the nasal and oral cavities, paranasal sinuses, larynx, or trachea, as well as focal lesions scattered throughout the lung parenchyma. These areas are generally surrounded by a zone of fibroblastic proliferation with giant cells and leukocytic infiltrate, creating a more than superficial resemblance to a tubercle (Fig. 12–20). These lesions undergo progressive fibrosis and organization. The lesions in the lung are usually small,

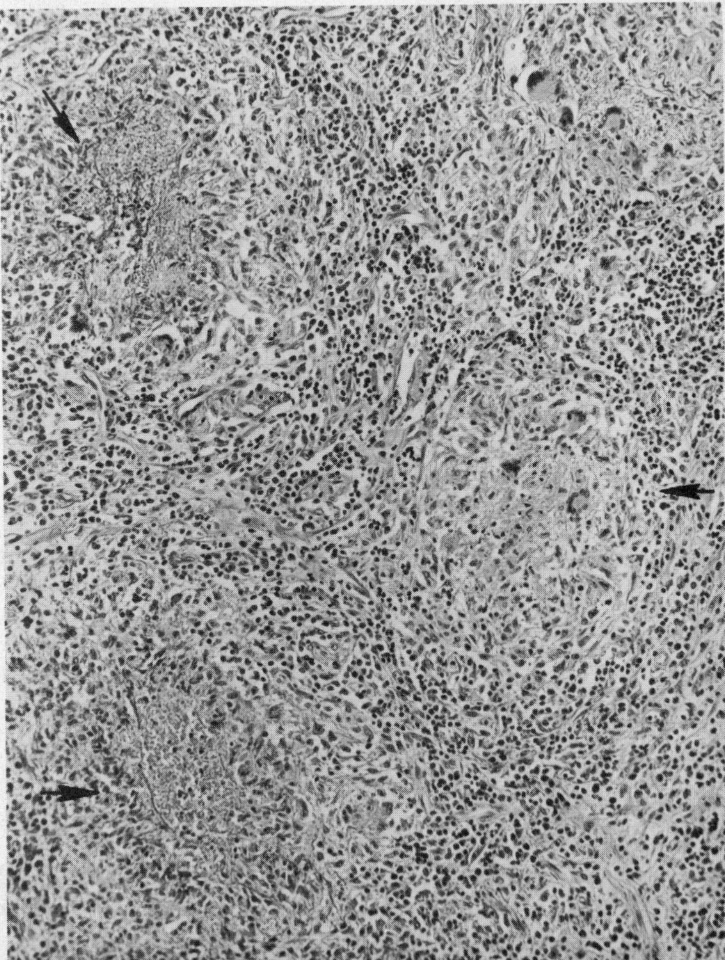

Figure 12–20. Multiple granulomas in lungs in Wegener's granulomatosis *(arrows)*. Note central necrosis and multinucleate giant cells.

but occasionally take the form of large (5- to 6-cm) foci of consolidation, which may also become cavitary. The vasculitis affects small arteries and veins and has been described in virtually every vessel and organ of the body, favorite sites being the respiratory tract, kidneys, and spleen. These lesions are almost identical with those of the acute phase of polyarteritis nodosa (Fig. 12–21), but often contain granulomas, which may be within, adjacent to, or clearly separated from the vessel wall.

The renal lesions are of two types: in milder forms, or early in the disease, there is acute focal proliferation and necrosis in the glomeruli, with thrombosis of isolated glomerular capillary loops. This **focal necrotizing glomerulonephritis** (p. 1018) may resolve with therapy or may progress rapidly to the second type, in which there is diffuse proliferation and necrosis of the glomerulus, together with the formation of many glomerular crescents. Patients with focal lesions may have hematuria and proteinuria, whereas those with crescentic glomerulonephritis develop rapidly progressive renal failure.

Because of its striking resemblance to polyarteritis nodosa and serum sickness, it is thought that the disease represents some form of hypersensitivity, possibly to an inhaled infectious or other environmental agent, but no etiologic agent has been identified. Immune complexes have been seen in the glomeruli and vessel walls in occasional patients. The dramatic response to cyclophosphamide also strongly suggests an immunologic mechanism, perhaps of the cell-mediated type. Because of the excellent response to therapy, a correct diagnosis of Wegener's granulomatosis is imperative. If necessary, the diagnosis should be confirmed by biopsy of the lung or nasopharyngeal lesions.

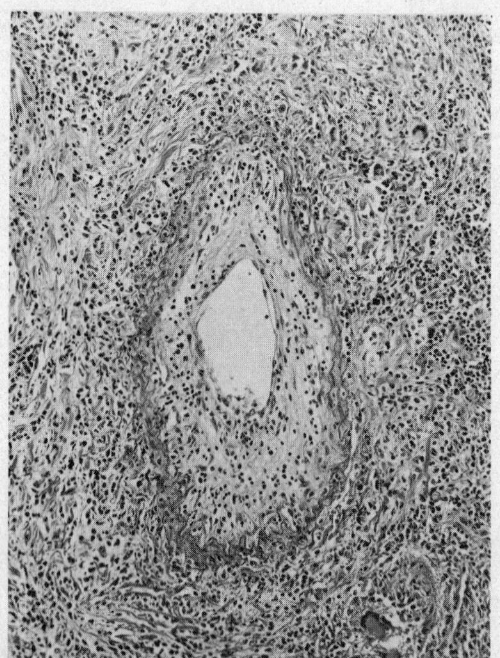

Figure 12–21. Small artery in lung in Wegener's granulomatosis. The wall is markedly thickened, fibrotic, and infiltrated with white cells.

Lymphomatoid granulomatosis[86] is an obscure entity that resembles Wegener's granulomatosis but does not exhibit the triad of respiratory tract granulomas, vasculitis, and glomerulonephritis. It is characterized by pulmonary infiltration by nodules of lymphoid and plasmacytoid cells, often with cellular atypia. These infiltrates invade vessels, giving the histologic appearance of a vasculitis. The condition is initially localized to the lungs, but about one-third of patients eventually show similar lesions in the kidneys, liver, brain, and other organs, and from 10 to 50% develop malignant lymphoid tumors, most commonly non-Hodgkin's lymphoma.

GIANT CELL (TEMPORAL) ARTERITIS

Temporal arteritis is a focal granulomatous inflammation of arteries of medium and small size that affects principally the cranial vessels, especially the temporal arteries in older individuals.[87] In the more severe expressions of this disorder, lesions have been found in arteries throughout the body, and in some cases the aortic arch has been involved to produce so-called *giant cell aortitis.* Women are slightly more often affected than men. This disease is rare under age 50, and the average age at onset is 70. In contrast, polyarteritis nodosa, which bears some morphologic resemblance to disseminated giant cell arteritis, and Takayasu's disease, which also involves the aortic arch, both tend to affect younger individuals.

Temporal arteritis is the most common of the vasculitides, its prevalence increasing significantly with age to about 850 per 100,000 population aged 80 years and over. Almost half of all patients with manifestations of temporal arteritis, such as headache, tenderness over the artery, visual loss, and facial pain, have systemic involvement and the syndrome of polymyalgia rheumatica, described later. However, 40% of biopsies of the temporal artery[88] are negative in patients with classic manifestations of this disease, and it must be assumed that the lesions were focal and were missed on biopsy.

ETIOLOGY AND PATHOGENESIS. The cause of this relatively common disease remains a puzzle. The morphologic alterations seem to suggest some sort of immunologic reaction against a component of the arterial wall. Some support for such a conception is provided by the finding of cell-mediated immunity to arterial antigen in some patients and by the response that is almost always achieved by corticosteroid treatment. In addition, the recognition of systemic patterns of this disease with prominent involvement of muscles has raised the issue of whether this disorder may be a form of rheumatoid arthritis with arteritis (having a more firmly established immunologic basis). The absence of firm serologic evidence of rheumatoid arthritis, however, argues against the identity of rheumatoid disease and giant cell arteritis. Genetic predisposition, as evidenced by increased prevalence of some histocompatibility antigens, has been claimed by some workers but refuted by others. The granulomatous nature of the inflammatory response obviously led to the suspicion of an infectious agent. However, no microbiologic agent has been isolated from affected vessels, and so the puzzle persists.

MORPHOLOGY. The histologic changes in arteries are quite variable and fall into three general patterns: (1) granulomatous lesions replete with giant cells, often in relation to fragments of the internal elastic membrane (Fig. 12–22); (2) nonspecific white cell infiltration (neutrophils and occasional lymphocytes and eosinophils) throughout the arterial wall; and (3) intimal fibrosis, usually with no morphologically apparent disruption of the internal elastic lamina. Giant cells are present in only two-thirds of cases, and frequently many sections may have to be examined before one is detected. Thrombus formation commonly occurs in affected vessels and may be followed by either obliteration of the lumen or organization and recanalization. In healed phases, the artery is transformed into an obliterated fibrous cord. In addition to temporal arteries, involvement of vertebral and ophthalmic arteries is common, and some patients develop systemic lesions in any intermediate or large-sized muscular artery.

CLINICAL COURSE. The disease may be insidious and vague in onset or may be heralded by the sudden onset of headache. Often, the illness begins with general symptoms of weight loss, malaise, fever, anorexia, and nausea, followed by generalized muscular aching and stiffness in the shoulders and hips, manifestations that suggest a flulike syndrome. Such an onset would be characterized as *polymyalgia rheumatica.*[88] There is often severe throbbing pain along the course of the artery; tenderness, swelling, and redness in the overlying skin; and claudication of the jaw. Visual symptoms (blurred or double vision or transient partial blindness) occur in 40% of patients. Permanent complete blindness in one or both eyes is fortunately uncommon, but in some instances the progressive development of blindness is the only manifestation of the vascular disease. Involvement of visceral vessels may give rise to manifestations of myocardial ischemia, gastrointestinal disturbances, or neurologic derangements. When the aortic arch is involved, the symptomatology may be identical to that of Takayasu's or aortic arch syndrome, discussed next.

The diagnosis of this condition, as must be apparent, is treacherous. The erythrocyte sedimentation rate (ESR) is markedly elevated in 95% of cases but is a nonspecific finding. Biopsy may be diagnostic but may be negative in otherwise characteristic clinical syndromes. Careful palpation of arteries in the hope of identifying a focal area of tenderness or nodularity is most important in securing an appropriate biopsy specimen. As mentioned, however, histologic changes may be present in clinically normal vessels. In the absence of morphologic confirmation, it is often necessary to institute therapy on clinical grounds alone. In some instances, the disease is of acute and almost calamitous onset, and corticosteroid therapy must be instituted promptly to prevent visual impairment. Fortunately, the response to steroids is excellent, with subsidence of headache, myalgia, and visual symptoms and return to normal of the ESR within a few days. In a small proportion of cases with widespread systemic involvement, the course is progressively downhill with a fatal outcome.

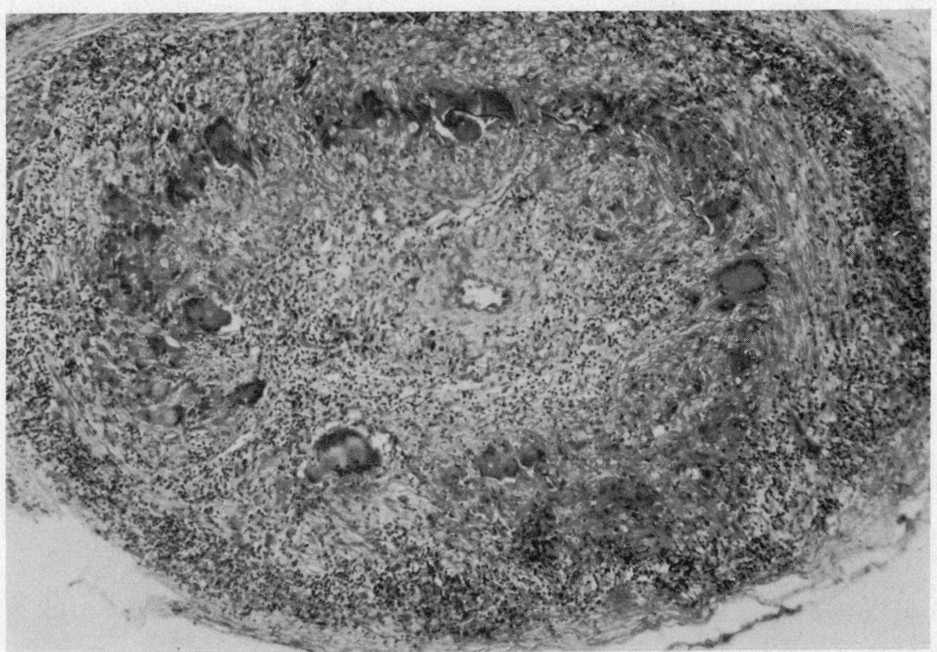

Figure 12–22. Temporal giant cell arteritis. Circumferential giant cells mark location of degenerated internal elastic membrane.

TAKAYASU'S ARTERITIS

A partial list of the descriptive terms by which this rare disorder has been known includes *aortic arch syndrome, pulseless disease, primary aortitis, aortitis syndrome, giant cell arteritis of the aorta, and nonsyphilitic aortitis.* The multiplicity of terms indicates the initial state of confusion about the precise nature of this disorder, and its differentiation from atherosclerotic or syphilitic involvement of the aortic arch. The entity, however, is now firmly established,[89, 90] and named after Takayasu, who in 1908 brought to attention a *clinical syndrome characterized principally by ocular disturbances and marked weakening of the pulses in the upper extremities. He related these findings to fibrous thickening of the aortic arch with narrowing or virtual obliteration of the origins of the great vessels arising in the arch.* A significant number of well-studied cases have since been reported from Japan, Korea, South Africa, Thailand, Sweden, England, and Mexico, with surprisingly few examples from the United States and Canada. The illness is seen predominantly in the 10- to 50-year old age group; children 3 to 4 years old can be affected, and 90% of patients are under the age of 30. There is a striking predilection for females, in the range of 80 to 90%.

ETIOLOGY AND PATHOGENESIS. Early studies called attention to a positive tuberculin test and pulmonary tuberculosis in a large proportion of cases, a finding confirmed in a large series in Mexico.[89] However, neither tubercle bacilli nor other microorganisms have been identified in the lesions. Circulating antiartery antibodies have been identified in some cases, raising the possibility of an immunologic causation, but these antibodies could represent a secondary response to some primary form of arterial injury. Other features suggest a relationship to the connective tissue diseases of presumed immunologic etiology, such as the predilection for younger females, occasional positive tests for the rheumatoid and LE cell factors, and hyperglobulinemia. Genetic factors are suggested by increased incidence of some haplotypes (e.g., HLA-B5) in affected individuals and reports of the disease in monozygotic twins. But at present the disorder is best considered as idiopathic.

MORPHOLOGY. Although Takayasu's arteritis classically involves the aortic arch, in 32% of cases it also affects the remainder of the aorta and its branches, and in 12% it is limited to the descending thoracic and abdominal aorta. The gross morphologic changes comprise, in most cases, irregular thickening of the aortic wall with intimal wrinkling. When the aortic arch is involved, the orifices of the major arteries to the upper portion of the body may be markedly narrowed or even obliterated, accounting for the designation **pulseless disease.** In approximately 50% of cases the pulmonary artery is also affected. Histologically, the early changes consist of an adventitial mononuclear infiltrate with perivascular cuffing of the vasa vasorum, changes similar to those of syphilitic aortitis. However, unlike the luetic lesion, the adventitial changes are accompanied by a diffuse mononuclear infiltration in the media. In some cases, granulomatous changes appear within the media, replete with Langhans' giant cells and central necrosis, producing more than a casual similarity to tuberculosis or giant cell arteritis. Later stages show extensive fibrosis of the media and marked acellular collagenous thickening of the intima. The fibrosing reaction thickens the wall of the aorta and extends into the proximal segments of the aortic branches, reducing their lumina to tiny, slitlike orifices.

CLINICAL COURSE. The salient clinical features include weakening of the pulses of the upper extremities; a marked drop in blood pressure in the upper extremities, often accompanied by elevation in the pressure in the lower extremities (sometimes inappropriately referred to as "reversed coarctation"); ocular disturbances including visual defects, retinal hemorrhages, and total blindness; and various neurologic deficits, ranging from dizziness and focal weaknesses to complete hemiparesis. In two-thirds of these patients, the vascular manifestations are preceded by a long prodrome of nonspecific malaise, low-grade fever, weight loss, polyarthralgia, muscle pains, and nausea lasting for a period of weeks to months. Hypertension is not infrequent and may well be due to involvement of the mouths of the renal arteries. The most common cause of death is heart failure, or it may be termed an unexplained sudden death, the latter probably related to rupture of aortic aneurysms in patients with hypertension. The course of the disease is quite variable, and if the patient survives the first year or two of illness, the fibrotic quiescent stage may ensue and permit long survival, albeit with distressing neurologic and visual impairments.

KAWASAKI'S DISEASE (MUCOCUTANEOUS LYMPH NODE SYNDROME)

This acute illness of young children and infants is manifested by fever, conjunctival and oral erythema and erosions, a skin rash, and enlargement of lymph nodes. In 1 to 2% of patients, death is caused by severe vasculitis involving the coronary arteries.[92] The disease is of epidemic prevalence in Japan, but has also been reported in Hawaii and is being described in increasing numbers in the United States. A viral etiology is suspected, but no definite agent is incriminated (p. 291). Although up to 70% of children may show clinical evidence of cardiac involvement, including coronary aneurysms (shown by angiography), the illness is self-limited in the vast majority of patients. Fatalities are all due to coronary arteritis with superimposed thrombosis or ruptured coronary artery aneurysm. Histologically the vasculitis resembles PAN, consisting of necrosis and pronounced inflammation affecting the entire thickness of the vessel wall.[93] Iliac and other large arteries are involved less frequently.

THROMBOANGIITIS OBLITERANS (BUERGER'S DISEASE)

This is a distinctive disease characterized by segmental, thrombosing, obliterative, acute and chronic inflammation of intermediate and small arteries and veins of the extremities that occurs almost exclusively in men who are heavy cigarette smokers.[94] It must be differentiated from the other more common causes of peripheral vascular disease, such as atherosclerosis, thromboembolism, and diabetic vascular disease.[95] Buerger's disease begins before the age of 35 years in most patients and before 20 years in some. In many it affects the arms as well as the legs. Remission and relapses correlate with cessation or resumption of smoking. Patients experience excruciating pain out of proportion to that found in other forms of peripheral vascular disease.[95] In many it is associated with migratory thrombophlebitis, but it is not associated with diabetes mellitus, hypercholesterolemia, or heart disease that might be the source of emboli.

ETIOLOGY AND PATHOGENESIS. The relationship to cigarette smoking is one of the most consistent aspects of this disease. Most patients are heavy smokers, and most are benefited when they stop smoking. Several possibilities have been postulated for this association. Some tobacco products (carbon monoxide) may be directly toxic to vessels, mainly endothelial cells; cigarette smoking may affect catecholamine metabolism and thus cause vasoconstriction, which predisposes to vascular injury; carbon monoxide may affect oxygen dissociation from the hemoglobin in peripheral tissues and lead to vascular ischemia; and a hypercoagulable state may lead to thrombosis. Of interest is the recent demonstration of cell-mediated immune hypersensitivity to types II and III collagen in these patients,[96] raising the question of immunologic factors in the pathogenesis of this disease.

The disease is rare in the U.S. and Europe, but more common in Israel, Japan, and India. Genetic predisposition is further suggested by the increased prevalence of HLA-A9 and HLA-B5 in patients with Buerger's disease.[97] It may be, then, that exposure of susceptible genotypes to tobacco is the precipitating cause of this disorder, that cellular hypersensitivity to collagen contributes to vascular damage, and that hormonal influences explain the marked predilection for men.

MORPHOLOGY. The lesions are sharply segmental and usually begin in arteries of small and medium size. It should be noted that, in contrast to atherosclerosis, Buerger's disease predominantly affects the medium and small arteries and only occasionally the larger arteries. Both upper and lower extremities are affected, in contrast to AS, which usually spares the upper extremities. After the arterial involvement, the accompanying veins and adjacent nerves are often secondarily affected, leading to progressive fibrous encasement of these three structures.

Only relatively few early lesions have been available for study because most of the pathologic specimens have been obtained from extremities amputated after a long chronic course of the disease. The acute involvements of either artery or vein are characterized by polymorphonuclear infiltration of all coats of the vessel wall, together with mural or occlusive thrombosis of the lumen. **Small microabscesses within the thrombus create a pattern quite distinct from the bland thrombosis of AS** (Fig. 12–23). These abscesses have a central focus of polymorphonuclear leukocytes surrounded by a fibroblastic, epithelioid-cell granulomatous enclosing wall that often contains Langhans'-type giant cells. In time, the thrombus undergoes organization and recanalization, and the small microabscesses are replaced by fibrosing granulomas.

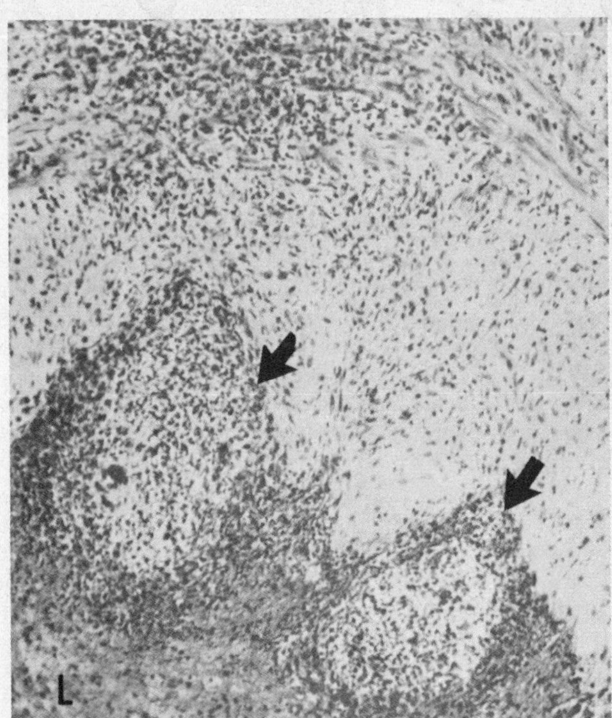

Figure 12–23. Thromboangiitis obliterans. Vessel lumen (L) *(left lower corner)* is occluded by a thrombus containing two abscesses *(arrows)*. Vessel wall *(above)* is infiltrated with leukocytes.

CLINICAL COURSE. The anatomic changes have many etiologic and clinical implications. The impression cannot be escaped that Buerger's disease begins in young males as an inflammatory process within the thrombus rather than within the arterial wall. It is true, of course, that over the years of recurrence of Buerger's disease, AS may develop in such vessels and may make differentiation of Buerger's disease from AS difficult. These patients suffer from vascular insufficiency that often leads to gangrene of the extremities.[97] Severe pain is common in the affected parts, in contrast to the relative painlessness of atherosclerotic occlusion. Abstinence from cigarette smoking is mandatory for these patients.

VASCULITIS ASSOCIATED WITH OTHER UNDERLYING DISORDERS

Vasculitis may sometimes be associated with an underlying disorder, such as an immunologic connective tissue disease, or a remote malignancy, or such systemic illnesses as mixed cryoglobulinemia and Henoch-Schönlein purpura. The vasculitis is usually of the hypersensitivity angiitis pattern (p. 522), but may resemble classic PAN in some cases.

Of the *connective tissue disorders*, rheumatoid arthritis and SLE most commonly manifest a vasculitis. *Rheumatoid vasculitis* affects small and medium-sized arteries in multiple organs and may result in life-threatening visceral infarction. It occurs predominantly after long-standing rheumatoid arthritis in patients who also exhibit rheumatoid nodules, hypocomplementemia, and high titers of rheumatoid factor. Vasculitis in SLE is usually confined to smaller vessels of the skin, although immunoglobulin deposits can be demonstrated in vessels of many organs (see also p. 183). *Malignancies* associated with vasculitis are most commonly of the lymphoproliferative type.

In concluding this discussion of the necrotizing vasculitides, it is obvious that they represent a heterogeneous group of syndromes that have in common, besides the vascular involvement, strong evidence for an immunologic basis. There is a great deal of overlap in morphologic and clinical manifestations among the disorders. Overlapping cases are sometimes referred to simply as "systemic necrotizing vasculitis." It may well be that the differences in specific organs involved, the size of the vessel affected, and the histologic picture reflect the nature of the antigen, the degree and chronicity of antigen exposure, the relative contribution of immune complex– versus cell-mediated mechanisms of injury, and the genetic variability among patients. Nevertheless, proper recognition of some of the subsets of vasculitis is of therapeutic import, as exemplified by the dramatic response of Wegener's granulomatosis to specific therapy with cyclophosphamide. Table 12–4 provides salient features of the major forms of vasculitis.

INFECTIOUS ARTERITIS

Most instances of this condition are caused by the direct invasion of bacteria from a neighboring infection. These lesions are associated with necrotizing inflammation and are frequently encountered in bacterial pneumonia, adjacent to caseous tuberculous reactions, in the neighborhood of abscesses, and in the superficial cerebral vessels in cases of meningitis. Much less commonly, they arise from the hematogenous spread of bacteria, a pathway that presumably accounts for the seeding of the aortic wall in cases of septicemia or infective vegetative endocarditis. The resultant inflammation in this circumstance is specifically designated as infective endaortitis. Such lesions may cause rupture or produce weakening of the aortic walls in the formation of a *mycotic aneurysm*.

The vascular inflammation is completely nonspecific in character, with edema, fibrin precipitation, and leukocytic infiltration in the affected arterial wall. Exudate may layer the endothelial surface and predispose to intravascular thrombosis or even rupture of the artery. The inflammatory involvement usually extends into the perivascular tissues. If the inflammatory reaction is prolonged, fibroblastic scarring may eventually cause narrowing and sometimes total obliteration of the vascular lumen.

Clinically, infectious arteritis may be important on several counts. By inducing thrombosis, it adds an element of infarction to tissues that are already the seat of inflammatory reaction and may therefore materially worsen the initial infection. In bacterial meningitis, for example, inflammation of the superficial vessels of the brain may predispose to vascular thromboses, with subsequent infarction of the brain substance and extension of the subarachnoid infection into the brain tissue. In tuberculous meningitis, it is the vascular involvement that leads to the most serious sequelae. However, although such arterial lesions undoubtedly occur commonly in any type of infectious disease, they usually involve small rather than large arteries and are of little consequence except in the occasional case.

Syphilitic vasculitis may take one of many forms. During the tertiary stage of syphilis, aortitis and aneu-

Table 12–4. CHARACTERISTICS OF SOME SYSTEMIC VASCULITIDES

Angiitides	Vessels Involved	Organ or Tissue Affected	Principal Morphologic Features
Polyarteritis nodosa	Muscular arteries	Gastrointestinal tract, mesentery, liver, gallbladder, kidney, pancreas, lung, muscles, other sites	Lesions of varying ages; all layers of vessels with acute fibrinoid necrosis and extensive periarterial inflammation
Hypersensitivity angiitis	Small venules, capillaries, arterioles	All organs and tissues (skin, muscles, heart, kidneys, lungs)	Acute necrotizing vasculitis with fibrinoid necrosis of entire wall; often thrombosis of lumen
Giant cell arteritis (temporal arteritis)	Muscular arteries	Usually temporal, ophthalmic and cranial arteries; may be systemic	Disruption of elastic lamina with most intense reaction in intimal medial layers; giant cells engulf elastic fiber fragments; occasionally thrombosis of lumen
Wegener's granulomatosis	Small arteries and veins	Lungs, kidneys, upper respiratory tract; occasionally systemic	Acute necrotizing vasculitis with fibrinoid necrosis of vessel wall; often proximate to granulomas in tissues
Buerger's disease	Arteries, veins, nerves	Extremities, viscera uncommonly	Thrombosis with microabscesses; acute inflammation permeates wall artery, but preserves underlying architecture

rysm formation may develop (p. 531). In a much more rare form of aortitis, known as gummatous aortitis, gummas develop within the wall of the aorta, usually in the ascending portion of the arch. Small vessel lesions (*obliterative endarteritis*) may also occur and may develop in any stage of acquired or congenital lues. This vasculitis consists of an *adventitial inflammation, which is classically characterized by lymphocytic and plasma cell perivascular cuffing of the vasa vasorum.* Although spirochetes must be present, they are extremely scant. Syphilitic vasculitis in the small vessels of the meninges may cause serious brain damage.

RAYNAUD'S DISEASE AND RAYNAUD'S PHENOMENON

Raynaud's disease is a *functional vasospastic disorder affecting the small arteries and arterioles of the extremities, occurring primarily in young, apparently healthy women.* It affects the small arteries and arterioles of the extreme periphery of the body (acral parts), most commonly the fingers and hands but occasionally the tip of the nose and the feet. Cold and emotional stimuli trigger the response, and the fingers become white, then blue, and finally red. The disease usually follows a benign course, but in long-standing, chronic cases trophic changes develop causing atrophy of the skin, subcutaneous tissue, and muscles. Ulceration and frank ischemic gangrene are rare. The etiology is unknown but is postulated to be related to some form of hyperlability of the autonomic innervation of the affected vessels. *The symptoms are due to vasoconstriction; thus, true organic changes within the vessel wall are absent.* In long-standing cases, secondary intimal thickening and endothelial proliferation may occur.

It is important to distinguish Raynaud's disease from Raynaud's phenomenon. The latter is also characterized by cold sensitivity pain, and color changes in the skin, but it is *always secondary to some underlying, often serious disorder causing an organic lesion in the arterial wall.* Raynaud's phenomenon is most often associated with arteriosclerosis, connective tissue diseases (scleroderma and SLE being the most common), thromboangiitis obliterans (Buerger's disease), cryoglobulinemia, ingestion of drugs (such as the ergotamine preparations), lead poisoning, occupational and industrial exposure to vibratory tools, primary pulmonary hypertension, and (rarely) cases of occult carcinoma. Raynaud's phenomenon may be the first manifestation of such underlying diseases. Trophic changes, ulcerations, and gangrene may develop.[98]

The relationship of Raynaud's phenomenon to *scleroderma* deserves emphasis. Raynaud's phenomenon may precede the skin changes by months or even years. In some of these patients, Raynaud's phenomenon is associated with sclerosis of the fingers, together with ulceration developing on the digital pulp or along the side of the nail. This condition is called *acrosclerosis*, a form of *localized scleroderma* (p. 193). However, about 20% of these patients eventually develop systemic scleroderma.

AORTIC ANEURYSMS

One of the most striking results of all forms of vascular disease is the formation of an aneurysm.[99] An *aneurysm* is a *localized abnormal dilatation of any vessel.* Aneurysms may occur in any artery or vein of the body, but are most common and most significant in the aorta. Aortic aneurysms produce serious clinical disease and often cause death by rupture.

Aneurysms may be classified by their location, etiology, or gross appearance. According to *location*, an aneurysm should be listed as arterial or venous, indicating the specific vessel affected (e.g., splenic artery or popliteal vein), and, when possible, further localized to the precise site (e.g., the transverse portion of the arch of the aorta, the descending thoracic aorta, or the lower abdominal aorta). With respect to *etiology*, aneurysms may be classified according to, when known, the specific nature of the vascular damage that leads to the aneurysmal dilatation. Virtually any vascular disease discussed here may, under special circumstances, predispose to aneurysmal dilatation of arteries or veins; however, the *three most important causes are arteriosclerosis, syphilis, and cystic medial necrosis,* the last to be described under the heading "dissecting aneurysm." These disorders are responsible for almost all aortic aneurysms. Less commonly, aneurysms of smaller vessels are caused by polyarteritis nodosa; trauma leading to arteriovenous aneurysm; a congenital defect, such as that producing berry aneurysms in the brain; and infections that significantly weaken vascular walls, causing so-called *mycotic aneurysms.*

The classification of aneurysms by *gross appearance* attempts to characterize the macroscopic shape and size of the aneurysmal dilatation. A *berry* aneurysm refers to a small, spherical dilatation rarely exceeding a diameter of 1 to 1.5 cm. A *saccular* aneurysm might be described as a giant berry aneurysm. These dilatations usually are essentially spherical and vary in size up to huge structures 15 to 20 cm in diameter. In their more usual distribution, saccular aneurysms are frequently 5 to 10 cm in diameter. The aneurysmal sac is connected to the vessel lumen by a mouth that varies in size but may have the same diameter as the aneurysmal dilatation. Characteristically, these aneurysms are partially or completely filled by thrombus. Usually the thrombus is laid down in progressive layers and is thus clearly laminated (*lines of Zahn*). In many, the oldest region is adjacent to the vessel wall and the freshest accretion is on the surface. In some cases, the thrombus may be poorly attached to the vessel wall and, by the contraction of the blood clot, may produce a thin, cleftlike space between the clot and the vessel into which fresh blood seeps so that the oldest portion of the thrombus is in contact with the flow of blood.

In *fusiform* aneurysm there is gradual, progressive dilatation of the vessel lumen. These aneurysms then take on a spindle shape, and the aneurysmal lumen is in direct continuity with the vascular lumen. Frequently these fusiform dilatations are eccentric so that one aspect of the wall is more severely affected. The fusiform aneurysm varies in diameter (up to 20 cm) and in length; many involve the entire ascending and transverse portions of the aortic arch, while others may extend over large segments of the abdominal aorta. *Dissecting aneurysm* refers to the condition in which blood enters the wall of the artery, dissecting between its layers and creating a cavity within the vessel wall (p. 532).

On the basis of these classifications, it is possible to characterize an aneurysm fairly specifically as, for example, a congenital berry aneurysm of the anterior cerebral artery or an arteriosclerotic fusiform aneurysm of the lower abdominal aorta.

Attention may now be turned to a more detailed consideration of arteriosclerotic, syphilitic, and dissecting aneurysms of the aorta.

ARTERIOSCLEROTIC (ATHEROSCLEROTIC) ANEURYSMS

With the decreasing incidence of tertiary syphilis, this type of aortic aneurysm has replaced the syphilitic aneurysm as the most common form. Such aneurysms rarely develop before the age of 50 and are much more common in males, in the ratio of 5 to 1. They usually occur in the abdominal aorta or common iliac arteries, but they occasionally affect the ascending arch and descending parts of the thoracic aorta. Luetic aneurysms are extremely infrequent in the abdominal aorta, and *all fusiform, cylindroid, or saccular aneurysms of the abdominal aorta should be considered to be arteriosclerotic until proved otherwise.*

Arteriosclerotic aneurysms are usually positioned below the renal arteries and above the bifurcation of the aorta (Fig. 12–24). Not infrequently, they are accompanied by smaller fusiform or saccular dilatations of the iliac arteries (Fig. 12–25). The genesis of these aneurysms is severe atherosclerosis, with consequent thinning and destruction of the media. With this severe atherosclerosis, it is very common to find atheromatous ulcers within the aneurysm, covered by mural thrombi. Sometimes the entire aneurysmal dilatation is filled with thrombus. Such mural thrombi are prime sites for the formation of emboli that lodge in the vessels of the lower extremity.

Occasionally the aneurysm may affect the take-offs of the renal, superior, and inferior mesenteric arteries, either by producing direct pressure on these vessels or by narrowing or occluding their ostia with mural thrombi. Aneurysms give rise to clinical symptoms by various secondary effects: (1) rupture into the peritoneal cavity or retroperitoneal tissues, with massive or fatal hemorrhage; (2) impingement upon an adjacent structure, such as compression of a ureter or erosion of vertebrae; (3) occlusion of a vessel by either direct pressure or mural thrombus formation, particularly the vertebral branches that supply the spinal cord; (4) embolism from the mural thrombus; and (5) presentation as an abdominal mass that simulates a tumor.

All reports agree that large arteriosclerotic aneurysms materially shorten longevity. Most fatalities result from rupture, a danger directly related to the size of the aneurysm. Patients with aneurysms less than 6 cm in diameter rarely die of rupture, whereas 50% of those with aneurysms 6 or more cm in diameter suffer fatal rupture within a ten-year period of follow-up. On this basis, most workers agree that, when discovered, large aneurysms should be replaced with prosthetic grafts. For abdominal aortic aneurysms, operative mortality for unruptured aneurysms is only 5%, whereas emergency surgery *after* rupture carries a mortality rate of more than 50%.

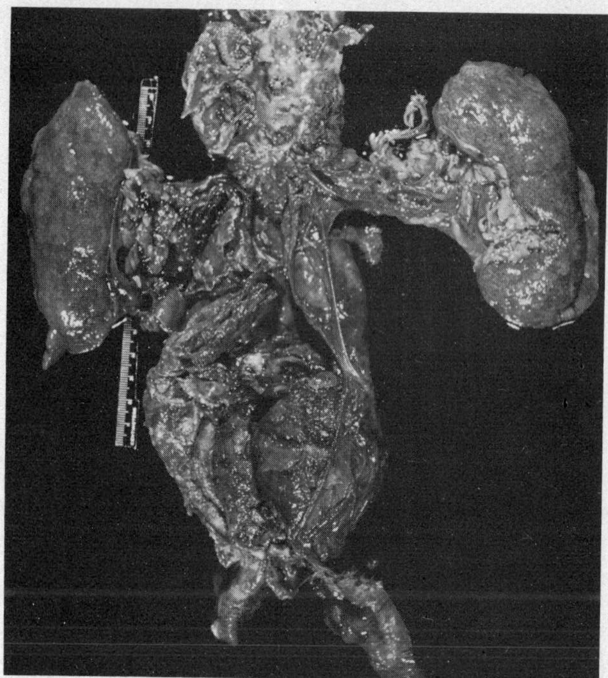

Figure 12–24. Atherosclerotic aneurysm of abdominal aorta situated below renal arteries and above iliac bifurcation. Atherosclerosis throughout aorta is far advanced. Some mural thrombus layers back wall of aneurysm.

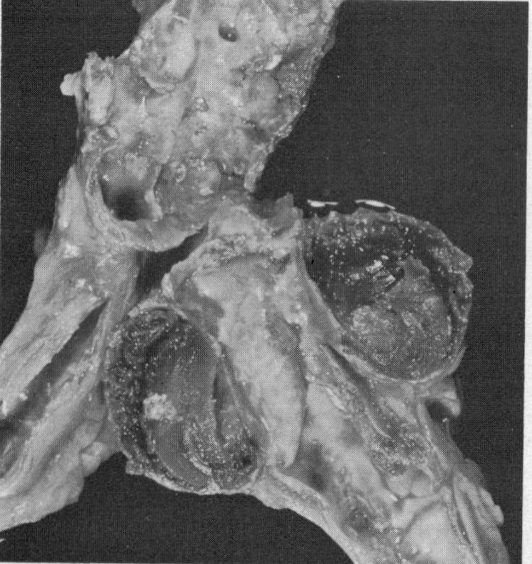

Figure 12–25. Arteriosclerotic saccular aneurysm of common iliac artery filled with laminated thrombus.

SYPHILITIC (LUETIC) ANEURYSMS AND HEART DISEASE

Syphilitic (luetic) aneurysms are almost always confined to the thoracic aorta and usually involve the arch. The ascending and transverse portions of the arch are favored sites, but the dilatation may extend distally to the level of the diaphragm and, even more important, proximally to the level of the aortic valve. By virtue of dilatation of the ring, the aortic valve may become incompetent, leading to luetic heart disease. At one time, lues accounted for the majority of aneurysms of the thoracic aorta, but with the decline in cases of tertiary lues, atherosclerosis and cystic medial necrosis now predominate. Unhappily, the increased incidence of syphilis in the past two decades may result in a resurgence of cases in the future. As discussed on page 337, cardiovascular involvement appears during the tertiary stage of syphilis.

Syphilitic aneurysms vary in gross appearance to encompass the saccular, fusiform, and cylindroid types (Fig. 12–26.) Many times the aneurysmal masses achieve a diameter of 15 to 20 cm or even larger. Their development is based on the medial destruction characteristic of tertiary luetic aortitis. The inflammatory involvement begins in the adventitia of the aorta, particularly involving the vasa vasorum with the production of obliterative endarteritis rimmed by an infiltrate of lymphocytes and plasma cells. The narrowing of the lumina of the vasa causes ischemic injury to the aortic media, with patchy uneven loss of the medial elastic fibers and muscle cells followed by inflammatory scarring and vascularization of the damaged media (Fig. 12–27). The focal areas of scarring may appear as subintimal or intimal pearly-gray plaques that tend to encircle the mouths of exiting small aortic branches, e.g., the coronaries and intercostals. Contraction of fibrous scars may lead to wrinkling of intervening segments of aortic intima, producing what has been called "tree-barking." Luetic involvement of the aorta favors the development of superimposed atherosclerosis, inducing sometimes florid atheromatosis of the aortic root (rarely seen in the absence of luetic aortitis).

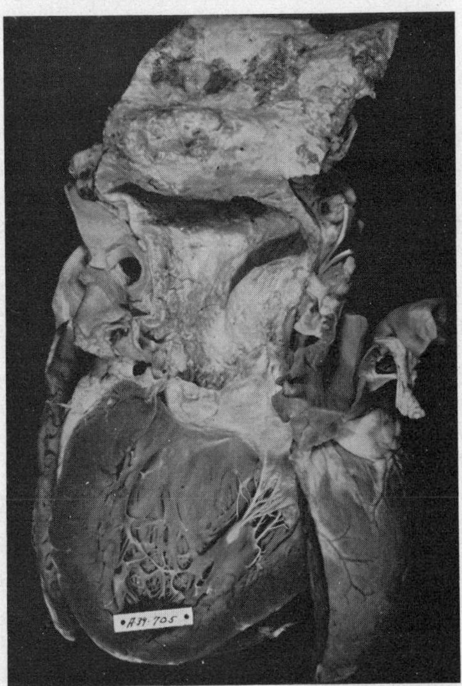

Figure 12–26. Advanced atherosclerosis superimposed on luetic aortitis. The ascending arch is widened and thrown into irregular folds by aneurysm dilatation.

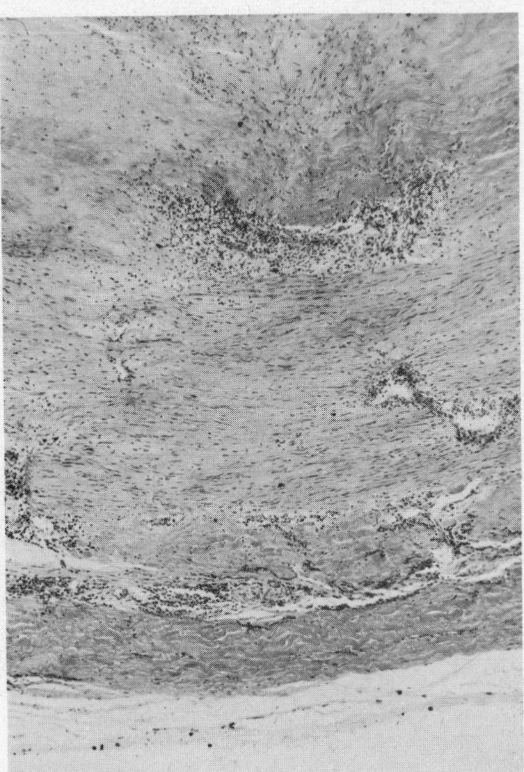

Figure 12–27. Luetic aortitis with scarring and vascularization of media.

When luetic aortitis involves the aortic valve ring, it dilates, causing valvular insufficiency. The circumferential stretching of the valve leaflets narrows them and widens the interleaflet commissures. Over the course of time, the regurgitant turbulence produces thickening and rolling of the free margins, worsening the valvular incompetence (Fig. 12–28). As a consequence, the left ventricular wall undergoes volume overload hypertrophy, sometimes producing a massively enlarged heart (600 to 1000 gm), descriptively referred to as "cor bovinum."

There are many potential sequelae to syphilitic aortitis and heart disease. The expansile pulsating aneurysms may cause erosion of ribs and vertebral bodies. Involvement of the aortic valve may lead to congestive heart failure. Death may be caused by sudden rupture of the aneurysm into the pericardial sac, pleural cavities, bronchi, trachea, or esophagus, or may be due to cardiac failure.

Thoracic aneurysms are much more prone to be associated with striking clinical manifestations than are the arteriosclerotic abdominal aneurysms. Within the confined space of the thoracic cage, these enlargements give rise to signs and symptoms referable to (1) encroachment on mediastinal structures, (2) respiratory difficulties due to encroachment on the lungs and air-

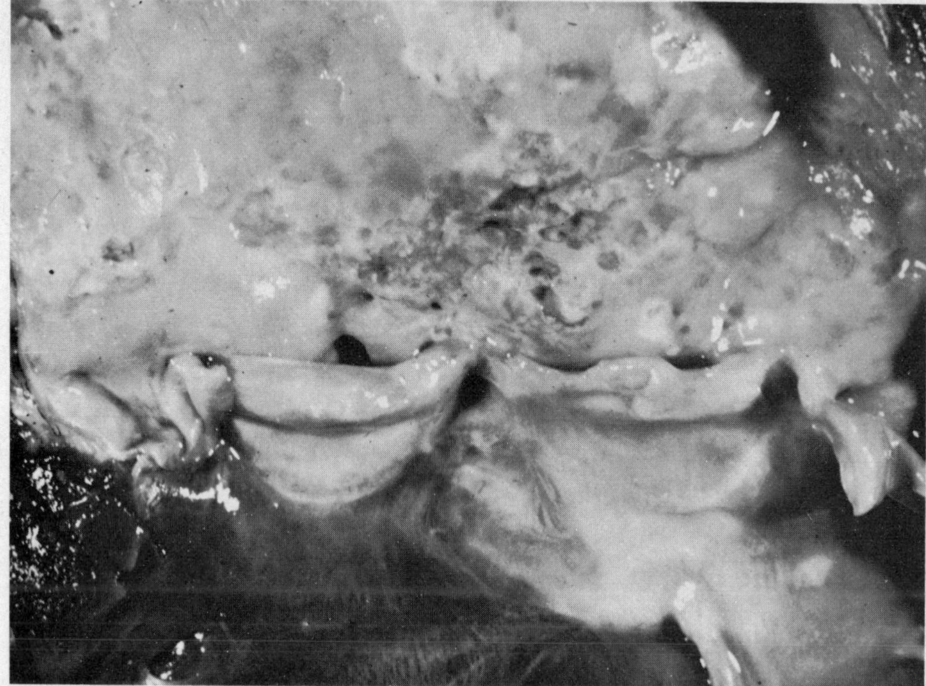

Figure 12–28. Luetic involvement of aorta and aortic valve. Opaque white plaques in aorta are intimal scars. Valve leaflets are rolled and thickened.

ways, (3) difficulty in swallowing due to compression of the esophagus, (4) persistent cough due to irritation of or pressure on the recurrent laryngeal nerves, (5) pain caused by erosion of bone (i.e., ribs and vertebral bodies), and (6) cardiac disease as the aneurysm leads to dilatation of the aortic valve or narrowing of the coronary ostia. Many patients with luetic aneurysms die of cardiac decompensation secondary to the luetic involvement of the aortic valve, unless the incompetent valve is surgically replaced.

DISSECTING ANEURYSMS (AORTIC DISSECTION OR DISSECTING HEMATOMA)

Once thought to be rare, dissecting aneurysm is now considered to be the most common catastrophic illness involving the aorta, being two or three times more frequent than ruptured abdominal aortic aneurysm.[99A] At least 2000 new cases per year are reported in the United States, but the condition is often unrecognized, so that the true prevalence must be substantially higher.[100] It is a dramatic illness in which, if untreated, the risk of death is 35% within 15 minutes after onset of symptoms and 75% by one week. Happily, these figures have improved considerably with early recognition and treatment.

As the name implies, these aneurysms are characterized by dissection of blood along the laminar planes of the aortic media, with the formation of a blood-filled channel within the aortic wall.[100A] *They differ from the luetic and atherosclerotic aneurysms in that they are not usually associated with marked dilatation of the aorta.* For this reason, the terms "aortic dissection" or "dissecting hematoma" are preferable. The condition most commonly occurs in the 40- to 60-year age group and is two or three times more frequent in men within this group. However, below age 40 the male/female distribution is equal, owing principally to the occurrence of dissections in women during pregnancy. Hypertension is almost invariably an antecedent (in 94% of cases) and may well play an important role in initiating the intramural hemorrhage.

The hemorrhage in dissecting hematomas occurs quite characteristically between the middle and outer thirds of the media (Fig. 12–29). The intimal tear, presumably the origin of dissection, is found in the ascending portion of the arch in 90% of cases, usually within 10 cm of the aortic valve. The tears are usually transverse or oblique, 4 to 5 cm in length, and have sharp and clean but jagged edges (Fig. 12–30). The dissection then extends proximally toward the heart, as well as distally along the aorta to variable distances, sometimes all the way into the iliac and femoral arteries (Fig. 12–31). In some instances, the blood reruptures into the lumen of the aorta, producing a **second or distal intimal tear.** The site of such reentry is most often the iliac vessels, followed by neck vessels. **Five to 10% of dissecting aneurysms, however, do not have an obvious intimal tear,** either proximally or distally.

Many times the dissection extends into the great vessels of the neck and, in other instances, into the coronary, renal, mesenteric, and iliac arteries (Fig. 12–32). The extravasation may completely encircle the aorta or may extend along one segment of the circumference. Infrequently the dissection is very short, and the extravasation almost directly penetrates the entire thickness of the aorta to cause immediate rupture.

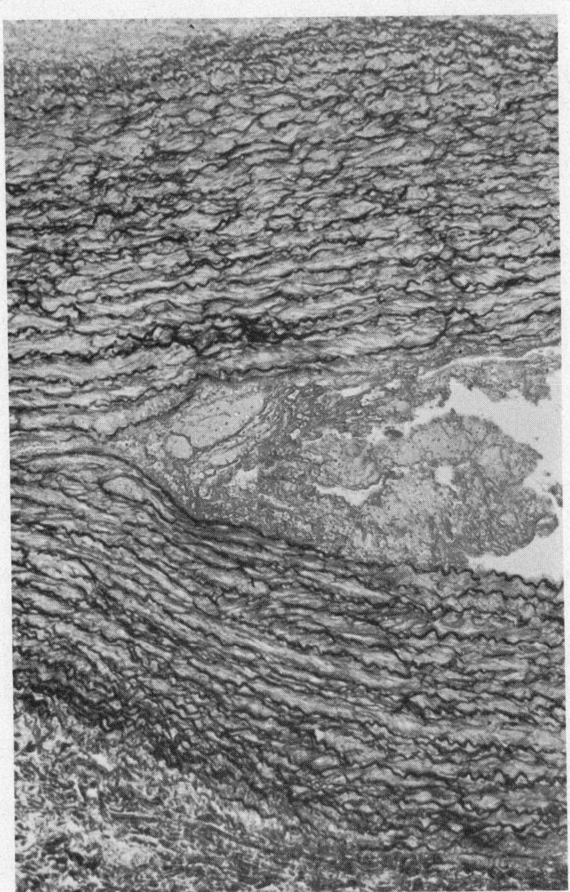

Figure 12–29. Dissecting aneurysm of aorta. The advancing dissection is cleaving laminar planes of media.

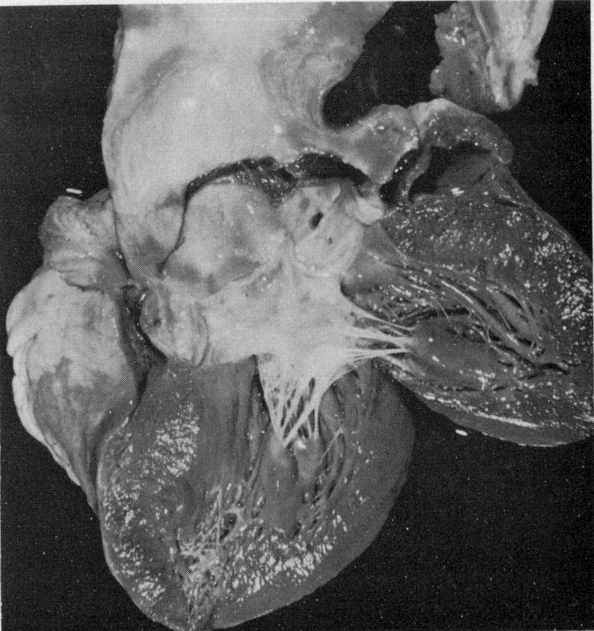

Figure 12–30. Irregular, jagged transverse tear in intima in a dissecting aneurysm.

Eventually, **in almost all fatal dissections, external hemorrhage occurs into the periadventitial tissues or into surrounding structures or cavities.**

At postmortem examination, the most common precipitating cause of death is rupture of the dissection into any of the three body cavities, i.e., pericardial, pleural, or peritoneal. Quite rarely, cases are discovered in which a new vascular channel has apparently been formed within the media of the aortic wall that connects the proximal and distal intimal tear. It is assumed that in these **double-barreled aortas,** the two intimal tears have permitted the establishment of a through-and-through blood flow and thus averted a fatal extra-aortic hemorrhage. In the course of time, such false channels may become endothelialized, and such favored and unusual patients may die of completely unrelated causes.

DeBakey and associates[101] initially divided these aneurysms into three types, on the basis of the extent of dissection, but most workers now use a two-type classification (Fig. 12–31); (1) *Type A or proximal dissections* involve the ascending aorta or the ascending and descending aorta (Types I and II of DeBakey's classification) and are the most common and lethal type; (2) *Type B or distal dissections* do *not* involve the ascending aorta and usually begin just distal to the subclavian artery, extending only downward into the descending and abdominal aorta.

Pathogenesis. Two questions arise concerning the pathogenesis of dissecting aneurysms. First, what causes the media of the aorta to weaken, allowing blood to dissect into the wall; second, what causes the hemorrhage and intimal tears?[99A, 100]

In most patients with dissecting aneurysm, the media shows a variety of histologic changes that could

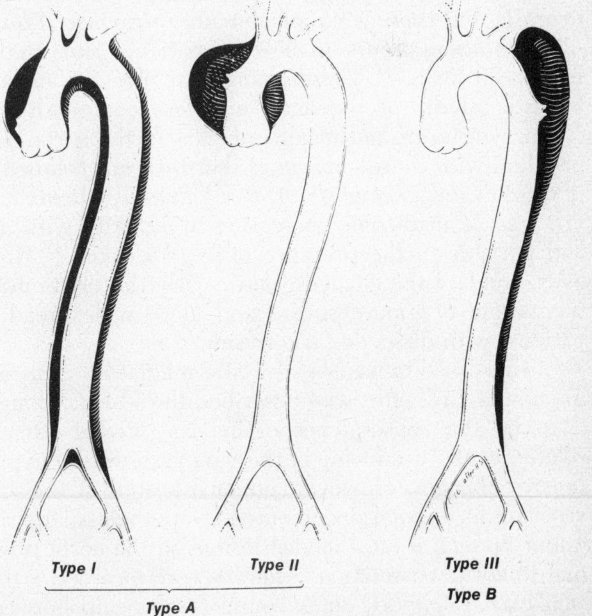

Figure 12–31. DeBakey classification of dissections into Types I, II, and III, respectively, from left to right. In the newer classification, Types I and II are combined into Type A (involving ascending aorta) and Type III is designated Type B *not* involving ascending aorta. (From Anagnostopoulos, C. E.: Acute Aortic Dissections. Baltimore, University Park Press, 1975.)

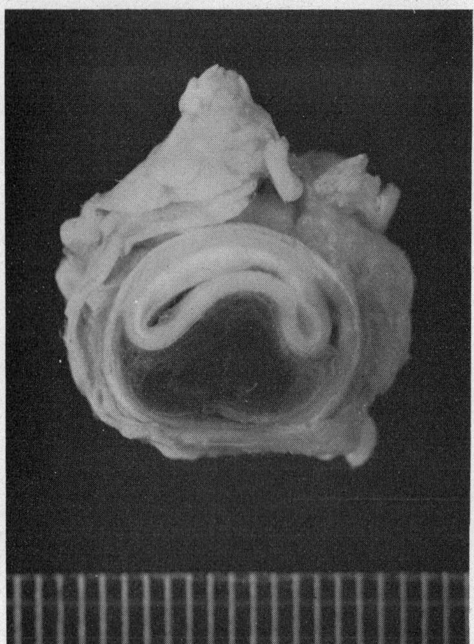

Figure 12–32. Cross section of common carotid with extension of a dissecting aneurysm and collapse of vessel lumen.

conceivably weaken the wall, but controversy exists about the specificity of these lesions and their role in causing dissection.[102] The most widely known lesion is so-called *cystic medial necrosis or Erdheim's mucoid degeneration,* which consists of the accumulation of basophilic amorphous material in the media, often with formation of cystlike mucoid pools. The media in these focal areas may show loss of cells, hence the term necrosis, but there is no inflammatory response. *Elastic fragmentation* occurs in 95% of patients and medial fibrosis in 60%.[102A] These changes involve the musculoelastic media of the aorta and less commonly the coronary arteries and major branches of the aorta. The problem with these changes is that *they are frequently present as a chance postmortem finding in patients who are free of dissection,* increasing in severity with age and possibly in the presence of hypertension.[103] However, some of the changes, particularly the elastic fragmentation, are more severe and more widespread in patients with dissecting aneurysm.

The cause or causes of cystic medial necrosis are unknown. Erdheim, who described the lesion, thought it to be the consequence of hypoxic medial damage related to the narrowing of the vasa vasorum by hypertensive changes. However, no such lesions in the vasa vasorum have been documented. Nonetheless, the frequent finding of focal medial lesions in the aorta proximal to aortic coarctation, where severe local hypertension exists, supports some causal relationship between hypertension and the development of lesions. Other explanations propose biochemical defects in the synthesis or maintenance of the proteoglycans, collagen, and elastic fibers of the tunica media. *The relatively high incidence of cystic change and dissecting aneurysm in patients with the hereditary disorder Marfan's syndrome* supports such notions. As described earlier (p. 137), these patients have a defect in chemically stable collagen cross-links,[104] structural defects involving the suspensory ligaments of the lens and the capsules of joints, excessive height, retinal detachment, and aortic regurgitation. The biochemical defect might also be due to exogenous influences. Foods rich in beta-aminopropionitriles derange the normal synthesis of collagen in the laboratory animal, and lead to the experimental syndrome known as *lathyrism.* These compounds act by inhibiting lysyl oxidase, one of the enzymes responsible for cross-linkages that form the basis of the structural stability of collagen. Rats fed on a sweet pea meal rich in propionitriles often develop a variety of structural defects including medial necrosis, and sometimes die of dissecting aneurysms. Turkeys also acquire medial necrosis when treated with estrogens, and it is of interest that dissecting aneurysms are more common in women during pregnancy. Experimental copper deficiency also leads to medial necrosis, and patients with Wilson's disease (a metabolic disorder characterized by an excess accumulation of copper) treated with a copper-chelating agent such as penicillamine sometimes develop medial necrosis.

Granted that ischemic, biochemical, or hydrodynamic factors could possibly weaken the vessel wall, what causes the intramural aortic hemorrhage? It was once thought that the initial hemorrhage occurred in the media, from the vasa vasorum, but this seems unlikely on morphologic and physiologic grounds.[100] *Favored today is the hypothesis that an intimal tear occurs owing to hemodynamic factors accentuated by the hypertension.* The intima overlying areas weakened by the medial degeneration *buckles into the lumen,* with the oncoming pressure wave creating a tendency for the buckled wall to be subjected to greater shearing force, thus inducing a luminal tear. Once the tear has occurred, the increased blood pressure present in most of these patients enhances dissection into the wall. Indeed, as discussed later, aggressive antihypertensive therapy is often effective in limiting dissection.

MORPHOLOGY. The gross morphology was described earlier. The characteristic microscopic lesion of **cystic medial necrosis** is that of focal separation of the elastic and fibromuscular elements of the tunica media by small cleftlike or cystic spaces filled with ground substance. In the individual foci, the normal lamellar pattern of the elastic media is destroyed and is replaced by a poorly defined area of increased, slightly basophilic, amorphous material resembling the ground substance of connective tissue (Fig. 12–33). These foci are referred to as cystic, but there are no well-defined enclosing walls or sharp delineations. The lesions are haphazardly distributed throughout the thickness of the media. Elastic tissue stains are desirable to highlight focal areas of apparent destruction or separation of the normal lamellae of the medial wall. In addition to the mucoid cystic change, fragmentation of elastic tissue lamellae is frequently present, even outside areas of well-defined mucoid change. **Indeed, the severity of elastic fragmentation correlates more consistently with the presence of dis-**

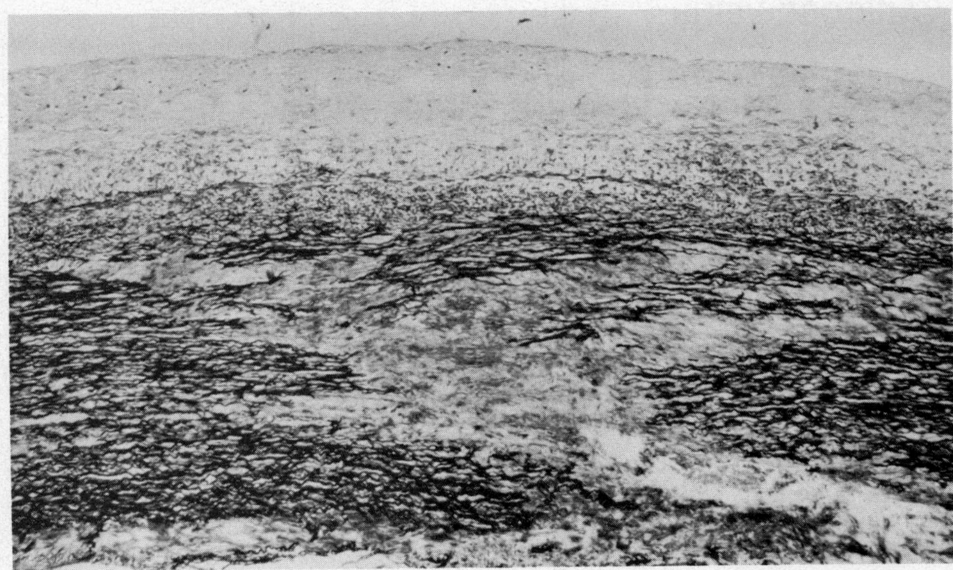

Figure 12–33. Cystic medial necrosis. Large defect in elastic lamellar pattern of media is highlighted by elastic tissue stain.

section than do the mucoid alterations. Focal fibrosis of the media is a third type of histologic change, the significance of which is not well understood.

The clinical manifestations of a dissecting aneurysm derive from (1) the dissection itself and (2) problems consequent upon occlusion of the arteries arising from the aorta. The classic features related to the dissection are the sudden onset of excruciating pain, usually beginning in the anterior chest, radiating to the back, and moving downward as the dissection progresses. The intensity of this pain is readily confused with that of acute myocardial infarction. Helpful in this differentiation is the fact that, although patients with acute dissection may appear to be in shock, they generally have normal or elevated systemic arterial pressures in counterdistinction to the hypotension usually associated with myocardial infarction. About 15% of patients have no pain and present with sudden onset of congestive heart failure associated with aortic valvular incompetence resulting from aneurysmal dilatation of the aortic valve ring. Such a presentation is characteristic of Type A. Unequal pulses and blood pressure between right and left extremities, neurologic manifestations, and renal failure reflect involvement of the origins of aortic branches.

The antemortem diagnosis of dissecting aneurysm and the differentiation of the types are based largely on aortic angiography. In some centers, premortem diagnosis is now possible in close to 90% of cases.[105]

At one time, the disease was almost invariably fatal, but the prognosis has markedly improved in recent years. Two major advances in treatment have been achieved: *the development of surgical procedures involving plication of the aortic wall, and the early institution of intensive antihypertensive therapy.*[99, 105] At present, immediate surgery is advocated in nearly all Type A dissections, while hypotensive therapy is reserved for noncomplicated Type B dissections and as an adjunct to surgery. Understandably, the prognosis of Type A dissections is much worse. Nevertheless, with these regimens, early recognition and treatment permit salvage of 65 to 75% of all dissections for two to four years, a remarkable achievement compared with the 5% one-year survival attained 20 years ago.

VEINS

Although diseases of veins are extremely common clinical problems, comparatively few entities are responsible for this high incidence. Varicose veins and phlebothrombosis together account for at least 90% of clinical venous disease. In general, the diseases of veins are clinically significant on two accounts. First, most of these disorders predispose to intravascular thrombosis and potential embolism, and since the systemic veins are most often affected, pulmonary embolism and infarction are the potential serious sequelae. Second, intravascular thrombosis, narrowing, or abnormal dilatation of veins with subsequent incompetence of the venous valves all cause venous stasis. A fairly constant clinical pattern follows with passive congestion of the affected area accompanied often by dusky cyanosis and edema. In many cases, venous drainage is restored by the opening of collateral bypasses. Often, however, the collateral channels create new clinical problems, well exemplified by the production of varices in the esophagus when the portal vein is obstructed. The possibility of rupture of the esophageal varices is of far greater clinical importance than the underlying cause of the portal vein obstruction. On these two scores, diseases of veins take on great clinical significance.

VARICOSE VEINS

Varicose veins are abnormally dilated, tortuous veins produced by prolonged, increased intraluminal pressure. Although any vein in the body may be affected, the superficial veins of the leg are the preponderant site of involvement. One special type of varicosity is an important clinical problem; portal hypertension (usually due to cirrhosis of the liver) leads to varices in the esophageal and hemorrhoidal veins (p. 917).

INCIDENCE. It is estimated that 10 to 20% of the general population eventually develop varicose veins in the lower legs. It is much more common in the age groups over 50, in which the incidence may reach a figure of 50%. Over the age of 30, females are affected four times more commonly than males, a reflection of the venous stasis in the lower legs caused by pregnancy. In younger individuals there is no striking sex preponderance.

PATHOGENESIS. Veins are frail structures that depend for their integrity on a thin media and the support of surrounding structures. A *familial tendency* toward the development of varicosities is postulated to be due to defective development of the walls of veins. *Obese* persons have a greater tendency to develop varicosities, probably because of the poor tissue support offered by the large accumulations of subcutaneous fat. The increase in the incidence of varicose veins with *age* is at least in part attributable to the loss of tissue tone, atrophy of muscles, and senile degenerative changes within the wall of the veins.

The most important influence on intraluminal venous blood pressure is posture. When the legs are dependent for long periods of time, venous pressures in these sites are markedly elevated (the increase has been measured to be ten times the normal). Therefore, occupations that require long periods of standing and long rides frequently lead to marked venous stasis and pedal edema, even in normal individuals with essentially normal veins (*simple orthostatic edema*). Any condition that compresses or obstructs veins may cause marked increases of venous pressure distally, so that pregnancy, intravascular thrombosis, and tumor masses that compress or narrow veins all promote the development of varicosities.

Varicose veins occur principally in the superficial veins of the body, especially those of the lower extremities. The lower extremities are most commonly affected because, in the erect position, these vessels are subject to the greatest increases of pressure. The affected veins are dilated, tortuous, and elongated. There is marked variation in the thickness of the wall, with thinning at the points of maximal dilatation. When the disease is long-standing, compensatory hypertrophy of the medial muscle and fibrosis of the wall may produce a thick, opaque vessel wall.

Intraluminal thrombosis and valvular deformities (thickening, rolling, and shortening of the cusps) are frequently discovered when these vessels are opened. These valvular changes contribute materially to venous stasis and further the development of varicosities and edema. Microscopically, the changes consist of variation in the thickness of the wall of the vein caused by dilatation on the one hand, and by hypertrophy of the smooth muscle and subintimal fibrosis on the other hand. Frequently, there is degeneration of the elastic tissue in the major veins and spotty calcifications within the media **(phlebosclerosis).**

CLINICAL COURSE. Varicose dilatation of veins renders the valves incompetent and leads to venous stasis, congestion, edema, and thrombosis. In the legs the distention of the veins is often painful, but most patients have no symptoms until marked venous stasis and edema develop. *Some of the most disabling sequelae are the development of persistent edema in the extremity and trophic changes in the skin that lead to stasis dermatitis and ulcerations* (Fig. 12–34). Because of the impaired circulation, the tissues of the affected part are extremely vulnerable to injury. Wounds and infections heal slowly or tend to become chronic *varicose ulcers. Although varicose veins frequently thrombose, embolization to the lungs from these superficial small vessels is uncommon.*

PHLEBOTHROMBOSIS AND THROMBOPHLEBITIS

According to current thought, phlebothrombosis and thrombophlebitis are two designations for a single entity caused by thrombus formation in veins. Thrombosis within a vein inevitably leads to inflammatory changes within the vein wall, hence the synonym thrombophlebitis.

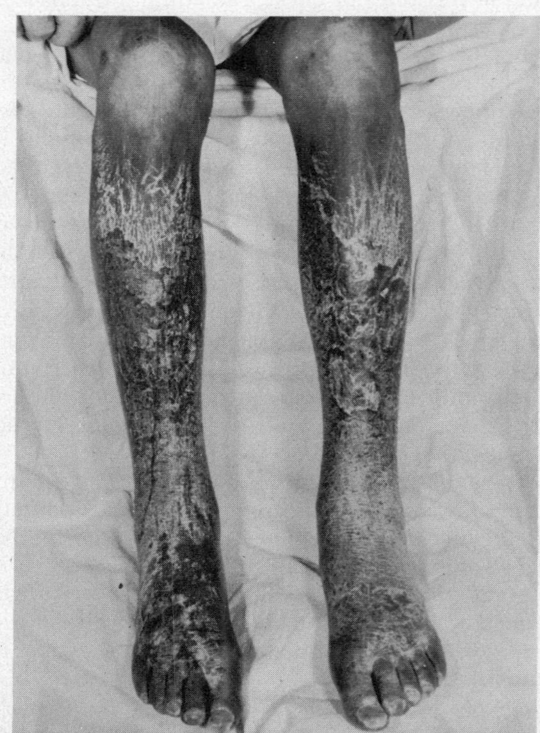

Figure 12–34. Stasis dermatitis in varicose veins of lower extremity.

The factors that predispose to venous thrombosis and the settings in which it is most often encountered have already been considered in the general discussion of thrombosis (p. 91). It need simply be reemphasized now that *cardiac failure* (particularly that associated with slowed venous return), *neoplasia, pregnancy, the postoperative state, and prolonged bed rest or immobilization are the five most important clinical settings predisposing to venous thrombosis.* The role of contraceptive pills in thrombosis was discussed earlier (p. 447). Phlebothrombosis is also commonly encountered in superficial varicose veins of the lower extremity. Such lesions are painful and sometimes somewhat disabling, but do not have the significance of thromboses within the deep veins, since they rarely are the origin of emboli.

The deep leg veins account for over 90% of cases of thrombophlebitis. Specific mention should be made of the periprostatic plexus in the male and the pelvic veins in the female as additional moderately common sites for the appearance of thrombi. The large veins in the skull and the dural sinuses are possible sites of thrombosis when these channels become inflamed by bacterial infections of the meninges, middle ears, or mastoids. Inflammatory diseases in these locations are in close physical and vascular continuity with the dural sinuses and provide ready pathways for the spread of infection. Similarly, infections in the abdominal cavity, such as peritonitis, acute appendicitis, acute salpingitis, and pelvic abscesses, may lead to inflammation and thrombosis of the portal vein or its tributaries.

CLINICAL COURSE. Thrombi in the legs tend, on the whole, to arise insidiously and to produce in the early stages few, if any, signs or symptoms. The local manifestations consist of edema distal to the occluded vein, dusky cyanosis, and dilatation of superficial veins. Sometimes local heat, tenderness, redness, swelling, and pain occur. However, even these signs may be absent, for when the patient is bedridden and the leg remains elevated, edema and congestion may be minimal or totally absent. Usually, however, in overt cases pain can be elicited by pressure over affected veins. In involvement of the lower extremities, squeezing the calf muscles or forced dorsiflexion of the foot evokes discomfort or pain. Because of the insidiousness of such vascular disease, it is necessary to examine vulnerable bedridden patients daily for any indications of venous occlusion. There are now several noninvasive methods (^{125}I-labeled fibrinogen; ultrasound; plethysmography) that aid in the diagnosis, but venous angiography may have to be performed in some cases to establish the presence of deep vein thrombosis.

Not infrequently, the first manifestation of thrombophlebitis is the development of an embolic episode. Indeed, pulmonary embolism is one of the most common clinical problems, particularly in hospitalized patients. At least 50,000 deaths annually in the United States can be attributed to pulmonary embolism.[106]

The gravity of the possible consequence of phlebothrombosis strongly influences the management of all cardiac, postpartal, and postoperative cases. All such patients are urged to move about constantly in bed, perform muscle exercises to stimulate the venous flow in the legs, and become ambulatory as soon as is clinically feasible. In particularly vulnerable individuals, such as those with varicose veins and in the older age groups, anticoagulant therapy may be administered when long-term bed rest is mandatory.

Bacterial infection of a thrombus may be a source of bacteremia and septic emboli. In the dural sinuses, such intravascular infections may spread to cause meningitis or abscess formations in the contiguous regions of the brain. Phlebitis of the portal veins may seed the liver with bacteria and produce multiple liver abscesses.

PHLEGMASIA ALBA DOLENS AND MIGRATORY PHLEBITIS

There are two special variants of primary phlebothrombosis, both of obscure nature. One is known as phlegmasia alba dolens and the other as migratory phlebitis. *Phlegmasia alba dolens* (painful white leg) refers to iliofemoral venous thrombosis occurring usually in pregnant women in the third trimester or immediately following delivery. Because of its association with pregnancy, this condition has also been called *"milk leg."* Classically, marked painful swelling of the lower extremity results, but experimental evidence suggests that venous stasis alone does not produce such severe edema. It is postulated that the thrombus initiates a secondary phlebitis, and the perivenous inflammatory response induces lymphatic blockage also. The predisposition to thrombosis here is attributed to the stasis of flow caused by the pressure of the gravid uterus and to the development of a hypercoagulable state during pregnancy.

Migratory thrombophlebitis is a term given to the appearance of venous thrombi, often multiple, which classically disappear at one site only to reappear elsewhere. This curious disorder is usually encountered in patients having a deep-seated visceral cancer. This association was brought to the attention of the medical world by Trousseau, who ironically developed migratory phlebitis himself as the first manifestation of his fatal pancreatic cancer. With considerable justice, then, migratory thrombophlebitis in patients having cancer is referred to as *Trousseau's sign.* It may be encountered with cancer of any viscus in the body, for example, in the pancreas, lung, stomach, colon, or kidney. The basis of this predisposition to thrombosis has been discussed earlier (p. 98).

LYMPHATICS

Because of their widespread distribution and important role as drainage channels, involvement of the lymphatics is almost inevitable in all inflammations and whenever tumors metastasize through these vessels. In most of these instances, the lymphatic lesions are so small and focal as to have no significance. However, in some cases these secondary lesions represent serious complications that sometimes overshadow the primary disease.

LYMPHANGITIS

Bacterial infections may spread into and through the lymphatics to create acute inflammatory involvements in these channels. The most common etiologic agents are the group A beta-hemolytic streptococci, although any virulent pathogen may be responsible for an acute lymphangitis. Anatomically, the affected lymphatics are dilated and filled with an acute leukocytic exudate, chiefly neutrophils and histiocytes. The inflammation usually extends through the wall into the perilymphatic tissues. Sometimes the surrounding reaction is so extensive as to convert the process into a cellulitis or into multiple focal abscesses. The lymph nodes of drainage are almost inevitably involved, with changes characteristic of acute lymphadenitis.

Clinically, lymphangitis is recognized by painful subcutaneous red streaks that extend along the course of lymphatics, with painful enlargement of the regional lymph nodes. If the lymph nodes fail to block the spread of the bacteria, the infective material may eventually drain into the venous system and initiate a bacteremia or septicemia.

LYMPHEDEMA

Any occlusion of lymphatic vessels is followed by the abnormal accumulation of interstitial fluid in the affected part, referred to as *obstructive lymphedema.* The most common causes of such lymphatic blockage are (1) spread of malignant tumors with obstruction of either the lymphatic channels or the nodes of drainage; (2) radical surgical procedures with removal of regional groups of lymph nodes, e.g., the axillary dissection of radical mastectomy; (3) postradiation fibrosis; (4) filariasis; and (5) postinflammatory thrombosis and scarring of lymphatic channels. The morphologic changes within the lymphatics consist of dilatation proximal to the points of obstruction, accompanied by increases of interstitial fluid. Persistence of the edema leads to an increase of interstitial fibrous tissue, most evident subcutaneously. Enlargement of the affected part, "peau d'orange" appearance of the skin, skin ulcers, and brawny induration are sequelae to such lymphedema. *Chylous ascites, chylothorax,* and *chylopericardium* are caused by rupture of obstructed dilated lymphatics into the peritoneum, pleural cavity, and pericardium. Almost invariably, this is due to obstruction of lymphatics by an infiltrating tumor mass.

Other rare types of lymphedema not secondary to any known obstructive disorder also occur, including those discussed below.

Lymphedema Praecox. This is an extremely uncommon condition affecting chiefly females between the ages of 10 and 25, characterized by the progressive onset of edema in one or both feet. The edema may remain localized to the feet or ankles or, with increasing severity of the condition, progress up the extremity into the lower trunk or other regions of the body. The edema is unremitting and slowly accumulates throughout life. The etiology is entirely obscure. The involved extremity may increase to many times its normal size, and the skin may become thickened and resemble orange peel. In some cases, ulcerations develop in the affected skin areas.

Milroy's Disease. Milroy's disease resembles lymphedema praecox but is present from birth and is inherited as a mendelian trait. The condition is presumed to be caused by faulty development of lymphatic channels, possibly with poor structural strength, permitting abnormal dilatation and incompetence of the lymphatic valves. In classic Milroy's disease, the lower extremities are the major, and frequently the only, site of involvement.

Simple Congenital Lymphedema. This disorder is distinguished from Milroy's disease by the fact that it affects only one member of the family, but it is present from birth. The anatomic distribution, histologic findings, and clinical significance are identical to those of Milroy's disease.

TUMORS

Neoplasms of blood vessels present complexities in classification and significance. Most of these center on three points: (1) Are small vascular lesions, so commonly found in infants at birth, true tumors or merely anomalous hamartomas? As many as 70% of benign, focal, well-differentiated vascular lesions—hemangiomas and lymphangiomas—are present from birth (p. 496). Some grow rapidly and regress, others grow slowly and commensurately with the growth of the child. Are these true neoplasms or merely congenital anomalies? (2) How does one differentiate tumorous vascular proliferation from non-neoplastic vasoproliferations such as are encountered in inflammatory states? Recall that granulation tissue consists in part of actively budding, growing capillaries. Sometimes this vascularization is so abundant that it may be difficult to differentiate tumor from inflammation. Such is the case with the entity designated as *granuloma pyogenicum,* which resembles both exuberant overgrowth of granulation tissue and capillary hemangioma. (3) How can vascular-derived tumors be recognized when the tumors are too undifferentiated to form vascular channels?

Vascular neoplasms are divided into benign and malignant on the basis of two major anatomic characteristics: (1) the degree to which the neoplasm is composed of well-formed vascular channels and (2) the

Table 12–5. TUMORS AND TUMOR-LIKE CONDITIONS OF BLOOD VESSELS

1. Benign
   - Hemangioma
     - Capillary
     - Cavernous
     - Epithelioid
     - Granuloma pyogenicum
     - Deep soft tissue hemangiomas
   - Glomus tumor
   - Vascular ectasias
2. Intermediate
   - Hemangioendothelioma
   - Epithelioid hemangioendothelioma
3. Malignant
   - Angiosarcoma
   - Hemangiopericytoma
   - Kaposi's sarcoma

abundance and regularity of the endothelial cell proliferation. In general, benign neoplasms are made up largely of well-formed vessels with a significant amount of regular endothelial cell proliferation, while on the opposite end of the spectrum, the frankly malignant tumors are solidly cellular and anaplastic and reproduce scant numbers of only abortive vascular channels. The endothelial nature of neoplastic proliferations that do not form distinct vascular lumina can sometimes be uncovered by finding the endothelial specific Weibel-Palade bodies via electron microscopy, or Factor VIII-related antigens by immunofluorescence or immunoperoxidase techniques.[107]

Table 12–5 lists the main types of vascular tumors.[108] Only the more important ones will be described.

BENIGN TUMORS AND TUMOR-LIKE CONDITIONS

HEMANGIOMA

Hemangiomas are extremely common tumors, making up 7% of all benign tumors, and are most common in infancy and childhood. There are several histologic and clinical variants.

Capillary Hemangioma

Capillary hemangiomas are so designated because *they are composed of blood vessels that, for the most part, conform to the caliber of normal capillaries.* Although any organ or tissue may be involved, they usually occur in the skin, subcutaneous tissues, and mucous membranes of the oral cavity and lips. They may also occur in internal viscera, such as the liver, spleen, and kidneys. They are, for the most part, small lesions that vary from a few millimeters up to several centimeters in diameter. Characteristically, they are bright red to blue, on a level with the surface of the skin or slightly elevated. Occasionally, pedunculated lesions are formed attached by a broad-to-slender stalk (Fig. 12–35). The covering epithelium is usually intact, but in exposed positions, traumatic ulceration of the overlying epithelium may create a weeping, oozing lesion that bleeds on slightest trauma. The "*strawberry type*" of capillary hemangiomas (juvenile hemangiomas) of the skin of newborns grow rapidly in the first few months, begin to fade when the baby is 1 to 3 years old, and regress completely by age 5 in 80% of cases.[109]

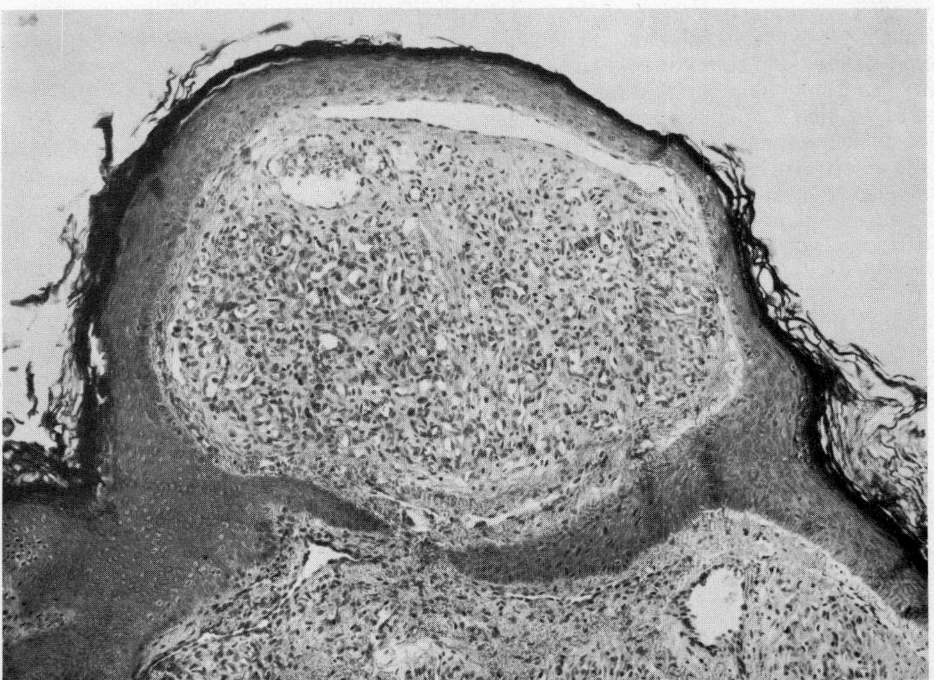

Figure 12–35. Capillary hemangioma of skin.

On section, the red-blue lesions are usually *well defined but unencapsulated.* Small, finger-like projections may extend into surrounding tissue spaces and planes of cleavage. This form of growth may create the appearance of invasiveness, but clinical experience has shown that this pattern of growth is produced by extension along planes of least resistance rather than malignant aggressiveness. Histologically, they are made up of closely packed aggregations of thin-walled capillaries, separated by scant connective tissue stroma. The channels are lined by endothelial cells and are usually filled with fluid blood. Many times, the lumina are partially or completely thrombosed and organized. Rupture of vessels causes further scarring and also accounts for the hemosiderin pigment found in occasional instances.

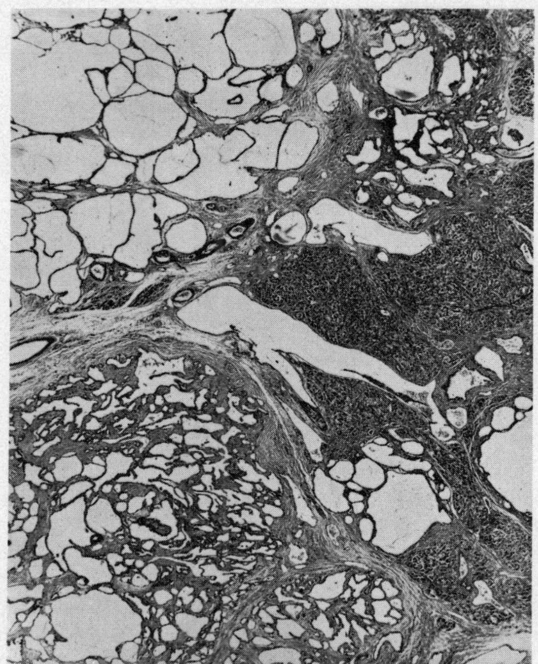

Figure 12–36. Cavernous hemangioma of liver.

Cavernous Hemangioma

Cavernous hemangiomas are distinguished by the formation of *large, cavernous, vascular channels.* Frequently, numerous small, capillary-like lumina are dispersed among the cavernous channels. The term cavernous hemangioma should be reserved for those lesions that are preponderantly composed of vascular channels considerably larger than those of capillary size. These hemangiomas often occur on the skin and mucosal surfaces of the body but are also found in many viscera, particularly the liver, spleen, pancreas, and occasionally in the brain. In one rare entity, *Lindau–von Hippel disease,* cavernous hemangiomas occur within the cerebellum or brain stem and eye grounds, along with similar angiomatous lesions or cystic neoplasms in the pancreas and liver, as well as other visceral neoplasms (p. 139).

Grossly, the usual cavernous hemangioma is a red-blue, soft, spongy mass 1 to 2 cm in diameter. On section, the lesions are sharply defined and compressible and exude blood. Quite rarely, giant forms occur that affect large subcutaneous areas of the face, extremities, or other regions of the body. Histologically, the mass is sharply defined, but not encapsulated, and made up of large, cavernous, vascular spaces, partly or completely filled with fluid blood separated by a scant connective tissue stroma (Fig. 12–36). Intravascular thrombosis or rupture of channels may modify the histologic appearance.

In most situations, the tumors are of little clinical significance, although, when present in the brain, they are potential sources of increased intracranial pressure or hemorrhage.

Granuloma Pyogenicum (Granulation Tissue–Type Hemangioma)

Although the neoplastic nature of this lesion is uncertain, it is currently classified as a polypoid form of capillary hemangioma.[108] The tumors appear as exophytic red nodules on the skin and gingival or oral mucosa, and are often ulcerated. One-third of lesions develop after trauma, growing rapidly to reach a maximum size of 1 to 2 cm within a few weeks. Histologically, the proliferating capillaries are separated by extensive edema and an acute and chronic inflammatory infiltrate. Thus, the lesions bear a striking resemblance to exuberant granulation tissue. They are benign and most do not recur after excision.

Pregnancy tumor (granuloma gravidarum) is a granuloma pyogenicum occuring in the gingiva of 1 to 5% of pregnant women. The lesions regress after delivery, and thus there is doubt whether they are true neoplasms.[107]

GLOMUS TUMOR (GLOMANGIOMA)

A glomangioma is a benign tumor that arises from the modified smooth muscle cells of the glomus body. The normal glomus is a neuromyoarterial receptor that is sensitive to variations in temperature and regulates arteriolar flow. The glomus has an afferent artery, arteriovenous anastomosis, and efferent veins. Glomus bodies may be located anywhere in the skin but are *most commonly found in the distal portion of the fingers and toes,* especially under the nails.[110] It is no surprise, then, that these are the common sites of glomus tumors (especially the fingers). These lesions can be almost positively identified by their extreme painfulness.

Grossly, the lesions are usually under 1 cm in diameter, and many are less than 3 mm in diameter. Tumors have been described that are productive of significant pain although they are smaller than the head of a pin! When present in the skin, they are slightly elevated, rounded, red-blue, firm, exquisitely painful nodules. Under the nail, they appear as minute foci of fresh hemorrhage. Histologically, **two components are present:** branching vascular channels separated by a connective tissue stroma that contains the second element—**aggregates, nests, and masses of the specialized glomus cells.** The individual cells are usually quite regular in size, round or cuboidal, with well-defined cell membranes separating their scant cytoplasm (Fig. 12–37). On electron microscopy, they have features typical of smooth muscle cells.[111]

Clinically, these tumors are readily recognized by the combination of their distinct color and exquisite painfulness. Excision produces prompt relief. Typical glomus tumors also occur in the stomach and nasal cavity.

VASCULAR ECTASIAS (TELANGIECTASES)

The term telangiectasis designates a group of abnormally prominent capillaries, venules, and arterioles that create small focal red lesions, usually in the skin and mucous membranes of the body. These dilatations probably represent congenital anomalies or acquired exaggerations of preexisting vessels, and are therefore not true neoplasms. They are included, however, under the category of tumors since they appear as small, tumor-like masses that require differentiation from true neoplasms.

Nevus Flammeus

This is a sophisticated name for the ordinary birthmark! The lesions are most common on the head and neck, range in color from light pink to deep purple, and are ordinarily flat. Histologically, they show only dilatation of vessels in the dermis. The vast majority ultimately fade and regress.

A special form of nevus flammeus, the so-called *port-wine stain,* may grow proportionately with the child, thicken the skin surface, and become unsightly. In addition, port-wine stains in the distribution of the trigeminal nerve may be associated with the *Sturge-Weber syndrome* (also called *encephalotrigeminal angiomatosis*). This is an extremely uncommon congenital disorder attributed to faulty development of certain mesodermal and ectodermal elements. It is characterized by venous angiomatous masses in the leptomeninges over the cortex and by ipsilateral port-wine nevi of the face, and is often associated with mental retardation, seizures, hemiplegia, and radioopacities in the skull. The importance of this entity lies in the recognition that a large vascular malformation in the face may well be more than a coincidence in a child who exhibits some evidence of mental deficiency.

Spider Telangiectasia

The spider telangiectasis consists of a focal minute network of subcutaneous small arteries or arterioles arranged in a radial fashion about a central core. It is usually found on the upper parts of the body, particularly the face, neck, and upper chest, and is most common in *pregnant women* or in patients with liver disease, particularly *cirrhosis of the liver.* It is believed that the hyperestrinism found in these two conditions in some way evokes these vascular changes. Grossly,

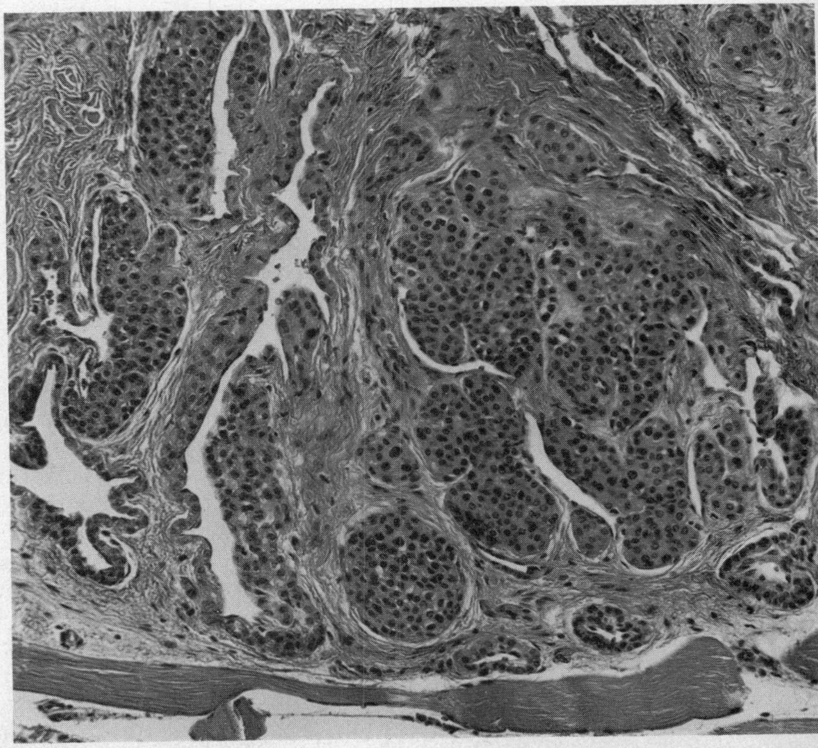

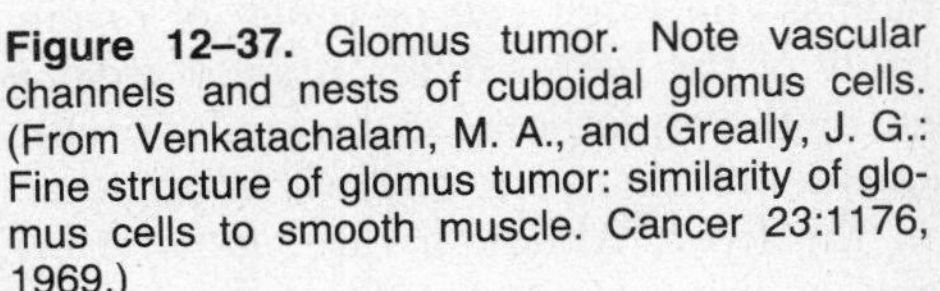

Figure 12–37. Glomus tumor. Note vascular channels and nests of cuboidal glomus cells. (From Venkatachalam, M. A., and Greally, J. G.: Fine structure of glomus tumor: similarity of glomus cells to smooth muscle. Cancer *23*:1176, 1969.)

the lesions are minute areas of redness, 2 to 5 mm in diameter, which on close inspection have the spider-like radiations described. Histologically, only abnormally dilated vessels are found. Because these are composed of arterial vessels, they frequently pulsate, a useful diagnostic feature.

Hereditary Hemorrhagic Telangiectasia (Osler-Weber-Rendu Disease)

This entity is characterized by multiple small aneurysmal telangiectases distributed over the skin and mucous membranes, present from birth and apparently of hereditary origin. It is an extremely uncommon disorder, transmitted as a *dominant mendelian trait by either the male or the female and affecting both sexes equally.* However, about 20% of cases lack a family history.

Grossly, the lesions are found directly beneath the skin or mucosal surfaces of the oral cavity, lips, alimentary tract, respiratory tract, and urinary tract, as well as in the liver, brain, and spleen. The individual lesions are usually small, less than 5 mm in diameter, but coalescent lesions may produce larger, red-blue masses. Microscopically, the lesions consist of thin-walled, dilated capillary and venular channels.

Nosebleeds and bleeding into the intestinal, urinary, or respiratory tracts are common clinical manifestations. This hemorrhagic tendency becomes more pronounced with increasing age. Some patients exhibit gastrointestinal bleeding without skin manifestations. There is frequent hepatomegaly, most often caused by focal fibrovascular lesions throughout the liver lobules, but these patients are also prone to develop viral hepatitis-B due to transfusion therapy. Usually, hemorrhages are readily controlled, and patients with this condition have a normal life expectancy.

BORDERLINE TUMORS

HEMANGIOENDOTHELIOMA

This term is used to denote a true neoplasm of vascular origin composed predominantly of masses of endothelial cells growing in and about vascular lumina. *The hemangioendothelioma represents an intergrade between the well-differentiated hemangiomas and the frankly anaplastic, totally cellular hemangiosarcomas.* It follows the pattern of distribution of the hemangiomas and is most frequently encountered in the skin, but may affect viscera, particularly the spleen and liver. Histologically, vascular channels are evident, but in addition there may be dominant masses and sheets of spindle-shaped cells. Occasionally, plump, somewhat larger cells and mitotic figures are encountered, producing a slight pleomorphism to the cell pattern. Frank anaplasia is not present.

The tumor's chief importance lies in its differentiation from the more ominous angiosarcoma. The clinical setting is critical. Borderline lesions that are present at birth often mature eventually, but in the setting of chronic lymphedema (p. 538) they should cause concern.

Epithelioid hemangioendothelioma is a unique vascular tumor occurring around medium-sized and large veins in the soft tissue of adults. Well-defined vascular channels are inconspicuous and the tumor cells are plump, often cuboidal, thus resembling epithelial cells. They may occur in the lung as a so-called "intravascular bronchioalveolar tumor." These tumors can thus be misdiagnosed as metastatic carcinomas. Their endothelial origin is confirmed by the presence of Weibel-Palade bodies and Factor VIII–associated antigens.[108] Their clinical behavior is variable. Most respond to excision, but up to 30% may recur or metastasize.

MALIGNANT TUMORS

HEMANGIOSARCOMA (ANGIOSARCOMA)

As the name indicates, this tumor is a malignant neoplasm of vascular origin, characterized by masses of endothelial cells displaying the cellular atypicality and anaplasia found in all malignancies. It occurs in both sexes at all ages. It may be found anywhere in the body, but most often in the skin, soft tissue, breast, and liver. Grossly, cutaneous angiosarcomas may begin as deceptively small, sharply demarcated, asymptomatic red nodules, which may be multiple, but eventually most angiosarcomas become large, fleshy masses of pale gray-white, soft, encephaloid tissue.[112] The margins blend imperceptibly with surrounding structures. Areas of central softening, necrosis, and hemorrhage are frequent.

Microscopically, *all degrees of differentiation of these tumors may be found,* from those that are largely vascular with plump, anaplastic but recognizable endothelial cells to tumors that are quite undifferentiated, produce no definite blood vessels, and are markedly atypical (Fig. 12–38). In this more malignant variant, pleomorphism, tumor giant cells, and mitoses are characteristic. These sarcomas may be similar in their cytologic detail to other connective tissue sarcomas. It is therefore sometimes difficult to determine in these spindle cell sarcomas the exact cell or tissue of origin, and careful scrutiny of the better differentiated areas is necessary to identify the endothelial and vascular origin.

There is considerable current interest in angiosarcomas arising in the liver. Although rare, *hepatic angiosarcomas* have been associated with at least three chemical carcinogens: arsenic (exposure to arsenical pesticides), Thorotrast (a radioactive contrast medium widely used in radiology between 1928 and 1950), and polyvinylchloride (widely used in plastics).[113] The increased frequency of angiosarcomas among workers in the polyvinylchloride industry is one of the truly well-documented instances of chemical carcinogenesis in man.[114] With all three agents, there is a very long latent period between exposure and the development of tumors, and there may be a premalignant phase in which there are diffuse sinusoidal hyperplasia and cytologic

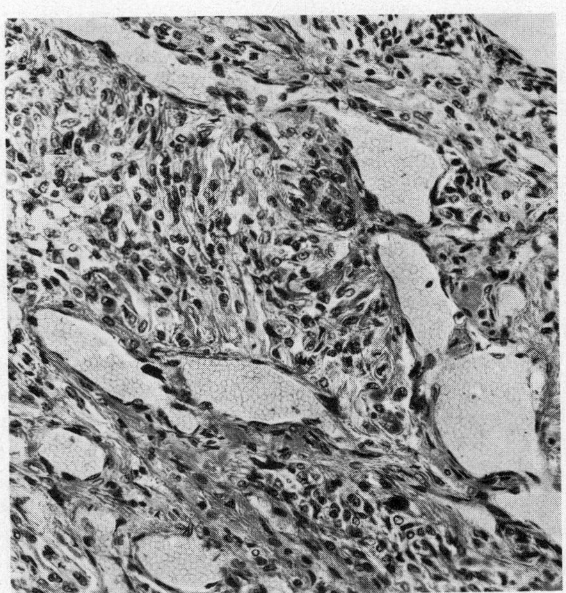

Figure 12–38. Hemangiosarcoma of low malignancy and only moderate anaplasia.

abnormalities in sinusoidal lining cells. The tumors are often multicentric and may arise concomitantly in the spleen.

Clinically, angiosarcomas have all the usual significance of a malignancy, with local invasion and distal metastatic spread. Some patients survive only weeks to months, whereas others may live for many years.

HEMANGIOPERICYTOMA

This rare neoplasm may occur anywhere on the body but is most common in the lower extremities and retroperitoneum.[115] Electron microscopic studies clearly trace the origin of these tumors to pericytes, which are cells present in the walls of capillaries and venules, external to endothelial cells and enveloped by basement membrane.[115] Most of these neoplasms are small, but rarely they achieve a diameter of 8 cm. They consist of numerous capillary channels surrounded by and enclosed within nests and masses of spindle-shaped cells, which can be occasionally ovoid or even round. Silver impregnations can be used to confirm that these cells are outside the basement membrane of the endothelium and hence are pericytes rather than endothelial cells. The tumors may recur, and as many as 50% metastasize to lungs, bone, and liver. Regional nodes are sometimes affected. They should be differentiated from the more benign glomus tumor. *Unlike the glomus tumor, they are rarely painful or multiple, frequently invade and metastasize,* and, as mentioned, are composed of pericytes rather than smooth muscle cells.

KAPOSI'S SARCOMA

Long considered to be an obscure, relatively rare tumor of unknown histogenesis, Kaposi's sarcoma has recently come to the forefront. This is mainly due to reports of near-epidemics of the disease among young homosexual males, intravenous drug users, female prostitutes, Haitian natives and immigrants to the United States, and hemophiliacs, in whom it occurs in association with the acquired immunodeficiency syndrome (AIDS, p. 208). In addition, Kaposi's sarcoma is recognized to be endemic in some parts of Central Africa.[118] The suspicion is strong that Kaposi's sarcoma is one of those *virus-associated tumors* whose etiology and pathogenesis may soon be uncovered: "an oncologic looking-glass."[117] In its sporadic form (not associated with AIDS), the disease affects males almost exclusively (90%) and has its highest incidence in the sixth or seventh decades.

It begins with multiple blue-red skin nodules, usually in the lower extremities, which slowly increase in size and number and spread to more proximal sites. The tumors frequently remain localized to skin and subcutaneous tissue, but widespread visceral involvement may occur. Histologically, the early lesions are composed of proliferating capillaries with plump endothelial cells, spindle-shaped perivascular cells, and interstitial inflammatory cells and extravasated red cells (with hemosiderin deposition), a picture difficult to distinguish from granulation tissue. As the lesions progress, the inflammatory component subsides, the perivascular spindle-shaped cells increase in number and may become pleomorphic, and the angiomatous elements tend to decrease and blend imperceptibly with the neoplastic spindle cells (Fig. 12–39).[108] Thus, the lesions may resemble angiosarcomas or fibrosarcomas. On the basis of ultrastructural and cytochemical studies, most of the tumor cells appear to be of endothelial origin.[107]

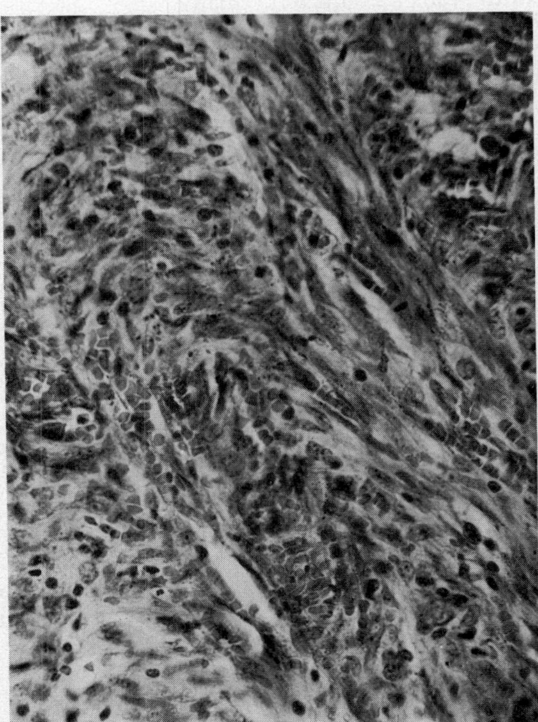

Figure 12–39. Kaposi's sarcoma. Medium-power view of highly cellular, vascular spindle cell sarcoma.

The prognosis depends on the extent of disease. In the sporadic form, patients with nodules confined to the skin have excellent survival rates; in those with locally aggressive disease, there is a 35% mortality rate as a result of the tumor; and all those with visceral dissemination die of the disease. Kaposi's sarcoma associated with AIDS appears to be a more virulent disease. It is frequently disseminated at first diagnosis or soon thereafter. Indeed, this generalized form may represent multicentric involvement rather than metastasis from a primary nodule. Approximately 40% of patients with AIDS/Kaposi's sarcoma die after one year, often in association with opportunistic infections (*Pneumocystis carinii*, fungi, unusual bacteria, viruses).

Another unfortunate aspect of Kaposi's sarcoma is that about one-third of patients subsequently develop a second malignancy, usually lymphoma, leukemia, or myeloma.[120] These considerations, as well as the association with AIDS and the increased frequency in immunocompromised hosts, suggest an interplay between viral infection and deficient immune regulation in the pathogenesis of this disorder.

TUMORS OF LYMPHATICS

LYMPHANGIOMA

Lymphangiomas are the lymphatic analog of the hemangiomas of blood vessels. These tumors may be present at birth but may be so small as to be missed. Growth occurs along with the development of the infant and produces lesions that become macroscopically visible. Both sexes are affected equally.

Simple (Capillary) Lymphangioma: These masses are composed of small lymphatic channels. They tend to occur subcutaneously in the head and neck region as well as in the axilla. Rarely, they are found in the trunk, within internal organs, or in the connective tissue in and about the abdominal or thoracic cavities.

On body surfaces, they are slightly elevated or sometimes pedunculated lesions, 1 to 2 cm in diameter. In internal structures, they are sharply circumscribed, compressible, gray-to-pink lesions. Histologically, they are composed of a network of endothelium-lined lymph spaces that can be *differentiated from capillary channels only by the absence of blood cells.* Sometimes the lining cells hypertrophy, become cuboidal, and take on the appearance of glandular epithelium. A scant fibrous tissue stroma, which occasionally contains aggregates of lymphocytes or small lymphoid nests, separates the small channels. In addition, fat or muscle cells or hemangiomatous portions may be present. A *lymphangiomyoma* is a variant that exhibits abundant smooth muscle in the wall of the lymphatic channels. These tumors are completely benign clinically.

Cavernous Lymphangioma (Cystic Hygroma): These benign lymphatic tumors are composed of cavernous lymphatic spaces, and therefore are analogous to the cavernous hemangioma. They almost invariably occur in the neck or axilla, and only occasionally retroperitoneally. Unlike the cavernous hemangioma, they are not necessarily limited to small lesions but occasionally achieve considerable size, up to 15 cm in diameter. Such large masses may fill the axilla or produce gross deformities in and about the neck. On section, they reveal a soft, compressible, spongelike, red-pink tissue that freely exudes a watery fluid to reveal the underlying loose-textured pattern of the mass. The tumors are made up of hugely dilated cystic spaces lined by endothelial cells and separated by a scant intervening connective tissue stroma. The margins of the tumor are not discrete and these lesions are not encapsulated. Their removal is therefore difficult, and when bits of tumor are left in surgical resections, recurrence may be expected. Because of their large size, they may not only disfigure but compress adjacent structures, such as blood vessels and even the trachea and esophagus.

LYMPHANGIOSARCOMA

Lymphangiosarcoma is a rare tumor that develops after prolonged lymphatic obstruction and lymphedema. Most cases occur in the edematous arms of patients treated with radical mastectomy for carcinoma of the breast.[121] Clinically, the edematous arm may undergo acute swelling followed by the appearance of subcutaneous nodules, hemorrhage, and skin ulceration. The nodules are frequently multiple, but they later become confluent, forming a large mass. On the average, they appear about ten years after the mastectomy and have a very poor prognosis. They may also develop after prolonged lymphedema in the lower legs. Histologically, the tumor is composed of channels lined by anaplastic endothelial cells, and resembles hemangiosarcoma, especially if hemorrhage has occurred. Indeed, some authors classify these tumors as *lymphedema-associated angiosarcoma*.

1. Schwartz, C.J., et al. (eds.): Structure and Function of the Circulation. Vol. 1. New York, Plenum Press, 1980.
2. Weibel, E.R., and Palade, J.E.: New cytoplasmic components in arterial endothelium. J. Cell Biol. *23*:101, 1964.
3. Jaffe, E.A. (ed.): The Biology of Endothelial Cells. The Netherlands, Martinus Nijhoff, 1983.
4. Hüttner, I., and Gabbiani, G.: Vascular endothelium: Recent advances and unanswered questions. Lab. Invest. *47*:409, 1982.
5. Gimbrone, M.A.: Vascular endothelium and atherosclerosis. *In* Moore, S. (ed.): Vascular Injury and Atherosclerosis. New York, Marcel Dekker, 1981, pp. 25–52.
6. Cotran, R.S.: The endothelium and inflammation. *In* Majno, G., and Cotran, R.S. (eds.): Current Topics in Inflammation and Infection. Baltimore, Williams & Wilkins Co., 1982, pp. 18–37.
7. Fishman, A.P. (ed.): Endothelium. Ann. N.Y. Acad. Sci. *401*:1, 1982.
8. Ross, R., and Kariya, B.: Morphogenesis of vascular smooth muscle in atherosclerosis and cell culture. *In* Bohr, D. (ed.): Handbook of Physiology: Circulation Vascular Smooth Muscle. New York, American Physiological Society, 1980, pp. 69–96.
9. Report of the Working Group on Arteriosclerosis of the National Heart, Lung and Blood Institute: Arteriosclerosis, 1981. Vol. 2. Public Health Service N.I.H. Publication No. 82-2035, 1981.
10. McGill, H.C., Jr.: Geographic Pathology of Atherosclerosis. Baltimore, Williams & Wilkins Co., 1968.

11. Strong, J.P., et al.: Coronary and aortic atherosclerosis in New Orleans. II. Comparison of lesions by age, sex and race. Lab. Invest. *39*:364, 1978.
12. McGill, H.C., Jr., and Stern, M.P.: Sex and atherosclerosis. Atheroscler. Rev. *4*:157, 1979.
12A. Neufeld, H.N., and Goldbourt, V.: Coronary heart disease. Genetic aspects. Circulation *67*:943, 1983.
13. Kannel, W.B.: et al.: A general cardiovascular risk profile. The Framingham study. Am. J. Cardiol. *38*:46, 1976.
14. Castelli, W.P., et al.: HDL, cholesterol and other lipids in coronary heart disease: The cooperative lipoprotein phenotyping study. Circulation *55*:76, 1977.
15. Eder, H.A., and Gidez, L.I.: The clinical significance of high density lipoproteins. Med. Clin. North Am. *66*:431, 1982.
16. Brook, J.G., et al.: HDL subfractions in normolipidemic patients with coronary atherosclerosis. Circulation *66*:923, 1982.
17. Editorial: Diet and ischaemic heart disease—agreement or not. Lancet *2*:317, 1983.
18. Glueck, C., et al.: Diet and coronary heart disease: Another view. N. Engl. J. Med. *298*:1471, 1978.
19. Wissler, R.W.: Principles of the pathogenesis of atherosclerosis. *In* Braunwald, E. (ed.): Heart Disease. A Textbook of Cardiovascular Medicine. Philadelphia, W.B. Saunders Co., 1984, pp. 1183–1204.
20. Levy, R.I., and Feinleib, M.: Risk factors for coronary artery disease and their management. *In* Braunwald, E. (ed.): Heart Disease. A Textbook of Cardiovascular Medicine. Philadelphia, W.B. Saunders Co., 1984, pp. 1205–1234.
21. Pooling Project Research Group: Relationship of blood pressure, serum cholesterol, smoking habits, relative weight and ECG abnormalities to incidence of major coronary events: Final report of the pooling project. J. Chronic Dis. *31*:201, 1978.
22. Multiple Risk Factor Intervention Trial Research Group: Risk factor changes and mortality results. J.A.M.A *248*:1465, 1982.
23. Hubert, H.B., et al.: Obesity as an independent risk factor for cardiovascular disease. Circulation *67*:969, 1983.
24. Review Panel on coronary-prone behavior and coronary heart disease. A critical review. Circulation *63*:1199, 1980.
25. Haynes, S.G., and Feinleib, M.: Type A behavior and the incidence of coronary artery disease in the Framingham Heart Study. Adv. Cardiol. *29*:85, 1982.
26. McGill, H.C.: Atherosclerosis: Problems in pathogenesis. Atheroscler. Rev. *2*:27, 1977.
27. Haust, D.: The natural history of human atherosclerotic lesion. *In* Moore, S. (ed.): Vascular Injury and Atherosclerosis. New York, Marcel Dekker, 1981, pp. 1–24.
28. Gerrity, R.G.: Transition of blood-borne monocytes into foam cells in fatty lesions. Am. J. Pathol. *103*:181, 1981.
29. Schaffner, T., et al.: Arterial foam cells with distinctive immunomorphologic and histochemical features of macrophages. Am. J. Pathol. *100*:57, 1980.
30. Mahley, R.W.: Atherogenic hyperlipoproteinemia. The cellular and molecular biology of plasma proteins altered by dietary fat and cholesterol. Med. Clin. North Am. *66*:375, 1982.
31. Roberts, W.C.: The coronary arteries in ischemic heart disease: Facts and fancies. Triangle *16*:77, 1977.
32. Montenegro, M.R., and Eggen, D.A.: Topography of atherosclerosis in the coronary arteries. Lab. Invest. *18*:586, 1968.
33. Moore, S., et al.: Evolution of fatty streak to fibrous plaque in injury-induced atherosclerosis. Fed. Proc. *34*:875, 1975.
34. Tejada, C., et al.: Distribution of coronary and aortic atherosclerosis by geographic location, race and sex. Lab. Invest. *18*:509, 1968.
35. Wissler, R.W., and Vesselinovitch, D.: Regression of atherosclerosis in experimental animals and man. Mod. Conc. Cardiovasc. Dis. *46*:27, 1977.
36. Smith, E.B.: Molecular interactions in human atherosclerotic plaques. Am. J. Pathol. *86*:665, 1977.
37. Velican, C., and Velican, T.: Intimal thickening in developing coronary arteries and its relevance to atherosclerotic involvement. Atherosclerosis *23*:345, 1976.
38. Fry, D.L.: Responses of arterial wall to certain physical factors. Ciba Found. Symp. *12*:93, 1974.
39. Chandler, A.B., et al. (eds.): The Thrombotic Process in Atherogenesis. New York, Plenum Press, 1978.
40. Moore, S. (ed.): Vascular Injury and Atherosclerosis. New York, Marcel Dekker, 1981.
41. Ross, R., and Glomset, J.A.: The pathogenesis of atherosclerosis. N. Engl. J. Med. *295*:369 and 420, 1976.
42. Ross, R.: Atherosclerosis: A problem of the biology of arterial wall cells and their interactions with blood components. Arteriosclerosis *1*:293, 1981.
43. Mahley, R.W.: Development of accelerated atherosclerosis: Concepts derived from cell biology and animal model studies. Arch. Pathol. Lab. Med. *107*:393, 1983.
44. Thomas, W.A., and Kim, D.N.: Atherosclerosis as a hyperplastic and neoplastic process. Lab. Invest. *48*:245, 1983.
45. Steinberg, D.: Lipoproteins and atherosclerosis. A look back and a look ahead. Arteriosclerosis *3*:283–301, 1983.
46. Duguid, J.B.: Pathogenesis of atherosclerosis. Lancet *2*:925, 1949.
47. Goldstein, J.L., and Brown, M.S.: Familial hypercholesterolemia. *In* Stanbury, J.B., et al. (eds.): The Metabolic Basis of Inherited Disease. 5th ed. New York, McGraw-Hill Book Co., 1983, pp. 672–712.
48. Goldstein, J.L., et al.: Defective lipoprotein receptors and atherosclerosis. Lessons from an animal counterpart of familial hypercholesterolemia. N. Engl. J. Med. *309*:288, 1983.
49. Havel, R.J., et al.: Lipoproteins and lipid transport. *In* Bondy, P.K., and Rosenberg, L.E. (eds.): Metabolic Control and Disease. 8th ed. Philadelphia, W.B. Saunders Co., 1980, pp. 393–494.
50. Brown, M.S., and Goldstein, J.L.: Lipoprotein metabolism in the macrophage: Implications for cholesterol deposition in atherosclerosis. Ann. Rev. Biochem. *52*:223, 1983.
51. Schechter, I., et al.: The metabolism of native and malondialdehyde-altered low-density lipoproteins by human monocyte-macrophages. J. Lipid Res. *22*:63, 1981.
52. Henricksen, T., et al.: Interactions of plasma lipoproteins with endothelial cells. Ann. N.Y. Acad. Sci. *401*:102, 1983.
53. Mahley, R.W., et al.: Cholesteryl ester synthesis in macrophages. Stimulation by beta-VLDL from cholesterol-fed animals of various species. J. Lipid Res. *21*:970, 1980.
54. French, J.E.: Atherosclerosis in relation to the structure and function of arterial intima with special reference to the endothelium. Int. Rev. Pathol. *5*:253, 1966.
55. Minnick, R.: Synergy of arterial injury and hypercholesterolemia in atherogenesis. *In* Moore, S. (ed.): Vascular Injury and Atherosclerosis. New York, Marcel Dekker, 1981, pp. 149–174.
56. Stemerman, M.B., and Ross, R.: Experimental arteriosclerosis: I. Fibrous plaque formation in primates: An electron microscopic study. J. Exp. Med. *136*:769, 1972.
57. Minick, C.R.: Immunologic arterial injury in atherogenesis. Ann. N.Y. Acad. Sci. *275*:210, 1976.
58. Harker, L., et al.: Homocystine-induced arteriosclerosis: The role of endothelial cell injury and platelet response in its genesis. J. Clin. Invest. *58*:731, 1976.
59. Ross, R., and Harker, L.: Hyperlipidemia and atherosclerosis. Science *193*:1094, 1976.
60. Wiener, J., and Giacomelli, F.: Morphogenesis of hypertensive vascular disease. *In* Kaley, G., and Altura, B.M. (eds.): The Microcirculation. Baltimore, University Park Press, 1979.
61. Gerrity, R.G., et al.: Endotoxin-induced endothelial injury and repair. I. Endothelial cell turnover in the aorta of the rabbit. Exp. Mol. Pathol. *24*:59, 1976.
62. Fabricant, C.G., et al.: Virus-induced atherosclerosis. J. Exp. Med *148*:335, 1978.
63. Gerrity, R., et al.: Endothelial cell morphology in areas of in vivo Evans Blue uptake in the aorta of young pigs. Am. J. Pathol. *89*:313, 1977.
64. Stemerman, M.B.: Effects of moderate hypercholesterolemia on rabbit endothelium. Arteriosclerosis *1*:25, 1981.
65. Gerrity, R.G., et al.: Dietary-induced atherogenesis in swine: Morphology of the intima in pre-lesion stages. Am. J. Pathol. *95*:775, 1979.
66. Florentin, R.A., et al.: Increased 3H-thymidine incorporation into endothelial cells of swine fed cholesterol for 3 days. Exp. Mol. Pathol. *10*:250, 1969.
67. Ross, R., and Vogel, A.: The platelet-derived growth factor. Cell *14*:203, 1978.
68. Heldin, C.-H., et al.: Platelet-derived growth factor. Isolation by a large scale procedure and analysis by subunit composition. Biochem. J. *193*:907, 1981.
69. Martin, B.M., et al.: Stimulation of human monocyte/macrophage-derived growth factor (MDGF) by plasma fibronectin. J. Immunol. *111*:369, 1983.
70. Gajdusek, C., et al.: An endothelial cell-derived growth factor. J. Cell Biol. *85*:467, 1980.
71. Schwartz, S.M., et al.: Vessel wall growth control. *In* Nossel, H.L., and Vogel, H.J. (eds.): Pathobiology of the Endothelial Cell. New York, Academic Press, 1982, pp. 63–78.
72. Benditt, E.P., and Benditt, J.M.: Evidence for a monoclonal origin of human atherosclerotic plaque. Proc. Natl. Acad. Sci. U.S.A. *70*:1753, 1973.
73. Thomas, W.A., et al.: Population dynamics of arterial cells in atherogenesis. *In* Moore, S. (ed.): Vascular Injury and Atherosclerosis. New York, Marcel Dekker, 1981, pp. 111–129.
74. Martin, G.M., et al.: Senescence of vascular disease. *In* Cristofalo, V.J., et al. (eds.): Explorations in Aging. New York, Plenum Press, 1976.
75. Castellot, J.J., Jr., et al.: Cultured endothelial cells produce a heparin-like inhibitor of smooth muscle cell growth. J. Cell Biol. *90*:372, 1981.
76. Guyton, J.R., et al.: Inhibition of rat arterial smooth muscle cell proliferation by heparin. Circ. Res. *46*:625, 1980.
77. McCluskey, R.T., and Fienberg, O.: Vasculitis in primary vasculitides,

granulomatoses, and connective tissue diseases. Hum. Pathol. *14*:305, 1983.

78. Cupps, T.R., and Fauci, A.S.: The vasculitic syndromes. Adv. Intern. Med. *27*:315, 1982.
79. Cupps, T.R., and Fauci, A.S.: The Vasculitides. Philadelphia, W.B. Saunders Co., 1981.
80. Duffy, J., et al.: Polyarthritis, polyarteritis and hepatitis. Medicine *55*:19, 1976.
81. Zeek, P.M.: Periarteritis nodosa. A clinical review. Am. J. Clin. Pathol. *22*:777, 1952.
82. Lochkin, M.D., and Sergent, J.S.: Necrotizing vasculitis in HBs antigenemia. *In* Hughes, G.R.V. (ed.): Modern Topics in Rheumatology. London, Heinemann, 1976.
83. Alarçon-Segovia, D.: The necrotizing vasculitides. Med. Clin. North Am. *61*:24, 1977.
84. Godman, J.C., and Churg, J.: Wegener's granulomatosis. Pathology and review of literature. Arch. Pathol. *58*:533, 1954.
85. Fauci, A.S., et al.: Wegener's granulomatosis: Prospective clinical and therapeutic experience with 85 patients for 21 years. Ann. Intern. Med. *98*:76, 1983.
86. Katzenstein, A.A., et al.: Lymphomatoid granulomatosis. A clinicopathologic study of 152 cases. Cancer *43*:360, 1979.
87. Bengtsson, B.A., and Malmvall, B.E.: Giant cell arteritis. Acta Med. Scand. (Suppl.) *658*:1982.
88. Allsop, C.J., and Gallagher, P.J.: Temporal artery biopsy in giant cell arteritis. A reappraisal. Am. J. Surg. Pathol. *5*:317, 1981.
89. Lupi-Herrera, E., et al.: Takayasu's arteritis. Study of 107 cases. Am. Heart J. *93*:94, 1977.
90. Ishikawa, K.: Natural history and clarification of occlusive thromboaortopathy (Takayasu's disease). Circulation *57*:27, 1978.
91. Cairun, S., and Oleesky, S.: Takayasu's disease and giant cell arteritis—a single disease? Br. Med. J. *2*:127, 1977.
92. Kawasaki, T., et al.: A new infantile acute febrile mucocutaneous lymph node syndrome (MCNS) prevailing in Japan. Pediatrics *54*:271, 1974.
93. Melish, M.E.: Kawasaki's syndrome (the mucocutaneous lymph node syndrome). Annu. Rev. Med. *33*:569, 1982.
94. Buerger, L.: Thromboangiitis obliterans: A study of the vascular lesions leading to pre-senile gangrene. Am. J. Med. Sci. *136*:567, 1908.
95. McKusick, V.A., et al.: Buerger's disease: a distinct clinical and pathologic entity. J.A.M.A. *181*:5, 1962.
96. Adar, R., et al.: Cellular sensitivity to collagen in thromboangiitis obliterans. N. Engl. J. Med. *308*:1113, 1983.
97. McLoughlin, G.A., et al.: Association of HLA-A9 and HLA-B5 with Buerger's disease. Br. Med. J. *2*:1165, 1976.
98. Brinstingl, M.: The Raynaud syndrome. *In* Harcus, A.W., et al. (eds.): Arteries and Veins. Edinburgh, Churchill Livingstone, 1975, p. 32.
99. Slater, E. E., and De Sanctis, R.W.: Diseases of the aorta. *In* Braunwald, E. (ed.): Heart Disease. A Textbook of Cardiovascular Medicine. Philadelphia, W.B. Saunders Co., 1984, pp. 1540–1571.
99A. Doroghazi, R.M., and Slater, E.E. (eds.): Aortic Dissection. New York, McGraw-Hill Book Co., 1983.
100. Anagnostopoulos, C.E.: Acute Aortic Dissections. Baltimore, University Park Press, 1975.
100A. Roberts, W.C.: Aortic dissection: Anatomy, consequences and causes. Am. Heart J. *101*:195, 1981.
101. DeBakey, M.E., et al.: Surgical management of dissecting aneurysms of the aorta. J. Thorac. Cardiovasc. Surg. *49*:130, 1965.
102. Hirst, A.E., and Gore, I.: Is cystic medial necrosis the cause of dissecting aneurysm? Circulation *53*:915, 1976.
102A. Klima, T., et al.: The morphology of ascending aortic aneurysms. Hum. Pathol. *14*:810, 1983.
103. Schlatmann, T., and Becker, A.: Pathogenesis of dissecting aneurysm of aorta. Comparative histopathologic study of significance of medial changes. Am. J. Cardiol. *39*:21, 1977.
104. Boucek, R., et al.: The Marfan syndrome: A deficiency in chemically stable collagen cross-links. N. Engl. J. Med. *288*:804, 1982.
105. Collins, J.J., et al.: Common aortic aneurysms. When to intervene? J. Cardiovasc. Med. *8*:245, 1983.
106. Standness, E., et al.: The present status of acute deep vein thrombosis. Coll. Rev. Surg. Gynecol. Obstet. *145*:433, 1977.
107. Ordóñez, N.G., and Batsakis, J.G.: Comparison of *Ulex europaeus* I lectin and factor VIII–related antigen in vascular lesions. Arch. Pathol. Lab. Med. *108*:129, 1984.
108. Enzinger, F.M., and Weiss, S.W.: Soft Tissue Tumors. St. Louis, C.V. Mosby Co., 1983, pp. 379–501.
109. MacCollum, D.W., and Martin, L.W.: Hemangioma in infancy and childhood. A report based on 6479 cases. Surg. Clin. North Am. *36*:1647, 1957.
110. Carroll, R.E., and Berman, A.T.: Glomus tumors of the hand. J. Bone Joint Surg. *54*:691, 1972.
111. Venkatachalam, M.A., and Greally, J.G.: Fine structure of glomus tumor: Similarity of glomus cells to smooth muscle. Cancer *23*:1176, 1969.
112. Maddox, J.C., and Evans, H.L.: Angiosarcoma of skin and soft tissue. Cancer *14*:1186, 1981.
113. Popper, H., et al.: Development of hepatic angiosarcoma in man induced by vinyl chloride, Thorotrast, and arsenic: Comparison with cases of unknown etiology. Am. J. Pathol. *92*:349, 1978.
114. Makk, L., et al.: Clinical and morphologic features of hepatic angiosarcoma in vinyl chloride workers. Cancer *37*:149, 1976.
115. Enzinger, F.M., and Smith, B.H.: Hemangiopericytoma. An analysis of 106 cases. Hum. Pathol. *7*:61, 1976.
116. Daimont, W.E., et al.: The ultrastructure of vascular tumors: Additional observations and a review of the literature. Pathol. Annu. *12*(Part 2):279, 1977.
117. Groopman, J.E., and Gottlieb, M.S.: Kaposi's sarcoma: An oncologic looking-glass. Nature *299*:103, 1982.
118. Slavin, G., et al.: Kaposi's sarcoma in mainland Tanzania. A report of 117 cases. Br. J. Cancer *23*:349, 1979.
119. Acquired immunodeficiency syndrome. Editorial. Lancet *1*:162, 1983.
120. Safai, B., et al.: Association of Kaposi's sarcoma with second primary malignancies. Cancer *45*:1472, 1980.
121. Woodward, A.M., et al.: Lymphangiosarcoma arising in chronic lymphedematous extremities. Cancer *30*:149, 1976.

THE HEART* 13

*With gratitude to Dr. Frederick J. Schoen, Brigham and Women's Hospital, for many helpful suggestions and for Figures 13–3, 13–6 to 13–9, 13–11, 13–13, 13–14, 13–20, 13–21, 13–23, 13–27, 13–32, and 13–41.

This chapter opens with the two ends of the cardiac spectrum: certain normal aspects of morphology and a brief review of congestive heart failure, which is the final destination of most pathways of serious cardiac disease.

NORMAL

ANATOMY. Determination of the size and gross configuration of the heart is of great clinical and pathologic importance. In the female, the average weight of the heart is 250 to 300 gm, and in the male, 300 to 350 gm, varying with height and skeletal structure. Normally the thickness of the wall of the right ventricle is 3 to 5 mm, and that of the left ventricle 1.3 to 1.5 cm. Ventricular thicknesses greater than these levels indicate hypertrophy and enlargement; measurements below these normal ranges imply dilatation. However, these measurements must be interpreted with reference to heart weight and chamber size. An apparently normal left ventricular thickness may be found in a markedly heavy, hypertrophied heart that has undergone cardiac dilatation during a period of congestive failure prior to death.

The anatomy of the cardiac valves is particularly important in assessing pathologic alterations of the heart. On gross inspection, the valve leaflets (cusps) should be delicate, translucent, and without apparent vascularity. When commissural fusion or vascularization occurs, it implies a previous inflammatory process. All act as loose flap valves that balloon out in a parachute-like fashion under the impact of the regurgitant blood to abut on each other and thus close the valvular orifice. They are apposed or come in contact with each other at a line of closure marked by a linear thickening most evident in the semilunar (pulmonic and aortic) leaflets. The centers of each of these linear thickenings are occupied usually by small fibrous nodules, the corpora arantii. Round-to-oval fenestrations, 1 to 3 mm in diameter, frequently occur in the semilunar cusps, close to the commissures. The normal chordae tendineae are thin cords that originate from the papillary muscles and divide progressively into fine, delicate strands that insert into the free margins of the atrioventricular (tricuspid and mitral) leaflets. Thickening of these chordae is often one of the conspicuous features of postrheumatic endocarditis. Estimation of the function of a valve from its postmortem anatomy is frequently difficult and may be misleading, since proper valve function is dependent not only on structure but also on the dynamics of the heart.

Normally, the pericardium contains up to 30 ml of clear fluid. As a serosal membrane, it reacts to inflammatory and neoplastic diseases in the same fashion as do the linings of the pleural and peritoneal cavities.

Histologically, the epicardium and parietal pericardium are mesothelium attached to an underlying typical fibrofatty tissue. The myocardium consists of cardiac myocytes, interstitial connective tissue, and blood vessels. The internal structure of the myocardial fiber differs from the skeletal striated muscle fiber (p. 1304) in its branching characteristics and central nuclei. At the point where branching fibers meet, the intercalated disc separates individual fibers. The myofibrils in the heart muscle cell are traversed by the usual A bands and I bands found in skeletal muscle, the I band having the characteristic centrally located Z line. A sarcomere is that portion of the cell contained between two Z lines. The A band is created by thick myosin filaments in register. The I bands have only the thin actin filaments, which are attached on either end of the sarcomere to the Z lines and extend centrally between the myosin filaments into the A band. Contraction of the sarcomere and myocardial cell is accomplished by the thin actin filaments sliding between the thick myosin filaments toward the center of the sarcomere. The myocardial fiber is especially rich in mitochondria—approximately one-third the cell volume—reflecting the high oxidative metabolic level of these cells. In addition to having a branching network of anastomosing tubules of sarcoplasmic reticulum (the counterpart of endoplasmic reticulum), the cardiac fiber is traversed across its long axis at the level of the Z lines by T tubules. This specialized structure found only in cardiac and skeletal muscle is essentially an invagination of the sarcolemma, so the lumina of the T tubules are continuous with the extracellular space. Thus, no point in the muscle fiber is more than 2 to 3 μ from the extracellular space. This unique arrangement provides an effective means of rapid flux of calcium, sodium, and potassium ions between muscle fiber and interstitial fluid, so critical to the contraction of cardiac muscle fibers. In the normal heart, the nuclei are fairly uniform in size and bear a fairly constant relationship to the mass of the individual cells. Significant disturbance in this nuclear-cytoplasmic ratio suggests some underlying derangement such as atrophy, hypertrophy, or previous inflammatory disease. Grossly, the endocardium itself is thin and usually inapparent. It consists of a layer of endothelial cells and scant subendothelial connective tissue.

BLOOD SUPPLY TO HEART. *Functionally, the right and left coronaries behave as end arteries, although anatomically there are numerous intercoronary anastomoses in most normal hearts.* You will recall that the ostia of the coronary arteries lie within the sinuses of Valsalva behind the aortic valve leaflets. Thus, these ostia are protected somewhat during systole from the Venturi effect of the rapid passing flow of blood during systolic contraction. Most of the coronary artery filling occurs during diastole. Knowledge of the area of supply of the three major coronary trunks helps to explain the correlation between vascular lesions and myocardial infarctions. The anterior descending branch of the left coronary artery supplies most of the apex of the heart, the anterior surface of the left ventricle, the contiguous third of the anterior wall of the right ventricle, and the anterior two-thirds of the interventricular septum. In most hearts the right coronary artery supplies the remainder of the anterior surface of the right ventricle, the posterior aspect of the right ventricle, the adjacent half of the posterior wall of the left ventricle, and the posterior third of the interventricular septum. To the circumflex branch of the left coronary artery remains only a small portion of the lateral aspect of the left ventricle extending slightly anteriorly and posteriorly. *Thus, occlusions of the right as well as the left coronary artery and their major branches may cause left ventricular damage.* The atria are supplied by branches from the arteries on the corresponding side. At the cellular level, individual muscle fibers are almost uniformly accompanied by individual capillaries. This distribution may be important in hypertrophied hearts in which it is postulated that enlarged fibers may become so thick as to outgrow their blood supply.

It is now amply documented that *in all or virtually all human hearts, there are numerous intercoronary anastomotic channels up to 40 μm in diameter.* In the normal heart, little blood courses through these channels because the blood pressure on both ends of a channel is the same and there is no flow gradient. However, when one trunk is narrowed, a pressure gradient develops, blood flows from the high to the low pressure system, and simultaneously the channels enlarge.[1] Thus, these anastomoses may play a role in supporting the blood flow to deprived areas of the myocardium, but, alas, they are not capable of compensating for sudden loss of a major coronary artery.

CONGESTIVE HEART FAILURE (CHF)

CHF will be considered at the outset since it is the potential end point of all forms of serious heart disease. *CHF can be defined as the pathophysiologic state resulting from impaired cardiac function rendering the heart unable to maintain an output sufficient for the metabolic requirements of the tissues and organs of the body.*[2] *CHF occurs either because of a decreased myocardial capacity to contract or because an increased pressure-stroke-volume load is imposed on the heart.* Most instances of heart failure are the consequence of progressive deterioration of the myocardial contractile function (systolic dysfunction). Sometimes the increased pressure load is caused by an inability of the heart to expand sufficiently during diastole to accommodate the ventricular volume (diastolic dysfunction). Uncommonly, acute heart failure may occur with basically normal myocardial function, as, for example, with sudden catastrophic rupture of a valve cusp or the chordae tendineae. Whatever its basis, CHF is characterized by diminished cardiac output (sometimes called forward failure) and/or damming back of blood in the venous system (so-called backward failure).

Although we speak of diminished myocardial contraction as the cause of heart failure, there is no clear understanding at the biomolecular level of the basis for the contractile failure.[3] In some instances—myocardial infarction, necrotizing inflammations—there is obvious death of myocytes and loss of vital elements of the "pump." In the absence of such acute losses, other mechanisms have been proposed, but none established. One such mechanism is reduced adrenergic drive. Recently a reduction in beta-adrenergic receptor density has been reported in severe chronic heart failure,[4] but this change may be a late and secondary event. Other proposed pathophysiologic mechanisms include decreased calcium availability, which is important in excitation-contraction coupling; impaired mitochondrial function; decreased ATPase function; and microcirculating spasm. In the last analysis, we still do not understand why chronically overtaxed hearts eventually decompensate.

Compensatory mechanisms come into play with the onset of failure. A fundamental defect in the failing heart is a reduction of ventricular stroke volume relative to the metabolic needs of the peripheral tissues. An increased heart rate (tachycardia) may, to an extent, buffer the reduction in stroke volume. With diminished contraction, the heart dilates and, according to the Frank-Starling mechanism, the increased end-diastolic ventricular volume permits the ejection of a larger stroke volume. By poorly understood mechanisms, the cardiac dilatation leads to myocardial hypertrophy, providing a larger contractile mass. Other mechanisms support this cardiac adaptation; there is an increased output of catecholamines by the adrenal medulla, which augments myocardial contractility. Simultaneously the renin-angiotensin-aldosterone system leads to sodium and water retention, with an increase in blood volume and ventricular stroke volume. Vital tissues are protected by adrenergic-mediated redistribution of blood flow, with shunting of blood from the skin and splanchnic beds to the heart and brain. In addition, there is increased oxygen extraction from the blood, to some extent compensating for the reduced vascular flow,[5] and a reduction in the affinity of hemoglobin for oxygen, facilitating oxygen transfer to the tissues.

The compensatory mechanisms, initially adaptive, ultimately constitute an added burden. The myocardial hypertrophy may become detrimental because of the increased metabolic requirements of the enlarged muscle mass. Increased blood volume, which supports the cardiac output in the short term, also imposes an additional load on the failing heart. Ultimately, the primary cardiac disease and the superimposed compensatory burdens further encroach on the myocardial reserve until the cardiac dilatation transgresses the point at which adequate myocardial tension can be generated. Then begins the downward slide of the stroke volume and cardiac output that often terminates in death. Thus, at autopsy the heart is often dilated and usually hypertrophied, but the extent of these changes varies from one patient to the next.

It is impossible from morphologic examination of the heart to differentiate the damaged but compensated organ from one that has decompensated. The amount of hypertrophy and dilatation does not permit a judgment nor does the extent of the primary cardiac disease. *Many of the significant morphologic changes encountered in CHF are distant from the heart and are produced by the hypoxic and congestive effects of the failing circulation upon other organs and tissues.* It is important to recall that hypoxic and/or congestive changes may be produced in peripheral tissues and organs by states of circulatory insufficiency of noncardiac origin, e.g., hemorrhagic or septic shock. During shock, many organs suffer hypoxic injury because of hypoperfusion. Moreover, circulatory congestion may arise because of hypervolemia (salt and water retention) secondary to chronic renal failure in the absence of significant disturbances in cardiac function. In time the heart may secondarily suffer and decompensate. It is clear that circulatory derangements may arise from extracardiac sources and induce tissue changes similar to those induced by CHF.

Although the heart is a single organ, to some extent it acts as two distinct anatomic and functional units. Under various pathologic stresses, one side or, rarely, even one chamber may fail before the other(s) so that, from the clinical standpoint, left-sided and right-sided failure may occur separately. Since the vascular system is a closed circuit, failure of one side cannot exist for long without eventually producing excessive strain upon the other, terminating in total heart failure. The clearest understanding of the pathologic physiology is derived from a consideration of failure of each side separately.

LEFT-SIDED HEART FAILURE

As will be discussed, left-sided heart failure is most often caused by (1) ischemic heart disease, (2) hypertension, (3) aortic and mitral valvular diseases (rheumatic heart disease, calcific aortic stenosis), and (4) myocardial diseases. Except with obstruction at the mitral valve or other processes that restrict the size of the left ventricle, this chamber is usually dilated, sometimes quite massively. With left ventricular restrictive disorders and particularly with mitral stenosis, the dilatation is confined to the left atrium. The distant effects of left-sided failure are manifested most prominently in the lungs, although the function of the kidneys and brain may also be markedly impaired.

LUNGS. With the progressive damming of blood within the pulmonary circulation, pressure in the pulmonary veins mounts and is ultimately transmitted to the capillaries. Pulmonary congestion and edema result, as described in detail on page 710. It is sufficient to note here that the congestion first leads to the development of a perivascular transudate—"cuffing"—followed by progressive edematous widening of the alveolar septa, and in time by the accumulation of edema fluid, perhaps admixed with some red cells (related to microhemorrhages) in the alveolar spaces. Not infrequently, transudate accumulates within the pleural spaces, particularly on the left, producing a gross pleural effusion.

These anatomic changes produce striking clinical manifestations. *Dyspnea* (breathlessness) is usually the earliest and the cardinal complaint of patients in left-sided heart failure, and is an exaggeration of the normal breathlessness that follows exertion. The pathophysiology of the dyspnea involves reduction of the vital capacity by the accumulation of fluid and blood within the air spaces, increased stiffness of the lungs related to the intraseptal edematous thickening, and air trapping secondary to obstructive fluid in the smaller airways. *Orthopnea* is dyspnea on lying down that is relieved by sitting or standing. Thus, the orthopneic patient employs several pillows and indeed may spend the night in a chair. Orthopnea results from increased venous return to the heart in the recumbent position because of reduced pooling of fluid in the usually dependent portions of the body. This overloads the failing pump and exaggerates the pulmonary congestion and edema. *Paroxysmal nocturnal dyspnea*, also known as *paroxysmal cardiac dyspnea*, is an extension of orthopnea that consists of attacks of extreme dyspnea bordering on suffocation; these usually occur at night and force the patient to sit upright struggling for breath. Often the patient in panic opens a window in the hope of relieving the breathlessness. There is no clear understanding of the origins of paroxysmal nocturnal dyspnea but depressed nocturnal respiratory drive, reduced adrenergic stimulation to the left ventricle during sleep, and increased venous return to the heart and lungs in the recumbent position all contribute. *Cough* is a common accompaniment of left-sided failure, and in severe cases may raise frothy, blood-tinged sputum.

KIDNEYS. With left-sided heart failure, the decreased cardiac output causes a reduction in renal perfusion, which has a number of consequences. The renin-angiotensin-aldosterone system is activated, inducing retention of salt and water with consequent expansion of the interstitial fluid volume and blood volume. This compensatory reaction contributes to the pulmonary edema in left-sided heart failure. In kidneys already suffering from hypoperfusion, whether related to the shock state or to hypertensive arteriolar narrowing, the reduced cardiac output may lead to ischemic acute tubular necrosis (p. 1027). If the perfusion deficit of the kidney becomes sufficiently severe, impaired excretion of nitrogenous products may cause azotemia, known as *prerenal azotemia*.

BRAIN. Cerebral hypoxia may give rise to many symptoms, such as irritability, loss of attention span, and restlessness, and may even progress to stupor and coma. These symptoms, however, are encountered only in far-advanced congestive heart failure.

RIGHT-SIDED HEART FAILURE

Right-sided heart failure occurs in pure form in only a few diseases. Usually it is a consequence of left-sided failure, because any increase in pressure in the pulmonary circulation incident to left-sided failure must inevitably produce an increased burden on the right side of the heart. The causes of right-sided failure, then, must include all those that create left heart failure, particularly lesions such as mitral stenosis or congenital left-to-right shunts, which produce great increases in pulmonary pressure.

Pure right-sided failure most often occurs with *cor pulmonale*, i.e., right ventricular strain produced by intrinsic disease of the lungs or pulmonary vasculature. In these cases, the right ventricle is burdened by increased resistance within the pulmonary circulation. Dilatation of the heart is confined to the right ventricle and atrium. Other and less common causes of right-sided heart failure include the various forms of cardiomyopathy and diffuse myocarditis, which appear to affect the right ventricle more often than the left for reasons to be presented later. Rarely, right-sided failure is caused by tricuspid or pulmonic valvular lesions. Clinically, constrictive pericarditis simulates right-sided failure by damming blood back into the systemic venous system, although the right ventricle itself may be normal.

The major morphologic and clinical effects of pure right-sided failure differ from those of left-sided failure in that pulmonary congestion is minimal, while engorgement of the systemic and portal systems is more pronounced. It should be remembered, however, that in both instances the twin problems of systemic venous congestion and impaired cardiac output remain qualitatively the same. The major organs affected by right-sided heart failure are the liver, spleen, kidneys, subcutaneous tissues, and brain and the entire portal area of venous drainage.

LIVER. The liver is usually slightly increased in size and weight and on sectioning displays a prominent "nutmeg" pattern (Fig. 13–1), described in greater detail

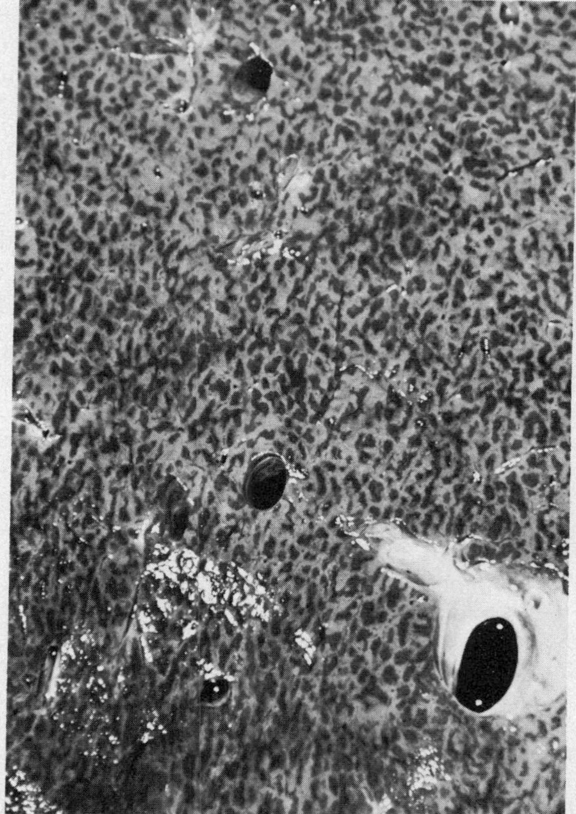

Figure 13–1. Close-up view of transected surface of liver with marked chronic passive congestion—the so-called nutmeg pattern.

on page 897. In essence, it comprises congestive red accentuation of the centers of the liver lobules surrounded by the paler, sometimes fatty, peripheral regions. The liver cells in the central region may become somewhat atrophic as a result of the congestive hypoxia related to the stagnant flow in the centrilobular sinusoids. Together, these changes are called *chronic passive congestion* (CPC) of the liver. If the right-sided failure is severe and rapidly developing, the passive congestion and circulatory failure may lead to necrosis of the centrilobular liver cells accompanied by rupture of sinusoids, producing *central hemorrhagic necrosis*. A 1981 study relates the centrilobular necrosis more to the ischemia associated with reduced arterial flow than to the sinusoidal congestion.[6] If the patient does not die of the severe cardiac failure, the central areas in time become fibrotic, creating so-called *cardiac sclerosis*.

SPLEEN. Congestion produces an enlarged spleen that is tense and cyanotic. On section, blood freely exudes and the tissue collapses so that the capsule becomes wrinkled. Microscopically, there may be marked sinusoidal dilatation, accompanied by areas of recent hemorrhage and possibly deposits of hemosiderin pigment. With long-standing congestion, the enlarged spleen may achieve a weight of 500 to 600 gm (normal, 150 gm), and the long-standing edema may produce fibrous thickening of the sinusoidal walls. The areas of previous hemorrhage are now transformed to hemosiderin deposits, to create the firm, meaty organ characteristic of *congestive splenomegaly* (p. 700).

KIDNEYS. Congestion and hypoxia of the kidneys are more marked with right-sided heart failure than with left, leading to greater fluid retention, peripheral edema, and more pronounced prerenal azotemia.

SUBCUTANEOUS TISSUES. Some degree of peripheral edema of dependent portions of the body occurs regularly. Indeed, ankle edema may be considered a hallmark of CHF. In severe or long-standing cases, edema may be quite massive and generalized, a condition termed *anasarca*. Of probable significance in the perpetuation of edema is the diminished clearing of plasma aldosterone by the congested liver. This contributes to the elevated levels of this hormone.

PLEURAL SPACES. Effusions may appear, particularly on the right.

BRAIN. Symptoms essentially identical to those described in left-sided failure may occur, representing venous congestion and hypoxia of the central nervous system.

PORTAL SYSTEM OF DRAINAGE. Splenic congestion has already been described. In addition, abnormal accumulations of transudate in the peritoneal cavity may give rise to *ascites*. Congestion of the gut may cause intestinal disturbances.

In summary, right-sided heart failure presents essentially as a venous congestive syndrome, with hepatic and splenic enlargement, peripheral edema, pleural effusions, and ascites. In contrast to left-sided failure, respiratory symptoms may be absent or quite insignificant. *The consideration of heart failure has been divided into two functional units. In the usual case of frank chronic cardiac decompensation, however, these early stages have already passed. Thus, the patient presents with the picture of full-blown CHF, encompassing the clinical syndromes of both right and left heart failure.*

TYPES OF HEART DISEASE

Heart disease is the predominant cause of disability and death in all industrialized nations. In the United States it accounts currently for about 335 deaths per 100,000 population (approximately 40% of the total mortality), overshadowing cancer, which follows with 183 deaths per 100,000. Since the turn of the century death rates from heart disease in the U.S. reveal some remarkable and most welcome trends. In 1900, heart disease occupied fourth place among the ten leading causes of death with a mortality rate of approximately 140. A steady climb ensued over the decades to reach a peak of 375 in 1963. Just when it seemed that the climb would never end, the rate began to fall to the current level. The rate of decline has, in fact, been accelerating; about 60% of the total reduction occurred between 1970 and 1980.[7] This most "heartening" trend is attributable largely to a decline in mortality from ischemic heart disease, as pointed out on page 506.

Four categories of cardiac disease account for about 85 to 90% of all cardiac deaths: (1) ischemic heart disease, (2) hypertensive heart disease and pulmonary hypertensive heart disease (cor pulmonale), (3) valvular disease, and (4) congenital heart disease. Since ischemic heart disease is responsible for the great majority of these deaths, this paramount condition is considered first, followed by the other three categories. The remaining disorders are grouped into myocardial diseases and pericardial diseases, with a miscellany at the end.

ISCHEMIC HEART DISEASE (IHD)

IHD is the generic designation for a spectrum of disorders resulting from imbalance between the myocardial need for oxygen and the adequacy of the supply. Because reduction in coronary blood flow is almost always the cause of the imbalance, IHD for years has been called *coronary heart disease*, under which rubric it still may be found in many textbooks. However, the most recent revision of the International Classification of Diseases prefers the term *ischemic heart disease*, and so we bow to authority in this presentation, while frequently reverting to past practice.

In 90 to 95% of cases the reduction in coronary blood flow is related to atherosclerotic narrowing of the subepicardial coronary trunks. Coronary vasospasm alone or superimposed on atherosclerotic narrowing may contribute to the reduction in flow.[8, 9] Often, thrombotic occlusion provoked by a complicated atheroma or a focus of vasospastic narrowing suddenly worsens the reduction in coronary flow. In a minority of cases the reduced coronary flow has other origins—coronary embolism; osteal stenosis in luetic aortitis; dissecting aortic aneurysm that extends back into the walls of the coronary arteries; direct trauma to the coronary vessels inducing thrombosis, disruption, or dissection; or some form of arteritis (e.g., polyarteritis nodosa, rheumatic and temporal arteritis, Kawasaki's disease). Even more uncommonly, IHD may be related to anomalous origin of the left coronary artery from the pulmonary trunk, reduction of oxygen transport of the blood related to either anemia or carbon monoxide poisoning, a defect in oxyhemoglobin dissociation, inadequate perfusion of the myocardium in hypotensive crises and shock. It is important to note that increased myocardial oxygen demands may exceed the level of supply of even a relatively normal coronary circulation and assuredly worsen any preexisting imbalance. Despite all these potential mechanisms, *until proved otherwise, IHD is caused by atherosclerotic narrowing of the coronary arteries (fixed obstruction), possibly aggravated by superimposed vasospasm (dynamic obstruction).* Depending on the rate of development of the arterial narrowing(s) and its ultimate severity, four basic clinicopathologic syndromes may result: (1) myocardial infarction, (2) angina pectoris, (3) chronic ischemic heart disease, and (4) sudden cardiac death, which may be superimposed on any of the preceding three conditions. As might be expected, there is considerable overlap among them. The classical patterns will be briefly characterized here, followed by a more complete discussion of each, along with the intermediate patterns that fall in the interfaces.

1. *Myocardial infarction* (MI) is the catastrophic, frequently fatal form of IHD that usually results from precipitous reduction or arrest of a significant portion of the coronary flow. One of two patterns of myocardial ischemic necrosis may appear: (a) a confluent left ventricular lesion, usually greater than 2.5 cm in longest dimension, which extends from the subendocardium to the subepicardium—the *transmural infarct*; or (b) multifocal areas of ischemic necrosis limited to the inner one-third to one-half of the thickness of the left ventricular wall, so-called *subendocardial infarct* or *subendocardial ischemic necrosis*. In both forms, severe atherosclerotic narrowing, possibly associated with thrombotic occlusion, is almost always present in one or more of the major coronary arterial trunks. The contribution of vasospasm is difficult to elucidate at postmortem because it is a transient phenomenon usually demonstrable only in the living patient.

2. *Angina pectoris* (AP) is a symptom complex consisting of severe paroxysmal chest pain resulting from transient ischemia that falls precariously short of inducing infarction. Three clinical patterns have been delineated: (a) stable angina, (b) Prinzmetal's variant angina, and (c) unstable angina (all detailed on p. 555). Underlying all are variable combinations of atherosclerotic coronary narrowing and vasospasm. Sometimes thrombotic occlusion of smaller coronary branches is superimposed. By definition, myocardial infarction is not present.

3. *Chronic ischemic heart disease (CIHD)*, sometimes also inappropriately called ischemic cardiomyopathy (p. 596), refers to the pattern of cardiac damage caused by long-term ischemia (years to decades). It is marked principally by general myocardial atrophy and foci of scarring. The scars may be small and numerous, related to isolated myofiber necrosis or the death of clusters of myocardial cells. However, in addition they may be punctuated by large areas of fibrosis resulting from past episodes of acute infarction. Generally, CIHD is the consequence of slow, progressive atherosclerotic narrowing of the coronary trunks that occurs over a span of years to decades; superimposed on such a course may be acute MIs that permit survival. Thus, CIHD may lead to death by progressive slow reduction of the myocardial reserve, but alternatively it may be terminated abruptly by an intercurrent acute MI or sudden cardiac death. These patients often have angina pectoris and/or CHF and are obviously at high risk of suffering a fatal acute event.

4. *Sudden cardiac death* is basically a clinical syndrome that accounts for over half of all the mortality related to IHD. Death occurs within minutes to hours of onset of an arrhythmia, usually ventricular fibrillation. In most cases, no recent coronary thrombosis or acute MI can be identified as the trigger event, and so there is often no obvious morphologic change to explain the fatal arrhythmia. Most likely preexistent IHD, whatever the morphologic pattern, induces changes leading to electrical instability. Ventricular fibrillation may then develop with any sudden imbalance between myocardial supply and needs.

It is evident that the patterns of IHD are closely interrelated. A long history of repeated attacks of anginal pain frequently precedes the development of an acute MI. Analogously, CIHD is a fertile soil for the development of angina pectoris and/or MI, and all three morphologic patterns may without notice be acutely terminated by sudden cardiac death. Thus, the individual patient may suffer from one or more of the clinicopathologic patterns of IHD.

INCIDENCE. IHD in its various forms accounts for about 60 to 75% of all deaths caused by heart disease. It is the leading cause of death in the United States and other industrialized nations. In 1979 it was responsible for approximately 600,000 deaths in the U.S., representing about 30% of the total mortality. *Alone, IHD causes over 200,000 more deaths annually in the U.S. than all forms of cancer and infection, collectively.* Awesome as these data may be, a ray of light has appeared. In the past two decades, the mortality from IHD has declined in the U.S. by about 25 to 35%.[7, 10] Other countries have enjoyed similar good fortune—Canada, Australia, Finland, Japan, Switzerland, Italy, and France—but not all to the same degree.[11] A recent autopsy study relates this trend to a general reduction in the severity of coronary atherosclerosis.[12] Speculations are rife as to the reasons for the control of this atherosclerotic epidemic. Favored notions include more vigorous control of hypertension; reduction in cigarette smoking; lowered consumption of cholesterol-containing foods; a shift in consumption from saturated animal fats to polyunsaturates; a growing awareness of the benefits of weight reduction and regular physical exercise; and improved medical management of threatened and overt IHD. The relative importance of each of these variables is a subject of vigorous debate.

Because of the dominating importance of coronary atherosclerosis, the distribution of IHD in the population of the U.S. follows that of atherosclerosis in general (discussed on p. 507). Since MI is the most important form of IHD, these data are detailed later (p. 557), but a few geographic differences merit mention. There is striking variation in the prevalence of IHD among the nations of the world. High-risk countries include Finland, the United Kingdom, the United States, New Zealand, Australia, and Canada. Enjoying a significantly lower risk are Japan, Switzerland, and Italy, as well as developing nations (where statistical data are reasonably complete). Indeed, the death rate for coronary heart disease in 1977 was about tenfold greater in Finland and almost sevenfold greater in the U.S. than in Japan. These geographic variations are thought to reflect environmental influences believed to influence the predisposition to atherosclerosis.[13]

PATHOGENESIS. *At the most fundamental level, IHD is caused by an imbalance between the myocardial blood flow and the metabolic demand of the heart.* Underlying the imbalance is either an absolute reduction in coronary blood flow, usually as a consequence of atherosclerotic disease, or an inability to increase the flow adequately when demand rises. Three factors are involved: (1) the adequacy of coronary arterial flow, (2) the level of myocardial metabolic demands, and (3) the available oxygen content of the blood. Of these three, the first is overwhelmingly the most important.

Reduced Coronary Flow. *Reduction in coronary arterial flow is almost always related to progressive stenosing, complicated atherosclerosis, sometimes worsened by superimposed events such as vasospasm, thrombosis, or circulatory changes leading to hypoperfusion.* The following general comments about the arterial involvement are applicable to all forms of IHD.[14]

1. The genesis of coronary atherosclerosis is identical to that of systemic atherosclerosis (discussed on p. 513), and the same "risk factors" apply.

2. There is surprisingly little difference in the extent and severity of coronary atherosclerosis among the clinical patterns of IHD.

3. With rare exceptions, in fatal IHD, at least one, usually two, or all three of the major coronary epicardial trunks have many stenoses that reduce the cross-sectional area of the lumen by more than 75% (Fig. 13–2). *As the terms are used here, stenosis refers to narrowing of the lumen, whereas occlusion implies total obstruction.* The degree of narrowing is critical. Resistance to flow is normally maximal at the level of the coronary arterioles. It requires more than a 75% reduction of the cross-sectional area of the lumen of an epicardial trunk to restrict the volume flow to the arteriolar bed. Lesser degrees of narrowing have little or no effect on myocardial perfusion.

4. The severe narrowings occur throughout the length of the three epicardial major trunks.[15] Infrequently the left main stem is stenosed proximal to its bifurcation.

5. Almost always, functionally significant narrowings are caused by so-called complicated plaques (p. 511). Often they are ulcerated and have an overlying thrombus or an intraplaque hemorrhage, with ballooning and rupture of the lesion.

6. Thromboses (recent or old) may be present in all three forms of IHD. They are more likely with acute MI but may be absent. Intercoronary anastomoses may prevent infarction despite thrombosis, and, conversely, infarction may occur in the absence of thromboses as with a hypotensive crisis and narrowed coronary arteries. Thus, *coronary artery thrombosis is not synonymous with acute MI.*

7. *In summary, advanced coronary atherosclerosis is usually present in all forms of IHD. Usually, there are narrowings greater than 75% of the lumen, but superimposed thromboses may or may not be present even with acute MI. It is impossible to gauge the severity or nature of the myocardial lesions from an examination of the coronary arteries.*

Hemodynamic alterations may compromise coronary flow, particularly in vessels already narrowed. In the normal state, the effective perfusion pressure depends on the pressure differential between the ostia and the coronary sinus. Since myocardial blood flow is maximal during diastole, coronary perfusion is dependent on the aortic diastolic pressure. Systolic contraction of the heart exerts a compressive effect on the intramyocardial ramifications of the major coronary trunks, increasing resistance to flow. Moreover, during systole, the rapid flow of ejected blood past the coronary orifices has a Venturi effect and so further reduces the perfusion pressure. The subendocardial region of the left ventricular myocardium is more vulnerable to a perfusion deficit than the outer zone of the myocardium. The inner myocardial cells must shorten more with each systolic contraction than those in the outer layers; thus, they have a higher metabolic demand, they exert a greater compressive force on the vascular bed, and the subendocardial vessels (for uncertain reasons) have a lower vascular tone and therefore a more limited reserve for dilatation. Marginal perfusion deficits thus may damage the subendocardial region while sparing the outer zone.

The most important hemodynamic cause of reduced coronary perfusion is a significant drop in blood pressure. Thus, shock or a hypotensive episode, as may occur during surgery, in an individual with preexisting fixed narrowings may precipitate acute myocardial ischemia and infarction. Any elevation in pressure in the right atrium and coronary sinus, as occurs with marked tricuspid regurgitation, reduces coronary perfusion by lowering the differential in pressure across the coronary system. Stenosing fibrocalcific disease of the aortic valve may also impact on coronary perfusion by extension into the root of the aorta to directly narrow the ostia. The increased resistance to ventricular outflow also raises intraventricular pressure and the compressive systolic pressures on the intramyocardial vascular bed. Analogously, aortic regurgitation affects the coronary circula-

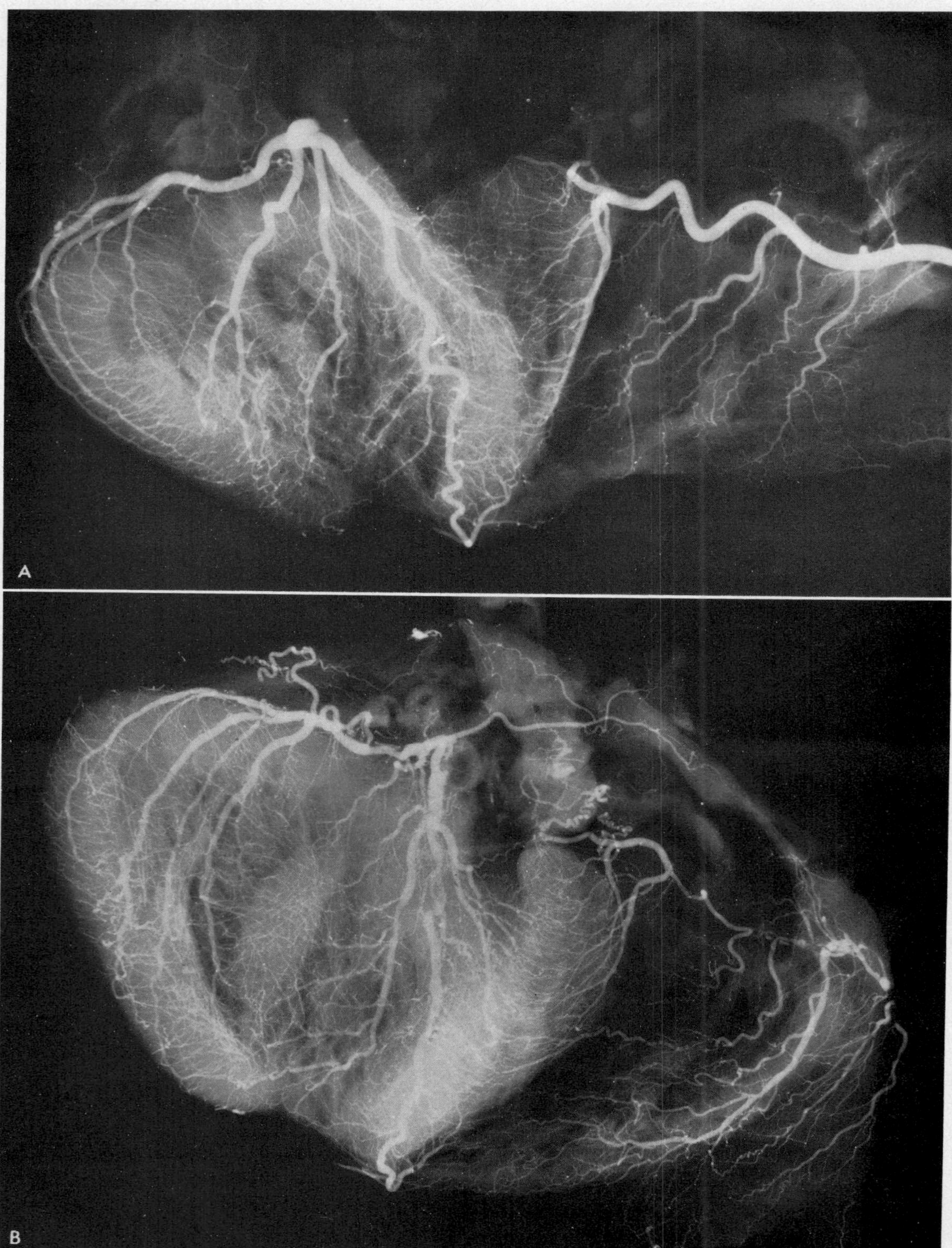

Figure 13–2. *A,* Angiogram of opened heart with normal coronary arteries filled with radiopaque mass. On right is the horizontal main right coronary artery with small descending twigs. On left is visualized the major left descending ramus and the horizontal major left circumflex ramus. Between these two are several large accessory branches. The vessels show progressively diminishing lumina with no irregular narrowings or obstruction. *B,* Angiogram of an opened heart with severely narrowed and occluded atherosclerotic coronaries. The right coronary artery fails to fill over much of its length. The twigs of this vessel are filled by retrograde anastomotic collaterals. There is uneven narrowing and tortuosity of the left descending ramus and left circumflex ramus. Compare with *A.*

tion adversely. Not only does it lower the diastolic pressure, but also, in the aortic valvular regurgitation of syphilitic heart disease, the leaflets are shortened and so the coronary take-offs are exposed to the forward flow of blood, heightening the Venturi effect mentioned earlier. Any of these incursions on the perfusion of the heart may become critically significant when superimposed on already compromised coronary flow related to atherosclerotic narrowings, especially in a hypertrophied heart.

Increased Myocardial Demand. *Myocardial ischemia is a relative term involving demand as well as supply.* Increased myocardial demand such as occurs during exercise, infection, pregnancy, hyperthyroidism, and other states causing tachycardia or hypermetabolism are obvious bases for the development of an imbalance. Too frequently we read of older individuals who drop dead while shoveling snow, presumably in relation to an acute cardiac ischemic event. Acceleration of the heart rate—tachycardia—both increases the metabolic demands of the heart and simultaneously diminishes the total amount of diastolic time per minute during which the most effective perfusion occurs. Myocardial hypertrophy, whatever its origins (e.g., hypertension, valvular disease, coarctation of the aorta), significantly increases the metabolic demand and is particularly dangerous because it simultaneously increases the compressive forces on the intramyocardial vessels. All of these influences may be superimposed on severe coronary atherosclerosis.

Availability of Oxygen in Blood. *Any disorder that diminishes the oxygen-carrying capacity of the blood may unfavorably alter the balance between supply and demand.* Anemia, the formation of carboxyhemoglobin in carbon monoxide poisoning, reduction of the blood Po_2 in pulmonary disease, and abnormal right-to-left shunting of blood (as typically occurs in certain forms of congenital heart disease) all render reduced levels of arterial flow even more threatening.

It is evident that many influences impinge on the balance between myocardial blood supply and myocardial needs. Although atherosclerotic narrowing of the epicardial coronary trunks is the dominating one, additional mechanisms may conspire with it to "do in" the heart and its owner. With this overview of IHD, we may turn to its various patterns.

ANGINA PECTORIS (AP)

Angina pectoris is a symptom complex of IHD characterized by paroxysmal attacks of chest pain, usually substernal or precordial, caused by myocardial ischemia that falls precariously short of inducing infarction. Although transient reversible myocardial injury (and sometimes spotty irreversible necroses) may occur, it is basically a clinical syndrome, and so our consideration of it can be relatively brief. It merits attention, not only because it is disabling and raises the "red alert" of serious myocardial ischemia, but also because its pathogenesis sheds light on the mechanisms underlying the more serious MI.

Three overlapping patterns of AP have been characterized: (1) stable angina, (2) variant or Prinzmetal's angina, and (3) unstable angina. These are not totally distinct subsets, since individual patients may manifest features of one or more patterns concurrently or at different times, and intergrades are not infrequent.[16] All are caused by fixed coronary narrowings and vasospasm in varying proportions, and although either one of these causes of ischemia may make a greater contribution than the other in a particular subset, both participate to some degree in all forms of AP. The three subsets, then, are best viewed as variations on a common theme.

Stable angina is the most common form and is therefore also called "typical AP." Usually, stable AP induces electrocardiographic ST-segment depression because the ischemia is most intense in the subendocardial region of the left ventricular myocardium. *It is characterized by paroxysms of pain related to exertion and relieved by rest.* Severe stenosing coronary atherosclerosis of the major trunks is almost always present. In addition, Blumgart and colleagues demonstrated that frequently there were occlusions of small epicardial atherosclerotic branches of one of the main coronary trunks.[17, 18] Presumably, intercoronary anastomoses prevented acute infarction, but the occlusive lesions may further compromise the adequacy of coronary flow and induce spotty myocardial necroses. Thus, individuals with this form of angina often have numerous small myocardial fibroses typical of chronic ischemic heart disease, and sometimes large fibrous scars of past acute MIs. *The effort-induced pain denotes that increased myocardial metabolic demand related to increased heart rate, myocardial contractility, or blood pressure (or all three) beyond the supply capacity of the severely atherosclerotic coronary arteries underlie this form of angina.* In some instances the attack of pain follows a level of exertion that would ordinarily be readily tolerated. Moreover, the pain can usually be alleviated by such vasodilators as nitroglycerin. It is possible therefore that coronary vasospasm may contribute, at least to a small degree, to the production of some of the episodic imbalances between supply and demand.

In 1959, Prinzmetal and co-workers described a form of angina that classically occurred at rest, which since has been designated Prinzmetal's or variant AP.[19] They postulated that it was caused by reversible spasm superimposed on atherosclerotic lesions. Subsequent angiographic studies have confirmed that individuals with Prinzmetal's variant angina have a spectrum of coronary findings ranging from near-normal coronary arteries to severe stenoses. Since variant angina typically occurs at rest, it is believed that *vasospasm with reduction of blood flow, rather than increase in myocardial demand, and fixed coronary disease is the major mechanism of the ischemia*; hence the frequently used synonym "vasotonic angina."[20] However, the atherosclerotic narrowing undoubtedly makes a contribution, albeit one of less importance than the vasospasm. In contrast to stable angina, Prinzmetal's variant angina is characterized by ST-segment elevation during the vasospastic attack, reflecting transmural ischemia, and total to near-total reduction of blood flow through a major coronary artery. However, other attacks in the same patient may be characterized by ST-segment depression typical of stable AP.

Unstable angina, the third pattern, is the most ominous and has been called "preinfarction angina," "acute coronary insufficiency," and "accelerated angina." These patients are at great risk of suffering a myocardial infarction. Clinically, unstable AP is characterized by prolonged pain, the onset of pain at rest in an individual with stable angina, or significant worsening of the pain of stable exertional angina. Most often these manifestations are accompanied by ST-segment depression. On angiography there almost always is severe stenosing coronary atherosclerosis. The fact that some attacks of unstable angina occur at rest and are associated with ST-segment elevation, both characteristic of Prinzmetal's angina, makes evident the variable contribution of vasospasm to the causation of this form of angina.

By definition, in AP, whatever the clinical pattern, there are no large acute lesions of ischemic myocardial necrosis, but there may well be small foci of fibrous scarring, scattered subendocardial myocardial vacuolization, and sarcoplasmic resorption (myocytolysis) as evidence of significant ischemia or large scars of past episodes of myocardial infarction. Electrocardiographic and serum enzyme analyses (detailed on p. 564) further suggest that during an acute attack these patients often have *acute* myocardial injury that in large part is reversible. Biopsies obtained during cardiac surgery (coronary artery bypass grafting) reveal areas of reversible ultrastructural changes as well as, frequently, death by myocytolysis (p. 561) of scattered individual myofibers.[21] AP is thus of importance on two scores. It warns of serious myocardial ischemia and also makes clear that vasospasm is a potent contributor to coronary insufficiency.

MYOCARDIAL INFARCTION (MI)

Myocardial infarction is overwhelmingly the most important form of IHD and, indeed, cardiac disease in the United States and other industrialized nations. In 1979 about 60% of the deaths caused by IHD (p. 551) in the U.S. were attributable to MI. The remainder were caused by chronic ischemic heart disease, marked frequently by large myocardial scars from past episodes of MI. In the aggregate, then, MI accounts for 20 to 25% of all fatalities in atherosclerosis-prone societies. To place these deaths in some perspective, they exceed by many thousands those related to all forms of neoplasia collectively.

Mortality data do not tell the whole story. Each day in the U.S about 3400 individuals suffer a "heart attack" (myocardial infarct). In more personal terms, a North American male has a one in five chance of having an MI or dying suddenly from an acute ischemic event before reaching the age of 65 years. It is painfully evident that MI is the number one cause of death and clinical challenge in affluent societies.

In the great majority of cases, widespread severe coronary atherosclerosis of the coronary arteries underlies MI. In addition, some sudden event such as coronary thrombosis must unfavorably alter the precarious balance (Fig. 13–3). Excessive exercise and increased myocardial demands can be documented in less than 15% of instances. Alternatively, the myocardial supply can be suddenly reduced by a superimposed occlusive thrombosis or by vasospasm, but the precise frequency of these events is still uncertain. *Whatever the sequence of events, the imbalance between myocardial needs and supply induces an episode of acute myocardial ischemia having one of four possible consequences: (1) it may only induce an attack of angina; (2) more severe ischemia may result in myocardial necrosis limited to the inner one-third to one-half of some portion or the entire circumference of the left ventricular wall to produce multiple subendocardial foci of ischemic necrosis, also called a "subendocardial infarct"; (3) the ischemic necrosis may more or less traverse the entire thickness of some portion of the left ventricular wall, creating a "transmural infarct"; or (4) the acute ischemic event*

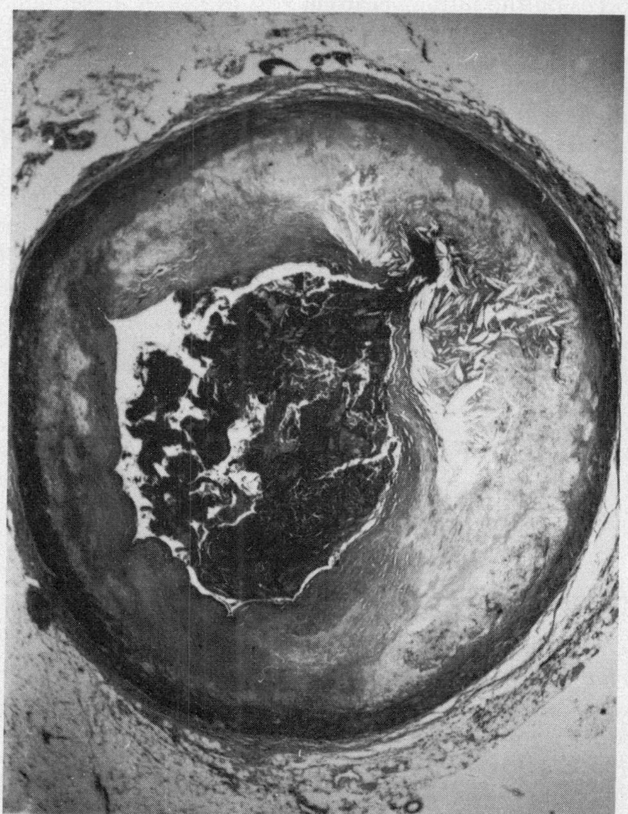

Figure 13–3. Cross section of a coronary artery narrowed by atherosclerosis. Rupture of a plaque at 2 o'clock has extruded atheromatous debris and initiated an occlusive thrombus within the lumen.

may cause "sudden cardiac death" within a few hours. Many of these sudden deaths are attributable to ischemia-provoked ventricular arrhythmias.

EPIDEMIOLOGY. Because of the dominating importance of coronary atherosclerosis in its pathogenesis, the epidemiology of MI is the epidemiology of atherosclerosis (p. 506). The striking geographic differences and the declining frequency in the United States and elsewhere in the mortality from ischemic heart disease, discussed earlier (p. 552), of necessity apply to MI, the principal cause of death from IHD. Whites are affected more often than blacks in the U.S., but for unknown reasons blacks tend to die of MI at an earlier age. *The incidence of fatal MI progressively rises with age* to peak in the 55- to 64-year-old group in males and in the eighth decade in females. Approximately 90% of all male deaths occur between the ages of 35 and 64. MI may occur in the very elderly, however, as well as in younger individuals, even in the third decade of life, particularly when such predispositions to atherosclerosis as hypertension, diabetes mellitus, familial hypercholesterolemia, and other causes of hyperlipoproteinemia are present. Virtually throughout life, males are at significantly greater risk than females, the differential progressively declining with advancing age. In the decade from 35 to 44 years, the death rate for white men is six times that for white women. In the next decade (45 to 54 years) there is a four- to fivefold difference, which falls to a twofold difference at ages 65 to 74.[22] *Except for those having some predisposing atherogenic condition, women are remarkably protected against MI during reproductive life.* However, there is now substantial evidence that the use of oral contraceptives, *as formulated in the past*, increases the risk of MI. The general data were presented on page 447. Up to the time of the studies, users who are 35 to 49 years of age have about a three- to fourfold greater risk than nonusers, and this increased risk does not appear to be related to duration of use.[23] For past users 40 to 49 years of age, the magnitude of the increased risk is related to duration of use. With less than five years of past use there is no persistent increased risk, but with long-term past use (five years or more) the risk is increased about twofold. In addition, oral contraceptives have been found to multiply the effects of other risk factors for MI such as cigarette smoking, which alone increases the risk 10- to 20-fold among young women.[24, 25] A recent report emphasizes that the risk of contraceptives may well have been exaggerated because of the difficulty in segregating their effects from other concurrent risk factors.[26] Cigarette smoking has a comparable effect among men.[27]

A number of other variables influence the risk and, therefore, the epidemiology of MI, but all must be categorized as somewhat controversial. Principal among these are personality structure, regular exercise, and alcohol consumption. A number of studies have claimed that so-called type A individuals—hard-driving, impatient, competitive, compulsive—are coronary prone. However, a recent panel concluded that the findings to date, although strongly suggestive, are not conclusive.[28] Equally uncertain is the value of exercise in the prevention of coronary heart disease and, in particular, MI.[29] Several reports contend that exercise conditioning, when regularly employed, reduces the rate of fatal heart attacks.[30] These epidemiologic studies have been buttressed by the demonstration that moderate conditioning exercise of monkeys on an atherogenic diet reduces the severity of coronary atherosclerosis. Whether the physical activity in humans acts in a similar fashion or instead increases the capacity of the coronary arterial supply or its anastomoses is still uncertain. It is relevant that the level of high-density lipoprotein (HDL) is increased with exercise, which, as discussed on page 514, is inversely correlated with atherogenesis. Physical conditioning may also augment the fibrinolytic response and thereby provide a potential protective mechanism against the development of thrombi within coronary arteries.[31] So it well may be that the joggers shall inherit the earth. Moderate alcohol consumption, which is also associated with increased HDL levels, has likewise been accorded a protective role. Attractive as this last notion may be to sedentary authors, the putative beneficial effect of moderate alcohol consumption is far from proven.

PATHOGENESIS. Consideration of the pathogenesis of MI involves analysis of the sequence of events leading to the critical imbalance between the myocardial perfusion and demands. It has already been pointed out (p. 552) that severe acute ischemic episodes may have one of four consequences: (1) angina pectoris, (2) a subendocardial infarct, (3) a transmural infarct, or (4) sudden death. The first of these has already been discussed (p. 555). The remaining three require separate consideration since they have somewhat different origins.

There is general agreement that subendocardial infarction is the consequence of global myocardial hypoperfusion secondary to severe stenosing atherosclerosis of at least two, and more often all three, major coronary trunks.[32] There is further agreement that an occlusive thrombus is present in less than 10 to 20% of cases (some say rarely).[14, 33] You may recall that the subendocardial region of the myocardium works harder and is less well perfused than the outer layers (p. 553). It is proposed, therefore, that with severe stenosing bi- or tri-vessel disease, a state of chronic marginal blood flow exists. Further reduction in flow, as might occur with episodes of congestive heart failure, hypotension, cardiac arrhythmia, or any increase in myocardial demand from exercise or disease-induced tachycardia, would then tip the balance to induce irreversible damage. The extent of the subendocardial necrosis about the ventricular circumference would depend on the severity of narrowing of each of the major coronary trunks. Thus, if one vessel were relatively free of disease, the subendocardial necrosis might not encircle the ventricle.

The *pathogenesis of transmural MI* is much more controversial. The basic question is the precise nature of the trigger event leading to the critical ischemic imbalance. Two views are equally ardently proposed. *The classic view holds that the dominating cause of acute MI is thrombotic occlusion of a coronary artery. Progressive atherosclerosis presumably leads in time to rupture or ulceration of an atheroma or an intraplaque hemorrhage as the trigger events inducing the thrombosis. More recently, the possibility has been raised that thrombosis is not necessary for infarction.* Conceivably, vasospasm or other mechanisms (detailed later) might cause the infarct and possibly be followed by thrombosis, or the vasospasm might initiate thrombosis. There is, however, agreement that in at least 90% of cases there is severe multivessel stenosing atherosclerosis with at least one, usually several, narrowings greater than 75% of the lumen.[34] Moreover, there is general agreement that infrequently increased myocardial demand or hypotension in the presence of severely narrowed coronary arteries may induce an acute infarct even in the absence of thrombosis. But what transpires with most transmural infarcts?

In support of the classic view, *many studies document thrombosis in 80 to 95% of acute myocardial infarcts overlying a stenosing complicated atheromatous plaque.*[33, 35, 36] Moreover, the thrombus is located at a site and in the vessel appropriate for the area of ischemic necrosis, suggesting cause and effect. Further support comes from a coronary angiographic study of patients within four hours of the onset of an apparent MI.[37] A totally occluded coronary artery was found in 87%, and proved to be caused by a thrombus in the great majority. When angiography could not be performed until 12 to 24 hours after the onset of symptoms, a total occlusion was found in only 65% of patients. This decreased frequency could imply lysis or disruption of a preexisting thrombus or, alternatively, release of vasospasm at the site of a thrombus, relieving the total occlusion.[37] These observations in living patients buttress the contention that thrombosis is usually the critical event in the production of a transmural infarct.

Arguments, however, have been presented against the critical role of thrombosis in the pathogenesis of MI. Many studies report finding thrombi in less than 55% (some would say only about 35%) of acute infarcts.[38, 39] If thrombosis is not requisite for the initiation of an acute transmural infarct, what is the trigger event inducing the necrosis? Only some plausible scenarios can be suggested. Vasospasm might be a mechanism, as pointed out in the discussion of angina pectoris (p. 555).[40–42] MI has been observed in relatively young males with no angiographically demonstrable coronary artery disease—not even stenoses.[43, 44] Infarcts have developed during or immediately following coronary angiography in locations appropriate for the segmental vasospasm observed during the angiography.[45] Moreover, thrombosis is sometimes found later at postmortem examination at the site of the spasm. Surprisingly, even atherosclerotic vessels may further narrow under the influence of vasospasm. There is, in addition, evidence that platelet activation and the release of vasoconstrictor substances such as thromboxane A_2 and possibly serotonin may contribute to the vasospasm.[46] Platelet activation might also result in microthrombi, which, in the aggregate, could significantly reduce coronary flow.[47] *The following sequence of events can thus be proposed. An episode of vasospasm known to be transient and unpredictable from the study of many patients with Prinzmetal's angina causes a critical reduction in coronary flow or damages a large atheroma, exposing collagen and activating platelets. Platelet aggregation may reduce myocardial perfusion, or the release of vasoconstrictors (e.g., thromboxane A_2) from the activated platelets might worsen vasospasm. By any of these pathways an infarct results and, with or without a superimposed arrhythmia, reduces coronary perfusion, potentiating the formation of a thrombus, logically at the site of vasospasm or possibly at a critical stenosis.*

As pointed out earlier, sudden cardiac death (SCD) may follow any form of IHD, but study of these patients sheds some light on the possible pathogenesis of acute MI. The deaths are attributable to the sudden onset of some fatal arrhythmia, usually ventricular fibrillation. Presumably some acute ischemic event precipitated the arrhythmia in a heart already having precarious electrical instability. A study of 923 individuals who were unconscious and pulseless when medical assistance arrived revealed that most of the victims were in ventricular fibrillation or asystole.[48] Fewer than 50% of the patients (some say as few as 13 to 28%) who are resuscitated after virtual SCD later have detectable acute MI.[49] But even when an infarct is later found, the question arises, did it initiate the arrhythmia, or was it precipitated by it? The frequency of *acute* thrombi in individuals who were temporarily rescued is related to duration of survival following the onset of symptoms, and ranges from 10% to about 50% of cases.[50] Despite the usual absence of a major thrombotic occlusion, there frequently are platelet aggregates and microthrombi in the intramural coronary branches.[51] Moreover, *in over 90% of cases there is extensive coronary atherosclerosis in at least one, and sometimes all three, coronary trunks, more severe on the average than in controls.* In addition, about one-half of the patients have evidence of an old MI. It therefore is now believed that *most SCDs occur in individuals having severe coronary atherosclerosis, often an old MI but only infrequently an acute MI. Significantly, most have no acute major coronary occlusion, but instead platelet-fibrin microthrombi. Thus, it appears that SCD, related to an arrhythmia, is caused by some acute ischemic event* that is not necessarily initiated by a thrombotic occlusion of a major coronary vessel.[52] It is possible, therefore, that a similar process, more severe or more prolonged, might lead to an acute MI.

We can go no further in unraveling the precise sequence of events. *Although in all likelihood coronary thrombosis is the major cause, it seems best to consider an acute transmural MI a multifactorial disorder related to influences acting singly or in combination that increase myocardial demand or decrease coronary per-*

fusion.[53] The issue of the precise event that initiates an MI is more than academic. If thrombosis is the initiating event, anticoagulation therapy might be of benefit to high-risk patients such as those with a previous infarct or unstable angina. Even if thrombosis were a secondary event, its prevention might speed the rate of healing of the myocardial lesion or even limit or reduce its size. Moreover, efforts to lyse thrombi during the early hours of MI by the intracoronary infusion of such thrombolytic agents as streptokinase might be of benefit. If vasospasm makes a substantial contribution, other therapeutic approaches are open. The same speculation could be offered for platelets. So it is that we are still struggling to understand the origins of acute MI, a disease that has been well characterized for over half a century and is the number one cause of death in many countries.

MORPHOLOGY. Acute myocardial infarcts may take one of two forms—transmural infarction or subendocardial infarction—with occasional overlaps. The classic transmural infarct will be described first, followed by a brief characterization of the subendocardial infarct.

Virtually all transmural infarcts involve the left ventricle (including the interventricular septum). When they affect the posterior free wall and posterior portion of the septum, they extend into the adjacent right ventricular wall in about 15 to 30% of cases.[54] Isolated infarction of the right ventricle is extremely uncommon. Either the thicker-walled left ventricle carrying the brunt of the cardiac work load is more vulnerable to hypoxia than the thinner-walled right ventricle, or the critical narrowing of the right coronary rarely occurs sufficiently proximal to affect the blood supply to the right ventricle. Atrial infarction is even more infrequent than right ventricular infarction. Most often it occurs in conjunction with a large posterior left ventricular infarct that extends into the right ventricle and into one or both of the atria. Rarest of all is isolated atrial infarction, most often on the right. Atrial infarctions are worthy of note because they are almost always followed by mural thrombosis within the affected chamber and sometimes by cardiac rupture.[55]

The **transmural infarct** as the term implies, extends from the endocardium to the epicardium. By agreed definition, the area of ischemic necrosis must be at least 2.5 cm in greatest diameter. It may be massive in size and sometimes may involve the entire circumference of the left ventricle. Usually infarcts range from 4 to 10 cm in longest dimension. The correlation between myocardial pathology and coronary artery pathology is imperfect. Infrequently, an acute transmural MI is encountered in the absence of significant coronary atherosclerosis; thus, it is presumed that the causal mechanism was vasospasm. Similarly, a thrombus may or may not be present, as already pointed out. Despite these inconstancies, severe stenosing coronary atherosclerosis is generally present and the frequencies of critical narrowing (and possibly thrombosis) of each of the three main arterial trunks and the associated myocardial lesions are as follows:

Left anterior descending coronary artery (40 to 50%)	Anterior wall of left ventricle near apex; anterior two-thirds of interventricular septum.
Right coronary artery (30 to 40%)	Posterior wall of left ventricle; posterior one-third of interventricular septum
Left circumflex coronary artery (15 to 20%)	Lateral wall of left ventricle

Other locations are sometimes encountered, such as the left main stem coronary artery. As pointed out earlier (p. 553), the stenoses may be located throughout the entire epicardial length of each of the three trunks. One virtually never encounters stenosing atherosclerosis or thrombosis of a penetrating intramyocardial ramification of the epicardial trunks. Occasionally, a thrombus is present in the absence of an MI, or the converse may be true, as already stressed. Occlusive thrombosis may not cause infarction when functioning intercoronary collaterals or anastomoses are adequate to maintain sufficient flow. Multiple severe stenoses or thromboses may be present with only a single transmural infarct. Here it must be assumed that collateral circulation was adequate, despite the initial arterial lesion to maintain the viability of the dependent myocardium, but that eventually the second arterial narrowing or occlusion rendered the anastomotic flow inadequate. Thus, it is possible for a severe stenosis or thrombosis of the right coronary artery to cause an infarction in the area of supply of the left anterior descending. Presumably, marked narrowing of the left anterior descending led to the development of collateral circulation from the right coronary artery. Subsequently, progressive encroachment or sudden occlusion of the right coronary flow resulted in infarction of the myocardium sustained by the collateral circulation. Such a phenomenon is referred to as **infarction at a distance** or **paradoxic infarction.**

Although most transmural infarcts occur singly, it is not infrequent to find several of varying age in the same heart. The patient may survive the initial insult only to succumb to a second weeks to years later. Indeed, recurrent infarctions are commonplace. Alternatively, expansion of an infarct may lead to lesions of varying age. Examination of the heart in such cases often reveals a central zone of infarction that is days to weeks older than a peripheral margin of more freshly ischemic necrosis. An initial infarct may expand because of retrograde propagation of a thrombus, more proximal vasospasm, impaired cardiac contractility that renders more proximal stenoses critically insufficient, the development of platelet-fibrin microemboli, or the appearance of an arrhythmia. Such a sequence of events is called **progressive infarction.**

Depending on the length of survival of the patient, the transmural infarct undergoes a progressive sequence of macroscopic changes.[56] Because of the time required for biochemical reactions to effect morphologic changes, myocardial infarcts **less than six to 12 hours old** are usually inapparent on gross examination. A slight pallor may be present. It is sometimes possible to highlight the gross area of ischemic necrosis within the first three to six hours by histochemical techniques. Because oxidative enzymes are depleted in the area of ischemia, immersion of tissue slices in a solution of triphenyl-tetrazolium chloride imparts a red-brown color to noninfarcted myocardium where oxidative enzymes are preserved, revealing the infarcted areas as an unstained pale zone.[57, 58] **By 18 to 24 hours** the infarct, even in the unstained heart, is usually more clearly anemic and gray-brown, contrasting with the surrounding normal red-brown myocardium. The consistency is still unaltered. Between the **second and fourth days,** the necrotic focus becomes more sharply defined with a hyperemic, quite irregular border owing to the interdigitating pattern of vascular supply. The central portion is distinctly yellow-brown and soft, owing to the onset of fatty change. Between the **fourth and tenth days,** the infarct is easily distinguished and varies from yellow-gray to bright yellow with the pro-

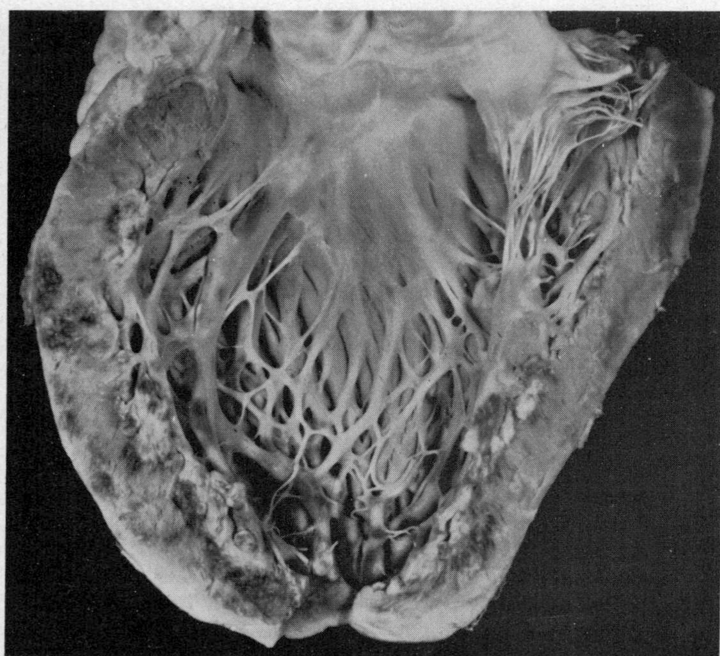

Figure 13–4. Myocardial infarction. A transmural infarct of approximately one week's duration. The necrotic muscle is pale and is rimmed by darker increased vascularization.

gression of fatty change. The central necrotic tissue is maximally soft and often contains areas of hemorrhage. The margins are intensely red and highly vascularized (Fig. 13–4). Becoming grossly apparent at approximately the **tenth day,** there is progressive replacement of the necrotic muscle by the ingrowth of fibrous, vascularized scar tissue. In most instances, this scarring is well advanced by the end of the sixth week, but the time required for total replacement depends on the size of the original infarct.

There are many complications associated with transmural MIs. **The anterolateral or, more often, the posteromedial papillary muscle may undergo infarction** when the contiguous free wall is affected. The resultant loss of papillary muscle contraction may acutely induce incompetence of the mitral valve that can persist with fibrous healing of the infarct. Even worse, the **acutely infarcted papillary muscle may rupture transversely** to cause catastrophic gross incompetence of the mitral valve. A **fibrinous** or **fibrinohemorrhagic pericarditis** usually develops about the second or third day. This may be localized to the region overlying the necrotic area or it may be generalized. With healing of the infarct, the pericarditis usually resolves, but occasionally it organizes to produce permanent **fibrous adhesions.** Involvement of the ventricular endocardium often results in **mural thrombosis,** which produces a risk of **peripheral embolism**, and later dense fibrous thickening (Fig. 13–5). **Rupture of the infarct** occurs in 1 to 5% of cases. The median time to rupture is four to five days when the ischemic focus is maximally soft.[59] However, rupture may occur within a day of infarction or, in other instances, as late as the end of the second week. Most ruptures lead to massive pericardial hemorrhage and **cardiac tamponade.** Rupture of the interventricular septum produces a left-to-right shunt.[60] With large infarcts, the developing fibrous scar may undergo progressive ballooning in the course of months to years, eventually to produce a **ventricular aneurysm** (Fig. 13–5). Mural thrombosis is common in such aneurysms.

The histopathologic changes also pursue a more or less predictable progression.[56, 61] The irreversibly injured cells undergo typical ischemic coagulative necrosis (Fig. 13–6). Under the light microscope **with routine tissue stains the coagulative necrosis is not detectable for the first four to eight hours.** However, a number of more subtle changes may be seen at this time. There may be slight separation of the myocardial fibers by edema fluid. **Stretching and waviness of the myocardial fibers at the border of the infarct may appear an hour after the onset of ischemia.**[62] It is thought that these changes result from the forceful systolic tugs by the viable fibers immediately adjacent to the noncontractile dead fibers, stretching and buckling them (Fig. 13–7). There may be some elongation of the nuclei in the wavy fibers and sometimes an increased eosinophilia of the

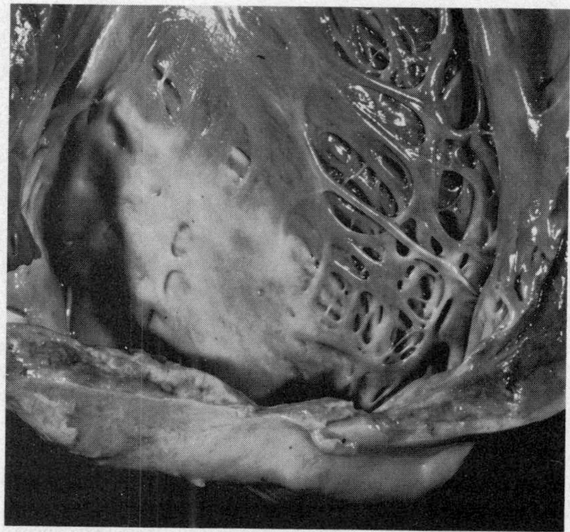

Figure 13–5. Healed myocardial infarction. Myocardium of apical region is thinned and pale gray, with some aneurysmal dilatation. Subendocardial fibrosis is apparent as pale gray thickening of endocardium.

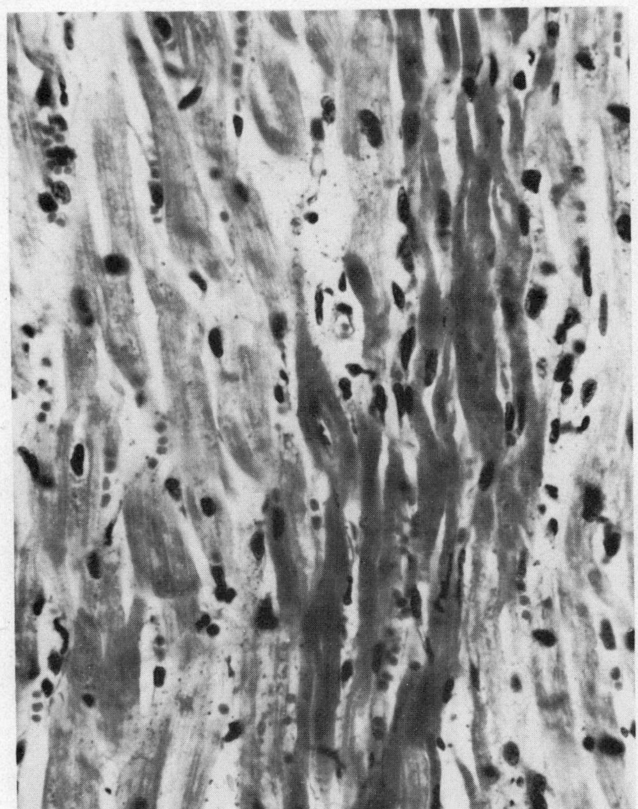

Fig. 13–6

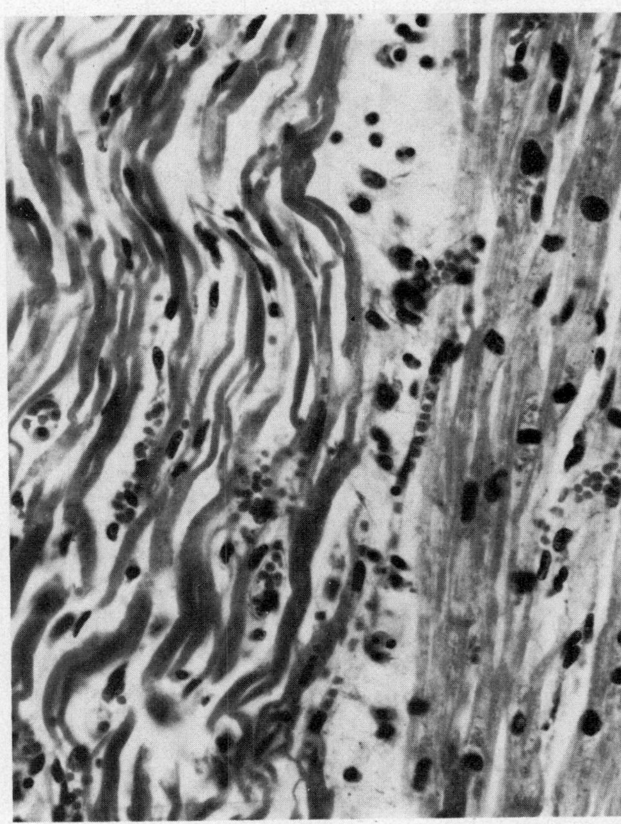

Fig. 13–7

Figure 13–6. A small focus of acute infarction (two days old) on margins of a large infarct. Dark coagulated myofibers with preserved outlines contrast with surrounding viable normal myocardial cells.

Figure 13–7. "Wavy fibers" in a two-day-old infarct showing coagulative changes, elongation, and narrowing as compared with normal fibers to right. Widened spaces between the dead fibers contain edema fluid and scattered neutrophils.

cytoplasm. However, wavy fibers are not present in many cases and, moreover, they have been identified in other forms of heart disease in the absence of myocardial necrosis; thus, they are not pathognomonic of infarction. Usually within 24 hours the morphologic changes have evolved sufficiently to be evident (in routine tissue stains) as classic coagulative necrosis. The necrotic fibers have increased eosinophilia, granularity of the cytoplasm, and nuclear pyknosis or karyolysis. Cross striations are usually visible even in coagulated fibers, although they may be blurred, but they progressively disappear over the ensuing few days. Usually within the first day, interstitial edema, fresh hemorrhage, and scant neutrophilic exudation appear in the margins of the infarct. During the second day, the neutrophilic exudation becomes more marked, the dead fibers more distinctly coagulated, and all nuclei begin to disappear. Some cells undergo progressive lysis of myofibrils **(myocytolysis),** producing clear vacuolation of the sarcoplasm and eventually leaving only empty sarcolemmal sheaths. Over subsequent days, the neutrophils are progressively replaced by macrophages and the coagulated cytoplasm becomes filled with finely dispersed fat droplets. Removal of the necrotic cytoplasm occurs by two mechanisms: release of lysosomal enzymes and phagocytosis by scavenger macrophages. Fibrovascular ingrowth becomes evident in the margins toward the end of the first week and usually completely replaces the area of necrosis by six weeks, although in very large infarcts central islands of persistent necrotic muscle may be present, even months after the acute event (Fig. 13–8).

The margins of the irreversibly coagulated cells may disclose a second pattern of acute ischemic cell injury, namely **contraction band necrosis.** While the central coagulated cells become arrested in a relaxed state, at the edges of the infarct there is some marginal reperfusion and the cells may eventually die in a hypercontracted state, producing intensely eosinophilic bands that span the width of the myofiber (Fig. 13–9).[63] Ultrastructural studies confirm marked shortening of sarcomeres, approximation of I bands, and calcium matrix densities within mitochondria. This distinctive pattern of contraction band injury and necrosis is not limited to the margins of acute infarcts but is also seen following temporary severe ischemia followed by reflow, and so is frequently encountered in patients undergoing coronary artery surgery, and is also seen in shock and following exposure to high levels of catecholamines and cardiotoxic drugs. The margins of a transmural infarct have also attracted a great deal of attention because of the hope that precariously viable border zones might be saved by acute intervention to reduce the size of the lesion.[64] Even in transmural infarcts there is usually a very narrow zone, only a few cells thick, of preserved subendocardial and subepicardial muscle. Presumably these cells are maintained by

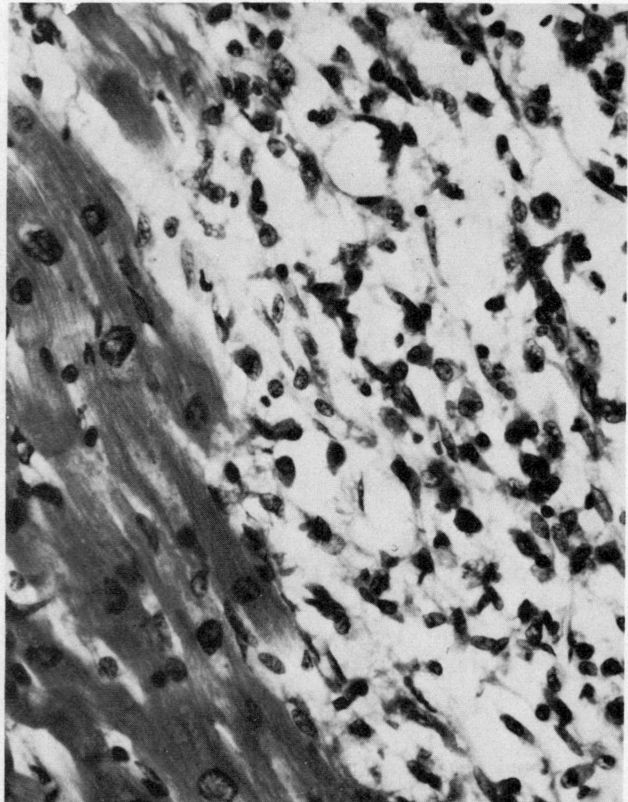

Figure 13–8. Healing margin of a ten-day infarct. Loose fibrovascular connective (granulation) tissue has totally replaced the infarcted myofibers.

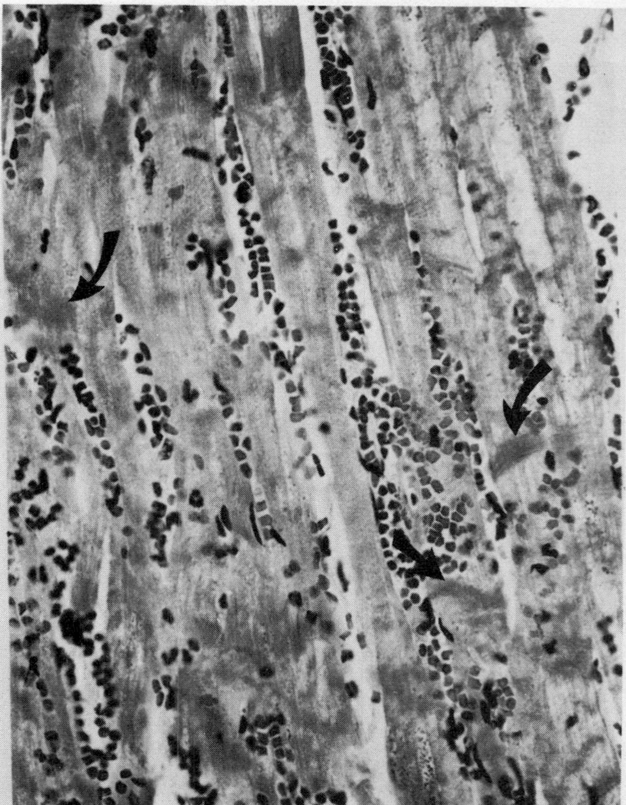

Figure 13–9. Contraction band necrosis *(arrows)* visible as dark bands spanning the myofibers. There is hemorrhage and neutrophilic infiltration between the fibers.

imbibition and collateral subepicardial vessels. More at issue are the lateral borders. Although opinions vary, most studies do not find a significant margin of reversibly injured myocardium when infarcts have evolved sufficiently to reveal unmistakable evidence of myofiber necrosis.[65, 66] This, however, does not preclude the possibility that in the early hours after an acute event there may be a perimeter of injured but salvageable tissue that, over the subsequent four to eight hours, either completely recovers or dies. Prompt interventions in the first three to four hours, therefore, might favorably influence the size of the infarct.[64]

Early histologic recognition of acute MIs continues to be a problem of considerable importance, as in the individual who dies within minutes to a few hours of a possible acute ischemic event. Depletion of glycogen granules, slight swelling of mitochondria, slight margination of nuclear chromatin, and focal dilatation of sarcoplasmic reticulum can be seen by electron microscopy after 10 to 15 minutes of coronary occlusion in the dog. Similar changes are believed to take place in infarcted human myocardium. With increasing duration of ischemia (20 to 60 minutes), mitochondrial swelling increases and amorphous densities appear within the mitochondrial matrix.[67] The matrix densities are composed of calcium phosphate and probably imply loss of normal membrane permeability and irreversible injury. With the passage of time, the clumping of chromatin at the periphery of the nuclei becomes more marked and is accompanied by swelling of the endoplasmic reticulum and the entire cell. Vacuoles sometimes appear within the cytoplasm and under the sarcolemmal membrane, and in three to six hours rupture of sarcolemmal membranes marks the cell as dead. Regrettably, autolytic changes mimic many of these alterations, severely limiting their usefulness in the usual postmortem examination of the heart. Biochemical analysis provides a promising approach. Within 10 to 15 minutes after an ischemic event, potassium is lost and sodium is increased in the infarcted area.[68] Thus, a **clear-cut decrease in the potassium-sodium ratio, as compared with the normal myocardium,** marks an area as infarcted, but this technique is of limited value in mapping the outlines of an infarct, and sometimes is not definitive. Histochemical techniques demonstrate reduced levels of succinic and isocitrate dehydrogenase, cytochrome oxidase, and phosphorylases within one to three hours following the onset of infarction. Depletion of glycogen within infarcted cells, as demonstrated by the periodic acid–Schiff (PAS) reaction, begins to appear in the experimental animal within five minutes of coronary ligation and is well developed in human lesions thought to be 30 to 60 minutes old. Still other techniques have been explored but none are completely reliable, and so identification of very early infarcts continues to be a problem.

The morphologic changes in transmural infarcts are summarized in Table 13–1, which attempts to correlate the various investigative modalities.

We can now turn to a brief characterization of the **subendocardial infarct, also referred to as subendocardial ischemic necrosis.** As mentioned, these are typically multifocal areas of necrosis confined to the inner one-third to one-half of the left ventricular wall. The focal lesions are less sharply demarcated than the classic transmural infarct and may be sufficiently subtle to be difficult to establish at gross examination. The tetrazolium staining technique facilitates the delineation of the necrotic areas (Fig. 13–10). Often they fan out widely over a large subendocardial zone.

Table 13–1. SEQUENCE OF CHANGES IN MYOCARDIAL INFARCTION

Time	Electron Microscope	Histochemistry	Light Microscope	Gross Changes
0–2 hr	Mitochondrial swelling; distortion of cristae; matrix densities; relaxation of myofibrils; margination of nuclear chromatin	↓ Dehydrogenases ↓ Oxidases ↓ Phosphorylases ↓ Glycogen ↓ K and ↑ Na^{+} and Ca^{++}	? Waviness of fibers at border	
4–12 hr	Margination of nuclear chromatin		Beginning coagulation necrosis; edema; hemorrhage; beginning neutrophilic infiltrate	
18–24 hr			Continuing coagulation necrosis (pyknosis of nuclei; shrunken eosinophilic cytoplasm); marginal contraction band necrosis	Pallor
24–72 hr			Total coagulative necrosis with loss of nuclei and striations; heavy interstitial infiltrate of neutrophils	Pallor, sometimes hyperemia
3–7 days			Beginning fatty change in dead myofibers and resorption of sarcoplasm by macrophages; onset of marginal fibrovascular response	Hyperemic border; central yellow–brown softening
10 days			Well-developed fatty changes; prominent fibrovascular reaction in margins	Maximally yellow and soft; vascularized margins; red-brown and depressed
7th wk				Scarring complete

The foci of ischemic necrosis do not evolve through the sequence of macroscopic changes described for the transmural infarct. Rather, at the early stages they appear as somewhat paler or redder areas, not more than 1 cm in diameter, separated by bridges of preserved myocardium.[32] The genesis of this pattern of damage is poorly understood, but must relate to the interdigitating distribution of the blood vessels derived from different sources of supply. As small areas of cell death, they are transformed to progressively more discrete foci of redness in the course of the first week, undergo more rapid vascularization in the reparative phase, and then undergo pale, fibrous scarring. Although mural thrombi may supervene over the endocardial surface of these lesions, pericarditis, ventricular aneurysms, and rupture rarely follow. Infrequently, a subendocardial infarct assumes the confluent, well-defined appearance of the trans-

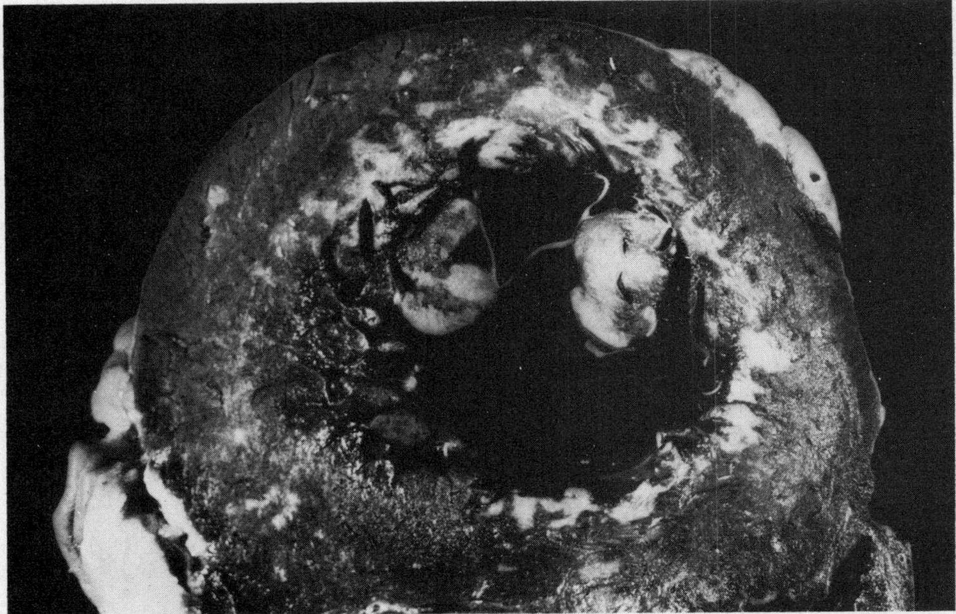

Figure 13–10. Subendocardial infarct. This slice of left ventricle has been stained for lactic dehydrogenase enzyme by the tetrazolium test. Infarcted subendocardial myocardium, which has lost the enzyme, is unstained.

mural infarct, and may then pursue the same evolving sequence of macroscopic and microscopic changes described for the transmural lesion.

Following the description of the transmural infarct and the subendocardial infarct, it is necessary to point out that, on occasion, both patterns are found in a heart. Typically, subendocardial infarction is present, involving a fairly large segment of the circumference with transmural extension in a more localized area. There is no way of ascertaining whether the transmural involvement followed on the heels of the subendocardial infarction, since both lesions often appear to be at the same stage of evolution. However, the possibility of a temporal sequence separated by a brief interval of time cannot be excluded. In some dogs, ligation of a coronary artery for 40 minutes produces subendocardial necrosis at first, but with increasing duration of coronary occlusion, the infarct tends to become transmural—referred to as the **"wavefront phenomenon."**[69] It is possible, therefore, that transmural infarcts begin with subendocardial necrosis that extends in some instances, depending on the severity and duration of the ischemia.

Clinical Course. The clinical diagnosis of acute MI is mainly based on three sets of data: (1) symptoms, (2) electrocardiographic (ECG) changes, and (3) elevations of specific serum enzymes, although other diagnostic modalities are available, e.g., radioisotope scanning. Typically, the onset is sudden and devastating with severe, constricting, crushing, burning, substernal or precordial pain that often radiates to the left shoulder, arm, or jaw. It is often accompanied by sweating, nausea, vomiting, or breathlessness. Occasionally, the clinical manifestations are much less specific and consist of burning substernal or epigastric discomfort that is interpreted as "indigestion" or "heartburn." In about one-third of patients the onset is entirely asymptomatic and the disease is only discovered later by routine ECG changes.

The ECG changes usually become evident from the outset of the attack, although they may be nondiagnostic in 20 to 25% of patients, depending on the location of the infarct, its size, and the number of ECG leads examined. The precise changes that may be encountered are too complex to be discussed here in detail, but basically they consist of new Q waves associated with evolving ST-segment and T-wave changes in transmural infarction, or only ST-segment and T-wave changes in the subendocardial infarct. As the infarct evolves, the ST segment normalizes and the T waves invert. A variety of arrhythmias also may be present, as will soon be pointed out. These may be present from the outset or appear in the course of the next few hours.

Alterations of serum enzymes are more sensitive and reliable indicators of myocardial infarction than ECG changes. Serum glutamic-oxaloacetic transaminase (SGOT), lactic dehydrogenase (LDH), and creatine kinase (CK) levels are generally elevated following an infarct. All are soluble cytoplasmic enzymes that leak out of damaged myocardial cells. However, the diagnostic specificity of these enzymes is compromised because increased levels may be observed with noncardiac lesions, e.g., elevations of SGOT with pulmonary infarction and of LDH with hepatic necrosis. Much greater specificity can be achieved with the use of particular isoenzymes. There are five isoenzymes of LDH, identified as 1 through 5. In the normal individual the serum levels of LDH_1 are lower than those of LDH_2. A reversal of this ratio is usually apparent about 12 hours after the onset of an MI, and peaks in 48 to 72 hours. This reversal has been found to be about 90% sensitive and 95% specific for acute MI, and moreover it may persist for up to six days and can thus be useful in instances of recent post infarction. However, false-positive results may be encountered from in vivo and in vitro hemolysis or renal cortical necrosis. The most specific indicator of myocardial necrosis is elevation of the MB isoenzyme of CK.[70] This isoenzyme is found in significant concentrations only in heart muscle; normally, it cannot be detected in the serum or is present in minute amounts. Thus, significant elevations are variously reported in 85 to 95% of patients following an acute MI when samples are taken at the appropriate time. The mean appearance time of this isoenzyme is about seven hours post infarction (peak levels occur at about 19 hours) and it is eliminated in about 48 hours. The level of the elevation has been used as a parameter of the size of the infarct. With all enzyme determinations, the analytic techniques and time of sampling are critical.

Radioisotope scanning techniques have added another approach to the diagnosis of myocardial infarction. Although only used in special instances, they provide a method of mapping the infarct and therefore estimating its size. Most widely used are technetium^{99m}, pyrophosphate, and thallium-201. Technetium-labeled pyrophosphate apparently binds to the calcium phosphate in the matrix densities accumulating in the mitochondria of irreversibly damaged myocardial cells. Thallium, on the other hand, distributes in the heart in proportion to the myocardial perfusion. Thus, highest concentrations appear in normal myocardium while the infarct remains "cold." Both of these scintigraphic techniques yield false-positive and false-negative results and are considerably less widely used than isoenzyme determinations. Nonetheless, a totally normal scan is strong evidence against the diagnosis of acute MI.

After the onset of an acute ischemic event, one of several pathways may be followed. Regrettably, one is very brief and marked by SCD (25% of patients).[71] Indeed, SCD accounts for about 70% of all deaths caused by IHD. However, mobile coronary care units and effective resuscitation teams now "rescue" many of these victims. If the patient develops an acute MI and reaches the hospital, the spectrum can be presented as follows:*

1. Uncomplicated cases (10 to 20%).
2. Complicated cases (80 to 90%).
   A. Cardiac arrhythmias including conduction defects (90%).

*Modified from Yu, P. N.: The acute phase of myocardial infarction. Cardiovasc. Clin. 7:45, 1975.

B. Left ventricular congestive failure with mild-to-severe pulmonary edema (60%).
C. Cardiogenic shock (10 to 15%).
D. Rupture of free wall, septum, papillary muscle (1 to 5%).
E. Thromboembolism (15 to 20%).

Cardiac arrhythmias may appear at once and undoubtedly are responsible for many sudden deaths. Often they take the form of heart block, sinus bradycardia, sinus tachycardia, ventricular tachycardia, or ventricular premature contractions. Ventricular fibrillation is the most lethal, but prompt intervention by mobile and hospital coronary care units has succeeded in controlling this form of arrhythmia in about one patient in four or five.

The next most important clinical problem in terms of both survival and frequency is left ventricular dysfunction, which varies from little or no contractile incompetence to severe "pump failure"—cardiogenic shock. Most often there is some degree of left ventricular failure with hypotension, pulmonary vascular congestion and transudation into the interstitial pulmonary spaces. This mild failure may be transient, but in others it progresses to a serious threat when intra-alveolar pulmonary edema causes marked respiratory embarrassment and even cyanosis. The most severe extreme degree of "pump failure" usually becomes manifest when more than 40% of the left ventricle is infarcted. This is marked by a profound drop in cardiac output and blood pressure and the development of cardiogenic shock. Despite all heroic efforts to improve and sustain the circulation in these patients, the mortality rate is near 80%.

Were these hazards not enough, patients still confront the risk of myocardial rupture and mural thrombosis with peripheral embolization (Fig. 13–11). As pointed out, rupture may occur through the left ventricular free wall to produce massive hemopericardium, cardiac tamponade, and sudden death. Rupture through the interventricular septum may yield grave pulmonary consequences. Rupture of the papillary muscle and valvular dysfunction is another mechanism for severe congestive failure or cardiogenic shock. The prevention of peripheral embolism by anticoagulation is usually instituted but incurs the risk of bleeding (hemopericardium, hematemesis, hematuria).

It is difficult to express a prognosis for acute MI because of many modifying influences, e.g., age of patient, previous cardiovascular status, size and site of infarct, and manner of treatment.[72, 73] Only some generalities can be offered. As pointed out, some patients rescued from SCD are later found to have had an acute MI. Thus, some of the mortality related to acute infarction is "buried" within the category of SCD. Of those who are spared this catastrophe, about 10 to 15% succumb, usually in a hospital during the first four weeks. An additional 10% die during the first year, mostly of recurrent MI or cardiac failure. There is a continued three- to fourfold excess mortality in subsequent years, related to recurrent MI and cardiac failure.

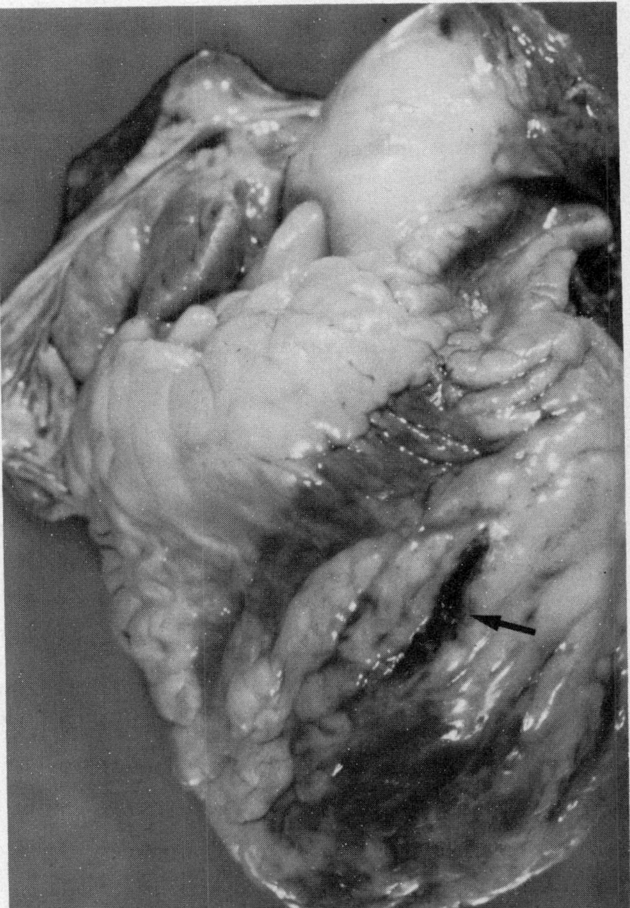

Figure 13–11. External surface of a heart with a three-day-old infarct. Dark linear tear *(arrow)* communicates with a rupture of anterior free wall of left ventricle.

Many efforts have been made to lower the incidence of MI in patients known to already have advanced coronary artery disease by reducing the major risk factors for coronary atherosclerosis (hypertension, hypercholesterolemia, and cigarette smoking). The results to date of these "secondary prevention" programs have been disappointingly equivocal. However, a very recent "primary prevention" study has been completed of men not having had any previous acute coronary events.[73A] It was focused only on lowering the hypercholesterolemia when it was above the level of 265 mg per dl of blood. Modest restriction in dietary cholesterol intake was instituted combined with cholesterol-lowering drugs (e.g., cholestyramine) and the incidence of nonfatal and fatal MIs was reduced by 20% compared with a carefully matched control group. This result is the first striking demonstration that the attack rate of MI can be lowered.

A substantial effort is also being made to improve the outlook by reducing or limiting the size of MIs with acute interventions. A variety of approaches have been used: (1) direct infusion of fibrinolytic agents, e.g., streptokinase, into the coronary arteries during the early hours after infarction to lyse thrombi;[74] and (2) agents to beneficially effect coronary perfusion, myofiber integrity, or myocardial metabolism, e.g., hyaluronidase, beta blockers, glucose-insulin-potassium, or corticosteroids.[75, 76] A major difficulty has been proof of reduction in infarct size in the living patient. Nonetheless, improvement in immediate postinfarction survival has been demonstrated.

The long-term prognosis has also been materially improved by regimens to reduce the frequency of SCD and recurrent MI in patients during the year or two following acute infarction.[77] The many approaches in current use can be only briefly mentioned—beta-adrenergic blockage (e.g., propranolol, timolol); calcium-channel blockers that, in addition to their negative inotropic and chronotropic effects, induce vasodilation (e.g., nifedipine, verapamil); anticoagulant therapy; and antiplatelet aggregating agents (aspirin, sulfinpyrazone). Significant reductions (on the order of 25 to 50%) have been achieved in the mortality from SCD and recurrent MI.[78] Still controversial is the bypass of coronary occlusions with venous grafts in an attempt to improve perfusion and prevent primary or recurrent infarction.[79] Coronary artery bypass grafts are subject to progressive intimal fibrosis, occasional thrombosis, and even atherosclerosis, but at least 60 to 80% remain patent for five or more years. It is clear that patients with ischemic heart disease are victims of an all-too-common and all-too-fatal disease, but at the same time the beneficiaries of intensive efforts to improve their outlook.

CHRONIC ISCHEMIC HEART DISEASE (CIHD)

Slow, progressive atherosclerotic encroachment on the blood supply to the myocardium may induce the insidious onset of CHF in the elderly. Frequently, one or more MIs have punctuated this course. This pattern of IHD is characterized anatomically by diffuse myocardial atrophy, loss of myocardial cells (singly and in clusters), diffuse myocardial fibrosis, and sometimes one or more large areas of scarring from past episodes of infarction. In the past, this entity has been known by a variety of terms—"aging" heart disease, atherosclerotic heart disease, and ischemic cardiomyopathy—but all are unsatisfactory. It is not the inevitable consequence of advancing years. The term "atherosclerotic heart disease" logically would also include acute infarction and AP. Cardiomyopathies, by definition, exclude myocardial damage related to coronary atherosclerosis, so the term CIHD is currently favored.

Chronic ischemic heart disease is a major cause of cardiac failure and death. It is responsible for about 40% of the mortality related to IHD, and in 1979 caused almost 250,000 deaths in the United States. In the absence of attacks of AP or acute infarction, this condition may remain entirely unsuspected until slow, progressive cardiac decompensation appears. There is an unfortunate tendency to ascribe cardiac failure to CIHD when other causes for heart failure cannot be identified. It is a distinctive form of cardiac involvement, having well-defined morphologic changes.

The heart in this condition may be normal, smaller than normal in size, or even hypertrophied. The pericardial surface is unaffected, but there may be some atrophy of subepicardial fat commensurate with the loss of subcutaneous adipose tissues encountered in very aged individuals. Almost invariably, there is moderate-to-severe stenosing atherosclerosis of the coronary arteries. There may even be foci of total occlusion, possibly resulting from organized thrombi. The myocardium is often browner than usual or may be of normal color. Scars may be grossly visible, but typically they are not more than 0.5 to 1.0 cm in diameter, almost always confined to the left ventricle. Occasionally there is an obvious well-healed infarct. The left ventricle is usually dilated. The left ventricular wall will vary in thickness, depending on the duration of failure and the extent of the myocardial adaptive changes. The mural endocardium is generally unremarkable, but there is often slight fibrous thickening of the valves of the left side of the heart sufficient to make the leaflets lose their normal translucence. The chordae tendineae of the mitral valve may be comparably thickened but are not fused or significantly shortened, as is characteristic of healed rheumatic heart disease. Heavy calcification of the mitral annulus behind the valve leaflets and piled-up masses of calcium within the sinuses of the aortic leaflets may both be present, but these valvular changes are accompaniments of the aging process and are not clearly related to ischemic injury.

The major microscopic findings are myocardial atrophy, myocytolysis of single cells or clusters of cells, and diffuse small scars, particularly about vessels (Fig. 13–12).[80] The overall decrease in size of the myocardial cells is difficult to appreciate but is made most apparent by a subtle, intercellular fibrosis and the increase in yellow-brown perinuclear lipofuscin—"aging"—pigment. Some myofibers may be en-

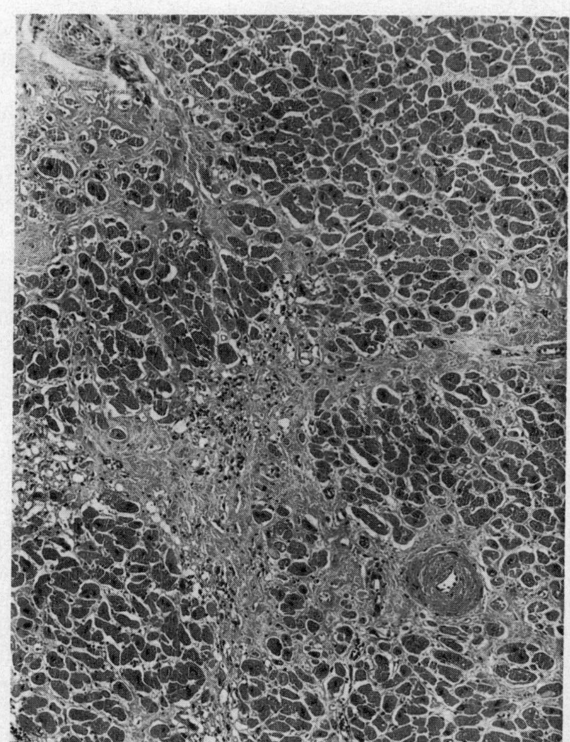

Figure 13–12. Patchy fibrous scarring principally about blood vessels of myocardium in CIHD.

larged owing to compensatory hypertrophy. Myocytolysis with resorption of sarcoplasm creates clear cytoplasmic large vacuoles or empty sarcolemmal sheaths. Collapse of the empty sheaths contributes to the appearance of the diffuse fibrosis. Large, healed myocardial scars may be present as the result of earlier episodes of acute infarction. **It is the concurrence of atherosclerotic narrowing of the coronary arteries, spotty myocytolysis, diffuse and small myocardial scars, and the changes of cell atrophy that delineates the diagnosis of CIHD.**[32]

CLINICAL COURSE. This form of heart disease is completely asymptomatic until its presence becomes manifest by the insidious appearance of cardiac decompensation, as the cardiac reserve is depleted fiber by fiber. Often it is discovered only as an incidental finding at autopsy. Some patients, however, have had attacks of angina or remote episodes of MIs. Occasionally the onset of congestive failure is more sudden and follows a precipitating illness such as pneumonia or some other form of debilitating disease. Failure, when it becomes manifest, is initially left-sided but ultimately leads to right-sided cardiac decompensation as well.

The clinical diagnosis of CIHD is made largely by the insidious onset of failure in patients who have had past episodes of MI or anginal attacks. In the absence of such evidence of severe coronary atherosclerosis, the diagnosis must rest on the exclusion of other forms of cardiac involvement in patients of advanced age.

The electrocardiographic changes merely confirm diffuse myocardial disease, sometimes with conduction bundle-branch blocks. Such murmurs as may be present are more likely related to left-sided ventricular dilatation with subsequent valvular regurgitation or to concurrent but unrelated calcific valvular changes. Generally, the congestive failure progresses slowly over the course of many years. However, a serious cardiac arrhythmia or an infarction may supervene and cause death. Patients with this condition may die of entirely unrelated causes before the cardiac involvement becomes symptomatic. It must be appreciated that in this geriatric group, patients rarely have one disease, and most often the manifestations of CIHD are intermixed with those related to all the other problems of these "not-so-golden years."

HYPERTENSIVE HEART DISEASE (HHD)

The minimal criteria for the diagnosis of HHD are (1) left ventricular hypertrophy in the absence of other cardiovascular pathology that might reasonably induce it and (2) a history of hypertension. Straightforward as this may sound, there are complexities. Hypertension strongly predisposes to atherosclerosis, and so most patients with elevated blood pressure have significant coronary atherosclerosis. It is difficult then, if not impossible, to segregate the contributions of ischemic injury with compensatory hypertrophy from those of hypertension in the induction of the cardiac enlargement. Equally bothersome is the concurrence of hypertension and some other form of heart disease in an individual with cardiac enlargement. By definition, *the diagnosis of HHD cannot be made when there is some other cause for hypertrophy,* such as aortic valvular stenosis, yet the hypertension may have contributed significantly to the hypertrophy and cardiac failure. Another problem, the definition of hypertension, is better left to clinicians and statisticians. Suffice it to note that the World Health Organization has designated 160/95 mm Hg as the dividing line, but these levels may be too high. In the Framingham Study, subjects having blood pressure readings between 140/90 and 160/95 had twice as much cardiovascular disease over the subsequent 18 years as the control group.[81]

Complexities notwithstanding, HHD is today the second most common cause of cardiac death, albeit totally overshadowed by IHD. In the United States in 1978 it caused about 7000 deaths. However, it should be noted that hypertension-accelerated coronary atherosclerosis contributes significantly to many of these deaths. About 30 to 50% of untreated hypertensives die of heart disease, and the remainder of stroke, hypertensive renovascular disease, and vascular complications (e.g., atherosclerotic aneurysms), in descending order. The mortality from hypertension and HHD over the past decades has declined in the U.S., and more among whites than among blacks. Much of this decline can reasonably be attributed to improved case finding and treatment of hypertension, but it is of interest that the decline began before effective methods of antihypertensive therapy came into wide use. Nonetheless, hypertension remains a major health problem. In the mid-1970s it was estimated that about 50% of blacks and 35% of whites in the U.S. over the age of 55 had a systolic blood pressure of at least 160 or diastolic pressure of at least 95.

PATHOGENESIS. The etiology and pathogenesis of hypertension are considered on page 1041. Here we are concerned with its effect on the heart. The blood pressure level is governed by the cardiac volume output and outflow resistance. The major components of the latter are peripheral arteriolar resistance, compliance of the large arteries, and the viscosity and inertia of the blood, all of which create resistance to the systolic ejection of blood from the left ventricle. High blood pressure places a so-called pressure overload on the left ventricle (much like aortic stenosis; aortic regurgitation, by contrast, imposes a volume overload). It does so largely by increasing the resistance to left ventricular outflow, mostly by widespread arteriolar vasoconstriction;[82] hence, the effectiveness of vasodilators in the reduction of elevated blood pressure. Once initiated, the increased blood pressure tends to rise progressively. Hypertension accelerates the development of atherosclerosis, reducing large vessel compliance, and induces thickening of the walls of small arteries and arterioles (see arteriolosclerosis, p. 518). The vascular disease in turn increases peripheral resistance and viscosity-related frictional drag. The heart, then, must maintain a normal cardiac output against this increased peripheral resistance and can accomplish this only by hypertrophy of myofibers, and so comes about the cardiac enlargement of HHD. However, thickening of the left ventricular wall imposes new burdens. The oxygen demand is increased and the left ventricular compliance reduced. The almost inevitably present coronary atherosclerosis undoubtedly adds another unfavorable element. Moreover, in aged hosts or when the stress is severe, the hypertrophied myofibers lack normal contractility.[83] Despite these problems, as long as the hypertrophy of the heart maintains a normal cardiac output, compensation may exist. Eventually, however, dilatation of the failing heart ushers in decompensation.

It is characteristic of HHD that cardiac failure usually begins insidiously and without apparent provocation. Why it commences at some point in time is a mystery, as is the precise genesis of the failure at the level of the myofiber, as already discussed (p. 548). The hypertension-induced myofiber enlargement may be pathologic with reduced contractility.[83] Another theory suggests that, with cardiac hypertrophy and increase in the size of myocardial fibers, the diffusion distance for oxygen increases and ultimately adversely affects the myofiber metabolism and function.[84] The arteriosclerosis mentioned earlier might further impair perfusion of the capillary beds.[82] Hypoxia or increased myocardial wall stress might lead to an increase in intercellular collagen, interfering with ventricular compliance and function.[85] Equally controversial is a putative reduction in the number of capillaries relative to the number of myofibers per unit volume of ventricular wall.[86] All these theories are highly speculative, and so the basis for myocardial and cardiac failure in HHD remains a mystery.

MORPHOLOGY. The principal morphologic evidences of HHD are left ventricular thickening with accompanying increases in size and weight of the heart (Fig. 13–13). It should be noted that **the anatomic diagnosis of HHD can be made only in the absence of other cardiac abnormalities, such as valvular lesions, congenital abnormalities, and diseases of the aorta, which of themselves may be productive of pressure or volume overload** and consequent myocardial hypertrophy. Such abnormalities make the anatomic diagnosis of HHD impossible, although, admittedly, concomitant hypertension may have contributed to the myocardial hypertrophy.

During the stages of compensated HHD, the hypertrophy principally affects the left ventricle. The hypertrophy may thicken the left ventricular wall to more than 2.5 cm and increase the total weight of the heart to 500 to 700 gm. Thickening of the left ventricular wall occurs at the expense of the volume of the left ventricular chamber, and is referred to as **concentric hypertrophy**. At this stage, the overall size of the heart measured by chest radiograph would not be excessive. In contrast with volume overload, as in aortic regurgitation, the hypertrophy is referred to as eccentric because the left ventricular chamber size (and heart) enlarge along with the increased thickness of the left ventricular wall.

With the onset of decompensation, dilatation of the left ventricle occurs, and the overall dimensions of the heart may then be considerably enlarged. It may be only at this time that cardiac enlargement is sufficiently prominent to be demonstrable on x-ray or clinical examination. The stretching of the heart wall decreases the thickness of the myocardium and may thus mask the preexistent thickening. Incomplete emptying of the failing left ventricle throws an increased burden through the atria and pulmonary circulation onto the right side of the heart, with resultant hypertrophy and dilatation of all cardiac chambers. Valvular deformities and pathologic involvement of the epicardium and endocardium are absent. Although coronary atherosclerosis is not an intrinsic feature of HHD, it is frequently found in such hearts because of the causal relationship mentioned previously.

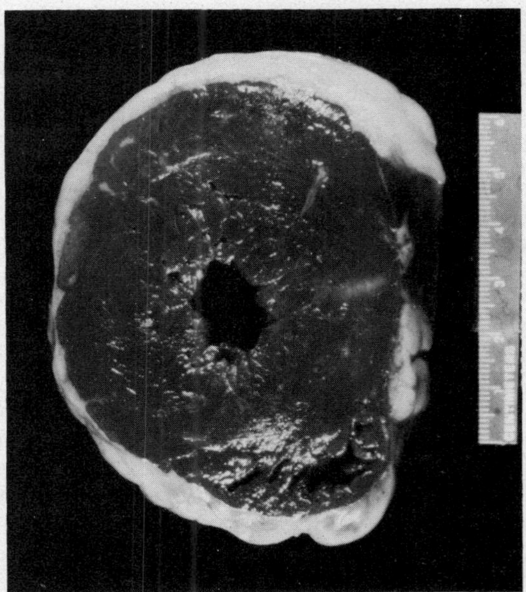

Figure 13–13. Hypertensive heart disease. Transection of heart revealing concentric marked thickening of left ventricular wall with reduction of lumen. Transected right ventricle is barely evident on lower right.

Microscopically, the changes in HHD are subtle, inconstant, and readily missed on routine examination. The myofibers may appear to be essentially normal, but micrometric analyses reveal an increase in myofiber volume and mean diameter that is more marked in the subepicardial region than in the subendocardial. The upper limit of normal myofiber diameter is generally accepted to be 12 to 13 μm. In HHD the diameters may double.[85] Nuclei in some cells are hyperchromatic and enlarged and sometimes become somewhat rectangular with squared ends, in contrast to the tapering conformation of normal myofiber nuclei. Occasionally they assume bizarre shapes and are vesicular. There may or may not be an apparent increase in interstitial collagen, but at most it is extremely subtle. In the normal heart, in appropriate planes of section a capillary can be found interposed between adjacent myofibers. No alteration in the number or distribution of capillaries is usually detectable in the hypertensive heart. However, the intramyocardial arterioles are usually thickened as a reflection of the hypertension (p. 518).

Electron microscopy of cardiac hypertrophy secondary to aortic stenosis has revealed a multiplicity of ultrastructural changes. Although it is not certain that these observations apply to hypertension-induced hypertrophy in both settings, the ultimate basis of the myofiber change is pressure overload. In mildly altered cells there is focal myofibrillar lysis with preferential loss of thick (myosin) filaments as well as proliferation of sarcoplasmic reticular tubules. More severely degenerated cells disclose more complete loss of myofibrils and degeneration of T tubules.[87] Reduction in the volume fraction of myofibrils relative to other organelles could account for poor myofiber performance.[88]

CLINICAL COURSE. Compensated HHD is asymptomatic and consists merely of cardiac enlargement without signs or symptoms of circulatory insufficiency. The patient, however, may have other symptoms of hypertension, such as palpitation, headaches, and poorly defined asthenia. Abnormalities of the retinal vessels and eye grounds, known as hypertensive retinopathy, may appear. These ocular changes are associated with extremely severe hypertension.

Symptoms of cardiac decompensation predominantly reflect left ventricular congestive failure. Diagnosis of this condition is based on the finding of systemic hypertension and clinical, roentgenologic, or electrocardiographic evidence of cardiomegaly. Other causes for the cardiac enlargement must be ruled out. In particular, cardiac hypertrophy in the absence of valvular defects may appear in certain forms of cardiomyopathy, as discussed on page 597. This possibility must be borne in mind in the clinical, and indeed the pathologic, diagnosis of HHD.

It is virtually impossible to express a course for HHD since it is dependent on the severity and progression of the elevation of blood pressure, and concurrent complications of hypertension such as hypertensive renal disease and cerebrovascular disease, and it is significantly altered by antihypertensive therapy. Although the hypertension may have been mild at the outset, there is a well-defined tendency for it to become progressively more severe when uncontrolled by therapy. With severe uncontrolled hypertension, cardiac decompensation is usually followed by death within a year. Even modest elevations of blood pressure, untreated, shorten longevity by as much as ten years.[138] It is significant that therapy for even mild hypertension significantly lowers the incidence of cardiovascular complications when other risk factors for IHD are present, e.g., hypercholesterolemia, cigarette smoking, or diabetes.[89]

COR PULMONALE (PULMONARY HEART DISEASE)

Most simply, cor pulmonale can be defined as right ventricular enlargement resulting from disorders that affect either the structure or function of the lungs. To this definition the following essentials should be added: (1) pulmonary arterial hypertension is the sine qua non responsible for the right ventricular hypertrophy or dilatation; (2) the pulmonary hypertension may result from intrinsic disease of the pulmonary parenchyma or vessels, inadequate function of the chest bellows, or inadequate ventilatory drive from the respiratory centers; (3) the cardiac involvement is confined predominantly but not exclusively to the right ventricle; and (4) right ventricular hypertrophy or dilatation resulting from congenital heart disease or acquired disease of the left side of the heart is not included under the designation cor pulmonale.[90]

Two forms of cor pulmonale are seen: acute and chronic. *Acute cor pulmonale refers to the right ventricular dilatation* that follows massive pulmonary embolization.

Chronic cor pulmonale usually implies right ventricular hypertrophy, although in time with cardiac decompensation, dilatation may follow (Fig. 13–14). The vascular lesions leading to chronic cor pulmonale are varied. Repeated small pulmonary embolizations or any form of diffuse pulmonary vascular involvement, such as is encountered in systemic hypersensitivity states and Wegener's granulomatosis, will cause pulmonary hypertension. Intrapulmonary shunts between the systemic bronchial arteries and the pulmonary arterial system sometimes arise in chronic inflammatory processes in the lung, such as bronchiectases, lung abscesses, and chronic pneumonitis imposing the systemic blood pres-

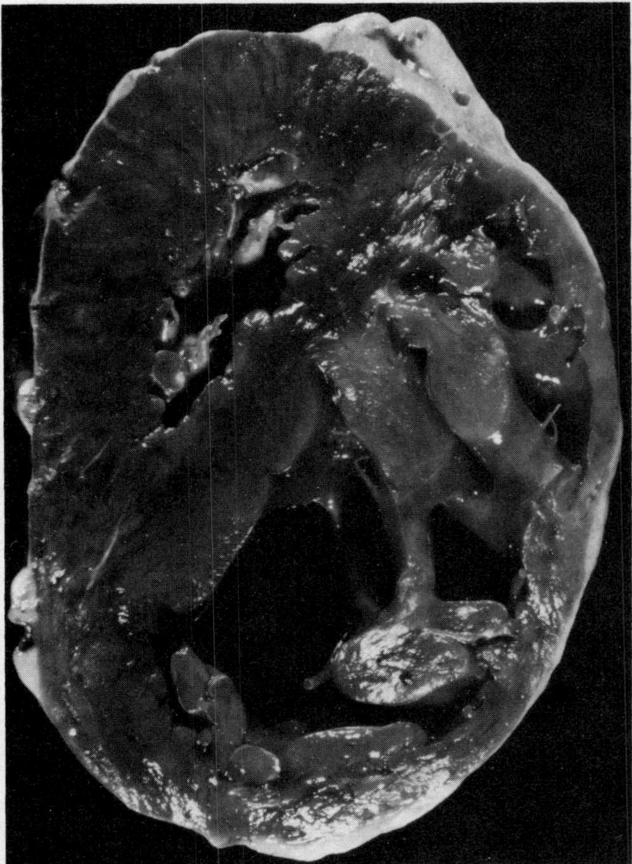

Figure 13–14. Chronic cor pulmonale. Transection of heart revealing a markedly dilated right ventricle below with thickened free wall and hypertrophied trabeculae. Transected left ventricle above has been compressed and dwarfed by right ventricular enlargement.

sure on the pulmonary pressure. Rarely, the pulmonary vascular changes are idiopathic and are termed primary pulmonary hypertension (p. 713).

Any chronic lung disease may lead to cor pulmonale, either by increasing pulmonary vascular resistance or by the induction of intrapulmonary vascular shunts. Included in this category are chronic obstructive pulmonary disease (chronic bronchitis and primary emphysema), the pneumoconioses, idiopathic interstitial fibrosis, bronchiectasis, extensive tuberculosis, and sarcoidosis. Pulmonary or mediastinal tumors that compress the vessels constitute additional causes of this form of heart disease. It is important to recognize that, *in all of these pulmonary parenchymal disorders, the polycythemia and vasoconstrictive effects of hypoxemia and respiratory acidosis contribute significantly to the development of the pulmonary hypertension.*[91]

Infrequently, chronic cor pulmonale is caused by skeletal or neuromuscular derangements that interfere with the bellows function of the chest, such as severe kyphoscoliosis, poliomyelitis, the neuromuscular dystrophies, and the pickwickian syndrome (marked obesity with inadequate thoracic excursion). Presumably, these act by the induction of hypoxemia, acidosis, and pulmonary vasoconstriction. The chronic hypoxemia, furthermore, leads to polycythemia, adding increased viscosity to the blood.

The pulmonary hypertension must usually be present for months to years before it induces right ventricular hypertrophy. During this long evolution, the cardiac changes evoke no symptoms until right-sided CHF ensues. Until then, the clinical manifestations are entirely those of the primary disorder. The diagnosis is made most often by radiography, cardiac catheterization, electrocardiography, and echocardiography.

VALVULAR HEART DISEASE

A number of acquired disorders are characterized principally by valvular involvement and dysfunction: rheumatic fever; mitral valve prolapse; aortic valve stenosis; mitral annular calcification; carcinoid heart disease; and three other conditions, characterized by the formation of valvular vegetations—infective endocarditis, nonbacterial thrombotic endocarditis, and Libman-Sacks endocarditis. The valvular cardiac ramifications of syphilis, have already been discussed on page 531. Before these disorders are presented, a few general principles are in order.

Stenosis implies failure of a valve to open completely, thereby preventing forward flow. Isolated aortic stenosis and isolated mitral stenosis account for approximately half of all valve lesions encountered. *Insufficiency* or *regurgitation, in contrast, results from failure of a valve to close completely,* thereby allowing reversed flow. Stenosis and insufficiency often coexist in the same valve, but one of these defects usually predominates. More than one valve may be involved (combined disease). These dysfunctions vary in degree from slight and physiologically unimportant to severe and rapidly fatal. The degree of tolerable stenosis or insufficiency varies from valve to valve and with the rate of development. At one end of the spectrum, sudden destruction of an aortic valve cusp by infection (infective endocarditis) may cause rapidly fatal cardiac failure. In contrast, hemodynamically significant mitral stenosis usually is remarkably well tolerated over the several decades it takes to develop. Depending on degree, duration, and etiology, valvular stenosis or insufficiency may produce secondary changes in the heart, blood vessels, and other organs, both proximal and distal to the valvular lesion. The abnormalities of flow also produce abnormal sounds (murmurs).

Valvular abnormalities may be caused by congenital disorders or a variety of acquired diseases. *Although valvular insufficiency may result from either intrinsic disease of the valve cusps or damage to the supporting structures (e.g., the aorta, mitral annulus, chordae tendineae, papillary muscles, etc.) without primary changes in the cusps; valvular stenosis almost always is due to a primary abnormality of the cusps.* The most important causes of heart valve dysfunction are summarized in Table 13–2 and are discussed in the specific sections below.

Frequently, diseased heart valves are surgically replaced by prostheses. Four major designs of cardiac valvular substitutes have been widely used—caged-ball, caged-disk, tilting-disk, and tissue valves (usually a tanned pig aortic valve mounted on a rigid frame). In addition to the perioperative deaths, there are fatalities (up to 50% of late deaths in some series) after cardiac valve replacement, induced by the prosthesis.[92] The

Table 13–2. MAJOR ETIOLOGIES OF ACQUIRED VALVULAR HEART DISEASE

Mitral Valve Disease	Aortic Valve Disease
Mitral Stenosis	***Aortic Stenosis***
Postinflammatory scarring	Postinflammatory scarring
(rheumatic heart disease)	(rheumatic heart disease)
(infective endocarditis)	Senile calcific aortic stenosis
	Calcification of congenitally deformed valve
Mitral Regurgitation	***Aortic Regurgitation***
Abnormalities of leaflets and commissures	Intrinsic valvular disease
Postinflammatory scarring	Postinflammatory scarring (rheumatic heart disease)
Infective endocarditis	Infective endocarditis
Floppy mitral valve	Aortic disease
Abnormalities of tensor apparatus	Syphilitic aortitis
Rupture of papillary muscle	Ankylosing spondylitis
Papillary muscle dysfunction (fibrosis)	Rheumatoid arthritis
Rupture of chordae tendineae	Marfan's syndrome
Abnormalities of left ventricular cavity and/or annulus	
LV enlargement (myocarditis, congestive cardiomyopathy)	
Calcification of mitral ring	

most frequent fatal prosthesis-related complications are either thrombotic occlusion of the artificial valve or distant embolization from the valvular thrombus. Valvular malfunction may result from a small thrombus or tissue fragment impairing movement of the occluder, or from degradation of materials. Partial dehiscence (separation) of the suture line anchoring the valve occasionally occurs, leading to a paravalvular leak (regurgitation of blood around the prosthesis). Destruction of blood components on passage through the prosthesis, especially a degraded valve, or around the device when there is a paravalvular leak, leads to destruction of erythrocytes and may cause severe anemia (see hemolytic microangiopathic anemia, p. 629). Infective endocarditis on the valve prosthesis is a devastating and often fatal complication. Although each type of prosthesis is subject to any of the problems cited above, the nature of the materials used and the mechanisms of action of the various prostheses lead to marked differences in frequency and type of complication. With this overview, the most important acquired diseases that affect the heart valves can be described.

RHEUMATIC FEVER (RF) AND RHEUMATIC HEART DISEASE (RHD)

Rheumatic fever is an acute, recurrent inflammatory disease, principally of children but also of adults, that usually follows a pharyngeal infection with group A beta-hemolytic streptococci. Although questions persist, *it most likely is the result of a cross reaction between the immune response to streptococcal antigens and tissue antigens, principally in the heart.* Previous infections anywhere in the body with specific strains of group A streptococci may cause acute glomerulonephritis. Thus, both RF and acute glomerulonephritis are poststreptococcal diseases, but the two conditions concur only by chance, probably because the nephritogenic strains of streptococci lack the specific antigens responsible for the cross reactions of RF.

Rheumatic fever is a systemic disease characterized principally by (1) migratory polyarthritis of the large joints, (2) carditis, (3) erythema marginatum of the skin, (4) subcutaneous nodules, and (5) Sydenham's chorea—a neurologic disorder with involuntary, purposeless, rapid movements. Uncommonly, the arteries, lungs, and periarticular tissues are also affected. During the acute attack a myocarditis may develop that tends to involve principally the interstitial connective tissue, largely close to small blood vessels; thus, RF (like RHD) is sometimes referred to as a "connective tissue" or "collagen vascular" disease. It is the late sequelae of the acute carditis (RHD), however, that are most threatening. Chronic or "healed" RHD is marked principally by deforming, postinflammatory, fibrocalcific valvular disease (particularly mitral and/or aortic stenosis), which produces permanent dysfunction and severe, sometimes fatal, cardiac failure decades later. The arthritis, although incapacitating during the acute attack, resolves without sequelae, and so it is often said: "rheumatic fever licks the joints but bites the heart."

EPIDEMIOLOGY. The incidence, morbidity, and death rate from RHD has steadily declined in most developed countries. In 1940, the mortality rate in the United States was 20.6 per 100,000, which fell to 3.4 in 1979. A number of factors have contributed to this gratifying trend. One is the possibility that the virulence of the streptococci has declined. In addition, RF is more common following epidemic outbreaks of streptococcal pharyngitis than it is following endemic sporadic infections. Improved public health measures, earlier diagnosis of infections, and more adequate methods of treatment have virtually eradicated epidemics. Equally important has been the early diagnosis and prompt treatment of sporadic streptococcal pharyngitis, since *the likelihood of RF is strongly correlated with the severity and duration of the pharyngitis and the magnitude of the immune response.*[93] Thus, RF and RHD are more frequently encountered today among the poor who live in crowded conditions and especially among those with large families—factors that favor cross infection and less than adequate medical attention. The incidence of acute RF peaks between the ages of 6 and 16 years and thereafter declines with advancing age. However, about one-fifth of first attacks occur in adults, sometimes in advanced life. There is no sex preponderance.

ETIOLOGY AND PATHOGENESIS. Although other theories persist, the weight of evidence implicates post-streptococcal immunity as the cause of RF and RHD.

1. There is a well-defined association between streptococcal pharyngitis and initial and recurrent attacks of RF. Although throat cultures at the time of the rheumatic attack are usually negative, elevated titers of antistreptolysin O (ASO), antihyaluronidase, antistreptokinase, anti-NADase, or antideoxyribonuclease B are present in all but 5 to 10% of patients.
2. Direct bacterial invasion can be ruled out since the tissue lesions are sterile. Moreover the latent period between pharyngitis and the onset of RF favors a causal role for an immune response.
3. The more severe the streptococcal infection, the stronger the antibody response, and the greater the likelihood of RF. When the organism is still recoverable after 21 days of acute pharyngitis there is an attack rate of approximately 3%, whereas those free of organisms at this time have a rate of only 0.3%.[94]
4. Most convincing, initial attacks of RF can virtually be eradicated by prompt antibiotic therapy of streptococcal throat infections, and recurrences almost totally prevented by long-term antibiotic prophylaxis.

Despite all the circumstantial evidence, many uncertainties persist. Skin infections (impetigo) caused by group A streptococci are rarely followed by RF. Why does RF mainly follow throat infections when acute glomerulonephritis may be induced by a group A streptococcal infection anywhere in the body? Equally puzzling is why only a small fraction of individuals with pharyngeal infections by rheumatogenic streptococci develop RF. Here, the issue of host factors and specific immune response genes has been raised.[95] It is speculated that only certain hosts are vulnerable to an immune reaction conducive to the development of RF.

Four distinct families of streptococcal antibodies have been identified that cross-react with the following four cellular and tissue targets: (1) cardiac myofiber–smooth muscle antigens, (2) heart valve fibroblast antigens, (3) neuronal antigens in subthalamic and caudate nuclei, and (4) heart valve and other connective tissue antigens.[96] Most consistently present (in about 80% of patients) are antibodies that bind to the sarcolemma and subsarcolemmal sarcoplasm of myofibers, to the smooth muscle cells in vessel walls and endocardium, and to foci of altered interstitial connective tissue.[96] The specific streptococcal antigens thought to evoke these antibodies are M proteins, a family of antigens found in the streptococcal cell wall.[97, 98] However, it should be noted that these antibodies are lacking in some patients with RHD, and conversely they may be present in the absence of carditis or other clinical manifestations of RF. The other antibodies mentioned above are of uncertain significance; they have been identified in patients who have recovered from streptococcal pharyngitis but who do not have RF, and, moreover, unmistakable RHD may develop in their absence. Thus, despite the plethora of antibodies, the role they play in the induction of RF and RHD is still far from clear. Significantly, the centers of Aschoff bodies—foci of apparent maximal tissue injury in acute RF—often lack concentrations of these antibodies.

Attention has turned to cell-mediated immunity since mononuclear cells are often present in the lesions of RF and RHD. Plasma cells and sensitized T cells have been found in chronic rheumatic heart valves. In experimental models, T cells sensitized to streptococcal antigens lyse heart cells in vitro,[99] but comparable evidence has not been derived from humans with active carditis. Despite the abundance of immunologic findings, the understanding of the pathogenesis of poststreptococcal RF is still far from complete.

MORPHOLOGY. The most distinctive anatomic feature of RF is the Aschoff body. These are foci of injury that pass through three phases: (1) a nondistinctive exudative phase, (2) a pathognomonic cellular lesion, and (3) the final stage of progressive fibrosis. Classic Aschoff bodies are found in the heart, but somewhat less distinctive variants are also encountered in the synovia of joints; in and about joint capsules, tendons, and fasciae; and less often in serosal membranes and subcutaneous tissues. Typically, Aschoff bodies are found in the interstitial connective tissue of the myocardium, usually in perivascular locations, but they may also occur in the subendocardial connective tissue and only rarely in the subepicardium. Histologically distinctive lesions are rare within the valves. **The earliest visible change is focal pooling of ground substance with separation of collagen fibers. The collagen appears swollen and smudged and has a deep eosinophilia attributable to deposits of plasma proteins on the collagen fibers (fibrin, globulins), creating what is classically referred to as "fibrinoid change" or "fibrinoid necrosis."** The accumulation of fibrinoid, you will recall, is typical of immunologic injury and is encountered in other so-called "connective tissue" or "collagen-vascular" diseases (p. 180). The focus of fibrinoid change is often surrounded by a scanty lymphocyte, plasma cell, and macrophage infiltrate. **As the lesion evolves into its classic phase, it is transformed into a round-to-oval aggregation of cells enclosing a central focus of irregular deposits of fibrinoid** (Fig. 13–15). The cellular rim contains plump mesenchymal cells called variously "Anitschkow cell," "Aschoff cell," or "cardiac histiocyte." These cells have one or several nuclei that are vesicular, with the chromatin disposed in the center of the nucleus in the form of a slender, wavy ribbon that resembles a caterpillar with fine, leglike projections; hence, the often-used term "caterpillar cells." When the chromatin is viewed on cross section it appears as a central nucleolus surrounded by a cleared halo, creating an "owl-eyed" appearance. When these histiocytes become multinucleated and enlarged, they are sometimes referred to as "Aschoff giant cells." Scattered among these cardiac histiocytes are lymphocytes, plasma cells, and, occasionally, neutrophils and mast cells. **It is these cellular, sometimes called proliferative, Aschoff bodies that are pathognomonic of RHD.** In time, Aschoff bodies undergo progressive fibrosis and so are much less frequently present in the late chronic stages of RHD. Although typically associated with the acute stage of an attack, they have been reported to be present in over 50% of hearts having chronic RHD.[100] However, Roberts and Virmani, using extremely rigorous criteria, found Aschoff bodies in only 2 to 3% of **autopsies** on patients over 14 years of age with chronic RHD and **only in hearts having chronic mitral valvulitis (mitral stenosis).**[100] Thus, Aschoff bodies apparently persist for some time after an acute attack and do not necessarily mean "active disease." With this consideration, we can turn to the general anatomic changes.

Heart. Carditis develops in about 50 to 75% of children between the ages of 2 and 16 years, but in only about 35%

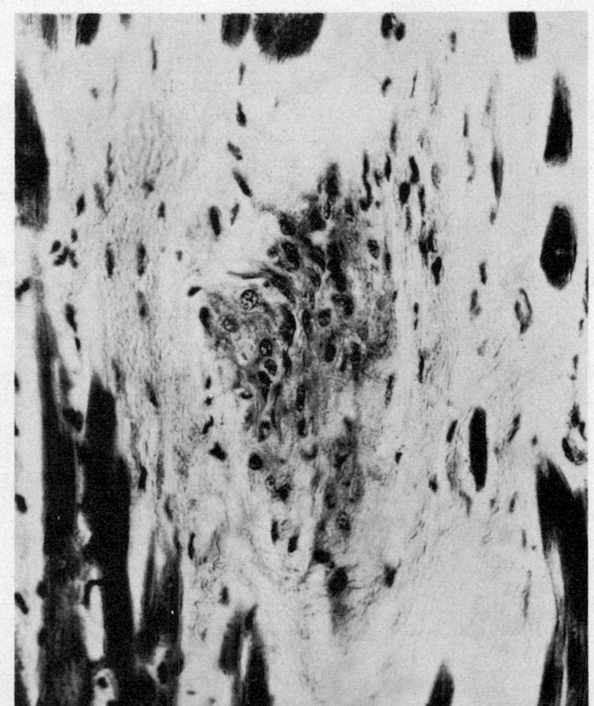

Figure 13–15. Aschoff body at medium power.

of adults having a single acute attack of RF.[101] Recurrences in adult life, however, are not uncommon, and with each recurrence there is a greater likelihood of progressive cardiac damage. Any of the three layers of the heart—pericardium, myocardium, or endocardium—may be involved singly or in combination. Most often, all three layers are affected simultaneously (pancarditis). Depending on the stage of the disease, the heart may exhibit the features of acute rheumatic carditis, chronic or so-called healed rheumatic carditis, or, in some cases, chronic carditis with superimposed active carditis when the patient has experienced recurrent attacks.

During the acute stage, the pericarditis takes the form of a diffuse, nonspecific fibrinous or serofibrinous inflammatory reaction described as a "bread and butter" pericarditis (Fig. 13–16). As with all fibrinous exudations, the pericarditis may either resolve or become organized, usually resulting in only delicate violin-string adhesions or plaquelike thickenings of the pericardial surfaces that do not impair cardiac function. Aschoff bodies may be seen in the subserosal fibrofatty tissue in fulminant cases.

Myocardial involvement with Aschoff bodies localized principally in the connective tissue stroma of the myocardium is responsible for most of the deaths during the acute, active phase of the disease. The myocarditis may be inapparent on gross inspection, save possibly for some dilatation, pallor, and flabbiness of the heart muscle. The extent of the myocardial involvement becomes evident only on histologic examination with the identification of Aschoff bodies. Later, as mentioned, the Aschoff bodies become fibrosed. Although myocarditis may exist alone, it is usually accompanied by endocarditis.

Endocardial involvement is the most ominous aspect of RF and is responsible for the chronic disability due to valvular scarring, usually several decades after the acute disease has subsided. The mitral valve alone is affected in 40 to 50% of cases; the aortic valve alone in 15 to 20%; the aortic and mitral valves together in 35 to 40%; and trivalvular disease (when combined with the tricuspid) in 2 to 3%. Tricuspid disease alone is rare and the pulmonary valve is virtually never affected. With all valves the involvement may induce either stenosis, insufficiency, or both. Early, the acutely affected valves are red, swollen, and thickened. This is usually most marked toward the free margins of the cusps. These changes may be accompanied by a precipitate of fibrin or extrusion of ground substance that produces tiny (1- to 2-mm) friable vegetations **(verrucae)** along the lines of closure of the leaflets (Fig. 13–17). These verrucae appear as irregular warty projections, and probably result from the precipitate of fibrin at sites of erosion or ulceration of inflamed endocardial surfaces along the lines of closure where the leaflets impinge upon each other. They occur on the surfaces exposed to the forward flow of blood and are distributed either along the entire line of closure or in small clusters with uninvolved intervening areas. At the commissures, they may cause interadherence of leaflets. Similar verrucae may sometimes be seen along the chordae tendineae. On histologic examination, these lesions may be nonspecific, revealing only precipitation of fibrinoid with an underlying, nonspecific, leukocytic infiltrate. However, plump fibroblasts and cells resembling the Anitschkow myocytes are occasionally found rimming the base of the vegetation. Recognizable Aschoff bodies are rarely present in these acute valvular lesions.

It is believed, but not definitely established, that acute rheumatic valvulitis may resolve without residuals, but in most instances it leads to fibrous scarring and permanent deformity. As organization of the endocardial inflammation takes place, the valvular leaflets become thickened, fibrotic,

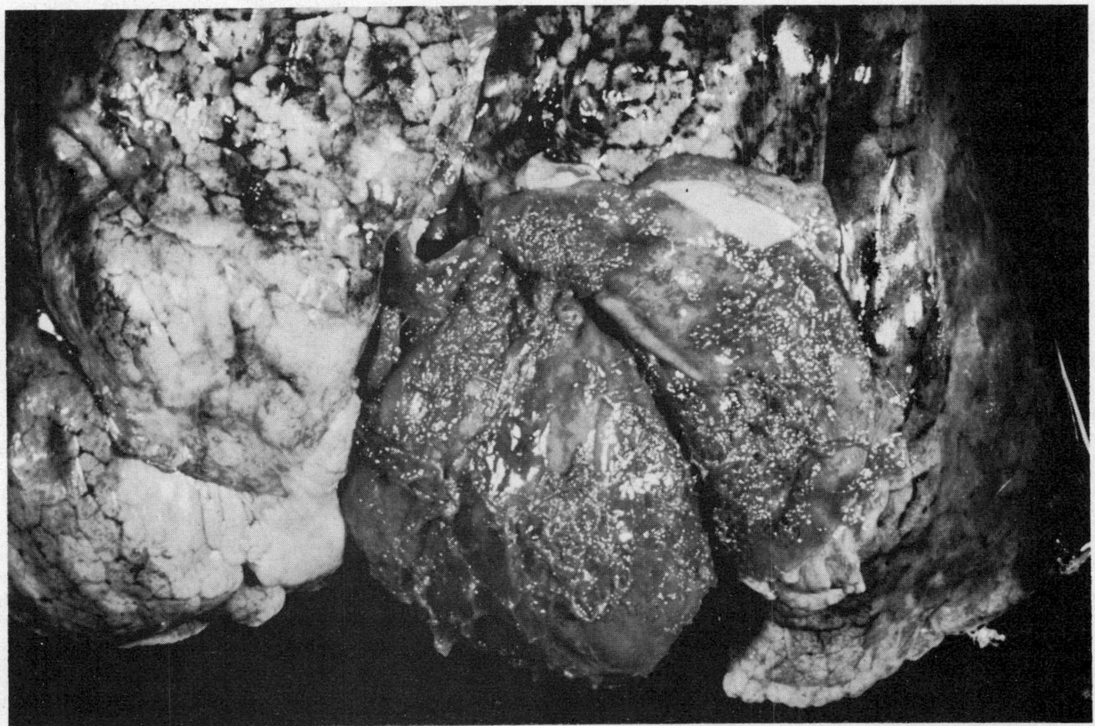

Figure 13–16. Acute rheumatic fibrinous pericarditis. Visceral pericardium (seen in center) and parietal pericardium to its right are shaggy. The lungs, still attached, are at left and right.

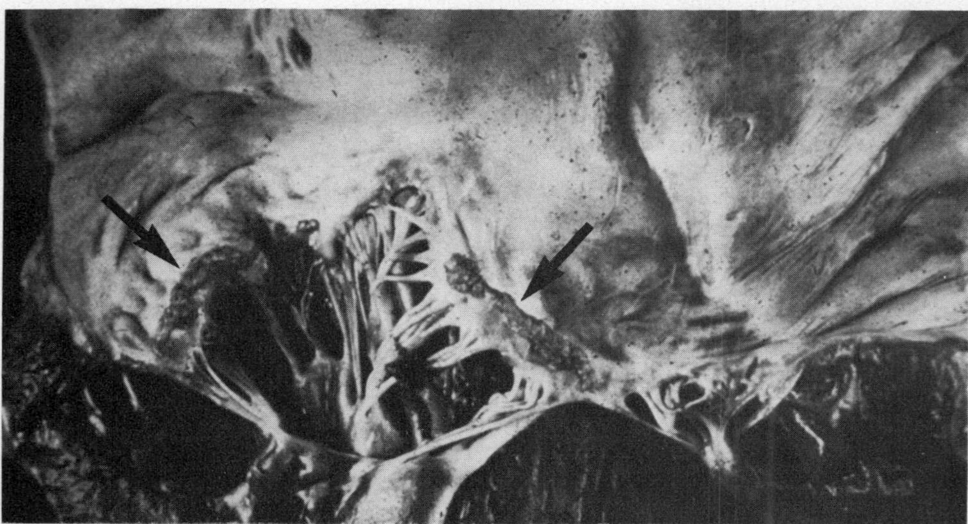

Figure 13–17. Acute rheumatic valvulitis superimposed on chronic mitral valvulitis. Rows of tiny beaded fresh vegetations *(arrows)* are seen along lines of closure of slightly deformed mitral leaflets. (Courtesy of Dr. J. Titus, Baylor College of Medicine).

shortened, and blunted (Fig. 13–18). Fibrous bridging across the valvular commissures often produces a rigid **"fish-mouth"** or **"button-hole" stenotic deformity of the mitral valve** (Fig. 13–19). The chordae tendineae simultaneously become thickened, fused, and shortened. When the tricuspid valve is involved, the changes resemble those of the mitral, but they are almost never as marked. In the aortic valve, the fibrosis also produces interadherence and stenoses as well as prominent nodular calcifications in the sinuses of Valsalva behind the leaflets. For unknown reasons, mitral stenosis tends to be more severe in females, whereas aortic stenosis is more severe in males. With a tight mitral stenosis, the left atrium, and sometimes also the right, progressively dilate. The long-standing congestive changes in the lungs (p. 569) may lead in time to right ventricular hypertrophy. Often, thrombi form within the auricular appendages. The mural endocardium in the left atrium may develop maplike thickenings called **MacCallum's plaques.** These are thought to represent subendocardial aggregations of Aschoff bodies accompanied by pooling of ground substance. In time, these plaques may undergo fibrosis, leaving only an irregular area of endocardial wrinkling. It is to be emphasized that in the late healed stage of endocarditis, histologic changes are generally those of nonspecific healed inflammation since all Aschoff bodies may have disappeared. **The recognition of healed rheumatic valvulitis is, therefore, more dependent on characteristic gross appearances than on histologic changes.**

Joints. The likelihood of **acute arthritis** increases with age, appearing in about 90% of adults and less commonly in children. The large joints, such as the knees, are most often affected, but sometimes also the small joints of the hands and feet. Few histologic observations are available on the joints since the changes are transitory and resolve without sequelae. Histologically, there is a nonspecific mononuclear inflammatory infiltrate with edema, focal deposits of fibrinoid, and sometimes lesions resembling Aschoff bodies. The synovial membranes do not become ulcerated and the articular cartilage is unaffected. When changes appear on the radiograph or there is persistent joint deformity, intercurrent disease such as rheumatoid arthritis must be suspected.

Skin. Lesions of the skin take the form of **subcutaneous nodules** or **erythema marginatum** and are present in 10 to 60% of cases, more often in children. The **subcutaneous nodules** are essentially giant Aschoff bodies with a large central area of fibrinoid enclosed by a cell population similar to that found in the cardiac lesions. The nodules are most often located overlying the extensor tendons of the extremities at the wrists, elbows, ankles, and knees. They sometimes are deeply situated over bony prominences, and rarely are located near the occiput. **Erythema marginatum** tends to have a bathing-suit distribution but may also occur over the thighs, lower extremities, and face. These lesions, which are quite distinctive for RF, begin as flat-to–slightly elevated, slightly reddened maculopapules that progressively enlarge. At the same time, the centers clear and may undergo slight pigmentation, but the peripheries continue to be reddened and elevated to create prominent erythematous margins.

Arteries. **Rheumatic arteritis** has been described in the coronary, renal, mesenteric, and cerebral arteries as well as in the aorta and pulmonary vessels during the height of an attack. The morphologic alterations are characteristic of hypersensitivity angiitis and were described on page 522.

Lungs. **Rheumatic pneumonitis** and **pleuritis** are rare complications of the acute disease. The pulmonary changes consist largely of an interstitial reaction resembling viral pneumonitis (p. 737), sometimes accompanied by fibrinoid changes and an acute angiitis. A nonspecific serofibrinous pleuritis may be present. In the late chronic stages of RHD with mitral stenosis, congestive changes or dense interstitial fibrosis with siderotic nodules often appear.

CLINICAL COURSE. The onset of RF, following by several weeks a streptococcal pharyngitis, may be quite

Fig. 13–18

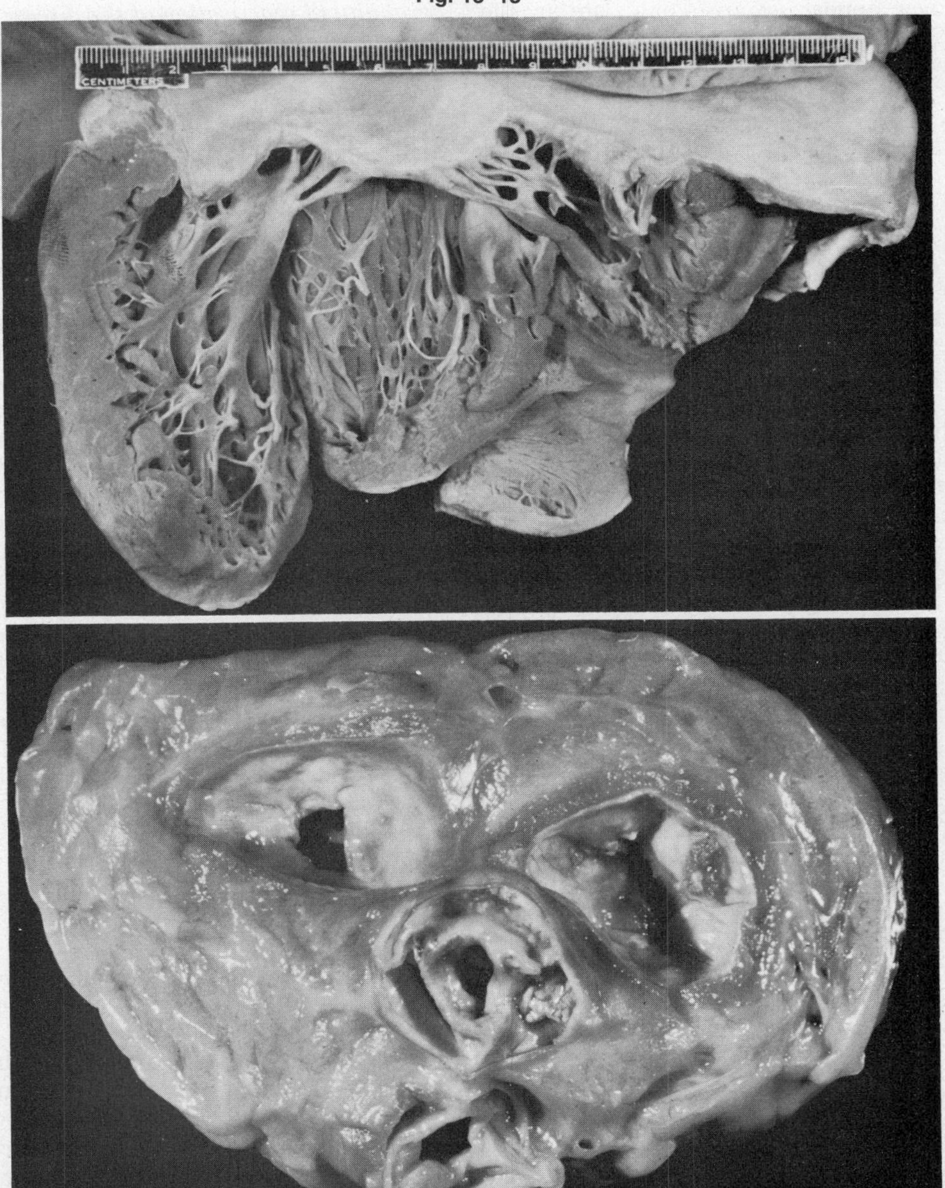

Fig. 13–19

Figure 13–18. Healed rheumatic mitral valvulitis illustrating fibrous thickening of leaflets; commissural fusion between leaflets; and fusion, thickening, and shortening of chordae tendineae.

Figure 13–19. Healed trivalvular rheumatic valvulitis as viewed from above with the atria cut off. Aortic valve is in mid-center field, mitral in upper right, and tricuspid in upper left. All three valves are stenotic, fibrosed, and markedly deformed.

abrupt with fever, tachycardia, and painful swollen joints, or it may be exceedingly subtle and insidious with vague malaise and mild fever. Sometimes fever and chorea (purposeless involuntary movements of hands, feet, arms, legs, tongue, and face) are the initial manifestations of an acute attack, but in other instances chorea may never appear or arise only late in the disease. There are no specific symptoms or signs and the diagnosis usually rests on the concurrence of two or more of "Jones' criteria," listed in Table 13–3. A diagnosis of RF is said to require at least two of the major, or one major and two minor, criteria. Although the arthritis is the most consistent finding, the most feared aspect of RF is the development of carditis. *With increasing age the relative frequency of polyarthritis increases, and that of carditis, subcutaneous nodules, and erythema marginatum decreases.* Typically, the arthritis produces pain and swelling that resolve within a week or two as other joints become involved. There may be manifestations referable to involvement of the pericardium, myocardium, or valves. Should a pericardial friction rub appear, it usually clears in the course of days to weeks and leaves no sequelae. During the initial acute attack it is the myocarditis that is most threatening, causing arrhythmias, particularly atrial fibrillation and prolongation of the electrocardiographic P-R interval. With fibrillation, auricular thrombi are prone to develop, constituting potential sources of emboli. Significant myocarditis may lead to cardiac dilatation and murmurs of insufficiency, principally of the mitral valve, but following the acute attack the insufficiency may resolve if there has been no direct damage to the valve leaflets. The prognosis for the primary attack is generally good and only 1% of patients die from fulminant RF.

Following an initial attack, there is increased vulnerability to reactivation of the disease with subsequent streptococcal pharyngeal infections, and the same manifestations are likely to appear with each recurrent attack. Thus, once carditis develops during the initial attack it is likely to be reactivated and to worsen with each recurrence. Conversely, if the heart is spared during the initial attack it may well go unscathed despite recurrences of RF. In the absence of cardiac involvement the patient may be entirely free from residuals and, spared recurrences, may live a normal life. However, because of the threat of recurrent disease it is now standard practice to administer prophylactic long-term antistreptococcal therapy to anyone who has had RF. When carditis has occurred, the outlook depends on the severity of the chronic valvular deformity. As mentioned, females appear to be more vulnerable to mitral valve stenosis than males. The heart, even with damaged valves, may remain compensated for the duration of a long life, but usually, over the span of decades, decompensation and eventual full-blown cardiac failure develop. However, this course can now be altered by surgical replacement of damaged valves. Other hazards include embolization from mural thrombi within the atrial appendages and infective endocarditis superimposed on chronically deformed valves. It should not be forgotten that recurrent or primary attacks may occur even in the advanced years of life, and therefore acute RF continues to be a cause of death even in adults.

Table 13–3. JONES' CRITERIA (REVISED) FOR GUIDANCE IN THE DIAGNOSIS OF RHEUMATIC FEVER*

Major Manifestations	***Minor Manifestations***
Carditis	*Clinical*
Polyarthritis	Previous rheumatic fever or rheumatic heart disease
Chorea	Arthralgia
Erythema marginatum	Fever
Subcutaneous nodules	*Laboratory*
	Acute phase reactions
	Erythrocyte sedimentation rate, C-reactive protein, leukocytosis
	Prolonged P-R interval

Supporting Evidence of Streptococcal Infection
Increased titer of streptococcal antibodies
ASO (antistreptolysin O)
Other antibodies
Positive throat culture for group A streptococcus
Recent scarlet fever

*The presence of two major criteria, or of one major and two minor criteria, indicates a high probability of the presence of rheumatic fever. Evidence of a preceding streptococcal infection greatly strengthens the possibility of acute rheumatic fever. Its absence should make the diagnosis doubtful (except in Sydenham's chorea or long-standing carditis).

These criteria, originally proposed by T. Duckett Jones in 1944, were revised by the Council on Rheumatic Fever and Congenital Heart Disease of the American Heart Association.

From Stollerman, G. H., et al.: Committee report. Circulation *32*:664, 1965. Revised, 1967. By permission of The American Heart Association, Inc. © 1967.

MITRAL VALVE PROLAPSE

In this curious valvular abnormality, one or both "floppy" enlarged mitral leaflets prolapse, or balloon back, into the left atrium during systole. On auscultation only a midsystolic click or clicks may be heard, corresponding to snapping or tensing of an everted cusp, scallop, or chordae tendineae. Often, however, the valve becomes incompetent and the mitral regurgitation induces an accompanying late systolic or sometimes holosystolic murmur. Hence, this condition is also referred to as the "midsystolic click syndrome," "midsystolic click, late-systolic murmur syndrome," or variations on this theme. Other names based on anatomic changes include "billowing," "ballooning," "hooding," and "myxomatous" degeneration of the mitral valve. More florid is the designation "parachute" mitral valve. Whatever its name, this is an extremely common condition found at any age in 5 to 7% of the general population, most often in young women (average age 32 years).[102] Usually it is an incidental finding on physical examination, but it may have serious import.

MORPHOLOGY. The essential anatomic characteristics of mitral valve prolapse are either excessively large leaflets (or portions of leaflets), excessively long chordae tendineae, or both. Most common is enlargement of entire leaflets. The posterior leaflet is always involved; the anterior, less frequently (Fig. 13–20). The excess may be the consequence of an increase in the transverse or commissure-to-commissure dimension or an increase in the base-to-distal margin length of the leaflet. Occasionally, prolapse is related to excessive length of the chordae tendineae or sometimes just a few of them, but generally there is concomitant abnormality in the leaflets themselves (Fig. 13–21). Rarely, the tricuspid valve is also affected. In the early stages the leaflets are delicate and transparent and sometimes look gelatinous. This appearance is related to myxomatous thickening of the central spongiosa layer that encroaches upon the outer fibrous layers that normally impart the structural strength to the mitral leaflets.[103] The myxomatous tissue is rich in acid mucopolysaccharide. Ultrastructural studies also disclose fragmentation, splitting, and distortions in the collagen fibrils of the outer fibrous layers that may be more important in reducing tensile strength than the myxomatous change.[104] At a later stage, the leaflets become more fibrotic, principally the atrial surfaces, and thickened, probably secondary to long-standing frictional trauma. Similarly, the chordae may become thickened by fibrous tissue, presumably the consequence of friction and organization of layered fibrin. The thickened chordae sometimes fuse. Although in the late stages the gross appearance may resemble that of a postrheumatic mitral valve, in myxomatous degeneration there is neither commissural fusion nor inflammatory neovascularization of the cusps.

A number of secondary anatomic changes may appear: (1) calcification of the basal portions of the affected leaflets, simulating calcified mitral annulus; (2) superimposed infective endocarditis; and (3) rupture of the chordae tendineae, either "spontaneously" or secondary to infective endocarditis.

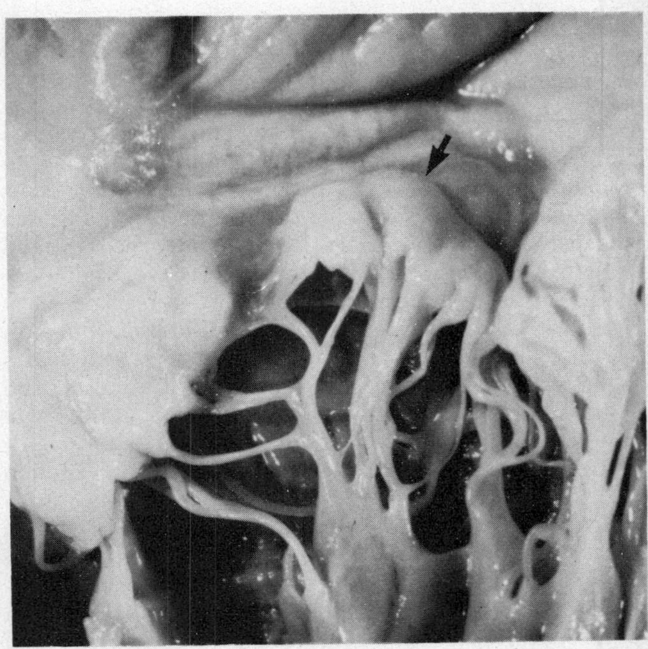

Figure 13–21. The same mitral valve, when opened, revealing parachute-like enlargement of posterior leaflet *(arrow)* on right as compared with relatively normal anterior leaflet on left.

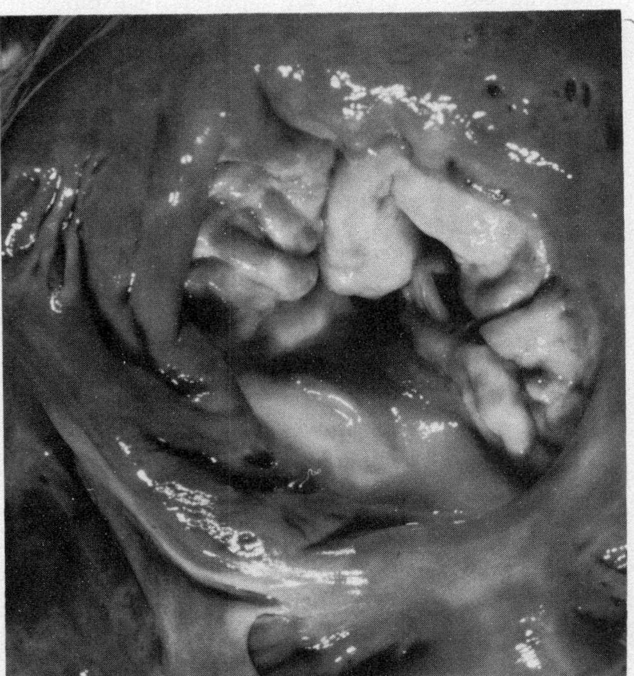

Figure 13–20. Mitral valve prolapse. Billowy posterior mitral leaflet (9 to 4 o'clock) is viewed from atrial surface as redundant membranous folds. Anterior leaflet below is not affected.

The etiology of the "floppy" mitral valve is unknown. It is a common feature of Marfan's syndrome and, in one series, was present in 90% of affected individuals.[105] Thus, it has been suggested that mitral valve prolapse without the other changes of Marfan's syndrome may represent a forme fruste of the hereditary disorder. Prolapse has also been encountered within families, apparently transmitted by mendelian dominant inheritance. Recently an association has been noted among mitral valve prolapse, low body weight, and low blood pressure, raising speculations about some inherited systemic defect in connective-tissue metabolism.[106] On the basis of these observations, some investigators consider it to be a form of congenital heart disease, which would make it the most common congenital cardiac anomaly. Infrequently, prolapse occurs in Turner's syndrome, hypertrophic cardiomyopathy, coronary artery disease, and postrheumatic fever, and in association with secundum atrial defects. However, most cases have no well-defined associations, underscoring the likelihood that the changes are congenital in origin. There is an alternative view, not widely held, that the leaflet prolapse is initiated by some ventricular myocardial abnormality, such as a cardiomyopathy. Impaired papillary muscle function might place undue strain on the leaflets, causing them to undergo abnormal stretching.

CLINICAL COURSE. As pointed out, mitral valve prolapse may only come to attention because of abnormal findings on physical examination. Some patients have only a midsystolic click or clicks. Echocardiography in such cases will usually reveal the mitral valve prolapse. To this group of individuals, making up the majority, the designation "normal" mitral valve prolapse has been applied. A minority of patients present with palpitations, dyspnea, fatigability, syncope, or chest pain, sometimes mimicking angina pectoris. In such instances, the systolic clicks are frequently accompanied by late or holosystolic murmurs related to regurgitation. Thus, it would appear that mitral valve prolapse may not be associated with significant regurgitation, but with more severe involvement of the valve; or possibly with progression of the condition, regurgitation appears. The latter category has been called "pathologic" mitral valve prolapse, having more ominous consequences. Heart failure may develop in those with gross regurgitation and may be initiated precipitously by rupture of chordae tendineae.[107] In major medical centers this is now the most common cause of isolated mitral regurgitation sufficiently severe to require valvular replacement. Infective endocarditis is a well-recognized hazard, and in one series mitral valve prolapse was present in 25% of a series of patients with infective endocarditis.[108] Embolism, particularly to the brain secondary to the development of thrombi on the deformed leaflets, is another serious complication. And finally, ventricular arrhythmias, particularly ventricular tachycardia and fibrillation, may appear and cause sudden death in some cases. Despite all these threats to life, most individuals are unaware of the valvular abnormality and live a normal life span without restriction.

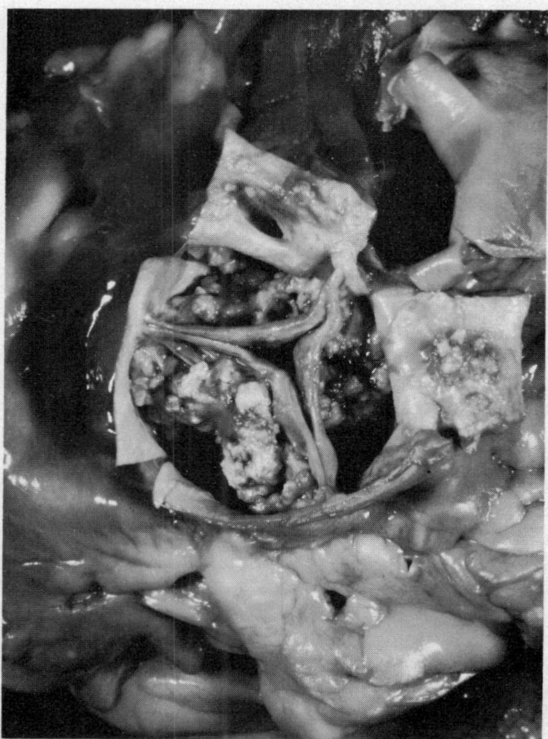

Figure 13–22. Degenerative calcific aortic stenosis in a 72-year-old woman. Granular masses of calcium are heaped up within sinuses of Valsalva (view looking down at valve). Note that commissures are not fused and free edges are not thickened as in postrheumatic aortic valve disease.

AORTIC VALVE STENOSIS

Although aortic stenosis (with or without regurgitation) may occur as an isolated valvular involvement in chronic rheumatic carditis (p. 573), there is substantial evidence that most isolated calcific aortic stenoses are nonrheumatic in origin.[109] There is no rheumatic history in the great majority of instances, neither are stigmata of RF (e.g., Aschoff bodies) present. In addition there is an increasing frequency of calcific aortic stenosis with advancing age. Most important, there is often an underlying congenital malformation of the aortic valve, particularly a bicuspid valve, which prior to the calcification induced no stenosis.[104, 110] It is hypothesized that "wear and tear" of such a congenitally abnormal valve may lead to fibrosing stenosis and calcification even in the relatively young, whereas with a normally formed aortic valve, calcific stenosis does not appear until the advanced years of life (Figs. 13–22, 13–23). The calcification occurring in bicuspid aortic valves is of the dystrophic type, but is identical to that which may occur in a normally formed valve.[111] The narrowed sinuses of Valsalva become filled with moundlike excrescences of calcium covered by a thin layer of endothelium (Fig. 13–22). Frequently, the fibrosis and calcification so overwhelm the aortic valve as to make difficult the identification of the preexisting architecture of the leaflets. Indeed, in the evolution of calcific aortic stenosis one of the commissures may be obliterated before the remaining two, to create an apparent bicuspid aortic valve, but usually some vestige of the commissural raphe remains in acquired bicuspid disease. Gross commissural fusion or vascularization of cusps indicates previous rheumatic or other inflammatory disease, such as infective endocarditis. The possibility cannot be ruled out that some calcific aortic stenoses represent healed infective endocarditis, prone to occur on bicuspid aortic valves, but such a pathway could account for only a relatively few cases.

The *obstruction to left ventricular outflow* leads to a pressure gradient between the left ventricle and aorta during systolic ejection *(pressure overload)*, which gradually increases over the course of many years. The left ventricular output is maintained by the development of *left ventricular hypertrophy*. A large pressure gradient may exist for many years without a reduction of cardiac output, or left ventricular dilatation, or the development of symptoms. As the severity of the stenosis increases, the left ventricular systolic pressure continues to rise (it may reach 300 mm Hg), increasing the myocardial burden. *Once symptoms appear, however, the prognosis is poor,* with a median survival of only two to three years. Critical obstruction constitutes a two-thirds reduction in valve area or a pressure gradient of 50 mm Hg. Although cardiac failure is the usual sequel, 10 to 20% of adults with this valvular disease die suddenly; thus, valvular replacement is urgent when possible.

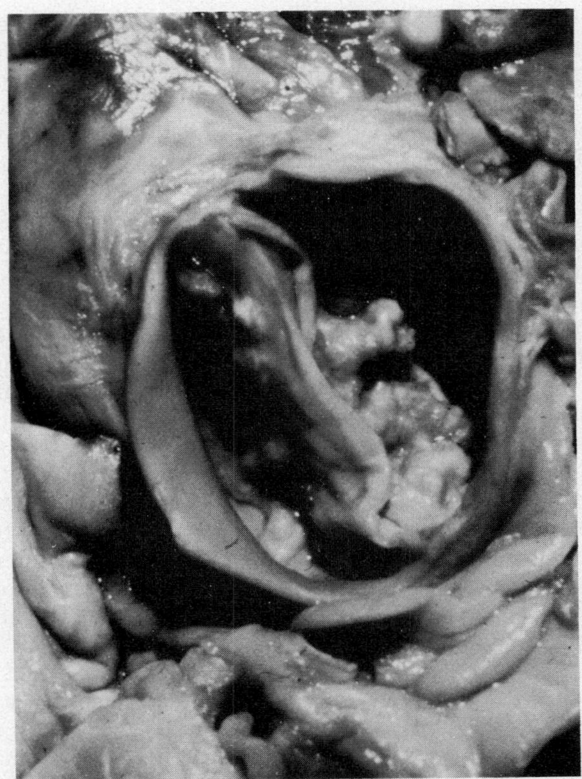

Figure 13–23. Degenerative calcific aortic stenosis superimposed on a bicuspid valve in a 52-year-old man.

CALCIFICATION OF MITRAL ANNULUS

In elderly individuals calcific deposits develop, often in association with ischemic heart disease, in the annulus of the mitral valve without significantly affecting the leaflets. It can often be visualized on gross inspection as an irregular, stony hard beading (2 to 5 mm in thickness) that lies behind the leaflets. There is virtually never any associated inflammatory change and it has been postulated without proof that the calcium deposition reflects the degenerative changes of aging. It generally does not affect valvular function, but sometimes narrows the valvular lumen. Occasionally, the calcium deposits may penetrate sufficiently deeply to impinge on the conduction system and produce arrhythmias, and infrequently it provides a site for infective endocarditis.[112] Heavy calcific deposits are sometimes visualized on echocardiography or seen as a distinctive, ringlike opacity on chest films.

CARCINOID HEART DISEASE

Involvement of the heart, principally the endocardium and valves of the right side, is one of the major features of the *carcinoid syndrome.* It is characterized in its entirety by *distinctive episodic flushing of the skin, and cramps, nausea, vomiting, and diarrhea in almost all patients; bronchoconstrictive episodes resembling asthma in about one-third of cases; and cardiac lesions in about one-half.* These clinical findings relate to the elaboration by argentaffinomas (carcinoid APUDomas) of a variety of bioactive products, including serotonin (5-hydroxytryptamine), 5-hydroxytryptophane, kallikrein that releases bradykinin, histamine, prostaglandins, and sometimes other hormones or hormonelike substances (p. 842). However, which of the secretory products produces the various features of the syndrome is still not clear. The carcinoid syndrome is generally encountered with gastrointestinal neoplasms only when there are metastases to the liver, because there is rapid deamination of polypeptides in the portal circulation during traversal of the liver. In contrast, argentaffinomas primary in organs outside of the portal system of venous drainage, e.g., in the ovary or lung, may induce the carcinoid syndrome without antecedent hepatic metastases.

The cardiovascular lesions associated with the carcinoid syndrome are unlike those produced by any other form of cardiac disease. In the majority of cases, plaquelike thickenings composed of an unusual type of fibrous tissue are superimposed on the endocardium of the cardiac chambers and valvular cusps, **mainly on the right side of the heart.** Occasionally, left-sided lesions are encountered, but they rarely induce valvular dysfunction. Even more rarely, both the right and left sides of the heart are involved, with extension of the changes onto the intima of the great veins and arteries. Typically, the plaques are deposited on the arterial aspect of the pulmonary valve, but both sides of the cusps may be affected, thickening and fusing the cusps to create inelastic stenoses. Similar thickening and fusion of the tricuspid valve leaflets may occur and may extend onto the chordae tendineae. Sometimes the mural endocardium in the right ventricle bears sclerotic plaques. Ultrastructural studies show that the thickenings are largely composed of smooth muscle cells embedded in a stroma rich in acid mucopolysaccharides, collagen, and microfibrils.[113] Elastic fibers are not present. The smooth muscle cells are thought to be derived from primitive mesenchymal cells that are normally present in the subendocardial-subendothelial space. Some of the cells have the ultrastructural features of myofibroblasts. The endothelium over the plaques is usually intact.

The pathogenesis of the cardiac lesions is uncertain, but they are most widely attributed to elevated blood levels of serotonin. However, 5-hydroxytryptophan or bradykinin may be involved, at least in the production of some of the cardiac changes. The argument for serotonin is based on the following: (1) it can induce inflammatory edema by increasing capillary permeability, leading, in time, to a fibroblastic reaction; (2) a somewhat similar cardiac lesion is encountered with endomyocardial fibrosis, most commonly seen in areas of Africa where serotonin-containing plantain and bananas are staples of the diet; and (3) somewhat similar heart lesions have been produced in guinea pigs by long-term administration of large quantities of serotonin. However, attempts to produce these changes by chronic infusion of serotonin in rats have failed.[114] Bradykinin, too, alters capillary permeability, and so might contribute to the inflammatory edema. The fact that the cardiac changes are largely right-sided is explained by inactivation of both serotonin and bradykinin in the blood during passage through the lungs by the monamine oxidase found in the pulmonary vascular endothelium. Incomplete inactivation of high blood levels might underlie the occasional occurrence of left-sided lesions.

Clinical diagnosis is made on the basis of the physical findings mentioned earlier. Usually, murmurs of both pulmonic stenosis and tricuspid insufficiency are also present. Confirmation of the diagnosis can be achieved by the demonstration of increased urinary excretion of 5-hydroxyindolacetic acid, a metabolite of serotonin. The clinical course of carcinoid heart disease depends entirely on the severity of the right-sided valvular lesions. In some patients, murmurs are present without cardiac decompensation; in others, the natural progression of the metastatic neoplasm is interrupted by the onset of marked congestive failure, leading to death. In other individuals, death results from hepatic failure or complications associated with the tumor growth.

INFECTIVE ENDOCARDITIS (IE)

Infective endocarditis, one of the most serious of all infections, is characterized by colonization or invasion of the heart valves or the mural endocardium by a microbiologic agent, leading to the formation of friable vegetations laden with organisms—so-called infective vegetations. A similar phenomenon may occur within the aorta (infective endaortitis), aneurysmal sacs, or other vessels. *Although normal hearts may be affected, IE is more often associated with a preexisting cardiac anomaly such as acquired valvular disease or some form of congenital heart disease.* Virtually every form of microbiologic agent has at one time or another been responsible for these infections, principally certain bacteria. IE has particular clinical importance because prompt diagnosis and effective treatment significantly alters the outlook for the patient.

On clinical grounds IE has been classified into acute and subacute forms. This subdivision expresses the range of severity of the disease and its tempo, conditioned in large part by the virulence of the infecting microorganism and the underlying cardiac status of the patient. A destructive, tumultuous infection with a highly virulent organism leads to death within days to weeks of 50–60% of patients.[115] On the other hand, with organisms of low virulence the disease may appear insidiously and, even untreated, pursue a protracted course of many months. Following appropriate therapy for such infections, most patients recover. There is, however, no clear clinical delineation between acute and subacute IE; they are points along a spectrum. Analogously, the morphologic lesions make up a spectrum. Acute disease tends to be associated with necrotizing, ulcerative, invasive valvular infections, whereas in subacute disease the vegetations are less destructive and often have evidence of healing. However, *the vegetations found in the heart in both clinical variants of the disease are often more alike than different.* Nonetheless, the microbial flora and the pathogenetic influences responsible for the two clinical subdivisions are somewhat different.

EPIDEMIOLOGY AND ETIOLOGY. The decline in the incidence of acute RF and RHD, the surgical correction of many congenital malformations, and the availability of a range of powerful antibiotics might have been expected to reduce significantly the frequency of IE, but there is no clear indication of such a trend. Perhaps predisposing influences have counterbalanced any gains that might have been made. Chronic alcoholism; intravenous drug abuse; cardiac surgery; insertion of "foreign bodies" such as substitute heart valves; and intravascular and intracardiac catheters, pacemakers, and other devices with their potential for providing portals of entry and causing endothelial injury; all are more prevalent now than ever before and all are significant predisposing circumstances. These influences and the decline in the incidence of RHD have altered the age distribution of IE. Whereas, in the past, underlying chronic RHD encountered largely in young adults was a major subsoil for IE, today it accounts for only a small minority of cases. Thus, the average age of patients with IE has increased; currently, over 90% are over the age of 20, with the peak incidence in the fourth and fifth decades of life. The male:female ratio is approximately 1.5:1.[116] About 50 to 75% of patients have preexisting cardiac abnormalities—chronic RHD, congenital malformations (e.g., aortic stenosis, bicuspid aortic valve, ventricular septal defects, and tetralogy of Fallot), mitral valve prolapse, acquired aortic stenosis, and, in particular, cardiac surgery, especially valvular replacement.[117] In one large survey, one-quarter of the patients had previously undergone cardiovascular surgery; when prosthetic valves had been implanted the infection appeared soon after surgery in about one-third, within one to five years after surgery in one-third, and more than five years later in the remainder.[118] Drug addicts represent 5 to 15% of patients in most large studies. *In 25 to 50% of cases of IE there is no apparent underlying cardiac disease or recognized cardiovascular predisposing influence.*

Myriad organisms have been isolated from these patients. At least 95% are bacteria, but exotic causes such as rickettsia, chlamydia, and (more frequently in the recent past) fungi are also implicated. In most analyses that include both acute and subacute disease, the following organisms predominate:[118–120]

Organism	Approximate Frequency (%)
Streptococcus viridans	50
Staphylococcus aureus	approx. 20
Enterococci	5–7
Other staphylococci *(albus, epidermidis)*	2–5
Pneumococci	2–5
Gram-negative rods	2–5
Culture-negative	5–10

Less common offenders still encountered sufficiently often to merit mention include gonococci, diphtheroids, *Hemophilus influenzae*, parainfluenzae, *Candida*, and sometimes several microbial agents together. It should be noted that, in about 5 to 10% of cases, no microbial agent can be identified despite multiple blood cultures. This well-recognized problem may reflect difficulty in culturing the etiologic agent if it is microaerophilic or fastidious in its growth requirements, or failure to use special methods for fungal isolation or previous antibiotic therapy.

There are some differences in the cardiac setting and microbiologic flora of acute IE and subacute IE, but these differences are not inviolate.

Acute IE tends to have the following associations:

1. The hearts are likely to be normal or to have had previous cardiac surgery.

2. Drug addiction and chronic alcoholism.

3. The organisms are likely to be highly virulent—*S. aureus* far outnumbering *S. viridans*. Other agents tending to cause acute IE are pneumococci, gonococci, beta-hemolytic streptococci, coliforms, *Candida*, and *Aspergillus*.

4. A well-defined extracardiac focus of infection is often present, particularly when *S. aureus* is involved on a normal valve.[121]

Drug addicts make up a distinctive subset of acute IE. The endocarditis tends to affect previously normal *right-sided valves*, particularly the tricuspid.[122, 123] Only occasionally is *S. viridans* involved; the most frequent infecting organism is *S. aureus*, with a disproportionate frequency of pneumococci and *Candida*.[124] Patients who have had previous cardiac surgery are another distinctive subset. The causative organisms in "early" infections (developing within two months of the surgical procedure) differ from those in "late"-acquired infections. Early infections are generally due to skin and airborne organisms introduced perioperatively, including *S. aureus*, *S. epidermidis*, diphtheroids, *Corynebacterium*, and aerobic gram-negative bacilli. The widespread use of antibacterial prophylaxis before, during, and after the operation has reduced the frequency of such infections, but may be responsible for the fact that fungi such as *Candida* and *Aspergillus* as well as other opportunists are now responsible for almost 15% of "early" infections. In "late" infections, occurring perhaps years after surgery, the microbiologic flora is very similar to that encountered in patients with underlying valvular lesions, and so *S. viridans*, staphylococci, and enterococci species become important. The organisms responsible for these "late" infections are generally antibiotic sensitive, providing an opportunity to control these unhappy sequelae.

In subacute IE the following should be noted:

1. Most of the hearts have underlying cardiac disease.

2. The involved organisms tend to be of relatively low virulence, unlikely to assume etiologic significance in the absence of previous cardiac damage.

3. The preponderance of cases are caused by *S. viridans* and, much less often, enterococci. However, *S. aureus* occasionally is associated with subacute IE.

4. A well-defined infection elsewhere is seldom identified, but occasionally there is a possible dental or urinary tract focus (e.g., dental work, catheterization, cystoscopy).

PATHOGENESIS. Four factors have been postulated as having importance in the development of *subacute* IE, but have not been clearly related to *acute* IE: (1) deranged blood flow producing regurgitant and jet streams, (2) the formation of sterile platelet-fibrin deposits, (3) seeding of these deposits by blood-borne organisms, and (4) agglutinating antibodies producing clumps of organisms.[115] Regurgitant and jet streams create "low-pressure sinks" at their peripheries that favor the deposition of fibrin and clumps of agglutinated organisms. Thus, in rheumatic mitral stenosis there is inevitably regurgitation of blood during systole, creating the conditions for the localization of infected vegetations on the atrial surface of the damaged valve close to the margins of the regurgitant orifice. With aortic stenosis and regurgitation the ventricular surface becomes the "low-pressure sink" during diastolic regurgitation. Moreover, jet streams may induce endocardial injury, which helps to explain why small ventricular septal defects associated with jet streams are much more frequently the site of IE than interatrial communications. It is understandable, then, that even organisms of relatively low virulence such as *S. viridans*, when blood borne, may become implanted at the site of an acquired or congenital cardiac defect.

The events surrounding the development of acute IE are less well understood. Sometimes there are well-defined predispositions such as intravenous drug abuse with frequent introduction of all kinds of microbial contamination (addicts have been known to use water from the toilet to prepare their "fix"). The suture material and prostheses used in cardiac surgery are obvious foreign bodies inviting the localization of blood-borne agents. However, such special circumstances may not be necessary when the blood is seeded by highly virulent organisms such as *S. aureus*. Moreover, the resistance of the host is also an important factor in the equation. Thus, IE is a well-recognized hazard in hospitalized patients who already have some debilitating disease, even in the absence of previous cardiac surgery. Nosocomial infections are often caused by antibiotic-resistant or opportunistic organisms. Similarly, immunosuppressed individuals have a greater risk of IE and an acute fulminating course whatever the infecting agent.

MORPHOLOGY. The anatomic changes in IE are usually quite spectacular and readily evident. First, some generalizations applicable to both acute and subacute forms will be made, followed by some possible points of difference. The diagnostic findings are the friable, bulky, usually bacteria-laden vegetations, most commonly on the heart valves (Fig. 13–24). They may occur singly or multiply on one or more

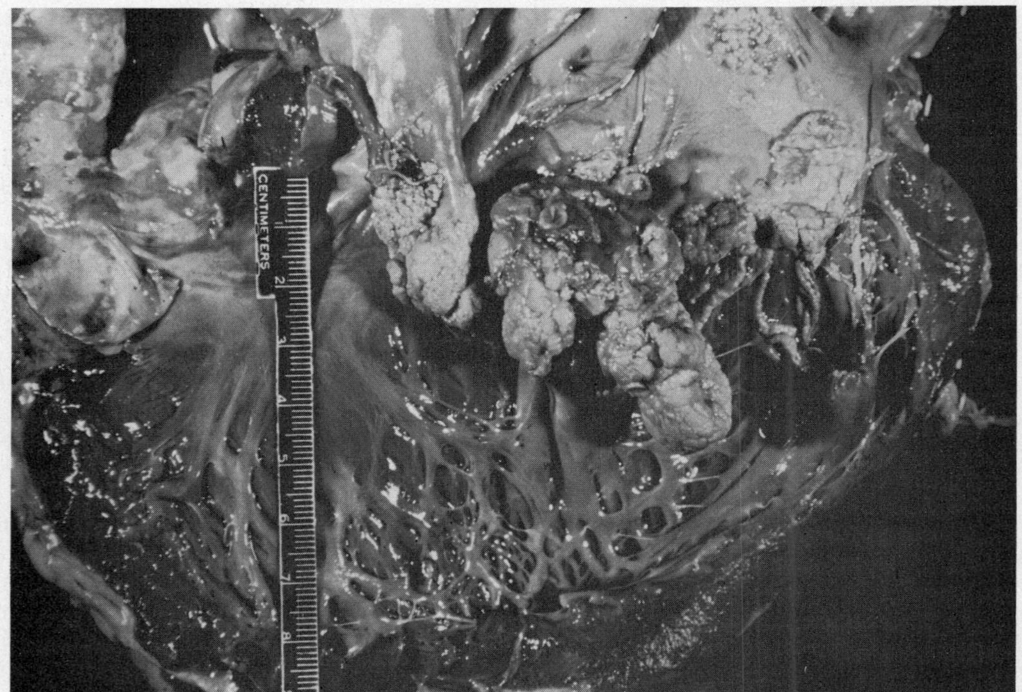

Fig. 13–24

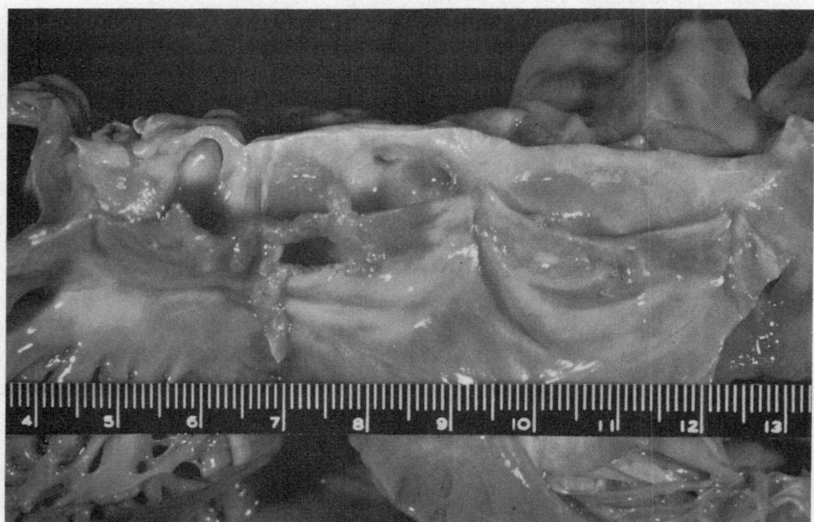

Fig. 13–25

Figure 13–24. Infective endocarditis (bacterial) of mitral valve with extensive friable vegetations, destruction of valve leaflets, and extension of vegetations to atrial endocardium.

Figure 13–25. Acute infective endocarditis of aortic valve with through-and-through perforation of one of the cusps.

valves. The mitral valve alone is affected in 25 to 30% of cases; aortic valve alone in 25 to 35%; mitral and aortic valves in 10%; tricuspid valve alone in 10%; heart valve prosthesis in 10%; and congenital defects in 10%.[124] The individual vegetations are often several centimeters in greatest dimension but may be small, measuring only a few millimeters. At the time of postmortem examination, they generally pile up on or hang from the free margins of the leaflets as friable, irregular masses. Classically, they do not encircle the entire free margins of the leaflets as do those in rheumatic fever. Usually the vegetations in acute endocarditis are bulkier (reflecting rapid microbial proliferation) than those in the subacute form of the disease, which can be small enough to be missed on casual inspection. Moreover, in acute endocarditis the vegetations more often occur on previously normal valves, cause perforation of the underlying valve leaflet, and sometimes erode into the underlying myocardial or vessel wall (Fig. 13–25). In the subacute form, the vegetations are generally superimposed on previously damaged valves, as already mentioned. From these sites of origin the vegetations may extend to the surface of the leaflet or to the adjacent endocardium, or they may burrow through the valve to invade the ventricular wall or one of the great vessels entering or leaving the heart.

The above description refers to the appearance of the disease in its florid, active stage. More and more often, cases are now identified with heaped-up, focal fibrotic or calcified masses along the free margins of one of the valve leaflets, suggesting a preexistent endocarditis. Indeed, the history occasionally confirms this. It is, therefore, now appreciated that these vegetations may undergo progressive fibrosis and organization and eventually become calcified. Such a happy outcome is, however, more frequent in patients with the subacute disease in which the causative organism is more likely to be amenable to therapeutic control.

Histologically, there is little to be seen in the vegetations save for the irregular, amorphous, tangled mass of fibrin strands, platelets, and blood cell debris that, along with the masses of organisms and inflammatory cells, compose the vegetation. The underlying leaflet shows the anticipated vascularization and nonspecific inflammatory response (Fig. 13–26). The bacteria or fungi may be extremely difficult to identify and are often deeply buried within the vegetation, which explains the difficulty in controlling these infections by antibiotic therapy. An important part of the examination of these vegetations is the identification of the organism by direct smear and culture. The tissue section morphology may provide a general clue to the type of organism, but ultimately cultural identification is required.

There may be a number of sequelae.[125] Congestive heart failure is the most common serious complication and the leading cause of death in patients with endocarditis. The vegetations may fragment and embolize, more often with the large friable vegetations in the acute form of the disease. The four principal sites of embolization are brain, spleen, coronary arteries, and kidneys, in that order, but other sites may also be affected. Almost always, these septic infarcts become converted to abscesses. Suppurative pericarditis may result from direct penetration of the heart wall or by lymphatic permeation. The burrowing infection may produce a valvular ring abscess, whose consequences depend on location. Erosion of the valve leaflets or of the chordae tendineae may cause sudden valvular insufficiency and acute cardiac decompensation. Seeding of the aorta may give rise to a bacterial endaortitis. The bacteremia may seed any organ in the body, but the kidney, spleen, and brain are

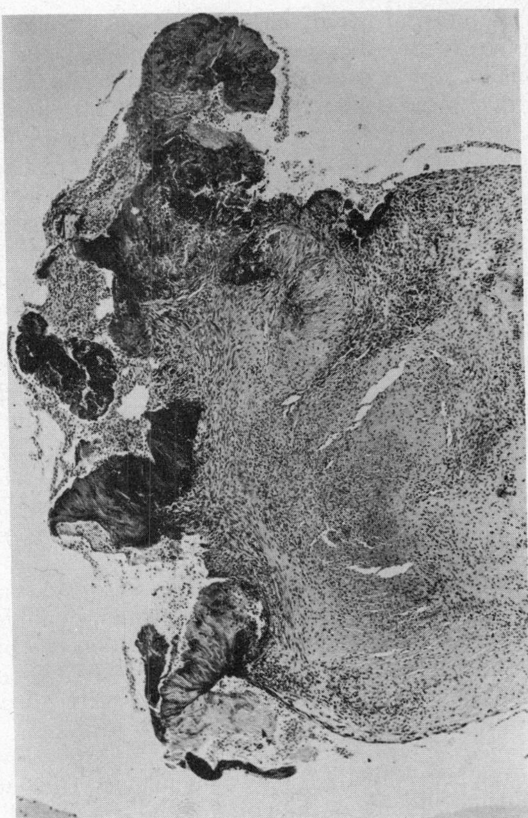

Figure 13–26. Low-power view of a bacterial vegetation illustrating marked inflammatory infiltration. Black masses on surface are bacteria in colony formation.

the most common sites of secondary infection. This sequence is more characteristic of the virulent organisms causing acute IE. The myocardium itself may exhibit scattered metastatic abscesses. Small linear hemorrhages or even microabscesses may appear in the skin or nailbeds from direct bacterial seeding and/or immune complex–induced acute vasculitis. Acute splenitis is so common as to be virtually a part of the disease. Renal complications have become somewhat uncommon, perhaps because persistent untreated infections are now less frequent. The renal involvement takes many forms, including metastatic abscesses, infarctions (usually septic), focal glomerulitis or glomerulonephritis (formerly called focal embolic glomerulonephritis) (p. 1022), and diffuse proliferative glomerulonephritis (p. 1007). Both forms of glomerulopathy are now considered to be immunologic in origin rather than due to direct embolization of bacteria.

CLINICAL COURSE. The subacute and acute forms of IE produce very different clinical syndromes. *Subacute disease is usually insidious in onset* and surreptitiously becomes apparent because of progressive weakness, weight loss, anemia, fever, and sometimes night sweats. Chills are uncommon. The presenting symptoms, deceptively, may be headache or arthralgia. Occasionally, the first manifestation relates to an embolic episode to the brain, heart, spleen, or kidneys. There may be a host of other manifestations, including focal skin or mucosal hemorrhages (sometimes having pale, infective centers); linear splinter hemorrhages under the nails; and (occasionally) tender, subcutaneous nodules (Osler's nodes) in the palms, soles, or fingertips. These changes may relate to specific microemboli, but immune complex–mediated vasculitis is more likely.[126] The physical examination at times can be deceptively negative early in the course of subacute disease. A cardiac murmur is generally present, but may relate to the preexisting cardiac abnormality. Only infrequently do the murmurs change in character, secondary to the build-up and fragmentation of vegetations. More important, murmurs are absent from a minority of cases in both the early and late stages of subacute IE. The spleen is frequently enlarged and may be tender. Sometimes clubbing of the fingers develops with prolonged disease. A variety of other manifestations may appear related to embolization, bacteremic seeding of organisms, and renal involvement, as detailed by Pelletier and Petersdorf.[116]

The diagnosis can be strongly suspected in an individual with unexplained embolizations and fever, but ultimately it rests with the identification of a blood-borne microbial agent. Blood cultures, when repeated sufficiently often, are positive in about 90% of cases. Culture-negative cases present serious problems since the choice of antibiotic, based on the sensitivity of the organism, critically influences the outcome. The outlook depends on the age of the patient, the susceptibility of the agent to antibiotic control, the duration of the disease prior to the institution of therapy, and the former cardiac status of the patient. Because of these variables, survival with subacute disease ranges from about 60% to 90% (with *S. viridans*). In resistant infections, increasing resort is being made to replacement of involved valves by prostheses, more often in acute destructive IE than in the subacute disease. The major causes of death in the subacute disease, in approximate descending order of frequency, are congestive heart failure, embolic MI, embolic cerebral infarction, arrhythmias, and renal failure. No longer do many patients with subacute IE die of uncontrolled sepsis.

Acute IE generally declares itself by the abrupt onset of high fever, shaking chills, and profound weakness. Splenomegaly may occur but often is not as prominent as in the subacute disease. Embolic manifestations appear relatively early, along with skin and mucosal petechiae. Murmurs are present in about two-thirds of these patients when vegetations involve the left side of the heart, and are more likely to change over the course of time as the vegetations build up and fragment. However, murmurs are not infrequently absent, particularly with involvement of the right side of the heart. Painful nodules of the palms, soles, and fingertips are uncommon. Cardiac decompensation appears relatively early and is prone to worsen suddenly as the valves erode or chordae tendineae rupture. Aortic ring abscesses may produce conduction disturbances or interventricular septal defects. Metastastic sites of infection are more frequent with acute IE than with the subacute pattern and positive blood cultures are generally more readily obtained with the highly virulent causative organisms. The outlook is largely dependent on the virulence of the infecting agent and its susceptibility to antimicrobial therapy modified by the age of the patient and the clinical setting in which the endocarditis has developed. Thus, it is most grave in those having previous cardiac surgery and prosthetic valves. When infections by resistant strains of *S. aureus*, gram-negative rods, and fungi are superimposed on prosthetic valves, the mortality rate may reach 70%. In other instances, however, significantly better results have been achieved with aggressive antibiotic therapy coupled with surgical intervention (débridement or valve replacement). The major causes of death are CHF primarily due to valve dysfunction, fatal embolism, arrhythmias, mycotic aneurysm formation with rupture, and uncontrolled sepsis. Failures with antibiotic therapy are largely related to inappropriate treatment when organisms cannot be isolated for sensitivity testing, wall abscesses, the presence of prosthetic devices, and resistant organisms. Unfortunately, the patient who survives an attack of subacute or acute IE often sustains permanent valvular damage and so remains at increased risk of recurrent infection with the same or a new organism.

NONBACTERIAL THROMBOTIC ENDOCARDITIS (NBTE), MARANTIC ENDOCARDITIS

This disorder is characterized by the precipitation of small masses of fibrin and other blood elements upon the valve leaflets of either side of the heart. In contrast to IE, the vegetations in this condition are sterile and tend to be small (1 to 5 mm). They resemble those of acute rheumatic endocarditis and Libman-Sacks disease much more closely. In NBTE, the vegetations may occur singly or multiply to form a small row along the line of closure of the leaflet (Fig. 13–27). Less often, they occur at other sites on the leaflets and even on the pulmonic and tricuspid valves. In some instances, the affected leaflets have some form of previous damage, such as old inflammatory rheumatic changes or degenerative alterations due to vascular heart disease. Histologically, the vegetations are bland thrombi and there is no significant accompanying inflammatory reaction or organization. Consequently, they are only loosely attached to the underlying valve.

The significance and interpretation of these lesions are controversial. In most instances, the patients have died of some protracted debilitating disease such as metastatic cancer, renal failure, chronic sepsis, or some other form of disease.[127] Sometimes they occur concomitantly with venous thromboses or in patients with pulmonary embolization, suggesting a common origin in a hypercoagulable state perhaps related to the underlying disease, such as cancer. Endocardial trauma as from an indwelling pulmonary artery (Swan-Ganz) catheter is a well-recognized predisposing condition. It

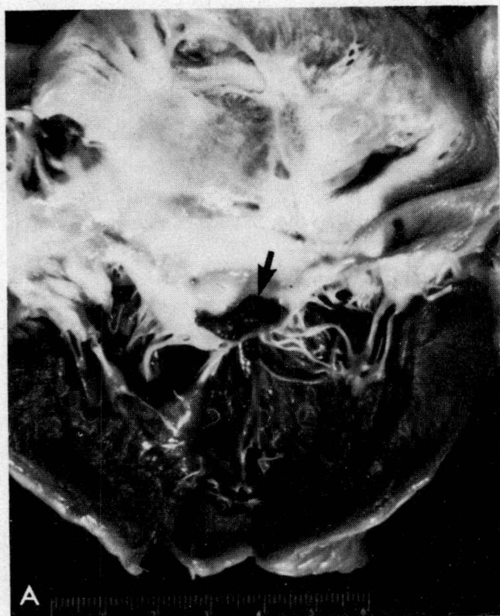

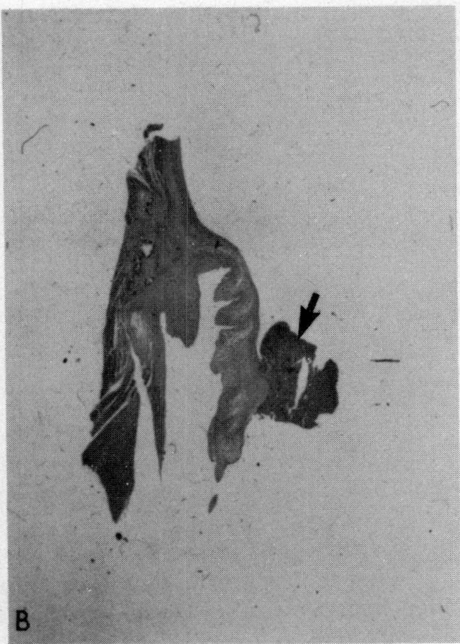

Figure 13–27. *A*, Nonbacterial thrombotic endocarditis. A solitary dark vegetation *(arrow)* is seen on posterior mitral leaflet. *B*, Bland dark vegetation on low power *(arrow)* sits on top of noninflammatory leaflet, as seen on a transection of the valve.

should be noted, however, that *this form of thrombotic endocarditis has occurred in young individuals, even children, and sometimes in patients who are well nourished and distinctly not marantic.*[128] Although the local effects on the valves are unimportant, the cardiac vegetations may be significant clinically because they are sometimes productive of emboli and infarctions in the brain, heart, kidneys, and lungs and elsewhere.[128] In addition, these bland vegetations are believed to provide a soil for the implantation of microorganisms to yield IE (p. 581).

NONBACTERIAL VERRUCOUS ENDOCARDITIS (LIBMAN-SACKS DISEASE)

In disseminated lupus erythematosus, mitral and tricuspid valvulitis is occasionally encountered. This form of endocardial involvement is one of the important components of this systemic immunologic disorder.[129] The connective tissue of the valves may become the site of mucoid pooling, fibrinoid necrosis, and subsequent collagenous fibrosis. Frequently, this type of valvulitis leads to the formation of small vegetations on the valve leaflets that sometimes can be confused with the much larger, friable vegetations of IE or with nonbacterial thrombotic endocarditis. The characteristics and significance of Libman-Sacks disease have already been discussed (p. 187).

CONGENITAL HEART DISEASE

Congenital heart disease is most simply defined as a structural abnormality of the heart, present from birth. The more severe anomalies may be incompatible with intrauterine survival. When they permit live birth they may produce manifestations soon thereafter, owing to the change from fetal to postnatal circulatory patterns. In some instances, the anomaly evolves postnatally: for example, a coarctation (narrowing) of the aorta may become more pronounced when the ductus arteriosus closes after birth. Some anomalies do not become evident until adult years. Thus, congenital heart disease, although usually the realm of the pediatrician, is also a cause of cardiac malfunction in adults. The disorders that normally do not cause cardiac malfunction until adult life, such as the mitral prolapse or "floppy mitral valve" syndrome, and hypertrophic cardiomyopathy, will not be included in our present consideration, nor the cardiovascular abnormalities encountered in a host of specific genetic disorders such as Marfan's, Ehlers-Danlos, and Hunter-Hurler syndromes, many of which are covered elsewhere.

INCIDENCE. Congenital heart disease is the most common type of heart disease among children, and fortunately most forms are now amenable to surgical correction. Although figures vary, a generally accepted incidence of congenital heart disease is 6 to 8 per 1000 live-born, full-term births. This prevalence does not include perhaps the two most common cardiac abnormalities, bicuspid aortic valve and mitral valve prolapse, which often do not constitute functionally significant derangements in the early years of life.[130] There are even wider discrepancies in the reported frequencies of specific forms of congenital heart disease. The ten most common, accounting for 90% of cases with approximate frequencies, are presented in Table 13–4, which is drawn from several sources.[131–133] These more common anomalies will be described after some brief comments

Table 13–4. FREQUENCY (%) OF TYPES OF CONGENITAL CARDIAC DEFECTS IN CHILDREN

Diagnosis	Percentage
Ventricular septal defect	20–30
Patent ductus arteriosus	10–20
Coarctation of aorta	10–15
Atrial septal defect	5–15
Tetralogy of Fallot	5–15
Transposition of great vessels	5–15
Pulmonary stenosis or atresia	5–15
Aortic atresia or stenosis	5–15
Tricuspid atresia	2
Mitral atresia	2
Others	5–10

on etiology and clinical correlations. For the less common lesions, reference may be made to specialized texts.[134, 135]

ETIOLOGY. In over 90% of instances the etiology of congenital heart disease is unknown. However, multifactorial inheritance with both genetic and environmental inputs is suspected.[136] About 5% of cases are associated with chromosomal abnormalities. The specific karyotypes often having cardiac anomalies are trisomies 21, 18, 13, 22, 9 (mosaic), and +14q− and Turner's Syndrome. About 2 to 3% of cardiovascular abnormalities are related to gene defects in a wide variety of autosomal dominant, autosomal recessive, and sex-linked hereditary syndromes, e.g., Ehlers-Danlos, Marfan's, mucopolysaccharidoses, muscular dystrophies, and glycogenoses. Probably less than 1% can be clearly attributed to environmental influences. Best documented is maternal rubella in the first trimester of pregnancy, which may result in patent ductus arteriosus, pulmonic valvular and/or arterial stenosis, and ventricular septal defect, either singly or in combination, and sometimes also cataracts, deafness, and microcephaly. A large number of other cardiac teratogenic influences have been identified in animals, such as hypoxia, ionizing radiation, and various drugs, but in humans, in addition to maternal rubella, there is substantial evidence implicating thalidomide, trimethadione, and excessive alcohol consumption. Excessive cigarette smoking is also suspect.

The belief that the great majority (about 90%) of structural cardiac anomalies are multifactorial in origin is largely inferential.[137] With most monozygotic twins, when one has a congenital cardiac defect, the other more often is free of it, indicating that, in general, the defect is not simply of genetic origin. On the other hand, about one-third of those with congenital malformations of the heart have one or more relatives with congenital heart disease, and there is a two- to fivefold increased risk of congenital heart disease when first-degree relatives (parents or siblings) are affected; sometimes the relatives have the same type of congenital defect. There is, in addition, a well-defined sex preponderance for certain specific defects. Patent ductus arteriosus and atrial septal defects are more common in females, while valvular aortic stenosis, coarctation of the aorta, tetralogy of Fallot, and transposition of the great arteries are more frequent in males. Overall, males are more often involved. Thus, there are many hints of genetic influence, but the twin studies make clear that environmental influences, although rarely identifiable, must also contribute.

Several important observations relevant to genetic counseling should be mentioned at this point. The basic development of the heart occurs between the second and eighth weeks of embryogenesis. Environmental insults, then, must occur during this vulnerable period to cause congenital heart disease. Most cardiovascular abnormalities clearly of genetic origin are associated with well-defined multisystem syndromes. The chromosomal syndromes, e.g., the trisomies, are largely the consequence of errors in gametogenesis and so most often are not familial. Only the cardiovascular abnormalities related to mutant genes, e.g., Marfan's, Ehlers-Danlos, and the mucopolysaccharidoses, are hereditary and familial. With these exceptions, parents of an affected child can be reassured that, while there is a somewhat increased risk for subsequent children, it is small (below 5%), and with a live-born infant the defect may well be amenable to surgical correction. However, when more than one member of a family is affected, the risk rises sharply.

CLINICAL CONSEQUENCES. Each of the myriad structural anomalies produces its own somewhat distinctive secondary effects on the heart and body. However, certain threads are common to many.

Cyanosis is a prominent manifestation of many forms of congenital heart disease. It appears whenever the blood contains more than 3 to 5 gm per dl of reduced hemoglobin. The cyanosis when less severe may affect only the peripheral parts of the body—fingers, toes, nose, earlobes (so-called "peripheral cyanosis") or it may be much more generalized and severe ("central cyanosis"). In general, peripheral cyanosis occurs with congenital or acquired cardiac defects that reduce the cardiac output, such as severe mitral stenosis and pulmonary stenosis, as well as in cardiac failure, whatever the cause. Central cyanosis, in contrast, arises either because of inadequate oxygenation of the blood in the lungs or (of particular interest here) with any cardiac anomaly that induces a right-to-left shunt. It may be present with congenital cardiac anomalies from birth, as seen with transposition of the great vessels in which the aorta arises from the right ventricle. However, it sometimes may appear after birth, possibly years later *(cyanose tardive)*. For example, an infant born with an atrial or ventricular septal defect has at first a left-to-right shunt without cyanosis, but in time the pressure and volume overload of the right side of the heart causes reversal of flow, producing cyanose tardive. *Clinical findings frequently associated with severe, long-standing cyanosis are clubbing of the tips of the fingers and toes, hypertrophic osteoarthropathy* (p. 1333) *and polycythemia.*

Pulmonary vascular disease is a serious consequence of all forms of congenital heart disease that increase pulmonary blood flow or pressure, such as atrial and ventricular septal defects, patent ductus arteriosus, and transposition of the great vessels.[130] Although described in some detail on page 713, it basically comprises medial, and sometimes intimal, thickening of the walls of the pulmonary arteries of medium and small size, and sometimes thrombosis and obliteration of the lumens of the small peripheral branches.[139] The increased resistance to flow constitutes a serious impairment of pulmonary function, and thus fear of this consequence of certain forms of congenital heart disease dictates early surgical treatment.[138]

Enlargement of the heart or of a particular chamber occurs with many types of congenital heart disease, and is produced by volume or pressure overloads. Right atrial dilatation occurs with an atrial septal defect. Left ventricular hypertrophy or dilatation is particularly prominent with aortic stenosis, coarctation of the aorta, patent ductus arteriosus, and aortic regurgitation. The right ventricle is similarly affected by the increased pressure resulting from pulmonary stenosis or the increased volume delivered by an atrial or ventricular septal defect.

Feeding difficulties and impaired growth and development are common in many cyanotic and, to a lesser extent, acyanotic disorders. In most instances, such compromised infants and children have congestive heart failure, which of course is the ultimate consequence of all uncorrected defects that seriously impinge on cardiac function.

A variety of other problems may arise with a congenital heart disorder. Cerebral thrombosis sometimes occurs in very young children having some form of cyanotic heart disease, presumably related to polycythemia and increased blood viscosity. Often the thrombotic episode is triggered by a febrile illness that leads to dehydration. Paradoxical embolus and brain abscess (if the embolus is infected) may arise with right-to-left shunts that bypass the normal filtration action of the lungs. Infective endocarditis is another hazard seen most often with tetralogy of Fallot, ventricular septal defect, aortic stenosis, and patent ductus arteriosus. It may also follow reparative cardiac surgery with the introduction of prosthetic conduits, patches, or valves. Finally, all children with significant congenital cardiac defects are at greater risk of developing any disease of childhood, giving added impetus to the recognition and, when possible, the surgical correction of all functionally significant anomalies.

CLASSIFICATION. There are as many classifications of congenital heart disease as there are writers on the subject. Widely used is the following framework:

1. Abnormal communications between the systemic and pulmonary circulations without cyanosis (left-to-right shunts).
2. Valvular and vascular obstructive lesions encompassing the right-to-left (cyanotic) shunts and the purely obstructive anomalies.
3. Transpositions.
4. Malpositions of the heart.

COMMUNICATIONS BETWEEN SYSTEMIC AND PULMONARY CIRCULATIONS WITHOUT CYANOSIS (LEFT-TO-RIGHT SHUNTS)

Atrial Septal Defect (ASD)

With the exception of mitral valve prolapse (p. 576) and bicuspid aortic valve (p. 591), ASD is the most common congenital cardiac anomaly first recognized in adults, more frequent in females than in males. It usually passes unnoted in infants and children, only becoming manifest when reversal of flow through the shunt (due to development of increased pulmonary arterial pressure) induces cyanosis, or right-sided heart failure develops. *There are three types of ASD: ostium primum, ostium secundum, and sinus venosus.*[140] Normally, at the end of the third or the beginning of the fourth week, the common atrial canal is divided by a septum primum contributed by the sinus venosus and endocardial cushion tissue. Two openings are left in the septum primum: a foramen primum, low and posteriorly in the neighborhood of the atrioventricular valve, and a foramen secundum, approximately where the foramen ovale will later be situated. At about the fifth week of embryogenesis, growth of the septum primum abolishes the low foramen primum. The foramen secundum, however, is partially closed by a newly-formed septum secundum derived from the medial wall of the right atrium, which lies to the right of the septum primum. However, since this secondary septum is itself not complete, an aperture is left, known as the foramen ovale, which is juxtaposed to a more or less intact region of the septum primum lying to its left. Thus, a flaplike membrane covers the foramen ovale. As long as pressure in the right atrium is higher than that in the left, the oxygenated blood in the right atrium flows into the left atrium. However, with birth and opening of the pulmonary circulation the pressure relationships are reversed, but flow from left to right is prevented by the flap valve covering the foramen ovale. Fusion of the membrane over the foramen normally follows. A nonfunctional oblique slit may persist, known as a *patent foramen ovale*, which permits little or no flow because of the flap valve arrangement.

Ostium primum anomalies represent only about 5% of ASDs. They occur low in the atrial septum adjacent to the atrioventricular valves, and are sometimes associated with deformities of these valves. This type of ASD is common in Down's syndrome.

Ostium secundum occurs at the location of the foramen ovale because of juxtaposed defects in the primary and secondary septa. This pattern represents approximately 90% of all ASDs. It is sometimes associated with other defects—patent ductus arteriosus, ventricular septal defect, pulmonary stenosis, transposition of the great arteries, and tetralogy of Fallot. The atrial aperture may be of any size: single, multiple, or sometimes fenestrated. A very large ostium secundum creates essentially a single atrial chamber.

Sinus venosus defects are located high in the atrial septum near the entrance of the superior vena cava. They account for about 5% of ASDs and are sometimes accompanied by anomalous connections of pulmonary veins from the right lung to the superior vena cava or right atrium.

ASDs are very well tolerated if small (less than 1 cm in diameter). Even larger defects do not constitute serious problems during the first decades of life when the flow is from left to right. A murmur is often present; it arises at the pulmonic valve as a result of excessive flow through the valve. Eventually, however, reversal of flow may occur as the right atrium and right ventricle hypertrophy, and pulmonary hypertension and arterial changes develop. Cyanosis, respiratory difficulties, and cardiac failure then ensue progressively. Rarely, a rheumatic, acquired mitral stenosis combines with an ASD (Lutembacher's syndrome) to greatly raise the left-sided pressure and hasten the development of pulmonary hypertension. Some would extend Lutembacher's syndrome to include the combination of ASD and pulmonary hypertension, whatever its cause, e.g., multiple pulmonary emboli or diffuse pulmonary vascular disease. Infective endocarditis is rare with ASDs because of the low pressure gradients and sluggish flow (see p. 581), but paradoxical embolism or brain abscess may appear.

Ventricular Septal Defect (VSD)

As pointed out earlier, VSD is the most common congenital cardiac anomaly. Frequently it is associated with other structural defects, particularly tetralogy of Fallot, but also with pulmonary stenosis, coarctation of the aorta, transposition of the great arteries, and tricuspid atresia.[140] Depending on the size of the defect, it may produce difficulties virtually from birth or, with smaller lesions, may not be recognized until later. Spontaneous closure of small defects sometimes occurs within the first three years of life. In normal cardiac development between the fifth and sixth weeks of embryonic life, the common ventricular canal is divided by a septum. The basal portion of the septum close to the atrioventricular valves is membranous and derived from endocardial cushion tissue and the conal ridges from the bulbus cordis. The remaining largest part of the septum is muscular and derived from the medial wall of the expanding ventricles.

VSDs vary enormously in size and location. They range from probe patencies to lesions sufficiently large to create virtually a single ventricle (cor triloculare biatriatum). Van Praagh and colleagues point out that univentricular hearts are not always the result of failure of development of the interventricular septum but may have other origins, e.g., aplasia of the right or left ventricle.[141] Ninety per cent of VSDs are located in the membranous portion of the interventricular septum (Fig. 13–28). Sometimes such defects are accompanied by prolapse of a defective or maldeveloped aortic valve. Most often single, though occasionally multiple, defects are found. In the course of time the left-to-right shunt induces right ventricular hypertrophy and sometimes, with small defects, focal endocardial thickenings where the jet stream impinges (jet lesions).

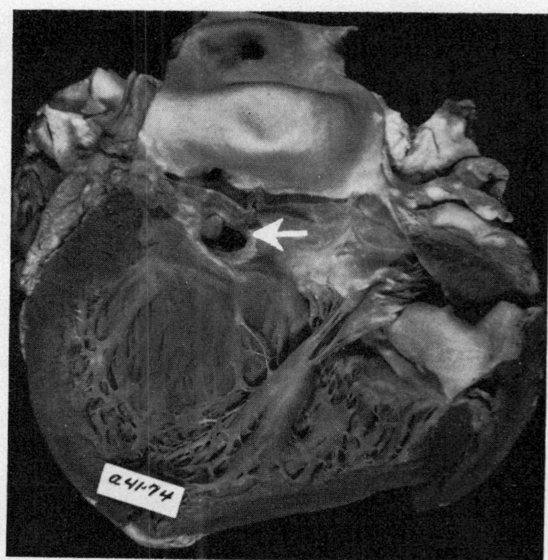

Figure 13–28. Ventricular septal defect high in membranous septum with fibrous thickening of margins of patency *(arrow)*.

The functional significance of a VSD depends on the size of the defect, level of pulmonary vascular resistance, and absence of pulmonary stenosis. Small defects (less than 0.5 cm in diameter) are generally well tolerated for years. However, they induce a loud murmur heard throughout systole, sometimes accompanied by a systolic thrill. Over the span of time the small defect may close. If it remains patent and permits a significant left-to-right flow (usually with diameters greater than 1 cm), right ventricular enlargement and pulmonary hypertension develop with reversal of flow and cyanose tardive, clubbing, and polycythemia. Large defects may become manifest virtually at birth because of signs of cardiac failure accompanying the murmur. There is, thus, a wide range in the behavior of VSD from spontaneous closure to fulminant cardiac failure.[142] A particular risk in those with small or moderate-sized defects is superimposed infective endocarditis, rarely encountered with large defects. Surgical closure of incidental VSDs is generally not attempted during infancy because of both the possibility of spontaneous closure and the operative mortality rate. However, correction is indicated in older children and adults when there is a moderate-to-large left-to-right shunt, before significant increased pulmonary vascular disease develops.

Patent Ductus Arteriosus

The ductus arteriosus is a normal vascular channel during intrauterine life that courses between the bifurcation of the pulmonary artery and the aorta, just distal to the origin of the left subclavian artery. In a healthy, full-term newborn, *functional* closure due to muscular contraction occurs within the first day of postnatal life, but anatomic closure by intimal proliferation and fibrosis may not occur for several months. Delay in functional closure often occurs in premature infants. The stimulus to closure is poorly understood, but the fact that any hypoxic condition such as the respiratory distress syndrome predisposes to delay suggests that arterial oxygen tension plays a role. Even in utero the patency of the ductus may depend on the elaboration of vasodilators, among them prostaglandins.[143] Thus, formation of specific vasodilating prostaglandins may also contribute to delayed closure of the ductus. Whatever the mechanism, persistence of a functional lumen greater than 2 mm in diameter after the first week of life is generally considered to be abnormal. In many analyses, patent ductus arteriosus is the second most frequent functional cardiovascular malformation in infancy and childhood, more common in females than in males. Although it may occur as the sole defect, it is sometimes accompanied by other malformations such as coarctation of the aorta, aortic stenosis, pulmonic stenosis, and VSD. Indeed, continued patency of the ductus may be lifesaving in the presence of severe pulmonic stenosis or atresia.

The length and diameter of the ductus vary widely. Sometimes it virtually consists of only a defect between closely approximated pulmonary artery and aorta. In other instances, it is several centimeters in length. The diameter may range up to 1 cm. Commonly, the left ventricle is hypertrophied and the pulmonary artery dilated. In older children and adults, right ventricular hypertrophy appears when pulmonary hypertension supervenes.

Most often, patent ductus arteriosus does not produce functional difficulties at birth. Indeed, a narrow ductus may have no effect on growth and development during childhood. However, its existence can generally be detected by a continuous harsh murmur described as machinery-like. Often it is accompanied by a systolic thrill. Since the shunt is at first left-to-right, there is no cyanosis. However, pulmonary hypertension and pulmonary vascular disease eventually ensue, with ultimate reversal of flow and all its associated consequences—right ventricular hypertrophy, cyanosis, clubbing, and polycythemia. Since the ductus empties into the aorta distal to the origin of the left subclavian artery, the cyanosis may affect the toes and lower extremities, but not the fingers. Elective surgical ligation is generally indicated because it carries a low morbidity and mortality, abolishes the abnormal shunt, and prevents the development of superimposed infective endoaortitis and pulmonary complications.

Coarctation of Aorta

Coarctation—narrowing or constriction—of the aorta ranks high in frequency among the common structural anomalies. Males are affected two to three times more often than females, although females with Turner's syndrome (p. 132) frequently have a coarctation. In the past, the narrowings have been subdivided into "infantile" and "adult" forms, but there is little utility to this separation since clinical manifestations depend almost entirely on the location of the narrowing and its severity. Although coarctation may occur as the sole defect, in 75% of instances it is accompanied by other anomalies—patent ductus arteriosus, bicuspid aortic valve, congenital aortic stenosis, ASD, VSD, mitral regurgitation, and berry aneurysms of the circle of Willis.

Narrowing of the aorta may occur anywhere along its length, even below the diaphragm, but most coarctations are located just distal or (less often) proximal to the ductus arteriosus or its obliterated ligamentum arteriosum. They may represent sharp, membrane-like constrictions, or narrowings several centimeters in length. The encroachment on the aortic lumen is also variable, sometimes leaving only a very small channel or, at other times, producing only minimal narrowing. With preductal coarctation, the ductus arteriosus is almost always open; in the postductal group, less than half have a patent ductus arteriosus (Fig. 13–29).

Preductal coarctation usually leads to manifestations early in life, and indeed it may cause signs and symptoms immediately after birth. Many infants with this anomaly do not survive the neonatal period. Much depends on the patency of the ductus arteriosus and its ability to supply sufficient blood to the aorta to sustain the circulation to the lower part of the body. With preductal coarctation, right ventricular hypertrophy develops in utero, and congestive heart failure may appear very early. In such cases the delivery of unsaturated blood through the ductus arteriosus produces cyanosis in the lower half of the body, while the head and arms are unaffected since their blood supply derives from vessels having origins proximal to the ductus.

The outlook is much brighter with *postductal coarctation*, unless very severe. Most of the children are asymptomatic and the disease may go unrecognized until well into adult life. Typically, there is hypertension in the upper extremities, but weak pulses and a lower blood pressure in the lower extremities associated with manifestations of arterial insufficiency, i.e., claudication

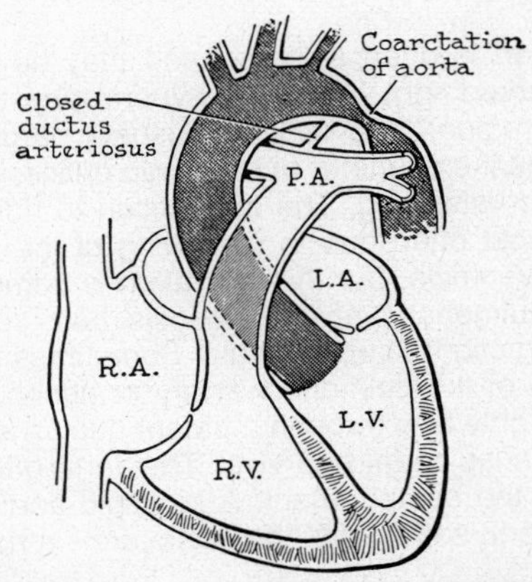

Figure 13–29. Diagram of major vessels showing a postductal coarctation of aorta.

and coldness. Particularly characteristic in adults is the development of collateral circulation between the precoarctation arterial branches and the postcoarctation arteries. Thus, the intercostals may become enlarged and palpable. Radiographically visible erosions ("notching") of the inner surfaces of the ribs may be produced by abnormally dilated internal mammary arteries. The axillary arteries may also become dilated and obviously pulsatile.

With all significant coarctations, murmurs are often present throughout systole, and sometimes a thrill. Similarly, there is cardiomegaly. Ultimately, aortography is definitive. With uncomplicated coarctation, surgical resection and end-to-end anastomosis or replacement of the affected aortic segment by a prosthetic graft yields excellent results. Untreated, the mean duration of life is about 40 years. Deaths are caused by congestive heart failure, intracranial hemorrhage, infective aortitis at the point of narrowing, and rupture of the precoarctation aorta related to the hypertension and the development of cystic medial necrosis (p. 534). Rarely, it should be noted, coarctation may occur in the proximal aorta prior to the origin of the major arteries to the head and neck and upper extremities, reducing the blood pressure and arterial supply of the entire body, or it may be located in the distal aorta and thus not be accompanied by any of the characteristic findings mentioned.

Tetralogy of Fallot

The four features of this disorder are (1) ventricular septal defect, (2) an aorta that overrides the ventricular defect, (3) obstruction to the right ventricular outflow, and (4) right ventricular hypertrophy (Fig. 13–30). The tetralogy is the most common form of cyanotic congenital heart disease that, even untreated, permits survival for more than a few years. Indeed, in an analysis of a large series of patients with this condition who died without ever having had cardiac surgery, about 10% were alive at 20 years and 3% at 40 years.[144] It is more frequent in males than in females. The severity of the clinical manifestations are directly related to the degree of obstruction to right ventricular outflow.

The heart is often enlarged and may be boot shaped owing to marked right ventricular hypertrophy, particularly of the apical region. The VSD is usually large and often approximates the diameter of the aortic orifice. It often abuts on the aortic valve ring. The obstruction to right ventricular outflow is most often due to narrowing of the infundibulum of the right ventricle, but this alteration is sometimes associated with pulmonary valvular stenosis. Less commonly, the outflow obstruction is supravalvular. Sometimes there is complete atresia of the pulmonary artery or absence of a main branch, and only flow through a patent ductus and/or dilated bronchial arteries permits survival. The aortic origin overrides or straddles the septal defect. A bicuspid aortic valve may be present, and sometimes the aortic arch is right-sided.

It is evident from the anatomic malformations that pulmonary flow is reduced, sometimes markedly, and so a large volume of unoxygenated right ventricular blood is shunted through the septal defect. Thus, cyanosis appears very early, although it may not be apparent at birth with milder obstruction. In time, even infants born without cyanosis often develop it as the right ventricular outflow obstruction progressively worsens. Dyspnea, underdevelopment, clubbing, and polycythemia accompany the appearance of cyanosis. A murmur is frequently present that may not be distinguishable from one caused by a VSD. It is produced by the pulmonary outflow obstruction and its intensity is *inversely* proportional to the severity of the obstruction. The diagnosis is frequently apparent from the clinical findings along with radiologic evidence of reduced pulmonary vascular markings. However, it may require selective angiocardiography with right ventricular injection to document the cardiac anomalies of both form and function. Surgical correction is indicated in almost all patients; untreated, less than one-quarter of those affected live for ten years.[145] Moreover, surgery is indicated as early in life as the condition of the patient permits because the infundibular narrowing increases with time. The causes of death are usually hypoxia and cardiac failure, sometimes aggravated by respiratory infections. Common complications are polycythemia with a thrombotic diathesis, infective endocarditis, paradoxic embolism, cerebral infarction, and cerebral abscess.

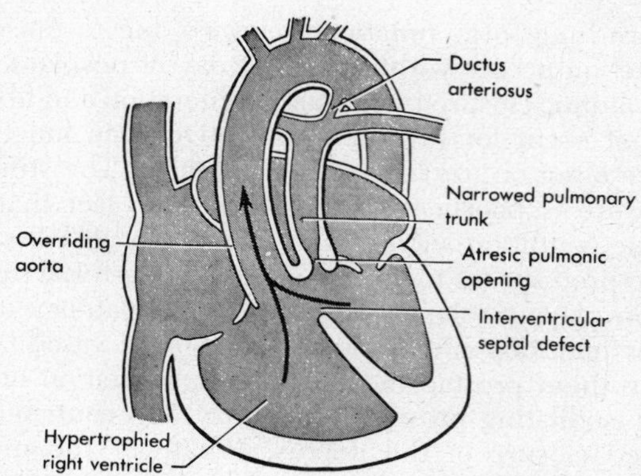

Figure 13–30. Diagram of heart and major vessels showing tetralogy of Fallot. *Note:* Origin of pulmonary artery has been schematically displaced to left to call attention to its stenosis.

VALVULAR AND VASCULAR OBSTRUCTIVE LESIONS

Tricuspid Atresia

Complete absence of the tricuspid valve is known as atresia. It is almost always associated with underdevelopment of the right ventricle and an ASD. The circulation is maintained by a right-to-left shunt through the interatrial communication. Often the tricuspid atresia is associated with hypoplasia of the pulmonary artery and atresia or stenosis of the pulmonary valve. A VSD also is frequently present. Cyanosis is present virtually from birth and there is a high mortality in the first weeks or months of life. Palliative surgery may be possible, depending on the severity and number of associated anomalies.

Pulmonary Stenosis or Atresia with Intact Interventricular Septum

This is a relatively uncommon cardiac malformation. When the valve is entirely atretic it is commonly associated with a hypoplastic right ventricle and an ASD. With atresia, there is no communication between the right ventricle and lungs, and so flow bypasses the right ventricle through an interatrial septal defect, thence entering the lungs through a patent ductus. Pulmonary stenosis, on the other hand, may be mild to severe. It is usually caused by fusion of the cusps creating a dome-shaped structure surmounted by the valvular orifice. Mild stenosis may be asymptomatic and compatible with long life. The smaller the valvular orifice, the more severe is the cyanosis and the earlier its appearance. The prognosis obviously depends on the severity of the pulmonary valvular narrowing and associated malformations. Isolated valvular stenosis is easily corrected with surgery. When associated with right ventricular hypoplasia, the outlook is poor. It should be noted that obstruction to the pulmonary flow may be due also to subvalvular or supravalvular narrowings, or sometimes there are multiple sites of stenosis.

Aortic Stenosis and Atresia

A relatively rare developmental anomaly, aortic atresia is incompatible with neonatal survival. Aortic stenosis, however, is compatible with survival, depending on its severity. There are two types, valvular and subvalvular. With valvular stenosis there is maldevelopment of the cusps to create essentially a thickened, fibrous diaphragm having a lumen of varying diameter. The subvalvular pattern comprises a thickened fibrous ring below the level of the cusps. With the exception of coarctation of the aorta and occasionally patent ductus arteriosus, other associated anomalies are uncommon. However, left ventricular hypertrophy frequently develops as a consequence of the pressure overload. Sometimes, poststenotic dilatation of the aortic root develops. A prominent systolic murmur is usually detectable and sometimes a thrill. It should be noted that there are other causes of obstruction to the left ventricular outflow such as an unusually proximal coarctation (supravalvular obstruction) and hypertrophic cardiomyopathy (idiopathic hypertrophic subaortic stenosis) (p. 597). In general, congenital stenoses are well tolerated unless very severe. Mild stenoses can be managed conservatively with antibiotic prophylaxis and avoidance of strenuous activity, but the threat of sudden death with exertion always looms. Surgical correction is usually indicated, however, with both mild and severe stenosis for hemodynamic reasons and to lessen the chance of infective endocarditis.

Bicuspid Aortic Valve

This malformation is one of the most common (1 to 2% of the population), but is of no functional significance at the outset. Over the span of years to decades, however, it is prone to become fibrotic and calcified and thus give rise to calcific aortic stenosis (p. 578). The bicuspid valve is also a favored site for the development of infective endocarditis.

Hypoplastic Left Heart Syndrome

This designation refers to a constellation of very similar congenital anomalies all marked by (1) underdevelopment of the left cardiac chambers, (2) atresia or stenosis of one or both of the left-sided valves, and (3) hypoplasia of the aorta. Commonly, there is endocardial fibroelastosis (p. 599) in the left chambers. The route of blood flow is from the lungs into the small left atrium, thence through a patent foramen ovale into the right heart and out the pulmonary artery to traverse a patent ductus arteriosus and thus reach the aorta. However, the cardiac output is markedly reduced, and most infants manifest cardiac failure from birth and die within days as the ductus begins to narrow postnatally. Even when the condition is recognized by catheterization, attempts at corrective or palliative surgery have generally been to no avail.

TRANSPOSITIONS

Transposition of Great Arteries and Veins

Transpositions are a complex group of malformations in which there may be inversion of the aorta and pulmonary artery with respect to the ventricles, inversion of the atria with respect to the ventricles, ventricular inversion relative to the atria, inversion of the atria and ventricles together, or origin of both great vessels from a single ventricle. Only the most common form will be described, along with a few comments on two other variants. More details are available elsewhere.[146, 147] *In the most common pattern, the aorta arises from the morphogenetic right ventricle and lies anteriorly to the pulmonary artery and toward the midline, while the pulmonary artery arises from the morphogenetic left ventricle (Fig. 13–31).* This malformation has a male-to-female ratio of 3:1 and is particularly common in offspring of diabetic mothers. During intrauterine life, the patency of the foramen ovale and ductus arteriosus provide sufficient "mixing" of venous and systemic blood to permit survival. Postnatal survival requires continued "mixing," otherwise two separate circulations would exist, with the aorta receiving unoxygenated blood from the systemic return and the pulmonary artery recycling oxygenated blood. Virtually all patients who survive the neonatal period have an interatrial communication; patent ductus is present in about 60% and a VSD in 30%. Right ventricular hypertrophy usually develops with survival for any period of time.

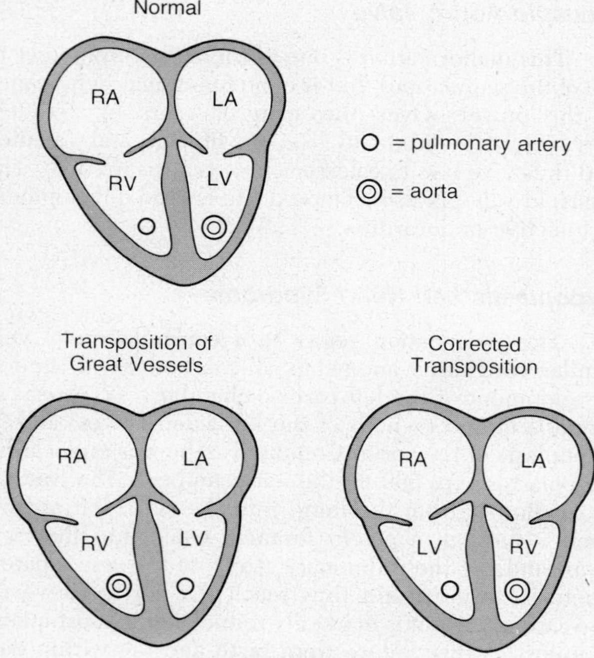

Figure 13–31.

This pattern of transposition is one of the common forms of cyanotic congenital heart disease and is a major cause of death in the first two months of life. Recognition of this entity requires correct differentiation of the morphogenetic, finely trabeculated left ventricle from the coarsely trabeculated right ventricle.

The outlook for infants with transposition of the great vessels depends on the degree of "mixing" of the blood, the magnitude of the tissue hypoxia, and the ability of the morphogenetic right ventricle to maintain the aortic outflow and systemic circulation. Without surgery, most patients die within the first months of life. Rare survivals into young adult life have been reported, usually when there is an associated large interatrial defect, a VSD with some pulmonic stenosis, or a single ventricle.

A variety of surgical approaches have been devised for increasing the intracardiac communication of the systemic and pulmonary circulations.

In so-called *"corrected" transposition* the ventricles are inverted relative to the atria. Thus, the morphogenetic right atrium communicates with the morphogenetic left ventricle that supplies a transposed pulmonary artery. On the other side of the heart, the left atrium communicates with the morphogenetic right ventricle that ejects into the transposed aorta (Fig. 13–31). In the absence of other associated malformations, a functionally normal circulation would exist save that the systemic arterial supply is maintained by a morphogenetic right ventricle that usually undergoes marked hypertrophy. However, other malformations are usually present, particularly of the atrioventricular valves, and so a satisfactory physiologic circulation is rarely achieved.[148]

Another variant is the *Taussig-Bing malformation.* In this condition, the aorta comes off the right ventricle and there is a VSD directly beneath an "overriding" pulmonary artery that is situated in front of the aorta. Frequently, an associated coarctation of the aorta is present.

MALPOSITIONS OF HEART

Positional anomalies are, fortunately, uncommon. Some are extraordinary and are encountered in teratologic monsters such as when the heart is situated outside of the body (ectopia cordis) or within the abdomen with a diaphragmatic hernia. Other malpositions, such as dextrocardia, are of importance only as clinical diagnostic curiosities imposed upon unsuspecting medical students. In dextrocardia, the apex of the heart points to the right and is in the right hemithorax. Dextrocardia may be accompanied by inversion of all of the viscera in the recessively inherited condition "situs inversus totalis," thus creating a mirror image of the anatomic location of all viscera. The left-sided appendix and gallbladder can cause confusion to the unwary surgeon. Sometimes the situs inversus is accompanied by sinusitis and bronchiectasis, thus constituting *Kartagener's syndrome.* The basis for this curious complex of abnormalities is discussed on page 729. In most instances, the heart is otherwise normal and the individual may not even be aware of being a "walking medical curiosity." However, other cardiac malformations may be present.

Dextrocardia may not be accompanied by inversion of other viscera—isolated dextrocardia. Such hearts are almost always abnormal. Particularly common associations are transposition of the atria relative to the ventricles, or transposition of the great arteries, as has been described. Conversely, the viscera may be inverted with the heart in its normal position.[149] There is a well-defined association of asplenia or polysplenia with malpositions of the heart.

MYOCARDIAL DISEASE

Myocardial disease occurs in many of the major forms of heart disease, such as MI, rheumatic heart disease, and hypertensive heart disease, already discussed. Here our consideration is limited to two broad categories of myocardial involvement: (1) myocarditis, characterized by morphologic changes indicative of an inflammatory reaction, usually to some microbiologic agent; and (2) noninflammatory myocardial disease (possibly postinflammatory disease of uncertain cause), excluding the well-defined causes discussed earlier, i.e., ischemic heart disease, pulmonary and systemic hypertension, and valvular and congenital heart disease. The noninflammatory involvements are further subdivided into cardiomyopathies of unknown cause and "specific heart muscle diseases" in which the clinical setting makes known the basis of the myocardial changes. Some authors would classify all forms of heart muscle disease as cardiomyopathy, identifying myocarditis as an infectious form of cardiomyopathy and the specific heart muscle diseases as secondary cardiomyopathies. These taxonomic issues are not of great importance, but it is useful to segregate myocarditis from cardiomyopathy from the specific heart muscle diseases for clinical reasons. The last-mentioned category usually presents with some well-defined systemic disease, as pointed out later (p. 601). Myocarditis, on the other hand, is often a primary heart disease. It is usually of sudden onset and often produces acute cardiac failure. It is generally characterized by a prominent inflammatory reaction, with necrosis of isolated cells or small groups of myocardial fibers, and it tends to pursue a course of varying length. In many instances, the prognosis is good. If the patient survives, it resolves, sometimes leaving little or no residual myocardial scarring. In contrast, in the idiopathic cardiomyopathies, the myocardial alterations are associated with little inflammatory reaction. Most run a protracted course, and many never remit. For long periods of time, they usually evoke no symptoms until, for mysterious reasons and apparently without provocation, cardiac failure insidiously sets in. Such a clear separation into myocarditis or cardiomyopathy is not always possible, and many cases must be classified arbitrarily. However, endomyocardial biopsies obtained at cardiac catheterization promise to broaden our understanding of the nature and course of the conditions.[150]

MYOCARDITIS

Myocarditis is an important form of heart disease because it may occur at any age, even in infancy, and occasionally with unexpected suddenness may induce cardiac failure or cause sudden death by arrhythmia. It is difficult to be certain of the precise clinical incidence of this condition because often the diagnosis is based on indirect evidence, e.g., fever and sudden appearance of ECG changes indicative of a diffuse myocardial lesion in the absence of other definable causes. It has been said to be present in from 1 to 4% of routine autopsies. In many of these cases, however, it was an incidental and chance finding, imparting in all likelihood an overestimate of the frequency of the clinically significant disease.[151-153]

The causes of myocarditis are legion and include virtually every known microbiologic agent, various forms of immunologically mediated damage, hypersensitivity reactions, and reactions to physical agents. The more important etiologies are present in Table 13–5, and a few comments are in order about some of these.

Over one-half of all cases of well-documented myocarditis are of viral origin. Infants, immunosuppressed individuals, and pregnant women are particularly vulnerable. The most frequently implicated agents are Coxsackie A and B, ECHO, polio, and influenza viruses. In most instances the cardiac involvement follows some days to a few weeks after a primary viral infection elsewhere, as in the lungs, upper respiratory tract, or neuromuscular system (in poliomyelitis). Occasionally, the myocarditis is the sole or, at least, major focus of infection and so is referred to as *primary myocarditis.* The documentation of a viral etiology is almost always difficult. Direct isolation of the virus from the heart is not generally possible except from endomyocardial biopsies or necropsy specimens, and then is only likely to be productive when done during the early days of the illness. Isolation of virus from noncardiac sources does not necessarily imply that the same agent is implicated in causing the cardiac changes. Visualization of viral particles in myofibers by electron microscopy or immunofluorescent techniques, although suggestive, is not proof of causality. Most often, recourse is made to serologic demonstration of a rising antibody titer in the serum. However, such evidence is indirect, and again does not prove a viral etiology for the myocarditis.

There is still uncertainty about the mechanisms involved in the production of cardiac damage by viral agents. Two possibilities exist.[154] There may be direct viral cytotoxicity. Alternatively, the specific agent may evoke a cell-mediated immune reaction, which then damages the cardiac myofibers harboring virus or viral-dictated antigens. The weight of evidence favors the latter mechanism. Infiltration of the myocardium by lymphocytes and macrophages is characteristic of most viral involvements of the myocardium. There is often a delay of days to a few weeks between the onset of an extracardiac viral infection and the appearance of the myocarditis. Immunoglobulins can often be demonstrated by immunofluorescent methods along the sarcolemmal sheaths of myofibers. In addition, activated T cells and a defect in suppressor T-cell activity have been reported.[155]

Among the bacteria, myocardial involvement is most commonly encountered with diphtheritic, meningococcal, and leptospiral infections. You recall from an earlier discussion (p. 317) that the exotoxin of the diphtheria bacillus causes cardiac damage by inhibiting protein synthesis, since it specifically interferes with a translocating enzyme involved in the delivery of amino acids to elongating polypeptide chains. The toxin also interferes with the metabolism of carnitine and so inhibits the oxidation of long chain fatty acids, causing triglycerides to accumulate in myofibers with the development of fatty change. Myocarditis is sometimes seen in individuals having fulminating meningococcemia, such as is characteristic of the Waterhouse-Friderichsen syndrome. Leptospiral Weil's disease is often marked by inflammatory myocardial changes related to the systemic dissemination of the organisms. Similarly, the myocardium may be affected in any bacterial infection when the causative agent is blood borne, as, for example, with salmonellosis or any form of bacterial endocarditis.

Myocarditis may be encountered with any of the systemic mycoses and is increasingly seen as an opportunistic disease with aspergillosis and candidiasis, particularly in immunosuppressed patients. Toxoplasmosis in the newborn is typically characterized by myocardial involvement. *A particularly important form of infection is that caused by* Trypanosoma cruzi *producing Chagas' disease.* Although uncommon in the northern hemisphere, Chagas' disease affects up to one-half of the population in endemic areas of South America, and myocardial involvement is found in approximately 80% of infected individuals. Approximately 10% of patients may die during an acute attack, or they may enter a chronic phase and develop progressive signs of cardiac insufficiency 10 to 20 years later. The importance of this cause of myocarditis is evident from the fact that it causes about 25% of all deaths in persons between the ages of 25 and 44 in endemic areas.[156] Trichinosis is the most common helminthic disease associated with localization of the causative agent in the heart muscle, as pointed out on page 379.

It is evident from Table 13–5 that *there are noninfectious causes of myocarditis.* Some are associated with systemic diseases of immune origin such as rheumatic fever and systemic lupus erythematosus. In other instances, hypersensitivity to a particular agent appears to be involved, as is the case with myocarditis related to allergic reactions to penicillin, sulfonamides, and other drugs. Heat stroke or chest radiography for lung or breast cancers may produce myocardial cell necrosis, and the products of the necrotic cells may then evoke inflammatory myocardial changes.

Several forms of myocarditis are of idiopathic origin. Cardiac lesions were found at autopsy in about 20% of patients with sarcoidosis.[157] Although in many of these instances the involvement was of little clinical significance, sarcoidosis may cause sufficient myocardial damage to produce cardiac decompensation and arrhythmias, sometimes leading to sudden death. Another idiopathic disorder is so-called giant cell myocarditis. Morphologically and clinically it closely resembles yet another form of myocarditis—Fiedler's. Both merit attention because they are often fatal.[158] The distinctive pathologic features of these entities are described later. Against this background we can turn to the anatomic changes seen in the various forms of myocarditis.

Table 13–5. MAJOR CAUSES OF MYOCARDITIS

Viruses
Coxsackie A and B
ECHO virus
Influenza
Poliomyelitis
Viral hepatitis
Epstein-Barr virus (infectious mononucleosis)
Cytomegalovirus
Chlamydia
C. psittaci
Rickettsia
R. typhi (typhus fever)
R. tsutsugamushi (scrub typhus)
Bacteria
Diphtheria
Salmonella
Tuberculosis
Streptococci (beta-hemolytic)
Meningococcus
Leptospira (Weil's disease)
Borrelia (relapsing fever)
Fungi and Protozoa
Trypanosoma (Chagas' disease)
Aspergillus
Blastomyces
Cryptococci
Candida
Coccidioidomyces
Metazoa
Echinococcus
Trichinella
Hypersensitivity Reactions
Poststreptococcal (rheumatic fever)
Systemic lupus erythematosus
Systemic sclerosis
Methyldopa
Sulfonamides
Penicillin
Para-aminosalicylic acid
Streptomycin
Physical Agents
Radiation
Heat stroke
Unknown
Sarcoidosis
Giant cell (Fiedler's) myocarditis

MORPHOLOGY. During the active phase of myocarditis the hearts are usually enlarged with dilatation of all chambers, but sometimes only the left or right ventricle. The lesions may be diffuse or patchy. The ventricular myocardium is typically flabby, and often mottled by either pale foci or minute hemorrhagic lesions. The endocardium and valves are unaffected except that mural thrombi may be present in any chamber. At some later date when the acute phase has passed, the heart may appear entirely normal or there may be residual hypertrophy. In other instances, small foci of fibrosis may be evident throughout the myocardium. Occasionally the involvement is most severe in the inner third of the myocardium, to induce diffuse subendocardial fibrosis with some flattening and atrophy of the columnae carneae, mimicking fibroelastosis (p. 599) or endomyocardial fibrosis (p. 599). Such hearts are often hypertrophied.

The histologic changes are even more varied and, as would be expected, vary with the specific causative agent. Only some generalizations can be offered. During active disease, isolated myofiber lysis (myocytolysis) or patchy foci of necrosis are present and are accompanied by an inflammatory cell infiltrate. **With viral myocarditis there is a tendency for isolated fiber necrosis. The infiltrate is usually mononuclear—lymphocytes, macrophages, and occasional plasma cells—and is accompanied by an interstitial edema that separates the individual myofibers** (Fig.13–32). This pattern is sometimes called "lymphocytic myocarditis" because in many instances it is impossible to be certain of its cause. Infrequently, with the poliomyelitis or influenzal viruses there is necrosis of a larger number of myofibers accompanied by a prominent neutrophilic infiltration. The histologic pattern of reaction to bacterial invasion depends on the specific causative organism, but, in general, mirrors the changes produced by the same organism in extracardiac localizations. Thus, **pyogens induce more of a patchy, focal, suppurative reaction, and sometimes microabscesses with less prominence of the diffuse interstitial component.** In contrast, the salmonelloses are

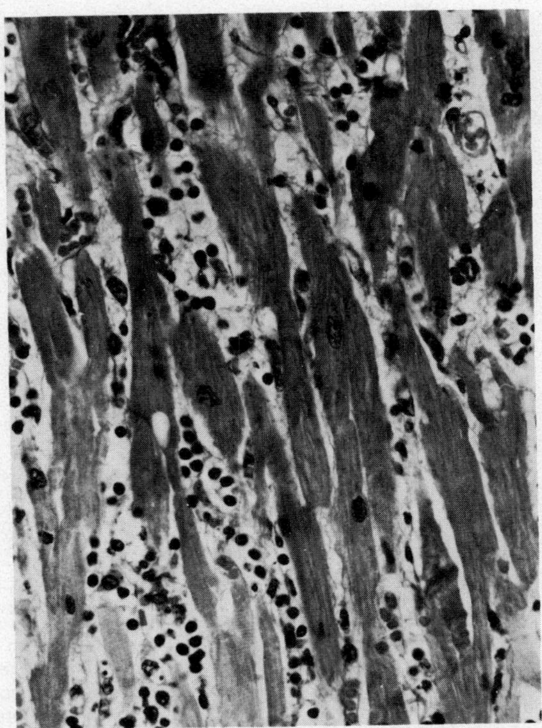

Figure 13–32. Viral myocarditis with marked interstitial edema and lymphocytic infiltration.

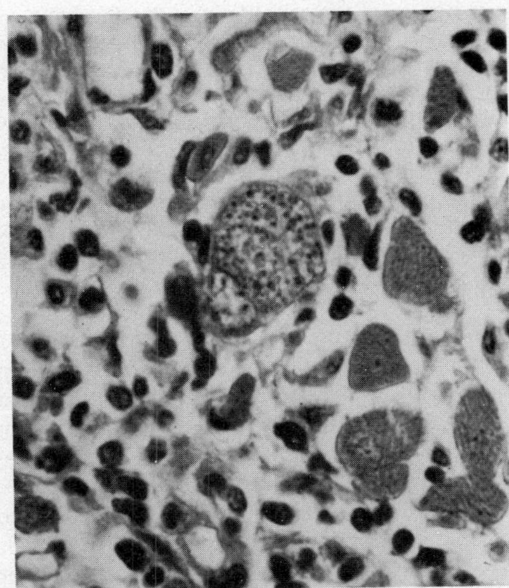

Figure 13–33. Chagasic myocarditis. A myocardial fiber *(center)* is filled with parasites. Surrounding fibers have been destroyed and replaced by a leukocytic infiltrate.

marked by a mononuclear focal, histiocytic reaction. Analogously larger parasites produce their typical tissue reactions within the heart muscle. You recall that, **in trichinosis, although the parasite often invades the heart, it rarely encysts within its myofibers.** Usually, therefore, only focal infiltrates of lymphocytes and eosinophils can be identified in foci of myocytolysis, but only rarely are larvae or fragments of larvae visible.[159] **The myocarditis of Chagas' disease is rendered distinctive by parasitization of scattered myofibers by trypanosomes accompanied by an inflammatory infiltrate of neutrophils, lymphocytes, macrophages, and occasional eosinophils** (Fig. 13–33). The protozoa may produce so-called pseudocysts in the more protracted infections, surrounded by a mononuclear and eosinophilic infiltration. Eventually, fibrosis ensues.

Hypersensitivity reactions that involve the myocardium induce interstitial infiltrates that are principally perivascular, composed of lymphocytes, plasma cells, macrophages, and eosinophils. Occasionally, acute vasculitis can be seen similar to the small vessel lesions in hypersensitivity reactions within noncardiac tissues.

The study of myocarditis by immunofluorescent and immunoperoxidase techniques is still in its infancy but a few observations are possible. Immunoglobulins, particularly IgG and C_3, are present in many cases of infectious origin and almost invariably in those related to hypersensitivity reactions. The immunoglobulins and C_3 are deposited principally along sarcolemmal membranes and in the walls of small vessels, but surprisingly are not confined to foci of obvious injury. Their presence in viral myocarditis argues strongly for immunologic mediation of the myofiber damage, as pointed out earlier.

There remain two morphologically distinctive forms of myocarditis—**Fiedler's** and **idiopathic giant cell myocarditis.** Both are characterized by focal necroses associated with a granulomatous reaction containing multinucleate giant cells interspersed with lymphocytes, eosinophils, plasma cells, and macrophages (Fig. 13–34).[100] There is a strong likelihood that both entities are, in fact, a single disease of unknown origin. A viral etiology is suspected, but the gran-

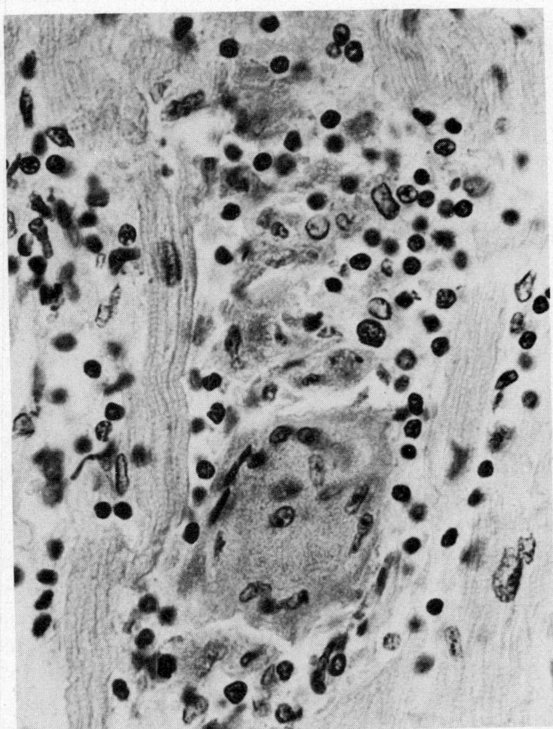

Figure 13–34. Giant cell myocarditis. The focus of myofiber necrosis is populated by macrophages, lymphocytes, occasional plasma cells, and a prominent multinucleate giant cell. (From Rabson, A., et al.: Hum. Pathol., in press.)

ulomatous nature of the reaction and the frequent presence of eosinophils suggest immune mediation.[158]

Whatever the pattern of histologic changes during the acute phase of the disease, all inflammatory lesions either resolve, leaving no residuals, or undergo progressive fibrosis, as mentioned earlier. Often the persistent connective tissue is sufficiently scattered and subtle to be virtually inapparent at a later date. With more severe damage, focal minute scars may remain; in extremely florid cases, they may become confluent and thus be grossly visible, particularly when subendocardial.

All forms of myocarditis evoke remarkably similar clinical manifestations that vary more in severity than in type. At one end of the clinical spectrum the disease is entirely asymptomatic and only suspected when ECG changes, particularly abnormalities of the ST segment and T wave, point to a diffuse myocardial lesion. At the other end of the spectrum the myocarditis announces itself by the sudden onset of congestive heart failure. In such cases, systolic murmurs related to dilatation of the atrioventricular valve rings may appear, and sometimes arrhythmias. Between these extremes are the many involvements associated with such symptoms as fatigue, dyspnea, palpitations, and precordial discomfort, sometimes accompanied by mild fever when the myocarditis is of infectious origin. Many patients recover completely without sequelae. The rare severe attack may pursue a rapidly downhill course to death in cardiac failure. Such fulminant progression is particularly characteristic of the giant cell myocarditides. Occasionally, a more protracted chronic course is followed and years later, when the attack of myocarditis is forgotten, the patient is diagnosed as having congestive cardiomyopathy of unknown cause. Endomyocardial biopsy is proving of great value in establishing the diagnosis and severity of the various forms of myocarditis.

CARDIOMYOPATHY (CMP)

The definition and classification of CMP is riddled with controversy. Some cardiologists would include any form of heart failure caused by myocardial insufficiency, including ischemic heart disease, nutritional deficiency such as beriberi, and myocarditis.[161] Others hew to the more generally accepted view that specifically excluded are ischemic heart disease, pulmonary and systemic hypertension, valvular and congenital heart disease, and all forms of "specific heart muscle disease" mentioned later (p. 601); hence, the objection to the term "ischemic cardiomyopathy." When a task force of "cardiomyopathists" was convened, agreement was reached on the following definition: "*cardiomyopathies are heart muscle diseases of unknown cause*."[162] Thus, myocardial dysfunction of known inflammatory origin (myocarditis) is excluded as is that associated with disorders of other systems, now referred to as "specific heart muscle disease" although such involvements have in the past been called "secondary CMP." The classification of

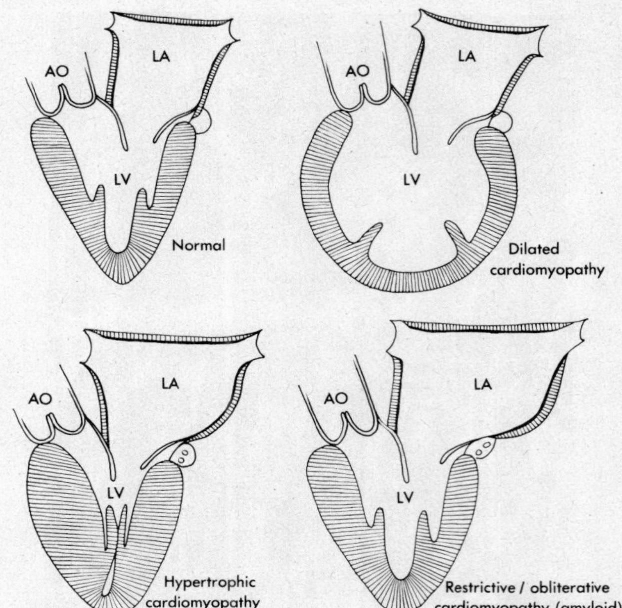

Figure 13–35. Various types of cardiomyopathies compared with normal heart. In dilated type, largest circumference of left ventricle is not at its base but midway between apex and base. In hypertrophic type, left ventricular cavity is small, and in restrictive-obliterative variety, as in amyloidosis, left ventricular cavity is of normal size. (Modified from Roberts, W. C., and Ferrans, V. J.: Pathologic anatomy of the cardiomyopathies. Hum. Pathol. *6*: 289, 1975.)

CMP (Fig. 13–35) as just defined has been greatly simplified, as follows:[163]

1. Dilated (congestive) CMP.
2. Hypertrophic CMP.
3. Restrictive/obliterative CMP.

Dilated (Congestive) CMP

Dilated or congestive CMP is characterized by dilatation of the left or right ventricles, or both. Although secondary hypertrophy usually supervenes, ventricular contraction is impaired, leading to low ejection fractions, high end-systolic volumes, and, often, congestive heart failure. The pathogenesis of the dilatation and poor ventricular function is unknown. Very likely, this entity has many origins and so represents a common outcome of a variety of forms of myocardial injury excluding that associated with coronary heart disease, systemic or pulmonary hypertension, or valvular or congenital heart disease. In most analyses of this condition, no significant genetic influence has been observed, although a small number of familial cases have been reported. Genetic modes of transmission have been proposed for such cases, but it is not possible to rule out coincidence or obscure environmental influences to which the entire family may have been exposed.

Occasionally, cardiac failure has appeared without an identifiable etiology in the last month of pregnancy or in the first five postpartum months in the absence of demonstrable previous heart disease. To this condition the designation "peripartum CMP" has been applied as a subset of dilated/congestive CMP.[164] Commonly, multiparity and malnutrition are associated, and it seems likely that the peripartal period merely stresses some underlying myocardial derangement, possibly even an unrecognized myocarditis.[164A]

The role of chronic alcoholism in the causation of dilated CMP is controversial.[165, 166] Although alcohol can clearly injure other organs and tissues, the point at issue is whether it is also a cardiotoxic agent by itself; if so, it should rightfully be considered a form of "specific heart muscle disease." In view of uncertainty about the etiologic importance of this agent with respect to the heart, it is considered here. On the one hand, there is evidence that in humans ethanol infusion induces cardiac myofiber ultrastructural alterations, including fatty change.[167] Moreover, the constellation of changes is alleged to be specific. On the other hand, there is no significantly increased incidence of congestive CMP in individuals with a history of heavy alcoholic intake, nor any correlation between survival and level of alcohol consumption, and withdrawal of alcohol has not always effected hemodynamic improvement. Moreover, most experts do not believe the morphologic changes to be specific for alcohol. However, such negative evidence cannot be considered as definitive, and on balance alcohol is generally considered to be detrimental to the heart and a possible cause of dilated CMP.[168]

Some instances of dilated CMP may have their origins in past, possibly subclinical, episodes of myocarditis, particularly those of viral origin, or conceivably in previous hypertension that is no longer present at the time of onset of the congestive failure. Dilated CMP is, then, in a sense, a wastebasket into which are placed all patients having CHF that cannot be related to well-defined origins at the time the dilated heart is first recognized.

The hearts are always increased in weight (up to 900 gm), but dilatation of the ventricles may neutralize preexistent thickening of the ventricular walls (Fig. 13–36). The poor cardiac contraction and stasis of blood in the cardiac chambers often leads to mural thrombi in the left ventricle, right ventricle, right atrial appendage, and left atrial appendage, in order of frequency.[169] The cardiac valves are usually normal, and most often the coronary arteries are normal or have minimal-to-moderate atherosclerosis compatible with the patient's age.

Histologic examination of hearts at necropsy and of endomyocardial biopsies discloses only vague and nonspecific changes. Indeed, there may be no significant alterations in as many as one-quarter of the cases.[170] Hypertrophy of occasional myocardial cells, atrophy of others, and occasionally some increase in interstitial fibrous tissue reminiscent of a past episode of viral myocarditis are the most common changes.[171] Sometimes there is mild-to-moderate endocardial thickening, principally in the ventricles. Small interstitial foci of mononuclear inflammatory cells are sometimes observed. Neither the electron microscope nor histochemistry has contributed to the specificity of the changes, revealing only regressive alterations.[169]

As is already obvious, dilated CMP is characterized clinically by progressive cardiac failure. Atrial fibrillation and systemic or pulmonary embolism may punctuate the course. Whatever its basis, it is a serious disorder, which to date has only been palliated with the usual forms of cardiac therapy. In a few instances, desperation has led to cardiac transplantation.

Hypertrophic CMP

This form of CMP is also known by such terms as asymmetric septal hypertrophy (ASH), idiopathic hypertrophic subaortic stenosis (IHSS), and hypertrophic obstructive cardiomyopathy. However, the name hypertrophic CMP seems preferable because the cardiac changes are not always obstructive and the hypertrophy is not always subaortic or asymmetric. It is, however, characterized by a heavy muscular *hyper*contracting heart in striking contrast to the flabby, *hypo*contracting heart of dilated CMP. The etiology and pathogenesis of this condition are unknown, and so hypotheses abound.[172] There is reasonably good evidence that, at least in some instances, it may constitute a heritable disorder. Studies using echocardiography for case identification reveal patterns of transmission compatible with autosomal dominant inheritance.[173] Further evidence of a genetic background is the increased prevalence of HLA-B12 in whites and -B5 in blacks, both loci being located on chromosome 6.[174] Whether there is also a

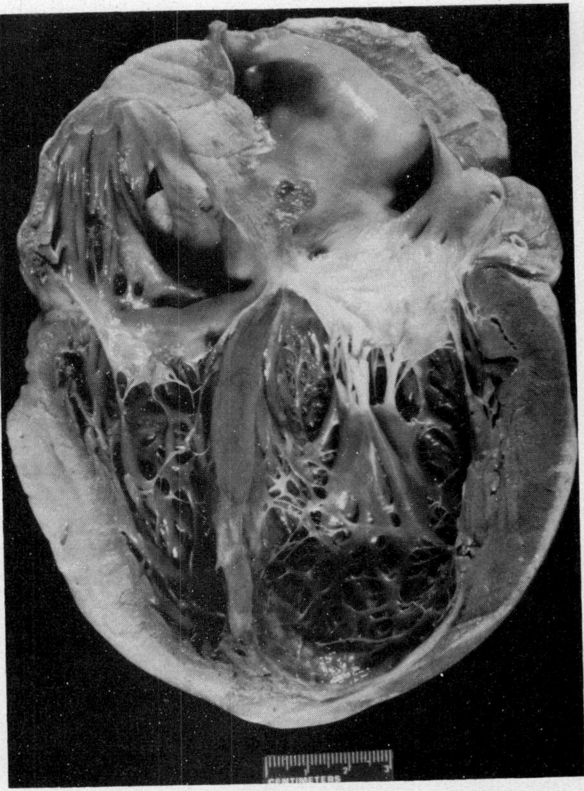

Figure 13–36. Congestive dilated cardiomyopathy with expansion of all chambers, particularly the ventricles. Slight thickening of chordae tendineae of mitral valve (seen on right) was of no functional significance clinically and may represent minimal healed rheumatic heart disease or hemodynamic alterations.

sporadic nongenetic form of the disease remains uncertain.

The morphologic features of hypertrophic CMP have been well summarized by Roberts.[169] Most distinctive are: (1) disproportional hypertrophy of the ventricular septum (95%); (2) disarray of myofibers in the ventricular septum (100%), but sometimes also in the left ventricular free wall; (3) reduction in the volume of the ventricular cavities (90%); (4) endocardial thickening or mural plaque formation in the left ventricular free outflow tract (75%); (5) mitral valve thickening (75%); (6) dilated atria (100%); and (7) abnormal intramural coronary arteries (50%).

Disproportional hypertrophy of the septum and diminution in the size of the left ventricular cavity are the two most important features of this condition. In adults the maximal thickness of the interventricular septum averages 3.0 cm, while the left ventricular free wall averages about 1.8 cm. **The thickest portion of the septum in patients with apparent obstructive symptoms is toward the base of the heart behind the mitral leaflet, whereas in those without obstructive symptoms it is located more apically, and therefore does not contribute to mitral valve dysfunction, as explained below.** Microscopically, in addition to the changes seen in myofibers in all forms of hypertrophy (p. 568), there is disarray of myofibers so that they are oriented in a haphazard pattern rather than in the usual parallel array, both in the ventricular septum and in the free wall (Fig. 13–37). Some reports contend that the disarray is more prominent in the septum than in the free wall, particularly in patients with obstructive manifestations, but recent analyses find no significant difference.[175] There is also disarray of myofibrils and myofilaments within individual cells. However, it is important to note that similar changes may occur with "ordinary" hypertrophy, but usually are less marked.[176] Another striking histologic change is a marked accumulation of glycogen within myofibers. Some fibrous thickening of the anterior mitral leaflet, particularly at its contact surface with the chamber wall, may be present, probably related to chronic impingement on the thickened ventricular septum and free wall. The remaining valves are normal and the coronary arteries unremarkable. Although none of these features alone is diagnostic of hypertrophic CMP, collectively they add up to considerable specificity.

Clinically, hypertrophic CMP, when symptomatic, presents manifestations of inadequate left ventricular outflow such as dizziness and syncope, or sometimes angina. In some patients the disease first becomes apparent with the onset of left ventricular failure. A prominent systolic murmur is present, which is due both to outflow obstruction to the left ventricle and to mitral regurgitation. *However, it is important to note that many patients with hypertrophic CMP documented by echocardiography and angiography do not have obstructive symptoms; moreover, obstructive symptoms can often be alleviated by drugs that decrease myocardial contractility, or sometimes the apparent obstruction spontaneously disappears as the heart fails.* Although at one time the obstruction was attributed to narrowing

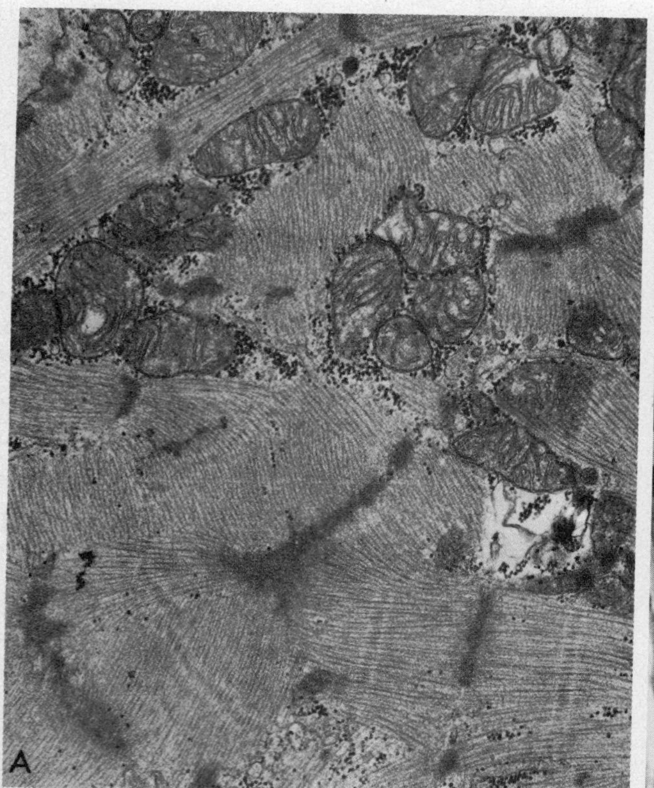

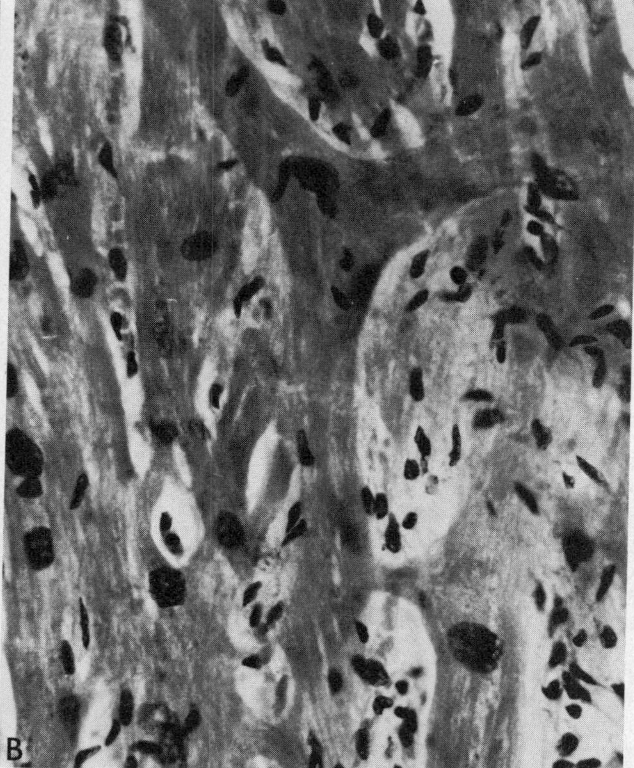

Figure 13–37. Electron micrograph *(A)* (courtesy of William C. Roberts, M.D., National Heart and Lung Institute, Bethesda, MD) and light microscopic section *(B)* of asymmetric septal hypertrophy revealing disarray and abnormal orientation of myofibers.

of the aortic outflow tract by septal hypertrophy, it is now clear that it has more complex origins. During systole there is some delay in closure of the mitral valve, and the anterior leaflet approaches the septum in a "pinch-cock" fashion, causing obstruction to outflow and at the same time mitral regurgitation. *Thus, septal hypertrophy located behind the mitral leaflet is more likely to contribute to obstructive disease than that situated closer to the apex. Another major contributor to reduced cardiac output is the reduced volume of the left ventricle and its noncompliance.* Paradoxically, then, dilatation of the heart with impairment of systolic contractile function improves the situation and apparently accounts for the spontaneous improvements seen with this condition.

The course of hypertrophic CMP is extremely variable. Many patients remain the same over years of observation. A significant fraction improve, and only a minority become worse. Major problems are atrial fibrillation with mural thrombus formation, embolization from the mural thrombi, infective endocarditis on the mitral valve, intractable cardiac failure, and sudden death. With the recognition that obstructive symptoms are not due solely to thickening of the ventricular septum, thinning of the septum by surgery is done increasingly less often. Most patients can be significantly helped by medical therapy alone.

Restrictive/Infiltrative CMP

Restrictive/infiltrative CMP is both rare and diverse, having as a common denominator restriction of ventricular filling. A number of disparate entities induce this form of CMP, including cardiac amyloidosis, sarcoidosis (discussed elsewhere, p. 390), endocardial fibroelastosis, endomyocardial fibrosis, and Loeffler's endocarditis. Cardiac amyloidosis (p. 203), you recall, may appear along with systemic amyloidosis, or may affect only the heart, particularly in the aged (so-called senile isolated cardiac amyloidosis). Indeed, senile cardiac amyloidosis has been identified in over 50% of individuals over the age of 70.[177] Although often an incidental finding, it may induce arrhythmias or restrictive CMP. Only brief comments about the last three entities follow.

Endomyocardial fibrosis and *Loeffler's endocarditis* (also called fibroplastic parietal endocarditis with blood eosinophilia) are rare entities that have sufficient morphologic features in common to raise the possibility that they are a single disorder at different stages of development.[178] *Endomyocardial fibrosis is principally a disease of children and young adults in Africa, characterized by fibrosis of the ventricular endocardium that extends from the apex toward the inflow tract of the right or left ventricle, or both.* Although largely subendocardial, the scarring may extend into the inner third of the myocardium. Varying degrees of inflammatory infiltrate, sometimes including eosinophils, may be found at the junction between the scarring and preserved myocardium. The fibrosis may also involve the tricuspid and mitral valves. Occasionally the fibrous tissue undergoes calcification, leading to fibrocalcific distortion of the tricuspid and mitral valves. Contraction of the fibrous tissue markedly diminishes the volume of affected chambers and so induces a restrictive CMP.[179] Ventricular mural thrombi sometimes develop and, indeed, there is a suggestion that the fibrous tissue results from the organization of mural thrombi. The etiology of this condition is unknown and, in addition to the usual speculations about viral infection, malnutrition, and autoimmune disease, heavy consumption of bananas and plantain has been implicated. These fruits are rich in serotonin, thought to induce the fibrotic changes similar to those of carcinoid heart disease (p. 579).

Loeffler's endocarditis is also marked by endomyocardial fibrosis similar to that seen in the African disease. The original cases of this condition were confined to the temperate zones, but subsequently Loeffler's endocarditis has been reported in Africa and endomyocardial fibrosis in Scandinavia and Europe. Large mural thrombi are typically present in Loeffler's endocarditis. In addition to the cardiac changes there is frequently (1) an eosinophilic leukocytosis, (2) infiltration of various organs (especially the heart) by eosinophils, and (3) a rapidly fatal downhill course.[180] Sometimes, frank eosinophilic leukemia is present. In other cases there is no peripheral eosinophilia, and some form of cardiac hypersensitivity reaction to drugs, for example, is postulated.[163] The histologic evolution of Loeffler's endocarditis begins with foci of myocardial necrosis accompanied by an eosinophilic infiltrate that is most prominent in the inner third of the myocardium. It is followed by scarring of the necrotic areas and layering of the endocardium by thrombus. Organization of the thrombus produces the final stage of endomyocardial fibrosis. Unanswered is the question: Do the eosinophils in some way cause the myofiber necrosis or are they merely a reaction to injury of other origins? It is evident that there are many overlaps in the geographic distribution and morphologic changes of the African disease and Loeffler's disease.

Endocardial fibroelastosis is an uncommon heart disease of obscure etiology characterized by focal or diffuse, cartilage-like fibroelastic thickening of the mural endocardium. Most often only the left side of the heart is affected, but it occasionally involves both sides or (least commonly) only the right side. When we speak of EFE as an entity, there is the strong possibility that the cardiac changes are the final common outcome of a variety of forms of cardiac damage. This condition occurs in all age groups but is far more common in the first two years of life. From the pathogenetic standpoint, cases have been reported in identical twins, triplets, and siblings. The pattern of transmission is still uncertain, and both autosomal dominant inheritance with incomplete penetrance and autosomal recessive inheritance have been proposed as the genetic basis for the cardiac changes.[181] Not infrequently, congenital malformations are also present in the heart or elsewhere in the body, supporting the notion of some genetic disturbance. However, the overwhelming majority of cases occur in individual siblings, and so the concept that EFE is a hereditary malformation can at most apply to only a very few cases.

The former practice of dividing EFE into primary and secondary forms is now discarded because such terms have unwarranted etiologic implications. Primary EFE was equated with congenital disease unassociated with other cardiac malformations. Secondary EFE implied multiple congenital defects or some acquired cardiac disorder, and so might appear later in life. Although such categorization has been discontinued in about one-third of 835 cases analyzed, there were concomitant congenital malformations and lesions in the heart as shown in Table 13–6.[182] Not specified in this compilation are how many of the aortic or mitral stenoses were components of the hypoplastic left heart syndrome commonly associated with EFE.

Table 13–6. ENDOCARDIAL FIBROELASTOSIS

Associated Cardiac Lesions	Number of Cases
Foramen ovale: Patent	167
Closed	200
Ductus arteriosus: Patent	173
Closed	190
Anomalous left coronary artery	27
Aortic stenosis	151
Aortic insufficiency	6
Mitral stenosis	120
Mitral insufficiency	16
Coarctation of aorta	51
Interventricular defect	17
Myocarditis	142
Myocardial scars	229
Myocardial calcification	15

*Modified from Schryer, M. J. P., and Kamauchow, P. N.: Endocardial fibroelastosis. Etiologic and pathogenetic considerations in children. Am. Heart J. *88*:557, 1974.

Fibroelastosis of the endocardium appears as a diffuse or patchy opaque thickening of the mural endocardium predominantly of the left ventricle. However, the left auricle, right ventricle, and right auricle, in order of frequency, may also be involved (Fig. 13–38). The thickening appears as a pearly-white, diffuse lining, sometimes having a depth ten times normal. It is usually covered by an intact endocardium. Mural thrombi overlying the fibrotic endocardium are present in a small percentage of cases. The trabeculae carneae are often flattened. Aortic stenosis, mitral stenosis, or both are present in some cases. The valves on the right are rarely affected. The aortic valve involvement is usually most severe and takes the form of diffuse thickening, rigidity, and nodularity of the cusps. Cardiac enlargement is usually present, due mainly to left ventricular hypertrophy, dilatation, or both.

On histologic examination, the endocardial thickening can be resolved as a marked increase of collagenous and elastic fibers on the endocardial surface. This fibroelastic layer extends sometimes into the immediate subjacent myocardium. In a few cases there are focal necroses in the myocardium immediately subjacent to the fibrotic endocar-

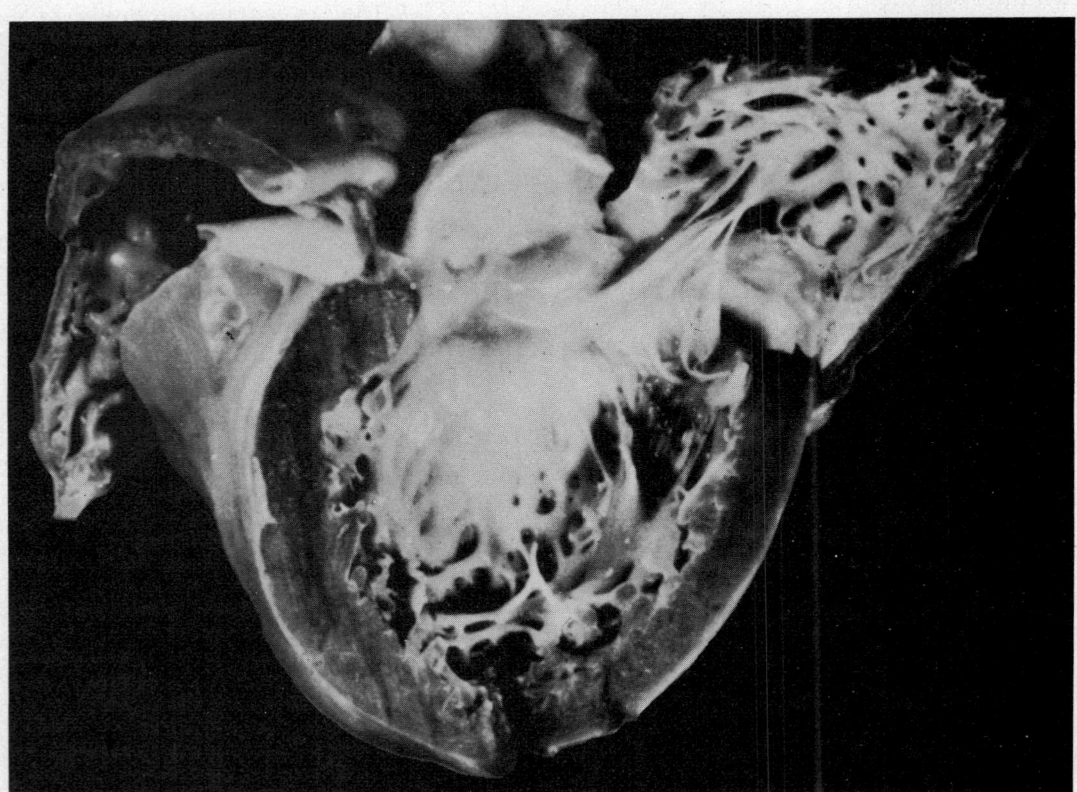

Figure 13–38. Marked fibroelastic thickening of entire left ventricular lining with involvement of aortic valve in a 6-year-old who died of heart failure.

dium, but it is not certain whether these necroses antedate the development of the endocardial thickening or, more likely, are a consequence of impaired vascular supply to the contiguous muscle fibers.

The numerous theories of causation of EFE can be categorized as follows: (1) hypoxia (e.g., anomalous origin of coronary arteries from the pulmonary arteries); (2) hemodynamic pressure overload with excessive endocardial tension (e.g., septal defects, coarctation of the aorta); (3) myocardial metabolic or enzymatic defect; (4) autoimmune connective tissue disease; (5) congenital malformation; (6) lymphatic obstruction; and (7) fetal endomyocarditis, most likely viral. All are so speculative as not to merit further comment, but at present the concept of intrauterine viral infection would seem most attractive. Histologic evidence of myocarditis and/or myocardial scars is present in about one-third of the cases, and in the remainder the infection may have left only the fibroelastosis as a residual.

The significance of this lesion depends on the extent of involvement. When focal, it may have no functional importance and permit normal longevity. When diffuse, it may be responsible for cardiac decompensation and death. In infants, the cardiac failure may be rapid, progressive, and even fulminating. In older children and adults, however, there usually are signs and symptoms of cardiac decompensation for months to years, and death is occasioned by emboli arising in the mural thrombi or by chronic cardiac failure and its superimposed complications.

Table 13–7. MAJOR ASSOCIATIONS OF SPECIFIC HEART MUSCLE DISEASE

Toxic
Alcohol
Cobalt
Catecholamines
Carbon monoxide
Lithium
Hydrocarbons
Arsenic
Cyclophosphamide
Doxorubicin (Adriamycin)
Daunorubicin
Metabolic Disease
Hyperthyroidism
Hypothyroidism
Hypokalemia
Hyperkalemia
Nutritional deficiency—thiamine, protein, other avitaminoses
Hemochromatosis
Neuromuscular Disease
Friedreich's ataxia
Muscular dystrophy
Congenital atrophies
Storage Disorders
Hunter-Hurler syndrome
Glycogen storage disease
Fabry's disease
Sandhoff's disease
Infiltrative
Leukemia
Carcinomatosis
Sarcoidosis

SPECIFIC HEART MUSCLE DISEASE

This somewhat unsatisfactory designation refers to a constellation of myocardial involvements of presumed known etiology or associated with well-defined systemic diseases formerly called "secondary cardiomyopathies." The major etiologies and clinical associations are cited in Table 13–7. The myocardial lesions related to systemic and pulmonary hypertension, coronary artery disease, valvular heart disease, and congenital defects are excluded. For our purposes, the various forms of inflammatory myocarditis are also omitted since they were discussed earlier (p. 593). The morphologic changes found in most of the entities mentioned in Table 13–7 have been presented along with the parent condition. Only some comments on the toxic patterns not covered elsewhere are necessary.

Alcohol, as a cause of specific heart muscle disease, is somewhat controversial, as noted earlier (p. 597), but the weight of evidence favors its being a cardiotoxic agent.[168] Some of the uncertainty derives from the difficulty in segregating the possible cardiotoxicity of alcohol per se from the deleterious influences that commonly accompany chronic alcoholism. For example, in industrialized nations, beriberi heart disease (p. 413) related to thiamine deficiency is sometimes encountered among chronic alcoholics subsisting on grossly inadequate diets. Cobalt cardiotoxicity came to attention among beer drinkers who suddenly developed heart failure. Investigation disclosed that cobalt was included in a secret formula used by several breweries to stabilize the foam on the beer. Cobalt was shown to block the oxidation of pyruvate to acetyl-CoA and of alpha-ketoglutarate to succinyl-CoA, thereby impairing myofiber metabolism. In severe cases of toxicity a variety of regressive morphologic changes were seen, including hydropic and lipid vacuolization, necrosis of isolated myofibers, and disturbances in the intracellular organelles. In time, diffuse or patchy interstitial fibrosis ensued. This brewing practice has been discontinued but industrial exposure to cobalt continues to be a hazard.[183]

Myocardial foci of apparent ischemic necrosis are frequently observed in patients having a pheochromocytoma with its elaboration of catecholamines. Similar changes have appeared in association with the administration of large doses of vasopressor agents such as epinephrine. The mechanism of cardiotoxicity is uncertain, but appears to relate to vasomotor constriction in the myocardial circulation in the face of an increased heart rate. The fact that aspirin, which blocks the cyclooxygenase of the arachidonic acid synthetic pathway, appears to offer some protection suggests that prostaglandins and platelets may contribute to the myocardial ischemia and cell death. Many other drugs, especially anthracycline derivative, have been implicated in causing myofiber degeneration and atrophy, particularly doxorubicin (Adriamycin) and daunorubicin. The hazard is dose dependent and attributed to lipid peroxidation of myofiber membranes.[184]

Common threads running throughout the cardiotoxicity of all chemicals and drugs (including diphtheria exotoxin) are myofiber swelling, fatty change, individual cell lysis (myocytolysis), and sometimes patchy foci of necrosis. Electron microscopy has revealed a variety of mitochondrial abnormalities, swelling and fragmentation of the endoplasmic reticulum, and lysis of myofibrils. With survival, these changes may completely resolve, leaving no apparent sequelae, but sometimes a subtle, interstitial fibrosis remains or, at most, small focal replacement scars.

PERICARDIAL DISEASE

Pericardial lesions are almost always associated with, or secondary to, some external disease (in other portions of the heart or in the surrounding structures) or a systemic disorder. Rarely, pericardial involvements may occur as primary, isolated processes. Despite the large number of etiologies of pericardial disease there are relatively few anatomic forms of pericardial involvement.[185]

ACCUMULATIONS OF FLUID IN PERICARDIAL SAC

Pericardial Effusion. The term "pericardial effusion" is restricted to accumulations of noninflammatory fluids in the pericardial sac, as distinguished from collections of inflammatory exudate or blood (discussed later). Normally, there is about 30 to 50 ml of thin, clear, straw-colored, translucent fluid in the pericardial space. Under a variety of circumstances, effusions rarely larger than 500 ml may appear. The various types of effusion and their common causes are:

Serous—congestive heart failure; hypoproteinemia (renal, hepatic, nutritional).

Serosanguineous—following blunt chest trauma; following cardiopulmonary resuscitation.

Chylous—lymphatic obstruction (benign or malignant mediastinal neoplasms).

Cholesterol—myxedema; idiopathic.

Most common is serous effusion in cardiac failure. The fluid is completely clear, watery, or straw-colored, and sterile. The serosal surfaces remain smooth and glistening. Since the fluid accumulates slowly it is usually without clinical significance save for producing a characteristic enlargement of the heart shadow on x-ray film. Rarely a large volume may embarrass diastolic filling of the heart, requiring withdrawal. Serosanguineous and chylous effusions—containing lipid droplets—rarely achieve sufficient volume to have clinical significance. Cholesterol effusions are exceedingly rare and are distinguished by the appearance of cholesterol crystals within the accumulated fluid. They are sometimes associated with myxedema, but more often are of unknown origin. It is speculated that breakdown of red cells in the past, with release of membrane lipids, may be the source of the crystals.

Hemopericardium. The term hemopericardium should be limited to the accumulation of pure blood in the pericardial sac, and should be differentiated from hemorrhagic pericarditis, a condition in which there is an inflammatory exudate containing blood mixed with pus.

Hemopericardium is almost invariably due to traumatic perforation of the heart, rupture of the heart wall secondary to MI, or rupture of the intrapericardial aorta. Quite rarely, it may follow penetration of a myocardial abscess or tumor. Small, usually insignificant amounts of blood may extravasate from the trauma sometimes sustained during cardiopulmonary resuscitation. Rarely, however, marked hemorrhage occurs, clearly emphasizing the hazard entailed in such therapy. Hemorrhages in the bleeding diatheses, such as scurvy, leukemia, or thrombocytopenia, are rare causes of this condition.

The blood that escapes because of rupture of the heart or aorta rapidly fills the sac under greatly increased pressure and produces cardiac tamponade (Fig. 13–39). As little as 200 to 300 ml may be sufficient to cause death. Although intracardiac injections may cause leakage of blood, death is usually already imminent when such measures are attempted and, under these circumstances, only small amounts of blood-tinged fluid appear in the pericardial sac.

PERICARDITIS

Inflammations of the pericardium are usually secondary to disorders in or about the heart, but sometimes they are caused by systemic disorders or by metastases from neoplasms arising in remote sites. Primary pericarditis is a rarity and almost always of viral origin. The major causes are presented in Table 13–8.

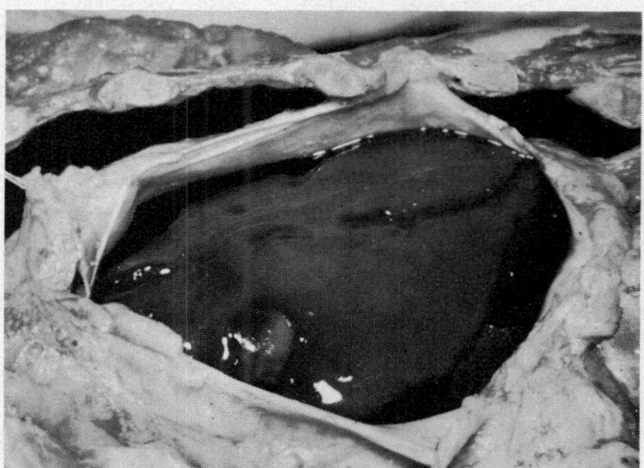

Figure 13–39. Hemopericardium. A pericardial sac in situ opened to expose the clotted blood that caused death after rupture of a myocardial infarct.

Table 13–8. CAUSES OF PERICARDITIS

Infectious Agents
Viral
Pyogenic bacteria
Tuberculous
Fungal
Other parasites
Presumably Immunologically-mediated
Rheumatic fever
Systemic lupus erythematosus
Scleroderma
Postcardiotomy
? Postmyocardial infarction
Drug-hypersensitivity reaction
Miscellaneous
Myocardial infarction
Uremia
Cardiotomy
Neoplasia
Trauma
Radiation

The various etiologies cited usually evoke an acute pericarditis, but a few, such as tuberculosis and fungi, produce chronic reactions. The acute and chronic reactions are morphologically nonspecific. Since many etiologies evoke identical anatomic changes and since it is usually impossible from pathologic examination to determine the etiologic basis for the reaction, a morphologic classification will follow, dividing the pericarditides into acute and chronic forms, and further subdividing the acute reactions on the basis of the character of the exudate. Sometimes, however, there is overlap among the categories. These subdivisions also have clinical relevance; to an extent, each induces somewhat distinctive signs and symptoms.

Acute Pericarditis

SEROUS PERICARDITIS. Serous inflammatory exudates are characteristically produced by nonbacterial inflammations, such as rheumatic fever, systemic lupus erythematosus, systemic scleroderma, tumors, and uremia. Similar effusions are also frequently encountered in the early stages of any form of bacterial pericarditis. Occasionally, a tuberculous infection of the pericardial sac or infections in the tissues contiguous to the pericardium evoke an inflammatory exudation that is principally serous in the early stages. For example, a bacterial pleuritis may cause sufficient irritation of the parietal pericardial serosa to cause a sterile serous effusion. In time, however, infection may extend across the anatomic barrier and the serous exudate is transformed into a frank suppurative reaction.

Occasionally, the Coxsackie A or B virus, adenovirus, or virus of influenza, ECHOvirus type 8, and mumps, as well as others, is isolated from a serous exudate. In some instances a well-defined viral infection elsewhere—upper respiratory tract, pneumonia, parotitis—antedates the pericarditis to serve as the primary focus of infection. Infrequently, a viral pericarditis, most often related to Coxsackie and ECHO agents, occurs as an apparent primary involvement, usually in young adults. However, in many instances the etiology of apparent primary serous pericarditis remains unknown.

Morphologically, whatever the cause, there is an inflammatory reaction in the epi- and pericardial surfaces with scant numbers of polymorphonuclear leukocytes, lymphocytes, and histiocytes. Sometimes bacterial organisms or malignant tumor cells may be identified in the fluid, thus providing an indication of the etiology. Usually the volume of fluid is not large and varies between 50 and 200 ml. Because it represents a purely exudative phenomenon, it occurs slowly and therefore rarely produces sufficient increase in pressure to encroach upon the cardiac function. The fluid resorbs when and if the underlying disease remits. Organization or fibrous adhesions rarely develop.

FIBRINOUS AND SEROFIBRINOUS PERICARDITIS. These two anatomic forms are considered together because they represent essentially similar processes in which there is a more or less serous fluid mixed with a fibrinous exudate. This is the most frequent type of pericarditis. Common causes include MI, uremia, radiation to the chest, rheumatic fever, SLE, and trauma.[185] Bacterial, viral, and occasionally obscure myocardial inflammations may produce similar changes. Just as pneumonia or suppurative infections in the pleural cavities may produce serous pericarditis, in more severe cases they may cause the outpouring of fibrin. Fibrinous exudation may also follow cardiac surgery.

The gross morphologic alterations have already been described on page 65.

As is the case with all inflammatory exudates, *the fibrin may be digested with resolution of the exudate, or may become organized.* Organization and fibrous interadherence result sometimes in complete obliteration of the pericardial sac. This fibrosis yields a delicate, stringy type of adhesion, called *adhesive pericarditis,* which only rarely hampers or restricts cardiac action. With this type of pericarditis, the organization rarely extends to surrounding contiguous structures, such as the thoracic wall, diaphragm, or lungs, and therefore results only in obliteration of the space. In some cases, organization merely produces plaquelike fibrous thickenings of the serosal membranes.

From the clinical standpoint, *the development of a loud pericardial friction rub is the most striking characteristic of fibrinous pericarditis.* A collection of serous fluid may obliterate the rub by separating the two layers of the pericardium. Pain, systemic febrile reactions, and signs suggestive of cardiac failure may accompany the pathognomonic friction rub.

Fibrinous or serofibrinous pericarditis rarely leads to serious sequelae.

PURULENT OR SUPPURATIVE PERICARDITIS. This form of pericardial inflammation almost invariably denotes the presence of bacterial, mycotic, or parasitic invasion of the pericardial space by organisms. It is most frequent in young males (male-to-female ratio, 3:1) between 10 and 40 years old. These organisms infect the pericardial cavity by (1) direct extension from neighboring inflammations, such as an empyema of the pleural cavity, lobar pneumonia, mediastinal infections, or, with infective endocarditis, bacterial invasion from the myocardium through the epicardium; (2) seeding from the blood; (3) lymphatic extension; or (4) direct introduction during cardiotomy. Immunosuppressive therapy potentiates all these pathways.

Quite rarely, a serosuppurative exudate may be produced by sterile inflammations, such as result from a MI or uremia. Rarely, severe viral infections of the heart, such as influenza or poliomyelitis, may cause suppurative pericarditis.

Morphologically, the exudate ranges from a thin to a creamy pus ranging up to 400 to 500 ml in volume. The serosal surfaces are reddened, granular, and coated with the exudate. Microscopically, there is a banal, acute, inflammatory reaction. Sometimes the inflammatory process extends into surrounding structures to induce a so-called *mediastinopericarditis*.

The clinical findings are essentially the same as those present in fibrinous pericarditis, but although a friction rub may be present, it is not usually so prominent as in the fibrinous variety. On the other hand, the signs of systemic infection are more marked: for example, spiking temperatures, chills, and fever.

Organization is the usual outcome of this inflammatory process, with resolution being infrequent. Because of the greater intensity of the inflammatory response, the organization produces *constrictive pericarditis*. Thus, suppurative pericarditis may lead to disabling consequences.

HEMORRHAGIC PERICARDITIS. Hemorrhagic pericarditis denotes an exudate composed of blood mixed with a fibrinous or suppurative effusion. It is most commonly caused by tuberculosis or by malignant neoplastic involvement of the pericardial space, most often related to spread of lung and breast carcinomas, melanocarcinomas, lymphomas, and leukemias. It may also be found in bacterial infections or in cases of pericarditis occurring in patients with some underlying bleeding diathesis. Hemorrhagic pericarditis must be differentiated from hemopericardium in which the fluid is purely blood of noninflammatory origin.

If the underlying cause is a tumor, neoplastic cells may be present in the effusion or in the pericardial or epicardial tissues. The clinical significance is that of a suppurative pericarditis, and resolution or organization with or without calcification is the eventual outcome.

Caseous Pericarditis

Caseation within the pericardial sac is, until proved otherwise, tuberculous in origin. Infrequently, mycotic infections evoke a similar pattern. The tubercle bacilli usually involve the pericardium by direct spread from tuberculous foci within the tracheobronchial nodes. Often such direct continuity cannot be identified at postmortem and the possibility of lymphatic or of hematogenous dissemination from a noncontiguous focus cannot be excluded. The anatomic changes are typical of tuberculous infections elsewhere and need no further description. Caseous pericarditis is the most frequent antecedent of disabling fibrocalcific, chronic constrictive pericarditis.

Chronic or Healed Pericarditis

The term chronic pericarditis is a misnomer, since it refers in reality to a healed stage of one of the forms of pericardial inflammation already described. One pattern comprises the formation of pearly, thickened, nonadherent, epicardial plaques ("Soldier's plaque"). Alternatively, thin, delicate adhesions may develop, which are termed diffuse or focal obliterative pericarditis according to their pattern. These rarely cause impairment of cardiac function, but occur fairly frequently at autopsy and are often of obscure origin.

Two forms of healed pericarditis are of clinical importance: adhesive mediastinopericarditis and constrictive pericarditis.

ADHESIVE MEDIASTINOPERICARDITIS. This form of pericardial fibrosis may follow a suppurative or caseous pericarditis, but can also be the consequence of previous cardiac surgery. Sometimes this pericardial reaction follows heavy irradiation to the mediastinum, as in radiotherapy for lymphomas or Hodgkin's disease. Only rarely is it a sequel to simple fibrinous exudation. The pericardial sac is obliterated, and adherence of the external aspect of the parietal layer to surrounding structures produces a great strain on cardiac function. With each systolic contraction, the heart is pulling not only against the parietal pericardium, but also against the attached surrounding structures. Systolic retractions of the rib cage and diaphragm, pulsus paradoxicus, and a variety of other fairly pathognomonic findings may be observed clinically. *The increased workload causes cardiac hypertrophy and dilatation, which may be quite massive in more severe cases.*

CONSTRICTIVE PERICARDITIS. The heart may be encased in a dense, fibrous, or fibrocalcific scar that limits diastolic expansion and seriously restricts cardiac output. Sometimes there is a well-defined history of a previous suppurative or caseous pericarditis, but more often the cause is buried in the remote past (idiopathic).[186] Fibrinous or serofibrinous inflammatory reactions rarely lead to this form of damage. In constrictive pericarditis, the pericardial space not only is obliterated but is transformed into a dense layer of scar or calcification, many times 0.5 to 1.0 cm thick, which resists dissection. In extreme cases, it appears as if the heart were enclosed within a plaster mold (*concretio cordis*). In less severe instances, only irregular calcific plates are produced.

Although the signs of cardiac failure may resemble those produced by mediastinopericarditis, the local findings in the heart are quite different. *Cardiac hypertrophy and dilatation cannot occur because of the dense enclosing scar*, and as a consequence the heart is described as a small, quiet heart with reduced minute volume output and reduced pulse pressure. Constriction of the venae cavae during the fibrotic process may block the venous return to the right side of the heart, simulating severe right heart failure.

RHEUMATOID HEART DISEASE

Rheumatoid arthritis is mainly a disorder of the joints, but many nonarticular involvements, e.g., subcutaneous rheumatoid nodules, acute vasculitis, and Felty's syndrome (p. 1355) may accompany the joint changes.[187] Recently, increasing attention has been drawn to cardiac lesions in patients having rheumatoid arthritis. These heart involvements are, however, uncommon and in a large series of 100 patients with generalized arthritis, only five instances of recognizable rheumatoid lesions were found in the heart.

The diagnostic features of rheumatoid heart disease consist of foci of fibrinoid necrosis within the valves, myocardium, or pericardium surrounded by a collar of radial, palisaded fibroblasts, accompanied by a diffuse, nonspecific chronic inflammation. Myocardial, valvular, and pericardial fibrosis may follow acute involvements.

TUMORS OF THE HEART

Primary tumors of the heart are extremely rare. They may involve any one or all of the three layers of the heart. Those of the pericardium may be primary (lipomas, mesotheliomas, hemangiomas), but these curiosities are much less common than metastases to the pericardial cavity.[188] Myocardial neoplasms are also rarities, but are of great clinical interest since they are more often benign than malignant and are often attached by slender stalks that make them amenable to surgical removal. In the past, they were very difficult to diagnose clinically because of their rarity and because they often presented as a mysterious cause of cardiac decompensation.[189] However, with present-day techniques of echocardiography, radionuclide imaging, and computerized tomography (CT scans), they can be diagnosed clinically, permitting sometimes life-saving surgical removal. Some idea of their frequency can be obtained by the incidence of primary cardiac tumors in necropsy series ranging from 0.0017 to 0.33%.[190, 191] About 80% of primary cardiac tumors are benign, and half of these are myxomas.

BENIGN

As pointed out, *myxomas* are the most common primary tumor of the heart. Although they may arise in any of the four chambers or, rarely, on the heart valves, about 90% are located in the atria with a left-to-right ratio of approximately 4:1.[192] The tumors are almost always single, rarely multiple, in several chambers. The region of the fossa ovalis is a favored site of atrial origin. They range from small (less than 1 cm) to large (up to 10 cm) sessile or pedunculated masses (Fig. 13–40). In general, sessile lesions are globular, hard, mottled with hemorrhage, and easily confused with an organizing mural thrombus. Pedunculated myxomas tend to be soft, translucent, papillary, or villous lesions having a myxoid appearance. All are usually covered by an intact endocardium, but fragmentation and embolization of papillary lesions is sometimes encountered. The sessile pattern, when unfortunately located, and particularly the pedunculated form, is frequently sufficiently mobile to move into or sometimes through the atrioventricular valves during diastole. Sometimes such mobility exerts a "wrecking ball" effect on the valve leaflets. Histologically, they are composed of stellate or globular myxoma cells, endothelial cells, macrophages, mature or immature smooth muscle cells, and a variety of intermediate forms embedded within an abundant acid mucopolysaccharide ground substance (Fig. 13–41). Numerous small blood vessels, sometimes having well-developed muscular walls, course through these lesions, and often hemosiderin pigment and macrophages laden with hemosiderin granules are present as stigmata of microhemorrhages. Ultrastructurally, the most prominent feature is an abundance of fine cytoplasmic fibrils similar to those of smooth muscle cells.[193] It has long been questioned whether cardiac myxomas are hamartomatous or organized thrombi, but the weight of evidence is on the side of benign neoplasia. All the cell types present are thought to derive from variable differentiation of primitive mesenchymal cells.

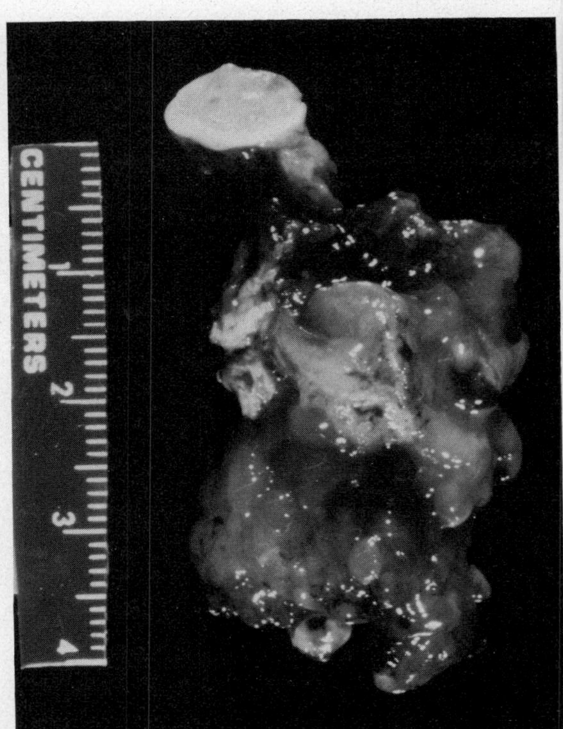

Figure 13–40. Excised myxoma of heart revealing slender stalk above and irregular, lobulated gelatinous mass.

These neoplasms may be encountered at any age, even in infants, with a predominance in females. Be-

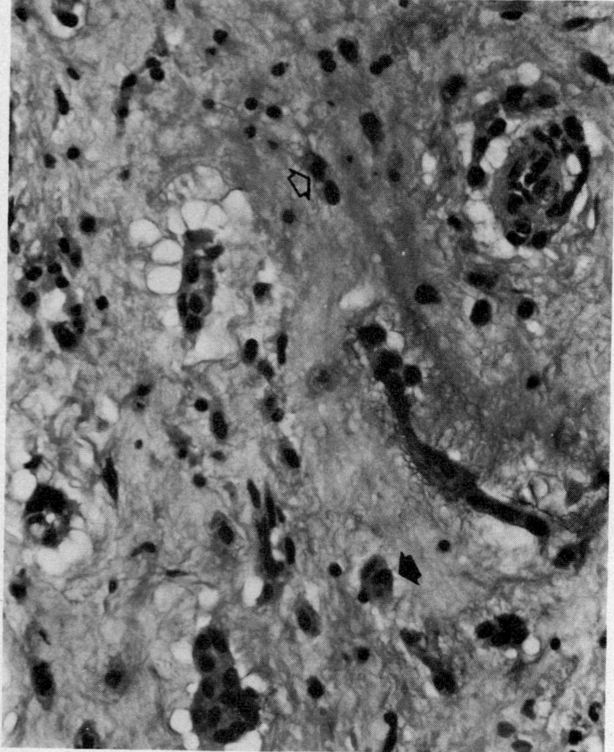

Figure 13–41. Atrial myxoma disclosing abundant ground substance in which are scattered mononuclear leukocytes, abnormal vascular formations, and a few myxoma cells *(solid arrow)*, one with stellate processes *(open arrow)*.

cause they may create ball-valve obstructions, they sometimes cause unanticipated syncopal attacks, cardiac insufficiency, and even sudden death, in apparently healthy young children and adults. Sometimes embolization, particularly to the brain, kidneys, or lungs, calls attention to these lesions. Present diagnostic techniques provide the opportunity to diagnose these masses, but differentiation from a mural thrombus is sometimes difficult despite all the newer diagnostic modalities. Surgical removal is usually curative, although sometimes the neoplasm recurs months to years later.

Rhabdomyomas, although the second most frequent primary tumor of the heart, are much more rare than the already uncommon myxoma.[194] These appear generally as multiple, sometimes single, circumscribed, pale gray masses, usually within the left or right ventricular walls. Histologically, they are composed of large, rounded, or polygonal cells that have one or two nuclei and abundant cytoplasm having numerous large, glycogen-laden vacuoles. Myofibrils are present in some cells and occasionally typical muscle cross striations can be seen. The nature of these lesions is still in some doubt, specifically whether they are derived from neoplastic striated muscle cells or instead are hamartomatous in nature. Most of the reported cases have occurred in infants and children, often in association with tuberous sclerosis, suggesting a malformational origin.

A wide variety of other benign neoplasms may arise in the heart, including so-called papillary fibroelastomas, lipomas, and angiomas, but all are exotic rarities.

PRIMARY SARCOMAS

Primary sarcomas of the heart are about half as common as benign tumors. In one of the largest experiences the following neoplasms, in descending order of frequency, were encountered: angiosarcoma, rhabdomyosarcoma, mesothelioma, lymphoma, and other even greater rarities.[195] All these cancers are generally so advanced at the time of discovery that it is difficult to be certain of their site of origin. They may be predominantly intrapericardial, intramural, intracavitary, and right-sided or left-sided, but most often they present all these characteristics. Histologically, they are identical to their counterparts arising in extracardiac locations. All ages may be involved but malignant tumors preponderantly occur in adults. They cause a variety of manifestations ranging from nonspecific fever, malaise, and weight loss to various cardiac abnormalities, often congestive heart failure. Despite all attempts at control, survival for more than a year is rare.

SECONDARY TUMORS

Metastatic involvement of the heart, more often of the pericardium than of the myocardium, may occur in any widely disseminated malignancy. A great many of these secondary lesions result from spread of bronchogenic carcinomas and lymphomas arising in the mediastinal nodes. However, there are many undoubted instances of blood- or lymphatic-borne metastases from carcinoma of the kidney, stomach, lungs and breast, and melanocarcinoma. On occasion the secondary involvement of the heart is important when the metastases evoke pericardial hemorrhagic effusions that produce cardiac tamponade, or by involvement of the myocardium induce arrhythmias.

1. Newman, P.E.: The coronary collateral circulation: Determinants in ischemic heart disease. Am. Heart J. *102*:431, 1981.
2. Braunwald, E.: Pathophysiology of heart failure. *In* Braunwald, E. (ed.): Heart Disease: A Textbook of Cardiovascular Medicine. Philadelphia, W. B. Saunders Co., 1980, p. 453.
3. Willerson, J.T.: What is wrong with the failing heart? N. Engl. J. Med. *307*:243, 1982.
4. Bristow, M.R., et al.: Decreased catecholamine sensitivity and β-adrenergic receptor density in failing human hearts. N. Engl. J. Med. *307*:205, 1982.
5. Weber, K.T., and Janicki, J.S.: The metabolic demand and oxygen supply of the heart. Am. J. Cardiol. *44*:722, 1979.
6. Arcidi, J.M., et al.: Hepatic morphology in cardiac dysfunction. A clinicopathologic study of 1000 subjects at autopsy. Am. J. Pathol. *104*:159, 1981.
7. Levy, R.I., and Moskowitz, J.: Cardiovascular research: Decades of progress, a decade of promise. Science *217*: 121, 1982.
8. Brown, B.G.: Coronary vasospasm. Observations linking the clinical spectrum of ischemic heart disease to the dynamic pathology of coronary atherosclerosis. Arch. Intern. Med. *141*:716, 1981.

9. Erlebacher, J.A.: Transmural myocardial infarction with "normal" coronary arteries. Am. Heart J. *98*:421, 1979.
10. Walker, W. J.: Changing U.S. life style and declining vascular mortality—a retrospective N. Engl. J. Med. *308*:649, 1983.
11. World Health Statistics Annuals. World Health Organization, Geneva, 1965–77.
12. Strong, J.P., et al.: Is coronary atherosclerosis decreasing in the USA? Lancet *2*:1294, 1979.
13. Glueck, C.J., et al.: Diet and coronary heart disease, another view. N. Engl. J. Med. *298*:1471, 1978.
14. Roberts, W.C.: The coronary arteries in ischemic heart disease: Facts and fancies. Triangle *16*:77, 1977.
15. Roberts, W.C., and Jones, A.A.: Quantification of coronary arterial narrowing at necropsy in acute transmural myocardial infarction. Analysis and comparison of findings in 27 patients and 22 controls. Circulation *61*:786, 1980.
16. Hillis, L.D., and Braunwald, E.: Coronary-artery spasm. N. Engl. J. Med. *299*:695, 1978.
17. Blumgart, H.L., et al.: Studies on the relation of angina pectoris, coronary thrombosis and myocardial infarction to the pathologic findings (with particular reference to the significance of collateral circulation). Am. Heart J. *19*:1, 1940.
18. Blumgart, H.L., et al.: Angina pectoris, coronary failure and acute myocardial infarction. The role of coronary occlusions and collateral circulation. J.A.M.A. *116*:91, 1941.
19. Prinzmetal, M., et al.: Angina pectoris. I. A variant form of angina pectoris. Am. J. Med. *27*:375, 1959.
20. Maseri, A., et al.: "Variant" angina: One aspect of continuous spectrum of vasospastic myocardial ischemia: Pathogenetic mechanisms, estimated incidence and clinical and coronary arteriographic findings in 138 patients. Am. J. Cardiol. *42*:1019, 1035, 1978.
21. Laguens, R.P., et al.: Ultrastructural and morphometric study of the human heart muscle cell in acute coronary insufficiency. Hum. Pathol. *10*:695, 1979.
22. Editorial: Coronary heart disease in young women. Lancet *2*:282, 1977.
23. Slone, D., et al.: Risk of myocardial infarction in relation to current and discontinued use of oral contraceptives. N. Engl. J. Med. *305*:420, 1981.
24. Stadel, B.V.: Oral contraceptives and cardiovascular disease. N. Engl. J. Med. *305*:612, 672, 1981.
25. Royal College of General Practitioners Oral Contraceptive Study: Further analyses of mortality in oral contraceptive users. Lancet *1*:541, 1981.
26. Population Reports, Population Information Program: OC's—Update on Usage, Safety, and Side Effects. Johns Hopkins University, Series A, No. 5, Jan., 1979.
27. Bain, C., et al.: Cigarette consumption and deaths from coronary heart disease. Lancet *1*:1087, 1978.
28. Review Panel on Coronary-Prone Behavior and Coronary Heart Disease: A critical review. Circulation *63*:1199, 1981.
29. Bruce, R.A.: Primary intervention against coronary atherosclerosis by exercise conditioning. N. Engl. J. Med. *305*:1525, 1981.
30. Froelicher, V.F.: Exercise and the prevention of coronary atherosclerotic heart disease. Cardiovasc. Clin. *9*:13, 1978.
31. Williams, R.S., et al.: Physical conditioning augments the fibrinolytic response to venous occlusion in healthy adults. N. Engl. J. Med. *302*:987,1980.
32. Geer, J.C., et al.: Subendocardial ischemic myocardial lesions associated with severe coronary atherosclerosis. Am. J. Pathol. *98*:663, 1980.
33. Woolf, N., and Davies, M.J.: Morphological variants of acute myocardial necrosis and their relationship to coronary artery thrombosis. Acta Med. Scand. (Suppl.) *642*:92, 1980.
34. Buja, L.M., and Willerson, J.T.: Clinicopathologic correlates of acute ischemic heart disease syndromes. Am. J. Cardiol. *47*:343, 1981.
35. Davies, M.J., et al.: Pathology of acute myocardial infarction with particular reference to occlusive coronary thrombi. Br. Heart J. *38*:659, 1976.
36. Brosius, F.C., III, and Roberts, W.C.: Significance of coronary arterial thrombus in transmural acute myocardial infarction. Circulation *63*:810, 1981.
37. DeWood, M.A., et al.: Prevalence of total coronary occlusion during the early hours of transmural myocardial infarction. N. Engl. J. Med. *303*:897, 1980.
38. Silver, M.D., et al.: The relationship between acute occlusive coronary thrombi and myocardial infarction. Studies in 100 consecutive patients. Circulation *61*:219, 1980.
39. Baroldi, G.: Coronary thrombosis and fatal myocardial ischemia. Circulation *49*:1, 1974.
40. Maseri, A.: The revival of coronary spasm. Am. J. Med. *70*:752, 1981.
41. Hillis, L.D., and Braunwald, E: Coronary-artery spasm. N. Engl. J. Med. *299*:695, 1978.
42. Buja, L.M., et al.: The role of coronary arterial spasm in ischemic heart disease. Arch. Pathol. Lab. Med. *105*:221, 1981.
43. Brest, A.N.: Myocardial infarction without demonstrable coronary artery disease. Cardiovasc. Clin. *7*:303, 1975.
44. Erlebacher, J.A.: Transmural myocardial infarction with normal coronary arteries. Am. Heart J. *98*:421, 1979.
45. Engel, H.J.: Coronary artery spasm as the cause of myocardial infarction during coronary arteriography. Am. Heart J. *91*:501, 1976.
46. Brown, B.G.: Coronary vasospasm. Observations linking the clinical spectrum of ischemic heart disease to the dynamic pathology of coronary atherosclerosis. Arch. Intern. Med. *141*:716, 1981.
47. Mehta, P., and Mehta, J.: Platelet function studies in coronary artery disease. V. Evidence for enhanced platelet microthrombus formation activity in acute myocardial infarction. Am. J. Cardiol. *43*:757, 1979.
48. Baum, R.S., et al.: Survival after resuscitation from out-of-hospital ventricular fibrillation. Circulation *50*:1231, 1974.
49. Lie, J.T., and Titus, J.L.: Pathology of the myocardium and the conduction system in sudden coronary death. Circulation (Suppl. III) *51/52*:41, 1975.
50. Weinberg, M.: Sudden cardiac death. Yale J. Biol. Med. *51*:207, 1978.
51. El-Maraghi, N., and Genton, E.: The relevance of platelet and fibrin thromboembolism of the coronary microcirculation with special reference to sudden cardiac death. Circulation *62*:936, 1980.
52. Myerburg, R.J., et al.: Clinical, electrophysiologic and hemodynamic profile of patients resuscitated from prehospital cardiac arrest. Am. J. Med. *68*:568, 1980.
53. Oliva, P.B.: Pathophysiology of acute myocardial infarction, 1981. Ann. Intern. Med. *94*:236, 1981.
54. Ratliff, N.B., and Hackel, D.B.: Combined right and left ventricular infarction: Pathogenesis and clinicopathologic correlations. Am. J. Cardiol. *45*:217, 1980.
55. Gardin, J.M., and Singer, D.H.: Atrial infarction: Importance, diagnosis and localization. Arch. Intern. Med. *141*:1345, 1981.
56. Mallory, G.K.: The speed of healing of myocardial infarction. A study of the pathologic anatomy in 72 cases. Am. Heart J. *18*:747, 1939.
57. Lie, J.T., et al.: Macroscopic enzyme-mapping verification of large homogenous experimental infarcts of predictable size and location in dogs. J. Thorac. Cardiovasc. Surg. *69*:599, 1975.
58. Fallon, J.T.: Post Mortem Histochemical Techniques in Myocardial Infarction. Measurement and Intervention. *In* Wagner, G. S. (ed.). The Hague, Martinus Nijhoff Publishers, 1981, p. 373.
59. Bates, R.J., et al.: Cardiac rupture—challenge in diagnosis and management. Am. J. Cardiol. *40*:429, 1977.
60. Radford, M.J., et al.: Ventricular septal rupture: A review of clinical and physiologic features and an analysis of survival. Circulation *64*:545, 1981.
61. Fishbein, M.C., et al.: The histopathologic evolution of myocardial infarction. Chest *73*:843, 1978.
62. Bouchardy, B., and Majno, G.: Histopathology of early myocardial infarcts. Am. J. Pathol. *74*:301, 1974.
63. Hutchins, G.M., and Bulkley, B.H.: Correlation of myocardial contraction band necrosis and vascular patency. A study of coronary artery bypass graft anastomoses at branch points. Lab. Invest. *36*:642, 1977.
64. Hearse, D.J., and Yellon, D.M.: The "border zone" in evolving myocardial infarction: Controversy or confusion? Am. J. Cardiol. *47*:1321, 1981.
65. Factor, S.M., et al.: The histologic border zone of acute myocardial infarction—islands or peninsulas? Am. J. Pathol. *92*:11, 1978.
66. Janse, M.J., et al.: The "border-zone" in myocardial ischemia. An electrophysiological, metabolic, and histochemical correlation in the pig heart. Circ. Res. *44*:576, 1979.
67. Jennings, R.B., and Ganote, C.E.: Structural changes in myocardium during acute ischemia. Circ. Res. (Suppl. III)*34–35*:156, 1974.
68. Zugibe, F.T., et al.: Determination of myocardial alterations at autopsy in the absence of gross and microscopic changes. Arch. Pathol. *81*:409, 1966.
69. Reimer, K.A., and Jennings, R.B.: The "wavefront phenomenon" of myocardial ischemic cell death. II. Transmural progression of necrosis within the framework of ischemic bed size (myocardium at risk) and collateral flow. Lab. Invest. *40*:633, 1979.
70. Roberts, R., and Sobel, B.E.: Creatine kinase isoenzymes in the assessment of heart disease. Am. Heart. J. *95*:521, 1978.
71. Rissanen, V.: Sudden coronary death and coronary artery disease: A clinicopathologic appraisal. Cardiology *64*:289, 1979.
72. Buckley, B.H.: Site and sequelae of myocardial infarction. N. Engl. J. Med. *305*:337, 1981.
73. Kannel, W.B., et al.: Prognosis after initial MI: The Framingham Study. Am. J. Cardiol. *44*:53, 1979.
73A. Levy, R.: Lipid Research Clinics Program: The Lipid Research Clinics primary prevention trial results. 1. Reduction of incidence of coronary heart disease, and 2. The relationship of reduction in incidence of coronary heart disease to cholesterol lowering. J.A.M.A. *251*:365, 1984.
74. Markis, J.E., et al.: Myocardial salvage after intra-coronary thrombolysis

with streptokinase in acute myocardial infarction; assessment by intracoronary thallium-201. N. Engl. J. Med. *305*:777, 1981.

75. Saltissi, S., et al.: Effects of early administration of a highly purified hyaluronidase preparation (GL enzyme) on myocardial infarct size. Lancet *1*:867, 1982.
76. Braunwald, E., et al.: Role of beta-adrenergic blockade in the therapy of patients with myocardial infarction. Am. J. Med. *74*:113, 1983.
77. Rapaport E.: Prevention of recurrent sudden death. N. Engl. J. Med. *306*:1359, 1982.
78. Anturane Reinfarction Trial Policy Committee: The Anturane reinfarction trial: Reevaluation of outcome. N. Engl. J. Med. *306*:1005, 1982.
79. Braunwald, E.: Effects of coronary-artery bypass grafting on survival: Implications of the randomized coronary-artery surgery study. N. Engl. J. Med. *309*:1181, 1983.
80. Schlesinger, M.J., and Reiner, L.: Focal myocytolysis of the heart. Am. J. Pathol. *31*:443, 1955.
81. Kannel, W.B., and Sorlie, P.: Hypertension in Framingham. *In* Paul, O. (ed.): Epidemiology and Control of Hypertension. Miami, Symposia Specialists, 1975, p. 553.
82. Webb, R.C., and Bohr, D.F.: Recent advances in the pathogenesis of hypertension. Consideration of structural, functional and metabolic vascular abnormalities resulting in elevated arterial resistance. Am. Heart J. *102*:251, 1981.
83. Grossman, W.: Cardiac hypertrophy: Useful adaptation or pathologic process? Am. J. Med. *69*:576, 1980.
84. Henquell, L., et al.: Intercapillary distance and capillary reserve in hypertrophied rat hearts beating in situ. Circ. Res. *41*:400, 1977.
85. Hess, O.M., et al.: Diastolic function and myocardial structure in patients with myocardial hypertrophy. Circulation *63*:360, 1981.
86. Pearlman, E.S., et al.: Quantitative histology of the hypertrophied human heart. Fed. Proc. *40*:2042, 1981.
87. Maron, B.J., and Ferrans, V.J.: Ultrastructural features of hypertrophied human ventricular myocardium. Prog. Cardiovasc. Dis. *31*:207, 1978.
88. Schwarz, F., et al.: Reduced volume fraction of myofibrils in myocardium of patients with decompensated pressure-overload. Circulation *63*:1299, 1981.
89. Freis, E.D.: Should mild hypertension be treated? N. Engl. J. Med. *307*:306, 1982.
90. Fishman, A.P.: Chronic cor pulmonale. Am. Rev. Respir. Dis. *114*:775, 1976.
91. Ferrer, I.: Cor pulmonale (pulmonary heart disease): Present-day status. Am. Heart J. *89*:657, 1975.
92. Schoen, F.J., et al.: Bioengineering aspects of heart valve replacement. Ann. Biomed. Eng. *10*:97, 1982.
93. Kaplan, M.H.: Rheumatic fever, rheumatic heart disease and the strep connection: The role of streptococcal antigens cross-reactive with heart tissue. Rev. Infect. Dis. *1*:988, 1979.
94. Stollerman, G.H.: A global view of rheumatic fever today. *In* Russek, H.I. (ed.): Cardiovascular Problems, Perspectives and Progress. Baltimore, University Park Press, 1976, p. 381.
95. Williams, R.C.: Host factors in RF and heart disease. Hosp. Pract. *16*:725, 1982.
96. Kaplan, M.H.: Induction of autoimmunity to heart in rheumatic fever by streptococcal antigen(s) cross-reactive with heart. Fed. Proc. *24*:109, 1965.
97. Kaplan, M.H.: Cross-reaction of group A streptococci and heart tissue: Varying serologic specificity of cross-reactive antisera and relation to carrier-hapten specificity. Transplant. Proc. *1*:976, 1969.
98. van DeRihn, I., et al.: Group A streptococcal cross-reaction with myocardium. Purification of heart-reactive antibody and isolation and characterization of the streptococcal antigen. J. Exp. Med. *146*:579, 1977.
99. Yang, L.C., et al.: Streptococcal-induced cell-mediated destruction of cardiac myofibers in vitro. J. Exp. Med. *124*:661, 1979.
100. Roberts, W.C., and Virmani, R.: Aschoff bodies at necropsy in valvular heart disease. Evidence from an analysis of 543 patients over 14 years of age that rheumatic heart disease, at least anatomically, is a disease of the mitral valve. Circulation *57*:803, 1978.
101. Chen, S., et al.: Rheumatic fever in children. A follow-up study with emphasis on cardiac sequelae. Jap. Heart J. *22*:167, 1981.
102. Procacci, P.M., et al.: Prevalence of clinical mitral valve prolapse in 1169 young women. N. Engl. J. Med. *294*:1086, 1976.
103. Guthrie, R.B., and Edwards, J.E.: Pathology of the myxomatous mitral valve. Nature, secondary changes and complications. Minn. Med. J. *59*:637, 1976.
104. Roberts, W.C.: Congenital cardiovascular anomalies usually "silent" until adulthood: Morphologic features of the floppy mitral valve, valvular aortic stenosis, discrete subvalvular aortic stenosis, hypertrophic cardiomyopathy, sinus of Valsalva aneurysm and the Marfan syndrome. Cardiovasc. Clin. *10*:407, 1979.
105. Brown, O.R., et al.: Aortic root dilatation and mitral valve prolapse in Marfan's syndrome. Circulation *52*:651, 1975.
106. Devereux, R.B.: Association of mitral-valve prolapse with low body weight and low blood pressure. Lancet *2*:792, 1982.
107. Barritt, D.W.: Mitral valve prolapse. J. R. Coll. Physicians *15*:193, 1981.
108. Clemens, J.D.: A controlled evaluation of the risk of bacterial endocarditis in persons with mitral valve prolapse. N. Engl. J. Med. *307*:776, 1982.
109. Roberts, W.C.: Anatomically isolated aortic valvular disease. The case against its being of rheumatic etiology. Am. J. Med. *49*:151, 1970.
110. Roberts, W.C.: The congenitally biscuspid aortic valve. A study of 85 autopsy cases. Am. J. Cardiol. *26*:72, 1970.
111. Fenoglio, J.J., et al.: Congenital bicuspid aortic valve after age 20. Am. J. Cardiol. *39*:164, 1977.
112. Fulkerson, P.K., et al.: Calcification of the mitral annulus: Etiology, clinical associations, complications and therapy. Am. J. Med. *66*:967, 1979.
113. Ferrans, V.J., and Roberts, W.C.: The carcinoid endocardial plaque, an ultrastructural study. Hum. Pathol. *7*:397, 1976.
114. Jager, R.M., and Polk, H.C., Jr.: Carcinoid APUDomas. *In* Hickey, R.C. (ed.): Current Problems in Cancer. Chicago, Year Book Publishers, 1977, p. 1.
115. Durack, D.T., and Beeson, P.B.: Pathogenesis of infective endocarditis. *In* Rahimtoola, S.H. (ed.): Infective Endocarditis. New York, Grune & Stratton, 1978, p. 1.
116. Pelletier, L.L., Jr., and Petersdorf, R.G.: Infective endocarditis: A review of 125 cases from the University of Washington Hospital, 1963–72. Medicine *56*:287, 1977.
117. Editorial: Infective endocarditis. Br. Med. J. *282*:677, 1981.
118. Kaplan, E.L., et al.: A collaborative study of infective endocarditis in the 1970's. Emphasis on infections in patients who have undergone cardiovascular surgery. Circulation *59*:327, 1979.
119. Schnurr, I.P., et al.: Bacterial endocarditis in England in the 1970's: A review of 70 patients. Q. J. Med. *46*:499, 1977.
120. von Reyn, C.F., et al.: Infective endocarditis and analysis based on strict case definitions. Ann. Intern. Med. *94*:505, 1981.
121. Weinstein, L., and Schlesinger, J.J.: Patho-anatomic, pathophysiologic and clinical correlations in endocarditis. N. Engl. J. Med. *291*:837, 1974.
122. Watanakunakorn, C.: Changing epidemiology and newer aspects of infective endocarditis. Adv. Intern. Med. *22*:21, 1977.
123. Banks, T., et al.: Infective endocarditis in heroin addicts. Am. J. Med. *55*:444, 1973.
124. Roberts, W.C.: Characteristics and consequences of infective endocarditis (active or healed or both) learned from morphologic studies. *In* Rahimtoola, S.H. (ed.): Infective Endocarditis. New York, Grune & Stratton, 1978, p. 55.
125. Wilson, W.R., et al.: Management of complications of infective endocarditis. Mayo Clin. Proc. *57*:162, 1982.
126. Kauffman, R.H.: The clinical implications and the pathogenetic significance of circulating immune complexes in infectious endocarditis. Am. J. Med. *71*:17, 1981.
127. Rosen, P., and Armstrong, D.: Nonbacterial thrombotic endocarditis in patients with malignant neoplastic diseases. Am. J. Med. *54*:23, 1973.
128. Young, R.S.K., and Zalneraitis, E.L.: Marantic endocarditis in children and young adults: Clinical and pathological findings. Stroke *12*:635, 1981.
129. Moschcowitz, E.: Essays on the biology of disease: Libman-Sacks disease. J. Mount Sinai Hosp. N.Y. *13*:143, 1946–47.
130. Higgins, I.T.: The epidemiology of congenital heart disease. J. Chronic Dis. *18*:699, 1965.
131. Ober, W.B., and Moore, T.E., Jr.: Congenital cardiac malformations in the neonatal period. An autopsy study. N. Engl. J. Med. *253*:271, 1955.
132. Storstein, O., et al.: Congenital heart disease in a clinical material. An analysis of 1,000 consecutive cases. Acta Med. Scand. *176*:195, 1964.
133. Jimenez, M.Q.: Ten common congenital cardiac defects. Paediatrician *10*:3, 1981.
134. Nadas, A.S., and Fyler, D.C.: Pediatric Cardiology. 3rd ed. Philadelphia, W. B. Saunders Co., 1972.
135. Friedman, W.F.: Congenital heart disease in infancy and childhood. *In* Braunwald, E. (ed.): Heart Disease. A Textbook of Cardiovascular Medicine. Philadelphia, W. B. Saunders Co., 1980, p. 967.
136. Nora, J.J., and Nora, A.H.: The evolution of specific genetic and environmental counseling in congenital heart diseases. Circulation *57*:205, 1978.
137. Nora, J.J., et al.: Etiologic aspects of cardiovascular disease and predisposition detectable in the infant and child. *In* Friedman, W.F., Lesch, M., and Sonnenblick, E.H. (Eds.): Neonatal Heart Disease. New York, Grune & Stratton, 1973, p. 279.
138. Hoffman, J.I.E., et al.: Pulmonary vascular disease with congenital heart lesions: Pathologic features and causes. Circulation *64*:873, 1981.
139. Rabinovitch, M., et al.: Early pulmonary vascular changes in congenital heart disease studied in biopsy material. Hum. Pathol. *11*(Suppl.):499, 1980.

140. Shankar, P.S.: Congenital heart disease. Q. Med. Rev. *32*:1, 1981.
141. Van Praagh, R., et al.: Single ventricle. Pathology, embryology, terminology and classification. Herz *4*:113, 1979.
142. Hoffman, J.I.E., and Rudolph, A.M.: The natural history of ventricular septal defects in infancy. Am. J. Cardiol. *16*:634, 1965.
143. Friedman, W.F., and Malony, D.: Prostaglandins and the perinatal period. Adv. Pediatr. *25*:141, 1978.
144. Bertranou, E.G., et al.: Life expectancy without surgery in tetralogy of Fallot. Am. J. Cardiol *42*:458, 1978.
145. Editorial: Tetralogy of Fallot in adults. Lancet *1*:74, 1980.
146. Lev, M., et al.: Pathologic anatomy of complete transposition of the arterial trunks. Pediatrics *28*:293, 1961.
147. Elliot, L.P., et al.: Complete transposition of the great vessels. I. An anatomic study of 60 cases. Circulation *27*:1105, 1963.
148. Van Praagh, R.: What is congenitally corrected transposition? N. Engl. J. Med. *282*:1097, 1970.
149. Haroutunian, L.M., and Neill, C.A.: Dextrocardia: Analysis of 100 cases and family study of 40 cases. Circulation *24*:951, 1961.
150. Fenoglio, J.J., et al.: Diagnosis and classification of myocarditis by endomyocardial biopsy. N. Engl. J. Med. *308*:12, 1983.
151. Wenger, N.K.: Infectious myocarditis. Postgrad. Med. *44*:105, 1968.
152. Saphir, O.: Myocarditis: General reviews with an analysis of 240 cases. Arch. Pathol. *32*:1000, 1941; *33*:88, 1942.
153. Gore, I., and Saphir, O.: Myocarditis: A classification of 1402 cases. Am. Heart J. *34*:827, 1947.
154. Woodruff, J.F.: Viral myocarditis: A review. Am. J. Pathol. *101*:425, 1980.
155. Editorial: Virus, immunology and the heart. Lancet *2*:1111, 1979.
156. Fejfar, Z.: Cardiomyopathy: An international problem. Cardiologia (Basel) *52*:9, 1968.
157. Roberts, W.C., et al.: Sarcoidosis of the heart. A clinicopathologic study of 35 necropsy patients (Group I) and review of 78 previously described necropsy patients (Group II). Am. J. Med. *63*:86, 1977.
158. Davies, M.J., et al.: Idiopathic giant-cell myocarditis—a distinctive clinicopathological entity. Br. Heart J. *37*:192, 1975.
159. Edwards, J.J., et al.: Studies on the pathogenesis of cardiac and cerebral lesions of experimental trichinosis in rabbits. Am. J. Pathol. *40*:711, 1962.
160. Pyun, K.S., et al.: Giant cell myocarditis. Light and electron microscopic study. Arch. Pathol. *90*:181, 1970.
161. Johnson, R.A., and Palacios, I.: Dilated cardiomyopathies of the adult. N. Engl. J. Med. *307*:1051, 1082.
162. Report of the WHO/ISFC Task Force on the Definition and Classification of Cardiomyopathies. Br. Heart J. *44*:672, 1980.
163. Olsen, E.G.J.: The pathology of cardiomyopathies. A critical analysis. Am. Heart J. *98*:385, 1979.
164. Demakis, J.G., and Rahimtoola, S.H.: Peripartum cardiomyopathy. Circulation *44*:964, 1971.
164A. Melvin, K.R., et al.: Peripartum cardiomyopathy due to myocarditis. N. Engl. J. Med. *307*:731, 1982.
165. Brigden, W.: Alcoholic cardiomyopathy. Br. J. Hosp. Med. *18*:122, 1977.
166. Goodwin, J.F.: Alcohol and the heart: Alcoholic cardiomyopathy. J.R. Coll. Physicians *12*:5, 1977.
167. Klein, H., and Harmjanz, D.: Effect of ethanol infusion on the ultrastructure of human myocardium. Postgrad. Med. *51*:325, 1975.
168. Rubin, E.: Alcoholic myopathy in heart and skeletal muscle. N. Engl. J. Med. *5*:28, 1979.
169. Roberts, W.C.: Cardiomyopathy and myocarditis; morphologic features. Adv. Cardiol. *22*:184, 1978.
170. Olsen, E.G.J.: Special investigations of COCM: Endomyocardial biopsies (morphological analysis). Postgrad. Med. *54*:486, 1978.
171. Baandrup, U., and Olsen, E.G.J.: Critical analysis of endomyocardial biopsies from patients suspected of having cardiomyopathy. Br. Heart J. *45*:475, 1981.
172. Perloff, J.K.: Pathogenesis of hypertrophic cardiomyopathy. Hypotheses and speculations. Am. Heart J. *101*:219, 1981.
173. Clark, C.E., et al.: Familial prevalence and genetic transmission of idiopathic hypertrophic subaortic stenosis. N. Engl. J. Med. *289*:709, 1973.
174. Darsee, J. R., et al.: Hypertrophic cardiomyopathy and human leukocyte antigen linkage. Differentiation of two forms of hypertrophic cardiomyopathy. N. Engl. J. Med. *300*:877, 1979.
175. Maron, B.J., et al.: Quantitative analysis of the distribution of cardiac muscle cell disorganization in the left ventricular wall of patients with hypertrophic cardiomyopathy. Circulation *63*:882, 1981.
176. Dingemans, K.P., and Backer, A.E.: Specificity of cellular and myofibrillar disorientation in hypertrophic obstructive cardiomyopathy. Arch. Pathol. Lab. Med. *101*:493, 1977.
177. Westermark, P., et al.: Senile cardiac amyloidosis: Evidence of two different amyloid substances in the aging heart. Scand. J. Immunol. *10*:303, 1979.
178. Baandrup, U.: Loeffler's endocarditis and endomyocardial fibrosis—a nosologic entity. Acta Pathol. Microbiol. Scand. *85*:869, 1977.
179. Olsen, E.G.: Endomyocardial fibrosis and Löffler's endocarditis parietalis fibroplastica. Postgrad. Med. J. *53*:538, 1977.
180. Solley, G.O., et al.: Endomyocardiopathy with eosinophilia. Mayo Clin. Proc. *51*:697, 1976.
181. Westwood, M., et al.: Heredity in primary endocardial fibroelastosis. Br. Heart. J. *37*:1077, 1975.
182. Schyrer, M.J.P., and Kamauchow, P.N.: Endocardial fibroelastosis. Etiologic and pathogenetic considerations in children. Am. Heart. J. *88*:557, 1974.
183. Kennedy, A., et al.: Fatal myocardial disease associated with industrial exposure to cobalt. Lancet *1*:412, 1981.
184. Ferrans, V.J.: Overview of cardiac pathology in relation to anthracycline cardiotoxicity. Cancer Treat. Rep. *62*:955, 1981.
185. Roberts, W.C., and Spray, T.L.: Pericardial heart disease. Curr. Probl. Cardiol. *2*:1, 1977.
186. Kamaras, J., and Zaborszky, B.: Chronic constrictive pericarditis in children—etiology, clinical picture and treatment. A report of 20 cases. Cor Vasa *23*:66, 1981.
187. Hollingsworth, J.W., and Saykaly, R.J.: Systemic complications of rheumatoid arthritis. Med. Clin. North Am. *61*:217, 1977.
188. Adenle, A.D., and Edwards, J.E.: Clinical and pathologic features of metastatic neoplasms of the pericardium. Chest *81*:166, 1982.
189. Goldberg, H., and Steinberg, I.: Primary tumor of the heart. Circulation *11*:963, 1955.
190. Straus, R., and Merliss, R.: Primary tumors of the heart. Arch. Pathol. *39*:74, 1945.
191. Griffiths, G.C.: A review of primary tumors of the heart. Prog. Cardiovasc. Dis. *7*:465, 1965.
192. Wold, L.E., and Lie, J.T.: Cardiac myxomas. A clinicopathologic profile. Am. J. Pathol. *101*:219, 1980.
193. Feldman, P.S., et al.: An ultrastructural study of 7 cardiac myxomas. Cancer *40*:2216, 1977.
194. Fenoglio, J.J., et al.: Cardiac rhabdomyoma: A clinicopathologic and electron microscopic study. Am. J. Cardiol. *38*:241, 1976.
195. McAllister, H.A., and Fenoglio, J., Jr.: Tumors of the cardiovascular system. Atlas of Tumor Pathology AFIP, Washington, D.C., 1977, p. 1.

14 DISEASES OF RED CELLS AND BLEEDING DISORDERS*

*With gratitude to Dr. Jose Hernandez, Department of Pathology, Southwestern Medical School, Dallas, Texas for many helpful suggestions.

The bone marrow, lymph nodes, and spleen are all involved in hematopoiesis. Traditionally, these organs and tissues have been divided into *myeloid tissue,* which includes the bone marrow and the cells derived from it, i.e., erythrocytes, platelets, granulocytes, and monocytes, and *lymphoid tissue,* consisting of thymus, lymph nodes, and spleen. This subdivision is artificial both with respect to the normal physiology of hematopoietic cells and the diseases affecting them. For example, although bone marrow is not the site where most of the mature lymphoid cells are found, it is the source of lymphoid stem cells. Similarly, leukemias, which are neoplastic disorders of the leukocytes, originate within the bone marrow but involve the lymph nodes and spleen quite prominently. Some red cell disorders (hemolytic anemias) result from the formation of autoantibodies, signifying a primary disorder of the lymphoid tissues. Thus, it is not possible to draw neat lines between diseases involving the myeloid and lymphoid tissues. Recognizing this difficulty, we have somewhat arbitrarily divided diseases of the hematopoietic tissues into two chapters. In the first, we will consider diseases of red cells and those affecting hemostasis. In the second, we will discuss diseases affecting the leukocytes, the lymph nodes, and disorders affecting primarily the spleen.

NORMAL

A complete discussion of normal hematopoiesis is beyond our scope, but certain features are helpful to an understanding of the diseases of blood.

NORMAL DEVELOPMENT OF BLOOD CELLS

In the human embryo, clusters of stem cells, called "blood islands," appear in the yolk sac in the third week of fetal development. At about the third month of embryogenesis some of these cells migrate to the liver, which then becomes the chief site of blood cell formation until shortly before birth, although the spleen, lymph nodes, and thymus make a small contribution during the last two trimesters. Beginning in the fourth month of development, hematopoiesis commences in the bone marrow. At birth, all the marrow throughout the skeleton is active and is virtually the sole source of blood cells. In the full-term infant, hepatic hematopoiesis has dwindled to a trickle but may persist in widely scattered small foci, which become inactive soon after birth. Up to the age of puberty, all the marrow throughout the skeleton is red and hematopoietically active. Usually by 18 years of age only the vertebrae, ribs, sternum, skull, pelvis, and proximal epiphyseal regions of the humerus and femur retain red marrow, the remainder becoming yellow, fatty, and inactive. Thus, in adults, only about one-half of the marrow space is active in hematopoiesis.

Several features of this normal sequence should be emphasized. By the time of birth, the bone marrow is virtually the sole source of all forms of blood cells and a major source of lymphocyte precursors. In the premature infant, foci of hematopoiesis are frequently evident in the liver, rarely in the spleen, lymph nodes, or thymus, but significant postembryonic extramedullary hematopoiesis is abnormal in the full-term infant. With an increased demand for blood cells in the adult, the fatty marrow may become transformed to red, active marrow. Moreover, this is accompanied by increased productive activity throughout the marrow. These adaptive changes are capable of increasing red cell production (erythropoiesis) seven- to eightfold. Thus, if the marrow precursor cells are not destroyed by metastatic cancer or irradiation, for example, and necessary substrate is available (e.g., adequate amounts of iron, protein, requisite vitamins, and so forth), such loss of red cells as may occur in hemolytic disorders produces anemia only when the marrow compensatory mechanisms are outstripped. Under these circumstances, extramedullary hematopoiesis may reappear, first within the liver and then in the spleen and lymph nodes. For unknown reasons, the thymus never resumes this embryonic function.

ORIGIN AND DIFFERENTIATION OF HEMATOPOIETIC CELLS

There is little doubt that the formed elements of blood—erythrocytes, granulocytes, monocytes, platelets, and lymphocytes—have a common origin in a totipotent hematopoietic stem cell. This common precursor then gives rise to lymphoid stem cells and the pluripotent myeloid stem cells, which are committed to produce lymphocytes and the myeloid cells, respectively (Fig. 14–1). The lymphoid stem cell, which has not been identified definitively, is believed to be the origin of precursors of T cells (pre–T cells) and B cells (pre–B cells), which differentiate into mature T cells and B cells under the inductive influence of the thymus and bursa, respectively. The details of lymphoid differentiation will not be discussed here, but it is worth pointing out that, unlike myeloid differentiation, there are no distinctive, morphologically recognizable stages. For definition, reliance must be placed on the detection of differentiation specific antigens by monoclonal antibodies (p. 159). From the pluripotent myeloid stem cell arise at least four types of unipotential, *committed stem cells* capable of differentiating along the erythroid, megakaryocytic, eosinophilic, and granulocyte/macrophage pathways. Recent advances in cell culture techniques have made it possible to grow these committed stem cells in vitro with the production of colonies of differentiated progeny. Thus, the committed stem cells have been called colony-forming units (CFU). As indicated in Figure 14–1, granulocytes and macrophages have a common precursor, and hence colonies derived from CFU-G/M (colony-forming unit–granulocyte/macrophage) have a mixture of neutrophils and macrophages. In the erythroid pathway, two distinct committed stem cells can be recognized. Based on the morphology of the colonies, the more primitive of the two stages is called BFU-E (bursa-forming unit–erythroid) and the later stage is called CFU-E (colony-forming unit–erythroid). From all these various committed stem cells, intermediate stages are derived, and ultimately the morphologically recognizable precursors of the differentiated cell lines, i.e., proerythroblasts, myeloblasts, megakaryoblasts, monoblasts, and eosinophiloblasts. These in turn give rise to mature progeny. Since the mature blood elements have a finite life span, it follows that their numbers must be constantly replenished. This can be realized if the stem cells possess the capacity not only to differentiate but also to renew themselves. *Thus, self-renewal is an important property of stem cells.* The totipotent stem cells have the greatest capacity of self-renewal, but normally most of them are not in cell cycle. As commitment proceeds, self-renewal ability becomes limited, but a greater fraction of the stem cells are found to be in cycle. For example, very few pluripotent myeloid stem cells are normally in cell cycle, but up to 50% of CFU-G/M are synthesizing DNA. This suggests that normally the pool of differentiated cells is replenished mainly by the proliferation of restricted stem cells. It is interesting to note that, although the earliest recognizable precursors (e.g., myeloblasts or proerythroblasts) are in active cell division, they cannot self-replicate, i.e., they differentiate and "die." By definition, then, they are not stem cells. Since most forms of marrow failure or neoplastic disorders (e.g.,

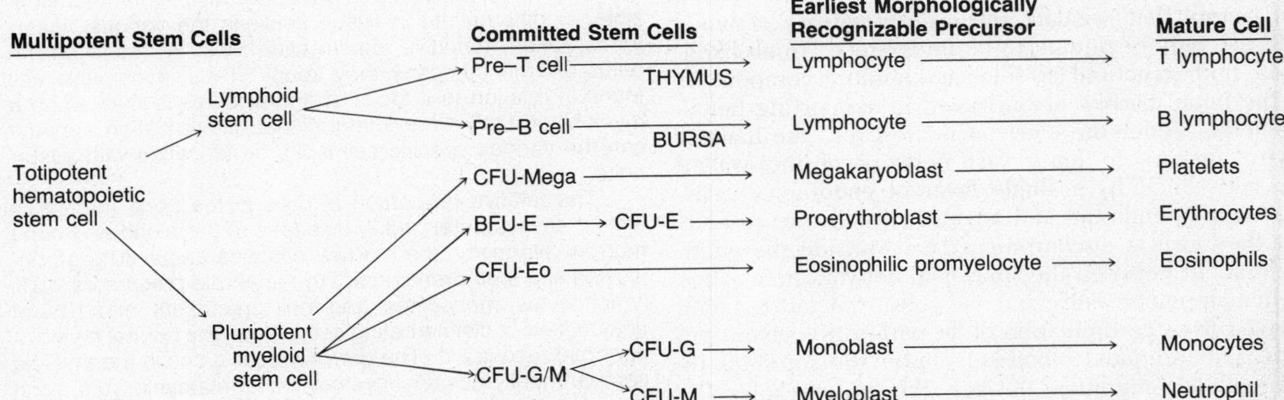

Figure 14–1. Differentiation of hematopoietic cells. (Modified from Wintrobe, M. M., et al.: Clinical Hematology. 8th ed. Philadelphia, Lea & Febiger, 1981, p. 43.)

aplastic anemias, leukemias, polycythemia) are disorders of stem cells, much interest is centered on the physiologic mechanisms that regulate the proliferation and differentiation of progenitor cells. Little is known about the factors that affect the proliferation of the most primitive stem cells, since clonal assays for their detection in vitro have not been fully developed. However, several regulatory factors that affect the committed stem cells have been identified. Most well characterized are colony-stimulating factor (CSF), which acts on CFU-G/M to produce granulocyte/macrophage colonies, and erythropoietin, which is essential for the differentiation of erythroid precursors. Thrombopoietin, which acts on CFU-Meg, is less well characterized at present. CSF is derived from macrophages and T cells, and exists in several molecular forms. Erythropoietin is derived from the kidney but can also be produced by the liver. There is some evidence that differentiation of BFU-E also requires T cells or their products. It seems, therefore, that the versatile T cells may have yet another role! Recall that before the advent of modern immunology, lymphocytes were believed to be "trephocytes" (feeders of other cells). This discredited theory may indeed have a grain of truth. Although it has not been possible to develop an in vitro assay for the totipotential stem cell, recent attempts to develop an assay for the pluripotential myeloid stem cells have met with success. It has been possible to obtain mixed colonies containing erythroblasts, megakaryocytes, granulocytes, and macrophages, which could have arisen only from a multipotent stem cell. These exciting new developments are interesting not only for developmental biologists but also for pathology students, since the pathogenesis of several hematologic disorders, including aplastic anemias, polycythemia, and leukemias, has already begun to be unraveled by the use of stem cell cultures.

NORMAL ANATOMY AND MORPHOLOGY OF BONE MARROW. The bone marrow not only is a reservoir of stem cells, but also provides a unique microenvironment in which the orderly proliferation and differentiation of precursor cells takes place. In addition, it regulates the release of fully differentiated cells into the circulation. The nature of the bone-marrow microenvironment and the factors that regulate the orderly release of blood cells are only beginning to be understood. In all likelihood, both structural (stromal) and humoral components of the bone marrow are involved in supporting hematopoiesis. Under the electron microscope, the marrow cavity appears to be a vast network of thin-walled sinusoids lined by a single layer of endothelial cells. Basement membrane and adventitial cells are present but they form a discontinuous layer outside the endothelium. In between the sinusoidal network lie clusters of hematopoietic cells and fat cells, the latter being derived from accumulation of fat within the adventitial cells. Differentiated blood cells enter the sinusoids by transcellular migration through the endothelial cells. That this process is finely regulated is attested to by the fact that when hematopoiesis takes place at extramedullary sites, e.g., the spleen (p. 686), the peripheral blood contains all forms of abnormal as well as primitive blood cells that do not enter the blood in normal medullary hematopoiesis.

Two recent developments have highlighted the role of marrow microenvironment in the maintenance of hematopoiesis. First, in some forms of marrow failure affecting all the myeloid cell lines (e.g., one variant of aplastic anemia, p. 639), the defect appears to lie in the microenvironment rather than in the stem cells, since transplantation of histocompatible bone marrow stem cells fails to benefit these patients. Second, for years experimental hematologists have been frustrated in their attempts to study hematopoiesis in vitro because the multipotent stem cells could not be maintained in culture flasks. However, Dexter has overcome this major hurdle by devising a technique that allows the maintenance of the bone marrow stroma (endothelial cells, fat cells, and adventitial cells) in vitro.[1] With the so-called Dexter technique, not only do the myeloid stem cells survive in vitro, but they can self-replicate for several months. This technique can now be applied to dissect the role of bone marrow stromal environment in both health and disease.

Although the morphology of the hematopoietic cells within the bone marrow is best studied in smears of marrow aspirates, useful information can also be obtained by studying the histology of bone marrow biopsies. For example, a reasonable estimate of marrow activity may be obtained by examining the ratio of fat cells to hematopoietic elements in bone marrow biopsies. In normal adults this ratio approaches 1:1, but with marrow hypoplasia (e.g., aplastic anemia) the proportion of fat cells is greatly increased and, conversely, fat cells may virtually disappear in diseases characterized by increased hematopoiesis (e.g., leukemias). When subjected to fixatives and tissue staining methods, the cells of the bone marrow and peripheral blood differ in appearance from those in air-dried Giemsa- or Wright-stained preparations. The maturational sequence of various cell types and their specific names are described in specialized texts.[2] The earliest identifiable myeloid cells, i.e., pronormoblasts, myeloblasts, and monoblasts, are all moderately large (10 to 20 μ in diameter), having abundant, deeply basophilic cytoplasm; round nuclei with coarsely clumped chromatin; and prominent nucleoli. It is extremely difficult, if not impossible, to differentiate in tissue sections the various "blast" forms. Often, tentative identification must be made on the basis of "the company they keep." Thus, a primitive cell found in relation to a focus of granulocytes is likely to be a myeloblast. Only when maturational differentiation appears can the various specific cell types be identified with assurance.

The relative proportion of cells in the bone marrow is almost always deranged in diseases of the blood and bone marrow. Normally, the marrow contains about 60% granulocytes and their precursors; 20% erythroid precursors; 10% lymphocytes, monocytes, and their precursors; and 10% of unidentified or disintegrating cells. Thus, the normal myeloid/erythroid ratio is 3:1. The dominant cell types in the myeloid compartment include myelocytes, metamyelocytes, and granulocytes. In the erythroid compartment the dominant forms are polychromatophilic and orthochromic normoblasts.

Under conditions of normal iron metabolism, approximately 30 to 40% of the normoblasts contain scattered ferritin granules, which are best visualized by special stains for iron (Prussian blue). Such cells are called **sideroblasts.** The ferritin granules presumably represent a reserve of iron on which the cell can draw for the synthesis of heme. The production of heme by the insertion of iron into protoporphyrin by heme synthetase and the production of globin are precisely balanced. When synthesis of either product is depressed, for whatever reason, excessive amounts of ferritin accumulate in sideroblasts (as occurs in sideroblastic anemia). With progressive accumulation of iron, mitochondria, the loci of heme synthetase, become stuffed with iron and rupture, producing distinctive **ring sideroblasts.** Thus, the state of iron reserves can be judged by the number of sideroblasts and their content of iron. If sideroblasts cannot be identified in the marrow, it signifies iron deficiency. However, an excess of sideroblasts, in particular ring sideroblasts, connotes an iron overload or the inability to utilize normal amounts of iron.

We now turn to consider the various disorders of the red blood cells.

PATHOLOGY

ANEMIAS

The function of red cells is the transport of oxygen into tissues. In physiologic terms, therefore, anemia may be defined as a reduction in the oxygen transport capacity of the blood. Since in most instances the reduced oxygen-carrying capacity of blood results from a deficiency of red cells, *anemia may be defined as a reduction below normal limits of the total circulating red cell mass.* This value is not easily measured, however, and therefore anemia has been defined as a reduction below normal in the volume of packed red cells, as measured by the hematocrit, or a reduction in the hemoglobin concentration of the blood. It hardly needs pointing out that fluid retention may expand plasma volume and fluid loss may contract plasma volume, creating spurious abnormalities in clinically used values.

Innumerable classifications of anemia have been proposed. A highly acceptable one based on the underlying mechanism is presented in Table 14–1. Whatever the nature of anemia, the reduction in red cell mass and oxygen transport, when sufficiently severe, leads to certain changes throughout the body.

Table 14–1. CLASSIFICATION OF ANEMIA ACCORDING TO MECHANISM OF PRODUCTION

I. Blood Loss
- A. Acute: Trauma
- B. Chronic: Lesions of GI tract, gynecologic disturbances

II. Increased Rate of Destruction (Hemolytic Anemias)
- A. Intrinsic (intracorpuscular) abnormalities of red cells
  - *Hereditary*
    - 1. Red cell membrane disorders
      - a. Disorders of membrane cytoskeleton: Spherocytosis, elliptocytosis
      - b. Disorders of lipid synthesis: Selective increase in membrane lecithin
    - 2. Red cell enzyme deficiencies
      - a. Glycolytic enzymes: Pyruvate kinase deficiency, hexokinase deficiency
      - b. Enzymes of hexose monophosphate shunt: G6PD, glutathione synthetase
    - 3. Disorders of hemoglobin synthesis
      - a. Deficient globin synthesis: Thalassemia syndromes
      - b. Structurally abnormal globin synthesis (hemoglobinopathies): Sickle cell anemia, unstable hemoglobins
  - *Acquired*
    - 1. Membrane defect: Paroxysmal nocturnal hemoglobinuria
- B. Extrinsic (extracorpuscular) abnormalities
  - 1. Antibody mediated
    - a. Isohemagglutinins: Transfusion reactions, erythroblastosis fetalis
    - b. Autoantibodies: Idiopathic (primary), drug-associated, SLE, malignancies, Mycoplasma infection
  - 2. Mechanical trauma to red cells
    - a. Microangiopathic hemolytic anemias: Thrombotic thrombocytopenic purpura, DIC
    - b. Cardiac traumatic hemolytic anemia
  - 3. Infections: Malaria
  - 4. Chemical injury: Lead poisoning
  - 5. Sequestration in mononuclear phagocytic system: Hypersplenism

III. Impaired Red Cell Production
- A. Disturbance of proliferation and differentiation of stem cells: Aplastic anemia, pure red cell aplasia, anemia of renal failure, anemia of endocrine disorders
- B. Disturbance of proliferation and maturation of erythroblasts
  - 1. Defective DNA synthesis: Deficiency or impaired utilization of vitamin B_{12} and folic acid (megaloblastic anemias)
  - 2. Defective hemoglobin synthesis
    - a. Deficient heme synthesis: Iron deficiency
    - b. Deficient globin synthesis: Thalassemias
  - 3. Unknown or multiple mechanisms: Sideroblastic anemia, anemia of chronic infections, myelophthisic anemias due to marrow infiltrations

MORPHOLOGY. The pattern and severity of tissue changes depend, to a considerable extent, on the suddenness and quantity of blood loss and the duration of anemia. With sudden severe hemorrhage, red cells and circulating blood volume are lost proportionally, with the possible development of shock and its attendant clinical and morphologic changes (p. 112). When blood loss is slow, when red cell destruction outpaces production, or when some other impairment of red cell formation leads to an anemia, the resultant tissue hypoxia is characteristically reflected in certain morphologic alterations.

The skin is pale and usually becomes thin and inelastic as the epidermis and dermis atrophy. Frequently, the nails become brittle and lose their normal convexity to assume a concave spoon-shape (koilonychia), particularly in iron deficiency anemia. Cells that are particularly vulnerable to hypoxia may undergo fatty change or even ischemic necrosis. Such damage is most frequently encountered in the muscle cells of the myocardium, the epithelial cells of the proximal convoluted tubules of the kidney, the centrilobular hepatic cells, and the sensitive ganglion cells of the cortex and basal ganglia (p. 1389).

The increased demand for erythropoiesis in anemia

causes the fatty marrow to become active and red if the marrow is capable of response. In some anemic states, such as aplastic anemia, the marrow cannot react. When the need is great, extramedullary hematopoiesis ensues, reverting to the fetal patterns of blood formation. Other more specific changes may also appear, determined by the particular type of anemia.

Clinical Features. Attendant on the deranged physiology and morphologic alterations described, many nonspecific clinical signs and symptoms are seen in patients with anemia. Classically, these patients are pale and many have the nail deformity described. Weakness, malaise, and easy fatigability are common complaints. The lowered oxygen content of the circulating blood leads to dyspnea on mild exertion. If the fatty changes in the myocardium are sufficiently severe, cardiac failure may develop and compound the respiratory difficulty caused by reduced oxygen transport. Occasionally, the myocardial hypoxia manifests itself by angina pectoris, particularly when a preexisting vascular disease has already rendered the myocardium partially ischemic. With acute blood loss and shock, oliguria and anuria may develop in the shock kidney. Central nervous system hypoxia may be evidenced by headache, dimness of vision, and faintness. Splenomegaly and hepatomegaly sometimes can be found, especially in infants with increased hematopoiesis in these organs. However, the most characteristic features of the anemia become evident only from laboratory studies of the peripheral blood.

ANEMIAS OF BLOOD LOSS

Acute Blood Loss

The clinical and morphologic reactions to blood loss depend on the rate of hemorrhage and whether the blood is lost externally or internally. With acute blood loss, the alterations reflect principally the loss of blood volume rather than the loss of hemoglobin. Shock and death may follow. If the patient survives, the blood volume is rapidly restored by shift of water from the interstitial fluid compartment. Restoration of blood fluid volume, which begins at once, reaches its full effect within 48 to 72 hours when hematocrit values reach their lowest level and the full extent of the anemia becomes evident. Reduction in the oxygenation of tissues triggers the production of erythropoietin, and the marrow responds by increasing erythropoiesis. When the blood is lost internally, as into the peritoneal cavity, the iron can be recaptured, but if the blood is lost externally, the adequacy of the red cell recovery may be hampered by iron deficiency when insufficient reserves are present.

Soon after the acute blood loss the red blood cells appear normal in size and color (normocytic, normochromic). However, as the marrow begins to regenerate, changes occur in the peripheral blood. Most striking is an increase in the reticulocyte count, reaching 10 to 15% after seven days. The reticulocytes are seen as polychromatophilic macrocytes in the usual blood smear. These changes of red cell regeneration can sometimes be mistaken for an underlying hemolytic process. Mobilization of platelets and granulocytes from the marginal pools leads to thrombocytosis and leukocytosis in the period immediately following acute blood loss.

Chronic Blood Loss

Chronic blood loss induces anemia only when the rate of loss exceeds the regenerative capacity of the erythroid precursors or when iron reserves are depleted. In addition to chronic blood loss, any cause of iron deficiency such as malnutrition, malabsorption states, or an increased demand above the daily intake as occurs in pregnancy will lead to an identical anemia, discussed later (p. 635).

HEMOLYTIC ANEMIAS

The hemolytic anemias are all characterized by (1) shortening of the normal red cell life span, i.e., premature destruction of red cells; (2) accumulation of the products of hemoglobin catabolism; and (3) a marked increase in erythropoiesis within the bone marrow, in an attempt to compensate for the loss of red cells. These and some other general features will be briefly discussed before we describe the features of specific hemolytic anemias.

As is well known, the physiologic destruction of senescent red cells takes place within the mononuclear phagocytic cells of the spleen. In hemolytic anemias, too, the premature destruction of red cells occurs predominantly within the mononuclear phagocyte system (extravascular hemolysis). Only in a few cases does lysis of red cells within the vascular compartment (intravascular hemolysis) predominate.

Intravascular hemolysis occurs when normal erythrocytes are damaged by mechanical injury (p. 629). For example, prosthetic cardiac ball valves and thrombi within the microcirculation (disseminated intravascular coagulation, DIC) may disrupt erythrocytes and produce a form of hemolytic anemia referred to as microangiopathic hemolytic anemia (p. 629). Another major mechanism of intravascular hemolysis involves complement-induced lysis. Complement binding and activation may be mediated by antibodies, as occurs in a mismatched blood transfusion, or complement may lyse erythrocytes in the absence of antibody, in the rare disorder known as paroxysmal nocturnal hemoglobinuria (p. 627).

Whatever the mechanism, *intravascular hemolysis is manifested by (1) hemoglobinemia, (2) hemoglobinuria, (3) methemalbuminemia, (4) jaundice, and (5) hemosiderinuria.* When hemoglobin escapes into the plasma it is promptly bound by an α_2 globulin (haptoglobin) to produce a complex that prevents excretion into the urine, since the complexes are rapidly cleared by the reticuloendothelial system. *A decrease in serum haptoglobin level is characteristically seen in all cases of intravascular hemolysis.* When the haptoglobin is depleted, the unbound or free hemoglobin is in part rapidly oxidized to methemoglobin, and both hemoglobin and methemoglobin are excreted through the kidneys, imparting a red-brown color to the urine—hemoglobinuria and methemoglobinuria. Should the excretory capacity of the kidneys be exceeded, the free heme group derived from the retained methemoglobin complexes with albumin to produce methemalbuminemia, imparting a red-brown color to the blood. The renal proximal tubular cells may reabsorb and catabolize much of this filtered hemoglobin, but some passes out with the urine. Within the tubular cells, iron released from the hemoglobin produces hemosiderosis of the renal tubular epithelium, and shedding of such cells into the urine (where they can be identified by iron stains) constitutes the basis of the *hemosiderinuria.* Concomitantly, the heme groups derived from the complexes are catabolized within the mononuclear phagocyte system, leading ultimately to jaundice. In hemolytic anemias, the serum bilirubin is unconjugated (p. 89) and the level of hyperbilirubinemia depends on the functional capacity of liver as well as the rate of hemolysis. With a normal liver, the jaundice is rarely severe. Excessive bilirubin excreted by the liver into the gastrointestinal tract leads eventually to increased formation and fecal excretion (p. 888) of urobilin.

Extravascular hemolysis takes place whenever red cells are injured, are rendered "foreign," or become less deformable. For example, in hereditary spherocytosis an abnormal membrane cytoskeleton decreases the deformability of the red cell. Analogously, in sickle cell anemia, the abnormal hemoglobin "gels" or "crystallizes" within the erythrocyte, deforming it and reducing its plasticity. Since extreme alterations in shape are required for red cells to navigate the splenic sinusoids successfully, reduced deformability makes the passage difficult and leads to sequestration within the cords, followed by phagocytosis (Fig. 14–2). This is believed to be an important pathogenetic mechanism of extravascular hemolysis in a variety of hemolytic anemias.[3] With extravascular hemolysis it is obvious that hemoglobinemia, hemoglobinuria, and the related intravascular changes do not appear. However, the catabolism of erythrocytes in the phagocytic cells induces anemia and jaundice that are otherwise indistinguishable from those caused by intravascular hemolysis. Furthermore, since some hemoglobin manages to escape from the phagocytic cells, plasma haptoglobin levels are invariably reduced. The morphologic changes that follow are identical to those in intravascular hemolysis, except that the erythrophagocytosis generally causes hypertrophy of the reticuloendothelial cells and this may lead to splenomegaly.

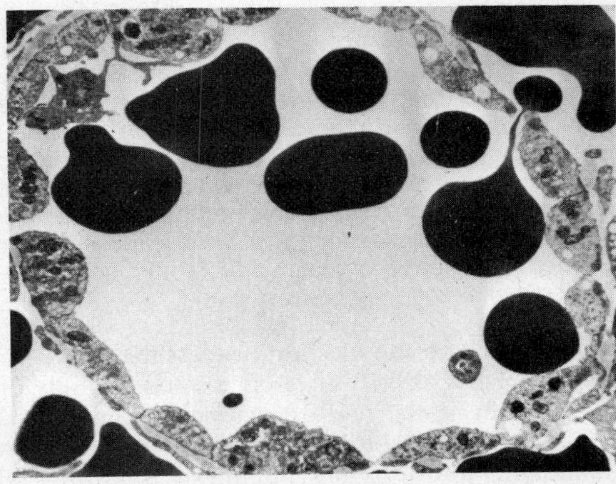

Figure 14–2. Splenic sinus (electron micrograph). An erythrocyte is in process of squeezing from cord into sinus lumen. Note degree of deformability required for red cell to pass through wall of sinus. (From Enriquez, P., and Neiman, R. S.: The Pathology of the Spleen: A Functional Approach. Chicago, The American Society of Clinical Pathologists, 1976, p. 7. Used by permission.)

Certain morphologic changes are standard in the hemolytic anemias, whether caused by intravascular or extravascular mechanisms. The anemia and lowered tissue oxygen tension stimulate increased production of erythropoietin, leading to an expansion of the erythron with markedly increased numbers of normoblasts in the marrow (Fig. 14–3); sometimes the expansion leads to extramedullary hematopoiesis. Unless there is some block in the formation of globin or heme, the accelerated compensatory erythropoiesis leads to a prominent reticulocytosis in the peripheral blood. Concomitantly, the expanded volume of the bone

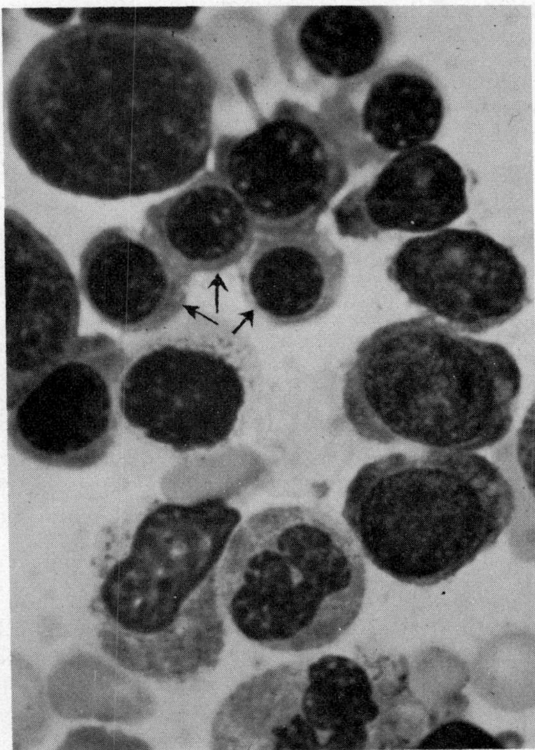

Figure 14–3. Marrow smear from one of the hemolytic anemias illustrating a proerythroblast *(upper left)* and normoblasts in various stages of differentiation. Arrows show late polychromatic normoblasts.

marrow causes pressure atrophy of the inner table of the cortical bone, resulting in neo-osteogenesis on the outer table. Such osseous changes are usually most evident in the ribs, facial bones, and calvaria. The elevated levels of bilirubin, when excreted through the liver, promote the formation of pigment gallstones (cholelithiasis). With chronicity, the phagocytosed red cells or hemoglobin will eventually lead to hemosiderosis, usually confined to the mononuclear phagocyte system. Thus, whatever the basis of the hemolysis, when sufficiently chronic, a common sequence of morphologic changes may be anticipated.

The hemolytic anemias can be classified in a variety of ways. One has already been suggested, namely division into intravascular and extravascular hemolytic disorders. However, since the number of disorders with predominantly intravascular hemolysis is limited, this classification is not entirely satisfactory. A pathogenetic classification could be based on whether the underlying cause of red cell destruction is extrinsic (extracorpuscular mechanism) or a defect inherent in the red cell (intracorpuscular defect). These anemias can also be divided into hereditary and acquired disorders. *In general, hereditary disorders are due to intracorpuscular defects and the acquired disorders to extrinsic factors such as autoantibodies.* Each of the classifications has value, but here we will follow the intrinsic-extrinsic outline given in Table 14–1, limiting consideration only to the more common entities.

Hereditary Spherocytosis (HS)

This autosomal dominant disorder is characterized by an intrinsic defect in the red cell membrane that renders erythrocytes spheroidal, less deformable, and vulnerable to splenic sequestration and destruction. The prevalence of HS is highest in people of North European extraction, in whom rates of one in 5000 have been reported. Although most cases are related to autosomal dominant inheritance, approximately 20% of patients have unaffected parents, suggesting that the mutation often arises de novo.

PATHOGENESIS. The pathogenesis of the spheroidal shape of the erythrocyte is still somewhat uncertain, but recent studies come close to proposing a mechanism.[4] It appears that the fundamental defect is in the skeleton of the red cell membrane. Spectrin is the major skeletal protein of the basic filamentous framework.[4A] It consists of two polypeptide chains, alpha and beta, which are intertwined (helical) dimers, lying "flat" on the cytoplasmic aspect of the cell membrane (Fig. 1–32). The individual spectrin dimers are like segments of an extensive cable network that are linked to each other head to head to form tetramers. Lateral connections between spectrin tetramers are established through two additional proteins, actin and protein 4.1. The two-dimensional spectrin cable meshwork so formed is tethered to the inner surface of the cell membrane by yet another protein called ankyrin, which forms a bridge between spectrin and the cell membrane protein 3.[5] Together these proteins are responsible for maintenance of the normal shape, strength, and flexibility of the red cell membrane. Although a deficiency of any one of the membrane skeletal proteins could adversely affect the red cells, the amounts of these proteins are normal in most patients with HS.[5] On the other hand, a qualitative defect in red cell spectrin molecules has been found in several affected families.[4] The defect, expressed as reduced binding to protein 4.1, appears to involve approximately 50% of the spectrin molecules in heterozygotes. Conceivably, *the weakening of protein 4.1-spectrin bonds results in reduced "pull" exerted on the cell membrane, permitting the cells to assume the smallest possible diameter for a given volume, namely, a sphere.* It should be noted that defective protein 4.1-spectrin interaction may not be the underlying defect in all cases of HS, and at present the proportion of HS patients with this defect is not known. A variety of other biochemical abnormalities, notably reduced phosphorylation of spectrin, increased permeability to passive sodium influx, and decreased membrane lipids, have been described in HS, but it is not clear whether they represent the cause or the effect of spherocytosis.[5]

Although much remains to be learned about the molecular defects in HS, the travails of the red cells resulting from spheroidal transformation are fairly well defined. In the life of the "portly" (and therefore inflexible) spherocyte, the spleen acts as the villain. As discussed earlier, the spleen serves as a watchdog ready to weed out the less-than-perfect erythrocytes as they traverse the red pulp. To enter the venous sinuses, normal red cells deposited into the cords of Billroth have to undergo extreme degrees of deformation (p. 615). Because of their spheroidal shape and reduced membrane plasticity, spherocytes have great difficulty in leaving the cords. The few, less affected cells that do manage to squeeze through the sinusoidal walls succeed at the expense of a portion of their cell membrane. These "bruised" red cells, called microspherocytes, are smaller and even less deformable, and are readily trapped in the cords when they enter the spleen subsequently. As more and more spherocytes are detained, the already sluggish circulation of the cords stagnates further and the environment around the cells becomes progressively more hostile. Lactic acid accumulates and the extracellular pH falls, which in turn inhibits glycolysis and generation of ATP. Loss of ATP impairs the ability to extrude sodium, adding an element of osmotic injury. Stagnation in the cords also promotes contacts with macrophages, which are plentiful, and eventually the hapless spherocytes fall prey to the appetite of phagocytic cells. *The cardinal role of the spleen in the premature demise of the spherocytes is proved by the invariably beneficial effect of splenectomy. The spherocytes persist but the anemia is corrected.*

MORPHOLOGY. Perhaps the most outstanding morphologic feature of this disease is the spheroidal shape of the red cells, apparent on smears as abnormally small cells lacking their central zone of pallor (Fig. 14–4). Spherocytosis, although distinctive, is not pathognomonic since it is also seen in autoimmune hemolytic anemias. In addition to

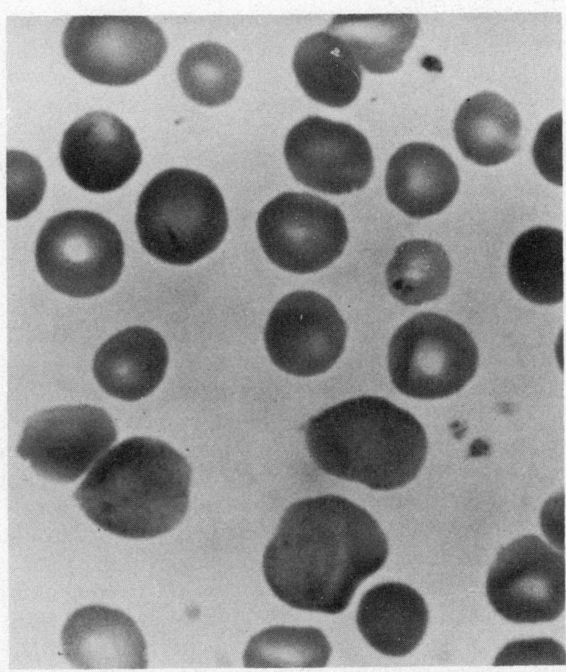

Figure 14–4. Peripheral blood smear from a patient with hereditary spherocytosis. Note the anisocytosis and several dark-appearing spherocytes with no central pallor. (Courtesy of Dr. Jose Hernandez, Department of Pathology, Southwestern Medical School, Dallas, Texas.)

reticulocytosis and the general features of all hemolytic anemias, as previously detailed (p. 615), certain alterations are fairly distinctive. Moderate splenic enlargement is characteristic of hereditary spherocytosis (500 to 1000 gm); in few other hemolytic anemias is the spleen enlarged as much or as often. It results from marked congestion of the cords of Billroth, leaving the sinuses virtually empty. Erythrophagocytosis can be seen within the congested cords. Typically present are the associated changes found in all hemolytic anemias, including expansion of the erythron, bone changes, and hemosiderosis, as well as cholelithiasis (pigment stones) in 50 to 85% of cases.

CLINICAL COURSE. The characteristic clinical features are anemia, splenomegaly, and jaundice. The severity of the disease varies greatly from one patient to another. It may make its appearance at birth with marked jaundice, requiring exchange transfusion. In others, the mild red cell destruction is readily compensated for by expansion of the erythron. Only when this compensatory reaction is outpaced do symptomatic patients have a chronic hemolytic anemia, usually of mild-to-moderate severity. However, this more or less stable clinical course may be punctuated by "crises" of two kinds, often triggered by intercurrent infections. A *hemolytic crisis* may develop, characterized by the sudden onset of a wave of massive hemolysis accompanied by fever, abdominal pain, nausea, vomiting, jaundice, low blood pressure, tachycardia, and even shock. During active hemolysis, the patient classically becomes markedly jaundiced. Alternatively, an *aplastic crisis* may appear, characterized by temporary suppression of red cell production, manifested by sudden worsening of the anemia, and the disappearance of reticulocytes from the peripheral blood. Transfusions may be necessary to support the patient, but eventually both of these crises remit in most instances. Enlargement of the spleen, which is often progressive, is seen in 75 to 95% of the adults. Gallstones, found in many patients, may also produce symptoms (p. 944). Diagnosis is based on family history, hematologic findings, and laboratory evidence of spherocytosis, expressed as increased osmotic fragility. The spherocytes are particularly vulnerable to osmotic lysis, induced in vitro by solutions of hypotonic salt, since there is little margin for expansion of red cell volume without rupture.

Hemolytic Disease Due to Erythrocyte Enzyme Defects: Glucose-6-Phosphate Dehydrogenase Deficiency

The erythrocyte and its membrane are vulnerable to injury by exogenous and endogenous oxidants. Normally, intracellular reduced glutathione (GSH) inactivates such oxidants. *Abnormalities in the hexose monophosphate shunt or in glutathione metabolism resulting from deficient or impaired enzyme function reduce the ability of red cells to protect themselves against oxidative injuries and lead to hemolytic disease.* The most important of these enzyme derangements is a hereditary deficiency of glucose-6-phosphate dehydrogenase (G6PD) activity involved in the hexose monophosphate shunt pathway.[6] Millions of people throughout the world have such a deficiency. More than 100 G6PD genetic variants have been identified, but fortunately most evoke no clinical disorder or hemolytic anemia. Two variants, designated G6PD A− and G6PD Mediterranean, lead to clinically significant hemolysis. The A− type is present in about 10% of American blacks; G6PD Mediterranean, as the name implies, is found largely in populations in the Middle East. The basis of G6PD deficiency is somewhat different in the two genetic variants. In the A− type of deficiency, a normal amount of the enzyme is synthesized in the red cell precursors, but it is more rapidly catabolized or inactivated during the life span of the red cell, so that older red cells become progressively more deficient in enzyme activity. Exposure to an oxidant, therefore, tends to induce hemolysis of older red cells but not the younger ones, and so the drop in hematocrit is mild or moderate. G6PD Mediterranean, on the other hand, is associated with markedly reduced activity throughout the entire life span of the red cell, suggesting that, in addition to rapid catabolism, impaired synthesis of the enzyme may also be involved. In these individuals, the hemolytic crisis may produce profound drops in hematocrit and hemoglobin levels.

Inheritance of the mutant gene is X-linked. Thus, the defect is expressed in all erythrocytes of the affected male. In the heterozygous female, two populations of red cells, some deficient, others normal, are present owing to random inactivation of the X chromosomes. It follows that males are more vulnerable to oxidant injury than females, who usually have a smaller fraction of enzyme-deficient red cells. Only those carrier females who have an unusually large fraction of vulnerable red cells ("unfavorable lyonization") are susceptible to hemolytic anemia. It might be noted that the prevalence of such deleterious genes has in part been maintained because a deficiency of G6PD is thought to protect against malaria due to *Plasmodium falciparum*.

Numerous oxidant drugs may trigger hemolytic crises, principally the antimalarials—primaquine and quinacrine (Atabrine)—in addition to sulfonamides, nitrofurans, and others.[6] Even more important are infections that presumably act by the generation of free radicals in macrophages. The free radicals exert oxidant effects on G6PD-deficient erythrocytes. Owing to the extremely low levels of G6PD, persons with the Mediterranean type of G6PD have chronic hemolysis, even in the absence of exposure to an oxidant drug. They also develop an explosive acute hemolytic disorder after ingestion of fava beans. It appears that two genes are involved in the genesis of this peculiar reaction, one responsible for G6PD deficiency and the other for an abnormal enzyme that causes the catabolism of a fava bean product into a highly oxidant derivative.

The pathophysiology of hemolysis seems to involve the following sequence. Exposure to the drug causes oxidation of GSH to glutathione, presumably through the production of H_2O_2. Since the regeneration of GSH is impaired in G6PD-deficient cells, hydrogen peroxide accumulates and injures other red cell constituents. Hemoglobin seems to be attacked on two fronts: oxidation of heme leading to formation of methemoglobin and, independently, oxidation of the sulfhydryl groups of the globin chains. The latter is particularly devastating since it leads to denaturation of hemoglobin and formation of precipitates (Heinz bodies) within the cell. When attached to the cell membrane, Heinz bodies decrease erythrocyte deformability, thus rendering them susceptible to sequestration in the spleen. A remarkable phenomenon also follows: as the red cells pass through the splenic cords, phagocytic cells, principally macrophages, pluck out the Heinz bodies, a process referred to as pitting. The loss of membrane induces further membrane damage and simultaneously induces the formation of spherocytes. All these changes predispose the red cells to become trapped in splenic cords and destroyed by erythrophagocytosis.

The clinical features of G6PD deficiency may be surmised from our discussion. Persons with the deficient enzyme do not have hemolysis unless exposed to the oxidant injuries alluded to above. After a variable lag period of two to three days, an acute hemolytic episode characterized by hemoglobinemia, hemoglobinuria, and deceased hematocrit levels is triggered. In patients with the G6PD A– variant, since only the senescent red cells are lysed, the episode is self-limited and hemolysis stops when only the younger red cells remain in the circulation (despite continued administration of the oxidant drug). In contrast the hemolytic episodes with the G6PD Mediterranean variant are much more severe, lasting for the duration of the oxidant injury. The peripheral blood smear shows Heinz bodies within the red cells as dark inclusions, when stained with crystal violet. The recovery phase is heralded by reticulocytosis, as in the case of other hemolytic anemias. Since hemolytic episodes related to deficiencies of G6PD occur only on exposure to particular drugs, the morphologic changes encountered in most chronic hemolytic anemias are rarely present.

Sickle Cell Disease

Sickle cell disease is the classic prototype of a *hereditary hemoglobinopathy*. It results from a point mutation in the genetic code such that a single amino acid is substituted for another in one of the polypeptide chains of hemoglobin, transforming HbA into HbS. About 300 variant hemoglobins have been identified in which there is either an amino acid substitution or a deletion in one of the globin chains. Hemoglobin, as you recall, is a tetramer of four globin chains, comprising two pairs of similar chains, each with its own heme group. The hemoglobin in the adult is composed of 96% HbA ($\alpha_2\beta_2$), 3% hemoglobin A_2 ($\alpha_2\delta_2$), and 1% fetal hemoglobin (HbF, $\alpha_2\gamma_2$). The clinically significant variant hemoglobins involve β-chain abnormalities, among which the archetype is sickle hemoglobin (HbS). *Substitution of valine for glutamine at the sixth position of the β chain produces HbS*. About 8% of black Americans are heterozygous for hemoglobin S. If an individual is homozygous for the genetic mutation, almost all the hemoglobin in the erythrocyte is HbS. In the heterozygote, only about 40% is HbS, the remainder being normal hemoglobins. Where malaria is endemic, as many as 30% of black Africans are heterozygous. This frequency may be related in part to the slight protection against falciparum malaria afforded by HbS.

The HbS molecules upon deoxygenation undergo aggregation and polymerization, leading ultimately to distortion of the red cells, which acquire a sickle or holly-leaf shape (Figs. 14–5 and 14–6). *Sickling of the red cells has two major consequences: (1) a chronic hemolytic anemia; and (2) occlusion of small blood vessels, resulting in ischemic tissue damage.*[7]

PATHOGENESIS. When exposed to low oxygen tensions, polymerization of HbS takes place in several stages. Initially, small aggregates (nuclei) containing approximately 30 HbS molecules are formed, which on further polymerization are organized into long tubular fibers with a diameter of 150 to 200 Å. In the final step (crystallization), the fibers align themselves into parallel bundles seen under the electron microscope to run along the long axis of the sickled cells. The net effect of polymerization is to convert HbS from a freely flowing liquid to a viscous gel that is responsible for the distortion and reduced plasticity of the red cells.

A number of factors that affect the rate and degree of sickling impact on the clinical expression of this disease. *Perhaps the most important of all is the amount*

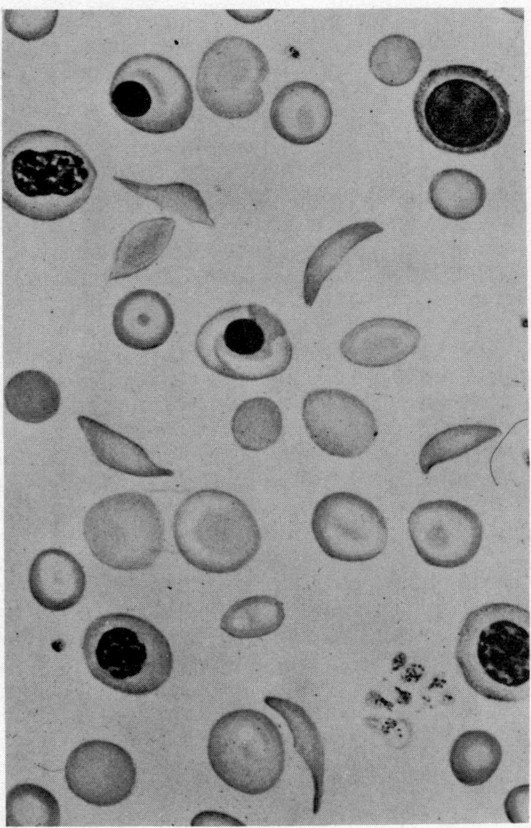

Fig. 14–5

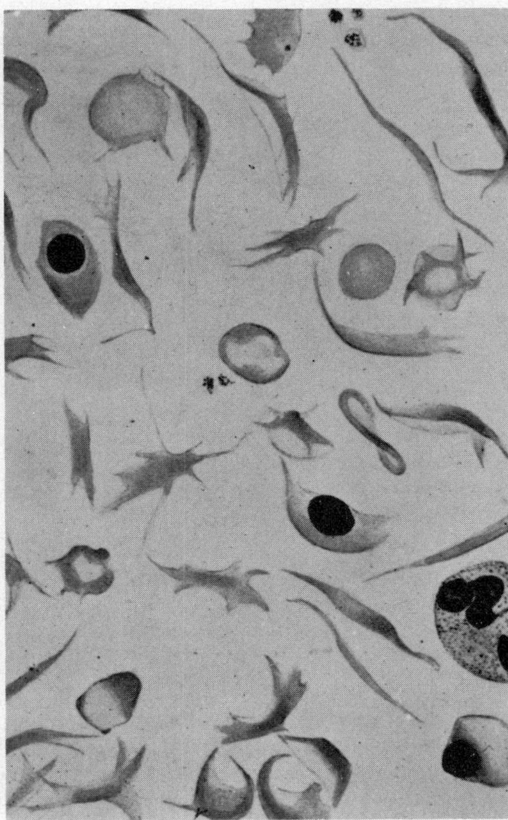

Fig. 14–6

Figure 14–5. In vivo sickling in a patient with sickle cell anemia (compare with Fig. 14–6). Drawing courtesy of Edith Piotti, Harvard Medical School.)
Figure 14–6. In vitro sickle cell preparation from same blood as illustrated in Figure 14–5 to highlight augmentation of sickling induced by low oxygen tension.

of HbS and its interaction with the other hemoglobin chains in the cell. In heterozygotes approximately 40% of the hemoglobin is HbS, the rest being HbA, which interacts only weakly with HbS during the processes of gelation. Therefore, the heterozygote has little tendency to sickle, except under conditions of severe hypoxia. Such an individual is said to have *sickle cell trait,* and unless exposed to significant hypoxia has no hemolysis of red cells, nor an anemia. In contrast, the homozygote with virtually undiluted hemoglobin of the S type has full-blown *sickle cell anemia.* β-Globin chains other than the normal HbA and other non-α globins influence the crystallization of HbS and the severity of sickle cell anemia. For example, fetal hemoglobin (HbF) with its γ-globin chains does not interact with HbS, and hence newborns do not manifest the disease until they are 1 to 2 years of age, when the amount of HbF in the cells falls to adult levels. The modulating effect of β-globin chains is seen also with other mutant hemoglobins such as HbC and HbD. Either of these may be present along with HbS in red cells of a double heterozygote for HbS and the variant globin gene. When HbC is present along with HbS, the clinical features are milder, since HbS copolymerizes with HbC to a lesser extent than with other HbS molecules. *The rate of HbS polymerization is also significantly affected by the hemoglobin concentration per cell,* i.e., the MCHC. The higher the HbS concentration within the cell, the greater are the chances of contact and interaction between HbS molecules. Thus, *dehydration, which increases the MCHC, greatly facilitates sickling* and may trigger occlusion of small blood vessels (vaso-occlusive crisis). The hypertonic environment of the renal medulla can also initiate local sickling and infarction. Conversely, for a given amount of HbS per cell, conditions that decrease the MCHC would be expected to ameliorate the disease severity. This seems to be the explanation for the recent observation that, in patients with homozygous sickle cell anemia, the coexistence of thalassemia lessens the severity of the anemia.[8] Thalassemia is characterized by reduced synthesis of globin chains (p. 622) which limits the total hemoglobin concentration per cell. Finally, *a fall in pH,* by reducing the oxygen affinity of hemoglobin, can increase sickling since it would enhance the amount of deoxygenated HbS.

Sickling of red cells is initially a reversible phenomenon; with oxygenation, HbS returns to the depolymerized state. However, with repeated episodes of sickling and unsickling, membrane damage ensues. Sickled cells lose potassium and water and at the same time gain calcium, which normally is rigorously excluded. The latter is considered particularly important in the genesis of *irreversibly sickled cells* (ISC),[9] which retain their abnormal shape even when fully oxygenated and despite the deaggregation of HbS. Irreversibly sickled cells have very rigid and nondeformable cell membranes, and therefore have the same difficulty in negotiating the splenic sinusoids as do the spherocytes (p. 616). The sickled cells become sequestered in the spleen, where they are destroyed by the mononuclear phagocyte system. Some intravascular hemolysis may also occur owing to increased mechanical fragility of the severely damaged cells. The average red cell survival correlates with the percentage of ISC in circulation and is shortened to approximately 20 days.[10] This finding supports the concept that the hemolysis results primarily from the lysis of ISC.

The pathogenesis of microvascular occlusions, a clinically important component of sickle cell anemia, is much less certain. The well-known "vicious viscous" or kinetic hypothesis is based on the increase in blood viscosity brought about by the relative inelasticity of the sickled red cells. This results in retardation of blood flow, particularly in the microcirculation. As the capillary transit times are prolonged, the red cells are exposed to a longer period of relative hypoxia, which favors further sickling of cells upstream, leading finally to complete vascular occlusion and infarction. Although this scheme is plausible and probably correct in its basic tenets, an important question remains unanswered. Why is there no correlation between the frequency of ISC (which contributes to viscosity) and severity of organ involvement? Two studies address this issue. By using very sensitive techniques, Noguchi and Schechter found that in sickle cell anemia a small amount of polymerized HbS is present even in normal-appearing red cells exposed to 96 to 98% oxygen saturation.[11] Sickling, according to these authors, occurs only in those cells that have a very large amount of the polymer, while deformability and plasticity is impaired even with lesser amounts of polymerized HbS. According to this view, the amount and properties of the HbS polymer within normal-looking red cells, rather than the obviously sickled red cells, are the major determinants of abnormal flow, and therefore lack of correlation between the frequency of ISC and the incidence of vascular occlusion is not entirely surprising. Other explanations have concentrated on the possibility that vascular occlusion may be initiated by adhesions between red cells and capillary endothelial cells.[9] Increased adherence of normal-looking red cells from patients with sickle cell anemia and endothelial cells has been reported in culture, but the in vivo significance of this phenomenon remains to be established.

MORPHOLOGY. The anatomic alterations are based on the following three characteristics of sickle cell anemia: increased destruction of the sickled red cells with the development of anemia, increased release of hemoglobin and formation of bilirubin, and capillary stasis and thrombosis. Sickling of the red cells may be identified in tissue sections, particularly those fixed in formalin, because under these conditions anaerobiosis develops before complete fixation. However, sickling may not be evident when the section is quickly fixed. The consequences of the increased red cell destruction and anemia have already been detailed in the general consideration of all hemolytic anemias. Briefly, these involve pallor of the skin; systemic iron overload; and fatty changes in the heart, liver, and tubules of the kidney. Rarely, the erythrostasis in the liver leads to so-called sickle cell cirrhosis. The bone marrow is hyperplastic, with activation of fatty marrow. This increased activity is due to expansion of normoblasts. The white cells and megakaryocytes are unaffected. The expansion of the marrow may lead to resorption of bone, with secondary new bone formation to produce the roentgenographic appearance in the skull of the "crew haircut." Extramedullary hematopoiesis may appear in the spleen or liver, and rarely in other sites.

In children, during the early phase of the disease, the spleen is commonly enlarged up to 500 gm. Histologically, there is marked congestion of the red pulp, due mainly to the trapping of sickled red cells in the splenic cords. However, sickling of cells may also occur in the sinuses, sometimes creating large lakes of red cells, sickled and jammed together in distended sinuses (Fig. 14–7). This erythrostasis in the spleen may lead to thrombosis and infarction or at least to marked tissue hypoxia. Sometimes the resulting focal fibrous scars contain deposits of hemosiderin and calcium, so-called **Gandy-Gamna bodies.** Continued scarring over the course of years causes progressive shrinkage of the spleen so that, in long-standing adult cases, only a small nubbin of fibrous tissue may be left; this is called **autosplenectomy** (Fig. 14–8). Infarctions secondary to vascular occlusions and anoxia may occur also in the liver, brain, kidney, and bone marrow.

Thrombotic occlusions have also been described in the pulmonary vessels, and many patients have cor pulmonale. Vascular stagnation in the subcutaneous tissue leads to leg ulcers in approximately 50% of adult patients, but is rare in children. The increased release of hemoglobin leads to pigment gallstones in some individuals, and all patients develop hyperbilirubinemia during periods of active hemolysis.

CLINICAL COURSE. *From the description of the disease to this point, it is evident that these patients are beset with problems stemming from (1) severe anemia, (2) vaso-occlusive complications, (3) predisposition to infections, and (4) chronic hyperbilirubinemia.* In infants, there is impairment of growth and development and an increased tendency to serious infections. In adults, the chronic hemolytic disease induces a fairly severe anemia, with hematocrit values ranging between 18 and 30%. The chronic hemolysis is associated with striking reticulocytosis and hyperbilirubinemia. Irreversibly sickled cells can usually be seen in the peripheral smear. This protracted course is frequently punctuated by a variety of "crises." *Vaso-occlusive crises,* also called *painful crises,* represent episodes of hypoxic injury and infarction. Usually no predisposing causes can be identified, although an association with infection, dehydration, and acidosis (all of which favor sickling) has been noted. The pain can be extreme and may be referred to the abdomen, chest, or joints, depending on the site of vascular insufficiency. Sites most commonly

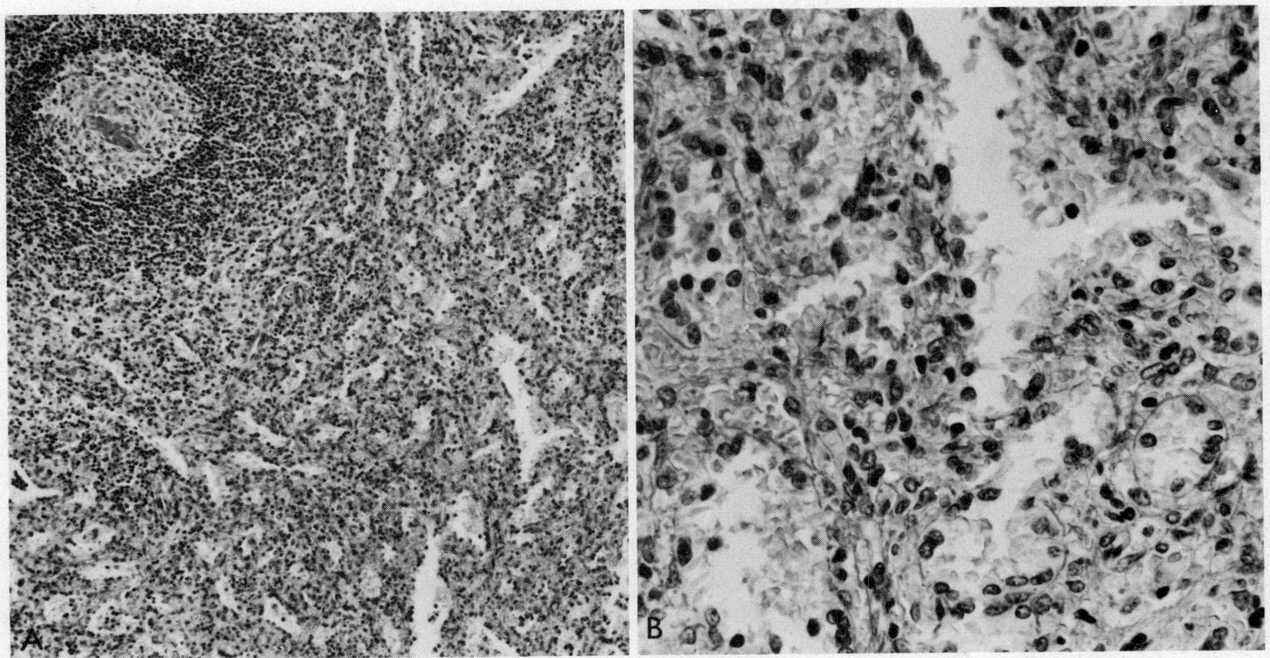

Figure 14–7. *A,* Spleen in sickle cell anemia (low power). White pulp on upper left is normal. Red pulp with its cords and sinusoids is markedly congested. *B,* Under high power, splenic cords are prominent owing to trapping of sickled red cells, which can also be seen in sinusoids. (Courtesy of Dr. Jose Hernandez, Department of Pathology, Southwestern Medical School, Dallas, Texas.)

involved by vaso-occlusive episodes are the bones, lungs, liver, brain, spleen, and penis. In children, painful bone crisis is extremely common and often difficult to distinguish from acute osteomyelitis. Similarly, chest pain may be confused with infections that are also common. Central nervous system hypoxia may produce manifestations of a seizure or stroke. Although such crises are frequently reversible, they may be fatal. Leg ulcers are an additional reflection of the vaso-occlusive tendency. An *aplastic crisis* represents a temporary cessation of bone marrow activity and it may be triggered by infections, folic acid deficiency, or both. Reticulocytes disappear from the peripheral blood and there is sudden and rapid worsening of anemia. A so-called *sequestration crisis* may appear in children with splenomegaly and sometimes in adults whose spleens have not undergone autoinfarction. Massive sequestration of deformed red cells leads to rapid splenic enlargement, hypovolemia, and sometimes shock. With transfusion, this can be reversed. Male patients may suddenly develop painful priapism owing to vascular engorgement of the penis.

For reasons that are not clear, but possibly related to erythrophagocytosis and blockade of the mononuclear phagocyte system, splenic function in children is impaired even though splenomegaly is present. Later, splenic infarctions may significantly reduce the size and function of this organ. The *"functional splenectomy"* predisposes to blood-borne infections and, for unknown reasons, particularly predisposes to Salmonella osteomyelitis. These individuals are also unusually prone to infections caused by pneumococci, possibly related to an impairment of the alternate complement pathway normally activated by bacterial polysaccharides such as

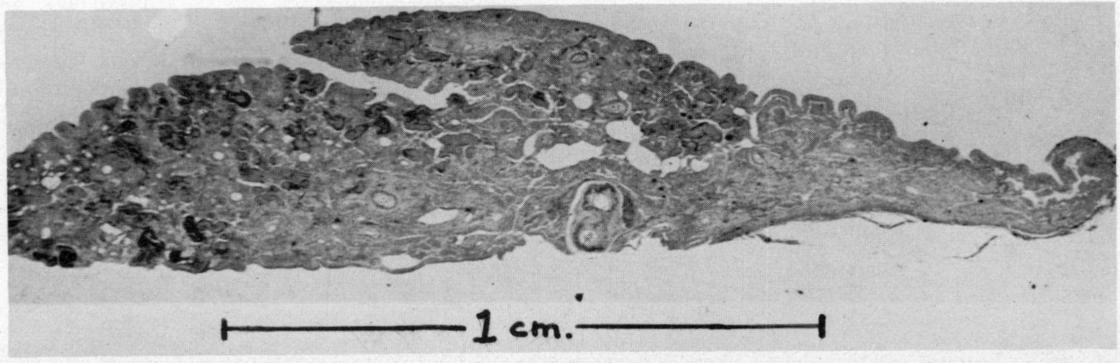

Figure 14–8. Sickle cell anemia. Cross section of a totally fibrotic spleen—autosplenectomy.

those produced by pneumococci. The infections in turn predispose to vaso-occlusive and aplastic crises.

In the course of the disease, chronic hypoxic organ damage may affect the spleen, heart, and lungs. The bones and joints are also favored sites of ischemic injury; microinfarctions may appear; or sometimes aseptic necrosis of the femoral head develops. Ocular lesions in the form of retinal infarcts, retinitis proliferans, and retinal detachment sometimes appear. Ischemic injury to the renal medulla may lead to loss of renal concentrating ability. The hyperbilirubinemia causes pigment stones in the gallbladder.

Diagnosis usually is readily made from the clinical findings and the appearance of the peripheral blood smear. It can be confirmed by diagnostic tests for sickling that, in general, are based on mixing a blood sample with an oxygen-consuming reagent such as metabisulfite to induce sickling. Hemoglobin electrophoresis can also demonstrate hemoglobin S on the basis of specific mobility. Despite improvements in therapy, sickle cell anemia still markedly shortens longevity; many patients die before the age of 30. However, with supportive measures an increasing number survive well into adult life. Detection of heterozygotes and genetic counseling are obviously most important in this condition. Recent advances in recombinant DNA technology have made it possible to diagnose sickle cell anemia antenatally (p. 122). The test uses DNA derived from amniotic fluid cells, and is based on the ability to cut DNA at specific nucleotide sequences by enzymes called restriction endonucleases. One such enzyme cuts the normal β-globin DNA at the sequences corresponding to the sixth amino acid position, which is the site of the sickle mutation (p. 618). If the mutation has occurred with alteration of nucleotide sequence, the enzyme fails to cleave the DNA at this specific site, producing a pattern of DNA fragments that is different from normal. This exciting new technique can identify both heterozygotes and homozygotes.[12]

Thalassemia Syndromes

The thalassemia syndromes are a heterogeneous group of mendelian disorders, all characterized by a lack of or decreased synthesis of either the α- or β-globin chain of hemoglobin A ($\alpha_2\beta_2$). *β-Thalassemia is characterized by deficient synthesis of the β chain, whereas α-thalassemia is characterized by deficient synthesis of the α chain. The hematologic consequences of diminished synthesis of one globin chain derive not only from the low intracellular hemoglobin (hypochromia) but also from the relative excess of the other chain.* For example, in β-thalassemia there is an excess of α chains. As a consequence, free α chains tend to aggregate into insoluble inclusions within erythrocytes and their precursors, causing premature destruction of maturing erythroblasts within the marrow *(ineffective erythropoiesis)* as well as lysis of mature red cells in the spleen *(hemolysis)*.

It should be emphasized that, in contrast to hemoglobinopathies that are characterized by the production of structurally abnormal globins at a normal rate, the thalassemia syndromes are characterized by reduced rates of synthesis of structurally normal globin chains. This observation is central to an understanding of the molecular lesions in thalassemias. Since the small amounts of globin chains synthesized are normal in amino acid composition, it follows that the genetic lesions responsible for thalassemias are likely to be *regulatory mutations that affect the normal expression of the globin structural genes* rather than mutations affecting the coding sequences. In cases with complete absence of globin chain synthesis, actual deletion of the structural gene must also be considered. These two categories of genetic defects (regulatory mutations or deletions) have now been proved responsible for most cases of thalassemias. To understand these, we must first review the normal structure and expression of human globin genes. Only the salient features will be pointed out here; more details are available in several reviews.[13, 14]

As is well known, the human hemoglobin molecule consists of two identical pairs of globin chains. The major adult human hemoglobin, HbA, contains two α chains and two β chains. All other normal embryonic, fetal, and adult hemoglobins also have two α-like chains and two β-like chains. A pair of α-globin genes is situated on each of the two number 16 chromosomes. In other words each individual possesses four α-chain genes, all of which are functional (Fig. 14–9). The β-globin family of genes includes the β-chain gene, the δ-chain gene, and two γ-chain genes. They are located on chromosome 11, in close linkage (Fig. 14–9).

A major change in thinking about the organization of eukaryotic genes has been brought about by the isolation and molecular cloning of the human globin genes. In each globin gene (as well as most other human genes), the nucleotide sequences that code for the polypeptide chains are not continuous but are interrupted by sequences not found in the mature cytoplasmic messenger RNA (mRNA). The sequences represented in cytoplasmic mRNA are called *exons,* whereas those in between the exons are called *intervening sequences* or *introns* (Fig. 14–10). Two intervening

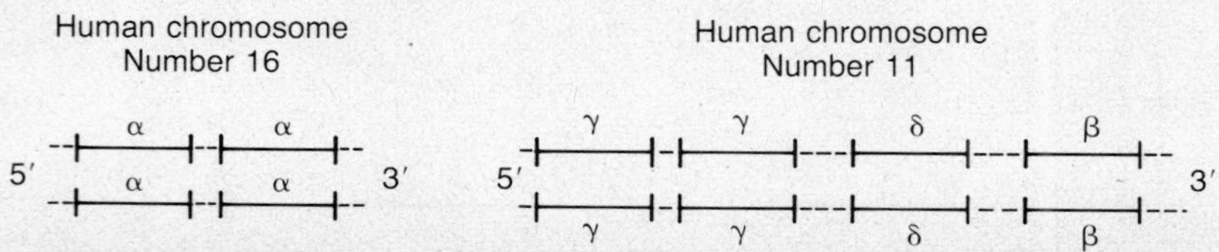

Figure 14–9. Number and chromosomal arrangement of human globin genes.

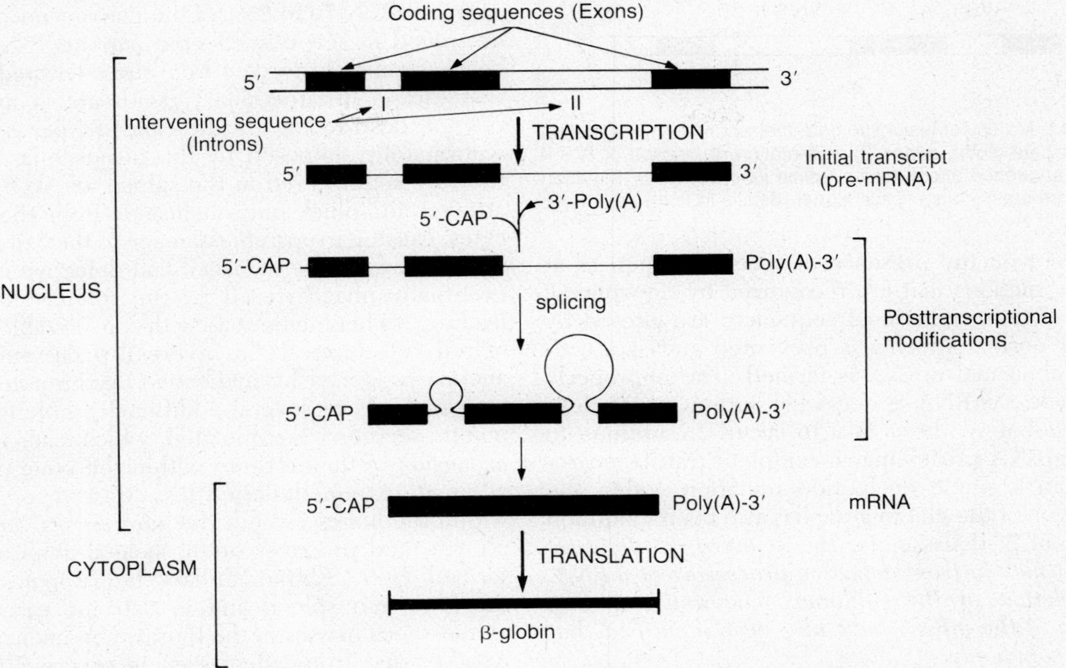

Figure 14–10. Human globin gene expression. (Modified from Benz, E.J., Jr., and Forget, B.G.: The thalassemia syndromes: Models for molecular analysis of human disease. Annu. Rev. Med. *33*:363, 1982.)

sequences (I and II) interrupt the coding sequences of globin genes into three separate blocks (exons). The process of transcription and translation of the β-globin gene is illustrated schematically in Figure 14–10. It may be noted that initially the entire gene (exons and introns) is transcribed to a large mRNA precursor within the nucleus. The mRNA precursor undergoes several important posttranscriptional modifications before it is converted into mature cytoplasmic mRNA, ready for translation. In the first step following transcription, both ends of the nuclear mRNA are modified. A methyl guanosine triphosphate residue is added to the 5′ end (called "capping"), whereas several adenosine residues are added to the 3′ end ("the poly-A tail"). The next step in posttranscriptional modification is called processing and involves cutting out the introns so that the exons are joined into a continuous sequence. Splicing is brought about by enzymes that recognize certain specific nucleotide sequences present at the junctions between exons and introns. The modified and spliced mature mRNA is then transported to the cytoplasm for translation. The pathway of α-globin gene expression is very similar. With this background we can proceed to discuss the molecular pathology, pathophysiology, and clinical features of thalassemias. The two major forms, α- and β-thalassemia, will be discussed separately, since each has distinctive features.

BETA-THALASSEMIA

The abnormality common to all β-thalassemias is a total lack or a reduction in the synthesis of structurally normal β-globin chains with unimpaired synthesis of α chains. However, the clinical severity of the anemia as well as the biochemical and genetic basis of β-globin chain deficiency are quite varied. We will begin our discussion with the molecular lesions in β-thalassemia and then integrate the clinical variants with the underlying molecular defects.

MOLECULAR LESIONS IN BETA-THALASSEMIA. Three genetic variants of β-thalassemia have been recognized: (1) β^0-*thalassemia*, characterized by total absence of β globin in the homozygous state; (2) β^+-*thalassemia*, associated with reduced β-globin synthesis in the homozygote (the most common form); and (3) *Hb Lepore*, an unusual variant in which there is reduced synthesis of a structurally abnormal β-like chain—this uncommon type will not be discussed further.

The molecular lesions underlying β^0- and β^+-thalassemias are heterogeneous and not completely known. In β^0-thalassemia a partial deletion of the 3′ end of the β-globin gene has been described in some families. As indicated in Figure 14–11①, this deletion removes one coding sequence and part of the intervening sequence II (IVS II), and therefore β-globin synthesis cannot occur.[15] Except for this reported example, deletion as a cause of β-thalassemia seems to be uncommon. *Since the β-globin gene is present in most cases, but the gene product is missing, defects in transcription, mRNA processing, or translation have been sought.* In some cases of β^0-thalassemia, defective processing of nuclear mRNA results from a mutation that alters the normal junction between IVS II and the middle exon (Fig. 14–11②).[13] As discussed earlier, normal excision of introns

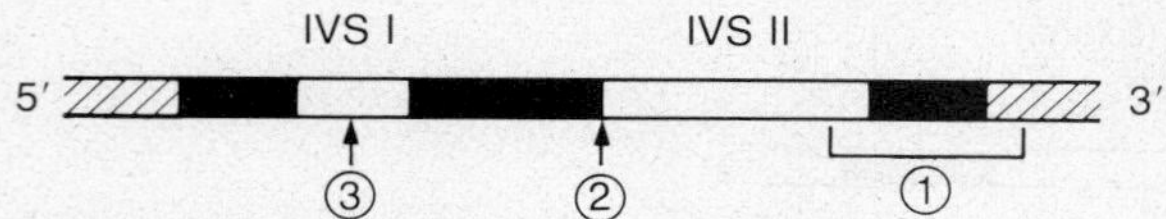

Figure 14–11. Molecular lesions in beta-thalassemia ① = Deletion of 3′ end of beta-globin gene; ② = Mutation at junction of IVS II and coding sequence alters normal splice junction; ③ = Mutation within IVS I creates a false splice signal (details in text).

is dependent on the presence of specific sequences at the splice junctions that are recognized by the splicing enzymes. If these junctional sequences are altered by mutations, normal splicing is prevented and as a consequence abnormal mRNA is formed. The improperly spliced nuclear mRNA is degraded within the nucleus and thus globin synthesis fails to occur. In addition to defective mRNA processing, incomplete translation resulting from a single nucleotide mutation within the coding region of the globin gene has also been identified as a cause of β^0-thalassemia. *In summary, β^0-thalassemias result mainly from defective processing of mRNA. Partial deletion of the β-globin gene and impaired translation of the mRNA have also been identified, but much less commonly.*

Much less is known about the molecular lesions in β^+-thalassemia, but defects in mRNA processing are suspected. In some cases, a mutation *within* an intron that produces a site resembling a normal splice junction has been noted (Fig. 14–11③). During processing the splicing enzymes cut the nuclear mRNA within the intron at the site corresponding to the mutation. The improperly spliced mRNA with a portion of IVS still attached, is unstable, and cannot be used for β-globin synthesis. Since the normal junction between IVS I and the middle exon is not altered by the mutation, some normal splicing also occurs, giving rise to small amounts of mature cytoplasmic mRNA and β-globin chains. These lesions represent only a few of the defects in β-thalassemias. Many more remain to be discovered, but with modern methods of gene cloning we can be sure that most common mutations will be identified in the near future.

PATHOPHYSIOLOGY OF ANEMIA. Two factors contribute to the pathogenesis of anemia in β-thalassemia. Reduced synthesis of β-globin chains leads to lack of adequate HbA formation, so that the overall concentrations of Hb (MCHC) in the cells is lower and the cells are hypochromic. Much more important, especially with severe impairment of β-globin synthesis, are the effects of imbalance between α- and β-chain synthesis. Since synthesis of α-globin chains continues unimpaired, most of the chains produced cannot find complementary β chains to bind. The free α chains form highly unstable aggregates that precipitate within the red cell precursors in the form of insoluble inclusions. *A variety of untoward effects follow, the most important being cell membrane damage leading to a loss of K^+ and impaired DNA synthesis. The net effect is destruction of the red cell precursors within the bone marrow, a phenomenon called ineffective erythropoiesis.* It is estimated that approximately 70 to 85% of the marrow normoblasts are destroyed in severely affected patients. The inclusion-bearing red cells derived from the nucleated precursors that escape intramedullary death are at an increased risk of destruction in the spleen. Because of poor deformability imposed by the intracellular aggregates, they are sequestered in the spleen where macrophages attempt to "pluck out" inclusions from these erythrocytes, causing irreparable damage to the cell membranes in some cases. The damaged and defective red cells are eventually phagocytosed by the splenic macrophages, leading to a hemolytic state with considerable shortening of red cell survival. In severe β-thalassemia, marked anemia produced by ineffective erythropoiesis and hemolysis leads to several additional problems. Erythropoietin secretion is stimulated, which leads to extensive expansion of the erythron within the bone marrow and often at extramedullary sites. Massive erythropoiesis within the bones invades the bony cortex, impairs bone growth, and produces other skeletal abnormalities described later. Extramedullary hematopoiesis involves the liver and spleen and in extreme cases produces extraosseous masses in the thorax, abdomen, and pelvis. Another disastrous effect seen in severe β-thalassemia (as well as other causes of ineffective erythropoiesis) is excessive absorption of dietary iron. Coupled with the iron accumulation due to repeated blood transfusions required by these patients, a severe state of iron overload develops. Secondary injury to parenchymal organs, particularly the iron-laden liver, often follows (p. 924).

CLINICAL SYNDROMES. The clinical classification of β-thalassemias is based on the severity of the anemia, which in turn is based on the type of genetic defect (β^+ or β^0) as well as the gene dosage (homozygous or heterozygous). In general, individuals who are homozygous for the β-thalassemia genes (β^+ or β^0), have very severe, transfusion-dependent anemia and are said to have *β-thalassemia major*. The presence of one normal gene in the heterozygotes usually leads to enough normal β-globin chain synthesis so that the affected individuals are usually asymptomatic with only a mild anemia. This condition is referred to as *β-thalassemia minor* or *β-thalassemia trait*. A third clinical variant is characterized by an intermediate degree of severity, the so-called *β-thalassemia intermedia*. These patients have severe anemia, but not enough to require regular blood transfusions. Genetically they are heterogeneous and include mild variants of homozygous β^+-thalassemia, some severe variants of heterozygous β-thalassemia (β^0/β or β^+/β) and double heterozygotes for the β^+ and β^0 genes (genotype β^+/β^0). The clinical and morphologic features of thalassemia intermedia will not be described separately but may be surmised from the following discussions of thalassemia major and minor.

Thalassemia Major. The β-thalassemia genes are most frequent and thalassemia major is most common in Mediterranean countries and parts of Africa and Southeast Asia. In the United States, the incidence is highest in migrants from these areas. As indicated in Table 14–2, the genotype of these patients is usually

Table 14–2. CLINICAL AND GENETIC CLASSIFICATION OF THALASSEMIAS

Clinical Nomenclature	Genotype	Disease	Molecular Genetics
A. Beta-Thalassemias			
I. Thalassemia major	1. Homozygous β^0-thalassemia (β^0/β^0)	Severe, requires blood transfusions regularly	1. Rare gene deletions in β^0/β^0
	2. Homozygous β^+-thalassemia (β^+/β^+)		
II. Thalassemia intermedia	β^0/β β^+/β^+	Severe, but does not require regular blood transfusions	2. Defects in processing or translation of β-globin mRNA in β^0 as well as β^+ forms.
III. Thalassemia minor	β^0/β β^+/β	Asymptomatic with mild or absent anemia; red cell abnormalities seen	
B. Alpha-Thalassemias			
I. Silent carrier	$-\alpha/\alpha\alpha$ (heterozygous α-thal-2)	Asymptomatic; no red cell abnormality	
II. Alpha-thalassemia trait	1. $--/\alpha\alpha$ (Asian) (heterozygous α-thal-1) 2. $-\alpha/-\alpha$ (Black African) (homozygous α-thal-2)	Asymptomatic, like β-thalassemia minor	Gene deletions mainly
III. HbH disease	$--/-\alpha$ (double heterozygous: α-1 thal/α-thal-2)	Severe, resembles β-thalassemia intermedia	
IV. Hydrops fetalis	$--/--$ (homozygous α-thal-1)	Lethal in utero	

β^+/β^+ or β^0/β^0. In some cases it is β^0/β^+ (double heterozygotes, if the two parents are carriers of β^+ and β^0 genes). With all these genotypes the anemia is very severe and first becomes manifest six to nine months after birth, as hemoglobin synthesis switches from HbF to HbA. In untransfused patients, Hb levels range between 3 and 6 gm per dl. The peripheral blood smear shows severe abnormalities; there is marked anisocytosis (variation in size) with several small and virtually colorless (hypochromic, microcytic) red cells. Abnormal forms, including target cells (so-called because the small amount of hemoglobin collects in the center), stippled red cells, and fragmented red cells are common. Inclusions representing aggregated α chains are usually not seen unless the spleen has been removed. Reticulocyte count is elevated but to an extent less than would be predicted from the severity of anemia. Variable numbers of normoblasts are usually seen in the peripheral blood. The red cells contain either no HbA at all (β^0/β^0 genotype) or very small amounts (β^+/β^+ genotype). HbF is markedly increased and indeed constitutes the major hemoglobin of red cells. HbA_2 levels are variable, ranging from normal to moderately elevated.

The major morphologic alterations, in addition to those characteristic of all hemolytic anemias, involve the bone marrow and spleen. In the typical patient there is striking expansion of the red marrow, virtually to the fetal level. The dominant change is a striking increase in the number of primitive nucleated erythroid precursors. The expansion of the marrow leads to thinning of the cortical bone, with new bone formation on the external aspect (Fig. 14–12). These changes are particularly evident in the maxilla and frontal bones of the face, sparing the mandible since it usually contains little marrow. The long bones, vertebrae, and ribs are similarly affected, and occasionally are rendered vulnerable to fracture. Marked splenomegaly and hepatomegaly result both from reticuloendothelial cell hyperplasia secondary to active erythrophagocytosis and from extramedullary hematopoiesis. The spleen may increase up to 1500 gm in weight.

Hemosiderosis and even sometimes secondary hemochromatosis appear related to a number of factors. Many of these patients have received numerous transfusions, providing a ready explanation for the iron overload. Ineffective erythropoiesis and possibly the chronic tissue hypoxia leads to increased intestinal absorption of iron. In any event, the hemosiderosis may have secondary consequences when the iron pigment accumulates in the myocardium, liver, or pancreas to induce organ injury.

The clinical course of β-thalassemia major is generally brief because, unless supported by transfusions, children suffer from growth retardation and die at an early age from the profound effects of anemia. Blood transfusions not only improve the anemia, but also suppress secondary features related to excessive erythropoiesis. With transfusions, survival into the second and third decades of life is possible, but the overall outlook is grim. The clinical manifestations can largely be deduced from the hematologic and morphologic changes. In those who survive long enough the face becomes overlarge and somewhat distorted. Since the mandible is unaffected there is often malocclusion. Hepatosplenomegaly is usually present; the tissue hy-

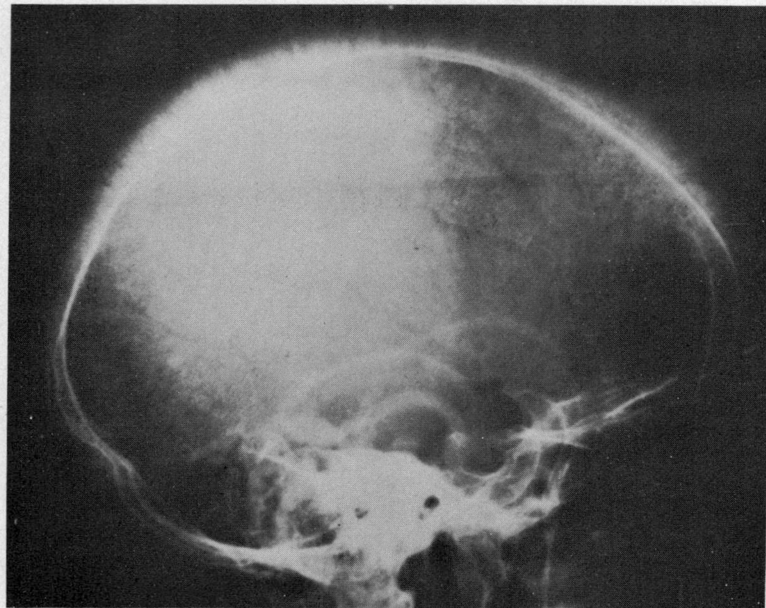

Figure 14–12. Thalassemia. X-ray of skull to show new bone formation on outer table producing perpendicular radiations characterized as a "crew haircut."

poxia and systemic hemosiderosis may lead to delayed sexual development secondary to regressive changes in the gonads and other endocrine organs. Cardiac disease resulting from progressive iron overload and secondary hemochromatosis (p. 924) is an important cause of death even in patients who can otherwise be supported by blood transfusions. To reduce the amount of iron overload, most patients also receive iron-chelators. Nevertheless, the average age at death is 17 years. It is hoped that the recent remarkable success in cloning of globin genes will pave the way for gene therapy and eventual cure of these patients in the future.

Thalassemia Minor. This is much more common than thalassemia major and understandably affects the same ethnic groups. In most cases these patients are heterozygotes for the β^+ or β^0 gene. Thalassemia trait is believed to offer resistance against falciparum malaria, accounting for its prevalence in those parts of the world where malaria is endemic. Almost invariably, individuals with the thalassemia trait are asymptomatic and anemia is very mild, if present. The peripheral blood smear usually shows some abnormalities affecting the red cells including hypochromia, microcytosis, basophilic stippling, and target cells. Mild erythroid hyperplasia is seen in the bone marrow. The red cell survival may be slightly shortened or normal. A characteristic finding on hemoglobin electrophoresis is an increase in HbA_2, which may constitute 4 to 8% of the total hemoglobin (normal 2.5 ± 0.3 %). HbF levels may be normal or slightly increased. Recognition of β-thalassemia trait is important on two counts: (1) its differentiation from the hypochromic microcytic anemia of iron deficiency and (2) genetic counseling. The importance of differentiating thalassemia trait from iron deficiency lies in the fact that the latter is benefited by iron therapy whereas the former may be worsened. In β-thalassemia trait there is a slight increase in iron absorption due to modest ineffective erythropoiesis, and therefore iron administration contributes to possible iron overload during later years. The distinction can usually be made by measurement of serum iron, total iron-binding capacity, and serum ferritin (p. 636). Hemoglobin electrophoresis is also helpful.

ALPHA-THALASSEMIAS

These disorders are characterized by reduced synthesis of α-globin chains. Since there are normally four α-globin genes, the severity of the clinical syndromes shows a great variation, depending on the number of defective α-globin genes. As in the case of β-thalassemias, the anemia stems both from lack of adequate hemoglobin and from the effects of excess unpaired non-α chains (β, γ, δ). However, the situation is somewhat complicated by the fact that normally different non-α chains are synthesized at different times of development. Thus, in the newborn with α-thalassemia, there is an excess of unpaired γ-globin chains, resulting in the formation of γ_4-tetramers called Hb Barts, whereas in adults the excess β-globin chains aggregate to form tetramers called HbH. Since the non-α chains in general form more soluble and less toxic aggregates than those derived from α chains, the hemolytic anemia and ineffective erythropoiesis tend to be less severe than with β-thalassemias of similar degree of chain imbalance. All these factors make α-thalassemias somewhat distinctive, and we will briefly consider these below.

MOLECULAR PATHOLOGY. Unlike β-thalassemia in which gene deletion has been detected only infrequently, the most common cause of reduced α-chain synthesis seems to be deletion of α-globin genes. As we shall discuss, one or all four of the α-globin genes may be deleted, giving rise to a wide range of clinical severities. Two other less common causes of reduced α-globin synthesis have also been recognized.[16] One nondeletional form resembles β-thalassemia in that the α-globin genes are present but they fail to be processed and expressed normally. In another variant, a larger-than-normal portion of mRNA is translated owing to a mutation in the terminator codon, leading to the formation of an abnormal α globin called Hb Constant Spring. However, the mRNA of Hb Constant Spring is unstable, and only a very small amount of the abnormal α-globin chain is synthesized.

CLINICAL SYNDROMES. These are classified on the basis of the number and position of the α-globin genes deleted, which in turn determine the clinical syndrome. It will be useful at this point to recall that α-globin genes occur in linked pairs on each of the two chromosomes 16 (Fig. 14–9). Each α gene normally contributes approximately 25% of the α-globin chains and may be deleted independently of the other α-globin genes. The terminology of α-thalassemias is varied and at times confusing, and is best considered along with Table 14–2, in which clinical terms and their genetic equivalents are presented along with the salient clinical features. Capsule descriptions follow.

Silent Carrier State. This is characterized by the deletion of a single α-globin gene and barely detectable reduction in α-globin chain synthesis. These individuals carrying three normal α-globin genes are completely asymptomatic and do not have anemia. They can, however, transmit the mutation to their offspring, who could develop a symptomatic form of α-thalassemia if the other parent also carries one or more α-globin mutations.

Alpha-Thalassemia Trait. This is characterized by deletion of two α-globin genes. The involved genes may be from the same chromosome (with the other chromosome carrying the two normal genes), or one α-globin gene may be deleted from each of the two chromosomes (see Table 14–2). The former genotype is more common among Asian populations, whereas the latter is seen in those of African origin. Both these genetic patterns produce similar quantitative deficiencies of α-globin chains and therefore are identical clinically, but the position of deleted genes makes a big difference to the likelihood of severe α-thalassemia (HbH disease or hydrops fetalis) in the offspring. As is evident from Table 14–2, in black African populations where the two α genes are deleted from two separate chromosomes, mating of two individuals with the α-thalassemia trait would not result in progeny with HbH disease or hydrops fetalis.

The clinical picture in α-thalassemia trait is identical to that described for β-thalassemia minor, i.e., minimal or no anemia and no abnormal physical signs. The peripheral blood shows microcytic hypochromic red cells. Clinically it has to be distinguished from β-thalassemia minor and iron deficiency anemia. Unlike β-thalassemia trait, hemoglobin electrophoresis fails to show elevated HbA_2 and HbF. In the newborn with α-thalassemia trait, some Hb Barts (γ tetramers) may be detected in the red cells, but this disappears in the adult. The diagnosis therefore is made mainly by exclusion and is important for genetic counseling as well as for avoiding unnecessary iron therapy.

Hemoglobin H Disease. This is associated with deletion of three of the four α-globin genes. As already discussed, HbH disease is seen mainly in Asian populations and rarely in those of African origin. With only one normal α-globin gene the synthesis of α chains is markedly suppressed and unstable tetramers of excess β globin are formed. These tetramers, called HbH, are considerably more soluble than the α-chain tetramers found in β-thalassemia. As such, the manifestations of HbH disease are milder than those of homozygous β-thalassemia and clinically resemble β-thalassemia intermedia. The hemoglobin value ranges from 7 to 10 gm per dl and the red cell abnormalities are similar to those in the other thalassemic syndromes. Inclusions of HbH can be demonstrated by incubation of red cells with brilliant cresyl blue in vitro. Oxidized HbH is precipated by this procedure since it is unable to withstand oxidative stress. This property of HbH is the major cause of anemia, since older red cells with precipitates of oxidized HbH are removed by the spleen. Since the senescent red cells are the ones most likely to be affected, ineffective erythropoiesis is not a significant factor in the pathogenesis of anemia. HbH, which forms 5 to 30% of the hemoglobin, can be detected as a fast-moving band in electrophoresis.

Hydrops Fetalis. This is the most severe form of α-thalassemia, resulting from the deletion of all four α-globin genes. In the fetus, excess γ-globin chains form tetramers (Hb Barts) that have extremely high oxygen affinity but are unable to deliver the oxygen to tissues. Severe tissue anoxia associated with this condition invariably leads to intrauterine fetal death. The fetus shows severe pallor, generalized edema, and massive hepatosplenomegaly similar to that seen in erythroblastosis fetalis (p. 487).

Paroxysmal Nocturnal Hemoglobinuria (PNH)

This rare disorder of unknown etiology is characterized by chronic intravascular hemolysis that tends to get worse during the night. The basic mechanism causing hemolysis seems to be unusual sensitivity of the red blood cells to complement-mediated lysis. To explain this exquisite susceptibility, some defect in the red cell membrane has been proposed, but it has not been possible to find any distinctive biochemical or morphologic abnormality in PNH red cells. Recent evidence suggests that the membrane defect in PNH is not restricted to red blood cells, since platelets and granulocytes are also more sensitive to lysis by complement. In addition, nonlytic interactions between their cell membranes and complement produce functional abnormalities manifested by a striking predisposition to intravascular thromboses and infections.[17] In light of these findings, PNH is now considered to be a disorder of pluripotent myeloid stem cells resulting from the proliferation of an abnormal clone of cells. This hypothesis is supported by the occasional transformation of PNH into other disorders of myeloid stem cells, including aplastic anemia (p. 638) and acute leukemia. The initiating event in all these cases may be a somatic mutation but the nature of the mutagenic event remains mysterious. The association of PNH with aplastic anemia suggests that marrow injury by drugs or chemicals may be involved.

Patients classically have intravascular hemolysis, which is paroxysmal and nocturnal only in 25% of cases. Most of the remaining patients have chronic hemolysis without dramatic hemoglobinuria. Over the long course of the disease, hemosiderinuria with loss of iron leads eventually to iron deficiency (Fig. 14–13). The other clinical manifestations include multiple episodes of venous thromboses in the hepatic, portal, or cerebral veins, which are fatal in 50% of cases. Infection related to granulocytopenia or abnormal leukocyte functions is also prominent. The course of this disease is chronic, with a median survival of ten years.

Table 14–3. CLASSIFICATION OF AUTOIMMUNE HEMOLYTIC ANEMIAS

I. *Warm antibody AHA.* Here the antibody is of the IgG type, does not usually fix complement, and is active at 37°C
   - A. *Primary* or idiopathic
   - B. *Secondary* to:
     1. Lymphomas and leukemias
     2. Other neoplastic diseases
     3. Autoimmune disorder (particularly SLE)
     4. Drugs

II. *Cold agglutinin AHA.* Here the antibodies are IgM and are most active in vitro at 0–4°C. The antibody fixes complement at warmer temperatures, but agglutination of cells by IgM and complement only occurs in the peripheral cool parts of the body. Antibodies dissociate at 30°C or above
   - A. *Acute* (mycoplasma infection, infectious mononucleosis)
   - B. *Chronic*
     1. Idiopathic
     2. Associated with lymphoma

III. *Cold hemolysins* (paroxysmal cold hemoglobinuria). In this condition, IgG antibodies bind to red cells at low temperature, fix complement and cause *hemolysis* when the temperature is raised to 30°C

Autoimmune Hemolytic Anemias (AHAs)

Hemolytic anemias in this category are caused by extracorpuscular mechanisms. Although commonly referred to as autoimmune hemolytic anemias (AHAs), many prefer the designation *immunohemolytic anemias,* because in some instances the immune reaction is initiated by drug ingestion. They may occur as primary disorders in the absence of an underlying disease or may be secondary to some predisposing condition such as lymphoma, carcinoma, viral infection, or drug ingestion. In all instances, however, the hemolysis is related to the appearance of anti–red cell antibodies.[18] These immunohemolytic disorders have been classified in various ways but most commonly on the basis of the specific nature of antibody involved (Table 14–3).

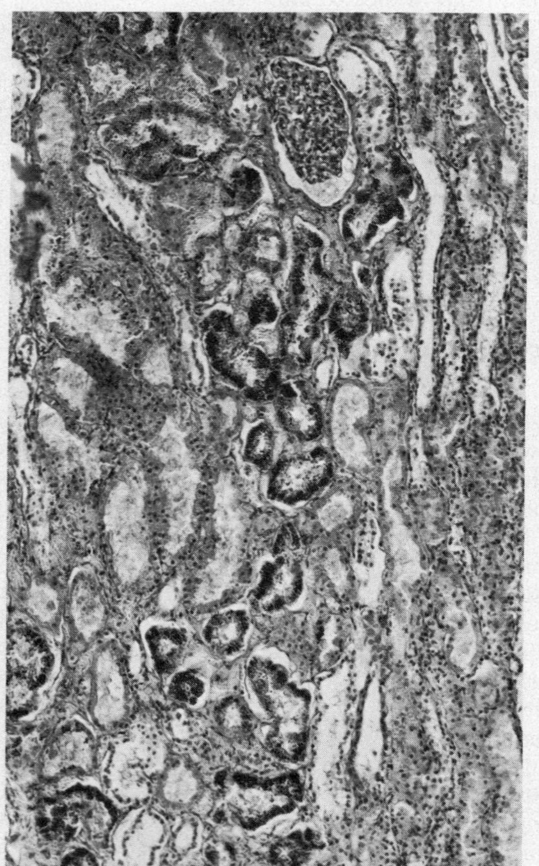

Figure 14–13. Paroxysmal hemoglobinuria. Dark renal tubules are heavily laden with hemosiderin in a 37-year-old patient with multiple recurrent hemolytic episodes.

Whatever the antibody, the differentiation of AHA from other forms of hemolytic anemia depends on demonstration of the existing antibodies. The major diagnostic criterion is the *Coombs antiglobulin test,* which relies on the capacity of the antibodies prepared in animals against human globulins to agglutinate red cells if these globulins are present on red cell surfaces. The temperature dependence of the autoantibody would further help specify the type of antibody. Quantitative immunologic methods to measure these autoantibodies directly are now available.

WARM ANTIBODY AHA

In about two-thirds of patients, the condition is idiopathic and primary. In the remaining one-third, there is an underlying predisposing condition, as mentioned in Table 14–3, or some drug exposure to thus produce a secondary form of AHA. Although autoantibodies are present in both groups (mainly IgG although occasionally IgA) and may cause hemolysis within the bloodstream when present in high titers, most of the red cell destruction in this form of hemolytic disease is not due simply to red cell lysis. Indeed, exposure of normal red blood cells to IgG antibodies and complement does not lead to hemolysis in vitro. In vivo, however, IgG-coated red cells are bound to Fc receptors on monocytes and splenic macrophages, and undergo spheroidal transformation.[19] This process results from a partial loss of the red cell membrane by attempted phagocytosis of the IgG-coated cell. The ability to cause this interaction is greatest with IgG of subclasses 1 and 3 (the most common subclasses). *The spherocytes are then sequestered and removed in the spleen, the major site of red cell destruction in this disorder. Thus, moderate-to-severe splenomegaly is characteristic of this form of AHA.*

A number of theories have been proposed to explain the appearance of red cell–directed antibodies. One theory postulates that an antigenic change in the red cell membrane initiates the immune reaction. Another suggests loss of self-recognition by the immune system owing to mechanisms discussed earlier for other autoimmune disorders (p. 177). Best documented is the manner by which certain drugs induce AHA. Three different immunologic mechanisms have been implicated.[20]

Hapten Model. The drug—exemplified by penicillin—may act as a hapten, and combine with the red cell membrane to produce antibody directed against the red cell–drug complex, resulting in the destructive sequence cited above.

Immune Complex Model. The drug serving as a hapten binds to a plasma protein and the drug-protein complex evokes antibodies. The resultant immune complexes nonspecifically attach to the red blood cell membrane, fixing complement and causing severe intravascular lysis. Here the red cells are "innocent bystanders." The red cell destruction, however, may also be extravascular. In the extravascular mechanism the immune complexes bind to monocytes and macrophages through Fc receptors, and spherocytosis and splenic sequestration ensue. Thus, the immune complexes lead to red cell destruction through one of two mechanisms, or possibly both. Quinidine and phenacetin are prototype drugs responsible for this form of hemolysis.

Autoantibody Model. The drug, such as the antihypertensive agent α-methyldopa, in some manner initiates the production of antibodies that are directed aginst intrinsic red cell antigens, in particular the Rh blood group antigens. A typical positive IgG Coombs test without evidence of activation of complement makes these patients identical with those having the idiopathic, so-called autoantibody variety of AHA. In essence, the drug initiates an autoantibody reaction.

COLD AGGLUTININ AHA

This form of immune hemolytic anemia is caused by IgM antibodies that have enhanced activity at temperatures below 30°C. Cold agglutinins occur *acutely* during the recovery phase of certain infectious disorders such as Mycoplasma pneumonia and infectious mononucleosis. In the former, the antibodies are directed against the I antigen (closely related to the ABO antigens). In the latter, the antibodies are mainly targeted on the i allelic antigen. This form of AHA is self-limited and rarely induces clinical manifestations of hemolysis. *Chronic* cold agglutinins occur with lymphoproliferative disorders and as an idiopathic condition. The antibodies produced are usually monoclonal, suggesting that the underlying basis is similar to that of other monoclonal gammopathies (p. 688). The clinical symptoms result from an in vivo agglutination of red cells and fixation of complement in distal body parts where the temperature may drop to below 30°C. The antibody exerts its hemolytic effect predominantly by fixation of C′3 to the red blood cell surface, making them more susceptible to phagocytosis.[21] For some obscure reason, the liver is more efficient in recognizing and sequestering the C′3-coated red cells than the spleen; thus, splenomegaly is uncommon in this condition. The hemolytic anemia usually is not severe, but vascular obstruction by red cell agglutinates results in pallor, cyanosis of the body parts exposed to cold temperatures, and Raynaud's phenomenon.

COLD HEMOLYSIN AHA

Destruction of red cells in this variant occurs within the intravascular compartment. These autoantibodies are characteristic of the disease *paroxysmal cold hemoglobinuria* (PCH), which is noted for acute intermittent massive hemolysis, frequently with hemoglobinuria, following exposure of the afflicted patient to cold. Lysis is clearly complement dependent. The autoantibodies are IgG in nature and are directed against the P blood group antigen; they attach to the red cells and bind complement at low temperatures. When the temperature is elevated, the hemolytic action is mediated by the complement sequence, through activation of the lytic C′5–9 complex. The antibody is also known as the Donath-Landsteiner (DL) antibody, previously associated with syphilis. Today, most cases of PCH follow various infections such as mycoplasma, measles, mumps, and some ill-defined viral and "flu" syndromes. Some cases are idiopathic. Attacks are associated with hemoglobinuria, muscular pain, and fever, which disappear when the infections resolve. The idiopathic variety has a prolonged benign course, the patients being asymptomatic between attacks. The mechanisms responsible for the production of such autoantibodies are unknown.

Hemolytic Anemia Resulting from Trauma to Red Cells

Fragmentation of red blood cells when exposed to physical trauma may be severe enough to give rise to significant intravascular hemolysis. Clinically important are the hemolytic anemias associated with insertion of valve prostheses and diffuse deposition of fibrin in the microvasculature. In addition to immediate rupture, a wide variety of erythrocytic abnormalities are produced and are recognized in the peripheral blood film as burr cells, helmet cells, and triangle cells, as well as fragments of erythrocytes (schistocytes). *Hemolysis due to narrowing or obstructions in the microvasculature is called microangiopathic hemolytic anemia.* This form of anemia is encountered in disseminated intravascular coagulation (DIC), thrombotic thrombocytopenic purpura (TTP), the hemolytic-uremic syndrome, malignant hypertension, renal cortical necrosis, systemic lupus erythematosus (SLE), and metastatic adenocarcinoma. The common denominator is the presence of some vascular lesion. In DIC, the microthrombi constitute the point of impaction. In malignant hypertension, it is the markedly narrowed arterioles. In SLE, it is the necrotizing arteritis and arteriolitis. In patients with prosthetic heart valves, the red cells are damaged by the shear stress resulting from the turbulent blood flow and abnormal pressure gradients caused by artificial heart valves.[22]

In most of these settings, the hemolysis is only a minor part of the clinical problem, and these patients rarely exhibit the morphologic changes encountered in the more chronic hemolytic diseases discussed earlier.

ANEMIAS OF DIMINISHED ERYTHROPOIESIS

It is astonishing to realize that in man approximately 9 billion red cells are normally destroyed hourly! Unless erythropoiesis can maintain this pace, anemia must develop. Diminished erythropoiesis can occur under a number of conditions. A major category constitutes a deficiency of some vital substrate that may lead to impaired proliferation or maturation of the erythroid cells. Included in this group are iron deficiency anemias in which heme synthesis is impaired, and anemia of vitamin B_{12} and folate deficiency characterized by defective DNA synthesis (megaloblastic anemias). Another major category of decreased erythropoiesis can be loosely termed "marrow stem cell failure," which embraces such conditions as aplastic anemia, pure red cell aplasia, and anemia of renal failure. Aplastic anemias are associated with marrow hypoproliferation, but in nutrient deficiency anemias, even though the marrow is functionally hypoactive, it may be very cellular, as documented in the following discussion.

Megaloblastic Anemias

The following discussion will attempt first to characterize the major features of these anemias and then to discuss the two principal types of megaloblastic anemia: (1) pernicious anemia (PA), the major form of vitamin B_{12} deficiency anemia; and (2) folate deficiency anemia.

The megaloblastic anemias constitute a diverse group of entities, having in common a typical morphologic pattern in the blood and bone marrow. As the name implies, the erythroid precursors and erythrocytes are abnormally large, thought to be related to impairment of cell maturation and division. The peripheral blood reveals marked variation in the size and shape of red cells (anisocytosis), which are nonetheless normochromic. *Many erythrocytes are macrocytic and oval shaped (macro-ovalocytes) with mean corpuscular volumes (MCVs) over 100 μ^3 (normal 82 to 92).* Because they are thicker than normal and well filled with hemoglobin, most macrocytes lack the central pallor of normal red cells. The reticulocyte count is lower than normal and, occasionally with severe anemia, nucleated red cells appear in the circulating blood. *Neutrophils too are larger than normal (macropolymorphonuclear) and are hypersegmented, i.e., have five to six or more nuclear lobules.* The marrow is hypercellular and the megaloblastic change is detected in all stages of red cell development. The most primitive cells (promegaloblasts) are large, with a deeply basophilic cytoplasm and a distinctive fine chromatin pattern in the nucleus (Fig. 14–14). As these cells differentiate and begin to acquire hemoglobin, the nucleus retains its finely distributed chromatin and thus fails to undergo the chromatin clumping typical of the normoblast. Indeed, the development of a dense pyknotic nucleus, which occurs in the normal sequence of erythropoiesis, is delayed or fails to occur, creating an apparent *asynchronism* or *dissociation* between the cytoplasmic maturation and nuclear maturation. Analogously, the granulocytic precursors also reveal nuclear-cytoplasmic asynchrony, yielding giant metamyelocytes and band forms and hypersegmentation of the neutrophils, previously mentioned. Megakaryocytes, too, may be abnormally large and have bizarre, multilobate nuclei, but sometimes they appear relatively normal. With increased cellularity, much or all of the normally fatty marrow may be converted to red marrow. The erythroid/myeloid ratio, normally 1:3, may be transformed to 1:1. Nuclear-cytoplasmic asynchrony becomes apparent in all cells having a relatively rapid turnover, so megaloblastic and atypical cytologic alterations appear in the mucosal epithelium of the gastrointestinal tract, principally within the stomach.

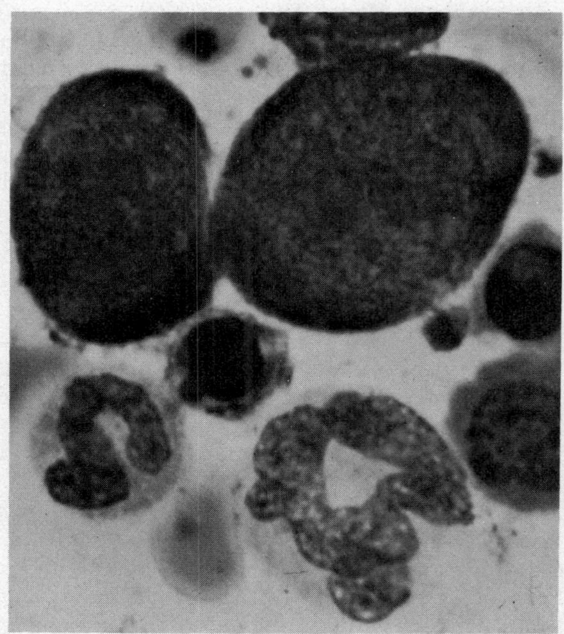

Figure 14–14. Marrow smear from a patient with pernicious anemia. Two megaloblasts are seen above and a "macropoly" below.

PATHOPHYSIOLOGY. The fundamental causes of the megaloblastic change, or (to paraphrase Kass) why the megaloblast is a megaloblast at all and why a deficiency of B_{12} or folate should cause cells to enlarge and result in anemia, are still unanswered questions.[23] Later we shall consider some of the metabolic role of B_{12} and folate, but for here it suffices that vitamin B_{12} and folic acid are coenzymes in the DNA synthetic pathway. A deficiency of these vitamins or impairment in their utilization results in deranged or inadequate synthesis of DNA. The synthesis of RNA and protein is unaffected, however, so there is cytoplasmic enlargement not matched by DNA synthesis, which appears to delay or block mitotic division. Two consequences stem from this cytologic derangement: (1) *ineffective erythropoiesis* and (2) *the production of abnormal erythrocytes prone to hemolytic destruction.*

Ineffective erythropoiesis may have several origins. The delay in nuclear maturation would reasonably be expected to slow production of red cells. In addition, there is intramedullary destruction of megaloblasts, which undergo autohemolysis more readily than normoblasts and are more vulnerable to phagocytosis by reticuloendothelial cells in the marrow than normal erythroid precursors. Premature destruction of granulocytic and platelet precursors also occurs, resulting in leukopenia and thrombocytopenia. The basis of the increased extramedullary hemolysis of the erythrocytes is not entirely clear. Both an intracorpuscular defect, related perhaps to the defective red cells and a poorly characterized plasma factor, are believed to contribute. As in other hemolytic states, accelerated destruction of the red cells may lead to anatomic signs of mild-to-moderate iron overload after several years (p. 924).

The major causes of megaloblastic anemia are listed in Table 14–4.

It is evident that there are many bases for vitamin B_{12} deficiency, as pointed out on page 418. Inadequate diet is obvious but must be present for many years to deplete the reserves. Gastrectomy removes the source of intrinsic factor (IF). Ileal resection or diffuse ileal disease would remove or damage the site of IF-B_{12} complex absorption. Tapeworm infestation, by competing for the nutrient, could induce a deficiency state. Under some circumstances, e.g., pregnancy, hyperthyroidism, and disseminated cancer, the demand for vitamin B_{12} might be so great as to produce a relative deficiency, even with normal levels of absorption. *The feature that sets pernicious anemia apart from the other vitamin B_{12} deficiency megaloblastic anemias is the cause of the B_{12} malabsorption: a lack of intrinsic factor* (IF).

PERNICIOUS ANEMIA (PA)

The basis of the defective absorption of vitamin B_{12} in this form of megaloblastic anemia is *chronic atrophic gastritis (p. 810) with failure of production of IF.* In childhood, "juvenile" pernicious anemia is not related to atrophic gastritis. The designation "pernicious" anemia is somewhat misleading, since the present availability of synthetic B_{12} makes possible treatment and, to a large extent, control of this disease. Nonetheless, long

Table 14–4. CAUSES OF MEGALOBLASTIC ANEMIA

Vitamin B_{12} Deficiency	
Decreased intake	Inadequate diet
	Impaired absorption
	Intrinsic factor deficiency
	Pernicious anemia
	Gastrectomy
	Malabsorption states
	Diffuse intestinal disease—lymphoma, scleroderma, etc.
	Ileal resection, ileitis
	Competitive parasitic uptake
	Fish tapeworm infection
	Bacterial overgrowth in blind loops and diverticula of bowel
Increased requirement	Pregnancy, hyperthyroidism, disseminated cancer
Folic Acid Deficiency	
Decreased intake	Inadequate diet—alcoholism, infancy
	Impaired absorption
	Malabsorption states
	Intrinsic intestinal disease
	Anticonvulsants, oral contraceptives
	Hemodialysis
Increased requirement	Pregnancy, infancy, disseminated cancer, markedly increased hematopoiesis
Impaired utilization	Folic acid antagonists
Unresponsive to Vitamin B_{12} or Folic Acid Therapy	
	Metabolic inhibitors, e.g., mercaptopurines, fluorouracil, cytosine, etc.
	Unexplained disorders
	Pyridoxine and thiamin-responsive megaloblastic anemia
	Erythremic myelosis (Di Guglielmo's syndrome)

Modified from Beck, W. S.: Megaloblastic anemias. I. Vitamin B_{12} deficiency. *In* Beck, W. S. (ed.): Hematology. 2nd ed. Cambridge, Mass., M. I. T. Press., 1977, p. 71.

historic usage and the need to set PA apart from the other B_{12} deficiency states justifies the continued use of this name. It is well to discuss first the economy of vitamin B_{12} in the body, to place PA in perspective relative to the other forms of vitamin B_{12} deficiency anemia.

Vitamin B_{12} is a complex organometallic compound containing a cobalt atom within a corrin ring (very similar to the porphyrin ring) trivially known as cobalamin. The therapeutic synthetic form of vitamin B_{12} is a stable cyanocobalamin that must be converted to the biologically active forms before it can enter into reactions. Since B_{12} cannot be synthesized in the human body, it must be derived from the diet, principally in meat and dairy foods. The daily requirement of this nutrient is 2 to 3 μg; the normal diet contains considerably larger amounts. The total body pool is 2 to 5 mg, and hence, even with grossly inadequate diets, several years must elapse before the reserves are depleted. Absorption of vitamin B_{12} requires IF, which is secreted by the parietal cells of the fundic mucosa along with HCl. After peptic digestion of vitamin B_{12}-containing foods, the liberated vitamin is bound to IF, creating a stable complex that resists peptic digestion and passes to the ileum. Evidence indicates that, in addition to IF, other B_{12}-binding proteins within the gastric juice (R binders) may also play a role in the intraluminal transport of vitamin B_{12}.[24] It is suggested that some or all of the vitamin B_{12} is bound first to R proteins in the stomach and then released in the duodenum by pancreatic proteases. It is here that IF-B_{12} complex is formed, which is then carried to the ileum. In the ileum the mucosal receptors bind the complex and, by mechanisms that are still uncertain, B_{12} traverses the plasma membrane to enter the mucosal cell. It is picked up from the cell by a plasma protein, transcobalamin II, which is capable of delivering it to the liver and cells of the body, particularly the rapidly proliferating pool in the bone marrow and mucosal lining of the gastrointestinal tract. Other plasma-binding proteins, known as transcobalamin I and transcobalamin III, have been identified, but their role is still somewhat unclear.

There are only two reactions in man known to need B_{12}. *Methylcobalamin is an essential cofactor for the enzyme N^5-methyltetrahydrofolate-homocysteine methyltransferase involved in the conversion of homocysteine to methionine* (Fig. 14–15). In the process, methylcobalamin yields its methyl group and is regenerated from N^5-methyltetrahydrofolic acid (N^5-methyl-FH_4), the principal form of folic acid in plasma, which is thus converted to tetrahydrofolic acid (FH_4). The FH_4 is crucial since it is required (through its derivative $N^{5,10}$-methylene FH_4) for the conversion of deoxyuridine monophosphate (dUMP) to deoxythymidine monophosphate (dTMP), which is an immediate precursor of DNA. It has been postulated that the fundamental cause of impaired DNA synthesis in B_{12} deficiency is the reduced availability of FH_4, since most of it is "trapped" as N^5-methyl-FH_4. Although the *methyltetrahydrofolate trap hypothesis* is supported by some experimental

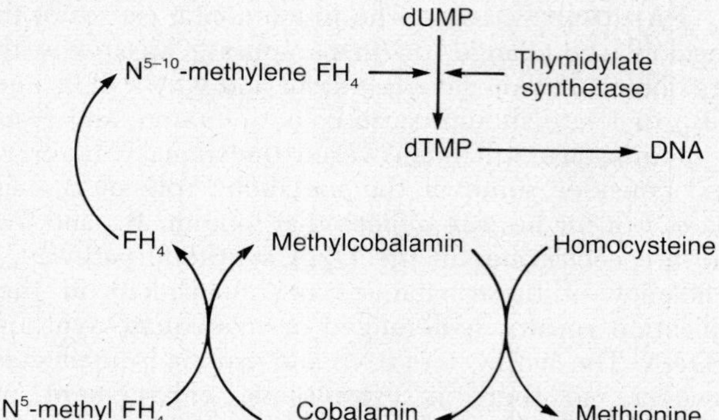

Figure 14–15. Relationship between vitamin B_{12} and folic acid metabolism in synthesis of DNA.

evidence, this issue is not resolved. Other investigators have suggested an alternative explanation that can best be dubbed the formate starvation hypothesis.[25] According to this view, the "internal" folate deficiency resulting from the lack of vitamin B_{12} is not primarily due to trapping of tetrahydrofolate but to failure to synthesize the metabolically active polyglutamate forms of folates. The synthesis of folate polyglutamates requires the single carbon formate groups derived from methionine, which in turn is generated by a B_{12}-dependent reaction (Fig. 14–15). In the formate starvation hypothesis, the importance of vitamin B_{12} is shifted from its role in the generation of FH_4 to the formation of methionine, which acts as the source of formate. Since the formation of both FH_4 and methionine are dependent on the availability of vitamin B_{12}, the two hypotheses are not mutually exclusive, but their relative contributions to the origins of megaloblastic anemia remain to be established.

Neurologic complications appear with vitamin B_{12} deficiency but are an even greater enigma. Since the administration of folic acid, which relieves the megaloblastic anemia of B_{12} deficiency, fails to improve the neurologic deficit, internal folate deficiency must not be involved. It was stated earlier that only two reactions in man are known to require B_{12}. In addition to the transmethylation reaction discussed above, cobalamin is involved in the *isomerization of methylmalonyl coenzyme A to succinyl coenzyme A, requiring adenosyl cobalamin as a prosthetic group on the enzyme methylmalonyl-coA mutase*. A deficiency of B_{12} thus leads to increased levels of methylmalonate, excreted in the urine as methylmalonic acid. Interruption of the succinyl pathway with the buildup of increased levels of methylmalonate and propionate (a precursor) could lead to the formation of abnormal fatty acids that may be incorporated into neuronal lipids. This biochemical abnormality may predispose to myelin breakdown and thereby produce some of the neurologic complications of B_{12} deficiency (p. 1421). An alternative explanation is suggested by some recent experiments in which monkeys exposed to N_2O developed a neuropathy clinically resembling the neuropathy of vitamin B_{12} deficiency in man.[26] N_2O inactivates an enzyme required for methionine synthesis, and therefore exposed animals can be protected from developing the neural changes by addition of methionine to their diet. Since vitamin B_{12} is an essential cofactor in the generation of methionine, it is postulated that deficiency of methionine or its products may be the common denominator responsible for neurologic changes in pernicious anemia and in experimental animals exposed to N_2O.

INCIDENCE. Although somewhat more prevalent in Scandinavian and "English-speaking" populations, PA occurs in all racial groups. It is slightly more common in males than in females and generally is diagnosed in the fifth to eighth decades of life. Whether or not there is a genetic predisposition to this disease is still unclear. Familial clusterings have been noted, but no definable genetic pattern of transmission has been discerned. An increased frequency of HLA-DR-2 and -DR-4 antigens has been reported, suggesting a possible immunologic basis for the development of pernicious anemia, discussed below.[27]

PATHOGENESIS. Chronic atrophic gastritis underlies the adult form of pernicious anemia, but its origin is still unknown. The mucosal atrophy is marked by a loss of parietal cells, a prominent infiltrate of lymphocytes and plasma cells, and megaloid and atypical nuclear changes in the mucosal cells similar to those found in the bone marrow. A number of immunologic reactions are associated with these morphologic changes. *Three types of antibodies are present in many, but not all, patients with PA.* About 75% of patients have an antibody that blocks B_{12}-IF binding, referred to as a *blocking antibody.* In the serum these are predominantly IgG, but may also be IgA. These are also found in the gastric juice, but here IgA antibodies predominate.[28] A second type, known as *binding antibody,* reacts with both IF or IF-B_{12} complex and is found in about 50% of patients. It is present in the serum and gastric juice and can also be identified by immunofluorescent techniques in plasma cells in the gastric mucosa. It does not occur in the absence of the blocking antibody. The third type of antibody present in 85 to 90% of patients localizes in the microvilli of the canalicular system of the gastric parietal cell, sometimes referred to as *parietal canalicular antibody.*[29] However, some patients with PA have none of these antibodies, and this has directed attention to possible cell-mediated immune reponses. Although in some patients there is evidence of T-cell reactions to IF (i.e., blast transformation and positive migration-inhibition tests), the frequency of these findings has not been established.

The meaning of the immunologic changes and their origin in patients with PA remain unestablished. You recall that up to 25% of patients with PA may not have any one of the two IF antibodies. *Yet it is rare to find antibodies to IF in the presence of completely normal B_{12} absorption.*[30] The fact that these antibodies can be synthesized in the gastric mucosa and that they can inhibit the absorption of B_{12}, when present in the gastric juice, suggests that they may play a role in the pathogenesis of vitamin B_{12} malabsorption. The parietal canalicular antibodies conceivably could cause the critical loss of parietal cells. Although detected in most patients, these antibodies are much less specific since they can be found in up to 50% of elderly patients with idiopathic chronic gastritis not associated with PA. It is tempting to propose that the immunologic abnormalities are causally related to the impaired absorption of vitamin B_{12}, but it could be argued that the gastric atrophy is primary and of unknown cause, and that the immunologic changes are merely reactions to gastric mucosal injury. Favoring their primacy is the significant association between PA and autoimmune diseases affecting the thyroid and adrenal glands. *Furthermore, an increased frequency of serum antibodies to intrinsic factor has also been reported in patients with other autoimmune diseases, particularly autoimmune thyroiditis and adrenalitis.*[31] The great majority of these patients do not have PA, although some may develop the hematologic disorder in time.

MORPHOLOGY. The major specific changes in PA are found in the bone marrow, alimentary tract, and central nervous system. Widespread nonspecific alterations incident to the generalized tissue hypoxia and abnormal hemolysis of blood may be present.

The bone marrow of untreated pernicious anemia is soft, red, jelly-like, and extremely hypercellular. It extends into the areas formerly occupied by fatty marrow. Sometimes this expansion extends to extramedullary hematopoiesis in the spleen and liver. Histologically, there is marked erythropoietic hypercellularity in which the erythroid elements sometimes equal or even outnumber the myeloid elements. **The most striking characteristic is the appearance of nests of megaloblasts** (Fig. 14–16). The earliest cells (promegaloblasts) are larger than pronormoblasts and have an abundant, deeply basophilic cytoplasm and a finely granular dispersion of chromatin within the nuclei. The nucleoli are large. As the megaloblasts differentiate, the immaturity of the nuclei contrasts with the apparent maturity of the cytoplasm. For example, **orthochromatic megaloblasts have a large amount of pink, well-hemoglobinized cytoplasm but the nucleus, instead of becoming pyknotic, remains relatively large and immature.** There may be a relative increase in the number of leukopoietic elements, but more striking is the presence of mature, large, polymorphonuclear leukocytes, the "macropolys." These cells characteristically have large nuclei, sometimes with six to seven individual lobes. Megakaryocytes may have similar changes.

With therapy, the megaloblasts, macrocytes, and macropolys disappear. Normal maturation and erythropoiesis reappear and are reflected in a great increase in the number of normoblasts and their descendants, as well as reticulocytes in the peripheral blood.

In the **alimentary system,** abnormalities are regularly found in the tongue and stomach. The tongue is shiny, glazed, and "beefy" **(atrophic glossitis).** The changes in the stomachs of adults are those of atrophic gastritis (p. 810). These atrophic changes are usually completely **absent** from juvenile patients with pernicious anemia. In the atrophic stomach, the submucosal vessels are readily visible and so produce a shiny red mucosal surface. The most characteristic histologic alteration is the atrophy of the fundic glands, affecting both chief cells and parietal cells. The parietal cells are virtually absent. The glandular lining epithelium is

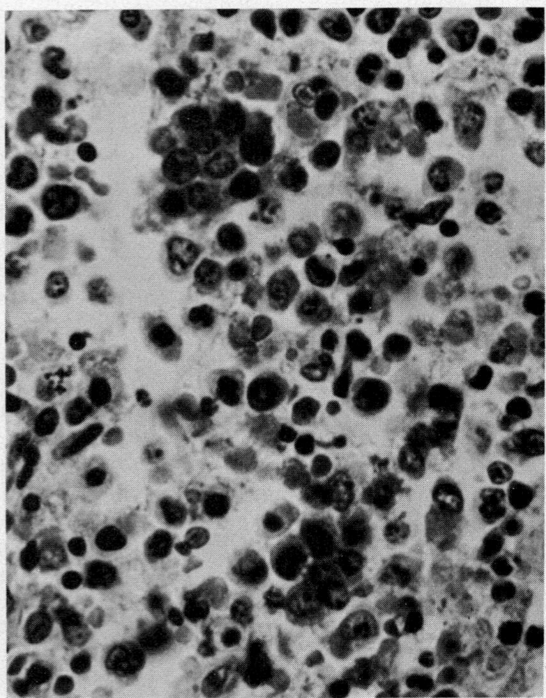

Figure 14–16. Pernicious anemia. Two nests of darkly stained megaloblasts in bone marrow.

metaplastically replaced by mucus-secreting goblet cells that resemble the lining of the large intestine, a change referred to as **intestinalization.** Some of the cells as well as their nuclei may increase to double the normal size. Presumably, these enlargements reflect the megaloid alterations discussed earlier. As will be seen, patients with pernicious anemia have a higher incidence of gastric cancer. It may be that these cellular alterations underlie the predisposition to malignancy.[32, 33]

Although parenteral administration of cyanocobalamin will correct the bone marrow changes in pernicious anemia, the gastric atrophy and achlorhydria persist unaffected. This exception is entirely compatible with the thesis that the gastric changes are primary and not the effect of the B_{12} deficiency.

Central nervous system lesions are found in approximately three-quarters of all cases of fulminant pernicious anemia. **The principal alterations involve the spinal cord where there is myelin degeneration of the dorsal and lateral tracts,** sometimes followed by loss of axons. Less frequently, degenerative changes occur in the ganglia of the posterior roots and in the peripheral nerves (p. 1421). Degenerative myelin changes are evident rarely within the brain, and in advanced cases may lead to death of neurons.

In addition to these fairly distinctive lesions, fatty degenerative changes in the heart, liver, and kidneys may be present secondary to the systemic hypoxia. Because of the hemolytic tendency and ineffective erythropoiesis in all megaloblastic anemias, hemosiderosis may be found in the liver, spleen, and bone marrow and in other elements of the mononuclear phagocyte system, but the spleen and liver usually are not significantly enlarged. The skin in severe relapse has a peculiar, lemon-yellow hue, not linearly related to the usually slightly elevated bilirubin levels in the plasma.

CLINICAL COURSE. Pernicious anemia is characteristically insidious in onset, so that by the time the patient seeks medical attention the anemia is usually quite marked. The usual course is progressive unless halted by therapy.

Diagnostic features include (1) a moderate-to-severe megaloblastic anemia, sometimes with hematocrit or hemoglobin levels reduced to 30% or less of normal; (2) leukopenia with hypersegmented granulocytes; (3) mild-to-moderate thrombocytopenia; (4) neurologic changes related to involvement of the posterolateral spinal tracts, as well as possibly to the brain; (5) achlorhydria even after histamine stimulation; (6) decreased vitamin B_{12} absorption; (7) low serum levels of vitamin B_{12}; (8) excretion of methylmalonic acid in the urine; and (9) most critically, a striking reticulocytic response and improvement in hematocrit levels following parenteral administration of vitamin B_{12}.

The cytologic aberrations in the gastric mucosa lead to a well-defined (threefold) increased incidence of gastric cancer. In addition, cardiac failure incident to hypoxic injury to the myocardium and intercurrent infections are hazards. However, with parenteral vitamin B_{12} the anemia can be cured and the peripheral neurologic changes reversed, or at least halted in their progression. Obviously, death of brain cells cannot be reversed. Overall longevity may be restored virtually to normal.

"JUVENILE" PERNICIOUS ANEMIA. Childhood PA differs from the adult type inasmuch as there is no associated gastric abnormality. The mechanism of vitamin B_{12} deficiency is not well understood and may be related to several hereditary derangements: (1) congenital inability to elaborate intrinsic factor, (2) synthesis of a biologically ineffective IF, and (3) some defect in the ileal mucosal receptors for the intrinsic factor B_{12} complex. Autosomal recessive inheritance has been identified within some families.

ANEMIA OF FOLATE DEFICIENCY

A deficiency of folic acid, more properly pteroylmonoglutamic acid, results in a megaloblastic anemia having the same characteristics as those encountered in vitamin B_{12} deficiency. However, the neurologic changes seen in B_{12} deficiency do not occur. Folic acid deficiency, not always severe enough to produce anemia, is surprisingly common. Inadequate serum folate levels were found in 47% of patients admitted to a municipal hospital in the U.S.[34] and are even more common in underprivileged societies. *The prime function of folic acid, specifically tetrahydrofolate (FH_4) derivatives, is to act as intermediates in the transfer of one-carbon units such as formyl and methyl groups to various compounds* (Fig. 14–17). In this process, FH_4 acts as an acceptor of one-carbon fragments from compounds such as serine and formiminoglutamic acid (FIGlu), and the FH_4 derivatives so generated donate the acquired one-carbon fragments for the synthesis of biologically active molecules. FH_4, then, may be viewed as the biologic "middle

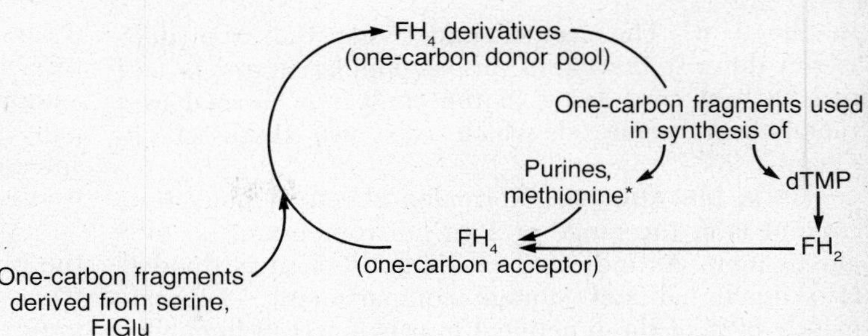

Figure 14–17. Schematic illustration of role of folate derivatives in transfer of one-carbon fragments for synthesis of biologic macromolecules. FH_4 = tetrahydrofolic acid; FH_2 = dihydrofolic acid; FIGlu = formiminoglutamate; dTMP = deoxythymidylate monophosphate; *synthesis of methionine also requires vitamin B_{12}.

man" in this trade. The most important metabolic processes dependent on such one-carbon transfers are (1) the synthesis of purines; (2) the synthesis of methionine from homocysteine, a reaction that also requires vitamin B_{12} (p. 632); and (3) the synthesis of deoxythymidylate monophosphate (dTMP). In the first two reactions, FH_4 is regenerated from its one-carbon carrier derivatives and is available to accept another one-carbon fragment and reenter the donor pool. In the synthesis of thymidylate, a dihydrofolate is produced that has to be reduced by dihydrofolate reductase to FH_4 to reenter the pool. The reductase step is significant since this enzyme is susceptible to inhibition by various drugs. Among the biologically active molecules whose synthesis is dependent on folates, thymidylate is perhaps the most important. As discussed earlier in relation to pernicious anemia (p. 632), dTMP is required for DNA synthesis. It should be apparent from our discussion that suppressed synthesis of DNA, the common denominator of folic acid and B_{12} deficiency, is the immediate cause of megaloblastosis. A clinically insignificant biochemical effect of folate deficiency is the failure to metabolize formiminoglutamic acid (FIGlu), a breakdown product of histidine. With a deficiency of folate, FIGlu piles up and is excreted in the urine, providing a useful clinical indicator of folate deficiency.

The dietary source and absorption of folates were considered in an earlier chapter (p. 417). Here we need discuss only the three major causes of folic acid deficiency: (1) decreased intake, (2) increased requirements, and (3) impaired utilization (Table 14–4).

Decreased intake can result from either a nutritionally inadequate diet or impairment of intestinal absorption. A normal daily diet contains folate in excess of the minimal daily adult requirement of 10 to 50 μg. Inadequate dietary intakes are almost invariably associated with grossly deficient diets, particularly lacking vitamins, such as those in the "B group." Such dietary inadequacies are most frequently encountered in chronic alcoholics, the indigent, and the very elderly. In alcoholics with cirrhosis, other mechanisms of folate deficiency such as trapping of folate within the liver, excessive urinary loss, and disordered folate metabolism have also been implicated. Under these circumstances, the megaloblastic anemia is often accompanied by general malnutrition and manifestations of other avitaminoses, including cheilosis, glossitis, and dermatitis. Malabsorption syndromes such as nontropical and tropical sprue may lead to inadequate absorption of this nutrient. Similarly, diffuse infiltrative disease of the small intestine, e.g., lymphoma, may impair intestinal absorption. In addition, certain drugs, particularly the anticonvulsant phenytoin and oral contraceptives, impair absorption.

Despite adequate intake of folic acid, a *relative deficiency* can be encountered in states of increased requirement, such as pregnancy, infancy, hematologic derangements in which appropriate therapy induces marked hyperactive hematopoiesis, and disseminated cancer. In all these circumstances, the demands of active DNA synthesis render normal intake inadequate.

Folic acid antagonists, such as methotrexate, 6-mercaptopurine, and cyclophosphamide, inhibit dihydrofolate reductase and lead to a deficiency of FH_4. With inhibition of folate function, all rapidly growing cells are affected, thus leading to ulcerative lesions within the gastrointestinal tract as well as megaloblastic anemia. Owing to their growth-inhibitory actions, these antimetabolites are used in cancer therapy.

As mentioned at the outset, *the megaloblastic anemia resulting from a deficiency of folic acid is identical to that encountered in B_{12} deficiency, both in terms of the alterations in the circulating blood and in the marrow precursors.* Thus, the recognition of folate deficiency requires the demonstration of (1) decreased folate levels in the serum or red cells and (2) increased excretion of FIGlu after an administered dose of histidine. The absence of neurologic changes and methylmalonic acid in the urine also rules against vitamin B_{12} deficiency as the cause of changes in the blood. Although prompt hematologic response heralded by the appearance of a reticulocytosis follows the administration of folic acid, it should be cautioned that, even in patients with a B_{12} deficiency anemia, a similar reticulocytosis may be produced by folic acid therapy. However, folic acid has no effect on the progression of the neurologic changes typical of the B_{12} deficiency states, and therefore the hematologic response to folate therapy cannot be used to rule out vitamin B_{12} deficiency.

Iron Deficiency Anemia

Deficiency of iron is probably the most common nutritional disorder in the world. Although the prevalence of iron deficiency anemia is higher in the developing countries, this form of anemia is also common in the U.S. The factors underlying the iron deficiency differ somewhat in various population groups and can be best considered in the context of normal iron metabolism, some of which was also discussed in Chapter 9.[35–37]

IRON METABOLISM. Normally, the total body iron content is in the range of 2 gm in women and up to 6 gm in men. As indicated in Table 14–5, it is divided into functional and storage compartments. Approximately 80% of the functional iron is found in hemoglobin; myoglobin and iron-containing enzymes such as catalase and the cytochromes contain the rest. The storage pool represented by hemosiderin and ferritin contains approximately 15 to 20% of total body iron. It should be noted that even healthy young females have substantially smaller stores of iron than do males. They are therefore in much more precarious iron balance and are accordingly more vulnerable to excessive losses or increased demands associated with menstruation and pregnancy.

All storage of iron is in the form of either ferritin or hemosiderin. *Ferritin is essentially a protein-iron complex* about which much is both known and unknown. The protein—known as apoferritin—is a spherical shell composed of approximately 24 subunits, each of molecular weight 18,500 to 19,000, giving a total molecular weight for apoferritin of approximately 450,000. This shell is perforated by six channels through which iron uptake and release occur.[38] The core of the apoferritin shell contains as many as 4500 iron atoms in the form of ferric oxyhydride.

Ferritin can be found in all tissues but particularly in liver, spleen, bone marrow, and skeletal muscles. In the liver, most of the ferritin is stored within the parenchymal cells, whereas in other tissues, such as spleen and bone marrow, it is mainly in the mononuclear phagocytic cells. The iron within the hepatocytes is derived from plasma transferrin, whereas the storage iron in the mononuclear phagocytic cells, including that in the Kupffer cells, is obtained largely from the breakdown of red cells. Within cells, ferritin is located both in the cell sap and in lysosomes where the protein shells of the ferritin are degraded and iron aggregated into *hemosiderin* granules. With the usual cellular stains, hemosiderin appears in tissues as golden-yellow granules that vary somewhat in size and shape, presumably because of variation in the number of incorporated ferritin molecules. The iron is chemically reactive, and when hemosiderin is exposed to potassium ferrocyanide (Prussian blue reaction) in tissue sections, the granules turn blue-black. With normal iron stores only trace amounts of hemosiderin are found in the body, principally in reticuloendothelial cells in the bone marrow, spleen, and liver. In iron-overloaded cells, most of the iron is stored in the form of hemosiderin.

Table 14–5. IRON DISTRIBUTION IN HEALTHY YOUNG ADULTS (mg)

	Men	Women
Total	3450	2450
Functional		
Hemoglobin	2100	1750
Myoglobin	300	250
Enzymes	50	50
Storage		
Ferritin, hemosiderin	1000	400

Very small amounts of ferritin normally circulate in the plasma. *Since the plasma ferritin is largely derived from the storage pool of body iron, its level is a good indicator of the adequacy of body iron stores.* Each microgram per liter of plasma ferritin is estimated to represent 8 mg of storage iron. In iron deficiency, serum ferritin is always below 12 μg per liter, whereas in iron overload very high values approaching 5000 μg per liter may be obtained. It should be noted, however, that the relationship between the degree of overload and serum ferritin levels is not linear. There are three circumstances under which serum ferritin cannot be used as a measure of body iron stores: in liver damage, in inflammatory states, and with some tumors. In these states, serum ferritin levels may be extremely high despite normal body iron stores. The physiologic importance of the storage iron pool is that it is readily mobilizable in the event of an increase in body iron requirements, as may occur following loss of blood.

Iron is transported in the plasma by an iron-binding protein called transferrin. It is a β globulin, synthesized in the liver, having a molecular weight of 76,000 with two iron-binding sites. The major function of plasma transferrin is to deliver iron to the cell surface receptors on immature erythroid cells. In the normal individual, transferrin is about 33% saturated with iron, yielding serum iron levels that average 120 μg per dl in men and 100 μg per dl in women. Thus, the total iron-binding capacity of serum is in the range of 300 to 350 μg per dl.

The absorption of iron and its regulation are complex and poorly understood. Some of the factors that affect iron absorption were discussed in an earlier chapter (p. 422). Here we will concentrate on the mucosal uptake of iron. The most active site of iron absorption is the duodenum, but the stomach, ileum, and colon may also participate to a small degree. The precise mechanism of iron uptake is still poorly understood, although evidence is accumulating that a mucosal transferrin distinct from plasma transferrin is secreted in the lumen of the gut, where it binds iron and then transports it across the brush border of the mucosal cell.[39] Normally, a fraction of the iron that enters the mucosal cell is rapidly delivered to plasma transferrin. Most, however, is deposited as ferritin within these cells, some to be transferred more slowly to plasma transferrin, and some to be lost with exfoliation of mucosal cells. The extent to which the mucosal iron is distributed along these various pathways depends largely on the body's iron requirements. When the body is replete with iron, formation of ferritin within the mucosal cells is maximal, whereas in iron deficiency transport into plasma is enhanced.

Since body losses of iron are limited, iron balance

is maintained largely by regulating the absorptive intake (mucosal block). The factors that regulate the absorption of available iron into the mucosal cell are largely unknown. It is, however, known that the rate and level of absorption is dependent on total body iron content and erythropoietic activity, more specifically the iron needs of the erythron. As body stores rise the percentage of iron absorbed falls, and vice versa. Some signal must be delivered to the mucosal cell modifying its uptake and transfer of iron, and although there are many hypotheses, the nature of the signal remains unknown.[40] Most attractive is the proposal that the iron content of the individual tissues itself is the regulating factor. It is assumed that there is a labile pool of iron in all the tissues, from which iron can be donated to plasma transferrin. The size of this labile pool in the individual tissues, particularly the reticuloendothelial cells and the gut mucosa, is proportionate to the total iron stored within that tissue (Fig. 14–18). Iron donated to the plasma is removed from plasma transferrin predominantly by the developing erythroid cells. A decrease in storage iron within the reticuloendothelial cells reduces their contribution to the plasma transferrin iron pool, which is compensated for by an increased entry of iron from the gut. Similarly, an increased drain by the erythron produces a "stimulus" for increased contribution to the plasma iron pool by the various donor sites, including the gut mucosa. This in turn causes a greater proportion of the iron absorbed into the mucosal cell to be transferred into the plasma. Although some experimental evidence supporting this hypothesis has been obtained,[41] in the final analysis the mechanism by which exchange of iron between donor tissues and plasma transferrin is regulated remains poorly understood.

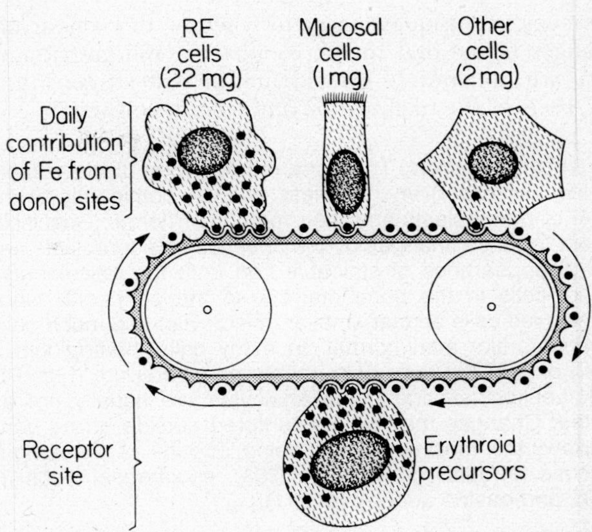

Figure 14–18. Regulation of internal iron exchange. Plasma iron turnover is visualized as a conveyer belt driven by uptake of transferrin iron by erythroid precursors. Amount of iron released at any one time from donor sites onto transferrin is dependent on amounts of iron being removed by erythroid precursors. (From Bothwell, T. H., et al.: Idiopathic hemochromatosis. *In* Stanbury, J. B., et al.: Metabolic Basis of Inherited Disease. 5th ed. New York, McGraw-Hill Book Co., 1982, p.1276. Copyright © 1982 by McGraw Hill, Inc. Used by permission of McGraw-Hill Book Company.)

ETIOLOGY. With this background of normal iron metabolism, we can discuss the causes and effects of iron deficiency. The consequences of excess iron accumulation (iron overload) are considered on page 924. Negative iron balance and consequent anemia may result from (1) low dietary intake, (2) poor absorption, (3) excessive demand, or (4) chronic blood loss. The daily iron requirement for adult males is 5 to 10 mg and for adult females 7 to 20 mg (p. 422). Since the average daily dietary intake of iron in the Western world approximates 15 mg, most men ingest more than adequate iron, whereas many women consume just enough or marginally adequate iron. It is not surprising, therefore, *that iron deficiency resulting solely from poor dietary intake is rarely seen in the U.S.;* even in women who have lower iron reserves and greater iron losses, other factors usually coexist. The situation is quite different in underdeveloped countries where low intake as well as poor bioavailability of the iron exist, owing to a lack of meats and to predominantly vegetarian diets from which iron is poorly absorbed. *Malabsorption* of iron may occur in association with generalized malabsorption syndromes such as sprue and celiac disease, or after gastrectomy. The latter affects iron absorption by decreasing hydrochloric acid and the transit time through the duodenum, the major site of iron absorption. *By far the most important cause of iron deficiency anemia in the Western world is chronic blood loss.* This may occur from the gastrointestinal tract (e.g., peptic ulcers, colonic cancer, hemorrhoids, hookworm disease, chronic aspirin ingestion) or the female genital tract (e.g., menorrhagia, maligancy). At the outset of chronic blood loss or other states of negative iron balance, the reserves in the form of ferritin and hemosiderin may be adequate to maintain normal hemoglobin and hematocrit levels as well as normal serum iron and transferrin saturation. Progressive depletion of these reserves will eventually lower the serum iron and transferrin saturation levels, but still may not be reflected in abnormalities in the erythron. Up to this stage of blood loss there is increased erythroid activity in the bone marrow and expansion of the erythron, but progressive disappearance of sideroblasts from the marrow. Thereafter, anemia will appear when all iron stores are depleted, now accompanied by low levels of serum iron and transferrin saturation as well as low serum ferritin. Pregnancy and infancy are two states that may be associated with iron deficiency owing to *increased demands* not met by normal dietary intake. *Whatever the basis, iron deficiency induces a hypochromic microcytic anemia.* Simultaneously, depletion of essential iron-containing enzymes in cells throughout the body may cause other changes, including koilonychia, alopecia, atrophic changes in the tongue and gastric mucosa, and intestinal malabsorption. Uncommonly, esophageal webs (p. 799) may appear to complete the triad of major findings in the *Plummer-Vinson syndrome:* (1) microcytic hypochromic anemia, (2) atrophic glossitis, and (3) esophageal webs. There is, however, some question as to whether the concurrent changes in the oral cavity, esophagus, and gastric mucosa are not merely coincidental or instead constitute the basis of the malnutriton and iron deficiency.

MORPHOLOGY. The bone marrow may disclose more or less increased erythropoietic activity, dominantly at the level of normoblasts and their maturation forms. Specificity is lent to these changes by the absence of sideroblasts and the disappearance of stainable iron from the reticuloendothelial cells in the bone marrow. In the peripheral blood smear, red cells appear smaller (microcytic) and much paler (hypochromic) than normal. In many cells, hemoglobin is seen only in the form of a narrow peripheral rim (Fig. 14–19). Leukocytes and megakaryocytes are usually not affected. Changes may be encountered outside of the bone marrow, the most important being atrophy of the tongue mucosa (atrophic glossitis) (p. 784), esophageal webs (p. 799), and gastric atrophy (p. 811).

The clinical manifestations related to the anemia are nonspecific and were detailed on page 613. Frequently, the dominating signs and symptoms relate to the underlying cause of the anemia, e.g., gastrointestinal or gynecologic disease, malnutrition, pregnancy, malabsorption, and so forth. The atrophic glossitis may be responsible for difficulty in swallowing. Gastrointestinal disturbances may be present associated with the disorder that led to the chronic blood loss (e.g., bleeding peptic ulcer or gastric carcinoma, diverticulitis, colonic cancer) or may emanate from the development of the atrophic gastritis.

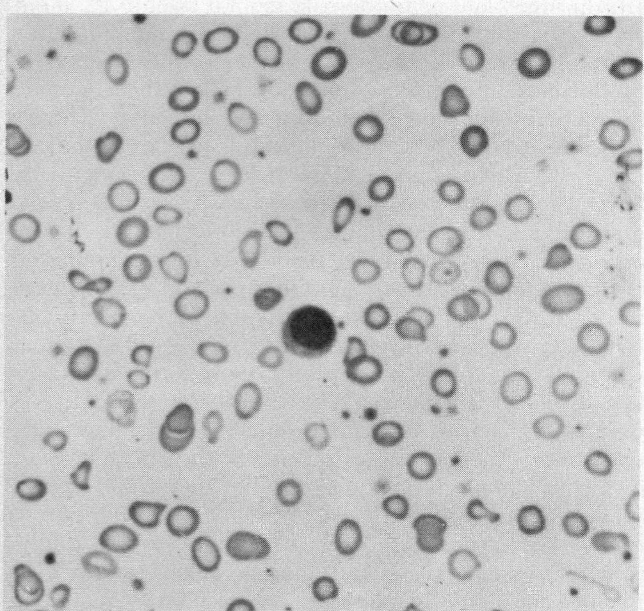

Figure 14–19. Hypochromic microcytic anemia of iron deficiency. Note that most red cells are smaller than lymphocyte nucleus seen in midfield. The small amount of hemoglobin is seen as a narrow rim at periphery of red cells. (Courtesy of Dr. Jose Hernandez, Department of Pathology, Southwestern Medical School, Dallas, Texas.)

The diagnosis of iron deficiency anemia ultimately rests upon laboratory studies. Both hemoglobin and hematocrit are depressed, usually to moderate levels, and are associated with hypochromia, microcytosis, and some poikilocytosis. As mentioned, the serum iron, serum ferritin, and transferrin saturation levels are typically low. Reduced heme synthesis leads to elevation of free erythrocyte protoporphyrin. Usually the leukocytes and platelets are not affected. The alert clinician who investigates an unexplained iron deficiency anemia occasionally discovers an occult lesion or cancer and thereby saves a life.

Aplastic Anemia

This somewhat misleading term is applied to pancytopenia, characterized by (1) anemia, (2) neutropenia, and (3) thrombocytopenia.[42] The basis for these changes is thought to be a failure or suppression of pluripotent myeloid stem cells, with inadequate production or release of the differentiated cell lines. Less commonly, the stem cell defect is limited to the committed precursors, giving rise to pure red cell aplasia, or selective suppression of the white cell series. These will be considered later. The bone marrow in aplastic anemia is almost always markedly hypocellular, with a striking reduction in the precursors of red cells, granulocytes, and platelets.

ETIOLOGY. The major circumstances under which aplastic anemia may appear are listed in Table 14–6.

Most cases of aplastic anemia of so-called "known etiology" follow exposure to chemicals and drugs. With some agents the marrow damage is predictable, dose related, and, in most instances, reversible when the use of the offending agent is stopped. Best documented as

Table 14–6. MAJOR CAUSES OF APLASTIC ANEMIA

- **A. Acquired**
  - I. Idiopathic
  - II. Chemical agents
    - Dose related
      - Alkylating agents
      - Antimetabolites
      - Benzene
      - Chloramphenicol
      - Inorganic arsenicals
    - Idiosyncratic
      - Chloramphenicol
      - Phenylbutazone
      - Organic arsenicals
      - Methylphenylethylhydantoin
      - Streptomycin
      - Chlorpromazine
      - Insecticides: e.g., DDT, parathion
  - III. Physical agents (whole-body radiation)
  - IV. Paroxysmal nocturnal hemoglobinuria
  - V. Infections
    - Viral hepatitis
    - Dengue
    - Infectious mononucleosis
  - VI. Miscellaneous
    - Infrequently, many other drugs and chemicals
- **B. Inherited**—Fanconi's anemia

known myelotoxins are benzene, chloramphenicol, alkylating agents, and antimetabolites, e.g., 6-mercaptopurine, vincristine, busulfan, etc. In other instances, the pancytopenia appears as an apparent idiosyncratic reaction to either very small doses of known myelotoxins, e.g., chloramphenicol, or following the use of such drugs as phenylbutazone, methylphenylethylhydantoin, streptomycin, and chlorpromazine, which are generally without effect in other individuals. In such idiosyncratic reactions the aplasia may be severe and sometimes irreversible and fatal.

Whole-body *irradiation* is an obvious mechanism for destruction of hematopoietic cells. The effects of irradiation are dose related. Persons at risk are those who receive therapeutic irradiation, radiologists, and individuals exposed to nuclear explosions.

Paroxysmal nocturnal hemoglobinuria, discussed earlier as a form of hemolytic anemia, is believed to be an acquired clonal disorder of pluripotent stem cells, which in some cases evolves into aplastic anemia (p. 627).

Although aplastic anemia may appear in a variety of *infections*, it most commonly follows viral hepatitis of the non-A, non-B type.[43, 43A] Why certain individuals develop this hematologic complication in the course of their infection is not understood but it is not related to the severity of infection. Direct injury to stem cells could be postulated, but there are reasons for doubting such a simplistic explanation.

Fanconi's anemia is a rare familial form of aplastic anemia. In these patients the marrow hypofunction becomes evident early in life and is accompanied by multiple congenital anomalies such as hypoplasia of the kidney and spleen and hypoplastic anomalies of bone, particularly involving the thumbs or radii. Some of these individuals develop leukemia if they survive the hazards of the marrow hypofunction.

Despite all these possible causal influences, in fully two-thirds of the cases no provocating factor can be identified, and hence most cases of aplastic anemia are lumped into the *idiopathic* category.[44]

PATHOGENESIS. Although we speak of myelotoxic chemicals, drugs, and infections as causes of aplastic anemia, the precise mechanism of stem cell injury in these settings is poorly understood. Idiopathic cases are even more mysterious, and therefore numerous hypotheses have sprouted. Some of the most important clues regarding pathogenetic mechanisms have been obtained by evaluating various forms of treatment. The remarkable efficacy of bone marrow transplantation in the treatment of aplastic anemia suggests that *most cases of aplastic anemia result from defects in the number or function of stem cells.* With marrow transplants, defective stem cells are replaced by infusion of normal cells from HLA-matched donors. Much attention has also focused on the possibility that *marrow failure may result from immunologically mediated suppression of hematopoiesis.* In support of the suppressor cell hypothesis is cited the ability of lymphocytes from aplastic patients to inhibit the in vitro growth of normal myeloid (CFU-G/M) or erythroid stem cells (BFU-E) obtained from healthy individuals. The recovery of autologous marrow in some cases by administration of immunosuppressive therapy is also consistent with an immunologic causation of aplastic anemia.[45] Yet another theory points the finger to possible *defects in the "marrow microenvironment."* According to this view, the stem cells, at least in some cases, are intrinsically normal but their milieu is unfavorable for hematopoiesis. This may very well be the mechanism of aplastic anemia in those patients who fail to benefit from bone marrow transplantation. Although much remains to be known, it is clear that aplastic anemia is not a single disease, but a group of pathogenetically distinct disorders.

MORPHOLOGY. The bone marrow is markedly hypocellular and is composed largely of empty marrow spaces populated by fat cells, fibrous stroma, and scattered or clustered foci of lymphocytes and plasma cells (Fig. 14–20). In less extreme instances, scattered primitive precursor cells are found. Megakaryocytes are either absent or scant in number. A number of additional morphologic changes may accompany these marrow failures. Fatty changes may result from the anemia. Also evident may be the pathology of bacterial infections or hemorrhagic diatheses secondary to the granulocytopenia or thrombocytopenia, respectively (p. 654). The toxic drug or agent may injure not only the bone marrow but also the liver, the kidneys, and other structures. Benzene, for example, may cause fatty changes in the liver and kidneys. In some instances, especially those with multiple tranfusions, systemic hemosiderosis is present.

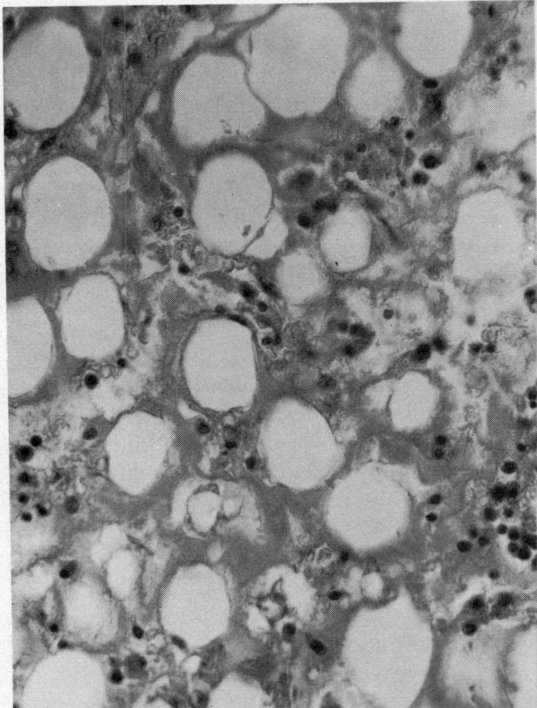

Figure 14–20. Aplastic anemia—bone marrow. Bone marrow is hypocellular. Most of the nucleated forms present are lymphocytes and scattered plasma cells.

Clinical Course. Aplastic anemia may occur at any age and in both sexes. Usually the onset is gradual, but in some instances the disorder strikes with suddenness and great severity. Patients may first become aware of their disease by the progressive onset of weakness, fatigability, and pallor. The thrombocytopenia may produce bleeding manifestations. At other times, the granulocytopenia is called to attention by repeated bacterial infections that are apparently more severe than would be anticipated in the normal individual. Splenomegaly is so uncommon that its presence should arouse the suspicion of alternative diagnoses such as "aleukemic" leukemia (p. 675).

Diagnosis rests largely upon examination of the peripheral blood and marrow biopsy. In most patients, the red cells are normochromic and normocytic. *Signs of erythropoiesis such as polychromatophilia or reticulocytosis are characteristically absent.* The white cell and platelet counts are also depressed. Serum iron is almost always elevated, frequently with 100% saturation of the total iron-binding capacity.

Bone marrow biopsy discloses an aplastic or hypocellular marrow, which also helps to rule out other causes of depressed marrow function such as metastatic cancer, leukemia, or some underlying bone disease that has replaced the marrow space to produce a myelophthisic anemia.

The prognosis in aplastic anemia is quite unpredictable. When associated with viral hepatitis it is extremely grave. If the toxic factor can be identified and further exposure avoided, the marrow production may recover. If idiopathic, the disease tends to be more prolonged and outlook is less favorable. In rare instances, leukemia later appears. The recent introduction of bone marrow transplantation offers new hope; a 60% five-year survival can be expected with this form of therapy.[43]

Pure Red Cell Aplasia (PRCA)

Pure red cell aplasia is a rare form of marrow failure resulting from a specific aplasia of erythroid elements while granulopoiesis and thrombopoiesis remain normal.[46] It may occur in an acute form as an aplastic "crisis" during the course of some form of preexisting hemolytic anemia or as a drug- or infectious disease–related disorder. PRCA may also appear insidiously in a chronic form, sometimes without apparent provocation, and at other times in patients having a thymoma. The latter association raises the question of some thymic-related immunologic mechanism and, indeed, in about half of the patients resection of the primary tumor is followed by hematologic improvement. Humoral or cellular autoimmunity against erythroid precursors can be demonstrated in some cases, and in such patients immunosuppressive therapy may be beneficial. In refractory cases, plasmapheresis has also been used with success.[47]

Other Forms of Marrow Failure

Space-occupying lesions that destroy significant amounts of bone marrow or perhaps disturb the marrow architecture depress its productive capacity. This form of marrow failure is referred to as *myelophthisic anemia.* As would be anticipated, all the formed elements of the blood are concomitantly affected. However, characteristically immature forms of the red and white cells appear in the peripheral blood, a phenomenon attributed to a poorly defined "irritation effect." The most common cause of myelophthisic anemia is metastatic cancer arising from a primary lesion in the breast, lung, prostate, thyroid, or adrenals. Multiple myeloma, leukemia, osteosclerosis, and lymphomas are less commonly implicated. Myelophthisic anemia has also been observed with myelofibrosis, a diffuse fibrosis of the marrow. Such cases are probably variants of the myeloproliferative syndrome (p. 686).

Diffuse liver disease, whether it be toxic, infectious, or a form of cirrhosis, is for obscure reasons often associated with an anemia attributed to bone marrow failure. Other contributing factors include folate deficiency and iron deficiency due to gastrointestinal blood loss (varices, hemorrhoids). In most of these instances, there is a pure erythropoietic depression; in about half the cases the red cells are normocytic, and in the other half they are macrocytic. Occasionally the red cell morphology is very much like that of pernicious anemia. Depression of the white cell count and platelets has been described, but is infrequent.

Chronic renal failure, whatever its cause, is almost invariably associated with anemia that tends to be roughly proportional to the severity of the uremia. The basis of the anemia is multifactorial. There is evidence of an extracorpuscular defect inducing chronic hemolysis. Concomitantly, there is reduced red cell production. In some cases this may be related to advanced destruction of the kidneys with inadequate formation of erythropoietin. Alternatively, some patients have an iron deficiency secondary to the bleeding tendency often encountered in uremia. Whatever the basis, if the uremia can be controlled by dialysis or other forms of therapy, the anemia is usually reversible.

Significant chronic microbiologic infections and chronic inflammatory states such as rheumatoid arthritis and rheumatic fever are often associated with a mild-to-moderate normocytic normochromic anemia, although sometimes the red cells may be hypochromic and microcytic. The underlying mechanism is poorly understood, but there is evidence for a hemolytic component with a shortened red cell survival time and some impairment in iron utilization. The hemolysis may be related to nonspecific stimulation of reticuloendothelial cells. With respect to the iron metabolism, the serum iron levels are low as is saturation of the iron-binding capacity, and concomitantly, hemosiderosis is present in reticuloendothelial cells. This paradoxic combination has led to the speculation that some impediment exists in the transfer to the erythroid precursors in the blood of iron from reticuloendothelial cells involved in normal red cell destruction. Whatever the pathophysiology of the anemia, it is reversible when the primary disease is controlled.

Endocrine disorders, particularly those affecting the

thyroid, pituitary, and adrenal, may be associated with anemia. Myxedema stands out as the most important disorder in this category. In some of these cases the anemia is normocytic, but in many it is macrocytic. Impaired absorption of vitamin B_{12} has been implicated in some cases of thyroid hypofunction, which may produce, therefore, a pattern similar to that of pernicious anemia. Alternatively, it is possible that the decreased metabolic activity of the body concomitantly slows marrow production. Supporting such a concept is the prompt recovery of marrow function following the administration of thyroid extract. Addison's disease (p. 1235) and hypofunction of the anterior lobe of the pituitary are sometimes associated with a normocytic anemia. The mechanisms here are obscure. In all these endocrine disorders, the bone marrow usually provides no morphologic clue to its physiologic hypoactivity.

POLYCYTHEMIA

Polycythemia refers to an increase in the concentration of red cells above the normal level, usually with a corresponding increase in hemoglobin level. Such an increase may be *relative* when there is hemoconcentration, or *absolute* when there is an increase in total red cell mass. It may occur as an idiopathic primary disorder, e.g., polycythemia vera, or as a secondary response to appropriate or inappropriate increased elaboration of erythropoietin.[48]

Relative Polycythemia

Relative polycythemia may occur when there is a loss of plasma volume without a corresponding loss in red cells, or when there is abnormal sequestration of a large volume of blood in the low-hematocrit capillary compartment of the circulation. Under these circumstances there is an apparent increase in the number of red cells within the circulation. The causes of such relative polycythemia include (1) deprivation of water; (2) loss of body fluids from vomiting, diarrhea, and sweating; (3) loss of electrolytes with corresponding loss of plasma volume, as occurs with adrenocortical insufficiency; (4) loss of plasma volume, as in burns and shock; and (5) an obscure condition sometimes referred to as *stress polycythemia* or *Gaisböck's syndrome.* The last condition is typically encountered in males in the fifth decade of life who are moderately overweight, hypertensive, tense, and heavy cigarette smokers. The basis for the relative polycythemia in this setting is unknown.

Polycythemia Vera (Primary Polycythemia, Erythremia)

Polycythemia vera is an insidious disease of unknown cause characterized by elevation of the total red cell mass, sometimes to double the normal value. As a consequence, the red cell count and hemoglobin levels are elevated. Although excessive proliferation of the erythroid stem cells is responsible for the increase in red cell mass, involvement of pluripotent myeloid stem cells is indicated by concomitant elevations of the granulocyte and platelet counts.

PATHOGENESIS. Several clues regarding the pathogenesis of polycythemia vera have been obtained from its natural history. It has been noted that a small but statistically significant fraction of patients, after a period of years with polycythemia vera, have insidiously become anemic with hypocellular fibrotic marrows, for completely mysterious reasons. Massive splenomegaly may then appear owing to extramedullary hematopoiesis, giving rise to the syndrome known as *myeloid metaplasia* (p. 686). Much less commonly, patients beginning with polycythemia vera later develop chronic granulocytic (myelogenous) leukemia. In explanation of these and other possible changeovers, Dameshek[49] proposed the concept of the *myeloproliferative syndrome.* He postulated that in some patients hemopoietic stem cells might become abnormally active or virtually neoplastic, and the particular stem line principally affected might change with time. Theoretically, the abnormal proliferation might initially involve mainly the erythrocytic, granulocytic, or megakaryocytic populations within the marrow. If the erythrocytic line predominated, presumably the patient would develop polycythemia vera. Granulocytic overgrowth would lead to chronic myelogenous leukemia. Excessive overgrowth of megakaryocytes might lead to primary thrombocythemia. Moreover, it was proposed that one of the end stages of the various expressions of the myeloproliferative syndrome was myelofibrosis resulting in anemia and, along with it, extramedullary myeloid metaplasia (p. 686). At one time, the proliferating fibroblasts in the marrow were believed to be the progeny of the neoplastic stem cells, but subsequent evidence indicates that the fibrosis is reactive.[50] It must be emphasized that the myeloproliferative syndrome is not a specific disease but rather a concept that appears to fit observed clinical phenomena. Within this context, polycythemia vera represents one variant of a larger group of myeloproliferative syndromes.

Current evidence strongly suggests that polycythemia vera arises as a monoclonal apparent neoplastic disorder of pluripotent myeloid stem cells. Using the approach of the X-linked G6PD enzymes as markers, it has been shown that females who are heterozygous for G6PD variant enzymes (having two populations of cells, each bearing one or the other variant enzymes) have only a single G6PD enzyme in the majority of their red cells, granulocytes, and platelets.[48] The same type of evidence has been used to show the monoclonal origin of such solid tissue tumors as leiomyomas. Additional support for the involvement of the myeloid stem cells in polycythemia vera has been obtained by the recently available techniques of hematopoietic cell culture.[51] In the bone marrow of patients with polycythemia vera there is an increase in the number of actively dividing myeloid stem cells that seem to require extremely small amounts of erythropoietin for erythroid differentiation. Although these abnormal erythropoietin-hypersensitive stem cells predominate, a small number of normal stem cells (which require much more erythropoietin) are also present. For reasons not entirely clear, their proliferation and differentiation is suppressed, and normal red cells therefore constitute a minority in the peripheral blood. It could be that the erythrocytosis induced by the proliferation of the abnormal (neoplastic) stem cells suppresses the production of erythropoietin, thereby keeping the normal erythroid stem cells inactive. Indeed, serum levels of erythropoietin are extremely low in polycythemia vera, perhaps enough only to keep the neoplastic stem cells going. The number of normal stem cells seems to decline as the disease progresses. This observation has potential clinical significance, since remission requires not only suppression of the neoplastic clones but the reemergence of the residual normal stem cells. The granulocytic and megakaryocytic precursors derived from the neoplastic clone of stem cells are also abnormal. They seem to be unresponsive to as yet unidentified signals that regulate their normal counterparts.

MORPHOLOGY. The major anatomic changes stem from the increase in red cell mass, the increase in total blood volume, and the increase in viscosity of the blood.

Plethoric congestion of all organs and tissues is characteristic of polycythemia vera. The major vessels are uniformly distended with a thick viscous blood, which because of the sluggish circulation may not be totally oxygenated. The liver is enlarged and frequently contains foci of myeloid metaplasia. The spleen is enlarged in over 75% of cases and usually weighs 250 to 350 gm. The splenic sinuses are packed with red cells, as are all the vessels within the spleen. Hematopoiesis sometimes can be identified within the red pulp.

Consequent to the increased viscosity and vascular stasis, thromboses and infarctions are common, affecting most often the heart, brain, spleen, and kidneys.

The active bone marrow is the primary site of alteration and is characteristically so increased in size that it floods into the fatty marrow. It has a soft, dark-red succulence. Histologically, this is due to striking hyperplasia of all the erythropoietic forms while the intervening fat cells disappear. Normoblastic proliferation is usually predominant, but there is also some increase in megakaryocytes and granulocytic precursors. The expanding marrow may encroach upon the cancellous bone as well as the cortical shafts. If the disease changes its course, the marrow pattern reflects this alteration and thus may become aplastic, fibrotic, or even leukemic.

Hemorrhages occur in many patients, probably as a result of distention of blood vessels and abnormal platelet function. These affect most often the gastrointestinal tract, urinary tract, oropharynx, and brain. The hemorrhages may be spontaneous, but more often they follow some minor surgical procedure or trauma. Peptic ulceration has been described in about 20% of these patients.

CLINICAL COURSE. Males, usually between the ages of 40 and 60, are affected somewhat more often than females. The condition is more common in whites but also occurs among blacks. The major clinical features of polycythemia vera stem from the increased blood volume, vascular stasis, thrombotic tendency, hemorrhagic diathesis, and transmutation into anemia or leukemia. About 30% of the patients die from some thrombotic complication, affecting usually the brain or the heart. An additional 10 to 15% die from a hemorrhagic condition. Approximately 15 to 20% of cases develop progressive fibrosis of the marrow accompanied by massive splenomegaly, along with other features characteristic of myelofibrosis (p. 686). A small number of patients develop acute leukemia, but the exact incidence is not known. It is clear, however, that the frequency of leukemic transformation is significantly increased in those treated with radioactive phosphorus or myelosuppressive drugs when compared with patients treated with phlebotomy alone. With most forms of therapy, a median survival of 10 to 12 years can be expected. Owing to the high cell turnover, symptomatic gout is seen in 5 to 10% of cases.

Classically, patients with polycythemia are plethoric or even cyanotic. Complaints such as headache, dizziness, gastrointestinal symptoms, hematemesis, and melena are common. Splenic or renal infarction may produce abdominal pain. The bleeding tendency may manifest itself as skin purpura or ecchymoses. Hypertension is a consequence of the increased blood volume. Only when the abnormal increase in the number of red cells is discovered does the basis for these symptoms and signs become apparent, and so the diagnosis is usually made by laboratory studies. The red cell counts range from 6,000,000 to 10,000,000, with hematocrit values of 60% or more. The white cell and platelet counts are elevated frequently, sometimes to levels several-fold above the normal range. Granulocyte alkaline phosphatase is increased in most cases, a point of distinction from chronic granulocytic leukemia (p. 679). Defects in platelet functions, including poor adhesiveness and aggregation, have also been noted.

Secondary Polycythemia

In contrast to primary polycythemia or polycythemia vera, secondary polycythemia refers to an absolute increase in red cell mass secondary to increased levels of erythropoietin. The elaboration of erythropoietin may be an appropriate response to tissue hypoxia, or it may be inappropriately synthesized by a variety of neoplasms.

The polycythemic influences causing appropriate erythropoietin secretion are:

1. Living at high altitudes with low oxygen tensions in the ambient air.
2. Respiratory disease impairing alveolocapillary exchange of oxygen, e.g., chronic obstructive pulmonary disease, chronic left ventricular failure, the pneumoconioses.
3. Abnormal right-to-left shunts in the circulation (cardiac septal defects and arteriovenous aneurysms).
4. Inadequate tissue perfusion as in some forms of shock and low-output cardiac failure.
5. Abnormalities in hemoglobin impairing oxygen dissociation, e.g., variant hemoglobins, methemoglobin.

Inappropriate elaboration of erythropoietin is encountered with a variety of neoplasms—renal cell carcinoma, cerebellar hemangioblastoma, hepatoma, adrenal adenoma, and uterine leiomyoma. It is also seen with hydronephrosis and renal cysts. When found in association with neoplasms, the erythropoietin apparently represents an ectopic secretory product. When seen in association with renal non-neoplastic diseases, it may result from disturbances in intrarenal flow, inducing local tissue hypoxia.

As expected, removal of the implicated tumor or control of the underlying disease is followed promptly by a reversion of the blood count to normal. In contrast to polycythemia vera, the secondary forms of polycythemia usually are not accompanied by any significant elevation in white cell or platelet counts. Moreover, the red cell counts usually are not as markedly elevated as in the primary form of the disease.

BLEEDING DISORDERS—HEMORRHAGIC DIATHESES

It is logical at this point to consider all the significant hemorrhagic disorders, whether they be related to platelet abnormalities or not. All have in common a tendency to spontaneous bleeding and excessive bleeding following trauma or a surgical procedure. Spontaneous bleeding usually takes the form of numerous small hemorrhages (petechiae, purpura) into the skin, mucous membranes, internal organs, joint spaces, or other tissues. Excessive bleeding following trauma may be triggered by such trivial provocations as bumping into the corner of a table or taking a misstep, followed by massive bleeding into the knee joint.

The causes of hemorrhagic diatheses can be divided into (1) increased fragility of vessels, (2) platelet deficiency or dysfunction, (3) derangements in the coagulation mechanism, and (4) combinations of these. Each of these categories is treated in successive sections.

HEMORRHAGIC DIATHESES RELATED TO INCREASED VASCULAR FRAGILITY

Disorders within this category, sometimes called nonthrombocytopenic purpuras, are relatively common but do not usually cause serious bleeding problems. Most often, they induce petechial and purpuric hemorrhages in the skin or mucous membranes, particularly the gingivae. On occasion, however, more significant hemorrhages may occur into joints, muscles, and subperiosteal locations or take the form of menorrhagia, nosebleeds, gastrointestinal bleeding, or hematuria. The platelet count, bleeding time, and coagulation time are usually normal. Sometimes, accompanying abnormalities in either platelet numbers or function contribute to the vascular instability by loss of the endothelial homeostatic role of platelets.

The varied clinical conditions in which hemorrhages can be related to abnormalities in the vessel wall include the following:

Many *infections* induce petechial and purpuric hemorrhages, but especially implicated are meningococcemia, other forms of septicemia, severe measles, and several of the rickettsioses. The involved mechanism is presumably microbiologic damage (vasculitis) to the microvasculature or DIC (p. 649).

Drug reactions sometimes induce abnormal bleeding. In many instances the vascular injury is mediated by the formation of drug-induced antibodies and the deposition of immune complexes in the vessel walls, with the production of a hypersensitivity vasculitis (p. 522).

Scurvy and the Ehlers-Danlos syndrome represent examples of predisposition to hemorrhage related to impaired formation of the collagenous support of vessel walls. Essentially the same mechanism may be encountered in the very elderly in whom atrophy of collagen is implicated. Similar is the predisposition to skin hemorrhages in *Cushing's syndrome*, in which the protein-wasting effects of excessive corticosteroid production cause loss of perivascular supporting tissue.

Henoch-Schönlein purpura is a systemic hypersensitivity disease of unknown cause characterized by a purpuric rash, colicky abdominal pain (presumably due to focal hemorrhages into the gastrointestinal tract), polyarthralgia, and acute glomerulonephritis (p. 1022). All these changes are thought to result from the deposition of circulating immune complexes within vessels throughout the body and within the glomerular mesangial regions. A generalized vasculitis occurs, accompanied by an acute glomerulonephritis. With immunofluorescent techniques, deposits of IgA, C′3, and fibrin can be seen within the mesangial regions of glomeruli. The trigger of the immunologic reaction is unknown, but there is some evidence suggesting activation of the alternate complement pathway because properdin is sometimes found in the glomeruli. In any event, the predisposition to hemorrhage resides in a hypersensitivity vasculitis.

In most of these conditions, the hemorrhagic diathesis does not cause massive bleeding but more often calls attention to the underlying disorder.

HEMORRHAGIC DIATHESES RELATED TO REDUCED PLATELET NUMBER: THROMBOCYTOPENIA

Reductions in platelet number constitute an important cause of generalized bleeding. Depletion of the number of circulating platelets (thrombocytopenia) must be quite severe, to levels of the order of 10,000 to 20,000 platelets per mm^3 (normal range = 150,000 to 300,000 per mm^3) before the hemorrhagic tendency becomes clinically evident.

The important role of platelets in hemostasis was discussed in an earlier chapter (p. 93). It hardly needs reiteration that they are vital to hemostasis in that they form temporary plugs and participate in the clotting reaction. Thus, thrombocytopenia is characterized principally by bleeding, most often from small vessels. The common sites of such hemorrhage are the skin and mucous membranes of the gastrointestinal and genitourinary tracts, where the bleeding is usually associated with the development of small petechiae. Intracranial bleeding is another danger in thrombocytopenic patients with markedly depressed platelet counts.

The many causes of thrombocytopenia are cited in Table 14–7.

A few comments about the rare causes are in order before we turn to the more common forms of thrombocytopenia. *Generalized diseases of bone marrow* may compromise the function or number of megakaryocytes. Thus, thrombocytopenia is seen in aplastic anemia, in the megaloblastic anemias of vitamin B_{12} and folate deficiency, and in the myelophthisic anemias related to metastatic cancer, leukemia, and diffuse myelofibrosis.

Thrombocytopenia apparently due to defective function of megakaryocytes may be encountered in rare congenital disorders such as Fanconi's anemia as well as in infections and drug reactions. In the Wiskott-Aldrich syndrome, a hereditary immunologic deficiency state (p. 208), there is also abnormal megakaryopoiesis.

As with hemolytic anemias, thrombocytopenia may be an acquired disorder related to increased destruction of platelets following infections or drug ingestion. The drugs most commonly involved are quinine, quinidine, chloramphenicol, alkylating agents, antimetabolites, and thiazide diuretics. Immune reactions are implicated in these drug reactions that are essentially similar to those underlying drug-induced hemolytic anemias (p. 629).

Just as red cells may be destroyed by *mechanical injury* in microangiopathic hemolytic anemia, so platelets may be destroyed by prosthetic heart valves, the narrowed microcirculation in malignant hypertension, and arterial disease associated with significant roughening of the endothelial surface.

Thrombocytopenia may appear unpredictably in any patient who has marked splenomegaly, or what has been referred to as *hypersplenism* (p. 699). Normally the spleen sequesters 30 to 40% of the mass of circulating platelets and, when enlarged, sequestrates as much as 90% of all platelets. Should the thrombocytopenia constitute an important part of the clinical problem, it can be cured by splenectomy.

Massive *transfusions* may produce a dilutional thrombocytopenia. Blood stored for longer than 24 hours contains virtually no viable platelets; thus, plasma volume and red cell mass are reconstituted by transfusion, but the number of circulating platelets is relatively reduced.

All these forms of thrombocytopenia are uncommon, compared with the following conditions.

Table 14–7. CAUSES OF THROMBOCYTOPENIA

- Decreased production of platelets
  - Generalized diseases of bone marrow
    - Aplasia, congenital and acquired
    - Invasive disease: leukemia, carcinoma, disseminated infection
    - Deficiency states: folate or vitamin B_{12} deficiency
  - Diseases affecting megakaryocytes specifically
    - Congenital
      - Deficiency of a thrombopoietin-like substance
      - Reduced or absent megakaryocytes, sometimes in association with other congenital defects
      - Normal numbers of megakaryocytes; defective platelets produced
    - Acquired
      - Infection
      - Drugs: cytotoxic drugs, chloramphenicol, thiazides
- Increased destruction of platelets
  - Immunologic
    - Autoimmune (ITP)
    - Isoimmune: neonatal and posttransfusion
    - Drug associated
  - Infection
  - Other drugs: alcohol; gold
  - Increased utilization: disseminated intravascular coagulation
  - Mechanical injury
    - Prosthetic heart valves
    - Thrombotic thrombocytopenic purpura
    - Hemolytic-uremic syndrome
- Sequestration of platelets: large spleen syndrome
- Dilution of platelets: massive transfusions

From Zieve, P. D., et al.: Thrombocytopenia. *In* Zieve, P. D., and Levin, J.: Disorders of Hemostasis. Philadelphia, W. B. Saunders Co., 1976, p. 26.

Neonatal and Posttransfusion (Isoimmune) Thrombocytopenia

Both these disorders are examples of the development of antibodies directed against a specific platelet isoantigen. In addition to HLA and ABO antigens, platelets possess several antigenic determinants not present in other blood cells.[52] These include the Duzo, PL, and Bak antigen systems. Neonatal thrombocytopenia develops in a fashion exactly parallel to the hemolytic reaction in erythroblastosis fetalis (p. 486). A PL^{A1} antigen–negative mother carrying an antigen-positive fetus develops IgG antibodies against the PL^{A1} antigen and the resulting antibodies cross the placenta to cause thrombocytopenia in the newborn. Anti-PL^{A1} antibodies are also believed to be responsible for the purpura associated with posttransfusional thrombocytopenia. In most cases the patient is PL^{A1}-negative and has been sensitized to PL^{A1}-positive blood by either a previous transfusion or pregnancy. When transfused with blood containing PL^{A1}-positive platelets, the anti-PL^{A1} antibody present in the recipient destroys not only the transfused PL^{A1}-positive platelets but also the autologous PL^{A1}-negative platelets, giving rise to thrombocytopenia. How the patient's own PL^{A1}-negative platelets are destroyed is not clear since the anti-PL^{A1} antibody cannot react with them directly. It has been postulated that immune complexes containing anti-PL^{A1} antibody and PL^{A1} antigen eluted from the donor platelets damage the PL^{A1}-negative platelets as "innocent bystanders." Alternatively, PL^{A1}-positive and -negative platelets may share a closely related antigenic determinant with which the anti-PL^{A1} antibody can cross-react. Proof, however, is lacking for either of these hypotheses.

Idiopathic Thrombocytopenic Purpura (ITP)

There is a growing tendency to refer to ITP as autoimmune thrombocytopenia. However, the designation "idiopathic" seems more appropriate for the present time because it is not certain that the cause of the platelet destruction in all cases is autoimmune in origin. Nevertheless, there is general agreement that the thrombocytopenia is mediated by immunologic mechanisms, involving in most cases humoral antibodies or antigen-antibody complexes. Traditionally, ITP has been divided into acute and chronic forms, both of which are associated with increased platelet destruction and normal or increased megakaryocytes in the bone marrow. However, the pathogenesis of reduced platelet survival in the acute and chronic forms is probably quite distinct.

Acute ITP is a self-limited disorder seen most often in children following a viral infection, e.g., rubella, cytomegalovirus, viral hepatitis, and infectious mononucleosis. It is assumed without definite proof that the infection in some way stimulates an immune response that leads to platelet destruction. It may well be that antigen-antibody complexes directed against the virus are adsorbed onto platelets, predisposing to phagocytosis in the mononuclear phagocyte system. Thus, acute ITP as currently understood does not represent direct antiplatelet, antibody-mediated thrombocytopenia.

Chronic ITP occurs most often in adults, particularly in women of childbearing age. It may appear as a primary disease but sometimes is associated with another immunologic disorder such as autoimmune hemolytic anemia or SLE, or occasionally with some form of lymphoproliferative disease.

PATHOGENESIS. There is a great deal of indirect evidence that most patients with chronic ITP have autoantibodies directed against platelets:[53, 54] (1) infants born to mothers with ITP are often thrombocytopenic; (2) the plasma of patients with ITP causes a rapid fall in platelet count when transfused into normal recipients; (3) the serum factor responsible for thrombocytopenia can be localized to the 7 S γ-globulin fraction of plasma and absorbed specifically to human platelets; (4) normal platelets are rapidly destroyed when administered to patients with ITP; and (5) ITP is sometimes encountered in patients with other forms of autoimmune disease such as SLE, autoimmune thyroiditis, and others. Nonetheless, direct evidence for the presence of circulating autoantibodies has been difficult to obtain, since conventional techniques for antibody detection such as agglutination are not easily adaptable for detection of antiplatelet antibodies. With some recently introduced refinements, however, it has been possible to detect and quantitate *platelet-associated immunoglobulins (PAIgG)*, which are elevated in more than 90% of the patients with ITP. More important, the levels of PAIgG are inversely related to the platelet count and the platelet survival, suggesting a pathogenetic role for these antibodies.[55] However, it should be pointed out that the detection of PAIgG in a patient with thrombocytopenia does not necessarily imply that the platelets are coated by autoantibodies. In certain clinical settings (e.g., drug-induced thrombocytopenia), the PAIgG may represent IgG-containing immune complexes bound to the platelet surface through its Fc-IgG receptor.

The exact nature of platelet antigens against which autoantibodies are formed in ITP has not been determined, nor is it clear what triggers autoantibody formation. One or more of the factors discussed previously in the general discussion of autoimmunity may be relevant (p. 177). The increased frequency of HLA-DRW2 and the occurrence of ITP in monozygotic twins suggest that there may be an underlying genetically determined disorder of immune regulation.[53, 56]

The mechanism of platelet destruction is similar to that seen in autoimmune hemolytic anemias (p. 629). Opsonized platelets are rendered susceptible to phagocytosis by the cells of the mononuclear phagocytic system. Lysis by complement fixation seems not to play a major role. About 75 to 80% of patients are remarkably improved or sometimes cured following splenectomy, which suggests that the spleen is the major site of removal of sensitized platelets. Since it is also the major site of autoantibody synthesis, the beneficial effects of splenectomy may in part derive from removal of the source of autoantibodies.

MORPHOLOGY. The principal morphologic lesions of thrombocytopenic purpura are found in the spleen and bone marrow. The secondary changes related to the bleeding diathesis may be found in any tissue or structure in the body.

The **spleen** may be slightly larger than normal but otherwise is grossly within normal limits. Histologically, there is congestion of the sinusoids and hyperactivity and enlargement of the splenic follicles, manifest by the formation of prominent germinal centers. In many instances, megakaryocytes are found within the sinuses and sinusoidal walls. However, in most cases of thrombocytopenic purpura the splenic findings are not distinctive, and in all instances can hardly be considered as pathognomonic of this disorder.

The alterations in the bone marrow are equally disappointing. Most often the bone marrow appears quite normal and contains the usual numbers and types of erythropoietic and leukopoietic cells. An increased number of megakaryocytes is usually seen. Some are apparently immature with large, nonlobulated, single nuclei. These findings are not characteristic of ITP, but merely represent accelerated thrombopoiesis. As such, they are seen in most forms of thrombocytopenia resulting from increased platelet destruction. The importance of the bone marrow examination is to rule out thrombocytopenias resulting from bone marrow failure. A decrease in the number of megakaryocytes virtually rules out the diagnosis of ITP.

The secondary changes relate to the hemorrhages that are dispersed throughout the body. The skin, serosal linings of the body cavities, epicardium and endocardium, lungs, and mucosal lining of the urinary tract are favorite sites for such petechial and ecchymotic hemorrhage (Fig. 14–21). Hemorrhages are also prone to occur in the brain, joint spaces, nasopharynx, and gastrointestinal tract.

The clinical manifestations of this disease are quite variable. Occasionally, the disease begins with a sudden shower of petechial hemorrhages into the skin without apparent antecedent injury or disease. More frequently, there is a long history of easy bruising, nosebleeds, bleeding from the gums, and extensive hemorrhages

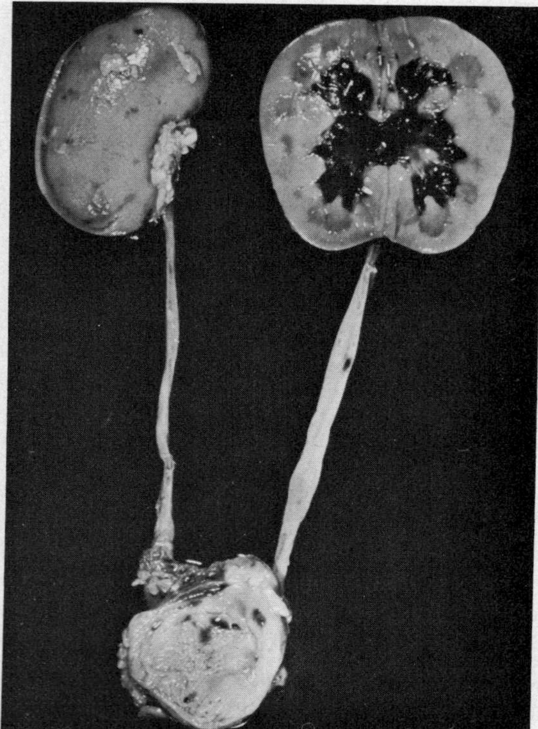

Figure 14–21. Thrombocytopenic purpura. Urinary tract with intrapelvic hemorrhages in kidneys and focal mucosal hemorrhages in urinary bladder.

into soft tissues from relatively minor trauma. Also, the disease may become manifest first by the appearance of melena, hematuria, or excessive menstrual flow. Subarachnoid hemorrhages and intracerebral hemorrhages are serious consequences of thrombocytopenic purpura, but are fortunately rare in patients treated with steroids. Occasionally the development of thrombocytopenia calls attention to the existence of an underlying autoimmune disease (e.g., SLE) or a lymphoproliferative disorder.

The diagnosis can be only suspected in any case characterized by spontaneous or excessive hemorrhages, and must be confirmed by demonstration of thrombocytopenia with normal or increased megakaryocytes in the bone marrow. Accelerated thrombopoiesis also leads to the formation of abnormally large platelets (megathrombocytes) detected easily in a blood smear. The prolongation of the bleeding time and the normal or relatively normal clotting time confirm the presence of thrombocytopenia. *A diagnosis of ITP, however, should be made only after all the possible overt causes for platelet deficiencies, such as those listed in Table 14–7, have been ruled out.*

Thrombotic Thrombocytopenic Purpura (TTP)

This rare disorder of obscure nature is characterized mainly by *thrombocytopenia, microangiopathic hemolytic anemia, fever, transient neurologic deficits, and renal failure.* Underlying most of these clinical manifestations are widespread microthrombi in the arterioles, capillaries, and venules throughout all organs and tissues in the body. The intravascular thrombi are composed primarily of loose aggregates of platelets that become consolidated into amorphous plugs and are eventually replaced by fibrin.[57]

The condition occurs more commonly in females than in males, and usually in young adults. At one time it was regarded as almost invariably fatal, but it is now clear that with appropriate therapy (corticosteroids, splenectomy, platelet aggregation inhibitors, and, most recently, exchange transfusions) many patients survive.

The pathogenesis of this disorder is still a puzzle.[58] Unlike DIC (p. 649), activation of the clotting sequence is not of primary importance. There are many suggestions that TTP is immunologically mediated. Complement components and immunoglobulins can be demonstrated in the vascular lesions. An IgG antibody cytotoxic for cultured human endothelial cells has been reported in some cases.[59] Thus, it has been proposed that this condition involves, for still unknown reasons, an immunologic reaction against endothelial cells predisposing to the aggregation of platelets. Alternatively, it has been proposed that the primary defect is formation of platelet aggregates in the circulation, which then lodge in the microcirculation. It is postulated that these patients synthesize abnormal forms of factor VIII complex, which cause pathologic aggregation of platelets.[59A] Factor VIII, as discussed later, is normally involved in the interaction of platelets with the subendothelial tissues (p. 648). A deficiency of prostacyclin, which normally prevents platelet aggregation, has also been suggested. At our present state of ignorance we can probe no farther into the pathogenesis of this condition. Only two facts seem reasonably clear: the development of myriad platelet aggregates induces the *thrombocytopenia*, and the intravascular thrombi provide a rational explanation for a *microangiopathic form of hemolytic anemia.* These clinicopathologic features are shared by two closely related conditions, the hemolytic-uremic syndrome (p. 1048) and DIC (p. 649). Although the three may have diverse etiologies and somewhat differing patterns of organ involvement, common to all of them is widespread occlusion of the microvasculature due to deranged hemostasis.

HEMORRHAGIC DIATHESES RELATED TO DEFECTIVE PLATELET FUNCTIONS

Qualitative defects of platelet function may be congenital or acquired. Several congenital disorders characterized by prolonged bleeding time and normal platelet count have been described. The significance of these rare diseases lies mainly in the fact that they provide excellent model systems for investigating the molecular mechanisms of platelet functions.[60] On the basis of the predominant functional abnormality, congenital disorders of platelet function may be classified into three groups: (1) *defects of adhesion,* (2) *defects of aggregation,* and (3) *disorders of platelet secretion (release reaction).* Bleeding resulting from defective adhesion of platelets to the subendothelial collagen is best illustrated by the autosomal recessive *Bernard-Soulier syndrome*. In this disorder there is an inherited deficiency of certain platelet membrane glycoproteins that are required for platelet-collagen interaction. Since adhesion of platelets to collagen also requires von Willebrand factor (p. 92), a similar defect is also seen in von Willebrand's disease (p. 648). However, unlike the latter, the prolonged bleeding time in the Bernard-Soulier syndrome cannot be corrected by infusion of plasma containing von Willebrand's factor since the defect is intrinsic to the platelet cell membrane. Bleeding due to *defective platelet aggregation* is exemplified by *thrombasthenia,* which is also transmitted as an autosomal recessive. Thrombasthenic platelets fail to aggregate with ADP, collagen, epinephrine, or thrombin, possibly owing to a deficiency of two membrane glycoproteins that are involved in binding fibrinogen. In normal platelets these glycoproteins favor aggregation, presumably by creating fibrinogen "bridges" between adjacent platelets. *Disorders of platelet secretion* are characterized by normal initial aggregation with collagen or ADP, but the subsequent responses, such as secretion of prostaglandins and release of granule-bound ADP, are impaired. The underlying biochemical defects are varied, complex, and beyond the scope of our discussion.

Among the *acquired defects* of platelet function, two are clinically significant. The first is related to ingestion of aspirin, which may significantly prolong the bleeding time. As you may recall, aspirin is a potent inhibitor of the enzyme cyclooxygenase and can suppress the synthesis of prostaglandins (p. 55), which are known to be involved in platelet aggregation and the subsequent platelet release reaction (p. 94). In approximately 10% of healthy normal subjects, ingestion of even 1 gm of aspirin may prolong the bleeding time significantly and lead to increased bruisability. Clinically, significant postoperative oozing may occur in such patients if aspirin is used as an analgesic. It is suspected that these individuals have minor platelet function defects that are magnified by the intake of aspirin. *Uremia* (p. 997) is the other condition that exemplifies an acquired defect in platelet functions. Although the pathogenesis of bleeding in uremia is complex and poorly understood, recent studies suggest that defective platelet function plays a role possibly related to impaired membrane interaction with von Willebrand factor.[61]

HEMORRHAGIC DIATHESES RELATED TO ABNORMALITIES IN CLOTTING FACTORS

A deficiency of every one of the known clotting factors has been reported at one time or another as the cause of a bleeding disorder. The bleeding in these conditions differs somewhat from that encountered in platelet deficiencies. The apparent spontaneous appearance of petechiae or purpura is uncommon. More often the bleeding manifests as the development of large ecchymoses or hematomas following an injury or prolonged bleeding after a laceration or any form of surgical procedure. Bleeding into the gastrointestinal and urinary tracts, and particularly into weight-bearing joints, is a common manifestation. Typical stories describe the patient who continues to ooze for days following a tooth extraction or who develops a hemarthrosis after a relatively trivial stress on a knee joint. History may well have been changed by the presence of a hereditary coagulation defect in the intermarried royal families of Great Britain and Europe. Clotting abnormalities may occur as acquired defects, or, as mentioned, be hereditary in origin.

Acquired disorders are usually characterized by multiple clotting abnormalities. Vitamin K deficiency (p. 412) results in depressed synthesis of factors II, VII, IX, and X. Since the liver makes virtually all of the clotting factors except for factor VIII, severe parenchymal liver disease may be associated with a hemorrhagic diathesis. DIC (p. 649) produces a deficiency of multiple coagulation factors.

Hereditary deficiencies have been identified for each of the clotting factors. Deficiency of factor VIII (classic hemophilia) and factor IX (Christmas disease) are transmitted as sex-linked recessive disorders. Most of the others follow autosomal patterns of transmission. *Typically, these hereditary disorders involve a single clotting factor.*

The details of the diagnostic tests used to identify the specific clotting factor deficiency are beyond our scope and are readily available in specialized texts.[62] In most cases, four screening procedures will localize the hemostatic abnormality: (1) the prothrombin time (PT), (2) the partial thromboplastin time (PTT), (3) the thrombin time (TT), and (4) assay of fibrin split products. Against this background we can turn to the more common of the coagulation disorders.

Deficiencies of Factor VIII Complex

Until recently, classic hemophilia was the only disorder known to be caused by a deficiency of factor VIII, the antihemophilic globulin. Subsequent observations make clear, however, that greater complexities exist. Factor VIII is no longer considered a single protein but a complex whose components are differentially affected in hemophilia and von Willebrand's disease. It is best, therefore, to begin our discussion with a review of the structure and functions of factor VIII.[63]

Currently, *plasma factor VIII is considered to be a complex made up of two components that can be distinguished by functional, biochemical, immunologic, and genetic criteria.* One component, which is required for the activation of factor X in the intrinsic coagulation pathway, is designated factor VIII:C, because of its role in the coagulation cascade. It is this component that has been referred to as factor VIII in the past and is deficient in classic hemophilia. Through noncovalent bonds, factor VIII:C is complexed to another, much larger component, called factor VIII–related protein (VIII:R). This latter component, which is required for the interaction of platelets with the subendothelium, is reduced in von Willebrand's disease, and hence is also called *von Willebrand's factor*. Although they circulate together in the form of a complex, the two functional components of factor VIII have distinct antigenic determinants, which are identified as factor VIII:CAg and factor VIII:RAg. Von Willebrand's factor (VIII:R) can also be detected in vitro by its ability to promote platelet aggregation induced by ristocetin (an antibiotic). Although ristocetin has no clinical usefulness as an antibiotic, it serves as a valuable tool for the detection of factor VIII:R in the laboratory. This in vitro function has earned yet another name for von Willebrand's factor, namely, *ristocetin cofactor (VIIIR:RC)*. The two components of factor VIII complex (VIII:C and VIII:R) appear to be products of separate genes, a concept supported by the distinct patterns of inheritance of hemophilia and von Willebrand's disease. Since hemophilia characterized by deficiency of factor VIII:C is inherited as a sex-linked recessive, it can reasonably be concluded that the gene coding for the procoagulant protein resides on the X chromosome. On the other hand, the gene (or genes) coding for von Willebrand's factor appear to be located on one or more autosomes, since von Willebrand's disease is inherited as an autosomal dominant. The site where factor VIII:C is synthesized is not yet certain, but the liver seems to be the favored organ. With respect to factor VIII:R, there is good evidence for synthesis by endothelial cells and possibly by megakaryocytes. *In summary, the two components of factor VIII complex (synthesized at separate sites) come together and circulate in the plasma as a complex molecule, which serves to promote clotting as well as platelet–vessel wall interaction necessary to ensure hemostasis.* With this background, we can discuss hemophilia and von Willebrand's disease, the two most common inherited disorders of bleeding.

HEMOPHILIA

This disease, also called hemophilia A or classic hemophilia, results from a reduced amount or activity of factor VIII:C. In keeping with sex-linked recessive inheritance, this condition occurs preponderantly in males and is usually transmitted by either affected fathers or carrier heterozygous mothers. Rarely, a female heterozygote with extremely unfavorable lyonization (i.e., inactivation of the normal X chromosome in the majority of cells) may also manifest hemophilia. It is important to note that at least 25% of the patients do not have a family history of hemophilia, suggesting a fairly high frequency of de novo mutations. A practical implication of this observation is that a negative family history cannot be used to rule out hemophilia.[64] As mentioned earlier, patients with hemophilia have reduced factor VIII procoagulant activity, but factor VIII:RAg and ristocetin cofactor are normal. The difference in levels of the two components of factor VIII is a fairly sensitive index, which can be used for the diagnosis of hemophilia as well as for detection of carriers. There is wide variation in the degree of factor VIII:C deficiency, the levels ranging from less than 1% of normal in severe cases to 5 to 50% in mildly affected cases. This variation is best explained by assuming that more than one type of mutation is involved. In most patients, factor VIII:CAg level is reduced in parallel with the decrease in functional procoagulant activity, but in approximately 10% of patients, factor VIII:CAg levels are normal even though coagulant activity is low. To account for this disparity, the theory has been invoked of a mutation that causes the synthesis of a nonfunctional but antigenically normal protein.

The clinical severity of hemophilia reflects the degree of factor VIII:C deficiency. Approximately 20% of patients who have mild disease rarely suffer bleeding episodes and come to attention only after dental or surgical procedures. Another 25% have moderately severe disease and bleed profusely even after minor trauma; however, spontaneous hemorrhage is not seen. Unfortunately, the majority (55%) have severe disease with frequent severe spontaneous hemorrhages, particularly in weight-bearing joints, giving rise to serious arthropathy in childhood. Such disabling complications can be reduced by replacement therapy in the form of cryoprecipitates or lyophilized factor VIII concentrates obtained from normal plasma. Therapy, however, is not without its problems. Recent reports point to the development of acquired immunodeficiency syndrome (AIDS, p. 208) in some hemophiliacs.[65] *Those who receive lyophilized preparations of factor VIII seem to be at particular risk.* How AIDS and therapy with lyophilized factor VIII are related is not known but transmission of an unidentified infectious agent is strongly suspected. The higher risk associated with transfusion of lyophilized factor VIII preparations may be related to the fact that these preparations (unlike cryoprecipitates) are derived from the pooled plasma of 2000 to 5000 donors; understandably, the multiplicity of donors increases the chance that one or more of the plasma donors may be an unsuspected carrier of the AIDS "agent."

VON WILLEBRAND'S DISEASE

This complex hemorrhagic disorder is characterized clinically by spontaneous bleeding from mucous membranes, menorrhagia, excessive bleeding from wounds, and a prolonged bleeding time.[63, 66] In most cases it is transmitted as an autosomal dominant, but rare autosomal recessive forms have also been described.

The underlying cause of von Willebrand's disease appears to be qualitative or quantitative defects of factor VIII:R. Recall that this component of factor VIII complex is required for the adhesion of platelets to subendothelial collagen. Thus, a deficiency of factor VIII:R results in a qualitative platelet defect, although the platelets themselves are intrinsically normal (in contrast with the Bernard-Soulier syndrome, p. 647). Deficiency of factor VIII:R can be detected by impaired ristocetin-induced platelet aggregation and reduced levels of factor

VIII:R antigen. Quite unexpectedly, *levels of factor VIII:C, the procoagulant component of factor VIII complex, are also reduced.* Even more puzzling is the observation that infusion of factor VIII:C–deficient (hemophilic) plasma causes an increase in the level of procoagulant activity. This observation, taken with the autosomal pattern of inheritance, suggests that these patients have the genetic capacity to synthesize factor VIII:C. Why factor VIII:C levels are low, then, is not clear. It has been postulated that normal factor VIII:R either protects the procoagulant component (VIII:C) from degradation or influences its synthesis and release in some undefined manner. *To summarize, in the most common form, called "classical" von Willebrand's disease, there is a deficiency of factor VIII:R manifested by reduced factor VIII:RAg and VIIIR:RC (ristocetin cofactor) accompanied by a secondary deficiency of factor VIII:C.* There is thus a compound defect involving both platelet functions and the coagulation pathway. Several much less common variant forms of von Willebrand's disease have also been described. In some of these, the level of factor VIIIR:Ag is normal but the ristocetin cofactor (VIII R:RC) is reduced, suggesting the synthesis of an antigenically normal but nonfunctional factor VIII:R. Although all these new findings might be considered a "tempest in a teapot," recent studies point out that von Willebrand's factor may also be important in other diseases. Thus, it may be involved in the pathogenesis of atherosclerosis, possibly by enhancing platelet adhesion to sites of endothelial injury. For now, we must leave it that von Willebrand's disease manifests as an inherited hemorrhagic diathesis that may be more common than has been appreciated.

Factor IX Deficiency (Christmas Disease, Hemophilia B)

Factor IX deficiency can be briefly characterized as a more rare but more severe form of hemophilia. The interesting designation Christmas disease has no festive connotation; it refers to the name of the original patient identified with this disorder. Two distinctive forms have been recognized, one with apparently normal levels of inactive protein and another with deficient levels of the coagulant factor. Both are transmitted by sex-linked recessive inheritance similar to the mode of transmission of classic hemophilia. Rarely, factor IX deficiency is encountered in patients having severe forms of protein-losing glomerulopathies. The bleeding in Christmas disease is usually severe and, when it affects joints, frequently leads to crippling deformities.

DISSEMINATED INTRAVASCULAR COAGULATION (DIC, CONSUMPTION COAGULOPATHY)

Disseminated intravascular coagulation is an acquired thrombohemorrhagic disorder occurring as a secondary complication in a variety of diseases. It is characterized by activation of the coagulation sequence that leads to the formation of microthrombi throughout the microcirculation of the body, but often in a quixotically uneven distribution. Sometimes the coagulopathy is localized to a specific organ or tissue. *As a consequence of the thrombotic diathesis, there is consumption of platelets, fibrin, and coagulation factors and, secondarily, activation of fibrinolytic mechanisms* (p. 96). Thus, DIC may present as an acute complication with signs and symptoms relating to tissue hypoxia and infarction caused by the myriad microthrombi, or as a hemorrhagic disorder related to depletion of the elements required for hemostasis (hence the term *consumption coagulopathy*). Activation of the fibrinolytic mechanism aggravates the hemorrhagic diathesis. Because of the consumption and secondary lysis of fibrin, DIC is also called *defibrination syndrome*

ETIOLOGY AND PATHOGENESIS. At the outset it must be emphasized the DIC is not a primary disease. It is a coagulopathy that occurs in the course of a variety of clinical conditions. In discussing the general mechanisms underlying DIC, it would be useful to review briefly the normal process of blood coagulation and clot removal discussed earler (p. 91). It suffices here to recall that clotting may be initiated by either of two pathways: (1) the *extrinsic pathway*, which is triggered by the release of tissue thromboplastin; and (2) the *intrinsic pathway*, which involves the activation of factor XII by surface contact with collagen or other negatively charged substances. Both pathways, through a series of intermediate steps, result in the generation of thrombin, which in turn converts fibrinogen to fibrin. This process is regulated by *clot-inhibiting influences*, which include the activation of fibrinolysis involving generation of plasmin, and the clearance of activated clotting factors by the reticuloendothelial system or by the liver. From this brief review, it may be concluded that DIC may result from pathologic activation of the extrinsic and/or intrinsic pathways of coagulation or impairment of clot-inhibiting influences. Since the latter rarely constitute primary mechanisms of DIC, we will focus our attention on the abnormal initiation of clotting.[67]

There are two major mechanisms by which DIC may be triggered: (1) release of tissue thromboplastin or thromboplastic substances into the circulation; (2) widespread injury to the endothelial cells. Tissue thromboplastins initiate the extrinsic pathway and may be derived from a variety of sources, such as placenta in obstetric complications (Table 14–8) and the granules of leukemic cells in acute promyelocytic leukemia (p. 684). Mucus released from certain adenocarcinomas can also act as a thromboplastic substance by directly activating factor X, independent of factor VII. In gram-negative sepsis, bacterial endotoxins can cause release of thromboplastic substances contained within the lysosomes of granulocytes and monocytes. Endothelial injury, the other major trigger, can initiate DIC by causing platelet aggregation and by activating the intrinsic coagulation pathway. Widespread endothelial injury may be produced by deposition of antigen-antibody complexes

Table 14–8. MAJOR DISORDERS ASSOCIATED WITH DIC

1. Obstetric Complications
Abruptio placentae
Retained dead fetus
Septic abortion
Amniotic fluid embolism
Toxemia
2. Infections
Gram-negative sepsis
Meningococcemia
Rocky Mountain spotted fever
Histoplasmosis
Aspergillosis
Malaria
3. Neoplasms
Carcinomas of pancreas, prostate, lung, and stomach
Acute promyelocytic leukemia
4. Massive Tissue Injury
Traumatic
Burns
Extensive surgery
5. Miscellaneous
Acute intravascular hemolysis, snakebite, giant hemangioma, shock, heatstroke, vasculitis, aortic aneurysm, liver disease

(e.g., SLE), temperature extremes (e.g., heat stroke, burns), or microorganisms (e.g., meningococci, rickettsiae).

Several disorders associated with DIC are listed in Table 14–8. Of these, DIC is most likely to follow *obstetric causes, malignancy, sepsis,* and *major trauma.* The initiating factors in these conditions are often multiple and interrelated. For example, in *infections,* particularly those caused by gram-negative bacteria, endotoxins released by the bacteria may activate both the intrinsic and extrinsic pathways by producing endothelial cell injury and release of thromboplastins from inflammatory cells. Endothelial cell damage may also be produced directly by meningococci, rickettsiae, and viruses. Antigen-antibody complexes formed during the infection can activate the classic complement pathway, and the complement fragments can secondarily activate both platelets and granulocytes. Endotoxins as well as other bacterial products are also capable of directly activating factor XII. In *massive trauma, extensive surgery,* and *severe burns,* the major mechanism of DIC is believed to be autoinfusion of tissue thromboplastins. In *obstetric* conditions thromboplastins derived from the placenta, dead retained fetus, or amniotic fluid may enter the circulation. However, hypoxia, acidosis, and shock, which often coexist with the surgical and obstetric conditions, can also cause widespread endothelial injury. Supervening infection may complicate the problems further. Among *cancers,* acute promyelocytic leukemia and carcinomas of the lung, pancreas, prostate, and stomach are most frequently associated with DIC.[68] These tumors are associated with the release of a variety of thromboplastic substances including tissue factors, proteolytic enzymes, mucin, and other undefined tumor products.

The consequences of DIC are twofold. First, there is widespread deposition of fibrin within the microcirculation. This may lead to ischemia of the more severely affected or more vulnerable organs, and to a hemolytic anemia resulting from fragmentation of red cells as they squeeze through the narrowed microvasculature (microangiopathic hemolytic anemia, p. 629). Second, a hemorrhagic diathesis may dominate the clinical picture. This results from consumption of platelets and clotting factors as well as activation of plasminogen. Plasmin can not only cleave fibrin but also digest factors V and VIII, thereby reducing their concentration further. In addition, fibrinolysis leads to the formation of fibrin degradation products, which inhibit platelet aggregation and fibrin polymerization, and have antithrombin activity. All these influences lead to the hemostatic failure seen in DIC (Fig. 14–22).

MORPHOLOGY. In general, thrombi are found in the following sites in decreasing order of frequency: brain, heart, lungs, kidneys, adrenals, spleen, and liver.[69] However, no tissue is spared and occasionally thrombi are found in only one or several organs without affecting others. In giant hemangiomas, for example, they are localized to the neoplasm. In this condition they are believed to result from local stasis and recurrent trauma to the poorly supported blood vessels. Sometimes they affect only the kidneys and here may induce only focal tubular cell necrosis, but in severe cases microinfarcts or even bilateral renal cortical necrosis may result. Numerous fibrin thrombi may be found in the alveolar capillaries, sometimes associated with pulmonary edema and exudation of fibrin, to create "hyaline membranes." In the central nervous system, microinfarcts may be caused by the fibrin thrombi, occasionally complicated by simultaneous fresh hemorrhage. Such changes are the basis for the bizarre neurologic signs and symptoms sometimes observed in this syndrome. Microthrombi may appear in the myocardium, but only rarely are they associated with infarction. The manifestations of DIC in the endocrine glands are of considerable interest. In meningococcemia, the massive adrenal hemorrhages of the Waterhouse-Friderichsen syndrome (p. 1236) are probably related to fibrin thrombi within the microcirculation of the adrenal cortex. Similarly, Sheehan's postpartum pituitary necrosis (p. 1198) may be one of the expressions of DIC. In toxemia of pregnancy (p. 1155), the placenta exhibits widespread microthrombi, providing a plausible explanation for the premature atrophy of the cytotrophoblast and syncytiotrophoblast encountered in this condition.

The bleeding manifestations of DIC are not dissimilar to those encountered in the hereditary and acquired disorders affecting the hemostatic mechanism discussed above.

CLINICAL COURSE. The onset may be fulminating, as in endotoxic shock or amniotic fluid embolism, or it may be insidious and chronic, as in cases of carcinomatosis or retention of a dead fetus. Overall, about 50% of individuals with DIC are obstetric patients having complications of pregnancy. In this setting, the disorder tends to be reversible with delivery of the fetus. About 33% of the patients have carcinomatosis. The remaining cases are associated with the very varied entities previously listed. The myriad manifestations may be slight or climactic and depend on whether circulatory obstruc-

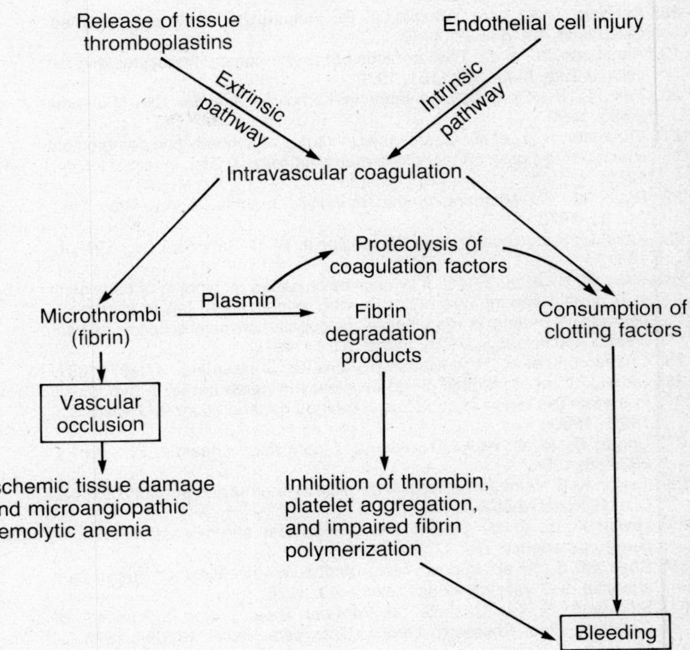

Figure 14–22. Pathophysiology of DIC.

tion or bleeding tendencies predominate and where the intravascular coagulation strikes. It is almost impossible to detail all the potential clinical presentations, but a few common patterns may be cited. A microangiopathic hemolytic anemia may appear. Respiratory symptoms such as dyspnea, cyanosis, and extreme respiratory difficulty may predominate. Neurologic signs and symptoms represent another pattern including convulsions and coma. Renal changes such as oliguria and acute renal failure may dominate. Circulatory failure and shock may appear suddenly or develop progressively. In general, *acute DIC, associated for example with obstetric complications or major trauma, is dominated by bleeding diathesis, whereas chronic DIC such as may occur in a patient with cancer tends to present initially with thrombotic complications.* But in all instances the signs and symptoms may change during the course of the disease as thrombotic manifestations are replaced by hemorrhagic complications, or vice versa. Accurate clinical observation and laboratory studies are necessary for the diagnosis. It is usually necessary to monitor the following: fibrinogen, platelets, prothrombin time, thrombin time, partial thromboplastin time, and fibrin degradation products.

The prognosis is highly variable and depends, to a considerable extent, on the underlying disorder. The management of these cases requires meticulous maneuvering between the Scylla of the thrombotic tendency and the Charybdis of the bleeding diathesis. Thus is posed the dilemma of whether to attempt to block coagulation or to control bleeding by the administration of coagulants. Each patient must be treated individually and, depending on the clinical picture, potent anticoagulants such as heparin and antithrombin III or coagulants in the form of fresh-frozen plasma may be administered. Platelet transfusions may sometimes be necessary. DIC is another of the therapeutist's nightmares.

---

1. Dexter, T. M.: Stromal cell associated hemopoiesis. J. Cell Physiol. (Suppl 1):87, 1982.
2. Wintrobe, M. M., et al.: Clinical Hematology. 8th ed. Philadelphia, Lea & Febiger, 1981.
3. Mohandas, N., et al.: Red blood cell deformability and hemolytic anemias. Semin. Hematol. *16*:95, 1979.
4. Wolfe, L. C., et al.: A genetic defect in the binding of protein 4.1 to spectrin in a kindred with hereditary spherocytosis. N. Engl. J. Med. *307*:1367, 1982.

4A. Marchesi, V. T.: The red cell membrane skeleton: Recent progress. Blood *61*:1, 1983.

5. Lux, S. E.: Disorders of the red cell membrane skeleton: Hereditary spherocytosis and hereditary elliptocytosis. *In* Stanbury, J. B., et al. (eds.): Metabolic Basis of Inherited Disease. 5th ed. New York, McGraw-Hill Book Co., 1982, p.1573.
6. Beutler, E.: Glucose-6-phosphatase dehydrogenase deficiency. *In* Stanbury, J. B., et al. (eds.): Metabolic Basis of Inherited Disease. 5th ed. New York, McGraw-Hill Book Co., 1982, p.1629.
7. Dean, J., and Schechter, A. N.: Sickle cell anemia: Molecular and cellular bases of therapeutic approaches. N. Engl. J. Med. *299*:752, 804, 863, 1978.
8. Schechter, A. N., and Bunn, H. F.: What determines severity in sickle cell disease? N. Engl. J. Med. *306*:295, 1982.
9. Eaton, J. W., and Hebbel, R. P.: Pathogenesis of sickle cell disease. Pathobiol. Annu. *11*:31, 1981.
10. McCurdy, P. R., and Sherman, A. S.: Irreversibly sickled cells and red cell survival in sickle cell anemia. A study with both $DF^{32}P$ and ^{51}Cr. Am. J. Med. *64*:253, 1978.
11. Noguchi, C. T., and Schechter, A. N.: The intracellular polymerization of sickle hemoglobin and its relevance to sickle cell disease. Blood *58*:1057, 1981.
12. Chang, J. C., and Kan, Y. W.: A sensitive prenatal test for sickle cell anemia. N. Engl. J. Med. *307*:30, 1982.
13. Benz, E. J., and Forget, B. G.: The thalassemia syndromes: Models for molecular analysis of human disease. Annu. Rev. Med. *33*:363, 1982.
14. Benz, E. J., and Forget, B. G.: Pathogenesis of the thalassemia syndromes. Pathobiol. Annu. *10*:1, 1980.
15. Orkin, S. H., et al.: Cloning and direct examination of a structurally abnormal human beta^0-thalassemia globin gene. Proc. Natl. Acad. Sci. U.S.A. *77*:3558, 1980.
16. Steinberg, M. H., and Adams, J. G.: Thalassemia: Recent insights into molecular mechanisms. Am. J. Hematol. *12*:81, 1982.
17. Rosse, W. F.: Paroxysmal hemoglobinuria: Present status and future prospects. West. J. Med. *132*:219, 1980.

18. Axelson, J. A., and LoBuglio, A. F.: Immune hemolytic anemia. Med. Clin. North Am. *64*:597, 1980.
19. Abramson, N., et al.: The interaction between human monocytes and red cells. J. Exp. Med. *132*:1191, 1970.
20. Petz, L. D.: Drug-induced immune hemolytic anemia. Clin. Hematol. *9*:455, 1980.
21. Kurlander, R. J., et al.: Quantitative influence of antibody and complement coating of red cells on monocyte-mediated lysis. J. Clin. Invest. *61*:1309, 1978.
22. Brain, M. C.: Microangiopathic hemolytic anemia. Annu. Rev. Med. *21*:133, 1970.
23. Kass, L.: Pernicious Anemia. Philadelphia, W. B. Saunders Co., 1976, p. 186.
24. Allen, R. H., et al.: Effect of proteolytic enzymes on binding of cobalamin to R protein and intrinsic factor. In vitro evidence that failure to partially degrade R protein is responsible for cobalamin malabsorption in pancreatic insufficiency. J. Clin. Invest. *61*:47, 1978.
25. Chanarin, I., et al.: How vitamin B_{12} acts. Br. J. Haematol. *47*:487, 1981.
26. Dinn, J. J., et al.: Methyl group deficiency in nerve tissue: A hypothesis to explain the lesion of subacute combined degeneration. Ir. J. Med. Sci. *149*:1, 1980.
27. Ungar, B., et al.: HLA-DR patterns in pernicious anaemia. Br. Med. J. *282*:768, 1981.
28. Taylor, K. B.: Immune aspects of pernicious anemia and atrophic gastritis. Clin. Hematol. *5*:497, 1976.
29. Lewin, K. J., et al.: Gastric morphology and serum gastrin levels in pernicious anemia. Gut *17*:551, 1976.
30. Rose, M. S., et al.: Intrinsic factor antibodies in absence of pernicious anaemia. 3–7 year follow-up. Lancet *2*:9, 1970.
31. Strickland, R. G.: Gastritis. *In* Van der Reis, L. (ed.): Frontiers of Gastrointestinal Research. Immune Disorders. Basel, Karger, 1975, p. 12.
32. Magnus, H. A.: A reassessment of the gastric lesion in pernicious anaemia. J. Clin. Pathol. (Lond.) *11*:289, 1958.
33. Payne, R. W.: Pernicious anaemia and gastric cancer in England and Wales. Br. Med. J. *1*:1807, 1961.
34. Leevy, C. M., et al.: Incidence and significance of hypovitaminemia in a randomly selected municipal hospital population. Am. J. Clin. Nutr. *17*:269, 1965.
35. Conrad, M. E., and Barton, J. C.: Factors affecting iron balance. Am. J. Hematol. *10*:199, 1981.
36. Finch, C. A., and Heubers, H.: Perspectives in iron metabolism. N. Engl. J. Med. *306*:1520, 1982.
37. Aisen, P.: Current concepts in iron metabolism. Clin. Hematol. *11*:241, 1982.
38. Harrison, P. M., et al.: Ferritin structure and function. *In* Jacobs, A., and Worwood, M. (eds.): Iron in Biochemistry and Medicine. II. London, Academic Press, 1981, p. 131.
39. Heubers, H. A., et al.: The significance of transferrin for intestinal iron absorption. Blood *61*:283, 1983.
40. Powell, L. W., and Halliday, J. W.: Iron absorption and iron overload. Clin. Gastroenterol. *10*:707, 1981.
41. Rosenmund, A., et al.: Regulation of iron absorption and storage iron turnover. Blood *56*:30, 1980.
42. Appelbaum, F. R., and Fefer, A.: The pathogenesis of aplastic anemia. Semin. Hematol. *4*:241, 1981.
43. Camitta, B. M., et al.: Aplastic anemia. N. Engl. J. Med. *306*:645, 1982.
43A. Zeldis, J. B., et al.: Aplastic anemia and non-A, non-B, hepatitis. Am. J. Med. *74*:64, 1983.
44. Gale, R. P., et al.: Aplastic anemia: Biology and treatment. Ann. Intern. Med. *95*:477, 1981.
45. Champlin, R., et al.: Antithymocyte globulin treatment in patients with aplastic anemia: A prospective randomized trial. N. Engl. J. Med. *308*:113, 1983.
46. Krantz, S. B.: Pure red cell aplasia. N. Engl. J. Med. *291*:345, 1975.
47. Messner, H. A., et al.: Control of antibody mediated pure red cell aplasia by plasmapheresis. N. Engl. J. Med. *304*:1334, 1981.
48. Golde, D. W., et al.: Polycythemia: Mechanism and management. Ann. Intern. Med. *95*:71, 1981.
49. Dameshek, W.: The myeloproliferative disorders. *In* Clark, W. J. (ed.): Myeloproliferative Disorders of Animals and Man. Washington, D.C., U.S. Atomic Energy Commission, 1970, p. 413.
50. Jacobson, R. J., et al.: Agnogenic myeloid metaplasia. A clonal proliferation of hematopoietic stem cells with secondary myelofibrosis. Blood *51*:189, 1978.
51. Ash, R. C., et al.: In vitro studies of human pluripotent hematopoietic progenitors in polycythemia vera. Direct evidence of stem cell involvement. J. Clin. Invest. *69*:1112, 1982.
52. Klein, C. A., and Blajchman, M. A.: Alloantibodies and platelet destruction. Semin. Thromb. Hemost. *8*:105, 1982.
53. Karpatkin, S.: Autoimmune thrombocytopenic purpura. Blood *56*:329, 1980.
54. Kelton, J. G., and Gibbons, S.: Autoimmune platelet destruction: idiopathic thrombocytopenic purpura. Semin. Thromb. Hemostas. *8*:83, 1982.
55. Kernoff, L. M., et al.: Influence of the amount of platelet-bound IgG on platelet survival and site of sequestration in autoimmune thrombocytopenia. Blood *55*:730, 1980.
56. Laster, A. J., et al.: Chronic immune thrombocytopenic purpura in monozygotic twins: Genetic factors predisposing to ITP. N. Engl. J. Med. *307*:1495, 1982.
57. Pisciotta, A., et al.: Clinical features of thrombotic thrombocytopenic purpura. Semin. Thromb. Hemostas. *6*:330, 1980.
58. Brain, M. C., and Neame, P. B.: Thrombotic thrombocytopenic purpura and the hemolytic uremic syndrome. Semin. Thromb. Hemostas. *8*:186, 1982.
59. Burns, E. R., and Zucker-Franklin, D.: Pathologic effects of plasma from patients with thrombotic thrombocytopenic purpura on platelets and cultured vascular endothelial cells. Blood *60*:1030, 1982.
59A. Moake, J. L., et al.: Unusually large plasma factor VIII: von Willebrand factor multimers in chronic relapsing thrombotic thrombocytopenic purpura. N. Engl. J. Med. *307*:1432, 1982.
60. Weiss, H. J.: Congenital disorder of platelet function. Semin. Hematol. *17*:228, 1980.
61. Carvalho, A. C. A.: Bleeding in uremia: A clinical challenge. N. Engl. J. Med. *308*:38, 1983.
62. Handin, R. I., and Rosenberg, R. D.: Hemorrhagic disorders. III. Disorders of primary and secondary hemostasis. *In* Beck, W. S. (ed.): Hematology. 2nd ed. Cambridge, MA, MIT Press, 1977, p. 547.
63. Hoyer, L.W.: The factor VIII complex: Structure and function. Blood *58*:1, 1981.
64. Aledrot, L. M.: Current concepts in diagnosis and management of hemophilia. Hosp. Pract. *17*:78, 1982.
65. Desforges, J.: AIDS and preventive treatment in hemophilia. N. Engl. J. Med. *308*:94, 1983.
66. Bloom, A. L.: The von Willebrand syndrome. Semin. Hematol. *17*:215, 1980.
67. Ockelford, P. A., and Carter, C. J.: Disseminated intravascular coagulation: The application and utility of diagnostic tests. Semin. Thromb. Hemostas. *8*:198, 1982.
68. Bell, W. R.: Disseminated intravascular coagulation. Johns Hopkins Med. J. *146*:289, 1980.
69. Kim, H.-S., et al.: Clinical unsuspected disseminated intravascular coagulation. Am. J. Clin. Pathol. *66*:31, 1976.

DISEASES OF WHITE CELLS, LYMPH NODES, AND SPLEEN* 15

White Cells and Lymph Nodes

*With gratitude to Dr. Jose Hernandez, Southwestern Medical School, Dallas, Texas, for a critical review of this chapter.

NORMAL

The origin and differentiation of white cells (granulocytes, monocytes, and lymphocytes) were briefly discussed in Chapter 14 along with the other formed elements of blood. Lymphocytes and monocytes not only circulate in the blood and lymph, but also accumulate in discrete and organized masses, the so-called lymphoreticular system. Components of this system include lymph nodes, thymus, spleen, tonsils, adenoids, and Peyer's patches. Less discrete collections of lymphoid cells also occur in the bone marrow, lungs, and gastrointestinal tract and other tissues. Lymph nodes are the most widely distributed and easily accessible component of the lymphoid tissue and are therefore frequently examined for the diagnosis of lymphoreticular disorders. It would therefore be advantageous to review the normal morphology of lymph nodes.

Lymph nodes, in general, are discrete structures, ovoid in shape, that vary from a few millimeters to 1 to 2 cm in length. Their consistency is soft and their cut surface is gray-white. They are surrounded by a capsule composed of connective tissue and a few elastic fibrils, perforated at various points by afferent lymphatics that empty into the peripheral sinus subjacent to the capsule. Branches of the sinus extend into the nodes and terminate at the hilus, where the efferent lymphatics emerge. All lymphatics are lined with reticuloendothelial cells. Situated in the cortex or peripheral portion of the node are spherical aggregates of lymphoid tissue, the so-called primary follicles, which represent the B-cell areas. Upon antigenic stimulation, the primary follicles enlarge and develop pale-staining germinal centers composed of follicular center cells (lymphocytes in varying stages of activation, described on p. 663). Surrounding these germinal centers are mantles of small unchallenged B cells. The T cells occupy the parafollicular regions (p. 158). The medullary cords, occupying the central portion of the node, contain predominantly plasma cells and some lymphocytes. A delicate reticulin that connects peripherally with the capsule is the predominant supporting structure within the lymph nodes.

The morphologic description of the lymph node just given is highly idealized and falsely static. The size and morphology of lymph nodes are modified by stress, thyroid and adrenal function, and immune responses. As secondary lines of defense, they are constantly responding to stimuli, even in the absence of clinical disease. Trivial injuries and infections effect subtle changes in lymph node histology. More significant bacterial infections inevitably produce enlargement of nodes and sometimes leave residual scarring. For this reason, lymph nodes in the adult are almost never "normal," since they usually bear the scars of previous events, rendering the inguinal nodes particularly inappropriate for evaluative biopsies. Except in the child, it is difficult to find a "normal" node, and in histologic evaluations it is often necessary to distinguish changes secondary to past experience from those related to present disease.

PATHOLOGY

Disorders of white cells may be classified into two broad categories, *proliferative* and those characterized by a deficiency of leukocytes, i.e., *leukopenias*. Proliferations of white cells and lymph nodes may be reactive or neoplastic. Since their major function is host defense, reactive proliferation in response to an underlying primary, often microbial disease is fairly common. Neoplastic disorders, although less frequent, are much more important. In the following discussion, we will describe first the leukopenic states and summarize the common reactive disorders, and then consider in some detail malignant proliferations of the white cells that in many instances arise in the nodes.

LEUKOPENIA

The number of circulating white cells may be markedly decreased in a variety of disorders. An abnormally low white cell count *(leukopenia)* may occur because of decreased numbers of any one of the specific types of leukocytes, but most often involves the neutrophils *(neutropenia, granulocytopenia)*. *Lymphopenias* are much less common, and in addition to the congenital immunodeficiency diseases (p. 205) they are associated with specific clinical syndromes (e.g., Hodgkin's disease, nonlymphocytic leukemias, following corticosteroid therapy, and occasionally in chronic diseases). Only the more common leukopenias involving granulocytes will be discussed here.

Neutropenia—Agranulocytosis

Reduction in the number of granulocytes in the peripheral blood—*neutropenia*—may be seen in a wide variety of circumstances. Frequently it is transient and of trivial significance. Sometimes the reduction in circulating neutrophils is marked and has serious consequences by predisposing to infections. When of this magnitude, it is referred to as *agranulocytosis*. The lymphocytes are not affected, so the percentage of lymphocytes is increased (relative lymphocytosis).

PATHOGENESIS. Considering first the broad topic of neutropenia, whatever its severity, a reduction in circulating granulocytes will occur if (1) granulopoiesis fails to keep pace with the normal turnover rate of neutrophils or (2) there is accelerated removal of neutrophils from the circulating blood. You recall that the neutrophil is a very short-lived cell having a half-life of only six to seven hours. Any impairment of granulopoiesis can therefore induce a neutropenia within hours to a few days.

Inadequate or ineffective granulopoiesis may be encountered with (1) suppression of pluripotent myeloid stem cells, as occurs in aplastic anemia (p. 638) and a variety of leukemias and lymphomas (p. 683)—in these conditions, granulocytopenia is accompanied by anemia and thrombocytopenia; (2) suppression of the committed granulocytic precursors, which occurs after exposure to certain drugs, as discussed below; (3) megaloblastic anemias, due to vitamin B_{12} or folate deficiency (p. 630), in which defective DNA synthesis produces abnormal granulocytic precursors, rendering them susceptible to intramedullary death (ineffective granulopoiesis). Marrow granulopoiesis is increased but the number of mature neutrophils entering the blood is decreased.

Accelerated removal or destruction of neutrophils is encountered with (1) immunologically mediated injury to the neutrophils, which may be idiopathic with no other abnormality, associated with a well-defined immunologic disorder (e.g., Felty's syndrome, p. 1355), or produced by exposure to drugs; (2) splenic sequestration in which excessive destruction occurs secondary to enlargement of the spleen (p. 699), associated also with excessive destruction of red cells and platelets.

Among the many associations mentioned, *the most significant neutropenias (agranulocytoses) are produced by drugs.*[1] Certain drugs, such as alkylating agents and antimetabolites used in cancer treatment, produce agranulocytosis in a predictable, dose-related fashion. They cause a generalized suppression of the bone marrow, and therefore other cells are also affected (aplastic anemia). Agranulocytosis may also be encountered as an idiosyncratic reaction to a large variety of agents. The roster of implicated drugs includes aminopyrine, chloramphenicol, sulfonamides, chlorpromazine, thiouracil, and phenylbutazone. Although the mechanism of agranulocytosis here is obscure, both decreased production and increased destruction have been implicated. The neutropenia induced by chlorpromazine and related phenothiazines is of slow onset and is believed to result from the suppression of granulocytic precursors in the bone marrow. Chlorpromazine can inhibit DNA synthesis of marrow cells in vitro, and therefore it is postulated that certain individuals unusually sensitive to this effect develop agranulocytosis. Neutrophil production gradually becomes normal after the cessation of drug therapy. Agranulocytosis following administration of aminopyrine, thiouracils, and certain sulfonamides is believed to result from immunologically mediated destruction of mature neutrophils. Antibodies reactive against a complex between the drug or its metabolite (acting as the hapten) and leukocyte proteins may evoke a Type II hypersensitivity reaction. Alternatively, neutrophils may be damaged as innocent bystanders by the adsorption of drug-antibody complexes on the surface and the subsequent activation of complement. In many cases, no antecedent cause of neutropenia can be detected but autoimmunity is suspected, since serum antibodies directed against neutrophil-specific antigens can be detected.

MORPHOLOGY. The anatomic alterations in the bone marrow depend on the underlying basis of the neutropenia. When it is caused by excessive destruction of the mature neutrophils, the marrow may be hypercellular with increased numbers of immature granulocytic precursors. Hypercellularity is also seen with ineffective granulopoiesis, as occurs in megaloblastic anemias. Agranulocytosis caused by agents that affect the committed granulocytic precursors are understandably associated with hypocellular marrow, resulting from greatly decreased leukopoietic elements. Erythropoiesis and megakaryocytes usually remain at normal levels, but with certain myelotoxic drugs all marrow elements may be affected. Occasionally, increased numbers of plasma cells and lymphocytes are found in the marrow, particularly as the marrow becomes acellular.

Infections are a characteristic feature of agranulocytosis. Ulcerating necrotizing lesions of the gingiva, floor of the mouth, buccal mucosa, pharynx, or anywhere within the oral cavity (agranulocytic angina) are quite characteristic of agranulocytosis (Fig. 15–1). These ulcers are typically deep, undermined, and covered by gray to green-black necrotic membranes from which numbers of bacteria or fungi can be isolated. Similar ulcerations may occur in the skin, vagina, anus, or gastrointestinal tract, but these sites are much less frequently involved. Severe necrotizing infections are also encountered, but less prominently, in the lungs, urinary tract, and kidneys. All these sites of infection are characterized by massive growth of bacteria (or other agents) with relatively poor leukocytic response. In many instances, the bacteria grow in colony formation (botryomycosis) as though they were cultured on nutrient media. The regional lymph nodes draining these infections are enlarged and inflamed. The spleen and liver are rarely enlarged.

Clinical Course. Agranulocytosis tends to follow a fairly characteristic clinical pattern. The initial symptoms are often malaise, chills, and fever, followed in sequence by marked weakness and fatigability, symptoms that stem from the severe infections characteristic of this disorder. In severe agranulocytosis with virtual absence of neutrophils, these infections may become so overwhelming as to cause death within a few days. Less extreme depression of the marrow may appear insidiously and come to light only during the investigation of frequent and persistent minor infections.

Characteristically, the total white cell count is reduced to 1000 cells per mm^3 of blood and, in certain instances, to levels as low as 200 to 300 cells. Usually there is no associated anemia, save that caused by the infections, nor is there thrombocytopenia.

The prognosis is very unpredictable. Before the advent of antibiotics, the mortality rate ranged between 70 and 90%. At present the antibiotics and supportive measures such as neutrophil transfusions allow better survival since, in many instances, the adverse effects of the toxic drug are discovered early and the depression of white cells eventually remits. The idiopathic form, too, may spontaneously remit or may progressively worsen, leading to death.

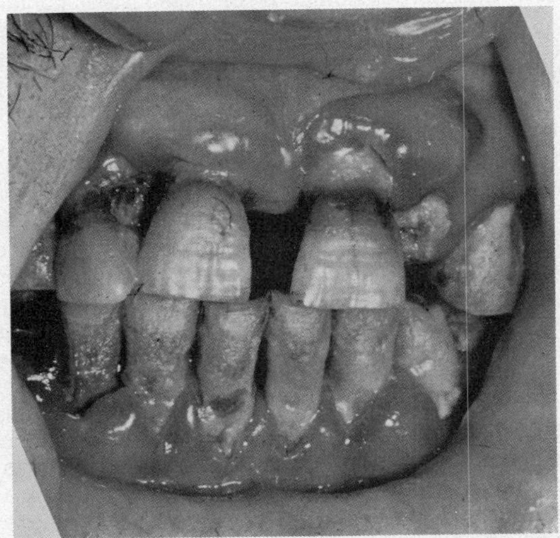

Figure 15–1. Granulocytopenia. Gingival margins show chronic suppurative necrotizing infection due to loss of protective white cells in circulation.

REACTIVE (INFLAMMATORY) PROLIFERATIONS OF WHITE CELLS

Leukocytosis

Leukocytosis is a common reaction in a variety of inflammatory states. The particular white cell series affected varies with the underlying cause. In Chapter 2 we discussed *polymorphonuclear leukocytosis* (granulocytosis), which accompanies acute inflammation. Pyogenic infections are common causes of neutrophilic leukocytosis, but it may also result from nonmicrobial stimuli such as tissue necrosis caused by burns or myocardial infarction. In patients with severe, life-threatening sepsis, in addition to leukocytosis there may be morphologic changes in the neutrophils such as toxic granulations, Döhle bodies, and cytoplasmic vacuoles. *Toxic granules* are coarse and darker than the normal neutrophilic granules. Although their precise origin is not entirely clear, they are believed to represent abnormal forms of azurophilic granules. *Döhle bodies* are pale blue, round or oval inclusions that represent aggregates of the rough endoplasmic reticulum.

Eosinophilic leukocytosis is characteristic of allergic disorders such as bronchial asthma, hay fever (p. 727), parasitic infections, and some diseases of the skin. The latter include pemphigus, eczema, and dermatitis herpetiformis, all of which are probably immunologic in origin. *Elevations in monocyte count* may be seen in several chronic infections including tuberculosis, bacterial endocarditis, brucellosis, rickettsiosis, and malaria. Certain collagen vascular diseases such as systemic lupus erythematosus (SLE) and rheumatoid arthritis are also associated with monocytosis. *Lymphocytosis* may accompany monocytosis in chronic inflammatory states such as brucellosis and tuberculosis, representing in these instances a sustained activation of the immune response. The lymphocyte count may also be increased in acute viral infections such as viral hepatitis, in cytomegalovirus infections, and particularly in infectious mononucleosis (p. 288).

In most instances, reactive leukocytosis is easy to distinguish from neoplastic proliferation of the white cells (i.e., leukemias) by the rarity of immature cells in the blood. However, in some inflammatory states, many immature white cells may appear in the blood and a picture of leukemia may be simulated *(leukemoid reaction)*. The distinction from leukemias may then be difficult, as discussed on page 680.

Infections and other inflammatory stimuli may not only cause leukocytosis but also involve the lymph nodes, which act as defensive barriers. The infections that lead to lymphadenitis (described below) are so numerous and varied that it is impossible to detail each, since it would be a virtual catalog of all systemic microbiologic diseases. Moreover, in most instances the lymphadenitis is of a banal variety and is entirely nonspecific, designated acute or chronic nonspecific lymphadenitis.

Acute Nonspecific Lymphadenitis

Lymph nodes undergo reactive changes whenever challenged by microbiologic agents or their toxic products, or by cell debris and foreign matter introduced into wounds or into the circulation, as in drug addiction.

Acutely inflamed nodes are most commonly caused by direct microbiologic drainage, and are seen most frequently in the cervical area in association with infections of the teeth or tonsil, or in the axillary or inguinal regions secondary to infections in the extremities. Similarly, acute lymphadenitis is found in those nodes draining acute appendicitis, acute enteritis, or any other acute infections. Generalized acute lymphadenopathy is characteristic of viral infections and bacteremia, particularly in children. The nodal reactions in the abdomen—mesenteric adenitis—may induce acute abdominal symptoms closely resembling acute appendicitis, a differential diagnosis that plagues the surgeon.

Macroscopically, the nodes become swollen, gray-red, and engorged. The capsules are generally intact, but permeation of infection may lead to inflammatory changes in the perinodal tissues. Histologically there is prominence of the lymphoid follicles and large germinal centers containing numerous mitotic figures. Histiocytes often contain particulate debris of bacterial origin or derived from necrotic cells (Fig. 15–2). When pyogenic organisms are the cause of the reaction, the centers of the follicles may undergo necrosis; indeed, the entire node may sometimes be converted into a suppurative mass. With less severe reactions, there is sometimes a neutrophilic infiltrate about the follicles, and numerous neutrophils can be found within the lymphoid sinuses. The cells lining the sinuses become hypertrophied and cuboidal and may undergo hyperplasia.

Clinically, nodes with acute lymphadenitis are enlarged because of the cellular infiltration and edema. As a consequence of the distention of the capsule, they are tender to touch. When abscess formation is extensive, they become fluctuant. The overlying skin is frequently red, and sometimes penetration of the infection to the skin surface produces draining sinuses, particularly when the nodes have undergone suppurative necrosis. With control of the infection, the lymph nodes may revert to their normal appearance or scarring may follow the more destructive disease.

Chronic Nonspecific Lymphadenitis

Chronic reactions assume one of three patterns, depending on their causation. Most chronic infections caused by organisms that represent B-cell antigens induce follicular hyperplasia. Microbiologic agents or antigens that stimulate T cells produce a second type of pattern, called paracortical lymphoid hyperplasia. Drugs such as the anticonvulsant Dilantin (phenytoin) serving

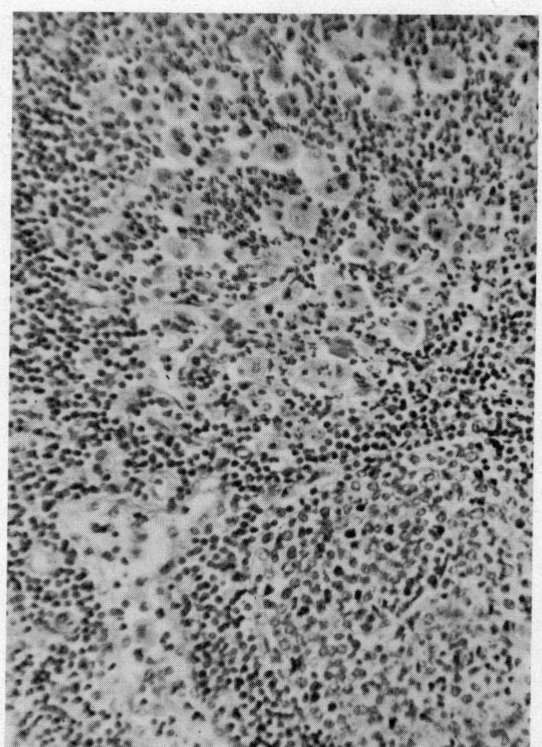

Figure 15–2. Acute lymphadenitis. High-power detail of germinal centers with large histiocytic cells showing phagocytic activity.

as haptens may induce this pattern of parafollicular hyperplasia. A third nonspecific pattern, referred to as sinus histiocytosis, is encountered in regional nodes draining a site of cancer.

Follicular hyperplasia is distinguished by prominence of the large germinal centers, which appear to bulge against the surrounding collar of small B lymphocytes (Fig. 15–3). The follicular enlargement may be readily mistaken for nodular lymphoma (p. 658). Prominent within these germinal centers are lymphocytes in varying stages of "blast" transformation and large numbers of histiocytes containing phagocytized debris of bacterial or cellular origin. Plasma cells, histiocytes, and occasionally neutrophils or eosinophils may be found in the parafollicular regions, and there generally is striking hyperplasia of the reticuloendothelial cells lining the lymphatic sinuses.

Paracortical lymphoid hyperplasia is characterized by reactive changes within the T-cell regions of the lymph node, which encroach on, and sometimes appear to efface, the germinal follicles. In these regions the T cells undergo progressive transformation to immunoblasts. These large cells, when viewed within a sea of smaller lymphocytes, impart a mottled appearance to the T-cell zones. In addition, there is hypertrophy of the sinusoidal and vascular endothelial cells and a mixed cellular infiltrate, principally of macrophages and sometimes of eosinophils. The striking increase in the number of immunoblasts may produce a pseudolymphomatous pattern, sometimes referred to as pseudolymphomatous lymphadenitis. Such changes are encountered particularly often in immunologic reactions induced by drugs (especially Dilantin) or following smallpox vaccination. Similar reactions have been described after the use of other vaccines.

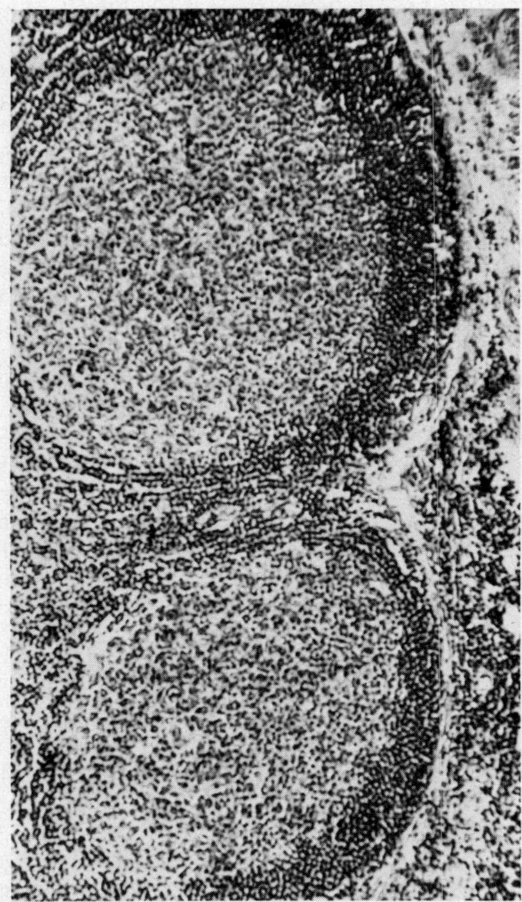

Figure 15–3. Chronic follicular hyperplasia, demonstrating marked enlargement and prominence of germinal follicles.

Sinus histiocytosis refers to distention and prominence of the lymphatic sinusoids, encountered in lymph nodes draining cancers, particularly carcinoma of the breast. The lining endothelial cells are markedly hypertrophied, and the sinuses may be virtually engorged with histiocytes (Fig. 15–4). This pattern of reaction has been thought to represent an immune response on the part of the host to the tumor or its products. According to some, the presence of sinus histiocytosis is a sign of a favorable prognosis, but this issue is debatable.

Although the three patterns of reaction have been described separately, frequent combinations and intergrades are encountered. Characteristically, lymph nodes in chronic reactions are not tender, because they are not under increased pressure. Chronic reactions are particularly characteristic of inguinal and axillary nodes. Both groups drain relatively large areas of the body and so are frequently challenged, for which reason these lymph nodes are inappropriate as biopsy specimens in the study of hematologic and lymphomatous disorders.

NEOPLASTIC PROLIFERATIONS OF WHITE CELLS

Malignant proliferative diseases constitute the most important of white cell disorders. The several categories of these diseases can be briefly defined as follows:

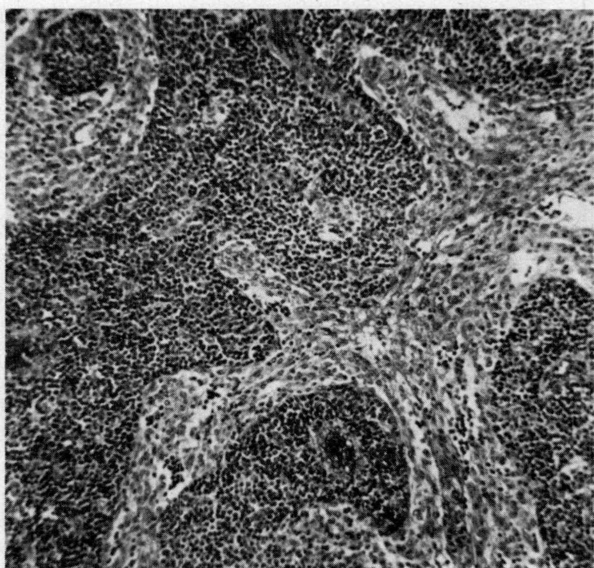

Figure 15–4. Sinus histiocytosis in an axillary node from a female patient with carcinoma of breast.

1. *Malignant lymphomas* take the form of cohesive tumorous lesions composed mainly of lymphocytes and rarely of histiocytes that arise in lymphoid tissue anywhere in the body, most commonly within lymph nodes.
2. *Leukemias* are systemic leukoproliferative disorders arising in the bone marrow that secondarily flood the circulating blood and other organs with leukemic cells.
3. *Plasma cell dyscrasias and related disorders* usually arising in the bones take the form of localized or disseminated proliferations of antibody-forming cells. Thus, this category is marked by the appearance in the peripheral blood of abnormal levels of immunoglobulins or the light or heavy chains of the immunoglobulins. Hence, these disorders are sometimes called gammopathies or dysproteinemias.
4. The *histiocytoses* represent proliferative lesions of tissue macrophages or histiocytes. There is unfortunately much confusion in the terminology of histiocytic disorders. First, as indicated above, the rare neoplastic proliferations of histiocytes originating within the lymphoid tissue are grouped with the malignant lymphomas. Second, there is no evidence that some of the tumor-like proliferations—the so-called histiocytoses X, which are traditionally listed under this category—are indeed neoplastic. Finally, there seem to be no clearly defined boundaries of histiocytoses since some investigators include clearly non-neoplastic, metabolic storage diseases in this category. These complexities will be discussed further on page 694.

As can be seen, the neoplastic disorders of the white cells are extremely varied. In the following sections, each of the categories is treated separately.

MALIGNANT LYMPHOMAS

Lymphomas are malignant neoplasms characterized by the proliferation of cells native to the lymphoid tissues, i.e., lymphocytes, histiocytes, and their precursors and derivatives. Like other neoplasms, all lymphomas are of monoclonal origin, as can be documented by isoenzyme and cell markers. The term lymphoma is something of a misnomer, since these disorders are lethal unless controlled or eradicated through therapy. In the past, the term lymphosarcoma was applied to some of these disorders, but to so many that, although it revealed their ominous nature, it lost any specific meaning.

Within the broad group of malignant lymphomas, *Hodgkin's disease* (Hodgkin's lymphoma) is segregated from all other forms, which constitute the *non-Hodgkin's lymphomas.* Although both have their origin in the lymphoid tissues, Hodgkin's disease is set apart by the presence of a distinctive unifying morphologic feature, the Reed-Sternberg giant cells. In addition, there is a variable component of non-neoplastic inflammatory cells, which in the past raised questions about the neoplastic nature of Hodgkin's disease. Therefore, we will discuss non-Hodgkin's lymphomas and Hodgkin's disease separately.

Non-Hodgkin's Lymphomas (NHL)

The usual presentation of NHL is as a localized or generalized lymphadenopathy. However, in about one-third of cases it may be primary in other sites where lymphoid tissue is found, e.g., in the oropharyngeal region, gut, bone marrow, and skin. Lymph node enlargement due to lymphomatous disease must be differentiated from that caused by the more frequent infectious and inflammatory disorders. Lymphomatous involvement often produces marked nodal enlargement, which is almost always nontender. Although variable, all forms of lymphoma have the potential to spread from their origin in a single node or chain of nodes to other nodes, and eventually to disseminate to the spleen, liver, and bone marrow. Some, after becoming widespread, spill over into the blood, creating a leukemia-like picture in the peripheral blood. In such blood-borne dissemination, all lymph nodes throughout the body become flooded with lymphomatous cells. It may therefore be impossible to determine from microscopic examination of a lymph node alone whether it represents primary lymphomatous disease with involvement of the bone marrow and blood, or nodal changes incident to leukemia. This problem is encountered more often with certain cytologic forms of lymphoma than with others.

Classification of NHL

Neoplastic proliferation of any one of the cell lines indigenous to lymphoid tissue can give rise to a lymphoma. Thus, theoretically it should be possible to classify them on the basis of cell types. Optimally, the classification should (1) provide categories that have clinical significance in terms of responsiveness to therapy and the outlook for the patient and (2) be based on morphologic criteria sufficiently distinctive to be generally applicable when interpreted by different observers. Regrettably, even among expert "lymphomaniacs" there are varying approaches to classification. Some use strictly morphologic criteria; others use morphologic criteria combined with functional features, e.g., immunologic markers and enzyme content of cells. Moreover, there are varying histogenetic interpretations of cell types. For example, when is a cell that looks like a histiocyte in reality a histiocyte and not a modified lymphocyte? What has emerged are more classifications than there are experts on the subject, or, to the "mere mortal," a veritable Augean stable in which the experts appear to have agreed to disagree. No attempt will be made to present all the current classifications.[2] Instead, two currently in favor in the United States—the Rappaport and Lukes-Collins classifications—will be discussed in some detail. Thereafter, brief comments will be made on the recent working formulation proposed by a panel of international experts.[3] Moreover, many of the potentially bewildering details of taxonomy to be found in the numerous references will be omitted, lest the forest get lost among the trees.

Rappaport Classification

Proposed in 1966 and subsequently modified in 1978, this approach is based on two criteria: (1) the cytologic characteristics of the lymphomatous cells in routinely employed stains; and (2) separation of the lymphomas into two growth patterns—a nodular form in which the lymphomatous cells are clustered into identifiable nodules within the lymph nodes, and a diffuse form in which the cells diffusely infiltrate the entire lymph node, without any definite organized pattern.[4]

The *nodular* pattern is characterized by cohesive aggregates of neoplastic cells that somewhat resemble the germinal centers of the lymph node follicles; hence, this architecture is sometimes referred to as *follicular lymphoma.* The lymphomatous nodules are dispersed throughout the cortex and the medulla of the node and therefore efface the normal nodal architecture (Fig. 15–5). In many instances the capsular and pericapsular tissue is infiltrated by neoplastic cells, sometimes with the formation of nodules outside the capsule. This nodular or follicular pattern of lymphoma may be confused morphologically with the reactive follicular hyperplasia (lymphadenitis) of inflammatory states.[5] It is beyond our scope to go into all the subtle morphologic features in this differential, but several points may be noted. Favoring reactive follicular hyperplasia are (1) restriction of the follicles to the cortical region of the node, (2) *a mixed cell population of lymphocytes in different stages of differentiation and histiocytes within the germinal centers—lymphomatous nodules are monomorphic, reactive follicles pleomorphic;* and (3) evidence of cellular phagocytic activity in the germinal centers.

Approximately 50% of all NHLs in adults are of the nodular variety. On the basis of cytology, nodular lymphomas are divided into three subtypes (Table 15–

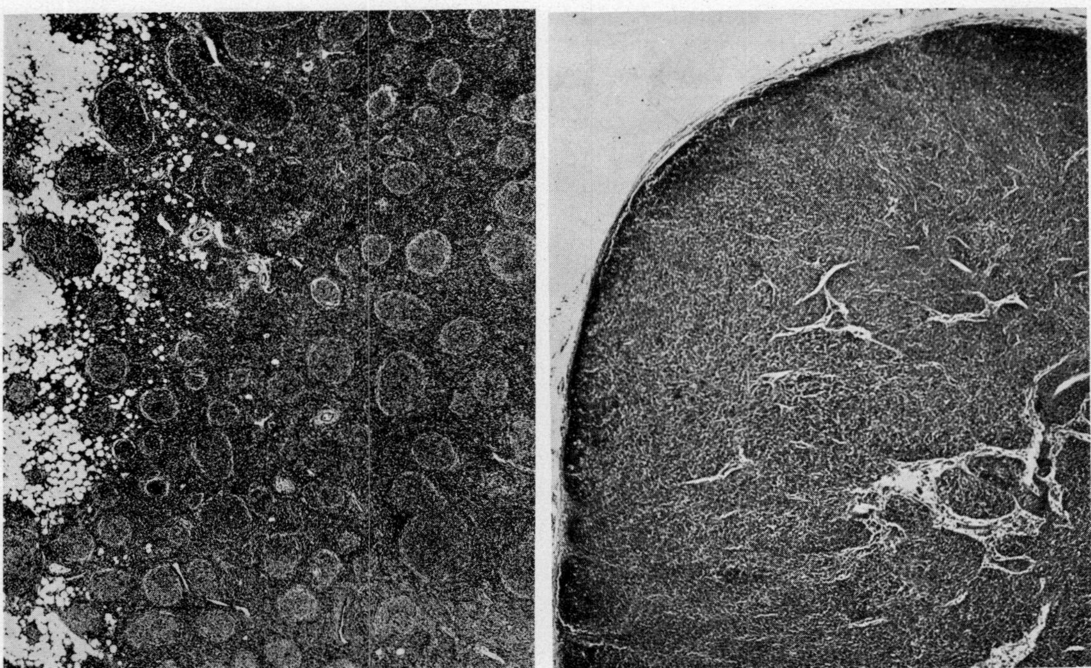

Fig. 15–5 Fig. 15–6

Figure 15–5. Non-Hodgkin's lymphoma, nodular pattern. Nodular aggregates of lymphoma cells are present throughout lymph node and in perinodal fat. (From Jackson, H. J., Jr., and Parker, F. Jr. (eds.): Hodgkin's Disease and Allied Disorders. New York, Oxford University Press, 1947.)
Figure 15–6. Non-Hodgkin's lymphoma, diffuse. Nodal architecture is replaced by a diffuse sea of neoplastic lymphoid cells.

1). Since the cytologic features of nodular lymphomas overlap with those of the diffuse type, these will be described later. *The nodular lymphomas have distinctive clinical features: (1) they occur predominantly in older individuals (rarely persons under 20 years of age); (2) they affect males and females equally; and (3) despite the common finding of involvement of many or all nodes as well as possibly extranodal sites at the time of diagnosis, they have a much better prognosis than diffuse lymphomas.*[6]

The *diffuse lymphomas* are characterized by flooding of the nodal architecture by a monotonous sea of cells (Fig. 15–6). All underlying architecture, such as the distinction between cortex and medulla and the sinusoidal morphology, is totally obscured. The capsule of the node and the extracapsular tissue are often heavily infiltrated. The diffuse lymphomas are more heterogeneous with regard to cell type (Table 15–1) and clinical behavior. Since some diffuse lymphomas are cytologically identical to their nodular counterparts, they are considered to represent progression of the disease from a nodular to a diffuse pattern. Indeed, the coexistence of nodular and diffuse patterns and the documented transformation over time of nodular to diffuse pattern in a small number of cases does support this concept. However, it should be emphasized that *there is no critical evidence that all diffuse lymphomas are preceded by nodular lesions.* Indeed, as will be discussed, some variants such as the well-differentiated lymphocytic lymphoma are not encountered as nodular lesions. *More-*

Table 15–1. RAPPAPORT CLASSIFICATION

Diffuse Lymphomas	% All Cases*	Nodular Lymphomas	% All Cases*
Lymphocytic, well differentiated	5		
Lymphocytic, poorly differentiated	16	Lymphocytic, poorly differentiated	24
Lymphoblastic†			
Histiocytic	28	Histiocytic	3
Mixed, lymphocytic-histiocytic	6	Mixed, lymphocytic-histiocytic	12
Undifferentiated (Burkitt's and non-Burkitt's)	6		

*Percentages based on references 3 and 4.
†Recently added category to Rappaport classification; comprises approximately half of the cases previously included under lymphocytic, poorly differentiated diffuse group.

over, nodular lymphomas may persist in the individual over the span of years and may disseminate throughout the body to cause death while retaining the distinctive nodular architecture.

In addition to the "nodular" and "diffuse" categorization, all NHLs are further subdivided into cytologic subsets. When Rappaport first presented the classification of NHLs, the immunologic typing of lymphoid cells was in its infancy, and so subdivision in the Rappaport scheme is based entirely on morphology. It takes into account first the apparent similarity of tumor cells to various normal cell types. Thus, terms such as lymphocytic and histiocytic lymphomas are used, to imply similarity and presumed derivation from normal lymphocytes or histiocytes. Second, within a cytologic category it further segregates tumors on the basis of degree of differentiation as judged by nuclear and cell size, nuclear configuration, chromatin pattern, and the presence or absence of nucleoli. The combined use of these two criteria permits differentiation of the following patterns.

Well-Differentiated Lymphocytic Lymphoma (WDLL). This pattern makes up approximately 5% of all NHLs and occurs only in the diffuse form; nodular variants have not been identified. The cell type consists of compact, small, apparently unstimulated lymphocytes with dark-staining round nuclei, scanty cytoplasm, and little variation in size (Fig. 15–7). Mitotic figures are very rare, and there is little or no cytologic atypia. *Diffuse WDLL may occur without involvement of the blood and bone marrow, but in about 40% of cases it may seed the blood, evoking a chronic lymphocytic leukemia–like blood picture.*[7] Conversely, in patients with the primary diagnosis of chronic lymphocytic leukemia (CLL), the nodes are invariably flooded with well-differentiated lymphocytes. Thus, it is impossible from a lymph node biopsy alone to differentiate CLL from WDLL. Their clinical features are also similar. Both occur primarily in the older age groups. Typically, these patients have generalized lymphadenopathy with mild-to-moderate enlargement of the liver and spleen; the associated symptoms are mild and prolonged survival is usual. Some patients with a histologic picture closely resembling WDLL also have monoclonal IgM immunoglobulin in the serum and a distinctive clinical syndrome called Waldenström's macroglobulinemia (p. 692). In these patients the lymph nodes often contain variable numbers of plasma cells or "plasmacytoid lymphocytes," in addition to the well-differentiated lymphocytes described above. As discussed later, WDLL, CLL, and Waldenström's macroglobulinemia represent different manifestations of the neoplastic proliferation of B lymphocytes, and as such are closely related to each other.

Poorly Differentiated Lymphocytic Lymphoma (PDLL). The tumor cells in PDLL consist of atypical lymphocytes, which may appear in nodular or diffuse patterns. The cells are somewhat larger than those seen in WDLL (but smaller than the nuclei of benign endothelial cells or histiocytes, which are used as a reference when evaluating size). *Much more distinctive are the nuclei, which are irregular, with marked indentations and angularity* (Fig. 15–8). The chromatin is coarse and condensed, and mitoses are rare. The nodular and diffuse patterns of PDLL together account for approximately 30% of all NHLs. Some cases of PDLL may spill over into the blood and produce a leukemic picture, the so-called acute lymphosarcoma cell leukemia. The precise incidence of leukemia in PDLL is not known. However, leukemic spread is definitely less common than in WDLL. Patients with PDLL are usually middle-aged to elderly and present commonly with generalized disease involving multiple lymph nodes, liver, spleen, and bone marrow. Despite the presence of extensive disease, the prognosis is relatively favorable, especially in nodular PDLL. The prognosis in diffuse PDLL is poorer, as is the case with most diffuse lymphomas.

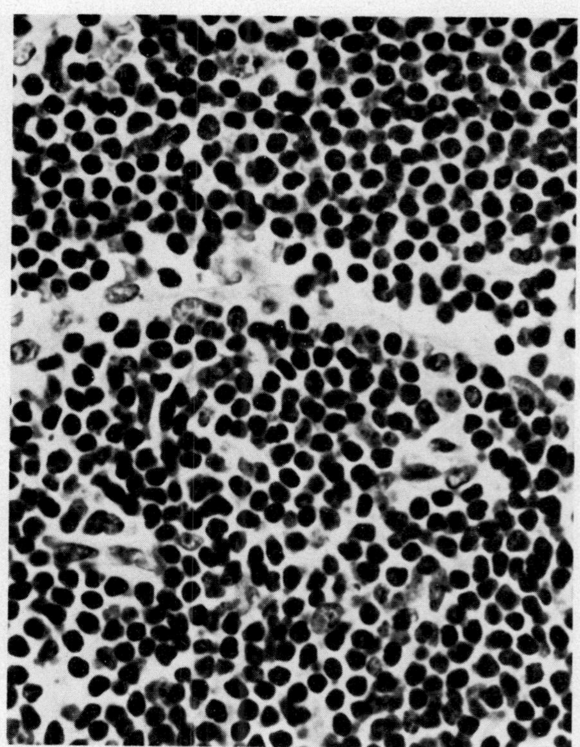

Figure 15–7. Non-Hodgkin's lymphoma, well-differentiated lymphocytic type. Cytology is that of mature, uniform, unstimulated lymphocyte. (Courtesy of Dr. Jose Hernandez, Department of Pathology, Southwestern Medical School, Dallas, Texas.)

Histiocytic Lymphoma (HL). *Characteristic of this form of NHL is the large size of tumor cells.* They are two to three times larger than normal lymphocytes and their nuclei are larger than those of benign tissue histiocytes or endothelial cells. As compared with WDLL and PDLL, the nuclei in HL not only are larger but also are more vesicular and usually have more prominent nucleoli (Fig. 15–9). The nuclear shape, however, is quite variable: it may be round and smooth, or irregular with marked indentations and lobulations. *Several cytologic subtypes can be recognized, ranging from a monotonous proliferation of large cells to ex-*

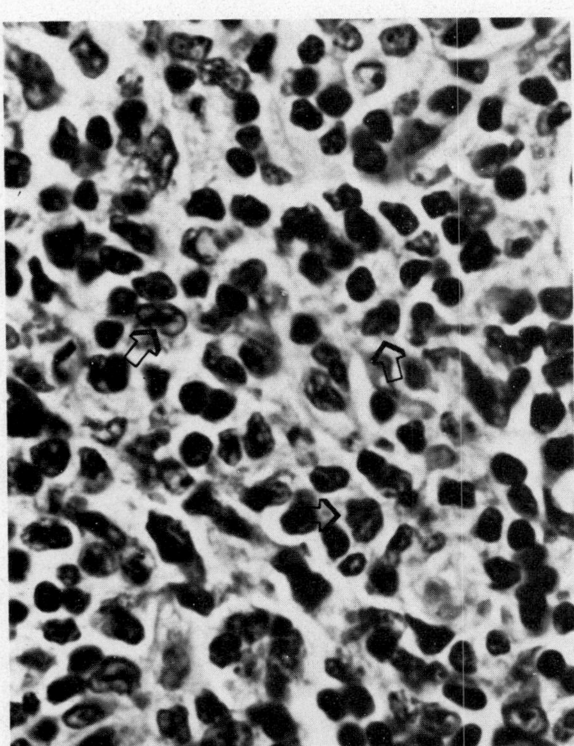

Figure 15–8. Non-Hodgkin's lymphoma, poorly differentiated lymphocytic type. Nuclei are irregular with indentations *(arrows)* and marked angularity. (Courtesy of Dr. Jose Hernandez, Department of Pathology, Southwestern Medical School, Dallas, Texas.)

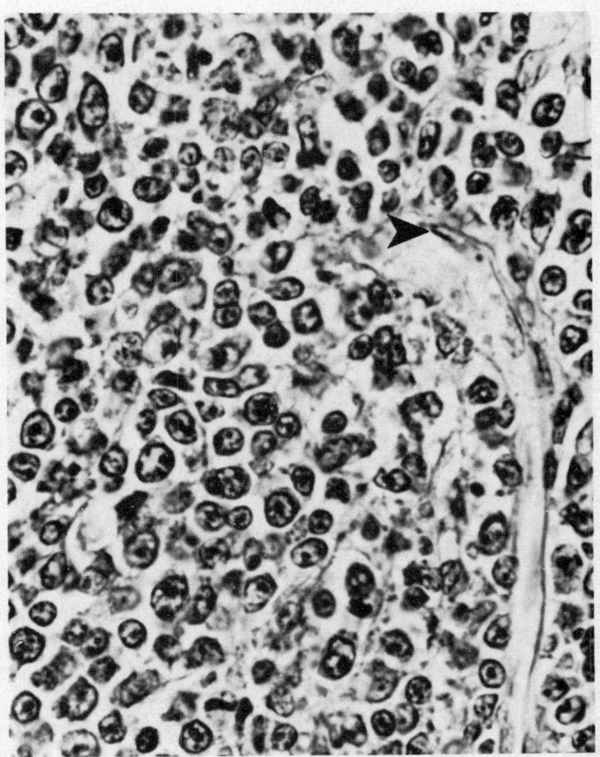

Figure 15–9. Non-Hodgkin's lymphoma, diffuse histiocytic type. Tumor cells in this example have large nuclei (compare with endothelial cell nucleus at tip of arrow) and prominent, centrally placed nucleoli. Nuclear pleomorphism is not marked. (Courtesy of Dr. Jose Hernandez, Department of Pathology, Southwestern Medical School, Dallas, Texas.)

tremely pleomorphic tumors with bizarre cells. Although HL can occur in both the nodular and diffuse forms, the latter is much more frequent and constitutes one of the most common forms of NHL (Table 15–1). The few cases of nodular HL tend to progress rapidly into the diffuse form and have the worst prognosis among nodular lymphomas. Diffuse histiocytic lymphomas are associated with somewhat distinctive clinical presentations. As compared with lymphocytic lymphomas, involvement of extranodal sites is more frequent; indeed, involvement of the gastrointestinal tract, skin, bone, or brain may be the presenting, and in some cases the only, feature, suggesting extranodal origin. When nodal involvement is the main presentation, it is usually restricted to one side of the diaphragm. Involvement of liver and spleen is not common at the time of presentation, but when it occurs the lymphoma cells form large, destructive tumorous masses. In contrast, for example, involvement of the liver and spleen in PDLL is associated with the formation of uniform discrete miliary nodules throughout these organs. Leukemic manifestations are distinctly uncommon, and when present indicate a very poor prognosis. HL is an aggressive disease, and the prognosis for the group as a whole is poor. However, several recent studies have indicated that up to 60% of patients with HL can achieve sustained clinical remission with combination chemotherapy, which may lead to long-term survival.[8]

MIXED LYMPHOCYTIC-HISTIOCYTIC LYMPHOMA. In this variant, cells of the PDLL type as well as large cells (histiocytic) are present. In general, a tumor is classified as mixed if the large cells constitute 30 to 50% of the total number of cells. This cytologic pattern is seen more commonly in the nodular form. As for most other nodular lymphomas, the prognosis is good.

LYMPHOBLASTIC LYMPHOMA. This is a relatively new addition to the Rappaport classification.[9] Previously, these cases were included under diffuse PDLL, but recent studies indicate that lymphoblastic lymphoma is a distinct clinicopathologic entity closely related to T-cell acute lymphoblastic leukemia (ALL) (p. 676). This variant is seen most commonly in adolescents or young adults, although any age group may be involved.[10] In affected males, there is a suggestion of bimodal age distribution, the two peaks being in the second and seventh decades. Overall, males are affected two to three times as often as females, but in the early peak encountered in the second decade, the male-to-female ratio is 6:1. *A very characteristic clinical feature, particularly in young males, is the presence of a mediastinal mass (50 to 70% of cases) at the time of diagnosis, suggesting a thymic origin.* This disease is rapidly progressive, and early dissemination to the bone marrow, blood, and central nervous system leads to the evolution of a picture resembling ALL.

The histologic pattern of the tumor is always diffuse

and the tumor cells resemble the lymphoblasts of ALL. They are fairly uniform in size, with scanty cytoplasm and nuclei that are somewhat larger than those of small lymphocytes. The nuclear chromatin is delicate and finely stippled, and nucleoli are either absent or inconspicuous. In many, but not all, cases the nuclear membrane shows deep subdivision, imparting a convoluted (lobulated) appearance. In keeping with its aggressive growth, the tumor shows a high rate of mitoses and, as with other tumors having a high mitotic rate (e.g., Burkitt's lymphoma), a "starry sky" pattern is produced by the interspersed benign macrophages. In the past, when this tumor was treated as diffuse PDLL, the survival was dismal, average life expectancy being less than one year. However, with the realization that lymphoblastic lymphoma is biologically more akin to ALL, treatment protocols employed for ALL have been utilized with much greater success, with a median survival in excess of 71 months in one series of adults.[11]

UNDIFFERENTIATED LYMPHOMA. This type is so termed because the cells do not have any morphologic evidence of "maturation" toward lymphocytes or histiocytes. Within this category, *two clinically distinct subgroups have been recognized: Burkitt's type and non-Burkitt's type.*

The *undifferentiated Burkitt's-type lymphoma* was described initially in Africa, where it is endemic in some parts, but it also occurs sporadically in nonendemic areas including the United States, where it has been called American Burkitt's lymphoma. Histologically, the African and the nonendemic American cases of Burkitt's lymphoma are identical, although there are some clinical and virologic differences. The relationship of these disorders to the Epstein-Barr virus (EBV) is discussed on pages 245 and 669. These tumors consist of a sea of strikingly monotonous cells, 10 to 25 μm in diameter, with round or oval nuclei containing two to five prominent nucleoli. The nuclear size approximates that of benign macrophages within the tumor. There is a moderate amount of faintly basophilic or amphophilic cytoplasm, which also is intensely pyroninophilic and often contains small, lipid-filled vacuoles (better appreciated on stained imprints of the tumor). A high mitotic index is very characteristic, as is cell death, accounting for the presence of numerous tissue macrophages with ingested nuclear debris. Since these benign macrophages, which are diffusely distributed among the tumor cells, are often surrounded by a clear space, they create a "starry sky" pattern (Fig. 15–10), which can also be seen in other lymphomas, such as the lymphoblastic type, with a high mitotic rate. Both the African and non-African cases are found largely in children or young adults. In both forms, the disease rarely arises in the lymph nodes. In African cases, involvement of the maxilla or mandible is the common mode of presentation (Fig. 15–11), whereas abdominal tumors (bowel, retroperitoneum, ovaries) are more common in cases seen in America. Leukemic transformation of Burkitt's lymphoma is uncommon, especially in African cases. These tumors respond well to aggressive chemotherapy, and long

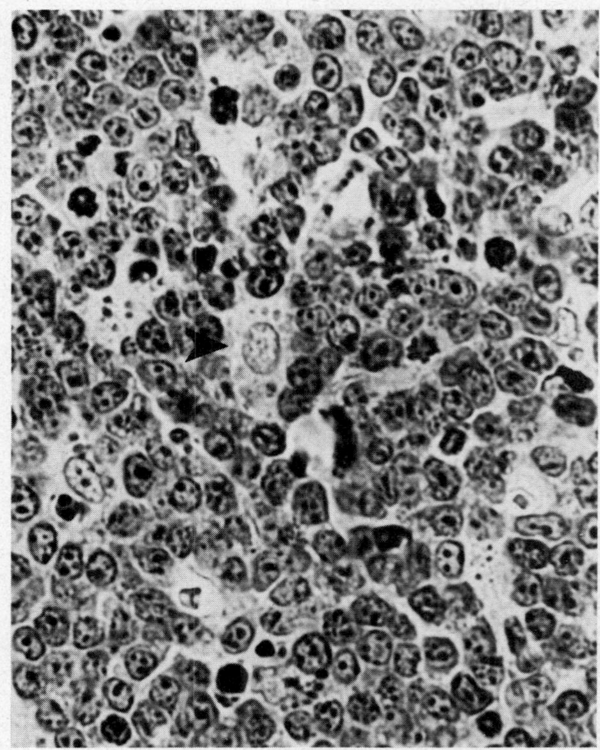

Figure 15–10. Burkitt's lymphoma. Tumor cells have multiple small nucleoli and high mitotic index. Lack of significant variation in nuclear shape and size lends a monotonous appearance interrupted by pale-staining, benign tissue macrophages *(arrow)*, which impart a "starry sky" appearance better appreciated at a lower magnification. (Courtesy of Dr. Jose Hernandez, Department of Pathology, Southwestern Medical School, Dallas, Texas.)

remissions have been reported. Although a relapse occurs in many cases, a 50% long-term survival rate can be expected with present methods of treatment.

The undifferentiated, non–Burkitt's-type lymphoma differs from the Burkitt's tumor both clinically and histologically.[12] This disease more commonly affects adults (median age 34 years) and is somewhat less responsive to treatment. There is no known clinical or virologic association with EBV. Histologically, the nuclei are approximately the same size as in Burkitt's tumor, but they show much greater variation both in shape and size, and occasional multinucleate cells are also seen. The nuclear chromatin is delicate and there is usually a single prominent eosinophilic nucleolus. Because of the nuclear appearance, this tumor has also been called undifferentiated, pleomorphic lymphoma. The cytoplasm is pale and scanty. The general view that this tumor is distinct from Burkitt's lymphoma has been challenged.[13] Since the frequency of these neoplasms is very low, more studies will be required to resolve this issue satisfactorily.

LUKES-COLLINS CLASSIFICATION

On the premise that the malignant lymphomas are neoplasms of the immune system, Lukes and Collins

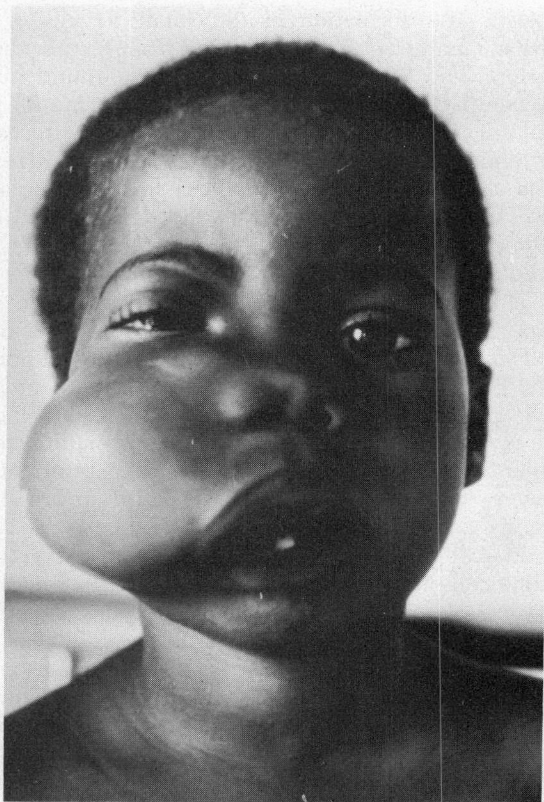

Figure 15–11. Burkitt's lymphoma in a 9-year-old child. The maxillary tumor mass is a characteristic presentation of this disease.

have classified the non-Hodgkin's lymphomas on the basis of their origins from T or B lymphocytes or histiocytes.[14] This classification proposes that lymphomas develop through either a block or a "switch-on" (derepression) in transformation of either B cells or T cells. Correlations are drawn between the cytologic patterns in lymphomatous nodes and those evoked by antigenic challenge or mitogen stimulation of lymphocytes.

In the germinal centers of the follicles, four distinctive morphologic stages could be identified in the process of transformation of the unchallenged B lymphocyte into an immunoblast. *These stages include (1) small cleaved cells, (2) large cleaved cells, (3) small noncleaved cells, and (4) large noncleaved cells*, as depicted in Figure 15–12. First, the small, round B cell in and about the follicle changes into a slightly larger cell having an angulated, a folded, or (as Lukes and Collins refer to it) a cleaved nucleus. The term "cleaved" refers to sharp infoldings of the nuclear membrane. Further transformation produces larger cleaved cells. In both these cell forms, the cytoplasm is scanty and the nuclear chromatin is slightly more dispersed than in the resting lymphocyte, and the nucleoli are inconspicuous. Up to this point in the sequence there is little evidence of mitotic activity. In the next stage of transformation, nuclear cleavage disappears as the nucleus becomes round or oval, the nuclear chromatin is finely dispersed, and one to three nucleoli appear along with a readily visible peripheral rim of pyroninophilic cytoplasm. Pyroninophilia (increased affinity for the pyronin stain) results from increased amounts of cytoplasmic RNA as cells become active in protein (antibody) synthesis. Numerous mitotic figures now appear. The fourth stage in B-cell transformation involves the continued enlargement of the noncleaved cell up to four or more times the size of the original small lymphocyte. Simultaneously, one to two nucleoli become prominent in the large, round vesicular nucleus, along with an increase in the quantity of the cytoplasm. Mitotic figures are frequent in these cells. *All four of these cell types are referred to as follicular center cells (FCC) and all are of B-cell origin.* The noncleaved cells are the dividing FCC, whereas the cleaved cells are the nondividing but morphologically altered FCC. It is the large noncleaved cells that ultimately undergo further enlargement to become immunoblasts. The immunoblasts have more marked pyroninophilia, larger and more vesicular nuclei, and prominent centrally located nucleoli. They also tend to show plasmacytoid features. Further proliferation of immunoblasts provides daughter cells that eventually either become plasma cells or revert to the dormant state as small memory lymphocytes. The small T cells in the T-cell regions of the lymph node may

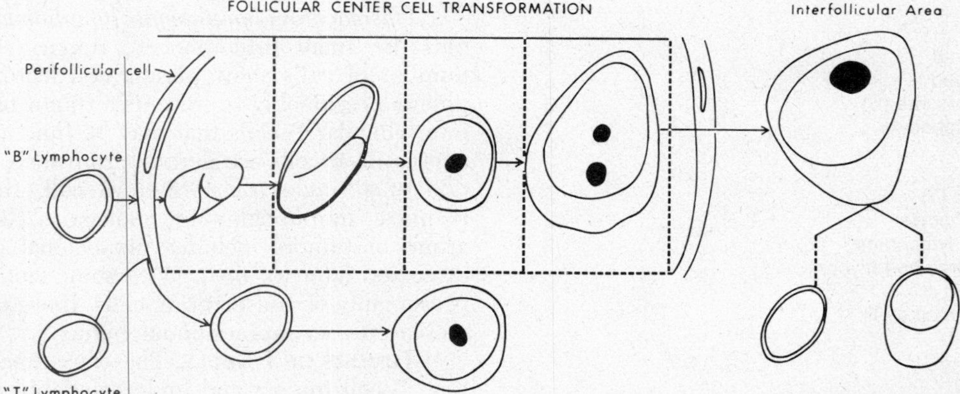

Figure 15–12. Schematic representation of normal transformation of follicular center B cells in comparison with transformation of T cells. (From Lukes, R. J., and Collins, R. D.: New approaches to the classification of the lymphomata. Br. J. Cancer *31*(Suppl. 2):7, 1975.)

undergo a parallel "blast" transformation without showing nuclear cleavage. From such studies, Lukes and Collins concluded that most cells interpreted as histiocytes in the Rappaport classification were actually neoplastic FCC. Lukes and Collins recognize true histiocytic lymphomas, but consider them rare, and cell marker techniques have supported this view.

Since *the Lukes-Collins classification is based on the concept that the various cytologic subtypes of malignant lymphomas arise by neoplastic transformation of the normal components of the immune system,* it divides NHL into three functional categories: B-cell tumors, T-cell tumors, and tumors of histiocytes (macrophages). A fourth undefined cell category includes tumors that cannot be assigned to the three functional categories by any of the presently available criteria. As seen in Table 15–2, B-cell tumors are the most common,. and true histiocytic tumors are rare. *Although this classification divides NHL into functional groups, Lukes and associates have repeatedly emphasized that "the classification of cases is based entirely on the morphologic features."*[14] Implicit in this view is the assertion that the cytologic features are distinctive enough to define immunologically homogeneous entities without requiring cytochemical and immunologic methods, except in those few cases in which morphology is not distinctive. We will examine the validity and practical implications of this view after a description of the morphologic features of NHL, according to the Lukes-Collins system.

TUMORS OF B LYMPHOCYTES. The great preponderance of NHLs are of B-cell origin (Table 15–2). Within this group, they are subclassified on the basis of the morphologic features characteristic of the different stages of normal B-cell differentiations, as depicted in Figure 15–12.

The *small B-cell lymphoma* apparently results from neoplastic transformation of the small B cells of the follicular mantle, which are blocked from further differentiation. The tumor cells have uniform round nuclei with compact chromatin and a narrow rim of pale cytoplasm, resembling normal lymphocytes. Mitoses are rare. Since the tumorous B cells are apparently arrested in this early stage, they fail to form follicles or plasma cells. This category conforms to the diffuse WDLL of the Rappaport classification and the closely related CLL.

Follicular center cell (FCC) lymphomas, like the normal follicles, are comprised of four cytologic subtypes, which are segregated on the basis of the similarity of cell size and nuclear characteristics to those of normal FCCs (Fig. 15–12 and Table 15–2). Since the neoplastic FCCs apparently retain their ability to form follicles, there is usually some degree of follicle formation (recall nodular architecture). The degree of follicle formation, however, varies with the state of B-cell transformation. Thus, FCC lymphomas of small cleaved cells and large cleaved cell types that are composed of less actively dividing cells are more frequently associated with follicle formation, whereas the rapidly proliferating small and large noncleaved cell tumors exhibit the follicular pattern in only 10% of cases. Most FCC lymphomas are of the small cleaved type, but in some cases a mixture of cell types is present. Such tumors are usually classified on the basis of the predominant cell type. (Fig. 15–8, representing PDLL according to the Rappaport classification, would be classified as small cleaved FCC lymphoma in the Lukes-Collins scheme.) Burkitt's tumor is believed to represent a form of small noncleaved FCC lymphoma; although these usually have a diffuse architectural pattern, in some cases there are follicles supporting their origin from the FCC.

Immunoblastic sarcoma of B cells is believed to arise from transformed interfollicular B cells; it therefore does not form follicles. The tumor cells resemble the large noncleaved FCCs, but have more abundant pyroninophilic cytoplasm and plasmacytoid features. In 30% of cases this aggressive tumor of transformed B lymphocytes is associated with a previous history of an immunologic disorder such as Sjögren's syndrome, SLE, or Hashimoto's thyroiditis or with states of immunosuppression.

Plasmacytoid lymphocytic lymphoma closely resembles the small B-lymphocyte tumors, but a variable number of cells show plasma cell features. This lymphoma presumably represents a tumor of differentiated interfollicular B cells that may be functional. Since the neoplastic B cells are derived from the clonal proliferation of a single transformed B cell, they all secrete identical immunoglobulin molecules. Therefore, this group of tumors includes monoclonal gammopathies, discussed later (p. 688). With some tumors, composed presumably of nonsecreting cells, there is no associated increase in serum immunoglobulins.

TUMORS OF T CELLS. These are much less frequent than B-cell tumors and understandably much less well defined. Four types have been recognized: small lymphocytic T-cell lymphoma, convoluted T-cell lymphoma,

Table 15–2. LUKES-COLLINS CLASSIFICATION*

	Percentage	
B Cell	65	
Small lymphocyte (B)		9
Follicular center cell		
Small cleaved		28
Large cleaved		5
Small noncleaved		7
Large noncleaved		6
Immunoblastic sarcoma (B)		3
Plasmacytoid lymphocyte		7
T Cell	20	
Small lymphocyte (T)		2
Convoluted lymphocyte		10
Cutaneous T-cell lymphoma (Sézary syndrome and mycosis fungoides)		2
Immunoblastic sarcoma (T)		4
Histiocytes	0.2	
U (Undefined) Cell	14.8	

*Adapted from reference 12.

the cutaneous T-cell lymphomas (mycosis fungoides Sézary syndrome), and immunoblastic sarcoma of T cells.

Small lymphocytic T-cell lymphoma is extremely rare, making up only 10 out of 425 cases in one large series.[14] The cells resemble small B lymphocytes, from which they cannot be easily differentiated morphologically. They may be associated with the uncommon T-cell CLL (p. 676).

Convoluted T-cell lymphoma in the Lukes-Collins classification is essentially identical to the lymphoblastic lymphoma of the Rappaport classification (p. 661); therefore, only brief additional comments will be offered. As mentioned earlier, in most cases of lymphoblastic lymphoma the tumor cells have markedly convoluted nuclei, an appearance said to resemble "chicken footprint." Those few cases that do not have the typical nuclear convolutions are excluded from this group in the Lukes-Collins classification. Recent studies with monoclonal antibodies, however, indicate that most tumor cells (with or without nuclear convolutions) express OKT10, a marker of primitive intrathymic T cells, and that nuclear configuration does not affect the clinical course. This, then, is a tumor of *immature intrathymic T cells,* and understandably no morphologic counterpart of the convoluted T cells is found in normal lymph nodes.

Cutaneous T-cell lymphomas include a spectrum of disorders, of which mycosis fungoides and Sézary syndrome are the best characterized.[16] Involvement of skin is a hallmark of the tumors within this group. Clinically, the cutaneous lesions of *mycosis fungoides* show three somewhat distinct stages, discussed later (p. 1271). Briefly, mycosis fungoides presents with an inflammatory premycotic phase and progresses through a plaque phase to a tumor phase. *Histologically, there is infiltration of the epidermis and upper dermis by neoplastic T cells, which have an extremely unusual cerebriform nucleus.* This appearance results from marked and complex infolding of the nuclear membrane. In most patients with progressive disease, extracutaneous manifestations, characterized by nodal and visceral dissemination, appear. *Sézary syndrome* is a related condition in which skin involvement is manifested clinically as a generalized exfoliative erythroderma, but *in contrast with mycosis fungoides, the skin lesions rarely proceed to tumefaction.* Instead, there is an associated leukemia of "Sézary" cells that have the same cerebriform appearance noted in the tissue infiltrates of mycosis fungoides. Circulating Sézary cells can also be identified in up to 25% of cases of mycosis fungoides in the plaque or tumor phase, indicating that the two diseases have much in common. Fundamentally, both these disorders result from clonal proliferations of T cells, presumably in the lymphoid tissues, followed by migration into the skin.[17] In most cases, Sézary-mycosis cells bear markers of helper T cells ($OKT4^+$), but $OKT8^+$ tumor cells have also been detected in some patients. Although the prognosis in a given case depends on the extent of disease at the time of diagnosis, a median survival rate of eight to nine years is not unusual.[18]

Immunoblastic sarcoma of T cells is the most poorly characterized category in the Lukes-Collins classification. Intended to include lymphomas derived from the transformed T lymphocytes in the paracortical area, this group contains tumors that have a mixture of small lymphocytes and many large transformed cells. The latter have round or oval nuclei with fine chromatin, and one or more small but distinctly eosinophilic nucleoli. Absence of plasmacytoid features and pyroninophilia are considered helpful in distinguishing them from B immunoblasts. However, this definition of T-immunoblastic sarcomas is extremely hazy and at present no distinct clinical or morphologic entity has emerged.[15]

Tumors of Histiocytes. True histiocytic lymphomas, i.e., those that can be cytochemically and immunologically confirmed to have arisen from macrophages, are extremely rare. Most tumors classified as histiocytic lymphomas in the Rappaport classification are accommodated in the B-cell category of the Lukes-Collins classification.

U-Cell (Undefined) Group. This group includes lymphomas that cannot be classified into a definite category either by morphologic or currently available immunocytochemical markers. These may indeed be tumors of very primitive T cells, B cells, or macrophages, or the so-called "null" cells.

Rappaport and Lukes-Collins Classifications—Comments and Comparisons

The basic purpose of a classification is to provide guidance in the clinical management of patients; i.e., it should define groups that are relatively homogeneous with respect to response to therapy and prognosis. Ideally, such a classification should also be scientifically accurate, highly reproducible, and readily learned by the practicing pathologist. It is by these criteria that we should assess the classifications of NHL.

Separation of NHL into nodular and diffuse categories has been a major contribution of the Rappaport classification, since nodular architecture is associated with a prognosis significantly superior to that of the diffuse pattern.[3,4] Furthermore, the histologic distinction between nodular and diffuse NHL is easily learned and therefore highly reproducible. In addition to the lymph node architecture, the cytologic categories defined by Rappaport also influence the clinical course,[19] but the identification of various cytologic subtypes (based on subtle differences in cell size and nuclear characteristics) is not very reproducible. Overall, the Rappaport classification has the virtue of long use, good clinical correlations, and a fair degree of reproducibility. However, the recent awareness of the remarkable morphologic transformation of lymphocytes in different stages of activation has shed new light on the histogenetic origins of various forms of lymphomas, particularly those classified as histiocytic by Rappaport. It is now evident from the studies of Lukes and Collins that approximately 76% of the so-called histiocytic or large-cell lymphomas are tumors of "transformed" (activated) B lymphocytes—some immunoblastic sarcomas (e.g., Fig. 15–9), others large cleaved and noncleaved cell types.[14, 20] Of those remaining, 8% are T-cell lymphomas, 11% cannot be defined by presently available immunocytochemical techniques, and only 5% are true histiocytic tumors. It is obvious, therefore, that histiocytic lymphomas in the Rappaport classification are not homogeneous with respect to their origin. Grouping of histogenetically diverse tumors purely on morphologic grounds is considered scientifically inaccurate and a major weakness of the Rappaport classification.

Conceptually, the Lukes-Collins classification is much more acceptable, since it places various lymphoid tumors into well-defined functional categories based on their origin from specific normal cell types. However, are the immunologically homogeneous categories associated with uniform clinical behavior? At present there are no clear answers, and disagreement persists regarding the clinical utility of an immunologically based classification of NHL.[21, 22] Another important difference between the Lukes-Collins and Rappaport classifications relates to the significance of nodular versus diffuse pattern. Recall that, according to Rappaport, nodular growth pattern is associated with an indolent disease. According to Lukes and Collins, however, when patients are stratified into groups based on the cell of origin, differences between nodular and diffuse lymphomas become biologically minimal. It is claimed, for example, that the observed superior survival of patients with nodular lymphomas is related to the fact that the nodular pattern is seen most often with small cleaved cell tumors, which are the least aggressive of the FCC lymphomas. Although this issue is not completely resolved, most published studies continue to support the notion that the nodular growth pattern, independent of the cytologic subtype, is associated with a better prognosis.[3]

In addition to clinical utility, we must also ask whether the Lukes-Collins classification is practical and reproducible. Although its authors contend that the functional classification can be applied by using only morphologic criteria, others have failed to achieve more than 60% accuracy in classifying the cell of origin on the basis of histologic examination.[23] Therefore, it has been advocated that markers that characterize various immune cells (Table 15–3) be routinely utilized as an adjunct to morphology. With this refinement, it is claimed that meaningful correlations can be made between the immunologic type and the clinical behavior

Table 15–3. TECHNIQUES USED FOR IDENTIFICATION OF T CELLS, B CELLS, AND HISTIOCYTES

	T Cells	B Cells	Histiocytes Monocytes	Comments
Rosette methods*				Cytocentrifuge preparations of value in evaluating lymphomas
Spontaneous sheep erythrocyte (E) receptor	+	–	–	Present on all peripheral T cells
Complement (EAC) receptor	(+)	+	+	Convoluted T-cell lymphomas are observed with complement receptors; normal T cells negative
Fc (EA) receptor	(+)	+	+	Present only on some T-cell subsets
Surface immunoglobulin	–	+	(+)	By immunofluorescence; monocytes may mark because of Fc receptors
Cytoplasmic immunoglobulin	–	+	–	Immunoperoxidase more useful than immunofluorescence in lymphomas because it can be used on paraffin sections
Monoclonal antibodies OKT3, OKT11	+	–	–	Present on all peripheral T cells; OKT11 is antibody to sheep red blood cell (E) receptor
OKT10	+	–	–	Present only on intrathymic T cells and tumors of immature T cells
Anti–HLA-DR	(+)	+	+	Present only on activated T cells; seen also on Langerhans' cells and dendritic cells
Cytochemistry				
α-Naphthyl butyrase (NSE)†	(+)	–	+	Focal staining reported in T cells; specificity for T cells is not proved
Acid phosphatase	(+)	–	–	Reported in convoluted T-cell lymphomas and T-cell ALL
Tartrate-resistant acid phosphatase	–	(+)	–	Present in hairy cell leukemia
Muramidase (lysozyme)	–	–	+	Immunoperoxidase method on paraffin sections or imprints
TdT	(+)	(+)	–	Present only in primitive T and B cells

*A rosette is identified as a nucleated cell surrounded by a cluster of appropriately treated sheep erythrocytes. Spontaneous sheep erythrocyte (E) receptor is detected by use of unsensitized sheep red cells. For detection of complement receptors, sheep erythrocytes (E) are coated with IgM antierythrocyte antibody (A) and sublytic amounts of complement (C); Fc receptors are detected by rosetting with erythrocytes (E) coated with IgG antierythrocyte antibody (A).

†NSE = nonspecific esterase.

Parentheses indicate that the presence of the marker is not characteristic or specific for that cell type, as explained under comments.

Table 15–4. A WORKING FORMULATION OF NON-HODGKIN'S LYMPHOMAS FOR CLINICAL USAGE (EQUIVALENT OR RELATED TERMS OF RAPPAPORT AND LUKES-COLLINS CLASSIFICATIONS ARE SHOWN)

Working Formulation	Rappaport Classification	Lukes-Collins Classification
Low-Grade		
A. Small lymphocytic	Lymphocytic, well differentiated	Small lymphocyte and plasmacytoid lymphocytic
B. Follicular, predominantly small cleaved cell	Nodular, poorly differentiated lymphocytic	FCC, small cleaved
C. Follicular, mixed small cleaved and large cleaved cell	Nodular, mixed lymphocytic histiocytic	FCC, small cleaved and large cleaved
Intermediate-Grade		
D. Follicular, predominantly large cell	Nodular, histiocytic	FCC, large cleaved and/or non-cleaved
E. Diffuse, small cleaved cell	Diffuse, poorly differentiated lymphocytic	FCC, small cleaved diffuse
F. Diffuse, mixed large and small cell	Diffuse, mixed lymphocytic and histiocytic	FCC, small cleaved, large cleaved, or large noncleaved
G. Diffuse, large cell	Diffuse histiocytic	FCC, large cleaved or noncleaved
High-Grade		
H. Large cell, immunoblastic	Diffuse histiocytic	Immunoblastic B- or T-cell type
I. Lymphoblastic	Lymphoblastic lymphoma	Convoluted T-cell lymphoma
J. Small noncleaved cell	Undifferentiated, Burkitt's and non-Burkitt's	FCC, small noncleaved
Miscellaneous		

of various NHLs.[24] It must be admitted, however, that the complex immunocytochemical procedures presently available have not yet been widely applied to the routine diagnostic evaluation of lymph node biopsies.

In summary, it appears that, with respect to prognostication or patient management, the superiority of the Lukes-Collins approach to that of Rappaport has not yet been proved beyond reasonable doubt. The major contribution of the Lukes-Collins classification has been that it has significantly advanced our understanding of the histogenesis of NHL and has provided an impetus for improving the existing classifications.

A Working Formulation of NHL for Clinical Usage

In addition to the two discussed above, four other well-described classifications are currently used in different parts of the world.[3] Of these, the Kiel classification, used widely in Europe, is similar to the Lukes-Collins in being based partly on functional concepts. The others are purely morphologic. The existence of many classifications not only has resulted in much confusion and controversy, but also has made it impossible to compare effectively the results of clinical studies utilizing different systems. To resolve this, the National Cancer Institute of the U.S.A., in collaboration with several international experts, has suggested a new Working Formulation for Clinical Usage (Table 15–4).[3] As the name indicates, this classification has a strong clinical bias. NHLs are divided into three major prognostic groupings based on survival statistics, each group containing several morphologic categories. *The five-year survival rate for the tumors classified as low grade ranged from 50 to 70%, and for tumors of intermediate and high grade from 35 to 45% and 23 to 32%, respectively.* The descriptive terminology is somewhat similar to that of the Lukes-Collins classification, but there is no attempt to segregate lymphomas on the basis of the presumed cell of origin. The histologic appearance of the tumors within the working formulation may be surmised from the equivalent terms in the Rappaport and Lukes-Collins classification (Table 15–4). Detailed comparisons with the other classifications are available in the report.

Morphology. The precise categorization of lymphomas rests heavily on the cytologic details already presented, but without doubt immunocytochemical methods greatly increase diagnostic accuracy. Required for diagnosis are representative samples (usually excised nodes) of the lymphoma, which should be promptly transferred to the diagnostic laboratory unfixed, so that "touch imprints" of fresh cut surfaces and special immunologic and cytochemical procedures can be performed. Obviously the best possible histologic tissue sections are also necessary.

Most lymphomas are characterized by lymphadenopathy and, as the disease advances, splenomegaly, hepatomegaly, and eventually involvement of other viscera. At first only one or a single chain of nodes is involved. In an analysis of a large series of cases, the cervical chain (either side) was the primary site of involvement in approximately 30 to 40% of cases, and the axillary nodes in approximately 20%, followed in order by the inguinal, femoral, iliac, and mediastinal nodes.[25] In approximately one-third of cases, extranodal disease may be the presenting feature. This is seen most frequently with histiocytic (large-cell) lymphomas. In all forms of lymphoma, affected nodes are variably enlarged, sometimes up to massive size (10 cm in diameter). They are generally soft and fleshy and are usually discrete without adherence to surrounding structures. On cut surfaces, the nodular forms may present foci of nodularity barely apparent to the naked eye. Nodes with diffuse disease are homoge-

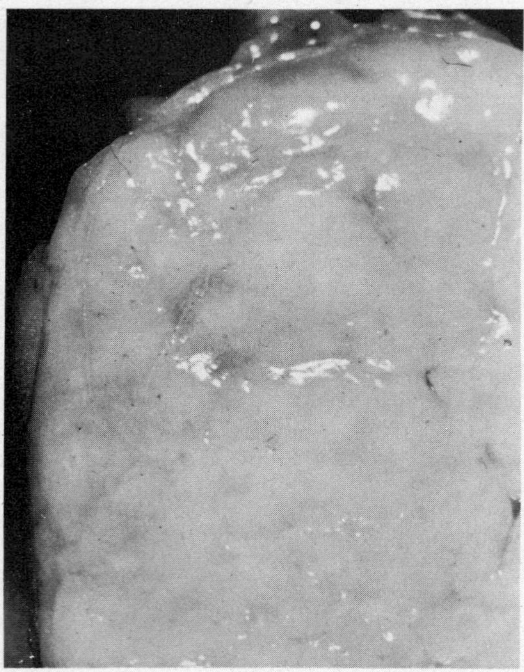

Figure 15–13. Cut surface of a lymph node with diffuse involvement with non-Hodgkin's lymphoma. The surface is homogeneous gray with total loss of nodal architecture.

neously gray and have the appearance of fish flesh (Fig. 15–13). Necrosis, hemorrhage, and foci of cystic softening are uncommon. With advance of the disease, progressively more nodes are affected, and the tumorous tissue may permeate the capsule of the node and extend into the pericapsular tissues to produce interadherence and matted, nodular tumorous masses (Fig. 15–14). Such a gross appearance is characteristic of the diffuse patterns of lymphoma. Lymphomatous spread to the spleen, liver, or other viscera may be inapparent macroscopically or may induce hepatosplenomegaly, sometimes without grossly visible lesions, but more often minute to moderate-sized tumorous nodules resembling metastases can be seen.

Etiology and Pathogenesis. The etiology and pathogenesis of NHLs is as mysterious as that of all cancers. However, since lymphomas are neoplasms of the immune system, certain special features that apply to these tumors will be discussed here. It is well-known that the proliferation of lymphocytes is a normal consequence of their exposure to antigens and that this physiologic response is kept in check by a variety of regulatory mechanisms. *It is postulated that malignant lymphomas develop when there is failure of immunoregulation in the face of a persistent stimulus for lymphocyte proliferation.* Several observations support such a hypothesis. Human recipients of organ transplants (e.g., kidney or heart), patients with congenital immune deficiency syndromes, and those with certain autoimmune diseases have an unusually high incidence of NHLs.

In the case of *allograft recipients,* the antigens of the graft provide persistent strong antigenic stimulus to the host lymphocytes, while feedback regulation of lymphoproliferation is impaired by simultaneous immunosuppressive therapy. In *autoimmune diseases,* chronic antigenic stimulation is provided by the constant exposure to self-antigens. In this clinical setting there is a genetically determined impairment of immunoregulation (p. 179), and immunosuppressive therapy with cytotoxic drugs further disturbs the regulatory networks. The greatly increased incidence of lymphomas with Sjögren's disease was mentioned earlier (p. 190); an increased risk is also noted with rheumatoid arthritis

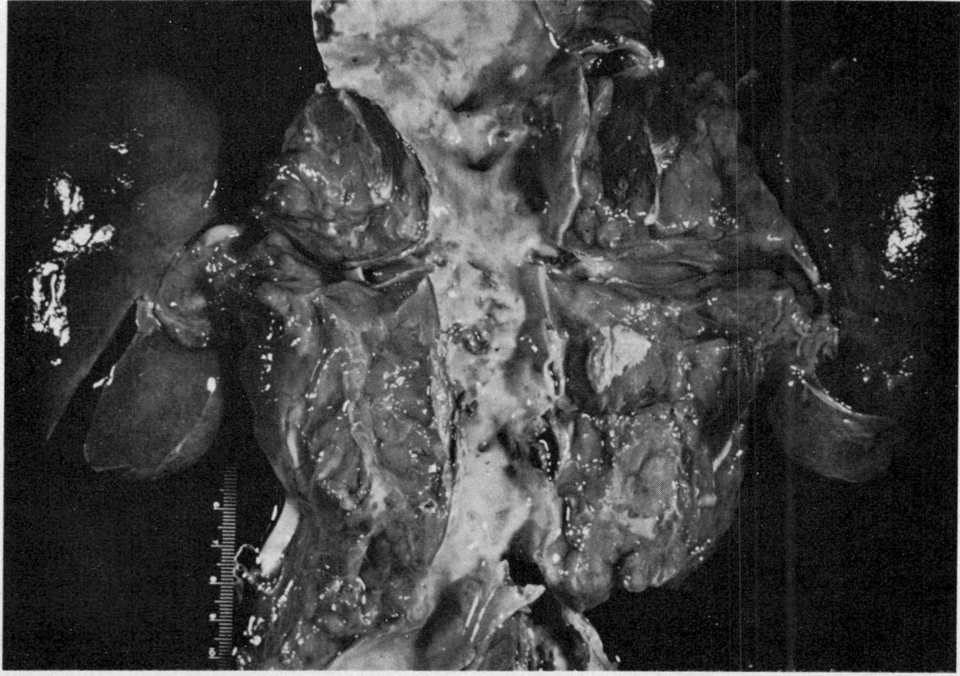

Figure 15–14. Lymphoma involving periaortic nodes.

and SLE. In *primary immunodeficiency syndromes,* recurrent infections are the obvious source for antigenic stimulation. Many of these disorders are also associated with abnormalities in T-suppressor cells (p. 205). One form of immunodeficiency, the X-linked lymphoproliferative syndrome (XLP), is of particular interest. Unlike patients with the generalized immunodeficiency states in whom there is predilection for a wide variety of bacterial and viral infections, those with XLP have specific defects in immune responsiveness to EBV.[26] As might be expected with any X-linked disorder, only males are affected, who develop a variety of progressive and rapidly fatal disorders following exposure to EBV in early childhood. You may recall that in infectious mononucleosis the EBV-induced B-cell proliferation is contained by the activation of immunoregulatory T cells, and the disease is therefore self-limited (p. 288). By contrast, in patients with the XLP syndrome, infection with EBV may lead to fatal infectious mononucleosis or a malignant B-cell lymphoma, because they are unable to mount T-cell surveillance against the virus.[27] Paradoxically, in some patients abnormal and excessive T-suppressor cell response to the EBV infection may shut down normal hematopoiesis or immunoglobulin synthesis, leading to aplastic anemia or hypogammaglobulinemia, respectively.

The studies cited above have provided an alternative explanation of the well-known association between EBV and Burkitt's lymphoma. According to this view, the pathogenesis of Burkitt's lymphoma is a three-step process. In the *first step,* the EBV acts as a B-cell mitogen and initiates a polyclonal B-cell proliferation. In most individuals the lymphoproliferation is arrested at this stage owing to the activation of immunoregulatory T cells, and there is either no clinical disease or a self-limited episode of infectious mononucleosis (p. 288). A congenital (e.g., XLP syndrome) or acquired (e.g., immunosuppression in allograft recipients) defect in the T-cell response to EBV leads to the *next step,* characterized by sustained polyclonal B-cell proliferation, which in some cases may present as acute severe infectious mononucleosis. Although usually fatal, this condition does not represent a true neoplasm since the proliferating B cells are not monoclonal. In other patients, the polyclonal B-cell proliferations may be chronic, setting the stage for the *third and final step,* lymphomagenesis—the emergence of a truly neoplastic clone of B cells. What brings about such a transition is not clear, but it seems reasonable to assume that the rapidly proliferating B cells are at a greatly enhanced risk of acquiring cytogenetic aberrations (such as translocations), some of which may offer growth advantage to the affected cell. In due course, the progeny of the cell with the translocated chromosome would replace all other B cells, resulting in a monoclonal B-cell neoplasm. Recall that the tumor cells in Burkitt's lymphoma frequently show a nonrandom t(8;14) chromosomal translocation (p. 245). This translocation may so derange cellular regulation that the cells become autonomous. *According to this view, then, EBV itself is not directly oncogenic but, by acting as a B-cell mitogen, it creates an environment for the oncogenic event involving some critical gene rearrangements.* Evidence for the stepwise transition from polyclonal to monoclonal B-cell proliferation has been observed, not only in cases with the XLP syndrome, but also in angioimmunoblastic lymphadenopathy, an unusual disorder described later in this chapter (p. 696). Although this scheme is derived largely from the study of Burkitt's lymphoma, it is not essential to invoke EBV in the causation of other malignant lymphomas. Sustained polyclonal proliferation of lymphocytes, an essential ingredient of this hypothesis, may derive from any one of the causes of chronic antigenic stimulation discussed earlier. It is interesting to note in this context that many distinctive nonrandom chromosomal abnormalities (mostly translocations) have been identified with a high frequency in several B-cell lymphomas other than Burkitt's tumor.[28] In most of these, chromosome 14 is involved in the translocation and the breakpoint is almost always at the same band, i.e., q32. There is no satisfactory explanation for this remarkable constancy of the breakpoint, but it has been suggested that genes close to band q32 on chromosome 14 are somehow capable of affecting the proliferative state of the affected cells, as discussed on pages 249 and 677.

In closing, it should be pointed out that in the great majority of patients with NHLs there is no overt immunologic abnormality. However, this does not preclude the possibility that subtle disturbances in immune regulation not easily detected by present-day techniques may underlie most cases of NHL.

STAGING. A staging system of Hodgkin's disease is described on page 674. Like NHL, Hodgkin's disease usually arises within lymph nodes and then disseminates more widely. A rigorous protocol has been devised to express the extent and distribution of Hodgkin's disease within the patient, employing meticulous physical examination, blood studies, lymphangiography, laparotomy, liver biopsy, and splenectomy. Unlike Hodgkin's disease, however, staging is of limited value in deciding therapy or offering prognosis for patients with NHL. This stems from the fact that in NHL the histologic type influences prognosis much more profoundly than does the extent of disease. For example, nodular lymphomas have the best prognosis despite disseminated (Stage IV) disease at the time of diagnosis. Staging is most valuable in the diffuse histiocytic lymphomas, since they often present with localized disease. However, staging is essential in order to compare different modalities of treatment within a given histologic category.

CLINICAL COURSE. Non-Hodgkin's lymphomas are most often diagnosed in adults, usually in the fifth to sixth decades of life, but may occur in children. *Childhood lymphomas* differ in many respects from those in adults. In general, extranodal (abdominal, mediastinal) disease is much more common and nodular lymphomas are rare. Lymphoblastic lymphoma and undifferentiated lymphomas constitute the two most common histologic types. Although these are aggressive lesions, they respond well to therapy and approximately 50% are curable.[29]

Typically, lymphomas present with the insidious

onset of peripheral, painless nodal enlargement. In some patients, these tumors come to attention as mediastinal masses, as gastrointestinal lesions, or as causes of splenomegaly or hepatomegaly. Rarely, they present as a bone tumor, tonsillar enlargement, or the cause of an anemia or leukemia. The range of clinical presentations is almost limitless, since they may be primary in any site bearing lymphoid tissue. Wherever they present, unless controlled by therapy, more and more nodes become involved over the span of months, along with the spleen and liver as well as other tissues and organs. Unlike Hodgkin's disease, the spread is not predictable. With more advanced disease, fever, sweats, and weight loss may appear. The hepatosplenomegaly may be quite massive. When the lymphomatous cells spill into the peripheral blood, a leukemia-like pattern of disease is created with lymphomatous seeding of all organs of the body.

As expected, the prognosis varies with the extent of the dissemination, the specific form of lymphoma, and the therapeutic modalities employed. Radiation alone may be used in the earlier stages of these diseases, but in the later stages, chemotherapy or combined radiation and chemotherapy are generally employed. The range of cytotoxic and cytostatic drugs used alone and in variable combinations is now quite large and beyond our scope. These diseases once cast a hopeless pall, but some have yielded remarkably to therapy, to the point at which it is now possible to speak of "long remissions" lasting for years of some of these once rapidly progressive disorders.

Hodgkin's Disease (Hodgkin's Lymphoma)

Hodgkin's disease has been segregated from NHL for many reasons. First, it is characterized histologically by the presence of neoplastic giant cells called Reed-Sternberg cells admixed with a variable inflammatory component. Second, its spread is almost always by contiguity—from one chain of nodes to the adjacent groups. Finally, it almost never has a leukemic component.

Several histologic variants of Hodgkin's disease have been recognized. The *one common denominator among all forms is the presence of a distinctive tumor giant cell known as the Reed-Sternberg (RS) cell.* It is considered to be the essential neoplastic element in all forms of Hodgkin's disease, and its identification is essential for the histologic diagnosis. *Classically, it is a large cell (15 to 45 μm in diameter), most often binucleate or bilobed with two halves often appearing as mirror images of each other (Fig. 15–15). At other times there are multiple nuclei, or the single nucleus is multilobate and polypoid. The nucleus is enclosed within an abundant amphophilic cytoplasm. Prominent within the nuclei are large, inclusion-like, "owl-eyed" nucleoli generally surrounded by a clear halo.* In typical RS cells the nucleoli are acidophilic or, at the least, amphophilic, and react strongly with RNA stains. Giant cells are sometimes found that have all the characteristics of the

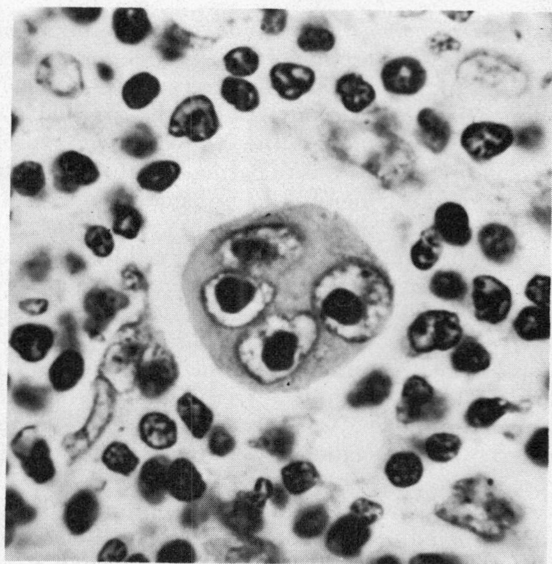

Figure 15–15. Reed-Sternberg cell. (From Neiman, R. S.: Current problems in histopathologic diagnosis and classification of Hodgkin's disease. Pathol. Annu. *13*:289, 1978.)

multinucleate cell just described and that contain only a single nucleus replete with large nucleolus. Although such cells may be biologic variants of the RS cell, they are not diagnostic of Hodgkin's disease. Other cells, uninucleate or multinucleate, may not have a nucleolus; these, too, are nondiagnostic. One additional variant, the so-called *lacunar cell,* is encountered primarily within one of the distinctive patterns of Hodgkin's disease called nodular sclerosis.

It is somewhat anticlimactic to report that cells closely simulating or identical with RS cells have been identified in conditions other than Hodgkin's disease. Lukes et al.[30] have reported RS-like cells in infectious mononucleosis, and Rappaport and colleagues[31] have observed cells that resemble the RS cell in solid tissue cancers, mycosis fungoides, lymphomas, and other conditions.[32] Thus, to quote Rappaport et al., "we believe that a definitive diagnosis of Hodgkin's disease cannot be rendered in the absence of Sternberg-Reed cells, but that the diagnosis depends upon the total histologic picture."[31] Stated another way, *the RS cell is necessary but not sufficient for the diagnosis.* Thus, we are faced with the dilemma that a histologic diagnosis of Hodgkin's disease cannot be made without identifying RS cells, but RS cells cannot be identified unless they are present in Hodgkin's disease. Recognizing this difficulty, we can turn to a characterization of the morphologic forms of Hodgkin's disease.

CLASSIFICATION. It is heartening that unlike the situation with NHLs, there is nearly universal acceptance of a single, well-characterized classification—the Rye.[33] Four distinctive patterns have been defined that vary in their gravity. The essential morphologic feature that separates three of the four subgroups (lymphocytic predominance, mixed cellularity, and lymphocytic depletion) is the frequency of the RS cells, relative to the number of lymphocytes, representing the host response. The frequency of lymphocytes seems to have a direct bearing on the spread and prognosis of Hodgkin's disease. The fourth variant, nodular sclerosis, which has distinctive histologic as well as clinical features, is believed to represent a special expression of the disease. In most series, nodular sclerosis is the most common variant (40 to 75%) followed by mixed cellularity (20 to 40%). The two polar groups, i.e., lymphocyte predominance and lymphocytic depletion groups, are the least common (5 to 15% each).

Lymphocyte-predominance Hodgkin's disease is characterized by a diffuse or sometimes vaguely nodular infiltrate of mature lymphocytes admixed with variable numbers of benign histiocytes. Scattered among these cells are the distinctive RS cells, but these are almost always few in number (Fig. 15–16). Variants that lack the large "owl-eye" nucleoli are somewhat more common, but are not diagnostic. However, they serve as useful clues since their presence warrants a careful search for typical RS cells. Without the identification of RS cells, the lymphocyte-predominance pattern could be readily mistaken for one of the lymphocytic forms of NHL. There usually is little fibrosis and no evidence of areas of necrosis.

Mixed-cellularity Hodgkin's disease is marked by a diffuse infiltrate of lymphocytes, histiocytes, eosinophils, and plasma cells. Classic RS cells are usually plentiful and lymphocytes are much less numerous than in the lymphocyte-predominance form. Small areas of necrosis and fibrosis may be present, but are not as prominent as in the lymphocyte-depletion form. Mixed cellularity disease occupies an intermediate position in clinical gravity between the lymphocyte-predominant and lymphocyte-depletion patterns.

The *lymphocyte-depletion pattern shows a paucity of lymphocytes and a relative abundance of RS cells or their atypical pleomorphic variants.* Since the ratio of the neoplastic elements to the reactive lymphocytes is tilted in favor of tumor cells, this pattern constitutes the most ominous form of Hodgkin's disease. It presents a somewhat broad range of morphologic changes, sometimes subdivided into *diffuse fibrosis* and *reticular variants.* In the diffuse-fibrosis variant, the hypocellular node is largely replaced by a proteinaceous fibrillar material that represents a disorderly, nonbirefringent connective tissue. Scattered within this background are lymphocytes, pleomorphic (atypical) RS cells, and a few typical RS cells (Fig. 15–17). The reticular variant is much more cellular and is composed of a diffuse infiltrate of highly anaplastic, large, pleomorphic cells, which may simulate RS cells but which lack all their classic features. Only a few typical RS cells can be identified.

The *nodular-sclerosis* pattern of this disease is described last because in many respects it appears to represent a distinct entity having a different biologic significance and epidemiology from the other three variants. Clinically, it is the only form more common in women and it has a striking propensity to involve mediastinal, supraclavicular, and lower cervical nodes. It is characterized morphologically by two features: (1) *birefringent, well-defined bands of collagen that traverse the lymph node, enclosing nodules of normal or abnormal lymphoid tissue (Fig. 15–18);* (2) *a tendency for the RS cells to assume the lacunar morphology.* The lacunar cells have a single hyperlobated nucleus with multiple small nucleoli and an abundant, pale-staining cytoplasm with well-defined borders. In formalin-fixed tissue, the pale cytoplasm of these cells often retracts, giving rise to the appearance of the nuclei lying in a clear space or a "lacuna" (Fig. 15–19). Classic RS cells are infrequent. In some cases the fibrosis is abundant, leaving only suggestive islets of lymphoid tissue. Within the lymphoid nodules the pattern may take the form of lymphocyte predominance, may show mixed cellularity, or at times may be composed almost entirely of lacunar cells. In other instances the fibrosis is quite scant, and diagnosis rests on the numerous lacunar cells.

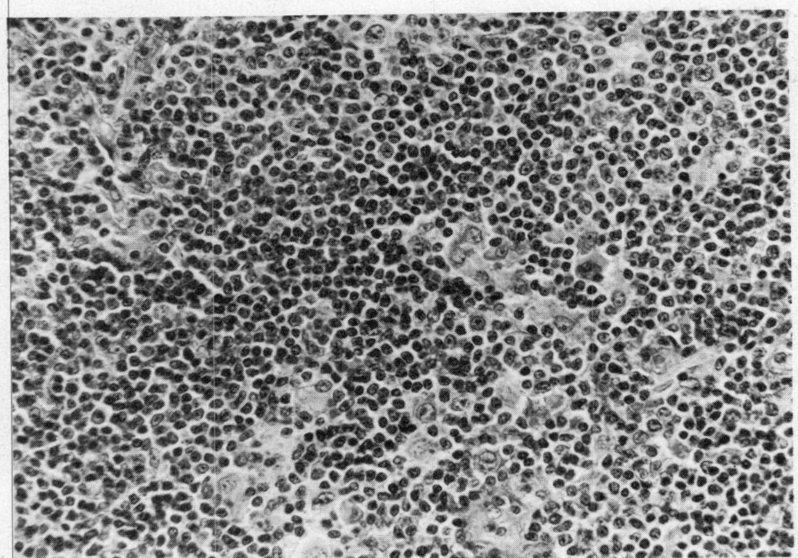

Figure 15–16. Lymphocyte-predominance Hodgkin's disease. (From Neiman, R. S.: Current problems in histopathologic diagnosis and classification of Hodgkin's disease. Pathol. Annu. *13*:289, 1978.)

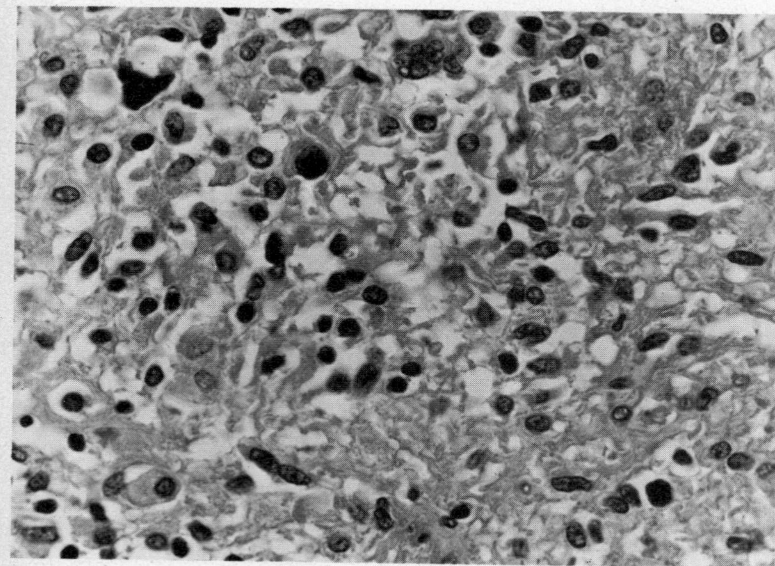

Figure 15–17. Lymph node in diffuse-fibrosis Hodgkin's disease. All cellular elements are greatly diminished, and granular, proteinaceous interstitial material is prominent. A few highly atypical polyploid cells that lack the cytologic features of Reed-Sternberg cells are present. (From Neiman, R. S.: Current problems in histopathologic diagnosis and classification of Hodgkin's disease. Pathol. Annu. *13*:289, 1978.)

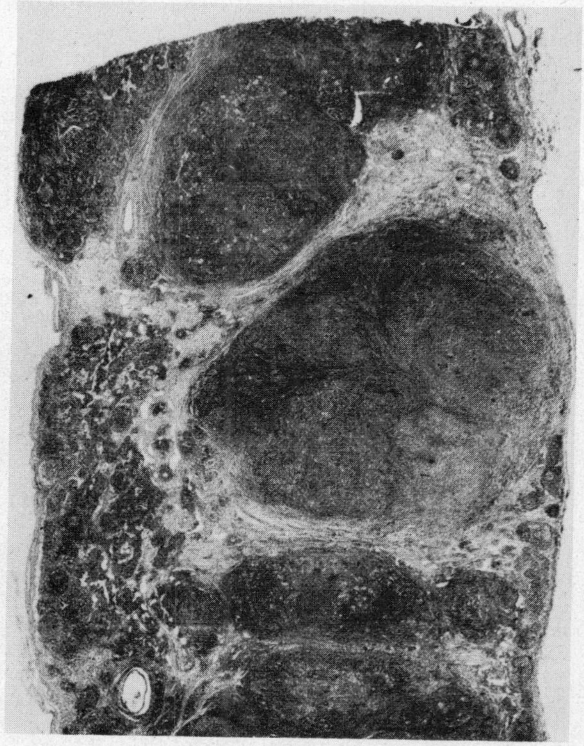

Figure 15–18. Hodgkin's disease—nodular sclerosis. This low-power view shows well-defined bands of collagen enclosing nodules of abnormal lymphoid tissue. On left, some compressed remnants of normal lymph node can be seen under capsule. (Courtesy of Dr. Jose Hernandez, Department of Pathology, Southwestern Medical School, Dallas, Texas.)

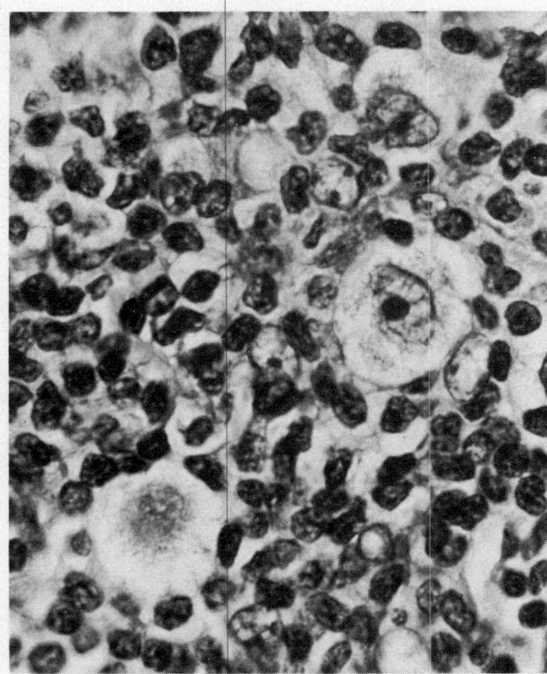

Figure 15–19. Hodgkin's disease—lacunar cells.

MORPHOLOGY. Hodgkin's disease almost always begins in a single node or chain of nodes, but occasionally it arises within the thymus or spleen. The nodular-sclerosis pattern most often arises in the mediastinum, suggesting a thymic origin, but it too may first appear in a node in the clavicular or neck region. Over the course of time the disease spreads to contiguous chains of nodes, a feature considered quite characteristic of Hodgkin's disease.

The gross appearance of involved nodes depends on the particular histologic pattern. With the lymphocyte predominance pattern, the nodes have a soft, uniform, fish-flesh appearance and are not distinguishable from nodes involved by the diffuse NHLs. With the mixed-cellularity pattern, foci of pale, opaque, yellow-white necrosis may be evident on the cut surface. With nodular sclerosis and the more fibrous lymphocyte-depletion patterns, the involved nodes may be tough and gray-white, as would be expected. In such instances, groups of nodes are often firmly matted together. As the disease extends, particularly in the more aggressive patterns, it may penetrate the nodal capsules to involve the perinodal tissue and to produce matted chains of nodes. Involvement of the spleen, liver, bone marrow, and other organs and tissues may appear in due course, taking the form of irregular, tumor-like nodules of tissue resembling that present in the nodes. At times, the spleen is greatly enlarged and the liver is moderately enlarged by these nodular masses. At other times, the involvement is more subtle and becomes evident only on microscopic examination.

The histologic details of the four variants of Hodgkin's disease have already been presented. **No morphologic variant can be diagnosed without identification of the distinctive, albeit not pathognomonic, RS cells.** This is particularly important to remember since some forms of Hodgkin's disease with an abundance of inflammatory cells (eosinophils, neutrophils, histiocytes, and plasma cells) come deceptively close to simulating a reactive inflammatory process, whereas others (such as the reticular form of lymphocyte-depletion Hodgkin's disease) can easily be mistaken for non-Hodgkin's, histiocytic lymphoma.

ETIOLOGY AND PATHOGENESIS. The origins of Hodgkin's disease are unknown. The question of etiology is especially complex since several fundamental issues have not been resolved. What is the derivation of the neoplastic RS cells? Do the various histologic variants of Hodgkin's disease represent a single disorder with a common etiology? Are some forms of Hodgkin's disease caused by an infectious agent? Central to many of these issues is a large body of epidemiologic data.[34] Hodgkin's disease has a bimodal age-incidence curve, with one early peak at 15 to 34 years and a second peak after the age of 45 years. In the younger age group there is an increased risk associated with smaller families, better housing, and higher education. These factors are known to be associated with late exposure to a variety of common childhood infections, including poliomyelitis. Therefore, it has been suggested that Hodgkin's disease, like paralytic poliomyelitis, may be a rare consequence of delayed infection with a common agent—possibly the EB virus. Some indirect evidence supports the viral hypothesis. In young adults with infectious mononucleosis, there is a two- to threefold higher incidence of Hodgkin's disease. Furthermore, relative to healthy controls, patients with Hodgkin's disease have a higher titer of antibody to EBV capsid antigen. However, none of this evidence can be considered conclusive. The role of EBV in the etiology of Hodgkin's disease is not supported by the reported absence of EBV nucleic acid sequences in cultured RS cells.[35] Thus, it could very well be that the epidemiologic association between EBV infection (or infectious mononucleosis) and Hodgkin's disease reflects a common population at risk for both the diseases. Several earlier reports suggested clustering of Hodgkin's disease in young adults, thus implicating a horizontal transmission of an infectious agent, but this hypothesis has not yet received wide support. In contrast with the younger age group, viral infection has not been implicated in the pathogenesis of Hodgkin's disease in older patients.

There are also clinical and histologic differences in the two age groups. In the younger patients, the male-to-female ratio is about equal, and most of the cases have the nodular-sclerosis pattern. In the older group, the male-to-female ratio is higher and there is greater frequency of the mixed-cellularity pattern. Whether these differences are truly indicative of two distinct etiologic forms of Hodgkin's disease remains to be proved. At present, the possibility cannot be excluded that the bimodal age incidence as well as other differences may reflect variation in host response to a single unknown causative agent.

A major hurdle to an understanding of the nature of Hodgkin's disease has been the mystery surrounding the genealogy of the "transformed" neoplastic cells. *It is now widely accepted that RS cells or their variant forms represent the tumorous element.*[36] However, there are disagreements over whether they are T cells, B cells, or histiocytes. Since patients with Hodgkin's disease have a marked impairment of T cell–mediated immunity, manifested by cutaneous anergy and increased susceptibility to various fungal and opportunistic infections, it has been suggested that RS cells represent transformed T cells. However, no T-cell markers have been detected on the RS cells, and moreover the impairment of T-cell immunity seems to be caused by activation of suppressor cells rather than loss of function due to neoplastic transformation of T cells.[37] Several workers have observed immunoglobulins either within or on the surface of RS cells, implicating a possible B-cell origin. However, recent studies with monospecific light-chain antisera indicate that both kappa and lambda light chains are present within the cytoplasm of RS cells. Since an individual B cell can produce only one kind of light chain, the intracytoplasmic immunoglobulins in the RS cells must derive from passive internalization rather than endogenous synthesis. Attention, therefore, is now focused on macrophages as the candidates for neoplastic transformations. This possibility is supported by some recent histochemical and cell culture techniques. RS cells are positive for two macrophage-associated enzymes, acid phosphatase and nonspecific esterase, but the staining pattern is weaker than that observed in normal histiocytes. Yet another possibility exists. A monoclonal antibody reactive against permanent cell lines obtained from Hodgkin's tissue seems to cross-react with a very small population of cells in the parafollicular areas of normal lymph nodes, suggesting an origin from the so-called "interdigitating reticulum cells" found in this site.[38] These cells are believed to represent a special type of histiocyte.[39] Thus, the mist that surrounds the origins of Hodgkin's disease seems about to clear, but we still await the clear light.

STAGING. The staging of Hodgkin's disease is of great importance since its extent and distribution influence the clinical course, choice of therapy, and prognosis (Table 15–5).

A rigorous protocol has been established to determine the extent of spread of the lymphoma within the patient. It comprises (1) meticulous physical examination with particular attention to all lymph nodes, spleen, and liver; (2) a bipedal lymphangiogram (i.e., injection of a radiopaque dye into lymphatic channels of the feet) to visualize possible involvement of iliac and para-aortic nodes; (3) computed tomography (CT scan), especially to visualize involved upper abdominal and thoracic lymph nodes; (4) laparoscopy to assess possible splenic and hepatic involvement; and (5) in many clinics, a staging laparotomy, which includes biopsies of the liver and intra-abdominal lymph nodes, and removal of the spleen. With such an approach, it has been shown that in about one-third of the cases the staging laparotomy materially alters previous assessments about the extent of disease. However, splenectomy, although it allows accurate staging, predisposes to severe fatal septicemias, and therefore the utility of this procedure in the management of Hodgkin's disease is being reevaluated.

CLINICAL COURSE. At the outset there is painless enlargement of a single node or group of nodes. With

Table 15–5. CLINICAL STAGES OF HODGKIN'S AND NON-HODGKIN'S LYMPHOMAS (Ann Arbor Classification)*

Stage	Distribution of Disease
I	Involvement of a single lymph node region (I) or involvement of a single extralymphatic organ or site (I_E).
II	Involvement of two or more lymph node regions on the same side of the diaphragm alone (II) or with involvement of limited contiguous extralymphatic organ or tissue (II_E).
III	Involvement of lymph node regions on both sides of the diaphragm (III), which may include the spleen (III_S) and/or limited contiguous extralymphatic organ or site (III_E, III_{ES}).
IV	Multiple or disseminated foci of involvement of one or more extralymphatic organs or tissues with or without lymphatic involvement.

*All stages are further divided on the basis of the absence (A) or presence (B) of the following systemic symptoms: significant fever, night sweats, and/or unexplained weight loss of greater than 10% of normal body weight.

From Carbone, P. T., et al.: Symposium (Ann Arbor): Staging in Hodgkin's disease. Cancer Res. *31*:1707, 1971.

spread, symptoms such as fever, night sweats, weight loss, pruritus, and anemia may appear. The extent of the dissemination and the presence or absence of systemic symptoms are expressed by the clinical staging system (Table 15–5). As might be expected, most patients with lymphocyte-predominance disease are first diagnosed in clinical Stage I-A or II-A, whereas those with the lymphocyte-depletion variant are more apt to be in Stage III-B or IV-B. The mixed-cellularity pattern falls intermediate between these extremes. With nodular sclerosis, the great majority of individuals are in clinical Stages I-A and II-A, but occasionally some fall into II-B or III-B and rarely into IV-B.

It is impossible at this time to express a prognosis for the various forms of Hodgkin's disease because of the rapidly changing and ever more effective modes of therapy. Before the introduction of current treatment protocols employing high voltage irradiation of lymph nodes and chemotherapy, there was a marked influence of the specific morphologic variant on the outlook. However, in the very recent past, much more aggressive modes of therapy have largely obliterated these differences. *Currently, the extent of disease appears to be the most important prognostic indicator.* Five-year survival of patients with Stages I and II-A is now close to 100%, and most can expect to be cured. With advanced (Stages III and IV) disease, approximately 50% can achieve long-term, relapse-free survival. It is evident that the outlook for this disease has dramatically improved. However, progress has created a new set of problems. Long-term survivors of combined chemotherapy and radiotherapy have an increased risk of developing acute leukemia or some form of NHL. The many therapeutic steps forward, in the light of this unhappy byproduct, may require a few steps backward.

LEUKEMIAS

The leukemias are best viewed as *malignant neoplasias of white blood cell precursors, characterized by*

(1) diffuse replacement of the bone marrow with proliferating leukemic cells; (2) abnormal numbers and forms of immature white cells in the circulating blood; and (3) widespread infiltrates in the liver, spleen, lymph nodes, and other sites throughout the body. The term leukemia ("white blood") was first used by Virchow to denote the tendency to reverse the usual ratio of red cells to white cells in the circulation. The white cell count in the peripheral blood may achieve staggering levels of over 500,000 cells/mm³, but in some cases, the count is less than 10,000 cells/mm³. Instances in which the white count is abnormally low have sometimes been referred to as *aleukemic* or *leukopenic leukemia*. However, it should be emphasized that the peripheral white count is merely the tip of the iceberg, having little to do with the ultimately fatal nature of leukemia. *It is the anemia, thrombocytopenia, and loss of normally functioning leukocytes incident to the suppression of normal marrow elements by leukemic cells as well as the infiltrates of the various tissues and organs in the body that give these disorders their ominous aspect.*

CLASSIFICATION. Inevitably, the classification of leukemias has become increasingly complex. They are first divided into acute and chronic forms. The acute forms are characterized by a rapidly fatal course when untreated (on the order of two to four months from the time of diagnosis) and by the appearance in the blood of poorly differentiated cells, called "blasts." The initial white count is subnormal in about one-third of the cases but is above 100,000 cells/mm³ in 20% of cases. The chronic forms permit longer survival even when untreated (two to six years in many cases) and are associated with more mature circulating leukocytes. The peripheral white count may be subnormal but is more often markedly elevated into the hundreds of thousands (Fig. 15–20).

The leukemias are then subclassified according to the particular type of white cell involved into (1) lymphocytic and (2) myelocytic or myelogenous. A rudimentary classification therefore has four patterns of leukemia: acute lymphocytic (lymphoblastic) (ALL), chronic lymphocytic (CLL), acute myelocytic (myeloblastic) (AML), and chronic myelocytic (CML). Regrettably, difficulties arise with the acute leukemias, which are extremely heterogeneous both morphologically and with respect to cell surface markers. In the widely accepted French-American-British (FAB) classification,[40] the acute leukemias are subclassified on the basis of morphology, apparent differentiation, and histochemistry. In Table 15–6 a brief characterization of cell types is given along with each category, but more details are provided in the later section on morphology. It should be noted, however, that monocytic leukemia and acute erythroleukemia (Di Guglielmo's syndrome), which were previously classified separately, are now included in the AML category. This change reflects a greater understanding of the origins of these variants, discussed later (p. 676). In addition to the FAB morphologic subgrouping, ALLs are also classified immunologically on the basis of cell markers.[41] In 65% of ALL the

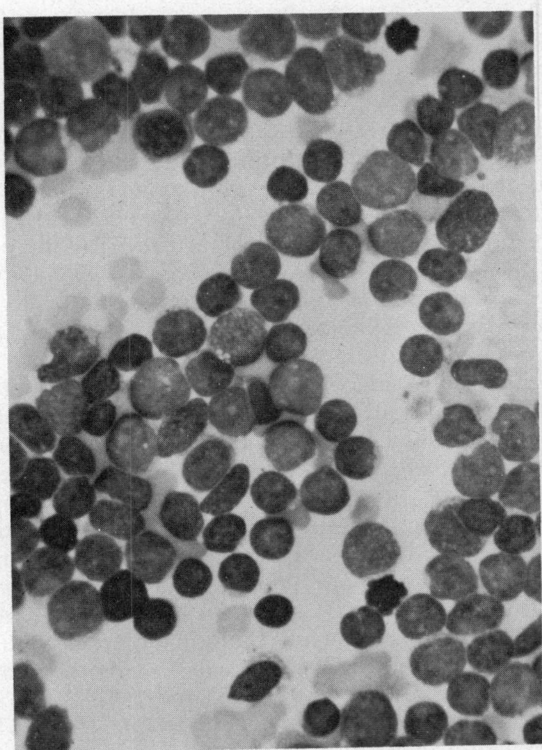

Figure 15–20. Peripheral blood smear from a patient with chronic lymphocytic leukemia who had a WBC count of 120,000.

Table 15–6. FRENCH-AMERICAN-BRITISH (FAB) CLASSIFICATION OF ACUTE LEUKEMIAS

Lymphocytic Acute (Lymphoblastic) (ALL)	
L1	Small cells predominate but may vary, with some cells up to twice diameter of small lymphocytes. Nuclei are generally round and regular with occasional clefts. Nucleoli often are not visible. Cytoplasm is scanty. Cell population is homogeneous.
L2	Cells are heterogeneous in size, and share in features of both L1 and L3. Nuclei often show clefts. Nucleoli are often present.
L3	There is a homogeneous population of large cells (3 to 4 times the diameter of small lymphocytes). Nuclei are round-to-oval with prominent nucleoli. Cytoplasm is abundant and deeply basophilic.
Acute Myelocytic (Myeloblastic) (AML)	
M1	Myeloblastic leukemia without maturation—cells are dominantly blasts without Auer rods or granules.
M2	Myeloblastic leukemia with maturation—many blasts but some maturation to promyelocytes or beyond.
M3	Hypergranular promyelocytic leukemia—mostly promyelocytes with cytoplasm packed with peroxidase-positive granules. Many Auer rods.
M4	Myelomonocytic leukemia—both myeloid and monocytic differentiation. Myeloid element resembles M2.
M5	Monocytic leukemia—both "monoblasts" and monocytes, the former having large round nuclei with lacy chromatin and prominent nucleoli. Diagnosis must be confirmed by fluoride-inhibited esterase reaction.
M6	Erythroleukemia—erythropoietic elements make up more than 50% of cells in marrow and have bizarre multilobate nuclei. May also be present in circulating blood, along with an admixture of myeloblasts and promyelocytes.

lymphoblasts *lack surface immunoglobulin, do not form E rosettes,* or react with monoclonal anti–T-cell antibodies (non-T, non-B group). The leukemic cells in the non-T, non-B group express the common ALL (CALLA) antigen, and therefore this group is referred to as common ALL (cALL). In approximately 20% of cases of cALL, the lymphoblasts have *cytoplasmic Ig,* suggesting that they represent immature (pre–B) cells. ALL, with the mature B-cell phenotype characterized by the presence of *surface Ig,* is quite uncommon (5%). T-cell ALL makes up 15 to 20% of all cases and is similar to the lymphoblastic lymphoma, already discussed (p. 661). The remaining cases (10 to 15%) do not bear any distinctive cell surface markers and hence cannot be classified at present. This immunologic subclassification has not only shed light on the origins of ALL, but is prognostically meaningful and hence widely accepted.

INCIDENCE. Leukemia is a common form of neoplasia. In 1983, it was expected to be the sixth leading cause of cancer death in the United States. It is particularly devastating in children under the age of 15, among whom it is the dominant cause of cancer death. ALL is the most frequent type in children under 15, and its peak incidence occurs at about age 4. AML dominates in the 15- to 39-year age range, and both AML and CML are encountered at ages 40 to 59. Thus, AML predominates in adults under 60. CLL predominates in adults over 60. Males are affected somewhat more often than females in all types of leukemia, the sex ratio reaching approximately 2:1 in CLL of the elderly. Overall 60% of leukemias are acute, of which 60% are classified as AML according to the FAB terminology and the remainder as ALL. Approximately 40% of cases are chronic, about two-thirds being CLL and one-third CML. Varying incidences have been reported from countries around the world, but there is some question whether these data reflect real differences or are the spurious results of differing levels of medical care and case-finding. There is, however, one example of a striking "racial" difference—the great rarity of CLL among the Japanese and other oriental populations.[42] Although the survivors of atomic bomb blasts in Japan later showed a marked increase in the other forms of leukemia, there was no observable increase in the incidence of CLL.

ETIOLOGY AND PATHOGENESIS. The origins of leukemia are shrouded in the mysteries of all forms of cancer. No single etiologic or pathogenetic factor is likely to be applicable to all forms. The complex issues relating to leukemogenesis include (1) the cell of origin in various leukemias, (2) the nature of proliferative defect in the transformed cells, (3) changes in the genome responsible for the expression of leukemic phenotype, and (4) etiologic factors responsible for initiating the genomic alterations.

All leukemias have their origin in neoplastic monoclonal proliferations of hematopoietic stem cells. The evidence that they are clonal disorders comes from the study of chromosomal markers such as the Philadelphia (Ph^1) chromosome (p. 232 and below) and analysis of the glucose-6-phosphate dehydrogenase (G6PD) isoenzymes (p. 221). The specific stem cells involved in different forms of leukemias have not been established with certainty, but progress has been made. In patients with the common form of acute lymphoblastic leukemia (cALL), the leukemic cells do not bear surface markers of T cells or B cells, but they contain the enzyme terminal deoxynucleotidyl transferase (TdT), which is presumed to be a marker of primitive lymphoid cells. Study of the immunoglobulin genes in the cALL leukemic cells suggests that in many cases they are genetically committed to B-cell differentiation.[43] Thus, it may be that in most cases cALL originates from very primitive B cells that have not yet acquired cytoplasmic or surface Ig. In the other major form of ALL, surface markers of intrathymic T cells are present, suggesting origin from cells committed to the T-cell differentiation pathway. These cells are also positive for TdT. *Thus, TdT, which is present in most cases of ALL, can be of help in differentiating ALL from other acute leukemias.*

The acute myelogenous leukemias are also of diverse origins. In some cases the leukemic transformation seems to occur at the level of pluripotent myeloid stem cells, whereas in others the committed granulocyte-macrophage stem cells are involved (Fig. 14–1). The transformation of myeloid stem cells is responsible for the presence of common cytogenetic abnormalities in the myeloid as well as the erythroid precursors, even though myeloblasts commonly dominate the blood and bone marrow. Less often, the dominant cells may be erythroblasts or monoblasts, giving rise to acute erythroleukemia (FAB, M6), or acute monocytic leukemia (FAB, M5). In *chronic myeloid leukemia,* the involvement of platelets, erythroid precursors, and granulocytic cells points to an origin from the pluripotent myeloid stem cells.[44] Some evidence, however, indicates that B cells and possibly T cells may also be a part of the neoplastic clone, suggesting that CML may result from transformation of the most primitive totipotential stem cells (p. 611).[45] With regard to CLL, most cases are of B-cell origin; in the individual patient all leukemic cells express identical immunoglobulins, confirming the monoclonality of the disease. This form of leukemia is closely associated with and sometimes indistinguishable from well-differentiated lymphocytic lymphoma (p. 660). CLL, arising from T cells, is extremely rare.

Relative to the nature of the proliferative defect in leukemia, all *acute* leukemias are characterized by a paucity of mature white cells and an excess of immature precursors. The accumulation of primitive cells could result from (1) defective maturation with a larger population of immature cells capable of self-replication, (2) a prolonged life span due to delayed senescence, or (3) a shortened generation time with an increased rate of cell production. In acute leukemia *the pool of actively proliferating cells is expanded but the cells have a prolonged rather than a shortened generation time.* When normal stem cells divide, one of the daughter cells becomes committed to a differentiation pathway, whereas the other remains an uncommitted stem cell with ability to self-replicate; thus, the normal ratio of stem cells to committed cells is maintained close to 1:1. When leukemic stem cells divide, this ratio is altered owing to a block in maturation, yielding an increased proportion of stem cells. Thus, *in acute leukemia there is an accumulation of leukemic cells resulting from a failure of maturation into functional end cells rather than hyperproliferation of neoplastic stem cells.*[46] This concept has important therapeutic implications, since in principle it may be possible with therapy to induce differentiation of the leukemic stem cells. The situation is quite different with CML, in which *there is a 10- to 20-fold increase in myeloid stem cells, but the accumulation is not due to a block in maturation.* The leukemic stem cells continue to differentiate, as evidenced by the presence of vast numbers of mature cells in the peripheral blood and by the ability of the leukemic cells to form colonies of differentiated progeny in vitro. Moreover, cell kinetic studies reveal that the leukemic myeloid stem cells do not divide more rapidly than normal stem cells.[47] Instead, the evidence points to some failure of leukemic stem cells to respond to physiologic growth regulators such as colony-stimulating factor (p. 612) and/or prostaglandins. The pathogenesis of *CLL* seems to involve an accumulation of mature-looking but immunologically incompetent B lymphocytes (Fig. 15–21). The turnover of leukemic B cells in CLL is extremely slow, since most of the cells are fairly long-lived and recirculate for several months.

Although the precise derangements that affect growth and differentiation of leukemic cells have not yet been identified, much interest is centered on defining the genetic alterations responsible for expression of the leukemic phenotype. Most exciting are the recent observations implicating chromosomal rearrangements as critical events in leukemogenesis. It has been known for several years that CML is characterized by a unique chromosomal abnormality, the Ph^1 (Philadelphia) chromosome. *In approximately 95% of patients with CML, the Ph^1 chromosome, usually representing a reciprocal translocation from the long arm of chromosome 22 to another chromosome (usually the long arm of chromosome 9), can be identified in all the dividing progeny of pluripotent myeloid stem cells (p. 611).* More recently, high-resolution techniques have allowed the detection of several nonrandom chromosomal abnormalities in acute leukemias as well. Some of these were discussed earlier (p. 231), but several points are worth reiterating. *Two specific translocations are consistently associated with particular subtypes of AML:* a translocation involving the long arm of chromosome 8 and 21 t(8q−, 21q+), hich is seen with AML-M2 in the FAB classification, etween 15 and 17 t(15q+, 17q−), which ute promyelocytic leukemia (AML-M3 fication).[48] A third group of patients ted with Ph^1 chromosome similar to addition, monosomy or partial es 5 or 7 and a trisomy of en in several cases. These and malities can be readily demonstrated in 50% of cases, but reports suggest that, with improved methods, subtle deletions and rearrangements can be found in virtually every patient with AML.[49] *Specific karyotypic changes have also been seen in ALL, although less frequently.* These include t(4q−; 11q+) in cALL; t(8q−; 14q+), similar to the translocation seen in Burkitt's lymphoma, in B-cell ALL; and, surprisingly, t(9q+; 22q−), i.e., the Ph^1 chromosome, in approximately 25% of adults with ALL.[50]

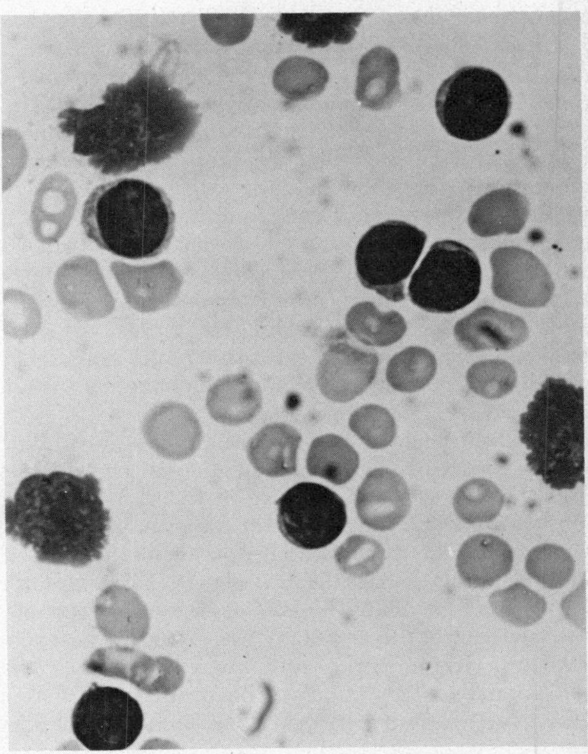

Figure 15–21. Peripheral blood smear from a patient with chronic lymphatic leukemia. Most leukemic cells have the appearance of unstimulated small or medium-size lymphocytes. Owing to excessive fragility, the neoplastic lymphocytes are often damaged, giving rise to several "smudge" cells. (Courtesy of Dr. Jose Hernandez, Department of Pathology, Southwestern Medical School, Dallas, Texas.)

Although the idea that specific chromosomal abnormalities may be associated with certain cancers is not new, the significance of the cytogenetic changes has been far from clear until recently. The current flurry of excitement in this area stems from convergence of the research on oncogenes and chromosomal abnormalities.[51] Recall that Burkitt's lymphoma is associated with t(8q−; 14q+), and a cellular oncogene has been mapped close to the breakpoint on chromosome 8. With translocation, the oncogene is shifted close to the gene coding for immunoglobulin heavy chain on chromosome 14 (p. 249). More recently, it has been discovered that the formation of Ph^1 chromosome is associated with the translocation of a cellular oncogene present on chromosome 9 to the proximity of immunoglobulin light chain gene on chromosome 22.[52] *It seems remarkable that in both instances the oncogenes are translocated close to genes that are actively transcribed in the process of normal immunoglobulin synthesis. It could be speculated, therefore, that oncogenes may be "turned on" at their new chromosomal locations owing to the influence of promoter sequences in the adjacent immunoglobulin genes.* The enhanced transcription and translation of oncogenes may alter growth regulation so as to produce an autonomous cell. Shifting of genes may also contribute to the well-known association between the chromosomal instability syndromes (ataxia telangiectasia, Bloom's syndrome, and Fanconi's anemia, p. 241) and leukemias and other neoplasms (p. 264). In trisomy 21 (Down's syndrome), the 10- to 20-fold increased risk of leukemia may result from disturbances caused by changes in the gene dosage.

In addition to their significance in unraveling the possible mechanisms of leukemogenesis, certain karyotypic changes are also valuable in the clinical management of leukemia. It is known, for example, that Ph^1-negative patients with CML respond poorly to chemotherapy and have a significantly shorter survival. On the other hand, in acute leukemias the presence of an abnormal karyotype is usually associated with a poorer prognosis. However, this notion may have to be revised if additional studies confirm the observation that virtually every patient with AML has an abnormal karyotype.[49]

We come finally to the possible etiologic factors that initiate leukemogenesis. The increased incidence of leukemia following exposure to *ionizing radiation* (p. 242) and *chemicals* such as benzene (p. 237) is well-known. More recently, the combined use of irradiation and alkylating agents for the treatment of Hodgkin's disease has been found to increase severalfold the incidence of AML in survivors.[53] A *viral causation* of human leukemias has long been suspected, but it is only recently that solid evidence has begun to accumulate.[54] The candidate retrovirus has been designated human T-cell leukemia virus (HTLV) owing to its association with certain forms of T-cell leukemias and lymphomas.[55] Much of the evidence linking HTLV to leukemogenesis was presented on page 243. A few summarizing observations follow. HTLV has been isolated from cultured neoplastic cells of a variety of T-cell malignancies, including cutaneous T-cell lymphoma (mycosis fungoides and Sézary syndrome), T-cell lymphomas arising in lymph nodes, and most consistently from the adult T-cell leukemia endemic in some parts of Japan and the Caribbean countries (p. 685). Hybridization and related studies reveal that HTLV is unique and is only distantly related to the other known mammalian retroviruses. HTLV proviral sequences are present in the DNA of neoplastic T cells but not in the DNA of non-neoplastic B cells of the same patient, indicating that HTLV is acquired by infection and not transmitted in the germ line. Over 90% of patients with adult T-cell leukemia in the endemic areas have HTLV antibodies in their serum. In Japan, 48% of the patients' relatives and some normal individuals also possess anti-HTLV antibodies. Although these serologic data are strongly suggestive of horizontal spread, the precise mechanism of HTLV transmission is still unknown, as are many other aspects of the HTLV puzzle. Nonetheless, the evidence obtained so far has electrified this area of research.

MORPHOLOGY. The morphologic features of leukemia fall into two categories: (1) the specific cytologic features of the particular type of leukemia, and (2) the gross alterations common to all forms of leukemia. Turning first to the specific cytologic details, identification of the specific form of leukemia requires an accurate assessment of the cell types found in the peripheral blood and bone marrow. Identification of individual cell types is best performed on Romanowsky-stained (Wright's, Giemsa) preparations (Fig. 15–22). Cytochemical stains are of particular value in the subcategories of acute myelogenous leukemia. Granulocytes possess two types of granules—azurophil and specific. During differentiation of neutrophils the azurophil granules are produced early, at the promyelocyte level of differentiation. These granules are primary lysosomes and contain various enzymes such as acid phosphatase and β-glucuronidase, common to all lysosomal granules (including those in lymphocytes) as well as myeloperoxidase specific to the granulocytic series. The specific granules that develop later (at the myelocyte stage) contain alkaline phosphatase, lactoferrin, and lysozyme. Esterases are found in granulocytic and monocytic cells. Thus, it is possible to differentiate the various myeloid cells by the battery of cytochemical techniques presented in Table 15–7. In addition, myeloblasts or promyelocytes contain rod-

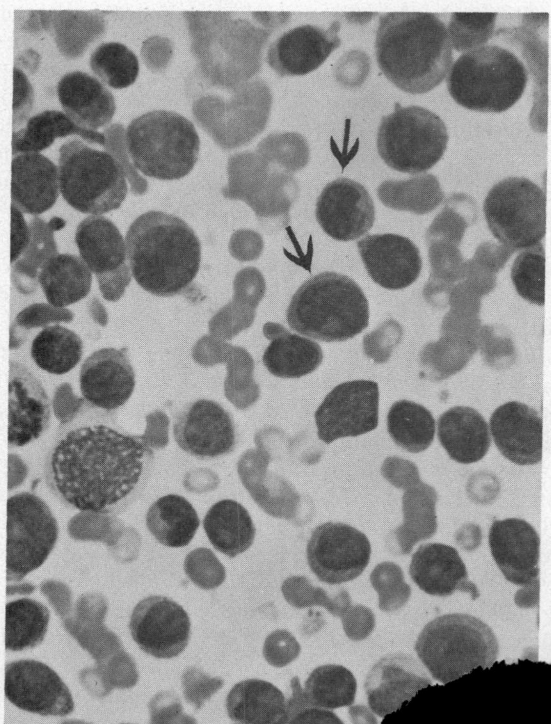

Figure 15–22. Peripheral blood smea[illegible]
myelomonocytic leukemia (FAB, M4)[illegible]
monocytes and earlier blast forms, [illegible]
reniform indented nuclei are visible [illegible]
46,000—42% monocytes and mo[illegible]

Table 15–7. CYTOCHEMICAL STAINING IN THE ACUTE MYELOID LEUKEMIAS

Cytochemical Stain	Acute Leukemia		
	Myelogenous (FAB, M1–3)	***Myelogenous-Monocytic (M4)***	***Monocytic (M5)***
Peroxidase	+	+	−
α-Naphthyl acetate esterase (ANE)	−	+	+
Naphthyl AS-D chloroacetate esterase (NCE)	+	+	−
Naphthyl AS-D acetate esterase (NAE) + fluoride inhibition	−	+	+
Sudan Black B	+	+	±

shaped, reddish structures called **Auer bodies or rods.** These are abnormal lysosomal structures found principally in myelocytic, but occasionally in monocytic, cells, which aid in their identification. Immature blasts lack these distinctive features and are therefore extremely difficult to identify unless there are also some more differentiated cell forms. Another cytochemical feature to be noted is that the **leukemic cells in CML usually have greatly reduced or no alkaline phosphatase.** This feature is helpful in distinguishing CML from nonleukemic elevations of the white cell count (p. 655). In acute erythroleukemia (FAB, M6), primitive erythroid cells, particularly proerythroblasts, dominate the bone marrow. Often these immature erythroid forms are extremely atypical and have distorted nuclear shapes, megaloblastic features, multiple nuclei, and all forms of bizarre conformations (Fig. 15–23). In keeping with the stem-cell origin of AML, variable numbers of myeloblasts (with Auer rods) and promyelocytes are also to be found in the bone marrow.

Identification of the cell types in lymphocytic leukemias may be aided by the use of rosetting and immunocytochemical techniques, as detailed in the consideration of NHL (p. 666). Also, as stated earlier, the enzyme terminal deoxynucleotidyl transferase is present in the leukemic cells of most cases of ALL. This enzyme is also found in some cases of CML in "blast crisis" (p. 685).

The shared gross alterations found in the various types of leukemia can be conveniently divided into **primary changes that are directly related to the abnormal numbers of white cells, and secondary changes that stem from the destructive effects of the cellular infiltrates and overgrowths as they seed various organs and tissues.** Macroscopic changes are much more prominent in the chronic leukemias. All, however, are characterized by abnormal flooding or infiltration of the bone marrow, lymph nodes, spleen, liver, and kidney. Any other tissue of the body may be involved, but with less frequency and usually less severely than the organs just cited. Leukemic cells more or less resemble their normal counterparts in the marrow or lymph nodes, save perhaps for a greater tendency to immaturity and the possible development of some anaplastic atypicality in individual scattered cells.

Primary Changes. The **bone marrow** in the full-blown case has a muddy red-brown to gray-white color as normal hematopoiesis is overrun by masses of white cells. The marrow replacement begins focally but, as the disease progresses, becomes generalized to affect all the normally active red marrow. It sometimes extends into areas of previously fatty marrow (Figs. 15–24 and 15–25). As the disease advances, the native marrow cells are progressively replaced. These neoplastic cells encroach upon and erode the cancellous and cortical bone. All the bones of the skeletal system are affected, but the process usually is first evident and most florid in the vertebral bodies, sternum, ribs, and pelvis. Sometimes the bony or soft tissue infiltrates in AML become tumorous masses called **chloromas** or granulocytic sarcomas. These may arise within the bone or subperios-

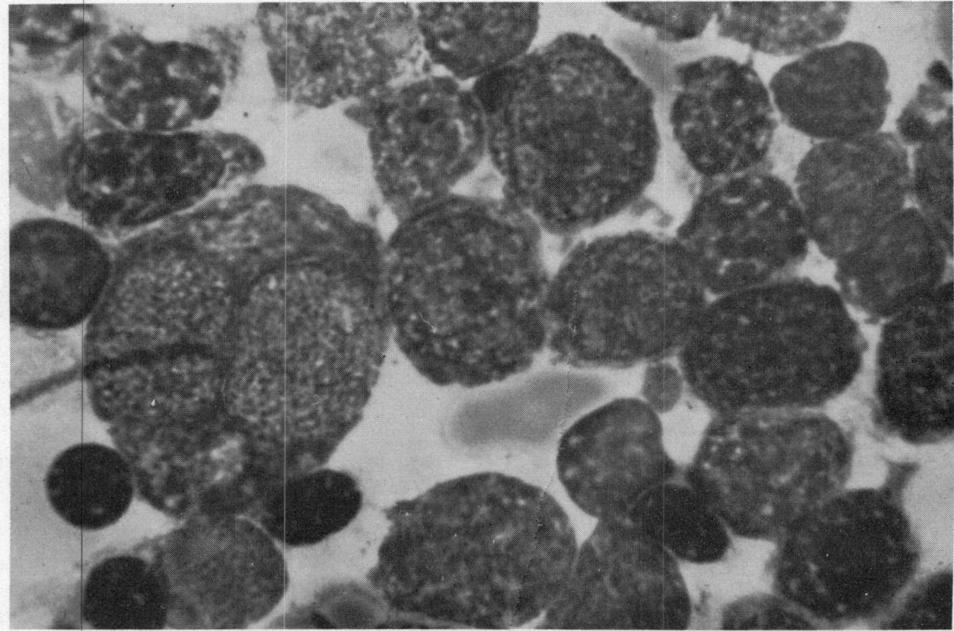

Figure 15–23. Marrow smear from a patient with acute erythroleukemia (Di Guglielmo's syndrome, FAB, M6) crowded with proerythroblasts.

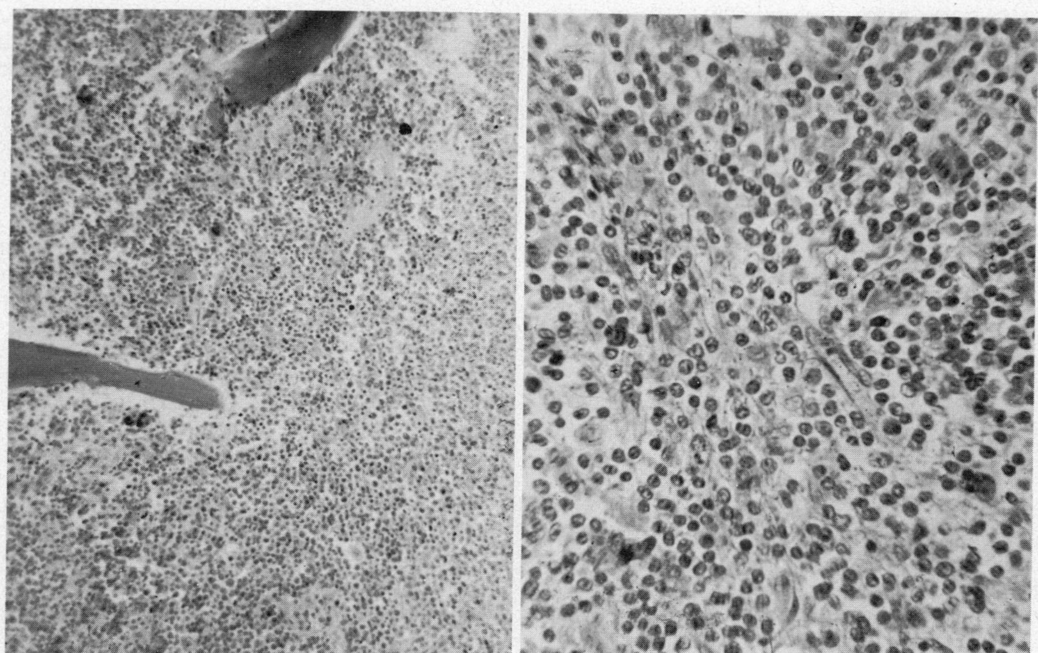

Fig. 15–24

Fig. 15–25

Figure 15–24. Chronic lymphocytic leukemia. Low-power view of marrow flooded by uniform leukemic cells.

Figure 15–25. Chronic lymphocytic leukemia. Medium-power view of same marrow as in Figure 15–24, to illustrate monotony of lymphocytes.

teally in any portion of the skeleton, but more often they affect the skull. Owing to the presence of myeloperoxidase the tumors are a distinctive evanescent green when first examined, but rapidly fade as the pigment oxidizes. The color can be restored by the use of such reducing agents as hydrogen peroxide and hyposulfite. As variants of the myelogenous infiltrates, these tumors are interesting but have no specific clinical significance.

The lymph nodes throughout the body may be enlarged in all forms of leukemia. There is, however, a marked difference in the degree of enlargement in various forms. Since lymphocytic leukemias arise within lymphoid tissue, they are associated with the most striking degrees of lymphadenopathy (4 to 5 cm in diameter), particularly in CLL (Fig. 15–26). The nodal enlargement of myelogenous leukemia is usually less prominent except in the monocytic variant (M5). In all the leukemias, involved lymph nodes characteristically remain discrete, rubbery, and homogeneous, features that distinguish these enlargements from the matted, sometimes soft fluctuance of inflammatory involvement. The cut section is soft and gray-white and tends to bulge above the level of the capsule. When the enlargement is extreme, areas of hemorrhage or infarction may appear. Not all nodes in the body are uniformly affected, and the distribution of lymphadenopathy is quite variable from one case to another.

On histologic examination, the nodes are partially or completely flooded by the neoplastic cell type to an extent that is roughly proportional to the enlargement of the node and the stage of advancement of the leukemia. Eventually, the sinuses are flooded and all structures, including the germinal follicles, are obliterated. The leukemic cells may invade the capsule of the node and infiltrate into the surrounding tissues. Such total flooding of nodes is quite characteristic of lymphocytic leukemia but less so of myelogenous leukemia.

The **spleen** is enlarged to a variable degree in almost all instances. CML produces the most striking splenomegaly; splenic weights of 5000 gm or more are not unusual. Such spleens may virtually fill the whole abdominal cavity and extend into the pelvis (Fig. 15–27). Infarcts due to leukemic infiltration and obstruction of vessels are frequent in CML (Fig. 15–28). In lymphocytic leukemias, the spleen rarely exceeds 2500 gm in weight. In monocytic leukemia, it is uncommon for the spleen to exceed 1000 gm. In all instances, the capsule becomes somewhat thickened. Frequently, fibrous adhesions to surrounding structures develop.

On section, the splenic substance is usually more firm than normal and has a muddy gray appearance. In extreme splenomegaly, the normal splenic follicles become indistinct and the tissue assumes a homogeneous appearance. Histologically, the leukemic infiltrations of the spleen follow the patterns described in the lymph nodes. They vary from focal to diffuse involvement to progressive obliteration of the underlying architecture in the areas affected.

The **liver** is commonly enlarged in all forms of leukemia but not to the same degree as the spleen. Hepatomegaly tends to be somewhat more striking in CLL than in the other forms, but rarely does the liver weight exceed 2500 gm. Hepatic involvement is usually diffuse in nature and therefore does not cause any striking alterations in the cut surface. Occasionally, however, patchy aggregates about portal areas may cause a diffuse, fine mottling that is visible on gross inspection (Fig. 15–29). Massive foci of infiltration of gray-white tissue sometimes appear that closely resemble metastatic patterns of other forms of cancer. The hepatic infiltrates tend to follow certain microscopic patterns that are somewhat distinctive for each form of leukemia. The infiltrates of myelogenous leukemia are not well defined and are present throughout the lobule (Fig. 15–30). Some aggregates of cells may be found in the portal triads but, in

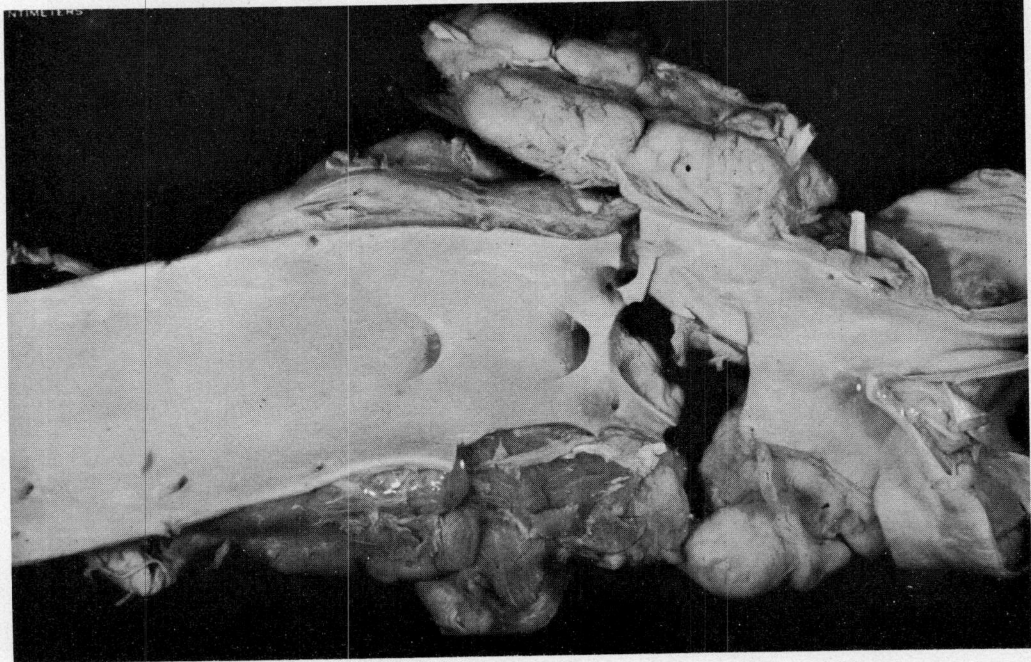

Figure 15–26. Periaortic lymph node enlargement in chronic lymphocytic leukemia.

Figure 15–27. Viscera in a patient with chronic myelogenous leukemia. Note massive hepatosplenomegaly, pale leukemic infiltrates in liver, and hemorrhages in subepicardial fat as manifestations of depression of platelet formation. This case of CML was unusual in that it occurred in an 8-year-old child.

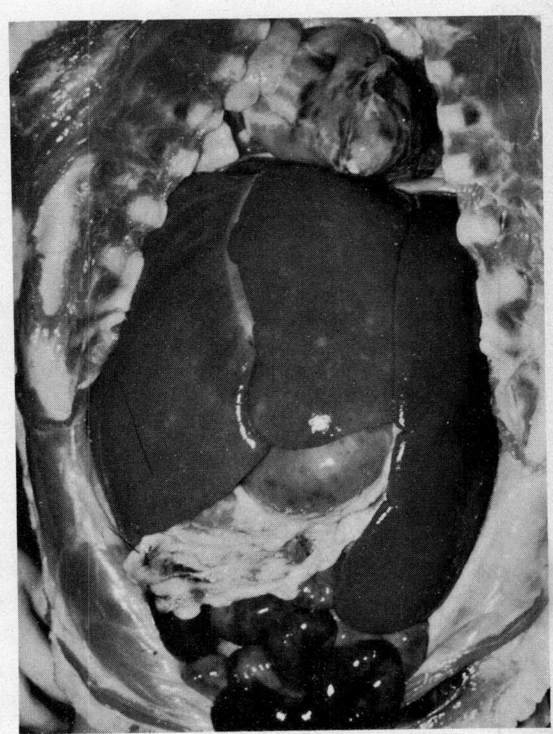

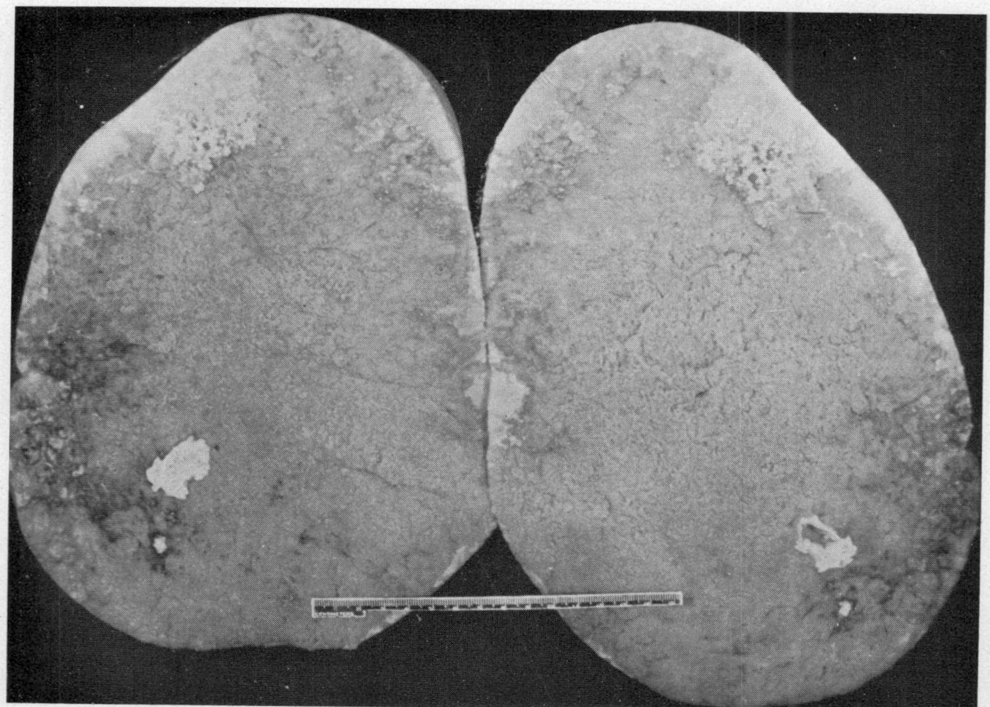

Figure 15–28. Spleen in chronic myelogenous leukemia. The massive enlargement dwarfs the 15-cm rule. Numerous small infarcts are dispersed through the cut surface.

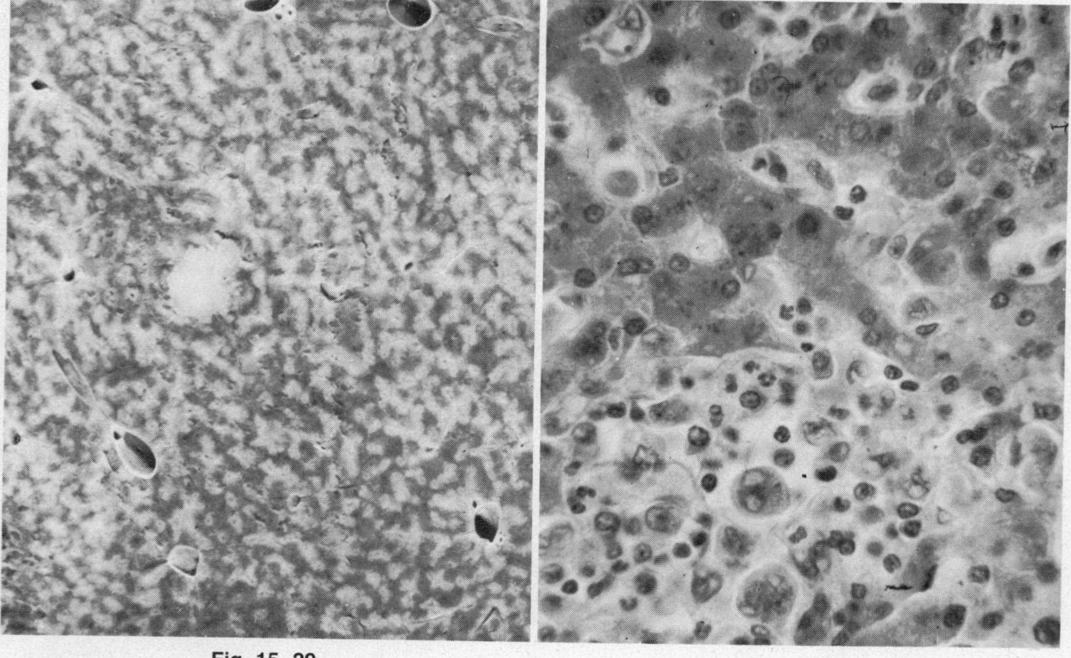

Fig. 15–29

Fig. 15–30

Figure 15–29. Chronic lymphocytic leukemia in liver. Close-up of cut surface of liver to illustrate unusually prominent leukemic infiltration producing a fine regular mottling.

Figure 15–30. Acute myelogenous leukemia in liver. Microscopic detail to illustrate scattered "polys" and immature myeloid cells through sinusoids.

addition, cells are dispersed along the liver cords subjacent to the vascular sinusoidal walls. The infiltrates are characteristically localized to the portal areas in lymphocytic leukemia (Fig. 15–31). The central regions of the liver lobule are relatively spared in this dyscrasia. The hepatic infiltrates of the monocytic variant are least prominent and are very often absent. When present, they tend to follow the pattern described in myelogenous leukemia.

In addition to these organ involvements, leukemic infiltrates are frequently found in the kidneys, adrenals, thyroid, and myocardium and in many other body tissues. Of particular importance is the infiltration of the central nervous system by the leukemic cells; this occurs most commonly in ALL. Protected by the blood-brain barrier, cells infiltrating the meninges may escape the effects of systemically administered drugs and eventually initiate a relapse. In all affected tissues, the infiltrates begin as small perivascular aggregates that progressively diffuse through the stroma of the affected organ. As the cells accumulate in sufficient number, they may compress and destroy adjacent parenchymal structures. When the infiltrates become large enough, they may produce macroscopically visible, pale-gray areas of infiltration. However, these infiltrates are usually different from ordinary metastases. They tend to be less sharply circumscribed and are more diffusely infiltrated, so that they do not wipe out the underlying architecture as completely as do the metastases of other types of cancer (Fig. 15–32).

Special mention should be made of the leukemic infiltrates of the skin and mucous membranes of the gingiva. On occasion, abnormal cells accumulate in the dermal and subcutaneous connective tissue **(leukemia cutis).** These cause variable forms of elevated-to-flat, pale-to-red skin macules or papules and are common in leukemias of T cells. Infiltrates in the gingiva are particularly characteristic of the monocytic variant of AML. Swelling and hypertrophy of the gingival margins occur, and frequently the soft tissues involved freely ooze blood, or secondary bacterial infection develops, forming superficial necrotic ulcerations.

Secondary Changes. By secondary changes are meant those lesions that stem from the destructive, erosive effects of the aggressive leukemic infiltrates and from the functional incompetence of leukemic cells. **Anemia and thrombocytopenia are characteristic secondary consequences of leukemic involvement of the bone marrow.** The marrow failure results not only from replacement of the hemopoietic cells but also from the inhibition of normal stem-cell function by leukemic cells or their products. The anemia may become quite profound and lead to systemic and local tissue hypoxia. A hemorrhagic diathesis results from the thrombocytopenia, and abnormal bleeding is one of the most characteristic manifestations of acute leukemias. Purpura and ecchymoses may occur in the skin, with or without leukemic infiltrates. Hemorrhages into the gingivae as well as hemorrhagic foci in the urinary bladder, the mucosa of the renal pelves and calyces, the serosal membranes lining the body cavities, and the serosal coverings of the viscera (particularly of the heart and lungs) are standard features in advanced leukemia. Not uncommonly, intraparenchymal hematomas develop, most frequently in the brain. Many times, this widespread hemorrhagic tendency is the most obvious anatomic postmortem finding in these cases. In acute promyelocytic leukemia (FAB, M3), the release of procoagulant substances from the granules often leads to DIC and the attendant hemorrhagic diathesis (p. 649).

Although the total white cell count is usually elevated in leukemia, the circulating abnormal white cells have little

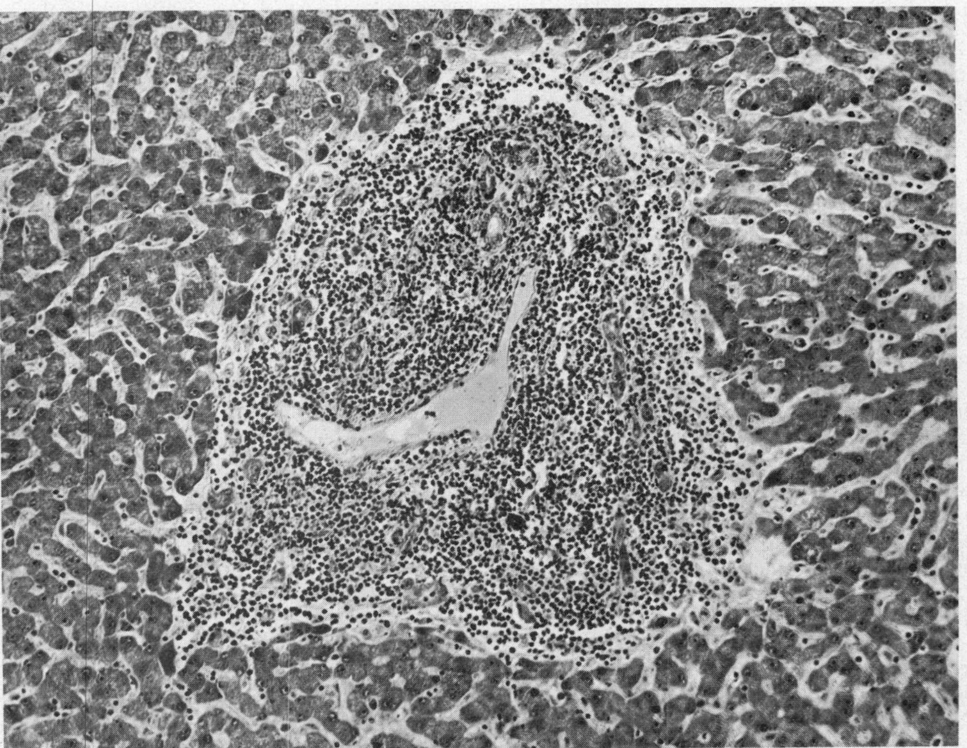

Figure 15–31. Chronic lymphocytic leukemia in liver. High-power detail of a periportal infiltrate. (From Jackson, H. J., Jr., and Parker, F., Jr. (eds.): Hodgkin's Disease and Allied Disorders. New York, Oxford University Press, 1947.)

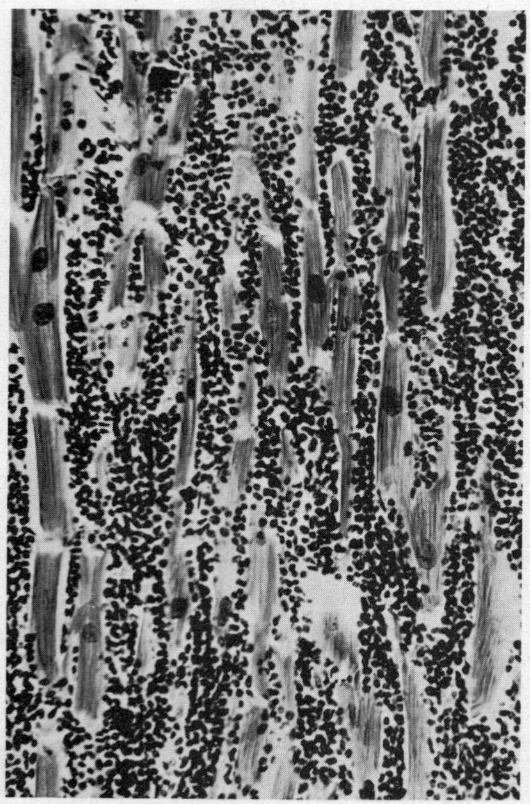

Figure 15–32. Chronic lymphocytic leukemia infiltrates in heart muscle. (From Jackson, H. J., Jr., and Parker, F., Jr. (eds.): Hodgkin's Disease and Allied Disorders. New York, Oxford University Press, 1947.)

defensive capacity, resulting in an enhanced susceptibility to bacterial infection. The morphologic changes of these infections may be found in any organ or site in the body but are particularly common in the oral cavity, skin, lungs, kidneys, urinary bladder, and colon. The bacterial infections of leukemia resemble, to a great extent, those found in granulocytopenia, since both have in common a deficiency of functioning leukocytes.

The leukemic proliferation in the bone marrow causes expansion of the marrow spaces, encroachment upon the cancellous and cortical bone, and resultant osteoporosis with increased radiolucency. The infiltrates within other tissues and organs remain confined for the most part to the interstitial connective tissue. The parenchymal elements are thus spread apart but usually are not severely damaged. For this reason, hepatic, renal, or cardiac failure is extremely uncommon in these cases. Only rarely does enlargement of the portahepatic nodes encroach sufficiently upon the extrahepatic biliary ducts to cause obstructive jaundice.

Therapy may significantly modify the anatomic changes. The use of cytotoxic drugs before death may virtually destroy all viable cells. It is not uncommon to find, post mortem, a striking paucity of preserved leukemic cells and indeed of all forms of marrow cells in patients who received intensive radiation therapy and chemotherapy in the terminal stages of their disease. Thus, the pathologist is sometimes confronted with the paradox of a patient having a clinically well-documented leukemia without anatomic changes to permit confirmation of the diagnosis.

Clinical Course. Acute leukemias have an almost totally different clinical presentation from chronic leukemias. *Chronic leukemias appear insidiously, but the acute disorders have a sudden, often stormy onset.* You recall that ALL is a disease of childhood, whereas AML usually appears in adult life. Symptoms, when they appear, are related to depression of normal marrow function and include (1) fatigue due mainly to anemia; (2) fever, usually reflecting an infection; and (3) bleeding (petechiae, ecchymoses, epistaxis, and gingival bleeding) secondary to thrombocytopenia. Generalized lymphadenopathy, splenomegaly, and hepatomegaly, the results of organ infiltration by leukemic cells, are characteristic of ALL but usually are not prominent with AML. The marrow involvement in both disorders leads to subperiosteal bone infiltration, marrow expansion, and bone resorption, often resulting in bone pain and tenderness on palpation. CNS manifestations may appear with leukemic infiltration of the meninges, producing headache, nausea, vomiting, papilledema, cranial nerve palsies, and sometimes seizures and coma. More acute CNS complications may arise, such as intracerebral or subarachnoid hemorrhages. Occasionally, DIC punctuates the course of the promyelocytic form of AML (p. 649), especially when cell lysis caused by therapy result in the release of thromboplastic substances from the granules.

Both forms of acute leukemia are characterized by distinctive laboratory findings. Anemia is almost always present. The white count in about half the patients is less than 10,000 cells/mm^3 of blood, whereas in about 20% it is elevated above 100,000 cells/mm^3. Much more important is the finding of immature white cells, including "blast" forms, in the circulating blood and the bone marrow, where they make up 60 to 100% of all the cells. The platelet count is almost always depressed and in a great majority of cases is less than 100,000/mm^3. Although not linearly related, the danger of bleeding manifestations progressively increases as the platelet count falls. Without treatment, the course of the acute leukemias is usually progressively downhill, ending in death in two to four months.

The onset of the chronic leukemias is so insidious that they are sometimes discovered only during a routine physical examination. Symptoms, when they appear, are related to the hypermetabolism of the leukemic cells and include low-grade fever, night sweats, weight loss, weakness, and easy fatigability. The profound anemia causes considerable exertional dyspnea. In some cases the patient first becomes aware of a heavy dragging sensation in the abdomen produced by the splenomegaly. In other instances, lymphadenopathy calls attention to the underlying condition. Frequently, generalized lymphadenopathy, splenomegaly, and hepatomegaly are already present at the time of diagnosis. *Generalized lymphadenopathy is most typical of CLL, whereas marked splenomegaly is most characteristic of CML.* Bleeding manifestations may dominate the clinical presentation, particularly as marrow failure develops. *CLL, characterized by accumulation of immunoincompetent*

B cells, is often associated with hypogammaglobulinemia and increased susceptibility to infections. Paradoxically, some patients develop anti–red cell antibodies and hemolytic anemia.

As with acute leukemias, anemia is usually present in chronic leukemias, but the critical laboratory finding is the presence of abnormal immature leukocytes in the peripheral blood, accompanied by an elevated white cell count. In chronic leukemias the white cell count ranges from 50,000 to 500,000 cells/mm^3 of blood. In CML the circulating white cells are predominantly neutrophils and metamyelocytes, but more immature forms are also present. An increased number of basophils is quite typical of CML, helping to distinguish it from *leukemoid reactions*, which may produce a peripheral blood picture deceptively similar to that of leukemia (p. 655). *Other features that help to differentiate leukemoid reactions from CML are the absence of the Ph^1 chromosome and the increased level of leukocyte alkaline phosphatase*. In CLL the peripheral white cells are largely mature lymphocytes, but some immature forms are also found. In both forms of chronic leukemia, platelets are depressed with advanced disease, but in the early course of CML the platelet count may be above normal.

The prognoses for each of the various forms of acute and chronic leukemia are best considered individually, since they differ so much. Remarkable advances in therapy bring fresh gains yearly, rendering data out of date by the time they are set to paper. In particular, the outlook for children with ALL is spectacularly improved. Intensive chemotherapy and the use of corticosteroids now induce a remission in almost all children. With prophylactic irradiation and intrathecal chemotherapy for CNS involvement, over 50% are living after five years, many apparently free of disease. In these fortunate young ones, a much more prolonged remission or even a cure is not beyond hope. The adult with ALL fares less well and, although remissions can be achieved, the average survival is for two to three years.

The outlook for patients with AML is more grim. Remissions can be achieved with chemotherapy in over half the patients, but these are generally transient and only 15 to 20% are alive after three years. In view of such a grim prognosis, bone marrow transplantation has been attempted in some centers. Early results are promising, with 50% long-term remissions, but this form of treatment is not yet widely available.

The course of the chronic leukemias is one of slow progression, and even without treatment permits survivals of two to three years. In CML, therapy may induce remissions, but there is little improvement in overall survival. Death in most cases is heralded by an acute phase known as a blast crisis during which a picture resembling acute leukemia develops. In about 25% of cases, blasts contain the enzyme TdT and thus represent lymphoblasts; the remaining cases have a myeloblastic crisis. Recent studies indicate that the blast cells found in the lymphoblastic crises belong to the B-cell lineage;[55A] this observation supports the thesis that CML represents a disease of totipotential stem cells (p. 611). CLL is the most indolent of the leukemias, and with therapy the median survival is four to six years. Unlike CML, blast crisis is rare and most patients die of infections, progressive leukemic infiltration, or causes unrelated to leukemia.

Unusual Types of Leukemias and Lymphomas

HAIRY CELL LEUKEMIA. This is an uncommon but distinctive form of chronic leukemia involving an unusual cell, which shows several features of B lymphocytes. The disorder derives its picturesque name from the appearance of the leukemic cells, which have fine "hairlike" cytoplasmic projections best recognized under the phase-contrast microscope or scanning electron microscope, but also visible in routine blood smears. The genealogy of the transformed cells has proved extremely baffling. In most cases the pathognomonic hairy cells synthesize surface immunoglobulins of restricted light-chain type, a feature characteristic of monoclonal B-cell proliferations. On the other hand, some relationships to the monocyte-macrophage lineage and T cells have also been described.[56] Confusingly, the markers may fluctuate from those of B cells to those of T cells during the course of the disease or in culture.[57] Without delving into further complexities, *hairy cell leukemia may be said to result from the neoplastic transformation of a poorly characterized cell with features most strongly suggestive of B cells; however, origin from a totipotent stem cell (p. 611) with some differentiation along the T-cell or monocyte pathway cannot be ruled out at present.* Mercifully, there is one cytochemical feature that is quite characteristic of hairy cell leukemia, i.e., the presence of tartrate-resistant acid phosphatase (TRAP). The exceptions to this observation are so few that positive TRAP staining in leukemic cells endowed with "hair" is considered virtually diagnostic of hairy cell leukemia in the appropriate clinical setting.

Hairy cell leukemia occurs mainly in older males and *its manifestations result largely from infiltration of bone marrow liver and spleen. Splenomegaly*, often massive, is the most common and sometimes the only abnormal physical finding. *Hepatomegaly* is less common and not as marked, and lymphadenopathy is distinctly rare. *Pancytopenia*, resulting from marrow failure and splenic sequestration, is seen in over half the cases. *Leukocytosis* is not a common feature, being present in only 25% of patients. Hairy cells can be identified in the peripheral blood smear in most cases. The course of this disease is chronic with no satisfactory treatment; the median survival is four years.

ADULT T-CELL LEUKEMIA-LYMPHOMA. This uncommon T-cell neoplasm has gained much prominence owing to its association with human T-cell leukemia virus (p. 243). Most of the initial cases were described from the southern part of Japan, where it is endemic,[58] but similar cases have now been found in the West Indies and sporadically in several other countries, including the U.S. *Characteristic clinical features of adult T-cell leukemia include generalized lymphadenopathy, hepatosplenomegaly, frequent skin involvement, severe hypercalcemia, and a poor prognosis.*[59] The tumor cells are usually OKT4-positive, a feature shared with the closely related cutaneous T-cell lymphomas. These disorders, along with T-cell chronic lymphocytic leukemia and the T-cell lymphomas involving lymph nodes (p. 665), represent the spectrum of differentiated *T-cell neoplasms*. In contrast, T-cell ALL and lymphoblastic lymphoma (convoluted T-cell lymphoma) represent tumors of *immature T cells*.

Histiocytic Medullary Reticulosis (Malignant Histiocytosis). This disease is widely believed to represent a malignant tumor of mature and immature histiocytes with diffuse invasion of the viscera and bone marrow. For mysterious reasons, however, it usually is not included among histiocytic lymphomas. Earlier it was classified into a poorly defined category called histiocytoses, which also included the "histiocytoses X," discussed later (p. 694). It derives its name from the infiltration of the medullary zone of lymph nodes by the histiocytes, which by no means is a diagnostic feature.

Masses of histiocytes and their precursors may be seen in the skin, bone marrow, lymph nodes, spleen, and liver. The levels of cellular maturation differ, but in most instances the cells are immature and variable in size and shape, with large round nuclei and an abundant amphophilic or slightly basophilic cytoplasm. The nuclear chromatin is lacy and the nucleoli are prominent. In other cases, the cells may closely resemble mature histiocytes, with oval-to-reniform nuclei, small nucleoli, and abundant amphophilic cytoplasm. It is impossible to differentiate these cell types from those encountered in histiocytic lymphoma. Sometimes these cells appear to fill the sinuses of lymph nodes. In the various organ involvements the infiltrates may be difficult to differentiate from histiocytic lymphoma with systemic dissemination. However, **characteristic of histiocytic medullary reticulosis is prominent erythrophagocytosis,** not seen in histiocytic lymphoma. The neoplastic histiocytes may also contain other phagocytized material, including leukocytes and platelets, all of which contribute to the pancytopenia associated with this disease.

The major clinical features of histiocytic medullary reticulosis include (1) lymphadenopathy, (2) hepatosplenomegaly, (3) anemia or pancytopenia, (4) fever, and sometimes (5) skin infiltrates. Leukemic spread to the blood has been reported, but is rare. It is a rapidly progressive and fatal disease. Survival for more than 15 months is unusual, the average being six months.

Agnogenic Myeloid Metaplasia (Myeloid Metaplasia with Myelofibrosis)

Agnogenic myeloid metaplasia, along with polycythemia vera, chronic granulocytic leukemia, and idiopathic thrombocythemia, belongs to the group of *myeloproliferative syndromes*. As discussed earlier, these disorders arise from the clonal, neoplastic proliferation of the pluripotent myeloid stem cells (p. 641). Although the dominant differentiated cell line differs in the various myeloproliferative diseases, all the myeloid cell types (i.e., granulocytes/macrophages, erythroid cells, and platelets) can be demonstrated to be monoclonal. Some cases of polycythemia vera and CML may ultimately evolve into a stage characterized by marrow fibrosis and extramedullary hematopoiesis in the spleen *(myeloid metaplasia)*. In many patients, however, splenic myeloid metaplasia and the accompanying marrow fibrosis arise insidiously without an identifiable preceding syndrome; hence, the term agnogenic (idiopathic) myeloid metaplasia.

The cause of marrow fibrosis in agnogenic myeloid metaplasia is not clear. In the initial formulation of the concept of myeloproliferative diseases, it was assumed that marrow fibroblasts were derived from the hematopoietic stem cells, and therefore proliferation of fibroblasts was considered but one manifestation of the stem-cell disorder. Several subsequent studies do not support this view. First, it is established that fibroblasts within the marrow do not arise from the hematopoietic stem cells, and second, studies with G6PD isoenzymes clearly indicate that the marrow fibroblasts in myelofibrosis do not belong to the neoplastic hematopoietic clone.[60] Thus, *fibrosis of the bone marrow appears to be a reactive phenomenon*. However, no cause for marrow destruction or scarring can be demonstrated, a feature that distinguishes myeloid metaplasia with myelofibrosis from myelophthisic anemia (p. 640). It has been suggested that the proliferation of marrow fibroblasts is triggered by the release of a platelet-derived growth factor (PDGF), which is a normal component of platelet alpha granules.[60] PDGF is known to be mitogenic for fibroblasts and a variety of other mesenchymal cells, but it is not clear why or how it is released in the marrow of patients with myelofibrosis. In one study, circulating immune complexes were detected in most patients, and it was suggested that interaction of the IgG in the complexes with the Fc IgG receptors on the platelets may lead to the release of PDGF.[61] It is also conceivable that the inappropriate release of PDGF is due to an intrinsic defect of the platelets, which are a part of the abnormal clone of myeloid cells. Attractive as these theories may be, they are entirely hypothetical.

Morphology. The principal anatomic change is striking extramedullary hematopoiesis. The principal site of this is the spleen, which is usually moderately to markedly enlarged, sometimes up to 4000 gm (Fig. 15–33). The capsule is unaffected but occasionally shows underlying small infarcts. On section the spleen is firm, red to gray, and not dissimilar from that seen in CML. However, the lymphoid follicles are usually preserved, implying that there has been no neoplastic obliteration of the native architecture. Occasionally, small red masses of hematopoietic tissue can be discerned grossly. Histologically, the extramedullary hematopoiesis seems to be largely confined to the red pulp. Intrasinusoidal proliferation of normoblasts and immature granulocytic cells is present, sometimes in small aggregates. Megakaryocytes are also prominent in the sinuses. These myeloid elements may diffuse into the splenic cords. Usually

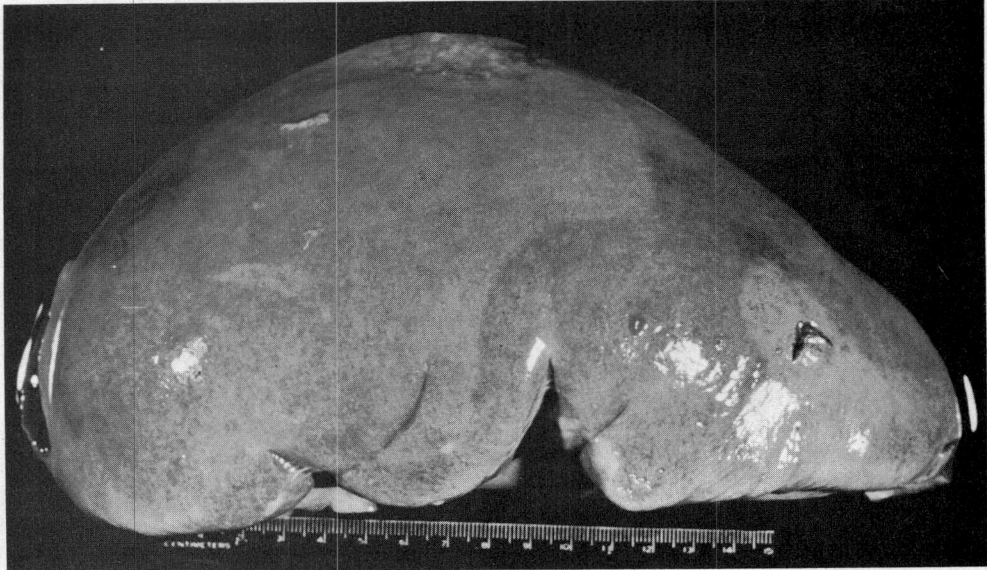

Figure 15–33. Myeloid metaplasia with myelofibrosis. Spleen is markedly enlarged and dwarfs the 15-cm rule. Irregular shading of capsule is an artifact.

the hematopoiesis is orderly, with relatively normal proportions of maturing red cells, white cells, and platelets, but certain cases show a disproportional activity in any one of these three major lines. Most readily visualized are the nests of normoblasts and megakaryocytes.

The liver is often moderately enlarged, with foci of extramedullary hematopoiesis. The lymph nodes are only rarely the site of blood formation and usually are not enlarged.

The classic bone marrow finding is diffuse fibrosis with obliteration of the normal myeloid elements (Fig. 15–34). On occasion, however, marrow biopsy discloses hypercellularity with proliferation of all the myeloid elements and sometimes prominent abnormal-looking megakaryocytes. Even in the early cellular phase, a tell-tale finding of the more extensive fibrosis to come is a delicate deposition of reticulin, only evident on special stains. Moreover, sequential studies have shown that the fibrosis appears first in centrally located bones, whereas the large bones of the extremities contain hyperplastic marrow.

Clinical Course. Myeloid metaplasia is uncommon in individuals under 50 years of age. Except when preceded by polycythemia vera or CML, it usually comes to clinical attention because of either progressive anemia or marked splenic enlargement, producing a dragging sensation in the left upper quadrant. Some patients are asymptomatic. Most striking are the laboratory findings. There is usually a moderate-to-severe normochromic normocytic anemia. Red cells show all manner of variation in size and shape, but *particularly characteristic are teardrop-shaped erythrocytes (poikilocytes).* In addition, numerous normoblasts and basophilic stippled red cells appear in the peripheral blood. The white cell count may be normal, leukopenic, or markedly elevated (80,000 to 100,000/mm^3), with a shift to the left. Typically, myeloblasts, myelocytes, and metamyelocytes constitute a small fraction of the white cell population on peripheral smear. The platelet count is usually elevated at the time of diagnosis, but thrombocytopenia supervenes as the disease progresses. Morphologic abnormalities of the platelets (giant forms) are frequent, and sometimes fragments of megakaryocytes may be detected in the peripheral blood. Biopsy of the marrow to detect the early deposition of reticulin or the more advanced fibrosis is essential for diagnosis. The differential diagnosis of CML frequently arises in these

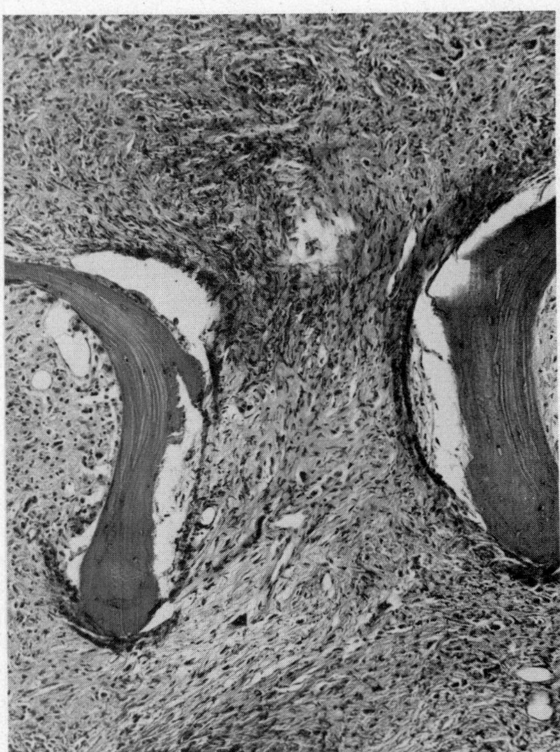

Figure 15–34. Myelofibrosis. Marrow cavity is virtually replaced by fibrous tissue, totally obliterating normal hematopoietic elements.

patients. In myeloid metaplasia, leukocyte alkaline phosphatase levels are often elevated, or at least normal, whereas in CML these levels are low or absent. Moreover, most patients with CML disclose the Ph^1 chromosome, which is absent in agnogenic myeloid metaplasia. An equally difficult differential diagnosis is myelophthisic anemia secondary to an identifiable cause of marrow injury. In such cases the diagnosis of agnogenic myeloid metaplasia can be established only by careful history-taking to elicit the cause of marrow injury, or by morphologic detection of the underlying cause (e.g., cancer) in the marrow biopsy.

The course of this disease is difficult to predict. Despite weight loss attributed to the increased metabolism of the hyperproliferating cells, most patients can survive for years with transfusions. Sometimes the course is punctuated by episodes of acute left upper quadrant pain arising from splenic infarctions. Secondary gout may appear as a manifestation of the rapid turnover of blood cells. Threats to life are intercurrent infections, thrombotic or hemorrhagic crises related to the thrombocytosis, and in some cases (10%) conversion to acute leukemia.

PLASMA CELL DYSCRASIAS AND RELATED DISORDERS

This rather vague title refers to a diverse group of conditions having in common: *(1) uncontrolled proliferation of plasma cells or closely related cell types, and (2) abnormally high levels in the blood and/or urine of a monoclonal homogeneous immunoglobulin or one of its constituent polypeptide chains.* In essence these conditions are neoplasms of B cells. They differ, however, from the B-cell lymphomas discussed earlier by virtue of the fact that in plasma cell dyscrasias the neoplastic B cells are differentiated enough to secrete immunoglobulins or their components. In the individual patient the immunoglobulin belongs to a single class, subclass, and type and is indistinguishable in structure from a normal immunoglobulin. Thus, there are IgG, IgM, IgA, IgD, and rarely IgE dyscrasias. It would appear, then, that the plasma cell proliferation in the individual patient is monoclonal in origin. The immunoglobulin as identified in the blood is referred to as a complete M component in reference to *M*yeloma. Since complete M components have molecular weights of 160,000 or higher, they are largely restricted to circulating plasma and extracellular fluid. However, they may appear in the urine when there is some form of glomerular damage with heavy proteinuria. In some of these dyscrasias, excess light (L) or heavy (H) chains are also synthesized along with complete immunoglobulins, but the polypeptide chains are always identical to those found in the complete immunoglobulin, and thus the L chains are either kappa or lambda (never both) or the H chains of a single class (e.g., either alpha, gamma, or mu, etc.), depending on the particular class of Ig. Occasionally only L chains or H chains are produced but no complete Ig. The *free L chains, known as Bence Jones proteins*, are sufficiently small in size to be rapidly excreted in the urine, and so may be totally cleared from the blood or persist only at very low levels. However, with renal failure or massive synthesis, they may appear in the blood in significant concentrations. Thus, *the common thread throughout this diverse group of entities is the appearance of excessive levels of complete or incomplete immunoglobulins in the plasma and/or urine. Hence, a variety of alternative designations have been applied to these dyscrasias, such as gammopathies, monoclonal gammopathies, dysproteinemias, and paraproteinemias.* It is of interest that, of the innumerable M components studied to date, no two have been structurally identical.

A variety of clinicoanatomic patterns, listed below, can be differentiated among these gammopathies.

1. *Multiple myeloma (plasma cell myeloma)* is the most important and most common syndrome. It is characterized by multiple neoplastic tumorous masses of more or less mature plasma cells, haphazardly scattered throughout the skeletal system and sometimes in soft tissues (Fig. 15–35). *Solitary myeloma or solitary plasmacytoma* is an infrequent variant consisting of a solitary neoplastic mass of plasma cells found in bone or some soft tissue site. Some, but not all, patients with solitary lesions eventually develop multiple myeloma, suggesting that the solitary lesions represent an early stage of the disseminated disease.

2. *Waldenström's macroglobulinemia* has been separated from the other gammopathies by virtue of the fact that it is characterized by the synthesis, usually of IgM and rarely IgG or IgA, and a diffuse infiltrate throughout the bone marrow, as well as extramedullary lymphoid tissues of plasma cells, plasmacytoid lymphocytes, and lymphocytes. The lytic bone lesions typical of myeloma are not present in this condition.

3. *Heavy-chain disease* is a rare gammopathy distinguished by neoplastic medullary and extramedullary infiltrates of plasma cells, and precursors that synthesize only heavy chains.

4. *Primary or immunocyte-associated amyloidosis* is also an expression of plasma cell dyscrasia. It may be recalled that this form of amyloidosis results from a monoclonal proliferation of plasma cells, with excessive production of free light chains that are deposited as amyloid (p. 197).

5. *Lymphoproliferative disease with dysproteinemia* refers to those uncommon cases of CLL and NHL in which the neoplastic B cells are differentiated enough to produce monoclonal immunoglobulins.

6. *Monoclonal gammopathy of undetermined significance (MGUS)* refers to instances in which M components are identified in the blood in patients having no symptoms or signs of any of the better characterized monoclonal gammopathies. At one time this condition was termed benign monoclonal gammopathy, but this designation is misleading because some of these patients develop symptomatic multiple myeloma or other plasma cell dyscrasias after a variable interval.[62]

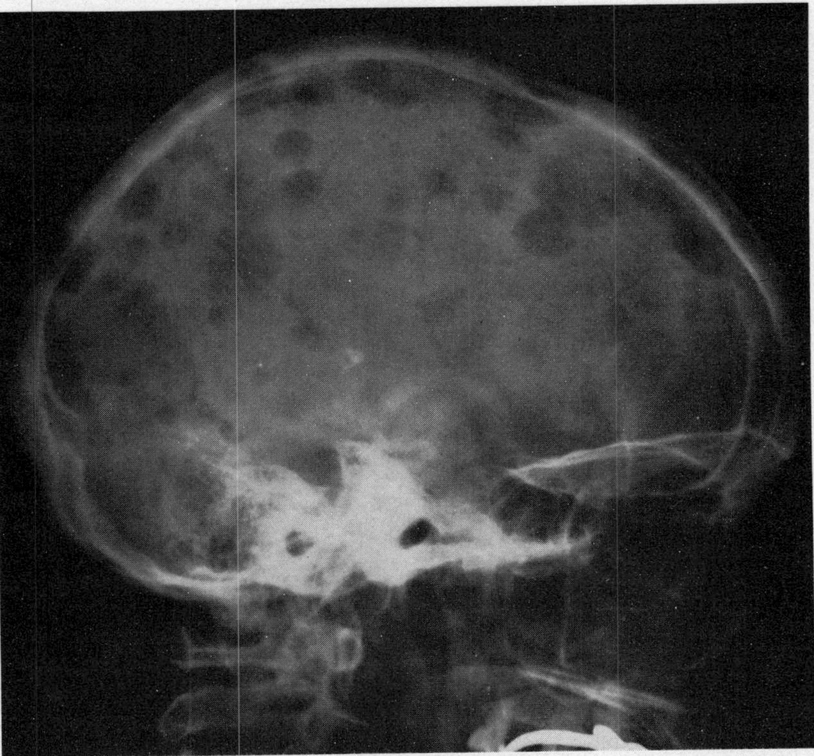

Figure 15–35. Radiograph of skull extensively involved by focal, sharply punched-out lesions of plasma cell myeloma.

Against this background we can turn to some of the specific clinicoanatomic entities not discussed elsewhere in this text.

Multiple Myeloma (Plasma Cell Myeloma)

Multiple myeloma is basically a multifocal plasma cell cancer of the osseous system that in the course of its dissemination may involve many extraosseous sites. As pointed out, the neoplastic plasma cells synthesize complete and/or incomplete immunoglobulins. It is the most common of the gammopathies and represents approximately 60%. Most patients are symptomatic when diagnosed. Clinical manifestations stem from the effects of (1) infiltration of organs, particularly the bones, by tumorous masses of plasma cells; and (2) the abnormal immunoglobulins secreted by the tumor cells.

In 99% of patients with multiple myeloma, electrophoretic analysis will disclose increased levels of one of the immunoglobulin classes in the blood and/or light chains in the urine (Bence Jones protein). In approximately 60% of patients, the M component is IgG, in 15 to 20% IgA, and rarely IgM, IgD, or IgE. In the remaining 15 to 20% of cases, Bence Jones proteinuria alone without serum M components is present. However, Bence Jones proteins are present in the urine along with plasma M components in 60 to 80% of all myeloma patients.[63] *Identification of these proteins in the blood and urine constitutes one of the most important diagnostic features of this disease.* Electrophoresis of the serum or urine (paper, agar, cellulose, acetate) is the most readily available and reliable procedure. When the serum electrophoretic pattern is analyzed, the homogeneous M component yields a high spike, referred to as an M protein or M-component "spike." Immunoelectrophoresis, using appropriate monospecific antisera directed against the various heavy and light chains, is essential to establish the monoclonal nature of the M component. Bence Jones proteins in the urine are similarly detected by immunoelectrophoretic techniques.

PATHOGENESIS. Some workers believe that long-persisting antigenic stimulation of B cells may in time provide the opportunity for spontaneous mutation or the activation of a latent oncogenic virus, leading eventually to neoplastic transformation.[64, 65] This proposition is supported by the increased frequency of plasma cell neoplasms in patients with long-standing chronic infections such as osteomyelitis, tuberculosis, cholecystitis, and pneumonitis.[66] Experimentally, plasma cell tumors have been induced in mice by the intraperitoneal injection of a variety of irritant substances, including Freund's adjuvant, mineral oil, and plastic. In recent years, these tumors have been widely utilized to produce monoclonal antibodies by the hybridoma technology (p. 159). Despite the association between persistent antigenic stimulation of B cells and plasma cell neoplasms, the cause-and-effect relationship is still uncertain.

MORPHOLOGY. Despite the abundance of abnormal biochemical findings, the ultimate diagnosis of plasma cell dyscrasias rests on the morphologic identification of the abnormal aggregates of plasma cells (Fig. 15–36). In most cases these cells make up more than 15%, and sometimes up to 90%, of all marrow cells. In many instances the neoplastic cells appear as mature plasma cells, but all ranges of immaturity may be encountered, including undifferentiated cells resembling lymphoid precursors as well as lymphocyte–plasma cell intermediates. It may be difficult to identify the neoplastic nature of the well-differentiated plasma cell lesions from the cytology of the individual cells; more important is their abnormal aggregation or evidence of their destructive potential in the form of infiltration, invasion, and erosion. Sometimes bi- or even trinucleate cells are seen in these lesions, essentially reproducing cancerous giant cells (Fig. 15–37). Electron microscopy has disclosed, in the myeloma cell, a highly developed endoplasmic reticulum, often stuffed with amorphous material compatible with immunoglobulin aggregates.[67] Under the light microscope, the protein aggregates may appear as acidophilic inclusions known as **Russell bodies.** These, however, are not pathognomonic of myeloma, since they can also be seen in reactive plasma cells that are actively synthesizing immunoglobulins.

Multiple myeloma presents as multifocal destructive bone lesions throughout the skeletal system. The bone resorption results from the activation of osteoclasts by an osteoclast-activating factor secreted by the myeloma cells. Although any bone may be affected, the following distribution obtains in large series of cases—vertebral column, 66%; ribs, 44%; skull, 41%; pelvis, 28%; femur, 24%; clavicle, 10%; and scapula, 10%. These focal lesions generally begin in the medullary cavity, erode the cancellous bone, and progressively destroy the cortical bone. On section, the bony defects are filled with red, soft, gelatinous tissue. **Radiographically, the lesions appear as punched-out defects,** usually ranging between 1 and 4 cm in diameter. In the late stages of multiple myeloma, plasma cell infiltrations of soft tissues may be encountered in spleen, liver, kidneys, lungs, and lymph nodes or more widely.

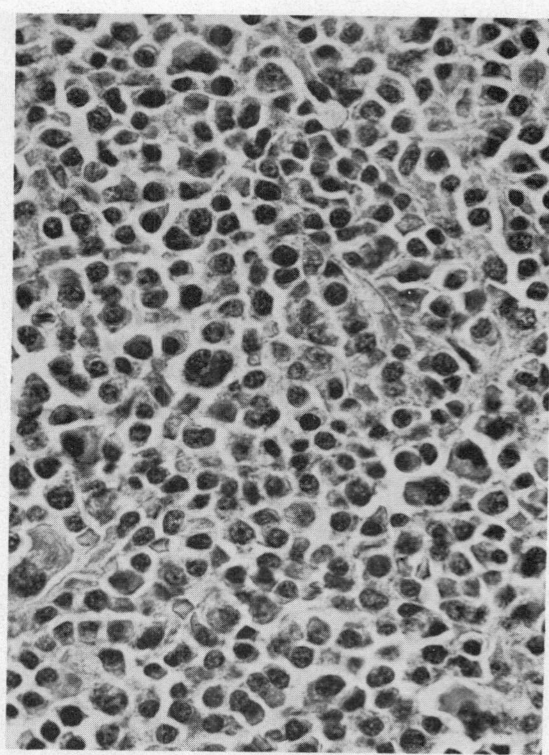

Figure 15–37. Multiple myeloma to show masses of plasma cells, mostly mature, but some with anaplasia and forming tumor giant cells.

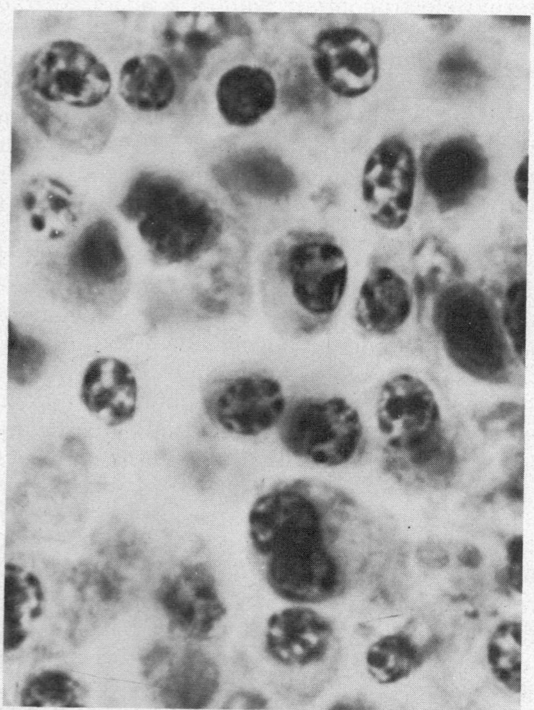

Figure 15–36. Multiple myeloma. High-power detail of tumor composed of mature characteristic plasma cells.

Renal involvement, generally called **myeloma nephrosis,** appears in 60 to 80% of cases. Grossly, the kidneys may be normal in size and color, slightly enlarged and pale, or shrunken and pale because of interstitial scarring. The most distinctive features are microscopic.[68] Interstitial infiltrates of abnormal plasma cells or chronic inflammatory cell infiltrates may be encountered. However, the most prominent lesions are found in the distal convoluted and collecting tubules, which contain protein casts (Fig. 15–38). The casts are homogeneous and eosinophilic or polychromatic. Sometimes they are lamellar or granular. On immunofluorescent microscopy the casts reveal albumin, all classes of immunoglobulins, kappa and lambda light chains, as well as Tamm-Horsfall protein.[69] In some cases the casts have the tinctorial and birefringent characteristics of amyloid (p. 201). The fact that amyloid fibrils can be produced in vitro by the proteolytic digestion of human Bence Jones protein makes this morphologic finding not so surprising.[70] The casts are usually surrounded by multinucleated giant cells, which were previously thought to be formed by the fusion of tubular epithelial cells. More recent studies suggest that the giant cells are derived from macrophages that migrate into the area through discontinuities in the tubular basement membrane. The tubular atrophy associated with these lesions is accompanied by an increase of interstitial fibrous tissue. A number of other intercurrent changes may be present, including metastatic calcifications as a reflection of bone destruction and secondary hypercalcemia, pyelonephritis incident to the predisposition to infection in these patients, and systemic amyloidosis. All of these contribute to renal insufficiency.

A myeloma neuropathy may develop owing to tumorous infiltrations of nerve trunk roots. Vertebra fractures and compression of roots may add to these neurologic complications. Occasionally, a form of neuropathy occurs in the absence of obvious causes and may represent the nonspecific carcinomatous polyneuropathy discussed on page 1432. Pathologic fractures are sometimes produced by the plasma cell lesions; they are most common in the vertebral column but may affect any of the numerous bones suffering erosion and destruction of their cortical substance.

Systemic amyloidosis occurs in about 10% of patients. When this complication supervenes, it may introduce all the morphologic changes associated with the widespread deposits of amyloid described in an earlier chapter (p. 195).

In most cases, infiltrates of neoplastic plasma cells may be found in the spleen, liver, lymph nodes, and other locations.

CLINICAL COURSE. The peak age incidence of multiple myeloma is between 50 and 60 years. Both sexes are affected equally. As previously stated, the *clinical features of myeloma stem from the effects of (1) infiltration of organs, particularly bones, by the neoplastic plasma cells; and (2) the production of excessive immunoglobulins, which lack antibody activity and often have abnormal physicochemical properties.* Infiltration of bones is manifested by pain and pathologic fractures.

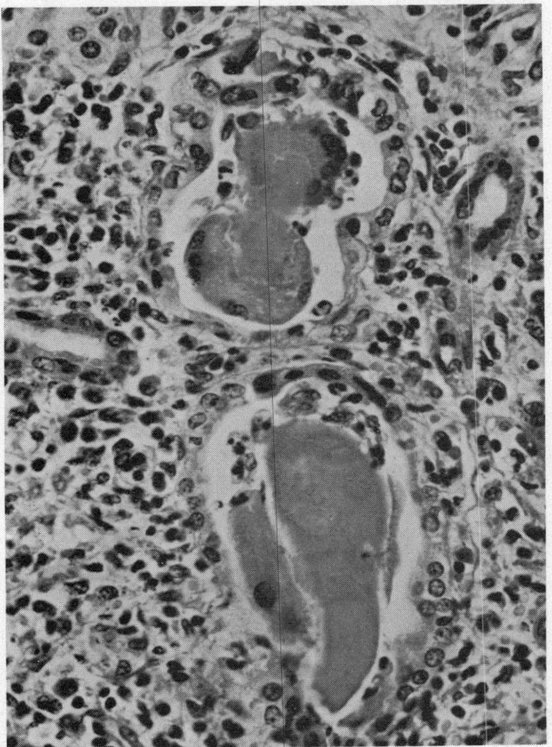

Figure 15–38. Proteinaceous casts surrounded by multinucleate giant cells in collecting tubules of kidney in myeloma nephrosis.

Hypercalcemia resulting from bone resorption may give rise to neurologic manifestations such as confusion, weakness, lethargy, constipation, and polyuria. It also contributes to renal disease. Recurrent infections with encapsulated bacteria (e.g., pneumococci) resulting from severe suppression of normal immunoglobulins pose a major clinical problem. Cellular immunity is relatively unaffected. To explain the loss of normal immunoglobulins it is postulated that the myeloma cells secrete a factor capable of activating suppressor macrophages, which in turn inhibit normal B cells.[71] Excessive production and aggregation of myeloma proteins may lead to the hyperviscosity syndrome in approximately 7% of patients. Those with the IgA myeloma are particularly prone to this complication because of the tendency of IgA molecules to form polymers. Manifestations of the hyperviscosity syndrome including retinal hemorrhages, prolonged bleeding, and neurologic changes are much more common with Waldenström's macroglobulinemia and are therefore discussed later (p. 693). Amyloidosis of the AL type results from excessive imbalanced production of immunoglobulin light chains (p. 197). Of great significance is *renal insufficiency,* which is second only to infections as a cause of death. Renal failure develops in two different settings. In the more common form it develops insidiously and usually progresses slowly over a period of months or years. Another form occurs suddenly in the absence of obvious previous renal impairment and is manifested by acute renal failure. The pathogenesis of renal failure, which may occur in up to 50% of patients, is multifactorial and is discussed in Chapter 21 (p. 1040). The most important factor appears to be Bence Jones proteinuria, since the excreted light chains are believed to be directly toxic to the tubular epithelial cells.[72] In addition to these specific symptoms, some patients may present with unexplained anemia or weakness.

The clinical diagnosis of multiple myeloma rests on radiographic and laboratory findings and ultimately on biopsy of a lesion to reveal the tumorous aggregates of plasma cells. The radiographic changes are so distinctive that a reasonably certain diagnosis can usually be made. Classically, the individual lesions appear as sharply punched-out defects, having a rounded soap-bubble appearance on x-ray film, but generalized osteoporosis may also be seen. Almost all patients have a normochromic normocytic anemia, sometimes accompanied by moderate leukopenia and thrombocytopenia due to marrow failure. Rarely, neoplastic plasma cells flood the peripheral blood, giving rise to *plasma cell leukemia.* The hyperglobulinemia leads to rouleaux formation on blood smear and an increased erythrocyte sedimentation rate. Hypercalcemia is frequently present. Most confirmatory of the diagnosis are M-protein spikes on blood or urine analysis. Quantitative analyses usually disclose more than 3 gm of Ig per 100 ml of serum and more than 6 mg of Bence Jones proteins per 100 ml of urine. The presence of the latter generally implies a graver prognosis.[73] As the disease progresses and the total mass of plasma cells expands, the level of M proteins increases. It should be remembered, however, that rarely elevated serum immunoglobulins are absent in this disease (nonsecretory myeloma). Perhaps one-third of the patients lack Bence Jones light chains. On the other hand, sometimes only Bence Jones proteins are present without increased serum gamma globulins (in so-called "light-chain disease").

The prognosis for this condition depends on the stage of advancement at the time of diagnosis. Patients with multiple bony lesions, if untreated, rarely survive for more than six to 12 months. Chemotherapy in the form of alkylating agents induces remission in 50 to 70% of patients, but the median survival is still a dismal two to three years. For reasons not entirely clear, these patients have an increased incidence of nonplasmacytic cancers, particularly acute myelogenous leukemias. It is unknown whether these are induced by alkylating agents used in therapy, or whether disordered immune surveillance underlies this predisposition to superimposed malignant neoplasia.

SOLITARY MYELOMA (PLASMACYTOMA)

About 3 to 5% of monoclonal gammopathies consist of a solitary plasmacytic lesion, in either bone or soft tissue. The bony lesions tend to occur in the same location as in multiple myeloma. Extraosseous lesions are often located in the lungs, oronasopharynx, or nasal sinuses. Wherever they arise, they have the fleshy, red-brown appearance characteristic of the lesions in multiple myeloma. The cytologic detail is also similar. Elevated levels of M proteins in the blood or urine are found in approximately 25% of cases, but when present they are not as extreme as with multiple myeloma.[74] When patients with such localized disease are followed, *progression to classic multiple myeloma becomes manifest in most patients with osseous plasmacytoma, whereas extraosseous primaries rarely disseminate.* It appears that the solitary plasmacytoma involving the bones is an early stage of multiple myeloma, but in some individuals it may be present for many years without progression.[75] Extraosseous plasmacytomas, particularly those involving upper respiratory tracts, represent limited disease that can usually be cured by local resection.

Waldenström's Macroglobulinemia

This dyscrasia, constituting about 5% of monoclonal gammopathies, *is marked by a diffuse, leukemia-like infiltrate of the bone marrow by lymphocytes, plasma cells, and hybrid forms that synthesize a structurally and antigenically homogeneous IgM immunoglobulin, leading to macroglobulinemia.* When first described, it was thought that the immunoglobulin was always of the IgM class, but it is now known that in some patients it may be IgG or IgA.[76] Approximately half the patients have lymphadenopathy, hepatomegaly, or splenomegaly, alone or in combination. This disease may best be viewed as a cross between multiple myeloma and well-differentiated lymphocytic lymphoma. As in myeloma, the neoplastic B cells secrete a monoclonal immunoglobulin. However, unlike myeloma but resembling lymphoma, the tumor cells diffusely infiltrate the lymphoid tissues including bone marrow, spleen, and lymph nodes.

MORPHOLOGY. Typically there is a diffuse, sparse-to-heavy infiltrate of the bone marrow by lymphocytes, plasma cells, lymphocytoid plasma cells, and other variants on this theme (Fig. 15–39). The infiltrate is rarely as heavy as that encountered in leukemia and does not occur in tumorous masses that are characteristic of plasma cell myeloma. Thus, there is no bone erosion or characteristic radiographic finding. Abnormal plasma cells are sometimes found. For example, "flame" cells have diffuse, intensely eosinophilic-staining cytoplasm. Thesaurocytes (storage cells) contain both cytoplasmic and intranuclear inclusions, which stain intensely with PAS (Fig. 15–40). The inclusions represent IgM or IgA, having the highest content of carbohydrate among the immunoglobulins. These cells are not diagnostic of Waldenström's macroglobulinemia and are sometimes encountered in other gammopathies, such as IgA myeloma. An increased number of mast cells may also be present.

A similar infiltrate may be present in the lymph nodes, spleen, or liver in patients having disseminated disease. Infiltration of the nerve roots, meninges, and cerebral substance by proliferating cells has also been reported.[77]

CLINICAL COURSE. Waldenström's macroglobulinemia is a disease of old age, rarely presenting before

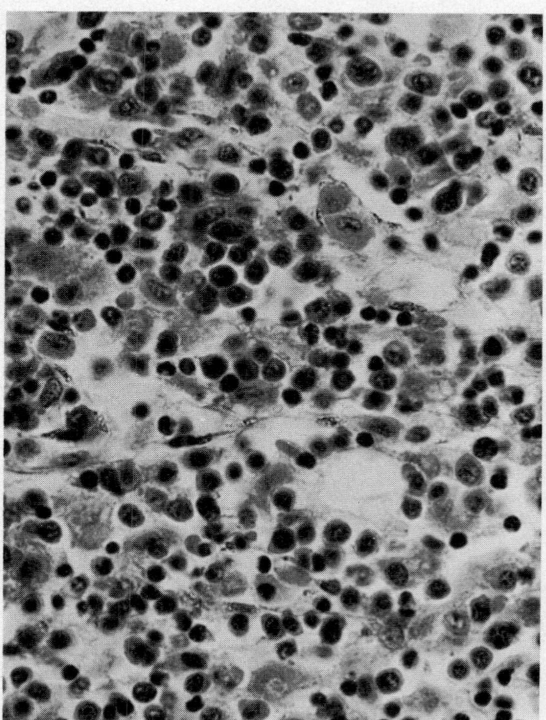

Figure 15–39. Waldenström's macroglobulinemia. Detail of marrow with pleomorphic cellularity containing recognizable lymphocytes, and plasma cells admixed with many hybrid forms. (From Cabot Case Record 26–1964. N Engl. J. Med. *270*:1190, 1964. Reprinted by permission from The New England Journal of Medicine.)

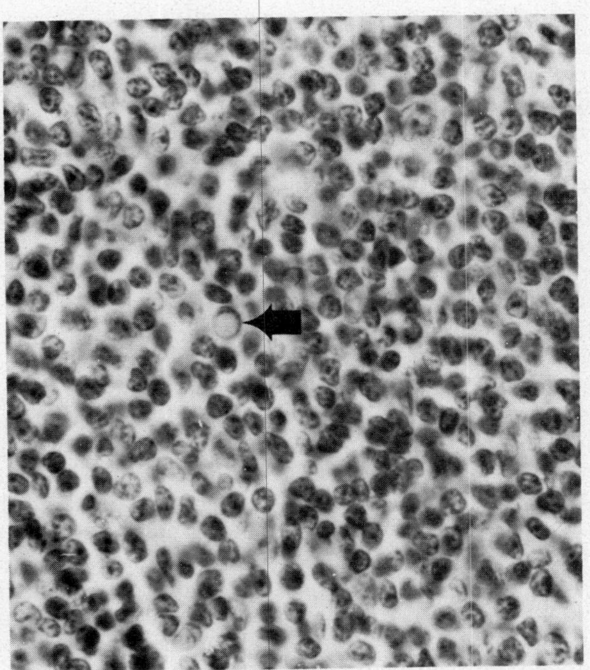

Figure 15–40. Waldenström's macroglobulinemia. High-power detail of infiltrate disclosing an intracellular inclusion *(arrow)* made up of macroglobulins. (H and E stain.) (Courtesy of Dr. Jose Hernandez, Department of Pathology, Southwestern Medical School, Dallas, Texas.)

the seventh decade. The dominant presenting complaints are weakness, fatigability, and weight loss—all nonspecific symptoms.[78] As pointed out, lymphadenopathy, hepatomegaly, and splenomegaly may be present. The specific complaints stem largely from the abnormal physicochemical properties of the macroglobulins. Because of their large size and increased concentration in blood, these paraproteins tend to form large aggregates that greatly increase the viscosity of blood. The resulting *hyperviscosity syndrome is characterized by visual impairment, neurologic signs, and excessive oozing from wounds.* The visual disturbances are related to the striking tortuosity and distention of retinal veins, with narrowing at arteriovenous crossings, producing what has been likened to a "sausage-link" pattern. Sometimes, retinal hemorrhages and exudates result from venous distention. The neurologic symptoms stemming from sluggish blood flow and sludging are protean; they include headache, dizziness, deafness, and even stupor in some cases. Excessive bleeding is related not only to hyperviscosity but also to interference in platelet function, as well as inhibition of clotting factors by macroglobulins. In some cases the abnormal globulins precipitate at low temperatures, giving rise to symptoms of *cryoglobulinemia* such as Raynaud's phenomenon and cold urticaria.

Despite the numerous clinical findings, diagnosis rests heavily on laboratory data. Unlike myeloma, there are no distinctive radiologic findings. Classically, the electrophoretic analysis of the serum discloses an M-protein spike, which is identified as IgM by immunoelectrophoresis. Associated Bence Jones proteinuria occurs in 20 to 30% of cases; for unknown reasons, however, renal damage is much less common than in multiple myeloma. A variety of other laboratory findings are present but are of less value diagnostically. These include anemia, an increased sedimentation rate, rouleaux formation, hyperviscosity, and cryoglobulinemia. Ultimately, *diagnosis rests on the typical bone marrow findings along with an M-protein spike, usually due to IgM, in the serum.* Differentiation of Waldenström's macroglobulinemia from malignant lymphoma is sometimes difficult. Since most lymphomas also have a B-cell origin, clinical forms intermediate between them and Waldenström's are not entirely unexpected. Differentiation, then, becomes largely a matter of semantics and is usually based on the predominant clinical symptoms.

The average survival in this disease is two to five years with appropriate chemotherapy.

Heavy-chain Disease

These extremely rare monoclonal gammopathies will be discussed only briefly. Three variants have been described, each characterized by elevated levels in the blood or urine of a specific heavy chain of immunoglobulins.[79] *Gamma-chain disease,* encountered most often in the elderly, resembles a malignant lymphoma more than a multiple myeloma. The manifestations consist of lymphadenopathy, anemia, and fever often accompanied by malaise, weakness, and hepatomegaly or splenomegaly. Immunoelectrophoresis with monospecific antisera discloses gamma chains in the serum or urine. Histologic study reveals an infiltrate of plasma cells and lymphocytes admixed with eosinophils and histiocytes. Lytic bone lesions are not present. Because levels of normal immunoglobulins are low, patients with this condition are susceptible to infection. In some instances the disease appears in association with tuberculosis, rheumatoid arthritis, and various autoimmune diseases, but no causal relationship has been established. The course can be rapidly downhill to death within a few months, or may be protracted for years.

Alpha-chain disease, the most common in this group, may be viewed as a disorder of IgA-producing cells involving mainly the sites of normal IgA synthesis. It occurs mainly in young adults in two clinical patterns. One, seen most commonly in the Mediterranean area, is characterized by massive infiltration of the lamina propria of the intestine and abdominal lymph nodes by lymphocytes, plasma cells, and histiocytes. Villous atrophy and severe malabsorption with diarrhea, steatorrhea, and hypocalcemia are consequences of the infiltrate. With progression, the infiltrate may be replaced by large neoplastic cells and transform into an immunoblastic sarcoma of B cells (p. 664). This abdominal form of alpha-chain disease is now designated "immunoproliferative small intestinal disease."[79A] The other clinical variant marked by a similar infiltrate limited to the respiratory tract is much less common.[80] Required for the diagnosis of both conditions is the demonstration of alpha-chain protein in the serum. Occasionally, small amounts of alpha-chains appear in the urine.

Mu-chain disease is the rarest of these entities, most often encountered in patients having chronic lymphocytic leukemia.[81] Characteristic are vacuolated plasma cells in the marrow. Immunoelectrophoresis reveals an excess of mu chains in the blood, and sometimes also kappa-type light chains in the urine. Hepatomegaly and splenomegaly are usually present, but in contrast to the usual case with CLL, peripheral lymphadenopathy is inconspicuous.

Monoclonal Gammopathy of Undetermined Significance

When large numbers of individuals above the age of 50 are screened by electrophoresis for M-protein serum spikes, about 1 to 3% are found to have elevated levels of IgG, IgA, or IgM, despite the fact that they are completely asymptomatic and clinical investigation does not disclose any of the well-defined immunoglobulin-producing diseases. *To this dysproteinemia without associated disease, the term "monoclonal gammopathy of undetermined significance" (MGUS) is applied.* MGUS is much more common than previously appreciated; in one large study, over two-thirds of the cases with a monoclonal serum protein belonged to this category.[62] Contrary to previous beliefs, the course of MGUS is not entirely benign. In a ten-year follow-up of 241 patients with MGUS, 18% developed a well-defined plasma cell dyscrasia (myeloma, macroglobulinemia, amyloidosis, or lymphoma). In another 9%, no overt disease appeared but a significant increase in the serum monoclonal protein suggested expansion of the abnormal plasma cell mass.[62] In general, patients with MGUS have less than 2.0 gm per dl of monoclonal protein, no Bence Jones proteinuria, and fewer than 5% plasma cells in the bone marrow. However, none of these criteria is absolutely reliable, and therefore the *diagnosis of MGUS requires careful exclusion of all the other specific forms of monoclonal gammopathies.* Whether a given patient with MGUS will follow a benign course, as most do, or develop a well-defined plasma cell neoplasm cannot be predicted, and hence periodic assessment of serum M component levels and Bence Jones proteinuria is warranted.

HISTIOCYTOSES

Several classifications of these disorders have been proposed. Some are based on segregation into reactive and neoplastic categories, others on the level of maturation of the histiocyte-macrophages involved. Still others include the histiocytic proliferations encountered in storage diseases such as Gaucher's and Niemann-Pick disease. Regardless of the nosologic scheme employed, it is relatively easy to segregate the clearly neoplastic proliferations such as the monocytic leukemias, the rare histiocytic lymphomas (p. 665), and histiocytic medullary reticuloses from the clearly reactive proliferations exemplified by tuberculosis and other infectious granulomas. Problems occur in trying to find a niche for certain rare proliferative disorders often described as *histiocytosis X. This term includes generalized histiocytosis (Letterer-Siwe syndrome), multifocal eosinophilic granuloma (Hand-Schüller-Christian disease), and unifocal or solitary eosinophilic granuloma.* These three conditions are believed to represent different clinicoanatomic patterns of the same basic disorder. Generalized histiocytosis, which behaves like a disseminated malignant tumor, lies at one end of the spectrum, whereas unifocal eosinophilic granuloma with its benign course represents the other end. In between lies multifocal eosinophilic granuloma, with intermediate prognosis. Although these disorders differ from each other with respect to the extent of organ involvement and the prognosis, they are unified by the presence in the lesions of large, histiocyte-like cells that bear several similarities to Langerhans' cells. These cells, you may recall (p. 160), are normally present within the epidermis and are believed to be related to the mononuclear phagocyte system. They have Fc receptors, bear HLA-D/DR antigens, and react with anti-OKT6 antibody, which also binds to thymocytes but not to peripheral T cells. These immunologic markers are also present on the so-called histiocytosis X cells (HXC) that infiltrate the organs involved by these disorders.[82] The similarity between Langerhans' cells and HXC extends also to the ultrastructural level. The cytoplasm of HXC contains characteristic inclusions called histiocytosis X (HX) bodies, which resemble Birbeck granules found in Langerhans' cells (Fig. 15–41).[83] *The HX body is seen as a pentalaminar, rodlike tubular structure with characteristic periodicity and sometimes a dilated terminal end (tennis-racquet appearance).* Thus, histiocytosis X is viewed currently as a proliferative disorder of Langerhans' cells or their marrow precursors, and hence the term "Langerhans' cell granulomatosis" has also been applied to them.[84] Although the cell of origin seems to be reasonably well established, the pathogenesis of histiocytosis X is still mysterious. Diffuse histiocytosis behaves like a malignant tumor, whereas eosinophilic granulomas, whether solitary or multifocal, appear to be non-neoplastic, rarely causing death. It is conceivable that they are all reactive disorders of variable severity, responding to unknown inciting agents.

Generalized Histiocytosis (Letterer-Siwe Syndrome)

This condition constitutes essentially an acute or subacute progressive systemic proliferation of mature and immature histiocytes. Classically, infants and young children under 3 years of age are affected. Sometimes the disease is present from birth. Occasional reports suggest that a closely similar disorder may also occur in adults.[85] In the very young the onset is marked by fever, sometimes related to a localized infection such as otitis

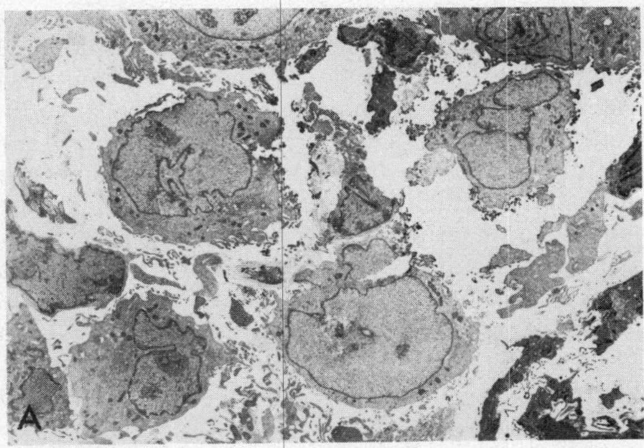

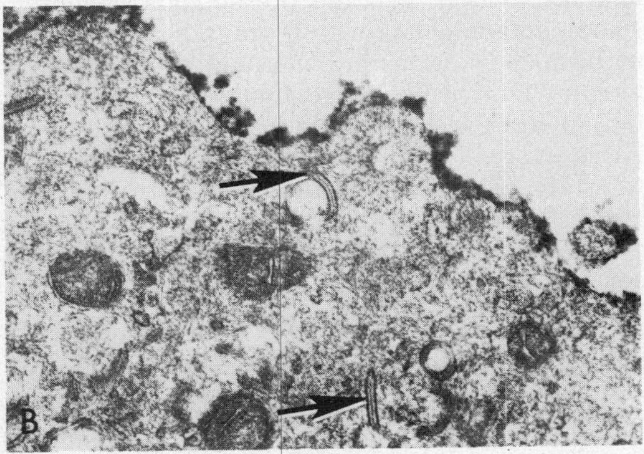

Figure 15–41. Histiocytosis X. Infiltrate is composed of large, rounded cells containing reniform and infolded nuclei (A). At higher power (B), characteristic Birbeck granules *(arrows)* and membrane reactivity for thymocyte differentiation antigen T6 (dense deposits along cell membrane) are observed. These features are also present in normal Langerhans' cells. (Courtesy of Dr. George Murphy, Harvard Medical School, Boston, MA.)

media or mastoiditis, followed soon by a diffuse maculopapular eczematous or purpuric skin rash and subsequent enlargement of the spleen, liver, and lymph nodes throughout the body. Cystic, rarefied lesions may become apparent radiographically in the skull, pelvis, and long bones. Anemia, thrombocytopenia, and leukopenia are frequently present as manifestations of flooding of the bone marrow by proliferating histiocytes. The clinical picture of diffuse histiocytosis shows several similarities to acute leukemia, histiocytic medullary reticulosis, and a variety of infectious processes. These must be clearly excluded by morphologic and other appropriate criteria before diagnosis is made.

Morphology. The characteristic microscopic feature of this disorder is an apparent neoplastic proliferation of histiocytes throughout virtually all the organs and tissues of the body. The cells have abundant, often vacuolated cytoplasm, which is amphophilic-to-acidophilic, and vesicular oval, reniform, or indented nuclei. Nucleoli, when present, are small. Occasionally, multinucleated giant histiocytes are present, and in some cases, especially those involving adults, there may be some atypia and variation in histiocyte size and shape. With electron microscopy, occasional histiocytes can be seen to contain HX bodies (Fig. 15–41), described earlier. The proliferating histiocytes sometimes disclose evidence of phagocytic activity in the form of inclusions of nuclear debris or occasional red cells, but striking erythrophagocytosis, such as is seen in histiocytic medullary reticulosis, is not present. The histiocytic infiltrates can be seen in the skin lesions, lymph nodes, spleen, and liver and particularly within the bone marrow, where they may cause erosive defects visible on x-ray film. In fatal cases, many other organs and tissues are affected, including the lungs, kidneys, gastrointestinal tract, and meninges.

The course of this condition is somewhat variable and appears to be related to age of onset. Up to the recent past, infants under 6 months of age generally pursued a rapid course to death within six months, and older children rarely survived more than one to two years. Intensive chemotherapy has remarkably improved this gloomy outlook. Lahey, in an analysis of a varied group of children with histiocytic disorders, cited "complete to good" remission in about two-thirds of infants under the age of 2 years with the use of several chemotherapy programs.[86] Several immunologic abnormalities, including a deficiency of T-suppressor cells, have been described in some patients. Administration of calf thymic extract has reversed some abnormal responses and also induced clinical remission, suggesting that deranged immunity may be an integral component of this disorder.[87] Thus, there is new hope in this previously grim situation. Death is usually related to intercurrent infections and progressive anemia and debility.

Eosinophilic Granuloma—Unifocal and Multifocal

The distinctive morphologic lesions of both the unifocal and multifocal variants consist of expanding, erosive accumulations of histiocytes usually within the medullary cavities of bones. Frequently, a few to many of the histiocytes are foamy and vacuolated. These are variably admixed with eosinophils, lymphocytes, plasma cells, and neutrophils (Fig. 15–42). Occasionally, there are areas of necrosis within these infiltrates, rimmed by a more intense infiltration of neutrophils and sometimes multinucleated histiocytes, resembling foreign body–type or Langhans' giant cells. The eosinophilic component ranges from scattered mature cells to sheetlike masses of cells. The foam cells, too, may be massed in some lesions, but since they merely reflect phagocytosis of lipid debris, they have no particular significance. Rod-shaped HX bodies may sometimes be present in the histiocytes within these lesions, similar to those described in the generalized histiocytoses. Although virtually any bone in the skeletal system may be involved, favored localities are the calvarium, ribs, and femurs. Thus, in a series of 50 cases of unifocal eosinophilic granuloma, approximately 60% of the lesions occurred in one of these three skeletal sites.[88] Similar lesions are sometimes found in the skin, lungs, or stomach, either as unifocal lesions or as components of the multifocal disease.

Unifocal eosinophilic granuloma is a benign disorder that occurs in children and young adults, especially males. The solitary lesions may be asymptomatic, or

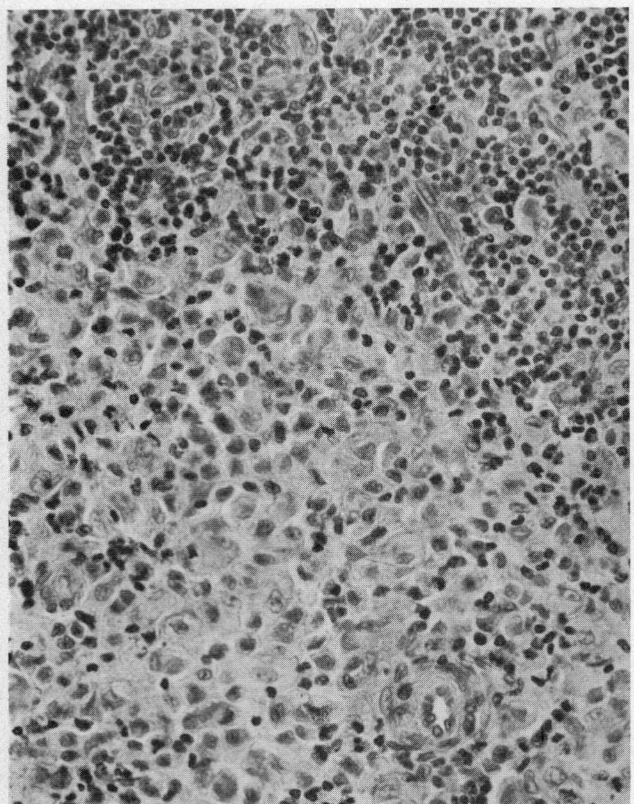

Figure 15–42. Eosinophilic granuloma. The typical round and oval macrophages are most numerous below and are interspersed with scattered lymphocytes, plasma cells, and eosinophils.

may cause pain and tenderness as the lesion erodes the bone and in some instances leads to pathologic fractures. There are usually no systemic manifestations, such as fever, nor involvement of the blood or viscera. Diagnosis is based on roentgenologic demonstration of a focal destructive bone lesion arising within the marrow cavity and on the characteristic morphologic findings. In some cases, spontaneous fibrosis and healing occur, usually in the span of a year or two. In other instances, curettage, excision, or local irradiation leads to a cure. Occasionally, individuals with an apparent unifocal lesion are encountered in whom, over the course of time, multiple lesions in bones or soft tissues develop. Whether such a sequence implies conversion of unifocal eosinophilic granuloma to the multifocal disease, or instead represents a single overt lesion presenting first in a patient with disseminated disease, is unknown. In any event, it is clear that patients with unifocal eosinophilic granuloma must be carefully followed for years.

Multifocal eosinophilic granuloma is a more disabling disease, with onset usually before the age of 5 years. *This syndrome was formerly called Hand-Schüller-Christian disease.* (p. 694). Typically, patients have fever; a diffuse, scaly, seborrhea-like eruption, particularly on the scalp and in the ear canals; and frequent bouts of otitis media, mastoiditis, and upper respiratory infections as well as gingival inflammations. Mild lymphadenopathy, hepatomegaly, and splenomegaly due to infiltrates may be present. Pneumonitis with diffuse radiographic pulmonary opacities are sometimes present, perhaps related to granulomatous involvement of the lungs or to intercurrent microbiologic infections. About half the patients have granulomatous involvement of the posterior pituitary stalk or hypothalamus leading to diabetes insipidus. Orbital granulomas induce exophthalmos in about one-third of patients. *The combination of calvarial bone defects, diabetes insipidus, and exophthalmos are referred to as the Hand-Schüller-Christian triad.* However, only a minority of patients with multifocal eosinophilic granuloma have the complete triad. It may be evident that the presentation of multifocal eosinophilic granuloma with fever, skin rash, and multiple histiocytic lesions in bones and viscera bears considerable resemblance to generalized histiocytosis, accounting for the belief that the two syndromes are variable expressions of a single disorder. However, in contrast to generalized histiocytosis, the prognosis in multifocal eosinophilic granuloma is good. In half the patients the lesions spontaneously resolve, and in the other half chemotherapy induces ultimate recovery.

ANGIOIMMUNOBLASTIC LYMPHADENOPATHY

This entity, sometimes also called "angioimmunoblastic lymphadenopathy with dysproteinemia," is an uncommon systemic disorder marked principally by generalized lymphadenopathy.[89] Seen principally in elderly individuals, it is characterized by fever, weight loss, generalized lymphadenopathy (present in all cases), hepatosplenomegaly, maculopapular rash, polyclonal hypergammaglobulinemia, and Coombs'-positive hemolytic anemia. A history of drug ingestion—penicillin, sulfonamides, aspirin, halothane, phenytoin sodium, griseofulvin, allopurinol, and methyldopa—is sometimes present and may precipitate the disease.

In addition to the involvement of the lymph nodes, less characteristic anatomic changes are encountered in the spleen, liver, bone marrow, skin, and lung.[90] The lymph nodes are generally 2 to 3 cm in diameter, soft, movable, nonmatted, and sometimes tender. *The histopathologic diagnosis rests on the following triad: (1) a pleomorphic cellular infiltrate of small and large lymphocytes, immunoblasts, and plasma cells that infiltrates the capsule and effaces the nodal architecture; (2) an arborizing vascular proliferation accompanied by endothelial cell hyperplasia; and (3) interstitial deposits of an amorphous, eosinophilic, PAS-positive material thought to be cellular debris (Fig. 15–43).* Immunofluorescent and immunoperoxidase techniques reveal cytoplasmic inclusions of immunoglobulins in many of the lymphoid cells.[91] Less characteristic pleomorphic infiltrates may be found in the other organs mentioned, sometimes with marked erythrophagocytosis in the spleen (accounting for the hemolytic anemia).

The nature of this entity is obscure, but the clinical

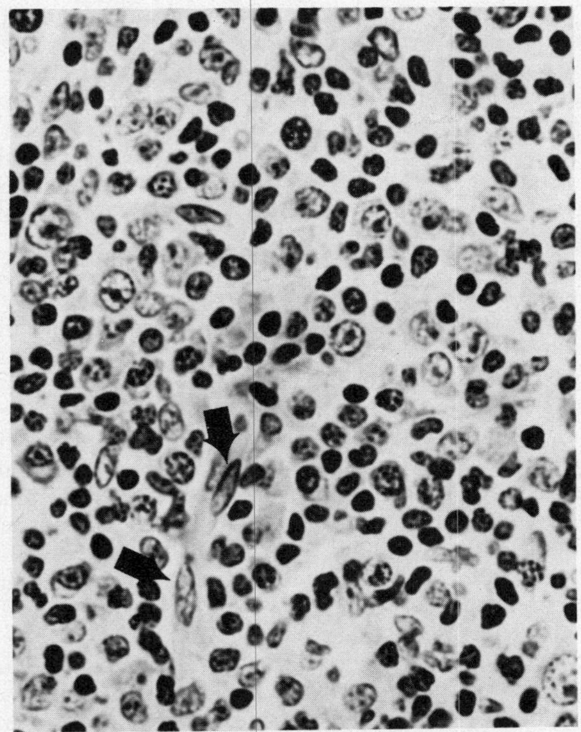

Figure 15–43. Angioimmunoblastic lymphadenopathy. Note pleomorphic infiltrate consisting of small dark cells (lymphocytes), plasma cells, and large cells with vesicular nuclei (immunoblasts). The elongated nuclei *(arrows)* represent endothelial cells, which are usually quite prominent owing to vascular proliferation. (Courtesy of Dr. Jose Hernandez Department of Pathology, Southwestern Medical School, Dallas, Texas.)

and anatomic findings are most consistent with chronic antigenic stimulation inducing non-neoplastic proliferation of B lymphocytes. The frequent, but not invariable, history of drug ingestion raises the possibility that these agents precipitate the immune response. Indeed, the anatomic changes in angioimmunoblastic lymphadenopathy are very similar to those encountered in lymph nodes in so-called "drug reactions," except that vasculitic lesions are often present in the latter. In patients without a history of drug ingestion, an autoimmune reaction is postulated, but no definite triggering agents have been identified. A variety of immunologic derangements including a deficiency of T-suppressor cells, cutaneous anergy, or the presence of suppressor monocytes have been described in patients with this disorder. However, there is no characteristic or constant immunologic abnormality, which suggests that angioimmunoblastic lymphadenopathy may evolve by several distinct mechanisms.

The course of this disorder is extremely variable. About one-half of the patients survive two to four years, some (25%) without any treatment, others (25%) with treatment (steroids, combination chemotherapy). In the remainder, the disease progresses rapidly, regardless of the treatment given. Most deaths are caused by severe infection, possibly related to immunologic incompetence, but some patients have developed immunoblastic sarcomas. In such cases, it is postulated that one of the several hyperactive B cells becomes autonomous and neoplastic. Thus, a monoclonal B-cell neoplasm, associated with a change from polyclonal to monoclonal hypergammaglobulinemia, may emerge (see also the discussion on p. 668).[92]

In this condition, confusion stems from two sources: (1) it is frequently misdiagnosed histologically as a lymphoma, particularly Hodgkin's disease, because of the pleomorphic cellular infiltrate; and (2) the presence in about 40% of patients of a pruritic, generalized, maculopapular rash, interpreted as a dermal drug reaction, may direct attention away from the potentially serious underlying systemic disorder.

Spleen

NORMAL

The spleen is to the circulatory system as the lymph nodes are to the lymphatic system. Among its functions are filtration from the bloodstream of all "foreign" matter including obsolescent and damaged blood cells, and participation in the immune response to all blood-borne antigens. Designed ingeniously for these functions, the spleen is a major repository of mononuclear phagocytic cells in the red pulp and of lymphoid cells in the white pulp. Normally in the adult it weighs about 150 gm and measures some 12 cm in length, 7 cm in width, and 3 cm in thickness. It is enclosed within a thin, glistening connective tissue capsule that appears slate gray and through which the dusky-red, friable parenchyma of the splenic substance can be seen. In man, unlike some animals, there is little if any smooth muscle in the capsule and therefore virtually no contractile function. The cut surface of the spleen is dotted with gray specks, the splenic or malpighian follicles that constitute the white pulp. In three dimensions this white pulp forms periarterial sheaths of lymphoid cells around the arteries, most abundant about the larger branches and progressively more attenuated as the arterial supply penetrates the splenic substance. A cross section of such an arrangement reveals a central artery surrounded eccentrically by a collar of T lymphocytes, the so-called periarteriolar lymphatic sheath. At intervals the lymphatic sheaths become expanded, usually on one side of the artery to form lymphoid nodules composed principally of B lymphocytes. Upon antigenic stimulation, typical germinal centers form within these B-cell areas (p. 656). Eventually the arterial system terminates in fine penicilliary arterioles, which at first are enclosed within a thin mantle of lymphocytes but which then enter the red pulp, leaving behind their "fellow-travelers."

The red pulp of the spleen is traversed by numerous thin-walled vascular sinusoids, separated by the splenic cords or "cords of Billroth." The endothelial lining of the sinusoid is of the open or discontinuous type, providing passage of blood cells between the sinusoids and cords. The splenic cords are spongelike and consist of a labyrinth of macrophages loosely connected through long dendritic processes to create both a physical and a functional filter through which the blood can slowly seep.

It is widely believed that the blood, as it traverses the red pulp, takes two routes to reach the splenic veins. Some of the capillary flow is into the splenic cords and is then gradually filtered out into the surrounding splenic sinusoids to reach the veins; this is the so-called "open circulation," which is functionally the slow compartment. The other pathway involves direct passage from the capillaries to the splenic veins without the intervening stage of passage through the cords. This, the "closed circuit," is understandably the more rapid compartment. According to current views, only a small fraction of the blood entering the spleen at any given time pursues the "open" route. Nevertheless, during the course of a day the total volume of blood passes through the filtration beds of the splenic cords, where it is exposed to the remarkably sensitive and effective phagocytic macrophages, which are able to screen the blood.

Most anatomic disorders of the spleen are secondary to some systemic disorder and thus are the consequence of normal splenic function. These can be segregated into four categories.

1. *Filtration of unwanted elements from the blood* by phagocytosis in the splenic cords is a major function of the spleen. As you know, 1/120th of all red cells are destroyed daily by phagocytosis in the reticuloendothelial system. Engulfment by splenic macrophages accounts for approximately half this removal of obsolescent red cells from the circulation. The splenic phagocytes are also remarkably efficient in "culling" damaged red cells and leukocytes, red cells rendered foreign by antibody coating, as well as the abnormal red cells encountered in several of the anemias (e.g., hereditary spherocytosis, sickle cell anemia). As discussed earlier (p. 615), the red cells have to undergo extreme degrees of deformation during passage from the cords into the sinusoids. In several hemolytic anemias, the reduced plasticity of the red cell membrane leads to trapping of the abnormal red cells within the cords and subsequent phagocytosis by the cordal macrophages. In addition to removal of the red cells, splenic macrophages are also involved in "pitting" of red cells by which inclusions such as siderotic granules, Heinz bodies, and Howell-Jolly bodies are neatly excised without destruction of the erythrocytes. The phagocytes are also active in removal of other particulate matter from the blood, such as bacteria, cell debris, or abnormal macromolecules produced in some of the inborn errors of metabolism (e.g., Gaucher's disease, Niemann-Pick disease).

2. A second function of the spleen relates to its role as a *major secondary organ in the immune system.* The reticular network in the periarterial lymphatic sheaths traps antigen, permitting it to come into contact with effector lymphocytes. Both T and B cells are present in the lymphoid tissue of the spleen, and thus it contributes to both humoral and cell-mediated immune responses.

3. The spleen is a *source of lymphoreticular cells and sometimes hematopoietic cells.* As you recall, splenic hematopoiesis normally ceases before birth, but in severe anemia, extramedullary splenic hematopoiesis may be reactivated. Lymphocyte and macrophage production normally occurs in the spleen throughout life, becoming progressively attenuated with increasing age.

4. Because of its rich vascularization and phagocytic function, the spleen also *constitutes a reserve pool and storage site.* In humans, the normal spleen harbors only about 30 to 40 ml of erythrocytes, but with splenomegaly this reservoir is greatly increased. The normal spleen also stores approximately 30 to 40% of the total platelet mass in the body. With splenomegaly this platelet storage may markedly increase, sometimes to up to 80 to 90% of the total platelet mass. Similarly, the enlarged spleen may trap a sufficient number of white cells to induce leukopenia. In addition to the blood elements, as mentioned, the spleen is a major storage site of red cell iron and macromolecular products of abnormal metabolism.

In view of all these functions it is no wonder that the spleen becomes secondarily involved in a wide variety of systemic disorders.

PATHOLOGY

As the largest unit of the reticuloendothelial system, the spleen is involved in all systemic inflammations and generalized hematopoietic disorders, and many metabolic disturbances. It is rarely the primary site of disease. When the spleen is involved in systemic disease, splenic enlargement usually develops, and therefore splenomegaly is a major manifestation of disorders of this organ.

SPLENOMEGALY

Splenic enlargement may be an important diagnostic clue to the existence of an underlying disorder, but the condition itself may cause problems. When sufficiently enlarged, the spleen may cause a dragging sensation in the left upper quadrant and, through pressure on the stomach, cause discomfort after eating. In addition, its storage function may lead to the sequestration of significant numbers of blood elements, giving rise to a syndrome known as *hypersplenism* (described below). A listing, by no means exhaustive, of the disorders associated with splenomegaly is provided in Table 15–8.

HYPERSPLENISM

Hypersplenism is encountered in only a minority of patients with splenic enlargement. In essence, this syndrome is characterized by the triad of (1) splenomegaly usually caused by one of the disorders listed in Table 15–8 (secondary hypersplenism), but sometimes of unknown etiology (primary hypersplenism); (2) a reduction of one or more of the cellular elements of the blood, leading to anemia, leukopenia, thrombocytopenia, or any combination of these, associated with hyperplasia of the marrow precursors of the deficient cell type; and (3) correction of the blood cytopenia(s) by splenectomy. The precise cause of this syndrome is still uncertain, but increased sequestration of the cells and the consequent enhanced lysis by the splenic macrophages seem to be the likely explanation for the cytopenias. In most cases there is a reasonable basis (underlying disease) for the splenomegaly, represented by the term secondary hypersplenism. In a minority of cases, however, the splenomegaly is of unknown origin and the syndrome is designated primary hypersplenism. In such cases, what caused the splenomegaly? Moreover, primary hypersplenism has also been diagnosed in patients having *no* apparent splenomegaly, in which case it must be assumed that sequestration was not operative. It is apparent that there are still many gray areas requiring explication. For now, it seems best to consider the diagnosis of hypersplenism to be appropriate only when there is splenic enlargement, however mild, and to view primary hypersplenism as covering those instances in which the systemic disease causing the splenomegaly has remained undiscovered.

The splenomegaly in virtually all the conditions previously mentioned has been discussed elsewhere. There remain only a few causes that require consideration.

CONGENITAL ANOMALIES

Complete absence of the spleen is rare and is usually associated with other congenital abnormalities. *Hypoplasia* is a more common finding.

Table 15–8. DISORDERS ASSOCIATED WITH SPLENOMEGALY

I. Infections
- Nonspecific splenitis of various blood-borne infections (particularly infective endocarditis)
- Infectious mononucleosis
- Tuberculosis
- Typhoid fever
- Brucellosis
- Cytomegalovirus
- Syphilis
- Malaria
- Histoplasmosis
- Toxoplasmosis
- Kala-azar
- Trypanosomiasis
- Schistosomiasis
- Leishmaniasis
- Echinococcosis

II. Congestive States Related to Portal Hypertension
- Cirrhosis of liver
- Portal or splenic vein thrombosis
- Cardiac failure (right-sided)

III. Lymphohematogenous Disorders
- Hodgkin's disease
- Non-Hodgkin's lymphomas
- Histiocytoses
- Multiple myeloma
- Myeloproliferative syndromes (chronic myelogenous leukemia, polycythemia vera, agnogenic myeloid metaplasia)
- Chronic lymphocytic leukemia
- Acute leukemias (inconstant)
- Hemolytic anemias (autoimmune hemolytic anemia, hereditary spherocytosis, hemoglobinopathies)
- Splenic neutropenia
- Thrombocytopenic purpura

IV. Immunologic-inflammatory Conditions
- Rheumatoid arthritis
- Felty's syndrome
- Systemic lupus erythematosus

V. Storage Diseases
- Gaucher's disease
- Niemann-Pick disease
- Mucopolysaccharidoses

VI. Miscellaneous
- Infarctions
- Amyloidosis
- Primary neoplasms and cysts
- Secondary neoplasms

Abnormal lobulations, either shallow or deep, are another form of anomaly. These must be distinguished from depressed healed infarcts.

Accessory spleens (spleniculi) are common and have been encountered singly or multiply in one-fifth to one-third of all postmortem examinations. They are usually small spherical structures that are histologically and functionally identical with the normal spleen, reacting to various stimuli in the same manner. They are generally situated in the gastrosplenic ligament or the tail of the pancreas, but are sometimes located in the omentum or mesenteries of the small or large intestine. Accessory spleens may have great clinical importance. In some hematologic disorders such as hereditary spherocytosis, thrombocytopenic purpura, and hypersplenism, splenectomy is a standard method of treatment. If a large accessory spleen is overlooked, the benefit from the removal of the definitive spleen may be lost.

NONSPECIFIC ACUTE SPLENITIS

Enlargement of the spleen, sometimes also called "acute splenic tumor," occurs in any blood-borne infection. The nonspecific splenic reaction in these infections may be caused not only by the microbiologic agents themselves but also by the products of the inflammatory disease. Obviously, acute splenitis is also encountered in many specific infections, but these histologic changes usually provide some clue to the nature of the infection, as for example the striking reticuloendothelial hyperplasia and erythrophagocytosis in typhoid fever or the characteristic "mononucleosis cells" in infectious mononucleosis. In nonspecific acute splenitis it is impossible to identify the causative agent from the splenic changes.

Morphologically the spleen is enlarged (up to 200 to 400 gm) and soft. The color of the cut surface varies from grayish-red to deep red; the white pulp is usually obscured. The splenic substance is often diffluent and may be sufficiently soft literally to flow out from the cut surface. Microscopically, the major change is acute congestion of the red pulp, which may encroach on and sometimes virtually efface the lymphoid follicles. Reticuloendothelial hyperplasia and numerous free macrophages are prominent within the sinusoids, and these phagocytic cells are often filled with viable and disintegrating bacteria as well as amorphous debris. An infiltrate of neutrophils, plasma cells, and occasionally eosinophils is sometimes present throughout the white and red pulp. At times there is acute necrosis of the centers of the splenic follicles, particularly when the causative agent is a hemolytic streptococcus. Rarely, abscess formation occurs. Infarcts, either bland or septic, may be present in those cases associated with infective endocarditis.

REACTIVE HYPERPLASIA OF SPLEEN

This rather vague designation refers to the splenic changes encountered in chronic inflammatory states, systemic antigenemia, immunologic-inflammatory conditions (rheumatoid arthritis, Felty's syndrome, bacterial endocarditis, SLE), systemic viremias (infectious mononucleosis, herpes simplex), and chronic graft rejections. In all these situations, the spleen along with the lymph nodes reacts as a component of the immune system, and so the spleen in these settings has been referred to by Enriquez and Neiman as an "activated spleen."[93]

The spleen is enlarged, sometimes up to 1000 gm, and generally is moderately firm. The splenic capsule is unaffected. The red pulp may be unusually congested, and on cut surface the splenic follicles are often prominent. Microscopically, the dominant changes are hyperplasia of the splenic follicles and marked reticuloendothelial hyperplasia, sometimes filling the sinusoids with phagocytic cells showing phagocytosis of debris (Fig. 15–44). Large germinal centers may be seen in the follicles, with prominent mitotic activity and transformation of many of the follicular center cells into "blasts." Macrophages, eosinophils, and numerous plasma cells are often present in both white and red pulp.

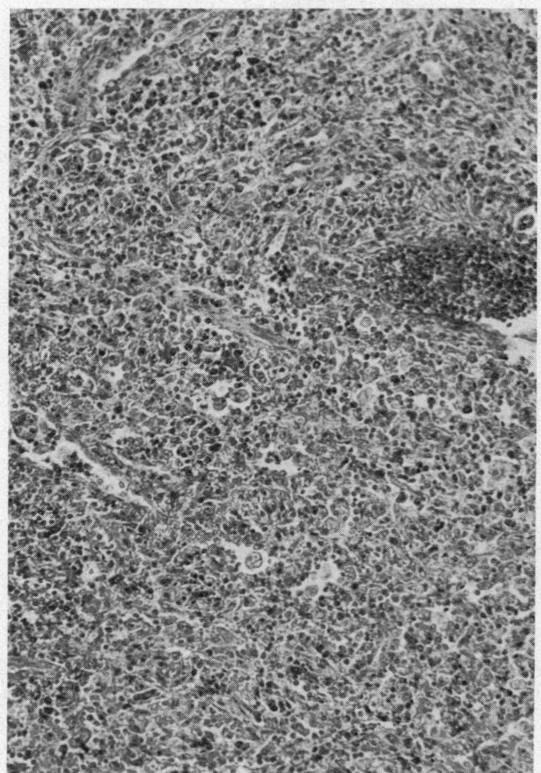

Figure 15–44. Chronic reactive hyperplasia of spleen. View of spleen substance. Sinuses are filled with macrophages and other white cells so that the low-power architecture is suffused with cells.

Should the underlying condition causing the splenic changes be amenable to control, the spleen in time generally reverts to normal or near-normal size.

CONGESTIVE SPLENOMEGALY

Persistent or chronic venous congestion may cause enlargement of the spleen referred to as *congestive splenomegaly*. The venous congestion may be systemic in origin, may be caused by intrahepatic derangement of portal venous drainage, or may be due to obstructive venous disorders in the portal or splenic veins. All these disorders ultimately lead to portal or splenic vein hypertension. *Systemic or central venous congestion* is encountered in cardiac decompensation involving the right side of the heart, and therefore is found in any type of long-standing cardiac decompensation. It is particularly severe in tricuspid or pulmonic valvular disease and in chronic cor pulmonale. In systemic venous stasis there are accompanying congestive changes in the liver and intestines, and frequently associated ascites and peripheral edema. Such systemic passive congestion produces only moderate enlargement of the spleen, so that it rarely exceeds 500 gm in weight.

The most common causes of striking congestive splenomegaly are the various forms of cirrhosis of the liver. The diffuse fibrous scarring of alcoholic cirrhosis and pigment cirrhosis evokes the most extreme enlargements. Less commonly, other forms of cirrhosis are implicated. In these conditions, there is sufficient impingement on the venous drainage through the liver to cause marked stasis within the portal system. At the same time, portohepatic artery shunts develop in the hepatic scars to raise the portal and splenic venous pressures even further. Only infrequently does tumorous obstruction of the vasculature of the liver give rise to congestive changes in the spleen. It is therefore uncommon for diffuse metastatic seeding of the liver to produce significant portal hypertension. Primary hepatic carcinoma may be an exception when it invades the major hepatic vessels.

Congestive splenomegaly is also caused by obstruction to the extrahepatic portal vein or splenic vein. The venous obstruction may be due to *spontaneous portal vein thrombosis.* Such thrombosis is usually associated with some intrahepatic obstructive disease, or may be initiated by inflammatory involvement of the portal vein *(pylephlebitis)* such as follows intraperitoneal infections. Thrombosis of the splenic vein itself may be initiated by the pressure of tumors in neighboring organs, e.g., carcinoma of the stomach or pancreas. Less often, it occurs as a splenic thrombophlebitis resulting from suppurative peritonitis, or as a bland thrombosis secondary to upper abdominal surgery or some disorder that predisposes to systemic venous thromboses.

Long-standing congestive splenomegaly produces marked enlargement of the spleen (1000 gm or more); the organ is firm and becomes increasingly so the longer the congestion lasts. The weight may reach 5000 gm. The capsule may be thickened and fibrous but is otherwise uninvolved. The cut surface has a meaty appearance and varies from gray-red to deep red, depending on the amount of fibrosis. Often the malpighian corpuscles are indistinct. Small gray-to-brown firm nodules scattered throughout the red pulp constitute the so-called **Gandy-Gamna** nodules described below. Microscopically, the pulp is suffused with red cells during the early phases but becomes increasingly more fibrous and cellular with time. The increased portal pressure causes deposition of collagen in the basement membrane of the sinusoids, which appear dilated owing to the rigidity of their walls (Fig. 15–45). The resulting impairment of blood flow from the cords to the sinusoids prolongs the exposure of the blood cells to the cordal macrophages, resulting in excessive destruction (hypersplenism).[94] Foci of recent or old hemorrhage may be present with deposition of hemosiderin in histiocytes. It is the organization of these focal hemorrhages that gives rise to the Gandy-Gamna nodules—foci of fibrosis containing deposits of iron and calcium salts encrusted on connective tissue and elastic fibers. The trabeculae are thickened and fibrous. In long-standing splenic congestion, foci of hematopoiesis appear, presumably as a response to the local vascular stasis and hypoxia.

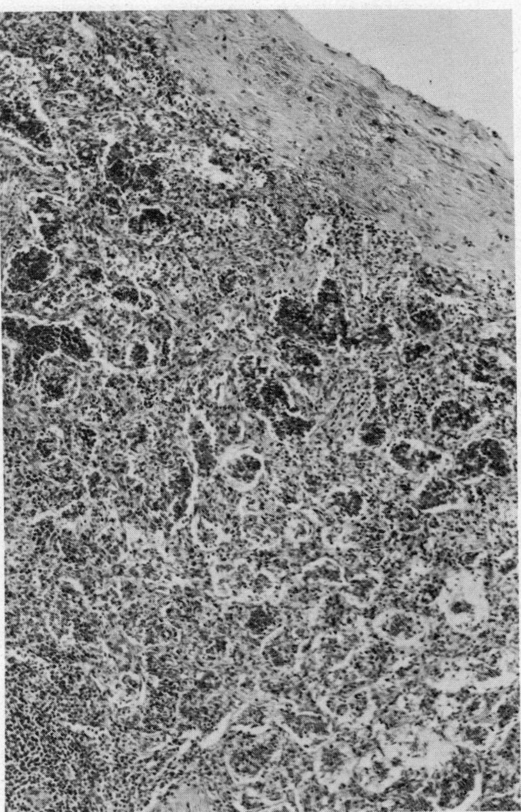

Figure 15–45. Congestive splenomegaly. Congestion of sinuses, fibrosis and widening of walls of sinuses, and fibrosis of capsule are the dominant features shown.

SPLENIC INFARCTS

During the acute stages, infarcts of the spleen may cause enlargement, depending on the size and number of the lesions. The splenomegaly, however, is at most slight, and as the infarcts undergo fibrosis the spleen returns to normal size. Indeed, in the late stages, multiple splenic infarcts may cause loss of splenic substance. Splenic infarcts are comparatively common lesions. Caused by occlusion of the major splenic artery or any of its branches, they are almost always due to emboli that arise in the heart. The spleen, along with kidneys and brain, ranks as one of the most frequent sites of localization of systemic emboli. The infarcts may be small or large, multiple or single, or sometimes may involve the entire organ. They are usually of the bland, anemic type. Septic infarcts are found in infective endocarditis of the valves of the left side of the heart. Much less often, infarcts in the spleen are caused by local thromboses, especially in the myeloproliferative syndromes, sickle cell anemia, polyarteritis nodosa, Hodgkin's disease, and bacteremic diseases.

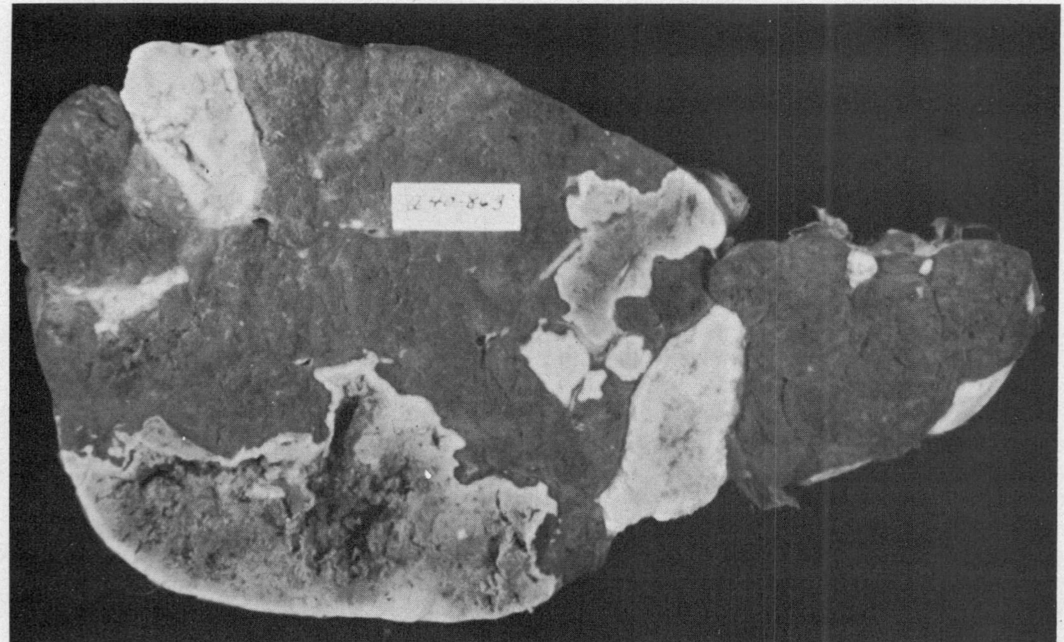

Figure 15–46. Splenic infarcts. Multiple wedge-shaped lesions are present, the largest having developed cystic softening.

Infarcts are characteristically pale and wedge-shaped, with their bases at the periphery where the capsule is often covered with fibrin (Fig. 15–46). Septic infarction modifies this appearance as frank suppurative necrosis develops. In the course of healing of these splenic infarcts, large, depressed scars may occur. The uncommon pattern of scattered in situ thromboses is characterized as the "spotted spleen" or "fleckmilz." It is usually produced by acute infectious diseases that initiate acute vasculitis and thromboses of splenic vessels. In this condition, the splenic substance is dotted by minute infarctions that vary from 1 to 5 mm in diameter.

Splenic infarcts are an important clinical consideration in older cardiac patients who suddenly complain of left upper quadrant pain. This clinical accident is not an unusual accompaniment of bacterial infective endocarditis. Occasionally in these cases, the fibrinous perisplenitis leads to friction rubs that can be heard in the left upper quadrant. The destruction of splenic substance is not critically significant, and the major importance of these infarcts is their differentiation from other more serious intra-abdominal diseases that cause left upper quadrant pain: e.g., rupture of the spleen, perforation of the stomach or intestines, or rupture of an intra-abdominal aneurysm.

NEOPLASMS

Neoplastic involvement of the spleen, whether primary or secondary, may induce splenomegaly.

PRIMARY LESIONS

In general, primary tumors, either benign or malignant, are rare.

BENIGN. The following types of benign tumors may arise in the spleen: fibromas, osteomas, chondromas, lymphangiomas, and hemangiomas. The last-named two are the most common and are often cavernous in type. Undoubtedly, some of the hemangiomas are better classified as hamartomas than as neoplasms.

MALIGNANT. Any of the types of non-Hodgkin's lymphomas or Hodgkin's disease primary in the lymph nodes (p. 657) may be primary in the spleen, and in this organ they have the same characteristics as in the lymph nodes. In addition to these lesions, hemangiosarcomas with metastases, especially to the liver, do occur (p. 542).

SECONDARY LESIONS

Whether to call involvement of the spleen in systemic Hodgkin's disease or disseminated non-Hodgkin's lymphomas a secondary lesion is largely a semantic issue; however, as you recall, splenic involvement in these conditions is by no means uncommon. Metastases of other types of tumors to the spleen have been reported to be rare, or present in 50% of cases when assiduously sought. In either event, metastases appear in the spleen only when the primary lesion has disseminated widely, and are of little clinical consequence since the patients are almost always in a terminal stage.

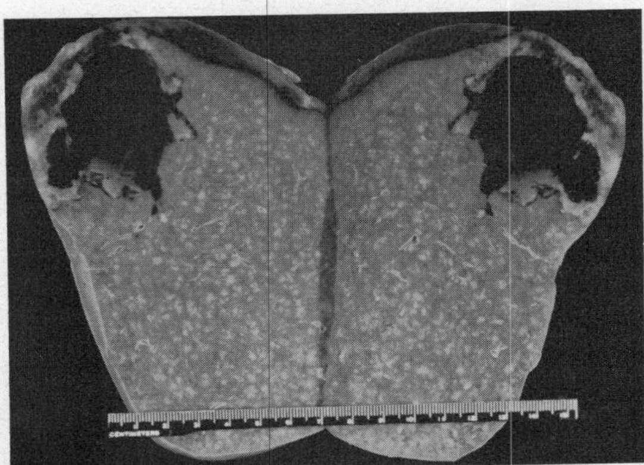

Figure 15–47. Large spontaneous hemorrhage into spleen of a 27-year-old patient with infectious mononucleosis. Hematoma ruptured through capsule and caused massive intraperitoneal hemorrhage.

RUPTURE

Rupture of the spleen is usually caused by a crushing injury or severe blow. Much less often, it is encountered in the apparent absence of trauma: this event is designated as spontaneous rupture. It is a clinical maxim that the normal spleen never ruptures spontaneously. In all instances of apparent nontraumatic rupture, some underlying condition should be suspected as the basis for the enlargement or weakening of this organ. Spontaneous rupture is encountered most often in infectious mononucleosis, malaria, typhoid fever, leukemia, and the other types of acute splenitis (Fig. 15–47). Rupture is usually followed by extensive, sometimes massive, intraperitoneal hemorrhage. The condition usually must be treated by prompt surgical removal of the spleen to prevent death from loss of blood and shock. In rare instances, clotting staunches the flow of blood. In some cases, following rupture, spleniculi may be found either localized or scattered throughout the peritoneal cavity, apparently transplants of splenic substance.

1. Young, G.A.R., and Vincent, P.C.: Drug-induced agranulocytosis. Clin. Hematol. *9*:483, 1980.
2. Nathwani, B.N.: A critical analysis of the classification of non-Hodgkin's lymphoma. Cancer *44*:347, 1979.
3. National Cancer Institute: Sponsored study of classifications of non-Hodgkin's lymphomas. Summary and description of a Working Formulation for Clinical Usage. Cancer *49*:2112, 1982.
4. Nathwani, B.N., et al.: Non-Hodgkin's lymphomas. A clinicopathologic study comparing two classifications. Cancer *41*:303, 1978.
5. Rappaport, H.: Follicular lymphoma, a reevaluation of its position in the scheme of malignant lymphoma based on a survey of 253 cases. Cancer *9*:792, 1956.
6. Mann, R.B., et al.: Malignant lymphomas—a conceptual understanding of morphologic diversity. A review. Am. J. Pathol. *94*:105, 1979.
7. Pangalis, G.A., et al.: Malignant lymphoma, well-differentiated lymphocytic: Its relationship with chronic lymphocytic leukemia and macroglobulinemia of Waldenström. Cancer *39*:999, 1977.
8. Fisher, R.I., et al.: Diffuse aggressive lymphomas: Increased survival after alternating flexible sequences of ProMACE and MOPP chemotherapy. Ann. Intern. Med. *98*:304, 1983.
9. Nathwani, B.N., et al.: Malignant lymphoblastic lymphoma. Cancer *38*:964, 1976.
10. Nathwani, B.N., et al.: Lymphoblastic lymphoma. A clinicopathologic study of 95 patients. Cancer *48*:2347, 1981.
11. Levine, A.M., et al.: Successful therapy of convoluted T-lymphoblastic lymphoma in the adult. Blood *61*:92, 1983.
12. Miliauskas, J.R., et al.: Undifferentiated non-Hodgkin's lymphoma (Burkitt's and non-Burkitt's types). The relevance of making this histologic distinction. Cancer *50*:2115, 1982.
13. Grogan, T.M., et al.: A comparative study of Burkitt's and non-Burkitt's "undifferentiated" malignant lymphoma: Immunologic, cytochemical, ultrastructural, cytologic, histopathologic, clinical and cell culture features. Cancer *49*:1817, 1982.
14. Lukes, R.J., et al.: Immunologic approach to non-Hodgkin's lymphomas and related leukemias. Analysis of the results of multiparameter study of 425 cases. Semin. Hematol. *15*:322, 1978.
15. Collins, R.D.: T-cell neoplasms. Am. J. Surg. Pathol. *6*:745, 1982.
16. Edelson, R.L.: Cutaneous T cell lymphoma. J. Dermatol. Surg. Oncol. *6*:358, 1980.
17. Miller, R.A., et al.: Sézary syndrome: A model for migration of T lymphocytes to skin. N. Engl. J. Med. *303*:89, 1980.
18. Broder, S., and Bunn, P.A., Jr.: Cutaneous T cell lymphomas. Semin. Oncol. *7*:310, 1980.
19. Byrne, G.E.: Rappaport classification of non-Hodgkin's lymphomas. Histologic significance. Cancer Treat. Rep. *61*:935, 1977.
20. Stein, R.S., et al.: Correlations between immunologic markers and histopathologic classifications—clinical implications. Semin. Oncol. *7*:244, 1980.
21. Whitcomb, C.C., et al.: Subcategories of histiocytic lymphoma: Association with survival and reproducibility of classification. The Southeastern Cancer Study Group. Cancer *48*:2464, 1981.
22. Nathwani, B.N., et al.: The clinical significance of the morphologic subdivision of diffuse "histiocytic" lymphoma. A study of 162 patients treated by Southwest Oncology Group. Blood *60*:5, 1982.
23. Jaffe, E.S., et al.: Predictability of immunologic phenotype by morphologic criteria in diffuse aggressive non-Hodgkin's lymphomas. Am. J. Clin. Pathol. *77*:46, 1982.
24. Rudders, R.A.: Surface markers in non-Hodgkin's lymphomas. Hosp. Pract. *18*:161, 1983.
25. Banfi, A., et al.: Preferential sites of involvement and spread in malignant lymphomas. Eur. J. Cancer *4*:319, 1968.
26. Purtillo, D.T., et al.: Epstein-Barr virus induced disease in boys with the X-linked lymphoproliferative syndrome (XLP). Update on studies of the registry. Am. J. Med. *73*:49, 1982.
27. Bird, A.G., and Britton, S.: The relationship between Epstein-Barr virus and lymphoma. Semin. Hematol. *19*:285, 1982.
28. Yunis, J.J., et al.: Distinctive chromosomal abnormalities in histologic subtypes of non-Hodgkin's lymphomas. N. Engl. J. Med. *307*:1231, 1982.
29. Murphy, S.B.: Classification, staging and end results of treatment of childhood non-Hodgkin's lymphomas: Dissimilarities from lymphomas in adults. Semin. Oncol. *7*:332, 1980.
30. Lukes, R.J., et al.: Reed-Sternberg–like cells in infectious mononucleosis. Lancet 2:1003, 1969.
31. Rappaport, H., et al.: Report of the committee on histopathological criteria contributing to staging of Hodgkin's disease. Cancer Res. *31*:1864, 1971.
32. Strum, S.B., et al.: Observation of cells resembling Sternberg-Reed cells in conditions other than Hodgkin's disease. Cancer *26*:176, 1970.
33. Lukes, R.J., et al.: Report of the nomenclature committee. Cancer Res. *26*:1311, 1966.
34. Gutensohn, N.M.: Social class and age at diagnosis of Hodgkin's disease: New epidemiologic evidence for the "two disease hypothesis." Cancer Treat Rep. *66*:689, 1982.
35. Gallo, R.C., and Gelmann, E.P.: In search of a Hodgkin's disease virus. N. Engl. J. Med. *304*:169, 1981.
36. Kaplan, H.S.: Hodgkin's disease: Biology, treatment, prognosis. Blood *57*:813, 1981.
37. Fisher, R.I.: Implications of persistent T cell abnormalities for the etiology of Hodgkin's disease. Cancer Treat. Rep. *66*:681, 1982.
38. Schwab, U., et al.: Production of a monoclonal antibody specific for Hodgkin's and Sternberg-Reed cells of Hodgkin's disease and a subset of normal cells. Nature *299*:65, 1982.
39. Kadin, M.E.: Possible origin of the Reed-Sternberg cell from an interdigitating reticulum cell. Cancer Treat. Rep. *66*:601, 1982.
40. Bennett, J.M., et al.: Proposals for the classification of the acute leukaemias. French-American-British (FAB) Cooperative Group. Br. J. Haematol. *33*:45, 1976.
41. Foon, K.A., et al.: Surface markers on leukemia and lymphoma cells: Recent advances. Blood *60*:1, 1982.
42. Tomonaga, M.: Statistical investigation of leukaemia in Japan. N.Z. Med. J. *65*:863, 1966.
43. Cossman, J., et al.: Induction of differentiation in a case of common acute lymphoblastic leukemia. N. Engl. J. Med. *307*:1251, 1982.
44. Goldman, J.M., and Lu, D.: New approaches in chronic granulocytic leukemia—origin, prognosis and treatment. Semin. Hematol. *19*:241, 1982.
45. Greaves, M.M.: "Target cells," cellular phenotypes, and lineage fidelity in human leukemia. J. Cell Physiol. (Suppl. 1):113, 1982.

46. Editorial: Leukaemogenesis and differentiation. Lancet *1*:33, 1983.
47. Koeffler, H.P., and Golde, D.W.: Chronic myelogenous leukemia—new concepts. N. Engl. J. Med. *304*:1201, 1981.
48. Lawler, S.D.: Significance of chromosomal abnormalities in leukemia. Semin. Hematol. *19*:257, 1982.
49. Yunis, J.J., et al.: All patients with acute non-lymphocytic leukemia may have chromosomal defect. N.Engl. J. Med. *305*:135, 1981.
50. Yunis, J.J.: Specific fine chromosomal defects in cancer: An overview. Hum. Pathol. *12*:503, 1981.
51. Marx, J.L.: The case of the misplaced gene. Science *218*:983, 1982.
52. Rowley, J.D.: Human oncogene locations and chromosomal aberrations. Nature *301*:290, 1983.
53. Bjergaard, J.P.: Incidence of acute non-lymphocytic leukemia, preleukemia and acute myeloproliferative syndrome up to 10 years after treatment of Hodgkin's disease. N. Engl. J. Med. *307*:965, 1982.
54. Editorial: Gallo on T-cell leukaemia-lymphoma virus. Lancet *2*:1083, 1982.
55. Blayney, D.W., et al.: The human T-cell leukemia/lymphoma virus, lymphoma, lytic bone lesions, and hypercalcemia. Ann. Intern. Med. *98*:144, 1983.
55A. Bakhshi, A., et al.: Lymphoid blast crises of chronic myelogenous leukemia represent stages in the development of B-cell precursors. N. Engl. J. Med. *309*:826, 1983.
56. Cawley, J.C., et al.: Hairy cell leukemia. Recent Results Cancer Res. *72*:58, 1980.
57. Worman, C.P., et al.: Alterations in the phenotype of hairy cells during culture in the presence of PHA: Requirement for T cells. Blood *59*:895, 1982.
58. Uchiyama, T., et al.: Adult T cell leukemia: Clinical and hematologic features of 16 cases. Blood *50*:481, 1977.
59. Shimoyama, M., et al.: Comparison of clinical, morphologic and immunologic characteristics of adult T-cell leukemia-lymphoma and cutaneous T-cell lymphoma. Jpn. J. Clin. Oncol. *9*(Suppl.):357, 1979.
60. Groopman, J.E.: Editorial—Pathogenesis of myelofibrosis in myeloproliferative disorders. Ann. Intern. Med. *92*:857, 1980.
61. Cappio, F.C., et al.: Idiopathic myelofibrosis: A possible role for immune complexes in the pathogenesis of bone marrow fibrosis. Br. J. Haematol. *49*:17, 1981.
62. Kyle, R.A.: Monoclonal gammopathy of undetermined significance (MGUS): A review. Clin. Hematol. *11*:125, 1982.
63. Solomon, A.: Bence Jones Proteins: Malignant or benign. N. Engl. J. Med. *306*:605, 1981.
64. Salmon, S.E., and Seligmann, M.: B-cell neoplasia in man. Lancet *2*:1230, 1974.
65. Isobe, T., and Osserman, E.F.: Pathologic conditions associated with plasma cell dyscrasias. A study of 806 cases. Ann. N.Y. Acad. Sci. *190*:507, 1972.
66. Baitz, T., and Kyle, R.A.: Solitary myeloma in chronic osteomyelitis. Arch. Intern. Med. *113*:872, 1964.
67. DePetris, S., et al.: Localization of antibodies in plasma cells by electron microscopy. J. Exp. Med. *117*:849, 1963.
68. Zlotnick, A., and Rosenmann, E.: Renal pathologic findings associated with monoclonal gammopathies. Arch. Intern. Med. *135*:40, 1975.
69. Cohen, A.H., and Border, M.D.: Myeloma kidney. An immunomorphogenetic study of renal biopsies. Lab Invest. *42*:248, 1980.
70. Glenner, G.G., et al.: Amyloidosis. Its nature and pathogenesis. Semin. Hematol. *10*:65, 1973.
71. Ullrich, S., and Zolla-Pazner, S.: Immunoregulatory circuits in myeloma. Clin. Hematol. *11*:87, 1982.
72. Defronzo, R., et al.: Renal function in patients with multiple myeloma. Medicine (Balt.) *57*:151, 1978.
73. Ritzmann, S.E.: Idiopathic (asymptomatic) monoclonal gammopathies. Arch. Intern. Med. *135*:95, 1975.
74. Bataille, R.: Localized plasmacytomas. Clin. Hematol. *11*:113, 1982.
75. Conklin, R., and Alexanian, R.: Clinical classification of plasma cell myeloma. Arch. Intern. Med. *135*:139, 1975.
76. Tursz, T.: Clinical and pathologic features of Waldenström's macroglobulinemia in 7 patients with serum monoclonal IgG or IgA. Am. J. Med. *63*:499, 1977.
77. Dutcher, T.F., and Fahey, J.L.: The histopathology of the macroglobulinemia of Waldenström. J. Natl. Cancer Inst. *22*:887, 1959.
78. Krajny, M., et al.: Waldenström's macroglobulinemia: Review of 45 cases. Can. Med. Assoc. J. *114*:899, 1976.
79. Seligmann, M., et al.: Heavy-chain diseases: Current findings and concepts. Immunol. Rev. *48*:145, 1979.
79A. Khojasteh, A., et al.: Immunoproliferative small intestinal disease. A "third world lesion." N. Engl. J. Med. *308*:1401, 1983.
80. Stoop, J.W., et al.: Alpha-chain disease with involvement of the respiratory tract in a Dutch child. Clin. Exp. Immunol. *9*:625, 1971.
81. Franklin, E.C.: Mu-chain disease. Arch. Intern. Med. *135*:71, 1975.
82. Murphy, G.F., et al.: Distribution of cell surface antigens in histiocytosis X cells. Quantitative immune electron microscopy using monoclonal antibodies. Lab Invest. *48*:90, 1983.
83. Corrin, B., and Basset, F.: A review of histiocytosis X with particular reference to eosinophilic granuloma of the lung. Invest. Cell Pathol. *2*:137, 1979.
84. Nezelof, C.: Histiocytosis X: A histologic and histogenetic study. Perspect. Pediatr. Pathol. *5*:153, 1979.
85. Wolfson, W.L., et al.: Systemic giant cell histiocytosis; report of a case and review of the adult form of Letterer-Siwe disease. Cancer *38*:2529, 1976.
86. Lahey, M.E.: Histiocytosis X—comparison of three treatment regimens. J. Pediatr. *87*:179, 1975.
87. Osband, M., et al.: Histiocytosis X. Demonstration of abnormal immunity, T cell histamine H-2 receptor deficiency, and successful treatment with thymic extract. N. Engl. J. Med. *304*:146, 1981.
88. Lieberman, P.H., et al.: A reappraisal of eosinophilic granuloma of bone, Hand-Schüller-Christian syndrome and Letterer-Siwe syndrome. Medicine *48*:375, 1969.
89. Berris, B., et al.: Immunoblastic lymphadenopathy: Report of four new cases and review of the disease. Can. Med. Assoc. J. *127*:389, 1982.
90. Pruzanski, W.: Lymphadenopathy associated with dysgammaglobulinemia. Semin. Hematol. *17*:44, 1980.
91. Neiman, R.S., et al.: Angioimmunoblastic lymphadenopathy. An ultrastructural and immunologic study with review of the literature. Cancer *41*:507, 1978.
92. Boros, L., et al.: Monoclonal evolution of angioimmunoblastic lymphadenopathy. Am. J. Clin. Pathol. *75*:856, 1981.
93. Enriquez, P., and Neiman, R.S.: The Pathology of the Spleen, A Functional Approach. Chicago, American Society of Clinical Pathologists, 1976, p. 11.
94. Bishop, M.B., and Lansing, L.S.: The spleen: A correlative overview of normal and pathologic anatomy. Hum. Pathol. *13*:334, 1982.

THE RESPIRATORY SYSTEM 16

LUNG

NORMAL

The lungs are ingeniously constructed to carry out their cardinal function, the exchange of gases between inspired air and the blood. The present consideration of the normal lung is confined to reemphasizing those features of the anatomy that are particularly pertinent to an understanding of the pathology of this organ.[1–3]

The normal adult lung weighs approximately 300 to 400 gm. Sometimes forgotten is the surface presentation of the various lobes of the lungs. The two lower lobes present almost entirely on the posterior aspect of the thoracic cavity, whereas the upper lobes and right middle lobe present almost entirely on the anterior aspect. However, because the apical portions of the lower lobes are thin, pathologic processes throughout most of the upper lobes yield clinical signs that can be detected both anteriorly and posteriorly. The right middle lobe is separated from the posterior chest wall by a thick mass of lower lobe. Disorders in the middle lobe, then, are clinically reflected chiefly by signs confined to the right anterior lower thorax.

The right main stem bronchus is more vertical and more directly in line with the trachea than is the left. As a consequence, aspirated foreign material, such as vomitus, blood, and foreign bodies, tends to enter the right lung rather than the left.

In the trachea and major bronchi, the cartilage takes the form of C-shaped plates, leaving the posterior membranous portion free of cartilage. Smooth muscle is present only in the membranous portion. However, as the main bronchi enter the lungs, this organization changes; discontinuous plates of cartilage and muscle now encircle the entire wall. Thus, only in the lung, where the muscle extends around the entire circumference of the bronchi, does bronchial constriction result in total obstruction of the airway lumen. Progressive branching of the bronchi forms *bronchioles*, which are differentiated from bronchi by the lack of cartilage and submucosal glands within their walls. Further branching of bronchioles leads to the *terminal bronchioles*, which are less than 2 mm in diameter.

The part of the lung distal to the terminal bronchiole is called the *acinus*, or the *terminal respiratory unit;* it is approximately spherical in shape, with a diameter of about 7 mm. Acini contain alveoli and are thus the site of gas exchange (Fig. 16–1). An acinus is composed of (1) *respiratory bronchioles* (emanating from the terminal bronchiole), which give off from their sides several alveoli; these bronchioles then proceed into (2) the *alveolar ducts*, which immediately branch and empty into (3) the *alveolar sacs*—the blind ends of the respiratory passages, whose walls are formed entirely of alveoli. It is important to note that the alveoli open into the ducts through large mouths. In the correct plane of section, therefore, all alveoli are open and have incomplete walls. This alveolar mouth is sometimes mistakenly interpreted as a defect caused by a rupture of an alveolar wall.

A cluster of three to five terminal bronchioles, each with its appended acini, is usually referred to as the

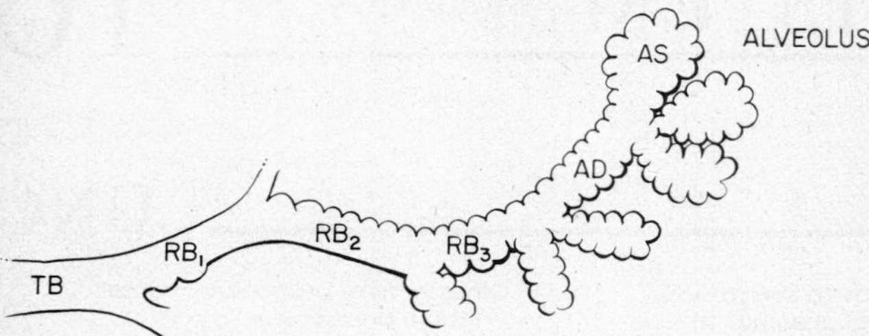

Figure 16–1. This diagrammatic representation of an acinus shows a terminal bronchiole (TB); respiratory bronchioles of first (RB_1), second (RB_2), and third (RB_3) orders; an alveolar duct (AD); and an alveolar sac (AS). The acinus is the part of the lung distal to a terminal bronchiole, and emphysema is defined in terms of the acinus. (From Thrulbeck, W. M.: Chronic Airflow Obstruction in Lung Disease. Philadelphia, W. B. Saunders Co., 1976.)

pulmonary *lobule*. As will be seen, this lobular architecture assumes importance in differentiation of the major forms of emphysema. Lobules are separated from each other by connective tissue septa, which are somewhat less well defined in humans than in animals.

Attention should be called to the double arterial supply to the lungs, i.e., the pulmonary and bronchial arteries. In the absence of significant cardiac failure, the bronchial arteries of aortic origin can sustain the vitality of the pulmonary parenchyma when pulmonary arterial supply is shut off, as by emboli.

From the microscopic standpoint, it is well to remember that except for the vocal cords, which are covered by stratified squamous epithelium, the entire respiratory tree, including the larynx, trachea, and bronchioles, is lined by pseudostratified, tall, columnar, ciliated epithelial cells, heavily admixed with mucus-secreting goblet cells. The mucinous secretion and cilia have important functions. The mucus moistens the inspired air, prevents drying of the delicate alveolar walls, and traps dust and particulate matter. The cilia aid in the removal of foreign material by constant beating wavelike motions that propel this material back into the larger bronchi and trachea where the cough reflex completes the expulsion.

The bronchial mucosa also contains neuroendocrine cells,[4] the bronchial counterparts of the argentaffin or *Kulchitsky* cells of the gastrointestinal tract. These cells exhibit neurosecretory-type granules; contain serotonin, calcitonin, and gastrin-releasing peptide (bombesin); and are important as precursors of the carcinoid tumors and small cell carcinomas of the lung. Numerous submucosal, mucus-secreting glands are dispersed throughout the walls of the trachea and bronchi but not the bronchioles.

The microscopic structure of the alveolar walls (or alveolar septa) consists, from blood to air, of the following (Fig. 16–2):[5, 6]

1. The *capillary endothelium* lining the intertwining network of anastomotic capillaries.

2. A *basement membrane and surrounding interstitial tissue* separating the endothelial cell from the alveolar lining epithelial cell. In thin portions of the alveolar septum, the basement membranes of epithelium and endothelium are fused, whereas in thicker portions they are separated by an interstitial space *(the pulmonary interstitium)*, containing fine elastic fibers, small bundles of collagen, ground substance, a few fibroblast-like interstitial cells, smooth muscle cells, mast cells, and rare lymphocytes and monocytes.

3. The alveolar epithelium, a continuous layer made up of two principal cell types: flattened, platelike pavement *Type I pneumocytes* (or membranous pneumocytes), covering 95% of the alveolar surface, and rounded, granular *Type II pneumocytes* (or granular pneumocytes), which exhibit surface microvilli and contain osmiophilic lamellated inclusion bodies. Type II cells are important for at least two reasons: (a) they are the source of *pulmonary surfactant* and (b) they are the main cell type involved in the repair of alveolar epithelium after destruction of Type I cells. Loosely attached to the epithelial cells or lying free within the alveolar spaces are the *alveolar macrophages*. These are derived from blood monocytes and belong to the mononuclear phagocyte system. Often they are filled with carbon particles and other phagocytosed materials. The alveolar walls are not solid but are perforated by numerous *pores of Kohn*, which permit the passage of bacteria and exudate between adjacent alveoli.

Adjacent to the alveolar cell membrane is the glycoprotein-containing cell coat upon which is a thin film of phospholipid, mostly phosphatidylcholine (lecithin), the *pulmonary surfactant*.[7] Lecithin is critical to the alveolar wall, since it serves to lower the surface tension of alveolar lining and maintain the stability of the alveoli. Indeed, about half the normal compliance of the lung is due not to its elastic tissue but to these surface tension–lowering forces. Surfactant is synthesized in Type II cells and stored in the osmiophilic lamellated bodies of such cells. Loss of surfactant activity is believed to play a role in the respiratory distress syndromes of infants (p. 482) and adults (p. 714).

The structure of bronchioles (especially those less than 2 mm in diameter) is of special interest, since alterations in these "small airways" are assuming increased importance in the pathogenesis of chronic bronchitis and emphysema (p. 725). The structure of bronchioles differs in several respects from that of the alveolus on one hand and larger bronchi on the other. *The bronchiolar surface is covered with cilia, which are surrounded by a water-protein layer rich in lysozyme and immunoglobulins, but unlike the alveoli, the surface layer contains no surfactant and, unlike the bronchi, no mucus.* Indeed, there are no mucous cells in the walls of the bronchioles. Instead, nonciliated granulated *Clara cells* secrete the mucus-poor lining protein. In some inflammatory conditions of bronchioles, there is goblet cell metaplasia of the bronchiolar lining with an increase in mucus production and a diminution in the number of Clara cells.

The all-important respiratory function of the lungs can be divided into two aspects: *ventilation*, concerned with the movement of air into the alveolar spaces, and

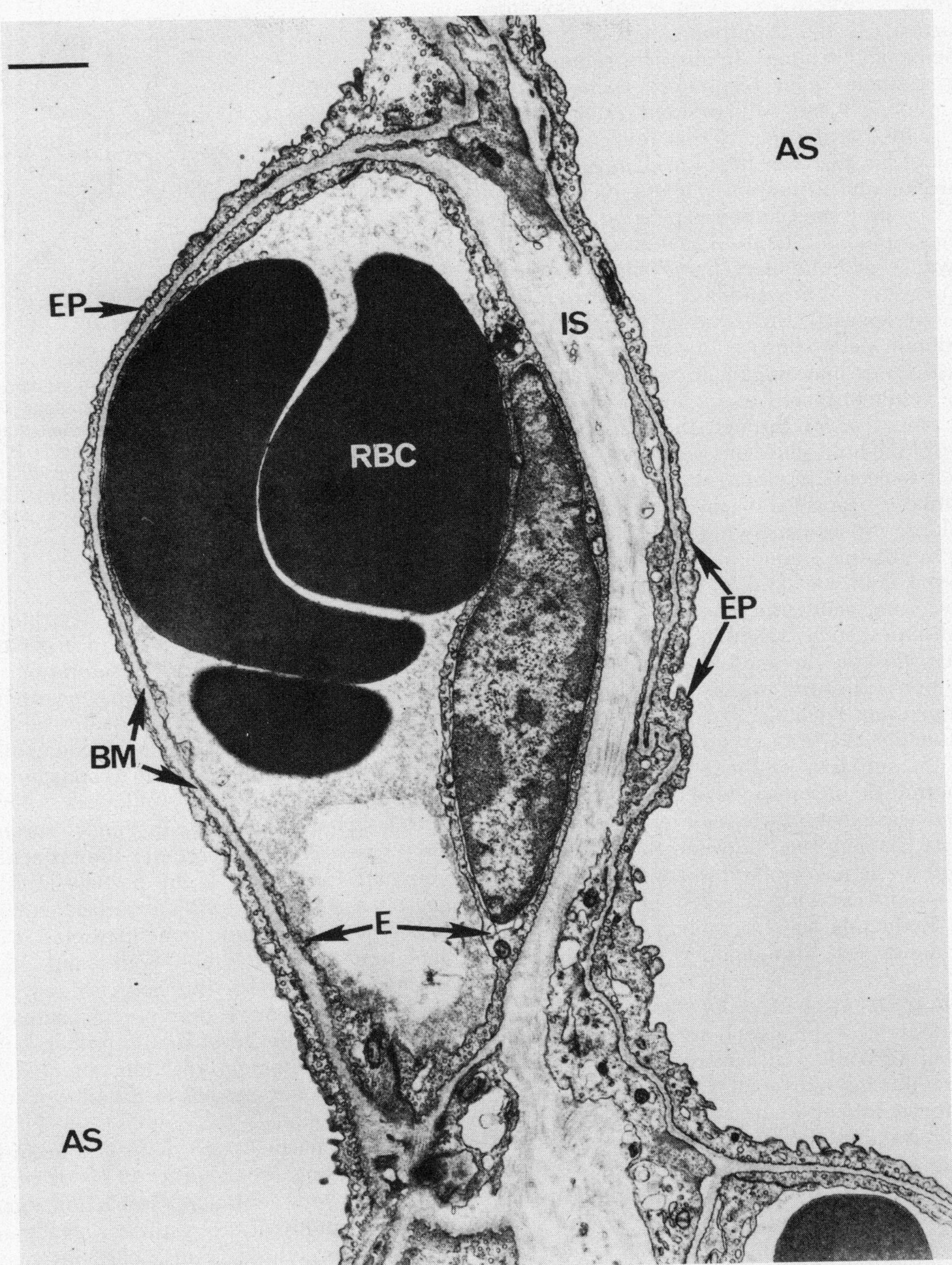

Figure 16–2. Electron photomicrograph of a transverse section through capillaries in interalveolar septum. Surface of septum facing alveolar spaces (AS) is lined by continuous Type I epithelium (EP). Capillary containing red blood cells (RBC) is lined by endothelium (E). Both layers rest on basement membranes (BM) that appear fused over "thin" portion of membrane and are separated by an interstitial space (IS) over "thick" portion of membrane. Horizontal bar = 1 μ. ($\times$ 11,500. Courtesy of Dr. Ewald R. Weiber.) From Murray, J. F.: The Normal Lung. Philadelphia, W. B. Saunders Co., 1976.

respiratory gas exchange, involving the diffusion of oxygen and carbon dioxide across the alveolar capillary membrane.

Ventilation is largely a function of the respiratory muscles, particularly the diaphragm, and of the volumetric capacity of the lungs. It must be remembered that during a single quiet respiratory cycle approximately 500 ml of air is moved in and out (tidal volume). However, the total lung capacity that reflects the maximal amount of air that can be moved in and out by forced inspiration and expiration is about 4000 ml (vital capacity). Even after such forced expiration, there is a residual volume of about 1200 ml that accounts for the normal buoyancy of pulmonary tissue when the lungs are floated in water. When there is abnormal collapse of the lungs (atelectasis), this residual volume may be sufficiently diminished to destroy this normal lung buoyancy. Disease states may impair normal ventilation by reducing the volume capacity of the lung or by obstructing the movement of air through the respiratory passages. Filling of the lung alveolar spaces by inflammatory exudate, such as occurs in various types of pneumonia, reduces ventilatory capacity by lowering vital capacity and tidal volume. Space-occupying fluid or tumors will also reduce ventilatory function. Compression of the lung by pleural fluid, exudate, or thoracic deformities acts similarly. Lung ventilation may also be reduced by obstructive diseases, such as asthma, and neuromuscular disorders that weaken the muscles of respiration and therefore do not permit full expansion of the lungs.

Respiratory gas exchange is the second aspect of pulmonary function. It is to a considerable extent dependent on the integrity of the alveolar wall and its capacity to permit the interchange of oxygen and carbon dioxide. Any disease that interposes edema fluid, fibrous tissue, exudate, or neoplasm between the air spaces of the alveoli and the septal capillaries hampers respiratory exchange by producing what is called an "alveolocapillary block." Reduction in the rate of flow of blood through the lungs will also hamper such respiratory exchange.

PULMONARY DEFENSE MECHANISMS.[2, 8, 9] Each day, the respiratory airways and alveoli are exposed to about 10,000 liters of air containing hazardous dusts, chemicals, and infectious microorganisms. However, the normal lung is sterile, and although residents of most cities inhale several hundred grams of particles over their lifetimes, their lungs at autopsy show only a few grams of mineral ash. This is the result of efficient filtering and clearing mechanisms, as follows (Fig. 16–3):

(1) *Nasal clearance.* Particles deposited near the front of the airway on the nonciliated epithelium are normally removed by sneezing and blowing, while those deposited posteriorly are swept over the mucus-lined ciliated epithelium to the nasopharynx, where they are swallowed.

(2) *Tracheobronchial clearance.* This is accomplished by mucociliary action: the beating motion of cilia moves a film of mucus continuously from the lung toward the oropharynx; particles deposited on this film are eventually either swallowed or expectorated.

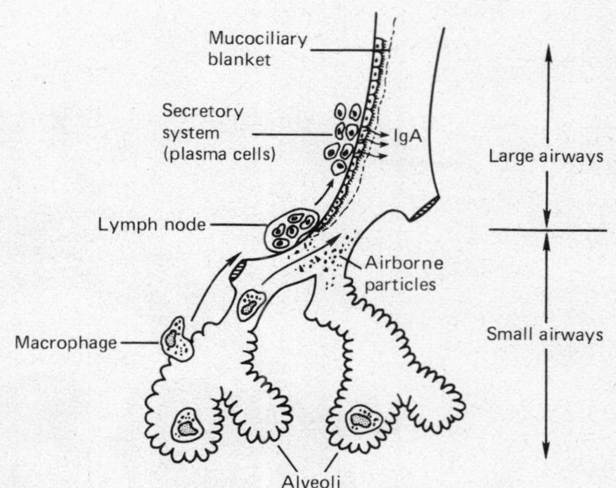

Figure 16–3. Components of lungs' defenses: mucociliary escalator in proximal bronchi and alveolar macrophages in distal airways. Arrows indicate possible routes alveolar macrophages may take in eliminating airborne particles. (From Daniele, R. P.: Immune defenses of the lung. *In* Fishman, A. P. (ed.): Pulmonary Diseases and Disorders. New York, McGraw-Hill Book Co., 1980. Copyright © 1980 by McGraw-Hill, Inc. Used by permission of McGraw-Hill Book Company.)

(3) *Alveolar clearance.*[10] Bacteria or solid particles deposited in the alveoli are phagocytosed by *alveolar macrophages,* which then eliminate the particle either by digesting it or by carrying it along to the ciliated bronchioles. From here the macrophage is propelled to the oropharynx and then swallowed. Alternatively, the particle-laden macrophage may move through the interstitial space and either reenter the bronchioles or enter lymphatic capillaries. If the particle load is heavy and macrophage transport via the surface and alveolar pathways is overwhelmed, some particles may eventually reach the regional lymph nodes and, via the bloodstream, elsewhere in the body. Massive exposure to noxious particles or virulent organisms that overwhelms the capacity of the alveolar macrophages may result in an acute inflammatory reaction, after which polymorphonuclear leukocytes aid in the phagocytic and bactericidal functions.

Inhaled particles are deposited according to their size, depending on the interaction of certain physical properties (sedimentation, impaction, and diffusion) with the anatomy of the respiratory tract and the host's pattern of breathing. Thus, particles over 10 μ are deposited largely in the turbulent air flow of the nose and upper airways; particles of 3 to 10 μ lodge in the trachea and bronchi by impaction; and smaller particles, about the size of most bacteria, 0.5 to 3.0 μ, are deposited in the terminal airways and alveoli. *Ineffective clearance of particles from these three sites is believed to be crucial to the pathogenesis of pulmonary infections and of the slowly developing pneumoconioses* (p. 431).

PATHOLOGY

It is impossible to overemphasize the importance of lung disease in the overall perspective of pathology and clinical medicine. Primary respiratory infections, such as bronchitis, bronchopneumonia, and other forms of pneumonia, are commonplace in clinical and pathologic practice. In this day of cigarette smoking and air pollution, emphysema has become rampant, affecting large segments of the total population. Moreover, the lungs are secondarily involved in almost all forms of terminal disease, so that at virtually every autopsy some degree of pulmonary edema, atelectasis, or bronchopneumonia is found. Malignancy of the lungs has risen steadily in incidence, until it is now the most common form of visceral malignancy in the male. In the present consideration of the lung, emphasis will be placed on primary diseases that affect this organ. Systemic disturbances that secondarily involve the lung, such as lupus erythematosus, will be largely omitted, since they receive consideration elsewhere as basic systemic processes. For detailed descriptions of pulmonary pathology, the reader is referred to comprehensive books of pulmonary diseases.[11–14]

CONGENITAL ANOMALIES

Developmental defects of the lung[5, 11] include (1) agenesis or hypoplasia of both lungs, one lung, or single lobes; (2) tracheal and bronchial anomalies; (3) intralobar and extrapulmonary lobar sequestrations (p. 729); (4) congenital lobar overinflation (emphysema, p. 724); (5) vascular anomalies; and (6) congenital cysts. *Congenital cysts* represent an abnormal detachment of a fragment of primitive foregut, and consist of *bronchogenic* (central) cysts and *pulmonary* (peripheral) cysts.

Bronchogenic cysts are usually central but may occur anywhere in the lungs as single or, on occasion, multiple cystic spaces from microscopic size to over 5 cm in diameter. They are usually adjacent to bronchi or bronchioles and may or may not have demonstrable connections. Histologically, they are lined by ciliated, mucus-secreting respiratory columnar epithelium, based on a thin layer of connective tissue (Fig. 16–4). In the uncomplicated case, the cavities are filled either with mucinous secretion or, if there is an orifice draining the secretions, with air. Infection of the secretions leads to suppuration, often associated with progressive metaplasia of the lining epithelium or even total necrosis of the wall of the cysts to create a lung abscess.

Peripheral pulmonary cysts are usually multiple and may affect both lungs. They rarely communicate with the main bronchi. Infection is frequent. Rupture of these cysts into the pleural cavity may cause pneumothorax and collapse the lung. Less often, the increase in intrapleural pressure compresses and partially blocks the respiratory tree, causing progressive expiratory obstruction. Under these circumstances, the cysts are blown up like a balloon with each aspiration.

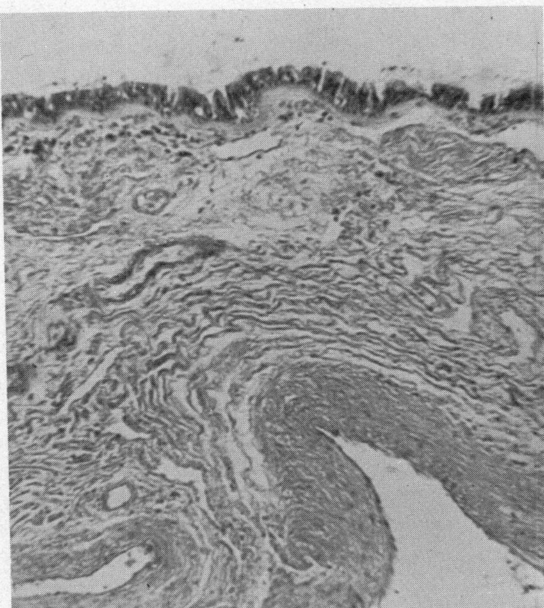

Figure 16–4. Bronchogenic cyst of lung. A microscopic detail of wall illustrating respiratory lining epithelium.

Congenital cysts are of clinical importance because (1) they may compress or displace sufficient lung volume to decrease the vital capacity and produce ventilatory insufficiency; (2) they are prime sites for the development of infection, which may then lead to the formation of lung abscesses, bronchopleural fistulas, and sometimes empyema; (3) through progressive cystic dilatation, vessels may be ruptured, causing hemorrhage and hemoptysis; and (4) rupture of the cysts into the pleural cavities may cause pneumothorax or dissection of air into connective tissue septa of the lung to produce interstitial pulmonary emphysema.

ALTERATIONS IN LUNG EXPANSION

ATELECTASIS

Atelectasis refers either to incomplete expansion of the lungs or to the collapse of previously inflated lung substance. This disorder may be present at birth, may arise during the first days of postnatal life, or may occur anytime thereafter. Whenever it occurs, it is characterized by areas of relatively airless pulmonary parenchyma. The term atelectasis should be applied only when the affected alveoli are structurally normal and therefore capable of reexpansion if the underlying cause can be removed.

Atelectasis in the newborn (atelectasis neonatorum) is divided into primary and secondary forms and is discussed in Chapter 11.

PATHOGENESIS. Acquired atelectasis, encountered principally in adults, may be divided into *obstructive*, *compressive*, *contraction*, and *patchy atelectasis*.

Obstructive atelectasis is the consequence of complete obstruction of an airway, which in time leads to absorption of the oxygen trapped in the dependent alveoli, followed by their collapse. Some air may percolate through the pores of Kohn, but does not compensate for the airway blockage or prevent collapse of the alveolar spaces. Obstructive-absorptive collapse implies total blockage of the affected airway but continued blood flow through the affected alveolar walls. The lung volume is diminished, and if a sufficient amount of parenchyma is affected the mediastinum shifts toward the atelectatic lung.

Compressive atelectasis results whenever the pleural cavity is partially or completely filled by fluid exudate, tumor, blood clot, or air (the last-mentioned constituting *pneumothorax*, p. 759). Similarly, abnormal elevation of the diaphragm such as follows peritonitis, subdiaphragmatic abscesses, and abdominal carcinomatosis will induce basal atelectasis. With compressive atelectasis, the mediastinum shifts away from the affected lung.

Contraction atelectasis occurs when localized fibrotic changes increase recoil in a local area of the lung. *Patchy atelectasis* develops when there is loss of pulmonary surfactant, as in the newborn and adult respiratory distress syndromes, discussed elsewhere.

MORPHOLOGY. Acquired atelectasis may involve all lobes (massive collapse), which is usually incompatible with life. In the massive collapse that follows rupture of blebs or penetrating wounds of the chest cavity, the entire lung may be folded against the mediastinum as pneumothorax develops. Most often, it is lobar or segmental. In the most common pattern, caused by elevated diaphragms or the accumulation of fluid within the pleural cavities, it is basal and bilateral. The collapsed lung parenchyma is shrunken below the level of the surrounding lung substance and is red-blue, rubbery, and subcrepitant with a wrinkled overlying pleura. In subtotal atelectasis of a portion of a lobe, the adjacent parenchyma often becomes overinflated, erroneously termed **compensatory emphysema.** Histologically, the collapsed alveoli become slitlike, and the lung appears to have "too much tissue and too little air" (Fig. 16–5). Occasionally, segmental atelectasis of the basal portions of the upper lobes follows surgery, presumably because of obstructive secretions in the bronchi. These segmental lesions create horizontal linear radiographic shadows to which the descriptive term **plate atelectasis** is applied.

Obstructive atelectasis is principally caused by excessive secretions or exudate within the second order and smaller bronchi, and is therefore most often found in bronchial asthma, chronic bronchitis, bronchiectasis, and postoperative states and with aspiration of foreign bodies. Bronchial neoplasms are additional important causes of atelectasis, although in most instances they cause subtotal obstruction and produce emphysema. Secretions may also produce atelectasis in the airways of the comatose patient.

The compressive form of atelectasis is most commonly encountered in patients in cardiac failure who develop hydrothorax and in neoplastic effusions within the pleural cavities. It is also seen with rupture of a thoracic aneurysm causing hemothorax and in spontaneous or induced pneumothorax. Elevated diaphragms, as mentioned, are important causes of basal atelectasis, particularly in seriously ill postoperative patients. Their recumbent position with abdominal distention causing pressure against the diaphragm, their tendency to limit respiratory motions because of pain, and their voluntary suppression of the cough reflex with resulting accumulation of secretions all contribute to the development of basal atelectasis and to serious respiratory embarrassment.

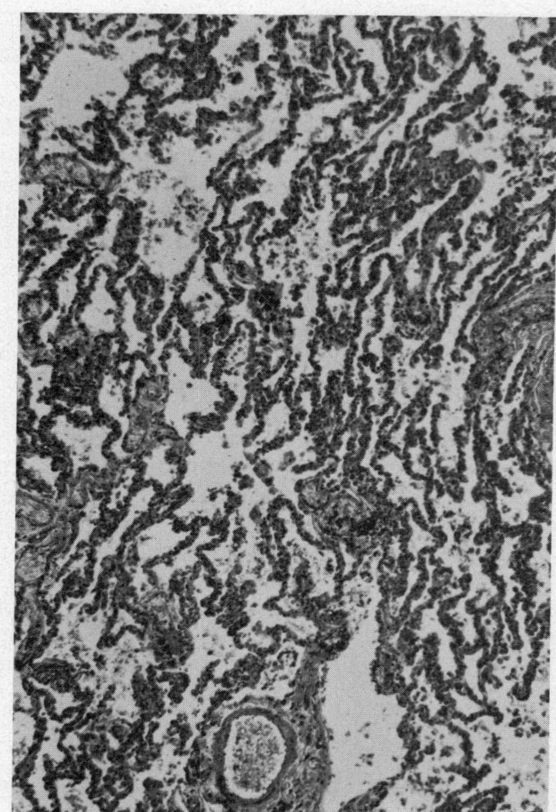

Figure 16–5. Atelectasis. Alveoli are partially collapsed, producing slitlike spaces.

Since the collapsed lung parenchyma can be reexpanded, atelectasis is a reversible disorder that should not be permitted to contribute significantly to a fatal outcome. Even if respiratory embarrassment is not marked, the atelectatic parenchyma is prone to develop superimposed infections.

DISEASES OF VASCULAR ORIGIN

PULMONARY CONGESTION AND EDEMA

A general consideration of edema is on page 85, and pulmonary congestion and edema were described briefly on page 88. Pulmonary edema can result from *hemodynamic* disturbances or from direct *increases in capillary and alveolar permeability.*[15, 16]

The most common *hemodynamic* mechanism of pulmonary edema is that due to *increased hydrostatic pressure,* as occurs in congestive heart failure. Accumulation of fluid in this setting can be accounted for by Starling's law of capillary interstitial fluid exchange (p. 43). In short, the forces that move fluid out of the vessel wall are the mean intracapillary pressure and the small oncotic pressure of the interstitial fluid, and the forces moving fluid from the interstitium into the vessel lumen are the mean interstitial fluid pressure and the oncotic pressure of the plasma. In heart failure, there is an increase in pulmonary venous and capillary pressure and therefore in the forces moving fluid into the interstitium of the lung. Simultaneously the interendothelial junctions stretch, are widened, and allow the increased movement of both fluid and macromolecules into the interstitium.[17] This results first in a marked increase in pulmonary lymphatic flow, which serves to drain off the accumulated fluid. *Only after lymphatic drainage has been increased by about tenfold does fluid accumulate.* At this stage, edema is purely "interstitial." It is only when critical elevations in interstitial pressure are reached or increased pressure is prolonged that the tight junctions between alveolar lining epithelial cells break and *alveolar edema* results.

Hemodynamic factors producing an imbalance in Starling forces also account for the pulmonary edema associated with volume overload and hypoalbuminemia (e.g., the nephrotic syndrome). In the latter setting the principal derangement is a decrease in plasma oncotic pressure. Blockage of lymphatic drainage by tumors or inflammation is yet another mechanism leading to the accumulation of fluid within the lung owing to hydrostatic alterations.

Whatever the clinical setting, pulmonary congestion and edema are characterized by heavy, wet, subcrepitant lungs. Fluid accumulates in the basal regions of the lower lobes. Histologically, the alveolar capillaries are engorged and an intra-alveolar granular pink precipitate is seen (Fig. 16–6). Alveolar microhemorrhages and hemosiderin-laden macrophages (heart failure cells) are present. In long-standing cases of pulmonary congestion, such as those seen in mitral stenosis, hemosiderin-laden macrophages are abundant, and fibrosis and thickening of the alveolar walls cause the soggy lungs to become firm and brown **(brown induration,** chronic passive congestion). Changes such as these not only impair normal respiratory function but also predispose to infection, termed **hypostatic bronchopneumonia.** Thus, bronchopneumonia often terminates long-term congestive heart failure.

The second mechanism leading to pulmonary edema is *injury to the alveolocapillary membrane.* Here the pulmonary capillary hydrostatic pressure need not be elevated, and hemodynamic factors play a secondary role. The edema is initiated by injury to the vascular endothelium and frequently also to alveolar epithelial cells, resulting in leakage of fluids and proteins first into the interstitial space and, in more severe cases, into the alveoli. This is clearly the mechanism of locally occurring edema in bacterial or viral pneumonias. When it remains

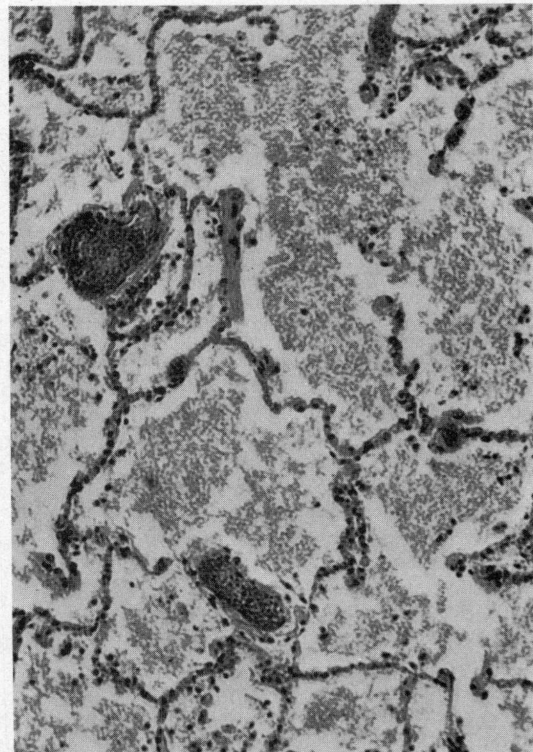

Figure 16–6. Pulmonary edema. Granular precipitate within alveolar spaces represents constituents of edema fluid.

localized, as it does in most forms of pneumonia, the edema is overshadowed by the manifestations of infection. When diffuse, however, alveolar edema is an important contributor to a serious and often fatal syndrome—the *adult respiratory distress syndrome*—discussed on page 714.

PULMONARY EMBOLISM, HEMORRHAGE, AND INFARCTION

Occlusions of the pulmonary arteries by blood clot are almost always embolic in origin. In situ thromboses are rare and develop only in the presence of pulmonary hypertension and pulmonary atherosclerosis. However, thrombosis superimposed on a nonocclusive embolus may complete the arterial obstruction. The usual source of these emboli (thrombi in the deep veins of the leg) and the magnitude of the clinical problem were discussed on page 102, where the awesome frequency of pulmonary embolism and infarction was emphasized. Suffice it to say here that pulmonary embolism causes more than 50,000 deaths in the United States each year. Its incidence at autopsy has varied from 8% in the general population of hospital patients to 30% in patients dying after severe burns, trauma, or fractures and to 65% of hospitalized patients in one study in which special techniques were applied to discover emboli at autopsy.[18] It is the sole or major contributing cause of death in 10 to 15% of adults dying in acute wards in general hospitals.

MORPHOLOGY. The morphologic consequences of embolic occlusion of the pulmonary arteries depend on the size of the embolic mass and the general state of the circulation. Large emboli may impact in the main pulmonary artery or its major branches or lodge astride the bifurcation as a **saddle embolus** (Fig. 16–7). Sudden death often ensues, owing to the block of blood flow through the lungs. Death may also be occasioned by acute dilatation of the right heart **(acute cor pulmonale).** In such sudden deaths, there may be no significant alterations in the lungs. Smaller emboli travel out into the more peripheral vessels where they may or may not cause infarction. **In patients with an adequate cardiovascular circulation, the bronchial artery supply can sustain the lung parenchyma despite obstruction to the pulmonary arterial system. Under these circumstances hemorrhages occur, but there is no infarction of the underlying lung parenchyma; less than 10% of human emboli actually cause infarction.** While the underlying pulmonary architecture may be obscured by the suffusion of blood, **hemorrhages are distinguished by the preservation of the native pulmonary substance.** Resorption of the blood permits reconstitution of the preexisting architecture.

Pulmonary emboli cause infarction when the circulation is already inadequate, namely, in patients with heart or lung disease. It is for this reason that infarctions tend to be uncommon in the young. About three-fourths of all infarcts affect the lower lobes, and in over one-half they occur multiply. They vary in size from lesions barely visible to the naked eye to massive involvement of large parts of an entire lobe. Characteristically, they extend to the periphery of the lung substance with the apex pointing toward the hilus of the lung. The pulmonary infarct is classically **hemorrhagic** and appears as a raised, red-blue area in the early stages (Fig. 16–8). Often the apposed pleural surface is covered by a fibrinous exudate. If the occluded vessel can be identified, it will be found near the apex of the infarcted area. The red cells begin to lyse within 48 hours, and the infarct becomes paler and eventually red-brown as hemosiderin is produced. With the passage of time, fibrous replacement begins at the margins as a gray-white peripheral zone and eventually converts the infarct into a scar that is contracted below the level of the lung substance. Histologically, **the diagnostic feature of pulmonary infarction is the ischemic necrosis of the lung substance** within the area of hemorrhage. Such necrosis affects the alveolar walls, bronchioles, and vessels.

If the infarct is caused by an infected embolus, the infarct is modified by a more intense neutrophilic exudation and more intense inflammatory reaction. Such lesions are referred to as **septic infarcts**, and indeed some convert to abscesses.

CLINICAL COURSE. Pulmonary embolism and infarction are principally complications of patients already suffering from some underlying disorder such as cardiac disease or cancer, or who are immobilized for long periods. Younger women have an increased risk of suffering embolism to the lung and possibly infarction in late pregnancy, following delivery, and with the use of "contraceptive pills" containing excesses of estrogens over progesterone (p. 447).

The significance of pulmonary embolism depends on the size of the occluded vessel, the number of emboli, and the general status of the cardiovascular system. Emboli result in two main pathophysiologic consequences: *respiratory compromise* due to the nonperfused, though ventilated obstructed segment, and *hemodynamic compromise* due to increased resistance to pulmonary blood flow engendered by the embolic ob-

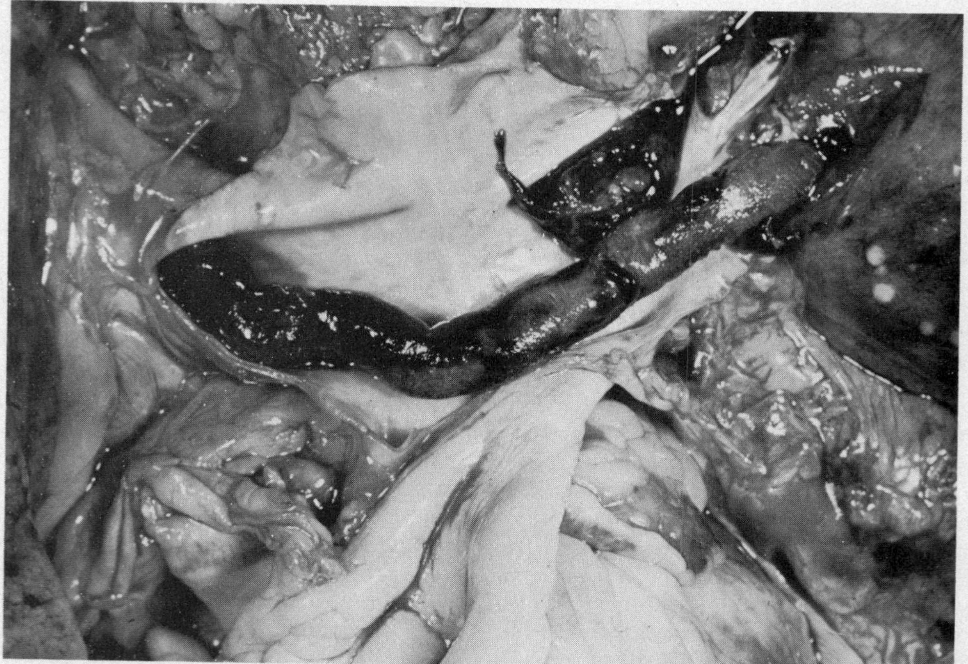

Figure 16–7. Large embolus from femoral vein lying astride main left and right pulmonary arteries.

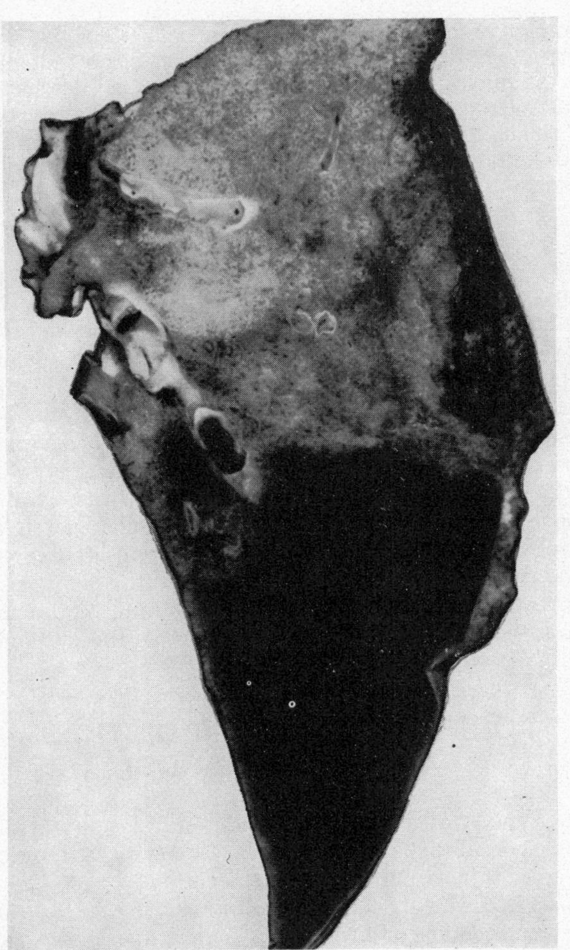

Figure 16–8. Cross section of a pulmonary infarct of several days' duration. The well-demarcated, wedge-shaped area of red-blue infarction appears densely black in the photograph.

struction. The latter leads to pulmonary hypertension and acute failure of the right ventricle. *Large emboli are one of the few causes of virtually instantaneous death.* If death occurs less suddenly, the clinical syndrome may mimic myocardial infarction with severe chest pain, acute dyspnea, shock, elevation of temperature, and increased levels of serum LDH (further mimicking myocardial infarction). Although the extent of embolic obstruction is a critical factor in survival, smaller emboli sometimes cause acute right heart failure either by stimulating reflex vasoconstriction of pulmonary vessels or by releasing vasoconstrictor agents (e.g., thromboxane) from platelets.[19]

In persons with a normal cardiovascular system, small emboli induce only transient chest pain and cough or possibly pulmonary hemorrhages without infarction. Only in the predisposed in whom the bronchial circulation itself is inadequate will they cause small infarcts. Such patients manifest dyspnea, tachypnea, fever, chest pain, cough, and hemoptysis. An overlying fibrinous pleuritis may produce a pleural friction rub.

The chest radiograph may disclose a pulmonary infarction, usually 12 to 36 hours after it has occurred, as a wedge-shaped infiltrate. In the absence of infarction, however, the changes produced by the pulmonary embolus are subtle, and a normal chest x-ray by no means rules out the diagnosis. A widely used technique to search for pulmonary emboli is pulmonary perfusion scintiphotography (photoscans) after parenteral injection of radionuclides such as iodine-131 or technetium-99.[20] The lung photoscan outlines the distribution of blood flow, and zones of decreased radioactivity provide diagnostic support in a patient suspected of having a pulmonary embolus. Although the technique has limitations (since other diseases also cause anomalies of blood flow distribution), it has proved invaluable because of its simplicity and safety. Pulmonary angiography is the most definitive diagnostic technique, but this modality entails more risk than do photoscans.

Emboli often resolve after the initial acute insult. The embolus contracts, as do all blood clots; fibrinolytic activity may then further reduce its size, and remarkable resolution with total lysis of the clot may follow. This happy outcome is the rule, rather than the exception, particularly in the relatively young. When unresolved, multiple small emboli over the course of time may lead to pulmonary hypertension, pulmonary vascular sclerosis, and chronic cor pulmonale. Perhaps most important is the fact that the small embolus may presage a larger one. In the presence of an underlying predisposing factor, patients with a pulmonary embolus have a 30% chance of developing a second embolus. The overall mortality rate in treated patients with pulmonary thromboembolism is about 8 to 12%.

Prevention of pulmonary embolism constitutes a major clinical problem for which there is no easy solution. Prophylactic therapy includes early ambulation in postoperative and postpartum patients, elastic stockings and isometric leg exercises for bedridden patients, and preventive anticoagulation in high-risk individuals. It is sometimes necessary to resort to insertion of a screen ("umbrella") or ligation of the inferior vena cava—no small procedures in an already seriously ill patient.

PULMONARY HYPERTENSION AND VASCULAR SCLEROSIS

As should be well-known, the pulmonary circulation is one of low resistance and pulmonary blood pressure is only about one-eighth of systemic blood pressure. Pulmonary hypertension is caused largely by an increase in pulmonary vascular resistance, and (as reviewed in the discussion of cor pulmonale, p. 569) is most frequently *secondary* to (1) chronic obstructive or interstitial lung diseases, (2) recurrent pulmonary emboli, or (3) antecedent heart disease. Uncommonly, pulmonary hypertension is encountered in patients in whom all known causes of increased pulmonary pressure are excluded, and this is referred to as *primary* or *idiopathic pulmonary hypertension*. Distinction of primary hypertension from that caused by recurrent thromboembolism may be particularly difficult without morphologic examination, but has been aided by angiography and radioisotope scanning.

PATHOGENESIS. Since the causes of secondary pulmonary vascular hypertension have already been considered (p. 569), we are here concerned with the pathogenesis of primary pulmonary hypertension. Many theories have been proposed, which is another way of saying the problem is still unsettled.[21] One older theory proposes that multiple small repeated silent pulmonary emboli are the cause of the pulmonary hypertension, and that their organization and incorporation within the arterial walls may be the cause of arterial thickening. Most current theories, however, postulate neurohormonal vascular hyperreactivity as a central mechanism, in which chronic vasoconstriction induces pulmonary hypertension and, in time, intimal and medial vascular hypertrophy. This concept is supported by the fact that patients with primary pulmonary hypertension often suffer from vasospastic disorders such as Raynaud's phenomenon (p. 529). In addition, pulmonary vascular resistance can be rapidly decreased in these patients with vasodilators. Such hyperreactivity in turn, is initiated by several postulated mechanisms. One holds that the vascular lesions are a form of immune collagen-vascular disease, since both Raynaud's phenomenon and pulmonary hypertension occur in other such disorders (scleroderma, SLE, rheumatoid arthritis); this is also in keeping with the prevalence of the disease in young women and its occasional occurrence in families.

Another theory implicates dietary or medicinal agents in pulmonary hypertension.[21] A leguminous plant, *Crotalaria spectabilis,* indigenous to the tropics and subtropics and used medicinally in "bush tea," causes pulmonary hypertension in animals. Well-documented cases of pulmonary hypertension have been associated in Europe with the ingestion of the appetite depressant agent aminorex. In man it has been suggested that such substances may cause subtle injury to the endothelium, which then fails to inactivate the vasoconstrictor substances that may be brought to the lungs. Vasoconstriction would then cause pulmonary hypertension, as described earlier.

MORPHOLOGY. A variety of vascular lesions occur in all forms of pulmonary hypertension, whether primary or secondary, but few are specific. The presence of many organizing or organized thrombi or the coexistence of diffuse pulmonary fibrosis favors secondary pulmonary hypertension. The vessel changes involve the entire arterial tree from the main pulmonary arteries down to the arterioles. In the main elastic arteries, the changes take the form of atheromatous deposits resembling atherosclerosis in the systemic arteries. However, they are rarely as marked as those found in advanced cases of atherosclerosis of the systemic arteries and are not often calcified or ulcerated. The medium-sized muscular arteries have striking medial hypertrophy (Fig. 16–9). In milder cases, there are only intimal thickening and fibrosis and some adventitial fibrosis. In both medium- and small-sized arteries, the internal and external elastic membranes often undergo thickening and reduplication (Fig. 16–10). The arterioles and small arteries (40 to 300 μ) are most prominently affected, with striking increases in the thickness of the media, sometimes narrowing the lumina to pinpoint channels. These changes are present in all forms of pulmonary vascular sclerosis, but are best developed in the primary form.[22, 23] A distinctive arteriolar lesion (referred to as the **plexiform lesion**) and consisting of cellular intraluminal angiomatous tufts, is considered by some pathologists to be sufficiently diagnostic of primary hypertension to justify the designation "plexogenic pulmonary arteriopathy" for this disease.

CLINICAL COURSE. Although secondary forms can occur at any age, primary pulmonary hypertension is most common in women of 20 to 40 years. Clinical signs and symptoms of both the primary and secondary forms of vascular sclerosis become evident only with advanced arterial disease. In cases of primary disease, the presenting features are dyspnea and fatigue, although occasionally syncopal attacks are the initial complaint. Some patients have chest pain of the anginal type and, indeed, develop severe respiratory distress and cyanosis. In the course of time, right ventricular hypertrophy occurs, and death from decompensated cor pulmonale usually ensues within two to eight years. However, continuous therapy with some of the more modern vasodilators appears to improve the outcome.

ADULT RESPIRATORY DISTRESS SYNDROME (ARDS)

Synonyms for ARDS include adult respiratory failure, shock lung, diffuse alveolar damage (DAD), acute alveolar injury, and traumatic wet lungs.

ARDS and its many synonyms are descriptive terms for a syndrome characterized clinically by the rapid onset of severe life-threatening respiratory insufficiency, tachycardia, cyanosis, and severe arterial hypoxemia that is refractory to oxygen therapy. In most patients there is evidence of severe pulmonary edema. Lung compliance is decreased, and chest radiographs usually show a diffuse alveolar infiltration.[24]

The syndrome received particular attention during the Vietnam war as a complication of nonthoracic trauma with shock (hence the term shock lung), but it is now a well-recognized complication of numerous other conditions seen in nonmilitary medicine.[25, 26] The latter include (1) septic shock; (2) shock associated with trauma, hemorrhagic pancreatitis, burns, and complicated abdominal surgery; (3) *diffuse* pulmonary infections, mostly viral; (4) oxygen toxicity; (5) inhalation of toxins and other irritants (e.g., nitrogen dioxide); (6) narcotic overdose; (7) hypersensitivity reactions to organic solvents; (8) cardiac surgery involving extracorporeal cardiac pumps; and (9) aspiration pneumonitis. In many cases, a combination of the above conditions—shock, oxygen therapy, and sepsis—is present.[27]

PATHOGENESIS. ***Concept of Diffuse Alveolar Damage.*** ARDS is best viewed as the clinical and morphologic end result of acute alveolar injury caused by a variety of stimuli and probably initiated by different mechanisms. The initial and basic lesion is *diffuse damage to the alveolar wall;*[12, 28] this is followed by a

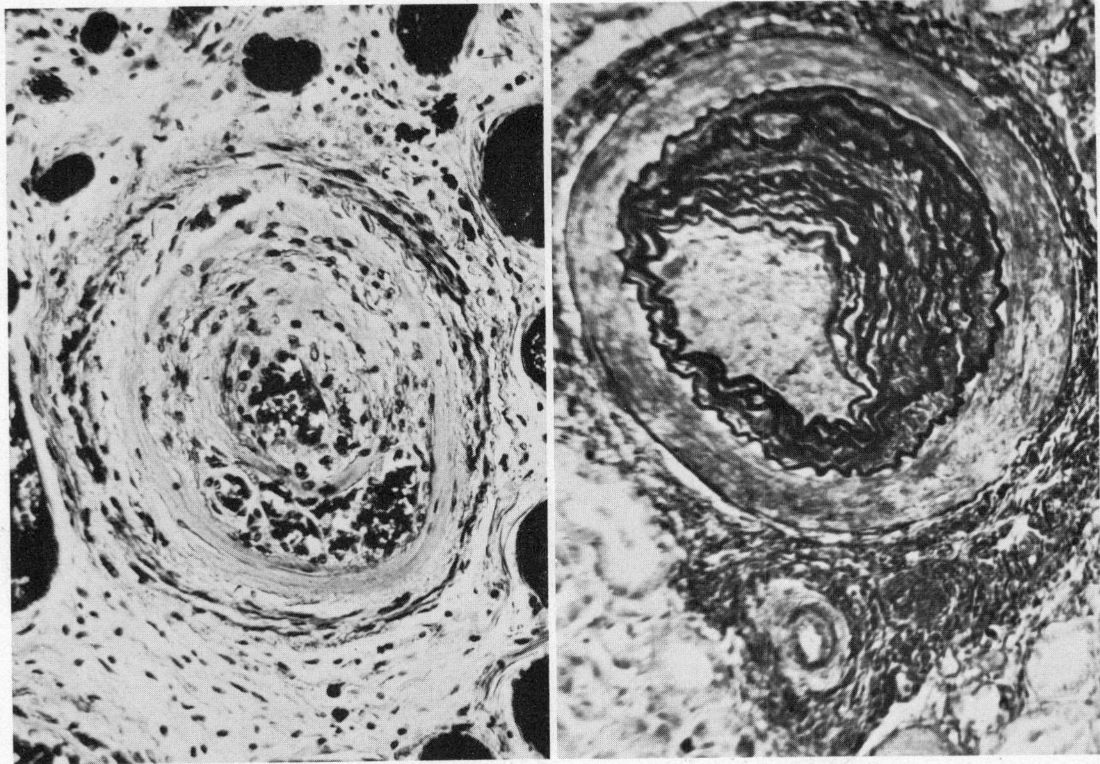

Figure 16–9. Pulmonary hypertension. Histologic detail of a thickened artery to illustrate medial hypertrophy.

Figure 16–10. Pulmonary hypertension with an elastic tissue stain showing elastic thickening of intima and duplication of internal elastic membrane.

rather nonspecific and usually predictable series of morphologic and physiologic alterations leading to respiratory failure (Fig. 16–11A). There is some uncertainty whether the initial injury is to capillary endothelium, alveolar epithelium, or both. In the most severe cases, both endothelium and epithelium are clearly affected. Of interest is that Type I epithelial cells are more vulnerable to most types of injury than are Type II cells. Cellular damage leads to increased capillary permeability, interstitial and intra-alveolar edema, fibrin exudation, and the formation of hyaline membranes.

What initiates endothelial or epithelial damage in these diverse conditions? The precise answer is unknown, but it seems likely that there is more than one initiating mechanism. For example, in toxicity induced by exposure to high concentrations (70 to 100%) of oxygen *(oxygen toxicity)*, the injurious agents are almost certainly oxygen-derived free radicals (superoxide, hydroxyl ion, singlet oxygen), which directly affect cell membranes. Such may also be the case in ARDS induced by other toxins, such as the weed killer paraquat. Indeed, experimental oxygen toxicity can mimic most of the morphologic and functional features of ARDS.[27]

The most obscure mechanisms are those that initiate ARDS in septic shock or shock following trauma and burns. Currently, the evidence points to *pulmonary intravascular aggregation of leukocytes*, principally neutrophils, as an important early event in the process. Infusion of *E. coli* endotoxin in experimental animals causes intrapulmonary leukocyte aggregation, pulmonary edema, and a syndrome analogous to ARDS.[29] A similar picture can be induced by injections of activated complement components (e.g., C5a) that cause leukocyte aggregation.[30] Stimulated neutrophils secrete at least three classes of agents that may contribute to the alveolar injury: oxygen-derived free radicals, lysosomal enzymes, and products of arachidonic acid metabolism (see p. 51). The scenario that emerges[31] is that ARDS may be initiated by *complement activation*, a known consequence of sepsis, endotoxin injection, trauma, cardiopulmonary bypass surgery, and other predisposing factors. This generates C5a, which induces leukocyte aggregation and activation in the lung. The liberated oxygen free radicals injure endothelium, causing increased permeability, and also probably epithelium, inducing alveolar edema. The liberated proteases destroy structural proteins, such as elastin and collagen.[32] In addition, as discussed in Chapter 2, neutrophil enzymes may further promote local injury by activating the kinin and clotting systems. Products of arachidonic acid metabolism, such as thromboxane, are thought to result in the pulmonary vasoconstriction that also char-

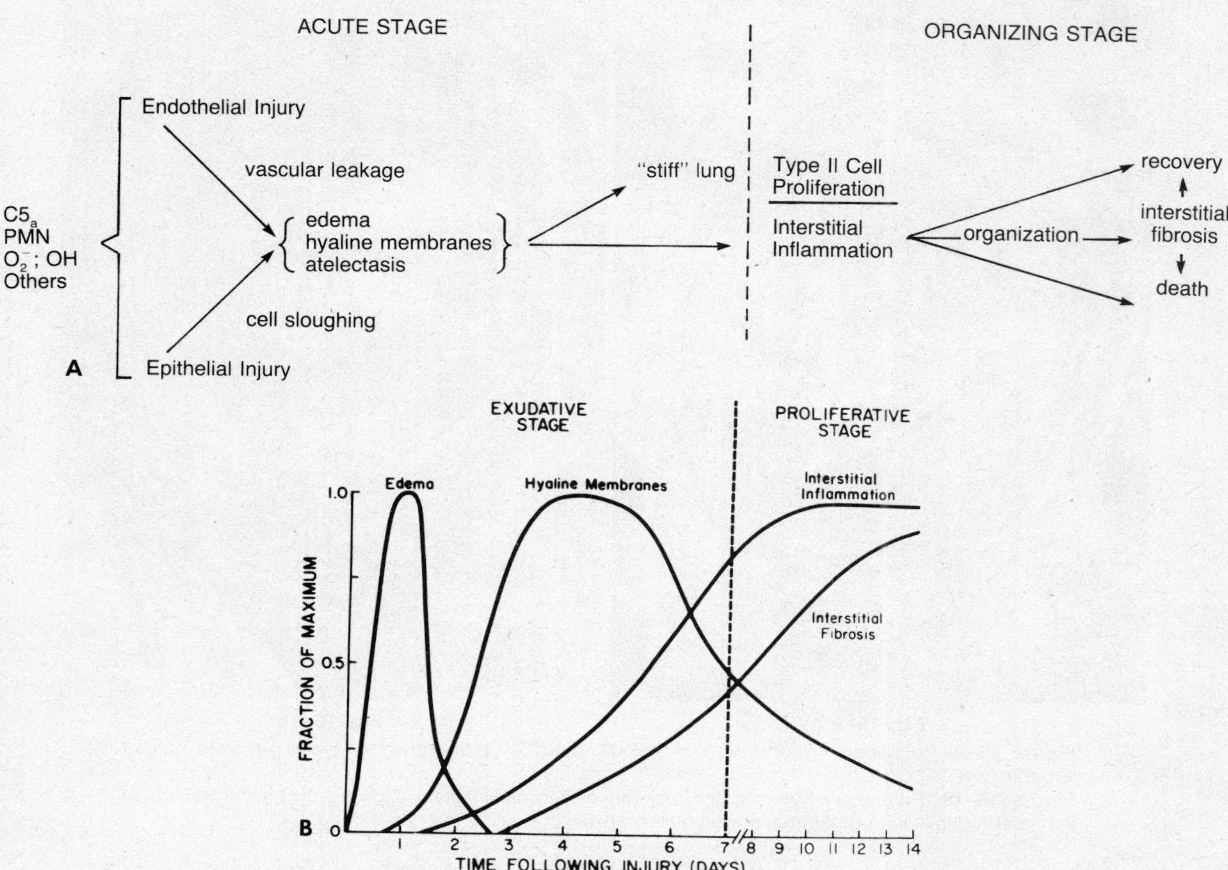

Figure 16–11. *A,* Pathogenesis of acute respiratory distress syndrome—a consequence of diffuse alveolar damage. *B,* Schematic representation of time course of evolution of diffuse alveolar damage. The times after injury (X-abscissa) vary considerably from patient to patient. (Modified from Katzenstein, A-L.A., and Askin, F. B.: Surgical Pathology of Non-Neoplastic Lung Disease. Philadelphia, W. B. Saunders Co., 1982, p. 30.)

acterizes ARDS.[31] Additional mechanisms postulated to play secondary roles in ARDS include platelet aggregation and release of their vasoactive products and intravascular coagulation.

The subsequent sequence of events[12, 33] is shown in Figure 16–11A. In addition to the congestion, edema, and fibrin deposition, the alveolar walls become lined with waxy *hyaline membranes* such as are seen in hyaline membrane disease of neonates (p. 482). Such membranes consist of protein-rich, fibrin-rich edema fluid admixed with the cytoplasmic and lipid remnants of necrotic epithelial cells; they always reflect substantial epithelial cell injury. Loss of surfactant leads to atelectasis, and the combination of pulmonary edema and atelectasis result in the stiff (noncompliant) lung characteristic of ARDS. Subsequently, Type II epithelial cells undergo proliferation, in an attempt to regenerate the alveolar lining. There then is organization of the fibrin exudate, with resultant intra-alveolar fibrosis. Marked thickening of the alveolar septa ensues, caused by proliferation of interstitial cells and deposition of collagen. Not all patients follow this course. Recovery may take place at any stage, with resorption of the edema fluid and reexpansion of atelectatic areas. However, the sequence leading from acute alveolar damage to fibrosis is an important one to keep in mind, as it also underlies most of the diffuse chronic interstitial diseases to be discussed later in this chapter.[12, 27]

MORPHOLOGY. In the acute exudative stage, the lungs are heavy, firm, red, and boggy. They exhibit congestion, interstitial and intra-alveolar edema and inflammation, fibrin deposition, necrosis of epithelial cells with formation of hyaline membranes, focal intra-alveolar hemorrhage, and patchy atelectasis (Fig. 16–11*B*). In fatal cases there is usually terminal bronchopneumonia. In the later proliferative or organizing stages, alveolar spaces become lined by cuboidal or columnar Type II epithelial cells, and there are variable degrees of interstitial and intra-alveolar fibrosis and inflammation.

CLINICAL COURSE. Patients who develop ARDS are usually hospitalized for one of the predisposing conditions listed earlier, and initially have no pulmonary symptoms. ARDS is heralded by profound dyspnea and tachypnea, but the chest radiograph is initially normal. Subsequently there is increasing cyanosis and hypoxemia, respiratory failure, and the appearance of diffuse bilateral infiltrates on x-ray examination. Hypoxemia then becomes unresponsive to oxygen therapy, and respiratory acidosis develops. Progression from one phase to the next does not occur in all patients, and some recover completely. However, despite recent improvements in supportive respiratory therapy, the mortality rate among the 150,000 cases seen yearly in the United States is still about 50%.

OBSTRUCTIVE VS. RESTRICTIVE PULMONARY DISEASE

Pulmonary physiologists have popularized the classification of *diffuse* pulmonary diseases into two categories: (1) *obstructive disease* (or *airway disease*), characterized by an increase in resistance to air flow due to partial or complete obstruction at any level—from the trachea and larger bronchi to the terminal and respiratory bronchioles; and (2) *restrictive disease*, characterized by reduced expansion of lung parenchyma, with a decreased total lung capacity. Although many pathologic conditions have both obstructive and restrictive components, distinction of the two patterns of pulmonary dysfunction has proved useful in correlating the results of pulmonary function tests with the radiologic appearance of the lungs and the histologic findings in individual patients.

The major obstructive disorders (excluding tumor or inhalation of a foreign body) are *emphysema*, *chronic bronchitis*, *bronchiectasis*, and *asthma*. In patients with these diseases, pulmonary function tests show increased pulmonary resistance and limitation of maximal expiratory flow rates during forced expiration. It is important to note that expiratory air flow obstruction may result either from *anatomic airway narrowing*, such as is most classically observed in asthma, or from *loss of elastic recoil* of the lung, which characteristically occurs in emphysema.

In contrast, restrictive diseases are identified by a reduced total lung capacity. The restrictive defect occurs in two general conditions: (1) *chest wall disorders in the presence of normal lungs* (e.g., neuromuscular diseases such as poliomyelitis, severe obesity, pleural diseases, and kyphoscoliosis with abnormal architecture of the rib cage) and (2) *interstitial and infiltrative diseases affecting primarily the alveoli*. The classic acute infiltrative disease is ARDS. Chronic restrictive diseases include the dust diseases or pneumoconioses, granulomatous diseases such as sarcoidosis, and most of the interstitial fibrosing conditions, to be discussed later (p. 742).

CHRONIC OBSTRUCTIVE AIRWAY DISEASE (CHRONIC OBSTRUCTIVE PULMONARY DISEASE)

The terms chronic obstructive pulmonary disease (COPD) or chronic obstructive airway disease (COAD) refer to a group of conditions—emphysema, chronic bronchitis, bronchial asthma, and bronchiectasis—that are accompanied by chronic or recurrent obstruction to air flow within the lung. Because of the increase in environmental pollutants, cigarette smoking, and other noxious exposures, the incidence of COPD has increased dramatically in the past two decades, and it now represents one of the major causes of morbidity and mortality in the Western world.

EMPHYSEMA

The American Thoracic Society and most American experts define emphysema as a condition of the lung characterized by *abnormal permanent enlargement of the air spaces distal to the terminal bronchiole, accompanied by destruction of their walls.*[1, 34] Enlargement of air spaces unaccompanied by destruction is termed *overinflation;* for example, the distention of air spaces in the opposite lung following unilateral pneumonectomy would be termed compensatory overinflation rather than emphysema. The compelling reason for including the factor of destruction of the alveolar wall in this anatomic definition is that it corresponds more closely to the *clinical* syndrome of emphysema and can be recognized more easily by the pathologist. Most British authors, however, generally do not require tissue destruction in their definition of emphysema[11, 35] and instead recognize two categories of the condition: (1) dilatation of air spaces alone and (2) dilatation with destruction.

The relationship between chronic bronchitis and emphysema is complicated, but fortunately the use of precise definitions has helped bring some order to what was once chaos. The definition of emphysema, as we have seen, is a morphologic one. Chronic bronchitis, on the other hand, is a disease that is defined in *clinical* terms as the condition characterized by chronic or recurrent excess mucus secretion in the bronchial tree. Indeed, the precise definition of chronic bronchitis states that "the sputum must be produced on most days for at least three months of the year and for at least two years."[34]

Emphysema and chronic bronchitis are best viewed as a spectrum.[36] Some patients, e.g., those with alpha-1-antitrypsin deficiency, have almost pure emphysema with lungs full of enlarged air spaces caused by destruction of alveolar walls. Others have virtually pure bronchitis with abundant sputum production and no alterations in the airways that cause organic obstruction. For the middle of the spectrum, mixtures of the two are the rule, partly because the same pathogenetic mechanisms, e.g., cigarette smoking, are common to both. Although the clinical features and functional abnormalities in both conditions also overlap, it is often possible to distinguish between patients with predominant emphysema and those with predominant bronchitis, as shown in Table 16–1.[36]

TYPES OF EMPHYSEMA. Not only is emphysema defined in terms of the *anatomic* nature of the lesion, but it is also further classified according to its *anatomic*

Table 16–1. EMPHYSEMA AND CHRONIC BRONCHITIS

	Predominant Bronchitis	Predominant Emphysema
Appearance	"Blue bloater"	"Pink puffer"
Age	40–45	50–75
Dyspnea	Mild; late	Severe; early
Cough	Early; copious sputum	Late; scanty sputum
Infections	Common	Occasional
Respiratory insufficiency	Repeated	Terminal
Cor pulmonale	Common	Rare; terminal
Airway resistance	Increased	Normal or slightly increased
Elastic recoil	Normal	Low
Chest radiograph	Prominent vessels; large heart	Hyperinflation; small heart

distribution within the lobule.[1, 35] Recall that the lobule is a cluster of acini, the alveolated terminal respiratory units. Although the term emphysema is sometimes loosely applied to diverse conditions, there are four types: (1) centriacinar, (2) panacinar, (3) paraseptal, and (4) irregular. Of these, the first two are the most important clinically.

Centriacinar (Centrilobular) Emphysema. The distinctive feature of this type of emphysema is the pattern of involvement of the lobules; **the central or proximal parts of the acini, formed by respiratory bronchioles, are affected, while distal alveoli are spared** (Fig. 16–12). Thus, both emphysematous and normal air spaces exist within the same acinus and lobule (Fig. 16–13). The lesions are more common and usually more severe in the upper lobes, particularly in the apical segments. The walls of the emphysematous spaces often contain large amounts of black pigment. Inflammation around bronchi and bronchioles and in the septa is common. In severe centriacinar emphysema, the distal acinus may be involved, and differentiation from panacinar emphysema becomes difficult. Further, centriacinar and panacinar emphysema may coexist in some patients. Mild degrees of centriacinar emphysema are common at autopsy in the absence of a history of lung disease. In symptomatic patients, however, moderate-to-severe degrees of emphysema occur predominantly in male smokers, often in association with chronic bronchitis. In addition, so-called coal workers' pneumoconiosis (p. 431) bears a striking resemblance to centriacinar emphysema. These points suggest an important role for tobacco products and coal dust in the genesis of this type of emphysema.

Panacinar (Panlobular) Emphysema. In this type the **acini are uniformly enlarged from the level of the respiratory bronchiole to the terminal blind alveoli** (Fig. 16–14). It is important to emphasize that the term *pan* refers to the entire acinus but not to the entire lung (Fig. 16–15). In contrast to centriacinar emphysema, panacinar emphysema tends to occur more commonly in the lower zones and in the anterior margins of the lung, and is usually most severe at the bases. Panacinar emphysema occurring by itself is not a common cause of chronic obstructive disease. However, it is the type of emphysema associated with **alpha-1-antitrypsin deficiency** (p. 721). In addition, postobstructive emphysema is usually panacinar rather than centriacinar.

Paraseptal (Distal Acinar) Emphysema. In this type the **proximal portion of the acinus is normal but the distal part is dominantly involved** (Fig. 16–16). The emphysema is more striking adjacent to the pleura, along the lobular connective tissue septa, and at the margins of the lobules. This localization accounts for the synonymous labels for this condition: **superficial, paraseptal, periacinar.** It commonly occurs adjacent to areas of fibrosis, scarring, or atelectasis and is usually more severe in the upper half of the lungs. The characteristic findings are of multiple, continuous, enlarged air spaces from less than 0.5 mm to more than 2.0 cm in diameter, sometimes forming cystlike structures. This type of emphysema probably underlies many of the cases of spontaneous pneumothorax in young adults[1] (p. 759).

Irregular Emphysema. **Irregular emphysema, so named because the acinus is irregularly involved, is almost invariably associated with scarring** (Fig. 16–17). Thus, it may be the most common form of emphysema, since careful search of most lungs at autopsy would show one or more scars. Adjacent to such scars there is usually irregular enlargement of acini accompanied by destructive changes. In most instances, these foci of irregular emphysema are asymptomatic. Extensive irregular emphysema occurs as a result of healing of tuberculosis, long-standing sarcoidosis, and other granulomatous diseases of the lung. Inflammatory scars are also frequent in the lungs of patients with chronic bronchitis;[35] these may cause irregular emphysema in addition to the centrilobular emphysema commonly found in patients with chronic bronchitis. Irregular emphysema is the only type of emphysema in which the pathogenesis seems to be clear. It is thought that the adjacent scarring increases the elastic pull on the alveoli and that the bronchiolar narrowing caused by fibrosis and inflammation results in **air trapping,** which may contribute to further distention of the alveoli and destruction of the walls.

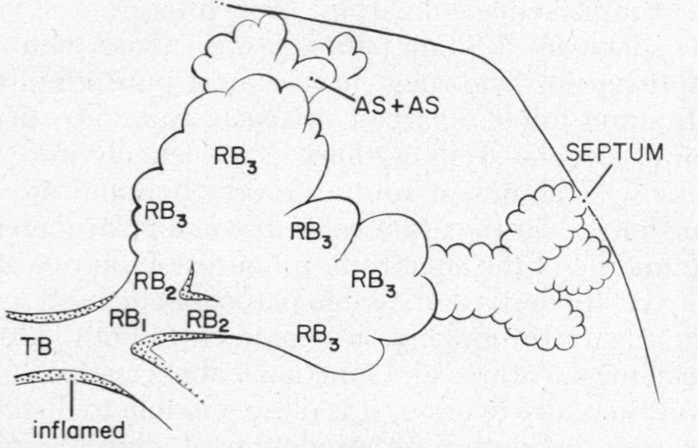

Figure 16–12. In centriacinar (proximal acinar) emphysema, respiratory bronchioles are selectively and dominantly involved. Abbreviations as in Figure 16–1. (From Thurlbeck, W. M.: Chronic Airflow Obstruction in Lung Disease. Philadelphia, W. B. Saunders Co., 1976.)

INCIDENCE. In considering the prevalence or incidence of emphysema, it must be remembered that it is an anatomic entity, that there are geographic differences in its incidence, and that there are subjective differences in interpretation of emphysematous changes at autopsy. Thurlbeck reports a 50% incidence of panacinar and centriacinar emphysema combined in the average autopsy population. He considers the pulmonary disease to be responsible for the death of 6.5% of these patients.[1]

Emphysema, especially the centriacinar type, is much more common and more severe in men than in

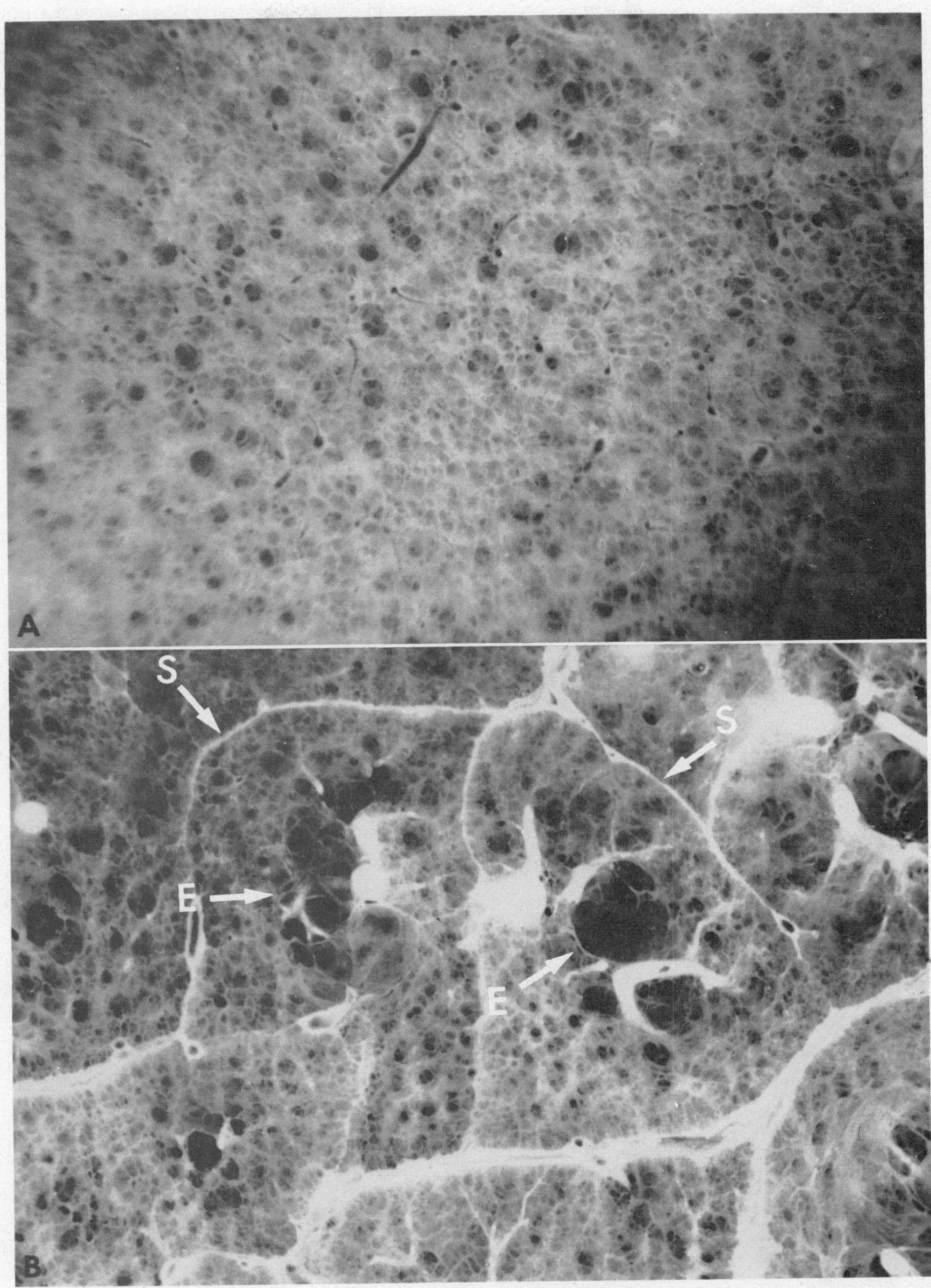

Figure 16–13. *A,* Normal lung as viewed through a dissecting microscope after fixation in inflation: magnification × 10. *B,* Centriacinar emphysema: magnification × 5.1. The pulmonary arteries contain a barium-gelatin injection mass. S = septum; E = emphysematous foci. (From Bates, D. V., et al.: Respiratory Function in Disease. 2nd ed. Philadelphia, W. B. Saunders Co., 1971.)

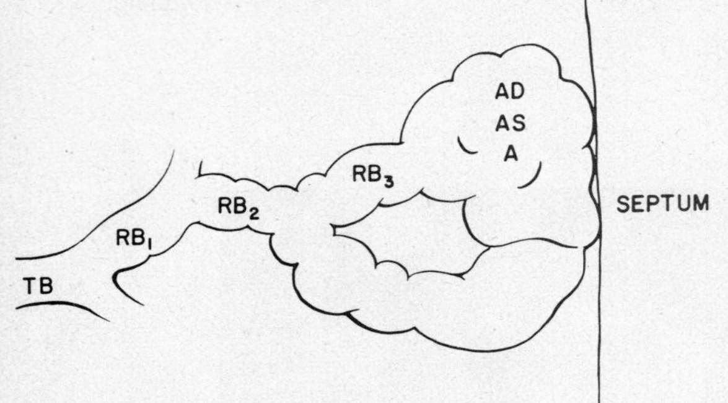

Figure 16–14. In panlobular (panacinar) emphysema, the enlargement and destruction of air spaces involve the acinus more or less uniformly. Abbreviations as in Figure 16–1. (From Thurlbeck, W. M.: Chronic Airflow Obstruction in Lung Disease. Philadelphia, W. B. Saunders Co., 1976.)

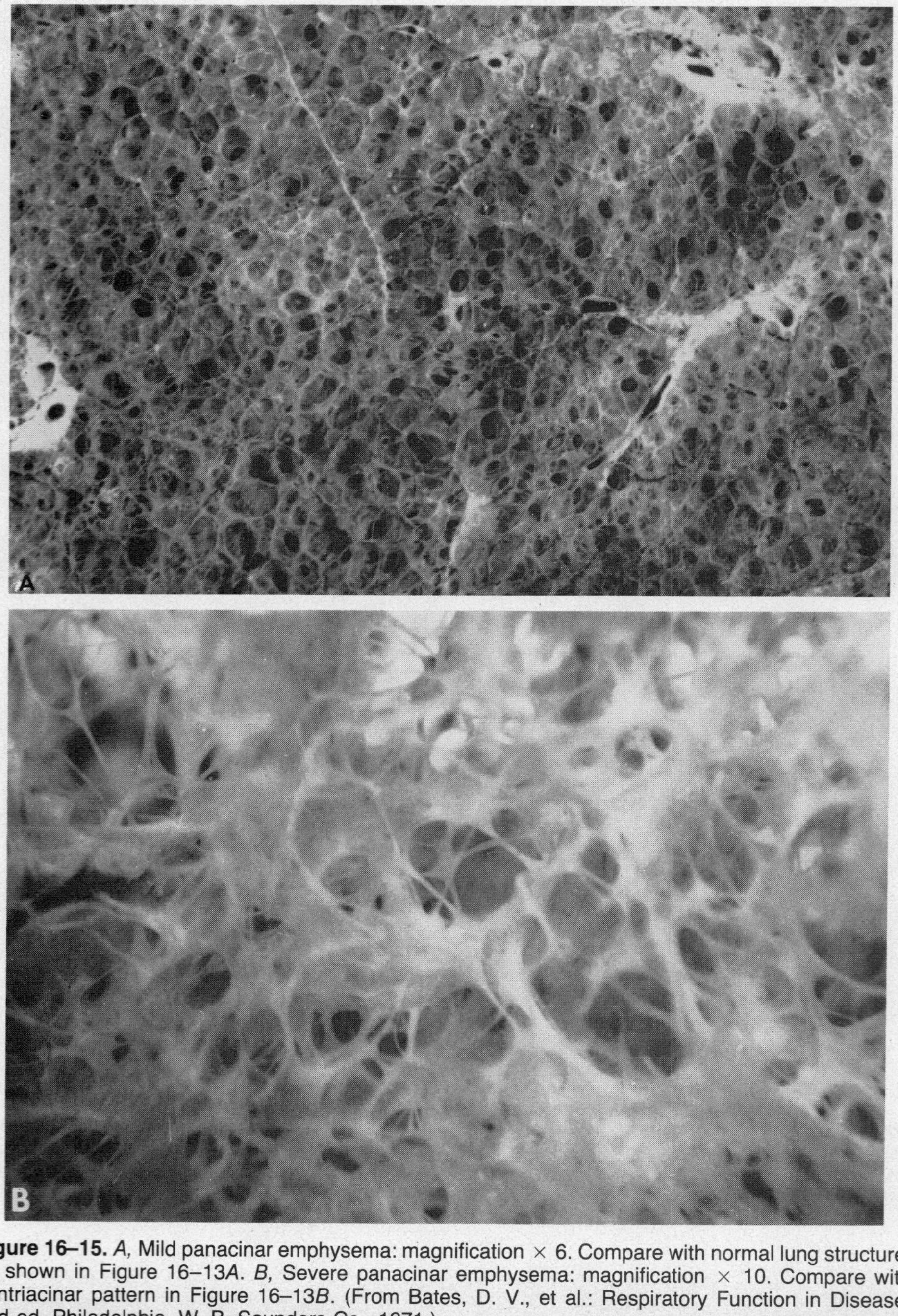

Figure 16–15. *A,* Mild panacinar emphysema: magnification × 6. Compare with normal lung structure, as shown in Figure 16–13*A*. *B,* Severe panacinar emphysema: magnification × 10. Compare with centriacinar pattern in Figure 16–13*B*. (From Bates, D. V., et al.: Respiratory Function in Disease. 2nd ed. Philadelphia, W. B. Saunders Co., 1971.)

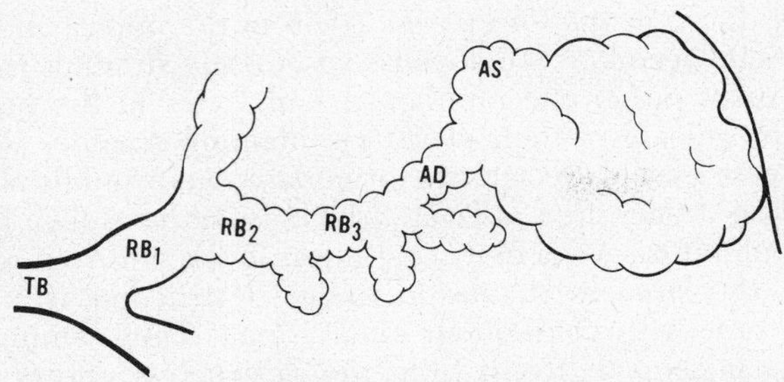

Figure 16–16. In paraseptal (distal acinar) emphysema, peripheral part of acinus (alveolar ducts and sacs) is dominantly or selectively involved. (From Thurlbeck, W. M.: Chronic Airflow Obstruction in Lung Disease. Philadelphia, W. B. Saunders Co., 1976.)

women. *There is clear-cut association between heavy cigarette smoking and emphysema,* and the most severe type occurs in males who smoke heavily. Although emphysema does not become disabling until the fifth to eighth decades of life, it is well known clinically that ventilatory deficits may make their first appearance decades earlier in those destined to develop the full-blown disease.[38] Indeed, emphysematous changes were found in the lungs of teenagers dying of accidental causes, who had been exposed to environmental air pollution.[39] Certain genetic and familial predispositions have been identified, as discussed below.

Chronic obstructive pulmonary disease, including emphysema, is the most common form of pulmonary disease in man. Death rates are said to be doubling every five years, and today COPD is probably responsible for more deaths than carcinoma of the lung, ranking among the leading causes of death in the industrialized world. It is responsible for 7% of all disability payments by the Social Security Administration in the United States, exceeded only by heart disease with respect to economic cost.

PATHOGENESIS. The genesis of the two common forms of emphysema—centriacinar and panacinar—is unsettled, and there is no reason why several etiologic and pathogenetic factors may not be involved. The three critical questions that need answers are: (1) what is the cause of alveolar wall destruction, the sine qua non of emphysema?; (2) what is the role of smoking or other pollutants in such destruction?; and (3) what is the relationship of emphysema to chronic bronchitis when both coexist?

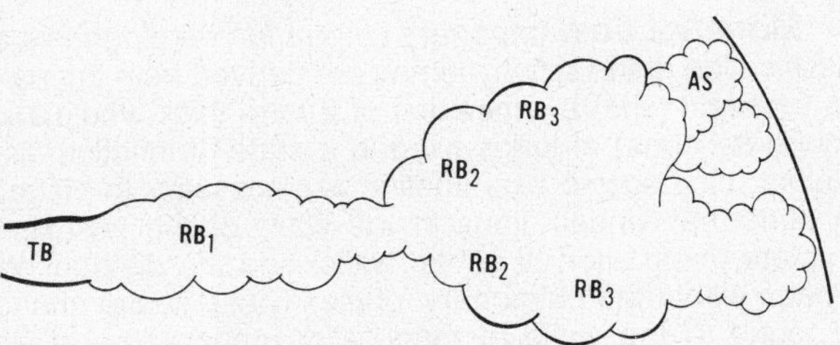

Figure 16–17. In irregular emphysema, acinus is irregularly involved. This form is often accompanied by scarring in lung. (From Thurlbeck, W. M.: Chronic Airflow Obstruction in Lung Disease. Philadelphia, W. B. Saunders Co., 1976.)

Whether chronic bronchitis (admittedly sometimes so mild as not to merit a clinical diagnosis) initiates the lesion in the air spaces or follows the development of emphysematous changes is a controversial issue. The oldest hypothesis holds that chronic bronchitis results in partial obstruction of the airways, particularly in the respiratory bronchioles, which then leads to air trapping, progressive overdistention of alveolar spaces, squeezing of septal capillaries, loss of blood supply, and secondary damage to alveolar walls.[40] In this scenario, the initiating influences for airway inflammation may be air pollutants, particularly tobacco smoke. Secondary bacterial infection of the retained mucus secretions compounds the problem. Loss of the septal walls adds to the bronchial and bronchiolar narrowings, since the normal pulmonary substance is elastic and tends to maintain the patency of the airways. Thus, a vicious cycle is created in which partial obstruction leads to increased expiratory effort, which in turn induces further obstruction.[41]

In support of this view, it is pointed out that emphysematous foci are often pigmented with carbon dust, particularly in centriacinar emphysema. Presumably, the coal dust and other noxious airborne particles (silicates, trace metals, and organic residues) collect in the bronchioles and initiate the bronchiolitis, leading to the chain of events cited. As we shall see later, there is indeed evidence that bronchiolar alterations (small airway disease, p. 725) may be the first manifestations of airway disease in heavy smokers.

There is, however, a substantial amount of evidence that destruction of alveolar walls is the *primary event.* In some cases, no bronchitis can be found even on morphologic examination. Such instances are sometimes designated *primary emphysema.* Conversely, severe chronic bronchitis is not necessarily associated with emphysematous destruction.[42] So the question has been raised: Does the destructive process in the septal walls itself deprive the bronchioles and bronchi of their tissue support, leading in turn to narrowing, mucus retention, secondary infection, and development of chronic bronchitis and bronchiolitis? If the emphysematous changes are indeed primary, what are the possible mechanisms of alveolar wall destruction? It is regarding this last issue that the discovery of the association of a genetic condition—alpha-1-antitrypsin deficiency—with emphysema has made the most significant impact on our understanding of the pathogenesis of emphysema.

The Protease-Antiprotease Hypothesis (The Enzyme Inhibitor Hypothesis). In 1963, Laurell and Eriksson called attention to a hereditary deficiency of serum *alpha-1-globulin* in certain families with a high incidence of emphysema.[43] The alpha-1-globulin fraction was shown to be a potent inhibitor of proteinases, especially of trypsin; these families had markedly diminished antitryptic serum activity, and thus the condition became known as alpha-1-antitrypsin (α1-AT) deficiency. α1-AT is encoded by two independent alleles at a single locus, resulting in an autosomal codominant mode of inheritance. Patients with very low levels of enzyme activity are homozygotes, whereas those with intermediate levels are heterozygotes.[44] There are multiple molecular variants of α1-AT, determined by at least 25 alleles on the Pi (proteinase inhibitor) locus. The common normal allele is PiM, and the normal Pi type is homozygous MM. The most common variant with α1-AT deficiency in the U.S. and Europe is PiZ; in the U.S., about one in every 3630 subjects is homozygous PiZZ, and 2 to 5% are heterozygous PiMZ.

The homozygous PiZZ state confers a greatly enhanced susceptibility to pulmonary emphysema, which is compounded by smoking. Thus, 60 to 75% of nonsmokers and up to 95% of homozygous smokers develop chronic lung disease. In these individuals the disease is characteristically of early onset, usually becoming evident before the fourth decade. The emphysema tends to be severe and panacinar, with accentuation in the lower lobes. Whether heterozygotes with intermediate levels of α1-AT are also at increased risk is a matter of controversy.[45] In some studies, cigarette smoking significantly increases the susceptibility of heterozygotes to the development of COPD.

The discovery of α1-AT deficiency, followed by the demonstration that intratracheal administration of the proteolytic enzyme papain causes emphysema in experimental animals, eventually led to the so-called *protease-antiprotease theory of emphysema*, for which there is now considerable support (Fig. 16–18).[46-49] The theory holds that alveolar wall destruction results from an imbalance between proteases (mainly elastases), and antiproteases in the lung. Anything that decreases antielastase or increases elastase tips the balance in favor of proteolytic destruction of elastin, and the formation of emphysema. The principal antielastase activity in serum and interstitial tissue is α1-AT (other protease inhibitors are serum α1-macroglobulin and inhibitors in bronchial mucus), and the principal endogenous elastase activity is derived from neutrophils (other elastases are formed by macrophages, pancreas, and bacteria). Neutrophil elastase is capable of digesting human lung, and this digestion can be inhibited by α1-AT. Such elastase induces emphysema when instilled into the trachea of experimental animals.[50] Thus, the following sequence is postulated to explain the effect of α1-AT deficiency on the lung: neutrophils are normally sequestered in the lung (more in the lower zones than in the upper) and a few gain access to the alveolar space. Any stimulus that increases either the number of leukocytes in the lung or the release of their elastase-containing granules will increase elastolytic activity. Stimulated neutrophils also release oxygen-free radicals, which as we have seen (p. 58) inhibit α1-AT activity. With low levels of serum α1-AT, the process of elastic tissue destruction is unchecked, with consequent emphysema. Thus, emphysema is seen to result from the destructive effects of high protease activity in subjects with low antiprotease activity.

The protease-antiprotease hypothesis also explains the deleterious effect of cigarette smoking, since both increased elastase availability and decreased antielastase activity occur in smokers (Fig. 16–18).[46-49] Smokers have greater numbers of neutrophils within their alveolar fluid, and smoke condensates stimulate neutrophils to release their elastase in vitro. The recruitment of neutrophils into the lung appears to occur, at least in part, by the release from activated alveolar macrophages of a *neutrophil chemotactic factor*, this release being stimulated by smoking.[52] Smoking also enhances elastase activity in macrophages; macrophage elastase is not inhibited by α1-AT, and indeed can proteolytically digest this enzyme.[51] Decreased antielastase activity in smokers results from the inhibition of elastolytic activity of α1-AT by oxidants in cigarette smoke, and by the oxygen-derived free radicals secreted by neutrophils and macrophages when these cells are stimulated by smoke. It has thus been suggested that impaction of smoke particles in the small bronchi and bronchioles, with the resultant influx of neutrophils and macrophages, increased elastase and decreased α1-AT activity, cause the centriacinar emphysema seen in smokers, as contrasted with the panacinar emphysema of patients with generalized α1-AT deficiency. These concepts also explain the additive influence of smoking and α1-AT deficiency in inducing serious obstructive airway disease.

Although there are still numerous gaps in our knowledge of the pathogenesis of emphysema, the basic observations on the protease-antiprotease events are sufficiently well established to have stimulated exploration of therapeutic measures, either by α1-AT replacement or by the administration of synthetic elastase inhibitors.

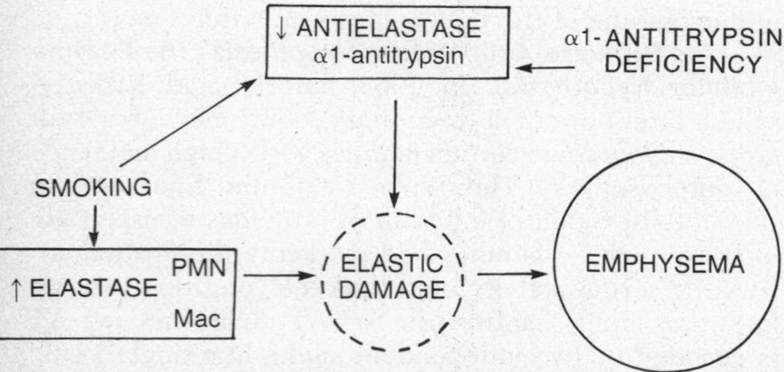

Figure 16–18. Protease antiprotease mechanism of emphysema. PMN = polymorphonuclear leukocytes; Mac = alveolar macrophages.

MORPHOLOGY. Important criteria for the diagnosis and classification of the emphysemas are derived from the naked eye (or hand lens) examination of 2 mm–thick whole slices (Gough sections) of lungs fixed in a state of inflation. More detailed microscopic examination is necessary to visualize the abnormal fenestrations in the walls of the alveoli, the complete destruction of septal walls, and the distribution of damage within the pulmonary lobule. These septal changes are found in the walls of respiratory bronchioles, alveolar ducts, and alveolar spaces. Enlargement of defects or coalescence of multiple adjacent ones can result in destruction of an entire septum, perhaps leaving only a strand of residual tissue, usually harboring a small blood vessel. In microscopic section, such a strand will appear as a "free-floating" island of tissue. With advance of the disease, adjacent alveoli fuse to produce even larger abnormal air spaces and possibly blebs or bullae. Often the respiratory bronchioles and vasculature of the lung are deformed and compressed by the emphysematous distortion of the air spaces (Fig. 16–19), and, as mentioned, there may or may not be evidence of bronchitis or bronchiolitis.

The differentiation of centriacinar from panacinar emphysema is made on the basis of the distribution of the septal destruction within the pulmonary lobule. As mentioned, in centriacinar emphysema, the central air spaces are primarily involved and the peripheral alveoli are generally spared and are essentially normal. In contrast, in panacinar emphysema, there is total involvement of the entire lobule. In both major forms of this disorder, there is remarkably little evidence of inflammatory change within the affected septa or air spaces.

The gross appearance of emphysematous disease depends on the form of emphysema and its severity. Panacinar emphysema, when well developed, produces voluminous lungs, often overlapping the heart and hiding it when the anterior chest wall is removed. The pulmonary tissue is diffusely hypercrepitant and pillowy to palpation, and the involvement usually extends out to the pleural surfaces. The emphysematous lobes are uniformly pale, owing to compression of the blood supply. The macroscopic features of centriacinar emphysema are less impressive. The lungs may not appear particularly pale or voluminous unless the disease is well advanced. Generally, the upper two-thirds of the lungs are more severely affected. The lesions become evident only on sectioning of the lung, since usually a narrow rim of subpleural lung parenchyma is spared. Large apical blebs or bullae are more characteristic of irregular emphysema secondary to scarring.

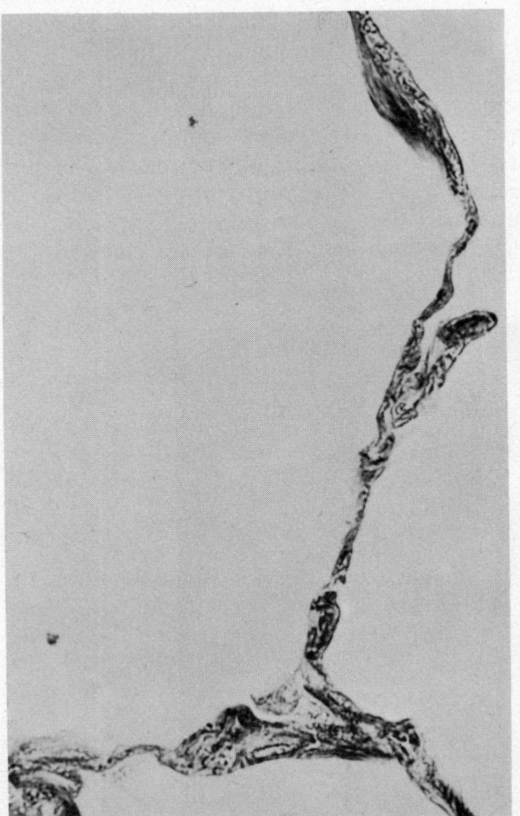

Figure 16–19. Panacinar emphysema in high-power detail, illustrating avascularity of septa.

Clinical Course. The clinical manifestations of emphysema do not appear until at least one-third of the functioning pulmonary parenchyma is incapacitated. The panacinar form tends to be the most disabling because all alveoli are more or less affected. Dyspnea is usually the first symptom and may appear with or without significant cough. In some patients, cough or wheezing is the chief complaint, easily confused with asthma. Typically, the dyspnea begins insidiously but is steadily progressive. Cough and expectoration are extremely variable and depend on the extent and severity of the associated bronchitis. Weight loss is common and may be so severe as to suggest a hidden malignant tumor. The physical findings are also variable. Classically, the patient is barrel-chested and dyspneic, with obviously prolonged expiration, and sits forward in a hunched-over position, attempting to squeeze the air out of his lungs with each expiratory effort. These unfortunates have a pinched face and breathe through pursed lips. Hyperresonance related to the emphysematous changes may be present but is unreliable as a diagnostic finding, since it is also caused by simple hyperinflation without the destructive changes of emphysema. Similarly, chest films showing large, translucent lungs with low, flattened diaphragms are not diagnostic. *The only reliable and consistently present finding on physical examination is slowing of forced expiration.* A variety of other physiologic abnormalities can be demonstrated, as detailed in textbooks on pulmonary disease.

The differentiation of chronic airway disease originating in chronic bronchitis from that due to emphysema may be a difficult clinical problem requiring a variety of diagnostic procedures. At the risk of oversimplification: with severe anatomic emphysema, cough is often slight, overdistention is severe, diffusing capacity is low, and blood gases are relatively normal. Such patients may overventilate and remain well oxygenated, and therefore are euphoniously if somewhat ingloriously designated as "*pink puffers*" (Table 16–1). Patients with chronic bronchitis more often have a history of recurrent acute inflammatory episodes, persistent abundant purulent sputum, hypercapnia, and severe hypoxemia, prompting the equally inglorious designation of "*blue bloaters.*" A hazard in severe emphysema, in addition to the respiratory difficulties, is the development of cor pulmonale and eventual congestive heart failure. Death of most of these patients is due to (1) right-sided heart failure, (2) respiratory acidosis and coma, and (3) massive collapse of the lungs secondary to pneumothorax.

Other Types of Emphysema. Now we come to some of the less stringent usages of the term "emphysema" and to some closely related conditions.

Compensatory Emphysema. This term is sometimes used to designate dilatation of alveoli in response to loss of lung substance elsewhere. It is best exemplified in the hyperexpansion of the residual lung parenchyma that follows surgical removal of a diseased lung or lobe. In most instances, this constitutes compensatory *hyperinflation*, since there is no accompanying destruction of septal walls.

Senile Emphysema. Senile emphysema refers to the overdistended, sometimes voluminous lungs found in the aged. This is a misnomer, because actual morphometric studies have shown that the alveolar surface area *decreases* progressively after age 30, at the rate of about 4% each decade. Nevertheless, the lung appears overinflated on histologic sections and grossly. This apparent discrepancy is explained by the fact that *alveolar ducts and respiratory bronchioles enlarge with age, whereas the alveoli proper become shallower and smaller.* The latter is probably due to loss of the alveolar capillary bed. At any rate, there is alteration of the internal geometry of the lung—*larger alveolar ducts* and *smaller alveoli.*[1] Primary functional changes consist of increased compliance and decreased elasticity, but careful analyses have failed to disclose any significant quantitative loss of elastic tissue, even in advanced age. Changes in the skeletal system (especially the spinal column) of the elderly probably also play a role in the lung alterations of senile emphysema. Displacement of the rib cage results in an increase in anteroposterior diameter of the chest (barrel chest). This increases the negative intrapleural pressure and the pull on the lungs, leading to a form of *compensatory hyperinflation.* Since there is no destruction of lung substance, and the respiratory deficit is usually minimal, a better designation for such aging lungs would be *senile hyperinflation.*

Obstructive Overinflation. *Obstructive overinflation refers to the condition in which the lung expands because air is trapped within it.* A common cause is subtotal obstruction by a tumor or foreign object. A classic example is *congenital lobar overinflation of infants.* This is a congenital anomaly, probably due to hypoplasia of bronchial cartilage, and is sometimes associated with other congenital cardiac and lung abnormalities. It can be a life-threatening emergency, since the affected portion extends sufficiently to compress the remaining normal lung. Overinflation in obstructive lesions occurs either (1) because of a ball-valve action of the obstructive agent, so that air enters on inspiration but cannot leave on expiration; or (2) because the bronchus may be totally obstructed, but ventilation through "collaterals" may bring in air from behind the obstruction. These collaterals are represented by the *pores of Kohn* and other direct accessory *bronchioloalveolar connections* (the canals of Lambert).

Bullous Emphysema. Bullous emphysema refers merely to any form of emphysema that produces large subpleural blebs or bullae. Bullae are defined as emphysematous spaces more than 1 cm in diameter in the distended state (Fig. 16–20). They represent localized accentuations of one of the four forms of emphysema, are most often subpleural, and occur near the apex, sometimes in relation to old tuberculous scarring. They result from progressive destruction of septal walls, which floods over to encompass many contiguous pulmonary lobules. Occasionally, they are present with minimal widespread emphysema. Insufficient lung substance is affected to induce increased resistance to air flow, but on occasion rupture of the bullae may give rise to pneumothorax (p. 759). Radiologically, bullae appear as avascular translucent areas that may be demarcated by a white line.

Interstitial Emphysema. *The entrance of air into the connective tissue stroma of the lung, mediastinum, or subcutaneous tissue is designated interstitial emphysema.* Interstitial emphysema is distinct, both anatomically and clinically, from the forms of pulmonary emphysema previously described. In most instances, alveolar tears in pulmonary emphysema provide the avenue of entrance of air into the stroma of the lung, but rarely a wound of the chest that sucks air or a fractured rib that punctures the lung substance may underlie this disorder. Alveolar tears usually occur when

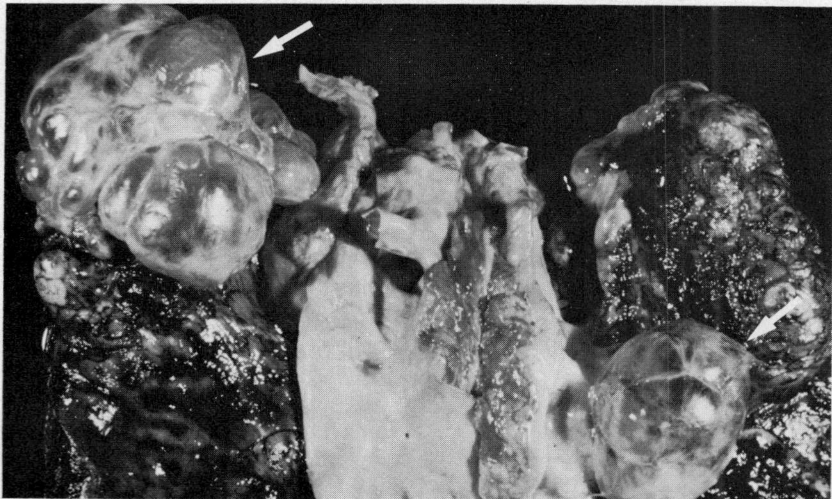

Figure 16–20. Bullous emphysema with large apical and marginal subpleural bullae *(arrows).*

there is a combination of coughing plus some bronchiolar obstruction, producing sharply increased pressures within the alveolar sacs. Children with whooping cough and bronchitis, adults with diphtheritic membranes, instances of obstruction to the airways (by blood clots, tissue, or foreign bodies), and individuals who suddenly inhale irritant gases are classic examples. Instrumentation of the airways, artificial resuscitation, and positive-pressure anesthesia are less common antecedents.

In all these circumstances, the tear is presumably widened by dilatation of the full inhalatory effort, but as the lung collapses in expiration, the tear closes and blocks the escape of air. In this pumplike fashion, there is progressive accumulation of air that dissects through the fibrous connective tissue of the alveolar walls and into and along the fibrous septa of the lung to reach the mediastinum, and thence possibly the subcutaneous tissues. If the collection of air is small, it usually has no clinical importance. However, extensive insufflation of the lung may encroach upon the small blood vessels to create serious impairment of blood flow through the lungs. These patients may therefore have marked respiratory difficulty and severe cyanosis, occasionally terminating in death. When the interstitial air treks into the subcutaneous tissues, the patient may literally swell up into an alarming, although usually harmless, "Michelin tire–ad" appearance, with marked swelling of the head and neck and crackling crepitation all over the chest. In most instances such air is resorbed promptly as soon as the point of entrance is sealed.

CHRONIC BRONCHITIS

This disorder, so common among habitual smokers and inhabitants of smog-laden cities, is not nearly so trivial as was once thought. When persistent for years, it may (1) cause chronic obstructive airway disease, as discussed earlier; (2) lead to cor pulmonale and heart failure; and (3) cause atypical metaplasia and dysplasia of the respiratory epithelium, providing a possible soil for cancerous transformation. The widely accepted definition of chronic bronchitis is the clinical one—*chronic bronchitis is present in any patient who has persistent cough with sputum production for at least three months in at least two consecutive years*. The condition can be further characterized as *simple chronic bronchitis*, in which the sputum is mucoid and uninfected; *mucopurulent chronic bronchitis;* and *obstructive chronic bronchitis*, in which there is physiologic evidence of airway obstruction. Both sexes and all ages may be affected, but it is most frequent in middle-aged men. Ten to 25% of the urban adult population may have chronic bronchitis;[1] country dwellers have a lower incidence.

PATHOGENESIS. Two sets of factors are important in the genesis of chronic bronchitis: (1) chronic irritation by inhaled substances and (2) microbiologic infections. Cigarette smoking remains the paramount influence. Chronic bronchitis is four to ten times more common in heavy smokers irrespective of age, sex, occupation, and place of dwelling.

The hallmark and earliest feature of chronic bronchitis is *hypersecretion of mucus*,[37] which starts in the large airways and is associated with *hypertrophy of the submucosal glands* in the trachea and bronchi. These changes contribute to excessive mucus production but not to airway obstruction. As chronic bronchitis persists, there is also an increase in the number of goblet cells in the surface epithelium of large bronchi, and, more important, a marked increase in goblet cells of small airways—small bronchi and bronchioles. It is this excessive mucus production by goblet cells in small airways that contributes to airway obstruction. It is thought that both the submucosal gland hypertrophy and the increase in goblet cells are caused by tobacco smoke or other pollutants (for example, sulfur dioxide, nitrogen dioxide); similar changes can be produced experimentally by inhalation of a variety of irritants. Submucosal glands are under vagal control, and both pilocarpine and isoproterenol increase the size of submucous glands and the number of goblet cells experimentally. It is thus possible that airway irritants cause mucus hypersecretion by stimulation of neurohormonal pathways.[46]

Concept of Small Airway Disease. Although mucus hypersecretion in large airways is the cause of sputum production in chronic bronchitis, it is now thought that *alterations in the small airways of the lung* (small bronchi and bronchioles, less than 2 to 3 mm in diameter) are the *physiologically important and perhaps earliest manifestations of chronic airway obstruction*.[53–56] These airways are in a critical position, forming the connecting link between the air-conducting system of bronchi and the air-exchanging alveoli. However, under normal conditions the total resistance of these airways is so small that it contributes little to overall airway resistance. Thus, half the bronchioles of this size could close in random fashion without increasing by more than 15% the overall resistance measurable at the mouth by standard pulmonary function tests.[57] However, specialized physiologic techniques, such as the so-called closing volume test, can reliably detect small-airway dysfunction, and such tests have shown distinct abnormalities in young smokers *before* the development of overt symptoms of respiratory obstruction. Histologic studies in the lungs of such young smokers disclose goblet cell metaplasia with mucous plugging of the bronchiolar lumen; clustering of pigmented alveolar macrophages; inflammatory infiltration; and (in a somewhat older group of patients) fibrosis of the bronchiolar wall.[58, 59] In one study there was good correlation between the structural changes in small airways and pulmonary function tests for small-airway obstruction. It is thus postulated that this respiratory *bronchiolitis* is the precursor of chronic obstructive airway changes. Of interest is that many of these alterations, such as intrabronchial mucous plugging and inflammation, are potentially reversible.[56, 59] Thus, the underlying pathologic process, if detected, can be either modified or reversed before the classic symptoms of chronic obstructive disease appear.

The role of infection appears to be secondary. It is not responsible for the initiation of chronic bronchitis, but is probably significant in maintaining it and may be critical in producing the acute exacerbations. The most common bacteria recovered are *Hemophilus influenzae*, the pneumococci, and *Streptococcus viridans*. Cigarette smoke probably predisposes to infection in more than one way: it interferes with ciliary action of the respiratory epithelium, may cause direct damage to airway epithelium, and inhibits the ability of bronchial and alveolar leukocytes to clear bacteria. Viruses such as adenovirus and respiratory syncytial rhinovirus can also cause exacerbations of chronic bronchitis.

Following a review of the pathogenesis of both emphysema and chronic bronchitis, reference should be made to Figure 16–21, which attempts to follow the evolution of both conditions into chronic obstructive airways disease.

MORPHOLOGY. Grossly, there may be hyperemia, swelling, and bogginess of the mucous membranes, frequently accompanied by excessive mucinous to mucopurulent secretions layering the epithelial surfaces. Sometimes, heavy casts of secretion and pus fill the bronchi and bronchioles.

The characteristic histologic feature of chronic bronchitis is enlargement of the mucus-secreting glands of the trachea and bronchi. Although goblet cells increase slightly, the **major increase is in the size of the mucous glands** (Fig. 16–22). This increase can be assessed by the ratio of the relative thickness of the mucous gland layer compared with the thickness of the wall between the epithelium and the cartilage (Reid index). The Reid index is increased in chronic bronchitis usually in proportion to the severity and duration of the disease.[37] The bronchial epithelium may exhibit squamous metaplasia and dysplasia. The changes in small bronchi and bronchioles have received particular attention. Morphometric studies clearly show a marked narrowing of these airways caused by goblet cell metaplasia, mucous plugging, inflammation, and fibrosis. In the most severe cases there may be obliteration of lumina **(bronchiolitis fibrosa obliterans).** As discussed earlier, these bronchiolar changes probably account for the obstructive features in bronchitic patients.

The clinical sine qua non of chronic bronchitis is a persistent cough productive of copious sputum. For many years, no other respiratory functional impairment is present, but eventually dyspnea on exertion develops. With the passage of time, COPD may appear, accompanied by hypercapnia, hypoxemia, and mild cyanosis. Differentiation of this form of obstructive lung disease from that associated with emphysema can be made in the classic case (Table 16–1), but, as mentioned, many such patients have both conditions. Long-standing severe chronic bronchitis commonly leads to cor pulmonale and possible cardiac failure. Death may also result from further impairment of respiratory function incident to acute intercurrent bacterial infections.

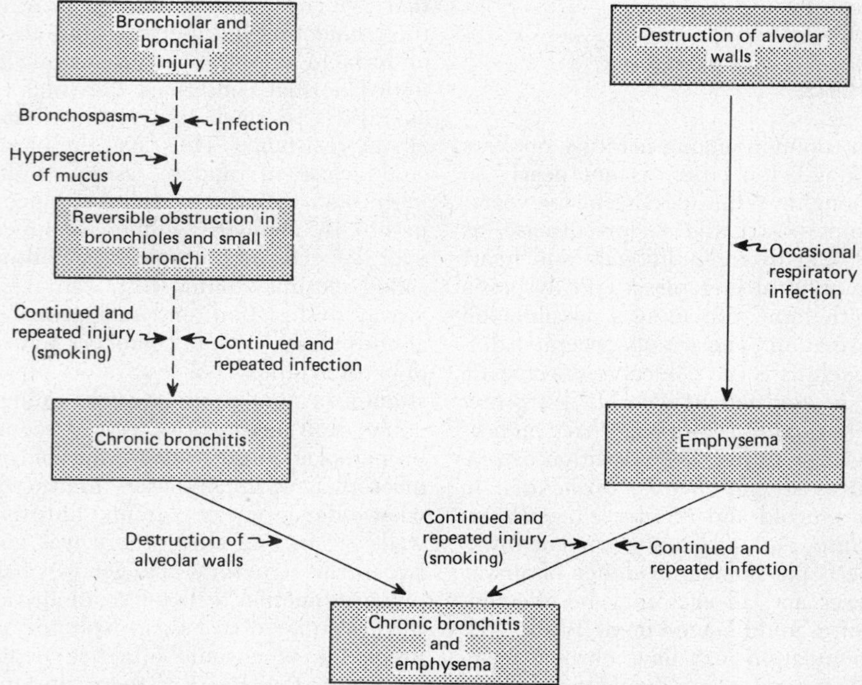

Figure 16–21. Schematic representation of evolution of chronic bronchitis *(left)* and of emphysema *(right)*. Although both can culminate in chronic bronchitis and emphysema, the pathways are different, and either one may predominate. Dashed arrows on left indicate that, in the natural history of chronic bronchitis, it is not known whether there is a predictable progression from obstruction in small airways to chronic (obstructive) bronchitis. (From Fishman, A. P.: The spectrum of chronic obstructive disease of the airways. *In* Fishman, A. P. (ed.): Pulmonary Diseases and Disorders. New York, McGraw-Hill Book Co., 1980, p. 463. Copyright © 1980 by McGraw-Hill, Inc. Used by permission of McGraw-Hill Book Company.)

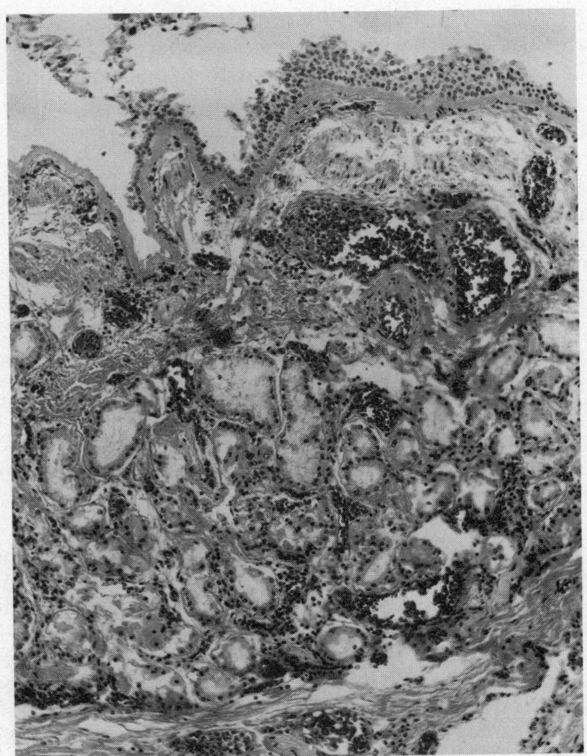

Figure 16–22. Chronic bronchitis. Lumen of bronchus is above. Note slight desquamation of mucosal epithelial cells and marked thickening of mucous gland layer (approximately twice normal). Vascular congestion is evident.

BRONCHIAL ASTHMA

Asthma is a disease characterized by increased irritability of the tracheobronchial tree, potentiating paroxysmal narrowing of the bronchial airways, which may reverse spontaneously or as a result of treatment.

It is a particularly distressing disease because those afflicted unpredictably experience disabling attacks of severe dyspnea and wheezing triggered by sudden episodes of bronchospasm. Between the attacks patients may be virtually asymptomatic, but in some individuals chronic bronchitis or cor pulmonale often supervenes. Rarely, a state of unremitting attacks *(status asthmaticus)* proves fatal; usually such unfortunate patients have had a long history of asthma. In some cases, the attacks are triggered by exposure to an allergen to which the patient has previously been sensitized, but often no clear evidence of an allergic trigger can be identified.

TYPES AND PATHOGENESIS. Asthma has traditionally been divided into two basic types—extrinsic (allergic, reagin-mediated, atopic) and intrinsic (idiosyncratic)—to which was added a third, mixed pattern in which both intrinsic and extrinsic factors are operative. However, it is probably more useful to classify the types of asthma according to the principal stimuli that provoke the attacks. The listing of the various groups shown in Table 16–2 presents the precipitating factors and the possible mechanisms involved in each group.[60]

Table 16–2. TYPES OF ASTHMA

Types of Asthma	Precipitating Factors*	Mechanism or Immunologic Reaction
Atopic (allergic)	Specific allergens	Type I (IgE) immune reaction
Nonreaginic	Respiratory tract infection	Unknown; hyperreactive airways
Aspirin sensitive	Aspirin	Decreased prostaglandins, increased leukotrienes
Occupational	Chemical challenge	Types I and III immune reactions
Allergic bronchopulmonary aspergillosis	Antigen (spores) challenge	Types I and III immune reactions

*All types may be precipitated by cold, stress, exercise. All have hypereactive airways.

The largest group is so-called *atopic* or *allergic asthma.* In these patients the disease is triggered by environmental antigens such as dusts, pollens, animal dander, and foods, but potentially any antigen is implicated. A positive family history of atopy is common, and asthmatic attacks are often preceded by allergic rhinitis, urticaria, or eczema. Serum IgE levels are usually elevated. A skin test with the offending antigen results in an immediate wheal-and-flare reaction, and *it is now clear that this type of asthma is a classic example of Type I IgE-mediated hypersensitivity reaction.*[61] You will recall that exposure of presensitized IgE-coated mast cells to the same or cross-reacting antigen stimulates the release of chemical mediators from these cells. In the case of airborne antigens, the reaction occurs first on sensitized mast cells *on the mucosal surface*; the resultant mediator release opens the mucosal intercellular tight junctions, and enhances penetration of antigen to the more numerous submucosal mast cells. In addition, direct stimulation of *subepithelial vagal* (parasympathetic) *receptors* provokes reflex bronchoconstriction. As detailed on page 163, the mediators of IgE-triggered reactions include both primary and secondary mediators. Of the primary mediators, histamine causes bronchoconstriction by direct and cholinergic reflex actions, increases venular permeability, and increases bronchial secretions. It is probably important in the first few minutes of an asthmatic attack. Eosinophilic (ECF-A) and neutrophilic (NCF) chemotactic factors selectively attract eosinophils and neutrophils. The secondary mediators include (1) *leukotriene* C_4, D_4, *and* E_4,[62, 63] extremely potent mediators that cause prolonged bronchoconstriction as well as increased vascular permeability; (2) *prostaglandin* D_2 *(*PGD_2*)*, which elicits bronchoconstriction and vasodilation; and (3) *platelet activating factor (PAF)*, the acetyl glyceryl ether phosphocholine (AGEPC), which causes aggregation of platelets and release of histamine and serotonin from their granules. In addition, PAF has direct vasomotor and other inflammatory effects (p. 57).

It is now thought that these mediators produce an intense local bronchoconstriction and increased permeability, followed by a phase of chronic reactivity. The recruitment of platelets, leukocytes, and eosinophils by the chemotactic factors, and of humoral substances caused by the increased permeability, set the scene for further inflammatory responses after the initial IgE-mediated response.

The second large group is the *nonatopic* or *nonreaginic* variety of asthma, which is most frequently triggered by respiratory tract infection. Viruses (e.g., rhinovirus, parainfluenza virus) rather than bacteria are the most common provokers. A positive family history is uncommon, serum IgE levels are normal, and there are no other associated allergies. In these patients, skin tests are usually negative, and although hypersensitivity to microbial antigens may play a role, present theories place more stress on hyperirritability of the bronchial tree. It is thought that virus-induced inflammation of the respiratory mucosa lowers the threshold of the subepithelial vagal receptors to irritants, possibly by opening the mucosal tight junctions.

Aspirin-sensitive asthma is a rather fascinating type occurring in patients with recurrent rhinitis and nasal polyps. These individuals are exquisitely sensitive to very small doses of aspirin, and experience not only asthmatic attacks but also urticaria. It is probable that aspirin triggers asthma in these patients by inhibiting the cyclooxygenase pathway of arachidonic acid metabolism without affecting the lipoxygenase route, thus tipping the balance toward elaboration of the bronchoconstrictor leukotrienes (see Fig. 2–13, p. 55).

Occupational asthma is stimulated by fumes (epoxy resins, plastics), organic and chemical dusts (wood, cotton, platinum), gases (toluene), and other chemicals (formaldehyde, penicillin products).[64] Very minute quantities of chemicals are required to induce the attack, which usually occurs after repeated exposure. The mechanisms vary according to stimulus and include Type I IgE-mediated reactions, Type III immune complex responses, direct toxic reactions, and hypersensitivity responses of unknown origin.

Allergic bronchopulmonary aspergillosis[65] is a special but well-studied type of asthma caused by the spores of *Aspergillus fumigatus*. When challenged with antigen intradermally or by inhalation, these patients develop *both an immediate Type I IgE-induced reaction and a four- to six-hour Type III IgG-mediated response*. It is thus thought that Aspergillus-induced, IgE-mediated mast cell degranulation causes bronchoconstriction and increased vascular permeability. The latter allows anti-Aspergillus antibodies to enter bronchi, combine with antigen, form immune complexes, and trigger inflammation and pulmonary damage.

Asthma can also be precipitated by cold, exercise, and emotional stress, but it is likely that these are nonspecific factors producing a spasm in bronchi that have been rendered hyperirritable by allergy or infection. Indeed, *an important feature of patients with asthma of all types—immunologic or otherwise—is the hyperreactivity of the airways to nonspecific irritants and bronchoconstrictor agents*. The airways of asthmatics, for example, become obstructed after inhalation of histamine at under 1/100th of the concentration required to cause bronchoconstriction in normals.[66] Several explanations have been advanced to explain such hyperirritability, including a decrease in the firing threshold of vagal (cholinergic, bronchoconstrictor) receptors in the subepithelial layer, or conversely an insensitivity to beta-adrenergic (bronchodilator) stimulation. Neither of these explanations accounts for all the findings in asthmatic patients and so the search goes on.

The role of *eosinophils* in asthma deserves brief mention. These cells are attracted by chemotactic factors (ECF-A) released by mast cells, and apparently serve to inhibit the allergic reaction by releasing enzymes capable of inactivating histamine and leukotrienes. Eosinophils also release the basic major protein (MBP) of their granules, and MBP has been shown to be toxic to respiratory epithelium and to accumulate in the lungs and sputum of patients with asthma.[67]

MORPHOLOGY. The morphologic changes in asthma have been described principally in patients dying of status asthmaticus, but it appears that the pathology in nonfatal cases is similar. Grossly, the lungs are overdistended because of overinflation, and there may be small areas of atelectasis. **The most striking macroscopic finding is occlusion of bronchi and bronchioles by thick, tenacious mucous plugs.** About 20% of patients also have small areas of saccular bronchiectasis, most commonly in the upper lobe. Histologically, the mucous plugs contain whorls of shed epithelium, which give rise to the well-known **Curschmann's spirals.** Numerous eosinophils and **Charcot-Leyden crystals** are present; the latter are collections of crystalloids made up of eosinophil membrane protein. The other characteristic histologic findings of asthma include (1) thickening of the basement membrane of bronchial epithelium; (2) edema and an inflammatory infiltrate in the bronchial walls, with prominence of eosinophils, which form 5 to 50% of the cellular infiltrate; (3) an increase in size of the submucosal mucous glands; and (4) hypertrophy of the bronchial wall muscle, a reflection of the prolonged vasoconstriction (Fig. 16–23). Emphysematous changes sometimes occur, and if chronic bacterial infection has supervened, bronchitis (described above) may appear.

CLINICAL COURSE. On the basis of the previously described changes, one can anticipate that an attack of asthma is characterized by the onset of respiratory difficulty with wheezing respiration, made particularly distinctive by prolongation of the expiratory phase. The victim labors to get air into his lungs and then cannot get it out, so that there is progressive hyperinflation of the lungs. The air gets trapped behind the mucous plugs. In the classic case, the acute attack lasts one to several hours and is followed by prolonged coughing; the raising of copious mucous secretions provides considerable relief of the respiratory difficulty. In some patients, these symptoms persist at a low level all the time. In its most severe form, *status asthmaticus*, the severe acute paroxysm persists for days and even weeks and, under these circumstances, the ventilatory function may be so impaired as to cause severe cyanosis and even death. The clinical diagnosis is aided by demon-

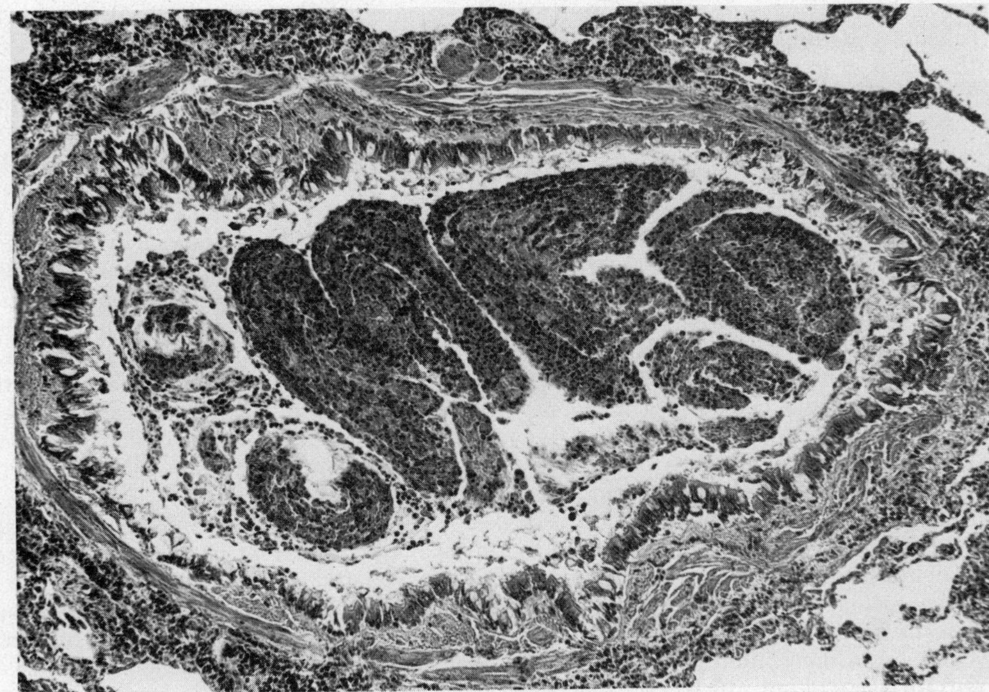

Figure 16–23. Bronchial asthma. A small bronchus containing plugs of mucin secretion as well as inflammatory cells within lumen. Note hypertrophy of mucin-secreting lining cells, hypertrophy of smooth muscle, and the peribronchial inflammatory infiltrate.

stration of an elevated eosinophil count in the peripheral blood and the finding of eosinophils, Curschmann's spirals, and Charcot-Leyden crystals in the sputum.

In the usual case, with intervals of freedom from respiratory difficulty, the disease is more discouraging and disabling than lethal. With appropriate therapy to relieve the attacks, these patients are able to maintain a productive life. However, in the more severe forms, the progressive hyperinflation may eventually produce emphysema. Superimposed bacterial infections may lead to chronic persistent bronchitis, bronchiectasis, or pneumonia that may ultimately cause death. In other cases, cor pulmonale and heart failure eventually develop.

BRONCHIECTASIS

Bronchiectasis is a chronic necrotizing infection of the bronchi and bronchioles leading to or associated with abnormal dilation of these airways. It is manifested clinically by cough, fever, and the expectoration of copious amounts of foul-smelling, purulent sputum. To be considered bronchiectasis, the dilatation should be permanent, since reversible bronchial dilatation often accompanies viral and bacterial pneumonia. In the latter case, the radiologic appearance may be the same as in bronchiectasis, but the changes are completely reversible within six weeks. Bronchiectasis has many origins and usually develops in association with the following conditions:

1. *Bronchial obstruction.* Common causes are tumor, foreign bodies, and occasionally mucous impaction. Under these conditions, the bronchiectasis is localized to the obstructed lung segment. Bronchiectasis can also complicate diffuse obstructive airway diseases, most commonly atopic asthma and chronic bronchitis.
2. *Congenital or hereditary conditions.* These include:
   a. *Congenital bronchiectasis.* This is caused by a defect in the development of bronchi and usually affects a whole lobe or entire lung.
   b. *Cystic fibrosis* (p. 493). Widespread severe bronchiectasis in this condition is a reflection of the generalized defects in exocrine gland secretion.
   c. *Intralobar sequestration of the lung.* In this condition a part of the lung, usually in the left lower lobe, is supplied with blood not by a branch of the pulmonary artery but directly from one of the systemic arteries. The affected part becomes infected and its airways dilate. Characteristically, the airways in the sequestered bronchiectatic lung tissue are separate from those in the adjacent normal lung.
   d. *Immunodeficiency states* (p. 205). These are associated with heightened susceptibility to repeated bacterial infections and localized or diffuse bronchiectasis.
   e. *Kartagener's and the immotile cilia syndromes.* A fascinating explanation for bronchiectasis is that which accounts for a curious disease called *Kartagener's syndrome* (bronchiectasis, sinusitis, and

situs inversus). Patients with this syndrome have a *defect in ciliary motility, most commonly associated with absent or irregular dynein arms*—the structures on the microtubular doublets of cilia that are responsible for the generation of ciliary movement (Fig. 16–24).[68, 69] The lack of ciliary activity interferes with bacterial clearance, predisposes the sinuses and bronchi to infection, and also affects cell motility during embryogenesis, resulting in the situs inversus. Males with this condition tend to be infertile, owing to ineffective motility of the sperm tail. About half the patients with defective cilia have no situs inversus. The immotile cilia syndrome is inherited as an autosomal recessive gene and occurs at a frequency of 1:20,000 among whites.

3. *Necrotizing pneumonia*. Bronchiectasis occasionally follows necrotizing or suppurative pneumonias caused by the tubercle bacillus or staphylococcal or mixed infections; in past years it was considered to be a sequel to childhood necrotizing infections complicating measles, whooping cough, and influenza. This form of *postinfective bronchiectasis*, however, is no longer common in the United States.

ETIOLOGY AND PATHOGENESIS. *Obstruction* and *infection* are the most frequent influences associated with bronchiectasis, and it is likely that both factors are necessary for the development of the full-fledged bronchiectatic lesions. After bronchial obstruction (such as by tumors or foreign bodies), air is resorbed from the airways distal to the obstruction, with resultant atelectasis. With atelectasis, the elastic forces within the lobe disappear, so that the airways are no longer taut and they "relax," resulting in dilatation of the walls of those airways that are patent. It is thought that these changes are reversible and that an airless lobe may reexpand. *However, the changes will become irreversible* (1) *if the obstruction persists,* especially during periods of growth, because the airways will not be able to develop normally; and (2) *if there is added infection.* Infection plays a role in the pathogenesis of bronchiectasis in two ways: (a) it produces bronchial wall inflammation, weakening, and further dilatation; and (b) the extensive bronchial and bronchiolar damage causes endobronchial obliteration, with atelectasis distal to the obliteration and subsequent bronchiectasis around atelectatic areas, as described above.

These mechanisms—infection and obstruction—are most readily apparent in the severe form of bronchiectasis associated with cystic fibrosis of the pancreas. In these patients, there is squamous metaplasia of the normal respiratory epithelium with impairment of normal mucociliary action, infection, necrosis of the bronchial and bronchiolar walls, and subsequent bronchiectasis. In younger children, the changes take the form of bronchiolitis (occlusion of the bronchioles by granulation tissue), but older children tend to develop full-blown bronchiectasis.

A variety of organisms can be cultured from bronchiectatic lungs, including staphylococci, streptococci, pneumococci, and enteric organisms as well as anaerobic and microaerophilic organisms. Which of these are pathogenic in any one case and which are saprophytic invaders is unknown. *Hemophilus influenzae* is thought by some to play an important role in the continued infection in bronchiectasis, as it seems to in chronic bronchitis.

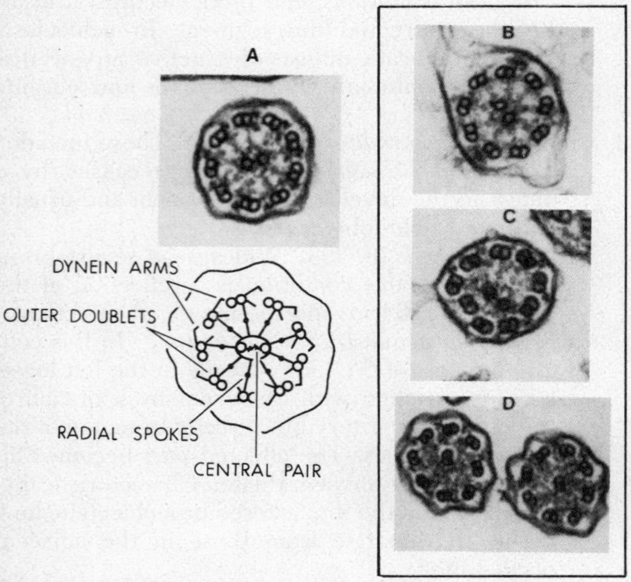

Figure 16–24. Ultrastructural abnormalities of cilia in immotile cilia syndromes. *A,* Normal cilium. *B,* Patient with Kartagener's syndrome. The dynein arms are absent. *C,* Radial spoke defect. *D,* transposition of microtubules. There are only eight peripheral doublets. The other peripheral pair of tubules has been transposed to center of cilium. The central pair is absent. Patients B, C, and D have immotile or poorly motile cilia. (From Katzenstein, A-L. A., and Askin, F. B.: Surgical Pathology of Non-Neoplastic Lung Disease. Philadelphia, W. B. Saunders Co., 1982, p. 397. Courtesy of Dr. Jennifer Sturgess et al., Toronto, Ontario, Canada.)

MORPHOLOGY. Bronchiectatic involvement of the lungs usually affects the lower lobes bilaterally, particularly those air passages that are most vertical. When tumors or aspiration of foreign bodies leads to bronchiectasis, the involvement may be sharply localized to a single segment of the lungs. Usually the most severe involvements are found in the more distal bronchi and bronchioles. **The airways are dilated, sometimes up to four times normal size.** These dilatations may produce long, tubelike enlargements **(cylindroid bronchiectasis)** or, in other cases, may cause **fusiform** or even sharply saccular distention **(saccular bronchiectasis).**

Characteristically, the bronchi and bronchioles are sufficiently dilated so that they can be followed, on gross examination, directly out to the pleural surfaces. By contrast, in the normal lung, the bronchioles cannot be followed by ordinary gross dissection beyond a point 2 to 3 cm removed from the pleural surfaces. The lumina of the affected bronchi are filled with a suppurative exudate that, when removed, exposes edematous, frequently ulcerated mucosa. In more severe involvements, the dilatation may produce an almost cystic pattern to the cut surface of the lung (Fig. 16–25*A*).

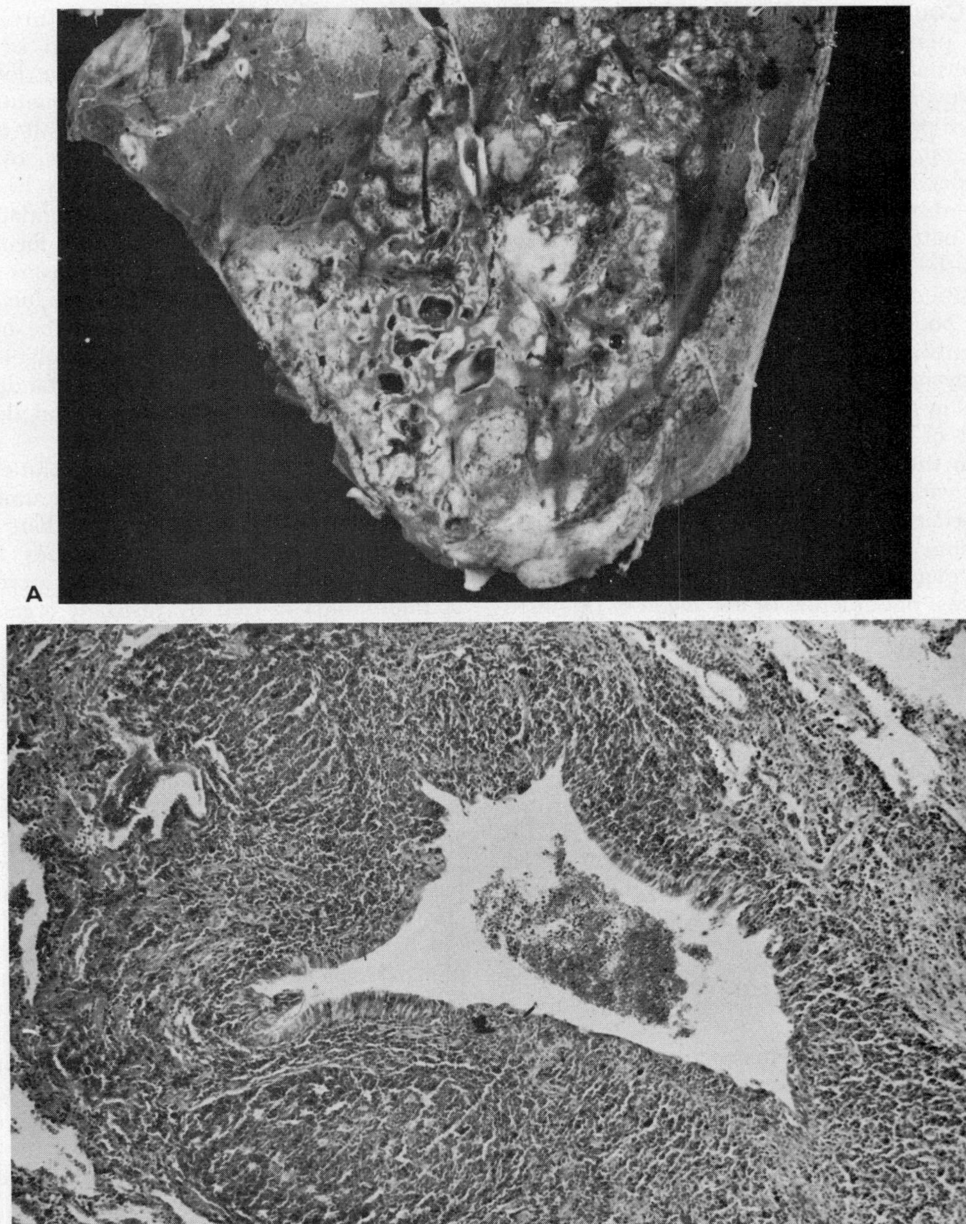

Figure 16–25. Bronchiectasis. *A,* Cut surface of basal region, showing transected, markedly distended peripheral bronchi. *B,* Bronchus is surrounded by an intense leukocytic infiltrate, and lining epithelium is eroded at 9 to 12 o'clock.

In clinically significant cases, the lung parenchyma shows patchy emphysema and atelectasis. When the infection extends to the pleura, it evokes a fibrinous or suppurative pleuritis.

The histologic findings vary with the activity and chronicity of the disease. In the full-blown, active case, there is an intense acute and chronic inflammatory exudation within the walls of the bronchi and bronchioles, associated with desquamation of the lining epithelium and extensive areas of necrotizing ulceration (Fig. 16–25*B*). There may be pseudostratification of the columnar cells or squamous metaplasia of the remaining epithelium. In some instances, the necrosis completely destroys the bronchial or bronchiolar walls and forms a lung abscess. Fibrosis of the bronchial and bronchiolar walls and peribronchiolar fibrosis develop in the more chronic cases.

When healing occurs, there may be complete regeneration of the lining epithelium. However, there usually has been so much injury that abnormal dilatation and scarring persist. In such healed cases, it may be impossible to distinguish preexistent bronchiectasis from bronchogenic congenital cysts.

CLINICAL COURSE. The clinical manifestations consist of severe, persistent cough; expectoration of foul-smelling, sometimes bloody sputum; and dyspnea and orthopnea in severe cases. A systemic febrile reaction may occur when powerful pathogens are present. These symptoms are often episodic and are precipitated by upper respiratory infections or the introduction of new pathogenic agents. In the full-blown case, the cough is paroxysmal in nature. Such paroxysms are particularly frequent when the patient rises in the morning, and the changes in position lead to drainage into the bronchi of the collected pools of pus. In the full-blown case, obstructive ventilatory insufficiency leads to marked dyspnea and cyanosis. Clubbing of the fingers sometimes develops in these patients.

The effect of bronchiectasis on life span is quite variable. When the disease is acquired in adult life, it is compatible with fairly long survival. However, it materially shortens life in young people with cystic fibrosis or immune deficiency. These cases with an early onset may develop one of several complications, such as lung abscesses, pneumonia, or extension of the infection through the pleura to produce bronchopleural fistulas and exudative inflammation of the pleural cavity, known as empyema. In some cases, small infected thrombi break off and are carried to the brain, producing metastatic abscesses or meningitis. Amyloidosis is a further hazard in cases of long duration. When the disease is widespread in the lungs, chronic fibrosis may encroach on the pulmonary vascular bed and, in the course of years, may lead to the development of cor pulmonale. All these complications are relatively uncommon.

PULMONARY INFECTIONS

Respiratory infections are more frequent than infections of any other organ and account for the largest number of workdays lost in the general population. The vast majority are upper respiratory infections caused by viruses, but infections of the lung (pneumonias, bronchopneumonias, lung abscesses, and tuberculosis—viral, mycoplasmal, bacterial, and fungal) still account for an enormous amount of morbidity and rank among the major immediate causes of death.[70] Many of these infections have been described in detail in Chapter 8. Here we shall review only those aspects of the pathology of pulmonary infections that need further discussion.

BACTERIAL PNEUMONIA

Bacterial invasion of the lung parenchyma evokes exudative solidification (consolidation) of the pulmonary tissue known as bacterial pneumonia. Many variables, such as the specific etiologic agent, the host reaction, and the extent of involvement, determine the precise form of pneumonia. Thus, classification may be made according to etiologic agent (e.g., pneumococcal or staphylococcal pneumonia), the nature of the host reaction (suppurative, fibrinous, and so forth), or the anatomic distribution of the disease (lobular [bronchopneumonia], lobar, or interstitial pneumonia). The anatomic classification is often difficult to apply in the individual case, since patterns often overlap considerably. The lobular involvement may become confluent to produce virtually total lobar consolidation; in contrast, effective antibiotic therapy for any form of pneumonia may limit involvement to a subtotal consolidation. Moreover, the same organisms may produce lobular pneumonia in one patient, whereas in the more vulnerable individual a full-blown lobar involvement develops. Most important, from the clinical standpoint, are identification of the causative agent and determination of the extent of disease.

PATHOGENESIS. Although antibiotics have reduced the mortality rate from bacterial pneumonia, the disorder remains one of the major immediate causes of death in the terminal phase of many diseases. In addition, the use of antibiotics has resulted in an increased incidence of pneumonia caused by resistant organisms, which is usually difficult to treat and cure.

Before we describe the various types of pneumonia, it is useful to discuss some of the pathogenetic factors that pertain to all types and that help to explain the frequent development of pneumonia in susceptible groups of patients. Recall first that the normal lung is free of bacteria and possesses a number of potent defense mechanisms that clear or destroy any bacteria inhaled with air or fortuitously deposited in the airway passages (p. 708). These defense mechanisms include (1) the filtering function of the nasopharynx, (2) the mucociliary action of the lower air passages, and (3) phagocytosis and elimination by the alveolar macrophages. In addition, immune mechanisms play a role in eliminating bacteria that reach the alveoli either through respiration or via the bloodstream. *Thus, pneumonia may result whenever these defense mechanisms are impaired or whenever the resistance of the host in general is lowered.*

The clearing mechanisms can be interfered with by many factors such as the following:

1. *Loss or suppression of the cough reflex*, as a result of coma, anesthesia, neuromuscular disorders, drugs, or chest pain. This may lead to *aspiration* of gastric contents.

2. *Injury to the mucociliary apparatus*, by either impairment of ciliary function or destruction of ciliated epithelium. Cigarette smoke, inhalation of hot or corrosive gases, viral diseases, and genetic disturbances (e.g., the immotile cilia syndrome) all have this effect.

3. *Interference with the phagocytic or bactericidal action of alveolar macrophages*. Many factors have been shown to have this effect, including alcohol, tobacco, anoxia, and oxygen intoxication.

4. *Pulmonary congestion and edema.* The mechanism by which this interferes with the clearing action is not known, but edema is one of the most common predispositions to terminal bronchopneumonia in pa-

tients with congestive heart failure or in debilitated patients with hypostatic pulmonary edema.

5. *Accumulation of secretions* in conditions such as cystic fibrosis and bronchial obstruction.

Factors that affect resistance in general include chronic diseases, immunologic deficiency, treatment with immunosuppressive agents, leukopenia, and unusually virulent infections.

Several other points need to be emphasized. One is the frequency with which one type of pneumonia predisposes to another, especially in debilitated patients. It is known, for example, that the most common cause of death in serious influenza epidemics is bacterial pneumonia. It is likely that viral diseases predispose to pneumonia by affecting both the clearing mechanism and the host's general defense and immune mechanisms. Second, although the portal of entry for most pneumonias is the respiratory tract, hematogenous spread from one focus to other foci can occur, and secondary seeding of the lungs may be difficult to distinguish from primary pneumonia. Finally, many patients with chronic diseases acquire terminal pneumonias while hospitalized. Thus, one must keep in mind the potential risks of nosocomial infection: bacteria common to the hospital environment may have acquired resistance to antibiotics, opportunities for spread are increased, invasive procedures such as catheterizations and injections are common, and bacteria may contaminate apparatus used in respiratory care units.

Bronchopneumonia (Lobular Pneumonia)

Patchy consolidation of the lung is the dominant characteristic of bronchopneumonia. This parenchymal infection usually represents an extension of a preexisting bronchitis or bronchiolitis. It is an extremely common disease that tends to occur in the more vulnerable two extremes of life—infancy and old age. In the young, there is little previous experience with pathogenic organisms, rendering these patients susceptible to organisms of even low virulence. Resistance likewise falls in the aged, particularly in those already suffering from some serious disorder. Bronchopneumonia thus frequently provides the period at the end of a long sentence of progressive heart failure or disseminated tumor. On this account, it is a common finding on postmortem examinations.

Etiology. Although virtually any pathogen may produce these lung infections, the common agents are staphylococci, streptococci, pneumococci, *Hemophilus influenzae*, *Pseudomonas aeruginosa*, and the coliforms. Fungi (particularly Candida, Aspergillus, and Mucor) are sometimes the responsible agents, particularly in the predisposed or immunocompromised patient.

Morphology. Foci of bronchopneumonia consist of consolidated areas of acute suppurative inflammation. The consolidation may be patchily distributed through one lobe but is more often multilobar and frequently bilateral and basal, because of the tendency for secretions to gravitate into the lower lobes. Often, these areas are more easily palpated than visualized at postmortem examination. Well-developed lesions are slightly elevated, dry, granular, gray-red to yellow, and poorly delimited at their margins. They vary in size up to 3 to 4 cm in diameter (Fig. 16–26). Confluence of these foci occurs in the more florid instances, producing the appearance of total lobar consolidation. When caused by such pyogenic organisms as staphylococci, small abscesses can be seen.

Histologically, the reaction usually comprises a suppurative exudate that fills the bronchi, bronchioles, and adjacent alveolar spaces (Figs. 16–27 and 16–28). Neutrophils are

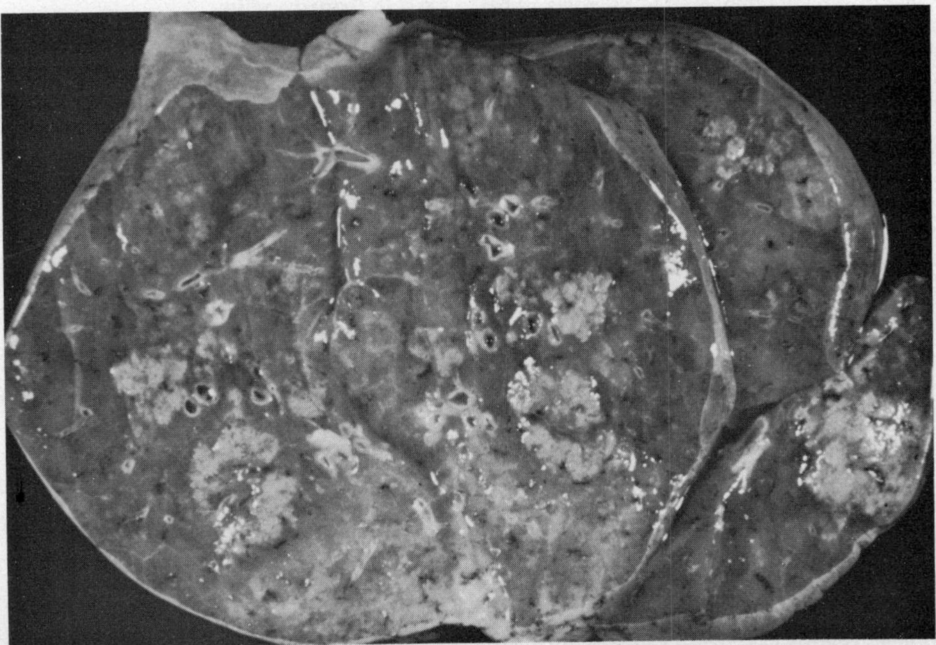

Figure 16–26. Bronchopneumonia. Foci of consolidation appear pale and gray.

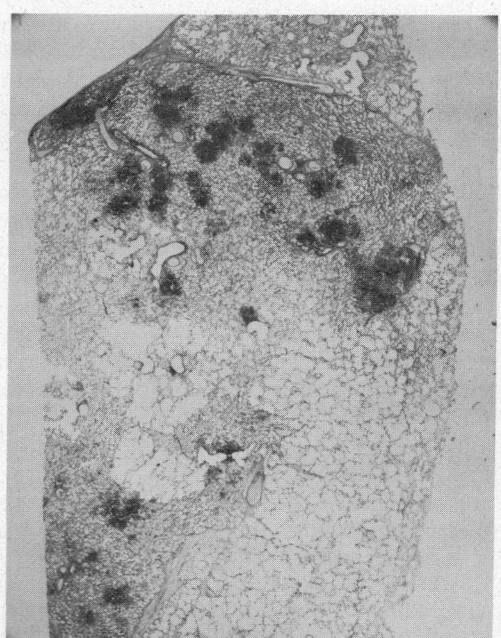

Fig. 16–27

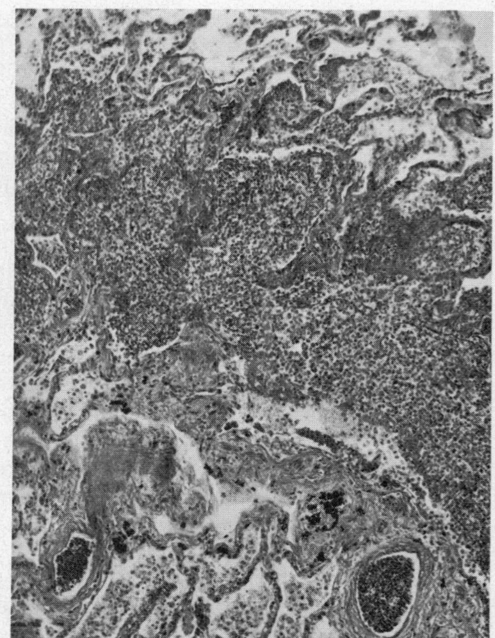

Fig. 16–28

Figure 16–27. Bronchopneumonia. Very low-power view of a large histologic section to illustrate patchiness of inflammatory reaction.

Figure 16–28. Bronchopneumonia. Histologic detail of exudative consolidation of focus of inflammation.

dominant in this exudation. Generally it is difficult to identify bacteria histologically. This standard pattern of reaction may be modified by a number of variables. Any blood disorder that lowers the white cell count, such as leukemia or agranulocytosis, or any influence that suppresses the immune response, such as hypo- or agammaglobulinemia or steroid or immunosuppressive therapy, may render the patient particularly vulnerable to bacterial or mycotic growth, and may permit bacterial overgrowth within the areas of exudation. Extremely aggressive organisms may lead to necrosis of the central regions of the lung lesions, to produce abscesses. Organization of the exudate may yield masses of fibrous tissue that constitute permanent residuals. Under happier circumstances, the exudate resolves, restoring the lung to its former state.

Particularly in infancy, the bacterial bronchopneumonia may remain interstitial within the alveolar septa, to produce an inflammatory reaction confined to the alveolar walls with little exudate in the air spaces. (This interstitial pattern is typical for viral pneumonia.) **E. coli** and group B hemolytic streptococci are the most common causes for such a pattern.

CLINICAL COURSE. The clinical signs and symptoms of bronchopneumonia depend on the virulence of the invading agent and the extent of pneumonic involvement. The patient, usually elderly, has a temperature of 38° to 39.5°C, along with cough, expectoration, and expiratory rales in one or more lobes. Often there is a previous history of confinement to bed, malnutrition, some underlying serious disorder, aspiration of gastric contents, or an upper respiratory infection. Respiratory difficulty may be present but is usually not prominent. When the pneumonia is caused by antibiotic-sensitive organisms, infection is readily controlled in patients not already mortally ill from some other cause.

The complications of bronchopneumonia are (1) the formation of lung abscesses; (2) spread to the pleural cavities, producing empyema; (3) spread to the pericardial cavity, producing suppurative pericarditis; or (4) the development of bacteremia with metastatic abscess formation in other organs and tissues in the body.

Lobar Pneumonia

This is an acute bacterial infection of a large portion of a lobe or of an entire lobe, which tends to occur at any age but is relatively uncommon in infancy and in late life. Males are affected more often than females in the ratio of about 3 or 4 to 1. Classic lobar pneumonia is now encountered much less often, owing to the effectiveness with which antibiotics abort these infections and prevent the development of full-blown lobar consolidation.

ETIOLOGY. Ninety to 95% of all lobar pneumonias are caused by pneumococci. Most common are types 1, 3, 7, and 2. Type 3 causes a particularly virulent form of lobar pneumonia. Occasionally, *Klebsiella pneumoniae*, staphylococci, streptococci, *Hemophilus influenzae*, and (in this day of antibiotic resistance) some of the gram-negatives, such as the Pseudomonas and Proteus bacilli, are also responsible for this lobar distribution of involvement.

PATHOGENESIS. The most common portal of entry is the air passages. The pathogenesis of a lobar distribution appears merely to be a function of the virulence of the organism and the vulnerability of the host. Heavy contamination by virulent pathogens may evoke this pattern in healthy adults, whereas organisms of lower virulence may accomplish the same in the predisposed patient. In lobar pneumonia there is more extensive exudation that leads to spread through the pores of Kohn. Moreover, the copious mucoid encapsulation produced by the pneumococci protects the organisms against immediate phagocytosis, and thus favors their spread.

MORPHOLOGY. The histologic changes are presented first, since they make the gross alterations understandable.

Lobar pneumonia consists, in essence, of a widespread fibrinosuppurative consolidation of large areas and even whole lobes of the lung. In its evolution, the pneumonic involvement follows the basic pattern of all inflammations and begins with serous exudation and accompanying vascular engorgement, followed by a fibrinocellular exudation, culminating ultimately in either resolution of the exudate or, less happily, its organization.

Four stages of the inflammatory response have classically been described: congestion, red hepatization, gray hepatization, and resolution. But present-day effective antibiotic therapy frequently telescopes or halts the progression, so that often at autopsy the anatomic changes do not conform to the older classic stages.

The first **stage of congestion** represents the developing bacterial infection and lasts for about 24 hours (and thus is rarely seen histologically). It is characterized by vascular engorgement, intra-alveolar fluid with few neutrophils, and often the presence of numerous bacteria. Grossly, the involved lobe is heavy, boggy, red, and subcrepitant.

The **stage of red hepatization** that follows is characterized by increasing numbers of neutrophils and the precipitation of fibrin to fill the alveolar spaces (Fig. 16–29). The massive confluent exudation obscures the pulmonary architecture. Extravasation of red cells causes the coloration seen on gross examination. In many areas, the fibrin strands stream from one alveolus through the pores of Kohn into the adjacent alveolus. The white cells contain engulfed bacteria. An overlying fibrinous or fibrinosuppurative pleuritis is almost invariably present. On gross examination, the lobe now appears distinctly red, firm, and airless with a liver-like consistency, hence the term hepatization (Fig. 16–30).

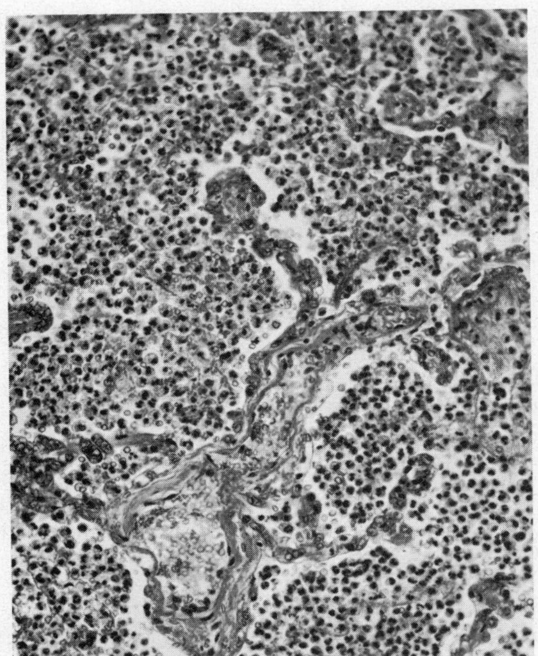

Figure 16–29. Lobar pneumonia. The stage of early red hepatization with congested septal capillaries and extensive white cell exudation into alveoli. Fibrin nets have not yet formed.

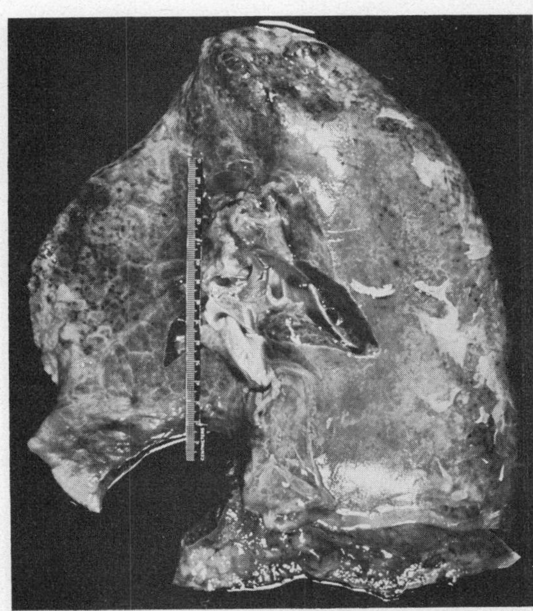

Figure 16–30. Lobar pneumonia. The stage of red hepatization. Lung is viewed from external aspect to show voluminous lower lobe, "plaster cast" of pleural cavity, and fibrinosuppurative pleuritis.

The **stage of gray hepatization** follows with a continuing accumulation of fibrin associated with the progressive disintegration of inflammatory white cells and red cells. This exudate, composed of deteriorating white cells, fibrin, and red cells, contracts somewhat to yield a clear zone adjacent to the alveolar walls. In the usual case, the alveolar septa are preserved. The pleural reaction of fibrin and white cells at this phase is more advanced. Sometimes, when the bacterial infection extends into the pleural cavity, the intrapleural suppuration produces what is known as **empyema.** The progressive disintegration of red cells and the persistence of fibrinosuppurative exudate gives the gross appearance of a grayish-brown, dry surface (Fig. 16–31).

The final **stage of resolution,** which in untreated cases occurs at eight to ten days, follows in the great preponderance of cases with a favorable outcome. The consolidated exudate within the alveolar spaces undergoes progressive enzymic digestion to produce a granular, semifluid debris that is either resorbed, ingested by macrophages, or coughed up. In such favorable cases, the normal lung parenchyma is restored to its normal state. The pleural reaction may similarly resolve, but more often it undergoes organization, leaving fibrous thickening or permanent adhesions.

Many **complications** may supervene during this classic evolution. (1) The type 3 pneumococcus and the Klebsiella bacillus characteristically produce an **abundant mucinous secretion,** so that on cut section stringy, turbid exudate clings to the knife and is readily scraped off. (2) These same organisms and the staphylococci frequently cause **abscess formations,** producing foci of necrosis in the otherwise solidified lung substance. (3) **Organization of the exudate**

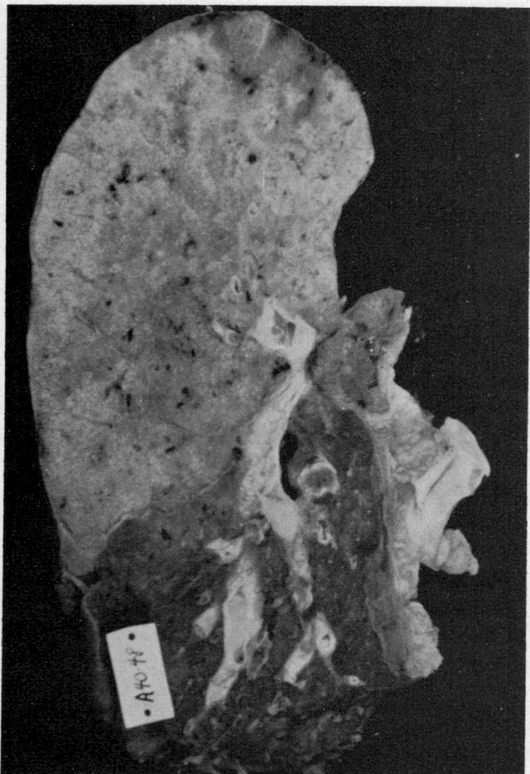

Figure 16–31. Lobar pneumonia of left upper lobe. The stage of gray hepatization with fairly sharp delimitation of pneumonic process at interlobar fissure.

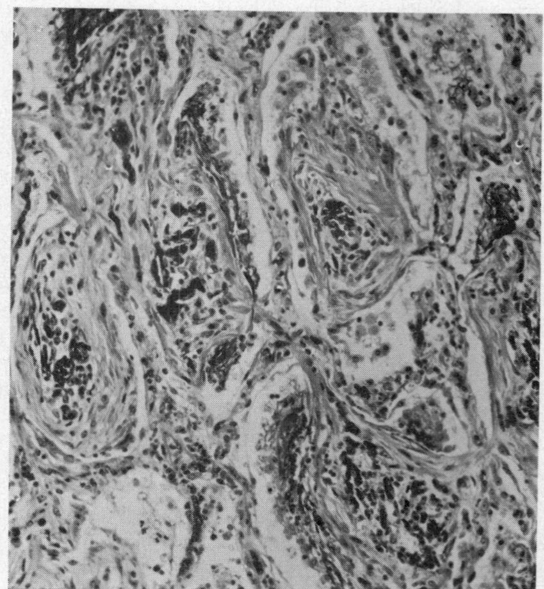

Figure 16–32. Organization of lobar pneumonia. Alveolar spaces are virtually filled with connective tissue that can be seen in areas to be streaming through pores of Kohn.

may convert the lung into a solid tissue (Fig. 16–32). (4) **Bacteremic dissemination** to the heart valves, pericardium, brain, kidneys, spleen, and joints may cause metastatic abscesses, endocarditis, meningitis, or suppurative arthritis.

CLINICAL COURSE. In the classic pattern, the pneumococcus attacks otherwise healthy adults 30 to 50 years of age, whereas type 3 and *Klebsiella pneumoniae* occur most often in the elderly, diabetics, and chronic alcoholics. In all, the onset of the disease is sudden, with malaise, chills, and fever. Cough appears with expectoration of at first a slightly turbid, watery sputum indicative of the stage of congestion, followed by a frankly purulent, hemorrhagic, so-called "rusty" sputum characteristic of the stage of red hepatization. The temperature elevation is very marked, frequently up to 40° or 41°C, and this elevation is usually maintained during the initial four to seven days of the full-blown classic stages of consolidation if treatment is not instituted. Chills are characteristic and sometimes so severe that they actually make the bed shake. These chills are presumed to represent episodes of bacteremia, and thus mark the most favorable time to take blood cultures. If the causative organism is the type 3 pneumococcus or Klebsiella bacillus, the sputum has the same tenacious, mucinous quality as does the exudate in the lungs. Shortness of breath, orthopnea, and cyanosis may appear when there has been encroachment upon the vital capacity of the lung parenchyma. The fibrinosuppurative pleuritis is accompanied by pleuritic pain and pleural friction rub.

The physical findings vary with the stage of pneumonia. Within the first few days, limitation of breath sounds and fine crepitant rales herald the development of the stage of congestion. Two or three days after onset, more fully developed dullness, increased tactile and vocal fremitus, and bronchial breath sounds reflect the solidification of the lung. As resolution occurs, moist rales reappear, the dullness diminishes, and the bronchial breath sounds and tactile and vocal fremitus gradually subside. The characteristic radiologic appearance is that of a radiopaque, usually well-circumscribed lobe.

This classic progressive symptom complex is, however, totally modified by the administration of antibiotics. Treated patients may be relatively afebrile with few clinical signs 48 to 72 hours after the initiation of antibiotics. For this reason, the classic "crisis" of lobar pneumonia, in which the temperature suddenly breaks and begins to fall, along with improvement in the patient's clinical condition, is now rarely encountered.

The identification of the organism and the determination of its antibiotic sensitivity are the keystones to appropriate therapy. Less than 10% of patients with lobar pneumonia now succumb and, in most such instances, death may be attributed either to a complication such as empyema, meningitis, endocarditis, or pericarditis or to some predisposing influence such as debility or chronic alcoholism.

PNEUMONIA IN IMMUNOCOMPROMISED HOST

The appearance of a pulmonary infiltrate and signs of infection (e.g., fever) is fast becoming one of the most

Table 16–3. CAUSES OF PULMONARY INFILTRATES IN IMMUNOCOMPROMISED HOSTS

Diffuse Infiltrate	Focal Infiltrate
Common	***Common***
Cytomegalovirus	Gram-negative rods
Pneumocystis carinii	*Staphylococcus aureus*
Drug reaction	Aspergillus
	Malignancy
Uncommon	***Uncommon***
Bacteria	Cryptococcus
Aspergillus	Nocardia
Cryptococcus	Mucormycosis
Malignancy	*Pneumocystis carinii*
	Legionella pneumophila

Modified from Fanta, C. H., and Pennington, J. L.: Fever and new lung infiltrates in the immunocompromised host. Clin. Chest Med. 2:19, 1981.

common and serious complications of patients whose immune and defense systems are suppressed by disease, chemotherapy for organ transplants and tumors, or irradiation.[71] A wide variety of infectious agents, many of which rarely cause infection in normal hosts, can cause these pneumonias, and often more than one agent is involved.[72] Mortality from these opportunistic infections is as high as 60% in some series. Table 16–3 lists some of the agents according to their prevalence and to whether they cause local or diffuse pulmonary infiltrates. It is well to remember that such infiltrates may also be due to drug reactions or to involvement of the lung by tumor. The specific infections are discussed in Chapter 8, and their morphologic expressions are well described in Myerowitz's recent book.[73]

VIRAL AND MYCOPLASMA PNEUMONIA (PRIMARY ATYPICAL PNEUMONIA)

The term primary atypical pneumonia (PAP) is applied to an acute febrile respiratory disease characterized by inflammatory changes in the lungs, largely confined to alveolar septa and pulmonary interstitium. The term "atypical" denotes the lack of alveolar exudate, but a much more accurate designation is *interstitial pneumonitis*. In about 40% of cases, the etiology remains undetermined. The largest group of known etiology are caused by *Mycoplasma pneumoniae*,[74, 75] which, although endemic, may cause epidemics of PAP in populations living in crowded, inadequate conditions. Viruses cause the remaining cases of PAP of known etiology, including influenza types A and B, the respiratory syncytial viruses (RSV), and rhinoviruses. RSV is the most common cause of atypical pneumonia in infants, accounting for up to 30% of cases. Other agents that may cause a similar picture include the Coxsackie and ECHO viruses, rickettsiae (Q fever), Chlamydia (psittacosis), and occasionally the viruses of rubeola and varicella.

Any one of these agents may cause merely an upper respiratory infection, recognized as the common cold, or a more severe lower respiratory infection. The circumstances that favor such extension of the infection are often mysterious but include malnutrition, alcoholism, and underlying debilitating illnesses.

MORPHOLOGY. All causal agents produce essentially similar morphologic patterns. Because the mild cases recover, our understanding of the anatomic changes is necessarily based on the more severe, fatal expressions of these infections. The pneumonic involvement may be quite patchy or may involve whole lobes bilaterally or unilaterally. The affected areas are red-blue, congested, and subcrepitant. On section, there is a slight ooze of red, frothy fluid, but since most of the reaction is interstitial, little of the inflammatory exudate escapes on transection of the lung substance. There is no obvious consolidation such as is encountered in lobar pneumonia. The pleura is smooth, and pleuritis or pleural effusions are infrequent.

The histologic pattern, too, depends on the severity of the disease. Predominant is the interstitial nature of the inflammatory reaction, virtually localized within the walls of the alveoli. The alveolar septa are widened and edematous and usually have a mononuclear inflammatory infiltrate of lymphocytes, histiocytes, and occasionally plasma cells. In very acute cases, neutrophils may also be present. The alveoli may be free of exudate, but in many patients there are intra-alveolar proteinaceous material, a cellular exudate, and characteristically a pink hyaline membrane lining the alveolar walls, similar to that seen in hyaline membrane disease of infants (Fig. 16–33). These changes reflect **alveolar damage** similar to that seen diffusely in the adult respiratory distress syndrome (p. 714).

Superimposed bacterial infection modifies the histologic picture by causing ulcerative bronchitis and bronchiolitis, and may yield the anatomic changes already described under bacterial pneumonia. Subsidence of the disease is followed by reconstitution of the native architecture.

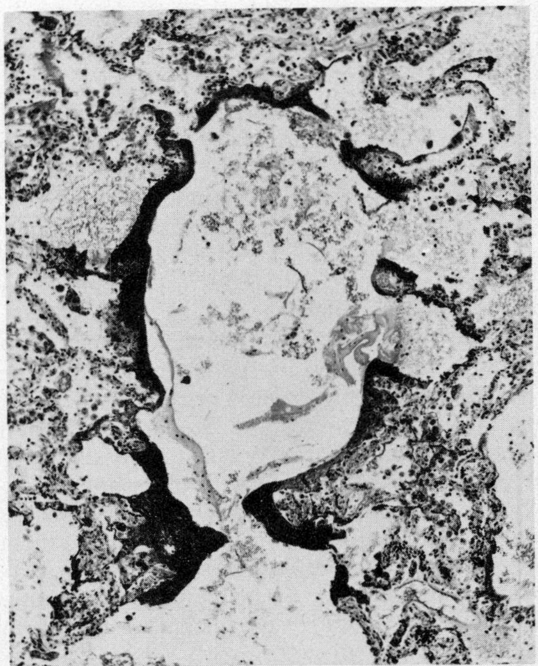

Figure 16–33. Primary atypical (viral) pneumonia with prominent hyaline membranes and interstitial inflammatory infiltration.

Some viruses such as herpes simplex, varicella, and adenovirus may be associated with necrosis of bronchial and alveolar epithelium and acute inflammation. Epithelial giant cells with intranuclear or intracytoplasmic inclusions may be present in cytomegalic inclusion disease. Other viruses produce cytopathic changes, as described in Chapter 8.

CLINICAL COURSE. As indicated, the clinical course is extremely varied. Many cases masquerade as severe upper respiratory infections or as "chest colds." Even cases with well-developed atypical pneumonia have few localizing symptoms. Cough may well be absent, and the major manifestations may consist only of fever, headache, muscle aches, and pains in the legs. Cough, when present, is characteristically dry, hacking, and unproductive of sputum. The edema and exudation are both strategically located to cause an alveolocapillary block and thus evoke symptoms out of proportion to the scanty physical findings. One of the useful laboratory aids in differentiating viral atypical pneumonia from the *M. pneumoniae* form is the detection of elevated cold agglutinin titers in the serum. These are present in 40% of patients with Mycoplasma and in 20% of adenovirus infections, and are absent in other viral pneumonias. Isolation of the causative agent, whether viral or Mycoplasma, requires fairly fastidious technical methods.

The ordinary sporadic form of the disease is usually mild with a low mortality rate, below 1%. However, interstitial pneumonia may assume epidemic proportions with intensified severity and greater mortality, as all too grimly documented in the highly fatal influenzal pandemics of 1915 and 1918. Secondary bacterial infection by staphylococci or streptococci is common in these situations.

LUNG ABSCESS

The term pulmonary abscess describes a local suppurative process within the lung characterized by necrosis of lung tissue. Lung abscesses may develop at any age and are especially frequent in young adults. Oropharyngeal surgical procedures, sinobronchial infections, dental sepsis, and bronchiectasis play important roles in their development. Males are affected somewhat more often than females.

ETIOLOGY AND PATHOGENESIS. Although under appropriate circumstances any pathogen may produce an abscess, the commonly isolated organisms include aerobic and anaerobic streptococci, *Staphylococcus aureus*, and a host of gram-negative organisms. Mixed infections occur very often because of the important causal role that inhalation of foreign material plays. *Anaerobic organisms* normally found in the oral cavity, including members of the Bacteroides, Fusobacterium, and Peptococcus species, are the exclusive isolates in about 60% of cases.[76, 77] The causative organisms are introduced by the following mechanisms:

1. *Aspiration of infective material* (the most frequent cause). This is particularly common in acute alcoholism, coma, anesthesia, sinusitis, gingivodental sepsis, and debilitation in which the cough reflexes are depressed. Aspiration of gastric contents is serious because the gastric acidity adds to the irritant role of the food particles, and, in the course of aspiration, mouth organisms are inevitably introduced.

2. *Antecedent primary bacterial infection.* Postpneumonic abscess formations are usually associated with *Staphylococcus aureus*, *Klebsiella pneumoniae*, and the type 3 pneumococcus. Fungus infections and bronchiectasis are additional antecedents to lung abscess formation.

3. *Septic embolism.* Infected emboli from thrombophlebitis in any portion of the systemic venous circulation or from vegetative bacterial endocarditis on the right side of the heart are trapped in the lung.

4. *Neoplasia.* Secondary infection is particularly common in the bronchopulmonary segment obstructed by a primary or secondary malignancy. This sequence is typical of bronchogenic carcinoma in which impaired drainage, distal atelectasis, and aspiration of blood and tumor fragments all contribute to the development of sepsis.

5. *Miscellaneous.* Direct traumatic penetrations of the lungs; spread of infections from a neighboring organ, such as suppuration in the esophagus, spine, subphrenic space, or pleural cavity; and hematogenous seeding of the lung by pyogenic organisms may all lead to lung abscess formation.

When all these causes are excluded, there are still many cases (25%) in which no reasonable basis for the abscess formation can be identified. These are referred to as *"primary cryptogenic"* lung abscesses.

MORPHOLOGY. Abscesses vary in diameter from a few millimeters to large cavities of 5 to 6 cm. They may affect any part of the lung and be single or multiple. Pulmonary abscesses due to aspiration are more common on the right (the more vertical main bronchus) and are most often single. Abscesses that develop in the course of pneumonia or bronchiectasis are usually multiple, basal, and diffusely scattered. Septic emboli and pyemic abscesses, by the haphazard nature of their genesis, are multiple and may affect any region of the lungs. Sometimes, solitary pulmonary abscesses occur in the subapical and axillary portions of the upper lobes and the apical portion of the lower lobes, particularly on the right. This distribution appears to be in conflict with the presumed aspiration theory of their pathogenesis. However, for postoperative patients remaining recumbent for long periods of time, dependent portions of the lungs are not the bases.

At the time of examination, the cavity may or may not be filled with suppurative debris, depending on the presence or absence of a communication with one of the air passages. When such communications exist, the contained exudate may be partially drained to create an air-containing cavity. Superimposed saprophytic infections are prone to flourish within the already necrotic debris of the abscess cavity. These alter the appearance because their proteolytic action provides a favorable soil for the primary pathogen, which then assumes an increased virulence to cause rapid spread of the infection. This sequence leads to large, fetid, green-black, multilocular cavities with poor margination, designated

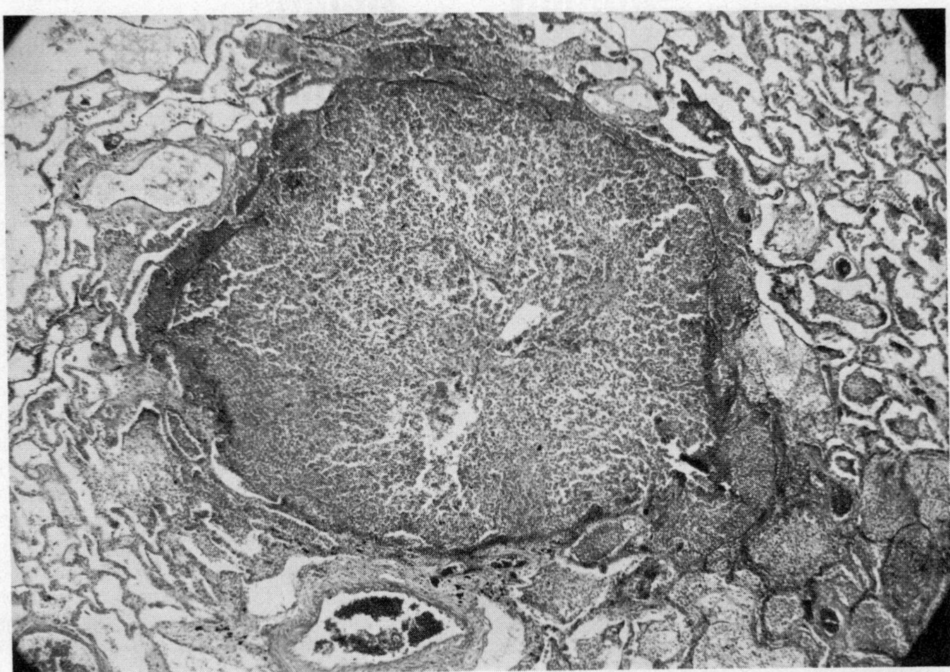

Figure 16–34. Pyemic lung abscess with complete destruction of underlying parenchyma within focus of involvement.

as **gangrene of the lung.** The **cardinal histologic change is suppurative destruction of the lung parenchyma within the central area of cavitation** (Fig. 16–34). In chronic cases, considerable fibroblastic proliferation produces a containing fibrous wall.

CLINICAL COURSE. The manifestations of pulmonary abscesses are much like those of bronchiectasis and are characterized principally by cough, fever, and copious amounts of foul-smelling purulent or sanguineous sputum. Characteristically, these patients have paroxysmal coughing as changes in position initiate sudden drainage of fluid exudate. If the abscess is solitary, respiratory difficulty may be minimal. Fever, chest pain, and weight loss are common. Clubbing of the fingers and toes may appear within a few weeks after onset of an abscess.

Diagnosis of this condition can only be suspected from the clinical findings and must be confirmed by roentgenography and bronchoscopy. Often the fluid levels can be demonstrated by x-rays. Whenever an abscess is discovered, it is important to suspect an underlying carcinoma, since these are present in 10 to 15% of cases.

The course of abscesses is quite variable. With antimicrobial therapy, over 75% resolve with no sequelae. For the remainder, the outlook depends entirely on the amount of lung tissue affected and the chronicity of the disease. If untreated, the process may cause invalidism of the patient through ventilatory malfunction. Complications include extension of the infection into the pleural cavity, the development of *brain abscesses* or *meningitis* from septic emboli, and (rarely) secondary amyloidosis.

PULMONARY TUBERCULOSIS

A general discussion of tuberculosis is on page 341. Here we shall only briefly describe the effects of this infection on the lungs.[78–80]

As indicated earlier, the overwhelming preponderance of tuberculous infections affect the lungs and, indeed, begin there. Pulmonary involvement is still the major cause of tuberculous morbidity and mortality. The prevention and control of these pulmonary infections accounts for tuberculosis being a relatively uncommon cause of death today, although a leading cause in 1900 in the United States. The present U.S. death rate from tuberculosis is about 2 per 100,000 population as compared with a death rate of 200 in 1900. Regrettably, in many parts of the world, underprivileged populations still suffer from death rates 20 times those of other industrialized nations.

Primary Pulmonary Tuberculosis

Except for the rare intestinal (bovine) tuberculosis, and the even more uncommon skin, oropharyngeal, and lymphoidal primary sites, the lungs are the usual location of primary infections. As detailed earlier (p. 342), the initial focus of primary infection is the *Ghon complex,* which consists of (1) a parenchymal subpleural lesion, either just above or just below the interlobar fissure between the upper and lower lobes; and (2) enlarged caseous lymph nodes draining the parenchymal focus (Fig. 16–35).

The course and fate of this initial infection are variable, but in most cases patients are asymptomatic

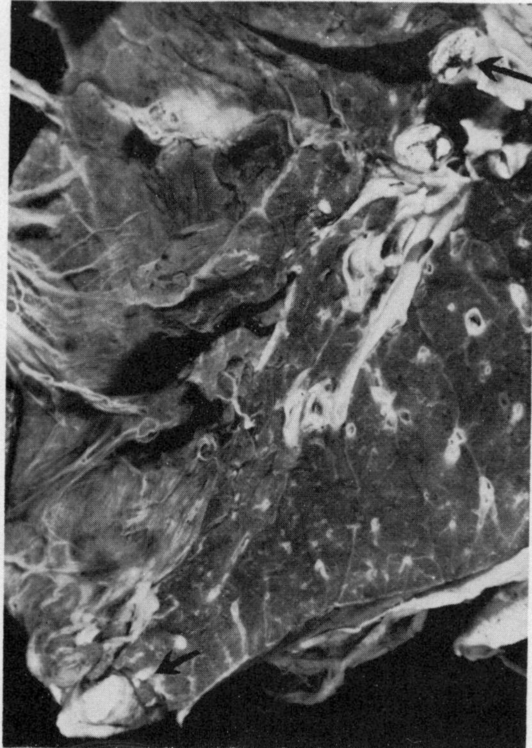

Figure 16–35. Primary pulmonary tuberculosis. Parenchymal focus of white caseation is present in lower left corner *(arrow),* and caseated lymph nodes of drainage can be seen in upper right *(arrow).*

and the lesions undergo fibrosis and calcification. Exceptionally, particularly in infants and children or immunodeficient adults, *tuberculous pneumonia or miliary tuberculosis* may follow a primary infection. However, even in these progressive cases the infection may be halted at any stage, followed by fibrous encapsulation, scarring, and calcification, leaving only fibrocalcific residues.

Secondary Pulmonary Tuberculosis (Chronic Pulmonary Tuberculosis)

Most cases of secondary pulmonary tuberculosis represent reactivation of an old, possibly subclinical infection. You will recall that during primary infection bacilli may disseminate, without producing symptoms, and establish themselves in sites with high oxygen tension, particularly the lung apices. Reactivation in such sites occurs in no more than 5 to 10% of cases of primary infection. However, secondary tuberculosis tends to produce more damage to the lungs than does primary tuberculosis. The contributions of immunity as opposed to hypersensitivity to the development of lesions have been discussed earlier.[81]

Although most adult forms of pulmonary tuberculosis begin as apical lesions, the presentation may be atypical in elderly persons. In epidemics of tuberculosis in nursing homes, the involvement may be in the lower or middle lobes.[79] The subsequent course of the infection is totally unpredictable and may lead to widespread exudative, proliferative, cavitated, and calcified lesions throughout the lungs. Many attempts have been made to subdivide these anatomic lesions into categories based on the nature and extent of the lesions. However, the disease refuses to follow these arbitrary subdivisions. It is therefore better to discuss the changes that constitute the full spectrum of pulmonary tuberculous lesions.

MORPHOLOGY. The **secondary pulmonary tuberculosis lesion** is located in the apex of one or both lungs. It begins as **a small focus of consolidation, usually less than 3 cm in diameter.** Less commonly, initial lesions may be located in other regions of the lung, particularly about the hilus. In almost every case of reinfection, the regional nodes develop foci of similar tuberculous activity. In the favorable case, the initial parenchymal focus develops a small area of caseation necrosis that does not cavitate, because it fails to communicate with a bronchus or bronchiole. The usual course is one of progressive fibrous encapsulation, leaving only fibrocalcific scars that depress and pucker the pleural surface and cause focal pleural adhesions. Sometimes these fibrocalcific scars become secondarily blackened by anthracotic pigment. In many instances a dense, collagenous, fibrous wall may totally enclose inspissated, cheesy, caseous debris that never resolves and remains as a granular lesion at postmortem examination.

Histologically, coalescent granulomas are present, composed of epithelioid cells surrounded by a zone of fibroblasts and lymphocytes that usually contains one or more Langhans' giant cells. Some caseation is usually present in the centers of these tubercles, the amount being entirely dependent on the sensitization of the patient and the virulence of the organisms (Fig. 16–36).

As the lesion progresses, more tubercles coalesce to create a confluent area of consolidation. In the favorable case, either the entire area is eventually converted to a fibrocalcific scar, or the residual caseous debris becomes totally and heavily walled off by hyaline collagenous connective tissue. In these late lesions, the multinucleate giant cells tend to disappear. Tubercle bacilli can be demonstrated by appropriate methods in the early exudative and caseous phases, but it is usually impossible to find them in the late fibrocalcific stages. However, it cannot be assumed that their absence in histologic sections is tantamount to their total destruction, since in many of these instances culture of the lesions or inoculation of this material into guinea pigs yields the organisms.

Late Progressive Pulmonary Tuberculosis

A variable, undetermined number of early lesions continue to progress over a period of months to years, causing further pulmonary and even distant organ involvements.

MORPHOLOGY. Apical, fibrocaseous tuberculosis with cavitation fairly well describes this stage of disease. By erosion into a bronchiole, drainage of the caseous focus transforms it into a cavity. Growth and multiplication of the tubercle bacilli are favored by the increased oxygen tensions. At the same time, the local accumulations of inhibitory organic acids are drained and the significantly acid caseous material is partially removed, further improving the environment for bacterial multiplication.

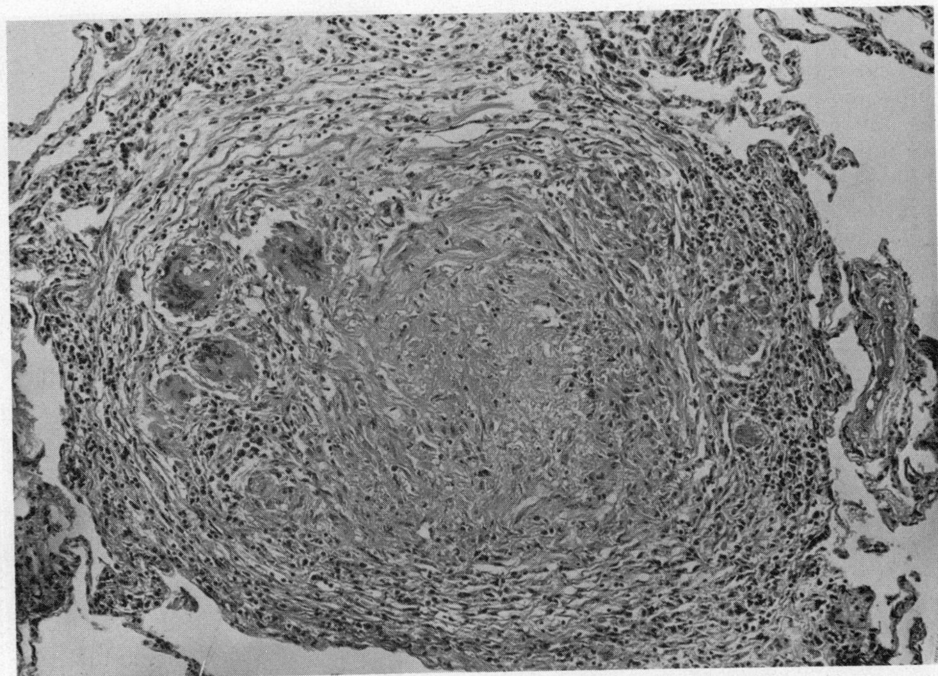

Figure 16–36. A characteristic tubercle in detail to illustrate central granular caseation and epithelioid and giant cells.

The cavity is lined by a yellow-gray caseous material and is more or less walled off by fibrous tissue. Not uncommonly, thrombosed arteries may traverse these cavities to produce apparent fibrous bridging bands. This tendency for tuberculosis to incite thrombosis is beneficial, since it prevents the hematogenous dissemination of bacilli and the erosion of large vessels. On the other hand, thrombosis many times does not occur, accounting for the hemoptysis associated with open cases. When such cavitation occurs in the apices, the pathways for further dissemination of the tuberculous infection are prepared. The infective material may now disseminate through the airways to other sites in the lung or upper respiratory tract. Spread may also occur to the lymph nodes via the lymphatics, and thence retrogressively through other lymphatics to other areas of the lung or other organs. Miliary dissemination through the blood is a further hazard.

Advanced fibrocaseous tuberculosis with cavitation may affect one, many, or all lobes of both lungs in the form of isolated minute tubercles, confluent caseous foci, or large areas of caseation necrosis. In some far-advanced cases of pulmonary tuberculosis that have ended in death, postmortem examination reveals the lung converted to a mass of honeycombed cavities separated only by scant areas of scarring or compressed atelectasis.

In the progress of this disease, the pleura is inevitably involved and, depending on the chronicity of the disease, serous pleural effusions, frank tuberculous empyema, or massive obliterative fibrous pleuritis may be found. In the course of extensive fibrocaseous tuberculosis, it is almost inevitable that tubercle bacilli become implanted on the mucosal linings of the air passages, and that **endobronchial and endotracheal tuberculosis** develop. These lesions may later become ulcerated to produce irregular, ragged, necrotic, mucosal ulcers. Accompanying the endobronchial tuberculosis, **laryngeal seeding and intestinal tuberculosis are common.**

Lymphohematogenous dissemination may give rise to miliary tuberculosis, confined only to the lungs or involving other organs also. The distribution of miliary lesions depends on the pathways of dissemination. Tuberculous infection may drain via the lymphatics through the major lymphatic ducts into the right side of the heart, and thence spread into a diffuse, blood-borne pattern throughout the lungs **alone.** Since most of the bacilli are filtered out by the alveolar capillary bed, the infective material may not reach the arterial systemic circulation. However, such limitation to the lungs usually is not complete, and some bacilli pass through the capillaries to enter the systemic circulation and produce distant organ seedings. In other circumstances, a tuberculous focus may erode directly into a pulmonary **artery** and thence be spread only in the pattern of supply of this single vessel to produce a localized miliary dissemination within the alveolar parenchyma. On the other hand, extension into a pulmonary **vein** is likely to be followed by disseminated miliary tuberculosis throughout the body or isolated organ tuberculosis.

In all instances of the miliary type of distribution, the individual lesions vary from one to several millimeters in diameter and are distinct, yellow-white, firm areas of consolidation that usually do not have grossly visible central caseation necrosis or cavitation at the time of examination (Fig. 16–37). Histologically, however, these present the characteristic pattern of individual or multiple confluent tubercles having microscopic central caseation.

In the highly susceptible, highly sensitized individual, the tuberculous infection may spread rapidly throughout large areas of lung parenchyma to produce a **diffuse bronchopneumonia,** or lobar exudative consolidation, at one time descriptively referred to as "galloping consumption"

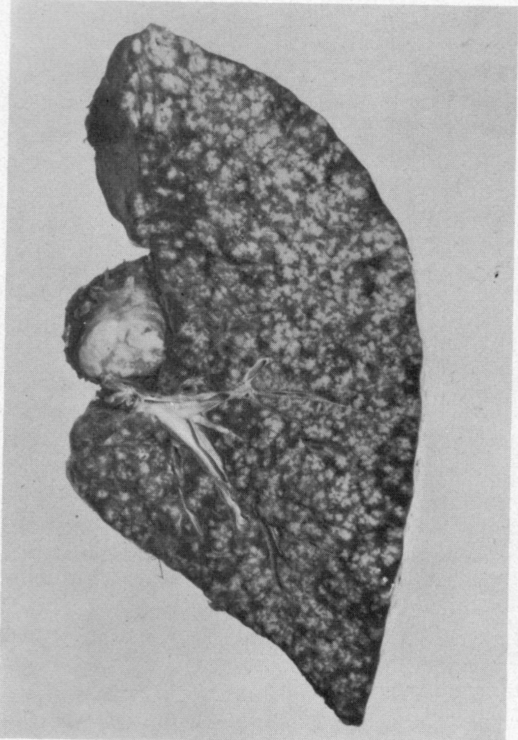

Figure 16–37. Advanced miliary tuberculosis lung. Foci of caseation have coalesced to produce large nodules of consolidation.

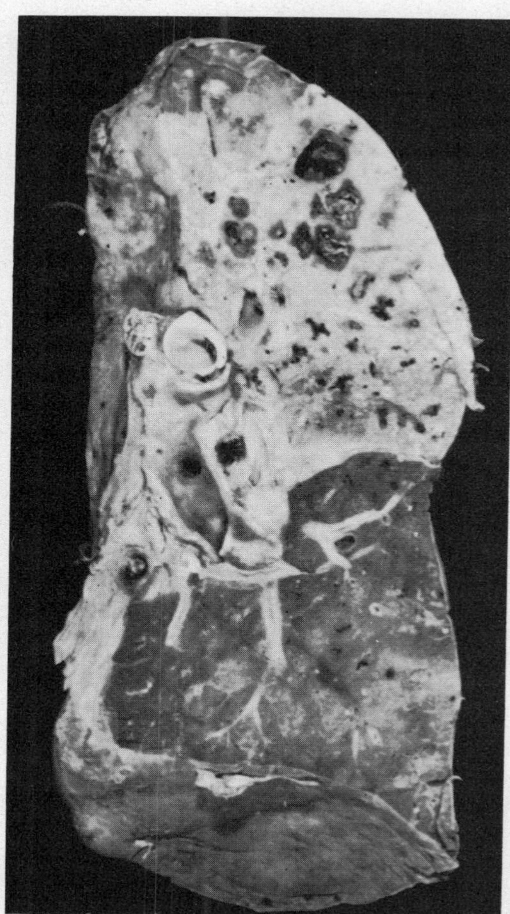

Figure 16–38. Tuberculous pneumonia of upper lobe viewed on cut section of lung.

(Fig. 16–38). Sometimes, with such overwhelming disease, well-developed tubercles do not form, and it may be difficult to establish on histologic grounds the tuberculous nature of the pneumonic process. However, numerous bacilli are usually present in such exudates.

CLINICAL COURSE. In all cases of suspected tuberculous tissue changes, acid-fast smears, cultures, and guinea pig inoculation to identify the bacilli should be employed before a diagnosis of such clinical importance is made.

The clinical course of pulmonary tuberculosis depends entirely on the activity, extent, and pattern of distribution of the tuberculous pulmonary infection and is too heterogeneous to describe here. Reference should be made to page 346, where the principal clinical manifestations are noted.

It is also impossible to make meaningful generalities about the prognosis in tuberculosis, since there are so many variables involved. The great majority of cases respond to present-day chemotherapeutic measures unless the disease is very advanced or intercurrent problems such as diabetes mellitus complicate the outlook. It should be recalled that amyloidosis may appear in long-standing chronic tuberculosis.

DIFFUSE INTERSTITIAL (INFILTRATIVE, RESTRICTIVE) DISEASES OF LUNG

This heterogeneous group of diseases is characterized predominantly by diffuse and usually chronic involvement of the pulmonary connective tissue, principally the most peripheral and delicate interstitium in the alveolar walls. Recall that the interstitium consists of the basement membrane of the endothelial and epithelial cells (fused in the thinnest portions), collagen fibers, elastic tissue, proteoglycans, fibroblasts, mast cells, and occasionally lymphocytes and monocytes.

There is no uniformity regarding terminology and classification of these diseases.[82] Many of the entities are of unknown etiology and pathogenesis, some have an intra-alveolar as well as an interstitial component, and there is frequent overlap in histologic features among the different conditions. Nevertheless, their similar clinical signs, symptoms, radiologic alterations, and pathophysiologic changes justify their consideration as a group. These disorders account for about 15% of noninfectious diseases seen by pulmonary physicians.

In general, the clinical and pulmonary functional changes are those of *restrictive rather than obstructive lung disease* (p. 717). Patients have dyspnea, tachypnea, and eventual cyanosis, without wheezing or other evidence of airway obstruction. The classic physiologic features are reductions in oxygen-diffusing capacity, lung volumes, and compliance. Chest radiographs show diffuse infiltration by small nodules, irregular lines, or "ground-glass" shadows (Fig. 16–39). Eventually, right-sided failure with cor pulmonale may result. Although

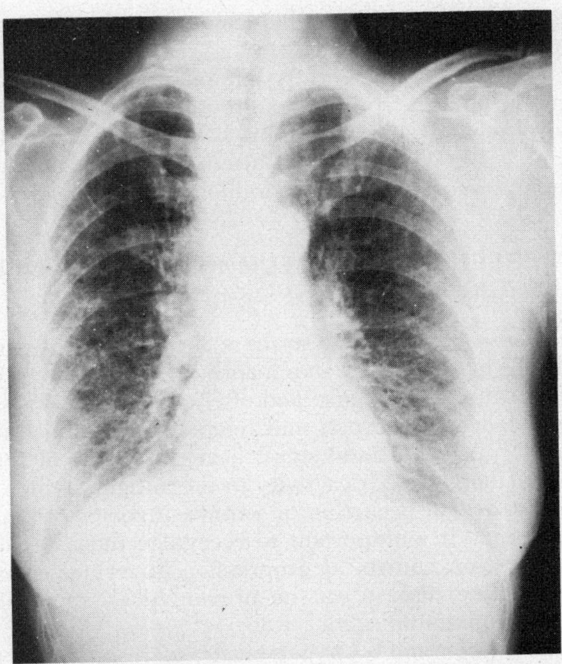

Figure 16–39. Diffuse interstitial pneumonitis. Note bilateral ground glass densities. (Courtesy of Dr. G. Balikian, Brigham and Women's Hospital, Boston.)

the entities can often be distinguished in the early stages, the advanced forms are hard to differentiate, since they result in scarring and gross destruction of the lung, often referred to as "end-stage lung" or "honeycomb lung."

CLASSIFICATION. Diffuse infiltrative disease can be divided into two broad categories (Table 16–4): those with known causes and those of unknown etiology, some of which can be defined either as clinicopathologic syndromes or as having characteristic histology.[83, 84] Most of these entities are discussed in other sections of this book. Here we shall briefly review current concepts of pathogenesis that may be common to all, and discuss those in which lung involvement is the primary or major problem. In terms of frequency, the most common conditions are environmental diseases (24%), sarcoidosis (20%), idiopathic pulmonary fibrosis (15%), and the collagen-vascular diseases (8%). The remainder have over 100 different etiologic agents.[82]

PATHOGENESIS. It is now thought that regardless of the type of interstitial disease or specific etiology, the earliest common manifestation of the interstitial diseases is *alveolitis*,[83, 85] i.e., an accumulation within the alveolar structure of inflammatory and immune effector cells (Fig. 16–40). Under normal conditions these cells account for no more than 7% of the total lung cell population, and consist of macrophages (93%), lymphocytes (7%), and neutrophils and eosinophils (less than 1%). In alveolitis there is a marked increase in the number of these cells, and a change in their relative proportions. This causes progressive derangement of alveolar structures, with increasing fibrocellular thickening of alveolar walls. The final result is an end-stage fibrotic lung in which the alveoli are replaced by cystic spaces separated by thick bands of connective tissue interspersed with inflammatory cells. This is the picture of the "end-stage lung" in which there is widespread loss of function of alveolocapillary units.

Let us briefly examine the various components of the scheme shown in Figure 16–40. The initial stimuli for the alveolitis are as heterogeneous as the causes outlined in Table 16–4. Some of these stimuli, such as oxygen-derived free radicals and some chemicals, are directly toxic to endothelial cells, epithelial cells, or both. But beyond direct toxicity, the critical event appears to be the *recruitment and/or activation of inflammatory and immune effector cells.* Neutrophil recruitment can be caused by complement activation in some immune-mediated disorders,[87] but in addition the alveolar macrophages, which increase in number in all interstitial diseases, release a *chemotactic factor* that is relatively specific for neutrophils (NCF). Asbestos particles and immune complexes (through the Fc receptor on the macrophage) stimulate the release of NCF. NCF also "activates" the neutrophils, causing them to secrete proteases and toxic oxygen free-radicals, which contribute further to tissue damage and provide a mechanism for maintenance of the alveolitis. In diseases such as sarcoidosis, *cell-mediated* immune reactions result in

Table 16–4. DIFFUSE INFILTRATIVE LUNG DISEASES

Known Etiology	Unknown Etiology
1. Occupational and environmental inhalants	1. Sarcoidosis (p. 390)
a. Inorganic dusts (silicosis, asbestos, coal workers' pneumoconiosis (Chapter 10)	2. Associated with collagen-vascular disorders and vasculitis (e.g., rheumatoid arthritis, SLE, Wegener's granulomatosis)
b. Organic dusts (hypersensitivity pneumonitis)	3. Goodpasture's syndrome
c. Gases, fumes, aerosols (oxygen toxicity, sulfur dioxide, toluene)	4. Idiopathic pulmonary hemosiderosis
2. Drugs and toxins	5. Eosinophilic pneumonia
Chemotherapeutic agents (busulfan, bleomycin)	6. Histiocytosis X (p. 694)
Antibiotics (nitrofurantoin)	7. Alveolar proteinosis
Other drugs (gold, penicillamine)	8. Desquamative interstitial pneumonitis
Toxins (paraquat)	9. Idiopathic pulmonary fibrosis
3. Infections	
Viral (influenza, cytomegalovirus)	
Bacterial (widespread tuberculosis)	
Fungal	
Parasitic *(Pneumocystis carinii)*	

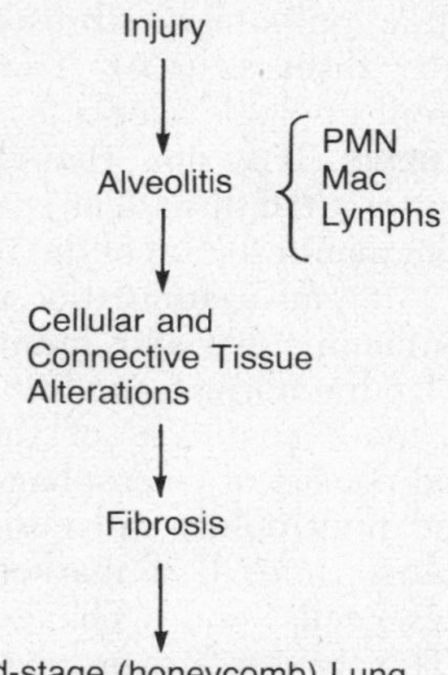

Figure 16–40. Pathogenesis of chronic interstitial lung diseases. Current concepts are that there is some type of initial injury and a resulting alveolitis. Unchecked, the alveolitis will become chronic and cellular, and connective tissue alterations will develop. The final common pathway is the end-stage lung. PMN = polymorphonuclear leukocytes; Mac = alveolar macrophages. (Modified from Fulmer, J.: An introduction to the interstitial lung diseases. Clin. Chest Med. *3*:458, 1982.)

the accumulation of monocytes and T lymphocytes, and formation of granulomas. It is thought that interactions among the inflammatory cells and the release of lymphokines and monokines may be responsible for the slowly progressive pulmonary fibrosis that ensues. As reviewed in the discussion of chronic inflammation (p. 76), macrophages (including alveolar macrophages)[88] elaborate factors that promote fibroblast growth; the production of these factors is enhanced by interactions with silica particles, immune complexes, and lymphokines. There is also evidence that neutrophils, lymphocytes, and macrophages are all involved in the changes in composition and distribution of the connective tissue components of the lung (collagen, elastin, fibronectin, proteoglycans) that occur in the progression to end-stage fibrosis, but the precise sequence of events and the biochemical mechanisms are still poorly understood.

It must be obvious at this juncture that some of the initiating mechanisms that result in interstitial fibrosis—e.g., accumulation and activation of neutrophils and macrophages—may be similar to those that lead to emphysema, as discussed earlier (p. 717). Is there a relationship between the two sequences of events? The answer is unclear, but experiments[89] show that the same toxic agent (cadmium chloride) that causes fibrosis in hamster lungs induces bullous emphysema if the animals are also given beta-aminoproprionitrile, an inhibitor of collagen and elastin cross-linking. Such studies suggest that divergent responses—emphysema and fibrosis—to similar injurious agents may depend on host metabolic factors.

PNEUMOCONIOSIS

This term designates a disease of the lungs caused by the inhalation of dust. Policard defines it far more elegantly: "The conflict of living matter with the mineral world: the pneumoconioses."[82]

The variety of clinically and anatomically described pneumoconioses appears to grow with each year. As environmental diseases, they have been covered in Chapter 10, with principal attention to coal workers' pneumoconiosis, silicosis, berylliosis, and asbestosis.

HYPERSENSITIVITY PNEUMONITIS (EXTERNAL ALLERGIC ALVEOLITIS)

These two terms describe a spectrum of immunologically mediated, predominantly interstitial lung disorders caused by intense and often prolonged exposure to inhaled organic dusts and related occupational antigens.[90, 91] Affected individuals have an abnormal sensitivity or heightened reactivity to the antigen, which, in contrast to that occurring in asthma, involves primarily the *alveoli.* It is important to recognize these diseases early in their course, as progression to serious chronic fibrotic lung disease can be prevented by removal of the environmental agent.

Most commonly, hypersensitivity results from the inhalation of organic dust containing antigens made up of spores of thermophilic bacteria, true fungi, animal proteins, or bacterial products. Numerous euphemistically named syndromes are described, depending on the occupation or exposure of the individual. *Farmers' lung* results from exposure to material generated from harvested, humid, warm hay that permits the rapid proliferation of the spores of thermophilic actinomycetes. *Pigeon breeders' lung* (bird fanciers' disease) is provoked by proteins from serum, excreta, or feathers of the birds. *Humidifier* or *air-conditioner lung* is caused by thermophilic bacteria in heated water reservoirs. There is also a mushroom pickers' lung, a maple bark disease, and duck fever (from duck feathers).

The clinical manifestations are varied. Acute attacks, which follow inhalation of antigenic dust in sensitized patients, consist of recurring attacks of fever, dyspnea, cough, and leukocytosis. Diffuse and nodular infiltrates appear in the chest radiograph, and pulmonary function tests show an acute restrictive effect. Symptoms usually appear four to six hours after exposure. If exposure is continuous and protracted, a chronic form of the disease supervenes that no longer features the acute exacerbations on antigen reexposure. Instead, there are signs of progressive respiratory failure, dyspnea, and cyanosis and a decrease in total lung capacity and compliance—a picture hard to differentiate from other forms of chronic interstitial disease.

Histologic descriptions come from biopsies of patients with subacute and chronic forms, rather than from those with acute attacks. The alterations include interstitial pneumonitis consisting primarily of lymphocytes, plasma cells, and macrophages (some of the latter having a foamy cytoplasm); interstitial fibrosis; obliterative bronchiolitis; and outright granuloma formation. In over half the patients there is also evidence of an intra-alveolar infiltrate.

The evidence from experimental and human studies strongly suggests a Type III immune complex pathogenesis for the early lesions, followed by a Type IV delayed hypersensitivity reaction for the granulomatous components. Why only a small percentage of those exposed actually develop the disease is still a mystery. Genetic studies have not detected consistent differences in the frequency of specific HLA antigens between patients and control populations.

Byssinosis is an occupational lung disease of textile workers that is apparently induced by the inhalation of airborne fibers of cotton, linen, and hemp. Acute effects include cough, wheezing, and airway obstruction, a picture that resembles bronchial asthma. Prolonged exposure leads to disabling chronic lung disease characterized by chronic bronchitis, emphysema, and interstitial granulomas. The agent in dust that provokes the disease is unknown, but gram-negative rod endotoxin has been implicated in some cases. Evidence for an immunologic hypersensitivity in this disorder is not as clear as in the other conditions described under this heading.

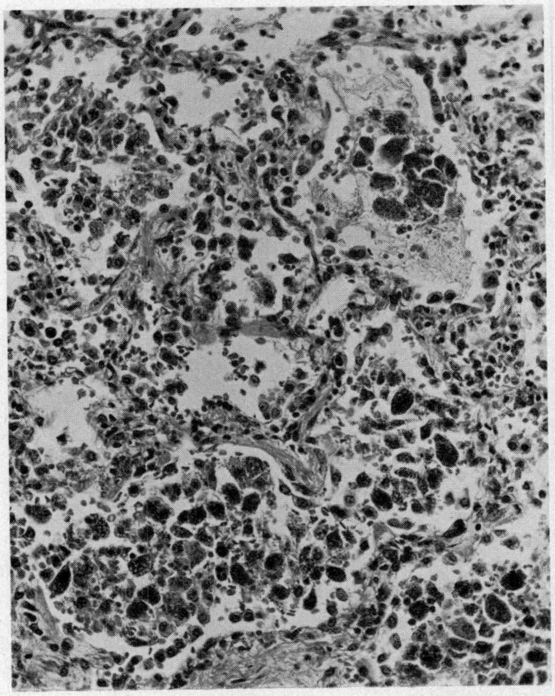

GOODPASTURE'S SYNDROME*

Hemorrhage from the lung is a dramatic complication of some interstitial lung disorders. Among these so-called *pulmonary hemorrhage syndromes*[92] are (1) Goodpasture's syndrome; (2) idiopathic pulmonary hemosiderosis; and (3) vasculitis-associated hemorrhage, which is found in conditions such as hypersensitivity angiitis and Wegener's granulomatosis.

Goodpasture's syndrome is an uncommon but intriguing condition characterized by the *simultaneous appearance of a form of proliferative, usually rapidly progressive glomerulonephritis and a necrotizing hemorrhagic interstitial pneumonitis.* The evidence is quite substantial that the renal and pulmonary lesions are the consequence of antibodies evoked by antigens common to the glomerular and pulmonary basement membranes.[93] Most cases begin clinically with respiratory symptoms, principally hemoptysis, and radiographic evidence of focal pulmonary consolidations. Very soon, manifestations of glomerulonephritis appear, leading to rapidly progressive renal failure. The common cause of death is uremia. Cases have been reported in females, but there is a striking preponderance among males. Most cases occur in the second or third decade of life.

In the classic case, the lungs are heavy and contain focal areas of red-brown apparent consolidation. Histologically, there are acute focal necroses of alveolar walls associated with intra-alveolar hemorrhages, fibrous thickening of the septa, and hypertrophy of lining septal cells. Depending on the duration of the disease, there may be organization of blood in the alveolar spaces. Often the alveoli contain hemosiderin-laden macrophages (Fig. 16–41). Immunofluorescent studies reveal linear deposits of immunoglobulins along the basement membranes of the septal walls. The kidneys reveal the characteristic findings of focal proliferative glomerulonephritis in the early cases or crescentic glomerulonephritis in those with rapidly progressive glomerulonephritis (p. 1009). Immunofluorescence reveals linear deposits of immunoglobulins and complement along the glomerular basement membranes, similar to those seen in the alveolar septa.

Figure 16–41. Lung in Goodpasture's syndrome. Alveolar walls are thickened with focal areas of necrosis. Alveolar spaces contain hemosiderin-laden macrophages secondary to intra-alveolar hemorrhages.

Although it is clear that antibasement antibodies are associated with this disease, the trigger initiating this immune disorder in man is still unknown. One hypothesis proposes the development of autosensitization to normal glomerular basement membrane antigens, which then cross-react with the alveolar basement membrane. Trace amounts of these antigens are normally excreted in the urine. Any mild injury to the kidney would expose these antigens to immunocompetent lymphocytes, initiating antibody formation. Because most cases begin with pulmonary symptoms, it is more likely that the initial antibody is to lung basement membrane, which then cross-reacts with the kidney. Virus infection and exposure to hydrocarbon solvents (used in the dry-cleaning industry) have been implicated as a trigger of the syndrome in some patients;[94, 94A] these compounds might act by altering the basement membrane, rendering it antigenic. Most cases, however, give no history of such exposure.

The once dismal prognosis for this disease has been markedly improved by intensive *plasma exchange.*[95] This procedure is thought to be beneficial by removing

*See also page 1010.

circulating antibasement membrane antibodies as well as chemical mediators of immunologic injury. Simultaneous immunosuppressive therapy inhibits further antibody production. Both the lung hemorrhage and the glomerulonephritis appear to improve with this form of therapy.

IDIOPATHIC PULMONARY HEMOSIDEROSIS

This uncommon pulmonary disease of obscure nature usually presents with an insidious onset of productive cough, hemoptysis, and weight loss associated with diffuse pulmonary infiltrations. However, it tends to occur in younger adults and children and, unlike Goodpasture's syndrome, shows no striking male preponderance.[96] The etiology and pathogenesis is unknown. Studies directed toward showing some immunologic derangement have been equivocal.

The lungs are moderately increased in weight, with focal areas of consolidation that are usually red-brown to red. The cardinal histologic features of pulmonary hemosiderosis are reported as "striking degeneration, shedding and hyperplasia of alveolar epithelial cells, and marked localized alveolar capillary dilatation." There are varying degrees of pulmonary interstitial fibrosis; hemorrhage into the alveolar spaces; and hemosiderosis, both within the alveolar septa and in macrophages lying free within the pulmonary alveoli.

In contrast to Goodpasture's syndrome, idiopathic pulmonary hemosiderosis runs the gamut from mild to severe disease. Some patients have recurrent, not severe episodes of hemoptysis with intervening periods of good health and may have a normal life span. Some develop progressive pulmonary fibrosis and run an erratic progressive course with advancing cardiac failure; others may die suddenly of massive pulmonary hemorrhage. Most patients follow a chronic remittent course over a period of years, and then improve spontaneously or with treatment and have no further recurrences.

PULMONARY ALVEOLAR PROTEINOSIS

This is a disease of obscure etiology and pathogenesis, characterized radiologically by diffuse pulmonary opacification and histologically by accumulation in intra-alveolar spaces of a dense granular, strongly PAS-positive material that contains abundant lipid. Although this entity is discussed here among the interstitial and restrictive diseases, its histologic alterations are intra-alveolar and it does not usually progress to chronic fibrosis. Patients, for the most part, present with nonspecific respiratory difficulty of insidious onset, cough, and abundant sputum that often contains chunks of gelatinous material.[97] Some have symptoms lasting for years, often with febrile illnesses. Progressive dyspnea, cyanosis, and respiratory insufficiency may occur, but some patients tend to have a benign course, with eventual resolution of the lesions.

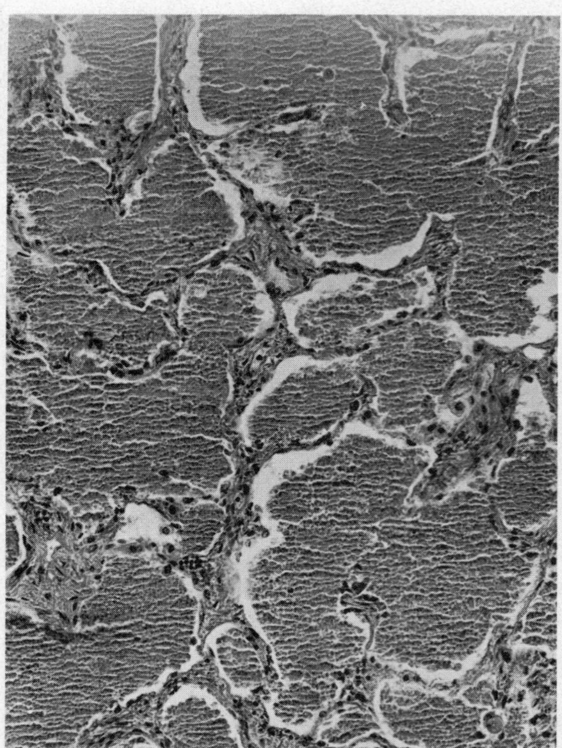

Figure 16–42. Pulmonary alveolar proteinosis. Alveoli are filled with a dense amorphous protein-lipid granular precipitate.

Morphologically, the disease is characterized by a peculiar, homogeneous, granular precipitate within the alveoli, causing focal-to-confluent consolidation of large areas of the lungs (Fig. 16–42). On section, turbid fluid exudes from these areas. As a consequence, there is a marked increase in size and weight of the lung. The alveolar precipitate is PAS-positive and also contains finely divided lipid. Biochemically, the material is rich in protein and phospholipids. The latter are chemically similar to surfactant but fail to show surfactant properties. By electron microscopy, the alveolar contents consist of necrotic alveolar macrophages and Type II pneumocytes, amorphous precipitate, with considerable numbers of lamellar osmiophilic bodies morphologically resembling surfactant material. The involved alveoli are often lined with hyperplastic pneumocytes, and focal areas of necrosis of these cells are seen with the light microscope. Within the amorphous alveolar precipitate, there also are occasionally concentric laminated bodies and long, needle-like crystalline spaces closely resembling cholesterol clefts. There is usually a surprising absence of any inflammatory reaction in the affected alveoli.

Some patients suffering from this disease may have an occupational exposure to irritating dusts (including silica dust) and other chemicals. The disease also occurs in immunosuppressed patients.[99] Theories of pathogenesis suggest either excessive production of surfactant-like material by hyperplastic type II epithelial cells, or a defect in the macrophage clearance of intra-alveolar accumulations. Current opinion favors the latter mechanism.[7, 98]

DESQUAMATIVE INTERSTITIAL PNEUMONITIS (DIP)

This is a rare disease characterized anatomically by an interstitial fibrosing pneumonitis accompanied by aggregation of mononuclear cells within the alveoli, presumably desquamated from the alveolar walls.[82, 100] These patients usually present with the slow development of cough and dyspnea, eventually leading to marked respiratory embarrassment, cyanosis, and clubbing of the fingers. Classically, the radiologic picture is that of bilateral lower-lobe ground-glass infiltrates.

The most striking finding is the accumulation in the air spaces of a large number of mononuclear cells (Fig. 16–43). Often there is accompanying hyperplasia of the septal lining epithelial cells and desquamation of these cells into the air spaces. Electron microscopy has shown that approximately 90% of the desquamated cells are macrophages, many of which contain lipid vacuoles and PAS-positive granules. Some of these macrophages contain lamellar bodies within phagocytic vacuoles, presumably derived from necrotic Type II pneumocytes. There is often an associated interstitial pneumonitis.

The etiology of this disorder is unknown. Patients are benefited by steroid therapy, which often leads to clearing of the lungs. Some patients with DIP have or subsequently develop significant interstitial fibrosis resembling the usual type; for this reason, many authors object to the term DIP and consider the entity an early stage of idiopathic interstitial fibrosis, discussed later.[101] Nevertheless, some long-term studies indicate that patients with a pronounced desquamative component to the lesion have a better prognosis and response to steroid therapy than do those with the usual interstitial fibrotic pattern.[102] Whether this represents different etiologic agents or pathogenetic mechanisms is unknown.

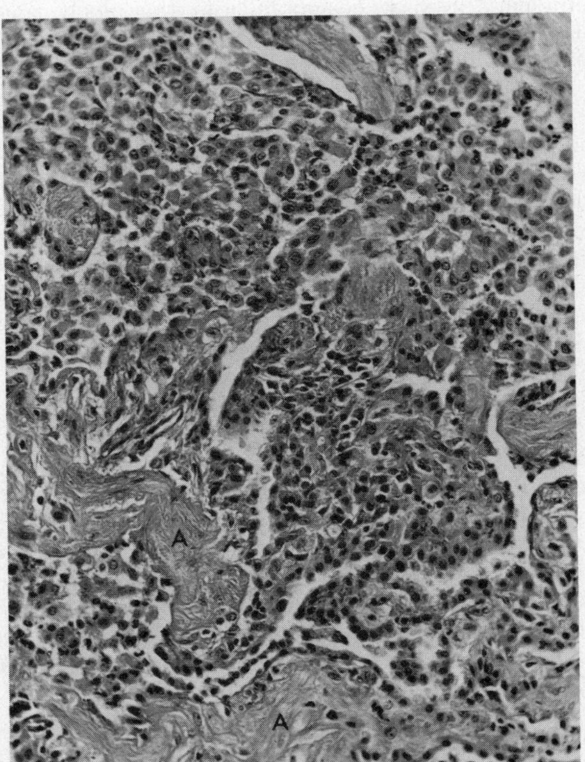

Figure 16–43. Desquamative interstitial pneumonitis. High-power detail of lung to demonstrate fibrous thickening of alveolar walls (A) and accumulation of large numbers of mononuclear cells within alveolar spaces.

DIFFUSE IDIOPATHIC PULMONARY FIBROSIS (CHRONIC INTERSTITIAL PNEUMONIA, FIBROSING ALVEOLITIS, HAMMAN-RICH SYNDROME)

These terms refer to a poorly understood pulmonary disorder characterized histologically by diffuse interstitial fibrosis and inflammation, which in the advanced case results in severe hypoxemia and cyanosis. There are at least 20 synonyms for this entity, and in Britain it is known as *diffuse* or *cryptogenic* (i.e., *idiopathic*) *fibrosing alveolitis*. Liebow coined the term *usual interstitial pneumonitis (UIP)* to differentiate this condition from the desquamative type (DIP) described earlier and from other rarer examples of so-called giant cell and lymphocytic interstitial pneumonitis.[103] It should be stressed that similar pathologic findings may occur as the result of well-defined entities, such as the pneumoconioses, hypersensitivity pneumonitis, oxygen toxicity pneumonitis, scleroderma, and irradiation injury. In about half the cases, however, there is no known underlying disease, and the term *idiopathic* is applied.

Males are affected more often than females, and although the disease may occur at any age, most patients are between 30 and 50 years old.

It is now thought that this disorder represents a stereotyped inflammatory response of the alveolar wall to injuries of different types, durations, and intensities. The proposed sequence of events, described earlier, begins with some form of alveolar wall injury, which results in interstitial edema and accumulation of inflammatory cells (alveolitis). It is thought that the Type I membranous pneumocyte is particularly susceptible to injury. Subsequently there is hyperplasia of Type II pneumocytes in an attempt to regenerate the alveolar epithelial lining. Fibroblasts then appear, and progressive fibrosis and collagenization of both the interalveolar septa and the intra-alveolar exudate result in obliteration of normal pulmonary architecture with the formation of what is termed "honeycomb" lung, the end stage of this chronic process.

Immune mechanisms may trigger this sequence of events.[101] There are high levels of circulating immune complexes or cryoimmunoglobulins in the serum of patients with idiopathic interstitial pneumonia, particularly in cases in which biopsy showed significant cellular infiltration rather than interstitial fibrosis.[104] Granular deposits of IgG can be seen in the alveolar walls, suggesting that immune complexes may play a pathogenetic role, but the nature of the antigens within the complexes is unknown.

The morphologic changes vary according to the stage of the disease. In early cases, the lungs grossly are firm in consistency and microscopically show pulmonary edema, hyaline membranes, and infiltration of the alveolar septa with mononuclear cells. There is hyperplasia of Type II pneumocytes, which appear as cuboidal or even columnar cells lining the alveolar spaces. With advancing disease, there is organization of the intra-alveolar exudate by fibrous tissue, as well as thickening of the interstitial septa due to fibrosis and variable amounts of inflammation. At this stage the lungs become solid, with alternating areas of fibrosis and more normal-appearing lung. In the end stages of the disorder, the lung consists of spaces lined by cuboidal or columnar epithelium and separated by inflammatory fibrous tissue (Fig. 16–44). This gives the typical appearance of the honeycomb lung. Small cysts are often seen, and there is also intimal thickening of the pulmonary arteries and lymphoid hyperplasia. As mentioned earlier, this advanced picture can result from any of the disorders listed on page 743. Thus it is necessary to exclude the known causes of interstitial fibrosis by clinical, radiologic, or serologic means before the diagnosis of idiopathic interstitial fibrosis is made.

As would be expected, patients exhibit varying degrees of respiratory difficulty and, in advanced cases, hypoxemia and cyanosis. The septal fibrosis constitutes a significant physiologic alveolocapillary block. Cor pulmonale and cardiac failure may result. The progress in the individual case is unpredictable. In some patients the disease remits spontaneously. In a few the process progresses very rapidly, leading to fibrosis in a matter of weeks, whereas in others it develops over many years. In most cases, death occurs in about two years.

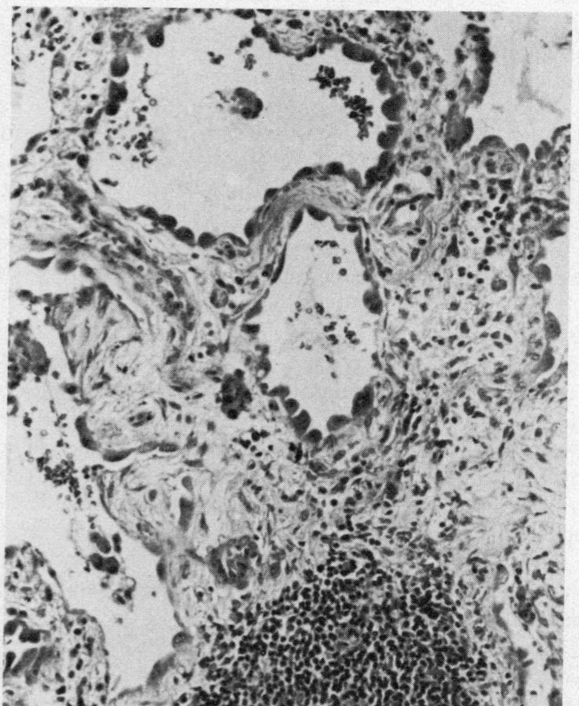

Figure 16–44. Diffuse interstitial fibrosis. Note marked interstitial fibrosis, focal chronic inflammation, and dilated spaces lined by cuboidal Type II epithelial cells.

PULMONARY EOSINOPHILIA (PULMONARY INFILTRATION WITH EOSINOPHILIA)

A number of clinical and pathologic pulmonary entities are characterized by an infiltration of eosinophils. The etiology and pathogenesis of these disorders are diverse. They have been divided into the following categories:[105, 106] (1) *simple pulmonary eosinophilia*, or Loeffler's syndrome; (2) *tropical eosinophilia*, caused by infection with *microfilariae* (p. 519); (3) *chronic pulmonary eosinophilia* (which occurs in a number of parasitic, fungal, and bacterial infections; in hypersensitivity pneumonitis; in drug allergies; and in association with asthma, allergic bronchopulmonary aspergillosis, or polyarteritis nodosa); and (4) so-called idiopathic *chronic eosinophilic pneumonia*. The mechanisms that lead to eosinophilia in these conditions are almost certainly immunologic, although the sequence of events for each is far from clear.

Loeffler's syndrome is characterized by transient pulmonary lesions, eosinophilia in the blood, and a rather benign clinical course. Roentgenograms are often quite striking, with shadows of varying size and shape in any of the lobes suggesting irregular intrapulmonary densities. The illness is dominated clinically by dyspnea, and pulmonary function tests usually show both restrictive and obstructive defects. It is thought that the syndrome results from a Type I allergic reaction, common inciting agents being Ascaris and Strongyloides parasites. In true simple eosinophilia[107] the lungs show alveoli whose septa are thickened by an infiltrate composed of eosinophils and occasional interspersed giant cells. There is also focal hyperplasia of the alveolar epithelial lining cells, but no vasculitis, fibrosis, or necrosis.

Chronic eosinophilic pneumonia is characterized by focal areas of cellular consolidation of the lung substance distributed chiefly in the periphery of the lung fields. Prominent in these lesions are heavy aggregates of lymphocytes and eosinophils within both the septal walls and the alveolar spaces.[108] Clinically there is high fever, night sweats, and dyspnea, all of which respond to corticosteroid therapy. Obviously, this rare entity can be diagnosed only when other causes of chronic pulmonary eosinophilia are excluded.

PULMONARY INVOLVEMENT IN COLLAGEN-VASCULAR DISORDERS

These diseases are discussed in other chapters but are listed here, since they can lead to a picture of chronic interstitial fibrosis.[109,110]

Diffuse interstitial fibrosis occurs classically in progressive systemic sclerosis *(scleroderma),* discussed on page 190. Less commonly, patchy and transient parenchymal infiltrates are noted in *lupus erythematosus,* and occasionally severe lupus pneumonitis may occur and may be one of the major clinical problems in such patients. In *rheumatoid arthritis,* pulmonary involvement is common and may occur in one of five forms:[111] (1) chronic pleuritis, with or without effusion; (2) diffuse interstitial pneumonitis and fibrosis; (3) intrapulmonary rheumatoid nodules; (4) rheumatoid nodules with pneumonoconiosis (Caplan's syndrome); and (5) pulmonary hypertension. Thirty to 40% of patients with classic rheumatoid arthritis have abnormalities in pulmonary function. In certain patients the disorder progresses to end-stage lung disease. Lung involvement is also common in the vasculitides[112] (p. 519), particularly in allergic angiitis and granulomatosis (the Churg-Strauss syndrome).

Wegener's granulomatosis, considered on page 523, represents an acute necrotizing vasculitis with granuloma formation, affecting particularly the lungs, kidneys, and upper respiratory tract. In the lung, there are necrotizing granulomas and a prominent vasculitis. *Lymphomatoid granulomatosis* is a disorder characterized by lymphoid proliferation, vasculitis, and granuloma formation. Although it may remain confined to the lung, the disease often evolves into a malignant lymphoma.[113]

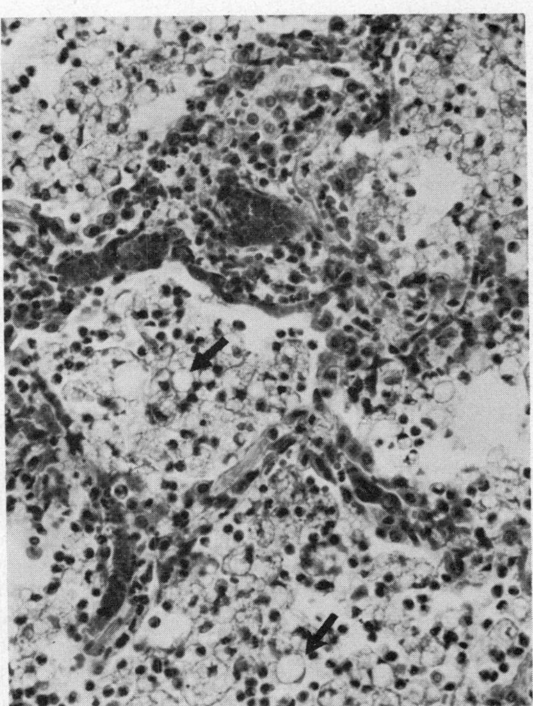

Figure 16–45. Lipid pneumonia. Alveoli contain the characteristic lipid-laden macrophages with large, clear cytoplasmic vacuoles *(arrows).*

OTHER FORMS OF PULMONARY DISEASE

LIPID PNEUMONIA

Patchy or diffuse consolidation of the lung may be caused by the aspiration of a variety of oils. This is usually encountered in infants and children who are forced to swallow mineral oil; in small, weak infants; and in those with congenital malformations in whom the swallowing reflex may be deranged. In adults, lipid pneumonia usually follows the protracted use of mineral oil as a laxative or the use of oily nose drops or sprays. Rarely, lipid pneumonia follows the use of radiopaque oil for x-ray visualization of the respiratory tree.

In general, the more unsaturated the oil, the greater is its toxicity. Some of the most reactive oils are those found in lard and peanuts and in chaulmoogra seeds. By contrast, corn and sesame oils are bland. Mineral oil is quite bland but acts as an inert foreign body in tissues. When aspirated, even milk and cream are capable of evoking an inflammatory response.

MORPHOLOGY. The extent of pneumonic reaction depends largely on the quantity and chemical nature of the oil implicated. In general, the lesions are bilateral, but tend to affect the right lung more than the left because of the direct drainage path of the right main stem bronchus. The aspirated oil is emulsified once it reaches the alveoli, and the fine droplets are phagocytized by large numbers of macrophages called out in response to this foreign material. In the early stages, the affected alveoli are partially or totally filled with aggregates of distended, occasionally multinucleate macrophages that contain large, clear, spherical, intracytoplasmic vacuoles (Fig. 16–45). With progression of the lesion, fibroblasts invade the cellular lipid exudate and eventually organize the macrophagic inflammatory response. Multinucleate giant cells may develop within the alveolar organization, to form granulomas that may resemble those found in tuberculosis and sarcoidosis.

Grossly, patchy foci (1 to 3 cm in diameter) or segmental involvements vary from gray to bright yellow and are dry and granular. The lesions are fairly sharply circumscribed and slightly elevated above the level of the cut lung surface. The anatomic diagnosis can only be suspected grossly and must be verified by means of histologic examination and lipid stains.

Lipid pneumonia may be discovered as an incidental finding at autopsy. However, symptomatic manifestations may be occasioned by superimposed bronchitis, bronchiolitis, bronchiectasis, and bronchopneumonia. If the areas affected become sufficiently extensive, pulmonary dysfunction may occur.

TUMORS OF LUNG

A variety of benign and malignant tumors may arise in the lung, but the vast majority (90 to 95%) are bronchogenic carcinomas.[114] About 5% are bronchial carcinoids, and 2 to 5% are mesenchymal and other miscellaneous neoplasms. The term "bronchogenic" is used for most lung cancers, but it is somewhat misleading in that it implies a bronchial origin for all lung cancers, despite the fact that adenocarcinomas, which are peripheral in location, are most often bronchiolar in derivation.

BRONCHOGENIC CARCINOMA

In industrialized nations, public enemy number one among cancers is bronchogenic carcinoma. It is the most common visceral malignancy in males; it alone accounts for approximately one third of all cancer deaths in males and 1/20th of all deaths in both sexes. Although females are affected less frequently, the incidence is increasing dramatically and lung cancer is about to pass breast carcinoma as a cause of cancer death in women.[115]

INCIDENCE. There is no longer any doubt that the rising incidence of lung cancer is real and not the spurious consequence of an aging population, better case findings, and more accurate diagnosis. The annual number of deaths from lung cancer in the United States increased from 18,000 in 1950 to an estimated 121,000 in 1984.[115] The age-adjusted death rate from cancer of the lung since 1950 has more than trebled in males, rising from 19.9 to an outstanding 70 per 100,000 population. The death rate in females since 1950 has risen from 4.5 to 19 per 100,000. Cancer of the lung now accounts for 22% of all cancers in males and 9% in females. In 1984 there were an estimated 139,000 new cases of lung cancer. These data on bronchogenic carcinoma must be viewed within the context of other forms of cancer. Death rates from cancer of the stomach and uterus in the U.S. have steadily fallen since 1950, and there has been no appreciable change in the death rates for colorectal, prostatic, breast, and urinary bladder cancers over this time span.

Cancer of the lung occurs most often between ages 40 and 70, with a peak incidence in the sixth or seventh decade. Only 2% of all cases appear before the age of 40.[116] The male:female death rate ratio for lung cancer among whites reached a peak of approximately 7:1 in 1960, but in 1984 it had fallen to 3:1—almost certainly the delayed consequence of increased cigarette smoking among women.

ETIOLOGY AND PATHOGENESIS. ***Tobacco Smoking.*** The evidence establishing a positive relationship between tobacco smoking and lung cancer is well-nigh incontrovertible. Most of the monumental documentation may be found in the reports of the Royal College of Physicians[117] and the United States Surgeon General.[118] The collective evidence is of three kinds: statistical, clinical, and experimental.[119]

Statistical evidence is most compelling.[120, 121] In numerous retrospective studies of patients who died of bronchogenic carcinoma compared with controls, there was an invariable statistical association between the frequency of lung cancer and (1) the amount of daily smoking, (2) the tendency to inhale, and (3) the duration of the smoking habit. Reduced lung cancer rates are found among ex-smokers. Compared with nonsmokers, average smokers of cigarettes have an approximately nine- to tenfold increase in the risk of developing lung cancer, and heavy smokers (over 40 cigarettes per day for several years) have at least a 20-fold risk increase. Ex-smokers who had smoked 20 or more cigarettes daily have, after 10 years of not smoking, a death rate from lung cancer similar to that of nonsmokers. The epidemiologic studies also show an association between cigarette smoking and the following cancers, in decreasing order of frequency: lip, tongue, floor of mouth, pharynx, larynx, esophagus, urinary bladder, and pancreas.[122] The exclusive smoking of *filter cigarettes* appears to reduce cancer risk; however, no decreased risk is seen among heavy smokers 50 to 69 years of age who shift to filter cigarettes for less than five years. Most studies in the United States have also associated cigar and pipe smoking with lung cancer, but the association has been less strong than that observed in some European countries.

Clinical evidence has dealt largely with changes in the lining epithelium of the respiratory tract in smokers and nonsmokers. In a systematic study of bronchial epithelium of smokers, Auerbach and colleagues[123] quantitated three histologic characteristics: (1) loss of bronchial cilia; (2) basal epithelial hyperplasia; and (3) nuclear abnormalities, sometimes approaching carcinoma in situ. The concurrence of these three types of changes was never seen in histologic specimens from nonsmokers but was seen in about 10% of smokers, 1 to 2% of those smoking filter-tipped cigarettes, and 15% of sections of patients who died of lung cancer; 96.7% of cigarette smokers showed some atypical cells in the bronchial tree, whereas 0.9% of controls had similar cells.[124]

The *experimental work* has focused mainly on attempts to induce cancer in experimental animals with extracts of tobacco smoke. Over 1200 substances have been counted in cigarette smoke and many of these are potential carcinogens. These include both initiators (polycyclic aromatic hydrocarbons, such as benzo[*a*]pyrene) and promoters such as phenol derivatives. Radioactive elements may also be found (polonium-210, carbon-14, potassium-40) as well as other contaminants, such as arsenic, nickel, molds, and additives. Protracted exposure of mice to these additives induces skin tumors. However, efforts to produce lung cancer by exposing animals to tobacco smoke or to tobacco smoke combined with air pollutants, viruses, and other possible carcinogens have given negative results. The few cancers that have been produced have been bronchioloalveolar carcinomas, a type of human tumor not associated with smoking in man. In 1967, Wynder and Hoffman concluded that, to that date, (1) there was no carefully controlled model of bronchogenic carcinoma produced by exposure to tobacco smoke alone in experimental animals and (2) those experimental lung tumors that had been produced probably resulted from complex carcinogenic consequences.[125] These conclusions remain largely true today.

Industrial Hazards. Certain industrial exposures increase the risk of development of lung cancer. Of historical interest is the account of lung cancer in the

Schneeberg mines in Saxony. In 1420, shortly after the opening of the mines (known for their richness in various metals, but also for *radon*), Paracelsus described the *Bergkrankheit*, or mountain sickness, in miners. It was not until 1879 that the malignant nature of the disease was recognized and not until 1913 that the accurate diagnosis of lung carcinoma was established for this illness. All types of radiation may be carcinogenic. There was an increased incidence of lung cancer among survivors of the Hiroshima and Nagasaki atomic bomb blasts.[126] *Uranium* is weakly radioactive, but lung cancer rates among nonsmoking uranium miners are four times higher than those of the general population, and among smoking miners they are about ten times higher. Many of these cancers in uranium miners are small cell carcinomas.

Asbestos has now become a universally recognized carcinogen.[127] The mean risk of bronchogenic carcinoma among nonsmoking asbestos workers is about five times greater than among the general population. The latent period before the development of lung cancer is between 10 and 30 years. Among asbestos workers, one death out of five is due to bronchogenic carcinoma, one out of ten to pleural or peritoneal mesotheliomas (p. 760), and one out of ten to gastrointestinal carcinomas. Tobacco is an important cofactor in asbestos carcinogenesis; the risk of bronchogenic carcinoma for heavy smokers exposed to asbestos is 92 *times greater* than for nonsmokers not exposed to asbestos. Asbestos hazards are discussed further on page 438.

There is also an increased risk of the development of respiratory cancer among individuals who work with *nickel, chromates, coal, mustard gas, arsenic, beryllium,* and *iron* and in newspaper workers, African gold miners, and haloether workers.[116, 119]

Air Pollution. Unquestionably, we all "swim" in a sea of carcinogens, and it is conceivable that atmospheric pollutants may play some role in the increased incidence of bronchogenic carcinoma today. However, there is difference of opinion as to whether there is an increased risk in urban as opposed to rural areas *after* populations are corrected for tobacco usage. Although most authorities acknowledge the existence of a small *urban factor* in lung cancer incidence,[128] the main culprit, far and away, is cigarette smoking.

Genetic Factors. Occasional familial clustering has suggested a genetic predisposition to lung cancer, as has the variable risk even among very heavy smokers. However attempts at defining markers of genetic susceptibility have proved elusive. At one time it was proposed that patients with lung cancer had genetically higher cellular levels of the enzyme aryl-hydrocarbon-hydroxylase (AHH), which converts noncarcinogenic polycyclic hydrocarbons to carcinogenic intermediates. This hypothesis has not withstood the test of time.[129] Decreased immunologic responsiveness occurs in some patients with lung cancer, but whether this is the cause or the effect of carcinomas is unclear.

Scarring. Finally, some lung cancers arise in the vicinity of pulmonary scars and are termed "scar cancers." Histologically, these tumors are usually adenocarcinomas. Among the scars incriminated are old infarcts, metallic foreign bodies, wounds, and granulomatous infections such as tuberculosis.

HISTOLOGIC CLASSIFICATION. Numerous histologic classifications of bronchogenic carcinoma have been proposed, but the currently popular ones, based on classifications of the World Health Organization (Table 16–5),[130] divides these tumors into four major categories: squamous cell carcinoma, making up 35 to 50%; adenocarcinoma, 15 to 35%; small cell carcinoma, 20 to 25%; and large cell carcinoma, 10 to 15%.[131] The range of incidences reflects different populations (autopsy or surgical series), and the use of varying histologic criteria among different pathologists. In addition, there may be overlap in the histologic pattern, even in the same cancer.[132] Thus, combined types of squamous and adenocarcinoma or of small cell and squamous carcinoma are not infrequent. Nevertheless, the histologic differentiation is useful, since there are differences among the types in terms of epidemiology, distribution in the lung, response to various forms of therapy, and prognosis. For example, squamous cell and small cell carcinomas are predominantly associated with smoking, adenocarcinomas are more often peripherally located in the lung, and small cell carcinomas have by far the poorest prognosis.

From a histogenetic point of view, it seems most likely that all histologic variants of bronchogenic carcinoma, as well as bronchial carcinoid to be described later, are derived from endoderm—a view consistent with the frequency of tumors with mixed histologic patterns.[131] The small cell carcinomas and bronchial carcinoids are derived from the endodermal-neuroendocrine cells and are examples of neuroendocrine tumors.

MORPHOLOGY.[131] Bronchogenic carcinomas arise most often in and about the hilus of the lung. About three-fourths of the lesions take origin from first-, second-, and third-order bronchi. A small percentage have a more peripheral origin but are still not located far out near the pleura. A small number of primary carcinomas of the lung arise in the periphery of the lung substance from the alveolar septal cells or terminal bronchioles. These are predominantly adenocarcinomas, including those of the bronchioloalveolar type, to be discussed separately.

In its development, **carcinoma of the lung begins as**

Table 16–5. HISTOLOGIC CLASSIFICATION OF BRONCHOGENIC CARCINOMA

- Squamous cell (epidermoid) carcinoma
- Adenocarcinoma
  - Bronchial derived
    - (acinar; papillary; solid)
  - Bronchioloalveolar
- Small cell carcinoma
  - Oat cell (lymphocyte-like)
  - Intermediate cell (polygonal)
  - Combined (usually with squamous)
- Large cell carcinoma
  - (Undifferentiated; giant cell; clear cell)
- Combined squamous cell carcinoma and adenocarcinoma

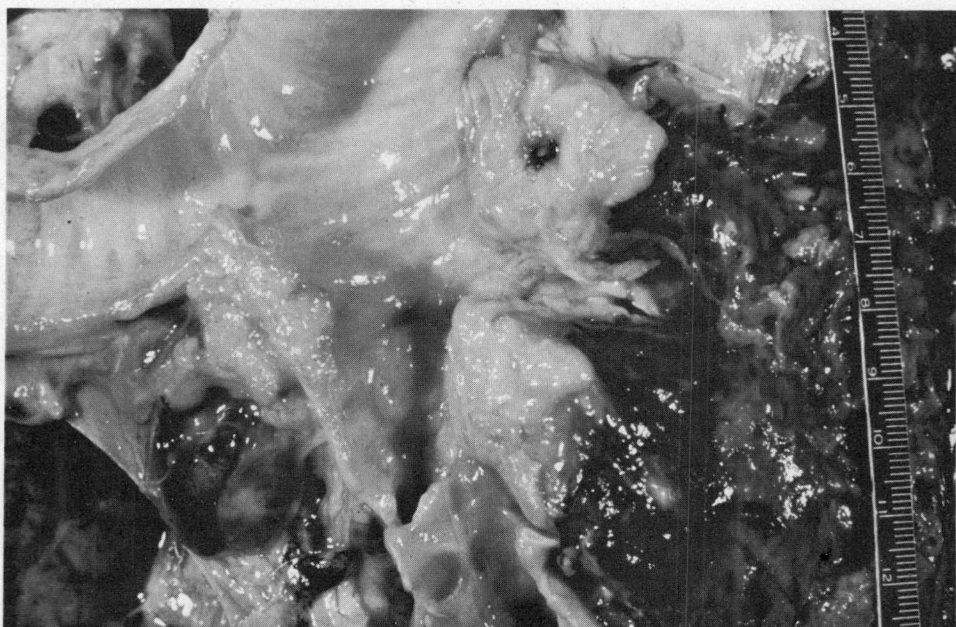

Figure 16–46. Early stage of a bronchogenic carcinoma arising at bifurcation of trachea. Nodular neoplasm invades wall of trachea and right main stem bronchus at several points.

an area of in situ cytologic atypia that, over an unknown interval of time, yields a small area of thickening or piling up of bronchial mucosa. With progression, this small focus, usually less than 1 cm in area, assumes the appearance of an irregular, warty excrescence that elevates or erodes the lining epithelium (Figs. 16–46 and 16–47). The tumor may then follow one of a variety of paths. It may continue to fungate into the bronchial lumen to produce an intraluminal mass. At other times, it rapidly penetrates the wall of the bronchus to infiltrate along the peribronchial tissue (Fig. 16–48) into the adjacent region of the carina or mediastinum. It may extend in this fashion into or about the pericardium. In other instances, the tumor grows along a broad front to produce a cauliflower intraparenchymal mass that appears to push lung substance ahead of it. In almost all patterns, the neoplastic tissue is gray-white and firm to hard. Especially when the tumors are bulky, focal areas of hemorrhage or necrosis may appear to produce yellow-white mottling and softening. Sometimes these necrotic foci cavitate. Extension may occur to the pleural surface and then within the pleural cavity.

Despite this variable behavior, certain characteristics remain uniform. **In most instances, a primary mucosal lesion may be found within the bronchus if sought for with sufficient diligence.** Spread to the tracheal, bronchial, and mediastinal nodes can be found in most cases. The frequency of such nodal involvement varies slightly with the histologic pattern, but averages over 50%. The scalene nodes are affected in about half the cases, providing a valuable clinical means (biopsy) of diagnosing these lesions.

More distant spread of bronchogenic carcinoma occurs through both lymphatic and hematogenous pathways. These tumors have a distressing habit of spreading widely throughout the body and often at a very early stage in their evolution. Often the metastasis presents as the first manifestation of the underlying occult bronchogenic primary lesion. Many craniotomies for brain tumor or explorations of a bone tumor have been performed only to discover metastatic bronchogenic carcinoma. It has been proposed that it may require as long as nine years of growth for a squamous cell bronchogenic carcinoma to achieve a size of 2 cm in diameter. No organ or tissue is spared in the spread of these lesions, but the adrenals, for obscure reasons, are involved in over half the cases. The liver (30 to 50%), brain (20%), and bone (20%) are additional favorite sites of metastases.

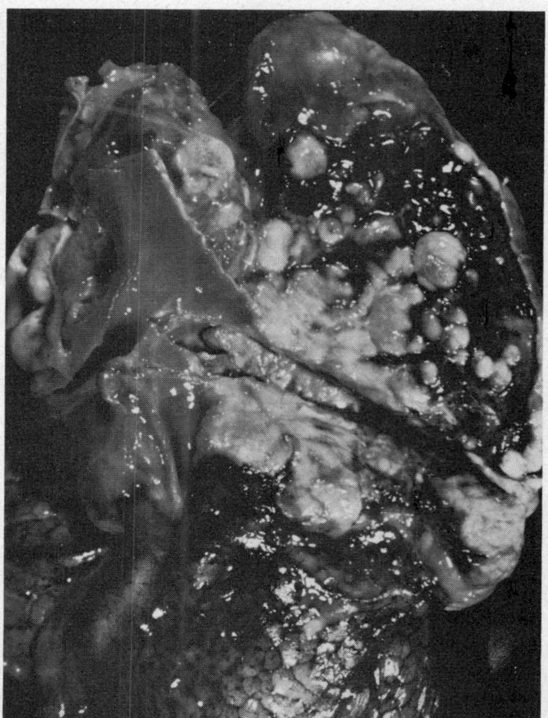

Figure 16–47. Invasive bronchogenic carcinoma with a piling up of tumor within bronchial lumen.

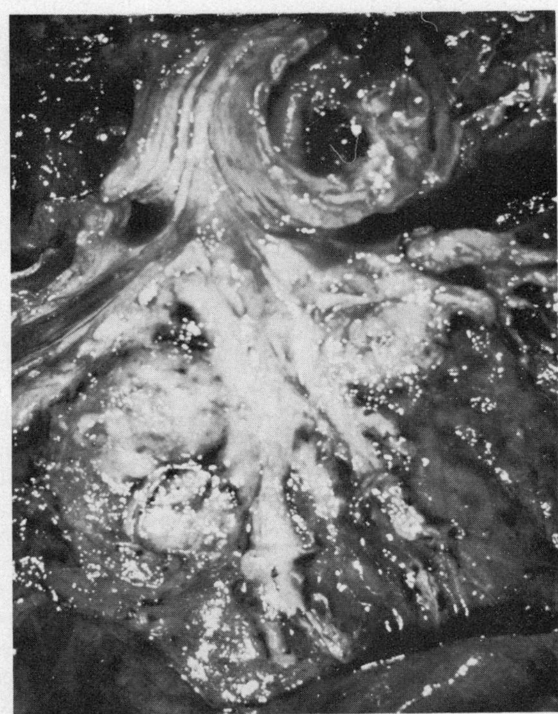

Figure 16–48. Bronchogenic carcinoma infiltrating peribronchial lung substance.

Squamous Cell Carcinoma. This type is most commonly found in men. It is the form most closely correlated with a smoking history. The microscopic features are familiar in the form of production of keratin and intercellular bridges in the well-differentiated forms, but many less well-differentiated squamous cell tumors are encountered that begin to merge with the undifferentiated large cell pattern. This tumor tends to metastasize locally and somewhat later than the other patterns, but its rate of growth in its site of origin is usually more rapid than that of other types. Squamous metaplasia, epithelial dysplasia, and foci of frank carcinoma in situ are regularly present in bronchial epithelium adjacent to the tumor mass.

Adenocarcinoma. Various histologic classifications of adenocarcinomas include at least two forms: (1) the usual bronchial-derived adenocarcinoma; and (2) a somewhat distinctive type termed **bronchioloalveolar carcinoma,** which probably arises from terminal bronchioles or alveolar walls. There may be overlap between these two forms, but the bronchioloalveolar carcinoma has sufficiently distinctive gross, microscopic, and epidemiologic features to be discussed separately.

The regular bronchial adenocarcinoma occurs with about equal frequency in males and females, unlike the small cell or squamous carcinomas, in which there is a preponderance among males. The lesions are usually more peripherally located; tend to be smaller; and vary histologically from well-differentiated tumors with obvious glandular elements to papillary lesions resembling other papillary carcinomas, to solid masses with only occasional mucin-producing glands and cells. About 80% contain mucin when examined with mucin stains. Adenocarcinomas grow more slowly than squamous cell carcinomas. It has been suggested that the adenocarcinoma requires virtually 25 years to reach a size of 2 cm. Peripheral adenocarcinomas are sometimes associated with areas of scarring (scar carcinoma), but it may be difficult to determine whether the scar preceded or followed the cancer. Adenocarcinomas are less frequently associated with a history of smoking than are squamous cell carcinomas.

Small Cell Carcinoma. This is a highly malignant tumor of a rather distinctive cell type. The epithelial cells are generally small, have little or no distinct cytoplasm, and are round or oval, occasionally lymphocyte-like (though about twice the size of a lymphocyte). This is the classic "oat cell" (Fig. 16–49). Other small cell carcinomas have spindle-shaped or polygonal cells and may be thus classified (spindle or polygonal small cell carcinoma). The tumor grows in clusters that exhibit neither glandular nor squamous organization.

Electron microscopic studies show dense-core neurosecretory granules in some of these tumor cells.[4,131] The granules are similar to those found in the argentaffin (Kulchitsky) cells in the gastrointestinal tract; such endocrine cells are present in fetal and neonatal human bronchial epithelium, although they are rare in the adult. The presence of neurosecretory granules in small cell carcinomas, and the ability of some of these tumors to secrete a variety of polypeptide hormones, are characteristics that these tumors share with other neuroendocrine tumors of the so-called APUD type.[4] As described elsewhere (p. 842), cells of this series are known to produce polypeptide hormones and have the ability to take up precursor amines (such as 5-hydroxytryptophan) and convert them to the corresponding peptides. Although a neural crest origin was once surmised for these bronchial cells, they are now thought to be endodermal in origin.

Small cell carcinomas have a strong relationship to cigarette smoking. Most often hilar or central, they are the most aggressive of lung tumors, metastasize widely, and are essentially incurable by surgical means. They are the most common tumor associated with ectopic hormone production.

Large Cell Carcinoma. These anaplastic carcinomas have larger, more polygonal cells and vesicular nuclei. They probably represent those squamous carcinomas and adenocarcinomas that are so undifferentiated that they can no

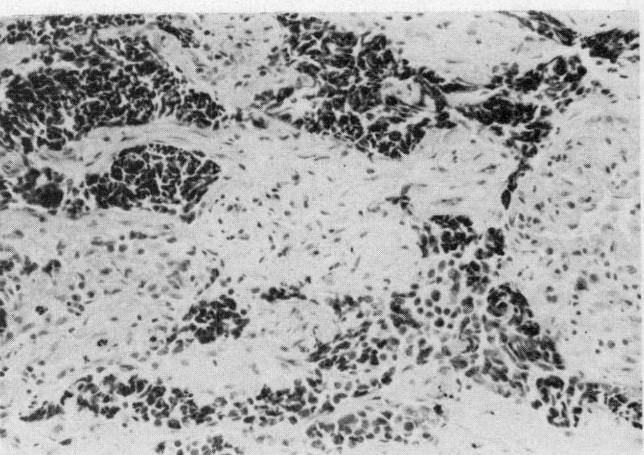

Figure 16–49. Small cell carcinoma. Note islands of small, round, oval or spindly, deeply basophilic cells (Courtesy of Dr. Marcel Seiler, Boston.)

longer be recognized. Some of these large cell carcinomas contain intracellular mucin, some exhibit large numbers of multinucleate cells **(giant cell carcinoma),** some have a clear cytoplasm and are termed **clear cell carcinoma,** and some have a distinctly spindly histologic appearance **(spindle cell carcinoma).**

Secondary Pathology. Bronchogenic carcinomas cause related anatomic changes in the lung substance distal to the point of bronchial involvement. **Partial obstruction may cause marked focal emphysema; total obstruction may lead to atelectasis.** The impaired drainage of the airways is a common cause for **severe suppurative** or **ulcerative bronchitis** or **bronchiectasis. Pulmonary abscesses** sometimes call attention to a silent carcinoma that has initiated the chronic suppuration. Compression or invasion of the superior vena cava may lead either to marked venous congestion or to the full-blown **superior vena caval syndrome.** Extension to the pericardial or pleural sacs may cause **pericarditis** or **pleuritis** with significant effusions.

STAGING. A uniform system for staging cancer according to its anatomic extent at the time of diagnosis is extremely useful for many reasons, chiefly for comparing treatment results from different centers.[133] Despite some lack of agreement on a staging system for lung cancer, the following TNM classification has widest acceptance:

Tumor.

TX: Demonstrable only by cytology of bronchopulmonary secretions.

T1: 3-cm diameter or less; distal-to-lobar bronchus.

T2: Any size extending to hilar region, or >3-cm diameter.

T3: Any size within 2 cm of the carina or invading adjacent structures (e.g., the mediastinum or diaphragm).

Nodes.

N0: None.

N1: Ipsilateral hilar nodes.

N2: Mediastinal nodes.

Metastases.

M0: None.

M1: Distant metastases including to scalene nodes or contralateral hilar nodes.

These data are combined to describe lung cancer as follows:

Occult. Bronchopulmonary secretions contain malignant cells, but there is no other evidence of lung cancer (TX N0 M0).

Stage I. A tumor classified as T1 with or without involvement of the ipsilateral hilar nodes, or a tumor classified as T2 without any nodal involvement (T1 N0 M0, T1 N1 M0, or T2 N0 M0).

Stage II. A tumor classified as T2 with involvement of the ipsilateral hilar nodes (T2 N1 M0).

Stage III. Any tumor with involvement of the mediastinal nodes or with distant metastases, or any tumor more extensive than T2 (N2 with any T or M, M1 with any T or N, or T3 with any N or M0).

CLINICAL COURSE. Lung cancer is one of the most insidious and aggressive neoplasms in the whole realm of oncology.[133] In the usual case, it is discovered in a male in the sixth decade of life whose symptoms are of approximately seven months' duration. The major presenting complaints are cough (75%), weight loss (40%), chest pain (40%), and dyspnea (20%). Not infrequently, the tumor is discovered by its secondary spread in the course of investigation of an apparent primary neoplasm elsewhere. Despite all efforts at early diagnosis by frequent radioscopic examination of the chest, the use of the Papanicolaou smears on sputum and bronchial washings, and the many improvements in thoracic surgery, the overall five-year survival rate is in the order of 9%.[134] In many large clinics, not more than 20 to 30% of lung cancer patients have lesions sufficiently localized even to permit an attempt at resection. In general, the adenocarcinoma and squamous cell patterns tend to remain localized longer and have a slightly better prognosis than the undifferentiated cancers, which usually are invasive lesions by the time they are discovered. In an analysis of almost 4000 cases, the overall five-year survival rate of males was approximately 10% for squamous cell carcinoma and adenocarcinoma, but only 3% for undifferentiated lesions. Surgical resection for *small cell carcinoma* is so ineffective that this diagnosis is said to preclude operative attempts at treatment; instead, radiotherapy and chemotherapy are instituted. Untreated, the survival time for small cell cancer is six to 17 weeks. With treatment, the mean survival after diagnosis is about one year.[135]

Despite this discouraging outlook, it must never be forgotten that many patients have been cured by lobectomy or pneumonectomy, emphasizing the continued need for early diagnosis and adequate prompt therapy. Indeed, *for localized solitary tumors less than 4 cm in diameter* (T1 and T2, N0, M0), *total surgical resection results in up to 50% five-year survival,* except in cases of small cell carcinoma and some larger cell anaplastic tumors.[136]

One of the most intriguing clinical aspects of bronchogenic carcinoma is its association with a series of hormonal and systemic syndromes (paraneoplastic syndromes, p. 255), some of which may antedate the development of a gross pulmonary lesion.[137] The hormones or hormone-like factors elaborated include (1) *antidiuretic hormone,* inducing hyponatremia due to inappropriate ADH secretion; (2) *ACTH,* producing Cushing's syndrome; (3) *parathormone and or prostaglandin E,* inducing hypercalcemia; (4) *calcitonin,* causing hypocalcemia; (5) *gonadotropins,* causing gynecomastia; and (6) *serotonin,* associated with the carcinoid syndrome. Any one of the histologic types of tumors may occasionally produce any one of the hormones, but tumors producing ACTH and ADH are predominantly small cell carcinomas, whereas those producing hypercalcemia are mostly squamous cell tumors. The carcinoid syndrome is associated rarely with oat cell carcinoma but is more common with the bronchial carcinoids, described later.

Other systemic manifestations of bronchogenic carcinoma include a *myopathy,* characterized by muscle weakness; *peripheral neuropathy,* usually purely sensory; dermatologic abnormalities, including *acanthosis nigricans* (p. 1274); hematologic abnormalities such as *leukemoid reactions;* and finally a peculiar abnormality of connective tissue called *hypertrophic pulmonary osteoarthropathy,* associated with clubbing of the fingers.

Apical lung cancers in the superior pulmonary sulcus tend to invade the neural structures around the trachea, including the cervical sympathetic plexus, and produce a group of clinical findings that includes severe pain in the distribution of the ulnar nerve and *Horner's syndrome* (enophthalmos, ptosis, miosis, and anhidrosis) on the same side as the lesion. Such tumors are also referred to as *Pancoast's tumors.*

There is much yet to be learned about the biology of these neoplasms, but most important is an understanding of their causation. Until we know more, cigarette smoking must stand indicted as the major villain.

BRONCHIOLOALVEOLAR CARCINOMA

As the name implies, this form of lung cancer occurs well out in the pulmonary parenchyma in the terminal bronchioloalveolar regions.[138, 139] It represents, in various series, 1.1 to 9.0% of all lung cancers. Changes are very similar histologically to an apparently infectious disease of South African sheep known as *jagziekte.* However, numerous efforts to identify an infectious agent in man or to transmit the disease to sheep with cell-free extracts of human carcinoma have been unavailing.

Histologically, the tumor is characterized by distinctive, tall, columnar-to-cuboidal epithelial cells that line up along alveolar septa and project into the alveolar spaces in numerous branching papillary formations (Fig. 16–50). The tumor cells often contain abundant mucinous secretions. Many times the columnar cells desquamate into the alveolar spaces, virtually filling them, and, in the more anaplastic lesions, masses of cytologically atypical epithelial cells fill the alveoli. Occasional large multinucleated giant cells are produced. The degree of anaplasia is quite variable, but most tumors are well differentiated and tend to preserve the native septal wall architecture. Ultrastructurally, bronchioloalveolar carcinomas are a heterogeneous group, consisting of mucin-secreting bronchiolar cells, Clara cells (most commonly), or (rarely) Type II pneumonocytes.

Macroscopically, the tumor almost always occurs in the peripheral portions of the lung either as a single nodule, or more often as multiple diffuse nodules that sometimes coalesce to produce a pneumonia-like consolidation. The parenchymal nodules have a mucinous gray translucence when secretion is present and otherwise appear as solid gray-white areas, which can be confused with pneumonia on casual inspection. Because the tumor does not involve major bronchi, atelectasis and emphysema are infrequent accompaniments. Metastases are not widely disseminated or large, nor do they occur early, but they eventually appear in up to 45% of cases.

Clinically, these tumors occur in patients of all ages from the third decade to advanced years of life. They are equally distributed among males and females. The symptomatology, which usually appears late, is much like that of bronchogenic carcinoma, with cough, hemoptysis, and pain the major presenting findings. Occasionally they may produce a picture of diffuse interstitial pneumonitis (p. 743). The overall five-year survival rate is about 25%.

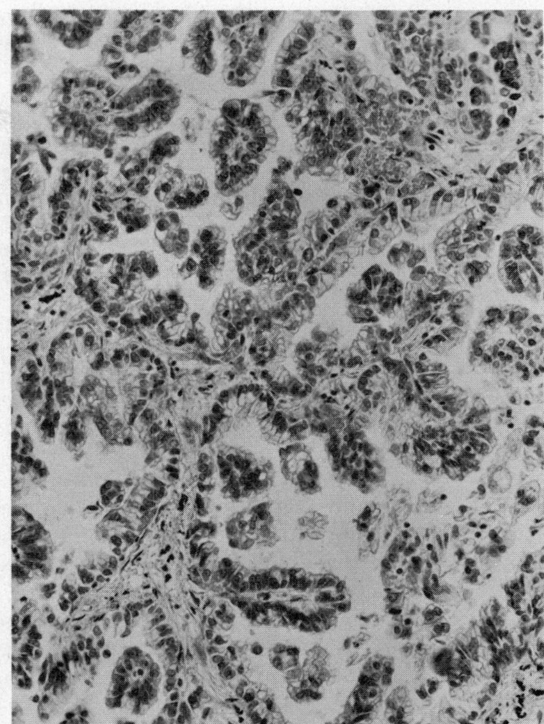

Figure 16–50. Terminal bronchiolar (alveolar) carcinoma with characteristic tall columnar cell papillary growth.

BRONCHIAL CARCINOID

Bronchial carcinoids represent about 5% of all lung tumors.[140] They make up over 90% of a group of bronchial tumors formerly classified as "bronchial adenoma," but now known to be often locally invasive or occasionally capable of metastasis. The remaining 10% of the group includes adenoid cystic carcinoma and mucoepidermoid carcinoma—tumors with histologic patterns reminiscent of similar tumors in salivary glands (p. 793). Most patients with carcinoid tumors are under 40 years of age, and the incidence is equal for both sexes. There is no known relationship to cigarette smoking or other environmental factors. Bronchial carcinoids arise from the neuroendocrine argentaffin cells of the bronchial mucosa (Kulchitsky) and resemble intestinal carcinoids, described in detail on page 842. They contain dense-core neurosecretory granules in their cytoplasm, secrete hormonally active polypeptides, and occasionally occur as part of multiple endocrine neoplasia (p. 988).

Histologically, the tumor is composed of nests, cords, and masses of cells separated by a delicate fibrous stroma. In common with the lesions of the gastrointestinal tract, the individual cells are quite regular and have uniform round nuclei and infrequent mitoses (Fig. 16–51). Occasional carcinoid adenomas display variation in the size and shape of cells and nuclei and, along with this pleomorphism, tend to demonstrate a more aggressive and more invasive behavior. On electron microscopy the cells exhibit the dense-core granules characteristic of other neuroendocrine tumors (Fig. 18–33, p. 842).

On gross examination, the tumors grow as finger-like or spherical polypoid masses that commonly project into the lumen of the bronchus and are usually covered by an intact mucosa. They rarely exceed 3 to 4 cm in diameter. Most are confined to the main stem bronchi. Others, however, produce little intraluminal mass but instead penetrate the bronchial wall to fan out in the peribronchial tissue, producing the so-called "collar-button" lesion. The parenchymal infiltration often forms a cohesive sphere apparently pushing the lung substance ahead of it (Fig. 16–52). This sharp line of delineation is more apparent than real, since microscopic examination usually indicates local infiltration and no encapsulation.

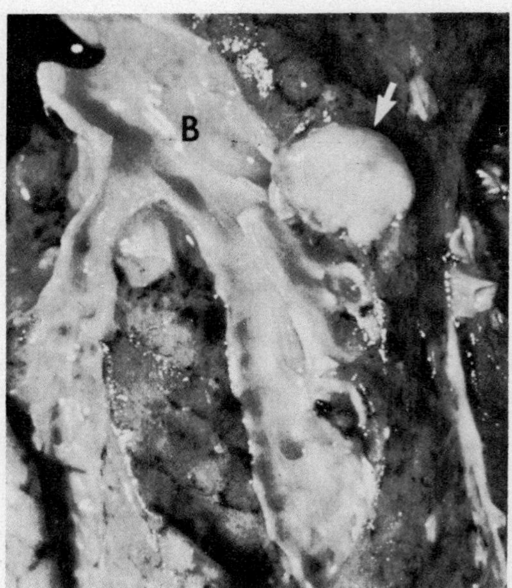

Figure 16–52. Bronchial carcinoid growing as a spherical pale mass *(arrow)* apparently external to lumen of bronchus (B).

The clinical manifestations of bronchial carcinoids emanate from their intraluminal growth, their capacity to metastasize, and the ability of some of these lesions to elaborate vasoactive amines. Persistent cough, hemoptysis, impairment of drainage of respiratory passages with secondary infections, bronchiectasis, emphysema, and atelectasis are all by-products of the intraluminal growth of these lesions.

About 40% of these tumors metastasize to regional nodes and cause enlargement of the hilar nodes; 5 to 10% also metastasize to the liver to produce hepatomegaly. Most interesting, however, are those functioning lesions of the argentaffinoma pattern capable of producing the classic carcinoid syndrome, i.e., intermittent attacks of diarrhea, flushing, and cyanosis (p. 844). It has, in fact, been possible to isolate 5-hydroxytryptamine (serotonin) from some lesions. In addition, bradykinin, a potent vasodilator, is released during flushes, probably by the action of kallikrein from tumors on the plasma globulin kininogen. Overall, most bronchial carcinoids do not have secretory activity and do not metastasize, but follow a relatively benign course for long periods and are therefore amenable to resection.

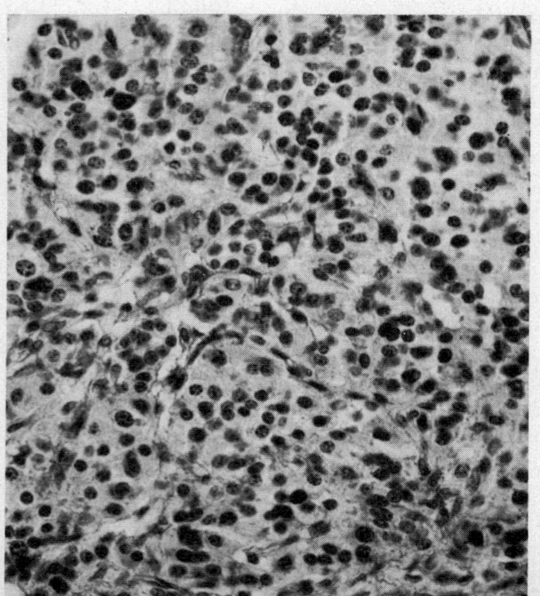

Figure 16–51. Bronchial carcinoid.

MISCELLANEOUS TUMORS

The complex category of benign and malignant mesenchymal tumors, such as fibroma, fibrosarcoma, leiomyoma, leiomyosarcoma, lipoma, hemangioma, and chondroma, may occur but they are rare. Benign and malignant lymphoreticular tumors and tumor-like conditions, largely similar to those described in other organs may also affect the lung, either as an isolated lesion or more commonly as part of a generalized disorder.[113] These include non-Hodgkin's and Hodgkin's lymphoma, lymphomatoid granulomatosis, pseudolymphoma, and plasma cell granuloma.

The relatively common *hamartoma* merits a brief description. It is usually discovered as an incidental, rounded focus of radiopacity on a routine chest film, giving rise to what the roentgenologist calls a "coin lesion." These neoplasms are rarely over 3 to 4 cm in diameter and are principally composed of mature hyaline cartilage. Occasionally, the cartilage contains cystic or cleftlike spaces, and these may be lined by characteristic respiratory epithelium. At other times, there are admixtures of fibrous tissue, fat, and blood vessels, making it clear that these lesions probably represent a hamartoma of the lung.

Tumors in the mediastinum either may arise in mediastinal structures or may be metastatic from the lungs or other organs. They may also invade or compress the lungs. Table 16–6 lists the most common tumors in the various compartments of the mediastinum. Specific tumor types are discussed in appropriate sections of this book.

Table 16–6. MEDIASTINAL TUMORS

Superior Mediastinum	Posterior Mediastinum
Lymphoma Thymoma Thyroid lesions Metastatic carcinoma Parathyroid tumors	Neurogenic tumors (schwannoma; neurofibroma) Lymphoma Gastroenteric hernia
Anterior Mediastinum	**Middle Mediastinum**
Thymoma Teratoma Lymphoma Thyroid lesions Parathyroid tumors	Bronchogenic cyst Pericardial cyst Lymphoma

METASTATIC TUMORS OF LUNG

The lung is more often affected by metastatic growths than it is by primary neoplasms. Both carcinomas and sarcomas arising anywhere in the body may spread to the lungs via the blood or lymphatics or by direct continuity. Growth of contiguous tumors into the lungs occurs most often with esophageal carcinomas and mediastinal lymphomas.

The pattern of metastatic growth within the lungs is quite variable. In the usual case, multiple discrete nodules are scattered throughout all lobes (Fig. 16–53). These discrete lesions tend to occur in the periphery of the lung parenchyma rather than in the central locations of the primary bronchogenic carcinoma.

As a second macroscopic variant, metastatic growths may confine themselves to peribronchiolar and perivascular tissue spaces, presumably when the tumor has extended to the lung through the lymphatics. Here the lung septa and connective tissue are diffusely infiltrated with the gray-white tumor. Least commonly, the metastatic tumor is totally inapparent on gross examination and only becomes evident on histologic section as a diffuse intralymphatic dissemination dispersed throughout the peribronchial and perivascular channels. The subpleural lymphatics may be outlined by the contained

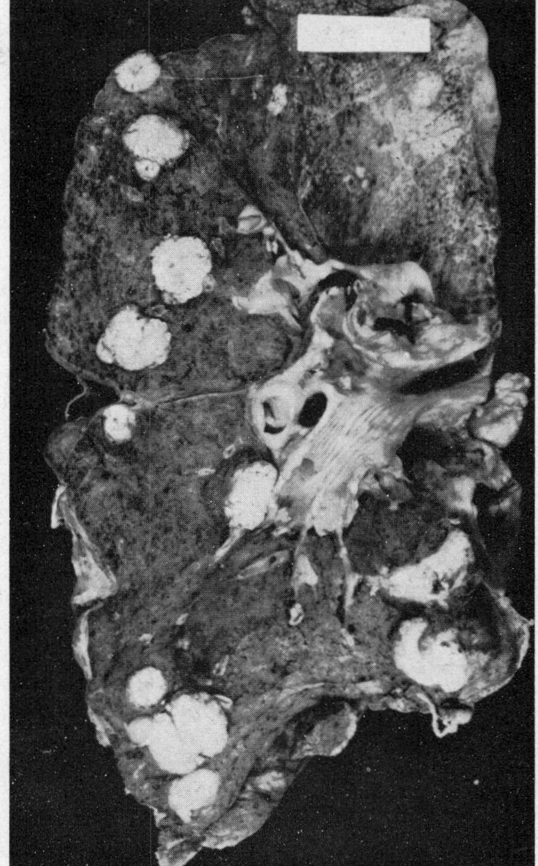

Figure 16–53. Metastases in lung from a breast carcinoma in a 56-year-old woman.

tumor, producing an anatomic pattern referred to as *lymphangitis carcinomatosa*. In certain instances, microscopic tumor emboli fill the small pulmonary vessels and may result in life-threatening pulmonary hypertension.

Pleura

Pathologic involvement of the pleura is, with rare exceptions, a secondary complication of some underlying disease. The only primary disorders that are reasonably common are (1) primary intrapleural bacterial infections that imply seeding of this space as an isolated focus in the course of a transient bacteremia and (2) a primary neoplasm of the pleura—mesothelioma. With these exceptions, pleural diseases usually follow some underlying disorder, most often pulmonary. Secondary infections are extremely common, however, and pleural adhesions or other forms of pleural involvement are present in at least two-thirds of all postmortem cases. Occasionally, the secondary pleural disease assumes a dominant role in the clinical problem, as occurs in bacterial pneumonia with the development of empyema.

Pleural effusion is a common manifestation of both primary and secondary pleural involvements.[141] Normally, no more than 15 ml of serous relatively acellular clear fluid lubricates the pleural surface. Increased accumulation of pleural fluid occurs under five settings: (1) increased hydrostatic pressure, as in congestive heart failure; (2) increased vascular permeability, as in pneumonia; (3) decreased oncotic pressure, as in nephrotic syndrome; (4) increased intrapleural negative pressure, as in atelectasis; and (5) decreased lymphatic drainage, as in mediastinal carcinomatosis. The character of the pleural effusion under these circumstances is variable, as we shall see.

Diseases of the pleura can be divided for convenience into inflammations, noninflammatory pleural effusions, and neoplasms.

INFLAMMATIONS

Inflammations of the pleura (pleuritis), depending on their stage and causative agent, can be divided on the basis of the character of the resultant exudate into serous, fibrinous, serofibrinous, suppurative (empyema), and hemorrhagic pleuritis.

SEROFIBRINOUS PLEURITIS

Serous, serofibrinous, and fibrinous pleuritis are all caused by essentially the same processes. Fibrinous exudations generally reflect a later and more severe exudative reaction that, in an earlier developmental phase, might have presented as a serous or serofibrinous exudate.

The common causes of such pleuritis are inflammatory diseases within the lungs, such as tuberculosis, pneumonia, lung infarcts, lung abscess, and bronchiectasis. Rheumatoid arthritis, disseminated lupus erythematosus, uremia, the diffuse systemic infections, and other systemic disorders also cause serous or serofibrinous pleuritis. Occasionally, metastatic involvement of the pleura produces a pure serous or serofibrinous pleuritis. The pleura is almost invariably affected in tuberculosis, and the pleural reaction in the early stages tends to remain as a serous or copious serofibrinous exudation, designated *pleurisy with effusion.* Irradiation used in therapy of tumors in the lung or mediastinum often causes a serofibrinous pleuritis.

It is frequently important to differentiate an exudate of inflammatory origin from a transudate of circulatory origin, particularly in older individuals suffering from cardiac failure, in whom pulmonary infection may be suspected. In general, the inflammatory effusions consist of relatively clear, limpid, straw-colored fluid in which, occasionally, small strands of opaque, yellow-white fibrin may be found floating. The specific gravity tends to be greater than 1.016 to 1.020, and scattered lymphocytes, macrophages, and polymorphonuclear neutrophils, as well as the ever-present mesothelial cells, can frequently be found within the sediment after centrifugation. In contrast, the transudates are clear and watery fluids with a specific gravity less than 1.012. Only mesothelial cells are present in the sediment, with possibly a few scattered lymphocytes.

In most instances the inflammatory reaction is only minimal, and the fluid exudate is resorbed with either resolution or organization of the fibrinous component. Since the exudative responses may sometimes cause the accumulation of up to several liters in each pleural cavity, they may be responsible for considerable encroachment upon lung space and give rise to respiratory distress.

SUPPURATIVE PLEURITIS (EMPYEMA)

A purulent pleural exudate usually implies bacterial or mycotic seeding of the pleural space. Most commonly, this occurs by contiguous spread of organisms from intrapulmonary suppuration, but occasionally it occurs by lymphatic or hematogenous dissemination from a more distant infection. Rarely, suppurative infections below the diaphragm, such as the subdiaphragmatic or liver abscess, may extend by continuity through the diaphragm into the pleural spaces, more often on the right side.

Empyema is characterized by yellow-green creamy pus that may accumulate in large volumes (up to 500 to 1000 ml), but usually in smaller amounts than the serous reactions described. The exudate is made up of masses of polymorphonuclear neutrophils admixed with other leukocytes. Although it may be difficult to visualize microorganisms on smears of the exudate, it should be possible to demonstrate them by cultural methods. Empyema may resolve, but this fortunate outcome is less common than organization of the exudate, with the formation of dense, tough fibrous adhesions that frequently obliterate the pleural space. Sometimes a thick, dense connective tissue layer is formed that envelops the lungs and seriously embarrasses pulmonary expansion. Calcification may occur in this scar tissue. Massive calcification is particularly characteristic of tuberculous empyema.

HEMORRHAGIC PLEURITIS

True sanguineous inflammatory exudates must be differentiated from bloody or traumatic contamination of serous or serofibrinous exudates. The slight bleeding that often occurs in the course of fluid withdrawal is the most frequent cause of confusion. Hemorrhagic exudates are infrequent and are found in hemorrhagic diatheses, rickettsial diseases, and neoplastic involvement of the pleural cavity. The sanguineous exudate must be differentiated from whole blood that may fill the pleural cavity when an aneurysm ruptures. When hemorrhagic pleuritis is encountered, careful search should be made for the presence of exfoliated tumor cells.

NONINFLAMMATORY PLEURAL EFFUSIONS

HYDROTHORAX

Noninflammatory collections of serous fluid within the pleural cavities are called hydrothorax. The fluid is clear and straw-colored and has the other characteristics already mentioned. Hydrothorax may be unilateral or bilateral, depending on the underlying etiology. The most common cause of hydrothorax is cardiac failure, and for this reason it is usually accompanied by pulmonary congestion and edema. In cardiac failure, hydrothorax is usually, but not invariably, bilateral. Transudations may collect in any other systemic disease associated with generalized edema, and are therefore found in renal failure and cirrhosis of the liver.

In most instances, hydrothorax is not loculated, but, in the presence of preexistent pleural adhesions, local collections may be found walled off by bridging fibrous tissue. Except for these localized collections, the fluid usually collects basally, when the patient is in an upright position, and causes compression and atelectasis of the inundated regions of the lung. If the underlying cause is alleviated, hydrothorax may be resorbed, usually leaving behind no permanent alterations. In many instances, highly satisfying relief of respiratory distress is accomplished by the withdrawal of large pleural transudates.

HEMOTHORAX

The escape of blood into the pleural cavity is known as hemothorax. It is almost invariably a fatal complication of a ruptured aortic aneurysm. Pure hemothorax is readily identifiable by the large clots that accompany the fluid component of the blood. Since this calamity almost invariably leads to death within minutes to hours, it is uncommon to find any response within the pleural cavity. Rarely, leakage of smaller amounts may not prove fatal promptly and provides a stimulus to organization and the development of pleural adhesions.

CHYLOTHORAX

Chylothorax is an accumulation of milky fluid, usually of lymphatic origin, in the pleural cavity. Chyle is milky white because it contains finely emulsified fats. When it is allowed to stand, a creamy, fatty, supernatant layer separates. True chyle should be differentiated from turbid serous fluid, which does not contain fat and does not separate into an overlying layer of high fat content. Chylothorax may be bilateral but is more often confined to the left side. The volume of fluid is variable but rarely assumes the massive proportions of hydrothorax.

Chylothorax is most often encountered in malignant conditions arising within the thoracic cavity, usually malignant lymphomas that cause obstruction of the major lymphatic ducts. More distant cancers may metastasize via the lymphatics and grow within the right lymphatic or thoracic duct to produce obstruction. Presumably obstruction causes rupture of these ducts, with the escape of the milky-white chylous fluid.

PNEUMOTHORAX

Pneumothorax refers to air or gas in the pleural cavities, and may be spontaneous, traumatic, or therapeutic. Spontaneous pneumothorax may complicate any form of pulmonary disease that causes rupture of an alveolus. An abscess cavity that communicates either directly with the pleural space or with the lung interstitial tissue may also lead to the escape of air. In the latter circumstance, the air may dissect through the lung substance or back through the mediastinum, eventually to enter the pleural cavity. Pneumothorax is most commonly associated with emphysema, asthma, and tuberculosis. Traumatic pneumothorax is usually caused by some perforating injury to the chest wall, but sometimes the trauma pierces the lung to provide two avenues for the accumulation of air within the pleural spaces. Therapeutic pneumothorax was once a commonly practiced method of deflating the lung to favor the healing of tuberculous lesions. Such induced pneumothorax slowly subsides, however, because of absorption of the introduced air, and requires constant replenishment. The same is true for spontaneous and traumatic pneumothorax, provided the original communication seals itself.

Of the various forms of pneumothorax, the one that attracts greatest clinical attention is so-called *spontaneous idiopathic pneumothorax*. This entity is encountered in relatively young people; appears to be due to rupture of small, peripheral, usually apical subpleural blebs; and usually subsides spontaneously as the air is resorbed. Recurrent attacks are common and may be quite disabling.

Pneumothorax can be identified anatomically only by careful opening of the thoracic cavity under water to detect the escape of gas or air bubbles. This technique is best performed by creating a pocket of a skin flap that can be filled with water before the thorax is opened. By puncturing the pleural cavity with some instrument under water, it is possible to note the escape of bubbles. Pneumothorax may have as much significance as a fluid collection within the lungs, since it also causes compression, collapse, and atelectasis of the lung and may be responsible for marked respiratory distress. Occasionally, the lung collapse is marked: when the defect acts as a flap valve and permits the entrance of air during inspiration, but fails to permit its escape during expiration, it effectively acts as a pump that creates tension pneumothorax.

TUMORS OF PLEURA

The pleura may be involved in primary or secondary tumors. Secondary metastatic involvement is far more common than are primary tumors. The most frequent metastatic malignancies arise from primary neoplasms of the lung and breast. Advanced mammary carcinomas frequently penetrate the thoracic wall directly to involve the parietal and then the visceral pleura. They may also reach these cavities through the lymphatics and, more rarely, the blood. In addition to these cancers, malignancy from any organ of the body may spread to pleural spaces. Ovarian carcinomas are the major offenders, since these tumors tend to cause widespread implants in both the abdominal and the thoracic cavities. In most of these metastatic involvements, a serous or serosanguineous effusion follows that may contain desquamated neoplastic cells. For this reason, careful cytologic examination of the sediment is of considerable diagnostic value.

MESOTHELIOMA

These are rare tumors that arise from either the visceral or the parietal pleura.[142, 143] Although distinctly uncommon, they have assumed great importance in the past few years because of the increased incidence of malignant mesothelioma among persons with a heavy exposure to asbestos.[142] In coastal areas with shipping industries in the United States and Britain, or in Canadian and South African mining areas, up to 90% of reported mesotheliomas are asbestos related. The lifetime risk of the development of mesothelioma in heavily exposed individuals is as high as 7 to 10%. There is a long-latent period of 25 to 45 years for the development of asbestos-related mesothelioma, and there seems to be no increased risk in asbestos workers who smoke. This is in contrast to asbestos-related bronchogenic carcinoma, in which the risk of cancer rises sharply within ten years of asbestos exposure and is markedly magnified by smoking. Thus, for asbestos workers (particularly those who are also smokers), the risk of dying of lung carcinoma far exceeds that of developing mesothelioma.

Asbestos bodies are found in the lungs of up to 100% of patients with mesothelioma, and mesotheliomas can be induced readily in experimental animals by intrapleural injections of asbestos.[144] There is thus little doubt about the carcinogenicity of asbestos; the mechanisms of cancer induction are discussed on page 440.

There are two types of mesotheliomas:

1. The benign, localized mesothelioma (also called pleural fibroma) is a localized growth that is often attached to the pleural surface by a pedicle. The tumors may be small (1 to 2 cm in diameter) or may reach an enormous size, but always remain confined to the surface of the lung. These tumors do not usually produce a pleural effusion. Grossly, they consist of dense fibrous tissue with occasional cysts filled with viscid fluid; microscopically, the tumors show whorls of reticulin and collagen fibers among which are interspersed spindle cells resembling fibroblasts. For this reason, these mesotheliomas are also termed "fibromas." In some instances, the mesothelial cells acquire a cuboidal appearance and line papillary processes. The benign mesothelioma has no relationship to asbestos exposure.

2. The malignant mesothelioma is a diffuse lesion that spreads widely in the pleural space and is usually associated with extensive pleural effusion and direct invasion of thoracic structures. The affected lung is ensheathed by a thick layer of soft, gelatinous, grayish-pink tumor tissue (Fig. 16–54). Microscopically, malignant mesotheliomas consist of a mixture of two types of tissues, one of which might predominate in an individual case. Mesothelial cells have the potential to develop as either mesenchymal stromal cells or epithelium-like lining cells. The mesenchymal type of mesothelioma appears as a spindle cell sarcoma, resembling fibrosarcoma **(sarcomatoid type)**, whereas the papillary type consists of cuboidal, columnar, or flattened cells forming a tubular and papillary structure **(epithelial type)**, resembling adenocarcinoma (Fig. 16–55). Indeed, epithelial mesothelioma may at times be difficult to differentiate from pulmonary adenocarcinoma. Special features that favor mesothelioma include:

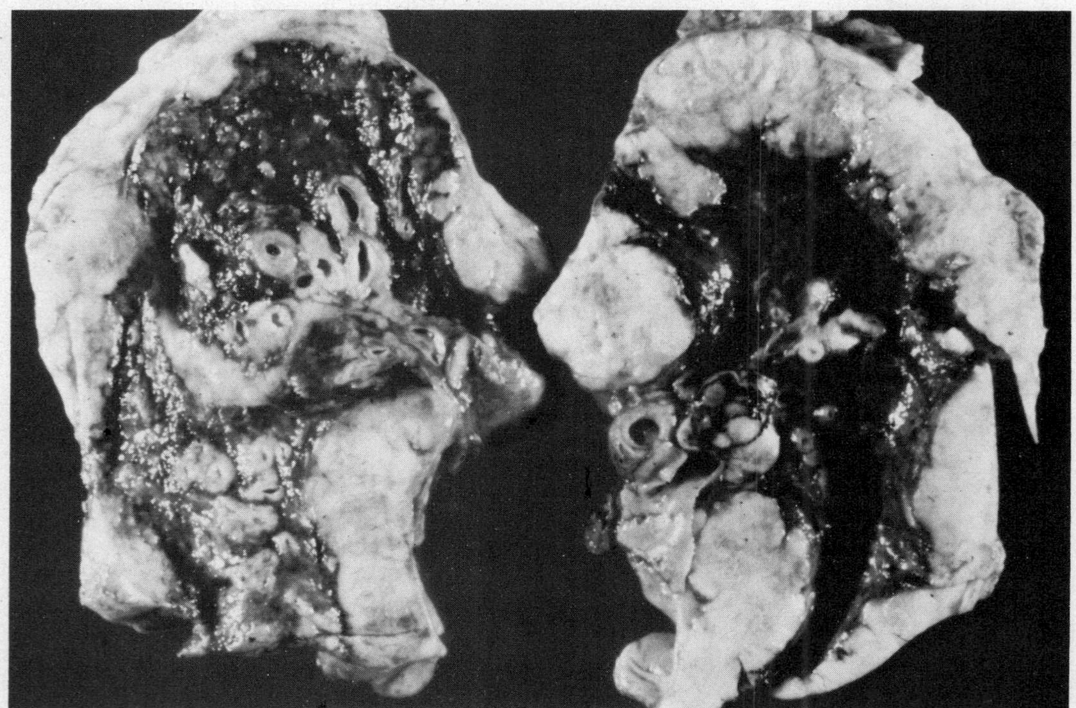

Figure 16–54. Malignant mesothelioma. Note thick, firm, white, pleural tumor tissue that ensheathes this bisected lung. (Courtesy of Dr. Marcel Seiler, West Roxbury Veterans Administration Hospital.)

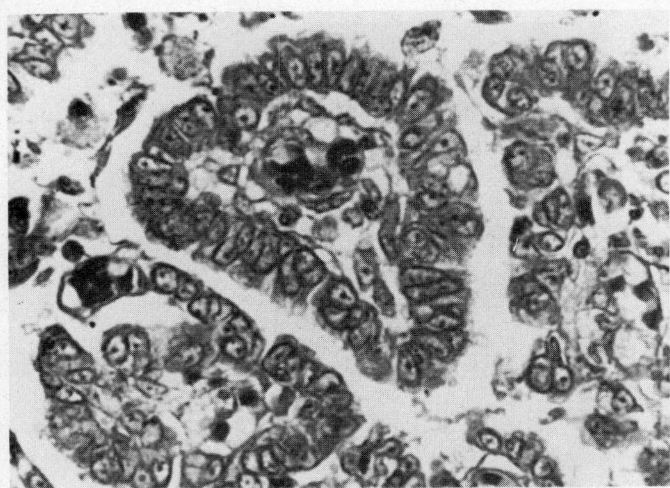

Figure 16–55. Mesothelioma, papillary epithelial type. Note resemblance to papillary adenocarcinoma. (Courtesy of Dr. John Godleski, Brigham and Women's Hosptal, Boston)

positive-staining for acid mucopolysaccharide, which is inhibited by previous digestion by hyaluronidase; strong staining for keratin proteins, with accentuation of perinuclear rather than peripheral staining; and, on electron microscopy, the presence of long microvilli and abundant tonofilaments, but absent microvillous rootlets and lamellar bodies.[143] The mixed type of mesothelioma contains both epithelial and sarcomatoid patterns.

The presenting complaints are chest pain, dyspnea, and, as noted, recurrent pleural effusions.[145] Concurrent pulmonary asbestosis (fibrosis) is present in only 20% of patients with pleural mesothelioma. Fifty per cent of those with pleural disease die within 12 months of diagnosis, and very few survive longer than two years. The lung is invaded directly, and there is metastatic spread to the hilar lymph nodes and eventually to liver and other distant organs.

Mesotheliomas also arise in the peritoneum, pericardium, tunica vaginalis, and genital tract (benign adenomatoid tumor, see p. 1098). *Peritoneal mesotheliomas* are particularly related to very heavy asbestos exposure; 50% of such patients also have pulmonary fibrosis. Although in about 50% of cases the disease remains confined to the abdominal cavity, intestinal involvement frequently leads to death from intestinal obstruction or inanition.

Larynx

INFLAMMATIONS

There are only two reasonably common forms of disease of the larynx: inflammation and neoplasms. Inflammation of the larynx, laryngitis, usually occurs as a part of inflammatory disorders of the lungs and lower respiratory air passages. Occasionally, most often in heavy smokers, the larynx is affected alone without involvement of the lower air passages. However, the larynx may also be affected in many systemic infectious diseases, such as tuberculosis, syphilis, and diphtheria, and it may also be secondarily involved in inflammations that begin in the oral cavity, such as streptococcal sore throat, thrush, or any of the nonspecific bacterial disorders of the oral cavity or accompanying lymphoid structures. Laryngeal inflammation, although usually of trivial clinical significance, may at times be serious, particularly in infancy or childhood when the marked exudation or edema may cause laryngeal obstruction. The severe edema of allergic origin that may follow inhalation or ingestion of an allergen or that sometimes arises after a bee or insect bite may cause sudden alarming, but usually transitory, distress.

TUMORS OF LARYNX

Neoplasms of the larynx are, on the whole, uncommon. These tumors may be either benign or malignant, and the malignant forms are almost invariably squamous cell carcinomas.[146]

BENIGN NEOPLASMS

The benign neoplasms run the gamut of every cell type found within this structure, and accordingly include polyps and papillomas, chondromas, and leiomyomas, corresponding to the native cellular structure of this organ. With the exceptions of the polyp and the papilloma, the benign tumors are extremely uncommon and follow the identical pattern of growth of these tumors situated anywhere in the body.

Polyps of the larynx are smooth, rounded, sessile, or pedunculated nodules that rarely exceed 1 cm in diameter and occur most often on the true vocal cords. They usually are totally covered by squamous epithelium that may become ulcerated when the nodules are exposed to the trauma of the opposing vocal cord. Microscopically, the polyp is composed largely of a core or stroma of connective tissue, varying from a loose myxomatous network to a dense, collagenous, hyaline, scarlike mass. Usually, the nonulcerated and noninfected polyp has only scattered inflammatory white cells within the stroma. Frequently, the stroma is intensely vascularized.

Polyps occur chiefly in adults and predominantly in males. They are more often found in heavy smokers or in individuals who impose great strain upon their larynx. Polyps are frequently found in singers and are sometimes designated *"singers' nodes."* Because of their strategic location, they characteristically cause modification of the character of the voice and progressive hoarseness.

The *papilloma* is a true neoplasm that grows as a soft, succulent, raspberry-like, friable excrescence or nodule, usually on the true vocal cords. These rarely exceed 1 cm in diameter, are frequently ulcerated because of their fragility, and bleed readily on manipulation. As papillomas, they are composed of multiple finger-like projections barely discernible on gross inspection. On histologic inspection, these papillae are composed of a central core of fibrous tissue covered by stratified squamous epithelium. In many cases, protracted trauma to these masses produces marked epithelial atypicality and proliferation. It is therefore not uncommonly difficult to distinguish the benign papilloma from a malignant squamous cell carcinoma, and in fact it is believed that these benign neoplasms have the potential of undergoing malignant transformation.

These lesions occur at any age and, although usually single in adults, may be multiple in children. The multiple juvenile papillomas often regress at puberty; they are now known to be caused by one of the human papilloma viruses (HPV II).[147] These childhood tumors are responsible for progressive hoarseness and, if large, encroachment upon the airway, with respiratory difficulty. Malignant transformation is rare and almost always occurs after irradiation of these lesions.

MALIGNANT TUMORS

Although any type of malignancy, carcinomatous or sarcomatous, may arise in the larynx from the native cell population, all are extremely uncommon save for carcinomas arising in the surface epithelium. The carcinomas are usually found in adults beyond the fourth decade of life and are considerably more common in males than in females, in the ratio of approximately 7 to 1. The basis for this sex relationship is not clear, but it is certain that cigarette smoking and other environmental factors play a role. An increased incidence of exposure to asbestos has been reported in patients with laryngeal cancer.

Most carcinomas of the larynx occur directly on the vocal cords, but they may also be found above and below the cords, on the epiglottis and aryepiglottic folds, and in the piriform sinuses. Those arising within the larynx are termed intrinsic; those that extend or arise outside are designated extrinsic. These begin as in situ lesions that later yield pearly gray wrinkling and thickening of the epithelium to become plaquelike lesions, which then ulcerate, fungate, and extend centrifugally. They may, therefore, vary in size from small involvements less than 1 cm in diameter to ulcerating, friable masses that involve large regions of the larynx, totally destroy one or both vocal cords, and infiltrate widely into the perilaryngeal structures (Fig. 16–56). Histologically, 95% are squamous cell carcinomas. The rare adenocarcinomas are presumed to originate in the mucus-secreting glands. The degree of anaplasia of the squamous cell pattern is quite variable, and very striking undifferentiation and anaplasia with massive tumor giant cells and multiple bizarre atypical mitotic figures are occasionally encountered in the more rapidly growing lesions.

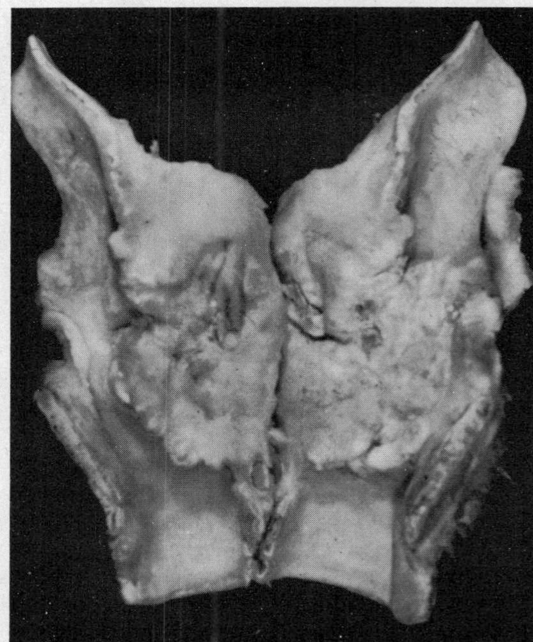

Figure 16–56. Invasive carcinoma of larynx, transected to illustrate intraluminal growth of neoplasm.

Clinically, cases usually first become apparent with the onset of resistant, progressive hoarseness, followed possibly by pain, difficulty in swallowing, hemoptysis, and eventually even respiratory distress. Because the lesions are ulcerated, secondary infection may modify the clinical symptom complex by the appearance of fever and other systemic reactions. Irradiation, often combined with laryngectomy, has increased the five-year survival rate of such patients to over 50%. The tumors kill by direct extension associated with ulceration, secondary bacterial infection, and resultant debilitation; by widespread metastasis; and by leading to secondary bacterial infections of the lower respiratory air passages and lungs.

Nasal Cavities and Accessory Air Sinuses

Inflammatory diseases are the most common disorders to affect the nose and accessory nasal sinuses. These inflammations are as frequent and as commonplace as the "common cold." Most are more discomforting than serious. However, occasionally persistent bacterial infections give rise to clinically significant disease, and in these instances spread of the infection may lead to dangerous sequelae. Not to be forgotten is the occasional instance of destructive inflammatory nasal disease, which represents one facet of the systemic entity Wegener's granulomatosis (p. 523). A clinically similar but histologically distinct lesion is the *idiopathic midfacial granuloma*, which is related to lymphomatoid granulomatosis (p. 749). Tumors may arise in either the nasal cavity or the sinuses, but these are infrequent. *The familiar nasal "polyp" is not a true neoplasm. These polyps represent focal accumulations of edema fluid accompanied by some hyperplasia of the submucosal connective tissue and a variable inflammatory infiltrate consisting of eosinophils, plasma cells, and lymphocytes.* As such, they are not neoplastic but rather inflammatory in nature.

RHINITIS AND SINUSITIS

Rhinitis is the designation given to inflammation of the nasal cavities. The etiology of rhinitis is based on the interplay of viruses, bacteria, and allergens. Acute rhinitis is almost invariably initiated by one of the many viruses now proved to cause upper respiratory infections. Several of the better studied adenoviruses (ARD, RI, APC) produce nasopharyngitis, pharyngotonsillitis, and many other clinical variants that are all included under the category of the "common cold" or upper respiratory infection.

These viral agents usually evoke a profuse catarrhal discharge that is familiarly recognized as the beginning of a cold. In other instances, the acute rhinitis may be initiated by sensitivity reactions to one of a large group of allergens, perhaps most commonly the plant pollens. Bacterial infections become superimposed upon either the viral or the allergic acute phase. In either case, staphylococci, streptococci, *Hemophilus influenzae*, and pneumococci are commonly isolated. In the interplay of these various etiologic agents, it may well be that the catarrhal exudation evoked by viruses and allergens injures the normal protective ciliary action of the nasal mucosa and thus prepares the soil for the seeding of bacteria. Changes in temperature, exposure, inhalation of dust or chemical irritants, and excessive dryness of the atmosphere may all contribute to this ciliary injury and thus predispose to rhinitis. Rarely, in the debilitated patient, such mycotic infections as candidiasis are encountered.

During the initial acute stages of the rhinitis, the nasal mucosa is thickened, edematous, and red. The nasal cavities are narrowed. The turbinates are enlarged. The mucosal surfaces are covered by a thin, watery-to-mucoid discharge, which is relatively clear in the developmental stages. Infection modifies the character of the discharge and produces an essentially mucopurulent to sometimes frankly suppurative exudate. Focal enlargements of the mucosa give rise to nasal *"polyps,"* which are merely inflammatory hypertrophic swellings but not true neoplasms. Recurrent allergic nasal polyps can reach dimensions of over 5 cm in diameter (Fig. 16–57).

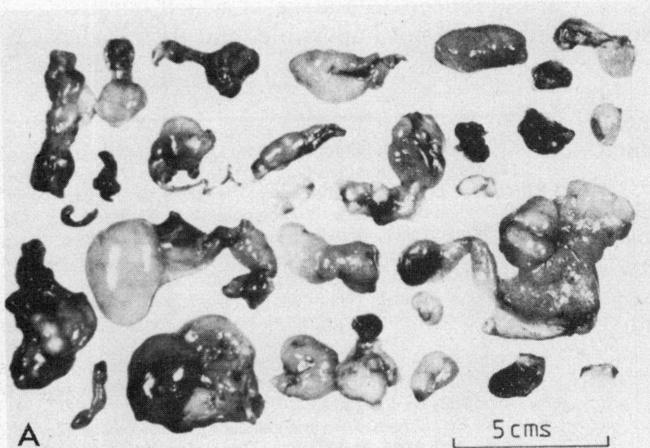

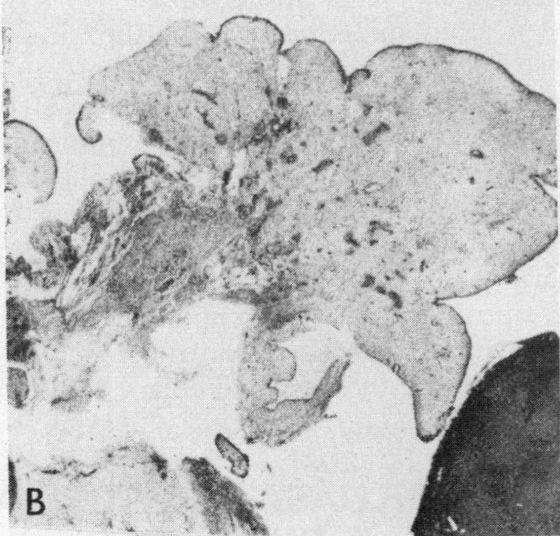

Figure 16–57. *A,* Multiple benign allergic polyps removed from nose of an old man. *B,* Low-power histology of an allergic polyp exhibiting marked submucosal edema. (Both from Friedman, I., and Osborn, D. A.: Pathology of Granulomas and Neoplasms of the Nose and Paranasal Sinuses. New York, Churchill Livingstone, 1982, p. 30. Reproduced with permission.)

Histologically, during the initial phases, the reaction is one of extreme edema. The tissue takes on a loose myxomatous appearance and is sparsely infiltrated with neutrophils, lymphocytes, plasma cells, and eosinophils. This edema is more marked in the polyps. The number of eosinophils is accentuated in some cases, presumably those of allergic origin. There is secretory hyperactivity of the mucus-secreting submucosal glands. In the stages of frank bacterial infection, the leukocytic infiltrate is considerably augmented and becomes predominantly neutrophilic.

In long persistence of an acute suppurative rhinitis, fibrous scarring of the subepithelial connective tissue may occur. In some of these instances, the epithelium becomes atrophic, and foci of squamous metaplasia may develop. In these cases, the progressive submucosal fibrosis causes atrophy of the mucus-secreting glands. These histologic changes result in a dry, glazed, shiny appearance to the nasal mucosa with total loss of mucinous secretion, sometimes designated *atrophic rhinitis* or *rhinitis sicca*.

The major significance of these disorders relates to their possible sequelae. The swelling of the nasal mucosa may obstruct the orifices of the accessory air sinuses and lead to *sinusitis*. The bacterially infected cases infrequently progress to osteomyelitis, cavernous sinus thrombophlebitis, epidural or subdural abscess, meningitis, or brain abscess. These complications, in light of the great frequency of these nasal inflammations, are rare.

Sinusitis is closely related to rhinitis. Almost invariably, acute inflammatory involvement of the nasal cavities precedes and leads to infections and inflammations of the air sinuses by obstructing the drainage orifices of the sinuses. The edema of the lining epithelium may completely obstruct the drainage orifice of the sinus and, if the sinus fills up with mucus, may lead to a *mucocele*. In the stages of secondary bacterial or mycotic infection, frank suppuration replaces the watery discharge. The accumulation of such pus is sometimes designated an *empyema* of the sinus.

Suppurative infections within the sinuses are of somewhat greater significance than those in the nose because of the close relationship of these structures to the cranial vault. The spread of these infections is more prone to produce osteomyelitis and the intracranial infections listed in the above discussion of rhinitis. A serious fungal infection by the *mucormycoses* (p. 354) is particularly seen in patients with diabetic acidosis. Chronic sinusitis is also a component of *Kartagener's syndrome*, which (together with bronchiectasis and situs inversus) is caused by defective ciliary action (p. 730).

TUMORS OF NASAL CAVITIES AND SINUSES

Tumors in these locations are extremely infrequent but may include the entire category of mesenchymal and epithelial neoplasms. Brief mention may be made of somewhat distinctive types. *Isolated plasmacytomas* may arise in the lymphoid structures adjacent to the nose and sinuses. These may protrude within these cavities as polypoid growths, varying from 1 cm to several centimeters in diameter, covered usually by an intact overlying mucosa. The histology is that of a malignant plasma cell tumor and is identical to that described on page 689. Only rarely do these lesions result in myeloma. *Olfactory neuroblastomas* (esthesioneuroblastomas) are malignant tumors resembling other neuroblastomas (p. 1247) and are exquisitely sensitive to radiation therapy. *Nasopharyngeal angiofibroma* is a highly vascular tumor that occurs almost exclusively in adolescent males. Despite its benign nature, it may cause serious clinical problems because of its tendency to bleed profusely during surgery. The *inverted papilloma* is a benign but locally aggressive neoplasm occurring in both the nose and the paranasal sinuses. If not adequately excised, it has a high rate of recurrence, with the potentially serious complication of invasion of the orbit or cranial vault; rarely, frank carcinoma may also develop in a papilloma.

Carcinomas in these locations are keratinizing or frequently nonkeratinizing squamous cell carcinomas. They are insidious malignant lesions that produce the characteristic ulcerating, fungating growth typical of these tumors elsewhere. Some are closer in histologic detail to *transitional cell carcinoma*, characterized by strands and masses of polygonal-to-spindle cells growing within a fibrous stroma. The cell boundaries are poorly defined, and often the masses of cells take on the appearance of a syncytium. In many of these growths, there is an abundant lymphoid infiltrate within the fibrous stroma, designated *lymphoepithelioma*. The Epstein-Barr virus has been identified in many of these tumors. All these malignancies progressively invade and destroy, spread to cervical nodes, and, in late cases, metastasize to distant areas, i.e., lungs, pleural cavities, liver, and remote chains of lymph nodes. As a group, these malignancies produce symptoms only when they are advanced to a stage at which curative resection is difficult, if not impossible, and the prognosis is poor.

1. Thurlbeck, W.M.: Chronic Airflow Obstruction in Lung Disease. Philadelphia, W.B. Saunders Co., 1976.
2. Murray, J.F.: The Normal Lung: The Basis for Diagnosis and Treatment of Pulmonary Disease. Philadelphia, W.B. Saunders Co., 1976.
3. Richardson J.B., and Ferguson, C.C.: Morphology of the airways. *In* Nadel, J.A. (ed.): Physiology and Pharmacology of the Airways. New York, Marcel Dekker, 1980, pp. 1–30.
4. Gould, V.E., et al.: Neuroendocrine components of the bronchopulmonary tract: Hyperplasias, dysplasia, and neoplasms. Lab. Invest. *49*:519, 1983.
5. Weibel, E.R.: Design and structure of the human lung. *In* Fishman, A.P. (ed.): Pulmonary Diseases and Disorders. New York, McGraw-Hill Book Co., 1980, pp. 224–271.
6. Kuhn, C.: Ultrastructure and cellular function in distal lung. *In* Thurlbeck, W.M., and Abell, M.R. (eds.): The Lung: Structure, Function and Disease. Baltimore, Williams & Wilkins Co., 1978, pp. 1–20.
7. Kikkawa, Y., and Smith, F.: Cellular and biochemical aspects of pulmonary surfactant in health and disease. Lab. Invest. *49*:122, 1983.
8. Muir, D.C.F.: Deposition and clearance of inhaled particles. *In* Muir, D.C.F. (ed.): Clinical Aspects of Inhaled Particles. London, Heinemann, 1972, pp. 1–20.

9. Brain, J.D., et al. (eds.): Respiratory Defense Mechanisms. New York, Marcel Dekker, 1977.
10. Green, G.M., et al.: Defense mechanisms of respiratory membranes. Am. Rev. Respir. Dis. *115*:495, 1977.
11. Spencer, H.: Pathology of the Lung Excluding Pulmonary Tuberculosis. 3rd ed. New York, Pergamon Press, 1977.
12. Katzenstein, A-L.A., and Askin, F.B.: Surgical Pathology of Non-Neoplastic Lung Disease. Philadelphia, W.B. Saunders Co., 1982.
13. Fishman, A.P. (ed.): Pulmonary Diseases and Disorders. New York, McGraw-Hill Book Co., 1980; Fishman, A.P. (ed.): Update: Pulmonary Diseases and Disorders. New York, McGraw-Hill Book Co., 1982.
14. Dunnill, M.S.: Pulmonary Pathology. Churchill Livingstone, 1982, p. 496.
15. Staub, N.C.: Pulmonary edema due to increased microvascular permeability to fluid protein. Annu. Rev. Med. *32*:291, 1981.
16. Ayres, S.M.: Mechanisms and consequences of pulmonary edema. Am. Heart J. *103*:97, 1982.
17. Pietra, G.G.: The basis of pulmonary edema with emphasis on ultrastructure. *In* Thurlbeck, W.M., and Abell, M.R. (eds.): The Lung: Structure, Function and Disease. Baltimore, Williams & Wilkins Co., 1978, pp. 215–234.
18. Freiman, D.G., et al.: Frequency of pulmonary thromboembolism in man. N. Engl. J. Med. *272*:1278, 1965.
19. Utsunomiya, T., et al.: Thromboxane mediation of cardiopulmonary effects of embolism. J. Clin. Invest. *70*:361, 1982.
20. Bell, W.R., and Simon, T.L.: Current status of pulmonary thromboembolic disease: Pathophysiology, diagnosis, prevention, and treatment. Am. Heart J. *103*:239, 1982.
21. Fishman, A.P., and Pietra, G.G.: Primary pulmonary hypertension. Annu. Rev. Med. *31*:421, 1980.
22. Edwards, W.D., and Edwards, J.E.: Recent advances in the pathology of the pulmonary vasculature. *In* Thurlbeck, W.M., and Abell, M.R. (eds.): The Lung: Structure, Function and Disease. Baltimore, Williams & Wilkins Co., 1978, pp. 235–261.
23. Wagenvoort, E.A., and Wagenvoort, E.: Pathology of Pulmonary Hypertension. New York, John Wiley & Sons, 1977.
24. Fein, A.M., et al.: Adult respiratory distress syndrome. Br. J. Anaesth. *54*:723, 1982.
25. Petty, T.L.: Adult respiratory distress syndrome: Definition and historical perspective. Clin. Chest Med. *3*:3, 1982.
26. Hudson, L.D.: Causes of the adult respiratory distress syndrome: Clinical recognition. Clin. Chest Med. *3*:195, 1982.
27. Pratt, P.C.: Pathology of adult respiratory distress syndrome. *In* Thurlbeck, W.M., and Abell, M.R. (eds.): The Lung: Structure, Function and Disease. Baltimore, Williams & Wilkins Co., 1978, pp. 43–57.
27A. Balentine, J.D.: Pathology of Oxygen Toxicity. New York, Academic Press, 1983.
28. Rinaldo, J.E., and Rogers, R.M.: Adult respiratory distress syndrome. Changing concepts of lung injury and repair. N. Engl. J. Med. *306*:900, 1982.
29. Meyrick, B., and Brigham, K.L.: Acute effects of *Escherichia coli* endotoxin on the pulmonary microcirculation of anesthetized sheep. Lab. Invest. *48*:458, 1983.
30. Fantone, J.C., and Ward, P.A.: Role of oxygen-derived free radicals and metabolites in leukocyte-dependent inflammatory reactions. Am. J. Pathol. *107*:395, 1982.
31. Brigham, K.L.: Mechanisms of lung injury. Clin. Chest Med. *3*:9, 1982.
32. McGuire, W.W., et al.: Studies on the pathogenesis of the adult respiratory distress syndrome. J. Clin. Invest. *69*:543, 1982.
33. Bachofen, M., and Weibel, E.R.: Structural alterations of lung parenchyma in the adult respiratory distress syndrome. Clin. Chest Med. *3*:35, 1982.
34. American Thoracic Society: Chronic bronchitis, asthma, and pulmonary emphysema. Statement by the Committee on Diagnostic Standards for Non-tuberculous Respiratory Disease. Am. Rev. Respir. Dis. *85*:762, 1962.
35. Reid, L.: The Pathology of Emphysema. London, Lloyd-Luke Medical Books, Ltd., 1967.
36. Fishman, A.: The spectrum of chronic obstructive diseases of the airways. *In* Fishman, A.P. (ed.): Pulmonary Diseases and Disorders. New York, McGraw-Hill Book Co., 1980, pp. 458–470.
37. Reid, L.: Chronic obstructive lung diseases. *In* Fishman, A.P. (ed.): Pulmonary Diseases and Disorders. New York, McGraw-Hill Book Co., 1980, pp. 503–535.
38. Diener, C.F., and Burrows, B.: Further observation on the course and prognosis of chronic obstructive lung disease. Am. Rev. Respir. Dis. *111*:719, 1975.
39. Kleinerman, J., et al.: The occurrence and incidence of emphysematous lesions in men from 15 to 44 years of age. Am. Rev. Respir. Dis. *98*:152, 1968.
40. Leopold, T.G., and Gough, J.: The centrilobular form of emphysema and its relation to chronic bronchitis. Thorax *12*:219, 1957.
41. Farber, S.M., and Wilson, R.H.L.: Chronic obstructive emphysema. Ciba Clin. Symp. *20*:35, 1968.
42. Pratt, P.C., and Kilburn, K.H.: A modern concept of the emphysemas based on correlations of structure and function. Hum. Pathol. *1*:443, 1970.
43. Laurell, C.B., and Eriksson, S.: The electrophoretic alpha-1-globulin pattern of serum in alpha-1-antitrypsin deficiency. Scand. J. Clin. Lab. Invest. *15*:132, 1963.
44. Tobin, M.J., and Hutchison, D.C.S.: An overview of the pulmonary features of alpha-1-antitrypsin deficiency. Arch. Intern. Med. *142*:1342, 1982.
45. Morse, J.O.: Alpha-1-antitrypsin deficiency. N. Engl. J. Med. *299*:1045 and 1099, 1978.
46. Snider, G.L.: Pathogenesis of emphysema and chronic bronchitis. Med. Clin. North Am. *65*:647, 1981.
47. Bignon, J., and de Cremoux, H.: Pathological and pathogenetic aspects of chronic obstructive lung disease. Bull. Eur. Physiopathol. Respir. *16*(Suppl.):13, 1980.
48. Cohen, A.B., and Kneppers, F.: Pathogenesis of emphysema. *In* Fishman, A.P. (ed.): Update: Pulmonary Diseases and Disorders. New York, McGraw-Hill Book Co., 1982, pp. 112–122.
49. Wewers, M., and Bone, R.C.: Emphysema and chronic bronchitis. Pulmonary Dis. Rev. *3*:229, 1983.
50. Senior, R.M., et al.: The induction of pulmonary emphysema with human leukocyte elastase. Am. Rev. Respir. Dis. *116*:469, 1977.
51. Werb, Z., et al.: Elastases and elastin degradation. J. Invest. Dermatol. *79*(Suppl.):154s, 1982.
52. Hunninghake, G.W., et al.: Human alveolar macrophage derived chemotactic factor for neutrophils. J. Clin. Invest. *66*:473, 1980.
53. Hogg, J.C., et al.: Site and nature of airway obstruction in chronic obstructive lung disease. N. Engl. J. Med. *278*:1355, 1968.
54. Hogg, J.C.: The pathophysiology of small airways. *In* Sadoul, P., et al. (eds.): Small Airways in Health and Disease. Amsterdam, Excerpta Medica, 1979.
55. Ranga, V., and Kleinerman, J.: Structure and function of small airways in health and disease. Arch. Pathol. Lab. Med. *102*:609, 1978.
56. Thurlbeck, W.M.: A pathologist's approach to chronic bronchitis and emphysema. *In* Fishman, A.P. (ed.): Update: Pulmonary Diseases and Disorders. New York, McGraw-Hill Book Co., 1982, pp. 137–148.
57. McFadden, E.R., et al.: Small airway disease: An assessment of the test of peripheral airway function. Am. J. Med. *57*:171, 1974.
58. Cosio, M., et al.: The relations between structural changes in small airways and pulmonary-function tests. N. Engl. J. Med. *298*:1277, 1978.
59. Niewoehner, D., and Cosio, M.G.: Chronic obstructive lung disease: The role of airway disease, with special emphasis on the pathology of small airways. *In* Thurlbeck, W.M., and Abell, M.R. (eds.): The Lung: Structure, Function and Disease. Baltimore, Williams & Wilkins Co., 1978, pp. 160–179.
60. Hogg, J.C.: Bronchial asthma. *In* Thurlbeck, W.M., and Abell, M.R. (eds.): The Lung: Structure, Function and Disease. Baltimore, Williams & Wilkins Co., 1978, pp. 180–191.
61. McFadden, E. R., Jr., and Austen, K. F.: Asthma. *In* Harrison's Principles of Internal Medicine. 10th ed. New York, McGraw-Hill Book Co., 1983, p. 1512.
62. Samuelsson, B.: Leukotrienes: Mediators of immediate hypersensitivity reactions and inflammation. Science *220*:568, 1983.
63. Weissman, G.: The eicosanoids of asthma. N. Engl. J. Med. *308*:454, 1983.
64. Butcher, B.T., and Hendrick, D.J.: Occupational asthma. Clin. Chest Med. *4*:43, 1983.
65. Schuyler, M.R.: Allergic bronchopulmonary aspergillosis. Clin. Chest Med. *4*:15, 1983.
66. Griffin, M., et al.: Effects of leukotriene D on the airways in asthma. N. Engl. J. Med. *308*:436, 1983.
67. Filley, W.V., et al.: Identification by immunofluorescence of eosinophil granule major basic protein in lung tissues of patients with bronchial asthma. Lancet *2*:11, 1982.
68. Eliasson, R., et al.: The immotile cilia syndrome—a congenital ciliary abnormality as an etiologic factor in chronic airway infections and male sterility. N. Engl. J. Med. *297*:1, 1977.
69. Mossberg, B.: Immotile-cilia syndrome: Clinical features. Eur. J. Respir. Dis. *118*(Suppl.):111, 1982.
70. Reynolds, H.Y. (ed.): Pulmonary Infections. Clin. Chest Med. *2*:1, 1981.
71. Fanta, C.H., and Pennington, J.E.: Fever and new lung infiltrates in the immunocompromised host. Clin. Chest Med. *2*:19, 1981.
72. Rubin, R.: Pneumonia in the immunocompromised host. *In* Fishman, A.P. (ed.): Update: Pulmonary Diseases and Disorders. New York, McGraw-Hill Book Co., 1982, pp. 1–26.
73. Myerowitz, R.L.: The Pathology of Opportunistic Infections with Pathogenetic, Diagnostic, and Clinical Correlations. New York, Raven Press, 1983.
74. Murray, H.W., et al.: The protean manifestations of *Mycoplasma pneumoniae* infection in adults. Am. J. Med. *58*:229, 1975.
75. Cherry, J.D.: *Mycoplasma pneumoniae* infections and exanthems. J. Pediatr. *87*:369, 1975.
76. Johanson, W.G., et al.: Aspiration pneumonia, anerobic infections and lung abscess. Med. Clin. North Am. *64*:385, 1980.

77. Bartlett, J.G., et al.: The bacteriology of aspiration pneumonia. Am. J. Med. *56*:202, 1974.
78. Stead, W.W., and Dutt, A.K. (eds.): Tuberculosis. Clin. Chest Med. *1*:1, 1980.
79. Stead, W.W., and Dutt, A.K.: What's new in tuberculosis? Am. J. Med. *71*:1, 1981.
80. Sbarbaro, J.A.: Tuberculosis. Med. Clin. North Am. *64*:417, 1980.
81. Collins, F.M.: The immunology of tuberculosis. Am. Rev. Respir. Dis. *125*:42, 1982.
82. Carrington, C.B., and Gaensler, E.A.: Clinical-pathological approach to diffuse infiltrative lung disease. *In* Thurlbeck, W.M., and Abell, M.R. (eds.): The Lung: Structure, Function and Disease. Baltimore, Williams & Wilkins Co., 1978, pp. 58–87.
83. Fulmer, J.D.: An introduction to the interstitial lung diseases. Clin. Chest Med. *3*:457, 1982.
84. Flint, A.: The interstitial lung diseases: A pathologist's view. Clin. Chest Med. *3*:491, 1982.
85. Crystal, R.G., et al.: Interstitial lung diseases of unknown cause: Disorders caused by chronic inflammation of the lower respiratory tract. N. Engl. J. Med. *310*:154, 1984.
86. Crystal, R.G., et al.: Interstitial lung disease: Current concepts of pathogenesis, staging and therapy. Am. J. Med. *70*:542, 1981.
87. Henson, P.M., et al.: Immune complex injury of the lung. Am. Rev. Respir. Dis. *124*:738, 1981.
88. Bitterman, P.B., et al.: Mechanisms of pulmonary fibrosis: Spontaneous release of the alveolar macrophage derived growth factor. J. Clin. Invest. *72*:1801, 1983.
89. Niewoehner, D.E., and Hoidal, J.R.: Lung fibrosis and emphysema: Divergent responses to a common injury? Science *217*:359, 1982.
90. Reynolds, H.Y.: Hypersensitivity pneumonitis. Clin. Chest Med. *3*:503, 1982.
91. Stankus, R.P., and Salvaggio, J.E.: Hypersensitivity pneumonitis. Clin. Chest Med. *4*:55, 1983.
92. Bradley, J.D.: The pulmonary hemorrhage syndromes. Clin. Chest Med. *3*:593, 1982.
93. Wilson, C.: Immunologic diseases of lungs and kidney. *In* Fishman, A.P. (ed.): Pulmonary Diseases and Disorders. New York, McGraw-Hill Book Co., 1980, pp. 699–707.
94. Beirne, J.B.: Goodpasture's syndrome and exposure to solvents. J.A.M.A. *222*:51, 1972.
94A. Churchill, D.N. et al.: Association between hydrogen exposure and glomerulonephritis. An appraisal of the evidence. Nephron *33*:169, 1983.
95. Lockwood, C.M., et al.: Plasma exchange in nephritis. *In* Hamburger, J., et al. (eds.): Advances in Nephrology. Vol. 8. Chicago, Year Book Medical Publishers, 1979, pp. 383–418.
96. Morgan, P.G.M., and Turner-Warwick, M.: Pulmonary haemosiderosis and pulmonary haemorrhage. Br. J. Dis. Chest *75*:225, 1981.
97. Altose, M.D.: Pulmonary alveolar proteinosis. *In* Fishman, A.P. (ed.): Pulmonary Diseases and Disorders. New York, McGraw-Hill Book Co., 1980, pp. 1341–1347.
98. Smith, F.B.: Alveolar proteinosis: Atypical pulmonary response to injury. N.Y. State J. Med. *80*:1372, 1980.
99. Bedrossian, C.W.M., et al.: Alveolar proteinosis as a consequence of immunosuppression. A hypothesis based on clinical and pathologic observations. Hum. Pathol. *11*:527, 1980.
100. Liebow, A.A., et al.: Desquamative interstitial pneumonia. Am. J. Med. *39*:369, 1965.
101. Jackson, L.K.: Idiopathic pulmonary fibrosis. Clin. Chest Med. *3*:579, 1982.
102. Carrington, C.B., et al.: Natural history and treated course of usual and desquamative interstitial pneumonia. N. Engl. J. Med. *298*:801, 1978.
103. Liebow, A.A., and Carrington, C.B.: The interstitial pneumonias. *In* Simon, M., et al. (eds.): Frontiers in Pulmonary Radiology. New York, Grune & Stratton, 1969.
104. Dreisin, R.B., et al.: Circulating immune complexes in idiopathic interstitial pneumonias. N. Engl. J. Med. *298*:353, 1978.
105. Schatz, M., et al.: Eosinophils and immunologic lung disease. Med. Clin. North Am. *65*:1055, 1981.
106. Spry, C.J.F., and Kumaraswami, V.: Tropical eosinophilia. Semin. Hematol. *19*:107, 1982.
107. Bedrossian, C.W., et al.: Ultrastructure of the lung in Loeffler's pneumonia. Am. J. Med. *58*:438, 1975.
108. Mayock, R.L., and Saldana, M.J.: Eosinophilic pneumonia. *In* Fishman, A.P. (ed.): Pulmonary Diseases and Disorders. New York, McGraw-Hill Book Co., 1980, pp. 926–939.
109. Eisenberg, H.: The interstitial lung diseases associated with collagen-vascular disorders. Clin. Chest Med. *3*:564, 1982.
110. Hunninghake, G.W., and Fauci, A.S.: Pulmonary involvement in the collagen vascular diseases. Am. Rev. Respir. Dis. *119*:471, 1979.
111. Petty, T.L., and Wilkins, M.: The five manifestations of rheumatoid lung. Dis. Chest *49*:75, 1966.
112. Dreisin, R.B.: Pulmonary vasculitis. Clin. Chest Med. *3*:607, 1982.
113. Colby, T.V., and Carrington, C.B.: Lymphoreticular tumors and infiltrates of the lung. Pathol. Annu. *18*:27, 1983.
114. Carter, D., and Eggleston, J.C.: Tumors of the lower respiratory tract. Atlas of Tumor Pathology. Second Series. Fascicle 17. Washington, D.C., Armed Forces Institute of Pathology.
115. Silverberg, E.: Cancer statistics. CA *34*:7, 1984.
116. Israel, L., and Chahinian, A.: Lung Cancer: Natural History, Prognosis, and Therapy. New York, Academic Press, 1976.
117. Royal College of Physicians: Smoking and Health. London, Pitman, 1962.
118. U.S. Surgeon General Reports on the Health Consequences of Smoking, 1964, 1979, 1982.
119. Frank, A.L.: The epidemiology and etiology of lung cancer. Clin. Chest Med. *3*:219, 1982.
120. Hammond, E.C., and Horn, D.: Smoking and death rates: Report on 44 months of follow-up of 187,783 men. J.A.M.A. *166*:1159 and 1294, 1958.
121. Hammond, E.C.: Smoking in relation to the death rate of one million men and women. Natl. Cancer Inst. Monogr. *19*:127, 1966.
122. Wynder, E.L., and Stellman, S.D.: The impact of long term filter cigarette usage on lung and larynx cancer: A case control study. J. Natl. Cancer Inst. *62*:471, 1979.
123. Auerbach, O., et al.: Changes in bronchial epithelium in relation to sex, age, residence, smoking and pneumonia. N. Engl. J. Med. *267*:111, 1962.
124. Auerbach, O.: Changes in bronchial epithelium in relationship to cigarette smoking, 1955–1960 vs. 1970–1977. N. Engl. J. Med. *300*:381, 1979.
125. Wynder, E.L., and Hoffman, D.: Tobacco and Tobacco Smoke: Studies in Experimental Carcinogenesis. New York, Academic Press, 1967.
126. Cihak, R.W.: Radiation and lung cancer. Hum. Pathol. *25*:25, 1971.
127. Selikoff, I.J., et al.: Asbestos-associated disease in United States shipyards. Ann. N.Y. Acad. Sci. *330*:295, 1979.
128. Wynder, E.L., and Hoffmann, D.: Tobacco. *In* Schottenfeld, D., and Fraumeni, J.F. (eds.): Cancer Epidemiology and Prevention. Philadelphia, W.B. Saunders Co., 1982, pp. 277–292.
129. Paigen, B., et al.: Questionable relation of aryl hydrocarbon hydroxylase to lung cancer risk. N. Engl. J. Med. *297*:346, 1977.
130. Yesner, R., et al. (eds.): International Histological Classification of Tumors. No. 1: Histological Typing of Lung Tumors. 2nd ed. Geneva, World Health Organization, 1982.
131. Yesner, R., and Carter, D.: Pathology of carcinoma of the lung: Changing patterns. Clin. Chest Med. *3*:257, 1982.
132. Vincent, R., et al.: The changing histopathology of lung cancer. A review of 1,682 cases. Cancer *39*:1647, 1977.
133. Cohen, M.H.: Natural history of lung cancer. Clin. Chest Med. *3*:229, 1982.
134. Jett, J.R., et al.: Lung cancer: Current concepts. CA *33*:74, 1983.
135. Carney, D.N., and Minna, J.D.: Small cell cancer of the lung. Clin. Chest Med. *3*:389, 1982.
136. Margolese, R.G., et al.: Recent advances in management of lung cancer. Adv. Surg. *15*:189, 1981.
137. Ayvasian, L.F.: Extrapulmonary manifestations of tumors of the lung. Postgrad. Med. *63*:93, 1978.
138. Edgerton, F., et al.: Bronchio-alveolar carcinoma. A clinical overview and bibliography. Oncology *38*:269, 1981.
139. Bolen, J.W., and Thorning, D.: Histogenetic classification of pulmonary carcinomas. Peripheral adenocarcinomas studied by light microscopy, histochemistry, and electron microscopy. Pathol. Annu. *17*:77, 1982.
140. Salyer, D.C., and Eggleston, J.C.: Bronchial carcinoid tumors. Cancer *36*:15, 1975.
141. Sahn, S.A.: Pleural manifestations of pulmonary disease. Hosp. Pract. *16*:73, 1981.
142. Kannerstein, M., et al.: Asbestos and mesothelioma. Pathol. Annu. *13*(Part I):81, 1978.
143. Antman, K.H., and Corson, J.M.: Benign and malignant mesothelioma. *In* Moosā, A.R., et al. (eds.): Comprehensive Textbook of Oncology. Baltimore, Williams & Wilkins Co., in press, 1984.
144. Churg, A., and Golden, J.: Current problems in the pathology of asbestos-related disease. Pathol. Annu. *17*:33, 1982.
145. Antman, C.: Malignant mesothelioma. N. Engl. J. Med. *303*:200, 1981.
146. Batsakis J.G.: Tumors of the Head and Neck. 2nd ed. Baltimore, Williams & Wilkins Co., 1979.
147. Howley, P.: The human papilloma viruses. Arch. Pathol. Lab. Med. *106*:429, 1982.
148. Friedman, I., and Osborn, D.A.: Pathology of Granulomas and Neoplasms of the Nose and Paranasal Sinuses. New York, Churchill Livingstone, 1982.

THE ORAL CAVITY, JAWS, AND SALIVARY GLANDS

17

GERALD SHKLAR, D.D.S., M.S.*

*Charles A. Brackett Professor of Oral Pathology and Head, Department of Oral Medicine and Oral Pathology, Harvard School of Dental Medicine, Boston, Massachusetts.

All too often the physician, in carrying out a physical examination, looks *through* the mouth at the oropharynx and tonsillar region rather than examining the oral tissues. A careful examination of the mouth may yield significant information concerning localized disease as well as possible oral manifestations of systemic disease. The oral mucosa can be affected by a variety of traumatic lesions; by viral, mycotic, and bacterial infections; by benign and malignant tumors; by developmental malformations; and by autoimmune, genetic, and psychosomatic diseases. The oral tissues may also reveal evidence of nutritional deficiencies, hematologic disturbances, and endocrinopathies. Oral lesions may accompany disease states affecting various organ systems; for example, they are found in such diverse conditions as Crohn's disease, ulcerative colitis, cystic fibrosis, Raynaud's disease, and Sjögren's syndrome. Diseases of the jaws and salivary glands may also be manifested by morphologic alterations in the mouth.

Examination of the mouth may also provide some insight into the patient's personal habits. Neglect of oral hygiene and dental care are obvious indicators, but the oral tissues may also reveal evidence of neurotic habits, such as ulceration of tissue or abrasion or excessive wear of tooth surfaces. In addition, there is a wide range of hysterical symptomatology such as "burning" tongue and altered taste perception that requires careful oral examination in order to rule out the possibility of somatic disease.

A knowledge of oral pathology and routine examination of the mouth provide important clues to the patient's general condition and, more important, result in early diagnosis of and successful therapy for serious oral lesions, such as cancer. A patient's complaints related to the head and neck area must also be evaluated in relation to possible oral disease. Difficulty in swallowing, for example, may be caused by a carcinoma of the tongue and floor of the mouth rather than of the oropharynx, esophagus, or larynx.

DISEASES OF TEETH

Diseases of the teeth consist of dental caries and a large variety of developmental malformations. The developmental malformations may involve a single tooth, multiple teeth, or the entire dentition. They may be of inflammatory or traumatic origin, reflect a variety of systemic disturbances occurring during tooth formation, or represent genetic disorders. The resultant abnormalities may take the form of abnormal development of enamel, abnormal calcification, pathologic pigmentation, or gross aberrations in form.

Teeth essentially develop as skin appendage–type structures and are of ectodermal origin. The tooth germs or enamel organs arise as small buds or pouches from the fetal oral epithelium, and gradually assume the appearance of spheres with invaginated undersurfaces that remain attached to the oral epithelium by thin stalks (Fig. 17–1*A*). The epithelium of the enamel organ undergoes a morphologic alteration so that, unlike the oral epithelium, which is stratified squamous, it appears as surface columnar epithelium enclosing a stellate reticulum in the central portion of the evolving structure. The stellate reticulum is of ectodermal origin, as is the columnar epithelium. The inner enamel organ epithelium (the invaginated surface) develops into the highly specialized or differentiated ameloblast layer, the function of which is to produce enamel matrix. Mesenchymal cells from the adjacent connective tissue line up along the ameloblasts and become the highly specialized odontoblasts, which produce predentin or dentinal matrix. Thus, dentin is produced against enamel in the shape of the tooth crown that is genetically determined for each tooth (Fig. 17–1*B*). As the enamel and dentin matrices become established, they undergo calcification.

When the crown of the tooth is developed, root formation begins, and the tooth moves toward the oral epithelium and erupts by piercing the oral mucosa of the infant, an event that is generally painful for both mother and child. Root formation is mediated entirely by connective tissue cells, with odontoblasts forming the inner dentin and cementoblasts forming the outer surface of cementum. The cementoblasts are derived from the fibroblasts of adjacent connective tissue. As the tooth crown is formed, the enamel organ atrophies and remains attached to the enamel surface of the tooth as a thin membrane or cuticle. Some cells of the enamel organ at the base of the crown join with the oral mucosa, as the tooth erupts, and form the epithelial attachment that unites the gingival mucosa to the tooth surface at the cementoenamel junction, the demarcation of the crown of the tooth from the root. The epithelial attachment on the tooth forms a shallow trough or space between tooth and gingiva, referred to as the gingival sulcus or gingival crevice.

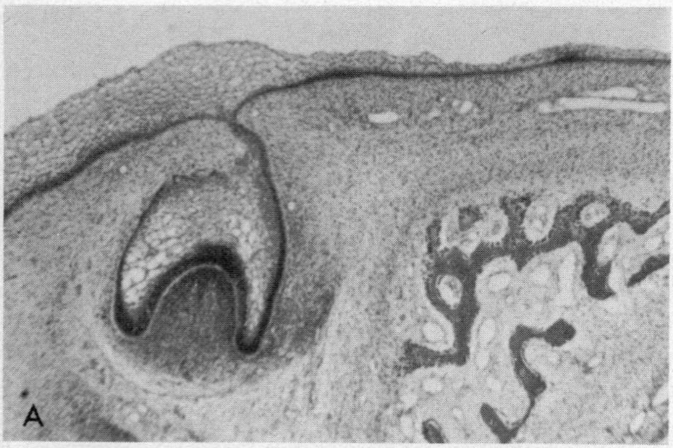

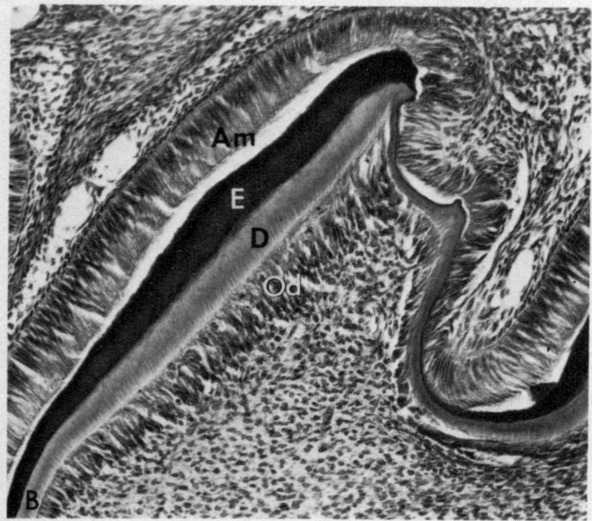

Figure 17–1. *A*, A tooth germ developing from fetal oral epithelium (×80). *B*, Ameloblasts (Am) and odontoblasts (Od) forming enamel (E) and dentin (D) matrices (×200).

There are two phases of tooth development. A set of 20 deciduous teeth begins to develop in utero and erupts in specific sequence during the first few years of life. A set of 32 permanent teeth begins to develop after birth and erupts in sequence from ages 6 to 13 years, with third molars ("wisdom teeth") erupting at approximately 17 to 22 years of age.

From the brief survey of normal tooth formation and eruption, it can be understood that many possibilities exist for abnormal development. If a tooth germ does not form initially, the tooth will be absent (anodontia). If an extra tooth germ develops, a supernumerary tooth will form. If the tooth germ should take on an unusual morphologic configuration, the developing tooth will be of an unusual shape. If ameloblasts lose their normal function temporarily, because of a systemic disturbance affecting the child, there will be bands of hypoplastic or defective enamel formed during that period of time. The entire dentition may develop with defective enamel or dentin if genetic disease impairs the function of ameloblasts or odontoblasts (amelogenesis imperfecta, dentinogenesis imperfecta).

It must be understood that developmental abnormalities of teeth can occur only during their development. Once the teeth have been completely formed, they can be affected only through destructive processes such as dental caries or acid etching of enamel. Root resorption can occur in unusual cases, in a process analogous to bone resorption. Pigmentation of the crowns of teeth must occur during tooth formation. Neither tetracycline nor bilirubin can stain the enamel once it has been formed, since these substances must be incorporated into the developing enamel to produce a permanent endogenous stain. Cementum can be stained throughout life, since this tissue undergoes active metabolism, but the cementum of the tooth is not normally visible in the mouth.

DEVELOPMENTAL MALFORMATIONS

Anodontia refers to the absence of one or more teeth. Failure of development of a single tooth could be the result of trauma or infection affecting the tooth germ. When a single tooth is missing from the permanent dentition, the cause is likely to be an odontogenic infection during tooth development at the apex of the deciduous tooth. Bilateral pairs of missing teeth are more likely to be of genetic origin. Total anodontia is often found in severe genetic disease affecting ectodermal tissues (ectodermal dysplasia).

Fusion refers to the joining of two adjacent tooth germs so that the two teeth develop as one large toothlike structure. A common site is the maxillary incisor area with lateral and central incisors fused. Two separate root canals indicate the fusion of separate tooth germs. *Gemination* presents a somewhat similar gross picture of a double tooth (Fig. 17–2*A*), but results from the invagination or splitting of a single tooth germ or the union of a tooth germ with a supernumerary tooth germ in the area. The usual adjacent tooth is present, and the large tooth usually presents a single root with a single root canal, although double root canals may be present.

Concrescence is a term used to indicate a union of adjacent teeth through attachment of roots by cementum. The crowns present a normal appearance, and the abnormality is perceived only on radiographs.

Supernumerary teeth develop from extra tooth germs and take on the appearance of the adjacent normal tooth. A common site for supernumerary teeth is the mandibular anterior region, where the only deformity perceived may be crowding of the teeth and malocclusion. Developing supernumerary teeth may become impacted if space is not sufficient for their complete formation and eruption. Cysts may develop around such impacted supernumerary teeth. Supernumerary teeth may also appear as additions to normally positioned teeth if both tooth germs develop in close proximity (Fig. 17–2*B*).

Dens in dente refers to an unusual malformation of a single tooth resulting from invagination of the outer enamel epithelium of the tooth germ. A toothlike structure appears to form within the developing tooth. Grossly, the tooth appears large and deformed (Fig. 17–2*C*), and a radiograph presents the characteristic pulpal abnormality (Fig. 17–2*D*).

Enamel hypoplasia refers to abnormal or insufficient enamel formation through inadequate function of the ameloblasts. It usually appears as a group of horizontal bands of brown, pitted, defective enamel on various teeth. Since the crowns of different teeth develop at different times, the hypoplastic bands affect

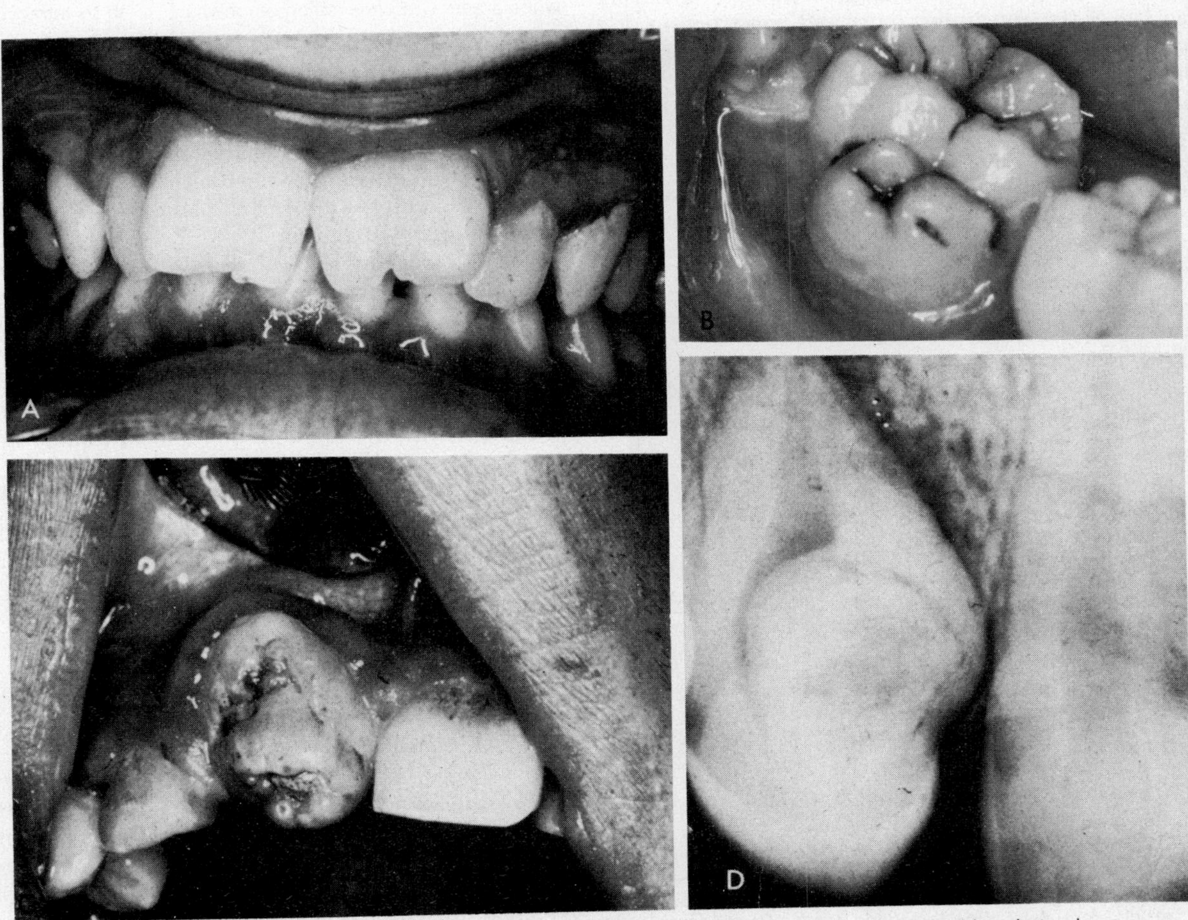

Figure 17–2. *A*, Gemination of maxillary central incisor teeth on both right and left sides. Lateral incisors are present. *B*, Supernumerary molar tooth joined to mandibular molar. *C*, Dens in dente. *D*, Radiograph of dens in dente showing invaginated structure.

only those teeth forming enamel at the time of ameloblastic malfunction, and the bands vary in position on the crowns of affected teeth, reflecting the developmental sequence (Fig. 17–3*A*). The width of the hypoplastic bands depends on the duration of the ameloblastic malfunction. Among systemic influences producing enamel hypoplasia are infections (exanthematous diseases, syphilis), nutritional deficiencies (of vitamins A, C, and D), endocrine disorders (hypoparathyroidism, hypothyroidism), toxic chemicals (fluoride in high concentrations), gastrointestinal disturbances, and renal disturbances. Enamel hypoplasia of a single tooth can be caused by trauma to the developing crown or localized infection in the area.

When the entire dentition is affected by hypoplasia of tissues, the etiology is genetic. Several *genetic diseases*, inherited as autosomal dominant traits with variable penetrance, uniquely affect the teeth. In *amelogenesis imperfecta* there is a hypoplastic form, a hypocalcified form, and a combined form. In the hypoplastic form, the teeth are brown, with an abnormal conical shape, and the enamel is normal but thin. In the hypocalcified form, the crown shape is normal, but the enamel is brown, soft, and defective (Fig. 17–3*B*). When this condition is severe, the crowns of the teeth are rapidly worn down to the gingival margin, requiring extraction of the remaining roots and construction of a denture for the child. In the combined form, there are features of both enamel hypoplasia and enamel hypocalcification, and the involvement tends to be severe, with early tooth loss.

Dentinogenesis imperfecta, also termed *hereditary opalescent dentin*, is also inherited as an autosomal dominant trait. It may be localized to the dentition or may appear with the generalized genetic disease of bone, osteogenesis imperfecta. The crowns of the teeth are normal in shape but purple-brown in color. Enamel is normal but dentin is defective, and the dentin-enamel junction lacks cohesion, so that the enamel can easily separate from the underlying dentin. Restoration of such teeth is difficult because of the abnormal structure and calcification of the dentin.

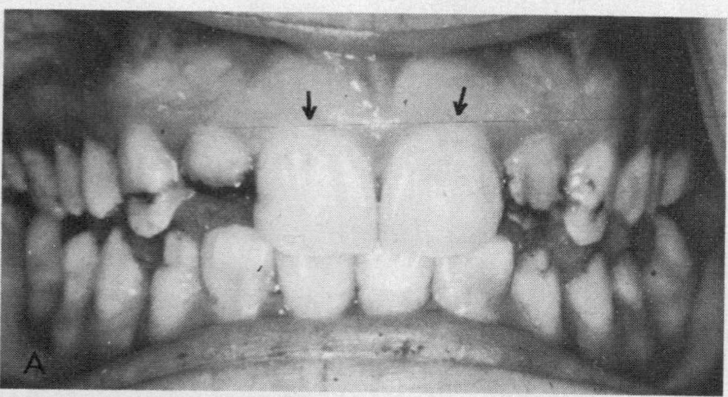

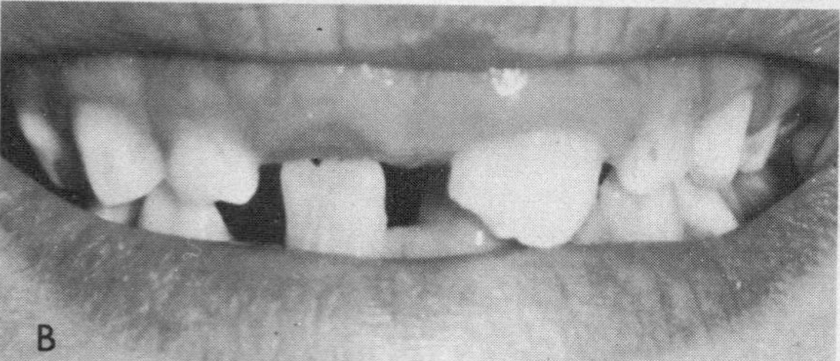

Figure 17–3. *A*, Enamel hypoplasia in a child. Note hypoplastic bands at different levels in deciduous teeth. Permanent teeth (*arrows*) are unaffected. *B*, Amelogenesis imperfecta. Note misshapen crowns and dull surfaces of teeth.

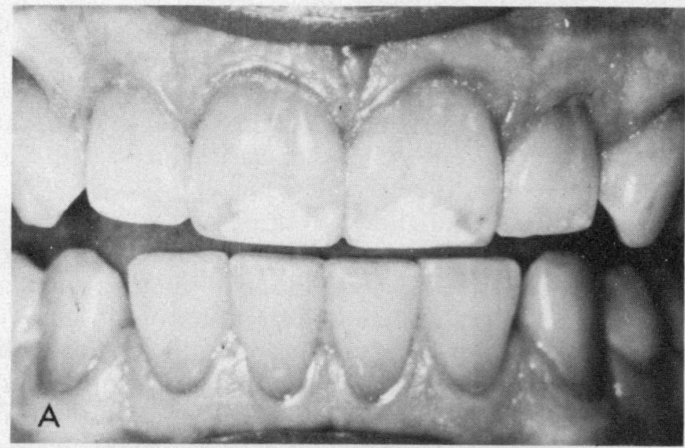

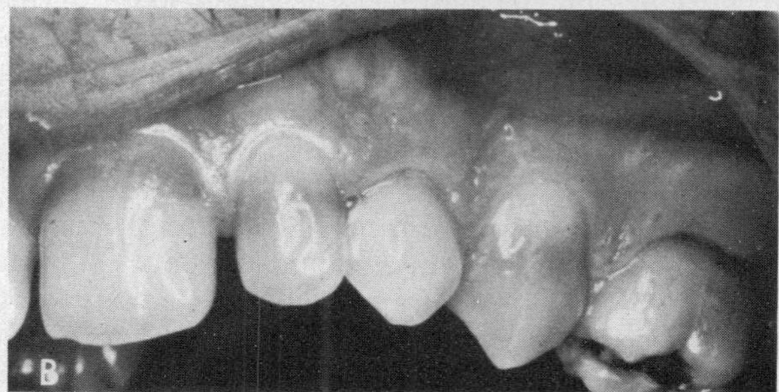

Figure 17–4. *A*, Hypocalcification defects of enamel appearing as white areas. *B*, Pigmentation of crowns of teeth by tetracycline.

Teeth may also show chalk-white areas representing *hypocalcification* or imperfect calcification. These defects appear opaque and are easily discerned in contrast to the normal translucence and off-white color of enamel (Fig. 17–4*A*).

Pigmentation of developing teeth is an endogenous condition, with the pigment being incorporated into the developing crown and remaining as a permanent stain. Once the crown has been formed it can no longer become pigmented except by superficial stains that can easily be removed. Pigments that can enter the developing crown are bilirubin (in hemolytic anemias), bile pigments (in biliary atresia or biliary tract disease), and pigmented pharmacologic agents such as tetracycline (Fig. 17–4*B*).

DENTAL CARIES

Dental caries refers to resorption or destruction of the calcified structure of the tooth, caused basically by bacterial action. It is the most widespread and common disorder of man and existed in prehistoric times. Principally implicated is *Streptococcus mutans*, but other bacteria and fungi may participate. This mixed bacterial-mycotic structure, termed *dental plaque*, proliferates in food residue on the tooth surface.[1] The consequence of the bacterial growth is proteolysis of the organic framework of the enamel by bacterial enzymes and acid decalcification of the enamel rods. The critical role of bacteria in the etiology of caries can be confirmed by the absence of carious lesions in germ-free animals.[2] Fluorides, the major caries-control agent in current use, render the enamel surface of the tooth more resistant to bacterial activity, and simultaneously act against microorganisms as a metabolic poison.

Prevention of the formation of dental plaque significantly protects against the development of caries. Microorganisms require a carbohydrate substrate for their metabolic activity. Refined carbohydrate increases the caries rate, but it must cling to the tooth surface for a significant effect. Caramel was shown to act in this manner in the well-controlled Vipehölm study.[3] Tooth brushing reduces the caries rate by removing food debris after meals and preventing the build-up of plaque. Saliva, with its mucolytic enzymes and immunoglobulins, also serves to cleanse the tooth surface and simultaneously controls bacterial growth. A significant decrease in salivary flow results in increased caries. For this reason, therapeutic irradiation to the oral cavity with resultant atrophy of salivary glands and xerostomia may induce so-called "radiation caries."

Microscopically, early caries of enamel appears as a loss of inter-rod organic material and an increased prominence of individual enamel rods. Gradually there is demineralization at the ends of the rods and penetration of bacteria. A brown pigmentation also appears in the early lesion. As the decalcification proceeds, the enamel rods lose their structure, and the carious lesion takes on a triangular configuration, with the apex pointed at the dentin-enamel junction (Fig. 17–5). As the enamel rods finally disintegrate, there is a break in the continuity of the enamel surface, and a gross clinical lesion appears that can be probed with an instrument. Carious attack is commonly seen in the pits and fissures of teeth as well as on smooth surfaces that are not self-cleansing, where food debris tends to accumulate. Once the carious lesion reaches the dentin, bacteria penetrate along the organic material of the dentin-enamel junction and gradually invade the dentinal tubules, causing breakdown of dentinal walls and the formation of clefts. Odontoblasts of the dental pulp, stimulated by degeneration of their elongate protoplasmic processes (Tomes' fibrils), react by forming a layer of protective or secondary dentin. However, if untreated, the carious lesion eventually penetrates through the dentin and secondary dentin, and infection enters the dental pulp, initiating pulpitis.

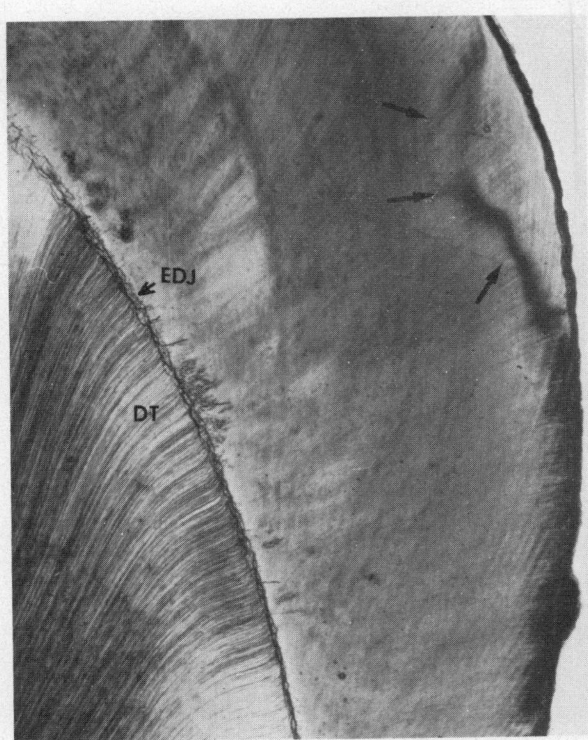

Figure 17–5. Early caries of enamel as seen on unstained section of tooth. Note triangular shape of lesion (*arrows*) with apex pointed toward enamel-dentinal junction (EDJ). Some dentinal tubules (DT) appear dark and may represent early dentinal irritation preceding the carious process.

ODONTOGENIC INFECTIONS

PULPITIS

Inflammation of the dental pulp may be caused by chemical, thermal, and physical irritation as well as by bacteria when any of these agents gains access to the pulp through a deep carious lesion. Opening of the dental pulp is referred to as pulp exposure, and this may be caused by deep instrumentation during evacuation of carious dentin as well as by the carious process itself. When microorganisms penetrate the pulp, acute purulent inflammation results. The process may be localized, creating a pulp abscess (acute partial pulpitis), or may involve the entire pulp and result in complete destruction of pulpal tissue (acute total pulpitis). Host resistance determines the extent of the pulpal reaction to infection. In the young child, with high tissue resistance, the infection is usually localized and the remainder of the pulp is essentially normal (Fig. 17–6), in which case surgical pulpotomy or pulpectomy can be utilized. When the entire pulp is involved, total extirpation is required (root canal therapy), and the entire pulp space is filled with an inert material and sealed. In pulpotomy or pulpectomy, the healthy pulp is covered and sealed.

Thermal injury to the pulp through improper cavity preparation can result in acute pulpitis. Chronic pulpitis results from mild but continuous irritation, such as a large, unlined metal filling transmitting heat and cold from the patient's mouth, or from irritation by a filling material that releases some acid, alkali, or other noxious chemical during its solidification.[4] In chronic pulpitis there is a lymphocytic and histiocytic infiltrate. The symptoms of pulpitis vary. Acute pulpitis causes extreme pain—the classic toothache, or odontalgia—when intense inflammation causes pressure on the many pain receptors in the pulp. Pain is relieved when the pulp is

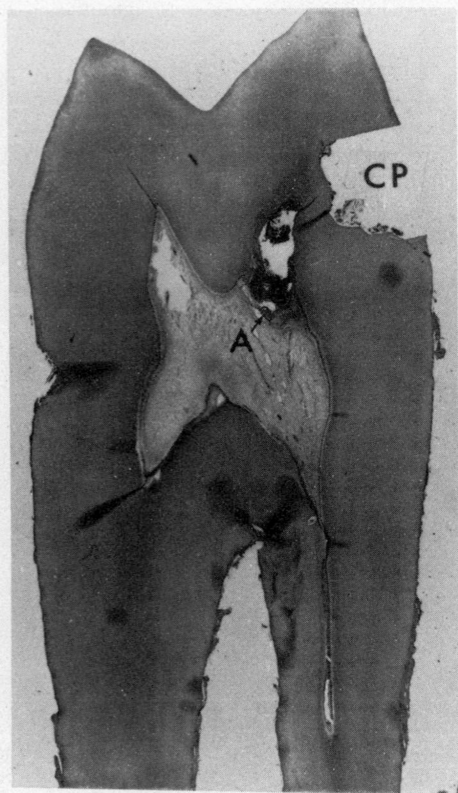

Figure 17–6. Acute partial pulpitis or pulp abscess (A) following caries and cavity preparation (CP) in tooth. Remainder of pulp is relatively normal.

opened to allow adequate drainage. Chronic pulpitis produces less intense discomfort.

PERIAPICAL DISEASE

Untreated pulpitis, particularly of infective origin, eventually involves the apical periodontium of the tooth and the surrounding apical alveolar bone. Three types of lesions may develop: (1) the apical or alveolar abscess, (2) the periapical granuloma, and (3) the epitheliated granuloma or radicular cyst.

The *apical* or *alveolar abscess* develops when pathogenic bacteria enter the apical periodontium from an acute pulpitis. The lesion is intensely painful as pressure develops, owing to the nonspecific inflammatory reaction. The affected tooth is slightly extruded from its alveolar socket and therefore is further traumatized. The abscess eventually drains by creating a fistulous tract through alveolar bone and erupting at the labial, lingual, or palatal gingiva as a "gumboil" (Fig. 17–7). The infection can be treated by antibiotics, drainage, and eventual root canal therapy of the affected tooth. In unusual cases, acute apical infection may spread widely along fascial planes and result in an extensive cellulitis rather than a localized alveolar abscess. This serious sequel of an apical infection tends to occur when a virulent organism challenges poor host resistance. Cellulitis arising from a mandibular tooth may involve the floor of the mouth and neck (Ludwig's angina), or cavernous sinus thrombosis can occur when a maxillary tooth is involved.

Chronic periapical lesions are referred to as *periapical granulomas*. These appear microscopically as granulation tissue with a dense infiltrate of lymphocytes, plasma cells, and histiocytes. Alveolar bone is gradually resorbed at the apex of the tooth, resulting in a well-demarcated spherical lesion that appears radiolucent on radiographs. A periapical granuloma may be asymptomatic or may present some discomfort or hypersensitivity of the involved tooth. The size of the lesion may remain relatively stable over a long period, representing a balance between local irritation and host response. A chronic periapical granuloma can evolve into an abscess if virulent organisms enter the region, or it can be transformed into a cyst if proliferating epithelium seals off part of the lesion.

The periapical region often contains islands of epithelium (rests of Malassez) that can be stimulated by the inflammatory lesion to proliferate into a network of stratified squamous epithelium penetrating throughout the periapical granuloma. It may now be termed an *epitheliated granuloma*, from which may arise a *radicular cyst*. The proliferating epithelial network eventually surrounds and completely encloses the central portion of the inflammatory lesion, which then no longer receives a blood supply (Fig. 17–8). The cellular material in the central area degenerates into a clear fluid, rich in protein and lipid (cholesterol). The epithelial lining of the cyst acts as a semipermeable membrane, and the difference in osmotic pressure draws more fluid into the cystic cavity, gradually enlarging the cyst and resorbing the surrounding bone. Occasionally, cholesterol may precipitate into a crystalline form within the cyst cavity or in the cyst wall, evoking a foreign body reaction. The cyst may become infected with virulent organisms, and the cyst wall may then undergo necrosis, yielding a

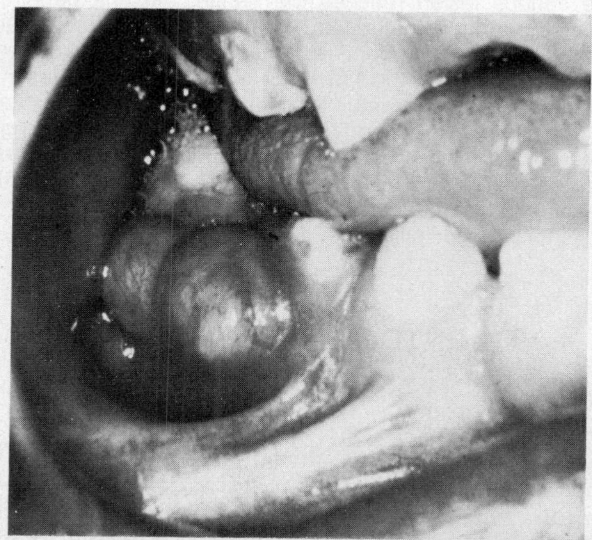

Figure 17–7. Gingival abscess.

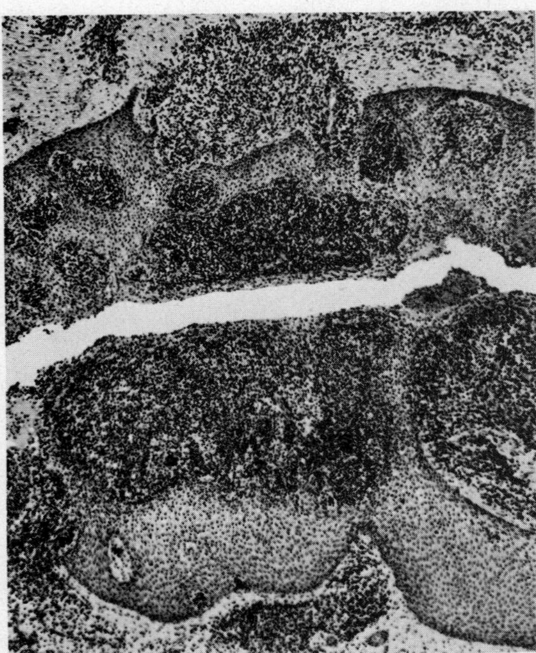

Figure 17–8. Radicular cyst showing ulceration of stratified squamous epithelial lining, inflammation of connective tissue capsule, and purulent exudate in central cavity.

granuloma or an abscess. It can be seen that these various periapical lesions represent a number of stages, or transitional lesions, of a basic disease process.

PERIODONTAL DISEASE

Periodontal disease is an inclusive term commonly used to describe inflammatory disease of the gingiva *(gingivitis)* or, in more severe cases, inflammation of the gingiva with extension of the disease to underlying tissues of the periodontium *(periodontitis)*. The major etiologic factor in both conditions is the oral bacterial and mycotic flora that colonizes the surface of the tooth within and above the gingival sulcus or crevice.[5] The microorganisms, including *Streptococcus mutans* and various filamentous groups, attach to the tooth surface as dental plaque (Fig. 17–9). As plaque accumulates at the gingival crevice together with food debris, it may become calcified, resulting in *calculus* or *tartar*. The calculus develops both above the gingival crevice, where it is visible and is termed supragingival calculus, and within the crevice, where it is hidden from view and is termed subgingival calculus. Calculus is both a mechanical and biologic irritant, with the microorganisms acting on gingival tissues by means of toxic metabolic products and probable immunologic mechanisms secondary to antigenic components of the bacteria. Microscopically, calculus is composed of an organic framework of bacterial and mycotic organisms, desquamated epithelial cells, leukocytes, and food debris in which calcium phosphate is deposited in the form of a hydroxyapatite crystalline structure.

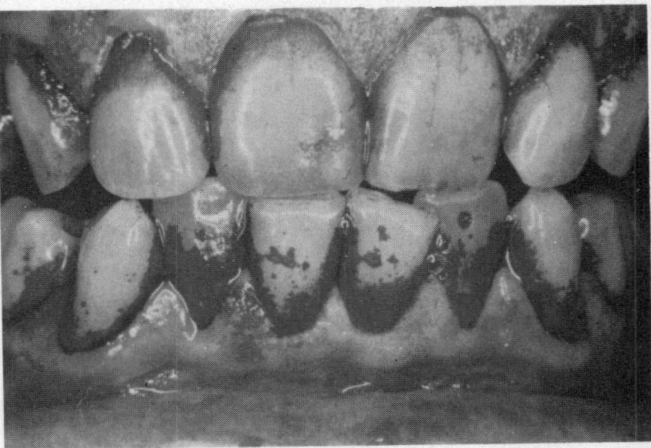

Figure 17–9. Dental plaque on teeth as demonstrated by a disclosing solution (1% basic fuchsin).

The progression from gingivitis to periodontitis depends to a large extent on the host's resistance to the local irritants. When there is a systemic predisposing condition, severe and rapid periodontal destruction may occur, particularly in young patients (periodontosis, juvenile periodontitis).[6] Thus, periodontal disease comprises a spectrum of severities ranging from basically local irritation to extensive destructive disease. In gingivitis or periodontitis of primarily local cause, the disease state can be successfully treated by mechanical removal of the tooth deposits (scaling) and the institution of a regimen of good oral hygiene to prevent accumulation of plaque and calculus. Other local irritational factors such as occlusal stresses can be corrected by selective reduction of tooth surfaces. In periodontitis associated with a predisposing systemic condition, such as diabetes, therapy requires continuous periodontal care for removal of local irritants, and the end results may still be poor if the underlying systemic disease cannot be adequately controlled. The interaction of local and systemic factors in the etiology of periodontal disease was first postulated by Znamensky[7] and confirmed by the experimental studies of Glickman[8] and others.[9]

GINGIVITIS. *Gingivitis is a chronic inflammation of the gingival margin, resulting from* local irritants (Fig. 17–10). Clinical manifestations include discomfort and

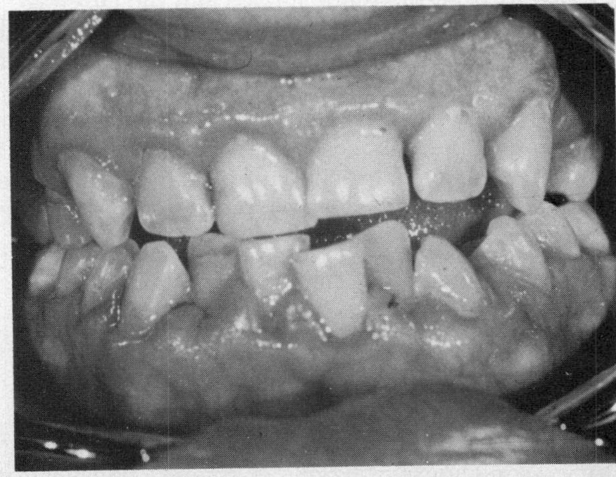

Figure 17–10. Gingivitis with erythema and inflammatory enlargement of gingiva.

bleeding upon tooth brushing. The course and severity of the disease can depend on a variety of metabolic and hormonal conditions that serve to exaggerate the gingival inflammatory response to the plaque or calculus. *This exaggerated gingival response is seen at puberty, during pregnancy, and in a number of nutritional and hematologic disturbances, such as scurvy, leukemia, and thrombocytopenia.* In addition to erythema, there may be considerable inflammatory hyperplasia of the gingiva in these conditions, often with notable vascular proliferation. For example, the so-called *"pregnancy tumor"* is an angiogranuloma of the gingiva, usually occurring in an area of gingivitis caused by the overhanging margin of a filling or crown or by a malposed tooth with extensive calculus deposition. Presumably, the altered hormonal homeostasis during pregnancy is further aggravated by the local irritant favoring the appearance of such a lesion.

PERIODONTITIS. *Periodontitis is an extension of gingivitis to the underlying periodontal tissues—the periodontal membrane, alveolar bone, and cementum of the teeth.* Clinical manifestations include, in addition to gingivitis, a pathologically deepened gingival crevice or periodontal pocket, suppuration within the periodontal pocket, tooth mobility resulting from resorption of alveolar bone, and gradual recession of the gingiva to expose the roots of the teeth (Fig. 17–11). The pathogenesis involves migration or proliferation of the epithelial attachment toward the root of the tooth and the creation of a deep gingival pocket, as the epithelium separates from the tooth during the migration. As calculus develops within the pocket, the epithelial surface ulcerates, and the bacteria cause suppuration. The older term for chronic periodontal disease was *pyorrhea* or *alveolar pyorrhea,* describing the purulent flow from the gingival sulcus. The eventual result of the chronic or subacute inflammation is resorption of tooth-supporting alveolar bone, mobility of teeth, and gradual loss of teeth. If the purulent exudate in the deep periodontal pocket cannot drain to the surface, a periodontal abscess may develop, with pointing and drainage through the alveolar bone and attached gingiva.

The therapy of periodontitis involves removal of the calculus from the tooth surface and the curettage or surgical removal of the epithelial attachment. When the irritants are removed, the gingiva reattaches to the tooth surface with gradual recession of the inflamed gingival tissue. The periodontal pocket is reduced, but the destroyed periodontal tissue is rarely restored to its original height, and the patient must accept the recession of the gingival tissues, with exposed visible roots of the teeth.

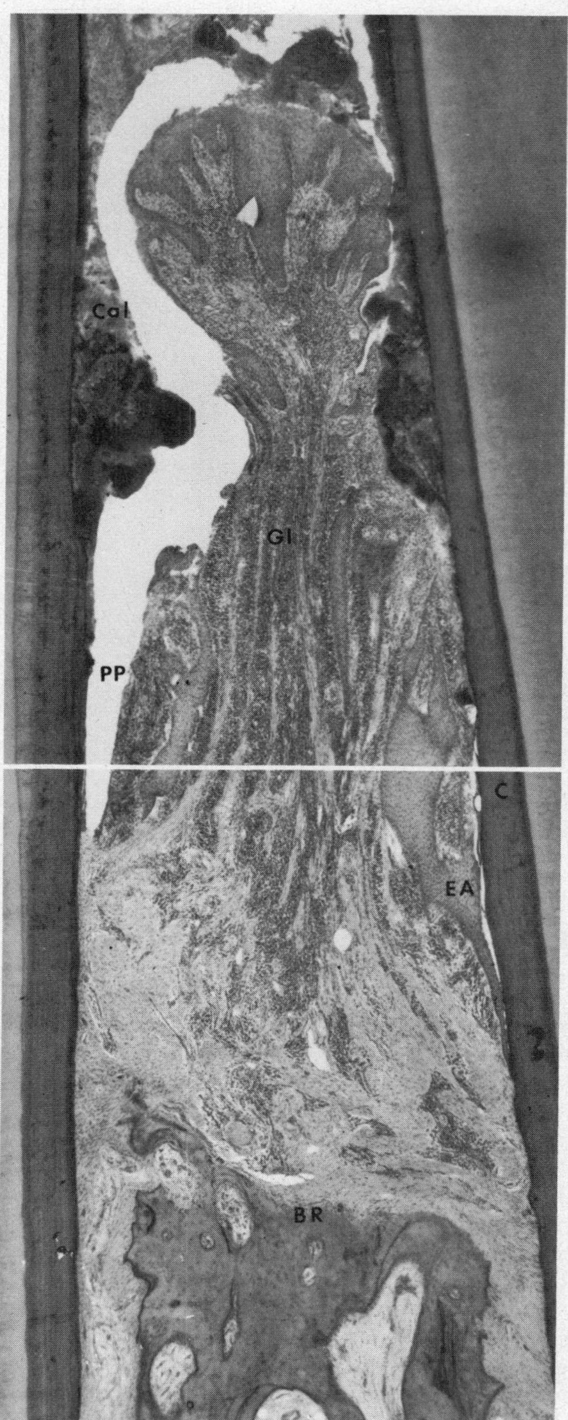

Figure 17–11. Periodontitis showing apical migration of epithelial attachment (EA) along cementum of root (C), gingival inflammation and its extension (GI), periodontal pocket formation (PP), calculus deposition (Cal), and alveolar bone resorption (BR).

DISEASES OF ORAL MUCOSA

DEVELOPMENTAL MALFORMATIONS

Normal oral mucous membrane is composed of stratified squamous epithelium overlying a dense fibrous connective tissue. The epithelium is either nonkeratinized (buccal mucosa) or lightly keratinized (tongue, gingiva). Skin appendages are absent, and the epithelium is composed of three layers (germinativum, spinosum, and corneum) rather than the five layers seen in skin. Occasionally a stratum granulosum appears if there is significant hyperkeratosis. Numerous mucous glands lie beneath the epithelium and release their secretions through narrow ducts that open on the mucosal surface. These glands are particularly prominent on the palate and lower lip.

Common developmental malformations of the oral mucosa include sebaceous glands beneath the buccal mucosa (Fordyce granules), hyperplasia of mucous glands (adenomatosis oris), fissures on the dorsal surface of the tongue (Fig. 17–12), and a fibrotic lingual frenum (tongue-tie, ankyloglossia). Less common malformations are clefts and fissures of the lips, macroglossia, and fibrous attachments between labial or buccal mucosa and the gingiva. Some of these malformations may occur in association with other craniofacial deformities in a variety of genetic syndromes.

TRAUMATIC LESIONS

The oral mucosa is not easily traumatized, since it is tough and flexible, but through no fault of its own it is forced to contend almost daily with all manner of attack, ranging from sharp fragments of food to imperfectly fitting dental appliances. Neurotic habits (cheek or tongue biting, gouging of mucosa with a pencil or sharp instrument) may produce severe ulceration suggestive of malignant neoplasia until a history is obtained. Occasionally, if the type of trauma remains undisclosed, biopsy is necessary to rule out malignancy. The traumatic ulcer is nonspecific microscopically and normally heals without scarring in 10 to 14 days. Since it is mechanically induced, its shape may be linear rather than round. Ulcers caused by dentures are easily interpreted and will heal once the sharp ridge or border of the appliance is reduced.

Chemical burns of the mucosa are unusual, but are sometimes seen in adults who place aspirin tablets against the gingiva for relief of toothache and in children who "sample" acid or alkaline kitchen cleansers. Electrical burns are occasionally seen in children who bite electrical wires, and thermal burns are seen in rare instances related to hot melted cheese (pizza lovers take note) or hot liquids such as coffee, tea, or soup.

BACTERIAL INFECTIONS

The oral mucosa is highly resistant to infection by the normal oral bacterial-mycotic flora. It is protected by the various antibacterial constituents of saliva. The elaboration of immunoglobulins, particularly secretory IgA, by local lymphocytes and plasma cells further protects the mucosa against the possible pathogenic effects of the endogenous oral flora, which consists of more than 20 different groups of organisms. Such antibacterial activity also protects the oral mucosa against "foreign" pathogens. Thus, the oral lesions of syphilis, gonorrhea, and the like are relatively rare, despite obvious exposure. The normal oral flora may, however, exaggerate the clinical features of other oral lesions such as traumatic ulcers, ruptured herpetic vesicles, or ruptured bullae of pemphigus. Moreover, if the patient's resistance is lowered because of systemic disease, nutritional deficiency, or emotional stress, or if antibiotic therapy alters the balance of microorganisms, the oral flora may become pathogenic and produce diseases such as necrotizing gingivitis or candidiasis. Immunodeficiency, in particular, predisposes to infections in the oral cavity. Both necrotizing gingivitis (fusospirochetal infection) and candidiasis are thus common complications following radiation therapy and chemotherapy.

NECROTIZING GINGIVITIS (ACUTE NECROTIZING ULCERATIVE GINGIVITIS, ANUG). This is an uncommon infection of the gingiva caused by the oral fusospirochetal complex of organisms. It is characterized by necrosis of the marginal gingiva and interdental papillae (Fig. 17–13). In some cases the infection extends from the gingival lesions to the oral mucosa, indicating poor host resistance. This is seen most often in children with Down's syndrome, leukemia, or immunodeficiency disease. With tissue resistance markedly lowered, the fusospirochetal flora may spread widely and invade deeply to produce the *noma* or *gangrenous stomatitis*

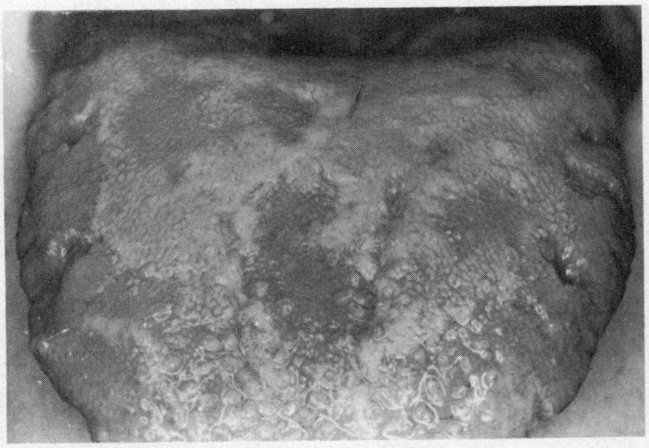

Figure 17–12. Congenital fissuring of tongue together with areas of papillary atrophy (geographic tongue).

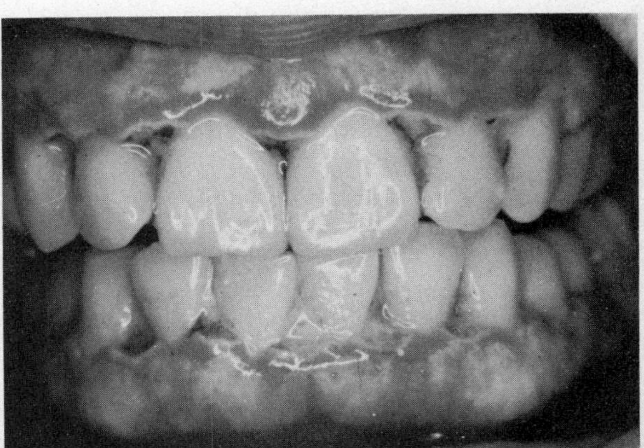

Figure 17–13. Necrotizing gingivitis, showing necrosis of tissue at gingival margin and in interdental areas.

seen in children suffering from parasitic diseases or kwashiorkor in underdeveloped countries. Emotional stress is considered to be a systemic predisposing influence[10] and may explain the occasional occurrence of the disease in groups of young people in the army or in college dormitories. An old World War I term for the infection was "trench mouth." Necrotizing gingivitis is not contagious, since the bacteria are normally present in all mouths. Local predisposing factors such as preexisting periodontal disease, malocclusion and poor oral hygiene exaggerate the infection.

ORAL CAVITY LESIONS OF SYPHILIS, TUBERCULOSIS, AND LEPROSY

Oral lesions occur in all stages of *syphilis.*[11] Chancres of the lip may appear as nonhealing large ulcers (p. 336). Biopsy to rule out cancer is necessary. In secondary syphilis the oral lesions take the forms of a maculopapular eruption analogous to the skin rash and/or the mucous patch seen on the genital mucosa. Tertiary syphilis may be marked by a gumma (p. 337) of the palate or by smooth atrophic luetic glossitis. The atrophy of filiform and fungiform papillae renders the tongue more susceptible to the development of leukoplakia. Prenatal syphilis may be associated with hypoplastic teeth of unique shape (hutchinsonian incisors, mulberry molars) as well as gummatous defects and atrophic glossitis.

Tuberculous lesions of the mouth are rare and appear as ulcers or raised nodular lesions. The histologic changes were described on p. 345. Tuberculous lesions may also extensively involve labial and perioral regions (tuberculosis cutis orificialis).

Oral lesions of *leprosy* are difficult to diagnose if skin lesions are absent. As pointed out in the earlier discussion of this disease (p. 347), when the reaction is granulomatous, the acid-fast organisms may not be present in the lesion.

VIRAL INFECTIONS

Two common viral diseases affecting the mouth are *herpetic stomatitis* and *herpangina. Herpetic stomatitis* represents the major primary disease response to herpesvirus type I infection (p. 284). Characteristic clinical features are acute gingivitis, vesicular eruption, nonspecific coated tongue,[12] and sometimes local lymphadenopathy (Fig. 17–14). The vesicles rupture early, leaving ulcers, but usually heal within two weeks. Microscopic features of the vesicular lesions are epithelial degeneration and the presence of virally modified cells with large multilobed hyperchromatic nuclei. Although common in childhood, herpetic stomatitis frequently occurs in young adults.[13] *Herpes labialis* represents recurrent disease caused by herpesvirus type I. The virus is known to survive in nerve ganglia and can leave the nerves to produce labial vesicular lesions if host resistance is

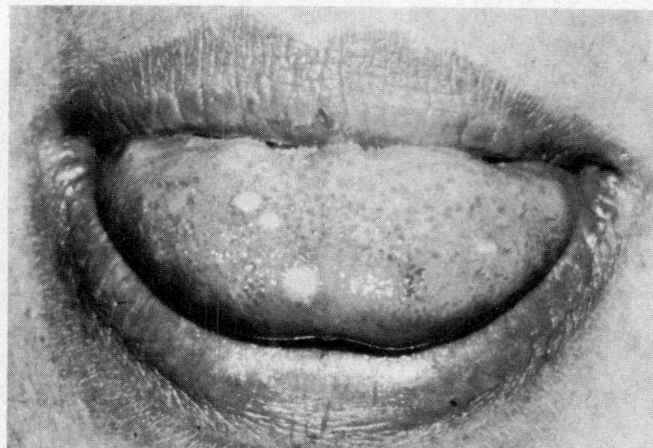

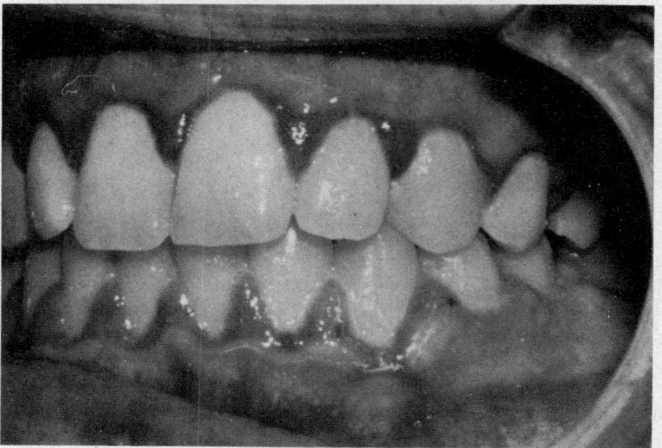

Figure 17–14. Coated tongue and vesicles (*above*) and acute gingivitis (*below*) in herpetic stomatitis.

lowered by trauma, fever, or emotional stress. Immunosuppressed patients may suffer recurrent attacks of *primary* herpetic stomatitis.

Herpangina caused by Coxsackie A virus presents a similar microscopic appearance but a different clinical appearance. There is an acute oropharyngitis[14] with vesicular lesions on the palate and other posterior oral tissues. The course is seven to ten days when immunity develops, but can be much longer in immunosuppressed patients. Several variant strains of Coxsackie A, notably A16, cause hand-foot-and-mouth disease, with clinical features similar to herpangina together with papular and vesicular lesions of the palms of the hands and soles of the feet.[15, 16]

The varicella-zoster virus can affect the mouth in the primary disease, *chickenpox*, and in the recurrent disease, *herpes zoster*. The lesions are vesicular and, in the latter, unilateral and follow the distribution of nerves (Fig. 17–15*A*). The virus survives in nerve ganglia and invades epithelial tissue. Microscopic features are similar to the lesions of herpetic stomatitis and other epithelial viral diseases, with the production of large, multilobed nuclei in epithelial cells (Fig. 17–15*B*). *Warts* of viral origin can be found in the mouth but are rarely seen, and usually represent lesions transferred from the skin or genitalia.

MYCOTIC INFECTIONS

The oral mucosa can develop such rare mycotic infections as actinomycosis, blastomycosis, mucormycosis, coccidioidomycosis, and histoplasmosis (Chap. 8). These conditions appear as nonhealing ulcerations; the diagnosis can be made only by ruling out more common diseases and by appropriate microscopic and cultural studies. The only fungus infection commonly seen in the mouth is *candidiasis* (thrush). It usually appears as an opportunistic infection in debilitated or immunosuppressed patients, since *Candida albicans* is a normal oral inhabitant. It is a common complication in patients receiving extensive chemotherapy for malignant tumors or leukemia, and in organ transplant patients receiving immunosuppressive agents. The frequency of oral candidiasis as a complication of antibiotic therapy has been exaggerated; it usually requires several different antibiotics over a period of time, and in these cases patients are often debilitated by the underlying disease. Candidiasis is also seen in young babies; the mouth is sterile at birth and Candida may become pathogenic while the oral bacterial-mycotic flora is becoming established. The clinical features are white patches (Fig. 17–16*A*) that rub off, leaving raw, ulcerated areas. Microscopic examination reveals the invading mycelia of Candida and epithelial destruction (Fig. 17–16*B*).

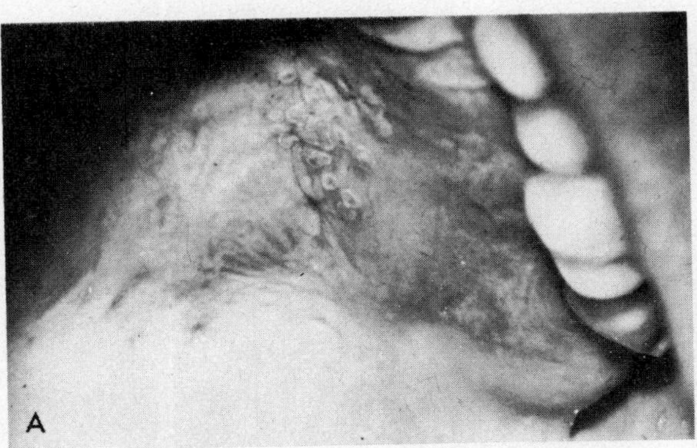

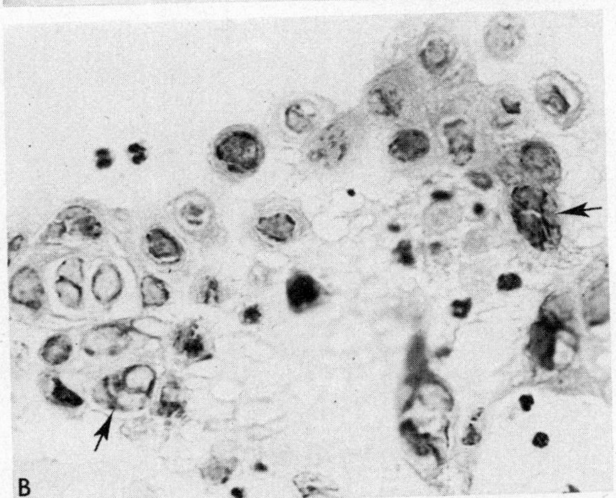

Figure 17–15. *A*, Herpes zoster developing on left side of palate. *B*, High-power view of base of a herpetic vesicle, revealing virally modified multilobed epithelial cells (*arrows*).

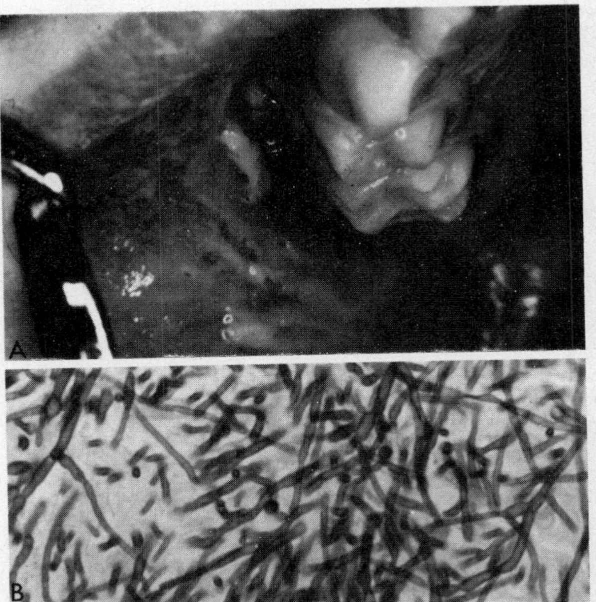

Figure 17–16. *A*, Candidiasis of oral mucosa showing numerous white lesions. *B*, Biopsy specimen of oral candidiasis showing invasion of tissue by mycelia of *Candida albicans*.

APHTHOUS STOMATITIS (RECURRENT APHTHOUS ULCERS)

Although clinical and experimental data suggest that aphthous stomatitis (canker sores) has a psychosomatic component,[17, 18] there is evidence to suggest that it is autoimmune in origin.[19, 20] The disease consists of recurrent episodes of painful oral ulcers (Fig. 17–17*A*), often attaining large size with considerable tissue destruction (Fig. 17–17*B*). Microscopically, the lesions present nonspecific ulceration with a marked vascular response in the deeper connective tissue. There may be thrombosis of these vessels and perivascular lymphocytic infiltration.[21, 22] Thus, small localized areas of infarction contribute to the expansion and persistence of these ulcers. Oral aphthous ulcers together with conjunctival and genital lesions may appear in Behçet's syndrome.[23, 24]

KERATOTIC DISEASES

Lichen planus is a common oral disease of uncertain etiology. Although many etiologic agents have been considered, a psychosomatic and/or autoimmune origin is currently favored. Oral lichenoid reactions can also occur as a systemic drug reaction. The histopathology and clinical lesions are quite characteristic in this disease. A papular eruption results in white, lacelike or reticulate lesions, usually on the buccal mucosa and tongue (Fig. 17–18*A* and *B*). Plaquelike, erosive, ulcerative, atrophic, and bullous lesions may also appear. The microscopic features consist of parakeratosis,

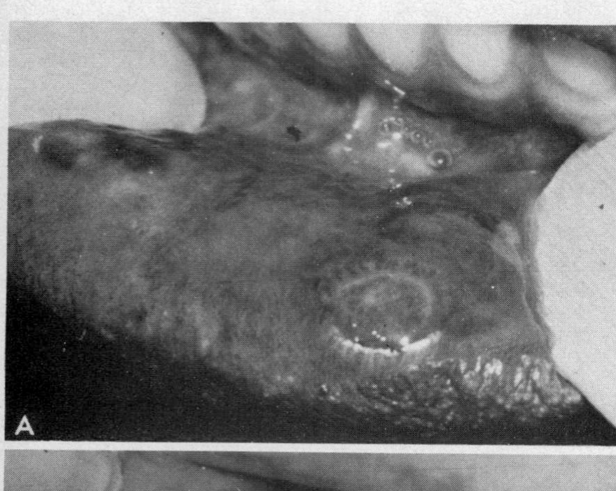

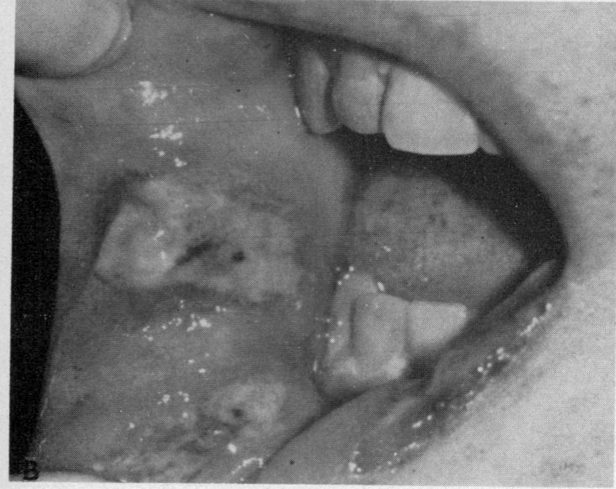

Figure 17–17. Aphthous stomatitis. *A,* Discrete round ulcer. *B,* Large necrotic lesions.

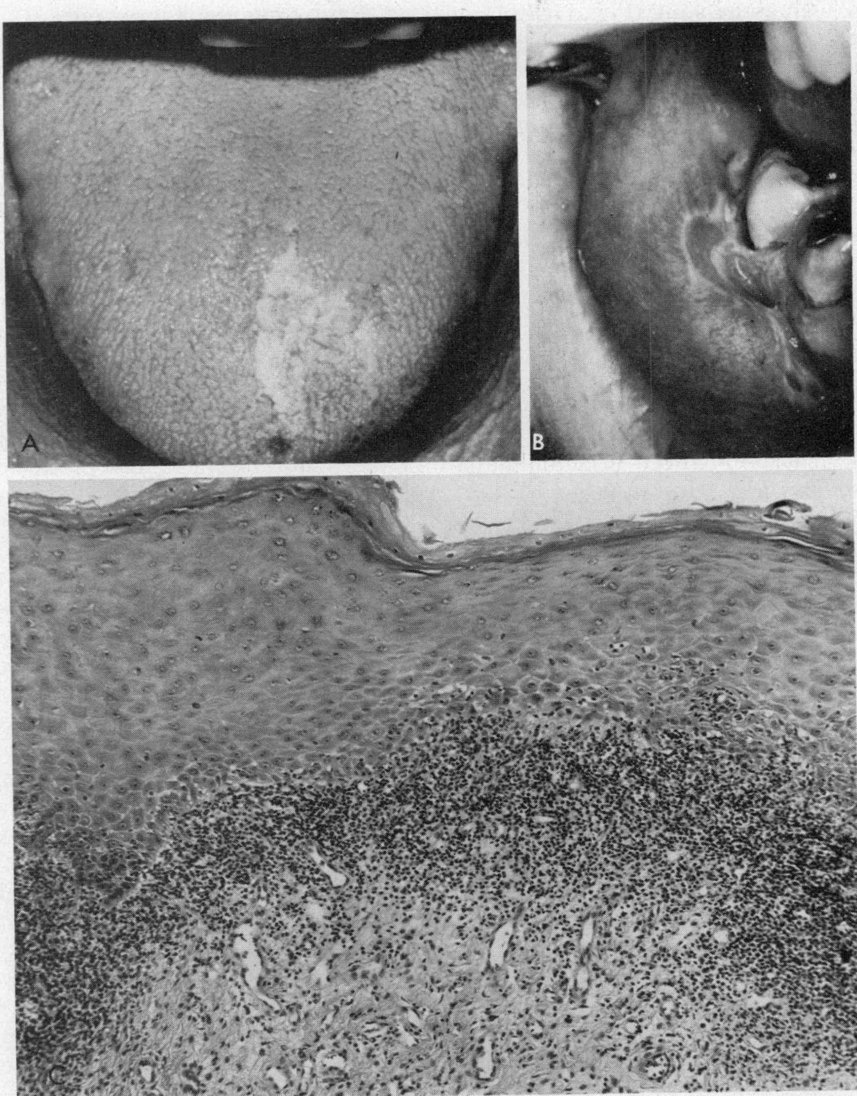

Figure 17–18. Lichen planus. *A,* Plaquelike white lesions on dorsum of tongue. *B,* Reticulate white lesions of buccal mucosa. *C,* Biopsy specimen of reticulate oral lichen planus showing parakeratosis and lymphocytic infiltrate beneath basal layer.

hydropic degeneration of the basal layer of epithelium, and a lymphocytic infiltration in the upper corium (Fig. 17–18*C*). The epithelial degeneration may be sufficiently severe so that the epithelium lifts off the connective tissue as a vesicle[25] or degenerates to form an ulcer. Lesions may be present on the skin as well as on the oral mucosa (see Chapter 27).

Leukoplakia is a clinical term signifying a white, plaquelike lesion on the mucosa.[26] The oral lesion is a reaction to irritation such as smoking (Fig. 17–19*A* and *B*).[27] *In 90% of cases, microscopic examination reveals a hyperkeratosis and varying amounts of submucosal chronic inflammatory infiltration (Fig. 17–19C). In 10% of cases there is also epithelial dysplasia, and these lesions are considered precancerous.* Many are transformed into carcinoma in situ and gradually become invasive epidermoid carcinomas (Fig. 17–19*D*). Genetic factors may determine whether a leukoplakic lesion will be of simple keratotic or dysplastic type. The simple keratotic type does not appear to develop into the dysplastic or precancerous variety.

AUTOIMMUNE DISEASES

The oral mucosa may be involved in autoimmune disease such as *systemic lupus erythematosus* (SLE). There are no characteristic oral lesions in SLE, but nonspecific ulceration may occasionally occur as a manifestation of the generalized debilitated status of the patient. In *pemphigus*, another disorder of probable immunologic origin, the mouth is invariably involved (Fig. 17–20*A*), and the oral vesiculobullous lesions precede the skin lesions. Early diagnosis facilitates therapy, and definitive diagnosis can be made from an oral tissue biopsy. The characteristic acantholysis is diagnostic.[28] Acantholysis refers to intraepithelial vesiculation caused by loss of desmosomes and separation of epithelial cells in the stratum spinosum.[29] The basal layer remains attached to the underlying corium (Fig. 17–20*B*). A high percentage of cases of pemphigus respond positively to direct immunofluorescent tests, but occasionally the test is negative in the early stage of the disease. In the direct immunofluorescent technique, a biopsy specimen from the oral mucosa is incubated with fluorescein-labeled IgG from the patient's serum. In a positive test for pemphigus, the immunofluorescent immunoglobulin is localized in the intercellular spaces between epithelial cells (p. 1294).

Mucous membrane pemphigoid may resemble oral pemphigus but is differentiated by the fact that the vesicles and bullae arise at the junction of the epithelium and corium. Pemphigoid affects the mouth and occasionally other mucosal sites, such as the conjunctiva. The etiology is possibly autoimmune. Bullous lesions may appear in the mouth in addition to a desquamative type of gingivitis.[30] Microscopic examination of the lesions reveals *subepithelial* vesiculation. Ultrastructural studies have demonstrated a split in the basal membrane.[31] In occasional cases, basement membrane antibodies can be demonstrated by immunofluorescence (p. 1295).[32]

In *chronic discoid lupus erythematosus* there may be oral lesions consisting of white plaques or areas of ulceration. Microscopic examination reveals four characteristic histologic features: parakeratosis, hydropic degeneration of the basal layer, a perivascular lymphocytic infiltration in the corium, and collagen degeneration. Basement membrane antibodies can often be demonstrated by immunofluorescence.

DRUG REACTIONS

Local reactions to drugs (stomatitis venenata) are rare. Occasional allergic responses to lipstick, toothpastes, mouthwashes, and denture material are reported.[33] Oral reactions to systemic drugs are common and of various types, and the clinical manifestations can be extremely variable. *Allergic reactions* usually appear as vesiculobullous eruptions, urticarial reactions, or fixed drug eruptions. Direct *toxic reactions* are more damaging and appear as erosions and ulcers. *Idiosyncratic reactions* can be unusual, such as the gingival hyperplasia seen as a frequent response to phenytoin. Iodides and bromides may produce granulomatous oral lesions. *Black tongue* may be caused by antibiotics, resulting from the proliferation of resistant chromogenic bacteria on the lingual papillae.

Erythema multiforme (p. 1284) is of unknown etiology, although many cases represent a drug reaction, and some appear to be a response to systemic infections or emotional stress. The mouth is usually affected, often severely, with the labial mucosa tending to be the site of major involvement. Lesions are vesiculobullous, with ulceration and secondary crusting on the lips (Fig. 17–21*A*). Typical target lesions may appear on the skin, characterized by concentric bands of erythema with a vesicle or ulcer in the center. A severe hemorrhagic variant of erythema multiforme is the *Stevens-Johnson syndrome*, with extensive involvement of mouth, skin, conjunctiva, and genitalia.[34] The histopathologic picture is relatively characteristic. There is a striking degeneration of the upper epithelium as well as inflammation and subepithelial vesiculation (Fig. 17–21*B*).[35]

Angioneurotic edema of the lips is an occasionally observed urticarial reaction. As discussed in Chapter 5 (p. 210), it is caused by a genetic deficiency in C1 inhibitor.

GENETIC DISEASES

Genetic diseases affecting the oral mucosa are rare. White, folded stomatitis or *white sponge nevus* is inherited as an autosomal dominant trait and appears as multiple white, plaquelike lesions. Microscopically there is extensive spongiosis or intracellular edema. Systemic genetic diseases affecting the oral mucosa include von Recklinghausen's neurofibromatosis (p. 138)

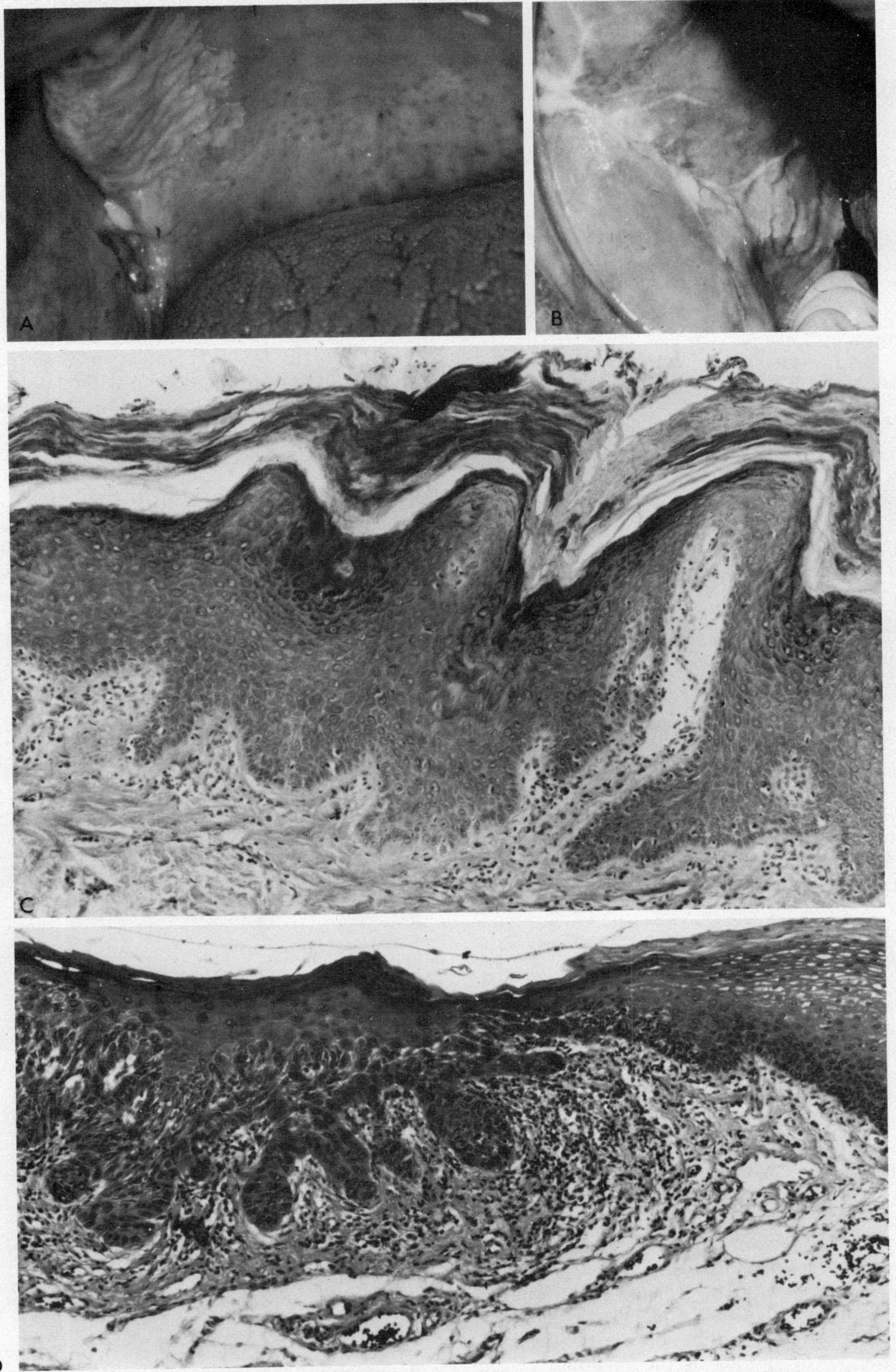

Figure 17–19. *A,* Leukoplakia of palate in a heavy smoker. *B,* Leukoplakia of buccal mucosa in a smoker. *C,* Microscopic appearance of simple leukoplakia showing hyperkeratosis. *D,* Microscopic appearance of dysplastic leukoplakia showing cellular pleomorphism and hyperchromatism (carcinoma in situ).

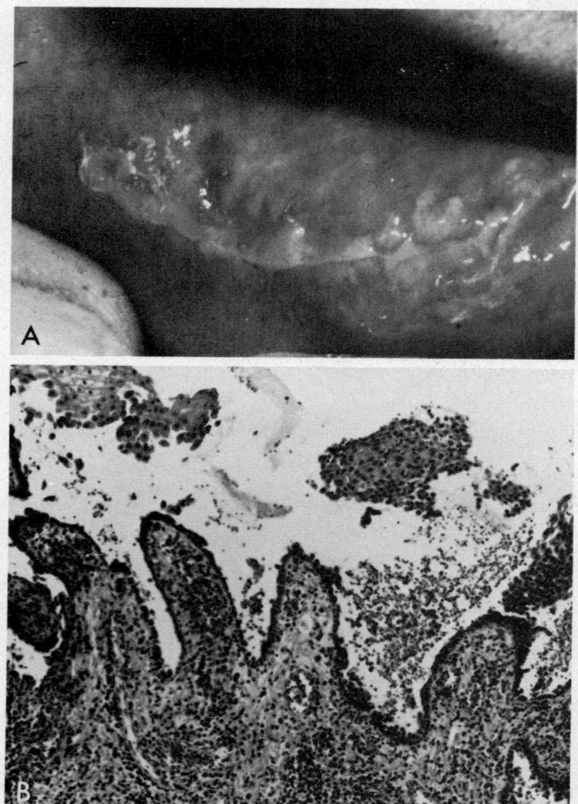

Figure 17–20. *A*, Bullous lesions confined to the mouth in a patient with pemphigus. *B*, Biopsy specimen of oral pemphigus lesion showing acantholysis.

and Osler-Weber-Rendu disease (hereditary hemorrhagic telangiectasia, p. 542). Cleft lip and cleft palate may occur either as developmental malformations or as part of a genetic disease syndrome.

TUMOR-LIKE LESIONS

Numerous tumor-like lesions develop in the mouth. *Mucocele* is a cystic lesion arising in distended mucosal mucous glands. As the glands distend, they often rupture. Since there is rarely a true cyst wall with an epithelial lining, the term "mucous cyst" is out of favor.[36] "Mucous extravasation phenomenon" is often used as a histopathologic diagnosis.[37] A large mucocele of the floor of the mouth, usually with a true epithelial lining, is often referred to as a *ranula* because of its thin, transparent covering and vascular network resembling a frog skin.

Dermoid cyst is an unusual cystic lesion that can develop either above or below the mylohyoid muscle, so that it can appear either as a tumor-like mass in the floor of the mouth or as a midline mass in the neck just inferior to the lower border of the mandible.[38] The dermoid cyst represents a developmental malformation derived from rests of multipotential cells. It is somewhat similar to those of the ovary (p. 1149).

Pyogenic granuloma is a common oral lesion constituting, in essence, a vasoproliferative inflammatory response.[39, 40] Thus, it is sometimes termed an angiogranuloma. If the epithelial surface is ulcerated and suppuration is evident, the preferred term is pyogenic granuloma. The so-called "pregnancy tumor," discussed earlier, is an angiogranuloma or pyogenic granuloma.

The peripheral (gingival) *giant cell granuloma* is another unusual tumor-like lesion thought to be of inflammatory origin.[41, 42] It appears as a 1- to 1.5-cm localized mass protruding from the gingiva (Fig. 17–22*A*). The lesion appears microscopically as a mass of multinucleate giant cells scattered throughout a fibroangiomatous matrix (Fig. 17–22*B*). Despite its inflammatory origin, the lesion is similar microscopically to the giant cell lesions of hyperparathyroidism (p. 1330) and giant cell tumors of bone (p. 1345). The term *epulis* has been used for this lesion.

BENIGN TUMORS

So-called "benign tumors" are very common in the mouth, particularly fibromas and hemangiomas. They are currently interpreted as hamartomatous lesions

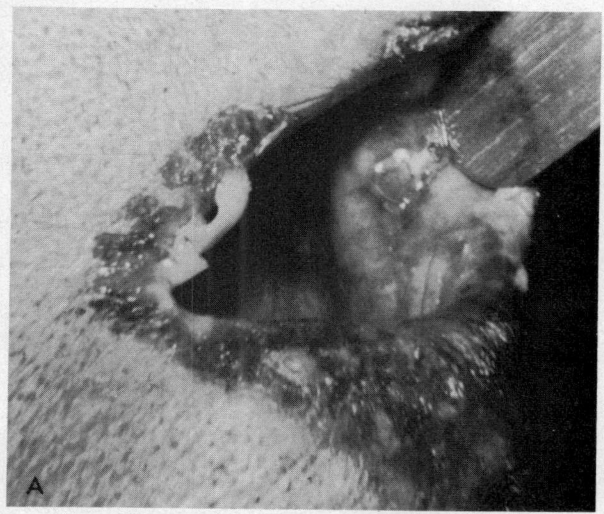

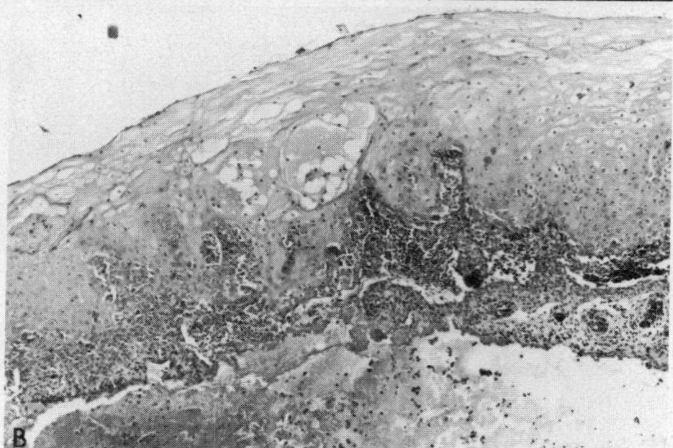

Figure 17–21. *A*, Erythema multiforme showing severe involvement of lips and bullous lesions on oral mucosa. *B*, Oral lesion of erythema multiforme showing subepithelial vesiculation and severe degeneration of upper layers of epithelium.

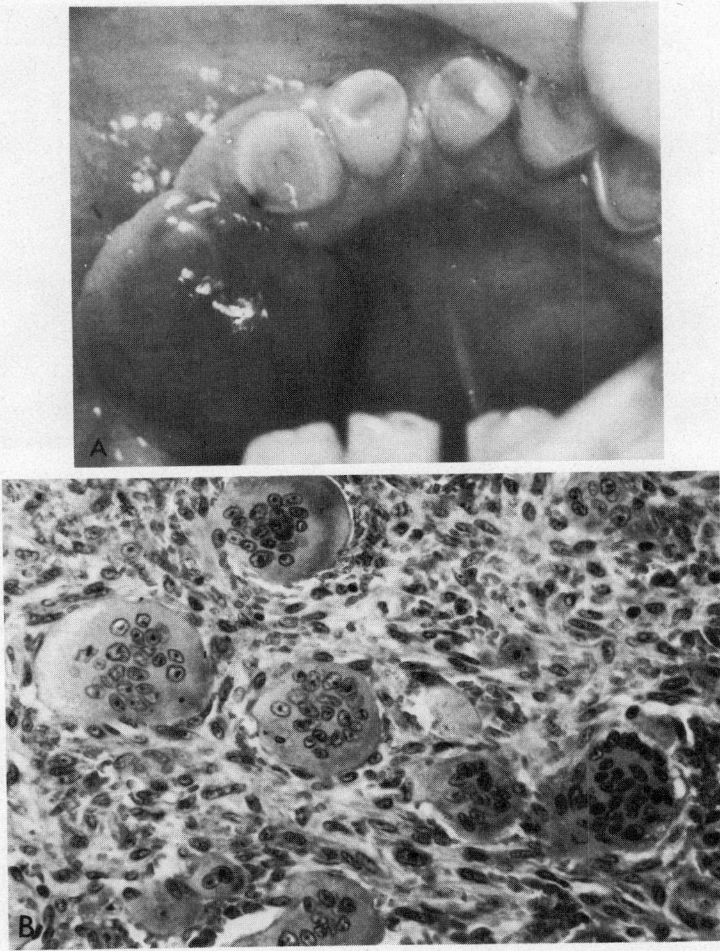

Figure 17–22. *A,* Giant cell granuloma of gingiva. *B,* Biopsy specimen of giant cell granuloma showing multinucleate giant cells and fibroangiomatous stroma.

rather than true neoplasms. Their size varies considerably; an entire tongue may be involved by an extensive angioma, resulting in macroglossia with numerous surface lesions. The terms angiomatosis[43] and fibromatosis are often used in describing very large and extensive lesions. Other benign tumors found in the oral cavity are papilloma, lymphangioma, lipoma, adenoma, pleomorphic adenoma (mixed tumor), neurofibroma, schwannoma, and nevus. An unusual type of oral benign tumor is the so-called granular cell myoblastoma, found most often in the tongue. Morphologically, this is identical to myoblastomas occurring elsewhere (p. 1316). Microscopically the tumor is composed of large cells with granular cytoplasm, and the overlying epithelium invariably demonstrates pseudoepitheliomatous hyperplasia. The histogenesis of these lesions is uncertain, but currently a neurogenic origin is favored.[44, 45] A rare lesion similar to myoblastoma microscopically is found on the gingiva of infants and is referred to as congenital epulis.[46] Other rare lingual tumors are chondroma[47] and osteoma.[48]

MALIGNANT TUMORS

Although every type of malignant tumor has been found in the mouth, only epidermoid (squamous cell) carcinoma can be considered reasonably common. When one speaks of oral cancer, one means epidermoid carcinoma, since this form of neoplasia represents approximately 97% of oral malignant tumors. Oral cancer accounts for 5% of all malignant tumors in the body and constitutes a serious problem. In a study of 14,253 cases of oral carcinoma, Krolls and Hoffman found the following distribution of tumors: lower lip (38%), tongue (22%), and floor of mouth (17%). Much less frequently involved were the gingiva (6%), palate (5.5%), tonsillar area (5%), upper lip (4%), and buccal mucosa (2%). Most patients were between the ages of 40 and 70 (74.5% of cases). Less than 10% of cases occurred in females and less than 10% in blacks.[49] Clinically, oral cancer may appear as a papillary, ulcerative, or (rarely) deeply infiltrative lesion (Fig. 17–23). Early diagnosis of oral cancer should be relatively simple, since the

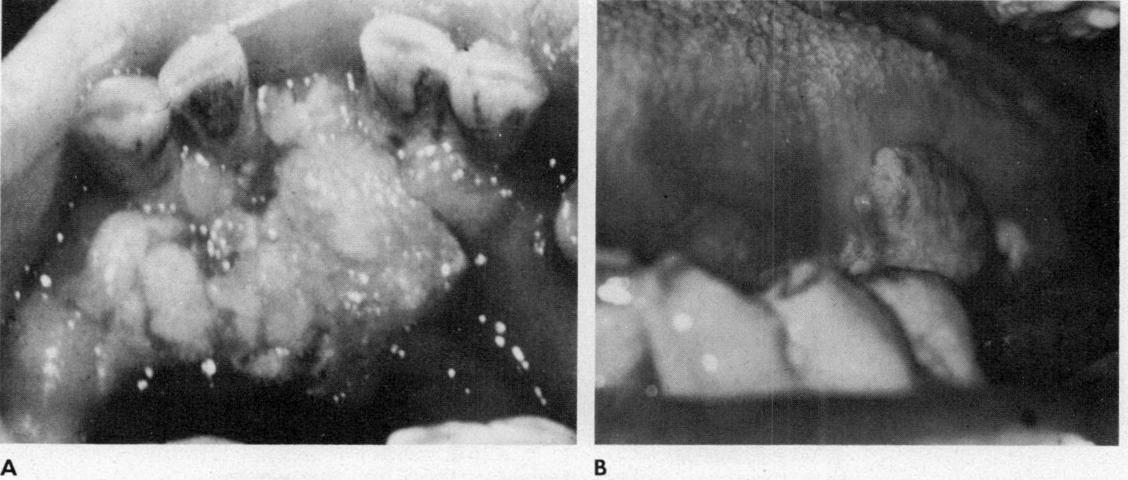

A B

Figure 17–23. *A*, Fungating epidermoid carcinoma arising in gingiva. *B*, Ulcerated and raised lesions of epidermoid carcinoma of lateral border of tongue.

region is easily accessible to visualization, palpation, and biopsy. However, current therapy for oral cancer is not highly successful, since most lesions are not discovered and treated in their early stages of development. A number of risk factors in oral cancer have been documented. Heavy tobacco use is a major etiologic factor in mouth cancer, and alcohol use has been found to be an additional risk.[49A, B]

Microscopically, oral epidermoid carcinoma varies in its degree of differentiation. Lesions of the lower lip tend to be well differentiated, whereas lesions of the tongue tend to be anaplastic or poorly differentiated. For this reason, cancer of the tongue and other areas such as the floor of the mouth have a poorer prognosis than lesions of the lip. The accuracy of initial biopsy in the diagnosis of oral epidermoid carcinoma has been shown to be close to 100% in a large series of cases studied,[50] but the accuracy of oral cytology was found to be approximately 85% in a controlled study.[51] Exfoliative examination of oral cavity secretions is not reliable, since saliva, with its proteolytic enzymes, rapidly destroys the cellular morphology as the cells are digested. Oral cytologic techniques require scraping of the surface of a suspicious lesion and smearing of the material onto a microscopic slide for fixation and staining. Oral cytology is widely used as a screening procedure but not as a diagnostic test, since biopsy is more reliable.

The only other intraoral malignant tumors seen with some degree of frequency are adenocarcinomas arising in submucosal salivary glands.[52-54] They occur on the palate and represent about 2 to 3% of oral malignant tumors. A variant is the mucoepidermoid carcinoma. The prognosis is guarded in all forms of oral adenocarcinoma because deep invasion of contiguous tissues and metastasis to regional lymph nodes are common with these lesions. Other oral malignancies, such as malignant melanoma, are extremely rare, representing less than 1% of cases of oral cancer. The melanocarcinoma usually presents as a darkly pigmented lesion within the oral mucosa, which histologically resembles its counterpart of the skin (p. 1279).[55]

ORAL MANIFESTATIONS OF SYSTEMIC DISEASES AND METABOLIC DISTURBANCES

Since the time of Osler, the mouth has been said to mirror the state of health of the individual. Although the concept has been somewhat exaggerated, there are a number of diseases and abnormal metabolic states that induce oral manifestations.[56] A smooth, atrophic tongue, resulting from atrophy of filiform and fungiform papillae,[57] is seen in iron deficiency anemia (Plummer-Vinson syndrome), pernicious anemia, sprue, vitamin B deficiency, and tertiary syphilis (Fig. 17–24*A*). Unusual hemorrhage from the gingiva suggests scurvy, thrombocytopenia, or other hemorrhagic diseases. Enlarged, red, boggy gingiva may occur in pregnancy, leukemia, polycythemia, or scurvy. Extensive oral and labial melanotic pigmentation may appear in Addison's disease, Peutz-Jeghers syndrome,[58] and possibly Albright's syndrome (polyostotic fibrous dysplasia) (Fig. 17–24*B*). An enlarged tongue with areas of yellow discoloration may be an early manifestation of amyloidosis. Blanching of the tongue may be observed in Raynaud's disease.[59] Oral mucous glands are affected as part of the generalized gastrointestinal glandular involvement in cystic fibrosis, and a labial biopsy may be useful in effecting a definitive diagnosis. Regional ileitis (Crohn's disease) may present small nodular or ulcerative granulomatous lesions in the mouth.[60] Patients with ulcerative colitis may also have small ulcerations in the mouth as well as a pyostomatitis vegetans, with papillary suppurative lesions.[61] Lesions of the oral mucosa have also been described in unusual dermatologic disorders such as Darier's disease.[62]

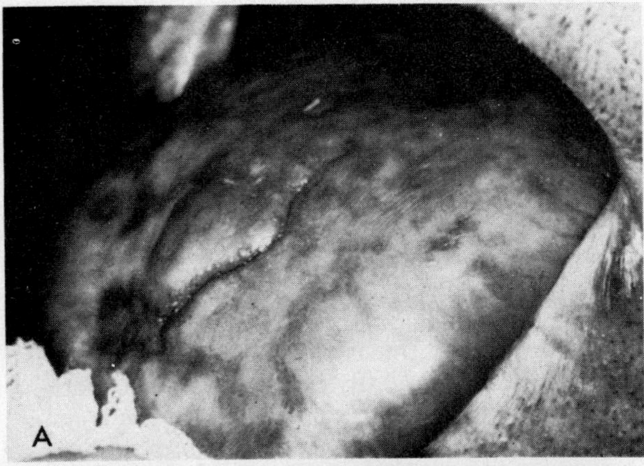

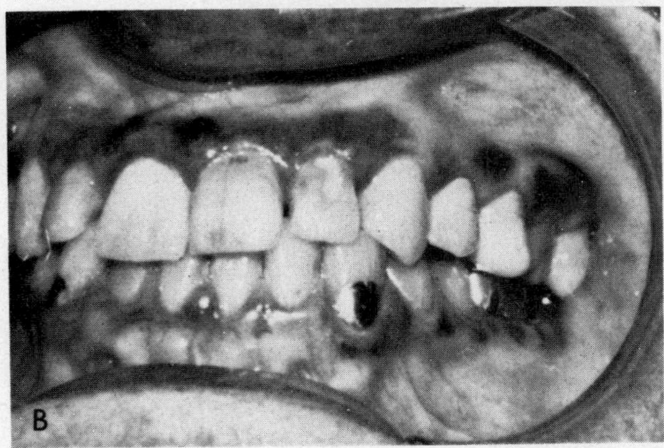

Figure 17–24. *A*, Severe atrophic glossitis with ulceration in pernicious anemia. *B*, Melanotic pigmentation of gingiva in Addison's disease.

DISEASES OF JAWS

The mandible and maxilla are affected by generalized skeletal diseases and develop infections and neoplasms similar to those in other parts of the skeletal system. However, there are a number of unique lesions related to the development of the tooth germs and to the embryonic development of the jaws.

DEVELOPMENTAL MALFORMATIONS

Cleft palate is the most common of the severe malformations affecting the upper jaw. Its frequency of occurrence is 1 in 2500 live births. It may involve only the palate and be midline, or it may affect the alveolus (tooth-bearing part of the jaws) and be unilateral or bilateral (Fig. 17–25*A*). Cleft palate may occur as a localized malformation or may be associated with a number of other developmental malformations in genetic conditions such as Apert's or Down's syndromes. Genetic diseases may also result in severe malocclusion due to developmental micrognathia or hypoplasia of jaws. Among minor developmental malformations of the jaws are localized, bony, tumor-like protuberances on the palate or on the mandibular alveolus, referred to as torus palatinus or torus mandibularis (Fig. 17–25*B*). Developmental lesions of the jaws also include a variety of developmental cysts, and a group of tumor-like hamartomatous lesions composed of dental tissues and referred to as odontomas.

OSTEOMYELITIS

Osteomyelitis is a rare infection of the jaws. Acute osteomyelitis was a common problem before the development of antibiotic drugs and represented extension of infection from a dental alveolar abscess. Chronic, nonspecific osteomyelitis is seen occasionally as a response to a chronic or subacute periapical infection. Specific forms of osteomyelitis such as tuberculous, syphilitic, or actinomycotic osteomyelitis are extremely rare, and represent hematogenous infection or entrance of the infection through a tooth extraction socket or through an exposed and infected dental pulp. The microscopic appearance of osteomyelitis of the jaws is similar to that of osteomyelitis affecting other parts of the skeletal system (p. 1323).

CYSTS

Cysts of the jaws are extremely common. Most frequently seen is the radicular cyst (already described), the origin of which is inflammatory. Others may be

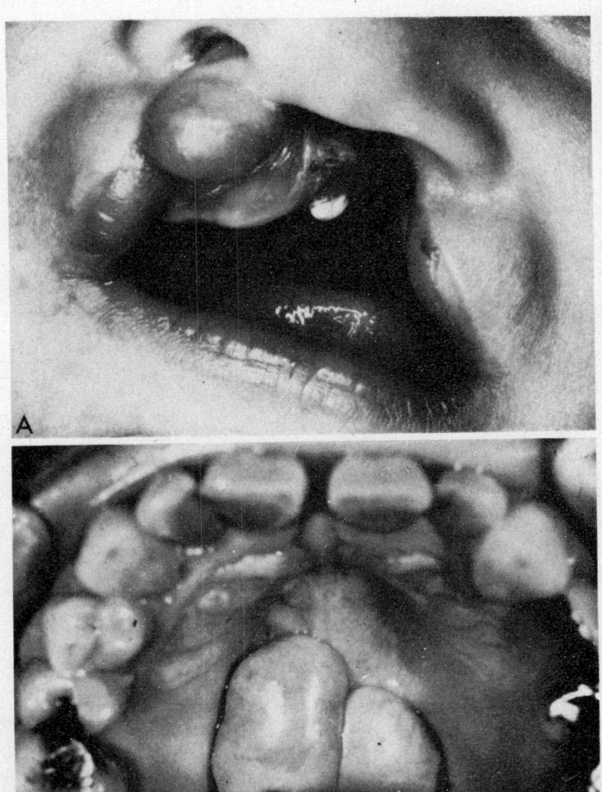

Figure 17–25. *A*, Cleft lip and palate, *B*, Torus palatinus.

termed developmental cysts, and arise from either the tooth germs (dental follicle) or multipotential cell rests that have remained in the suture areas of the jaws (where the primordial jaw processes unite during embryologic development to form the mandible and maxilla). Those cysts arising from the dental organ may be termed *odontogenic developmental cysts* or *follicular cysts* (arising from the dental follicle). Those arising in suture regions are termed *fissural cysts* and are usually described by their area of origin—globulomaxillary cyst, median mandibular cyst, nasopalatine cyst, etc. The globulomaxillary cyst always arises between the maxillary lateral incisor and cuspid teeth. This is the suture region between the embryonic maxillary and globular processes.

Follicular cysts arise in any region of the alveolus. A tooth may be absent, suggesting that the cyst arose from its follicle and prevented its normal development. If all teeth are present, it can be assumed that the cyst arose from the follicle of a supernumerary tooth. If the follicular cyst develops once the tooth has started to form, the tooth or its crown may be part of the cyst wall and may penetrate into the cystic cavity. This type is referred to as a *dentigerous* cyst (Fig. 17–26*A*). All cysts of the jaws have a cyst wall composed of dense fibrous connective tissue lined with epithelium. The epithelium is usually nonkeratinizing stratified squamous (Fig. 17–26*B*). In maxillary cysts, it may be pseudostratified columnar. Rarely, it may be simple columnar or cuboidal, or the stratified squamous epithelium may develop keratin. The term epidermoid cyst is used if the epithelium is of the keratinizing variety.

ODONTOGENIC TUMORS

Out of all proportion to their incidence, odontogenic tumors have received considerable attention over the years.[63, 64] *Odontomas* are to be regarded as hamartomatous lesions rather than true tumors. They represent abnormal development of dental tissues. The classifications of odontomas have been unnecessarily detailed, since they merely describe minor variations in structure. Most calcified or hard odontomas contain all dental tissues and are observed radiographically as circumscribed lesions in the jaws. The dental tissues may form small teeth (compound composite odontoma) or may be arranged haphazardly (complex composite odontoma). Soft odontomas are usually composed of loose mesenchymal connective tissue (odontogenic fibromyxoma) and may contain islands of ameloblastic epithelium (ameloblastic fibroma) (Fig. 17–27*A* and *B*). An unusual type of calcifying epithelial odontogenic tumor was first described by Pindborg.[65] The tumor is composed of sheets of pleomorphic epithelial cells and a stroma of connective tissue. Eosinophilic spherical bodies that undergo calcification are seen among the groups of epithelial cells and in the stroma.

Ameloblastoma is a true neoplasm, comparable in appearance and activity with the basal cell tumor of

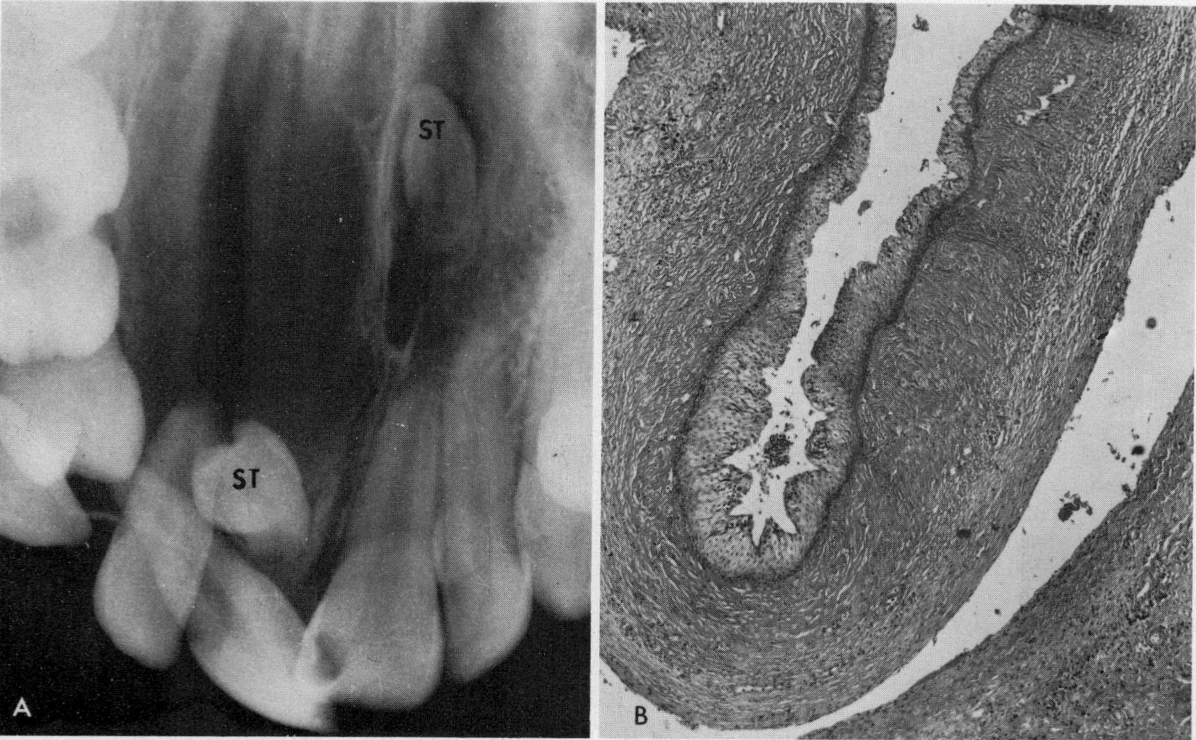

Figure 17–26. *A,* Dentigerous cyst of maxilla with two supernumerary teeth (ST). *B,* Biopsy specimen of dentigerous cyst.

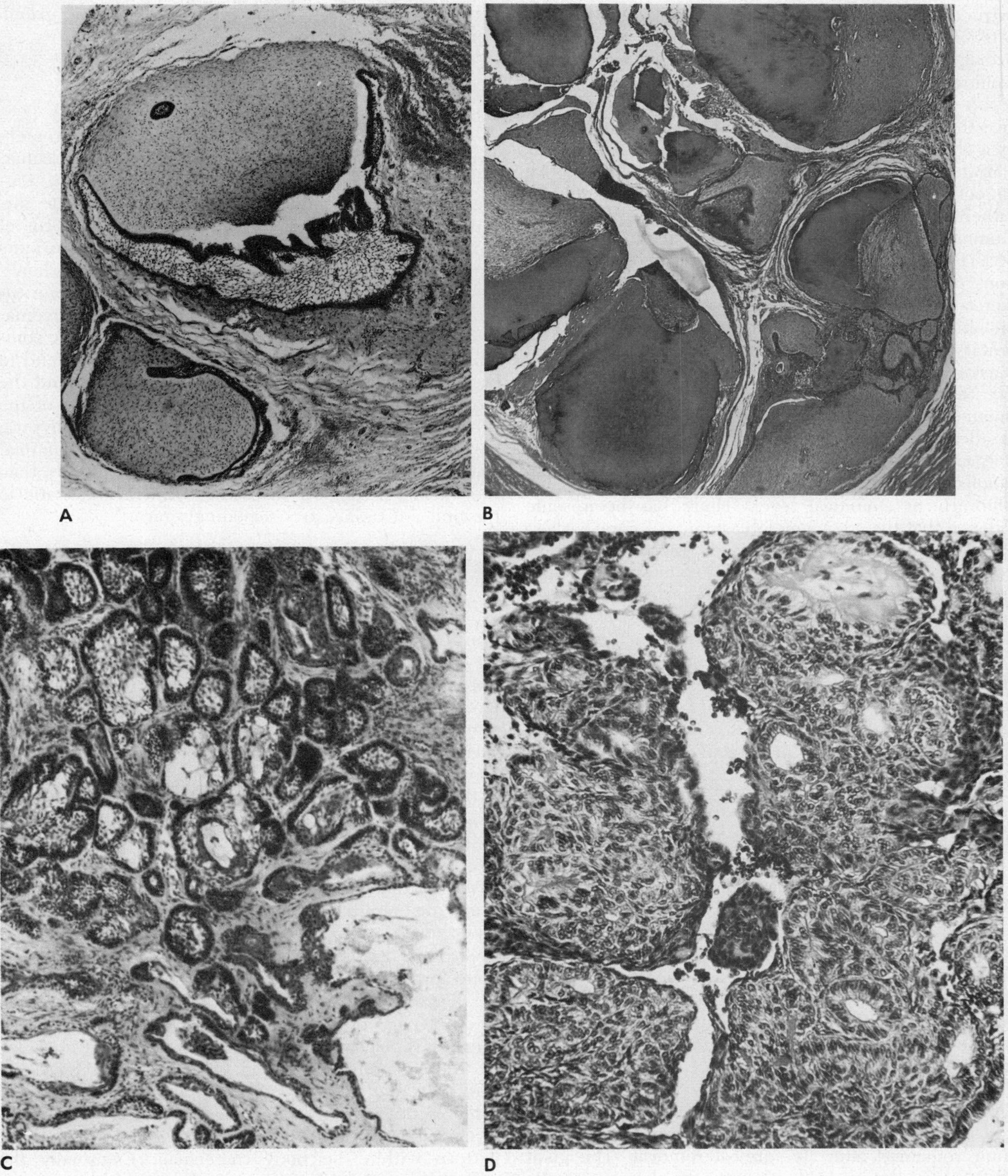

Figure 17–27. *A,* Odontoma consisting of structures resembling tooth buds. *B,* Odontoma composed of a variety of dental tissues, often in a disorganized pattern (complex composite odontoma). *C,* Ameloblastoma showing nests of epithelial cells within a fibrous connective tissue stroma. Varying stages of cystic development are seen. *D,* Odontogenic adenomatoid tumor showing the formation of structures resembling ducts or acini.

skin. It occurs most often in the mandible in the areas of the molars and ramus and is a locally invasive, highly destructive tumor that does not metastasize. Most reports of metastatic ameloblastoma represent original misdiagnoses, the tumor being a carcinoma or adenocarcinoma rather than an ameloblastoma. The older term for this tumor, adamantinoma, has now been discarded, since the tumor does not form enamel. Ameloblastoma has a characteristic microscopic appearance with cords or nests of ameloblastic epithelium lying in a dense connective tissue stroma. The nests of ameloblastic epithelium are composed of peripheral cuboidal or columnar cells and a central stellate reticulum (Fig. 17–27*C*). The central reticulum often undergoes degeneration, creating microcysts that may eventually reach macroscopic size to form a polycystic tumor. In some ameloblastomas, the stellate reticulum undergoes rudimentary keratinization, and this histologic variant is occasionally termed acanthomatous ameloblastoma.[66] The stellate reticulum may disappear, leaving an adenomatoid appearance (adenoameloblastoma).[67, 68] The classification of ameloblastomas based on minor histologic variations is of little value, since it has not been demonstrated that the different histologic types behave differently at a clinical level. There has been some evidence that the adenoameloblastoma is somewhat less aggressive clinically than the more typical forms of this neoplasm,[67, 68] and the term odontogenic adenomatoid tumor[69] has been suggested in order to differentiate these lesions from ameloblastomas (Fig. 17–27*D*).

An unusual melanotic tumor found in the maxilla of infants, often described as a melanoameloblastoma or retinal anlage tumor, is now considered to be of neural crest origin[70] and is termed melanotic neuroectodermal tumor of infancy.[71] The tumor may be locally invasive, but is benign and does not recur following surgical removal.

NONODONTOGENIC BENIGN TUMORS

Benign tumors of the jaws include such entities as hemangioma, myxoma, fibroma, neurofibroma, and true giant cell tumor (as distinct from reparative giant cell granuloma). These neoplasms are identical to their counterparts occurring elsewhere. All benign tumors of the jaws expand in size relatively slowly, but their configuration is not spherical. Their margins extend into the intertrabecular spaces of bone for some distance, so that curettage of the tumor may not completely remove all tissue at the margins, and for this reason the tumor may recur. Recurrence does not signify malignancy or aggressive behavior but merely that remnants of the tumor remained after its surgical removal. The giant cell tumor of the jaws, like that of other bones, may be a benign lesion that may recur after surgical therapy. However, some giant cell tumors are locally aggressive, and bone and even the roots of teeth are resorbed as the lesion expands. *It should be noted that all intraosseous giant cell lesions are not true giant cell tumors, since central giant cell reparative granulomas occur in hyperparathyroidism; indeed, some workers interpret all giant cell lesions of the jaws as reparative granulomas.*[72]

NONODONTOGENIC MALIGNANT TUMORS

Primary malignant tumors of the jaws are extremely rare.[73, 74] In order of frequency they are fibrosarcoma, osteogenic sarcoma, chondrosarcoma, lymphoma, neurogenic sarcoma, angiosarcoma, and ameloblastic sarcoma as well as rarer variants. An unusual form of lymphoma affecting the jaws is known as Burkitt's lymphoma,[75] a distinctive neoplasm described earlier.

The jaws are also involved in multifocal bone tumors such as multiple myeloma[76] and Ewing's sarcoma. Malignant tumors *metastatic* to the jaws are more common than are primary malignant tumors. They tend to be carcinomas, and various surveys[77, 78] have found the most frequent primary lesions to be carcinoma of the breast, lung, kidney, rectum or colon, prostate, thyroid, stomach, and salivary glands and malignant melanoma. The mandible is involved much more frequently than the maxilla (over 85% of cases). Tumors metastatic to the oral soft tissues are exceedingly rare.[78]

METABOLIC BONE DISEASES

The jaws are affected by metabolic diseases such as *fibrous dysplasia*, *Paget's disease of bone*, *histiocytosis X*, *hyperparathyroidism*, and *osteoporosis*. Monostotic fibrous dysplasia tends to occur more commonly in the jaws than does polyostotic disease. Because of its microscopic similarity, cementoma, a common lesion of bone seen at the apices of the teeth, is now considered to be a localized form of fibrous dysplasia. In fibrous dysplasia of the jaws (described more completely on p. 1333), the bone initially is replaced by active fibrous connective tissue. Gradually, trabeculae or islands of dense, relatively acellular bone develop within the connective tissue and may result in a relatively calcified lesion that is opaque on radiographs.[79] Fibrous dysplasia of the jaws may remain localized to a small region or may increase in size and gradually expand beyond the cortex of the bone, producing gross deformity of the jaw or face.

Paget's disease may affect the maxilla in addition to other parts of the skeletal system (p. 1331). Initially there is replacement of marrow spaces and trabeculae by fibrous connective tissue. Gradually the typical picture of active Paget's disease appears, with increased osteoblastic as well as increased osteoclastic activity. Irregular resorption and appositional lines form a mosaic pattern within the bony trabeculae. Eventually the disease becomes inactive and sclerotic as osteoblastic activity predominates.[80] Radiographic studies of the maxilla present radiolucency in the lytic phase, a ground-glass appearance in the active phase, and radiopacity in the inactive phase. Unique features of Paget's disease in the maxilla are hypercementosis of the roots of the teeth, with occasional ankylosis to bone, and progressive malocclusion and spreading of teeth as the maxilla expands.

The jaws can be involved in multifocal eosinophilic granuloma (Hand-Schüller-Christian disease) and Letterer-Siwe disease, but these conditions are extremely rare. However, eosinophilic granuloma is occasionally seen as a solitary lesion of the mandible or maxilla, and presents the typical microscopic picture of eosinophils lying within a background of histiocytes (p. 695).[81]

DISEASES OF SALIVARY GLANDS

Generalized disease of the salivary glands affects the production of saliva, and significantly decreased salivary flow results in a dry mouth (xerostomia) leading to irritation, erosion, and ulceration of the oral mucous membrane as well as enhanced susceptibility to periodontal disease and dental caries. Generalized diseases of salivary glands also tend to involve the mucous glands of the oral mucosa, and characteristic histopathologic alterations may be observed in a simple biopsy specimen of labial mucosa, obviating biopsy of the parotid gland. Localized lesions of the major salivary glands and their ducts usually do not affect the mouth significantly, but result in swelling, pain, and discomfort in the parotid and submandibular regions. The sublingual glands are rarely affected by localized disease such as neoplasia.

XEROSTOMIA

Xerostomia may be caused by physiologic mechanisms such as the use of sympathomimetic drugs, by emotional disturbances, by anticholinergic organic nervous system disease, by degeneration of glands following radiation to the area, by atrophic changes in aging, and by diseases such as sarcoidosis or Sjögren's disease.[82] Acute infections such as mumps (epidemic parotitis) run a brief course and rarely result in permanent glandular disease, but produce a temporary xerostomia. Obstruction of a duct by lithiasis or traumatic scar may decrease the amount of saliva, but the remaining glands usually maintain adequate function. Likewise, a neoplasm affects salivary flow but only to a minor extent. Sjögren's disease of probable autoimmune etiology,[83] described earlier (p. 189), is a major cause of xerostomia.

GLANDULAR DUCTAL OBSTRUCTION

Obstruction of Stensen's or Wharton's ducts by inflammatory fibrosis or lithiasis results in glandular distention that is usually painful. The ductal obstruction predisposes to retrograde spread of oral bacteria, thus inducing sialadenitis. Such retrograde migration of infection is rare in the absence of ductal obstruction but occasionally occurs during general anesthesia, and is known as "postsurgical parotitis."

NEOPLASMS

In view of their relatively undistinguished normal morphology, the salivary glands give rise to a surprising variety of benign and malignant tumors. Approximately 75 to 85% occur in the parotids, 10 to 20% in the submandibular glands, and the remaining 5 to 15% in the minor salivary glands (mainly palatal). The considerable variability of the histologic appearance and clinical behavior of both the benign and malignant forms has resulted in complex and differing classifications.[84-86] Table 17–1 presents a classification developed by the World Health Organization along with the approximate frequency of the specific forms of neoplasms. Several points should be noted:

1. This compilation refers only to epithelial tumors; mesenchymal lesions such as hemangiomas, lipomas, and others may arise in these glands but account for only about 5% of all tumors.[87]

2. The ratio of benign to malignant differs among the neoplasms of the various salivary glands as follows: parotid, 3–5:1; submandibular, 2:1; palatal glands, 1:1.[88] It is evident that a neoplasm within a minor salivary gland is much more likely to be malignant than one in the parotid.

3. For reasons that are unclear, carcinomas of the salivary glands as a group tend to pursue a slow course characterized by local recurrences, invasion of adjacent structures, late metastases, and death. Thus, only 10- to 20-year survival data have any validity in terms of therapy.

Irrespective of the histologic pattern, all neoplasms of the major salivary glands tend to present

Table 17–1. EPITHELIAL TUMORS IN THE PAROTID AND SUBMANDIBULAR GLANDS*

	Parotid	Submandibular
Adenomas		
Pleomorphic adenoma	53 to 76%	29 to 68%
Monomorphic adenoma		
Adenolymphoma	5 to 15%	0 to 2%
Oxyphilic adenoma	0.5 to 1%	0 to 0.5%
Other types (basal cell adenoma, trabecular adenoma, tubular adenoma, sebaceous lymphadenoma, etc.)	0 to 2%	0%
Mucoepidermoid tumors	2 to 6%	0 to 7%
Acinic cell tumors	1 to 3%	0 to 0.5%
Carcinomas		
Adenoid cystic carcinoma	2 to 3%	11 to 17%
Adenocarcinoma	1 to 7%	0 to 11%
Epidermoid carcinoma	0.5 to 6%	3 to 11%
Undifferentiated carcinoma	3.5 to 4%	7 to 9%
Carcinoma in pleomorphic adenoma (malignant mixed tumor)	1.5 to 4%	2%

*Data compiled from Skolnik, E. M., et al.: Tumors of the major salivary glands. Laryngoscope *87*:843, 1977; Eneroth, C. M.: Salivary gland tumors in the parotid glands, submandibular gland, and the palate region. Cancer 27:1415, 1971; Thackray, A. C., and Lucas, R. B. (eds.): Tumors of the Major Salivary Glands. Washington, D. C., Armed Forces Institute of Pathology, 1974, p. 14.

clinically in a somewhat standard fashion. Both benign and malignant tumors present as palpable masses, dominantly in the parotid glands, sometimes in the submandibular glands, and rarely in other salivary glands. However, it should not be overlooked that enlargement of the salivary glands is less often due to a tumor than to such non-neoplastic conditions as inflammations and ductal obstruction. Parotid lesions usually produce distinctive swellings in front of and below the ear (Fig. 17–28). Sometimes, tumors arising in the anterior portion of the parotid appear surprisingly far removed from the ear, while others arising in the lower regions of the gland masquerade as cervical masses. Some parotid tumors situated deep to the course of the facial nerve do not become palpable until they are moderately advanced. When diagnosed, adenomas are generally 2 to 6 cm in diameter and are mobile upon palpation. They enlarge very slowly, do not invade or metastasize, and are painless. Malignant lesions often present in a similar manner and are of similar size when diagnosed. However, they tend to enlarge more rapidly. Most significantly, because of their close relationship to the facial nerve, invasive malignant tumors may induce pain, numbness, paresthesias, or facial nerve paralysis when the nerve becomes involved. The usual age of all patients with benign tumors is 45, but those with malignant parotid tumors are, on the average, only slightly older. The average duration of symptoms with benign tumors is approximately 24 months as compared with nine to ten months for malignant tumors. However, a significant number of patients with malignant tumors have a long history of a mass and some for more than ten years before diagnosis. Ultimately, the only reliable means of differential diagnosis of these lesions is excisional biopsy and morphologic analysis.[89]

Benign

PLEOMORPHIC ADENOMA. This most common tumor of the major salivary glands is distinctive by virtue of its marked histologic diversity. It is characterized principally by epithelial and myoepithelial components distributed in varied patterns through an abundant matrix of mucoid, myxoid, or chondroid supporting tissue. Islands of well-formed cartilage, bone, and occasionally squamoid and/or sebaceous epithelial cells may also be present. This heterogeneity gave rise in the past to the designation "mixed tumor of salivary glands" in the belief that the lesion arose from epithelial and mesenchymal anlage. There is now general agreement that the apparent mesenchymal components are all derived from either the epithelial or myoepithelial cells, accounting for the currently accepted designation "pleomorphic adenoma," but the precise contribution of myoepithelial cells remains unclear.[90]

Grossly, these tumors are encapsulated, somewhat lobulated masses ranging from 1 to 6 cm in diameter. They may be buried within the salivary gland substance or protrude superficially beneath the glandular capsule. The cut surface is yellow-white and basically soft and fleshy, but often there are blue-gray translucent areas of increased consistency caused by the chondroid foci and other regions where the neoplasm is mucoid and gelatinous.

Microscopic examination reveals the heterogeneity previously mentioned. Some tumors are predominantly cellular and composed of epithelial and myoepithelial elements, whereas others are dominantly made up of apparent mesenchymal components with only a scattering of epithelial cells (Fig. 17–29*A*). Some importance is attached to the proportions of these two basic components on the grounds that cellular, predominantly epithelial neoplasms are more likely to grow rapidly and recur following resection than those made up largely of mesenchymal-appearing components.[91] However, within an individual tumor there is considerable variability from one microscopic field to another. The range of patterns can best be encompassed by describing the individual elements that may be present. The epithelial cells may be dispersed throughout the stromal background in small strands or sheets, or may form ducts, acini, irregular tubules, or microcysts. The cells may be cuboidal or columnar and sometimes have mucin-containing vacuoles. Squamous differentiation may occur in the form of intercellular bridges or keratin pearls. The myoepithelial cells are smaller and darker and tend to be polygonal, with an eccentric nucleus and hyalin eosinophilic cytoplasm, giving rise to such terms as "plasmacytoid" or "hyaline" cells.[92] Sometimes the myoepithelial cells are spindle shaped or show squamous differentiation (Fig. 17–29*B, C,* and *D*). Surrounding this epithelial component, sometimes dispersing it, are areas of myxoid tissue with abundant basophilic ground substance that is metachromatic with toluidine blue stain and is PAS negative. Distinctive is the imperceptible blending of the epithelial and mesenchyma-like elements at their interface. Islands of chondroid material may be present having the appearance of true cartilage, but the margins of these islands also merge imperceptibly with the surrounding myxoid or cellular areas. Foci of bone may also be present in the myxoid stroma. The histologic range is almost limitless, but it is precisely this variation that characterizes the pleomorphic adenoma.

As the name implies, pleomorphic adenoma is a benign lesion. However, when located in the parotid gland close to the facial nerve, it is sometimes difficult, despite the encapsulation, to enucleate completely. Adding to the difficulty, the capsule may at points be thinned and somewhat deficient, and therefore difficult to define surgically. At such foci of capsular deficiency, small pseudopods of tumor may protrude and be left behind in the enucleation. Thus, recurrences following resection are reported to occur in 5 to 50% of cases, with a higher incidence in tumors of the minor salivary glands.[93] Sometimes these recurrences do not become apparent until one to two decades later. Because of the wide scattering of the pseudopods that are left behind, recurrent lesions tend to be multifocal, in contrast to primary tumors, which are almost always unifocal. Despite such behavior, the recurrent tumors are almost always benign, but their multicentricity makes secondary resection increasingly difficult if facial nerve injury is to be avoided. Later, it will be pointed out that carcinomas may arise in pleomorphic adenomas. The issue of whether previous surgery or long persistence contributes to such malignant transformation is contro-

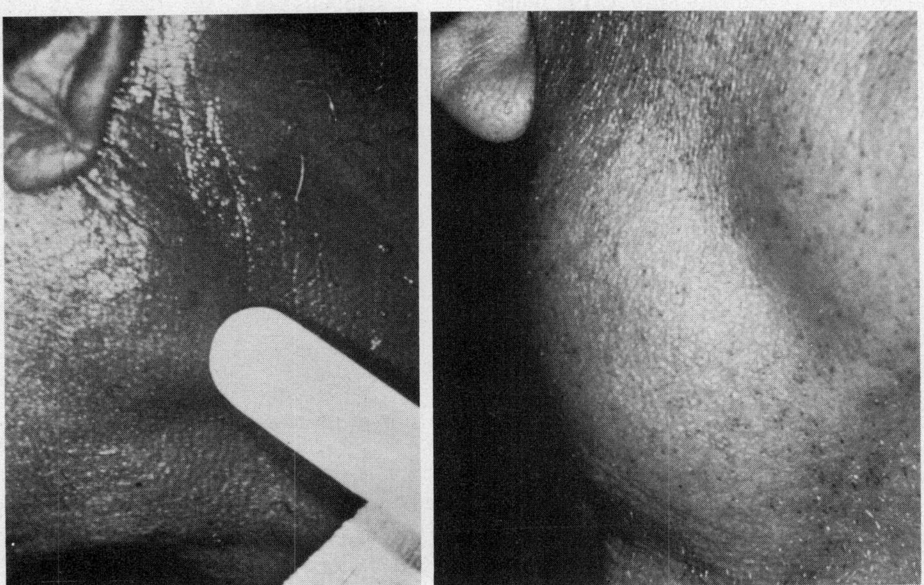

Figure 17–28. Pleomorphic adenomas of parotid gland.

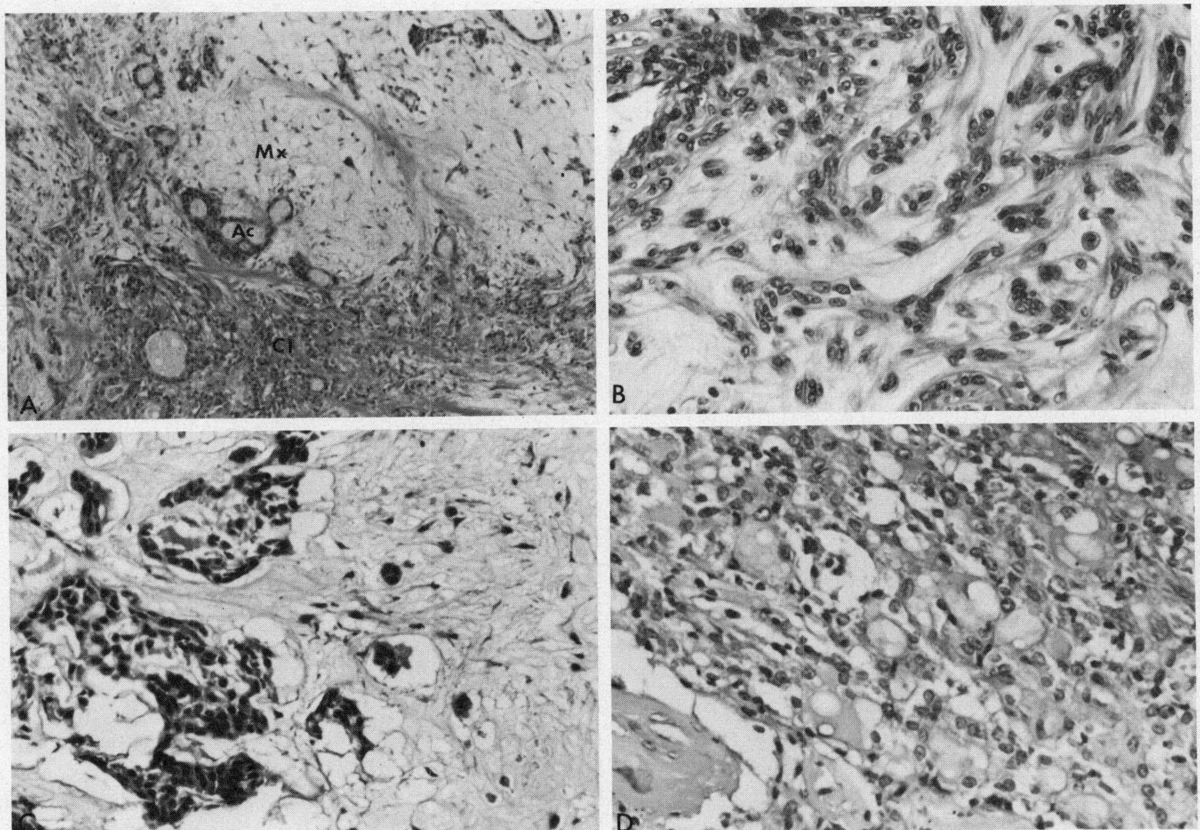

Figure 17–29. *A*, Low-power view of a pleomorphic adenoma showing myxoid (Mx) and cellular (Cl) components. Acinar (Ac) formations are scattered throughout. *B*, Pleomorphic adenoma showing strands of myoepithelial cells. *C*, Pleomorphic adenoma showing myoepithelial cell clusters with deeply staining nuclei and myxoid stroma. *D*, Pleomorphic adenoma showing a glandular secretory pattern and mucoid material.

versial, but current opinion holds that the great preponderance of benign tumors remain benign even when recurrent.

ADENOLYMPHOMA (LYMPHADENOMA). This tumor is composed of cystic or glandular spaces lined by columnar epithelium overlying an abundant lymphoid tissue harboring germinal centers. Although the term adenolymphoma is firmly entrenched, the older terms lymphadenoma, papillary cystadenoma lymphomatosum, or Warthin's tumor may be preferable since they do not suggest that the lymphoid component is malignant. According to current best evidence, these neoplasms are basically of epithelial origin and the lymphoid component is viewed as either a reactive or bystander element. One intriguing hypothesis holds that the epithelial parenchyma is derived from ductal anlagen entrapped during embryogenesis within intra- and periparotid lymph nodes.[94] Newer studies on the lymphoid cells reveal a mixture of B and T cells in a ratio and pattern identical to that in normal or reactive lymph nodes, lending support to the entrapment hypothesis.[95]

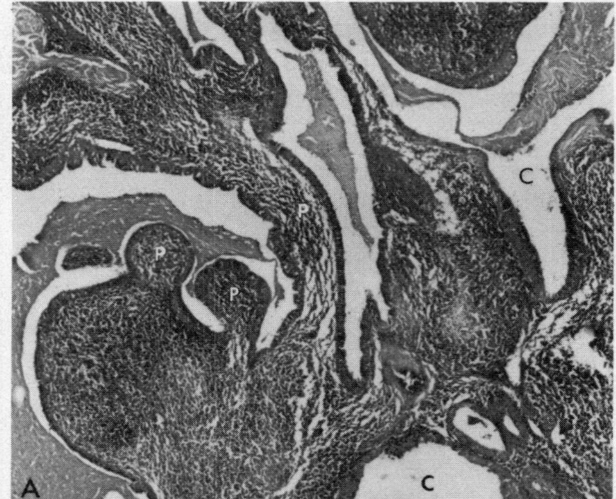

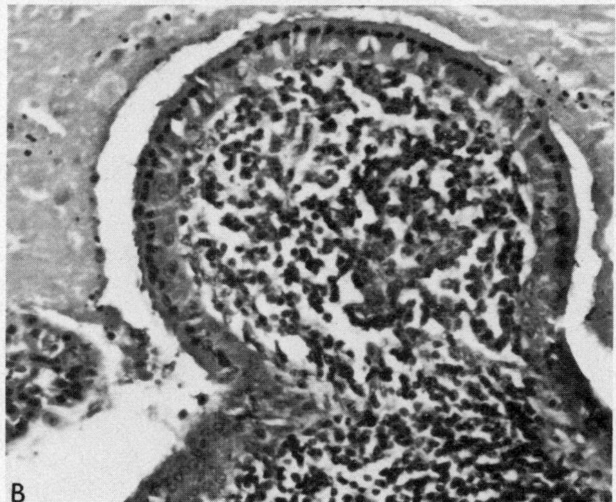

Figure 17–30. *A,* Low-power view of adenolymphoma (Warthin's tumor) showing cystic spaces (C) and papillary projections (P). *B,* High-power view of papillary projection showing double-layered epithelium (best seen to left) and lymphoid tissue in central portion.

Most Warthin's tumors occur in the lower portion of the parotid overlying the angle of the mandible. Infrequently, there are bilateral tumors. The neoplasms are firm, spherical, often coarsely lobulated, encapsulated gray-tan masses, sometimes containing grossly visible clefts or cystic spaces from which a cloudy, serous, or tenacious fluid escapes. Histologically, these cystic or cleftlike spaces are narrowed by many papillary projections and are lined by a double-layered epithelium in which the surface cells are strikingly tall and eosinophilic, while the cells of the underlying layer are polygonal or pyramidal and often not easily identified (Fig. 17–30). The cells with eosinophilic cytoplasm somewhat resemble oxyphilic oncocytes, which often appear in ducts and acini as the cells undergo aging changes. Ultrastructurally, the eosinophilic cytoplasm can be seen to contain large numbers of mitochondria with cristae of unusual conformations as well as crystalloid inclusions. The epithelium is supported by a rich lymphoid tissue, often containing large germinal centers. The lymphoid tissue fills the centers of the coarse, papillary projections that extend into the cystic spaces, sometimes converting them into irregular or stellate cleftlike conformations. Often the cystic spaces contain granular precipitate, sometimes with cholesterol crystal clefts. Occasionally, cyst contents that have extravasated into the lymphoid tissue induce granulomatous reactions, sometimes enclosing needle-shaped cholesterol deposits. **The inflammatory reaction may induce squamous metaplasia of the columnar epithelial cells.**

These neoplasms represent about 5 to 15% of parotid tumors. For unknown reasons they occur preponderantly in males (5:1). Almost all are benign and readily removed by adequate resection. Very rarely (less than 1%) they are malignant.

OTHER ADENOMAS. A variety of monomorphic adenomas have been described, including some composed virtually solely of oxyphils (oxyphilic adenomas), others having lacelike conformations of basal cells (basal cell adenomas), tumors in which the epithelium produces glandular and tubular patterns (tubular adenomas), rare variants in which the myoepithelial cells form tubular and glandular patterns surrounded by hydropically vacuolated myoepithelial cells (clear cell adenoma), and still other variations. All are well described by Thackray and Lucas.[96] These monomorphic adenomas assume importance only insofar as they are recognized as benign neoplasms and differentiated from the more ominous neoplasms, described next.

Malignant

The World Health Organization's classification of salivary gland neoplasms[97] divided the epithelial tumors into benign and malignant categories. Interpolated between them were the mucoepidermoid tumor and acinic cell tumor (see Table 17–1) because some pursue a benign course whereas others recur, invade aggressively, and metastasize. Unfortunately, the biologic behavior is difficult to predict from the histology. It seems best to consider all these tumors as having the potential for malignant behavior, but the ambiguities have led to the terms mucoepidermoid tumor and acinic cell tumor.

MUCOEPIDERMOID TUMOR. These neoplasms are composed of variable mixtures of squamous cells, mucus-secreting cells, and cells having intermediate differentiation. They account for 2 to 7% of all salivary gland neoplasms, occurring preponderantly in the parotids and much less frequently in the submandibular glands. However, they may also arise in minor salivary glands where they represent the second most common form of malignant neoplasm.

Grossly, these present as poorly defined masses that usually are partially but not completely encapsulated. They are not larger than the usual salivary gland neoplasms described. On cross section they may be solid, cystic, or semicystic. The fluid within the cystic spaces ranges from clear, thin mucus to thick, tenacious, turbid secretion. Histologically, the basic pattern is that of cords, sheets, or cystic conformations of squamous, mucous, or intermediate cells. The hybrid cell types often have squamous features in which small-to-large mucus-filled vacuoles are present, best brought out by PAS or mucicarmine stains (Fig. 17–31). The cytology ranges from well-differentiated cells with small regular nuclei to less well-differentiated cells with variably sized nuclei, hyperchromatism, and occasional mitotic figures. The squamous elements may show intercellular bridges, or areas of keratin pearl formation. A common pattern is one in which well-defined squamous cells about the periphery of a nest of cells merge imperceptibly into well-defined mucus-secreting cells within the center of the nest. The intermediate zone contains the expected transitional forms. The fibrous connective tissue stroma enclosing these epithelial elements is nondistinctive.

The difficulty in judging the clinical behavior of an individual neoplasm from the degree of differentiation of the epithelial cells has already been pointed out. Nonetheless, in a large series of cases there is some concordance between the clinical course and the histologic appearance of the tumor.[98] In general, the less aggressive neoplasms, representing about 40% of all cases, have a preponderance of mucus-secreting cells with well-defined cyst formations. It must be emphasized that even these better differentiated lesions may metastasize. Poorly differentiated tumors are generally solid and consist preponderantly of epidermoid and intermediate cells, which exhibit nuclear pleomorphism and mitoses. Often there is infiltration through the tumor capsule with lymphatic and perineurial invasion. Such features are clearly suggestive of a worse prognosis.

ACINIC CELL TUMOR. This uncommon tumor gets its name from the fact that histologically it is composed of cells similar to those making up the serous acinar cells of the parotid gland. It occurs most commonly in the parotids, although it may also arise in the submandibular or minor salivary glands.[99] Despite the similarity of the tumor cells to serous acinar cells, the origin of these neoplasms is now thought to be multipotential intercalated duct cells.[100]

The gross morphology of these lesions is indistinguishable from that of many pleomorphic adenomas. They are usually well encapsulated and sometimes contain areas of necrosis or hemorrhage.

Microscopically the acinic cells are generally disposed in glandular patterns, sometimes producing a remarkable resemblance to the normal parotid architecture. At other times the groupings take the forms of solid cords or diffuse sheets. Occasionally there are microcystic spaces into which papillary fronds project. The individual cells may be polyhedral or rounded with small, regular nuclei and basophilic granular cytoplasm—features found in normal acinar cells. The granules are PAS positive and ultrastructurally are characteristic of secretory granules. Secretion may accumulate within the cytoplasm to produce small-to-large vacuoles, sometimes with virtual clearing of the cytoplasm (Fig. 17–32). Mitoses are generally infrequent, but in more aggressive lesions there may be some loss of differentiation. In some neoplasms there is a prominent stromal lymphoid infiltrate.

Overall, the prognosis after resection of these tumors is good, and five-year survival rates of 70 to 85%

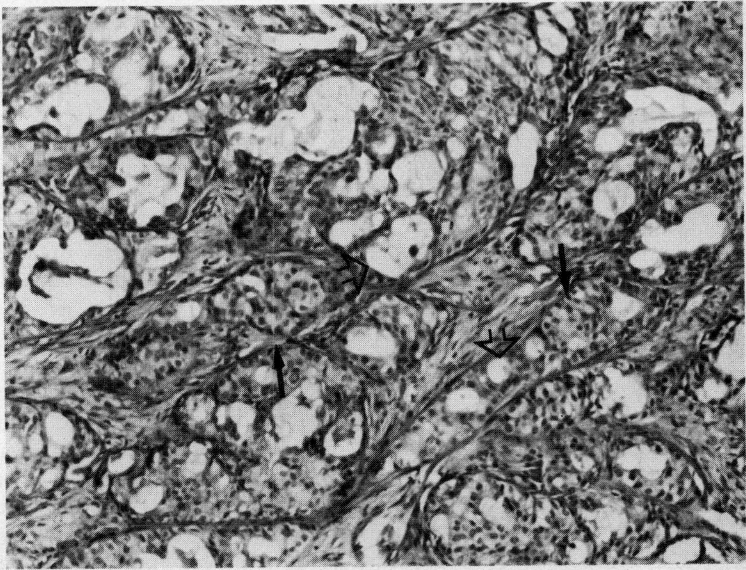

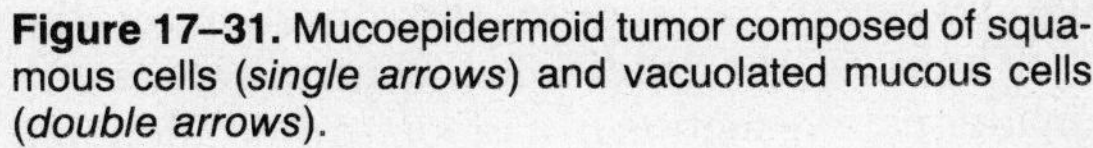

Figure 17–31. Mucoepidermoid tumor composed of squamous cells (*single arrows*) and vacuolated mucous cells (*double arrows*).

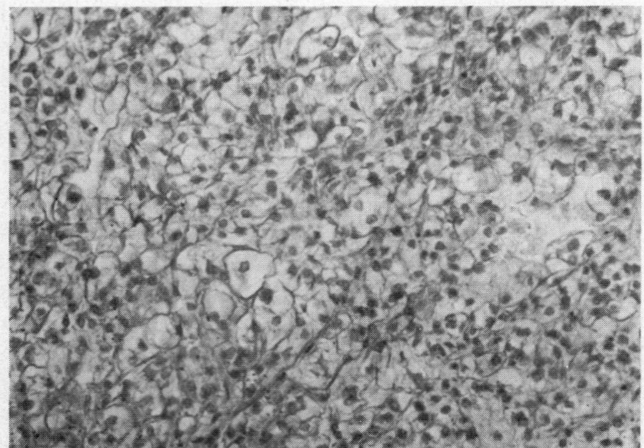

Figure 17–32. Acinic cell carcinoma composed almost entirely of clear cells.

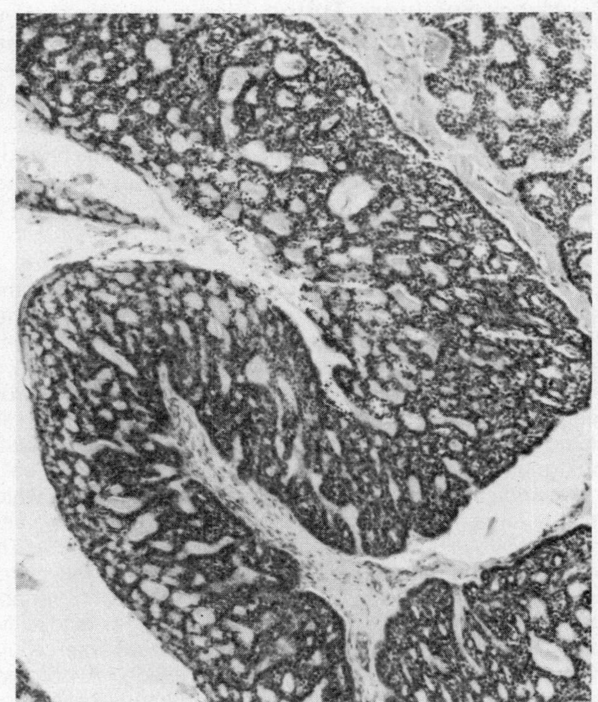

Figure 17–33. Adenoid cystic carcinoma of salivary glands showing cribriform pattern.

have been achieved. However, late recurrences and metastases lower the cure rate to approximately 65% at 10 years and 45% at 15 years.[101]

Adenoid Cystic Carcinoma. These clearly malignant neoplasms of salivary glands are also known as cylindromas. They arise most frequently in the parotids. In the submandibular glands they represent a higher proportion of all neoplasms (approximately 20%). They are also the most common malignant tumor of minor salivary glands, with a particular predilection for those of the palate.

Grossly, these are obviously infiltrative lesions that invade the surrounding glandular substance and sometimes the overlying skin. Rarely, they ulcerate through the skin. The cut surface is typically gray-white and firm.

Histologically, there is a wide range of patterns that can best be characterized as tubular, cribriform, or solid.[102] These architectural patterns are made up of either duct-lining secretory cells or possibly myoepithelial cells. The tubular lesion exhibits numerous branching and anastomosing tubules, often having a double layer of lining epithelial cells. The cribriform pattern is most distinctive of adenoid cystic carcinoma, appearing as lacelike reticulated strands of cells, sometimes completely or incompletely encircling cystic spaces filled with a granular or stringy precipitated secretion (Fig. 17–33). Occasionally, broad sheets of cells are perforated by closely packed glandular or microcystic spaces. Both the microcystic spaces and the region directly adjacent to the cribriform nests may contain strikingly hyalinized eosinophilic material that corresponds ultrastructurally and histochemically to reduplicated basement membrane. The third histologic variant, referred to as solid, is least common and consists of masses and sheets of small compact cells.

As locally invasive lesions, these tumors infiltrate the surrounding normal gland substance and classically extend into perineurial spaces. Metastases may occur to regional lymph nodes and sometimes even more widely to viscera, but aggressive local extension is more characteristic of these cancers. Thus, involvement of the facial nerve sometimes occurs, rendering resection of the tumor difficult. The prognosis is best for the tubular pattern, worst for the solid pattern, and intermediate with the cribriform lesions. Of patients who eventually died of their neoplasms, those having tubular lesions had an average survival of nine years, whereas those with solid tumors survived for an average of five years.

Carcinoma in Pleomorphic Adenoma. From 2 to 10 per cent of pleomorphic adenomas (with an average figure in reported data of approximately 5%) are cancerous and so are called *malignant mixed salivary gland tumors*. Often, residual benign pleomorphic adenoma can be found in or about the carcinomatous lesion. There is considerable controversy over the interpretation of such findings. In some instances there is a long history of a salivary gland mass that, following resection, is discovered to be a malignant tumor. Implied is the existence of a pleomorphic adenoma that in time was transformed into a cancer. Thus, some experts believe that few carcinomas would arise if benign adenomas were adequately removed soon after they appeared.[103] On the other hand, some believe that these lesions begin in chance latent foci of in situ change in preexisting benign lesions unrelated to the duration of the disease.[104] There is the additional controversy as to whether inadequate resection of a pleomorphic adenoma followed by recurrence predisposes to malignant transformation. But the preponderant view is that benign pleomorphic adenomas remain benign when the confounding variable of duration is taken into account. Resolution of these issues cannot be achieved at present, but about all that can be said with certainty is that many patients with malignant mixed tumors have a short duration of symptoms and are younger in age than those with a pleomorphic adenoma. Both features suggest that, at least in some instances, these neoplasms are malignant from the outset. Generally, the malignant focus consists of poorly differentiated adenocarcinoma, although a cylindromatous pattern similar to that of adenoid cystic lesions may be encountered. As carcinomas, they are frequently recurrent following local resection, and about one-third of patients die from local or distant spread of the tumor within five years.

Other Carcinomas of Salivary Glands. *Little need be said about adenocarcinomas, epidermoid carcinomas, and undifferentiated carcinomas since all are extremely rare and their histologic characteristics are those expected according to their designations.* In addition, cancers of extrasalivary origin may also metastasize to the parotid gland, in particular cutaneous squamous cell carcinoma and malignant melanoma on the face. For details on these rarities, reference may be made to the review by Thackray and Lucas.[96]

Staging of Salivary Gland Cancers. On the basis of a comprehensive retrospective study of 861 patients, a clinical staging system has been proposed. It is based on the TNM system and so incorporates the following features: (1) size and local extension of the primary tumor (T), (2) palpability and suspicion of regional lymph nodes (N), and (3) presence or absence of distant metastases (M).[105]

NECROTIZING SIALOMETAPLASIA

Necrotizing sialometaplasia is a benign condition involving the palate that clinically, and often histologically, may resemble a malignant neoplasm.[106, 107] Clinically, the lesion may present as a unilateral or bilateral nonhealing ulceration of the palate. Histologically, there is necrosis of mucous gland acini and replacement by connective tissue and granulation tissue. A notable squamous metaplasia of ducts and mucous acini presents an appearance suggestive of an invasive oral cancer or mucoepidermoid tumor. Careful analysis of cellular detail and overall pattern are necessary for a correct diagnosis. The etiology of necrotizing sialometaplasia is not clear, but localized infarction has been suggested,[108] followed by unusual glandular activity. Infection may play an additional role.

1. Gibbons, R. J., and van Houte, J.: Bacterial adherence in oral microbial ecology. Annu. Rev. Microbiol. *29*:19, 1975.
2. Orland, F. J., et al.: Use of the germfree animal technic in the study of experimental dental caries. I. Basic observations on rats reared free of all microorganisms. J. Dent. Res. *33*:147, 1954.
3. Gustafsson, B. E., et al.: Vipehölm dental caries study; the effect of different levels of carbohydrate intake on caries activity in 436 individuals observed for 5 years. Acta Odontol. Scand. *11*:232, 1954.
4. Kapur, K., et al.: The response of human dental pulp to various physical and chemical agents; a correlated clinical and histopathologic study. Oral Surg. *17*:640, 1964.
5. Löe, H., et al.: Experimental gingivitis in man. J. Periodontol. *36*:177, 1965.
6. Carranza, F. A.: Glickman's Clinical Periodontology. 5th ed. Philadelphia, W. B. Saunders Co., 1979, pp. 201–207.
7. Znamensky, N. N.: Alveolar pyorrhoea—its pathologic anatomy and its radical treatment. J. Br. Dent. Assoc. *23*:585, 1902.
8. Glickman, I., et al.: The systemic influence upon bone in periodontoclasia. J. Am. Dent. Assoc. *31*:1435, 1944.
9. Shklar, G.: Systemic influences in the etiology of periodontal disease—animal models. J. Periodontol. *45*:567, 1974.
10. Goldhaber, P. S., and Giddon, D. B.: Present concepts concerning the etiology and treatment of acute necrotizing gingivitis. Int. Dent. J. *14*:468, 1964.
11. Meyer, I., and Shklar, G.: The oral manifestations of acquired syphilis. Oral Surg. *23*:45, 1967.
12. Shklar, G.: Oral reflections of infectious diseases. I. Viral infections. Postgrad. Med. *49*:87, 1971.
13. Silverman, S., and Beumer, J.: Primary herpetic gingivostomatitis of adult onset. Oral Surg. *36*:496, 1973.
14. Zahorsky, J.: Herpangina, a specific infectious disease. Arch. Pediatr. *41*:181, 1924.
15. Lennett, E. H., and Magoffin, R. L.: Virologic and immunologic aspects of major oral ulcerations. J. Am. Dent. Assoc. *87*:1055, 1973.
16. Magoffin, R. L., et al.: Vesicular stomatitis and exanthem: A syndrome associated with Coxsackie virus type A16. J.A.M.A. *175*:441, 1961.
17. Ship, I. I.: Epidemiologic aspects of recurrent aphthous ulcerations. Oral Surg. *33*:400, 1972.
18. Sircus, W., et al.: Recurrent aphthous ulcerations of the mouth: A study of the natural history, etiology and treatment. Q. J. Med. *26*:235, 1957.
19. Dolby, A. E.: Recurrent aphthous ulcerations. Effect of sera and peripheral blood lymphocytes upon oral epithelial tissue culture cells. Immunology *17*:709, 1969.
20. Lehner, T.: Immunologic aspects of recurrent oral ulcers. Oral Surg. *33*:80, 1972.
21. Lehner, T.: Pathology of recurrent oral ulceration and oral ulceration in Behçet's syndrome: light, electron and fluorescence microscopy. J. Pathol. *97*:481, 1969.
22. Stanley, H. R.: Aphthous lesions. Oral Surg. *33*:407, 1972.
23. Behçet, H.: Ueber rezidivierende, apthose, durch ein Virus verursachte Geschwure am Mund, am Auge und an den Genitalien, Dermatol. Wochenschr. *105*:1152, 1937.
24. Francis, T. C.: Recurrent aphthous stomatitis and Behçet's disease. A review. Oral Surg. *30*:476, 1970.
25. Shklar, G.: Erosive and bullous oral lesions of lichen planus; histologic studies. Arch. Dermatol. *97*:411, 1968.
26. Waldron, C. A., and Shafer, W. G.: Leukoplakia revisited: A clinicopathologic study of 3,256 oral leukoplakias. Cancer *36*:1386, 1975.
27. Pindborg, J. J., et al.: Role of smoking in floor of the mouth leukoplakia. J. Oral Pathol. *1*:22, 1972.
28. Shklar, G., and Cataldo, E.: Histopathology and cytology of oral lesions of pemphigus. Arch. Dermatol. *101*:635, 1970.
29. Hashimoto, K.: Electron microscopy and histochemistry of pemphigus and pemphigoid. Oral Surg. *33*:206, 1972.
30. Shklar, G., and McCarthy, P. L.: Oral lesions of mucous membrane pemphigoid: A study of 85 cases. Arch. Otolaryngol. *93*:354, 1971.
31. Susi, F. R., and Shklar, G.: Histochemistry and fine structure of oral lesions of mucous membrane pemphigoid. Arch. Dermatol. *104*:244, 1971.
32. Dabelsteen, E., et al.: Demonstration of basement membrane autoantibodies in patients with benign mucous membrane pemphigoid. Acta Derm. Venereol. (Stockh.) *54*:189, 1974.
33. Giunta, J., and Zablotsky, N.: Allergic stomatitis caused by self-polymerizing resin. Oral Surg. *41*:631, 1976.
34. Stevens, A. M., and Johnson, F. C.: Eruptive fever with stomatitis and ophthalmia. Am. J. Dis. Child. *24*:526, 1922.
35. Shklar, G.: Oral lesions of erythema multiforme. Histologic and histochemical observations. Arch. Dermatol. *92*:495, 1965.
36. Cataldo, E., and Mosadomi, A.: Mucoceles of the oral mucous membrane. Arch. Otolaryngol. *91*:360, 1970.
37. Standish, S. M., and Shafer, W. G.: The mucous retention phenomenon. J. Oral Surg. *17*:15, 1959.
38. Meyer, I.: Dermoid cysts (dermoids) of the floor of the mouth. Oral Surg. *8*:1149, 1955.
39. Shklar, G., and Meyer, I.: Vascular tumors of the mouth and jaws. Oral Surg. *19*:335, 1965.
40. Bhaskar, S. N., and Jacoway, J. R.: Pyogenic granuloma—clinical features, incidence, histology and result of treatment: Report of 242 cases. J. Oral Surg. *24*:391, 1966.
41. Cooke, B. E. D.: The giant cell epulis: histogenesis and natural history. Br. Dent. J. *93*:13, 1952.
42. Giansanti, J. S., and Waldron, C. A.: Peripheral giant cell granuloma: Review of 720 cases. J. Oral Surg. *27*:787, 1969.
43. Giunta, J., et al.: Diffuse angiomatosis of the tongue. Arch. Otolaryngol. *93*:83, 1971.
44. Aparicio, S. R., and Lumsden, C. E.: Light- and electron-microscope studies on the granular cell myoblastoma of the tongue. J. Pathol. *97*:339, 1969.
45. Fust, J. A., and Custer, R. P.: On the neurogenesis of so-called granular cell myoblastoma. Am. J. Clin. Pathol. *19*:522, 1949.

46. Bhaskar, S. N., and Akamine, R.: Congenital epulis (congenital granular cell fibroblastoma). Oral Surg. *8*:517, 1955.
47. Bruce, K. W., and McDonald, J. R.: Chondroma of the tongue. Oral Surg. *6*:1281, 1953.
48. Cataldo, E., et al.: Osteoma of the tongue. Arch. Otolaryngol. *85*:202, 1967.
49. Krolls, S. O., and Hoffman, S.: Squamous cell carcinoma of the oral soft tissues: A statistical analysis of 14,253 cases by age, sex and race of patients. J. Am. Dent. Assoc. *92*:571, 1976.
49A. Keller, A. Z.: Alcohol, tobacco and age factors in the relative frequency of cancer among males with and without liver cirrhosis. Am. J. Epidemiol. *106*:194, 1977.
49B. Graham, S., et al.: Dentition, diet, tobacco, and alcohol in the epidemiology of oral cancer. J. Natl. Cancer Inst. *59*:1611, 1977.
50. Giunta, J., et al.: Accuracy of biopsy in the diagnosis of oral cancer. Oral Surg. *28*:552, 1969.
51. Shklar, G., et al.: Reliability of cytologic smear in the diagnosis of oral cancer: A controlled study. Arch. Otolaryngol. *91*:158, 1970.
52. Chaudhry, A. P., et al.: Intraoral minor salivary gland tumors. An analysis of 1,414 cases. Oral Surg. *14*:1194, 1961.
53. Frable, W. J., and Elzay, R. P.: Tumors of minor salivary glands. A report of 73 cases. Cancer *25*:932, 1970.
54. Luna, M. A., et al.: Minor salivary gland tumors of the oral cavity. A review of sixty-eight cases. Oral Surg. *25*:71, 1968.
55. Chaudhry, A. P., et al.: Primary malignant melanoma of the oral cavity. A review of 105 cases. Cancer *11*:923, 1958.
56. Shklar, G., and McCarthy, P. L.: The Oral Manifestations of Systemic Disease. Boston, Butterworth's, 1976.
57. Afonsky, D.: Oral lesions in niacin, riboflavin, pyridoxine, pantothenic acid and folic acid deficiencies in adult dogs. Oral Surg. *8*:207, 313, and 867, 1955.
58. Jeghers, H., et al.: Generalized intestinal polyposis and melanin spots of the oral mucosa, lips and digits. A syndrome of diagnostic significance. N. Engl. J. Med. *241*:993 and 1031, 1949.
59. Giunta, J. L.: Raynaud disease with oral manifestations. Arch. Dermatol. *111*:78, 1975.
60. Eisenbud, L., et al.: Oral manifestations in Crohn's disease. Oral Surg. *34*:770, 1972.
61. McCarthy, P. L., and Shklar, G.: A syndrome of pyostomatitis vegetans and ulcerative colitis. Arch. Dermatol. *88*:281, 1963.
62. Weathers, D. R., and Driscoll, R. M.: Darier's disease of the oral mucosa: Report of five cases. Oral Surg. *37*:711, 1974.
63. Gorlin, R. J., et al.: Odontogenic tumors. Classification, histopathology and clinical behavior in man and domesticated animals. Cancer *14*:73, 1961.
64. Thoma, K. H., and Goldman, H. M.: Odontogenic tumors. A classification based on observations of the epithelial, mesenchymal and mixed varieties. Am. J. Pathol. *22*:433, 1946.
65. Pindborg, J. J.: Calcifying epithelial odontogenic tumor. Cancer *11*:838, 1958.
66. Robinson, H. B. G.: Histologic study of the ameloblastoma. Arch. Pathol. *23*:664, 1937.
67. Abrams, A. M., et al.: Adenoameloblastoma. A clinical pathologic study of ten new cases. Cancer *22*:175, 1968.
68. Bhaskar, S. N.: Adenoameloblastoma; its histogenesis and report of 15 new cases. J. Oral Surg. *22*:218, 1964.
69. Giansanti, J. S., et al.: Odontogenic adenomatoid tumor (adenoameloblastoma). Survey of 111 cases. Oral Surg. *30*:69, 1970.
70. Shafer, W. G., and Frissel, C. T.: The melanoameloblastoma and retinal anlage tumors. Cancer *6*:360, 1953.
71. Borello, E. D., and Gorlin, R. J.: Melanotic neuroectodermal tumor of infancy; a neoplasm of neural crest origin. Cancer *19*:196, 1966.
72. Waldron, C. A., and Shafer, W. C.: The central giant cell reparative granuloma of the jaws. An analysis of 38 cases. Am. J. Clin. Pathol. *45*:437, 1966.
73. Garrington, G. E., et al.: Osteosarcoma of the jaws. Cancer *20*:377, 1967.
74. Steg, R. F., et al.: Malignant lymphoma of mandible and maxillary region. Oral Surg. *12*:128, 1959.
75. Burkitt, D.: A sarcoma involving the jaws in African children. Br. J. Surg. *46*:218, 1958.
76. Bruce, K. W., and Royer, R. Q.: Multiple myeloma occurring in the jaws. A study of 17 cases. Oral Surg. *6*:729, 1953.
77. Clausen, F., and Poulsen, H.: Metastatic carcinoma to the jaws. Arch. Pathol. Microbiol. Scand. *57*:361, 1963.
78. Meyer, I., and Shklar, G.: Malignant tumors metastatic to mouth and jaws. Oral Surg. *20*:350, 1965.
79. Glickman, I.: Fibrous dysplasia in alveolar bone. Oral Surg. *1*:895, 1948.
80. Tillman, H. H.: Paget's disease of bone; a clinical, radiological and histopathological study of twenty-four cases involving the jaws. Oral Surg. *15*:1225, 1962.
81. Shklar, G., et al.: Oral lesions of eosinophilic granuloma; histologic and clinical considerations. Oral Surg. *19*:613, 1965.
82. Bertram, U.: Xerostomia. Clinical aspects, pathology and pathogenesis. Acta Odontol. Scand. 25(Suppl. 49):1967.
83. Shearn, M. A.: Sjögren's syndrome. Med. Clin. North Am. *61*:271, 1977.
84. Buxton, R. W., et al.: Surgical treatment of epithelial tumors of the parotid gland. Surg. Gynecol. Obstet. *97*:401, 1953.
85. Foote, F. W., and Frazell, E. L.: Tumors of the major salivary glands. Cancer *6*:1065, 1953.
86. Morgan, M. N., and Mackenzie, D. H.: Tumours of salivary glands. A review of 204 cases with 5-year follow-up. Br. J. Surg. *55*:284, 1968.
87. Nussbaum, M., et al.: Parotid space tumors of non-salivary origin. Ann. Surg. *183*:10, 1976.
88. Eneroth, C. M.: Salivary gland tumors in the parotid gland, submandibular gland and the palate region. Cancer *17*:1415, 1971.
89. Skolnick, E. M., et al.: Tumors of the major salivary glands. Laryngoscope. *87*:843, 1977.
90. Dardick, I., et al.: Histiogenesis of salivary gland pleomorphic adenoma (mixed tumor) with an evaluation of the role of the myoepithelial cells. Hum. Pathol. *13*:62, 1982.
91. Ryan, R. E., et al.: Cellular mixed tumors of the salivary glands. Arch. Otolaryngol. *104*:451, 1978.
92. Lomax-Smith, J. D., and Azzopardi, J. G.: The hyaline cell: A distinctive feature of "mixed" salivary tumours. Histopathology *2*:77, 1978.
93. Lucas, R. B.: Pathology of Tumours of Oral Tissue. 3rd ed. Edinburgh, Churchill Livingstone, 1976.
94. Thompson, A. S., and Bryant, H. C., Jr.: Histiogenesis of papillary cystadenoma lymphomatosum (Warthin's tumor) of the parotid salivary gland. Am. J. Pathol. *26*:807, 1950.
95. Diamond, L. W., and Braylen, R. C.: Cell surface markers on lymphoid cells from Warthin's tumors. Cancer *44*:580, 1979.
96. Thackray, A. C., and Lucas, R. B.: Tumors of the Major Salivary Glands. Fascicle 10, Atlas of Tumor Pathology, Second Series. Washington, D.C., Armed Forces Institute of Pathology, 1974.
97. Thackray, A. C., and Sobin, L. H.: Histological typing of salivary gland tumors. Geneva, WHO International Histologic Classification of Tumors, No. 7, 1972.
98. Spiro, R. H., et al.: Mucoepidermoid carcinoma of salivary gland origin. A clinicopathologic study of 367 cases. Am. J. Surg. *136*:461, 1978.
99. Chen, S. Y., et al.: Acinic cell adenocarcinoma of minor salivary glands. Cancer *42*:678, 1978.
100. Abrams, A. M., et al.: Acinic cell adenocarcinoma of the major salivary glands. A clinicopathologic study of 77 cases. Cancer *18*:1145, 1965.
101. Perzin, H. K., and LiVolsi, V. A.: Acinic cell carcinoma arising in salivary glands. A clinicopathologic study. Cancer *44*:1434, 1979.
102. Perzin, K. H., et al.: Adenoid cystic carcinomas arising in salivary glands: A correlation of histologic features and clinical course. Cancer *42*:265, 1978.
103. Spiro, R. H., et al.: Malignant mixed tumor of salivary origin. A clinicopathologic study of 146 cases. Cancer *39*:388, 1977.
104. LiVolsi, V. A., and Perzin, K. H.: Malignant mixed tumors arising in salivary glands. I. Carcinomas arising in benign mixed tumors: A clinicopathologic study. Cancer *39*:2209, 1977.
105. Levitt, S. H., et al.: Clinical staging system for cancer of the salivary gland. Cancer *47*:2712, 1981.
106. Abrams, A. M., et al.: Necrotizing sialometaplasia: A disease simulating malignancy. Cancer *32*:130, 1973.
107. Fechner, R. E.: Necrotizing sialometaplasia: A source of confusion with carcinoma of the palate. Am. J. Clin. Pathol. *67*:315, 1977.
108. Dunley, R. E., and Jacoway, J. R.: Necrotizing sialometaplasia. Oral Surg. *47*:169, 1979.

THE GASTROINTESTINAL TRACT 18

Esophagus

NORMAL

An awareness of certain features of the normal structure and function of the esophagus is helpful to an understanding of its diseases, but there are still gaps in our knowledge. This muscular tube, which connects the pharynx to the stomach, is lined by stratified squamous epithelium; has a well-developed submucosa, a muscularis of striated muscle in the upper third, and smooth muscle in the lower two-thirds; and lacks a serosa. The absence of a serosa and the inadequacy of its own blood supply facilitate the spread of infection and render surgery difficult. The transition between the squamous epithelium of the esophagus and the glandular mucosa of the stomach is quite abrupt in most normal individuals and takes the form of interdigitating tongues of the two types of epithelia. Occasionally, isolated islands or significant sections of the lower esophagus are lined by columnar secretory epithelium. Whether such changes are congenital malformations or acquired alterations will be discussed later. The esophagus narrows slightly at three levels—the cricoid cartilage, the bifurcation of the trachea, and the diaphragmatic hiatus—creating three loci vulnerable to trauma, abnormal dilatation, and perforation by foreign bodies. Motor studies indicate that there is an upper esophageal sphincter at about the level of the fifth to sixth cervical bodies and a lower esophageal sphincter (also marked by subtle specialized morphologic features), which lies below the diaphragm in the abdomen and guards against reflux of stomach contents into the esophagus.

The functions of the esophagus, as is well-known, are to conduct food and fluids from the pharynx to the stomach and to prevent reflux of gastric contents into the esophagus. These functions require coordinated motor activity, namely, a wave of peristaltic contraction in response to swallowing or esophageal distention; relaxation of the lower esophageal sphincter in anticipation of the peristaltic wave; and closure of the lower esophageal sphincter after the swallowing reflex. The mechanisms governing this motor function are surprisingly complex and still imperfectly understood. It suffices for our purposes that they involve both extrinsic and intrinsic innervation, myogenic properties, and circulating humoral substances.[1] On swallowing, neural impulses are initiated in the dorsal vagal nuclei and are transmitted through the vagus nerve to the intrinsic myenteric (Auerbach's) plexus situated in the muscularis of both the striated and smooth muscle portions of the esophagus. The plexus comprises nests of ganglion cells from which postsynaptic fibers are distributed to the muscle cells. Distention of the esophagus may also initiate peristalsis through stretch receptors in the muscle fibers. The esophagus also contains receptors for many neurohumoral substances, and so the amplitude of peristalsis in the smooth muscle portion of the esophagus is augmented by cholinergic stimulation, alpha-adrenergic drugs, and histamine. Conversely, anticholinergic drugs reduce the amplitude of peristalsis in the smooth muscle of the esophagus but do not affect the orderly propagation of the wave of contraction.

The control of lower esophageal sphincter (LES) function is poorly understood. LES relaxation in anticipation of a peristaltic wave may be mediated by adenosine triphosphate or vasoactive intestinal peptide, but is dependent on one intact vagal trunk to the esophageal plexus. Maintenance of sphincteric closure of the LES is necessary to prevent reflux of gastric contents, which, relative to the esophagus, are under positive pressure. Many substances increase LES tone, e.g., gastrin, acetylcholine, serotonin, prostaglandin $F_{2\alpha}$, motilin, substance P, histamine, and pancreatic polypeptide. Which of these agents are of importance in the normal physiologic function of the LES is uncertain, but at present gastrin is accorded only a minimal role.[2] The rather banal anatomy of the esophagus and the LEF belies their complex physiology.

PATHOLOGY

Lesions of the esophagus run the gamut from highly fatal cancers to less life-threatening, but nonetheless disabling, neuromuscular disturbances, inflammations, and vascular abnormalities. Because they are lethal, carcinomas of the esophagus are the most important disorders of this level of the gut, making up about 10% of all cancers of the alimentary tract. Second in importance are esophageal varices, which are mostly associated with portal hypertension and cirrhosis. Their rupture is frequently followed by massive hematemesis (vomiting of blood) and exsanguination. Other lesions such as achalasia, webs, esophagitis, and hiatus hernias are more frequent but less threatening to life. Distressing to the gastroenterologist is the fact that all disorders of the esophagus tend to produce similar symptoms. Dysphagia (subjective difficulty in swallowing) and "heartburn" are major symptoms of all forms of esophageal pathology. Pain and hematemesis are sometimes evoked, particularly by those lesions associated with ulceroinflammatory changes in the esophageal wall. The clinical differential diagnosis of disorders of the esophagus is difficult and often requires specialized procedures such as cineradiography, manometry, and esophagoscopy.

CONGENITAL ANOMALIES

Developmental defects in the esophagus are uncommon. Because they cause immediate regurgitation when feeding is attempted, they are usually discovered soon after birth. They must be corrected early, since they are incompatible with life.

ATRESIA AND FISTULAS

Absence (agenesis) of the esophagus is extremely rare and may affect the entire length or only a portion of it. Much more common are atresia and fistula formation. In embryologic development, *the gut and respiratory tract begin as a single tube; thus, it is no surprise that developmental anomalies may affect and interconnect both tracts.* In atresia, a segment of the esophagus is represented by only a thin, noncanalized cord with the resultant formation of an upper blind pouch connecting with the pharynx and a lower pouch leading to the stomach. Most commonly, the atresia is located at or near the tracheal bifurcation. *In about 80 to 90% of cases, the lower pouch communicates through a fistulous tract with the trachea or main stem bronchi.* Much less commonly, a fistulous communication exists between the blind upper esophageal pouch and the respiratory tree.

Excessive salivation, vomiting, coughing from regurgitated aspirated mucus, or paroxysmal suffocation from food that passes directly from the upper pouch into the respiratory tree are the prominent clinical manifestations. Even cyanosis and asphyxia may result. When the lower pouch communicates with the respiratory tract, the stomach tends to fill with air. Reconstructive surgery can effect cures, but if the condition is not recognized promptly, death may occur from asphyxia, aspiration pneumonia, and fluid and electrolyte imbalances. Often associated with such anomalies are congenital heart disease and malformations of the small intestine, rectum, and anus.

STENOSIS

Abnormal narrowing of the esophagus with the persistence of a constricted lumen may occur as a developmental defect, or may be an acquired lesion resulting from involvement of the esophagus in scleroderma or inflammatory scarring incident to esophagitis (p. 801). The narrowing may be quite limited or may involve up to 10 cm of the esophagus. When present as a congenital defect, stenosis is manifested by feeding difficulty from birth.

Acquired stenoses usually first become manifest in adult life. The anatomic changes are nonspecific and consist of fibrous thickening of the esophageal wall associated with atrophy of the muscularis. The fibrosis of scleroderma is described on page 191. Secondary to esophagitis, it is generally accompanied by chronic inflammatory infiltrates, principally in the submucosa and periesophageal fibrous tissue. The lining epithelium is usually thin and sometimes ulcerated. The extent and location of such changes depend on the initial disorder giving rise to the fibrotic reaction. In severe acquired stenoses, virtually total obstruction may result.

LESIONS ASSOCIATED WITH MOTOR DYSFUNCTION

Dysphagia is encountered both with derangements in motor function of the esophagus and with diseases that narrow or obstruct the lumen, such as fibrous stenoses or cancerous lesions. True dysphagia can be mimicked by the psychologic disturbance *globus hystericus,* which produces the sensation of uncomfortable fullness or "a lump in the throat" not necessarily associated with swallowing. In this section our attention is directed to four entities that are caused by or induce motor dysfunction of the esophagus: achalasia, esophageal rings and webs, hiatal hernias, and lacerations of the esophagus.

ACHALASIA

This uncommon disorder of esophageal motility is characterized clinically by progressive dysphagia and regurgitation, which usually become manifest in young adulthood but may appear in infancy or childhood. The term *cardiospasm* was once in vogue because the motor dysfunction was thought to arise from abnormal spasm of the lower esophageal sphincter (LES). *The currently used name, achalasia, literally means failure of relaxation, implying a defect in relaxation of the esophageal musculature in advance of the propulsive wave of peristalsis.* Both terms have validity because three functional abnormalities have been identified: (1) aperistalsis, (2) partial or incomplete relaxation of the LES, and (3) increased basal tone of the LES.[3]

The pathogenesis of these motor dysfunctions is still not understood, but they would appear to involve some derangement in the innervation of the esophagus and its lower sphincter. However, the locus of the neural defect is uncertain because anatomic studies have yielded inconstant findings. *Most studies, but not all, reveal a loss of myenteric ganglion cells in the body of the esophagus.*[4] *There is less agreement as to whether the ganglion cells in the lower sphincter are normal, reduced, or absent.* However, abnormalities in the vagus nerve and all the way back to the dorsal motor nucleus in the brain have also been reported, as well as hyperresponsiveness of the lower sphincter to the hormone gastrin.[5] Thus, the locus and nature of the neural derangement is still somewhat unsettled.

The etiology of the neural changes is totally obscure. Arguing against a congenital defect is the fact that the disease usually becomes manifest in young adult life. Nutritional deficiencies or infection with a neurotropic virus have been proposed but without convincing evidence. In only one situation is the etiology of achalasia known, namely, Chagas' disease caused by *Trypanosoma cruzi.* This quite common infection in South America causes destruction of the myenteric plexus. However, in Chagas' disease the esophageal achalasia is frequently accompanied by trypanosomal infection and neural disturbances in other sites leading to megaloureter, megaduodenum, and megacolon. These extraesophageal involvements are not seen in the nontrypanosomal cases of achalasia.

Classically, in the usual sporadic form of achalasia there is progressive dilatation of the esophagus above the level of the lower sphincter. It may become elongated and tortuous and assume a "sigmoid" appearance. The wall of the esophagus may be of normal thickness, thicker than normal owing to hypertrophy of the muscularis, or thinned out by dilatation. The myenteric ganglia are usually absent from the body of the esophagus but may or may not be reduced in number in the region of the lower sphincter. There have been reports of degeneration of the myelin sheaths and breaks in the axons of the intraesophageal ramifications of the vagus nerve, but these changes have been denied by others. The lining of the esophagus may be unaffected, but sometimes ulceroinflammatory lesions with fibrotic thickening are seen just above the lower sphincter. Leukoplakia may appear in the inflammatory regions, and rarely these mucosal thickenings progress to cancer.

The classic clinical symptom of achalasia is progressive dysphagia. Gradual in onset, and at first intermittent and precipitated by emotional stress, the difficulty in swallowing later becomes more persistent and disturbing. Regurgitation of undigested food may occur at night and be aspirated, leading possibly to aspiration pneumonia. The most serious aspect of this condition is the hazard of development of carcinoma of the esophagus, said to occur in 2 to 7% of affected patients. These cancers usually appear at a younger age than in individuals without this disease, sometimes as early as the third decade of life.

ESOPHAGEAL RINGS AND WEBS

Annular narrowings of the esophagus, sometimes comprising circumferential mucosal folds, are uncommon lesions encountered in a variety of clinical circumstances. *Those lesions in the upper esophagus (above the aortic arch) are often designated "webs" to differentiate them from lower esophageal "rings."* Most patients are over the age of 40 years. Webs are generally, although not exclusively, seen in women. In the past, much emphasis was placed on the fact that these women often had a concomitant iron deficiency anemia and sometimes hypochlorhydric chronic gastritis as well. Thus was created the *Plummer-Vinson or Paterson-Kelly syndrome,* being the triad of esophageal web, iron deficiency anemia, and hypochlorhydria. Recent studies indicate, however, that esophageal webs may be seen without an associated anemia and that the concurrence of webs, anemia, and hypochlorhydria is probably coincidental, because chronic gastritis and anemia are by themselves very common in older women.

Lower esophageal (Schatzki's) rings usually occur close to the squamocolumnar junction and are not associated with iron deficiency anemia nor confined to women. The gastroenterologic literature suggests that they are more frequent than pathologic studies would indicate. Undoubtedly, they might be missed by the pathologist, since normal LES tone contributes to their prominence and, once the esophagus is opened, they could virtually disappear. About 15% of patients with this anatomic condition have an accompanying hiatal hernia.

Well-developed esophageal webs appear as smooth mucosal ledges in the opened esophagus. Virtually all lower rings are found in the caudal 5 cm and mostly at the squamocolumnar junction. They rarely protrude into the lumen more than 5 mm and have a thickness of 2 to 4 mm. Histologically, the upper surface is covered by stratified squamous epithelium and the undersurface by columnar gastric-like epithelium. The central core is composed of a vascularized fibrous tissue often containing scattered inflammatory cells.

Dysphagia, usually provoked when an individual bolts solid food, is the main symptom associated with esophageal rings or webs. Pain is infrequent. Often the discomfort is episodic, with long, symptom-free intervals. In some patients, the discomfort progressively worsens with years and is elicited even by soft food; in others, the condition constitutes only a nonprogressive annoyance that persists throughout life.[6]

HIATAL HERNIA

Hiatal hernia is a disorder of the gastroesophageal junction that results in a saclike dilatation of the stomach protruding above the diaphragm.

Two anatomic patterns can be recognized, but only with difficulty because relaxation of tissue tone after death obscures both forms of hiatus hernia. In the first, the esophagus ends above the diaphragm, creating a symmetric, bell-like dilatation of that portion of the stomach within the thoracic cavity. The dilatation is bounded below by the diaphragmatic narrowing. This abnormality may result from a congenitally short esophagus or may be an acquired defect secondary to long-standing fibrous scarring of the esophagus. Whatever the basis, traction on the stomach pulls a portion of it into the thorax. About 90% of all hiatal hernias are of this type.[7] The supradiaphragmatic herniation of the stomach is accentuated by muscular contraction of the esophagus during the act of swallowing, and so this traction pattern is also called a **sliding hernia.**

The second pattern is designated "paraesophageal hiatal hernia." A portion of the cardiac end of the stomach dissects alongside the esophagus through a defect in the diaphragmatic hiatus to produce an intrathoracic sac. It is usually small and is found alongside the normally positioned lower end of the esophagus. Because the stomach rolls up alongside the esophagus, this form is sometimes called a **rolling hernia.** Less than 10% of hiatal hernias are of this type. More extreme forms of paraesophageal hernia are encountered following traumatic rupture of the diaphragm.

It is important to differentiate these two forms; only the paraesophageal is vulnerable to strangulation and infarction.

Enthusiastic roentgenologists report hiatal hernias in 4 to 7% of otherwise normal individuals,[8] over half of whom have no symptoms whatsoever. Only about 9% (usually those with a sliding hernia) suffer from such disturbances as retrosternal burning pain ("heartburn") and sometimes regurgitation of gastric juices into the mouth. These manifestations are attributed to incompetence of the esophagogastric sphincter and are accentuated by positions favoring reflux, e.g., bending forward or lying supine. Such symptoms are more common in elderly, obese women and it is not certain that they are related to the hiatal hernia. It should be cautioned that gastroesophageal reflux or heartburn can occur without a hiatal hernia; conversely, hiatal hernia can be present without these symptoms. Bleeding is sometimes seen but very likely is associated with the development of secondary esophagitis or gastritis.[9]

LACERATIONS (MALLORY-WEISS SYNDROME)

Small tears in the esophagus are fairly uncommon lesions that usually occur as a result of prolonged vomiting. Some are said to occur without antecedent vomiting. These lesions are encountered most commonly, but not exclusively, in chronic alcoholics with a history of hematemesis following a bout of excessive vomiting. Normally, a reflex relaxation of the musculature of the gastrointestinal tract precedes the antiperistaltic wave of contraction. One pathogenetic concept speculates that during episodes of prolonged vomiting, this reflex relaxation fails to occur.[10] The refluxing gastric contents suddenly overwhelm the contraction of the sphincter of the cardia, and massive dilatation and tearing of the esophageal wall ensue at the esophagogastric junction. Since these tears also occur in persons who have no history of vomiting, other mechanisms must exist. Several studies have related these tears to underlying inapparent hiatal hernias. It is postulated that the inadequate diaphragmatic support provides an area of weakness that potentiates abnormal dilatation when subjected to increased intragastric pressure. This view contends that lacerations do not occur in the absence of these hiatal defects.

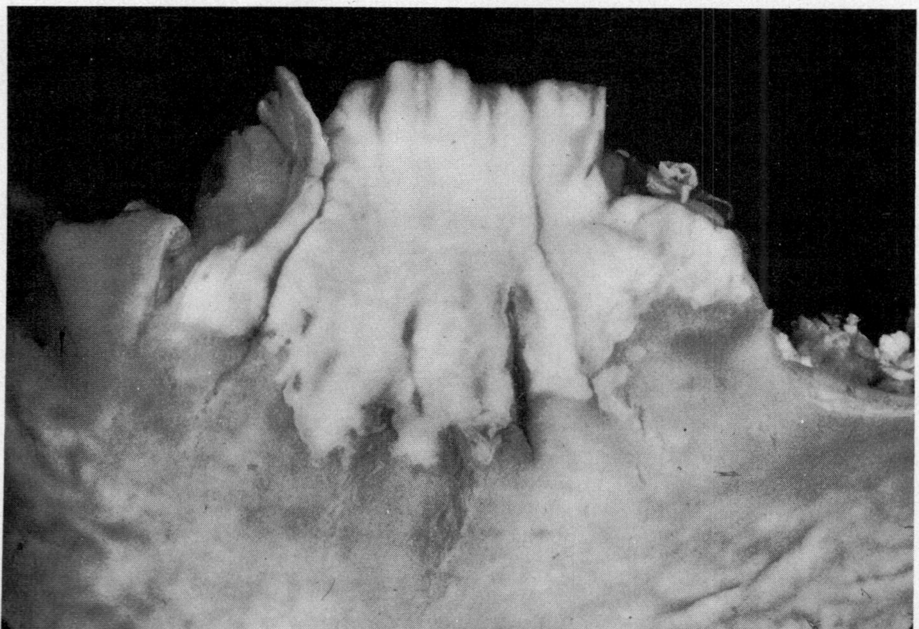

Figure 18–1. Esophageal laceration. Gross view demonstrating a longitudinal laceration extending from esophageal mucosa into stomach mucosa.

The linear irregular lacerations are oriented in the axis of the esophageal lumen and are several millimeters to several centimeters in length. **They usually are found astride the esophagogastric junction or in the proximate gastric mucosa** (Fig. 18–1). The tears may involve only the mucosa or may penetrate deeply enough to perforate the wall.

The histology is not distinctive. The early lesion is a nonspecific traumatic defect accompanied by fresh hemorrhage into the margins of the defect. A nonspecific inflammatory response follows. Infection of the defect may lead to an inflammatory ulcer or to mediastinitis.

Esophageal lacerations account for 5 to 10% of all cases of massive hematemesis, but more often the bleeding is not profuse and ceases without surgical intervention; supportive therapy such as vasoconstrictive medications and transfusions, or sometimes balloon tamponade, are usually all that is required.[11] Clinical evidence suggests that complete healing may occur, since a previous episode may leave no residuals.

INFLAMMATIONS

Inflammatory lesions of the esophagus are relatively common autopsy findings, but only rarely do they cause clinical symptoms. Indeed, in most cases they represent agonal changes appearing within the last days of life, presumably reflecting profound debility and deranged sphincteric control mechanisms at the cardioesophageal junction. Significant inflammation is encountered in a wide variety of clinical circumstances, and may be responsible for disturbing symptoms and even death.

ESOPHAGITIS

The following are the more important circumstances under which inflammations of the esophagus (esophagitis) may appear:

1. Reflux of gastric contents, so-called reflux esophagitis.
2. Prolonged gastric intubation.
3. Ingestion of irritants such as alcohol, corrosive acids or alkalis (in suicide attempts), excessively hot fluids such as tea, and heavy smoking.
4. Uremia.
5. Bacteremia or viremia with direct infection of the esophageal wall or contiguous structures. Herpes simplex virus and cytomegalovirus are the more common offenders.
6. Fungal infections (moniliasis, mucormycosis, aspergillosis) in debilitated patients, in those with an immunologic deficiency or receiving immunosuppressive therapy, and in association with broad-spectrum antibiotic therapy.
7. Radiation.
8. Cytotoxic anticancer therapy, with or without superimposed fungal infection.
9. In association with such systemic desquamative dermatologic conditions as pemphigoid and epidermolysis bullosa.
10. Graft-versus-host disease.

PATHOGENESIS. Among these associations, reflux of gastric contents is the first and foremost cause of esophagitis. The origins of reflux esophagitis are more obscure than the term would imply. Reflux of small amounts of acid-peptic gastric juice is a common event in normal individuals and is not productive of esophagitis. *The development of inflammatory changes in the esophagus is thought to require multiple concurrent influences:*[12] (1) *frequent and protracted reflux is requisite*—thus, incompetence of the lower esophageal sphincter is an important predisposition; (2) *disordered esophageal motility* permits the refluxed gastric contents to remain in contact longer with the esophageal mucosa; (3) *elevated acid-peptic levels of the regurgitated fluid as well as of bile acids and lysolecithin* derived from regurgitated duodenal contents are additional contributing factors.

There are many other origins of esophagitis, as has been indicated. With some, such as intubation, radiation, and direct microbial seeding, the cause of injury is obvious. *Monilial esophagitis* has increased in frequency with the growing use of immunosuppressive, broad-spectrum antibacterial and antineoplastic drugs. The monilial infections are usually encountered in terminally ill patients, who become particularly vulnerable to fungal opportunists. *Exogenous damaging influences* such as smoking and consumption of alcohol and excessively hot fluids may also play causal roles. Esophagitis is more frequent among chronic alcoholics and heavy cigarette smokers. In Northern Iran, where alcohol is not consumed, the drinking of copious quantities of hot tea is suspected; esophagitis was observed in 86% of the population.[13] But often the pathogenesis is obscure, as it is with uremia.

MORPHOLOGY. The anatomic changes depend on the causative agent, and the duration and severity of the exposure. Simple hyperemia may be the only alteration. More severe degrees of injury result in edema and thickening of the wall, sometimes pseudomembrane formation, or areas of superficial necrosis and ulceration. Typically, moniliasis produces large, gray-white inflammatory pseudomembranes or ulcerative lesions teeming with the causative fungus. If the inflammatory process has been severe, fibrosis and stricture formation may follow. Histologically, the reaction depends on the intensity of the injury. Thickening of the epithelium, largely by widening of the basal layer; thinning of the surface layers so that submucosal pegs reach the lumen; and submucosal inflammatory cell infiltrates have been recorded.[14]

In patients with persistent gastroesophageal reflux, the distal esophagus may become lined with columnar secretory epithelium rather than the usual stratified squamous epithelium. In 1957 Barrett referred to this morphologic change as **lower esophagus lined by columnar epithelium**.[15] Although this designation has gained wide acceptance, the entity is more often referred to as **Barrett's esophagus.** The transformed epithelium may be of congenital origin but is more likely an upgrowth of gastric glandular epithelium that, in most instances, undergoes metaplasia. A mosaic of cells appear—surface mucous, goblet, absorptive, mucous, neck, and neuroendocrine—typical of intestinal and gastric mucosa.[16] The significance of Barrett's esophagus lies in the facts that, in addition to indicating reflux, characteristic peptic ulcerations may appear in this columnar-lined esophagus (sometimes leading to fibrosing strictures), and there is an increased risk of cancer. In a survey of 130 cases, there were 12 instances of superimposed adenocarcinoma.[17]

Clinical Course. The clinical manifestations of esophagitis consist principally of dysphagia, retrosternal pain, and sometimes hematemesis or melena.

Esophagitis must be differentiated from agonal or postmortem digestion—*esophagomalacia.* Characteristically, these postmortem lesions produce superficial discolorations or autolysis of the esophageal wall, which are brown-black owing to acid digestion of hemoglobin. A spotted or bizarre maplike pattern, often called "leopard spotting," is produced. The ultimate criterion of the nature of such postmortem lesions is the absence of an inflammatory response.

MISCELLANEOUS LESIONS

DIVERTICULA

Esophageal diverticula comprise usually small (2 to 4 cm) outpouchings of the esophageal wall. In some, the outpouching dissects between the muscle fibers and so is composed principally of mucosa, submucosa, and some investing fibrous tissue; in others, however, the muscularis yields and becomes distended along with the inner layers of the esophageal wall. Diverticula occur in three principal areas: *(1) immediately above the upper esophageal sphincter (Zenker's diverticulum), (2) near the midpoint of the esophagus, and (3) immediately above the lower esophageal sphincter.* Classically it has been taught that lesions in the upper and lower esophagus result from increased intraluminal pressure, creating pulsion diverticula, whereas those occurring in the midesophagus result from the pull of inflammatory adhesions, thus creating traction diverticula (Fig. 18–2). Manometric studies, however, suggest that all are due to yielding of the esophageal wall to increases in intraluminal pressure.

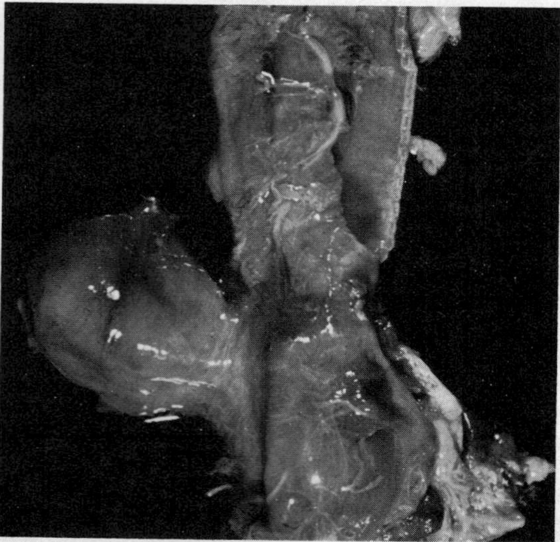

Figure 18–2. Diverticulum of esophagus.

Diverticula may cause no symptoms when they are small and may be discovered only incidentally. However, they may induce dysphagia, regurgitation when overdistended with food, pulmonary aspiration, or a sense of fullness in the neck. Persistent stasis of food may lead to ulcerations and hematemesis. Fortunately, such ulcerations perforate extremely rarely, leading to mediastinitis.

SYSTEMIC SCLEROSIS (SCLERODERMA)

Involvement of the esophagus in the systemic disease scleroderma is usually accompanied by involvement of other levels of the gut and other internal organs also. Because these visceral components exist, scleroderma is now more appropriately termed systemic sclerosis. The major consideration of this disease has already been presented (p. 190). The esophageal and lower intestinal lesions consist of submucosal fibrosis, followed by fibrous overgrowth and atrophy of the smooth musculature. Concomitantly, the overlying mucosa becomes atrophic and sometimes develops large ulcerations. In far-advanced cases, extreme rigidity and narrowing of the esophagus develop. Similar narrowing occurs in the affected small and large bowel. When such visceral lesions develop in the course of scleroderma, the prognosis worsens.

VASCULAR LESIONS

VARICES

Regardless of cause, portal hypertension, when sufficiently prolonged or severe, induces the formation of collateral bypass channels wherever the portal and caval systems interdigitate. The pathogenesis of portal hypertension and the locations of these bypasses are considered in some detail on page 917. Here we are concerned with the bypasses that develop in the region of the lower esophagus when portal flow is diverted through the coronary veins of the stomach into the plexus of esophageal submucosal veins, thence into the azygous veins, and eventually into the systemic circulation. The increase in pressure in the esophageal plexus produces dilated tortuous vessels called varices. *Portal hypertension is most commonly caused by cirrhosis,* although rarely it may be produced by portal vein thrombosis, hepatic vein thrombosis (Budd-Chiari syndrome), pylephlebitis, or *tumorous compression or invasion of the major portal radicles.* Varices occur in approximately two-thirds of all cirrhotic patients and are most often associated with alcoholic cirrhosis, sometimes called fatty nutritional cirrhosis. They are less commonly

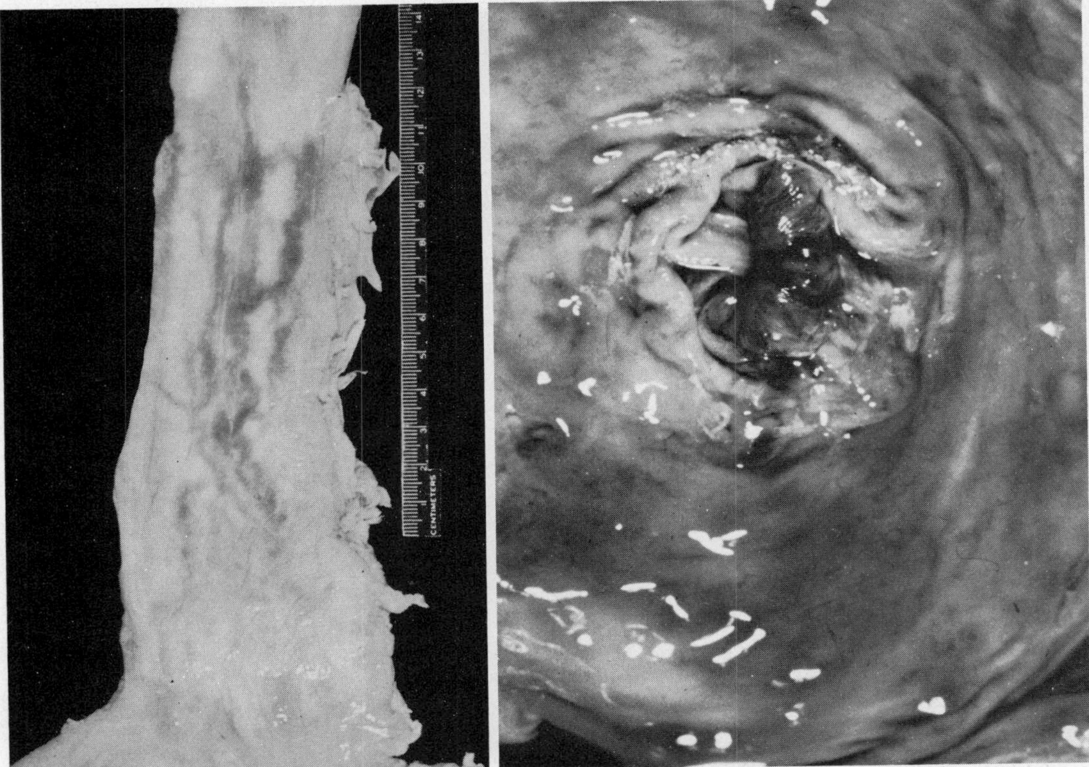

Fig. 18–3

Fig. 18–4

Figure 18–3. Esophageal varices. Gross view demonstrating tortuous dilated submucosal varices in middle and lower thirds of esophagus.
Figure 18–4. Esophageal varices. View from below of unopened cardia showing remarkable similarity between varices of esophagus, as they protrude into stomach, and their rectal counterparts, hemorrhoids.

found in association with pigment cirrhosis and postnecrotic scarring of the liver and are rarely produced by biliary or cardiac cirrhosis. Very infrequently, varices are encountered in systemic amyloidosis and sarcoidosis. Furthermore, rare cases have been described without evident cause for the portal hypertension.

Varices are difficult to visualize in surgical or postmortem material, because when the veins are transected and drained, the varices collapse. Under optimal conditions, they appear as tortuous dilated veins in the long axis of the bowel that protrude directly beneath the mucosa or are found in the periesophageal tissue (Figs. 18–3 and 18–4). Varices are most commonly seen in the distal third of the esophagus but are occasionally found in the middle third.

When the varix is unruptured, the overlying mucosa may be normal, but often it is eroded and inflamed because of its exposed position. If rupture has occurred in the past, thrombosis or superimposed inflammation may be seen (Fig. 18–5).

Varices produce no symptoms until they rupture, and then calamitous massive hematemesis usually ensues. Among patients with advanced cirrhosis of the liver, half the deaths result from rupture of a varix. Some patients die as a direct consequence of the hemorrhage and others of hepatic coma triggered by the hemorrhage. Once begun, the hemorrhage rarely subsides spontaneously. Rupture of the varix may occur without an apparent triggering event, usually when there has been silent inflammatory erosion of the overlying thinned mucosa. On the other hand, in many of these patients, vomiting with presumed increase of hydrostatic pressure within the varix is the antecedent to the rupture. It is clinically important that even when varices are present, they account for only half of all episodes of massive hematemesis. In the remainder the bleeding arises from concomitant gastritis, esophageal laceration, or peptic ulcer. However, when varices bleed, 40% of patients die after the first episode. In those who survive, rebleeding occurs in about half, with an approximate 40% mortality rate following each episode.

TUMORS OF ESOPHAGUS

BENIGN

A variety of benign tumors occur in the esophagus. These are usually small, rarely over 3 cm in diameter, and occur mostly as intramural, solid, gray submucosal

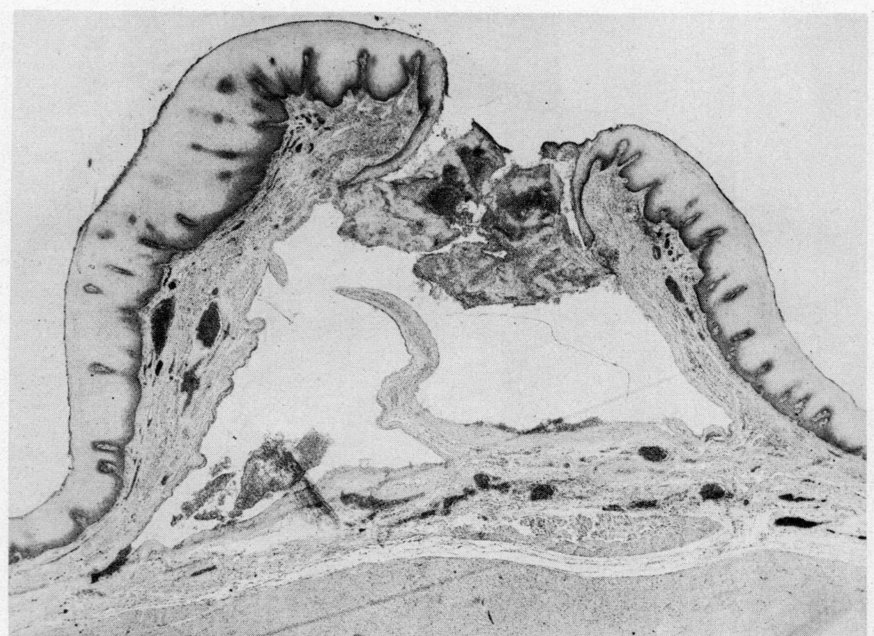

Figure 18–5. Esophageal varix. Low-power cross section of a dilated submucosal varix that has ruptured through the mucosa. A small amount of thrombus is present within the point of rupture.

masses. The most common is the leiomyoma, but fibromas, lipomas, hemangiomas, neurofibromas, lymphangiomas, and squamous papillomas may also arise in this location. They are usually chance findings at postmortem and are rarely large enough to cause symptoms.

MALIGNANT

The great preponderance of cancers in the esophagus are squamous cell carcinomas of variable levels of differentiation. About 5 to 10% are adenocarcinomas and an equal percentage are undifferentiated carcinomas. Sarcomas (leiomyosarcoma and fibrosarcoma) and melanocarcinoma are so rare as to be medical curiosities. The following discussion relates to the various forms of carcinoma (excluding melanocarcinomas, which are identical to those occurring in other locations).

Carcinomas

In the United States, carcinomas of the esophagus represent about 10% of all cancers of the gastrointestinal tract, but they cause a disproportionate number of cancer deaths. They remain asymptomatic during much of their development and so are often discovered too late to permit cure. Most in the U.S. occur in adults over the age of 50; children are seldom affected.

EPIDEMIOLOGY. Global epidemiologic data on the incidence of this form of cancer are both intriguing and baffling. The U.S. incidence rates per 100,000 population are about four for white males and one for white females. For unknown reasons, blacks throughout the world are more vulnerable than whites, and in the U.S. both black males and females have a roughly fourfold greater incidence than whites. In three areas of the world—Northeast Iran, the Transkei in South Africa, and North China—esophageal carcinoma is very common, having incidence rates 10- to 25-fold greater than those of the U.S.[18] In Northeast Iran, esophageal cancer is one of the most common causes of death in adults. Globally, this form of neoplasia is generally more common in males than in females, but in Iran the reverse obtains. The incidence of this form of cancer in the Transkei has risen 100-fold in the past 50 years.

ETIOLOGY AND PATHOGENESIS. Not surprisingly, we do not understand the origins of this form of cancer but there are many strong suggestions that preexistent esophageal disease and environmental factors play important roles. *The incidence of carcinoma is higher among those with esophagitis, achalasia, lye strictures, esophageal diverticula, and esophageal webs than in control groups.* Esophagitis in particular increases the risk: witness the 10% incidence of adenocarcinomas in those with a "Barrett esophagus" in association with reflux esophagitis (p. 802). Analogously, esophagitis is found in over 80% of the population where esophageal cancer is very frequent in Iran and China.[19] It seems plausible that any type of esophageal disease associated with mucosal injury, regeneration, and dysplasia, and also possibly with impaired transport exposing the mucosa longer to environmental influences, might predispose to cancer. Environmental influences are thus thought to contribute to causing this form of cancer, particularly alcohol, smoking, and irritants such as excessively hot and spicy foods, but even with these, enigmas remain. Epidemiologic surveys in the United

States indicate a 25-fold increased risk among heavy drinkers and a six- to sevenfold increased risk among habitual smokers of cigarettes, cigars, or pipes.[20, 21] However, in the high-incidence areas of China and Iran, smoking and alcohol consumption are not implicated. Indeed, in certain regions of Iran the frequency of this form of cancer is extremely low and surveys comparing high-risk with low-risk regions disclose no differences in alcohol or smoking practices.[22] Copious consumption of hot foods and beverages has been proposed as a causative influence; hot tea drinking, for example, has been shown to raise intraesophageal temperatures to potentially damaging levels. Conceivably, local injury to the mucosal cells disrupts intracellular junctions, thereby inducing increased shedding of cells and consequently more rapid proliferation of basal elements. Long-standing regenerative efforts might lead in time to neoplastic transformation. However, other studies point out that the diet in high-incidence areas of Iran is based on bread, tea, and sheep's milk, whereas in low-incidence areas it consists mainly of rice and tea with a high intake of fruits and vegetables. No significant differences could be identified in consumption of tea or other hot foods;[13] thus, the role of these irritant foods has been challenged but not ruled out. In the Transkei contamination of food by aflatoxins is suspected, and in North China silica fragments from coarse grains.[23] Conceivably, there are many influences that can injure the mucosa and set up esophagitis and mucosal dysplasia, but much is speculative at present.

MORPHOLOGY. Like squamous cell carcinomas arising in other locations, those of the esophagus begin as inapparent in situ lesions. When they become overt, about 50% of these tumors are located in the middle third, 30% in the lower third, and 20% in the upper third of the esophagus. Early overt lesions are usually discovered accidentally and appear as small, gray-white, plaquelike thickenings or elevations of the mucosa. These extend with time along the long axis of the bowel and, in months to years, encircle the lumen. From this point, three morphologic patterns may evolve. **The most common one (60%) is that of a polypoid fungating lesion that protrudes into the lumen. The second gross pattern (25%) is a necrotic cancerous ulceration that excavates deeply into surrounding structures** and may erode into the respiratory tree and the aorta, or permeate the mediastinum and pericardium (Fig. 18–6). **The third morphologic variant is a diffuse infiltrative form that tends to spread within the wall of the esophagus, causing thickening, rigidity, and narrowing of the lumen** with ulceration of the mucosa (Fig. 18–7).

Histologically, about 60 to 70% are either poorly or well-differentiated squamous cell carcinomas; about 5 to 10% are adenocarcinomas that originate either from the esophageal mucous glands or from changes previously referred to as Barrett esophagus (p. 801); and the remainder are undifferentiated tumors. Some of these undifferentiated neoplasms are composed of large, pleomorphic anaplastic cells. A few are so-called "oat cell" carcinomas, composed of small uniform cells that have deeply chromatic nuclei. These oat cell lesions are probably derived from endocrine cells and so belong to the family of APUDomas capable of secreting a variety of amine and polypeptide hormones (p. 842).[24]

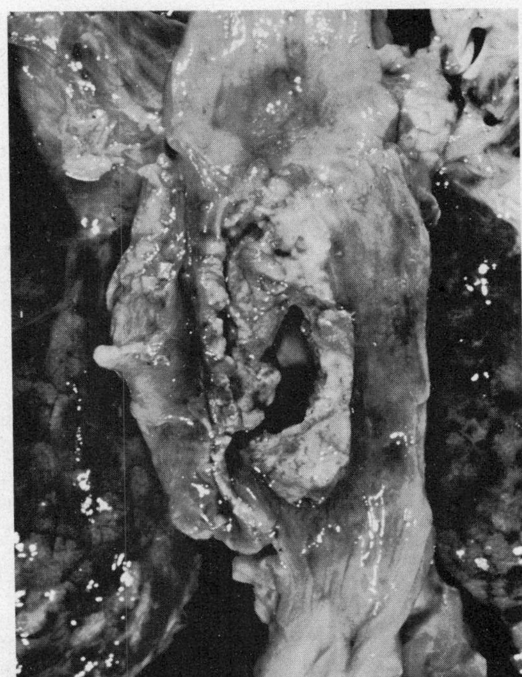

Figure 18–6. Carcinoma of esophagus viewed from esophageal aspect, showing a large defect in central necrotic portion. Tumor has directly invaded trachea to produce an esophagotracheal fistula.

All esophageal cancers tend to spread by direct continuity, but they also metastasize. Upper-third lesions tend to spread to the cervical nodes, middle-third to the tracheobronchial nodes, and lower-third to gastric and celiac nodes.

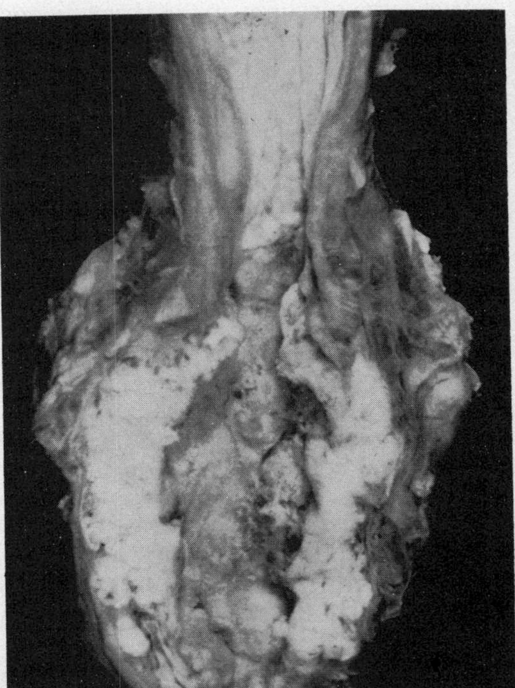

Figure 18–7. Cancer in lower third of esophagus, far advanced with central ulceration and extension into periesophageal tissue.

Visceral metastases most often involve the liver and lungs; direct spread is to the larynx, trachea, thyroid glands, recurrent laryngeal nerves, and pericardium.

Carcinoma of the esophagus has been staged as follows:

Stage I Limited to esophagus; less than 5 cm in length.

Stage II Limited to esophagus; greater than 5 cm in length, with resectable nodes.

Stage III Lesion greater than 10 cm in length; extension through esophagus into adjacent structures; inoperable nodes or inoperable lesion.

Stage IV Lesion as in Stage III; evidence of perforation, fistula, or distant metastases.

CLINICAL COURSE. Esophageal carcinoma is insidious in onset and produces dysphagia and obstruction gradually and late. Patients subconsciously adjust to their increasing difficulty in swallowing by progressively altering their diet from solid to liquid foods. Extreme weight loss and debilitation result from both the impaired nutrition and the effects of the tumor itself. Hemorrhages and sepsis may accompany the ulcerative changes. Occasionally, the first alarming symptom is the aspiration of food that enters the respiratory tree through a cancerous tracheoesophageal fistula. It should be noted that such fistula formation is almost always caused by carcinoma of the esophagus. Bronchogenic carcinoma rarely invades the esophagus and hence rarely produces fistulous tracts. Metastasis occurs as a relatively late phenomenon. The insidious invasive growth of these neoplasms usually leads to large lesions by the time a diagnosis is established, making resection difficult if not impossible. Generally, resection is possible in less than half the cases. Even with standard methods of therapy, such as surgical resection or supervoltage irradiation, 70% of patients are dead within one year of the diagnosis, and the five-year survival rate is 5 to 10%.

Stomach

NORMAL

Certain normal features of the structure and function of the stomach merit brief review because they are highly relevant to later discussions.

The stomach is divided into the following anatomic regions:

1. The *cardia,* which represents the region proximate to the esophagogastric junction. The glands here are entirely mucin-secreting and contain no parietal (acid-secreting) cells or zymogenic chief (pepsin-secreting) cells.

2. The *fundus,* which is the bulbous subdiaphragmatic region of the stomach, is located to the left of the esophagus and cephalad to the entrance of the esophagus into the stomach. The glands within the mucosa of the fundus are similar to those in the body of the stomach.

3. The *body (corpus),* which is the largest anatomic region interposed between the fundus and the more caudad antrum. The beginning of the antrum is demarcated by a vertical line drawn through the incisura angularis of the lesser curvature of the stomach. The mucosa of the body and fundus of the stomach contains the gastric glands where the parietal and chief cells are found.

4. The *antrum,* which extends from the body of the stomach to the pyloric sphincter. Sometimes the narrow 2.5-cm segment of the antrum lying just proximal to the pylorus is designated the prepyloric canal. The antral glands do not elaborate acid-peptic secretion but are the major site of gastrin formation.

Histologically, distinctive gland patterns having specific secretory functions are found in the various anatomic regions—cardiac glands in the cardia, gastric (oxyntic) glands in the fundus and body of the stomach, and pyloric glands in the antrum. All these glands are more or less test tube–shaped and several of them empty into so-called gastric pits or foveolae.

The entire mucosal surface as well as the linings of the gastric pits are composed of so-called surface cells that are tall, columnar, and mucin-secreting. They have basal nuclei and crowded small, relatively clear mucigen-containing granules in the supranuclear regions. With appropriate fixation the mucigen granules can be stained with mucicarmine or the PAS reaction. Ultrastructurally, the surface mucous cells have short microvilli and a thin coating of fine filamentous glycocalyx on their free surfaces. Deep within the gastric pits where the various glands empty into these pits the surface epithelial cells are somewhat modified into so-called *neck cells.* Mucigen granules are scant in these cells and restricted to only a thin layer immediately beneath the cell surface. These neck cells are thought to be the progenitors of both the surface epithelium and the cells of the gastric glands. Mitoses are extremely common in these neck cells since, as you recall, the entire gastric mucosal surface is totally replaced every two to six days.

The *cardiac* glands in the gastric cardia are lined by cells indistinguishable from the neck cells of the gastric glands. Scattered individual argentaffin cells (described below) may be present among the mucous cells.

The *gastric (oxyntic) glands* in the body and fundus of the stomach are composed in their upper regions of mucous neck cells, below which are chief cells that elaborate pepsinogen. Acid-secreting parietal cells, which also elaborate *intrinsic factor*, are scattered among the chief cells. The chief cells are rendered distinctive by their large, pale, zymogen granules, most prominent apically. The parietal cells are quickly recognized in H and E preparations by their bright eosinophilia. Ultrastructurally they reveal numerous mitochondria and prominent intracellular canaliculi into which the gastric acid is secreted.

Pyloric glands, which are the major site of gastrin secretion, are found within the antral region of the stomach. They are made up largely of cells resembling those of the neck regions of the gastric glands. They may contain granules similar to those found in the chief cells or the surface epithelium. Numerous endocrine cells producing gastrin are also present.

Endocrine cells are dispersed widely throughout the glands of the various regions of the stomach. Indeed, they are dispersed throughout the entire gut and, in terms of their aggregate number, make the gut the largest endocrine organ in the body. These endocrine cells can be recognized in tissue sections by a variety of histochemical procedures. Some are capable of reducing soluble silver salts and depositing metallic silver; these are referred to as *argentaffin cells*. Since they also give a positive chromaffin reaction, they are also called *enterochromaffin cells*. Other endocrine cells lack strong reducing properties but are able to take up prereduced silver; these are referred to as *argyrophil cells*. Still others do not bind silver salts. Ultrastructurally, all endocrine cells in the gut, like those in other endocrine glands, contain distinctive secretory granules. The specific size and shape of the granules permit segregation of these cells into subsets that to an extent correlate with the synthesis of particular gut hormones.[25] We need not delve into the details of the various subsets since it suffices for our purposes that collectively the endocrine cells in the stomach produce a variety of amine and peptide hormones, the best characterized of which are serotonin (5-hydroxytryptamine), gastrin, somatostatin, substance P, vasoactive intestinal peptide, bombesin, and possibly glucagon. Details on the function of these various hormones are available in the review of Bloom and Polak.[26] All the gut endocrine cells belong to the larger category of APUD cells (p. 842) (an acronym for *a*mine *p*recursor *u*ptake and *d*ecarboxylation). These characteristics confer the ability to synthesize the amine and peptide hormones just mentioned.[27] Neoplasms and hyperplasias of the endocrine cells produce clinically important endocrinopathies, discussed later in this chapter.

The process of gastric acid secretion is relevant to the later consideration of peptic ulcer disease. The capacity to secrete hydrochloric acid is directly proportional to the total number of parietal cells in the glands of the body and fundus of the stomach, i.e., *the parietal cell mass*. The most important physiologic stimulus to these cells is food in the stomach, but its effect is mediated by humoral and neural mechanisms. *The secretory process is best considered by dividing it into its three traditional phases—cephalic, gastric, and intestinal*. The *cephalic phase* is initiated by the sight, taste, smell, chewing, and swallowing of palatable food. This phase is largely mediated by direct vagal stimulation of parietal cells but may also involve vagal stimulation of gastrin release. In animals, the cephalic phase of acid secretion can also be initiated by agents that induce glucopenia in the brain either by decreasing the supply of glucose or interfering with its utilization; this process has not been clearly established in humans, however. The *gastric phase* involves stimulation of mechanical and chemical receptors in the gastric wall. Mechanical stimulation occurs with gastric distention and appears to be mediated by vagal impulses. The chemical stimuli, the most important of which are digested proteins and amino acids, induce the release of gastrin, the most potent mediator of acid secretion. Fat and glucose in the stomach do not stimulate gastric acid secretion. Gastrin, as you know, is synthesized by so-called G cells within the pyloric antrum. A small amount of gastrin may also be elaborated in the proximal duodenum. Gastrin is, in fact, a family of polypeptides that vary chiefly in amino-acid-chain length. The two most important forms of this hormone are so-called "little gastrin," having 17 amino acids (G-17), and "big gastrin," having 34 amino acids (G-34). Other smaller and larger gastrins have also been identified. G-34 has the longest half-life in the circulation and so is the major form present in the blood. However, G-17, having a much shorter circulating half-life, is the most potent stimulus to gastric acid secretion. These details make it clear why assay of the gastrin level in the blood may not accurately reflect the acid secretory drive unless radioimmunoassay is employed using antibodies specific for the G-17 form of gastrin, which do not cross-react with smaller and larger peptides. The *intestinal phase* is initiated when food containing digested proteins enters the proximal small intestine. The stimulation of acid secretion that occurs at this time is thought to be related to the elaboration in the small intestine of polypeptide quite distinct from gastrin.

Although histamine, when administered, is a potent acid secretagogue, the role of endogenous histamine elaborated mainly by mast cells in the gastric wall (possibly also by endocrine cells) is still somewhat uncertain. However, the irrefutable evidence that antagonists to histamine H_2 receptors, such as cimetidine, inhibit acid secretion argues strongly that histamine plays an important role in the secretory process. Cimetidine inhibits basal acid secretion as well as the secretory response to feeding, gastrin, histamine, and vagal stimulation. It must be concluded that in some way histamine acts along with gastrin and vagal activity to stimulate parietal cells. Possibly it plays a "permissive" role, serving as the final mediator of gastrin and vagal action.

How does the normal stomach resist the corrosive

effects of the acid-peptic-gastric secretion? At maximal secretory rates the intraluminal concentration of hydrogen ion in the stomach is three million times greater than that of the blood and tissues. Most important is the so-called "gastric mucosal barrier." Normally, the mucosal luminal epithelial cells are bound to each other by intercellular tight junctions, and so the intact surface epithelial layer provides a barrier to backdiffusion of hydrogen ions. Adding to this barrier is secretion of acid buffer by the surface cells, since there is a pH gradient across the layer of mucous secretion attached to the surface cells. Any impairment of this mucosal barrier permits penetration of hydrogen ions into the mucosa, which ironically stimulates further secretion of gastric acid and pepsinogen. Thus, while acid is diffusing into the mucosa, the luminal hydrogen ion concentration is simultaneously rising. *A number of agents have been shown to damage the mucosal barrier, including alcohol, cigarettes, bile acids, lysolecithin, and particularly aspirin.* All disrupt the continuity of the epithelial surface and so induce increased shedding of surface cells, to contribute possibly to the development of gastric mucosal erosions or ulcers. A variety of other influences, all imperfectly understood, conduce to the protection of the gastric mucosa, at least in animals.[28] Adequate mucosal blood flow, normal levels of carbonic anhydrase in mucosal cells (which participates in the formation of bicarbonate and so protects cells to an extent against excessive drops in pH), and prostaglandins all serve to defend the mucosa against the erosive action of acid-peptic secretion.[29] Gastric mucin must play some role in protection of the mucosa; therapeutic agents that stimulate mucus output have been shown to favor the healing of peptic ulcers and protect against recurrences.[30] Dilution and neutralization of gastric acid by protein foods and refluxed bicarbonate from the duodenum also make some contribution. Imperfect as our understanding of the defensive mechanism(s) may be, it is obviously a physiologic marvel, or our gastric walls would suffer the same fate as a piece of swallowed meat.

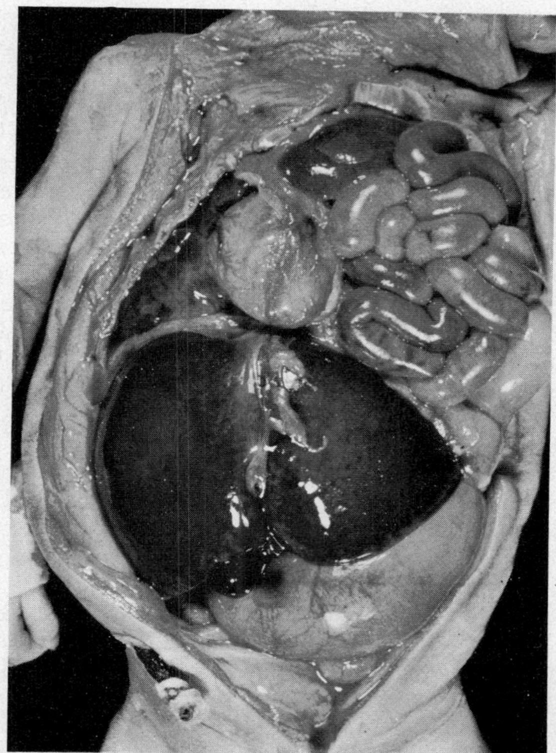

Figure 18–8. In situ view of opened trunk of an infant with a diaphragmatic hernia. Numerous loops of small bowel and portions of the colon are evident in the left pleural cavity. The markedly displaced lung can be seen at the very apex of the cavity.

PATHOLOGY

The stomach is an important segment of the alimentary tract from the standpoint of its diseases. Peptic ulcers have become almost a hallmark of so-called "civilized life" and are found in up to 10% of the general population in North America. In this day of cigarette smoking, alcohol consumption, and stress, gastritis is one of the everyday causes of "indigestion." Gastric carcinoma remains an important cause of cancer death in the United States although its incidence has decreased, for reasons discussed later.

CONGENITAL ANOMALIES

DIAPHRAGMATIC HERNIAS

Weakness or partial-to-total absence of a region of the diaphragm, usually on the left, may permit the abdominal contents to herniate into the thorax. These hernias differ from hiatal hernias only insofar as the defect in the diaphragm does not involve the hiatal orifice. The hernial wall in these lesions is most often composed only of peritoneum and pleura. Usually, the stomach or a portion of it insinuates into the pouch, but occasionally small bowel and even a portion of the liver accompany it (Fig. 18–8).

Sometimes these hernias are asymptomatic and are discovered only by x-ray or by the identification of intestinal sounds within the chest. However, large protrusions, particularly in infants, may lead to respiratory embarrassment or vomiting.

PYLORIC STENOSIS

Narrowing of the pyloric lumen may be encountered in infants as a congenital defect or in adults as an acquired disease secondary to inflammatory fibrosis or tumorous invasion. Rarely, in adults, the condition represents a previously unrecognized congenital defect.

Congenital hypertrophic pyloric stenosis is an apparently familial malformation characterized by hypertrophy and hyperplasia of the circular muscle of the muscularis propria of the pylorus. The narrowing may lead to edema or inflammatory changes within the mucosa and submucosa, which aggravate the narrowing. It is reported to occur in from one in 300 to one in 900 live births. The disease is much more common in males than in females, in a ratio of 4:1. The genetic mode of transmission is not firmly established but appears to be multifactorial inheritance. Monozygotic twins have a high rate of concordance for the condition.

Infants with hypertrophic pyloric stenosis are apparently well during the first week of life. Regurgitation of food and vomiting usually do not appear until the second or, more often, the third week. Often it is possible to see visible peristaltic contractions on examination of the abdomen, and almost invariably a firm ovoid mass is readily palpable. The mass is composed of hypertrophied pyloric musculature, sometimes accompanied by mucosal edema. A muscle-splitting incision down to the mucosa usually results in a prompt and effective cure and, with it, the slow disappearance of the hypertrophic muscle.

Acquired pyloric stenosis is one of the long-term risks of patients with antral gastritis or peptic ulcers close to the pylorus. Carcinomas of the pylorus or head of the pancreas or lymphomas are more ominous causes of acquired disease. Whatever the cause, resection of the involved segment of bowel or some form of bypass procedure may be necessary as a curative or palliative measure.

MISCELLANEOUS LESIONS

Gastric diverticula are rare and generally inconsequential lesions. They tend to occur in two locations: (1) in the cardia, unassociated with contiguous disease; and (2) in the antrum, often associated with a healing ulcer or periantral inflammation. The diverticular wall may or may not have a muscularis component, and sometimes it is composed only of mucosa and submucosa invested by either serosa or perigastric fibrosis.

Gastric dilatation may arise because of organic or functional obstruction of the pylorus. The organic bases were alluded to in the discussion of pyloric stenosis. The functional basis appears to be atony of the stomach and intestines (paralytic ileus), which may appear in patients with generalized peritonitis. The stomach may contain as much as 10 to 15 liters of fluid. Not only is it enormously expanded, but the wall is markedly thinned, even to the point of translucency. The distention may be serious, since it causes elevation of the diaphragms and adds an element of respiratory embarrassment in patients already seriously ill.

Gastric rupture is a rare but devastating event. It may follow blunt trauma to the abdomen; has rarely followed consumption of enormous quantities of beer (medical students please take note), with apparent release of sufficient carbon dioxide to bring the beer-drinking spree to an unhappy end; and may complicate cardiac resuscitation with mouth-to-mouth breathing and inflation of the stomach when external cardiac massage is applied. Gastric rupture has also been associated with the strain of labor. Whatever the basis, it is a calamitous event followed rapidly by shock or death, unless immediately recognized and treated surgically.

INFLAMMATION

GASTRITIS

Although gastritis is an unquestioned clinical and anatomic disorder, it is a much abused medical term. It is commonly used to explain such transient or seemingly trivial complaints as "sour stomach," "dyspepsia," and "indigestion" without substantiating clinical or anatomic evidence. On the other hand, gastritis may be present anatomically without inducing clinical symptoms. Thus, gastritis is both an overused term and an underdiagnosed clinical condition.

There is no general agreement on a classification of the various forms of gastritis. Basically there are two categories—acute and chronic. However, within each of these a range of subvarieties has been established. *Depending on the amount of desquamation or destruction of the gastric mucosa, acute involvements have been subdivided into acute gastritis, acute hemorrhagic gastritis, acute erosive gastritis, and acute stress erosions (stress ulcers).* These terms encompass an anatomic continuum with no well-defined delineations between one pattern and the next. Accordingly, here we shall retreat to the simple designation *acute gastritis* and describe the range of changes encountered up to acute stress ulcers, which are discussed in a later section (p. 813).

Chronic gastritis has also been subdivided into a number of variants, the most important being fundal gastritis and antral gastritis.[31] Justification for this subdivision derives both from direct visual gastroscopic findings and from apparent differences in the clinical associations of these two variants, as detailed later. Both forms have been further subdivided somewhat arbitrarily into chronic superficial gastritis, atrophic gastritis, and gastric atrophy. There are no clear-cut morphologic lines of delineation between these variants of chronic gastritis and so they can all be considered together.

There are, in addition, several uncommon forms of gastritis that merit only brief mention later: hypertrophic gastritis, granulomatous gastritis, and eosinophilic gastritis.

Acute Gastritis

Acute gastritis, as the term implies, is an acute mucosal inflammatory process, usually of transient nature. The inflammation may be accompanied by hemorrhage into the mucosa, and, in more severe instances, by concomitant erosions to produce what has been called acute erosive or acute hemorrhagic erosive gastritis. The severe erosive form of the disease is an important cause of acute gastrointestinal bleeding, which may be massive and alarming.

PATHOGENESIS. The pathogenesis of these lesions is poorly understood. Clinical (and some experimental) data indicate that acute gastritis frequently is associated with (1) chronic use of aspirin; (2) excessive alcohol consumption; (3) heavy smoking; (4) treatment with cancer chemotherapeutic drugs; (5) uremia; (6) systemic infections (e.g., salmonellosis); (7) staphylococcal food poisoning; (8) severe stress, such as extensive burns, trauma, and surgery; (9) shock; and (10) gastric irradiation or freezing. *One or more of the following influences are thought to be operative in these varied settings: increased acid secretion with backdiffusion; decreased production of bicarbonate buffer; reduced blood flow, which permits acid ions to accumulate; and damage to the barrier itself.* Reference has been made earlier to the important role of the intact mucosa (p. 808) in preventing backdiffusion of hydrogen ion. It was pointed out that aspirin breaks this mucosal barrier and causes increased turnover of surface mucosal cells. A significant number of patients with rheumatoid arthritis who take aspirin regularly have at least minor degrees of occult gastric bleeding. Is this related solely to the aspirin or could the arthritic disease contribute in some obscure manner? Unfortunately, there are no data on the comparable use of aspirin in the absence of arthritis or other diseases (presumably some underlying condition must be present to call for the chronic use of this agent). Alcohol also damages the mucosal barrier. Could it be a contributor in habitual users of aspirin? Increased backdiffusion has also been demonstrated in critically ill patients and in animals subjected to hemorrhagic shock, so stress alone may play some role.

Mucosal hypoperfusion is the other major contributory mechanism leading to mucosal injury. Diminished blood flow to the mucosa would reasonably be expected in any form of shock and might also occur from the vasoconstrictive effects of nicotine with heavy smoking. The acute gastritis following gastric irradiation or freezing might also, at least in part, be mediated by mucosal hypoperfusion. Concomitantly, the mucosal ischemia would impair the barrier function of the mucosa. Thus, ischemic injury would synergize the deleterious effects of backdiffusion of hydrogen ions. Other mucosal insults have been identified in experimental animals, such as regurgitation of bile acids and lysolecithin, and inadequate mucosal synthesis of prostaglandins, but what role these play in the acute gastritis of humans is unknown.[28] Although the gastric mucosa is capable of regeneration following an acute injury, persistence of any of the deleterious influences cited could well lead to the morphologic changes described below.

MORPHOLOGY. Depending on the severity of the insult, the mucosal response may vary from only moderate edema and slight hyperemia to hemorrhagic erosion of the gastric mucosa. In the milder forms, the surface epithelium may be intact and the lamina propria may contain only occasional scattered leukocytes. In the extreme pattern, best referred to as **acute hemorrhagic erosive gastritis**, there is superficial sloughing of the mucosa, accompanied by hemorrhage into the lamina propria and an acute inflammatory leukocytic infiltrate. Large areas of the gastric mucosa may be denuded, but the involvement, as stated, is superficial and rarely affects the entire depth of the mucosa, sparing the underlying wall. Such gastric erosions are but one step removed from the more deeply penetrating "stress ulcers" described later.

CLINICAL COURSE. The wide range of morphologic changes embraced by the term "acute gastritis" is paralleled by the range of clinical manifestations. Undoubtedly, minor involvements occur that produce no symptoms. At the other end of the spectrum are the cases with massive hematemesis and acute abdominal pain. In between are those cases manifested by epigastric pain, nausea, and vomiting. In some instances, the first indication of gastritis is the sudden onset of hematemesis or melena. In Great Britain, 25% of all cases of hematemesis and melena arise in severe gastritis related to the widespread use of aspirin.[32]

Chronic Gastritis—Fundal and Antral

The unqualified term chronic gastritis encompasses a range of lesions extending from superficial gastritis to atrophic gastritis to gastric atrophy. These forms are poorly delineated from each other since *they make up a morphologic continuum of increasingly intense inflammatory infiltration of the mucosa accompanied by progressively more marked atrophy of the mucosal glands.* The glandular atrophy is often accompanied by metaplasia, dysplasia, and atypia of the surface epithelium. These changes underlie the major clinical consequences of chronic gastritis: (1) the possible loss of parietal cells and their synthesis of intrinsic factor (IF), resulting in inadequate absorption of vitamin B_{12} and pernicious anemia (PA); (2) an increased predisposition to gastric carcinoma; and (3) its possible contribution to peptic ulceration (p. 817).

Chronic gastritis may involve the entire stomach or be patchily distributed without regard for anatomic regions. Often, however, only the fundus and body or only the antrum is affected, giving rise to the subsets of chronic fundal gastritis and chronic antral gastritis. *There are reasons, detailed below, for suspecting that fundal and antral gastritis represent more than morphologic variations of a single disease, since they may have different origins as well as differing clinical significances.*

PATHOGENESIS. With regard to the origins of chronic gastritis in general, only this much can be said with any degree of assurance—there is *no* evidence that aspirin, alcohol and smoking are etiologic factors, and it is not preceded by acute gastritis. On the other hand, long-term observation of patients with chronic superficial gastritis has disclosed that in some the mucosal lesion improves with time, whereas in a significant number it progresses into the atrophic forms.[33] Thus, it would seem that superficial gastritis is the initial stage of the more severe patterns of mucosal involvement.

Fundal gastritis is encountered in two distinct population subsets: (1) in adults of any age having PA and (2) in an older age group not having PA. In the first group with PA, the fundal gastritis appears to be autoimmune in origin. Typically, these patients have severe mucosal damage, i.e., chronic atrophic gastritis or gastric atrophy with complete or near-complete loss of parietal cells and consequent severe hypochlorhydria or achlorhydria. Three distinctive autoantibodies against gastric parietal cell antigens are present in these individuals,[34] as discussed on page 633. Two are targeted on IF, which, as you recall, is elaborated in humans by parietal cells. It suffices to note here that they block the absorption of vitamin B_{12} and so lead to PA, as noted on page 418. *Whenever either antibody is identified in the circulation, it may be inferred that the patient has PA or is at risk of developing it.* The third autoantibody is directed against gastric parietal cells (GPC). GPC antibodies are present in 80 to 90% of patients with PA, but can also be identified in about 60% of elderly individuals with atrophic gastritis but no apparent PA. There is still some uncertainty whether GPC antibodies are cytotoxic in man[35] and are responsible for the loss of parietal cells seen in the atrophic gastritis of PA. For this reason, the possibility has been raised of a role for cell-mediated immunity in the production of the mucosal changes, perhaps in concert with the antibodies. Whatever the mechanism, patients with PA usually have titers of IF and GPC antibodies, and virtually always have severe atrophic gastritis or gastric atrophy involving the fundus and body of the stomach with marked or total destruction of parietal cells. *According to this conception, the atrophic gastritis of classic PA in adults is an autoimmune disease with immunologic destruction of parietal cells.* Several observations are relevant to this autoimmune thesis. About 30% of first-degree relatives of patients with PA have detectable GPC antibodies in their sera, suggesting genetic predisposition. In addition, there is a well-documented association between PA and other autoimmune diseases, such as Hashimoto's thyroiditis, thyrotoxicosis, idiopathic hypoadrenalism, idiopathic hypoparathyroidism, and insulin-dependent diabetes mellitus. A lingering doubt must be expressed—could the immune reactions be epiphenomena related to mucosal damage of other origins?

Chronic fundal gastritis may also appear in an older age group not having PA. About 60% of these individuals have antibodies to GPC but not to IF. Some have an iron deficiency anemia, but the association may be merely coincidental. Other instances of chronic fundal gastritis are seen in relatives of patients with PA but in the complete absence of autoantibodies. Thus, the basis for chronic fundal gastritis in these older individuals is completely unknown.

Chronic antral gastritis appears to have totally different origins from those of fundal gastritis. In a minority of instances, autoantibodies to gastrin-producing cells are present.[36] *More often there are no autoantibodies, but instead the patients have concurrent gastric peptic ulcers or, less frequently, gastric carcinomas.* Sometimes, duodenitis is present. The association of gastric ulcers with antral gastritis raises the possibility that dysfunction of the pyloric sphincter and regurgitation of bile acids and possibly lysolecithin may play a causal role for both, as discussed on page 816.

MORPHOLOGY. The morphologic changes in chronic gastritis may affect most of the stomach or only patchy areas, or may be limited to the fundus and body (fundal gastritis) or to the antrum (antral gastritis). Whatever the distribution, in the **chronic superficial variant** there may be some flattening of the mucosa but it is generally not marked. An inflammatory infiltrate of lymphocytes and plasma cells is typically present within the lamina propria, usually limited to the upper third of the gastric mucosa (Fig. 18–9). In **chronic atrophic gastritis,** whether fundal, antral, or more dispersed, the mucosa is more obviously thinned and flattened with extension of the infiltrate in the lamina propria to the deeper layers about the glands. It may appear reddened as the submucosal vessels become more apparent. There is often atrophy of the glands and a variety of cytologic changes in the surface epithelial cells, as described below. In chronic fundal gastritis the gastric glands are atrophic; those that persist often undergo cystic dilatation and are lined by gastric mucous cells or metaplastic intestinal cells. There is a conspicuous paucity of parietal cells. The antral mucosa is relatively spared in pure forms of chronic fundal gastritis. Conversely, in chronic atrophic antral gastritis the inflammatory and glandular changes are largely limited to the antrum but, save for location, resemble those already described in fundal gastritis.

The morphologic alterations of **chronic gastric atrophy** are an extension of the atrophic changes encountered in atrophic gastritis. Rugal folds are flattened or absent and the mucosa takes on a shiny, glazed appearance. The glandular atrophy is now almost complete save for scattered, shortened, sometimes cystically dilated glands. The surface epithelium, as well as that lining the gastric pits, takes the form of mucous-secreting goblet cells interspersed with cells characteristic of intestinal epithelium bearing microvilli. Occasionally, abortive, villous-like projections may appear. **In**

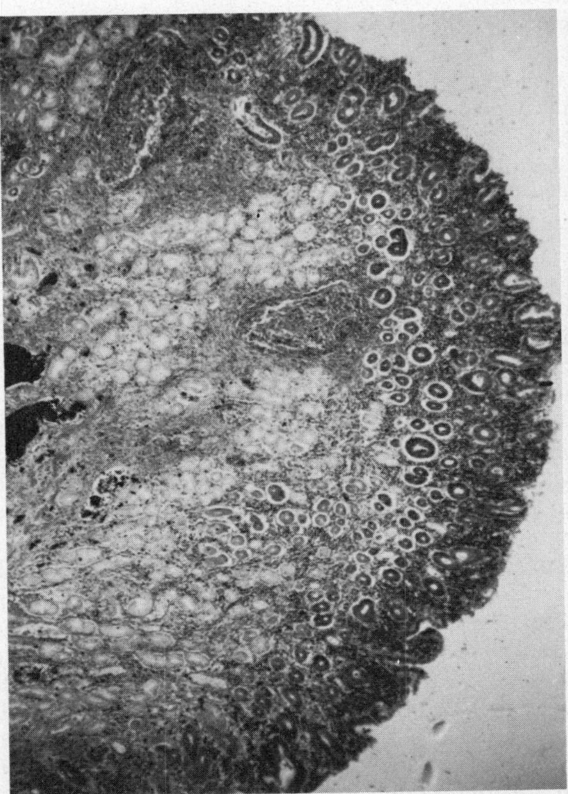

Figure 18–9. Chronic superficial gastritis with an intense inflammatory infiltrate and some disorganization of glands involving upper one-third of gastric mucosa.

the fundal variant associated with PA, parietal cells are almost totally absent from such atrophic glands as persist. In contrast, in the antral pattern the parietal cells in the body and fundus of the stomach persist. **Whatever the distribution of the mucosal involvement, the surface epithelium undergoes a variety of metaplastic and dysplastic alterations** including variation in size, shape, and orientation of the epithelial cells, often accompanied by nuclear enlargement and atypicality. The interpretation of these cellular alterations is unclear and may merely reflect the persistence of damaging influences responsible for the development of the gastric mucosal atrophy. The cellular atypia tends to be most marked in chronic fundal gastric atrophy associated with PA. In this setting, it is tempting to speculate that the deficient absorption of vitamin B_{12} impairs DNA synthesis and so inhibits cell replication with the formation of abnormally large atypical cells, as discussed on page 630. Whatever their origin, the cytologic changes may become so severe as to mimic in situ carcinoma; indeed, they probably account for the increased incidence of gastric cancer in atrophic forms of gastritis, particularly in association with PA.

CLINICAL COURSE. Chronic gastritis may cause no symptoms referable to the gastrointestinal tract. However, it is vulnerable to superimposed acute gastritis and then is associated with epigastric discomfort, pain, nausea, vomiting, and sometimes bleeding. Most often the atrophic variants of fundal gastritis come to attention because the patient is discovered to have PA or in the course of investigating the cause of hypochlorhydria in an individual. The severity of the acid deficiency depends on the severity of the gastric atrophy. With atrophic fundal gastritis there is usually hypochlorhydria, whereas fundal gastric atrophy is likely to produce achlorhydria. However, serum gastrin levels are high because the uninvolved antrum is not subject to the inhibitory control of gastric acid. As indicated previously, autoantibodies to IF or parietal cells may be present.

In chronic antral gastritis, even when marked, acid secretion may be normal or low, depending on the extent of loss of gastrin production. Antibodies to gastrin-secreting cells can be demonstrated in some instances. Particularly important is the relationship of this form of gastritis to gastric peptic ulcer. Most patients with a gastric peptic ulcer have antral gastritis, but the reverse is not true. When the two conditions coexist it is not certain which comes first, but since healing of the ulcer may occur with persistence of the antral gastritis, it is believed that the gastritis is primary and plays a role in the development of the ulcer (p. 817). Note that both atrophic gastritis and gastric atrophy constitute precancerous lesions. The risk is seen with both fundal and antral patterns, but is greatest with the fundal gastritis associated with PA. Over the span of decades, about 7 to 10% of individuals with PA develop a gastric carcinoma.[37] Although hematologic improvement of the anemia can be achieved by vitamin B_{12} therapy, the gastric atrophy persists and, with it, the predisposition to cancer [38]

Hypertrophic Gastritis

This designation encompasses a group of uncommon conditions, all characterized by giant cerebriform enlargement of the rugal folds of the gastric mucosa (Fig. 18–10). The term hypertrophic gastritis, although firmly fixed in medical practice, is a misnomer since the rugal enlargement is caused by neither inflammatory gastritis nor hypertrophy, but by hyperplasia of the mucosal epithelial cells. *Three variants are recognized: (1) Ménétrier's disease related to hyperplasia of the surface mucous cells, (2) hypersecretory gastropathy associated with hyperplasia of the parietal and chief cells within the gastric glands, and (3) gastric gland hyperplasia secondary to the excessive gastrin-secretion of a gastrinoma in the Zollinger-Ellison syndrome (p. 987).* The first two may be variations of a single entity differing only in the amount of parietal and chief cell hyperplasia and, therefore, in the levels of gastric acid secretion. All three conditions are uncommon but are of clinical importance because on x-ray examination or

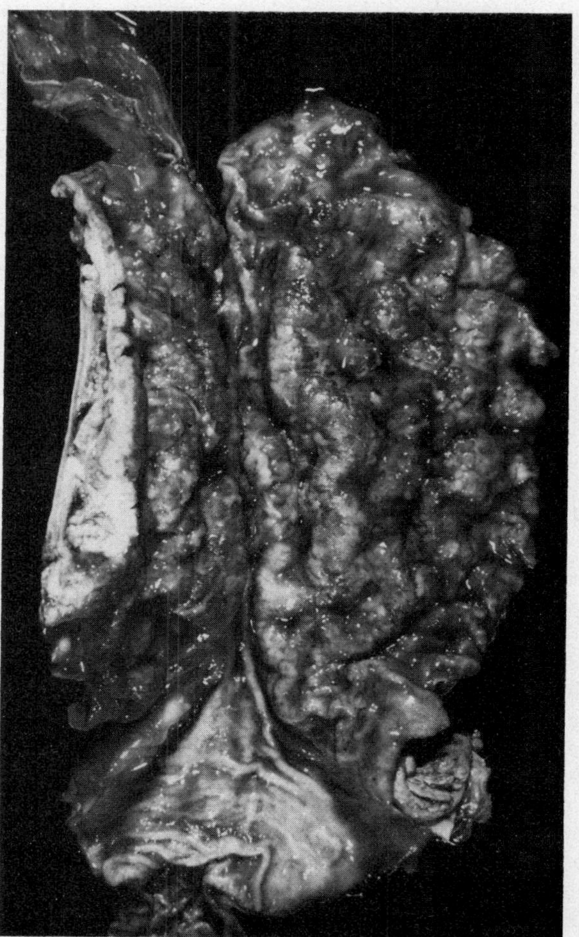

Figure 18–10. Hypertrophic gastritis of stomach, sparing antral region below. Marked thickening of rugal folds simulates diffuse neoplastic infiltration.

endoscopy they mimic infiltrative cancer or lymphoma of the stomach. They may also be associated with significant clinical morbidity.

Ménétrier's disease, most often encountered in men in their fourth to sixth decades, is of unknown cause. As was pointed out, the exaggerated rugal folds are produced by hyperplasia of the surface mucous cells, which often produces enlargement and tortuosity as well as cystic dilatation of the gastric pits. Sometimes the cysts become sufficiently large to penetrate into the gastric submucosa. This involvement may be diffuse or affect principally the greater curvature of the stomach. Although the condition may be asymptomatic and be discovered only on radiography, it often produces epigastric pain, nausea, vomiting, and sometimes bleeding related to superficial rugal erosions. As would be expected, the gastric secretions contain excessive mucus and in many instances little or no hydrochloric acid when the parietal cells undergo atrophy. In some patients, there is excessive protein loss in the gastric secretion sufficient to produce hypoalbuminemia and peripheral edema, thus constituting a form of *protein-losing gastroenteropathy.* Infrequently the mucosal hyperplasia becomes metaplastic to provide a soil for the development of gastric carcinoma.

Hypersecretory gastropathy may well be a variant of Ménétrier's disease that differs only in the amount of parietal and chief cell hyperplasia, thereby producing high-normal or excessive levels of gastric acid. Most patients with this condition have a duodenal ulcer and, therefore, ulcer symptoms. Protein loss may occur but is less characteristic of this variant than of Ménétrier's disease.

Rugal hyperplasia associated with gastrinoma is only one feature of the Zollinger-Ellison syndrome, and so is discussed on page 987.

Other Forms of Gastritis

A *granulomatous gastritis* may occur in patients with sarcoidosis and regional enteritis, but more often appears as an isolated disorder. This last pattern of involvement is uncommon. The distinction between these three variants depends on the demonstration of extragastric diseases in the first two, leaving the third variant by exclusion. Moreover, isolated granulomatous gastritis tends to occur in persons 40 years of age or older, whereas the other two variants generally are found in younger individuals.

Another rare variant is *eosinophilic gastritis.* Here there is prominent infiltration of the mucosa and sometimes of the deeper layers of the stomach wall by eosinophils. This distinctive infiltrate may be accompanied by granuloma formation (allergic granulomatosis) and occasionally by acute vasculitis of the small arteries within the stomach wall (reminiscent of the changes in the allergic granulomatosis of Churg and Strauss, p. 522). This uncommon constellation of morphologic changes is generally thought to reflect some type of hypersensitivity reaction that may also involve other organs and tissues in the body.[39] Occasionally these patients have other forms of allergic disease such as asthma.

ACUTE GASTRIC EROSION AND ULCERATION

Focal, acutely developing gastric mucosal defects may appear following severe stress, whatever its nature—hence, the often used designation *stress ulcers.* Whether other agents such as aspirin, ethanol, smoking, corticosteroids, indomethacin, and phenylbutazone are also implicated is controversial. Generally, there are multiple lesions located mainly in the stomach, but occasionally also involving the duodenum. They range in depth from mere shedding of the superficial epithelium to deeper lesions that penetrate into or through the mucosa but rarely deeper. The shallow erosions are then, in essence, an extension of acute erosive gastritis (p. 810). The deeper lesions comprise well-defined ulcerations, but are not precursors of chronic peptic ulcers and have a totally different pathobiology.

Stress erosions and ulcers are most commonly encountered in patients with shock, extensive burns, sepsis, severe trauma; in any intracranial condition that raises intracranial pressure, e.g., trauma, brain tumors; and following intracranial surgery. The mucosal lesions associated with intracranial problems are referred to as *Cushing's ulcers,* while those seen with burns are known as *Curling's ulcers.* The genesis of the acute mucosal defects in these varied clinical settings is poorly understood. Acid-peptic secretions are requisite for their appearance, but hypersecretion of gastric acid is clearly documented only with Cushing's ulcers. Here, direct stimulation of vagal nuclei by increased intracranial pressure is proposed, and indeed the acid hypersecretion can be blocked by parenteral administration of anticholinergic drugs.

In contrast, low-to-normal levels of gastric acid are present in the other clinical settings associated with stress lesions. Mucosal hypoxia, related either to neurogenic or catecholamine-induced vasoconstriction, is perhaps the leading pathogenetic hypothesis for such lesions. The ischemic hypoxia may: (1) damage the mucosal barrier and permit backdiffusion of hydrogen ions, rendering the mucosa more vulnerable to acid-peptic attack; or (2) directly injure mucosal cells by oxygen or metabolic deprivation.[40] Systemic acidosis, a common finding in shock states, may also contribute to erosive lesions in the stomach, presumably by lowering the intracellular pH levels of mucosal cells already rendered hypoxic by stress-induced vasoconstriction. Whatever the mechanism may be, there is substantial evidence that it is mediated, at least in part, by blood-borne influences. In an ingenious experiment, one of a pair of parabiotic rats was stressed by being immobilized to a small skateboard. The other parabiont was free to move at will, towing its restrained, but "free-wheeling," partner. When the immobilized rat developed stress lesions, so did the other.[41]

A number of exogenous agents such as alcohol, smoking, caffeine, and certain drugs—aspirin, corticosteroids, indomethacin, and phenylbutazone—are widely thought to be ulcerogenic and might potentiate the appearance of stress ulcers. Best documented is the damaging effect on the mucosa of unbuffered aspirin, as pointed out on page 808, but what role it plays in the induction of acute stress ulcers is uncertain.[42] Chronic ethanol consumption and smoking may induce gastric hypersecretion and injure the mucosal barrier, but it is not certain that they produce mucosal defects. Similarly, corticosteroids and indomethacin have been associated with gastric complaints and even evidence of gastric bleeding, and although they may potentiate stress ulceration, their pathogenetic role is far from clear. In the last analysis, the pathogenesis of acute gastric stress lesions in man is unknown. Very likely they are multifactorial in origin; one influence may suffice in some cases, whereas in others several may be required.

MORPHOLOGY. The morphologic differentiation between an acute erosion and an acute stress ulcer is poorly defined. The term erosion is applied to those lesions confined to the upper levels of the gastric or duodenal mucosa. When they penetrate the full mucosal depth or muscularis mucosae, they are called acute gastric or stress ulcers. They may occur singly or, more often, multiply throughout the stomach and rarely in the duodenum. Typically they are found anywhere in the stomach and do not have the predilection for the antral region and lesser curvature exhibited by chronic peptic ulcers. Circular and small, they are usually less than 1 cm in diameter. The ulcer base is frequently stained a dark brown by the acid digestion of the accompanying bleeding (Fig. 18–11). The margins, which rarely show significant hyperemic reaction, are poorly defined because the ulcer is superficial in nature. The rugal pattern is not affected, and the margins and base of the ulcer are not indurated.

Depending on the duration of the ulceration, there may be some inflammatory infiltration in the margins and base. Red blood cells and fibrin often coat the base. There is usually conspicuous absence of underlying scarring or thickening of blood vessel walls such as is seen in the more chronic forms. Healing with complete reepithelialization occurs after the causative factors are removed. This regrowth of epithelium may be quite active and demonstrate many mitotic figures. The time required for complete healing varies from days to several weeks.

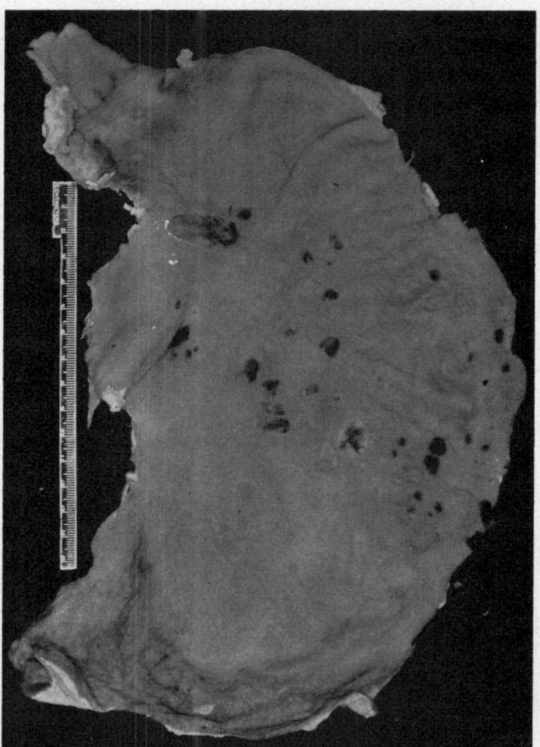

Figure 18–11. Acute gastric ulcers occurring in a patient dying of severe burns. The dark brown staining is produced by digestion of exuded red cells.

Acute gastric erosions and ulcerations are common in severely stressed patients. Over half of all those with extensive burns or major injuries develop these complications. Usually the first clinical evidence of their presence is painless, sometimes massive gastrointestinal bleeding. Obviously, the severely stressed patient already gravely ill is little able to cope with heavy blood loss. A strong case has been made, therefore, for preventive treatment of high-risk patients with antacids and cimetidine on the basis that, whatever their precise origins, acid-peptic activity is requisite for the development of these lesions.

PEPTIC ULCERS

Peptic ulcers are chronic, most often solitary, lesions that occur in any level of the gastrointestinal tract exposed to the aggressive action of acid-peptic juices. They are so common in industrialized nations that they virtually represent "stigmata of civilization." Characteristically, peptic ulcers occur in one of the following six sites, in descending order of frequency: (1) the duodenum, principally the first portion; (2) the stomach, principally the antrum; (3) the esophagus in glandular mucosa, e.g., Barrett's esophagus; (4) the margins of the stoma of a gastroenterostomy; (5) a Meckel's diverticulum of the ileum with heterotopic gastric mucosa; and (6) anywhere in the stomach or small intestine down to the ligament of Treitz in the Zollinger-Ellison syndrome. Approximately 98 to 99% of peptic ulcers occur in either the duodenum or the stomach in a ratio of about 4:1. About 10 to 20% of patients with a gastric ulcer have a concurrent duodenal lesion.

Wherever they occur, chronic peptic ulcers have a fairly standard, virtually diagnostic gross and microscopic appearance (Fig. 18–12). Despite this uniform morphology, gastric and duodenal ulcers may represent two somewhat distinctive diseases. Different influences

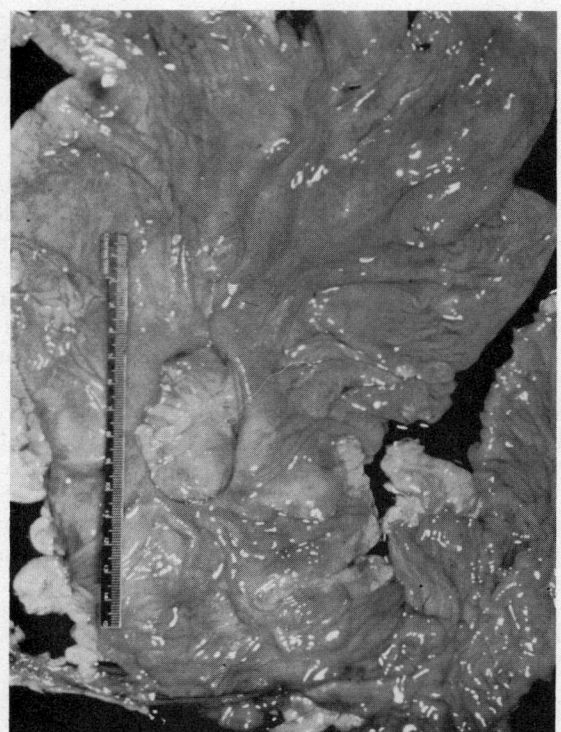

Figure 18–12. A large, deeply excavated peptic ulcer occurring in prepyloric region of stomach along lesser curvature.

are thought to be involved in their pathogenesis and there are further contrasts in their genetic linkages. Nonetheless, gastric and duodenal ulcers will be considered together, highlighting these variables.

EPIDEMIOLOGY. Peptic ulcers are remitting-relapsing lesions that are most often diagnosed in middle-aged to older adults, but they may first become evident in young adult life. They often appear without obvious precipitating influences and may then, after a period of weeks to months of active disease, heal with or without therapy. However, "once a peptic ulcer patient, always a peptic ulcer patient." Thus, it is difficult to express accurate data on the frequency of active disease. The best estimates of gastroduodenal ulcer frequency from autopsy studies and surveys of patients indicate a range of 6 to 14% for men and 2 to 6% for women.[43] The male:female ratio for duodenal ulcers is about 3:1, and for gastric ulcers more nearly 1.5 or 2:1. Women are most often affected at, or after, the menopause. In more individual terms it is estimated that an adult male in the United States has about 1 chance in 10 of developing an ulcer before the age of 65. It is of interest that a half-century ago, duodenal ulcer was much more common; the reasons for its decline are obscure, and no similar welcome trend has been observed for the gastric ulcer.[44]

Genetic influences are important in the predisposition to duodenal ulcer but appear to play no role with gastric ulcer. Duodenal ulcers are about three times more common in first-degree relatives of ulcer patients than in the general population. A 50% concordance for duodenal ulcers has been observed in monozygotic twins as compared with 14% in dizygotic twins.[45] Individuals of blood group O are about 37% more likely to develop these lesions than those of other blood groups. Another genetic trait is the capacity to secrete mucopolysaccharide blood group substances into salivary and gastrointestinal secretions. "Nonsecretors" are 50% more prone to duodenal ulcer than "secretors." An increased incidence of HLA-B5 antigen has also been identified in white males with duodenal ulcer.[46] An elevated serum level of immunoreactive pepsinogen I has been observed in several kindreds having multiple members with duodenal ulcers.[47] This genetic trait segregates as an autosomal dominant; it is hailed as a "marker" of a predisposition to duodenal ulcer. The lack of similar genetic findings in patients with gastric ulcers underscores the previously expressed suspicion that duodenal and gastric ulcers may represent different diseases sharing in common only "a hole in the gastroduodenal mucosa."

Duodenal ulcer is more frequent in patients with alcoholic cirrhosis, chronic renal failure, chronic obstructive pulmonary disease, and hyperparathyroidism. Numerous explanations have been offered to explain these associations but all are tenuous. All that can be said with any certainty is that increased serum calcium levels, whatever the cause, stimulate gastrin secretion and, therefore, acid secretion in the stomach.

PATHOGENESIS. The old aphorism—"the greater the volume of writing, the less certain the conclusions"—assuredly applies to the still unknown pathogenesis of peptic ulcer. Nonetheless, certain observations are well established.

1. *Some level of acid-pepsin secretion is requisite for the development of duodenal and gastric ulcers—"no acid, no ulcer."*[48]
2. *All peptic ulcerations probably arise because of an imbalance between the aggressive action of acid-pepsin secretion and the normal defenses of the gastroduodenal mucosa.*
3. *For duodenal ulcers the major causal influence appears to be exposure of the duodenal mucosa to excessive amounts of acid and pepsin.*
4. *For gastric ulcers the major causal influence appears to be some breakdown in gastric mucosal defenses against acid and pepsin.*

It would be simplistic, however, to ascribe duodenal ulcerogenesis solely to excessive gastric acid, and gastric ulcers solely to impaired defenses. Both sides of the equation are probably relevant for all peptic ulcers. Moreover, other influences must exist to explain the facts that peptic ulcers are usually focal solitary lesions and have a predilection for specific locations within the duodenum and stomach. Peculiarly, localized forces must be at work, but their nature is unknown. Within this framework of uncertainty we can turn first to a consideration of duodenal ulcer.

Duodenal Ulcers. There is a large body of evidence documenting that, in general, *duodenal ulcer patients have (1) an increased capacity to secrete acid and pepsin, (2) increased responsiveness to stimuli of acid secretion, and (3) more rapid gastric emptying.*[49] It should be noted, however, that not all these characteristics are present in every patient, and occasionally none are.

In general, duodenal ulcer patients have a higher mean basal acid output and maximal acid output than normal controls, and significantly higher levels than are present in patients with gastric ulcers. However, in almost half the patients with duodenal ulcer the hypersecretion is not very marked, and there is considerable overlap between the duodenal ulcer and normal groups. The acid hypersecretion can be directly correlated with an increased parietal cell mass, on average twice normal.[50] Here again, there is overlap with both normals and gastric ulcer patients. The basis for the elevated number of parietal cells is unknown. It could be congenital in origin and merely represent one end of the normal distribution in the population. On the other hand, the fact that individuals with the Zollinger-Ellison syndrome caused by hypergastrinemia also have an increased parietal cell mass indicates that it may be an acquired change. That an excessive level of acid is ulcerogenic is well brought out by the Zollinger-Ellison syndrome (p. 987), characterized by gastrin-producing neoplasms (or, less frequently, diffuse hyperplasia) of gastrin-secreting cells, hypersecretion of gastric acid and pepsin, and peptic ulcers in 90 to 95% of these individuals. In some instances, multiple ulcers develop concurrently and sometimes in aberrant locations, e.g., the upper jejunum. This "experiment of nature" underscores the importance of "too much" gastric acid. The pepsin levels in patients with duodenal ulcers correlate with the acid secretion.

Increased responsiveness to all known stimuli of gastric acid secretion is usually present in patients with duodenal ulcers.[51] This is not merely a function of their greater parietal cell mass, since the maximal secretory output is disproportionate to the basal acid output. The mechanism of this increased responsiveness is unknown. It does not appear to be due to increased vagal tone since vagotomy reduces the acid secretion in duodenal ulcer patients no more than in those with gastric ulcers. The weight of evidence points to increased gastrin drive, but what form it takes and why remain uncertain. Alkaline duodenogastric reflux may increase the sensitivity of parietal cells to gastrin.[52] The antral mucosa is held to be less susceptible to inhibition of gastrin release by hydrogen ions than is the case in normal controls.[53] Another possibility is that, although the serum levels of gastrin are normal, the gastrin-producing G cells in duodenal ulcer patients may elaborate larger amounts of G-17 gastrin relative to G-34, and (as pointed out on p. 807) the smaller molecule is a much more potent secretogogue. Whatever its basis, there is increased acid output in response to secretory stimuli.

Abnormally rapid gastric emptying is another frequent finding in patients with duodenal ulcer. As a consequence, gastric contents are emptied into the duodenum before the buffering capacity of a meal has effectively neutralized the gastric acidity. Thus, the duodenal mucosa is exposed to a greater acid load.[51]

Many more pathogenetic influences have been reported but all are of uncertain significance. Viral infection, possibly by herpes simplex, has been implicated on serologic grounds and on the basis of the similarity between herpetic mucosal ulceration and the duodenal lesions.[54] Deficient neutralization of gastric acid, because of insufficient pancreatic secretion of bicarbonate or inadequate elaboration of secretin in the small intestine, has been proposed. Since women have a low incidence of ulcers before the menopause, estrogens are vaguely suspected of being protective, but if this is so the mechanism is unknown. Similarly, the prevailing wisdom that ulcers, both duodenal and gastric, tend to occur in individuals having certain personalities—hard-driving, achievement-oriented "ulcer types"—can be neither confirmed nor denied. There are, however, numerous instances in which stress, anxiety, and fatigue have reactivated or perpetuated ulcer disease. Concern has been expressed about the ulcerogenic potential of cigarette smoking, corticosteroids, and certain drugs (principally unbuffered aspirin), but substantial evidence is lacking that they induce duodenal ulceration. These agents have also been incriminated in the reactivation of duodenal ulcer, but once again the evidence is unconvincing.

In conclusion, most of the accumulated data support the hypothesis that *the production of a duodenal ulcer is the consequence of excess exposure of the duodenal mucosa to the aggressive actions of gastric acid-pepsin that overwhelm the normal defenses.* The fact that most ulcers occur in the first portion of the duodenum might relate to the heavier burden of unbuffered acid in this segment. But it remains unexplained why a focal lesion, often 1 cm in diameter, results.

Gastric Ulcers. More is known about what is *not* involved in the pathogenesis of gastric ulcers than about what is involved. The older concept that poor gastric emptying (gastric stasis) with excessive release of gastrin and acid is responsible for their appearance is now fairly well ruled out. On the average, *patients with gastric ulcers have low-to-normal levels of gastric acid* but, as already emphasized, never true achlorhydria.[55] *Most of the accumulated data favor the existence of some primary defect in gastric mucosal resistance.*[49] Two influences have been observed with some regularity that might explain the lowered resistance: (1) an increased tendency to backdiffusion of hydrogen ions suggesting some derangement in the gastric mucosal barrier; and (2) the frequent association of chronic antral gastritis with the ulcer. Instillation of acid into the stomach or exposure of the mucosa to such agents as aspirin, bile salts, lysolecithin, and ethanol produces significantly more backdiffusion of hydrogen ions in patients with gastric ulcer than in controls or duodenal ulcer patients.[56] It has been possible in a few patients to confirm that such increased backdiffusion persists despite healing of the ulcer.

In 60 to 80% of instances, gastritis is present in association with gastric ulcerations. It invariably involves the antrum (chronic antral gastritis) but sometimes also the body of the stomach. It is significant that in most cases the gastritis persists after the ulcer heals, suggesting that it is primary and the ulcer secondary.[57] When we come to the issue of what initiates the gastritis, the ice becomes thin. *A favored theory proposes pyloric sphincter incompetence and reflux of bile acids and possibly lysolecithin.* Lower basal sphincter pressure has been observed in patients with gastric ulcer than in normal individuals or those with duodenal ulcers. Moreover, the sphincter pressure apparently does not increase in response to such normal stimuli as secretin, cholecystokinin, or intraduodenal amino acids or fat. Cigarette smoking also decreases the resting sphincter pressure and thus increases bile reflux. Thus, it is possible that bile acids and possibly lysolecithin diffuse back into the stomach, damage the mucosal barrier, and thus lead to chronic gastritis and simultaneously to increased acid production, with its ulcerogenic potential.[52] Attractive as this proposal may be, bile acid reflux cannot be seen in all patients with gastric ulcer, nor is antral gastritis always present.

Chronic exposure to exogenous damaging agents such as unbuffered aspirin, alcohol, and certain drugs has been invoked as another possible basis for gastric ulceration. *The minority of patients who do not have gastritis often are habitual users of aspirin.* It is proposed, then, that aspirin-induced backdiffusion (discussed on p. 808) may cause ulceration without producing gastritis, but this remains to be proved.[58] As pointed out earlier, most studies deal with patients on long-term aspirin therapy for rheumatoid arthritis, introducing the variable of another disease.[59] Chronic ethanol consumption, corticosteroids, indomethacin, and phenylbutazone have also been implicated in the development of gastric peptic ulcers, but solid evidence has not yet been presented. Nonetheless, most clinicians would avoid the use of corticosteroids, indomethacin, phenylbutazone, and other anti-inflammatory drugs in patients having any evidence of gastric disease or discomfort because of the concern that "where there is smoke, there must be a fire."

Yet another postulation for the pathogenesis of gastric ulcer invokes some deficiency—quantitative or qualitative—in gastric mucus. The supportive evidence derives largely from the healing effects of a variety of drugs that promote mucus output.[30] *There is the suggestion, then, that gastric mucus is protective, and lowering of this defense favors gastric ulceration.*

If one accepts the concept of lowered gastric mucosal resistance, the problem remains—why are ulcerations almost always solitary with specific preferential localizations? *Most gastric ulcers occur in the antral mucosa adjacent to the acid-secreting fundic mucosa.* Furthermore, they are almost always located in an area crossed by a broad band of circular muscle.[60] It is speculated that in this location peristaltic muscular contractions reduce mucosal blood flow, and thus lower defenses in the non–acid-secreting antral mucosa against the load of acid elaborated by the body and fundus.

In summary, the favored current theory for the causation of gastric ulcerations is as follows. *Ulcer subjects, for unknown reasons, are prone to mucosal injury by virtue of a defective mucosal barrier to backdiffusion of hydrogen ions. They are also predisposed to pyloric reflux and the development of chronic antral gastritis. In some, exogenous agents (in particular, unbuffered aspirin) may produce a level of mucosal damage that would not occur in normal individuals having normal mucosal barriers. Mucosal ischemia governs the localization of the ulcer when these injury-producing influences are present.*

MORPHOLOGY. The gross appearance of a chronic peptic ulcer, whether gastric or duodenal, is quite characteristic. Most can be recognized on sight—a fact of great importance, since occasionally the surgeon is called on to make this judgment at the operating table. As mentioned, in at least 80% of cases they are solitary lesions. In about 10 to 20% of patients with gastric ulceration there is a coexistent duodenal ulcer. Moreover, in the Zollinger-Ellison syndrome (p. 987) multiple ulcerations are occasionally present, sometimes in such aberrant locations as the jejunum. About 90% of duodenal ulcers occur in the first portion of the duodenum, generally within a few centimeters of the pyloric ring. The anterior wall of the first portion of the duodenum is more often affected than is the posterior wall. Gastric ulcers are predominantly found as mentioned in the antrum, and in one series about 95% occurred within 2 cm of the border zone, between the acid-secreting mucosa of the corpus and the antral mucosa. The most common site within this region is the lesser curvature. Nonetheless, chronic gastric ulcers may occur on the anterior or posterior walls of the stomach, as well as on the greater curvature. It used to be said that greater curvature ulcers are highly suspect of being ulcerative gastric cancers, but **as many as 14% of benign gastric ulcers occur on or in contact with the greater curvature.**

Peptic ulcers are usually small; well over 50% are less than 2 cm in diameter, and 75% are less than 3 cm. However, about 10% of benign ulcers are greater than 4 cm in diameter. Almost all these larger lesions occur in the stomach. Some carcinomatous ulcers are less than 4 cm in diameter. **Size, therefore, does not differentiate a benign from a malignant ulcer.**

The classic peptic ulcer is a round-to-oval, sharply punched-out defect with relatively straight walls perpendicular to the base. The mucosal margin may overhang the base slightly, particularly on the upstream portion of the circumference. The margins are usually level with the surrounding mucosa or are only slightly elevated (Fig. 18–13). Heaping up or beading of these margins is extremely rare in the benign ulcer but is characteristic of the malignant lesion. The depth of the ulcer varies from superficial lesions, involving only the mucosa, down to deeply excavated penetrating ulcers having their base in the muscularis. Penetration of the entire wall may occur, and occasionally the base of the ulcer may be formed by the adjacent pancreas, omental fat, or adherent liver. The base of all peptic ulcers is smooth and clean, owing to peptic digestion of any exudate. At times, thrombosed or even patent vessels that provided the source of a fatal hemorrhage project into the base. In most chronic peptic ulcers, underlying scarring causes puckering of the surrounding mucosa, so that the mucosal folds radiate out from the crater in spokelike fashion. Such a mucosal pattern provides a valuable clue to the location of the lesion for surgeon, pathologist, and radiologist alike. The gastric mucosa surrounding an ulcer is somewhat edematous and may be reddened, owing to the almost invariable gastritis.

The histologic appearance varies with the activity,

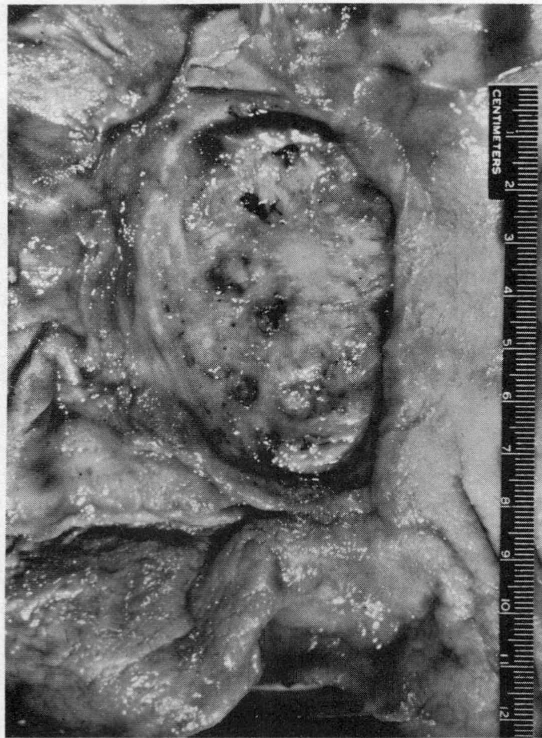

Figure 18–13. A large, benign peptic ulcer illustrating sharply defined margins, which overhang on proximal aspect (*right*) and shelve on distal aspect. Note absence of beading of margin and apparent absence of necrotic tissue in clean-appearing base. Despite the 8-cm diameter, no malignancy is present.

chronicity, and amount of healing. In the stage of active necrosis, four zones are classically demonstrable: (1) the base and margins have a superficial thin layer of necrotic fibrinoid debris not visible to the naked eye; (2) beneath this layer is the zone of active nonspecific cellular infiltrate with neutrophils predominating; (3) in the deeper layers, especially in the base of the ulcer, there is active granulation tissue infiltrated with mononuclear leukocytes; and (4) the granulation tissue rests on a more solid fibrous or collagenous scar (Figs. 18–14 and 18–15). The scarring characteristically fans out widely and may extend to the serosal surface. To be particularly noted are the mucosal margins, which bear the brunt of epithelial regeneration and inflammatory change. Often these glands contain goblet cells, a change referred to as "intestinalization." If carcinomatous transformation were to occur, these areas would provide the first histologic clue. The vessel walls within the scarred area are characteristically thickened by the surrounding inflammation and occasionally are thrombosed. The lamina propria of the mucosa surrounding the gastric ulcer is almost always infiltrated by plasma cells, lymphocytes, and a few neutrophils. The infiltrate may involve the entire antrum and in some cases may extend into the body of the stomach. When the gastritis is severe there may be some atrophy of the gastric glands.

Peptic ulcers will heal to varying degrees, depending on their chronicity and their size. The typical lesions without massive underlying scarring may completely reepithelialize to leave no residual trace. As the scarring becomes more intense, regeneration of the mucosa is less perfect and healing is retarded, presumably because blood supply is impaired.

CLINICAL COURSE. Gastric and duodenal ulcers represent chronic and recurrent lesions. They may heal, but there is always the risk of recurrence in the exact same focus or of the development of another ulcer elsewhere. Some ulcer patients are virtually asymptomatic, but much more often they experience pain, usually epigastric, which is variably described as burning, gnawing, or boring. The pain is intermittent; with duodenal ulcers, it classically begins 90 minutes to three

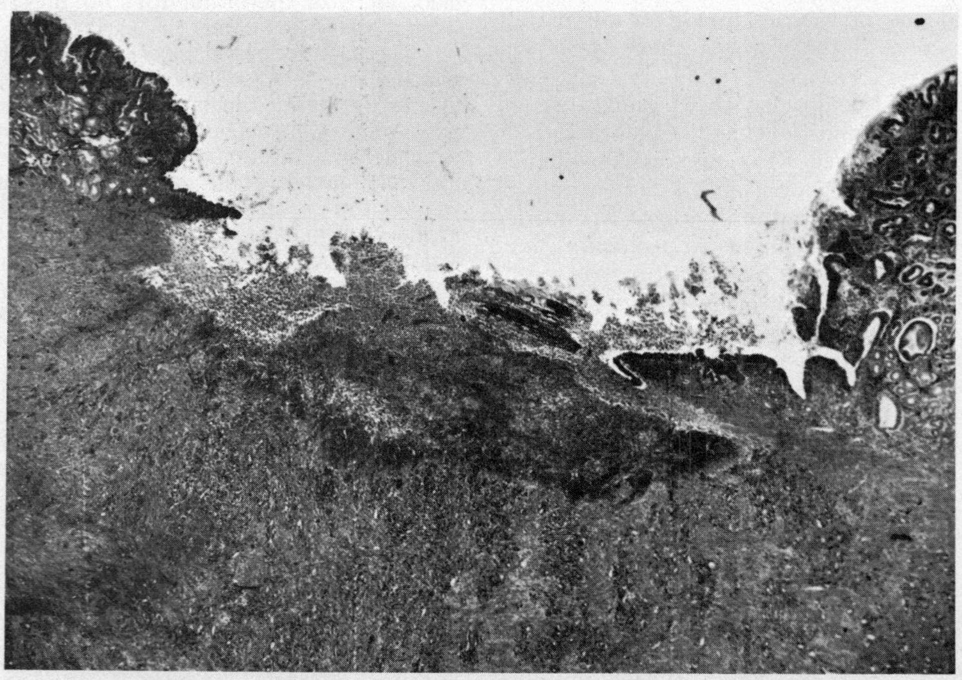

Figure 18–14. Low-power view of a peptic ulcer to illustrate depth of lesion.

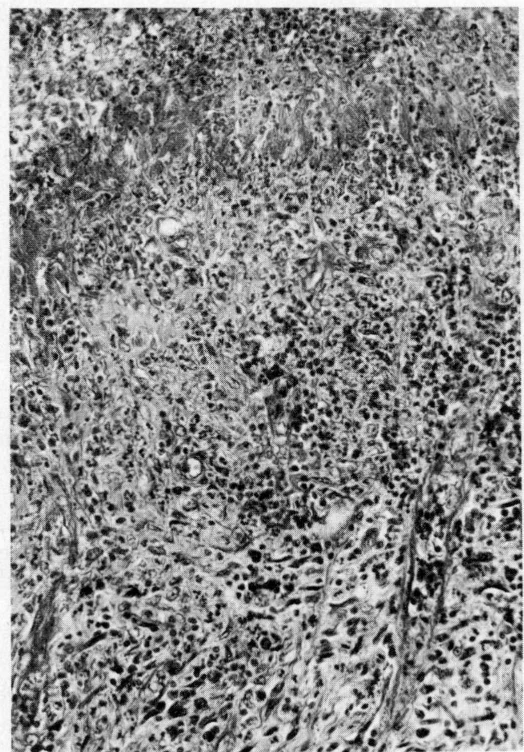

Figure 18–15. High-power detail of base of an ulcer demonstrating some of the zones that constitute the inflammatory response. The zone of fibrinoid necrosis is above.

hours after a meal and is relieved by eating (especially milk or other protein-rich foods), antacids, or vomiting. With gastric ulcers, about one-fifth of patients experience pain within the first 30 minutes after eating, and some get no relief from eating. Similarly, about half the patients with either gastric or duodenal ulcer have pain or discomfort one to two hours after going to bed. Ironically, such pain is more likely to occur in patients who eat a bedtime snack. Occasionally with penetrating duodenal ulcers, particularly those on the posterior wall, the pain may be steady, severe, and referred to the back or right upper quadrant, whereas with penetrating gastric ulcers the pain is more often referred to the left upper quadrant, thorax, and back. Uncommonly, the first manifestation of an ulcer is hematemesis. The "bleed" may be small and recurrent or may be massive, sometimes leading to shock. Other less common symptoms include anorexia, nausea, and vomiting. Weight loss is not uncommon with benign peptic ulcers, perhaps related to self-imposed dietary restrictions, and it should thus be noted that weight loss does not necessarily signify ulcerative cancer.

Under appropriate management such as regulated diet, antacids, and drugs to reduce acid secretion (e.g., cimetidine) or to increase mucus output, the pain abates and indeed may not recur if the ulcer heals. However, a recurrence of symptoms may follow at any time (weeks to years), often triggered by dietary indiscretions or stress. Whether patients with an ulcer should receive long-term cimetidine therapy to prevent recurrence is a moot question. A few instances of gastric carcinoma have been reported with such regimens, but the neoplasms may have been present at the outset unrecognized.[61] A major concern in the management of gastric ulcers is their differentiation from an ulcerative cancer, a concern that does not apply to duodenal ulcers since cancers almost never arise in this segment of the intestines. In one study of gastric ulcers, the incidence of unexpected cancer after thorough initial assessment was almost 4%.[62]

The diagnosis and localization of peptic ulcers involves a variety of techniques, including gastric analyses for acidity; upper gastrointestinal radiographic studies; endoscopy; and cytologic examinations of gastric aspirate or brushings to confirm the absence of exfoliated tumorous cells. The diagnosis of duodenal ulcer can usually be made readily by radiographic studies. With gastric peptic ulcers it is more difficult, because the lesion may be small and difficult to visualize in the capacious stomach. In most reported series, roentgenologic examination detects 90% of all gastric lesions and correctly interprets approximately 90% of detected lesions. The same data apply to gastroscopy, but x-ray studies and gastroscopy together accurately detect and diagnose 95 to 98% of gastric lesions.

The complications of peptic ulcer disease are (1) bleeding, (2) perforation or penetration into an adjacent viscus, (3) obstruction from edema or from scarring of the pylorus or duodenum, and (4) malignant transformation. Bleeding, sometimes massive, is the most common of these complications. It is estimated that one-fourth to one-third of peptic ulcers give rise to significant bleeding; indeed, massive hematemesis may be the first sign of existence of the ulcer in a previously asympto-

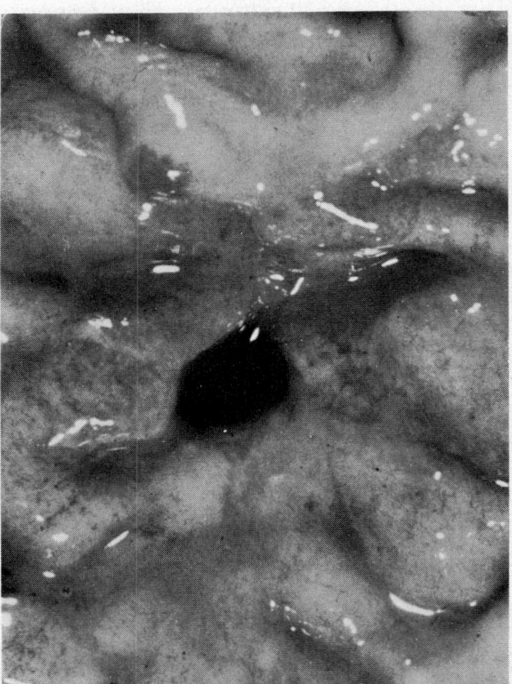

Figure 18–16. Close-up view of a small, completely penetrating duodenal ulcer. Diameter of mucosal defect is approximately 1 cm, the perforation being of almost equal size.

matic patient. The mortality rate in these bleeding patients ranges from 3 to 10%. Fatal hematemesis is responsible for about one-fourth of all deaths attributable to peptic ulcer disease. Although perforation of an ulcer is infrequent, occurring in only about 5% of patients, it is a grave complication and accounts for about 65% of all deaths in these patients (Fig. 18–16). Incredibly, perforation may be the first indication of the existence of the ulcer. Obstruction is encountered only in ulcers occurring within either the pyloric canal or the duodenum, and although it may produce serious vomiting and fluid-electrolyte disturbances, it rarely is a threat to life. As stated previously, malignant transformation of an ulcer is almost unknown with duodenal lesions. The frequency with which gastric ulceration leads to cancer is still debated. Although older reports have stated that 5 to 10% of gastric ulcers may be expected to give rise to a carcinoma, it is now clear that this occurs in 1% of cases or less. Sufficient evidence has now been accumulated to permit the statement that "cancers commonly ulcerate, but ulcers rarely cancerate." Despite these complications, most patients with peptic ulcers die *with* their disease rather than *of* it.

TUMORS OF STOMACH

BENIGN

Benign gastric tumors have variously been reported to be present in 5% to almost 25% of autopsies, which must reflect differences in the vigor and enthusiasm devoted to their quest.[63, 64] However, they are very uncommon *clinical* problems since most are incidental curiosities discovered at autopsy. They comprise leiomyomas, polyps, lipomas, neurogenic tumors, fibromas, hemangiopericytomas, hemangiomas, granular cell tumors, and heterotopic pancreatic rests. Only three lesions—leiomyoma, polyp, and aberrant pancreatic rest—occur with sufficient frequency to merit further consideration.

Leiomyomas and polyps are the two most common benign gastric tumors. Leiomyomas are well-demarcated, firm nodules (almost always less than 2 cm in diameter) arising within the muscularis. Thus, they are submucosal and, being small, do not erode the overlying mucosa. Morphologically, they exactly resemble their counterparts in other locations (p. 1136). Rarely, they grow to larger size (up to 5 cm in diameter) and produce hemispheric elevation of the mucosa with ulceration over the dome of the tumor. Such larger lesions may produce symptoms resembling those of peptic ulcer, particularly bleeding, sometimes massive. Most often, discovery before death is incidental to radiographic or endoscopic examination of the stomach for other reasons.

Polyps are the other most common benign neoplasm of the stomach but they are nonetheless rarities, found in about 0.5% of autopsies. Although they can be histologically classified into a number of subcategories, *the great preponderance are either hyperplastic (inflammatory) polyps or adenomas (some papillary), which differ greatly in their clinical significance.*[65, 66] About 80 to 90% of all gastric polyps belong to the hyperplastic category. Grossly, these are soft, pale gray, elevated lesions, seldom over 3 cm in diameter. Smaller ones tend to be sessile; larger ones may be pedunculated and have hemorrhages and ulcerations on their bulbous tips. Most often they occur singly, but rarely multiple polyps are present (Fig. 18–17). Located anywhere in the stomach, classically they are oval or round, smooth-surfaced lesions arising from the crest of a rugal fold. Microscopically, they appear to be composed predominantly of hyperplastic glands lined by cells similar to those in the gastric pits. Tubules and microcysts are formed, which are lined by a single layer of regularly arrayed cells. The intervening stroma often has a chronic inflammatory infiltrate. *Hyperplastic polyps are regenerative non-neoplastic lesions having no relationship to gastric carcinoma since they very rarely undergo transformation.* Generally asymptomatic, when they are discovered incidentally, simple polypectomy provides a cure. Often they are found in stomachs removed for carcinoma, but the association is probably coincidental.[67]

In contrast, *gastric polypoid adenomas* are true neoplasms, and carcinomatous transformation has been reported in 18 to 75% (average 50%) of these lesions.[68] Most are larger than hyperplastic polyps (averaging 4 cm in diameter); about 80% are greater than 2 cm in diameter. Sessile and flat or attached by a broad stalk with irregular, cauliflower-like heads, they are composed of gray-to-hemorrhagic firm tissue. Microscopi-

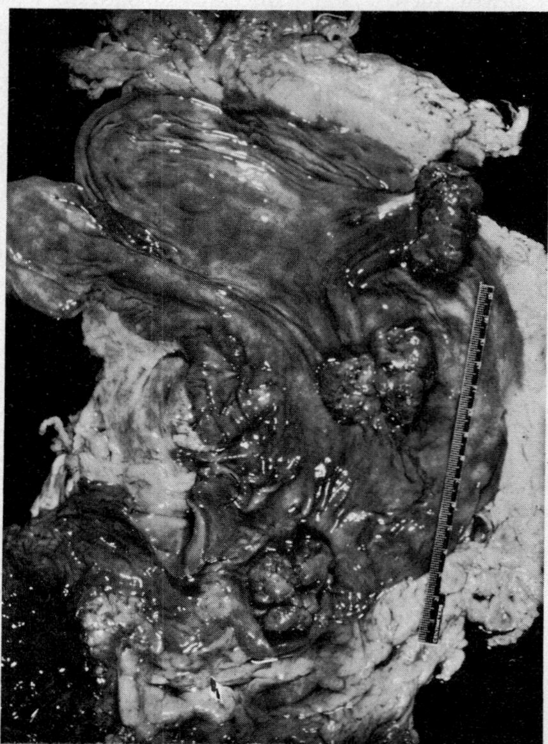

Figure 18–17. Multiple benign pedunculated polyps of stomach, 3 to 4 cm in diameter.

cally, they display the range of cellular dysplasia and atypia characteristic of tubulovillous or villous adenomas of the colon, described in detail on pages 866 and 865. Simple polypectomy is not sufficient in their treatment since carcinomatous glands may invade the cores of these lesions and extend into the underlying wall. Indeed, 10 to 15% of frank carcinomatous lesions have metastasized by the time of discovery. A gastric carcinoma may be present along with an adenoma, raising the possibility that it too was once a polyp.

Infrequently, multiple polyps occur in the stomach as part of the diffuse gastrointestinal polyposis of familial multiple polyposis (p. 867) or the Peutz-Jeghers syndrome (p. 868).

Submucosal rests of aberrant pancreatic tissue may be located in the stomach. Usually less than 1 cm in diameter, these intramural or submucosal rests may elevate the mucosa to produce sessile polypoid lesions sometimes visible in barium studies of the stomach. Their significance lies in their not being mistaken for a more ominous neoplasm.

MALIGNANT

Among the malignant tumors that occur in the stomach, carcinoma is overwhelmingly the most important and the most common (approximately 90 to 95%). Next in order of frequency, but far less common, are the lymphomas (3%) and leiomyosarcomas (2%). In addition, argentaffinomas (now often referred to as gastrointestinal endocrine tumors) may arise in this segment of the gut. Collectively, these four forms of neoplasia account for 95 to 99% of all cancers in the stomach.

Carcinoma

It is pleasant to note that the death rate from gastric carcinoma in the United States has been declining for many decades. The same can be said of Finland, Australia, and many other Western nations. Once at or near the top among the "cancer killers," gastric carcinoma is no longer a leading cause of cancer mortality in the U.S.[69] The current U.S. death rate from this form of cancer is about seven to eight per 100,000 population; in 1930 it was 33 per 100,000. The reasons for this welcome trend are not known but changing environmental influences are suspected. However, gastric carcinoma remains a disease to be reckoned with, being responsible for about 8000 deaths annually in the U.S. Indeed, in Japan it causes approximately one-half of all cancer deaths and is the leading cause of cancer mortality among adult males.

EPIDEMIOLOGY. As pointed out, there is striking variation among countries in the death rate from gastric carcinoma; Japan, Chile, Iceland, and Finland have rates about five to six times higher than those in the United States, Australia, and New Zealand.[70] First-generation migrants from high-risk countries to low-risk areas continue to suffer the rate of their country of origin even though they may have migrated early in life, suggesting that the causative mechanisms, whatever they may be, exert their effects in childhood. Subsequent generations, however, acquire the mortality rate of their new environment. In low-risk countries, most tumors are discovered in the fifth to seventh decades of life: only 5% of patients are under the age of 40. However, in high-risk countries the peak incidence is somewhat earlier. In all countries, whether high- or low-risk, there is an overall male preponderance. In the U.S. the male:female ratio is close to unity in young adults, rises to a peak of 2:1 in the sixth decade, and then declines to 1.5:1 in older individuals.

ETIOLOGY AND PATHOGENESIS. Although genetic factors may play some role in the predisposition to gastric carcinoma, most of the evidence suggests that environmental influences are of overriding importance. A family history of gastric carcinoma increases the risk, but it exerts only a small influence: only 4% of patients with a gastric carcinoma have a family history of this form of neoplasia. A slightly greater concordance has been noted for monozygotic twins than for dizygotic twins. Gastric cancer may be slightly more common in individuals of blood group A, but some analyses point to blood group O. Thus, whatever the genetic factors may be, they make at most a small contribution.

Most epidemiologists believe that *environmental influences underlie the origins of gastric cancer.* The range of implicated factors to be found in various reports is bewildering and includes diet, low socioeconomic class, urban dwelling, background irradiation, trace metals in the soil, and occupation. Greatest interest centers on the role of diet, since this would provide the most plausible explanation for the intercountry differences, but the search for specific causative dietary items has led only to confusion. Rice has been implicated in Japan, fried foods in Wales, grain products in Finland, and spices in Java, to name only a few. To date, no one has yet indicted marshmallows! However, agreement is developing on a few dietary correlations. A high intake of vegetables and fruits rich in vitamin C is alleged to exert a protective influence. On the other hand, nitrosamines and nitrosamides are suspected of causing gastric cancer. The source of these carcinogens in the diet was discussed on page 426; it is adequate here to recall that nitrites may be directly added as a preservative to foods such as smoked meats, sausages, and frankfurters. The declining incidence of gastric cancer in many countries might then be related to wider availability of refrigeration, which reduces the need for nitrite preservatives and simultaneously inhibits the reduction of nitrates to nitrites in stored foods. It is pertinent that this reduction reaction is also inhibited in vivo by vitamin C.

In addition to hereditary and environmental influences, *certain disorders impose an increased risk of gastric carcinoma:* (1) intestinal metaplasia of the gastric epithelium as occurs in chronic atrophic gastritis, and (2) gastric adenomas (polyps). As pointed out, atrophic gastritis or gastric atrophy, particularly when marked (as in patients with pernicious anemia), is frequently characterized by metaplastic and dysplastic epithelial changes leading to a long-term, 7 to 10% risk of gastric carcinoma. Somewhere between 18 and 75% of adenomas of the stomach undergo carcinomatous transformation. Fortunately, this type of gastric polyp is uncommon. Ménétrier's disease and hyperplastic secretory gastropathy impose a slightly increased risk. Common to all these "precancerous" conditions are epithelial intestinal metaplasia and dysplasia, producing what has been referred to as a "restless soil" predisposed to malignant transformation.[70] There is also histologic evidence to support the concept of a dispersed "restless soil"; many gastric cancers arise in discrete multicentric foci that coalesce as the tumor grows larger. Moreover, many gastric carcinomas are composed of intestine-like cells presumably arising in the metaplastic epithelium. It appears that intestinal metaplasia has a significant predisposition to cancer induction or is a forerunner.

Without knowledge of its etiology, the only hope for improving the outlook for patients with gastric carcinoma is earlier diagnosis while curative resection is still possible. It has been found that all gastric carcinomas arise as in situ lesions confined to the mucosal epithelium alone. The in situ lesion may represent a solitary focus, but in about one-half of the cases multiple foci, perhaps closely adjacent, arise simultaneously. The in situ lesion then progressively invades the lamina propria of the mucosa and eventually the submucosa, and, with time, ultimately the deeper layers. Metastases may appear at any stage of this evolution. *When the local lesion is still limited to the mucosa and submucosa, without penetration of the muscularis propria, it is now referred to as "early gastric carcinoma" (EGC).*[71] Thus, EGC is not congruent with in situ carcinoma. It is important to note that, as the term EGC is used, the cancer may, have metastasized to regional lymph nodes, as reported in about 5% of cases. Nonetheless, most of the time EGC is a potentially resectable curable lesion. Elaborate classifications of the gross morphology of EGC have been developed, dividing them into protruding, flat, and depressed categories, as well as others.[72] However, here it sufficies to note that in most instances EGC produces sufficient alteration of the mucosa to allow recognition of the lesion on barium study or endoscopy permitting confirmatory biopsy. In Japan (where gastric carcinoma is a major cause of death), remarkable results were achieved when these diagnostic procedures were included in annual clinical examinations of middle-aged to older adults. Whereas EGC in 1961 accounted for about 6% of all resectable cancers, recently it represented 35%. The five-year survival rates for patients with EGC after surgical resection is 60 to 95%, in comparison with 5 to 15% in the usual case mix.[73] Ample opportunity exists for discovery of early gastric carcinomas because they evolve very slowly and, in some instances, have been found to take eight years to become more invasive.[72]

MORPHOLOGY. Gastric carcinomas have been divided into a bewildering array of subsets based on gross patterns, extent of invasion, and histogenesis. Remarks here will be restricted to the major categories. The localization of tumors within the stomach is as follows: pylorus and antrum, 50 to 60%; cardia, 10%; whole organ, 10%; and the remainder in other areas. The lesser curvature is involved in about 40%, the greater curvature in 12%, and the entire circumference in about 25% of instances; the remainder are found on the anterior or posterior walls. Thus, a favored location is the lesser curvature of the pyloroantrum. Ulcerative lesions in this location may closely mimic, both radiographically and on inspection, chronic peptic ulcers that have a predilection for this same site. By contrast, a pyloroantral ulcerative lesion on the greater curvature is more likely to be malignant; once again, however, it can be benign. Carcinomas at the time of discovery range from relatively small tumors (about 10% are less than 2 cm in diameter) to lesions that involve virtually the entire stomach; about 80% are between 2 and 10 cm in diameter on discovery. They have been segregated into five gross patterns.

Early gastric carcinoma (10 to 35%). The frequency of this pattern is obviously dependent on the intensity of the diagnostic effort to uncover asymptomatic disease. The term **superficial carcinoma** is sometimes used as a synonym and may in fact be preferable, since the term early gastric carcinoma has in the past been applied to any form of gastric carcinoma amenable to curative resection. When used appropriately, early gastric carcinoma can only be defined histologically. It appears as flat areas of mucosal thickening and induration, more readily appreciated by palpation than inspection, or the lesions may be polypoid, ulcerated, or excavated. Some cover large areas, presumably because of multicentric origins. Typically the lesions can be displaced by lateral pressure over the underlying muscularis because, as mentioned, by definition they do not penetrate below the submucosa. Ultimate proof that such changes do indeed represent early gastric carcinomas rests with histologic examination.

Fungating carcinoma (about 30%). These are usually large intraluminal masses that project many centimeters above the surrounding gastric wall. They are generally infiltrative both laterally and in depth. Occasionally the tumor appears somewhat polypoid, merging with what will be described as the polypoid pattern (Fig. 18–18).

Ulcerated-infiltrative carcinoma (about 30%). This pattern may be difficult to differentiate on radiologic or endoscopic examination from chronic peptic ulcer. Characteristically, the tumor presents as a deeply excavated ulcer 2 to 8 cm in diameter, having irregularly beaded margins that overhang the crater base. The marginal, heaped-up beading is in contrast to the nonelevated, almost perpendicular wall of the margin of the benign ulcer. A further contrast is the relatively clean base of the peptic ulcer, whereas the carcinomatous ulcer typically has a shaggy, necrotic base. Moreover, the gastric wall about the crater is almost always infiltrated and thickened, but the lateral spread may be limited, rendering the differential diagnosis more difficult (Fig. 18–19). With limited lateral spread the rugal folds may extend virtually up to the margins of the tumorous ulcer.

Polypoid carcinoma (about 10%). This tumor appears as a very large sessile polyp that protrudes into the gastric lumen. The surface of the cancer may have some irregular superficial erosion or ulceration. The cauliflower-like mass may achieve a diameter of 6 to 8 cm. Tumor infiltration of the underlying wall is usually present but lateral spread is not prominent. Occasionally there is sufficient mucinous secretion to create a gelatinous appearance and consistency, giving rise to the term colloid carcinoma. This variant may arise in a previous adenoma.

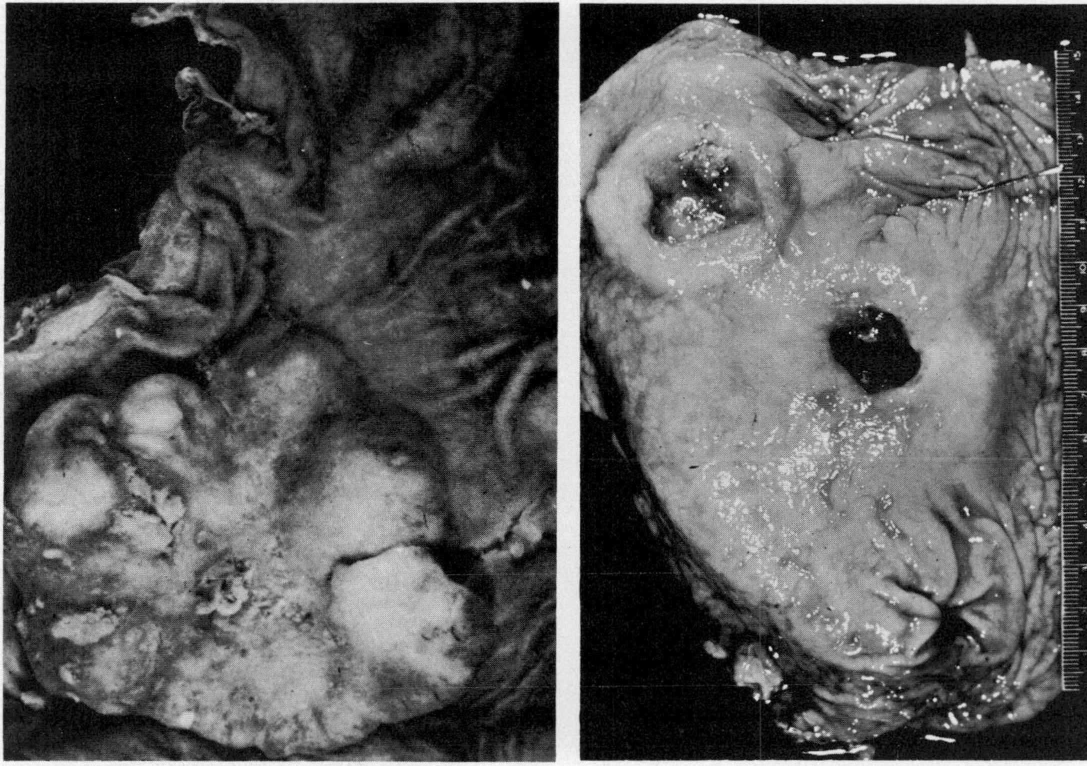

Fig. 18–18 Fig. 18–19

Figure 18–18. Fungating cancer of stomach showing beginning central necrosis and excavation.
Figure 18–19. Ulcerative pattern of gastric carcinoma. Late stage with diffuse infiltration of wall and two distinct crater formations, one to left with typical beaded overhanging margins, and one to right with deep excavation.

Diffusely infiltrative carcinoma (about 10%). This tumor extends widely, sometimes throughout the entire gastric wall, without forming a large intraluminal mass. The wall of the stomach, where involved, is typically thickened up to 2 to 3 cm and has a leathery, inelastic consistency. The rugal folds are generally flattened or totally obliterated. On transection there is obvious spreading apart of the layers of the stomach wall by gray-white infiltrative tissue, which is most prominent in the submucosal and subserosal regions. As will be seen, the infiltrative tissue is in part epithelial, and in part the consequence of a striking desmoplastic reaction. It is to this pattern that the older designations "leather-bottle" stomach and linitis plastica were applied (Fig. 18–20).

More recently, dissatisfaction has been expressed with this descriptive classification on the grounds that it does not have biologic significance. An alternative classification simply divides them into (1) expanding carcinomas and (2) infiltrative carcinomas.[74] **Expanding carcinomas** are characterized by an apparently cohesive mass of tumor cells that grow along broad fronts, creating a "pushing" invasive margin. With this type of invasion the extent of the lateral spread can generally be appreciated by the surgeon, to permit adequate margins of resection. In the more ominous **infiltrative pattern**, the tumor cells do not appear to be cohesive and so penetrate individually and in small clusters, resulting in poorly defined invasive margins and generally more diffuse involvement of the stomach. The correlation of the classic morphologic patterns with this newer pathobiologic schema is presented in Table 18–1.

Histologically, all gastric carcinomas are composed of basically two cell types: metaplastic intestinal cells or gastric mucous cells. Sometimes, mixtures of these cell types are found. The metaplastic intestinal cells contain large apical vacuoles (goblets) of mucus that usually can be shown to be, in part, acidic intestinal mucin but sometimes neutral gastric mucin. Microvillous striated borders may be found along the luminal surface of some cells. In addition, these cells contain alkaline phosphatase, amino peptidase, and beta-glucuronidase—enzymes not usually observed in normal gastric mucosal cells. In contrast, the gastric mucous cells resemble those found on the surface and in the pits of the gastric mucosa. Here the mucin is disposed in fine droplets in the apical one-half of the cell. In well-differentiated tumors, these two types of cells are readily identified, but with loss of differentiation and progressive anaplasia, both mucin secretion and distinctive cell characteristics disappear.

Either cell type may form well-defined neoplastic glands (adenocarcinomas), occasionally with papillary ingrowths (papillary adenocarcinomas). In less well-differentiated neoplasms, the cells tend to be disposed in disorderly masses, islands, or small clusters, or sometimes singly. In addition, the amount of mucin secretion varies, irrespective of the cell type. Numerous mucin vacuoles may distend cells or may coalesce and compress the flattened nucleus against the plasma membrane to create "signet-ring cells" (Fig. 18–21). In other instances, the mucus may lie within neoplastic glands. Sometimes, large lakes of secretion, in which isolated tumor cells or glands appear to float, literally dissect

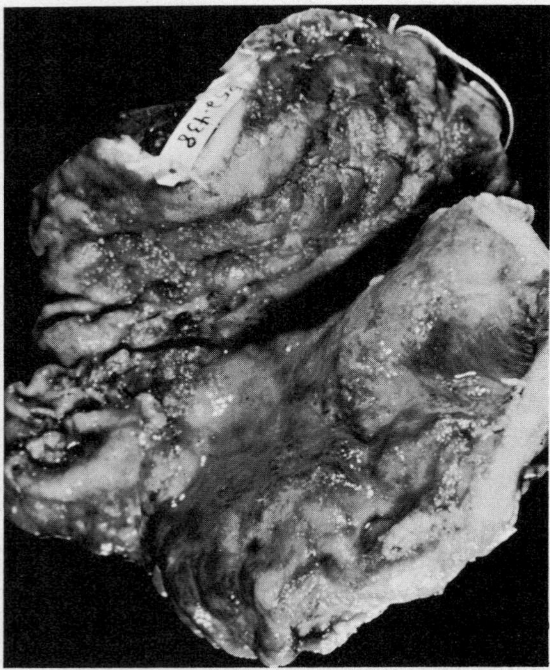

Figure 18–20. Gastric carcinoma infiltrative pattern (linitis plastica). Anterior wall is diffusely thickened, with flattening of rugal folds.

through cleavage planes. In diffuse infiltrative cancers the tumor cells are often accompanied by an abundant fibrous stroma. This desmoplasia accounts for much of the thickening of the gastric wall and it may be so florid as to render identification of the cancerous cells difficult.

Gastric cancers have also been divided by some experts into "intestinal-type" and "gastric-infiltrative" categories based on the predominant cell type in the neoplasm.[75] It is argued that this subdivision has pathogenetic and clinical significance. Intestinal-type lesions are more often of the expanding type, associated with chronic gastritis and the consequent intestinal metaplasia seen in chronic gastritis. This pattern has a somewhat better prognosis than the gastric infiltrative type and appears to be more closely correlated with environmental influences; it is the form predominantly encountered in high-incidence locales and countries. Perhaps the control of environmental influences accounts for the reduction in frequency and therefore the decline in mortality from gastric cancer in the United States and elsewhere.[76] However, the correlation between this histologic classification and the expanding and infiltrative patterns is at best imperfect, and indeed some neoplasms are composed of mixed-cell patterns probably arising from multiple foci of origin.

One additional variant of gastric carcinoma merits mention: a so-called undifferentiated carcinoma composed of sheets of small cells with round-to-ovoid, deeply hyperchromatic nuclei. Cytoplasmic secretory granules are evident on electron microscopy in these cells and some are argentaffin positive. Such tumors are presumably derived from endocrine cells found in the gastric mucosa as well as throughout the gut.[77] Because these neoplasms are capable of elaborating a variety of amine or polypeptide hormones, e.g., histamine, 5-hydroxytryptamine, and ACTH, they belong to the category of APUDomas (discussed on p. 842).

Infiltrative gastric carcinomas progressively penetrate the gastric wall to appear as small, gray-white subserosal nodules. They extend laterally, sometimes to invade the entire stomach and occasionally the duodenum. Interestingly, the duodenal invasion is generally subserosal, without involvement of the mucosa. Metastases to regional lymph nodes are present in 80 to 90% of specimens obtained from total gastrectomy. Widespread peritoneal seedings and metastases to the liver or lungs, as well as to other organs, are encountered in 20 to 40% of necropsies on patients who have died of this disease. One pattern of metastatic dissemination deserves special citation. Dissemination of tumor cells to the ovaries is encountered in about 10% of fatal cases of gastric carcinoma. The ovarian masses have been called **Krukenberg tumors.** These are discussed more

Table 18–1. PERCENTAGE OF TUMOR TYPE IN EACH GROSS FORM OF GASTRIC CARCINOMA

Gross Form	Expanding Carcinoma	Infiltrative Carcinoma
Polypoid	100%	0%
Superficial	100%	0%
Ulcerated	57%	43%
Fungating	96%	4%
Diffuse	9%	91%

From Ming, S.-C.: Gastric carcinoma. A pathobiological classification. Cancer *39*:2479, 1977.

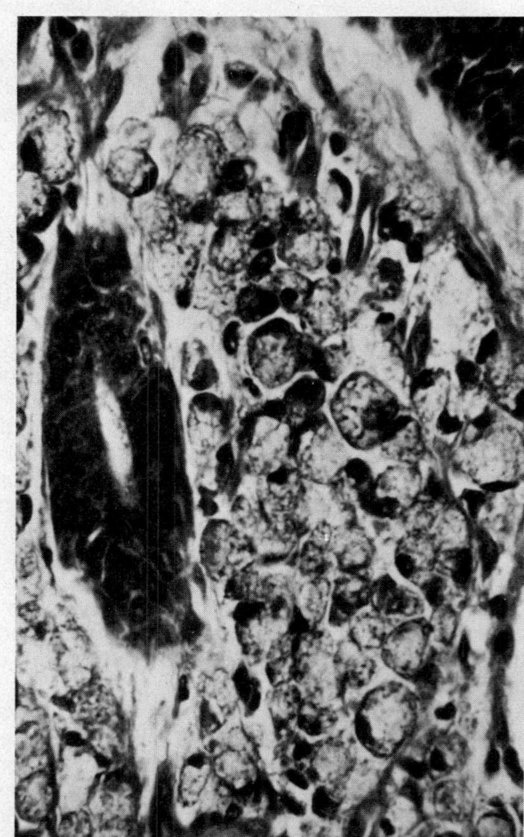

Figure 18–21. High-power detail of a gastric adenocarcinoma. The well-formed gland *(left, center)* contrasts with mucin-laden tumor cells, in some of which the nucleus is compressed against the membrane to create "signet-ring cells."

Table 18–2. CLINICAL FEATURES OF BENIGN AND MALIGNANT ULCERS

	Benign Ulcer	Malignant Ulcer
Age of patient	Tends to occur in younger individuals	Tends to occur in older individuals
Duration of symptoms	Varies from weeks to many years	Varies from weeks to months but rarely for years
Sex	Marked male preponderance	Slight male preponderance
Gastric acidity	May be normal or increased—anacidity rare	Usually normal levels but can be totally absent
Location of lesion	Usually lesser curvature of pyloric or prepyloric region—however, may be on greater curvature or anterior or posterior wall	Greater curvature of pyloric and prepyloric regions—however, may be on lesser curvature or in other sites in stomach
Size of lesion	Usually is less than 2 cm in diameter and rarely over 4 cm	Usually greater than 4 cm in diameter but may be smaller
Response to medical therapy	Usually shows prompt evidence of healing on adequate treatment	May respond to medical therapy but usually is refractory
X-ray	Demonstrates a small punched-out niche without involvement of surrounding wall	Demonstrates defect with irregular or heaped-up margins and possible involvement of surrounding wall and mucosa

completely on page 1155, but we might note here that Krukenberg tumors of the ovaries may also arise by spread to the ovary of other abdominal neoplasms such as carcinomas of the pancreas and gallbladder. Typically, the enlarged ovaries contain signet-ring, mucin-secreting cells in an abundant fibrous stroma. There have been remarkable cases in which clinical recognition of the ovarian mass(es) led to the identification of the primary gastric cancer, and at the time of laparotomy there was no evidence of metastases in other organs.

CLINICAL COURSE. Gastric carcinoma is an insidious disease that is generally asymptomatic until late in its course. At present the five-year survival rate for gastric cancer in the United States ranges between 5 and 15%, and this prognosis has not improved in the last 40 years.[78] The discovery of "early gastric carcinoma," having a much better prognosis, is totally dependent on its early recognition by endoscopy and radiographic barium studies. In individuals with more advanced cancer, the frequency of symptoms is as follows:

Symptom	*% of Cases*
Weight loss	80
Abdominal pain	72
Anorexia	57
Vomiting	44
Changed bowel habit	35
Dysphagia	14
Anemic symptoms	12
Hemorrhage	10

As can be seen, most of these symptoms are not very specific, rendering the diagnosis of this form of cancer very difficult. The abdominal pain is usually referred to the epigastrium but is often vague and intermittent. Occult bleeding is frequent, sometimes producing "coffee grounds" vomitus, but more often associated only with guaiac-positive stools. Some patients (10%) experience massive hematemesis, sufficient to cause shock. Achlorhydria or hypochlorhydria is present in about half the patients. Abnormally low levels of gastric acid are infrequent in young individuals and those with superficial carcinoma. When the achlorhydria is histamine- or pentagastrin-fast, one can assume that an ulcerative lesion is cancerous.

In view of the nonspecific presentation of this form of cancer, the diagnosis and, in particular, the differentiation of a benign from a malignant ulcer require careful evaluation, involving radiographic, endoscopic, cytologic, and finally biopsy studies (Table 18–2).

All too often the primary lesion comes to attention because of metastatic disease. Hepatomegaly due to metastases is already present at the time of first diagnosis in about 10% of cases. It may be accompanied by ascites and, less frequently, jaundice. Spread to remote lymph nodes sometimes heralds the existence of the gastric primary. *For uncertain reasons, the supraclavicular (Virchow's) nodes and scalene nodes are often involved and enlarged relatively early in the course of the disease.* Metastases to the ovaries *(Krukenberg tumors)* are sometimes discovered on pelvic examination, even before gastric symptoms appear. The tumor mass may seed the peritoneal cul-de-sac, producing a so-called "rectal shelf" on rectal examination. Thus, the prognosis for this disease to date has been bleak. On the basis of past practices of case finding, only about half the lesions at the time of discovery are sufficiently localized to permit an attempt at resection, accounting in large part for the overall five-year survival rate of 5 to 15%.[79]

Endocrine Cell Tumors (Argentaffinomas, Carcinoids)

Although these stomach lesions are rare, they tend, like those in the small and large intestine, to be infiltrative, aggressive tumors that metastasize in about one-third of cases. These are described in detail on page 842.

Gastrointestinal Lymphomas

Lymphomas in the course of their systemic dissemination may secondarily involve any segment of the gastrointestinal tract, but they may also arise as primary neoplasms anywhere in the lymphoid elements found normally throughout the gut. Irrespective of site of origin, they have similar morphologic characteristics and thus are all considered here as a group. Most arise in the stomach and small intestine. The gastric primaries represent only 3 to 5% of all stomach cancers. The next most favored sites, in order, are the ileum, large intestine, and appendix. Generally, in primary involvements, the lesion is localized to one site or at least one level of the gastrointestinal tract. In contrast, lymphomas primary in the mesenteric or retroperitoneal lymph nodes, or indeed primary outside the abdomen, typically affect multiple foci.[80] To a large extent, the primary lesions conform to the cytologic patterns encountered in lymph node disease (p. 658). Thus, in analyses of large series of cases using the Rappaport classification, diffuse histiocytic lymphoma constituted about 60%.[81, 82] Lymphocytic lymphomas, nodular or diffuse, well or poorly differentiated, were the next most common category. The remainder of the cases in one series included rare instances of primary Hodgkin's disease of the gastrointestinal tract. However, even the expert "lymphomaniacs" disagree about the interpretation of some lesions. Plasma cells are found in the background of other cell types in a significant number (20 to 40%) of small intestinal lymphomas.[80] This has led to these lesions being called plasmacytomas, plasmacytoid lymphocytic lymphomas, or Mediterranean-type lymphomas (because they were originally described in Israel).[83] We need not enter into this nosologic quagmire except to note that they are now called immunoproliferative small intestinal lymphomas, and some elaborate specific immunoglobulins, particularly alpha heavy chains, as do plasmacytomas arising elsewhere.[84] In contrast, in another series of gastrointestinal lymphomas, none were interpreted as these lesions.[85]

Primary lymphomas assume a variety of gross appearances. In most cases only one segment of the gut is involved. Infiltrative lesions with raised margins, often having ulceration of the overlying mucosa, constitute the most frequent macroscopic pattern. Next most common are polypoid, often multilobate masses that project into the lumen and sometimes have surface ulcerations. Occasionally, particularly in the stomach, the tumor infiltrates widely, producing giant rugal folds (Fig. 18–22) to thereby mimic hypertrophic gastritis (p. 812). All patterns are softer, grayer, and more rubbery than the usual carcinoma. Central necrosis may lead to perforation of the gut. In about half the cases the tumor is restricted to the gastrointestinal tract; regional lymph nodes are already affected at the time of diagnosis in an additional third. In the remainder there is widespread dissemination both to abdominal lymph nodes and viscera and to extra-abdominal sites.

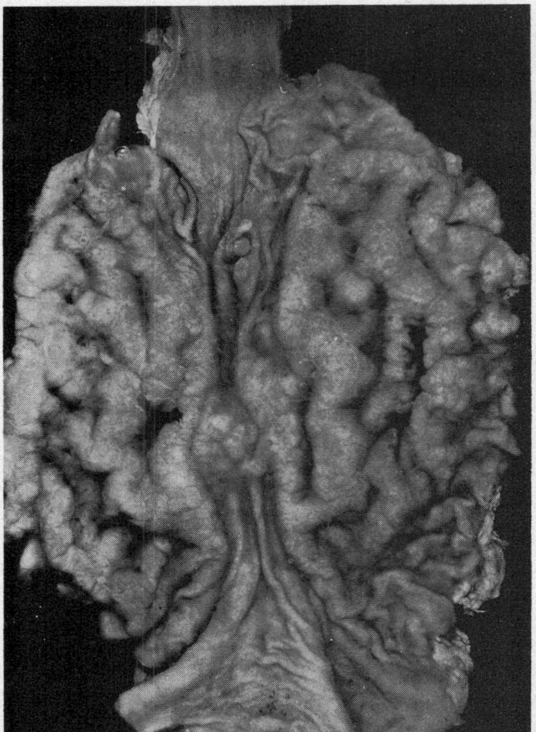

Figure 18–22. Lymphoma of stomach showing marked accentuation of rugal folds produced by diffuse infiltrative type of growth.

Histologically, the lesions replicate the cytologic features found in lymphomatous disease primary in the lymph nodes (p. 657).

Although children may be affected, gastrointestinal lymphoma is predominantly a disease of the middle-aged of either sex. Primary gastric involvement is often called to attention because of ulcer-like symptoms. Tumors arising in the small intestine most often produce manifestations of intestinal obstruction accompanied by pain, hemorrhage, and, rarely, perforation. When they involve large segments of the small intestine, they can lead to the malabsorption syndrome (p. 846). Lymphomas in general have a much better prognosis than carcinoma, and many are resectable with cure. Chemotherapy, radiation, or both often induce long remissions in nonresectable cases. The reported five-year survival rate ranges from 30 to 55%. The prognosis is chiefly dependent on the extent of the involvement, and does not appear to be affected by the histologic type. Several additional details are worthy of note. There is a reported association of gastrointestinal lymphoma with ulcerative colitis, Crohn's disease, and celiac disease.[86] There is also a greater-than-chance concurrence of carcinomas in patients with gastrointestinal lymphoma. Most of these carcinomas have arisen in the stomach in close proximity to gastric lymphomas, but some have been primary in extraintestinal sites.[87]

It is important to caution that chronic gastritis and chronic peptic ulcer may lead to massive inflammatory infiltrates into the stomach wall, creating more than a casual resemblance, both grossly and microscopically, to a true lymphoma. Such inflammatory lesions have been designated "pseudolymphoma." These non-neoplastic infiltrates differ histologically from true lymphomas by having well-developed lymphoid germinal cell centers as well as polymorphic infiltrative cells including lymphocytes, histiocytes, plasma cells, and fibroblasts. Lymphomas, in contrast, are typically monomorphic. Moreover, at the margins of the pseudolymphomatous lesions there is usually sufficient fibrosis to suggest an inflammatory origin. The use of immunohistochemical techniques to identify cell markers and cell-related immunoglobulins has greatly facilitated differentiation of the many cell types to be found in pseudolymphomas from the monoclonality of lymphomas.[88]

Sarcomas

The most frequent sarcomas in the stomach are leiomyosarcomas, fibrosarcomas, and endothelial sarcomas. Both individually and collectively they are rare. Among these, only the leiomyosarcoma and the closely related leiomyoblastoma occur sufficiently often to merit brief comment.

Leiomyosarcomas may appear at any age and in either sex. Grossly, either they produce large, bulky, intramural masses, which eventually fungate and ulcerate into the gastric lumen, or they project subserosally. On cross section they have the typical soft, fish-flesh appearance of all sarcomas and frequently contain areas of hemorrhage, necrosis, or cystic softening. Histologically they resemble leiomyosarcomas found elsewhere (p. 271). Because they tend to grow as cohesive masses without the diffuse infiltrative characteristics of gastric carcinomas, many are amenable to surgical removal, yielding a 50 to 60% five-year survival rate. Metastases, however, are present in about one-third of cases.

Leiomyoblastomas are uncommon gastric tumors that rarely arise elsewhere. Nonetheless, their recognition is important because, despite their ominous gross and microscopic appearance, many are biologically benign. Their malignant potential is intermediate between that of the leiomyoma and that of the leiomyosarcoma. Grossly, they are usually large, fairly well-circumscribed intramural masses that project into the gastric lumen, sometimes with ulceration of the gastric mucosa over the dome of the mass. On cross section they may closely resemble the leiomyosarcoma. Microscopically they are characterized by large pleomorphic cells having central nuclei that are variable in size and shape. The cells have an abundant eosinophilic or clear cytoplasm that sometimes leaves distinct, clear, perinuclear halos. Ultrastructural studies in some cells reveal microfilaments typical of smooth muscle cells, which, with the immunoperoxidase technique, can be shown to be myosin. Special stains for reticulin (silver, gold techniques) disclose an abundant reticulum that encloses individual cells. Mitoses may be scant or abundant and the biologic behavior appears to be related to the number of mitoses. When five or more are present in ten high-power fields, the neoplasm is very likely to be malignant and have metastatic potential. In several analyses 5 to 30% have metastasized.[89]

Metastatic Carcinoma

Metastatic involvement of the stomach is a rarity. Although such spread may be produced by carcinomas arising elsewhere, particularly breast carcinomas and malignant melanoma, the most common sources of gastric metastases are generalized lymphomatosis and leukemia. Most lesions are multiple, and differ from primary tumors in that they usually affect the submucosa and muscularis primarily, and only secondarily invade the mucosa. Central ulceration of these masses may occur.

Small Intestine

NORMAL

Certain features of the normal structure and function of the small intestine have particular clinical significance. The adult human small intestine ranges from 12 to 20 feet in length and, unfortunately, is prey to as many diseases as its footage would imply. The duodenum, which is the first portion of the small intestine, is the widest and most fixed section and is shaped like the letter C. The head of the pancreas nestles in the concavity of the C. The common bile duct, ampulla of Vater, and pancreatic ducts, and the proximity to the liver, gallbladder, and colon, make this short segment the most critical area for lesions in the entire small intestine.

There is no sharp demarcation between the jejunum and ileum. Customarily, the proximal two-fifths is considered jejunum. The diameter of the proximal jejunum is virtually twice that of the distal ileum. The arterial supply of the small intestine is largely derived from the superior mesenteric artery, which progressively divides as it approaches the gut. A small lesion, then, in the root of the mesentery may compromise the vascular integrity of yards of small intestine. However, the arterial branches are richly interconnected by arching arcades. Thus, obstructive lesions of a secondary branch of the superior mesenteric artery may be without effect. When vascular lesions occur close to the gut in the small terminal "end arteries," small ischemic lesions result. Since the lymphatic drainage essentially parallels the vascular supply but does not have the intricate patterns of arcades, involvement of a small focus of lymph nodes or lymphatics produces a rather large segment of intestinal lymphedema.

The histologic identification of the small bowel rests on the recognition of villi. They are most numerous and leaflike in the duodenum, and become progressively less well defined and finger-like toward the terminal ileum. Between their bases and extending into the deeper levels of the mucosa are the pitlike crypts. The height of the villi is three times greater than the depth of the crypts, a point of some importance in the interpretation of small bowel biopsies. Distinctive of the duodenum are the elaborately branched Brunner's glands, which penetrate the muscularis mucosae into the submucosa. The lamina propria in the small intestine contains not only phagocytic cells but also lymphocytes (in great abundance in the ileal Peyer's patches) as well as plasma cells. Immunoglobulins, particularly IgA, are synthesized by these cells and probably serve an important protective function against bacterial invasion.

The epithelium lining the crypts differs from that covering the villi. Four types of crypt epithelial cells have been identified: (1) Paneth cells, (2) undifferentiated cells, (3) goblet cells, and (4) endocrine cells.[90] *Paneth cells* have a basophilic cytoplasm that contains large secretory granules, but the nature of their secretion is unclear. Studies suggest that these cells contain lysozyme, IgG and IgA.[91] *Undifferentiated cells* are the most numerous in the crypts. They take up IgA from the lamina propria, conjugate it with a secretory component, and secrete water and electrolytes. They also contain small secretory granules that are best visualized in PAS stains, but the nature of the secretion is not known. *Goblet cells* are packed with mucigen granules, creating large apical vacuoles that, when seen in the light microscope, give these cells some fanciful resemblance to brandy goblets. The goblet cells are obviously the source of the mucus secretion of the small intestine. In the adult, *there are at least nine distinct populations of endocrine cells* separable by ultrastructural and immunohistochemical features.[92] All contain well-defined secretory granules, and at least one subset is argentaffin and chromaffin positive. The argentaffin cells are discussed later in the consideration of argentaffinomas. The endocrine cells secrete gastrointestinal hormones such as secretin, cholecystokinin, and serotonin, as well as a kallikrein-like enzyme that may participate in the formation of bradykinin. Excessive secretion of some of these products by argentaffinomas accounts for the carcinoid syndrome (p. 842).

The surface covering of the villi is made up of three types of cells, principally absorptive cells interspersed with goblet cells and a few endocrine cells. These are fused together by "tight junctions" that maintain a virtually impermeable barrier between the luminal contents and the subepithelial lamina propria. All molecules save the smallest, such as sodium, chloride, and water, which diffuse to some degree between cells, must pass through the surface mucosal cells. The absorptive cells are highly specialized on their luminal surface by microvilli (seen only in electron micrographs), expanding their luminal surfaces perhaps 30-fold. Microvilli are remarkably uniform, tall, straight, and regularly spaced over the villi but become shorter, blunter, and more irregular in the crypts (Fig. 18–23). They in turn are covered by a firmly attached, filamentous-appearing glycoprotein coat that is secreted by the absorptive cells. This microvillous, membrane-fuzzy coat complex provides an ideal milieu for the terminal digestion of foodstuffs by amylases and proteases. The microvillous membrane also contains disaccharidases and certain peptidases involved in the terminal degradation of saccharides and polypeptides to their monosaccharide and amino acid residues, as well as other enzymes and carrier proteins involved in sugar and amino acid transport.[93] The membrane also possesses specific receptors, such as those in the ileum for intrinsic factor–vitamin B_{12} complexes.

The regenerative capacity of the small intestinal epithelium is remarkable. Cellular proliferation is confined to the basal portions of the crypts; from here, by some extraordinary process, the cells slide along the crypt and villous surface to be shed at the tip of the villus within six to seven days. Thus, the entire epithelial covering of the small intestine is replaced every week. During this migration the cells undergo differentiation with the progressive acquisition of intramembrane particles (probably representing membrane-associated enzymes) and the development of the tight junctions, which are better organized in villous cells than in crypt cells.[94] The looser junctions in the crypts suggest that this region is more involved in secretion of ions and water than the surface of the villi. The rapid renewal of the small intestinal epithelium provides a remarkable capacity for repair, but in another sense renders the small intestine particularly vulnerable to agents that interfere with cell replication, as, for example, radiation or cancer chemotherapeutic drugs.

PATHOLOGY

The principal types of pathologic conditions in this segment of the gut are inflammatory disorders and derangements that lead to malabsorption. Because the

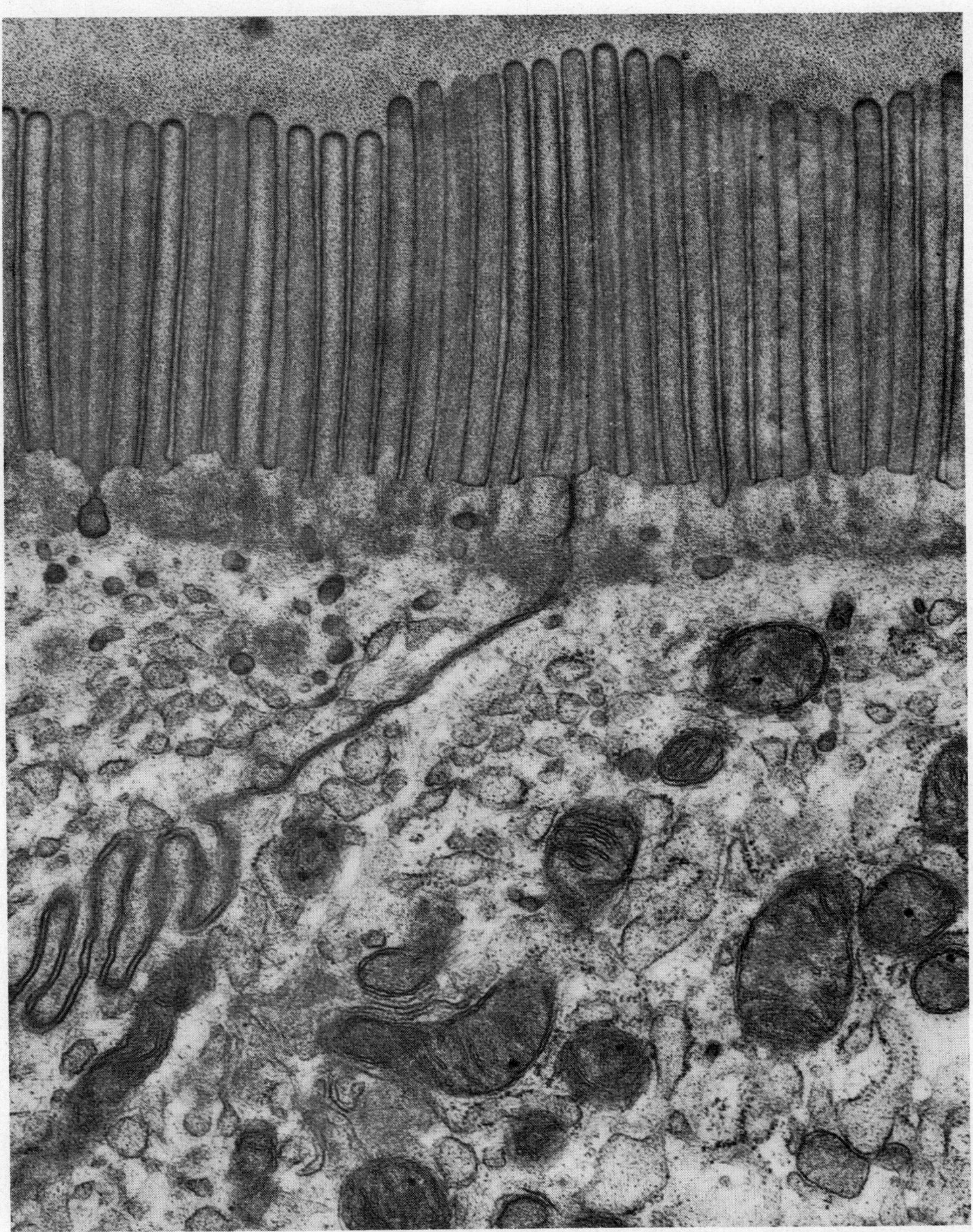

Figure 18–23. High-power detail of tip of a villus of normal mouse duodenal mucosa with elegant microvilli. Mitochondria, endoplasmic reticulum, and interlocking cell borders are evident. (Courtesy of Dr. L. Gottlieb, Mallory Institute of Pathology.)

lumen is narrow, intestinal obstruction is a frequent complication of some of the lesions. In contrast to those of the stomach and colon, primary tumors are extremely rare in the small intestine.

CONGENITAL ANOMALIES

Numerous developmental defects of rotation and reduplication occur in the small intestine, but they are rare. Four other anomalies are encountered sufficiently often to merit description.

CONGENITAL ATRESIA AND STENOSIS

In atresia, either a segment of the bowel is entirely missing, leaving a proximal segment with a blind end separated at some distance from the distal bowel, or the upper and lower segments are united by a solid fibrous cord. Stenosis, on the other hand, implies narrowing that may be either mild and of little consequence or severe and obstructive. Atresias and stenoses may occur singly or multiply (approximately 5 to 10% of patients), involving any level of the jejunum or ileum. Obviously, atresias and severe stenoses cause intestinal obstruction that leads to persistent vomiting, usually within the first two weeks of life. Early surgical intervention to prevent serious fluid, electrolyte, and nutritional problems is curative. However, other more serious developmental anomalies may also be present, prejudicing survival in these patients.

DIVERTICULA OF DUODENUM, JEJUNUM, AND ILEUM

In the muscular wall of the jejunum and ileum, the points where mesenteric vessels and nerves enter provide loci of weakness where the mucosa and submucosa may herniate into the mesentery. Such diverticula occur about one-tenth as often as duodenal diverticula and are therefore exceedingly rare. They are more frequent in older individuals, perhaps owing to the role played by continued intraluminal pressure in their causation. Because they dissect into the fat of the mesentery, they are easily missed at autopsy. Histologically, the muscular coats of the diverticula are absent or thinned, leaving only the mucosa and submucosa. In rare instances, intestinal stasis within their lumina has led to considerable overgrowth of bacteria that use excessive amounts of vitamin B_{12}, producing a pernicious anemia–like syndrome. Under these circumstances, the diverticula produce an analog of the blind-loop macrocytic anemia of experimental animals. Very rarely, the diverticula are the sites of intestinal bleeding or inflammatory perforation.[95] Those of the duodenum may impinge on the biliary and pancreatic ducts.

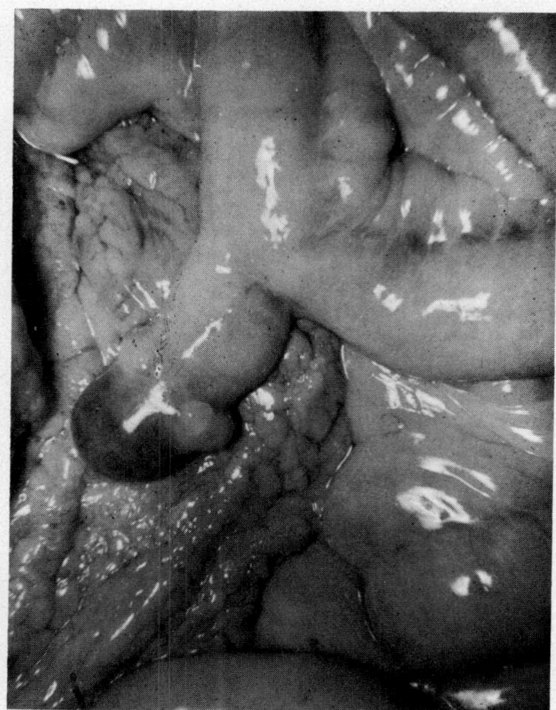

Figure 18–24. Meckel's diverticulitis. Tip of diverticulum is reddened because of peptic ulceration secondary to a rest of gastric epithelium.

MECKEL'S DIVERTICULUM

Persistence of a vestige of the omphalomesenteric duct may give rise to a solitary diverticulum, usually within 12 inches of the ileocecal valve. Rarely, it occurs in more proximal locations, sometimes up to 2 to 3 feet from the ileocecal valve.

These diverticula vary in conformation from a fibrotic cord to a pouch having a lumen greater than that of the ileum and a length as much as 5 to 6 cm. The composition of the wall is similar to that of the small bowel, but there are several points of difference. Heterotopic rests of gastric mucosa are found in about one-half of all Meckel's diverticula. Peptic ulceration sometimes occurs in the mucosa of the diverticulum adjacent to the island of gastric mucosa (Fig. 18–24). Mysterious intestinal bleeding or symptoms resembling an acute appendicitis may result. Rarely, perforation occurs, or the inflammatory disease causes adhesion to surrounding loops of bowel with resultant intestinal obstruction. Infrequently, pancreatic rests may occur in Meckel's diverticula.

PANCREATIC RESTS

Foci of essentially normal pancreatic tissue, appearing as small mucosal polyps, occur anywhere in the small bowel, least often in the jejunum. They are of chief interest to the surgeon and endoscopist, since they should not be confused with a primary tumor of the bowel. They usually are not more than 1 or 2 cm in diameter and present, on cut surface, the typical yellow, lobulated appearance of normal pancreatic tissue. These rests usually are freely movable and are not attached to the underlying muscularis.

ISCHEMIC BOWEL DISEASE

The small intestine alone, the colon alone, or sometimes both may sustain hypoxic injury related to various causes of vascular compromise. Collectively, all these lesions are designated acute mesenteric ischemias. The lesions of the colon are sometimes referred to as ischemic colitis.[96] Depending on the severity of the reduction in blood flow, three morphologic patterns are somewhat arbitrarily segregated: (1) *infarction or gangrene of the bowel,* implying transmural ischemic necrosis related to total or near-total reduction in blood flow; (2) *hemorrhagic gastroenteropathy,* characterized by hemorrhage and necrosis limited to the mucosa and submucosa with sparing, usually of the deeper layers, related to less extreme reduction in blood flow; and (3) *chronic ischemia* leading in time to fibrotic narrowing of affected bowel. Classically, these categories have implied that infarction is the result of total mesenteric occlusion by a thrombus or embolus; hemorrhagic gastroenteropathy follows acute nonocclusive hypoperfusion; and chronic ischemia is the consequence of severe organic vascular narrowing inducing a persistent perfusion deficit. However, chronic ischemic fibrosis related to ischemia is difficult to segregate from fibrotic narrowing secondary to bacterial injury. Because there is no sharp line dividing infarction from severe hemorrhagic enteropathy, a more descriptive simplified terminology has been proposed: (a) *transmural infarction;* (b) *mural infarction*—if the injury extends from the mucosa into the submucosa and muscularis; and (c) *mucosal infarction*—if the lesion extends no deeper than the muscularis mucosae.[97] Here we shall adopt the newer terminology.

TRANSMURAL INTESTINAL INFARCTION

Transmural infarction is more common in the small intestine than in the large intestine, probably because of differences in the patterns of blood supply. The small intestine is totally dependent on its mesenteric vessels, but the large intestine throughout much of its course is closely applied to the posterior abdominal wall from which it may derive accessory blood supply and venous drainage. Transmural infarction usually involves one (often long) segment of gut, although rarely several discontinuous areas are affected.

The basic patterns of transmural infarction are *thromboses or embolism of the superior mesenteric artery* affecting only the small bowel (about 50% of acute mesenteric ischemia); *mesenteric venous thromboses* involving the small or large bowel or both (25% of cases); and *partial narrowing of arteries or veins with superimposed reduced flow* affecting the small or large bowel or both (25% of cases).

Arterial thromboses are most often triggered by advanced atherosclerosis. The superior mesenteric artery is commonly involved, close to its origin, but sometimes also the celiac axis and/or the inferior mesenteric artery. Because of the rich anastomotic communications between these three major arterial trunks, critical reduction of flow may require compromise of at least two. Sometimes cardiac failure or a hypotensive crisis in a patient with marked atherosclerotic narrowing (without total occlusion) may suffice to cause infarction. Vasospasm of uncertain cause superimposed on vascular narrowing is another potential pathogenetic mechanism.[98] Other causes of arterial narrowing, usually with superimposed thrombosis, include dissecting aortic aneurysm, tumorous invasion of the root of the mesentery, and *fibromuscular hyperplasia of the intestinal arteries.* The last-mentioned refers to vascular narrowing caused by hyperplastic thickening of the intima and media of the terminal straight portions of the mesenteric arteries just before they enter the bowel.[99] Most individuals with this form of vascular disease are elderly, have cardiac failure, and are on digitalis therapy. Digitalis toxicity or a sensitivity reaction to the drug may play some role in the induction of the vascular lesions. Arterial thrombosis has also been reported in association with the use of oral contraceptives having a high estrogenic content. More often, oral contraceptives induce venous thromboses. Acute arteritis, such as may be encountered in polyarteritis nodosa, systemic lupus erythematosus, and rheumatoid disease, is a rare cause of arterial thrombosis.

Embolic arterial occlusion involves most often the branches of the superior mesenteric artery, but sometimes one of the other major trunks. The origin of the inferior mesenteric artery from the aorta is oblique, and therefore may spare it somewhat from embolic occlusion. The emboli arise from intracardiac mural thrombi, infective endocarditis, nonbacterial thrombotic endocarditis, thrombi superimposed on valvular prostheses, atrial myxomas, or ulcerated atherosclerotic plaques, particularly during intra-aortic diagnostic or therapeutic procedures (angiography, balloon pumping). As with thromboses, the embolus must lodge in the proximal segments of the arteries to induce sufficient restriction of the blood supply to cause ischemic injury. More distal lodgement may be compensated for by anastomotic channels.

Venous thrombosis accounts for a minority of bowel infarctions. Some instances follow upper abdominal surgery. Venous thromboses may also be associated with cardiac failure, polycythemia, portal stasis, external pressure on veins by tumors or aneurysms, and the hypercoagulable state. Ischemic lesions of the bowel secondary to venous thrombosis have also been encountered in young women using oral contraceptives, but the causal relationship is still in some doubt.[100]

Gangrene of the bowel may also result from occlusion of arterial or venous vessels by strangulated hernias, torsions, and intestinal adhesions. Despite the multiplicity of possible causes, there remains a significant percentage of cases in which no well-defined underlying or antecedent basis for the vascular insufficiency can be demonstrated.[101]

MORPHOLOGY. Transmural infarction of the small bowel may involve only a short segment, but more often a substantial portion of the total length. Colonic infarction tends to occur at the splenic flexure, which represents the watershed between the distributions of the superior and inferior mesenteric arteries. Regardless of whether the arterial or venous side is occluded, the infarction always appears grossly hemorrhagic.[102] In the early stages, the segment of bowel appears intensely congested, dusky to purple-red, with small and large foci of subserosal and submucosal ecchymotic discoloration (Fig. 18–25). Later the wall becomes edematous, thickened, rubbery, and hemorrhagic. Commonly at this stage, the lumen contains sanguineous mucus or frank blood. In arterial occlusions the demarcation from normal bowel is usually sharply defined, but in venous occlusions the area of dusky cyanosis fades gradually into the adjacent segments of normal bowel, leaving no clear-cut definition between viable and nonviable bowel. Within approximately 24 hours, a fibrinous or fibrinosuppurative exudate appears on the serosa, making it dull or granular. The associated inflammatory reaction depends on the duration of the disorder. If death occurs within 24 hours, little cellular response may be demonstrable. Later, lesions may show characteristic inflammatory infiltrations and ulcerations. Ulceration of the mucosa, complicated by inevitable secondary bacterial contamination, and perforation of the wall are likely to occur within three to four days. However, most patients do not live long enough to develop such complications. Identification of the vascular occlusion is often difficult, and indeed may be impossible when the critical ischemia is caused by spasm combined with a low perfusion state.

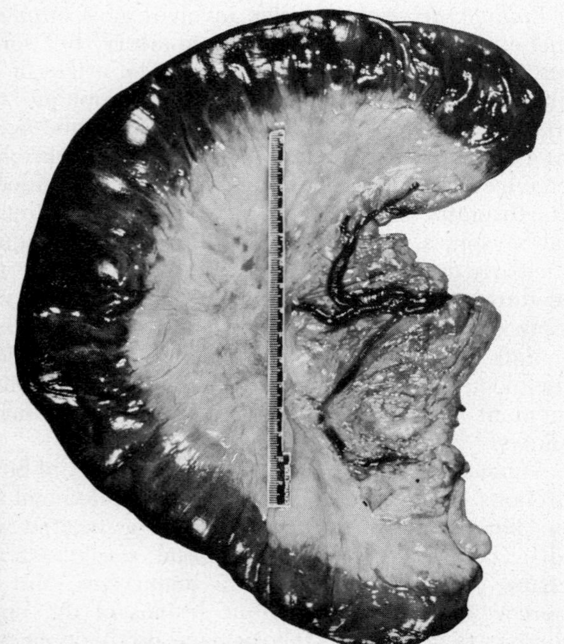

Figure 18–25. A loop of infarcted small intestine showing dark hemorrhagic discoloration. A large branching thrombus is evident in the arterial supply.

CLINICAL COURSE. Bowel infarction is an uncommon but grave disorder that imposes a 50 to 75% mortality rate. Constant awareness of the possibility of this catastrophe in high-risk individuals must be maintained because prompt diagnosis and immediate surgery offer the only hope of cure. This condition tends to occur in older individuals, usually in their fifth and sixth decades, when cardiac and vascular diseases are most prevalent. Older diabetics are at particular risk. There is no particular sex predilection. Preexistent intra-abdominal disease with the potential of adhesions or torsion also increases the risk. The onset is heralded by the development of signs and symptoms clinically indistinguishable from those encountered in all "acute abdomens," whatever the cause. Characteristically, there is sudden onset of severe abdominal pain, nausea, vomiting, or sometimes diarrhea that may progress rapidly (within 24 to 48 hours) to frank shock. Soon after, peristaltic sounds diminish or disappear, and spasm to boardlike rigidity of the abdominal wall becomes evident secondary to the development of acute peritonitis, as bacteria permeate the necrotic bowel wall.[103] Because there are far more common causes for these manifestations, such as acute appendicitis, perforated peptic ulcer, and acute cholecystitis, the diagnosis of intestinal gangrene is frequently delayed or missed. With the development of suppurative peritonitis, the downward course is extremely fulminating. Unless the condition is treated within the first 48 hours, death may follow from blood loss and shock, overwhelming infection, or perforation of the intestine.

MUCOSAL AND MURAL INFARCTION

These patterns of ischemic injury have in the past been called *acute hemorrhagic gastroenteropathy.*

Any level of the gut from stomach to anus may be involved. Freiman emphasizes that, unlike outright infarction, the ischemic injury appears to relate to hypoperfusion, damaging only the inner layers of the gut, while sparing the deeper levels of the muscularis and the serosa.[104]

The lesions may be widely distributed but strangely focal or segmental throughout the gastrointestinal tract, with a predilection for the small and large bowel. Before opening, affected segments of bowel may appear dark red or purple owing to the accumulated luminal hemorrhage. Notable, however, is the absence of hemorrhage, necrosis, or inflammatory exudation involving the serosal surface, changes that are more typical of transmural infarction of the bowel wall. On opening the bowel lumen, there is hemorrhagic, edematous thickening of the mucosa, sometimes with superficial ulceration. Edema and hemorrhages may in some cases penetrate more deeply into the submucosa and muscular layers. As expected, the histologic findings range from vascular dilatations, associated with a few extravasated red cells, to hemorrhagic necrosis of the mucosa, more often

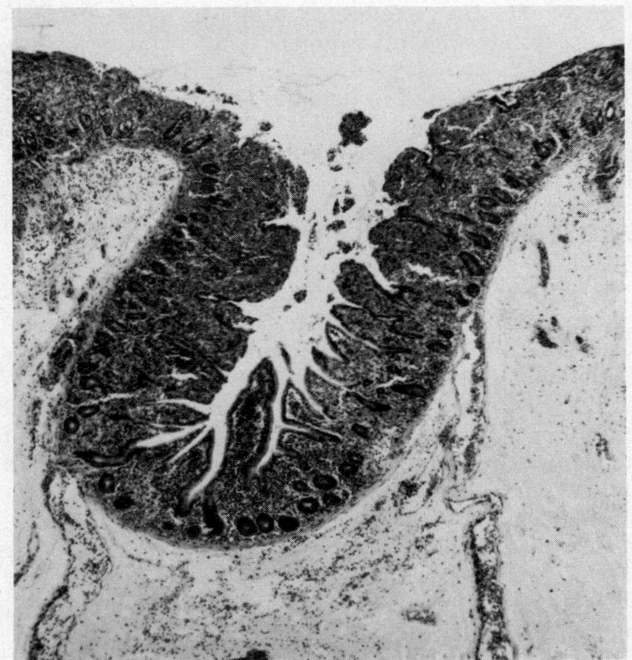

Figure 18–26. Mucosal infarction of small intestine with hemorrhagic suffusion of lamina propria and superficial sloughing of surface at upper left. There is marked edema but no hemorrhage in noninfarcted submucosa.

superficial, but sometimes extending into the submucosa and superficial muscularis.

As the terms "mucosal" and "mural infarction" are used here, the hypoxic damage may extend deeply, but by definition the serosa is spared (Fig. 18–26). Bacterial superinfection and the formation of enterotoxic bacterial products (p. 862) may induce superimposed pseudomembranous inflammation, particularly in the colon.[105] Thus, the anatomic changes of mucosal and mural infarction, in some cases, may mimic ulceroinflammatory enterocolitis (p. 835) or pseudomembranous enterocolitis (p. 862) of nonvascular origins.

The pathogenesis of mucosal and mural infarction involves nonocclusive hypoperfusion of the intestinal tract. Why the resultant lesions are segmental and patchy remains unexplained. Shock, with its splanchnic vasoconstriction, is the most important underlying cause. Cardiac failure is another major cause. The common denominator in these settings is a reduction in the effective circulating blood volume, with shunting of blood to vital organs and away from the splanchnic bed. Infections may contribute by inducing vasomotor changes such as have been described in endotoxic shock (p. 113). Many patients have received digitalis and norepinephrine, and since both agents have vasoconstrictive effects, they may contribute to the perfusion deficit. In some cases, minute intramural thrombi have been found, possibly representing causative mechanisms. Alternatively, these vascular thromboses may be only secondary to the surrounding inflammatory reaction.

The clinical onset is marked by abdominal pain, cramps, and bloody diarrhea, often with worsening of the shock state. Although, up to now, most diagnoses of this condition were made at autopsy, it is now being recognized clinically. Should the low perfusion state be correctable, the acute mucosal and mural infarction is reversible and complete restoration of the bowel wall can occur, as evidenced by failure to find residual changes at a later date.

INFECTIVE ENTEROCOLITIS

Inflammatory diarrheal diseases of the bowel make up a veritable Augean stable of entities. Some are caused by microbiologic agents, including bacteria, viruses, fungi, protozoa, and helminths. Noninfectious causes such as ischemia, irradiation, uremia, cytotoxic drugs, and heavy metal poisoning may produce mucosal changes and diarrhea. In addition, such important idiopathic conditions as Crohn's disease and ulcerative colitis also cause severe ulceroinflammatory disease. Our consideration here is limited to those inflammations of the bowel caused directly by specific infective agents. To be considered later in separate discussions are Crohn's disease, ulcerative colitis, and so-called pseudomembranous enterocolitis, which, according to present evidence, is usually if not always caused by an exotoxin derived from *Clostridium difficile*.

Insights have been gained recently from the study of mechanisms by which coliform enteropathogens cause diarrhea. Three attributes are of importance: (1) the capacity to invade; (2) enterotoxins, some of which are heat labile while others are heat stable; and (3) an adherence mechanism providing for binding of organisms to the mucosal lining. Whereas in many enteropathogens these capabilities are transmitted by chromosomal DNA, with *Escherichia coli* they are encoded within plasmids, as detailed on page 318. Invasive organisms often induce mucosal ulcerations accompanied by white cells or pus in the stools. Organisms such as particular strains of *E. coli* or *Vibrio cholerae* that release toxins cause diarrhea by activation of membrane-associated adenylate cyclase stimulating fluid and electrolyte secretion, inducing the time-honored "rice-water" stools. With organisms capable of adherence, the pathogenesis of the diarrhea is obscure, but electron microscopy reveals a virtual carpeting of the mucosal surface by the causative agent. It is possible, therefore, to divide the diarrheal syndromes into two large pathogenetic categories: (1) those associated with enteroinvasive organisms in which mucosal ulcerations often occur; and (2) those resulting from enterotoxins that, despite the functional derangement, are not associated with invasive mucosal ulcerations.

Some of the microbial causes of diarrhea principally affect the small intestines (enteritis) and others principally the colon, but in most instances there is considerable overlap. Whatever the main localization, the intestines respond with a limited range of reactions. Thus, many microbiologic agents produce nondistinctive morphologic changes that can be characterized as ulceroinflammatory, with the exception of the enterotoxigenic agents (serotypes of *E. coli* and *V. cholerae*). *Morphologic examination of the lesions, then, is of limited value in establishing the specific etiology.* From the clinical standpoint also, virtually all forms of inflammatory disease of the bowel produce similar manifestations, principally diarrhea, some with associated fever, while others are afebrile. Although a history of travel to some endemic focus of particular agents may raise leads for investigation, *the establishment of the specific cause of a diarrheal inflammatory disease of the intestines requires a battery of diagnostic methods—bacterial and viral isolations; direct examination of exudate in stools and from lesions; radiographic studies; sigmoidoscopy and/or colonoscopy; and sometimes biopsy—to identify the causative agent. Indeed, only when all known causes of inflammatory bowel disease have been ruled out can the diagnosis of Crohn's disease or ulcerative colitis be entertained.* Further, identification of a specific enteropathogen is clinically important because they respond best to particular antibiotics, and because in many instances the use of antispasmodic drugs with slowing of the bowel transit time may aggravate the problem.

Bowel infections may occur in previously healthy individuals, but are particularly serious in patients already suffering from some disorder that lowers the normal defenses and thus predisposes to intestinal colonization by organisms of even low virulence. Common settings are uremia, hypoperfusion states such as shock and cardiac failure, nonenteric infections requiring broad-spectrum antibiotic therapy, cancer under treatment by radiation or cytotoxic drugs, or some conditions requiring immunosuppressive therapy. The premature infant also is often predisposed to its own intestinal flora. Although in otherwise healthy adults these infections are disturbing but not usually threatening incursions on the "joie de vivre," in the predisposed they may lead to disseminated lesions in other organs and even death.[106]

The major microbiologic offenders are listed in Table 18–3. With some the bowel disease is only one component of a systemic disorder. In other instances the gastrointestinal involvement is the primary feature, sometimes having systemic ramifications. All these agents are discussed in detail in Chapter 8 and so only some general comments are offered, followed by a survey of the morphologic lesions.

Table 18–3. MICROBIAL CAUSES OF DIARRHEAL DISEASE

Bacterial invasive enterocolitis
Campylobacter jejuni
Escherichia coli (particular serotypes)
Salmonella
Shigella
Tuberculosis
Yersinia enterocolitica
Aeromonas hydrophila
Bacterial toxigenic enterocolitis
Vibrio cholerae
E. coli (particular serotypes)
Viral (nonbacterial) enterocolitis
Fungal enterocolitis
Moniliasis
Mucormycosis
Enterocolitis caused by protozoa and metazoa
Entamoeba histolytica
Giardia lamblia
Schistosoma mansoni
Cryptosporidia

BACTERIAL ENTEROCOLITIS

At the outset, food poisonings related to the ingestion of preformed bacterial toxins should be differentiated from enteric infections. Improperly stored foods contaminated by *Clostridium botulinum* and *Staphylococcus aureus* permit the elaboration in vitro of potent enterotoxins that, when ingested, may cause a violent and sometimes fatal gastroenterocolitis or a self-limited mild disease, depending on dosage. Although the mucosal inflammatory changes can mimic the early invasive stage of bacterial infections, *they are extremely acute intoxications.* Usually they are not accompanied by ulcerations and promptly regress if the subject survives. Somewhat analogous enterotoxigenic bacteria that colonize the gut may induce acute, sometimes severe, diarrheal syndromes despite the absence of mucosal defects. Among the invasive organisms, *Campylobacter jejuni* has emerged in the recent past as a major cause of enterocolitis. In one analysis of patients hospitalized for diarrheal disease, *C. jejuni* was identified in about 8% of cases.[107] Outbreaks of this infection in humans have mainly arisen from ingestion of contaminated food or water.[108] The reservoir of infection is the gastrointestinal tract of wild and domesticated animals that man either eats, or contacts directly or indirectly. The severity of the disease ranges from a self-limited mild enterocolitis to severe recurrent disabling diarrhea that may mimic ulcerative colitis or Crohn's disease.

Specific serotypes of *E. coli* cited on page 318 have been identified as causes of diarrhea in infants and in adults who are exposed to organisms during foreign travel (traveler's diarrhea) to which they have not developed immunity. Specific serotypes possess one or more of the three pathogenetic capabilities mentioned earlier.[109] Certain serotypes have receptors permitting them to adhere to epithelial cells and induce diarrhea without the elaboration of toxins or invasion of the mucosa.[110] These organisms penetrate the surface glycocalyx, disrupt the microvillous brush border, and may cause blunting of the villi as well as a mild histiocytic infiltrate in the lamina propria, but it is not clear whether the diarrheal disorder is functional or due to damage to surface epithelial cells. Other "gram-negative" enteropathogens are the well-known Salmonella and Shigella. These are all food- and water-borne infections that are frequently characterized by marked involvement of the small and large intestine. They are discussed in detail on page 319.

Tuberculosis may involve the bowel as a primary gastrointestinal infection from ingestion of contaminated milk or milk products where control of bovine tuberculosis is not rigorous. More often, enteric infections are secondary to the swallowing of organisms coughed up from a caseating pulmonary focus. The organisms invade the intestinal lymphoid tissues to produce, eventually, ulcerations, as discussed on page 345. Although the granulomatous nature of the inflammation may strongly suggest the diagnosis, other disorders such as Crohn's disease may also produce granulomas, and so it is necessary to identify the acid-fast bacilli in lesions or by cultural studies to establish the diagnosis solidly.

Yersinia enterocolitica is a gram-negative coccobacillus that uncommonly produces enteric disease, principally in infants and children, which is very severe and potentially lethal.[111] Extraintestinal sites of infection may appear with the enteric involvement such as pharyngitis, pericarditis, and peritonitis.

With invasive organisms, all levels of the bowel from the stomach to the anus may develop ulceroinflammatory lesions requiring isolation of the specific offending agent for identification of the specific etiology. Some pathogens preferentially involve the small intestine, others the colon, and still others both levels. The macroscopic alterations with all enteric pathogens are extremely variable and range from focal areas of mucosal, edematous hyperemia to enlargement of lymphoid tissues to excavated ulcerations (Fig. 18–27). Sometimes the inflammation is marked by pseudomembrane formations that range from yellow-gray to more hemorrhagic exudates to thus mimic clostridial pseudomembranous enterocolitis (p. 862). The distribution of such focal lesions is extremely variable. On occasion, only one rather long segment of bowel is affected. More often, there are multiple scattered lesions with intervening areas of uninvolved mucosa. The ulcerations may therefore be dispersed or sometimes virtually coalescent to denude large areas, reminiscent of severe ulcerative colitis (p. 860). The serosal surfaces juxtaposed to these lesions may be entirely normal or covered by serous, fibrinous, or hemorrhagic exudate.

Some subtle microscopic differences may be noted among the various causative agents, but basically all induce acute-to-chronic inflammatory changes. Tubercle bacilli, as you know, evoke a characteristic granulomatous reaction. Salmonella are associated with striking hypertrophy of mononuclear phagocytes within lymphoid aggregates that sometimes reveal phagocytized red cells. Campylobacter tends to produce granulomatous stellate ulcers. Nonetheless, more evidence must be derived from identification of the offending pathogen by culture of the stool or tissue lesions. Such substantiation is even more important since **nonmicrobiologic agents may also produce inflammation and ulceration of the bowel mucosa. Radiation enteritis** may be associated with mucosal changes indistinguishable from those caused by bacteria. Ischemia leading to mucosal and mural infarction may at times mimic bacterial infection. Pseudomembranous enterocolitis is yet another entity that must be included in the differential diagnosis. And finally, the two major ulceroinflammatory disorders of the bowel—Crohn's disease and ulcerative colitis—must be brought into consideration. The differential diagnosis is almost as difficult anatomically as it is clinically.

On occasion the ulceroinflammatory changes are confined to the anorectal region; this pattern of proctitis is particularly common among male homosexuals. The causative agents include *Treponema pallidum,* gonococci, chlamydia, and herpes simplex. The enteric disease is distinctive by virtue of its localization, but Crohn's disease also may induce only proctitis without involvement of more proximal levels of the gut.

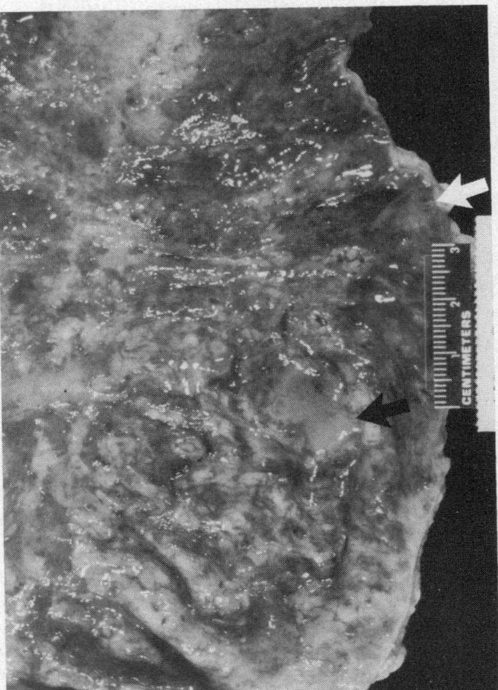

Figure 18–27. Infective enterocolitis. Segment of colon showing pale granular inflamed mucosa with patches of coagulated exudate (*black arrow*). Compare with relatively normal mucosa (*white arrow*).

NONBACTERIAL GASTROENTEROCOLITIS

Microbiologic agents other than bacteria—viruses, fungi, protozoa, and helminths—may induce clinical gastroenteric diseases, some of which are very common in underdeveloped parts of the world (e.g., schistosomiasis).[112] *Viral gastroenteritis* is said to be second only to the common cold as a cause of illness in the United States. Only a few comments about these diseases are offered here to serve as a reminder of their existence; the specific offending agents are treated in greater detail in other sections of this book. Several groups of viral enteric pathogens are responsible for what is clinically termed *acute infectious nonbacterial gastroenteritis.* Parvovirus-like agents may produce disease in adults and reovirus-like agents in infants. More recently, the rotavirus has emerged as another cause of diarrheal disease, principally in infants and children, in whom rotaviral infection is so severe that strenuous efforts are being made to develop a preventive vaccine.[113] Although viral diarrheal diseases are generally transient and only temporarily incapacitating, they may be more serious and indeed fatal in infants and the malnourished, particularly when concomitant bacterial or protozoal enteric infections are also present.

Knowledge of the viral-induced morphologic changes is derived largely from biopsy studies of otherwise healthy individuals, since fatal illnesses are usually complicated by bacterial infections. In nonfatal cases, frank necrosis and ulceration of the mucosa have not been observed. The major findings consist of shortening of the villi of the small intestine accompanied by an inflammatory infiltrate of neutrophils and mononuclear cells within the lamina propria. The surface absorptive cells have revealed a variety of abnormalities including vacuolation, shortening or loss of microvilli, and accumulation of increased numbers of lysosomes. Viral particles have not been identified within affected tissues in infections caused by the parvovirus-like agent, but they have been seen in disease caused by the reovirus-like agent.[114]

Fungi—candida and mucormycetes—may invade the mucosa of the small or large intestine, but almost always as a consequence of fungemia in a terminally ill patient either immunosuppressed or dying of some debilitating disease. Wherever the organisms localize they induce focal to sometimes segmental areas of hyperemia, edema, superficial necrosis, deep ulcerations, and sometimes pseudomembranes. Further details of these agents are offered in Chapter 8.

The *protozoa—Entamoeba histolytica* and *Giardia lamblia*—are well-known causes of intestinal disease, also discussed in Chapter 8. In particular, amebiasis may induce extensive ulcerations, mainly in the large bowel, which require differentiation from nonspecific ulcerative colitis and bacteria-induced ulcerations. The much larger *Schistosoma mansoni* may also induce intestinal lesions, as pointed out on page 388.

It is evident that the bowel is the reluctant host to a large number of injury-producing agents, the full roster of which must be kept in mind in evaluating any patient or specimen with enteric inflammatory or diarrheal disease.

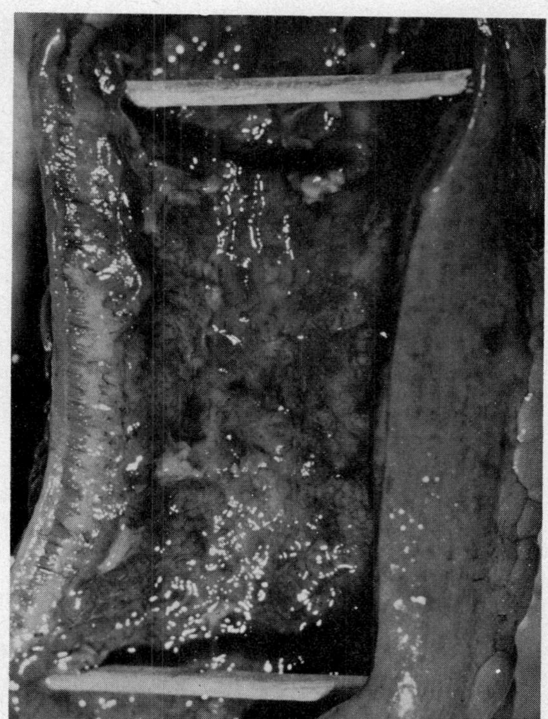

Figure 18–28. Crohn's disease of ileum. Close-up of a segment of thickened bowel wall. Note wooden pegs required to keep lumen exposed.

CROHN'S DISEASE (REGIONAL ENTERITIS)

Crohn's disease is perhaps best described as a recurrent granulomatous, fibrosing inflammatory disorder that usually affects the terminal ileum or colon, but may occur at any level in the gastrointestinal tract from mouth to anus (Fig. 18–28). Although primarily an enteric disorder, it appears to be systemic in distribution. Lesions of Crohn's disease have been observed in the skin, femur, striated muscle, and lung.[115] Moreover, many complications may accompany the bowel involvement such as arthritis (particularly sacroiliitis and ankylosing spondylitis), uveitis, erythema nodosum, various inflammatory changes in the liver, gallstones, and other extraintestinal changes.[116] These complications often improve or clear following resection of the diseased bowel, strongly suggesting a common etiology. Could immune complexes be involved? When first described in 1932 by Crohn and colleagues, it was thought that the bowel involvement was limited to the terminal ileum, and it was thus designated *terminal ileitis*. Later it was appreciated that sharply delineated segmental areas of the small bowel might be affected, leaving intervening, unaffected ("skip") segments—hence the designation *regional enteritis*. Since that time it has become apparent that any level of the enteric tract may be involved. Indeed, there is epidemiologic evidence that the intestinal distribution of the disease is shifting with increased involvement of the large bowel.[117] Analyses of large series of patients reveal that the terminal ileum is affected in 65 to 75% of cases, with concurrent involvement of the colon in half of these. The colon alone is involved in 20 to 30% of cases.[118, 119] The colonic involvement is often referred to as *granulomatous colitis* to distinguish it from ulcerative colitis, which is rarely, if ever, associated with a granulomatous inflammation.

As will become clear, Crohn's disease bears many similarities to ulcerative colitis, and a strongly held current view proposes that the two disorders are in reality a single "inflammatory bowel disease" with variable tissue reactivity to a common etiologic agent. Typically, Crohn's disease is characterized by a granulomatous inflammatory reaction with through-and-through involvement of the thickness of the bowel wall. In approximately 40% of cases, however, granulomas are either poorly developed or totally absent. In contrast, ulcerative colitis is a nonspecific inflammatory response limited largely to the colonic mucosa and submucosa. Nonetheless, the two conditions have in common the following features::

1. The colon is frequently affected in Crohn's disease and is invariably involved in ulcerative colitis.

2. Rarely, patients with total colonic involvement in ulcerative colitis may develop a so-called "backwash

ileitis." Thus, both conditions may cause changes in the small intestine.

3. Patients with Crohn's disease often have close relatives with ulcerative colitis, and vice versa.[115]

4. When there is no granulomatous reaction in Crohn's disease of the colon, the two lesions may resemble each other, not only clinically but also pathologically.

5. There are many epidemiologic similarities between the two diseases, including age, race, sex, and geographic distribution.

6. The same extraintestinal complications (already mentioned) occur in both conditions.

7. The cause or causes of both ulcerative colitis and Crohn's disease are unknown, but current studies suggest many possible etiologic parallels.

8. Both conditions are associated with an increased frequency of colonic carcinoma.

For these many reasons, the two conditions are often referred to by the generic designation inflammatory bowel disease, an unfortunate (but historically sanctified) practice since, as you know, there are many other forms of inflammatory bowel disease (p. 833). However, the putative etiologic parallels justify consideration of the origins of Crohn's disease and ulcerative colitis together.

EPIDEMIOLOGY. Crohn's disease occurs throughout the world. There are, however, striking differences in incidence; for example, it is much more frequent in the United States, Britain, and Scandinavia than in Japan, the U.S.S.R., and the South American nations. Moreover, the incidence is on the increase in high-risk countries. It occurs at any age but most often is first detected in the second decade of life. A minor peak occurs in the elderly. Females are affected slightly more often than males. Whites develop the disease two to five times more often than nonwhites, but diagnostic facilities and case finding may play some role. In the U.S., regional enteritis occurs three to five times more often among Jews than among non-Jews.

Because there are many hints that immunologic mechanisms play a role in the initiation or perpetuation of Crohn's disease (and ulcerative colitis), an intensive search has been made for genetic markers that might identify individuals having a particular immunoconstitution rendering them more vulnerable. The results, on the whole, have been confusing. In about 15 to 40% of cases, multiple members of a family have Crohn's disease, or sometimes ulcerative colitis.[120] There are occasional instances of disease in both monozygotic twins.[121] No well-defined HLA associations have been identified.[122] An older observation that patients with Crohn's disease complicated by a form of vertebral arthritis known as ankylosing spondylitis have an increased frequency of HLA-B27 is now recognized to relate to the ankylosing spondylitis alone. The most provocative finding to date derives from a kindred study containing five pairs of siblings affected with regional enteritis: four shared both haplotypes and one shared only one haplotype.[123] Immunologic vulnerability might then be linked to specific immunoregulatory genes. In summary, there are hints of genetic predisposition but the findings are inconclusive. Virtually identical statements will be made about ulcerative colitis.

ETIOLOGY AND PATHOGENESIS. Since the origins of Crohn's disease and ulcerative colitis have revealed a great many similarities, it is reasonable to consider the etiology and pathogenesis of both conditions together, employing the commonly used term "inflammatory bowel disease" (IBD).

Theories about the origins of IBD can be divided into three groups: (1) those invoking an infectious agent; (2) those contending that immunologic mechanisms initiate or perpetuate the condition; and (3) an assortment of concepts implicating psychosomatic, dietary, vascular, traumatic, hormonal, and other mechanisms. Currently favored theories fall with the first two groups.

Many microorganisms have been hailed as putative causes of IBD, but to date none has been confirmed. The volumes of writing on this line of investigation permit only an overview, but excellent reviews are available.[115, 124, 125] Impetus for a microbiologic etiology was provided by a report in 1970 that cell-free filtrates prepared from Crohn's tissue, when inoculated into the footpads of mice, would induce granulomas.[126] The same investigators then reported that filtrates from either Crohn's disease or ulcerative colitis, when inoculated into the abdominal cavity of rabbits, would induce inflammatory bowel disease, suggesting an organ specificity for the causative agent.[127] It appears likely, however, that the inflammatory reactions are secondary to xenotropic tissue antigens, since inoculation of rabbits with *normal* human bowel homogenate has been shown to produce inflammatory changes resembling the granulomas of Crohn's disease. However, such studies do not rule out a putative transmissible agent, and indeed a number of organisms have been implicated, so many as to cast doubt on all.

Viruses—rotavirus, Epstein-Barr virus, cytomegalovirus, and uncharacterized RNA intestinal cytopathic viruses—continue to be favored candidates.[128] Without reviewing all the evidence, it suffices to note that ultrafiltrates of tissue of Crohn's disease and ulcerative colitis are cytopathic when introduced into tissue cultures of mucosal epithelial cells, and virus-like particles have been observed in the dying cells.[129] Attempts to isolate the cytopathic agent suggest that in Crohn's disease it is a small RNA virus variously classified as ECHO-27, reovirus, rotavirus, or uncertain. Electron and immune electron microscopic studies, however, have failed to reveal viral particles in lesions,[130] and attempts to culture viruses from diseased bowel have largely failed or revealed merely passenger agents. Bacteria have also been implicated in the causation of the IBD, including Pseudomona-like organisms, enteric anaerobes, cell wall–defective *Mycobacterium kansasii*, chlamydia, and *Yersinia enterocolitica*, but proof of their roles is still lacking.[124, 131] The search for an infectious etiology for IBD continues, but at present no organism has been substantially implicated.

A mountain of evidence points to immunologic derangements in IBD, but whether they are causal or

secondary phenomena is unclear. Antibody-mediated mechanisms, cell-mediated reactions, and immunologic deficiencies all have their champions. At one time there was great enthusiasm for the notion of antibody against *E. coli*—particularly 014—lipopolysaccharide antigens, which cross-reacted with intestinal cell antigens to thus cause damage. However, efforts to demonstrate such cross-reacting antibodies in the lesions themselves have largely been unsuccessful. A specific anticolon antibody that does not cross-react with *E. coli* has been described in diseased tissues, and increased synthesis of IgG has been documented in mucosal lymphoid cells derived from diseased segments of bowel.[132, 133] However, there does not appear to be any clear correlation between the level of these antibodies and the activity of the underlying disease. Moreover, IBD may occur in individuals with agammaglobulinemia, and ultimately none of these antibodies is regularly with effect in tissue culture.

Attempts to relate circulating immune complexes to the intestinal lesions have also been discouraging. However, they may play some role in the causation of the extraintestinal lesions associated with IBD. Attention has also been directed to the possibility that an anaphylactoid hypersensitivity reaction mediated by IgE might release vasoactive substances from mast cells in the bowel wall, and thus cause edema of the bowel wall to impair the normal barrier function of the mucosa. An increasing number of mast cells and basophils in specimens of Crohn's disease have been described.[134] However, IgE concentrations in serum are not consistently elevated, and immunofluorescent counts of IgE-containing immunocytes in diseased segments of bowel have yielded extremely variable results ranging from decreased to increased numbers.[135] The case for antibody- or immune complex-mediated mechanisms is at best not strong.

Cell-mediated immunologic damage is an attractive hypothesis because lymphocytes and macrophages are so numerous in the lesions of IBD. Various studies have documented circulating T cells sensitized to a number of colonic and bacterial antigens, but it remains to be proved that the T cells are cytotoxic to bowel epithelium.[136] Collaboration between humoral antibodies and K cells might induce so-called antibody-dependent cellular cytotoxicity (ADCC). Indeed, it has been shown that K cells are cytotoxic in vitro to colonic epithelial cells when the IgM fraction of serum from patients with colitis is introduced into the culture. However, there is poor correlation between antibody-dependent cellular cytotoxicity and the activity of the disease. A slightly different approach suggests that some immunologic deficiency leads to uncontrolled exaggerated reactions to a variety of bowel antigens resulting in mucosal damage. Indeed, there are hints of some immunodeficiency with Crohn's disease, such as impaired synthesis of IgA in the bowel mucosa or macrophage incompetence.[137] The litany regarding immune mechanisms could be extended almost indefinitely, but the reasonable conclusion to be drawn from all the evidence has been well summarized by Sachar:[124] "We can conclude that (IBD) probably induces immune aberrations in the host and that the inflammatory reactions may even be mediated in part via immune effector pathways. To date, however, the case for the primary pathogenetic role of immunologic factors in IBD remains unproved."

The many other etiologic theories are all too poorly substantiated to merit detailed mention. Psychosomatic factors have long been invoked because certain personality types—immature, dependent, passive—often suffer from a so-called "irritable colon." But there is no evidence that such emotional bowel disturbances lead to organic disease. Food allergies, primary vascular disease within mural small arteries or arterioles, and chronic trauma have all received their share of attention but at present are not given credence as pathogenetic mechanisms. Prostaglandins have come to the forefront with reports of elevated PGE_2 levels in colonic venous blood and rectal mucosa in patients with ulcerative colitis.[138] However, prostaglandins are known to be mediators of inflammatory reactions, and thus increased levels might merely be epiphenoma. Therefore, despite the plethora of theories, the causation of IBD remains unknown.

MORPHOLOGY. Although there are many morphologic similarities between the two conditions, Crohn's disease differs sufficiently from ulcerative colitis (discussed on p. 859) to merit separate consideration.

One of the most distinctive macroscopic features of Crohn's disease is the **sharp demarcation of the segmental bowel involvement, which may occur, as mentioned, in any level of the enteric tract.** In its classic form, 15 to 25 cm of the terminal ileum is affected. Sometimes, several sharply demarcated diseased segments are separated by normal bowel, producing what are called "skip" lesions, a distribution not found in ulcerative colitis. The usual distribution of these involvements in the small and large intestine was cited earlier, but first the small intestinal changes will be described. Early Crohn's disease is marked by rubbery, edematous, hyperemic thickening of the small intestinal wall. At this stage the mucosa may show only minute hyperemic ("aphthoid") ulcerations closely resembling canker sores.[139] As the disease evolves to the classic stage, **the diseased segment becomes thickened and inflexible and has been likened to a lead pipe or rubber hose.** The serosal surface is granular and dull gray, and often the mesenteric fat "creeps up" over the bowel surface, so that the gut may seem virtually buried. The mesentery of the involved small intestinal segment is also thickened, edematous, and sometimes fibrotic. The striking inflexibility and fibrosis of the bowel wall tend to maintain the cylindrical shape even after the bowel is opened, so that it must be propped open for inspection. The lumen is almost always narrowed; this is evidenced on x-ray as the "string-sign," a thin stream of barium. Close examination of the opened bowel reveals separation of the usual anatomic layers by gray, gritty, fibrous tissue, which classically involves mainly the submucosal and subserosal zones. Varying degrees of mucosal edema, ulceration, and sloughing are found. Commonly, the ulcers are long and serpentine (Fig. 18–29). **Often they are extremely narrow fissures** and can be virtually hidden between the folds of the mucosa. In chronic cases, the ulcers or fissures may penetrate deeply to form fistulous tracts with other loops of bowel. In other instances, penetra-

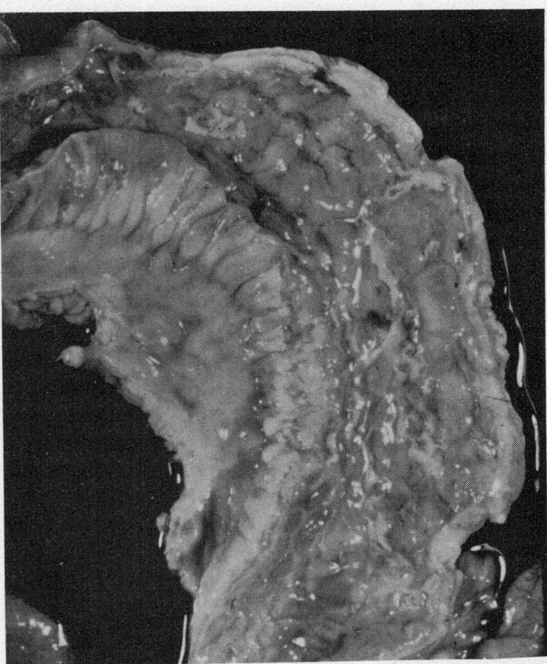

Figure 18–29. Regional enteritis of distal ileum demonstrating fibrosis and thickening of wall as well as long, serpentine, pale ulcerations of mucosa.

tion of the wall of the small intestine may create abscesses, either within the peritoneal cavity or within the mesenteric fat.

When present, the distribution of the colonic involvement, referred to as **granulomatous colitis,** is extremely variable.[140] Most often the cecum and a portion of the right colon are affected in continuity with ileal involvement. In other instances, isolated or multiple segments are diseased, sometimes producing "skip" lesions similar to those in the small bowel. The colitis may be limited to the descending colon, sometimes extending into the sigmoid. It should be particularly noted that the rectum is diseased in about half of all patients with colonic involvement—either in continuity with left-sided colitis or sometimes as a "skip" lesion. In a small percentage of patients the involvement is restricted to the anorectal region, and in the most severe expression of granulomatous colitis the entire large bowel is affected. It is obvious that virtually any distribution may be encountered. Typically, the macroscopic changes are almost identical with those described in the small intestine, complete with transmural fibrosing inflammation, linear fissures, thickening of the bowel wall, and sometimes narrowing of the lumen. **It is the "skip" lesions, the thickening of the bowel wall, and the tendency for the ulcerations to form fissures that most sharply distinguish granulomatous colitis from ulcerative colitis, macroscopically.** However, in some instances there is less fibrotic thickening and the inflammation is more limited to the mucosa and submucosa, closely mimicking ulcerative colitis. Indeed, most experts concede that in 10 to 20% of cases it is impossible to discriminate granulomatous from ulcerative colitis.[141] Whatever the gross appearance, the colonic changes in Crohn's disease may be complicated by perforation, fistulas, pericolonic abscesses, and perianal and perirectal sepsis.

The most characteristic histologic features of Crohn's disease are (1) transmural inflammation (in the form of chronic inflammatory infiltrates and fibrosis) affecting all layers to the serosa, (2) noncaseating granulomas resembling those of sarcoidosis, (3) dilatation or sclerosis of lymphatic channels, and (4) lymphoid aggregates (sometimes with germinal centers) in all levels of the bowel wall. The granulomas, however, are absent or not well developed in approximately 40% of cases. From the inside out, there is variable ulceration and destruction of the mucosa, marked submucosal fibrosis with chronic inflammatory reaction, relative preservation of the muscularis, and, again, marked subserosal fibrosis with chronic inflammatory changes (Fig. 18–30). The inflammatory response in the mucosal ulcerations is entirely nonspecific and is largely composed of neutrophils, lymphocytes, macrophages, and plasma cells.[142] The preserved mucosa between the ulcers often shows a diffuse nonspecific inflammation with flattening of the villi and active goblet cell secretion (Fig. 18–31). More important, atypical metaplasia and dysplasia of epithelial cells may be present not only close to ulcerations, but also in intervening areas. Within the submucosal and subserosal zones, the inflammatory foci of mononuclear cells are often aggregated into lymphoid follicles, and some of these contain well-formed, sarcoid-like granulomas (Fig. 18–32). The resemblance to sarcoid is complete with the production of multinucleated giant cells, some of which contain Schaumann bodies. However, even when these granulomas are missing from some cases, regional enteritis must still be diagnosed histologically on the basis of the other changes described. Similar chronic

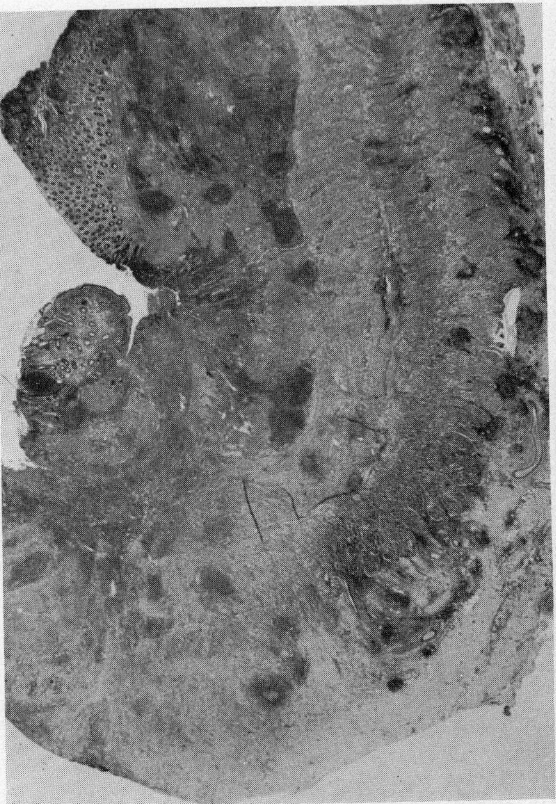

Figure 18–30. Low-power view of marked inflammation, thickening, and ulceration caused by regional enteritis. Foci of inflammatory cells are evident at points distant from the ulceration. Note width of submucosa.

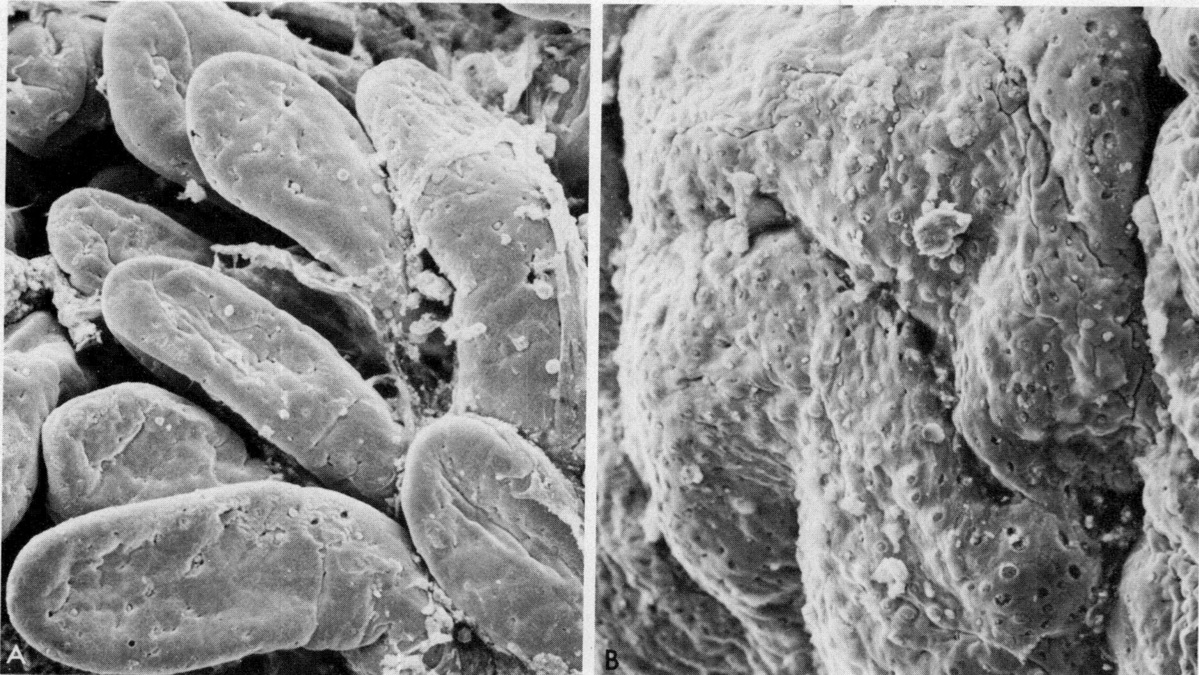

Figure 18–31. *A*, Scanning electron micrograph of normal ileal mucosa with thin, finger-shaped villi and mucus secretion exuding from goblet cell orifices. *B*, Uninvolved, nonulcerated mucosa of Crohn's disease with complete flattening and fusion of surface villi. More goblet cell orifices are visible, actively secreting mucus. (Courtesy of Dr. A. M. Dvorak, Beth Israel Hospital, Boston.)

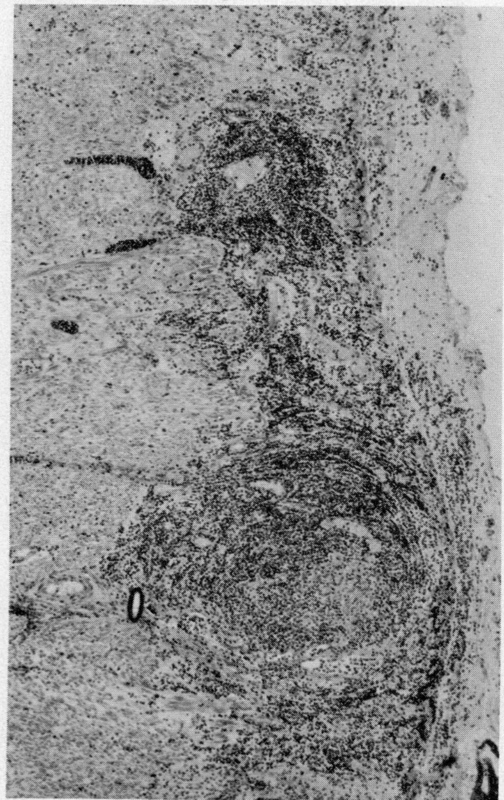

Figure 18–32. Serosal surface of a segment of bowel involved by regional enteritis, illustrating foci of chronic inflammatory cells, which sometimes contain central granulomatous responses resembling sarcoid.

inflammatory changes, often replete with granulomas, affect the regional nodes of drainage. The precise stimulus to this granuloma formation remains unclear. It is logical to assume that it reflects some form of T-cell hypersensitivity, and increased levels of lysosomal enzymes have been found in these foci, suggesting released cellular antigens as the immunologic trigger.[143]

A variety of additional nonspecific structural and ultrastructural changes have been described. Villi are shortened, thickened, and fused, and the microvilli often show budding of their tips along with necrosis of individual epithelial cells. These same changes may appear in contiguous, apparently uninvolved bowel. An increased number of mast cells, some degranulated, can often be observed sometimes in proximity to eosinophils, suggesting some role for vasoactive and immunologic mechanisms in the production of the lesions. There is active mucus secretion in both involved and uninvolved mucosa.[144]

The histologic changes in granulomatous colitis conform to those cited previously. Fibrosis and thickening tend to be less severe and do not cause the marked stenosis seen in the small intestine. This difference in macroscopic appearance may merely reflect differences in the size of the lumina and in the vascular and lymphatic supply of these two levels of the gut. Sarcoid-like granulomas, complete with multinucleated giant cells, are also present in the colon, justifying the designation granulomatous colitis.[145] Anal lesions may take the form of an indolent ulcer or fissure, which sometimes penetrates deeply to produce a fistula. Here again, the histologic changes are those seen in the upper levels of the gut, including granuloma formations sometimes enclosing multinucleated giant cells.

CLINICAL COURSE. The clinical manifestations of Crohn's disease are extremely variable. The disease usually begins with intermittent attacks of relatively mild diarrhea, fever, and right lower quadrant or sometimes periumbilical abdominal pain. These attacks are spaced by asymptomatic periods lasting for weeks to many months. In those with colonic involvement, the pain may be localized to the left lower quadrant or lower abdomen. The manifestations are often present for several years before the diagnosis is established. Often the attacks are precipitated by periods of physical or emotional stress. As pointed out earlier, emotional influences are not thought to have any role in the initiation of the disease, but they may contribute to flareups. Occult or overt (in those with colonic involvement) blood in the stool may lead to anemia over the span of time, but massive bleeding is uncommon. In about one-fifth of the patients the onset is more abrupt, with acute right lower quadrant pain, fever, and diarrhea sometimes suggesting acute appendicitis or an acute bowel perforation.

Whatever the onset, the course of the disease includes progressive fluid and electrolyte losses, weight loss, and weakness. *A number of problems may appear during this lengthy, chronic disease. Fibrosing strictures,* particularly of the terminal ileum, may lead to intestinal obstruction. *Fistulas*—to other loops of the bowel, to the urinary bladder, perirectal, or into a peritoneal abscess—develop in about 10 to 15% of cases. *Extensive mucosal involvement may cause marked loss of albumin (protein-losing enteropathy); generalized malabsorption; specific malabsorption of vitamin B_{12}, with consequent pernicious anemia; or malabsorption of bile salts, leading to steatorrhea.* Migratory polyarthritis, sacroiliitis, ankylosing spondylitis, erythema nodosum, or clubbing of the fingertips may appear, sometimes even before bowel symptoms appear. Uveitis, nonspecific mild hepatic pericholangitis, and renal disorders secondary to trapping of the ureters in the inflammatory process sometimes develop. An increased incidence of gallstones has also been noted in these patients. Rarely (1%), systemic amyloidosis is a late consequence. Overshadowing all these complications is the now well-documented increased incidence of cancer of the gastrointestinal tract in patients with Crohn's disease. Most of these cancers arise in diseased segments of the gut probably from dysplastic epithelial cells.[146] Similarly, the incidence of colorectal cancer in patients with granulomatous colitis is several times greater than in a control population. Mysteriously, however, there is an excess of cancers of the gastrointestinal tract in areas not involved with Crohn's disease and sometimes quite remote from affected segments of the bowel, such as the oral cavity, esophagus, and stomach.[147] Whether there is an excess of extraintestinal cancer is not clear at present. The risk of complicating gastrointestinal cancer appears to be correlated with the duration of the disease, but it begins to become evident within ten years of onset. However, it is much less substantial than with chronic ulcerative colitis. Thus, Crohn's disease, although primarily affecting the gut, emerges as a systemic disorder with wide-ranging implications, including a predisposition to cancers of the entire enteric tract.

TUMORS OF SMALL INTESTINE

It is one of the enigmas of medicine that tumors of the small intestine, both benign and malignant, are such rarities. Although the small bowel represents 75% of the length of the entire gastrointestinal tract, neoplasms in this location account for only 3 to 6% of all gastrointestinal tumors. Numerous explanatory theories—all speculative—have been proposed, including: rapid transit-time, permitting only brief exposure of the mucosa to possible carcinogens; low mechanical irritation because of the fluidity of small intestinal contents; a high concentration of IgA, which might maintain a level of immunosurveillance; and a low bacterial population, resulting in the formation of fewer carcinogenic compounds.[148, 149] Neoplasms of the small intestine are usually difficult to diagnose clinically because they are so uncommon and because the fluidity of the intestinal contents prevents obstructive symptoms. In most series, malignant tumors are slightly more common than benign, in a ratio approximating 1.5:1.

BENIGN

Most benign tumors of the small intestine are discovered only at postmortem examination, or incidentally in the course of radiographic studies of the small bowel for other reasons. However, large lesions may produce partial or intermittent obstruction, bleeding, intussusception, and volvulus. *Leiomyomas are generally the most common form, followed in descending order of frequency by lipomas, adenomas (polyps), angiomas, and fibromas.* Since most of these neoplasms are identical to their counterparts in other locations, they require no further description. Only adenomatous polyps justify a few words. They may occur singly or multiply, most often in the duodenum and ileum. Morphologically, they resemble those occurring in the stomach and colon (p. 864), and range from pedunculated adenomas to sessile villous adenomas with the full spectrum of intergrades.[150] The larger adenomas, particularly those having villous features like those in the colon, often undergo malignant transformation; in one series of 51 pedunculated and sessile adenomas, 33 contained foci of carcinoma.[150] Thus, sporadic polyps of the small intestine, although rarities, are ominous lesions. Multiple pedunculated polyps may appear in the small intestine in familial multiple polyposis (p. 867) and in the Peutz-Jeghers syndrome (p. 868).

MALIGNANT

As stated earlier, cancers are very uncommon in the small intestine, but they are more prevalent than benign tumors. More than half arise in the ileum.[151, 152] Either endocrine cell tumors (argentaffinomas) or lymphomas are the most frequent forms of cancer in the small intestine, followed in order by adenocarcinomas and leiomyosarcomas. Rhabdomyosarcomas, liposarcomas, angiosarcomas, fibrosarcomas, and neurogenic sarcomas are all exceedingly uncommon. Lymphomas in the small intestine are identical both morphologically and clinically to those encountered in other segments of the gastrointestinal tract, and are described on page 826.

Endocrine Cell Tumors (Argentaffinomas, Carcinoids)

Argentaffinomas, as they have been called for some time, may arise in such diverse sites as the breast, thymus, liver, gallbladder, lung, ovary, and urethra, but most are primary in the gastrointestinal tract anywhere from mouth to anus. In all sites of origin they have a remarkably constant banal histologic appearance, but nonetheless many invade and metastasize. Because it takes years for such cancerous behavior to be expressed, they have been called "malignant neoplasms in slow motion" or carcinoma-like—hence the name "carcinoids."[153] They arise from endocrine cells in the gut, known as Kulchitsky cells or enterochromaffin cells (because of an affinity for chrome salts). With this endocrine origin, the neoplastic cells of carcinoids usually contain secretory granules that have an affinity for soluble silver salts and are readily visualized in electron micrographs (Fig. 18–33). The cells in some neoplasms can directly deposit soluble silver salts to which they are exposed—hence the designation "argentaffinoma." Sometimes an exogenous reducing agent is required; such neoplasms are referred to as *argyrophilic.* However, some tumors, perhaps because they are less well-differentiated, are both argentaffin and argyrophil negative.[154] *Most of these neoplasms are capable of elaborating a variety of amine and peptide products*—histamine, serotonin, 5-hydroxytryptophan, ACTH, kallikrein, and sometimes prostaglandins. Some of these products may induce systemic manifestations known as the *carcinoid syndrome.* The ability of the cells to synthesize, store in secretory granules, and secrete polypeptides and amines has led to the inclusion of these neoplasms in the larger family of APUD tumors, to which our attention must now be directed.

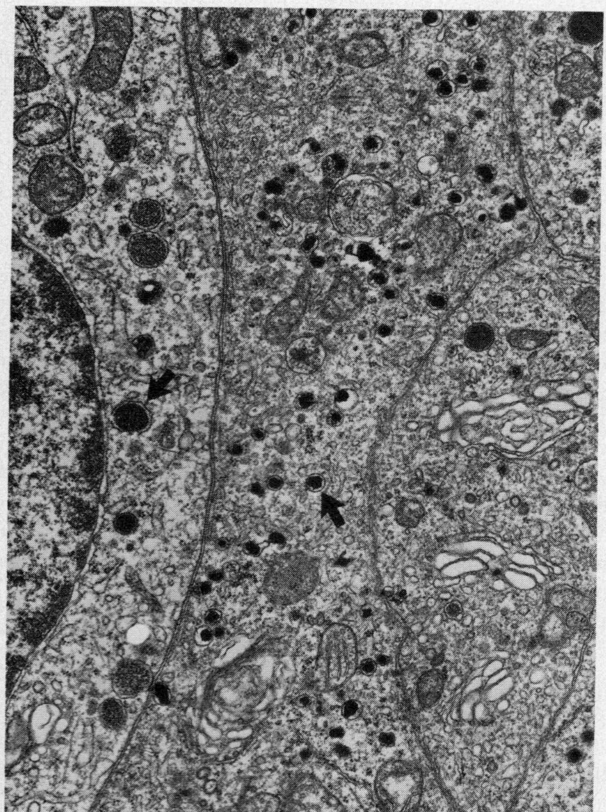

Figure 18–33. Electron micrograph of several cells in an endocrine cell tumor (argentaffinoma) revealing prominent membrane-bound dense-core neurosecretory granules *(arrows)* (approximately 6000×). (Courtesy of Dr. John Godleski, Brigham and Women's Hospital, Boston.)

Pearse, in 1969, was the first to recognize that a widely distributed system of interrelated endocrine cells all shared common cytochemical, ultrastructural, and biosynthetic features, and he further proposed that all had similar embryologic origins.[155] *The principal distinguishing feature of these cells is their capacity for amine precursor uptake and decarboxylation (APUD cells) with the synthesis of bioactive amines or polypeptide hormones.* Approximately 40 different cell types, distributed throughout many organs, share this biosynthetic function, and so belong to the APUD system. Major sites of localization of these cells are the hypothalamus, pituitary, adrenal medulla, and C cells of the thyroid, as well as the endocrine cells of the gastrointestinal tract, pancreatic islets, and lung.[156] Tumors derived from these cells are currently called APUDomas, whether benign or malignant (Table 18–4). Because hyperplasia of these cells also produces similar endocrinopathies, they too are somewhat inappropriately termed APUDomas.[157] Thus, endocrine cell tumors or argentaffinomas are often designated "carcinoid APUDomas."

Central to the conception of the APUD system was the belief that all the dispersed cells were derived from neuroendocrine-programmed epiblast that migrated during early embryogenesis to the various widely scattered sites. In support of this concept was the evidence that APUD cells elaborated many of the polypeptides produced by ganglion cells in the brain and peripheral ganglia as well as adrenal medullary cells.[158] Additional supportive cytochemical evidence is the presence of neuron-specific enolase (a glycolytic enzyme of neurons) in cells of all types of APUDomas.[159] However, many have challenged this unitary concept and contended that some neuroendocrine cells of the gut, pancreas, and lung are of endodermal origin, and further that not all tumors elaborating polypeptide hormones are necessarily of neuroendocrine origin—recall the well-known capabilities of neoplasms to elaborate ectopic hormones.[160, 161] Thus, the controversy continues to bubble, but the APUD concept is useful to explain a group of neoplasms having many cytochemical and secretory similarities whatever their origins.[162]

Just as the number of cells included within the APUD system has vastly expanded, so has the concep-

Table 18–4. APUD CELLS, APUDOMAS, AND ECTOPIC POLYPEPTIDE HORMONES PRODUCED BY APUDOMAS

Cell	Putative Tumor	Ectopic Hormone
Hypothalamic neurosecretory	None identified	
Pinealocyte	Pinealoma	Unknown
Adenohypophyseal*	Pituitary adenoma	Unknown
Autonomic neuron	Neurocytoma†	ACTH; vasoactive intestinal peptide (VIP)
Chromaffin	Pheochromocytoma	ACTH; follicle-stimulating hormone; calcitonin (CT); insulin
Carotid-body and other para-ganglion cells	Paraganglioma; chemodectoma	ACTH; CT
Thyroid C	Medullary carcinoma of thyroid	ACTH; insulin
Bronchial Kulchitsky	Bronchial carcinoid; oat cell carcinoma	ACTH; ADH; CT; glucagon; insulin; growth hormone; prolactin
Gastrointestinal endocrine	Intestinal carcinoid	ACTH; ADH
Pancreatic islet	Islet cell tumor	ACTH; ADH; VIP
Melanocyte	Melanoma	ACTH; gastrin

*ACTH, melanocyte-stimulating, somatotropic, and prolactin cells.
†Neuroblastoma, ganglioneuroblastoma, and ganglioneuroma.
From Tischler, A. S., et al.: Neuroendocrine neoplasms and their cells of origin. N. Engl. J. Med. *296*:920, 1977, by permission of The New England Journal of Medicine.

tion of the physiology of the APUD system.[160] *It now appears that APUD cell-derived peptides play important roles in diverse metabolic processes. Some may function as neural transmitters, and others have important systemic effects on the vascular system.* For example, insulin, glucagon, growth hormone, and epinephrine, all derived from APUD cells, play roles in glucose metabolism. At least seven of these peptide hormones have been identified in the central and gut nervous systems—substance P, somatostatin, vasoactive intestinal peptide, enkephalin, bombesin, neurotensin, and cholecystokinin-gastrin. Some of these hormones, such as vasoactive intestinal peptide, long thought to be only a gastrointestinal hormone, may also function as neurotransmitters.[163] Conversely, the brain neurotransmitters—enkephalin, bombesin, and neurotensin—have been discovered to be present in the gut and pancreas.[164] Such observations help to explain why a patient with a glucagonoma of the pancreas developed severe neurologic involvement, which responded to chemotherapy for the pancreatic lesion.[165] It is highly unlikely that the full complexity of the APUD system has yet emerged. Against this background, we can return to the endocrine cell tumors.

MORPHOLOGY. In an analysis of a large series of patients with these neoplasms, the distribution was as follows: appendix, 35%; small bowel, 25%; rectum and rectosigmoid, 12%; colon (except appendix), 7%; esophagus and stomach, 2%; lungs and bronchi, 14%; and other sites, 5%.[166] Multiple endocrine cell tumors have been variously reported as occurring rarely or in as many as 20 to 30% of these patients. Most often, multiple primaries are all located within the small intestine, presumably related to the large number of endocrine cells scattered throughout this segment of the gut. Within the gastrointestinal tract, extra-appendiceal carcinoids usually appear as small, round, or plaquelike submucosal elevations up to 4 to 5 cm in diameter, but commonly under 3 cm (Fig. 18–34). The overlying mucosa is usually intact, and in many instances the lesion is deceptively mobile and unattached to the underlying muscularis. Some are obviously bound to the underlying muscularis. Rarely, they become large, ulcerating, or polypoid growths. Sometimes, penetration of the bowel wall can be discerned, with extension into the mesentery of the small intestine or perirectal tissue. Appendiceal carcinoids, in contrast, are generally small nodules situated near the tip, 1 to 2 cm in diameter. These, too, may extend through the muscularis to the appendiceal serosa. Classically, all gastrointestinal carcinoids are yellow-gray on transsection, but they may not be distinctive from other types of neoplasms. For reasons that are unclear, **appendiceal carcinoids rarely metastasize, but extra-appendiceal lesions may spread to regional nodes, liver, lungs, and bones.**

Histologically, the typical pattern is that of solid nests of cells separated by a delicate, connective tissue framework. Occasionally, there is a tubular, acinar, or rosette-like arrangement of cells. **The individual cells have a striking resemblance to each other, with a monotony of cell and nuclear size and shape** (Figs. 18–35 and 18–36). The nuclei are round to oval and deeply chromatic with fine stippling throughout. Abundant cytoplasmic secretory granules are usually present and stain red with eosin, yellowish-brown with chrome salts, black with iron-hematoxylin, and sometimes metallic black with silver salts.[153] As mentioned earlier, reactivity with silver salts when present is a distin-

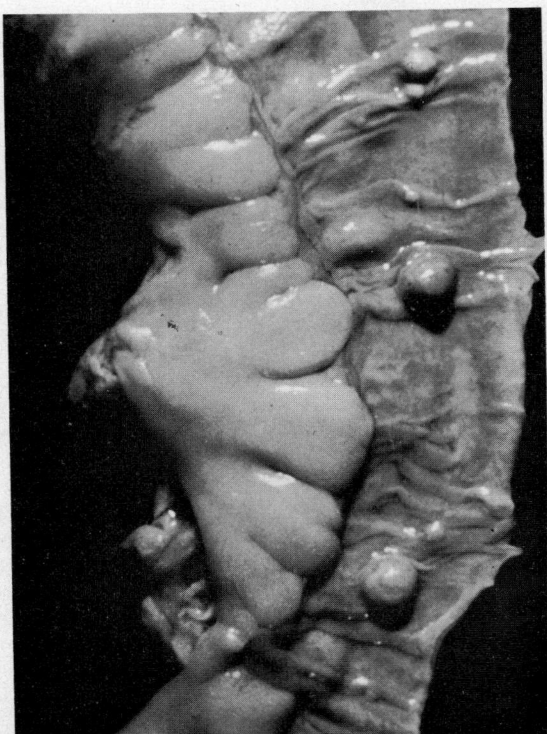

Figure 18–34. Multiple small polypoid endocrine cell tumors in small intestine.

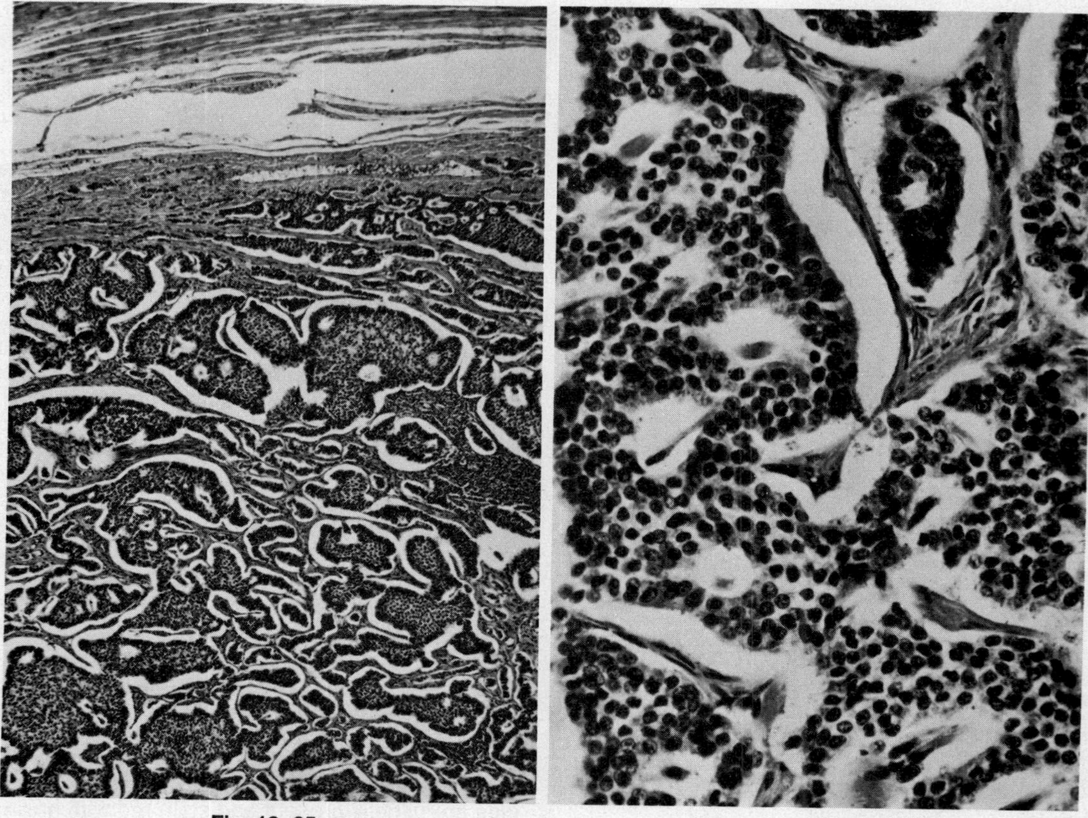

Fig. 18–35

Fig. 18–36

Figure 18–35. Endocrine cell tumor of appendix. Low-power view taken from one margin of tumor in contact with muscularis. Characteristic pattern of growth and invasion of wall is evident.
Figure 18–36. Close-up of cellular detail to show uniformity of nuclear size and shape and growth pattern.

guishing feature of endocrine cell tumors, but it is extremely variable. In general, foregut tumors (bronchus, stomach, biliary system, and pancreas) are either argyrophilic or nonreactive. Midgut lesions (small bowel, appendix, cecum, and right colon) are usually argentaffin positive and hence also argyrophil positive, whereas hindgut lesions (left colon, sigmoid, and rectum) yield variable results with both argentaffin and argyrophil reactions. With the electron microscope, the secretory granules can be seen to contain a dense core of variable shape separated from the granule membrane by a clear halo. The granules vary widely in size but average 150 to 200 nm in diameter.[167] Giant cells, anaplasia, and mitoses are rarely seen in carcinoids. Nonetheless, despite this innocent cytologic appearance, **most tumors (both appendiceal and nonappendiceal) invade the submucosa and muscularis and sometimes penetrate the bowel wall.**

The cytologic uniformity of carcinoids makes it impossible to estimate their metastatic potential on microscopic examination. Tumor size, however, appears to be important with extra-appendiceal lesions. Most small bowel carcinoids greater than 2 cm and large bowel lesions greater than 5 cm in diameter are associated with metastases.[168] In contrast, as pointed out earlier, the incidence of metastasis with appendiceal carcinoids is in the range of 0.2%.

CLINICAL COURSE. Endocrine cell tumors may appear at any age. Extra-appendiceal gastrointestinal lesions are most often encountered in the sixth decade, whereas appendiceal carcinoids are more common in the fourth (perhaps because appendectomies are more frequent in young adults). There is no sex predilection. Appendiceal lesions are almost always asymptomatic. Those located elsewhere in the gastrointestinal tract may also be silent for some time, but eventually they are likely to produce clinical manifestations in one of two ways—as a consequence of their local invasive growth or by virtue of their secretory products. In one study, abdominal pain was the dominant local presenting symptom.[169] Other presenting complaints included weight loss, anorexia and nausea, weakness, rectal bleeding, and diarrhea. Only rarely do endocrine cell tumors produce partial or complete intestinal obstruction, and this complication is largely limited to small bowel primaries. Sometimes they first come to attention because of metastatic nodular enlargement of the liver.

Far more distinctive is the development of a *carcinoid syndrome* related to the elaboration of secretory products:

1. *Vasomotor disturbances—distinctive episodic flushing of the skin and "cyanosis" (in almost all patients).*
2. *Intestinal hypermotility—diarrhea, cramps, nausea, and vomiting (in almost all patients).*

3. *Bronchoconstrictive attacks—cough, dyspnea, and wheezing resembling asthma (in about one-third of cases).*

4. *Right-sided cardiac involvement—valvular thickening and stenosis with endocardial fibrosis (in about one-half of cases).*

5. *Hepatomegaly—related to hepatic metastases (apparent only in some cases).*

It is important to emphasize that this symptom complex is seen only in patients having either extensive liver metastases or tumors whose venous drainage bypasses the immediate deamination of the liver—for example, primaries located in the ovary or lung. Only about 5 to 10% of patients with gastrointestinal carcinoids (most often primary in the small intestine) develop the carcinoid syndrome; a heavy burden of hepatic metastases must be present and the neoplasm must elaborate sufficient amounts of secretory products.[170]

The pathophysiology of the carcinoid syndrome is poorly understood. As APUDomas, the endocrine cell tumors or argentaffinomas produce a large variety of peptide hormones as well as other bioactive substances. Most important, with respect to the carcinoid syndrome, are serotonin (5-hydroxytryptamine—5-HT), histamine, kallikrein, and prostaglandins. In addition, however, individual case reports point to ACTH, calcitonin, insulin, gastrin, antidiuretic hormone, vasoactive intestinal peptide, and other products as possible contributors to the syndrome.[153] *The major secretion of carcinoid APUDomas is serotonin* derived by the hydroxylation of tryptophan to 5-hydroxytryptophan followed by its decarboxylation to serotonin (5-HT). Elaborated into the bloodstream by the liver metastases, 98% is degraded to 5-hydroxyindoleacetic acid (5-HIAA) in a single pass through the pulmonary circulation. For this reason, serotonin is proposed as the factor responsible for the right-sided valvular lesions, since the left heart is protected by the catabolism of serotonin in the lungs. However, attempts to produce heart lesions by chronic infusion of serotonin in rats have failed. The origin of the cutaneous flushing is less clear. It may be related to bradykinin formed secondary to the release of kallikrein by the APUDoma, or alternatively to 5-HT or prostaglandins. The diarrhea has also been related to these three products. The respiratory symptoms have been attributed to 5-HT, bradykinin, or histamine, all of which can cause bronchospasm. Whatever the origin of the clinical manifestations, identification of 5-HIAA in the urine provides an important diagnostic marker of the syndrome.

Surgical excision remains the only method of cure of this disease. Appendiceal carcinoids are usually discovered incidentally after the appendix has been removed and are cured by the appendectomy, save in the rare instance in which metastasis has occurred. In contrast, five-year survivals after surgical therapy range from 50% with neoplasms of the midgut to 80% with those of the rectum.[160] *A major consideration in the clinical management of patients with argentaffinomas is the associated increased incidence of other malignant neoplasms, some in extraintestinal sites.* These are found in about 15% of patients with carcinoids of the appendix, 10% of those with carcinoids of the rectum, and about 30% of those with carcinoids of the small intestine.[171, 172] About half of these concurrent cancers occur in the gastrointestinal tract. It is requisite, therefore, that a careful surgical exploration be done during excision of a gastrointestinal carcinoid to rule out the possible presence of another malignant neoplasm.

Carcinoma

Adenocarcinomas, despite the rapid turnover of the small intestinal mucosa, are very uncommon. They grow in a napkin-ring encircling pattern and rarely as polypoid fungating masses, recapitulating in a sense left-sided and right-sided colonic cancers (p. 869), respectively (Fig. 18–37). Crampy pain, nausea, vomiting, and weight loss are the common presenting signs and symptoms but, as pointed out, such manifestations generally appear late in the course of these cancers. Thus, most have already penetrated the bowel wall, invaded the mesentery or other segments of the gut, spread to regional nodes, and sometimes metastasized to the liver and more widely by the time of diagnosis. Despite these problems, wide "en bloc" excision of these cancers yields about a 70% five-year survival rate.[173]

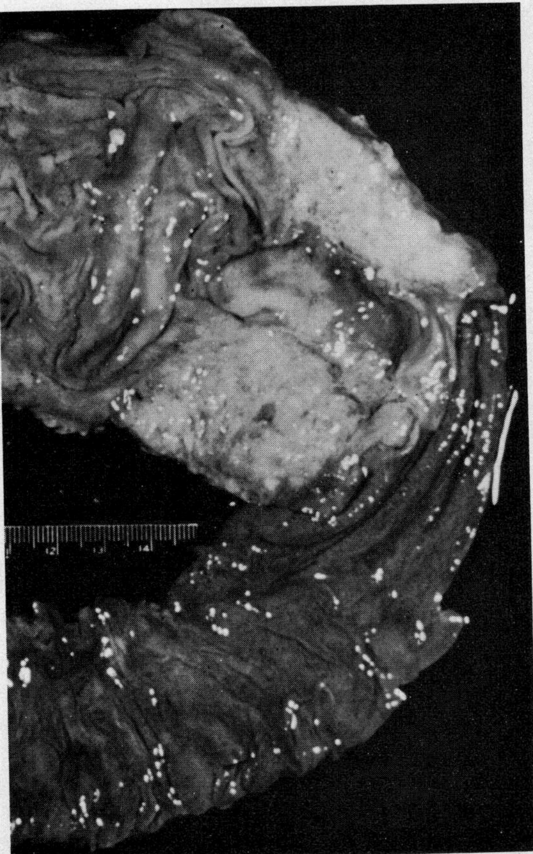

Figure 18–37. Carcinoma of small intestine growing in an annular encircling fashion.

Sarcoma

As in all levels of the bowel, sarcomas (leiomyosarcoma, rhabdomyosarcoma, liposarcoma, angiosarcoma, fibrosarcoma, and neurogenic sarcoma) may arise from the various mesenchymal elements of the wall of the small gut. They are all rare, producing the bulky, soft, hemorrhagic necrotic masses typical of sarcomas with their characteristic histologic picture. Most of these neoplasms are quite large at the time of discovery and have already metastasized through the bloodstream.

MALABSORPTION

The malabsorption syndrome is characterized by abnormal fecal excretion of fat (steatorrhea) and variable malabsorption of fats, fat-soluble vitamins, other vitamins, proteins, carbohydrates, minerals, and water. At the most basic level, it is the result of a disturbance in most cases of at least one of three functions: (1) digestion of nutrients to smaller molecules able to be absorbed or transported across the intestinal mucosal cell; (2) a reduction in the absorptive capacity of the bowel, principally the small intestine; or (3) transport of absorbed products. You recall that most of the digestive process begins in the stomach, with its content of acid and pepsin, and continues in the small intestine, under the influence of bile and the pancreatic and small intestinal enzymes. Absorption, although it may occur throughout the small intestine and, indeed, to a minimal amount in the colon as well, takes place chiefly in the upper small intestine, namely the duodenum and jejunum. Vitamin B_{12} and bile acids are notable exceptions and are absorbed in the lower small intestine. The absorptive surface of the small intestine is enormously expanded by the villi and the microvilli, which are estimated to number 2×10^8 per cm^2. Any disorder reducing the absorptive surface of the gut will lead to malabsorption.

The diseases and disorders causing malabsorption are both numerous and variably classified. First, an all-inclusive classification prepared by Sleisenger and Brandborg is presented in Table 18–5, from which it is apparent that malabsorption may be caused by a number of dissimilar mechanisms. Some affect mainly intraluminal digestion of nutrients. Others involve principally the transport and absorption of foodstuffs across the intestinal mucosal cell. Still others, such as lymphatic obstruction, impinge principally on the transport of fats once they have traversed the mucosal cell membrane. However, in many of the categories mentioned the basis for the malabsorption is poorly understood, or is a consequence of multiple defects. Each of these various mechanisms induces its own somewhat distinctive clinical signs and symptoms, but it is frequently necessary to resort to a number of diagnostic tests to differentiate among them, as, for example, stool fat determinations, measurement of xylose absorption, and gastrointestinal x-ray studies; perhaps most definitive is small intestinal biopsy. It is now possible with the use of peroral suction biopsy techniques to obtain specimens from the small intestinal mucosa that permit elegant evaluation of mucosal changes, particularly those affecting villous structure.[174] Some concept of the usefulness of intestinal biopsy can be gained from Table 18–6, which presents some of the typical findings and their specificity in many of the malabsorptive conditions.

Clinically, all the malabsorption syndromes resemble each other more than they differ. Particularly com-

Table 18–5. CLASSIFICATION OF MALABSORPTION SYNDROMES

Category I: Defective Intraluminal Hydrolysis or Solubility

- A. Primary pancreatic insufficiency
- B. Secondary pancreatic insufficiency
- C. Deficiency of conjugated bile salts, including intestinal resection
- D. Bacterial overgrowth (bile salt deconjugation)
  1. Blind loops
  2. Multiple strictures and jejunal diverticula
  3. Fistulas
  4. Postgastrectomy
  5. Scleroderma and pseudo-obstruction

Category II: Mucosal Cell Abnormality and Inadequate Surface

- A. Primary mucosal cell disorders
  1. Disaccharidase deficiency and monosaccharide malabsorption
  2. Abetalipoproteinemia
  3. Vitamin B_{12} malabsorption
  4. Cystinuria and Hartnup's disease
- B. Small bowel disease
  1. Celiac disease
  2. Whipple's disease
  3. Allergic and eosinophilic gastroenteritis
  4. Nongranulomatous ileojejunitis
  5. Crohn's disease (transmural enteritis)

Category III: Lymphatic Obstruction

- A. Lymphoma
- B. Tuberculosis and tuberculous lymphadenitis
- C. Lymphangiectasia

Category IV: Multiple Defects

- A. Subtotal gastrectomy
- B. Distal ileal resection, disease, or bypass
- C. Radiation enteritis

Category V: Unexplained

- A. Hypogammaglobulinemia
- B. Carcinoid syndrome
- C. Diabetes mellitus
- D. Mastocytosis
- E. Hyperthyroidism, hypothyroidism, hypoadrenocorticism, and hypoparathyroidism

Category VI: Infection

- A. Tropical sprue
- B. Acute infectious enteritis
- C. Parasitoses

Category VII: Drug-induced Malabsorption

- A. Cholestyramine
- B. Colchicine
- C. Irritant laxatives
- D. Neomycin
- E. *p*-Aminosalicylic acid
- F. Phenindione

From Sleisenger, M. H., and Brandborg, L. L.: Malabsorption. Vol. 13. Major Problems in Internal Medicine. Philadelphia, W. B. Saunders Co., 1977, p. 130.

Table 18–6. MALABSORPTION SYNDROMES—ABNORMALITIES IN SMALL INTESTINAL BIOPSIES

Disorders with Characteristic Findings

1. *Celiac and tropical sprue:* Blunted or absent villi, abnormal surface epithelium, lengthened crypts, increased mononuclear cell infiltrate in lamina propria
2. *Whipple's disease:* Lamina propria stuffed with glycoprotein-containing macrophages, villous abnormality of variable severity, bacilli demonstrable in macrophages during active disease in ultrathin sections or on electron microscopy
3. *Abetalipoproteinemia:* Mucosal absorptive cells vacuolated by lipid inclusions, villous structure normal
4. *Agammaglobulinemia:* Flattened or absent villi, absence of plasma cells, increased lymphocytic infiltrate
5. *Amyloidosis:* Demonstration of amyloid in and about vessels of lamina propria with Congo red staining and birefringence
6. *Regional enteritis:* Noncaseating granulomas
7. *Parasitic infections:* Identification of parasite in biopsy sections, e.g., giardiasis, strongyloidiasis, schistosomiasis, histoplasmosis, cryptosporidiosis
8. *Mastocytosis:* Mast cell infiltrates of lamina propria
9. *Intestinal lymphoma:* Possible foci of malignant lymphoid cells in lamina propria, villous abnormality of variable severity
10. *Allergic and eosinophilic gastroenteritis:* Infiltrates of excessive numbers of eosinophilic leukocytes, lesion patchy, villous structure may be normal or severely deranged
11. *Tuberculosis and tuberculous lymphadenitis:* Chance finding of caseating granuloma or margin of tuberculous ulcer

Disorders in which Biopsy may be Abnormal but is Not Necessarily Diagnostic

1. *Folate deficiency:* Shortened villi, megalocytes in blood vessels, decreased mitoses in crypts
2. *Vitamin B_{12} deficiency:* Similar to folate deficiency
3. *Radiation enteritis:* Similar to folate deficiency
4. *Systemic scleroderma:* Increased fibrosis in lamina propria, possible derangement in villous structure
5. *Lymphangiectasia:* Dilated lacteals and lymphatics in lamina propria, blunted and clubbed villi

mon are weight loss, anorexia, abdominal distention, borborygmi, muscle wasting, and passage of abnormal stools, which are in many instances light yellow to gray and greasy or frothy. Often there are frequent bowel movements, but occasionally there is only one stool per day. More specific manifestations appear in particular categories of malabsorption. When there is inadequate protein absorption, edema and ascites may become superimposed. Severe disturbances of fat absorption may lead to signs and symptoms of avitaminosis A, avitaminosis K, and avitaminosis D. In turn, absorption of calcium is hampered, contributing to skeletal changes. Thus, bone pain and predisposition to fracture may be encountered in patients with malabsorption of vitamin D and calcium. Sometimes, hypocalcemia appears and results in paresthesias or even tetany, convulsions, and coma. Inadequate absorption of folate and vitamin B_{12} produces its own set of signs and symptoms related to the resultant megaloblastic anemia. When the malabsorption syndrome is associated with profuse diarrhea, there may be significant loss of fluids and electrolytes, sometimes leading to severe acid-base, fluid, and electrolyte imbalances. Losses of fluids, sodium, and potassium may be life threatening.

Among the many disorders that may give rise to such syndromes, those most commonly encountered in the United States are celiac disease, regional enteritis, and chronic pancreatitis. To this group should be added viral enteritis, discussed earlier (p. 835). Although malabsorption is not often found with this type of involvement, the frequency of the infection, particularly in the pediatric age group, makes it a common cause of absorptive dysfunction. A second category of importance would include Whipple's disease, small intestinal diverticulosis, tropical sprue, disaccharidase deficiency, abetalipoproteinemia, amyloidosis, intestinal scleroderma, postgastrectomy states, and blind-loop syndromes (related to surgical procedures or congenital reduplication of the ileum).[175] Many of these more or less common entities have been discussed elsewhere; only a few remain to be considered.

CELIAC SPRUE

This condition is known by a variety of names—*gluten-sensitive enteropathy, nontropical sprue, and adult and childhood celiac disease.* It is related to dietary gluten, very likely an immune reaction to a constituent of this protein. Celiac disease is characterized by a striking loss of villi in the small intestine and, with it, a marked reduction in the absorptive surface area. Although the disease is usually diagnosed in early childhood, it may not be detected until years later. Females are affected more frequently than males. There are many suggestions pointing to a hereditary background. Familial clustering has been noted; as many as 80% of patients are HLA-B8, and over 90% D/DR3 or D/DR7, which may have relevance to the pathogenesis of this condition in terms of inherited specific immune response genes.[176]

There is now unmistakable evidence that celiac

disease can be cured by placing patients on a gluten-free diet. Gluten and the derivative gliadin are proteins found particularly in wheat, barley, and rye grains. *The preponderance of data points to a hypersensitivity reaction to antigenic determinants within gliadin as the cause of the intestinal changes.*[177] The small intestinal mucosa, when exposed to gluten, accumulates a large number of B cells sensitized to gliadin.[178] Circulating antibodies to gliadin are present in all patients under 2 years of age and in many who are older. It would appear that with antigenic challenge by gliadin there is local synthesis of immunoglobulins in the small bowel mucosa.[179] On gluten-free diets the titers of circulating antibodies fall or disappear.[180] However, antibodies cannot be demonstrated in all patients with this condition, and moreover there is often a poor correlation between the severity of the disease and the level of the antibodies.

Substantial as all the immunologic changes may be, the possibility cannot be ruled out that they are secondary phenomena. Conceivably, other mechanisms for injury of bowel mucosa permit the entry of antigenic fractions contained in food, thus accounting for the appearance of immunoglobulin-secreting cells in the mucosa. The antigliadin antibodies may then have no greater significance than the antibodies to nongluten milk proteins that can also be identified in some individuals with this condition. Thus, the older and still not invalidated "toxic" theory cannot be totally discounted.[181] Although the weight of evidence favors an immunologic basis for this condition, the etiology must still be considered uncertain.

The characteristic anatomic finding in celiac disease is marked atrophy of the villi diffusely throughout the jejunum with flattening of the mucosal surface. The villi become severely blunted and distorted and may even disappear (Fig. 18–38). There is an accompanying increase in depth of the crypts and in the number of mitoses within the crypt epithelium. Particularly prominent is a marked chronic inflammatory reaction in the lamina propria composed of lymphocytes and plasma cells with occasional eosinophils. With the immunoperoxidase technique, large numbers of immunocytes bearing IgA antigliadin antibodies are present in the small bowel mucosa, with some increase in IgM-bearing cells. The surface epithelial cells become cuboidal and stain poorly, and their nuclei assume irregular positions within the cell rather than the regular basal orientation.[174] Electron microscopy discloses that the microvilli are markedly distorted and shortened, while the mitochondria have unusual sizes and shapes and show changes in their cristae. The ribonucleoprotein granules are abnormally abundant. Although these changes are characteristic of celiac sprue, they are not pathognomonic since they can be mimicked by tropical sprue and other conditions.

The symptoms and signs of celiac disease are essentially those shared by all malabsorption syndromes (p. 847). Elevated titers of circulating IgA antigliadin antibodies are frequently present, but ultimately the diagnosis rests on the characteristic findings in the intestinal biopsy and the response to a gluten-free diet.[182] In some patients the histologic appearance of the small bowel mucosa returns to normal remarkably promptly following avoidance of gluten-containing foods, whereas in others the recovery is delayed for months or even a year. Indeed, in some patients, although an appropriate diet permits some restoration of the normal architecture, the mucosa may never totally revert to normal.

Individuals with long-term untreated celiac sprue may suffer a number of complications. Faulty absorption of nutrients may lead to anemia, probably secondary to a deficiency of iron and possibly of folate. Impaired calcium absorption may cause paresthesias, muscle cramps, and tetany, and if sufficiently prolonged may induce osteomalacia and osteoporosis (p. 1327). A variety of neurologic symptoms may appear in the forms of cerebellar atrophy and patchy demyelination of the spinal cord with sensory losses and ataxia. It is tempting to attribute these to malabsorption of thiamine, riboflavin, and pyridoxine, but administration of these vitamins does not correct the neurologic abnormalities. The most unpleasant consequence of long-term celiac disease is a 10 to 15% chance of developing cancer within eight to ten years. Over half are gastrointestinal lymphomas, now referred to as B-cell lymphomas, and the remainder are carcinomas distributed throughout the gastrointestinal tract disproportionately in the small intestine.[183] Still unknown is whether strict adherence to a gluten-free diet reduces the hazard particularly of lymphomas.

TROPICAL SPRUE

Tropical sprue is somewhat inappropriately named. Save for the similarity of the mucosal changes to those of nontropical sprue (celiac disease), there is little commonality between these two entities. Tropical sprue is of unknown etiology, although there are suggestions that it may be caused by enterotoxigenic *E. coli.*[184] It has a curious geographic distribution: although common in the Caribbean, it has not been reported from Jamaica, and it does not occur in Africa, south of the Sahara. Travelers to endemic areas may not become symptomatic until months or years after returning to their homes in temperate climates. Occasionally, the disease occurs in epidemics, but even these cases do not always have identifiable enteric pathogens. Thus, no specific causal microbiologic agent has been clearly associated with tropical sprue, although specific strains of *E. coli* are currently favored candidates. Despite the etiologic uncertainties, most patients are benefited or cured by long-term broad-spectrum antibiotic therapy.

Intestinal changes are extremely variable. In some patients the mucosal histology is not abnormal, whereas in others the changes are similar to those of celiac disease.[185]

WHIPPLE'S DISEASE

This uncommon multisystem disease is intriguing and frustrating. *Apparent rod-shaped bacilli can be*

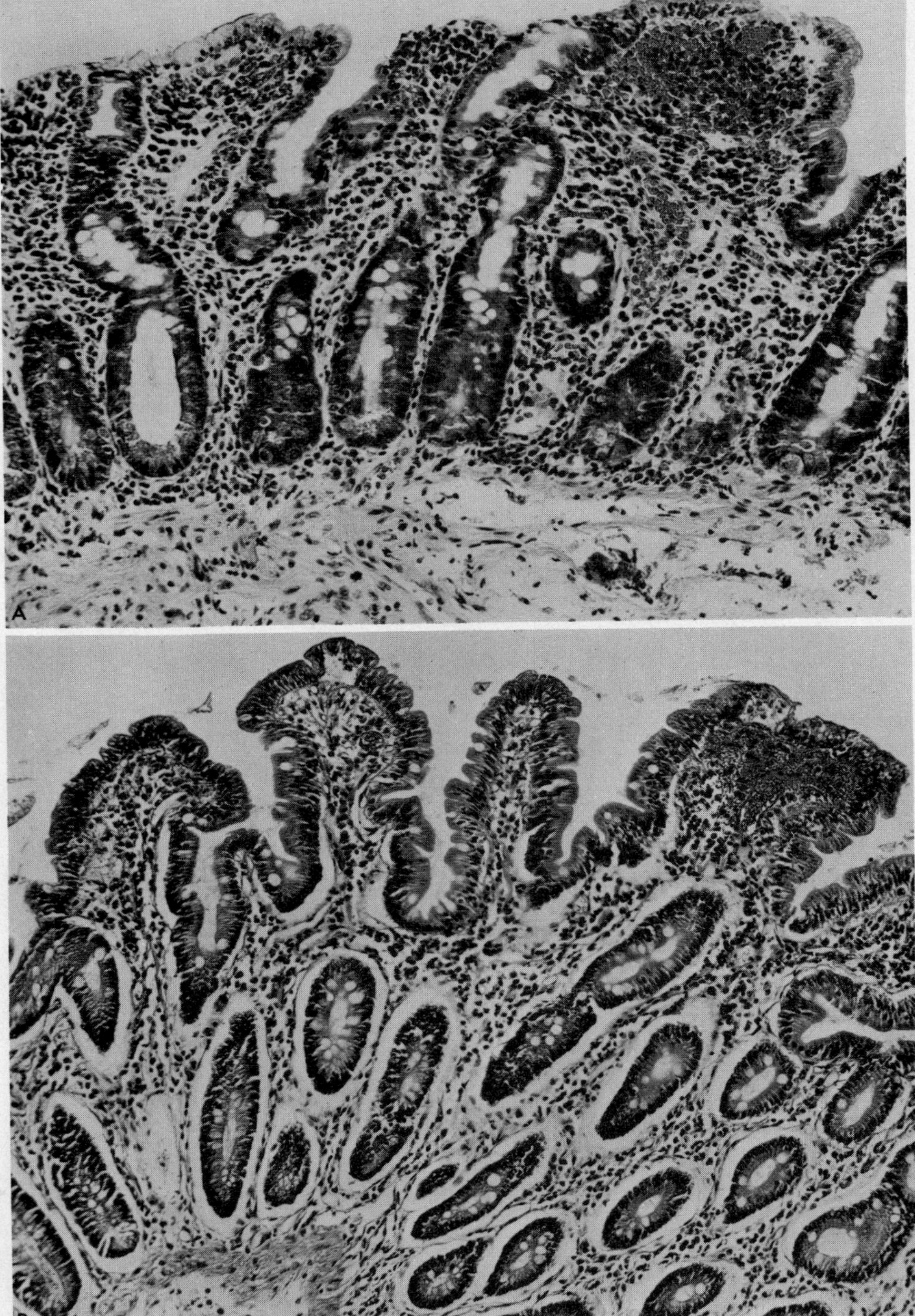

Figure 18–38. *A*, Celiac disease—a jejunal peroral biopsy of gluten enteropathy with atrophy and blunting of villi and an inflammatory infiltrate in lamina propria. *B*, Celiac disease—same patient as in *A* after five days on a gluten-free diet.

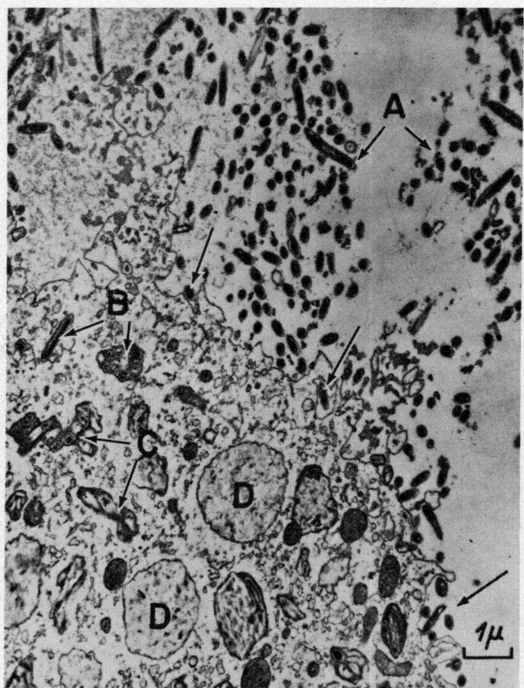

Figure 18–39. Electron micrograph of an involved histiocyte in Whipple's disease. A = bacilliform bodies outside cell with arrows pointing to loci where they appear to be penetrating cell boundaries. B and C = distorted forms. D = uninvolved lysosomes.

readily visualized under the electron microscope within and between glycoprotein-laden PAS-positive macrophages in many organs throughout the body, principally the small bowel mucosa, but it cannot be isolated and so no specific agent has yet been identified. The bacilli are approximately 2.50 × 0.15 μ in size (Fig. 18–39). The PAS-positive glycoprotein granules within the macrophages are thought to be bacterial products. Numerous microbiologic studies of patients with Whipple's disease have yielded over 25 different microorganisms, many not bacilliform.[186] Immunologic and histochemical studies of lesions have been equally frustrating, yielding positive results with antisera for streptococcus groups A, B, C, and G and *Shigella flexneri*.[187] Superimposed on all these complexities is the lack of an inflammatory response at the sites of localization of the apparent bacilli in the various tissues. Nevertheless, Whipple's disease responds promptly and dramatically to antibiotic therapy, often with permanent remission. The tangle is yet to be unraveled, however.

Whipple's disease was once thought to be solely an intestinal disorder characterized by malabsorption, but it is now apparent that it is systemic in distribution, involving not only the small intestine but also the skin, central nervous system, joints, heart, blood vessels, kidney, lung, serosal membranes, lymph nodes, spleen, and liver.[188] Indeed, a migratory polyarthritis is often the presenting manifestation. Occasionally, patients develop neurologic disturbances without manifestations of intestinal disease.[189] This condition has also presented as cardiac disease before intestinal, articular, or systemic involvement was apparent.[190] Whether intestinal involvement would eventually have developed with these unusual presentations is not clear.

MORPHOLOGY. The hallmark of this condition is the macrophage laden with PAS-positive granules and occasional rod-shaped organisms. In the classic case these cells crowd the lamina propria of the small intestine and mucosa (Fig. 18–40). In untreated cases the bacillary bodies may also be seen lying free in the interstitial spaces in the lamina propria of the small bowel, in neutrophils, and sometimes within the mucosal epithelial cells. Thus, the organism has the capacity to invade cells. Accompanying all these changes within the intestinal mucosa is dilatation of the lymphatics, which sometimes contain lipid droplets, suggesting some lymphatic obstructive process. Occasionally, rupture of these channels may give rise to lipogranulomas. The draining mesenteric lymph nodes of affected segments of the gut reveal the same microscopic changes. Characteristic macrophages containing bacillary bodies may be found in other levels of the gastrointestinal tract as well as in various other organs. For example, they can be found in the synovial membranes of affected joints, but damage to the articular surface is rarely present. They may also diffusely infiltrate the central nervous system, sometimes collecting into focal aggregates. PAS-positive macrophages containing bacilli have also been seen within cardiac valves, subendocardium, and myocardial interstitial tissue.[186] With antibiotic therapy

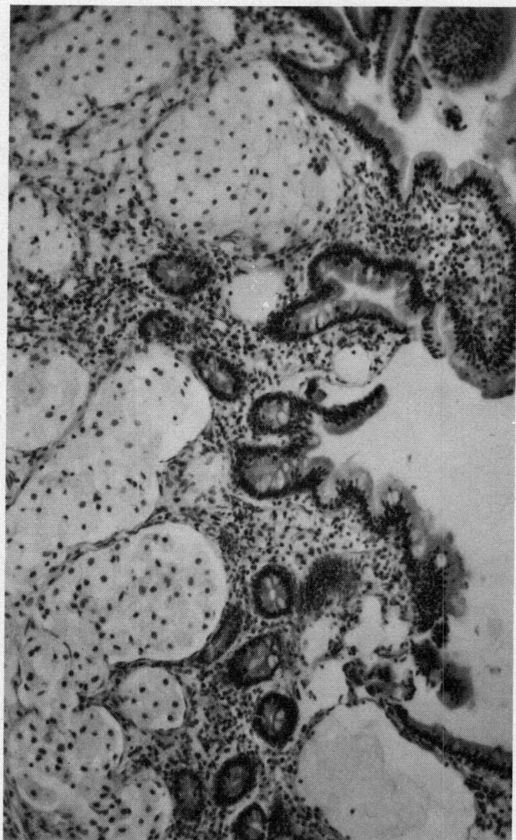

Figure 18–40. Whipple's disease with clusters of distended macrophages lying within lamina propria of intestinal mucosa.

the bacillary bodies disappear, only to reappear if the patient suffers a relapse.

Macroscopically, in the typical case, there is thickening of the wall of the small intestine, dulling of the serosa, and some thickening and induration of the mesentery. Fine, lacelike patterns of lymphatics can often be seen on the serosal surface. **The intestinal villi are distended and blunted by the phagocytic macrophages, sometimes giving to the mucosa the appearance of a shaggy bearskin rug** (Fig. 18–41). Mucosal thickening and pallor may be found in the large bowel and stomach, but less consistently than the changes in the small intestine. The involvements of other organs and sites rarely produce macroscopically apparent lesions.

CLINICAL COURSE. Whipple's disease usually presents as a form of malabsorption with diarrhea, steatorrhea, abdominal cramps, distention, fever, and marked weight loss. It is principally encountered in Caucasians in the fourth to fifth decades of life, with a strong male predominance in the ratio of 10:1. As pointed out, atypical presentations are quite frequent; indeed, Whipple's disease must be suspected, even in the absence of intestinal symptomatology, as a cause of polyarthritis, obscure CNS complaints, focal hyperpigmentations of the skin, and numerous other symptom complexes related to specific organ involvements. The diagnosis rests on light microscopic recognition of PAS-positive macrophages in appropriate biopsies that can be shown to contain rod-shaped organisms under the electron microscope. This once usually fatal condition can now be cured promptly by appropriate antibiotic therapy, and thus its recognition is crucial.

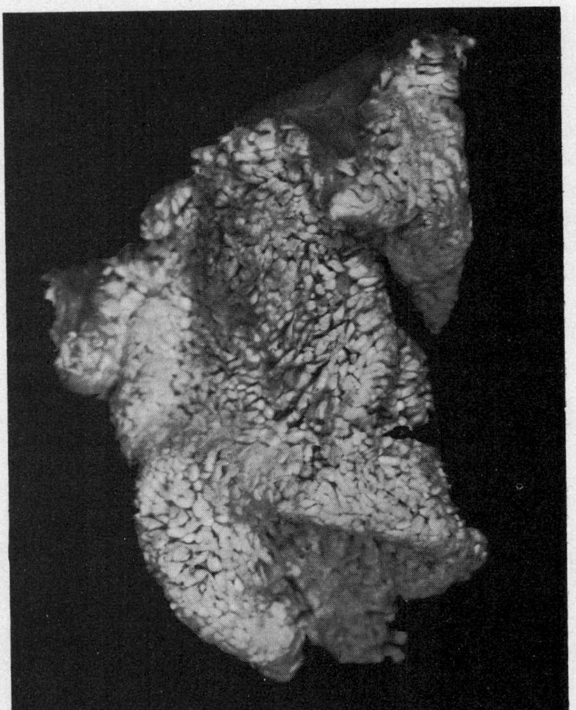

Figure 18–41. Whipple's disease of small intestine. The hugely distended villi resemble the pile of a shaggy rug.

DISACCHARIDASE DEFICIENCY

The disaccharidases, of which the most important clinically is lactase, are localized to the apical cell membrane of villous absorptive epithelial cells. Congenital lactase deficiency is a very rare condition, but acquired lactase deficiency is common, particularly among North American blacks. With insufficient lactase, the disaccharide lactose cannot be broken down into its monosaccharides, glucose and galactose. The unabsorbed lactose exerts an osmotic pull, leading to watery diarrhea and malabsorption. A deficiency of this enzyme may occur as a familial inborn error of metabolism or may apparently develop in adult life as an acquired disorder. When hereditary, malabsorption becomes evident with the initiation of milk feeding. The infants develop explosive, watery, frothy stools and abdominal distention. When exposure to milk or milk products is terminated, the malabsorption is promptly corrected.

In the adult, lactose intolerance may appear with viral and bacterial infections of the gastrointestinal tract as well as in other disorders of the gut. Despite the clinical manifestations, neither light nor electron microscopy has disclosed abnormalities of the mucosal cells of the bowel in either the hereditary or the acquired forms of the disease.

The diagnosis can be suspected with the breath hydrogen test. Bacterial fermentation of the unabsorbed sugars leads to the production of increased amounts of hydrogen, which can be measured readily by gas chromatography.[181]

ABETALIPOPROTEINEMIA

This form of malabsorption is familial and transmitted by autosomal recessive inheritance. It fundamentally constitutes an inborn error of metabolism, characterized by an inability to synthesize apoproteins required for the export of lipoproteins from mucosal cells. As a consequence, triglycerides are stored within them, creating lipid vacuolation, which is readily evident under the light microscope, particularly with special fat stains. Concomitantly, there is severe hypolipidemia related largely to depressed levels of chylomicrons, prebetalipoproteins (VLDL), and betalipoproteins (LDL). The disease becomes manifest in infancy and is dominated by failure to thrive, diarrhea, and steatorrhea.

OBSTRUCTIVE LESIONS

Obstruction of the gastrointestinal tract may be caused by lesions at any level, but the narrow lumen of the small intestine makes obstruction most common at this location. The causes of such obstruction may be classified as follows:

1. Mechanical obstruction:
   a. Strictures, congenital and acquired; atresias.
   b. Meconium in mucoviscidosis.

c. Imperforate anus.
d. Obstructive gallstones, fecaliths, foreign bodies.
e. Adhesive bands or kinks.
f. Hernias.
g. Volvulus.
h. Intussusception.
i. Neurogenic paralytic ileus.
j. Tumors.

2. Vascular obstruction:
a. Bowel infarction.

Tumors and infarction, although the most serious, account for only about 10 to 15% of small bowel obstructions. Four of the entities—hernias, intestinal adhesions, intussusception, and volvulus—account collectively for 80%.

HERNIAS

A weakness or defect in the wall of the peritoneal cavity may provide an area where persistent intraperitoneal pressure will eventually push out a pouchlike, serosal lined sac called a hernial sac. The usual sites of such weakness in the anterior abdominal wall are the areas of the inguinal and femoral canals, at the umbilicus, and in surgical scars. More rarely, similar retroperitoneal defects occur in the posterior wall of the abdominal cavity, chiefly about the ligament of Treitz. Hernias are of chief interest because segments of viscera may become trapped in them. This circumstance is more apt to occur in inguinal than in femoral hernias, since the former tend to have narrow orifices and large sacs. If the small bowel is involved, partial or complete obstruction to the lumen may follow. Pressure by the neck of the pouch may impair the venous drainage of the trapped viscus. A vicious cycle then develops whereby the edema produced by the venous stasis increases the bulk of the contents of the hernial sac, so that the intestinal loops are permanently trapped or *incarcerated.* The increased volume causes further increase of pressure on the collapsible blood vessels, and in time the venous and possibly the arterial supply may be cut off *(strangulation),* thus producing infarction of the trapped segment (Fig. 18–42).

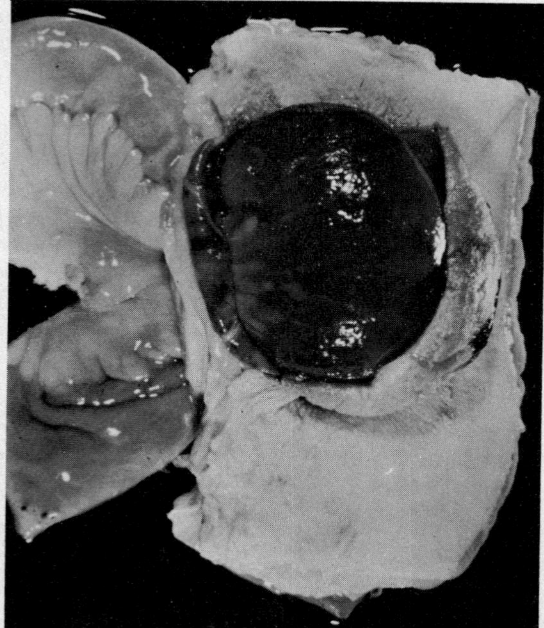

Figure 18–42. A knuckle of small intestine trapped in an inguinal hernial sac is demonstrated en bloc with encircling skin of inguinal region in situ. Sac has been opened to demonstrate hemorrhagic condition of contents.

If strangulation does occur, the gross and microscopic picture of the affected gut exactly resembles that previously described under bowel infarction. Not only the small bowel but portions of the omentum, and sometimes also segments of the large bowel, tend to become trapped in these hernial sacs. When the right side of the colon is loosely attached, or when there are large redundant sigmoid flexures, these segments of bowel may enter a hernial sac. Even ovary, fallopian tube, and segments of urinary bladder have been identified in such sacs. All these structures may suffer the same fate described for the small bowel—incarceration or strangulation with infarction. However, involvement of the small bowel is most serious, since it may cause intestinal obstruction or perforation.

INTESTINAL ADHESIONS

As peritonitis (an inflammatory reaction of the peritoneal serosa) heals, adhesions may develop. These fibrous bridges can create closed loops through which other viscera may slide and eventually become trapped, just as in a hernial sac. Intestinal obstruction, partial or complete, ensues and may be complicated by infarction of the trapped segment of bowel. This sequence of events is found most commonly in postoperative patients who develop peritoneal adhesions to the wound in the abdominal wall and within the operative site. Quite rarely, adhesions may occur without previous peritoneal inflammation from fibrous bands arising as congenital defects. Intestinal obstruction and strangulation must be considered, then, even without a previous history of peritonitis or surgery.

INTUSSUSCEPTION

This is an uncommon disorder, most often encountered in infants and children, in which one segment of small intestine, constricted by a wave of peristalsis, suddenly becomes telescoped into the immediately distal segment of bowel. Once trapped, the invaginated segment is propelled by peristalsis farther into the distal segment, pulling its mesentery along behind it (Fig. 18–43). The trapped bowel is referred to as the intussusceptum, and the segment that envelops it is known as the intussuscipiens. The pathogenesis of this lesion in children and infants is obscure. There is usually no

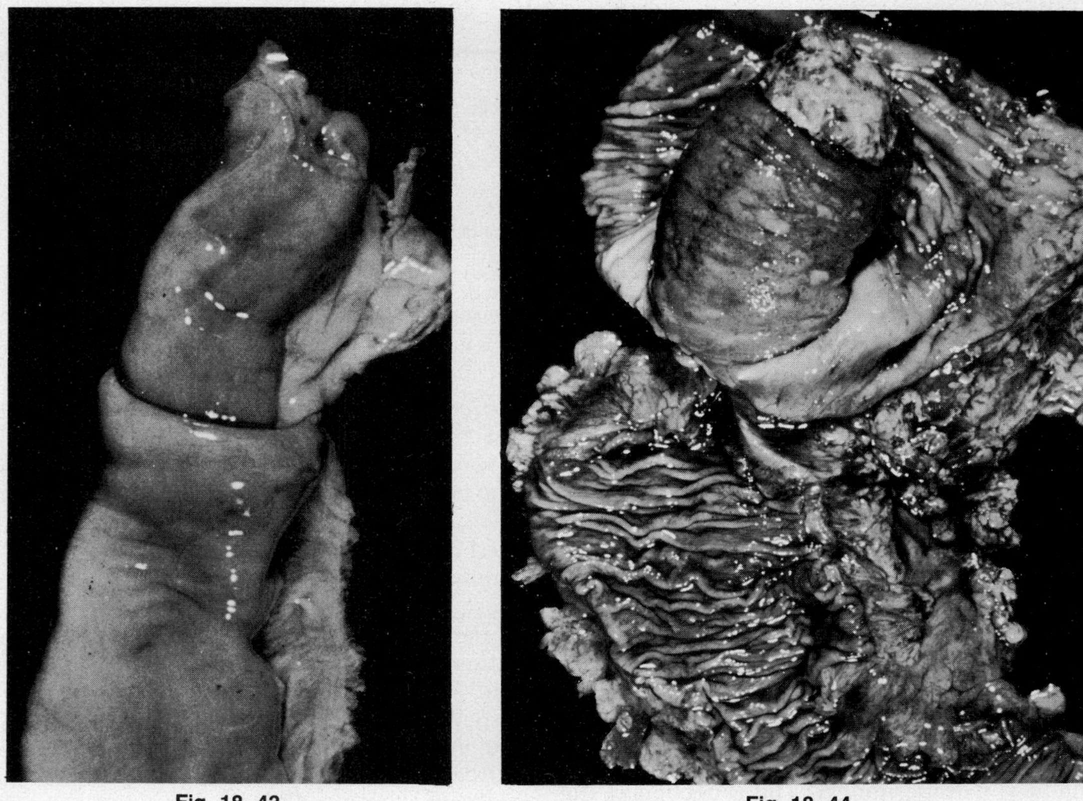

Fig. 18–43

Fig. 18–44

Figure 18–43. Intussusception of small intestine viewed from external aspect.
Figure 18–44. Intussusception of small intestine. Bowel has been opened to demonstrate necrotic tip of intussusceptum.

underlying anatomic lesion or defect in the bowel to explain such an occurrence. However, intussusception also occurs in adults, and in this age group some intraluminal mass or tumor serves as a point of traction that pulls out the base of attachment and segment of gut along with it. In both the spontaneous infantile and the adult cases, not only does intestinal obstruction ensue, but the trapped mesenteric blood supply may eventually become compressed and produce infarction (Fig. 18–44). In the infantile variety, the disorder, if discovered before infarction has occurred, is readily reduced, usually by simple administration of a barium enema. In the adult, surgical exploration is necessary, not only to determine the cause but also to deliver the trapped loop.

VOLVULUS

Complete twisting of a loop of bowel about its mesenteric base of attachment provides another mechanism for producing intestinal obstruction and infarction. This lesion occurs most often in the small bowel; however, large redundant loops of sigmoid are sometimes involved. Recognition of this seldom encountered lesion demands a constant awareness of its possible occurrence. If the bowel is not obviously strangulated, a hasty manual exploration at surgery or autopsy may miss the twisted loop. In most cases, obvious signs of obstruction or infarction develop and require further therapy.

Colon

NORMAL

The colon in man is a storage and absorptive organ. It is not essential for life. The subdivisions of the large bowel into the cecum, ascending colon, transverse colon, and descending colon are well-known. Perhaps somewhat less well understood are the exact limits of the sigmoid colon and rectum. The former begins at the pelvic brim, includes the sigmoid flexures, and connects below with the rectum at approximately the level of the third sacral vertebra. The rectum is that portion distal to the sigmoid. It is approximately 6 inches long; the proximal portion is within the peritoneal cavity and the distal segment is extraperitoneal. The reflection of the peritoneum from the rectum over the pelvic floor produces a cul-de-sac known as the "pouch of Douglas." This space is a favored site for the implantation of spreading intra-abdominal tumors, which produce a perirectal mass called a "rectal shelf." These masses are within 3 inches of the anus and are therefore within reach of the examining finger.

The blood supply to the right side of the colon up to the midportion of the transverse colon is derived from the superior mesenteric artery. Occlusion of the superior mesenteric artery therefore causes infarction not only of the small bowel but also of the ascending colon. Almost the entire remainder of the intra-abdominal colon is supplied by the inferior mesenteric artery. The lower rectum receives its supply from the hemorrhoidal branches of the internal iliac or internal pudendal artery; the upper level is supplied by the superior hemorrhoidal branch of the inferior mesenteric. The venous drainage follows essentially the same distribution. Therefore, within the rectal vasculature there is an anastomotic capillary bed between the superior hemorrhoidal veins draining through the portal system and the inferior hemorrhoidal veins, which drain through the inferior vena cava. In portal hypertension, these capillaries can become distended and provide a bypass for portal venous obstruction. Throughout most of its extent, the colon is a fixed retroperitoneal organ. Therefore, it derives considerable accessory blood supply and lymphatic drainage from a wide area of the posterior abdominal wall, making infarction and obstructive lymphedema most uncommon in this level of intestine.

Microscopically, in contrast to the small intestine, the colon has no villi. The absorptive surface itself is flat but is punctuated by numerous straight tubular crypts that extend into the underlying lamina propria. The crypts are lined mainly by goblet mucous cells with occasional endocrine cells. The mucosal surface is covered mainly by absorptive cells that bear on their luminal surfaces microvilli that are less abundant than those found in the small intestine. Intimately attached to these microvilli is an elaborate fibrillar glycoprotein extraneous coat similar to that found in the small intestine. Paneth cells, found mostly in the lower crypts, are dispersed throughout the right colon. Scattered within the mucosa are lymphoid foci covered by somewhat flattened cells that are thought to engulf and transfer antigens to the underlying immunocytes. Cell renewal in the colon and rectum essentially follows the pattern described in the small intestine, with most of the cell replication occurring in the base of the crypts. Once formed, the cells migrate upward from the crypt to the surface in about two to six days. The mitotically active epithelial cells are vulnerable to radiation and cancer chemotherapeutic drugs. However, they provide the potential for rapid repair. The intrinsic innervation of the colon comprises Auerbach's plexus, located between the circular and longitudinal muscle layers, and Meissner's plexus, situated in the submucosa. Both comprise nests of ganglion cells interconnected by unmyelinated postganglionic fibers that extend through the thickness of the bowel wall to provide communications between the plexuses.

PATHOLOGY

Certain lesions that affect the colon constitute some of the most frequently encountered diseases in clinical practice, particularly surgical practice. Cancer of the large bowel is the second most common cause of cancer death in man. The extremely common hemorrhoid, a comparatively trivial lesion, may produce in the aggregate more clinical discomfort than almost any other lesion to which man is subject. In addition, inflammatory disorders such as ulcerative colitis and functional derangements such as spastic and mucous colitis are by no means uncommon. In terms of clinical and pathologic importance, then, the colon and the stomach are two areas of major importance in the gastrointestinal tract.

CONGENITAL ANOMALIES

Congenital anomalies of the colon are encountered infrequently. *Malrotations* may occur in which the cecum fails to descend to its definitive adult position in the right lower quadrant. Such malpositioning may confuse the diagnosis of acute appendicitis. *Reduplications* of the colon have been described rarely with the occasional formation of entire double large bowels. The most frequently occurring and clinically important anomalies of the colon are megacolon (Hirschsprung's disease) and imperforate anus.

MEGACOLON

Marked dilatation of the colon, or megacolon, occurs both as a congenital and as an acquired disorder. Although the mode of transmission of congenital megacolon, also known as Hirschsprung's disease, is unclear, about 4% of siblings of an index patient may be expected to have the disease. It is ten times more frequent in patients with Down's syndrome than in the general population and is often associated with a host of other congenital anomalies.

The origin of congenital megacolon is a failure during embryogenesis of development of Meissner's and Auerbach's plexuses. Normally, neuroblasts migrate in a cephalocaudal direction in the gut to reach the rectum at about 12 weeks of development. If the migration falls short, some portion of the distal colon lacks ganglion cells and there is a consequent functional loss of peristalsis and, in effect, a colonic obstruction. Thus, in all patients, ganglion cells are lacking at the anorectal junction, but the extent of more proximal involvement depends on the severity of the migratory defect. In the vast majority of patients the proximal border of the aganglionic segment is located within the rectum or sigmoid. In only 10 to 20% of patients is a longer segment affected, and only very rarely the entire colon (aganglionosis of the colon). However, neural trunks from more proximal ganglion cells may extend into the aganglionic segment, and it has been proposed that these contribute to spasm within the aganglionic segments, worsening the functional obstruction.[191]

MORPHOLOGY. **Hirschsprung's disease is characterized by the absence of ganglion cells and proliferation of nonmyelinated nerve fibers in the submucosal and intermuscular levels of the nondilated segment of colon.** Whatever the extent of the involvement, the rectum is always affected and thus provides a site for biopsy. However, the distal 2 to 3 cm should be avoided since ganglia are normally sparse here. Since both Meissner's and Auerbach's plexuses develop more or less contemporaneously in the embryo, colonoscopic biopsies that include only the mucosa and submucosa are usually sufficient to reveal ganglion cells if they are present.[192] However, if they are not found, transmural biopsy at the time of surgery may be necessary to confirm their absence.

In the common pattern in which both rectum and rectosigmoid are affected, the descending colon undergoes dilatation and hypertrophy first. Eventually, however, the entire colon may become involved, and indeed the functional obstruction may cause dilatation of the small intestine. The appendix, too, may become dilated and in some cases has perforated. In far-advanced cases the colon may appear as a huge, elongated balloon (Fig. 18–45). The wall of the dilated bowel may undergo hypertrophy and thickening. Sometimes, however, the distention outruns the hypertrophy, leading to thinning and potentiating rupture, particularly of

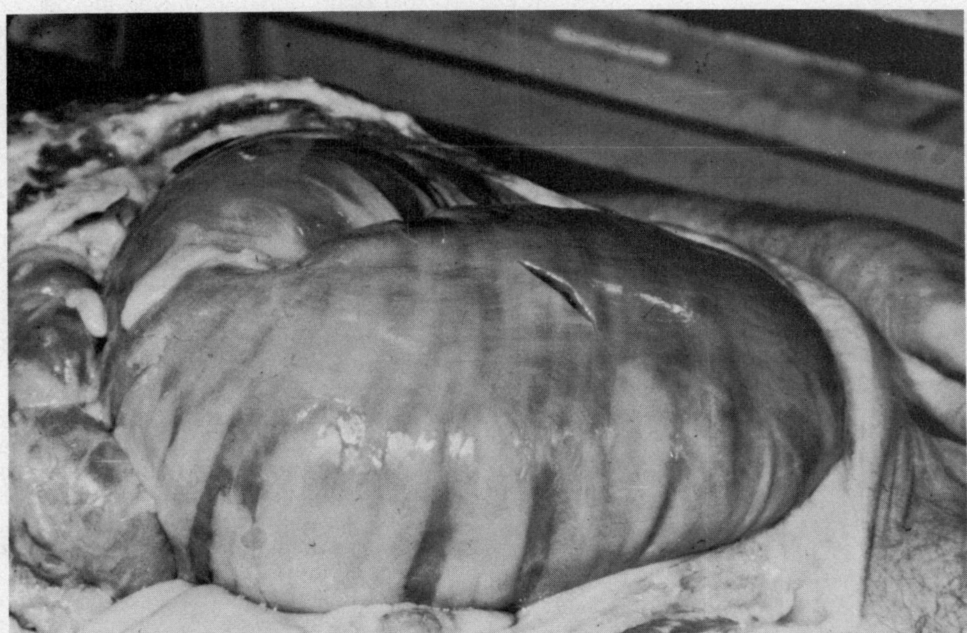

Figure 18–45. Megacolon. Hugely distended bowel viewed in situ just after abdomen has been opened in a postmortem examination. Bowel has been accidentally nicked.

the distended cecum, which has the thinnest wall. The mucosal lining may be intact throughout, but the functional obstruction may predispose to an inflammatory enterocolitis, or impacted feces may induce stercoral ulcerations.

CLINICAL COURSE. Hirschsprung's disease usually makes itself known in the immediate neonatal period by failure of passage of meconium followed by obstructive constipation. Vomiting soon follows. In some instances, when only a short segment of the rectum is affected, the build-up of pressure may permit occasional passage of stools, or even intermittent bouts of diarrhea. Abdominal distention (when a sufficiently large segment of colon is involved) confirms the presence of an intestinal obstruction. The diagnosis can be suspected on the basis of the clinical findings, but it is firmly established on histologic examination of a biopsy documenting the absence of ganglion cells in the nondilated colon. X-rays of the abdomen and barium enema studies may not be helpful early in the condition before significant bowel dilatation has developed. The major threats to life in this disorder are superimposed enterocolitis with fluid and electrolyte disturbances, and perforation of the colon or appendix with peritonitis.[193]

Acquired megacolon is encountered either in circumstances of chronic organic obstruction, such as narrowing of the bowel due to the inflammatory disease or neoplasia, or as an apparent functional disorder. Emotional problems may underlie some of these functional disturbances, but in other instances there appears to be a motility dysfunction also found in asymptomatic relatives. Nevertheless, the intrinsic innervation of the bowel is normal. Generally the entire colon, including the rectum, is dilated, but only rarely is the dilatation as massive as that encountered in the congenital form.

IMPERFORATE ANUS

Imperforate anus results when the membrane that separates the entodermal hindgut from the ectodermal anal dimple fails to perforate. An intact membranous septum may completely close the anal canal. This type of anomaly is said to occur in one in 5000 births. Many times the occlusion is more serious than a simple membranous covering and takes the form of agenesis, atresia, or stenosis of the rectal canal. In a significant number of these developmental failures, fistulous communications occur with the genital tract in the female or with the urinary tract in either sex.

IDIOPATHIC DISORDERS

DIVERTICULAR DISEASE

Numerous saccular outpouchings of the colon, particularly in the rectosigmoid, are prone to develop with advancing age and are referred to as "diverticular disease." At one time this condition was called "diverticulosis" and was thought to be of importance principally because it predisposed to the development of inflammatory changes in and about the diverticula, creating "diverticulitis." It is now clear that diverticulosis in the absence of inflammatory changes may produce lower abdominal discomfort with intermittent crampy pain or sometimes continuous pain indistinguishable from the symptomatology of diverticulitis. Moreover, in about half of the instances, diverticulitis is not associated with fever or leukocytosis.[194] It therefore is frequently impossible to differentiate diverticulosis and diverticulitis clinically; hence, the use of the term "diverticular disease." It is noteworthy that, in one study, one-third of referral center patients operated on for presumed diverticulitis had no inflammatory changes in the resected bowel.[195]

The prevalence of this condition in Western societies has risen remarkably since the turn of the century. In 1910 diverticular disease was found in about 5 to 10% of autopsies in the United States, United Kingdom, and Australia.[196] Currently the prevalence in these countries approaches 30 to 50%. It is much less frequent in nonindustrialized tropical countries and in Japan. It has been said, therefore, that diverticular disease is a disorder of Western civilization.[197] Environmental influences are thought to underlie this epidemiology, as will be explained. Another important influence on prevalence is age. Diverticula are rare in persons under 30 years of age; in those over the age of 60 the prevalence is about 50% in high-risk locales. Thus, a progressive rise in the mean age of certain populations may explain at least some of the increased frequency of this condition. The pathogenesis of diverticular disease is best considered after the morphology.

MORPHOLOGY. Most diverticula are located in the sigmoid colon (95%). However, the descending colon and indeed the entire colon may also be affected. Hypertrophy of the musculature of affected segments of colon is present in about 50 to 70% of specimens. The teniae coli are unusually prominent and have an almost cartilaginous consistency. The circular muscles are also thicker than normal and may impart a corrugated appearance to the gut as viewed from the serosal surface. In most specimens, small flasklike or spherical outpouchings, usually 0.5 to 1 cm in diameter, can be identified along the margins of the teniae. In the absence of secondary inflammation they are elastic, compressible, and easily emptied of fecal contents. Characteristically, these sacs dissect into the appendices epiploicae and may therefore be missed on casual inspection. They often have slitlike communications with the bowel lumen, which sometimes escape detection.

A "prediverticular state" has been described in which there is muscular thickening and luminal narrowing, but no outpouchings. The validity of this state is open to challenge because, as mentioned, many specimens with overt diverticula do not have muscular hypertrophy, and there is no way of knowing whether hypertrophy will always lead to the formation of diverticula.

When inflammatory changes supervene they tend to extend about the diverticula, producing peridiverticulitis, and to dissect into the immediately adjacent pericolic fat. Perforation of diverticula usually initiates the inflammatory process. Over the course of time the numerous foci of inflammatory reaction may cause marked fibrotic thickening in and about the colonic wall, producing sufficient narrowing to resemble remarkably a colonic cancer. Extension of the infection may lead to pericolic abscesses, sinus tracts, and sometimes pelvic or generalized peritonitis.

Histologic examination of uninflamed diverticula discloses a remarkably thin wall composed of a flattened or atrophic mucosa, compressed submucosa, and attenuated or totally absent muscularis (Fig. 18–46). The lack of muscularis is significant with respect to the pathogenesis of these outpouchings. The inflammatory reaction, when present, is nonspecific and may be attended by considerable fibrosis in and about the bowel wall. Bacterial cultures usually yield a mixed flora, with *E. coli* predominating.

PATHOGENESIS. The morphology of diverticula strongly suggests that *two factors are important in their genesis: (1) foci of muscular weakness in the colonic wall, and (2) intraluminal pressure.*[198] Thus, *diverticula represent herniations of the mucosa and submucosa at points of muscular weakness.* Angiographic studies indicate that such weaknesses occur wherever the arterial vasa recta penetrate the muscularis to ultimately ramify in the submucosa and mucosa. The connective tissue sheaths that surround these perforating vessels provide avenues devoid of muscularis for the development of herniations. The largest vasa recta are located along the margins of the teniae, conforming in most cases to the distribution of the diverticula. The fact that diverticula appear in some children with Marfan's syndrome, and the association of these lesions with aging, suggests that loss of tensile strength of collagen favors their development.

Whether especially high intraluminal pressure is requisite for the formation of these herniations remains controversial.[199] To explain the epidemiologic data cited earlier, it has been proposed that diets low in fiber content (resulting from the increased use of white flour, refined sugar, and meat) reduce the stool bulk. This, in turn, leads to increased peristaltic activity, particularly within the sigmoid colon.[200] Hyperplasia of the muscularis, as, for example, in the prediverticular stage of the disease, would favor bandlike contractions that might isolate short segments of the bowel (so-called segmentation) in which elevated pressures might develop. According to this hypothesis, diverticular disease is the consequence of disordered motility in the colon. Subsequent studies have challenged this sequence. It has been shown that asymptomatic patients with diverticula do not necessarily have increased intraluminal pressure or decreased stool weight.[201] However, it is important to note that *exaggerated peristaltic contractions and segmentation of the sigmoid colon are correlated with symptomatic disease whether inflammation is present or not.* Moreover, augmentation of the fiber content of the diet, say with bran, is usually effective in abatement of the pain. Thus, we may conclude that *a low-fiber diet, hyperactive peristalsis with segmentation, and increased intraluminal pressure is not requisite for the development of diverticula; however, such deranged motility accounts for most of the symptomatology of this condition.* There is no substantial evidence that a high-fiber diet prevents the development of diverticular disease.

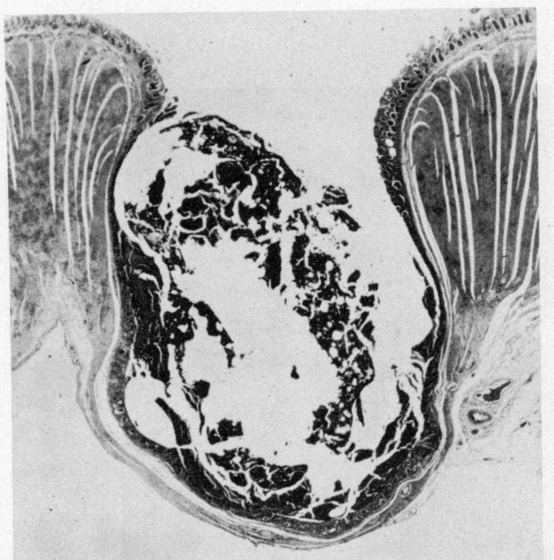

Figure 18–46. Low-power view of diverticulum of colon indicating marked thinning of wall and absence of muscularis.

CLINICAL COURSE. Most individuals with diverticular disease remain asymptomatic throughout their lives. Indeed, the lesions are most often discovered as incidental findings during barium studies for other reasons or at postmortem. Only about 20% of those affected ever develop manifestations. These are intermittent, crampy, or sometimes continuous lower abdominal discomfort; constipation; distention; and a sensation of never being able to empty the rectum completely. Sometimes there is alternating constipation and diarrhea. Patients with this condition may have minimal chronic or intermittent bleeding or sometimes massive hemorrhages, but before such blood loss is attributed to diverticular disease, other more likely causes must be excluded. When inflammatory changes supervene they may or may not be associated with fever, leukocytosis, and, in chronic cases, the development of a palpable sausage-shaped mass in the left lower quadrant. As emphasized earlier, it may not be possible on clinical grounds to distinguish inflammatory from noninflammatory disease.

Longitudinal studies have shown that diverticula can regress in the early stages of their development or, conversely, become more numerous with time. Whether a high-fiber diet prevents such progression or protects against superimposed diverticulitis is still unestablished. In most instances patients live comfortably with their diverticula, although some require high-fiber diets such as supplementation with unprocessed bran—leading one improved but revolted patient to grumble: "The treatment may be worse than the disease."[202] Even when diverticulitis supervenes, as judged by an increase in pain, fever, and leukocytosis, it most often resolves spontaneously. Only about 20% of patients with sufficiently severe symptomatic disease to lead them to seek hospitalization require surgery for obstructive or inflammatory complications.

MELANOSIS COLI

This curious brown-black discoloration of the mucosa, involving either a large segment or the entire large bowel, is of anatomic interest alone since it never produces clinical symptoms. The mucosal surface is intact and unaltered other than for the pigmentation, which histologically is associated with brown-black pigment granules within large mononuclear cells or macrophages in the lamina propri. The granules can be resolved as lysosomes under the electron microscope.[203] Histochemical studies indicate that the pigment has some of the characteristics of both melanin and lipofuscin. Even more obscure than the nature of the pigment is its origins. It has been attributed to the use of cathartics of the anthracene type, including cascara sagrada, senna, aloe, and rhubarb, and indeed can be induced in individuals by the chronic use of these agents. The pigmented lysosomal granules might then represent phagocytized debris of mucosal cells damaged by the toxic action of the cathartics. However, such speculation fails to account for the fact that the pigmentation stops abruptly at the ileocecal junction. What spares the small intestine? The incidence of carcinoma in such colons is no higher than in less colorful colons.

VASCULAR LESIONS

ISCHEMIC INJURY

Ischemic injury to the colon, often somewhat inappropriately referred to as "ischemic colitis," was discussed on page 831. There, it was pointed out that, to an extent, the large bowel is protected from such damage because of its double blood supply, i.e., mesenteric vessels as well as accessory vessels from the posterior abdominal wall. Nonetheless, vascular insufficiency infrequently induces one of three patterns of injury, referred to as (1) transmural infarction, (2) mural infarction, and (3) mucosal infarction. The meaning of transmural infarction is clear. The terms mural infarction and mucosal infarction are applied to ischemic injuries that involve the inner layers of the colon but spare the deeper levels, i.e., the muscularis and serosa. In the past, this pattern of ischemic injury has been referred to as "hemorrhagic enteropathy."

HEMORRHOIDS

Hemorrhoids are variceal dilatations of the anal and perianal venous plexuses. These extremely common lesions affect about 5% of the general population and are rarely encountered in persons under the age of 30, except in pregnant women. They develop secondary to persistently elevated venous pressure within the hemorrhoidal plexus. Although any cause of consistent venous congestion may be responsible, the most frequent predisposing influences are constipation with straining at stool and the venous stasis of pregnancy. The latter state is related to the overall congestion in the pelvis as well as the pressure of the enlarged uterus upon the iliac vessels. More rarely, but much more importantly, hemorrhoids may reflect collateral anastomotic channels that develop as a result of portal hypertension. On this basis, the appearance of hemorrhoids may be a clue to the existence of some diffuse hepatic disease or portal vein occlusion.

The varicosities may develop in the inferior hemorrhoidal plexus and be located below the anorectal line (external hemorrhoids), or they may develop from dilatation of the superior hemorrhoidal plexus and produce internal hemorrhoids (Fig. 18–47). Commonly, both plexuses are affected, and the varicosities are referred to as combined hemorrhoids.

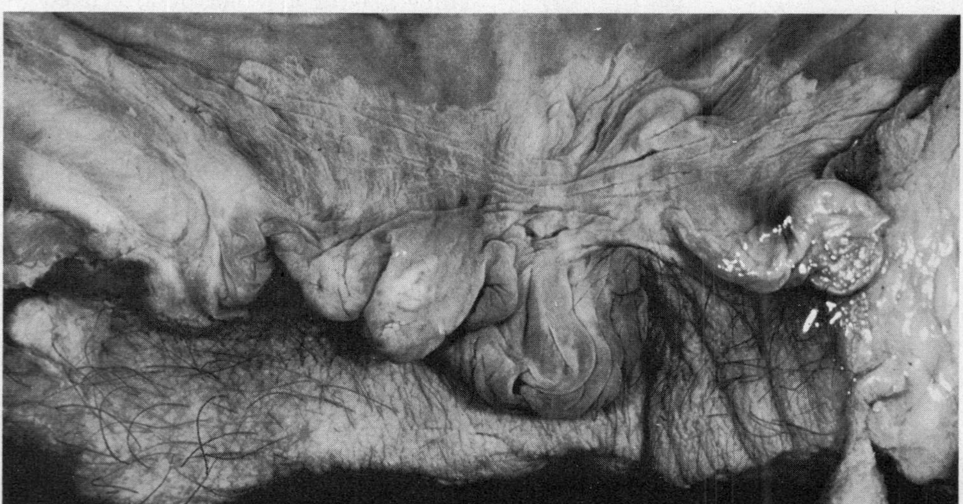

Figure 18–47. Hemorrhoids. External mucosal protrusions containing markedly dilated veins.

Histologically, these lesions consist only of thin-walled, dilated, typical varices that protrude beneath the anal or rectal mucosa. In their exposed, traumatized situation, they tend to become thrombosed and, in the course of time, canalized. Occasionally, internal hemorrhoids may protrude through the anal sphincter and become strangulated by the contraction of the sphincter about their bases. Superficial ulceration, fissure formation, and hemorrhagic infarction with strangulation complicate the histologic picture and clinical problem.

ANGIODYSPLASIA (VASCULAR ECTASIA) OF RIGHT COLON

Tortuous, abnormal dilatations of the submucosal veins in the cecum and ascending colon are a recently recognized frequent cause of lower gastrointestinal bleeding in the aged. These vascular lesions have escaped detection in the past because they were so hard to identify clinically with the then available diagnostic methods.[204] Barium studies do not reveal the vascular dilatations since they are almost entirely intramucosal. The pathologist, too, may miss them as the blood drains out during dissection. Only when colonoscopy and selective mesenteric angiography became available was it possible to identify these lesions.

Angiodysplasia is most often located within the cecum, but the right colon may also be affected. The vascular alterations range from small, focal, mucosal, vascular ectasias to large, dilated, tortuous, submucosal veins associated with extensive dilatation of thin-walled mucosal venules and capillaries.[205] Rupture of one or more of these abnormal vessels accounts for the colonic bleeding.

The incidence of this condition is not known but it has been referred to as one of the major causes of unexplained anemia or gastrointestinal bleeding in the aged.[206] Although it is possible that the lesions represent congenital malformations or are neoplastic, most believe that they are acquired vascular ectasias that rarely appear before the seventh decade of life. Partial, intermittent obstruction of the submucosal veins where they traverse the muscularis may underlie their development. According to Laplace's law, tension in the wall of a cylinder is a function of intraluminal pressure and diameter. Because the cecum has the widest diameter of the colon, it develops the greatest wall tension, predisposing to intermittent occlusion of thin-walled veins where they pass through the muscularis, raising pressures in the submucosal and mucosal tributaries. Presumably, decades of intermittent obstruction are required, which explains the restriction of this condition to the aged. Vascular degenerative changes related to aging may play some role.

INFLAMMATIONS

The many forms of colitis caused by specific infectious agents were considered together with the involvements of the small intestine on page 833, since inflammations of the small bowel and colon are so closely related and have similar causes. There remain to be considered only idiopathic ulcerative colitis and pseudomembranous colitis.

IDIOPATHIC ULCERATIVE COLITIS

This form of colitis is a recurrent acute and chronic ulceroinflammatory disorder of unknown etiology affecting principally the rectum and left colon, but sometimes the entire large bowel.[115] Like Crohn's disease, ulcerative colitis is in reality a systemic disorder associated in some patients with migratory polyarthritis, sacroiliitis, ankylosing spondylitis, uveitis, various forms of hepatic involvement, and skin lesions. As mentioned previously, there are many other similarities between the two conditions (see p. 836). Most important, Crohn's disease may also involve the colon.[207] Indeed, in about 30 to 35% of cases of Crohn's disease the large and small intestine are affected concurrently, and in an additional 20 to 30% the colon alone is involved.[118] Thus, there is a growing tendency to refer to both as a single entity—"inflammatory bowel disease" (IBD). However, unlike the granulomatous inflammatory changes in Crohn's disease (hence the term *granulomatous colitis*), well-developed granuloma formation rarely, if ever, appears in ulcerative colitis. Other distinguishing features between the two conditions have already been mentioned in the consideration of Crohn's disease, but will be emphasized in the later discussion (p. 861). In our present state of confusion and ignorance, it seems best to consider them as separate entities.

EPIDEMIOLOGY. Ulcerative colitis is global in distribution despite previous misconceptions that it was principally a disease of Western nations. In the United States, Great Britain, and Scandinavia the incidence is about four to six per 100,000 population. It is much less common in the U.S.S.R., Japan, and the South American nations. The incidence of this condition in high-risk locales has risen significantly in the past few decades.[208] In the U.S. it is more common among whites than among blacks. Females are affected more often than males. The onset of the disease peaks between the ages of 20 and 25 years, but the condition may arise in both younger and considerably older individuals. It was thought that Jews were affected more often than non-Jews, but studies from Israel contradict this. As with Crohn's disease there are hints of genetic influences. About 25% of families of patients have other members with ulcerative colitis and/or Crohn's disease.[120] Individuals with both ulcerative colitis and ankylosing spondylitis have an increased frequency of HLA-B27, but this association is now clearly related to the spondylitis and not to the ulcerative colitis. Other HLA associations have been recorded, but none are impressive.[115]

ETIOLOGY AND PATHOGENESIS. The current state of confusion about the origins of the two forms of IBD—ulcerative colitis and Crohn's disease—was discussed on page 837.

MORPHOLOGY. Ulcerative colitis invariably begins in the rectum and spreads proximally in continuity. "Skip" lesions such as occur in Crohn's disease are not found. Sometimes one segment of the colon shows active inflammatory ulceration while another segment may be healing, creating the false impression of discontinuous lesions. In severe expressions of ulcerative colitis, with involvement of the entire colon, a "backwash ileitis" may develop in about 10% of cases, but the small intestinal involvement is not readily confused with fully evolved regional enteritis.[140]

An acute and chronic phase can be recognized. In acute ulcerative colitis the bowel wall is neither significantly thickened nor inelastic, and the serosa is unaffected. The hyperemic, edematous mucosa at this stage may reveal a lack of the usual mucous secretions. More apparent in the acute disease is the development of small focal mucosal hemorrhages, many of which develop suppurative centers (crypt abscesses) that may give rise to small ulcerations. With chronicity the suppuration extends laterally in the submucosa to undermine the mucosal margins, thus producing numerous so-called aphthous ulcers, often closely spaced. Typically they are round or oval. With progression these small ulcers coalesce to become irregular in shape, but rarely do they replicate the linear serpentine fissuring of Crohn's disease (Fig. 18–48). In the usual acute-to-chronic disease the ulcerations are confined to the mucosa and submucosa and do not erode the muscularis. Often the undermined edges of adjacent ulcers interconnect to create tunnels covered by tenuous mucosal bridges (Fig. 18–49). Expansion and coalescence of the ulcers can denude large tracts of the involved colon, and sometimes in severe cases they become deeper to extend into the muscularis. Virtually the entire mucosa may be destroyed, often leaving residual islands of edematous hyperemic mucosa. Swollen, inflammatory tags of mucosa may bulge upward to create "pseudopolyps." Sometimes, in the very acute severe disease, there is marked "toxic" dilatation of the colon. Indeed, the inflammatory process may create microfissures to penetrate the colonic wall, producing pericolic abscesses, but gross fistulous tracts such as are seen in Crohn's colitis are very rare. In the absence of such penetration, the serosa does not appear to be affected.

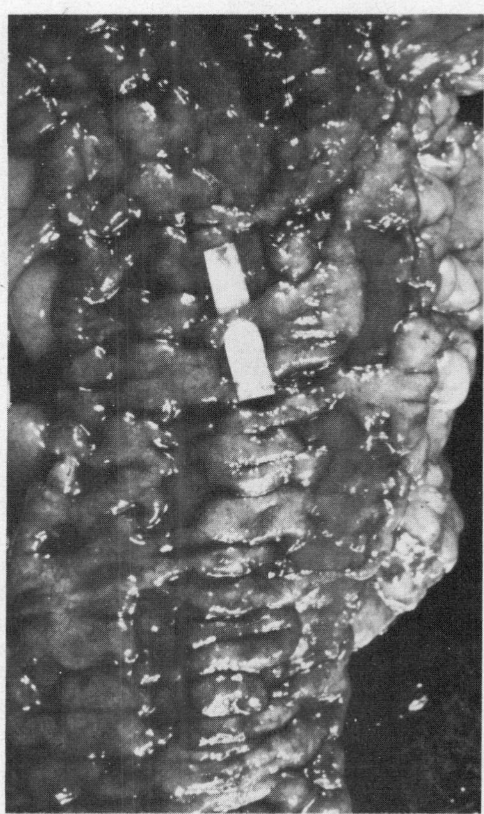

Figure 18–49. Chronic nonspecific ulcerative colitis. The irregular, elongated, seemingly smooth-based ulcers are separated by transversely corrugated strands of persisting mucosa. Coalescence of undermined margins of closely adjacent ulcers has left a bridge of mucosa, seen over the central paper tab.

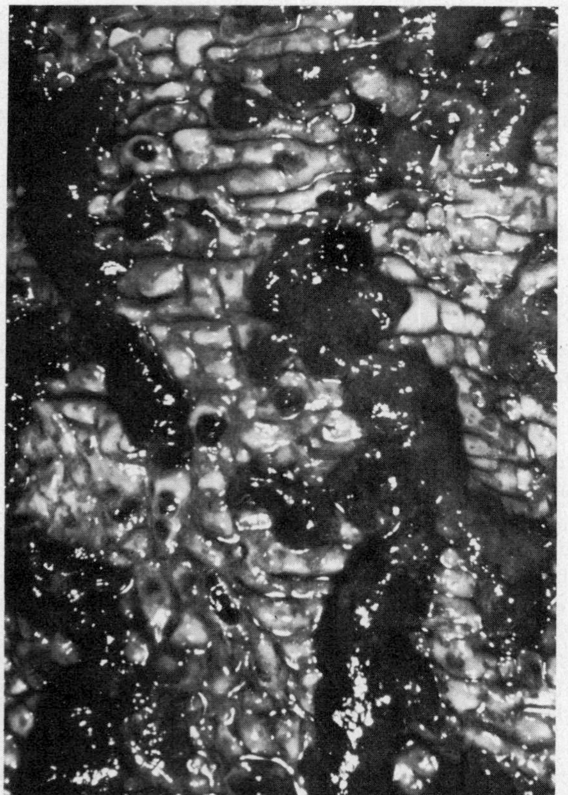

Figure 18–48. Ulcerative colitis. The dark, irregular pattern comprises ulcerations that have in many instances coalesced, leaving virtual islands of residual, paler mucosa. A tendency toward pseudopolyp formation is already evident.

Over the long chronicity of recurring attacks, the ulceroinflammatory disease leads to fibrosis and thickening of the bowel wall, but rarely to the same degree as in granulomatous colitis. The fibrosis does narrow the lumen, but rarely sufficiently to cause obstruction. With remission, the ulcers heal, but the pseudopolyps may remain, as well as such residual fibrosis and thickening of the wall as have developed. Particularly important is the possible superimposition of colonic carcinoma, as discussed later.

Histologically, the active phase of the disease is characterized by crypt abscesses and ulcerations extending down to the muscularis and surrounded by a

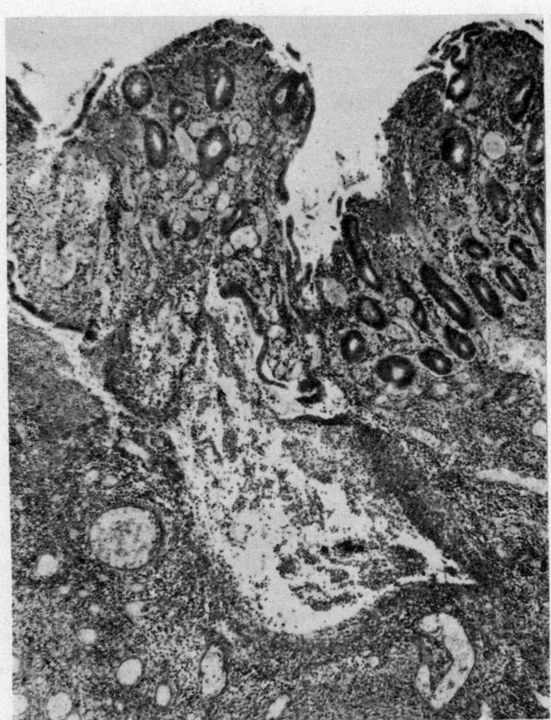

Figure 18–50. A deeply situated mucosal abscess in early developmental stage of acute ulcerative colitis.

prominent mucosal infiltrate of inflammatory cells (Fig. 18–50). The inflammatory process appears to begin within the depths of scattered crypts; as the disease continues and becomes chronic, rupture of the crypts into the lamina propria and into the submucosa permits the process to expand laterally. In this way the surrounding mucosa is undermined and sloughs to produce an ulceration. The remaining lamina propria is heavily infiltrated with neutrophils, lymphocytes, plasma cells, and occasionally mast cells. Sometimes the small vessels immediately underlying an ulceration disclose acute vasculitis, raising the possibilities that the ulcerations are the consequence of ischemic necrosis of the mucosa followed by secondary infection, and that the basic process in ulcerative colitis is an immunologically mediated diffuse vasculitis. Important features that help to differentiate ulcerative colitis from Crohn's colitis are as follows: (1) the ulcerations rarely extend significantly into the muscularis, and hence there rarely is fistula formation; (2) the inflammatory reaction is nonspecific and there is no granuloma formation; (3) there are no "skip" lesions as in Crohn's disease; and (4) the inflammatory tags of mucosa, the pseudopolyps, are not seen in Crohn's disease.

Particularly significant in this condition are the cytologic changes in the epithelium of the inflamed segment of colon, as well as in the pseudopolyps, collectively referred to as low- to high-grade dysplasia to overt carcinoma. Sometimes these cytologic changes are present in uninflamed mucosa, some distance from active disease. They have been elaborately subdivided into various grades of dysplasia ranging from mild to severe, becoming transformed too frequently into carcinoma.[209] The severity of the dysplasia and risk of carcinoma are directly related to the extent of the disease in the colon and the duration. With extensive involvement or so-called universal (entire colon) involvement, the incidence of carcinoma is about 1% under 10 years, 3.5% at 15 years, 10 to 15% at 20 years, and over 30% at 30 years.[210] With only left or right-sided colitis, the risk with long-standing disease is in the range of 3 to 5%. When the involvement is limited to the rectum, there is less danger of cancer. Ulcerative colitis is typically a recurrent disease. During remissions the mucosa may regenerate, often with the production of a more primitive epithelium lining cystically dilated and atypical glands. The precancerous epithelial changes may persist, however, as does the risk, and so the statement "10 years' duration" does not necessarily imply unremitting active disease.

Although repeated reference has been made to anatomic features that help to differentiate ulcerative colitis from Crohn's disease, experts point out that in about 10 to 20% of resected colonic specimens the colitis is "indeterminate."[139] Some of the overlaps and differential features are summarized in Table 18–7.

Clinical Course. Ulcerative colitis typically presents as a remitting, relapsing disorder marked by attacks of bloody mucoid diarrhea that may persist for days, weeks, or months and then subside, only to recur after an asymptomatic interval of months to years or even decades. In the fortunate patient, the first attack is the last. At the other end of the spectrum, the explosive initial attack may lead to such serious bleeding and fluid and electrolyte disturbance as to constitute a medical emergency. In most patients, bloody diarrhea containing stringy mucus, lower abdominal pain, and cramps, usually relieved by defecation, are the first manifestations of the disease. These appear insidiously but become progressively worse. Often this first attack is preceded by a stressful period in the patient's life. Persistence of the manifestations for even a short time is usually followed by fever and weight loss. Sponta-

Table 18–7. RELATIVE FREQUENCY OF MORPHOLOGIC FINDINGS IN ULCERATIVE COLITIS (UC) vs. CROHN'S DISEASE OF COLON (CD)

Gross Features	UC	CD
Total colonic involvement	+ + +	+
Distal predominance	+ + + +	+
Right colon predominance	0	+ + +
"Skip" lesions	0	+ + +
Broad-based ulcers	+ + +	+
Serpentine fissures	+	+ + + +
Transmural fibrous thickening	+	+ + + +
Pseudopolyps	+ + +	0 to +
Microscopic Features		
Granulomas	0	+ +
Nonspecific acute and chronic inflammation	+ + + +	+ +
Crypt abscesses	+ + + +	+
Transmural inflammation	+	+ + +

Modified from Yardley, J. H., and Donowitz, M.: Colorectal biopsy in inflammatory bowel disease. *In* Yardley, J. H., et al. (eds.): The Gastrointestinal Tract. Baltimore, Williams & Wilkins Co., 1977, p. 50.

neously, or more often after appropriate therapy, these symptoms abate in the course of days to weeks. An asymptomatic interval of varying length follows, after which stress (emotional or physical) may typically cause a flareup of the clinical manifestations. Sometimes, concurrent intraluminal growth of *Clostridium difficile* with its enterotoxin provokes the recurrent attack. Sudden cessation of bowel function with production of toxic dilatation of the colon, called "toxic megacolon," may appear with any acute attack.

As mentioned earlier, with chronic disease, extragastrointestinal manifestations are quite common: ankylosing spondylitis in 5 to 15%, arthritis of large joints in another 6%, and uveitis in 11% as well as nonspecific hepatitis, pericholangitis, and skin lesions (principally erythema nodosum and pyoderma gangrenosum). Some of these systemic problems, indeed, may precede the onset of the bowel disease and persist after colectomy.

The outlook for patients with this condition depends on two factors: (1) the severity of the disease and (2) its duration. About 60% of patients have what can be called "mild disease." In these individuals, the bleeding and diarrhea are not severe, and systemic signs and symptoms are absent. Medical management is usually effective in controlling the manifestations, and the development of colonic cancer is much less frequent than in the severe forms of the disease. About 25% of patients have "fulminant ulcerative colitis." The sudden onset may be characterized by intractable diarrhea, severe bleeding, high fever, and serious electrolyte and fluid disturbances. This toxic form of the disease, unless controlled, can lead to death soon after its onset.

As must now be obvious the most feared long-term complication is cancer.[211] Depending on the duration and extent of the disease, it is now standard practice to monitor closely the possible appearance of dysplastic changes or carcinoma with colonoscopy and multiple mucosal biopsies at regular intervals. When carcinomas develop in these patients they tend to be more infiltrative, and multiple cancers are more frequent than in those without preexisting colitis. Moreover, the underlying inflammatory disease tends to mask the symptoms and signs of carcinoma, so that these cancers are extremely insidious and inoperable twice as often as those in patients without colitis.[212]

PSEUDOMEMBRANOUS COLITIS (PMC)

This entity (also described on p.327) constitutes an acute form of colitis characterized by pseudomembrane formation overlying sites of mucosal injury. It is usually, if not always, caused by the toxin of *Clostridium difficile*, a normal gut commensal. However, this brief characterization requires qualification. Infrequently, the small intestine is involved, and so the condition sometimes is truly "pseudomembranous enterocolitis." Pseudomembrane formation is not restricted to *Cl. difficile;* it may result from ischemic injury or other enteric infections with staphylococci, Shigella, and sometimes Candida. *Cl. difficile* has also been implicated in initiating relapses of chronic IBD such as Crohn's disease and idiopathic ulcerative colitis.[213] *More often, however, it appears as an acute diarrheal colitis in patients without a background of chronic enteric disease who have received broad-spectrum antibiotics, particularly clindamycin and lincomycin.*[214] Thus, the condition is sometimes referred to as "antibiotic-associated colitis." However, it may appear in the absence of antibiotic therapy typically after surgery or superimposed on some chronic debilitating illness. It has also been recorded as a spontaneous infection in young adults without predisposing influences.[215]

Fully evolved PMC is marked by patchy areas of mucosal inflammation in the large intestine to which are attached dirty gray-yellow membranous coagula constituting the pseudomembranes. The underlying mucosal surface may reveal very shallow to well-defined ulcerations of the mucosa. Milder expressions may reveal only hyperemia, edema, and thickening of the mucosa without pseudomembrane formation. Microscopically, the pseudomembrane is composed of a coagulum of fibrin and mucin containing recognizable inflammatory cells, as well as a potpourri of cellular debris derived from leukocytes and mucosal epithelial cells. Typically, the fibrinomucinous exudate appears to erupt in volcano-like fashion from the crypts in the mucosa. There is an intense infiltrate of neutrophils admixed with mononuclear cells in the lamina propria of affected areas.

The diagnosis can be established clinically by identification of the toxin in the stools. Recognition of this condition is paramount since it can be promptly cured by vancomycin administration.

LYMPHOPATHIA VENEREUM

The primary site of origin of this disease in the female is the cervix or vagina (p. 294). Drainage of the infection in this sex occurs to the lymph nodes about the rectum. In the male, with the external genitalia as the primary site, only the inguinal nodes are affected. Therefore, in females, inflammation may extend from the neighboring nodes to involve the rectal wall. Although basically a perirectal process, at a far advanced stage it produces sufficient inflammation, fibrosis, and scarring of the rectum to cause narrowing of the bowel. Trauma to the wall by the passage of solid feces through the point of narrowing occasionally produces mucosal ulcers. Lymphopathia must therefore be considered in the differential diagnosis of rectal obstruction in the female.

TUMORS OF COLON

The colon (as used here taken to include the rectum) is the segment of the gastrointestinal tract most frequently affected by tumors. Bronchogenic cancer "holds the grisly trophy" for being the leading cancer killer, but colonic carcinoma is second; the respective number of deaths in the United States in 1984 were estimated at 121,000 and 59,500. Benign tumors such as lipomas, leiomyomas, angiomas, and mesenchymal lesions may occur here (Fig. 18–51), but the great majority of benign tumors are epithelial polyps. These are even more common than cancers and are present in as many as 25 to 50% of older adults.[216] Many are non-neoplastic and are referred to as hyperplastic polyps. However, some are true neoplasms and are called "adenomatous polyps." The adenomatous lesions have great importance because of the growing body of evidence that they represent precursors of colonic cancer.[217] Both adenomatous polyps and colonic carcinomas represent a challenge to clinical medicine since diagnostic modalities are widely available for their early discovery and cure can be achieved by resection. Thus, deaths from colonic cancer in the U.S. must each be viewed as a preventable tragedy.

POLYPS

A polyp of the colon may be defined as any lesion that protrudes above the surface of the surrounding mucosa. Although a large variety of benign neoplasms—leiomyomas, fibromas, lipomas, as well as cancers—may take the form of polyps, the great majority are mucosal in origin and fall into two broad categories: hyperplastic and adenomatous. The latter are true neoplasms and sometimes harbor foci of carcinoma, whereas the former are best viewed as benign, controlled proliferations. *Adenomatous polyps can be subdivided further into three histologic types: tubular (glandular), tubulovillous, and villous.* There is, in general, a correlation between type and size. Hyperplastic polyps are the smallest, tubular adenomas are next in size, and the villous adenoma is generally the largest. There is also a correlation between the size of a lesion and its likelihood of harboring cancer. There is general agreement that *hyperplastic polyps almost always are benign.* There is equal unanimity that somewhere between 25% and 50% of villous adenomas harbor carcinomas. It is the intermediate-sized tubular adenomas that are the center of a major controversy. Some experts contend that they rarely give rise to cancer; others are less confident, particularly of the larger lesions. Fenoglio, for example, holds to the latter view, as the following excerpt indicates:[218]

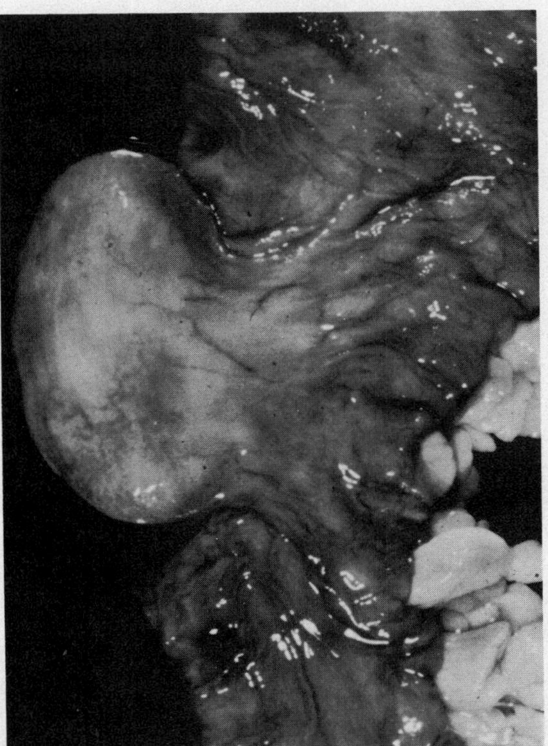

Figure 18–51. Submucosal lipoma in colon, which has been pedunculated by traction of intestinal peristalsis.

> Hyperplastic polyps [not having cancerous potential] are at least ten times more frequent than adenomas. Adenomas smaller than 1.5 cm are ten times more frequent than larger adenomas; thus, large adenomas represent about 1% of all large-bowel polyps. Let us consider a population of 1000 occurring in the colorectum. Of these 1000 polyps, 900 will be the small, non-neoplastic, hyperplastic polyps. The remaining 100 will be adenomas. Of these 100 adenomas, 90 will be small adenomas, less than 1.5 cm in diameter, and focal carcinoma will be very rare. The remaining 10 polyps will be large adenomas, and of these, one will contain a focus of invasive carcinoma. Thus, if one considers all polyps, the incidence of invasive carcinoma is 0.1%. However, if you consider only the larger adenomas, that is, greater than 1.5 cm, then 10% of these polyps will contain invasive cancer.
>
> Thus, we see that the likelihood of developing cancer in any polyp, which is randomly chosen from all polyps without regard for the histologic type or the size, is very small. However, if one considers the subgroup, that is, larger adenomas, the chance of developing carcinoma is significant and indeed the larger adenomas may be considered precancerous lesions.

We will return to the adenoma-carcinoma controversy after a description of the various histologic types of epithelial polyps. But first, a few words are in order about their biologic origins. All epithelial polyps arise from the cells deep in the crypts of the colonic mucosal glands. *Normally, cell division in the colonic mucosa is restricted to the deepest third of the crypt.* Presumably in the formation of epithelial polyps the controlling mechanisms of cell divisions are deranged, leading to hyperplastic polyps or adenomatous lesions.[219] Thus, it is proposed that *some loss of growth control in a slightly expanded zone of crypt cells leads to a hyperplastic polyp. A more complete loss of controls along the entire crypt results in a neoplastic polyp.* In the course of such changes, the cells along the entire depth of the crypt (including the upper two-thirds) retain their capacity to divide, as can be shown by their ability to incorporate thymidine and synthesize DNA. It would appear that the mechanisms that normally shut off DNA synthesis in the upper two-thirds of the crypt are to a greater or lesser extent lost. The ultimate size of the neoplastic polyp may be a function of time, the extent of loss of growth controls, the adequacy of the blood supply, or other factors still unknown.

Hyperplastic Polyps

Although hyperplastic polyps represent 90% of all epithelial polyps in autopsy surveys, they account for only 15 to 20% of surgically removed polyps because most are asymptomatic and only removed when discovered in the course of investigations for other reasons. They may arise at any age, but are usually diagnosed in the sixth and seventh decades when other disorders calling for sigmoidoscopy, colonoscopy, and radiography (e.g., colonic cancer) are also particularly prevalent.

About 60 to 80% are located in the rectosigmoid, 20% in the ascending colon, and the remainder in other colonic locations.[220] Typically, they are smooth, moist, round to finger-like, tan, sessile lesions sitting on top of a mucosal fold. They may occur singly, but multiple polyps are very frequent. In autopsies 90% are less than 5 mm in diameter, but surgical specimens tend to be larger because with enlargement they are more likely to produce bleeding and be discovered. Among surgical specimens they represent less than half of all polyps smaller than 5 mm in diameter since they are outnumbered by small tubular adenomas. Larger lesions may have a short broad stalk and so can resemble the pedunculated tubular adenoma. Histologically, they are composed of well-formed glands and crypts lined by non-neoplastic epithelial cells, most of which show differentiation into either mature goblet or absorptive cells. Owing to infoldings of the crowded epithelial cells, the linings often develop a serrate or sawtooth luminal profile. The glands and crypts are separated by connective tissue resembling the lamina propria. Larger hyperplastic polyps sometimes develop foci of adenomatous change, described below.

The major clinical significance of these lesions is their differentiation from the more ominous adenomatous polyps. The small, sessile moist lesions are reasonably distinctive. The rare hyperplastic polyp with a stalk may be discriminated only by anatomic study. There is general agreement that by themselves hyperplastic polyps have no cancerous potential. Still unanswered is the question whether the hyperplastic polyp would in time be transformed into neoplastic adenoma;[221] the fact that a small minority contain adenomatous foci suggests such a possibility.

Tubular Adenoma (Pedunculated Polyp)

About 75% of all adenomatous polyps are tubular adenomas. Because of this predominance they are sometimes referred to as "adenomatous polyps," an unfortunate practice since tubulovillous and villous adenomas are also adenomatous. Tubular adenomas occur sporadically in the general population but are also encountered in certain well-defined hereditary syndromes such as familial multiple polyposis. The following remarks are limited to the sporadic lesions; the familial patterns will be discussed later. In one large series, the average age of patients having sporadic tubular adenomas was 60 years, with a male preponderance of 2:1.[222] Their frequency progressively increases after 30 years of age. These are the lesions that sit in the center of the "adenoma-carcinoma sequence" controversy.

MORPHOLOGY. Tubular adenomas are found mainly in the left colon, including the rectum (75%). About 50 to 60% arise in the rectosigmoid, accessible to sigmoidoscopic examination. More than 50% of sporadic tubular adenomas occur singly. In about 30 to 40% of cases two or more are present simultaneously, and one-sixth of patients have more than five.[223] In practical clinical terms, when a single tubular adenoma is present there is a 20% chance of finding an additional one or more within five years, which increases to 40% when multiple polyps are present. Most often they have slender stalks and raspberry-like heads, hence the term **pedunculated adenomas** (Fig. 18–52). Occasionally they are sessile, ovoid, or hemispheric lesions or, rarely, flat and plaquelike. The heads of the pedunculated lesions range in size from a few millimeters to many centimeters in diameter, and the stalks from 1 to several centimeters in length.[224] Transsection discloses a central core of fibrovascular tissue that arises in the submucosa and extends in continuity through the center of the stalk and head. The stalk is usually covered with normal colonic mucosa, but in the head of the lesion the polypoid epithelium is considerably thicker.

Histologically the adenomatous epithelium in the bulbous head is composed of closely aggregated, elongated tubules and glands separated by a scant connective tissue stroma. The epithelial cells lining these configurations show poor differentiation into the two normal cell types, although scattered goblet cells may persist. **The lack of differentiation into specialized cell types most clearly separates neoplastic adenomatous polyps from hyperplastic polyps.** The cells are tall and crowded and have pseudostratified nuclei, giving the appearance of a "picket fence."

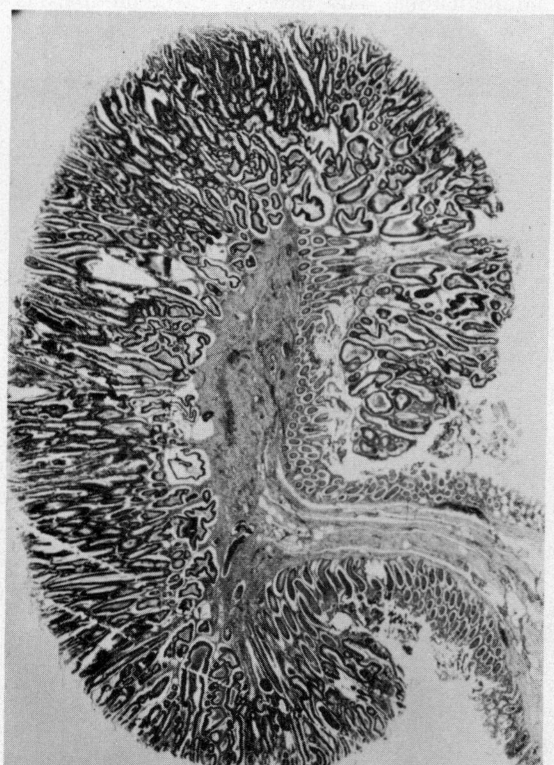

Figure 18–52. Low-power view of a slender-stalked colonic polyp indicating increased chromaticity and height of glands covering head of lesion.

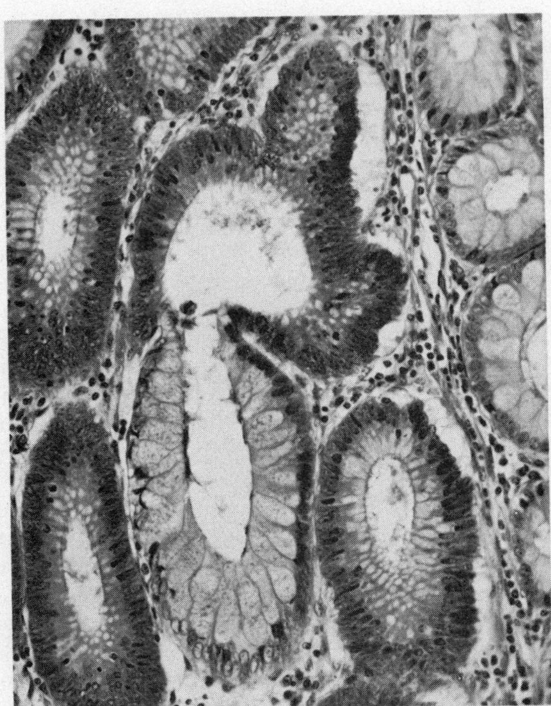

Figure 18–53. High-power detail of a junctional group of glands at point of transition between normal colonic mucosa and polypoid atypicality. A striking comparison is evident between regular, columnar, mucus-secreting epithelium and atypical, but not cancerous, polypoid epithelium.

Marked nuclear hyperchromasia and an increase in the nuclear-cytoplasmic ratio are usually present. A range of dysplasia and atypia is encountered. At one end of the spectrum the cells lining the tubules and glands are arrayed in orderly palisades. In such lesions the individual cells may show occasional mitoses and some hyperchromasia, but anaplasia is absent (Fig. 18–53). As would be expected of a benign lesion, there is no evidence of penetration of glands or cells into the central fibrovascular core. From this clearly innocent end of the spectrum all degrees of cytologic atypia and dysplasia may be encountered, to the extreme of unmistakable anaplasia indicative of carcinoma. Glands and crypts tend to be more closely packed and sometimes "back to back." Cell crowding and increase in nuclear size as well as hyperchromasia become progressively more marked; the cells lose their normal palisaded array and pile up upon one another. Mitotic figures become more numerous and abnormal. The atypical epithelium may remain restricted within the glandular basement membranes (carcinoma in situ) or invade the fibrovascular core. Whether the invasion must penetrate the muscularis mucosae, or more deeply into the core of the polyp to constitute a biologically significant carcinoma, or merely be superficial above the muscularis mucosae is still in dispute. However, there is no disagreement over the fact that tubular adenomas may contain villous areas. **By generally accepted convention, tubular lesions having up to 20 to 25% of villous growth are still referred to as tubular adenomas.** In most instances when carcinomatous change arises in a tubular adenoma it is located within such villous foci.[222]

The diagnosis of carcinoma in a tubular adenoma can be treacherous and, ultimately, is subjective, accounting for the great variability in the reported frequencies of cancer in tubular adenomas. **Clear-cut invasion of the fibrovascular core, particularly when it extends through the muscularis mucosae, is the most reliable criterion.** The following generalizations are relevant. Pure tubular adenomas having no villous component very rarely have either carcinoma in situ or invasive carcinoma. The risk is directly related to the proportion of the villous growth, which in turn is correlated with size. **Tubular adenomas less than 1 cm in diameter have a 1% chance of containing a focus of cancer, which in many instances has not penetrated the muscularis mucosae and so is not biologically significant.**[225] In those 1 to 2 cm in size, the risk of cancer rises to 5 to 10% in parallel with the proportion of villous architecture.[226] When a tubular adenoma is greater than 2 cm in diameter, the risk of cancer is even higher and is usually associated with a significant villous component. Overall, when tubular adenomas of all sizes are included, the incidence of carcinoma is about 3 to 5%.[227]

Tubular adenomas are most often discovered as incidental lesions at autopsy, or during endoscopic or barium enema studies performed for investigation of some other intestinal problem. Occasionally, however, they come to clinical attention because of bleeding. Rarely, large pedunculated lesions may be the leading point of an intussusception. Their major significance relates to their biologic potential, as has already been made clear. According to best available evidence, the presence of in situ or intramucosal carcinoma requires no further treatment of a stalked polyp other than its excision. With submucosal invasion of sessile lesions, segmental resection of the colon is necessary, since residual tumor is likely in 15 to 20% of cases.[221] The dilemma arises with stalked lesions having some invasion of the stalks. Although opinions vary widely, the prevailing practice is segmental resection if the invasion extends into the base of the stalk.

Villous Adenoma

Any colonic adenoma more than 50% (some would say 75%) villous in architecture is called a villous adenoma. These are the least common, the largest, and the most ominous of the epithelial polyps. In most series they represent about 10 to 15% of resected adenomatous polyps.[225] These lesions usually are first identified in patients 60 to 65 years of age; uncommonly they occur under the age of 50. Males and females are affected almost equally.

The localization of villous adenomas is as follows: rectum, 50 to 55%; sigmoid, 30%; descending colon, 10%; and the remainder distributed throughout the more proximal levels of the large bowel. These neoplasms therefore predominantly arise within reach of the sigmoidoscope; tubular adenomas are not as heavily clustered in the rectosigmoid. They range in size from less than 1 cm to 8 to 10 cm in diameter. The great preponderance are broad sessile, slightly lobular, or velvety gray-tan, nonpedunculated lesions projecting along a broad front about 1 to 3 cm above the surrounding mucosa (Fig. 18–54). Focal areas of hemorrhage or surface ulcerations are sometimes present. Infrequently, they have a broad, short stalk.

Histologically, at least half of the villous adenoma is composed of finger-like, or sometimes branching, papillae covered by polypoid epithelium. The residual portion of the polyp may present tubular features. There is an almost linear correlation between the size of the polyp and its proportion of villous features.[228] Each papilla is composed of fibrovascular core covered by epithelium ranging (among the various lesions) from a single layer of regularly aligned, tall columnar cells to unmistakably anaplastic cells having a disorderly multilayered arrangement. Sometimes the anaplastic cells form closely-packed aggregates or anaplastic glands (Fig. 18–55). The individual cells have large hyperchromatic nuclei, and mitoses may be numerous. Carcinoma in situ without invasion of the underlying fibrovascular core or submucosa of the colon is present in about 10% of villous adenomas, with frank invasive carcinoma in an additional 25 to 40% (average among series, 30%).[227]

Villous adenomas are symptomatic much more frequently than are the other adenomatous polyps. Most commonly they cause rectal bleeding, but in addition they infrequently may hypersecrete copious amounts of mucoid material that is sufficiently rich in protein to produce hypoproteinemia, particularly hypoalbuminemia, constituting in effect a protein-losing enteropathy. In addition, the mucous secretion contains large amounts of potassium, sometimes causing hypokalemia. Rarely, the villous lesions may induce persistent diarrhea and significant loss of fluid and other electrolytes.

There is no dispute that *villous adenomas are precancerous lesions that harbor invasive cancers in about one-third of cases.* Thus, diagnosis at the earliest possible moment and adequate resection are imperative.

Tubulovillous Adenoma

Tubulovillous adenomas, as the name implies, combine features of both tubular and villous adenomas. By definition, the villous component ranges between 20 and 50%. As already noted, lesions with less than 20% villous architecture are defined as tubular adenomas, and those with more than 50% as villous adenomas. With their proportion of villous elements, the malignant potential of tubulovillous adenomas is about halfway between the other two types.

The distribution of these lesions in the colon is the same as that of tubular adenomas. They range in diameter from 0.5 to 5 cm and thus are intermediate between tubular and villous adenomas. Most have a stalk and are macroscopically indistinguishable from tubular adenomas, but they have a slightly greater tendency to sessile growth. The histologic appearance covers a wide spectrum from that of the clearly benign tubular adenoma to all levels of atypia and anaplasia, extending to invasive carcinoma in the villous areas. Differentiation of tubulovillous lesions from the other two forms can be accomplished only microscopically.

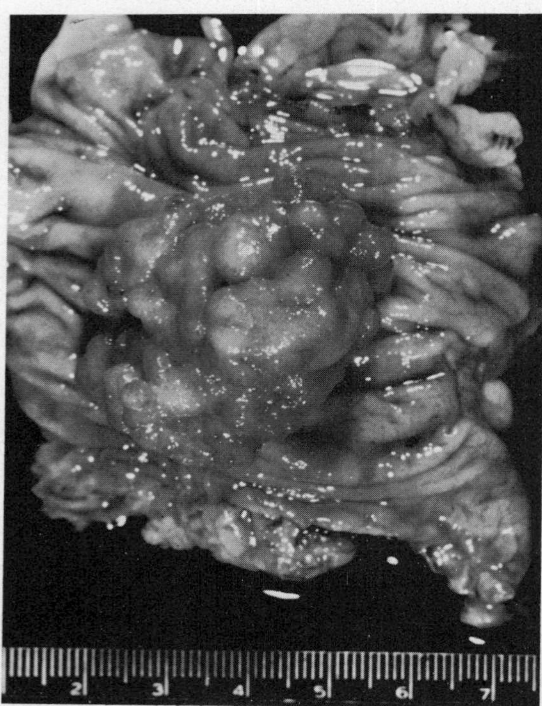

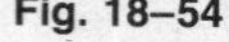

Fig. 18–54

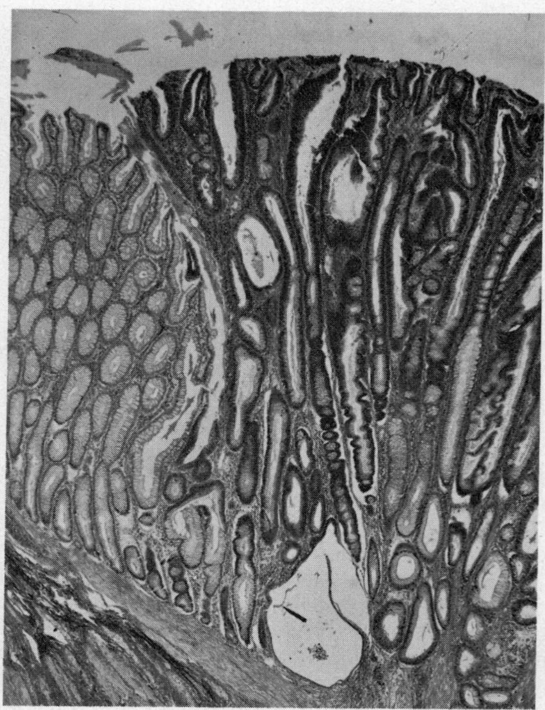

Fig. 18–55

Figure 18–54. Close-up of villous sessile polyp of colon that, on histologic examination, proved to be benign.

Figure 18–55. Junction between normal colonic mucosa on left and sessile polyp on right. Polypoid area reveals crowded papillae covered by hyperchromatic epithelium with loss of mucus secretion, sometimes containing cross sections of glands representing a tubuloadenomatous component.

Relationship of Adenomatous Polyps to Carcinoma

It has already been emphasized that all adenomatous polyps have malignant potential, greatest with the villous adenoma and least with the pure tubular adenoma. One correlate is sufficiently important for reiteration—*there is a relationship between the size of the adenoma (whatever its histologic type) and its likelihood of containing carcinoma.* The incidence of cancer in polyps under 1 cm in diameter is very low indeed; between 1 and 2 cm the incidence rises to about 5 to 10%; those above this size are cancerous in up to 30 to 40% of the instances, correlated with their size. *As stated before, the increasing risk of cancer is directly related to the proportion of the adenoma represented by villous elements.* Thus, some experts see cancer formation as a biologic sequence beginning with controlled hyperplasia and then passing progressively through the stages of uncontrolled neoplastic tubular growth into villous growth, terminating in carcinoma.[224] On the other hand, some take the position that tubular polyps are biologically distinct from villous adenomas and rarely (1% or less of cases) give rise to "biologic cancer."[229, 230] In this view, foci of cancer within the head of a stalked polyp are not considered to be precursors to invasive cancer. *While the controversy continues, the weight of evidence favors the position that biologically significant cancers may arise in neoplastic adenomatous and villous epithelial polyps.*

Three difficult questions must be raised: (1) do all adenomatous polyps with sufficient time become cancerous?; (2) what is the time frame for the adenoma-carcinoma sequence?; (3) do all colonic carcinomas arise in preexisting adenomas? Only tentative answers can be offered.

It is highly unlikely that all adenomas will become transformed into carcinoma. Were this true, one might expect a much higher incidence of colonic cancer, given the much greater prevalence of adenomatous polyps than of colonic cancers. More direct is the evidence drawn from studies of patients with familial multiple polyposis. In this condition, the large bowel and sometimes higher levels of the gut are literally peppered by hundreds or thousands of adenomatous polyps, most tubular, but some villous. It is currently believed that almost all these individuals will inevitably develop colonic cancer unless total colectomy is performed.[231] Typically, one carcinoma emerges, presumably from one of the larger polyps. Infrequently, two or three cancers develop simultaneously. Thus, during the time span that it took for one or a few of the adenomas to become cancerous, the overwhelming majority (over 99%) remain benign. Another point in evidence: even benign villous adenomas that have recurred after resection have been observed to remain benign for decades.[232] It can therefore be concluded, but only tentatively, that all adenomatous polyps are not inevitably destined to become cancerous—at least within the time span of the remaining years of the patient's life.

Turning to the question of how long it takes for an adenoma destined to become malignant to evolve into a carcinoma, it can be said tentatively: at least years, possibly decades. In one series, the average age at diagnosis of multiple familial polyposis without cancer was about 27 years, and for polyposis with cancer about 39 years.[182] In the days before total colectomy was performed for familial multiple polyposis, among 59 patients with this condition, 12% developed cancer within five years, 25% in 10 years, 30% within 15 years and over 50% at 20 years. The data are not conclusive, but they at least strongly suggest that the adenoma-carcinoma sequence takes place over a period of years to decades.

The question whether all colonic carcinomas arise in preexisting adenomatous polyps remains moot despite impassioned writings supporting both affirmative and negative viewpoints. On the one hand it is pointed out that certain very small cancers less than 1 cm in diameter contain no evidence of having arisen in a preexisting adenoma. On the other hand are the epidemiologic studies demonstrating a parallel in various countries between a high incidence of colonic cancer and a high incidence of adenomas. For example, there is a low incidence of colonic cancer in Japan and a correspondingly very low frequency of villous adenomas of the colon.[233] It is further argued that even a 1- to 2-cm carcinoma may have overgrown and obliterated all trace of a preexisting adenoma.[218] There is, indeed, an inverse relation between the persistence of recognizable adenomatous tissue and the size of the cancer.[234] When large groups of individuals were periodically studied by sigmoidoscopy and all mucosal protrusions removed, the anticipated incidence of rectosigmoid carcinoma was reduced by 85%.[235] There are, therefore, a number of "suggestoid" observations in favor of the view that all or most colonic cancers arise in preexisting adenomas, but the evidence can hardly be called definitive.

We must leave these controversies in this unsatisfactory state, but *from a practical standpoint, to ignore the existence of a polyp, however small, is in some measure a gamble.*

Familial Polyposis

In a few instances, the tendency to develop polyps of the colon is familial, having most often an autosomal dominant mode of transmission.[236] In many cases, the polyps are associated with developmental abnormalities outside the intestinal tract. Six distinctive syndromes have been described by McKusick.[237] The four more important of this group are familial multiple polyposis of the colon, Peutz-Jeghers syndrome, Gardner's syndrome, and Turcot's syndrome.

Familial multiple polyposis of the colon is made distinctive by the myriad neoplastic polyps, which may cover virtually the entire mucosa of the colon and sometimes extend into the upper levels of the intestinal tract, including the stomach. Although the disease is hereditary, transmitted as an autosomal dominant, polyps do not appear before the second and third decades of life. A member of an involved family who has not developed polyps by age 40 is not likely to develop them later.

The individual polyp is usually a small pedunculated tubular adenoma 1 cm in diameter. When closely packed, the polyps may impart a furry appearance to the mucosal surface (Fig. 18–56). In histologic detail, these adenomas are indistinguishable from the tubular lesions already described. Occasionally, polyps may be of the villous sessile pattern.

There is a high incidence of malignant transformation of the polyps in this hereditary disorder. It is not uncommon to find certain adenomas larger and presumably more actively growing than the remainder. Such lesions may develop into cancer. Multiple polyps may become cancerous concurrently. Malignancy is more likely if the disease is of long duration, and unless the diseased colon is removed, *multiple polyposis inevitably develops into cancer*, which appears in retrospective surveys about 12 years following the diagnosis of the polyposis.[234] Diagnosis can be readily made by either sigmoidoscopic or barium enema study. The adenoma-carcinoma sequence in this hereditary disorder is used as strong evidence by those who regard all sporadic neoplastic polyps as precancerous lesions.

The *Peutz-Jeghers syndrome* is an autosomal dominant disorder characterized by polyps of the entire gastrointestinal tract, particularly in the small intestine, associated with melanin pigmentation of the buccal mucosa, lips, palms of the hand, fingers, and soles of the feet.[238] The individual polyp may resemble the pedunculated tubular adenoma of familial multiple polyposis or the nonhereditary tubular adenoma, but more often they are hemispheric or finger-like protrusions from the mucosal surface. Histologically, instead of the neoplastic aggregation of tubules and glands seen in tubular adenomas, the polyps in the Peutz-Jeghers syndrome consist of hamartomas having dilated, mucin-filled cysts lined by normal-looking, mucin-secreting epithelial cells. *These polyps do not undergo malignant transformation.* Thus, unlike familial multiple polyposis, the Peutz-Jeghers syndrome incurs no increased risk of cancer. However, individuals with this familial condition may develop neoplastic adenomas and cancers, the latter not only in the gastrointestinal tract, but also in extraintestinal sites.[239]

Gardner's syndrome refers to the association of polyposis in the colon with desmoid tumors (p. 1312) and neoplasms elsewhere. The risk of cancer in the colon is as high in this syndrome as in familial multiple polyposis and approaches 100%. The extracolonic neoplasms have occurred in the skin, subcutaneous tissue, and bone. A systemic derangement in the genetic repressor mechanisms that control cell growth is postulated but not established.

Turcot's syndrome combines polyps of the colon with brain tumors. In contrast to the other entities mentioned, it is transmitted as an autosomal recessive trait. There is some increased risk of carcinoma of the colon, but the magnitude of the risk is still uncertain.

Miscellaneous Polyps

The whole gamut of mesenchymal tumors may occur in the colon. These include leiomyomas, fibromas, lipomas, hemangiomas, and neurofibromas that are not

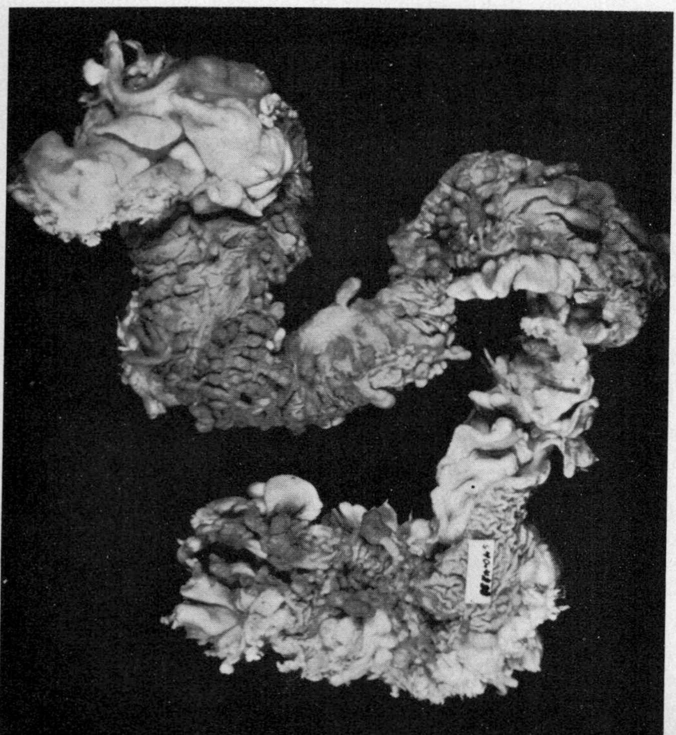

Figure 18–56. Heredofamilial polyposis of colon. Bowel is studded with numerous small polyps.

distinctive from the same lesions occurring elsewhere (Fig. 18–51). When small, they may present as intramural lesions, but as they enlarge they tend to become polypoid. Only rarely are these benign lesions of clinical significance. Two other polypoid lesions merit brief mention. Polyps are sporadically found in the colons of children, most frequently in the rectosigmoid; these differ in appearance from the polyps of pedunculated and villous adenoma and are designated *juvenile polyps*. They may be quite large and pedunculated. Histologically, they are made distinctive by a very abundant loose fibrovascular stroma containing widely spaced glands, some sufficiently dilated to constitute cysts. These lesions are thought to develop from congenitally malformed glands that give rise to mucous retention cysts. A scant leukocytic infiltrate is often present in the stroma. Malignant transformation and recurrence are extremely rare if they occur at all.

Lymphoid polyps are an additional rare form of benign tumor consisting of aggregates of lymphoid tissue covered usually by a fairly regular, although sometimes atrophic, colonic mucosa. The lymphoid architecture may be quite regular, with prominent lymphoid follicles in a stroma of mature lymphocytes. The pattern resembles that of the nodular lymphoma, and some workers have considered these to be true lymphomas occurring in the bowel. The preponderant opinion, however, is that these lesions are foci of striking submucosal lymphoid hyperplasia rather than neoplasms.[240] In almost all cases, local resection is curative. Occasionally, true neoplastic lymphomatous involvement occurs in the rectum as a primary lesion or a systemic dissemination of a lymphoma, and this differential must be borne in mind in the interpretation of these lesions.

MALIGNANT TUMORS

Carcinoma

Virtually 98% of all cancers in the large intestine are carcinomas. They represent one of the prime challenges to the medical profession, because they produce symptoms relatively early and at this stage are generally curable by resection. Too often these early symptoms are largely ignored by the patient and sometimes insufficiently investigated by the physician. Colorectal cancer was responsible for about 60,000 deaths in the United States in 1983 and was superseded only by lung cancer, which caused about 117,000 deaths.

EPIDEMIOLOGY. The epidemiology of colorectal (including rectal) cancer has provided some significant insights into its possible causation and has led to the strong conviction that environmental influences are of great importance. In general, the incidence of colonic carcinoma is highest in Northwest Europe, North America, and other Anglo-Saxon areas and is lowest in South America, Africa, and Asia. It would appear that it occurs most frequently in populations with the highest standards of living. Yet Japan, with its high standard of living, has one of the lowest prevalences of this form of cancer. Moreover, among populations enjoying relatively similar standards of living, there are striking differences. The mortality rate in Denmark is more than twice that in Finland.

Some interesting but poorly understood trends have emerged over the past three or four decades.[241] Although the mortality rate for this form of neoplasia for whites in the United States has remained the same over this time span, i.e., about 20 per 100,000 population (an improved prognosis has counterbalanced the 50% increase in incidence), the mortality rate for blacks has doubled. For the first time since data have been available, colorectal cancer may be relatively more common among blacks than among whites. There are other puzzling comparisons, such as striking differences in mortality rates in different regions of the same country. There is a well-defined higher mortality rate for colorectal cancer in urban areas than in rural areas in the U.S. and many other countries. This is most striking in Africa, where colonic cancer is extremely rare in rural blacks and is two to three times more frequent in urban blacks. Migrants from one country to another over the span of several generations assume the mortality rate of their new home. Japanese immigrants to the U.S. have a mortality rate three to four times higher than that of their forebears in their native land.[242] It is small wonder that dietary factors have come under suspicion.

Despite all these national and racial differences, there is no evidence that genetic factors play a large role in the generality of colorectal cancers. There are, however, a minority of cases in which hereditary factors undoubtedly contribute. There is some evidence of an increased incidence of colonic or rectal cancer in relatives of patients with the disease.[243] There are, in addition, well-defined hereditary syndromes associated with an increased frequency of cancer of the large bowel, as cited below. Some genotypes, then, are at increased risk, but most neoplasms occur in individuals having no apparent familial predisposition; hence, varying incidence rates are thought to be due largely to environmental influences.

Carcinoma of the large bowel has its peak incidence in the seventh decade of life. Less than 20% of cases are diagnosed in persons under the age of 50 and undoubtedly some of these younger patients are accounted for by the hereditary syndromes just mentioned. In such individuals the tumor may appear as early as the third or fourth decade of life. When the neoplasm occurs in the rectum, there is a male:female ratio of approximately 2:1; in more proximal levels of the large bowel there is no sex predominance.

ETIOLOGY AND PATHOGENESIS. With regard to the roles of nature and nurture in predisposing to colorectal cancer, (1) certain precancerous and dysplastic disorders are of probable importance[244] and (2) dietary factors are of uncertain significance. It is established that villous adenomas, ulcerative colitis, Crohn's colitis, familial polyposis, Gardner's syndrome, and a cancer-family syndrome (in which colonic and other forms of cancer are common) are all associated with a well-defined, increased risk of colorectal cancer, the magnitude of which has already been discussed with each of the more common conditions. It seems reasonable to call tubular and tubulovillous adenomas precancerous lesions, but this is a vexed issue, as amply delineated earlier (p. 867).

The role of diet is much more controversial, but is believed by many to be very significant. It is thought to underlie the striking differences previously cited in the prevalence of colonic cancer around the world. Principally implicated are: (1) the level of dietary animal fat and protein and (2) the fiber content of the diet. Other dietary items have also come under scrutiny, but have not proved meaty.

The thesis that a high consumption of meat, principally beef, with its accompanying fat predisposes to colorectal cancer proposes in essence the formation of carcinogens from neutral sterols or from the increased level of bile acids called forth by the burden of dietary fat. The high-animal-fat diet not only increases the level of neutral sterols and bile acids in the fecal stream but also modifies the bacterial flora, leading to a relative increase in the number of anaerobes, particularly clostridia and/or bacteroides.[245] These organisms are able to convert bile acids or cholesterol into metabolites capable of promoting or initiating neoplasms.[246] A number of epidemiologic studies detailed in an earlier discussion (p. 427) have supported or challenged this theory, but in the last analysis it must be considered as interesting but unproven.

The tenuous argument ascribing a pathogenetic role to low fiber and consequent slowing of bowel transit time was detailed on page 427. Greater opportunity for the endogenous production of carcinogens and longer exposure of the intestinal wall to the carcinogen would then follow.[247] The decreased stool bulk would also reduce the *dilution* or binding of carcinogens. This line of argument derives from the epidemiologic observations that Bantus who live on a fiber-rich diet have a much lower rate of colon cancer than urban Africans with their low-fiber diets. However, unequivocal evidence is lacking that a high-fiber diet always shortens transit time. It may, at least in part, be a genetic characteristic, rather than solely dependent on diet.[248] Moreover, low-fiber diets are frequently a consequence of reduced consumption of fruits and vegetables containing vitamin A, C, or E. Could lower levels of these vitamins, which are thought to reduce the risk of cancer, be of importance rather than the fiber content? Analogously cruciferous vegetables—cabbage, broccoli, Brussels sprouts, cauliflower, and turnips—are said to inhibit tumor production (demonstrable in experimental systems) not by virtue of their fiber content but by inducing increased levels of aryl hydrocarbon hydroxylase activity in the intestine.[249] This enzyme facilitates the degradation of carcinogenic hydrocarbons and so might exert a protective effect in vivo. It is evident that other aspects of a low-fiber diet may be more important than merely stool bulk.

Thus, although there is evidence that dietary factors predispose to colorectal cancer, the precise carcinogenic influence (if any) has not been identified.

MORPHOLOGY. About 70 to 75% of colorectal carcinomas are located in the rectum, rectosigmoid, or sigmoid colon. The remainder are fairly evenly distributed all the way back to the cecum. Infrequently, multiple carcinomas arise concurrently, most often in patients with familial multiple polyposis or ulcerative colitis.

Although all colorectal cancers must begin as in situ lesions, when discovered they usually assume one of two patterns: carcinomas of the left side and those of the right. **Carcinomas of the left side tend to grow in an annular encircling fashion. They produce a so-called "napkin-ring" constriction of the bowel with early symptoms of obstruction** (Fig. 18–57). These lesions may begin as sessile or plaquelike masses, but over the span of time they grow to infiltrate and encircle the circumference. **On the right side, the lesions tend to grow as polypoid fungating masses that extend along one wall of the more capacious cecum and ascending colon. Obstruction is uncommon.** Thus, from the standpoint of morphology and clinical behavior, carcinomas of the left and right colon behave as two distinct tumor types.

The **early lesion on the left side** appears as a small elevated button or as a small polypoid mass. As the tumor grows, it forms a flat plaque that continues to increase in size (Fig. 18–58). It eventually extends circumferentially to encircle the wall, and it has been estimated that it takes approximately one to two years for such a lesion to encircle the lumen totally. The deeper layers are invaded slowly, and for a long time the neoplasm tends to remain superficial. Eventually, ulceration takes place in the middle of the ring as penetration of the bowel wall encroaches on the blood supply. At this time, the annular constriction characteristically shows heaped-up margins with a central ringlike ulceration or excavation. Infrequently, leftsided lesions produce little luminal growth but, instead, infiltrate the bowel wall and cause flattening and small ulcerations of the mucosa. Extension of the tumor through the bowel wall into the pericolic fat and regional lymph nodes occurs as these lesions progress. The penetration of bowel wall may, on occasion, produce pericolic abscesses or even peritonitis. Eventually these cancers metastasize to the liver, lungs, bone marrow, and other distant organs but not before a considerable period of growth. Rarely, right-sided lesions assume this annular pattern.

The **cancers in the right colon** begin as sessile lesions similar to those of the left but progressively assume a polypoid fungating appearance (Fig. 18–59). They frequently become bulky, cauliflower-like masses or large, irregular spreading papillomatous plaques that protrude into the lumen. Plaquelike or ulcerative lesions of the right side occur but very infrequently. These right-sided lesions eventually penetrate the wall and extend to the mesentery, regional nodes, and more distant sites. Because the lesions occur in the capacious cecum and do not cause obstruction, they may remain clinically silent for long periods of time. Quite uncommonly, colonic carcinomas of the right side grow in an invasive, infiltrating fashion with mucosal flattening and ulceration without luminal projections.

Unlike the gross pathology, the microscopic characteristics of right- and left-sided colonic carcinomas are similar. **Ninety-five per cent of all carcinomas of the colorectum are adenocarcinomas,** many of which produce mucin (Figs. 18–60 and 18–61). Commonly this mucin is secreted extra-

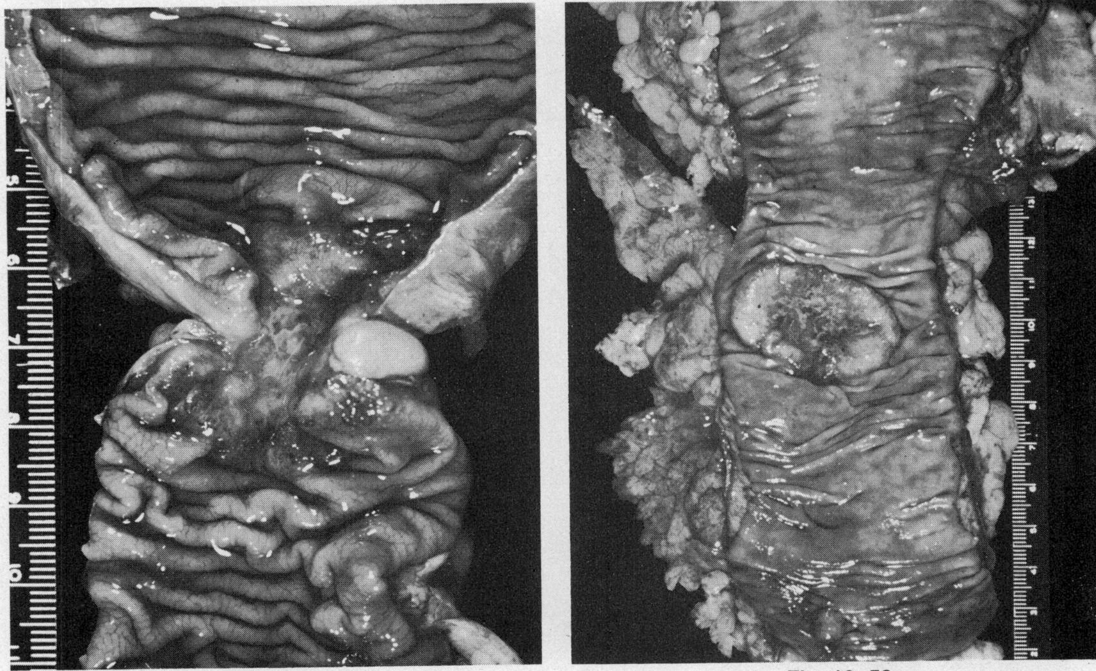

Fig. 18–57 Fig. 18–58

Figure 18–57. Carcinoma of left colon that has completely encircled lumen. Dilation of proximal bowel lumen is evident.
Figure 18–58. An elevated, plaquelike adenocarcinoma of colon.

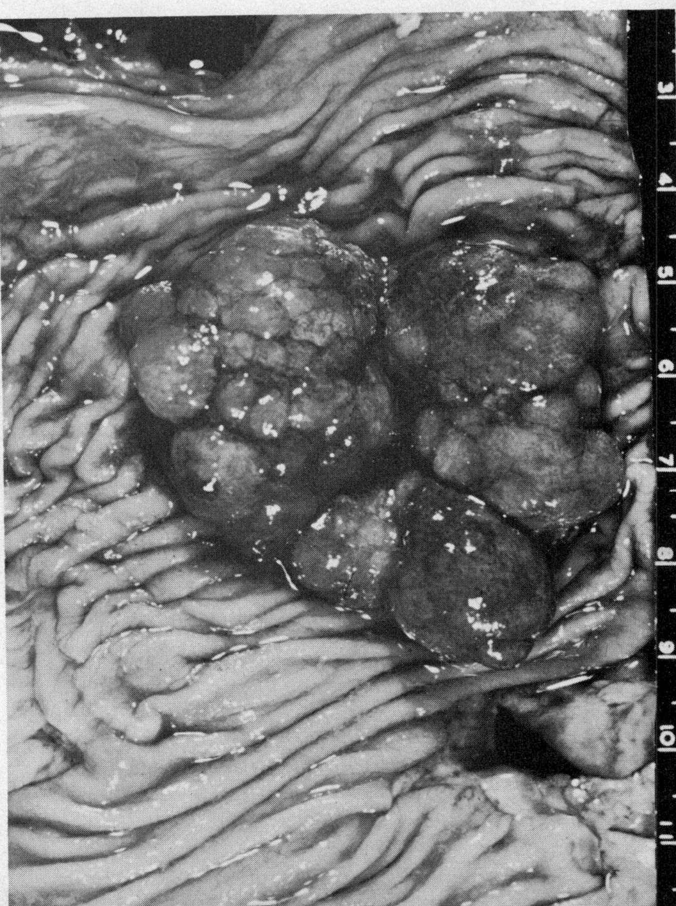

Figure 18–59. A polypoid fungating carcinoma of right colon in a 56-year-old male.

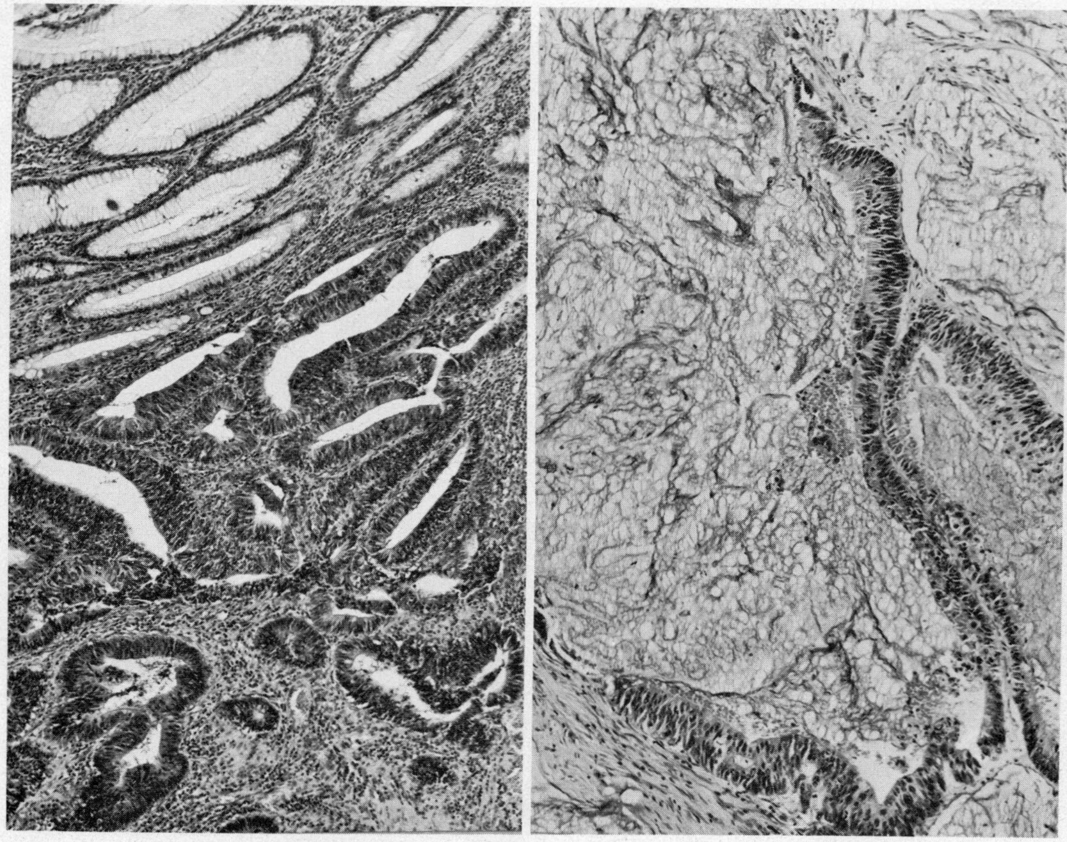

Fig. 18–60 Fig. 18–61

Figure 18–60. Transition zone between anaplastic glands of an adenocarcinoma of colon and the normal colonic epithelium.

Figure 18–61. Low-power field of an invasive cancer of colon illustrating extensive mucin formation, which appears in the illustration as stringy coagulated material.

cellularly either within gland lumina or within the interstitium of the gut wall. Because this secretion dissects the wall, it aids the extension of the malignancy and worsens the prognosis.

Certain exceptions to the general pattern should be cited. Some cancers, particularly in the distal colon, have foci of squamous cell differentiation to create **adenoacanthomas.** Another infrequent variant is the small cell undifferentiated carcinoma presumably arising from endocrine cells. Such neoplasms, as you may surmise, elaborate a variety of hormonal or bioactive secretory products. Another variant is the infiltrative, poorly differentiated carcinoma that tends to produce long, tapered strictures. It may occur in the absence of ulcerative colitis but is particularly associated with inflammatory bowel disease. The lack of exophytic growth renders radiographic identification difficult, particularly when it is against a background of ulcerative colitis.

CLINICAL COURSE. It is now appreciated that carcinoma of the colorectum is present for a considerable time before it produces clinical symptoms. Whether one subscribes to the adenoma-carcinoma sequence theory or not, rectal bleeding and/or change in bowel habit are present for many months, perhaps years, before diagnosis. In theory, the chance for early discovery and successful removal should be greater with lesions of the left side because these patients usually have prominent disturbances in bowel function such as melena, diarrhea, and constipation. It would be suspected, therefore, that rectosigmoid lesions would yield a better survival rate. However, cancers of the rectum and sigmoid tend to be more infiltrative than those of the proximal levels of colon, and this characteristic is apparently responsible for a somewhat poorer prognosis for these lesions. Cecal and right colonic cancers are most often called to clinical attention by the appearance of weakness, malaise, weight loss, and unexplained anemia. These lesions bleed readily, and the investigation of occult melena sometimes leads to their discovery at an early stage.[250]

All colorectal tumors spread by direct extension into adjacent structures and by metastasis through the lymphatics and blood vessels. In order of preference, the favored sites of metastatic spread are the regional lymph nodes, liver, lungs, and bones, followed by many other sites including the serosal membrane of the peritoneal cavity, brain, and others. In general, the disease

Table 18–8. MODIFIED DUKE'S CLASSIFICATION OF CARCINOMA OF THE COLON AND ITS PROGNOSTIC SIGNIFICANCE

Duke's Type	% of Five-Year Survival	Stage of Neoplasm
A	100.0	Limited to mucosa
B1	66.6	Extending into muscularis propria but not penetrating through it with uninvolved nodes
B2	53.9	Through entire wall with uninvolved nodes
C1	42.8	Limited to the wall with involved nodes
C2	22.4	Through all layers of the wall with involved nodes

From Astler, V. B., and Coller, F. A.: The prognostic significance of direct extension of carcinoma of the colon and rectum. Ann. Surg. *139*:846, 1954.

has spread beyond the range of curative surgery in 25 to 30% of patients.

The diagnosis of colorectal cancer relies on a large variety of techniques, including tests for blood in the stool, digital examination, proctoscopy, sigmoidoscopy, colonoscopy, contrast radiographic studies, and CT scans. Colonic cancers produce a variety of tumor antigens that can be detected in the blood and provide potential methods of diagnosis. In longest use as a diagnostic aid is carcinoembryonic antigen (CEA), but many other new markers are under study.[25] The serum levels of CEA are directly related to the size of the primary tumor and its extent of spread. Thus, in early favorable lesions, CEA "positivity" is found in 19 to 40% of patients. In contrast, in those with large metastatic neoplasms, there is virtually 100% CEA positivity. Overall, in an unselected series of preoperative patients, the test is positive in 60 to 70%.[252] More valuable is the use of CEA levels to assess the patient following resection of the primary tumor. If total removal has been accomplished, the CEA levels disappear. Return of CEA positivity is a highly reliable indicator of recurrence of the primary neoplasm. Similarly, the CEA test can provide a rough quantitation of the effectiveness of chemotherapy. It must be cautioned that positive CEA tests may also be produced by cancers of the lung, breast, ovary, urinary bladder, and prostate as well as a number of non-neoplastic disorders, including alcoholic cirrhosis, pancreatitis, and ulcerative colitis.

The prognosis for patients with colorectal carcinoma, as might be expected, is dependent on (1) the extent of bowel involvement, (2) the presence or absence of spread to lymph nodes or more distant sites, (3) the histologic differentiation of the lesion, and (4) to some extent its location within the colon. Among these variables, the extent of the neoplasm and its potential metastases clearly are of greatest importance. Several staging systems are now in use. The modified Duke's proposal with five-year survivals is presented in Table 18–8. It is, however, a postoperative staging system based on morphologic examination of the specimen. The American Joint Committee (AJC) for Cancer Staging and End-Result Reporting has come forward with a classification of use clinically, based on the TNM system (Table 18–9).[253] Overall, if all patients, even those whose lesions prove to be inoperable, are included, the five-year survival rate is in the range of 35 to 40%. These data are particularly discouraging in light of the earlier remarks about the potential for early diagnosis and cure of this disease.

Squamous Cell Carcinoma

These tumors are largely limited to the anal region. They produce plaquelike thickenings that eventually fungate and ulcerate, as do squamous cell carcinomas that occur elsewhere. They tend to be locally invasive, and to metastasize eventually to the regional nodes of drainage and then to more distant sites.

Adenoacanthoma

Adenoacanthomas, mentioned earlier, having a mixed squamous adenocarcinomatous histology are rare cancers of the large intestine that may arise at any level of the colorectum. Despite their histologic characteristics, they behave as the usual adenocarcinoma and have the same gross features and clinical significance.

Table 18–9. AJC POSTSURGICAL PATHOLOGIC ASSESSMENT

Primary tumor (T)	
TX	Depth of penetration not specified
T0	No clinically demonstrable tumor
TIS	Carcinoma in situ (no penetration of lamina propria as shown by biopsy or histological examination of the resected specimen)
T1	Clinically benign lesion or lesion confined to the mucosa or submucosa
T2	Involvement of muscular wall or serosa; no extension beyond
T3	Involvement of all layers of colon or rectum, with extension to immediately adjacent structures or organs; no fistula present
T4	Fistula present along with any of the above degrees of tumor penetration
T5	Tumor spread by direct extension, beyond the immediately adjacent organs or tissues
( )T	Multiple primary carcinoma
Regional nodal involvement (N)	
NX	Nodes not assessed or involvement not recorded
N0	Nodes not believed to be involved
N1	Regional nodes involved (distal to origins of the ileocolic, right colic, middle colic, and inferior mesenteric arteries)
Distant metastasis (M)	
MX	Not assessed
M0	No (known) metastasis
M1	Distant metastasis present (including extra-abdominal nodes, intra-abdominal nodes proximal to mesocolon and inferior mesenteric artery, peritoneal implants, liver, lungs, and bones)

From Stearns, M. W., Jr.: Staging colonic and rectal cancer. Int. Adv. Surg. Oncol. *4*:189, 1981.

Sarcoma

Sarcomas, principally leiomyosarcoma, angiosarcoma, liposarcoma, and fibrosarcoma, rarely arise in the large bowel. These tumors produce large fleshy masses that exactly resemble their counterparts elsewhere, spread to regional nodes, and may metastasize widely.

Lymphoma

Lymphomas are infrequent in the large intestine relative to their occurrence in the stomach and small intestine. They have the same morphologic and clinical characteristics as those in the upper segments of the bowel, described earlier (p. 826).

Endocrine Cell Tumors (Argentaffinomas, Carcinoids)

These neoplasms occur in all levels of the gastrointestinal tract, including the appendix. Their gross and microscopic features have been presented (p. 842), and here it need be emphasized only that neoplasms of the colon are infrequently argentaffin positive, and even the metastasizing carcinoids rarely give rise to the carcinoid syndrome.

Melanocarcinoma

Melanocarcinomas may arise in the pigmented areas of the anus but are extremely uncommon (p. 1279).

Appendix

NORMAL

The appendix in man is a mysterious structure with no known function. There are speculations that it may be the analog of the immunologically important bursa of Fabricius in avians. It varies greatly in size, having an average diameter of 0.5 to 1.0 cm. It is usually a mobile structure, having a short mesentery called the mesoappendix, which carries the blood, nerve, and lymphatic supply. It generally lies directly at the extremity of the anterior tenia of the cecum. On occasion, it lies behind the colon in a so-called retrocecal position. It is sometimes enveloped in congenital fibrous bands that may produce torsion, kinking, or sharp angulation. These malpositions alone, under certain clinical situations, may cause pain, since the angulated lumen may distend with feces or gas and cause colicky pain. With developmental malrotation of the colon, the cecum and appendix are rarely located in the right upper quadrant (not simplifying the diagnosis of acute appendicitis).

Histologically, the appendix has the same four layers as the remainder of the gut. The distinguishing feature of this organ is the extremely rich lymphoid tissue present in the mucosa and submucosa, which, in young individuals, forms an entire layer of germinal follicles and lymphoid pulp. This lymphoid tissue underlying the mucosal epithelium and glands undergoes progressive atrophy during life to the point of complete disappearance in advanced age. In the elderly the appendix, particularly the distal portion, sometimes undergoes fibrous obliteration.

PATHOLOGY

Diseases of the appendix loom large in surgical practice. Appendicitis is the most common acute abdominal condition the surgeon is called on to treat. It is, under different conditions, one of the best recognized clinical entities and one of the most difficult diagnostic problems that confront the clinician. A differential diagnosis of this disease must include virtually every acute process that can occur within the abdominal cavity as well as some of the emergencies that affect the organs of the thorax.

INFLAMMATIONS

ACUTE APPENDICITIS

Acute appendicitis is mainly a disease of adolescents and young adults, but may occur in the very young and very elderly. Males are affected more often than females in a ratio of about 1.5:1.

Almost a half-century ago, Wangensteen and coworkers demonstrated that obstruction to the appendiceal lumen predisposed to the development of acute appendicitis.[254] Obstruction, usually in the form of a fecalith and, less commonly, a calculus, tumor, or ball of worms (oxyuriasis vermicularis), can be demonstrated in 50 to 80% of inflamed appendices. It should be comforting to grape addicts that seeds have not yet been implicated. Presumably, with obstruction and continued secretion of mucinous fluid the intraluminal pressure builds up in the obstructed segment to cause eventual collapse of the veins of drainage. Ischemic injury then favors bacterial invasion to add an element of inflammatory edema and exudation, further embarrassing the blood supply. Thus, a vicious cycle is created leading to inflammatory changes in the appendix related to both bacterial invasion and ischemic injury. However, a significant minority of inflamed appendices have no demonstrable luminal obstruction. A number of possibilities exist, all admittedly speculative. Sharp angulation of the appendix, as may be produced by external adhesions, fibrous bands, or retrocecal location, could occlude the lumen. Lymphoid hyperplasia in response to viral systemic infection might contribute to luminal obstruction. For example, in measles, the appendix often undergoes striking lymphoid hyperplasia. Here, characteristic measles giant cells (Warthin-Finkeldey cells) sometimes appear, permitting the astute surgical pathologist to tell the physician that his patient is about to develop the rash of measles. Similar lymphoid hyperplasia may occur with other forms of viral infection. It has further been proposed that, in the course of such viral involvement, superficial mucosal ulcerations may develop, providing avenues for bacterial invasion.[255] Other valiant attempts to explain nonobstructive appendicitis invoke predisposition to bacterial infection, vaguely attributed to progressive atrophy of the lymphoid tissue encountered with aging or interference with the vascular supply to the appendix.[256] It is evident that the basis for appendiceal inflammation in the absence of obvious obstruction is not known.

MORPHOLOGY. The inflammatory changes seen in developing appendicitis will be presented, beginning with the early alterations and then proceeding to the subsequent, more marked reactions as the process progressively worsens. In the earliest recognizable acutely inflamed appendix, there is usually a scant neutrophilic exudation throughout the mucosa, submucosa, and muscularis. Occasionally, the mucosal involvement is most prominent. At this phase of the reaction, the subserosal vessels are congested and contain marginated neutrophils, and often there is scant, perivascular, neutrophilic emigration. This serosal reaction transforms the normal glistening serosa into an injected, dull, granular, red membrane. This external appearance is recognized by the surgeon as **early acute appendicitis.** At a later stage, the neutrophilic exudation through the wall is more advanced, with numerous polymorphonuclear leukocytes within the muscularis and a layered fibrinopurulent reaction over the serosa (Figs. 18–62 and 18–63). As the inflammatory process worsens, there are abscess formations within the wall, along with ulcerations and foci of suppurative necrosis in the mucosa. At this stage, the serosa usually is heavily layered with fibrinosuppurative exudate, and the state of the appendix might be termed **acute suppurative appendicitis.** Further worsening of the reaction leads to large areas of hemorrhagic green ulceration of the mucosa, along with similar green-black gangrenous necrosis throughout the wall, extending to the serosa. This level of severity is the immediate antecedent to rupture of an **acute gangrenous appendicitis.** When fecaliths or calculi become impacted, there is distention of the appendix distal to the obstruction, with almost invariably enhanced inflammatory reaction in this obstructed segment.

The histologic criterion for the diagnosis of acute appendicitis is **polymorphonuclear leukocytic infiltration of the muscularis.** Usually, neutrophils and ulcerations are

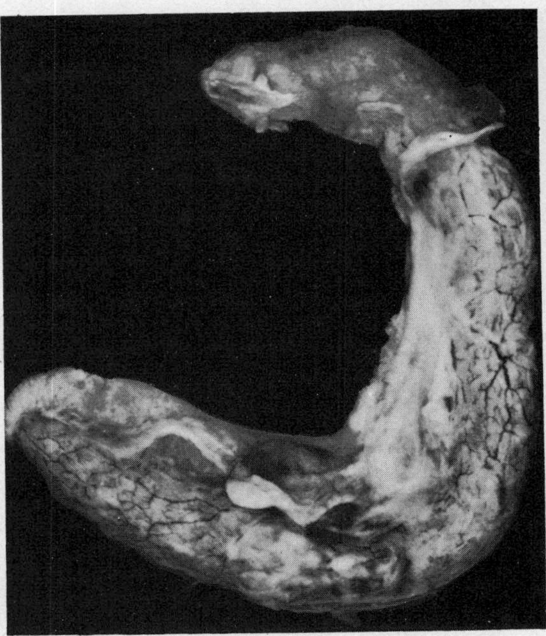

Fig. 18–62

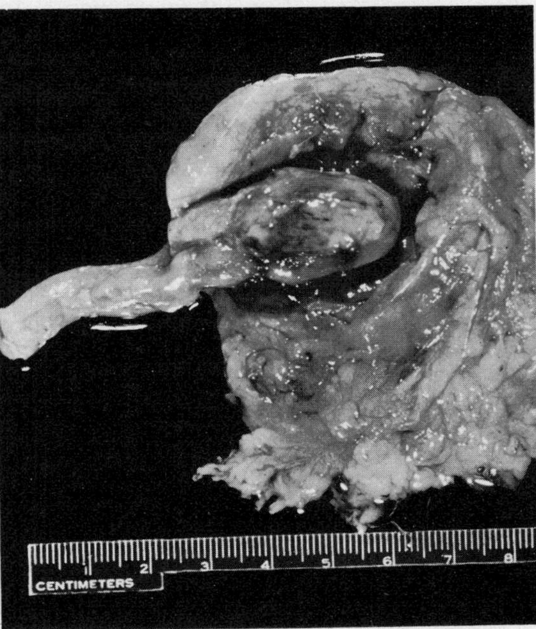

Fig. 18–63

Figure 18–62. A suppurative exudate covering serosa of appendix. Uneven dilatation is produced by impacted fecaliths.

Figure 18–63. Acute inflammation of distal third of appendix together with segment of omentum that had become applied to inflammatory focus.

also present within the mucosa. Since drainage of an exudate into the appendix from a focus of infection in a higher level of bowel may also induce some scant neutrophilic infiltrate in the mucosa, it is usually believed that evidence of the inflammation within the muscularis is requisite for diagnosis. The progressively worsening stages of acute appendicitis with suppuration and gangrenous necrosis require no further description, since these are entirely nonspecific and follow the pattern of inflammatory reactions in other tissues. The possibility of acute vasculitis or inflammatory thrombosis of the blood vessels in the mesoappendix must always be borne in mind. Such vascular involvement may lead to pylephlebitis or pyemic liver abscesses.

Classically, acute appendicitis produces the following, in the sequence given: (1) pain, at first periumbilical but then localizing to the right lower quadrant; (2) nausea and/or vomiting; (3) abdominal tenderness, particularly in the region of the appendix; (4) mild fever; and (5) an elevation of the peripheral white cell count up to 15,000 to 20,000 cells/mm^3. Regrettably, this classic presentation is more often absent than present. The pain, nausea, and vomiting are most consistently present, but tenderness may be deceptively absent or maximal in atypical locations, e.g., right flank or midline pelvis. The white cell count may not be elevated, or at other times may be so high as to suggest alternative diagnoses. These nonclassic presentations are encountered more often in young children and the very elderly. Indeed, in the latter, inflammatory disease may be present with few, if any, manifestations. Thus, the diagnosis of acute appendicitis requires a high index of suspicion and the willingness to explore an abdomen on slender intuitions. There is general agreement that highly competent surgeons make about 10 to 30% false-positive diagnoses of acute appendicitis.[257] The most common conditions that mimic acute appendicitis are mesenteric lymphadenitis, usually secondary to an enterocolitis (often unrecognized) caused by Yersinia or some virus; a systemic viral infection; acute salpingitis; ectopic tubal pregnancy; "mittelschmerz" (pain caused by trivial pelvic bleeding at time of ovulation); and Meckel's diverticulitis. But most often, when the abdomen is explored and the appendix is uninvolved, no disease of any kind is found, leaving the surgeon mumbling such vagaries as "cecitis" or "appendiceal colic." The penalty for undue delay is perforation followed by a periappendiceal abscess and/or peritonitis. Other potential but uncommon complications of appendicitis include pylephlebitis with thrombosis of the portal venous drainage, liver abscess, and bacteremia. *The discomfort and risks associated with an exploratory laparotomy and discovery of "no disease" are far outweighed by the morbidity and mortality (about 2%) associated with perforation.*

CHRONIC INFLAMMATION

True chronic inflammation of the appendix is rare. Much more frequently, recurrent acute attacks may be inappropriately referred to as "chronic appendicitis." In some patients, the appendix from birth is a mere fibrous cord. It must not be assumed, therefore, that extensive fibrosis of the appendiceal architecture implies a chronic inflammatory reaction or the end stage of a previous inflammation.

MUCOCELE OF APPENDIX AND PSEUDOMYXOMA PERITONEI

Dilatation of the appendiceal lumen by mucinous secretion is designated *mucocele* (Fig. 18–64). Traditionally in the past two forms of mucocele were described: (1) obstructive and (2) neoplastic. The former proposal was that obstruction of the appendiceal lumen by a fecalith did not inevitably lead to inflammatory changes, but instead permitted mucinous secretions to accumulate in the sequestered lumen, leading to mucocele formation.[258] Plausible as this sequence may be, an evaluation of a large number of appendiceal mucoceles failed to reveal a single instance of obstructive mucocele, presumably because luminal obstruction usually is followed by inflammation or, in time, pressure-induced atrophy of the mucus-secreting epithelium. Instead, three patterns of epithelial proliferation were observed: (1) mucosal hyperplasia remarkably similar to the changes seen in hyperplastic polyps of the colon, (2) mucinous cystadenoma (by far the most common form), and (3) mucinous cystadenocarcinoma.[259]

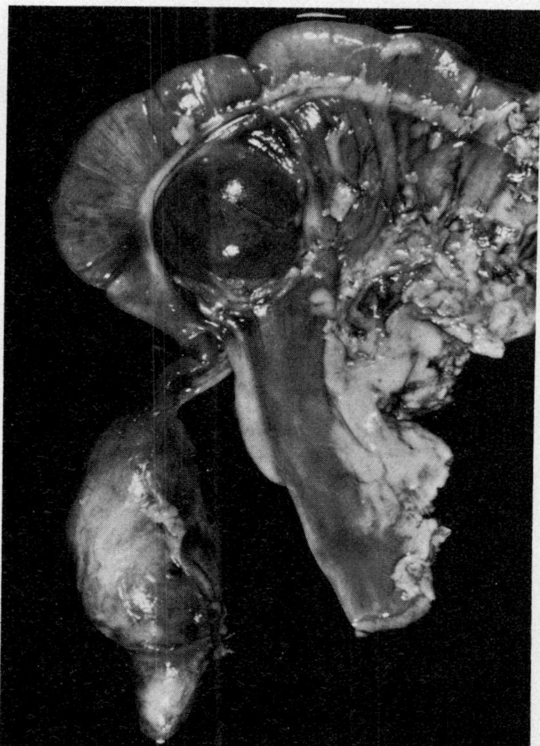

Figure 18–64. Mucocele of appendix shown still attached to terminal ileum and cecum.

Morphology. The histologic features of cystadenomas and cystadenocarcinomas closely mimic their ovarian counterparts, as described on page 1146. All three lesions were associated with appendiceal dilatation secondary to mucinous secretions, but with mucosal hyperplasia there was no evidence of appendiceal rupture or of peritoneal mucinous implants. With **cystadenomas** the luminal dilatation was more striking and associated with appendiceal perforation in 20% of instances, and in such cases **localized collections of mucus** were present, either attached to the serosa of the appendix or lying free in the peritoneal cavity. Histologic examination of the mucus revealed **no neoplastic cells.** Follow-up of these patients after removal of the appendix, and sometimes the right colon, documented that none had any complications related to the appendiceal lesion or the extravasated mucus. **Mucinous cystadenocarcinomas** were one-fifth as common as cystadenomas. Macroscopically, they produced mucin-filled cystic dilatation of the appendix indistinguishable from that associated with the benign tumors. However, **penetration of the bowel wall by neoplastic cells and spread beyond the appendix in the form of peritoneal implants was frequently present.** In its fully developed state the peritoneal cavity becomes distended with tenacious, semisolid mucin—**pseudomyxoma peritonei**—in which anaplastic cystadenocarcinomatous cells can be found.[260] The feature that differentiates pseudomyxoma peritonei from mucinous spillage is the presence of cancerous cells within the mucin, not seen with the nonmalignant lesions producing mucocele.[261] Thus, in reality, **pseudomyxoma peritonei is a form of intraperitoneal spread of a mucin-secreting cancer.** Spread of the neoplasm above the diaphragm or invasion of abdominal viscera is exceptional. Ovarian mucinous cystadenocarcinomas may produce an identical picture (p. 1146).

TUMORS OF APPENDIX

Tumors of the appendix such as those described above are very rare. The most common is the endocrine cell tumor (argentaffinoma), which was discussed on page 842 along with similar lesions of the entire gut. Only a capsule characterization is provided here. The tumor most frequently involves the distal tip of the appendix, where it produces a solid bulbous swelling 2 to 3 cm in diameter, which on section is yellow and firm. The lumen and architecture of the wall are obliterated in the area of involvement. Histologically, these tumors have the same appearance as those described in the small intestine. The same uniformity of cells and nuclear size and shape is present. Giant cells, anaplasia, and mitoses are virtually absent but, despite the benign cytologic appearance, the tumor invades deeply throughout the muscularis and sometimes out to the serosa. These tumors virtually never metastasize, and although regional node involvement may occur, it is very uncommon. It is extremely rare for these small lesions to produce the carcinoid syndrome.

CARCINOMA

On rare occasions, non–mucin-producing carcinomas of the appendix may produce a typical neoplastic enlargement of the organ. The mucin-secreting lesions may produce a mucocele (see opposite page). Metastases may follow the pattern of other intestinal carcinomas or may induce pseudomyxoma peritonei.

MISCELLANEOUS TUMORS

Benign and malignant mesenchymal growths in this organ are reported as medical curiosities. These neoplasms resemble their counterparts in other areas.

Peritoneum

INFLAMMATION

Peritonitis is an inflammatory process that may be due to either bacterial invasion or chemical irritation. It is therefore here divided into sterile and bacterial types.

STERILE PERITONITIS

The most common causes of sterile peritonitis in order of frequency are described below.

Bile

Perforation or rupture of the biliary system evokes a highly irritating peritonitis. In the early stage, it is usually limited to the right upper quadrant, and on examination the peritoneal exudate will be bile-stained. Later the biliary discoloration is masked by the progressive suppuration that ensues concomitantly with superimposed bacterial contamination. Any type of acute inflammatory disease or obstruction within the gallbladder or bile ducts may produce perforation or rupture, and spill bile into the peritoneal cavity. Not uncommonly, the bile may gain access to the peritoneal cavity through a perforated peptic ulcer. In almost all these conditions that predispose to the soiling of the peritoneum by bile, bacterial contamination is present and thus places the peritonitis in another category.

Pancreatic Enzymes

Acute hemorrhagic pancreatitis is a calamitous disorder characterized by hemorrhage and necrosis of the pancreas (p. 963). Concomitantly, pancreatic enzymes leak into the peritoneal cavity. These proteolytic and lipolytic ferments evoke a striking peritoneal reaction and, at the same time, digest lipid tissue. With the release of fatty acids, saponification (formation of soaps) produces chalky white precipitates in focal areas of fat wherever it is exposed to these enzymes. At the same time, globules of free fat may be found floating in the peritoneal fluid that accumulates. Both these features, the formation of soaps and fat globules, are virtually diagnostic of the peritonitis produced by pancreatic necrosis. After 24 to 48 hours, however, bacterial permeation of the bowel wall usually leads to a frank suppurative exudation.

Surgically Introduced Foreign Material (Particularly Talcum Powder)

The reaction to such agents is usually localized and minimal. No clinical symptoms may result, and the only significance of such disease lies in the possible development of chronic inflammatory granulomas, followed by fibrosis and adhesions, which may eventually lead to intestinal obstruction or strangulation of the bowel.

BACTERIAL PERITONITIS

Bacterial peritonitis is almost invariably secondary to extension of bacteria through the wall of a hollow viscus or to rupture of a viscus. The common primary disorders leading to such bacterial disseminations are *appendicitis, ruptured peptic ulcer, cholecystitis, diverticulitis, strangulation of bowel, and acute salpingitis.* Virtually every bacterial organism has been implicated as a cause of peritonitis, most commonly *E. coli*, alpha-hemolytic and beta-hemolytic streptococci, *Staphylococcus aureus*, enterococci, "gram-negative rods," and *Clostridium perfringens*. This last organism is a frequent inhabitant of the gut and therefore a frequent component of peritonitis. However, it rarely causes true gas gangrene in the abdominal cavity. Next to the secondary forms of bacterial peritonitis in frequency is the so-called "spontaneous bacterial peritonitis" that appears in about 10% of cirrhotics. The usual causal agent is *E. coli*, but the manner by which it invades the peritoneal cavity is unknown (possibly blood-borne). Seldom encountered today are gonococcal and tuberculous peritonitis, the former arising from an acute salpingitis and the latter secondary to tuberculosis of the intestinal tract or hematogenous dissemination from a primary pulmonary focus. Spontaneous pneumococcal peritonitis is a curiosity occasionally encountered in children with renal disease. Both the source of the organism and the mode of spread are obscure.

Depending on the duration of the peritonitis, the membranes show the following changes. Approximately two to four hours after involvement, the membrane loses its gray, glistening quality and becomes dull and lusterless. There is, at this time, a small accumulation of essentially serous or slightly turbid fluid. Later the exudate becomes creamy and obviously suppurative. In some cases, it may become extremely thick and plastic and even inspissated, especially in dehydrated patients. The volume of such exudate varies enormously. In many cases, it may be **localized** by the omentum and viscera to a small area of the peritoneal cavity, particularly as in an appendiceal abscess; or it may become **generalized** to involve the entire abdominal cavity. In generalized peritonitis, it is important to remember that exudate may accumulate under and above the liver to form **subhepatic and subdiaphragmatic abscesses.** Collections in the lesser omental sac may likewise create residual persistent foci of infection.

The inflammatory process is typical of an acute bacterial infection anywhere and produces the characteristic neutrophilic infiltration with a fibrinopurulent exudate. The reaction usually remains superficial and does not penetrate deeply into the visceral structures or abdominal wall. Tuberculous peritonitis tends to produce a plastic exudate studded with minute pale granulomas.

These inflammatory processes can heal either spontaneously or with therapy. In the course of healing, the following results may be obtained: *(1) the exudate may be totally resolved, leaving no residual fibrosis; (2) residual, walled-off abscesses may persist, eventually to heal or serve as foci for new infection; or (3) organization of the exudate may occur, with the formation of fibrous adhesive bands termed adhesions.* On occasion, these adhesions may be responsible for later symptoms or pathologic findings, forming potential sources of obstruction to the lumen of the bowel or strangulation of a segment of gut.

SCLEROSING RETROPERITONITIS

Dense fibromatous overgrowth of the retroperitoneal tissues may sometimes develop, as described on page 1064. This occurrence is designated sclerosing retroperitonitis or retroperitoneal fibromatosis. In some instances the mesentery is also involved. The fibrous overgrowth is entirely nondistinctive and, although infiltrative, does not display frank anaplasia. There is usually an accompanying inflammatory infiltrate of lymphocytes, plasma cells, and neutrophils, suggesting inflammatory rather than neoplastic disease. The fibrosis is particularly important because it often encroaches on the ureters and may produce hydronephrosis. The fibrous tissue insinuates itself into the retroperitoneal fat and about the retroperitoneal organs, and in some ways is the analog of the desmoid tumor. Distant metastasis or regional node involvement is not encountered. The origin of this condition is obscure, as pointed out in the more complete discussion of this entity.

MESENTERIC CYSTS

Large-to-small cystic masses are sometimes found within the mesenteries in the abdominal cavity or attached to the peritoneal lining of the abdominal wall. These cysts are usually of obscure nature and origin, but sometimes offer difficult clinical diagnostic problems because they present on palpation as abdominal masses. Many classifications have been proposed that attempt to designate groups according to common pathogenetic origins. On this basis, it has been suggested that mesenteric cysts be divided into (1) those arising from sequestered lymphatic channels; (2) those derived from pinched-off enteric diverticula that usually arise during the early development of the fore- and hindgut; (3) those derived from the urogenital ridge or its derivatives, i.e., the urinary tract and male and female genital tracts; (4) those derived from walled-off infections or postpancreatitis, more properly called pseudocysts; and (5) those of malignant origin.

Usually these cysts are single, but occasionally multiple loculations are found either attached to or dispersed throughout the abdominal cavity. They vary from small, 1- to 2-cm nodules to massive structures, 15 to 20 cm in diameter. The fluid content in those of lymphatic origin is chylous; in the remainder it is fairly nondescript and may be either serous or mucinous, varying in color from pale yellow to muddy red-brown. Considerable turbidity may be imparted by necrotic tissue or old blood in the pseudocysts. Histologically, the wall is composed of fibrous tissue and may have such specialized cytologic detail as permits identification of the derivation of the cyst. The principal anatomic feature of importance in these cysts is the clear separation of the non-neoplastic from the very rare cystadenocarcinomas. Since most are non-neoplastic and since they usually are fairly mobile or at most are loosely attached structures, surgical resection is the treatment of choice and permits cure.

TUMORS OF PERITONEUM

Virtually all tumors of the peritoneum are malignant and can be divided into primary and secondary forms.

Primary tumors of the peritoneum are extremely rare and are called mesotheliomas. These exactly duplicate the tumors found in the pleura and the pericardium. Like the supradiaphragmatic tumors, peritoneal mesotheliomas are associated with asbestos exposure in at least 80% of cases. How inhaled asbestos induces a peritoneal neoplasm is a mystery. Conceivably some is swallowed, but this is sheer speculation. Mesotheliomas all look alike and behave alike, regardless of their primary sites of origin. Thus, for further details, reference should be made to the discussion of the most common of these unusual forms of neoplasia, pleural mesotheliomas (p. 760).

Secondary tumors of the peritoneum are, in contrast, quite common. In any form of advanced cancer, penetration to the serosal membrane or metastatic seeding may occur. The most common tumors producing a diffuse serosal miliary implantation are ovarian or pancreatic carcinomas. However, it is seen in any type of intra-abdominal malignancy, and occasionally represents distant metastases from tumors in other locations within the body.

Additional mention might be made of the very uncommon tumors that may arise from retroperitoneal tissues, i.e., fat, fibrous tissue, blood vessels, lymphatics, nerves, and the lymph nodes alongside the aorta. These native structures may give rise to benign or malignant neoplasms called *retroperitoneal tumors* that resemble their counterparts arising elsewhere in the body.

---

1. Cohen, S.: Motor disorders of the esophagus. N. Engl. J. Med. *301*:184, 1979.
2. Cohen, S., et al.: Gastrointestinal motility. Int. Rev. Physiol. *19*:107, 1979.
3. Fisher, R., and Cohen, S.: Disorders of the lower esophageal sphincter. Annu. Rev. Med. *26*:373, 1975.
4. Adams, W. M., et al.: Ganglion cells in achalasia of the cardia. Virchows Arch. [Pathol. Anat.] *372*:75, 1976.
5. Cohen, S., et al.: The site of denervation in achalasia. Gut *13*:556, 1972.
6. Schatzki, R., and Gary, J. E.: The lower esophageal ring. Am. J. Roentgenol. *75*:246, 1956.
7. Hagarty, G.: A classification of esophageal hiatus hernia with special reference to sliding hernia. Am. J. Roentgenol. *84*:1056, 1960.
8. Editorial: Asymptomatic hiatus hernia. Lancet *1*:870, 1969.
9. Palmer, E. D.: Hiatus hernia and hemorrhage. Am. J. Med. Sci. *249*:417, 1963.
10. Weiss, S., and Mallory, G. K.: Lesions of cardiac orifice of the stomach produced by vomiting. J.A.M.A. *98*:1353, 1932.
11. Editorial: Mallory-Weiss through the endoscope. Lancet *1*:1294, 1978.
12. Dodds, W. J., et al.: Pathogenesis of reflux esophagitis. Gastroenterology *81*:376, 1981.
13. Crespi, M., et al.: Oesophageal lesions in Northern Iran: A pre-malignant lesion. Lancet *2*:217, 1979.
14. Behar, J., and Sheahan, D. C.: Histologic abnormalities in reflux esophagitis. Arch. Pathol. *99*:387, 1975.
15. Barrett, N. R.: The lower esophagus lined by columnar epithelium. Surgery *41*:881, 1957.
16. Thomson, J. J.: Barrett's metaplasia and adenocarcinoma of the esophagus and gastroesophageal junction. Hum. Pathol. *14*:42, 1983.
17. Naef, A. P., et al.: Columnar-lined lower esophagus, an acquired lesion with malignant predisposition: Report on 140 cases of Barrett's esophagus with 12 adenocarcinomas. J. Thorac. Cardiovasc. Surg. *70*:826, 1975.
18. Gilder, S. S.: Carcinoma of the esophagus. Ann. Intern. Med. *87*:494, 1977.
19. Muñoz, N., et al.: Precursor lesions of oesophageal cancer in high risk populations in Iran and China. Lancet *1*:876, 1982.
20. United States Department of Health, Education and Welfare: Public Health Service Review 1967. The health consequences of smoking. Public Health Service Publication, No. 1696, 1968, p. 150.
21. Mandard, A. M., et al.: Autopsy findings in 111 cases of esophageal cancer. Cancer *48*:329, 1981.
22. Joint Iran/IARC Study Group: Oesophageal cancer studies in the Caspian Littoral of Iran. Results of population studies—a prodrome. J. Natl. Cancer Inst. *59*:1127, 1977.
23. O'Neill, C., et al.: Silica fragments from millet bran on mucosa surrounding oesophageal tumours in patients in Northern China. Lancet *1*:1202, 1982.

24. Reid, H. A. S.: Oat cell carcinoma of the esophagus. Cancer *45*:2342, 1980.
25. Lechago, J.: Endocrine cells of the gastrointestinal tract and their pathology. Pathol. Annu. *13*:329, 1978.
26. Bloom, S. R., and Polak, J. M.: The new peptide hormones of the gut. Prog. Gastroenterol. *3*:109, 1977.
27. Gould, V. E., et al.: The APUD cell system and its neoplasms. Observations on the significance and limitations of the concept. Surg. Clin. North Am. *59*:93, 1979.
28. Kivilaakso, E., and Silen, W.: Pathogenesis of experimental, gastric-mucosal injury. N. Engl. J. Med. *301*:364, 1979.
29. Miller, T. A., and Jackobson, E. D.: Gastrointestinal cytoprotection by prostaglandins. Gut *20*:75, 1979.
30. Editorial: Acid reduction or mucosal protection for peptic ulcer? Lancet *2*:473, 1982.
31. Strickland, R. G., and Mackay, I. R.: A reappraisal of the nature and significance of chronic atrophic gastritis. Am. J. Dig. Dis. *18*:426, 1973.
32. Valman, H. B., et al.: Lesions associated with gastroduodenal haemorrhage in relation to aspirin intake. Br. Med. J. *4*:661, 1968.
33. Ihamaki, T., et al.: Long-term observation of subjects with normal mucosa and with superficial gastritis: Results of 23–27 years' follow-up examinations. Scand. J. Gastroenterol. *13*:771, 1978.
34. Chisholm, M.: Immunology of gastritis. Clin. Gastroenterol. *5*:419, 1976.
35. Strickland, R. G.: Gastritis. Front. Gastrointest. Res. *1*:12, 1975.
36. Vandelli, C., et al.: Autoantibodies to gastrin-producing cells in antral (Type B) chronic gastritis. N. Engl. J. Med. *300*:1406, 1979.
37. Zamcheck, N., et al.: Occurrence of gastric cancer among patients with pernicious anemia at the Boston City Hospital. N. Engl. J. Med. *252*:1103, 1955.
38. Bone, E. S., et al.: Pathogenesis of gastric cancer in pernicious anaemia. Lancet *1*:52, 1978.
39. Suen, K. C., and Burton, J. D.: The spectrum of eosinophilic infiltration of the gastrointestinal tract and its relationship to other disorders of angiitis and granulomatosis. Hum. Pathol. *10*:31, 1979.
40. Menguy, R.: The prophylaxis of stress ulceration. N. Engl. J. Med. *302*:461, 1980.
41. Tramp, A., and Gregg, R. V.: Transmittal of restraint-induced gastric ulcers by parabiosis in rats. Gastroenterology *66*:63, 1973.
42. Rees, W. D., and Turnberg, L. A.: Reappraisal of the effects of aspirin on the stomach. Lancet *2*:410, 1980.
43. Watkinson, G.: The incidence of chronic peptic ulcer found at necropsy. Gut *1*:14, 1960.
44. Mendeloff, A. I.: What has been happening to duodenal ulcer. Gastroenterology *67*:1020, 1974.
45. Eberhard, G.: Peptic ulcer in twins. A study in personality, heredity and environment. Acta Psychiatr. Scand. *44*(Suppl.): 205, 1968.
46. Rotter, J. I., et al.: HLA-B5 association with duodenal ulcer. Gastroenterology *73*:438, 1977.
47. Rotter, J. I., et al.: Duodenal-ulcer disease associated with elevated serum pepsinogen. I. An inherited autosomal dominant disorder. N. Engl. J. Med. *300*:63, 1979.
48. Grossman, M. I., et al.: Peptic diseases. Gastroenterology *69*:1071, 1975.
49. Chapman, M. L.: Peptic ulcer. A medical perspective. Med. Clin. North Am. *62*:39, 1978.
50. Cox, A. J.: Stomach size and its relation to chronic peptic ulcer. Arch. Pathol. *54*:407, 1952.
51. Fordtran, J. S., and Walsh, J. H.: Gastric acid secretion rate and buffer content of the stomach after eating. J. Clin. Invest. *52*:647, 1973.
52. Thomas, W. E. G.: Duodeno-gastric-reflux. A common factor in pathogenesis of gastric and duodenal ulcer. Lancet *2*:1166, 1980.
53. Walsh, J. H., et al.: pH dependence of acid secretion and gastrin release in normal and ulcer subjects. J. Clin. Invest. *55*:462, 1975.
54. Editorial: Viruses and duodenal ulcer. Lancet *1*:705, 1981.
55. Grossman, M. I.: A new look at peptic ulcer. Ann. Intern. Med. *84*:57, 1976.
56. Overholt, B., and Pollard, H.: Acid diffusion into the human gastric mucosa. Gastroenterology *54*:182, 1968.
57. Gear, M., et al.: Gastric ulcer and gastritis. Gut *12*:639, 1971.
58. Piper, D. W., et al.: Analgesic ingestion and chronic peptic ulcer. Gastroenterology *80*:427, 1981.
59. Silvoso, G. R., et al.: Incidence of gastric lesions in patients with rheumatic disease on chronic aspirin therapy. Ann. Intern. Med. *91*:517, 1979.
60. Oi, M., et al.: A possible dual control mechanism in the origin of peptic ulcer. Gastroenterology *57*:280, 1969.
61. Elder, J. B., et al.: Cimetidine and gastric cancer. Lancet *1*:1013, 1979.
62. Grossman, M. I.: The Veterans Administration cooperative study on gastric ulcer. 10. Résumé and comment. Gastroenterology *61* (Suppl. 2): 635, 1971.
63. Beard, R. J., et al.: Non-carcinomatous tumours of the stomach. Br. J. Surg. *55*:535, 1968.
64. Ming, S.-C.: Tumors of the esophagus and stomach. Atlas of Tumor Pathology, AFIP, Washington, D.C., Fascicle #7, 99, 1973.
65. Ming, S.-C., and Goldman, H.: Gastric polyps. A histogenetic classification and its relation to carcinoma. Cancer *18*:721, 1965.
66. Ming, S.-C.: The adenoma-carcinoma sequence in the stomach and colon. II. Malignant potential of gastric polyps. Gastrointest. Radiol. *1*:121, 1976.
67. Tomasuto, J.: Gastric polyps. Histologic types and their relationship to gastric carcinoma. Cancer *27*:1345, 1971.
68. Bone, G. E., and McClelland, R. N.: Management of gastric polyps. Surg. Gynecol. Obstet. *142*:933, 1976.
69. Silverberg, E.: Cancer statistics—1980. Cancer *30*:23, 1980.
70. Haenszel, W., and Correa, P.: Developments in the epidemiology of stomach cancer over the past decade. Cancer Res. *35*:3452, 1975.
71. Grundmann, E.: Early gastric carcinoma—today. Pathol. Res. Pract. *162*:347, 1978.
72. Fugita, S.: Biology of early gastric carcinoma. Pathol. Res. Pract. *163*:297, 1978.
73. Peter, H. R., et al.: Early gastric cancer. Gastroenterology *81*:247, 1981.
74. Ming, S.-C.: Gastric carcinoma. A pathobiological classification. Cancer *39*:2475, 1977.
75. Laruen, P.: The two histological main types of gastric carcinoma: Diffuse and so-called intestinal-type carcinoma. An attempt at a histoclinical classification. Acta Pathol. Microbiol. Scand. *64*:31, 1965.
76. Muñoz, N., and Connelly, R.: Time trends of intestinal and diffuse types of gastric cancer in the United States. Int. J. Cancer *8*:158, 1971.
77. Chejfec, G., and Gould, V. E.: Malignant gastric neuroendocrinomas. Ultrastructural and biochemical characterization of their secretory activity. Hum. Pathol. *8*:433, 1977.
78. Adashek, K., et al.: Cancer of the stomach. Review of consecutive 10-year intervals. Ann. Surg. *189*:6, 1979.
79. Dupont, J. B., Jr., et al.: Adenocarcinoma of the stomach: Review of 1,497 cases. Cancer *41*:941, 1978.
80. Henry, K., and Farrer-Brown, G.: Primary lymphomas of the gastrointestinal tract. I. Plasma cell tumours. Histopathology *1*:53, 1977.
81. Lewin, K. J., et al.: Lymphomas of the gastrointestinal tract: A study of 117 cases presenting with gastrointestinal disease. Cancer *42*:693, 1978.
82. Weingrad, D. N., et al.: Primary gastrointestinal lymphomas. Cancer *49*:1258, 1982.
83. Lewin, K. J., et al.: Primary intestinal lymphoma of "Western" and "Mediterranean" type, alpha chain disease and massive plasma cell infiltration. Cancer *38*:2511, 1976.
84. Selzer, G., et al.: Primary small intestinal lymphomas and alpha-heavy-chain disease. A study of 43 cases from a pathology department in Israel. Isr. J. Med. Sci. *15*:111, 1979.
85. Radaszkiewiez, T., and Dragosics, B.: Primary lymphomas of the gastrointestinal tract. Pathol. Res. Pract. *169*:353, 1980.
86. Holmes, G. K. T., et al.: Coeliac disease, gluten-free diet and malignancy. Gut *17*:612, 1976.
87. Shani, A., et al.: Primary gastric malignant lymphoma followed by gastric adenocarcinoma. Cancer *42*:2039, 1978.
88. Saraga, P., et al.: Lymphomas and pseudolymphomas of the alimentary tract. Hum. Pathol. *12*:713, 1981.
89. Smithwick, W., III, et al.: Leiomyoblastoma. Behavior and prognosis. Cancer *24*:996, 1969.
90. Trier, J. S.: Studies on small intestinal crypt epithelium. I. The fine structure of the crypt epithelium of the proximal small intestine of fasting humans. J. Cell Biol. *18*:599, 1963.
91. Rodning, C. B., et al.: Immunoglobulins within human small-intestinal Paneth cells. Lancet *1*:984, 1976.
92. Moxey, P. C., and Trier, J. S.: Endocrine cells in the human fetal small intestine. Cell Tissue Res. *183*:33, 1977.
93. Isselbacher, K. J.: The intestinal cell surface. Some properties of normal, undifferentiated and malignant cells. Ann. Intern. Med. *81*:681, 1974.
94. Madara, J. L., et al.: Structural changes in the plasma membrane accompanying differentiation of epithelial cells in human and monkey small intestine. Gastroenterology *78*:963, 1980.
95. Thomas, C. S., Jr., et al.: Jejunal diverticula as a source of massive gastrointestinal bleeding. Arch. Surg. *95*:89, 1967.
96. Ottinger, L. W.: Acute mesenteric ischemia. N. Engl. J. Med. *307*:535, 1982.
97. Swerdlow, S. H., et al.: Intestinal infarction. A new classification. (Letter.) Arch. Pathol. Lab. Med. *105*:218, 1981.
98. Boley, S. J.: Early diagnosis of acute mesenteric ischemia. Hosp. Pract. *16*:63, 1981.
99. Aboumrad, M. H., et al.: Intimal hyperplasia of small mesenteric arteries. Occlusive, with infarction of the intestine. Arch. Pathol. *75*:196, 1963.
100. Civetta, J. M., and Kolodny, M.: Mesenteric venous thrombosis associated with oral contraceptives. Gastroenterology *58*:713, 1970.
101. Jona, J., et al.: Recurrent primary mesenteric venous thrombosis. J.A.M.A. *227*:1033, 1974.

102. Kirschner, P. A.: Occlusion of the mesenteric arteries and veins with infarction of the bowel. J. Mt. Sinai Hosp. N.Y. *21*:307, 1954–55.
103. Ver Steeg, K. R., and Broders, W. C.: Gangrene of the bowel. Surg. Clin. North Am. *59*:869, 1979.
104. Freiman, D. G.: Hemorrhagic necrosis of the gastrointestinal tract. Circulation *32*:329, 1965.
105. Marshak, R. H., et al.: Ischemia of the colon. Mt. Sinai J. Med. *48*:180, 1981.
106. Editorial: Traveller's diarrhoea. Lancet *1*:777, 1982.
107. Colgan, T., et al.: *Campylobacter jejuni* enterocolitis. Arch. Pathol. Lab. Med. *104*:571, 1980.
108. Blaser, M. J., and Reller, L. B.: Campylobacter enteritis. N. Engl. J. Med. *305*:1444, 1981.
109. Guerrant, R. L.: Yet another pathogenic mechanism for *Escherichia coli* diarrhea. N. Engl. J. Med. *302*:113, 1980.
110. Ulshen, M. H., and Rollo, J. L.: Pathogenesis of *Escherichia coli* gastroenteritis in man—another mechanism. N. Engl. J. Med. *302*:99, 1980.
111. Bradford, W. B., et al.: Pathologic features of enteric infection with *Yersinia enterocolitica*. Arch. Pathol. *98*:17, 1974.
112. Trier, J. S.: The pathology of acute nonbacterial gastroenteritis. *In* Morson, B. C., and Abell, M. R. (eds.): The Gastrointestinal Tract. Baltimore, Williams & Wilkins Co., 1977, p. 36.
113. Kapikian, A. Z.: Approaches to immunization of infants and young children against gastroenteritis due to rotaviruses. Rev. Infect. Dis. *2*:459, 1980.
114. Suzuki, H., and Konno, T.: Reovirus-like particles in jejunal mucosa of a Japanese infant with acute infectious non-bacterial gastroenteritis. Tohoku J. Exp. Med. *115*:199, 1975.
115. Kirsner, J. B., and Shorter, R. G.: Recent developments in "non-specific" inflammatory bowel disease. N. Engl. J. Med. *306*:775, 837, 1982.
116. Greenstein, A. J., et al.: The extraintestinal manifestations of Crohn's disease and ulcerative colitis: A study of 700 patients. Medicine *55*:401, 1976.
117. Janowitz, H. D.: Crohn's disease—50 years later. N. Engl. J. Med. *304*:1600, 1981.
118. Janowitz, H. D., and Sachar, D. B.: New observations in Crohn's disease. Annu. Rev. Med. *27*:269, 1976.
119. Selby, W. S., et al.: Crohn's disease. A review of 122 cases. Aust. N.Z. J. Med. *9*:145, 1979.
120. Farmer, R. G., et al.: Studies of family history among patients with inflammatory bowel disease. Clin. Gastroenterol. *9*:271, 1980.
121. Sherlock, P., et al.: Familial occurrence of regional enteritis and ulcerative colitis. Gastroenterology *45*:413, 1963.
122. Strickland, R. G., and Sachar, D. B.: The immunology of inflammatory bowel disease. *In* Jerzy Glass, G. B. (ed.): Progress in Gastroenterology, Vol. III. New York, Grune & Stratton, 1977, p. 821.
123. Schwartz, S. E., et al.: Regional enteritis: Evidence for genetic transmission by HLA typing. Ann. Intern. Med. *93*:424, 1980.
124. Sachar, D. B.: Aetiologic theories of inflammatory bowel disease. Clin. Gastroenterol. *9*:231, 1980.
125. Kirsner, J. B.: Inflammatory bowel disease; considerations of etiology and pathogenesis. Am. J. Gastroenterol *69*:253, 1978.
126. Mitchell, D. N., and Rees, R. J. W.: Agent transmissible from Crohn's disease tissue. Lancet 2:168, 1970.
127. Cave, D. R., et al.: Experimental animal evidence of a transmissible agent in Crohn's disease. Lancet *2*:1120, 1973.
128. Gitnick, G. L.: Etiology of inflammatory diseases: Are we making progress? Gastroenterology *78*:1090, 1980.
129. Gitnick, G. L., et al.: Evidence for the isolation of a new virus from ulcerative colitis patients: Comparison with virus derived from Crohn's disease. Dig. Dis. Sci. *24*:609, 1979.
130. Dvorak, A. M., et al.: Absence of virus structures in Crohn's disease tissues studied by electron microscopy. Lancet *1*:328, 1978.
131. Gorbach, S. L.: Intestinal microflora in inflammatory bowel disease. *In* Kirsner, J. B., and Shorter, R. G. (eds.): Inflammatory Bowel Disease. Philadelphia, Lea & Febiger, 1980, p. 55.
132. Das, D. M., et al.: Isolation and characterization of colonic tissue-bound antibodies from patients with idiopathic ulcerative colitis. Proc. Natl. Acad. Sci. U.S.A. *9*:4528, 1978.
133. Bookman, M. A., and Bull, D. M.: Characteristics of isolated intestinal mucosal lymphoid cells in inflammatory bowel disease. Gastroenterology *77*:503, 1979.
134. Dvorak, A. M., et al.: Crohn's disease. Transmission electron microscopic studies. II. Immunologic inflammatory response. Alterations of mast cells, basophils, eosinophils and the microvasculature. Hum. Pathol. *11*:606, 1980.
135. O'Donoghue, D. P., and Kumar, P.: Rectal IgE cells in inflammatory bowel disease. Gut *20*:149, 1979.
136. Falchuk, Z. M., et al.: Human colonic lamina propria lymphocytes mediate mitogen-induced but not spontaneous cell-mediated cytotoxicity (abstr.). Gastroenterology *76*:1129, 1979.
137. Brooks, M.: Crohn's disease. A functional deficiency of IgA? Lancet *1*:158, 1981.
138. Gould, S. R., et al.: Increased prostaglandin production in ulcerative colitis. Lancet *2*:98, 1977.
139. Morson, B. C.: Pathology of inflammatory bowel disease. Gastroenterol. Jpn. *15*:184, 1980.
140. Price, A. B., and Morson, B. C.: Inflammatory bowel disease: The surgical pathology of Crohn's disease and ulcerative colitis. Hum. Pathol. *6*:7, 1975.
141. Lee, K. S., et al.: Indeterminate colitis in the spectrum of inflammatory bowel disease. Arch. Pathol. Lab. Med. *103*:173, 1979.
142. Sommers, S. C., and Korelitz, B. I.: Mucosal cell counts in ulcerative and granulomatous colitis. Am. J. Clin. Pathol. *63*:539, 1979.
143. Otto, H. F., and Gebbers, H. O.: Electron microscopic, ultracytochemical and immunohistological observations in Crohn's disease of the ileum and colon. Virchows Arch. [Pathol. Anat.] *391*:189, 1981.
144. Dvorak, A. M., and Dickerson, G. R.: Crohn's disease: Transmission electron microscopic studies. I. Barrier function: Possible changes related to cell coat, mucous coat, epithelial cells and Paneth cells. Hum. Pathol. *11*:561, 1980.
145. Tizes, R.: Granulomatous colitis. N. Engl. J. Med. *282*:1273, 1970.
146. Lightdale, C. J., et al.: Carcinoma complicating Crohn's disease. Report of 7 cases and review of the literature. Am. J. Med. *59*:262, 1975.
147. Gyde, S. N., et al.: Malignancy in Crohn's disease. Gut *21*:1024, 1980.
148. Garvin, P. J., et al.: Benign and malignant tumors of the small intestine. Curr. Probl. Cancer *3*:1, 1979.
149. Freund, H., et al.: Primary neoplasms of the small bowel. Am. J. Surg. *135*:757, 1978.
150. Perzin, K., and Bridge, M. F.: Adenomas of the small intestine: A clinicopathologic review of 51 cases and a study of their relationship to carcinoma. Cancer *48*:799, 1981.
151. Sager, G. F.: Primary malignant tumors of the small intestine, a 22-year experience with 30 patients. Am. J. Surg. *135*:601, 1978.
152. Wilson, J. M., et al.: Primary malignancies of the small bowel: A report of 96 cases and review of the literature. Ann. Surg. *180*:175, 1974.
153. Jager, P. N., and Polk, H. C., Jr.: Carcinoid APUDomas. Curr. Probl. Cancer *1*:1, 1977.
154. Wilander, E., et al.: Argentaffin and argyrophil reactions of human gastrointestinal carcinoids. Gastroenterology *73*:733, 1977.
155. Pearse, A. G.: The diffuse neuroendocrine system and the APUD concept: Related "endocrine" peptides in brain, intestine, pituitary, placenta, and anuran cutaneous glands. Med. Biol. *55*:115, 1977.
156. Gould, V. E., et al.: The APUD cell system and its neoplasms, observations on the significance and limitations of the concept. Surg. Clin. North Am. *59*:93, 1979.
157. Whitehead, R.: The APUD system—an update. Pathology *12*:333, 1980.
158. Friesen, S. R.: Tumors of the pancreas. N. Engl. J. Med. *306*:580, 1982.
159. Tapia, F. J., et al.: Neuron-specific enolase as produced by neuroendocrine tumours. Lancet *1*:808, 1981.
160. Temple, W. J., et al.: The APUD system and its APUDomas. Int. Adv. Surg. Oncol. *4*:255, 1981.
161. Stevens, R. E., and Moore, G. E.: Inadequacy of APUD concept in explaining production of peptide hormones by tumours. Lancet *1*:118, 1983.
162. Pearse, A. G.: Islet cell precursors are neurons. Nature *295*:96, 1982.
163. Bryant, M. G., et al.: Possible dual role for vasoactive intestinal peptide as gastrointestinal hormone and neurotransmitter substance. Lancet *2*:991, 1976.
164. Rayford, P. L., et al.: Secretin, cholecystokinin, and newer gastrointestinal hormones. N. Engl. J. Med. *294*:1093, 1157, 1976.
165. Khandekar, J. D., et al.: Neurologic involvement in glucagonoma syndrome. Response to combination chemotherapy with 5-fluorouracil and streptozotocin. Cancer *44*:2014, 1979.
166. Godwin, J. D., 2d.: Carcinoid tumors. An analysis of 2837 cases. Cancer *36*:560, 1975.
167. Capella, C., et al.: Gastric carcinoids of argyrophil ECL cells. Ultrastruct. Pathol. *1*:411, 1980.
168. Welch, J. P., and Malt, R. A.: Management of carcinoid tumors of the gastrointestinal tract. Surg. Gynecol. Obstet. *145*:223, 1977.
169. Thompson, J. F.: The carcinoid tumor. Aust. N.Z. J. Surg. *49*:317, 1979.
170. Beacon, H., et al.: Gastrointestinal carcinoids and the malignant carcinoid syndrome. Surg. Gynecol. Obstet. *152*:268, 1981.
171. Moertel, C. G., et al.: Carcinoid tumors of the vermiform appendix. Cancer *21*:270, 1968.
172. Moertel, C. G., et al.: Life history of the carcinoid tumor of the small intestine. Cancer *14*:901, 1961.
173. Coutsoftides, T., and Shibata, H. R.: Primary malignant tumors of the small intestine. Dis. Colon Rectum *22*:24, 1979.
174. Perera, D. R., et al.: Small intestinal biopsy. Hum. Pathol. *6*:157, 1975.
175. Cooke, W. T.: Common problems of malabsorption. Practitioner *216*:637, 1976.

176. Keuning, J. J., et al.: HLA-DW3 associated with coeliac disease. Lancet *1*:506, 1976.
177. Ashkenezi, A., et al.: An in vitro immunological assay for the diagnosis of coeliac disease. Lancet *1*:627, 1978.
178. Rosekrans, P. C., et al.: Long-term morphological and immunohistochemical observations on biopsy specimens of small intestine from children with gluten-sensitive enteropathy. J. Clin. Pathol. *34*:138, 1981.
179. Savilahti, E., et al.: IgA antigliadin antibodies: A marker of mucosal damage in childhood coeliac disease. Lancet *1*:320, 1982.
180. Congdon, P.: Small bowel mucosa in asymptomatic children with celiac disease. Am. J. Dis. Child. *135*:118, 1981.
181. Isselbacher, K. J.: Malabsorption syndrome including disease of pancreatic and biliary origin. Curr. Concepts Nutr. *9*:93, 1980.
182. McNeish, A. S., et al.: The diagnosis of coeliac disease. A commentary on the current practices and members of the European Society for Paediatric Gastroenterology and Nutrition (ESPGAN). Arch. Dis. Child. *54*:783, 1979.
183. Swinson, C. M., et al.: Coeliac disease and malignancy. Lancet *1*:111, 1983.
184. Klipstein, F. A., et al.: Enterotoxigenic intestinal bacteria in tropical sprue. Ann. Intern. Med. *79*:632, 1973.
185. Schenck, E. A., et al.: Morphologic characteristics of jejunal biopsies in celiac disease and tropical sprue. Am. J. Pathol. *47*:765, 1965.
186. Keren, D. F.: Whipple's disease. A review emphasizing immunology and microbiology. CRC Crit. Rev. Clin. Lab. Sci. *14*:75, 1981.
187. Kent, S. P., and Kirkpatrick, P. M.: Whipple's disease. Immunological and histochemical studies of 8 cases. Arch. Pathol. Lab. Med. *104*:544, 1980.
188. Bayless, T. M., and Knox, D. L.: Whipple's disease: A multisystem infection. N. Engl. J. Med. *300*:920, 1979.
189. Feurle, G. E., et al.: Cerebral Whipple's disease with negative jejunal histology. N. Engl. J. Med. *300*:907, 1979.
190. Bostwick, D. G., et al.: Whipple's disease presenting an aortic insufficiency. N. Engl. J. Med. *305*:995, 1981.
191. Weinberg, A. G.: Hirschsprung's disease—a pathologist's view. Perspect. Pediatr. Pathol. *2*:207, 1976.
192. Andrassy, R. J., et al.: Rectal suction biopsy for the diagnosis of Hirschsprung's disease. Ann. Surg. *193*:419, 1981.
193. Gryboski, J. D.: The enterocolitis of Hirschsprung's disease. J. Clin. Gastroenterol. *1*:248, 1979.
194. Larson, D. M., et al.: Medical and surgical therapy in diverticular disease: A comparative study. Gastroenterology *71*:734, 1976.
195. Morson, B. C.: The muscle abnormality in diverticular disease of the sigmoid colon. Br. J. Radiol. *36*:385, 1963.
196. Painter, N. S., and Burkitt, D. P.: Diverticular disease of the colon, a twentieth century problem. Clin. Gastroenterol. *4*:3, 1975.
197. Painter, N. S.: Diverticular disease of the colon—a disease of western civilization. DM, June 1970, p. 1.
198. Almy, T. P., and Howell, D. A.: Diverticular disease of the colon. N. Engl. J. Med. *302*:324, 1980.
199. Weinreich, J., and Anderson, D.: Intraluminal pressure of the sigmoid colon. II. Patients with sigmoid diverticula and related conditions. Scand. J. Gastroenterol. *11*:581, 1976.
200. Painter, N. S.: Diverticular disease of the colon: A bane of the elderly. Geriatrics *31*:89, 1969.
201. Eastwood, M. A., et al.: Colonic function in patients with diverticular disease. Lancet *1*:1181, 1978.
202. Editorial: Keep taking your bran. Lancet *1*:1175, 1979.
203. Steer, H. W., and Colin-Jones, D. G.: Melanosis coli: Studies of toxic effects of irritant purgatives. J. Pathol. *115*:199, 1975.
204. Editorial: Angiodysplasia. Lancet *2*:1086, 1981.
205. Mitsudo, S. M., et al.: Vascular ectasias of the right colon in the elderly. A distinct pathologic entity. Hum. Pathol. *10*:585, 1979.
206. Howard, O. M., et al.: Angiodysplasia of the colon; experience of 26 cases. Lancet *2*:16, 1982.
207. Bull, D. M., et al.: Crohn's disease of the colon. Gastroenterology *76*:607, 1979.
208. Garland, C. F., et al.: Incidence rates of ulcerative colitis and Crohn's disease in 15 areas of the U.S. Gastroenterology *81*:1115, 1981.
209. Riddell, R. H., et al.: Dysplasia in inflammatory bowel disease: Standardized classification with provisional clinical applications. Hum. Pathol. *14*:931, 1983.
210. Greenstein, A. J., et al.: Cancer in universal and left-sided ulcerative colitis: Factors determining risk. Gastroenterology *99*:290, 1979.
211. Sachar, D. B., and Greenstein, A. J.: Cancer in ulcerative colitis: Good news and bad news. Ann. Intern. Med. *95*:462, 1981.
212. Ritchie, J. K., et al.: Prognosis of carcinoma in ulcerative colitis. Gut *22*:752, 1981.
213. Bolton, R. P., et al.: Clostridium difficile–associated diarrhoea—a role in inflammatory bowel disease. Lancet *1*:383, 1980.
214. Bartlett, J. G., et al.: Antibiotic-associated pseudomembranous colitis due to toxin-producing clostridia. N. Engl. J. Med. *298*:531, 1978.
215. Moskovitz, M., and Bartlett, J. G.: Recurrent pseudomembranous colitis unassociated with prior antibiotic therapy. Arch. Intern. Med. *141*:663, 1981.
216. Chapman, I.: Adenomatous polyps of large intestine: Incidence and distribution. Ann. Surg., *157*:223, 1963.
217. Fenoglio, C. M., and Lane, N.: The anatomic precursor of colorectal cancer. Cancer *34*:819, 1974.
218. Fenoglio, C. M.: Symposium. Colonoscopy in 1977. Poly-cancer controversy updated. N.Y. State J. Med. *78*:1889, 1978.
219. Kaye, G. I., et al.: Comparative electron microscopic features of normal, hyperplastic and adenomatous human colonic epithelium. Gastroenterology *64*:926, 1973.
220. Estrada, R. G., and Spjut, H. J.: Hyperplastic polyps of the large bowel. Am. J. Surg. Pathol. *4*:127, 1980.
221. Goldman, H., and Antonioli, D. A.: Mucosal biopsy of the rectum, colon, and distal ileum. Hum. Pathol. *13*:981, 1982.
222. Spjut, H. J., and Estrada, R. G.: The significance of epithelial polyps of the large bowel. Pathol. Annu. *12*(Part 1):147, 1977.
223. Helwig, E. B.: Evolution of adenomas of the large intestine and their relation to carcinoma. Surg. Gynecol. Obstet. *84*:36, 1947.
224. Fenoglio, C. M., et al.: Defining the precursor tissue of ordinary large bowel carcinoma—implications for cancer prevention. Pathol. Annu. *12* (Part 1):87, 1977.
225. Panish, J. F.: State of the art: Management of patients with polypoid lesions of the colon—current concepts and controversies. Am. J. Gastroenterol. *71*:315, 1979.
226. Muto, T., et al.: The evolution of cancer of colon and rectum. Cancer *36*:2251, 1975.
227. Coutsoftides, T., et al.: Malignant polyps of the colon and rectum. A clinicopathologic study. Dis. Colon Rectum *22*:82, 1979.
228. Gillespie, P. E., et al.: Colonic adenomas—a colonoscopy survey. Gut *20*:240, 1979.
229. Spratt, J. S., Jr., and Ackerman, L. V.: Pathologic significance of polyps of the rectum and colon. Dis. Colon Rectum *3*:330, 1960.
230. Spratt, J. S., Jr., and Watson, F. R.: The rationale of practice for polypoid lesions of the colon. Cancer *28*:153, 1971.
231. Bussey, H. J. R.: Familial Polyposis Coli: Family Studies, Histopathology, Differential Diagnosis, and Results of Treatment. Baltimore, Johns Hopkins University Press, 1975.
232. Morson, B. C.: Polyps and cancer of the large bowel. *In* Yardley, J. H., et al. (eds.): The Gastrointestinal Tract. Baltimore, Williams & Wilkins Co., 1977, p. 101.
233. Segi, M., and Kurihara, M.: Cancer mortality for selected sites in 24 countries. No. 6. Tokyo, Japan Cancer Society, 1966–67.
234. Morson, B. C.: Factors influencing the prognosis of early cancers of the rectum. Proc. R. Soc. Med. *59*:607, 1966.
235. Gilbertsen, V. A.: Proctosigmoidoscopy and polypectomy in reducing the incidence of rectal cancer. Cancer *34* (Suppl.):936, 1974.
236. Veale, A. M. O.: Intestinal Polyposis. Cambridge, Cambridge University Press, 1965.
237. McKusick, V. A.: Genetic factors in intestinal polyposis. J.A.M.A. *182*:271, 1962.
238. Dormandy, T. L.: Gastrointestinal polyposis with mucocutaneous pigmentation (Peutz-Jeghers syndrome). N. Engl. J. Med. *256*:1093, 1141, and 1186, 1957.
239. McAllister, A. J., and Richards, K. F.: Peutz-Jeghers syndrome. Experience with 20 patients in 5 generations. Am. J. Surg. *134*:717, 1977.
240. Helwig, E. B., and Hansen, J.: Lymphoid polyps (benign lymphoma) and malignant lymphoma of rectum and anus. Surg. Gynecol. Obstet. *92*:233, 1951.
241. Annual Global Data on Mortality: Mortality by cause, sex and age. World Health Statistical Reports *22*:462, 1969.
242. Walker, A. R. P., and Burkitt, D. P.: Colon cancer epidemiology. Semin. Oncol. *3*:341, 1976.
243. Lynch, H. T., et al.: Familial cancer syndromes. A survey. Cancer *39*:1867, 1977.
244. Lev, R., and Grover, R.: Precursors of human colon carcinoma: A serial section study of colectomy specimens. Cancer *47*:2007, 1981.
245. Graham, S., and Mettlin, C.: Diet and colon cancer. Am. J. Epidemiol. *109*:1, 1979.
246. Bresnick, E.: Colon carcinogenesis. An overview. Cancer *45*:1047, 1980.
247. Burkitt, D. P., et al.: Effect of dietary fibre on stools and transit-times, and its role in the causation of disease. Lancet *2*:1408, 1972.
248. Glober, G. A., et al.: Bowel transit-times in two populations experiencing similar colon-cancer risks. Lancet *2*:80, 1974.
249. Graham, S., et al.: Need to pursue new leads in the epidemiology of colorectal cancer. J. Natl. Cancer Inst. *63*:879, 1979.
250. Gilbertsen, V. A.: Adenocarcinoma of the large bowel. J.A.M.A. *174*:1789, 1960.
251. Farrands, P. A., et al.: Radioimmunodetection of human colorectal cancer by an anti-tumour monoclonal antibody. Lancet *2*:297, 1982.

252. Zamcheck, N.: The present status of CEA in diagnosis, prognosis and evaluation of therapy. Cancer *36*:2460, 1975.
253. Stearns, M. W.: Staging colonic and rectal cancer. Int. Adv. Surg. Oncol. *4*:189, 1981.
254. Wangensteen, O. H., and Dennis, T.: Experimental proof of the obstructive origin of appendicitis in man. Ann. Surg. *110*:629, 1939.
255. Sisson, R. G., et al.: Superficial mucosa ulceration and the pathogenesis of acute appendicitis. Am. J. Surg. *122*:378, 1971.
256. Thorbjarnarson, B., and Loehr, W. J.: Acute appendicitis in patients over the age of 60. Surg. Gynecol. Obstet. *125*:1277, 1967.
257. Law, D., et al.: The continuing challenge of acute and perforated appendicitis. Am. J. Surg. *131*:533, 1976.
258. Woodruff, R., and MacDonald, J. R.: Benign and malignant cystic tumors of the appendix. Surg. Gynecol. Obstet. *71*:750, 1940.
259. Higa, E., et al.: Mucosal hyperplasia, mucinous cystadenoma, and mucinous cystadenocarcinoma of the appendix. Cancer *32*:1525, 1973.
260. Shanks, H. G.: Pseudomyxoma peritonei. J. Obstet. Gynaecol. Br. Commonw. *68*:212, 1961.
261. Sandenbergh, H. A., and Woodruff, J. D.: Histogenesis of pseudomyxoma peritonei. Review of 9 cases. Obstet. Gynecol. *49*:339, 1977.

19 THE LIVER AND BILIARY TRACT

Liver

NORMAL

The liver, quite rightly, has been called "the custodian of the milieu intérieur." Hepatic disorders, therefore, have far-reaching consequences on the body's homeostasis that are best understood from the perspective of normal structure and function. Only a few salient features can be reviewed. Enclosed within a delicate, fibrous, serosa-covered Glisson's capsule, the normal adult liver weighs 1400 to 1600 gm. In the right midclavicular line its upper border is usually at the fifth intercostal space and the lower border at or close to the costal margin. Enlargement of the liver with protrusion below the costal margin is often a signal of hepatic disease. Occasionally in normal individuals, and particularly in those with some intrathoracic disorder such as pleural fluid or emphysema, the lower border of the normal liver may protrude 1 to several centimeters below the costal margin, but nonetheless the normal edge is smooth, yielding, nonpulsatile, and unmarred by nodularity.

Microscopically and functionally, the liver has been subdivided classically into roughly hexagonal *lobules*, 1 to 2 mm in diameter, oriented about a central vein (a tributary of the hepatic vein). The lobules are poorly demarcated on the periphery by portal tracts situated approximately at the angles of the hexagon. The blood supply to the liver parenchyma flows from the portal triads to the central veins; about 30 to 40% is provided by the terminal ramifications of the hepatic artery and the remainder by the portal vein radicles. On this basis it is argued that the portal triads constitute the center of the functional unit, and the central veins mark the outer boundary of what is called a *portal* lobule. More recent studies point out that the functional unit of the liver, referred to as an *acinus*, is centered about portal vein and hepatic artery *branches* that leave the portal tracts at intervals and run along the sides of the classic hexagonal lobule to serve pie-shaped segments of contiguous lobules.[1] The parenchyma of the acinus is divided into three zones, zone 1 being closest to the arterial and portal supply, zone 3 abutting the central vein, and zone 2 being intermediate. This may explain why many forms of toxic injury to the liver are most severe in the periphery of the *classical lobule* but in zone 1 are exposed to the greatest concentration of blood-borne hepatotoxins. Analogously, hypoxic injury such as occurs with shock or cardiac failure, although referred to as "central necrosis," is actually located at the periphery of the acinus in zone 3 most remote from the arterial and portal supply. Despite the many virtues of the acinus conception, the classical lobule is an "old soldier" that will not die and so persists as the standard hepatic unit.

There is little disagreement about the internal architecture of the lobule or acinus. Oversimplified for the sake of brevity, it comprises cribriform, branching, or anastomosing sheets or plates of hepatocytes. In microscopic sections the plates appear as cords of cells radially disposed about the central vein, some of which terminate at the margin of the portal triads. The line-up of hepatocytes about the portal tracts is referred to as "the limiting plate." In the normal adult in middle life, there is relatively little variation in liver cell size and structure. The great preponderance of hepatocytes have single round nuclei and are remarkably uniform in size (Fig. 19–1). Variations in nuclear size and binucleate cells are exceedingly uncommon, and mitoses are rare to absent. In later life, atrophy and dropping out of isolated cells, followed by compensatory hypertrophy and regeneration, introduces some variation in size of

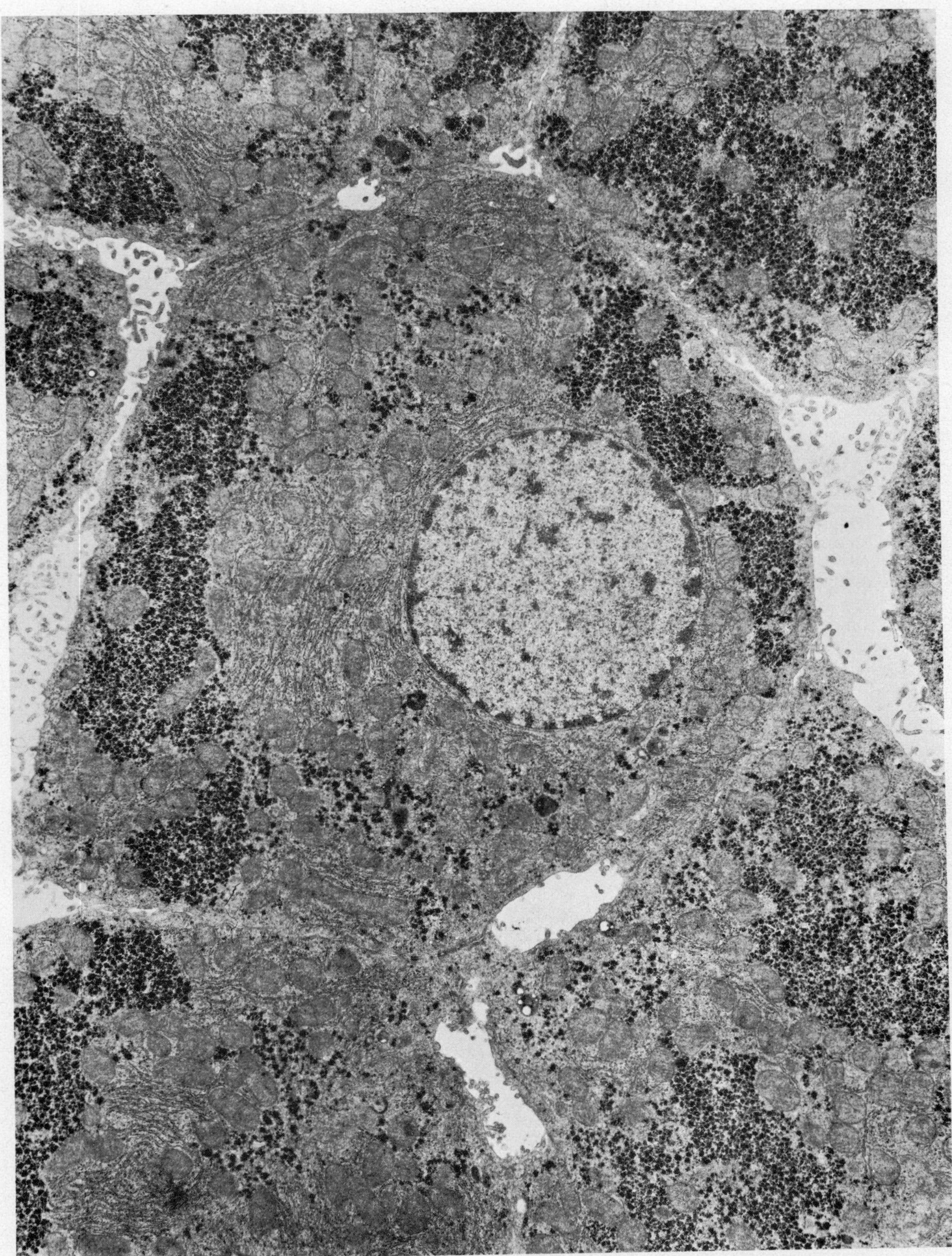

Figure 19–1. Low-power electron micrograph of normal rat liver cell. Dark granules are glycogen. The large lateral spaces are vascular sinusoids. Above and below are biliary canaliculi sandwiched between liver cells. Note microvilli in sinusoids and canaliculi. (Courtesy of Dr. H. D. Fahimi, Mallory Institute of Pathology.)

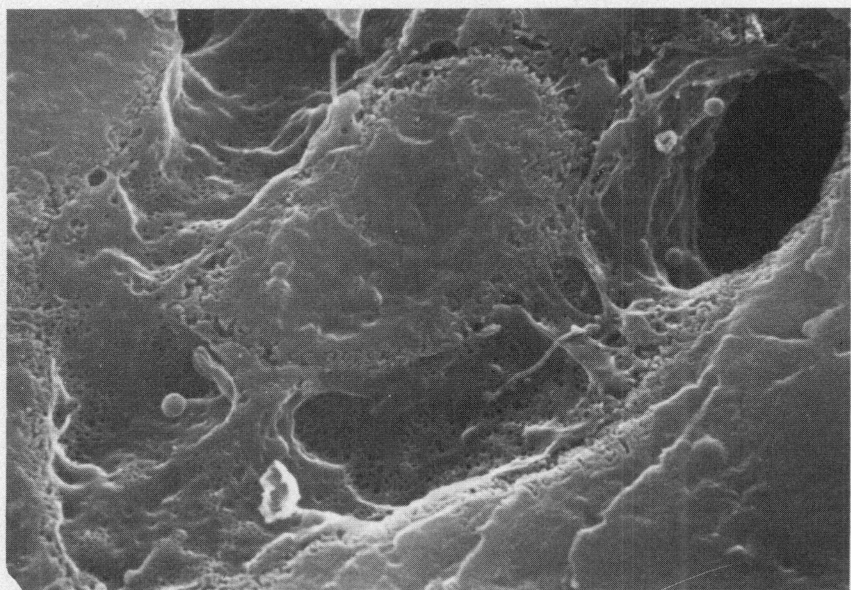

Figure 19–2. Scanning electron micrograph of mouse liver. Sinusoidal lining with typical fenestrations of endothelial cells. (Fixation by perfusion with glutaraldehyde; × 15,000.) (Courtesy of Drs. G. Stöhr and H. D. Fahimi, University of Heidelberg.)

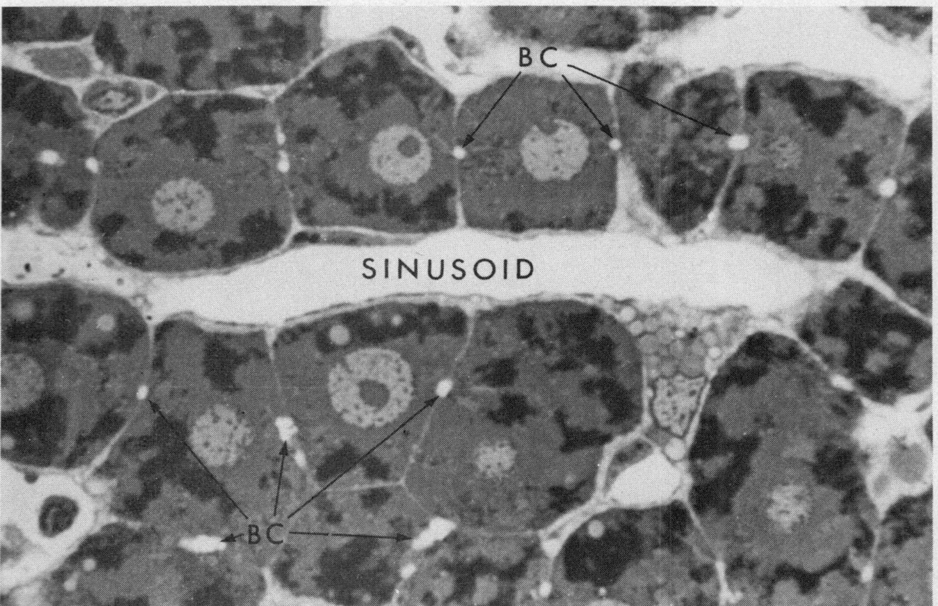

Figure 19–3. Low-power photomicrograph of liver fixed by vascular perfusion. Liver cords are oriented on both sides of vascular sinusoid. BC marks biliary canaliculi between adjacent liver cells. (Courtesy of H. D. Fahimi, M.D., University of Heidelberg. Reproduced with permission from Lab. Invest. *16*:736, 1967. Copyright 1967, The Williams and Wilkins Company, Baltimore.)

cells and nuclei and the appearance of binucleate forms, as well as rare mitotic figures. Changes such as these before later life strongly suggest previous parenchymal injury and regenerative activity. Interposed between the radial cords of hepatocytes are vascular sinusoids receiving blood from both the portal and arterial systems and draining into the central veins. The sinusoids are lined by fenestrated endothelial cells among which are scattered the Kupffer cells of the reticuloendothelial or monocyte phagocyte system. Between the sinusoids and liver cell cords are the narrow spaces of Disse into which protrude hepatocytic microvilli and in which are found scattered fat-containing lipocytes (Ito cells) of mesenchymal origin, thought to play some role in fat transport and storage of vitamin A.[2, 3] The endothelial fenestrations provide numerous interconnections between the spaces of Disse and the sinusoidal lumens (Fig. 19–2). The dual blood supply through the portal vein and hepatic artery provides a great deal of, but not total, protection against infarctions because both vascular systems, interconnected by numerous anastomoses, contribute to the sinusoidal flow. The hepatic artery, before entering the liver, gives off branches such as the right gastric and gastroduodenal arteries as well as anomalous vessels to structures in the right upper quadrant. Retrograde flow through these vessels, when the hepatic artery is accidentally or sometimes electively ligated (because of trauma to the liver), may prevent parenchymal ischemic necrosis.

The biliary system begins in the centrilobular regions as an elaborate network of canaliculi interposed between abutting hepatocytes (Fig. 19–3). These progressively join toward the periphery of the lobule, to drain eventually into the intermediate canals of Hering close to the portal tracts, which become the interlobular bile ducts within the portal triads. The interhepatocytic biliary canaliculi are channels, 1 to 2 μm in diameter, formed merely by grooves along the external surfaces of abutting liver cells. Thus, the walls of these channels are the plasma membranes of the liver cells punctuated by numerous microvilli that protrude into the lumens of the canaliculi (Fig. 19–4). Membrane-associated actin microfilaments within the hepatocytes are particularly abundant about the canalicular walls as well as in the microvilli. The microfilaments, as will be seen, are thought to play some role in transport of bile through the canaliculi.[4] It is within the canals of Hering that specialized, somewhat flattened bile duct epithelial cells first appear and become cuboidal and better defined in the ducts within the portal triads. Progressive anastomosis of the portal bile ducts gives rise to the major intrahepatic ducts and, finally, to the extrahepatic and common bile ducts.

The liver has an enormous reserve and regenerative capacity. When the remaining hepatic parenchyma is normal, patients have survived resection of about 80 to 90% of the liver. Reexploration or hepatic scan a year later has confirmed regeneration of the liver mass to approximately normal levels.[5] Among the numerous functions of the liver, only bilirubin metabolism and bile excretion will be briefly reviewed, to facilitate the understanding of hyperbilirubinemia.[6] A schema of normal bilirubin metabolism is offered in Figure 19–5. As indicated, the preponderance of bilirubin (80 to 85%) is derived from the extrahepatic breakdown of senescent red cells. About 15 to 20% comes mainly from the destruction of newly formed red cells in the bone marrow and a small fraction from the turnover, largely

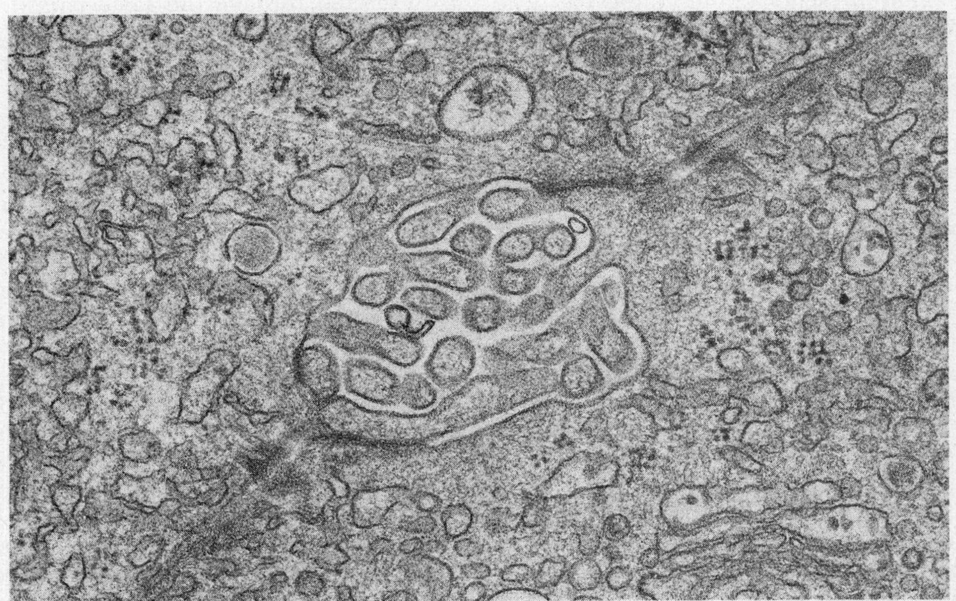

Figure 19–4. Electron micrograph of a biliary canaliculus in center field virtually filled by microvilli, many of which are cut in cross section (× 1600). (Courtesy of H. D. Fahimi, M.D. Reproduced with permission from Biol Cell. *34*:119, 1979.)

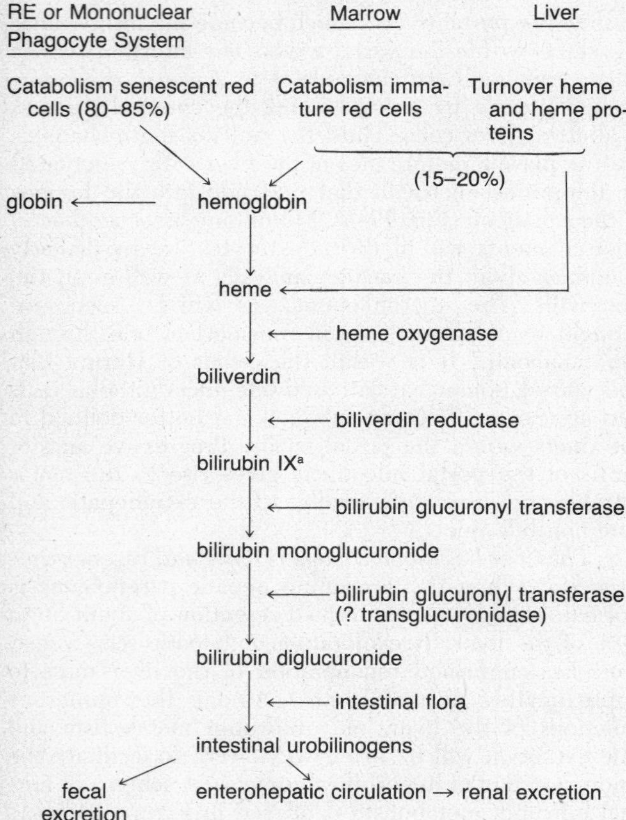

Figure 19–5. Normal bilirubin metabolism.

in the liver, of heme and heme proteins (e.g., myoglobin, cytochrome, heme-containing enzymes). These sources provide what is referred to as "early labeled bilirubin," since with isotopic studies it appears before the major fraction from senescent erythrocytes. The hemoglobin molecule is split and the heme, together with that derived from nonerythroid sources, is oxidatively cleaved within phagocytes by a microsomal heme oxygenase to yield biliverdin. The biliverdin is then converted to bilirubin IX[a] by a reductase and released into the plasma, where it is tightly bound to albumin for transport to the liver. This unconjugated bilirubin is toxic and liposoluble, but not water soluble. Because it is tightly bound to albumin, very little, if any, is excreted through the renal glomeruli. A very small fraction of unconjugated bilirubin is present in the plasma as a protein-free diffusible anion. This unbound bilirubin can cross the blood-brain barrier, more readily in the newborn than in the adult, particularly when it is rendered more permeable by systemic hypoxia that simultaneously interferes with albumin binding. Thus, when appropriate conditions prevail, as they do in hemolytic disease of the newborn and certain hereditary unconjugated hyperbilirubinemias, serious damage to the myelin-rich structures of the brain, known as kernicterus (p. 487), may be caused by the liposoluble unconjugated bilirubin. The further metabolism of unconjugated bilirubin takes place in the liver and involves three separable processes: (1) uptake by hepatocytes, (2) conjugation, and (3) secretion or excretion into bile. Most vulnerable to derangement by disease is the third.

Uptake of bilirubin by hepatocytes implies transport of the pigment from the blood across the plasma membrane of the liver cell. The precise events involved are still poorly understood. Presumably, close to or with the spaces of Disse, the albumin-unconjugated bilirubin complex is dissociated and the pigment traverses the cell membrane to be picked up by cytoplasmic proteins (ligandin and Z protein).[7] Many observations suggest that the transmembrane passage is mediated by receptors and carriers, but they have not been well characterized. Whatever the process of uptake may be, it is extremely rapid and effective, since the plasma bilirubin level is normally less than 1 mg/dl.

Conjugation is required to convert bilirubin into a water-soluble nontoxic pigment that can be secreted by the liver cell. Two steps are involved. First, utilizing glucuronic acid, a monoglucuronide is produced by bilirubin glucuronyl transferase, followed by the formation of a diglucuronide. The transferase is also involved in the formation of the diglucuronide but a plasma membrane-associated transglucuronidase may also participate. Normally, 85% of the bilirubin in bile is in the form of diglucuronide, the remainder being monoglucuronide.

Excretion or secretion of bilirubin into the bile is virtually limited to the conjugated form of the pigment. The precise details of the process are still unknown, but active secretory transport is involved and the process is saturable. *The secretion of bilirubin by the hepatocyte is the rate-limiting step in bilirubin metabolism.* With excess production of bilirubin, the secretory process may be overloaded. Other organic anions such as Bromsulphalein (BSP) and agents used for cholecystography are excreted through the same pathway, whereas bile acids pass through a totally independent pathway. When secretion is compromised, conjugated water-soluble bilirubin "regurgitates" from hepatocytes into the bloodstream, where most is loosely complexed to albumin and so is readily dissociated and filtered through the glomeruli. However, some of the conjugated bilirubin is tightly bound to albumin by covalent bonds.[7A] This so-called "third form of bilirubin" (the other two being unconjugated bilirubin and conjugated bilirubin loosely complexed to albumin) cannot pass the glomerular filter and so accounts for slow clearance of this form of conjugated hyperbilirubinemia. Because of its recent recognition, little is yet known about the full clinical or functional significance of this covalently bound bilirubin.

Conjugated bilirubin, whether loosely or tightly bound to albumin, once in the bile, passes eventually into the intestinal tract. Most is converted here into urobilinogen by the intestinal flora. A small amount of urobilinogen is excreted in the stool, but most is readily absorbed to be returned to the liver through the portal blood, only to be excreted again in the bile. During this enterohepatic circulation, a small amount is excreted through the urine.

To complete the consideration of bilirubin metabolism, bile formation and flow should be described. As formed within the liver, it is an isotonic fluid having an electrolyte composition similar to that of interstitial fluid. It contains a variety of inorganic electrolytes, mainly Na^+, Cl^-, and Ca^{++}, and organic components, principally conjugated bilirubin, bile acids (mainly cholic and chenodeoxycholic), and their salts, unesterified cholesterol and phospholipids (mainly lecithin). Cholesterol is virtually insoluble in water but is maintained in solution by incorporation into micelles with the bile acids and phospholipids. The concentration of cholesterol in the bile relative to that of the bile acids and phospholipids is critical to its solubility (detailed on p. 945). The bile acids are synthesized in the liver cell and are largely conjugated to taurine and glycine. Their transport across the hepatocytic plasma membrane is an active energy-dependent process (bile acid pump) totally independent of bilirubin transport. When the bile is excreted into the small intestine the micelles are dissociated and some of the bile acid is excreted with the intestinal contents, but most is reabsorbed, returned to the liver, and again secreted into the bile, making up a bile-acid enterohepatic circulation.

Particularly important for our later consideration of hyperbilirubinemia and jaundice are the forces that facilitate the flow of bile through the canaliculi. *Two processes appear to be involved: (1) osmotic forces and (2) mechanical forces. The osmotic force* is generated by the active pumping of two solutes into the lumen of the channel, bile acids by the so-called bile acid pump, and sodium under the influence of Na-K-ATPase (the bile acid–independent pump). Water then flows along the osmotic gradient to create a driving force. The *mechanical force* is less well defined. As you recall, microvilli and actin microfilaments are arrayed about the walls of the canaliculi. The microfilaments are thought to maintain the patency of the canaliculi and possibly to contribute contractile tone, which aids in the propulsion of the bile. In theory, then, *impaired bile flow could result from: (1) some derangement at the level of the canaliculi in bile acid transport or sodium transport or (2) alterations in the cytoskeleton of the canalicular walls or blockage of the canaliculi or ducts.* The relevance of these details of bilirubin and bile metabolism will become evident in the later consideration of the disorders that cause hyperbilirubinemia and, therefore, jaundice.

PATHOLOGY

Vulnerable to a wide variety of metabolic, circulatory, toxic, microbial, and neoplastic insults, the liver is one of the most frequently injured organs in the body. In some instances the disease is primary in the liver: for example, viral hepatitis and hepatocellular carcinoma. More often the hepatic involvement is secondary, often to some of the most common diseases of man, such as cardiac decompensation, disseminated cancer, alcoholism, and extrahepatic infections. Many liver disorders have already been discussed elsewhere and receive no further consideration here. A few examples follow for recall. Fatty change was discussed on page 18. It is a common alteration that appears with many forms of injury, notably in alcoholics. Excess accumulation of glycogen (p. 21) is seen principally in the diabetic and the glycogen storage diseases. With its rich content of Kupffer cells, the liver participates along with the remainder of the mononuclear-phagocyte system in the clearance of abnormal macromolecules circulating in the blood in a variety of inborn errors of metabolism, such as Gaucher's disease (p. 146), Niemann-Pick disease (p. 145), and the mucopolysaccharidoses (p. 150). Marked hepatic involvement is often seen with systemic amyloidoses (p. 203), sometimes with the production of striking hepatomegaly and even functional hepatic failure. Various forms of pigment may accumulate in the liver, the two most important being hemosiderin and lipofuscin. Both were described on page 23, and further details on hemosiderosis will be presented in the consideration of hemochromatosis. You may recall that the appearance of lipofuscin within cells is a marker of atrophy, and so is encountered in livers that have decreased in size and undergone what is called "brown atrophy." With these few reminders, further discussions can be limited to involvements not covered elsewhere.

Whether primary or secondary, all hepatic derangements tend to cause similar signs and symptoms; because of the liver's considerable reserve, however, manifestations appear only when the injury is significant and diffuse or strategically located so as to obstruct biliary outflow. Common presenting complaints are malaise, weakness, and loss of appetite. These nonspecific complaints are usually accompanied by clinical or laboratory evidence of deranged hepatic functions relating to synthesis of proteins and lipids, amino acid metabolism, energy generation, detoxification, and excretion of bilirubin and bile. Ultimately, hepatic failure may ensue. Because jaundice and hepatic failure are common to so many forms of liver disease, they will be discussed at the outset.

JAUNDICE

Jaundice, also called *icterus*, refers to yellow pigmentation of the skin or sclerae by bilirubin. It is particularly noticeable in the eyes because of the high scleral content of elastin, which has a special affinity for bilirubin. With deep jaundice the pigmentation may take on a green hue, since conjugated bilirubin is readily oxidized to biliverdin. *Jaundice always signifies hyperbilirubinemia*, but it does not become clinically evident until the serum bilirubin level exceeds 2 mg/dl (normal 0.5 to 1 mg). *The cause of hyperbilirubinemia can be categorized as (1) overproduction of bilirubin related to intravascular or extravascular hemolysis; (2) impaired liver cell uptake, conjugation, or secretion of bilirubin; and (3) inhibition of the outflow of bile (cholestasis).* On this basis jaundice is sometimes divided into hemolytic, hepatocellular, and cholestatic categories. The differentiation of these three categories is of major clinical importance, but first some details about cholestasis.

Cholestasis can be defined broadly as a reduction of canalicular bile flow. It is caused by a great many disorders that have in common either impairment of canalicular bile flow or obstruction of the bile ducts, usually the extrahepatic ducts. On this basis, cholestasis can be divided into extrahepatic and intrahepatic categories. Many clinicians restrict the term "cholestasis" to jaundice caused by intrahepatic disease, and refer to the extrahepatic form as "obstructive jaundice," but here the use of the term "cholestasis" embraces both categories.[8] *Extrahepatic cholestasis* may be produced in approximate order of frequency by (1) gallstones impacted within the right or left hepatic ducts, common bile duct, or ampulla of Vater; (2) carcinoma of the head of the pancreas; (3) obstructive carcinomas of the extrahepatic ducts or papilla of Vater; (4) acute and chronic pancreatitis; (5) inflammatory stenosing strictures sometimes related to previous surgery of the biliary apparatus; (6) congenital atresia of the major bile ducts; and (rarely) (7) inadvertent surgical interruption of a major extrahepatic duct. The *intrahepatic cholestatic category* must be divided into two subgroups: (a) cholestasis associated with diffuse parenchymal disease, referred to as *hepatocellular cholestasis;* and (b) cholestasis related to some disturbance in canalicular bile flow but unassociated with parenchymal disease, and thus called *"pure" cholestasis.* It will become evident that the distinction between these two subgroups can become blurred because, with persistent "pure" cholestasis, the retention of bilirubin and bile acids uncouples oxidative phosphorylation of hepatocytes and damages the P450 cytochrome enzymes, and the detergent action of the bile acids increases membrane permeability. Thus, with long-standing cholestasis, whatever its origins, parenchymal cell injury secondarily appears.[9, 10] Nonetheless, the two subsets usually can be differentiated, at least at the outset. *The major causes of hepatocellular cholestasis* are (1) some cases of viral hepatitis, often designated cholestatic or cholangiolitic viral hepatitis; (2) some cases of alcohol-induced fatty liver or hepatitis; and (3) some forms of chemical or drug-induced injury. *The subset associated with "pure" cholestasis includes* (1) "early" biliary cirrhosis; (2) fibrocystic disease of the pancreas; (3) the hereditary Dubin-Johnson and Rotor syndromes; (4) congenital atresia of the intrahepatic ducts; (5) the use of natural and synthetic sex hormones such as estrogens, oral contraceptives, and anabolic steroids such as methyltestosterone; (6) benign familial recurrent cholestasis; and (7) recurrent jaundice of pregnancy. Virtually all the extrahepatic and intrahepatic causes of cholestasis are described later. Only a few comments are required here on the last two uncommon entities.

Benign familial recurrent cholestasis is an obscure, nonprogressive form of jaundice that, as indicated, tends to run in families and usually has an early age of onset. For these reasons it is vaguely attributed to some congenital derangement in canalicular bile flow. There are no apparent histologic changes in the liver or obstructive lesions in the biliary apparatus, despite the persistence of the disease or the number of recurrences. *Recurrent jaundice of pregnancy* most often appears during the last trimester. The biochemical changes mimic those of extrahepatic obstructive disease, but they promptly clear after delivery and sometimes recur with subsequent pregnancies. The condition is thought to be related to some idiosyncrasy to increased levels of estrogens analogous to the jaundice caused in some individuals by exogenous female sex hormones.

The pathogenesis of the cholestasis with extrahepatic obstruction is obvious, but with the intrahepatic disorders it is still poorly understood. As pointed out earlier (p. 889), two mechanisms are thought to contribute to canalicular bile flow: (1) flow of water along the osmotic gradient created by the bile acid dependent– and bile acid independent–sodium "pumps" and (2) the canalicular contractile tone provided by the actin microfilaments. Without substantial proof, it is speculated that some derangement in one or both of these mechanisms produces intrahepatic cholestasis.[11] Alterations (to be described) in the pericanalicular actin microfilaments have been observed in association with cholestasis. In addition, reduced activity of membrane-associated ATPase and retention of bile acids is seen with cholestasis, and so injury to the "pumps" may also play a role.[12] Unfortunately, there is still some uncertainty about whether these changes are primary or the consequences of cholestasis.

The morphologic features of cholestasis depend somewhat on its severity, duration, and underlying cause. In general, the intrahepatic disorders tend to produce milder degrees of cholestasis than the extrahepatic disorders. **The most distinctive features of intrahepatic disorders are elongated green-brown plugs of bile in dilated canaliculi, most prominent toward the centers of the lobules, accompanied by droplets of pigment within liver cells and sometimes Kupffer cells** (Fig. 19–6). In "pure" cholestasis the liver cells at the outset appear morphologically normal by light microscopy, but ultrastructural examination reveals distortion or loss of microvilli, and an increase in number but disorganization of membrane-associated actin microfilaments in the region of the canaliculus.[4] The alterations in microvilli are thought to be secondary to the cholestasis,[12] but those of the microfilaments may be important, as has been noted. Similar changes appear in cholestasis associated with parenchymal disease, but are superimposed on those of the underlying disease. Hepatocytic swelling may contribute an obstructive element, but even with "pure" cholestasis the liver cells swell in time and undergo so-called "feathery" degeneration or necrosis. The cytoplasmic appearance is created by vacuoles containing dense lamellated membranes, probably representing liquid crystals of bile acids and phospholipids.[13] Distention of the cisternae of the Golgi complex and mitochondrial swelling and distortion are also evident with protracted cholestasis. Eventually **the canalicular bile stasis, whatever its origin, leads to**

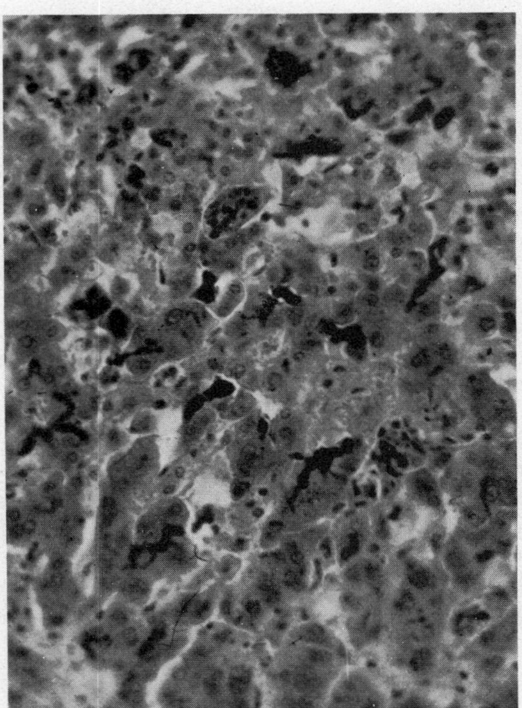

Figure 19–6. Liver-bile stasis. Bile canaliculi distended with inspissated bile. Kupffer cells contain phagocytized bile.

proliferation of intralobular ductules and portal tract bile ducts, sometimes accompanied by mild periportal fibrosis, mimicking biliary cirrhosis (p. 928).

In contrast to the intrahepatic cholestatic syndromes, **extrahepatic obstructions induce a pattern of cholestasis that begins with distention of the extrahepatic biliary apparatus by bile, with progressive retrograde extension of the bile stasis into the intrahepatic duct system.** The bile stasis in the duct radicles within the portal triads leads to proliferation of the epithelial lining cells, sometimes accompanied by an increase in surrounding fibrous tissue. Eventually the canaliculi become distended with bile, and pigment can be seen within liver cells and Kupffer cells, recapitulating the changes of intrahepatic cholestasis. **The most helpful differential feature of extrahepatic obstruction is rupture of canaliculi with extravasation of bile, producing so-called "bile lakes" surrounded by injured or necrotic liver cells.** Because stasis of bile predisposes to ascending bacterial infections, extrahepatic cholestasis may be complicated by ascending cholangitis and cholangiolitis marked by intraductal and intraductular accumulations of neutrophils.

Whatever the underlying disorder, cholestasis itself is regularly associated with distinctive clinical changes. Not only is there conjugated hyperbilirubinemia and jaundice but, even more characteristic, elevation of the serum level of bile acids, which produces one of the most distressing features of cholestasis—itching (pruritus). Often the rise in serum bile acids and the pruritus precede the appearance of jaundice. When the cholestasis is prolonged, most of the conjugated bilirubin becomes tightly bound to albumin by covalent bonds (the "third form of bilirubin") and so accounts for persistence of the jaundice long after bilirubinuria ceases.[13A] Hyperlipidemia also appears related, for poorly understood reasons, to impaired excretion of cholesterol into the bile, sometimes with formation of skin xanthomas. There is also increased synthesis of cholesterol by liver cells.[14] Another characteristic finding is an elevated serum level of alkaline phosphatases. This group of enzymes is normally present in many tissues including liver, bile ducts, bone, placenta, intestine, kidney, and leukocytes. Elevated serum levels of alkaline phosphatase are therefore encountered in a variety of conditions in addition to hepatobiliary cholestatic disease, including skeletal disorders associated with new bone formation, active normal growth, pregnancy, and certain cancers that elaborate the Regan isoenzyme (an alkaline phosphatase). The various isoenzymes can be segregated by electrophoretic analysis. The increased phosphatase levels found with cholestasis reflect increased enzyme synthesis rather than decreased biliary excretion, and are a more sensitive marker of cholestasis than hyperbilirubinemia, often preceding it. Many other changes may accompany the reduced bile flow into the intestines, including malabsorption of fat and fat-soluble vitamins, and so steatorrhea and manifestations related to a deficiency of vitamins A, D, or K sometimes develop, principally hypoprothrombinemia (vitamin K deficiency). *Thus come about the major clinical markers of cholestasis: conjugated hyperbilirubinemia, elevated levels of serum bile acids and alkaline phosphatase, hyperlipidemia, and hypoprothrombinemia with a consequent bleeding diathesis.*

With this overview of cholestasis, it is now possible to classify jaundice based on pathophysiologic mechanisms (Table 19–1). It is of great clinical importance to differentiate unconjugated from conjugated hyperbilirubinemia and, further, to identify the particular cause of the conjugated hyperbilirubinemia. Unconjugated hyperbilirubinemia is said to be present when 80 to 85% of the total serum bilirubin is unconjugated. The van den Bergh reaction can be used to differentiate these two types of hyperbilirubinemia. When the test is carried out in an aqueous medium, the water-soluble conjugated bilirubin reacts to give the so-called "direct" fraction. When carried out in methanol, both conjugated and unconjugated pigments react, giving the total bilirubin level. The difference between the total and direct levels represents the "indirect" or unconjugated fraction. A simple, valuable clinical marker of unconjugated hyperbilirubinemia is the absence of bilirubin from the urine, since the unconjugated pigment is tightly bound to albumin and is not filtered through the renal glomeruli. In contrast, conjugated bilirubin is water soluble, is less avidly bound to albumin, and therefore is filtered, producing a brown-green darkening of the urine. *The hemolytic anemias are the major causes of unconjugated hyperbilirubinemia*, but you will also note from Table 19–1 that there are other causes that usually produce only very mild jaundice: resorption of extravascular blood from infarcts, hematomas, gastrointestinal bleed-

Table 19–1. PATHOPHYSIOLOGIC CLASSIFICATION OF JAUNDICE*

I Predominantly Unconjugated Hyperbilirubinemia
- A. Overproduction
  - Intravascular hemolysis
    - Hemolytic anemias
  - Extravascular hemolysis
    - Resorption of blood from large hemorrhagic (e.g., pulmonary) infarcts, large hematomas, gastrointestinal bleeding
- B. Decreased hepatic uptake
  - Prolonged severe fasting
  - Sepsis
- C. Impaired bilirubin conjugation (decreased glucuronyl transferase activity)
  - Gilbert's syndrome
  - Crigler-Najjar syndrome
  - Jaundice in newborn
  - Diffuse advanced hepatocellular disease (e.g., hepatitis, cirrhosis)

II Predominantly Conjugated Hyperbilirubinemia
- A. Impaired hepatocellular secretion of bilirubin
  - Dubin-Johnson syndrome
  - Rotor's syndrome
- B. Cholestatic
  - Intrahepatic disorders
    - "Pure" cholestasis
      - Drug-induced (e.g., methyltestosterone, estrogens, oral contraceptives)
      - Recurrent jaundice of pregnancy
      - Recurrent familial jaundice
      - Early primary biliary cirrhosis
    - Cholestasis associated with hepatocellular injury
      - Viral hepatitis
      - Alcohol-induced injury
      - Drug toxicity or sensitivity
  - Extrahepatic lesions
    - Obstructive lesions of major excretory bile ducts
      - Gallstones
      - Carcinomas of common bile duct, ampulla of Vater, and head of pancreas
      - Inflammatory strictures of bile ducts
      - Atresia of bile ducts

*The disorders cited are illustrative and not a complete listing.

ing, and several hereditary conditions (the Gilbert and Crigler-Najjar syndromes). In addition, severe diffuse hepatocellular disease may so impair conjugating capacity as to cause a mixed conjugated and unconjugated hyperbilirubinemia.

It is much more difficult to identify the cause of conjugated hyperbilirubinemia. It is said to be present when more than 50% of the serum bilirubin is in the conjugated form. In particular, the differentiation of intrahepatic (so-called "medical") jaundice from that due to extrahepatic lesions (often referred to as "surgical" or sometimes "obstructive" jaundice) can be critical. Extrahepatic obstructive jaundice often can be surgically cured, particularly since it is most often produced by impaction of a gallstone in the common bile duct or ampulla of Vater. In contrast, intrahepatic "medical" jaundice cannot be benefited by surgery, and indeed the patient's condition may be worsened by operation. It is beyond our scope to delve into this difficult diagnostic problem except to point out that the level of elevation of the serum alkaline phosphatase may be helpful since extrahepatic obstruction induces, in general, higher rises than intrahepatic disease. The same can be said of serum bile acids. Abnormal liver function tests (some of which will be described in the consideration of hepatic failure), in contrast, point to "medical" jaundice. Unfortunately, long-standing cholestasis, whatever its origin, causes hepatocellular injury; thus, extrahepatic lesions, unless identified early, may also become associated with some parenchymal dysfunction with elevated serum levels of both unconjugated and conjugated bilirubin. The problem is further compounded because, with hepatocellular dysfunction, the glucuronyl transferase conjugating capacity decreases, favoring unconjugated hyperbilirubinemia. Thus, in many instances, laboratory tests alone do not permit a secure differentiation. Even such diagnostic adjuncts as cholecystography, cholangiography, ultrasonography, CT scan, and others do not yield a clear diagnosis, and so needle liver biopsy is performed in pursuit of a morphologic diagnosis. Ultimately, laparotomy may be required in the search for a surgically remediable lesion.

HEPATIC FAILURE

Like a sandcastle on the shore, the liver's functional capacity may crumble grain by grain as it dries, be more rapidly undermined by the oncoming tide, or be suddenly obliterated by a massive wave. Before we present some of the disorders that may lead to such liver damage, the clinical features of hepatic failure and its pathophysiology should be discussed. Hepatic failure has many dimensions because of the liver's varied functions, but certain signs, symptoms, and biochemical changes are fairly constant. *Jaundice is almost invariably present,* mainly related to conjugated hyperbilirubinemia, but, as described above, unconjugated hyperbilirubinemia may also contribute. There is often evidence of impairment of the liver's synthetic functions, leading sometimes to *hypoalbuminemia,* but it is not specific for hepatic failure since it may have other origins such as protein-losing glomerulopathies or enteropathies. Occasionally with liver failure there is, for poorly understood reasons, increased globulin synthesis, particularly with certain forms of liver injury, such as cirrhosis, which together with the hypoalbuminemia may produce reversal of the albumin-globulin ratio. Fibrinogen, prothrombin, and clotting factors V, VII, and X are synthesized in the liver, and so *bleeding tendencies may appear with hepatic failure.* Particularly vulnerable to liver injury is the synthesis of prothrombin, sometimes aggravated by a deficiency of vitamin K related to fat malabsorption. Thus, prolongation of the prothrombin time (PT) and partial thromboplastin time (PTT) are sensitive indices of impaired hepatic synthetic activity. *Leakage of cytoplasmic enzymes into the blood occurs with all forms of hepatocellular injury.* Although the serum levels of a variety of enzymes may be increased, including the relatively nonspecific lactic dehydrogenase

(LDH), the two most commonly evaluated are alanine aminotransferase (glutamic pyruvic transaminase—GPT) and aspartate aminotransferase (glutamic oxalacetic transaminase—GOT). GOT is also abundant in myocardium and skeletal muscle, and so diseases of these organs and tissues must be taken into consideration in the evaluation of elevated serum levels; GPT is much more specific for hepatobiliary disease. Several cautions must be noted about the interpretation of the serum levels of these enzymes. The level of rise is not linearly correlated with the severity of liver injury, but nonetheless a marked elevation generally means severe parenchymal damage. However, the levels may drop to normal or near normal if the evaluation is delayed for a few days after an episode of sudden massive hepatic necrosis. Moreover, sudden complete extrahepatic biliary obstruction also raises the serum level of these enzymes even before significant parenchymal damage develops. Serum transaminase levels must then be interpreted with caution.

A variety of clinical manifestations may appear, some more regularly than others. *Fetor hepaticus*, a rather characteristic musty odor of the breath and urine, is frequently noted with both acute and chronic hepatic failure. It is thought to be related to the production of mercaptans from methionine by the action of the gastrointestinal flora. With chronic liver failure, particularly that associated with cirrhosis of the liver, impaired degradation of estrogens may induce *gynecomastia* and *testicular atrophy*. *Palmar erythema* secondary to vasodilation of the dermal vessels and *"spider" angiomas of the skin* have also been attributed to hyperestrinism.

Decreased renal function is a relatively infrequent accompaniment of hepatic failure that may arise in a variety of circumstances. Hepatic and renal failure may be the consequence of toxic damage to both organs by drugs or chemicals such as carbon tetrachloride. Immune complex glomerulopathies (p. 1005) may appear in patients with hepatitis. Acute tubular necrosis may follow a massive gastrointestinal bleed and hypotensive crisis in patients with advanced cirrhosis. Disseminated intravascular coagulation (DIC) sometimes complicates hepatic failure and causes renal insufficiency. *In some instances the renal failure is caused by the hepatorenal syndrome*. Unfortunately, a great deal of confusion surrounds the use of this term, and so an attempt will be made to qualify it carefully.

There is a growing consensus that the hepatorenal syndrome should be restricted to patients with severe liver disease (most often advanced cirrhosis), and functional renal failure in the absence of morphologically overt renal damage. Preservation of structure is attested to by the normal function of the kidneys when they are used for transplantation[15] and the reversibility of renal failure following transplantation of a new liver into the patient.[16] Characteristic is azotemia and severe oliguria (urine output falls to 200 to 400 mg per day) with hyperosmolarity of the urine despite a low sodium output.[17] Specifically excluded from this conception of the hepatorenal syndrome are the various forms of renal damage previously mentioned. The interpretation of renal failure in patients undergoing surgery for biliary tract obstruction is more difficult. In some of these instances the renal insufficiency can be reasonably related to blood loss or hypotension incident to the surgery, thus casting it into the category of prerenal azotemia or acute tubular necrosis. Occasionally, however, no such well-defined precipitating factors can be identified, and so biliary tract obstruction with marked jaundice and renal insufficiency is still included within the limits of the hepatorenal syndrome.[18] Despite all these qualifications, the *term "hepatorenal syndrome" is still variously employed, but as used here it implies a renal functional derangement without anatomic changes except possibly for bile staining of tubular epithelial cells and bile-proteinaceous casts in the renal medulla.*

The pathogenesis of the hepatorenal syndrome is a mystery. It is known that there is reduction of renal blood flow due to generalized renal vasoconstriction that is more marked in the cortex than in the medulla.[19] However, the uncertainty as to the cause of the vasoconstriction is attested to by the numerous explanatory hypotheses. A deficiency of vasodilators such as prostacyclin or bradykinin has been proposed, but without convincing proof. A decrease in renal perfusion secondary to some reduction in "effective circulating volume" related to the large accumulations of ascitic fluid (when cirrhosis is present) would be followed by compensatory renal vasoconstriction. However, clinical and experimental studies have failed to confirm this mechanism even in cirrhotics, and, moreover, noncirrhotic settings do exist with the hepatorenal syndrome.[20, 21] Failure of the damaged liver to filter gut-derived endotoxins (potent vasoconstrictors) is an attractive theory that has been neither substantiated nor excluded.[22] Thus, the hepatorenal syndrome is as much a pathogenetic puzzle as it is a conceptual tangle.

Hepatic encephalopathy, also called *hepatic coma*, is another feared feature of acute and chronic liver failure, discussed on page 1422.[23] It may also appear with portosystemic shunting, and so is also referred to as *portal-systemic encephalopathy*. It is a metabolic disorder of the central nervous system with nonspecific electroencephalographic changes characterized by disturbed consciousness, drowsiness, fluctuating neurologic signs, and a distinctive "flapping tremor" known as asterixis that progresses finally to coma and often to death. Particularly characteristic is the *asterixis*, a series of nonrhythmic, rapid extension-flexion movements of the head and extremities best brought out when the arms are held in extension with dorsiflexed wrists. The genesis of the CNS manifestations is still uncertain but, whatever the causative agent, there is circumstantial evidence that it is produced in the intestines and probably derived from protein metabolism. Consistent with these beliefs is the development of the encephalopathy with portosystemic shunting, whether spontaneous in advanced cirrhosis or surgical (portacaval anastomosis), bypassing hepatic metabolism of putative toxins. In addition, a high protein intake worsens the encephalopathy and, conversely, a low protein diet is often beneficial. Analogously, gastrointestinal bleeding with resorption of the blood products may precipitate the syndrome. Antibiotics to reduce the intestinal flora are effective in treatment. Thus, the evidence points to a gut-derived protein metabolite.[24] *Ammonia has received a great deal of attention as the toxic agent.* In the normal liver ammonia is degraded to urea, but in patients with hepatic encephalopathy, high levels have been found in the blood and cerebrospinal fluid.[23] At the cell level, ammonia interferes with the transfer of NADH from cytoplasm to mitochondria, resulting in decreased production of ATP. However, hyperammonemia is not invariably present, and therefore other potential toxins have been proposed. The administration of methionine to patients and experimental animals with portosystemic shunts induces CNS changes that mimic hepatic encephalopathy. Thus, it is possible that mercaptans produced in the gut by bacterial action on sulfur-containing amino acids not only may result in *fetor hepaticus,* but also may contribute to the encephalopathy. A variety of other compounds including short-chain fatty acids, false neurotransmitters, and branched-chain amino acids have been implicated by one or another investigator.[25, 26] To date, there is no convincing evidence to indict any one of these toxins as the basic cause of the syndrome. Conceivably, several may act in concert, or each may be capable of inducing the neurologic syndrome in individual patients. Morphologic abnormalities may appear in the brain and are described on page 1422.

With this overview of the features of hepatic failure, we can turn to its clinical settings. *Only conditions that diffusely involve all or the largest part of the liver are likely to cause liver failure.* Thus, liver abscesses, metastases, and traumatic lesions (unless massive) infrequently destroy sufficient parenchyma to deplete the reserve. *The common disorders in North America and Europe leading to liver failure can be divided into three categories: (1) chronic progressive liver cell destruction, (2) ultrastructural lesions unassociated with overt liver cell necrosis, and (3) sudden massive necrotizing lesions (massive necrosis).*[27]

The two most common conditions in the United States causing slow progressive liver cell destruction are alcoholic cirrhosis and chronic active hepatitis. Alcohol-induced liver injury is much the more frequent, progressively depleting the liver reserve over the span of years (p. 917). Not infrequently superimposed on this chronic course are waves of acute destruction. Chronic active hepatitis, on the other hand, may lead to failure more rapidly in a few years or less. Intercurrent complications (to be described) may drastically worsen the picture.

Disorders capable of causing functional insufficiency in the absence of significant overt liver cell necrosis include Reye's syndrome in children, acute fatty liver of pregnancy, tetracycline toxicity, and (rarely) the massive fatty liver in chronic alcoholism.

Although many potential causes of *massive necrosis of the liver* will be cited later (p. 923), the great preponderance of cases are related to overwhelming viral hepatitis and toxic drug injury as by halothane. The liver functional insufficiency may appear within days of the acute assault and may occur despite the lack of preexisting liver damage.

A variety of forms of stress may precipitate the onset of failure, whatever the basic hepatic disorder. *Gastrointestinal bleeding* is particularly common in patients with cirrhosis of the liver because esophageal varices are prone to occur secondary to the portal hypertension. In addition, alcoholics have an increased incidence of peptic ulcer and acute gastritis. The bleeding may precipitate a hypotensive crisis and add an element of hypoxic injury to the underlying liver damage. Moreover, resorption of nitrogenous breakdown products of the blood may contribute to the encephalopathy. *Acute infections* through uncertain pathways are important precipitating factors. *Electrolyte disturbances,* particularly hypokalemic alkalosis caused by excessive vomiting or diuresis, may initiate the onset of hepatic encephalopathy. Indeed, *any form of severe stress,* such as major surgery, heart failure, and shock, may serve as the final straw when the hepatic functional reserve is already precarious. Unfortunately, there is no satisfactory treatment for hepatic failure and when it appears it is usually fatal.

HEREDITARY HYPERBILIRUBINEMIAS

A small group of familial disorders is characterized by jaundice, ranging from mild to severe, caused by specific hepatocellular defects in the metabolism of bilirubin. They extend in clinical significance from the common and fortunately trivial Gilbert's syndrome to the rare and uniformly fatal Type I Crigler-Najjar syndrome. All the hereditary hyperbilirubinemias are of interest on two scores: (1) they are experiments of nature that have helped dissect the process of normal bilirubin metabolism; and (2) they may mimic (some more than others) acquired hepatobiliary disease, and so must be taken into account in the differential diagnosis of jaundice. The salient features of the various syndromes are listed in Table 19–2, and thus only a few additional comments are necessary.

GILBERT'S SYNDROME

Also known as *constitutional hepatic dysfunction* and *asymptomatic familial unconjugated hyperbilirubinemia,* this benign, presumably autosomal dominant syndrome may represent a constellation of derangements associated with mild jaundice. Most commonly there is a defect in hepatocytic uptake of unconjugated bilirubin. However, in another subset there appears to be some deficiency in glucuronyl transferase, manifested mainly by decreased conversion of the monoglucuronide to the diglucuronide.[28] Almost half of the patients also

Table 19–2. THE HEREDITARY HYPERBILIRUBINEMIAS

	Unconjugated Hyperbilirubinemia			Conjugated Hyperbilirubinemia	
		Crigler-Najjar Syndrome (Congenital Nonhemolytic Jaundice)			
	Gilbert's Syndrome	***Type I***	***Type II***	***Dubin-Johnson Syndrome***	***Rotor's Syndrome***
Identified defects in bilirubin metabolism	(a) Decreased hepatic uptake (b) Decreased glucuronyl transferase activity	Absent glucuronyl transferase activity	Variably decreased or absent glucuronyl transferase activity	Impaired biliary excretion	Impaired biliary excretion
Plasma bilirubin concentration (mg/dl)	Total: ≤ 3 in absence of hemolysis or fasting Conjugated: ≤ 0.4	Total: 17–50 (usually >20) Conjugated: 0	Total: 6–45 (usually <20) Conjugated: 0–2	Total: 1–25 (usually <7) Conjugated: averages 60% of total	Total: 1–20 (usually <7) Conjugated: averages 60% of total
Bile pigment	Diglucuronide decreased and monoglucuronide increased compared with normal	Small amount of unconjugated bilirubin: trace monoconjugates	Predominantly monoglucuronide	Not studied	Not studied
Incidence	$\leq 7\%$ of population	Rare	Uncommon	Rare, up to 1:1300 in Iranian Jews	Rare
Inheritance	? Autosomal dominant	Autosomal recessive	? Autosomal dominant with variable penetrance	Autosomal recessive	Autosomal recessive
Age when hyperbilirubinemia recognized	Variable, usually by early adulthood (often during fasting)	1–3 days after birth	Usually during first year of life, occasionally later	Variable (birth to age 70), usually by early adulthood	Variable, usually in childhood
Physical findings	Occasional scleral icterus	Jaundice, findings of kernicterus in infants: seizures, myoclonus, athetosis, incoordination, retardation in young adults	Jaundice, findings of kernicterus only rarely present	Jaundice, occasional hepatomegaly	Jaundice
Routine liver tests	Normal	Normal	Normal	Usually normal, minor abnormalities reported	Usually normal
Liver — Macroscopic	Normal	Normal	Normal	Black	Normal
Liver — Microscopic	Normal, lipofuscin may be increased	Normal	Normal	Coarse dark pigment in centrilobular cells	Normal
Prognosis	Normal	Usually death in infancy: rarely, later onset of neurologic damage	Usually normal; kernicterus occurs only rarely	Probably good	Probably good

Modified from Scharsschmidt, B. F., and Gallan, J. L.: Current concepts of bilirubin metabolism and hereditary hyperbilirubinemia. Prog. Liver Dis. 6:187, 1979.

have mildly increased hemolysis stressing the metabolic dysfunction of the liver cell.[29] Because of this heterogeneity it has been suggested that Gilbert's syndrome is not a disease, but rather one end of the spectrum of the population having one or another mild impairment in bilirubin metabolism.[30] As noted, the major importance of this completely benign condition lies in the physician's awareness of its existence, so that more serious hepatobiliary disease is not diagnosed in error. There are no anatomic alterations in the liver save possibly for an increase of lipofuscin in centrilobular cells, and the individual is "more yellow than sick."

CRIGLER-NAJJAR SYNDROMES

The two variants of the Crigler-Najjar syndrome appear to be distinctive disorders rather than variable severities of a single condition. Affected families have one or the other variant, but not both. *Type I, with its complete or near-complete lack of glucuronyl transferase, is lethal usually in infancy* owing to the extensive brain damage (kernicterus, p. 487) caused by the severe unconjugated hyperbilirubinemia. It is an autosomal recessive disorder manifested by homozygotes, usually the product of consanguineous marriage. Because there is little or no conjugation, the hyperbilirubinemia is almost entirely due to unconjugated bilirubin. Only trace amounts of conjugated bilirubin, largely monoglucuronides, are secreted in the bile, and so it is virtually colorless. The only inconstant morphologic change in the liver is canalicular cholestasis.

The *Type II variant* appears to follow autosomal dominant transmission with variable penetrance.[31] A generally mild deficiency in hepatic glucuronyl transferase activity has been identified that varies in severity from one to another patient, and so there is some production of monoglucuronide. The unconjugated hyperbilirubinemia is generally mild, and thus kernicterus appears only rarely. Indeed, with milder deficiencies of the transferase, the longevity may be normal. Rarely, however, there is a greater deficiency of transferase and a commensurately more marked hyperbilirubinemia. Although there are many similarities between the milder expressions of Type II Crigler-Najjar syndrome and the subset of Gilbert's syndrome, having a lack of glucuronyl transferase, there is greater production of monoglucuronide in the Type II Crigler-Najjar disorder.[32] In passing, it might be noted that the Gunn rat, also deficient in glucuronyl transferase, constitutes an excellent animal model of the Type I disease. It, too, develops marked unconjugated hyperbilirubinemia and an encephalopathy very similar to the kernicterus seen in humans.

DUBIN-JOHNSON AND ROTOR'S SYNDROMES

These two heritable syndromes are both characterized by a defect in the secretion or excretion of bilirubin by the liver cell. There is no derangement in uptake or

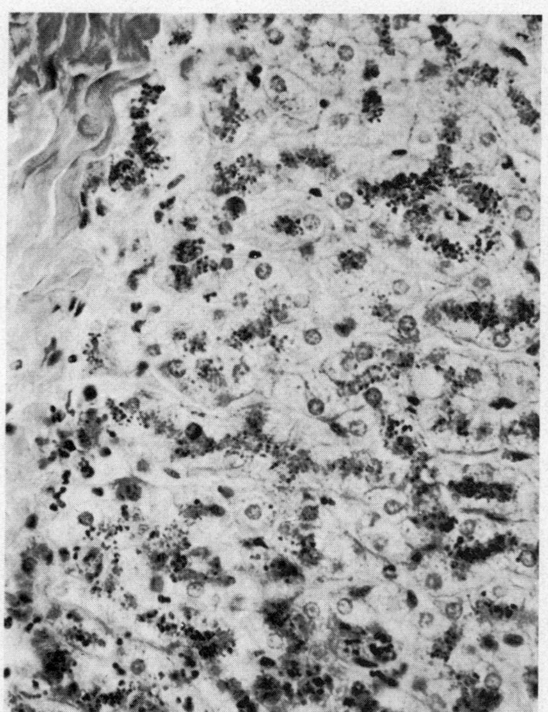

Figure 19–7. Dubin-Johnson disease, showing fine dustlike pigmentation of liver cells.

in conjugation, and thus a conjugated hyperbilirubinemia results. Concomitantly there is an inability to excrete other organic anions using the same secretory pathway, and so there is impaired excretion of BSP by the liver as well as oral dyes used in cholecystography, more complete in the Dubin-Johnson syndrome than in Rotor's.[33] The major difference between the two conditions is found in the hepatic morphology. *In the Dubin-Johnson syndrome the liver is macroscopically dark-brown to black, caused by a cytoplasmic accumulation of pigment* mainly within lysosomes (Fig. 19–7).[34] The nature of the pigment is not known; both lipofuscin and melanin have been suggested as possibilities, but the results of histochemical studies argue against melanin[35] and the evidence for lipofuscin is also shaky. However, a deficiency of superoxide dismutase has been observed in a few patients, providing a plausible basis for peroxidation of membrane lipids and the formation of lipofuscin residual bodies.[36] Apart from the pigmentation, the liver is morphologically normal and free of cholestasis because biliary flow is normal. *In Rotor's syndrome, on the other hand, there is no hepatic pigmentation* despite the similarity of the bilirubin excretory defect in the two syndromes. Corriedale sheep provide an almost identical animal model of the Dubin-Johnson syndrome, complete with the brown-black pigmentation of the liver.

CIRCULATORY DISORDERS

Disturbances in the vascular supply or venous drainage of the liver are extremely common findings at autopsy, but they are only infrequently productive of clinically significant liver dysfunction. The resultant hepatic changes range from the commonplace and usually trivial congestion incident to cardiac decompensation to the rare and frequently fatal hepatic vein thrombosis.

ACUTE AND CHRONIC PASSIVE CONGESTION (CPC) AND CENTRAL HEMORRHAGIC NECROSIS (CHN) OF LIVER

These hepatic alterations are considered together because they represent essentially a morphologic continuum.

Chronic passive congestion of the liver develops with cardiac decompensation, particularly right-sided failure (p. 550). It is more commonly present than absent in every postmortem examination, since with virtually every death there is an element of preterminal circulatory failure. Involved in its production are congestion of the central veins and centrilobular hepatic sinusoids accompanied by hypoxia incident to the stasis and reduction of arterial flow from the cardiac failure. However, the congestion falls short of rupturing centrilobular hepatic sinusoids, and the hypoxia falls short of causing overt necrosis of liver cells (typical of CHN).

The morphologic changes are dependent on the suddenness of onset of the congestion and its severity. With **acutely developing congestion** the liver is slightly enlarged, somewhat tense, and cyanotic with rounded edges. On transection blood freely exudes, relieving somewhat the purple-red centrilobular congestion that contrasts with the peripheral, more normal color of the liver lobules. With **CPC** slight liver enlargement may or may not be present, but it is less tense than in the acute disease. Here the centrilobular congestion is often surrounded by yellow-brown parenchyma because of the accumulation of microvacuolar fat in the surrounding hypoxic hepatocytes. Histologically, the central veins are prominent, somewhat distended, and associated with distended centrilobular sinusoids. Often, there is some atrophy of the hepatocytes due to compression and hypoxia. Minimal extrasinusoidal hemorrhages may be present but there is no significant necrosis of the adjacent liver cells. With more **severe CPC** the transection takes on the appearance of the cut surface of a nutmeg, hence the frequently used term **nutmeg liver** (Fig. 19–8). The centrilobular congestion now appears more irregular and sometimes stellate in shape, outlined by a racemose (cluster of grapes) pattern of pale, distinctly fatty parenchyma. Liver cell atrophy and extrasinusoidal microhemorrhages are somewhat more prominent.

Congestion, acute or chronic, rarely produces more than minimal hepatomegaly, but the lower edge of the liver may become palpable and sometimes pulsatile, with tricuspid incompetence. Often it is tender to palpation owing to distention of Glisson's capsule. Usually, congestive changes alone do not produce jaundice or clinically significant hepatic dysfunction, but intercurrent stress such as blood loss, systemic infections, or shock with hypoperfusion may tip the balance.

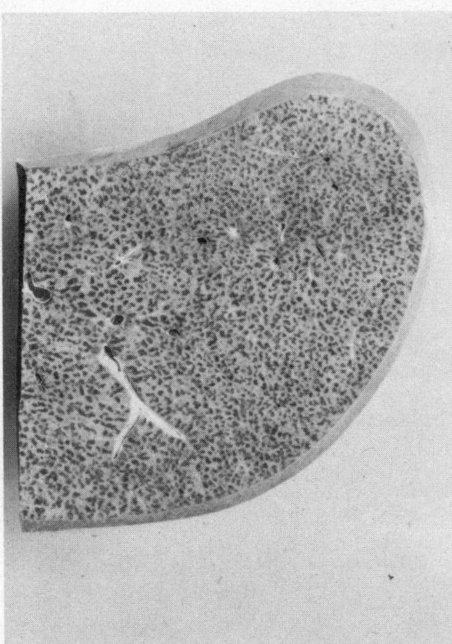

Figure 19–8. Cross section of liver with chronic passive congestion. Congestive bridges give nutmeg pattern.

Central hemorrhagic necrosis seen with more severe cardiac failure is essentially an extension of CPC of the liver. Although marked congestion may play a contributory causal role, studies implicate hypoxia secondary to arterial hypoperfusion as the main factor.[37] Thus, hepatic CHN may also be encountered with shock and even lesser degrees of systemic vascular collapse. Because hypoperfusion alone may induce the hepatic changes in the absence of venous congestion, some investigators prefer the designation *centrilobular necrosis*.

Grossly, the liver may not be distinguishable from that in marked CPC, but occasionally it is slightly reduced in size and may have a granularity to the surface best seen on reflected light owing to depression of the necrotic lobular centers. On transection the nutmeg appearance is accentuated, as are the subtle depressions of the centrilobular regions. **The distinctive features that differentiate CHN from CPC microscopically are (1) marked centrilobular sinusoidal dilatation with hemorrhages into the hepatic cords and (2) atrophy and overt necrosis of scattered hepatocytes about the central vein. In severe expressions, virtually all cells within the centers of the lobules are necrotic** (Fig. 19–9). Occasionally, bands of necrosis in adjacent lobules may interconnect or "bridge."[38] Neutrophilic infiltration may be evident in the periphery of the areas of necrosis, but it is usually scant and sometimes completely absent. When it is preceded by CPC there may be fatty change of the surviving liver cells at the periphery.

CHN is more likely to appear with marked right-sided failure, but may be caused by left-sided failure, shock, or any other basis for systemic hypoperfusion. Infrequently it is associated with hepatic vein thrombosis or any condition that severely impedes the venous

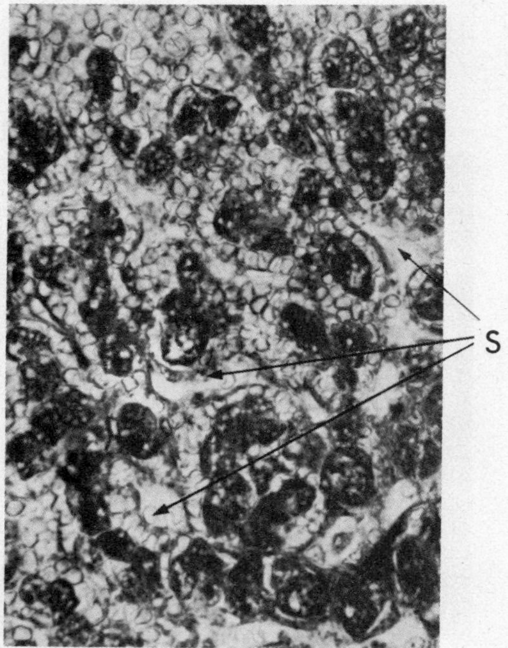

Figure 19–9. Central necrosis of liver. Microscopic detail revealing dark, shrunken hepatocytes in center of lobules and numerous red cells lying outside of sinusoids. S points to sinusoids.

return to the heart, such as constrictive pericarditis or cardiac tamponade. The parenchymal damage may be sufficient to induce elevated serum transaminases, mild-to-moderate jaundice, and other manifestations of hepatic insufficiency.

CARDIAC SCLEROSIS

This uncommon complication of severe cardiac failure basically represents the fibrosing reaction that follows long-standing severe CPC and/or centrilobular necrosis. Presumably the protracted central hypoxia prevents hepatocellular regeneration resulting in scarring. Sometimes this condition has been called *cardiac cirrhosis* but, as will be evident (p. 915), the pattern of liver fibrosis and damage rarely fulfills the accepted criteria for the diagnosis of cirrhosis.

The scarring of cardiac sclerosis is delicate, subtle, and easily missed on both gross and microscopic examination. Typically, the liver is slightly reduced in size and has a fine pigskin grain on its external surface. On transection there is a subtle depression of the centers of the lobules, creating a resemblance to CHN, but the congestive features are less prominent. There is often some increased resistance to finger-fracture of the hepatic substance. Microscopically, there is a subtle increase in fibrous tissue about the central veins from which delicate strands fan out into the surrounding liver substance. The fibrosis is often sufficiently subtle to require special stains to highlight the collagen, but may be marked (Fig. 19–10). Interconnection of the fibrous strands to produce tracts of fibrous tissue bridging with those of adjacent lobules (cardiac cirrhosis) is seen only in extreme examples, usually in association with tricuspid insufficiency.

The clinical consequences of cardiac sclerosis are either negligible or identical to those of CHN. The chronic liver damage rarely induces portal hypertension or the other accompaniments of well-defined cirrhosis of the liver.

INFARCTS OF LIVER

As noted earlier, the double blood supply to the liver undoubtedly accounts for the rarity of infarcts. Infrequently, however, thrombosis or compression of an intrahepatic branch of the hepatic artery caused by polyarteritis nodosa, embolism, neoplasia, or sepsis results in a localized infarct that is usually anemic or sometimes hemorrhagic when small (owing to suffusion of portal blood). It is often difficult to identify the arterial occlusion, and so it has been said that infarcts of the liver may occur in the apparent absence of arterial obstruction, merely as a result of shock and hypoperfusion.[39] It should be noted that occlusion of an intrahepatic branch of the portal vein does not cause ischemic infarction, but instead a sharply demarcated area of red-blue discoloration inappropriately referred to as an *infarct of Zahn*. Microscopically there is no necrosis, only hepatocellular atrophy secondary to marked sinusoidal congestion. Occasionally, thromboses are evident in the portal vein branches within the affected parenchyma.

As pointed out in the discussion of normal liver

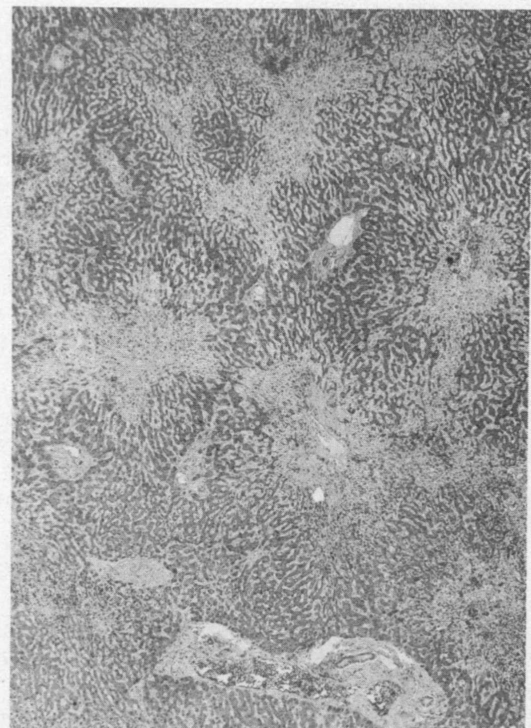

Figure 19–10. Marked cardiac sclerosis of liver, low power. Liver cells in centers of lobules have disappeared and are replaced by fibrous tissue.

structure, accidental or intentional interruption of the main hepatic artery does not always produce ischemic necrosis of the organ if the liver is otherwise normal and the point of arterial interruption is proximal to one of its major or large accessory branches. The retrograde arterial flow through these vessels, when coupled with the portal venous supply, may be sufficient to sustain the vitality of the liver parenchyma.

HEPATIC VEIN THROMBOSIS (BUDD-CHIARI SYNDROME)

Obstruction of the hepatic veins is a rare condition that may appear with catastrophic suddenness or insidiously over the course of many months.[40] The acute pattern is usually caused by thrombosis of the main hepatic vein or its major tributaries or the proximal inferior vena cava. The disorders initiating such thrombosis are: (1) intravascular invasion by primary or secondary cancers (hepatocellular, renal cell, adrenal carcinomas); (2) intrahepatic infections; (3) polycythemia vera with its thrombotic diathesis; (4) the myeloproliferative syndrome; (5) paroxysmal nocturnal hemoglobinuria;[41] and (6) intravascular webs or membranes, possibly related to closure of the ductus venosus (particularly common in Egyptian children). A number of cases of hepatic vein thrombosis have been related in the past to the use of oral contraceptives, but later analyses suggest that the association is merely coincidental.[42] The chronic form of the Budd-Chiari syndrome is related to fibrous narrowing of the intrahepatic venous channels or the main hepatic vein, seemingly caused by an endophlebitis. Radiation and herbal (bush) tea have been implicated. Superimposed thromboses sometimes suddenly aggravate the problem. After all these mechanisms have been excluded, about 25 to 30% of cases remain unexplained.

Whatever the precipitating condition, the liver is swollen and red-purple and has a tense capsule. On transection the appearance is that of severe centrilobular congestion and necrosis. There may be complete destruction of central cells, and the extravasation of blood may be accompanied by a fibrinous coagulum. Emphasis has been placed on distention and rupture of the spaces of Disse by blood.[43] Thrombi may or may not be evident within the central veins of the lobules but, as pointed out, they are sometimes present in the major outflow channels or main hepatic vein. In the endophlebitic pattern, there is fibrous thickening of the venous walls encroaching on the lumens of the central veins. This venous involvement may be followed into the larger outflow veins and sometimes the major hepatic vein. Because of the chronicity of this process, fiber strands may radiate out from the central veins, or sometimes the fibrosis may completely replace the centrilobular zones. In this chronic phase of the disease, organized thrombi may be evident within the veins.

The cardinal clinical manifestations of the Budd-Chiari syndrome are abdominal pain; enlarged, tender liver; and intractable ascites. These features may appear with sufficient rapidity to induce shock, may mimic other causes of an "acute abdomen," and may be followed by death within days. In the chronic pattern of the condition there is slow progression of abdominal distress, liver enlargement, ascites, and sometimes the development of superficial, dilated, collateral venous channels bypassing the hepatic obstruction. Portal hypertension (p. 916) develops in all forms of the condition and may eventually produce hematemesis from ruptured esophageal veins. Attempts at treatment, such as portacaval anastomosis and removal of webs or diaphragms when visualized by angiography, are largely unsatisfactory. Patients with the chronic syndrome usually die within months of the onset of symptoms from (1) hepatic failure, (2) inanition with secondary infections or electrolyte derangements, or (3) a gastrointestinal bleed.[44]

PORTAL VEIN OBSTRUCTION AND THROMBOSIS

Blockage of the portal vein is much better tolerated than obstruction of the hepatic vein. The occlusive process may arise within the extrahepatic course of the portal vein or within its intrahepatic distribution. *Extrahepatic causes* include (1) cancers arising within abdominal organs, (2) peritoneal sepsis initiating *pylephlebitis* within the portal vein itself or its major radicles with propagation into ever larger channels, (3) pancreatitis that initiates thrombosis within the splenic vein followed by propagation into the portal vein, and (4) postsurgical thromboses following upper abdominal procedures. Rarely, agenesis or aplasia of the portal vein is found. The most common *intrahepatic cause* is cirrhosis of the liver followed, in terms of frequency, by intravascular invasion by primary or secondary cancer in the liver.

Obstruction or thrombosis of the portal vein induces portal hypertension and related manifestations, notably splenomegaly. When it is unrelated to cirrhosis, there is little or no ascites. Unlike the situation in hepatic vein thrombosis, the liver is not enlarged or tender. When the condition is secondary to pylephlebitis, the infection may produce multiple abscesses by spread into the liver. Portal vein occlusion can often be managed by a splenorenal shunt, and is compatible with long survival unless the course is complicated by fatal bleeding from a ruptured esophageal varix.

INFECTIONS

The liver is almost inevitably involved in all bloodborne infections, whether systemic or arising in the abdominal cavity. Virtually all have been considered elsewhere, but some of the more common implicated infections are miliary tuberculosis, malaria, staphylococcal bacteremia, infectious mononucleosis, the salmoneloses, and amebiasis. Indeed, needle liver biopsy is often employed in occult infections for telltale evidence of the causative agent, particularly when miliary tuberculosis is suspected. There are, in addition, several primary hepatic infections that require detailed consideration: the important and common viral hepatitis, and the less common but distinctive cholangitis and liver abscess.

VIRAL HEPATITIS

Hepatitis may appear in the course of a number of systemic viral infections. A generally mild hepatic involvement is common during the acute phase of infectious mononucleosis caused by the Epstein-Barr virus. The cytomegalovirus may produce hepatitis that can be quite severe in the newborn or immunosuppressed adult. The yellow fever virus is a major and serious source of hepatitis in tropical countries. Infrequently and primarily in children, significant liver disease appears in the course of rubella, adenovirus, and enterovirus infections.[45] However, *unless otherwise specified, the term "viral hepatitis" is generally reserved for infection of the liver caused by any one of a small group of hepatotropic viruses.* Two of these agents—hepatitis A virus (HAV) and hepatitis B virus (HBV)—have been well delineated, but there is at least one agent, possibly several, known as non-A, non-B (NANBV), and yet another, recently identified as "delta agent," about which little is yet known. Hepatitis A is also sometimes referred to as *infectious hepatitis* or *short-incubation hepatitis,* and hepatitis B is sometimes called *serum hepatitis* or *long-incubation hepatitis.* All the viruses produce basically similar clinical patterns of acute hepatitis, which can be differentiated serologically. However, several agents have differing potentials for the causation of the carrier state, chronic and fulminating disease. First, the causative agents, their immunologic markers, and the epidemiology will be characterized, followed by a discussion of our present understanding of the pathogenesis of the hepatic injury. Thereafter, the varied patterns of clinical disease will be described.[46–48]

Causative Agents, Immunologic Markers, and Epidemiology

HEPATITIS A

The HAV usually causes a benign, self-limited, transiently infective, acute hepatitis. The incubation period between exposure and the onset of acute symptoms (if overt disease does develop) ranges from 15 to 45 days (average 2 to 4 weeks). *Only very rarely does this agent induce fulminating hepatitis, so that the overall mortality for hepatitis A infections is 0.1% or less. It does not produce chronic hepatitis, nor is it associated with a carrier state.* Although HAV has not been isolated, it can be transmitted to marmoset monkeys and chimpanzees and be serially propagated in a variety of subhuman primate cell lines.[49] The causative agent is an RNA virus closely resembling enterovirus that appears in the stools and hepatocytes of infected humans and monkeys as nonenveloped 27-nm icosahedral particles. Fecal infectivity is maximal during the prodrome and persists for up to one to two weeks into the illness. The viremia is transient, beginning during the prodrome and disappearing soon after the onset of symptoms.[50] When symptoms appear, usually accompanied by jaundice, anti-HAV antibodies of the IgM class can be detected in the serum (radioimmunoassay is most sensitive) even while fecal HAV shedding is still occurring. The titer of IgM antibody rises rapidly during the acute illness but disappears within months. As the acute phase begins to subside and during convalescence, the titer of IgG antibodies rises and remains elevated for a lifetime, conferring immunity to the HAV. The time relationship of these various markers is diagrammed in Figure 19–11.[51] The clinical differentiation of hepatitis A from other forms of viral hepatitis depends generally on the identification of HAV-specific IgM antibody in the serum as a marker of recent acute infection, and of IgG as a marker of recovery and past disease. There is no cross immunity between hepatitis A and the other hepatotropic viral infections.

The natural reservoir of HAV is humans. Transmission of hepatitis A is generally by the fecal-oral route. *The acute hepatitis accounts for about 45% of sporadic disease.* Transmission is favored by poor personal hygiene, close contact, and overcrowding. An increased incidence has been observed in homosexual males.[52] Spread within a family or within an institution, particularly among children, accounts for occasional localized epidemics of hepatitis A. Outbreaks have also occurred from contaminated food, water, milk, and shellfish, particularly among populations having no previous exposure to HAV, such as children and adults from higher socioeconomic groups. Mollusks such as clams, mussels, and oysters from polluted waters have been shown to concentrate the virus. For lovers of oysters, however, it has been estimated that the chance of so acquiring the infection is about one in 10,000; therefore, no more than 9999 of these delicacies should be consumed at one sitting![53] Only rarely is the virus spread percutaneously (including blood transfusion) because the viremia is so transient and there is no carrier state with hepatitis A.

Although HAV is endemic globally, there is wide variation in its prevalence among populations as judged by serologic markers. For example, over 80% of blood donors in Taiwan, Israel, Yugoslavia, and Belgium have anti-HAV antibodies.[54] In the United States the prevalence of antibodies in the 1970s was about 45% among urban adults, almost 80% in Orientals, and less than 10% among Jews. The great preponderance of these antibody-positive individuals had subclinical infections of which they were totally unaware.[55]

HEPATITIS B

In contrast to HAV, *HBV may cause a variety of clinical syndromes ranging from a carrier state (with or without underlying hepatic disease) to acute hepatitis that infrequently is fulminant, and to chronic hepatic disease that may be self-limited (chronic persistent hepatitis) or progressive and sometimes fatal (chronic active hepatitis).* It is evident that infection with HBV may be

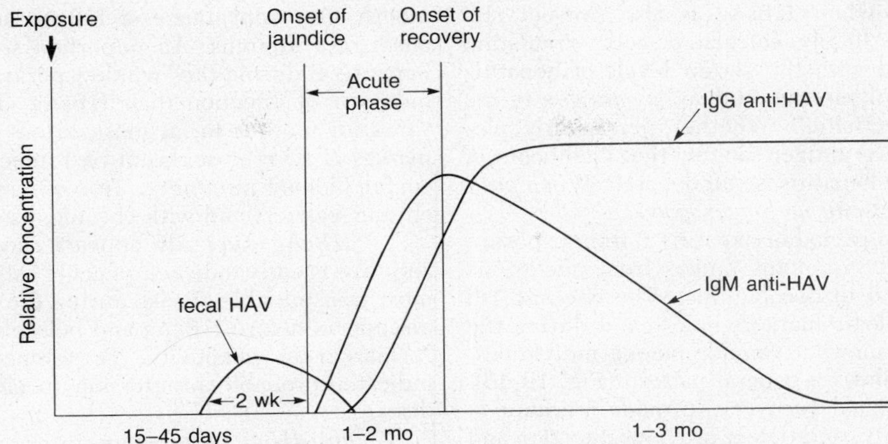

Figure 19–11. Sequence of serologic changes in acute hepatitis A.

much more serious than that caused by HAV. During active infection the causative agent can be visualized in liver cells, but rarely in the blood, as a 42-nm enveloped particle having an inner icosahedral core 27 nm in diameter surrounded by an outer coat. These complete virions are sometimes called *Dane particles* in recognition of the investigator who first described them.[56] The core is synthesized within the nuclei of hepatocytes and consists mainly of hepatitis B core antigen (HBcAg), double-stranded DNA, and DNA polymerase. An "e" antigen is also associated with the core. The protein-lipid envelope (coat) containing "surface antigen" (HBsAg) is synthesized in the liver cell cytoplasm.[57, 58] For unknown reasons, there is always excess production of coat material in the forms of spherules 22 nm in diameter or tubules of similar diameter and up to several hundred nanometers in length (Fig. 19–12). These particles possess HBsAg but no HBcAg. Naked core particles are rarely, if ever, found in the blood, but HBsAg particles abound during active viral replication, unique among viral infections. Indeed, it was the identification by Blumberg of this antigen in the blood of an Australian aborigine that paved the way for our present understanding of viral hepatitis.[59] *Thus, HBsAg is sometimes called Australia antigen. The HBsAg particles in the blood are not infective since they lack the critical viral core, but they nonetheless constitute the diagnostic hallmark of hepatitis B infection.* It has been shown that the antigen is so plentiful in the blood that it can be harvested to produce a vaccine.[60] Antigenic subtypes of HBsAg have been identified, but these are principally of value as epidemiologic markers and have no other clinical impact. This antigen evokes specific antibodies that confer immunity to the HBV. The antigenemia may be present despite a low level of anti-HBs. Circulating immune complexes may be formed and are responsible for a variety of extrahepatic manifestations, as will be detailed.

An "e" antigen is also associated with the core particle. It is immunologically distinct from both HBcAg and HBsAg. In fact, three subtypes of "e" antigen have been characterized, but they need not concern us further. The nature of the "e" antigen and its precise localization within the core are still uncertain. It appears to have the immunologic and physicochemical properties of an IgG-4 immunoglobulin.[61] HBeAg appears in the blood with acute infection but typically, only tran-

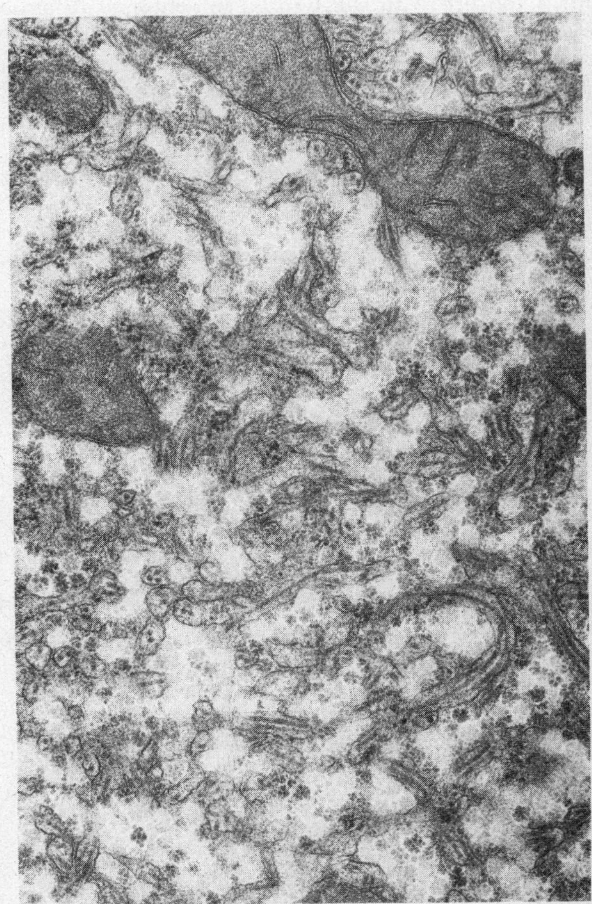

Figure 19–12. Electron micrograph of hepatitis B surface antigen in the form of spherules and tubules within hepatocytic cytoplasm (× 21500). (Courtesy of Drs. M. A. Gerber and S. N. Thung, Mount Sinai School of Medicine.)

siently, and only when HBsAg is also present. Its presence there is highly correlated with circulating Dane particles and with the serum levels of hepatitis B–specific DNA polymerase, and so *"e" antigen in the blood implies infectivity.*[62] Whether persistently elevated titers of this antigen augur the likelihood of developing chronic hepatitis is still debated. *When anti-HBe appears, infectivity no longer exists.*[63]

The incubation period of hepatitis B from exposure to onset of clinical symptoms ranges from one to six months (average 1.5 to two months). The rise and fall of the various serologic markers before and during the active disease is somewhat variable among individuals, but nonetheless follows a general pattern (Fig. 19–13). Certain markers signal recovery, provide warning of impending chronicity, and detect previous infection and immunity to the agent. They also identify the carrier state sometimes in individuals without a history of a previous apparent infection. The salient interpretations (best followed in the diagram) to be drawn from the serologic studies and applicable to 75 to 85% of cases are as follows:

– HBsAg: the earliest marker of acute infection. Serum titer begins to rise several weeks to months before symptoms appear, perhaps as early as one week after exposure.[64] In self-limited infection, it disappears several months later as biochemical indicators of liver damage, such as transaminases, return to normal levels. Titer may be low or undetectable in some cases. Persistence of HBsAg for over six months implies chronic disease.[65]

– *anti-HBs:* not detectable in blood until several weeks to months following disappearance of HBsAg. Time lag between disappearance of antigen and appearance of antibody is referred to as the "window period." A rising titer of anti-HBs following acute infection signals clinical recovery; it remains elevated for life and confers immunity. Not detectable in carriers.

– *anti-HBc:* first detectable approximately one month after appearance of HBsAg and at the time of onset of symptoms. An important serologic marker of hepatitis B during the "window period." More sensitive indicator of infection than HBsAg. Titer remains elevated for months to, at most, a few years, and thus is marker of current or recent past infection, but does not confer lifelong immunity. Titer remains elevated in all chronic carriers and with chronic disease.

– *HBeAg:* typically appears shortly after HBsAg, and thus is early indicator of acute active infection while most transmissible. Peaks during the acute disease and disappears before HBsAg and before onset of recovery. A marker of infectivity. Persistence of "e" antigen indicates probable progression to chronic active liver disease.

– *anti-HBe:* titer begins to rise as antigen disappears. Seroconversion from "e" antigen to "e" antibody signals resolution of acute infection and elimination of virus. A marker of recent acute disease during the "window period." In the absence of chronicity, titer slowly falls over the next one to two years. Does not confer immunity.

Individuals with any impairment of immunologic competence have increased vulnerability to infection by HBV, do not mount adequate antibody responses, tend to have higher titers of the antigens, and are prone to become carriers or develop chronic active disease.

Only humans and, experimentally, the unwilling chimpanzee are vulnerable to HBV. The main sources of infection are not individuals with acute disease, but rather the carriers in the world, over 100 million in number. *Transmission may occur through three routes—percutaneous, nonpercutaneous, and vertically (from mother to infant).* Because of the viremia and carrier state, blood transfusions and infusions of blood derivatives are obvious modes of spread, but meticulous screening of donors for HBsAg has substantially reduced this risk. It is now appreciated that HBV is responsible for only about 10% of posttransfusion hepatitis; most are

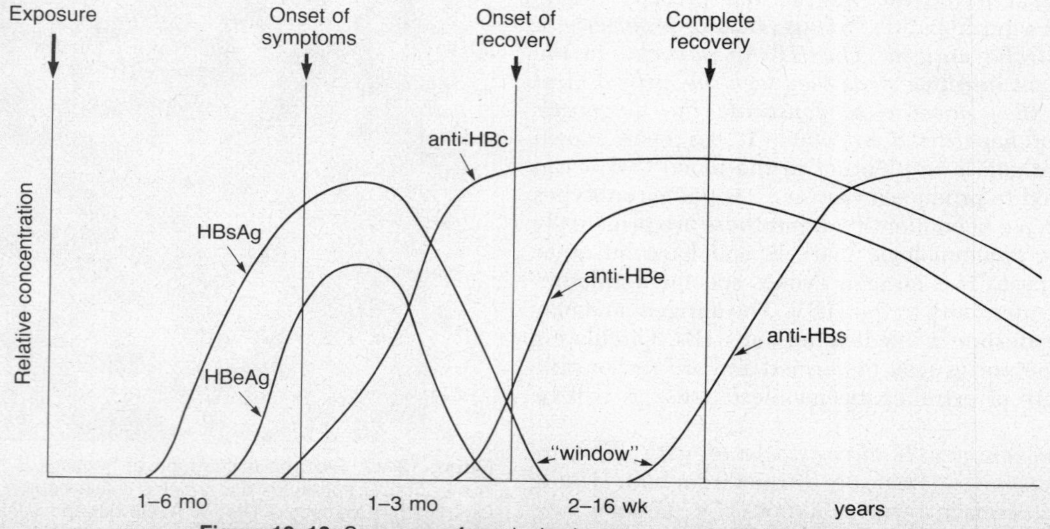

Figure 19–13. Sequence of serologic changes in acute hepatitis B.

related to the non-A, non-B virus(es). Transmission may also occur with hemodialysis, via transplantation, and through any break in the skin. Health care personnel (notably dentists), those employed in hemodialysis units, and handlers of infected primates are at particular risk. Not unexpectedly, serologic evidence of HBV is present in over 50% of drug addicts. In addition, nonpercutaneous transmission is now recognized as a major mode of spread. HBsAg, and presumably HBcAg, has been identified in feces, urine, saliva, vaginal secretions, semen, colostrum, and every other bodily secretion and fluid. Thus, high attack rates occur in spouses and sexual partners of affected patients, in family members of chronic carriers, among male homosexuals, and among institutionalized children, particularly those with Down's syndrome.[66] In addition, HBV may be transmitted vertically from mother to infant during the perinatal period (by contact with blood and/or secretions during delivery, or in the immediate postnatal period). The risk is greatest when the mother has acute hepatitis during the last trimester of pregnancy.[67] Carrier mothers may also infect their infants, and the level of risk appears to be correlated with the serum titer of HBeAg. Conversely, elevated levels of anti-HBe imply noninfectivity. Vertical transmission probably accounts for the high prevalence of this infection in Asian and African populations (up to 30 to 40%).[68] In the United States the prevalence of detectable HBsAg in the serum (in the normal population) is in the range of 0.1 to 1.5%. However, as many as 15% of immunocompromised individuals and those with Down's syndrome may harbor this antigen. Parenthetically, it may be noted that *persistence of HBV is suspected of causing hepatocellular carcinoma* (discussed more fully on p. 935).

Non-A, Non-B Hepatitis

At least one, very likely two, and possibly more non-A, non-B viruses (NANBV) are capable of causing infections remarkably similar clinically to hepatitis B.[69] The NANBV may induce a carrier state, acute hepatitis indistinguishable from that caused by the other hepatotropic viruses, chronic persistent or chronic active hepatitis, and sometimes fulminant disease.[70] Its clinical potential, therefore, parallels that of HBV. However, acute hepatitis caused by NANBV is more often followed by chronic hepatitis (about 30%) than is the case with HBV. NANBV is/are thought to be responsible for about 90% of cases of posttransfusion hepatitis. The percutaneous route probably also accounts for the development of infections in drug addicts, in transplant recipients, and within hemodialysis units. Nonpercutaneous spread is also highly likely because of transmission to family and occupational contacts as well as within institutions.[71]

We are still at the threshold of characterizing the causative agents of NANB hepatitis.[72] Inferential evidence points strongly to at least two different agents. The incubation period following exposure ranges from 14 to 180 days, with two distinct peaks suggesting two viruses. Repeated attacks of acute NANB hepatitis have been observed in drug addicts, suggesting immunologically distinctive agents. To date it has not been possible to isolate any agent, but the disease can be transmitted to chimpanzees by inoculation of blood from acute cases. No well-established serologic tests have so far been developed, but there have been several reports of identification of an antigen-antibody system in patients with NANB hepatitis.[73] In one, a single antigen-antibody system was present in all of 26 patients studied, a surprising finding relative to the evidence suggesting the existence of more than one virus.[74] Viral particles of such diversity have been observed in infected livers that their interpretation is uncertain. They have ranged from 22 to 100 nm in diameter, some cytoplasmic, others nuclear.[75] Best characterized is a 27-nm particle having some similarity to HAV.[76] However, it is by no means clear as yet whether any of the particles visualized are indeed the causative agents.[77]

Delta Hepatitis

Very recently a unique RNA virus has been described distinct from all the others that can cause either acute or chronic hepatitis.[77A] The agent appears to have a core of δ antigen encapsulated by HBsAg necessary for its replication. Delta hepatitis therefore occurs in only three circumstances: (1) as an acute disease along with acute hepatitis B, (2) as an acute hepatitis in a chronic carrier (p. 904) of HBV, and (3) as a chronic hepatitis in a chronic carrier of HBV. As far as is now known, the delta agent is uncommon in the U.S. but prevalent about the Mediterranean, and is only transmitted parenterally (e.g., transfusions, drug addiction). Time, however, may change our present understanding.

Pathogenesis. The mechanisms involved in the causation of liver injury by the various viruses are still uncertain. There is no documentation of direct cytotoxicity, but the short incubation period of hepatitis A raises this possibility. However, propagation of HAV in subhuman primate cell cultures is not associated with cell injury or death. In addition, the fact that asymptomatic carriers of HBV and NANBV having no evidence of liver damage may transmit the disease, and so harbor the virus, argues against cytotoxicity for these agents. *The favored theory invokes immunologically mediated mechanisms of injury (described later), although the supportive evidence is fragmentary.* It is not clear, however, whether humoral or cell-mediated responses, or both, participate. With HAV there is a temporal relationship between onset of the acute illness, associated hepatocyte injury, and the appearance of anti-HAV of the IgM class and depressed levels of serum complement. However, weak pointers to cell-mediated mechanisms are a concomitant peripheral T-cell lymphocytopenia and putative inhibitors of T lymphocytes in the serum at the time of acute liver injury. Conceivably, antibodies and immunocompetent cells both contribute to antibody-dependent cellular cytotoxicity.

The immunopathogenesis of hepatitis B is equally murky.[78] Inferential evidence suggests that immune mechanisms both eradicate the virus and destroy virus-infected hepatocytes. *Despite the presence of at least three specific types of antibodies in hepatitis B infections, the weight of evidence suggests that cell-mediated mechanisms play the major role, albeit one that is still poorly defined.* It has been shown that patients with acute hepatitis or those who have recovered usually have circulating T cells that undergo blast transformation and elaborate migration inhibition factor on exposure to HBsAg.[79] In contrast, asymptomatic carriers rarely have such sensitized T cells. More directly, lymphocytes from patients with acute viral hepatitis B are cytotoxic to hepatocytes in culture.[80] There is a concomitant peripheral T-cell lymphocytopenia, as mentioned above, but this may be the spurious consequence of circulating factors that inhibit their in vitro recognition. Free antigen or immune complexes might block antigen recognition sites; also, a factor has been identified in the serum of patients with hepatitis B (as well as hepatitis A and NANB hepatitis) that inhibits the E-rosette function of normal T cells.[81] Defective T-suppressor cell function also has been observed in those with chronic disease.[82] Conceivably, then, failure of immunoregulation or T-cell function plays some role in the hepatic injury and, as will be pointed out, may contribute to the development of chronic infections.

Humoral mechanisms must also participate in hepatitis B. *The development of an antibody response during the prodrome and early phase while there is an antigen excess results in the formation of circulating immune complexes, and without doubt these underlie the development of the extrahepatic manifestations* seen in a small fraction of patients with acute hepatitis B: namely, a serum sickness–like syndrome, urticaria, other rashes, polyarthritis, acute vasculitis resembling polyarteritis nodosa, cryoglobulinemia, and immune complex–mediated glomerulopathies.[83] Antibodies also clearly play some role in eradicating the virus. You may recall the disappearance of HBeAg from the circulation accompanied by loss of infectivity as the serologic titer of anti-HBe rises. A unifying theory has therefore been proposed: *antibodies participate mainly in the clearance of virus from the blood and the coating of virally infected liver cells while cell-mediated mechanisms play a major role in the destruction of hepatocytes bearing viral or modified antigens, possibly by antibody-dependent cellular cytotoxicity.* Although integral viral antigens may be the specific targets in hepatocytes, it has been suggested that a viral-modified hepatocyte membrane lipoprotein is the primary antigenic target.[84] Whatever the precise focus of attack, it could be theorized that *in the typical acute infection with HBV a normal effective immune response soon brings the virus under control, but at the cost of moderate hepatocyte destruction. However, the virus is eradicated and complete recovery follows. With a less adequate immune response, perhaps related to abnormal suppressor T-cell activity, the virus persists, as does viral modification of hepatocytes, leading to a low level of cell destruction for a long time, i.e., the development of chronic hepatitis. With a totally inadequate immune response, there is no liver cell destruction and persistence of the virus (the asymptomatic carrier). Conversely, with a hyperimmune response, there is massive necrosis but prompt eradication of the virus (fulminant hepatitis); thus, not unexpectedly, survivors rarely, if ever, become carriers.* Whether genetic or acquired factors condition the level of the immune response is not known. Little has yet been learned about NANBV.

CLINICAL SYNDROMES. As indicated, HAV causes only self-limited, acute hepatitis that very rarely is fulminant. In contrast, infection with HBV or NANBV may have a number of outcomes, which can be categorized as follows:

Carrier State

A. Without clinically apparent disease—asymptomatic
B. With chronic hepatitis

Acute Hepatitis

A. Icteric
B. Anicteric

Chronic Hepatitis

A. Chronic persistent hepatitis
B. Chronic active hepatitis

Fulminant Hepatitis

A. With massive-to-submassive hepatic necrosis

Each of these patterns is discussed separately.

Carrier State

There are individuals who harbor and transmit HBV or NANBV (rarely both) for years, possibly for a lifetime. Generally, when related to HBV they are discovered in routine screening of blood donors, but sometimes only as sources of infection already transmitted to someone else. With NANBV, carriers can be identified only as HBsAg-negative sources of viral infection, usually post-transfusion hepatitis. Whatever the agent, the carriers fall into one of two categories. Some provide no history of an acute attack of viral hepatitis and have neither clinical manifestations of infection nor elevated levels of transaminases to suggest liver disease. Such individuals are referred to as *asymptomatic* or *"healthy" carriers.* The second category has chronic liver disease, either chronic persistent or chronic active hepatitis, and so they are referred to as *liver disease carriers.* They may or may not have a history of overt antecedent acute hepatitis and may or may not be asymptomatic, but there is clear evidence of liver injury in the form of elevated transaminase levels as well as other possible stigmata of chronic disease, to be detailed later. Obviously, those with HBV disease have serologic markers.

There are no data on the prevalence of carriers of NANBV. About 0.1% of North Americans carry HBV; a significantly higher prevalence is found elsewhere, particularly in Africa and Asia.[85] The carrier state is most likely to develop in immunodeficient or immunosuppressed individuals, those on hemodialysis or receiving multiple transfusions, drug addicts, and persons with Down's syndrome.

In "healthy" carriers of hepatitis B, the liver biopsy reveals essentially normal morphology, except for occasional cells modified by their content of viral antigens. **Most nu-**

merous are clusters of "ground-glass" hepatocytes having uniform, finely granular eosinophilic cytoplasm with H and E staining (Fig. 19–17, p. 907). The granules are better seen after staining with orcein or aldehyde fuchsin.[86] Often, there is a clear peripheral halo of cytoplasm enclosing this region of change. With the electron microscope, the granularity can be resolved as spherules and filaments, which can be shown to be HBsAg by immunofluorescent and immunoperoxidase techniques. With these immunologic methods, HBcAg can sometimes be found in nuclei, and rarely in cells having the "ground-glass" change. **Nuclei bearing an abundance of HBcAg may take on a "sanded" appearance in H and E and orcein preparations.**[87] As pointed out before, the abundance of these viral antigens in "healthy" carriers having no liver damage supports the belief that the virus is not cytotoxic and that the hepatocyte injury is immunologically mediated.

Carriers having chronic liver disease in addition to the morphologic evidence of chronic infection, described later, also have "ground-glass" hepatocytes and "sanded nuclei" but only in widely scattered cells, rather than cell clusters. Immunodeficient or immunosuppressed patients with mild chronic hepatitis often have more numerous affected cells.[88] More details about chronic hepatitis follow, but it may be noted that there is an inverse relationship between the number of antigen-bearing hepatocytes and the severity of liver injury.

Because of the lack of systems to identify NANBV in histologic preparations, nothing is known about the anatomic changes in carriers. Carriers are the main reservoir of HBV and, despite screening programs, continue to be an important source of posttransfusion hepatitis. The HBV carrier state, even in the absence of liver damage, predisposes to the development of hepatocellular carcinoma, raising speculations about the oncogenicity of the virus.

Acute Viral Hepatitis

All the hepatotropic viruses cause essentially the same clinical and morphologic pattern of acute hepatitis, although that caused by HAV tends to be the mildest. The specific causative agent can be identified only by virologic or serologic tests. When no markers of HAV or HBV are present, it is assumed to be NANBV, although (as mentioned) an antigen-antibody system has been described that may be helpful in the future. All the viruses are widely endemic and most often cause sporadic disease. Most commonly implicated is HAV (approximately 45% of cases) followed by HBV. NANBV is responsible for only about 20 to 25% of sporadic disease. Posttransfusion hepatitis, on the other hand, is related to NANBV in 90% of cases, the remainder being almost entirely due to HBV. Only rarely is HAV involved. When an epidemic outbreak occurs it is highly likely to be due to HAV, but rarely (as mentioned) food and water contaminated by HBV has caused multiple concurrent, acute infections. Whatever the clinical setting, following exposure there is an incubation period that, as explained, is shortest in hepatitis A, longest in hepatitis B, and intermediate and quite variable in NANB hepatitis. The *earliest symptoms of the prodrome* are nonspecific and include malaise, fatigue, anorexia, nausea, vomiting, and sometimes arthralgias. These may be accompanied by a low-grade fever, and so the presentation is readily mistaken for "flu" or an upper respiratory infection. The clinical manifestations tend to appear more abruptly and the fever tends to be higher with HAV than with HBV. Thus, HBV infection begins more insidiously, and occasionally a serum sickness–like syndrome ushers in the acute attack. Whatever the specific agent, during the prodrome the patient may express a distaste for coffee or cigarettes. The first clue to the nature of the infection may be the development of abdominal discomfort, calling attention to an enlarged, tender liver. By this time the serum transaminases and LDH levels are elevated, pointing to parenchymal injury. Serologic studies at this time would very likely disclose markers of the causative agent were it HBV or HAV, as already detailed.

An *icteric phase follows in most patients after days to a week or more of the relatively nonspecific prodrome.* The jaundice, related to conjugated and unconjugated hyperbilirubinemia, slowly increases during the first two weeks to a maximal serum bilirubin level in the range of 5 to 20 mg/dl. Typically, the systemic constitutional symptoms abate as the jaundice appears, but even before this there may be darkening of the urine by bilirubin and lightening of the color of the stools because of functional obstruction. The liver enzymes are elevated and serologic markers are present. Also, the liver continues to be enlarged and tender. It is important to note at this juncture that, *in some instances of acute hepatitis, jaundice never appears—anicteric hepatitis.* On the other hand, particularly with HBV, the jaundice may be quite marked and associated with severe pruritus, reflecting retention of bile salts. An elevated alkaline phosphatase level frequently accompanies these obstructive manifestations. This pattern of disease is sometimes called *cholestatic or cholangiolitic viral hepatitis.*

After an icteric or anicteric febrile phase lasting two or more weeks (longest with HBV, shortest with HAV, and intermediate with NANBV), convalescence begins. The serum bilirubin and enzyme levels slowly return to normal, and the liver tenderness and enlargement begin to slowly abate. At or about this time, a rising serum titer of IgG anti-HAV or anti-HBc is present in most patients. Complete recovery, particularly the return of all biochemical test results to normal, may require many months. *If abnormalities persist for longer than six months without steadily progressive improvement, it is highly likely that one of the forms of chronic hepatitis has developed.* Rarely, in less than 1% of cases of acute hepatitis, the infection is fulminant with massive necrosis of the liver and a high fatality rate.

A variety of extrahepatic complications may appear in the course of acute hepatitis B. The prodromal phase may be marked by apparent serum sickness, urticaria, and other sensitivity eruptions, sometimes accompanied by polyarthritis, all reflections of circulating immune complexes. With prolonged antigenemia, cryoglobulinemia, acute vasculitis resembling polyarteritis nodosa, or membranous or membranoproliferative glomerulonephritis sometimes develop later in the course, also attributable to circulating immune complexes.

The morphologic changes in typical acute hepatitis are qualitatively the same irrespective of the particular causative agent. Although distinctive, they can be mimicked by other viral infections and reactions to drugs. As seen by laparoscopy, the liver is slightly enlarged during the acute phase, and more or less green depending on the level of jaundice.

Histologically, **the major findings are: (1) diffuse liver cell injury with lobular disarray; (2) necrosis of random, isolated liver cells; (3) reactive changes in Kupffer cells and sinusoidal lining cells; (4) an inflammatory infiltrate in the portal tracts; and (5) evidence of hepatocyte regeneration during the recovery phase.**[89] The liver cell injury is manifested by swelling, sometimes with partial clearing of the cytoplasm secondary to hydropic distention of endoplasmic reticulum, producing what is called **ballooning degeneration. Lobular disarray** results from the cellular swelling, necrosis, and regeneration producing compression of the vascular sinusoids and loss of the normal, more or less radial, arrangement of hepatocytes (Fig. 19–14*A*). Two patterns of isolated liver cell necrosis appear. Rupture of the plasma membrane of ballooned cells may cause them literally to disappear—**drop-out necrosis.** Often, there is a small cluster of lymphocytes, macrophages, and reactive Kupffer cells in the locus of the dead hepatocyte. Alternatively, single cells may undergo shrinkage and condensation with increased eosinophilia of the cytoplasm and eventual disappearance of the nuclei to produce rounded, refractile, **acidophilic or Councilman bodies.**[90] The acidophilic body may appear free in the sinusoidal space or space of Disse, but more often is engulfed by a Kupffer cell (Fig. 19–14*B*). The Councilman body may be a forerunner of so-called "apoptosis" or piecemeal necrosis, seen in chronic active hepatitis (p. 908). A prominent feature of acute viral hepatitis is the **marked hypertrophy and probable hyperplasia of Kupffer cells and sinusoidal lining cells,** both of which are often laden with lipofuscin pigment. The portal tracts are almost universally infiltrated with inflammatory cells, mainly lymphocytes admixed with macrophages and rare eosinophils and neutrophils. Plasma cells are uncommon in the usual case of acute viral hepatitis. The inflammatory infiltrate does not spill out through the limiting plate in classic acute disease. Eventually, during the recovery phase, bi- and trinucleate liver cells and mitotic figures become apparent as evidence of regeneration. Mentioned last, because of its inconstancy and variability, is bile stasis. It may be entirely absent in anicteric hepatitis. Conversely, a typical cholestatic picture may appear (p. 890) and be quite marked in cholestatic or cholangiolitic viral hepatitis, when it is often accompanied by inflammatory changes in the bile ducts within the portal triads. Characteristically, "ground-glass" hepatocytes bearing HBsAg or "sanded nuclei" bearing HBcAg are not present or, at most, are very infrequent in acute hepatitis B.

A number of changes suggest deviation from the usual benign, self-limited course of the disease. Necrosis of confluent areas of hepatocytes may merely reflect a severe attack of acute viral hepatitis, but may herald progression to fulminant hepatitis. These foci may interconnect with adjacent areas of necrosis, referred to as **bridging necrosis** (p. 908). Often accompanying this alteration is "piecemeal necrosis" of hepatocytes, particularly at the limiting plate. Both **bridging and piecemeal necrosis are characteristic of chronic active hepatitis** and so are described in more detail later. They are distinctly uncommon in uncomplicated acute hepatitis and, when present, raise the red alert for progressive disease—chronic active hepatitis leading to either hepatic failure or cirrhosis.[91] Analogously, an increase in the number of liver cells bearing HBV antigens is a portent of threatened evolution into chronic liver disease.[92]

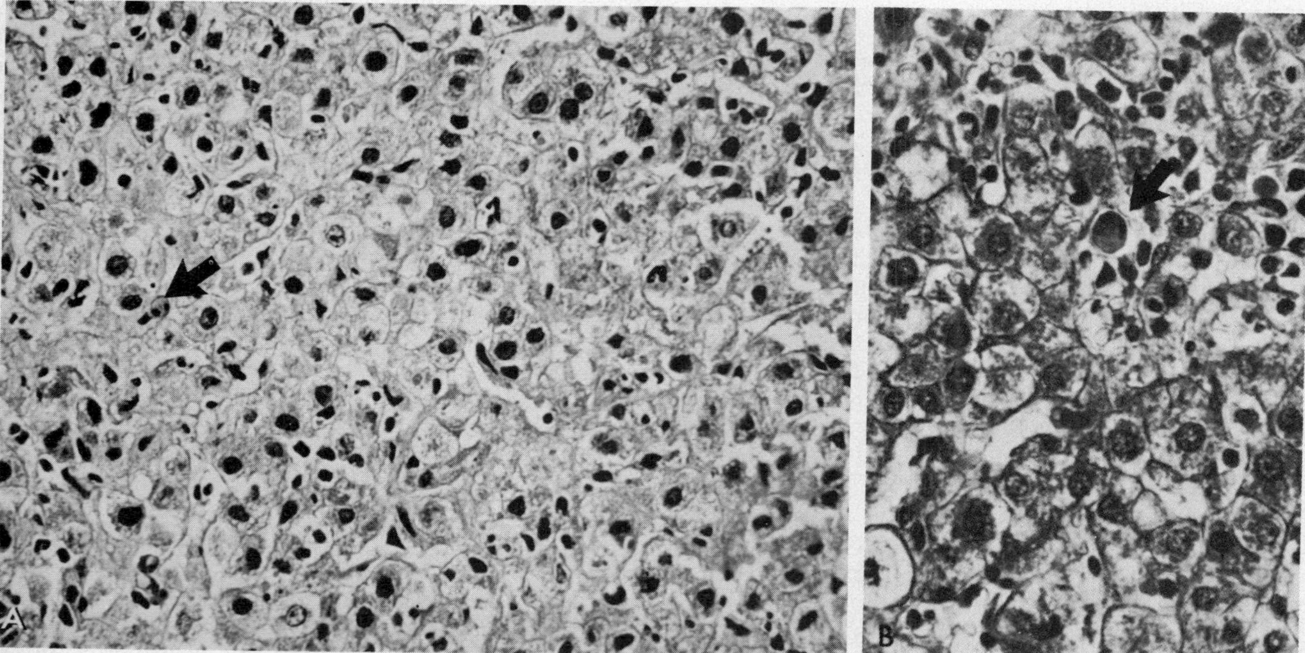

Figure 19–14. *A,* Acute viral hepatitis showing swelling of liver cells and lobular disarray. Arrow points to a developing acidophilic or Councilman body. *B,* Similar changes in hepatocytes with a well-developed Councilman body (*arrow*). (Courtesy of Dr. Hans Popper, The Mount Sinai Medical Center.)

Most patients with acute hepatitis (and virtually all with HAV infections) recover completely with restoration of normal liver architecture over the span of months. Fulminant hepatitis is very uncommon, particularly with HAV. Chronic hepatitis, as will become evident, is a greater threat in attacks caused by HBV or NANBV. With complete recovery from the acute attack, there is permanent immunity to the particular causative agent.

Chronic Hepatitis

Symptomatic or biochemical evidence of ongoing inflammatory hepatic disease for more than six months without steady improvement is generally interpreted as chronic hepatitis, although some experts accept a shorter time span. It follows about 5 to 10% of attacks of acute hepatitis B and in the range of 30 to 40% of acute infections by NANBV (more often with drug addiction than posttransfusion).[93, 94] HAV does not cause chronic hepatitis. *In about 60 to 75% of instances the chronicity represents chronic persistent hepatitis, which is generally benign and self-limited. The remaining cases are of chronic active hepatitis with progressive liver damage, leading often to cirrhosis, hepatic failure, and death.* Chronic active hepatitis may also have other than viral origins, discussed later.

Differentiation of chronic persistent hepatitis from chronic active hepatitis is of great importance because of their very different prognoses. It may be simple when clinical and laboratory data indicate serious advancing hepatic destruction. On the other hand, there are many intermediate cases in which even interpretation of the liver biopsy is difficult, particularly when the changes have been modified by treatment. The problem is compounded by the fact that a few cases of chronic persistent hepatitis may have episodes of apparent activation suggesting conversion to chronic active hepatitis, or, conversely, quiescent chronic active hepatitis may be misinterpreted as chronic persistent hepatitis.[95] Nonetheless, the differentiation can be made reliably with liver biopsy in the great majority of instances, providing welcome reassurance to a large number of patients.

There are no sure clinical criteria by which impending chronicity can be predicted during the acute phase of viral hepatitis. With HBV, markedly elevated titers of HBeAg or persisting titers for more than six to eight weeks after the acute phase have been associated with the development of chronic liver disease.[96] Persistence of circulating HBsAg/IgM complexes has also been reported to have significance.[97] None of these criteria has a high confidence level; the severity of the acute attack is of no value. In general, *chronic active hepatitis is most likely to develop in the very young and very elderly, in males, in association with immunoincompetence or immunosuppression, in Down's syndrome, in patients on hemodialysis, and in recipients of multiple transfusions.*

Chronic Persistent Hepatitis (CPH)

This sequel to acute hepatitis caused by HBV or NANBV is a relapsing, remitting condition that is usually benign and eventually self-limited. It is not associated with progressive liver damage. *In most instances, it can be viewed as delayed recovery from the acute episode, but it may take as long as several years to clear.*[98] During this long recovery period, the individual may be symptom free and the only evidence of persistent abnormality is an elevated serum transaminase level—hence, the facetious designation "transaminitis." However, fatigue, malaise, and loss of appetite may wax and wane, sometimes with bouts of mild jaundice. HBsAg is found in the serum of 20 to 60% of these patients, and the remaining cases are assumed to be related to NANBV.

The mild morphologic changes are not pathognomonic and can be summarized as **chronic triaditis.** An inflammatory infiltrate of lymphocytes and macrophages, with possibly a rare neutrophil or eosinophil, is present in the portal tracts, indistinguishable from that seen in acute hepatitis. Importantly, **the infiltrate is limited to the portal tracts and does not spill out into the hepatic parenchyma.** The liver architecture is usually well preserved but sometimes reveals vestiges of the acute disease. With CPH related to the HBV, "ground-glass" hepatocytes (p. 905) are sometimes present but are not numerous.[99] **Notably absent are significant hepatocyte necrosis or the important hallmarks of chronic active hepatitis (CAH), i.e., piecemeal necrosis of the liver cells at the limiting plate and bridging necrosis.** The alterations of CPH are then quite nonspecific and can be mimicked by drug injury, systemic infections, and early primary biliary cirrhosis.

In most cases, a ready diagnosis of CPH, as distinct from CAH, can be made on the basis of the hepatic changes described. Infrequently, however, the differential morphologic diagnosis is much more difficult. Occasionally, during a relapse, swollen and ballooned hepatocytes, spotty necrosis, acidophilic bodies, and even piecemeal necrosis may appear, suggesting either reactivation of the acute disease or evolving CAH. Indeed, there have been rare reports of transition from CPH to CAH.[100] Conversely, corticosteroid treatment of CAH has led to conversion of the liver biopsy to apparent CPH, but with cessation of the therapy the morphologic changes often revert.[101] Thus, persistent hepatitis and active hepatitis in a sense represent the two ends of a spectrum of chronicity; there are cases that swing one way or the other, depending apparently on the immunologic responsiveness of the host.

Chronic Active Hepatitis (CAH)

Chronic active hepatitis has been broadly defined as a chronic inflammatory and fibrosing hepatic lesion of varied etiology.[102] It is a serious progressive disorder that often results in cirrhosis or liver failure and death. As indicated, it follows about 5 to 10% of attacks of acute hepatitis B and is an even more frequent sequel to NANB hepatitis, but the exact frequency is uncertain. In one analysis, about 30 to 40% of patients with posttransfusion NANB hepatitis developed CAH.[103] In addition to its viral origin, *CAH may be observed in association with (1) drug toxicity or hypersensitivity, (2) chronic alcohol consumption, (3) Wilson's disease, (4) alpha-1-antitrypsin deficiency, and (5) evidence suggesting "autoimmunity," perhaps better called idiopathic.* The most common drugs implicated are oxyphenisatin, methyldopa, isoniazid, and acetaminophen. It should be noted that hepatitis A has not been known to lead to CAH.

It is not possible on histologic grounds to identify the specific etiology of CAH, except possibly with hepatitis B infection, in which "ground glass" cells are often present. Reliance must be placed on historical, clinical, and serologic evidence. *Only when all known causes have been excluded can the diagnosis of idiopathic CAH be made.* Often, in such circumstances, there are features that suggest autoimmunity. Typically, the patient is a perimenopausal female with some of the following: hypergammaglobulinemia, antinuclear antibodies, rheumatoid factor, a positive LE cell test, antimitochondrial or smooth muscle antibodies (more specifically antiactin antibodies), and defective suppressor T-cell function. Findings such as these gave rise to the designation of this condition as *lupoid hepatitis,* but there is now grave doubt about the validity of a truly autoimmune form of CAH since similar immunologic findings are sometimes present in patients having CAH related to specific etiologies. Better to admit ignorance than invent a "nondisease."[104]

The morphologic changes of CAH are superimposed on those of acute hepatitis, rendered distinctive by (1) a more pronounced portal inflammatory reaction that spills out of the portal tracts; (2) piecemeal necrosis of hepatocytes, principally in the periportal region; (3) bridging necrosis; and (4) progressive periportal fibrosis, leading possibly to cirrhosis.[105] In contrast to classic acute hepatitis, in which the inflammatory reaction is limited to the portal tract, in CAH it floods out into the periportal parenchyma (Fig. 19–15). It is composed mainly of lymphocytes but is heavily admixed with plasma cells (distinctly uncommon in acute hepatitis) and macrophages, with a scattering of neutrophils and eosinophils. Sometimes, lymphoid aggregates, with or without germinal centers, are present in this infiltrate. **Piecemeal necrosis** describes a liver cell undergoing condensation and fragmentation followed by engulfment of the fragments by Kupffer cells and possibly adjacent hepatocytes in which the fragments undergo dissolution. It is proposed that sensitized T cells or K cells on contact with the hepatocyte are responsible for this peculiar pattern of cell destruction, referred to as "apoptosis."[106] In this manner, the periportal hepatocytes are destroyed, giving a moth-eaten appearance to the limiting plate. **Bridging necrosis** is the consequence of destruction of confluent foci of liver cells in adjacent lobules with lysis of the necrotic cells. At first, only a collapsed empty reticulin network and dilated sinusoids remain. This pattern of confluent necrosis occurs most frequently in the central and midzonal regions of the lobule (zones 3 and 2 of the acinus), and by linking up to adjacent areas of necrosis may produce central-central bridging or central-portal bridging, or (rarely) may interconnect portal areas (Fig. 19–16).[107] **Scarring eventually appears; fibrous strands replace the condensed bands of reticulin, and in this manner a cirrhosis develops.** When

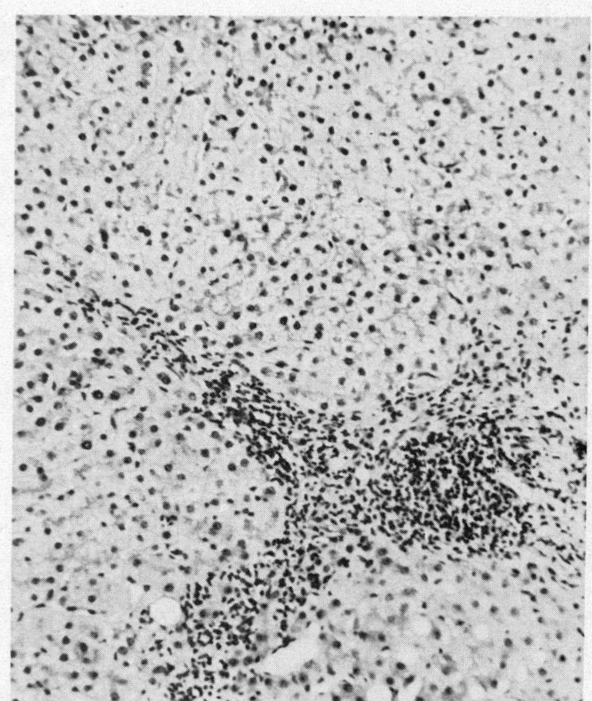

Figure 19–15. Periportal inflammatory infiltrate in developing chronic active hepatitis, spilling out into hepatic parenchyma. (Courtesy of Dr. Hans Popper, The Mount Sinai Medical Center.)

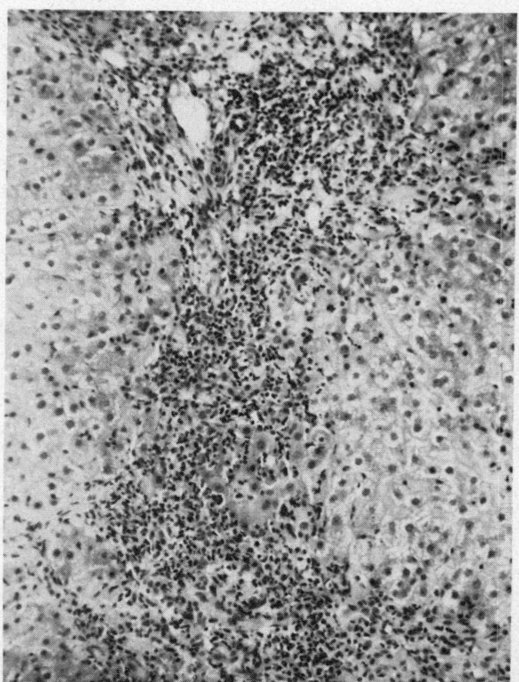

Figure 19–16. Chronic active hepatitis with bridging necrosis. (Courtesy of Dr. Hans Popper, The Mount Sinai Medical Center.)

related to HBV, "ground-glass" cells and "sanded nuclei" are present; their number is inversely related to the aggressiveness of the disease (Fig. 19–17). Additional changes may be present but are not requisite for the diagnosis of CAH. These include cholestasis, evidence of regeneration of liver cells, and hypertrophy and hyperplasia of Kupffer cells, which are often lipofuscin-laden. Sometimes, along with the cholestasis, prominent inflammatory changes appear in the interlobular bile ducts with reactive changes in the lining epithelium. This pattern may be referred to as cholangiolitic CAH.[108]

The clinical diagnosis of CAH is heavily dependent on the liver biopsy and the specific morphologic changes described. Clinical manifestations such as fatigue, malaise, anorexia, and low-grade fever are often not distinctive. However, there is almost always biochemical evidence of parenchymal disease, e.g., elevated serum LDH and transaminases, and sometimes also alkaline phosphatase. Jaundice may be absent, but when present is often mild, persistent, or remitting and relapsing. A history of an antecedent attack of acute hepatitis is obtained in only 30 to 50% of cases. When related to HBV, vasculitis, glomerulonephritis or arthritis may appear, mediated (as described) by circulating immune complexes. Sometimes, CAH only comes to attention when cirrhosis has already developed, by the appearance of ascites, bleeding esophageal varices, and liver failure.

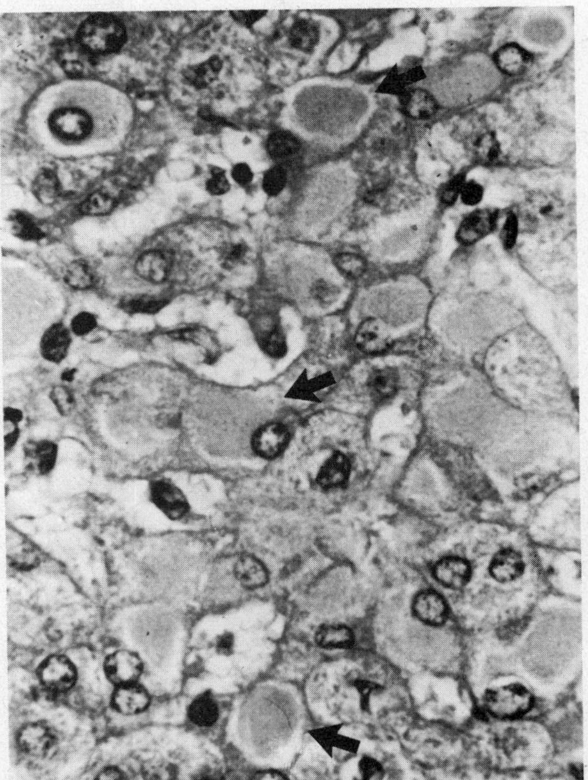

Figure 19–17. Ground-glass hepatocytes (*arrows*) in HBV infection (H and E). (Courtesy of Dr. Hans Popper, The Mount Sinai Medical Center.)

The course and prognosis of this condition is extremely variable and heavily dependent on the etiology and response to therapy. Overall, it tends to pursue a slow, progressive course over a 10- to 20-year period before cirrhosis or hepatic failure terminates it. On the other hand, some patients (spontaneously or with therapy) do much better, and others much worse. A substantial percentage of patients with apparent NANB posttransfusion CAH have improved spontaneously after a year or more. With idiopathic disease having prominent "autoimmune" features, corticosteroids have improved the defect in suppressor cell function and have arrested the condition.[109] The outlook is most uncertain for those with hepatitis B–related disease. When bridging necrosis is present in the liver biopsy, the five-year mortality rate reaches 50%. Whether therapy improves this outlook is still unclear. It should be noted that individuals with HBV-related CAH are at increased risk of hepatocellular carcinoma (p. 935).

SUBMASSIVE-TO-MASSIVE NECROSIS (FULMINANT HEPATITIS)

Submassive-to-massive necrosis of the liver, causing precipitous hepatic failure, is fortunately uncommon. In about 25% of cases it can be related to fulminant viral hepatitis (HBV or NANBV). Only rarely (in less than 1% of cases) is it related to HAV. The most common causes of submassive-to-massive necrosis, accounting for about 40% of cases, are hepatotoxic drugs (detailed later). The remaining cases are either idiopathic or related to exposure to various other hepatotoxins.

This hepatic catastrophe may be precipitated by exposure to carbon tetrachloride, trichloroethylene, yellow phosphorus, and mushroom poisoning (discussed on p. 452). The extent of liver destruction is extremely variable with all the etiologies. In the case of viral infections it appears to depend on the level of the immune response. Ironically, the stronger the immunologic reaction, the greater is the destruction. With drugs and other hepatotoxins the major determinants are intensity and duration of exposure. The previous condition of the liver and the patient's age are also important. Otherwise healthy young adults do better than the aged in whom an element of cardiac decompensation may superimpose hypoxic injury. Depending on these variables, the mortality rate ranges from 25 to 90%. In the usual case, soon after the onset of the necrotizing process hepatic function rapidly deteriorates with deepening jaundice, sometimes complicated by metabolic encephalopathy or renal failure (hepatorenal syndrome). Most ominous is rapid decrease in liver size. When related to viral infection, these manifestations may appear within days of onset of apparent acute hepatitis, but sometimes only weeks later. Even with massive necrosis, most patients survive for days to weeks. By clinical definition, when death occurs within eight weeks of onset of the acute event it is termed "fulminant hepatic failure.[110]

All the causative agents produce essentially identical morphologic changes that vary with the severity of the necrotizing process (submassive to massive) and duration of survival. With all, the pattern of distribution of liver destruction is extremely capricious. The entire liver may be involved or sometimes, for completely obscure reasons, only random asymmetric areas. Thus, the left lobe may be wiped out, curiously sparing the right lobe, or patchy large areas dispersed haphazardly throughout the liver may be affected. Basically, during the early phase there is progressive loss of liver substance. With massive involvement of the entire liver, it shrinks in size over the course of days to as little as 500 to 700 gm and is transformed into a red, limp organ covered by a wrinkled, too large capsule (Fig. 19–18). Blotchy green bile staining may be present. With patchy or asymmetric involvement, affected areas have a similar appearance and are depressed below the level of the spared parenchyma. These necrotic areas are often rimmed by yellow-green discoloration from the progressive accumulation of fat and bile pigment. On transection, necrotic areas have a muddy-red mushy appearance with patchy bile staining.

Histologically, the necrosis may wipe out entire lobules or be less extreme, with destruction of the central and midzonal regions sparing the periphery of the lobule. Presumably, the affected zones are most hypoxic and therefore most vulnerable to further insult. Occasionally, as with phosphorus intoxication, the peripheral zone is principally affected (zone 1 of the acinus), exposed most directly to the blood-borne toxin. **Most often, there is complete destruction of innumerable contiguous lobules with liquefaction of hepatocytes, leaving only collapsed reticulin framework and preserved portal tracts** (Fig. 19–19). Sometimes, for completely unknown reasons, islands of parenchyma are preserved despite massive necrosis of the surrounding liver substance. There may be surprisingly little inflammatory infiltrate with massive destruction, save possibly for an increase in lymphocytes, macrophages and occasional neutrophils within the portal tracts. A scanty inflammatory infiltrate is much more characteristic in the margins of patchy areas of necrosis. With loss of the hepatic parenchyma and shrinkage of the liver, the reticulin framework becomes more condensed and the portal tracts appear to converge.

A number of secondary changes appear when the patient survives for more than a week. Regenerative activity can be seen in surviving hepatocytes, sometimes producing disorganized nodules of parenchyma. With submassive zonal necrosis, the regeneration can be orderly and, in time, may restore the native architecture. Proliferating narrow cords of epithelial cells derived from the ducts of Hering (cholangioles) may appear in the periportal region. The Kupffer cells that survive the necrotizing process also undergo hypertrophy and hyperplasia, and in the course of time become laden with lipofuscin and cellular debris. **With massive necrosis there very often is little or no scarring;** either the patient succumbs or is kept alive by virtue of regeneration of surviving hepatocytes. Scarring is much more likely in those with a protracted course of submassive or patchy necrosis. When the massive necrosis is superimposed upon chronic active viral hepatitis, large tracts of fibrous tissue containing trapped portal triads replace the destroyed parenchyma. To anticipate a later discussion, massive necrosis is then an infrequent antecedent to postnecrotic cirrhosis.

The only happy aspect of this very grave clinical condition is that survivors of massive necrosis related to viral infections almost never become carriers and have lifelong immunity to recurrent infection.

PERICHOLANGITIS AND CHOLANGITIS

An increase in inflammatory cells within the portal tracts (principally about the bile ducts), when unaccom-

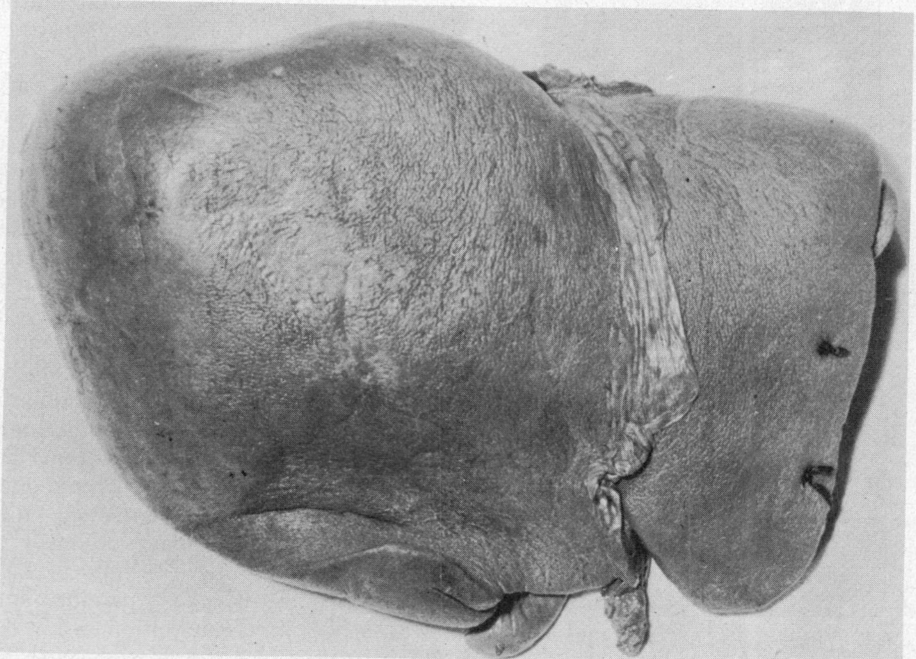

Figure 19–18. Massive necrosis. Liver is small (700 gm), pale, and soft in consistency. Capsule is wrinkled.

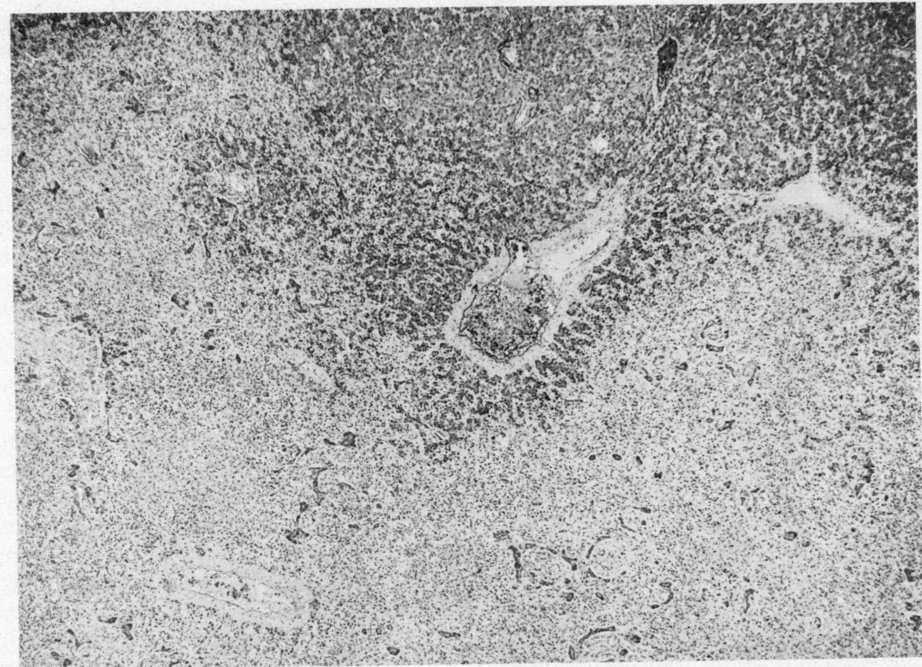

Figure 19–19. Massive necrosis. In lower portion of field, complete necrosis is apparent, with removal of all liver cells in many adjacent liver lobules.

panied by evidence of intraductal inflammatory or parenchymal injury, is referred to as *pericholangitis.* It consists solely of a portal triaditis marked principally by lymphocytes and macrophages with occasional plasma cells, neutrophils, and eosinophils. This is an extremely common anatomic finding and is usually of little or no clinical significance. Infrequently it is associated with fever, mild pruritus, mild jaundice, and modest elevations of alkaline phosphatase.

The genesis of *pericholangitis* is obscure. Its strongest clinical association is with inflammatory bowel disease.[111] It is also encountered in association with blood-borne infection, abdominal sepsis, and pancreatitis. In these settings it is natural to assume that drainage of bacteria, bacterial products, or other toxic substances through the portal system or peribiliary lymphatics underlies the inflammatory changes. The fact that in symptomatic patients antibiotic therapy is usually without benefit argues against direct bacterial infection. The anatomic changes have also been attributed to retention of bile acids, but without substantial evidence. The principal importance of this condition lies in an awareness of it as a possible explanation for mild jaundice and elevated alkaline phosphatase levels in patients with inflammatory bowel disease or significant extrahepatic infections.

Cholangitis implies intraductal inflammation of the extrahepatic or intrahepatic ducts, or more often both. It is marked anatomically by suppuration within the ducts, usually accompanied by bile stasis (Fig. 19–20). Almost always, it is related to some obstructive lesion within the major extrahepatic ducts, usually a gallstone impacted in the common bile duct. Infrequently, cholangitis complicates carcinomas arising in the extrahepatic bile ducts, papilla of Vater, or head of the pancreas; acute pancreatitis; and previous surgical procedures on the bile ducts. With these origins, infection by enteric organisms and, less frequently, staphylococci and strep-

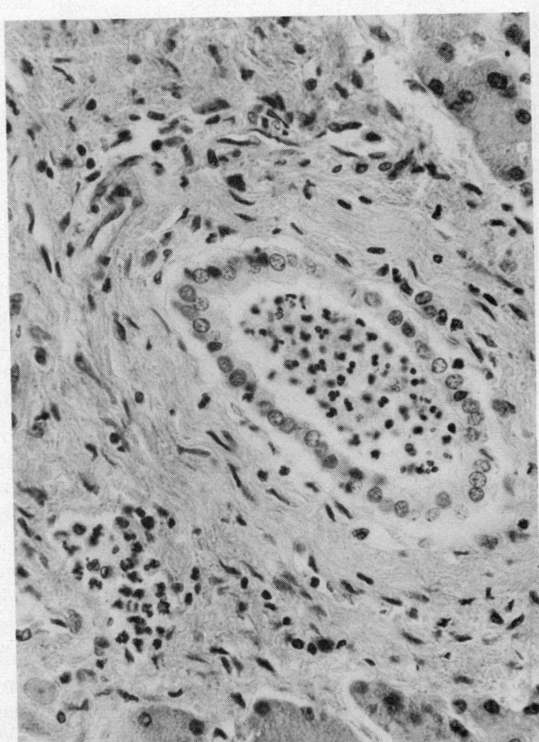

Figure 19–20. Acute cholangitis with neutrophils within a bile duct and in a focus on lower left outside of duct.

tococcal species are the usual causative agents. Almost always the infection begins in the common bile duct or hepatic ducts and progressively ascends into the intrahepatic ramifications *(ascending cholangitis)*. The patient typically has high fever, chills, jaundice, and often a marked peripheral neutrophilia. Surgical drainage of the duct system is often necessary for relief of symptoms, control of infection, and prevention of subsequent liver abscesses.

LIVER ABSCESS

In developed countries, with rare exceptions, liver abscesses are the result of seeding of the hepatic parenchyma by pyogenic organisms (pyogenic liver abscess). In less-developed locales, where parasitic infections are still very common, amebic, echinococcal, and (less commonly) other helminthic or protozoal infections are responsible for a larger percentage. These parasitic infections have already been discussed in Chapter 8. Further comments are limited to pyogenic abscesses. Virtually every known pyogen has, at one time or another, been involved. More often than not, there is a mixed flora.[112] The four most frequent offenders in published series are *E. coli*, Klebsiella, streptococcal species (*S. faecalis*, *S. viridans*, anaerobic, microaerophilic), and staphylococcal species, followed by bacteroides, Proteus species, Pseudomonas species, and fungi.[112] The flora of pyogenic liver abscesses appears to be changing, and at present anaerobes and microaerophilic organisms, particularly bacteroides, and fungi (notably Candida) are increasingly often implicated.[113] Among the many other possible offenders, mention should be made of the actinomyces because of their resistance to antibiotic control, dictating the need for surgical drainage when possible. Not infrequently, no causative agent can be identified, most often because of previous antibiotic therapy, but sometimes because the infection "burns out" or the organism (e.g., an anaerobe or fungus) is difficult to isolate.

The causative agent(s) may reach the liver through a number of pathways. The most common is ascending cholangitis with spread of the infection to the extraductal parenchyma. As indicated, obstruction or stasis within the extrahepatic ducts usually underlies this sequence of events. Next most common is blood-borne seeding of the liver, frequently secondary to acute bacterial endocarditis, but other extrahepatic sites of infection may be involved. In the days before effective antibiotics, intra-abdominal sepsis and pylephlebitis were important antecedents to liver abscesses, but currently they are less often implicated. The uncommon origins of pyogenic abscesses are direct penetration from a nearby infection (empyema of the gallbladder or subdiaphragmatic, subhepatic, and perinephric abscesses); trauma resulting from blunt or penetrating injuries with secondary infection; and preexisting lesions that predispose to bacterial seeding (partially necrotic cancers, echinococcal cysts, or developmental or neoplastic cysts and amebic abscesses).

Little need be said about the morphology of liver abscesses since they do not differ from those in other locations. It is necessary only to point out that in about half of the cases there is a solitary abscess, and in the other half there are multiple abscesses, frequently small and scattered through the liver. Sometimes with ascending cholangitis only one of the hepatic lobes is affected, and perhaps, because of its greater mass, the right more often than the left. Bacteremic spread, pylephlebitis, and biliary tract disease tend to produce multiple small abscesses, whereas trauma and direct penetration often cause solitary, or at most few, lesions that sometimes are very large (over 5 cm in diameter).

Liver abscesses are serious clinical problems and, in addition to producing symptoms and signs of systemic infection and sometimes jaundice, directly lead to death in about 40% of cases.[114] Contributing to the mortality is the nature of the underlying disease; the age of the patient (over 40); concomitant infection elsewhere; and impaired immunity (from immunosuppressive therapy following transplantation or antineoplastic drugs for leukemia or cancer). However, liver abscesses may occur at any age and against widely varying backgrounds. They may be amenable to antibiotic control, but in their lush havens the organisms are often difficult to eradicate, and resort must be made to drainage when the lesions are sufficiently large and not too numerous.[115] Among the many possible diagnostic approaches, ultrasonography, angiography, and CT scan have proved remarkably effective in the localization of lesions sometimes smaller than 2 cm in diameter.

DRUG-RELATED INJURY

Adverse drug reactions, as noted on page 443, have wide-ranging consequences, one of which is liver injury. Drug reactions are said to be responsible for about 2% of all cases of jaundice in general hospital populations[116] and for many more in hospitalized geriatric populations. Moreover, they grow ever more frequent; in one study in Japan, ten times as many cases of drug-related hepatic injury were reported in the years 1964 to 1973 as in the previous decade—perhaps the price that must be paid for medical progress.[117] No attempt will be made to provide a definitive compilation of implicated drugs. Instead, there follows an overview of the mechanisms of drug-related injury, the resultant morphologic patterns of hepatic reaction, and the most common agents implicated in their causation. Far more complete coverage is readily available.[118–120]

PATHOGENESIS. The hepatotoxicity of therapeutic agents is rarely the direct effect of the drug itself on the liver cell. Two independent but perhaps at times cooperative mechanisms are involved: (1) *biotransformation of the drug takes place in the liver with the formation of toxic metabolites; or (2) the drug or, more likely, one of its metabolites serves as a hapten to convert an intracellular protein into an immunogenic molecule.* The former pathway is said to be *"direct" hepatotoxicity*, and so the latter constitutes *"indirect" hepatotoxicity.*

The hepatotoxicity of certain therapeutic agents can be clearly related to one or the other of these pathways, but often the issue is unclear.[121] For example, there is substantial documentation that the toxic effects of acetaminophen and isoniazid on the liver are exerted directly by biochemical metabolites of the drugs. On the other hand, controversy still persists as to whether many agents, such as halothane, are direct hepatotoxins or whether they mediate their effects through a hypersensitivity reaction. It is not necessary to delve deeply into the details of the metabolic biochemical transformation, except to point out that most drugs are metabolized in the liver by the mixed-function oxidase system. The emergence of toxic metabolites involves the formation of potent alkylating or acylating agents that bind covalently to hepatocyte macromolecules critical to the viability of the cell. You may recall that this same enzyme system is involved in the metabolism of a variety of other substances such as alcohol, phenobarbital, carbon tetrachloride, and carcinogenic hydrocarbons. Thus, prolonged exposure to, say, alcohol or phenobarbital leads to an adaptive increase in the functional capacity of the enzyme system referred to as induction, enhancing possibly the formation of hepatotoxic metabolites. However, there may be competition for enzyme-binding sites in liver cells, and the competitive inhibition may slow the rate of metabolic biotransformation. Which of these two processes predominates is a function of level of drug and level of enzyme induction. Still another factor is important in "direct" hepatotoxicity. There is usually an abundant supply within the liver cell of substances such as glutathione capable of preferentially conjugating drug metabolites to render them nontoxic, water soluble, and excretable in the urine. Prolonged exposure to large doses of a drug-derived hepatotoxin or preexisting diffuse liver disease may deplete the glutathione supply and so enhance the injury-producing potential of an agent. Recognition of this detoxification mechanism has made possible the use of certain precursors of glutathione as an antidote, particularly for acetaminophen.[122] The amount of damage produced by direct hepatotoxic agents is thus influenced by many variables, but perhaps most important is intensity of exposure. *Direct-acting therapeutic agents, also referred to as "predictable hepatotoxins," are characterized by (1) dose dependency, (2) the causation of injury in more than 1% of recipients, (3) a relatively short interval between drug ingestion and the adverse reaction, and (4) the induction of similar hepatic changes in laboratory animals.*

The other possible mechanism of hepatic injury is the induction of an allergic or hypersensitivity reaction. Drugs in general are small molecules and are therefore likely to be antigenic only as haptens covalently bound to carrier-macromolecules. For the most part, the haptens are the electrophilic reactive metabolites capable of binding cellular macromolecules. Individual hypersensitivity plays a large role in this form of hepatotoxicity.[123] Characteristic of so-called "unpredictable hepatotoxins" are *(1) lack of dose dependency of the liver injury; (2) a delay between exposure and the hepatic reaction; (3) a low percentage (less than 1%) of recipients being affected; (4) frequency of other allergic manifestations, e.g., fever, skin rash, and eosinophilia; and (5) heightened reactivity with rechallenge by the agent.* However, there are many instances of unpredictable adverse reactions that do not fulfill all these criteria, and unpredictability does not necessarily prove hypersensitivity; thus, the concept of individual idiosyncrasy has been invoked. For example, the anesthetic halothane is a well-recognized hepatotoxin that sometimes causes massive liver necrosis.[124] The cited frequencies of such adverse reactions have ranged from one in 6000 to one in 110,000 exposures. In most instances the hepatotoxicity appeared after some delay on second or third exposure of the patient to the anesthetic, making it natural to assume sensitization. Lymphocytes derived from these patients have elaborated migration inhibition factor on exposure to liver homogenates that have been obtained from rabbits pretreated with halothane.[125] One brave anesthetist, who suspected personal sensitivity to the agent, intentionally reexposed himself to a very small amount of halothane and developed recurrent, but fortunately nonfatal, hepatic injury.[126] Despite all this documentation of presumed hypersensitivity, liver damage has occurred in patients within a few days of *first exposure;* thus, the monumental controversy continues—allergy or individual idiosyncrasy.[127] Unfortunately, not enough is known about most agents to determine the means by which they induce liver injury, but some clearly fall into the category of direct predictable hepatoxins, as will be seen.

Adverse drug reactions cause an astonishing range of hepatic lesions. They are cited in Table 19–3 together with the major implicated agents.[128] Certain agents are involved in a variety of morphologic reactions: halothane, isoniazid, and acetaminophen, for example, may cause spotty centrilobular or submassive-to-massive necrosis, depending on dosage and host vulnerability. Analogously, alpha-methyldopa may be responsible for acute-to-chronic hepatitis or sometimes massive necrosis. Even with the major offenders that would be characterized as predictable hepatotoxins—acetaminophen, isoniazid, methotrexate, methyldopa, and chlorpromazine—individual susceptibility is still involved. Thus, the dosage level required to induce an adverse hepatic reaction is extremely variable and cannot be foreseen. The term "predictable," then, serves only as a warning. The ingestion of about 10 gm of acetaminophen, for example, will quite reliably induce hepatic necrosis.

Only a few comments are necessary on the morphology of liver reactions since they replicate quite faithfully lesions of other origins. Uncomplicated "pure" cholestasis is produced by methyltestosterone, oral contraceptives, and estrogens; it is unaccompanied by hepatocyte injury or inflammatory changes. A variety of hepatotoxins may cause centrilobular necrosis (Fig. 19–21). The *fatty changes induced by tetracycline* are virtually identical to those seen in pregnancy and Reye's syndrome. The fat accumulates in cytoplasmic micro-

Table 19–3. DRUG-INDUCED HEPATIC DISEASE

Pattern of Reaction	Drug Implicated
"Pure" Cholestasis	C-17 alkylated steroids (anabolic, contraceptive) Estrogens
Cholestasis with Hepatocyte Injury	Chlorpromazine Erythromycin Some oral antidiabetics Some antithyroid drugs 6-Mercaptopurine ? Azathioprine Para-aminosalicylic acid Sulfonamides
Fatty Change (Steatosis)	Tetracycline Methotrexate (usually with hepatocyte necrosis)
Zonal (Centrilobular) Necrosis	Halothane Acetaminophen Salicylates Phenacetin Isoniazid
Submassive-to-Massive Necrosis	Halothane Isoniazid α-Methyldopa Acetaminophen Iproniazid
Acute Hepatitis	Halothane Isoniazid Iproniazid Phenytoin Salicylates
Chronic Persistent Hepatitis	α-Methyldopa Oxyphenisatin Isoniazid Salicylates
Chronic Active Hepatitis	α-Methyldopa
Cirrhosis	Drugs causing acute or chronic active hepatitis Methotrexate
Budd-Chiari Syndrome	? Oral contraceptives Pyrrolizidine alkaloids (bush tea) Urethane
Peliosis Hepatis	C-17 Alkylated steroids (anabolic, contraceptive)
Granulomas	Phenylbutazone Sulfonamides α-Methyldopa
Adenoma of Liver	C-17 Alkylated steroids (anabolic, contraceptive)
Focal Nodular Hyperplasia	Oral contraceptives
Hepatocellular carcinoma	C-17 Alkylated steroids (anabolic, contraceptive)

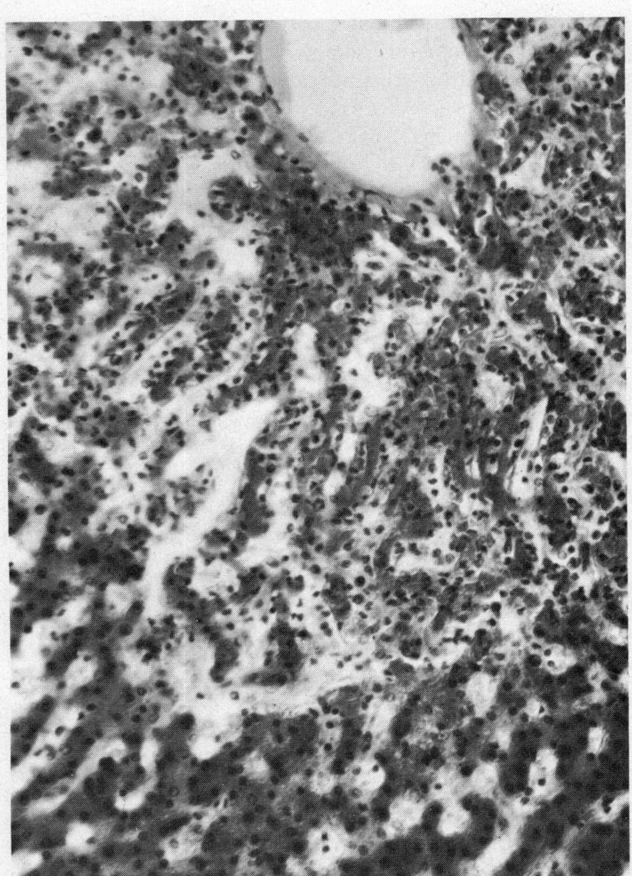

Figure 19–21. Central necrosis. Liver cells adjacent to central vein are necrotic and surrounded by polymorphonuclear infiltrate.

vacuoles throughout the hepatocyte, often without displacement of the nucleus (see Fig. 19–42).[129] Hepatocyte necrosis is rarely evident, but the rapid deterioration of liver function and poor prognosis underline the gravity of tetracycline toxicity. *Adverse drug reactions recapitulate the entire spectrum of liver disease associated with viral hepatitis.* Chlorpromazine may produce "pure" cholestasis (alone), but more often there is portal inflammation and spotty hepatocyte necrosis. Indeed, in some instances the changes are indistinguishable from those of acute viral hepatitis. *Peliosis hepatis* is an uncommon and distinctive lesion characterized by blood-filled spaces scattered randomly through the hepatic substance. The individual lesions range from 1 mm to 4 cm in diameter, and are lined by hepatocytes and occasionally spindled fibroblastic or endothelial cells. These strange abnormalities sometimes develop following chronic exposure to C-17 alkylated steroids, both anabolic and contraceptive.[130] Their genesis is unknown but it may involve aneurysmal sinusoidal dilatation. Although usually incidental, the blood-filled spaces have been known to rupture when superficial and cause massive, even fatal, hemoperitoneum.[130] As indicated in Table 19–3, focal nodular regeneration and benign and malignant tumors of the liver have also been associated with the use of therapeutic agents, although the evidence relating to tumors is somewhat controversial. It is clear that the possibility of an adverse drug reaction must be kept in mind with a variety of hepatic disorders lest the opportunity be missed to effect a cure by simple withdrawal of a drug.

CIRRHOSIS

Every physician knows what is meant by the term "cirrhosis," but there is no universally accepted definition. However, there is agreement that *cirrhosis is a generic term for a hepatic disease of varied etiology (e.g., alcohol abuse, iron overload, drugs, chronic active hepatitis)* having the following characteristics:[131]

1. The architecture of the *total* liver is disorganized by interconnecting fibrous scars formed in response to hepatocytic injury and loss.
2. The fibrosis may take the form of delicate bands (portal-central, portal-portal, or both) but may constitute broad scars replacing multiple adjacent lobules.
3. Parenchymal nodules are created by the regenerative activity and network of scars. The nodules vary in size, depending on causation, from micronodules (less than 3 mm in diameter) to macronodules (3 mm to several centimeters in diameter).
4. The parenchymal architecture is generally disorganized within micronodules, i.e., loss of central veins and single-cell parenchymal cords, but in the macronodular pattern recognizable lobules may persist.

A number of secondary changes follow. Usually there is some evidence of cholestasis. Abnormal vascular connections develop in the fibrous scars between the portal, arterial, and venous systems that, to an extent, bypass the hepatic parenchyma. A mononuclear inflammatory infiltrate is usual within the portal tracts and scars, but is of variable intensity among the different forms of cirrhosis. Depending on the particular type and duration of the cirrhosis, there may be proliferation of cholangioles.

Cirrhosis, most of it related to alcohol abuse, ranks among the ten leading causes of death in many countries of the Western world, including the United States. Among those 25 to 65 years of age in the U.S., it is the third leading cause of death.[132] All forms of cirrhosis, whatever their origins, are chronic progressive disorders, largely because the causation cannot be controlled in most instances. Most of the fatalities over the span of years result from liver failure or one of the consequences of portal hypertension related to the extensive scarring and nodularity. There is, however, experimental and some scanty clinical evidence that the collagenous scarring is not irreversible.[133] In all scars, collagen is in a constant state of turnover. With control of the underlying cause of the cirrhosis, regression of the fibrous septa has been reported, notably in the pigment cirrhosis caused by iron overload.[134] However, with few other forms of cirrhosis can the direct cause of the liver injury be controlled as effectively. It remains to be proved that abstinence from alcohol will stem the onward march of cirrhosis in chronic alcoholics once it has become established.

There is no satisfactory classification of cirrhosis. An etiologic approach suffers from a lack of knowledge about the precise causes of all forms of cirrhosis. The pathogenesis frequently is no longer evident at the time of examination. Moreover, the morphology is not always distinctive and undergoes change with progression of the condition. Thus, it has been proposed that *cirrhosis be divided simply into two large categories: (1) micronodular, in which the preponderance of parenchymal nodules are less than 3 mm in diameter; and (2) macronodular, in which most of the nodules exceed 3 mm in diameter.* Appealing as such simplification may be, it is purely descriptive and offers no guidelines for clinical management. Accordingly, resort will be made to the historically sanctified classification drawing on both putative etiologies and presumed pathogenesis. An approximate frequency of each category in the Western world is included.

Alcoholic cirrhosis	30–70%
Postnecrotic cirrhosis	10–50%
Biliary cirrhosis (primary and secondary)	10%
Pigment cirrhosis (in hemochromatosis)	5%
Cirrhosis associated with Wilson's disease	rare
Cirrhosis associated with alpha-1-antitrypsin deficiency	rare
Cryptogenic cirrhosis	15–60%

Not included in the above classification are the very infrequent types of cirrhosis associated with chronic right heart failure (cardiac cirrhosis); galactosemia; diffuse infiltrative cancers of the liver (carcinomatous cirrhosis); and syphilis (congenital and tertiary). Also not included is *Indian childhood cirrhosis*, encountered principally in India, Southeast Asia, and the Middle East, which partakes of the morphologic features of cirrhosis associated with chronic active hepatitis and alcoholic cirrhosis.[135] In passing, it might be noted that this obscure disorder has also been related to copper toxicity.[136]

All forms of cirrhosis may lead to certain clinical manifestations that are usually most marked in the alcoholic form. Palmar erythema, spider angiomas (usually most visible over the chest), gynecomastia, gonadal atrophy, amenorrhea, and changes in the distribution of body hair are all attributed to hyperestrinism secondary to impaired hepatic metabolism of estrogens. However, with chronic exposure to alcohol a direct effect on pituitary-gonadal function may also contribute.[137] Dupuytren's contracture of the palmar fascia and finger clubbing develop infrequently, for poorly understood reasons. When the liver disease is advanced there is not only impaired synthesis of albumin, but also fibrinogen, prothrombin, and coagulant factors V, VII, IX, and X. Although some of these changes may have serious consequences such as a bleeding diathesis, they are significant for the most part as clinical clues to the presence of advanced liver disease and cirrhosis. Sometimes renal failure (the hepatorenal syndrome) complicates the course. Were these problems not sufficient, the alcoholic with or without cirrhosis also has an increased frequency of acute gastritis and peptic ulcers. Portal hypertension, however, is the most serious consequence of cirrhosis of the liver, and plays an important role in the life or death of the patient.

PORTAL HYPERTENSION

Pressure in any vascular system can only be elevated by either an increase in blood flow or an increase in resistance to outflow. With rare exceptions, *portal hypertension is related to increased resistance to outflow.* The only significant cause of increased flow into the portal venous system is massive splenomegaly, such as is encountered in some of the hematologic disorders. Here the organ enlargement creates an arteriovenous fistula that shunts blood into the splenic vein. *The causes of increased resistance to flow fall into three categories: (1) posthepatic, (2) prehepatic, and (3) intrahepatic.* The *major posthepatic causes of portal hypertension* are severe right-sided heart failure, Budd-Chiari syndrome and constrictive pericarditis. The major *prehepatic origins* constitute thrombosis or narrowing (as by cancers) of the portal vein before it ramifies within the liver. The dominant *intrahepatic cause* is cirrhosis and, far less frequently, schistosomiasis, massive fatty change, and diffuse fibrosing granulomatous disease such as sarcoidosis and miliary tuberculosis. Despite all these possibilities, *unless proved otherwise, portal hypertension implies cirrhosis of the liver.* Although more complex explanations have been offered, the elevation of the portal pressure is mainly attributable to compression of sinusoids and central veins by the fibrous scarring and regenerative nodules, and the development of arteriovenous anastomoses within the scars bringing to bear hepatic arterial pressure on the portal circulation.[138] *Four major clinical consequences follow:* (1) *ascites;* (2) *the formation of portosystemic venous shunts, particularly in the submucosa of the esophagus and stomach (gastroesophageal varices);* (3) *progressive enlargement of the spleen—congestive splenomegaly; and* (4) *occasionally hepatic (metabolic) encephalopathy secondary to the diffuse parenchymal damage and portosystemic shunting.*

ASCITES. Ascites refers to the collection of excess fluid in the peritoneal cavity. It usually becomes clinically detectable when 500 ml has accumulated, but many liters may collect, causing abdominal distention. It is generally a serous fluid having less than 3 gm per 100 ml of protein (largely albumin) as well as the same concentrations of solutes, such as glucose, sodium, and potassium as the blood. Thus, withdrawal of large volumes of ascitic fluid for relief of symptoms invokes a substantial loss of protein and solutes. The fluid may also contain a scant number of mesothelial cells and mononuclear leukocytes. The presence of neutrophils suggests secondary infection; red cells, on the other hand, suggest other origins of the fluid such as disseminated intra-abdominal cancer. Sequestration of large volumes of fluid in the peritoneal cavity is often accompanied by peripheral edema and decreased urine volume.

The pathogenesis of ascites is complex and not entirely understood. Four factors contribute in varying degrees to its development:

(1) *Elevated pressure within the portal venous system.* The role of portal hypertension is curiously enigmatic. On the one hand, individuals with thrombosis of the main portal vein rarely develop ascites, but on the other hand, decompression of the portal system by a portacaval anastomosis often relieves the ascites. Most likely, portal hypertension together with decreased plasma colloid oncotic pressure increases the formation of interstitial fluid in the splanchnic bed, which is followed by seepage of fluid from overloaded lymphatics.

(2) *Decreased plasma colloid oncotic pressure.* Hypoalbuminemia often develops with cirrhosis because of hemodilution, impaired synthesis in the liver, and loss of albumin into the ascitic fluid. The lowered plasma colloid oncotic pressure contributes to the expansion of the interstitial fluid compartment, with secondary increased lymph flow and seepage.

(3) *Increased formation of hepatic lymph.* Distortion and blockage of the hepatic sinusoids and lymphatics along with the hypoalbuminemia accounts for a considerable amount of seepage of lymph fluid through the capsule of the liver. Thus, in contrast to portal vein thrombosis, hepatic vein thrombosis as well as cirrhosis is frequently marked by ascites.

(4) *Secondary hyperaldosteronism and sodium retention.* For uncertain reasons, although it is sometimes attributed to sequestration of a large volume of blood within the splanchnic bed, the effective circulating blood volume is reduced with decreased renal blood flow and secondary hyperaldosteronism (p. 1240). Impaired hepatic metabolism of aldosterone aggravates the situation. Thus comes about sodium retention and the train of sequelae described in the formation of edema (p. 86), with increased loss of fluid through the lymphatics and peritoneal surfaces.

PORTOSYSTEMIC SHUNTS (COLLATERAL CHANNELS). With the rise in pressure, portal vein bypasses develop wherever the systemic and portal circulations share common capillary beds. Principal sites are: veins around and within the rectum (hemorrhoids); the cardioesophageal junction (esophagogastric varices (Fig. 19–22)); the retroperitoneum; and the falciform ligament of the liver (periumbilical or abdominal wall collaterals). The hemorrhoids are indistinguishable from those encountered in noncirrhotic persons, but serve as a possible clinical clue to the liver disease. Hemorrhoidal bleeding may occur but is rarely massive or life threatening. Much more important are the esophagogastric varices (see p. 802) that appear in about 65% of patients with advanced cirrhosis of the liver, and cause massive hematemesis and death in about half of these. Abdominal wall collaterals appear as dilated subcutaneous veins that extend from the umbilicus toward the rib margins *(caput medusae).* These tortuous dilated channels constitute an important clinical hallmark of portal hypertension.

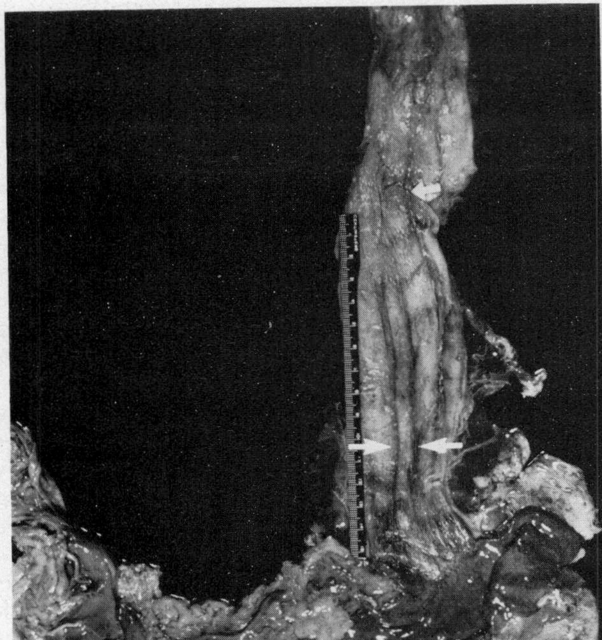

Figure 19–22. Esophageal varices. Dilated submucosal veins (*arrows*) in lower portion of esophagus in a patient with advanced alcoholic cirrhosis.

SPLENOMEGALY. Long-standing congestion may cause congestive splenomegaly (p. 700). The degree of enlargement varies widely up to 1000 gm and is not necessarily correlated with other features of portal hypertension. Massive splenomegaly may secondarily induce a variety of hematologic abnormalities attributed to hypersplenism (p. 699).

HEPATIC (METABOLIC) ENCEPHALOPATHY. This serious neurologic disorder has already been described (p. 893). Although it may appear with hepatic failure from any cause, it is particularly associated with advanced cirrhosis because of the diffuse parenchymal damage and portosystemic shunting.

After this general overview of the clinical consequences of cirrhosis we can turn to the specific types.

ALCOHOLIC LIVER DISEASE AND CIRRHOSIS

Chronic excessive consumption of ethanol may lead to fatty liver (steatosis), alcoholic hepatitis, and alcoholic cirrhosis (also known as Laennec's cirrhosis and cirrhosis of alcohol abuse). Any of these entities may be complicated by one or both of the other two and so may coexist in the liver, but *there is a growing conviction that fatty liver, alcoholic hepatitis, and alcoholic cirrhosis are separate and not necessarily interdependent entities.* Both short-term and long-term exposure to alcohol regularly induces a fatty liver, which, in time and with continued excessive intake of ethanol, may be followed by cirrhosis. However, fatty change by itself is a reversible condition with cessation of exposure to alcohol. It is relevant, for example, that the fatty liver of kwashiorkor, marked obesity, and diabetes is not followed by cirrhosis.[139] Thus, it is believed that the fat and the cirrhogenic process are separate independent consequences of chronic alcoholism. The place of alcoholic hepatitis in this spectrum is murkier. As the term implies, it represents an acute form of liver damage associated with spotty necrosis of hepatocytes as well as other changes (to be detailed later) that produce clinical manifestations reminiscent of acute viral hepatitis. The genesis of this condition is not clear but it is commonly associated with bouts of heavy drinking.[140] Although fat is often present in livers with alcoholic hepatitis, there is no known correlation between the fat and the acute hepatitis. More controversial is the role of the hepatitis in the development of cirrhosis.[141] Individuals with alcoholic cirrhosis may or may not have a history of overt bouts of acute hepatitis. Certainly, evidence of alcoholic hepatitis is more frequently absent than present in developed cirrhosis, and moreover does not appear during the evolution of alcohol-induced cirrhosis in baboons.[142] Thus, although episodes of hepatitis may contribute to the fibrous scarring of alcoholic cirrhosis, they are not thought to be requisite since there are other mechanisms of alcohol-related fibrogenesis. It seems best, then, to consider the three types of liver change as independent consequences of excessive exposure to ethanol.

EPIDEMIOLOGY. Alcoholic cirrhosis accounts for about 60 to 70% of all cirrhosis in North, South, and Central America as well as in many parts of Western Europe, notably France. It is much less frequent, at least presently, in other parts of the world. In the high-prevalence areas of the world it is one of the ten leading causes of death, climbing ever higher in rank order with the passing years. In the United States the number of deaths from cirrhosis increased more than 70% between 1950 and 1974, and a similar trend has been reported from Canada.[143] Although this condition was once preponderantly a disease of males, more females are now developing it, and the male:female ratio of deaths now stands at about 2:1. The peak incidence is in the fifth decade, but alcoholic liver disease and cirrhosis may appear in early adult life. Alcoholic abuse and liver disease are traditionally associated with lower socioeconomic status; in a recent report, however, alcoholism was four times more prevalent among Scottish doctors than in less well-educated members of the community.[144]

Numerous clinical and epidemiologic studies have attempted to establish a "safe" upper limit of daily alcohol consumption. At one time it was contended that up to 160 gm of alcohol per day incurred little or no risk (10 gm of alcohol is equivalent to 1 oz of 86-proof beverage). However, it is now thought that chronic daily intake in excess of 60 to 80 gm for men and 20 gm for women over a period of years incurs a significant risk of cirrhosis.[145] Most patients with alcoholic cirrhosis have consumed about 190 to 200 gm daily for over ten years, *yet only 10 to 20% of heavy drinkers develop alcoholic cirrhosis, about 30% develop alcoholic hepatitis, and half have no significant liver damage.*[146] Individual, possibly genetic, susceptibility must therefore exist. Associations between certain HLA profiles have been claimed, but they vary among geographic locales (B8 in Britain, B13 in Chile, and DW40 in Norway) and are of uncertain importance.[147] In the last analysis, the death rate from alcoholic cirrhosis in various populations correlates quite well with per capita alcohol consumption irrespective of the type of beverage used. Rationing of wine in France between 1941 and 1947 led to an 80% reduction in mortality from cirrhosis.

MORPHOLOGY. In view of the present belief that fatty liver, alcoholic hepatitis, and alcoholic cirrhosis do not necessarily constitute a continuum, they will be described separately, noting features of possible progression from one to the other.

Fatty liver (steatosis) is the earliest, almost inevitable consequence of alcoholism. At the outset, the accumulation of fat does not differ from that encountered in other clinical settings, as described on page 18. At first, the vacuoles are small and distributed throughout the cytoplasm. (Fig. 19–23). **With progressive accumulation, however, they coalesce, creating large cleared spaces that enlarge and virtually transform the cell into a lipocyte with compressed, peripherally displaced nucleus.** Concomitant retention of proteins normally secreted by hepatocytes adds to the cellular enlargement.[148] In the alcoholic patient, the accumulation of fat and protein may be considerable, creating massive, soft, yellow, greasy livers weighing up to 4 to 6 kg. Rupture and coalescence of adjacent expanded cells may produce so-called microscopic fatty cysts. Cholestatic changes may appear with bile droplets within hepatocytes and bile plugs within canaliculi.

Ultrastructural changes can be seen in the liver cells within two days in well-nourished, nonalcoholic human volunteers administered large amounts of ethanol for short periods of time (as detailed later) even before the first appearance of fat.[149] Most prominent are enlargement and distortion of mitochondria accompanied by vesiculation and reduplication of the smooth endoplasmic reticulum. After eight days, giant mitochondria develop as well as focal cytoplasmic degradation and autophagic vacuoles, but by this time there are also fat vacuoles. Similar changes are evident in ethanol-fed baboons.[150] **Despite the ultrastructural evidence of cell injury and even massive fat accumulation, the morphologic changes are entirely reversible if further exposure to alcohol ceases and a normal diet is resumed.**

Additional changes appear in some fatty livers, which have been interpreted as warnings of the possible onset of cirrhosis. These include (1) delicate fibrosis about central veins, sinusoids, and hepatocytic cords; (2) marked accumulation of fat in the Ito cells within the spaces of Disse; and (3) hypertrophy and hyperplasia of mononuclear sinusoidal cells. Among these changes, greatest significance is accorded the fibrosing reaction about the central veins. Serial liver biopsies of ethanol-fed baboons have revealed that cirrhosis develops only in those having perivenular sclerosis

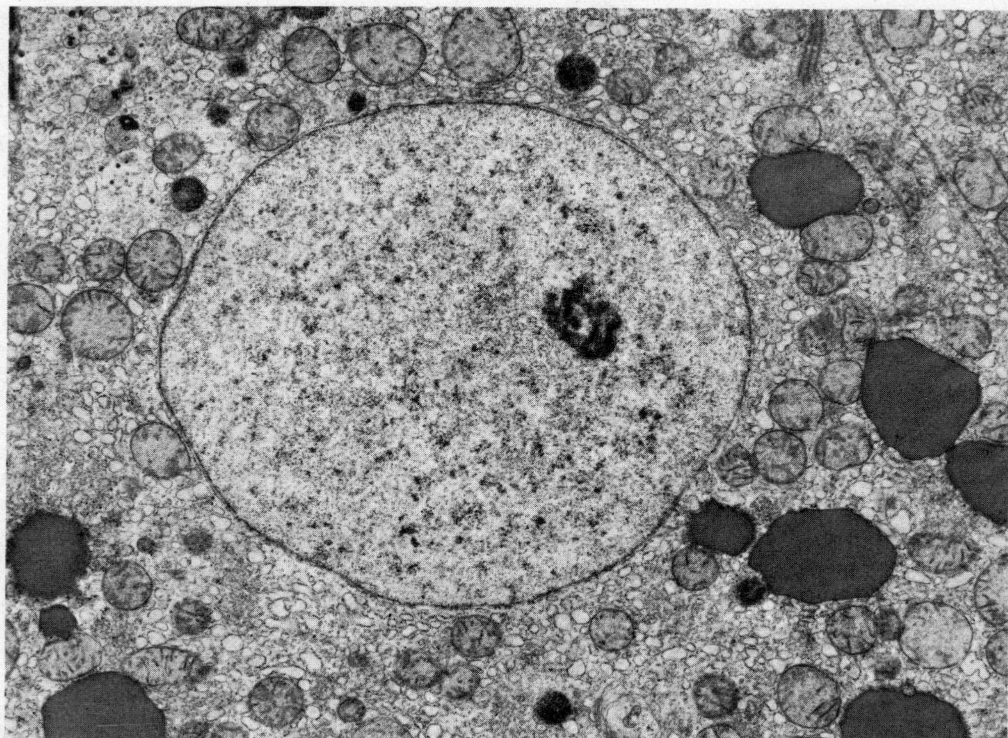

Figure 19–23. Liver cell in male rats maintained for seven days on nutritionally adequate diet in which ethanol isocalorically replaces sucrose up to 36% of total calories. Early changes comprise the appearance of fat vacuoles (dark inclusions), slight vesiculation of endoplasmic reticulum, and slight swelling of mitochondria. (Courtesy of Dr. O. Iseri, Mallory Institute of Pathology.)

in earlier biopsies.[150] A similar sequence has been observed in serial biopsies from chronic alcoholics. Thus, it is proposed (not without contention) that pericellular, perisinusoidal, and particularly perivenular delicate fibrosis constitute precirrhotic changes.[151]

Alcoholic hepatitis may appear in the precirrhotic or cirrhotic liver but almost always is accompanied by some fatty change. The hepatitis, initially centrilobular (zone 3 of the acinus), is marked principally by **(1) swelling of hepatocytes; (2) necrosis of single random cells; (3) infiltration of neutrophils about foci of necrosis; and (4) in most instances, alcoholic hyalin or Mallory bodies within swollen or necrosing liver cells.**[152] The enlargement of hepatocytes is related to hydropic distention of endoplasmic reticulum, the accumulation of fat, and the retention of proteins. Individual ballooned cells become necrotic and are often replaced by clusters of neutrophils, admixed with occasional lymphocytes and macrophages. **Alcoholic hyalin** (Mallory body) appears in swollen hepatocytes, sometimes in cells already partially or completely necrotic. In routine tissue stains it takes the form of cytoplasmic, eosinophilic, waxlike droplets that may coalesce to form tangled perinuclear skeins (Fig. 19–24). Ultrastructurally the hyalin is composed of closely aggregated, intermediate filaments yielding positive reactions to cytokeratin by immunocytochemical methods (Fig. 19–25).[153] The designation "Mallory body" may be preferable to "alcoholic hyalin" since it can also be seen in other forms of liver disease, including primary biliary cirrhosis, Wilson's disease, Indian childhood cirrhosis, hepatocellular carcinoma, and others.[154] The inflammatory necrotizing parenchymal injury is usually associated with prominent cholestasis. In severe cases the alcoholic hepatitis

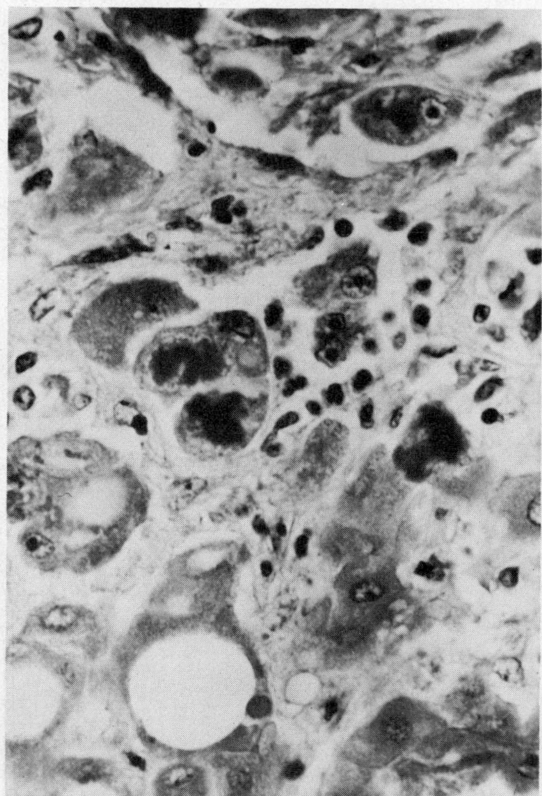

Figure 19–24. Alcoholic hepatitis. Numerous dark Mallory bodies are seen within both vital and disintegrating hepatocytes.

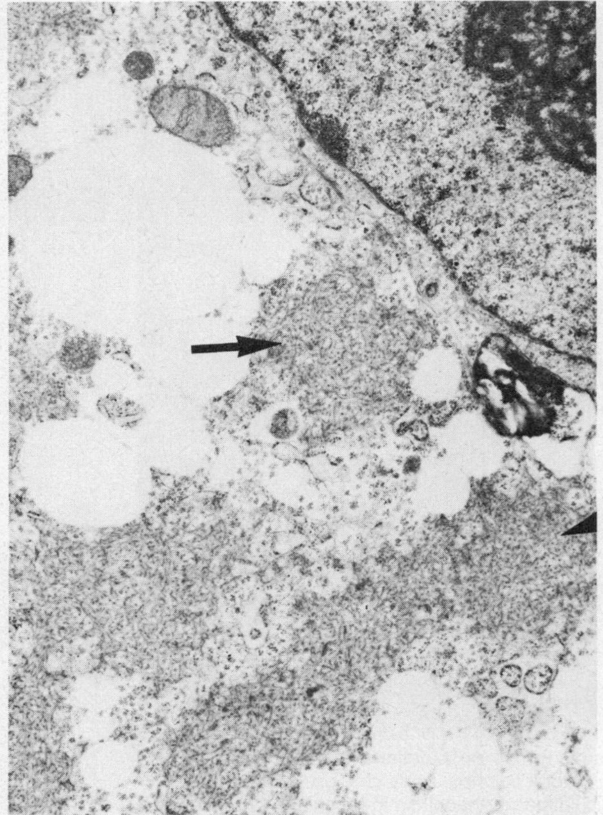

Figure 19–25. Electron microscopic detail of a liver cell revealing closely packed filaments of alcoholic hyalin (*arrows*) as well as large, cleared lipid vacuoles. (Courtesy of Dr. Marcel Seiler, Pathology Department, West Roxbury VA Hospital, Harvard Medical School, Boston.)

may extend throughout the lobule, with accentuation of the inflammatory infiltrate.

The relationship of alcoholic hepatitis to the later development of cirrhosis, as mentioned, is still controversial. Acute and recurrent bouts of hepatitis may subside with regeneration of lost cells, leaving no residuals. In one serial biopsy study, however, most patients with *persistent* alcoholic hepatitis and continuing chronic alcoholism later developed cirrhosis.[155] **Thus, on the one hand, protracted alcoholic hepatitis may predispose to the development of alcoholic cirrhosis, but on the other hand, cirrhosis may develop, as it does in alcohol-fed baboons, without the intervention of alcoholic hepatitis.**[142]

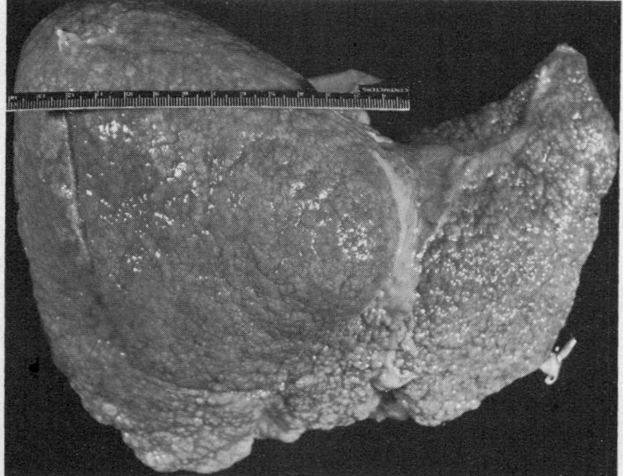

Figure 19–26. Alcoholic cirrhosis at an intermediate stage. Liver is enlarged, contains fat, and has a well-developed micronodular pattern.

Alcoholic cirrhosis begins as a large, fatty, micronodular liver (usually weighing over 2 kg) that is transformed over the span of years, into a shrunken, nonfatty, macronodular cirrhotic liver (sometimes less than 1 kg in weight) (Fig. 19–26). **There is generally an inverse relationship between the amount of fat and the amount of fibrous scarring.** Early in the course of the cirrhogenic process, a faintly perceptible nodularity is evident both on the surface and on transection. The fibrous septa are delicate and extend from central vein to portal regions as well as from portal tract to portal tract. Thus, individual lobules are dissected, which accounts for the micronodular pattern. The parenchyma within the nodules is extensively fatty and disorganized as regeneration transforms the normal liver cords into irregular aggregates. Because of their fat content, the nodules and the liver are tawny-yellow, from which the term "cirrhosis" derives. The changes of alcoholic hepatitis (in particular, liver cell necrosis and Mallory bodies) and bile stasis may or may not be present.

As the scarring increases with time, the nodularity becomes more prominent, and scattered nodules enlarge because of regenerative activity, creating a so-called "hobnail" appearance on the surface (Fig. 19–27). The amount of fat may be reduced but is still abundant. Now the fibrous septa are prominent and often have a modest infiltrate of lymphocytes with some reactive bile duct proliferation about the portal tracts (Fig. 19–28). The liver shrinks progressively in size, becomes more fibrotic, loses fat, and is converted into a macronodular pattern as parenchymal islands are engulfed by ever wider bands of fibrous tissue (Fig. 19–29). The parenchymal disorganization becomes more pronounced because of the irregular regeneration, and with disruption of the canaliculi, bile stasis often develops. The liver cells now contain no fat, and active cell necrosis and Mallory bodies are only rarely evident in this late stage. Thus, **end-stage alcoholic cirrhosis comes to resemble, both macroscopically and microscopically, postnecrotic cirrhosis (to be described).**

Pathogenesis. It is now generally accepted that alcohol, its metabolites, or its effects on hepatocyte metabolism is or are the cause of alcoholic liver disease and cirrhosis, unrelated to any concomitant malnutrition so commonly observed in chronic alcoholics. Ultrastructural changes (described earlier) appeared in hepatocytes of well-nourished nonalcoholic volunteers maintained on completely adequate diets two days after simulated "weekend" drinking of 245 to 270 gm alcohol daily.[149] Analogously, about 25% of baboons, maintained on nutritionally adequate diets containing alcohol as the carbohydrate, developed cirrhosis.[142] How, then, does alcohol exert its effects? The origin of fatty change was discussed on page 18; thus, it is sufficient to state only that alcohol reduces mitochondrial fatty acid oxidation, increases triglyceride formation from fatty acids, mobilizes peripheral fat depots, and impairs secretion of lipoproteins. However, the precise basis for the ethanol-

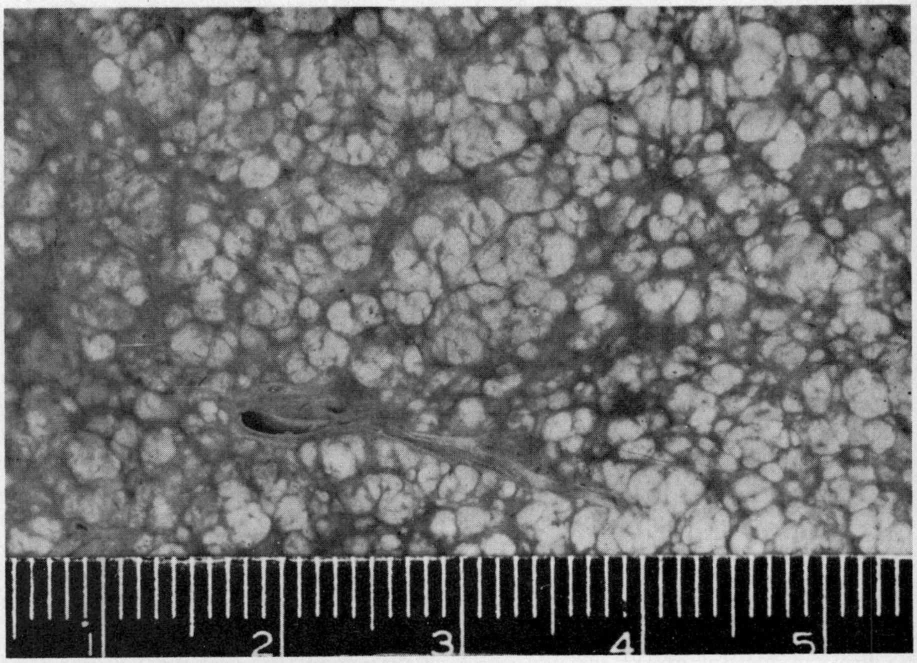

Figure 19–27. Alcoholic cirrhosis. Somewhat enlarged gross photograph to show variation in size of nodules and large amounts of intervening connective tissue.

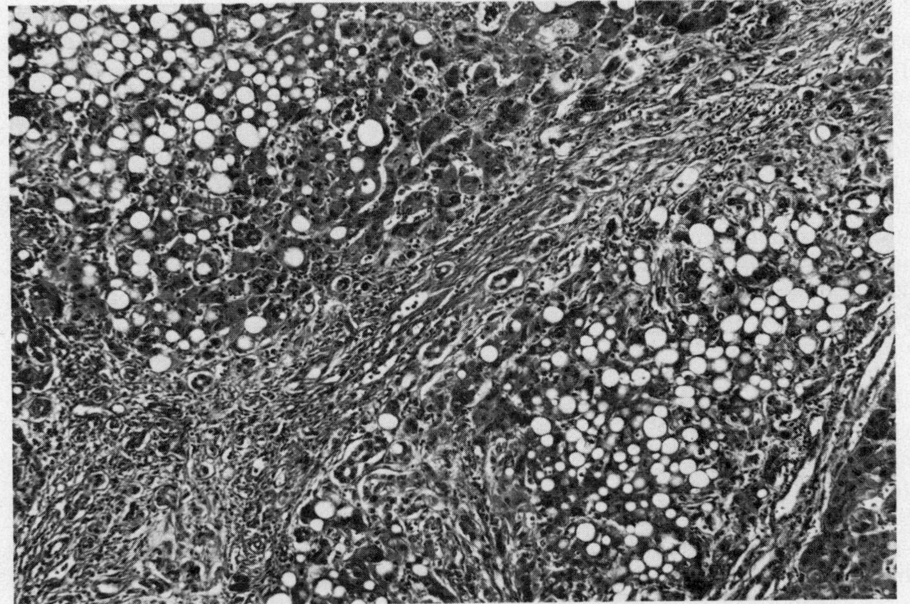

Figure 19–28. Alcoholic cirrhosis. Microscopic appearance of the liver seen in Figure 19–27 with fat and well-developed fibrous scarring.

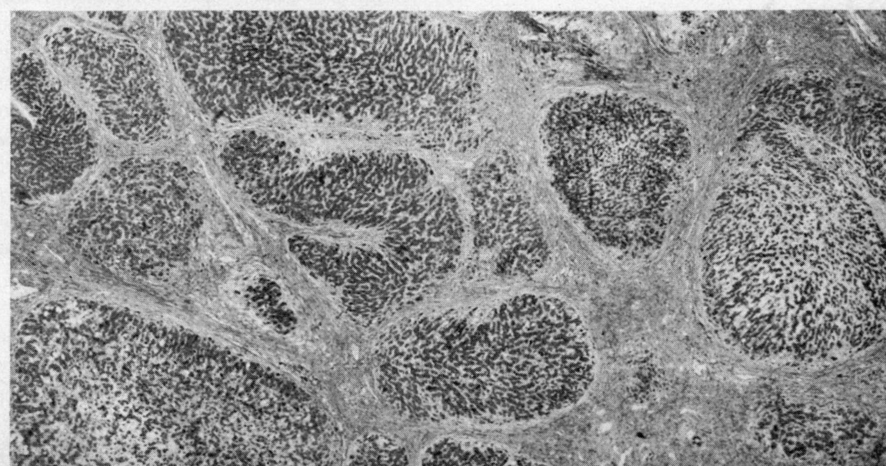

Figure 19–29. Alcoholic cirrhosis. Late stage with no fat and large amounts of fibrosis.

related liver cell necrosis is still unknown. A number of proposals have been made, including (1) mitochondrial injury and cellular hypoxia; (2) acetaldehyde toxicity; (3) superoxide formation and lipid peroxidation; and (4) cell-mediated or antibody-mediated cytotoxicity. There is little convincing evidence that mitochondrial injury and cellular hypoxia are important contributors.[156] The possibility that acetaldehyde, known to be a by-product of ethanol metabolism, is the hepatotoxin leading to alcoholic hepatitis continues to be seriously entertained, albeit not established.[145] Not only is it a very toxic metabolite, but reduced levels of hepatic acetaldehyde dehydrogenase leading to increased serum levels of acetaldehyde have been observed in alcoholics.[157] One study suggests that the lower enzyme level is not the result of alcohol-related injury, but is a primary genetic defect rendering certain individuals particularly vulnerable to the adverse effects of alcohol.[158] There is, nonetheless, a poor correlation between blood levels of acetaldehyde and the development of hepatitis or cirrhosis. Another possible mechanism may relate to the formation of free radicals in the course of degradation of acetaldehyde to acetate by xanthine oxidase.[159] Uncertainty about these pathways has inevitably led to immunologic proposals that gain support from the variable individual susceptibility to chronic alcoholism. A large number of immunologic abnormalities have been described in patients with alcoholic liver disease, including (1) antibody directed against liver cells, (2) immune complex formation with complement activation; (3) abnormal T-cell function; and (4) antibody-dependent cellular cytotoxicity.[160] However, proof is lacking that any of these mechanisms are the cause of the acute liver damage and are not merely secondary phenomena. Whether primary or secondary, they may contribute to fibrogenesis, as will become clear.

The mechanisms involved in the development of fibrosis are also uncertain. Some experts maintain that active liver cell necrosis and alcoholic hepatitis are requisite for, or at least very important contributors to, the fibrogenesis. The necrotic cells and inflammatory reaction may well lead to fibrous scarring. Activated lymphocytes, macrophages, and phagocytic sinusoidal cells involved in the inflammatory response to alcoholic hepatitis also may release fibrogenic factors.[161] A variant of this concept proposes that Mallory bodies serve as antigens for an autoimmune reaction with the secretion of a fibrogenic lymphokine.[162] Attractive as these proposals may be, not all patients with alcoholic cirrhosis have had known episodes of alcoholic hepatitis. Moreover, as pointed out, active hepatitis is consistently absent in the baboon model of cirrhosis. An alternative pathway was proposed by Popper and Kent,[163] who suggest that perivenular and perisinusoidal fibrosis, which first appears in the early fatty stage, progresses to produce fibrous septa that radiate from the central vein to eventually yield the network of scarring seen in alcoholic cirrhosis. Lipid-laden Ito cells (of mesenchymal origin) in the spaces of Disse may contribute to this fibrogenesis. Yet another possibility has been raised, namely, that ethanol directly stimulates collagen synthesis in vitro as well as in vivo.[164] There is no dearth of theories to explain the fibrous scarring, but at present all are conjectural.

Finally, the current theories of origin of the Mallory body should be mentioned. Abnormal keratinization secondary to a lack of vitamin A has been proposed in these malnourished individuals.[165] Another appealing hypothesis, which, however, has many opponents, invokes "microtubular failure." Alcohol might cause disassembly of tubulin and microtubules, leading to disarray of cytoplasmic organelles and aggregation of intermediate filaments into hyalin. The "microtubule failure" theory might also provide an explanation for the marked retention of proteins in alcoholic liver disease. Still another proposal regards the development of hyalin as a "preneoplastic" change.[154] It is clear that much remains to be learned, not only about the actions of alcohol on the liver but also about the origin of alcoholic hyalin.

CLINICAL COURSE. The clinical manifestations of alcohol-related liver disease vary widely, depending on the nature and stage of the hepatic pathology. At one end of the spectrum is the asymptomatic patient with marked fatty hepatomegaly. Only rarely is there jaundice, sometimes accompanied by minimal elevation of SGOT. On the other hand, alcoholic hepatitis is rarely asymptomatic; commonly, it presents as an acute viral hepatitis with fever, tender hepatomegaly, jaundice, and almost invariably some elevation of SGOT (frequently less than would be expected for the severity of the clinical manifestations). The alkaline phosphatase is also elevated, sometimes markedly in patients who have a cholestatic picture. These manifestations may be superimposed on those related to portal hypertension when cirrhosis is also present. With severe alcoholic hepatitis, hepatic failure, encephalopathy, and sometimes renal failure develop; indeed, each bout of hepatitis imposes a 10 to 20% mortality rate.

The characteristic features of developed cirrhosis with its accompanying portal hypertension have already been described. Particularly prominent are marked wasting, weakness, and ascites, sometimes producing a massively distended abdomen in a pathetically wasted body with skeletal extremities. In about 10% of cases, the cirrhosis is clinically silent until late in the course; sometimes it is discovered only at autopsy. Whatever the clinical presentation, massive hematemesis from ruptured gastroesophageal varices may punctuate the course or sometimes announce the existence of the underlying cirrhosis. The long-term outlook depends heavily on the level of continued exposure to ethanol. The natural progression of the disease can be arrested or significantly slowed with complete abstinence.[166] Approximately 90% of those who do not have jaundice, ascites, or hematemesis at diagnosis and who refrain from further drinking survive for five years, but with continued drinking the rate drops to about 50%. The major causes of death, in order, are (1) liver failure; (2) intercurrent infections; (3) massive gastrointestinal hemorrhage; and (4) hepatocellular carcinoma, which appears in about 5 to 10% of cases. Concurrent hepatitis B virus infection significantly increases the risk of superimposed cancer.[167]

POSTNECROTIC CIRRHOSIS

This is a macronodular pattern of cirrhosis of varied and sometimes unknown origin. In about 20 to 25% of cases it evolves from chronic active hepatitis B infection, as evidenced by positive serologic tests for HBsAg. How many additional cases are related to non-A, non-B chronic active hepatitis is not known. In a small number of instances there is a well-documented history of acute liver damage caused by some hepatotoxin such as phosphorus, carbon tetrachloride, mushroom poisoning, or a drug such as acetaminophen, oxyphenisatin, or alpha-methyldopa. Undoubtedly, some cases represent end-stage alcoholic cirrhosis readily misinterpreted as macronodular postnecrotic cirrhosis in the absence of a history of chronic alcoholism. After all these possibilities have been excluded, there remains a large residual of uncertain origin. *A single attack of massive hepatic necrosis only infrequently gives rise to postnecrotic cirrhosis,*[168] because either it is fatal or regeneration of the liver cells permits survival with little or no residual scarring. In other instances of repeated bouts of submassive necrosis, survival is possible but only with massive random scars, or perhaps with a shrunken lobe. Such livers are said to have *postnecrotic scarring* because they lack the overall nodularity and scarring necessary for the diagnosis of cirrhosis. Submassive necrosis, whether caused by viruses or other hepatotoxins, when it is zonal and reaches into most lobules, sometimes may indeed produce diffuse scarring, meriting the designation "postnecrotic cirrhosis."

MORPHOLOGY. From analyses of series of cases, it is possible to deduce the natural course of postnecrotic cirrhosis. At the outset the liver is normal in size and color, but has faintly perceptible nodularity created by narrow trabeculae of fibrous tissue. Characteristically, the nodules are of variable size; some exceed 3 mm and may even be more than 1 cm in diameter. With progression the liver shrinks, sometimes to less than 1 kg in weight. The fibrous septa become coarser and, in places, become confluent to produce broad tracts of connective tissue, and simultaneously the markedly irregular macronodularity becomes accentuated (Fig. 19–30). Microscopically, the fibrous scars are typically infiltrated with lymphocytes and macrophages and, in places where entire lobules have been destroyed, they may contain distorted portal triads along with irregular strands and nests of bile duct epithelium resulting from replication of bile ducts and cholangioles. Characteristically the portal triads are closely approximated where the hepatocytes of entire lobules have been destroyed with collapse of the reticular framework. The architecture within the parenchymal nodules is distorted by both cell loss and regeneration. In the end-stage disease, active liver cell necrosis is inconspicuous, except possibly at the margins of parenchymal islands where piecemeal necrosis may persist as a residuum of chronic active hepatitis. Fat may or may not be present within surviving hepatocytes, but it is rarely prominent and bile stasis is equally variable. **Ultimately, the diagnosis rests on ex-**

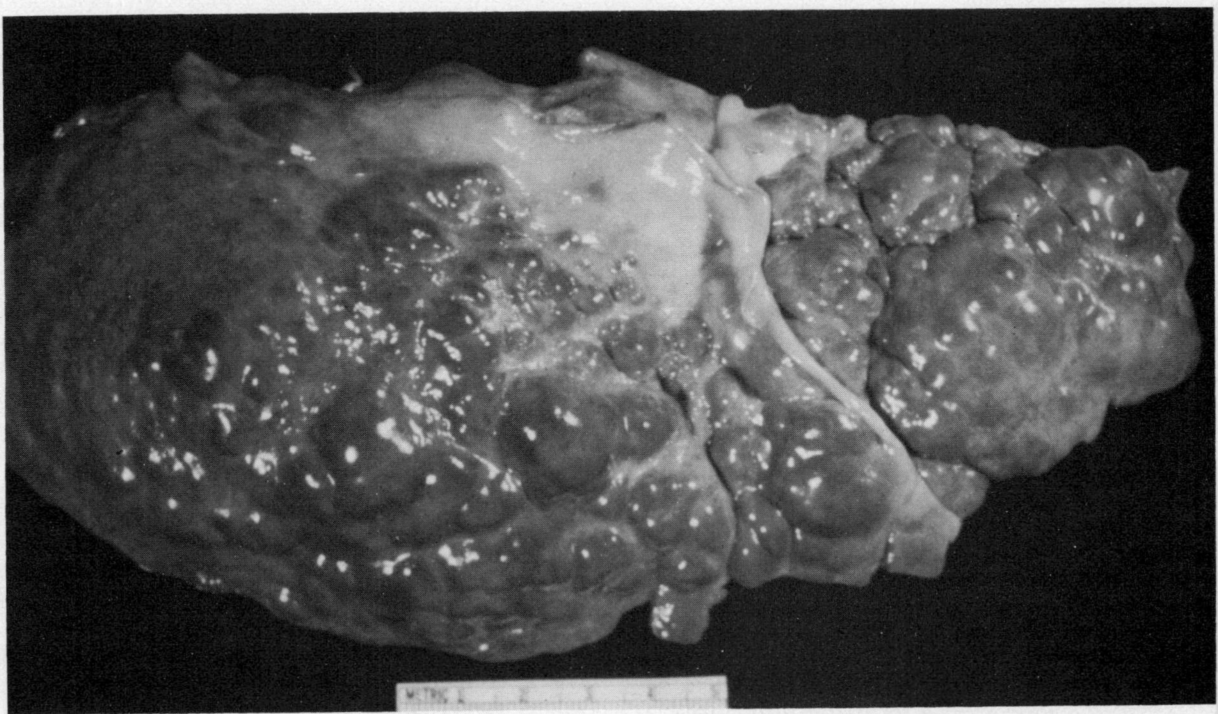

Figure 19–30. Postnecrotic cirrhosis. Scarring is very irregular and has become confluent at subdiaphragmatic surface of liver above. (Courtesy of Dr. Harvey Goldman, Pathology Department, Beth Israel Hospital, Harvard Medical School, Boston.)

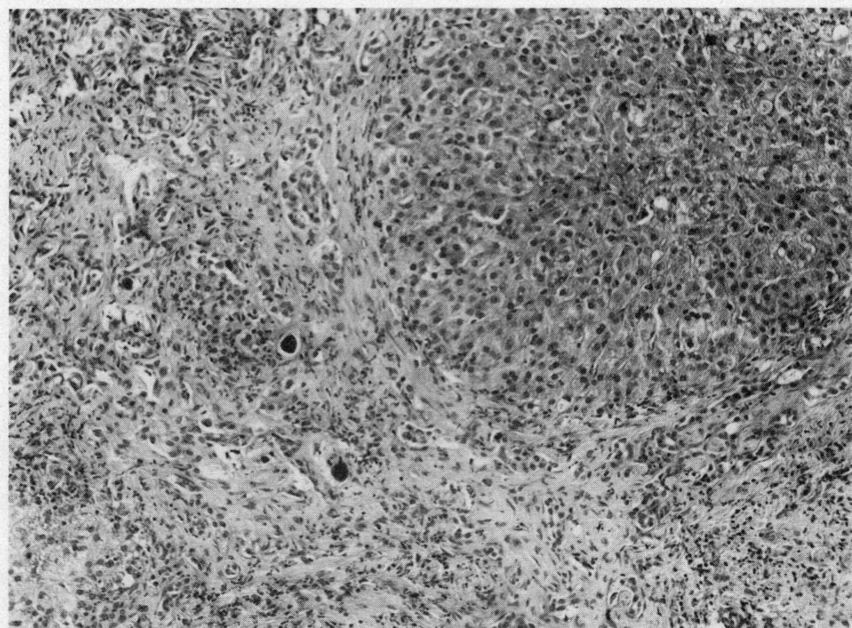

Figure 19–31. Postnecrotic scarring. An island of preserved parenchyma is visible at upper right. Remainder of field represents a broad area of scarring.

cluding other bases for a macronodular cirrhosis (e.g., end-stage alcoholic disease), the coarseness of the scars and the size and irregularity of the parenchymal nodules (Fig. 19–31).

The clinical course is as varied as the origins of this form of cirrhosis. In many cases the cirrhosis is asymptomatic and is only discovered at laparotomy or autopsy, or by the chance finding of abnormal liver function test results. Sometimes splenomegaly or other manifestations of portal hypertension, such as a massive gastrointestinal bleed or ascites, call attention to the hepatic involvement, or such stigmata of cirrhosis as spider angiomas, gynecomastia, or amenorrhea constitute the presenting features of the disease. Also, there may be prominent signs and symptoms suggestive of progressive chronic active hepatitis, described earlier (p. 907). In such instances the disease may pursue a relentless course to death within a year or more, but some patients have a more indolent, prolonged course. The ultimate cause of death is usually hepatic failure, sometimes with encephalopathy, or massive hemorrhage from a ruptured gastroesophageal varix. This form of cirrhosis, particularly when related to hepatitis B virus infection, often (15 to 25% of cases) leads to hepatocellular carcinoma, a frequency exceeded only by pigment cirrhosis.

PIGMENT CIRRHOSIS—HEMOCHROMATOSIS

Pigment cirrhosis is the dominant feature of the iron overload disorder known as hemochromatosis. It takes the form of a micronodular cirrhosis rendered distinctive by massive deposits of ferritin and hemosiderin, mainly in hepatocytes and Kupffer cells. Ferritin, as noted (p. 636), is found in the cell sap and lysosomes, and consists of micelles having an outer shell of apoprotein surrounding an iron-rich core in the form of ferric oxyhydroxide with a small amount of phosphate.[169] Hemosiderin represents aggregates of iron formed by degradation of the protein shells of ferritin micelles with coalescence of the iron cores (*endogenous hemosiderin*). Hemosiderin may also be formed by the deposition of iron oxide following parenteral administration of iron-containing drugs (*exogenous hemosiderin*).[170] In hemochromatosis the increase in total body iron is quite extraordinary and may reach a total of 80 gm (normal 3 to 5 gm). One sufferer is reported to have set off the metal detector alarms at airports! The liver bears the brunt of this accumulation but there is also deposition of hemosiderin in the parenchymal cells of the heart, pancreas, and other organs, often damaging these organs also. It is necessary, therefore, to characterize hemochromatosis and consider the origins of the iron overload.

The term hemochromatosis is the generic designation for all iron overload syndromes marked by (1) a progressive increase in total body iron stores; (2) the deposition of large quantities of iron in the form of ferritin and hemosiderin in the parenchymal cells of the liver, heart, pancreas, and other organs; and (3) both morphologic and functional damage to the organs and sites bearing the brunt of the iron deposition. In these terms, a number of forms of hemochromatosis can be distinguished on the basis of the cause of iron accumulation, as set out in Table 19–4. The basis for these various forms of hemochromatosis will become more clear when the pathogenesis of iron overload is considered. It is important, however, to note that *all forms of hemochromatosis are characterized by parenchymal cell*

Table 19–4. CAUSES OF HEMOCHROMATOSIS*

Idiopathic (primary, hereditary) hemochromatosis
Secondary hemochromatosis
Secondary to anemia and ineffective erythropoiesis
Thalassemia, major
Sideroblastic anemia
Secondary to liver disease
Alcoholic cirrhosis
Following portacaval anastomosis
Secondary to high iron intake
Prolonged ingestion of medicinal iron
Prolonged consumption of iron-laden wine, Kaffir beer, etc.
Multiple transfusions

*Based on Powell, L. W., et al.: Hemochromatosis: 1980 update. Gastroenterology *78*:374, 1980.

damage in organs, secondary to iron overload. Some iron may be present in RE cells, but it is overshadowed by the parenchymal deposition. Accumulations of reticuloendothelial iron from broken down red cells, such as occurs in hemolytic anemias or multiple transfusions, appear to be relatively innocuous and unassociated with parenchymal cell and organ injury; thus, this condition is referred to as *hemosiderosis.* Such terms as "systemic hemosiderosis," "hemolytic siderosis," and "transfusional siderosis" describe this pattern of iron accumulation. Convenient as this distinction may be, the line demarcating hemosiderosis from hemochromatosis may, at times, get blurred. For example, there is some question about the iron overload syndromes secondary to transfusions and oral intake of iron. Most of this iron accumulates in RE cells, but with massive reticuloendothelial hemosiderosis there may be shift of enough iron into parenchymal cells to induce some organ injury and usually a mild form of hemochromatosis. *It is best, therefore, to view hemosiderosis and hemochromatosis as the two ends of a spectrum of iron overload, recognizing that intergrades sometimes defy categorization.*

Pathogenesis—Iron Metabolism. The pathogenesis of iron overload and hemochromatosis requires an understanding of normal iron metabolism, already discussed on pages 422 and 636. For brief review, the normal total iron content is in the range of 2 to 5 gm in women and up to 6 gm in men. This amount is a closely guarded constant maintained by the regulation of intake to balance the very limited, almost fixed losses (at least in the male).[172] In men, the daily loss is about 1 mg per day, but in women it is much more variable because of fetal demands for iron during pregnancy (0.5 to 1 gm) and the losses of menstrual bleeding (10 to 20 mg per period), averaging 2 mg per day. The average adult, meat-rich Western diet provides about 10 to 20 mg of iron per day, mostly in the form of readily absorbed heme- and myoglobin-iron. It is apparent that not more than 10% of this daily supply can be taken in if overload is to be prevented.

Absorption of iron from the diet involves not only its absorbability but also intestinal mucosal cell uptake and then transfer across the cell into the plasma.[173] The most active site of absorption is the duodenum, but the stomach, ileum, and colon may also participate to a small degree. The precise mechanism of mucosal cell uptake of iron is still poorly understood, but (as discussed earlier, p. 636) involves two iron-binding proteins, mucosal cell ferritin and transferrin.[174] After uptake a fraction of the iron that enters the mucosal cell is rapidly delivered to the plasma transport protein—transferrin. Most, however, is deposited as ferritin within these cells, some to be transferred to plasma transferrin, and some to be slowly lost over the course of weeks with exfoliation of mucosal cells, referred to as postabsorption excretion. The level of such excretion may regulate the amount of iron absorbed. Although the factors governing the level of immediate transfer of iron across the mucosal cell and the amount to be lost slowly in postabsorption excretion remain a mystery, it is known that *the total uptake and transfer of iron is dependent on body iron content and erythropoietic activity, more specifically the iron needs of the erythron.* As body stores rise, the percentage of iron absorbed falls, and vice versa. For unknown reasons, increased erythropoiesis alone, as in the hemolytic anemias, rarely leads to iron overload. More critical appears to be ineffective erythropoiesis, such as occurs with thalassemia major and sideroblastic anemia. Some signal must be delivered then to the mucosal cell, regulating its uptake and transfer of iron by modifying the level of postabsorption excretion. There are many hypotheses, but the nature of this signal is still unknown.[175] One proposal holds that the level of saturation of plasma transferrin (serum ferritin) is central to the regulatory process. Serum ferritin is in constant flux with iron absorbed by the gut and with the ferritin pool in cells. There is some evidence that the RE cells, including the peripheral monocytes, are most important in this internal pool. A decrease in cellular iron or a greater drain by the erythron would lower the serum ferritin and lead to an increase in uptake and transfer of iron from the gut. When the serum ferritin level is above normal, more iron is held within mucosal cells to be shed with them, and absorption is inhibited. An alternative theory proposes that mononuclear phagocytes, particularly the peripheral monocytes with their heme- and non–heme-derived ferritin, constitute the primary circulating signal and not the level of plasma transferrin. Although additional refinements might be mentioned, *the essence of this hypothesis states that the level of iron within cells (perhaps mainly mononuclear phagocytes and intestinal mucosal cells) modifies iron absorption in the gut.*[176] However, it is important to note that with nonphysiologic levels of dietary iron, excessive amounts are rapidly transferred to the plasma.

It is now possible to revert to the various forms of hemochromatosis to consider the origins of the iron overload. *Idiopathic hemochromatosis is by far the most common and the most severe expression of the disease; it is clearly an inborn error of iron metabolism transmitted as an autosomal recessive with full expression of the derangement in homozygotes and sometimes partial expression in heterozygotes.*[177] Although a "bigenic" theory cannot be completely refuted, the weight of evidence favors a single mutant gene located close to the HLA region on chromosome 6 with fairly tight linkage to HLA-A3. Additional associations have been reported with HLA-B14 and -B7.[178] Argument has persisted for years about the nature of the metabolic fault in idiopathic hemochromatosis, but it has generated more heat than light.[175] Currently the favored proposals are (1) a defect in intestinal mucosal control of iron absorption, perhaps in the mechanism regulating post-absorption excretion;[179] (2) abnormal affinity of the liver for transferrin iron;[180] or (3) some abnormality in the monocytic-reticuloendothelial handling of iron.[181] Whatever the basis, the iron overload is far more extreme, as is the organ injury, in the primary idiopathic disease than it is in the secondary forms.

In *secondary hemochromatosis* the iron overload has many possible origins. It may result from increased absorption related to the demands of a hyperfunctioning, but ineffective, bone marrow (erythropoietic hemochromatosis). The development of hemochromatosis with alcoholic cirrhosis and portacaval anastomosis is less well understood. Alcohol appears to increase iron absorption. In some cases, consumption of iron-rich alcoholic beverages such as red wine may favor the overload. However, although there is some increase in stainable iron in the liver in most patients with alcoholic cirrhosis, it reaches the level of hemochromatosis in only a minority. The question arises—are iron-overloaded alcoholic individuals heterozygous for the mutant gene causing idiopathic hemochromatosis? The issue of high oral iron intake and hemochromatosis is more controversial, as mentioned earlier. South African Bantus who consume large quantities of alcoholic beverage fermented in vessels made of iron have developed what is called "Bantu siderosis," with moderate degrees of pigmentation and cirrhosis in the liver. In these individuals the excessive consumption of alcohol and iron appears to be responsible for a disorder having many resemblances to classic idiopathic hemochromatosis. Whether medicinal iron has the same potential is still being argued because, in the few reported cases of secondary hemochromatosis attributed to oral intake of iron-containing drugs, the possibility of an underlying hereditary defect cannot be excluded. The same question arises with patients who have received transfusions over a lifetime for, say, aplastic anemia, and have later developed hemochromatosis. Are they genetically predisposed, or does sufficient overload of the RE cells induce a shift of iron into parenchymal cells, with organ injury? Despite these uncertainties, there is a message: patients consuming or being administered large quantities of iron must be monitored for the possible development of hemochromatosis.

An estimate of the level of body iron stores can be made by the combined measurements of (1) serum ferritin, (2) plasma iron concentration, and (3) iron-binding capacity. Serum ferritin, an iron-binding beta globulin, is normally 10 to 200 ng/ml, but rises into the range of 800 to 6000 with hemochromatosis. Analogously, the plasma iron, which is normally 50 to 150 μg/dl, is elevated two- or threefold. There is also a fall in the plasma of the iron-binding capacity from 250 to 350 μg/dl to 200 to 300 μg/dl, reflecting the greater saturation of transferrin. An additional valuable test is increased excretion of iron in the urine following administration of the iron chelator desferrioxamine. Other more sophisticated measurements can be made and will be described later. Ultimately, however, liver biopsy is definitive when it reveals more than the normal barely detectable amounts of hemosiderin.

Granted that iron overload of parenchymal cells is fundamental to hemochromatosis, the question arises as to how the cellular damage and consequent fibrosis occur. The currently favored theory proposes that *the ultimate toxicity of iron derives from the formation of free radicals that induce peroxidation of membrane lipids*. Trump and colleagues have suggested that, with progressive iron overload, the cells' capacity to form innocuous ferritin is exceeded and the excess "free iron," in undergoing reduction from the ferric to the ferrous state, catalyzes the formation of free radicals from oxygen.[182, 183] Possibly contributing to the cellular damage is the release of lysosomal enzymes, presumably because of free radical–induced damage to lysosomal membranes. Other mechanisms have been proposed, such as the possibility of direct stimulation of collagen synthesis by excess iron, with the resulting fibrosis then producing parenchymal injury.[184] Another theory invokes a fundamental derangement in RE handling of

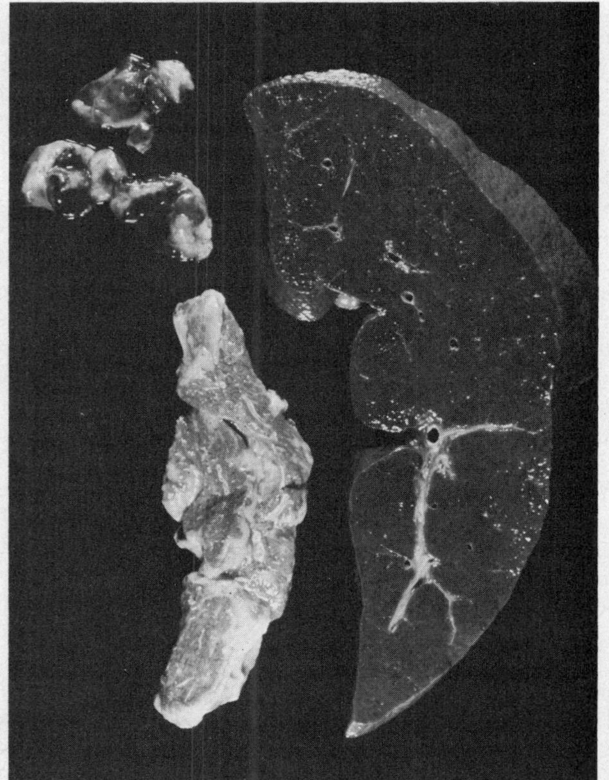

Figure 19–32. Hemochromatosis. Darkly pigmented micronodular liver is seen on right, slightly pigmented transected pancreas on lower left, and pigmented lymph nodes at upper left.

iron. In idiopathic hemochromatosis the RE system appears to be unable to store as much iron as usual, and so parenchymal cells are exposed to a greater load.[185] There is still much uncertainty about the pathogenesis of the parenchymal injury, but the evidence favors the free-radical theory.

MORPHOLOGY. Only the morphologic changes of idiopathic hemochromatosis will be described, because the changes in the various forms of secondary hemochromatosis are qualitatively the same but usually less marked. **The principal features of idiopathic hemochromatosis are: (1) excessive deposits of hemosiderin in the following organs in decreasing order of severity: liver, pancreas, myocardium, pituitary, adrenals, thyroid, parathyroids, joints, and skin; (2) micronodular pigment cirrhosis of the liver; and (3) atrophy and fibrosis of the pancreas** (Fig. 19–32). Despite the pigmentation, fibrosis is relatively scanty in organs other than the liver and pancreas.

The **liver** progressively develops a micronodular cirrhosis with hemosiderin-laden parenchymal cells, Kupffer cells, and bile duct epithelium. Sequential liver biopsies indicate that first there is deposition of the pigment, followed in time by the development of fibrous septa resembling in distribution those seen in evolving alcoholic cirrhosis. At this early stage the liver is characteristically slightly larger than normal and is dense and chocolate-brown. Over the span of years the progressive accumulation of pigment and the scarring become more prominent, as does the parenchymal nodularity. There is some reduction in liver size but rarely is it marked. The hemosiderin is readily evident in routine tissue stains but is highlighted by the Prussian blue reaction, when applied to whole organ or tissue slices, rendering them blue-black (Fig. 19–33). With death of hepatocytes or Kupffer cells, iron may be released into extracellular spaces and incorporated within the fibrous septa. Fat is usually strikingly absent as is active cell necrosis, but nonetheless cell death must have occurred followed by regeneration. As with all forms of cirrhosis, there is disorganization of the normal architecture within the parenchymal nodules. Carcinoma of the liver is a frequent complication of pigment cirrhosis and appears in 15 to 30% of cases.[186]

The **pancreas** is intensely pigmented, has a diffuse interstitial fibrosis, and may be somewhat decreased in size because of atrophy and loss of parenchymal cells. Hemosiderin is found in both the acinar and islet cells, and sometimes in the interstitial fibrous stroma. As will be seen, diabetes is a major clinical feature of idiopathic hemochromatosis, but there is poor correlation between the intensity of the iron deposits in the pancreatic islets and the occurrence and severity of the diabetes.

The **heart** is often enlarged and has hemosiderin granules within the myocardial fibers. The pigmentation may induce a striking brown coloration to the myocardium. A delicate interstitial fibrosis may or may not be present.

The **endocrine glands** (thyroid, parathyroid, pituitary, and, in particular, adrenals) also reveal a brownish coloration related to the accumulation of hemosiderin in the parenchymal cells.

The **skin** has increased pigmentation in 80 to 90% of patients. This is mainly due to increased amounts of melanin (seen with various forms of cirrhosis), which imparts a golden-brown color. There is also a distinctive, metallic, slate-gray pigmentation related to accumulation of hemosiderin in dermal macrophages and fibroblasts.

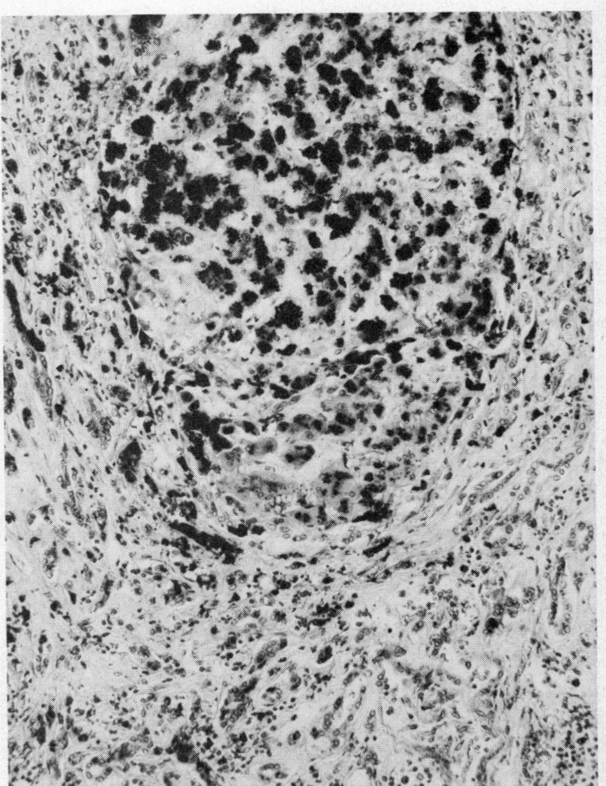

Figure 19–33. Pigment cirrhosis with well-developed scarring. The hemosiderin principally within hepatocytes appears black in Prussian blue reaction.

The **joint synovial linings** have hemosiderin pigmentation in 30 to 50% of cases. An acute synovitis may follow. There is also excessive deposition of calcium pyrophosphate, which damages the articular cartilage and sometimes produces disabling polyarthritis, referred to as "pseudogout."

The **testes** may be small and atrophic but are not usually significantly pigmented. It is thought that the atrophy is secondary to some derangement in the hypothalamic-pituitary axis.

CLINICAL COURSE. The clinical features of idiopathic hemochromatosis will be described; the findings in the secondary pattern are fundamentally the same but tend to be less well defined and more variable, depending on the severity of the iron overload and organ injury. Idiopathic hemochromatosis affects males more often than females in a ratio of 9:1. Protection of females is attributed to the losses of iron from menstruation and pregnancy. Most patients come to clinical attention between the ages 40 and 60, presumably the time required for accumulation of sufficient iron to cause organ injury. Mention has already been made of the close association between the so-called "susceptibility gene" and HLA-A3. Thus, individuals who possess this antigen and who require multiple transfusions or prolonged iron therapy are at particular risk.

The classic clinical triad of findings has traditionally been liver disease, diabetes, and skin pigmentation. To these must be added *cardiac manifestations* (*e.g.*, *congestive heart failure and/or arrhythmias) indistinguishable from other cardiomyopathies, joint symptoms resembling those of gout, and often impotence.* The liver disease—pigment cirrhosis—may be silent clinically except possibly for some SGOT elevation, but hepatomegaly is detectable in about 80% of patients and often the liver is unusually radiopaque. The reported frequency of diabetes mellitus ranges from about 30% to 80%.[187] The skin pigmentation (80 to 90% of patients) responsible for the older designation of "bronze diabetes" is, as was noted, a reflection of increased melanin as well as iron deposits. Neurologic symptoms such as somnolence, apathy, ataxia, and hearing loss are sometimes manifested despite the failure to identify pigmentary or other regressive alterations in the central nervous system. In some patients, cardiac abnormalities or arthritis first call attention to the underlying disease.

Although the diagnosis can be suspected on the basis of the clinical findings, it must be confirmed by evidence of inappropriate levels of iron accumulation in the blood, such as a marked increase in transferrin saturation, serum ferritin, and plasma iron, as discussed earlier. Other criteria of iron overload are increased hepatic density revealed by CT scan, as well as by magnetic measurements.[188] However, the level of iron stores is better judged by the amount excreted in the urine after an injection of desferrioxamine (usually more than 2 mg), and ultimately by the parenchymal iron overload and pigment cirrhosis in the liver biopsy. The major differential diagnosis is alcoholic cirrhosis accompanied by some iron loading, particularly when there is a history of consumption of large quantities of red wine. Moreover, chronic alcoholism can of course be seen in patients with idiopathic hemochromatosis.

More than with most forms of cirrhosis, early diagnosis in the precirrhotic phase and appropriate treatment have a great deal to offer. The use of iron chelators and frequent phlebotomies drains the iron stores and, according to clinical observations, may prevent or at least markedly delay progression to cirrhosis. Even more surprising, this regimen has reportedly caused reversal of the hepatic fibrous scarring (p. 915), ameliorated or cleared the diabetes, and relieved other signs and symptoms.[186] The five-year mortality rate in patients on intensive iron-draining therapy is about 10%, but is almost 70% in the untreated.[189] There is, therefore, a clear need for recognition of individuals at risk, particularly among family members. Relatives having the same HLA profile as the index case may incur the disease, and even heterozygotes sharing only one HLA haplotype often have somewhat elevated transferrin saturation, serum ferritin, and plasma iron and are at increased risk, particularly when normal iron metabolic balance is stressed by alcoholism, anemia, transfusions, or augmented oral intake. The major causes of death in untreated patients are cardiac failure or sudden cardiac death related to an arrhythmia, hepatic failure, complications of chronic diabetes mellitus (p. 972), and hepatocellular carcinoma. Although depletion of iron stores by the therapy has successfully prevented or corrected most of these fatal sequelae, it has not prevented the development of the cancers. Perhaps, however, the origin of these neoplasms dated back to prephlebotomy days. For obscure reasons, an increased incidence of other forms of cancer has also been reported in these patients—bronchial, pancreatic, cholecystic and rectal. In the absence of these neoplastic hazards, with current methods of therapy, many patients have remained well for 20 or more years without apparent progression of their disease.

BILIARY CIRRHOSIS

There are two distinctive forms of biliary cirrhosis. One, *primary biliary cirrhosis, is thought to be an autoimmune disorder focused on interlobular bile ducts and cholangioles, and so is best remembered as destructive sclerosing cholangitis and cholangiolitis. The other variant, secondary biliary cirrhosis, results from obstruction to the major extrahepatic ducts.* Both forms, however, are characterized morphologically by a micronodular cirrhosis resulting from fibrous septa that emanate from the portal tracts to eventually enclose individual lobules.

Secondary biliary cirrhosis is the simpler to characterize. It follows any of the disorders discussed earlier (p. 890) that cause prolonged extrahepatic obstructive jaundice. The outflow obstruction produces bile stasis throughout the entire biliary tree until eventually the inspissated impacted bile damages the interlobular bile ducts and cholangioles. A secondary inflammatory reaction initiates the scarring, leading to the cirrhosis. Secondary bacterial infection (ascending cholangitis and cholangiolitis) may contribute to the damage. Sometimes an ascending infection, even in the absence of marked bile stasis, produces a so-called infectious variant of secondary biliary cirrhosis. Enteric organisms such as coliforms and enterococci are the common culprits. With this form of secondary biliary cirrhosis, there may be little or no bile stasis.

Primary biliary cirrhosis is of less certain origin and has evoked much speculation. It has many features of an autoimmune disease and, indeed, has some similarities to the immune reactions following liver transplantation.[190] Moreover, there is a greater-than-chance association between primary biliary cirrhosis and other autoimmune diseases such as rheumatoid arthritis, Hashimoto's thyroiditis, and Sjögren's disease.[191] Most of those affected are middle-aged women known to have an increased frequency of autoimmune disease. *Numerous abnormalities of both humoral and cell-mediated immunity have been detected in these patients.* Antimitochondrial antibody is present in 90 to 100% of patients and, less frequently, smooth muscle antibody, antinuclear antibodies, and rheumatoid factor. Hyperglobulinemia, particularly of the IgM class, is characteristic and has been related to a failure of the immune response to convert from IgM to IgG antibody synthesis.[192] Circulating immune complexes are often found and are associated with activation of the classic and alternate complement pathways.[193] The finding of IgM and complement in areas of damaged bile ducts and cholangioles raises the possibility of humoral mechanisms in the production of the injury.[194] An equal number of observations point to the participation of cell-mediated immunity. As will be seen, *there is a prominent mononuclear inflammatory reaction in areas of scarring frequently marked by granuloma formation*, typically a manifestation of delayed hypersensitivity. T-cell sensitization to biliary antigens and liver-specific proteins has been demonstrated, as well as peripheral T-cell cytotoxicity for liver cells.[195] Paradoxically, these patients often have cutaneous anergy and an impaired T-cell response to such nonspecific mitogens as phytohemagglutinin. Despite all the immunologic findings, there is no satisfactory construct to relate them to the liver damage. Conceivably, biliary antigens evoke a humoral response with activation of lytic fractions of complement. A fundamental defect in T cells has been proposed, either in the form of cytolytic T cells or a lack of suppressor-cell function, contributing to a hyperreactive humoral response.[196] Antibody-dependent cellular cytotoxicity has also been invoked. Yet another theory emphasizing the similarity of the granulomas in the liver to those of sarcoidosis raises the possibility that primary biliary cirrhosis is a variant of sarcoidosis (itself of unknown origin).[197]

Other etiologies are still being considered. The liver in primary biliary cirrhosis has a high concentration of copper, which has been incriminated in the production of the cirrhosis of Wilson's disease (discussed below). Since this metal is excreted in the bile, elevated hepatic levels would not be unanticipated with prolonged bile stasis. Penicillamine (a copper chelator), known to be effective in Wilson's disease, has been reported to have beneficial effect in primary biliary cirrhosis. However, such therapy also reduces the circulating levels of immunoglobulins and immune complexes, making interpretation of its therapeutic effectiveness (if any) uncertain. The plethora of pathogenetic theories makes clear that the cause of primary biliary cirrhosis is still unknown.

MORPHOLOGY. Early in the course of all forms of biliary cirrhosis the liver is slightly enlarged with a regular, delicate micronodular scarring and deep-green bile pigmentation. Very rarely, when there is ascending infection in the absence of significant obstruction, the bile staining may be minimal or absent. As the disease advances the micronodularity becomes more evident, the scarring becomes more prominent but still fine, and the liver may shrink somewhat in size, but at most only slightly (Fig. 19–34). Important in the macroscopic examination is the identification or exclusion of disease—obstructive or infectious—in the extrahepatic ducts.

Microscopically, there are significant differences between the secondary and primary forms of biliary cirrhosis. However, **both are characterized by prominent periportal fibrosis that extends out from and interconnects portal triads, thus demarcating one lobule from the next.** The regularity of the scarring is a distinctive feature of this form of cirrhosis. There is usually a prominent mononuclear infiltrate within the scars as well as reduplication of bile ducts and ductules. Bile stasis within hepatocytes and canaliculi, as well as within Kupffer cells, are prominent features of most cases. Here the similarity ends. **Secondary biliary cirrhosis is associated with bile stasis in hepatocytes with prominent plugging of the interlobular bile ducts and canaliculi with inspissated bile, sometimes accompanied by intraductal neutrophils. Accumulations of bile pigment (referred to as "bile lakes") with local necrosis of hepatocytes may be present within the parenchyma.** As implied earlier, in rare cases of secondary biliary cirrhosis the intraductal changes may be largely confined to a heavy neutrophilic inflammation without significant bile stasis, either within the ducts or hepatic parenchyma. In contrast, **primary**

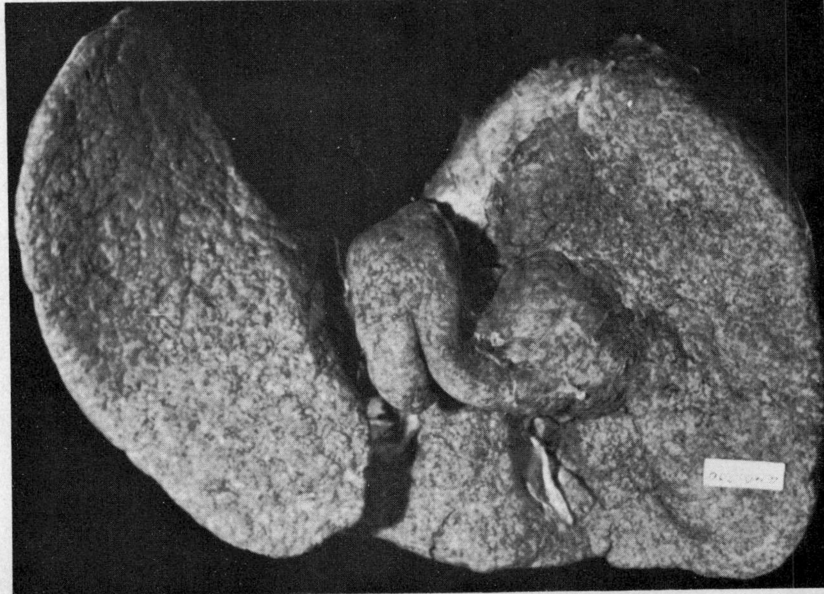

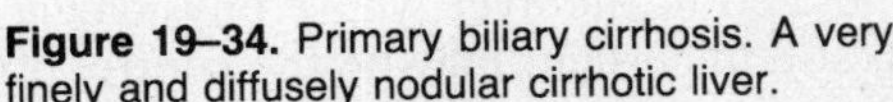

Figure 19–34. Primary biliary cirrhosis. A very finely and diffusely nodular cirrhotic liver.

biliary cirrhosis consists of a "nonsuppurative, destructive, sclerosing cholangitis and cholangiolitis." The brunt of the change is borne by the cholangioles, which are converted to tangled knots or strands of cells devoid of lumens (Fig. 19–35). Although necrosis of bile duct epithelium must have occurred, it is not a prominent feature at the time of autopsy and is replaced by regenerative activity. The interlobular ducts may be similarly affected or, at times, are better preserved but lack the prominent bile stasis and neutrophilic exudation seen in the secondary variants. The mononuclear infiltrate in the periportal regions in primary biliary cirrhosis is composed largely of lymphocytes with numerous plasma cells and macrophages. Sometimes lymphoid follicles appear in the inflammatory response as well as nests of foamy histiocytes. **In about 50% of cases, well-developed granulomas are associated with the inflammatory infiltrate**, and when present have been associated with an improved outlook for the patient.[198] In about 25% of cases, Mallory bodies are seen within hepatocytes similar to those described in alcoholic hepatitis (p. 919). Their significance is obscure and their number does not correlate with the severity or progression of the liver disease. As already emphasized, in primary biliary cirrhosis there is no evidence of obstructive or infectious disease in the major extrahepatic bile ducts.

Clinical Course. The signs, symptoms, and laboratory findings of both secondary and primary biliary cirrhosis are those of protracted obstruction to bile flow, i.e., progressive jaundice, pruritus, and elevated alkaline phosphatase levels. Whereas the secondary variants are likely to begin with jaundice, in the primary form the pruritus related to retention of bile acids often antedates the appearance of jaundice. Accompanying the obstructive jaundice are bilirubinuria, decolorization of stools, and steatorrhea with associated findings related to malabsorption of fats. Fever, right upper quadrant pain, and marked leukocytosis may be prominent with secondary infectious biliary cirrhosis. In the primary pattern, marked hypercholesterolemia may lead to skin xanthomas, florid atherosclerosis, and an increased risk of myocardial infarction.

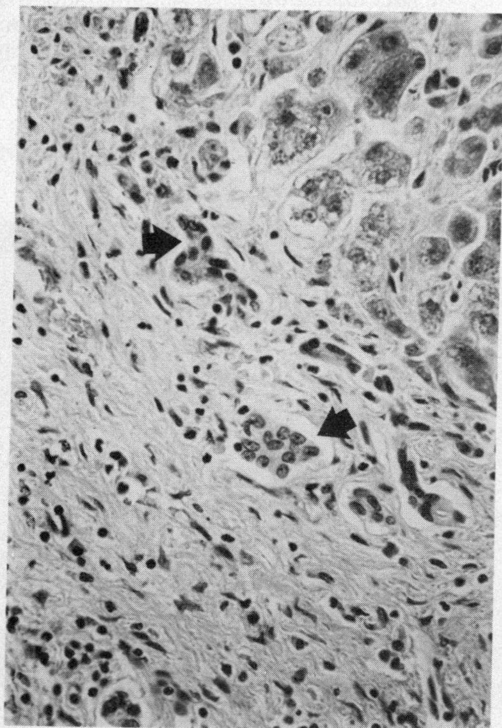

Figure 19–35. Primary biliary cirrhosis. A fibrous scar traversing liver (hepatocytes at upper right). Note tangled knots of bile duct epithelial cells (*arrows*) within scar.

Differentiation of the two basic patterns of the disease may be very difficult clinically and even with liver biopsy. As mentioned, primary biliary cirrhosis is predominantly a disease of middle-aged women. However, secondary disease is also encountered more often in women, in whom it is probably related to the increased frequency of obstructive gallstones. Demonstration of obstruction of the major extrahepatic bile ducts by cholangiography or CT scan would strongly favor the diagnosis of secondary disease.[199] Support for the diagnosis of primary biliary cirrhosis would be provided by elevated levels of IgM, immune complexes, and antimitochondrial antibodies in the serum. Often, however, resort must be made to liver biopsy. The outlook for the patient depends heavily on the amount of scarring found in the biopsy.[200]

In contrast to many other forms of cirrhosis, hepatic failure and portal hypertension are found infrequently early in the course of the disease. Generally the patient has a slow, progressive course of worsening jaundice, abnormal liver function test results, and manifestations related to malabsorption of fat over the span of 10 to 15 years, until eventually manifestations of liver failure (the usual cause of death) appear. At this late stage, splenomegaly, ascites, palmar erythema, spider angiomas, and other manifestations common to all the cirrhoses may develop. Only infrequently does hepatocellular carcinoma supervene.

CIRRHOSIS ASSOCIATED WITH ALPHA-1-ANTITRYPSIN (A1AT) DEFICIENCY

The association of A1AT deficiency with pulmonary disease and the nature and inheritance of A1AT have already been discussed on page 721. It is sufficient to recall that this major serum protease inhibitor is a glycoprotein synthesized in the liver whose physiologic function, although still uncertain, may be the control of proteases released at sites of cell injury and inflammation. At least 26 protease inhibitor (Pi) codominant alleles, labeled alphabetically, have been identified. The common, normal phenotype is homozygous for the M allele (Pi MM) resulting in normal plasma A1AT levels. The "classical" deficiency state is designated Pi ZZ, having 10 to 15% of the normal plasma level. Pi MZ heterozygotes have an intermediate deficiency of A1AT, as do Pi SS homozygotes. A rare variant, termed Pi null, characterized probably by a gene deletion, has no detectable A1AT in the plasma. *With a deficiency of A1AT, round-to-oval cytoplasmic globular inclusions appear within hepatocytes that immunocytochemical methods confirm are antigenically similar or identical to A1AT* (Fig. 19–36). In routine tissue stains, such as H and E, the globules are acidophilic and indistinctly demarcated from the surrounding cytoplasm. However, they are strongly PAS positive (and diastase resistant), which enhances their visualization. Characteristically, these inclusions are scattered throughout the cytoplasm and do not displace the nucleus but, when numerous, may coalesce into a single, large globule pushing the nucleus to one side. By electron microscopy they lie within smooth, and sometimes rough, endoplasmic reticulum.[201] The globules are most numerous in the Pi ZZ phenotype, but are also present in diminished size and number in heterozygous MZ patients and others with intermediate deficiency states.

The hepatic syndromes associated with A1AT deficiency are extremely varied and enigmatic. They range from neonatal hepatitis to childhood cirrhosis to cirrhosis that only becomes apparent late in life when the liver scarring is well advanced.[202] It is puzzling that many Pi ZZ neonates never develop liver disease. With the remainder the involvement ranges from overt hepatitis with cholestatic jaundice, either beginning at birth or only three to four months later, to subclinical hepatitis to merely laboratory evidence of abnormal liver function.[203] The hepatitis may subside with apparent complete recovery or may lead to cirrhosis.[204] Often the hepatic involvement is not discovered until cirrhosis has already developed. In adults the association between specific Pi phenotypes and liver disease is even less clear. Chronic hepatitis or cirrhosis (negative for hepatitis B surface antigen, but positive for the characteristic inclusions) was identified in adults having ZZ, MZ, SZ, MS, and even MM phenotypes.[205] It appears, therefore, that not only the Pi ZZ but also heterozygous deficiency states are vulnerable to this form of liver injury, as is the rare MM individual with apparent normal levels of A1AT.

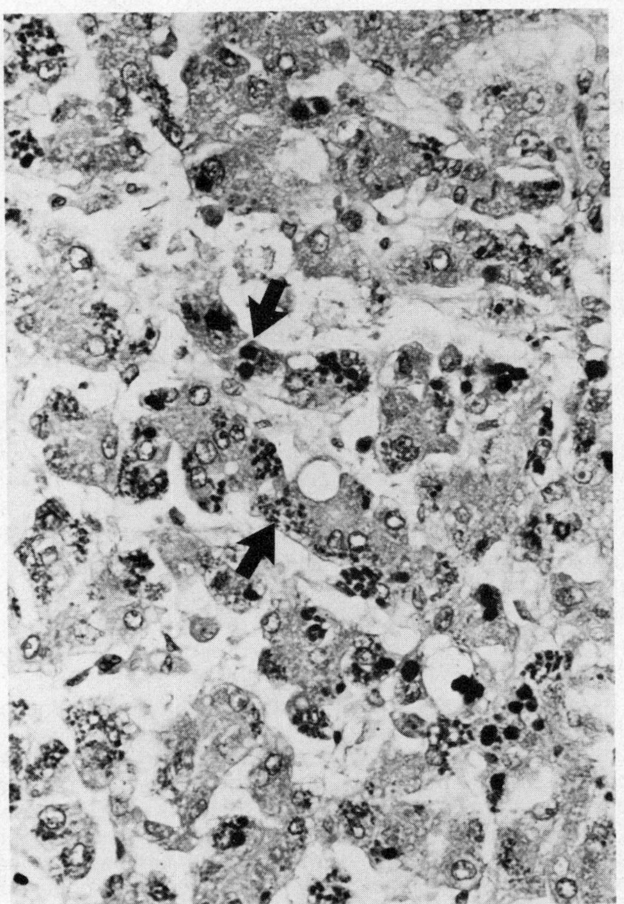

Figure 19–36. Alpha-1-antitrypsin deficiency. PAS stain of liver. The characteristic cytoplasmic granules (*arrows*) vary markedly in size. (Courtesy of Dr. R. A. DeLellis, Pathology Department, Tufts Medical School, Boston.)

Neonatal hepatitis is described later (p. 940) and it is sufficient to note that the histologic manifestations vary from active inflammatory disease to a form of almost "pure" cholestasis resembling biliary tract obstruction.[206]

Childhood cirrhosis, as noted, may appear with or without an antecedent history of neonatal hepatitis. It takes the form of a micronodular cirrhosis, but in a few cases, with progression of the condition, a macronodular pattern has emerged. The diagnostic feature is the characteristic presence of A1AT globules within hepatocytes.

Adult cirrhosis may be micronodular, but in most cases, presumably with progression of the disease, a macronodular pattern appears. The fibrous scarring is irregular, expanding and interconnecting portal tracts, sometimes isolating individual lobules or at other times enclosing many adjacent lobules. Frequently, piecemeal necrosis reminiscent of hepatitis B can be identified in the periportal regions where the globules are most prominent. Infrequently, fatty change and Mallory bodies are present. Rarely, hepatocarcinoma complicates the liver disease in adults.[207]

The role of the deficiency and subsequent accumulation of A1AT in the induction of the liver disease is not clear. It is significant that patients who are Pi null have no detectable A1AT in the plasma and no characteristic globules within hepatocytes, and show no clinical, laboratory, or histopathologic evidence of liver disease. Although this would suggest that the accumulation of antiprotease within hepatocytes is damaging, numerous inclusions may be present in completely viable cells, arguing against direct cytotoxicity. Contrariwise, globules may not be evident in individuals with a deficiency state and well-developed hepatic disease. Moreover, hepatic A1AT inclusions may be present in marked deficiency states, without detectable liver disease. An attractive, although still unproved, hypothesis suggests that inflammatory reactions resulting from gut-derived bacteria or from hepatotoxins may be exaggerated with deficiencies of protease inhibitors to thus ascribe to the liver cell globules and deficiency state only a potentiating role.[208]

CIRRHOSIS OF WILSON'S DISEASE (HEPATOLENTICULAR DEGENERATION)

Wilson's disease is an inherited autosomal recessive disorder of copper metabolism. The fundamental defect appears to be an impairment in the hepatic excretion of the metal, which leads to the accumulation of toxic levels. *The major anatomic and clinical consequences are (1) liver damage in the form of either active hepatitis or cirrhosis; (2) degenerative changes in the brain, particularly in the lenticular nuclei—hence, the synonym for this condition: hepatolenticular degeneration; and (3) a pathognomonic deposit of copper in the limbus of the cornea, producing a green-brown Kayser-Fleischer ring.* These changes rarely become evident in patients under 5 to 10 years, the time required for the accumulation of injurious levels of copper. About 50% of untreated patients remain asymptomatic until adolescence. The tissue accumulation of copper is most rapid in the liver, but eventually the brain and cornea become burdened. Thus, this condition comes to attention most often because of the liver involvement. Frequently its presence in childhood or adolescence as an acute, or even fulminating, lethal hepatitis is readily mistaken for viral hepatitis. More often there is the insidious onset of chronic active hepatitis, which directly progresses over the span of years to cirrhosis. On the other hand, the hepatitis may apparently remit and remain asymptomatic for years to decades only to be followed much later by cirrhosis. Indeed, in some instances, the cirrhosis is discovered in middle-to-later life without a previous history of hepatitis. Alternatively, the hepatic involvement may remain covert and the first manifestations are neurologic or psychiatric abnormalities, usually accompanied by Kayser-Fleischer rings.

PATHOGENESIS. Like iron, free copper has the potential of causing cell injury by the production of free radicals. *In Wilson's disease, toxic levels of copper accumulate primarily in the liver, brain, and cornea because absorption continues but excretion is impaired.* Although normally a small amount of copper is excreted in the urine, most is excreted in the bile, and some defect in biliary excretion is thought to underlie Wilson's disease. Thus, individuals with this condition are unable to balance output with intake. In a sense, then, the metabolic defect in Wilson's disease is diametrically opposed to that in idiopathic hemochromatosis, in which excessive intake underlies the accumulation of iron. Normally, copper absorbed from the upper gastrointestinal tract is transported to the liver loosely bound to albumin and perhaps to amino acids. These complexes are dissociated at the plasma membranes of hepatocytes and the copper is transferred into the cell where it is bound to copper-associated proteins, also known generically as heavy metal-binding metallothioneins, that allow safe storage of toxic heavy metals. Some is incorporated within hepatic enzymes, notably superoxide dismutase. Another copper-associated protein synthesized in the liver is an alpha-2-globulin known as apoceruloplasmin that, when bound to copper, forms ceruloplasmin. Ceruloplasmin is released into the plasma, accounting for 90 to 95% of total plasma copper, and is recycled to the liver, where it is degraded within lysosomes with release of the copper, which is then excreted in the bile. The remainder of the plasma copper is loosely bound to albumin and is sometimes called "free" copper. It is this fraction that is cytotoxic.

Against this background of normal metabolism, the following abnormalities have been observed in Wilson's disease: (1) the concentration of copper in the bile is significantly below normal; (2) there is a striking increase in the hepatic copper concentration, but it is often difficult to document by histochemical methods because the copper-protein complexes do not aggregate and become incorporated within lysosomes as visible granules;[209] (3) in most cases there is some reduction of the serum ceruloplasmin level below normal; (4) the amount of toxic "free" copper within the serum is increased, so that the total serum copper approaches the normal level; and (5) with expansion of the plasma free copper compartment, there is significantly increased urinary excretion of copper. Numerous attempts have been made to explain these abnormalities, including deficient synthesis of ceruloplasmin, or a lysosomal catabolic defect impairing cleavage and biliary excretion of copper, but both proposals fail to satisfy the observed findings. A new and intriguing concept invokes the production of a copper-associated protein or metallothionein, which has an abnormal avidity for copper.[210, 211] The following might then occur. Because of its high affinity for copper there is reduced transfer to ceruloplasmin, accounting for the characteristic low levels in the plasma. Metallothionein-copper complexes in hepatocytes might form insoluble aggregates that resist incorporation within lysosomes, which appears to be requisite for cleavage of the protein-copper complexes prior to biliary excretion. With accumulation, free copper may be released within the cytoplasm of the hepatocyte and simultaneously may leak into the blood. The toxic copper then produces free radicals that ultimately mediate the cell injury. Attractive as this proposition may be, it is still conjectural. It does not explain why lysosomal incorporation is critical to excretion nor why cell damage is limited to the liver, brain, and sometimes kidney. Thus, there is still much speculation about the origins of Wilson's disease but, whatever the defect may be, it has been corrected by liver transplant.

MORPHOLOGY. Three basic morphologic patterns of liver disease can be identified: (1) fatty change accompanied by mild portal inflammation and unicellular necrosis, (2) chronic active hepatitis, and (3) cirrhosis.[212] It seems reasonable to assume that these are merely stages in progression. Thus, it is believed that all patients with Wilson's disease, if they survive long enough, will develop cirrhosis. In the **presymptomatic phase** of the liver involvement, a dominant alteration is microvacuolar fatty change in the hepatocytes (resembling Reye's syndrome—p. 941), sometimes accompanied by ballooned nuclei filled with glycogen. In addition, there may be a minimal portal infiltrate of lymphocytes and swelling or necrosis of single random cells. Electron microscopic studies have revealed pleomorphic distortion of mitochondria, increased matrix density, and a curious separation of the inner and outer lamellae of the bounding membrane. Although increased amounts of copper can be identified biochemically, granular lysosomal aggregation of copper may or may not be evident by such histochemical techniques as rubeanic acid or rhodanine staining.

The **chronic active hepatitis of Wilson's disease** bears many resemblances to that of viral origin. Degeneration and necrosis of random hepatocytes; piecemeal necrosis most evident in the periportal region; marked inflammatory infiltration of the portal triads by lymphocytes, plasma cells, and occasional neutrophils with extension beyond the limiting plate; and progressive extension of fibrous tissue from the triads into the parenchyma, are all superimposed on the earlier morphologic changes. Cholestatic changes also are usually present but may be minimal. The earlier comments about increased copper in the liver are equally applicable to this phase of the disease.

The **cirrhosis may be micronodular, macronodular, or some hybrid of these two patterns.** It is likely that, like alcoholic cirrhosis, it begins as a micronodular disease and then with progression is converted into macronodular scarring reminiscent of postnecrotic cirrhosis. Whatever the pattern of nodularity, the color of the liver remains unchanged and its size may be near normal or may show a slight reduction in weight. Accompanying the scarring of variable intensity, there is a prominent portal inflammatory infiltrate, partly mononuclear and partly polymorphonuclear, along with proliferation of periportal cholangioles and minimal-to-moderate cholestasis. Vestiges of chronic active hepatitis such as piecemeal necrosis and fatty change may persist from earlier phases of the disease. The hepatocytes often contain marked amounts of lipofuscin. Mallory bodies can be identified in about half of the cases. At this stage the liver usually is heavily burdened by aggregated copper within lysosomes, which can usually be identified by special stains, principally in the periphery of the nodules.

If the liver disease does not prove fatal, brain involvement usually develops. The principal findings consist of cavitations in the lenticular nucleus, in the thalamus, and rarely in the dentate nucleus of the cerebellum. When cavitation is not present, there is often brownish discoloration and atrophy of the nuclear masses mentioned. Histologically, neuronal and astrocytic degeneration and death may be widely dispersed but are most prominent in the margins of the cavitated foci. Simultaneously, perhaps as a regenerative mechanism, there is an increase in the size and number of protoplasmic astrocytes throughout the brain, maximally in the lenticular nucleus, particularly in relation to the cavitations. The thalamus, red nucleus, and dentate nucleus of the cerebellum are similarly affected. Nerve fiber degeneration may appear in these same sites. Staining for copper may show an increased pericapillary deposition in loci of maximal injury.

The Kayser-Fleischer rings are the result of an accumulation of brown granules of copper in Desçemet's membrane close to the limbus of the cornea. These rings, which constitute one of the most distinctive clinical features of the disease, are usually readily evident to the naked eye but may require slit-lamp examination.

The renal tubules in some patients exhibit the changes described as nephrotoxic acute tubular necrosis on page 1027.

CLINICAL COURSE. The diagnosis of this condition may be readily evident when hepatic and neurologic disease are accompanied by the classic Kayser-Fleischer rings. However, the time sequence of these changes must be kept in mind. Earlier in the course there may only be manifestations related to liver involvement, or the hepatic lesion may be totally silent, with only neurologic or psychiatric signs and symptoms present. These manifestations are always accompanied, however, by the eye changes. With well-advanced cirrhosis, manifestations related to portal hypertension become evident and are often accompanied by the other clinical features of all forms of advanced cirrhosis, such as spider angiomas, gynecomastia, hypoprothrombinemia, and so forth. Whatever the clinical presentation, confirmation of a deficiency of serum ceruloplasmin, increased urinary excretion of copper, and, when all else is uncertain, an increase in chemically identifiable copper in the liver biopsy are necessary to establish the diagnosis.

The natural progression of this condition has been dramatically slowed and even stopped by the use of penicillamine for the remainder of the patient's life (increasing urinary excretion of the metal). The effectiveness of this therapy requires that all siblings and children of affected individuals, as well as blood relatives, be screened for the possible presence of early asymptomatic disease. Even heterozygotes retain excessive amounts of copper, albeit more slowly than homozygotes, and so carry an increased risk of developing Wilson's disease.[213]

OTHER FORMS OF CIRRHOSIS

Infrequently, cirrhosis appears in certain clinical settings not previously mentioned. *Infants and children with the inborn metabolic errors galactosemia and tyrosinosis may develop cirrhosis if they survive long enough.* Uncommonly, severe *cardiac sclerosis* (p. 898) becomes sufficiently marked to justify the designation "cardiac cirrhosis." Even more uncommonly, the desmoplastic reaction excited by a diffusely infiltrative cancer of the liver (primary or secondary) creates a *carcinomatous cirrhosis* or pseudocirrhosis disease. *Congenital syphilis*, happily now a rare disease, causes diffuse interstitial scarring of the liver that may mimic cirrhosis. In the adult, *multiple hepatic gummas in tertiary syphilis* may, in time, give rise to contracted scars that produce deep creases in the surface of the liver. This pattern of involvement is called *hepar lobatum*, but does not constitute a valid form of cirrhosis because the large tracts of intervening hepatic parenchyma are unaffected (Fig. 19–37). Infections caused by *Clonorchis sinensis* and other liver flukes, which preferentially invade the larger bile ducts within the liver, may cause sufficient obstruction to mimic or induce secondary biliary cirrhosis. Sometimes the portal venous branches are invaded by the periductal inflammatory reaction, adding an element of ischemia to the inflammatory process. *Cirrhosis has also been observed in patients with inflammatory bowel disease.* The genesis of this hepatic involvement is uncertain, but malnutrition, spread of organisms or bacterial antigens to the liver, and progressive pericholangitis have been implicated.

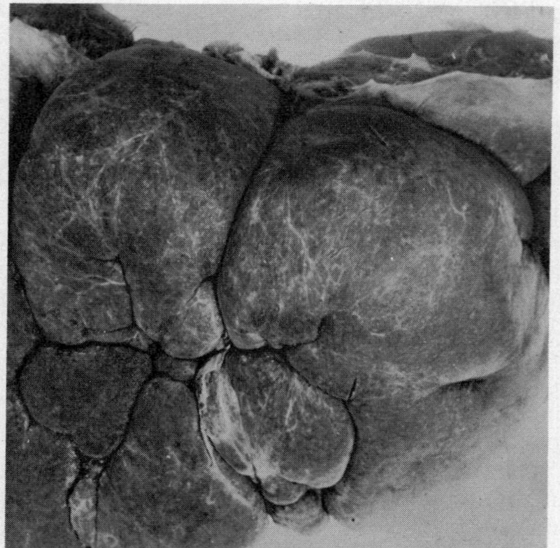

Figure 19–37. Hepar lobatum. Liver substance cut up into coarse lobes by deep furrows.

After all the major categories of cirrhosis and the rare instances of known causation have been excluded, there remain 15 to 60% of cases of completely obscure origin, referred to as *cryptogenic cirrhosis.*[214, 215] The magnitude of this "wastebasket" and its variable size in reported series speak eloquently to the differences in criteria employed in the categorization of diverse forms of cirrhosis and the general lack of understanding of the origins of many cases of cirrhosis.

BENIGN TUMORS AND NODULAR HYPERPLASIA

The various lesions embraced by this heading are all quite rare but have significance because of their possible confusion with primary cancer of the liver.

NODULAR HYPERPLASIA

These nontumorous nodules may occur singly, or multiply, sometimes in such profusion as to create an overall nodularity to the liver that may be readily mistaken for cirrhosis. It is likely that the solitary nodule represents a hamartoma, whereas the multiple nodules result from some curious multicentric regenerative hyperplasia.

The solitary nodule is also called *focal nodular hyperplasia,* despite the fact that it is probably a hamartomatous developmental defect. It occurs as a discrete, usually subcapsular, nodule ranging up to several centimeters in diameter that usually is clearly demarcated from the hepatic parenchyma by a thin rim of fibrous tissue. Typically, it has a fibrous, stellate center from which septa radiate out into the surrounding normal or slightly variable hepatocytes. The central connective tissue often contains scattered bile ductules and dilated vascular sinusoids supporting the hamartomatous nature of these lesions. More common in women than in men, at one time they were associated with the use of oral contraceptives, but the fact that they have not increased in incidence since the advent of this form of contraception undermines this relationship.[216]

Multiple nodules within the liver, whether few or many, are designated *nodular regenerative hyperplasia.* They vary in size from a few millimeters to several centimeters in diameter. Typically they are composed of essentially normal cords of hepatocytes separated by vascular sinusoids that differ from normal only in the loss of the symmetric radial array. The nodules are not enclosed by fibrous tissue and are demarcated only by a thin rim of collapsed reticular framework resulting from compression and atrophy of adjacent hepatocytes.[217] The etiology of this curious change is entirely obscure. Once again, an association has been noted with the long-term use of oral contraceptives and anabolic androgenic steroids, but the evidence is less than convincing.[218] For unknown reasons, almost half of all reported cases have appeared in patients with Felty's syndrome (p. 1355). When the liver is diffusely involved, this condition may give rise to portal hypertension, sometimes leading to massive bleeding from gastroesophageal varices. It is difficult to establish the diagnosis of nodular regenerative hyperplasia with needle liver biopsy because the architecture within the nodules is so banal, and often the condition is more apparent macroscopically than microscopically.

LIVER CELL ADENOMA

The incidence of these benign tumors, once curiosities, has increased since the advent of oral contraceptive pills, but not sufficiently to remove them from the rare category.[219] Estrogens, you recall, may serve as promoters in the induction of at least certain forms of malignant neoplasia in both humans and animals. They are also enzyme inducers. Whether either of these activities has any relevance to the induction of liver cell adenomas is unknown.

Adenomas are pale yellow-white, frequently bile-stained nodules, found anywhere in the hepatic substance but often beneath the capsule. They range from several centimeters up to 30 cm in diameter. Although they are usually well demarcated, encapsulation may not be grossly evident. On occasion, peripheral pseudopods project into the normal liver substance, creating the false impression of malignant invasion. Histologically adenomas are composed of sheets and cords of cells that may be entirely normal in appearance or have some variation in cell and nuclear size. Sometimes the cells have cleared cytoplasm. Prominent in these tumors are abnormally disposed, dilated vascular sinusoids, but bile ducts are usually absent. A capsule that ranges from delicate collapsed reticulin to well-defined connective tissue usually separates the lesion from the surrounding normal parenchyma, but it may be deficient in places and indeed be entirely lacking in some adenomas.

Adenomas have clinical significance for two reasons: (1) when they present as an intrahepatic mass they are readily mistaken for more ominous hepatocellular carcinomas; and (2) subcapsular adenomas have a tendency to rupture, particularly during pregnancy, and cause severe intraperitoneal hemorrhage.[220]

OTHER BENIGN TUMORS

Several generally insignificant lesions merit brief mention. *Cavernous hemangiomas*, identical to those occurring in other parts of the body, sometimes produce discrete, red-blue, soft nodules, usually less than 1 to 2 cm in diameter. They are readily mistaken for small foci of hemorrhage, particularly when subcapsular. *Bile duct adenomas* are firm, pale, discrete nodules, rarely over 1 cm in diameter. Unlike the liver cell adenoma, they are almost never bile stained. Histologically they are composed of epithelial-lined channels or ducts separated by a scant-to-abundant connective tissue stroma. Since they often lack well-developed capsules, many consider them to be hamartomas. *Cysts* may occur singly or multiply. The single cyst, interpreted as a benign neoplasm, may achieve a diameter of 5 to 10 cm. They contain clear serous fluid and are lined by flattened, atrophic, bile duct–like epithelial cells that can become sufficiently attenuated to be inapparent. More often there are multiple developmental smaller cysts ranging up to 3 to 4 cm in diameter (Fig. 19–38). The cuboidal lining is generally more apparent in such lesions and resembles that of bile ductules. Some contain brown-green concretions, possibly representing inspissated bile. It is likely that polycystic liver disease is developmental in origin, borne out by its well-defined association with polycystic kidney disease.

MALIGNANT TUMORS

The liver and lungs share the dubious distinction of being the visceral organs most often involved in the metastatic spread of cancers. Thus, the overwhelming majority of cancers in the liver are metastases, most commonly from carcinomas of the breast, lung, and colon. By contrast, primary carcinomas of the liver are relatively uncommon in North America and Western Europe. However, these primary malignant neoplasms are very prevalent in other countries and, on a global basis, primary carcinoma of the liver is probably the most common visceral malignant tumor in males.[221]

PRIMARY CARCINOMA OF LIVER

There are basically two types of primary carcinoma of the liver: one is of the hepatocyte line and is called *hepatocellular carcinoma* (HCC) or *liver cell carcinoma;* the other, composed of bile duct epithelium, is designated *cholangiocarcinoma.* Very infrequently a neoplasm appears to share characteristics of both lines—the hepatocholangiocarcinoma—possibly because it arises in more primitive cells capable of differentiating in both directions. HCC, grievously sometimes still called a hepatoma, accounts for about 90% of all primary liver cancers. Virtually all the remaining 10% are cholangiocarcinomas; the mixed pattern is very uncommon. There has been a recent upsurge of interest in HCC for several reasons: (1) the striking differences in its worldwide distribution; (2) the existence of new insights into potential causative influences; and (3) the possibility that interventions now available could reduce the incidence of this form of cancer. There is now substantial evidence that, in addition to a well-defined association with cirrhosis of the liver, there is an even closer connection between the hepatitis B virus (HBV) and liver cell

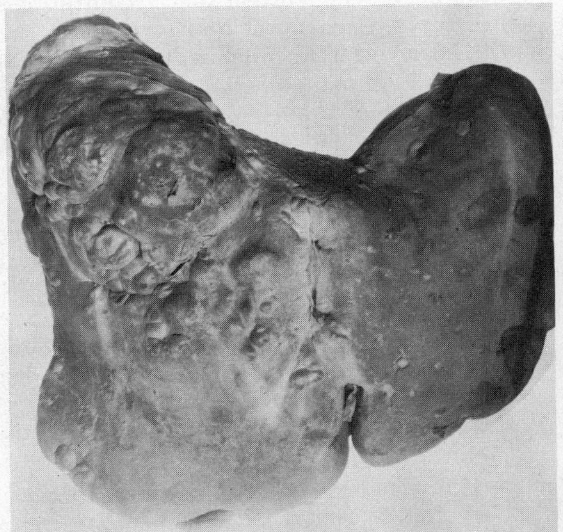

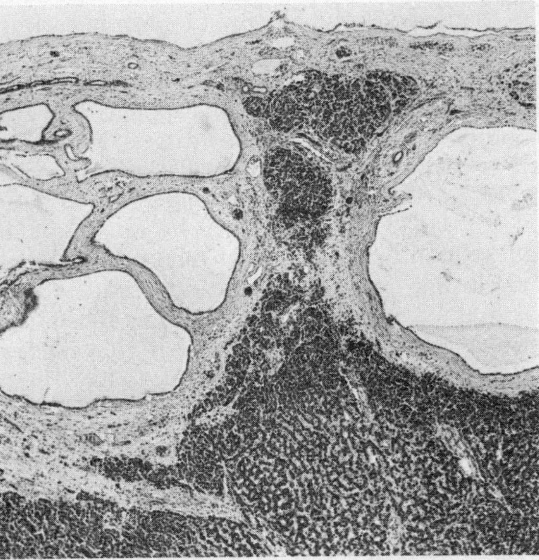

Figure 19–38. *A,* Congenital cysts of liver, showing numerous subcapsular cysts. *B,* Microscopically, cysts are surrounded by fibrous tissue and lined by cuboidal epithelium.

carcinoma. Thus, the hope arises that immunization with hepatitis B vaccine may be preventive.

EPIDEMIOLOGY. The disparity in the frequency of HCC between high-risk and low-risk countries can only be described as dramatic (30- to 40-fold). It is the most frequent type of cancer in many parts of Asia and Africa: Mozambique, 70% of all carcinomas; Senegal, 67%; Bantus in South Africa, 50%; India, China, Taiwan, and the Philippines, each 20%.[222] In contrast, HCC in the United States, Canada, and Western Europe represents about 2 to 3% of all carcinomas. There is a remarkable concordance in high-risk areas between the prevalence of HCC and infection by HBV. In such locales, markers of HBV are almost always present in patients with the neoplasm. Moreover, the disease tends to be fulminant and to occur in those under the age of 40, and the male:female ratio is approximately 3:1. In contrast, in low-risk areas such as the U.S. and Western Europe, markers for HBV are found in less than half of the patients, the neoplasm tends to occur in cirrhotic elderly men (male:female ratio about 9:1), and it runs a subacute course.[223] In low-risk countries there is a very much smaller peak in HCC incidence in children who usually have otherwise normal livers.

ETIOLOGY AND PATHOGENESIS. One cannot look at the epidemiologic data without strongly suspecting a causal role for HBV infection in the genesis of liver cell carcinoma. The supporting evidence is voluminous and can only be sampled here. There is the concordance in high-risk locales between the prevalence of the two diseases and the extremely high frequency (approaching 90%) of serologic viral markers such as HBV surface antigen (HBsAG) or antibody to core antigen in patients with the cancer. The presence of HBsAG implies persistent infection such as is characteristic of carriers and chronic active hepatitis.[224] In high-incidence locales, many chronic carriers derive their infection vertically in the perinatal period from carrier mothers. Infection so early in life might reasonably contribute to the neoplasm's appearance at a younger age in such populations. More direct evidence is the finding in chronic carriers of HBV surface antigen in both normal liver cells and cancer cells, and (significantly) viral DNA sequences in the genome of these cells.[225, 226] It thus appears that this virus, like other known oncogenic viruses, is able to integrate all or part of its genetic information into a host cell. Were all this evidence not enough, there is an animal model of HCC that appears to be caused by an agent closely related to HBV. Woodchucks have a high frequency of chronic active hepatitis and hepatocellular carcinomas; viral particles closely resembling those seen in humans with HBV infection have been identified in some of the neoplasms; and viral sequences have been identified in the DNA of the tumor cells in two neoplasms. The viral core and surface antigens in the two species have antigenic cross reactivity.[227] As a further test for the causal role of HBV infection, a large series of asymptomatic chronic carriers are now being followed for the possible development of hepatocellular carcinoma.[228] After three to five years of follow-up, 61 cases of HCC have appeared among 3400 chronic carriers, but only one tumor among 19,000 noncarriers. The evidence implicating HBV grows stronger every day.

The dominating importance of HBV infection does not preclude a role for cirrhosis in the development of HCC. In low-risk locales such as the U.S. where persistent HBV infection is relatively infrequent, *about 80 to 90% of liver cell carcinomas arise in cirrhotic livers.* The risk with certain forms of cirrhosis is extremely variable, but is particularly high in chronic active hepatitis B converting to postnecrotic cirrhosis (15 to 25%) and pigment cirrhosis (15 to 30%). It is considerably lower in alcoholic cirrhosis (3 to 5%), perhaps because the natural course of this disease is relatively short. Overall, in countries where infection with HBV is relatively infrequent, the conversion rate of cirrhosis is in the range of 5 to 15%. Where HBV infection is near universal, the rate of conversion of cirrhosis to cancer approaches 50%.[229] This contrast in conversion rates may relate to the fact that chronic active viral hepatitis is the most frequent cause of cirrhosis where the HBV is prevalent, whereas alcoholic cirrhosis predominates in Western cultures. The reason why cirrhosis and particularly certain types predispose to HCC is not clear. Chronic regenerative activity may be involved, but it is equally likely that the damaged liver is rendered more vulnerable to environmental carcinogens.[223] It should be noted, however, that about 10% of patients with hepatocellular carcinoma, particularly children, do not have cirrhosis.

Still other influences may contribute to the development of hepatocellular carcinoma. There are many reports of an increased incidence with the use of oral contraceptives and androgenic steroids.[230] Aflatoxin B_1, a documented hepatocarcinogen in rats, fowl, and fish, has long been suspected to contribute to the high prevalence of liver cell cancer in tropical parts of the world, where improperly stored grains and nuts are frequently contaminated by *Aspergillus flavus*. It has always been assumed that the mycotoxin or its metabolites serve as chemical initiators of the cancer.[231] In 1979, however, it was proposed that aflatoxin suppresses cell-mediated immunity and so favors the development of persistent HBV infections.[232] Other plant derivatives such as cycasin and pyrrolizidine, found in "bush tea," have been implicated without strong proof.

None of the influences related to HCC have any bearing on the development of cholangiocarcinoma. No association has been identified among cholangiocarcinoma and HBV, cirrhosis, or the exogenous putative carcinogens mentioned above. The only recognized causal influences for this form of cancer are previous exposure to Thorotrast (formerly used in radiography of the biliary tract) and invasion of the biliary tract by liver flukes, *Clonorchis sinensis* and its close relatives.

MORPHOLOGY. Any one of the histologic variants of primary liver carcinoma mentioned earlier—the HCC, cholangiocarcinoma, or the mixed pattern—may appear grossly as: (1) a **unifocal,** usually large mass; (2) **multifocal,**

apparently disconnected, widely distributed nodules; or (3) a diffusely **infiltrative** cancer, permeating widely or sometimes involving the entire liver.[223] All three patterns may cause liver enlargement (2000 to 3000 gm), particularly the unifocal massive and multinodular patterns, which also often produce clinically palpable irregularity of the liver edge. When discrete masses can be seen, they are basically yellow-white; when they are large they are often punctuated by areas of hemorrhage or necrosis (Fig. 19–39). The diffuse pattern may blend in deceptively with the cirrhotic background. **Hepatocellular carcinomas sometimes take on a green hue when composed of well-differentiated hepatocytes capable of secreting bile. Cholangiocarcinomas are rarely bile stained,** except possibly for peripheral diffusion of pigment from the surrounding hepatic substance, because differentiated bile duct epithelium does not synthesize bile. Infrequently with HCC, but very often with cholangiocarcinoma, the tumor substance is extremely firm and gritty, related to a dense desmoplasia. **All patterns of HCC have a strong propensity for invasion of vascular channels.** Sometimes the intravascular neoplasm extends in a long, snakelike mass into the portal vein or hepatic vein, and even into the inferior vena cava and right side of the heart.

The histology of **HCC** is given first. These cancers range from well-differentiated to highly anaplastic undifferentiated lesions. The well- and moderately well-differentiated forms are composed of tumor cells, recognizable as hepatocytic in origin (Fig. 19–40). There is the usual variation in cell and nuclear size, prominent nucleoli, and occasional mitotic figures. The cytoplasm basically resembles that of the normal hepatocyte and in some instances contains inclusions of bile pigment. The differentiated cells are disposed either in a trabecular (sinusoidal) or an acinar (tubular) pseudoglandular pattern. The trabeculae are made up of several layers of tumor cells, separated by vascular channels (bearing some resemblance to sinusoids) embedded within a connective tissue sheath. In the acinar or pseudoglandular pattern, the differentiated tumor cells are often disposed about lumens, creating the pseudoglandular pattern. Sometimes these lumens contain plugs of inspissated bile. An uncommon variant of the well- to moderately well-differentiated HCC is made up of "clear cells" because of the high content of cytoplasmic glycogen. Such tumors bear a strong resemblance to clear-cell renal carcinomas. Differentiated tumor cells often form abortive bile canaliculi, complete with microvilli.

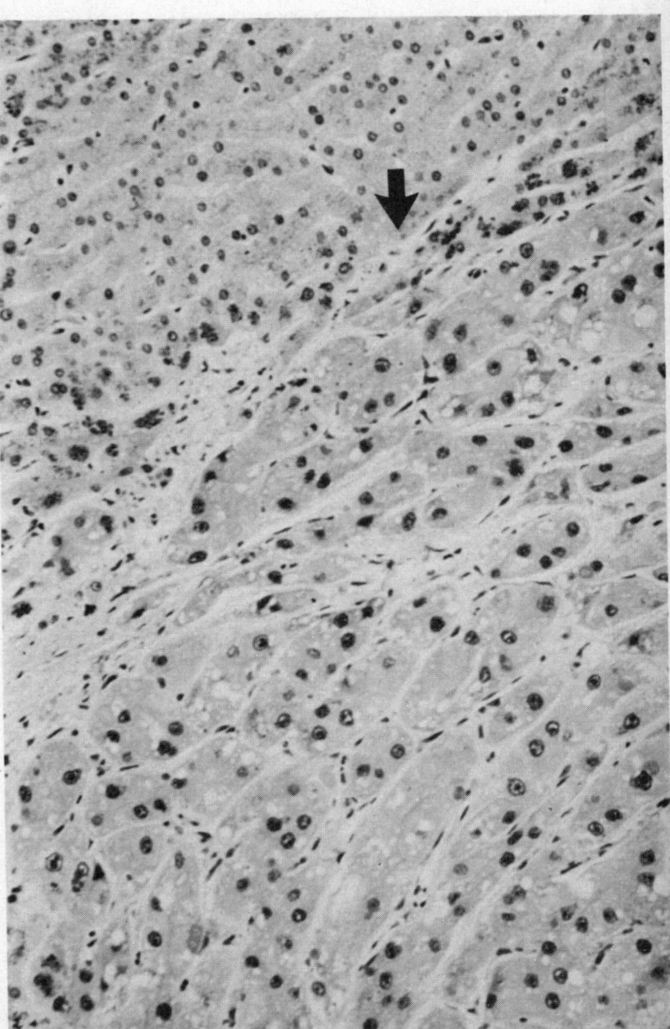

Figure 19–40. Hepatocellular carcinoma, moderately well-differentiated. Advancing margin of mass is indicated by arrow. Tumor cells have moderate variation in cell and nuclear size and shape but retain a remarkable resemblance to normal liver cells, seen at upper left.

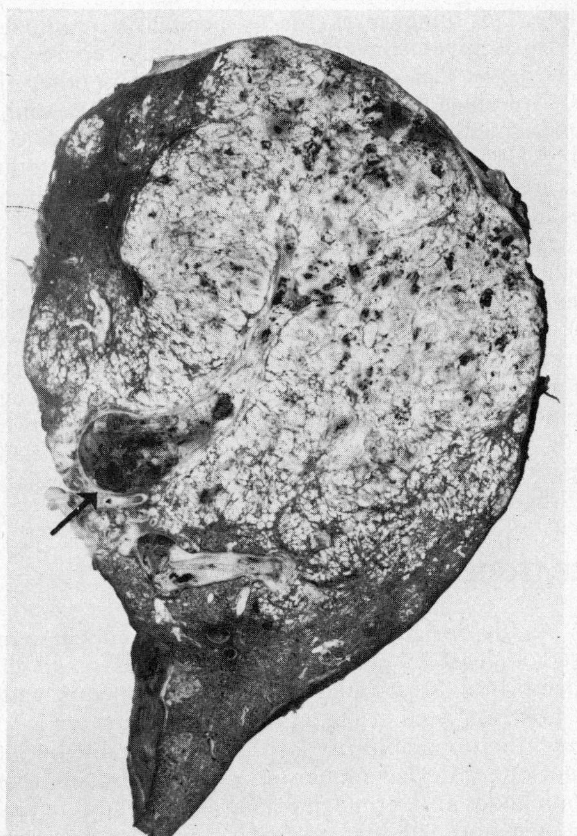

Figure 19–39. Hepatocellular carcinoma complicating pigment cirrhosis. Tumor thrombus in branch of portal vein (*arrow*).

Poorly differentiated forms of HCC present a wide range of histologic patterns that can be characterized as pleomorphic giant cell or small, completely undifferentiated cell or spindle cell. The giant cell neoplasm may be totally anarchic with sheets of wild-looking cells (having abundant cytoplasm) and often bearing multiple nuclei and atypical mitoses. Areas of ischemic necrosis are frequent in such lesions. The spindle cell variant may mimic a sarcoma, and indeed often has an abundant fibrous stroma separating the parenchymal cells. Sometimes the stroma is sufficiently vascularized to resemble an angiosarcoma. Bile formation in such undifferentiated lesions is uncommon. Vascular invasion is a common finding in all forms of HCC.

A number of additional features may be present in HCC, more often in the well-differentiated variants. Occasionally cytoplasmic inclusions, typical of Mallory's alcoholic hyalin, are found. When persistent hepatitis B infection is present, the tumorous hepatocytes may have ground-glass cytoplasm and contain (with immunofluorescent or immunoperoxidase techniques) large amounts of hepatitis B surface antigen. Immunohistochemical staining also reveals A1AT in tumor cells in 70 to 75% of cases despite the absence of an apparent A1AT deficiency state in the patient.[234] Alpha-fetoprotein (AFP) can be identified in 50 to 90% of tumors, and carcinoembryonic antigen in 30%. The most reliable features of HCC are bile pigment within tumor cells or, on electron microscopic examination, the formation of bile canaliculi.

Cholangiocarcinomas have a more limited histologic range. Most are well-differentiated sclerosing adenocarcinomas with clearly defined glandular and tubular structures lined by somewhat anaplastic cuboidal-to-columnar epithelial cells. These neoplasms are often desmoplastic, so that dense collagenous stroma separates the parenchymal elements. Occasionally, microcysts are formed into which may project branching papillary structures covered by epithelial cells. Mucus is frequently present within cells and the lumens, but not bile. Thus, in needle biopsies these neoplasms may be extremely difficult to differentiate from metastatic adenocarcinomas. Vascular invasion is less common with cholangiocarcinomas than with HCC and, when present, takes the form of lining of vessels by cancer cells rather than the solid cords of neoplasm seen with HCC. There is no association other than coincidence with preexisting cirrhosis, nor with HBV antigens or AFP.

The HCC and the cholangiocarcinoma differ somewhat in their patterns of spread. Hematogenous metastases to the lungs, bones (mainly vertebrae), adrenals, brain, or elsewhere are present at autopsy in about 50% of cases of cholangiocarcinoma. Hematogenous metastases are less frequent with HCC and may not be present despite clear evidence of venous invasion, attributed to the short survival with this form of cancer. Lymph node metastases to the perihilar, peripancreatic, and para-aortic nodes above and below the diaphragm are found in about half of all cholangiocarcinomas and less frequently with HCC. An even more distinctive difference is the tendency (about 5% of cases) for HCC to penetrate the liver capsule directly and extend into the diaphragm, right chest wall, and pleural and peritoneal cavities. This pattern of spread sometimes causes severe intraperitoneal bleeding.

Clinical Course. Hepatocellular carcinomas are rarely detected early in their development because so often their initial signs and symptoms merge into the background of preexisting chronic liver disease, such as chronic active hepatitis and cirrhosis. Indeed, survival after diagnosis is usually less than six months. There are, however, uncommon reports of successful resection of monofocal hepatocellular carcinomas and cholangiocarcinomas. When HCC comes to attention it is usually because of rapid enlargement of the liver, with pain or tenderness or rapid deterioration of liver function. Other characteristic findings are a friction rub or bruit over the liver and bloody ascites. Weight loss, fever, polycythemia (ectopic production of erythropoietin), and hypoglycemia related to extensive destruction of hepatic parenchyma are sometimes present. Occasional neoplasms, more often cholangiocarcinomas, have a more indolent course and are discovered because of pain or nodular enlargement of the liver. Some of these cancers announce themselves by massive intraperitoneal or gastrointestinal bleeding. Angiography, isotopic liver scans, and CT scans are highly useful in diagnosis, but cannot differentiate primary from secondary tumors, nor benign from malignant tumors. As mentioned, AFP is found in the serum of 50 to 90% of patients with HCC. Elevated serum levels of AFP are also encountered with cancers arising from yolk sac remnants, and less regularly with germ cell tumors of the testis and ovary and cancers of the stomach and pancreas. Moreover, elevated levels are also encountered with non-neoplastic conditions including cirrhosis, massive liver necrosis, chronic hepatitis, normal pregnancy, fetal distress or death, and fetal neural tube defects such as anencephaly and spina bifida. This tumor marker lacks specificity, but the level of rise is greatest with HCC. Although reports vary, most agree that only rarely do conditions other than HCC produce serum levels above 150 to 200 ng/ml. In contrast with HCC, the level often exceeds 2000 ng/ml.[235] HCC also rarely produces such ectopic products as carcinoembryonic antigen, chorionic gonadotropin, Regan isoenzyme, and erythropoietin.

Most patients with primary liver cancers die of hepatic failure or gastrointestinal bleeding from esophageal varices (probably related to the underlying cirrhosis). Other significant causes of death include cachexia, intercurrent infection, and intraperitoneal hemorrhage. The only ray of light in this otherwise dismal scene is the possibility of significantly reducing the incidence of HCC by immunization of high-risk populations against hepatitis B infection.[236] A vaccine has become available, but the results of early trials must be awaited.[237]

HEPATOBLASTOMA

As the designation implies, these tumors are composed at least in part of embryonic cells resembling hepatoblasts. Most often discovered in infants within the first two years of life and only very uncommonly in adults, their overall rarity justifies considerable brevity. About one-third have metastasized to lungs, brain, and lymph nodes at the time of diagnosis, but they generally pursue a more indolent course than primary carcinomas of the liver, permitting successful resection when recognized. However, differentiation of these masses from primary liver carcinomas (which also may arise in children) is difficult but facilitated by the following features: (1) frequent association with congenital abnormalities such as hemihypertrophy and renal malformations, (2) the visualization by x-rays of calcifications within some of the neoplasms, and (3) unusually high serum levels of AFP.

There are two types of hepatoblastoma. Both may appear as a single large mass or as multiple dispersed nodules.[238] The *epithelial type* has a uniform gray-white cut surface and is composed of varied proportions of embryonal and fetal cells. The embryonal cells are small, have scant cytoplasm, and are largely composed of round-to-ovoid dark nuclei. They are laid down in sheets, but often form rosettes or pseudorosettes analogous to those seen in the neuroblastoma. The fetal cells have more cytoplasm that may contain fat, glycogen, or bile, and may bear more resemblance to hepatocytes. The *mixed type* of hepatoblastoma has a more variegated, gray-tan, hemorrhagic, or bile-stained cut surface and often contains gritty foci of apparent calcification. Histologically, it consists of not only the epithelial elements described above but also foci of mesenchymal differentiation (osteoid, cartilage, striated muscle), and ductlike structures sometimes secreting mucin. Both variants of hepatoblastoma pursue similar courses and lead to death within about one year unless successfully resected.

ANGIOSARCOMA

This rare form of cancer may occur without known predisposing influences, but also is clearly associated with previous exposure to vinyl chloride, arsenic, and Thorotrast.[239] An increased incidence of this form of cancer has been reported in industrial workers making or using vinyl chloride[240] and in vineyard workers exposed to arsenic-containing insecticide sprays and dusts. Thorotrast was once used for radiographic visualization of the biliary tract. The interval between exposure and appearance of the neoplasm has ranged up to several decades. A sequence of preneoplastic liver changes has been seen in these individuals. It begins with areas of hyperplasia of hepatocytes associated with hyperplasia of sinusoidal and Kupffer cells and the deposition of perisinusoidal reticulin. Continued proliferation of the various cells eventually leads to the formation of blood-filled vascular channels lined by anaplastic endothelial-like spindled cells or by more plump anaplastic polyhedral cells separated by small-to-large trabeculae of similar cells.[241] *Critical to the diagnosis of angiosarcoma is the recognition that the vascular channels are formed by and lined by anaplastic tumor cells, rather than by mature endothelial cells.* Foci of hematopoiesis and variable amounts of lymphocytic infiltration are often present. Most of these neoplasms are highly aggressive; metastasize widely to the lungs, pleura, spleen, lymph nodes, bone, and elsewhere; and cause death within one year.

METASTATIC TUMORS

As indicated before, metastatic involvement of the liver is far more common than primary neoplasia. Although the most common primaries producing hepatic metastases are those of the breast, lung, and colon, any cancer in any site of the body may spread to the liver. Typically, multiple nodular implants are found that often cause striking hepatomegaly (Fig. 19–41). The liver weight may exceed several kilos. There is a tendency for metastatic nodules to outgrow their blood supply, producing central necrosis and umbilication when viewed from the surface of the liver. Infrequently a solitary metastasis is encountered, small or large, sometimes in the absence of apparent extrahepatic metastases. In such bizarre instances, resection may be attempted, but almost always there are occult foci of spread elsewhere, which appear later. It is neither possible nor necessary to attempt to characterize the range of morphologic patterns produced by the always unpredictable metastatic seeding. In general the metastases replicate the histology of the primary cancer, but not infrequently the secondaries are less well differentiated than the primary, since neoplastic clones having the potential for hematogenous dissemination tend to be more aggressive and less well differentiated. The converse is exceptional. The multiplicity of implants usually differentiates secondary from primary involvement, but there are multinodular primary liver carcinomas and rarely, as noted, unifocal metastases.

Always surprising is the amount of metastatic involvement that may be present in the absence of clinical or laboratory evidence of hepatic functional insufficiency. Often the only clinical telltale sign is hepatomegaly, sometimes with nodularity of the free edge. However, with massive or strategic involvement (obstruction of major ducts), jaundice and abnormal liver function tests may appear. Very useful in establishing

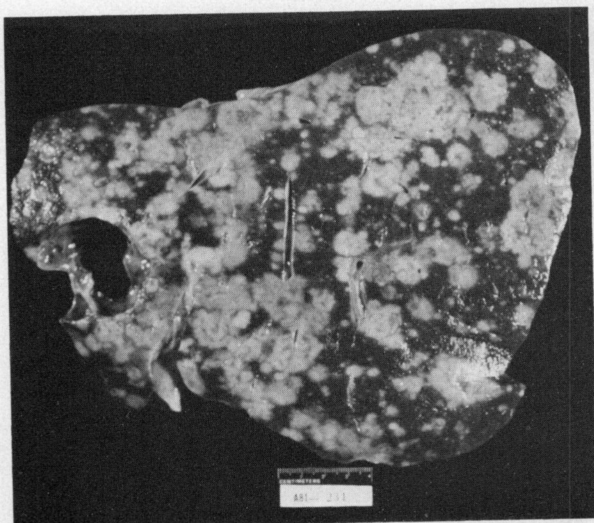

Figure 19–41. Multiple hepatic metastases from a primary gastric carcinoma.

the existence of metastases are scintiscans, celiac arteriography, ultrasonography, and CT scans, which in varying combinations yield correct diagnosis in about 95% of cases.[242] Blind liver needle biopsy yields positive results in approximately 50% of cases[243] and obviously depends on the extent of hepatic involvement. Despite heroic efforts at selective infusion of antitumor agents into the celiac axis, metastases within the liver usually spell death within one year.

MISCELLANEOUS DISORDERS

A few hepatic disorders do not fit well into any of the previous categories and so are included here.

NEONATAL HEPATITIS (INCLUDING BILIARY ATRESIA)

The term "neonatal hepatitis" is always used in a clinical sense to embody all the diseases that result in hepatocellular dysfunction or bile duct obstruction in the neonate.[244] Neonatal hepatitis, therefore, is not a specific morphologic entity. The major causative disorders are listed in Table 19–5. Justification for inclusion of all these disorders under the term "neonatal hepatitis" comes from the fact that all cause essentially identical conjugated hyperbilirubinemia, and all evoke a remarkably similar morphologic lesion resembling viral hepatitis characterized by obstructive and inflammatory changes accompanied by parenchymal injury. Even the metabolic or obstructive diseases in the neonate cause parenchymal and inflammatory reactions typical of hepatitis.

Table 19–5. CAUSES OF NEONATAL HEPATITIS

Infectious
Bacterial sepsis
Syphilis
Listeria monocytogenes
Hepatitis B
Rubella
Toxoplasmosis
Herpes simplex
Cytomegalovirus (CMV)
Coxsackie virus
Echovirus
Adenovirus
Metabolic/Genetic
Alpha-1-antitrypsin deficiency
Cystic fibrosis
Wilson's disease
Galactosemia
Fructosemia
Tyrosinemia
Biliary Tract Abnormalities
Extrahepatic atresia and hypoplasia
Choledochal cysts
Intrahepatic ductular atresia/hypoplasia
Others
Hemolytic disease of newborn
Familial intrahepatic cholestasis (Byler disease)

Most of the diseases producing neonatal hepatitis have been discussed elsewhere, and so only a few explanatory comments follow. Although hepatitis B can be transmitted perinatally, overt disease rarely appears at birth but usually between the ages of 2 and 5 months. It may be acute or even fulminant, but in most instances the infection results only in the "healthy" carrier state. Among the metabolic disorders, Wilson's disease, galactosemia, and fructosemia, when promptly recognized, permit the establishment of appropriate therapy with more or less complete restitution of normal liver structure and function. The biliary tract abnormalities present a special problem in interpretation. They may take the form of hypoplasia or marked atretic narrowing of the extrahepatic or intrahepatic ducts. In some instances, the abnormalities involve both ductal systems.[245] Debate continues as to whether these disorders constitute congenital or acquired anomalies.[246] Anatomic study of the ducts, whether extrahepatic or intrahepatic, often reveals marked inflammatory changes accompanied by fibrosis and narrowing.[247] The question arises—are such changes secondary to a developmental biliary tract defect or are they initiated by some form of infection causing, in turn, acquired narrowing or obstruction of the ducts? At present it seems impossible to resolve this uncertainty, and conceivably both processes may contribute. However, it should not be overlooked that when the extrahepatic ducts are involved without intrahepatic abnormalities, early surgical repair may prevent the development of biliary cirrhosis and death from hepatic failure. Despite the long list of implicated disorders, the basis of neonatal hepatitis is very often unknown.

The morphologic features common to all forms of neonatal hepatitis are: **(1) cholestasis; (2) a mononuclear infiltrate largely limited to the portal tracts; (3) parenchymal changes ranging from disorganization to random cell necrosis, and prominently the formation of multinucleate hepatocytic giant cells; and (4) proliferation of bile ductules in many instances.** A number of ancillary findings may be present depending on the underlying disorder: e.g., characteristic cytoplasmic inclusions of alpha-1-antitrypsin deficiency, viral inclusions in CMV, or fibrotic narrowing in the extrahepatic or intrahepatic ducts. With persistence of the cholestasis, the changes of biliary cirrhosis appear in all cases.

It is impossible to express a prognosis for such diverse derangements. On the one hand is intrahepatic bile duct atresia or hypoplasia, for example, with no form of curative therapy except possibly liver transplantation; death usually occurs in such instances within one year from progressive cirrhosis and liver failure. On the other hand are the fortunate cases of neonatal hepatitis caused by bacterial infection, in which cure and complete recovery can be expected. With unremitting neonatal hepatitis, cirrhosis and liver failure will follow within one year.

REYE'S SYNDROME

Reye's syndrome is an acute, sometimes catastrophic, systemic disorder seen predominantly in children between 6 months and 15 years of age. In full-blown cases, it is characterized by an edematous encephalopathy and striking fatty change in the liver. However, it is now apparent that milder expressions of the condition, called grade I Reye's syndrome, are much more frequent, are infrequently associated with neurologic impairment, are nonprogressive, and are almost always compatible with recovery.[247A] Typically, Reye's syndrome appears following a mild respiratory tract infection or other viral illness, most commonly influenza A or B or varicella. Recovery from the viral illness is complicated by the onset of severe vomiting and evidence of liver dysfunction such as elevated SGOT, prolongation of prothrombin time, hyperammonemia, and sometimes jaundice. In those with more severe involvements, progressive obtundation follows, leading to delirium, coma, and convulsions. Death occurs within a day or two in about 25 to 40% of cases with neurologic impairment, from progressive cerebral edema and brain herniations. Complete recovery follows in the remainder of the severe cases, but neurologic or psychiatric sequelae unfortunately persist in about one-half of the survivors.[248] The hepatic dysfunction is less threatening than the CNS involvement, and in survivors of mild and severe disease normal liver function is usually restored.

The search for the cause of this condition is now intense. Clearly there is some association with viral infection. Clusters of cases may erupt within a few months in a particular geographical locale, usually following an outbreak of respiratory viral infections, particularly influenza B or A. The sporadic cases occurring throughout the year are more often associated with other viral infections such as chickenpox. However, there is no correlation between the severity of the viral illness and the onset of Reye's syndrome, and in fact it is most often rather mild. Moreover, in fatal cases there are no stigmata in the brain pointing to viral encephalitis. Another line of study focuses on the possibility of deficiencies in urea-cycle enzymes, particularly ornithine transcarbamylase and carbamyl phosphate synthetase, which may explain the hyperammonemia and the neurologic changes that bear some resemblance to those of hepatic encephalopathy.[249] In rare cases the enzyme deficiencies are thought to represent hereditary inborn errors of metabolism, but the syndrome has also been associated with transient acquired deficiencies of the urea-cycle enzymes.[250] Epidemiologic data have also cast suspicion on insecticide-related chemicals, aflatoxin, and particularly aspirin. Conceivably, toxic reactions to any one of these agents could enhance the injurious effects of a virus.[251, 252] Without detailing all the evidence for and against each of these agents, it is sufficient to note the *growing consensus in the United States that "there is a high probability that the administration of aspirin contributes to the causation of Reye's syndrome."*[254] The evidence implicating aspirin (acetylsalicylate) is indirect but impressive. Changes remarkably similar to those of Reye's syndrome have been seen in fatal salicylate intoxication.[255] About 95 to 98% of persons affected have been exposed to aspirin during the viral infection immediately before the onset of Reye's syndrome, in contrast to only 60 to 70% of controls having similar viral infections uncomplicated by Reye's syndrome. There is no evidence of a direct dose relationship; indeed, in most instances, affected children have received only normal therapeutic levels. Thus, at the present time, *the favored view is that Reye's syndrome is of multifactorial origin related to a combination of microbiologic, genetic, and environmental factors. Conceivably, affected patients have lower toxicity thresholds to aspirin related to genetic influences or the preceding illness.* This hypothesis does not countermand the use of aspirin, which is near universal, but it does indicate the need for caution in the young following any viral infection, particularly influenza and chickenpox.

The morphologic changes in fatal cases are largely restricted to the brain and liver. There is striking cerebral edema (p. 1375) without evidence of an inflammatory infiltrate in either the substance of the brain or the meninges. Often the ultimate cause of death is herniation of the cerebellar tonsils and medulla into the foramen magnum as a consequence of the increased intracranial pressure. The liver has marked microvesicular fatty change without evidence of significant hepatocellular necrosis (Fig. 19–42). In

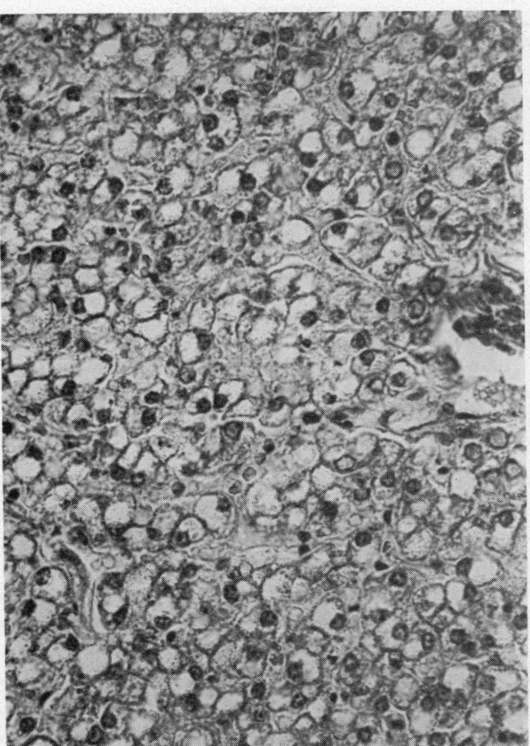

Figure 19–42. Reye's syndrome. Numerous small vacuoles of lipid are seen within liver cells having intact, apparently viable, nuclei. (Courtesy of Dr. Larry Weiss, Pathology Department, Brigham & Women's Hospital, Boston.)

both hepatocytes and neurons, distinctive mitochondrial abnormalities are seen by electron microscopy—expansion (megamitochondria), reduction in number, distortion, fragmentation of cristae, and flocculation of the matrix.[256, 257] These ultrastructural changes are apparently nonlethal since cell necrosis is not encountered even in fatal cases.

POSTMORTEM CHANGES

It is necessary to mention briefly the morphologic changes that may occur after death, to avoid confusion with antemortem liver disease. Depending on the adequacy and promptness of the methods used to preserve the body, such as refrigeration, the liver may undergo postmortem autolysis. Usually it begins to become evident about 24 hours after death, and produces progressive mushy softening and enzymic disintegration of cells in the complete absence of reactive inflammatory changes. The nuclei progressively fade and the cells fall away from the reticular framework. Often, bacterial proliferation can be seen within the autolytic parenchyma. In some instances, gas-forming organisms such as *Clostridium welchii* are borne from the gastrointestinal tract to the liver through the portal system during the agonal stage of life. Growth of these organisms and the release of gas may produce visible or palpable gaseous bubbles—*foamy liver*. Obviously, no inflammatory response accompanies the bacterial invasion.

Appropriately, the description of postmortem changes brings to an end the consideration of the liver.

The Biliary System

NORMAL

The extrahepatic ducts are critical to life, but the gallbladder is largely of use only to the surgeon. In its absence, man thrives and usually suffers no physiologic disturbance.

In the adult, the gallbladder is a conical, musculomembranous sac lying in a fossa in the undersurface of the right lobe of the liver. It is divided into three regions: (1) the fundus, the hemispheric blind end which may protrude below the liver edge; (2) the body, the portion between the fundus and the neck; and (3) the neck, a narrow, tubelike structure that tapers into the cystic duct. The relaxed gallbladder measures 7 to 10 cm in length and 2 to 3 cm in width, and has a capacity of about 30 to 50 ml. From each lobe of the liver, a hepatic duct emerges. These soon unite to form the common hepatic duct, which passes between the two layers of the lesser omentum for about 4 cm. It is joined at an acute angle by the cystic duct to create the common bile duct, having an approximate diameter of 0.5 to 0.7 cm. Dilatation of this duct often arises with obstruction. The common bile duct empties into the posterior wall of the second portion of the duodenum through the ampulla of Vater. It is therefore in close contact with, and sometimes buried within, the head of the pancreas. In approximately 60 to 70% of persons, the pancreatic duct joins with the common bile duct to drain through a common channel. In the remainder, the ducts enter separately. These anatomic details are of some interest in the pathogenesis of acute cholecystitis and pancreatic necrosis (p. 963). The ampullary orifice in the duodenum is marked by a 0.7- to 1.0-cm hemispheric protrusion of the duodenal mucosa known as the papilla of Vater.

Histologically, the gallbladder wall has four distinct layers. (1) The mucosa of the gallbladder is formed by a single layer of tall columnar cells that are thrown up into numerous interlacing tiny folds creating a honeycombed mucosal surface. Simple tubuloalveolar, mucus-secreting glands are present only in the neck, whereas the body and fundus have none. Similar lining epithelium and glands are found throughout the major extrahepatic biliary ducts. The mucosa of the gallbladder neck is thrown into a varying number of crescentic folds forming the spiral valves of Heister. The mucosal epithelium of the gallbladder and ducts is based on a delicate connective tissue stroma, but there is no well-developed submucosa in the gallbladder, a feature differentiating it from the intestines histologically. (2) Beneath the mucosa is a fibromuscular layer composed of smooth muscle cells and elastic fibrils. This layer provides contractility to the gallbladder. (3) A perimuscular layer of connective tissue and elastic fibers, often sparsely infiltrated with lymphocytes, is interposed between the muscular wall and the outer wall of the gallbladder. (4) A serous peritoneal layer covers all but the bare area of the hepatic bed.

Two common histologic variants merit mention here, and are so common as to constitute virtually normal details. Small, ductlike structures (*ducts of Luschka)*, lined by typical epithelial cells, are often found in the perimuscular connective tissue layer (Fig. 19–43). These do not communicate with the lumen, but are occasionally connected in the bile ducts and are assumed to represent aberrant supernumerary ducts. As sites for the inspissation of bile and stasis of bacteria and debris, they may contribute to the genesis of inflammatory disease. *Rokitansky-Aschoff sinuses* are small outpouchings of the mucosa of the gallbladder that extend into the underlying connective tissue and sometimes into the muscular layer. These obviously communicate directly with the lumen of the gallbladder. They are lined with typical columnar epithelium and are found occasionally in normal and often in diseased gallbladders (Fig. 19–44). Their higher incidence in inflamed gallbladders raises the possibility that preexisting injury to the wall may predispose to their development. However, their infrequent occurrence in completely normal gallbladders suggests that they may also represent a minor deviation from the norm—possibly attributable to the herniation of the mucosa through minute points of muscular weakness.

The blood supply to the extrahepatic biliary system is derived from the hepatic artery, the arterial branch to the gallbladder being known as a cystic artery. Many variable patterns of arterial supply are encountered that are of interest principally to the surgeon.

The extrahepatic biliary system has two main functions: storage and concentration of bile and the delivery of bile to the duodenum. Bile, as it is secreted by the liver, contains water, cholesterol, bile salts, bile acids, bilirubin, lecithin in micellar complexes, inorganic ions and mucoproteins secreted by the epithelium of the biliary tract. The primary bile acids are cholic and chenodeoxycholic acid which, with cations (abundant in bile) form the bile salts necessary for maintenance of cholesterol in solution. As secreted by the liver, bile is composed of about 3% solids, the remainder being water. One of the principal functions of the gallbladder is the concentration of this bile by selective absorption of water, inorganic ions (Na^+, Cl^-, HCO_3^-) and small amounts of bile salts to a volume possibly five to ten times smaller than the original hepatic secretion. Cholesterol is not soluble in the aqueous bile, but is maintained in solution by incorporation into micelles with the bile acids and phospholipids, as discussed later (p. 945).

The delivery of bile to the duodenum involves mechanisms that are still somewhat controversial. The sphincter of Oddi or some sphincteric mechanism (since there is doubt about the existence of an anatomic sphincter) is usually closed except when fatty food enters the duodenum and bile is thus diverted into the gallbladder. Contraction and partial emptying of the gallbladder occurs when foods (especially fatty ones) or other stimulants enter the duodenum. Gallbladder emptying is under neural (vagal) and hormonal control. The autonomic innervation appears to maintain gallbladder tone. Emptying is mediated through a hormone, cholecystokinin, which is released from the duodenum into the blood. At the same time, the sphincter of Oddi is

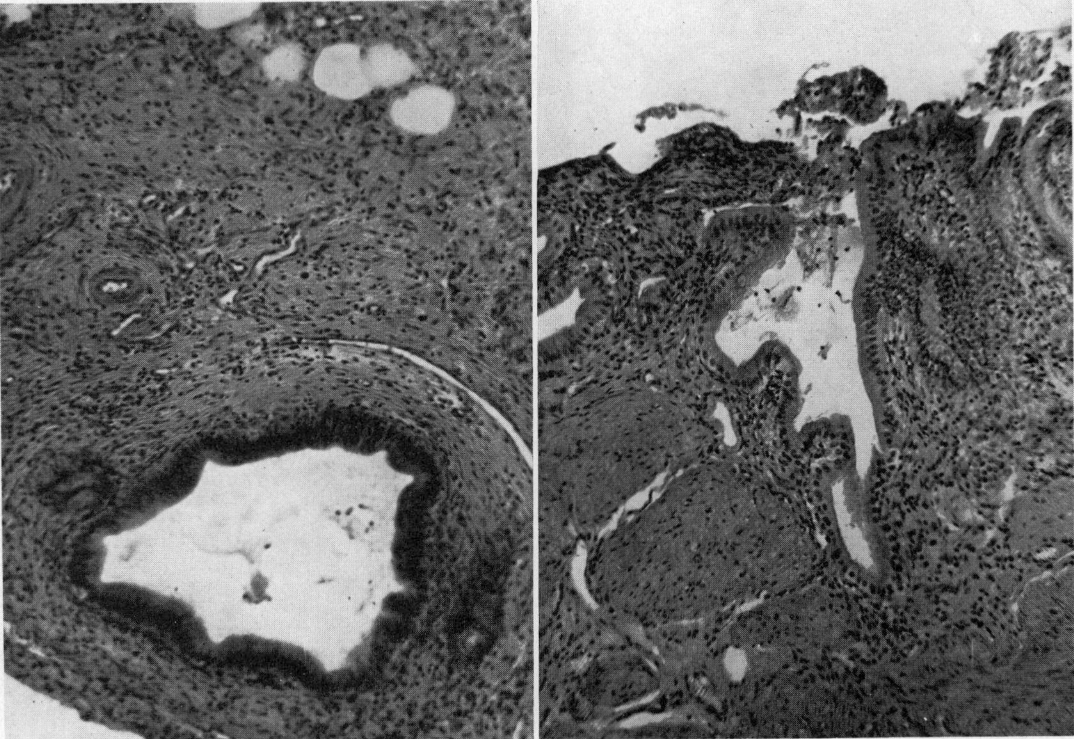

Fig. 19–43 Fig. 19–44

Figure 19–43. Duct of Luschka deep within wall close to serosa.
Figure 19–44. Rokitansky-Aschoff sinus in an inflamed gallbladder.

relaxed, thereby facilitating the passage of concentrated bile into the duodenum. Vasoactive intestinal peptide (VIP) may participate in the regulation of contraction by opposing the action of cholecystokinin.

The remarkable resorptive capacity of the gallbladder provides the basis for the radiographic diagnostic technique of cholecystography, the so-called *Graham-Cole test.* A variety of radiopaque substances, when taken orally or administered intravenously, are taken up by the liver and excreted in the bile, and so reach the gallbladder. Since they are not resorbed by the gallbladder, they become concentrated as the water in the bile is resorbed. Thus, levels are achieved that can be readily visualized roentgenographically. In this way, the outline of the gallbladder can be seen on x-ray examination, and the normal contractile response of the gallbladder to a fatty meal can be visualized. This diagnostic procedure sometimes also discloses the presence of radiolucent gallstones, seen as "holes" in the radiopaque shadow representing the gallbladder lumen.

PATHOLOGY

Although diseases of the biliary tract do not occupy a central place in medicine, some are very common (cholecystitis and cholelithiasis), and others are too often fatal (carcinomas) because they are generally silent until beyond cure. Thus, diseases of this system merit careful consideration.

CONGENITAL ANOMALIES

Developmental anomalies of the gallbladder and bile ducts take many forms and are of varied clinical significance. Most are chiefly of interest to the surgeon and embryologist and do not affect the patient's health. A few, mentioned below, have clinical importance. With respect to the gallbladder, there may be complete *agenesis, hypoplasia, hyperplasia, total reduplication* to form a double gallbladder, or subtotal division of the fundus and body to create a *bilobed* structure. The gallbladder may be abnormally located within the left lobe; is sometimes totally embedded within the liver substance (*intrahepatic*); or, at other times, is described as a *floating gallbladder*, having a long pendulous mesentery. Angulation, kinking, or a circumferential constriction of the body of the gallbladder gives rise to an apparently expanded bulbous end to the fundus, known as a *phrygian cap.* The bile ducts frequently do not conform to the classic anatomic form and have a variety of anomalous connections and patterns, the most important of which are total *agenesis of all or any portion of the hepatic or common bile ducts*, or *atretic narrowing* of these channels. Agenesis, or severe stenosis, is incompatible with life and is usually discovered shortly after birth by the progressive development of jaundice. Unless it is surgically corrected, death ensues within months to years.

CHOLELITHIASIS

Some concept of the frequency of cholelithiasis, better known as gallstones, is provided by the estimate that about 20 million Americans have them and 1 million develop them each year. Almost all form within the gallbladder, but rarely they arise within the extrahepatic or intrahepatic bile ducts. Their clinical significance varies. When confined to the gallbladder they are often asymptomatic (about 50%), despite the fact that mild, chronic inflammatory changes are almost always present in the gallbladder wall. The question as to which comes first is a time-hallowed controversy to be discussed presently. Should they pass into the cystic duct, they induce not only severe biliary colic, but also frequently acute cholecystitis. If they enter the common duct, they usually produce obstructive jaundice with the potentials of secondary ascending cholangitis or pancreatitis. Still a matter of dispute is the role of stones in the initiation of carcinoma of the gallbladder. There is considerable uncertainty whether all gallbladders containing even asymptomatic stones should be removed upon discovery.

Gallstones arise when a normally solubilized component of bile becomes supersaturated and precipitates to begin the formation of stones. The two major implicated constituents are cholesterol and bilirubin. Although there are well-defined ethnic and geographic differences, in the United States about 85% of stones are composed mainly of cholesterol and the remainder of bilirubin in the form of calcium bilirubinate (pigment). The preponderance of cholesterol stones also contain varying amounts of calcium salts such as carbonates, phosphates, or bilirubinates and so are referred to as "mixed"; only about 10% are "pure" cholesterol. Cholesterol is normally insoluble in aqueous bile and is held in solution in micelles also containing bile acids and phospholipids, principally lecithin. *Bile becomes lithogenic for cholesterol whenever there is excess secretion of cholesterol or a reduction in bile acids.* Like cholesterol, *unconjugated* bilirubin is largely insoluble in aqueous solution. Normally, however, at least 99% of bilirubin is in the form of the water-soluble conjugated pigment. Two factors are thought to contribute to pigment stone formation: (1) the presence of a glucuronidase probably derived from bacteria that deconjugates bilirubin diglucuronide; and (2) increased loading of the bile with bilirubin, as occurs with all forms of hemolytic disease. However, this traditional and perhaps too neat categorization and overview of the composition of gallstones has been shaken by a recent x-ray diffraction study of calculi from 152 patients.[258] Approximately 80% of the stones were made up of varying proportions of cholesterol and its derivatives, bile salts, bile pigments, and various inorganic salts of calcium. No pure stones were found. The remaining 20% were composed entirely of minerals, principally calcium salts, or, mysteriously, a new compound of oxides of silicon and aluminum. Further studies must confirm the general applicability of these findings; until then we will revert to traditional concepts.

INCIDENCE AND RISK FACTORS. There are marked variations in the incidence of cholelithiasis among countries, ethnic groups, and individuals. The major contributing factors are summarized in Table 19–6. Gallstones, mostly of cholesterol, occur in about 20% of women and 8% of men in the United States. They are much less frequent in Oriental and African countries, and two to three times more common in Sweden, in both women and men. Women are thought to be predisposed because of either increased synthesis of cholesterol or suppression of synthesis of bile acids by female sex hormones; hence, the greater frequency with the use of exogenous estrogens, pregnancy, and possibly multiparity. Similarly, the use of oral contraceptives has, in the past, been thought to increase the likelihood of stone formation, but a 1982 study casts doubt on this association.[259] Almost 70% of North and South American women of Indian extraction over the age of 30 have gallstones, but only 10% of black women. Age is also a factor, especially among men. The independent, but obviously interrelated variables of obesity and high-calorie diet predispose to gallstones, related in both instances to enhanced hepatic secretion of cholesterol. Clofibrate lowers serum lipid levels but roughly doubles the incidence of gallstones by increasing biliary cholesterol secretion.[260] In the rural Orient, pigment stones are more frequent than cholesterol stones, for reasons explained later. As mentioned, in all locales hemolytic diseases such as sickle cell anemia, spherocytosis, the hemolytic-uremic syndrome, and microangiopathic anemia predispose to the development of pigment stones attributed without proof to bilirubin loading of the bile. Obstructions or anomalies of the ducts predispose to their formation by favoring concentration of the bile. Cirrhosis—particularly alcoholic cirrhosis—also favors stone formation, for obscure reasons.

PATHOGENESIS. The formation of gallstones has been divided into three steps: *(1) bile supersaturation; (2) initiation of stone formation, i.e., nucleation; and (3) enlargement by accretion.*[261] The most is known about the first step, particularly as it relates to cholesterol stone formation. As pointed out, *bile can become supersaturated with cholesterol either as a result of increased cholesterol secretion or of decreased secretion of bile acids or phospholipids.* The rate-limiting enzyme for cholesterol synthesis within the liver is 3-hydroxy-3-methylglutaryl coenzyme A. Some studies have shown an increased activity of this enzyme with obesity and possibly also with the use of clofibrate.[262] Although cholesterol supersaturation is requisite, it must be followed by cholesterol crystallization for stone formation. Many individuals have no crystallization despite marked supersaturation, but the factors that regulate this phenomenon have not been elucidated.[263] Even without increased synthesis, *cholesterol supersaturation may develop with reduced levels of bile acids or phospholipids within the bile.* Decreased bile acid synthesis attributed to overactivity of feedback inhibition has been observed in both Indian and non-Indian patients with gallstones.[264] A reduction in the bile acid pool related to impaired reabsorption is encountered with severe intestinal disease and with major ileal resection or bypass. Although reduction in phospholipid synthesis could play a role, it remains as yet only theoretical.

Initiation or nucleation of cholesterol gallstones may begin with either crystallization of cholesterol or its precipitation about some "foreign" particulate matter such as bacteria, parasites, or fragments of detached mucosal epithelial cells. Various substances within bile, such as mucoproteins and calcium salts, also appear to serve as nucleating agents. Another important influence is the water content of bile, irrespective of the relative proportions of cholesterol, bile acids, and phospholipids. Other factors being equal, the more dilute the bile, the lower the tendency for cholesterol crystallization. Thus, obstructive biliary disease, which favors infection and permits greater concentration of the bile, predisposes to stone formation.

Table 19–6. RISK FACTORS FOR GALLSTONES

Cholesterol Stones
Demography: Northern Europe, North & South America—slightly less prevalent in Orient; American Indians; probable familial predisposition
Obesity
High-calorie diet
Clofibrate therapy
Gastrointestinal disorders; ileal disease, resection or bypass; cystic fibrosis with pancreatic insufficiency
Female sex hormones; women more than men, after puberty; oral contraceptives and other estrogenic medications
Age, especially among males
Probable but not well established: pregnancy, multiparity, diabetes mellitus, and polyunsaturated fats
Pigment Stones
Demography: oriental more than occidental; rural more than urban
Chronic hemolysis
Alcoholic cirrhosis
Biliary infection
Age

Modified from Bennion, L. J., and Grundy, S. M.: Risk factors for the development of cholelithiasis in man. N. Engl. J. Med. *299*:1161, 1221, 1978.

Once nucleation has occurred, accretion appears to be related to supersaturation of cholesterol with the progressive enlargement of the original nidus.

The details of *pigment stone formation* are not well understood.[265] It is known only that in patients with pigment stones, the bile is supersaturated with unconjugated bilirubin. Normally, less than 1% of the total bilirubin in bile is in the insoluble, unconjugated form. The enzyme beta-glucuronidase is thought to contribute to pigment stone formation by deconjugation of bilirubin, but whether this occurs within the liver before the bilirubin is secreted into the bile, or instead occurs within the biliary tract, is uncertain. Favoring the latter pathway is the predisposing influence of bacterial and parasitic infections of the biliary apparatus attributed to microbial release of the enzyme. This process is thought to account for the increased frequency of pigment stones in oriental countries in which infections by liver flukes such as *Clonorchis sinensis* are so common. However, the parasites may merely serve as nucleating agents. Chronic hemolysis presumably acts by increased bilirubin loading of the bile. In this connection, most pigment stones in Americans are related to chronic hemolysis and are found within the gallbladder, but are most commonly located within intrahepatic ducts in Orientals, in whom parasitic invasions prevail.

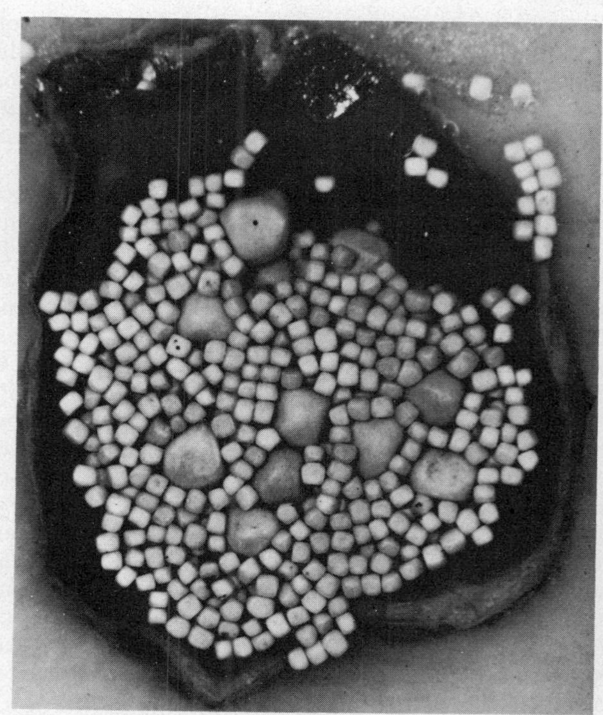

Figure 19–46. Opened gallbladder contains two families of gallstones: one, small, multifaceted, and remarkably uniform in size and shape; the other, considerably larger, showing some faceting and considerable variation in shape.

Pure cholesterol stones, representing 10% of all stones, tend to be solitary, round or ovoid, and usually 1 to 2 cm in diameter; sometimes they enlarge up to 6 cm in greatest dimension. Pale yellow in color, they may have a fine granular external surface, or when large, become polished in the gallbladder with a smooth eggshell surface (Fig. 19–45). Transection usually reveals a glistening, crystalline, radiating palisade. When composed of pure cholesterol or having little calcium content, they are radiolucent.

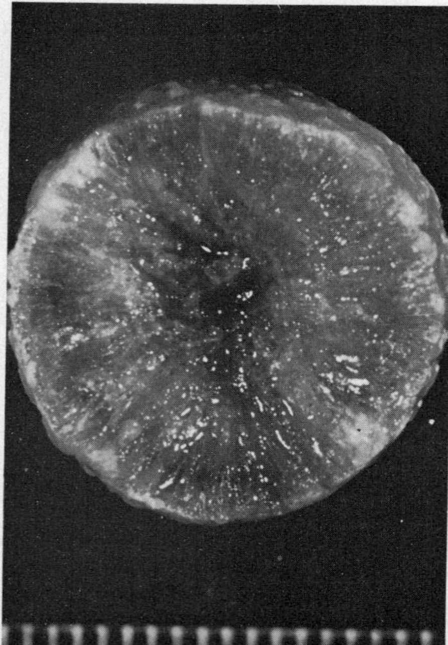

Figure 19–45. Cholesterol stone transected, showing translucence and radial crystalline pattern.

Pigment stones, when pure, usually take the form of jet-black jackstones ranging from 0.5 to 1 cm in diameter. Classically they occur in profusion and are all of a similar size, suggesting a single nucleating event. They almost never occur singly.

Mixed stones are the most common type and are almost invariably associated with chronic cholecystitis. They have a variable composition of cholesterol and calcium bilirubinate as well as other calcium salts. Such calculi are usually multiple and indeed may entirely fill the gallbladder and so develop faceting where adjacent stones impinge on each other. They range from gravel size up to 1 to 2 cm in diameter and vary from pale yellow-white to virtually black, depending on the bilirubin content (Fig. 19–46). Typically, they are laminated on transection.

CLINICAL COURSE. Gallstones that remain in the gallbladder are asymptomatic, so-called "silent." Only when they enter the ductal system to cause biliary pain ("colic"), become impacted within the cystic duct or neck of the gallbladder, and induce acute cholecystitis or obstruct the extrahepatic bile ducts do they evoke symptoms. There is the additional highly controversial issue (addressed later) as to whether stones predispose over the span of years to carcinoma of the gallbladder. Generally accepted data on the frequency of clinical complications versus "silent" stones are not available, but in one 15-year follow-up of 123 "healthy" individuals with stones discovered on cholecystographic screening, only 18% later developed pain or other complications;[266]

none developed carcinoma. Although minimal chronic inflammatory changes may appear in the gallbladder wall in such cases, and some patients have vague dyspepsia, neither feature has clinical significance. These data underlie the historic dilemma—should gallbladders containing asymptomatic stones be removed on discovery? Every clinician "marches to his own drum," but the conventional practice is cholecystectomy in those under 50 years of age when there are no other contraindications, because of possible later complications, and "watchful waiting" for those over 50. In those fortunate enough to have radiolucent stones presumably composed largely or entirely of cholesterol, dissolution may sometimes be accomplished with oral doses of ursodeoxycholic or chenodeoxycholic acid. Both agents are thought to act by decreasing the cholesterol saturation of bile by inhibiting hydroxymethylglutaryl coenzyme A involved in cholesterol synthesis. This form of therapy, however, is still somewhat controversial and not without undesirable side effects.[267]

Despite the fact that stones can be "silent," they cause problems in a minority of patients. Paradoxically, small stones are a greater hazard than large ones that remain confined to the gallbladder. Stones that obstruct the gallbladder neck or cystic duct are likely to produce biliary "colic" or acute cholecystitis. The term "colic" is something of a misnomer. The pain tends to be steady and severe, or take the form of aching or pressure in the epigastrium or right upper quadrant, often radiating to the interscapular area, right scapula or shoulder. It is frequently accompanied by nausea and vomiting. Traditionally the attacks of pain have been related to fatty foods (fat intolerance), but this association is now challenged. Acute cholecystitis and its sequelae are described subsequently, but they are major complications of cholelithiasis. Infrequently, obstruction of the gallbladder or cystic duct does not evoke acute symptoms; instead, over the span of time, the gallbladder becomes filled with a clear, mucinous secretion referred to as *"hydrops"* or *"mucocele of the gallbladder."*

Much more serious is the passage of a gallstone into the common bile duct (choledocholithiasis); this occurs in about 5% of cases of cholelithiasis, resulting in biliary colic and persistent obstructive jaundice with all of its consequences. Less frequently, ascending cholangitis or pancreatitis follows. Very rarely the intraductal inflammation and physical trauma permit the stone to erode through the ductal wall and then sometimes into an adherent loop of bowel to produce a choledochoenteric fistula. Large stones may then obstruct the small intestine—*gallstone ileus*. It is difficult to differentiate the obstructive jaundice caused by gallstones from that related to cancers (in the head of the pancreas, bile ducts, or papilla of Vater) or indeed sometimes from the nonobstructive jaundice caused by hepatocellular disease (p. 890). Obviously, identification of stones within the gallbladder suggests, but does not prove, calculous obstruction. Pain (colic) accompanying the jaundice favors the diagnosis of gallstones, but unfortunately some obstructive stones are painless and cancers may cause similar pain. The much talked about and, unfortunately, somewhat unreliable "Courvoisier's law" is sometimes of help: i.e., with calculous obstruction the gallbladder often is not distended and may even be smaller than normal because of the fibrotic changes of chronic cholecystitis and cholelithiasis, whereas neoplastic obstruction is more likely to be unassociated with inflammatory gallbladder disease, and thus undergoes progressive distention. Seductive as this postulate may be, other means are almost always necessary to distinguish calculous from neoplastic obstruction, as discussed later.

A large number of methods are now available for the diagnosis of cholelithiasis. Approximately 20% of gallstones contain sufficient calcium for visualization on plain film of the abdomen. Oral cholecystography provides a correct diagnosis in approximately 95% of patients. It depends on hepatic excretion into the bile of a radiopaque substance such as calcium ipodate, which is not reabsorbed and so permits visualization of the gallbladder as it undergoes concentration. Thus, nonopaque stones appear as radiolucent areas within the opacified bile. Additional diagnostic modalities include intravenous cholangiography, transhepatic cholangiography, endoscopic retrograde cholangiopancreatography (ERCP), and ultrasonography. The last-mentioned technique alone has an accuracy of approximately 95 to 97%, and so in combination these diagnostic methods can be expected to disclose the presence of stones in nearly 100% of patients with cholelithiasis.

ACUTE CHOLECYSTITIS

Acute cholecystitis in 90% of cases is initiated by impaction of a gallstone within the neck of the gallbladder or the cystic duct, referred to clinically as *calculous acute cholecystitis*. In the remaining minority of cases the acute inflammatory process is not associated with calculi—"acalculous acute cholecystitis."

Acute calculous cholecystitis is one of the major clinical presentations of cholelithiasis. The predisposition to this acute inflammatory condition understandably follows that of gallstones. Thus, it occurs in women, usually obese, three times more often than in men, and principally in middle-to-later life. The condition usually appears with remarkable suddenness and constitutes, in many instances, an acute surgical emergency because of its potential for rupture or spread of the infection (when present). The precise events leading to the acute inflammation are little understood. Only this much is known: it begins with calculous obstruction to the gallbladder. Bacteria—streptococci, staphylococci, *E. coli*, enterococci, Klebsiella, or Proteus—can be identified in the bile in about 75% of cases. This bacterial invasion is thought to be a secondary event since it is not present in the remaining 25%. At least in some instances, then, other factors must contribute to the acute reaction. Without substantial proof, increased intraluminal pressure with compromise of the blood supply, in concert with chemical irritation of bile acids, have been invoked. In a few cases, enzymes of pancreatic origin such as phospholipase have been identified within the bile that could release the toxic lysolecithin from membrane lipids. However, reflux of pancreatic secretions into the biliary tract has been identified even in normal individuals, but with obstruction of the gallbladder and concentration of the bile, the increased level of the enzymes could contribute to the injury. It is evident that much is speculative.

In **acute calculous cholecystitis,** the gallbladder is usually enlarged (two- to threefold) and tense, and often assumes a bright red or blotchy, violaceous to green-black discoloration, imparted by subserosal hemorrhages. The serosal covering is frequently layered by fibrin and, in the very intense reaction, by a definite suppurative, coagulated exudate. On being opened, the obstructive stone is present in the neck of the gallbladder or cystic duct. The gallbladder lumen, in addition to other possible gallstones, is tensely filled with a cloudy or turbid bile that may contain large amounts of fibrin and frank pus, as well as hemorrhage. When the contained exudate is virtually pure pus, the condition is referred to as **empyema of the gallbladder.** Gallstones are present in up to 80% of these cases, or a fine, sandy gravel is mixed in with the contained biliary contents. The gallbladder wall is thickened up to ten times normal and has a rubbery, yielding consistency. Edema fluid, exudate, and hemorrhage flow out from the cut surface. The mucosa may be merely patchily or totally hyperemic in the milder cases, transformed to a green-black necrotic surface in more severe cases **(gangrenous cholecystitis),** or have small-to-large ulcerations. In this fashion infections may penetrate the wall to give rise to pericholecystic abscesses or generalized peritonitis, or worse, the gallbladder may rupture.[268] Other possible complications are ascending cholangitis, liver abscess, subhepatic or subdiaphragmatic abscess, and septicemia.

Histologically, the inflammatory reactions are not distinctive and consist of the usual patterns of acute inflammation, i.e., edema, leukocytic infiltration, vascular congestion, frank abscess formation, or gangrenous necrosis, when vascular stasis complicates the edematous inflammatory response. As mentioned earlier, on the basis of the severity of the inflammatory reaction and the possible presence of vascular stasis, these acute reactions are divided into acute cholecystitis, suppurative cholecystitis, and acute gangrenous cholecystitis (Fig. 19–47).

The inflammatory reaction may subside and the neutrophils then are replaced by eosinophils to constitute the diagnostic features of subacute cholecystitis. Alternatively, in other cases, the deposition of calcium within the gallbladder wall gives rise to the so-called calcified gallbladder or **porcelain gallbladder.** It should be noted that this sequela of acute cholecystitis incurs a significantly increased risk of cancerous transformation. In an unknown number of instances, the subsidence of the acute response leads to chronic cholecystitis.

Acute calculous cholecystitis typically presents with marked right upper quadrant pain, tenderness, fever, and leukocytosis.[269] Attacks of biliary colic may have preceded or, less often, accompanied the acute inflammatory process. However, in about one-third of patients the acute cholecystitis is the first indication of the existence of cholelithiasis. The gallbladder may become sufficiently enlarged to be palpable below the liver edge, but in all cases deep inspiration during palpation of the right upper quadrant increases the tenderness. Liver function tests are usually normal but there may be slight elevation of serum transaminases and bilirubin. The natural course of this condition is totally unpredictable. In over half of the cases the symptoms resolve within two to three days after conservative management. Presumably, the obstructive stone either falls back into the gallbladder or passes through the ducts to relieve the obstruction. However, in the remainder the manifestations worsen as the inflammation progresses to *empyema* or *gangrenous necrosis of the gallbladder,* usually accompanied by signs of upper abdominal or generalized peritonitis unless, of course, cholecystectomy is performed earlier. Perforation or rupture is the most feared consequence; it may occur without warning in persons with progressive disease. Even with spontaneous resolution, recurrence can be anticipated in 25 to 60% of patients within five years if the gallbladder is not surgically removed.

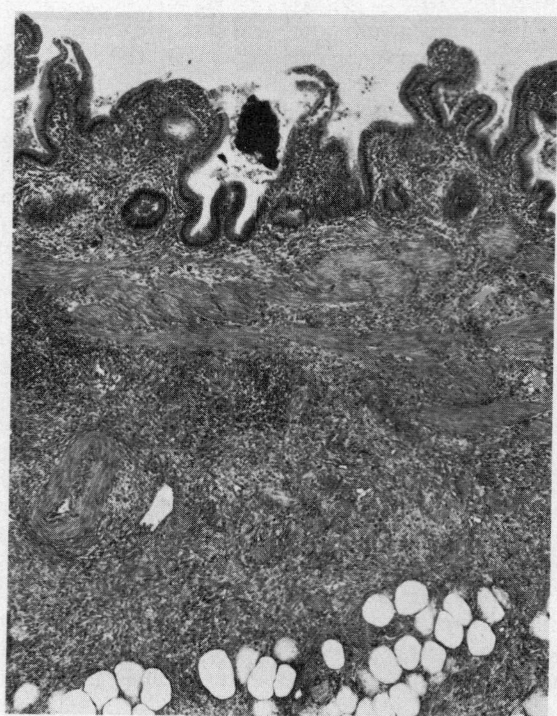

Figure 19–47. Acute cholecystitis with intense leukocytic infiltration of wall throughout all layers.

ACALCULOUS ACUTE CHOLECYSTITIS

As indicated above, only infrequently does acute cholecystitis develop in the absence of calculous obstruction. Notable associations are diabetes; systemic arteritis (particularly polyarteritis nodosa); bacterial and helminthic infections; trauma to the abdomen; burns; and abdominal and extra-abdominal surgery. In children, biliary tract anomalies may be present. There is no ready understanding of the pathogenesis of the acute involvement of the gallbladder in most of these settings, and differing mechanisms are very likely implicated. The diabetic's enhanced vulnerability to bacterial infection may play a role. In cases associated with diffuse arterial disease, necrotizing vasculitis has been observed within the wall of the gallbladder. Blood-borne spread of organisms could seed the gallbladder. Invasion of the gallbladder by *Ascaris lumbricoides* or liver flukes may be implicated in endemic locales. Except for the absence of calculi, the morphologic changes and clinical consequences are the same as those in calculous acute cholecystitis.

CHRONIC CHOLECYSTITIS

Chronic cholecystitis may be a sequel to acute cholecystitis, but in most instances it develops in the apparent absence of antecedent attacks of acute inflammation. *Virtually always it is associated with cholelithiasis and so is encountered most often in middle-aged and older obese females (female:male ratio, 3:1).* The evolution of chronic cholecystitis is even more obscure than that of acute cholecystitis. Although virtually always associated with gallstones, it is doubtful that they play a direct role in the initiation of inflammatory disease within the gallbladder wall. More likely, supersaturation of the bile predisposes to both the inflammation and the stone formation. Thus, bile acids and lysolecithin may cause chemical injury, but proof is lacking. Microorganisms, usually enteric bacteria, can be cultured from the bile in only about one-third of the cases. It is evident that the cause of chronic cholecystitis is little understood.

The morphologic changes in chronic cholecystitis are extremely variable. Generally the mere presence of stones within the gallbladder, in the absence of acute inflammation, is taken as sufficient justification for the diagnosis, and in such circumstances there may be only minimal evidence of mural chronic inflammation. The gallbladder may be contracted, normal in size, or enlarged. The size of the organ depends on the balance between the development of fibrosis in the wall and the element of obstruction in the genesis of the inflammation. The serosa is usually smooth and glistening, but often it is dulled by subserosal fibrosis. In other instances, dense fibrous adhesions may remain as sequelae of preexistent acute inflammation. On section, the wall is variably thickened, rarely to more than three times normal. It has an opaque gray-white cut section and may be less flexible and translucent than normal. In the uncomplicated case, the lumen usually contains fairly clear, green-yellow, mucoid bile. Stones are present in almost all cases (Fig. 19–48). The mucosa itself is usually preserved and has no loss of the usual mucosal folds that create the normal honeycombed pattern. In other instances, when the lumen of the gallbladder is partially or totally obstructed, the gallbladder contents may be under sufficient pressure to cause flattening of the mucosal folds and thinning and atrophy of the mucosa.

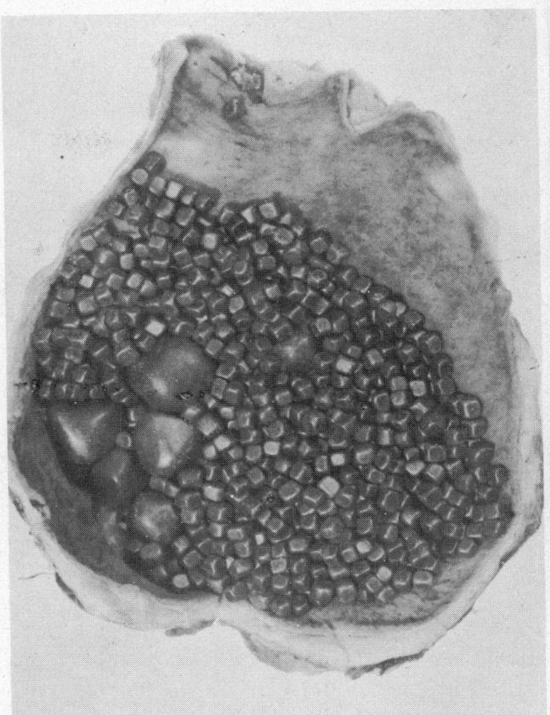

Figure 19–48. Chronic cholecystitis with cholelithiasis. Gallbladder wall is thickened, but mucosa is intact.

Histologically, the degree of inflammatory reaction is quite variable. In the mildest cases, only scattered lymphocytes, plasma cells, and macrophages are found beneath the columnar lining epithelium and in the subserosal fibrous tissue. In better developed cases, there is some increase of fibrous tissue subepithelially and subserosally, accompanied by a mononuclear cell infiltration (Fig. 19–49). In more extreme instances, the wall may be permeated by fibrous scar, with considerable obliteration of the smooth musculature. Rokitansky-Aschoff sinuses are found in up to 90% of these chronically inflamed gallbladders, presumably because the inflammatory damage to the wall predisposes to the herniation of the lining epithelium. Inflammatory proliferation of the mucosa and fusion of the mucosal folds may give rise to buried crypts of epithelium within the gallbladder wall, designated as **cholecystitis glandularis.** Dystrophic calcification within the gallbladder wall may yield a **"porcelain gallbladder"** identical to that which follows acute cholecystitis.

Sometimes the anatomic changes of acute cholecystitis are superimposed upon the chronic changes just described, implying acute exacerbation of a previously chronically injured gallbladder. This pattern of reaction is called **acute on chronic cholecystitis.**

Chronic cholecystitis is more a morphologic than a clinical entity. Such signs and symptoms as may appear relate entirely to the concomitant gallstones. Although heartburn, belching, intolerance to fatty foods, and vague epigastric discomfort are frequently attributed to chronic cholecystitis, these manifestations occur with equal frequency in patients having no gallstones and presumably no inflammatory involvement of the gall-

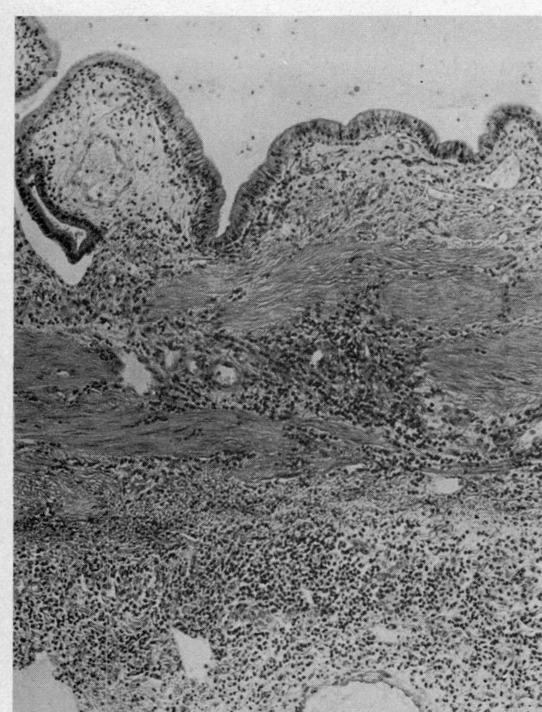

Figure 19–49. Chronic cholecystitis with increased subepithelial fibrosis and marked leukocytic infiltration. Mucosal folds are somewhat flattened.

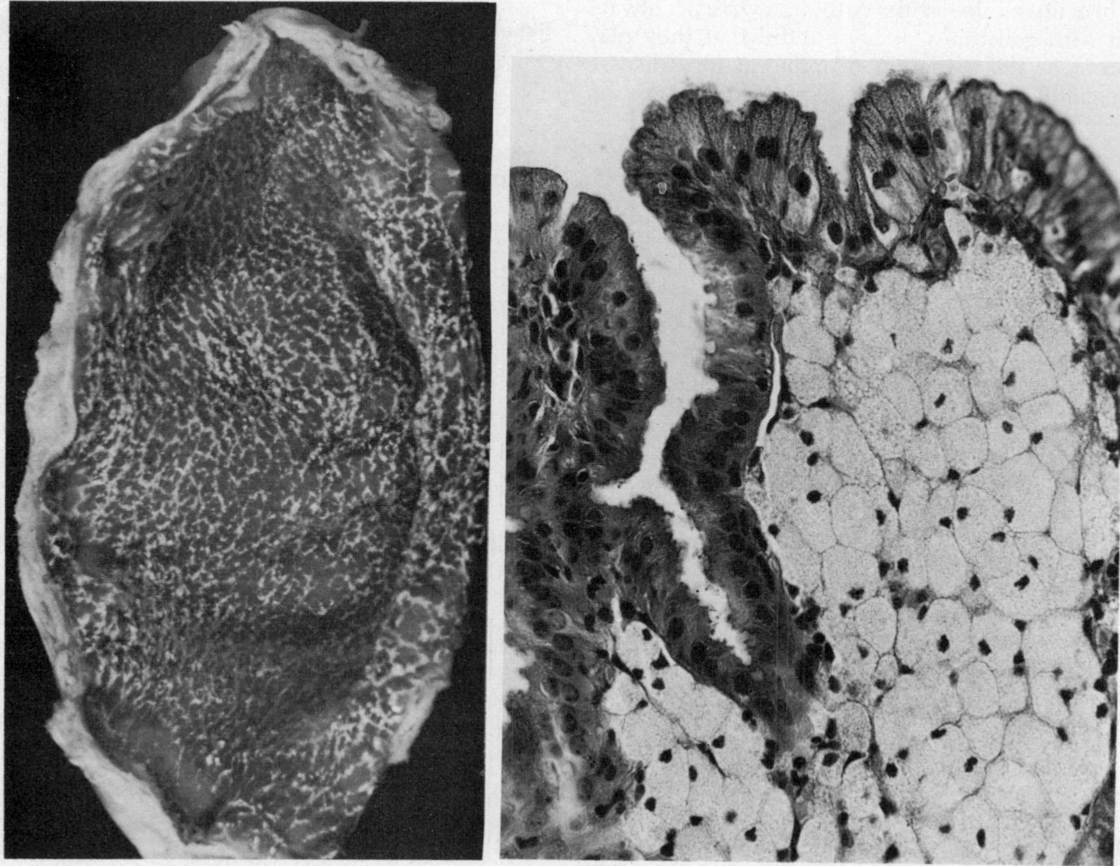

Fig. 19–50

Fig. 19–51

Figure 19–50. Cholesterolosis. Typical flecking of a "strawberry" gallbladder.

Figure 19–51. Cholesterolosis. Mucosal folds at their tips are stuffed by aggregates of lipid-laden histiocytes.

bladder. Nonetheless, the condition may be discovered in the course of the investigation of such complaints. Thus, chronic cholecystitis is a diagnosis that is made only after the gallbladder has been removed or at autopsy. Its clinical significance derives from the accompanying gallstones.

CHOLESTEROLOSIS

Cholesterolosis is also commonly designated as a "strawberry" gallbladder, because the focal deposits of lipid in the epithelium and subepithelial region of the gallbladder produce a likeness to the pale yellow-gray seeds that punctuate the surface of a strawberry.[269] Although this condition afflicts approximately 10% of the general autopsy population, cholesterolosis rarely causes clinical symptoms and therefore is not of great clinical significance. It does not, as far as we know, predispose to cholecystitis. The origin of this mucosal alteration is uncertain. The favored view is that it results from imbibition of cholesterol from the supersaturated bile. Support for this proposal comes from the commonly associated cholesterol-containing calculi. Local lymphatic and venous stasis may predispose to the accumulation of the absorbed cholesterol.

Whatever the mechanism, the *mucosa of the gallbladder is studded with minute yellow flecks*, imparting the strawberry appearance (Fig. 19–50). Usually, the intervening mucosa is yellow-green and intact, but accompanying cholecystitis occasionally modifies the macroscopic appearance.

Histologically, the diagnostic features are *enlargement and distention of the mucosal folds into club shapes by aggregations of round-to-polyhedral histiocytes* within these clubbed ends (Fig. 19–51). These cells have a foamy, reticulated, fat-laden cytoplasm and small, round, dark, prominent nuclei. When the deposit becomes more massive, these cells may die, and the release of lipids gives rise to the precipitation of cholesterol crystals in the subepithelial region and a subsequent inflammatory reaction of white cells, giant cells, and fibroblasts. This inflammatory pattern is, however, quite uncommon. It is not known whether the process is reversible, since it is asymptomatic and is discovered only incidentally at surgery or postmortem. When symptoms are present, they are usually due to accompanying cholelithiasis.

Infrequently, exaggerations of the focal accumulations of lipid produce sessile, so-called "*cholesterol polyps*," up to 4 mm in diameter. Clearly these lesions are not neoplastic, but nonetheless may mimic, on cholecystography, some of the benign tumors of the gallbladder to be described.

HYDROPS OF GALLBLADDER

Hydrops of the gallbladder is also known as *mucocele* of the gallbladder, referring to *distention of the gallbladder by a clear, watery, mucinous secretion*. This condition is invariably due to total obstruction of the cystic duct. Presumably, the trapped bile is resorbed, and the gallbladder becomes filled with a clear, mucinous secretion derived from the mucosal cells. Anatomically, the gallbladder is usually tense and enlarged and has a translucent appearance before being opened. The serosa usually is not involved; the wall is not thickened and, in fact, is often quite thin. When the gallbladder is opened, the clear mucinous contents disclose the nature of the condition (Fig. 19–52). Stones are usually present but are not intrinsic to the hydrops. When the condition is long-standing, the mucosa of the wall becomes atrophic or thinned out, and the lining may have a pale gray-red, smooth, glazed surface.

Histologically, depending on the severity of the condition, there is more or less atrophy of the epithelium so that, in far-advanced cases, no columnar or flattened cuboidal epithelial cells are present, and the wall of the gallbladder is composed only of an inner layer of connective tissue surrounded by the usual muscularis and other layers. As mentioned earlier, a prominent anatomic feature is demonstration of the underlying cause of the cystic obstruction, most often a stone, but less frequently neoplasia within the cystic duct or kinking of the duct (Fig. 19–53). The condition is usually asymptomatic, but occasionally there are manifestations of epigastric pain, discomfort, nausea, vomiting, and other features suggestive of nonspecific cholecystitis. No serious clinical sequelae attend this lesion.

TUMORS

Tumors of the biliary system range from benign to malignant and occur in all possible sites within the ducts and gallbladder.[270] Although fibromas, myomas, neuromas, hemangiomas, and the malignant counterparts of these lesions as well as carcinoids have been described in these organs, the only neoplasms of sufficient frequency and clinical importance to merit description are the papilloma, adenoma, and adenomyoma of the gallbladder; carcinoma of the gallbladder; and carcinoma of the bile ducts and ampulla of Vater.

PAPILLOMA, ADENOMA, AND ADENOMYOMA OF GALLBLADDER

Papillomas and adenomas of the gallbladder are very infrequent, benign epithelial tumors.[271] They both represent localized overgrowths of the lining epithelium, the papilloma growing as a pedunculated, complex, branching structure and the adenoma as a flat, sessile thickening. Although these lesions are small and easily missed unless careful inspection is carried out, there is a greater tendency to overdiagnose these conditions, since inflammatory hyperplasia or edema of the wall may create local projections that are often inter-

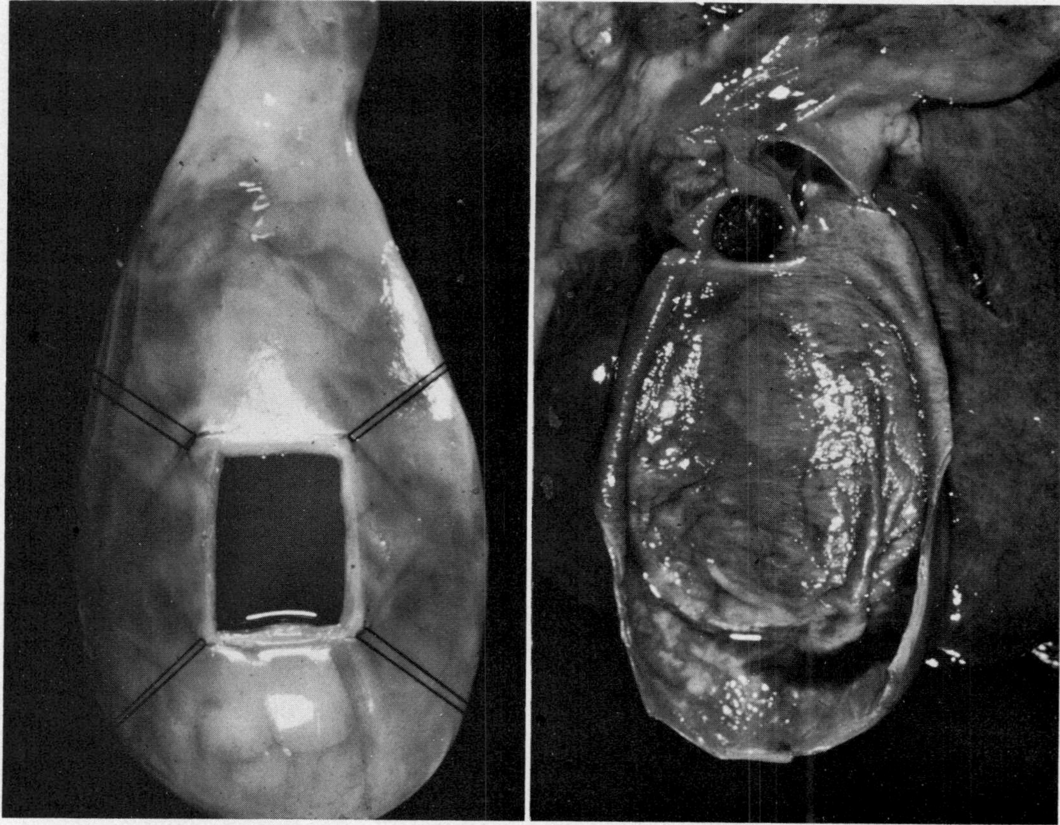

Fig. 19–52

Fig. 19–53

Figure 19–52. Hydrops of gallbladder. A window has been cut out to reveal the clear, translucent, mucoid contents.

Figure 19–53. Hydrops of gallbladder caused by stone impacted in cystic neck. Mucosa is atrophic and replaced by a shiny surface.

preted as benign neoplasms. The papilloma may occur singly or multiply as small, branching, pedunculated masses less than 1 cm in diameter that project into the lumen of the gallbladder. They are usually connected to the underlying wall by a slender stalk. In contrast, the adenoma is a broad-based, hemispheric elevation, again less than 1 cm in diameter, that is firmly attached to the underlying wall.

Both are composed histologically of a vascularized connective tissue stroma covered by a single layer of well-oriented, well-differentiated columnar lining epithelial cells. The adenoma also has contained glands in the stroma. Rarely, there is concomitant proliferation of the smooth muscle cells to create a leiomyomatous tumor enclosing cystic gland spaces lined by columnar epithelial cells—the so-called *adenomyoma*. In all macroscopic patterns, the cellular proliferation is regular, does not invade the underlying wall, and is entirely well differentiated. These lesions are only of clinical significance insofar as they may be detected on cholecystography and then require differentiation from more ominous malignancies. Papillomas, by fragmentation, may further provide a nidus for the formation of a gallstone. None of these benign lesions is believed to predispose to the development of a cancer.

CARCINOMA OF GALLBLADDER

Other forms of cancer may arise in the gallbladder, but carcinoma is much more frequent than all other types of malignancy together and, indeed, is considerably more common than benign tumors.[272] Although not one of the common cancers in humans, it is found in about one in 200 to 300 routine autopsies and accounts for about 5000 deaths annually in the United States. This form of neoplasia constitutes a major medical challenge; only rarely is it discovered at a resectable stage, and so the mean five-year survival (whether surgery is performed or not) has remained for many years at the disappointing level of about 3%. It is about two times more common in women than in men, and the risk increases steadily with age. The peak incidence is greatest in the eighth decade in men and the seventh decade in women. In Western countries, whites are affected more often than blacks.

A number of influences are thought to predispose to this form of cancer. Most important, but still poorly understood, are gallstones and the associated inflammation. Cholelithiasis and chronic cholecystitis are present in 75 to 90% of cases of carcinoma of the gallbladder.[273] Cancers have been reported to arise in 12 to 62%

of calcified (porcelain) gallbladders, underscoring the potential importance of long-standing chronic inflammation.[274] Conversely, carcinomas of the gallbladder are found in about 0.5% of patients with gallstones. However, it is not clear whether the stones and inflammation directly predispose to the carcinomatous change, or are the consequence of influences that also predispose to the development of cancer. It may be significant that derivatives of cholic acid are powerful experimental carcinogenic agents. Because of their association with stones, obesity, estrogen therapy, clofibrate therapy, ileal disease and bypass, and American-Mexican heritage all constitute predisposing factors. Also, workers in automotive, textile, rubber, and metal fabricating industries have been discovered to have an increased incidence of this cancer although the particular putative carcinogen(s) has/have not been identified.[275]

Morphologically, carcinomas of the gallbladder are usually divided into two gross patterns, infiltrating and fungating. The most common sites of involvement are the fundus and neck; about 20% involve the lateral walls. The **infiltrating type** is more common and usually appears as a poorly defined area of diffuse thickening and induration of the gallbladder wall that, when discovered, may cover several square centimeters or may involve the entire gallbladder or large portions of it (Fig. 19–54). These tumors are scirrhous and therefore have an extremely firm consistency. The luminal surface may be ulcerated, and often the tumor extends beneath the serosa in small, irregular, nodular projections or may directly penetrate the gallbladder wall to invade the liver bed. On cross section of the masses, the architecture of the wall is entirely obscured and replaced by a gritty, hard, white, solid tissue. Deep ulceration of the center of the mass may cause direct penetration of the gallbladder wall or fistula formation to adjacent viscera into which the neoplasm has grown.

The **fungating pattern** grows into the lumen as an irregular, small cauliflower mass, but at the same time invades the underlying wall. The luminal portion may be necrotic, hemorrhagic, and ulcerated. By the time these neoplasms are discovered, **most have invaded the liver centrifugally** and many have extended to the cystic duct and adjacent bile ducts and portahepatic lymph nodes (Fig. 19–55). This state of advancement is made possible by the fact that these neoplasms, in their developmental stages, are entirely asymptomatic and can thus grow for a long time until discovered by their extension into surrounding structures. If the cystic duct is occluded, the trapped bile is resorbed and replaced by mucinous secretion (white bile), creating hydrops of the gallbladder.

Histologically, five patterns can be identified. The most common is differentiated adenocarcinoma (approximately 40%) followed by poorly differentiated adenocarcinoma (30%) (Fig. 19–56). Papillary adenocarcinoma represents about 10% (Fig. 19–57). This histologic variant almost always takes the form of an exophytic fungating cancer. The least common are the adenosquamous or squamous cell carcinomas (5 to 10%), presumably originating in metaplastic epithelium. Not surprisingly, the poorly differentiated lesions

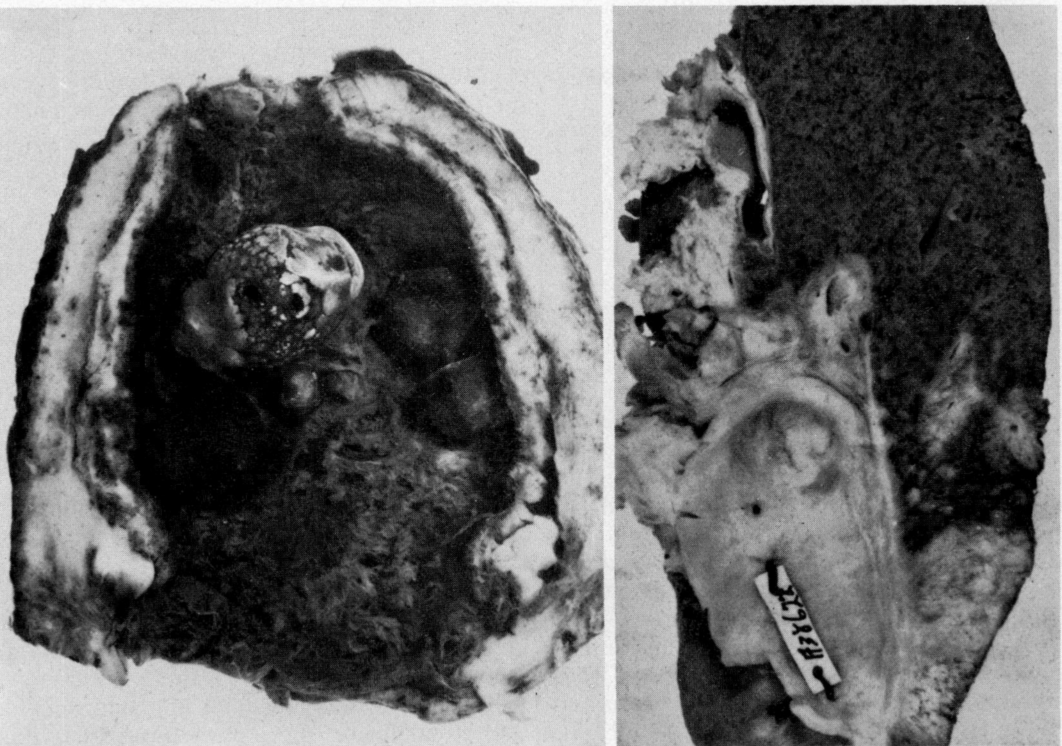

Fig. 19–54 **Fig. 19–55**

Figure 19–54. Carcinoma of gallbladder. Infiltrating pattern with diffuse, irregular thickening of gallbladder wall.

Figure 19–55. Gallbladder and its liver bed have been transected longitudinally to disclose direct permeation by carcinoma of contiguous liver substance.

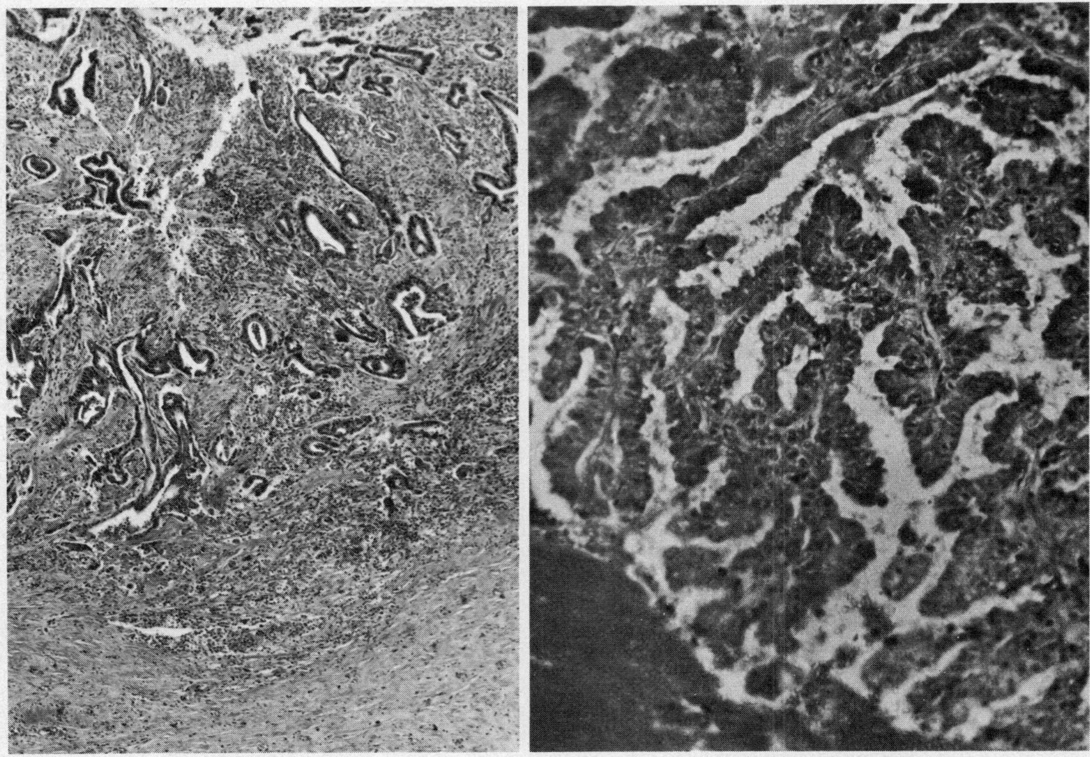

Fig. 19–56 Fig. 19–57

Figure 19–56. Adenocarcinoma of gallbladder with typical abundant fibrous stroma.
Figure 19–57. Papillary carcinoma of gallbladder.

tend to be associated with the widest metastatic dissemination; in contrast, those with squamous differentiation produce few metastases. Overall, the liver, perihilar and more distant lymph nodes, peritoneum, gastrointestinal tract, and lungs are the most frequent sites of seeding.

As mentioned, these carcinomas are extremely insidious and frequently asymptomatic until called to attention by their spread into the liver or into the cystic and common bile ducts. Occasionally, hepatic enlargement due to metastases is the first indication of the neoplasm. The most frequent presenting symptom is abdominal pain, but it is found in less than half of all cases. Other manifestations are jaundice, anorexia, weight loss, abdominal mass or swelling, nausea, and vomiting, but none of these manifestations is present in more than one-quarter of patients. Thus, a large number of neoplasms are found unexpectedly either at laparotomy for other disease or in gallbladders removed for cholelithiasis. The lucky symptomatic patient develops acute cholecystitis secondary to extension of the tumor into the cystic duct before it has spread elsewhere. The diagnosis rests largely on cholecystography documenting gallstones accompanied by abnormalities of the gallbladder wall profile. Ultrasonography to identify dilated bile ducts and CT scans are sometimes helpful. Neither radiation nor chemotherapy is effective in treatment. Surgical resection is rarely curative because of local or distant spread. Thus, there is the view that earlier cholecystectomy for gallstones would have prevented the development of this form of carcinoma in one patient in 200—but which one?!

CARCINOMA OF BILE DUCTS AND AMPULLA OF VATER

The designation carcinoma of the bile ducts is meant to include involvement of any of the extrahepatic bile ducts as well as the intraduodenal segment. The latter form is usually distinguished as *carcinoma of the ampulla of Vater*. Carcinomatous involvement of these ducts in the aggregate occurs somewhat less often than carcinoma of the gallbladder. However, these malignancies far outnumber in frequency all the other rather uncommon benign neoplastic (papilloma and adenoma) involvements of these structures. The same age range is affected as in carcinoma of the gallbladder but, although this last-mentioned neoplasm is more common in females, carcinomas of the bile ducts are slightly more frequent in males.[276] There is no convincing association between gallstones and bile duct cancer. On the other hand, there is a suggestion that chronic infection and inflammation within the ducts may constitute predisposing influences. In the Orient, infections by liver flukes—*Clonorchis sinensis*, and mainly *Opisthorchis viverrini*—are thought to constitute significant predispositions, but the frequency of such infections in the population raises the possibility that the concurrence may be coincidental. For unknown reasons, patients with ulcerative colitis are at slightly increased risk.

The sites of these tumors in order of frequency are: the periampullary region; the common bile duct, especially the lower end; the junction of the cystic hepatic and common ducts (sometimes called a Klatskin tumor); the hepatic ducts; and the cystic duct. Most neoplasms, when clinically discovered, are small because they give rise to obstructive symptoms early. Nonetheless, spread along the ductal system, to regional nodes, as well as hematogenous dissemination, too often precludes curative resection. Tumors arising at the junction of the hepatic ducts have been said to be more indolent and slower to metastasize. **The neoplasms take one of three forms: (1) papillary fungating, (2) intraductal nodules, and (3) diffuse infiltrative lesions of the wall of the ducts.** In the region of the papilla they generally take the form of small hemispheric masses narrowing the orifice and protruding into the duodenal lumen. Only rarely do they exceed 2 to 3 cm in diameter and 1 cm in height (Fig. 19–58). In most instances the overlying duodenal mucosa is intact, but occasionally permeation of the duodenal wall may cause ulcerations and, for this reason, is associated with melena. Whatever the location, obstruction may give rise to dilatation of the more proximal biliary structures. Cancers arising in the cystic duct may produce hydrops of the gallbladder.

Histologically, most of these neoplasms are adenocarcinomas that may or may not be mucin secreting. Some have papillary characteristics and, uncommonly, squamous metaplasia gives rise to squamous cell carcinomas or adenoacanthomas. For the most part, an abundant fibrous stroma accompanies the epithelial proliferation.

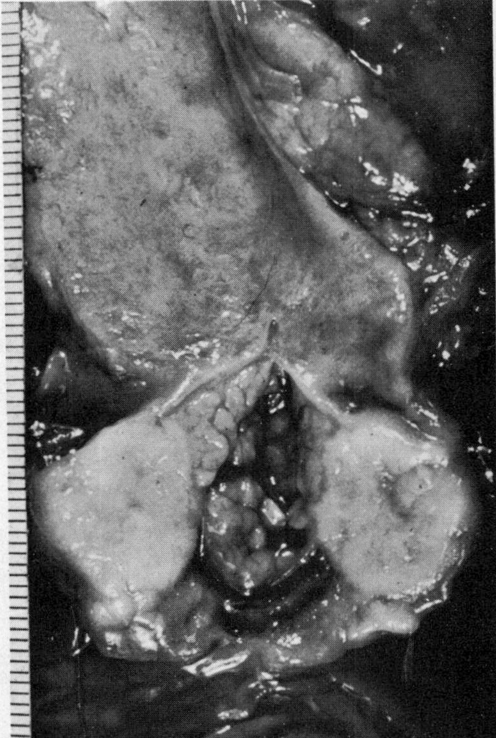

Figure 19–58. Carcinoma of papilla of Vater. Widened common bile duct comes down from above. Neoplasm has been split open to demonstrate 1.5 cm size of mass.

When symptoms appear with these neoplasms they are usually related to ductal obstruction (85 to 100% of cases), namely, obstructive jaundice, often preceded by pruritus and sometimes accompanied by weight loss. Associated changes are elevated levels of serum alkaline phosphatase, bile-stained urine, decolorized stools, and sometimes malabsorption of fats and fat-soluble vitamins. Regrettably, bile has detergent properties and thus can flow through minute orifices, so that obstructive symptoms only appear quite late. Classically, obstructive jaundice caused by impacted gallstones is often accompanied by pain, but carcinomas of the bile duct sometimes also cause pain.[277] Indeed, severe pain and fever occasionally constitute the presenting manifestations. The fever usually implies complicating ascending cholangitis. According to Courvoisier's law (p. 947), enlargement of the gallbladder would be anticipated with neoplastic obstruction, but it is present in only about one-half of the cases.

As pointed out in the discussion of gallstones (p. 947), the differentiation of obstructive jaundice due to neoplasia from calculous disease is a major clinical problem. In this differential diagnosis it is important to rule in or out the presence of stones in the gallbladder or ducts, using one of the many diagnostic modalities mentioned. However, the mere presence of gallstones does not preclude the existence of concomitant neoplasia. The cancers can sometimes be diagnosed by transhepatic or retrograde cholangiography, ultrasonography, and, in some cases, CT scan, but most often all that can be established is abnormal dilatation of ducts (ultrasonography is said to be 95% accurate).[278] Examination of duodenal drainage for tumor cells or for crystalline debris accompanying gallstones is sometimes of use in the differential diagnosis. Ultimately, however, surgical exploration may be necessary. Most of these ductal cancers are not surgically resectable at the time of clinical diagnosis and, therefore, the best that can be achieved is palliation in the form of relief of the ductal obstruction. The average postoperative survival is six months to one year. Cancer of the periampullary region, however, offers a somewhat better prognosis; a 20 to 40% five-year survival has been achieved by radical pancreaticoduodenectomy (Whipple's procedure).

1. Rapaport, A. M.: The structural and functional units of the human liver (liver acinus). Microvasc. Res. *6*:212, 1973.
2. Bronfenmajer, S., et al.: Fat-storing cells (lipocytes) in the human liver. Arch. Pathol. *82*:447, 1966.
3. Wake, K.: Sternzellen in the liver: Perisinusoidal cells with special reference to vitamin A. Am. J. Anat. *132*:429, 1969.
4. Adler, M., et al.: Pericanalicular, hepatocytic and bile ductular microfilaments in cholestasis in man. Am. J. Pathol *98*:603, 1980.
5. Pack, G. T., et al.: Regeneration of human liver after major hepatectomy. Surgery *52*:617, 1962.
6. Scharschmidt, B. F., and Gollan, J. L.: Current concepts of bilirubin metabolism and hereditary hyperbilirubinemia. Prog. Liver Dis. *6*:187, 1979.
7. Wolkoff, A. W., et al.: Role of ligandin in transfer of bilirubin from plasma into liver. Am. J. Physiol. *236*:E638, 1979.

7A. Lester, R.: Not two, but three bilirubins. N. Engl. J. Med. *309*:183, 1983.
8. Zimmerman, H. J.: Intrahepatic cholestasis. Arch. Intern. Med. *139*:1038, 1979.
9. Hutterer, F., et al.: Alteration of microsomal biotransformation in the liver in cholestasis. Proc. Soc. Exp. Biol. Med. *133*:702, 1970.
10. Seidel, D., et al.: On the metabolism of lipoprotein-X (LP-X). Clin. Chim. Acta *66*:195, 1976.
11. Erlinger, S.: Cholestasis: Pump failure, microvilli defect or both? Lancet *1*:553, 1978.
12. Kaplowitz, N.: Cholestatic liver disease. Hosp. Pract. *14*:83, 1978.
13. Popper, H., and Schaffner, F.: Pathophysiology of cholestasis. Hum. Pathol. *1*:1, 1970.
13A. Weiss, J. S., et al.: The clinical importance of a protein-bound fraction of serum bilirubin in patients with hyperbilirubinemia. N. Engl. J. Med. *309*:147, 1983.
14. McIntyre, N., et al.: The hypercholesterolemia of obstructive jaundice. Progress report. Gut *16*:379, 1975.
15. Koppel, M. H., et al.: Transplantation of cadaveric kidneys from patients with hepatorenal syndrome; evidence for the functional nature of renal failure in advanced liver disease. N. Engl. J. Med. *280*:1367, 1969.
16. Iwatsuki, S., et al.: Recovery from "hepatorenal syndrome" after orthotopic liver transplantation. N. Engl. J. Med. *289*:1155, 1973.
17. Editorial: Hepatorenal syndrome or hepatic nephropathy? Lancet *1*:801, 1980.
18. Wilkinson, S. P., et al.: Endotoxaemia and renal failure in cirrhosis and obstructive jaundice. Br. Med. J. *2*:1415, 1976.
19. Epstein, M., et al.: Renal failure in the patient with cirrhosis. The role of active vasoconstriction. Am. J. Med. *49*:175, 1970.
20. Reynolds, T. B., et al.: Functional renal failure with cirrhosis. Medicine *46*:191, 1967.
21. Levy, M.: Sodium retention and ascites formation in dogs with experimental portal cirrhosis. Am. J. Physiol. *233*:F572, 1977.
22. Wilkinson, S. P., and Williams, R.: Endotoxins and renal failure in liver disease. *In* Bartoli, E., and Chiandussi, L. (eds.): Hepato-renal Syndrome. Padua, Piccin Medical Books, 1979, p. 229.
23. Schenker, S., et al.: Hepatic encephalopathy: Current status. Gastroenterology *66*:122, 1974.
24. Treve, L., and Nicoloff, D. N.: Pathogenesis of hepatic coma. Annu. Rev. Med. *26*:143, 1975.
25. Fischer, J. E., and Baldessarini, R. J.: Pathogenesis and therapy of hepatic coma. *In* Popper, H., and Schaffner, F. (eds.): Progress in Liver Disease. Vol. 5. New York, Grune & Stratton, 1976, p. 363.
26. Zieve, F. J., et al.: Synergism between ammonia and fatty acids in the production of coma: Implications for hepatic coma. J. Pharmacol. Exp. Ther. *191*:10, 1974.
27. Popper, H.: Pathogenesis of hepatic failure. Kidney Int. *10*:S-225, 1976.
28. Goresky, C. A., et al.: Definition of a conjugation dysfunction in Gilbert's syndrome: Studies on the handling of bilirubin loads and of the pattern of bilirubin conjugate secreted in bile. Clin. Sci. Mol. Med. *55*:63, 1978.
29. Okolicsanyi, L. O., et al.: An evaluation of bilirubin kinetics with respect to the diagnosis of Gilbert's syndrome. Clin. Sci. Mol. Med. *54*:539, 1978.
30. Bailey, A., et al.: Does Gilbert's disease exist? Lancet *1*:931, 1977.
31. Odell, G. B., and Childs, B.: Hereditary hyperbilirubinemias. *In* Steinberg, A. G., et al. (eds.): Progress in Medical Genetics. Vol. IV. Philadelphia, W. B. Saunders Co., 1980, p. 103.
32. Gordon, E. R., et al.: Bilirubin secretion and conjugation in the Crigler-Najjar syndrome, Type II. Gastroenterology *70*:761, 1976.
33. Dubin, I. N.: Chronic idiopathic jaundice. A review of 50 cases. Am. J. Med. *24*:268, 1958.
34. Baba, N., and Ruppert, R. D.: The Dubin-Johnson syndrome. Electron microscopic observation of hepatic pigment—a case study. Am. J. Clin. Pathol. *57*:306, 1972.
35. Swartz, H. M., et al.: On the nature and excretion of the hepatic pigment in the Dubin-Johnson syndrome. Gastroenterology *76*:958, 1979.
36. Peters, T. J., and Seymour C. A.: The organella pathology and demonstration of mitochondrial superoxide dismutase deficiency in two patients with Dubin-Johnson-Sprinz syndrome. Clin. Sci. Mol. Med. *54*:549, 1978.
37. Arcidi, J. M., et al.: Hepatic morphology in cardiac dysfunction. A clinicopathologic study of 1,000 subjects at autopsy. Am. J. Pathol. *104*:159, 1981.
38. Buhac, I., et al.: Jaundice and bridging centrilobular necrosis of liver in circulatory failure. N.Y. State J. Med. *76*:678, 1976.
39. Chen, V., et al.: Hepatic infarction. Arch. Pathol. Lab. Med. *100*:32, 1976.
40. Parker, R. G. F.: Occlusion of the hepatic veins in man. Medicine *38*:369, 1959.
41. Grossman, J. A., and McDermott, W. V.: Paroxysmal nocturnal hemoglobinuria associated with hepatic and portal venous thrombosis. Am. J. Surg. *127*:233, 1974.
42. Reynolds, T. B., and Peters, R. L.: Budd-Chiari syndrome. *In* Schiff, L. (ed.): Diseases of the Liver. 5th ed. Philadelphia, J. B. Lippincott Co., 1982, p. 1622.
43. Leopold, J. G., et al.: A change in the sinusoid-trabecular structure of the liver with hepatic venous outflow block. J. Pathol. *100*:87, 1970.
44. Langer, B., et al.: Clinical spectrum of the Budd-Chiari syndrome and its surgical management. Am. J. Surg. *129*:137, 1975.
45. Soltis, R. D.: New concepts in viral hepatitis. Geriatrics *36*:62, 1981.
46. Rubin, E.: Acute and chronic viral hepatitis. Fed. Proc. *38*:2665, 1979.
47. Melnick, J. L., et al.: Viral hepatitis. Sci. Am. *237*:44, 1977.
48. Fitzgerald J. F., et al.: The hepatitis spectrum. Curr. Prob. Pediatr. *11*:1, 1981.
49. Dienstag, J. L.: Hepatitis A virus. Virologic, clinical and epidemiological studies. Hum. Pathol. *12*:1097, 1981.
50. Coulepsis, A. G., et al.: Detection of hepatitis A virus in the feces of patients with naturally acquired infections. J. Infect. Dis. *141*:151, 1980.
51. Dienhardt, F.: Medical perspective: Predictive value of markers of hepatitis viral infection. J. Infect. Dis. *141*:299, 1980.
52. Corey, L., and Holmes, K. K.: Sexual transmission of hepatitis A in homosexual men: Incidence and mechanism. N. Engl. J. Med. *302*:435, 1980.
53. Dienstag, J. L., et al.: Mussel-associated viral hepatitis, type A: Serological confirmation. Lancet *1*:561, 1976.
54. Szmuness, W., et al.: The prevalence of antibody to hepatitis A antigen in various parts of the world. A pilot study. Am. J. Epidemiol. *5*:392, 1977.
55. Szmuness, W., et al.: Distribution of antibody to hepatitis A antigen in urban adult populations. N. Engl. J. Med. *295*:755, 1976.
56. Dane, D. S., et al.: Virus-like particles in serum of patients with Australia antigen–associated hepatitis. Lancet *1*:695, 1970.
57. Yamada, G., et al.: Hepatitis B: Cytologic localization of virus antigens and the role of the immune response. Hum. Pathol. *9*:93, 1978.
58. Huang, S. N., and Neurath, A. R.: Immunohistologic demonstration of hepatitis B viral antigens in liver with reference to the significance in liver injury. Lab. Invest. *40*:1, 1979.
59. Blumberg, B. S., et al.: A "new" antigen in leukemia sera. J.A.M.A. *191*:541, 1965.
60. Szmuness, W., et al.: A controlled clinical trial of the efficacy of the hepatitis B vaccine (Heptavax B); a final report. Hepatology *1*:377, 1981.
61. Neurath, A. R., and Strick, N.: Host specificity of a serum marker for hepatitis B; evidence that "e antigen" has the properties of an immunoglobulin. Proc. Natl. Acad. Sci. U.S.A. *74*:1702, 1977.
62. Grady, G. F.: Relation of "e" antigen to infectivity of HBsAg-positive inoculations among medical personnel. Lancet *2*:1171, 1976.
63. Okada, K., et al.: "E" antigen and anti-"E" in the serum of asymptomatic carrier mothers as indicators of positive and negative transmission of hepatitis B virus to their infants. N. Engl. J. Med. *295*:746, 1976.
64. Krugman, S., et al.: Viral hepatitis, type B. Studies on natural history and prevention reexamined. N. Engl. J. Med. *300*:101, 1979.
65. Careoda, F., et al.: Persistence of circulating HBsAg-IgM complexes in acute viral hepatitis type B: An early marker of chronic evolution. Lancet *2*:358, 1982.
66. Perrillo, R. P., et al.: Hepatitis B "e" antigen, DNA polymerase activity and infection of household contacts with hepatitis B virus. Gastroenterology *76*:1319, 1979.
67. Aziz, M. A., et al.: Transplacental and postnatal transmission of the hepatitis-associated antigen. J. Infect. Dis. *127*:110, 1973.
68. Stevens, C. E., et al.: Vertical transmission of hepatitis B antigen in Taiwan. N. Engl. J. Med. *292*:771, 1975.
69. Holland, P. V., and Alter, J. H.: Non-A, non-B viral hepatitis. Hum. Pathol. *12*:114, 1981.
70. Tabor, E., et al.: Chronic non-A, non-B hepatitis carrier state. Transmissible agent documented in one patient over a six-year period. N. Engl. J. Med. *303*:140, 1980.
71. Stern, H., et al.: Non-A, non-B hepatitis in West London. Lancet *1*:982, 1982.
72. Dienstag, J.: Non-A, non-B hepatitis. Adv. Intern. Med. *26*:187, 1981.
73. Tabor, E., et al.: Detection of an antigen-antibody system in serum associated with human non-A, non-B hepatitis. J. Med. Virol. *4*:161, 1979.
74. Spertini, O., and Frei, P. E.: Demonstration of a single antigen-antibody in 26 patients with non-A, non-B viral hepatitis. Lancet *2*:899, 1982.
75. Marciano-Cabral, F., et al.: Chronic non-A, non-B hepatitis: Ultrastructural and serologic studies. Hepatology *1*:575, 1981.
76. Yoshizawa, H., et al.: Viruslike particles in a plasma fraction (fibrinogen) and in the circulation of apparently healthy blood donors capable of inducing non-A, non-B hepatitis in humans and chimpanzees. Gastroenterology *79*:512, 1980.
77. Robinson, W. S.: The enigma of non-A, non-B hepatitis. J. Infect. Dis. *145*:387, 1982.
77A. Hoofnagle, J. H.: Type A and type B hepatitis. Lab. Med. *14*:705, 1983.

78. Edgington, T. S., and Chisari, V.: Immunological aspects of hepatitis B virus infection. *In* Symposium on Viral Hepatitis. Washington, D.C., Natl. Acad. Sci., 1975.
79. Rubin, E.: Acute and chronic viral hepatitis. Fed. Proc. *38*:2665, 1979.
80. Geubel, A. P., et al.: Lymphocyte cytotoxicity and inhibition studied with autologous liver cells. Observations in chronic active liver disease. Gastroenterology *71*:450, 1976.
81. Chisari, F. V., et al.: Extrinsic modulation of human T-lymphocyte E-rosette function associated with prolonged hepatocellular injury after viral hepatitis. J. Clin. Invest. *59*:134, 1977.
82. Hatta, R.: Loss of suppressor T cell function and circulating immune complexes in chronic active liver diseases. Clin. Exp. Immunol. *46*:375, 1981.
83. Gocke, D. J.: Extrahepatic manifestations of viral hepatitis. Am. J. Med. Sci. *270*:49, 1975.
84. Hopf, U., et al.: Detection of liver-membrane autoantibody in HBsAg-negative chronic active hepatitis. N. Engl. J. Med. *294*:578, 1978.
85. Szmuness, W.: Recent advances in the study of the epidemiology of hepatitis B. Am. J. Pathol. *81*:629, 1975.
86. Kostich, N. D., and Ingram, C. D.: Detection of hepatitis B surface antigen by means of orcein staining of liver. Am. J. Clin. Pathol. *67*:20, 1977.
87. Bianchi, L., and Gudat, F.: Sanded nuclei in hepatitis B: Eosinophilic inclusions in liver cell nuclei due to excess in hepatitis B core antigen formation. Lab. Invest. *35*:1, 1976.
88. Camilleri, J. P., et al.: Immunohistochemical patterns of hepatitis B surface antigen (HBsAg) in patients with hepatitis, renal homograft recipients and normal carriers. Virchows Arch. [Pathol. Anat.] *376*:329, 1977.
89. Phillips, M. J., and Poucell, S.: Modern aspects of the morphology of viral hepatitis. Hum. Pathol. *12*:1060, 1981.
90. Ishak, K. G.: Light microscopic morphology of viral hepatitis. Am. J. Clin. Pathol. *65*:787, 1976.
91. Boyer, J. L., and Klatskin, G.: Pattern of necrosis in acute viral hepatitis. Prognostic value of bridging (subacute hepatic necrosis). N. Engl. J. Med. *283*:1063, 1970.
92. Wright, R.: Type B hepatitis: Progression to chronic hepatitis. Clin. Gastroenterol. *9*:97, 1980.
93. Koretz, R. L., et al.: The long-term course of non-A, non-B, post-transfusion hepatitis. Gastroenterology *79*:893, 1980.
94. Villa Rejos, V. M., et al.: Development of chronic non-A, non-B viral hepatitis. Gastroenterology *78*:1325, 1980.
95. Reynolds, T. B.: Chronic hepatitis: Current dilemmas. Am. J. Med. *69*:485, 1980.
96. Deinhardt, F.: Predictive value of hepatitis virus infection. J. Infect. Dis. *141*:299, 1980.
97. Careoda, F., et al.: Persistence of circulating HBsAg/IgM complexes in acute viral hepatitis, type B: An early marker in chronic evolution. Lancet *2*:358, 1982.
98. Dietrichson, O.: Chronic persistent hepatitis. A clinical, serologic and prognosis study. Scand. J. Gastroenterol. *10*:249, 1975.
99. Deodhar, K. P., et al.: Orcein staining of hepatitis B antigen in paraffin sections of liver biopsies. J. Clin. Pathol. *28*:66, 1975.
100. Celle, G., et al.: Morphologic evaluation of CAH with and without therapy. A two-year follow-up. Hepatogastroenterology *27*:283, 1980.
101. Czaja, A. J., et al.: Corticosteroid-treated chronic active hepatitis in remission. Uncertain prognosis of chronic persistent hepatitis. N. Engl. J. Med. *304*:5, 1981.
102. Bianchi, L., et al.: Acute and chronic hepatitis revisited. Review by an international group. Lancet *2*:914, 1977.
103. Rakela, J., and Redeker, A. G.: Chronic liver disease after acute non-A, non-B viral hepatitis. Gastroenterology *77*:1200, 1979.
104. Soloway, R. D., et al.: "Lupoid" hepatitis. A non-entity in the spectrum of chronic active liver disease. Gastroenterology *63*:458, 1972.
105. Scheuer, P. J.: Chronic hepatitis: A problem for the pathologist. Histopathology *1*:5, 1977.
106. Searle, J., et al.: Necrosis and apoptosis: Distinct modes of cell death with fundamentally different significance. Pathol. Annu. *17*:Pt. 2, 229, 1982.
107. Boyer, J. L., and Klatskin, G.: Pattern of necrosis in acute viral hepatitis. Prognostic value of bridging (subacute hepatic necrosis). N. Engl. J. Med. *283*:1063, 1970.
108. Shouval, D., et al.: Chronic active hepatitis with cholestatic features. Am. J. Gastroenterol. *72*:551, 1979.
109. Nour-Aria, K. T., et al.: Effect of corticosteroids on suppressor-cell activity in "autoimmune" and viral chronic active hepatitis. N. Engl. J. Med. *307*:1301, 1982.
110. Nachbauer, C. A., and Fischer, J. E.: The failing liver. Surg. Clin. North Am. *61*:221, 1981.
111. Dordal, E., et al.: Hepatic lesions in chronic inflammatory bowel disease. I. Clinical correlations with liver biopsy diagnoses in 103 patients. Gastroenterology *52*:239, 1967.
112. Pitt, H. A., and Ziudema, G. D.: Factors influencing mortality in the treatment of pyogenic hepatic abscess. Surg. Gynecol. Obstet. *140*:228, 1975.
113. Sabbaj, J., et al.: Anaerobic pyogenic liver abscess. Ann. Intern. Med. *77*:629, 1972.
114. Lazarchick, J., et al.: Pyogenic liver abscess. Mayo Clin. Proc. *48*:349, 1972.
115. Editorial: Pyogenic liver abscess—a continuing problem of management. Lancet *1*:1170, 1976.
116. Koff, R. S., et al.: Profile of hyperbilirubinemia in three hospital populations. Clin. Res. *18*:680, 1970.
117. Sameshina, Y., et al.: Clinical statistics on drug-induced liver injuries. Drug-induced liver injuries in Japan in the last thirty years. Jap. J. Gastroenterol *71*:799, 1974.
118. Zimmerman, H. J.: Hepato-toxicity. New York, Appleton-Century-Crofts, 1978.
119. Zimmerman, H. J., and Maddrey, W. C.: Toxic and drug-induced hepatitis. *In* Schiff, L.: Diseases of the Liver. (5th ed.) Philadelphia, J. B. Lippincott Co., 1982, p. 621.
120. Davis, M., Tredger, J. M., and Williams, R. (eds.): Drug Reactions and the Liver. London, Pitman Medical Ltd. 1981.
121. Ludwig, J.: Drug effects on the liver: A tabular compilation of drugs and drug-related hepatic disease. Dig. Dis. Sci. *24*:785, 1980.
122. Mitchell, J. R., and Lauterburg, B. H.: Drug-induced liver injury. Hosp. Pract. *13*:95, 1978.
123. Popper, H., et al.: Drug-induced liver disease. A penalty for progress. Arch. Intern. Med. *115*:128, 1965.
124. Sherlock, S.: Halothane hepatitis. Lancet *2*:364, 1978.
125. Vergani, D.: Sensitization to halothane-altered liver components in severe hepatic necrosis after halothane anaesthesia. Lancet *2*:801, 1978.
126. Klatskin, G., and Kimberg, D. V.: Recurrent hepatitis attributable to halothane sensitization in an anesthetist. N. Engl. J. Med. *280*:515, 1969.
127. Dienstag, J. L.: Halothane hepatitis: Allergy or idiosyncrasy? (editorial). N. Engl. J. Med. *303*:102, 1980.
128. Rubin, E.: Iatrogenic hepatic injury. Hum. Pathol. *11*:312, 1980.
129. Peters, R. L., et al.: Tetracycline-induced fatty liver in nonpregnant patients. Am. J. Surg. *113*:622, 1967.
130. Bagheri, S. A., and Boyer, J. L.: Peliosis hepatis associated with androgenic-anabolic steroid therapy. A severe form of hepatic injury. Ann. Intern. Med. *81*:610, 1974.
131. Anthony, P. P., et al.: The morphology of cirrhosis: Definition, nomenclature and classification. Bull. W. H. O. *55*:521, 1977.
132. Lieber, C. S.: Pathogenesis and early diagnosis of alcoholic liver injury. N. Engl. J. Med. *298*:888, 1978.
133. Perez-Tamayo, R.: Cirrhosis of the liver: A reversible disease. Pathol. Annu. *14*:183, 1979.
134. Powell, L. W., and Kerr, J. F. R.: Reversal of "cirrhosis" in idiopathic haemochromatosis following long-term intensive venesection therapy. Australas. Ann. Med. *19*:54, 1970.
135. Popper, H., et al.: Cytoplasmic copper and its toxic effects. Studies in Indian childhood cirrhosis. Lancet *1*:1205, 1979.
136. Tanner, M. S., et al.: Increased hepatic copper concentration in Indian childhood cirrhosis. Lancet *1*:1203, 1979.
137. Thiel, D. H., and Rogers, L.: Alcoholism: Its effect on hypothalamic-pituitary-gonadal function. Gastroenterology *71*:318, 1976.
138. Popper, H.: Pathologic aspects of cirrhosis. A review. Am. J. Pathol. *87*:228, 1977.
139. Christofferson, P., and Petersen, P.: Morphological features in non-cirrhotic livers from patients with chronic alcoholism, diabetes mellitus, or adipositas. A comparative study. Acta Pathol. Microbiol. Scand. (A) *86*:495, 1978.
140. Sherlock, S.: Alcohol and liver damage. Acta Med. Port. (Suppl. 2): 49, 1981.
141. Lieber, C. S.: Alcoholic fatty liver: Its pathogenesis and precursor role for hepatitis and cirrhosis. Panminerva Med. *18*:346, 1976.
142. Popper, H., and Lieber, C. S.: Histogenesis of alcoholic fibrosis and cirrhosis in the baboon. Am. J. Pathol. *98*:695, 1980.
143. Rankin, J. G.: The natural history and management of the patient with alcoholic liver disease. *In* Fisher, M. M., and Rankin, J. G. (eds.): Alcohol and the Liver. New York, Plenum Press, 1977, p. 365.
144. Murray, R. M.: Alcoholism amongst male doctors in Scotland. Lancet *2*:729, 1976.
145. Lieber, C. S.: Pathogenesis and early diagnosis of alcoholic liver injury. N. Engl. J. Med. *298*:888, 1978.
146. Lelbach, W. K.: Cirrhosis in the alcoholic and its relation to the volume of alcohol abuse. Ann. N. Y. Acad. Sci. *252*: 85, 1975.
147. Saunders, J. B., et al.: Accelerated development of alcoholic cirrhosis in patients with HLA-B8. Lancet *1*:1381, 1982.
148. Baraona, E., et al.: Alcoholic hepatomegaly: Accumulation of protein in the liver. Science *190*:794, 1975.

149. Rubin, E., and Lieber, C. S.: Alcohol-induced hepatic injury in nonalcoholic volunteers. N. Engl. J. Med. *278*:1869, 1968.
150. Rubin, E., and Lieber, C. S.: Fatty liver, alcoholic hepatitis and cirrhosis produced by alcohol in primates. N. Engl. J. Med. *290*:128, 1974.
151. Van Waes, L., and Lieber, C. S.: Early perivenular sclerosis in alcoholic fatty liver: An index of progressive liver injury. Gastroenterology *73*:646, 1977.
152. Gregory, D. H., and Levi, D. F.: The clinical-pathologic spectrum of alcoholic hepatitis. Am. J. Dig. Dis. *17*:479, 1972.
153. Phillips, M. J.: Mallory bodies and the liver. Lab. Invest. *47*:311, 1982.
154. French, S. W.: The Mallory body. Structure, composition and pathogen. Hepatology *1*:76, 1981.
155. Galambos, J. T.: Natural history of alcoholic hepatitis. III. Histological changes. Gastroenterology *63*:1026, 1972.
156. Editorial: How does alcohol damage the liver? Br. Med. J. *2*:1733, 1978.
157. Jenkins, W. J., and Peters, T. J.: Selectively reduced hepatic acetaldehyde dehydrogenase in alcoholics. Lancet *1*:628, 1980.
158. Thomas, M.: Role of hepatic acetaldehyde dehydrogenase in alcoholism: Demonstration of persistent reduction of cytosolic activity in abstaining patients. Lancet *2*:1058, 1982.
159. Lewis, K. O., and Paton, A.: Could superoxide cause cirrhosis? Lancet 2:188, 1982.
160. Hall, P. de la M., et al.: Alcoholic liver disease. A review. Pathology *11*:677, 1979.
161. Chen, T. S., and Leevy, C. M.: Collagen biosynthesis in liver disease of the alcoholic. J. Lab. Clin. Med. *85*:103, 1075.
162. Zetterman, R., et al.: Alcoholic hyalin and hepatic fibrosis. Clin. Res. *22*:559A, 1974.
163. Popper, H., and Kent, G.: Fibrosis in chronic liver disease. Clin. Gastroenterol. *4*:315, 1975.
164. Rojkind, M., and Dunn, M. A.: Hepatic fibrosis. Gastroenterology *76*:849, 1979.
165. Denk, H., et al.: Mallory bodies in experimental animals and man. Int. Rev. Exp. Pathol. *20*:77, 1979.
166. Powell, W. J., and Klatskin, G.: Duration of survival in patients with Lannec's cirrhosis, influence of alcohol withdrawal and possible effects of recent changes in general management of the disease. Am. J. Med. *44*:406, 1968.
167. Brechat, C., et al.: Evidence that hepatitis B virus has a role in liver cell carcinoma in alcoholic liver disease. N. Engl. J. Med. *306*:1384, 1982.
168. Popper, H., and Schaffner, F.: Chronic hepatitis: Taxonomic, etiologic and therapeutic problems. *In* Popper, H., and Schaffner, F. (eds.): Progress in Liver Disease. Vol. 5. New York, Grune & Stratton, 1976, p. 535.
169. Munro, H. N., and Linder, M. C.: Ferritin: Structure, biosynthesis, and role in iron metabolism. Physiol. Rev. *58*:317, 1978.
170. Richter, G. W.: The iron-loaded cell—the cytopathology of iron storage. A review. Am. J. Pathol. *91*:362, 1978.
171. Powell, L. W., et al.: Hemochromatosis: 1980 update. Gastroenterology *78*:374, 1980.
172. Finch, C. A., and Huebers, H.: Perspectives in iron metabolism. N. Engl. J. Med. *306*:1520, 1982.
173. Charlton, R. W., and Bothwell, T. H.: Iron absorption. Annu. Rev. Med. *34*:44, 1983.
174. Huebers, H. A.: Significance of transferrin for intestinal iron absorption. Blood *61*:283, 1983.
175. Powell, L. W., and Halliday, J. W.: Iron absorption and iron overload. Clin. Gastroenterol. *10*:707, 1981.
176. Bjorn-Rasmussen, E.: Iron absorption: Present knowledge and controversies. Lancet *1*:914, 1983.
177. Cartwright, G. E., et al.: Hereditary hemochromatosis. Phenotypic expression of the disease. N. Engl. J. Med. *301*:175, 1979.
178. Simon, M., et al.: The genetics of hemochromatosis. Prog. Med. Genet. *4*:135, 1980.
179. Bjorn-Rasmussen, E., et al.: Losses of ingested iron temporarily retained in the gastrointestinal tract. Scand. J. Haematol. *25*:124, 1980.
180. Batey, R. G., et al.: Hepatic iron clearance from serum in treated hemochromatosis. Gastroenterology *75*:856, 1978.
181. Bosset, M. J., et al.: Ferritin synthesis in peripheral blood monocytes in idiopathic haemochromatosis. J. Lab. Clin. Med. *100*:137, 1982.
182. Trump, B. F., et al.: The relationship of intracellular pathways of iron metabolism to cellular iron overload and the iron storage diseases. Am. J. Pathol. *72*:295, 1973.
183. Grace, N. D., and Powell, L. W.: Iron storage disorders of the liver. Gastroenterology *64*:1257, 1974.
184. Rojkind, M., and Dunn, M. A.: Hepatic fibrosis. Gastroenterology *76*:849, 1979.
185. Brink, B., et al.: Patterns of iron storage in dietary iron overload and idiopathic hemochromatosis. J. Lab. Clin. Med. *88*:725, 1976.
186. Bomford, A., and Williams, R.: Long-term results of venous section therapy in idiopathic haemochromatosis. Q. J. Med. (New Series) *45*:611, 1976.
187. Milder, M. S., et al.: Idiopathic hemochromatosis, an interim report. Medicine *59*:34, 1980.
188. Finch, C. A.: Detection of iron overload. N. Engl. J. Med. *307*:1703, 1982.
189. Galambos, J. T.: Hemochromatosis. Am. J. Gastroenterol. *64*:169, 1975.
190. Anthony-Jones, E.: Primary biliary cirrhosis and liver transplantation. N. Engl. J. Med. *306*:41, 1982.
191. Epstein, O., et al.: Primary biliary cirrhosis is a dry gland syndrome with features of chronic graft-versus-host disease. Lancet *1*:1166, 1980.
192. Thomas, H. C., et al.: Immune response to phi-X-174 in man. V. Primary and secondary antibody production in primary biliary cirrhosis. Gut *17*: 844, 1976.
193. Wands, J. R., et al.: Circulating immune complexes and complement activation in primary biliary cirrhosis. N. Engl. J. Med. *298*:233, 1978.
194. Anthony-Jones, E., et al.: Primary biliary cirrhosis and the complement system. Ann. Intern. Med. *90*:72, 1979.
195. Geubel, A. P., et al.: Lymphocyte cytotoxicity and inhibition studied with autologous liver cells: Observations in chronic active liver disease and the primary biliary cirrhosis syndrome. Gastroenterology *71*:450, 1976.
196. James, S. P., et al.: The role of the immune response in the pathogenesis of primary biliary cirrhosis. Semin. Liver Dis. *1*:322, 1981.
197. Fogan, E. A., et al.: Multiorgan granulomas and mitochondrial antibodies. N. Engl. J. Med. *308*:572, 1983.
198. Lee, R. G., et al.: Granulomas in primary biliary cirrhosis: A prognostic feature. Gastroenterology *81*:983, 1981.
199. Sherlock, S.: Primary biliary cirrhosis. Am. J. Med. *65*:217, 1978.
200. Roll, J., et al.: The prognostic significance of clinical and histologic features in asymptomatic and symptomatic primary biliary cirrhosis. N. Engl. J. Med. *308*:1, 1983.
201. Yunis, E. J., et al.: Fine structural observations of the liver in alpha-1-antitrypsin deficiency. Am. J. Pathol. *82:* 265, 1976.
202. Millward-Sadler, G. H.: Alpha-1-antitrypsin deficiency and liver disease. Acta Med. Port. Suppl to ii, 1981.
203. Sveger, T.: Liver disease in alpha$_1$-antitrypsin deficiency detected by screening of 200,000 infants. N. Engl. J. Med. *294*:1316, 1976.
204. Editorial: Alpha$_1$-antitrypsin deficiency and liver disease. Br. Med. J. *283*:807, 1981.
205. Hodges, J. R., et al.: Heterozygous MZ alpha$_1$-antitrypsin deficiency in adults with chronic active hepatitis and cryptogenic cirrhosis. N. Engl. J. Med. *304*:557, 1981.
206. Talbot, I. C., and Mowat, A. P.: Liver disease in infancy: Histological features and relationship to alpha-1-AT phenotype. J. Clin. Pathol. *28*:559, 1975.
207. Ericksson, S.: Liver disease and intermediate alpha$_1$-antitrypsin deficiency. Acta Med. Scand. *210*:241, 1981.
208. Sharp, H. L.: Alpha$_1$-antitrypsin deficiency. Hosp. Pract. *6*:83, 1976.
209. Evans, J., et al.: Observations on copper-associated protein in childhood liver disease. Gut *21*:970, 1980.
210. Editorial: Wilson's disease and copper-associated protein. Lancet *1*:644, 1981.
211. Evans, G. W., et al.: Wilson's disease: Identification of an abnormal copper-binding protein. Science *181*:1175, 1973.
212. Stromeyer, F. W., and Ishak, K. G.: Histology of the liver in Wilson's disease. Am. J. Pathol. *73*:12, 1980.
213. Gibbs, K., et al.: The urinary excretion of radiocopper in presymptomatic and symptomatic Wilson's disease, heterozygotes and controls: Its significance in diagnosis and management. Q. J. Med. (new series) *47*:349, 1978.
214. MacSween, R. N. M, and Scott, A. R.: Hepatic cirrhosis: A clinicopathologic review of 520 cases. J. Clin. Pathol. *26*:936, 1973.
215. Purtilo, D. T., and Gottlieb, L. S.: Cirrhosis and hepatoma occurring at Boston City Hospital (1917–1968). Cancer *32*:458, 1973.
216. Fechner, R. E.: Benign hepatic lesions and orally administered contraceptives. Hum. Pathol. *8*:255, 1977.
217. Pieterse, A. S., et al.: Nodular regenerative hyperplasia of the liver. Aust. N. Z. J. Med. *11*:268, 1981.
218. Klatskin, G.: Hepatic tumors: Possible relationship to use of oral contraceptives. Gastroenterology *73*:386, 1977.
219. Edmondson, H. A., et al.: Liver cell adenomas associated with use of oral contraceptives. N. Engl. J. Med. *294*:480, 1976.
220. Hayes, D., et al.: Hepatic cell adenoma presenting with intraperitoneal haemorrhage in the puerperium. Br. Med. J. *2*:1394, 1977.
221. London, W. T.: Primary hepatocellular carcinoma—etiology, pathogenesis, and prevention. Hum. Pathol. *12*:1085, 1981.
222. Neumayr, A., and Weiss, W.: Liver tumours—new aspects. Hepatogastroenterology *28*:1, 1981.
223. Sumithran, E., and MacSween, R. N. M.: An appraisal of the relationship between primary hepatocellular carcinoma and hepatitis B virus. Histopathology *3*:447, 1979.
224. Larouze, B., et al.: Forecasting the development of primary hepatocellular carcinoma by the use of risk factors: Studies in West Africa. J. Natl. Cancer Inst. *58*:1557, 1977.

225. Shafritz, D. A., and Kew, M. C.: Identification of integrated hepatitis B virus DNA sequences in human hepatocellular carcinomas. Hepatology *1*:1, 1981.
226. Shafritz, D. A., et al.: Integration of hepatitis B virus DNA into the genome of liver cells in chronic liver disease and hepatocellular carcinoma. N. Engl. J. Med. *305*:1067, 1981.
227. Summers, J., et al.: A virus similar to human hepatitis B virus associated with hepatitis and hepatoma in woodchucks. Proc. Natl. Acad. Sci. U.S.A. *75*:4533, 1978.
228. Beasley, R. P., et al.: The risk of hepatocellular carcinoma in hepatitis B virus infections: A prospective study in Taiwan presented at International Symposium of Viral Hepatitis, New York, 1981 (as reported by London, W. T.). Hum. Pathol. *12*:1085, 1981.
229. Anthony, P. P.: Carcinoma of the liver in man. Int. Pathol. *15*:29, 1974.
230. Shar, S. R., and Kew, M. C.: Oral contraceptives and hepatocellular carcinoma. Cancer *49*:407, 1982.
231. Linsell, C. A., and Peers, F. G.: Aflatoxin and liver cell cancer. Trans. R. Soc. Trop. Med. Hyg. *71*:471, 1977.
232. Lutwick, L. I.: Relation between aflatoxin hepatitis-B virus and hepatocellular carcinoma. Lancet *1*:755, 1979.
233. Lapis, K., and Johannessen, J. V.: Pathology of primary liver cancer. J. Toxicol. Environ. Health *5*:315, 1979.
234. Thung, S. N., et al.: Distribution of five antigens in hepatocellular carcinomas. Lab. Invest. *41*:101, 1979.
235. Maltz, C., et al.: Hepatocellular carcinoma. New directions in etiology. Am. J. Gastroenterol. *74*:361, 1980.
236. Blumberg, B. S., and London, W. T.: Hepatitis B virus and the prevention of primary hepatocellular carcinoma. N. Engl. J. Med. *304*:782, 1981.
237. W. H. O. Scientific Group: Prevention of primary liver cancer. Lancet *1*:463, 1983.
238. Ishak, K. G., and Glunz, P. R.: Hepatoblastoma and hepatocarcinoma in infancy and childhood. Cancer *20*:396, 1967.
239. Popper, H., et al.: Development of hepatic angiosarcoma in man induced by vinyl chloride, Thorotrast, and arsenic. Am. J. Pathol. *92*:349, 1978.
240. Center for Disease Control: M.M.W.R. *23*:210, 1974.
241. NIH Conference: Vinyl chloride–associated liver disease. Ann. Intern. Med. *84*:717, 1976.
242. Smith, I. E., et al.: Comparison of gray-scale ultrasound with other methods for the detection of liver metastases from breast carcinoma. Clin. Oncol. *2*:47, 1976.
243. Dixon, A. G., and Burns, W. A.: Liver biopsy in patients with malignancy: A postmortem study. Lab. Invest. *28*:405 (abstr.), 1973.
244. Watkins, J. B., et al.: Neonatal hepatitis: A diagnostic approach. Adv. Pediatr. *24*:399, 1977.
245. MacMahon, H. E., and Thannhauser, S. J.: Congenital dysplasia of interlobular bile ducts with extensive skin xanthomata: Congenital acholangic biliary cirrhosis. Gastroenterology *21*:488, 1952.
246. Landing, B. H.: Considerations of the pathogenesis of neonatal hepatitis, biliary atresia and choledochal cyst. *In* Bill, A. H., and Kasai, M. (eds): The Concept of Infantile Obstructive Cholangiopathy. Vol. 6. Pediatric Surgery. Baltimore, University Park Press, 1974, p.113.
247. Witzelben, C. L., et al.: Studies on the pathogenesis of biliary atresia. Lab. Invest. *38*:525, 1978.
247A. Lichtenstein, P. K., et al.: Grade I Reye's syndrome. N. Engl. J. Med. *309*:133, 1983.
248. Brunner, R. I., et al.: Psychological consequences of Reye's syndrome. J. Pediatr. *95*:706, 1979.
249. Snodgrass, P. J., and DeLong, G. R.: Urea-cycle enzyme deficiences and an increased nitrogen load producing hyperammonemia in Reye's syndrome. N. Engl. J. Med. *294*:855, 1976.
250. Brown, T., et al.: Transiently reduced activity of carbamyl phosphate synthetase and ornithine transcarbamylase in liver of children with Reye's syndrome. N. Engl. J. Med. *294*:861, 1976.
251. Crocker, J. F. S., et at.: Lethal interaction of ubiquitous insecticide carriers with a virus. Science *192*:1351, 1976.
252. Nelson, J. G., et al.: Aflatoxin and Reye's syndrome: A case control study. Pediatrics *66*:865, 1980.
253. Report of the Reye's Syndrome Working Group: Update: Reye's syndrome and salicylate usage. M.M.W.R. *31*:53, 61, 1982.
254. Fulginiti, V. A., et al.: Aspirin and Reye's syndome. Pediatrics *69*:810, 1982.
255. Starko, K. M., and Mullick, F. G.: Hepatic and cerebral findings in children with fatal salicylate intoxication: Further evidence for a causal relationship between salicylate and Reye's syndome. Lancet *1*:326, 1983.
256. Mitchell, R. A., et al.: Comparison of cytosolic and mitochondrial hepatic enzyme alterations in Reye's syndrome. Pediatr. Res. *14*:1216, 1980.
257. Partin, J. S., et al.: Brain ultrastructure in Reye's syndome. J. Neuropathol. Exp. Neurol. *37*:796, 1978.
258. Arnaud, J. P., et al.: The x-ray diffraction study of gallstones: Identification of pure mineral stones. Br. J. Surg. *65*:362, 1978.
259. Royal College of General Practitioners Oral Contraception Study: Oral contraceptives and gallbladder disease. Lancet *2*:957, 1982.
260. The Coronary Drug Project Research Group: Gallbladder disease is a side effect of drugs influencing lipid metabolism. N. Engl. J. Med. *296*:1185, 1977.
261. Bennion, L. J., and Grundy, S. M.: Risk factors for the development of cholelithiasis in man. N. Engl. J. Med. *299*:1161, 1221, 1978.
262. Salen, G., et al.: Hepatic cholesterol metabolism in patients with gallstones. Gastroenterology *69*:767, 1975.
263. Sedaghat, A., and Grundy, S. M.: Cholesterol crystals and the formation of cholesterol gallstones. N. Engl. J. Med. *302*:1274, 1980.
264. Mok, H. Y. I., et al.: Regulation of pool size of bile acids in man. Gastroenterology *73*:684, 1977.
265. Soloway, R. D., et al.: Pigment gallstones. Gastroenterology *72*:167, 1977.
266. Gracie, W. A., and Ransohoff, D. F.: The natural history of silent gallstones. The innocent gallstone is not a myth. N. Engl. J. Med. *306*:798, 1982.
267. Editorial: Gallstones in Basel. Lancet *2*:1083, 1982.
268. Hallendorf, L. C., et al.: Gangrenous cholecystitis: A clinical and pathologic study of 100 cases. Surg. Clin. North Am. *28*:979, 1948.
269. Feldman, M., and Feldman, J., Jr.: Cholesterolosis of the gallbladder. Gastroenterology *27*:641, 1954.
270. Babcock, J. R., and Eyerly, R. C.: A 5-year survey of 1055 consecutive patients with extrahepatic biliary tract disease. Surg. Gynecol. Obstet. *105*:711, 1957.
271. Shepard, V. D., et al.: Benign neoplasms of the gallbladder. Arch. Surg. *45*:1, 1942.
272. Illingworth, C. F. W.: Carcinoma of the gallbladder. Br. J. Surg. *23*:4, 1936.
273. Brandt-Rauf, P. W., et al.: Cancer of the gallbladder. A review of 43 cases. Hum. Pathol. *13*:48, 1982.
274. Polk, H. C., J.R.: Carcinoma and the calcified gallbladder. Gastroenterology *50*:582, 1966.
275. Krain, L. S.: Gallbladder in extrahepatic bile duct carcinoma: Analysis of 1,808 cases. Geriatrics *12*:111, 1972.
276. Fraumeni, J. F., Jr.: Cancers of the pancreas and biliary tract: Epidemiological considerations. Cancer Res. *35*:3437, 1975.
277. Van Heerden, J. A., et al.: Carcinoma of extrahepatic bile ducts. Am. J. Surg. *113*:49, 1967.
278. Bismuth, H., and Malt, R. A.: Carcinoma of the bilary tract. N. Engl. J. Med. *301*:704, 1979.

20 THE PANCREAS

The Exocrine Pancreas

NORMAL

In its posterior location in the upper abdomen, the pancreas is one of the "hidden" organs in the body. It is virtually impossible to palpate clinically. Diseases that impair its function only evoke signs or symptoms when far advanced, because there is such a large reserve of both endocrine and exocrine function. Some lesions are only manifested by encroachment on neighboring structures. For example, carcinoma of the pancreas may be discovered only when it invades the vertebral column, occludes the biliary system, or causes disturbances in the stomach or colon.

The pancreas arises from two duodenal buds that are referred to, respectively, as the dorsal and ventral pancreas.[1] Fusion of the two creates the adult organ, after which the two contributions can no longer be distinguished. The ductal drainage systems anastomose, and the major excretory duct of the dorsal pancreas, draining into the duodenum, persists as the duct of Wirsung. Usually, the duct of the ventral pancreas disappears, but if it persists it creates the accessory duct of Santorini. However, there is much variability in this ductal system. In two-thirds of adults the major pancreatic duct does not empty directly into the duodenum but into the common bile duct just proximal to the ampulla of Vater, thus providing a common channel to the pancreatic and biliary drainage.

In the adult the average pancreas is about 15 cm in length and weighs 60 to 140 gm. Its gross anatomic relationships include immediate proximity to the duodenum, ampulla of Vater, common bile duct, superior mesenteric artery, portal vein, spleen and its vascular supply, stomach, transverse colon, left lobe of the liver, and lower recesses of the lesser omental cavity. Inflammatory and neoplastic processes within the pancreas may cause secondary involvement of many adjacent structures that produces, in many cases, the characteristic signs and symptoms of pancreatic disease.

Histologically, the pancreas has two separate components, exocrine and endocrine glands. The endocrine pancreas is described on page 972. The exocrine portion, constituting 80 to 85% of the organ, is made up of numerous small glands (acini) aggregated into the lobules seen in the gross. These acini are separated by a scant connective tissue stroma. The epithelial cells are columnar to truncated pyramids radially oriented about the gland circumference. The central lumen of the acinus is extremely small in the normal state and may not even be visible. Small microvilli project from the apical surfaces of the secretory cells into the lumen. The exocrine secretory cells are deeply basophilic in routine tissue stains because of their abundance of granular endoplasmic reticulum and ribosomes. The Golgi complex is well developed in these cells and, along with the endoplasmic reticulum, appears to be oriented toward the basal region. The apical regions of the cells contain abundant membrane-bound sacs enclosing zymogen granules.

The ductal system of the pancreas is produced by progressive anastomosis of the extremely fine radicles that begin within the secretory acini. These small ducts eventually drain into the main pancreatic ducts. At first cuboidal, their lining epithelium becomes progressively higher to produce tall, columnar, regular aligned cells. This ductal epithelium is mucus secreting. About the larger ducts, there are numerous accessory branching ducts and mucous glands, which may be sufficiently agglomerated in the region of the duodenum to create the false impression of a well-differentiated glandular carcinoma.

It is hardly necessary here to reiterate the secretory functions of the pancreas and the regulatory mechanisms that control such activity. Several points, however, are directly pertinent to disease processes and merit reemphasis. The pancreas secretes 1.5 to 3 liters per day of an alkaline fluid containing enzymes and zymogens. Secretion is adjusted to the workload that it is called on to perform, i.e., the volume and character of the intestinal contents. The regulation of this secretion is a complex process that involves humoral and neural factors. The most important of these regulators are the hormones *secretin* and *cholecystokinin*, produced in the duodenum. The former stimulates water and bicarbonate secretion by duct cells, and the latter enhances the discharge of enzyme-containing zymogen granules by acinar cells. When the pancreas is stimulated to secretory activity, the zymogen granules, enclosed within

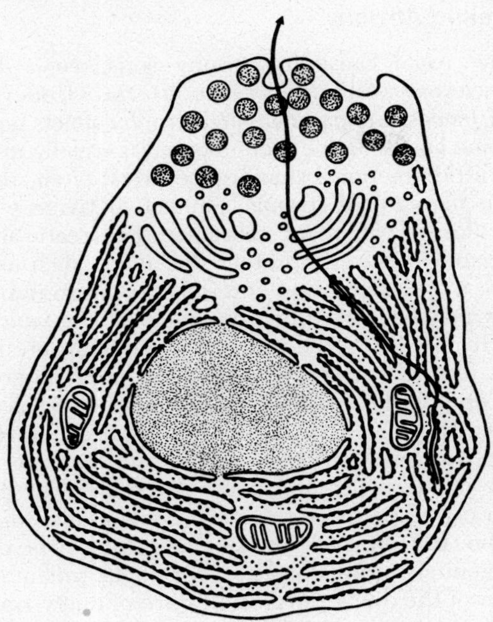

Figure 20–1. Schematic representation of pathway of protein secretion in an exocrine pancreas *(see text)*. (Modified from Jamieson, J. D.: Membranes and secretions. *In* Weissman, G., and Claiborne, R. (eds.): Cell Membranes: Biochemistry, Cell Biology and Pathology. New York, H. P. Publishing Co., 1975.)

membranous sacs originating from the Golgi complex, migrate to the apical region of the cell. Here the sac becomes attached to the plasma membrane, and rupture at the point of attachment releases the enzyme-rich zymogen granules into the acinus of the gland (Fig. 20–1). Fats and alcohol are particularly active stimulators of secretin production, and therefore indirectly of the pancreas.

A second point of interest relates to the elaboration of the proteolytic enzymes. These include trypsin, chymotrypsin, aminopeptidases, and elastase. In addition, the pancreas secretes amylases, lipases, and phospholipases. Self-digestion of the pancreas is prevented by two means: (1) these enzymes are elaborated as inactive precursors that are only activated in the duodenum and (2) protease inhibitors are normally present within acini and pancreatic secretion. One of the most important pancreatic diseases, acute hemorrhagic pancreatic necrosis, is initiated by activation of these enzymes within the pancreatic parenchyma.

PATHOLOGY

The most significant disorders of the exocrine pancreas are cystic fibrosis (p. 493), acute and chronic pancreatitis, and tumors.[3] It should be emphasized that, from the standpoints of both morbidity and mortality, diabetes mellitus (a disorder of endocrine metabolism) overshadows all the other pancreatic disorders. However, a knowledgeable alertness to exocrine pancreatic disease is most necessary, since almost all these disorders are difficult to diagnose because of the hidden position and large reserve function of this organ, and because they appear under such diverse guises as a catastrophic "acute abdomen" or the silent growth of a carcinoma.

CONGENITAL ANOMALIES

The pancreas is subject to a variety of congenital disorders that, with the exception of fibrocystic disease, are either quite uncommon or of little clinical significance.[2] The gland may be totally absent (agenesis). Complete agenesis is quite regularly associated with widespread severe malformations that are incompatible with life. The endocrine and exocrine elements may be *hypoplastic*. The gland may exist as two separate structures representing the persistence of the dorsal and ventral pancreas. The head of the pancreas may encircle the duodenum as a collar *(annular pancreas)* and sometimes may cause subtotal duodenal obstruction and consequent clinical symptoms. Two additional anomalies occur with sufficient frequency or have sufficient clinical significance to merit separate consideration.

ABERRANT PANCREAS

Aberrant, or ectopic, displaced pancreatic tissue is found in about 2% of all routine postmortems. The most favored sites for such ectopia follow the order of the descent of the intestinal tract; i.e., they are most common in the stomach and duodenum with about equal frequency, next in the jejunum, then in Meckel's diverticulum, and then in the ileum. Usually, the masses vary from a few millimeters to 3 to 4 cm in diameter. They appear as single or multiple, firm, yellow-gray nests within the wall of the gut subjacent to the mucosa, lying usually within the submucosa (Fig. 20–2). They

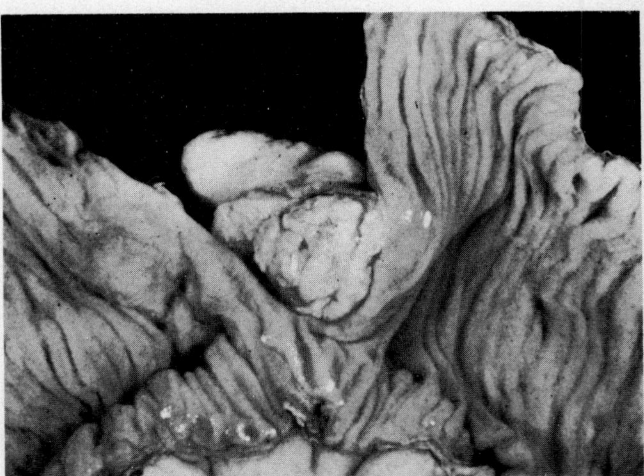

Figure 20–2. Aberrant pancreas. Mucosa of jejunum has been incised to disclose the rest of the pale yellow-white, submucosal, lobulated pancreatic tissue.

are composed histologically of glands that appear completely normal, and not infrequently islets of Langerhans are also present.

In such locations, they may be discovered accidentally in the course of a laparotomy, visualized radiographically as sessile lesions that project slightly into the lumen of the bowel, or seen on endoscopy in the course of studies for gastrointestinal symptoms. About 2% of islet cell tumors arise in ectopic pancreas.[4]

ANOMALIES OF DUCTS

Anomalies of the pancreatic duct represent a second type of congenital defect that is sometimes of clinical importance. The ducts of Wirsung and of Santorini may both persist as totally separate structures. The major excretory pancreatic duct, the duct of Wirsung, may drain into the common bile duct or may drain through an abnormally high orifice in the duodenum. These variations seem to be of little importance except for two considerations: (1) unless recognized, they may potentiate ligation or severance of ducts during surgery around the ampulla, causing serious sequelae; and (2) one of these anomalies, *pancreas divisum,* predisposes to recurrent pancreatitis (p. 966).

MISCELLANEOUS "REGRESSIVE" CHANGES

The pancreas is extremely labile and susceptible to a great variety of adverse influences. Following death, it undergoes postmortem autolysis almost as rapidly as the brain. It is likewise affected by any severe febrile or systemic toxic disorder and reacts by cell swelling and hydropic degeneration. For the most part, these cytologic alterations are of little clinical import. Certain so-called regressive changes, however, are of some significance. Most have already been discussed in the earlier sections of the book, but are briefly reiterated for emphasis.

Stromal Fatty Infiltration or Fatty Ingrowth

These alterations sometimes enlarge the apparent size of the pancreas by spreading apart the lobular structure, but much more commonly the pancreas is either normal in size or even smaller *(adipose atrophy).* The dispersion of the parenchyma may create the impression that the pancreas has been totally replaced by a mass of adipose tissue. However, the fat is confined to the interstitial stroma and does not disturb the parenchymal elements; if the fat is dissolved out, a normal amount of pancreatic substance can be recovered. It has been pointed out that the genesis of this condition is entirely obscure. Fatty ingrowth of the pancreas is unrelated to any apparent pancreatic dysfunction.

Pancreatic Atrophy

The usual cause of atrophy is *ischemia* due to atherosclerosis of the pancreatic arteries. Under these circumstances, the parenchymal atrophy affects both the endocrine and exocrine elements but is usually minimal and of little functional significance. Most often, there is only an increase of stromal connective tissue without obvious loss of pancreatic substance. Pancreatic atrophy also occurs in chronic protein deficiency such as kwashiorkor or protein-losing enteropathy. More important atrophy may be caused by *obstruction of the pancreatic ducts.* In this form, the islets of Langerhans are totally spared, but the exocrine glands undergo progressive disuse or pressure atrophy to the point of total disappearance (Fig. 20–3). The discovery that such exocrine atrophy with preservation of islets could be induced by ligature of the pancreatic ducts paved the way for the pioneer experiments on the extraction and identification of insulin. In man, such exocrine atrophy may be caused by congenital stenosis or atresia of ducts, inflammatory stenoses of the ducts, surgical ligature of ducts, obstructive pancreatic calculi, squamous metaplasia of the lining epithelium with piling up of epithelial debris, or neoplastic obstruction. Whatever the cause, the pancreas becomes reduced to a small, irregular, nodular, fibrous mass.

On section, only fibrous tissue can be identified, usually traversed by dilated ducts that are sometimes ballooned out into cystic enlargements. When the obstruction affects only tributaries of the main pancreatic duct, the atrophy involves only regional portions of the pancreas. The histologic identification of such atrophy

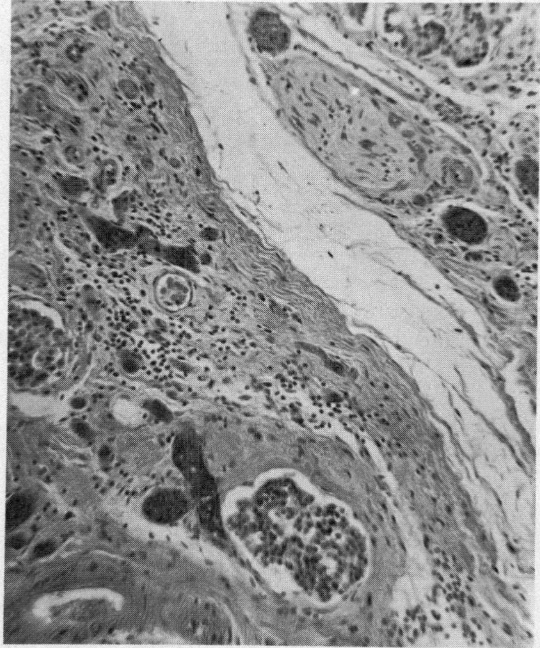

Figure 20–3. Pancreatic atrophy due to ductal obstruction. Acinar glands are totally replaced by fibrous tissue, but islets are preserved.

is readily made by the preservation of islets, with total disappearance and fibrofatty replacement of the acinar glands.

Agonal Changes

Not uncommonly, at postmortem examination focal or extensive areas of hemorrhage are found in the pancreas (pancreatic apoplexy). These hemorrhages are usually unassociated with either macroscopic or microscopic evidence of inflammatory reaction or tissue necrosis. The absence of inflammatory reaction indicates that such bleeding must have occurred in the agonal stages of life, probably influenced by shock and hypoxia (*shock pancreas*).

PANCREATITIS

Inflammation of the pancreas, almost always associated with acinar cell injury, is termed pancreatitis.[5, 6] Clinically and histologically, pancreatitis presents as a spectrum, dependent on duration and severity.[5] Acute pancreatitis includes a mild, self-limited form termed *interstitial or edematous pancreatitis*, and a more serious severe type, *acute hemorrhagic* (necrotizing) *pancreatitis*. In *chronic relapsing pancreatitis*, there is persistence or recurrence of episodes of active pancreatitis, eventually leading to chronic pancreatic insufficiency (*chronic pancreatitis*).

ACUTE HEMORRHAGIC PANCREATITIS

Acute hemorrhagic pancreatitis (acute pancreatic necrosis) refers to a sudden, more or less diffuse destruction of pancreatic substance caused by the escape of activated pancreatic enzymes into the parenchyma. These enzymes characteristically cause focal areas of fat necrosis in and about the pancreas and in other fatty depots in the abdominal cavity. They also lead to rupture of pancreatic vessels and relatively insignificant or massive hemorrhages into the parenchyma of this organ.

INCIDENCE. This condition occurs about once in every 500 to 600 medical and surgical admissions to a general hospital. Although by no means common, it is a dramatic, life-threatening illness. Acute pancreatitis occurs most often in middle life and is frequently associated with two conditions: *biliary tract disease* and *alcoholism*. Hemorrhagic pancreatitis often follows an alcoholic debauch or an excessively large meal. The male:female ratio for pancreatitis is 1:3 in those with biliary tract disease and 6:1 in those with alcoholism. A hereditary predisposition to pancreatitis has been identified in some families, transmitted apparently as an autosomal dominant trait.[7] However, such familial disease more commonly takes the form of chronic relapsing pancreatitis (p. 966) rather than acute pancreatitis. Although relatively rare, familial pancreatitis is the most common type encountered in children.

ETIOLOGY. As mentioned, the two leading conditions associated with acute pancreatitis are biliary tract disease (especially cholelithiasis) and excessive alcohol intake.[8] Gallstones are present in 35 to 60% of cases of pancreatitis, and about 5% of patients with gallstones develop pancreatitis. The proportion of cases of acute pancreatitis caused by alcoholism varies in different countries: it is 65% in the United States, but 20 to 25% in Sweden and 5% or less in southern France and England.[9] Other apparent but less common causes of pancreatitis include trauma; extension of inflammation from adjacent peptic ulcers or abdominal infections; blood-borne bacterial infections; viral infections such as mumps and hepatitis; acute ischemia induced by vascular thrombosis, embolism, polyarteritis nodosa, and shock;[10] hypothermia; and drugs (azathioprine, thiazides, sulfonamides, and oral contraceptives).[11] Pancreatitis also is occasionally associated with hyperlipoproteinemia (especially types I and V)[12] and with hyperparathyroidism and other hypercalcemic states.[13] In many patients the etiology of pancreatitis is obscure; in various studies this so-called *"idiopathic" pancreatitis* accounts for 9 to 50% of all patients with the disease.

PATHOGENESIS. The anatomic changes in this disease clearly indicate that the acute pancreatic necrosis is caused by the destructive effects of pancreatic enzymes, which run amuck within the pancreatic parenchyma.

It will be well to remember that the exogenous pancreas secretes at least 22 enzymes: 15 proteases (including elastase), three to six amylases, lipase, and phospholipase. These are normally present in the proenzyme form and need to be activated to fulfill their enzymatic potential. Proteolysis, lipolysis, and hemorrhage account for the three major morphologic features of this disorder. Thus, it would be natural to assume that proteases (trypsin, chymotrypsin), lipase, and elastase (which breaks down the elastic tissue of vessels) are the keys to such pancreatic destruction. *Trypsin could play a key role, as it is able to activate the majority of proenzymes taking part in the process of autodigestion*, such as proelastase and prophospholipase.[13] Indeed, reflux of proteases into the pancreatic ducts initiates pancreatic inflammation in the experimental animal.[14] Trypsin or chymotrypsin activity has been detected in human pancreatic juice or ascitic fluid in acute pancreatitis, and experimental studies show that significant amounts of trypsin, chymotrypsin, and elastase can be measured in the pancreas early in the disease.[15] Trypsin also converts prekallikrein to kallikrein, thereby activating the kinin system and indirectly, through activation of Hageman factor, the clotting and complement system (p. 53). These mediators then contribute to the local inflammation, thrombosis, tissue damage, and hemorrhage characteristic of acute hemorrhagic pancreatitis, as well as to systemic manifestations of the disease. Thus, *the activation of trypsinogen is an important triggering event in pancreatitis.*[16]

Two other enzymes that deserve mention are *elastase and phospholipase A. Elastase* is present in zymogen granules of acinous cells and in pancreatic secretions as an inactive precursor. It is activated by trypsin, causes dissolution of elastic fibers of blood vessels and ducts, and is a likely culprit in the production of hemorrhage. *Phospholipase A*, when activated, has two effects: destruction of cell membranes and conversion of lecithin in bile to lysolecithin. This latter compound is highly toxic and may be capable of damaging the ductal system of the pancreas.

But how are these enzymes activated and released within the pancreas? Theories abound, largely based on animal models, but facts on the human disease are scanty. It is likely that more than one pathway may lead to such activation. Some of the postulated mechanisms are listed below (Fig. 20–4).

1. *Acinar cell injury*. Viruses, endotoxin, toxic chemicals, ischemia, and trauma[17] result in direct acinar cell damage, with intrapancreatic activation and release of enzymes. This is the currently favored theory for pancreatitis not caused by biliary tract disease or alcoholism.

2. *Duct obstruction*. This presumably leads to leakage of enzymes from small ducts as a result of increased intraductal pressure. Since the main pancreatic duct joins the common bile duct in two-thirds of normal individuals, gallstones impacted in the ampulla of Vater cause pancreatic obstruction. Indeed, 70 to 85% of patients with gallstone-associated pancreatitis have evidence of gallstones either in the ampulla or in the stools.[18] However, experimental work indicates that obstruction alone is insufficient to cause hemorrhagic pancreatitis. Two additional factors that may contribute to pancreatic necrosis in this setting are *biliary reflux* and *duodenal reflux*. *Biliary reflux* into the pancreatic ducts allows delivery of the lecithin in bile into the pancreas, where it can be converted by phospholipase A to the highly toxic lysolecithin. *Duodenal reflux* may occur owing to damage of the sphincter of Oddi as a result of biliary disease, allowing duodenal contents to enter the pancreatic enzymes. Gallstones impacted in the common bile duct or duodenal papilla may also splint or dilate the sphincter, causing the same effect.

Alcohol may also induce partial pancreatic duct obstruction. It has been shown that chronic alcohol ingestion increases the protein concentration of pancreatic secretions, inducing inspissated protein plugs in ducts and focal pancreatic duct obstruction. This effect, however, is more important in the pathogenesis of *chronic* alcoholic pancreatitis.

3. *Hyperlipidemia*. Hypertriglyceridemia clearly

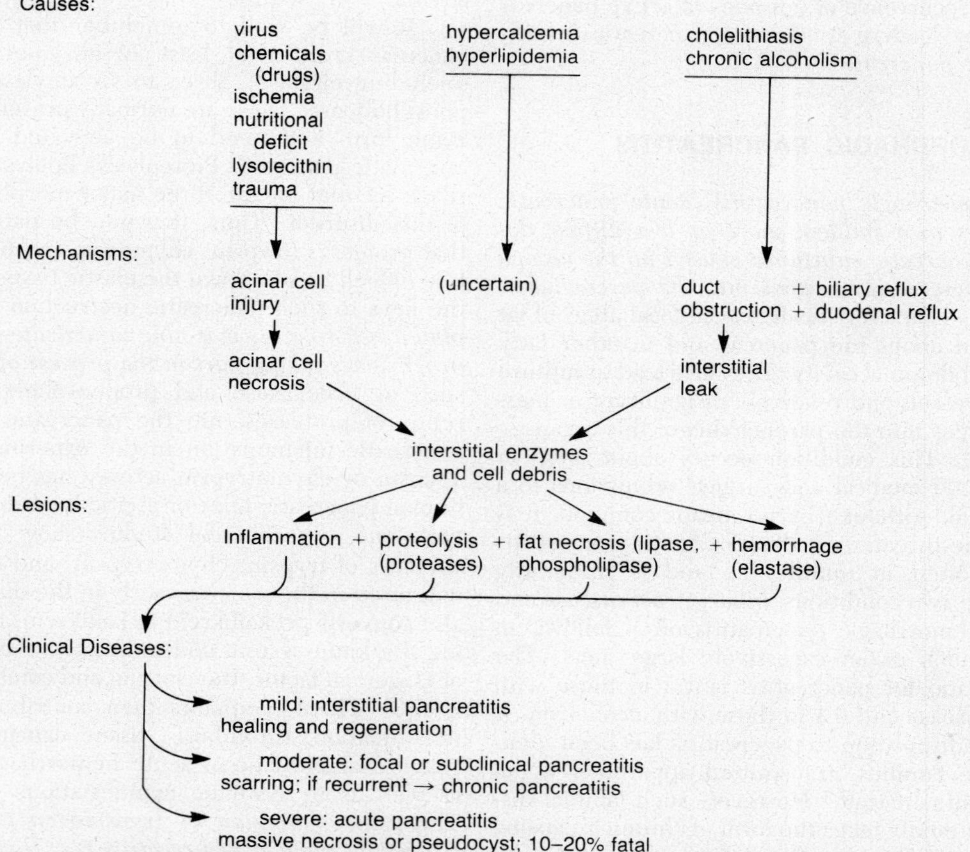

Figure 20–4. Etiology and pathogenesis of pancreatitis. (Modified from Longnecker, D. S.: Pathology and pathogenesis of diseases of the pancreas. Am. J. Pathol. *107*:103, 1982.)

contributes to the pathogenesis of acute recurrent pancreatitis in patients with types I and V hyperlipoproteinemia,[12] in females and males on estrogen therapy, and also probably in acute alcoholics. In the latter, serum triglycerides may rise to over 1000 mg/dl after a lipid meal.[22] The mechanism is not clear, but experimental studies suggest that lipolysis of triglycerides by pancreatic lipase in and around the pancreas leads to high local tissue levels of free fatty acids. These free fatty acids are presumably toxic to acinar cells and blood vessels.[23]

4. *Hypercalcemia*. Seven to 19% of patients with either a parathyroid adenoma or a parathyroid carcinoma develop acute pancreatitis.[13] The basis for this association is not entirely clear, but increased calcium concentrations are known to stimulate an increase in the autoactivation of trypsinogen.[24]

Figure 20–4 summarizes the proved or postulated mechanisms in the pathogenesis of pancreatitis.

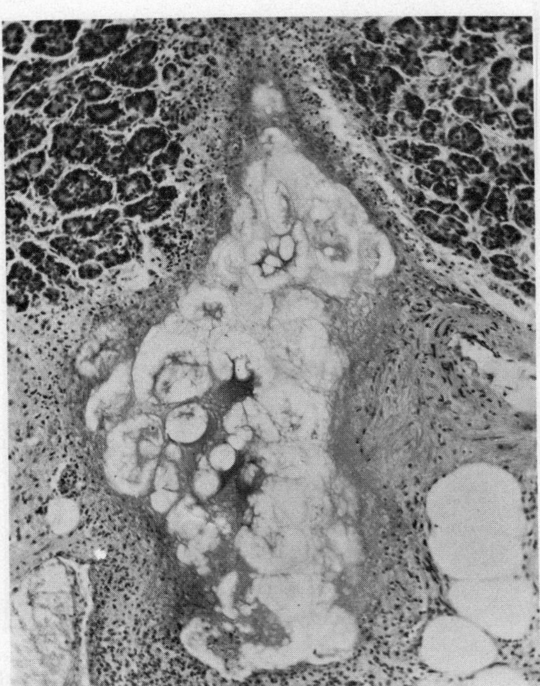

Figure 20–5. Acute pancreatic necrosis. Central focus of necrotic fat is surrounded by a rim of leukocytic infiltration.

MORPHOLOGY. The histologic changes are presented first because they can be predicted, to a considerable extent, from the presumed pathogenesis of this disease. The basic alterations are four in number: **proteolytic destruction of pancreatic substance, necroses of blood vessels with subsequent hemorrhage, necrosis of fat by lipolytic enzymes, and an accompanying inflammatory reaction.** The extent and predominance of each of these alterations depend on the duration and severity of the process. In the very early stages, a phase that has usually passed by the time the patient comes to postmortem examination, only interstitial edema is present. Soon after, focal and confluent areas of frank necrosis of endocrine and exocrine cells are found. The affected cells assume a glassy, clouded appearance and then progressively undergo granular coagulative necrosis. The accompanying neutrophilic inflammatory reaction is usually confined to the margins of the necrotic foci. Hemorrhagic extravasation may be minimal to extreme. In milder cases, the interstitium is suffused with red blood cells and fibrin clots; in severe instances, large areas of the pancreatic substance are virtually converted to a mass of blood clot.

Perhaps the most characteristic histologic alteration of acute pancreatic necrosis is the focal areas of fat necrosis that occur in the stromal, peripancreatic fat, and fat depots throughout the abdominal cavity (Fig. 20–5). These lesions consist of enzymatic destruction of fat cells, in which **the vacuolated fat cells are transformed to shadowy outlines of cell membranes filled with pink, granular, opaque precipitate.** Presumably, this contained granular material is derived from the hydrolysis of fat. The liberated glycerol is reabsorbed, and the released fatty acids combine with calcium (a process referred to as saponification, or the formation of soaps) to form insoluble salts that are precipitated in situ. Amorphous basophilic calcium precipitates may be visible within the necrotic focus.

Secondary bacterial invasion, a common occurrence after the passage of three to four days, may modify this picture by converting many areas into foci of characteristic suppurative necrosis or frank abscess formation. If the patient survives, the acute necrotizing damage may resolve slowly and be replaced by diffuse or focal parenchymal or stromal fibrosis, calcifications, and irregular ductal dilatations. Occasionally, liquefied areas are walled off by fibrous tissue to form small or large cystic spaces, known as **pseudocysts.**

Macroscopically, the dominant characteristics of acute pancreatic necrosis are **areas of gray-white proteolytic destruction of parenchymal substance, hemorrhage, and chalky white areas of fat necrosis.** In the typical case there is an extremely variegated, maplike patterning in the pancreas, with areas of blue-black hemorrhages and other areas of gray-white necrotic softening, alternating with sprinkled foci of yellow-white, chalky fat necrosis (Fig. 20–6).

Characteristically, there are accompanying changes in the remainder of the abdominal cavity. In most instances, the peritoneal cavity contains a serous and slightly turbid, brown-tinged fluid in which globules of oil can be identified (so called "chicken-broth" fluid). In late cases, this fluid may become bacterially infected to produce suppurative peritonitis. Additionally, foci of fat necrosis may be found in any of the fat depots, such as in the omentum, mesentery of the bowel, and properitoneal deposits. Occasionally, fat necrosis has been described in fat depots outside the abdominal cavity. Associated biliary tract disease, cholecystitis, and cholelithiasis have been reported in up to two-thirds of cases of acute pancreatic necrosis. The relationship between this biliary tract disease and pancreatitis has already been noted.

CLINICAL COURSE. Full-blown, acute pancreatic necrosis is a medical emergency of the first magnitude.[6] These patients usually have the sudden calamitous onset of an "acute abdomen" that must be differentiated from diseases such as acute appendicitis, perforated peptic ulcer, acute cholecystitis with rupture, and occlusion of mesenteric vessels with infarction of the bowel, to mention a few. Characteristically, the pain appears without prodromal symptoms, usually soon after a large

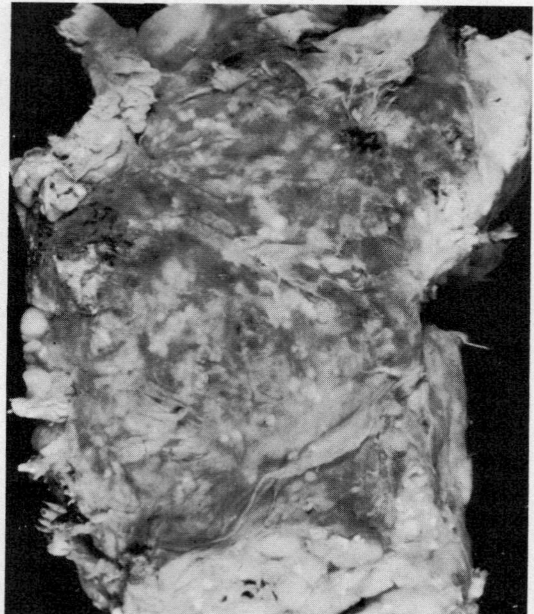

Figure 20–6. Acute hemorrhagic pancreatic necrosis. The destruction here is moderate in severity and consists principally of scattered foci of white necrotic fat with several darker areas of hemorrhage above.

meal or an alcoholic binge. The pain is constant and intense, and is often referred to the upper back. In many cases, the agonizing pain soon leads to peripheral vascular collapse and sometimes is followed by a profound shocklike state. Many explanations have been offered for this rapid development of shock. Loss of blood, when severe, and electrolyte disturbances clearly contribute to the hypotension. There is increasing evidence, however, that release of vasodilatory agents such as bradykinin and the prostaglandins may be the cause of shock in acute pancreatitis. Endotoxemia with complement activation has also been observed.[25]

Jaundice sometimes appears after the first day and is presumed to be due to edematous narrowing of the common bile duct. The laboratory may provide direct support for the diagnosis. Characteristically, there is an elevation of the serum amylase level within the first 24 hours and the serum lipase level somewhat later (72 to 94 hours). Both fall to basal levels two to five days after the acute phase passes. Elevated enzyme levels may also be produced by acute cholecystitis, perforated peptic ulcer, and other inflammatory conditions in the upper abdomen that impinge on the pancreas, but they rarely attain a value of five times normal, which so commonly occurs in primary acute pancreatitis. Elevated serum lipase is somewhat more specific for pancreatic disease, and there are now simple sensitive assays for this enzyme.

Glycosuria develops transiently in about 5 to 10% of cases, apparently as an expression of acute disturbance in islet cell function. In patients with fat necrosis, hypocalcemia is frequent, and if persistent is a poor prognostic sign.

Therapy for acute pancreatitis is supportive and aimed at "giving the pancreas a vacation," i.e., inhibition of pancreatic secretion. This is accomplished by stopping oral intake of food and fluids, withdrawal of gastric secretions by nasogastric suction, and intravenous fluid replacement. About 5% of these patients die from the acute effects of peripheral vascular collapse and shock during the first week of the clinical course. Acute adult respiratory distress syndrome (shock lung) and acute renal failure are particularly ominous complications. If patients survive this period, a variety of sequelae may follow, including *abscess*, *pseudocyst* (p. 968), and *duodenal obstruction.*

CHRONIC PANCREATITIS

This entity might be more appropriately termed *chronic relapsing pancreatitis* because it often represents progressive destruction of the pancreas by repeated flareups of a mild or subclinical type of acute pancreatitis.[27–29] The disease occurs in the same type of patient likely to develop acute pancreatitis—most commonly the alcoholic and, less frequently, the patient with biliary tract disease. Hypercalcemia and hyperlipidemia also predispose to chronic pancreatitis. Studies show that, in up to 12% of patients, recurrent pancreatitis is associated with *pancreas divisum,* a developmental anomaly of the pancreatic duct resulting from incomplete fusion of ventral and dorsal pancreatic anlage.[26] *However, chronic pancreatitis is not usually preceded by an attack of classic acute hemorrhagic pancreatitis,* and usually patients with acute hemorrhagic pancreatitis who recover develop "pseudocysts" rather than chronic fibrosing pancreatitis. The condition is more common in males than in females. Up to 40% of patients have no recognizable predisposing factor. There are relatively rare special forms of chronic pancreatitis, such as *nonalcoholic tropical pancreatitis* and *familial hereditary pancreatitis.* Familial pancreatitis begins in childhood and predisposes to the development of pancreatic carcinoma in later years.

The pathogenesis of chronic pancreatitis is as varied as that of acute pancreatitis. In chronic alcoholic pancreatitis, Sarles and colleagues[27] believe that chronic alcohol intake causes increased protein secretion by the pancreas, owing to increased cholinergic tone, and that the subsequent obstruction of ducts by protein-rich plugs contributes to the damage. Genetic factors appear to operate in certain cases. Protein-calorie malnutrition probably plays a role in the tropical pancreatitis present in southeast Asia and parts of Africa, where alcohol consumption is extremely low.

Morphologically, several types of chronic pancreatitis[27] have been described, but by far the most common is **chronic calcifying pancreatitis.** This type is seen most frequently in alcoholics.[20] The lesions have a lobular distribution, and all components of the involved lobule are affected. There is atrophy of the acini, marked increased in interlobular fibrous tissue, and a chronic inflammatory infiltrate around lobules and ducts (Fig. 20–7). The interlobular and intralobular ducts are dilated and contain protein plugs in their lumina. The ductal epithelium may be atrophied or hyperplastic, or may show squamous metaplasia (Fig. 20–8). The islets appear remarkably unaltered, even though they are enmeshed in sclerosed tissue or severely damaged lobules. **Grossly,** the gland is hard and exhibits foci of calcification and fully developed pancreatic calculi. Pancreatic calculi vary from concretions invisible to the naked eye to stones 1 cm to several centimeters in diameter. **Pseudocyst formation is common in this type of pancreatitis.**

A second morphologic form of pancreatitis is **chronic obstructive pancreatitis;** here, the distribution of lesions is not lobular, and the ductal epithelium generally is less severely damaged. There may be protein plugs in the ducts, but this is a rare finding, and calcified stones are exceptional. The most common cause of this type appears to be stenosis of the sphincter of Oddi associated with **cholelithiasis.** The lesions are more prominent in the head of the pancreas, and regress after sphincterotomy of the sphincter of Oddi. Any other obstructive lesion of the pancreatic ducts may result in this morphologic change, such as carcinoma or accidental ligation of the duct during gastrectomy.

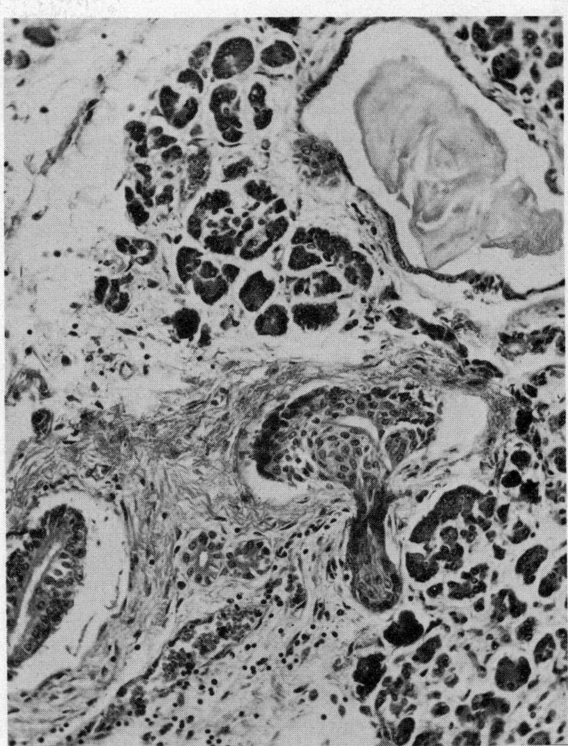

Figure 20–8. Pancreas with squamous metaplasia of one of the small ducts virtually obliterating its lumen. Note dilated duct above filled with inspissated secretion.

Both morphologic forms of the disease are characterized by recurrent attacks of pain at intervals of months or years. The intervals between episodes may shorten progressively until the attacks are almost constant. The attacks may be precipitated by alcohol abuse, overeating, or the use of opiates and other drugs. In an acute attack there may be mild fever and slight jaundice, upper abdominal tenderness, mild or moderate elevations of serum amylase, elevations of serum alkaline phosphatase, and, less commonly, hyperlipemia and hypocalcemia. Abdominal radiography may show calcification in the region of the pancreas. Diabetes, steatorrhea, and pancreatic pseudocysts occur so frequently that they may perhaps be considered late features rather than complications of chronic pancreatitis. Abnormal glucose tolerance or frank diabetes occurs in 14 to 90% of cases of pancreatitis, and steatorrhea in 25 to 35% of cases. Fat content of stools often exceeds that found in other disorders marked by steatorrhea, and a disturbing rectal leakage of oily material is almost pathognomonic. Profound weight loss and hypoalbuminemic edema are present in end-stage pancreatic insufficiency.

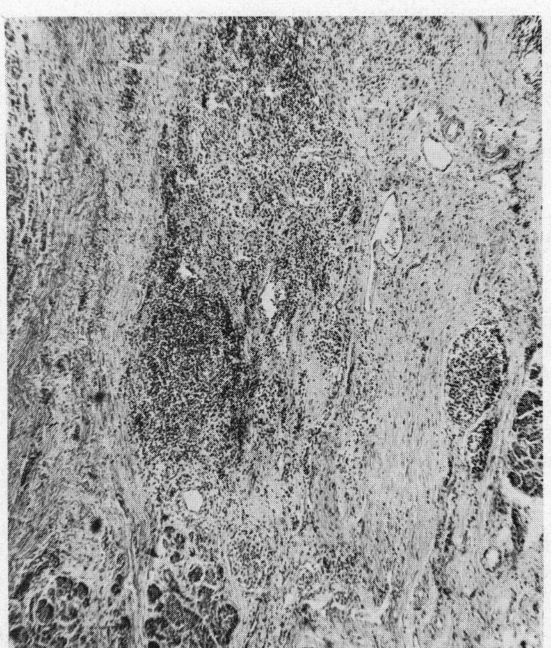

Figure 20–7. Chronic pancreatitis. Large fibrous scar with lymphocytic infiltration occupies center of field.

Between attacks during the early stages of the disease, patients may be entirely asymptomatic. For this reason and because of the wide spectrum of the clinical manifestations and the recurrent nature of this condition, chronic relapsing pancreatitis is a difficult diagnosis to make clinically. Ultrasound and CT scanning are most helpful in such settings; they can detect cysts, calcifications, and enlarged ducts and can exclude tumors.

TUMORS

The heading "tumors" is used to include a variety of non-neoplastic and neoplastic masses that involve this organ. The non-neoplastic masses almost invariably take the form of cysts, whereas the neoplasms are of both benign and malignant and primary and secondary types.

CYSTS

Cysts are infrequent findings in the pancreas, but are of considerable clinical significance since they may present as abdominal masses that are suspected of being malignant. Distinction among the several types of cysts described is of practical importance, since it affects their clinical management.

Congenital Cysts

Congenital cysts are believed to result from anomalous development of the pancreatic ducts. In the genesis of the pancreas, it is postulated, a succession of duct systems develop and degenerate until the adult definitive pattern is created. Persistence and segmentation of some of the primitive ducts may give rise to small sequestered nests of ductal secretory cells that fill up with fluid to create cysts. Congenital cystic disease of the pancreas, liver, and kidney not infrequently coexists. These cysts are usually multiple, but occasionally occur singly. They range in size from microscopic lesions to larger spaces up to 3 to 5 cm in diameter. They are lined by a smooth, glistening membrane that may, on histologic section, have total atrophy of the lining epithelial cells or may show preservation of flattened pavement or low cuboidal epithelial cells. They are usually enclosed in a thin fibrous capsule and are filled with a clear-to-turbid mucoid or serous fluid. Occasionally, hemorrhage or infection modifies the appearance of the lining epithelium and the cystic contents.

In one rare entity, *Lindau–von Hippel disease,* angiomas are found in the retina and cerebellum or brain stem in association with cysts in the pancreas, liver, and kidney.

Pseudocysts

This term is applied to a collection of fluid that arises from loculation of inflammatory processes, necroses, or hemorrhages.[30] *This type represents the overwhelming majority of clinically important cysts and is almost always associated with pancreatitis.* Pseudocysts may also follow traumatic injury to the abdomen with direct damage and hemorrhage in the pancreas. Acute pancreatitis or trauma precedes the clinical discovery of a pseudocyst in nine of ten cases. These cysts are usually solitary and are frequently quite massive, but most measure 5 to 10 cm in diameter. They may be situated within the pancreatic substance, but more often they are found adjacent to the pancreas, particularly in the region of the tail of the pancreas. Sometimes these pseudocysts are formed by the accumulation of fluid in the lesser omental sac adjacent to the tail. The cyst walls may be moderately thin, but are usually quite thick and fibrous (Fig. 20–9). Characteristically, they do not have an epithelial lining and have no connection or communication with surrounding ductal systems. There may be a marked inflammatory reaction in the fibrous capsule and often organizing blood clot, old blood pigment, precipitates of calcium, and cholesterol crystals. Usually, by the time the lesion is removed, the fluid contents have been transformed to a turbid serous fluid, and even though the initial lesion may have been bacterially infected, the bacterial contamination may have long since died out.

Pseudocysts may produce abdominal pain and intraperitoneal hemorrhage, and if infected may cause generalized peritonitis. However, their clinical significance lies in their being discovered as an abdominal mass in a location that strongly suggests a primary intra-abdominal malignancy.

In the past few years, ultrasonography has emerged as a safe, powerful procedure for the diagnosis of pancreatic cysts and their differentiation from other intra-abdominal cysts and tumors (Fig. 20–10). With ultrasound, pancreatic cysts are evident as sonolucent areas with relatively smooth, well-circumscribed outlines. Pseudocysts are usually unilocular; multiloculation suggests a neoplastic cyst. CT scanning adds to the specificity of ultrasound in this setting.

Neoplastic Cysts

These lesions are cystadenomas or cystadenocarcinomas. They are very uncommon tumors of the pancreas, presumed to arise as cystic neoplasms from the ducts. The neoplasms are usually solitary, 5 to 15 cm in diameter, and often multilocular. Histologically, they have a well-defined lining epithelium characteristically thrown up into numerous papillary projections that form branching villous processes.

In the benign form, the columnar epithelial lining cells are well oriented to their basement membrane, are regularly aligned, and have no evidence of anaplasia, piling up, or invasiveness. In the cystadenocarcinomatous varieties, however, the epithelium assumes the anaplasia of all malignancy, becomes piled up into irregular proliferative masses, and invades the underlying wall and adjacent structures.

CARCINOMA OF PANCREAS

The term "carcinoma of the pancreas" is meant to imply carcinoma arising in the exocrine portion of the gland. Although duct cells make up only 4% of all pancreatic cells, virtually all these cancers begin in the ductal epithelium; the acini themselves give origin to less than 1% of malignant tumors.[31, 32] Tumors that arise from the islets of Langerhans are specifically designated as islet cell tumors and will be considered later (p. 986).

Pancreatic cancer continues to be a depressingly difficult problem.[33] These highly fatal cancers have a deceptively silent growth habit, so that by the time they are diagnosed they are rarely curable. They account for 5% of all cancer deaths in the United States, with about 25,000 new cases and 22,000 deaths from the disease each year.[34] The incidence has increased threefold in

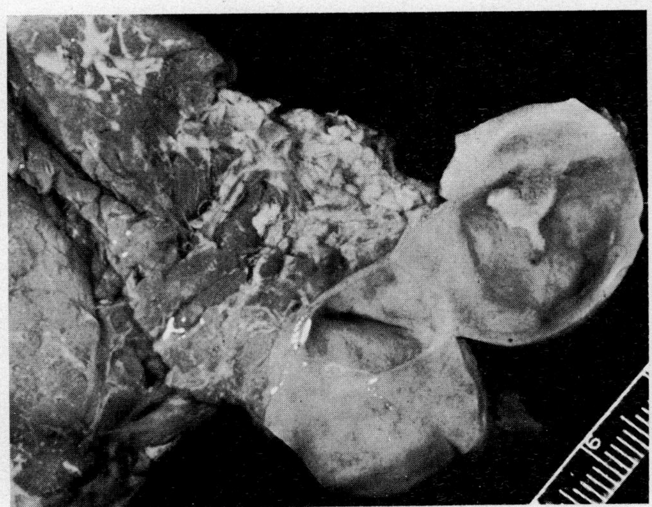

Fig. 20–9

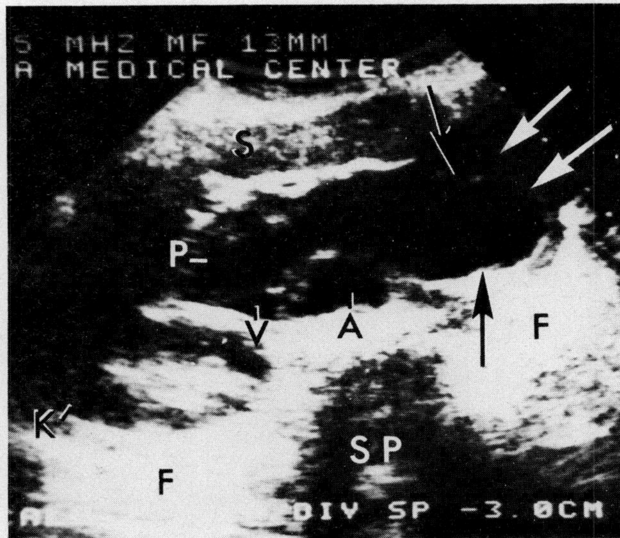

Fig. 20–10

Figure 20–9. Pseudocyst of pancreas. Cyst has been opened and the contents drained. A small plaque of white calcium is visible in wall.

Figure 20–10. Ultrasound of transverse section of abdomen showing a large pancreatic cyst *(arrows)*. Anterior abdominal wall is on top. A = aorta; V = inferior vena cava; SP = spine; K = kidney; F = fat; S = stomach; P = splenic vein–portal vein confluence. (Courtesy of Dr. T. Jones, Brigham and Women's Hospital, Boston.)

the last 40 years; this has been ascribed to smoking, diet, and chemical carcinogens.[35] The risk of pancreatic cancer among heavy smokers is about 2 to 2.5 times that of nonsmokers. There is also a positive but unexplained correlation between mortality from cancer of the pancreas and per capita consumption of fats, and possibly calories. There is a higher risk of pancreatic cancer among chemists, and particularly in those exposed to industrial agents such as beta-naphthylamine and benzidine. Both ductal and acinar cancers can be induced by chemicals (e.g., nitrosamines) in animals.[36] The increased risk ascribed to coffee drinking is controversial at present.[37] These tumors occur most often in the sixth, seventh, and eighth decades of life, although about 10% of patients are much younger. The incidence rates are higher in blacks than in whites, in males than in females, and in diabetics than in nondiabetics.

These lesions may arise anywhere in the pancreas, but most studies show a fairly standard distribution: head of pancreas, 60%; body of pancreas, 15% to 20%; and tail of pancreas, 5%.[33] In 20% the tumor is either diffuse or has spread so widely as to preclude localization of its site of origin. From the standpoints of their clinical significance, usual life history and manner of spread, carcinomas of the head of the pancreas differ strikingly from those of the body and tail. Tumors of the head of the pancreas are in a strategic location to impinge upon the ampulla of Vater, common bile duct, and duodenum and thus cause obstructive biliary symptoms relatively early in their life history. These lesions, therefore, tend to be discovered while still small and before widespread metastasis has occurred. In contrast, cancers in the body and tail may grow silently for longer periods and become manifest only by extension to adjacent structures and by metastatic dissemination.

Carcinoma of Head of Pancreas. Grossly, tumors in this region of the pancreas are fairly small lesions that frequently cause little or only moderate expansion of the head of the pancreas. Sometimes they are totally inapparent on external examination of the organ and create only the impression of some increased consistency and irregular nodularity. Other lesions create masses up to 8 to 10 cm in diameter. The gray-white, scirrhous, homogeneous tumor infiltrates and replaces the usual yellow lobular architecture. Characteristically, such lesions have poorly defined, obviously infiltrative margins with few, if any, foci of hemorrhage (Fig. 20–11). The tumor extends usually to the margin of the duodenum and invades the wall as well as the common bile duct. In a small percentage of cases, it extends directly through the wall either to produce a small fungating lesion within the duodenal lumen or, more often, to cause a shallow, irregular ulceration (Fig. 20–12). In this infiltrative growth, it surrounds and compresses, and less commonly directly invades, the common bile duct or ampulla of Vater, causing biliary obstruction. As a consequence, there is marked distention of the gallbladder in about 50% of patients. Those who die of carcinoma of the pancreas have intense bile stasis in the liver and other tissues, and may develop biliary cirrhosis.

Most carcinomas of the pancreas grow in more or less well-differentiated glandular patterns and are thus **adenocarcinomas** (Fig. 20–13). The tumors may be mucinous or non-mucin secreting. The glands are atypical, irregular, small, and bizarre, and are usually lined by anaplastic cuboidal-to-columnar epithelial cells. Other variants grow in an undifferentiated pattern. About 10% assume either an **adenosquamous pattern** or the uncommon pattern of extreme anaplasia with **giant cell formation**, numerous mitoses, and bizarre pleomorphism; 0.5% arise in cysts and are termed **cystadenocarcinoma.** Rarely, carcinomas arise in acini **(acinar cell carcinoma),** particularly in children.

Invasion of ducts, obliteration of ducts, destruction of islets, and invasion of lymphatics and vessels can often be

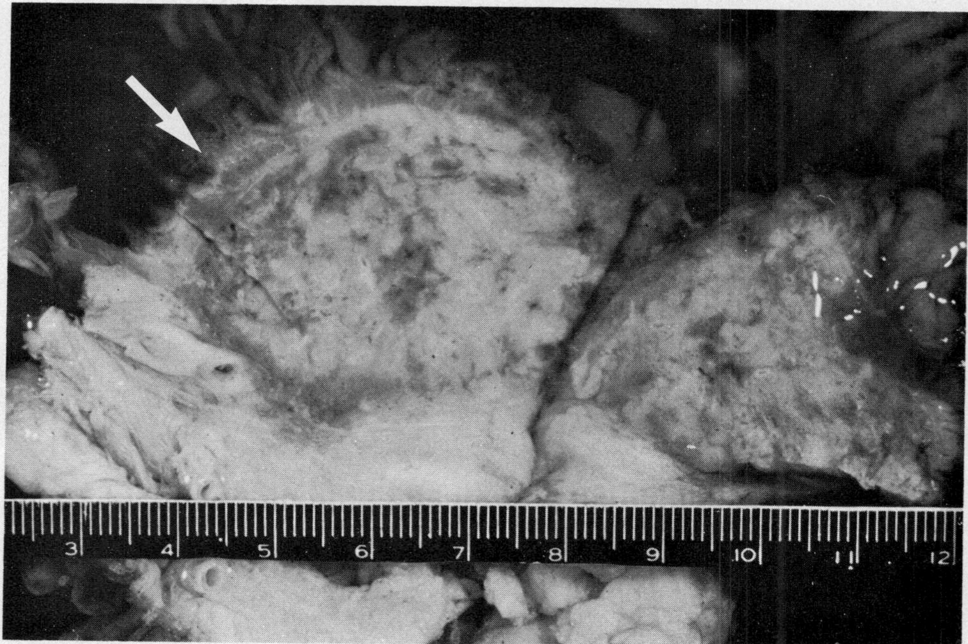

Figure 20–11. Carcinoma of head of pancreas. Mottled invasive lesion has grown into wall of duodenum, which appears at upper extent of tumor *(arrow)*.

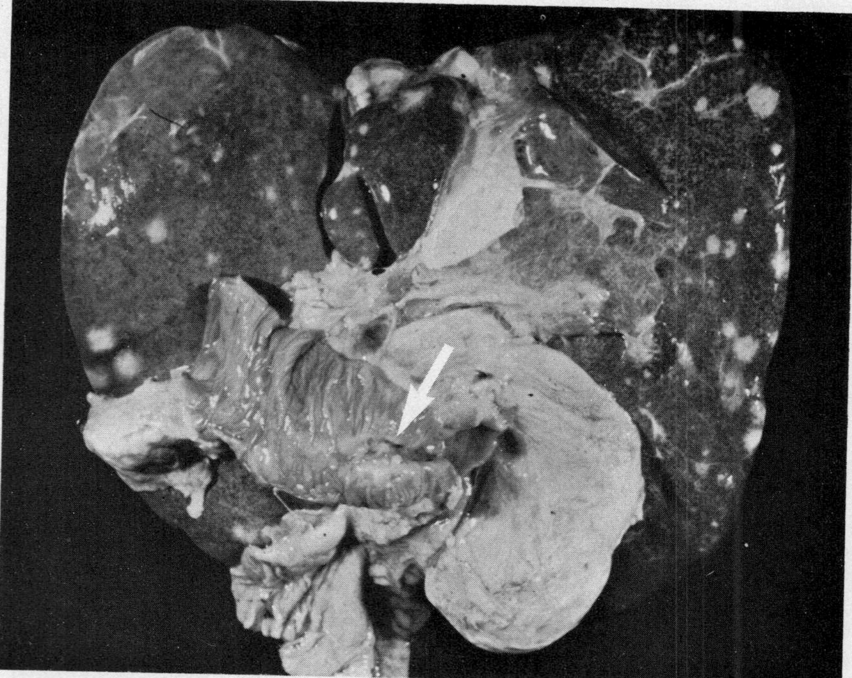

Figure 20–12. Carcinoma of head of pancreas with bile stasis and metastases in liver. Primary lesion has caused a small ulceration in exposed wall of duodenum *(arrow)*.

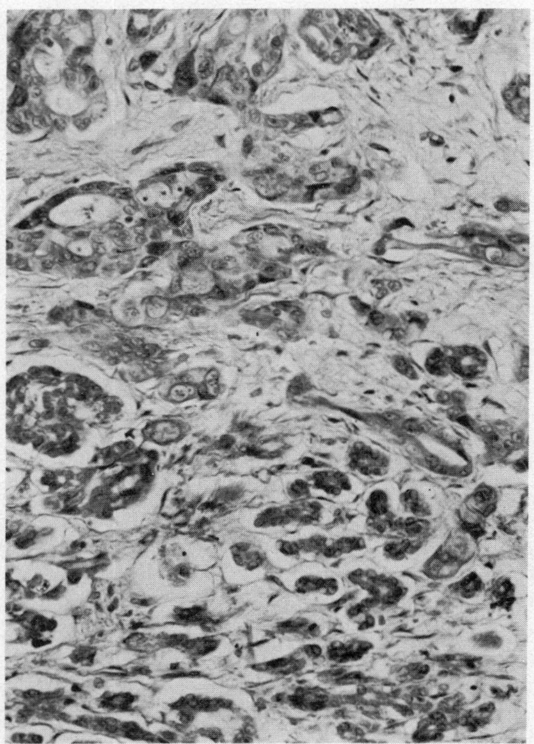

Figure 20–13. Adenocarcinoma of pancreas. Atypical glands are invading pancreatic substance seen at bottom of photograph.

identified. Notwithstanding this gross and microscopic evidence of invasiveness, carcinoma of the head of the pancreas is usually not a widely disseminated lesion when found at autopsy. Extension to peripancreatic and portohepatic nodes with isolated, small metastases in the liver is not uncommon. But because these tumors produce biliary tract obstruction and jaundice at an early date, they usually have not had a long life history before discovery, and patients die of their hepatobiliary dysfunction before the tumor has become widely disseminated.

Carcinoma of Body and Tail of Pancreas. These tumors are usually large, hard, irregular masses that may sometimes wipe out virtually the entire tail and body of the pancreas. On cross section, the tumors exactly resemble those of the head of the gland and, microscopically, the same cytologic and architectural patterns are repeated. In this location, **these carcinomas frequently extend more widely than those of the head.** They impinge upon the adjacent vertebral column, extend through the retroperitoneal spaces inferiorly and superiorly, and occasionally invade the adjacent spleen or adrenal. They may extend into the transverse colon or stomach. Peripancreatic, gastric, mesenteric, omental, and portohepatic nodes are involved, and the liver is strikingly seeded with tumor nodules to produce hepatic enlargement two to three times the normal size. Such massive hepatic metastases are quite characteristic of carcinoma of the tail and body of the pancreas, and are attributed to invasion of the splenic vein that courses directly along the margins of this organ.

CLINICAL COURSE. Carcinomas of the pancreas, even those of its head, are insidious lesions that undoubtedly are present for months and possibly years before they produce symptoms referable to their expansile growth. The major symptoms include weight loss (approximately 70%), abdominal pain (approximately 50%), back pain (approximately 25%), anorexia, nausea, vomiting and generalized malaise, and weakness. Carcinoma of the pancreas was often considered a painless disease until far advanced. It is classically held out as a cause of painless jaundice. It should, therefore, be specifically noted that most patients have pain. Jaundice is present in about 50% of patients with carcinomas of the head of the pancreas. There is an additional, widely prevalent misconception that jaundice, when it appears, is progressive and unremitting owing to the continued expansile growth of these tumors. However, necrosis of the tumor sometimes permits transient flow of the bile, and so there may well be fluctuations in the mounting serum bilirubin levels.

The symptomatic course of pancreatic carcinoma is typically brief and progressive. The average duration of symptoms until diagnosis is four months and that of diagnosis until death is three to five months. For these reasons, there is an active search for tumor markers that may provide a clue to the existence of these cancers early in their course. Among the currently promising methods is measurement of serum galactosyltransferase isoenzyme, which is elevated in patients with pancreatic (and other gastrointestinal) cancers.

The diagnosis and localization of pancreatic tumors can also be aided by ultrasonography, which can differentiate cysts from solid tumors. With this diagnostic modality, percutaneous needle biopsies from specifically localized tumors may obviate the need for exploratory laparotomy. CT scan of the pancreas has also become a most useful resource in patients suspected of having a pancreatic tumor (Fig. 20–14).

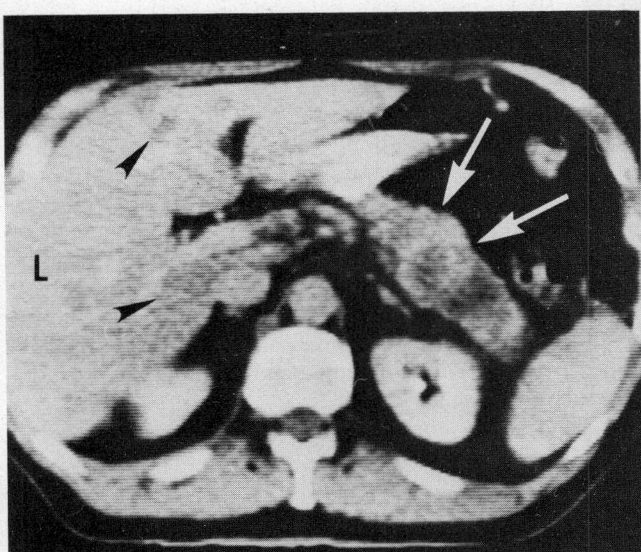

Figure 20–14. CT scan at mid-abdominal level demonstrating pancreatic carcinoma. Pancreatic tail is enlarged and heterogeneous *(long arrows)*. Liver (L) contains multiple focal lucencies, corresponding to metastatic deposits *(arrowheads)*. Stomach, spleen, and kidneys are also visible. (Courtesy of Dr. S. Seltzer, Brigham and Women's Hospital, Boston.)

Migratory thrombophlebitis known clinically as *Trousseau's sign* occurs in 10% of patients. Ironically, Trousseau diagnosed his own fatal disease as cancer of the pancreas when he developed migratory thrombophlebitis. These spontaneously appearing and disappearing thromboses are also encountered in other forms of cancer, but the two highest levels of correlation are with pancreatic and pulmonary neoplasms. Their pathogenesis was discussed on p. 98.

While surgical resection is attempted in the appropriate cases, the overall one-year survival is 10% and the three-year survival about 2%.

The Endocrine Pancreas

NORMAL

The endocrine pancreas consists of about 1 million microscopic cellular units—the islets of Langerhans—and a few scattered cells within the small pancreatic ducts.[41] In the aggregate the islets in the adult human weigh only 1 to 1.5 gm.

Embryologically islet cells are of endodermal origin, and form at many points along the pancreatic tubuloductal system. The first evidence of islet formation in the human fetus occurs at nine to 11 weeks, with the appearance, on H and E sections, of dark, deeply eosinophilic cells interspersed among the lighter duct cells. Insulin and glucagon, however, can be measured and visualized earlier immunocytochemically. The dark cells subsequently proliferate, forming clusters that evaginate and then detach from the tubuloductal system to form discrete islets. The islets are then invaded by capillaries that separate the cluster into the typical islet cell cords.

In the human adult, islets measure 50 to 250 μm and consist of four distinct cell types: *B (beta), A (alpha), D (delta), and PP (for pancreatic polypeptide) cells.*[41, 42] These make up about 70, 20, 5 to 10, and 1 to 2% of the islet cell population, respectively. They can be differentiated by their staining properties with certain dyes, by the ultrastructural morphology of their granules,[43, 44] and (most important) by their hormonal content. The availability of antibodies to specific hormones and the application of immunoperoxidase techniques to tissue has permitted localization of individual hormones to individual islet cells, and has greatly facilitated correlation of islet cell morphology with functional hormone production (Fig. 20–15).

The *B cell* (beta) (Fig. 20–16) has been studied most intensively because it produces *insulin*. The description of insulin secretion by beta cells is detailed in the discussion of diabetes (p. 977). The granules have rectangular profiles and a crystalline matrix, and are surrounded by a halo. Hyperplasia and neoplasia of these cells are responsible for the important clinical syndrome of hyperinsulinism. *A cells* (alpha) secrete *glucagon*, which induces hyperglycemia by its glycogenolytic activity in the liver. Alpha-cell granules are round with a closely applied membrane and a dense center (Fig. 20–17). *D cells* (delta) contain somatostatin,[45] which suppresses both insulin and glucagon release. Delta cells have large, pale granules with closely applied membranes (Fig. 20–17). *PP cells* have small, dark granules and are not only present in islets but also scattered in the exocrine pancreas. They contain a unique pancreatic polypeptide that exerts a number of gastrointestinal effects when injected in experimental animals (diarrhea, hypermotility), but its physiologic significance in humans is unknown. Other rare, less well-characterized cells (D1, G) have distinctive granules by electron microscopy but no definite hormone identifiable by immunochemistry. Small numbers of *serotonin-containing enterochromaffin cells* are the source of pancreatic tumors that induce the carcinoid syndrome.

We now turn to the two main disorders of islet cells: diabetes mellitus and islet cell tumors.

PATHOLOGY

Despite the minute size of the islets of Langerhans, even collectively, the endocrine pancreas is responsible for a disproportionate amount of morbidity and mortality. Diabetes mellitus alone ranks among the top ten causes of death in Western nations, and despite important improvements in its clinical management, to date it has not been possible to control significantly its lethal consequences. The various forms of neoplasia arising in the islets, although far less common, sometimes produce some fascinating, often difficult to diagnose endocrinopathies. The endocrine pancreas is therefore a major source of significant clinical disease.

DIABETES MELLITUS

Idiopathic or primary diabetes mellitus is a chronic disorder of carbohydrate, fat, and protein metabolism characterized in its fully expressed clinical form by an absolute or relative insulin deficiency, fasting hyper-

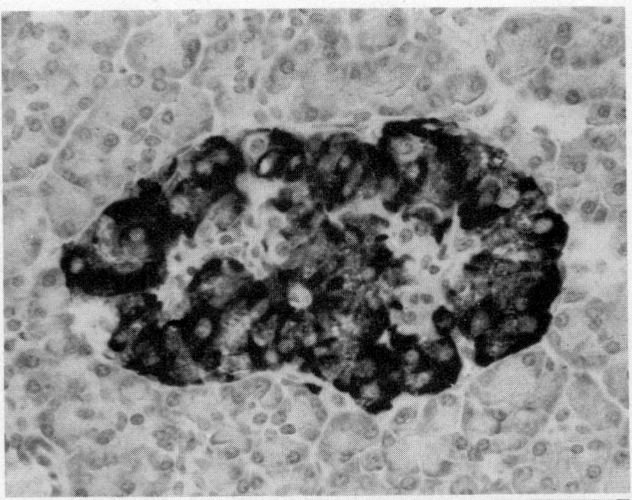

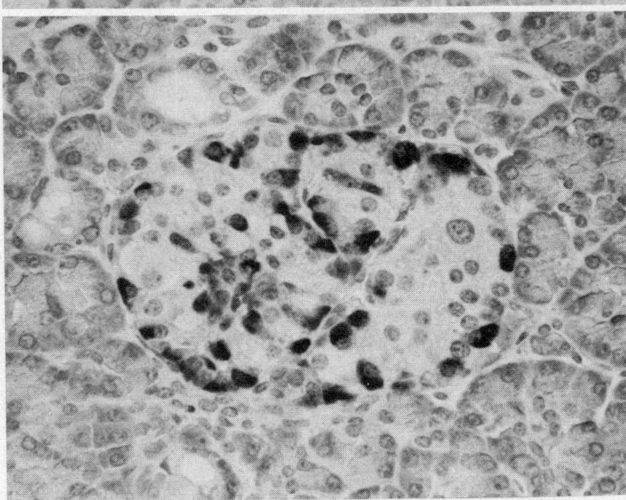

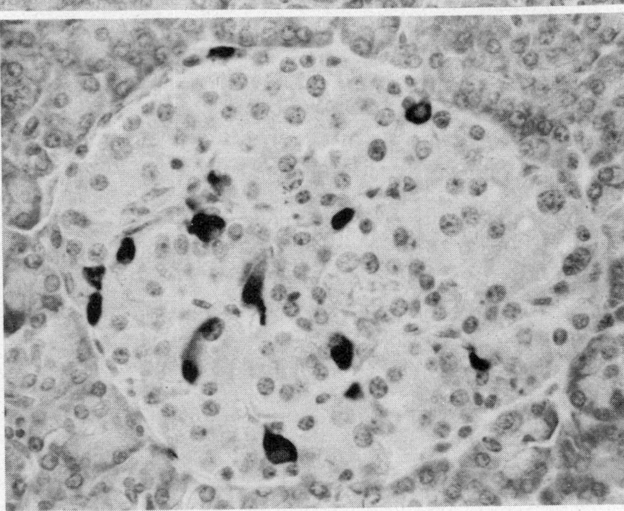

Figure 20–15. Islets stained by immunoperoxidase technique for insulin *(top)*, glucagon *(middle)*, and somatostatin *(bottom)*. The dark reaction product identifies beta, alpha, and delta cells, respectively. (Courtesy of Dr. A. Like, University of Massachusetts School of Medicine.)

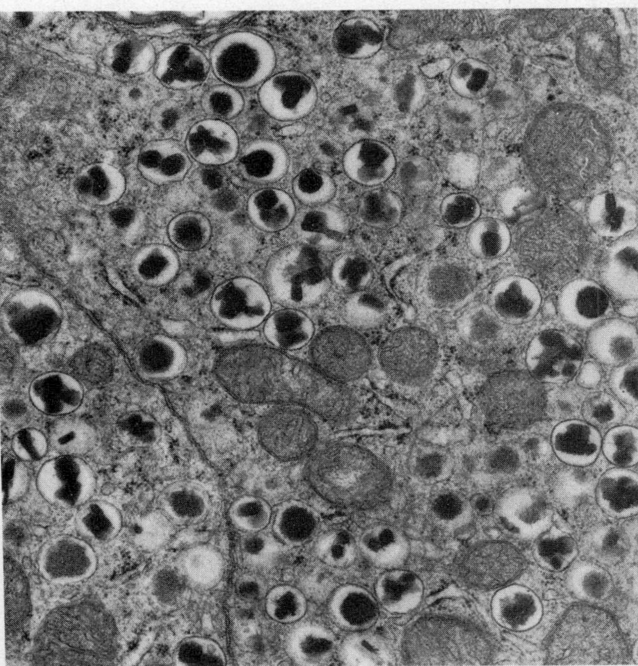

Figure 20–16. Electron micrograph of a portion of a beta cell with characteristic membrane-bound granules, each containing a dense, often rectangular core and a distinct halo. (Courtesy of Dr. A. Like, University of Massachusetts School of Medicine.)

glycemia, glycosuria, and a striking tendency toward development of atherosclerosis, microangiopathy, nephropathy, and neuropathy. To this brief characterization the following must be added:

1. *Underutilization of glucose is characteristic of all diabetic patients, but only some have a clearly defined severe insulin deficiency resulting from a loss of beta cells; the large remainder suffer from some impairment of insulin secretory response associated with a marked resistance to insulin in the peripheral tissues. Excessive glucagon secretion may also play a role.*

2. *Almost certainly, "idiopathic diabetes mellitus" embraces a heterogeneous group of disorders having in common disordered carbohydrate, fat, and protein metabolism. At least two major as well as several less common variants of the disease (too rare to merit description) have been identified. One major variant, insulin-dependent "juvenile-onset" ketosis-prone diabetes, accounts for about 10% of diabetics; non–insulin-dependent "maturity-onset" ketosis-resistant diabetes represents the remaining 90% of all diabetic patients. More will be said about this heterogeny later, but it should be stressed that the terms "juvenile-onset" and "maturity-onset" are misleading. Insulin-dependent diabetes mellitus (IDDM) (Type I) may appear in adult life, and non–insulin-dependent diabetes mellitus (NIDDM) (Type II) may occur in the young.*

3. *Hereditary influences contribute significantly to the development of both major variants of diabetes*

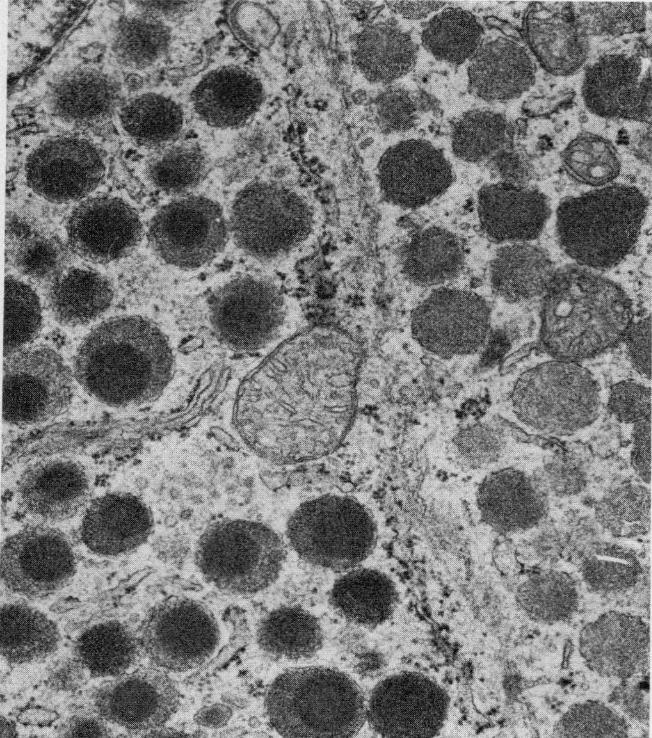

Figure 20–17. Portions of an alpha cell (*left*) and a delta cell (*right*). Granules in both cells have closely apposed membranes, but the alpha cell granule exhibits a dense, round center. (Courtesy of Dr. A. Like, University of Massachusetts School of Medicine.)

mellitus. Although the precise nature and mode of inheritance are still uncertain, and regrettably there are no genetic "markers," the risk of acquiring the several variants of the disease is related to the extent of the hereditary input, e.g., the number of affected relatives, the closeness of the relationships, and the severity of their disease.

4. *Environmental influences such as pregnancy, obesity, and infection contribute significantly to the expression of the diabetic state.*

5. *Idiopathic diabetes mellitus must be differentiated from the secondary types of diabetes or carbohydrate intolerance resulting from destruction of the pancreas by inflammation (pancreatitis), trauma, surgery, or tumor infiltration or that encountered in hemochromatosis or in association with certain endocrinopathies such as acromegaly, Cushing's syndrome, hyperthyroidism, pheochromocytoma, and the carcinoid syndrome. All these secondary forms are genetically unrelated to the primary disease(s), and whether they are associated with some tendency to the development of macro- and microvascular disease is still somewhat uncertain.*

6. *The metabolic derangements may be life-threatening, or even fatal in IDDM, but the major challenge today is the understanding and control of the frequently fatal long-term effects of both major variants of this disease on the large and small vessels, sometimes referred to as the "chronic vascular syndrome."*

Diabetic patients cover a wide spectrum of deranged carbohydrate metabolism, from those having mild or asymptomatic disease without fasting hyperglycemia to those having severe fasting hyperglycemia in the fully expressed clinical disease. *Although attention is focused on the disordered carbohydrate metabolism, we should not overlook the important fact that all pathways of intermediary metabolism are disrupted.* Insulin is a major anabolic hormone in the body. Derangement of insulin function affects not only glucose metabolism but also fat and protein metabolism.

The most profound deficiency of insulin, and therefore the most severe derangements in metabolism, are usually encountered in IDDM. The assimilation of glucose and other insulin-sensitive sugars into muscle and adipose tissue is sharply diminished or abolished. Not only does storage of glycogen in liver and muscle cease, but reserves are depleted by glycogenolysis. Fasting hyperglycemia may reach levels many times greater than normal, and when the level of circulating glucose exceeds the renal threshold, glycosuria ensues. The excessive glycosuria induces an osmotic diuresis and thus polyuria, causing a profound loss not only of water but also of electrolytes (Na, K Mg, P). This obligatory water loss combined with the hyperosmolarity resulting from the increased levels of glucose in the blood tends to deplete intracellular water, as, for example, in the osmoreceptors of the thirst centers of the brain. In this manner, intense thirst (polydipsia) appears. Through poorly defined pathways, increased appetite (polyphagia) develops, thus completing the classic triad of diabetic findings—*polyuria, polydipsia, and polyphagia.* With a deficiency of insulin, the scales swing from insulin-promoted anabolism to catabolism of proteins and fats. Proteolysis follows, and the glucogenic amino acids are removed by the liver and used as building blocks in gluconeogenesis, worsening the deranged carbohydrate metabolism. Nitrogen loss in the urine is excessive. There is concomitant excessive breakdown of fat stores, sometimes resulting in elevated levels of free fatty acids and hyperlipidemia. Oxidation of free fatty acids within the liver through acetyl CoA produces ketone bodies. The rate at which the ketone bodies are formed may exceed the rate at which acetoacetic acid and beta-hydroxybutyric acid can be utilized by muscles and other tissues. Ketogenic amino acids aggravate the derangements in lipid metabolism. Ketogenesis thus increases, leading to ketonemia and ketonuria. If the urinary excretion of "ketones" is compromised by dehydration, the plasma hydrogen ion concentration increases, and systemic metabolic ketoacidosis results. The combination of dehydration and breakdown of proteins and fats may indeed impart to these patients a wasted appearance, and growth and development in young children are stunted.

Although the metabolic derangements in NIDDM of adults may be as severe as those just described for the insulin-dependent form of the disease, they are extremely uncommon. In these patients, polyuria, polydipsia, and polyphagia may accompany the fasting hyperglycemia, but ketoacidosis is so rare that this form of diabetes is also called "ketosis-resistant."

CLASSIFICATION. As indicated earlier, diabetes mellitus embraces a heterogeneous group of disorders having in common an inability to utilize glucose. Until recently there were several classifications of diabetes, some using clinical features such as age of onset, others etiology, and some the presumed natural history. To add to this complexity, there were no uniform criteria for the diagnosis of diabetes, since the levels of blood glucose show a wide range with no obvious cut-off point between those who have symptoms of diabetes and other apparently normal individuals. To resolve these problems, two international groups of experts have proposed uniform guidelines for the diagnosis and classification of diabetes.[46]

The diagnosis of diabetes mellitus is relatively easy in patients who are *symptomatic and have unequivocal hyperglycemia, or in asymptomatic individuals with fasting plasma glucose greater than 140 mg/dl on more than one occasion.* If these criteria are not met and a diagnosis of diabetes mellitus is suspected, it is necessary to perform a provocative test called the oral glucose tolerance test (OGTT). For this procedure, the subject is given 75 gm of glucose orally, followed by venous blood sampling at 30-minute intervals for up to two hours. If the plasma glucose concentration in venous blood is equal to or exceeds 200 mg/dl at two hours, the patient has diabetes mellitus. According to some experts, one additional blood glucose value at some point in the two-hour test period should also be equal to or above 200 mg/dl to establish the diagnosis. Once diagnosed, diabetes mellitus can be subclassified into two major and several minor variants on the basis of criteria outlined in Table 20–1. This classification also proposes the creation of a new category of deranged carbohydrate metabolism called impaired glucose tolerance (IGT). *The criteria for the diagnosis of IGT are fasting blood glucose values of less than 140 mg/dl and between 140 and 199 mg/dl two hours after the oral glucose load:* in other words, glucose tolerance intermediate between normal and diabetic. In the past it was assumed that most individuals with the biochemical characteristics of IGT would eventually develop overt diabetes mellitus, and hence terms such as asymptomatic, chemical, or latent diabetes were used. It is now apparent that, although patients classified as having IGT are at a higher risk of developing diabetes, only 1 to 5% actually develop the disease within five to ten years. These risk estimates must be considered tentative, however, since few prospective long-term studies utilizing strict criteria for the diagnosis of IGT have been performed. *Gestational diabetes mellitus* is another special category in which diabetes or IGT is detected for the first time during pregnancy. *This group does not include diabetics who became pregnant.* Following childbirth, such women have to be reclassified according to the criteria defined above. *Two additional groups associated with normal glucose tolerance, but possible increased risk of developing diabetes mellitus, are also recognized.* These have been called previous abnormality of glucose intolerance (PrevAGT) and potential abnormality of glucose intolerance (PotAGT), as described in Table 20–1.

INCIDENCE. Diabetes mellitus is now the sixth leading cause of death from disease in the United States. The precise incidence and prevalence of diabetes are difficult to estimate since there are no "genetic markers," and therefore diagnosis is based on the presence of symptoms or the oral glucose tolerance test. According to recent estimates, diabetes mellitus may have been overdiagnosed in the past, since many patients now classified as having IGT were considered to be diabetics. With the new criteria for diagnosis, it is estimated that the prevalence of diabetes in the adult population is 1 to 2%.[47] Since aging is associated with increased carbohydrate intolerance, the prevalence rises to over 10% in the eighth decade. Overall, it is estimated that there are close to 2 million diabetics in the U.S., making diabetes one of the most common chronic diseases.

INHERITANCE. Although there is no doubt that diabetes mellitus is at least in part a genetic disorder, the task of unraveling the precise mode of inheritance has proved to be a "geneticist's nightmare." Part of the problem stems from the fact that until recently idiopathic diabetes mellitus was considered a homogeneous entity, and therefore attempts were made to find a single pattern of inheritance that would fit all cases. To make a difficult situation even worse, the lack of a genetic "marker" has made it impossible to trace accurately the transmission of "diabetogenic gene(s)" in families or populations.

It is now agreed that IDDM and NIDDM exhibit substantial genetic differences. Evidence in support of such a conclusion derives principally from twin studies. Among identical twins there was a concordance rate (both twins affected) of IDDM of about 50%, as contrasted with a concordance rate of over 90% for twins having NIDDM.[48] *Clearly, therefore, genetic factors play a much larger role in the induction of NIDDM than in that of IDDM.* Since discordance between identical twins is as frequent as concordance in IDDM, environmental factors must play a large role in its development (p. 977). Genetic difference between the two major variants of diabetes is also supported by the study of HLA antigens in diabetics. *IDDM shows strong association with certain HLA types, whereas there is no known relationship between NIDDM and histocompatibility antigens.* Among patients with IDDM, there is a significant increase in the frequency of HLA-B8, B15, B18, Dw3, Dw4, DR3 and DR4 antigens. The association with the D/DR antigens is considered primary, whereas others are believed to result from linkage disequilibrium between the D/DR- and B-region genes. Although the presence of any one of these antigens increases the risk of development of IDDM, the inheritance of two antigens, each with a positive association, has a more than additive effect on the relative risk. For example, the presence of Dw3 or Dw4 is associated

Table 20–1. CLASSIFICATION OF DIABETES MELLITUS AND OTHER CATEGORIES OF GLUCOSE INTOLERANCE*

Class	Former Terminology	Associated Factors	Clinical Characteristics
Clinical Classes			
Diabetes Mellitus (DM)			
Insulin-dependent type (IDDM)-Type 1	Juvenile diabetes Ketosis-prone diabetes Brittle diabetes	Associated with HLA-D/DR antigens and autoimmune reactions. Both genetic and environmental (viral) factors involved in etiology.	Absolute lack of insulin and dependent on injected insulin to prevent ketosis and preserve life. In most cases onset in youth but may occur at any age.
Non–insulin-dependent types (NIDDM)-Type II 1. Obese NIDDM 2. Nonobese NIDDM	Adult-onset DM Maturity-onset DM Ketosis-resistant DM	Probably multiple etiologies. Both genetic and environmental factors involved. Insulin resistance is an important pathogenetic factor. No association with HLA, viruses, or autoimmunity.	Serum insulin levels normal, elevated, or low. In most cases onset after age 40 but can occur at any age. 60–90% of patients are obese.
Other types include DM associated with other identifiable causes	Secondary DM	(1)Pancreatic disease; (2)hormonal diseases, e.g., Cushing's; (3)drug-induced; (4)insulin receptor abnormalities; (5)certain genetic syndromes.	Diabetes mellitus and associated clinical features.
Impaired Glucose Tolerance (IGT)	Asymptomatic DM Chemical diabetes Latent diabetes	Glucose intolerance mild; may be due to normal variation in a population. In some cases represents a stage in development of NIDDM. Majority remain in this class for years or return to normal glucose tolerance.	Glucose tolerance test (GTT) shows values between normal and diabetic. Some suggestion of increased risk for arterial disease but clinically significant renal and retinal lesions absent.
Gestational Diabetes (GDM)	Gestational diabetes	Glucose intolerance that has its onset and recognition during pregnancy. Complex metabolic and hormonal factors involved, including insulin resistance. Diabetics who become pregnant are not included. Associated with increased perinatal complications and with increased risk for progression to diabetes in 5–10 years after childbirth.	
Statistical Risk Classes			
Previous Abnormality of Glucose Tolerance (PrevAGT)	Latent diabetes Prediabetes	Persons who have normal glucose tolerance now but have previously demonstrated diabetic hyperglycemia or IGT either spontaneously or in response to an identifiable stimulus. Individuals with GDM who return to normal form a subclass of PrevAGT. Also includes obese diabetics in whom glucose tolerance has returned to normal after they have lost weight. Studies on patients with previous GDM indicate 30% will become overt diabetics in 5 to 10 yr. No data available on the course of other causes of PrevAGT but it is likely that the risk of these patients developing DM is higher.	
Potential Abnormality of Glucose Tolerance (PotAGT)	Prediabetes	Individuals who have never exhibited abnormal glucose tolerance but have a substantially increased risk for development of diabetes. Those at increased risk to develop IDDM are: persons with islet cell antibodies, monozygotic twin of a patient, sibling and offspring of IDDM diabetic. In the case of NIDDM, this category includes: monozygotic twin of a patient, first-degree relative, mother of a neonate weighing more than 9 lb, obese individuals, and certain ethnic groups. The degree of increased risk for most of these conditions is not well established.	

*Modified from National Diabetes Data Group: Classification and diagnosis of diabetes mellitus and other categories of glucose intolerance. Diabetes *28*:1039, 1979.

with relative risks of 2.6 and 4.8, respectively, whereas the presence of both Dw3 and Dw4 increases the relative risk to 9.4. These data strongly suggest that there are two or more susceptibility genes for IDDM that exist in close linkage to the HLA-D/DR region. In view of the fact that several immune response (Ir) genes map within the D/DR region, it is suspected that the diabetogenic genes may actually be Ir genes that regulate immune reactions directed against the pancreatic beta cells (p. 161).

Despite all the collective evidence supporting some role for genetic factors in both IDDM and NIDDM, we still do not know the modes of inheritance involved in each of these two major variants, nor whether each variant is indeed genetically homogeneous. *Virtually every pattern of inheritance has been invoked at one time or another, including autosomal dominant, autosomal recessive, and multifactorial.* The autosomal dominant mode seems to be involved with reasonable certainty only in a small subset of young individuals with NIDDM (the so-called "maturity-onset diabetes of the young"); in the overwhelming majority of diabetics, this pattern can be clearly excluded. Among the remaining possibilities, multifactorial inheritance is currently favored since it best fits the genetic analyses and also provides a role for environmental factors. However, autosomal recessive inheritance with reduced penetrance cannot be easily distinguished from the multifactorial pattern. It will remain difficult to resolve this problem until the products of the diabetogenic genes are identified.

ENVIRONMENTAL INFLUENCES. In individuals who carry the diabetogenic genes, a number of environmental factors such as body weight, pregnancy, infectious agents, and hormones significantly influence the risk of developing the disease. Among these, *obesity* plays a very important role in the pathogenesis of NIDDM (p. 979). Approximately 80% of patients with NIDDM are notably overweight (i.e., 25% over ideal weight). Even in normal subjects, significant weight gain induces carbohydrate intolerance, higher insulin levels, and insensitivity of muscle and fat tissue to insulin (a subject to which we shall return in the consideration of peripheral resistance). Weight loss corrects all the above changes and moreover, in the diabetic, notably improves the metabolic derangement (see PrevAGT, Table 20–1).

Pregnancy constitutes another major diabetogenic influence, for two reasons: (1) it increases the metabolic workload of the maternal pancreas and (2) it in some way induces a state of insulin resistance. In women without a genetic predisposition, pregnancy induces only mild carbohydrate intolerance, but in those with a hereditary predisposition, it significantly worsens glucose intolerance and may produce a picture of NIDDM.

Viruses are believed to be important in the pathogenesis of IDDM. Much evidence indicates that the loss of beta cells, a characteristic feature of IDDM, may be initiated by viral infection of the islets. This aspect of IDDM will be discussed in detail later (p. 978).

Any form of *stress* tends to unmask the diabetic tendency or worsen the diabetic state. *Infections* of all kinds constitute a major form of stress. Repeatedly it is observed that, when an infection prevails, the diabetic's dose of insulin or oral hypoglycemics must be increased. These stresses probably act through altered homeostasis, such as steroid-induced gluconeogenesis or increased secretion of catecholamines. In this connection, a variety of *endocrinopathies*—Cushing's disease, acromegaly, carcinoid syndrome, pheochromocytoma with epinephrine secretion or exogenously administered corticosteroids—all tend to induce carbohydrate intolerance.

PATHOGENESIS. ***Normal Insulin Metabolism.*** It is helpful to begin discussion of the pathogenesis of diabetes mellitus with a brief survey of the normal physiology of insulin. Insulin, as you may recall, is produced in the beta cell of the islets of Langerhans by enzymatic cleavage of the precursor polypeptide called proinsulin. It is then stored within membrane-bound cytoplasmic granules that are derived from the Golgi apparatus. The complex sequence of insulin secretion, involving the extrusion of the granule's contents from the beta cells, can be triggered by a variety of insulinogenic stimuli including glucose, various gut hormones, amino acids, and sulfonylureas. Glucose is the primary in vivo stimulus for insulin secretion. Among amino acids, arginine and leucine are the most potent insulin secretagogues.

Insulin release in response to glucose is a biphasic phenomenon, reflecting probably a two-pool system within the beta cell.[49] A prompt or immediate release involves insulin that is stored within secretory granules. A more delayed, chronically released pool could be derived from stored proinsulin, requiring conversion to insulin, as well as from activation of the ribosomal system, with synthesis of more proinsulin. *In contrast with glucose, other insulinogenic agents such as amino acids and sulfonylureas (used in the treatment of NIDDM) act only on the acutely releasable pool and have no effect on stimulating beta-cell synthesis of insulin.*[50]

The mechanism of action of insulin on cells has stubbornly resisted explication. It has been well established that insulin enhances the membrane transport of glucose, amino acids, and certain ions and also induces increased storage of glycogen, formation of triglycerides, and synthesis of protein, RNA, and DNA. Facilitation of the cellular uptake of glucose seems to occur by translocation of glucose transport units, synthesized within the cells, to the plasma membrane.[51] How insulin affects all these processes, however, is far from clear. Like several other polypeptide hormones, *insulin must first bind to specific receptors located on the cell membrane.* Since the amount of insulin bound to the cell is affected by the availability of receptors, their numbers are important in regulating the action of insulin. Insulin receptors have been found on a variety of cells including fat cells, monocytes, red cells, and fibroblasts,[52] but their concentration on various cells is not uniform. For example, adipocytes possess several hundred thousand receptors, whereas erythrocytes have much fewer binding sites. Moreover, the intrinsic level of receptors per cell is subject to dynamic regulation by several factors in the cells' environment. Quite interestingly, *insulin itself is a major downregulator of its own receptors.* In other words, increasing amounts of insulin reduce the receptor concentration per cell, a phenomenon of considerable importance in the pathogenesis of NIDDM (p. 980). Other modulators of insulin receptors include dietary composition, exercise, hormones such as cortisol, ions, ketones, and autoantibodies against receptors. Some of these may act indirectly by affecting the ambient insulin levels, whereas others act independently. Collectively, these factors may be relevant in the pathogenesis of not only NIDDM but also other clinical conditions characterized by impaired insulin action (*insulin resistance*).

Although the precise events triggered by the binding of insulin to its receptors have not yet been defined, it is strongly suspected that the postreceptor actions of insulin involve the formation of one or more intracellular mediators.[53] It seems that insulin binding to the cell initiates a limited proteolysis of certain membrane proteins, leading to the formation of several small peptides (molecular weight 1000–1500). These peptides are then believed to activate (or inactivate) a variety of insulin-sensitive enzymes such as pyruvate dehydrogenase and glycogen synthetase, and possibly other enzymes involved in the synthesis of glucose-transport units. *It is proposed, therefore, that the intracellular metabolic effects of insulin are mediated by a set of "second messengers" that are generated following the membrane perturbations initiated by the interaction of insulin with its membrane receptors.*[54]

With this brief characterization of insulin secretion and action, we can turn to the possible mechanisms involved in the pathogenesis of the two major variants of diabetes mellitus.

Theories of Genesis of Diabetes. The pathogenesis of diabetes mellitus is a veritable "no man's land," strewn with theories, each ardently supported by some and doubted by others. Some of the difficulties stem from past failures to recognize the possibility that the many variants of this disease do not necessarily have similar causations. In addition to the genetic data already reviewed, there is now an immense mass of immunologic, metabolic and clinical evidence, which indicates that IDDM and NIDDM have different etiologies and pathogeneses. Each of these variants, therefore, requires separate consideration.

The insulin-dependent, ketosis-prone form of diabetes mellitus (IDDM) is due to an absolute and severe lack of insulin. In the fully expressed condition, the pancreas contains little or no extractable insulin and has an overall reduction in beta-cell mass, resulting from loss of beta cells. Plasma insulin levels are low and respond poorly, if at all, to administration of glucose or other stimulators of insulin secretion, notably oral hypoglycemic agents. *These patients therefore require exogenous insulin administration to prevent ketoacidosis and death; hence, the term "insulin-dependent."* Although the presence of insulin deficiency is established, the etiology of beta-cell injury remains mysterious. On the basis of the genetic data (particularly twin studies) discussed earlier, it is obvious that environmental factors must be involved in the pathogenesis of IDDM. No definite environmental agent has been identified as yet, but viruses are considered to be the prime suspects.

For many years there have been sporadic reports of a close temporal association between common childhood viral infections such as mumps, measles, influenza, and Coxsackie B infections and the onset of IDDM.[55, 56] Seasonal variations in the diagnosis of new cases of IDDM corresponding to the prevalence of these viral infections have also been noted. New impetus was imparted to these epidemiologic observations by the isolation of Coxsackie B4 virus from the pancreas of a child who died of diabetic ketoacidosis after a flu-like illness.[57] Inoculation of mice with the human isolate led to infection of beta cells and hyperglycemia. Further strengthening the viral link is the demonstration that a diabetes-like disorder can be induced in certain strains of mice by the subcutaneous inoculation of the M variant of encephalomyocarditis virus. This microbiologic agent appears to localize specifically within the islets of Langerhans to produce direct viral damage to the beta cells.[58] Thus, there is evidence to support the notion that viral infections may injure beta cells in humans as well as in rodents. However intriguing these observations may be, overwhelming virus infection with direct beta-cell injury is not commonly associated with IDDM. More often, a history of virus infection, if present, relates to a relatively minor illness weeks to months before the detection of diabetes mellitus. Therefore, the exact role of viruses in the pathogenesis of human IDDM is not entirely clear. Two possibilities may be considered: (1) virus-induced beta-cell injury, mild in itself, may nevertheless trigger autoimmunity against the islet cell, as discussed later; or (2) the viral infection of the pancreatic islets may merely lead to a terminal decompensation of beta cells, whose mass has been gradually eroded over the proceeding years, by autoimmune reactions of unknown origin.[58A]

Whether initiated by viruses or by other unknown agents, there is much evidence for the presence of pancreatic autoimmunity in IDDM.[59] Most pervasive is the *frequent presence of antibodies directed against cytoplasmic as well as cell membrane components of the islet cells.* The islet cell antibodies (ICA) are organ specific for endocrine pancreas and include both complement-fixing and non–complement-fixing immunoglobulins. The complement-fixing ICA directed against the beta-cell membrane are cytotoxic in vitro and could conceivably damage the beta cells in vivo. ICA can be found in 60 to 90% of all newly diagnosed cases of IDDM. After five years, their prevalence falls to approximately 20%, and by ten years only 5–10% of the patients are ICA-positive. In addition to autoantibodies, sensitized T cells reactive against pancreatic beta cells have also been found in some patients.[59] The presence of pancreatic autoimmunity is also supported by the frequent presence of mononuclear cell infiltrate in the islets of young diabetics ("insulitis") (p. 982). What triggers the anti–self-reactions against the islets is not entirely clear. Current opinion favors an initial insult by a beta-cytotropic virus, resulting in the release of beta cell–specific antigens. Sensitization against these antigens may lead to the production of autoantibodies and autoreactive T cells. As more and more beta cells are damaged by these autoimmune reactions, further release of antigens would be expected to potentiate the ongoing autoimmune response and progressively increasing loss of beta cells. The presence of appropriate immune response genes (which regulate reactivity against islet cell antigens) may be crucial to the development of pancreatic autoimmunity. Thus, the association of IDDM with certain HLA-D/DR antigens may very well reflect the presence of HLA-linked Ir genes that facilitate anti–islet cell immune responses. According to this hypothesis, immune reactivity against the islets would be intense early in the course of IDDM. Over the years, as the mass of beta cells is progressively reduced, the antigenic stimulus would abate and the frequency of ICA-positive patients would be expected to decline. This prediction is upheld by the observed relationship between the frequency of ICA and the duration of IDDM, as discussed earlier.

Although in most cases an environmental agent is suspected to initiate the chain of events leading to the development of autoimmunity, it is postulated that, in a small subset of IDDM, autoimmune reactions arise spontaneously. These patients are characterized by concomitant autoimmunity against several other endocrine glands including thyroid and adrenals, and may also have gastric parietal cell antibodies. In these instances, ICA are often present before the onset of clinical diabetes and persist for several years after its onset. IDDM under these circumstances may be one manifestation of a broad range of anti–self-reactivity.

To summarize: in a few cases, IDDM may be caused by a direct, severe, virus-induced injury of the beta cells; in other rare cases, it may present as a component of polyendocrine autoimmunity; in the great majority of cases, however, it results from a complex interplay of environmental (possibly viral), genetic (HLA-linked), and immunologic factors.[60]

Uncertain as the causation of IDDM may be, the riddle of NIDDM is even more obscure. Unlike IDDM, the lack of insulin is not severe. Indeed, for several years the very existence of insulin deficiency in NIDDM was doubted and the derangement in glucose homeostasis was ascribed solely to impaired action of insulin, i.e., insulin resistance. It is now widely accepted, however, that both insulin deficiency and insulin resistance are involved in the pathogenesis of NIDDM, although their relative contributions to the metabolic abnormalities vary with the clinical severity of the disease. In the following discussion each of these two factors will be considered separately, beginning with the status of insulin secretion in NIDDM.[61]

For an evaluation of the adequacy of insulin response in NIDDM, two considerations are of utmost importance. *First,* insulin secretion in response to a load of glucose occurs in two phases: an initial rapid phase (within 0 to 10 min of an intravenous glucose challenge) followed by a delayed response (10 to 12 min after glucose infusion). Both of these have to be assessed independently. *Second,* the plasma insulin levels should be considered in the context of body weight, since obesity (a common accompaniment of NIDDM), even in the absence of diabetes, is associated with insulin resistance and hyperinsulinemia. To avoid the confusing variable introduced by obesity, we will first discuss insulin secretion in NIDDM without associated obesity.

In patients with mild NIDDM (fasting plasma glucose 115 to 200 mg/dl), the basal (fasting) plasma insulin levels are either normal or often moderately elevated, but there is *a significant reduction in the first-phase insulin response.*[62, 63] The second-phase insulin secretion is normal and the insulin levels may actually peak higher as compared with normal weight-matched controls. Despite the loss of early response to glucose, the acute responses to other secretagogues such as arginine and isoproterenol remain normal. It should be pointed out, however, that such responses cannot be considered completely normal since the elevated blood glucose levels (seen in these patients) are known to potentiate the effect of nonglucose stimuli on the pancreatic beta cells.[64] Although the second-phase insulin secretion is sufficient to restore plasma glucose levels to basal levels in these (mild) cases, impairment of the early secretion leads to prolonged postprandial hyperglycemia. In patients with more severe NIDDM (fasting plasma glucose 200 to 300 mg/dl), both the early and late glucose responses are blunted, indicating an absolute deficiency of insulin. Quite remarkably, the fasting plasma insulin levels are normal even in these more severely affected patients. It could be argued, however, that although the insulin levels are within the range for normal nondiabetics, they are low relative to the needs of the diabetic who has fasting hyperglycemia.

In the obese diabetic the picture becomes more complicated. Obesity (with or without associated NIDDM) is characterized by insulin resistance and hyperinsulinemia. Since most patients with NIDDM are obese, their plasma insulin levels are "elevated," and thus initially it was assumed that they did not have insulin deficiency. However, when obese NIDDM patients are compared with weight-matched nondiabetics, it appears that insulin levels of obese diabetics (although well above those of lean nondiabetics) are below those observed in obese nondiabetics, suggesting again a state of relative insulin deficiency. *We can conclude, therefore, that impaired beta-cell function manifested either as a delayed insulin response or as a relative or absolute state of insulin deficiency is observed in most patients with NIDDM. However, this insulin deficiency is milder than that of IDDM and is most clearly demonstrated in those who have significant fasting hyperglycemia.*

Since the metabolic derangements in NIDDM are

often disproportionately larger than would be predicted from the degree of insulin deficiency, there must be some impairment of insulin action. Indeed, in recent years an impressive body of data has accumulated that incriminates insulin resistance as the major factor in the pathogenesis of NIDDM with or without obesity.[65, 66] End-organ insensitivity to insulin is a complex phenomenon that could arise by at least three mechanisms: (1) synthesis of abnormal insulin, (2) circulating antagonists of insulin, and (3) defects in the target tissues of insulin. It is the last of these that seems to be involved in the pathogenesis of NIDDM. Before we discuss the cellular basis of insulin resistance in NIDDM, it should be pointed out that impairment of insulin action is not restricted to the diabetic syndrome. In both obesity and pregnancy (even in the absence of NIDDM), there is reduced tissue response to circulating insulin, but the pancreas compensates by secreting excessive amounts of insulin. These conditions, therefore, are associated with hyperinsulinemia and only a modest impairment of glucose tolerance. However, in persons with a genetically determined defect in insulin production, obesity would precipitate diabetes mellitus. In many obese diabetics, weight loss, by reducing the "stress" on the beta cells, may lead to a restoration of normal glucose tolerance. Although obesity is emphasized as a factor in insulin resistance, the latter is also encountered in nonobese diabetics.

The cellular basis for the tissue resistance to the action of insulin is not completely understood. Since binding to cell surface receptors is the first step in the action of insulin, one mechanism could be reduced binding of insulin to its target cells. *In patients with NIDDM, a decrease in the number of insulin receptors is seen in a variety of cells including monocytes, fat cells, red cells, and hepatocytes.* Cells from obese nondiabetics also show a reduction in receptor concentration, but obesity alone cannot explain the receptor defect in NIDDM, since nonobese diabetics also demonstrate reduced insulin binding. We mentioned earlier that insulin itself can downregulate its receptors in vitro (p. 978). Since basal (fasting) insulin levels are often elevated in patients with mild NIDDM and obese nondiabetics, it is believed that the reduced receptor concentration is the consequence of hyperinsulinemia. In the more severely affected patients who have fasting hyperglycemia, insulin binding is also reduced, but the full extent of insulin resistance cannot be explained solely on the basis of reduced receptor concentration. Therefore, postreceptor defects must also exist.[52, 62, 65] Indeed, *most of the recent evidence suggests that postreceptor defects are the major cause of the impaired insulin action associated with severe NIDDM.* Although the pathogenesis of the postreceptor defects has not been clarified, it is strongly suspected that insulin deficiency (which characterizes advanced NIDDM) is itself responsible for the impairment of the postreceptor pathways. This concept is supported by a preliminary report demonstrating that the beneficial effect of insulin therapy in NIDDM is due largely to a significant amelioration of the postreceptor defect.[67] *In summary, insulin resistance, a universal feature of NIDDM, may result from a decrease in insulin receptors and/or an impairment of the postreceptor effects of insulin. In mild NIDDM, the receptor defects predominate, whereas with severe disease, postreceptor defects are the major cause of insulin resistance.*

From the evidence reviewed above, it is clear that most cases of NIDDM have both impaired beta-cell function and insulin resistance. Which of the two defects is primary? According to one view, the basic problem is in the pancreatic beta cells, which are genetically vulnerable to injury, resulting in accelerated cell turnover and premature aging.[68] Early in the course of NIDDM, when the beta-cell defect is mild and manifested principally by impaired early secretion of insulin, there is no fasting hyperglycemia but there is an excessive and prolonged postprandial increase in plasma glucose levels (p. 979). This in turn provides a persistent stimulus to insulin secretion, which is successful in maintaining fasting euglycemia but gives rise to insulin resistance by downregulating the insulin receptors (Fig. 20–18). Thus, a vicious cycle is set up with progressive impairment of glucose utilization and increased need for insulin secretion. Over a period of time, excessive demands of insulin could lead to beta-cell "exhaustion," insulinopenia, fasting hyperglycemia, and the emergence of postreceptor defects. A very similar sequence of events could also be initiated by a primary defect in the insulin-mediated uptake of glucose at the level of peripheral tissues, as illustrated in Figure 20–18. In both the proposed pathways, insulin resistance plays a major role.

Extremely severe insulin resistance is also seen in a rare group of syndromes associated with somewhat unusual hyperpigmented verrucous skin lesions (*acanthosis nigricans*). In one variant, circulating anti–insulin receptor antibodies that arise spontaneously (i.e., without exogenous insulin administration) are responsible for impaired insulin binding; in others, there seems to be an intrinsic deficiency in the number of insulin receptors per cell.[52] These uncommon forms of diabetes mellitus are of interest largely because they provide useful models for the study of insulin action.

Despite all the evidence pointing toward a relative or absolute deficiency of insulin as a fundamental cause of diabetes mellitus, the controversial issue of concomitant alpha-cell dysfunction and hyperglucagonemia must be raised. Within the recent past, *the time-honored theory that some form of insulin derangement alone is the cause of diabetes mellitus has been challenged by assigning to glucagon the role of essential comediator of the disease.* The bihormonal theory ascribes to insulin deficiency the underutilization of glucose, but imputes to glucagon excess, either absolute or relative, most of the glucose overproduction.[69] This conception has been referred to as the "double-trouble" hypothesis. In almost every respect, glucagon has a metabolic effect directly opposite to that of insulin. Whereas insulin promotes the storage of glycogen in

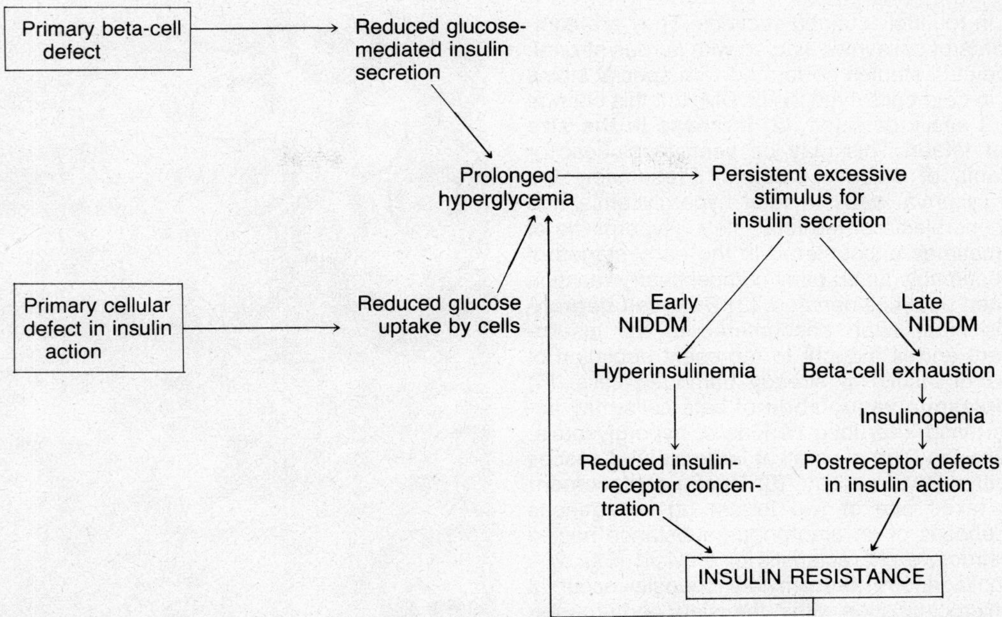

Figure 20–18. Pathogenesis of NIDDM. The central role of insulin resistance should be noted. (Modified from Defronzo, R. A., et al.: New concepts in the pathogenesis and treatment of non–insulin-dependent diabetes mellitus. Am. J. Med. *74*(Suppl.):52, 1983.)

liver and muscle, glucagon inhibits it; whereas insulin inhibits glycogenolysis in the liver, glucagon promotes it and also activates gluconeogenesis; whereas insulin inhibits lipolysis, glucagon stimulates it. Moreover, glucagon favors ketogenesis. Thus, a push-pull system is proposed for the maintenance of blood glucose levels by the opposing actions of glucagon and insulin. If this balance is disturbed, as may occur in diabetes, hyperglycemia results from hepatic overproduction of glucose (glucagon excess) and its simultaneous underutilization (insulin deficiency). Support for such a theory comes from several observations: (1) absolute or relative hyperglucagonemia can be demonstrated in both major variants of diabetes mellitus; (2) glucagon opposes several actions of insulin (as discussed above); (3) correction of hyperglucagonemia by infusion of somatostatin reduces the hyperglycemia. Nevertheless, *the role of glucagon as an essential comediator is not universally accepted.* For example, diabetes mellitus can be produced in dogs in the total absence of glucagon following pancreatectomy.[70] Without delving deeper into this controversy, we can state that, although excess glucagon does contribute significantly to the metabolic abnormalities of uncontrolled diabetes mellitus, there is insufficient evidence to incriminate it as an essential comediator. Most current evidence suggests that the abnormality in glucagon secretion itself is secondary to the lack of insulin, which in some manner regulates glucagon secretion by the A cells.

In concluding this discussion of the causation of diabetes, it should be noted that none of the theories so far discussed addresses the relationship between the metabolic changes and the major complications of diabetes—microangiopathy, atherosclerosis, renal disease, retinopathy, and neuropathy. This aspect of the pathogenesis of diabetes can best be considered with the description of the anatomic changes affecting various organs and tissues.

MORPHOLOGY. The diagnosis of diabetes mellitus on morphologic grounds alone can be made only in some patients on the basis of a few lesions that are for all practical purposes pathognomonic of the disease. Most patients have lesions that are only suggestive, and some have no anatomic changes that may not also be found in age-matched nondiabetics. The basis for this extreme variability is poorly understood, but five influences may contribute: (1) the age of the patient at the time of death, (2) the duration of the disease, (3) the severity of the metabolic derangement, (4) the rigidity of the therapeutic control, and (5) poorly defined genetic factors. Surprisingly, no consensus has been reached on the respective importance of each of these variables. In particular, the desirability of meticulous control of the disordered metabolism has long been disputed. In essence, the disagreement centers around whether "rigid" insulin control of glucose levels will decrease or prevent the appearance of some of the crippling and fatal long-term effects of the disease. The current consensus seems to be that the severity of the metabolic derangements is directly related to the occurrence of vascular and other complications. More about this later, but for now we can state that when the disease has been present for 10 to 15 years, regardless of the type of diabetes (IDDM or NIDDM), morphologic changes are likely to be found in the basement membranes, small vessels, arteries, pancreas, kidneys, retinae, nerves, and other tissues.

Pancreas. Surpisingly, lesions in the pancreas are neither constant nor necessarily pathognomonic.[71,72] They are more likely to be distinctive in IDDM than in NIDDM. One or more of the following alterations may be present: (1) **Reduction in the size and number of islets.** This is most often seen in IDDM, particularly with rapidly advancing disease. Most of the islets are small, inconspicuous, and not easily detected in routinely stained sections. They are composed of thin cords of cells intermingled with fibrous stroma. Careful morphometric studies performed with special stains show reduction in beta cells even in NIDDM, but this change is subtle and not easily detected. (2) **Increase in the size and number of islets.** This may be seen in diabetic or nondiabetic infants of diabetic mothers. Presumably the maternal hyperglycemia leads to fetal hyperglycemia and compensatory hyperplasia of the fetal islets. Hyperplasia of the islets is sometimes encountered in the early stages of IDDM, again presumably as an early compensatory reaction to some presumed beta-cell damage. (3) **Beta-cell degranulation.** This is most often encountered in the insulin-dependent variant and is thought to represent depletion of secretory stores of insulin in already damaged cells. (4) **Glycogen cytoplasmic vacuolation** of beta cells may appear in patients dying after long periods of hyperglycemia. The vacuoles take the form of small or large cleared spaces that yield a positive PAS reaction. (5) **Hyalin replacement of islets.** This takes one of two forms: (a) collagenous fibrosis or (b) deposits of an amorphous substance having the fibrillar substructure characteristic of amyloid (Fig. 20–19). Both the collagenous and amyloid deposits occur at first about the microcirculation within the islets and progressively extend to obliterate the surrounding cells. These changes may be found in IDDM but are more characteristic of the late chronic stages of NIDDM. Neither change is diagnostic of diabetes, since both are sometimes found in elderly nondiabetic patients with advanced atherosclerosis and presumably ischemic injury to islets.[73] (6) **Leukocytic infiltrations** may take one of two forms. The most common pattern is a heavy lymphocytic infiltrate within and about the islets, referred to as **insulitis**. Insulitis is most frequent in young diabetics with a brief history of symptomatic diabetes. The possible autoimmune significance of such an inflammatory infiltrate has already been discussed (p. 979). Eosinophilic infiltrates may also be found, particularly in diabetic infants who fail to survive the immediate postnatal period. These too are interpreted as an immunologic reaction.

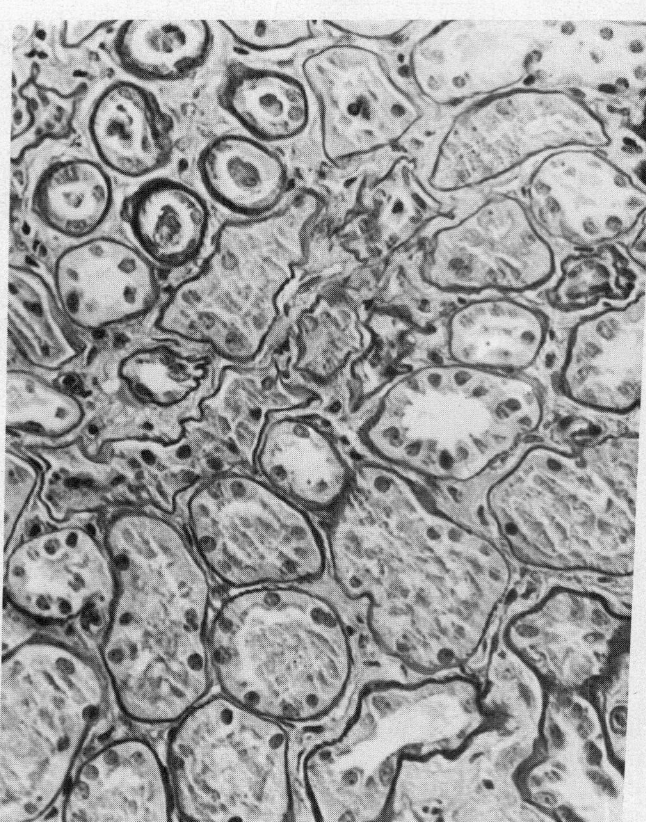

Figure 20–20. PAS stain of renal cortex showing thickening of basement membrane in a diabetic.

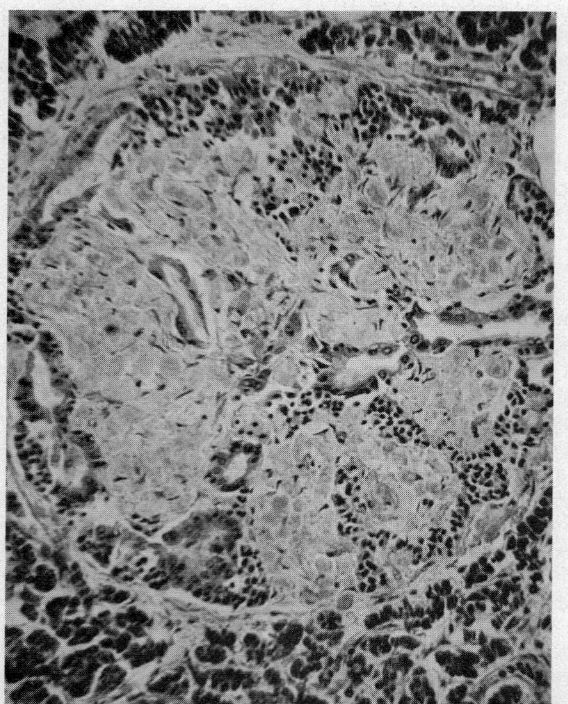

Figure 20–19. Hyalinization of an islet in pancreas in a diabetic.

Diabetic Microangiopathy and Basement Membrane Thickening. One of the most consistent anatomic features of diabetes is diffuse thickening of basement membranes. The thickening is most evident in the capillaries of the skin, skeletal muscles, retina, renal glomeruli, and renal medulla, giving rise to the characteristic diabetic microangiography of these organs. However, it may also be seen in such nonvascular structures as renal tubules, Bowman's capsule, peripheral nerves, and placenta. By light microscopy, the thickening appears as widening of the basement membrane by a homogeneous, sometimes multilayered hyaline substance, which is strongly positive with the PAS stain (Fig. 20–20). Under the electron microscope the thickening either may be homogeneous (Fig. 20–21) or, particularly in the skin, may consist of several laminated circumferential layers.[74] Despite the increased thickness of basement membranes, diabetic capillaries are more leaky to plasma proteins than normal.[75] As will be seen, the microangiopathy has far-reaching implications, inducing serious lesions in the renal glomeruli and retinae and possibly contributing to the increased vulnerability of the diabetic to neuropathy. The question of whether rigid control of diabetes delays or prevents the appearance of microangiopathy is a subject to which we will turn later. It should be noted that indistinguishable microvascular lesions can be found in aged nondiabetic patients, but rarely to the extent seen in those with longstanding diabetes.

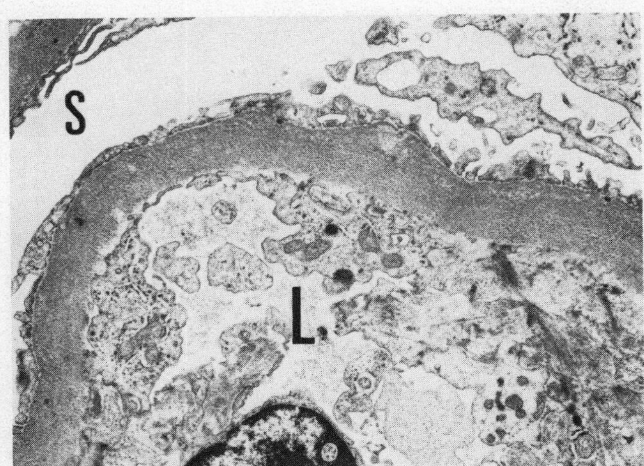

Figure 20–21. Markedly thickened glomerular basement membrane in a diabetic. L is the glomerular capillary lumen and S is the urinary space.

The pathogenesis of diabetic microangiopathy is still unknown, but several mechanisms are postulated and are not mutually exclusive.[76] As detailed later, it is now thought that persistent **hyperglycemia,** per se, is necessary for the full development of microangiopathy. There is also evidence that binding of the glucose molecule to the amino acid of proteins (nonenzymatic glycosylation) may be responsible for some of the metabolic defects of diabetes. Glycosylation may contribute to the microangiopathy in several ways. Increased vascular permeability may be due either to increased filtration of glycosylated plasma proteins, or to glycosylation of some critical proteins in vascular endothelium. Evidence for either of these events is not available, but there is some evidence of increased glycosylation of basement membranes in diabetics.[76] Other basement membrane alterations also occur. It will be recalled (p. 77) that basement membranes consist of collagen (mainly type IV), laminin, and anionic proteoglycans (including heparan sulfate).[75, 77] Several studies show increased amounts and increased synthesis of collagen type IV, and increased levels of laminin in diabetes.[75, 77] There is, however, a **decrease** in the amount and synthesis of proteoglycans.[78, 79] The latter may contribute to the increased permeability to cationic proteins, particularly in the kidney (p. 1024); one notion is that compensatory increased synthesis of basement membrane molecules, to correct the deficient filter, eventually generates the thickened basement membranes.[78] Two additional events may contribute to the basement membrane thickening. Vracko and Benditt[68] suggested that the multilayered thickening could be due to repeated episodes of endothelial cell degeneration and regeneration, each layer representing a new cycle of endothelial injury and repair. Finally, thickening may be caused in part by enhanced binding of filtered protein to the altered basement membrane.

Atherosclerosis. Atherosclerosis begins to appear in most diabetics, whatever their age, within a few years of onset of both IDDM and NIDDM. Less than 5% of nondiabetics as opposed to approximately 75% of diabetics below the age of 40 have moderate-to-severe atherosclerosis. In most diabetics, the vascular lesions, called atheromas, do not differ qualitatively from those found in nondiabetics (p. 506); however, diabetic lesions tend to be more numerous and florid and to undergo the constellation of changes leading to complicated lesions, i.e., ulceration, calcification, and superimposed thromboses (Fig. 20–22). Thus, relatively early in the diabetic's life, atherosclerosis may result in arterial narrowings or occlusions and attendant ischemic injury to organs; alternatively, it may induce aneurysmal dilatation, seen most often in the aorta, with the grave potential of rupture. **This large vessel disease accounts for the heavy toll exacted by myocardial infarction, cerebral stroke, and gangrene of the lower extremities in these patients.** Significant coronary atherosclerosis and myocardial infarction is up to five times more prevalent in diabetics than in the normal population. Whereas myocardial infarction is uncommon in nondiabetic females during reproductive life, it is almost as common in diabetic females as in diabetic males. Gangrene of the lower extremities is 100 times more common in diabetics than in nondiabetics.

The susceptibility of the diabetic to atherosclerosis is not well explained.[80] It has been loosely attributed to hyperlipidemia; however, many diabetics have normal or only minimally elevated serum triglyceride and cholesterol levels. Attention is, therefore, focused on the level of HDL, which, you will recall, has an inverse risk-relationship to atherosclerosis (p. 507). Since HDL levels are reduced in NIDDM, susceptibility to atherogenesis may be enhanced. Speculation exists as to whether deranged arterial metabolism is important. When glucose levels are high, sorbitol, a product

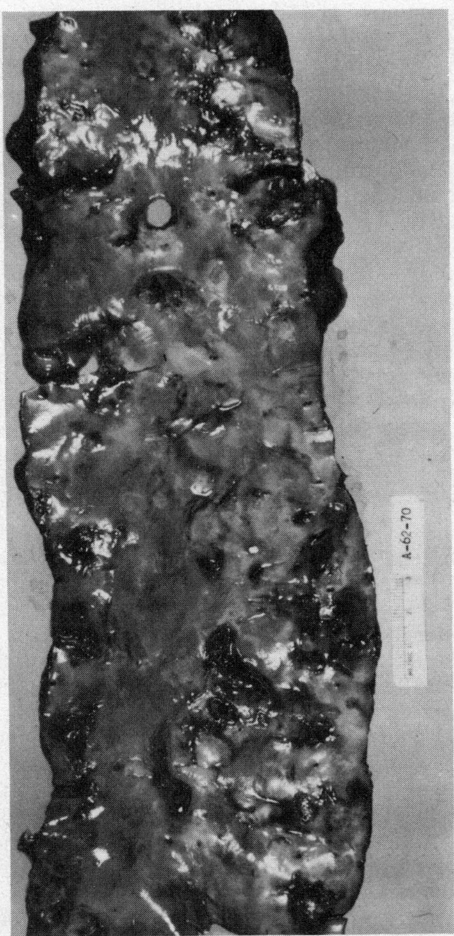

Figure 20–22. Advanced aortic atherosclerosis in a 53-year-old male with NIDDM of 21 years' duration.

of glucose metabolism, is enzymatically formed. Increased activity of the enzymes involved in sorbitol metabolism has been identified in the aortic wall, leading to changes in intimal metabolism. Most patients with NIDDM also tend to be obese and hypertensive, so that other contributing influences are present. Diabetics have increased platelet adhesiveness and response to aggregating agents. These changes are also likely to favor atherogenesis. For whatever reason, all diabetics who have had the disease for at least ten years, irrespective of the age of onset, are likely to have clinically significant atherosclerosis.

Arterioles. Thickening of arteriole walls (arteriolosclerosis) is not only more common among diabetics than normals but also tends to be more severe. Indistinguishable arteriolosclerosis can also be found in nondiabetic hypertensive patients (p. 1045); in the diabetic it may be found in the absence of hypertension.[81] The arteriolosclerosis affects all vascular beds, particularly those in the kidneys. The most common lesion encountered is hyaline arteriolosclerosis, described in detail on page 1045.

Kidneys. The kidneys are usually the most severely damaged organs in the diabetic. Renal failure, usually due to renal microvascular disease, accounts for many diabetic deaths in both juveniles and adults. Any one or any combination of the following major lesions may be found: (1) **glomerular involvement** with three distinctive patterns: diffuse glomerulosclerosis, nodular glomerulosclerosis, and exudative lesions—these result in proteinuria, and in time progress to chronic renal failure; (2) **arteriolosclerosis**, including so-called benign nephrosclerosis and frequently associated with hypertension; (3) bacterial urinary tract infection, with **pyelonephritis** and sometimes **necrotizing papillitis.**

The glomerular and arteriolar lesions are the most important and are intimately linked to the overall diabetic microangiopathy. Since diabetic renal disease is one of the major causes of renal morbidity and mortality, the subject will be discussed in detail in Chapter 21 (p. 1022).

Eyes. One of the most threatening aspects of diabetes mellitus is the development of visual impairment consequent to retinopathy, cataract formation, or glaucoma. Diabetic retinopathy is the fourth leading cause of all legal blindness (visual acuity of 20/200 or worse) in the United States today. In the development of diabetic retinopathy, the duration of disease appears to be a very important determinant. It has been estimated that if a patient is diagnosed as a diabetic at age 30, there is a 10% chance he will have some degree of diabetic retinopathy by age 37, a 50% chance by age 45, and a 90% chance by age 55. However, it should be appreciated that diabetic retinopathy does not always impose a visual handicap, depending on whether the macula is involved or not. **The retinopathy can be divided into nonproliferative and proliferative stages.**

Nonproliferative retinopathy, also called "background retinopathy," is characterized by the appearance of microaneurysms accompanied by edema, exudates, hemorrhages, and arteriolar and venous changes. The microaneurysms comprise globular or fusiform outpouchings from one side of the capillary wall, ranging from 10 to 200 μ in diameter (Fig. 20–23). When vascularized they appear as cherry-red spots in the retina, but thrombosis and organization may transform them to yellow-white lesions. Their origins are still somewhat uncertain. One theory suggests that initially there is loss of capillary pericytes, leading to focal weakening and dilatation of the capillary walls. Alternatively, the systemic microangiopathy and retinal edema may lead first to focal collapse of the capillary bed in the retina, followed by the development of dilated, circuitous capillary shunts. The tortuous capillaries kinked upon themselves may create the microaneurysm. However they develop, **retinal microaneurysms are generally thought to be virtually diagnostic of diabetes mellitus.** Although initially described in the retina, microaneurysms have also been reported in cardiac and glomerular capillaries.[82] It is of interest that approximately half the patients with retinal microaneurysms have nodular glomerular sclerosis. Conversely, if a patient has nodular glomerular sclerosis he is almost certain to have retinal microaneurysms. Retinal edema appears most evident in the macular region when the macroangiopathy in the capillaries induces increased vascular permeability. "Hard, waxy exudates" constitute localized accumulations of extravasated protein and lipid that form in the deep layers of the retina as a consequence of altered capillary permeability. "Cotton-wool spots" comprise, in essence, gray-white microinfarcts in the superficial retinal layers. Any or all of these changes are construed as manifestations of nonproliferative retinopathy.

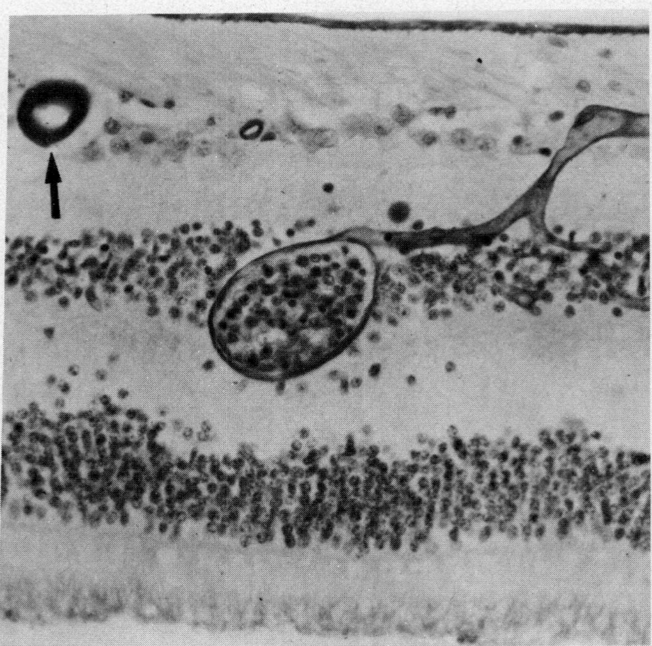

Figure 20–23. Cross section of a retinal microaneurysm. Note microangiopathy in upper left corner *(arrow)*. (Courtesy of Dr. Merle Legg, New England Deaconess Hospital, Boston.)

Much more ominous is the appearance of **proliferative diabetic retinopathy** characterized by neovascularization and fibrosis of the retina. This may progress over the span of a few years to create a vascular connective tissue mass over the retina and disc, causing severe visual impairment or total blindness. Adhesions between this fibrovascular tissue and the vitreous body may develop, leading to vitreous hemorrhages and/or retinal detachment, aggravating an already serious problem.[83]

Nervous System. Peripheral nerves, brain, and spinal cord may all be damaged in long-standing diabetes.[84] Most commonly encountered is **symmetric peripheral neuropathy** affecting both motor and sensory nerves of the lower extremities. It is characterized by Schwann cell injury, myelin degeneration, and also axonal damage. Damage to the Schwann cells or possibly axons is believed to be the primary event, but this issue is not settled (p. 1431).[85] The peripheral neuropathy is sometimes accompanied by disturbances in the neural innervation of the pelvic organs **(autonomic neuropathy)** leading to sexual impotence and bowel and bladder dysfunction.

The cause of the neuropathy is somewhat uncertain and several explanations have been offered. It may be related to diffuse microangiopathy affecting the nutritional maintenance of the peripheral nerve. This mechanism seems to be the most likely explanation for **diabetic mononeuropathies** affecting, for example, obturator, femoral, or sciatic nerves. Disordered glucose metabolism, rather than vascular insufficiency, is believed to be the cause of polyneuropathies. In experimental models of diabetes, a marked decrease in the nerve myo-inositol concentration has been noted in association with decreased neural conduction. It is postulated that hyperglycemia somehow alters the metabolic pathways responsible for maintaining the myo-inositol levels in the nerves. Much, however, remains to be known.[86] Neuronal degeneration in the brain and spinal cord may also appear. In addition, the diabetic has some predisposition to cerebral infarctions and brain hemorrhages, the latter related to the hypertension seen so often in these patients. It is worth noting that neurons are vulnerable to the hypoglycemia encountered in insulin reactions and to the ketoacidosis of the uncontrolled diabetic state.

Other Organs. A variety of skin lesions occur in long-term diabetics. Perhaps most common are skin infections, reflecting the diabetic's predisposition to infections. Localized collections of lipid-laden macrophages (foam cells or xanthoma cells) in the dermis and subcutaneous fat create so-called **diabetic xanthomas.** These appear as firm, yellow nodules directly beneath the epidermis, usually on the extensor surfaces of the elbows and knees and on the back and buttocks. Other distributions may also occur. Xanthomas are thought to result from the hyperlipemia of diabetes and are seen in other disorders associated with high blood lipid levels.

Clinical Course. It is difficult to sketch with brevity the diverse clinical presentations of idiopathic diabetes mellitus, because the disease may appear as silently as a cat or storm in like an enraged bull. Only a few stereotypical responses can be presented. IDDM, sometimes following a transient remission, is dominated largely by signs and symptoms emanating from the disordered metabolism (p. 974). Glucose intolerance is of the unstable or brittle type and is quite sensitive to administered exogenous insulin, deviations from normal dietary intake, unusual physical activity, infection, or other forms of stress. Inadequate fluid intake or vomiting may rapidly lead to significant disturbances in fluid and electrolyte balance. Thus, these patients are vulnerable on the one hand to hypoglycemic episodes and on the other to ketoacidosis. Fortunately, these hazards are more avoidable than the long-term sequelae of angiopathy, nephropathy, retinopathy, and neuropathy. However, in some children and adolescents the onset of IDDM is asymptomatic, detectable only by means of postprandial hyperglycemia or an abnormal glucose tolerance test.

NIDDM begins with few, if any, signs or symptoms. The disease may be discovered in these patients during routine examination revealing postprandial hyperglycemia or glycosuria, or because they have insidiously, and without its being diagnosed, developed vascular complications. Some of the many presentations of this insidious form of the disease include impairment of vision, susceptibility to skin infections, vulvar pruritus, a recalcitrant ulcerative lesion on the toe or foot unresponsive to the usual forms of therapy, gangrene of a toe or foot, loss of sensation, paresthesias, impotence related to neuropathy, or indeed the dramatic occurrence of a myocardial infarct or cerebral stroke in a relatively young person. At other times the patient is discovered to be diabetic because of the insidious onset of renal failure, producing unexplained anemia, excessive fatigue, or proteinuria. The glomerular changes in diabetes mellitus may induce a severe proteinuria, sometimes sufficient to cause the nephrotic syndrome (p. 1022). In addition, elevated blood pressure is found in up to 80% of patients with NIDDM, especially in those who are obese. Thus, the patient with NIDDM usually does not have the dramatic acute metabolic syndrome, but instead has a stable, frequently insidious form of glucose intolerance, often leading to the chronic vascular syndrome.

As mentioned earlier, there is still disagreement as to whether "rigid" control of the carbohydrate intolerance will delay or prevent the appearance and/or progression of the late complications of this disease.[87] Central to this important controversy is the question whether the microangiopathies and neuropathies are related directly to the high-glucose metabolic environment. Some reports suggest that the microangiopathy is not related to the metabolic derangement and represents a separate genetic predisposition that may appear in patients having little or no carbohydrate intolerance, such as in individuals in the PotAGT category (Table 20–1). On the other side of the fence is the *much more widely held opinion that there is a definite relationship between glucose intolerance and basement membrane thickening as well as neurologic complications.* This view is supported by the following observations: (1) Several clinical studies indicate a correlation between the degree of hyperglycemia and the appearance of retinal, renal, and neurologic changes. Some (but not all[87]) studies have shown arrest[88] or reversal[89] of basement membrane thickening by strict diabetic control. (2) In animal models of diabetes, if islet cell transplantation is performed soon after the induction of diabetes, microvascular lesions do not appear. If the islet cell transplantation is delayed, basement membrane thickening occurs. (3) When normal kidneys are transplanted into diabetic recipients, arteriolar and glomerular changes resembling spontaneous diabetic nephropathy appear in the transplanted kidney. (4) Conversely, when experimental or human diabetic kidneys have been tranplanted to nondiabetic recipients, reversal of the diabetic glomerular changes has occurred.[90]

The view that hyperglycemia is in some way related to the late complications of diabetes has received additional support from the recent observations that glucose can react nonenzymatically with several body proteins to form stable covalent linkages. For example, nonenzymatic glycosylation of HbA leads to the formation of HbA_{1c}, which normally constitutes about 4% of the red cell hemoglobin. The rate of nonenzymatic glycosylation is directly related to the degree of hyperglycemia, and therefore the red cell HbA_{1c} increases severalfold in uncontrolled diabetics. Since HbA_{1c} is formed continuously during the 120-day life span of the red cells, its blood level provides an index of the average blood glucose levels over the preceding 60 to 90 days. Although HbA_{1c} is the most widely studied glycosylated protein, nonenzymatic glycosylation of a variety of other proteins, including serum albumin, lens crystallin, collagen, and basic myelin protein, has also been detected. Glycosylation, it is postulated, can alter the structure and function of body proteins and thus contribute to the development of various late complications of diabetes. Even if future investigations substantiate this attractive hypothesis, metabolic abnormalities may not be the only factor in the genesis of diabetic microangiopathies. It is well known, for example, that, in a significant minority of patients with poorly controlled, long-standing diabetes, typical vascular complications such as retinopathy do not develop. Therefore, other factors, possibly genetic, are also involved.[91]

Life expectancy for the diabetic is shortened. In a general survey of diabetics in Iowa encompassing all ages and all forms of diabetes, the average estimated life expectancy at birth for diabetic males was approximately 60 years and for diabetic females approximately 70 years, representing a reduction of nine years for males and approximately seven years for females.[92] The age of onset of the disease appears to have a material effect on these figures. There is thus a significant excess mortality in diabetics, more marked with onset in youth. Nonetheless, some patients with IDDM are remarkably spared and have been shown to be relatively free of later sequelae, even after 40 years of disease.[93]

The causes of death in order of importance are myocardial infarction, renal failure, cerebrovascular disease, ischemic heart disease, and infections as well as a number of other possible complications, including gangrene of an extremity or mesenteric thrombosis. Special mention should be made of the diabetic's enhanced susceptibility to infections, collectively responsible for about 5% of all deaths. The basis for this is still imperfectly understood but may be related to impaired blood supply to tissues secondary to microangiopathy; in addition, decreased leukocyte chemotaxis and bactericidal activity have been demonstrated (p. 51). Thus, any infection in the diabetic is serious and may lead ultimately to death. A happy note in this otherwise sad litany is that hypoglycemia and ketoacidosis are rare causes of death today. Even happier is the breakthrough showing that diabetes in the experimental animal can be virtually *cured* by islet transplantation, since innovative techniques designed to overcome the histocompatibility barriers are being devised. It is hoped that some of the experimental protocols used to prolong islet cell transplants in animal models will become available for human use.

ISLET CELL TUMORS

Islet cell tumors[41] are rare in comparison with tumors of the exocrine pancreas. They are most common in adults and can occur anywhere along the length of the pancreas. They may be hormonally functional or entirely nonfunctional. The tumors may be single or multiple and benign or malignant, the latter metastasizing to lymph nodes and liver. When multiple, each tumor may be composed of a different cell type.

The three most common and distinctive clinical syndromes associated with hyperfunction of the islets of Langerhans are: (1) *hyperinsulinism and hypoglycemia,* (2) *the Zollinger-Ellison syndrome (gastrinoma), and* (3) *multiple endocrine neoplasia.* Each of these may be caused by (1) diffuse hyperplasia of the islets of Langerhans, (2) benign adenomas that occur singly or multiply, and (3) malignant islet tumors.[41, 94]

BETA-CELL TUMORS (HYPOGLYCEMIA)

Beta-cell tumors (insulinomas) are the most common of islet cell tumors and may be responsible for the elaboration of sufficient insulin to induce clinically significant hypoglycemia. There is a characteristic clinical triad resulting from these pancreatic lesions: (1) attacks of hypoglycemia occur with blood sugar levels below 50 mg/dl of serum; (2) the attacks consist principally of such central nervous system manifestations as confusion, stupor, and loss of consciousness and are clearly related to fasting or exercise; (3) the attacks are promptly relieved by the feeding or parenteral administration of glucose. There are other causes for hypoglycemia when a patient manifests this classic triad, but the cause should first be sought in the pancreas.

Analysis of pancreatic islet lesions inducing hyperinsulinism indicates that about 70% are solitary adenomas, approximately 10% are multiple adenomas, 10% are metastasizing tumors that must be interpreted as carcinomas, and the remainder are a mixed group of diffuse hyperplasia of the islets and adenomas occurring in ectopic pancreatic tissue.[95] The insulin-producing adenomas, often called **insulomas,** vary in size from minute lesions difficult to find even on the dissecting table to huge masses of over 1500 gm (Fig. 20–24). Most occur singly, as indicated earlier, but in about one case in seven, multiple adenomas are found scattered throughout the pancreatic substance. They are usually encapsulated, firm, yellow-brown nodules that, by expansile growth, compress the surrounding pancreatic substance. Histologically, they are composed of cords and nests of well-differentiated beta cells that do not differ from those of the normal islet (Fig. 20–25). On electron microscopy, the tumor cells resemble non-neoplastic beta cells and exhibit membrane-bound granules 150 to 200 μ in diameter, with a dense core, a halo, and a single-limiting membrane.[43] By immunohistochemistry, insulin can be readily visualized in tumor cells.

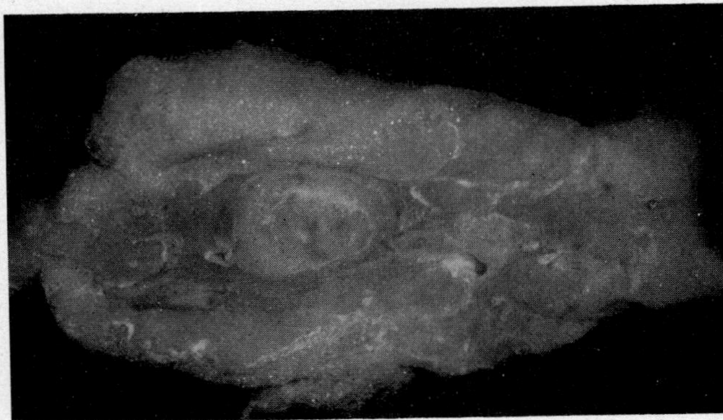

Figure 20–24. Islet cell adenoma of pancreas. Small, pale tumor is seen on transection of pancreas.

The malignant tumor displays little evidence of anaplasia and, in fact, it may be impossible from the histologic evaluation of the tumor to determine its biologic behavior. Rupture of the capsule and extension into the surrounding pancreatic substance are not reliable criteria of malignancy, and the diagnosis of carcinoma of the islets should not be made in the absence of unmistakable evidence of metastasis or local invasion beyond the substance of the pancreas. Although, with newer evaluation procedures, up to 80% of islet cell tumors may show excessive insulin secretion, the hypoglycemia is mild in all but 20%, and many never become clinically symptomatic.[94] Malignant tumors are more often hormonally active.

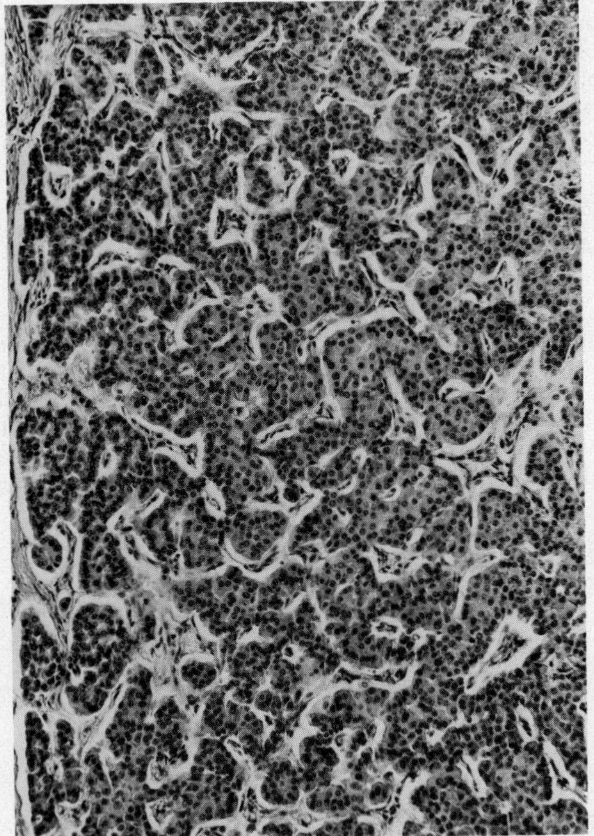

Figure 20–25. Islet cell adenoma of pancreas. The well-defined margin of an islet cell tumor. Note resemblance of tumor cells to normal islet cells.

Hyperinsulinism may also be caused by diffuse hyperplasia of the islets. This change is found occasionally in adults but is rather characteristic of infants born of diabetic mothers. Long exposed to the hyperglycemia of the maternal blood, the infant responds by an increase in the size and number of its islets. In the postnatal period, these hyperactive islets may be responsible for serious episodes of hypoglycemia.

The differential diagnosis of hypoglycemia must also include a consideration of a variety of functional and organic disorders in addition to the beta-cell lesions already discussed. Functional hypoglycemia is sometimes encountered quite mysteriously in patients without apparent underlying cause, and may here be referred to as idiopathic hypoglycemia. It is also found in so-called insulin-sensitivity states, early diabetes mellitus, after partial gastrectomy, in starvation, and in certain leucine-sensitive states. The organic causes for hypoglycemia include, in addition to the beta-cell lesions already described, diffuse liver disease, the glycogenoses, hypofunction of the anterior pituitary and adrenal cortex, and a variety of extrapancreatic neoplasms. The association of hypoglycemia with these extrapancreatic neoplasms has excited considerable interest in the effort to elucidate the underlying mechanisms. Fibromas and fibrosarcomas located in the retroperitoneal space adjacent to the diaphragm or in the thorax predominate among these interesting problems. Also responsible, although less commonly, are such varied tumors as hepatic, adrenal, gastric, and bile duct carcinomas. All these tumors generally are of large size and, although many have metastasized, there is no linear correlation between the production of hypoglycemia and the total mass of tumor. Several studies have identified elevations of a circulating insulin-like substance (nonsuppressible insulin-like activity, NSILA), probably somatomedin, in patients with these tumors.[96]

ZOLLINGER-ELLISON SYNDROME (GASTRINOMA; ULCEROGENIC ISLET CELL TUMOR)

Reference has previously been made, in the consideration of peptic ulcer, to the syndrome described by Zollinger and Ellison: the association of pancreatic islet cell tumors with gastric hypersecretion and peptic ulceration.[97] Fundamental to the peptic ulcerations is gastric hypersecretion. The stimulus to such hypersecretion has been clearly established as gastrin, so the tumor is also known as a *gastrinoma*. Gastrin has been demonstrated in these tumors by radioimmunoassay and has been elaborated in cultures of tumor cells. Although most common in the pancreas, 10 to 15% of gastrinomas occur in the duodenum.

A definitive gastrin-producing cell in the *normal* human pancreas has not been identified. However, gastrin-producing cells in some of the more well-differentiated islet cell tumors have ultrastructural features similar to those of normal intestinal and gastric G cells, the latter known to be the source of gastrin in these tissues.[41]

In an extensive review of 260 of these lesions, approximately 60% were malignant, two-thirds having metastasized at the time of discovery, and 40% were benign. Only spread to lymph nodes or metastases marks the tumors as malignant. Some of the benign adenomas occurred multiply and in association with endocrine adenomas elsewhere, justifying their being classified as examples of multiple endocrine neoplasia.[97] Seventy-five per cent of the ulcers occur in the usual sites within the stomach or, more often, in the first and second portions of the duodenum. Abnormally located peptic ulcers in the distal portions of the duodenum and jejunum occur in 25% of cases. In one of ten patients, there are multiple ulcerations. The stomach also shows hyperplasia of the acid-secreting parietal cells.[98]

Patients with the Zollinger-Ellison syndrome present formidable problems in clinical management. They have striking gastric hypersecretion, which presumably produces the intractable ulcers. In addition, diarrhea is often sufficiently extreme to cause serious problems in fluid and electrolyte control, and many patients develop malabsorption syndromes. Moreover, the lesions in the pancreas not only may be malignant but, even when benign, may be very small or multiple and difficult to discover at surgical exploration. It is not uncommon, therefore, for symptoms to be recurrent following removal of any apparent solitary lesion, with later discovery of additional lesions within the pancreas.

MULTIPLE ENDOCRINE NEOPLASIA (MEN) SYNDROMES

These fascinating syndromes, as first described, comprised the common association of "multiple endocrine adenomas" of the pituitary, pancreas, and parathyroid glands. Wermer[99] expanded this entity when he noted the frequent occurrence of peptic ulcers in these patients. He further postulated a familial distribution, now defined as an autosomal dominant mode of transmission with incomplete penetrance. Almost contemporaneously, the Zollinger-Ellison syndrome was described, associating some non–insulin-producing islet cell tumors of the pancreas with peptic ulcers. Since these original descriptions, the Zollinger-Ellison syndome has been noted in individuals with multiple endocrine tumors, and families have been identified in which one member had the Zollinger-Ellison syndrome while others had multiple adenomas. Currently, it is believed that multiple endocrine tumors and the Zollinger-Ellison syndrome are phenotypic variants of the same mutant gene. Because some of these tumors are malignant, the term multiple endocrine neoplasia (MEN) has replaced the older designation of multiple endocrine adenomatosis.[100]

The MEN syndromes have been further subdivided into several types, depending on the organs involved and the presence or absence of peptic ulcerations (Table 20–2). MEN I consists of tumors or hyperplasias of the parathyroid glands, pituitary, adrenal cortex, and pancreas; together with peptic ulcerations and gastric hypersecretion. In contrast, MEN II (Sipple syndrome) is characterized by multiple pheochromocytomas (tumors of the adrenal medulla), medullary carcinoma of the thyroid (p. 000), and parathyroid hyperplasia or adenoma, *but no pancreatic islet cell tumors or peptic ulceration*. In some families with MEN II, there is, in addition to the tumors described, a distinctive constellation of mucocutaneous lesions, including neuromas of the eyelids, tongue, lips, intestines, bronchus, and bladder. To these, the term MEN IIb or MEN III has been given, to differentiate them from MEN IIa, in which mucocutaneous neuromas are not present. Table 20–2 indicates the areas of overlap of MEN I and MEN II. It is evident that MEN I comprises, in essence, polyendocrine involvement associated with peptic ulcers. In contrast, MEN II is better remembered as the medullary carcinoma–pheochromocytoma syndrome not associated with peptic ulcers. Both patterns of MEN are familial. Other variants have been segregated, strongly suggesting a spectrum of familial disorders arising out of specific gene mutations or variable expressions of a common mutant gene.

It is impossible even to summarize the range of clinical presentations that may be encountered in MEN I and MEN II. In the individual patient, one or two of the functioning lesions usually overshadow the others. Among the more frequent presentations are: (1) intractable peptic ulcer disease; (2) evidence of hyperparathyroidism; (3) manifestations arising in the pancreatic islet lesions, such as hyperinsulinism; (4) Cushing's syndrome; and (5) hypertension related to the pheochromocytoma.

RARE ISLET CELL TUMORS

Alpha-cell tumors (glucagonomas) are associated with increased serum levels of glucagon and a syndrome consisting of mild diabetes mellitus, a characteristic migratory necrotizing skin erythema, and anemia. *Delta-cell tumors* (somatostatinoma) are associated with diabetes mellitus, cholelithiasis, steatorrhea, and hypochlorhydria and are exceedingly difficult to detect pre-

Table 20–2. MULTIPLE ENDOCRINE NEOPLASIA SYNDROMES

Lesions	MEN I	MEN IIa	MEN IIb or III
Pituitary	+ + + +	0	0
Medullary carcinoma of thyroid	+	+ + + +	+ + + +
Parathyroid	+ + + +	+ +	+
Adrenal cortex	+ + + +	+	+
Pheochromocytoma	0	+ + + +	+ + + +
Pancreas	+ + + +	0	0
Peptic ulcer	+ + + +	0	0
Mucocutaneous neuromas	0	0	+ + + +

operatively. Polypeptide-secreting islet cell tumors[102] are endocrinologically asymptomatic. *Vipoma* is an islet cell tumor that induces a characteristic syndrome of *watery diarrhea*, *hypokalemia*, and *achlorhydria* (the WDHA syndrome), and is caused by release of vasoactive intestinal peptide (VIP) from the tumor. Pancreatic *carcinoid tumors* producing serotonin and an atypical carcinoid syndrome are exceedingly rare.

Some pancreatic and extrapancreatic tumors produce two or more hormones, usually simultaneously and occasionally in sequence. In addition to insulin, glucagon, and gastrin, islet cell tumors produce ACTH, MSH, vasopressin, norepinephrine, and serotonin. These are called *multihormonal tumors* to distinguish them from the multiple endocrine neoplasias described earlier, in which a multiplicity of hormones are produced by several different glands.

---

1. Ermak, T. H., et al.: The pancreas. Anatomy, embryology, and developmental anomalies. *In* Sleisenger, M. H., and Fordtran, J. S. (eds.): Gastrointestinal Disease. Pathophysiology, Diagnosis, Management. 3rd ed. Philadelphia, W. B. Saunders Co., 1983, p. 1415.
2. Meyer, J. H.: Pancreatic physiology. *In* Sleisenger, M. H., and Fordtran, J. S. (eds.): Gastrointestinal Disease. Pathophysiology, Diagnosis, Management. 3rd ed. Philadelphia, W. B. Saunders Co., 1983, p. 1426.
3. Fitzgerald, P. J., and Morrison, A. B. (eds.): The Pancreas. Baltimore, Williams & Wilkins Co., 1980.
4. Douglas, H. D., et al.: The significance of pancreatic heterotopia in relation to cancer of the head of the pancreas. Gastroenterology *59*:860, 1970.
5. Longnecker, D. S.: Pathology and pathogenesis of diseases of the pancreas. Am. J. Pathol. *107*:103, 1982.
6. Paloyan, D. (ed.): Pancreatitis. New Hyde Park, New York Medical Examination Publishing, 1983.
7. Lebenthal, E.: Pancreatic function and disease in infancy and childhood. Adv. Pediatr. *25*:223, 1978.
8. Sarles, H., et al.: Observations on 205 cases of confirmed cases of pancreatitis. Gut *6*:545, 1965.
9. Hermon-Taylor, J.: An etiological and therapeutic review of acute pancreatitis. Br. J. Hosp. Med. *18*:546, 1977.
10. Warshaw, A. L., and O'Hara, P. J.: Susceptibility of the pancreas to ischemic injury in shock. Ann. Surg. *188*:197, 1978.
11. Mallory, A., and Kern, F.: Drug-induced pancreatitis: A critical review. Gastroenterology *78*:813, 1980.
12. Cameron, J. L., et al.: Acute pancreatitis with hyperlipidemia. Surgery *70*:53, 1971.
13. Bess, N. A., et al.: Hyperparathyroidism and pancreatitis. Chance or a causal association? J.A.M.A. *243*:246, 1980.
14. Schmidt, H., and Creutzfeldt, W.: Etiology and pathogenesis of pancreatitis. *In* Bockus, H. L. (ed.): Gastroenterology. 3rd ed. Vol. III. Philadelphia, W. B. Saunders Co., 1976, p. 1005.
15. Lombardi, B.: Pathogenesis of ethioinine-induced pancreatic necrosis. Panminerva Med. *18*:359, 1976.
16. Keith, R. G.: Symposium on pancreatitis. Can. J. Surg. *21*:56, 1978.
17. Longnecker, D. S.: Environmental factors and diseases of the pancreas. Environ. Health Perspect. *20*:105, 1977.
18. Kelly, T. R., and Swaney, P.: Gallstone pancreatitis: The second time around. Surgery *92*:571, 1982.
19. Sum, P. T., et al.: Pathogenesis of bile-induced acute pancreatitis in the dog. Am. J. Dig. Dis. *15*:637, 1970.
20. Sarles, H., and Sahel, J.: Pathology of chronic calcifying pancreatitis. Am. J. Gastroenterol. *66*:117, 1976.
21. Kelly, T. R.: Gallstone pancreatitis. Pathophysiology. Surgery *80*:488, 1976.
22. Cameron, J., et al.: A pathogenesis for alcoholic pancreatitis. Surgery *77*:754, 1975.
23. Saharia, P., et al.: Acute pancreatitis with hyperlipemia: Studies with an isolated perfused canine pancreas. Surgery *82*:60, 1977.
24. Goebell, H.: The role of calcium in pancreatic secretion and disease. Acta Hepatogastroenterol. (Stuttg.) *23*:151, 1976.
25. Foulis, A. K., et al.: Endotoxemia and complement activation in pancreatitis. Gut *23*:656, 1982.
26. Richter, J. M., et al.: Association of pancreatic divisum and pancreatitis, and its treatment by sphincteroplasty of the accessory ampulla. Gastroenterology *81*:1104, 1981.
27. Sarles, H., et al.: Chronic pancreatitis, relapsing pancreatitis, calcifications of the pancreas. Part 1: Pathology. *In* Bockus, H. L. (ed.): Gastroenterology. 3rd ed. Vol. III. Philadelphia, W. B. Saunders Co., 1976, p. 1040.
28. Vennes, J. A.: Chronic pancreatitis. Gastroenterology *82*:1471, 1982.
29. Grendell, J. H., and Cello, J. P.: Chronic pancreatitis. *In* Sleisenger, M. H., and Fordtran, J. S. (eds.): Gastrointestinal Disease. Pathophysiology, Diagnosis, Management. 3rd ed. Philadelphia, W. B. Saunders Co., 1983, p. 1485.
30. Winship, D., et al.: Pancreatitis: Pancreatic pseudocysts and their complications. Gastroenterology *73*:593, 1977.
31. Cubrilla, A., and Fitzgerald, P. J.: Pancreatic cancer. 1. Duct carcinoma. Pathol. Annu. *13*:241, 1978.
32. Moosa, A. R. (ed.): Tumors of the Pancreas. Baltimore, Williams & Wilkins Co., 1980.
33. Beazley, R. M., and Cohn, I.: Pancreatic cancer. CA *31*:346, 1981.
34. Silverberg, E.: Cancer statistics 1983. CA *33*:9, 1983.
35. Wynder, E. L., et al.: Epidemiology of cancer of the pancreas. J. Natl. Cancer Inst. *50*:645, 1973; Cancer Res. *35*:228, 1977.
36. Pour, P., et al.: Current knowledge of pancreatic carcinogenesis and its relevance to human disease. Cancer *47*:1573, 1981.
37. MacMahon, B., et al.: Coffee and cancer of the pancreas. N. Engl. J. Med. *304*:630, 1981.
38. Levin, D. C., et al.: Demographic characteristics of cancer of the pancreas: mortality, incidence and survival. Cancer *47*:1456, 1981.
39. Haubrick, W. S., and Berk, J. E.: Tumors of the pancreas. Part 1: Medical aspects of exocrine tumors. *In* Bockus, H. L. (ed.): Gastroenterology. 3rd ed. Vol. III. Philadelphia, W. B. Saunders Co., 1976, p. 1102.
40. Cohn, I., Jr., and Hasting, P. R. (eds.): Pancreatic Cancer. UICC Technical Report Series-Geneva, International Union Against Cancer, Vol. 57, No. 12, 1981.
41. Bloodworth, J. M. B., Jr., and Greider, M. H.: The endocrine pancreas and diabetes mellitus. *In* Bloodworth, J. M. B., Jr. (ed.): Endocrine Pathology. Baltimore, Williams & Wilkins Co., 1982, pp. 556–720.
42. Lacy, P. E.: Islet cell functional pathology. Pathol. Annu. *12*(part 1):1, 1977.
43. Larson, L. I.: Endocrine pancreatic tumors. Hum. Pathol. *9*:401, 1978.
44. Munger, B. L.: Morphological characterization of islet cell diversity. *In*: Cooperstein, S. J., and Watkins, D. (eds.): The Islets of Langerhans: Biochemistry, Physiology and Pathology. New York, Academic Press, 1981, p. 3.
45. Erlandson, S. E., et al.: Pancreatic islet cell hormones. Distribution of cell types in the islet and evidence for the presence of somatostatin and gastrin within the D cell. J. Histochem. Cytochem. *24*:883, 1976.
46. Bennett, P. H.: The diagnosis of diabetes: New international classification and diagnostic criteria. Annu. Rev. Med. *34*:295, 1983.
47. Foster, D. W.: Diabetes mellitus. *In* Stanbury, J. B., et al. (eds.): The Metabolic Basis of Inherited Disease. 5th ed. New York, McGraw-Hill Book Co., 1982, p. 101.
48. Barnett, A. H., et al.: Diabetes in identical twins: A study of 200 pairs. Diabetologia *20*:57, 1981.
49. Porte, D., Jr., and Pupo, A. A.: Insulin responses to glucose. Evidence for a two-pool system in man. J. Clin. Invest. *48*:2309, 1969.
50. Lebovitz, H. E.: Drugs enhancing insulin secretion. *In* Fajans, S. S. (ed.): Diabetes Mellitus. USDHEW Publication (NIH)76-854. Bethesda, National Institutes of Health, 1976, p. 327.
51. Karnieli, E., et al.: Insulin stimulated translocation of glucose transport system in the isolated fat adipose cell. Time course, reversal, insulin concentration dependency, and relationship to glucose transport activity. J. Biol. Chem. *256*:4772, 1981.
52. Flier, J. S.: Insulin receptors and insulin resistance. Annu. Rev. Med. *34*:145, 1983.
53. Larner, J.: Mediators of post-receptor action of insulin. Am. J. Med. *74*:Vol. 1A (Suppl.) 38, 1983.
54. Jarret, L., et al.: The chemical mediators of insulin action: Possible targets for post-receptor defects. Am. J. Med. *74*:1A (Suppl.) 31, 1983.
55. Craighead, J. E.: The role of viruses and the pathogenesis of pancreatic disease and diabetes mellitus. Prog. Med. Virol. *19*:161, 1975.
56. Menser, M. A., et al.: Rubella infection and diabetes mellitus. Lancet *1*:57, 1978.
57. Yoon, J., et al.: Virus induced diabetes mellitus. Isolation of a virus from the pancreas of a child with diabetic ketoacidosis. N. Engl. J. Med. *300*:1173, 1979.
58. Craighead, J. E.: Viral diabetes. *In* Volk, B. W., and Wellman, K. F. (eds.): The Diabetic Pancreas. New York, Plenum Press, 1977, p. 467.

58A. Srikanta, S., et al.: Type I diabetes mellitus in monozygotic twins: Chronic progressive beta cell dysfunction. Ann. Intern. Med. *99*:320, 1983.

59. Doniach, D., et al.: Etiology of type I diabetes mellitus: Heterogeneity

and immunologic events leading to clinical onset. Annu. Rev. Med. *23*:13, 1983.
60. Cahill, G. F., and McDevitt, H. O.: Insulin-dependent diabetes mellitus: The initial lesion. N. Engl. J. Med. *304*:1454, 1981.
61. Editorial. Type II diabetes: Towards improved understanding and rational therapy. Diabetes Care *5*:447, 1982.
62. Defronzo, R. A., et al.: New concepts in the pathogenesis and treatment of non–insulin-dependent diabetes mellitus. Am. J. Med. *74*:1A (Suppl.) 52, 1983.
63. Pfeifer, M. A., et al.: Insulin secretion in diabetes mellitus. Am. J. Med. *70*:579, 1981.
64. Weir, G. C.: Non–insulin-dependent diabetes mellitus: Interplay between beta-cell inadequacy and insulin resistance. Am. J. Med. *73*:461, 1982.
65. Kolterman, O. G., et al.: Insulin resistance in non–insulin-dependent diabetes mellitus: Impact of sulfonylurea agents *in vivo* and *in vitro*. Am. J. Med. *74*:1A (Suppl.) 82, 1983.
66. Olefsky, J. M., and Kolterman, O. G.: Mechanism of insulin resistance in obesity and non–insulin-dependent (type II) diabetes. *In* Skyler, J. S., and Cahill, G. F. (eds.): Diabetes Mellitus. New York, Yorke Medical Books, 1981, p. 73.
67. Scarlet, J. A., et al.: Insulin treatment reverses the insulin resistance of type II diabetes mellitus. Diabetes Care *5*:353, 1982.
68. Vracko, R., and Benditt, E. P.: Manifestations of diabetes mellitus—their possible relationships to an underlying cell defect. Am. J. Pathol. *75*:204, 1974.
69. Unger, R. H., and Orci, L.: Glucagon and the A cell: Physiology and pathophysiology. N. Engl. J. Med. *304*:1518, 1575, 1981.
70. Barnes, A. J., et al.: Persistent metabolic abnormalities in diabetes in the absence of glucagon. Diabetologia *13*:71, 1977.
71. Gepts, W., and LeCompte, P. M.: The pancreatic islets in diabetes. *In* Skyler, J. S., and Cahill, G. F. (eds.): Diabetes Mellitus. New York, Yorke Medical Books, 1981, p. 1.
72. Wellmann, K. F., and Volk, B.: Islets of Langerhans structure and function in diabetes. Pathobiol. Annu. *5*:105, 1980.
73. Bennett, P. H., et al.: Diabetes mellitus in American (Pima) Indians. Lancet *2*:125, 1971.
74. Vracko, R.: A comparison of the microvascular lesions in diabetes mellitus with those of normal aging. J. Am. Geriatr. Sco. *30*:201, 1982.
75. Martinez-Hernandez, A., et al.: The basement membrane in pathology. Lab. Invest. *48*:656, 1983.
76. Cohen, P. M., et al.: Nonenzymatic glycosylation of glomerular basement membrane. Renal Physiol. *4*:90, 1981.
77. Kefalides, N. A.: Basement membrane: Structure function relationships. Renal Physiol. 4:57, 1981.
78. Rohrbach, D. H., and Martin, G. R.: Structure of basement membrane in normal and diabetic tissue. Ann. N.Y. Acad. Sci. *401*:203, 1982.
79. Kanwar, Y. S., et al.: Decreased de-novo synthesis of glomerular proteoglycans in diabetes: Biochemical and autoradiographic evidence. Proc. Natl. Acad. Sci. U.S.A. *80*:2272, 1983.
80. Ganda, O. P.: Pathogenesis of macrovascular disease in the human diabetic. Diabetes *29*:931, 1980.
81. Bell, E. T.: Renal vascular disease in diabetes mellitus. Diabetes *2*:376, 1953.
82. Factor, S. M., et al.: Capillary microaneurysms in the human diabetic heart. N. Engl. J. Med. *302*:384, 1980.
83. Smith, M. E., and Becker, B.: Ocular complications in diabetes. *In* Fajans, S. S. (ed.): Diabetes Mellitus. USDHEW Publication (NIH)76-854.
Bethesda, National Institutes of Health, 1976, p. 213.
84. Colby, A. O.: Neurologic disorders of diabetes mellitus. Diabetes *14*:424, 1965.
85. Clements, R. S., Jr., and Bell, D. S. H.: Diabetic neuropathy: Peripheral and autonomic syndromes. Postgrad. Med. *71*:50, 1982.
86. Winegrad, A. I., et al.: Has one diabetic complication been explained? N. Engl. J. Med. *308*:152, 1983.
87. Siperstein, M. D.: Diabetic microangiopathy and the control of blood glucose. N. Engl. J. Med. *309*:1577, 1983.
88. Raskin, P., et al.: The effect of diabetic control on the width of skeletal-muscle capillary basement membrane in patients with type I diabetes mellitus. N. Engl. J. Med. *309*:1546, 1983.
89. Camerini-Davalos, R. A., et al.: Drug-induced reversal of early diabetic microangiopathy. N. Engl. J. Med. *309*:1551, 1983.
90. Abouna, G. M., et al.: Reversal of diabetic nephropathy in human cadaveric kidneys after transplantation into non-diabetic recipients. Lancet *2*:1274, 1983.
91. Doran, T. L., et al.: Genetic susceptibility to the development of retinopathy in insulin-dependent diabetics. Diabetes *31*:226, 1982.
92. Bale, G. S., and Entmacher, P. S.: Estimated life expectancy of diabetics. Diabetes *26*:434, 1977.
93. Oakley, W. G., et al.: Long-term diabetes. A clinical study of 92 patients after 40 years. Q. J. Med. *43*:145, 1974.
94. Freisen, S. R.: Tumors of the endocrine pancreas. N. Engl. J. Med. *306*:580, 1982.
95. Hoard, J. M., et al.: Hyperinsulinism and islet cell tumors of the pancreas (with 398 recorded tumors). Int. Abstr. Surg. *90*:417, 1950.
96. Plovnick, H., et al.: Non–beta-cell tumor hypoglycemia associated with increased nonsuppressible insulin-like protein (NSILP). Am. J. Med. *661*:154, 1979.
97. Ellison, E. H., and Wilson, S. D.: The Zollinger-Ellison syndrome: Reappraisal and evaluation of 260 registered cases. Ann. Surg. *160*:512, 1964.
98. Solcia, E., et al.: Pathology of the Ellison-Zollinger syndrome. Prog. Surg. Pathol. *1*:119, 1980.
99. Wermer, P.: Endocrine adenomatosis and peptic ulcer in a large kindred: Inherited multiple tumors and mosaic pleiotropism in man. Am. J. Med. *35*:205, 1963.
100. Sherwood, C. M., and Gould, U. E.: Ectopic hormone syndromes and multiple endocrine neoplasias. *In* DeGroot, L. (ed.): Endocrinology. New York, Academic Press, 1977.
101. Creutzfeldt, W.: Endocrine tumors of the pancreas *In* Fitzgerald, P., and Morrison A. (eds.): The Pancreas. Baltimore, Williams & Wilkins Co., 1980.
102. Tomita, T., et al.: Pancreatic polypeptide-secreting islet-cell tumors. A study of three cases. Am. J. Pathol. *113*:134, 1983.

THE KIDNEY 21

NORMAL

The story-teller of Isak Dinesen's *Seven Gothic Tales* defined man as an ingenious machine designed to turn, with "infinite artfulness, the red wine of Shiraz into urine." More accurately but less poetically, human kidneys serve to convert over 1700 liters of blood per day into about 1 liter of a highly specialized concentrated fluid called urine. In so doing, the kidney performs some of the most critical functions necessary for survival. It excretes the waste products of metabolism, precisely regulates the body's concentration of water and salt, maintains the appropriate acid balance of plasma, and serves as an endocrine organ, secreting such important hormones as erythropoietin, renin, and prostaglandins. The physiologic mechanisms that the kidney has evolved to carry out these functions require a high degree of structural complexity. An understanding of kidney diseases requires a thorough knowledge of its structure and the interrelationships and interdependence of its various components.

Embryologically, the adult kidney, or the metanephros, is formed after two primitive attempts have regressed—the pronephros and mesonephros.[1] The renal collecting system is derived from the main excretory duct of the earlier pronephros, now termed the *wolffian duct.* This duct branches, forming the renal calyces and the collecting tubules. The functioning nephrons derived from the metanephric anlage become attached to the growing ends of the collecting system. Thus, in developmental abnormalities, there may be developmental failure of the metanephric anlage, of the collecting system, or of both.

Each human adult kidney weighs about 150 gm. As the ureter enters the kidney at the hilus, it dilates into a funnel-shaped cavity, *the pelvis,* from which derive two to three main branches, the *major calyces;* the latter subdivide again into about three to four *minor calyces.* There are about 12 minor calyces in the human kidney. On cut surface, the kidney is made up of a *cortex* and a *medulla,* the former 1.2 to 1.5 cm in thickness. The medulla consists of *renal pyramids,* the apices of which are called *papillae,* each related to a calyx. Cortical tissue extends into spaces between adjacent pyramids as the *renal columns of Bertin.* From the standpoint of its diseases the kidney can be divided into four components: blood vessels, glomeruli, tubules, and interstitium.

BLOOD VESSELS. The kidney is richly supplied by blood vessels, and although both kidneys make up only 0.5% of the total body weight, they receive about 25% of the cardiac output. Of this, the cortex is by far the more richly vascularized, receiving 90% of the total renal circulation. In humans, the main renal artery divides into anterior and posterior sections at the hilus. From these, *interlobar arteries* emerge and course between lobes. As they reach the corticomedullary junction, they give rise to the *arcuate arteries,* which arch between cortex and medulla, in turn giving rise to the *interlobular arteries,* which run perpendicular to the cortical surface. From the interlobular arteries, *afferent arterioles* enter the glomerular tuft where they progressively subdivide into 20 to 40 capillary loops arranged in several units or lobules. Capillary loops ultimately merge together to exit from the glomerulus as *efferent arterioles.* From the efferent arterioles, the subsequent course of capillaries varies considerably. In general, efferent arterioles from superficial nephrons form a rich vascular network that encircles cortical tubules (*peritubular vascular network*), while deeper juxtamedullary glomeruli give rise to the *vasa recta,* which descend as straight vessels to supply the outer and inner medulla. These descending arterial vasa recta then make several loops in the inner medulla and ascend as the *venous vasa recta.*

The anatomy of renal vessels has several important implications. First, because the arteries are largely end arteries, occlusion of any branch results in infarction of the specific area it supplies. It must also be evident that glomerular disease that interferes with blood flow through the glomerular capillaries must have profound effects on the tubules, within both the cortex and the medulla, since all tubular capillary beds are derived from the efferent arterioles. The peculiarities of the blood supply to the renal medulla render them especially vulnerable to ischemia; the medulla is relatively avascular and the capillary loops in the medulla have a remarkably low hematocrit. Thus, any minor interference with the blood supply of the medulla may result in medullary necrosis. The renal cortex, on the other hand, is more vulnerable to hypertensive changes, since the normal pressure in glomerular capillaries is higher than in other capillary beds, and elevations of blood pressure in the aorta are transmitted to the afferent arterioles.

GLOMERULUS. The glomerulus is a vascular-epithelial organ designed for the ultrafiltration of plasma. Embryologically, it is formed by an invagination of a capillary-containing mesenchymal mass into an epithelium-lined sac, Bowman's space. The epithelium that invests the capillary network (visceral epithelium) is incorporated into and becomes an intrinsic part of the

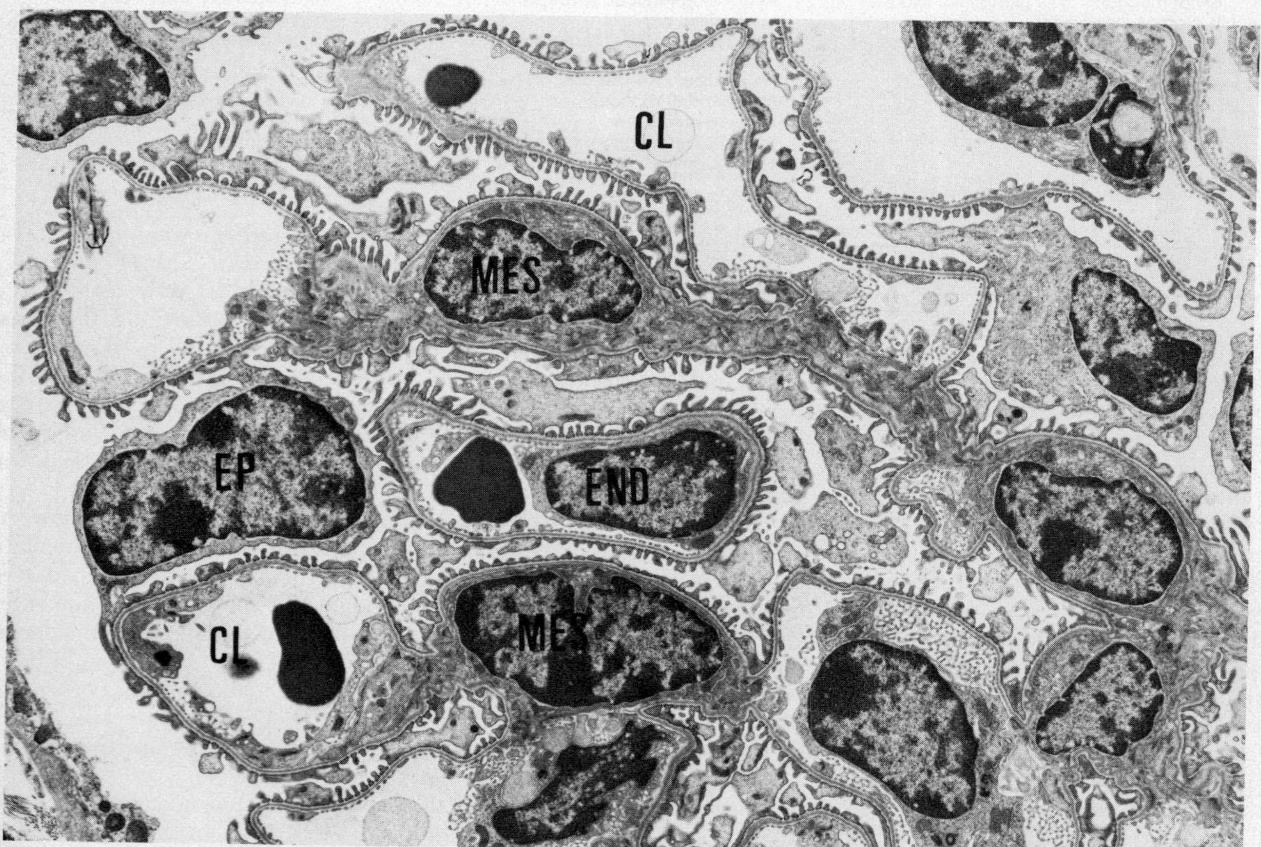

Figure 21–1. Low-power electron micrograph of mouse renal glomerulus. CL = capillary lumen; MES = mesangium; END = endothelium; EP = visceral epithelial cells with foot processes. (Courtesy of Dr. Vicki Kelley, Brigham and Women's Hospital.)

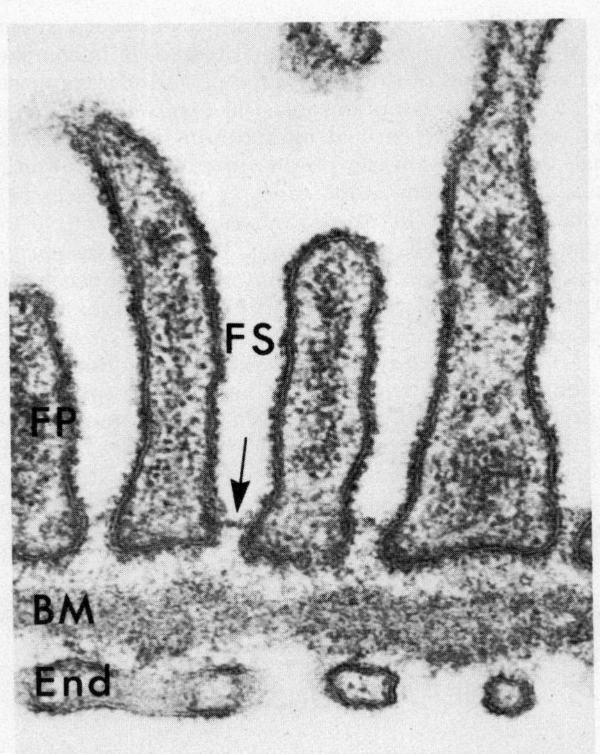

Figure 21–2. Glomerular filter consisting of fenestrated endothelium (End), basement membrane (BM), and foot processes (FP). FS = filtration slit. Arrow indicates the slit diaphragm.

filtration membrane, whereas the parietal epithelium lines Bowman's space, the cavity in which plasma filtrate first collects. From the capillary lumen to the urinary space (Figs. 21–1 and 21–2), the filtering membrane consists of:[2] (1) a thin layer of fenestrated *endothelial cells*, each fenestrum being about 70 to 100 nm in diameter; (2) a *glomerular basement membrane* (GBM) about 320 nm wide in the human adult, with a thick central electron-dense layer, the *lamina densa*, and peripheral thinner electron lucent layers, the *lamina rara interna and externa*; and (3) the *visceral epithelial cells* (podocytes). Podocytes are structurally complex cells that possess interdigitating processes embedded in and adherent to the lamina rara externa of the basement membrane. Adjacent *foot processes* (pedicels) are separated by 20 to 30 nm wide *filtration slits*, which are bridged by a thin diaphragm that, when viewed en face, exhibits an orderly structure with multiple repeating rectangular pores each about 4 by 14 nm, in the shape of a zipper.

Several biochemical components are present in the GBM (Fig. 21–2).[3] (1) *Collagen type IV* occupies all three layers and accounts for about 50% of dry weight of GBM; collagen is presumably responsible for the structural strength of the capillary wall. (2) *Laminin* is present throughout the GBM but concentrated in both laminae rarae; it probably plays a role in the adhesion and attachment of endothelial and epithelial cells to the matrix. (3) *Polyanionic proteoglycans*, particularly heparan sulfate, are distributed in clusters, spaced at 50- to 60-nm intervals, along both laminae rarae.[4] As we shall see, they are thought to account—at least in part—for the so-called *glomerular polyanion* responsible for the charge-dependent glomerular filtration barrier. (4) *Entactin* is a newly discovered glycoprotein of uncertain role. (5) *Fibronectin* is distributed in small amounts in the laminae rarae, but there is some question whether it represents filtered plasma fibronectin or an intrinsic component of the GBM.[3] In addition to these components, an anionic sialoglycoprotein layer coats the surface of endothelial and visceral epithelial cells.

The main function of the glomerulus is filtration. Two characteristics distinguish glomerular filtration from transcapillary exchange in other organs: (1) the glomerulus almost completely excludes plasma proteins of the size of albumin (M.W. ± 70,000, radius 3.6 nm) and larger from the filtrate; and (2) it exhibits an extraordinarily high permeability to water and small solutes. The latter can be accounted for by the highly fenestrated endothelium and the presence of the epithelial slits, both of which allow free passage of fluid.

Physiologic studies indicate that the filtration of macromolecules across the glomerulus decreases with increasing effective molecular radius, approaching zero at a radius of approximately 3.5 nm.[5] There is thus a *size-dependent permeability barrier in the glomerulus.* From studies that employ particles visible under the electron microscope (e.g., ferritin, peroxidases of differing molecular weights, and dextrans), it appears that the *GBM is the principal structure responsible for this size discrimination*, although admittedly a pore of appropriate dimensions (3.5 nm) has not been resolved.[6] Alterations in the structure and composition of the GBM are thus central to the leakage of proteins and blood cells characteristic of glomerular injury.

In addition to size, clearance studies using dextrans and protein molecules of different isoelectric points (pI) demonstrate that the *glomerulus can discriminate among molecules according to their charge*, allowing greater penetration of neutral and cationic molecules as compared with anionic molecules of the same size.[5, 7] This charge-dependent restriction is important in the virtually complete exclusion of albumin from the filtrate, since albumin is an anionic molecule of a pI ± 4.5. Charge selectivity is dependent on the presence of the negatively charged glomerular polyanions described above, including heparan sulfate proteoglycan.[6] It follows, therefore, that loss of glomerular polyanion may result in increased filtration of proteins.[8]

Another important component of the glomerulus is the *mesangium*, also called the centrilobular or axial region (Fig. 21–1).[8A] The mesangium forms a branching supportive framework around which the anastomosing capillaries of individual glomerular lobules ramify. It consists of stellate *mesangial cells* embedded in a basement membrane–like PAS-positive glycoprotein—the *mesangial matrix*. The mesangial matrix is composed of the same biochemical components as the GBM. Mesangial cells are clearly contractile;[9] by their contraction in response to neurohormonal agents they are thought to modulate intraglomerular blood flow under physiologic conditions. Mesangial cells are also endocytic and can serve to ingest macromolecules that may have leaked across the glomerulus. Small numbers of Ia-positive phagocytic cells are present in the normal rat glomerulus;[10] these may be involved in phagocytosis of larger particles and in local immune reactions within the glomerulus. In normal glomeruli the mesangial area is narrow and contains a small number of cells and scant matrix. However, mesangial cell hyperplasia, increased mesangial matrix, and infiltration of the mesangium by circulating leukocytes are seen in a variety of glomerular diseases.

TUBULES. The structure of renal tubular epithelial cells varies considerably at different levels of the nephron and, to a certain extent, correlates with the functional capacity of the tubular segment. For example, the highly developed structure of the *proximal tubular cells,* with their abundant long microvilli (which appear in histologic sections as the brush border), numerous mitochondria, apical canaliculi, and extensive intercellular interdigitations, may be correlated with its major functions: reabsorption of two-thirds of filtered sodium and water as well as glucose, potassium, phosphate, amino acids, and proteins. A sodium pump is thought to be located in the basal lateral labyrinth of the proximal tubular cells; operation of the pump is by the action of the membrane-bound Na^{+}-K^{+} ATPase and closely situated mitochondria, which supply energy through oxidative phosphorylation. It is thus no surprise that the proximal tubule is particularly vulnerable to ischemic damage. Furthermore, toxins are frequently reabsorbed by the proximal tubule, rendering it also susceptible to chemical injury.

A remarkable structure, the *juxtaglomerular apparatus* (JG),[11] snuggles closely against the glomerulus where the afferent arteriole enters it. The JG apparatus consists of (1) *the juxtaglomerular cells,* modified granulated smooth muscle cells in the media of the afferent arteriole that contain the hormone renin; (2) *the macula densa,* a specialized region of the distal tubule as the latter returns to the vascular pole of its parent glomerulus—here the tubular cells are more crowded and the cells are somewhat shorter and possess distinct patterns of interdigitation between adjacent membranes; and (3) *the lacis cells* or *nongranular cells,* which reside in the area bounded by the afferent arteriole, the macula densa, and the glomerulus. They resemble mesangial cells and appear to be continuous with them. The JG apparatus is a small endocrine organ, the JG cells being the principal source of renin production in the kidney. As we shall discuss (p. 1042), excessive renin production is implicated in the pathogenesis of several types of hypertension.

INTERSTITIUM. The renal *interstitium* is an important component of the kidney, since it appears to be the primary site of reactivity in a variety of renal diseases. In the normal cortex, the interstitial space is compact, being occupied by the fenestrated peritubular capillaries and a small number of fibroblast-like cells.[12] Any obvious expansion of the cortical interstitium is usually abnormal; this expansion can be due to edema or infiltration with acute inflammatory cells, as in acute interstitial diseases, or may be caused by accumulation of chronic inflammatory cells and fibrous tissue, as in chronic interstitial diseases. The amount of mucopolysaccharide in the interstitial tissue of the medulla increases with age and in the presence of ischemia.

The kidneys are *innervated* by both cholinergic and adrenergic fibers from the autonomic nervous system. Nerve endings are present in the smooth muscle cells of the vascular tree and near the tubules, but the glomeruli are not innervated. Sympathetic stimulation appears to be an important determinant of renin secretion (p. 1042).

PATHOLOGY

GENERAL CONSIDERATIONS

Disorders primary in the kidneys are responsible for a great deal of morbidity but fortunately are not major causes of mortality. To place the problem in some perspective, approximately 35,000 deaths are attributed yearly to renal disease in the United States, in contrast to about 750,000 to heart disease, 400,000 to cancer, and 200,000 to stroke. The mortality data do not give the whole picture, however; the morbidity is by no means insignificant. Millions of persons are affected annually by nonfatal kidney diseases, most notably infections of the kidney or lower urinary tract, kidney stones, and obstruction to the free flow of urine. Urinary infection constitutes the second most common bacterial disease in clinical practice; 20% of all women suffer from infection of the urinary tract or kidney at some time in their lives. At least 1% of the U.S. population develop renal stones during their lifetime. Similarly, dialysis and transplantation programs keep many patients alive who would formerly have died of renal failure, adding to the pool of renal morbidity.[13] The cost of such programs now exceeds 2 billion dollars annually. Renal disease also has special importance to the clinician because so many of the deaths occur in young people.

Traditionally, diseases of the kidney have been divided into those that affect the four basic morphologic components: glomeruli, tubules, interstitium, and blood vessels. This is generally a useful approach, since the early manifestations of disease affecting each of these components tend to be distinct. Further, some components appear to be more vulnerable to specific forms of renal injury; for example, *glomerular diseases are most often immunologically mediated, whereas tubular and interstitial disorders are more likely to be caused by toxic or infectious agents.* Nevertheless, the anatomic interdependence of structure in the kidney implies that damage to one almost always secondarily affects the others. Disease primary in the blood vessels, for example, inevitably affects all the structures dependent on this blood supply. Severe glomerular damage impairs the flow through the peritubular vascular system; conversely, tubular destruction, by increasing intraglomerular pressure, may induce glomerular atrophy. Thus, whatever the origin, there is a tendency for all forms of chronic renal disease ultimately to destroy all four components of the kidney, culminating in chronic renal failure and what has been called *end-stage contracted kidneys.* The functional reserve of the kidney is large, and much damage may occur before there is evident functional impairment. For these reasons, the early signs and symptoms are particularly important to the clinician.

Some suggestions for an approach to the morphologic diagnosis of renal disease may be worth detailing. In the *gross inspection* of the kidney, attention should be directed to its size; the presence of cortical scars; the presence of focal lesions such as abscesses, tumors, or cysts; and the integrity of the papillae and the pelvic and calyceal systems. Generally, except for polycystic kidney disease and sometimes amyloidosis and diabetes, chronic renal diseases produce scarred kidneys that are smaller than normal. The presence of necrotic papillae on gross examination limits the diagnosis to a small number of diseases—diabetes, obstruction, pyelonephritis, sickle cell disease, and analgesic nephropathy—and the presence of calyceal deformity almost always indicates chronic pyelonephritis.

In *histologic* examination of the kidney, each component requires individual attention. Glomeruli, tubules, interstitium, and vessels should be systematically surveyed serially, in preference to a random scanning of the kidney for general impressions. By this approach, it is usually possible, especially early in the disease, to distinguish the principal point of attack from the secondary or concomitant alterations.

The widespread use of renal biopsy has changed our concepts of renal disease, particularly of the various types of glomerulonephritis. A number of special stains and techniques are used to highlight morphologic and immunologic details in such biopsies. These include:

(1) The **periodic acid–Schiff stain** (PAS), which outlines the basement membranes of glomeruli and tubules and highlights the mesangial matrix.

(2) **Silver impregnation** stains, which also mark the glomerular and tubular basement membranes (Fig. 21–3).

(3) **Immunofluorescence and immunoperoxidase studies,** which localize various types of immunoglobulins, antigens, complement, fibrin-related compounds, and cell surface markers.

(4) **Electron microscopy**, which is frequently essential in resolving the fine details of glomerular lesions.

(5) **Other special stains**, such as those for fibrin, amyloid, and lipids.

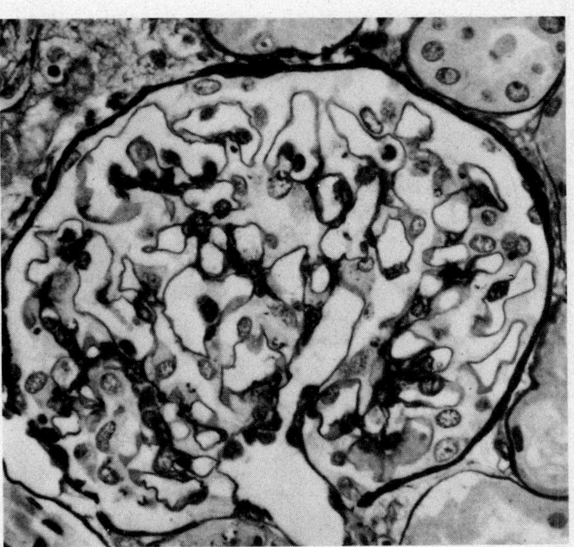

Figure 21–3. Glomerulus, stained with silver impregnation method. Note silver-positive (black) thin basement membranes of glomerulus and tubules.

CLINICAL AND PATHOPHYSIOLOGIC CONSIDERATIONS

THE MAJOR SYNDROMES

Clinical manifestations of renal disease vary according to the component of the kidney primarily affected, the acuteness of development of the disorder, and, to a certain extent, the mechanism of renal injury. In general, however, the clinical presentations can be grouped into ten reasonably well-defined syndromes.[14] Some of these are peculiar to glomerular diseases (p. 1003); others are present in diseases that affect any one of the components.

1. *Acute nephritic syndrome* is a glomerular syndrome dominated by the acute onset of usually grossly visible hematuria (red blood cells in the urine), mild-to-moderate proteinuria, and hypertension; it is the classic presentation of acute poststreptococcal glomerulonephritis (p. 1007).

2. *Rapidly progressive nephritis* is characterized by an acute or subacute onset dominated by hematuria and profound oliguria (reduced urine output), leading to renal failure in weeks (p. 1009).

3. *The nephrotic syndrome* is characterized by heavy proteinuria (over 3.5 gm per day), hypoalbuminemia, severe edema, hyperlipidemia, and lipiduria (lipid in the urine) (p. 1011).

4. *Asymptomatic hematuria, proteinuria,* or a combination of these two are usually manifestations of subtle or mild glomerular abnormalities.

5. *Chronic renal failure,* characterized by prolonged symptoms and signs of uremia (p. 996), is the end result of all chronic renal diseases.

6. *Acute renal failure* is dominated by oliguria or

anuria (no urine flow), with recent onset of azotemia (p. 1027).

7. *Hypertension* (p. 1041) may be either the result of several acute and chronic renal diseases or the direct cause of renal impairment (essential benign and malignant hypertension).

8. *Urinary tract infection* is characterized by bacteriuria and pyuria (bacteria and leukocytes in the urine). The infection may be *symptomatic* or *asymptomatic*, and may affect the kidney (*pyelonephritis*) or the bladder (*cystitis*) only (p. 1030).

9. *Nephrolithiasis* (renal stones) is manifested by renal colic, hematuria, and recurrent stone formation (p. 1052).

10. *Renal tubular defects* are dominated by polyuria (excessive urine formation), nocturia, and electrolyte disorders (e.g., metabolic acidosis). They are either the result of diseases directly affecting tubular structure (e.g., medullary cystic disease, p. 1001) or defects in specific tubular functions. The latter can be inherited (e.g., familial nephrogenic diabetes, cystinuria, renal tubular acidosis) or acquired (e.g., lead nephropathy).

In addition to these ten syndromes, *urinary tract obstruction* (p. 1051) and *renal tumors* (p. 1053) represent specific anatomic defects with often varied manifestations.

CHRONIC RENAL FAILURE

Acute renal failure implies a rapid and frequently reversible deterioration of renal function. As a characteristic syndrome with a complex pathogenesis, it is discussed separately on page 1027. Here we shall limit our discussion to chronic renal failure, which is the end result of a variety of renal diseases and is the major cause of death from renal disease.

Although the term *renal failure* appears quite explicit, implying renal function that is inadequate to maintain a normal internal milieu in both volume and composition, it has come to have a variety of interpretations. Some terminology must therefore be clarified. *Azotemia* is, strictly speaking, a biochemical abnormality that refers to an elevation of the blood urea nitrogen (BUN) and creatinine levels and is largely related to decreased glomerular filtration rate (GFR). Azotemia may, of course, be produced by many renal disorders, but it may also arise from extrarenal disorders. *Prerenal azotemia* is encountered when there is hypoperfusion of the kidneys, as occurs in congestive heart failure, shock, volume depletion, and hemorrhage, all of which impair renal function without parenchymal damage. Similarly, *postrenal azotemia* is seen whenever there is obstruction to urinary flow below the level of the kidney; if the obstruction is severe and protracted, it will inevitably produce renal lesions. Until such time, however, relief of the obstruction will be followed by prompt correction of the azotemia.

When azotemia becomes associated with a constellation of clinical signs and symptoms and biochemical abnormalities, it is termed uremia. Thus, uremia is a clinical syndrome, not merely a biochemical abnormality. It is characterized not only by failure of renal excretory function but also by a host of metabolic and endocrine alterations incident to renal damage. There are, in addition, secondary gastrointestinal, neuromuscular, and cardiovascular involvements, which are usually necessary for the diagnosis of uremia. Uremia is thus the sine qua non of symptomatic chronic renal failure.

Although exceptions abound, the evolution from normal renal function to symptomatic chronic renal failure may progress in stages as follows:

GFR 30 to 50% of normal: serum BUN and creatinine are normal and the patients are asymptomatic. However, they have *diminished renal reserve* and are more susceptible to develop azotemia with an additional renal insult.

GFR 20 to 35% of normal: azotemia appears, usually associated with anemia and hypertension. Polyuria and nocturia occur, as a result of decreased concentrating ability. Sudden stress (e.g., with nephrotoxins) may precipitate uremia.

GFR less than 20 to 25% of normal: overt uremia develops, associated with edema, metabolic acidosis, and neurologic, gastrointestinal, and cardiovascular complications.

GFR less than 5%: end-stage renal disease, the terminal stage of uremia.

The details of the pathophysiology of chronic renal failure are beyond our scope and are well covered in various nephrology texts.[14–17] Here we shall only briefly mention the principal clinical abnormalities and their presumed cause.

FLUID, ELECTROLYTE, AND ACID-BASE DISTURBANCES. These are directly related to the role of the kidney in volume and electrolyte homeostasis. *Dehydration* tends to appear early in the course of some forms of renal disease in which there is impairment of concentrating ability and consequent excretion of large volumes of water. With progression, glomerular filtration is ultimately impaired, with retention of both salt and water. Moreover, in most forms of chronic renal disease, an activated renin-angiotensin system leads to hyperaldosteronism, which further compounds the retention of salt and water and results in *edema*.

Metabolic acidosis is largely due to a reduction in NH_3 production, resulting in insufficient buffering of H^+ ions in the urine. There also is commonly a decreased serum bicarbonate level, a lowered blood pH, and variable degrees of compensatory hyperventilation. Occasionally, the sighing respiration through somewhat pursed lips demonstrates the classic *Kussmaul breathing*.

ABNORMALITIES IN CALCIUM PHOSPHATE AND BONE METABOLISM. Classically, the patient with chronic renal failure exhibits an increase in serum phosphate when the GFR falls below 25% of normal. This hyperphosphatemia enhances calcium entry into bones, causing hypocalcemia, which in turn leads to compensatory activity in the parathyroid glands, increased serum parathormone levels, and progressive hypertrophy and hyperplasia of the parathyroid glands (p. 1229). There are other causes for the hypocalcemia. The diseased kidney fails to synthesize 1,25-dihydroxyvitamin D_3, the active metabolite of vitamin D that normally enhances absorption of calcium from the gastrointestinal tract; thus, diminished calcium absorption by the gut contributes to hypocalcemia. In addition there is some evidence that parathormone fails to mobilize calcium salts from bone adequately in patients with chronic renal failure. Thus, in long-standing uremia, skeletal abnormalities characteristic of hyperparathyroidism and hypocalcemia may appear, sometimes referred to as *renal osteodystrophy*. Morphologically, these changes resemble those seen in *osteomalacia* or *osteitis fibrosa cystica*. Impaired bone growth in children and a tendency to spontaneous fractures are further manifestations of such renal osteodystrophy.

CARDIOPULMONARY ABNORMALITIES. Congestive heart failure, probably in part secondary to salt retention, is one of the most common manifestations. *Hypertension* is often present and is caused largely by the hypervolemia. There is also evidence of increased renin production in uremia (p. 1041). *Uremic pericarditis* is a frequent complication of chronic uremia. Characteristically, it takes the form of a marked fibrinous exudate and is sometimes accompanied by a fibrinous pleuritis. To the clinician, these are manifested as pericardial and pleural friction ribs. Both have been shown to clear with adequate dialysis, and only rarely do they give rise to significant fibrous adhesions. *Pulmonary edema* is usually secondary to congestive heart failure, or overhydration. Occasionally uremia is associated with the presence of hyaline membranes along alveolar walls (p. 716), suggesting a direct increase in pulmonary capillary permeability (*uremic pneumonitis*).

HEMATOPOIETIC MANIFESTATIONS. *Anemia* is generally normochromic and normocytic, but is sometimes hypochromic. The anemia is due to decreased production of erythropoietin by the diseased kidney, bone marrow depression caused presumably by uremic plasma, uremic hemolysis due to a poorly defined extracorpuscular defect, blood loss from gastroenteritis, and some degree of hypersplenism. Some uremic patients develop a *bleeding diathesis*. This is due in part to abnormal platelet aggregation and decreased platelet factor 3 release.

GASTROINTESTINAL SIGNS AND SYMPTOMS. These may consist of only nausea and vomiting, but some patients have gastrointestinal bleeding. The hemorrhage arises in diffuse or patchy ulcerations that may affect virtually any level of the gut, from the oral cavity to the anus. Uremic *esophagitis*, *gastritis*, and *colitis* are the more common localizations of the gastrointestinal lesions.

DERMATOLOGIC CHANGES. These consist principally of a peculiar sallow coloration to the skin and itching. The skin color is in part the consequence of anemia, but may also result from the accumulation in the skin of urinary pigment, principally urochrome (which normally gives urine its characteristic color). The origin of uremic itching remains unexplained, but it can be very distressing to the patient.

NEUROMUSCULAR DISTURBANCES. These are common manifestations of the uremic state that, although often mild, may sometimes be incapacitating. They include myopathy, encephalopathy, and peripheral neuropathy (p. 1429). Most of these are reversed by dialysis. Seizures, stupor, and coma are common in terminal uremia.

Having discussed the manifestations of uremia, we should ask what produced them. One observation appears to be well established: although the severity of uremic signs and symptoms correlates roughly with the blood concentration of urea, this product is not the prime cause. When uremic patients are dialyzed with fluid containing sufficient urea to prevent a fall in the concentration of urea in blood, the manifestations of uremia nevertheless clear. Other compounds suspected of causing the uremic syndrome are the guanidino compounds, urates and other metabolic end products of nucleic acid metabolism, aliphatic amines, and the so-called *"middle molecules."* The latter are polypeptides of 300 to 3500 daltons that produce prominent abnormal "uremic peaks" in uremic plasma subjected to a variety of chemical separation procedures. There is also evidence that elevated levels of *parathormone* may be directly toxic to cells, and may also contribute to uremic toxicity by augmenting catabolism and the resultant plasma accumulation of nitrogenous waste products. Interesting as these leads may be, the precise "uremic toxin"—the culprit responsible for all the far-ranging manifestations of uremia—is still at large.[18] Against this background of the clinical syndrome of chronic renal failure, we can turn to consider the renal diseases that cause it.

CONGENITAL ANOMALIES

About 10% of all persons are born with potentially significant malformations of the urinary system. Renal dysplasias and hypoplasias account for 20% of chronic renal failure in children. Polycystic kidney disease (a congenital anomaly that becomes apparent in adults) is present in one in 3000 hospital admissions and is responsible for 6 to 12% of chronic renal failure in humans. The frequency of congenital malformations should come as no surprise in view of the complex embryologic development of the kidney from three successive embryonic renal structures. Although the first two—pronephros and mesonephros—eventually regress, they have a vital role in the morphogenesis of the third—the metanephros—which eventually forms the infant kidney.

Congenital renal disease is most often a result of a developmental defect that arises during gestation and does not have a hereditary basis. However, some developmental defects, notably polycystic kidney disease and medullary cystic disease, are clearly hereditary. As a rule, developmental abnormalities involve structural components of the kidney and urinary tract. However, enzymatic or metabolic defects in tubular transport, such as cystinuria and renal tubular acidosis, also occur. Here we shall restrict the discussion to structural anomalies involving primarily the kidney. Anomalies of the lower urinary tract are discussed in Chapter 22.

Renal malformations are best discussed under three headings:[19] (1) *abnormalities in amount of renal tissue*, such as renal agenesis and hypoplasia; (2) *abnormalities of position, form, and orientation*, such as horseshoe kidneys; and (3) *abnormalities of differentiation*. The last-named are by far the most important in terms of renal morbidity, and almost all are associated with the formation of renal cysts.

ABNORMALITIES IN AMOUNT OF RENAL TISSUE

Agenesis of Kidney

Total bilateral agenesis of the kidneys is obviously incompatible with life and is encountered only in stillborn infants. Unilateral agenesis is an infrequent anomaly presumably due to the unilateral absence of a nephrogenic primordium or to a failure of the wolffian duct to make contact with the mesodermal mass, out of which the functioning nephrons develop. Occasionally, a small undifferentiated mass of connective tissue, 2 to 3 cm in size, may mark the site of the developmental failure. The renal artery and vein may be absent or rudimentary. The opposite kidney is usually enlarged (compensatory hypertrophy). Although unilateral agenesis is compatible with adequate renal function, some patients eventually develop progressive glomerular sclerosis in the remaining kidney, probably as a result of the adaptive hemodynamic changes in hypertrophied nephrons (p. 1007).

Hypoplasia

Renal hypoplasia refers to failure of the kidneys to develop to a normal size. This anomaly may occur bilaterally but is more commonly encountered as a unilateral defect (Fig. 21–4). True renal hypoplasia is extremely rare, most cases reported probably representing not an underlying developmental failure but acquired scarring due to vascular, infectious, or other parenchymal diseases. Differentiation between congenital and acquired atrophic kidneys may be impossible, but *a truly hypoplastic kidney possesses a reduced number of renal lobules and calyces:* five or fewer, in contrast with the normal complement of ten or more. In one form of hypoplastic kidneys, *oligomeganephronia,* the kidney is small but curiously the remaining nephrons are markedly hypertrophied. Persons with bilateral hypoplasia usually die in infancy or early childhood, often after the superimposition of another renal disease (infection, stone formation) that reduces renal function further.

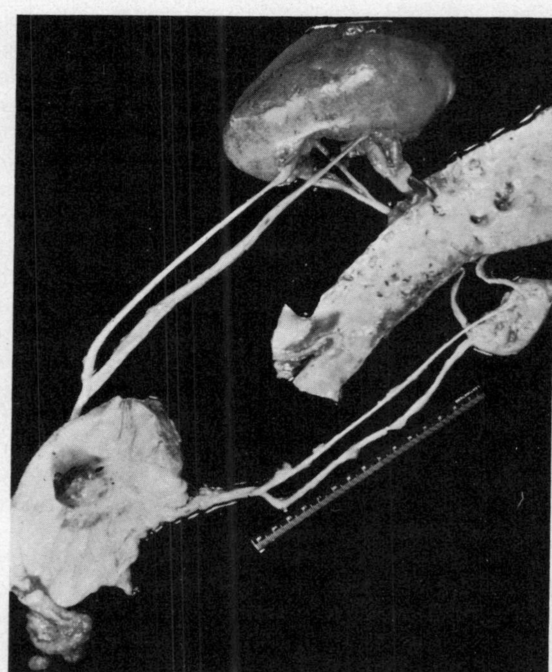

Figure 21–4. Multiple congenital anomalies of urinary tract. One kidney is hypoplastic. The ureters bilaterally are bifid (divided in their upper regions), and there are accessory anomalous renal arteries.

Other anomalies in the amount of renal tissue include nephromegaly (large kidney) and supernumerary kidneys.

ANOMALIES OF POSITION, FORM, AND ORIENTATION

Displacement of Kidneys

The development of the definitive metanephros may occur in ectopic foci, usually at abnormally low levels. These kidneys lie either just above the pelvic brim or sometimes within the pelvis. They are usually normal or slightly smaller in size, but otherwise are not remarkable. Because of their abnormal position, kinking or tortuosity of the ureters may cause some obstruction to urinary flow, which predisposes to bacterial infections. This anomaly may produce a palpable pelvic mass, which has at times been confused with a pelvic tumor.

Horseshoe Kidney

Fusion of the upper or lower poles of the kidneys produces a horseshoe-shaped structure continuous across the midline anterior to the great vessels. This anomaly is quite common and is found in about one in 500 to 1000 autopsies. The majority of such kidneys are fused at the lower pole, although approximately 10% are fused at the upper pole. In those that have a bridge at the lower pole, the ureters usually pass anterior to the renal parenchyma. These malformed kidneys are capable of normal function and are not more predisposed to renal disease than the normal. Renal calculi are said to be slightly more common, perhaps owing to angulation of the ureters with stasis of urinary flow through the ureters.

Miscellaneous Anomalies

There is a heterogeneous group of developmental anomalies that affect the kidney, most of which are of no clinical significance. A double or an extrarenal pelvis may occur with otherwise normal kidneys. These are of interest only insofar as they may produce modifications in the patterns of the pyelogram. Anomalous renal arteries may arise either directly from the aorta or as branches from the renal artery. Sometimes such vessels are of benefit, since they maintain the blood supply to a portion of the kidney if the main renal artery is occluded. However, some of these anomalous vessels to the lower pole may cause ureteral obstruction when they cross anterior to the ureter and compress it.

ANOMALIES OF DIFFERENTIATION—RENAL CYSTS

Although not all cysts of the kidney are congenital, all types of cysts are discussed here for convenience.

Cystic diseases of the kidney are a heterogeneous group comprising hereditary, developmental but non-hereditary, and acquired disorders. As a group, they are important for several reasons: (1) they are reasonably common and often represent diagnostic problems for clinicians, radiologists, and pathologists; (2) some forms, such as adult polycystic disease, are major causes of chronic renal failure; (3) they can occasionally be confused with malignant tumors. A useful classification of renal cysts, modified from that given by Bernstein,[20] is as follows:

1. Cystic renal dysplasia
2. Polycystic kidney disease
   a. Adult polycystic disease
   b. Childhood polycystic disease
3. Medullary cystic disease
   a. Medullary sponge kidney
   b. Nephronophthisis–uremic medullary cystic disease (UMCD) complex
4. Acquired (dialysis-associated) cystic disease
5. Simple renal cysts
6. Miscellaneous parenchymal renal cysts
   a. Associated with infection (tuberculous, echinococcal cyst)
   b. Associated with tumor (cystic degeneration of carcinoma)
   c. Traumatic intrarenal hematoma
7. Perihilar renal cysts (pyelocalyceal cysts, hilar lymphangitic cysts)

Only the more important types of cystic disease will be discussed.

Many theories have been suggested to explain the genesis of polycystic kidneys. Current studies, largely based on spontaneous and drug-induced cystic disease in animals, favor two mechanisms: (1) partial intratubular obstruction, causing dilatation proximal to obstructed sites;[21] and (2) a defect of the tubular basement membranes, causing loss of compliance of the tubular wall.[22] These mechanisms are not mutually exclusive, and both could indeed result from a primary defect in tubular cell metabolism.

Cystic Renal Dysplasia

This disorder is due to an abnormality in differentiation *characterized histologically by the persistence in the kidney of abnormal structures—cartilage, undifferentiated mesenchyme, and immature collecting ductules.* These structures presumably represent abnormal nephron development, and their presence is necessary to confirm a diagnosis of renal dysplasia. Renal dysplasia occurs as a sporadic disorder, without familial clustering.

Dysplasia can be unilateral or bilateral and is almost always cystic. Grossly, the kidney is enlarged, extremely irregular, and multicystic. The cysts vary in size from small microscopic structures to some that are several centimeters in diameter. They are lined by flattened epithelium. Histologically, although normal nephrons are present, many have immature ducts. **The pathognomonic feature is the presence of islands of undifferentiated mesenchyma or cartilage** (Fig. 21–5).

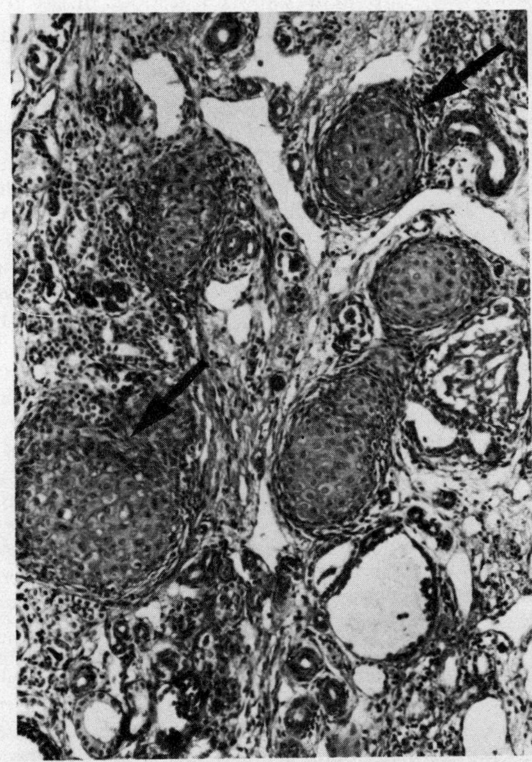

Figure 21–5. Renal dysplasia. Note disorganized architecture, dilated tubules, and islands of immature cartilage *(arrow).*

Renal dysplasia is frequently associated with obstructive abnormalities of the ureter and lower urinary tract, and indeed most authors hold that the dysplasia is caused by *intrauterine ureteral obstruction*. When unilateral, the dysplasia is discovered by the appearance of a flank mass that leads to surgical exploration and nephrectomy. Function in the opposite kidney is normal and such patients have an excellent prognosis after surgical removal of the affected kidney. In bilateral renal dysplasia, renal failure may ultimately result.

Polycystic Kidney Disease

This designation should be limited to kidneys so completely cystic that the intrarenal parenchyma appears virtually obliterated. The disease occurs in two forms, adult and childhood. These are completely separate disorders, with variable patterns of inheritance and distinct clinical and morphologic features.

ADULT POLYCYSTIC DISEASE.[23, 24] Adult polycystic kidney disease is a relatively common condition affecting roughly one of every 500 persons and accounting for 6 to 12%[13] of patients requiring renal transplantation or chronic dialysis. The pattern of inheritance is *autosomal dominant*, with very high penetrance, approaching 100% in those surviving through their 70s or 80s. The disease is universally bilateral; unilateral cases reported probably represent multicystic dysplasia. The cysts initially involve only portions of the nephrons, so that renal function is retained until about the third or fourth decade of life. In some patients, however, the first symptoms may appear in early childhood, in the teens, or as late as 70 or 80 years of age. In time, most patients develop hypertension or progress to chronic renal failure.[23]

Grossly, the kidneys are bilaterally enlarged and may achieve enormous sizes, weights up to 4 kg for each kidney having been reported. The external surface appears to be composed solely of a mass of cysts, up to 3 to 4 cm in diameter, with no intervening parenchyma (Fig. 21–6). However, microscopic examination reveals functioning nephrons dispersed between the cysts. The cysts may be filled with a clear serous fluid or, more usually, with turbid, red-to-brown, sometimes hemorrhagic fluid. As these cysts enlarge, they may encroach upon the calyces and pelvis to produce pressure defects. The cysts arise from the tubules throughout the nephron and therefore have variable lining epithelia. Occasionally, Bowman's capsules are involved in cyst formation, and glomerular tufts may be seen within the cystic space. Since the pressure of the expanding cysts leads to ischemia of the intervening renal substance, progressive atrophy narrows functional reserve. Superimposed bacterial infection and vascular disease due to concomitant hypertension are common, and these further encroach upon the already precarious renal reserve.

There is considerable evidence that tubules involved in the cystic change contribute to the final urine composition during the course of polycystic disease. Thus, both inulin and PAH can be recovered from the cyst fluids, suggesting both filtration and secretion. Further, there is evidence that the composition of cyst fluid within individual cysts reflects the type of epithelium lining these cysts—proximal or distal, indicating that the cyst epithelium has functional capacity.

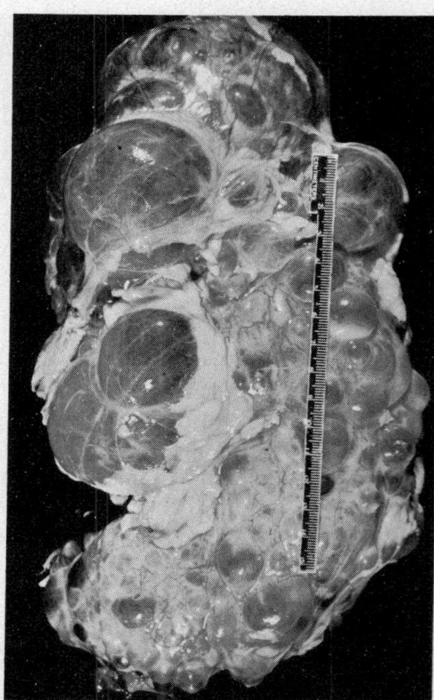

Figure 21–6. Adult polycystic kidney. Note its length of over 20 cm.

Clinically, many of these patients remain entirely asymptomatic until indications of renal insufficiency announce the presence of the underlying kidney disease. In others, hemorrhage or progressive dilation of cysts may produce pain. Excretion of blood clots may cause renal colic. The larger masses usually apparent on abdominal palpation may induce a dragging sensation. Occasionally, the disease begins with the insidious onset of hematuria, followed by other features of progressive chronic renal disease such as proteinuria (rarely more than 2 gm per day), polyuria, and hypertension. Patients with polycystic kidney disease also tend to have other congenital anomalies: *one-third have one to several cysts in the liver (polycystic liver disease) that are almost always asymptomatic*. Cysts occur much less frequently in the spleen, pancreas, and lungs. *Intracranial berry aneurysms in the circle of Willis are present in about one-sixth of patients*, and subarachnoid hemorrhages from these account for death in about 10% of patients. The clinical diagnosis is aided by intravenous or retrograde pyelography, which shows the elongated stretched pelves and calyces; ultrasonography and radioisotopic scanning can also demonstrate cysts in the kidneys and liver. This form of chronic renal failure is quite remarkable in that patients may survive for many years with azotemia slowly progressing to uremia. Ultimately, about one-third of adult patients die with renal failure; in another third, hypertension is responsible for death (cardiac disease, berry aneurysm); the remaining third die of unrelated causes.

CHILDHOOD POLYCYSTIC DISEASE. This rare developmental anomaly is genetically distinct from adult polycystic kidney disease, having an *autosomal recessive* type of inheritance.[23] Perinatal, neonatal, infantile, and juvenile subcategories have been defined, dependent on time of appearance and presence of associated hepatic lesions. The first two are most common; serious manifestations are usually present at birth, and the young infant may succumb rapidly to renal failure.

Kidneys are enlarged and have a smooth external appearance. On cut section, numerous small cysts in the cortex and medulla give the kidney a spongelike appearance. With the hand lens, it is possible to visualize dilated elongated channels at right angles to the cortical surface, completely replacing the medulla and cortex. Microscopically, there is saccular or, more commonly, cylindrical dilatation of all collecting tubules, together with some hypoplasia of such tubules. The cysts have a uniform lining of cuboidal cells, reflecting their origin from the collecting tubules. The disease is invariably bilateral. **In almost all cases, there are multiple epithelial-lined cysts in the liver as well as proliferation of portal bile ducts.**

The few patients with childhood polycystic kidney disease who survive infancy (infantile and juvenile form) develop a peculiar type of hepatic fibrosis characterized by bland periportal fibrosis and proliferation of well-differentiated biliary ductules, a condition now termed *congenital hepatic fibrosis*. In the juvenile form, the hepatic picture in fact predominates. Such patients may develop portal hypertension with splenomegaly. Curiously, congenital hepatic fibrosis sometimes occurs in the absence of childhood polycystic kidney and has been reported occasionally in the presence of adult polycystic kidney disease.

Cystic Diseases of Renal Medulla

Although the names used for the two major types of medullary cystic disease are confusing, it is important to differentiate between the two types since one, *medullary sponge kidney*, is a relatively common and usually innocuous structural change, whereas the other, *nephronophthisis–uremic medullary cystic disease* complex, is almost always associated with renal dysfunction, and is a relatively common cause of chronic renal failure in children.

MEDULLARY SPONGE KIDNEY. *The term medullary sponge kidney should be restricted to lesions consisting of multiple cystic dilatations of the collecting ducts in the medulla.* The condition occurs in adults and is usually discovered radiographically, either as an incidental finding or sometimes in relation to secondary complications. The latter include calcifications within the dilated ducts, infection, and urinary calculi. Renal function is usually normal. Grossly, the papillary ducts in the medulla are dilated and small cysts may be present. The cysts are lined by cuboidal epithelium or occasionally by transitional epithelium. Unless there is superimposed pyelonephritis, cortical scarring is absent. The pathogenesis of medullary sponge kidney is unknown.

NEPHRONOPHTHISIS–UREMIC MEDULLARY CYSTIC DISEASE (UMCD) COMPLEX. This is a group of progressive renal disorders that usually have their onset in childhood. The common characteristic is the presence of a variable number of *cysts in the medulla associated with significant cortical tubular atrophy and interstitial fibrosis.*[25] Although the presence of medullary cysts is important, the *cortical tubulointerstitial damage is the cause of the eventual renal insufficiency.* Four variants are recognized: (1) *sporadic, nonfamilial* (20%); (2) *familial juvenile nephronophthisis* (50%) inherited as a recessive disease; (3) *renal-retinal dysplasia* (15%), recessively inherited and associated with retinitis pigmentosa; and (4) *adult-onset medullary cystic disease,* dominantly inherited (15%). As a group this complex accounts for about 25% of cases of chronic renal failure in children and adolescents.

Affected children present first with polyuria and polydipsia, which reflect a marked tubular defect in concentrating ability. Sodium wasting and tubular acidosis are also prominent, findings consistent with initial injury to the distal tubules and collecting ducts. The expected course is progression to terminal renal failure over a period of five to ten years.

Grossly, the kidneys are small, have contracted granular surfaces, and show cysts in the medulla, most prominently at the corticomedullary junction (Fig. 21–7). Small cysts are

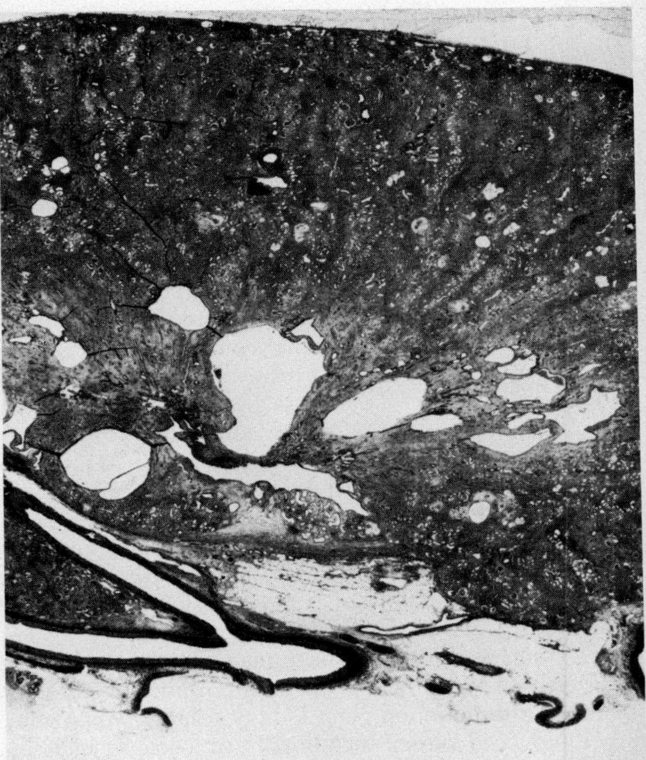

Figure 21–7. Uremic medullary cystic disease. Cut section of kidney showing cysts at corticomedullary junction and medulla.

also seen in the cortices. The cysts are lined by flattened or cuboidal epithelium and are usually surrounded by either inflammatory cells or fibrous tissue. In the cortex there is widespread atrophy and thickening of the basement membranes of proximal and distal tubules together with interstitial fibrosis. Some glomeruli may be hyalinized but, in general, glomerular structure is preserved.

There are few specific clues to diagnosis, since the medullary cysts may be too small to be visualized radiographically. The disease should be strongly considered in children or adolescents with otherwise unexplained chronic renal failure, a positive family history, and chronic tubulointerstitial nephritis on biopsy.

Acquired (Dialysis-Associated) Cystic Disease

The kidneys from patients with end-stage renal disease who have undergone prolonged dialysis sometimes exhibit numerous cortical and medullary cysts.[26] The cysts measure 0.5 to 2 cm in diameter, contain clear fluid, are lined by flattened tubular epithelium, and often contain calcium oxalate crystals. They probably form as a result of obstruction of tubules by interstitial fibrosis or by oxalate crystals. Tumors, usually of the renal adenoma type (p. 1053), may be present in the walls of these cysts, and occasionally the cysts bleed, causing hematuria.[27]

Simple Cysts

These occur as multiple or single cystic spaces that vary in diameter over wide limits. Commonly, they are 1 to 5 cm in size; translucent; lined by a gray, glistening, smooth membrane; and filled with clear fluid. Microscopically, these membranes are composed of a single layer of cuboidal or flattened cuboidal epithelium, which, in many instances, may be completely atrophic. These cells rest on an outer enclosing thin fibrous capsule. These cysts are usually confined to the cortex, but may sometimes occur in the medullary portion of the kidney, where they must be differentiated from hydronephrotic dilatation of the collecting system. It is apparent that, in the latter disease, connections with the pelvis and ureter can be demonstrated, whereas in the true cysts no such connection exists. Rarely, large massive cysts up to 10 cm in diameter are encountered.

Simple cysts are common postmortem findings without clinical significance. On occasion, hemorrhage into them may cause sudden distention and pain, and calcification of the hemorrhage may give rise to bizarre radiographic shadows. The main importance of cysts lies in their differentiation from kidney tumors, when they are discovered either incidentally or because of hemorrhage and pain during life. Radiologic studies show that, in contrast to renal tumors (p. 1054), renal cysts have smooth contours, are almost always avascular, and give fluid rather than solid signals on ultrasound.

GLOMERULAR DISEASES

Glomerular diseases constitute some of the major problems encountered in nephrology; indeed, chronic glomerulonephritis is the most common cause of chronic renal failure in man. The glomerulus plays a central role in renal anatomy and physiology. All else pivots on its structure and function, and damage to glomeruli will often impair other segments of the nephron. Thus, in most forms of glomerular disease, particularly in advanced stages, there is structural and functional damage to the other three major components of the kidney, i.e., the tubules, interstitium, and blood vessels.

Glomeruli may be injured by a variety of factors and in the course of a number of systemic diseases. Immunologic diseases such as systemic lupus erythematosus (SLE), vascular disorders such as hypertension and polyarteritis nodosa, metabolic diseases such as diabetes mellitus, and some purely hereditary conditions such as Fabry's disease often affect the glomerulus. These are termed *secondary glomerular diseases* to differentiate them from those in which the kidney is the only or predominant organ involved. The latter constitute the various types of *primary glomerulonephritis* (GN) or *glomerulopathy*. Here we shall discuss the various types of primary GN, and only briefly review the glomerular alterations in systemic diseases, which are covered in other parts of this book.

There are several types of glomerulonephritis, but no entirely satisfactory classification is available. Table 21–1 lists the most common forms that have reasonably well-defined morphologic and clinical characteristics. In reviewing the specific types of GN, it is useful to consider each in terms of (1) clinical presentation, (2) the morphology of the glomerular lesion, and (3) the etiology and pathogenesis. The response of the glomerulus in all forms of injury is remarkably limited histologically and clinically, and only a small number of

Table 21–1. GLOMERULAR DISEASES

Primary Glomerulonephritis
Acute diffuse proliferative glomerulonephritis (GN)
Poststreptococcal
Nonpoststreptococcal
Rapidly progressive (crescentic) glomerulonephritis
Membranous glomerulonephritis
Lipoid nephrosis (minimal change disease)
Focal segmental glomerulosclerosis
Membranoproliferative glomerulonephritis
Focal proliferative glomerulonephritis
IgA nephropathy
Chronic glomerulonephritis
Systemic Diseases
Systemic lupus erythematosus
Diabetes mellitus
Amyloidosis
Goodpasture's syndrome
Polyarteritis nodosa
Wegener's granulomatosis
Henoch-Schönlein purpura
Bacterial endocarditis
Hereditary Disorders
Alport's syndrome, Fabry's disease

pathogenetic mechanisms are known. These will be summarized briefly before the specific types of GN are discussed.

CLINICAL MANIFESTATIONS

The clinical manifestations of glomerular disease are clustered into the five major glomerular syndromes described in Table 21–2. Both the primary glomerulonephritides and systemic diseases affecting the glomerulus can result in these syndromes. Thus, a critical point in the clinical differential diagnosis is first to exclude the major systemic disorders, of which the major four are diabetes mellitus, SLE, vasculitis, and amyloidosis.

HISTOLOGIC ALTERATIONS

Various types of GN are characterized by one or more of four basic tissue reactions:

CELLULAR PROLIFERATION. This is reflected by an increase in the number of cells in the glomerular tuft due to proliferation of endothelial, mesangial, and epithelial cells. In certain diseases, there is also proliferation of the parietal epithelial cells that takes the form of a *crescent*, a histologic feature characteristic of diseases presenting clinically with rapidly progressive GN.

LEUKOCYTIC INFILTRATION. Neutrophils and monocytes infiltrate the glomerulus in some types of acute GN, and this is often accompanied by cellular proliferation.

GLOMERULAR BASEMENT MEMBRANE (GBM) THICKENING. By light microscopy, this change appears as thickening of the capillary walls best seen in sections stained with PAS. On electron microscopy such thickening can be resolved as either (1) thickening of the basement membrane proper, as occurs in diabetic glomerulosclerosis; or, more commonly, (2) deposition of amorphous electron-dense material representing plasma proteins, either on the endothelial or epithelial side of the basement membrane, or within the GBM itself. *By far the most common type of thickening is due to extensive subepithelial deposition, as occurs in membranous GN.* In most instances the deposits are thought to be immune complexes, although fibrin may also show as an electron-dense material.

HYALINIZATION AND SCLEROSIS. Hyalinization or hyalinosis, as applied to the glomerulus, denotes the accumulation of material that is homogeneous and eosinophilic by light microscopy. By electron microscopy the material is heterogeneous and consists of amorphous substance (probably precipitated plasma protein) as well as increased amounts of basement membrane or mesangial matrix. This change results in obliteration of structural detail of the glomerular tuft (sclerosis) and usually denotes irreversible injury as the end result of various forms of glomerular damage.

Additional alterations include fibrin deposition, intraglomerular thrombosis, or deposition of abnormal materials (amyloid, "dense deposits," lipid). Because many of the primary glomerulonephritides are of unknown etiology, they are often classified by their histology, as can be seen in Table 21–1. The histologic changes can be further subdivided into *diffuse*, involving all glomeruli and the entire glomerulus; *focal*, involving only a certain proportion of the glomeruli; *segmental*, affecting a part of each glomerulus; or *mesangial*, affecting predominantly the mesangial region. These terms are sometimes appended to the histologic classifications.

Table 21–2. THE GLOMERULAR SYNDROMES

Acute nephritic syndrome
Rapidly progressive glomerulonephritis
Nephrotic syndrome
Chronic glomerulonephritis (chronic renal failure)
Asymptomatic hematuria and/or proteinuria
A. Primary GN B. Part of systemic disease

PATHOGENESIS OF GLOMERULAR INJURY

Although much has yet to be learned, there has been considerable progress in our understanding of the pathogenesis of glomerular injury. It is best, for this discussion, to distinguish between (1) the primary immune and nonimmune mechanisms initiating glomerular injury and (2) the secondary mediators of glomerular damage. Regrettably, few of the *etiologic agents* triggering these events are known, and these will be noted in the discussion of the specific diseases.

Table 21–3 lists the various proved or postulated mechanisms of glomerular injury.

Immune mechanisms clearly underlie the majority of primary glomerulonephritides and many of the secondary glomerular involvements.[28–30] Experimentally, GN can be readily induced by classical antigen-antibody reactions, and glomerular deposits of immunoglobulins, often with various components of complement, are

Table 21–3. MECHANISMS OF GLOMERULAR INJURY

- **I. Immune Mechanisms**
  - A. Antibody-mediated
    - 1. In situ immune complex formation
      - a. Insoluble fixed (intrinsic) antigens
        - Anti-GBM nephritis (linear deposits)
        - Others (Heymann antigen; rabbit spontaneous nephritis antigen; ? human membranous GN [interrupted granular deposits])
      - a. Planted antigens
        - Endogenous (DNA, immunoglobulins, complexes)
        - Exogenous (lectins, infectious products, drugs)
    - 2. Circulating immune complex deposition
      - a. Endogenous antigens (e.g., DNA, thyroglobulin tumor antigens)
      - b. Exogenous antigens (infectious products)
  - B. ? Cell-mediated
  - C. Activation of alternate complement pathway
- **II. Loss of Glomerular Polyanion**
- **III. Hemodynamic Changes (Hyperfiltration)**

found in over 70% of human GN. Thus, antibody-mediated mechanisms of damage predominate, and these have received the greatest attention.

Two basic forms of such antibody-associated injury have been established by experimental work: (1) injury by antibodies reacting in situ within the glomerulus, either with *insoluble fixed* (intrinsic) glomerular antigens or with circulating antigens *planted* within the glomerulus; and (2) injury resulting from deposition of *soluble circulating antigen-antibody complexes* in the glomerulus. These pathways are not mutually exclusive, and in man both seem to play a role.

In Situ Immune Complex Formation

As noted, antibodies in this form of injury react directly with fixed or planted antigens in the glomerulus. The most well-established model for such type of mechanism is so called "classic" anti–glomerular basement membrane (anti-GBM) nephritis.

Anti–Glomerular Basement Membrane (Anti-GBM) Nephritis. *This term is now restricted to the type of injury in which antibodies are directed against fixed antigens in the glomerular basement membrane, which induce a linear pattern of localization by immunofluorescence microscopy.* Although relatively rare, this entity provided one of the first insights into immune mechanisms in nephritis. In 1934, Masugi showed that a GN similar to the human disease could be produced in rats by injections of anti–rat kidney antibodies prepared by immunizing rabbits with rat kidney tissue. This experimental disease is known as nephrotoxic or Masugi nephritis. The circulating antibodies bind along the entire length of the GBM, *resulting in a homogeneous, diffuse linear pattern as visualized by immunofluorescent techniques* (Fig. 21–8). This is contrasted with the granular lumpy pattern seen in other in situ models or after deposition of circulating immune complexes (Fig. 21–9). To come back to Masugi's model, it should be noted that the deposited immunoglobulin of the rabbit is foreign to the host and thus acts as an antigen eliciting antibodies in the rat. This rat antibody then reacts with the rabbit immunoglobulin within the basement membrane, leading to further glomerular injury. This is referred to as the *autologous phase* of nephrotoxic nephritis, to distinguish it from the initial *heterologous phase* caused by the anti-GBM antibody. *The fluorescence in both instances is linear.* Anti-GBM nephritis can also be induced by direct immunization of experimental animals with homologous or heterologous basement membrane preparations in Freund's adjuvant. The biochemical nature of the nephritogenic, so-called "classic" GBM antigen is not yet known, but it is thought to be a glycoprotein distinct from any of the GBM components such as collagen or laminin (p. 993).[29]

Anti-GBM nephritis accounts for less than 5% of human GN. It is well established as the cause of injury in Goodpasture's syndrome (p. 1010). Most instances of anti-GBM nephritis are characterized by very severe glomerular damage, with the development of rapidly progressive renal failure. It must be apparent, then, that anti-GBM disease is a form of *autoimmune GN*, and the question arises: why do such patients develop antibodies to their own basement membranes? Any one of the mechanisms postulated for other autoimmune diseases has been implicated (p. 178), but the precise answer is unknown.

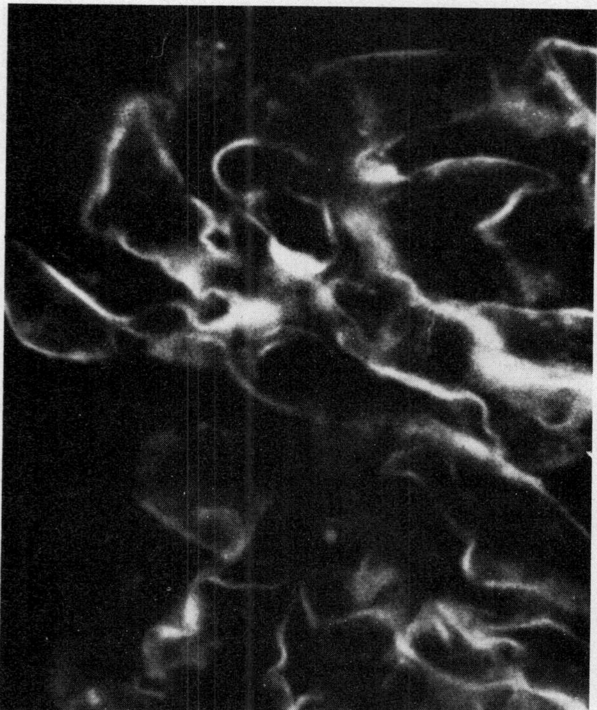

Figure 21–8. Linear fluorescence along GBM typical of classic anti-GBM disease. Compare with Figure 21–9.

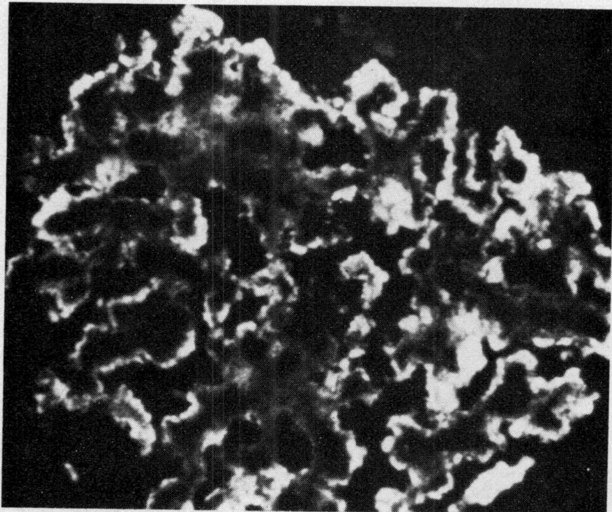

Figure 21–9. Immune complex glomerulonephritis showing granular immunofluorescent deposits along GBM. Compare with linear fluorescence in Figure 21–8.

Antibodies Against Other Fixed Antigens. Although classic anti-GBM disease is the one established form of immune injury to intrinsic antigen, two other fixed antigens have been identified experimentally that initiate in situ immune deposition. Both are distributed in a *discontinuous* pattern along the visceral epithelial cell foot processes; thus, the resultant pattern of immune deposition in the glomerulus is *granular* and interrupted, rather than diffuse linear (Fig. 21–9).[30] One of these is the so-called *Heymann* antigen. The Heymann model of rat GN is induced by immunizing animals with preparations of proximal tubular brush border in Freund's adjuvant. The rats develop antibodies to brush border antigens, and a membranous GN (p. 1012), closely resembling human membranous GN, develops. This is characterized on immunofluorescence by the deposition of immunoglobulins and complement in a granular (rather than linear) pattern along the GBM, and on electron microscopy by the presence of numerous electron-dense deposits (presumably immune reactants) along the subepithelial aspect of the basement membrane. Although it was once thought to be due to trapping of circulating immune complexes, it is now clear that the GN results from the reaction of anti–brush border antibody with a fixed but discontinuously distributed glomerular antigen present on the base of visceral epithelial cells, and cross-reactive with brush border antigen.[31] The Heymann antigen has since been isolated and largely purified.[32] A second nonlinear fixed antigen is responsible for a spontaneous form of GN in rabbits.[29] Unfortunately, despite the resemblance of these models to human membranous GN, there is no evidence as yet that the human disease is indeed caused by antibodies to some fixed glomerular antigen.

Antibodies Against Planted Antigens. More attractive is the possibility that antibodies react in situ with previously "planted" nonglomerular antigens. Such antigens may localize in the kidney by interacting with various intrinsic components of the glomerulus. There is increasing experimental support for such a mechanism.[30] Injections of *cationic* proteins, which bind to anionic sites in the GBM (p. 993), followed by passively administered or actively induced antibody, result in immune complex GN, before or in the absence of circulating immune complexes.[33, 34] Other planted antigens include lectins, which bind to capillary wall glycoprotein; DNA, which has an affinity for basement membrane components; bacterial products, such as endostreptosin, a protein of Group A streptococci (p. 1018); and large aggregated proteins (e.g., aggregated IgG), which deposit in the mesangium because of their size.[29] There is no dearth of other possible planted antigens, including viral, bacterial, and parasitic products and drugs. Finally, immunoglobulins, complement components, and immune complexes themselves may potentially serve as planted antigens, since they continue to have reactive sites for further interactions with free antibody, free antigen, or complement.[29] Most of these planted antigens induce a granular or heterogeneous pattern of immunoglobulin deposition by fluorescence microscopy, the pattern found also in circulating immune complex nephritis (see below).

Circulating Immune Complex Nephritis

Here the glomerular injury is caused by the trapping of circulating antigen-antibody complexes within glomeruli. The antigens are nonglomerular and thus the glomerulus is, in a sense, an innocent victim of its own filtration functions. The antibodies have no immunologic specificity for glomerular constituents, and the complexes localize within the glomeruli because of their physicochemical properties and the hemodynamic factors peculiar to the glomerulus. The immune complexes can be visualized by electron microscopy or by immunofluorescent techniques as granular deposits along the GBM.

The evocative antigens are of two origins: (1) *exogenous*, as occurs in human serum sickness nephritis and experimental foreign protein nephritis; and (2) *endogenous*, as in SLE, in which circulating DNA–anti-DNA complexes induce injury.

Serum sickness nephritis is the prototype of circulating immune complex disease. You will recall (p. 168) that injections of a large dose of a foreign protein, e.g., bovine serum albumin (BSA) in a rabbit, results in the formation of antigen-antibody complexes that deposit in the glomeruli, heart, joints, and blood vessels.[35] These complexes can be localized in the glomerulus by immunofluorescent microscopy as discrete granular (lumpy-bumpy) particles (Fig. 21–9) and with electron microscopy as electron-dense deposits on the subendothelial or subepithelial side of the GBM and within the mesangium. Serum complement activity is decreased and complement can be seen in the deposits. The amount of antibody formed in response to the antigen is critical to the development of nephritis.[36] Animals producing large amounts of antibody develop transient nephritis, since the large insoluble antigen-antibody aggregates formed in these animals are cleared by the reticuloendothelial system, and the glomerular injury is fleeting. At the other end of the spectrum are those animals with no immune response and which do not develop GN. Only in animals with a sufficiently weak antibody response, so that the ratio of antibody to antigen approaches equivalence or slight antigen excess, does significant GN develop. Well-studied examples of exogenous circulating immune complex nephritis in humans are the glomerular lesions of bacterial endocarditis, leprosy, syphilis, hepatitis B antigenemia, and malaria.[28] Endogenous antigens include DNA, thyroglobulin, and tumor-specific or tumor-associated antigens.

Factors affecting glomerular localization of antigen, antibody, or complexes deserve some discussion. The molecular charge and size of these reactants are clearly important. Highly cationic immunogens tend to cross the GBM, and the resultant complexes eventually achieve a subepithelial location.[34] Highly anionic macromolecules are excluded from the GBM and either are trapped subendothelially or may, in fact, not be nephritogenic at all. Molecules with more neutral charge and their complexes tend to accumulate in the mesangium. Very large circulating complexes are not usually nephritogenic since they are cleared by the reticuloendothelial system and do not enter the GBM in sufficient quantities. The pattern of localization is also affected by changes in glomerular hemodynamics, mesangial function, and integrity of the charge-selective barrier in the glomerulus. These influences, as well as possible affinities of immune reactant to intrinsic glomerular components, underlie the variable pattern of immune reactant deposition and histologic change in the glomerulus.[36]

It has been argued that trapping of circulating immune complexes rarely or never causes glomerular injury;[30] in humans there is little correlation between the presence or level of serum complexes and the severity of GN, and experimental injections of *preformed* complexes rarely produce renal lesions or proteinuria. In this view antibody-mediated nephritogenicity is ascribed solely to in situ complex formation. However, this seems to be too extreme a view at our current state of knowledge, since the in situ mechanism in man has actually been proved only for the rare form of classical anti-GBM (linear) disease. Further, immune complex trapping can either initiate or be superimposed on in situ formation, as discussed earlier.[29] It is best to consider, then, that *antigen-antibody deposition in the glomerulus is a major pathway of glomerular injury; and that in situ mechanisms, trapping of circulating immune complexes, interactions between these two events, and local hemodynamic and structural determinants in the glomerulus all contribute to the morphologic and functional expression of GN.*

Cell-mediated Immunity in Glomerulonephritis

There is no definite evidence that sensitized T-cells, as a reflection of cell-mediated immune reaction, can lead to glomerular injury.[38] The idea is an attractive one, since it may account for the many instances of progressive GN in which there are either no immune deposits, or the deposits do not correlate with the severity of damage. Clues to its occurrence in GN include the presence of macrophages in some forms of human and experimental GN, in vitro evidence of lymphocyte reactivity upon exposure to altered glomerular basement membrane antigen in progressive human GN, and a few successful attempts to transfer mild glomerular histological alterations by lymphocytes in experimental GN.[38, 39] Proteinuria and significant glomerular damage, however, have not been transferred with lymphocytes and the issue is still unsettled.

Activation of Alternate Complement Pathway

Alternate complement pathway activation clearly occurs in the clinicopathologic entity called *membranoproliferative glomerulonephritis* (MPGN) (p. 1016), sometimes independent of immune complex deposition, and also in some forms of proliferative GN. There is no a priori reason why such activation, if it occurred in the glomerulus, would not result in the same sequence of glomerular damage as activation by antigen-antibody reactions. However, it has not yet been possible to induce GN in experimental animals by this pathway. The issue is discussed further on page 1016.

Mediators of Immunologic Glomerular Injury

Once immune reactants have localized in the glomerulus, how does glomerular damage ensue? One well-established pathway is the *complement-neutrophil–mediated mechanism.* Activation of complement initiates the generation of chemotactic agents (mainly C5a) and the recruitment of neutrophils. The latter release proteases and other enzymes, which cause GBM degradations, as well as oxygen-derived free radicals, which cause cell damage (p. 10). Indeed, in some experimental models, depletion of neutrophils or complement inhibits both the proteinuria and the histologic change.[28] However, this mechanism applies only to some types of GN, since many types show few neutrophils in the damaged glomeruli. Some experimental models suggest *complement- but not neutrophil-dependent injury,* possibly owing to an effect of the C5-C9 lytic component (membrane-attack complex) of complement.[40, 41] Finally, injury may also occur in the absence of both complement and neutrophils.

Monocytes/macrophages infiltrate the glomerulus in many forms of human and experimental proliferative GN.[38, 42] Depletion of monocytes by irradiation or anti-macrophage serum prevents the proteinuria and histologic alterations in experimental nephritis. Activated macrophages release a vast number of biologically active molecules (Table 2–3, p. 58), and it is likely that some of these participate in the evolution of GN.

The *coagulation system* may also be a mediator of glomerular damage.[43] Fibrin and fibrin degradation products are frequently present in the glomeruli in GN, and fibrinogen may leak into Bowman's space, serving as a stimulus to cell proliferation. Pretreatment of animals with anticoagulants or defibrinating agents protects from the development of proliferative glomerular lesions in some experimental models of GN and this has led to the use of anticoagulant therapy in human GN. The beneficial effect, however, is by no means uniform either in experimental animals or in man. Nevertheless, on balance the evidence does indicate that intraglomerular coagulation plays a role in progressive renal damage in GN.

Many of the other mediator systems reviewed for acute or chronic inflammation have also been invoked in the mediation of glomerular injury; for example, arachidonic acid metabolites,[44] oxygen-derived free radicals, and platelet activating factor.[45]

Other Mechanisms of Glomerular Injury

Two other important mechanisms of glomerular damage have recently gained attention. Both were invoked to explain specific clinical or experimental observations, but may have general implications for many glomerular diseases.

LOSS OF GLOMERULAR POLYANION. You will recall (p. 993) that the glomerulus is rich in polyanionic sites (proteoglycans, sialoglycoproteins) that confer on the glomerular filter a charge-selective barrier, facilitating filtration of cationic proteins and restricting anionic molecules. Loss of such anionic sites results in loss of charge selectivity and leakage of anionic molecules such as albumin. Experimentally, infusion of polycationic molecules such as protamine sulfate, which neutralize anionic sites, leads to reversible albuminuria[46] and to structural changes in the visceral epithelium.[47] These changes are similar to those occurring in a common glomerular disease of obscure etiology called *lipoid nephrosis*, and there is now evidence of loss of charge selectivity in this condition.[5] Loss of anionic sites from the GBM may also lead eventually to defects in the size-selective barrier, resulting in leakage of larger proteins.[48] What brings about the loss of anionic sites is unknown, but the phenomenon seems also to occur in other glomerular disorders such as diabetic nephropathy and congenital nephrosis.[8]

"HYPERFILTRATION" AND PROGRESSIVE GLOMERULAR INJURY. It has been amply documented that once any renal disease, glomerular or otherwise, destroys sufficient functional nephrons to reduce the glomerular filtration rate (GFR) to about 30 to 50% of normal, progression to end-stage renal failure proceeds inexorably (though at variable rates), even if the initial cause of renal injury (e.g., infection, immune reaction) has been eliminated. Such kidneys show widespread glomerular hyalinization or sclerosis. Insight into the mechanism of such glomerular injury comes from experiments in rats subjected to ablation of renal mass by subtotal nephrectomy. Although compensatory hypertrophy of remaining nephrons serves to maintain renal function in these animals, proteinuria and focal glomerulosclerosis soon develop, leading eventually to total glomerular hyalinization,[49] and if the renal ablation is severe, death of the animals in uremia ensues. Micropuncture studies of remnant glomeruli of such animals show increases in single nephron GFR, glomerular blood flow, and capillary pressure, all well-known adaptive responses in hypertrophied glomeruli.[50] That these hemodynamic changes, conveniently abbreviated "hyperfiltration," are linked to the glomerular damage can be shown by subjecting subtotally nephrectomized animals to a low-protein diet. This diet blunts the increases in glomerular filtration, flow, and pressure; abrogates the proteinuria; and protects from progressive glomerulosclerosis.[51] Which of the three hemodynamic changes is the critical factor in inducing glomerular damage is unclear, but the sequence of events entails endothelial and epithelial cell injury, increased glomerular permeability to proteins, accumulation of proteins in the mesangial matrix, and, by some unknown mechanism, glomerular hyalinization.[51] This results in further reductions in nephron mass and a vicious cycle of progressive glomerulosclerosis (Fig. 21–10).[52] As we shall see, this mechanism may play a role in the progressive renal failure of chronic pyelonephritis, diabetic nephropathy, unilateral renal agenesis, and other disorders.

We now turn to a consideration of specific types of GN. For more detailed clinical and morphologic descriptions, refer to Heptinstall's comprehensive book, *Pathology of the Kidney*.[53]

ACUTE GLOMERULONEPHRITIS

Certain types of glomerular disease are characterized anatomically by inflammatory alterations in the glomeruli and clinically by a complex of findings classically referred to as *the syndrome of acute nephritis*. The nephritic patient usually presents with hematuria, red cell casts in the urine, azotemia, oliguria, and mild-to-moderate hypertension. The patient also commonly has proteinuria and edema, but these are not as severe as those encountered in the nephrotic syndrome, discussed later. The acute nephritic syndrome may occur in such multisystem diseases as SLE and polyarteritis nodosa. Typically, however, it is characteristic of acute proliferative GN.

Acute Poststreptococcal (Proliferative) Glomerulonephritis

This is a fairly common glomerular disease that usually appears one to two weeks after a streptococcal infection of the throat or occasionally of the skin. It occurs most frequently in children, but adults of any age can be affected. The onset is generally abrupt and is heralded by the manifestations of acute nephritis.

ETIOLOGY AND PATHOGENESIS. Only certain strains of group A beta-hemolytic streptococci are nephritogenic, over 90% being traced to types 12, 4, and 1,

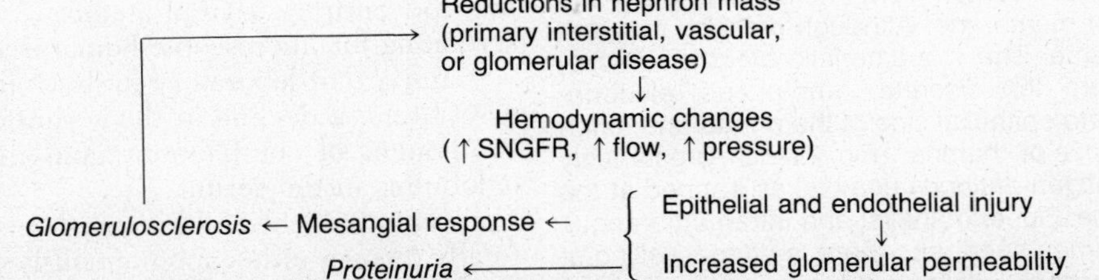

Figure 21–10. Progressive glomerulosclerosis due to hemodynamic alterations (hyperfiltration) (see text). SNGFR = single nephron glomerular filtration rate.

which can be identified by typing of M protein of the cell wall. Skin infections are responsible for two-thirds of cases in the southern United States and are commonly associated with overcrowding.

Poststreptococcal GN is an immunologically mediated disease. The latent period between infection and onset of nephritis is compatible with the time required for the building up of antibodies. Elevated titers to one or more of the streptococcal exoenzymes, e.g., anti-streptolysin-O (ASO), are present in a great majority of patients. Serum complement levels are low, compatible with involvement of the complement system as a mediator of the immune reaction. The presence of granular immune deposits of immunoglobulin and complement in the glomeruli suggest an immune complex–mediated mechanism, and so does the finding of electron-dense deposits seen under the electron microscope. The streptococcal antigenic component(s) responsible for the immune reaction has eluded identification for years, but recent work suggests that a cytoplasmic antigen called *endostreptosin* and several *cationic* streptococcal antigens[55] are present in affected glomeruli. Whether these represent "planted" antigens, are part of circulating immune complexes, or both is unknown. The absence in some cases of C1 and C4, the early components of complement in glomeruli, also suggests activation of the alternate complement pathway (p. 1018).

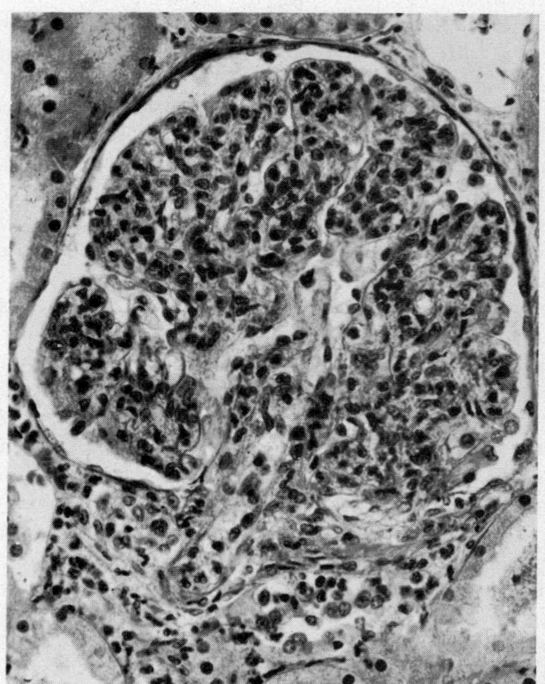

Figure 21–11. Poststreptococcal glomerulonephritis. Glomerular hypercellularity is due to an immigrant leukocytic infiltrate and proliferation of intrinsic glomerular cells. There is also an infiltrate of white cells in renal interstitium about glomerulus.

MORPHOLOGY. The macroscopic appearance of kidneys is rarely seen, since most patients survive the acute attack. In fatal cases, the cortical surface appears red-brown and smooth, often dotted by fine, punctate petechiae produced by acute inflammatory rupture of glomerular capillaries.

The classic diagnostic picture is one of enlarged, hypercellular, relatively bloodless glomeruli (Fig. 21–11). The hypercellularity is caused by (1) proliferation of endothelial and mesangial cells and, in many cases, epithelial cells; and (2) infiltration by leukocytes, both neutrophils and monocytes. The proliferation and leukocyte infiltration are diffuse, i.e., involving all lobules of all glomeruli. There is also swelling of endothelial cells, and the combination of proliferation, swelling, and leukocyte infiltration obliterates the capillary lumina. Small deposits of fibrin within capillary lumina and mesangium can be demonstrated by special stains. There may be interstitial edema and inflammation, and the tubules often contain red cell casts and may show evidence of degeneration. Focal proliferation of parietal epithelial cells and infiltration with monocytes may be present, causing crescents, but diffuse crescent formation is uncommon except in a small proportion of patients with rapidly progressive GN.

By **immunofluorescence microscopy** there are granular deposits of IgG and complement in the mesangium and along the basement membrane. Although present, they are often focal and sparse. The characteristic **electron microscopic findings** are the discrete, amorphous, electron-dense deposits on the epithelial side of the membrane, often having the appearance of "humps" (Fig. 21–12), presumably representing the antigen-antibody complexes trapped at the epithelial cell surface. Subendothelial and intramembranous deposits are sometimes seen, and there is often swelling of endothelial and mesangial cells, occasional rupture of the basement membrane (allowing red cells to leak), and fibrin deposits. In the great majority of cases the glomerular changes begin to subside approximately four to six weeks after the onset of disease. In some cases they may persist for months, however, and are accompanied by persistent hypercellularity in the mesangial area with excessive deposition of mesangial matrix. Persistence of such abnormalities for prolonged periods may augur progression to chronic GN.

CLINICAL COURSE. In the classic case, a young child abruptly develops malaise, fever, nausea, oliguria, and hematuria (smoky or cocoa-colored urine) one to two weeks after recovery from a sore throat. Red cell casts in the urine are one of the most diagnostic findings. Proteinuria is generally mild (less than 1 gm), although it may reach 3 gm or even nephrotic levels. Edema may be limited to the periorbital areas but may subsequently progress, and hypertension is usually mild to moderate. In adults, the onset is more apt to be atypical, with the sudden appearance of hypertension or edema, frequently with elevation of BUN. During epidemics caused by nephritogenic streptococcal infections, GN may be entirely asymptomatic, discovered only when screening for microscopic hematuria.

Important laboratory findings include elevations of ASO titers, a decline in the serum concentration of C3 component of complement, and the presence of cryoglobulins in the serum.

Over 95% of children with poststreptococcal GN totally recover either spontaneously or with conservative therapy aimed at maintaining sodium and water balance.

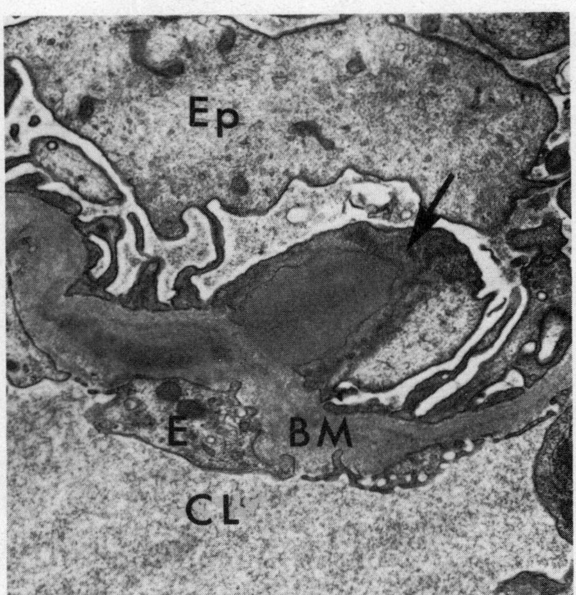

Figure 21–12. Poststreptococcal glomerulonephritis. Electron micrograph showing a hump-shaped electron-dense deposit *(arrow)* on epithelial side of basement membrane (BM). There is also a dense deposit within BM. CL = capillary lumen; E = endothelium; Ep = epithelium.

Microscopic hematuria, mild proteinuria, and histologic changes confined to the mesangium may persist in some patients for several weeks or months, but even then complete long-term recovery is the rule. A small minority of children (perhaps under 1%) do not improve, become severely oliguric, and develop a rapidly progressive form of GN (to be described later). Another 1 to 2% may undergo slow progression to chronic GN with or without recurrence of an active nephritic picture. Prolonged and persistent heavy proteinuria and abnormal GFR mark patients with an unfavorable prognosis.

In adults, the disease is probably less benign. Although the overall prognosis in epidemics is good, only about 60% of *sporadic* cases recover promptly. Some patients develop rapidly progressive GN. In the remainder the glomerular lesions fail to resolve quickly, as manifested by persistent proteinuria, hematuria, and hypertension. In some of these patients the lesions eventually clear totally, but others develop chronic GN. The factors leading to progression in some patients are unclear. They include adaptive hyperfiltration, leading to progressive glomerulosclerosis (p. 1007); hypertension; and cell-mediated reactions directed to GBM cross-reacting with or altered by streptococci.[58]

Although most patients with acute GN have poststreptococcal disease, a similar form has been reported sporadically in association with other bacterial infections such as staphylococcal endocarditis, infected atrioventricular shunts (for hydrocephalus), pneumococcal pneumonia, secondary syphilis, and meningococcemia. A number of viral diseases, such as hepatitis B, mumps, varicella, and infectious mononucleosis may also be associated with a similar disorder.[53] In all of these, granular immunofluorescent deposits and subepithelial humps characteristic of immune complex nephritis are present.

RAPIDLY PROGRESSIVE GLOMERULONEPHRITIS (RPGN)

This form represents a *clinicopathologic syndrome* in which glomerular damage is accompanied by rapid and progressive decline in renal function, frequently with severe oliguria or anuria, usually resulting in irreversible renal failure in weeks or months.[59, 60] *The syndrome is characterized histologically by accumulation of cells in Bowman's space in the form of "crescents."* Thus, the terms *crescentic* and *extracapillary GN* are used synonymously. Hematuria is a common finding, but proteinuria is variable and hypertension and edema may or may not be present.

RPGN may occur in the course of several groups of diseases that can affect the glomerulus (Table 21–4): (1) poststreptococcal or postinfectious RPGN, (2) GN associated with systemic diseases, and (3) primary or idiopathic RPGN. Here we shall discuss postinfectious RPGN, Goodpasture's syndrome as a prototype for the multisystem diseases causing RPGN, and idiopathic RPGN.

Postinfectious RPGN

Most patients with poststreptococcal or postinfectious GN recover, but in a small proportion intractable oliguria persists, anuria may ensue, and renal failure develops within weeks or months. This complication is rare in children but somewhat more common in adults. The initial clinical manifestations and pathogenetic mechanisms are similar to those of the diffuse proliferative GN: ASO serum titers are usually elevated, serum complement levels are reduced, and there is granular deposition of IgG and C3 in the glomeruli. Histologically, in addition to the diffuse proliferation and leukocyte infiltration, there is widespread crescent formation. Although all forms of RPGN have a dismal prognosis, the postinfectious type tends to fare better, and in some series up to 50% of patients may recover sufficient renal function to escape the necessity for long-term dialysis or transplantation.

Table 21–4. RAPIDLY PROGRESSIVE GLOMERULONEPHRITIS (RPGN)

1. Postinfectious RPGN
2. Systemic diseases
   a. Systemic lupus erythematosus
   b. Goodpasture's syndrome
   c. Polyarteritis nodosa
   d. Wegener's granulomatosis
   e. Henoch-Schönlein purpura
   f. Essential cryoglobulinemia
3. Idiopathic RPGN

Goodpasture's Syndrome

This is an acute, often fulminating disorder characterized by pulmonary hemorrhages and acute GN, commonly of the rapidly progressive type. It is seen mostly in young adults, principally males. The pulmonary involvement usually precedes the onset of nephritis and is, in fact, the dominant cause of morbidity and mortality (p. 745). Here our interest is in the glomerular involvement.

ETIOLOGY AND PATHOGENESIS. Although pulmonary hemorrhage and GN may coexist in a variety of other conditions, such as SLE, Wegener's granulomatosis, scleroderma, and polyarteritis nodosa, the term *Goodpasture's syndrome is used here, in the strictest sense, to denote a disease that is the result of damage by anti–glomerular basement membrane antibodies.*[61] Immunofluorescent studies in these patients reveal the characteristic continuous linear staining for IgG seen in experimental anti-GBM nephritis. When immunoglobulins are eluted from glomeruli, they react in vitro with GBM, and when they are injected into monkeys, glomerular disease with typical linear staining is found in glomeruli. Circulating anti-GBM antibodies can be readily detected in the serum of most patients with Goodpasture's syndrome, and IgG may also be present in a linear fashion along the alveolar basement membranes. Experimentally, anti-GBM antibodies induce renal lesions as well as lung hemorrhage, provided the lung is previously injured (e.g., by oxygen toxicity).[62] Thus, the renal and lung injury appears to be the result of antibodies against antigens to both basement membranes. What triggers the formation of these antibodies is unclear. Exposure of lung to viruses or hydrocarbon solvents (found in paints and dyes) has been implicated in some patients, as have been various drugs (e.g., rifampicin) and cancers, but most patients give no such history.[61] Antibody production is usually self-limited. There is a high prevalence of DRW2 haplotype in Goodpasture's syndrome,[63] a finding consistent with the genetic predisposition common to many of the autoimmune diseases.

MORPHOLOGY. In cases with mild renal involvement or early in the disease, there is focal and segmental proliferation with fibrinoid necrosis in glomerular tufts. **This lesion may be present early, but more often as renal involvement progresses the picture is soon dominated by striking formation of extracapillary crescents** (Fig. 21–13). As we shall see later, these crescents are formed by proliferating epithelial cells, often accompanied by monocytes and neutrophils. On electron microscopy the glomerulus discloses extensive fibrin deposition, epithelial and endothelial degeneration, and **characteristic focal disruptions of the GBM,** which may be filled with either fibrin or infiltrating leukocytes (Fig. 21–14). As mentioned earlier, immunofluorescent staining for immunoglobulins and complement reveal the uniform linear pattern characteristic of anti-GBM disease.

CLINICAL COURSE. The course may be dominated by recurrent hemoptysis or even life-threatening pulmonary hemorrhage (p. 745). Although milder forms of glomerular injury may subside, the renal involvement is usually progressive over a matter of weeks. When renal failure develops, dialysis support is necessary. Immunofluorescence or radioimmunoassays for circulating anti-GBM antibodies are helpful in the diagnosis, but severity of the disease does not correlate well with antibody titers. Dramatic remission may follow intensive plasmapheresis (plasma exchange) combined with steroids and cytotoxic agents.[65] This therapy appears to reverse both pulmonary hemorrhage and renal failure and is most beneficial when instituted before severe oliguria or anuria has developed. Plasma exchange

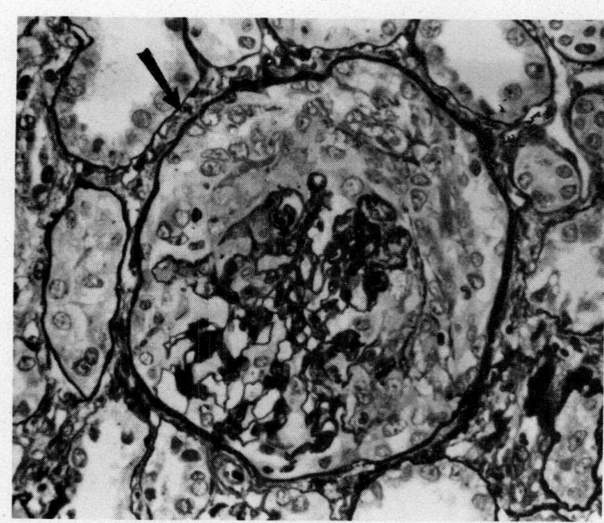

Figure 21–13. Rapidly progressive glomerulonephritis, with proliferation of cells and crescent formation (silver stain). Glomerular tuft is collapsed. Note that crescent is in Bowman's space *(arrow).*

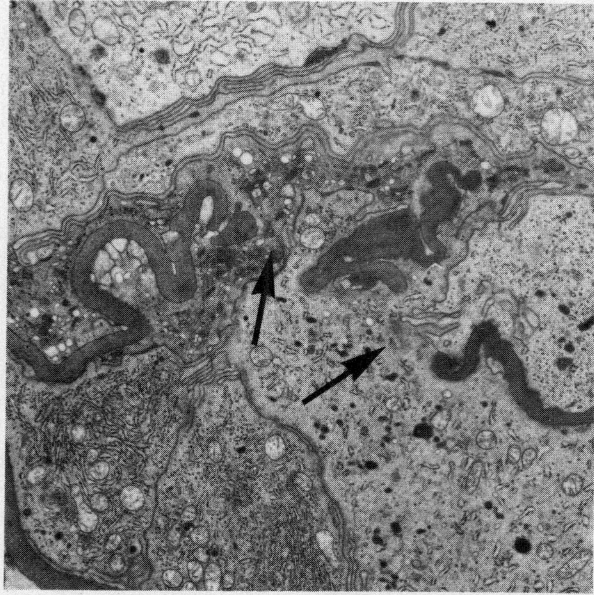

Figure 21–14. Rapidly progressive glomerulonephritis. Electron micrograph showing characteristic wrinkling of GBM with focal disruptions in its continuity *(arrows).*

presumably removes both the anti-GBM antibodies responsible for initiating the damage as well as secondary circulating mediators of the inflammatory response. Despite therapy, patients may eventually require chronic dialysis or transplantation. Transplantation is usually delayed for several months to reduce the small but definite risk of recurrence of the disease in the transplanted kidney.

Idiopathic RPGN

In about half the patients presenting with RPGN, the conditions cited in Table 21–4 can be excluded; such cases are referred to as idiopathic RPGN. A flulike syndrome may precede the onset, but most often the signs of azotemia (weakness, nausea, vomiting), oliguria, hematuria, and proteinuria herald the disease.

Immunofluorescence microscopy of glomeruli in such patients shows linear fluorescence in about one-fourth (anti-GBM disease), granular fluorescence in about one-fourth, and scanty or no immune deposits in about one-half of patients.[60] This is thus not a distinctive entity but is best viewed as an ominous pathway that may follow many types of GN of differing etiologies and pathogenesis and having in common severe glomerular damage.[66]

The kidneys are bilaterally and symmetrically enlarged and pale. Petechial hemorrhages are frequently evident on the cortical surface. By light microscopy, the glomeruli are hypercellular with varying degrees of proliferation of endothelial and mesangial cells, but characteristic is the striking crescent formation in Bowman's space throughout most glomeruli (Fig. 21–13). Sequential renal biopsies have indicated that these crescents form quite rapidly and may be fully developed within a few days of onset of nephritis. Crescents compress and distort the capillary lumina, and many of them occlude the opening into the proximal renal tubule. **Fibrin is universally present in these lesions, often deposited among the interstices of the crescent.** Electron microscopy discloses electron-dense deposits in those with granular fluorescence, but in those with linear or no fluorescence, deposits are absent. The GBM is focally disrupted (Fig. 21–14). There is usually marked interstitial edema and infiltration by inflammatory cells, and the tubules may show degenerative changes. With the advance of disease, there is organization of crescents to form collagen with eventual hyalinization of the glomeruli.

Untreated, the prognosis for most forms of RPGN is bleak, the vast majority of these patients eventually requiring long-term dialysis or transplantation. Uncontrolled therapeutic results from regimens employing high-dose corticosteroids or plasma exchange with immune suppression are encouraging, particularly when instituted in less severely oliguric patients early in the course.

The Nature of Crescents

It must be clear by now that crescent formation is not pathognomonic of any one disease but is a hallmark of severe glomerular damage. Traditionally, crescents have been thought to arise from proliferation of parietal epithelial cells, probably as a reaction to the leakage and deposition of fibrin and fibrin-related proteins into Bowman's space. The presence of focal disruptions in the basement membrane in relation to crescents (Fig. 21–13) and the finding of mitotic figures in parietal epithelial cells lend credence to these ideas.[67] Further, in some experimental models, crescent formation can be prevented by previous treatment of animals with either anticoagulants (heparin) or fibrinogenolytic agents (ancrod). Recent work, however, clearly shows that blood monocytes also emigrate across damaged glomerular walls into Bowman's space, transform into activated macrophages, and constitute part of the crescent. They can also be demonstrated in human crescents by a variety of techniques.[42] Thus, both parietal epithelial cells and macrophages contribute to crescent formation under various conditions; when present in large numbers, crescents are a poor prognostic sign.

NEPHROTIC SYNDROME (NS)

Certain glomerular diseases (membranous GN, lipoid nephrosis, focal sclerosis) virtually always produce the nephrotic syndrome. In addition, many other forms of primary and secondary GN discussed in this chapter may evoke it. It is convenient, therefore, before presenting the major causes of NS, to discuss this clinical complex.[68] NS comprises the following findings: (1) massive proteinuria with the daily loss of 3.5 gm or more of protein, (2) hypoalbuminemia with plasma albumin levels less than 3 gm per dl, (3) generalized edema, and (4) hyperlipidemia.

The syndrome is fundamentally the *result of excessive glomerular permeability to plasma proteins, and thus heavy proteinuria is its prime characteristic.* The biochemical and ultrastructural mechanisms underlying such increased protein leakage vary in the different diseases causing the syndrome and, to the extent that they are understood, will be discussed under the individual conditions. Whatever its cause, the heavy proteinuria leads to depletion of serum albumin levels below the compensatory synthetic abilities of the liver, with consequent hypoalbuminemia and a reversed albumin-globulin ratio. Increased renal catabolism is also an important contributor to the hypoalbuminemia. The generalized edema is, in turn, the consequence of the loss of colloid osmotic pressure of the blood and the accumulation of fluid in the interstitial tissues. There is also *sodium and water retention*, which aggravates the edema. This appears to be due to several factors, including compensatory secretion of aldosterone, mediated by the hypovolemia enhanced antidiuretic hormone secretion, stimulation of the sympathetic system, and a primary renal effect of uncertain nature. Edema is characteristically soft and pitting, most marked in the periorbital regions and dependent portions of the body. It may be quite massive with pleural effusions and ascites, a condition termed *anasarca*.

The largest proportion of protein lost in the urine

is albumin, but globulins are also excreted in some diseases. The ratio of low- to high-molecular-weight proteins in the urine in various cases of NS determines the so-called "selectivity" of proteinuria. A *highly selective proteinuria* consists mostly of low-molecular-weight proteins (albumin 66,000; transferrin 76,000), whereas a *poorly selective proteinuria* consists of larger-molecular-weight proteins in addition to albumin.

The genesis of the *hyperlipidemia* in the nephrotic syndrome is complex.[69] There is a close inverse relationship between the hyperlipidemia and the serum albumin levels. Low serum albumin or the diminished plasma osmotic pressure stimulates increased synthesis in the liver of cholesterol-rich lipoproteins, particularly low-density lipoproteins (LDL) and, in more severe nephrotics, triglyceride-rich low-density components (VLDL); there is also decreased catabolism of these lipids. Thus, these patients have hyperlipidemia and hypercholesterolemia (types IIa and IIb) (p. 515). *Lipiduria* follows the hyperlipidemia, since not only albumin molecules but also lipoproteins leak across the glomerular capillary wall. The lipid appears in the urine either as free fat or as "oval fat bodies" representing lipoprotein resorbed by tubular epithelial cells and then shed along with the degenerated cells. Whether associated hyperlipidemia increases the risk toward atherosclerosis and coronary heart disease is controversial. The conflicting data may be related to the high-density lipoprotein (HDL) level in the serum, which may be increased, normal, or decreased in nephrotics. You will recall that HDL levels are inversely related to coronary risk (p. 514).

These patients are particularly vulnerable to *infection*, especially with staphylococci and pneumococci. The basis for this vulnerability could be related to loss of immunoglobulins or low-molecular-weight complement components (e.g., Factor B) in the urine. *Thrombotic and thromboembolic complications* (p. 98) are also quite common. The hypercoagulable state is due in part to loss of anticoagulant factors (e.g., antithrombin III) and antiplasmin activity through the leaky glomerulus. There are also thrombocytosis and marked increases in serum factors V, VII, and VIII and fibrinogen. *Renal vein thrombosis*, once thought to be a cause of NS, is most often a consequence of this hypercoagulable state.[70]

A compilation of the forms of renal involvement that give rise to NS is presented in Table 21–5. Several features are noteworthy in this table. Among children, the great preponderance of cases of NS is the consequence of primary renal disease. The outstanding cause is lipoid nephrosis (65%), and membranous GN accounts for only 5%. In adults, primary renal disease is less predominant. Most important is membranous glomerulonephritis (40%). Systemic diseases such as diabetic glomerulosclerosis, amyloidosis, and lupus nephritis make a substantial contribution to the spectrum of NS in adults.

Table 21–5. CAUSES OF NEPHROTIC SYNDROME

Primary Glomerular Disease	Incidence*	
	Children	*Adults*
Lipoid nephrosis	65%	15%
Focal segmental glomerulosclerosis	10%	15%
Membranous GN	5%	40%
Membranoproliferative GN	10%	7%
Other proliferative (focal, "pure mesangial," IgA nephropathy)	10%	23%
Systemic Diseases		
Diabetes mellitus		
Amyloidosis		
Systemic lupus erythematosus		
Drugs (gold, penicillamine, "street heroin")		
Infections (malaria, syphilis, hepatitis B)		
Malignancy (carcinoma, melanoma)		
Miscellaneous (bee-sting allergy, hereditary nephritis)		

*Approximate incidence of primary disease = 95% in children, 60% in adults.

Approximate incidence of systemic disease = 5% in children, 40% in adults.

Membranous Glomerulonephritis (MGN)

Membranous glomerulonephritis, or membranous nephropathy, a major cause of the nephrotic syndrome, is characterized by the presence of electron-dense, immunoglobulin-containing deposits along the epithelial (subepithelial) side of the basement membrane.[71] Early in the disease, the glomeruli may appear normal by light microscopy, but well-developed cases show *diffuse thickening of the capillary wall.* Although children may suffer from this disease, it is most common in young adults and in middle life.

ETIOLOGY AND PATHOGENESIS. Because of the close similarity of the lesions of MGN to those seen in experimental chronic serum sickness, it is believed to be a form of chronic antigen-antibody–mediated disease. In particular, the immunofluorescence findings are of diffuse granular deposits of IgG and complement along the basement membrane, corresponding to the electron-dense deposits seen subepithelially with the electron microscope. MGN occurs in 10% of patients with SLE, presumably owing to DNA–anti-DNA complex deposition (p. 181). Other evidence is the association of MGN with certain infections (syphilis, malaria, hepatitis B virus), drugs (mercury, gold, penicillamine), and tumors (e.g., lung carcinoma, melanoma).[71] However, in only a small number of patients have specific antigens been identified in the deposits. In about 85% of patients with MGN, none of these associated conditions exist; the term "idiopathic" MGN is applied in such cases.[72]

A genetic component to the pathogenesis is suggested by the increased prevalence of HLA-DRW3 in European patients with MGN; in the United States there is a markedly increased incidence of a unique allotype BfF, of factor B of the alternate complement pathway, and new B-cell antigen system MT-2.[73] This suggests possible defects in immune regulation, and indeed an imbalance in T-helper and T-suppressor lymphocyte function has been reported in these patients.[74]

Circulating immune complexes are found in only 15 to 25% of cases, and thus an in situ immune reaction with a glomerular or planted antigen is postulated to account for the subepithelial immune deposits (as discussed earlier).[30] However, neither intrinsic nor planted antigens have been identified with any frequency in these deposits. Thus, the mechanism of immune deposition and the nature of the antigen(s) involved must remain speculative.

Begging the question of the nature of the immune deposits, how does the glomerular capillary wall become leaky? We simply do not know. In MGN there is loss of *size selectivity* of the GBM, allowing leakage of large-molecular-weight proteins, but the biochemical abnormality underlying this defect is unknown, as is the manner by which immune complexes cause the leakage in the apparent total absence of neutrophils, monocytes, or other putative mediators. Since complement is almost always present in glomeruli, one possibility is the direct action of the terminal components of complement, the membrane-attack complex.[40, 41]

MORPHOLOGY. The kidneys are large, swollen, and pale. By light microscopy, in fully developed cases **there is uniform, diffuse thickening of the glomerular capillary wall** (Fig. 21–15). By electron microscopy, irregular, dense deposits can be seen between the basement membrane and the overlying epithelial cells, the latter appearing swollen and having lost their foot processes (Fig. 21–16). Basement membrane material is laid down between these deposits, appearing as irregular spikes protruding from the GBM. In time, these spikes thicken to produce domelike protrusions; with progression of the disease, these eventually close over the immune deposits, burying them within a markedly thickened, irregular membrane. Progressive disintegration of the deposits creates a "moth-eaten" appearance, but eventually the holes fill in. Visualization of these membranous details requires either electron microscopy or, with light microscopy, silver impregnation stains. Immunofluorescence demonstrates that the many granular deposits contain both immunoglobulins and complement (Fig. 21–9). As the disease advances, the membranous thickening progressively encroaches upon the capillary lumina, and some proliferation and sclerosis of the mesangium may occur. Thus, the glomeruli become relatively sclerosed and, in the course of time, may eventually become totally hyalinized. The epithelial cells of the proximal tubules contain hyaline droplets, reflecting protein reabsorption. In the advanced stage of the

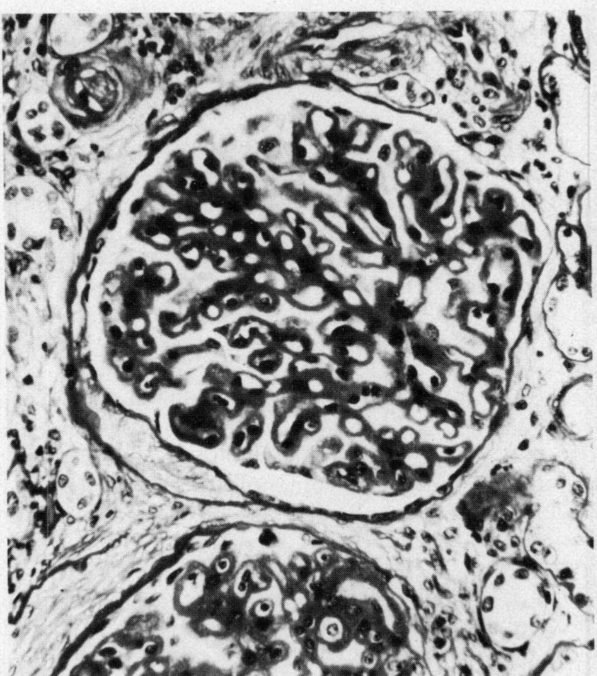

Figure 21–15. Membranous glomerulonephritis (PAS stain). Note diffuse thickening of capillary wall without increase in number of cells. Thickening is due to immune deposits on epithelial side of GBM.

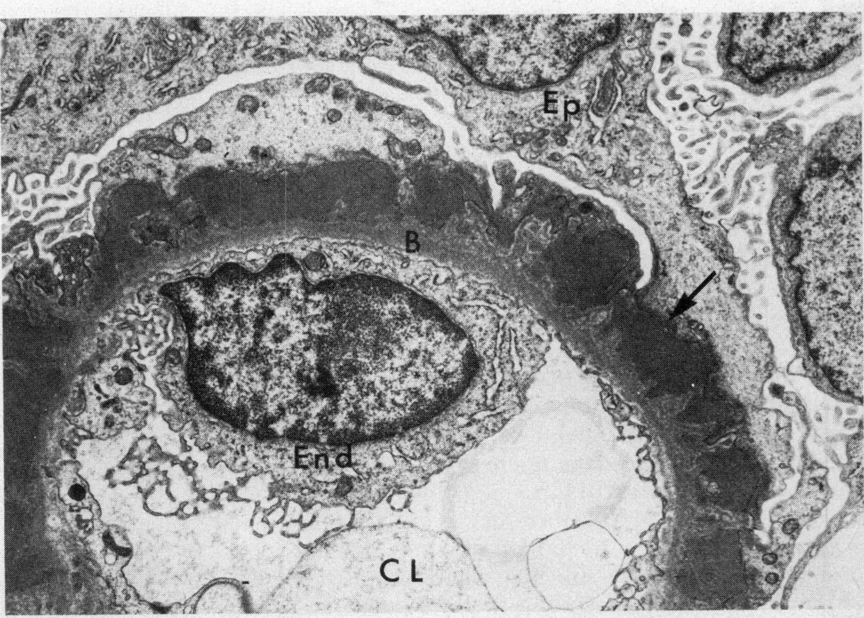

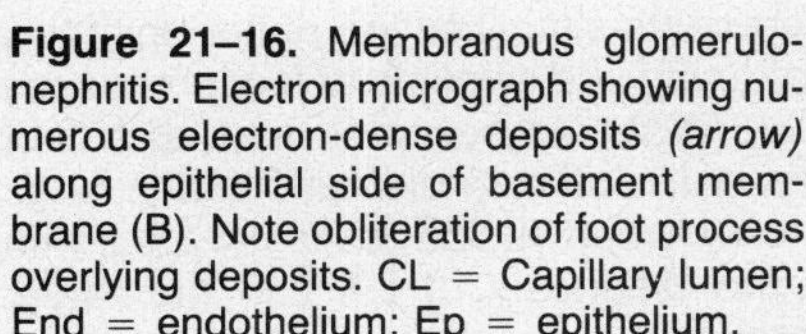

Figure 21–16. Membranous glomerulonephritis. Electron micrograph showing numerous electron-dense deposits *(arrow)* along epithelial side of basement membrane (B). Note obliteration of foot process overlying deposits. CL = Capillary lumen; End = endothelium; Ep = epithelium.

disease, tubular atrophy and interstitial fibrosis occur, and indeed the kidneys may become contracted, finely granular, and scarred, closely resembling other forms of chronic GN (p. 1019).

CLINICAL COURSE. In a previously healthy individual this disorder usually begins with the insidious onset of nephrotic syndrome or, in 15% of patients, with non-nephrotic proteinuria. Hematuria and mild hypertension are present in 15 to 35% of cases. MGN may occur in association with known disorders or etiologic agents,[71] which are well to bear in mind: malignant epithelial tumors, particularly carcinoma of the lung and colon, and melanoma; SLE (p. 180); exposure to inorganic (gold salts, mercury) or organic (penicillamine, captopril) drugs; infections (chronic hepatitis B, syphilis, schistosomiasis, malaria); and metabolic disorders (thyroiditis, diabetes mellitus). In some of these conditions, the exogenous (hepatitis B, syphilis) or endogenous (tumor products, thyroglobulin) antigens can be identified in glomeruli.

In most patients the condition is truly idiopathic. The course of the disease is notoriously irregular, but in 70 to 90% it is irreversible and progresses to renal failure over an unpredictable span of two to 20 years. Progression is associated with increasing sclerosis of glomeruli, rising BUN, relative reduction in the severity of proteinuria, and the development of hypertension. Perhaps 10 to 30% of patients have a more benign course, with partial or complete remissions. Renal vein thrombosis may occur as a reflection of the hypercoagulability.[70] Because of the variable course, it has been difficult to evaluate the effectiveness of steroids in controlling the disease, but studies suggest a significant beneficial effect of alternate-day steroid therapy in patients treated before the onset of renal insufficiency.[75]

Lipoid Nephrosis (LN) (Minimal Change Disease, Foot Process Disease, Nil Lesion)

These terms are used to describe a disorder in which the nephrotic syndrome is associated with diffuse loss of foot processes of epithelial cells in glomeruli that appear virtually normal by light microscopy. LN is the most common cause of NS in children (see Table 21–5). The peak incidence is in children between 2 and 3 years of age. The disease sometimes follows a respiratory infection (25% of cases) or routine prophylactic immunization (9%).[76] Its most characteristic feature is its dramatic and uniform response to corticosteroid therapy.

ETIOLOGY AND PATHOGENESIS. These are essentially unknown. By fluorescence microscopy there is no deposition of immunoglobulins or complement in glomeruli, and by electron microscopy no deposits are seen, excluding classical immune complex mechanisms. Nevertheless, several features of the disease point to an immunologic basis,[77] including: (1) the clinical association with respiratory infections and prophylactic immunizations; (2) the response to corticosteroid and immunosuppressive therapy; (3) the association with other atopic disorders (e.g., eczema, rhinitis); (4) the increased prevalence of HLA-B12 or HLA-DR7[73] in patients with minimal change disease associated with atopy (suggesting a possible genetic predisposition); (5) the increased incidence of LN in patients with Hodgkin's disease, in whom defects in T cell–mediated immunity are well recognized; and (6) the elaboration of lymphokine-like activity by lymphocytes of patients with LN cultured with renal tissue. Such findings have led to *speculations* that lipoid nephrosis involves some dysfunction of T-cell immunity, eventually resulting in the elaboration of a lymphokine-like circulating substance that increases the permeability of the glomerular wall.

Much more has been learned about the molecular basis of protein leakage and the pathogenesis of the characteristic loss of foot processes in this condition. An early event in LN and experimental aminonucleoside nephrosis (a model that mimics LN) appears to involve *loss of glomerular polyanion* (p. 1007). This reduction in negative charge is associated with two defects: (1) enhanced filtration of circulating polyanions, mainly albumin, resulting in proteinuria;[78] and (2) a change in epithelial cell shape leading to the familiar disappearance of foot processes.[46] The first seems to involve loss of heparan sulfate proteoglycan,[6, 8] and the second a reduction of the sialoglycoprotein cell coat.[47] How the glomerular polyanion loss is brought about, however, is mysterious. It could conceivably result from the action of circulating factor or of a metabolic defect that affects the ability of glomerular epithelial cells to elaborate these compounds, a notion consistent with the pronounced epithelial alterations in this disease.

MORPHOLOGY. The term **lipoid nephrosis** was initially coined because of the presence of lipid in tubules and fat bodies in the urine in the absence of glomerular changes. This lipid reflects glomerular leakage and reabsorption of lipoprotein. The protein reabsorption droplets appear as hyaline droplets or fatty vacuoles in the proximal convoluted tubules. The glomeruli appear normal; there is no thickening of basement membranes and no cellular proliferation (Fig. 21–17). By electron microscopy the basement membrane appears morphologically normal, and no electron-dense material is deposited. **The principal lesion is in the visceral epithelial cells, which show a uniform and diffuse loss of foot processes,** these being replaced by a rim of cytoplasm often showing vacuolization and swelling (Fig. 21–18). This change, often incorrectly termed "fusion" of foot processes, actually represents simplification of the epithelial cell architecture with flattening and swelling of foot processes rather than actual fusion. It should be noted that such foot process loss is also present in other proteinuric states (e.g., MGN, diabetes). It is only when fusion is associated with normal glomeruli that the diagnosis of LN can be made. Other changes in visceral epithelial cells include an increase in vacuoles and endoplasmic reticulum, as well as the formation of surface microvilli that are normally absent in this cell type. The visceral epithelial changes are completely reversible after corticosteroid therapy and remission of the proteinuria.

CLINICAL COURSE. Despite massive proteinuria, renal function remains good and there is usually no hypertension and no hematuria. The proteinuria usually

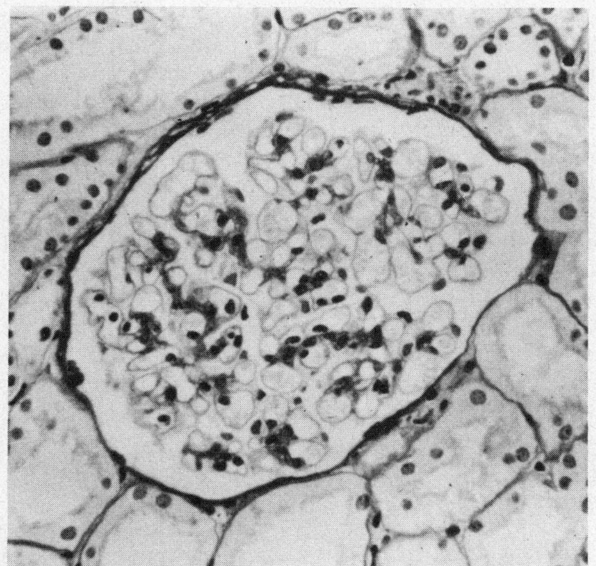

Figure 21–17. Lipoid nephrosis. Thin section of glomerulus stained with PAS. Note thin basement membrane and absence of proliferation. Compare with membranous glomerulonephritis in Figure 21–15.

is highly selective. It may be impossible, however, short of renal biopsy, to differentiate LN from MGN in the early stages of both diseases. The great majority of patients with LN exhibit a rapid response to corticosteroid therapy. Indeed, the absence of a response may indicate an error in diagnosis and the necessity to review the renal biopsy. However, the nephrotic phase may recur and some patients may become "steroid-dependent." Nevertheless, the long-term prognosis for patients is excellent, and even steroid-dependent disease resolves when the patient reaches puberty. In a series of 209 patients, followed up to ten years, 71% were in complete remission, 10% still exhibited the nephrotic syndrome, and only three had died of chronic renal insufficiency.[76] In adults, relapses are more frequent and the prognosis is generally less favorable.[79]

Focal Segmental Glomerulosclerosis (FSGS; Focal Sclerosis)

Although the morphologic lesion of focal sclerosis had long been recognized, the entity came to light only in 1970 in the course of an International Study on Childhood Lipoid Nephrosis.[80] It was noted that a small proportion of children responded poorly to corticosteroids, and in these the renal biopsies showed occasional glomeruli exhibiting an area of sclerosis confined to only one segment of the glomerulus (*thus, focal and segmental*). The morphologic entity has since been well defined and now accounts for 10 and 15% of cases of nephrotic syndrome seen among children and adults, respectively.[81, 82] About 80% of patients with this lesion have NS but differ from the usual patients with LN in the following respects: (1) they have a higher incidence of hematuria, reduced GFR, and hypertension; (2) their proteinuria is more often nonselective; (3) they respond

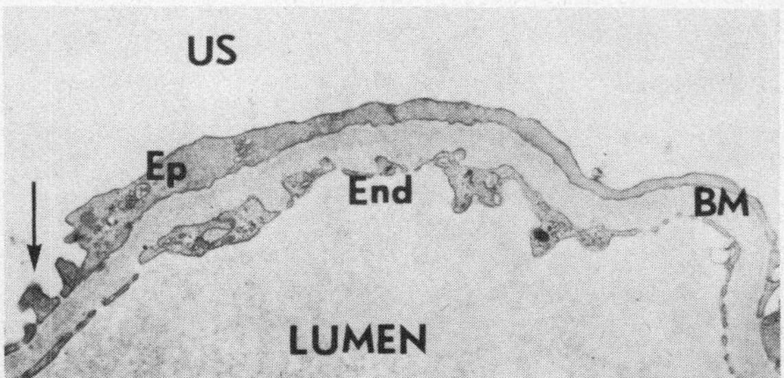

Figure 21–18. Lipoid nephrosis. Electron micrograph showing loss of characteristic epithelial cell foot processes. (Some relatively normal processes are seen [*arrow*]). Note absence of deposits along BM. End = endothelium; BM = basement membrane; Ep = epithelium; US = urinary space.

poorly or not at all to corticosteroid therapy; (4) many progress to chronic GN, at least 50% dying within ten years of diagnosis; (5) immunofluorescence microscopy shows deposition of IgM and C3 in the sclerotic segment; and (6) there is a high incidence of recurrence in transplant recipients (25 to 50% of cases).

MORPHOLOGY. As seen by light microscopy, the segmental lesions may involve only a minority of the glomeruli (Fig. 21–19) and may be missed if insufficient glomeruli are present in the biopsy. The lesions initially involve the juxtamedullary glomeruli, although they subsequently become more generalized. In the sclerotic segments there is collapse of basement membranes, increase in mesangial matrix, and deposition of hyaline masses **(hyalinosis),** often with lipoid droplets (Fig. 21–20). Glomeruli not exhibiting segmental lesions appear either entirely normal on light microscopy (as in LN) or may show increased mesangial matrix and mild mesangial proliferation. On electron microscopy, nonsclerotic areas show the diffuse loss of foot processes characteristic of LN, but in the sclerotic lesions there is also focal denudation of the epithelial cells. Masses of electron-dense amorphous material and lipoid granules are also present within the sclerotic areas. By immunofluorescence, nodular deposits of IgM and C3 are present within the hyaline masses in the sclerotic areas, but nonsclerotic glomeruli show either no staining or slight staining with IgM and C3.

In addition to the focal sclerosis, there is often rather pronounced hyaline thickening of afferent arterioles, foci of

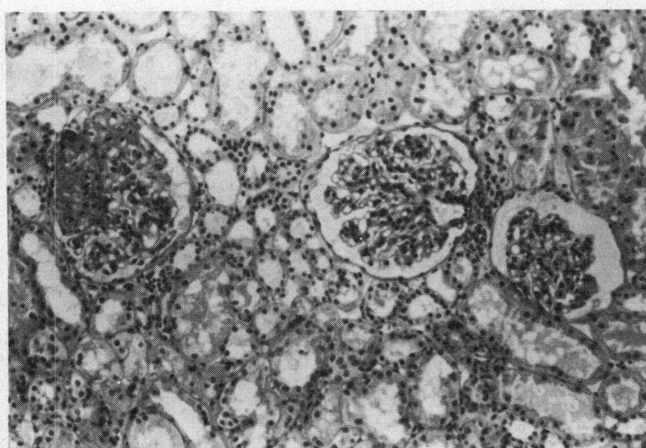

Figure 21–19. Focal and segmental glomerulosclerosis. Low-power view showing two normal glomeruli and one *(on left)* with a focus of sclerosis.

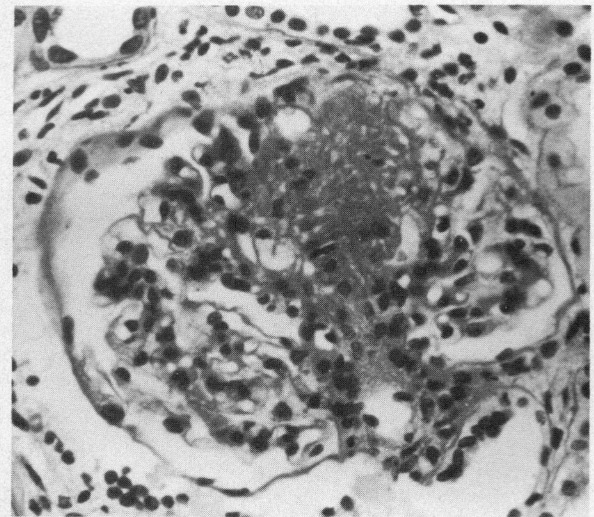

Figure 21–20. Focal and segmental sclerosis, high-power view. Only one portion of glomerulus shows an area of sclerosis. There is slight mesangial hyperplasia in rest of glomerulus.

interstitial fibrosis and tubular atrophy, and occasional glomeruli that are completely sclerosed (global sclerosis). With the progression of the disease, increased numbers of glomeruli become involved, sclerosis spreads within each glomerulus, and there is increase in mesangial matrix. In time this leads to total sclerosis of glomeruli with pronounced tubular atrophy and interstitial fibrosis. This advanced picture would be almost impossible to differentiate from other forms of chronic GN.

PATHOGENESIS. Whether FSGS represents a distinct disease or is simply a phase in the evolution of a subset of patients with LN is a matter of debate, most investigators favoring the latter possibility.[82, 83] The characteristic degeneration and focal disruption of visceral epithelial cells is thought to represent an accentuation of the diffuse epithelial cell change typical of LN. It is this pronounced epithelial damage that is the hallmark of FSGS. The hyalinosis and sclerosis represent entrapment of plasma proteins in extremely hyperpermeable foci and mesangial cell reaction to such deposited proteins. The recurrence of proteinuria in patients with focal sclerosis who receive renal allografts, sometimes within 24 hours of transplantation, suggests the existence of a circulating toxin as the cause of the epithelial damage, but no such toxin has yet been identified. It is worth noting that an identical lesion, associated with heavy proteinuria, occurs as a complication of other nonglomerular renal diseases causing reduction in functioning renal tissue, particularly reflux nephropathy (p. 1034),[84] chronic pyelonephritis (p. 1034), and unilateral agenesis (p. 998).[84] The lesions in the latter settings are almost certainly the result of "adaptive hyperfiltration," detailed earlier.[52] Whether the hemodynamic changes play a role in the idiopathic form of FSGS is at present unknown.

CLINICAL COURSE. As mentioned earlier, there is little tendency for spontaneous remission, and responses to corticosteroid therapy are infrequent. In general, children have a better prognosis than adults. Progression of renal failure occurs at variable rates. About 20% of patients follow an unusually rapid course (*malignant focal sclerosis*), with intractable massive proteinuria ending in renal failure within two years. Recurrences occur in 25% to 50% of patients receiving allografts.

Before we leave focal sclerosis, it is worth emphasizing that the histologic lesion of FSGS in itself is nonspecific, and can be present in glomeruli in some stages of other forms of GN. It is only when associated with NS (or at least heavy proteinuria) *and* the characteristic electron microscopic loss of epithelial foot processes that the entity has the implications discussed here.[82]

Membranoproliferative Glomerulonephritis (MPGN)

As the term implies, this group of disorders is characterized histologically by *alterations in the basement membrane and proliferation of cells.* Because the proliferation is predominantly in the mesangium, a frequently used synonym is mesangiocapillary GN.

The condition was first described in 1965 when a form of GN in children and young adults was found associated with low levels of the third component of complement. These patients had no evidence of poststreptococcal GN or SLE that would account for the hypocomplementemia. Subsequent observations showed that the latter was not invariably present, and further that the histologic lesion of MPGN may underlie different ultrastructural and immunofluorescent patterns.[85]

The clinical manifestations are variable. In two-thirds of patients NS is present and, indeed, MPGN accounts for 5 to 10% of cases of idiopathic NS in children and adults. Some patients present with only hematuria or proteinuria of non-nephrotic range, and others have a combined nephrotic-nephritic picture.

MORPHOLOGY. By light microscopy, the glomeruli are large and hypercellular, the latter condition being due to a prominent increase in mesangial cells (Fig. 21–21). The GBM is clearly thickened, often focally, most evident in the peripheral capillary loops. The glomerular capillary wall often shows a "double-contour" or "tram-track" appearance, especially evident in silver or PAS stains (Fig. 21–22). This is caused by "splitting" of the basement membrane because of the inclusion within it of processes of mesangial cells extending into the peripheral capillary loops, so-called **mesangial interposition.**

MPGN is divided into two main types according to the ultrastructural characteristics:[86, 87]

Type I MPGN (two-thirds of cases) is characterized by the presence of **subendothelial electron-dense deposits.** Mesangial and occasional subepithelial deposits may also be present (Fig. 21–23). By immunofluorescence, C3 is deposited in a granular pattern, and IgG and early complement components (C1q and C4) are often also present, suggesting an immune complex pathogenesis.

In the Type II lesion, the lamina densa of the GBM is

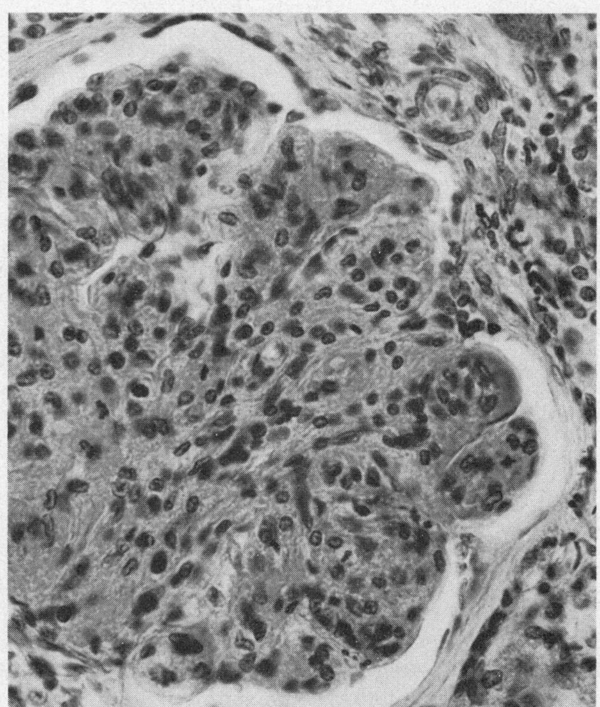

Figure 21–21. Membranoproliferative glomerulonephritis. Glomeruli are enlarged, and there is a marked increase in mesangial cells. Peripheral basement membrane (at 4 o'clock) is thickened.

transformed into an irregular, extremely electron-dense structure, due to the deposition of dense material of unknown compositing in the GBM proper, giving rise to the term **dense-deposit disease** (Fig. 21–24). In Type II, C3 is present in irregular granular-linear foci in the basement membranes on either side, but not within the dense deposits. C3 is also present in the mesangium in characteristic circular aggregates (mesangial rings). IgG is often absent, and the

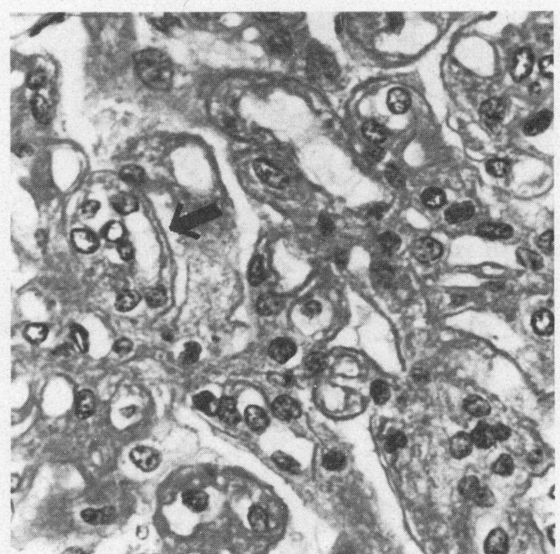

Figure 21–22. Detail of glomerular basement membrane in membranoproliferative glomerulonephritis (PAS stained). Note splitting of BM, giving characteristic "double-contour" or "tram-track" pattern *(arrow).*

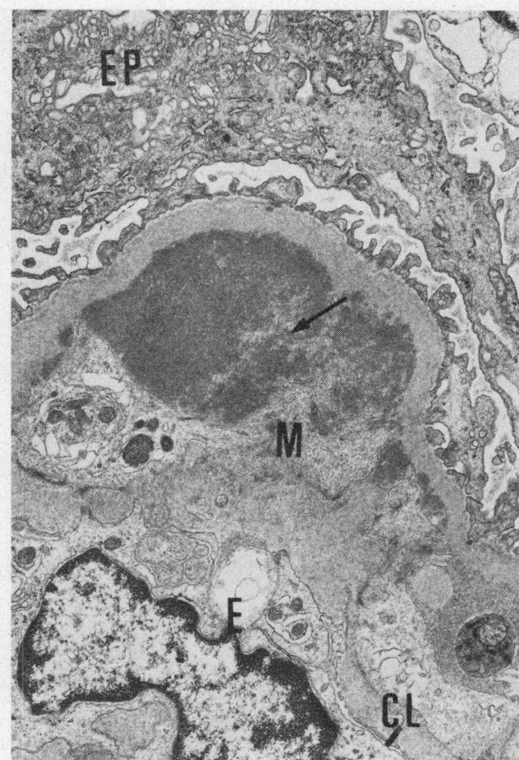

Figure 21–23. Membranoproliferative glomerulonephritis, type I. Note large subendothelial deposit *(arrow)* incorporated into mesangial matrix (M) through process of "mesangialization" (see text). E = endothelium; EP = epithelium; CL = capillary lumen.

early-acting complement components (C1q and C4) are usually absent from the deposits. **A rare variant (Type III)** is segregated because it exhibits both subendothelial and subepithelial deposits, associated with GBM disruption and reduplication. Its clinical features are similar to those of Type I.

Other histologic findings include neutrophilic and mononuclear infiltrates within the capillary walls; epithelial crescents in severe forms of the disease; vascular sclerosis; and variable degrees of interstitial inflammation, fibrosis, and tubular atrophy.

PATHOGENESIS. Although there are exceptions, most cases of Type I MPGN present evidence of immune complexes in the glomerulus and activation of both classic and alternate complement pathways.[86, 87] On the other hand, most patients with dense-deposit disease (Type II) have abnormalities that suggest *primary activation of the alternate complement pathway* (normal C1, C4; diminished factor B and properdin).[88] In the latter there is also deposition of C3 and properdin, but not C1q or C4 in the glomeruli. Recall that, in the alternate complement pathway, C3 is directly cleaved to C3b (Fig. 21–25) (see also Fig. 2–10, p. 52). The reaction depends on the initial interaction of C3 with such substances as bacterial polysaccharides, endotoxin, aggregates of IgA in the presence of factors B and $\overline{D}$, and magnesium. This leads to the generation of $\overline{C3bBb}$, the alternate pathway C3 convertase, which is equiva-

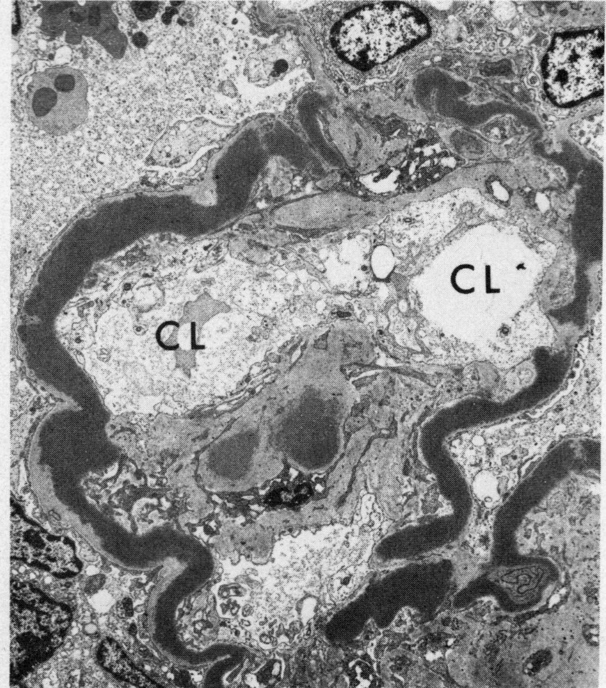

Figure 21–24. Type II MPGN, dense-deposit disease. There are markedly dense homogeneous deposits within basement membrane proper. CL = capillary lumen. (Courtesy of Dr. M. Federman, New England Deaconess Hospital, Boston, MA).

lent to the C3 convertase of the classic pathway, $\overline{C42}$. $\overline{C3bBb}$ is extremely labile but can be stabilized by properdin, which binds to the C3b moiety of $\overline{C3bBb}$, allowing the latter to cleave native C3. Almost all patients with dense-deposit disease have in their serum a factor, *termed C3 nephritic factor (C3NeF)*, which acts at the same step as properdin, helping to stabilize $\overline{C3bBb}$ by binding to it. *C3NeF is, in fact, immunoglobulin of the IgG class,*[89] *suggesting that it is an autoantibody to the alternate pathway C3 convertase* ($\overline{C3bBb}$). If this suggestion is correct, dense-deposit disease would be added to the category of *autoimmune diseases*. It is interesting that, in addition to increased consumption of C3, there is decreased C3 synthesis by the liver, further contributing to the profound hypocomplementemia.

How these complement defects are translated into glomerular injury is unclear. It has *not* been possible to induce glomerular damage in experimental animals by prolonged activation of the alternate complement pathway.[40] Could it be, instead, that the complement defects—either genetic or acquired—predispose to GN by limiting the patient's ability to deal with microbiologic agents and toxins or to clear complexes? Alternatively, could a product of complement activation be nephrotoxic only in certain otherwise genetically susceptible individuals? A genetic predisposition is indeed suggested by the presence of C3NeF activity in some patients with the genetically determined disease, *partial lipodystrophy*, some of whom develop Type II MPGN. The nature of the dense deposit in the GBM in Type II MPGN is unknown.

CLINICAL COURSE. Few remissions occur spontaneously in either type and the disease follows a slowly progressive but unremitting course. Some patients develop numerous crescents and a clinical picture of rapidly progressive GN. About 50% develop chronic renal failure within ten years. There is a high incidence of recurrence in transplant recipients, particularly in Type II disease.

It is worth noting that histologic alterations very similar to MPGN (mostly Type I) occur in GN associated with hepatitis B antigenemia, infected ventriculoatrial shunts, schistosomiasis, alpha$_1$-antitrypsin deficiency, and inherited deficiencies of C2.[53, 85]

FOCAL PROLIFERATIVE GLOMERULONEPHRITIS

Focal glomerulonephritis represents a histologic entity in which glomerular proliferation is restricted to segments of individual glomeruli and commonly involves only a certain proportion of glomeruli. The lesions are predominantly proliferative and should be differentiated from those of focal sclerosis. Focal necrosis and fibrin deposition within the lesions may occur (Fig. 21–26).

Focal GN occurs under two circumstances: (1) It may be an early or mild manifestation of a systemic disease that sometimes involves entire glomeruli; among these are lupus erythematosus, polyarteritis nodosa, Henoch-Schönlein purpura, Goodpasture's syndrome, subacute bacterial endocarditis, and Wegener's granulomatosis. (2) It can occur unrelated to any systemic disease and constitute a form of primary focal GN. The clinical manifestations may be subclinical, manifested by recurrent microscopic or gross hematuria or nonnephrotic proteinuria, but occasional cases present with nephrotic syndrome. One type of primary focal GN, IgA nephropathy, has sufficiently distinctive immunoflu-

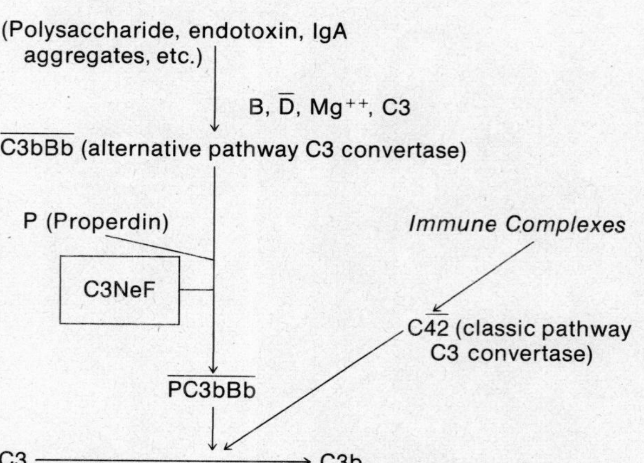

Figure 21–25. Alternate complement pathway (see text). C3NeF present in serum of patients with MPGN is an immunoglobulin that stabilizes $\overline{C3bBb}$ by binding to it, probably as an antibody, thus activating pathway. (See also Fig. 2–10.)

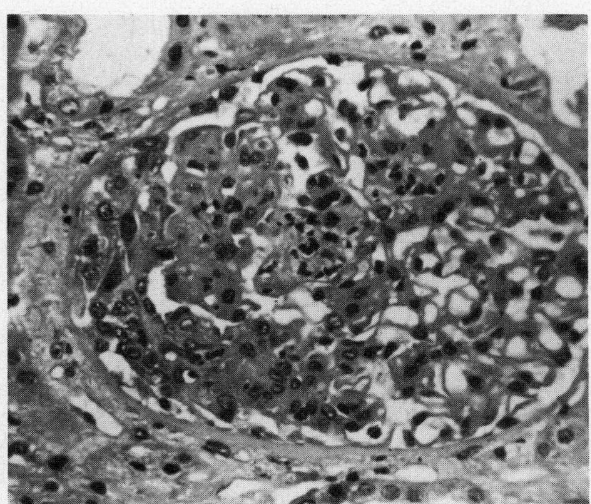

Figure 21–26. Focal glomerulonephritis in lupus erythematosus. There is segmental proliferation *(left)* and necrosis *(middle)*. In the necrotic area there are neutrophils and fragmented nuclei (nuclear dust).

orescent and clinical manifestations to warrant its discussion as a separate entity.

IgA Nephropathy (Berger's Disease)

First described by Berger, *this entity is characterized by the presence of prominent IgA deposits in the mesangial regions by immunofluorescence microscopy.*[90] The disease can be suspected by light microscopic examination, but diagnosis is made only by immunofluorescence microscopy (Fig. 21–27). IgA nephropathy is a common cause of recurrent gross or microscopic hematuria. Mild proteinuria is usually present, and occasionally NS may develop.[91] A rare patient may present with rapidly progressive crescentic GN. The disease affects children and young adults and may occur within a day or two of a nonspecific respiratory infection. Typically, the hematuria lasts for several days and then subsides, only to return every few months.

Histologically, the lesions vary considerably. The glomeruli may be normal or may show mesangial widening and segmental proliferation confined to some glomeruli (focal GN); diffuse mesangial proliferation (mesangioproliferative); or rarely, overt crescentic GN. The characteristic immunofluorescent picture is of **mesangial deposition of IgA** (Fig. 21–27), often with C3 and properdin and lesser amounts of IgG or IgM. Early complement components are usually absent. Electron microscopy confirms the presence of electron-dense deposits in the mesangium in the vast majority of cases. In some biopsies, prominent hyaline thickening of arterioles is present, a feature associated with a greater likelihood of progression to chronic renal failure.

The pathogenesis is unknown although there are several clues.[92] The exclusive mesangial deposition of IgA suggests entrapment of large circulating aggregates or complexes, and the absence of C1q and C4 in glomeruli point to activation of the alternate complement pathway. You may recall that aggregated IgA is a known activator of the alternate pathway. Circulating IgA immune complexes are present in some individuals. Up to 50% of patients have elevated IgA serum levels. A genetic influence in IgA nephropathy is suggested by its occasional occurrence in families and in HLA identical brothers, and its possible increased frequency in the HLA-BW35 (DR4) haplotype.[73] There is also evidence of defective phagocytic function of the mononuclear phagocyte system in such patients. Taken together, these and other findings suggest a primary (probably genetic) abnormality in regulation of IgA production and increased IgA synthesis in response to some environmental agent (? viruses, food proteins). IgA aggregates or complexes are then entrapped in the mesangium, where they activate the alternate complement pathway.[93] Defective phagocytic function, either inherited or acquired, may contribute by affecting the clearance of the complexes, either in the mesangium or in the mononuclear phagocyte system.[94]

Clinical Course. As noted above, IgA nephropathy is clinically a heterogeneous disease. Although most patients have an initially benign course, the disease appears to be slowly progressive: it is estimated that chronic renal failure develops in up to 50% of cases over a period of 20 years. Onset in old age, heavy proteinuria, hypertension, and the presence of vascular sclerosis or crescents on biopsy are clues to an increased risk of progression. Recurrence of IgA deposits in transplanted kidneys occurs in 50% of cases, but with seemingly limited clinical consequence in most of these.[95]

CHRONIC GLOMERULONEPHRITIS

Chronic glomerulonephritis is best considered an end-stage pool of glomerular disease fed by a number of streams of glomerulonephritis, most of which have been described earlier in this chapter. Poststreptococcal

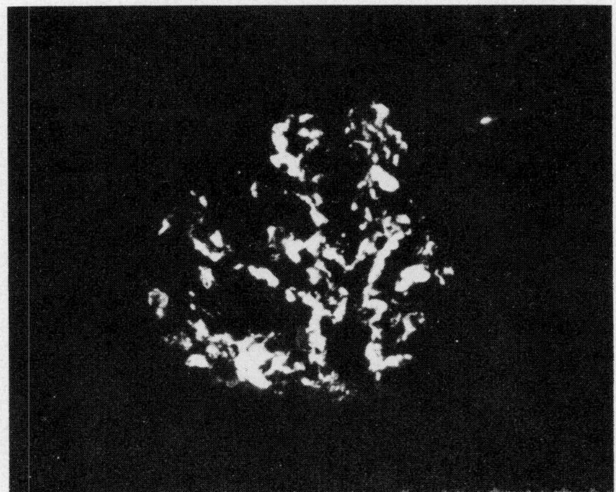

Figure 21–27. IgA nephropathy. Characteristic immunofluorescence deposition of IgA, principally in mesangial regions. Compare with Figures 21–8 and 21–9, in which fluorescent deposits are along GBM.

GN is a rare antecedent of chronic GN, except in adults. Patients with rapidly progressive GN, if they survive the acute episode, invariably end with chronic GN. Membranous, membranoproliferative glomerulonephritis and IgA nephropathy progress more slowly to chronic renal failure, whereas focal sclerosis often advances rather rapidly into chronic GN. *Nevertheless, in any series of patients with chronic GN, about one-fourth arise mysteriously with no antecedent history of any of the well-recognized forms of early GN.* These cases represent the end result of relatively asymptomatic forms of GN, either known or still unrecognized, that progress to uremia.

MORPHOLOGY. The kidneys are symmetrically contracted and have red-brown, diffusely granular, cortical surfaces. Each generally weighs in the range of 100 gm. Such symmetric contraction must be differentiated from that caused by chronic pyelonephritis, which generally shows more irregular and asymmetric contraction. On section, the cortex is thinned and there is increase in peripelvic fat. The glomerular histology depends on the stage of the disease. In early cases, the glomeruli may still show evidence of the primary disease, e.g., membranous or menbranoproliferative GN. However, there eventually ensues hyaline obliteration of glomeruli, transforming them into acellular eosinophilic PAS-positive masses (Fig. 21–28). The nature of the hyaline material is not well understood, but it appears to represent a combination of trapped plasma proteins, increased mesangial matrix, basement membrane–like material, and collagen. Cases seen in the end stage of advanced glomerular hyalinization provide no clues as to their origin. Because hypertension is an accompaniment of chronic GN, arterial and arteriolar sclerosis may be conspicuous. Marked atrophy of associated tubules, irregular interstitial fibrosis, and lymphocytic infiltration also occur. The secondary vascular, tubular, and interstitial changes in end-stage renal failure may make it difficult to determine that the primary disease was GN rather than an interstitial or vascular process.

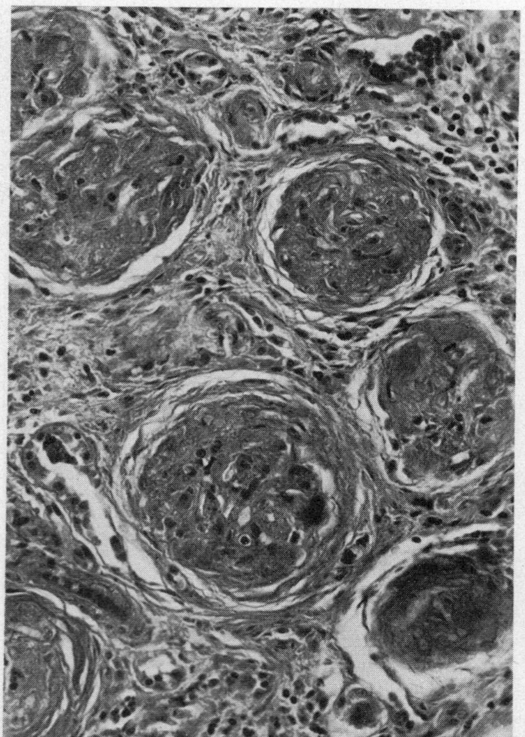

Figure 21–28. Chronic glomerulonephritis. Glomeruli are totally replaced by hyaline connective tissue.

Kidneys from patients with end-stage disease on long-term dialysis exhibit a variety of so-called "dialysis changes" that are unrelated to the primary disease.[53] These include arterial intimal thickening caused by accumulation of smooth muscle–like cells and a loose, proteoglycan-rich stroma; calcification, most obvious in glomerular tufts and tubular basement membranes; extensive deposition of calcium oxalate crystals in tubules and interstitium; acquired cystic disease (p. 1002); and increased numbers of renal adenomas and borderline adenocarcinomas.

Patients dying with GN also exhibit pathologic changes **outside** the kidney that are related to the uremic state and are also present in other forms of chronic renal failure (p. 996). Often clinically important, these include **uremic pericarditis, uremic gastroenteritis, secondary hyperparathyroidism with nephrocalcinosis and renal osteodystrophy, left ventricular hypertrophy due to hypertension, and pulmonary changes often ascribed to uremia (uremic pneumonitis).**

CLINICAL COURSE. In most patients, chronic GN develops insidiously and slowly progresses to death in uremia over a span of years or possibly decades. Not infrequently, patients present with such nonspecific complaints as loss of appetite, anemia, vomiting, or weakness. In some, the renal disease is suspected with the discovery of proteinuria, hypertension, or azotemia on routine medical examination. In others, the underlying renal disorder is discovered in the course of investigation of edema. *Most patients are hypertensive, and sometimes the dominant clinical manifestations are cerebral or cardiovascular.* In all, the disease is relentlessly progressive, although at widely varying rates. In some patients, the slow progression is punctuated by bouts of active nephritis with its attendant hematuria, red cell casts, and oliguria. In other instances, episodes of marked proteinuria may evoke the nephrotic syndrome, but in general, as the disease advances and the glomeruli become obliterated, the protein loss in the urine diminishes and so does the likelihood of nephrotic episodes. If such patients are not maintained on continued dialysis or if they do not receive a renal transplant, the outcome is invariably death.

Table 21–6 summarizes the main clinical and histologic features of the major forms of primary GN.

GLOMERULAR LESIONS ASSOCIATED WITH SYSTEMIC DISEASE

Many immunologically mediated, metabolic, or hereditary systemic disorders are associated with glomerular injury, and in some, e.g., SLE and diabetes mellitus, the glomerular involvement is a major clinical manifestation. Most of these diseases have been dis-

Table 21–6. SUMMARY OF MAJOR PRIMARY GLOMERULONEPHRITDES

Disease	Most Frequent Clinical Presentation	Pathogenesis	Pathology Light Microscopy	Pathology Fluorescence Microscopy	Pathology Electron Microscopy
Poststreptococcal glomerulonephritis	Acute nephritis	Antibody-mediated; circulating or planted antigen	Diffuse proliferation; leukocytic infiltration	Granular IgG and C3 in GBM and mesangium	Subepithelial humps
Goodpasture's syndrome	Rapidly progressive GN	Anti–GBM	Proliferation; crescents	Linear IgG and C3; fibrin in crescents	No deposits; GBM disruptions; fibrin
Idiopathic RPGN	Rapidly progressive GN	Mixed (see text)	Proliferation; focal necrosis; crescents	25% linear 25–50% granular IgG + C3 25–50% negative or equivocal	No deposits Deposits may be present No deposits
Membranous glomerulonephritis	Nephrotic syndrome	Antibody-mediated;? In situ	Diffuse capillary wall thickening	Granular IgG and C3; diffuse	Subepithelial deposits
Lipoid nephrosis	Nephrotic syndrome	Unknown, loss of glomerular polyanion	Normal; lipid in tubules	Negative	Loss of foot processes; no deposits.
Focal segmental glomerulosclerosis	Nephrotic syndrome; non-nephrotic proteinuria	Unknown	Focal and segmental sclerosis and hyalinosis	Focal; IgM and C3	Loss of foot processes; epithelial damage
Membrano-proliferative glomerulonephritis Type I Type II	Nephrotic syndrome Hematuria Chronic renal failure	(I) Immune complex (II) Immune complex; alternate complement pathway activation	Mesangial proliferation; basement membrane thickening; splitting	(I) IgG + C3; C1 + C4 (II) C3 ± IgG; no C1 and C4	(I) Subendothelial deposits; (II) Dense-deposit disease
IgA nephropathy	Recurrent hematuria and/or proteinuria	Unknown; see text	Focal proliferative GN; mesangial widening	IgA + IgG, M, and C3 in mesangium	Mesangial and paramesangial dense deposits
Chronic glomerulonephritis	Chronic renal failure	Variable	Hyalinized glomeruli	Granular or negative	——

cussed elsewhere in this book. Here we shall briefly recall some of the lesions and discuss only those not considered in other sections.

Systemic Lupus Erythematosus

The various types of lupus nephritis are described and illustrated in detail on page 184. As discussed, SLE gives rise to a heterogeneous group of lesions and clinical presentations.[96] The clinical manifestations include recurrent microscopic or gross hematuria, acute nephritis, the nephrotic syndrome, and hypertension. Histologically, glomerular changes have been separated by the World Health Organization (WHO) into five groups.

NO RENAL LESIONS (WHO CLASS I). This refers to glomeruli that are normal by light microscopy or show no mesangial deposits of immunoglobulin and complement by immunofluorescence microscopy. Such patients are usually asymptomatic.

MESANGIAL LUPUS NEPHRITIS (WHO CLASS II). This lesion occurs in 5 to 10% of biopsies. Patients may exhibit slight microscopic hematuria or proteinuria and normal renal function. The glomeruli are either normal (Class IIa) or show slight increase in mesangial cells, with mild diffuse mesangial prominence by light microscopy (Class IIb). However, all these biopsies show deposition of IgG and C3 in a granular fashion in the mesangium, even in glomeruli that appear normal by light microscopy. These deposits are also seen by electron microscopy.

FOCAL PROLIFERATIVE GLOMERULONEPHRITIS (WHO CLASS III). This type is observed in about one-third of patients on initial biopsy, and consists of focal and segmental proliferation (often in the mesangium). Fibrin, hyalin thrombi, and fragmented nuclei (nuclear dust) and necrosis may be present within the focal lesions, which in later stages undergo sclerosis and fibrosis. Clinically, patients with this lesion usually have microscopic hematuria and proteinuria. Although it was once thought that such patients have a benign course, many studies show that some progress to diffuse and/or chronic renal insufficiency.

DIFFUSE PROLIFERATIVE GLOMERULONEPHRITIS (WHO CLASS IV). This is the most frequent lesion, occurring in 50% of patients with SLE and characterized histologically by diffuse proliferation and leukocytic infiltration (Fig. 5–19, p. 185). Nuclear fragmentation, hyalin thrombi, fibrin deposits, and foci of necrosis are common. In some patients there is, in addition, membranous thickening; thus the lesion may resemble *membranoproliferative glomerulonephritis.* Fluorescence microscopy shows large nodular deposits of immunoglobulins and complement in the mesangium and the peripheral capillary loops. There is strong staining for C1q and C4. Electron microscopy shows the massive deposits in the mesangium, in the subepithelial region and particularly in the subendothelial space. *The subendothelial deposits are characteristic of active proliferative lupus nephritis and, indeed, cause the wire-loop lesions seen by light microscopy* (Fig. 5–21A, p. 186).

Patients with diffuse proliferative lupus GN usually have a symptomatic nephritic syndrome, with hypertension and reduction of GFR, but about 25% have either mild or no clinical renal abnormalities. This is a common and sometimes serious type of nephritis, especially when associated with signs of "activity" such as subendothelial deposits, fibrinoid change, and crescents. Therapy with corticosteroids and immunosuppressive agents has a beneficial effect, but recurrences occur. Progression to chronic renal failure is now much less common than in the past.

DIFFUSE MEMBRANOUS GN (WHO CLASS V). In this type, the lesions resemble those seen in membranous GN described earlier, and patients tend to have recurrent proteinuria or nephrotic syndrome. In the pure membranous type of lupus nephritis, subendothelial deposits are infrequent or absent. This type accounts for only 10% of lupus nephritis and generally has a much better prognosis than the diffuse proliferative GN. In one study only two of 28 patients developed progressive renal failure over a follow-up period of 12 years.

Although these types of lupus nephritis have been presented separately, one type occasionally may transform to another in the course of the disease in the same patient. In particular, focal proliferative GN transforms fairly often to the diffuse type.

Henoch-Schönlein Purpura

This syndrome consists of *purpuric skin lesions characteristically involving the extensor surfaces of arms and legs as well as buttocks; abdominal manifestations including pain, vomiting, and intestinal bleeding; nonmigratory arthralgia; and renal abnormalities.* Not all components of the syndrome need be present and individual patients may have purpura, abdominal pain, or urinary abnormalities as the dominant feature. The disease is most common in children 3 to 8 years old, but also occurs in adults, in whom the renal manifestations are usually more severe. There is a strong background of atopy in about one-third of patients. The onset often follows an upper respiratory infection. Renal manifestations occur in one-third of patients and include gross or microscopic hematuria, proteinuria, and nephrotic syndrome. A small number of patients, mostly adults, develop a rapidly progressive form of GN with many crescents.

Histologically, the renal lesions vary, according to the severity of the disease, from mild focal mesangial proliferation to diffuse mesangial proliferation to rather typical crescentic GN. Whatever the histologic lesions, the prominent feature by fluorescence microscopy is the *deposition of IgA, sometimes with IgG and C3 in the mesangial region* in a distribution similar to that described for IgA nephropathy.[97] This has led to the belief that Berger's disease and Henoch-Schönlein purpura are perhaps spectra of the same disease. The skin lesions consist of subepidermal hemorrhages and a necrotizing vasculitis involving the small vessels of the dermis. IgA is also present in such vessels. Vasculitis can also occur in other organs such as the gastrointestinal tract, but is rare in the kidney. Although the pathogenesis of Henoch-Schölein purpura is unknown, the same types of speculations presented for IgA nephropathy apply.

The course of the disease is quite variable, but recurrences of hematuria may persist for many years after onset. Patients with the more diffuse lesions or with NS have a somewhat poorer prognosis, and renal failure occurs in those with the crescentic lesions.

Bacterial Endocarditis

Glomerular lesions occurring in the course of subacute bacterial endocarditis have long been known and were termed "focal embolic GN." It is now clear, however, that these lesions are not embolic in nature and simply represent a type of immune complex nephritis initiated by bacterial antigen-antibody complex. Clinically, hematuria and proteinuria of various degrees characterize this entity, but an acute nephritic presentation is not uncommon, and even rapidly progressive GN may occur in rare instances. It must be apparent by now that the histologic lesions, when present, generally reflect these clinical manifestations. Milder forms have a focal and segmental necrotizing GN, whereas more severe ones exhibit a diffuse proliferative GN, and the rapidly progressive forms show large numbers of crescents. GN in acute endocarditis is rare, except in some patients with coagulase-positive *Staphylococcus aureus* endocarditis in whom a diffuse proliferative GN occurs (p. 1007).[53]

Diabetic Glomerulosclerosis and Diabetic Nephropathy

Diabetes mellitus is a major cause of renal morbidity and mortality. End-stage kidney disease occurs in up to 30% of juvenile diabetics and accounts for 20% of deaths in patients under age 40.[98] By far the most common lesions involve the glomeruli and are associated clinically with three glomerular syndromes, including non-nephrotic proteinuria, nephrotic syndrome, and chronic renal failure. However, diabetes also affects the arterioles, causing *arteriolar sclerosis*; increases susceptibility to the development of pyelonephritis, and particularly *papillary necrosis*; and causes a variety of tubular lesions. The term *diabetic nephropathy* is applied to the conglomerate of lesions that often occur concurrently in the diabetic kidney.

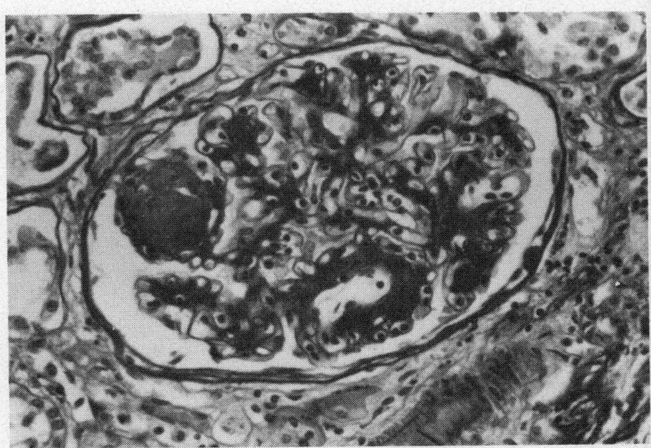

Figure 21–30. Diffuse and nodular diabetic glomerulosclerosis (PAS stain). Note diffuse increase in mesangial matrix and characteristic acellular PAS-positive nodule.

Diabetic Glomerulosclerosis

Proteinuria, sometimes in the nephrotic range, occurs in about 55% of juvenile- and 30% of adult-onset diabetics. It is usually discovered 12 to 22 years after the clinical appearance of diabetes, and (particularly in juvenile diabetics) often heralds the progressive development of chronic renal failure ending in death or end-stage disease within a period of four to five years. The morphologic changes in the glomeruli include (1) capillary basement membrane thickening, (2) diffuse diabetic glomerulosclerosis, and (3) nodular glomerulosclerosis.[99]

Morphology. ***Capillary Basement Membrane Thickening.*** Widespread thickening of the glomerular capillary basement membrane occurs in virtually all diabetics, irrespective of the presence of proteinuria, and is part and parcel of the diabetic microangiopathy described earlier (p. 982). Pure capillary basement membrane thickening can be detected only by electron microscopy. Careful morphometric studies demonstrate that this thickening begins as early as two years after the onset of juvenile diabetes, and by five years amounts to about a 30% increase.[100] The thickening continues progressively, and usually concurrently with mesangial widening (Fig. 20–21, p. 983). Simultaneously there is thickening of the tubular basement membranes.

Diffuse Glomerulosclerosis. This consists of diffuse increase in mesangial matrix with proliferation of mesangial cells, and is always associated with the overall thickening of the GBM described earlier. The increase in mesangial volume appears to lag slightly behind basement membrane widening, but becomes pronounced after ten to 20 years of diabetes. The matrix depositions are PAS positive. The changes almost always begin in the vascular stalk and sometimes seem continuous with the invariably present hyaline thickening of arterioles (Fig. 21–29). As the disease progresses, the mesangial areas expand further and obliterate the mesangial cells, gradually filling the entire glomerulus **(obliterative diabetic glomerulosclerosis).** Immunofluorescence microscopy often shows a linear pattern of staining for plasma proteins (both albumin and globulins), a reflection of the binding of these proteins to the diabetic GBM rather than of anti-GBM disease. Although the severity of diffuse glomerulosclerosis correlates well with proteinuria and progression to renal failure, the lesion is not pathognomonic of diabetes by light microscopy, as it may resemble some stages of glomerulonephritis.[53] However, the presence of dominant arteriolar hyalinization, the linear pattern of fluorescence for globulins and albumin, and the absence of granular immune reactants in the glomerulus aid in differentiating glomerulonephritis from diabetic glomerulosclerosis.

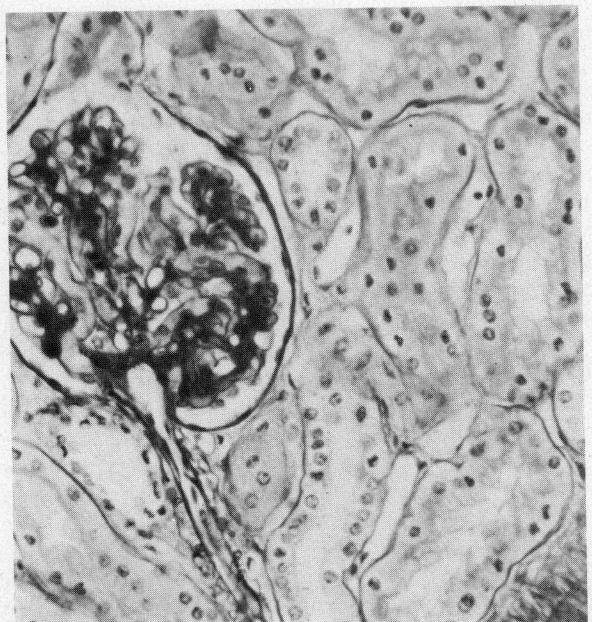

Figure 21–29. Early diffuse diabetic glomerulosclerosis with accentuation of axial framework of glomerular tuft. (Courtesy of Dr. Merle Legg.)

Nodular Glomerulosclerosis. This is also known as intercapillary glomerulosclerosis or Kimmelstiel-Wilson disease. The glomerular lesions take the form of ovoid or spherical, often laminated, hyaline masses situated in the periphery of the glomerulus. They lie within the mesangial core of the glomerular lobules and often are surrounded by peripheral patent capillary loops (Fig. 21–30). Usually, not all the lobules in the individual glomerulus are involved. **Uninvolved lobules and glomeruli all show striking diffuse glomerulosclerosis.** The nodules are PAS positive; contain lipids and fibrin; and have the same composition as the matrix deposits of diffuse glomerulosclerosis. Often they contain trapped mesangial cells. As the disease advances, the individual nodules enlarge and eventually compress and engulf capillaries, obliterating the glomerular tuft (Fig. 21–31). Eventually the entire glomerular structure assumes a hyaline, sclerotic appearance. As a consequence of the glomerular involvement, whether it be diffuse or nodular, the kidney suffers from ischemia, develops tubular atrophy and increased interstitial fibrosis, and undergoes overall contraction in size, accompanied by pallor and a fine granularity of the cortical surface.

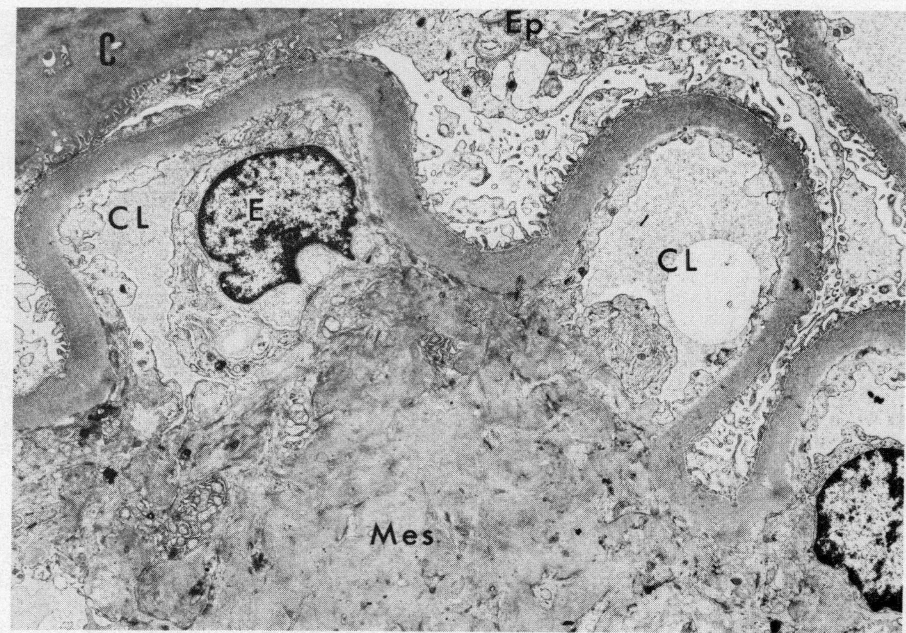

Figure 21–31. Electron micrograph of advanced diabetic glomerulosclerosis. Note massive increase in mesangial matrix (Mes) encroaching on glomerular capillary lumina (CL). GBM and Bowman's Capsule (C) are markedly thickened. Ep = epithelium; E = endothelium.

Although the relationship between nodular glomerulosclerosis and the diffuse lesion is still somewhat controversial, most workers believe them to be fundamentally similar lesions of the mesangium. The nodular lesion, however, is virtually pathognomonic of diabetes, if care is taken to exclude membranoproliferative (lobular) GN and the GN associated with light-chain nephropathy (p. 1026). Approximately 15 to 30% of long-term diabetics develop nodular glomerulosclerosis, and in most instances it is associated with renal failure. It is rarely encountered in those who have had diabetes for less than ten years, except perhaps in a few juvenile diabetics with rapidly advancing disease.[99]

Minor Lesions. "Exudative lesions" (fibrin caps and capsular drops) constitute another form of glomerular involvement seen in the diabetic. The **fibrin cap** appears as a homogeneous, brightly eosinophilic, crescentic deposit overlying a peripheral capillary of a lobule. With high resolution, the deposit is found to lie either trapped between the endothelial cells and the basement membrane of the capillary or outside the basement membrane under the visceral epithelial cells. It appears to represent a condensate of plasma proteins, and may be merely a reflection of the heavy proteinuria sometimes encountered in the diabetic as a consequence of widespread glomerular membrane alterations. Fibrin caps are also encountered in the nondiabetic. The **capsular drop** appears as an eosinophilic, focal thickening of the parietal layer of Bowman's capsule, which apparently hangs into the uriniferous space. The capsular drop is PAS positive and contains plasma proteins. Neither the fibrin cap nor the capsular drop has significance in terms of causing renal functional impairment, but the capsular drop, when identified in tissue sections, is characteristic of diabetes.

PATHOGENESIS OF DIABETIC GLOMERULOSCLEROSIS. The pathogenesis of diabetic glomerulosclerosis is intimately linked with that of the generalized diabetic microangiopathy, discussed on page 982. The principal points to remember are as follows:

1. Some investigators still believe that the basement membrane thickening and the metabolic disturbances are separate genetic defects in diabetics, but the bulk of the evidence suggests that diabetic glomerulosclerosis is caused by the metabolic defect, i.e., the insulin deficiency, or the resultant hyperglycemia, or some other aspects of glucose intolerance (p. 985).

2. Biochemical alterations in diabetic GBM have been described,[3, 102] including increased amount and synthesis of collagen type IV and decreased synthesis of proteoglycan heparan sulfate.[103] Theoretically, the latter can account for the loss of barrier function of the glomerulus[104] One recent speculation is that the actual thickening of the GBM and the accumulation of mesangial matrix are due to compensatory increased synthesis of defective GBM and mesangial matrix.[105]

3. Nonenzymatic glycosylation of proteins, known to occur in diabetics and exemplified by hemoglobin A1C (p. 983), may *theoretically* contribute to the glomerulopathy. Glycosylation of plasma proteins, or endothelial and epithelial cell membrane proteins, or any of the components of the GBM proper may explain both the increased glomerular permeability and the biochemical alterations to the GBM. These possibilities are being investigated currently.

4. One novel explanation for the initiation or modulation of diabetic glomerulosclerosis involves the "hyperfiltration" mechanism discussed earlier (p. 1007). It is well-known that early onset juvenile diabetics, particularly those with imperfectly controlled hyperglycemia,

have an increased GFR and an increase in filtration area in the glomerulus.[101] Hyperfiltration has been observed in experimental streptozotocin-induced diabetes in rats, where it is associated with proteinuria and can be reversed by diabetic control.[106] There is some experimental evidence that the contractile ability of mesangial cells is reduced by a hyperglycemic or insulin-deficient environment;[107] this could result in glomerular vasodilatation and an increase in intraglomerular plasma flow, filtration pressure, and hyperfiltration. Could it be that the subsequent morphologic alterations in the mesangium are somehow influenced by these hemodynamic changes, akin to the situation in the adaptive responses to reductions in renal mass described earlier?

Although the pathogenesis of diabetic glomerulopathy still eludes us, the recent interesting leads on nonenzymatic glycosylation, the biochemical GBM alterations, and the possible role of hyperfiltration may soon clarify at least parts of the puzzle.

OTHER MANIFESTATIONS OF DIABETIC NEPHROPATHY

Atherosclerosis and Arteriolosclerosis. Although generalized in the diabetic, these vascular changes often involve the kidneys more severely than other organs. Atheromas in the renal arteries or its major branches may cause either generalized ischemia and contraction or focal infarcts. Advanced hyaline arteriolosclerosis can affect not only the afferent but also the efferent arterioles. It is almost inevitably accompanied by diffuse glomerulosclerosis and clearly contributes to the progressive renal scarring seen in end-stage kidney disease. The frequency of hypertension is markedly increased in diabetics as opposed to nondiabetics.

Pyelonephritis. The incidence of acute pyelonephritis (p. 1030) at autopsy in diabetics is higher than that in nondiabetics, probably as a manifestation of the final illness. However, whether diabetics have a greater susceptibility to urinary tract infection than controls is questionable. One special pattern of acute pyelonephritis, known as **papillary necrosis** (p. 1032), is particularly prone to develop in diabetic patients. The acute bacterial infection within the renal pyramids, and the impaired circulation to the papilla engendered by the vascular sclerosis, induce an infarct-like necrosis of the distal segment. One or more papillae may be involved, unilaterally or bilaterally. When both kidneys are totally involved, the selective destruction of the collecting tubules almost always leads to acute renal failure and death in uremia. Less frequently, there is subtotal involvement, and the necrotic papillae may either slough off or appear for the first time at autopsy.

CLINICAL COURSE OF DIABETIC NEPHROPATHY. The clinical manifestations of diabetic nephropathy are linked to those of diabetes in general, as discussed on page 985. Glomerular involvement is associated with proteinuria, which may be mild and asymptomatic initially but gradually increases to nephrotic levels in some patients. The increased GFR typical in early-onset diabetics is then followed by progressive loss of GFR, leading to end-stage renal failure within a period of five years.

Associated with this progression is the development of hypertension, retinopathy, and neuropathy. The disease is more frequent, more severe, and more progressive in juvenile-onset (insulin-dependent) diabetics. Whether precise control of the blood sugar in diabetes will prevent the glomerulopathy is one of the unanswered questions in clinical medicine (p. 985). At present the vast majority of patients with end-stage diabetic nephropathy are maintained on long-term dialysis, and a few receive renal transplantation. Diabetic lesions may recur in the renal allografts, but whether these will eventually result in progressive loss of graft function is still unknown.

Amyloidosis

Disseminated amyloidosis, whether it conforms to the so-called primary or secondary pattern of distribution, may be associated with deposits of amyloid within the glomeruli (p. 202). The typical amyloid fibrils are present within the mesangium and subendothelium, and occasionally within the subepithelial space. Eventually, they obliterate the glomerulus completely. Recall that deposits of amyloid also appear in blood vessel walls and in the kidney interstitium. Amyloid can be detected on light microscopy by special stains, particularly by the characteristic birefringence after staining with Congo red. Patients with glomerular amyloid may present with heavy proteinuria or the nephrotic syndrome, and later, with destruction of glomeruli, die in uremia. Characteristically, kidney size tends to be either normal or slightly enlarged.

Other Systemic Disorders

Goodpasture's syndrome (p. 1010), polyarteritis nodosa (p. 520), and Wegener's granulomatosis (p. 523) are commonly associated with glomerular lesions and have been discussed earlier. Suffice it to say here that the glomerular lesions in these three conditions can be very similar. In the early or mild forms of involvement there are focal and segmental, sometimes necrotizing, GN and most of these patients will have hematuria with rather mild decline in GFR. In the more severe cases associated with rapidly progressive GN, there are also extensive necrosis, fibrin deposition, and the formation of epithelial crescents. It should be recalled, however, that these diseases have different pathogenetic mechanisms. Goodpasture's syndrome is mediated by anti-GBM antibodies and exhibits linear fluorescence of immunoglobulin and complement, whereas polyarteritis nodosa and Wegener's granulomatosis are of somewhat more obscure etiology, although immune complexes are frequently present in the former.

Essential mixed cryoglobulinemia is another rare systemic condition in which deposits of cryoglobulins composed principally of IgG–IgM complexes induce cutaneous vasculitis, synovitis, and focal or diffuse proliferative glomerulonephritis.[108]

Plasma cell dyscrasias (p. 688) may also induce

glomerular lesions. *Multiple myeloma* is associated with (1) amyloidosis, (2) deposition of monoclonal cryoglobulins in glomeruli, and (3) peculiar nodular lesions resembling nodular diabetic glomerulosclerosis and ascribed to the deposition of nonfibrillar light chains. This *light-chain nephropathy* also occurs in the absence of overt myeloma, usually associated with deposition of kappa chains in glomeruli.[109] The glomeruli show PAS-positive mesangial nodules, lobular accentuation, and mild mesangial hypercellularity and need to be differentiated from diabetic nodules and membranoproliferative GN. These patients usually present with proteinuria or the nephrotic syndrome, hypertension, and slowly progressive azotemia.

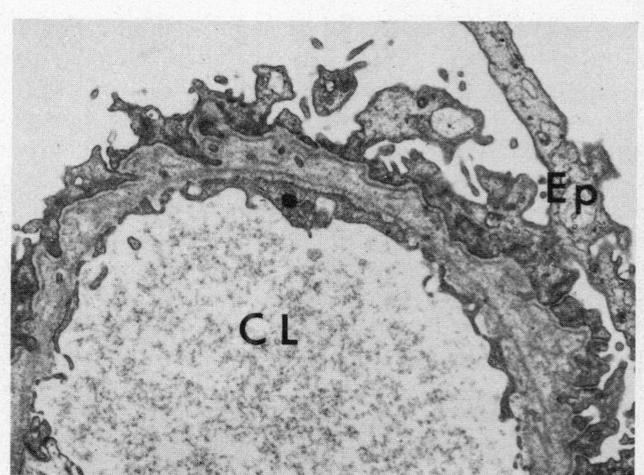

Figure 21–32. Hereditary nephritis. Electron micrograph of glomerulus with irregular thickening of basement membrane, lamination of lamina densa, and foci of rarefaction. Such changes may be present in other diseases but are most pronounced and widespread in hereditary nephritis. CL = capillary lumen; EP = epithelium.

HEREDITARY NEPHRITIS

Hereditary nephritis refers to a group of hereditary-familial renal diseases associated primarily with glomerular injury. The clinical, pathologic, and genetic features of the various types appear to be heterogeneous. The most well-studied entity is so-called *Alport's syndrome, the name usually given to the disease in which nephritis is accompanied by nerve deafness and various eye disorders, including lens dislocation, posterior cataracts, and corneal dystrophy.* Males tend to be affected more frequently and more severely than females and are more likely to progress to renal failure. Females, however, are not completely spared. The most common presenting sign is gross or microscopic hematuria, frequently accompanied by erythrocyte casts. Proteinuria may occur and, rarely, the nephrotic syndrome develops. Symptoms appear at ages 5 to 20 and the onset of overt renal failure is between ages 20 and 50.[110] The auditory defects may be subtle, requiring extensive testing. The mode of inheritance in most kindreds is autosomal dominant. In some families a sex-linked dominant mode of genetic transmission is seen.

Histologically, the glomeruli are always involved. The most common early lesion is segmental proliferation and/or sclerosis. There is increase in mesangial matrix, and in some patients the persistence of fetal-like glomeruli. In some kidneys, glomerular or tubular epithelial cells acquire a foamy appearance due to accumulation of neutral fats and mucopolysaccharides **(foam cells).** At one time these were thought characteristic of Alport's syndrome, but it is now known that they can be present in other glomerular diseases, particularly those associated with NS. As the disease progresses, there is increasing glomerulosclerosis, vascular narrowing, tubular atrophy, and interstitial fibrosis. With the electron microscope, characteristic basement membrane lesions are found in some (but not all) patients with hereditary nephritis. The basement membrane shows irregular foci of thickening or attenuation, with pronounced splitting and lamination of the lamina densa (Fig. 21–32). Similar alterations are found in the tubular basement membranes. Although such basement membrane changes may be seen focally in diseases other than hereditary nephritis, they are most widespread and pronounced in patients with this disorder.

The nature of the basement membrane defect is not clear, but it is most likely the result of a disturbance in the synthesis of some GBM component. Indeed, glomeruli of some patients with familial nephritis lack the "Goodpasture's" antigen; i.e., they fail to react with anti-GBM antibodies derived from patients with Goodpasture's syndrome.[111]

In addition to Alport's syndrome, other forms of familial and hereditary nephritides (without nerve deafness or ocular abnormalities) also occur with reasonable frequency, but genetic, clinical, and morphologic features in these are not well defined.

DISEASES OF TUBULES

Under this heading we will discuss *acute tubular necrosis* and a limited number of alterations that affect the proximal or distal tubular segments. In point of fact, most types of injury affecting the tubules also involve the interstitial tissue, and thus are discussed later under *tubulointerstitial diseases.*

ACUTE TUBULAR NECROSIS (ATN) AND ACUTE RENAL FAILURE

Acute tubular necrosis is a major cause of acute renal failure (ARF). The latter term refers to a syndrome associated with acute suppression of renal function, often accompanied by severe oliguria and, rarely, anuria. ARF can be caused by diverse clinical conditions that include the following:[53]

1. *Organic involvement of renal vessels.* ARF may be caused by diffuse involvement of the intrarenal vessels, such as in polyarteritis nodosa, malignant hypertension, and the hemolytic uremic syndrome. In rare instances, ARF may be due to bilateral occlusion of

renal arteries by thromboemboli or by external compression.

2. *Severe glomerular disease* such as rapidly progressive glomerulonephritis.

3. *Acute tubulointerstitial nephritis,* most commonly occurring as a hypersensitivity to drugs (p. 1036).

4. *Massive infection* (pyelonephritis), especially when accompanied by papillary necrosis (p. 1032).

5. *Disseminated intravascular renal coagulation* with cortical necrosis of the kidneys (p. 1050).

6. *Urinary obstruction* by tumors, prostatic hypertrophy, or blood clots (so-called postrenal acute renal failure).

7. *Acute tubular necrosis.*

Acute tubular necrosis (ATN) is the designation for all forms of acute renal failure associated with destruction of tubular epithelial cells. Two distinctive patterns were defined by Oliver in his classic studies.[112] (1) *Ischemic or tubulorrhectic ATN* occurs in cases that have in common a preceding hypotensive episode (shock), causing severe renal ischemia. (2) *Nephrotoxic ATN* results from the ingestion, injection, or inhalation of some toxic agent that directly damages tubular cells, principally those in the proximal segments of the nephron. It must be emphasized at the outset that, although morphologic evidence of tubular necrosis is obvious in the nephrotoxic form, it is quite focal, mild, and often subtle in ischemic ATN. Clinical recognition of ATN is of particular importance because it represents a reversible disorder compatible with full recovery of renal lesions and of the patient.

Ischemic ATN appears most often after an episode of shock produced by severe bacterial infections; large cutaneous burns; massive crushing injuries; or any medical, surgical, or obstetric event complicated by peripheral circulatory collapse. ATN is surprisingly uncommon when the shock is due to massive hemorrhage alone, e.g., following rupture of an aneurysm or laceration of a large artery. Mismatched blood transfusions or massive hemolysis from any cause may also lead to this form of renal tubular lesions. Hence, the ischemic pattern of ATN has also been called "shock kidneys" and "hemoglobinuric nephrosis."

Ischemic ATN is characterized by focal tubular necrosis at multiple points along the nephron, with large skip areas in between, often accompanied by rupture of basement membranes (tubulorrhexis) and occlusion of tubular lumina by casts (Fig. 21–33). Nephron microdissection studies show that relatively small lengths of tubules are affected.[112] The straight portion of the proximal tubule is especially vulnerable, but focal necrotic lesions may also occur in the distal nephron, often in conjunction with casts. Although tubular necrosis may be difficult to see in regular histologic sections, careful light microscopic studies show focal necrosis of single cells or small clusters of cells in over 90% of cases.[113] In the non-necrotic portions, the tubules either may be dilated or may show ultrastructural alterations such as loss of the microvilli of proximal tubules.

Eosinophilic hyaline casts, as well as pigmented granular casts, are extremely common, particularly in distal

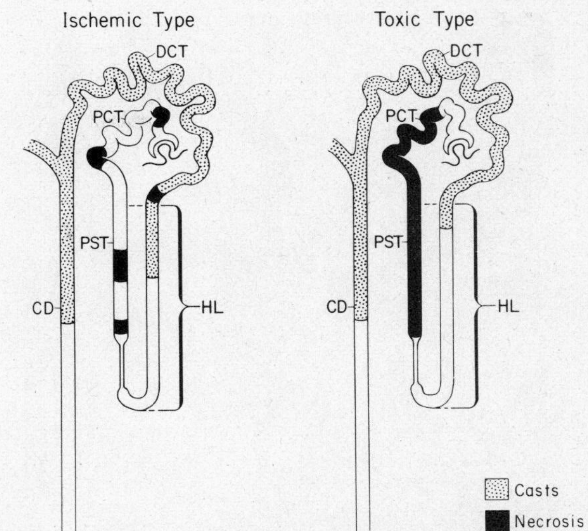

Figure 21–33. Patterns of tubular damage in ischemic and toxic ATN (adapted from microdissections by J. Oliver[112]). In ischemic type, tubular necrosis is patchy, relatively short lengths of tubules are affected, and straight segments of proximal tubules (PST) are most vulnerable. In toxic ATN, extensive necrosis is present along proximal tubule segments (PCT). In both types, lumina of distal convoluted tubules (DCT) and collecting ducts (CD) contain casts. HL = Henle's loop. (Courtesy of Dr. M. A. Venkatachalam, University of Texas at San Antonio.)

tubules and collecting ducts (Fig. 21–34). These casts consist principally of Tamm-Horsfall protein[114] (a specific urinary glycoprotein normally secreted by the cells of ascending thick limb and distal tubules) in conjunction with hemoglobin, myoglobin, and other plasma proteins. Other common findings in ischemic ATN are interstitial edema and accumulations of leukocytes within dilated vasa recta. In the absence of overt tubular necrosis, these latter two findings should raise the suspicion of ischemic acute renal failure. In patients who come to autopsy or who are biopsied after the first week of illness, there is often evidence of **epithelial regeneration:** flattened epithelial cells with hyperchromatic nuclei and mitotic figures are often present. In the course of time, this regeneration repopulates the tubules so that if survival occurs no residual evidence of damage can be seen. Glomeruli are remarkably normal, even by electron microscopy, although fibrin deposition and platelet thrombi have been reported in some cases.

Nephrotoxic ATN is caused by a wide variety of renal poisons, including heavy metals (mercury, lead, gold, arsenic, bismuth, chromium, uranium), organic solvents (carbon tetrachloride, chloroform, methyl alcohol), phenol, antibacterial agents (polymyxin, neomycin, sulfonamides, methicillin), anesthetics (methoxyflurane), mushroom poisoning, ethylene glycol, and pesticides.

Characteristic of toxic ATN is acute necrosis, most prominent in the proximal convoluted tubules (Figs. 21–33 and 21–35). The kidneys, when examined during the acute phase of the poisoning, are swollen and pale. Histologically, the tubular necrosis may be entirely nonspecific

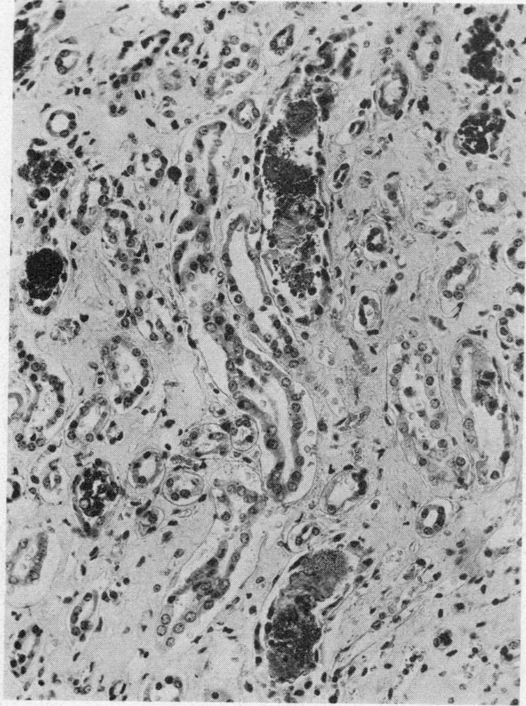

Figure 21–34. Ischemic ATN. Granular pigment casts are seen in collecting tubules. Some of the tubular epithelial cells in affected tubules are necrotic, whereas others are flattened, stretched out, and regenerating.

but is somewhat distinctive in poisoning with certain agents. With mercuric chloride, for example, severely injured cells not yet dead may contain large acidophilic inclusions. Later, these cells become totally necrotic, are desquamated into the lumen, and may undergo striking calcification. Carbon tetrachloride poisoning, in contrast, is characterized by the accumulation of large amounts of neutral lipids in injured cells but, again, such fatty change is followed by necrosis. Ethylene glycol produces marked ballooning and hydropic or vacuolar degeneration of proximal convoluted tubules. Calcium oxalate crystals are often found in the tubular lumina in such poisoning. Whatever the etiology, if the patient survives, epithelial regeneration occurs. In the course of time, this regeneration restores the tubules to their normal architecture.

Two features differentiate nephrotoxic ATN from the ischemic pattern: (1) the tubular basement membranes are preserved and (2) the distal tubular segments of the nephron are generally spared.

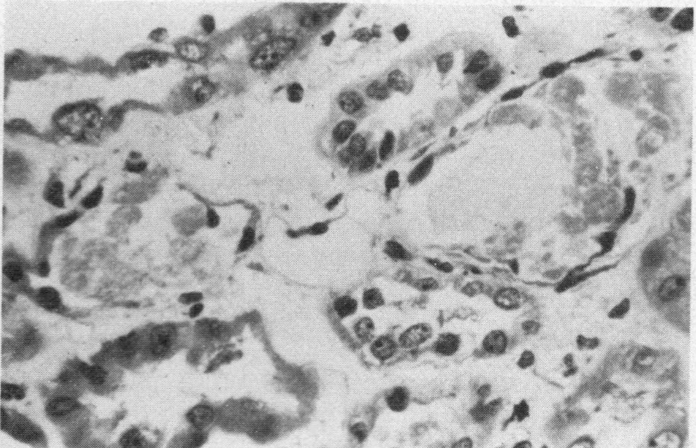

Figure 21–35. Toxic ATN. In center, two tubules show loss and desquamation of epithelial cells. (Courtesy of Dr. Kim Solez, Johns Hopkins University.)

PATHOGENESIS. The sequence of events leading to acute renal failure and oliguria in ischemic or toxic renal failure has been the subject of extensive study and controversy.[113] Four principal mechanisms have been proposed: (1) failure of glomerular filtration due to decreased renal perfusion pressure or *persistent preglomerular vasoconstriction,* possibly related to the activity of the renin-angiotensin system; (2) destruction of the tubular integrity with leakage of tubular fluid into the interstitium (*tubular back leak* or *tubular back flow*); (3) *tubular obstruction* by either interstitial edema or intratubular casts; and (4) a *direct effect* on the permeability properties of the glomerular capillary wall.

Evidence has been marshaled from numerous experimental studies in favor of one or the other of these hypotheses. A possible scheme incorporating some of these mechanisms is summarized in Figure 21–36. It is thought that both ischemia and nephrotoxins initially induce some type of tubular damage. The latter has at least three consequences, each of which contributes to the eventual development of oliguria. (1) *Arteriolar vasoconstriction.* This has been variously ascribed to activation of vasoconstrictive agents (angiotensin, thromboxane, catecholamines) or loss of vasodilator effects (prostaglandins, kallikrein), but how tubular damage triggers these events is unclear. Whatever the mechanism, vasoconstriction results in decreases in renal blood flow, glomerular filtration, tubular fluid flow, and oliguria. (2) The necrotic debris from tubular cells, together with proteinaceous material derived from either blood or tubular cells, results in cast formation. These casts increase proximal intratubular pressure and there-

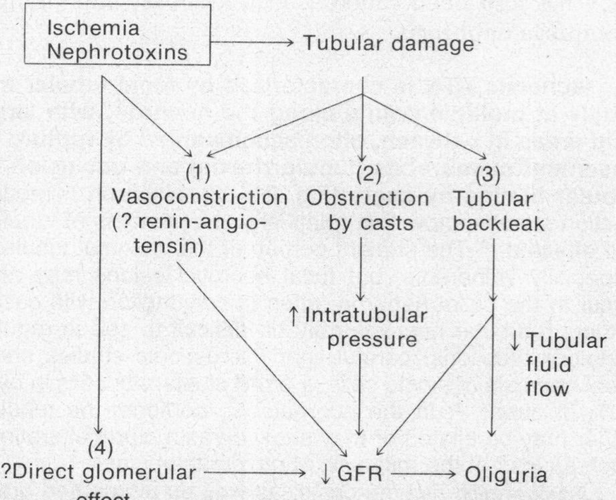

Figure 21–36. Possible pathogenetic mechanisms in acute renal failure. Sequence of events 1, 2, 3, and 4 are described in text.

fore further decrease GFR. (3) Back leak of tubular fluid into the interstitium, due to tubular damage, further decreases tubular fluid flow. The oliguria is thought to be the consequence of all these events. (4) Additionally, there is some evidence that ischemia or some toxins may directly affect glomerular ultrafiltration by some still unclear mechanism. Although some investigators argue for the primacy of one or the other of these mechanisms, it may be that a combination of all these effects in some individuals results in acute renal failure.[116] One or the other may predominate according to the inciting cause of ATN.

Clinical Course. The nephrotoxic and ischemic forms of ATN are important causes of acute and reversible renal failure. Although the course may be variable, four phases have been identified. *The stage of onset* lasting for about 36 hours is usually dominated by the inciting medical, surgical, or obstetric event, or in the case of toxins by the extrarenal toxic manifestations of such chemicals. Although hypotension or frank shock is often a part of the picture, many patients with no apparent drop in blood pressure indeed develop ATN. The *second* or *oliguric stage* is characterized by decreasing urine output to between 50 and 400 ml per day. Anuria is distinctly unusual except in the presence of obstruction or a vascular catastrophe. The symptoms of fluid overload and uremia dominate this phase, which may last any time from a few days to as long as three weeks. Hyperkalemia becomes a life-threatening problem requiring scrupulous clinical management. With appropriate attention to balance of water and blood electrolytes, including dialysis, the patient can be carried over this oliguric crisis. The *third* or *early diuretic phase* is heralded by a steady increase in urine volume that may reach up to 3 liters per day. The tubules are still damaged, so that large amounts of water, sodium, and potassium are lost in the urinary flood. Hypokalemia, rather than hyperkalemia, becomes a clinical problem. The serious electrolyte imbalances caused by deranged tubular function in the presence of marked diuresis account for death in this phase, commonly due to mismanagement of electrolyte balance. There is a peculiar increased vulnerability to infection at this stage. In the *late diuretic phase*, sometime in the third week, renal tubular function is restored with improvement in concentrating ability. At the same time, BUN and creatinine levels begin to return to normal. Subtle tubular functional impairment may persist for months, but most patients who reach the late diuretic phase eventually recover completely.

The prognosis of ATN depends on the clinical setting surrounding its development. In general, it is much better in the nephrotoxic form of the disease when the toxin has not caused serious damage to other organs such as the liver or heart or to other systems. In these instances, 95% recovery is expected. Conversely, in shock related to overwhelming sepsis or caused by extensive burns and obstetrical, surgical, or medical emergencies, the mortality rate may rise to 80%. In large part, the excessive mortality is attributable not to the acute renal failure per se but to the inability to control the underlying disease producing the shock state: e.g., massive myocardial infarction and cardiogenic shock or gram-negative sepsis.

It should be noted that about one-fifth of patients with ATN may have normal or increased urine volumes. So-called nonoliguric ATN occurs particularly often with nephrotoxins such as methoxyflurane, and generally tends to follow a more benign clinical course.

TUBULOINTERSTITIAL DISEASES

This group of renal diseases is characterized by histologic and functional alterations that involve predominantly the tubules and interstitium.[117] Glomerular and vascular abnormalities may also be present but either are mild or occur only in advanced stages of these diseases. The term interstitial nephritis is also commonly used for these disorders, since interstitial inflammation and fibrosis may be the major histologic changes. Whichever term one uses, the point to emphasize is that *the group of tubulointerstitial diseases have diverse etiologies and different pathogenetic mechanisms* (Table 21–7). It is an important group, however, because it is second only to chronic glomerulonephritis as a cause of chronic renal failure in man.

The *acute interstitial nephritides* (AIN) have an acute clinical onset and are characterized histologically by interstitial edema, often accompanied by leukocytic infiltration and focal tubular necrosis. In *chronic inter-*

Table 21–7. TUBULOINTERSTITIAL DISEASES

Infections
Acute bacterial pyelonephritis
Chronic pyelonephritis (including reflux nephropathy)
Other infections (viruses, parasites, etc.)
Toxins
Drugs
Acute hypersensitivity interstitial nephritis (e.g., methicillin)
Analgesic nephritis
Heavy metals
Lead, cadmium
Others
Metabolic Diseases
Urate nephropathy
Nephrocalcinosis (hypercalcemic nephropathy)
Hypokalemic nephropathy
Oxalate nephropathy
Physical Factors
Chronic urinary tract obstruction
Radiation nephritis
Neoplasms
Multiple myeloma
Immunologic Reactions
Transplant rejection
Tubulointerstitial disease associated with glomerulonephritis
Sjögren's syndrome
Vascular Diseases
Miscellaneous
Balkan nephropathy
Nephronophthisis–medullary cystic disease complex
Other rare diseases (sarcoidosis)
"Idiopathic" interstitial nephritis

stitial nephritis (CIN) there is infiltration with mononuclear cells, prominent interstitial fibrosis, and widespread tubular atrophy. When the etiologic agent is evident, the disorder is identified by cause or by associated disease (e.g., analgesic nephritis, irradiation nephritis). However, in some cases the etiologic agents are unknown and the term idiopathic tubulointerstitial nephritis is used.

Clinically, this group is distinguished from the glomerular diseases by the absence, in early stages, of such hallmarks of glomerular injury as persistent proteinuria or nephrotic syndrome and by the presence of defects in tubular function. The latter may be quite subtle and include impaired ability to concentrate urine, evidenced clinically by polyuria or nocturia; salt wasting; diminished ability to excrete acids (metabolic acidosis); or isolated defects in tubular reabsorption or secretion. The advanced forms, however, may be difficult to distinguish clinically from other causes of renal insufficiency.

Some of the specific conditions listed in Table 21–7 are discussed elsewhere in this book. In this section we shall deal principally with pyelonephritis and interstitial diseases induced by drugs and shall briefly touch on some of the immunologically mediated tubular interstitial disorders.

PYELONEPHRITIS (PN) AND URINARY TRACT INFECTION

Pyelonephritis is a renal disorder affecting tubules, interstitium, and renal pelvis and is one of the most common diseases of the kidney. It occurs in two forms. *Acute PN* is caused by bacterial infection and is the renal lesion associated with urinary tract infection. *Chronic PN* is a more controversial disorder: bacterial infection plays a dominant role, but other factors (vesicoureteral reflux, obstruction) are critically involved in its pathogenesis.

The term *urinary tract infection* (UTI) implies involvement of either the bladder (cystitis) or the kidneys and their collecting systems (pyelonephritis), or both. UTIs are extremely common disorders, second only to respiratory infections as causes of clinically significant morbidity due to infectious agents. It is important to realize, however, that bacterial infection of the urinary tract may be completely asymptomatic (asymptomatic bacteriuria) or may remain localized to the bladder without the development of renal infection. However, UTI always carries the potential of spread to the kidney, and it is often difficult clinically to distinguish between infection that is confined to the bladder and that which also affects renal tissue.

ETIOLOGY AND PATHOGENESIS. The dominant etiologic agents, accounting for over 85% of cases of UTI, are the gram-negative bacilli that are normal inhabitants of the intestinal tract.[118] By far the most common is *E. coli,* followed by Proteus, Klebsiella, and Enterobacter. These species have a low order of virulence for most other tissues in the body. *Streptococcus fecalis,* also of enteric origin, and staphylococci can also produce renal infection; rare etiologies extend to virtually every other bacterial and fungal agent. In general, the less common enteric organisms as well as the nonenteric forms are encountered in special circumstances, e.g., infections following antimicrobial therapy or instrumentation of the urinary tract, those acquired in hospitals, or those secondary to septicemia.

From serologic studies, it is known that *in most patients with UTI, the infecting organisms are derived from the patient's own fecal flora.* This is thus a form of endogenous infection. In the pathogenesis of PN, therefore, the questions to ask are: how do these relatively avirulent organisms reach the kidney and what are the factors that enhance their pathogenicity for renal tissue? Three routes of infection are theoretically possible: (1) the bloodstream (hematogenous infection); (2) the ureters, from the bladder (ascending infection); or (3) the lymphatics. There is little evidence for lymphatic spread.

Hematogenous Infection. Although hematogenous seeding of the kidney undoubtedly occurs under some circumstances, such as in the course of septicemia or endocarditis (e.g., staphylococcal endocarditis), the normal kidney is resistant to blood-borne infection, especially with *E. coli.* Experimentally, when *E. coli* are introduced into the bloodstream, only small numbers, about one of every 10,000 bacteria, are trapped in the kidney, and these are destroyed by antibacterial mechanisms within the kidney without causing injury. *If the kidney is injured in some way, however, such as by ligation of a ureter causing obstruction, blood-borne organisms will localize in the obstructed kidney, multiply, and produce a unilateral acute pyelonephritis,* without affecting the unobstructed kidney. Obstruction also predisposes to infection in man. Strictures of the urethra, tumors of the urinary bladder, calculi in the ureters, prostatic hypertrophy, and intrarenal scars all increase the likelihood of infection.

In the experimental animal, the stage of acute PN persists for one to two weeks. Subsequently, healing begins, and by six weeks the kidneys become sterile and the areas of acute inflammation are replaced by corticomedullary scars. This sequence appears to be true in uncomplicated human acute *E. coli* PN; i.e., *acute suppurative inflammation is followed by healing with a resultant corticomedullary scar.*

Ascending Infection. Abundant clinical evidence indicates that *the most common pathway of renal infection is ascension of bacteria up the urinary stream from the bladder cavity.*[119] Normal human bladder and bladder urine are sterile, and only saprophytic organisms are generally present in the distal part of the urethra and, in females, in the vaginal vestibule. In females susceptible to recurrent infection, however, coliform organisms colonize the distal urethra and vaginal vestibule and form the initial inoculation site for ascending infection. The reasons for this initial colonization are now under study. Current studies suggest that colonization is influenced by the ability of bacteria to adhere to vaginal or urethral mucosal cells. Increased *bacterial adherence* due to bacterial or host factors (p. 318) may initiate colonization and enhance the possibility of infection.[120] As discussed in Chapter 8, bacterial attachment by pili (or other determinants) to receptors on epithelia plays an important role in bacterial virulence.

How do these organisms then gain entrance into the bladder? *Urethral instrumentation* (as used in catheterization, cystoscopy, and urologic surgery) introduces organisms into the bladder; long-term catheterization, in particular, carries a high risk of infection. In the absence of instrumentation, *urinary infections are much more common in females and in the age group of 15 to 40, the ratio of females to males affected being 8:1.* This has been variously ascribed to the shorter urethra in females, the absence of antibacterial properties of prostatic fluid, hormonal changes affecting adherence of bacteria to the mucosa, and urethral trauma during sexual intercourse (the latter accounting for the well-recognized entity of "honeymoon cystitis"), or a combination of all these factors.[121]

Under normal conditions, organisms introduced into the bladder are cleared by the continual flushing of voiding and by other poorly understood antibacterial mechanisms.[121] However, in the presence of bladder obstruction or of an inability to empty the urinary bladder completely (residual urine volume), bacteria multiply and cystitis develops. Such is the case in patients with prostatic hypertrophy and bladder diverticula (Chapter 22).

Vesicoureteral Reflux. Once cystitis has occurred, it may remain localized in the urinary bladder for years without ascension to the kidney. In some individuals, however, bacteria reach the renal pelvis owing to a pathologic condition in which urine is actively propelled up one or both ureters during micturition. This so-called *vesicoureteral reflux* (VUR) is now well recognized as a serious condition that is the major cause of pyelonephritic damage, particularly in children.[122] Reflux can be documented radiologically by the *voiding cystourethrogram,* in which the bladder is filled with a radiopaque dye and the patient is instructed to void. In normal individuals the dye exits only through the urethra; VUR is prevented by virtue of the oblique insertion of the ureter in the bladder wall, so that the ureter is compressed during micturition (Fig. 21–37). In the presence of reflux, dye is seen clearly refluxing into the ureter, often all the way to the pelvis (Fig. 21–38). Reflux occurs in 30 to 50% of infants and children with recurrent UTIs, often in the first year of life. In *children,* reflux is due to a congenital absence or shortening of the intravesical portion of the ureter (Fig. 21–37*D*). In adults, VUR can be caused by bladder diverticula, and neurogenic factors, but its consequences are less serious than in children and infants. Mild grades of reflux (I and II) are innocuous and reversible, but more severe reflux (grades III and particularly IV) is associated with more or less permanent dilatation of ureters and renal pelvis.

In severe cases of reflux, 30 to 60% of untreated children eventually develop typical pyelonephritic scarring (p. 1034). In some children with moderate or severe forms of VUR, the dye also fills the collecting ducts of pyramids and fans out into the cortex in the shape of a V or U. This *intrarenal reflux* is the mechanism by which bacteria spread into the renal parenchyma, as has been well demonstrated in experimental VUR in

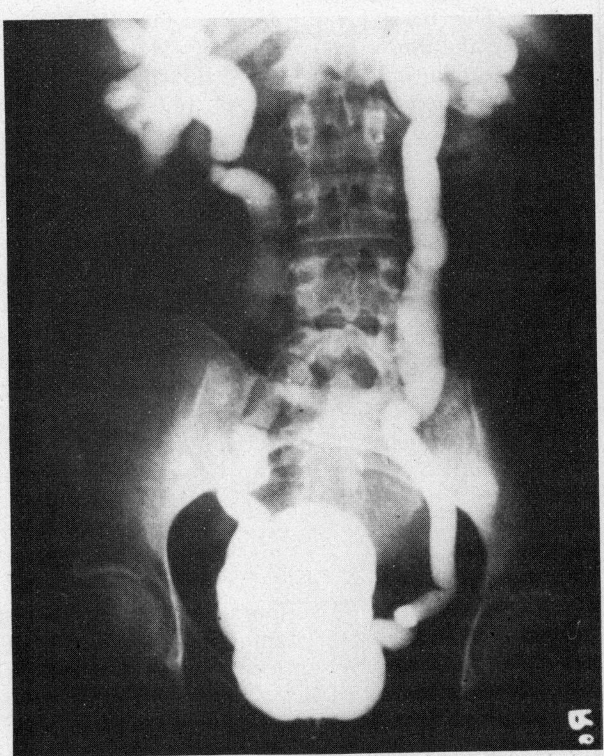

Figure 21–38. Vesicoureteral reflux demonstrated by a voiding cystourethrogram. Dye injected into bladder refluxes into both dilated ureters, filling pelvis and calyces. (Courtesy of Dr. Harry Mellins, Brigham and Women's Hospital, Boston.)

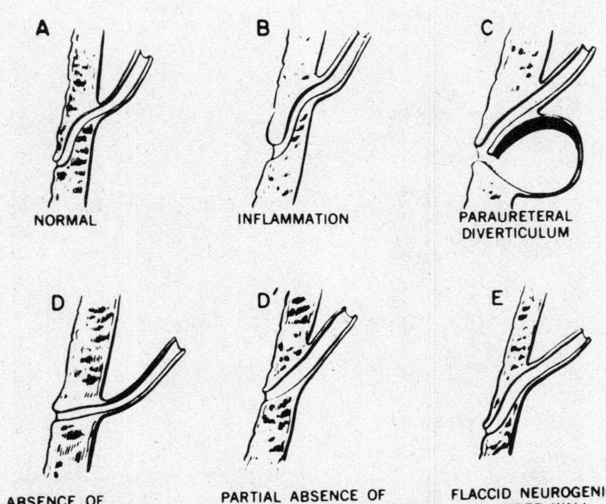

Figure 21–37. Intravesical position of ureter in normal person and in patients with vesicoureteral reflux. (Redrawn with permission from King, L. R., et al.: J.A.M.A. *203*:169, 1968.)

pigs.[124, 125] The basis for intrarenal reflux lies in the anatomic configuration of papillae.[126] Many "normal" papillae in human infants are not of the simple, convex, pointed type depicted in textbooks, but have concave or deeply indented tips with widened ducts of Bellini opening into the calyx. Such papillae are potentially refluxing, in that the orifices of their ducts cannot be occluded by a raised intrapelvic pressure. Two-thirds of normal kidneys possess at least one potentially refluxing papilla; they are located most often in the upper and lower poles of the kidneys, the usual sites of intrarenal reflux and pyelonephritic scars.

To summarize, VUR followed by intrarenal reflux is a major mechanism whereby bacteria can be delivered from the infected bladder into the renal parenchyma. Once in the parenchyma, bacterial multiplication and suppurative inflammation lead to a typical picture of PN.

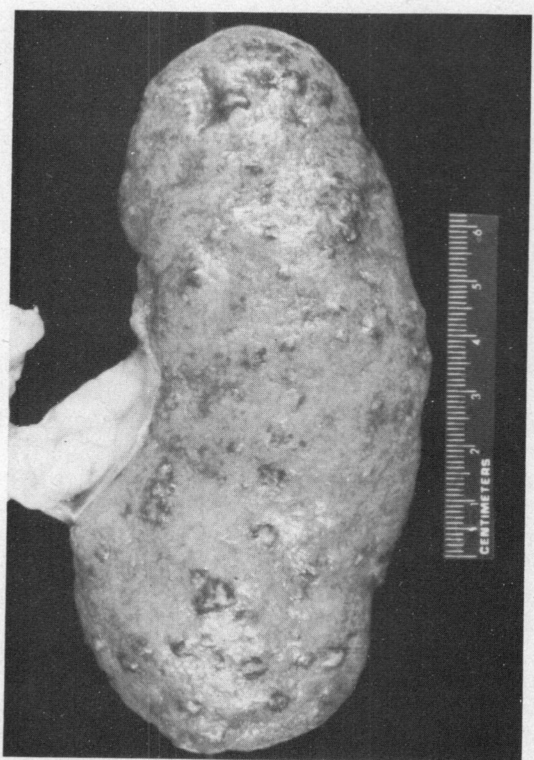

Figure 21–39. Acute pyelonephritis. Cortical surface is dotted with abscesses.

Acute Pyelonephritis

Acute PN is an acute suppurative inflammation of the kidney caused by bacterial infection—whether hematogenous and induced by septicemic spread, or ascending and associated with VUR.

MORPHOLOGY. The hallmarks of acute PN are **patchy interstitial suppurative inflammation and tubular necrosis.** The suppuration may occur as discrete focal abscesses involving one or both kidneys, or as large, wedge-shaped areas of coalescent suppuration (Fig. 21–39). The distribution of these lesions is unpredictable and haphazard, but in PN associated with reflux, damage occurs most commonly in the lower and upper poles.

Externally, the lesions consist of abscesses on the cortical surface, usually rimmed by narrow zones of hyperemia. On section, the inflammatory foci are generally distributed throughout the kidney and, although the medulla is usually involved, paradoxically the suppuration is often most evident in the cortex. Depending on the severity of involvement, the kidney may or may not be enlarged. Hyperemia, granularity of the pelvic mucosa, or even suppuration is occasionally present.

In the very early stages, the neutrophilic infiltration is limited to the interstitial tissue. By the time most kidneys are examined, however, the reaction has ruptured into tubules and produced a characteristic abscess with the destruction of the engulfed tubules (Fig. 21–40). Since the tubular lumina present a ready pathway for the extension of the infection, large masses of neutrophils frequently extend along the involved nephron into the collecting tubules. Characteristically, the glomeruli appear to be resistant to the infection, and often abscess formations surround glomeruli without actually invading them. Large areas of severe necrosis, however, eventually destroy the glomeruli, and fungal PN (e.g., Candida) often affects glomeruli.

Three complications of acute PN are encountered in special circumstances. **Necrotizing papillitis**, or **papillary necrosis**, is seen mainly in diabetics and in those with urinary tract obstruction. Necrotizing papillitis is usually bilateral but may be unilateral. One or all of the pyramids of the affected kidney may be involved. On cut section, the tips or distal two-thirds of the pyramids have gray-white to yellow necrosis that resembles infarction. The junction of the ne-

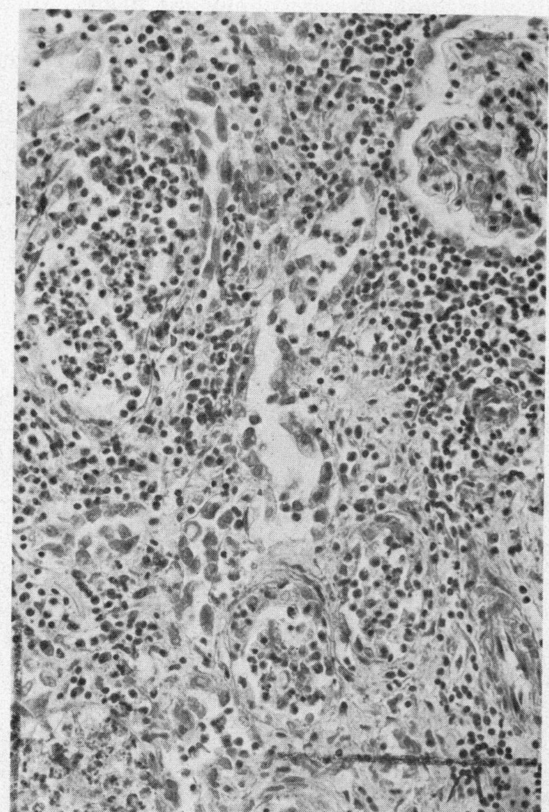

Figure 21–40. Acute pyelonephritis marked by an acute neutrophilic exudate within tubules and renal substance.

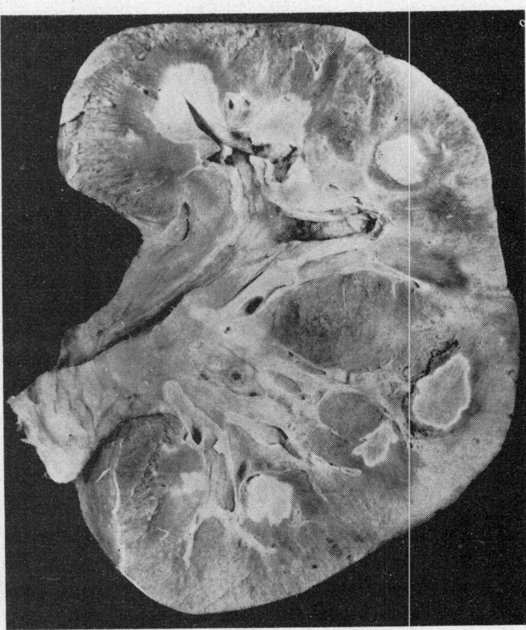

Figure 21–41. Necrotizing papillitis. Areas of pale gray necrosis are limited to papillae.

crotic papillae with the preserved proximal portion of the pyramid is usually sharply defined and outlined by a narrow zone of hyperemia (Fig. 21–41). Microscopically, the necrotic tissue shows characteristic coagulative infarct necrosis, with preservation of outlines of tubules. The leukocytic response is limited to the junctions between preserved and destroyed tissue. Large masses of proliferating bacteria are sometimes found within the acellular necrotic foci. Clinically, papillary necrosis is often associated with acute renal failure, commonly leading to death in uremia.

Pyonephrosis is seen when there is total or almost complete obstruction, particularly when it is high in the urinary tract. The suppurative exudate is unable to drain and thus fills the renal pelvis, calyces, and ureter, producing pyonephrosis. The kidney may be converted virtually to a sac of pus, as the renal damage characteristic of hydronephrosis (p. 1051) is added to that caused by the bacterial infection. **Perinephric abscess** implies extension of suppurative inflammation through the renal capsule into the perinephric tissue.

After the acute phase of PN, healing occurs. The neutrophilic infiltrate is replaced by one that is predominantly mononuclear with macrophages, plasma cells, and (later) lymphocytes. The inflammatory foci are eventually replaced by scars that can be seen on the cortical surface as fibrous depressions. Such scars are characterized microscopically by atrophy of tubules, interstitial fibrosis, and lymphocyte infiltrate and may resemble scars produced by ischemic or other types of injury to the kidney. **However, the pyelonephritic scar is almost always associated with inflammation, fibrosis, and deformation of the underlying calyx and pelvis,** reflecting the role of ascending infection and VUR in the pathogenesis of the disease.

CLINICAL COURSE. Acute PN is often associated with specific predisposing conditions, some of which were covered in the discussion of pathogenetic mechanisms. These include

1. *Urinary obstruction*, either congenital or acquired.
2. *Instrumentation* of the urinary tract, most commonly catheterization.
3. *VUR*.
4. *Pregnancy*. Four to 6% of all pregnant women develop bacteriuria sometime during pregnancy, and 20 to 40% of these eventually develop symptomatic urinary infection if not treated.[127]
5. *Patient's sex and age*. After the first year of life (when congenital anomalies are common in males) and up to around age 40, infections are much more frequent in females, and in the absence of obstruction and instrumentation, urinary infection in this age group is almost exclusively a disease of females. With increasing age, the incidence in males increases owing to the development of prostatic hypertrophy and frequent instrumentation.
6. *Preexisting renal lesions*. These cause intrarenal scarring and obstruction.
7. *Diabetes mellitus*. The higher incidence of urinary infection among diabetics reported in some, but not all, studies is probably caused by more frequent instrumentation, the general susceptibility to infection, and the neurogenic bladder dysfunction exhibited by such patients.

When acute PN is clinically apparent, the onset is usually sudden, with pain at the costovertebral angle and systemic evidence of infection, such as fever and malaise. There are usually indications of bladder and urethral irritation, such as dysuria, frequency, and urgency. The urine contains many leukocytes (pyuria) derived from the inflammatory infiltrate, but pyuria does not differentiate upper from lower urinary infection. The finding of leukocyte casts (pus casts) indicates renal involvement, since casts are formed only in tubules. The diagnosis of infection is established by quantitative urine culture. True infection can usually be differentiated from contamination by the presence of over 10^3 to 10^5 pathogenic organisms per milliliter in the urine. It is frequently difficult to differentiate cystitis alone from PN, since the symptoms referable to upper urinary infection may be absent. As mentioned earlier, pus casts, if present, always indicate kidney involvement. Several immunologic methods developed to aid with this distinction (such as the presence of antibody coating on bacteria in the urine) have not yet proved of widespread value.

Uncomplicated acute PN usually follows a benign course and the symptoms disappear within a few days after the institution of appropriate antibiotic therapy. Bacteria, however, may persist in the urine, the incidence of recurrence of infection with new serologic types of *E. coli* or other organisms being as high as 30% in some series. Such bacteriuria then either disappears or may persist sometimes for years. In the presence of unrelieved urinary obstruction, diabetes mellitus, and immunocompromised hosts, acute PN may be more serious, leading to repeated septicemic episodes. The superimposition of papillary necrosis leads to acute renal failure.

The significance of *asymptomatic bacteriuria* (defined as bacteriuria without pyuria or symptoms of infection) deserves comment. This is a frequent condition whose prevalence increases with age in both sexes, but at all ages females far outnumber males. Population screening studies have shown that 1.2% of girls between the ages of 5 and 9 and 3% of those between the ages of 12 and 16 have bacteriuria.[128] In the overall adult female population the prevalence range is between 3 and 6%. A certain proportion of these have some evidence of renal damage or VUR. However, the likelihood that adults with asymptomatic bacteriuria will develop progressive renal damage is extremely small. Conversely, there is significant danger of chronic PN developing in infants and young children with infection, especially in the presence of VUR or anomalies of the urinary tract.

Chronic Pyelonephritis (CPN) and Reflux Nephropathy

Although there is some controversy regarding terminology, CPN is considered here as a chronic tubulointerstitial renal disorder in which *renal scarring is associated with pathologic involvement of the calyces and pelvis* (Fig. 21–42). The criteria for the diagnosis of CPN include irregular scarring (if bilateral, asymmetric); inflammation, fibrosis, and deformity of the calyces underlying the parenchymal scars; and predominant tubulointerstitial histologic damage. These criteria are important in that virtually all the diseases listed in Table 21–7 produce chronic tubulointerstitial alterations, but excepting for CPN and analgesic nephropathy, none affects the calcyes. If these criteria are adhered to, bacterial infection, superimposed on VUR or obstruction, plays a role in most cases of CPN. CPN is an important cause of end-stage kidney disease. In various series, CPN is found in 11 to 20% of patients in renal transplant or dialysis units (40 to 60% of cases being caused by chronic GN).

CPN can be divided into two forms: chronic obstructive and chronic reflux–associated.

Chronic Obstructive PN. We have seen that obstruction predisposes the kidney to infection. Recurrent infections superimposed on diffuse or localized obstructive lesions lead to recurrent bouts of renal inflammation and scarring, resulting in a picture of CPN. In this condition, the effects of obstruction obviously contribute to the parenchymal atrophy, and indeed it is sometimes difficult to differentiate the effects of bacterial infection from those of obstruction alone. The disease can be bilateral, as with congenital anomalies of the urethra (posterior urethral valves), resulting in fatal renal insufficiency unless the anomaly is corrected; or unilateral, such as occurs with calculi and unilateral obstructive anomalies of the ureter.

Reflux Nephropathy (Chronic Reflux–Associated PN). This is by far the more common form of chronic pyelonephritic scarring. As discussed earlier, renal involvement in reflux nephropathy occurs early in childhood, as a result of superimposition of a urinary infection on congenital VUR and intrarenal reflux, the latter conditioned by the number of potentially refluxing papillae. Reflux may be unilateral or bilateral; thus, the resultant renal damage either may cause scarring and atrophy of one kidney, or may involve both and lead to chronic renal insufficiency. Whether VUR causes renal damage in the absence of infection (sterile reflux) is uncertain, since it is difficult clinically to rule out remote infection in a patient first seen with pyelonephritic scarring.

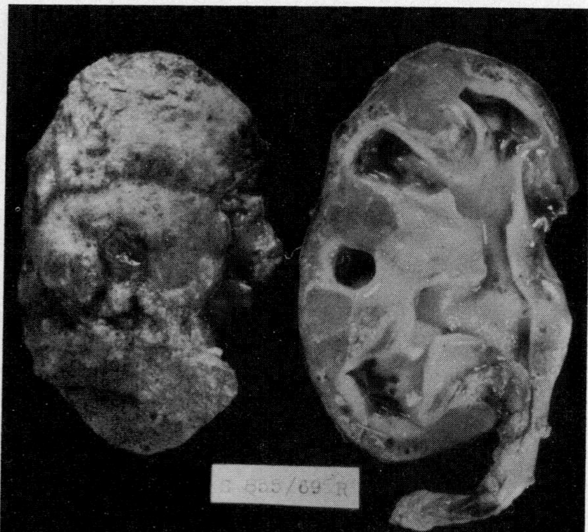

Figure 21–42. Chronic pyelonephritis. Surface *(left)* is irregularly scarred. Cut section *(right)* reveals characteristic dilatation and blunting of calyces. Ureter is dilated and thickened—a finding consistent with chronic vesicoureteral reflux.

MORPHOLOGY. It should be emphasized first that the **characteristic morphologic changes of CPN are seen on gross rather than on microscopic examination** (Fig. 21–42). The kidneys usually are irregularly scarred; if bilateral, the involvement is asymmetric. This contrasts with chronic glomerulonephritis, in which the kidneys are diffusely and symmetrically scarred. The hallmark of CPN is the coarse, discrete, corticomedullary scar overlying a dilated, blunted, or deformed calyx (Fig. 21–43). The scars can vary from one to several in number and many affect one or both kidneys. Most are in upper and lower poles, consistent with the frequency of reflux in these sites.

The microscopic changes predominantly involve tubules and interstitium (Fig. 21–44). The tubules show atrophy in some areas and hypertrophy in others, or dilatation. Dilated tubules may be filled with colloid casts, a pattern referred to as **thyroidization** (Fig. 21–45). There are varying degrees of chronic interstitial inflammation and fibrosis in the cortex and medulla. In the presence of active infection, there may be neutrophils in the interstitium and pus casts in the tubules. Arcuate and interlobular vessels disclose obliterative endarteritis in the scarred areas, and in the presence of hypertension hyaline arteriolosclerosis is seen in the entire kidney. There is often fibrosis around the calyceal mucosa as well as marked chronic inflammatory infiltrate. Lymphoid follicles may appear in the calyceal wall (Fig. 21–43). Glomeruli may appear normal except for periglomerular fibrosis, but a

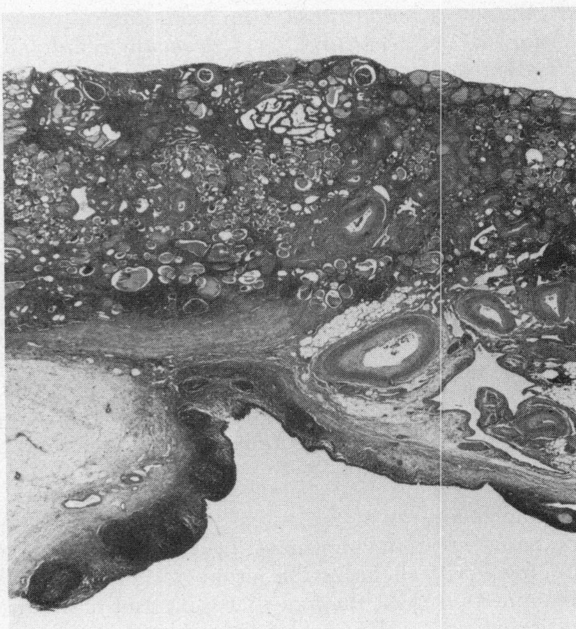

Figure 21–43. Chronic pyelonephritis. Low-power view to show corticomedullary renal scar with an underlying dilated deformed calyx. Note inflammatory infiltrate with lymphoid follicles around calyx.

variety of glomerular changes may be present, including ischemic fibrous obliteration as well as proliferation and necrosis ascribed to hypertension. Patients with CPN and reflux nephropathy who develop proteinuria in advanced stages exhibit **focal and segmental glomerulosclerosis**, similar to that seen in patients with focal sclerosis associated with nephrotic syndrome (p. 1015).

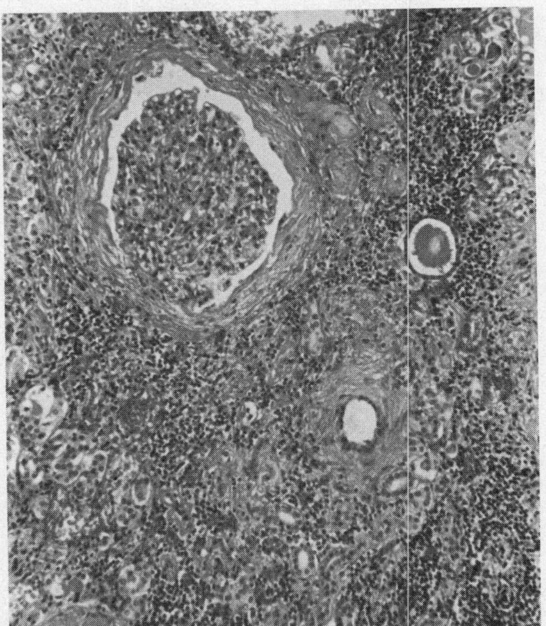

Figure 21–44. Cortex in CPN showing interstitial chronic inflammation, marked tubular atrophy, and occasional dilated tubules. Glomerulus is normal, but there is periglomerular fibrosis.

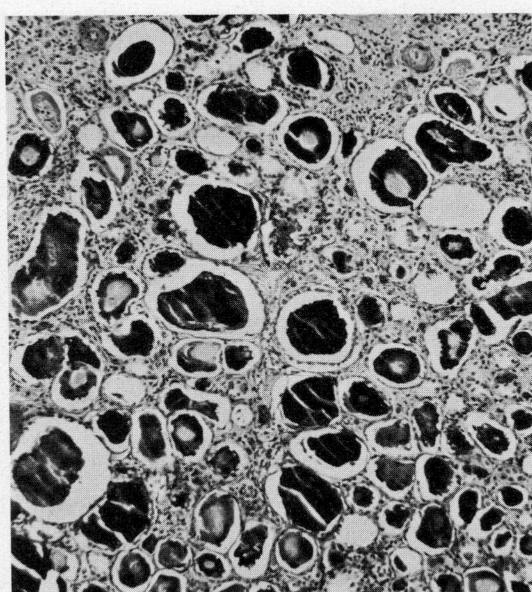

Figure 21–45. A large area of scarring with dilated, cast-filled tubules.

Xanthogranulomatous PN[129] is an unusual and relatively rare form of CPN characterized by accumulation of foamy macrophages intermingled with plasma cells, lymphocytes, polymorphs, and occasional giant cells. Often associated with Proteus infections and obstruction, the lesions sometimes produce large, yellowish-orange nodules that may be confused with renal cell carcinoma (p. 1054).

CLINICAL COURSE. Chronic obstructive PN may be insidious in onset or may present the clinical manifestations of acute recurrent PN with back pain, fever, frequent pyuria, and bacteriuria. CPN associated with reflux may have a silent insidious onset. These patients come to medical attention relatively late in the course of their disease because of the gradual onset of renal insufficiency and hypertension, or because of the discovery of pyuria or bacteriuria on routine examination. Reflux nephropathy is a common cause of hypertension in children. Loss of tubular function—in particular of concentrating ability—gives rise to polyuria and nocturia. Pyelography is required for the diagnosis. Pyelograms show the affected kidneys or kidney to be smaller than normal, often asymmetrically contracted, with characteristic coarse scars and blunting and deformity of the calyceal system. Significant bacteriuria may be present, but in the late stages it is sometimes absent. Some of these patients develop severe and intractable hypertension, which contributes to the progressive renal failure.

Although proteinuria is usually mild, some patients with pyelonephritic scars develop significant proteinuria, even in the nephrotic range, usually many years after the scarring has occurred and often in the absence of continued infection, persistent VUR, or hypertension.[84, 130] The appearance of proteinuria is a poor prognostic sign and many such patients proceed to chronic end-stage renal failure. Renal biopsies show focal segmental glomerulosclerosis superimposed on the tubulointerstitial damage caused by CPN. The pathogenesis of the glomerular lesions in this setting is now under study; the most plausible explanation is that they are due to glomerular "hyperfiltration" in nephrons adapting to loss of renal mass caused by pyelonephritic scarring (p. 1007).[84]

TUBULOINTERSTITIAL NEPHRITIS INDUCED BY DRUGS AND TOXINS

Several general points should be stressed with regard to the effects of drugs and toxins on the kidney. The kidney is especially susceptible to toxic injury because of its high blood supply, most of it to the metabolically active cortex. Normal physiologic processes may increase the local concentrations of certain toxins in various segments of the nephron. For example, toxins that are actively reabsorbed by the proximal tubules will cause predominant proximal damage, whereas those affected by the normal urinary concentrating mechanisms may reach high levels in the medulla, predisposing the medulla and papilla to injury. Toxins that are relatively insoluble in acid pH tend to precipitate in the distal tubules and collecting ducts, allowing for increased local concentrations and causing obstruction of tubular lumina.

Toxins can produce renal injury in at least three ways: (1) they may trigger an interstitial immunologic reaction, exemplified by the acute hypersensitivity nephritis induced by such drugs as methicillin; (2) they may cause acute renal failure (p. 1027) by direct tubular damage (such as in mercuric chloride poisoning) or by some other poorly understood mechanisms (e.g., the antibiotic aminoglycosides such as gentamicin); and (3) they may cause subtle but cumulative injury to tubules that takes years to become manifest, resulting in chronic renal insufficiency. The latter type of damage is especially treacherous, since it may be clinically unrecognized until significant renal damage has occurred. Such is the case with analgesic abuse nephropathy, which is usually detected only after the onset of renal failure.

Acute Drug-induced (Hypersensitivity) Interstitial Nephritis

This is now a well-recognized adverse reaction to a constantly increasing number of drugs. First reported after the use of sulfonamides, acute tubulointerstitial nephritis has occurred most frequently with synthetic penicillins (methicillin, ampicillin), but other synthetic antibiotics (rifampin), diuretics (furosemide, thiazides), nonsteroidal inflammatory agents (phenylbutazone), and miscellaneous drugs (phenindione, cimetidine) have also been implicated.[117, 132] The disease begins about 15 days (two to 40) after exposure to the drug and is characterized by fever, eosinophilia (which may be transient), hematuria, mild proteinuria, sterile pyuria, and a skin rash, the latter being present in about 25% of patients. A *rising serum creatinine level or acute renal failure with oliguria develops in about 50% of cases,* particularly in older patients. The azotemia typically resolves after withdrawal of the offending drug, although it may take several months for return of renal function to normal.

Grossly, the kidneys are usually slightly enlarged. Histologically, the abnormalities are in the interstitium, which shows pronounced edema and infiltration by mononuclear cells, principally lymphocytes and macrophages (Fig. 21–46). Eosinophils and neutrophils may be present, often in large numbers, and plasma cells and basophils in small numbers are sometimes found. With some drugs (e.g., methicillin, thiazides), interstitial granulomas with giant cells may be seen.[132] Variable degrees of tubular necrosis and regeneration are present.

Many features of the disease suggest an immunologic basis for its development. (1) Clinical evidence of hypersensitivity includes the latent period, the eosinophilia and skin rash, the fact that the onset of nephropathy is not dose related, and the recurrence of hypersensitivity following reexposure to the same or a cross-reactive drug. (2) Immunofluorescent studies in rare cases have disclosed linear staining for IgG and complement along the tubular basement membranes (TBM), and circulating antibody to tubular basement membranes has been found in the circulation in some pa-

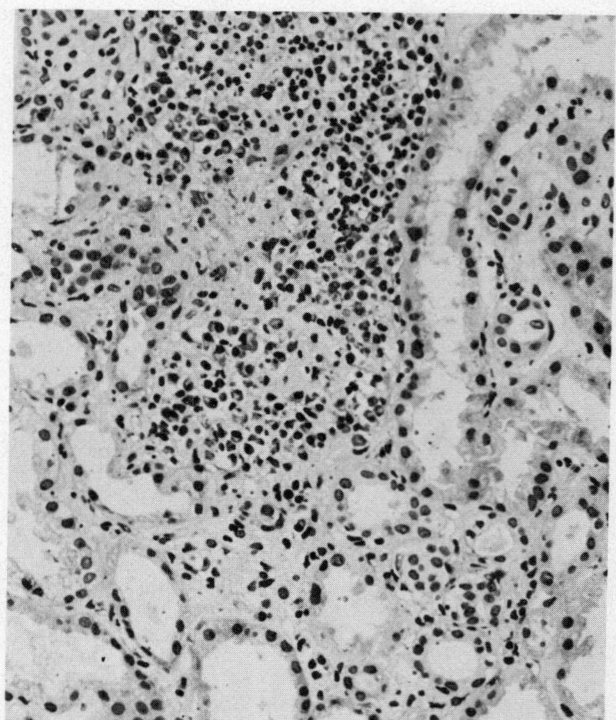

Figure 21–46. Acute drug-induced interstitial nephritis. Note interstitial inflammation and edema.

tients. This has led to the suggestion that in these individuals the drug hapten (the penicilloyl moiety in methicillin), which is secreted by the proximal tubules, conjugates with tubular basement membrane protein, thus stimulating the production of anti-TBM antibody, with resultant damage to the tubules and secondarily to the interstitium. This hypothesis is weakened by the fact that many patients in fact fail to show anti-TBM antibody. (3) IgE serum levels are increased in some patients, and IgE-containing plasma cells and basophils are sometimes present in the lesions, suggesting that a Type I IgE-mediated hypersensitivity may be involved in the pathogenesis. (4) Finally, the mononuclear or granulomatous infiltrate, together with positive skin tests to drug haptens, suggest a delayed-hypersensitivity type reaction (Type IV), but as yet there has been no experimental evidence for such a mechanism.

Thus, although an immunologic reaction is clearly involved, the precise type of reaction and the sequence of events leading to damage are still obscure. It is important to recognize drug-induced renal failure since withdrawal of the drug is followed by recovery, although irreversible damage may occur occasionally in older subjects.

Analgesic Nephritis (Analgesic Abuse Nephropathy)

This is a form of chronic renal disease caused by excessive intake of analgesic mixtures and characterized morphologically by chronic tubulointerstitial nephritis with renal papillary necrosis.

First reported in Switzerland in 1953, analgesic nephropathy is of world-wide distribution, and in some parts of Australia and Western Europe it ranks as one of the most common causes of chronic renal insufficiency.[133] The renal damage was first ascribed to phenacetin, but the analgesic mixtures consumed often contain, in addition, aspirin, caffeine, acetaminophen (a metabolite of phenacetin), and codeine. Patients who develop this disease usually ingest large quantities of analgesic mixtures,[134] and consumptions of up to 30 kg over a 30-year period have been recorded, the average being 10 kg over a mean period of 13 years. The minimal requirements for the development of renal damage are between 2 and 3 kg of phenacetin taken over a period of three years. The incidence of analgesic nephropathy in the United States is variable; it is low in the Northeast, accounting for 2% of patients with end stage renal failure. The highest incidence appears to be in the Southeastern U.S.; in one study, the disorder in 13% of patients with end-stage renal disease was attributed to analgesic abuse.[135]

PATHOGENESIS. Experimentally, phenacetin, aspirin, or acetaminophen alone can cause papillary necrosis, but only if given in very large doses. However, papillary necrosis is readily induced by a mixture of aspirin and phenacetin, usually combined with water depletion. Most patients consume phenacetin-containing mixtures,[136] and cases ascribed to ingestion of aspirin, phenacetin, or acetaminophen alone are uncommon. It is now clear that in the sequence of events leading to renal damage, *papillary necrosis occurs first and cortical tubulointerstitial nephritis is a secondary phenomenon.* It is not certain whether the initial injury is to the vasa recta or to the tubules in the inner medulla or to both. The phenacetin metabolite, acetaminophen, binds covalently to cellular proteins and depletes renal glutathione; it may injure cells by both covalent binding and oxidative damage. The ability of aspirin to inhibit prostaglandin synthesis suggests that this drug may induce its potentiating effect by inhibiting the vasodilatory effects of prostaglandin, thus predisposing the papilla to renal tissue ischemia. Thus, the papillary damage may be due to a combination of direct toxic effects of phenacetin metabolites as well as ischemic injury to both tubular cells and vessels, a notion consistent with the morphologic findings and with the synergistic effects of drug combinations.

MORPHOLOGY. Grossly, the kidneys are either normal or slightly reduced in size, and the cortex exhibits depressed and raised areas, the depressed areas representing cortical atrophy overlying necrotic papillae. On cut section, the papillae show various stages of necrosis, calcification, fragmentation, and sloughing. **This gross appearance contrasts with the papillary necrosis seen in diabetic patients, in which all papillae are at the same stage of acute necrosis.** Microscopically, the papillary changes may take one of several forms: in early cases there is patchy necrosis and widening of the interstitium, but in the advanced form the entire papilla is necrotic, often remaining in place as a structureless mass with ghosts of tubules and foci of dystrophic calcification (Fig. 21–47). If segments or entire portions of the papilla have been sloughed and excreted in the urine, the underlying calyx appears dilated, accounting for some of the diagnostic radiologic features of the disease.

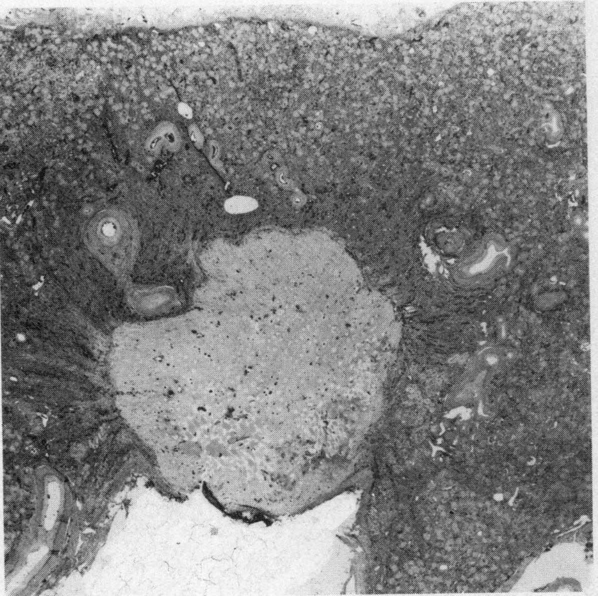

Figure 21–47. Analgesic nephropathy. Cortex is scarred and papilla is transformed to a necrotic, structureless mass.

The cortical changes consist of loss and atrophy of the tubules, and interstitial fibrosis and inflammation. These changes are mainly due to obstructive atrophy caused by the tubular damage in the papilla, but superimposed pyelonephritic changes may be present. **The cortical columns of Bertin are characteristically spared from this atrophy.** The glomeruli in the atrophic cortex may either be normal or show various degrees of hyalinization. A peculiar "analgesic microangiopathy" affects small vessels in the inner medulla, the papilla, and the submucosa of the urinary tract from pelvis to bladder.[137] It consists of a homogeneous, PAS-positive thickening of capillary walls ascribed to a thickened, multilayered basement membrane. Its pathogenesis is unknown, but it may represent successive episodes of endothelial necrosis and regeneration induced by toxic metabolites.

CLINICAL COURSE. Analgesic nephropathy occurs four times more commonly in women than in men and is particularly prevalent in women with recurrent headaches and muscular pain, in psychoneurotic women, and in factory workers. The clinical symptoms may be slight before the onset of chronic renal insufficiency, but if renal function tests are done, inability to concentrate the urine occurs early, as would be expected with lesions in the papilla. Acquired distal renal tubular acidosis and diminished citrate secretion may also contribute to the development of renal stones. Headache, anemia, gastrointestinal symptoms, and hypertension are common accompaniments of analgesic nephropathy. The anemia in particular is out of proportion to the renal insufficiency, owing to damage to red cells by the phenacetin metabolites. Pyuria is an early finding, occurring in almost 100% of patients; although the urine is often sterile, urinary tract infection occurs in about 50% of patients. Occasionally, entire tips of necrotic papillae are excreted, and these may cause gross hematuria or renal colic due to obstruction of the ureter by necrotic fragments. Necrotic papillae may appear in the urine sediment and aid in the diagnosis. Intravenous pyelography (IVP) will often disclose the characteristic picture of absent papillae, but if the papillae remain in place the IVP may be entirely normal. Progressive impairment of renal function may lead to chronic renal failure, but *with proper therapy of any infection and drug withdrawal, renal function may either stabilize or actually improve.* Thus, analgesic nephropathy may represent one of the few types of chronic renal failure from which recovery is possible.

Unfortunately, a serious complication sometimes occurs in patients with analgesic nephropathy who survived because of their discontinuance of the offending drugs,[138] namely, the development of *transitional papillary carcinoma of the renal pelvis.* Whether the carcinogenic effect is due to a metabolite of phenacetin or to some other component of the analgesic compounds is still unsettled.

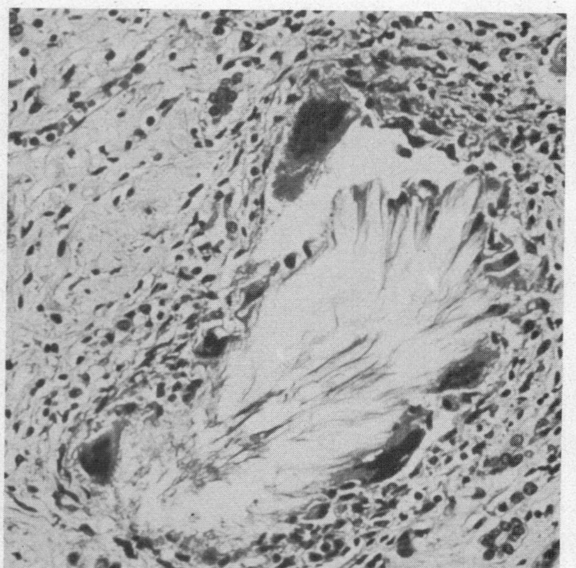

Figure 21–48. Urate crystals in renal medulla. Note inflammatory reaction with giant cells around needle-like crystals.

TUBULOINTERSTITIAL DISEASES CAUSED BY METABOLIC DISTURBANCES

Urate Nephropathy

Three types of nephropathy can occur in patients with hyperuricemic disorders (p. 1356).[139, 140] *Acute uric acid nephropathy* is caused by the precipitation of uric acid crystals in the renal tubules, principally in collecting ducts, leading to obstruction of nephrons and the development of acute renal failure. This type is particularly apt to occur in patients with leukemias and lymphomas who are undergoing chemotherapy; the latter increases the destruction of neoplastic nuclei and the elaboration of uric acid. Precipitation of uric acid is favored by the acidic pH in collecting tubules. The crystals are amorphous and doubly refractile and cause dilatation of the tubules proximal to the obstruction. Treatment with the uricosuric agent allopurinol before chemotherapy reduces the danger of this complication.

Chronic urate nephropathy or gouty nephropathy is a form of chronic tubulointerstitial nephritis occurring in patients with more protracted forms of hyperuricemia. The lesions are ascribed to the deposition of monosodium urate crystals in the acidic milieu of the distal tubules and collecting ducts, as well as in the interstitium. *These deposits have a distinct histologic appearance, in the form of birefringent, needle-like crystals present either in the tubular lumina or in the interstitium* (Fig. 21–48). The urates induce a *tophus* often surrounded by foreign body giant cells, other mononuclear cells, and a fibrotic reaction. Tubular obstruction by the urates causes cortical atrophy and scarring. Arterial and arteriolar thickening are also common in these kidneys, owing to the relatively high incidence of hypertension in patients with gout; in addition, there is sometimes a superimposed PN potentiated by the tubular obstruction. The resultant histologic picture may therefore disclose a mix of interstitial, tubular, and vascular lesions, but the characteristic feature of gouty nephropathy is the presence of large numbers of urate deposits in the medulla.

Clinically, urate nephropathy is a subtle disease associated with tubular defects that may progress slowly, but the condition should be suspected in patients with prolonged hyperuricemia. It has recently been claimed that patients with gout who actually develop a chronic nephropathy have evidence of increased exposure to lead (mostly by way of "moonshine" whiskey contaminated with lead), and that lead, rather than urates, is therefore the cause of the renal disease and hypertension in gouty nephropathy.[141]

The third renal syndrome in hyperuricemias is *nephrolithiasis*; uric acid stones are present in 22% of patients with gout and 42% of those with secondary hyperuricemia.

Hypercalcemia and Nephrocalcinosis

Disorders characterized by hypercalcemia, such as hyperparathyroidism, multiple myeloma, vitamin D intoxication, metastatic bone disease, or excess calcium intake (milk alkali syndrome), may result in the formation of calcium stones (p. 1052) and deposition of calcium in the kidney (nephrocalcinosis). Extensive degrees of calcinosis, under certain conditions, may lead to a form of chronic tubulointerstitial disease and renal insufficiency.[140] The first damage induced by the hypercalcemia is at the *intracellular level,* in the tubular epithelial cells, resulting in mitochondrial distortion and evidence of cell injury. Subsequently, calcium deposits can be demonstrated within the mitochondria, cytoplasm, and basement membrane. Calcified cellular debris then aids in obstruction of the tubular lumina and causes obstructive atrophy of nephrons with interstitial fibrosis and nonspecific chronic inflammation. Both proximal and distal tubules are involved by the calcification; in particular, the basement membranes of the proximal segments become heavily calcified. Atrophy of entire cortical areas drained by calcified tubules may occur and this accounts for the alternating areas of normal and scarred parenchyma seen in such kidneys. Vascular and glomerular calcification may also occur. Obstruction by calcium concretions predisposes to infection and thus an element of focal PN is frequently present in these kidneys.

The earliest functional defect is an inability to elaborate a concentrated urine, which appears to be related to decreased transport of chloride in the ascending thick segment. Other tubular defects, such as tubular acidosis and salt-losing nephritis, may also occur. With further damage, a slowly progressive renal insufficiency will develop. This is usually due to nephrocalcinosis, but many of these patients also have calcium stones and secondary PN. Renal calcification can be obvious radiologically and these patients often have calcifications in other organs and blood vessels.

Hypokalemic Nephropathy

Chronic potassium depletion is encountered clinically in gastrointestinal diseases (such as diverticulitis and regional enteritis) that cause potassium losses in diarrheic fluid; in adrenal overactivity; in certain renal diseases; and in patients treated with diuretics that cause potassium to be lost in the urine. Some of these patients develop disturbances of renal function dominated by impairment of concentrating mechanism, evidenced by polyuria and nocturia. The tubules show a remarkable coarse vacuolization of tubular cells, mainly in the proximal convoluted tubules. The vacuolization is coarser than that seen in the usual osmotic nephrosis (Fig. 21–49). Electron microscopy shows both intracytoplasmic vacuolization and dilatation of the intercellular spaces, with separation of the basal plasma membranes. The lesions are reversible, but increases in serum creatinine, associated with interstitial inflammation and fibrosis and tubular atrophy, occur in some patients.[142]

TUBULOINTERSTITIAL LESIONS CAUSED BY NEOPLASTIC DISEASES

Nonrenal malignant tumors, particularly those of hematopoietic origin, affect the kidneys in a number of ways (Table 21–8).[143] The most common involvements are tubulointerstitial, caused by complications of the tumor (hypercalcemia, hyperuricemia, obstruction of ureters) or therapy (irradiation, hyperuricemia, chemotherapy, infections in immunosuppressed patients). As

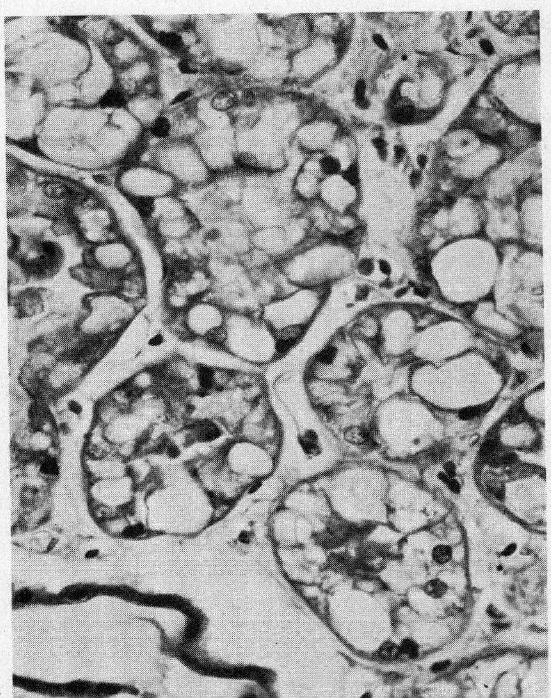

Figure 21–49. Vacuolar hypokalemic nephrosis. High-power detail of large clear vacuoles within proximal tubules.

Table 21–8. RENAL INVOLVEMENT BY NONRENAL NEOPLASMS

1. Direct tumor invasion of renal parenchyma
   Ureters → obstruction
   Artery → renovascular hypertension
2. Hypercalcemia
3. Hyperuricemia
4. Amyloidosis
5. Excretion of abnormal proteins (multiple myeloma)
6. Radiotherapy
7. Chemotherapy
8. Infection
9. Glomerulopathy
   Immune complex GN (carcinomas)
   Lipoid nephrosis (Hodgkin's disease)

the survival rate of patients with malignant neoplasms increases, so do these renal complications. Here we shall limit the discussion to the renal lesions in multiple myeloma that sometimes dominate the clinical picture in patients with this disease.

Multiple Myeloma (Myeloma Kidney)

Renal involvement is a common and sometimes ominous manifestation of multiple myeloma (p. 689), overt renal insufficiency occurring in half the patients with this disease.[143] The main cause of renal dysfunction is related to Bence Jones (light-chain) proteinuria, since renal failure correlates well with the presence and amount of such proteinuria and is extremely rare in its absence.[144] Two mechanisms appear to account for the renal toxicity of Bence Jones proteins. First, some of these light chains appear to be directly toxic to epithelial cells; second, Bence Jones proteins combine with the urinary glycoprotein (Tamm-Horsfall protein) under acidic conditions to form large, histologically distinct tubular casts that obstruct the tubular lumina and also induce a peritubular inflammatory reaction. Other factors that may contribute to renal failure include (1) vascular disease in the usually elderly population affected with myeloma; (2) hypercalcemia and hyperuricemia (p. 1039), which are often present in these patients; (3) amyloidosis, which occurs in 6 to 24% of patients with myeloma; and (4) urinary tract obstruction with secondary PN.

Grossly, the kidneys usually are normal but sometimes are shrunken and pale because of extensive interstitial scarring. The most prominent changes are histologic. The tubular casts appear as pink-to-blue amorphous masses, sometimes concentrically laminated, filling and distending the tubular lumina. Many of the casts are surrounded by multinucleate giant cells, derived from either reactive tubular epithelium or possibly mononuclear phagocytes (see Fig. 15–38, p. 691). The epithelium surrounding the cast is often necrotic, and the adjacent interstitial tissue usually shows a nonspecific inflammatory response. Occasionally, the casts erode their way from the tubules into the interstitium and here evoke a granulomatous inflammatory reaction. Sometimes, metastatic calcification occurs in these kidneys owing to the hypercalcemia commonly associated with disseminated multiple myeloma, and these kidneys are prone to develop amyloidosis, uric acid granulomas due to the hyperuricemia, and focal PN due to the obstructive lesions.

Clinically, the renal manifestations are of two main types. In the more common form, *chronic renal failure* develops insidiously and usually progresses slowly over a period of several months to years. Another form occurs suddenly, sometimes in the absence of obvious previous renal impairment, and is manifested by *acute renal failure* with oliguria.[145] ARF commonly occurs in patients with other precipitating factors, such as dehydration, hypercalcemia, acute infection, administration of nephrotoxic antibiotics, or intravenous pyelography. *Proteinuria* occurs in 70% of patients with myeloma; the presence of significant non–light-chain proteinuria (e.g., albumin) suggests secondary amyloidosis or light-chain glomerulopathy (p. 1026). Actual intrarenal infiltration by myeloma cells is rarely the cause of renal dysfunction.

OTHER TUBULOINTERSTITIAL DISORDERS

Immunologically Mediated Tubulointerstitial Disease

Immunologic tubulointerstitial reactions are involved in rejection of renal transplants (p. 174), and we have seen earlier that a hypersensitivity reaction is the cause of acute interstitial nephritis induced by drugs. In addition, tubulointerstitial damage may be induced by immunologic mechanisms similar to those involved in glomerulonephritis (i.e., *tubular immune complex disease and antitubular basement membrane antibody disease*).[146, 147]

Tubular immune complex disease is manifested by a characteristic immunofluorescent pattern of staining; granules containing immunoglobulin and complement are seen along the tubular basement membrane: In humans, immune complex tubular deposits are seen in patients with accompanying glomerulonephritis: 50% of patients with lupus nephritis and occasional patients with membranoproliferative glomerulonephritis, mixed cryoglobulinemia, and Sjögren's syndrome. It is thought that the complexes contribute to the tubulointerstitial damage in these conditions.

In antitubular basement membrane (anti-TBM) antibody disease, immunofluorescence discloses smooth, continuous linear accumulations of immunoglobulin and complement along the basement membrane of the proximal tubules of animals. In man, anti-TBM antibodies frequently occur in conjunction with anti-GBM nephritis in Goodpasture's syndrome and rapidly progressive GN, suggesting that cross-reactive autoantibodies to both glomerular and tubular basement membrane are formed in these conditions. More unusually, they occur in other types of GN, drug-induced hypersensitivity, and idiopathic interstitial nephritis.

Radiation Nephritis

This condition, which follows therapeutic irradiation of tumors in the regions of the kidneys,[148] is now an uncommon complication, since damaging radiation levels can be predicted and the kidneys appropriately shielded. Doses of greater than 2300 rads in less than five weeks are sufficient to cause renal damage. The clinical presentation may be acute, beginning six to 12 months after radiation, and characterized by edema, hypertension (often malignant), anemia, proteinuria, and renal insufficiency (*acute radiation nephritis*). Other patients present more than 18 months after irradiation with hypertension (benign or malignant) or proteinuria. Histologically, all renal structures are affected; there is glomerular hyalinization, severe interstitial fibrosis and inflammation, tubular atrophy, and sometimes striking vascular thickening. In some instances, tubulointerstitial damage is out of proportion to the vascular or glomerular damage, but in the presence of severe hypertension, fibrinoid necrosis and hyperplastic changes in arterioles are common.

Balkan Nephropathy

This is a most mysterious entity occurring in a limited geographic zone, about 40 kilometers wide and 100 kilometers long, which includes adjacent regions of Romania, Bulgaria, and Yugoslavia.[149] The clinical picture is one of insidious onset of progressive renal insufficiency, most patients succumbing within ten years of onset. Morphologically, there is interstitial fibrosis with a variable number of chronic inflammatory cells and widespread tubular loss. The nature of this disorder has been vigorously pursued but remains uncertain. Currently, fungal toxins contaminating local foodstuffs (mycotoxins) are thought to be possible etiologic agents.

DISEASES OF BLOOD VESSELS

Renal vessels are affected secondarily by virtually all forms of renal disease. Here we are concerned with those disorders in which the vascular lesions are the primary cause of disease and in particular those associated with hypertension. Within this group, benign and malignant nephrosclerosis are of preeminent importance. Because the kidney and its diseases are intimately related to hypertension, it is first necessary to review briefly the subject of hypertension.

HYPERTENSION

Elevated levels of blood pressure cause vascular changes throughout the body, particularly in the kidneys; conversely, kidney disease plays an important role in the causation of certain forms of hypertension. Ironically, there is no universally accepted definition of hypertension, but most investigators agree that a sustained diastolic pressure above 90 mm Hg is an essential feature. A sustained systolic pressure above 140 mm Hg may also constitute hypertension, but systolic elevations are generally thought less significant than elevations of the diastolic pressure. Ninety to 95% of hypertension is of uncertain origin and is called *primary or essential hypertension*. The remaining 5 to 10%, called *secondary hypertension*, is associated with a variety of renal, endocrine, neurologic, and vascular disorders (Table 21–9).

Essential hypertension is an extremely common condition, which through its cardiovascular complications remains a leading cause of morbidity and mortality in the Western world.[150] Females are affected more often than males, and blacks significantly more often than whites. The incidence of the disease rises with age and as much as 50% of the population over age 50 may have essential hypertension. In most instances, even if not treated, it is characterized by extremely slow, progressive elevation of blood pressure over the span of decades. It may eventually lead to cardiovascular and cerebrovascular disorders, but the rate of development of these complications is a function of the severity of blood pressure elevations. In many milder expressions it is readily controlled by antihypertensive therapy. In other words, the disorder is relatively benign and is sometimes referred to as *benign hypertension*. However, even benign hypertension is one of the major risk factors in the development of atherosclerosis and its complications (p. 507). In time, benign hypertension causes thickening of the walls of small arteries and arterioles in the kidney, but the renal ischemia rarely causes significant renal insufficiency. Even before the advent of effective antihypertensive therapy, only about 5% of patients with benign hypertension died of uremia; the remainder died largely of coronary or hypertensive heart disease, of cerebral vascular accidents, or of unrelated causes. As we shall see, some cases of essential hypertension pursue an accelerated malignant course

Table 21–9. TYPES OF HYPERTENSION

- **A. Primary or Essential Hypertension**
- **B. Secondary Hypertension**
  - Renal
    - Acute glomerulonephritis
    - Chronic renal disease
    - Renal artery stenosis
    - Renal vasculitis
    - Renin-producing tumors
  - Endocrine
    - Adrenocortical hyperfunction (Cushing's syndrome)
    - Oral contraceptives
    - Pheochromocytoma
    - Acromegaly
    - Myxedema
    - Thyrotoxicosis (systolic)
  - Vascular
    - Coarctation of aorta
    - Polyarteritis nodosa
    - Aortic insufficiency (systolic)
  - Neurogenic
    - Psychogenic
    - Increased intracranial pressure
    - Polyneuritis, bulbar poliomyelitis, others

(malignant hypertension), characterized by a rapidly mounting blood pressure, usually to diastolic levels over 110 mm Hg, with the systolic often well over 200 mm Hg and uniformly resulting in renal failure unless controlled with proper antihypertensive therapy.

Pathogenesis of Hypertension

The search for the origins of essential hypertension[150–152] has been most frustrating. Much more has been learned about the pathogenesis of the secondary forms of hypertension, and so we will review first the more well-established mechanisms that cause secondary hypertension.

As is well-known, the magnitude of the arterial pressure is dependent on two fundamental hemodynamic variables: total systemic blood flow (*cardiac output*) and the resistance offered by the blood vessels and blood to forward flow—*total peripheral resistance* (Fig. 21–50). Blood volume, through its effect on cardiac output, also influences blood pressure. For the most part, the total peripheral resistance is accounted for by resistance of the arterioles. This in turn is determined by the thickness of the arteriolar wall in relation to lumen size *and* the effects of neural and hormonal influences that either constrict or dilate these vessels. Vasoconstricting agents are angiotensin II, catecholamines thromboxane, and leukotrienes; the main vasodilators are the kinins and prostaglandins. These mediators act by binding to specific receptors on the surface of smooth muscle cells. Certain metabolic products, such as lactic acid, hydrogen ions, and adenosine, as well as hypoxia are also local vasodilators. An important property intrinsic to resistance vessels is *autoregulation*, a process by which increased blood flow to such vessels leads to vasoconstriction. This is an essentially adaptive mechanism designed to protect from hyperperfusion; the resultant vasoconstriction leads to increased cardiac overload, reduction of cardiac output, and correction of hyperperfusion. *Arterial hypertension can best be considered as a disease dependent on any factors that may alter the relationship between blood volume and total arteriolar resistance* (Fig. 21–50).

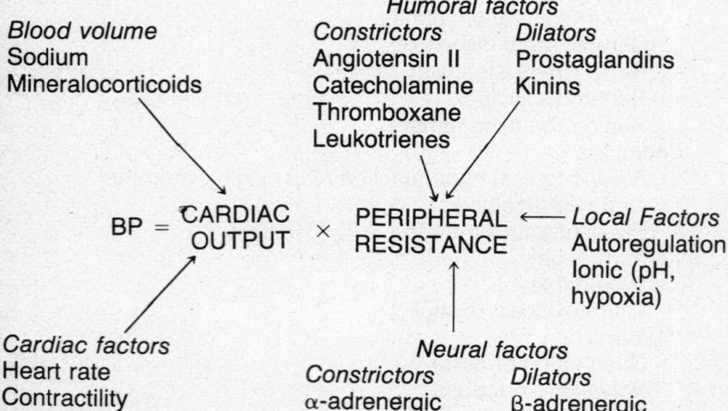

Figure 21–50. Blood pressure regulation. (Modified from Kaplan, N. M.: Systemic hypertension: mechanisms and diagnosis. *In* Braunwald, E. (ed.): Heart Disease. 2nd ed. Philadelphia, W. B. Saunders Co., 1984, p. 861.)

RENAL HYPERTENSION. The kidney participates in the control of blood pressure by affecting both peripheral resistance and blood volume. It is no surprise, therefore, that hypertension is common in a variety of renal disorders. It occurs, for example, in the course of acute poststreptococcal glomerulonephritis, in almost all chronic renal diseases such as chronic GN and PN, in the necrotizing vasculitides such as polyarteritis nodosa, and in renal artery stenosis.[153]

The renal mechanisms that control blood pressure and which, therefore, may be deranged in renal hypertension can be grouped under three headings: (1) *secretion by the kidney of vasoactive substances that have a pressor effect*, (2) *maintenance of extracellular fluid (ECF) and blood volume*, and (3) *elaboration by the kidneys of substances that normally lower blood pressure*. These three mechanisms are interrelated but will be discussed separately.

Renal Pressor Effects—The Renin-Angiotensin System. The renin-angiotensin system is the major renal humoral pressor mechanism (Fig. 21–51). Renin is released by the juxtaglomerular (JG) cells under many circumstances, of which the most important are (1) a decrease in pressure in the afferent arteriole sensed by stretch receptors within the vessel wall, (2) decreased sodium (or chloride) load delivered to the macula densa, and (3) direct stimulation of sympathetic nerves or beta-adrenergic agonists such as epinephrine.

Renin itself is not a pressor substance but acts on angiotensinogen, a liver-derived circulating apha-2-globulin, to produce the decapeptide angiotensin I; the latter is converted by converting enzyme to the octapeptide angiotensin II, a potent vasoconstrictor of renal and extrarenal arterioles. Renin also stimulates aldosterone secretion by the adrenal cortex, thus causing sodium retention. It should be appreciated that angiotensin II tends to increase arterial blood pressure in two ways: direct vasoconstriction increases vascular resistance, and aldosterone secretion causes sodium retention and increases blood volume.

Under normal conditions, the increased renin secretion is quickly corrected by negative feedback mechanisms that tend to suppress renin release and bring circulating renin levels back to normal. Thus, increased blood pressure diminishes stretch receptor stimulation in the afferent arteriole and therefore diminishes renin secretion; similarly, the increased ECF volume consequent to aldosterone secretion increases GFR, thus decreasing proximal sodium reabsorption, and through the sensors in the macula densa diminishes renin secretion. Increased arterial pressure also diminishes renal sympathetic nerve stimulation by a poorly understood autoregulatory mechanism, further decreasing renin secretion. Finally, angiotensin II itself appears to suppress JG-cell secretion directly. *Thus, in the presence of normal renal function, plasma renin values are restored to normal.*

Summarizing a large body of evidence, it seems

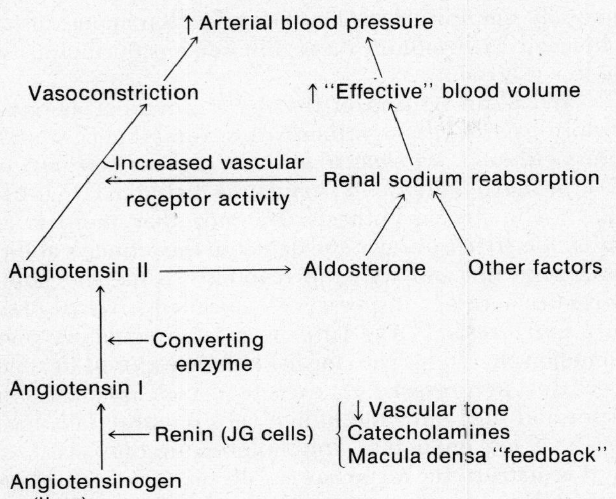

Figure 21–51. Renin-angiotensin mechanism and control of blood pressure.

likely that increased renin secretion plays a role in the following forms of renal hypertension:[155] (1) in unilateral renal artery stenosis (renovascular hypertension); (2) in malignant hypertension, in which extremely high levels of renin and aldosterone have been measured; (3) in the vasculitides; (4) in some patients with unilateral chronic PN or reflux nephropathy; (5) in renin-secreting JG cell tumors, renal cell carcinoma, or Wilms' tumors; and (6) in some patients with chronic renal failure of diverse etiology who have elevated serum renin levels. In the last-named group of patients it has been suggested that the elevated renin levels are due to failure of the feedback control mechanisms outlined earlier because (a) the patients are more likely to have sodium and water retention and (b) there is diminished inhibition of renin secretion in response to volume expansion.

Sodium Retention and Alterations in Blood Volume. As is well-known, total body sodium is the main determinant of ECF volume, and the latter in turn influences blood volume and cardiac output. The kidney is the principal organ responsible for such sodium homeostasis. The following renal factors appear to be most important in achieving such sodium homeostasis: (1) *Glomerular filtration rate.* A reduction in GFR decreases the filtered sodium load and increases proximal sodium reabsorption, serving to conserve body sodium stores, and vice versa; i.e., an increase in GFR with volume expansion will result in sodium loss (natriuresis). (2) *Aldosterone.* This hormone increases distal renal tubular reabsorption of sodium. (3) *A GFR-independent, aldosterone-independent mechanism.* In the presence of volume expansion, this mechanism tends to inhibit sodium reabsorption (causing natriuresis), probably at a distal tubular site. The nature of this "third" or natriuretic factor is still poorly understood. *Sodium retention due to failure of these homeostatic mechanisms is probably the most important factor responsible for hypertension in patients with end-stage renal failure.* Increased total exchangeable sodium and ECF volume are found in such patients, and there is marked improvement of blood pressure when these excesses are removed. Sodium retention is postulated to account also, at least in part, for the hypertension that occurs in acute GN.

Renal Antihypertensive Agents. The notion that renal hypertension is caused by deficient production of an agent that lowers blood pressure directly or inactivates a pressor substance is known under the rubric "renoprival hypertension." This mechanism is lent credence by the isolation of at least three groups of antihypertensive agents from the kidney.[157, 157A]

(1) *Prostaglandins* (PG) are synthesized in the kidney by medullary interstitial cells, papillary collecting tubules, cortical tubules, glomeruli, and afferent arterioles. In all likelihood, the cortical PGs induce vascular effects, while the medullary PGs control salt and water secretion. In most species, PGs decrease ECF volume, exert direct effects on vascular tone and reactivity, and blunt the renal vasoconstrictor and antidiuretic action of angiotensin II. Prostacyclin causes an increase in renal blood flow, increased GFR, diuresis, natriuresis, and vasodilatation—all being antihypertensive phenomena.

(2) *Kallikrein-kinin.* All elements involved in kinin formation and destruction (p. 53) are present in the kidney, including kininogen, the serum substrate; kallikrein, which converts kininogen to kinin; and kininases, which hydrolyze kinins to inactive peptides. Bradykinin causes generalized as well as renal vasodilatation and increases sodium excretion, both being pressure-reducing effects. Urinary kallikreins are decreased in some models of experimental hypertension, in spontaneously hypertensive rats, in essential hypertension with mild renal insufficiency, and in some hypertensives with parenchymal renal disease, lending credence to a role for this system in hypertension.

(3) A third antihypertensive agent produced by the interstitial cells of the renal medulla is a *neutral lipid factor*, which has been shown by Muirhead and coworkers to prevent experimentally induced hypertension in the dog and rabbit.[158] It is apparently distinct from PGs.

There are poorly understood but obviously important relationships among the three humoral systems operating in the kidney: renin-angiotensin, prostaglandins, and kallikrein-kinin.[157] PGs, for example, stimulate both the kallikrein-kinin and the renin-angiotensin systems, and inhibit the vasoconstrictive action of angiotensin II. It is possible, therefore, that the hypertensive and hypotensive factors elaborated by the kidney are involved in some delicately balanced feedback system controlling blood pressure. There is no dearth of possible mechanisms that can interfere with this balance and account for hypertension in renal disease, but the precise sequence of events is still far from clear.

The mechanisms of other secondary forms of hypertension are heterogeneous. In *primary aldosteronism,* the major cause is aldosterone-induced sodium retention causing increased blood volume; in *pheo-*

chromocytoma, the tumor in the renal medulla secretes epinephrine and norepinephrine, which cause vasoconstriction and increased cardiac contractility; *oral contraceptives*, a common cause of secondary hypertension, seem to activate the renin-angiotensin mechanism; and in *polyarteritis nodosa* there are marked increases in renin production.

ESSENTIAL HYPERTENSION. By definition, essential hypertension is idiopathic, *but it is believed that a combination of genetic and environmental factors together are responsible for the condition.*[150] Numerous epidemiologic studies have shown a rather high degree of concordance in levels of blood presure among twins, siblings, and families. The increased prevalence of hypertension among blacks, the recognition in hypertensive families of hypertension in infants and children, and the development by inbreeding of various strains of spontaneously hypertensive rats all point to a genetic predisposition. The inheritance appears to be polygenic.

Environmental factors clearly influence the development of hypertension. This is illustrated by the lower incidence of hypertension in Chinese people living in their native country as compared with the Chinese living in the United States. Although behavior patterns, stress, obesity, and the intake of oral contraceptives all have important implications, it is the relationship of *dietary sodium* to essential hypertension that has stimulated the most interest. Although the evidence is by no means unambiguous, most workers now agree that in those with a genetic predisposition, high sodium intake predisposes to or may lead to hypertension. People living in remote areas in Asia, South America, and Africa who have diets very low in sodium chloride show little evidence of essential hypertension or of a rise of blood pressure with advancing age. When some of these groups migrate to coastal towns where the salt intake is high, they begin to get their share of hypertension. The daily consumption of salt in such "civilized" areas as the U.S., Europe, and Japan is 8 gm or more and correlates with an 8 to 25% incidence of hypertension. Experimentally susceptible strains of rats develop hypertension when fed high-sodium diets, but remain normotensive on low-salt diets.

What can be said of the *pathogenesis* of essential hypertension? Although there are several theories, most stress either (1) *a primary defect in sodium excretion or* (2) *a primary increase in peripheral resistance* (Fig. 21–52).[159] The first hypothesis contends that there is an initial *nonstructural* genetic defect in the kidney's ability to excrete salt and water in response to the inevitable periodic increases in pressure—so-called *arterial pressure natriuresis.*[160] The latter is an autoregulatory phenomenon that helps the normal kidney exposed to small increases in pressure to excrete excess quantities of water and salt, until the individual's pressure falls back to a level low enough to stop the pressure diuresis. Loss of this natriuretic response results in increased blood and ECF volumes, and eventually increased peripheral vascular resistance and hypertension. Natriuretic hormone, which enhances sodium influx into vascular cells and increases vascular reactivity, is thought to mediate increased resistance. In time the vasoconstriction produces changes in the arteries and arterioles (smooth muscle hyperplasia and hypertrophy), which narrow the lumen and enhance the increase in peripheral resistance. The primacy of a sodium transport defect is supported by studies showing membrane transport alterations in the red cells[161] as well as early renal defects in "prehypertensive" offspring of hypertensive parents.[162] The second set of hypotheses implicates vasoconstrictive influences as the primary events. These could be due to (1) behavioral or neurogenic factors, as shown by the reduction of blood pressure that can be achieved by meditation (the relaxation response); (2) increased release of vasoconstrictor agents, e.g., renin and catecholamines; or (3) a primary increased sensitivity of arterioles possibly due to sodium transport defects. High sodium intake clearly influences blood pressure in both hypotheses.

These two hypotheses are not mutually exclusive,

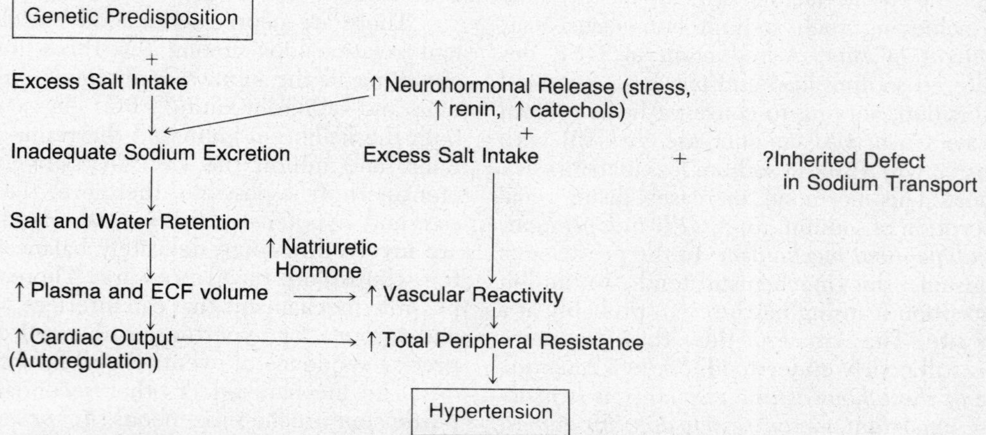

Figure 21–52. Hypothetical scheme for pathogenesis of essential hypertension (see text).

and Figure 21–52 depicts a sequence that is consistent with both events. Essential hypertension is thus a complex disorder that may have more than one cause. It may be initiated by a disturbance in any of the factors that control normal blood pressure, many of which are environmental (stress, salt intake, estrogens) but act in the genetically predisposed individual. In established hypertension, both increased blood volume and increased peripheral resistance contribute to the increased pressure.

We shall now examine some of the renal vascular disorders associated with hypertension.

Benign Nephrosclerosis and Benign Hypertension

Benign nephrosclerosis (BNS), the term used for the kidney of benign hypertension, is always associated with hyaline arteriolosclerosis. Some degree of BNS, albeit mild, is present at autopsy in many individuals over age 60. The frequency and severity of the lesions are increased in young age groups in association with hypertension and diabetes mellitus.[53]

Morphology. Grossly, the kidneys are either normal in size or moderately reduced to average weights between 110 and 130 gm. The cortical surfaces have a fine, even granularity that resembles grain leather (Fig. 21–53). On section, the loss of mass is mainly due to cortical narrowing. The reduction in size is usually equal on both sides.

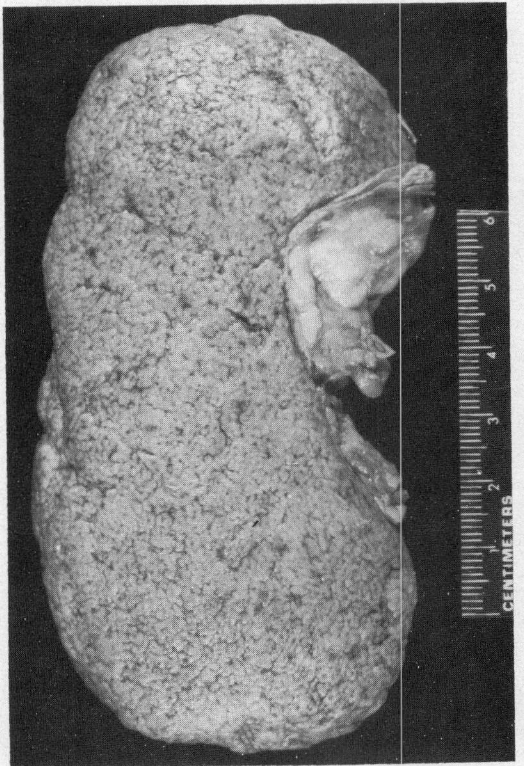

Figure 21–53. Benign nephrosclerosis illustrating fine granularity of surface.

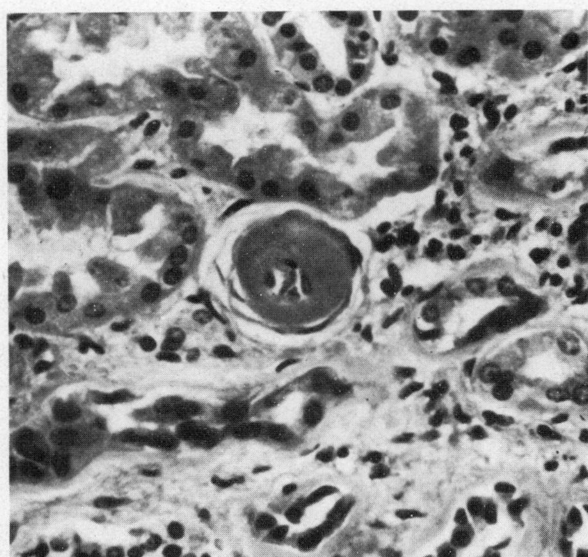

Figure 21–54. Hyaline arteriolosclerosis. Arteriolar wall is hyalinized and lumen is markedly narrowed. Note also interstitial fibrosis and tubular atrophy.

The primary histologic characteristic of BNS is narrowing of the lumina of arterioles and small arteries, caused by thickening and hyalinization of the walls (Fig. 21–54). Hyaline arteriolosclerosis occurs to some degree in normotensive individuals after the fifth decade, but, as mentioned earlier, it is more severe and frequent in patients with hypertension and diabetes mellitus. It is thought that the hyaline material is composed in large part of plasma proteins and lipids that have leaked out of the circulation, probably owing to endothelial injury, and precipitated in the vessel wall. In addition, there is deposition of intimal basement membrane material.

Consequent to the hyaline vascular narrowing, there is patchy ischemic atrophy, which consists of (1) foci of tubular atrophy and interstitial fibrosis and (2) a variety of glomerular alterations. The latter include collapse of glomerular basement membranes, deposition of collagen within Bowman's space, periglomerular fibrosis, and total sclerosis of glomeruli. In general, the severity of the ischemic atrophy parallels that of the vascular changes.

In addition to arteriolar hyalinization, the larger interlobular and arcuate arteries exhibit a characteristic lesion that consists of reduplication of the elastic lamina and increased fibrous tissue in the media, with consequent narrowing of the lumen. This change, called **fibroelastic hyperplasia,** often accompanies hyaline arteriolosclerosis and increases in severity with age and in the presence of hypertension. Little is known of its pathogenesis, but most workers include the changes together with those of smaller vessels.

It must be emphasized that renal biopsies of some patients with essential hypertension show no arteriolosclerosis. Thus, hyaline arteriolosclerosis cannot be the cause of hypertension. However, the possibility remains that the development of hyaline arteriolosclerosis may cause renal ischemia and may sustain or aggravate high blood pressure by activating the renin-angiotensin system.

Uncomplicated benign nephrosclerosis alone rarely causes renal insufficiency or uremia. There are usually moderate reductions in renal plasma flow, but the GFR may remain normal or be slightly reduced. Occasionally, there is moderate loss of concentrating power, with mild proteinuria. Patients with moderate degrees of benign nephrosclerosis appear to have lost an element of renal reserve and are thus more prone to develop azotemia in the face of volume depletion, surgical stress, or gastrointestinal hemorrhage. Renal failure and azotemia occur in 1 to 5% of patients with severe, prolonged benign nephrosclerosis and hypertension. In most patients with essential hypertension, renal failure results from the development of the malignant or accelerated phase of hypertension, discussed next.

Malignant Phase of Hypertension (Malignant Nephrosclerosis)

Malignant nephrosclerosis is the form of renal disease associated with malignant or accelerated phase of hypertension. This dramatic pattern of hypertension may occasionally develop in previously normotensive individuals, but more often is superimposed on preexisting benign hypertension, whether primary or secondary. Malignant nephrosclerosis may therefore appear as a new form of nephropathy, or it may be superimposed on an underlying chronic renal disease, particularly benign nephrosclerosis, GN, or PN. It is also a frequent cause of death from uremia in patients with scleroderma. Malignant hypertension is relatively uncommon, occurring in less than 5% of all patients with elevated blood pressure. In its pure form, it usually affects younger individuals, with a high preponderance in males and in blacks.

MORPHOLOGY. Grossly, the kidney size is dependent on the duration and severity of the hypertensive disease. Small, pinpoint petechial hemorrhages may appear on the cortical surface from rupture of arterioles or glomerular capillaries, giving the kidney a peculiar "flea-bitten" appearance. When superimposed on preexisting renal disease, the presence of malignant hypertension may be completely undetectable grossly.

Two histologic alterations characterize malignant hypertension. (1) **Fibrinoid necrosis of arterioles**. This appears as an eosinophilic granular change in the blood vessel wall, which stains positively for fibrin by histochemical or immunofluorescent techniques (Fig. 21–55*A*). In addition, there is often an inflammatory infiltrate within the wall, giving rise to the term **necrotizing arteriolitis.** (2) In the interlobular arteries and arterioles there is intimal thickening caused by a proliferation of elongated, concentrically arranged cells, probably smooth muscle cells, together with fine concentric layering of collagen. This alteration is known as **hyperplastic arteriolitis,** also referred to as "onionskinning" (Fig. 21–55*B*). The lesion correlates well with renal failure in malignant hypertension. Sometimes the glomeruli become necrotic and infiltrated with neutrophils, and the glomerular capillaries may thrombose **(necrotizing glomerulitis).** Rupture of these necrotic capillaries gives rise to hemorrhage into the glomerular spaces and adjacent tubules, providing the microscopic basis for the petechiae seen grossly. The arteriolar and arterial lesions result in considerable narrowing of all vascular lumina, with ischemic atrophy and infarction distal to the abnormal vessels.

When superimposed on an underlying benign nephro-

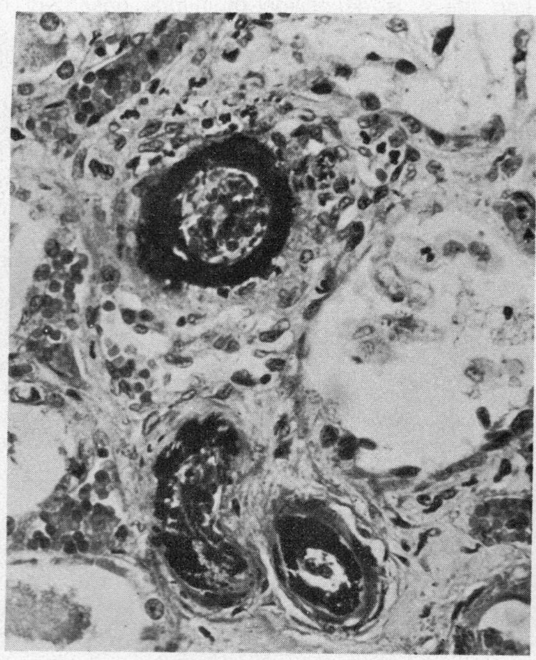

A

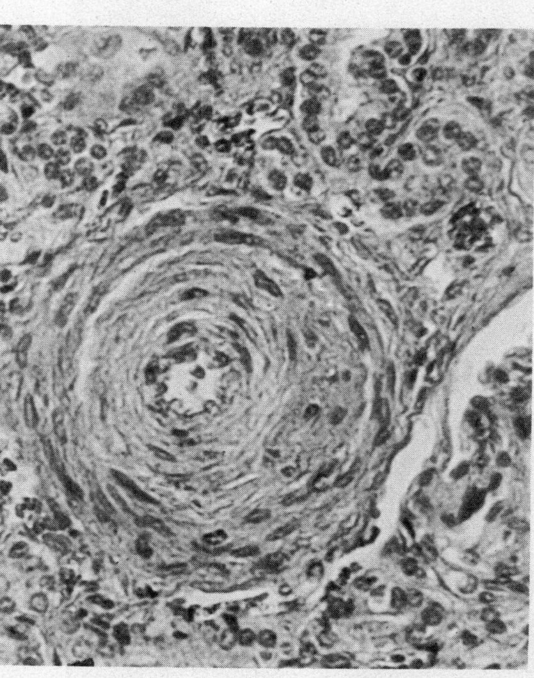

B

Figure 21–55. *A,* Necrotizing arteriolitis of malignant nephrosclerosis with fibrinoid degeneration of walls of arterioles and small arteries. *B,* Hyperplastic arteriolitis of malignant hypertension (onionskinning).

sclerosis, the arterioles and small arteries also show changes characteristic of benign hypertension and hyaline arteriolosclerosis.

PATHOGENESIS. The basis for the development of malignant hypertension is shrouded in the cause of essential hypertension. The rapidly mounting levels of arterial pressure often appear without any signs or symptoms or apparent cause. Malignant hypertension, however, is usually associated with remarkably high levels of renin, angiotensin, and aldosterone. Nonetheless, the initial stimulus for the hyperreninemia is obscure. It has been suggested that sodium retention as a consequence of prolonged benign hypertension or renal disease is the cause of the increased renin.[150] Whatever the initial stimulus for the hyperreninemia, experimental studies suggest that vasoconstriction and the severe increases in blood pressure accentuate the vascular necrosis that occurs in arterioles of the kidney and other organs. Such an increase in blood pressure causes endothelial injury, platelet thrombosis, and intravascular coagulation; by causing ischemia, these perpetuate the vicious cycle of hyperreninemia in malignant hypertension.[163] It is thought that the intimal proliferation characteristic of the onionskin lesion is due to organization of the deposits of fibrin. Alternatively, the intravascular coagulation may well *initiate* the malignant phase; this view is suggested by the observation that intravascular coagulation in patients with microangiopathic hemolytic disorders *precedes* the appearance of increased blood pressure (p. 1048). Whatever the mechanism of malignant hypertension, the cause of the renal insufficiency is the profound ischemic change resulting from the arteriolar and arterial narrowing.

CLINICAL COURSE. Usually the clinical manifestations of malignant hypertension appear abruptly, and initially are referable to the cardiovascular or central nervous systems. Cardiac decompensation, demonstrated principally as left ventricular failure, may be the first manifestation. Rarely, patients with malignant hypertension present in oliguric acute renal failure. More often, the early symptoms are related to increased intracranial pressure and include headaches, nausea, vomiting, and visual impairments, particularly the development of scotomas or spots before the eyes. "Hypertensive crises" are sometimes encountered, characterized by episodes of loss of consciousness or even convulsions. At the onset of rapidly mounting blood pressure, there is marked proteinuria and microscopic or sometimes macroscopic hematuria, but no significant alteration in renal function. Soon, however, renal failure makes its appearance. The syndrome is a true medical emergency requiring the institution of aggressive and prompt antihypertensive therapy before the development of irreversible renal lesions. Before introduction of the new antihypertensive drugs, malignant hypertension was associated with a 50% mortality rate within three months of onset, progressing to 90% within a year. At present, however, about 50% of patients will survive five years, and further progress is still being made. Ninety per cent of deaths are caused by uremia and others by cerebral hemorrhage or cardiac failure.

Renal Artery Stenosis

Unilateral renal artery stenosis is a relatively uncommon cause of hypertension, responsible for 2 to 5% of cases, but is of importance because it is the most common curable form of hypertension, surgical treatment being successful in 70 to 80% of carefully selected cases in humans. Further, much of our knowledge of renal mechanisms in hypertension has come from studies of experimental and human renal artery stenosis.

PATHOGENESIS. The classical experiments of Goldblatt in 1934[164] showed that constriction of one renal artery in dogs results in hypertension, and that the magnitude of the effect is roughly proportional to the amount of constriction. Later experiments in rats confirmed these results, and in time the importance of the renin-angiotensin system in renal hypertension was established. The bulk of the evidence now indicates that this system is responsible for renovascular hypertension.[165] Thus, renin is released in increased amounts from the experimentally ischemic kidney within minutes after renal artery constriction, and the elevated blood pressure can be prevented by previous treatment with agents that either block conversion of angiotensin I to angiotensin II or are antagonists of angiotensin II. Fifty per cent of patients with renovascular hypertension have elevated renin levels, and almost all show a reduction of blood pressure when given competitive antagonists of angiotensin II (e.g., saralasin). Additional explanations for the sustenance of long-term renovascular hypertension include sodium retention, inhibition of the prostaglandin and kinin systems, and increased vascular reactivity to subpressor levels of angiotensin.

The most common cause of renal artery stenosis is occlusion by an atheromatous plaque at the origin of the renal artery. This lesion occurs more frequently in males, the incidence increasing with advancing age and diabetes mellitus. The plaque is usually concentrically placed and superimposed thrombosis often occurs, precipitating hypertension by reducing the blood supply even further. The second type of lesion leading to stenosis is so-called **fibromuscular dysplasia** of the renal artery.[166] This is a heterogeneous group of lesions characterized by fibrous or fibromuscular thickening and may involve the initima, the media, or the adventitia of the artery. These lesions are thus subclassified into intimal, medial, and adventitial hyperplasia—the medial type being by far the most common (Fig. 21–56). In contrast to atherosclerosis, the lesions, as a whole, are more common in females and tend to occur in younger age groups, i.e., in the third and fourth decades. The lesions may consist of a single well-defined constriction or a series of narrowings, usually in the middle or distal portion of the renal artery. They may also involve the segmental branches and may be bilateral. Fibromuscular dysplasia can often be differentiated from atherosclerotic stenosis by arteriography, since lesions tend to be segmental, with alternating segments of thickening and thinning of the vessels. The pathogenesis of the dysplasia is unknown.

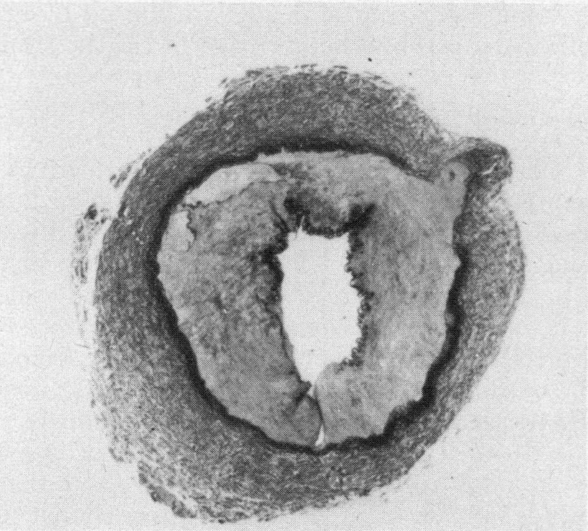

Figure 21–56. Fibromuscular dysplasia of renal artery, medial type (elastic tissue stain). Media shows marked fibrous thickening, and lumen is stenotic. (Courtesy of Dr. Seymour Rosen, Beth Israel Hospital, Boston.)

The ischemic kidney is usually reduced in size and shows signs of diffuse ischemic atrophy, with crowded glomeruli, atrophic tubules, interstitial fibrosis, and focal inflammatory infiltrate. The JG apparatus may disclose hyperplasia and increased granularity. The arterioles in the ischemic kidney are usually protected from the effects of high pressure, thus showing only mild arteriolosclerosis, in contrast to the contralateral nonischemic kidney, which may exhibit hyaline arteriolosclerosis, depending on the severity of the preceding hypertension.

CLINICAL COURSE. Few distinctive features suggest the presence of renal artery stenosis and, in general, these patients resemble those presenting with essential hypertension. Occasionally, a bruit can be heard on auscultation of the kidneys. *An intravenous pyelogram shows* (1) *a delay in the appearance of the contrast agent on the stenotic side,* owing to diminished blood flow and GFR; (2) *a small kidney*, owing to the ischemic atrophy and decreased blood volume; and (3) *delayed hyperconcentration of contrast material* caused by increased reabsorption of tubular fluid, thus enhancing the concentration of the nonreabsorbable contrast agent. Arteriography is required to localize the stenotic lesion. Increased renin activity in blood obtained from the renal vein on the stenotic side and an antihypertensive response to angiotensin antagonists favor a good outcome after surgical correction of the stenosis. In properly selected patients, the cure rate after surgery is about 90% in fibromuscular dysplasias and 60 to 75% in atherosclerotic stenosis.

RENAL DISEASE ASSOCIATED WITH MICROANGIOPATHIC HEMOLYTIC ANEMIA

A group of diseases with overlapping clinical manifestations are characterized morphologically by thrombosis in the interlobular arteries, afferent arterioles, and glomeruli together with necrosis and thickening of the vessel walls (Fig. 21–57), and clinically by microangiopathic hemolytic anemia, thrombocytopenia, renal failure, and manifestations of intravascular coagulation.[167] The morphologic changes are similar to those seen in malignant hypertension, but in these conditions they may precede development of hypertension or may be seen in its absence. The diseases include (1) childhood hemolytic uremic syndrome, (2) adult hemolytic uremic syndrome, (3) thrombotic thrombocytopenic purpura, and (4) scleroderma (p. 190). Although these disorders may have diverse etiologies, *endothelial injury* and/or *intravascular coagulation* appear to be shared pathogenetic mechanisms.

Childhood Hemolytic Uremic Syndrome

Although relatively uncommon, this is one of the main causes of acute renal failure in children. It is characterized by the *sudden onset, usually after a gastrointestinal or flulike prodromal episode, of bleeding manifestations* (especially hematemesis and melena), *severe oliguria, hematuria, a microangiopathic hemolytic anemia, and (in some patients) prominent neurologic changes.* Hypertension is present in about half the patients. Biochemical evidence of intravascular coagulation (e.g., fibrin split products, p. 649) is found in most cases.[168]

The most important findings are in the kidney. Grossly, the kidneys may show patchy or widespread renal cortical necrosis. Microscopically, the glomeruli show thickening of capillary walls, due largely to endothelial and subendothelial swelling or fibrin thrombi occluding their lumina. The mesangium and subendothelial areas are often filled with fibrillar material. Some of the material has the periodicity of fibrin on electron microscopy. Interlobular and afferent arterioles show fibrinoid necrosis and intimal hyperplasia and are often occluded by thrombi.

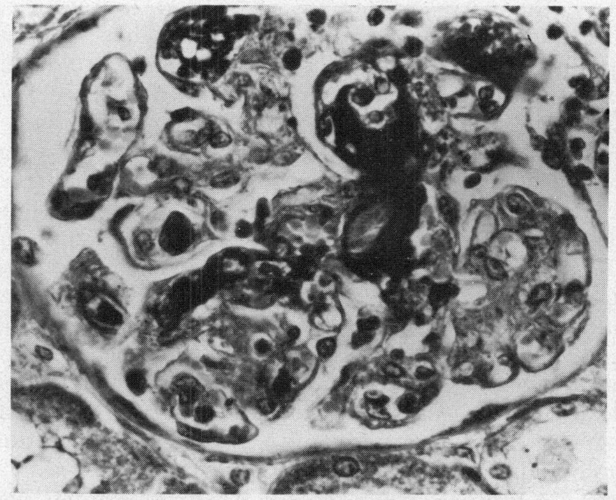

Figure 21–57. Thrombi in glomerular capillaries characteristic of intravascular coagulation and microangiopathic disorders.

If the renal failure is managed properly with dialysis, mortality is limited to 10 and 15%, most patients experiencing complete recovery. In some patients, organization of the thrombi leads to chronic ischemia, and these individuals develop chronic renal insufficiency and hypertension. The etiology is unknown, but the occurrence of epidemics in Argentina and California has suggested an infectious etiologic agent, either viral or rickettsial.

Adult Hemolytic Uremic Syndrome

A syndrome similar to that described above in children occurs in adults under a variety of settings:

1. In pregnant women with complications of pregnancy, such as hemorrhage or retained placental fragments.
2. In women in the postpartum period. This so-called *postpartum renal failure* usually occurs after an uneventful pregnancy, one day to several months following delivery, and is characterized by microangiopathic hemolytic anemia, oliguria, anuria, and mild or absent hypertension. The condition has a grave prognosis, although in milder cases recovery may occur.[169] The renal lesions are identical to those described in the childhood uremic syndrome.
3. In association with contraceptive agents. Women taking oral contraceptives have an increased risk of hypertension; in addition, both malignant nephrosclerosis and a typical hemolytic uremic syndrome develop with a greater frequency than in women not taking contraceptives.
4. In association with infection, such as typhoid fever, *E. coli* septicemia, viral infections, and shigellosis.

The clinical and morphologic features are more or less similar to those in children.

Thrombotic Thrombocytopenic Purpura

This entity, discussed earlier (p. 646), is manifested by fever, neurologic symptoms, hemolytic anemia, thrombocytopenic purpura, and the presence of thrombi in glomerular capillaries and afferent arterioles. The disease is more common in females, and most patients are under 40 years of age. The entity differs from hemolytic uremic syndrome in that central nervous system involvement is the dominant feature, whereas renal involvement occurs in only about 50% of patients. In addition, biochemical evidence of intravascular coagulation is uncommon. Histologically, eosinophilic granular thrombi are present predominantly in the terminal part of the interlobular arteries, afferent arterioles, and glomerular capillaries. The thrombi contain both platelets and fibrin and are found in arterioles of many organs throughout the body. The disease was once highly fatal, resulting in the death of 90% of patients. Recently, however, exchange transfusion or plasmapheresis coupled with corticosteroids has improved the outcome considerably.

Pathogenesis of Microangiopathic Disorders

The fibrin deposition in small vessels, the presence of microangiopathic hemolytic anemia, and the chemical evidence of coagulation disturbances all point to the importance of disseminated intravascular coagulation (DIC). The lesions bear a great resemblance to those found in the generalized Shwartzman phenomenon, in which intravascular coagulation appears to play an important role. Fibrin and fibrin products are present within the glomerular and vascular lesions. The clinical conditions associated with hemolytic uremic syndrome are those that predispose experimental animals to the Shwartzman phenomenon. For example, pregnancy can prepare an animal for the Shwartzman reaction, so that only a single injection of endotoxin is required to induce this lesion. The question whether the DIC is caused by some primary effect on the coagulation system or is secondary to endothelial injury is unanswered. It is possible, for example, that infectious agents that predispose to the hemolytic uremic syndrome do so by inducing endothelial damage, either directly or by eliciting antibody- or cell-mediated immunologic injury. Endotoxin appears to have a direct endothelial damaging effect and also interferes with normal hemostasis. There are reports of the presence of antiendothelial antibodies and cell-mediated immunity to endothelium in some patients. Finally, plasma from some patients inhibits prostacyclin production by endothelium; this presumably interferes with the antithrombotic role of endothelium and predisposes to thrombosis.[170]

ATHEROEMBOLIC RENAL DISEASE

Embolization of fragments of atheromatous plaques from the aorta or renal artery into intraparenchymal renal vessels occurs in elderly patients with severe atherosclerosis, especially after surgery on the abdominal aorta and aortography.[171] These emboli can be recognized in the walls of arcuate and interlobular arteries by their content of cholesterol crystals, which appear as rhomboid clefts. The clinical consequences of atheroemboli vary according to the number of emboli and the preexisting state of renal function. Frequently, they have no functional significance. However, acute renal failure is the result in elderly patients in whom renal function is already compromised, principally after abdominal surgery on atherosclerotic aneurysms. Fortunately, modified surgical techniques have diminished this surgical complication. Some workers also believe that chronic atheroembolization, with subsequent vascular fibrosis and narrowing, may induce a chronic type of renal failure, especially if superimposed on preexisting renal disease.

SICKLE CELL DISEASE NEPHROPATHY

Sickle cell disease in both the homozygous and heterozygous forms may lead to a variety of alterations in renal morphology and function, some of which, fortunately uncommonly, produce clinically significant abnormalities. The various manifestations are termed "sickle cell nephropathy" and have received considerable attention in recent years.[53]

The most common clinical and functional abnormalities are *hematuria* and a *diminished concentrating ability*. These are thought to be largely due to accelerated sickling in the hypertonic hypoxic milieu of the renal medulla, which increases the viscosity of the blood during its passage through the vasa recta, leading to plugging of vessels and decreased flow. Microangiographic studies of autopsied kidneys from patients with sickle cell disease disclose focal occlusions of the vasa recta, and functional studies show a diminished medullary blood flow. Patchy *papillary necrosis* may occur in both homozygotes and heterozygotes; this is sometimes associated with cortical scarring. Thus, sickle cell nephropathy should enter into the differential diagnosis of causes of papillary necrosis (together with diabetes mellitus, obstruction, pyelonephritis, and analgesic nephropathy). *Proteinuria* is also common in sickle cell disease, occurring in about 30% of patients. It is usually mild to moderate, but on occasion the overt nephrotic syndrome arises, associated with a membranoproliferative glomerular lesion.

DIFFUSE CORTICAL NECROSIS

This is an uncommon condition that occurs most frequently following an obstetric emergency such as abruptio placentae (premature serparation of the placenta), septic shock, or any medical/surgical or other calamity. When bilateral and symmetric it is uniformly fatal, but patchy cortical necrosis may permit survival. The cortical destruction has all the earmarks of ischemic necrosis. Glomerular and arteriolar microthrombi, suggesting intravascular coagulation, are found in some but by no means all cases; if present, they clearly contribute to the necrosis and renal damage. However, there are some who believe that the primary lesion is a functional vasospasm of arteries and arterioles and that the DIC is a secondary phenomenon. In support of this view are experimental studies showing that angiotensin II antagonists or alpha-adrenergic blocking agents protect against cortical necrosis. The two mechanisms, DIC and vasoconstriction, are not mutually exclusive and may act in concert or individually in specific cases.

The gross alterations of the massive ischemic necrosis are sharply limited to the cortex (Fig. 21–58). On external examination, the kidney is usually enlarged and the surface has a variegated color of marked congestion and hemorrhage, interspersed with pale, yellow-white, irregular geographic areas of massive infarction. On section, these changes are limited to the cortex and more or less completely spare the medulla. The histologic appearance is that of acute ischemic infarction. The lesions may be patchy, with areas of apparently better preserved cortex. At the deeper levels, in contact with the preserved medulla, there is usually a massive leukocytic infiltration. Intravascular and intraglomerular thrombosis may be prominent but are usually focal, and occasionally acute necroses of small arterioles and capillaries may be present. Hemorrhages occur into the glomeruli, together with the precipitation of fibrin in the glomerular capillaries.

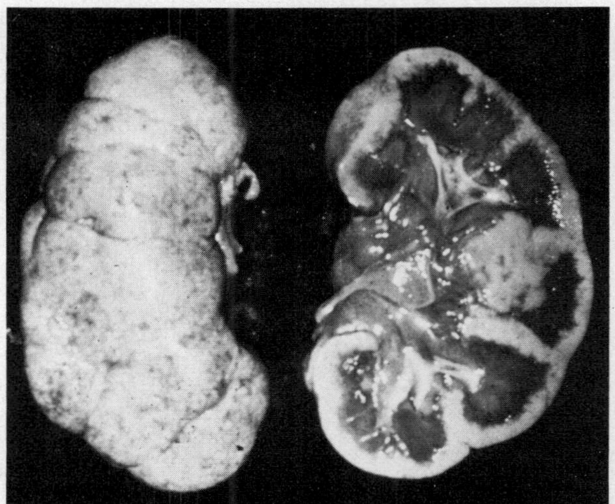

Figure 21–58. Diffuse cortical necrosis. Pale ischemic necrotic areas are confined to cortex and columns of Bertin.

Massive acute cortical necrosis is of grave significance since it gives rise to sudden anuria, terminating rapidly in uremic death. Instances of unilateral or patchy involvement are compatible with survival.

RENAL INFARCTS

The kidneys are favored sites for the development of infarcts, presumably because approximately one-fourth of the entire cardiac output passes through these organs. Although thrombosis in advanced atherosclerosis and the acute vasculitis of polyarteritis nodosa may occlude arteries, most infarcts are due to embolism. The major source of such emboli is the heart, more specifically mural thrombosis in the left atrium and mural thrombosis in the ventricle on the basis of myocardial infarction. Vegetative endocarditis and thrombosis in aortic aneurysms and aortic atherosclerosis are less frequent sites for the origin of emboli.

Because the arterial supply to the kidney is of the "end-organ" type, most infarcts are of the "white" anemic type. They may occur as solitary lesions or be multiple and bilateral. In the very early stages, anemic infarcts appear externally as slightly elevated, maplike areas that may show only slight congestive discoloration. Within 24 hours infarcts become sharply demarcated, pale, yellow-white areas that may contain small irregular foci of hemorrhagic discoloration. They are usually ringed by a zone of intense hyperemia.

On section, they characteristically assume a wedge shape, with the base against the cortical surface and the apex pointing toward the medulla (Fig. 21–59). Close inspection may disclose a very narrow rim of preserved

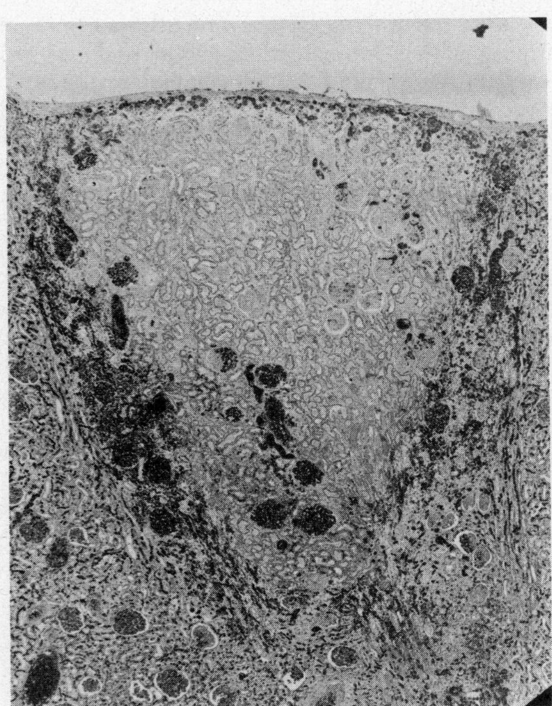

Figure 21–59. Renal infarction at low power, illustrating wedge shape, shadowy outlines of necrotic renal substances, and darker peripheral zone of leukocytic infiltration.

subcortical tissue that has been spared by the collateral capsular circulation. In time, these acute areas of ischemic necrosis undergo progressive fibrous scarring, giving rise to depressed, **pale, gray-white scars** that characteristically assume a V shape on section and are associated with wedge-shaped strands of fibrous tissue extending into the underlying kidney substance. Not infrequently, infarcts of varying ages are encountered in the same kidney, denoting recurrent embolic episodes. The histologic changes in renal infarction have already been covered in Chapter 3. It suffices for now to recall that, in common with all infarctions, there is at first progressive coagulative necrosis of cells, with preservation of shadowy cell outlines.

Many renal infarcts are clinically silent. Sometimes, pain and tenderness localized to the costovertebral angle occurs, and this is associated with the showers of red cells in the urine. Large infarcts of one kidney are a well-known basis for hypertension.

URINARY TRACT OBSTRUCTION (OBSTRUCTIVE UROPATHY)

Recognition of urinary obstruction is one of the most important priorities facing the nephrologist or urologist, *since obstruction increases susceptibility to infection and to stone formation and unrelieved obstruction almost always leads to permanent renal atrophy.* Fortunately, many causes of obstruction are surgically correctable or medically treatable.

Obstruction may be sudden or insidious and may occur at any level of the urinary tract from the urethra to the renal pelvis. The common causes of the obstruction are as follows:[172]

1. *Congenital anomalies:* posterior urethral valves and urethral strictures, meatal stenosis, bladder neck obstruction; ureteropelvic junction narrowing or obstruction; severe vesicoureteral reflux.
2. *Urinary calculi.*
3. *Benign prostatic hypertrophy.*
4. *Tumors:* carcinoma of the prostate, bladder tumors, contiguous malignant disease (retroperitoneal lymphoma), carcinoma of the cervix or uterus.
5. *Inflammation:* prostatitis, ureteritis, urethritis, retroperitoneal fibrosis.
6. *Sloughed papillae or blood clots.*
7. *Normal pregnancy.*
8. *Functional disorders:* neurogenic (spinal cord damage with bladder paralysis) and other functional abnormalities of the ureter, bladder, and urethra (often termed *dysfunctional obstruction*).

Hydronephrosis (Obstructive Atrophy)

This term is used to describe dilatation of the renal pelvis and calyces associated with progressive atrophy of the kidney due to obstruction to the outflow of urine. The urinary obstruction can exist at any level from the urethra up to the pelvis and may be partial or complete, intermittent or total, unilateral or bilateral. Even with complete obstruction, glomerular filtration persists for some time since the filtrate subsequently diffuses back into the renal interstitium and perirenal spaces, where it ultimately returns to the lymphatic and venous systems. Because of this continued filtration, the affected calyces and pelvis become dilated, often markedly so. The high pressure in the pelvis is transmitted back through the collecting ducts into the cortex, causing renal atrophy, but it also compresses the renal vasculature of the medulla, causing a diminution in the inner medullary plasma flow. The medullary vascular defects are reversible, but if protracted, obstruction will lead to functional disturbances. Accordingly, the initial functional alterations are largely tubular, manifested primarily by impaired concentrating ability. Only later does the GFR begin to diminish. Experimental studies indicate that serious irreversible damage occurs after about three weeks of complete obstruction and three months of incomplete obstruction.

MORPHOLOGY. Hydronephrosis may be unilateral or bilateral. When the obstruction is sudden and complete, the reduction of glomerular filtration usually leads to mild dilatation of the pelvis and calyces but sometimes to atrophy of the renal parenchyma. When the obstruction is subtotal or intermittent, glomerular filtration is not suppressed and progressive dilatation ensues. Depending on the level of urinary block, the dilatation may affect first the bladder or ureter and then the kidney. Usually, in low obstruction in which both kidneys are affected, uremia cuts short the development of far-advanced hydronephrotic changes.

Grossly, the kidney may have slight-to-massive enlargement. The earlier features are those of simple dilatation of the pelvis and calyces. Progressive blunting of the apices of the pyramids occurs, and eventually these become cupped. In far-advanced cases, the kidney may become transformed into a thin-walled cystic structure having a diameter of up to 15 to 20 cm (Fig. 21–60) with striking parenchymal atrophy, total obliteration of the pyramids, and thinning of the cortex.

CLINICAL COURSE. *Acute obstruction* may provoke pain attributed to distention of the collecting system or renal capsule. Most of the early symptoms are produced by the basic cause of the hydronephrosis. Thus, calculi lodged in the ureters may give rise to renal colic, and prostatic enlargements to bladder symptoms.

Unilateral, complete, or partial hydronephrosis may remain silent for long periods of time. The unaffected kidney can maintain adequate renal function, and unfortunately the hydronephrosis may remain silent and lead to progressive nephron atrophy and destruction of one kidney. Sometimes its existence first becomes apparent in the course of intravenous pyelography. It is regrettable that this disease tends to remain asymptomatic, since it has been shown that in its very early stages, perhaps the first few weeks, relief of such obstruction is compatible with reversion to normal function. *Ultrasound* has emerged as a very useful noninvasive technique in the diagnosis of obstructive uropathy.

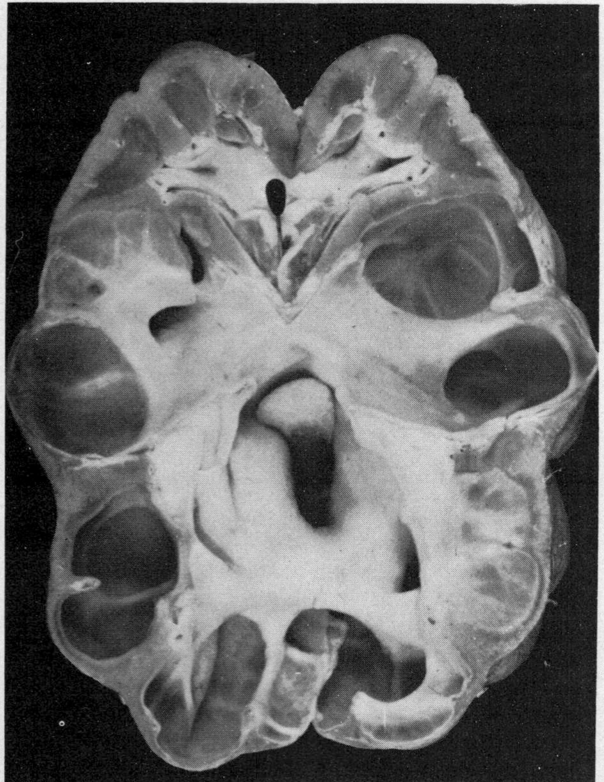

Figure 21–60. Hydronephrosis of kidney, with marked dilatation of pelvis and calyces and thinning of renal parenchyma.

In *bilateral partial obstruction,* the earliest manifestations are those of inability to concentrate the urine, reflected by polyuria and nocturia. Some patients will have acquired distal tubular acidosis, renal salt wasting, and secondary renal calculi, and a typical picture results of tubulointerstitial nephritis with scarring and atrophy of the papilla and medulla. Hypertension is common in such patients.

Complete bilateral obstruction results in oliguria or anuria and is incompatible with long survival unless the obstruction is relieved. Curiously, after relief of complete urinary tract obstruction, postobstructive *diuresis* occurs. This can often be massive, with the kidney excreting large amounts of hypotonic urine rich in sodium chloride. The diuresis is caused by (1) impairment of sodium chloride reabsorption in the proximal distal tubules by the increased intertubular pressure, (2) effects of retained urea that act as a poorly reabsorbable solute, (3) an impaired response to antidiuretic hormone, and (4) other poorly understood natriuretic factors.

UROLITHIASIS

Stones may form at any level in the urinary tract, but most arise in the kidney. Urolithiasis is a frequent clinical problem, with an incidence of 0.1 to 6% in the general population. From the clinical standpoint, it is said that one in every 1000 hospital admissions in the United States is for kidney stones. Males are affected somewhat more often than females and most patients are over age 30. Familial and hereditary predisposition to stone formation has long been known. Many of the inborn errors of metabolism, such as gout, cystinuria, and primary hyperoxaluria, provide good examples of hereditary disease characterized by excessive production and excretion of stone-forming substances.

ETIOLOGY AND PATHOGENESIS. *Most stones, about 75 to 85%, are calcium containing,* composed of calcium oxalate, or calcium oxalate mixed with calcium phosphate, and (less commonly) calcium phosphate alone. Another 15% are so-called "triple stones" or struvite stones, composed of magnesium ammonium phosphate; 6% are uric acid stones; and 1 to 3% are made up of cystine. An organic matrix of mucoprotein, making up 1 to 5% of the stone by weight, is also present. Although there are many causes for the initiation and propagation of stones, *the most important determinant is an increased urinary concentration of the stones' constituents.*

In the case of calcium-containing stones, about 10% of patients have both *hypercalciuria* and *hypercalcemia,* the latter occasioned by hyperparathyroidism, diffuse bone disease, vitamin D intoxication, sarcoidosis, the milk-alkali syndrome, renal tubular acidosis, or Cushing's syndrome. Over one-half have *hypercalciuria without hypercalcemia.* This so-called "idiopathic hypercalciuria" is thought to be caused by one of two mechanisms. The first, called *absorptive hypercalciuria,* involves hyperabsorption of calcium from the intestine, which, however, is promptly offset by an increased renal output without the development of hypercalcemia. The second, called *renal hypercalciuria*, is due to an intrinsic impairment in renal tubular reabsorption of calcium. Up to 20% of calcium-containing stones are associated with increased uric acid secretion (*hyperuricosuria*), with or without hypercalciuria. The mechanism of stone formation in this setting involves nucleation of calcium oxalate by uric acid crystals in the collecting ducts. *In 20% of patients with calcium stones, there is neither hypercalcemia nor hypercalciuria,* and stone formation remains unexplained (idiopathic calcium stone disease). The contribution of *hyperoxaluria* to calcium oxalate stones is small and is limited to patients with the rare hereditary disorder of primary hyperoxaluria, and to the acquired hyperoxalurias found in patients with intestinal disease and with pyridoxine deficiency. Although the solubility of calcium oxalate does not vary within the pH range of urine, calcium phosphate precipitates in alkaline urine.

Magnesium ammonium phosphate stones are formed largely following infections by urea-splitting bacteria (such as Proteus and some staphylococci), which convert urea to ammonia. The resultant alkaline urine causes the precipitation of magnesium ammonium phosphate salts. These form some of the largest stones, as the amounts of urea excreted normally are huge. Indeed, so-called *stag-horn calculi* are almost always associated with infection.

Uric acid stones are common in patients with hyperuricemia, such as gout, and diseases involving rapid cell turnover, such as the leukemias. However, more than half of all patients with urate calculi have neither hyperuricemia nor increased urinary excretion of uric acid. In this group, it is thought that an unexplained tendency to excrete urine of pH below 5.5 may predispose to uric acid stones, as uric acid is insoluble in relatively acidic urine. In contrast to the radiopaque calcium stones, uric acid stones are radiolucent. *Cystine stones* are associated with a genetically determined defect in the renal transport of certain amino acids, including cystine.

It can thus be appreciated that increased concentration of stone constituents, changes in urinary pH, or the presence of bacteria influence the formation of calculi. However, many calculi occur in the absence of these factors. It has, therefore, been postulated that changes in the urinary content of mucoproteins, which form the organic matrix of uroliths, may be important or, alternatively, that there is a deficiency in inhibitors of crystal formation in urine. The list of such inhibitors is long, including pyrophosphate, diphosphonate, magnesium, citrate, urea, polypeptides, and amino acids, but no consistent deficiency of any of these substances has been demonstrated in stone formers.

Stones are unilateral in about 80% of patients. The favored sites for their formation are within the renal calyces and pelves and in the bladder. If formed in the renal pelvis, they tend to remain small, having an average diameter of 2 to 3 mm. These may have smooth contours or may take the form of an irregular, jagged mass of spicules. Often, many stones are found within one kidney (Fig. 21–61). Occasionally, progressive accretion of salts leads to the development of branching structures known as stag-horn stones, which create a cast of the pelvic and calyceal system (Fig. 21–62).

Clinical Course. Stones are of importance when they obstruct urinary flow or produce ulceration and bleeding. They may be present without producing any symptoms or significant renal damage. In general, smaller stones are most hazardous, since they may pass into the ureters, producing pain referred to as colic (one of the most intense forms of pain) as well as ureteral obstruction. Larger stones cannot enter the ureters and are more likely to remain silent within the renal pelvis. Commonly, these larger stones first manifest themselves by hematuria. Stones also predispose to superimposed infection, both by their obstructive nature and by the trauma they produce.

TUMORS OF KIDNEY

Both benign and malignant tumors occur in the kidney. In general, the benign tumors are incidental findings at autopsy and rarely have clinical significance. Malignant tumors, on the other hand, are of great importance clinically and deserve considerable emphasis.[174–176] By far the most common of these malignant tumors is renal cell carcinoma, followed by Wilms' tumor, which is found in children, and finally urothelial tumors of the calyces and pelves.

BENIGN

Cortical Adenoma

Small, discrete adenomas having origin in the renal tubules are found rather commonly (7 to 22%) at autopsy.

These are usually under 2 cm in diameter. They are present invariably within the cortex and appear grossly as pale yellow-gray, discrete, seemingly encapsulated nodules. Microscopically, several variants are recognizable. Some tumors are composed of complex, branching, papillomatous structures with numerous complex fronds that project into a cystic space. Solid variants are found in which the cells grow in tubules, glands, cords, and totally undifferentiated masses of cells.

The cell type for all these growth patterns is quite regular and free of atypia. The cells are cuboidal to polygonal in shape with distinct cell membranes; round, regular small central nuclei; and a highly granular cytoplasm that may be partially or totally vacuolated. The vacuoles contain neutral fats and, in addition, anisotropic lipids, presumably cholesterol. Despite the apparent discrete margin there is no well-defined capsule histologically.

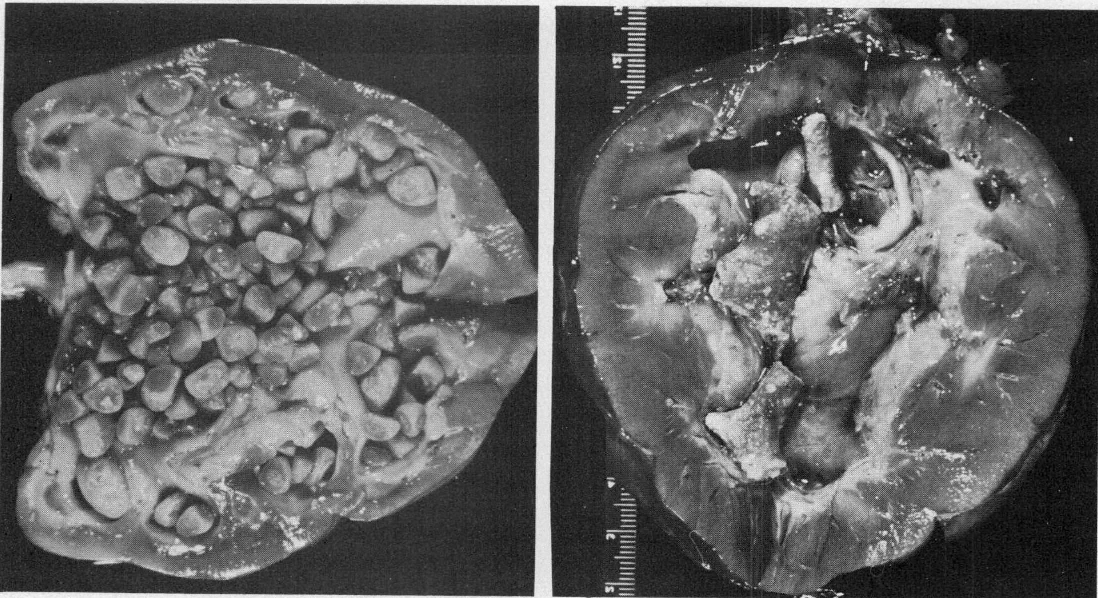

Fig. 21–61 Fig. 21–62

Figure 21–61. Nephrolithiasis. Multiple, somewhat rounded stones are present in expanded pelvis and calyces.
Figure 21–62. Nephrolithiasis. A fractured stag-horn calculus is present in somewhat dilated pelvis.

By histologic criteria, these tumors do not differ from renal cell adenocarcinoma. In this differential, the size of the tumor has been used as a diagnostic feature; tumors over 3 cm in diameter are likely to metastasize, whereas those under 3 cm rarely do. This is obviously useful as a rule of thumb only, since adenocarcinomas may arise from adenomas (see p. 1055). In addition, although most renal adenomas are incidental findings at autopsy, some of borderline size (2 to 3 cm) may be detected clinically during angiography (usually to rule out renal artery stenosis) or surgery. It seems appropriate to consider and treat those of borderline size as early cancers.[178]

Renomedullary Interstitial Cell Tumor (Renal Fibroma or Hamartoma)

Occasionally, at autopsy, small foci of gray-white firm tissue, usually under 1 cm in diameter, are found within the pyramids of the kidneys. Characteristically, they tend to occur at the junction of the distal and middle thirds of the pyramids. Microscopic examination of these discloses fibroblast-like cells and collagenous tissue. Ultrastructurally, the cells have features of renal interstitial cells. The tumors have no malignant propensities and, contrary to previous views, are not associated with hypertension.[179] Rarely, one finds small, gray, hamartomatous nodules within the renal substance, composed of abundant amounts of fibrous tissue, small cords of tubular cells, and prominent vessels.

Miscellaneous Benign Tumors

As might be anticipated, any other form of mesenchymal benign tumor may occur in the kidney, such as hemangioma and *angiomyolipoma.* The latter is thought to be a hamartomatous malformation consisting of vessels, smooth muscle, and fat. However, angiomyolipomas are *common in patients with tuberous sclerosis,* a disease characterized by lesions of the cerebral cortex that produce epilepsy and mental retardation, as well as a variety of skin abnormalities.

A rare but interesting tumor is the so-called *renin-producing juxtaglomerular cell tumor.* These tumors usually occur in younger individuals and are associated with hypertension. Histologically, they resemble *hemangiopericytomas* (p. 543), but granules similar to those in normal JG cells are seen with the electron microscope. Not all renin-secreting tumors are JG cell tumors, as *some renal cell carcinomas and Wilms' tumors have been shown to secrete renin.*

Oncocytoma is an epithelial tumor composed of large eosinophilic cells having small rounded benign appearing nuclei. The tumors are usually well encapsulated. However, they may achieve a large size (up to 12 cm in diameter) and thus should be differentiated from renal cell carcinomas.[180]

MALIGNANT

Renal Cell Carcinoma (Hypernephroma, Adenocarcinoma of Kidney)

Renal cell carcinomas represent about 1 to 3% of all visceral cancers and account for 85 to 90% of all renal cancers in adults. They occur most often in older individuals, usually in the sixth and seventh decades of life, showing a definite male preponderance in the ratio of 3:1. Because of their gross yellow color and the resemblance of the tumor cells to clear cells of the adrenal cortex, it was once thought that they arose from adrenal "rests," accounting for the term *hypernephroma*. It is now clear that these tumors arise from tubular epithelium and are therefore renal adenocarcinomas.

PATHOGENESIS. In laboratory animals, renal adenocarcinomas are readily induced by a variety of carcinogens, including chemical and viral agents, but few of these are potential carcinogens in humans. Epidemiologic studies show a significantly greater frequency of adenocarcinoma of the kidney in cigarette, pipe, and cigar smokers.[181] Genetic factors may play an important role. Nearly two-thirds of patients with the von Hippel-Lindau syndrome develop bilateral, often multiple renal cell carcinomas. Recently a family with a history of adenocarcinomas was reported to have a dominantly inherited chromosomal aberration involving a translocation between chromosomes 3 and 8.[182] The relationship of *renal cortical adenoma* to the development of renal carcinoma deserves comment. Tumors less than 3 cm in diameter have traditionally been regarded as adenomas because of their low frequency of metastases. However, large cortical adenomas have no histologic, histochemical, ultrastructural, or immunologic features that clearly distinguish them from well-differentiated adenocarcinomas. Some evidence suggests possible transition of a benign to a malignant growth. For these reasons, many workers believe that adenomas may form the subsoil from which the larger renal cell adenocarcinomas eventually develop.

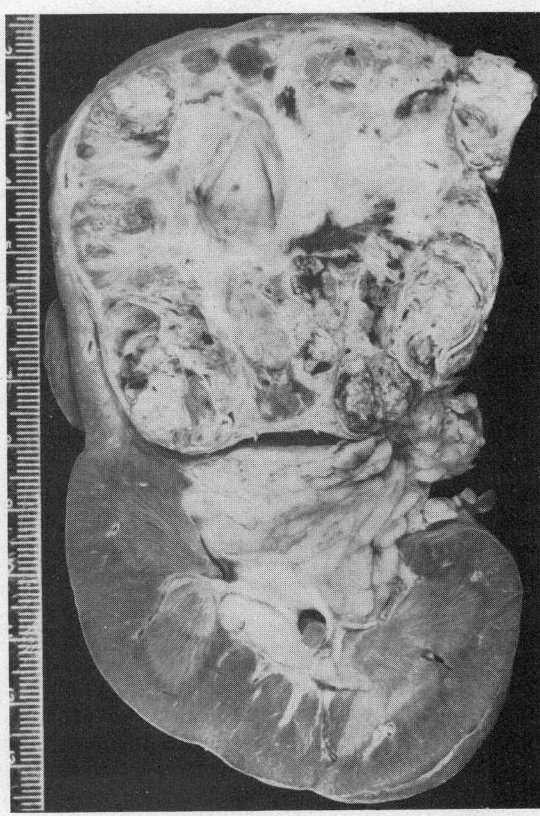

Figure 21–63. Renal cell carcinoma. Typical cross section of spherical neoplasm in one pole of kidney. Note necrosis and hemorrhages in tumor.

MORPHOLOGY. In its macroscopic appearance, the tumor is quite characteristic. It may arise in any portion of the kidney, but more commonly affects the poles, particularly the upper one. Usually these neoplasms occur as solitary unilateral lesions, but occasionally bilateral tumors have been said to have arisen simultaneously. They are spherical masses, 3 to 15 cm in diameter, composed of bright yellow-gray-white tissue that distorts the renal outline. Commonly there are large areas of ischemic, opaque, gray-white necrosis, foci of hemorrhagic discoloration and areas of softening. The margins are usually sharply defined and confined within the renal capsule, and deceptively give the appearance of encapsulation (Fig. 21–63). However, small satellite nodules are often found in the surrounding substance, providing clear evidence of the aggressiveness of these lesions. As the tumor enlarges, it may bulge into the calyces and pelvis, and eventually may fungate through the walls of the collecting system to extend even into the ureter. One of the striking characteristics of this tumor is its tendency to invade the renal vein and grow as a solid column of cells within this vessel. Further extension produces a continuous cord of tumor in the inferior vena cava and even in the right side of the heart. Despite this intravascular growth, however, discrete metastases may not occur. Occasionally, the tumor grows through the capsule to invade the adrenal and perinephric fat.

Histologically the growth pattern varies from papillary to solid, trabecular (cordlike), or tubular (resembling tubules).[183] In any single tumor, all variations in patterns of growth may be present. The most common tumor cell type is the **clear cell**, having a rounded or polygonal shape and abundant clear cytoplasm (Fig. 21–64); the latter on special stains contains glycogen and lipids. Twelve per cent of carcinomas consist of **granular** cells, which have a moderately eosinophilic cytoplasm, and 14% grow as spindle-shaped cells resembling mesenchymal tumors. Nuclear atypia is highly variable and shows some correlation with prognosis. Most tumors are either well differentiated (Grades I and II), but some (Grade IV) show marked nuclear atypia with formation of bizarre nuclei and giant cells (Fig. 21–65). The stroma is usually scanty, but highly vascularized. Hemorrhages, scars, blood pigment, and calcification are common additional histologic features.

CLINICAL COURSE. The three classic diagnostic features of costovertebral pain, palpable mass, and hematuria unfortunately appear in only 10% of cases. The most reliable of the three is hematuria, which eventually appears in about 90% of cases. However, the hematuria is usually intermittent and may be microscopic; thus, the tumor may remain silent until it attains a large size. At this time, it gives rise to generalized constitutional symptoms such as fever, malaise, weakness, and weight loss. This pattern of asymptomatic growth occurs in many patients, so that the tumor may have reached a diameter of over 10 cm when it is discovered.

Renal cell carcinoma is classified as one of the great "mimics" in medicine, since it tends to produce a diversity of systemic symptoms not related to the kid-

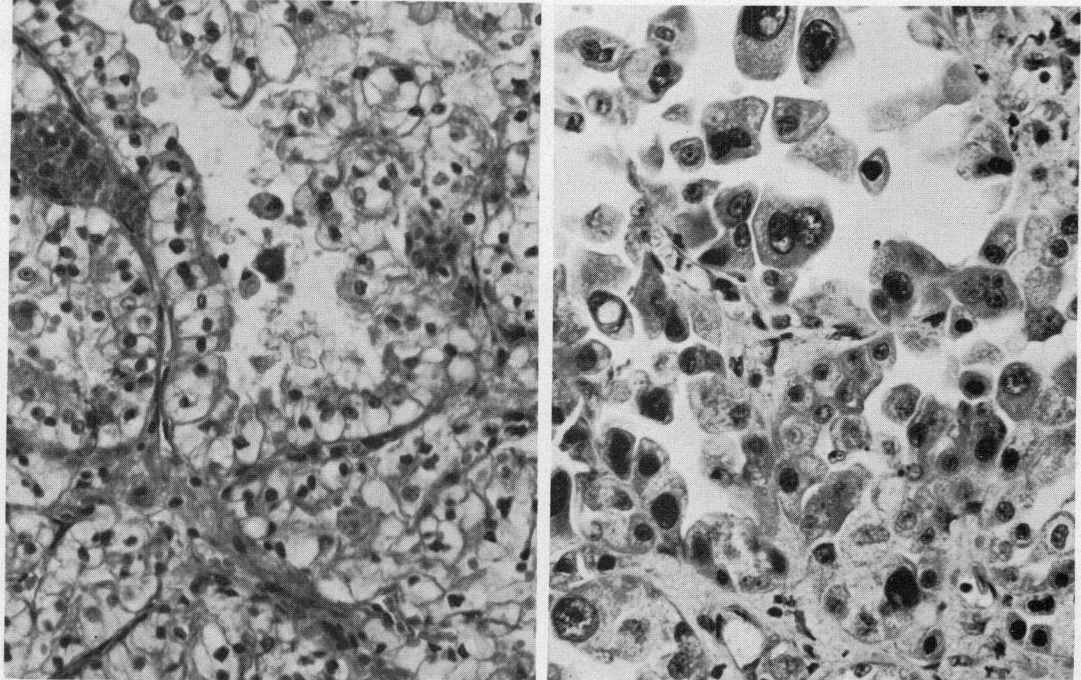

Fig. 21–64 Fig. 21–65

Figure 21–64. Renal cell carcinoma. Pathognomonic clear cell type.
Figure 21–65. Renal cell carcinoma. Solid cell anaplastic variant.

ney. In addition to the fever and constitutional symptoms mentioned earlier, renal cell carcinomas produce a number of manifestations ascribed to hormones and hormone-like substances. These include (1) *polycythemia,* seen in 5 to 10% of patients, due to erythropoietin production by tumor cells; (2) *hypercalcemia,* due to production of parathyroid-like hormone; (3) *hypertension,* caused by renin secretion; (4) *feminization* or *masculinization,* due to elaboration of gonadotropins; (5) *Cushing's syndrome,* caused by secretion of glucocorticosteroids; (6) *eosinophilia* and *leukemoid reactions;* and (7) *amyloidosis.*[184]

One of the common characteristics of this tumor is its *tendency to metastasize widely before giving rise to any local symptoms or signs.* In 25% of new patients with renal cell carcinoma, there is radiologic evidence of metastases when first seen. The histologic pattern of the excised lesion may disclose that it is, in reality, a metastatic site of latent renal carcinoma. The most common locations of metastasis are the lungs (over 50%) and bones (33%), followed in order by the regional lymph nodes, liver and adrenals, and brain. In 10 to 15% of cases, the primary tumor metastasizes across the midline to the opposite kidney. In addition to these favored sites, renal cell carcinoma has been described as having metastasized to virtually every organ and every site in the body, sometimes to such uncommon locations as the eye and vagina.

These tumors manifest some of the most bizarre growth behaviors in the realm of neoplasia. Sudden explosive growth with widespread metastasis is matched by slow, silent, asymptomatic growth for years. In a small number of cases, solitary metastases have occurred so that removal of the metastasis and the primary tumor has produced a cure. In still other instances, the metastases have mysteriously appeared in patients who have had nephrectomies 10 to 20 years before the discovery of the metastatic focus.

It is essential that renal cell carcinomas be diagnosed at the earliest possible stage, which is usually accomplished during the investigation of hematuria in a middle-aged or elderly patient. Renal ultrasonography, nephrotomography, CT scanning, and intravenous pyelography aid in the differential diagnosis of a simple cyst from a tumor. *The most characteristic diagnostic feature of the tumor is its vascular pattern, which can be appreciated by renal arteriography in over 95% of patients.* Urinary cytology may also be helpful in identifying tumor cells.

The average five-year survival of renal cell carcinoma is about 45%, and up to 70% in the absence of distant metastases. With renal vein invasion or extension into the perinephric fat, the figure is reduced to approximately 15 to 20%. Nephrectomy is the treatment of choice.

Wilms' Tumor (Nephroblastoma)

This tumor is one of the more common organ cancers in children under the age of 10. The tumor arises most frequently between the ages of 1 and 4 years, but rare cases have been reported in adults.

Histologically, the tumor consists of different cell types, including epithelium, muscle, bone, and cartilage, all derived from the mesonephric mesoderm. The tumor is characterized by a number of karyotypic[185] and congenital[186] associations, including deletions in the short arms of chromosome 11, and occasionally trisomy, hemihypertrophy, aniridia, and urogenital anomalies.

Grossly, these tumors are generally large, expansile, spherical masses that totally dwarf the kidney. In certain cases, they may grow so large as to produce distention of the abdomen and a readily observable mass on casual inspection. In a child, one is reported to have achieved the weight of 30 lb! They are usually unilateral but, in 5 to 10% of cases, bilateral tumors are encountered. On section, these tumors have a very variegated surface dependent on the tissue types produced. Myxomatous, soft, fish-flesh areas; solid gray, hyaline cartilaginous tissue; and areas of hemorrhagic necrosis are the common components. The aggressive nature of these neoplasms is manifested by their propensity to rupture through the renal capsule and extend locally into the perirenal tissues. Sometimes they invade the mesentery of the bowel. Although they may invade the adrenal, more often they tend to push it ahead of the advancing neoplasm.

Histologically, the characteristic features are primitive or abortive glomeruli with apparent or poorly formed Bowman spaces, and abortive tubules enclosed within a spindle cell stroma (Fig. 21–66). This combination of mesenchymal spindle cells and tubules has led to these tumors being called adenosarcomas and carcinosarcomas. In addition, striated muscle, smooth muscle, collagenous fibrous tissue, cartilage, bone, fat cells, and areas of necrotic tissue containing cholesterol crystals and lipid macrophages may all be seen. The most consistent of these various elements are the striated muscle cells. The ultimate histologic diagnosis rests on identification of the primitive organoid structures of the glomeruli and tubules as well as the strongly supportive evidence of striated muscle fibers. The degree of atypia in the stromal component generally correlates with prognosis.[187]

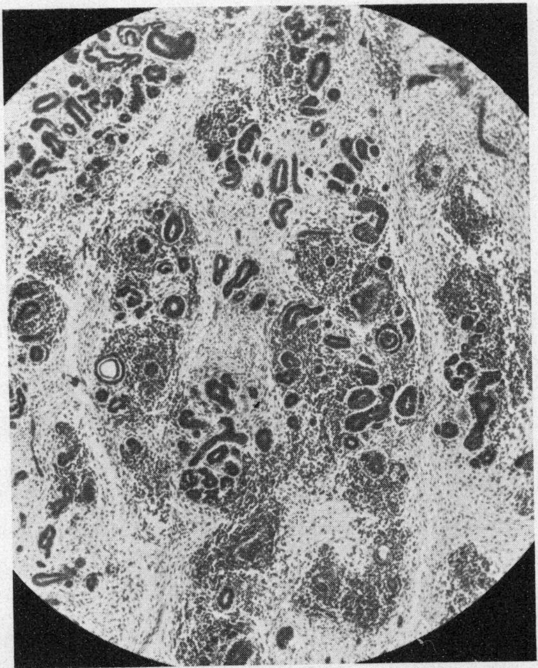

Figure 21–66. Wilms' tumor, illustrating tubule formation and abortive glomeruli in a loose fibrous stroma.

Most children with these neoplasms present with a large abdominal mass that may be unilateral or, when very large, may extend across the midline and down into the pelvis. Hematuria, pain in the abdomen following some hemorrhagic incident, intestinal obstruction, and the appearance of hypertension are other patterns of presentation. In a considerable number of these patients, pulmonary metastases are present at the time of primary diagnosis.

Up to the mid-1960s, the five-year survival of these patients was tragically low (10 to 40%), a tragedy rendered the more poignant because of the age of the patients. However, the combined use of chemotherapy, radiotherapy, and surgery has produced dramatic results in patients whose lesions were previously thought to be inoperable. Most large centers now report up to 90% long-term survivals if the tumors are available for primary treatment with the three modalities mentioned. Even recurrences can be successfully treated.

Urothelial Carcinomas of Renal Pelvis

Approximately 5 to 10% of primary renal tumors occur in the renal pelvis. These tumors span the range from apparently benign papillomas to frank papillary carcinomas but, as with bladder tumors, the benign papillomas are difficult to differentiate from the low-grade papillary cancers (p. 1070).

Renal pelvic tumors usually become clinically apparent within a relatively short time because they lie within the pelvis and, by fragmentation, produce noticeable hematuria. They are almost invariably small when discovered (Fig. 21–67). These tumors are almost never palpable clinically; however, they may block the urinary outflow and lead to palpable hydronephrosis and flank pain. Histologically, pelvic tumors are the exact counterpart of those found in the urinary bladder; for further details, reference should be made to that section (p. 1070).

Occasionally, urothelial tumors may be multiple, involving the pelvis, ureters, and bladder. In 50% of renal pelvic tumors there is a preexisting or concomitant bladder urothelial tumor.[188] Histologically, there are also foci of atypia or carcinoma in situ in grossly normal urothelium remote from the pelvic tumor.[189] All these facts point to a generalized "field" effect, caused by a carcinogenic influence on urothelium (p. 1072). As mentioned earlier, there is a strikingly increased incidence of urothelial carcinomas of the renal pelvis and bladder in patients with analgesic (and Balkan) nephropathy, but the precise carcinogen in these conditions is at present unknown.

Infiltration of the wall of the pelvis and calyces is common, and renal vein involvement likewise occurs. For this reason, despite their apparent small, decep-

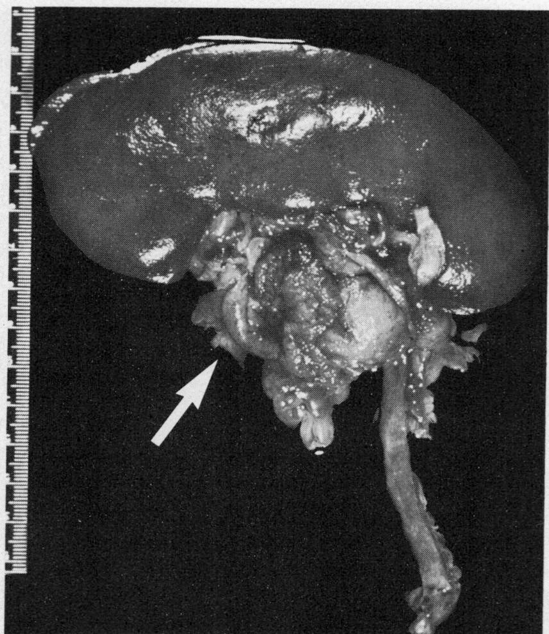

Figure 21–67. Urothelial carcinoma of renal pelvis. Pelvis has been opened to expose nodular irregular neoplasm *(arrow)*.

tively benign appearance, the prognosis for these tumors is not good. Five-year survivals vary from 50 to 70% for low-grade superficial lesions to 10% with high-grade infiltrating tumors.

1. Kissane, J.: Development of the Kidney. *In* Heptinstall, R. H. (ed.): Pathology of the Kidney. Vol. I. Boston, Little, Brown & Co., 1983, pp. 61–82.
2. Karnovsky, M. J.: The ultrastructural basis of glomerular permeability. *In* Churg, J., et al. (eds.): Kidney Disease—Present Status. Baltimore, Williams & Wilkins Co., 1979, pp. 1–41.
3. Martinez-Hernandez, A., and Amenta, P. S.: The basement membrane in pathology. Lab. Invest. *48*:656, 1983.
4. Kanwar, Y. S., and Farquhar, M. G.: Presence of heparan sulfate in the glomerular basement membrane. Proc. Natl. Acad. Sci. U.S.A. *76*:1303, 1979.
5. Deen, W. M., et al.: The glomerular barrier to macromolecules: Theoretical and experimental considerations. *In* Brenner, B. M., and Stein, J. H. (eds.): Nephrotic Syndrome. Contemporary Issues in Nephrology. Vol. 9. New York, Churchill Livingstone, 1982.
6. Farquhar, M. G., et al.: Current knowledge of the functional architecture of the glomerular basement membrane. *In* Kuehn, R., et al. (eds.): New Trends in Basement Membrane Research. New York, Raven Press, 1982, pp. 57–71.
7. Venkatachalam, M. A., and Rennke, H. G.: Structural and molecular basis of glomerular filtration. Circ. Res. *43*:337, 1978.
8. Cotran, R. S., and Rennke, H. G.: Anionic sites and the mechanisms of proteinuria. N. Engl. J. Med. *309*:1050, 1983.

8A. Michael, A. F., et al.: The glomerular mesangium. Kidney Int. *17*:141, 1981.

9. Ausiello, D., et al.: Contraction of cultured rat glomerular cells of apparent mesangial origins after stimulation with angiotensin II and vasopressin. J. Clin. Invest. *65*:754, 1980.
10. Schreiner, G., and Cotran, R. S.: Localization of an Ia-bearing glomerular cell in the mesangium. J. Cell Biol. *94*:483, 1982.
11. Barajas, L.: The juxtaglomerular apparatus: Anatomical considerations of feedback control of GFR. Fed. Proc. *40*:78, 1981.
12. Bohman, S-O.: The ultrastructure of the renal interstitium. *In* Cotran, R. S., et al. (eds.): Tubulo-interstitial Nephropathies. Contemporary Issues in Nephrology. Vol. 10. New York, Churchill Livingstone, 1983, pp. 1–34.
13. Krakaurer, H.: The recent US experience in the treatment of end-stage renal disease by dialysis and transplantation. N. Engl. J. Med. *308*:1558, 1983.
14. Brenner, B. M., and Rector, F. C. (eds.): The Kidney. 2nd ed. Philadelphia, W. B. Saunders Co., 1981.
15. Black, D. A. K. (ed.): Renal Disease. 4th ed. St. Louis, Blackwell, 1980.
16. Earley, L. E., and Gottschalk, C. W. (eds.): Strauss and Welt's Diseases of the Kidney. 3rd ed. Boston, Little, Brown & Co., 1979.
17. Massry, S. G., and Glassock, R. J. (eds.): Textbook of Nephrology. Baltimore, Williams & Wilkins Co., 1983.
18. Massry, S. G., and Kopple, J. D. (eds.): Symposium on uremic toxins. Semin. Nephrol. *3*:1, 1983.
19. Kissane, J. M.: Congenital malformations. *In* Heptinstall, R. H. (ed.): Pathology of the Kidney. Boston, Little, Brown & Co., 1983, pp. 83–140.
20. Bernstein, J.: A classification of renal cysts. *In* Gardner, K. D. (ed.): Cystic Diseases of the Kidney. New York, John Wiley & Sons, 1976, pp. 7–30.
21. Evan, A. P., et al.: Polypoid and papillary epithelial hyperplasia and potential cause of ductal obstruction in adult polycystic kidney disease. Kidney Int. *16*:743, 1979.
22. Kanwar, Y. S., and Carone, F. A.: Reversible tubular cell and basement membrane changes in drug-induced renal cystic disease. Kidney Int., *26*:35, 1984.
23. Gardner, K. D.: Cystic diseases of the kidney. *In* Massry, S. G., and Glassock, R. J. (eds.): Textbook of Nephrology. Baltimore, Williams & Wilkins Co., 1983, pp. 6.160–6.169.
24. Suki, W.: Polycystic kidney disease. Kidney Int. *22*:571, 1982.
25. Bernstein, J., and Gardner, K.: Hereditary tubulo-interstitial nephropathies. Contemp. Issues Nephrol. *10*:335, 1983.
26. Dunnill, M. S., et al.: Acquired cystic disease of the kidneys. A hazard of long-term intermittent hemodialysis. J. Clin. Pathol. *30*:868, 1977.
27. Hughson, M. D., et al.: Atypical cysts, acquired cystic disease and renal cell tumors in end-stage dialysis kidneys. Lab. Invest. *42*:475, 1980.
28. McCluskey, R. T.: Immunologic mechanisms in glomerular disease. *In* Heptinstall, R. H. (ed.): Pathology of the Kidney. Boston, Little, Brown & Co., 1983, pp. 301–387.
29. Neale, T. J., and Wilson, C. B.: Glomerular antigens in glomerulonephritis. Springer Semin. Immunopathol. *5*:221, 1982.
30. Couser, W. G., and Salant, D. J.: Immunopathogenesis of glomerular capillary wall injury in nephrotic states. *In* Brenner, B. M., and Stein, J. H. (eds.): Nephrotic Syndrome. Contemporary Issues in Nephrology. Vol. 9. New York, Churchill Livingstone, 1982, pp. 47–84.
31. Van Damme, B. J. C., et al.: Fixed glomerular antigens in the pathogenesis of immune complex glomerulonephritis. Lab. Invest. *38*:502, 1978.
32. Kerjaschki, D., and Farquhar, M.: Immunocytochemical localization of the Heymann nephritis antigen (GP330) in glomerular epithelial cells of normal Lewis rats. Kidney Int. *23*:184, 1983.
33. Border, W. A., et al.: Induction of membranous nephropathy in rabbits by administration of an exogenous cationic antigen: Demonstration of a pathogenic role for electrical charge. J. Clin. Invest. *69*:41, 1982.
34. Gallo, G. R., et al.: Nephritogenicity and differential distribution of glomerular immune complexes related to immunogen charge. Lab. Invest. *48*:353, 1983.
35. Germuth, F. G., and Rodriguez, E. (eds.): Immunopathology of the Renal Glomerulus. Boston, Little, Brown & Co., 1973.
36. Dixon, F. J., et al.: Experimental glomerulonephritis: The pathogenesis of a laboratory model resembling the spectrum of human glomerulonephritis. J. Exp. Med. *113*:899, 1961.
37. McCluskey, R. T.: Modification of glomerular immune complex deposits. Lab. Invest. *48*:241, 1983.
38. Schreiner, G. F., et al.: Macrophages and cellular immunity in experimental glomerulonephritis. Springer Semin. Immunopathol. *5*:251, 1982.
39. Fillit, H., and Zabriskie, J. B.: Cellular immunity in glomerulonephritis. Am. J. Pathol. *109*:225, 1982.
40. Madaio, M. P., et al.: Comparative study of *in situ* immune deposit formation in active and passive Heymann nephritis. Kidney Int. *23*:498, 1983.
41. Biesecker, G.: Membrane attack complex of complement as a pathologic mediator. Lab. Invest. *49*:237, 1983.
42. Atkins, R. C., et al.: Cellular immune mechanisms in human glomerulonephritis: The role of mononuclear leucocytes. Springer Semin. Immunopathol. *5*:269, 1982.
43. Andrassy, K., et al.: What is the evidence for activated coagulation in glomerulonephritis? Am. J. Nephrol. *2*:293, 1982.
44. Dunn, M. J.: The role of arachidonic acid metabolites in glomerulonephritis. *In* Bertani, T., and Remuzzi, G. (eds.): Glomerular Injury 300 Years After Morgagni. Milan, Wichtig Editors, 1983, pp. 75–88.
45. Camussi, G., et al.: Platelet activating factor–induced loss of glomerular anionic charges. Kidney Int., in press.
46. Vehaskari, V. M., et al.: Glomerular charge and urinary protein excretion: Effects of systemic and intrarenal polycation infusion in the rat. Kidney Int. *22*:127, 1982.

47. Seiler, M. W., et al.: Pathogenesis of polycation-induced alterations of glomerular epithelium. Lab. Invest. *36*:48, 1977.
48. Barnes, J. L.: Size and charge selective permeability defects induced in the glomerular basement membrane. Kidney Int., *25*:11, 1984.
49. Shimamura, T., and Morrison, A. B.: A progressive glomerulosclerosis occurring in partial five-sixths nephrectomized rats. Am. J. Pathol. *79*:95, 1975.
50. Hostetter, T. H., et al.: Hyperfiltration in remnant nephrons. A potentially adverse response to renal ablation. Am. J. Physiol. *10*:F85, 1981.
51. Olson, J. L., et al.: Altered glomerular permeability and progressive sclerosis following ablation of renal mass. Kidney Int. *22*:112, 1982.
52. Brenner, B. M., et al.: Dietary protein intake and the progressive nature of kidney disease. N. Engl. J. Med. *307*:652, 1982.
53. Heptinstall, R. H.: Pathology of the Kidney. 3rd ed. Boston, Little, Brown & Co., 1983.
54. Lange, K., et al.: Evidence for the *in situ* origin of poststreptococcal GN. Glomerular localization of endostreptosin. Clin. Nephrol. *19*:3, 1983.
55. Vogt, A., et al.: Cationic antigens in post-streptococcal glomerulonephritis. Clin. Nephrol. *20*:271, 1983.
56. Jennings, R. B., and Earle, D. P.: Post-streptococcal glomerulonephritis: Histopathologic and clinical studies of the acute, subsiding acute and early chronic latent phases. J. Clin. Invest. *40*:1525, 1961.
57. Baldwin, D. S.: Poststreptococcal glomerulonephritis: A progressive disease? Am. J. Med. *62*:1, 1977.
58. Baldwin, D. S.: Non-immunologic mechanisms of progressive glomerular damage. Kidney Int. *2*:109, 1982.
59. Cohen, A. H., et al.: Crescentic glomerulonephritis: Immune vs. nonimmune mechanisms. Am. J. Nephrol. *1*:78, 1981.
60. Couser, W. G.: Idiopathic rapidly progressive glomerulonephritis. Am. J. Nephrol. *2*:57, 1982.
61. Glassock, R. J.: Clinical aspects of acute, rapidly progressive and chronic glomerulonephritis. *In* Earley, L., and Gottschalk, C. (eds.): Diseases of the Kidney. Boston, Little, Brown & Co., 1979, pp. 691–763.
62. Downie, G. H., et al.: Experimental anti–alveolar basement membrane mediated injury. J. Immunol. *129*:2647, 1982.
63. Briggs, W. A., et al.: Antiglomerular basement membrane antibody-mediated glomerulonephritis and Goodpasture's syndrome. Medicine *58*:348, 1979.
64. Rees, A. J., et al.: Strong association between HLA-DRW2 and antibody-mediated Goodpasture's syndrome. Lancet *1*:996, 1978.
65. Simpson, I. J., et al.: Plasma exchange in Goodpasture's syndrome. Am. J. Nephrol. *2*:301, 1982.
66. Lewis, E. J., and Schwartz, M. M.: Idiopathic crescentic glomerulonephritis. Semin. Nephrol. *2*:193, 1982.
67. Cotran, R. S.: Monocytes, proliferation and glomerulonephritis. J. Lab. Clin. Med. *92*:837, 1978.
68. Brenner, B. M., and Stein, J. H. (eds.): Nephrotic Syndrome. *In* Contemporary Issues in Nephrology. Vol. 9. New York, Churchill Livingstone, 1982.
69. Bernard, D. B.: Metabolic abnormalities in nephrotic syndrome: Pathophysiology and complications. *In* Brenner, B. M., and Stein, J. H. (eds.): Nephrotic Syndrome. Contemporary Issues in Nephrology. Vol. 9. New York, Churchill Livingstone, 1982.
70. Wagoner, R. D., et al.: Renal vein thrombosis in idiopathic membranous glomerulopathy and nephrotic syndrome: Incidence and significance. Kidney Int. *23*:368, 1983.
71. Arnaout, M. A., et al.: Membranous glomerulonephritis. *In* Brenner, B. M., and Stein, J. H. (eds.): Nephrotic Syndrome. Contemporary Issues in Nephrology. Vol. 9. New York, Churchill Livingstone, 1982, pp. 199–236.
72. Noel, L.H., et al.: Long-term prognosis of idiopathic membranous GN. Study of 116 untreated patients. Am. J. Med. *66*:82, 1979.
73. Garovoy, M. R.: Immunogenetic associations in nephrotic states. *In* Brenner, B. M., and Stein, J. H. (eds.): Nephrotic Syndrome. Contemporary Issues in Nephrology. Vol. 9. New York, Churchill Livingstone, 1982, pp. 259–282.
74. Ooi, B. S., et al.: Diminished synthesis of immunoglobulin by peripheral lymphocytes of patients with idiopathic membranous glomerulonephritis. J. Clin. Invest. *65*:789, 1980.
75. Collaborative Study of the Adult Idiopathic Nephrotic Syndrome: A controlled study of short-term prednisone treatment in adults with membranous nephropathy. N. Engl. J. Med. *301*:1301, 1979.
76. Habib, R., and Kleinknecht, C.: The primary nephrotic syndrome of childhood: Classification and clinicopathologic study of 406 cases. Pathol. Annu. *6*:417, 1971.
77. Hoyer, J. R.: Idiopathic nephrotic syndrome with minimal glomerular changes. *In* Brenner, B. M., and Stein, J. H. (eds.): Nephrotic Syndrome. Contemporary Issues in Nephrology. Vol. 9. New York, Churchill Livingstone, 1982, pp. 145–174.
78. Michael, A. F., et al.: Glomerular polyanion: Alteration in aminomononucleoside nephrosis. Lab. Invest. *23*:649, 1970.
79. Coggins, C. L.: Minimal change nephrosis in adults. *In* Proceedings of VIIIth International Congress of Nephrology. Basel, S. Karger, 1981, pp. 336–341.
80. Churg, J., et al.: Pathology of the nephrotic syndrome in children. A report for the international study of kidney disease in children. Lancet *1*:1299, 1970.
81. Tisher, C. C., and Alexander, R. W.: Focal glomerular sclerosis. *In* Brenner, B. M., and Stein, J. H. (eds.): Nephrotic Syndrome. Contemporary Issues in Nephrology. Vol. 9. New York, Churchill Livingstone, 1982, pp. 175–198.
82. Goldzer, R. H., et al.: Focal segmental glomerulosclerosis. Annu. Rev. Med., *35*:429, 1984.
83. Rosen, S., et al.: Progress in human pathology: Glomerular disease. Hum. Pathol. *12*:964, 1981.
84. Cotran, R. S.: Glomerulosclerosis in reflux nephropathy. Kidney Int. *21*:528, 1982.
85. Donadio, J. V., and Holley, K. E.: Membranoproliferative glomerulonephritis. Semin. Nephrol. *2*:204, 1982.
86. Levy, M., et al.: New concepts of membrane-proliferative GN. *In* Kincaid-Smith, P., et al. (eds.): Progress in Glomerulonephritis. New York, John Wiley & Sons, 1979, pp. 177–203.
87. Kim, Y., et al.: Idiopathic membranoproliferative glomerulonephritis. *In* Brenner, B. M., and Stein, J. H. (eds.): Nephrotic Syndrome. Contemporary Issues in Nephrology. Vol. 9. New York, Churchill Livingstone, 1982, pp. 237–258.
88. Schreiber, R. D., and Muller-Eberhard, H. J.: Complement and renal disease. *In* Zabriskie, J. B., et al. (eds.): Clinical Immunology of the Kidney. New York, John Wiley & Sons, 1982, pp. 77–108.
89. Davis, A. E., et al.: Heterogeneity of nephritic factor and its identification as an immunoglobulin. Proc. Natl. Acad. Sci. U.S.A. *74*:3980, 1978.
90. Berger, J.: IgA glomerular deposits in renal disease. Transplant. Proc. *1*:939, 1969.
91. A multicenter study of IgA nephropathy in children. A report of the Southwest Pediatric Nephrology Group. Kidney Int. *22*:643, 1982.
92. Woodroffe, A. J., et al.: Mesangial IgA nephritis. Springer Semin. Immunopathol. *5*:321, 1982.
93. Emancipator, S. N., et al.: Experimental IgA nephropathy induced by oral immunization. J. Exp. Med. *157*:572, 1983.
94. Lawrence, S., et al.: Mesangial IgA nephropathy: Detection of defective reticulophagocytic function *in vivo*. Clin. Nephrol. *19*:280, 1983.
95. Porter, K. A.: Renal transplantation. *In* Heptinstall, R. H. (ed.): Pathology of the Kidney. Boston, Little, Brown & Co., 1983, pp. 1455–1548.
96. Hill, G. S.: Systemic lupus erythematosus and mixed connective tissue disease. *In* Heptinstall, R. H. (ed.): Pathology of the Kidney. Boston, Little, Brown & Co., 1983, pp. 839–906.
97. Levy, M., et al.: Anaphylactoid purpura nephritis in childhood: Natural history and immunopathology. Adv. Nephrol. *6*:183, 1976.
98. McCrary, R. F., et al.: Diabetic nephropathy: Natural course, survivorship and therapy. Am. J. Nephrol. *1*:206, 1981.
99. Bloodworth, J. M. B., Jr., and Greider, M. H.: The endocrine pancreas and diabetes mellitus. *In* Bloodworth, J. M. B. (ed.): Endocrine Pathology. Baltimore, Williams & Wilkins Co., 1982, pp. 556–722.
100. Osterby, R.: Early phases in the development of diabetic glomerulopathy. A quantitative electron microscopic study. Acta Med. Scand. *574*(Suppl.):1, 1975.
101. Mogensen, C. E.: Introduction: Diabetes mellitus and the kidney. Kidney Int. *21*:673, 1982.
102. Kefalides, N. A.: Basement membrane: Structure function relationships. Renal Physiol. *4*:57, 1981.
103. Kanwar, Y. S., et al.: Decreased *de novo* synthesis of glomerular proteoglycans in diabetes: Biochemical and autoradiographic evidence. Proc. Natl. Acad. Sci. U.S.A. *80*:2272, 1983.
104. Winetz, J. A., et al.: Glomerular function in advanced human diabetic nephropathy. Kidney Int. *21*:750, 1982.
105. Rohrbach, D. H., and Martin, G. R.: Structure of basement membrane in normal and diabetic tissue. Ann. N.Y. Acad. Sci. *401*:203, 1982.
106. Hostetter, T. H., et al.: Glomerular hemodynamics in experimental diabetes mellitus. Kidney Int. *19*:41a, 1981.
107. Kreisberg, J. I.: Insulin requirement for contraction of cultured rat glomerular mesangial cells in response to angiotensin II: A possible role for insulin in modulating glomerular hemodynamics. Proc. Natl. Acad. Sci. U.S.A. *79*:4190, 1982.
108. Hill, G. S.: Multiple myeloma, amyloidosis, Waldenström's macroglobulinemia, cryoglobulinemias and benign monoclonal glomerulopathies. *In* Heptinstall, R. H. (ed.): Pathology of the Kidney. Boston, Little, Brown & Co., 1983, pp. 993–1068.
109. Verroust, P., et al.: Renal lesions in dysproteinemias. Springer Semin. Immunopathol. *5*:333, 1982.
110. O'Neill, W. M., et al.: Hereditary nephritis: A re-examination of its clinical and genetic features. Ann. Intern. Med. *88*:176, 1978.
111. Jeraj, K., et al.: Absence of Goodpasture's antigen in male patients with familial nephritis. Am. J. Kidney Dis. *2*:626, 1983.

112. Oliver, J., et al.: The pathogenesis of acute renal failure associated with traumatic and toxic injury, renal ischemia, nephrotoxic damage and the ischemic episode. J. Clin. Invest. *30*:1307, 1951.
113. Solez, K.: The pathology and pathogenesis of acute tubular necrosis in man. *In* Solez, K., and Finckh, E. S. (eds.): Acute Renal Failure—Correlations Between Morphology and Function. New York, Marcel Dekker, 1983.
114. Venkatachalam, M. A.: Pathology of acute renal failure. *In* Brenner, B. M., and Stein, J. H. (eds.): Acute Renal Failure. Contemporary Issues in Nephrology. Vol. 6. New York, Churchill Livingstone, 1980, pp. 79–107.
115. Anderson, R. J., and Schrier, R. W.: Clinical spectrum of oliguric and nonoliguric acute renal failure. *In* Brenner, B. M., and Stein, J. H. (eds.): Acute Renal Failure. Contemporary Issues in Nephrology. Vol. 6. New York, Churchill Livingstone, 1980, pp. 1–16.
116. Oken, D. E.: Theoretical analysis of pathogenetic mechanisms in experimental acute renal failure. Kidney Int. *24*:16, 1983.
117. Cotran, R. S., et al.: Tubulo-interstitial nephropathies. *In* Brenner, B. M., and Rector, F. (eds.): The Kidney. Philadelphia, W. B. Saunders Co., 1984, in press.
118. Tolkoff-Rubin, N. E., and Rubin, R. H.: Urinary tract infection. *In* Cotran, R. S., et al. (eds.): Tubulo-interstitial Nephropathies. Contemporary Issues in Nephrology. Vol. 10. New York, Churchill Livingstone, 1983, pp. 49–82.
119. Stamey, T. A.: Pathogenesis and Treatment of Urinary Tract Infection. Baltimore, Williams & Wilkins Co., 1980.
120. Svanborg, E., et al.: Adhesion of *E. coli* in urinary tract infection. Ciba Found. Symp. *80*:161, 1981.
121. Schaeffer, A. J.: Bladder defense mechanisms against urinary tract infections. Semin. Urol. *1*:106, 1983.
122. Hodson, C. J., and Cotran, R. S.: Vesicoureteral reflux, reflux nephropathy, and chronic pyelonephritis. *In* Cotran, R. S., et al. (eds.): Tubulo-interstitial Nephropathies. Contemporary Issues in Nephrology. Vol. 10. New York, Churchill Livingstone, 1983, pp. 83–120.
123. Hodson, C. J., et al. (eds.): Reflux nephropathy. Update. Contrib. Nephrol. *39*:1, 1984.
124. Hodson, C. J., et al.: The pathogenesis of reflux nephropathy (chronic atrophic pyelonephritis). Br. J. Radiol. *48*:1, 1975.
125. Ransley, P. G., and Risdon, R. A.: The pathogenesis of reflux nephropathy. Br. J. Radiol. *14*(Suppl.):1, 1978.
126. Ransley, P. G., and Risdon, R. A.: The renal papilla, intrarenal reflux, and chronic pyelonephritis. *In* Hodson, C. J., and Kincaid-Smith, P. (eds.): Reflux Nephropathy. New York, Masson Publishing Co., 1979, pp. 126–133.
127. Norden, C. W., and Kass, E. H.: Bacteriuria of pregnancy: A critical appraisal. Annu. Rev. Med. *19*:431, 1968.
128. Kunin, C. M.: Detection, Prevention and Management of Urinary Tract Infections. 3rd ed. Philadelphia, Lea & Febiger, 1979.
129. Goodman, M., et al.: Xanthogranulomatous pyelonephritis (XGP): A local disease with systemic manifestations: Report of 23 patients and review of the literature. Medicine *58*:171, 1979.
130. Kincaid-Smith, P.: Glomerular lesions in atrophic pyelonephritis and reflux nephropathy. Kidney Int. *8*(Suppl.):81, 1975.
131. Appel, G. B., and Kunis, C. L.: Acute tubulo-interstitial nephritis. *In* Cotran, R. S., et al. (eds.): Tubulo-interstitial Nephropathies. Contemporary Issues in Nephrology. Vol. 10. New York, Churchill Livingstone, 1983, pp. 151–186.
132. Magil, A. B.: Drug-induced acute interstitial nephritis with granulomas. Hum. Pathol. *14*:36, 1983.
133. Kincaid-Smith, P.: Analgesic abuse and the kidney. Kidney Int. *17*:250, 1980.
134. Grimlund, K.: Phenacetin and renal damage at a Swedish factory. Acta Med. Scand. 405(Suppl.):*96*:3, 1963.
135. Gonwa, T. A., et al.: Chronic renal failure and end-stage renal disease in northwest North Carolina. Importance of analgesic-associated nephropathy. Arch. Intern. Med. *141*:462, 1981.
136. Dubach, U. C., et al.: Epidemiologic study of abuse of analgesics containing phenacetin: Renal morbidity and mortality (1968–1979). N. Engl. J. Med. *308*:357, 1983.
137. Mihatsch, M. J., et al.: Capillary sclerosis of the urinary tract and analgesic nephropathy. Clin. Nephrol. *20*:285, 1983.
138. Bengtsson, U., et al.: Malignancies of the urinary tract and their relation to analgesic abuse. Kidney Int. *13*:107, 1978.
139. Yu, T. F., and Berger, L. (eds.): The Kidney in Gout and Hyperuricemia. Mount Kisco, Futura Publishing Co., 1982.
140. Wedeen, R. P., and Batuman, V.: Tubulointerstitial nephritis induced by heavy metals and metabolic disturbances. *In* Cotran, R. S., et al. (eds.): Tubulointerstitial Nephropathies. Contemporary Issues in Nephrology. Vol. 10. New York, Churchill Livingstone, 1983, pp. 212–241.
141. Wedeen, R. R.: Lead and the gouty kidney. Am. J. Kidney Dis. *2*:559, 1983.
142. Riemenschneider, T., and Bohle, A.: Morphologic aspects of low-potassium and low-sodium nephropathy. Clin. Nephrol. *19*:271, 1983.
143. Pirani, C. L., et al.: Tubulo-interstitial disease in multiple myeloma and other nonrenal neoplasias. *In* Cotran, R. S., et al. (eds.): Tubulointerstitial Nephropathies. Contemporary Issues in Nephrology. Vol. 10. New York, Churchill Livingstone, 1983, pp. 287–334.
144. Hill, G. S., et al.: Renal lesions in multiple myeloma: Their relationship to associated protein abnormalities. Am. J. Kidney Dis. *2*:423, 1983.
145. Defronzo, R. A., et al.: Acute renal failure in multiple myeloma. Medicine *54*:209, 1975.
146. McCluskey, R. T.: Immunologically mediated tubulo-interstitial nephritis. *In* Cotran, R. S., et al. (eds.): Tubulo-interstitial Nephropathies. Contemporary Issues in Nephrology. Vol. 10. New York, Churchill Livingstone, 1983, pp. 121–150.
147. Brentjens, J. R., et al.: Immunologically-mediated lesions of kidney tubules and interstitium in laboratory animals and in man. Springer Semin. Immunopathol. *5*:357, 1982.
148. Arruda, J. A. L.: Radiation nephritis. *In* Cotran, R. S., et al. (eds.): Tubulo-interstitial Nephropathies. Contemporary Issues in Nephrology. Vol. 10. New York, Churchill Livingstone, 1983, pp. 275–286.
149. Hall, P. W., and Dammin, G. J.: Balkan nephropathy. Nephron *22*:281, 1978.
150. Kaplan, N. M.: Systemic Hypertension: Mechanisms and Diagnosis. *In* Braunwald, E. (ed.): Heart Disease. 2nd ed. Philadelphia, W. B. Saunders, 1984, pp. 849–901.
151. Laragh, J. H., et al. (eds.): Frontiers in Hypertension Research. New York, Springer Verlag, 1981.
152. Genest, J., et al. (eds.): Hypertension. Physiopathology and Treatment. 2nd ed. New York, McGraw-Hill Book Co., 1983.
153. Ferris, T. F.: The kidney and hypertension. Arch. Intern. Med. *142*:1889, 1982.
154. Kaplan, N.: Hypertension and the kidney. Semin. Nephrol. *3*:1, 1983.
155. Del Greco, F., et al.: The renin-angiotensin-aldosterone system in primary and secondary hypertension. Ann. Clin. Lab. Sci. *11*:497, 1981.
156. Hsueh, W. A.: Components of the renin system. An update. Am. J. Nephrol. *3*:109, 1983.
157. Smith, M. C., and Dunn, M. J.: Renal kallikrein, kinins, and prostaglandins in hypertension. *In* Brenner, B. M., and Stein, J. H. (eds.): Hypertension. Contemporary Issues in Nephrology. Vol. 8. New York, Churchill Livingstone, 1981, pp. 168–202.
157A. Dunn, M. J.: Renal prostaglandins. *In* Dunn, M. J. (ed.): Renal Endocrinology. Baltimore, Williams & Wilkins Co., 1983, pp. 1–74.
158. Muirhead, E.: Depressor functions of the kidney. Semin. Nephrol. *3*:14, 1983.
159. Cruz-Coke, R.: Etiology of essential hypertension. Hypertension *3*:191, 1982.
160. Guyton, A. C., et al.: A systems analysis approach to understanding long-range arterial blood pressure control and hypertension. Circ. Res. *35*:159, 1974.
161. Canessa, M., et al.: Na countertransport and cotransport in human red cells: Function, dysfunction, and genes in essential hypertension. Clin. Exp. Hypertens. *3*:783, 1981.
162. Bianchi, G., et al.: Renal dysfunction as a possible cause of essential hypertension in predisposed subjects. Kidney Int. *23*:870, 1983.
163. Kincaid-Smith, P.: Participation of intravascular coagulation in the pathogenesis of glomerular and vascular lesions. Kidney Int. *7*:242, 1975.
164. Gavras, H., and Gavras, I.: The renin-angiotensin system in hypertension. *In* Brenner, B. M., and Stein, J. H. (eds.): Hypertension. Contemporary Issues in Nephrology. Vol. 8. New York, Churchill Livingstone, 1981, pp. 65–99.
165. Dzau, V. J., et al.: Renovascular hypertension: An update on pathophysiology, diagnosis and treatment. Am. J. Nephrol. *3*:172, 1983.
166. McCormack, L. J.: Morphologic abnormalities of renal artery associated with hypertension. *In* Onesti, G., et al. (eds.): Hypertension: Mechanisms and Management. New York, Grune & Stratton, 1973, p. 707.
167. Pirani, C. L.: Coagulation and renal disease. *In* Bertani, T., and Remuzzi, G. (eds.): Glomerular Injury 300 Years After Morgagni. Milan, Wichtig Editors, 1983, pp. 119–138.
168. Lieberman, E.: Hemolytic uremic syndrome. J. Pediatr. *81*:2116, 1972.
169. Finkelstein, F. O., et al.: Clinical spectrum of postpartum renal failure. Am. J. Med. *57*:649, 1974.
170. Defreyn, G., et al.: Abnormal prostacyclin metabolism in the hemolytic uremic syndrome: Equivocal effect of prostacyclin infusions. Clin. Nephrol. *18*:43, 1982.
171. Kassirer, J. P.: Atheroembolic renal disease. N. Engl. J. Med. *280*:812, 1969.
172. Arruda, J. A. L.: Obstructive uropathy. *In* Cotran, R. S., et al. (eds.): Tubulo-interstitial Nephropathies. Contemporary Issues in Nephrology. Vol. 10. New York, Churchill Livingstone, 1983, pp. 243–274.
173. Coe, F., et al. (eds.): Nephrolithiasis. Contemporary Issues in Nephrology. Vol. 5. New York, Churchill Livingstone, 1980.

174. Mostofi, F. K.: Tumors of the kidney. *In* Churg, J., et al. (eds.): Renal Disease—Current Status. Baltimore, Williams & Wilkins Co., 1979, pp. 356–410.
175. Bannayan, G. A., and Lamm, D. C.: Renal cell tumors. Pathol. Annu. *15*:271, 1980.
176. Bennington, J. L., and Beckwith, J. B.: Tumors of the kidney, renal pelvis and ureters. Atlas of Tumor Pathology, Series 2, Fascicle 12. Washington, D.C., AFIP, 1975.
177. Skinner, D. G., and deKernion, J. B. (eds.): Genitourinary Cancer. Philadelphia, W. B. Saunders Co., 1978.
178. Skinner, D. G., and deKernion, J. B. (eds.): Clinical manifestations and treatment of renal parenchymal tumors. *In* Genitourinary Cancer. Philadelphia, W. B. Saunders Co., 1978, pp. 107–133.
179. Stuart, R., et al.: Renomedullary interstitial lesions and hypertension. Hum. Pathol. *7*:327, 1976.
180. Kay, S., et al.: Oncocytic tubular adenoma of the kidney. Prog. Surg. Pathol. *2*:259, 1980.
181. Bennington, J. L.: Cancer of the kidney—etiology, epidemiology and pathology. Cancer *32*:1017, 1973.
182. Recent Advances in Renal Cell Carcinomas. *In* Bollack, C. (ed.): Progress in Surgery. Vol. XVII. New York, S. Karger, 1983.
183. Colvin, R. B., and Dickersin, G. R.: Pathology of renal tumors. *In* Skinner, D. G., and deKernion, J. B. (eds.): Philadelphia, W. B. Saunders Co., 1978, pp. 84–106.
184. Vanatta, P. R., et al.: Renal cell carcinoma and systemic amyloidosis: Demonstration of AA protein and review of the literature. Hum. Pathol. *14*:195, 1983.
185. Yunis, J. J.: The chromosomal basis of human neoplasia. Science *221*:227, 1983.
186. Pendergass, T. W.: Congenital anomalies in children with Wilms' tumor. Cancer *37*:403, 1976.
187. D'Angio, G. J., et al.: Wilms' tumor—an update. Cancer *45*(Suppl.):1791, 1980.
188. McCarron, J. P., et al.: Tumors of the renal pelvis and ureter: Current concepts and management. Semin. Urol. *1*:75, 1983.
189. Nocks, B. N., et al.: Transitional cell carcinoma of the renal pelvis. Urology *19*:472, 1982.

22 THE LOWER URINARY TRACT

Ureters

NORMAL

The ureters arise as budlike outgrowths from the mesonephric or wolffian ducts. These buds elongate to produce the long, definitive tubular structures found in the adult. They grow into the metanephric anlage, which covers them in the form of a cap. Tubular projections from the blind end give rise to the collecting tubules. These eventually anastomose with the distal convoluted tubules of the renal nephron and thus provide drainage for the functioning nephron.

In the normal adult of average size, the ureters are approximately 30 cm in length and about 5 mm in diameter. They lie throughout their course in a retroperitoneal position. As they enter the pelvis, they pass anterior to either the common iliac or external iliac artery. In the female pelvis, they lie close to the uterine arteries and are therefore vulnerable to injury in operations on the female genital tract. There are three points of slight narrowing: at the ureteropelvic junction, where they enter the bladder, and where they cross the iliac vessels, all providing loci where renal calculi may become impacted when they pass from the kidney to the bladder.

On histologic section, ureters are composed of three distinct coats: an outer fibrous investment; a thick muscular coat with the fibers traveling, for the most part, in a circular fashion but with, however, a less well-developed longitudinal layer of muscle; and a lining mucosa of transitional epithelium (urothelium) resembling that found in the renal pelvis and bladder (p. 1065). This epithelium rests on a well-developed basement membrane. Active peristaltic waves propel urine through the ureters into the bladder. As the ureters enter the bladder, they pursue an oblique course, terminating in a slitlike orifice. This orifice is marked by a slight papilliform elevation in the floor of the bladder. The obliquity of this intramural segment of the ureteral orifice permits the enclosing bladder musculature to act as a sphincteric valve, blocking the upward reflux of urine even in the presence of marked distention of the urinary bladder. As discussed earlier, a defect in the intravesical portion of the ureter leads to vesicoureteral reflux (p. 1031).

PATHOLOGY

As a generalization, the processes in which the ureters become involved are most commonly primary in either the kidney or the bladder. Ureteral involvement, then, is usually overshadowed clinically and anatomically by the accompanying underlying disorders. The most important category of lesions to affect them falls under the heading of obstructive disease.

CONGENITAL ANOMALIES

Congenital anomalies of the ureters occur in about 2 or 3% of all autopsies. They are, for the most part, of only incidental interest and have little clinical significance. Rarely, certain anomalies may contribute to obstruction to the flow of urine and thus cause clinical disease. Anomalies of the ureterovesical junction, potentiating reflux, are discussed on p. 1031.

DOUBLE AND BIFID URETERS

Double ureters (derived from a double or split ureteral bud) are almost invariably associated either with totally distinct double renal pelves or with the anomalous development of a very large kidney, having a partially bifid pelvis terminating in separate ureters. Double ureters may pursue separate courses to the bladder, but commonly are joined within the bladder wall and drain through a single ureteral orifice. Separate ureteral orifices into the bladder are extremely unusual. More commonly with a double origin, they unite at some midway point to create a Y-shaped structure. Division of a proximally single ureter in the pelvis into two ureters, forming essentially an inverted Y, is a very infrequent occurrence. These anomalies are consistent with adequate function.

ABERRANT RENAL VESSELS

Occasionally an aberrant vein, but more usually an artery, is found supplying the lower pole of the kidney.

These aberrant vessels are derived from the major renal vessels or even from the aorta. When they cross anterior to the ureter, these vessels may compress the ureter, usually at the ureteropelvic junction, causing narrowing and sometimes obstruction of the ureteropelvic junction. Contrary to previous belief, however, aberrant vessels are uncommon causes of ureteropelvic obstruction. Most frequently the latter is due to a congenital anatomic abnormality of the junction itself, or to acquired periureteral inflammatory fibrous bands.

MISCELLANEOUS CONGENITAL ANOMALIES

Anomalous valves, narrowing or strictures, kinks, and torsions of the ureters usually occur at the level of the ureteropelvic junction. Although infrequent, they may be important as causes of obstruction. *Diverticula*, saccular outpouchings of the ureteral wall, are uncommon lesions. They appear as congenital or acquired defects and are of importance as pockets of stasis and secondary infections. Dilatation, elongation, and tortuosity of the ureters *(hydroureter)* may occur as congenital anomalies or as acquired defects. Congenital hydroureter is thought to reflect some neurogenic defect in the innervation of the ureteral musculature. The acquired form is seen in Chagas' disease, in low ureteral obstruction, or in pregnancy. In the last-named circumstance, pressure of the enlarged uterus and relaxation of the smooth muscle both contribute. Massive enlargement of the ureter is known as *megaloureter* and is probably due to a functional defect of ureteral muscle. These anomalies are sometimes associated with some congenital defect of the kidney. They are more frequently encountered in patients who die early in life from this associated renal disorder, but are sometimes found in adults with polycystic kidney disease. Megaloureter may cause some functional impairment of urinary flow and thus may secondarily lead to dilatation of the renal collecting system.

INFLAMMATION

Ureteritis may develop as one component of urinary tract infections, described on page 1030. The morphologic changes are entirely nonspecific. Only infrequently does such ureteritis make a significant contribution to the clinical problem.

Persistence of infection or repeated acute exacerbations may give rise to chronic inflammatory changes within the ureters.

In the more usual form, the chronic inflammatory changes comprise reddening and granularity of the ureteral mucosa, both of which are more marked than those found in acute inflammation. Superficial ulcerations or areas of sloughing necrosis may be present in the more virulent infections and merit the designation of **ulcerative gangrenous ureteritis.** Noteworthy is the possible causation of gangrenous ureteritis by irradiation of the abdomen and pelvis for the treatment of a malignancy.

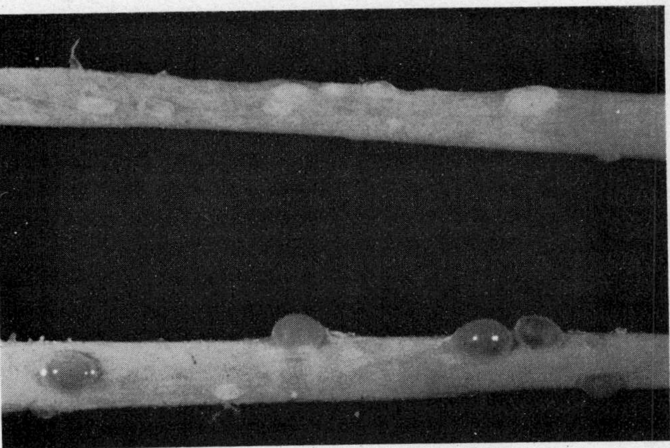

Figure 22–1. Ureteritis cystica.

In certain cases of long-standing chronic ureteritis, specialized reaction patterns are sometimes observed. The accumulation or aggregation of lymphocytes in the subepithelial region may cause slight elevations of the mucosa and produce a fine granular mucosal surface **(ureteritis follicularis).** At other times, the mucosa may become sprinkled with fine cysts varying in diameter from 1 to 5 mm **(ureteritis cystica).** Chronic urinary tract infection is the most common antecedent of this interesting lesion. Nests of epithelium become pinched off and buried in inflammatory reaction. These sequestered epithelial nests give rise to small submucosal cysts. The cysts appear on the surface of the mucosa as small (0.1 to 0.5 cm), clear, thin-walled (hemispheric) vesicles (Fig. 22–1). They may aggregate to form small, grapelike clusters. When they are opened, clear serous or slightly viscid fluid escapes. Histologic sections through such cysts demonstrate a lining of modified transitional epithelium with some flattening of the superficial layer of cells.

TUMORS

Primary neoplasia of the ureter is very rare; the most common forms are malignant. Metastatic seeding from other primary lesions occurs much more often than primary growths.

Small *benign tumors* of the ureter are generally of mesenchymal origin. They include the usual variety of neoplasms derived from fibrous tissue, blood vessels, lymphatics, and smooth muscle. These appear as well-encapsulated, submucosal nodules less than 1 cm in diameter, which are rarely of sufficient size to cause obstruction of the ureteral lumen.

The primary *malignant tumors* of the ureter follow the identical patterns of those arising in the renal pelvis, calyces, and bladder, because all these structures are lined by the same transitional epithelium (urothelium).[1] They are found most frequently during the sixth and seventh decades of life, and are sometimes multiple and occasionally concurrent with similar neoplasms in the bladder or renal pelvis.

OBSTRUCTIVE LESIONS

A great variety of pathologic lesions may obstruct the ureters and give rise to hydroureter, hydronephrosis, and sometimes pyelonephritis. Obviously, it is not the ureteral dilatation that is of significance in these cases, but the consequent involvement of the kidneys.[2] The latter has been detailed on page 1051. Here, some of the causes of ureteral obstruction will be discussed. These may be conveniently separated into intrinsic ureteral disease and extrinsic lesions that compress the ureters.

INTRINSIC OBSTRUCTIVE DISEASES

These will be mentioned in order of clinical importance.

CALCULI. Calculous obstruction of the ureters not only is the most frequent cause of obstruction but, at the same time, is the cause of one of the most intense forms of pain encountered in clinical practice—renal colic. Ureteral calculi almost invariably arise within the kidney and are more fully considered on page 1052. They vary from small, round-to-ovoid formations to irregular crystalline deposits, usually less than 0.5 cm in diameter. Stones larger than this do not enter the ureteropelvic junction, and therefore remain within the pelvis. The usual sites of impaction, as mentioned, are at loci of ureteral narrowing: the ureteropelvic junction; where the ureters enter the bladder; and where they cross the iliac vessels. Intrapelvic calculi are usually quite innocuous, except for the possible production of traumatic injury to the pelvic mucosa.

STRICTURES. Narrowing by strictures may occur from either congenital anomalous development or acquired deformities. Acquired strictures may be caused by operative trauma. Because of the close anatomic relationship of the ureter to the uterine arteries, ureteral damage occasionally occurs in pelvic surgery. Inclusion of the ureter into a surgical ligature or even transection of a ureter is encountered, fortunately rarely. Early recognition of this accident permits reconstructive procedures and restoration of normal urinary flow. Intrinsic inflammation or periureteral inflammatory reactions, occurring, for example, in chronic salpingitis, diverticulitis, sclerosing retroperitonitis, and adhesions following peritonitis, may also lead to narrowing or obstruction. Congenital strictures usually occur at the sites of physiologic narrowing, particularly the ureteropelvic junction and the entrance of the ureter into the urinary bladder. Other common causes of such narrowing are aberrant renal vessels, congenital valves, or stenosis.

TUMORS. Malignant tumors and, quite rarely, benign tumors may give rise to obstruction. The manner in which they produce impairment of urinary flow is twofold: first, by formation of an intraluminal mass, and second, by invasion and thickening of the underlying wall with consequent narrowing of the lumen.

BLOOD CLOT. Hematuria arising in the kidney or in a ureteral lesion may be sufficiently massive to permit the formation of clots, which may lodge and cause obstruction. This magnitude of bleeding is most often associated with calculi, tumors, or papillary necrosis. The hematuria associated with various forms of inflammatory and degenerative disease of the kidneys is usually sufficiently diluted by urine to prevent the formation of clots. Organization of the blood clot at its site of lodgement may anchor the obstruction and produce progressive narrowing of the constriction by the fibroblastic response.

EXTRINSIC OBSTRUCTIVE DISEASES

PREGNANCY. Ureteral dilatation is a frequent accompaniment of pregnancy. It is still not known whether the dilatation results from endocrine causes, physiologic relaxation of smooth muscle, or pressure upon the ureters at the pelvic brim. The greater tendency for the right than for the left ureter to be dilated suggests that the last explanation is more likely, since the uterine fundus twists slightly to the right with increase in size.

TUMORS. Malignant tumors of the rectum, prostate, bladder, and female pelvic organs, particularly endometrial and cervical carcinoma, are major causes of narrowing of the ureters, either by external pressure or by direct invasion of the ureteral wall. This sequence of events constitutes one of the major complications of advanced carcinoma of the cervix. Retroperitoneal sarcomas, including lymphomas, and metastatic involvement of periureteral lymph nodes all behave in a similar fashion.

INFLAMMATION. It has already been indicated that periureteral inflammations may involve the ureters secondarily and, in the course of healing, cause scarring that may give rise to significant narrowing.

SCLEROSING RETROPERITONITIS (RETROPERITONEAL FIBROMATOSIS). This entity of obscure origin is an uncommon cause of ureteral narrowing or obstruction, and comes to medical attention by causing hydronephrosis.

It is characterized by ill-defined fibrous masses that begin over the sacral promontory, encircle the lower abdominal aorta, and extend laterally through the retroperitoneum to enclose and encroach on the ureters. Microscopically, the otherwise banal inflammatory fibrosis is marked by a prominent inflammatory infiltrate of lymphocytes, plasma cells, and eosinophils. Sometimes, foci of fat necrosis, granulomatous inflammation of the walls of veins, and acute or chronic vasculitis are seen in and about the fibrosis.

The etiology of this condition is obscure. In some instances there is an underlying lymphoproliferative malignancy, a traumatic retroperitoneal injury, a visceral or intra-abdominal infection, or a history of intake of the drug methysergide, an ergot derivative used for migraine.[3] However, most cases have no obvious cause. Several cases have been reported with similar fibrotic changes in other sites in the body, such as mediastinal fibrosis, sclerosing cholangitis, and Riedel's (fibrosing) thyroiditis, suggesting that the disorder is systemic in distribution but preferentially involves the retroperitoneum. Thus, a systemic autoimmune reaction, possibly triggered by drugs, has been proposed.[3]

Bladder

NORMAL

Only those anatomic features that have pertinence to pathology will be mentioned here. The bladder exists almost entirely as an extraperitoneal structure situated deeply within the pelvis. It is in contact with the peritoneal cavity only in its most superior anterior aspect, where the peritoneum reflects from the anterior abdominal wall over the dome of the bladder. In the female, this peritonealized area is somewhat smaller than in the male, owing to the posteriorly situated uterus. The close relationship of the female genital tract to the bladder is of considerable significance. It makes possible the spread of disease from one tract to the other. In middle-aged and elderly females, relaxation of pelvic support leads to prolapse (descent) of the uterus, pulling with it the floor of the bladder. In this fashion, the bladder is protruded into the vagina, creating a pouch—*cystocele*—that fails to empty readily with micturition. Frequency, loss of sphincteric control with dribbling, and predisposition to urinary tract infections may follow. In the male, the seminal vesicles and prostate have similar close relationships, being situated just posterior and inferior to the neck of the bladder. Thus, enlargement of the prostate, so common in middle to later life, constitutes an important cause of urinary tract obstruction.

HISTOLOGY OF NORMAL UROTHELIUM.[4] The normal bladder is lined by a uniform transitional epithelium, which rests on a thin basal lamina. In humans the normal urinary mucosa is rarely more than seven to eight cells thick and consists of three zones (Fig. 22–2). The *superficial zone* consists of a single layer of large, flattened cells that cover relatively large areas, giving rise to the term "umbrella" cells. An *intermediate zone* contains four to five layers when the bladder is maximally stretched, and six to eight when it is fully contracted. The *basal zone* consists of a single layer of small cells that are cylindrical in contracted bladders and flattened in distended ones. Thickening (hyperplasia) of this mucosal layer and irregularity of the cell and nuclear size and shape are seen in inflammatory, preneoplastic, and neoplastic states. Indeed, cellular atypia is an almost invariable antecedent to the development of neoplasms. Ultrastructurally, bladder epithelium is characterized by unique scalloped, concave, rigid membrane plaques—the *asymmetric unit membrane* (AUM) plaque—present mostly on the luminal surface of such cells (Fig. 22–3). These plaques form one side of the *fusiform vesicles*, which are intracytoplasmic structures unique to urothelium. Bladder epithelium also contains numerous desmosomes, which increase in number from basal to superficial layers.

Several variants of this normal mucosal pattern may be encountered. Nests of urothelium or inbudding of the surface epithelium may be found occasionally in the mucosal lamina propria; these are sometimes referred to as *Brunn's nests*. Although in the past such changes have been thought to result from chronic inflammatory stimulation of the bladder mucosa, they may merely represent normal variations in morphology. Similarly, small cystic inclusions lined by cuboidal or columnar epithelium are sometimes found in the lamina propria.

PATHOLOGY

Diseases of the bladder, particularly inflammation (cystitis), constitute an important source of clinical signs and symptoms. Usually, however, these disorders are more disabling than lethal. Cystitis is particularly common in young women in the reproductive age and in older age groups of both sexes. Tumors of the bladder are an important source of both morbidity and mortality.

CONGENITAL ANOMALIES

DIVERTICULA

A bladder or vesical diverticulum consists of a pouchlike eversion or evagination of the bladder wall. Diverticula may arise as congenital defects or as acquired lesions from persistent urethral obstruction. The acquired forms are more frequent. Diverticula, of both congenital and acquired origin, are encountered in approximately 5 to 10% of the routine autopsy population of older individuals. They are uncommon in persons under the age of 50 and are more prevalent in males, presumably because of the causal role of enlargement of the prostate.

The *congenital form* may be due to a focal failure of development of the normal musculature or to some urinary tract obstruction during fetal development. Al-

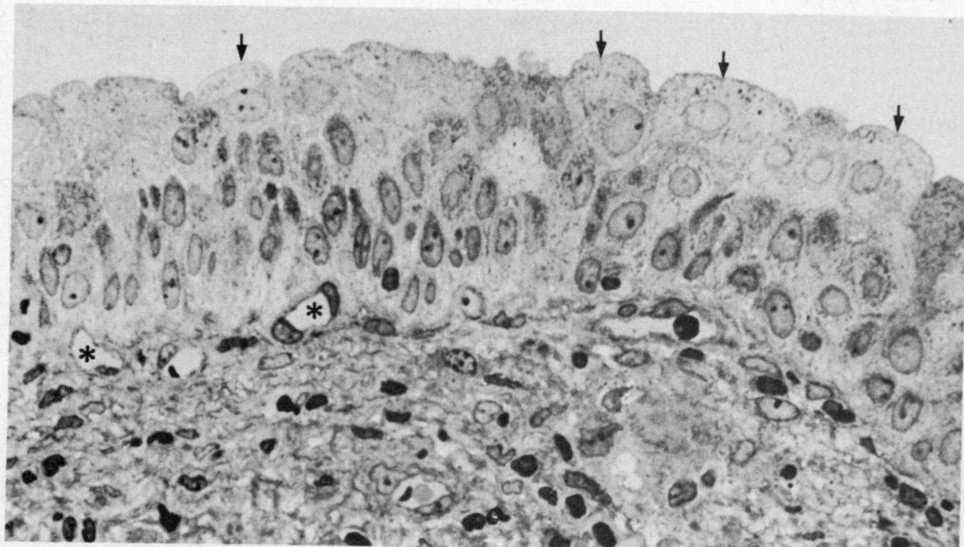

Figure 22–2. Human urinary bladder epithelium consists of superficial, intermediate, and basal zones. The superficial zone contains a single layer of large, so-called "umbrella" cells *(arrows)*. The intermediate zone is several cell layers thick. The basal zone is composed of a single layer of small, cylindrical cells. Submucosal capillaries in the contracted bladder characteristically invaginate into the subepithelial basement membrane *(asterisk)* (×530). (From Pauli, B. U., et al.: The ultrastructure and pathobiology of urinary bladder cancer. *In* Cohen, S., and Bryan, G. T. (eds.): The Pathology of Bladder Cancer. Boca Raton, CRC Press, 1984. Reprinted with permission. Copyright CRC Press, Inc. Courtesy of Dr. J. Alroy, Tufts New England Medical Center, Boston.)

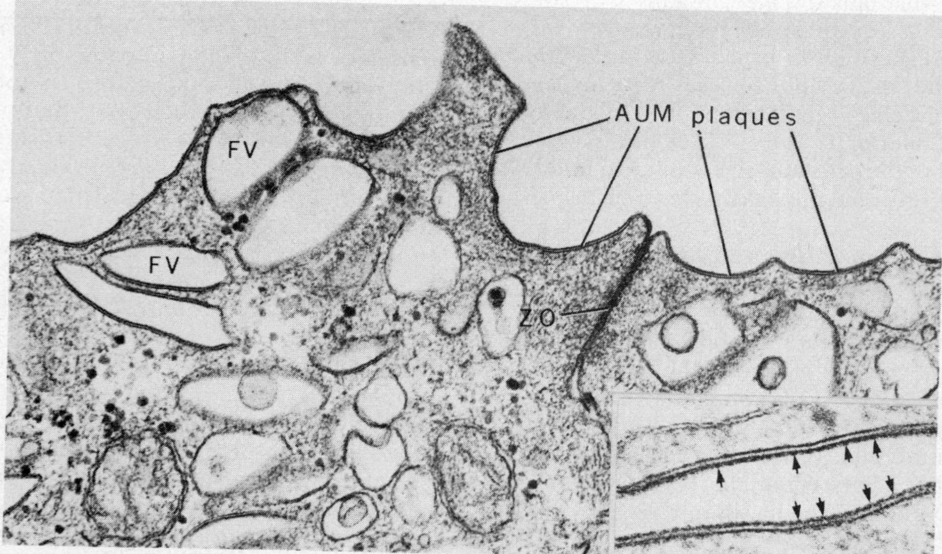

Figure 22–3. Luminal surface of two superficial cells of dog urinary bladder, joined by a zonula occludens intercellular junction (ZO). The luminal membrane has a scalloped appearance due to the presence of rigid, curved, AUM plaques alternating with short segments of symmetric unit membrane, which serve as "hinge" areas. Intracytoplasmic fusiform vesicles (FV) are lined by AUM plaques (×52,000). *Inset:* The thicker leaflets of the AUM plaque of fusiform vesicles face inward, lining the intravesicular space. This leaflet contains particulate membrane components *(arrows)* (×160,000). (From Alroy, J.: Ultrastructure of canine urinary bladder carcinoma. Vet. Pathol. *16*:693, 1979. Reprinted with permission.)

ternatively, diverticula may develop from budlike outgrowths of the fetal bladder. In any event, *some musculature is retained within the wall* of such diverticula, although it may be thinner than normal. These may occur as single defects or, at most, are few in number (Fig. 22–4).

The *acquired variety* implies the presence of a normal bladder at the time of birth, with consequent urethral obstruction causing pouchlike eversions at points of decreased resistance to pressure. The sequence of events can be set forth as follows: (1) urethral obstruction; (2) hypertrophy of the bladder muscle with trabeculation of the wall; (3) formation of small, primitive sacculations (cellules) between the muscle trabeculae; and (4) creation of large, saclike pouches that expand between muscle groups. The diverticula have markedly thinned musculature and, in the more advanced lesions, may have virtually *no intrinsic musculature* but only a mucosa with tunica propria. This form occurs as multiple lesions throughout the bladder (Fig. 22–5). In both forms, the diverticulum usually consists of a round-to-ovoid, saclike pouch that varies from less than 1 cm to 5 to 10 cm in diameter. The mucosal lining may show inflammation as well as glandular or squamous metaplastic changes.

Diverticula are of clinical significance because they constitute sites of urinary stasis that tend to become infected. The thinness of the wall predisposes to bacterial penetration or perforation and the possible development of perivesical infections or spread of infection into the peritoneal cavity. Urinary stasis in these structures also predisposes to the precipitation of calcium salts and the formation of bladder calculi.

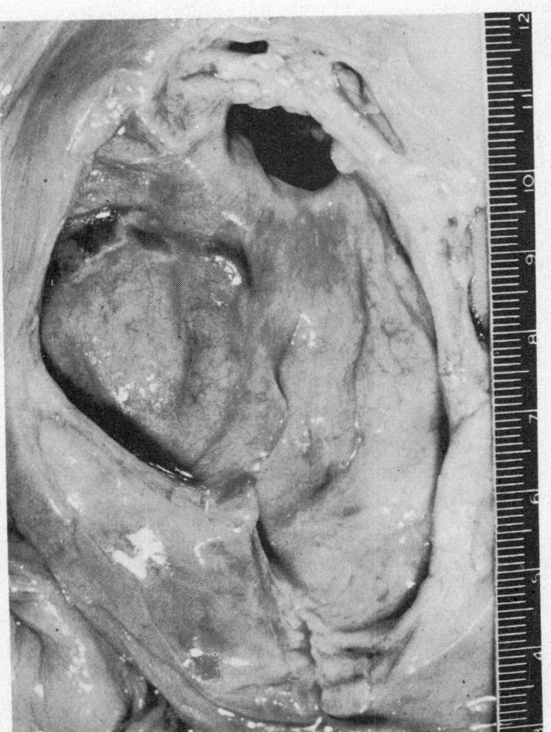

Figure 22–4. Mouth of a bladder diverticulum of congenital origin, situated high in dome of bladder.

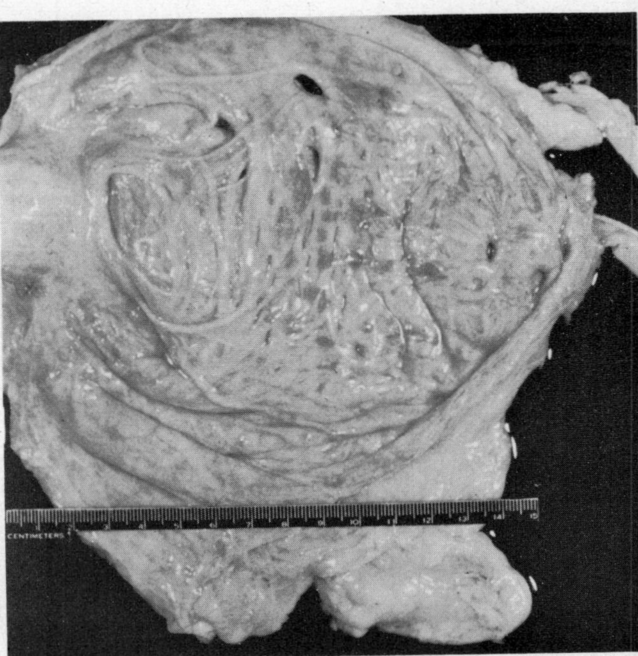

Figure 22–5. Acquired diverticula of bladder. Note bladder distention as indicated by 15-cm rule and trabeculation of wall.

EXSTROPHY OF BLADDER

Exstrophy of the bladder implies the presence of a developmental failure in the anterior wall of the abdomen and the bladder, so that the bladder either communicates directly through a large defect with the surface of the body or lies as an opened sac. It is believed to have its origin in the failure of downgrowth of the mesoderm over the anterior aspect of the bladder. The musculature of the bladder and adjacent abdominal wall never develops, and the bladder ruptures anteriorly to communicate with the skin surface. Exstrophy is associated not only with developmental defects in the musculature of the abdominal wall, but also with defective closure or formation of the symphysis pubis. This anomaly is rare. The exposed bladder mucosa is subject to the development of infections that often spread to upper levels of the urinary system. In the course of persistent chronic infections, the mucosa often becomes converted into an ulcerated surface of granulation tissue, and the preserved marginal epithelium becomes transformed into a stratified squamous type. There is an increased tendency toward the development of carcinoma, mostly adenocarcinoma. Although death from pyelonephritis or urinary failure is common, these lesions are amenable to surgical correction, and long-term survival is possible.

MISCELLANEOUS ANOMALIES

Vesicoureteral reflux is the most common and serious anomaly. As a major contributor to renal infection and scarring it is discussed in detail in Chapter 21.

Absence of the bladder and hypoplasia are very uncommon congenital defects. Occasionally, an incomplete transverse septum may create a so-called "hourglass" deformity. Abnormal connections between the bladder and the vagina, rectum, or uterus may create congenital vesicouterine fistulas.

Rarely, the *urachus* may remain patent in part or in whole. When it is totally patent, a fistulous urinary tract is created that connects the bladder with the umbilicus. At times, the umbilical end or the bladder end remains patent, while the central region is obliterated. A sequestered umbilical epithelial rest or bladder diverticulum is formed that may provide a site for the development of infection. At other times, only the central region of the urachus persists, giving rise to *urachal cysts*, lined by either transitional or metaplastic epithelium. Carcinomas, mostly adenocarcinomas, have been reported to arise in such cysts.

INFLAMMATIONS

ACUTE AND CHRONIC CYSTITIS

The pathogeneses of cystitis and the common bacterial and mycotic etiologic agents were already discussed in some detail in the consideration of urinary tract infections (UTI) on page 1030. As emphasized earlier, bacterial pyelonephritis is frequently preceded by infection of the urinary bladder, with retrograde spread of microorganisms into the kidneys and their collecting systems. The common etiologic agents of cystitis are the coliforms—*E. coli*, followed by Proteus, Klebsiella and Enterobacter. Less common offenders are *Streptococcus faecalis* and staphylococci. Thus, in the great preponderance of cases, the causative agents of cystitis are the patients' own fecal flora. Tuberculous cystitis is almost always a sequel to renal tuberculosis. Rarely, *Candida albicans* (monilia) and, much less often, cryptococcal agents cause cystitis, particularly in patients on long-term antibiotics. More is said about monilial infection on page 352. More rarely seen are trichomonal and schistosomal causations. Within the recent past, it has become apparent that viruses (e.g., adenovirus), chlamydia (p. 292), and mycoplasma may also be causes of cystitis. Patients receiving cytotoxic antitumor drugs and radiation may develop *noninfectious cystitis*.

MORPHOLOGY. The great majority of cases of cystitis take the form of nonspecific acute or chronic inflammation of the bladder.[6]

The first alteration, in the acute stage, is hyperemia of the mucosa. At this stage, the normal velvety character of the mucosa is preserved. In more advanced cases, hyperemia may become transformed to focal or diffuse hemorrhagic discolorations associated with the precipitation of gray-white to yellow suppurative exudate. As the inflammatory reaction progresses in severity, the normal mucosa is replaced by a friable, hemorrhagic, granular surface with many shallow, focal ulcers filled with exudate. When the hemorrhagic component is a dominant feature, it is designated **hemorrhagic cystitis.** This form of cystitis sometimes follows radiation injury or antitumor chemotherapy with cyclophosphamide[7] and is often accompanied by epithelial atypia. Adenovirus infection also causes a hemorrhagic cystitis. The accumulation of large amounts of suppurative exudate may merit the designation of **suppurative cystitis.** Progression of the infection may give rise to sloughing and ulceration of large areas of the mucosa, or sometimes the entire bladder mucosa; this is known as **ulcerative cystitis.** One variant of this condition is ulcerative interstitial cystitis (Hunner's ulcer), described later. In suppurative cystitis, coagulation of the exudate and necrotic mucosa may produce a **membranous cystitis.** This infection may extend into the underlying wall to cause deeply excavated ulcerations and intramural abscesses. Inflammatory edema may cause sufficient ischemia to produce **gangrenous cystitis.** Under these circumstances, the surface mucosa may appear green-black and totally necrotic. In far-advanced cases, when the organisms are particularly virulent, the infection may extend through the bladder to cause perivesical abscesses, perforation, sinus tracts to neighboring structures, and pelvic peritonitis.

Persistence of the infection leads to chronic cystitis, which differs from the acute form only in the character of the inflammatory infiltrate. There is more extreme heaping up of the epithelium with the formation of a red, friable, granular, sometimes ulcerated surface. Chronicity of the infection gives rise to fibrous thickening in the tunica propria and consequent thickening and inelasticity of the bladder wall.

The histologic findings of most of these variants of acute and chronic nonspecific cystitis are exactly those that can be anticipated in any such nonspecific inflammation (Fig. 22–6). Mention might be made of a special form of chronic inflammatory reaction, the aggregation of lymphocytes into lymph follicles within the bladder mucosa and underlying wall, creating a variant of chronic cystitis known as **cystitis follicularis.**

All forms of cystitis are characterized by a triad of symptoms: (1) frequency, which in acute cases may necessitate urination every 15 to 20 minutes; (2) lower abdominal pain localized over the bladder region or in the suprapubic region; and (3) dysuria—pain or burning on urination. Associated with these localized changes, there may be systemic signs of inflammation such as elevation of temperature, chills, and general malaise. In the usual case, the bladder infection does not give rise to such a constitutional reaction.

The local symptoms of cystitis may be disturbing but these infections are more important as antecedents to pyelonephritis. Cystitis is usually a secondary complication of some underlying disorder such as prostatic enlargement, cystocele of the bladder, or kidney infections. These primary diseases must be corrected before the cystitis can be relieved.

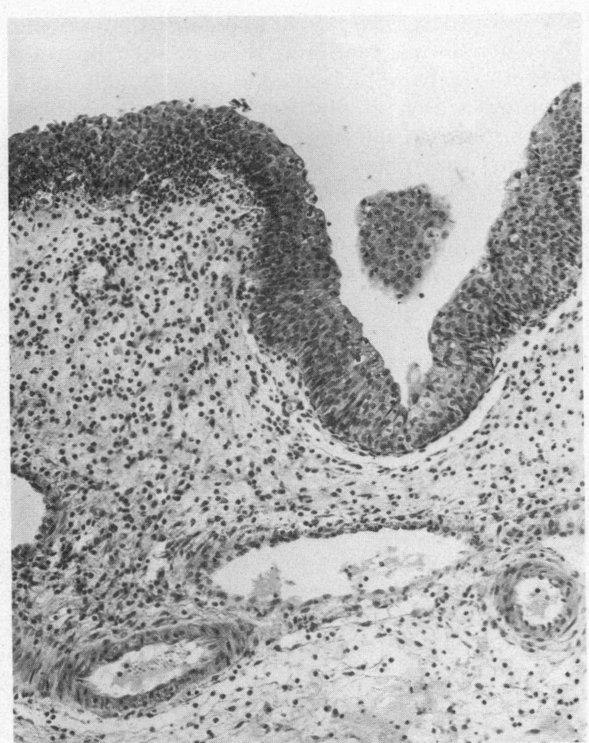

Figure 22–6. Chronic cystitis with a subepithelial mononuclear infiltrate and marked dilatation of blood vesssels.

SPECIAL FORMS OF CYSTITIS

There is a multiplicity of so-called special variants of cystitis that are distinctive by either their morphologic appearance or their causation.

ENCRUSTED CYSTITIS. This term is applied to those instances of nonspecific cystitis characterized by precipitation of urinary salts, particularly phosphates, upon the bladder surface. The crystalline, gray-white, granular precipitate creates a focal or diffuse encrustation of the bladder mucosa. Chronic cystitis with its attendant changes invariably underlies this condition. Usually, urea-splitting bacteria are found in such infections. These produce alkalinity of the bladder urine, and favor precipitation of magnesium or calcium ammonium phosphate stones.

ULCERATIVE INTERSTITIAL CYSTITIS (HUNNER'S ULCER). This is a persistent chronic cystitis occurring most frequently in women and associated with inflammation and fibrosis of all layers of the bladder wall. A localized ulcer is often present. The condition is of unknown etiology, but is often highly incapacitating and difficult to treat.[8]

EMPHYSEMATOUS CYSTITIS. This occurs most frequently in diabetics and is associated with gas bubbles in the submucosal connective tissue. It is presumably caused by gas-forming bacteria. Giant cells often surround the gas bubbles.

MALAKOPLAKIA. This designation refers to a *peculiar pattern of vesical inflammatory reaction characterized macroscopically by soft yellow, slightly raised, mucosal plaques 3 to 4 cm in diameter* (Fig. 22–7).[9] The surrounding mucosa is generally edematous, hyperemic, and inflammatory. Histologically, the plaques are made up of closely packed, large, foamy macrophages with occasional multinucleate giant cells and interspersed lymphocytes. The macrophages have an abundant granular cytoplasm. The granularity is PAS positive and due to phagosomes stuffed with particulate and membranous debris of bacterial origin. In addition, laminated mineralized concretions known as Michaelis-Gutmann (MG) bodies are typically present, both within the macrophages and between cells (Fig. 22–8). Similar lesions have been described in the colon, lungs, bones, kidneys, prostate, and epididymis.

The genesis of the malakoplakic lesion is still uncertain. Current opinion favors the hypothesis that the unusual-appearing macrophages and giant phagosomes result from a localized defect in macrophage function.[10] With a bladder infection, organisms would normally be engulfed and destroyed by phagocytic cells. Postulated is a malfunction of the cytoskeleton of the macrophages, impairing the movement of lysosomes to phagocytic vacuoles, and thus blocking lysosomal enzymic degradation of engulfed bacteria. Thus, the phagosomes become overloaded with bacteria. The MG bodies are thought to result from the deposition of calcium phosphate and other minerals on these overloaded, perhaps disintegrating phagosomes.

CYSTITIS CYSTICA. In long-standing chronic inflammation, nests of transitional bladder mucosa may become buried and give rise to small, cystic, mucosal inclusions. The accompanying gross and microscopic

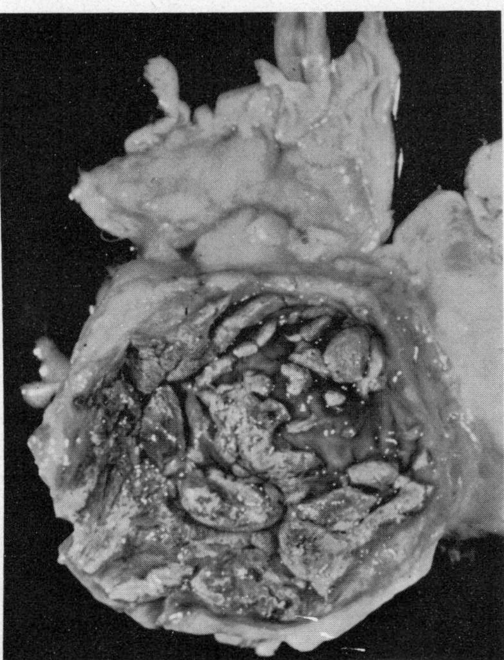

Figure 22–7. Malakoplakia of bladder, showing classic, broad, flat, inflammatory plaques.

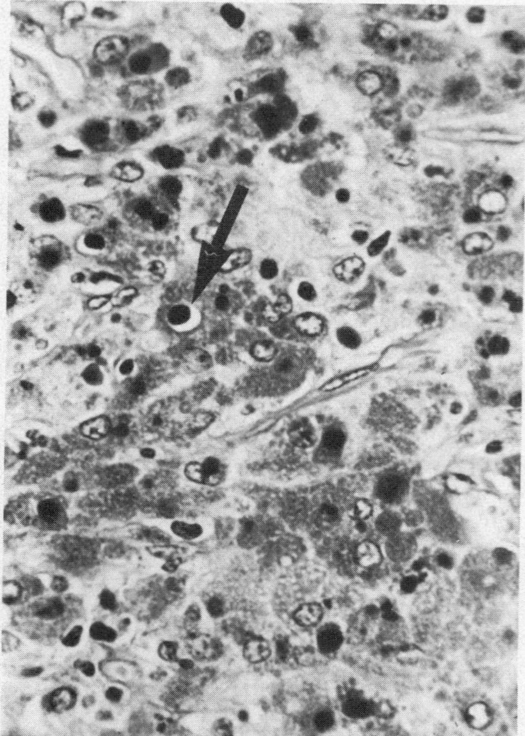

Figure 22–8. Malakoplakia, PAS stain. Note large macrophages with granular cytoplasm and round, dense Michaelis-Gutmann bodies *(arrow)*.

histologic features are identical with those already described in the renal pelvis and ureter. Occasionally, the epithelium is transformed by metaplasia to being mucus-secreting and columnar, producing *cystitis glandularis.* It should be recalled, however, that in the absence of accompanying inflammatory changes, buried nests of transitional cuboidal or columnar epithelia still may be found in the lamina propria as a normal variation.

EOSINOPHILIC CYSTITIS. This rare condition is characterized by a chronic cystitis with abundant eosinophils in the subepithelial connective tissue.[11] The etiology is unknown.

NEOPLASMS

EPITHELIAL TUMORS

Approximately 95% of neoplasms of the bladder are of epithelial (urothelial) origin; the remainder are largely mesenchymal tumors of myoblastic, fibroblastic, or endothelial origin, similar to those arising elsewhere in the body. The epithelial tumors, most of which are malignant, are of interest for many reasons. First, these are rather common tumors: there are some 38,000 new cases of bladder cancer each year in the United States, and 10,000 deaths from the disease. Second, as we shall see, there is now substantial evidence that a long prodrome of widely dispersed mucosal epithelial hyperplasia and progressive atypia antedates the appearance of these neoplasms, rendering them at least theoretically subject to early detection. Third, although many of these tumors are initially of low histologic grade, they are often multiple and recurrent. With each recurrence, the tumors may show greater atypia and worse prognosis. It is therefore difficult to manage these tumors and to predict the outcome. Finally, the bladder is especially vulnerable to environmental carcinogenic influences; the study of chemically induced bladder cancers in humans and experimental animals has greatly advanced our knowledge of the pathobiology of cancer.

Confusion persists with regard to the classification of bladder tumors. There are relatively "pure" forms of transitional cell carcinoma, squamous cell carcinoma, and adenocarcinoma, but occasional neoplasms have both transitional-cell and squamous-cell components, and others are mixtures of transitional cells and glandular patterns. Much more vexing is the segregation of the epithelial neoplasms into categories that express their probable future clinical course. Among the transitional cell neoplasms there are no easy histologic features for the differentiation of benign papillomas from very well-differentiated papillary transitional cell carcinomas. Even if this difficulty is surmounted, there are further problems in the staging of these neoplasms, i.e., in the determination of the presence or absence of invasion of the malignant neoplasms, on which much of their biologic significance rests. Thus, various classifications have been proposed in the attempt to encompass both histologic and staging features.[12–16] Table 22–1 presents a simplified classification consistent with most current views, and Table 22–2 summarizes the histologic differences among transitional cell tumors.

Papilloma

These mucosal neoplasms may arise anywhere within the bladder, most commonly on the lateral walls, with the trigone next in frequency. They are of importance for several reasons. Because they are delicate branching structures, fragmentation of papillomas may lead to painless intermittent or sometimes persistent hematuria. More important is the distinction between those that are truly benign and those that may be cancers. True papillomas, as distinct from Grade I

Table 22–1. CLASSIFICATION OF EPITHELIAL BLADDER TUMORS

Papilloma	
Transitional cell carcinoma	
Grade I	Invasive and noninvasive
Grade II	Invasive and noninvasive
Grade III	Invasive and noninvasive
Squamous cell carcinoma	
Adenocarcinoma	
Mixed carcinoma	
Undifferentiated carcinoma	
Carcinoma in situ	

Table 22–2. MORPHOLOGY OF UROTHELIAL TRANSITIONAL CELL TUMORS

	Hyperplasia (>7 Layers)	Superficial Cell Layer	"Clear" Cytoplasm	Pleomorphism	Nuclear Polarization	Nuclear Crowding	Chromatin	Mitoses
Papilloma	None	Preserved	Present	None	Normal	None	Normal	Rare
TCC-I*	Variable	Variable	Often absent	Variable	Slightly abnormal	Slight	Fine–regular	Uncommon
TCC-II	Variable	Absent	Often absent	Variable	Abnormal	Moderate	Fine–regular	Common
TCC-III	Prominent	Absent	Absent; vacuoles common	Prominent	Absent	Moderate	Coarse–usually irregular	Prominent

*TCC = transitional cell carcinoma—grades I, II, III.
From Murphy, W. M.: Current topics in the pathology of bladder cancer. Pathol. Annu. *18*:1, 1983. Reproduced with permission.

papillary carcinomas, are quite uncommon and represent less than 1% of papillary tumors of the bladder.[15]

Papillomas usually arise singly, but multiple and sequential lesions may occur at varied and random locations. The individual tumor is usually a small (0.5 to 2.0 cm), delicate, soft, branching structure, superficially attached to the mucosa by a short, sometimes elongated, slender stalk. When seen during cystoscopy, the mass virtually floats in the bladder urine and is covered by numerous frondlike delicate papillae. The individual finger-like papillae have a central core of loose fibrovascular tissue covered by layers of normal-appearing transitional cells. (Fig. 22–9). The cells recapitulate the normal architecture of transitional urinary tract epithelium. Sequential lesions are not infrequent. Rarely, the entire bladder mucosa is sprinkled with papillomas (a condition called papillomatosis), or concurrent lesions arise in several levels within the urinary tract.

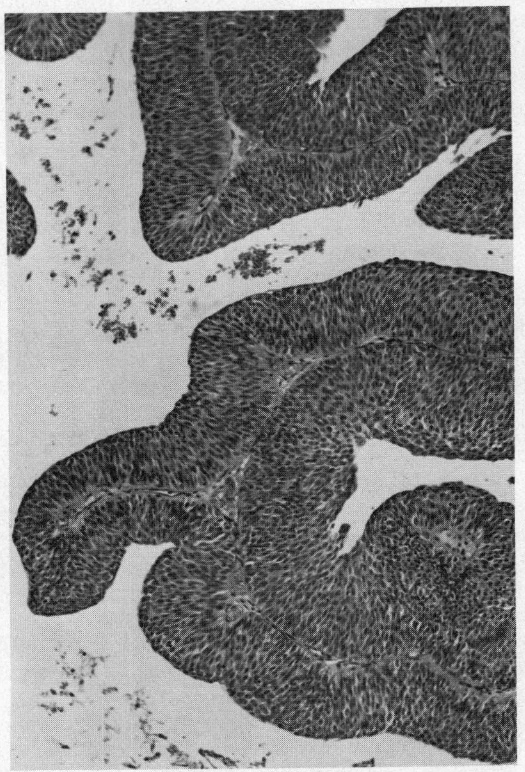

Figure 22–9. Low-power view of typical papillomatous growth of bladder. Note delicate axial stromal framework.

The usual papilloma is readily removed by transurethral resection since it is attached only to the mucosa. The frequency of recurrence is largely a function of the rigor employed in diagnosis of this form of neoplasia. In one series of 26 patients followed for five years, not a single recurrence was observed.[17] However, as pointed out earlier, there are numerous reported instances in which new growths appeared within one year. The regrowth may again be benign, but sometimes it exhibits more marked irregularity of the epithelial cells sufficient to merit the diagnosis of transitional cell carcinoma. Two questions arise: (1) Was the primary diagnosis correct? (2) Are these subsequent lesions true recurrences or de novo lesions arising in a "restless epithelium" prone to the development of multiple neoplasms, with an ever-greater chance of a malignant offspring with each passing year?[18] We have no answer to this vexatious problem, but it suffices that when properly diagnosed, the risk of the later development of another benign papilloma is high. However, the risk of a subsequent cancer is small, although greater than is the case in a patient with no previous history of bladder tumors.

Carcinoma

Bladder cancers account for 3% of cancer deaths in the United States.[19] Although the incidence of these cancers has steadily increased over the past three decades in the U.S., the death rate has remained relatively constant, probably as a result of improved methods of early diagnosis and treatment.

The three basic types are transitional cell carcinoma, squamous cell carcinoma, and adenocarcinoma. As mentioned earlier, however, some are mixed lesions. Because of the difficulties of histologic interpretation of these mixed lesions, it is understandable that analyses of series of cases have yielded varying data on the frequency of the several histologic forms.[15] It suffices for our purpose to note that approximately 90% are basically transitional cell carcinomas, 5% are squamous cell carcinomas, and 5% are mixed; adenocarcinomas are rare. Some reports suggest a higher incidence of squamous carcinomas. First, some comments will be made on the incidence and pathogenesis of all forms of bladder cancer.

INCIDENCE. The incidence of carcinoma of the bladder resembles that of bronchogenic carcinoma, being more common in males than in females, in industrialized nations than in developing nations, and in urban than in rural dwellers. The male:female ratio for transitional cell tumors is approximately 3:1, whereas for squamous cell tumors it approaches 3:2. Carcinoma of the bladder occurs most often in the fifth and sixth decades of life; however, about one-third of neoplasms arise in younger or older patients. These neoplasms occur frequently where bilharzial *(Schistosoma haematobium)* infections of the bladder are common. It has been estimated that 85% of Egyptians become infected with these parasites at some time in their lives. Most affected individuals do not develop vesical neoplasms, but a sufficient number do develop bladder cancer to account for the astounding fact that they are reported to represent 10 to 40% of all malignant tumors in Egypt. Although transitional cell cancers are preponderant in other populations, bilharzic cancers are almost always squamous cell lesions.

PATHOGENESIS. Much evidence suggests that the origins of bladder cancer are related to local influences, e.g., endogenous or exogenous constituents of the urine and/or irritative phenomena within the bladder or bladder wall.[4, 20] A number of chemical agents have been identified in the urine of patients who have developed bladder cancer, some of which have been clearly established as carcinogenic and others strongly suspected. *Occupational exposure to beta-naphthylamine, 4-aminobiphenyl, 4-nitrobiphenyl, and 4,4-diaminobiphenyl has been clearly demonstrated to be carcinogenic.* These compounds are intermediaries in the synthesis of a wide range of azo dyes and pigments used in textile, printing, plastic, rubber, and cable industries. Bladder cancers occur among workers after a mean exposure of approximately 23 years, accounting for up to a 50-fold increased incidence in those exposed. The common denominator among these agents appears to be the excretion and concentration in the urine of orthohydroxylated metabolites complexed to sulfates or glucuronic acid. The pH of urine is closer to optimal for beta-glucuronidase than is the pH of tissue or blood. Thus, the glucuronides are split in the urine, exposing the bladder epithelium to higher levels of the active carcinogens than any other tissue of the body. Herein may lie the explanation of the carcinogenic effect of these chemicals being limited to the bladder. Many other agents have been shown to be carcinogenic in animals, particularly *N*-[4-(5-nitro-2-furyl)-2-thiazolyl] formamide (FANFT), providing useful models for the study of chemically induced bladder neoplasms.

Nonoccupational or environmental exposure to potentially carcinogenic agents may also play a role in the induction of some vesical cancers. Are residents in the vicinity of factories synthesizing or using some of the carcinogenic chemicals exposed to dangerous levels of the carcinogens? Similarly, are users of rubber and plastic goods, cosmetics, or dyed textiles containing impurities of carcinogenic amines at increased risk? Such environmental exposures may explain some of the geographic differences in bladder cancer incidence.

Reference has already been made to the increased incidence of bladder cancer in patients harboring *Schistosoma haematobium* in their bladders. It is not certain whether the parasites elaborate a carcinogenic agent into the urine or instead cause local inflammation, irritation, and subsequent reparative, hyperplastic, and eventually neoplastic changes in the bladder mucosa. In either event, schistosomal cancers have a distribution within the bladder somewhat different from that seen in occupational exposure or spontaneous occurrence, arguing for a local effect.[21] As mentioned, most of these bladder tumors are squamous rather than transitional cell neoplasms.

Abnormal tryptophan metabolism has received intensive study as a factor in the causation of bladder cancer. It must suffice here to note that certain metabolites of tryptophan-kynurenine, and some of its closely related compounds, are excreted in increased amounts in patients with bladder cancer. L-Tryptophan enhances chemically induced carcinogenesis.[22] Tryptophan metabolites induce tumors in mice when incorporated in cholesterol pellets inserted into the bladder. In addition, *cyclophosphamide,* an immunosuppressive agent used in immune diseases, causes hemorrhagic cystitis and atypia in the urothelium, and increases the risk of bladder cancer.[23]

Smoking deserves special mention. Numerous studies point out that the risk of bladder cancer is two to four times greater among male cigarette smokers than among nonsmokers. Several prospective studies have confirmed this association. *Excessive alcohol consumption and artificial sweeteners have* also been implicated as possible contributors to this form of neoplasm, but the evidence is highly controversial. Happily, there is no good evidence implicating coffee, tea, or freshly squeezed orange juice, leaving for the faint of heart at least these pale forms of dissipation.

In conclusion, it is evident that certain occupational and microbiologic hazards are well-established causes of bladder cancer, and there is much suspicion that a number of other influences may also be important.

MORPHOLOGY. Before going into details of the major forms of bladder cancer, it is necessary to clarify the terminology used to describe the patterns of growth employed in the grading and staging of these neoplasms.

The gross appearance of all vesical cancers may be described or categorized as:

1. Papillary—exophytic polypoid lesions attached by a stalk to the mucosa. Penetration of the basement membrane by the neoplastic cells may or may not be present.
2. Noninvasive—thickening of the mucosa by proliferation of cells similar to those seen in carcinoma, but without penetration of the basement membrane.
3. Infiltrating or invasive—penetrating the mucosal basement membrane into the bladder wall, and possibly into contiguous structures.
4. Flat lesions—growing as plaquelike thickenings of the mucosa without the formation of well-defined papillary structures. The neoplasm may be in situ or invasive (more often the latter), and these neoplasms generally tend to be more anaplastic than the papillary lesions.

Grading

Grading of the transitional cell neoplasms (see Table 22–2) is based on the degree of atypia exhibited by the cancer cells. Some observers attempt to grade all three histologic patterns of bladder cancer, but no satisfactory definitions have been developed for squamous cell and adenocarcinomas.

Grade I

The tumor cells display some atypia but are well differentiated and closely resemble normal transitional cells. Mitoses are rare. There is a significant increase in the number of layers of cells, i.e., more than seven layers, but only slight loss of polarity (Fig. 22–10).

Grade II

The tumor cells are still recognizable as of transitional origin. The number of layers of cells is increased (often over ten), as is the number of mitoses, and there is greater loss of polarity. Greater variability in cell size, shape, and chromaticity is present.

Grade III

The tumor cells are barely recognizable as of transitional origin, and all the changes mentioned under Grade II are more aggravated. In particular, there is evident disarray of cells with loosening and fragmentation of the superficial layers of cells (Fig. 22–11).

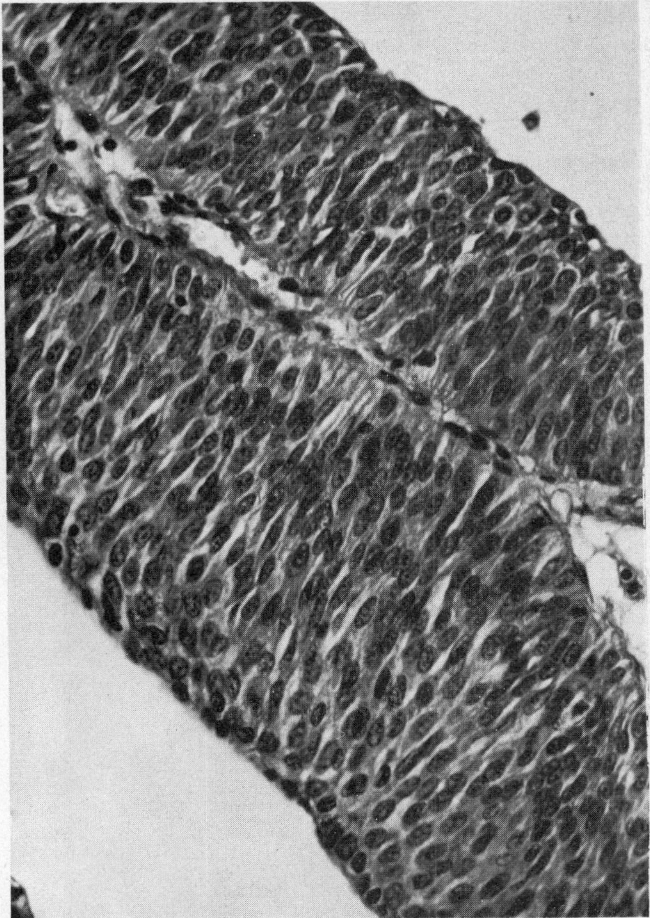

Figure 22–10. Papillary carcinoma of bladder, Grade I. Epithelium is hyperchromatic, slightly disorderly, and in some areas, over 7 cells thick. Compare well-differentiated transitional epithelium with lesion in Figure 22–11.

Staging

The staging of these cancers has become increasingly complex, and several classifications are now in current use.[24–26] The complete details of these staging systems are beyond our present scope, but the TNM classification is presented in somewhat abridged form here.

T = Primary Tumor. The suffix (m) may be added to the appropriate T category to indicate multiple tumors.

T1S: Carcinoma in situ. Definite anaplasia of surface epithelium without infiltration.

TX: The minimal requirements to assess fully the extent of the primary tumor cannot be met.

T0: No evidence of primary tumor.

T1: On bimanual examination a freely mobile mass may be felt (this should not be felt after complete transurethral resection of the lesion) and/or, microscopically, the tumor does not extend beyond the lamina propria.

T2: On bimanual examination, the bladder wall is mobile. There is no residual induration after complete transurethral resection of the lesion and/or there is microscopic invasion of superficial muscle.

T3: On bimanual examination, induration or a nodular mobile mass is palpable in the bladder wall that persists after transurethral resection of the exophytic portion of the lesion and/or there is microscopic invasion of deep muscle or extension through the bladder wall.

T4: Tumor fixed or invading neighboring structures and/or there is microscopic evidence of such involvement.

N = Regional and Juxtaregional Lymph Nodes. The regional lymph nodes are the pelvic nodes below the bifurcation of the common iliac arteries. The juxtaregional lymph nodes are the inguinal nodes and the common iliac and para-aortic nodes.

NX: The minimal requirements to assess the regional lymph nodes cannot be met.

N0: No evidence of involvement of regional lymph nodes.

N1: Involvement of a single homolateral regional lymph node.

N2: Involvement of contralateral or bilateral or multiple regional lymph nodes.

N3: There is a fixed mass on the pelvic wall with a free space between this and the tumor.

N4: Involvement of juxtaregional lymph nodes.

M = Distant Metastases

MX: The minimal requirements to assess the presence of distant metastases cannot be met.

M0: No evidence of distant metastases.

M1: Distant metastases present.

Against this background we can now turn to the individual types of tumors.

Transitional cell carcinomas range from noninvasive to invasive lesions, from flat to papillary, and from well-differentiated (Grade I) to highly anaplastic, aggressive can-

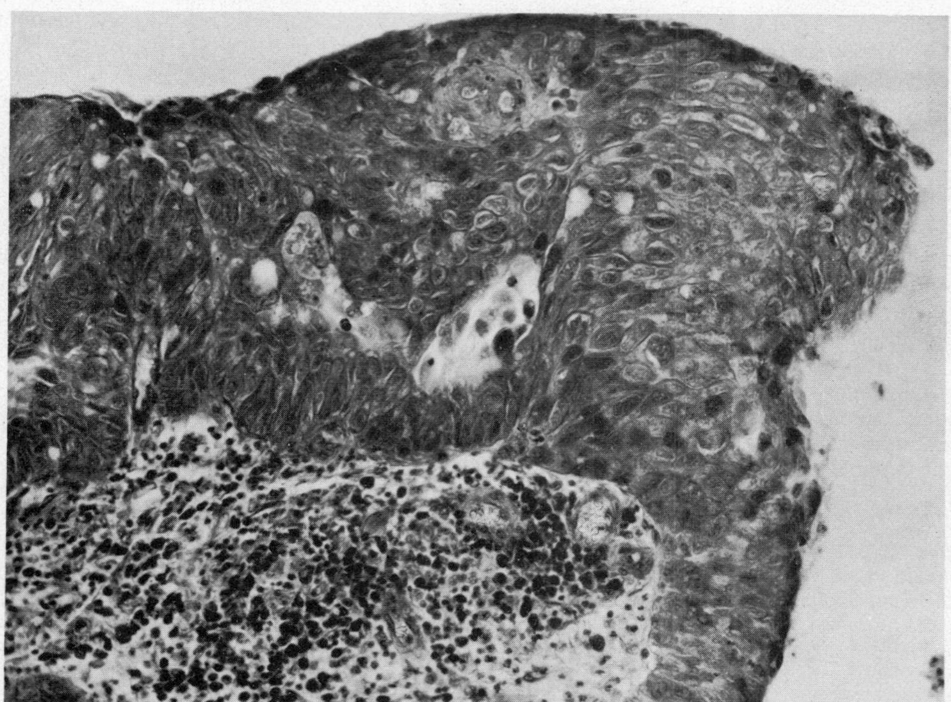

Figure 22–11. Papillary carcinoma of bladder, Grade III, for comparison with Figure 22–10. Note loss of orderly normal transitional growth.

cers (Grade III). Almost 70% are papillary, noninvasive, and of low cytologic grade (I); 25 to 30% are invasive and of variable grades of cytologic atypia.[4, 14, 15]

Papillary neoplasms have a complicated fernlike structure composed of a delicate connective tissue stalk, covered by transitional epithelium that ranges from Grade I (Fig. 22–10) to Grade III (Fig. 22–11). It may be impossible on gross inspection to differentiate these papillary cancers from benign papillomas. Only when the papillary cancer becomes invasive and causes thickening or induration of the underlying bladder wall, or adherence to surrounding structures, can the true malignant nature of the lesion be readily recognized on macroscopic examination. Most of these papillary lesions appear as small, red, elevated excrescences varying in size from less than 1 cm in diameter to large masses up to 5 cm in diameter. Multicentric origins may produce separate tumors (Fig. 22–12). The long, slender fronds often have a velvety consistency and, when viewed within the urinary bladder through the cystoscope, resemble aquatic grasses waving in water currents. Some Grade II and Grade III papillary cancers spread over wide areas of the bladder wall (Fig. 22–13). Fragmentation of the tips of the papillae, ulceration, necrosis, and hemorrhage may complicate the basic macroscopic appearance.

Grade I lesions are almost always papillary. Grade II neoplasms also are most often papillary but may be flat. Both the papillary and flat patterns may be invasive or noninvasive. The Grade III transitional cell carcinomas represent the other end of the spectrum of anaplasia. Some of these lesions retain a papillary configuration, but many are flat or fungating necrotic, sometimes ulcerative, tumors, which have unmistakably invaded deeply (Fig. 22–14). Papillary and flat noninvasive grade III lesions are rarely encountered; with this degree of anaplasia, invasion is the rule. Thus, in one series, 6% of Grade I, but 82% of Grade III tumors, were invasive.[28] However, **carcinoma in situ** (see later), a flat noninvasive transitional Grade III lesion, is often present in areas adjacent to carcinomas.[16] Invasive tumors may extend only into the bladder wall, but the more advanced stages invade the adjacent prostate, seminal vesicles, ureters, and retroperitoneum, and some produce fistulous communications to the vagina or rectum. About 40% of these

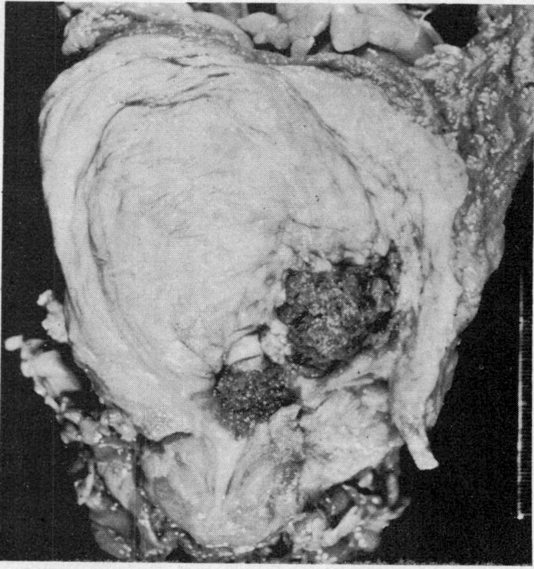

Figure 22–12. Papillary transitional cell carcinoma of bladder. Two discrete lesions in trigonal area.

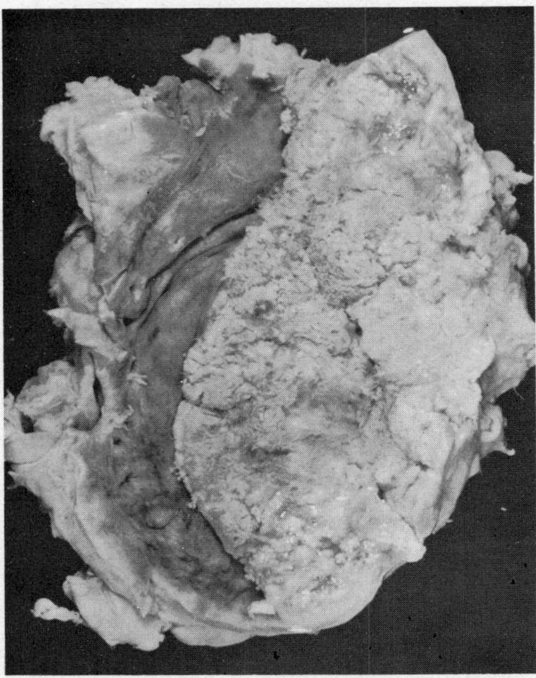

Figure 22–13. Transitional cell carcinoma, Grade II. Entire right side of bladder is overgrown by spreading lesion.

deeply invasive tumors metastasize to regional lymph nodes. Hematogenous dissemination, principally to the liver, lung, and bone marrow, generally occurs late, and only with highly anaplastic tumors.

After the description of the pure transitional cell pattern, it is necessary to emphasize that 50 to 80% of transitional cell neoplasms of Grades II and III develop small focal areas of squamous metaplasia not worthy of being designated "mixed cancers." Metaplastic changes are rarely encountered in the well-differentiated Grade I tumors. The squamous nests are quite well differentiated in most instances

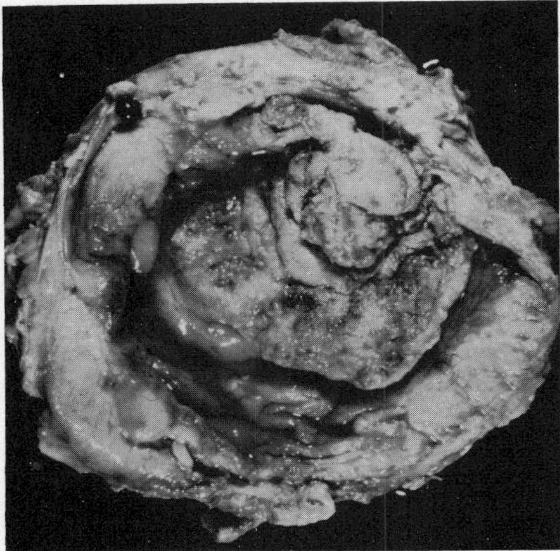

Figure 22–14. Infiltrative transitional carcinoma of bladder, Grade III, seen as a fungating ulcerative mass occupying almost the entire floor.

and do not influence the biology of these neoplasms. When such metaplasia becomes widespread, the neoplasm is termed **mixed**. For unknown reasons, certain transitional cell tumors develop foci of glandular metaplasia rather than squamous metaplasia.

The **squamous cell carcinoma** in pure form accounts for about 5% of all bladder carcinomas. Transitional cell carcinomas with areas of squamous metaplasia are much more frequent. Squamous cell carcinomas may be in situ but much more often are invasive, fungating tumors or infiltrative and ulcerative. True papillary patterns are almost never seen. The level of cytologic differentiation varies widely, from the highly differentiated lesions producing abundant keratohyaline pearls to very anaplastic giant cell tumors showing no evidence of squamous differentiation. Prognosis depends on the grade of anaplasia and the extent of infiltration and spread.

Adenocarcinoma of the bladder is rare. These tumors may arise from urachal remnants, from periurethral and periprostatic glands, from cystitis cystica, or from metaplasia of transitional epithelium. The glandular neoplastic components may secrete mucin, making it impossible to differentiate unmistakably such primary bladder neoplasms from those arising in adjacent structures such as the prostate or seminal vesicles, with secondary extension into the bladder. Rare variants are the highly malignant **signet cell carcinoma** and the relatively nonaggressive **mesonephric or nephrogenic adenoma.**

Carcinoma in situ and Precancerous Lesions

Studies of chemically induced bladder cancer in animals have shown that a series of progressive changes occur in bladder epithelium, culminating in the formation of bladder tumors.[4, 16] These include *hyperplasia*, *dysplasia* (atypical hyperplasia), and *carcinoma in situ*. Similar changes occur in humans,[27–29] usually in association with fully developed tumors, and there is great current interest in detecting such lesions and determining their malignant potential before full-fledged cancer has developed.

Hyperplasia is characterized by a significantly increased number of epithelial cell layers, beyond the seven found in normal bladder. The cells show some de-differentiation, in that they usually resemble the basal cells of epithelium. The change can be focal or multifocal or can involve large areas of the mucosa.

Atypical hyperplasia and dysplasia are associated with significant nuclear atypicalities, which may be mild, moderate, or severe; increased mitotic activity; and evidence of de-differentiation.

Carcinoma in situ is the best studied of these lesions in humans. The lesions are flat and consist of highly anaplastic, overtly malignant cells with numerous mitoses, confined to the mucosa. They are most frequently detected in patients with previous or simultaneous papillary and invasive tumors, being present in from 5% to as many as 90% of such patients (the latter high figure being derived from cystectomy specimens in which the entire mucosa is histologically "mapped"[30]). It is reasonable to assume that all overt cancers must have passed through an in situ phase, but the natural history of in situ lesions is still uncertain.[4, 16, 28–30] Is progression inevitable or may some in situ lesions remain static for decades? In the most thorough studies, about 55% of patients had developed invasive carcinoma within five years. However, some patients were alive and free from tumor for up to 12 years after the initial treatment. Could the treatment have eliminated the lesions? The answer is unknown, but there is fairly general agreement that in situ lesions rarely regress spontaneously.[16, 28] Most workers now believe that these lesions are part and parcel of the generalized influence of a putative carcinogen on urothelium, and further, that these flat lesions are the precursors of *invasive* cancer in patients who also harbor noninvasive transitional cell carcinomas of various grades. Although carcinoma in situ is almost certainly precancerous, the malignant potential of hyperplasia and dysplasia is unknown.

CLINICAL COURSE. All bladder tumors classically produce painless hematuria. This is their dominant and sometimes only clinical manifestation. Occasionally, frequency, urgency, and dysuria accompany the hematuria. When the ureteral orifice is involved, pyelonephritis or hydronephrosis may follow. The use of cytologic examination of urinary sediment for the desquamated tumor cells deserves special mention in regard to the clinical investigation of these patients.[31] Although a negative result does not exclude the presence of a tumor, it has been possible not only to identify anaplastic cells, dictating the need for cystoscopic or radiographic, studies, but also to grade the lesions.

All transitional cell cancers, whatever their grade, have a tendency to recur following excision, and usually the recurrence exhibits greater anaplasia. Overall, 60 to 80% of Grade I papillary carcinomas recur, whereas 80 to 90% of Grade III lesions do so. In many instances, the recurrence is seen at a different site and the question of a new primary tumor must be entertained. Transitional cell tumors seem to be prime examples of neoplasms arising in a "restless epithelium."

The prognosis depends on the histologic pattern of the neoplasm, on the histologic grade, and principally on the clinical stage when first diagnosed. There is a strong correlation between the grade and the stage of the lesion. Thus, most Grade I lesions are T1S, or at most T1, whereas most Grade III tumors are T2 or at a more advanced stage. For the benign papilloma there is good agreement that the five-year survival is over 90%, with a simple local resection or fulguration. Failure to achieve 100% survival relates to either misdiagnosis or recurrence. For the malignant lesions, the five-year survival data not only vary among reports but also are complicated by the choice of treatment—supervoltage irradiation or total cystectomy. Thirty to 80% five-year survival has been achieved for cancers that have not infiltrated more deeply than the superficial layers of the muscular wall of the bladder. With deeper invasion of the bladder wall, but no extension into surrounding structures, the five-year survival is only 10 to 30%. In general, the transitional cell cancers have a better prognosis than the squamous cell neoplasms. For the latter, approximtely 70% of patients are dead within one year. In all forms of bladder cancer, death is usually caused by either progressive infiltration of the ureters leading to bacterial and obstructive renal disease, or dissemination of the cancer.

The difficulty of predicting aggressive clinical behavior in tumors of seemingly similar histologic grades has led to a search for modern cytologic, biochemical, and ultrastructural markers for aggressive tumors.[4, 28] Tumors that are more likely to behave as malignant tumors (recur, invade, metastasize) have been shown to (1) lack blood group antigens on their cell surfaces,[4] (2) induce angiogenesis, (3) exhibit alterations in junctional complexes on electron microscopic examination, and (4) manifest highly abnormal karyotypes. The latter can be detected by automated flow cytometry of cells in bladder washings, providing a highly promising technique for the evaluation and follow-up of bladder tumors.[32, 33]

MESENCHYMAL TUMORS

BENIGN. A great variety of benign mesodermal tumors may arise in the bladder, including leiomyomas, rhabdomyomas, fibromyxomas, neurofibromas, xanthomas, hemangiomas, granular cell myoblastomas, lipomas, and osteomas. Individually and, indeed, collectively, they are rare. The most common is *leiomyoma.* They all tend to grow as isolated, intramural, encapsulated, oval-to-spherical masses, varying in diameter up to several centimeters. Occasionally, they assume submucosal pedunculated positions. They have the histologic features of their counterparts elsewhere. As a group they are somewhat more common in adults, but certain lesions such as the myxomas and angiomas tend to occur more frequently in children.

SARCOMAS. Sarcomatous growths may also involve the bladder. As a group, they tend to produce large masses (varying up to 10 to 15 cm in diameter) that protrude into the vesical lumen. Their soft, fleshy, gray-white gross appearance suggests their sarcomatous nature.

One form, rhabdomyosarcoma, which deserves special mention, takes one of two forms. The "adult" form occurs mostly in adults over 40 years of age and shows a range of histology similar to rhabdomyosarcomas of striated muscle (p. 1314). The other variant is the embryonal rhabdomyosarcoma, encountered chiefly in infancy or childhood. This type of neoplasm tends to grow in large, polypoid projections into the bladder lumen, producing grapelike clusters of soft, fleshy tissue. These malignancies, called *sarcoma botryoides*, are similar to those that occur in the female genital tract (p. 1121).

SECONDARY TUMORS

Secondary malignant involvement of the bladder may reach it by one of three pathways: (1) by direct extension from primary lesions in nearby organs; (2) by implantation from primary lesions within the upper urinary tract; or (3) by spread through lymphatics and blood from such primaries as the stomach, lungs, and breast and elsewhere. Direct extension is the most common form of secondary involvement, from carcinomas of the cervix, uterus, prostate, and rectum, in the order given. Since some of these carcinomas are squamous cell lesions of the cervix, they may, on casual inspection of the bladder, appear as primary squamous cell carcinomas of this organ. Hemorrhage, ureteral obstruction, and vesicovaginal fistulas are the common sequelae.

Endometrial carcinomas less commonly affect the bladder, but may produce essentially the same sequence of events. In the male, far-advanced prostatic carcinoma may extend into the bladder wall, but more usually affects the seminal vesicles and the perivesical connective tissue.

MECHANICAL LESIONS

OBSTRUCTION. Obstruction to the bladder neck is of major clinical importance, not only for the changes induced in the bladder, but also because of its eventual effect on the kidney. A great variety of intrinsic and extrinsic diseases of the bladder may narrow the urethral orifice and cause partial or complete vesical obstruction. In the male, the most important lesion is enlargement of the prostate gland due either to nodular hyperplasia or to carcinoma (Fig. 22–15). Vesical obstruction is somewhat less common in the female and is most often caused by cystocele of the bladder. The more infrequent causes can be listed as (1) congenital narrowings or strictures of the urethra; (2) inflammatory strictures of the urethra; (3) inflammatory fibrosis and contraction of the bladder following varying types of cystitis; (4) bladder tumors—either benign or malignant—when strategically located; (5) secondary invasion of the bladder neck by growths arising in perivesical structures, such as the cervix, vagina, prostate, and rectum; (6) mechanical obstructions caused by foreign bodies and calculi; and (7) injury to the innervation of the bladder causing cord bladder.

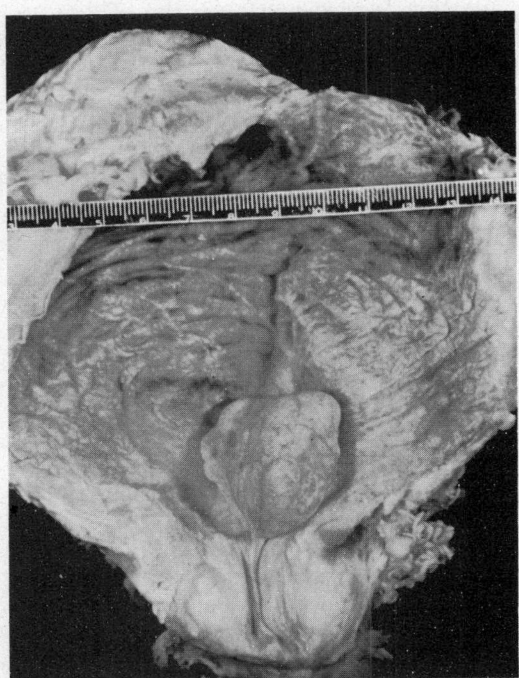

Figure 22–15. Hypertrophy and trabeculation of bladder wall secondary to polypoid hyperplasia of prostate.

In the early stages, there is only some thickening of the bladder wall, presumably due to hypertrophy of the smooth muscle. The mucosal surface at this time may be entirely normal. With progressive hypertrophy of the muscular coat, the individual muscle bundles greatly enlarge and produce trabeculation of the bladder wall. These submucosal, cordlike thickenings run in all directions and produce a crisscross pattern of mucosal ridging. Persistent obstruction leads to more marked trabeculation, and the prominent ridging produces cryptlike depressions between the interlacing bands that resemble small diverticula. In the course of time, these crypts may become converted into true acquired diverticula. The hypertrophy of smooth muscle is difficult to evaluate histologically and can only be surmised by an increase in the total thickness of the muscular layer of the bladder wall.

In some cases of acute obstruction or in terminal disease when the patient's normal reflex mechanisms are depressed, the bladder may become extremely dilated. The enlarged bladder may reach the brim of the pelvis or even the level of the umbilicus. In these cases, the bladder wall is markedly thinned and the trabeculation becomes totally inapparent.

MISCELLANEOUS LESIONS

CALCULI. Bladder calculi may either be of primary origin within the bladder or pass into the bladder from a renal or ureteral focus of origin. Most occur in adults over the age of 40, although younger persons may also be affected. The pathogenesis and chemical composition of these calculi are identical to those involved in the formation of renal calculi, discussed on p. 1052 (Fig. 22–16).

Vesical calculi usually merely reside within the capacious bladder lumen and remain entirely asymptomatic, since they are generally too large to enter the urethral orifice. They may cause symptoms by producing chronic irritation and inflammation of the bladder wall, or by becoming lodged in the neck of the bladder and producing urinary tract obstruction. Under these circumstances, frequency and urgency may be evoked by the partial obstruction, and dysuria, pyuria, and hematuria may be caused by the inflammatory changes in the mucosa. The diagnosis can only be suspected clinically and must be confirmed by cystoscopic or radiographic examination.

NEUROGENIC OR CORD BLADDER. A cord bladder may be defined as one in which normal vesical function

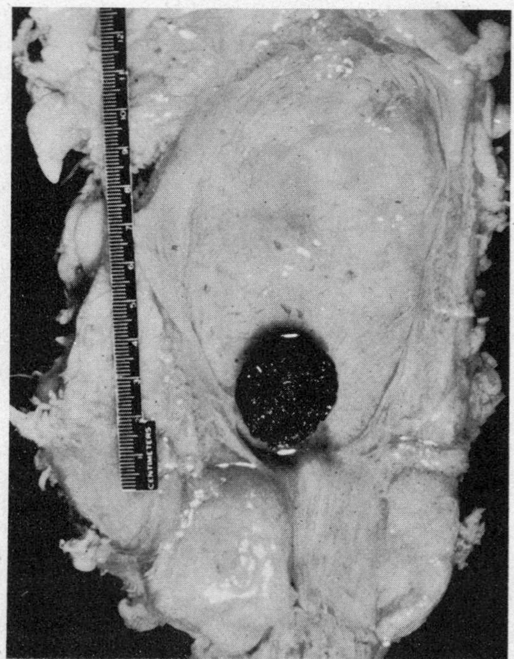

Figure 22–16. A relatively large solitary bladder calculus.

is disturbed by interruption of the neural pathways of the bladder. Depending on the level of cord injury, various types result. The understanding of this impaired function requires a knowledge of the normal neural connections that control bladder function. Two totally separate sets of pathways exist. *Voluntary micturition is under the control of the brain,* acting by way of somatic nerves that control the internal sphincter of the bladder. In addition to this volitional mechanism, there is an *automatic conditioned emptying reflex, actuated by autonomic nerve impulses that pass through a spinal reflex arc.* When the *connections with the brain* are severed, volitional control of the bladder function is lost, and totally automatic function ensues. Consequently, any form of injury to the spinal cord *above* the level of the spinal reflex arc causes an automatic cord bladder. Trauma, tumors, inflammations, and central nervous system degenerations may all cause such interruption of the pathways between the brain and the bladder. *Lower cord injuries to the corda equina and sacral plexus may destroy the automatic mechanism* so that reflex activity is abolished and *evacuation of the bladder occurs only by overflow (automatic neurogenic bladder).* Peripheral nerve lesions may also sever these pathways and produce total interruption of nervous control of vesical function. Depending on the level of the nerve lesion, the bladder may be either atonic or hypertonic, and consequently may show either contraction and thickening of the wall or marked dilatation and thinning of the wall.

Neurogenic dysfunction is an important disorder because of the vulnerability of such bladders to infection. Urinary stasis and the necessity for catheterization provide the appropriate circumstances for the introduction of bacterial contamination. Only meticulous attention to asepsis, irrigation of the bladder, and appropriate techniques of catheterization can stave off these complications.

FISTULAS. Abnormal fistulous tracts may occur between the bladder and the vagina, uterus, rectum, small intestines, or skin. The most common form is the *vesicovaginal fistula,* in which a communication between the bladder and vagina develops secondary to a carcinoma of the cervix or its irradiation. Less commonly, connections may exist to the uterus, known as *vesicouterine fistulas.* Neoplastic disease and postirradiation necrosis are the common antecedents. In both instances, the major presenting clinical finding is the escape of urine from the vaginal orifice. Abnormal communication may occur between the bladder and the rectum *(vesicorectal fistula)* and between the bladder and loops of small intestine *(vesicoenteric fistula).* These are most commonly caused by infections, tumors, and irradiation necrosis. It is obvious that infection immediately complicates the presence of such fistulous tracts, and severe acute and chronic cystitis invariably results. Gross intestinal and fecal contamination may cause the accumulation of foreign material within the bladder and may give rise to urethral obstruction. The most striking clinical finding is the passage of turbid urine, containing recognizable fecal contents.

Urethra

INFLAMMATIONS

Urethritis is classically divided into gonococcal and nongonococcal urethritis. As noted earlier, gonococcal urethritis is one of the earliest manifestations of this venereal infection. Nongonococcal urethritis is very common, and can be caused by a variety of bacteria, among which *E. coli* and other enteric organisms predominate. In females urethritis is often accompanied by cystitis and in males by prostatitis. In many instances bacteria cannot be isolated. Various strains of chlamydia (e.g. *C. trachomatis*) are the cause of 25 to 60% of

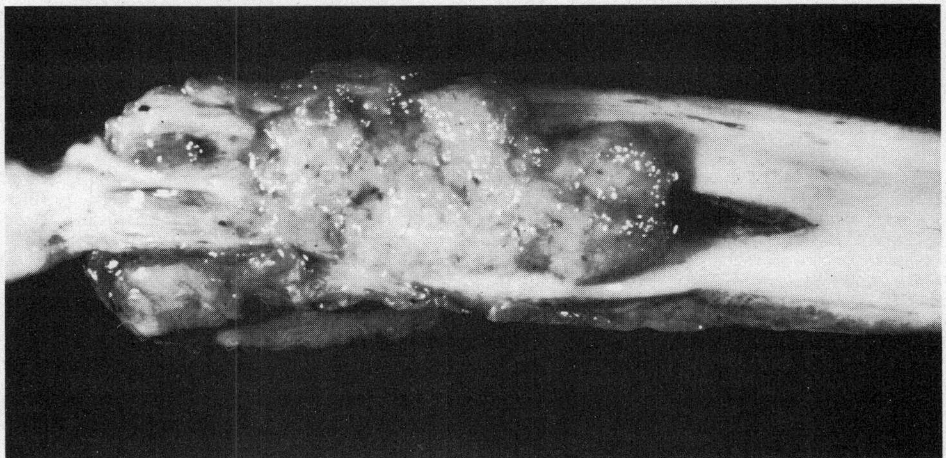

Figure 22–17. Carcinoma of urethra with typical fungating growth.

nongonococcal urethritis in males[34] and about 20% in females.[35] Mycoplasma (*Ureaplasma urealyticum*) also accounts for the symptoms of urethritis in many cases.[36] Urethritis is also one component of *Reiter's syndrome*, which comprises the clinical triad of arthritis, conjunctivitis, and urethritis.

The morphologic changes are entirely typical of inflammation in other sites within the urinary tract. The urethral involvement is not itself a serious clinical problem, but may cause considerable local pain, itching, and frequency, and may represent a forerunner of more serious disease in higher levels of the urogenital tract.

TUMORS

CARUNCLE

Urethral caruncle is the designation applied to small, red, painful masses that occur about the external urethral meatus in the female. They may be found at any age but are more common in later life. The lesion usually consists of a hemispherical, friable, 1- to 2-cm nodule that usually occurs singly, either just outside or just within the external urethral meatus. It may be covered by an intact mucosa, but is extremely friable, and the slightest trauma may cause ulceration of the surface and bleeding. Histologically, it is composed of a *highly vascularized, young, fibroblastic connective tissue, more or less heavily infiltrated with leukocytes.* The overlying epithelium, where present, is either transitional or squamous cell in type. When there is no ulceration, the white cell infiltration is considerably less prominent. The question of whether the urethral caruncle represents merely a mass of inflammatory granulation tissue or a capillary hemangioma has been disputed for years. The consistent failure of this lesion ever to grow beyond 1 to 2 cm in size argues strongly against a neoplastic origin. Surgical excision affords prompt relief and complete cure.

PAPILLOMA

Papillomas of the urethra occur usually just within or on the external meatus. In this location, they also fall within the scope of condylomas of the external genitalia, and are discussed in that section (p. 1082).

CARCINOMA

Carcinoma of the urethra is an uncommon lesion. It tends to occur in advanced age and, in most instances, begins about the external meatus or on the immediately surrounding structures, such as the glans penis, or the introitus in the female. Some apparently begin just inside the external meatus or even at a higher level within the urethra. Those that occur at and protrude from the external meatus appear as warty, papillary growths that at first resemble the sessile papillary carcinomas described in the bladder. As they progress, they tend to become ulcerated on their surfaces and to assume the characteristics of a fungating, ulcerating lesion (Fig. 22–17).

Most of these malignancies are squamous cell carcinomas. The papillary lesions that protrude from the external meatus are apt to show a transitional cell growth that further heightens their similarity to bladder carcinoma. Uncommonly, an adenocarcinomatous growth pattern is found.

1. McCarron, J. P., and Vaughn, E. D.: Tumors of the renal pelvis and ureter: Current concepts and management. Semin. Urol. *1*:75, 1983.
2. Arruda, J.: Obstructive uropathy. *In* Cotran, R. S., et al. (eds.): Contemporary Issues in Nephrology. Vol. 10. Tubulointerstitial Nephropathies. New York, Churchill Livingstone, 1983, pp. 243–273.
3. Mitchinson, M. J.: The pathology of idiopathic retroperitoneal fibrosis. J. Clin. Pathol. *23*:681, 1970.

3A. Lepor, H., and Walsh, P. C.: Idiopathic retroperitoneal fibrosis. J. Urol. *122*:1, 1979.

4. Pauli, B. U.: The ultrastructure and pathobiology of urinary bladder cancer. *In* Cohen, S., and Bryan, G. T. (eds.): The Pathology of Bladder Cancer. Boca Raton, CRC Press, 1984.

5. Engel, R. M., and Wilkinson, H. A.: Bladder extrophy. J. Urol. *104*:699, 1970.
6. Friedell, G. H., et al.: The renal pelvis, ureter, urinary bladder and urethra. *In* Silverberg, S. G. (ed.): Principles and Practice of Surgical Pathology. New York, John Wiley & Sons, 1983, pp. 1125–1145.
7. Lawrence, H. J., et al.: Cyclophosphamide and hemorrhage cystitis. J. Urol. *115*:191, 1976.
8. Smith, B. H., and Dehner, L. P.: Chronic ulcerating interstitial cystitis (Hunner's ulcer). Arch. Pathol. *93*:75, 1972.
9. Smith, B. H.: Malakoplakia of the urinary bladder. A study of twenty-four cases. Am. J. Clin. Pathol. *43*:409, 1965.
10. Abdou, N. I., et al.: Malakoplakia: Evidence for monocyte lysosomal abnormality correctable by cholinergic agonist *in vitro* and *in vivo*. N. Engl. J. Med. *297*:1413, 1977.
11. Rubin, L., and Pincus, M. B.: Eosinophilic cystitis. J. Urol. *112*:457, 1974.
12. Mostofi, F. K., et al.: Histological typing of urinary bladder tumors. Classification of Tumors *19*, WHO, Geneva, 1972.
13. Bergkvist, A., et al.: Classification of bladder tumours based on the cellular pattern. Preliminary reports of a clinicopathological study of 300 cases with a minimum follow-up of 8 years. Acta. Chir. Scand. *130*:371, 1965.
14. Koss, L. G.: Tumors of the urinary bladder. Atlas of Tumor Pathology II, Series 2. Washington, D.C., Armed Forces Institute of Pathology, 1975.
15. Friedell, G. H., et al.: Histopathology and classification of urinary bladder carcinoma. Urol. Clin. North Am. *3*:53, 1976.
16. Murphy, W. M.: Current topics in the pathology of bladder cancer. Pathol. Annu. *18*:1, 1983.
17. Miller, A., et al.: The Bristol bladder tumour registry. Br. J. Urol. *41* (Suppl.):1, 1969.
18. Skinner, D. G., et al.: The clinical significance of carcinoma *in situ* of the bladder and its association with overt carcinoma. J. Urol. *112*:68, 1974.
19. Silverberg, E.: Cancer statistics, 1983, CA *33*:9, 1983.
20. Matanoski, G. M., and Elliott, E. A.: Bladder cancer epidemiology. Epidemiol. Rev. *3*:203, 1981.
21. Khafagy, M. M., et al.: Carcinoma of the bilharzial urinary bladder; a study of the associated mucosal lesions in 80 cases. Cancer *30*:150, 1972.
22. Fukushima, S., et al.: Effect of L-tryptophan and sodium saccharin on urinary tract carcinogenesis initiated by *N*-(4-(5-nitro 2-furyl)-2-thiazolyl) formamide. Cancer Res. *41*:3100, 1981.
23. Plotz, P. H., et al.: Bladder complications in patients receiving cyclophosphamide for systemic lupus erythematosus or rheumatoid arthritis. Ann. Intern. Med. *91*:221, 1979.
24. Collins, W.E.: TNM classification of malignant tumours of the bladder, prostate, testis and kidney. Can. J. Surg. *18*:468, 1975.
25. Prout, G. R.: Classification and staging of bladder carcinoma. Semin. Oncol. *6*:189, 1979.
26. Cummings, K. B.: Diagnosis, staging and classification of bladder tumors. Semin. Urol. *1*:7, 1983.
27. Wolf, H., and Hojgaard, K.: Urothelial dysplasia concomitant with bladder tumours as a determinant factor for future new occurrences. Lancet *2*:134, 1983.
28. Koss, L. G.: Evaluation of patients with carcinoma *in situ* of the bladder. Pathol. Annu. *17*:353, 1982.
29. Utz, D. C.: Carcinoma *in situ* of the bladder. Cancer *45*:1842, 1980.
30. Koss, L. G.: Mapping of the urinary bladder: Its impact on the concepts of bladder cancer. Hum. Pathol. *10*:553, 1979.
31. Murphy, W. M., et al.: The diagnostic value of urine versus bladder washing in patients with bladder cancer. J. Urol. *126*:320, 1981.
32. Klein, F. A., et al.: Detection and follow-up of carcinoma of urinary bladder by flow cytometry. Cancer *50*:389, 1982.
33. Devonec, M., et al.: Flow cytometry of low-stage bladder tumors: Correlation with cytologic and cystoscopic diagnosis. Cancer *49*:109, 1982.
34. Berger, R. E.: Urethritis and epididymitis. Semin. Urol. *1*:138, 1983.
35. Fihn, S. D., and Stamm, W. E.: The urethral syndrome. Semin. Urol. *1*:121, 1983.
36. Bowie, W. R., et al.: Etiology of nongonococcal urethritis. Evidence for *Chlamydia trachomatis* and *Ureoplasma urealyticum*. J. Clin. Invest. *59*:735, 1977.

MALE GENITAL SYSTEM 23

EMBRYOGENESIS

The male genital tract is derived from the urogenital ridge. During the second month of fetal development, the genital ridge of mesenchyme differentiates into an outer, germinal epithelium and an inner, loosely arranged epithelial mass. To this point, there is no sex differentiation and the primitive gonad is intersexual. By differential rates of growth, and by more marked proliferation of the caudal end of this ridge, a recognizable intracelomic testis is produced. It comes to lie just above the pelvis by about the third month of fetal development, a process termed the *internal descent*.

The further passage of the testis into its definitive adult position in the scrotum occurs in the eighth to ninth months of fetal development and is designated the *external descent*. The internal structure of the testis develops during the third month of gestation. The external germinal epithelium differentiates into the tunica coverings of the testis. The inner epithelial mass or included totipotential cells give rise to the tubular structures of the testis including the rete testis. At the time of birth, a well-developed branching system of seminiferous tubules is present. These still lack a lumen and continue as solid cords until puberty. At puberty, the testis cords acquire lumina and mature. Differentiation of secondary spermatocytes into spermatids and spermatozoa, which begins at this age, characterizes the adult form of spermatogenesis, which continues throughout life into extreme old age.

It is during the early ambisexual period that aberrations of development may give rise to both male and female sex organs in the same individual, producing a true hermaphrodite, or to various intergrades of sexual differentiation that create pseudohermaphrodites (p. 133).

The external genitals begin to appear at about the sixth week of fetal life in the form of a conical protuberance in the midline of the body about midway between the umbilical cord and tail. This protuberance is designated the genital tubercle. In the course of time, it develops a shallow ventral groove with lateral ridges that fuse to create a urethral canal. Progressive growth of this tubercle creates a cylindrical phallus that gives rise to the penis in the male or the clitoris in the female. Later swellings are the first indication of the developing scrotum in the male or the labia in the female. As with the primitive gonad, the genital tubercle is a sexually undifferentiated structure that may give rise to either male or female external genitals. Aberration in its early development, therefore, accounts for the occurrence of intergrades between the definitive patterns of adult genital structure found in each sex.

Penis

NORMAL

The body of the penis is made up of three intimately attached erectile structures, two lateral penile corpora cavernosa and the medial corpus cavernosum urethrae, containing the penile urethra. The glans penis is molded over the distal extremities of these three longitudinal corpora. The penis is covered with pigmented skin, which is folded over at the distal extremity to form the prepuce. The prepuce is attached about the coronal sulcus. In the normal state it is readily retracted, but when this epithelial sheath is abnormally small it sometimes cannot be retracted. When forcibly retracted, it may be caught about the glans and impinge upon the urethra or even the blood supply to the tip of the penis.

The arterial supply to the penis is derived from the internal pubic arteries, which are branches of the hypogastrics. These vessels enter the erectile corpora at the penile base. Traumatic injuries and lesions in the pubic region may thus impair this arterial supply. The venous drainage of the penis joins the prostatic plexus. Conceivably, therefore, disease in the prostate may embarrass such venous drainage, but, for obscure reasons, this rarely occurs. Moreover, it is quite uncommon for disease processes to extend through these common vascular channels from one organ to the other. The lymphatic drainage of the penis and scrotum passes through the superficial inguinal and subinguinal lymph nodes. These nodes are often involved in inflammatory and neoplastic processes arising in the penis.

PATHOLOGY

The most important diseases of the penis consist of inflammations and tumors. The venereal infections, e.g., syphilis and gonorrhea, usually begin with penile lesions. Carcinoma of the penis, although not one of the more common neoplasms in the male, still accounts for about 1% of cancers in this sex. Despite the fact that this malignancy is readily apparent in its earliest stages, these cancers often are not brought to medical attention until they are well advanced and beyond cure. Penile cancer, therefore, is a significant cause of mortality.

CONGENITAL ANOMALIES

The penis is the site of many varied forms of congenital anomalies, some of which have some clinical significance. These range from congenital absence and hypoplasia to hyperplasia, duplication, and other aberrations in size and form. For the most part, these deviations in size and form are extremely uncommon and readily apparent on inspection. Certain other anomalies are more frequent and, therefore, have greater clinical significance.

HYPOSPADIAS AND EPISPADIAS

Malformation of the urethral groove and urethral canal may create abnormal openings either in the *ventral surface of the penis (hypospadias)* or in the *dorsal surface (epispadias).* Such anomalies are commonly associated with failure of normal descent of the testes and with malformations of the urinary bladder. Frequently, the penile anomalies are accompanied by other severe congenital defects that are incompatible with life. Even the isolated urethral defects may have clinical significance, because often the abnormal opening is constricted, producing partial urinary obstruction and an attendant hazard of spread of bacterial contamination from the obstructed penile urethra into the bladder and remainder of the urinary tract. Moreover, these anomalies may have more serious consequences. When the orifices are situated near the base of the penis, normal ejaculation and insemination are hampered or totally blocked. These lesions, therefore, are possible causes of sterility in the male.

PHIMOSIS

When the orifice of the prepuce is too small to permit its normal retraction, the condition is designated phimosis. Such an abnormally small orifice may result from anomalous development but may also be produced by inflammatory scarring of the prepuce. Phimosis is important since it interferes with cleanliness and permits the accumulation of secretions and detritus under the prepuce, favoring the development of secondary bacterial infections. When a phimotic prepuce is forcibly retracted over the glans penis, marked constriction and subsequent swelling may block the replacement of the prepuce, creating what is known as *paraphimosis.* This condition not only is extremely painful, but also may be a potential cause of urethral constriction and serious acute urinary retention.

INFLAMMATIONS

Inflammations of the penis almost invariably involve the glans and prepuce and include a wide variety of specific and nonspecific infections. The specific infections—syphilis, gonorrhea, chancroid, granuloma inguinale, lymphopathia venereum, genital herpes—are venereal and have been discussed in Chapter 8. Only the nonspecific infections causing so-called balanoposthitis need description here.

BALANOPOSTHITIS

Balanoposthitis is a nonspecific infection of the glans and prepuce caused by a wide variety of organisms, e.g., staphylococci, streptococci, coliform bacilli, and (less often) the gonococci. It is usually encountered in patients having phimosis or a large, redundant prepuce that interferes with cleanliness and predisposes to bacterial growth within the accumulated secretions and smegma. Such inflammations, if neglected, may lead to frank ulcerations of the mucosal covering of the glans (Fig. 23–1). If they persist and become chronic, they lead to further inflammatory scarring of the phimosis, with aggravation of the underlying condition. The inflammatory reaction in the urethral and periurethral glands in gonorrheal balanoposthitis is indistinguishable morphologically from the nonspecific forms of balanoposthitis, and correct identification of the specific agent requires bacterial smears and cultures.

TUMORS

Tumors of the penis are, on the whole, uncommon. The most frequent neoplasms of the penis are carcinomas arising in the covering epithelium. Benign tumors are exceedingly rare. However, in addition to the clearly defined benign and malignant categories, there are several conditions that fall into an intermediate zone commonly designated precancerous lesions.

BENIGN TUMORS

Although lipomas, neuromas, fibromas, and angiomas occur in the penis, they are so rare as to be medical curiosities.

Condyloma

Three types of condyloma occur on the penis: (1) the relatively frequent *condyloma acuminatum* of viral origin, related to the common wart (verruca vulgaris); (2) the rare *giant condyloma;* and (3) the *syphilitic condyloma lata,* described elsewhere (p. 337).

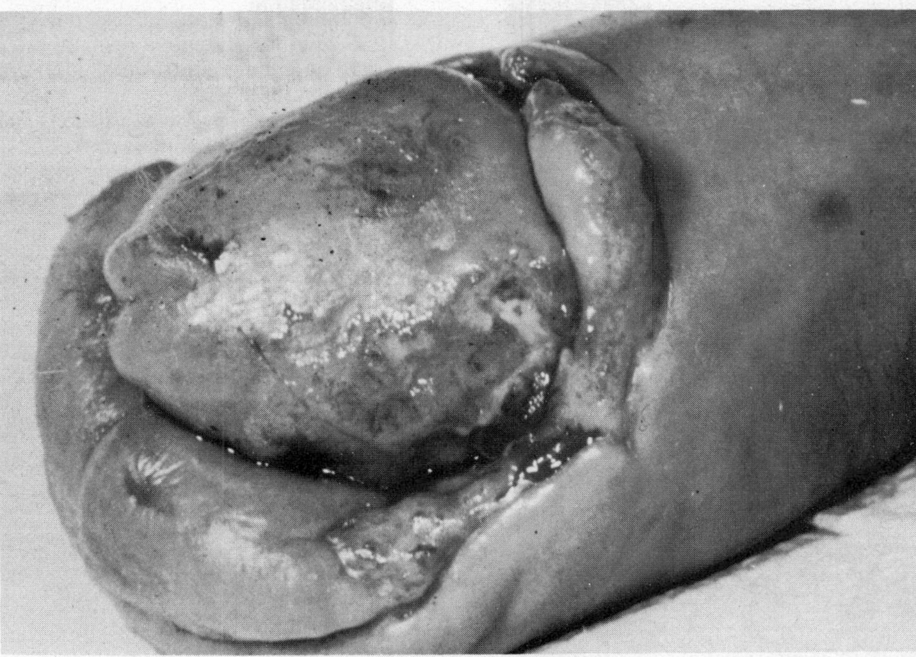

Figure 23–1. Balanoposthitis with acute ulcerative lesions of glans penis.

The condyloma acuminatum may occur on any moist mucocutaneous surface of the external genitals in both males and females, including the vaginal, anal, or urethral mucosa. On the penis, these lesions occur most often about the coronal sulcus and inner surface of the prepuce. They consist of sessile or pedunculated, red papillary excrescences that vary from minute lesions 1 mm to several millimeters in diameter up to large, raspberry-like masses several centimeters in diameter (Fig. 23–2). Histologically, a branching, villous, papillary connective tissue stroma is covered by a thickened hyperplastic epithelium that may have considerable superficial hyperkeratosis and thickening of the underlying epidermis (acanthosis) (Fig. 23–3). The normal orderly maturation of the epithelial cells is preserved, but may be slightly modified by increased mitotic activity in the basal layers and by some widening of the prickle cell layers. Clear vacuolization of the prickle cells may appear and is said to be characteristic of these lesions. The basement membrane is usually intact and there is no evidence of invasion of the underlying stroma. This lesion is caused by human papilloma virus type 6 (HPV-6), which is antigenically related to the common wart virus. HPV can be demonstrated within the lesions by the immunoperoxidase technique as well as by molecular hybridization.[1,2] As far as we know, these lesions remain benign throughout their course.

The rare **giant condyloma,** although it resembles somewhat its more innocuous "cousin," is not of viral origin, grows larger and covers wider areas, and may be ulcerative and invasive. Indeed, the giant condyloma may represent a form of well-differentiated squamous cell carcinoma, characterized by striking hyperkeratosis and a verrucal pattern of growth.[3] The term giant condyloma should be reserved, however, for those giant verrucous lesions that do not metastasize, as contrasted with carcinomas that have all the potentials of squamous cell cancers elsewhere. Although the true giant condyloma displays somewhat greater cellular pleomorphism than is seen in condyloma acuminatum, it usually does not present the atypia and anaplasia so typical of carcinomas, and moreover the downward growth is along a broad front rather than the crablike penetration of the cancer.

MALIGNANT TUMORS

With very rare exceptions, malignancy of the penis is virtually synonymous with squamous cell carcinoma. The rare exceptions, so infrequent as to barely merit citation, include malignant melanoma, hemangiosarcoma, and fibrosarcomas.

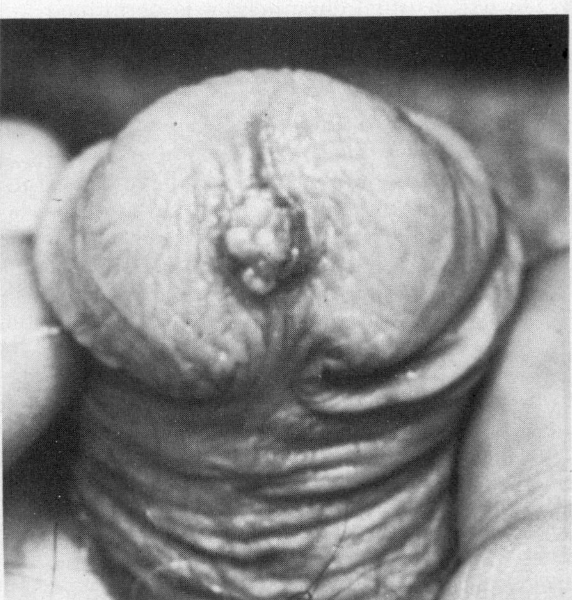

Figure 23–2. Condyloma acuminatum of penis.

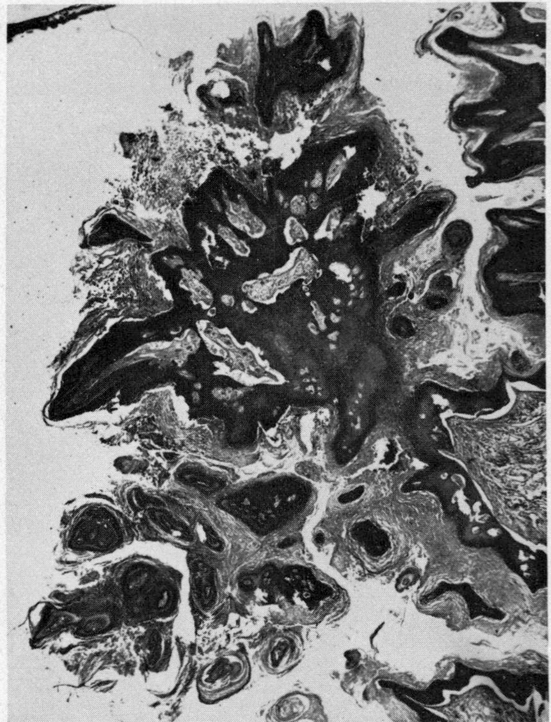

Figure 23–3. Condyloma of penis. Low-power view to illustrate papillary excrescence covered by epithelium.

Carcinoma

Squamous cell carcinoma of the penis represents about 1% of cancers in males in the United States. Since protection against this malignancy is apparently conferred by circumcision, the incidence among different population groups varies widely throughout the world. Carcinoma of the penis is virtually unknown among Jews, in whom ritual circumcision is performed in the first days of life. It is extremely rare among Mohammedans, in whom circumcision is performed before the tenth year of life. In other regions of the world where circumcision is not routinely practiced, carcinoma of the penis is correspondingly more common, so that it is reported to represent about 18% of all malignant tumors in the Orient. Presumably, circumcision protects against tumorigenesis by preventing the accumulation of smegma (carcinogenic in animals) and minimizing the tendency to irritation and infections. Carcinomas are usually found in patients between the ages of 40 and 70.

The lesion usually begins on the glans or inner surface of the prepuce near the coronal sulcus. The first observable changes are a small area of epithelial thickening accompanied by graying and fissuring of the mucosal surface. With progression, an elevated leukoplakic papule is produced that often ulcerates when a diameter of approximately 1 cm is reached. Despite the obviousness of such lesions, by the time most patients seek medical attention large characteristic malignant ulcers are present, having necrotic, secondarily infected bases with ragged, irregular, heaped-up margins (Fig. 23–4). In far-advanced lesions, the ulceroinvasive disease may have destroyed virtually the entire tip of the penis or large areas of the shaft.

A second pattern of macroscopic tumor growth is the papillary tumor that simulates the condyloma and progressively enlarges to form a cauliflower-like, fungating mass. As this tumor enlarges, it undergoes central ulceration and may become transformed to a pattern that resembles the ulcerative lesion just described.

Histologically, both the papillary and ulceroinvasive lesions are squamous cell carcinomas exactly resembling those that occur elsewhere on the skin surface.

Clinical Course. Carcinoma of the penis is a slowly growing, locally metastasizing lesion[4] which often has been present for a year or more before it is brought to medical attention. Such delay is occasioned sometimes by the existence of a phimosis that completely hides the developing lesion, but more often by unawareness of the significance of the developing papule. The lesions are nonpainful until they undergo secondary ulceration and infection. Frequently they bleed. At the time when most patients are first diagnosed, about 30 to 50% have enlarged inguinal nodes; approximately half of these harbor metastasis, whereas others represent reactive lymphadenitis.[5] Metastasis to local nodes characterizes the early stage, and widespread dissemination is extremely uncommon until the lesion is far advanced. The prognosis following surgical excision and regional node dissection is related to the stage of advancement of the tumor. In persons with limited lesions without invasion of the penile shaft, there is a 90 to 95% five-year survival rate, whereas tumors that invade the shaft of the penis and the regional lymph nodes yield only a 30 to 50% five-year survival rate.[5]

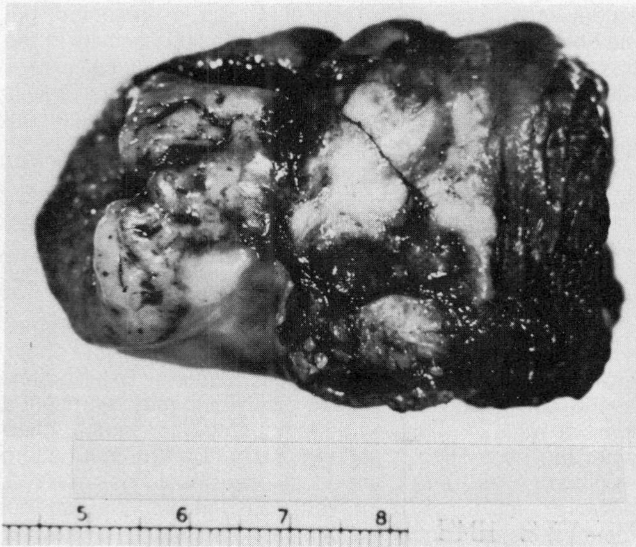

Figure 23–4. Squamous cell carcinoma of penis with typical shaggy fungating ulcerations. (Courtesy of Dr. Fred Silva, Department of Pathology, University of Texas Health Science Center, Dallas.)

PREMALIGNANT LESIONS

There is a group of hyperplastic, dysplastic epithelial lesions occurring on the penis that predispose to the genesis of frank malignancy. These entities are (1) pseudoepitheliomatous hyperplasia, (2) erythroplasia of Queyrat, and (3) Bowen's disease.

Pseudoepitheliomatous hyperplasia usually occurs in proximity to or overlying some inflammatory or ulcerative lesion. It is marked by epithelial hyperplasia, thickening the epidermal layer and prolonging the rete pegs. Sometimes there is hyperkeratosis of the surface layer, producing a pearly, leukoplakic macroscopic appearance. A chronic inflammatory infiltrate is almost always present in the dermis. The surface is rarely verrucose as in condyloma acuminatum. The tendency to carcinomatous change is slight, although definitely greater than that of the normal epidermis.

Erythroplasia of Queyrat is a form of epithelial dysplasia encountered principally on the penis, although rarely it affects the lips, oral mucosa, tongue, vulva, and glabrous skin. The penile lesion occurs at any age in adults, usually in the uncircumcised. It generally appears on the glans and prepuce as a red, soft plaque, generally about 1.0 to 1.5 cm in diameter. The plaque may be elevated and flat, sometimes papillary, or occasionally ulcerated.

Histologically, erythroplasia of Queyrat is characterized by a diminished keratin layer, irregular dysplastic acanthosis, and a dermal inflammatory infiltrate. The dysplasia is of variable severity, ranging from mild disorientation of epithelial cells with variable cellular pleomorphism to changes of carcinoma in situ.[6] Lesions at the carcinomatous end of this spectrum closely resemble Bowen's disease, but (as will be seen), erythroplasia of Queyrat is not suspected to be associated with an increased risk of visceral cancers, as is Bowen's disease. Nonetheless, about 5 to 10% of patients with erythroplasia of Queyrat eventually develop an overt squamous cell carcinoma.

Bowen's disease is a curious form of carcinoma in situ that has a possible association with visceral cancer (Fig. 23–5). The lesion occurs in the genital region of both males and females, usually in those over the age of 35 years, and in males it is prone to involve the shaft of the penis and the scrotum. Grossly it appears as a thickened, opaque plaque with shallow ulceration and crusting. Another pattern recognized in more recent years has been termed *bowenoid papulosis*.[7, 8] Such lesions may appear as innocent-looking papules or may even be verrucoid, being easily mistaken for condyloma acuminatum. Over the span of years, Bowen's disease may become invasive and transformed into a characteristic squamous cell carcinoma. The relationship of Bowen's disease to visceral cancers is controversial. On the one hand are those who contend that the association is well defined, involving most often the respiratory, gastrointestinal, and genitourinary tracts. About one-third

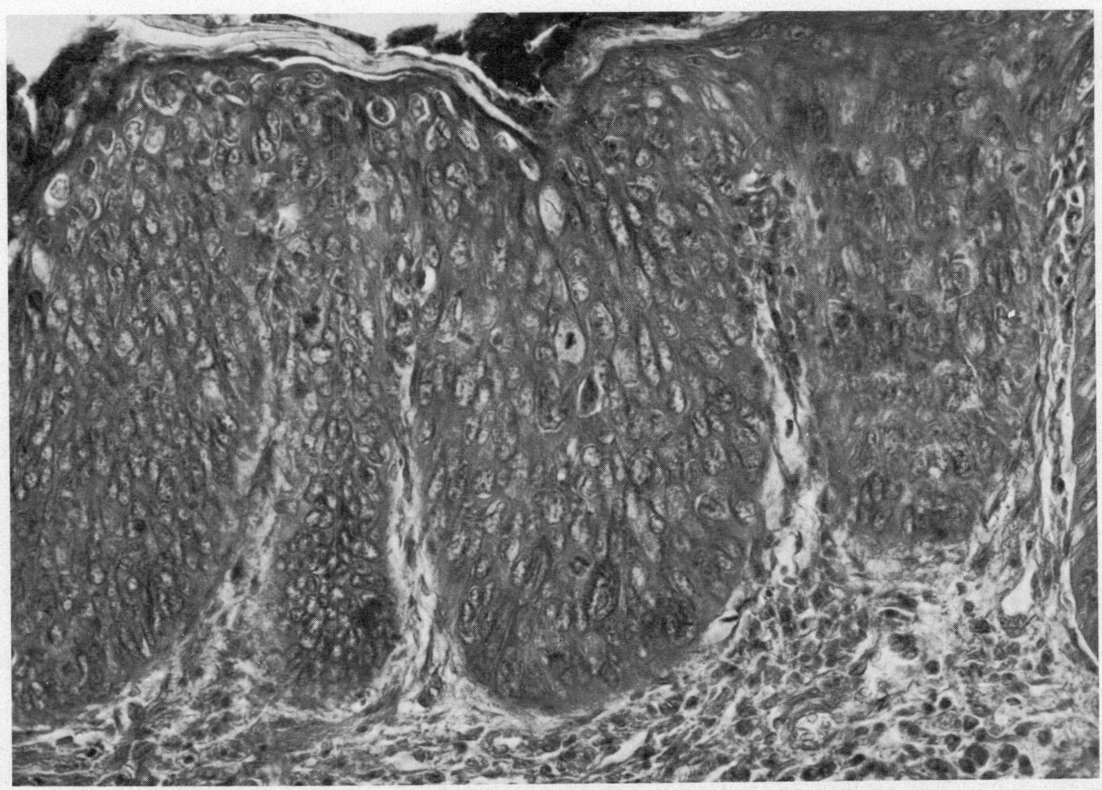

Figure 23–5. Bowen's disease illustrating dysplasia and anaplasia of epithelial cells.

of the patients are said to develop visceral cancers, often after a latent period of several years. However, this view has been challenged since others have failed to find a significant association between Bowen's disease and internal cancer. It has been suggested that the association with other malignancies, noted by some, may stem from exposure to a common carcinogenic agent such as arsenic. Thus, the relationship remains unresolved and with it the validity of a sharp differentiation of erythroplasia of Queyrat from Bowen's disease.

Testis and Epididymis

NORMAL

In the adult, the testis weighs approximately 12 gm and measures about 5 × 3 × 3 cm. It is covered by a serosal membrane, the visceral layer of the tunica vaginalis, which is reflected off the hilus of the testis to form an inner lining of the scrotal sac, the parietal tunica vaginalis. Thus, in the normal adult, there is a completely closed, serosa-lined potential space folded about the testes, much as Bowman's capsule envelops the glomerular tuft. The lining of this space is derived from the processus vaginalis of the peritoneum. Beneath the visceral tunica vaginalis there is the dense, white, fibrous tunica albuginea and deep to it a so-called tunica vasculosa, which is, in reality, merely a condensation of fibrous tissue and blood vessels on the inner surface of the tunica albuginea. All the arteries, veins, lymphatics, and nerves enter through the hilus. The epididymis is a crescentic tubular organ lying along the posterolateral border of the testis. The rete tubules of the testis drain into the collecting tubules of the head of the epididymis, and the tail of the epididymis communicates with the vas deferens.

Histologically, the testis consists of branching tubular cords separated from adjacent cords by a scant, loose, connective tissue stroma. These tubules have distinct basement membranes that increase in thickness with age. The testis is divided into many lobules by condensed fibrous septa that all radiate from the hilus of the testis. Within the testicular tubules are found the Sertoli supporting cells and the maturing germinal epithelium that has already been mentioned in the embryology of this organ. Within the stroma, there are scattered groups and nests of round-to-polygonal, epithelial-like Leydig cells having abundant acidophilic cytoplasm and large nuclei that contain coarse chromatin granules and a prominent nucleolus. In the cytoplasm of these cells are found lipofuscin; lipid granules; and long, slender, crystalline structures, the crystalloids of Reinke. These interstitial cells are a site of formation of androgens. The number of these Leydig cells bears an inverse ratio to the preservation and activity of the tubular germinal epithelium. In advanced age or acquired disease, with atrophy of the germinal epithelium, there is an accompanying proliferation of the Leydig cells.

The histology of the epididymis is composed essentially of a coiled, twisted, single duct formed by the agglomeration of the vasa efferentia. This duct is lined by extremely tall, pseudostratified, columnar, ciliated epithelium, having nuclei for the most part disposed basally, and luminal portions of the cells composed only of cytoplasm containing fat droplets, pigments, and fat vacuoles.

PATHOLOGY

The major pathologic involvements of the testis and epididymis are quite distinct. In the case of the epididymis the most important and frequent involvements are inflammatory diseases, whereas in the testis the major lesions consist of tumors. However, their close anatomic relationship permits the extension of any of these processes from one organ to the other.

CONGENITAL ANOMALIES

With the exception of incomplete descent of the testes (cryptorchidism), congenital anomalies are extremely rare and include absence of one or both testes, fusion of the testes (so-called *synorchism*), and the formation of relatively insignificant cysts within the testis.

CRYPTORCHIDISM

Cryptorchidism is synonymous with undescended testes and is found in approximately 0.28% of the adult male population. This anomaly represents a complete or incomplete failure of the intra-abdominal testes to descend into the scrotal sac. From the preceding description of embryogenesis of the male genital tract, it will be recalled that in the fetus the testis arises within the celomic cavity and then, by differential growth of the body as well as more rapid proliferation of the caudal end of the urogenital ridge, the testis comes to lie within the lower abdomen or brim of the pelvis, a process referred to as the internal descent. Following this, it descends through the inguinal canal into the scrotal sac: the external descent. On this basis, *malpositioned testes may be found at any point in this pathway of descent.* The precise cause of cryptorchidism is still poorly understood. In a small percentage of cases, it is believed to be a congenital, hereditary disturbance. In another small group, it is related to some hormonal imbalance with incomplete sexual development. In most cases, however, it represents an isolated, random, congenital anomaly or some mechanical obstruction to the complete external descent. A short spermatic cord, a narrow inguinal canal, inadequate development of the gubernaculum testis, and fibrous adhesions in the pathway of descent are all attributed causal significance. The condition is completely asymptomatic, and is found by the patient or the examining physician only when the scrotal sac is discovered not to contain the testis.

Cryptorchidism may be unilateral or bilateral. When unilateral, it is somewhat more common on the right side. When discovered before the age of puberty, the organ is essentially normal in size, shape, and consistency and is only malpositioned. However, at about the time of puberty, progressive atrophy ensues and the organ shows progressive decrease in size, progressive increase in consistency, and, on cut surface, an increased amount of fibrous tissue, apparently replacing the testicular substance (Fig. 23–6*A*). At this stage, the testicular tubules fail to string out as do the normal.

Histologically, the gross atrophy is accompanied by increasing hyaline thickening of the basement membranes of the tubules, with progressive increase of the interstitial connective stroma. Concomitantly, spermatogenic activity is diminished and then totally ceases. The germinal epithelium then undergoes significant atrophy until only a few primitive spermatogonia and Sertoli cells persist.[9] During this time, the basement membranes show increasing hyalinization and thickening, so that eventually the tubules become replaced by dense cords of hyaline connective tissue outlined by the prominent thickened basement membranes (Fig. 23–6*B*). There is a concomitant increase of interstitial stroma and usually some hyperplasia of the interstitial cells of Leydig. However, in certain cases these cells may appear to remain normal or even be decreased in number when pituitary insufficiency underlies the condition.

Cryptorchidism is of more than academic interest for many reasons. When the testis lies in the inguinal

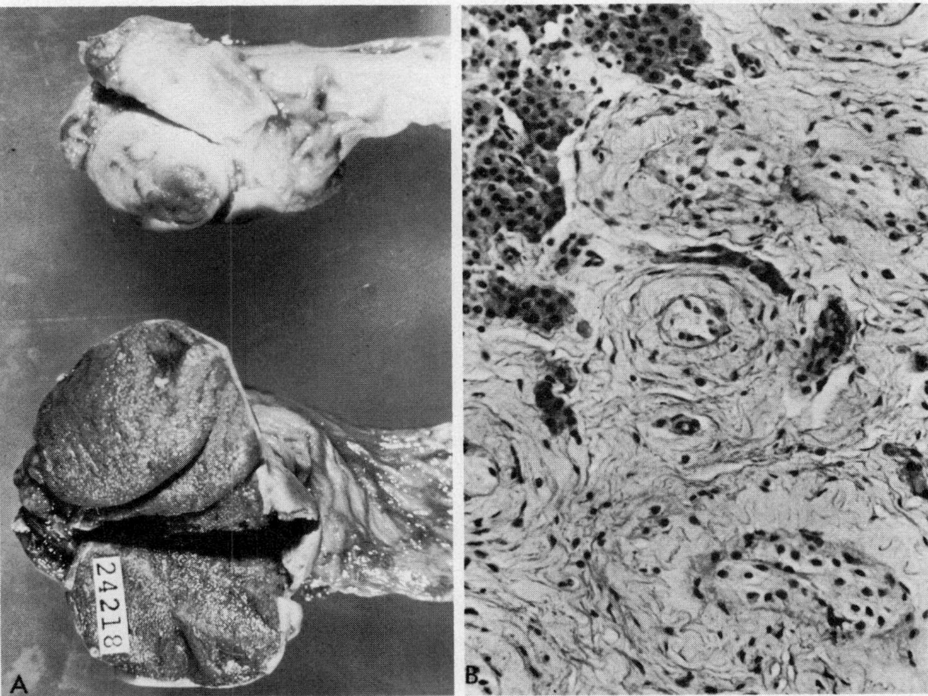

Figure 23–6. Testicular atrophy. *A,* The atrophic testis *(above)* is small and is replaced by white fibrous scars. Compare with cut surface of a normal testis *(below)*. *B,* Microscopically, the tubules are visible as shadowy structures with markedly thickened basement membranes. Note the prominence of Leydig cells in upper left corner. (Courtesy of Dr. Fred Silva, Department of Pathology, University of Texas Health Science Center, Dallas.)

canal, it is particularly exposed to trauma and crushing against the ligaments and bones. A concomitant inguinal hernia frequently accompanies such malposition of the testis. From the morphologic changes, it is apparent that bilateral cryptorchidism may result in sterility attributed to the higher temperature in the environment of the nonscrotal testis or to concurrent primary gonadal dysgenesis. Finally, there is now agreement that the risk of testicular cancer is 17 to 29 times greater in cryptorchid men than in the general male population.[10, 11] The incidence of tumors is four times greater in abdominal testes than in those located in the inguinal canal. The placement of the testis within the scrotum does not preclude the possibility of a cancer developing at a later date. Indeed, malignant change may occur in the contralateral, normally descended testis, suggesting that unilateral cryptorchidism may represent a generalized defect of testicular development.[12] The undescended testis demands surgical correction, both to lessen the risk of sterility and to facilitate detection of a tumor at an early stage.

REGRESSIVE CHANGES

ATROPHY

Atrophy is the only important regressive change that affects the scrotal testis, and may have a number of causes. These can be listed as (1) progressive atherosclerotic narrowing of the blood supply in old age; (2) the end stage of an inflammatory orchitis, whatever the etiologic agent; (3) cryptorchidism; (4) hypopituitarism; (5) generalized malnutrition, or cachexia; (6) obstruction to the outflow of semen; and (7) irradiation. (8) Prolonged administration of female sex hormones, such as is used in treatment of patients with carcinoma of the prostate, may lead to atrophy. (9) Exhaustion atrophy may follow the persistent stimulation produced by high levels of follicle-stimulating pituitary hormone. The gross and microscopic alterations follow the pattern already described for cryptorchidism. When the process is bilateral, as it frequently is, sterility results. Atrophy or sometimes improper development of the testes occasionally occurs as a primary failure of genetic origin. The resulting condition, called Klinefelter's syndrome, represents a sex chromosomal disorder that is discussed in detail on page 129 along with other cytogenetic diseases.

INFLAMMATIONS

Inflammations are distinctly more common in the epididymis than in the testis. It is classically taught that, of the three major specific inflammatory states, *gonorrhea and tuberculosis almost invariably arise in the epididymis, whereas syphilis affects first the testis.*

NONSPECIFIC EPIDIDYMITIS AND ORCHITIS

Epididymitis and possible subsequent orchitis are commonly related to infections in the urinary tract (cystitis, urethritis, genitoprostatitis), which presumably reach the epididymis and the testis through either the vas deferens or the lymphatics of the spermatic cord. Two sexually transmitted diseases, gonorrhea and nongonococcal urethritis (caused by *Chlamydia trachomatis*), are also important causes of epididymitis. The latter organism, in particular, is becoming an increasingly frequent cause of "idiopathic" epididymitis characterized by failure to isolate bacteria from urine or epididymal aspirates.[13] In one five-year study it was found that *E. coli* or Pseudomonas was isolated from most patients over 35 years of age, whereas *C. trachomatis* or (less often) gonococci was the most frequent pathogen in persons under 35 years.[14] Rarely, the testis or epididymis is seeded hematogenously from some other focus of infection.

The bacterial invasion sets up a nonspecific acute inflammation characterized by congestion, edema, and a white cell infiltration chiefly by neutrophils, macrophages, and lymphocytes. Although the infection, in the early stage, is more or less limited to the interstitial connective tissue, it rapidly extends to involve the tubules and may progress to frank abscess formation or complete suppurative necrosis of the entire epididymis (Fig. 23–7). Usually, having involved the epididymis, the infection extends either by direct continuity or through tubular channels or lymphatics into the testis to evoke a similar inflammatory reaction within the testis.

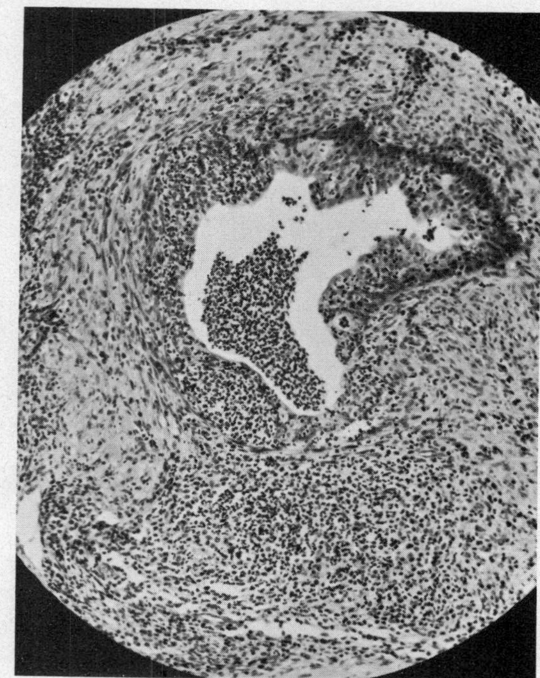

Figure 23–7. Nonspecific acute epididymitis. Inflammation has partially destroyed tubule and has caused metaplasia of lining epithelium.

Such inflammatory involvement of the epididymis and testis is often followed by fibrous scarring, which, in many cases, leads to permanent sterility. Sterility may result from inflammatory obstruction of the excretory pathways or may be due to the intense pressure placed on the blood supply of the testis by the development of edema within a tight, fibrous, enclosing tunica albuginea. Thus, even when suppurative necrosis has not occurred, extensive inflammations may be followed by considerable atrophy of spermatic tubules and loss of spermatogenesis. Usually the interstitial cells of Leydig are not totally destroyed and are believed to be capable of regeneration when partially injured, so that sexual activity is not disturbed. Any such nonspecific infection may become chronic.

GRANULOMATOUS (AUTOIMMUNE) ORCHITIS

Among middle-aged men, a rare cause of unilateral testicular enlargement is nontuberculous, granulomatous orchitis. Often, the testicular swelling develops after an interval of a week to months following trauma to the testis.[15] Histologically, the orchitis is distinguished by granulomas seen both within spermatic tubules and in the intertubular connective tissue. The lesions closely resemble tubercles but differ somewhat in having plasma cells and occasional neutrophils interspersed within the enclosing rim of fibroblasts and lymphocytes. The cause of these lesions remains unknown, but traumatic destruction of spermatocytes within tubules or rupture of tubules with extravasation of damaged sperm is postulated. Lipid extracts of human spermatozoa will induce granulomas in humans. Alternatively, spermatozoa may contain so-called sequestered antigens (p. 179), but the evidence for such is controversial. In any event, death of spermatozoa or rupture of tubules may be the trigger that initiates the inflammatory response.

SPECIFIC INFLAMMATIONS

Gonorrhea

Extension of infection from the posterior urethra to the prostate, seminal vesicles, and thence to the epididymis is the usual course of a neglected gonococcal infection. Inflammatory changes similar to those described in the nonspecific infections occur, with the development of frank abscesses in the epididymis, resulting in extensive destruction of this organ. In the more neglected cases, the infection may thence spread to the testis and produce a suppurative orchitis.

Mumps

About 25 to 30% of cases of mumps in males occur in persons 10 years of age or older. In this pubertal and postpubertal group, orchitis may develop and has been reported in aproximately 30% of male patients who sought the care of a physician. Obviously, this sample is biased by the undoubted fact that many cases of mumps without orchitis do not come to medical attention, and only the more severe cases, particularly those with testicular involvement, are likely to be included in reported surveys. Most often, the acute interstitial orchitis develops about one week following onset of swelling of the parotid glands. Rarely, cases of orchitis precede the parotitis.

In the acute stage, the inflammatory reaction is characterized by intense interstitial edema and mononuclear infiltration, consisting chiefly of lymphocytes, plasma cells, and macrophages. Neutrophils are usually not prominent but, in the more intense inflammatory responses, frank suppuration may develop and the tubular lumina may become filled with purulent exudate (Fig. 23–8). Since the process usually remains largely interstitial and is characteristically patchy and haphazard, healing of the inflammatory reaction may not be followed by any late residuals. However, when the edema has been intense, atrophy of the germinal epithelium may develop and give rise to sterility. Testicular neoplasms have arisen in such atrophic testes.

Tuberculosis

Tuberculosis almost invariably begins in the epididymis and may spread to the testis. On all but rare occasions, such lesions reflect a tuberculous infection elsewhere in the body, almost invariably in the lungs. Rarely, tuberculous epididymitis has followed apparently isolated renal tuberculosis. In many of these cases,

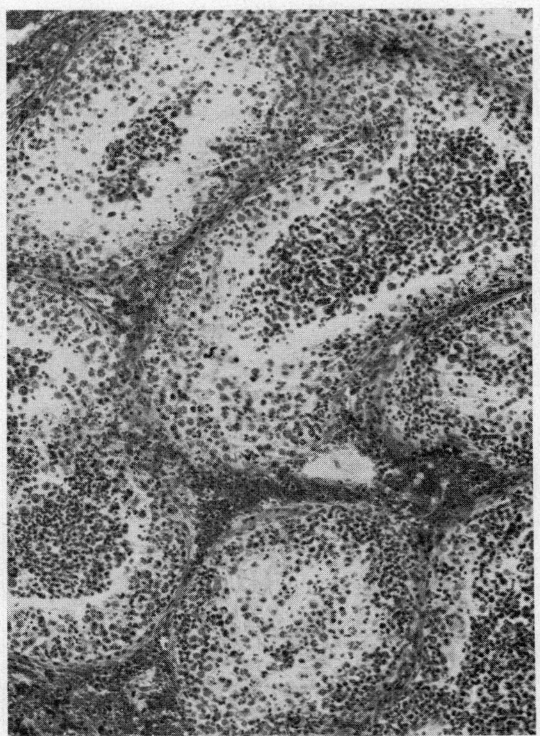

Figure 23–8. Acute severe mumps orchitis with extensive interstitial and intratubular exudation.

there is associated tuberculous prostatitis and seminal vesiculitis, and it is believed by some that epididymitis usually represents a secondary spread from these other involvements of the genital tract. However, the epididymal involvement as a metastatic dissemination through the blood cannot be excluded, even in those cases with involvement of the organs in the urogenital system.

The infection invokes the classic morphologic reactions of tuberculosis. Numerous tubercles become confluent to produce large caseous masses that, in the course of time, may obliterate the entire epididymal structure. By continuity or lymphogenous spread, such infections may extend into the adjacent regions of testis, but in most cases this organ is spared for long periods. The inflammatory involvement is followed, in the course of weeks or months, by progressive fibrous scarring and sometimes calcification. Infrequently, exudate accumulates within the tunica vaginalis and, equally rarely, tuberculous scrotal skin sinuses develop.

Syphilis

The testis and epididymis are affected in both acquired and congenital syphilis, but *almost invariably the testis is involved first by the infection.* In many cases, the orchitis is not accompanied by epididymitis.

The morphologic pattern of the reaction takes two forms: the production of gummas, or a diffuse interstitial inflammation characterized by edema and lymphocytic and plasma cell infiltration with the characteristic hallmark of all syphilitic infections, i.e., obliterative endarteritis with perivascular cuffing of lymphocytes and plasma cells. In the early case, the gummas cause a nodular enlargement and the characteristic yellow-white foci of necrosis. The diffuse reaction causes swelling and induration. In the course of time, whether or not the morphologic reaction is that of the already described gumma formation or diffuse inflammation, progressive fibrous scarring follows, which in turn leads to considerable tubular atrophy and, sometimes, sterility. Usually the testes shrink and become pale and fibrotic. The interstitial cells of Leydig are spared and sexual potency is not impaired. However, when the process is extremely advanced, the Leydig cells may be destroyed, resulting in loss of libido. Sterility occurs less often with the gumma than with the diffuse inflammation.

Miscellaneous Infections

The testis and epididymis are involved by hematogenous metastatic dissemination of organisms in a wide variety of infectious diseases, such as leprosy, typhoid fever, brucellosis, and meningococcal and rickettsial infections, and in some fungal diseases such as blastomycosis and actinomycosis. In all these instances, the testicular and epididymal involvement is only one small component of the systemic disorder, and the local inflammatory changes resemble those found in the systemic disease.

VASCULAR DISTURBANCES

TORSION

Twisting of the spermatic cord may cut off the venous drainage and the arterial supply to the testis. Usually, however, the thick-walled arteries remain patent so that intense vascular engorgement and venous infarction follow. The usual precipitating cause of such torsion is some violent movement or physical trauma. In most instances, however, there are predisposing causes, such as incomplete descent, absence of the scrotal ligaments or the gubernaculum testis, atrophy of the testis so that it is abnormally mobile within the tunica vaginalis, abnormal attachment of the testis to the epididymis, or other abnormalities.

Depending on the duration and severity of the process, the morphologic changes may be those of merely intense congestion to widespread extravasation of blood into the interstitial tissue of the testis and epididymis. In more extreme instances, hemorrhagic or even anemic infarction of the entire testis may occur (Fig. 23–9). In these late stages, the testis is markedly enlarged and is converted virtually into a sac of soft, necrotic, hemorrhagic tissue. The leukocytic reaction is very variable and depends on the free access of blood via the arterial system. Usually the blood flow is so impaired that leukocytic infiltration is not a prominent feature and the process essentially resembles one of pure coagulative necrosis without considerable inflammatory reaction.

TESTICULAR TUMORS

Testicular neoplasms span an amazing gamut of anatomic types. Approximately 95% arise from germ cells. Most of these germinal tumors are highly aggressive cancers capable of rapid and wide dissemination, although with current therapy the outlook for these patients has improved considerably. Many when limited to the testis can be cured, and even with disseminated tumors complete remissions can sometimes be achieved. Nongerminal tumors, in contrast, are generally benign, but some elaborate steroids leading to interesting endocrinologic syndromes.

CLASSIFICATION AND HISTOGENESIS. Classifications of the testicular tumors abound and, regrettably, vary widely. The major problems are the differing concepts of the histogenesis of these lesions and the endless variability in morphology among the various forms of neoplasms as well as within a single tumor. As one might guess, totipotential germ cells that become cancerous are not inhibited in their lines of differentiation. The most authoritative and readily understood classification in the United States has been offered by Mostofi. More recently the W.H.O. has presented a classification of testicular tumors (Table 23–1) that differs in only minor aspects from the Mostofi classification.[16]

The latter classification is based on the view that the vast majority of tumors in the testis arise from the

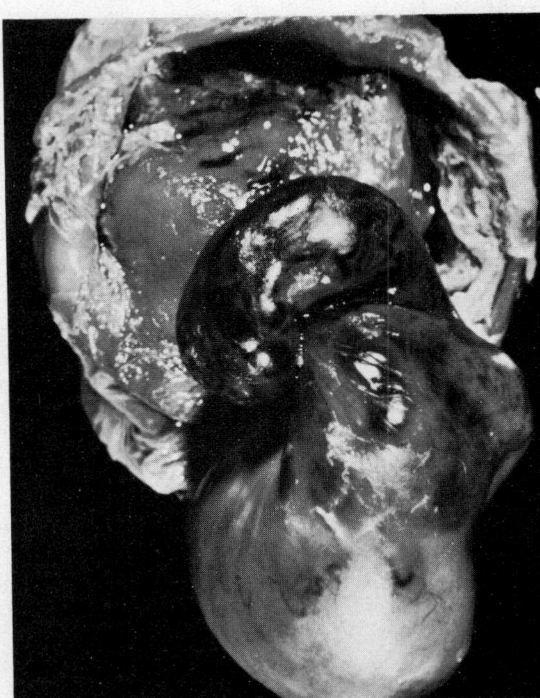

Figure 23–9. Torsion of testis.

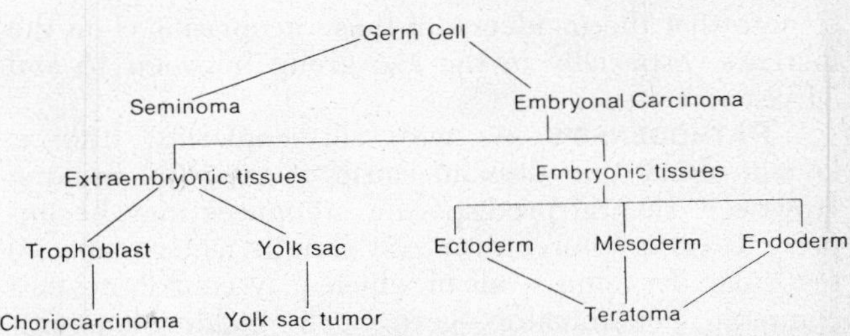

Figure 23–10. Histogenesis of testicular tumors. (Adapted from Pierce, G. B., Jr., and Abell, M. A.: Embryonal carcinoma of the testis. *In* Sommers, S. C. (ed.): Pathology Annual. New York, Appleton-Century-Crofts, 1970, p. 28.

testicular germ cells (Fig. 23–10).[17] The germ cells may give rise to seminoma, reflecting gonadal differentiation, or they may transform into totipotential tumor cells represented by embryonal carcinoma. According to this concept, embryonal carcinoma is the stem for all nonseminomatous germ cell tumors. Depending on the degree and line of differentiation of embryonal carcinoma cells, tumors with different histologic patterns result. The most undifferentiated state is represented by pure embryonal cell carcinoma, whereas choriocarcinoma and yolk sac tumor represent commitment of the tumor stem cells to differentiate into specific extraembryonic cell types. Teratoma, on the other hand, results from differentiation of the embryonic carcinoma cells along the lines of all three germ cell layers, and therefore teratomas contain the greatest variety of neoplastic cells and tissues. This scheme provides a rational explanation for the apparently bewildering array of histologic patterns and is supported by the following observations: (1) the frequent coexistence of embryonal carcinoma and teratoma in the testis; (2) the presence of teratoma or choriocarcinoma in the metastasis of a tumor, which in its primary site appears to be an embryonal carcinoma; (3) the ultrastructural similarity between seminoma cells and normal primitive germ cells; and (4) the in situ origin of seminoma, embryonal carcinoma, and choriocarcinoma within the seminiferous tubules.[18] The last-mentioned finding strengthens the concept of an intratubular germ cell origin for the great majority of testicular tumors. Furthermore, this scheme of the histogenesis of testicular tumors is also supported by murine models of testicular carcinoma.[19] Although this scheme is widely accepted, it should be pointed out that an alternative hypothesis, which forms the basis of the British system of classification, states that only seminomas arise from germ cells, whereas all others originate from blastomeres displaced early in embryonic development. According to this view, all the nonseminomatous tumors (excluding the stromal tumors) should be classified as teratomas with varying degrees of differentiation.[20]

Table 23–1. W.H.O. PATHOLOGIC CLASSIFICATION OF TESTICULAR TUMORS

I. Germ Cell tumors
- A. Tumors of one histologic type
  1. Seminoma
  2. Spermatocytic seminoma
  3. Embryonal carcinoma
  4. Yolk sac tumor (embryonal carcinoma infantile type)
  5. Polyembryoma
  6. Choriocarcinoma
  7. Teratomas
     - a. Mature
     - b. Immature
     - c. With malignant transformation
- B. Tumors showing more than one histologic pattern
  1. Embryonal carcinoma plus teratoma (teratocarcinoma)
  2. Choriocarcinoma and any other types (specify types)
  3. Other combinations (specify)

II. Sex Cord–Stromal Tumors
- A. Well-differentiated forms
  1. Leydig cell tumor
  2. Sertoli cell tumor
  3. Granulosa cell tumor
- B. Mixed forms (specify)
- C. Incompletely differentiated forms.

GERM CELL TUMORS

The incidence of testicular tumors in the United States is approximately two per 100,000 males. They cause about 0.5% of all male cancer deaths. In the 15- to 34-year age group, which is when these neoplasms have a peak incidence, they constitute the most common tumor of males and cause approximately 14% of all cancer deaths. Two smaller peaks of incidence are encountered in infancy and in later life. It is distressing to note that the incidence of these neoplasms is on the increase, especially in the age group between 15 and 34 years.[21]

PATHOGENESIS. As with all neoplasms, little is known about the ultimate cause of germinal tumors. However, several predisposing influences may be important: (1) cryptorchidism, (2) genetic factors, and (3) testicular dysgenesis, all of which may contribute to a common denominator—germ cell maldevelopment. Reference has already been made (p. 1087) to the increased incidence of neoplasms in *undescended testes.* It has been calculated that one in 20 abdominal testes and one in 80 inguinal testes will develop a tumor. Although clinical studies suggest a ten- to 40-fold higher risk of development of testicular cancer in undescended testes, more recent epidemiologic (case control) studies place the risk between 2.5 and 8.8.[21] The factors impinging on the cryptorchid that contribute to this increased risk of oncogenesis are not clear. It seems unlikely that the abnormal environment of the misplaced testis is related to the increased risk of carcinogenesis, since there is also an increased incidence of tumors in the contralateral, normally positioned testes. It seems more probable that there are common predisposing factors, possibly hormonal, associated with both testicular cancer and cryptorchidism.[22]

The putative risk factors must act early, since surgical correction of maldescent (orchiopexy), even when done several years before the age of peak tumor incidence, does not eliminate the increased risk.[21] Although orchiopexy before the age of 6 years is recommended, there are virtually no data to prove that it ensures a normal risk of testicular cancer.[23] Genetic predisposition also seems to be important, although no well-defined pattern of inheritance has been identified. In support, the striking racial differences in the incidence of testicular tumors can be cited. Blacks in Africa have an extremely low incidence of these neoplasms, which is unaffected by migration to the U.S. It is interesting to note that, in a study performed in Los Angeles county, there was not only a fourfold higher incidence of testicular cancer in white males than in black males, but also a threefold greater risk of undescended testis in whites,[22] pointing again to possible common factors in the pathogenesis of cryptorchidism and testicular cancer. Genetic influences may also underlie the incidence of testicular tumors in certain families. Moreover, a patient having a testicular tumor is at much greater risk of having a second tumor in the other testis, sometimes years later.[24] Testicular dysgenesis (p. 134) also seems to predispose to tumor development since malignant germ cell tumors develop in approximately 25% of dysgenetic testes.[23]

In summary, it appears that some abnormality in the development of germ cells may be the common denominator in predisposition to testicular cancer. Although such abnormalities are overt and severe only in some cases (e.g., cryptorchidism), more subtle aberrations may well underlie most cases. The changes may be genetically determined or perhaps may result from the interplay of genetic and endocrine factors.

With this background of histogenesis, we can discuss the morphologic patterns of germ cell tumors followed by the clinical features common to most germinal tumors. The student can take comfort in the fact that some of the tumors listed in Table 23–1 are sufficiently rare to justify exclusion from the following discussion.

Specific Types of Germinal Tumors

About 60% of germinal tumors are composed of a single cell type. These "pure" types will be described first, followed by some comments about the mixed patterns. Only then will the staging and clinical features common to most germ cell tumors be presented.

SEMINOMA

Seminomas are the most common type of germinal tumor (40%) and the type most likely to produce a uniform population of cells. They almost never occur in infants; they peak in the fourth decade, somewhat later than the collective peak.

Three histologic variants of seminoma are described: typical (85%), anaplastic (5 to 10%), and spermatocytic (4 to 6%). The last-mentioned has been segregated into a separate category in the W.H.O. classi-

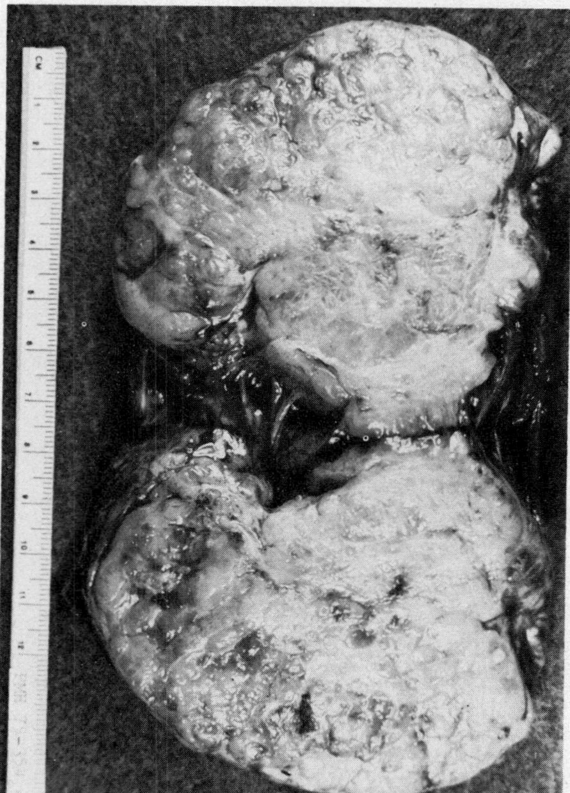

Figure 23–11. Seminoma. Testis is enlarged and virtually replaced by lobulated, homogeneous, gray-white tumor tissue. Hemorrhage and necrosis are not prominent. (Courtesy of Dr. Fred Silva, Department of Pathology, University of Texas Health Science Center, Dallas.)

fication and will be discussed later. All produce bulky masses, sometimes ten times the size of the normal testis.

The typical seminoma has a homogeneous, gray-white, lobulated, cut surface, usually devoid of hemorrhages or necroses (Fig. 23–11). In over half the cases, the entire testis is replaced. The anaplastic variant has a similar macroscopic appearance. Generally, the tunica albuginea is not penetrated, but occasionally extension to the epididymis, spermatic cord, or scrotal sac occurs.

Microscopically, the typical seminoma, presumably derived from the proliferation of primary germ cells, presents sheets of uniform, so-called "seminoma cells" divided into poorly demarcated lobules by delicate septa of fibrous tissue. The classic "seminoma cell" is large and round-to-polyhedral and has a distinct cell membrane, a cleared or watery-appearing cytoplasm, and a large, central hyperchromatic nucleus with one or two prominent nucleoli. Mitoses are infrequent. The cytoplasm contains varying amounts of glycogen and, rarely, lipid vacuoles. Tumor giant cells may be present as well as syncytial giant cells; the latter resemble the syncytiotrophoblast of the placenta both morphologically and in that they contain human chorionic gonadotropins (HCG). The amount of stroma varies greatly. Sometimes it is scant and at other times abundant. Usually, well-defined fibrous strands are present, creating lobules of neoplastic cells. The septa are infiltrated with lymphocytes in 80% of cases (Fig. 23–12). In about 20% of tumors, the septa also bear prominent granulomatous reactions, i.e., aggregates of histiocytes enclosed within a rim of fibroblasts, lymphocytes, and occasional foreign body giant cells. The lymphocytic and granulomatous reactions are believed to reflect an immune response, and there is evidence that the richer these features, the better is the prognosis.

The anaplastic seminoma, as the name indicates, presents greater cellular and nuclear irregularity with more frequent tumor giant cells and many mitoses. Most critical to the identification of this pattern are the size of the cells and the presence of three or more mitoses per high-power field. Well-developed lymphocytic and granulomatous reactions are infrequent.

SPERMATOCYTIC SEMINOMA

Although related by name, there is little in common between spermatocytic and classic seminomas. Both clinically and histologically, spermatocytic seminoma appears to be a distinctive tumor, and as such its separation from classic seminoma in the W.H.O. classification seems justified. It is an uncommon tumor, the reported incidence being approximately 4 to 6% of all seminomas. The age of involvement is much later than for most testicular tumors: affected individuals are mostly over the age of 65 years. Unlike classic seminoma, it is a slow-growing tumor that rarely if ever produces metastases, and hence the prognosis is excellent.

Grossly, spermatocytic seminoma tends to be larger than classic seminoma and presents with a pale gray, soft, and friable cut surface. As compared with classic seminoma, the cut surface is more often mucoid and areas of cystic degeneration are common. Spermatocytic seminomas have three cell populations, all intermixed: (1) medium-sized (15 to 18 μ), the most numerous, which contain a round nucleus and eosinophilic cytoplasm; (2) smaller cells (6 to 8 μ), with a narrow rim of eosinophilic cytoplasm resembling secondary spermatocytes; and (3) scattered giant cells (50 to 100 μ), either uni- or multinucleate. Thus, marked variation in tumor cell size is an important microscopic feature. Unlike classic seminomas, there are no lymphocytes in the tumor, and the mitoses are more common. Under the electron microscope, tumor cells show nuclear and cytoplasmic features of spermatocytic maturation, thus justifying the term spermatocytic seminoma.

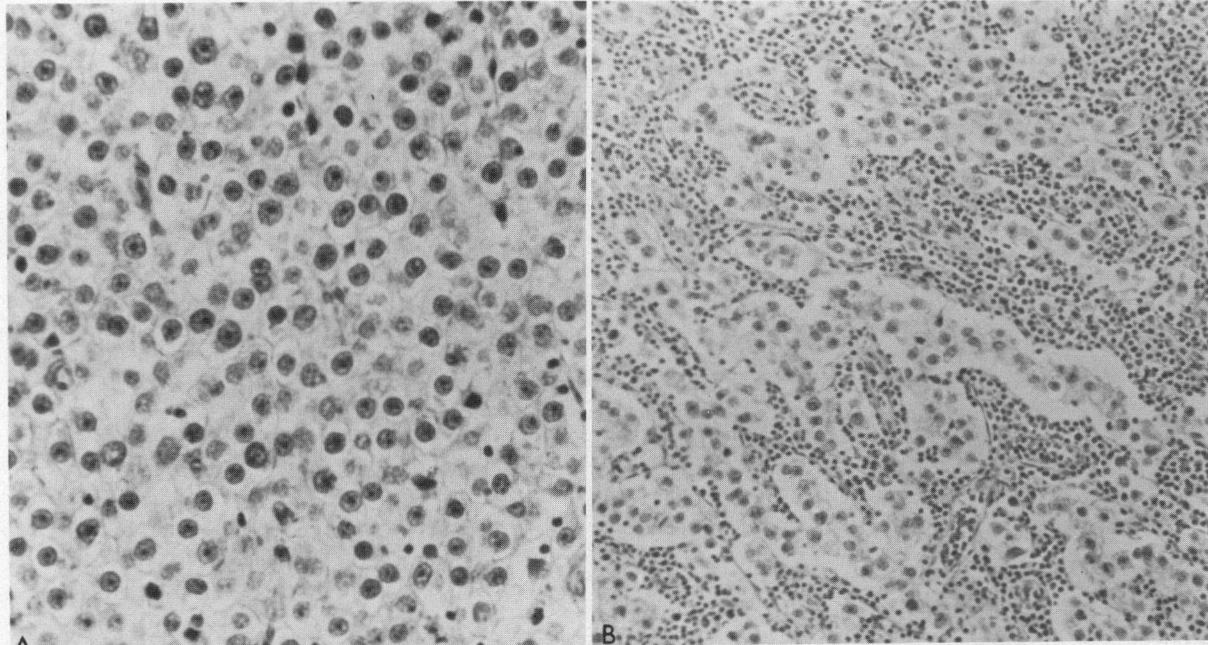

Figure 23–12. *A,* Microscopic detail of large, cleared seminoma cells. *B,* Seminoma with abundant lymphoid infiltrate.

EMBRYONAL CARCINOMA

Embryonal carcinomas represent approximately 20% of testicular tumors and occur mostly in the 20- to 30-year age group. Although considerable progress has been made in treating these tumors with chemotherapy, they are more aggressive and lethal than typical seminomas.

Grossly, the tumor is often a small lesion that does not replace the entire testes. Larger, bulky tumors may be found, but are the exception. On cut surfaces the mass is basically gray-white, but often variegated, poorly demarcated at the margins, and punctuated by foci of hemorrhage or necroses (Fig. 23–13). Extension into the epididymis or cord is not infrequent. **Histologically, the cells grow in glandular, alveolar, or tubular patterns, sometimes with papillary convolutions** (Fig. 23–14). **More undifferentiated lesions may present sheets of cells.** The neoplastic cells have an epithelial appearance and are large, anaplastic, and embryonic in aspect, with angry-looking hyperchromatic nuclei having prominent nucleoli. Unlike the case with seminoma, the cell borders are usually indistinct and there is considerable variation in cell and nuclear size and shape. Mitotic figures and tumor giant cells are frequent. Occasionally, syncytial giant cells are present, which then may contain HCG. Immunocytochemical studies also demonstrate the presence of alpha-fetoprotein (AFP) in the tumor cells.[25] The stroma may be scant or abundant, and loose or hyalinized; however, it does not contain lymphocytes as seen in seminomas.

YOLK SAC TUMOR

Also known as infantile embryonal carcinoma or endodermal sinus tumor, the yolk sac tumor is the most common testicular tumor in infants and children. In adults, the pure form of this tumor is rare; more often it occurs in combination with embryonal carcinoma.

Grossly, the tumor is nonencapsulated, and on cross section it presents a homogeneous, yellow-white, mucinous appearance. Characteristic on microscopic examination are spaces of varying size lined by flattened-to-cuboidal epithelial cells. In addition, papillary structures or solid cords of cells may be found. In some tumors the so-called endodermal sinuses may be seen: these consist of a mesodermal core with a central capillary and a visceral and parietal layer of cells resembling primitive glomeruli. More typically the tumor cells have vacuolated cytoplasm, and in some cases the vacuoles coalesce to form large cleared spaces. Present within and outside the cytoplasm are eosinophilic, hyaline-like globules in which AFP and alpha-1-antitrypsin can be demonstrated by immunocytochemical staining. The presence of AFP in the tumor cells is highly characteristic and it underscores their differentiation into yolk sac cells.

POLYEMBRYOMA

This tumor in its pure form is extremely rare. Most often it forms a component of embryonal carcinoma or teratoma. It consists of so-called "embryoid bodies" that may appear in the form of a disc, a cavity, or a tubular

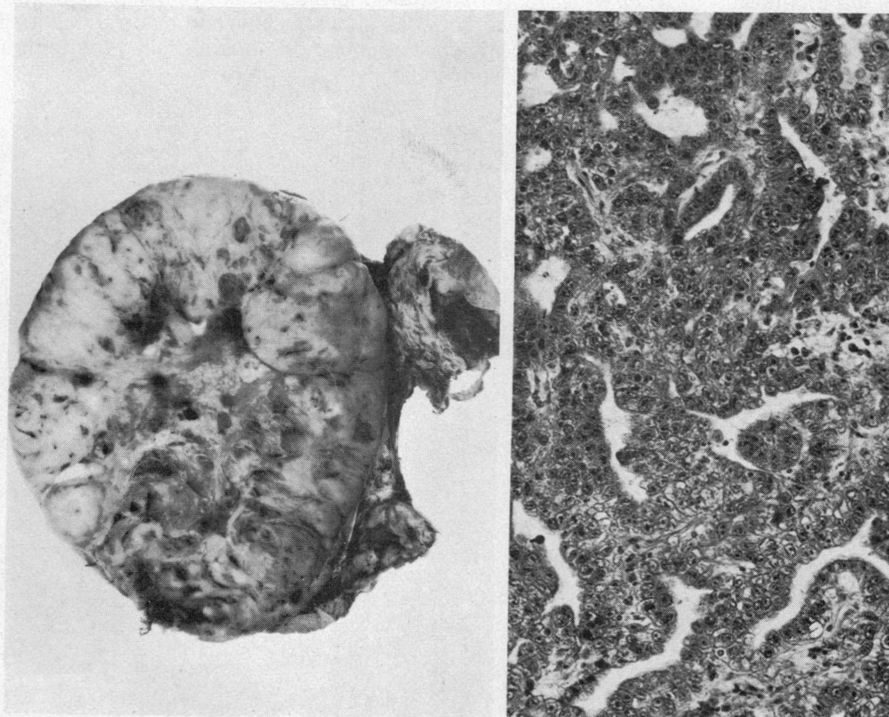

Fig. 23–13 Fig. 23–14

Figure 23–13. Embryonal carcinoma with extensive mottled necrosis and hemorrhage.
Figure 23–14. Embryonal carcinoma growing in glandular and papillary fashion.

structure. The disc resembles embryonic disc and is made up of undifferentiated, large epithelial cells; the cavity that represents the amniotic space is lined by flattened epithelial cells. These embryoid structures are surrounded by loose mesenchyme in which trophoblastic elements may be seen.

CHORIOCARCINOMA

This highly malignant form of testicular tumor is composed of both cytotrophoblast and syncytiotrophoblast; *both cell types must be present to enable the diagnosis to be made.* Identical tumors may arise in the placental tissue, ovary, or sequestered rests of totipotential cells, e.g., in the mediastinum or abdomen. Fortunately, in its "pure" form it is a rare testicular tumor. As emphasized later, foci of choriocarcinoma are much more common in mixed patterns.

Despite their aggressive behavior, pure choriocarcinomas are usually small lesions. **Often they cause no testicular enlargement and are detected only as a small palpable nodule.** Because they are rapidly growing, they may outgrow their blood supply, and sometimes the primary testicular focus is replaced by a small fibrous scar, leaving only widespread metastases. On the other hand, the primary lesion may be a hemorrhagic, large bulky mass of clotted blood in which tiny bits of gray tumor, or indeed no tumor, can be identified. It is the necrotic hemorrhagic appearance that is most characteristic of these neoplasms. Histologically, one must find the two cell types. The syncytiotrophoblastic cell is large and has many irregular or lobular hyperchromatic nuclei and an abundant eosinophilic vacuolated cytoplasm. As might be expected, HCG can be readily demonstrated in the cytoplasm of syncytiotrophoblastic cells. The cytotrophoblastic cells are more regular and tend to be polygonal with distinct cell borders and clear cytoplasm; they grow in cords or masses and have a single, fairly uniform nucleus. Often the syncytial cells cap a cluster of cytotrophoblastic cells, but well-formed placental villi are never seen. These viable tumor cells are generally scattered within large areas of hemorrhage or necrotic tumor, or both. More anatomic details are available in the discussion of these neoplasms in the female genital tract (p. 1151).

TERATOMA

The designation teratoma refers to a group of complex tumors having various cellular or organoid components reminiscent of normal derivatives from more than one germ layer. They may occur at any age from infancy to adult life. Indeed, teratomas are some of the more common tumors in infants and children; in adults they make up about 10% of testicular neoplasms. These tumors are derived from totipotential cells having the capacity to differentiate into elements representative of any of the three germ layers—ectoderm, mesoderm, and endoderm.

Histologically, three variants based on the degree of differentiation are recognized.[26]

Mature teratomas are composed of a heterogeneous, helter-skelter collection of differentiated cells or organoid structures such as neural tissue, muscle bundles, islands of cartilage, clusters of squamous epithelium, structures reminiscent of thyroid gland, bronchial or bronchiolar epithelium, and bits of intestinal wall or brain substance, all embedded in a fibrous or myxoid stroma (Fig. 23–15). All the elements are differentiated and present no evidence of potentially malignant, more embryonic cells. This mature variant occurs with relatively greater frequency in infancy and childhood. Similar tumors may occur in adults, but there is a far greater risk of small hidden foci of immature or malignant components that may escape detection despite rigorous sampling of the lesion. Thus, although teratomas may appear entirely mature and benign, such a diagnosis in an adult must be made with circumspection. Dermoid cysts, common in the ovary (p. 1149), are rare in the testis. They represent a special form of mature teratoma.

Immature teratomas can be viewed as intermediate between mature teratoma and embryonal carcinoma. Unlike the mature teratoma, elements of the three germ cell layers are incompletely differentiated and not arranged in organoid fashion. Even though the differentiation is incomplete, the nature of the embryonic tissue can be clearly identified; thus, poorly formed cartilage, neuroblasts, loose mesenchyme, and clusters of glandular structures may be seen lying helter-skelter. In some areas, more mature forms of these tissues may also be seen. Although these tumors are clearly malignant, the tissue elements may not show the cytologic features of malignancy. In contrast, the third variant—**teratoma with malignant transformation**–shows clear evidence of

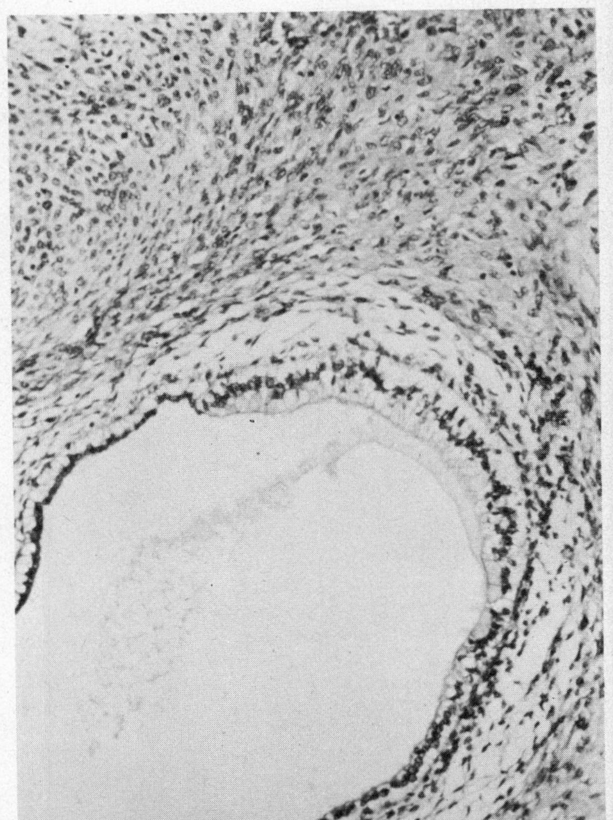

Figure 23–15. Mature teratoma with (1) a well-developed columnar-lined epithelial cyst *(below)* reminiscent of bronchial epithelium, (2) an island of immature chondroid tissue *(upper left),* and (3) a loose-to-compact fibrous stroma.

malignancy in derivatives of one or more germ cell layers. Thus, there may be a focus of squamous cell carcinoma, mucin-secreting adenocarcinoma, or a sarcoma. Immature and frankly malignant teratomas occur more commonly in adults.

Owing to the wide variety of tissues present in teratomas, the gross appearance is understandably variable. Teratomas, whether mature or immature, reveal on gross inspection a variegated cut surface with minute cysts, islands of translucent cartilage, and possibly foci of bone, all embedded within a gray-white solid matrix (Fig. 23–16). They often cause testicular enlargement, sometimes producing bulky masses.

In the child, differentiated mature teratomas may be expected to behave as benign tumors, and almost all these patients have a good prognosis. In the adult, it is difficult to be certain because, as pointed out, even apparently differentiated mature teratomas may harbor minute foci of cancer. It would require meticulous serial-sectioning of all these large neoplasms to uncover the small foci of cancer in some. Thus, some writers say that all teratomas in the adult should be considered malignant. Clinical experience has proved, however, that some solid mature teratomas are indeed benign and capable of local excision, with cure following orchiectomy.

MIXED TUMORS

About 40% of testicular tumors are composed of more than one of the "pure" patterns. The most common mixture is that of teratoma and embryonal carcinoma, which constitutes 25% of all testicular neoplasms to which the designation *teratocarcinoma* has been applied. Much less often, the teratoma has varying components of embryonal carcinoma, seminoma, or choriocarcinoma, as well as sarcomatous elements and sometimes several of these features together. Combinations of seminoma and embryonal carcinoma may also appear. These varied mixtures are indicated by the elements that they contain. In most instances the prognosis is worsened by the inclusion of more aggressive elements: e.g., the teratoma with a focus of choriocarcinoma has an outlook worse than that of pure teratoma, but better than that of pure choriocarcinoma. It is noteworthy that metastases of these mixed tumors may be composed of only one or more of the various neoplastic components, and indeed a new line of differentiation sometimes appears.

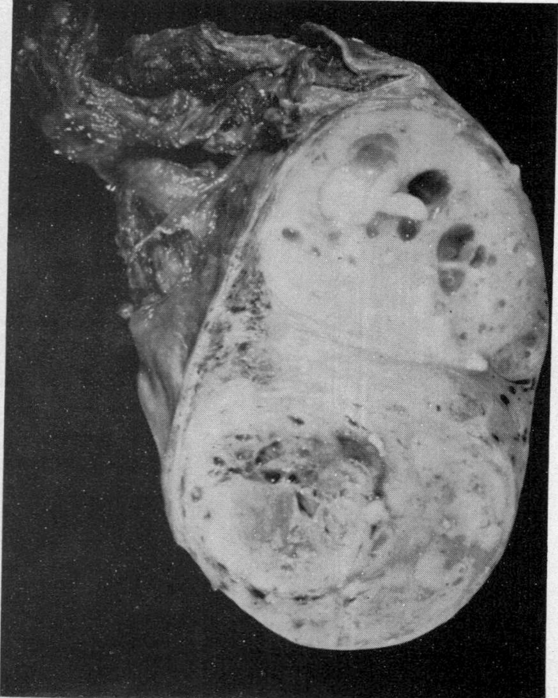

Figure 23–16. Teratoma of testis. The variegated cut surface reflects the multiplicity of tissue found histologically.

CLINICAL FEATURES. Testicular tumors present most often as *painless enlargement of the testis*. Indeed, any testicular mass should be considered neoplastic unless proved otherwise. Clinical differentiation between various types of germ cell tumors is at best imperfect since there are no distinctive clinical features to the testicular masses produced by these tumors. As mentioned earlier, the rare choriocarcinoma may not cause any testicular enlargement but instead may reveal its ominous nature by presenting with widespread metastasis. Only a small fraction of the other testicular tumors manifest initially with symptoms referable to distant metastasis. Tumors of the testis have a characteristic mode of spread, knowledge of which is helpful in clinical staging as well as treatment. In general, testicular tumors initially involve the common iliac and paraortic nodes, and later spread to mediastinal and supraclavicular lymph nodes. Tumors that extend to the epididymis may spread to the external iliac nodes. Seminomas typically spread via the lymphatic route after having remained localized for a long time. Visceral involvement with seminomas is usually a late event. In contrast, embryonal carcinomas not only metastasize earlier but also utilize the hematogenous route more frequently. Thus, lymph nodes, liver, and lungs may be involved. Choriocarcinoma, the most aggressive variant, spreads predominantly via the bloodstream, and therefore lungs and liver are involved early in virtually every case. Although most testicular tumors retain the morphologic appearance of the primary in the metastatic foci, the histology of metastases may sometimes be different from that of the testicular lesion. Such divergence could indeed result from inadequate sampling of the primary, but in some instances the difference is real. Thus, a mature teratoma may show foci of embryonal carcinoma or choriocarcinoma in the lymph nodes, and conversely embryonal carcinoma may present a teratomatous picture in the secondary deposits. As discussed earlier (p. 1090), if one accepts the view that all these tumors are derived from the neoplastic germ cells, the apparent "forward" and "backward" differentiation seen in different locations is not entirely surprising.

STAGING AND MARKERS OF GERM CELL TUMORS. Unfortunately, there is no uniformly accepted method of staging these tumors. Basically, two forms of staging classifications exist. The TNM classification is complex and not yet widely used.[27] Most others define three stages based on whether the tumor is confined to the testis (Stage I), has spread to the nodes below the diaphragm (Stage II), or has spread to distant sites (Stage III). One such scheme is presented in Table 23–2.[25]

Major advances in the diagnosis, staging, and management of testicular germ cell tumors have been made possible by the development of sensitive and specific assays for the detection of tumor-associated polypeptides.[25] Germ cell testicular cancers are associated with the production of AFP and HCG. AFP, a protein with a molecular weight of 70,000, is the major serum protein of the early fetus and is synthesized by the fetal gut, liver cells, and yolk sac. One year after birth, the serum levels of AFP fall to less than 16 ng per ml, which is undetectable except by the most sensitive assays. HCG is a glycoprotein consisting of two dissimilar polypeptide units called alpha and beta. It is normally synthesized and secreted by the placental syncytiotrophoblast. The beta subunit of HCG has unique sequences not shared with other human glycoprotein hormones, and therefore the detection of HCG in the serum is based on a radioimmunoassay using antibodies to its beta chain. As might be expected from the histogenesis and morphology, elevated levels of these markers are most often associated with nonseminomatous tumors. In one large series,[25] 7% of seminomas, 44% of teratomas, 88% of embryonal carcinomas, 86% of teratocarcinomas, and 75% of yolk sac tumors, and all cases of choriocarcinoma demonstrated elevated levels of serum HCG and/or AFP. Yolk sac tumors produce AFP exclusively, and choriocarcinomas elaborate only HCG, whereas most patients with teratoma, embryonal carcinoma, and teratocarcinoma (but not all) have elevations of both AFP and HCG simultaneously. Patients with nonseminomatous tumors who do not have increased levels of these tumor markers usually have minimal disease.[28] Studies of tumor markers, in addition to their value in diagnosis, are also helpful in staging and follow-up. For example, an elevated serum level following orchiectomy is a clear indication of Stage II disease; similarly, serial measurements of marker levels after therapy often can predict recurrences well in advance of clinical relapse.

Table 23–2 STAGING OF TESTICULAR TUMORS

Stage I Local Spread	
P1	Confined to testis
P2	Involvement of testicular adnexa
P3	Involvement of scrotal wall
Stage II Confined to Retroperitoneal Lymphatics	
N1	Microscopic
N2	Gross involvement without capsular invasion
N3	Gross involvement with capsular invasion
N4	Massive involvement of retroperitoneal structures
Stage III Beyond Retroperitoneum	
M1	Solitary metastasis
M2	Multiple metastasis

P = primary lesion

The presence of elevated serum HCG levels in some patients with seminoma is not fully understood. Could all the serum HCG be produced by the syncytial giant cells known to occur in some seminomas, or should one suspect a mixed tumor with elements of choriocarcinoma? Alternatively, one might suspect the presence of nonseminomatous metastasis, which admittedly is not common. Definite answers are not yet available, but some authorities believe that the presence of elevated serum HCG in a patient with seminoma calls for a more aggressive therapeutic approach.[25]

The therapy and prognosis of testicular tumors depend largely on clinical stage and to some extent on the histologic type. Seminoma, which is extremely radiosensitive and tends to remain localized for long periods, has the best prognosis. More than 90% of patients with Stage I and II disease can be cured. According to some investigators, the prognosis for anaplastic seminomas is similar to that of classic seminoma for the same stage of disease.[29] Others, however, consider the anaplastic variant to be a more aggressive tumor.[30] Among nonseminomatous tumors, the histologic subtype does not influence the prognosis significantly, and hence these are treated as a group. Although they do not share the good prognosis of seminoma, studies report considerable success in achieving significant remissions with aggressive chemotherapy.[31] Currently, a 75% to 90% two-year survival rate for Stage I disease, and 50% two-year survival rate for Stage II disease, is being reported.

TUMORS OF SEX CORD–GONADAL STROMA

As indicated in Table 23–1, these tumors are subclassified on the basis of their presumed histogenesis and differentiation. The two most important members of this group—Leydig cell tumors (derived from the stroma) and Sertoli cell tumors (derived from the sex cord)—are described here.

Leydig (Interstitial) Cell Tumors

Tumors of Leydig cells are particularly interesting because they may elaborate androgens or androgens and estrogens and, indeed, some tumors have also elaborated corticosteroids. As might be expected, the tumor cells are rich in enzymes and 11- and 17-beta-hydroxylases; 17-alpha-hydroxylase, as well as other steroidogenic enzymes normally found in interstitial and adrenal cortical cells, has been identified in these tumors. They make up about 2% of testicular tumors and may arise at any age. In children they may induce precocious masculinization or, less often, feminization. In adults the only hormonal influence detectable is gynecomastia.

These neoplasms range from small nodules less than 1 cm in diameter to bulky masses 10 cm in diameter. Bilateral neoplasms are encountered in 5 to 10% of patients. On cut surface they can often be recognized by a distinctive, uniform, yellow-brown hue.

Histologically, Leydig cells usually are remarkably similar to their normal forebears. They are large, round, or polygonal, and have an abundant granular eosinophilic cytoplasm and a round central nucleus. Cell boundaries are often indistinct. **The cytoplasm frequently contains lipid granules, vacuoles, or lipochrome pigment, but, most characteristically, rod-shaped crystalloids of Reinke occur in about half the tumors.** Although the cells are most often found in diffuse sheets or masses, sometimes cords or nests appear separated by a fibrous or hyaline stroma. As in the case of other endocrine tumors, they may display variability in cell and nuclear size and shape, often with bi- or multinucleate cells. These do not necessarily indicate that the tumor is malignant: most are benign; only 10% are invasive and produce metastases.

Sertoli Cell Tumors (Androblastoma)

These tumors may be composed entirely of Sertoli cells or may have a component of granulosa cells. Some induce endocrinologic changes. Either estrogens or androgens may be elaborated but only infrequently in sufficient quantity to cause precocious masculinization or feminization. Occasionally, as with Leydig cell tumors, gynecomastia appears.

These neoplasms may appear as firm, small nodules or rarely as bulky masses causing considerable testicular enlargement. On cross section the surface is homogeneous gray-white to yellow. Histologically, in the classic form the cells are quite distinctive and are either tall, columnar, or polyhedral, having abundant, usually vacuolated cytoplasm. Uniformity of cell size and shape is the rule, and mitoses and giant cells are rare. Quite distinctive is the tendency for these cells to grow in cords highly reminiscent of spermatic tubules. Variations on this theme may occur in the form of foci of spindled theca-like cells or areas of small cuboidal cells having a follicular arrangement reminiscent of granulosa cell tumors (p. 1152). The great majority of Sertoli cell tumors are benign, but occasional tumors (approximately 10%) are more anaplastic and pursue a malignant course.

TESTICULAR LYMPHOMA

Although not primarily a tumor of the testis, testicular lymphoma is included here since affected patients present with only a testicular mass. *Lymphomas account for 5% of testicular neoplasms and constitute the most common form of testicular cancer in elderly men.* In most cases, disseminated disease follows detection of the testicular mass, but in some the tumor remains confined to the testis.[32] The histologic pattern of the tumors is diffuse in *almost all* the cases and the predominant cell type is diffuse histocytic (in the Rappaport classification, p. 660). Less common tumors made up of other cell types, discussed on page 659, may also be seen. The prognosis is extremely poor, unless after appropriate staging procedures the disease is found to be confined to the testis.

ADENOMATOID TUMORS

These are benign, slow-growing nodules that arise in the epididymis. They usually have an encapsulated, firm, gray-white macroscopic appearance and are rarely larger than a few centimeters in size. On microscopic examination, they contain variable amounts of stroma and an admixture of cells that seem to have an epithelial origin. In some instances, these apparent epithelial cuboidal cells line cystic spaces. At other times, they form small apparent glandular patterns; at still other times, they are disposed in cords and nests. Occasionally, these cells contain vacuoles that do not react with the usual fat or glycogen stains. Tumors of identical gross and histologic appearance also occur on the serosal surface of the fallopian tubes and the uterus. The origin of these uncommon tumors is believed to be from the mesothelium, although other origins have been considered, including that from müllerian duct vestiges, endothelium, and mesonephric ducts.

MISCELLANEOUS LESIONS OF TUNICA VAGINALIS

Brief mention should be made of the tunica vaginalis. As a serosa-lined sac immediately proximal to the testis and epididymis, it may become involved by any lesion arising in these two structures. Clear serous fluid may accumulate from neighboring infections or tumors (*hydrocele*). Usually about 100 ml of fluid is found, but amounts of up to 300 ml, rarely larger, have been described. The tunica may fill up with fluids when there is systemic edema, as in cardiac failure or renal disease; at other times, when the processus vaginalis has failed to close completely, peritoneal fluid may seep in and

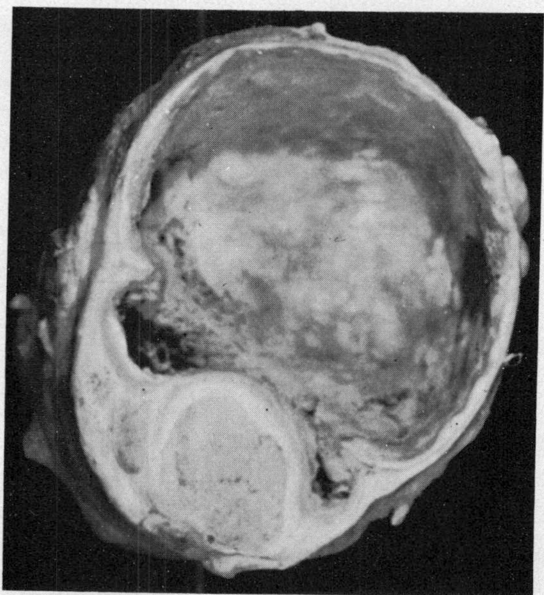

Figure 23–17. An infected hydrocele sac. The wall is thick and fibrous and has a shaggy lining.

accumulate. Considerable enlargement of the scrotal sac is produced, which can be readily mistaken for testicular enlargement. However, by transillumination it is usually possible to define the clear, translucent character of the contained substance, and many times the opaque testis can be outlined within this fluid-filled space. When infected, as in the course of a tap or by the extension of organisms directly from infections within the testis or epididymis or through the lymphohematogenous route, the serosa-lined membrane may be converted to a shaggy, thickened, fibrous wall and the serous fluid may be transformed to frank pus (Fig. 23–17). In the course of time, overgrowth of the organisms may halt their multiplication, and the process may undergo autosterilization with organization of the exudate and destruction of the original serosa-lined space.

Hematocele indicates the presence of blood in the tunica vaginalis. It is an uncommon condition usually encountered only when there has been either direct trauma to the testis or torsion of the testis with hemorrhagic suffusion into the surrounding vaginalis, or in hemorrhagic diseases associated with widespread bleeding diatheses. Tumorous invasion may evoke a hydrohematocele.

Chylocele refers to the accumulation of lymphatic fluid in the tunica and is almost always found only in patients with elephantiasis who have widespread and severe lymphatic obstruction. For clarity's sake, mention should be made of the *spermatocele* and *varicocele*, which refer respectively to small cystic accumulations of either semen or blood in the spermatic cord. In the spermatocele, the cyst usually represents a dilatation of one of the ducts in the head of the epididymis; in the case of varicocele, it might be more properly described as a cystic varix of one of the veins of the spermatic cord.

Prostate

NORMAL

In the normal adult, the prostate weighs approximately 20 gm. It is a retroperitoneal organ encircling the neck of the bladder and urethra and is devoid of a distinct capsule. Classically, the prostate has been divided into five lobes, to which are attributed distinctive significance in the development of tumors and benign enlargements. These five lobes include a posterior, middle, and anterior lobe and two lateral lobes. However, other investigators deny the clear definition of these five lobes and suggest that, in the course of development, the five become fused into only three distinct lobes—two major lateral lobes and a small median lobe, which presumably includes the classic posterior lobe. Cross section of the gland, however, fails to disclose well-defined lobes, and only two lateral masses can be found on either side of the urethra, as well as a much thinner median lobe, which forms the floor of the urethra. In the normal adult, the prostate has a homogeneous, pale gray, cut surface in which it is possible with a low-power lens to identify small, discrete, yellow-white, minute cystic areas representing prostatic glands from which may be extruded, by slight pressure, a milky fluid.

Histologically, the prostate is a compound tubuloalveolar gland, which, in one plane of section, presents small to fairly large glandular spaces lined by epithelium. Characteristically, the glands are lined by two layers of cells: a basal layer of low cuboidal epithelium covered by a layer of columnar mucus-secreting cells. Ultrastructurally, the usual organelles are present as well as electron-dense granules, which yield positive reactions for acid phosphatase.[33] In many areas, there are small villous projections or papillary inbuddings of the epithelium. These glands all have a distinct basement membrane and are separated by an abundant fibromuscular stroma. McNeal has called attention to two apparently distinct glandular divisions within the prostate:[34] (1) the central zone, which has its apex at the verumontanum and its base above and behind the bladder neck; and (2) a peripheral zone, which lies more caudally and more peripheral to the central zone and which partially encloses the apex of the latter (Fig. 23–18). Microscopically the central zone acini are large and have irregular contours with prominent intraluminal projections, whereas the acini in the peripheral zone are small, round, and simple. The central zone, which forms about 25% of the glandular mass, may be derived embryologically from the wolffian duct. McNeal also defines a transitional zone, which is a small wedge of tissue lying immediately lateral to the lower end of the pre-prostatic sphincter. This sphincter, you may recall, is a cylindrical sheath of smooth muscle surrounding the urethra between the bladder above and the verumontanum below. This division of the prostate into separate zones has some significance in the etiology of prostatic diseases. Thus, benign prostatic hyperplasia almost always begins in the transitional zone and the adjacent submucosal tissue of the periurethral gland region. The central zone seems to be immune from disease processes, whereas the peripheral zone is the site of prostatitis and, more important, prostatic cancer. Of interest

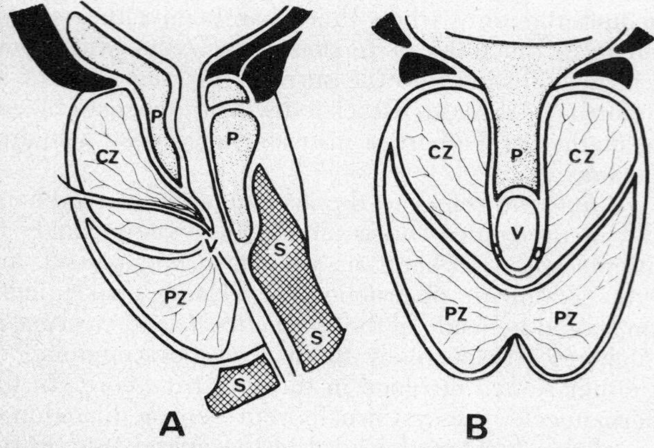

Figure 23–18. Diagrams of midline sagittal section through urethra *(A)* and coronal section behind urethra of human prostate *(B)*. P = pre-prostatic sphincter; S = striated sphincter of urethra and external sphincter; V = verumontanum or colliculus; CZ = central zone; PZ = peripheral zone. (From Blacklock, N. J.: Prostate cancer. Morphology in health and disease. Recent Results Cancer Res. *78*:22, 1981. Reproduced with permission.)

is the finding that the peripheral zone equivalent in primates has significantly greater androgen receptor sites.[35] Could this and other endocrine and/or metabolic differences among various zones be responsible for the difference in disease susceptibility? Future studies will tell.

The prostate is an endocrine-dependent organ. However, our knowledge of its endocrine relationships is still somewhat confused. Testicular androgens are clearly of prime importance in controlling prostatic growth since castration leads to atrophy of the prostate. There is some evidence that prolactin acts synergistically with androgens. In addition, normal prostate cells have cytoplasmic receptors for estrogens and progesterone, hinting at a possible influence of the female sex hormones. This is also suggested by the therapeutic effect of estrogen on the growth of prostatic cancer. It is beyond our scope to delve into the complexities of the hormonal effects and relationships in the normal prostate physiology; these may be found in a review by Coffey and Isaacs.[36]

PATHOLOGY

The only three pathologic processes that affect the prostate gland with sufficient frequency to merit discussion are inflammation, benign nodular enlargement, and tumors. Of these three, the benign nodular enlargements are by far the most common and occur so often in advanced age that they can almost be construed as a "normal" aging process. Prostatic carcinoma is also an extremely common lesion in the male and one, therefore, that merits careful consideration. The inflammatory processes are, for the most part, of much less clinical significance and can be treated briefly.

INFLAMMATIONS

Prostatitis may be divided into nonspecific acute and chronic prostatitis and granulomatous prostatitis.

NONSPECIFIC ACUTE AND CHRONIC PROSTATITIS

Acute prostatitis consists of an acute focal or diffuse suppurative inflammation in the prostatic substance. The bacteria responsible are similar in type and in incidence to those that cause urinary tract infections (UTI). Thus, most cases are caused by various strains of *E. coli.* Most of the remaining infections are due to Klebsiella, Proteus, Pseudomonas, Enterobacter, and Serratia. Among gram-positive bacteria, only Enterococcus is significant as a causative agent. These organisms become implanted in the prostate usually by direct extension from the posterior urethra or from the urinary bladder, but occasionally seed the prostate by the lymphohematogenous routes from distant foci of infection. Invasion from the rectum has also been proposed. One of the most common clinical sequences encountered is prostatitis following some surgical manipulation on the urethra or prostate gland itself, such as catheterization, cystoscopy, urethral dilatation, or resection procedures on the prostate.

Even more significant clinically than acute prostatitis is chronic prostatitis, because it is frequently recurrent and is probably the most common cause of relapsing UTI in men.[37] Two major types of chronic prostatitis are recognized: chronic bacterial prostatitis and abacterial prostatitis, sometimes called "prostatosis." These two patterns of the disease may mimic each other clinically, but only the bacterial variant predisposes to UTI.[37] The mode of development of chronic bacterial prostatitis is not well understood. In a minority of cases it represents a sequel to acute prostatitis. In some cases it follows urethral or prostatic manipulation, sometimes without a well-defined episode of acute inflammation. However, in the great majority of instances it appears insidiously and without obvious provocation. The implicated organisms are the same as those cited as causes of acute prostatitis. Chronic abacterial prostatitis is the most common form of prostatitis seen today.[38] Affected patients rarely have a preceding UTI and the causative organisms remain untracked. With the recognition that Ureaplasma species and *Chlamydia trachomatis* may give rise to nongonococcal urethritis (p. 1078), these two are considered the prime suspects in the causation of chronic abacterial prostatitis.

Acute prostatitis may appear as minute, disseminated abscesses; as large, coalescent focal areas of necrosis; or as a diffuse edema, congestion, and boggy suppuration of the entire gland. When these reactions are fairly diffuse, they cause an overall soft, spongy enlargement of the gland.

Histologically, depending on the duration and severity of the inflammation, there may be minimal stromal leukocytic infiltrate accompanied by increased elaboration of prostatic secretion or leukocytic infiltration within gland spaces (Fig. 23–19). When abscess formation has occurred, focal or large areas of the prostatic substance may become necrotic. Such inflammatory reactions may totally subside and leave behind only some fibrous scarring. These acute reactions may become chronic, particularly when the excretory ducts are plugged and the infection continues to smolder within walled-off minute abscesses in the prostatic substance.

Chronic prostatitis, when correctly diagnosed, should be restricted to those cases of inflammatory reaction in the prostate characterized by the aggregation of numerous lymphocytes, plasma cells, and macrophages, as well as neutrophils, within the prostatic substance. It should be pointed out that, in the normal aging process, aggregations of lymphocytes are prone to appear in the fibromuscular stroma of this gland. All too often, such nonspecific aggregates are diagnosed as chronic prostatitis, even though the pathognomonic inflammatory cells, i.e., the macrophages and neutrophils, are not present.

Chronic prostatitis is a much more common condition than the acute form. Both may cause local symptoms—low back pain, discomfort, dysuria, frequency, urgency, and prostatic enlargement and tenderness—but very often the chronic disease is asymptomatic. Their major significance derives from their seeding the urinary tract with organisms. Thus, any male patient with recurrent UTI, especially when it is caused by a single pathogen, must be evaluated for the possible presence of one of these forms of prostatic involvement.

GRANULOMATOUS PROSTATITIS

Two forms of granulomas are found in the prostate. Nonspecific granulomas may occur secondary to acute or chronic prostatitis. In these conditions, there may be inspissation of secretions, followed by surrounding focal aggregations of neutrophils, lymphocytes, histiocytes, and plasma cells, enclosed within a fibroblastic proliferative response. The granuloma production is further augmented by the appearance of foreign body giant cells. These granulomas do not have caseous centers, nor do they contain acid-fast bacilli. They are nonspecific inflammatory reactions to the accumulation of inspissated secretion or necrotic tissue. An autoimmune causation has also been postulated.

The other pattern of granulomatous prostatitis consists of tuberculosis of the prostate that almost invariably follows tuberculosis of some other region of the genitourinary tract, such as renal or urinary bladder tuberculosis. Less commonly, miliary spread to the prostate may occur from distant pulmonary tuberculosis. The microscopic appearance is usually dominated by extensive caseation necrosis along with the typical granulomatous reaction. In far-advanced cases, the process may destroy large areas of the prostate and extend into neighboring seminal vesicles. Considerable enlargement may attend such tuberculous prostatitis.

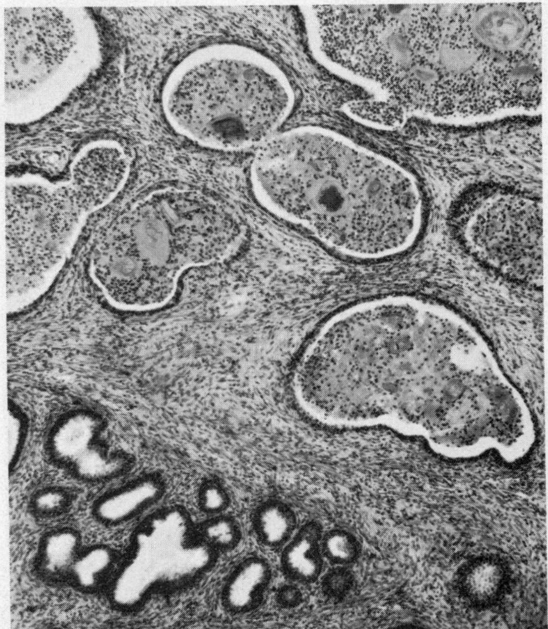

Figure 23–19. Acute prostatitis. Gland lumina are filled with neutrophils, and stroma contains a sprinkling of similar leukocytes.

BENIGN ENLARGEMENT

NODULAR HYPERPLASIA (BENIGN PROSTATIC HYPERTROPHY OR HYPERPLASIA)

Nodular hyperplasia, still referred to by the redundant term benign prostatic hyperplasia (all hyperplasias are benign), is an extremely common disorder in men over age 50. It is characterized by the formation of large, fairly discrete nodules in the periurethral region of the prostate. When sufficiently large, the nodules compress and narrow the urethral canal to cause partial, or sometimes virtually complete, obstruction of the urethra.

INCIDENCE. Although reports vary slightly, a careful survey of the prostate in an unselected series of postmortems disclosed nodular hyperplasia in approximately 50 to 60% of men 40 to 59 years of age and in more than 95% of those over age 70.[39] With this prevalence, it has been argued that nodular hyperplasia is not truly a disease but rather a normal aging process; this is a dilemma we can leave to the semanticists. Clinically significant nodular hyperplasia is much less prevalent. Not more than 5 to 10% of men with this condition require surgical treatment for relief of urinary tract obstruction; in the remainder the condition is of little clinical significance. For obscure reasons the disease appears about a decade earlier in blacks than in whites, and is somewhat more common in Protestants than in Jews and Catholics.

ETIOLOGY. Although the cause of nodular hyperplasia is still uncertain, the available evidence suggests that both androgens and estrogens are involved in its genesis.[40] Much evidence relating to the hormonal basis of nodular hyperplasia has been obtained in dogs, the only animal species that develops prostatic hyperplasia with aging. Both in humans and dogs, hyperplasia of the prostate develops only in the presence of intact testes. In castrated young dogs it is possible to induce prostatic hyperplasia by administration of androgens, an effect markedly enhanced by simultaneous administration of 17-beta-estradiol, thus pointing to possible synergism between androgens and estrogens. In humans as well as dogs, the content of dihydrotestosterone is markedly increased in the hyperplastic prostate. More important, its accumulation is selective in the periurethral region (where nodules arise) and within the nodules of prostatic hyperplasia. On the basis of these studies, it has been suggested that dihydrotestosterone may be the ultimate mediator of prostatic hyperplasia, but the events that lead to its accumulation are not entirely clear. Dihydrotestosterone within the prostate is derived from plasma testosterone, but there is no difference between levels of plasma testosterone in patients with prostatic hyperplasia and in age-matched controls; indeed, plasma testosterone levels decline after the age of 60 years. To explain this apparent paradox, it has been proposed that dihydrotestosterone accumulation in the hyperplastic gland results from increased binding to intracellular receptors and/or decreased catabolism.[40, 41] In dogs, administration of 17-beta-estradiol enhances the expression of cytoplasmic androgen receptors. Thus, the increase in the level of estrogens that occurs with aging may facilitate the accumulation of androgens within the prostate, even in the face of declining testicular output of testosterone. This hypothesis seems plausible and attempts to explain the role of androgens as well as the synergistic effects of estrogens, but formal proof is still lacking.[42]

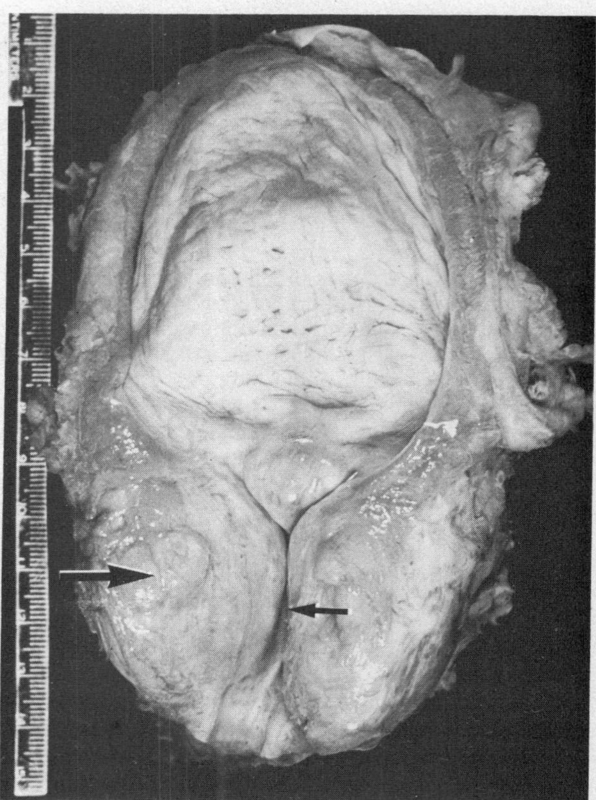

Figure 23–20. Nodular prostatic hyperplasia. Prostatic urethra and urinary bladder have been opened anteriorly to disclose enlarged prostatic gland that narrows urethral lumen to a slit *(small arrow)*. Note evident nodularity within prostatic gland *(large arrow)*. Urinary bladder is enlarged with hypertrophy of wall.

MORPHOLOGY. In the usual case of nodular enlargement, the prostatic nodules weigh between 60 and 100 gm. However, not uncommonly, aggregate weights of up to 200 gm are encountered, and even larger masses have been recorded. Careful studies by McNeal have demonstrated that nodular hyperplasia of the prostate originates almost exclusively in the pre-prostatic region. This area, which lies proximal to the verumontanum, includes the transitional zone described earlier, and the submucosal tissues of the periurethral gland region.[34] It corresponds to the "inner" periurethral portion of the classically defined middle and lateral lobes. From their origin in this strategic location, the nodular enlargements may encroach upon the lateral walls of the urethra to compress it to a slitlike orifice while, at the same time, nodular enlargement of the middle lobe may project up into the floor of the urethra as a hemispheric mass directly beneath the mucosa of the urethra (Fig. 23–20). At other times, the middle lobe enlargement may assume even a long, slender, delicate, polypoid appearance attached by a narrow neck; in many of these instances, it appears to act as a ball-valve obstruction to the mouth of the urethra.

On cross section of the affected prostate, the nodules usually are fairly readily identified because of the compression of the remainder of the prostatic tissue about the nodule (Fig. 23–21). As pointed out above they usually arise from the inner prostatic mass, and only rarely do they extend to

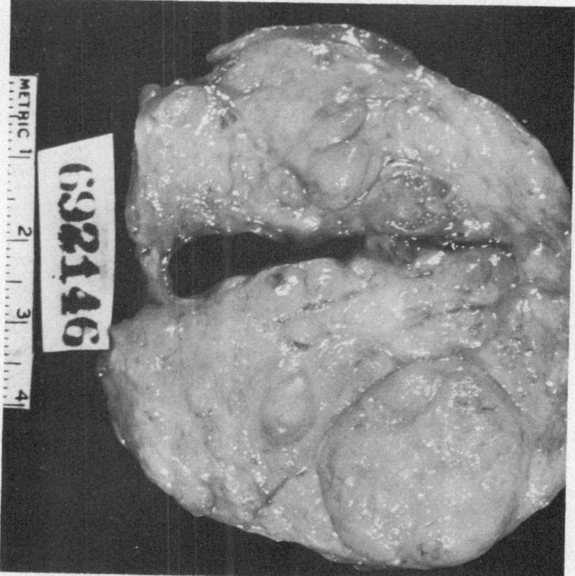

Figure 23–21. Nodular hyperplasia of prostate. Cut surface shows well-defined nodules of various sizes. (Courtesy of Dr. Fred Silva, Department of Pathology, University of Texas Health Science Center, Dallas.)

the outer perimeter of the gland. The nodule itself varies in color and consistency, depending, as will be shown, on whether it is primarily due to fibromuscular stromal hypertrophy and hyperplasia or to glandular proliferation. In those that are primarily glandular, the tissue has a yellow-pink soft consistency, which is fairly discretely demarcated from the more gray, glistening, firm, compressed prostatic capsule. Usually a milky-white prostatic fluid oozes out of these areas. In those primarily due to fibromuscular involvement, the nodule itself is also pale gray, tough, and fibrous; does not exude fluid; and is less clearly demarcated from the surrounding prostatic capsule.

Although the nodules do not have true capsules in the sense that benign neoplasms are encapsulated, the compressed surrounding prostatic tissue creates a plane of cleavage about them, utilized by the surgeon in the enucleation of prostatic masses in so-called suprapubic prostatectomies. A considerable amount of prostatic tissue remains behind so that, at a later date, it is entirely possible for recurrent nodules to develop or for the patient to develop a carcinoma.

Microscopically, **there are many patterns of nodular hyperplasia.** Ultimately, all are differentiated on the basis of whether the nodularity is due mainly to glandular proliferation or dilatation, or to fibrous or muscular proliferation of the stroma. All three elements are involved in almost every case although, in individual instances, one may predominate over the others. Usually the epithelial element predominates, and it takes the form of aggregations of small to large to cystically dilated glands, lined by two layers, an inner columnar and an outer cuboidal or flattened epithelium, based on an intact basement membrane (Fig. 23–22). The epithelium is characteristically thrown up into numerous papillary buds and infoldings, which are more prominent than in the normal prostate.

In certain cases, many small glands are formed that may simulate the pattern of adenocarcinoma. Usually the glandular size is sufficiently large to be visible on hand lens inspection of the tissue section. Frequently these glands contain inspissated secretion, granular desquamated epithelial cells, and numerous corpora amylacea. When the fibromuscular hypertrophy or hyperplasia predominates, it may produce aggregates of almost solid spindle cells, free of glands, that have sometimes been designated **fibrobromatous hyperplasia or leiomyomatous hyperplasia of the prostate.** However, such differentiation is probably not clinically useful. Not infrequently, aggregates of lymphocytes are found within the stroma, probably related to senile atrophic death of cells. Two other histologic changes are frequently found: (1) foci of squamous metaplasia and (2) small areas of infarction. The former tend to occur in the margins of the foci of infarction as nests of metaplastic, but orderly, squamous cells.

Clinical Course. Although nodular enlargement is an extremely common condition, it has been pointed out already that in only a small percentage of those

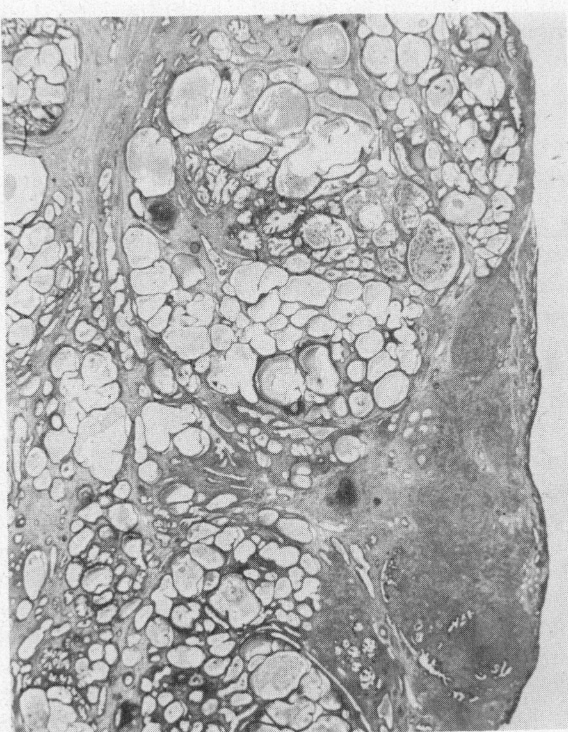

A

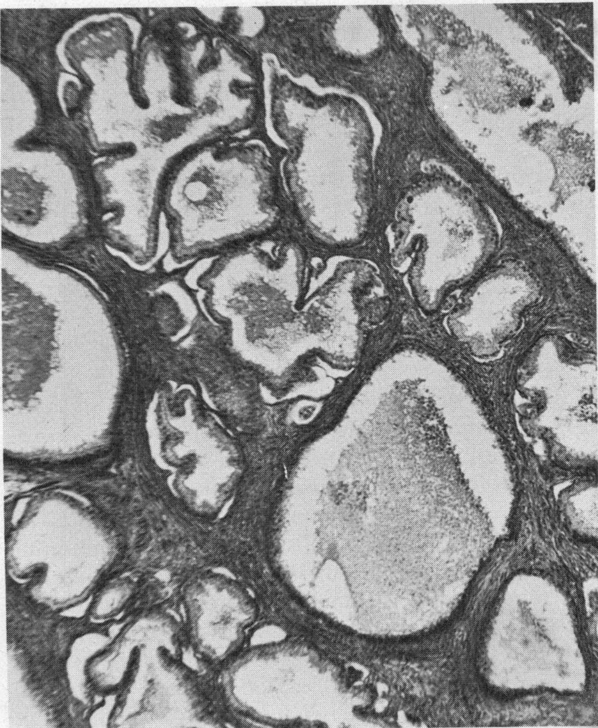

B

Figure 23–22. Nodular hyperplasia of prostate. *A,* Low-power view shows proliferation of glands, some cystically dilated, with formation of nodules. (Courtesy of Dr. Fred Silva, Department of Pathology, University of Texas Health Science Center, Dallas.) *B,* High-power view shows hyperplastic glands with single epithelial layer, thrown into small papillary folds.

affected does the lesion produce clinical symptoms. Symptoms, when produced, relate to two secondary effects: (1) compression of the urethra with difficulty in urination; and (2) retention of urine in the bladder with subsequent distention and hypertrophy of the bladder, infection of the urine, and the development of cystitis and renal infections.

These patients have frequency, nocturia, difficulty in starting and stopping the stream of urine, overflow dribbling, and dysuria (painful micturition). In many cases, sudden, acute urinary retention appears for unknown reasons and persists until the patient receives emergency catheterization. In addition to these difficulties in urination, prostatic enlargement results in the inability to empty the bladder completely. Presumably this is due to the raised level of the urethral floor so that, at the conclusion of micturition, a considerable amount of residual urine is left. This residual urine provides a static fluid that is vulnerable to infection. On this basis, catheterization or surgical manipulation provides a real danger of the introduction of organisms and development of pyelonephritis.

Many secondary changes occur in the bladder, such as hypertrophy, trabeculation, and diverticulum formation (p. 1067). Hydronephrosis or acute retention, with secondary UTI and even azotemia or uremia, may develop.

Finally, it should be noted that controversy persists as to whether nodular hyperplasia predisposes to cancer of the prostate. Most studies deny any association.[43] On the other hand, occasional reports suggest a higher than anticipated incidence of prostatic cancer in men with nodular hyperplasia.[44] It is impossible to reconcile these differences and the issue must be left with the opinion that the weight of evidence is against any causal relationship.

TUMORS

CARCINOMA

Carcinoma of the prostate is the second most common form of cancer in males and the third leading cause of cancer death. In addition to these lethal neoplasms, there is an even more frequent anatomic form of prostatic cancer in which the cancer is discovered as an incidental finding, either at postmortem examination or in a surgical specimen removed for other reasons, e.g., nodular hyperplasia. In almost all these instances, the lesions are small and sometimes comprise only microscopic foci. This form is sometimes called *latent cancer*. It has always been assumed, without proof, that these small lesions would in time become clinically significant, but, as discussed later, there is still some uncertainty about their natural history.

INCIDENCE. Cancer of the prostate is a disease of men over 50. The age-adjusted incidence in the United States is 69 per 100,000. Much more revealing, however, are the age-specific rates, which are 4.8 in the 45- to 49-year age group, but increase to a staggering 513 between the ages of 70 and 75.[45] The prevalence of latent prostatic cancer is even higher. In one series, approximately 30% of all the prostates removed at autopsy harbored a latent carcinoma.[46]

There are some remarkable and puzzling national and racial differences in the prevalence of this disease. Prostatic cancer is extremely rare in Orientals. The prevalence rate among Japanese is in the range of three to four, and for the Chinese in Hong Kong only one, as compared with a rate of 50 to 60 among whites in the U.S. The disease is even more prevalent among blacks, and indeed U.S. blacks not only have a markedly higher age-adjusted death rate from prostatic cancer than the white male population of the U.S. but also the highest rate among 24 countries having reasonably accurate mortality data.[47] Whites, in contrast, ranked fifteenth in the order. These differences are thought to be due to environmental influences, since in Japanese migrants to the U.S. the incidence of the disease seems to have risen, but not nearly to the level of that of native-born Americans.[48]

ETIOLOGY. Little is known about the causes of prostatic cancer. It is conventional to speak about three major factors—age, race, and the endocrine system.[49] To this triad a fourth might be added: environmental influences. The association of this form of cancer with advancing age and the enigmatic differences among race has already been mentioned. Could these be related to environmental influences? The tendency for the incidence of this disease to rise among those enjoying a low-incidence rate when they migrate to a high-incidence locale is consistent with environmental influences, but if such influences exist, they remain, with one exception, unidentified. It has been noted that workers in cadmium industries have an increased incidence of this disease.

The role of the endocrine system in the induction of prostatic cancer is also poorly understood, but one observation has been well established since the pioneer work of Huggins and Hodges.[50] The growth of metastatic prostatic cancer in men can usually be arrested or retarded for a time by castration, the administration of estrogens, or both. This leads to the assumption that androgens play a causal role. It has been impossible to document this hypothesis, however, and many studies have failed to establish a causal relationship between steroid hormone levels—estrogens, androgens, or adrenal steroids—in the blood or urine and the development of prostatic cancer.[51] It seems more likely that the role of hormones in the evolution of this tumor is essentially permissive. It could be that androgens are required for the maintenance of the prostatic epithelium, so that enough potential target cells for as yet undefined carcinogens exist.

As mentioned previously, *the role of nodular hyperplasia of the prostate as a precursor is still in dispute, but most experts do not believe that this benign lesion has any relationship to the development of cancer.*[43] Any concurrence of the two conditions could be a reflection of the prevalence of both diseases in aging men.

MORPHOLOGY. Carcinoma of the prostate arises in all but rare instances in the peripheral zone.[34] Areas of "atypical hyperplasia" that may be forerunners of prostatic cancer are also frequent in this zone. The origin may be multifocal but, by the time most lesions are discovered, the multiple foci have coalesced into a poorly delimited cohesive area of cancer (Fig. 23–23). Characteristically, on cross section of the prostate, **the neoplastic tissue is gritty and firm, but when embedded within the prostatic substance it may be extremely difficult to visualize and be more readily apparent on palpation.** It should be noted, however, that uncommonly prostatic cancers are not hard, particularly those lesions that do not evoke a stromal proliferative reaction. The tumor tissue is usually somewhat yellower than the surrounding tissues and is therefore distinctive, but at other times it is gray-white and therefore blends imperceptibly into the background. Only when the tumor invades the prostatic capsule, or has extended beyond the confines of the prostate to invade the seminal vesicles or the adjacent rectum or bladder, can it be unmistakably identified on gross inspection. Such extraprostatic extension ultimately occurs in almost all advanced, biologically aggressive lesions. In time, most prostatic cancers metastasize. Dissemination occurs via both lymphatics and bloodstream. Hematogenous spread occurs chiefly to the bones, particularly the vertebrae, but some lesions spread widely to viscera. Massive visceral dissemination is exceptional rather than the rule. The bony metastases may be osteolytic, but osteoblastic lesions are common and in males point strongly to prostatic cancer. Lymphatic spread occurs initially to the obturator nodes followed by hypogastric, iliac, presacral, and para-aortic nodes. Only recently has it been appreciated that lymph node spread occurs frequently and may precede spread to the bones. As we shall discuss later, metastases to the lymph nodes in apparently localized prostatic cancer have a significant impact on the prognosis.

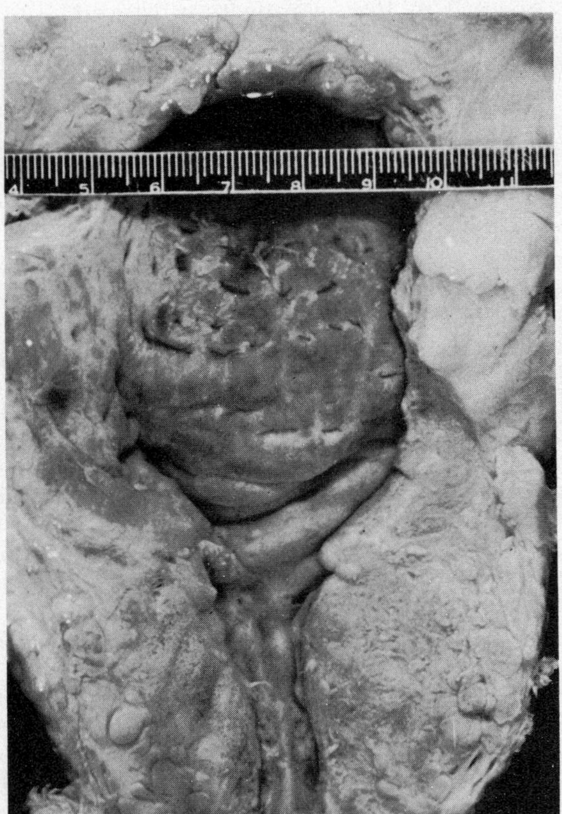

Figure 23–23. Carcinoma of prostate. Carcinomatous tissue cannot be distinguished within prostate itself but has invaded floor of urethra and infiltrated into vesicle neck.

Histologically most lesions are adenocarcinomas that produce well-defined, readily demonstrable gland patterns. In well-differentiated tumors the glands are either small or medium-sized with a single uniform layer of cuboidal or low columnar epithelium. Occasionally the glands are somewhat larger with a papillary or cribriform pattern. The cytoplasm of the tumor cells is pale and often granular, and the nuclei are round or oval and vesicular. Mitotic figures are extremely uncommon. When well-differentiated tumors occur in sharply delimited rounded masses, they have to be distinguished from nodular hyperplasia. In general, malignant acini are smaller and closely spaced, with little intervening stroma, and are lined by a single layer of cells. However, not all prostatic cancers are well differentiated. In some poorly differentiated tumors the glandular pattern is apparent only on careful examination; the tumor cells in such cases tend to grow in cords, nests, or sheets. Concomitantly, the cells display obvious cytologic features of malignancy with prominent acidophilic nucleoli and increased mitotic activity. Stromal production may be scant or quite extensive in certain lesions, producing a scirrhous-like consistency to the neoplasm.

The frequent uniformity of cells and lack of anaplasia contribute to the histologic difficulties of diagnosing carcinomas of the prostate. The most reliable hallmarks of malignancy are clear evidence of invasion of the capsule with its lymphatic and vascular channels and/or perineurial invasion (Fig. 23–24). The perineurial spaces, which are involved in most cases, are not lined by endothelium and they do not represent lymphatics, as formerly believed.

Epidermoid carcinoma, adenoid cystic carcinoma, and transitional cell carcinoma are rare forms of prostatic cancer.

GRADING AND STAGING. Carcinomas of the prostate, like most other forms of cancer, are graded and staged. Regrettably, several systems have been described, of which four are commonly used in the United States.[52] A discussion of all is beyond our scope. Suffice it to say that all grading systems attempt to define histologic criteria by which tumors of differing biologic behavior (metastatic potential, response to treatment, and survival) can be segregated. For example, the Gleason system is based on the degree of glandular differentiation and growth pattern of tumor in relation to the stroma. Well-differentiated tumors are assigned to Grade 1, whereas the most poorly differentiated tumors are classed as Grade 5. In the Gaeta system, on the other hand, only four grades are recognized on the basis of glandular differentiation as well as nuclear cytology. *Grading is of particular importance in prostatic cancer since there is in general an excellent correlation between the prognosis and the degree of differentiation.* Not surprisingly, therefore, there is also a good correlation between histologic grading and clinical staging.[53]

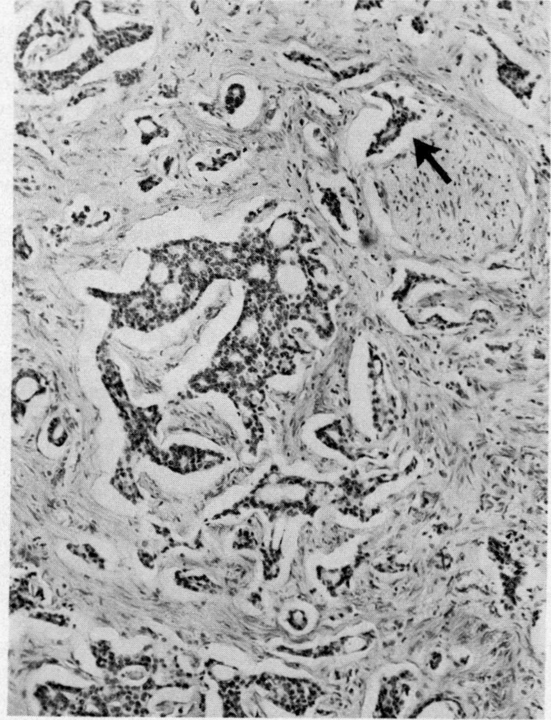

Figure 23–24. Carcinoma of prostate. Cords of tumor cells permeate stroma. Perineurial invasion is present *(arrow)*

Staging of prostatic cancer is very important in the selection of the appropriate form of therapy and in establishing a prognosis. Inevitably, two systems exist. The one proposed by the American Joint Committee is most widely used in the U.S. and is described below.[54] The other, proposed by the International Union Against Cancer (UICC), follows the TNM format.[55] The staging classification adopted by the American Joint Committee in its simplest form divides prostatic carcinoma into four clinical stages with subdivisions as follows:

Stage A. Latent cancer

A_1: Focal

A_2: Diffuse

Stage B. Tumor confined to the prostate

B_1: Lesion 1.5 cm in diameter or smaller, in one lobe

B_2: Tumor exceeds 1.5 cm in diameter or involves more than one lobe, not extending beyond the capsule

Stage C. Extracapsular extension, no nodal or distant metastases

C_1: No involvement of seminal vesicles; less than 70 gm

C_2: Involvement of seminal vesicles; greater than 70 gm

Stage D. Metastatic disease

D_1: Pelvic lymph node metastases or ureteral obstruction with hydronephrosis

D_2: Distant lymph node, bony or visceral metastases.

This staging classification, based solely on clinical features, has some obvious limitations. For example, many patients in Stages B and C have lymph node metastases that are discovered only during surgery or subsequent histologic examination. This is particularly relevant since nodal involvement is an important prognostic indicator.[56] Several radiologic techniques including lymphography and nuclear imaging can be employed to visualize the draining lymph nodes, but their utility in detecting microscopic metastases is limited. Even with these limitations, the current schema of staging provides a good estimate of prognosis and can be used as a guide for therapy.

CLINICAL COURSE. Approximately 30% of males over age 50 harbor Stage A cancer of the prostate.[46] These latent cancers are asymptomatic and are discovered incidentally at autopsy or in tissue removed for nodular hyperplasia of the prostate. The long-term significance of these lesions is still not entirely clear. It is generally accepted that most Stage A lesions (60 to 90%) will not progress to produce clinically manifest disease, but 10 to 40% of patients will eventually progress to develop extensive local or metastatic disease.[57, 58] Two subgroups have been proposed to distinguish between the clearly innocent (A_1) and potentially malignant (A_2) form of latent prostatic carcinoma. In making this distinction, both the extent (volume) and the histologic grade of the tumor are considered helpful. However, none of the criteria described for distinguishing A_1 and A_2 lesions have been tested extensively.[57]

About 5 to 10% of patients with overt prostatic cancer are discovered in Stage B. These patients do not have urinary symptoms and the lesion is discovered by the finding of a suspicious nodule on rectal examination. You recall that most prostatic cancers arise in a subcapsular location removed from the urethra and, therefore, urinary symptoms occur late. Most of these lesions are destined to progress unless eradicated by surgery or radiation. Although theoretically all these lesions are totally resectable, all patients are not cured. When treated by radical prostatectomy, patients with Stage B_1 disease are estimated to have an 85 to 90% five-year survival rate and 50% 15-year survival, whereas patients with Stage B_2 have a five- and 15-year survival of 20 and 1%, respectively.[59] It is estimated that up to 45% of patients classified in Stage B have microscopic metastases to the lymph nodes. As discussed earlier (p. 1105), lymph node metastases occur early and may precede bone metastases. Since lymphatic spread has an impact on both treatment and survival, some authors recommend extensive bilateral pelvic lymphadenectomy for more accurate surgical staging.[60]

Over 75% of patients with prostatic cancer present with Stages C or D. They come to clinical attention usually because of urinary symptoms such as difficulty in starting or stopping the stream, dysuria, frequency, or hematuria. Pain is a late finding reflecting involvement of capsular perineurial spaces. Some patients in Stage D come to attention because of back pain caused by vertebral metastases. *The finding of osteoblastic metastases in bone is virtually diagnostic of this form of cancer in males* (Fig. 23–25). The outlook for these

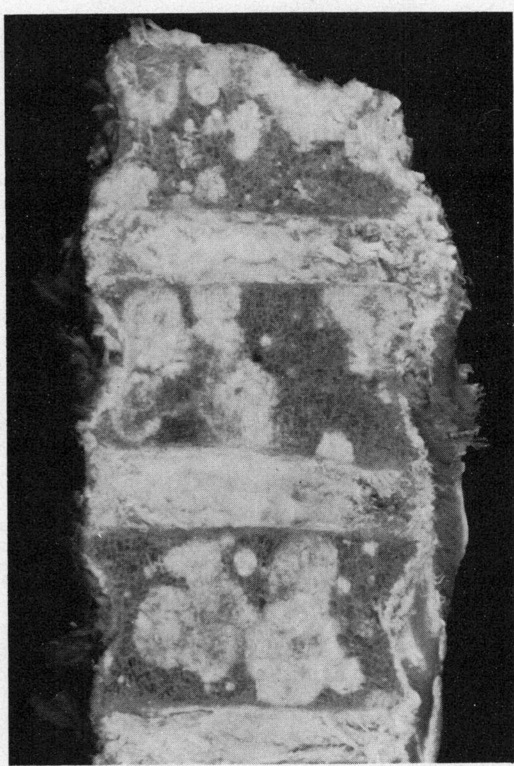

Figure 23–25. Metastatic osteoblastic prostatic carcinoma within vertebral bodies.

patients is bleak. Examination of lymph nodes in clinical Stage C shows metastases in 40 to 80% of cases.[58] In keeping with this finding, the ten-year survival rate is a dismal 36%. Disseminated prostatic carcinoma (Stage D) is clearly not amenable to surgery. Such cases are treated by orchidectomy and administration of estrogens. Less than 20% of patients survive five years and only a rare individual survives ten years. Death in these advanced cases is usually attributable to encroachment on the ureters, with resultant kidney disease, or to visceral and bone metastases.

Careful rectal digital examination is a very useful and direct method for detection of early prostatic carcinoma, since the posterior location of most tumors renders them easily palpable. A transperineal or transrectal biopsy can confirm the diagnosis. Other diagnostic approaches include cytologic examination of prostatic secretions, or detection of bony metastases by x-rays or by scintillation bone scanning, which is much more sensitive. Both the normal and malignant prostatic epithelium produce acid-phosphatase, which can be detected in the serum. *With the standard assay, elevations in serum enzyme levels are found only with cancer that has extended beyond the capsule or has metastasized, or both.* However, the traditional biochemical assay does not distinguish between the phosphatase isoenzymes of prostatic origin and those originating from nonprostatic tissue such as blood cells, liver, and spleen. Despite improvements in sensitivity and specificity (e.g., tartrate inhibition), the great preponderance of cases do not yield positive results until they are incurable. Since prostatic acid phosphatase is antigenically distinct from nonprostatic acid phosphatase, sensitive radioimmunoassays for prostatic acid phosphatase have been developed.[61] One report suggested that over 50% of patients with localized (intracapsular) prostatic cancer showed elevated levels of prostatic acid phosphatase if a radioimmunoassay was used.[61] Others doubt the utility of this assay in the diagnosis of localized prostatic cancer.[62] At the present the value of radioimmunoassay for prostatic acid phosphatase in the diagnosis of early localized (Stages A and B) prostatic cancer has not been fully established. Several newer screening and diagnostic tests, including the detection of a prostate tissue–specific antigen, are being currently evaluated.[63] The presence of prostate-specific antigen in metastases is very useful histologically in establishing prostatic origin. Significant progress in the treatment of this common cancer in men will depend heavily on our ability to detect the lesions in their earliest, curable stages.

---

1. Gissmann, L., et al.: Analysis of human genital warts (condylomata acuminata) and other genital tumors for human papilloma-virus type 6 DNA. Int. J. Cancer *29*:143, 1982.
2. Howley, P.: The human papillomavirus. Arch. Pathol. Lab. Med. *106*:429, 1982.
3. Smith, R. B., et al.: Verrucous carcinoma of the penis: Report of a case and review. Br. J. Urol. *41*:326, 1969.
4. Merrin, C. E.: Cancer of the penis. Cancer *45*:1973, 1980.
5. Droller, M. J.: Carcinoma of the penis: An overview. Urol. Clin. North Am. *7*:783, 1980.
6. Payne, R. A.: Erythroplasia of Queyrat. Br. J. Urol. *29*:163, 1957.
7. Wade, T. R., et al.: Bowenoid papulosis of the penis. Cancer *42*:1890, 1978.
8. Peters, M. S., and Perry, H. O.: Bowenoid papules of the penis. J. Urol. *126*:482, 1981.
9. Cohen, D. B.: Histology of the cryptorchid testis. Surgery *62*:536, 1967.
10. Wobbes, T. H., et al.: The relation between testicular tumors, undescended testes, and inguinal hernias. J. Surg. Oncol. *14*:45, 1980.
11. Fonger, J. D., et al.: Testicular tumors in maldescended testes. Can. J. Surg. *24*:353, 1981.
12. Batata, M. A., et al.: Testicular cancer in cryptorchids. Cancer *49*:1023, 1982.
13. Editorial. Epididymo-orchitis: Br. Med. J. *283*:627, 1981.
14. Berger, R. E., et al.: Etiology, manifestations and therapy of acute epididymitis. Prospective study of 50 cases. J. Urol. *121*:750, 1979.
15. Elecker, E. R., and Evans, A. T.: Granulomatous orchitis. J. Urol. *113*:199, 1975.
16. Mostofi, F. K., and Sobin, L. H.: International histological classification of testicular tumors (no. 16): International Histologic Classification of Tumors. Geneva, W.H.O., 1977.
17. Pierce, G. B., Jr., and Abell, M.A.: Embryonal carcinoma of the testis. *In* Sommers, S. C. (ed.): Pathology Annual. New York, Appleton-Century-Crofts, 1970, pp. 27–60.
18. Jacobsen, G. K., et al.: Carcinoma in situ of testicular tissue adjacent to malignant germ cell tumors: A study of 105 cases. Cancer *47*:2660, 1981.
19. Fraley, E. E., et al.: Germ cell testicular cancer in adults. N. Engl. J. Med. *301*:1370, 1979.
20. Pugh, R. C. B., and Cameron, K. M.: Teratoma. *In* Pugh, R. C. B. (ed.): Pathology of the Testis. Oxford, Blackwell Scientific Publications, 1976, pp. 199–244.
21. Schottenfeld, D., et al.: The epidemiology of testicular cancer in young adults. Am. J. Epidemiol. *112*:232, 1980.
22. Henderson, B. E., et al.: Risk factors for cancer of testis in young men. Int. J. Cancer *23*:598, 1979.
23. Kaplan, J. H., et al.: Testicular tumors of germ cell origin I. Epidemiology, pathogenesis, clinical presentation, and diagnosis. Postgrad. Med. *70*:114, 1981.
24. Peckham, M. J., and McElvain, T. J.: Testicular tumors. Clin. Endocrinol. Metab. *4*:665, 1975.
25. Javadpour, N.: Immunocytochemistry of testicular tumors. *In* Anderson, T. (moderator): Testicular germ cell neoplasms: Recent advances in diagnosis and therapy. Ann. Intern. Med. *90*:373, 1979.

26. Mostofi, F. K.: Classification of tumors of testis. Ann. Clin. Lab. Sci. *9*:455, 1979.
27. Collins, W. E.: TNM classification of malignant tumours of the bladder, prostate, testis, and kidney. Can. J. Surg. *18*:468, 1975.
28. Catalona, W. J.: Current management of testicular tumors. Surg. Clin. North Am. *62*:1119, 1982.
29. Jose, B., et al.: Anaplastic seminoma: An analysis of eight cases with literature review. J. Surg. Oncol. *18*:331, 1981.
30. Shulman, Y., et al.: Anaplastic seminoma. Urology *21*:379, 1983.
31. Drasga, R. E., et al.: The chemotherapy of testicular cancer. CA *32*:66, 1982.
32. Turner, R. R., et al.: Testicular lymphomas: A clinicopathologic study of 35 cases. Cancer *48*:2095, 1981.
33. Fisher, E. R., and Jeffrey, W.: Ultrastructure of human normal and neoplastic prostate; with comments relative to prostatic effects of hormonal stimulation in the rabbit. Am. J. Clin. Pathol. *44*:119, 1965.
34. McNeal, J.: Normal and pathologic anatomy of prostate. Urology *17*(Suppl. 3):11, 1981.
35. Blacklock, N. J.: Prostate: Morphology in health and disease. Recent Results Cancer Res. *78*:21, 1981.
36. Coffey, D. S., and Isaacs, J. T.: Control of prostate growth. Urology *17*(Suppl. 3):17, 1981.
37. Meares, E. M., Jr.: Prostatitis. Annu. Rev. Med. *30*:279, 1979.
38. Meares, E. M., Jr.: Prostatitis syndromes: New perspectives about old woes. J. Urol. *123*:141, 1980.
39. Harbitz, T. B., and Haugen, O. A.: Histology of the prostate in elderly men. A study in an autopsy series. Acta Pathol. Microbiol. Scand. *80*:756, 1972.
40. Wilson, J. D.: The pathogenesis of benign prostatic hyperplasia. Am. J. Med. *68*:745, 1980.
41. Isaacs, J. T., et al.: Changes in the metabolism of dihydrotestoterone in the hyperplastic human prostate. J. Clin. Endocrinol. Metab. *56*:139, 1983.
42. Trachtenberg, J., et al.: Androgen receptor content of normal and hyperplastic human prostate. J. Clin. Endocrinol. Metab. *54*:17, 1982.
43. Greenwald, P., et al.: Cancer of the prostate among men with benign prostatic hyperplasia. J. Natl. Cancer Inst. *53*:335, 1974.
44. Armenian, H. K., et al.: Relation between benign prostatic hyperplasia and cancer of the prostate. Lancet *2*:115, 1974.
45. Hutchinson, G. B.: Incidence and etiology of prostatic cancer. Urology *17*(Suppl. 3):4, 1981.
46. Guileyardo, J. M., et al.: Prevalance of latent prostate carcinoma in two U.S. populations. J. Natl. Cancer Inst. *65*:311, 1980.
47. Jackson, M. S., et al.: Characterization of prostatic cancer among blacks. A continuation report. Cancer Treat. Rep. *61*:167, 1977.
48. Haenzel, W., and Kurihara, M.: Studies of Japanese migrants. I. Mortality from cancer and other diseases among Japanese in the U.S. J. Natl. Cancer Inst. *40*:13, 1968.
49. Franks, L. M.: Etiology, epidemiology, and pathology of prostatic cancer. Cancer *32*:1092, 1973.
50. Huggins, C., and Hodges, C. V.: Studies of prostatic cancer. I. The effect of castration, of estrogen, and of androgen injections on serum phosphatase in metastatic carcinoma of the prostate. Cancer Res. *1*:203, 1941.
51. Harper, M. E., et al.: Prostate cancer: Hormonal relationships, receptors and tumor markers. Recent Results Cancer Res. *78*:44, 1981.
52. Murphy, G. P., and Whitmore, W. F.: A report of the workshops on the current status of the histologic grading of prostatic cancer. Cancer *44*:1490, 1979.
53. Gaeta, J. F.: Glandular profiles and cellular patterns in prostatic cancer grading. Urology *17*(Suppl. 3):33, 1981.
54. American Joint Committee for Cancer Staging and End Result Reporting. Manual for Staging for Cancer, 1978. New Jersey, Whiting Press, 1978, pp. 123–124.
55. Hendry, E. F.: Prostate cancer: Surgery. Recent Results Cancer Res., *78*:119, 1981.
56. Prout, G. R., et al.: Nodal involvement as prognostic indicator in prostatic carcinoma. Urology *17*(Suppl. 3):72, 1981.
57. Cantrell, B. B., et al.: Pathologic factors that influence prognosis in Stage A prostatic cancer: the influence of extent versus grade. J. Urol. *125*:516, 1981.
58. Klein, L. A.: Prostatic carcinoma. N. Engl. J. Med. *300*:824, 1979.
59. Droller, M. D.: Adenocarcinoma of the prostate: An overview. Urol. Clin. North Am. *7*:579, 1980.
60. McCullough, D. L.: Surgical staging of carcinoma of the prostate. Cancer *45*:1902, 1980.
61. Foti, A. G., et al.: Detection of prostatic cancer by solid-phase radioimmunoassay of serum acid phosphatase. N. Engl. J. Med. *297*:1357, 1977.
62. Watson, R. A., and Tang, D. B.: The predictive value of prostatic acid phosphatase as a screening test for prostatic cancer. N. Engl. J. Med. *303*:497, 1980.
63. Kuriyama, M., et al.: Multiple marker evaluation in human prostatic cancer with the use of tissue-specific antigens. J. Natl. Cancer Inst. *68*:99, 1982.

FEMALE GENITAL TRACT 24

NORMAL

EMBRYOLOGY. The many congenital anomalies of the female genital tract can be understood only from the standpoint of the embryology of this system. At about the sixth week of fetal development, invagination of the coelomic lining epithelium creates a groove whose lips later fuse to form the lateral *müllerian* (or *paramesonephric*) *ducts.* Müllerian ducts first become apparent high on the dorsal wall of the coelomic cavity and then progressively grow caudally to enter the pelvis where they swing medially to fuse. Further caudal growth brings these fused ducts into contact with the urogenital sinus. With relatively uncomplicated transformations, the unfused portions mature into the fallopian tubes, and the fused caudal portion into the uterus and the vagina. The upper portion of the vagina is generally held to be of müllerian origin, and the lower portion is probably derived from the urogenital sinus. *It is apparent that the entire lining of the uterus and tubes is derived from coelomic epithelium.* The embryogenesis here serves to explain the origin of such congenital anomalies as a bicornuate or totally septate uterus and a septate or double vagina. It also serves to explain the various histologic patterns of those ovarian tumors derived from coelomic epithelium, as we shall see.

Parallel to the müllerian ducts are the paired *wolffian* (or *mesonephric*) *ducts*, which in the male are destined to form the epididymis and the vas deferens. Normally, the mesonephric duct regresses in the female. Remnants, however, may persist into adult life as epithelial inclusions about the hilus of the ovary and mesosalpinx, designated respectively the epoophoron and paroophoron. If the caudal portions of this mesonephric anlage persist, they may appear as epithelial inclusions within the wall of the lower uterine segment and cervix and as epithelial rests in the lateral walls of the vagina. Sometimes in the vagina these rests produce cysts that are known as Gartner's duct cysts.

The ovary, like the testis, arises from a medial proliferation of the urogenital ridge specified as the genital ridge. At six weeks of fetal development, this sexless gonad has three components: a covering of differentiated *coelomic lining epithelium*, previously incorrectly designated as "germinal epithelium;" *an underlying undifferentiated stroma (the mesenchyme); and primitive germ cells.* Differentiation of the ovarian mesenchyme provides an origin for theca cells, and probably also for the granulosa cells of the follicle. It is generally believed that the germ cells are set aside as totipotential gametes in the earliest stage of formation of the embryonic disc. As the embryo develops, they migrate or are carried into the primitive mesenchyme destined to become the ovary. It is of interest that these divide during the first half of fetal development to reach a maximum number of 6 to 7 million, but subsequently some regress; thus, at birth approximately 1 to 2 million oocytes remain. None are formed after the fifth month of fetal development and, indeed, there is a progressive loss so that at puberty the number has dwindled into the hundreds of thousands, still more than needed to provide 12 per year during the woman's active reproductive life.

Certain details of the embryogenesis of the ovary assume importance in the histogenesis of ovarian tumors. The coelomic epithelium or inclusions of coelomic epithelium within the inner mesenchyme may be the cytologic origin of some of the epithelial cysts, cystadenomas, and carcinomas of the ovary. The concept that the mesenchyme may differentiate into both granulosal and thecal elements provides a reasonable origin for neoplasms such as the granulosa cell tumors and Sertoli-Leydig cell tumors, which synthesize estrogens, androgens, or both, and which span a morphologic range of epithelial and stromal patterns. The germ cell is the third type of cell giving rise to distinctive ovarian tumors.

MEASUREMENTS. Certain normal dimensions of the female genital tract are of value, since so much importance attaches to various diseases that cause enlargement of the ovaries and uterus. During active reproductive life, the ovaries measure about 4 cm in length, 2.5 to 3 cm in width, and 1 to 1.5 cm in thickness. It should be emphasized that in ovaries removed in the course of surgical procedures on the pelvic organs, small follicle cysts, to be described presently, are found so commonly as to represent virtually normal anatomic features. Postmenopausally the ovaries atrophy to wrinkled nodules 2.0 × 1.0 × 0.5 cm or smaller.

The uterus varies in size, depending on the age and parity of the individual. During active reproductive life, it weighs about 50 gm and measures 8 cm in length, 5 to 6.5 cm in breadth in the fundic region, and 3 cm in thickness (1.5 cm of anterior and posterior myometrium). Pregnancies may leave small residual increases in these dimensions (up to 70 gm in weight) since the uterus rarely involutes completely to its original size. Postmenopausally, the atrophic changes may cause diminution to 5 to 6 cm in length, 3 cm in width, and 1.5 to 2 cm in thickness.

HISTOLOGY. The *ovary* is divided into a cortex and a medulla. Ordinarily, the cortex comprises a layer of closely packed spindle cells that resemble plump fibroblasts separated by only a scant intercellular ground substance. The very outermost portion directly beneath the surface epithelium is compacted into a thin layer of relatively acellular collagenous connective tissue. Thickening of this layer may accompany ovarian dysfunction (p. 1142). By puberty, follicles and ova in varying stages of maturation are found within the outer cortex. Corpora lutea of varying ages as well as nodules of collagenous connective tissue, the corpora albicantia, are also present in the cortex of the adult.

The medulla of the ovary is made up of a more loosely arranged mesenchymal tissue. Occasionally, large, round-to-polygonal, epithelial-appearing cells are buried within the medulla in the hilar region. These "hilus" cells, presumed to be vestigial remains of the gonad from its primitive "ambisexual" phase, are steroid producing, and thus resemble the interstitial cells of the testis. Rarely, these cells give rise to masculinizing tumors.

In the *fallopian tube*, the mucosa is thrown up into numerous high, delicate folds that on cross section produce a papillary appearance. In the normal, these mucosal folds are not interadherent, and hence the folds form deep crypts. In the absence of fusion of these folds, no sequestered, buried, cystic, or follicle-like spaces are found. When glandlike or cystic patterns are produced, it can be assumed that inflammatory fusion of adjacent folds has occurred. The lining epithelium of the tube is made up of three cell types: ciliated columnar cells; nonciliated, columnar, secretory cells; and so-called intercalated cells that may simply represent inactive secretory cells.

The uterus has three distinctive anatomic and functional regions: the cervix, the lower uterine segment, and the corpus. The *cervix* is further divided into the vaginal portio and the endocervix (Fig. 24–1). The anatomic portio is that portion of the cervix visible to the eye on vaginal examination. It is covered by a stratified squamous nonkeratinizing epithelium reflected off the vaginal vaults onto the cervix. This squamous epithelium covers the entire anatomic portio and extends more or less up to the central dimple that comprises the external os. In the normal cervix of nulliparous women, this os is virtually closed. The endocervix is normally not exposed and is lined by columnar, mucus-secreting epithelium that dips down into the underlying stroma to produce crypts sometimes designated as endocervical glands.

The *squamocolumnar junction* is of considerable importance, since most cervical carcinomas arise at this site. The position of the junction is variable. The original anatomic junction is at the cervical os (Fig. 24–1, *left*). However, in virtually all adult women who have borne children, the columnar endocervical epithelium migrates downward from the cervical os and thus is visible to the naked eye. This is referred to as an *ectropion* or *eversion* (Fig. 24–1, *middle*). An ectropion appears red or pink on visual examination and is thus called an *erosion*, which is a misnomer since the mucosal layer is actually intact. Ectropions become gradually reepithelialized by squamous epithelium (squamous metaplasia or prosoplasia), producing the so-called *transformation* or *transition zone* (Fig. 24–1, *right*); in postmenopausal women, this zone is high, above the external os, and thus this critical area is not visible to the naked eye. As we shall see, it is this transformation zone that must be biopsied to exclude carcinoma or precancerous lesions.

The *lower uterine segment* has no clear delimitation. It is lined by columnar, mucus-secreting epithelium that progressively becomes transformed to non–mucus-secreting epithelium resembling the basal resting glands of the endometrium. It does not participate in the cyclic changes of the functional endometrium; hence, failure to recognize lower uterine segment mucosa in curettings leads to erroneous impressions that the endometrium is nonfunctional.

ENDOMETRIAL HISTOLOGY AND MENSTRUAL CYCLE. The endometrial changes that occur during the menstrual cycle are keyed to the rise and fall in the levels of ovarian hormones, and the student should be familiar with the complex but fascinating interactions among hypothalamic, pituitary, and ovarian factors underlying maturation of ovarian follicles, ovulation, and the menstrual cycle. Suffice it to say that under the influence of the pituitary follicle stimulating and luteotropic hormones (FSH and LH), development and ripening of a

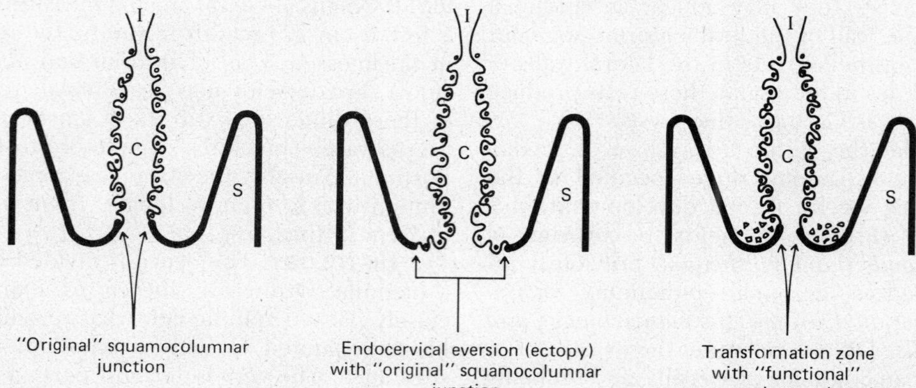

Figure 24–1. Schematic representation of "original" and "functional" squamocolumnar junctions and three basic types of portios. *Left,* Diagram of a portio completely covered with native squamous epithelium. Squamocolumnar junction is at external os. *Middle,* Denotes an endocervical eversion, with squamocolumnar junction located on exocervix below external os. *Right,* Indicates areas of eversion covered with squamous epithelium. This area is the cervical transformation zone. New or "functional" squamocolumnar junction of transformation zone is at external os. S = squamous epithelium; C = endocervical columnar epithelium; I = uterine isthmus. (From Blaustein, A. (ed.): Anatomy and histology of the cervix. *In* Pathology of the Female Genital Tract. 2nd ed. New York, Springer-Verlag, 1982. Reproduced with permission.)

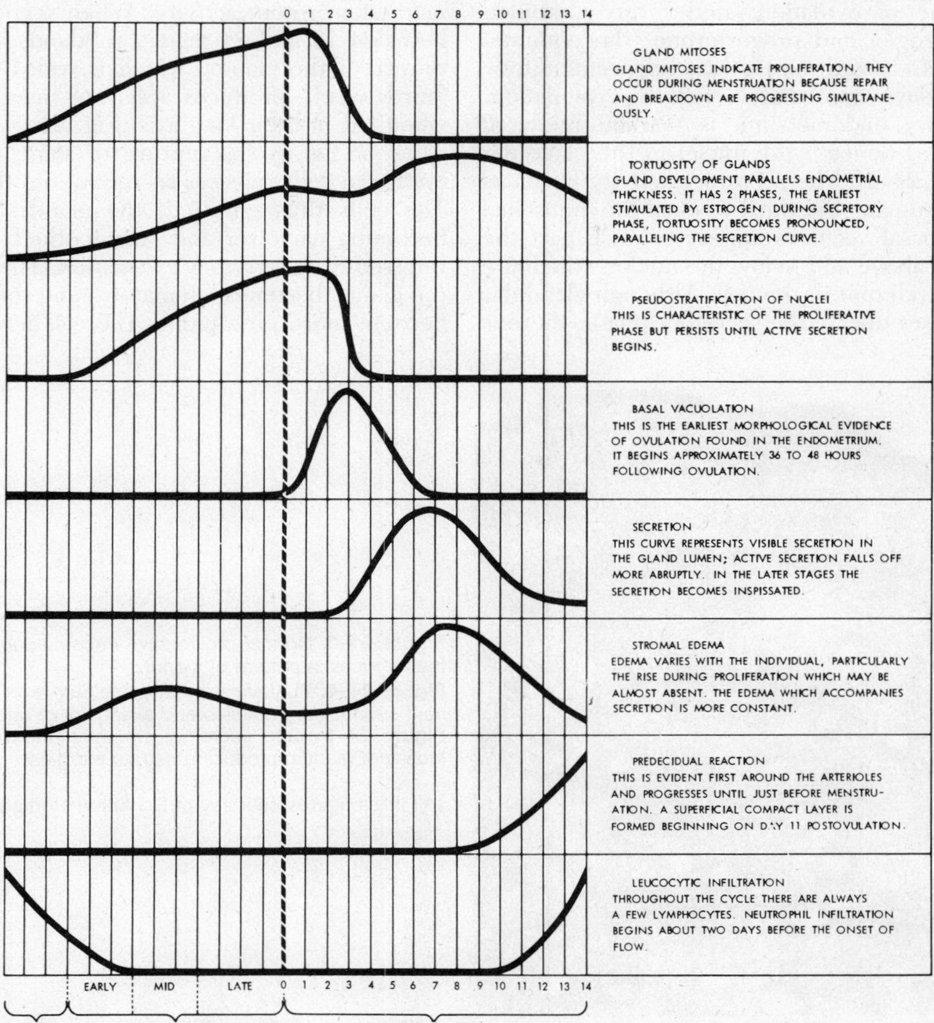

0 1 2 3 4 5 6 7 8 9 10 11 12 13 14
GLAND MITOSES
GLAND MITOSES INDICATE PROLIFERATION. THEY OCCUR DURING MENSTRUATION BECAUSE REPAIR AND BREAKDOWN ARE PROGRESSING SIMULTANEOUSLY.
TORTUOSITY OF GLANDS
GLAND DEVELOPMENT PARALLELS ENDOMETRIAL THICKNESS. IT HAS 2 PHASES, THE EARLIEST STIMULATED BY ESTROGEN. DURING SECRETORY PHASE, TORTUOSITY BECOMES PRONOUNCED, PARALLELING THE SECRETION CURVE.
PSEUDOSTRATIFICATION OF NUCLEI
THIS IS CHARACTERISTIC OF THE PROLIFERATIVE PHASE BUT PERSISTS UNTIL ACTIVE SECRETION BEGINS.
BASAL VACUOLATION
THIS IS THE EARLIEST MORPHOLOGICAL EVIDENCE OF OVULATION FOUND IN THE ENDOMETRIUM. IT BEGINS APPROXIMATELY 36 TO 48 HOURS FOLLOWING OVULATION.
SECRETION
THIS CURVE REPRESENTS VISIBLE SECRETION IN THE GLAND LUMEN; ACTIVE SECRETION FALLS OFF MORE ABRUPTLY. IN THE LATER STAGES THE SECRETION BECOMES INSPISSATED.
STROMAL EDEMA
EDEMA VARIES WITH THE INDIVIDUAL, PARTICULARLY THE RISE DURING PROLIFERATION WHICH MAY BE ALMOST ABSENT. THE EDEMA WHICH ACCOMPANIES SECRETION IS MORE CONSTANT.
PREDECIDUAL REACTION
THIS IS EVIDENT FIRST AROUND THE ARTERIOLES AND PROGRESSES UNTIL JUST BEFORE MENSTRUATION. A SUPERFICIAL COMPACT LAYER IS FORMED BEGINNING ON DAY 11 POSTOVULATION.
LEUCOCYTIC INFILTRATION
THROUGHOUT THE CYCLE THERE ARE ALWAYS A FEW LYMPHOCYTES. NEUTROPHIL INFILTRATION BEGINS ABOUT TWO DAYS BEFORE THE ONSET OF FLOW.
EARLY
MID
LATE
0 1 2 3 4 5 6 7 8 9 10 11 12 13 14
MENSES
PROLIFERATIVE PHASE
SECRETORY PHASE

Figure 24–2. Approximate quantitative changes in eight morphologic criteria found to be most useful in dating human endometrium. (From Noyes, R. W.: Normal phases of the endometrium. *In* Norris, H. J., et al. (eds.): The Uterus. Baltimore, Williams & Wilkins Co., 1973. Copyright © 1973, The Williams & Wilkins Company, Baltimore.)

single ovum occurs, and estrogen production by the enlarging ovarian follicle progressively rises during the first two weeks of the classic 28-day menstrual cycle. It reaches a peak, presumably just before ovulation, and then falls. Following ovulation, the estrogen levels again begin to rise to a plateau at about the end of the third week, but these levels are never as high as the preovulatory peak. The level of this hormone then progressively falls, beginning three to four days before the onset of menstruation. Progesterone, produced by the corpus luteum, rises throughout the last half of the menstrual cycle to fall to basal levels just before the onset of menstrual bleeding. By some poorly understood mechanism involving prostaglandins, vasospasm of the spiral arterioles of the endometrium leads to endometrial necrosis and consequent menstrual bleeding.

We can begin describing the endometrial changes with the shedding of the upper one-half to two-thirds of the endometrium during the menstrual period (Fig. 24–2). The basal third does not respond to the ovarian steroids and is retained at the conclusion of the menstrual flow. From this basal third the surface epithelium is regenerated during the first half of the menstrual cycle. During this preovulatory proliferative phase of the cycle, there is extremely rapid growth of both glands and stroma. The glands are straight, tubular structures lined by quite regular, tall, columnar cells. The nuclei in these cells are not aligned, mitotic figures are numerous, and there is no evidence of mucous secretion or vacuolation. The gland lumina are relatively tubular and devoid of secretion (Fig. 24–3). The endometrial stroma is composed of thickly compacted spindle cells that have very scant cytoplasm but abundant mitotic activity. Although one can readily identify a proliferative endometrium, there are no characteristic cell or architectural changes that permit precise dating of this phase of the menstrual cycle. The height of glands is an unreliable criterion.

At the time of ovulation, under the combined influence of estrogen and progesterone, the endometrium slows in its growth and ceases apparent mitotic activity within days immediately following ovulation. The postovulatory endometrium is marked by basal secretory vacuoles beneath the nuclei in the glandular epithelium (Fig. 24–4). The secretory activity becomes more prominent during the third week of the menstrual cycle, and the basal vacuoles appear to push past the nuclei to appear above and below the nuclei, which are thus aligned at midpoint in the cell. Although glandular proliferation ceases during the secretory phase, there is marked secretory activity. When secretion is maximal, between 18 and 24 days, the glands are dilated. Tortuosity of the glands, which is well developed by the fourth week, produces a serrate margin to the glands when cut in their long axis (Fig. 24–5). During the last week of the cycle, rupture of some of the columnar epithelial cells releases secretion into the gland lumina. The cells thus emptied, the glands begin to shrink, becoming narrower and "saw-toothed"—an appearance referred to as *secretory exhaustion*. The stroma between the glands becomes edematous, and the spiral arterioles become more prominent. There is now a considerable

Fig. 24–3

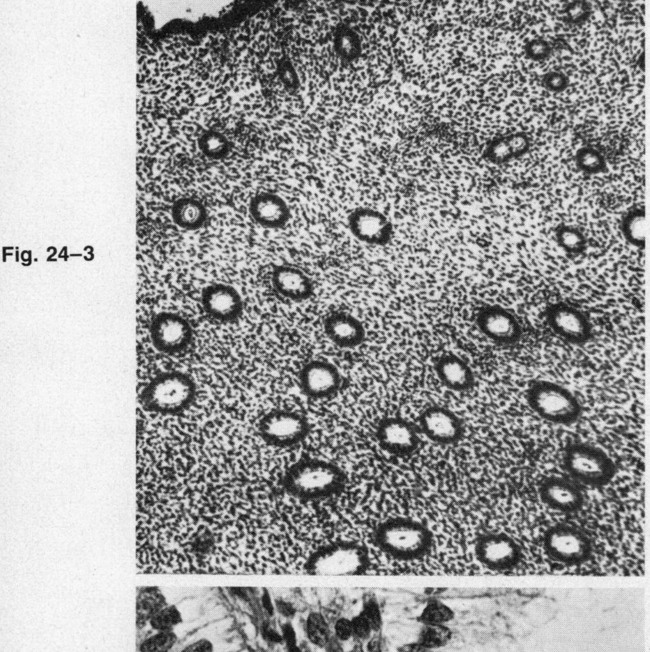

Figure 24–3. Normal proliferative endometrium, illustrating tubelike pattern of glands.

Figure 24–4. Postovulatory endometrium with prominent subnuclear vacuoles and alignment of nuclei.

Figure 24–5. Late secretory endometrium with tortuosity of glands, producing serrate margins.

(All three figures courtesy of Dr. Arthur Hertig.)

Fig. 24–4

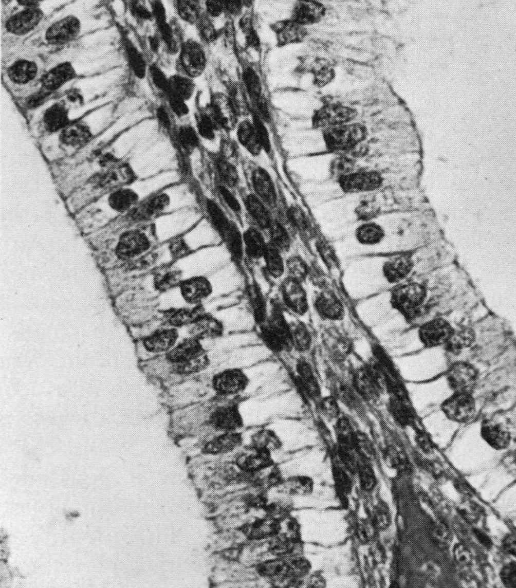

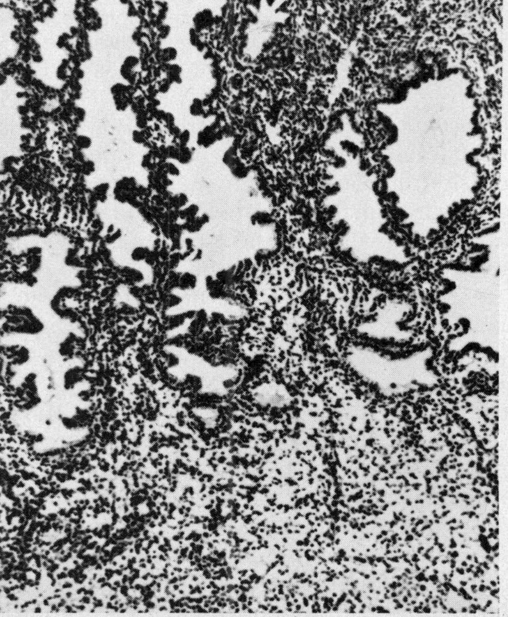

Fig. 24–5

increase in ground substance and edema between the stromal cells. In the nonpregnant state, three to four days before the menstrual flow, the stromal cells become hypertrophied and accumulate a considerable amount of pink cytoplasm to produce so-called predecidual changes. The escape of blood into the stroma marks the beginning of menstrual shedding. This stromal bleeding is apparently initiated by necrosis and rupture of the walls of the spiral arterioles. In the premenstrual and menstrual phases, the endometrial stroma contains scattered neutrophils and occasional lymphocytes. The normal presence of such leukocytes is to be particularly noted since these white cells are ordinarily considered to be indicators of an inflammatory reaction.

The proliferative phase should therefore be readily differentiated from the secretory phase. *The hallmark of the proliferative phase is mitotic activity in glandular and stromal cells. Ovulation should be fairly well denoted by the basal vacuolation of the columnar epithelial cells of the glands.* When ovulation fails to occur, there is no secretory vacuolation in the endometrial glands, and the characteristic stromal edema and later decidual transformation are absent. For these reasons, endometrial biopsy to determine ovulation should not be performed before the twentieth day and preferably on or about the twenty-fifth day, at which time it can be assumed that the secretory changes in glands and stroma are well developed.

PATHOLOGY

Diseases of the female genital tract are numerous and extremely common in clinical and pathologic practice. They include complications of pregnancy, inflammations, tumors, and hormonally induced defects. The following discussion presents the major entities that compose the majority of clinical problems. Details can be found in several books[2–6] and chapters in current volumes of surgical pathology.[7, 8]

Vulva

Congenital Anomalies
Inflammations
- Pelvic inflammatory disease (PID)
- Bartholin's adenitis and Bartholin's cyst
- Miscellaneous infections

Vulvar Dystrophies
- Atrophic dystrophy (lichen sclerosus)
- Hyperplastic dystrophy (with or without atypia)

Tumors
- Condyloma acuminatum
- Papillary hidradenoma
- Carcinoma
- Extramammary Paget's disease
- Malignant melanoma

Diseases of the vulva in the aggregate comprise only a small fraction of gynecologic practice. The great variety of inflammations that occur here are usually amenable to therapy and do not constitute significant threats to the patient. Only malignant neoplasms can be considered as diseases of major clinical significance.

CONGENITAL ANOMALIES

Of the various malformations of the vulva, only hypoplasia, duplication, and imperforate hymen merit mention. The *imperforate hymen* sometimes escapes recognition in the infant and remains uncorrected until the onset of menstruation. At this time, the absence of menstrual flow in association with pelvic pain and discomfort reflect the progressive accumulation of menstrual blood in the vagina (*hematocolpos*), in the uterus (*hematometra*), and in the tubes (*hematosalpinx*). If the condition persists long enough, the overflow of blood may spill into the pelvic cavity and produce signs of pelvic peritonitis. The accumulated blood may organize within the tubes, with resultant permanent sterility.

Duplication of the vulva is quite rare and is almost invariably accompanied by a septate double vagina and uterus.

Hypoplasia of the vulva or external female genitals may arise as a congenital developmental defect. More often, it implies a failure of normal growth response. The hypodevelopment may be due to an ovarian or pituitary insufficiency, or may reflect an end-organ unresponsiveness to normal levels of hormone. Such infantilism is usually accompanied by hypodevelopment of the remainder of the genital tract and by inadequate development of the secondary sex characteristics.

INFLAMMATIONS

Any dermatologic conditions that affect hair-bearing skin elsewhere on the body may also occur on the vulva, so that vulvitis may be encountered in psoriasis, eczema, and allergic dermatitis. The vulva is prone to skin infections, since it is constantly exposed to secretions and moisture. Nonspecific vulvitis is particularly likely to occur in the blood dyscrasias, uremia, diabetes mellitus, malnutrition, and the avitaminoses. Because itching is the most prominent feature of these conditions, secondary trauma from scratching complicates the clinical and histologic picture. Here we shall cover only entities that are either specific for or common in the vulva.

PELVIC INFLAMMATORY DISEASE (PID)

Pelvic inflammatory disease (PID) is considered here because it begins in the vulva or its accessory glands, but usually the infection spreads upward through the entire genital tract, involving more or less all the structures in the female genital system. Despite the availability of effective antibiotics, the gonococcus continues to be a common cause of PID, the most serious complication of gonorrhea in women. The basic biology of gonococcal infections was discussed earlier (p. 309). Besides gonorrhea, infections following spontaneous or induced abortions and normal or abnormal deliveries are important in the production of PID. Such postabortion and postpartum infections are caused by staphylococci, streptococci, coliform bacteria, and *Clostridium perfringens*. Species of *Mycoplasma*, *Chlamydia* and non–spore-forming anaerobic bacteria have also been implicated in cases of nongonococcal PID.[9]

Whatever the etiologic agent, the anatomic changes that result are similar. The pathway of spread of these various organisms, however, may differ. Gonococcal inflammation usually begins in Bartholin's glands and other vestibular glands, or Skene's ducts and periurethral glands, or sometimes the endocervical glands. From any of these loci, the organisms spread upward over the mucosal surfaces, eventually to involve the tubes and tubo-ovarian region. In such spread, the adult vagina is remarkably resistant. In the child, presumably because of a more delicate lining mucosa, vulvovaginitis may develop. The nongonococcal infections that follow induced abortion, dilatation and curettage of the uterus, and other surgical procedures on the female genital tract are thought to spread upward through the lymphatics or venous channels rather than on the mucosal surfaces. These infections therefore tend to produce less mucosal involvement but more reaction within the deeper layers.

With the gonococcus, approximately two to seven days after inoculation of the organism, nonspecific inflammatory changes appear in the affected glands. Wherever it occurs, gonococcal disease is characterized by an acute suppurative reaction accompanied by the copious outpouring of pus. The involved structures become hyperemic, edematous, and tense. The infection usually but not invariably affects both sides. Histologically, the reaction is nonspecific. In gonococcal infections, the inflammatory changes are largely confined to the superficial mucosa and underlying submucosa. Smear of the exudate should disclose the intracellular gram-negative diplococcus, but absolute confirmation requires cultural identification. In most acute cases, with therapy, the infection promptly subsides and does not involve the upper levels of the genital tract. If spread occurs, a gonorrheal endometritis may develop, but more often the endometrium is remarkably spared, for obscure reasons. Once within the tubes, an **acute suppurative salpingitis** ensues. The tubal serosa becomes hyperemic and layered with fibrin, the tubal fimbriae are similarly involved, and the lumen fills with purulent exudate that may leak out of the fimbriated end. In the course of days or weeks, the tubal fimbriae may seal or become plastered against the ovary to create a **salpingo-oophoritis.** Pus may collect in these sealed tubes to cause distention (*pyosalpinx*). So enclosed, the infection tends to smolder and becomes chronic for months and even years. In the course of time the infecting organisms may disappear. The pus then undergoes slow proteolysis and the contents of the tubes are transformed to a thin, serous fluid **(hydrosalpinx). Tubo-ovarian abscesses** may result from collections of exudate where the tube is sealed against the ovary. This process is not truly an ovarian abscess since the underlying ovarian substance is remarkably spared except for the most superficial layers.

PID caused by staphylococci, streptococci, and the other puerperal invaders tends to have less exudation within the lumina of the tube and less involvement of the mucosa, with correspondingly greater inflammatory response within the deeper layers. The infection tends to spread throughout the wall to involve the serosa, and may often track into the broad ligaments, pelvic structures, and peritoneum. Bacteremia is a more frequent complication of streptococcal or staphylococcal pelvic inflammatory disease than of gonococcal infections.

PID causes pelvic pain, dysmenorrhea, disturbance in intestinal function, menstrual abnormalities, and sometimes manifestations of an acute abdomen. The complications of PID include (1) peritonitis; (2) intestinal obstruction due to adhesions between the small bowel and the pelvic organs; (3) bacteremia, which may potentially induce endocarditis, meningitis, and suppurative arthritis; and (4) infertility, one of the most feared consequences of long-standing chronic PID.

In the early stages, gonococcal infections are readily controlled with antibiotics although, regrettably, penicillin-resistant strains have emerged. When the infection becomes walled off in suppurative tubes or tubo-ovarian abscesses, it is difficult to achieve a sufficient level of antibiotic within the centers of such suppuration to control these infections effectively. Postabortion and postpartum PID are also amenable to antibiotics but are far more difficult to control than the gonococal infections. Frequently, it becomes necessary to remove the organs surgically.

BARTHOLIN'S ADENITIS AND BARTHOLIN'S CYST

These vulvovaginal glands are frequently involved in gonorrheal infections, although at times other organisms may be responsible for the inflammatory reaction. Acute adenitis may result in abscess formation, which needs to be drained for relief. A chronic form, with asymptomatic intervals alternating with acute exacerbations, also occurs. If the main duct of the gland is blocked, a *Bartholin's cyst* results. This may become quite large, up to 3 to 5 cm in diameter. The lesion is fairly common and occurs at all ages. The cyst is lined by either the transitional epithelium of the normal duct or cells that are flattened by the increased intracystic pressure. The cysts produce pain and local discomfort but are otherwise of no systemic significance.

MISCELLANEOUS INFECTIONS

Syphilitic chancres, chancroid, granuloma inguinale, and lymphogranuloma inguinale all pursue virtually parallel courses in the male and female, and have already been adequately considered (Chap. 8). It is necessary here only to point out that, in the female, lymphogranuloma of the vulva tends to drain not only to the inguinal nodes but also to the deep nodes about the rectum. Intense scarring may follow and produce rectal strictures in the female. Such drainage does not occur in the male.

Herpes simplex infection of the vulva is common and is usually accompanied by infection involving the vagina and cervix. The frequency of genital herpes is increasing dramatically, particularly in teenagers and young women, and indeed, herpes simplex virus type II (HSV II) infection is now second only to gonorrhea as a sexually transmitted disease.[10] The lesions begin three to seven days after sexual relations and consist of painful red papules that progress to vesicles and then coalescent ulcers. Cervical and vaginal involvement causes severe leukorrhea. There may be systemic symptoms such as fever, malaise, and tender inguinal lymph nodes. The vesicles and ulcers contain numerous virus particles, accounting for the high transmission rate during active infection. The lesions heal spontaneously in one to three weeks but, as with herpetic infections elsewhere, the latent infection persists and about two-thirds of women suffer recurring relapses. Relapses are less painful and transmission is less likely after contact with asymptomatic carriers. As discussed later, these patients have an increased incidence of cervical dysplasias and carcinoma. In the pregnant mother, the risk of newborn infection with herpes is particularly high when the virus particles are present at the time of delivery. Herpetic vulvovaginitis is a difficult disease to prevent or cure, but topical or intravenous treatment with new antiviral agents (e.g., acyclovir) seem to shorten the duration of viral shedding and accelerate healing.[11]

Mycotic and *yeast infections* on the vulva also occur. About 10% of women are thought to be carriers of vulvovaginal fungi. Monilial vulvitis is by far the most common form of fungal infection (p. 352).

VULVAR DYSTROPHIES

A heterogeneous group of lesions of the vulva present as opaque, white, plaquelike mucosal thickenings that are sometimes pruritic and scaly. In the past, clinicians have used the term "leukoplakia" to designate these lesions—an unfortunate choice of words, since white plaques may underlie a variety of histologic patterns, some of which are clearly benign, whereas others are premalignant or malignant.[12] Indeed, when such "leukoplakic" lesions are biopsied, they are found to represent any one of the following conditions: (1) vitiligo (loss of pigment [p. 1274]); (2) an inflammatory dermatosis (e.g., psoriasis, chronic dermatitis [p. 1291]); (3) carcinoma in situ, Paget's disease, or even invasive carcinoma; or (4) a variety of alterations of unknown etiology that elude proper classification. Considerable confusion existed in the past because of imprecise and inconsistent terms used for this last group (e.g., kraurosis vulvae, leukoplakia, atrophic vulvitis), but a nomenclature developed by the International Society for the Study of Vulvar Disease now places the different lesions in this group under the single heading of "*dystrophy.*"[13]

There are three varieties of dystrophy: (1) *atrophic dystrophy* or *lichen sclerosus* (et atrophicus), a characteristic disorder manifested by epithelial atrophy and subepithelial fibrosis; (2) *hyperplastic dystrophy*, characterized by hyperplasia and hyperkeratosis of the lining epithelium; and (3) *mixed dystrophy*, in which these forms coexist in different areas of the same vulva. When atypical cellular changes are present in the hyperplastic area, these are labeled as mild, moderate, or severe atypia; *it is these atypical alterations that have the greatest relevance for the future development of carcinoma.* Although most of the dystrophic patches are benign and have no premalignant potential, the lesions are often multiple, making their clinical management particularly difficult.

ATROPHIC DYSTROPHY (LICHEN SCLEROSUS)

Lichen sclerosus (atrophic dystrophy) is a disorder of the skin that can occur anywhere on the body and in all age groups (p. 1290). It consists of yellowish-blue papules or macules that eventually coalesce into thin, gray, parchment-like areas. When they affect the vulva, these lesions are most common in women between 45 and 55 years of age. They become easily irritated and may lead to progressive shrinkage of the vulvar and perivulvar connective tissue. For this reason, the condition has also been termed "chronic atrophic vulvitis" and "kraurosis vulvae."

The skin becomes pale gray and parchment-like, the labia are atrophied, and the introitus is narrow. The entire vulvar area becomes smooth, with loss of the usual skin folds, and the skin may assume a glazed red appearance as the subcutaneous vessels become more apparent. Histologically, there is atrophy and thinning of the epidermis, with disappearance of the rete pegs and replacement of the underlying dermis by dense collagenous fibrous tissue (Fig. 24–6). A nonspecific mononuclear cell infiltrate about blood vessels may also occur. The avascular skin and mucosa are particularly susceptible to trauma and infections, and the lesions therefore are frequently complicated by chronic inflammatory changes, fissuring, ulceration, and even frank abscess formation.

Clinically, this disease occurs after the menopause and, on this basis, it has been postulated that it is caused by estrogen deficiency. However, lesions are occasionally encountered in women in active reproductive life. At all ages, the disorder tends to be slowly developing,

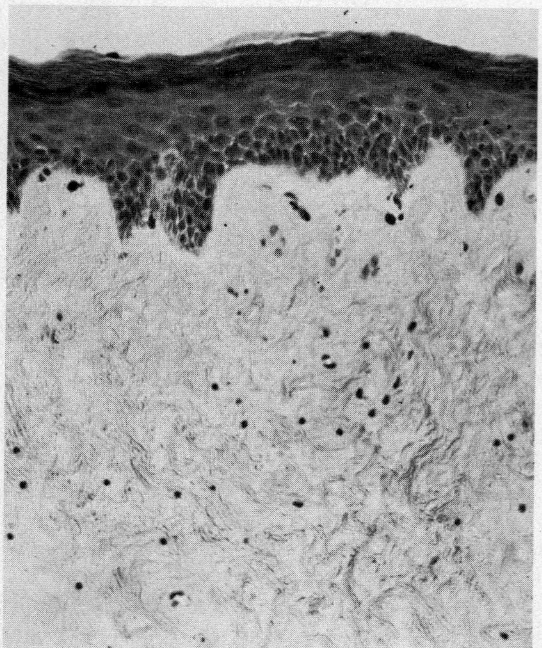

Figure 24–6. Lichen sclerosus illustrating atrophy of epidermis and dense sclerosis of dermis with total atrophy of dermal adnexal structures. (Courtesy of Dr. Arthur Hertig.)

insidious, and progressive. It causes considerable discomfort and predisposes to acute infection, but is usually of little systemic significance. Pure atrophic dystrophy rarely progresses to carcinoma and most (but not all[12]) authors do not consider it a precancerous lesion.[5, 15]

HYPERPLASTIC DYSTROPHY (WITH OR WITHOUT ATYPIA)

In hyperplastic dystrophy there is hyperplasia of the squamous epithelial lining, sometimes with varying degrees of atypia. The epithelium is thickened and may show increased mitotic activity in both the basal and prickle cell layers (Fig. 24–7). Frequently there is marked hyperkeratosis. The differentiation from basal to surface cell can be preserved, but in some cases there is dysplasia with variability of nuclear and cell size. The hyperplastic epithelial changes may be entirely benign or may show foci of atypia sometimes approximating intraepithelial carcinoma (Bowen's disease). Leukocytic infiltration of the dermis is often pronounced in these cases. In the absence of atypia, hyperplastic dystrophy does not progress to carcinoma, but a small proportion of those with atypia (1 to 5%) eventually develop invasive cancer.[14] It is important to remember, however, that lesions that appear clinically as white plaques may be benign without the propensity to develop carcinoma (e.g., vitiligo, chronic dermatitis), hyperplastic or atypical. Biopsy is therefore indicated in all lesions, even those that are remotely suspicious.

MIXED DYSTROPHIES. In 10 to 50% of cases of vulvar dystrophy, both forms (lichen sclerosus and hyperplastic dystrophy) may affect different areas of the same vulva at the same time, requiring multiple biopsies from various sites. These cases probably account for the apparent increased incidence of carcinoma developing in lichen sclerosus, reported by some authors.

TUMORS

Tumors of the vulva are the most important lesions to affect this region. Many types have been recorded, both benign and malignant, including fibromas, neurofibromas, angiomas, sweat gland tumors, carcinomas, malignant melanomas, and various types of mesenchymal sarcoma. All these forms are uncommon and, moreover, are histologically analogous to similar tumors occurring elsewhere in the body. Therefore, attention is focused on the more frequent tumors and other proliferative lesions distinctive of the vulva.

CONDYLOMA ACUMINATUM

Benign verrucous protuberances of the vulva occur in three forms. (1) By far the most common is the *condyloma acuminatum*, a virus-induced squamous papilloma also called "venereal wart." (2) A much rarer form is the usually discrete *squamous papilloma*, which may be indistinguishable from condyloma acuminatum but is usually single, occurs in older age groups, and is not venereally transmitted; these squamous papillomas may be the forerunners of carcinoma in a few cases. (3) The *syphilitic condyloma lata* is described on page 337.

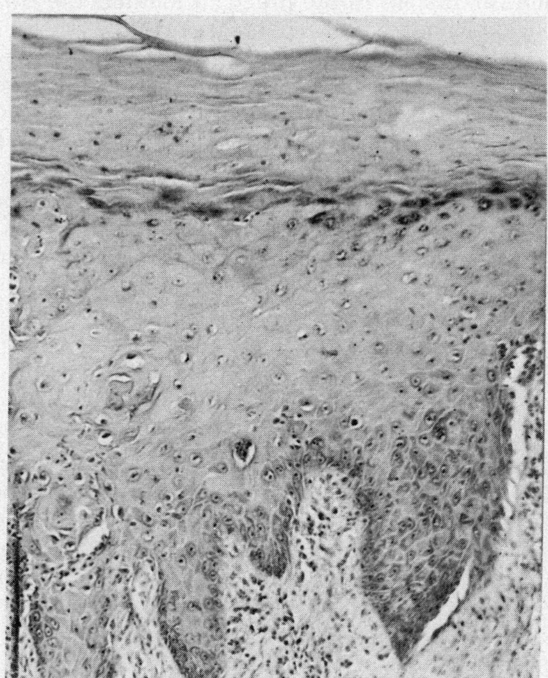

Figure 24–7. Hyperplastic vulvar dystrophy. Marked epithelial hyperplasia and hyperkeratosis, present clinically as leukoplakia. (Courtesy of Dr. Arthur Hertig.)

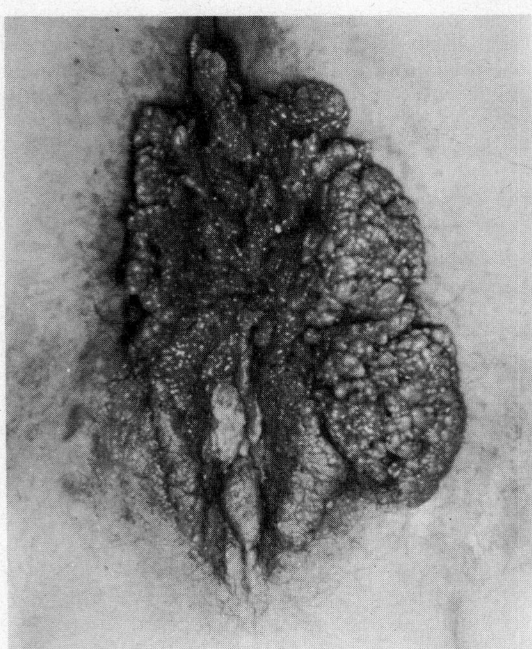

Figure 24–8. Numerous condylomas of vulva, almost obscuring labia minora. (Courtesy of Dr. Arthur Hertig.)

Condylomata acuminata have a distinctly verrucous gross appearance (Fig. 24–8), and although they may be solitary, they are more frequently multiple involving perineal, vulvar, and perianal regions; the vagina; and, rarely, the cervix. Histologically, they consist of a treelike proliferation of stratified squamous epithelium supported by a fibrous stroma (Fig. 24–9). Acanthosis, parakeratosis, hyperkeratosis, and a peculiar vacuolization of epithelium (called koilocytosis) are often present; there is usually a mild degree of atypicality of squamous cells, which is increased when the lesions are painted with podophyllin, the chemical often used to treat these lesions. The growth is induced by the human papilloma virus (HPV), which is similar to but antigenically different from the common wart virus. The virus has been recovered from the lesions, identified by molecular hybridization techniques,[16] and localized in epithelial cells by electron microscopy and with the immunoperoxidase technique.[17] The condition is transmitted by coitus, and the lesion is identical to that found on the penis and around the anus in males. The condyloma accuminatum itself is not considered to be a precancerous lesion, having diploid or polyploid rather than the aneuploid DNA content of precancerous cells.[18] However, condylomas sometimes *coexist* with areas of dystrophy, atypia, or carcinoma in situ,[19] a finding that may account for the reported cases of carcinomas arising from them.

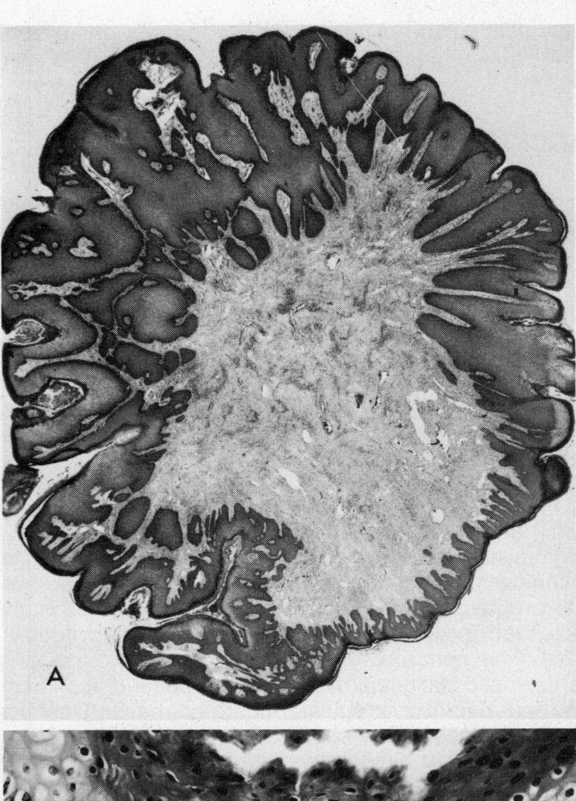

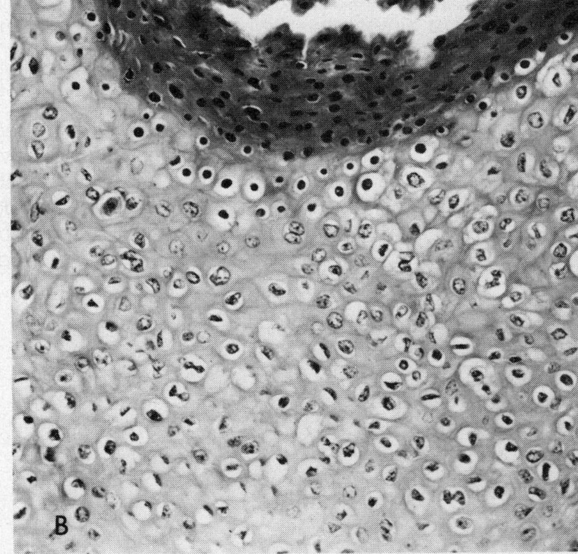

Figure 24–9. *A*, Condyloma acuminatum. Note "cauliflower" appearance of epidermal hyperplasia. *B*, High-power view of epithelial hyperplasia in condyloma acuminatum. Cytoplasmic vacuolization (koilocytosis) and oval nuclei in superficial layers are characteristic. (Courtesy of Dr. T. Kwan.)

PAPILLARY HIDRADENOMA

This benign tumor arises from the modified apocrine sweat glands of the vulva. It presents as a sharply circumscribed nodule, most frequently on the labia majora or interlabial folds. This rare tumor can be mistaken for carcinoma by the clinician because of its tendency to ulcerate, and by the pathologist because of its complex histologic appearance, which consists of tubular ducts lined by a single or double layer of nonciliated columnar cells, with a layer of flattened "myoepithelial cells" underlying the epithelium. These myoepithelial elements are characteristic of sweat glands and sweat gland tumors. Hidradenoma is a benign lesion, and when completely excised it does not recur.

CARCINOMA

Carcinoma of the vulva is an uncommon malignancy that represents about 3% of all genital cancers in the female.[20] It is rarely seen in those under the age of 60. In a considerable number of instances, these malignancies are preceded by atypical vulvar hyperplasias or dysplasias and, in a small percentage of cases, by benign papillomas and Bowen's disease (described later). 85% of malignant tumors of the vulva are squamous cell carcinomas, the remainder being basal cell carcinomas, melanomas, or adenocarcinomas.

Any region of the vulva may be affected and, in fact, a small percentage arise from the perineal skin about the rectum also. These tumors begin as small areas of epithelial thickening that resemble leukoplakia but, in the course of time, progress to create firm, indurated, elevated, maplike areas that become fissured and frequently secondarily infected. The central regions may ulcerate to produce the characteristic malignant ulceration with heaped-up, firm margins and necrotic, irregular, indurated base. Destructive ulceration wipes out all structures in its path. Histologically, these tumors are almost invariably squamous cell carcinomas, showing good differentiation with the formation of keratohyalin pearls and prickle cells (Fig. 24–10).

The tumors infiltrate locally for a period of weeks to months and tend to metastasize at a relatively early stage to the regional nodes.[20] In about 65% of cases, vulvar carcinoma has metastasized to the regional nodes at the time of discovery. The nodes affected are the inguinal nodes and the nodes within the pelvis, about the rectum, and about the iliac vessels and bifurcation of the aorta. Such nodal metastasis is correlated more with the size and duration of the lesion than with the degree of differentiation of the squamous cell growth. Ultimately, lymphohematogenous dissemination involves the lungs, liver, and other internal organs.

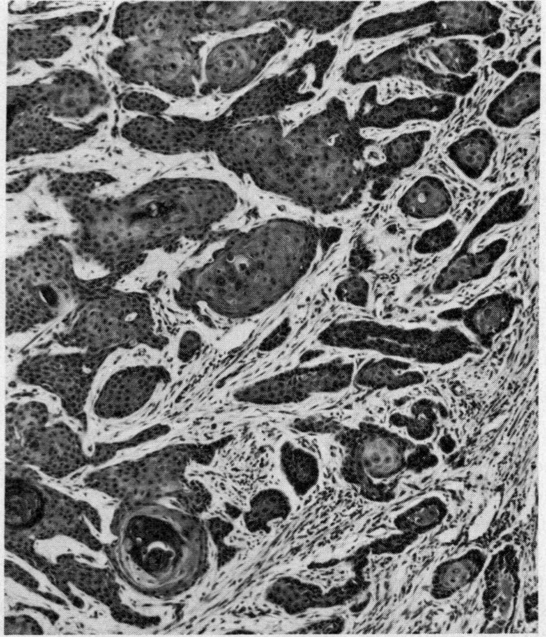

Figure 24–10. Carcinoma of vulva at medium power, illustrating typical invasive cords of squamous cell carcinoma.

Although these lesions are superficial tumors that are obviously apparent to the patient and the clinician, many are misinterpreted as dermatitis, eczema,or leukoplakia for long periods of time.

The clinical manifestations evoked are chiefly those of pain, local discomfort, itching, and exudation, since superficial secondary infection is common. If biopsies were performed on all questionable alterations of the vulva, many of these tumors would be discovered at an earlier date. Lesions less than 2 cm in diameter have a 60 to 80% five-year survival rate, with one-stage vulvectomy and lymphadenectomy; larger lesions with lymph node involvement yield a less than 10% five-year survival.

Carcinoma in situ of the vulva, or *Bowen's disease*, is an intraepithelial squamous cell carcinoma that presents clinically as leukoplakia. Identical lesions are encountered in the male (p. 1085). The disease is appearing with increasing frequency, and more commonly in women under the age of 40.[21] The lesions are sometimes multicentric[22] and may coexist with microinvasive or more deeply penetrating carcinomas. Twenty to 30% are also associated with in situ or invasive *cervical* or *vaginal* carcinoma, suggesting a field effect of a carcinogen. However, actual progression of an in situ cancer to invasive carcinoma occurs in only about 5% of patients, and then principally in those who are elderly or immunosuppressed.[23] Spontaneous regression of vulvar carcinoma in situ has also been observed, typically when these lesions occur in women in their late teens or twenties. Kaufman and colleagues[24] found herpes simplex virus type II antigens in 90% of patients with carcinoma in situ of the vulva, and preliminary studies have demonstrated the presence of HSV-specific DNA polymerase in invasive vulvar cancers and their metastases. As discussed later (p. 1125), the virus is also implicated in the causation of cervical carcinoma, but it is still unclear whether the presence of virus is important etiologically or simply reflects an opportunistic infection by a ubiquitous agent.[25]

Verrucous carcinoma is a special type of highly differentiated squamous cell carcinoma that presents as a large fungating tumor. It may resemble condyloma acuminatum histologically. Local invasion confirms the malignant nature of the lesion, but it rarely metastasizes and can be cured by wide excision.[26] It is particularly resistant to irradiation.

Basal cell carcinomas and adenocarcinomas, the latter arising in Bartholin's glands or sweat glands, also occur in the vulva but are uncommon.

EXTRAMAMMARY PAGET'S DISEASE

This curious and rare lesion of the vulva, and sometimes the perianal region, is similar in its skin

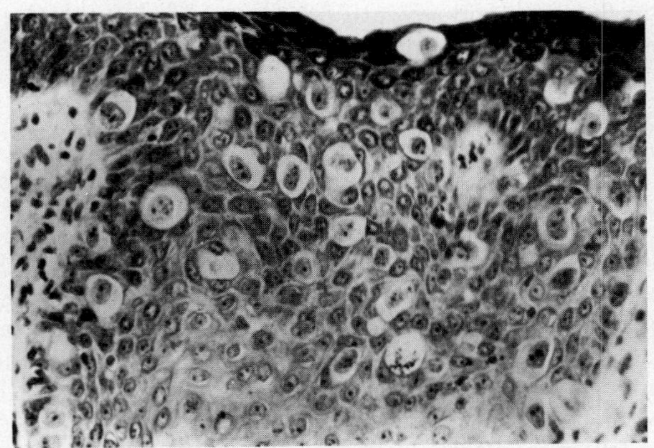

Figure 24–11. Paget's disease of vulva, with clusters of large clear tumor cells within squamous epithelium.

manifestations to Paget's disease of the breast (p. 1181). As a vulvar neoplasm it manifests itself as a red, crusted, sharply demarcated, maplike area, occurring usually on the labia majora.[27, 28] It may be accompanied by a palpable submucosal thickening or tumor. *The diagnostic microscopic feature of this lesion is the presence of large, anaplastic tumor cells lying singly or in small clusters within the epidermis, and its appendages.* These cells are rendered distinctive by a clear halo that sets them off from the surrounding epithelial cells (Fig. 24–11). The halo is due to a high content of cytoplasmic mucopolysaccharide, which can be visualized by such special stains as PAS, Alcian blue, or mucicarmine. The stains serve to differentiate Paget's disease from malignant melanoma—the intraepidermal clear cells in the latter are negative for mucopolysaccharides. Most electron microscopic studies indicate that Paget's cells are secretory glandular cells with apocrine or eccrine differentiation.[27] By immunohistochemistry they contain the so-called GCD protein 15 derived from gross cysts of the breast, which is characteristic of apocrine cells.[29]

In contrast to Paget's disease of the nipple, in which 100% of cases show an underlying ductal breast carcinoma, vulvar lesions are most frequently confined to the epidermis of the skin and adjacent hair follicles and sweat glands. The dermis may be invaded by Paget's cells in some cases, but an underlying or adjacent adenocarcinoma is distinctly uncommon; it is thus assumed that the Paget's cells arise de novo from primitive intraepithelial precursors.[27] The prognosis of Paget's disease is poor in the rare case with associated carcinoma, but intraepidermal Paget's disease may persist for many years, even decades, without the development of invasion, although recurrences may occur. Occasional untreated cases eventually become invasive.[30]

MALIGNANT MELANOMA

Melanomas of the vulva are uncommon, representing 5 to 10% of all vulvar cancers and 2% of all melanomas in women. Their peak incidence is in the sixth or seventh decade; they tend to have the same biologic and histologic characteristics as melanomas occurring elsewhere[31] and are capable of widespread metastatic dissemination. The overall survival rate is around 32%.[32]

Early in its evolution the melanoma is sometimes confined to the epithelium, where it may produce pagetoid cellular changes, described above. As already indicated, the differentiation of Paget's disease of the vulva from an intraepithelial superficial melanoma may require special stains for mucopolysaccharides.

Vagina

Congenital Anomalies
Inflammations
- Trichomonal vaginitis
- Monilial vaginitis
- Herpes simplex vaginitis

Tumors of Vagina
- Carcinoma
  - Squamous cell carcinoma
  - Adenocarcinoma
- Sarcoma botryoides

The vagina is a portion of the female genital tract that is remarkably free from primary disease. In the adult, inflammations often affect the vulva and perivulval structures and spread through the vagina to the cervix without significant involvement of the vagina. The major serious primary lesion of this structure is the seldom found primary carcinoma. The remaining entities can therefore be cited quite briefly.

CONGENITAL ANOMALIES

Atresia and total absence of the vagina are both extremely uncommon. The latter usually occurs only when there are severe malformations of the entire genital tract. Septate, or double, vagina is also a very uncommon anomaly that arises from failure of total fusion of the müllerian ducts. Congenital cysts, however, are relatively common defects that are innocuous and usually arise from *Gartner's ducts,* vestigial remnants of the wolffian ducts. Occasionally, these cysts arise from persistent inclusions of müllerian ductal epithelium.

Gartner's duct cysts are found along the lateral walls of the vagina, and commonly are 1- to 2-cm, fluid-filled cysts that occur submucosally. Rarely, they may enlarge up to 5 to 6 cm. The lining epithelium is at times cuboidal and at times columnar, or may even be transitional in form. Mixtures of these epithelial types are frequent. The cysts are of no consequence, save for their differentiation from more ominous tumor masses.

INFLAMMATIONS

Any vulvar inflammation may extend through the introitus and thus affect the vagina, but the only types of intrinsic vaginal inflammation of any consequence are gonorrheal vulvovaginitis in the child (already cited, p. 1114), trichomonal and monilial vaginitis that occur at any age, senile vaginitis in postmenopausal women, and herpes simplex infection of the vagina.

TRICHOMONAL VAGINITIS. Acute or chronic vaginal infections may be caused by *Trichomonas vaginalis*, a large, flagellated, ovoid protozoan measuring up to 30 microns in length and 10 to 15 microns in diameter. It is readily recognized by several tufted, elongated flagella at one end, matched usually by a solitary flagellum at the opposite pole. Infections with this organism may occur at any age, but are somewhat more common in postmenopausal women.

When the inflammation is well developed, the underlying vaginal and cervical mucosa has a characteristic brilliant fiery red, sometimes called "strawberry," appearance. Histologically, there is a suppurative inflammatory reaction, but it is usually quite superficial and involves only the vaginal mucosa and immediate subjacent lamina propria. This reaction may extend over the vulva and perineum into the urethra and even the urinary bladder.

MONILIAL VAGINITIS. As presented in Chapter 8, *Candida albicans* may implant on the mucosa of the vagina and produce its characteristic anatomic changes.

HERPES SIMPLEX VAGINITIS. Herpes simplex infection of the vagina accompanies vulvar infection. It is important in that it may be the source of neonatal infection during childbirth (p. 284).

TUMORS OF VAGINA

The malignant tumors of the vagina of clinical significance in terms of frequency and biologic behavior are carcinomas and sarcoma botryoides. However, benign neoplasms and non-neoplastic lesions that simulate tumors also arise in the vagina. Epithelial papillomas, fibromas, leiomyomas, and hemangiomas are uncommon and resemble their counterparts in other sites. Small red nodules of granulation tissue may simulate tumors in the vagina. These usually follow hysterectomy or long-standing chronic inflammation. Because these nodules bleed freely, they are often mistaken for hemangiomas. Foci of endometriosis may arise in the vagina and masquerade as a neoplasm (p. 1130). Gartner's duct cysts (p. 1191) and other epithelial inclusion cysts may also present as intravaginal masses.

CARCINOMA

Primary carcinoma of the vagina is an extremely uncommon cancer accounting for about 1% of malignant neoplasms in the female genital tract. Its peak incidence is in the sixth and seventh decades of life but, rarely, it occurs in younger women.

Squamous Cell Carcinoma

Over 95% of vaginal carcinomas are *squamous cell carcinomas*, usually of the well-differentiated type.[32]

Most often the tumor affects the upper posterior vagina, particularly along the posterior wall at the junction with the exocervix. It begins as a focus of epithelial thickening, progressing to a plaquelike mass that extends centrifugally and invades, by direct continuity, the cervix and perivaginal structures such as the urethra, urinary bladder, and rectum. The lesions in the lower two-thirds metastasize to the inguinal nodes, whereas upper lesions tend to involve the regional iliac nodes and, in late advanced stages, distant organs via the blood.

These lesions first come to the patient's attention by the appearance of irregular spotting or the development of a frank vaginal discharge (leukorrhea). At other times, they remain totally silent and only become clinically manifest by the onset of urinary or rectal fistulas.

Adenocarcinoma

Adenocarcinomas are rare but have received considerable attention because of the increased frequency of clear cell adenocarcinomas in young women whose mothers had been treated with diethylstilbestrol (DES) during pregnancy for a threatened abortion.[33] These tumors are usually discovered between the ages of 15 and 20 and are often composed of vacuolated, glycogen-containing cells; hence, the term clear cell carcinoma (Fig. 24–12). Since the initial description of six cases by Herbst and co-workers,[33] over 400 cases of adenocarcinoma of the vagina have been reported to an official registry for these tumors. Fortunately, less than 0.14% of DES-exposed pregnant women develop adenocarcinoma.[34] The tumors are most often located on the anterior wall of the vagina, usually in the upper third, and vary in size from 0.2 to 10 cm in greatest diameter.

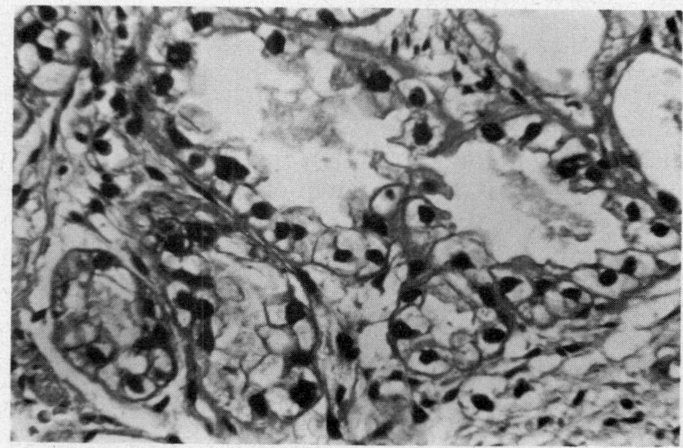

Figure 24–12. Clear cell adenocarcinoma of vagina, DES related, showing vacuolated tumor cells forming glands.

These cancers can also arise in the cervix; the ratio of vaginal to cervical carcinomas in the Registry is 7:3.[34]

A probable precursor of the tumor is *vaginal adenosis,* a condition in which glandular columnar epithelium of müllerian type either appears beneath the squamous epithelium or replaces it.[35] Adenosis presents clinically as red, granular foci contrasting with the normal pale pink, opaque vaginal mucosa. Microscopically the glandular epithelium may be either mucus-secreting, resembling endocervical mucosa, or so-called tuboendometrial, often containing cilia. Adenosis has been reported in 35 to 90% of the offspring of estrogen-treated mothers. Detailed histologic studies suggest that clear cell adenocarcinomas arise from the tuboendometrial areas of vaginal adenosis,[36] but, as mentioned earlier, such malignant transformation is extremely rare.

Because of its insidious, invasive growth, vaginal cancer (squamous and adenocarcinoma) is difficult to cure. With radiotherapy or radical surgery, the five-year survival rate for squamous carcinoma and adenocarcinoma not related to DES is on the order of 20 to 30%; the ten-year survival rate, about 15%. On the other hand, surgery and irradiation have successfully eradicated DES-related tumors in up to 80% of cases.

Extension of cervical carcinoma to the vagina is much more common than primary malignancies of the vagina. Accordingly, before a diagnosis of primary vaginal carcinoma can be made, a preexisting cervical lesion must be ruled out.

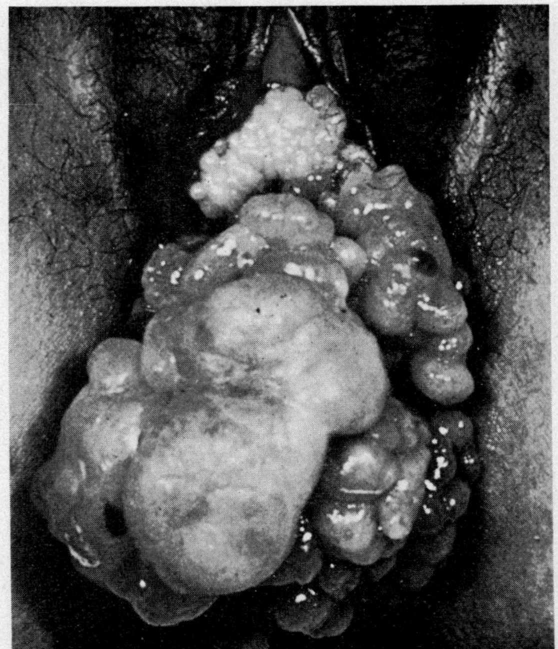

Figure 24–13. Sarcoma botryoides of vagina appearing as a polypoid mass protruding from vagina. (Courtesy of Dr. Arthur Hertig.)

SARCOMA BOTRYOIDES

Sarcoma botryoides is an interesting but very uncommon vaginal tumor most frequently found in infants and children under the age of 5. The tumor consists predominantly of malignant embryonal rhabdomyoblasts and is thus a type of rhabdomyosarcoma (p. 1314).[37]

Grossly, these tumors tend to grow as polypoid, rounded, bulky masses that sometimes fill and project out of the vagina; they have the appearance of grapelike clusters (hence the designation "botryoides," grapelike) (Fig. 24–13). They have a gelatinous friable consistency. Fragments may break off, with subsequent bleeding and secondary infection. Histologically, the tumor cells are small and have oval nuclei, with a small protrusion of cytoplasm from one end, resembling a tennis racket. Rarely, striations can be seen within the cytoplasm. Beneath the vaginal epithelium the tumor cells are crowded in a so-called "cambium" layer, but in the deep regions they lie within a loose fibromyxomatous stroma that is edematous and may contain many inflammatory cells. For this reason, the lesions can be mistaken for benign inflammatory polyps if care is not taken to sample sufficient sections, leading to unfortunate delays in diagnosis and treatment.

These tumors tend to invade locally and cause death by penetration into the peritoneal cavity or by obstruction of the urinary tract.[38] Radical surgery, unpleasant as it is for the young female, coupled with chemotherapy appears to offer the best results in cases diagnosed sufficiently early. Embryonal rhabdomyosarcoma, identical in gross and microscopic appearance, also occurs in the bile duct, urinary bladder, and eustachian tube.

Cervix

Lesions of the cervix are extremely common if one includes the great abundance of minor inflammatory changes designated as nonspecific cervicitis. In fact, excessive inflammatory vaginal discharge, referred to clinically as leukorrhea, constitutes one of the most common clinical complaints in gynecologic practice. However, in addition to these for the most part innocuous inflammatory lesions, the cervix is extremely vulnerable to the development of cancer. As will be re-emphasized presently, cervical carcinoma alone is responsible for about 5% of all cancer deaths in women.

CONGENITAL ANOMALIES

Hypoplasia of the cervix usually accompanies infantile development of the uterus and is frequently only one feature of general underdevelopment of the female genital tract. Duplication of the cervix almost invariably implies a septate, totally bifid uterus. Stenosis and atresia of the cervical os may occur as congenital developmental defects. In this condition, the narrowing may be so extreme as to represent a complete absence of the cervical canal. In most instances, the developmental narrowing is at least probe patent. Stenosis of the cervix is more commonly an acquired defect from chronic cervicitis, with subsequent fibrosis and scarring. Both the developmental and acquired stenoses may result in sterility and retention of menstrual blood and secretions.

INFLAMMATIONS

Inflammations of the cervix are extremely common. They are caused by a variety of bacteria, many of which compose the normal flora of the vagina. This form of banal inflammation is referred to as nonspecific cervicitis. However, it should not be inferred that all nonspecific cervicitis is without serious significance because, as will be pointed out, it may predispose to serious complications in a small percentage of cases. In addition to this commonplace type of cervicitis, there are many types of specific cervical inflammations, i.e., gonorrhea, syphilis, chancroid, and tuberculosis, described in Chapter 8.

ACUTE AND CHRONIC CERVICITIS

Depending on the histologic criteria selected for the establishment of this diagnosis, some degree of cervical inflammation may be found in virtually all multiparous and in many nulliparous adult women. It is extremely doubtful whether the minor involvements are of any clinical consequence.

ETIOLOGY AND PATHOGENESIS. Despite its commonplace occurrence, few data have been accumulated on the precise causes of this disorder. Specific infections by gonococci, *Trichomonas vaginalis*, *Candida albicans*, and herpes (mostly type II) are clearly responsible for many cases of either acute or chronic cervicitis. However, the most commonly identified organisms are streptococci, enterococci, *E. coli*, and a variety of staphylococci. The vagina and the cervix normally contain a mixed flora that includes similar organisms. Predisposing causes to infection must then be sought. Trauma of childbirth, instrumentation in the course of gynecologic treatment, hyperestrinism, hypoestrinism, intercourse, excessive secretion of the cervical glands, high alkalinity of the cervical mucus, and congenital eversion of the endocervical mucosa have all been cited as predisposing influences.

MORPHOLOGY. Cervicitis may be divided into an acute and a chronic phase.

Excluding gonococcal infections, *acute cervicitis* is most commonly encountered postpartally and is usually caused by either staphylococci or streptococci. Microscopically, there is stromal edema, infiltration by polymorphonuclear leukocytes, and frequently focal loss of the lining mucosa. In the more marked cases, the inflammatory infiltration extends to involve the endocervical mucosa and glands (endocervicitis).

Chronic nonspecific cervicitis is far more common than acute cervicitis. It begins or is most marked within the endocervix, in and about the external cervical os, or in the squamocolumnar junction. In its simplest form, chronic cervicitis appears as a slight reddening, swelling, and granularity limited to the margins of the external cervical os. With progression, the reddening and granularity extend to produce a progressively widening ring of inflamed mucosa (Fig. 24–14). Inflammatory stenosis of the cervical glands may yield cystic dilatations designated as **nabothian cysts.** The chronic inflammatory cells may accumulate into lymphoid follicles, **follicular cervicitis.** All these anatomic lesions are merely variations on the basic theme of nonspecific cervicitis.

Histologically, the inflammatory infiltrate is preponderantly mononuclear, but neutrophils may also be present. The infiltrate is usually limited to the superficial regions and extends about the endocervical mucus-secreting glands as well as into the gland lumina (Fig. 24–15).

The cervical and endocervical mucosa are sites of additional changes. The epithelium usually shows only mild-to-moderate hyperplasia. In more marked cases, these epithelial alterations may produce downgrowth of epithelial pegs into the inflammatory granulation tissue. In the course of these changes, the epithelial cells are depleted of their normal content of glycogen (Fig. 24–16). The loss of glyco-

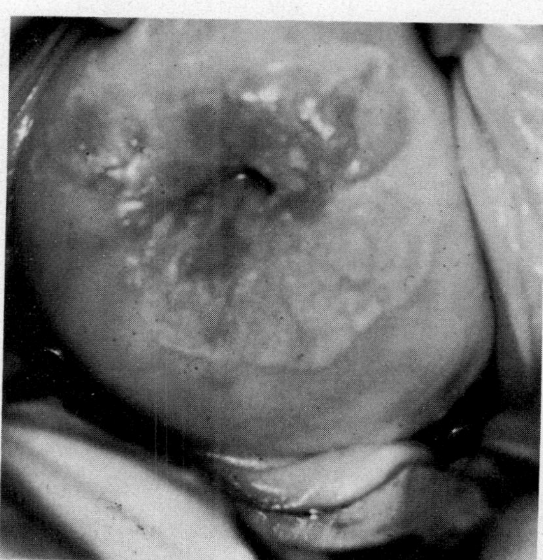

Figure 24–14. Chronic cervicitis as viewed through a speculum. The inflammatory area rims the external os. (Courtesy of Dr. Arthur Hertig.)

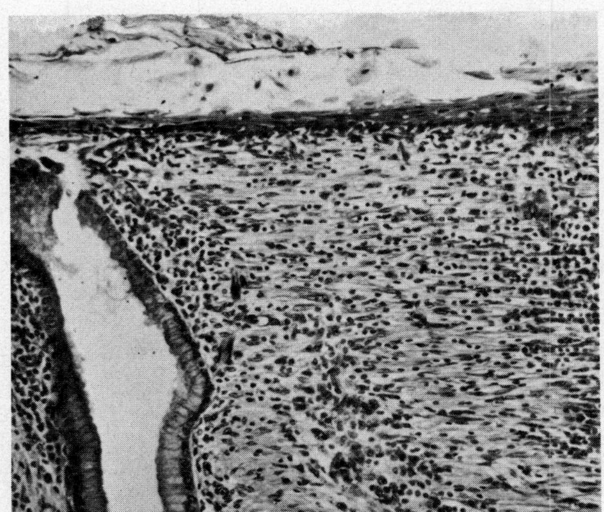

Figure 24–15. Chronic ulcerative cervicitis with previous loss and partial regrowth of surface epithelium. An inflammatory infiltrate is present in subjacent tissue.

gen is an important biochemical alteration, since it accounts for the failure of these areas to stain brown with Schiller's solution (an iodine preparation), as detailed on page 1126.

In certain cases, in the region of the external os, tongues of stratified squamous epithelium may extend down from the surface mucosa into the endocervical glands (Fig. 24–17). These changes are designated squamous metaplasia of endocervical glands. This form of epithelial alteration merits careful attention because it can be mistaken, on casual inspection, for the infiltrative growth of squamous cell carcinoma.

Clinical Course. Nonspecific cervicitis may be a completely banal, asymptomatic lesion that is discovered when the cervix is removed for other causes, in the course of routine gynecologic examination, or because of leukorrhea. Diagnosis may be made by simple visual examination of the cervix when the changes are well defined, but at times may be difficult to differentiate from the much more serious condition of cancer of the cervix. The cervical distortion, ulceration, and overgrowth of inflammatory tissue may sometimes make this lesion resemble a neoplasm. Colposcopy, which allows a magnified view of vaginal and cervical mucosa, has greatly facilitated follow-up or direct biopsy of suspicious lesions (p. 1128). Ultimately, the differentiation rests on histologic examination of biopsy specimens.

TUMORS OF CERVIX

Although the cervix may develop a wide variety of neoplasms, at least 95% of cervical tumors are represented by three lesions: carcinomas, polyps, and papillomas.

CARCINOMA

No form of cancer better documents the remarkable effects of early diagnosis and curative therapy on the mortality rate than cancer of the cervix. Fifty years ago, carcinoma of the cervix was the leading cause of cancer deaths in women in the United States, but the death

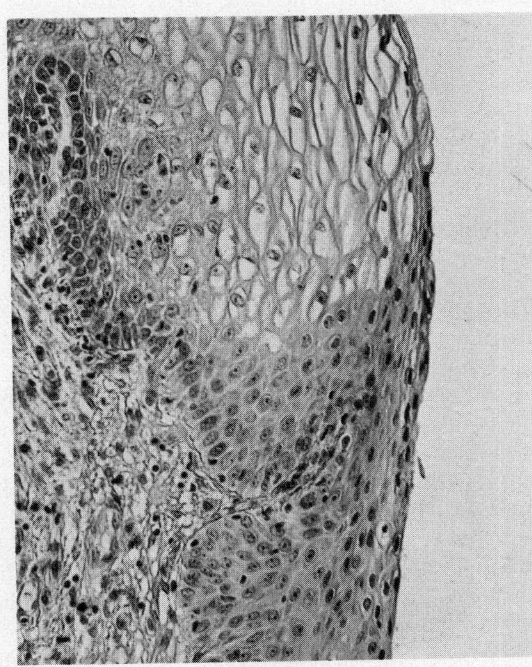

Fig. 24–16

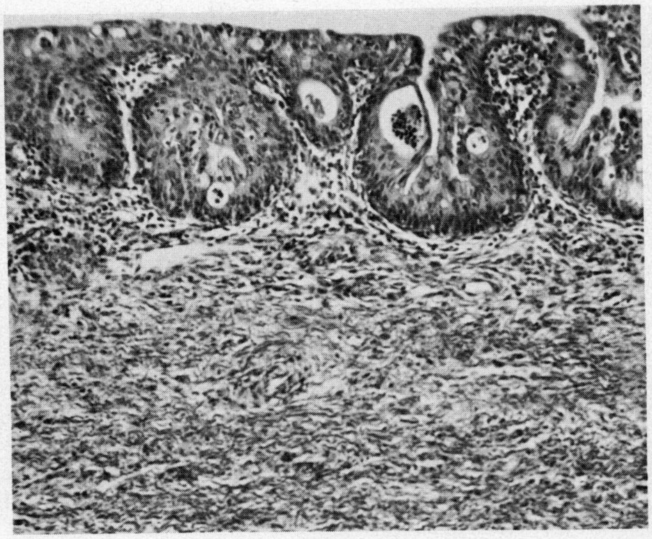

Fig. 24–17

Figure 24–16. Junction between normal glycogen-laden vacuolated epithelium *(above)* and glycogen-depleted cells *(below)*. (Courtesy of Dr. Arthur Hertig.)

Figure 24–17. Chronic cervicitis with squamous metaplasia that has obliterated the endocervical glands. Note marked subepithelial inflammation. (Courtesy of Dr. Arthur Hertig.)

rate has dropped remarkably to its present rank as the sixth cause of cancer mortality (behind breast, lung, colon, ovary, and pancreas).[39] Better cure of cervical cancer has reduced deaths due to uterine cancer from 27 per 100,000 female population in 1930 to eight per 100,000 in 1980. The trend continues. In the last decade alone, the estimated number of new cervical cancers and the estimated deaths from cervical cancers decreased by approximately 20%.[40] The low mortality rate reflects the earlier discovery of curable lesions. Today, about 50% of cervical cancers are detected when they are small localized lesions (Stages 0 and 1), whereas 20 years ago only 20% were discovered in these curable stages. Thanks for these impressive improvements are largely owed to the Papanicolaou cytologic test for detection of cancer (p. 265). However, the disease has not been conquered and still accounts for approximately 7500 deaths per year. The American Cancer Society estimates that there are 16,000 new patients with invasive cervical cancers each year, as well as 45,000 new patients with carcinoma in situ.[39] On the average, a woman under 40 years of age has a 2% risk of developing cervical cancer.[41]

More is known about the life history of this form of cancer than any other. Cervical cytology and the accessibility of the cervix to biopsy provide the opportunity for the early discovery and close follow-up of these lesions. Indeed, the entire concept of "in situ" cancer originated with studies of this neoplasm, and it is therefore appropriate to consider here in some detail the relationship of carcinoma in situ to overt clinical malignancy.

INCIDENCE. Carcinoma of the cervix may occur at any age from the second decade of life to senility. The peak incidence of invasive lesions occurs around 45 years of age, and of in situ lesions about 15 years earlier. The frequency of this form of cancer in young women appears to have risen significantly in the recent past. Many social and personal factors may be implicated in this trend. However, the overall incidence of *invasive* cervical carcinoma has declined by approximately 58% since 1947, almost certainly owing to the increased use of mass screening by cytology, which contributes to early detection and removal of precursor lesions.[42]

EPIDEMIOLOGY AND ETIOLOGY. Much of our insight into the etiology of cervical cancer comes from clinical or epidemiologic studies of risk factors for the development of these cancers. In the case of cervical carcinoma a high incidence, denoting increased risk, has been correlated with the following:[43]

1. Low socioeconomic class.[44]
2. Race. Black women have about twice the incidence of cervical cancer as do white women, this being related largely to socioeconomic influences.[44] Mortality and incidence are also greater in Spanish-Americans and American Indians.[45]
3. Early marriage and increased parity.
4. Age of onset of sexual relations, frequency of coitus, possibly the number of sexual partners, and early age at first pregnancy.[46, 47] There is a high incidence of cervical carcinoma in prostitutes and a low incidence in nuns.

Other risk factors either are subjects of debate or are yet to be confirmed. Cervical carcinoma is less frequent in Jews, Indian Moslems, and Parsees. However, the postulated role of early circumcision of males in protecting against cervical cancer in these groups has been challenged, since the negative association with circumcision is not observed in all populations.[48] Other factors are diethylstilbestrol therapy for pregnant mothers, use of contraceptive pills, and hormonal treatment of menopausal women.[49] Only 4.3% of partners of cervical cancer patients are vasectomized, compared with 19.4% of partners of matched controls, remotely suggesting a role for semen as a vehicle for a potential carcinogenic agent.[50] An association with cigarette smoking has been reported,[51] but there are so many complex interactions between smoking and other risk factors such as social class and early sexual activity that a direct relationship is hard to establish.[43]

What clues about causation can be inferred from the epidemiologic data? Obviously, the risk of developing this disease is strongly related to sexual practice. Reliable epidemiologic data on this subject are difficult to obtain. Nevertheless, attempts to evaluate each of these features separately indicate that a direct pathogenic role can be ascribed to two variables: *early onset of coitus, and possibly multiple sexual partners.* Most of the other factors, such as early and multiple marriage, early and multiple parity, and low socioeconomic status, can be almost entirely related to predisposing sexual practices. Thus, it would seem that carcinoma of the cervix involves some initiating agent transmitted at an early age from male to female—a one-way venereal disease, if you will. Multiple sexual partners would increase the likelihood of initially encountering this agent, as well as make possible repeated contact with it.

Viruses and Cervical Cancer. Two classes of viruses are currently suspected to play a role in the causation of cervical cancer: herpes simplex virus type II (HSV II) and the human papilloma virus (HPV).[52]

HERPES SIMPLEX VIRUS. A relationship between HSV II and cancer of the cervix is suggested by a large number of observations.[52, 53] The main findings can be summarized as follows:

1. Genital HSV II infection occurs in about 0.15% of the general female population, and there is an increased incidence of cervical dysplasia and carcinoma in patients with such infection. In one study, 23% of women with herpes infection had cervical dysplasia or cancer, whereas only 2.6% without infection had these conditions.[54] The prevalence of HSV II antibodies is significantly higher in women with cervical cancer or dysplasia than in controls.
2. Women with herpetic cervicitis have a four- to 16-fold greater risk of cervical cancer than those without disease.
3. Studies of antibodies to a specific herpesvirus protein antigen (AG4) show that 50 to 96% of patients

with dysplasia, carcinoma in situ, or active invasive cancer have positive titers, compared with 11.7% of controls, 7.7% of patients with cancer in other sites, and 7.4% of patients with treated invasive cancer.[55]

4. Cervical tumor cells have been shown to express viral messenger RNA and a variety of other viral proteins.[56] Viral DNA sequences corresponding to about 40% of the genome were found in the cervical tumor, and infectious HSV II was isolated from a lesion of a patient with carcinoma in situ.[57]

5. HSV and viral DNA have been shown to cause neoplastic transformation in culture, and the transforming sequences have been identified.

6. Finally, in preliminary reports, a proportion of monkeys vaginally or cervically infected with HSV II were shown to develop dysplasia five years after infection.

HUMAN PAPILLOMA VIRUS (HPV). As noted earlier (p. 1117), this virus is the known cause of the venereally transmitted vulvar and cervical condyloma acuminatum.[17] The same class of virus has been localized by immunoperoxidase techniques, electron microscopy, and DNA sequencing studies in patients with cervical dysplasia, a lesion considered to be precancerous.[57] The virally infected cells are identified histologically by the presence of highly vacuolated, ballooned cytoplasm, a change termed *koilocytosis* (Fig. 24–9, p. 1117). Koilocytotic cells, however, are frequent in the cervical epithelium of many women with benign condylomas or only mild dysplasia, but are uncommon (less than 10%) in carcinoma in situ or invasive carcinoma.[58] Recent studies suggest that HPV type 16 is closely associated with malignant lesions of the cervix, while types 6 and 11 are present in the benign condylomas.[59]

The possibility that either virus or both viruses (synergistically) play a role in cervical cancer is attractive, since it would explain many of the previously mentioned correlations, all of which might contribute to the possible spread of an infectious agent. However, the questions whether these infections and cervical cancer are merely independent consequences of promiscuity and are not biologically related, or whether they follow the development of the earliest precancerous lesion, remain unanswered.

RELATIONSHIP OF CERVICAL DYSPLASIA AND CARCINOMA IN SITU (CERVICAL INTRAEPITHELIAL NEOPLASIA) TO INVASIVE CARCINOMA. One of the most significant advances in the therapy of neoplasia has been the realization that cervical carcinoma arises from *precursor lesions.*[42, 60–63] Most authorities now agree that *cervical cancer is the end stage of a continuum of progressively more atypical changes in which one stage merges imperceptibly with the next.* The first and apparently earliest change is the appearance of atypical cells in the basal layers of the squamous epithelium, but nonetheless with persistence of the normal differentiation toward the prickle and keratinizing cell layers. *The atypical cells show changes in nucleocytoplasmic ratio, loss of polarity, increased mitotic figures, and pleomorphism*—in other words, all the hallmarks of malignant cells. As the lesion evolves, there is progressive involvement of more and more layers of the epithelium, until it is totally replaced by atypical cells, exhibiting no surface differentiation.

Precancerous squamous lesions of the cervix are classified by one or the other of two schemes, as shown in Figure 24–18.

1. The most widely used term is *dysplasia,* which literally means "bad molding" or, in more scientific terms, disordered development. Dysplasia is subdivided into very mild, mild, moderate, and severe, depending on the proportion of the thickness of squamous epithelium involved by atypical cells. When there is full-thickness involvement by atypical cells, the term carcinoma in situ is applied (Figs. 24–18 and 24–19).

2. The second approach emphasizes that the dysplastic changes represent a spectrum of the same basic change, i.e., cervical intraepithelial neoplasia (CIN).[61] There are three grades of CIN: Grade I represents less than one-third involvement of the thickness of epithelium; Grade II one-third to two-thirds involvement; and Grade III two-thirds to full-thickness involvement, thus including the classic carcinoma in situ of the dysplasia scheme terminology. Although the designation CIN has been criticized on the basis that the milder grades of atypicality may be reversible (and thus not *neoplasia*), it has been adopted by a number of authorities on

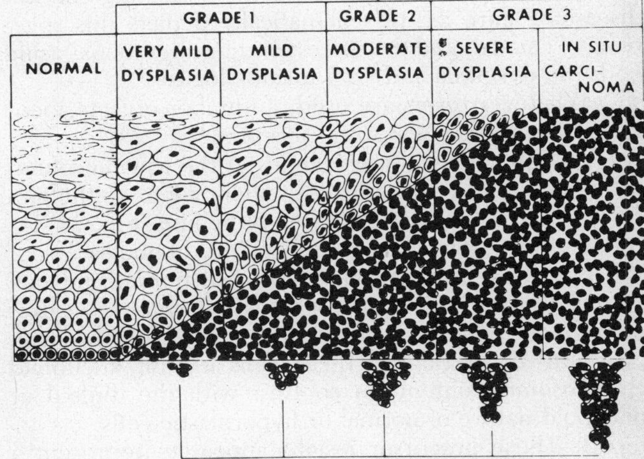

Figure 24–18. Schematic representation of cervical cancer precursors. CIN Grades 1, 2, and 3 correspond to traditional very mild–to-mild dysplasia, moderate dysplasia, and severe dysplasia–to-CIS, respectively. They are characterized by progressive increase in number of undifferentiated, malignant cells and decrease in superficial cell differentiation paralleling increasing severity of CIN. Schema also illustrates that microinvasion, although more commonly associated with a Grade 3 lesion, may also develop directly from any given stage of untreated CIN. The risk of developing microinvasion from different stages of CIN is not necessarily proportional to that illustrated in the schema, however. (From Ferenczy, A.: Cervical intraepithelial neoplasia. *In* Blaustein, A. (ed.): Pathology of the Female Genital Tract. 2nd ed. New York, Springer-Verlag, 1982. Reproduced with permission.)

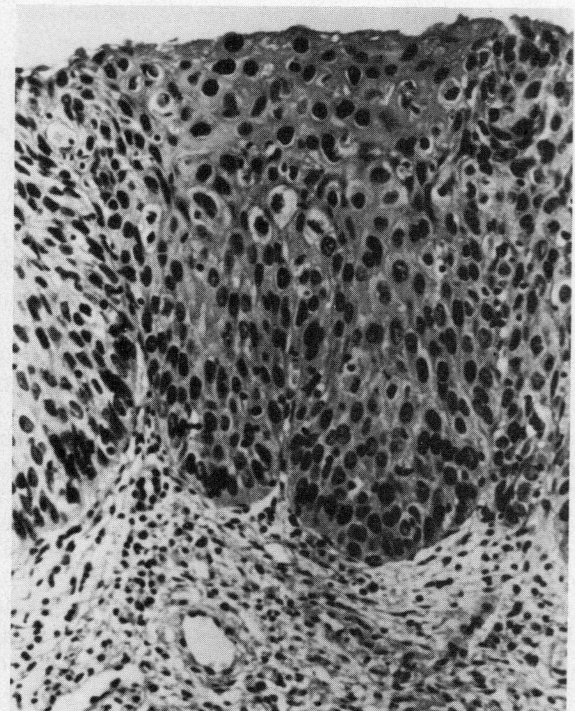

Figure 24–19. Focus of carcinoma in situ of cervix (CIN Grade III), showing markedly atypical cells occupying full thickness of epithelium. (Courtesy of Dr. D. Antonioli, Beth Israel Hospital, Boston.)

cervical neoplasia and clinical centers treating cervical disease. Figure 24–18 schematically depicts this spectrum of changes and the corresponding alterations, using both the dysplasia and CIN terminologies.[42]

Whatever terms are used, a number of facts about these alterations seem to be accepted:

1. CIN almost always begins at the squamocolumnar junction, in the transformation zone epithelium contiguous to the native portio epithelium (Fig. 24–1).

2. Physicochemical measurements of nuclear mass, DNA content, and chromosome distribution and cell kinetic studies indicate that the cell alterations in dysplasia and carcinoma are qualitatively similar and remain constant. In particular, these cells exhibit aneuploid chromosomal content, in contrast with the diploid or polyploid nature of normal or hyperplastic cells.

3. These precursor lesions appear to represent a continuum of changes when followed up in individual patients or when analyzed statistically in large populations: i.e., CIN Grade I may progress to the next higher grade during a ten-year follow-up period, Grade II may progress to III, and so on.[61, 63] All grades may progress or may persist without progression. In one study,[66] 6% of mild dysplasias, 13% of moderate dysplasias, and 29% of severe dysplasias ultimately evolved to carcinoma in situ. The more severe the grades of dysplasia, the shorter is the time span for the development of carcinoma in situ.[67] The rates of progression, however, are by no means uniform and, in general, it is difficult, if not impossible, for a clinician using any technique to predict who among those patients in a population being followed will remain static and who will progress. Whether true *regression* of these lesions occurs is debatable,[57] but they are particularly fragile and may be eradicated by biopsy, by drugs, or possibly even by physiologic trauma such as delivery.[62]

4. Carcinoma in situ or CIN Grade III is a precursor of invasive carcinoma. This conclusion is based on three pieces of evidence: (a) the finding of foci of carcinoma in situ and invasive carcinoma simultaneously in the same cervix, usually in adjacent areas; (b) the development of invasive carcinoma in patients followed without treatment after a diagnosis of carcinoma in situ has been made; and (c) the fact that most (but not all) new cases of invasive carcinoma originate from a population of women with previously proved dysplasia.

5. Several studies strongly suggest that detection and eradication of dysplasia and carcinoma in situ in a population will prevent the development of invasive cervical carcinoma and lead to a fall in death rate from that disease.[68]

6. As in the case of cervical cancer, these precursor lesions are confined almost exclusively to women who have had sexual intercourse, and a high relative index risk is associated with early sexual experience and promiscuity.

Before leaving the question of dysplasia, it is important to emphasize that there is a wide variety of alterations in the cervical epithelium that are abnormal in appearance but are benign lesions and not precancerous. For example, following trauma, biopsy, or surgery, the epithelium undergoes a reparative process, with regeneration and hyperplasia. In such epithelium, atypicality is minimal or nonexistent; the cell borders are well defined; there are one or more single large nucleoli; and the nuclei are, in general, regular. The hyperplasia that accompanies chronic cervicitis has the same features. Finally, the benign squamous metaplasia of endocervical glands should be clearly differentiated from precancerous lesions; in these, the abnormal cytologic features required for a diagnosis of dysplasia are absent.

MORPHOLOGY. Carcinoma of the cervix begins at or close to the squamocolumnar junction of the exocervical os. Carcinomas rarely if ever arise from the more lateral regions of the exocervix. **In situ carcinoma** of the cervix consistently produces no recognizable alteration to the naked eye. The diagnosis can be suspected only by the Schiller test, the Papanicolaou smear, or colposcopy. The Schiller test involves painting the cervix with a solution of iodine and potassium iodide. The normal cervical epithelium is rich in glycogen and stains a mahogany brown. The cancerous focus, because it is depleted of glycogen, fails to stain. It should be cautioned that this method may yield false-positive results since areas of inflammation may also fail to stain with the Schiller solution. The changes seen on colposcopy are detailed later (p. 1128).

At the stage of carcinoma in situ, one sees characteristic cellular anaplastic changes within the cervical mucosa without invasion of the stroma. Atypical cells and mitotic figures can be seen in the entire thickness of epithelium. Sometimes the anaplastic changes extend along the surface into the underlying endocervical glands, but such superficial spread should not be construed as invasion since the basement membranes of these glands are not penetrated.

Invasive cervical carcinoma presents in three somewhat distinctive macroscopic patterns: **fungating (or exophytic), ulcerating, and infiltrative cancer.** The most common variant is the fungating tumor, which produces an obviously neoplastic mass that projects above the surrounding mucosa (Fig. 24–20). In the ulcerating pattern, the progressive epithelial thickening leads to sloughing necrosis of the surface of the tumor with the production of a necrotic neoplastic ulceration. The infiltrative pattern is the least common variant in which the tumor grows downward into the underlying stroma of the cervix, causing only irregular thickening of the mucosal surface without ulceration or fungation. In the course of time, all cervical carcinomas infiltrate the underlying cervix, obliterate the external os, grow up into the endocervical canal and lower uterine segment, and eventually extend into the wall of the fundus.

Advanced cervical carcinoma extends by direct continuity to involve every contiguous structure including the peritoneum, urinary bladder, ureters, rectum, and vagina. Local and distant lymph nodes are also involved. The paracervical, hypogastric, obturator, and external iliac nodes are affected in about half the cases and more distant periaortic nodes in about the same number. Distant metastasis occurs to the liver, lungs, bone marrow, and other structures.

The histology of 75 to 90% of carcinomas of the cervix is that of a typical squamous cell carcinoma of varying differentiation and growth rate. Some of the tumors are extremely well differentiated, producing keratohyalin, epithelial pearls, and prickle cells, whereas others are composed of more undifferentiated squamous cells. The majority (over 60%) are nonkeratinizing, moderately well differentiated, and composed of large cells. It is usually possible to identify in situ carcinoma in the margins of overt invasive lesions.

Many systems of classifying these carcinomas have been devised, but all include essentially either histologic grading of the degree of differentiation of the neoplasm or expression of its clinical extent in stages. As would be suspected, the better differentiated tumors generally yield a better survival rate than the anaplastic undifferentiated lesions. With comparable radiation therapy, differentiated lesions of similar clinical stage yielded a 51% five-year survival rate as compared with 28% for anaplastic tumors. The most widely accepted classification of staging is the 1976 modification of the International Federation of Gynecology and Obstetrics (FIGO) classification:

Stage 0. Carcinoma in situ or intraepithelial carcinoma.

Stage I. Includes carcinoma that is strictly confined to the cervix. It may be subdivided into:

Ia. Carcinoma in situ with early stromal invasion (microinvasive carcinoma).

Ib. Clinically invasive carcinoma confined to cervix.

Ib (Occult). Histologically invasive carcinoma of the cervix that could not be detected at routine clinical examination but was diagnosed on a biopsy or cone biopsy.

Stage II. The carcinoma extends beyond the cervix but has not extended onto the pelvic wall. The carcinoma involves the vagina, but not the lower third.

Stage III. The carcinoma has extended onto the pelvic wall. On rectal examination, there is no cancer-free space between the tumor and the pelvic wall. The tumor involves the lower third of the vagina.

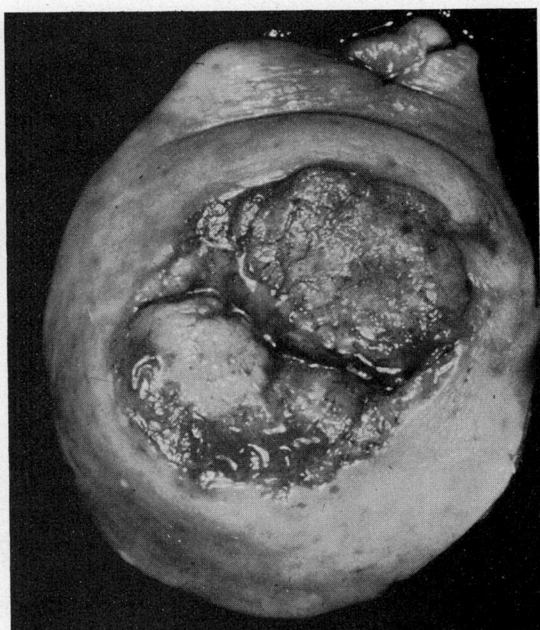

Figure 24–20. Carcinoma of cervix, well advanced.

Stage IV. The carcinoma has extended beyond the true pelvis or has involved the mucosa of the bladder or rectum. This stage obviously includes those with metastatic dissemination.

The term microinvasive carcinoma (Stage Ia) deserves some comment. This refers to a tumor in which the lesion is in situ, but in which there might be small, microscopic foci or tongues of neoplastic epithelium invading beyond the basement membrane. The W.H.O. International Committee could reach no agreement as to the depth of invasion beyond which the tumor could be classified as frankly invasive (1b). Various groups use 1, 3, and 5 mm as the depth beyond which the tumor should be classified as frankly invasive cancer, Stage 1b, and treated by means of radical surgery.[69]

The remaining 10 to 25% of cervical carcinomas constitute **adenocarcinomas, adenosquamous carcinomas, undifferentiated carcinomas,** or other rare histologic types. The **adenocarcinomas** presumably arise in the endocervical glands. Rarely, such adenocarcinomas may arise in remnants of the mesonephric ducts. These look and behave as do the squamous cell lesions. They arise, however, in a slightly older age group. The **adenosquamous carcinomas** have mixed glandular and squamous patterns and are thought to arise from the reserve cells in the basal layers of the endocervical epithelium. They are distinguishable from the more common squamous cell lesions only by histologic examination, but tend to have a less favorable prognosis than squamous cell carcinoma of similar stage. Clear cell adenocarcinomas of the cervix in DES-exposed women are similar to those occurring in the vagina (p. 1120).

CLINICAL COURSE. It is apparent from the preceding discussion that cancer of the cervix evolves slowly over the course of many years. The peak incidence of invasive carcinoma is in the fifth and sixth decades; that of in situ lesions is in the early to late thirties. With the sexual revolution, the disease sometimes appears in much younger women. During the long evolution, the

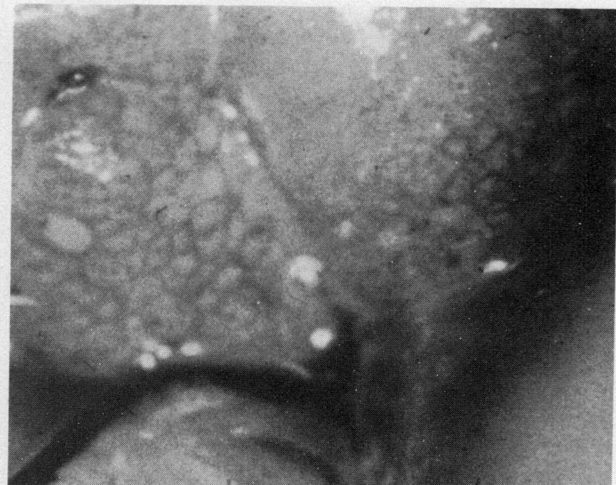

Figure 24–21. Colposcopic view of cervical mucosa showing characteristic mosaic pattern of cervical dysplasia. (Courtesy of Dr. D. Antonioli, Beth Israel Hospital, Boston.)

cytologic abnormalities produce no clinical manifestations. Such nonspecific symptoms as increased vaginal discharge may be present. For these reasons, it is generally acknowledged that periodic Papanicolaou smears should be performed on all women after they become sexually active, since these examinations afford an excellent opportunity to detect these incipient cancers when they can be eradicated with almost complete certainty. Cytologic examination merely detects the possible presence of a cervical cancer; it does not make an absolute diagnosis, which requires histologic evaluation of appropriate biopsy specimens. Ultimately, when these cancers become clinically overt, they usually produce irregular vaginal bleeding, leukorrhea, pain on coitus, and dysuria as the dominant clinical manifestations.

Colposcopy provides a well-lighted, magnified, stereoscopic view of the cervix, including the transformation zone in which intraepithelial neoplasia most frequently occurs.[70] The alterations that accompany dysplasia include areas of white epithelium and abnormal patterns referred to as "mosaic or punctuation" patterns (Fig. 24–21). These are by no means diagnostic of cervical neoplasia, but their presence has been correlated with disease in many cases. Highly abnormal vascular patterns regularly accompany invasive cervical cancer.

The treatment of carcinoma of the cervix depends on the stage of the neoplasm. For invasive carcinoma, three therapeutic modalities—surgical excision, radiation alone, or combined surgery and radiation—are sponsored equally ardently by various clinicians. Reports of end results indicate that, for Stages I and II, there is little difference in five-year survival rates with all three forms of therapy.

The prognosis and survival of these patients depends largely on the stage at which cancer is first discovered.[71] If these lesions are discovered at Stage 0, 100% cure should be effected. With current methods of treatment, there is a five-year survival rate of about 80 to 90% with Stage I, 75% with Stage II, 35% with Stage III, and 10 to 15% with Stage IV disease.[72] Most patients with Stage IV cancer die as a consequence of local extension of the tumor—e.g., into and about the urinary bladder and ureters, leading to ureteral obstruction, pyelonephritis, and uremia—rather than of metastatic disease.

As for the treatment of dysplasia and carcinoma in situ, there is no need for hasty radical surgery for these lesions. Years usually elapse before in situ lesions become invasive. Simple hysterectomy is clearly curative for severe dysplasia or carcinoma in situ, and indeed is advocated by many clinicians for women no longer wishing to conceive. However, many preinvasive lesions can be localized by colposcopy and eradicated by freezing (cryotherapy), electrocoagulation, or at the most conization (removal of a cone of cervical mucosa and submucosa). As long as the patient can be followed by means of periodic Papanicolaou smears or colposcopy, much can be gained from a conservative and individualized approach. Thus, Richart and colleagues noted a recurrence rate of less than 1% in almost 3000 patients with CIN treated with cryosurgery and followed for more than five years.[73]

POLYPS

Endocervical polyps are common, relatively innocuous, inflammatory tumors that occur in 2 to 5% of adult women, usually in the fourth and fifth decades of life. They are frequently associated with chronic cervicitis, although it is doubtful that the two conditions have a causal relationship. Perhaps the major significance of

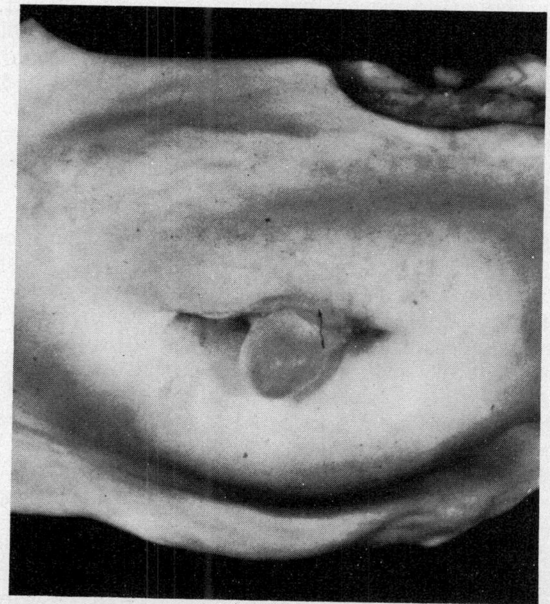

Figure 24–22. Endocervical polyp, protruding through external os.

polyps lies in their production of irregular vaginal "spotting" or bleeding that arouses suspicion of some more ominous lesion.

Polyps may occur singly (approximately 90%) or multiply. Most arise within the endocervical canal and vary from small, hemispheric, sessile projections several millimeters in diameter to large, 5-cm bulbous masses that are pedunculated and may protrude or prolapse through the cervical os (Fig. 24–22). All are soft, almost mucoid, and histologically are composed of a loose fibromyxomatous stroma harboring hypertrophied or cystically dilated, mucus-secreting endocervical glands. Ulceration and chronic inflammation may lead to squamous metaplasia or considerable inflammatory epithelial alterations.

In almost all instances, simple curettage or surgical excision effects a cure, although formation of an additional polyp may occur.

Microglandular Endocervical Hyperplasia

This benign cervical lesion occurs in women receiving progestogen-containing oral contraceptive agents.[74] Clinically the lesion resembles a cervical polyp, and histologically it is composed of a mass of tightly packed proliferating glands or tubules, with occasional focal squamous metaplasia. At times the epithelium may show atypical changes. Occasionally the lesions occur in the absence of ingestion of contraceptive drugs.[75] The importance of the lesions lies in their possible confusion with endocervical adenocarcinoma.[75]

PAPILLOMA

Several types of papilloma arise on the cervix. They take one of three forms: (1) The cockscomb papilloma or polyp almost invariably occurs during pregnancy and regresses following delivery. It is a small, red lesion that projects above the surrounding mucosa and has a resemblance to a cockscomb. (2) The condylomata acuminata are similar to those lesions occurring in the vulva. As pointed out, they are caused by human papilloma virus. (3) The rare solitary, true neoplastic papillary proliferations of the cervical mucosa usually arise from the squamocolumnar junction. As proliferative lesions, this form of papilloma may, rarely, convert to a squamous cell cervical cancer.

Body of Uterus and Endometrium

The uterus, stimulated continually by hormones, denuded monthly of its endometrial mucosa, and inhabited periodically by fetuses, is subject to a variety of disorders, the most common of which result from endocrine imbalances, complications of pregnancy, and neoplastic proliferation. Together with the lesions that affect the cervix, the lesions of the corpus of the uterus and the endometrium account for the great preponderance of gynecologic practice.

CONGENITAL ANOMALIES

Hypoplasia of the uterus is encountered in a variety of endocrine disorders. Such small uteri are referred to clinically as infantile. Most are due to ovarian or pituitary hypofunction. Strictly speaking, such failure of growth is not a congenital anomaly but an acquired defect.

Various anomalies may derive from the imperfect fusion of the primitive müllerian ducts. These consist of many patterns that vary from simple notching of the fundus to a partial septum that divides the fundus but not the cervix, to total division of the uterus by a septum into two endometrial cavities, a *septate uterus.* The most extreme anomaly is a completely *double uterus with double cervix,* each organ receiving only one tube. Such anomalies are perfectly compatible with normal fertility and normal menstrual cycles, but sometimes result in interesting and confusing clinical problems. Pregnancy in one half of a septate uterus may be accompanied by bleeding from the unaffected half or by a second conception. Pregnancy may occur in one half of the uterus after the other half has already developed a pregnancy, so-called superfetation.

INFLAMMATIONS

The endometrium and myometrium are relatively resistant to infections. Acute endometritis and myometritis are thus uncommon clinical problems. Acute reactions are virtually limited to bacterial infections that arise following delivery or miscarriage. Retained products of conception are the usual predisposing influence. The most common causative agents are the group A hemolytic streptococci, although the staphylococci and other bacteria are sometimes involved. The inflammatory response is chiefly limited to the interstitium and is entirely nonspecific in nature. Removal of the retained gestational fragments by curettage is promptly followed by remission of the infection.

CHRONIC ENDOMETRITIS. Chronic inflammation of the endometrium occurs in the following settings:[76] (1) in patients suffering from chronic PID (p. 1114); (2) in tuberculosis, either from miliary spread or more commonly from drainage of tuberculous salpingitis (Fig. 24–23); (3) in postpartal or postabortal endometrial cavities, usually due to retained gestational tissue; and (4) in patients with intrauterine contraceptive devices (IUD). In the last-named case, the endometritis is sometimes caused by actinomycetes.[77] The chronic endometritis in all these cases represents a secondary disease, and under these circumstances there is a plausible cause for the endometrial inflammation.

In about 15% of cases no such primary cause is present, yet plasma cells are found in the endometrium. It will be remembered that, in the normal menstrual cycle, the endometrial mucosa is suffused with neutrophils, lymphocytes, and histiocytes during the menstrual phase. Therefore, only one type of inflammatory cell, the plasma cell, is not a normal inhabitant of the endometrium. Some women with this so-called "nonspecific" chronic endometritis have such gynecologic complaints as abnormal bleeding, pain, discharge, or infertility. It would appear to be justified to accept the entity of nonspecific (or idiopathic) chronic endometritis when plasma cells alone are present, even though we fail to understand the cause of the changes.

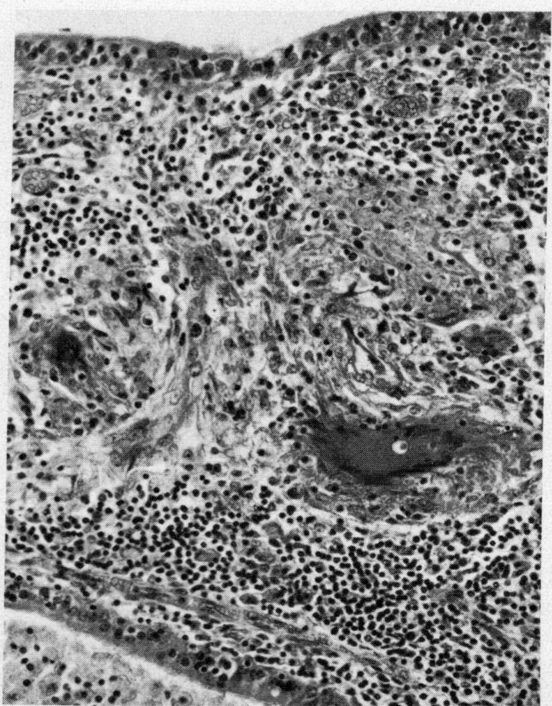

Figure 24–23. Tuberculous endometritis.

ADENOMYOSIS

Adenomyosis refers to the presence of nests of endometrium in the myometrium of the uterine wall. It is currently believed to represent an abnormal growth activity of the endometrium, reflecting a downgrowth of the basal zone of the endometrium into the myometrium.[77] It is found at postmortem examination in 10 to 15% of uteri, depending on the criteria used for the diagnosis and the zeal with which it is sought.

Adenomyosis usually causes symmetric uterine enlargement, although in some cases the uterus is normal in size. The uterine wall is often thickened to 2 to 2.5 cm, sometimes irregularly, but otherwise appears unremarkable in most cases. In some cases the included endometrium is functional, menstruates, and therefore produces small nests of red-brown blood pigmentation within the myometrium (Fig. 24–24A).

The histologic diagnosis of adenomyosis rests on the identification of buried endometrial stroma or glands, or both, between the muscle bundles of the myometrium. In most instances, the nests are composed of typical glands enclosed within a spindle cell stroma (Fig. 24–24*B*). Occasionally, the nests are composed only of stroma, designated as **benign stromal nodules.** For a justifiable diagnosis of adenomyosis, the endometrial nests should be one low-power field or more (2 to 3 mm) below the endomyometrial junction. In those few instances in which the glands function, blood accumulates within the ectopic foci to cause local hemosiderosis.

Patients with adenomyosis frequently have menorrhagia, colicky dysmenorrhea, dyspareunia, and pelvic pain, particularly during the premenstrual period.

ENDOMETRIOSIS

Endometriosis is the term used to describe the presence of endometrial glands or stroma in abnormal locations outside the uterus.[78] It occurs in the following sites in descending order of frequency: (1) ovaries, (2) uterine ligaments, (3) rectovaginal septum, (4) pelvic peritoneum, (5) laparotomy scars, and rarely in the umbilicus, vagina, vulva, and appendix.

INCIDENCE. This disorder is principally a disease of women in active reproductive life, most often in the third and fourth decades. It practically never arises in women over 50. There is a higher incidence of this condition in women in the higher economic groups who tend to marry later in life, having fewer children, and have a lower fertility rate than lower income groups. Microscopically proved endometriosis was found in 33% of patients undergoing surgery for the assessment of infertility.[79]

PATHOGENESIS. The derivation of the nests of aberrant endometrium has long been argued. The *metaplastic theory* holds that endometriosis represents an abnormal differentiation of coelomic epithelium. The *regurgitation* or *implantation theory* proposes that endometrium is regurgitated through the fallopian tubes

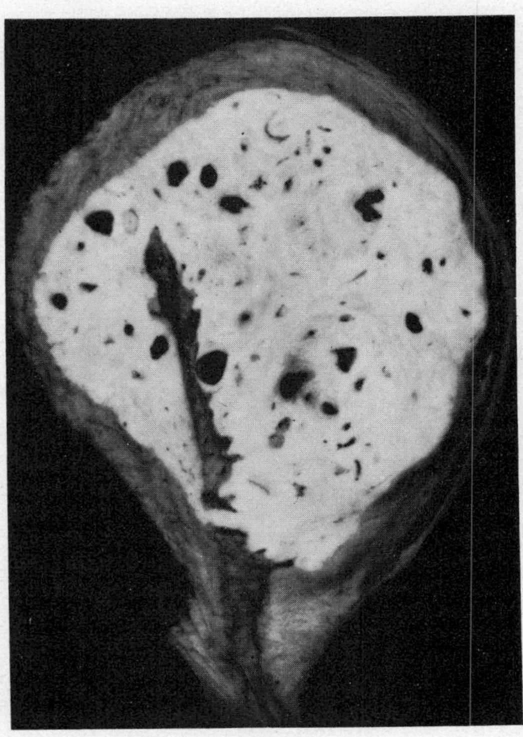

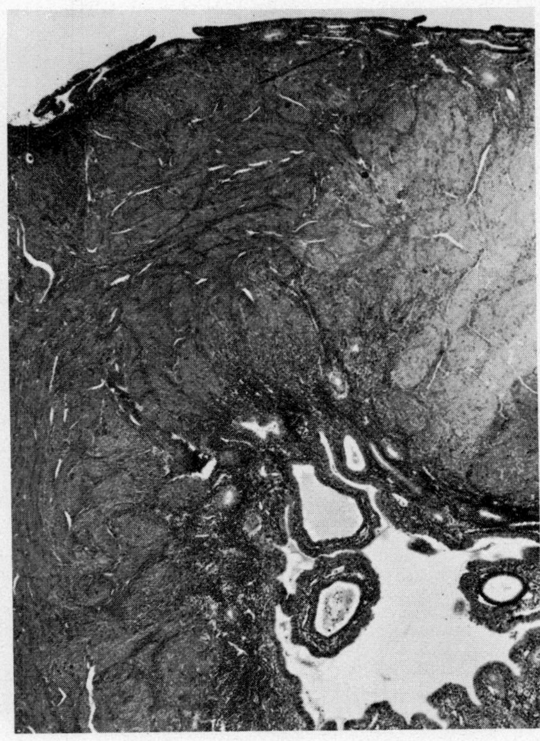

A B

Figure 24–24. Adenomyosis. *A,* An unusual variant with function of endometrial nests producing foci of hemorrhage within uterine wall. *B,* Nest of typical endometrium within uterine wall, well below endometrial surface *(at top).*

at the time of the normal menstrual period and spills out through the fimbriated ends to become implanted in various sites. Regurgitation can indeed be demonstrated during menstruation, particularly when the cervix is stenotic or narrowed. Moreover, the tendency for endometriosis to be localized within the pelvis further fits the implantation theory. However, it obviously does not suffice to explain the development of endometriosis in the umbilicus or in sites removed from the pelvis. The *lymphatic* or *hematogenous dissemination theory* is advanced to explain endometriosis in lymph nodes and such rare sites as the nose and arm. The theories are not mutually incompatible, and endometriosis may encompass all three pathways described.

MORPHOLOGY. Endometriosis may present in many varied patterns. The foci of endometrium are almost invariably under the influence of the ovarian hormones and, therefore, undergo the cyclic menstrual changes with periodic bleeding. As a result, these foci appear as red-blue to yellow-brown nodules implanted on the serosal surfaces or apparently lying beneath the surface in the sites mentioned. They vary from microscopic lesions to 1 to 2 cm in diameter. Individual lesions may enlarge and coalesce. In time, these nodules may evoke a marked fibroblastic proliferation as the result of the irritative effect of the blood to produce dense fibrous nodules. When the accumulation of blood is extensive, its organization causes interadherence of structures, obliteration of the pouch of Douglas, distortion and total fibrosis in and about the tubes and ovaries, and sometimes a virtually frozen pelvis. The ovaries may become markedly distorted by large cystic spaces (3 to 5 cm in diameter) filled with brown blood debris to form so-called chocolate cysts (Fig. 24–25).

The histologic diagnosis of endometriosis is sometimes readily made (Fig. 24–26), but at other times may be most obscure. Paradoxically, the diagnosis is most difficult in advanced, florid, long-standing cases because, as the disease progresses, the fibroproliferative response to the retained blood progressively obliterates recognizable features. In late cases, then, it may be possible only to identify hemosiderin pigment and nests of macrophages containing green-brown granular debris within areas of dense fibrosis. A definite histologic diagnosis requires two of the three following features: glands, stroma, or hemosiderin pigment.

CLINICAL COURSE. The clinical manifestations of endometriosis are dependent on the distribution of the endometrial lesions and on their functional activity. It may therefore be present as an asymptomatic lesion. Clinical signs and symptoms usually consist of severe dysmenorrhea and pelvic pain due to the intrapelvic bleeding and periuterine adhesions. Dyspareunia may be present on the same basis. Pain on defecation reflects rectal wall involvement, and dysuria reflects involvement of the serosa of the bladder. Intestinal disturbances may appear when the small intestine is affected. Menstrual irregularities are common for obscure reasons. Infertility is the presenting complaint in 30 to 40% of women. As the tubes become embedded in fibrous

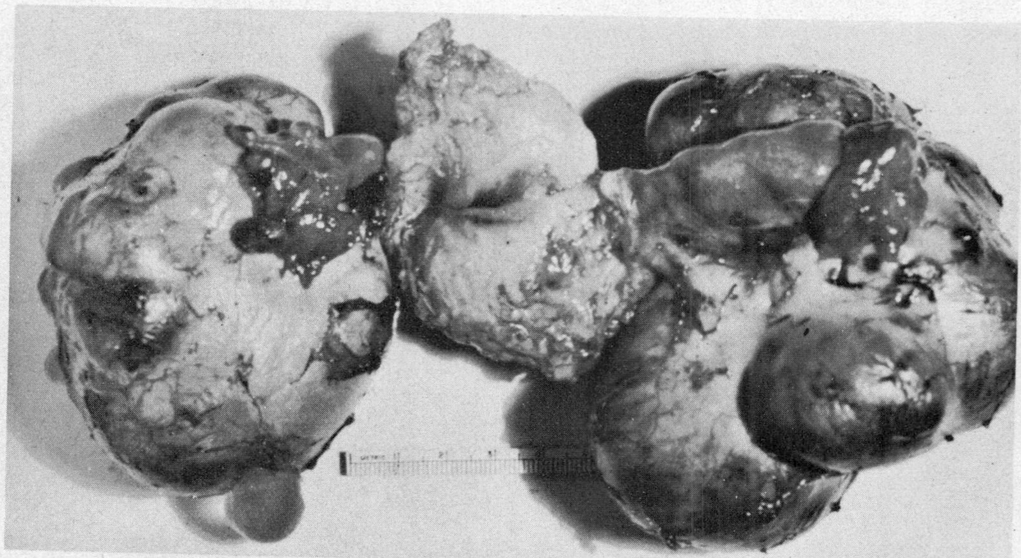

Figure 24–25. Endometriosis. Ovaries are converted into enlarged irregular masses by large "chocolate cysts." (Courtesy of Dr. Arthur Hertig.)

tissue and the ovaries are deformed by the bleeding process, sterility is a late serious complication. These clinical manifestations are similar to those that accompany chronic salpingitis. Accordingly, the diagnosis of pelvic endometriosis should be entertained when the physical findings suggest inflammatory involvement of pelvic viscera, or thickenings or masses in the cul-de-sac or tubo-ovarian regions.

FUNCTIONAL MENSTRUAL DISORDERS (DYSFUNCTIONAL UTERINE BLEEDING)

During active reproductive life, the normal monthly cyclic shedding and regrowth of the endometrium is a finely balanced mechanism. It is controlled by the rise and ebb of pituitary and ovarian hormones, not only in regulated, absolute amounts, but also in carefully integrated, relative levels. This finely adjusted proliferation of a new endometrial mucosa each month is subject to many aberrations that cause either hyperplasia or atrophy of the endometrium.

By far the most frequent problem facing the physician in gynecologic practice is the occurrence of excessive bleeding during or between menstrual periods. The causes of abnormal bleeding from the uterus are many and vary among women of different age groups (Table 24–1). In some instances, bleeding is the result of a well-defined organic lesion such as a leiomyoma, carcinoma, or polyp, but *the largest single group is so-called dysfunctional uterine bleeding.*[80] This is defined as abnormal bleeding in the absence of an organic lesion of the endometrium or uterus.

ANOVULATORY CYCLE. In most instances, dysfunctional bleeding is due to the occurrence of an *anovulatory cycle,* which results in excessive and prolonged estrogenic stimulation, without the development of the progestational phase that regularly follows ovulation. In a small percentage of patients, lack of ovulation is the result of (1) a known basic endocrine disorder, such as thyroid disease, adrenal disease, or pituitary tumors; (2) a specific primary lesion of the ovary such as functioning ovarian tumors (granulosa–theca cell tumors, p. 1152) or polycystic ovaries (p. 1142); or (3) certain generalized metabolic disturbances such as marked obesity, severe malnutrition, and any chronic systemic disease. In most patients, however, anovulatory cycles with dysfunctional uterine bleeding occur with no basic underlying meta-

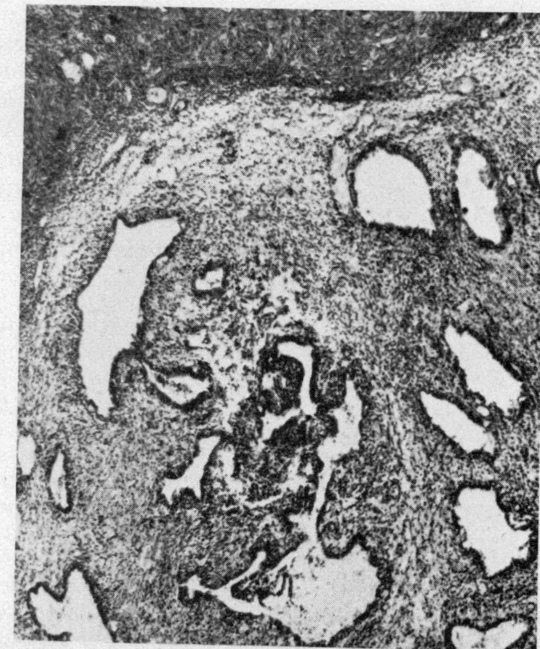

Figure 24–26. Classic diagnostic endometriosis of ovary with readily recognized, well-formed endometrium within ovarian stroma.

Table 24–1. CAUSES OF ABNORMAL UTERINE BLEEDING IN DIFFERENT AGE GROUPS

1. Prepubertal
   - Precocious puberty (hypothalamic, pituitary, or ovarian origin)
   - Trauma or foreign body (mostly of vaginal origin)
2. Adolescence
   - Anovulatory cycle
3. Reproductive age
   - Complications of pregnancy (abortion, trophoblastic disease, ectopic pregnancy)
   - Organic lesions (e.g., leiomyoma, adenomyosis, polyps, endometrial hyperplasia, carcinoma)
   - Anovulatory cycle
   - Ovulatory dysfunctional bleeding (e.g., inadequate luteal phase)
4. Perimenopausal
   - Anovulatory cycle
   - Irregular shedding
   - Organic lesions (carcinoma, hyperplasia, polyps)
5. Postmenopausal
   - Organic lesions (carcinoma, hyperplasia, polyps)
   - Endometrial atrophy

bolic or endocrine disorder, although certain contributing or precipitating factors such as physical or psychic stresses, febrile illness, and seasonal variations are encountered.

Failure of ovulation results in abnormal persistence of the graafian follicle; the endometrium is thus subjected to *prolonged and excessive action of estrogens,* with no evidence of the endometrial secretory activity normally evoked by the progesterone derived from the corpus luteum. The *nonsecretory endometrium* shows mild degrees of hyperplasia characterized histologically by mitotic activity and an increase in gland size. Anovulatory cycles are most common at the two extremes of menstrual life—at menarche and about the time of menopause (perimenopause)—but they can occur at any age and can be interspersed with ovulatory cycles. *Patients with endometrial carcinoma are more likely to have a history of repeated anovulatory cycles.*

INADEQUATE LUTEAL PHASE. Abnormal bleeding can also be associated with ovulatory cycles. The exact hormonal disturbances that underlie this type of bleeding are poorly understood, and the histologic alterations in an endometrial biopsy tend to be less specific. One such type is *inadequate luteal phase,* which refers to the occurrence of inadequate corpus luteum function and low progesterone output, with an irregular ovulatory cycle.[81] Clinically, the condition often manifests itself by infertility and either increased bleeding or amenorrhea. Endometrial biopsy performed at an estimated postovulatory date shows secretion and differentiates this type of bleeding from that seen in the anovulatory cycle.

IRREGULAR SHEDDING. This is another type of abnormal bleeding associated with ovulatory cycles. The syndrome is characterized by profuse menstrual flow, averaging nine to 15 days but occurring regularly. It is associated with normal progesterone secretion by the corpus luteum, but is apparently due to a delay in the involution of the corpus luteum and therefore to the persistent elevation of progesterone levels for a number of days after the onset of flow. If a biopsy is performed on the fourth or fifth day of menstruation, it shows the residual late secretory activity as well as proliferative changes *at a time when only early proliferative endometrium should be present.*

ENDOMETRIAL HYPERPLASIA

Endometrial hyperplasia is another cause of abnormal bleeding that differs from the functional endometrial disorders inasmuch as the origin of the bleeding is a variety of disordered glandular and stromal growth patterns. *Endometrial hyperplasia is important because of its special relationship to endometrial carcinoma.* Almost 40 years ago, Hertig and Sommers[82] proposed a progression of endometrial changes from hyperplasia through a spectrum of atypical changes leading eventually, in some cases, to endometrial carcinoma. Numerous studies have since largely confirmed the malignant potential of endometrial hyperplasia,[60, 83–87] and the concept of a continuum of atypical changes culminating in carcinoma.[88] Unfortunately, the relative risk of the development of cancer is still uncertain owing to the variable criteria and differing terms used for the diagnosis of these conditions, and the effects of therapeutic interventions on the natural history of hyperplasia.

Although it is relatively easy to recognize both ends of the spectrum of endometrial abnormality—benign hyperplasia on one end and frank adenocarcinoma on the other—there is little agreement among pathologists as to the terms or histologic criteria to be used for intermediate stages, or gray zones.[88a] The three most common terms for the variants of hyperplasia are *cystic hyperplasia, adenomatous hyperplasia,* and *atypical hyperplasia.* Because cystic and adenomatous patterns often coexist, Kurman and Norris[89] have proposed a more practical histologic classification of *mild, moderate,* and *atypical hyperplasia.*

Whatever terms one uses, these patterns are characterized by an excessive proliferation of both epithelial and stromal elements, accompanied by an increase in endometrial volume. Endometrial hyperplasia occurs around the time of, or after, menopause and is associated clinically with abnormal or excessive uterine bleeding. The hyperplasia in these patients results from an abnormally high and prolonged level of estrogenic stimulation with diminished or absent progestational activity. These conditions are encountered in states with absolute increases in estrogen production: e.g., the persistence of follicle cysts in the ovary, as may occur in the Stein-Leventhal syndrome (p. 1142); functioning granulosa and theca cell tumors of the ovary; excessive adrenocortical function; and prolonged administration of estrogenic substances. These are the same influences postulated to be of pathogenetic significance in endometrial carcinoma (p. 1138), a point that speaks to the precancerous potential of hyperplasia.

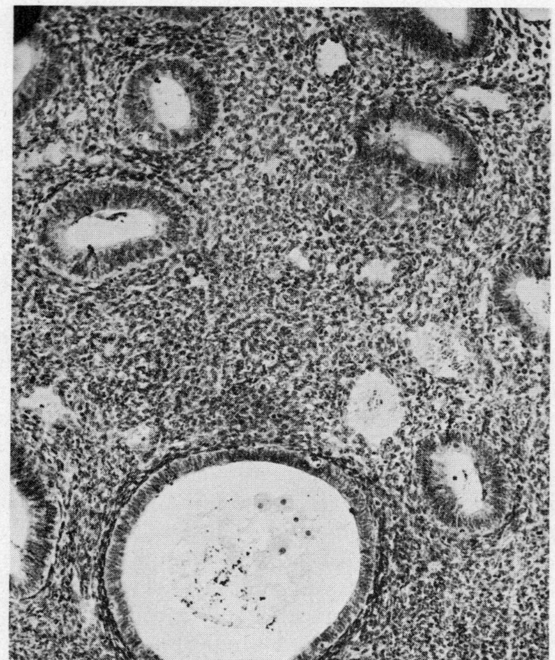

Figure 24–27. Cystic mild hyperplasia of endometrium with marked dilatation of only one gland. (Courtesy of Dr. Arthur Hertig.)

Mild hyperplasia (also known as cystic) is characterized by the presence of glands of various sizes, including many that are cystic (Fig. 24–27). The epithelial lining may be cuboidal or tall columnar and occasionally multilayered. Mitoses are scant, but typical proliferative endometrium may be admixed with the dilated glands. The stroma between glands also is frequently increased. When severe, cystic hyperplasia evokes a so-called "Swiss-cheese pattern." Cystic hyperplasia should be differentiated from senile cystic atrophy; in the latter, the stroma is atrophic and the dilated glands are lined by flattened epithelial cells.[84]

Moderate hyperplasia (also known as adenomatous) results in a thickened, gray, velvety endometrial mucosa. The mucosal surface may be irregular and may even have polypoid projections. There is an increase in the number and size of endometrial glands, but the characteristic feature is the disparity in the size of glands and their irregularity in shape. Some glands may be small, whereas others are large and cystic. Papillary buddings into the glands are formed, as are finger-like outpouchings into the adjacent endometrial stroma. The lining epithelium is hyperplastic, and there is frequent stratification of the epithelium surrounding the lumina (Fig. 24–28). The hyperplasia can be focal and there may be increased mitotic activity in the endometrial stroma.

Atypical hyperplasia is indistinguishable grossly from adenomatous hyperplasia. Histologically, however, there is severe crowding of the glands, as they are backed up to each other in apparent contact. The epithelial cells lining the glands are often no longer neatly palisaded. In addition to crowding, the distinguishing feature of atypical hyperplasia is the cellular atypia: loss of polarity, hyperchromatism, and prominence of nucleoli. Occasionally, large cells with abundant pale eosinophilic cytoplasm are prominent (Fig. 24–29). Mitotic figures are frequent. In the most severe forms, cytologic and architectural atypia may resemble frank adenocarcinoma, but the term **carcinoma in situ** suggested by some authors is now out of favor.

All types of hyperplasia produce abnormal bleeding in the form of either spotting between periods or excessive menstrual flow. Distressing as these are, the role of these lesions in the genesis of endometrial cancer is far more important. *The increased risk from mild or cystic hyperplasia is minimal or nonexistent. All workers agree, however, that moderate (adenomatous) and in particular atypical hyperplasia are potentially precancerous lesions.* In one study of untreated endometrial hyperplasias, 22% of the former and 57% of the latter progressed to carcinoma within two to 18 years.[86] Predictions cannot be made for the individual patient,[90] but in general, the more severe the atypia, the greater the risk. It is important, therefore, in any assessment of an endometrial hyperplastic lesion for the pathologist to indicate the type and degree of atypia in a manner clearly understandable by the clinician.[60]

MISCELLANEOUS ENDOMETRIAL CHANGES

Senile Cystic Endometrial Atrophy. In the postmenopausal woman, the endometrium normally atrophies and becomes a rudimentary layer composed only of the basal glands. For obscure reasons, in some women the glands, instead of undergoing atrophy, become cystically dilated. Grossly, the atrophic endometrium has a flat, thin, glazed, gray-red appearance, and histologically consists of compact endometrial stroma containing simple tubular, nonproliferative, nonsecretory resting glands. Against this background are scattered, large, cystically dilated glands lined by flattened or totally atrophic epithelial cells. Such cystic changes should not be confused with cystic hyperplasia in which the cystic glands are lined by proliferating as well as flattened cells, and the stroma is hyperplastic.

Oral Contraceptives and the Endometrium. As might be suspected, the use of oral contraceptives containing synthetic or derivative ovarian steroids induces a wide variety of endometrial changes. The precise pattern of morphologic change varies with the specific compound (its content, both absolute and relative, of estrogenic and progestational agents), the dosage, and the schedule of administration. A common reaction pattern can be best characterized as a discordance between glandular and stromal activity. Implied here is the presence of inactive, virtually atrophic glands lined by low, nonproliferative, nonsecretory cells surrounded by a lush stroma showing large cells with abundant cytoplasm and considerable mitotic activity. This morphologic pattern is reminiscent of the decidua of pregnancy. Indeed, when encountered in a curetting, the stromal changes might be confused with those of early pregnancy. The inactive glands, however, are inconsistent with such a diagnosis. In other instances, with other contraceptives employed on a different schedule, the glandular epithelial cells are sometimes vacuolated and embedded within a less reactive stroma, once again readily confused with pregnancy changes. When such therapy is discontinued, the endometrium

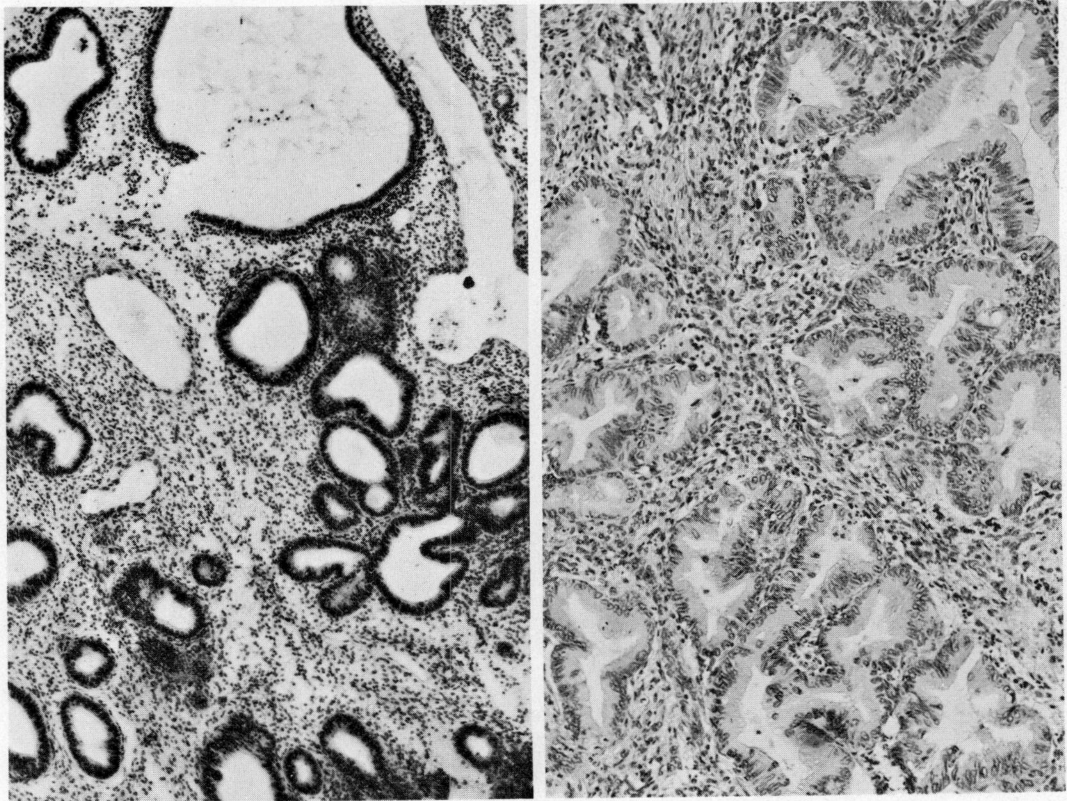

Figure 24–28. Moderate (adenomatous) hyperplasia of a nest of closely packed glands in right side of field.
Figure 24–29. Severe atypical hyperplasia. Note both marked crowding of glands and cellular atypia manifested by large, pale-staining cells.
(Figs. 24–28 and 24–29 courtesy of Dr. Arthur Hertig.)

eventually reverts to its normal pattern. *All these changes have been minimized since the introduction of low-dose contraceptive pills.* An increased risk of the development of endometrial carcinoma has been reported mainly with sequential contraceptive regimens using high doses of the most potent estrogens and weak progestin (Oracon);[92] these have been withdrawn from prescription use.

As noted earlier, the cervical epithelium also undergoes modifications with the use of oral contraceptives. Striking glandular proliferation is frequently seen in the region of the squamocolumnar junction, giving rise to so-called *microglandular endocervical hyperplasia*, which may be confused with a neoplasm. When oral contraceptive therapy is stopped, the changes apparently revert to normal, but during the height of the reaction they can be quite confusing to the unwary pathologist.

TUMORS OF UTERINE CORPUS

The uterine corpus, including its endometrium and myometrium, is affected by a great variety of neoplastic growths. These can be benign or malignant and arise from (1) the endometrial glands (endometrial polyp, endometrial carcinoma); (2) the endometrial stroma (endometrial stroma sarcoma); (3) the müllerian mesoderm differentiating into both glandular and stromal elements (mixed mesodermal tumors); or (4) the smooth muscle of the myometrium (leiomyoma, leiomyosarcoma).[93] The most common of these tumors are the endometrial polyps, leiomyomas, and endometrial carcinomas.

ENDOMETRIAL POLYPS

Endometrial polyps are small, mostly sessile masses that project into the endometrial cavity and are attached to the endometrium by a pedicle or stem. They may be single or multiple and usually are small, 0.5 to 3.0 cm in diameter, but occasionally are large and pedunculated (Fig. 24–30). They may occur at any age but are somewhat more common at or near menopause.[94] Smaller polyps are usually asymptomatic, incidental findings, whereas larger ones may ulcerate, degenerate, and cause clinical bleeding. Histologically, they are generally of two types, made up of (1) functional endometrium

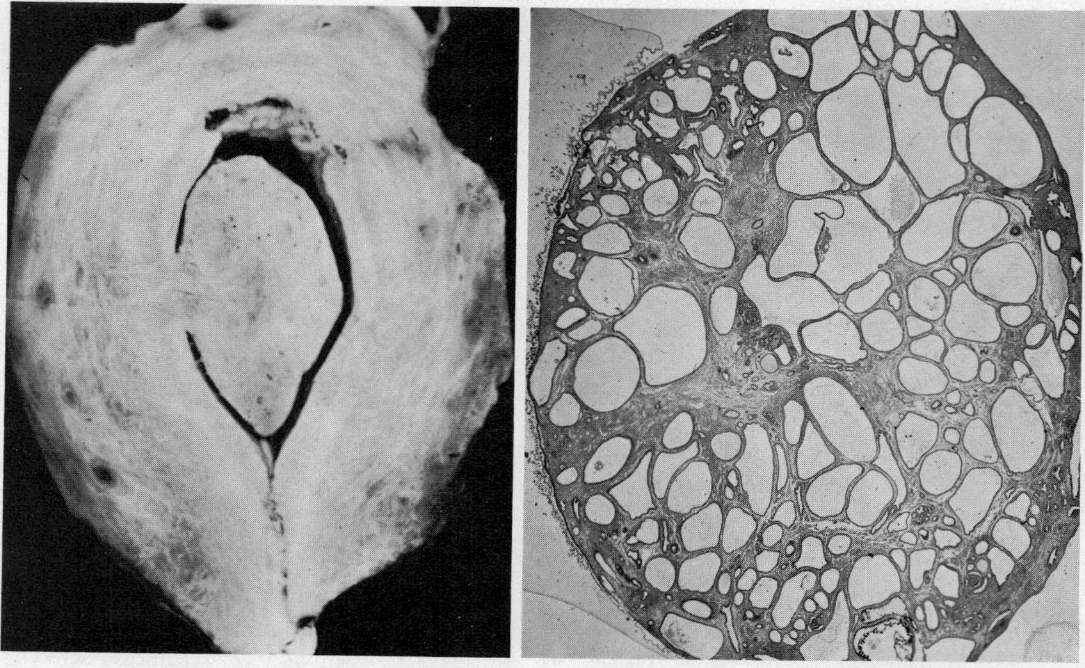

Fig. 24–30

Fig. 24–31

Figure 24–30. Large pedunculated polyp within endometrial cavity, viewed on cross section.
Figure 24–31. Cystic endometrial polyp at low power, illustrating cystic dilatation of glands. (Courtesy of Dr. Arthur Hertig.)

paralleling the cycle of the surrounding nonpolypoid endometrium and (2) more commonly, hyperplastic endometrium, mostly of the cystic variety, although an adenomatous pattern is sometimes seen. Such polyps may develop in association with generalized endometrial hyperplasia and are responsive to the growth effect of estrogen, but exhibit no progesterone response (Fig. 24–31). Malignant change in an initially benign endometrial polyp is extremely rare. It is to be emphasized, however, that frank carcinoma may be polypoid, and further that submucosal leiomyomas may be pedunculated and present as polypoid lesions.

LEIOMYOMA

Leiomyomas are benign tumors of smooth muscle origin. They are the most common tumors in women. They are also referred to as myomas and, in colloquial clinical usage, as "fibroids." The tumors are responsible for at least one-third of all gynecologic admissions to hospitals and are found in the general population in about one in four women in active reproductive life. Although most common in the third and fourth decades, they may persist and be discovered in advanced age. They are more common in blacks.

There is much controversy over the role of hyperestrinism in the production of these tumors. It is known that they shrink and become fibrosed and even calcified postmenopausally. They rarely arise following the menopause. Castration makes them atrophy premenopausally. Perhaps most important, during pregnancy there is sometimes a rapid increase in their size, accompanied by cellular proliferation. On all these bases, the tumors are thought to be caused by excessive estrogenic stimulation. Experimental proof in animals is still lacking, however, and there is no evidence that estrogen initiates their formation or does more than maintain the size. It is perhaps more accurate, then, to consider leiomyomas as endocrine-dependent lesions whose growth or size is dependent on estrogens.

Leiomyomas, wherever they occur, are sharply circumscribed, unencapsulated but discrete, usually round, firm, gray-white masses that have a characteristic whorled cut surface. Except in rare instances, they are found within the myometrium of the corpus. Only infrequently do they involve the uterine ligaments, lower uterine segment, or cervix. Descriptive terms have been applied to their various situations within the myometrial wall. Those embedded within the myometrium are referred to as **intramural.** When they occur beneath the covering serosa of the uterine corpus, they are called **subserosal.** Some occur in immediate proximity to the endometrium and are designated **submucous.** Frequently, the subserosal and submucosal masses protrude either from the outer contour of the uterus or into the endometrial cavity (Fig. 24–32). These may become pedunculated and appear as bulbous polyps having a firm, round head (Fig. 24–33).

Uncommonly, the pedunculated subserosal lesion may develop an extremely long, tenuous stalk and it is sometimes designated as a **wandering or migratory leiomyoma.** Occasionally, such tumors become adherent to surrounding structures or omentum, develop an auxiliary blood supply,

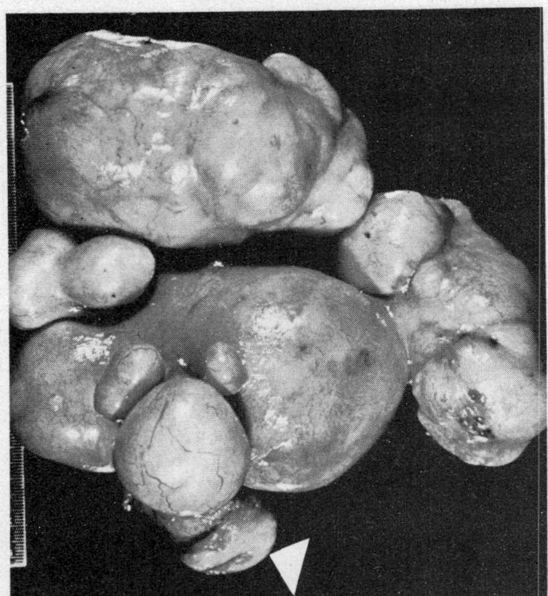

Figure 24–32. Multiple subserosal leiomyomas of uterus. Uterine body is "lost" in irregular mass, but cervix is visible as most dependent portion of specimen *(arrowhead)*.

and lose their original attachment to the uterus. They are then termed **parasitic leiomyomas.**

In the great majority of cases, multiple leiomyomas are present. They vary in size from barely visible, pale gray seedlings to massive tumors that may simulate a pregnant uterus. Although not encapsulated, they are sufficiently discrete to be readily shelled out. Whatever their size, the characteristic whorled pattern of smooth muscle bundles on cut section usually makes these lesions readily identifiable on gross inspection. Large tumors may develop areas of yellow-brown to red softening which may undergo proteolytic liquefaction to produce **cystic degeneration.** In advanced ages, the masses atrophy, tending to become more collagenous, firm, and sometimes partially or completely calcified.

Histologically, the leiomyoma is composed of whorling bundles of smooth muscle cells that resemble the architecture of the uninvolved myometrium (Fig. 24–34). Usually, the individual muscle cells are uniform in size and shape, and have the characteristic oval nucleus and long, slender bipolar cytoplasmic processes. Mitotic figures are scarce, and giant cells and anaplasia are not present. Tumors that occur in advanced age groups, as well as occasionally in younger individuals, may have an increase of the connective tissue with dense hyalinization of this stroma.

Leiomyomas of the uterus may be asymptomatic or may cause a variety of symptoms, the most important of which is profuse bleeding at the time of the menstrual period.[94] Abnormal, irregular vaginal bleeding may also occur, presumably from congestion of arcuate veins by the tumor. Pain, pressure on the urinary bladder causing urinary frequency, and impaired fertility are other clinical manifestations.

Leiomyomas frequently undergo rapid increase in size during pregnancy and, at this time, these tumors may have considerable hypertrophy of individual cells with some variability in nuclear and cell size, as well as some mitotic figures. Such changes are sometimes alarming as histologic observations, since they can be confused with malignant transformation. Myomas in pregnant women increase the frequency of spontaneous abortion, fetal malpresentation, uterine inertia, and postpartum hemorrhage. Malignant transformation is said to occur but is rare; it will be discussed in the consideration of leiomyosarcomas (p. 1140).

CARCINOMA

Carcinoma of the endometrium is becoming increasingly common. At one time, it was far less frequent

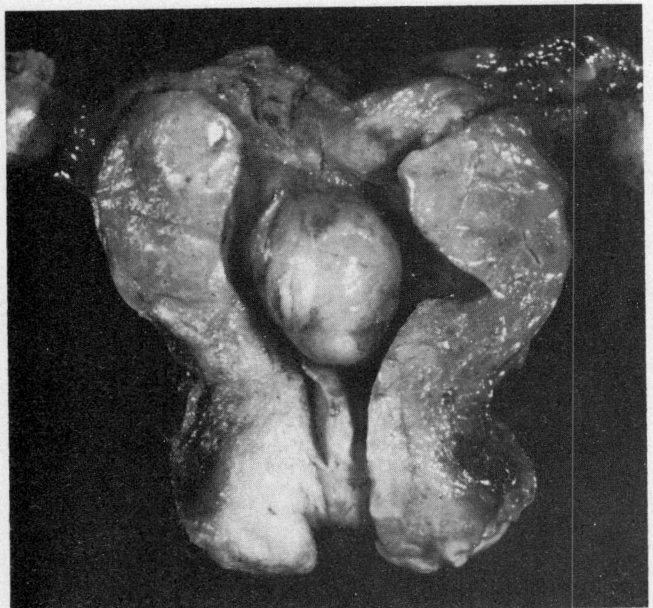

Figure 24–33. Submucosal leiomyoma appearing as a bulbous polyp, protruding into endometrial cavity.

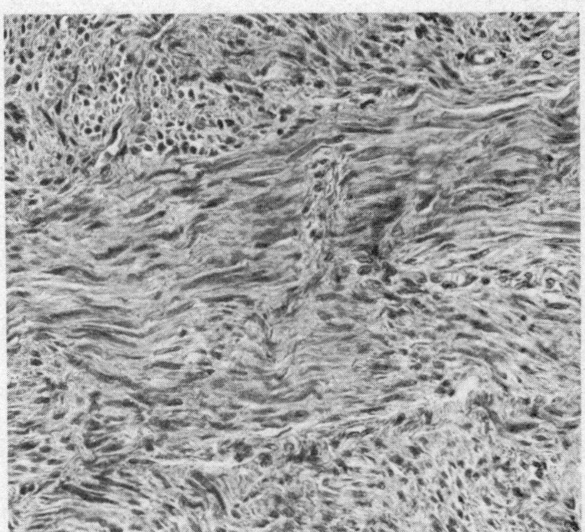

Figure 24–34. Leiomyoma showing bundles of well-differentiated, regular, spindle-shaped smooth muscle cells.

than cancer of the cervix, in a ratio of 1:4. Earlier detection and eradication of in situ cervical cancer has lowered its prevalence as a form of life-threatening cancer. The longer life expectancy has led to a real increase in endometrial carcinomas but in addition there has been an unexplained increase in younger age groups.[95] Thus, the ratio of endometrial to invasive cervical cancer is now approximately 2:1.[39] Carcinoma of the endometrium is fast becoming one of the most frequent forms of fatal cancer in women.

INCIDENCE. Carcinoma of the endometrium accounts for close to 10% of all cancer in women. The disease is predominantly seen in older women, 85% of cases occuring after menopause, with a peak frequency of 60 per 100,000 in the age group 55 to 65. Less than 10% occur in patients under age 40. A number of important constitutional and other factors correlate with the risk of developing endometrial carcinoma:[96] (1) *obesity*—50% of women with endometrial carcinoma weigh over 180 lbs; (2) *diabetes* is present in 5 to 11% of patients, while abnormal glucose tolerance is found in over 60%; (3) *hypertension* is found in 50% of patients; and (4) *infertility*—women who develop cancer of the endometrium tend to be single and nulliparous and to give a history of functional menstrual irregularities consistent with anovulatory cycles.

PATHOGENESIS. There is quite compelling evidence that carcinoma of the endometrium is caused or influenced by *prolonged estrogen stimulation.* The evidence can be summarized as follows:[97, 98] (1) patients with estrogen-secreting granulosa–theca cell tumors of the ovaries have a much higher incidence of this form of cancer than do age-matched controls; (2) endometrial cancer is extremely rare in women with ovarian agenesis or in those castrated early in life; (3) endometrial carcinoma is sometimes preceded by endometrial hyperplasia, which, as discussed (p. 1133), is related to hyperestrinism, and patients who develop endometrial carcinoma frequently have a past history of anovulatory cycles; (4) there is an association between carcinoma of the endometrium and carcinoma of the breast; (5) prolonged administration of large doses of diethylstilbestrol in rabbits and other laboratory animals has resulted in the production of endometrial polyps, hyperplasia, and carcinoma; (6) some studies suggest an increased risk of endometrial carcinoma in women treated with high doses of exogenous estrogens (principally estrone), usually for menopausal symptoms. The magnitude of the risk is uncertain, as it varies with the dose and duration of estrogen use, the concomitant cyclic administration of progesterone (which tends to decrease the risk), and the criteria used for the histologic diagnosis of carcinoma.[99] Oral contraceptives play no role.

The paradox of an increased incidence of endometrial cancer after menopause, a time when estrogen production is assumed to be decreasing, is explained by an increased synthesis of estrogens in body fats from adrenal and ovarian androgen precursors.[100] The amount of estrone thus produced is proportionate to total body weight, a finding that may partly explain the association of increased risk of endometrial cancer with age and obesity. There is, in addition, increased conversion of androgen to estrone in patients with endometrial cancer.

MORPHOLOGY. Grossly, endometrial carcinoma presents either as a localized polypoid tumor or as a diffuse tumor involving the entire endometrial surface. Both forms may in time fungate into the endometrial cavity, which becomes filled with a nodular, firm-to-soft, partially necrotic neoplasm (Fig. 24–35). When the myometrium is invaded by carcinoma the uterus may become enlarged but rarely more than twofold. Myometrial extension produces subserosal and serosal nodules, and eventually the tumor spreads to the periuterine structures by direct continuity. Spread into the broad ligaments may create a clinically palpable mass. Eventually dissemination to the regional iliac, aortic, inguinal, and hypogastric lymph nodes occurs and in the late stages the tumor may be hematogenously borne to the lungs, liver, bones, and other organs.

Histologically, most endometrial carcinomas (about 85%) are **adenocarcinomas** characterized by more or less well-defined gland patterns lined by malignant cuboidal or columnar epithelial cells (Fig. 24–36). They may be well differentiated (Grade 1) having a prominent, easily recognizable glandular pattern; moderately differentiated (Grade 2), where well-formed glands are mixed with solid sheets of malignant cells; or poorly differentiated (Grade 3) characterized by solid sheets of cells with barely recognizable glands and a great degree of nuclear atypia and mitotic activity.

Ten to 20% of endometrial carcinomas contain foci of squamous differentiation. Both adenomatous and squamous patterns are encountered within individual glands (Fig. 24–37). Squamous elements most commonly are histologically benign in appearance but may also be frankly malignant and poorly differentiated. Traditionally the terms used were **adenoacanthoma** for adenocarcinomas with benign or mature squamous epithelium, and **adenosquamous carcinoma** for those in which the squamous elements are malignant.[3] However, subsequent writings deemphasize these terms and advocate the simple term **adenocarcinoma with squamous differentiation**, which is graded as well differentiated,

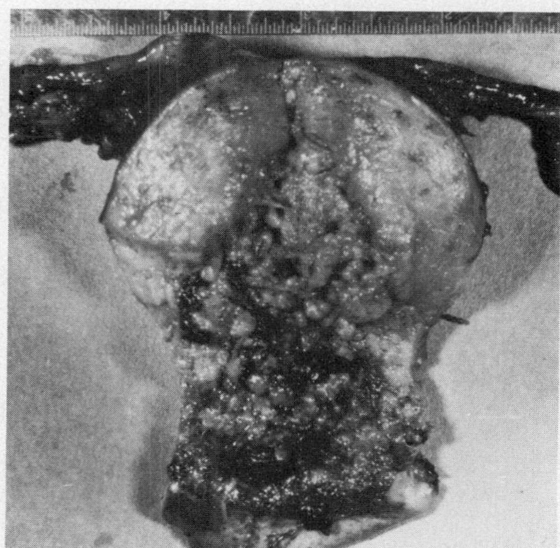

Figure 24–35. Endometrial carcinoma, presenting as a fungating mass in fundus of uterus.

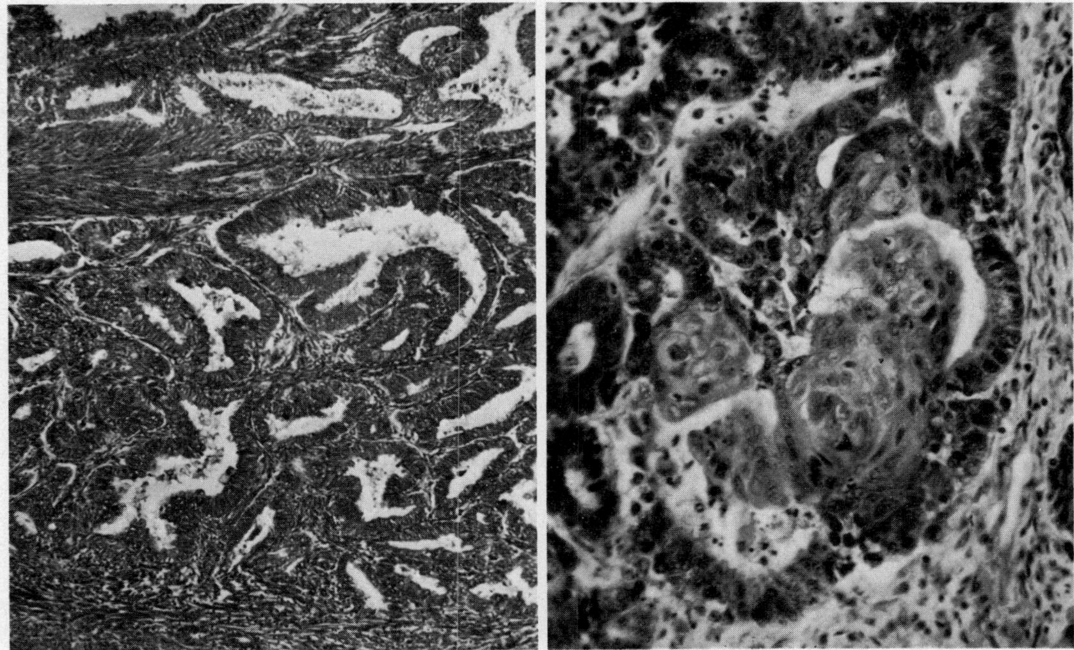

Fig. 24–36

Fig. 24–37

Figure 24–36. Endometrial carcinoma in classic "adeno" pattern.
Figure 24–37. Endometrial carcinoma with squamous differentiation.

moderately differentiated, or poorly differentiated according to usual criteria.[93] When both glandular and squamous elements are poorly differentiated, the prognosis is clearly grim.

Other rare histologic types of endometrial carcinoma are **clear cell carcinoma,**[101] **mucinous adenocarcinoma, secretory carcinoma**, and **papillary serous carcinoma.**[102] The latter, in particular, is a highly malignant form of uterine cancer.

Staging of Endometrial Adenocarcinoma. The Cancer Committee of the International Federation of Gynecology and Obstetrics proposed a plan of clinical staging for endometrial adenocarcinoma that is now used to compare end-result data of therapy.

Stage I. Carcinoma is confined to the corpus uteri itself.

Stage II. Carcinoma has involved the corpus and the cervix.

Stage III. Carcinoma has extended outside the uterus but not outside the true pelvis.

Stage IV. Carcinoma has extended outside the true pelvis or has obviously involved the mucosa of the bladder or the rectum.

Cases in various stages can also be subgrouped with reference to histologic type of adenocarcinoma as follows:

G1—Highly differentiated adenocarcinoma
G2—Differentiated adenocarcinoma with partly solid areas
G3—Predominantly solid or entirely undifferentiated carcinoma

Clinical Course. Carcinoma of the endometrium may be asymptomatic for a long time. The most common manifestation is irregular vaginal bleeding accompanied by excessive leukorrhea. This tumor may extend down through the endocervical canal and appear at the external os, but most often patients have a completely negative-appearing cervix. Uterine enlargement in the early stages may be deceptively absent. Cytologic examination of vaginal smears by competent observers is helpful, but ultimately the diagnosis must be established by curettage and histologic examination of the tissue.

As would be anticipated, the prognosis is heavily dependent on the clinical stage of the disease when discovered, and to a lesser degree also on the histologic grade. Fortunately the great majority of women (about 80%) have Stage I disease clinically, and histologically have well- or moderately well-differentiated lesions. Surgery alone, or in combination with irradiation, yields close to 90% five-year survival in Stage I disease. This rate drops to 30 to 50% in Stage II, and to less than 20% in any of the other more advanced stages of the disease.[7]

SARCOMA

Collectively, sarcomas[93, 104–107] make up 5% or less of uterine tumors; mixed mesodermal tumors, leiomyosarcomas, and endometrial stromal sarcomas are the most common variants.

MIXED MESODERMAL TUMORS (MIXED MÜLLERIAN TUMORS). These are malignant and relatively rare tumors of the endometrium, generally regarded as being derived from the müllerian mesoderm.[93] They are called mixed tumors because they consist of malignant glandular and stromal sarcomatous elements, and the latter tend to differentiate into a variety of mesodermal components, including muscle, cartilage, and even osteoid. Although a variety of tissues is present, the tumor is not a teratoma, since all elements are derived from one germ layer—the mesoderm. The tumor occurs in postmenopausal women and presents like the adenocarcinoma, with postmenopausal bleeding. Many of these patients give a history of previous radiation therapy. The tumors are highly malignant and have a five-year survival rate of 25 to 30%.

Grossly, such tumors are bulky and polypoid, and may protrude into the vagina. On histology, much of the tumor may consist of endometrial adenocarcinoma, which tends to be poorly differentiated, but the glandular elements are intermixed with anaplastic, spindle-shaped stromal cells that have bizarre nuclei and numerous mitoses. As mentioned, the sarcomatous part might differentiate into recognizable smooth or striated muscle cells, cartilage, adipose tissue, and bone. When these heterotopic structures are not present, the tumor consists simply of glands and malignant mesenchyme, and the terms **carcinosarcoma** or **homologous mixed tumors** are applied to such lesions. **Adenosarcoma** is a rare variant of mixed mesodermal tumors composed of benign glands and malignant stroma. Although recurrences are common (40%), distant metastases are relatively infrequent (15%).[108]

LEIOMYOSARCOMAS. These infrequent malignancies almost always arise directly from the myometrium. Their origin from a preexisting leiomyoma is a controversial issue, but the consensus holds that these cancers are extremely rare complications of the very common benign leiomyoma.

Leiomyosarcomas grow within the uterus in two somewhat distinctive patterns: bulky, fleshy masses that invade the uterine wall; or polypoid masses that project into the uterine lumen. Histologically, they show a wide range of atypia, from those that are extremely well differentiated to anaplastic lesions that have the cytologic abnormalities of wildly growing sarcomas (Fig. 24–38). Many of the borderline, well-differentiated sarcomas are difficult to delineate from cellular leiomyomas. Histologic features indicative of leiomyosarcoma include (1) more than ten mitoses per ten high-power fields (HPF), with or without cellular atypism; and (2) five to ten mitoses per ten HPF with cellular atypism. Lesions with zero to four mitoses per ten HPF and cytologic atypia are designated atypical or cellular leiomyomas, and those with five to ten mitoses per ten HPF and no atypia are described as of uncertain malignant potential.

Leiomyosarcomas are equally common pre- and postmenopausally, with a peak incidence at 40 to 60 years of age. Leiomyosarcomas have a striking tendency to recur after removal, and over half the cases eventually metastasize to distant organs such as lungs, bone, and brain. Dissemination throughout the abdominal cavity is also encountered. The five-year survival averages about 40%. The better differentiated lesions have a better prognosis than the anaplastic lesions, which have a very low five-year survival of about 10 to 15%.

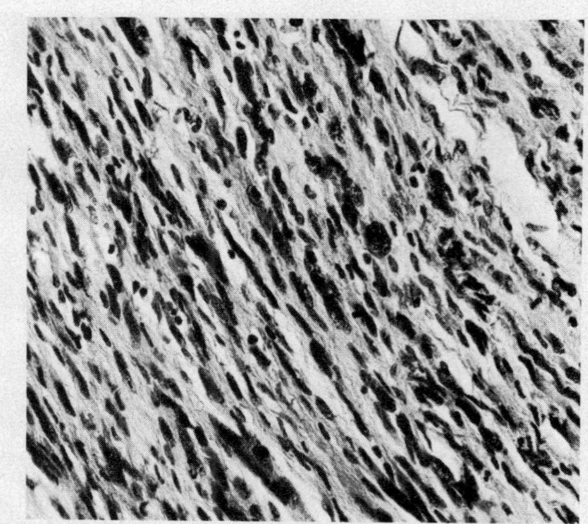

Figure 24–38. Leiomyosarcoma. Cells are large and irregular and have hyperchromatic nuclei.

ENDOMETRIAL STROMAL TUMORS. Strands and nests of more or less well-differentiated endometrial stroma are sometimes encountered in the myometrium. The cytologic differentiation of the stromal cells ranges from patterns virtually indistinguishable from the normal endometrial stroma to obviously sarcomatous anaplasia. These involvements have been divided into three categories: (1) *benign stromal nodules* (p. 1130), (2) *endolymphatic stromal myosis, and* (3) *endometrial stromal sarcoma.*

Low-grade stromal sarcoma or *endolymphatic stromal myosis* refers to the appearance of masses of well-differentiated endometrial stroma lying between muscle bundles of the myometrium, which can be differentiated from stromal nodules only by the tendency of the stromal nests to penetrate lymphatic channels (hence the term endolymphatic stromal myosis). Occasionally, blood vessels and the serosa are also invaded. About half of these tumors recur, sometimes after 10 to 15 years; distant metastases and death from tumor occur in about 15% of cases.

Endometrial stromal sarcoma is the overtly cancerous counterpart of endolymphatic stromal myosis. Here the neoplasm forms large fleshy tumor masses that project into the endometrial cavity and penetrate the underlying myometrium. Commonly, these cancers arise high in the fundus. The cells display a wide range of atypia from fairly well-differentiated stromal cells, which nonetheless present variability in size and shape and frequent mitoses, to highly undifferentiated lesions with wild pleomorphic tumor giant cells. Less anaplastic lesions are differentiated from endolymphatic stromal myosis by the number of mitotic figures; *more than ten mitoses per ten HPF usually indicates malignancy.* As with all sarcomas, these cancers invade vessels and are capable of widespread metastasis. Five-year survival averages 50%.

Fallopian Tubes

The most common disorders in these structures are inflammations, followed in frequency by ectopic (tubal) pregnancy (p. 1158) and endometriosis (p. 1130).

INFLAMMATIONS

SUPPURATIVE SALPINGITIS (PELVIC INFLAMMATORY DISEASE). Salpingitis may be caused by any of the pyogenic organisms, i.e., streptococci, staphylococci, coliforms, and gonococci. In spite of effective antibiotics, the gonococcus still accounts for over 60% of cases of suppurative salpingitis. In almost all instances, these tubular infections are a part of the pelvic inflammatory disease (PID) described on page 1114 (Fig. 24–39).

TUBERCULOUS SALPINGITIS. Another type of salpingitis encountered is almost invariably a secondary complication of a focus of tuberculosis elsewhere in the body. Presumably, the tubes are seeded hematogenously and then the process spreads to other organs in the genital tract, such as the endometrium, and to the peritoneal cavity. Tuberculous salpingitis is extremely uncommon in the United States and accounts for probably not more than 1 to 2% of all forms of salpingitis. However, it is more common in parts of the world where tuberculosis is frequent and is an important cause of infertility in these areas.

TUMORS OF FALLOPIAN TUBES

Only rarely do tumors arise within the fallopian tubes. The most common forms of tumor, which hardly merit such a designation, are minute, 0.1- to 2-cm, translucent cysts filled with clear serous fluid, found near the fimbriated end of the tube or in the broad ligaments, referred to as *parovarian cysts* or *hydatids of Morgagni*. Some of these cysts are presumed to arise in remnants of wolffian duct and are of little more than academic significance. Carcinoma of the fallopian tubes is rare. These tumors arise from the mucosal lining of the tubes (usually near the distal ends), grow as adenocarcinomas, spread by continuity to adjacent structures, and may metastasize in the late stages to distant organs such as the lungs and bones. The condition is so uncommon that the diagnosis can be made only at exploration, when an intrapelvic mass of obscure nature is found clinically. Equally rarely, adenomatoid tumors (mesotheliomas) occur subserosally on the tube or sometimes in the mesosalpinx. These small nodules are the exact counterparts of those already described in relation to the testes or epididymides (p. 1098) and are benign.

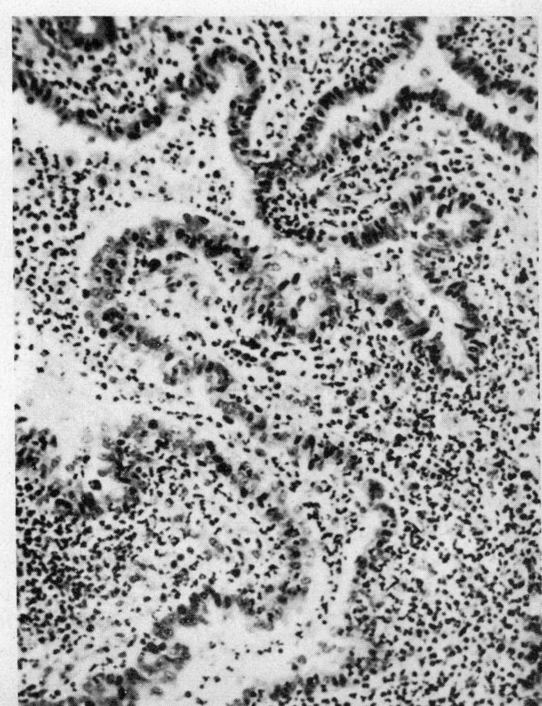

Figure 24–39. Acute salpingitis with a diffuse neutrophilic exudate within both the mucosal folds and the lumen.

Ovaries

Tumors are the most common type of lesion encountered in the ovary. With the exception of these neoplasms, the ovary appears remarkably resistant to disease. Intrinsic inflammations of the ovary are uncommon, and usually periovarian inflammations are secondary to involvement of the adjacent tube. Endometriosis does affect the ovary but usually in conjunction with the pelvic endometriosis described (p. 1130). Save for the important subject of tumors, only non-neoplastic cysts and polycystic ovaries merit separate treatment.

NON-NEOPLASTIC CYSTS

FOLLICULAR AND LUTEAL CYSTS

Follicle cysts in the ovary are so common as to be virtually physiologic. They originate in unruptured graafian follicles or in follicles that have ruptured and immediately sealed. These cysts may be single but are usually multiple. They rarely exceed 1 to 1.5 cm in diameter, are filled with a clear serous fluid, and are lined by a gray, glistening membrane. They are usually found within the cortex of the ovary immediately subjacent to the serosal covering. Histologically, granulosal lining cells can be identified when the intraluminal pressure has not been too great. But as the cysts increase in size, the lining cells atrophy under the pressure of contained fluid (Fig. 24–40). When the lining becomes totally atrophic, further secretion ceases and the cyst no longer enlarges. On this basis, these cysts always remain small and are of little clinical significance. Rarely, the increased production of estrogen stimulates endometrial hyperplasia.

Luteal cysts may be formed in much the same way, usually by the immediate sealing of a corpus hemorrhagicum. The liquid contents of the follicle are retained, and the corpus luteum cannot fill with hemorrhage and thus cannot become fibrosed. Clear serous fluid may accumulate to produce small cystic spaces up to 2 to 3 cm in diameter. These cysts are lined by a rim of bright yellow luteal tissue. Luteal cysts are much less common than follicle cysts but are of the same innocuous significance. When numerous, the aggregate production of hormone may induce endometrial hyperplasia.

POLYCYSTIC OVARIES

In 1935 Stein and Leventhal described a syndrome characterized by secondary amenorrhea, obesity, hirsutism, infertility, and *bilaterally enlarged polycystic ovaries.* Bilateral resection of wedges of ovary containing the multiple cysts restored normal fertility and menstrual cycles. This method of treatment remains successful today, but it has become apparent that the polycystic ovaries are associated with at least three types of clinical presentation: (1) the Stein-Leventhal syndrome described above, (2) abnormal bleeding associated with hypermenorrhea, and (3) virilism. These syndromes occur in young women in the second or third decade of life.

The three syndromes are associated with similar pathologic alterations in the ovaries. The ovaries are usually but not invariably enlarged, contain multiple cysts, and show a thick, tough, pearly white outer tunica ("large white ovary"). Microscopically there is extensive collagenization of the outer cortex; the cyst walls consist

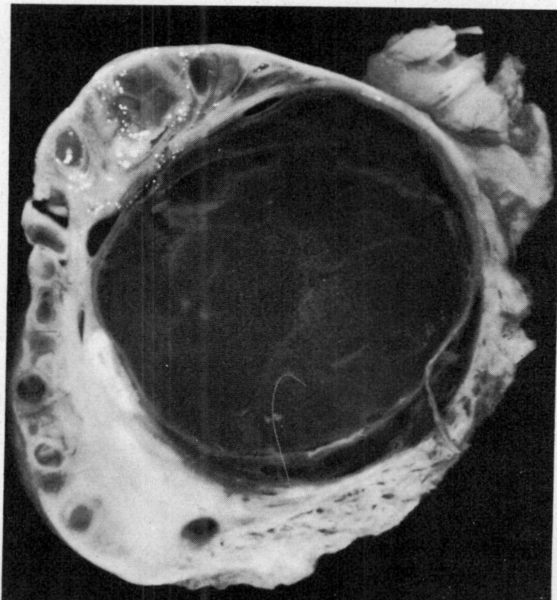

Figure 24–40. Follicular-luteal cysts of ovary, showing one large cyst and multiple subcortical smaller cavities.

of a granulosa cell layer with a luteinized theca interna. Except in extremely rare cases, infertility is absolute and corpora lutea are thus absent.

The pathogenesis of polycystic ovaries has received considerable attention. The evidence now suggests that in many patients with the syndrome there is a disturbance in the hypothalamic-pituitary mechanism, consisting of continuous abnormal stimulation of the ovary by both FSH and LH, instead of periodic, synchronized, and sequential stimulation. In the absence of a midcycle burst of LH to trigger ovulation, there is the formation of follicular cysts and luteinization of the theca interna of such cysts. It is thought that these luteinized theca cells produce predominantly androgenic hormones, accounting for the virilism. It is also thought that wedge resection removes some of the actively functioning follicular cysts with their luteinized theca cells; abnormal ovarian function is thus diminished, and in this way an opportunity is created for the return of normal hypothalamic-pituitary activity. With this procedure, normal menses follow in 80% of patients and pregnancy in 60 to 80%.

TUMORS OF OVARY

Tumors of the ovary are common forms of neoplasia in women.[109–111] Among cancers of the female genital tract, the incidence of ovarian cancer ranks below only carcinoma of the cervix and the endometrium. It accounts for 6% of all cancers in the female and is the fifth most common form of cancer in women in the U. S. (excluding skin cancer). In addition, because many of these ovarian neoplasms cannot be detected early in their development, they account for a disproportionate number of fatal cancers, being responsible for almost half of the deaths from cancer of the female genital tract. There are numerous types of ovarian tumors, both benign and malignant. About 80% are benign, and these occur mostly in young women between the ages of 20 and 45 years. The malignant tumors are more common in older age groups, between 40 and 65.

Risk factors for ovarian cancer are much less clear than for other genital tumors.[43, 112] Black women have about one-third less ovarian cancer than white women, mainly because they have a lower incidence of the epithelial carcinomas; rates for germ cell and sex cord–stromal cancers are slightly higher in blacks than in whites. Most case control studies agree on two risk factors: nulliparity and family history. There is a higher frequency of carcinoma in unmarried women and in married women with low parity. Estrogen therapy seems to have no effect. Indeed, there is decreased risk of developing ovarian cancer in women 40 to 59 years of age who have taken oral contraceptives.[113] Gonadal dysgenesis in children is associated with increased risk of ovarian cancer.

The classification of ovarian tumors given in Table 24–2 is a simplified version of the W.H.O. Histological Classification of Ovarian Tumors, which separates ovarian neoplasms according to the most probable tissue of origin.[109] It is now believed that tumors of the ovary arise ultimately from one of three ovarian components: (1) *the surface coelomic epithelium,* which embryologically has the potential of differentiating into epithelium that resembles closely that of fallopian tubes (ciliated, serous, columnar cells), the endometrial lining (nonciliated, columnar cells), or the endocervical glands (tall, mucus-secreting, nonciliated cells); (2) *the germ cells,* which migrate to the ovary from the yolk sac and are totipotential; and (3) *the stroma of the ovary,* which includes the sex cords, forerunners of the endocrine apparatus of the postnatal ovary. There is, as usual, a group of tumors that defy classification, and finally there are secondary or metastatic tumors, the ovary being a common site of metastases from a variety of other cancers.

Table 24–2. OVARIAN NEOPLASMS

Tumors of Surface Epithelium (75% of all ovarian tumors; 95% of malignant ovarian tumors)
- Serous tumors
  - Serous cystadenoma
  - Borderline serous tumor
  - Serous cystadenocarcinoma
  - Adenofibroma and cystadenofibroma
- Mucinous tumors
  - Mucinous cystadenoma
  - Borderline mucinous tumor
  - Mucinous cystadenocarcinoma
- Endometrioid carcinoma
- Clear cell adenocarcinoma
- Brenner tumor
- Undifferentiated carcinoma

Germ Cell Tumors (15% of all ovarian tumors; 1% of malignant ovarian tumors)
- Teratoma
  - Benign (mature, adult)
    - Cystic teratoma (dermoid cyst)
    - Solid teratoma
  - Malignant (immature)
  - Monodermal or specialized (e.g., carcinoid, struma ovarii)
- Dysgerminoma
- Endodermal sinus tumor
- Choriocarcinoma
- Others (embryonal carcinoma, polyembryoma, mixed germ cell tumors)

Sex Cord–Stromal Tumors (10% of all ovarian tumors; 2% of malignant ovarian tumors)
- Granulosa–theca cell tumors
  - Granulosa cell tumor
  - Thecoma
  - Fibroma
- Sertoli-Leydig cell tumor (androblastoma)
- Gonadoblastoma

Unclassified Tumors
Metastatic tumors

Although some of the specific tumors have distinctive features, the clinical characteristics of most ovarian tumors are similar. These tumors tend to produce relatively mild symptoms until they have reached a large size. In the case of malignant tumors, they have usually spread outside the ovary by the time a definitive diagnosis is made. Abdominal pain and distention, urinary and gastrointestinal tract symptoms due to compression by tumor or cancer invasion, and abdominal and vaginal bleeding are the most common symptoms. The benign forms may be entirely asymptomatic and occasionally are unexpected findings on abdominal or pelvic examination or during surgery.

TUMORS OF SURFACE (COELOMIC) EPITHELIUM

The great majority of primary neoplasms in the ovary fall within this category.[114] There are three major types of such tumors, depending on whether the epithelium is *serous*, mimicking the fallopian tube epithelium; *mucinous*, mimicking the endocervical epithelium; or *endometrioid*, recapitulating the endometrial lining. Mixtures of these epithelia occasionally occur in the same tumor. In some tumors, the epithelium is so undifferentiated that it is unclassifiable. Neoplasms composed of these three cell types range from clearly benign to frank cancers; however, between these two extremes fall a group of intermediate tumors that are best considered as low-grade cancer and are called tumors of "borderline malignancy" or carcinomas of low malignant potential.[115]

These neoplasms run the gamut from small to massive tumors that sometimes fill the pelvis and even the abdominal cavity. Many of the serous and mucinous varieties are cystic and thus the terms *cystadenoma* or *cystadenocarcinoma* is applied to these tumors. Solid areas are often interspersed. As one ascends the scale of aggressiveness, papillary projections into the cystic lumina become more prominent, multiloculation more complex, and solidification of cystic spaces more complete. In general, unilocular cysts with few papillary projections and no solid areas tend to be benign, whereas multiloculated cysts that are highly papillated with frequent solid areas are likely to be malignant.

Serous Tumors

These common *cystic neoplasms are lined by tall, columnar, ciliated epithelial cells and are filled with serous fluid,* the two distinctive features of these tumors. Together the benign, borderline, and malignant types account for about 30% of all ovarian tumors. In the overall spectrum of serous tumors, about 10% are benign, 30% borderline, and 60% malignant. Thus, the ratio of benign to malignant serous tumors is 1:9. The serous cystadenocarcinomas account for approximately 50% of all cancers of the ovary. As with all ovarian tumors, these serous lesions occur at any age, but are most common between the ages of 20 and 50, the malignant forms being seen later in life. They are quite uncommon before puberty.

The benign, borderline, and malignant variants are usually large, spherical, or ovoid cysts that average 10 to 15 cm in diameter but may be as large as 40 cm. The smaller masses usually have only a single cystic cavity, but as they enlarge they may become multilocular, and then they lose their symmetric external aspect (Fig. 24–41). In the cystadenoma, the serosal covering is smooth and glistening. The **cystadenocarcinomas** often have small, solid nodularities or irregular thickenings either directly beneath the serosa or protruding through it. Both benign and malignant forms are filled with a clear serous fluid in most instances, but occasionally there is mucinous content to the fluid because some tumors are mixed serous and mucin-secreting.

The character of the lining varies. The usual small (up to 10 cm), unilocular cyst has a smooth, glistening lining. Only infrequently are papillary formations or projecting intracystic masses identified in these small tumors.

As the tumors enlarge, they tend to develop multiloculation and papillary projections or large masses or thickenings of the wall that jut into the cystic cavities. It should be emphasized that the papillary tendency, the solid projecting masses, the presence of totally solid locules, and penetration or nodularity of the capsule are all important indicators of probable malignancy (Fig. 24–42). Only 20 to 30% of benign tumors occur bilaterally, but 40% of borderline tumors and approximately two-thirds of malignant forms affect both ovaries. Half of these bilateral borderline and malignant lesions remain confined to the female genital tract and are therefore amenable to surgical extirpation.

Histologically, the lining epithelium in the smooth areas of the cysts is composed of a single layer of tall columnar epithelium. The cells are ciliated, dome shaped, and serous secreting (Fig. 24–43). Microscopic papillae may be found. In the benign variants, these papillae have a delicate fibrous core covered by a single layer of well-oriented columnar cells. Typical psammoma bodies are often found in the stroma of these tumors, their exact significance being unknown.

There is no sharp line of demarcation between this histologic pattern in the cystadenoma and the progressive atypical changes that denote borderline or frank malignancy. The histologic features that denote malignancy consist of piling up of the epithelial lining into more than one layer; invasion of the underlying stroma or capsule of the cyst; the formation of large, solid, epithelial masses that usually represent the jutting areas described in the gross; and frank penetration or invasion of the cyst wall (Fig. 24–44). The individual tumor cells in the carcinomatous lesions display the usual features of all malignancy and, with the more extreme degrees of atypia, the cells may become quite undifferentiated. To express this range of differentiation, the malignant tumors may be classified as Grades I to III.

The histologic criteria for borderline tumors are obviously imprecise but include, in varying combinations, stratification of epithelial cells, apparent detachment of epithelial clusters from their site of origin, moderate mitotic activity, and nuclear atypia, **but lack of obvious invasion of the stroma.** Of these, stromal invasion appears to be the most consistent feature distinguishing carcinoma from borderline lesions.

All ovarian neoplasms derived from surface epithelium and/or ovarian stroma tend to produce similar clinical manifestations, which will be discussed later. Here it is important to cite some of the prognostic data for the borderline and cancerous lesions. The ten-year survival rate for the overt cancers is on the order of 10 to 20%, but for the borderline serous neoplasms is

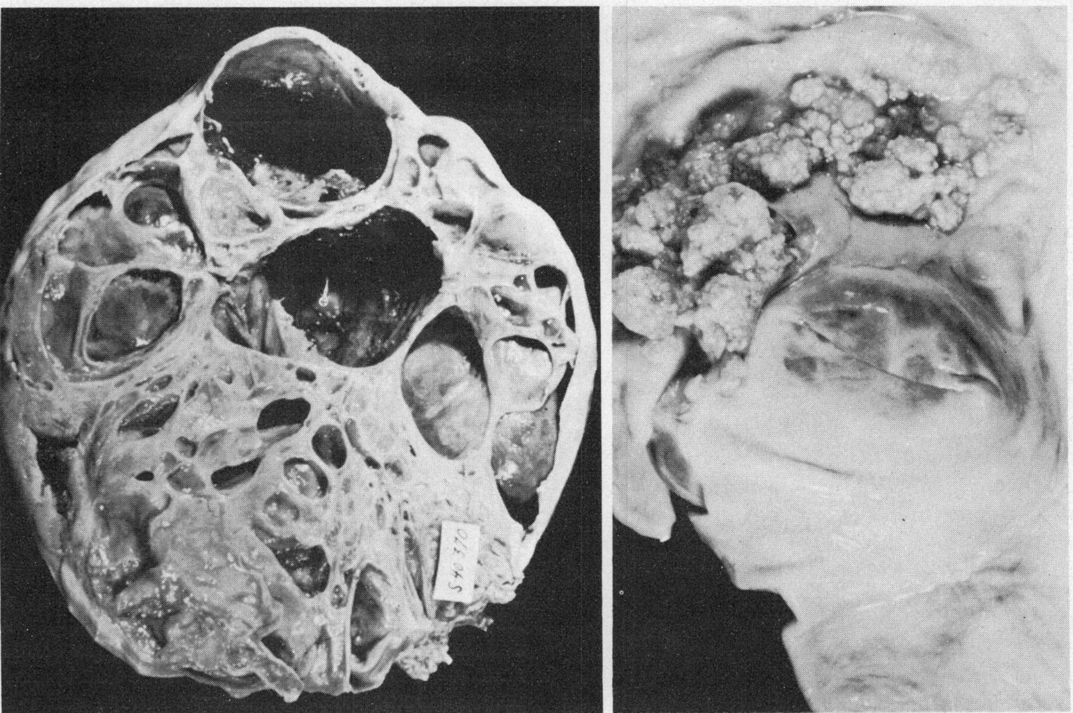

Fig. 24–41

Fig. 24–42

Figure 24–41. Multilocular serous cystadenoma of ovary on cross section.

Figure 24–42. Multilocular serous cystadenocarcinoma of ovary. Close-up of papillary excrescences that have penetrated covering serosa.

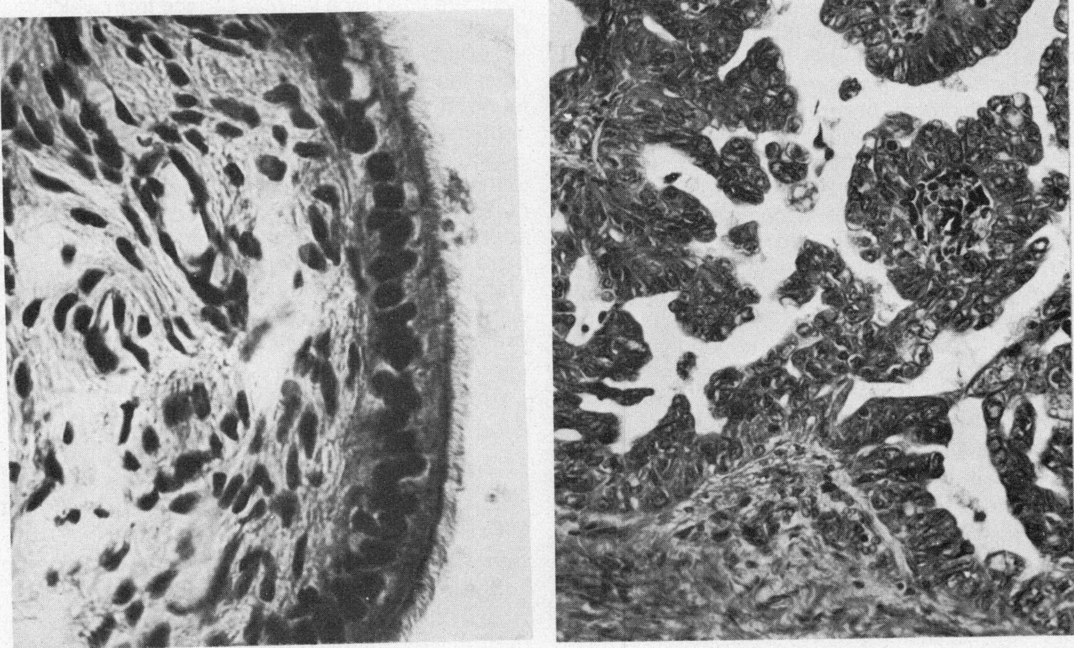

Fig. 24–43

Fig. 24–44

Figure 24–43. Histologic detail of classic ciliated columnar lining epithelial cells of a serous cystadenoma.

Figure 24–44. Papillary serous cystadenocarcinoma of ovary with loss of orientation and piling up of atypical epithelium.

approximately 75%. Even when borderline tumors give rise to extraovarian implants, surgery and radiation have yielded a ten-year survival rate of about 70%.

Mucinous Tumors

These tumors closely resemble their serous counterparts. They are somewhat less common than the serous forms and account for about 20% of all ovarian neoplasms. They occur principally in middle adult life and are rare before puberty and after menopause. The benign variants are much more common than the malignant in the ratio of approximately 7:1. Indeed, mucinous cystadenocarcinomas are uncommon and account for 5 to 10% of all ovarian cancers. You recall that, for serous neoplasms, the benign:malignant ratio is 1:9. The mucinous neoplasm differs from the serous in the character of the lining epithelium. It is composed of nonciliated, tall, columnar, mucus-secreting cells. The nuclei are disposed basally and the mucoid secretion is found in the luminal portion of the cell. The cystic spaces are filled with this sticky, slightly gelatinous fluid rich in glycoproteins.

Grossly, the mucinous tumors resemble the serous cystadenomas and cystadenocarcinomas. However, in contrast to serous tumors, the mucinous tumors are more apt to be unilateral. Approximately 5% of the benign forms and only 20% of the carcinomas are bilateral (contrasted with serous tumors in which up to 30% of benign tumors and 70% of carcinomas are bilateral). Mucinous tumors tend to produce larger cystic masses and some have been recorded with weights of over 25 kg! They tend to be more strikingly multiloculated and, on cross section, often present a honeycombed appearance (Fig. 24–45).

Metastases from these cystadenocarcinomas or rupture of a malignant tumor may give rise to a clinical condition designated **pseudomyxoma peritonei.** The peritoneal cavity becomes filled with a glairy mucinous material resembling the cystic contents. Multiple tumor implants are found on all the serosal surfaces, and extensive interadherence and adhesion of the viscera produces a complete matting together of all the abdominal contents (Fig. 24–46). This fortunately rare form of pseudomyxoma peritonei is a manifestation of malignant dissemination; it is similar in significance to the pseudomyxoma peritonei encountered in rupture of a carcinomatous mucocele of the appendix (p. 876).

Histologically, these mucinous tumors are identified by the apical mucinous vacuolation of the tall columnar lining epithelial cells and the absence of cilia (Fig. 24–47). Not uncommonly, however, mixtures of epithelium may be encountered that make it impossible clearly to distinguish serous from mucinous tumors. The same characteristics that applied to serous cystadenocarcinoma (i.e., piling up of epithelium, formation of papillae and complicated glandular structures, atypia of epithelial cells, invasion of the capsule, and formation of solid masses of tumor) also apply to the segregation of the mucinous variants into benign, borderline, and malignant tumors.

Because of the complexity of the loculation in mucinous tumors, it may be exceedingly difficult to differentiate histologically between benign, borderline, and malignant lesions. Hence, greater reliance must be placed on the level of differentiation of the epithelial components and, where the cells are quite regular and display only slight atypia, the borderline classification may be applied. In 5 to 10% of these mucinous tumors, nodules of a dermoid cyst or Brenner tumor are found in the wall of a cystic space.

The importance of differentiating between borderline and malignant mucinous tumors is made clear by the reported 68% ten-year survival rate in patients with borderline lesions, in contrast with a 34% rate for the overt carcinomas. With tumors localized to the ovary, ten-year survival for borderline lesions is 96%, compared with 60% for carcinomas.[117]

Endometrioid Tumors

These neoplasms account for approximately 20% of all ovarian cancers. *Although benign and borderline forms may occur, most are true carcinomas.*[118] They are distinguished from serous and mucinous tumors by the presence of tubular glands bearing a close resemblance to benign or malignant endometrium. For obscure reasons, 15 to 30% of endometrial carcinomas are accompanied by a carcinoma of the endometrium.[119] It is not thought that one represents metastatic spread from the other.

Although about 15% of cases with endometrioid carcinoma also harbor benign endometriosis, most endometrioid tumors are thought to arise de novo from ovarian coelomic epithelium.[120]

Grossly, endometrioid carcinomas present as a combination of solid and cystic areas. These tumors do not achieve the monstrous proportions of their mucinous cousins. The cysts are lined by a velvety surface from which may protrude polypoid masses or papillae.

Thirty to 50% of patients with endometrioid carcinoma have involvement of both ovaries. When such bilaterality is found, it usually, but not always, implies extension of the neoplasm beyond the female genital tract. Histologically, glandular patterns are seen bearing a strong resemblance to those of endometrial origin. In some cases, there are foci of squamous differentiation, recapitulating the pattern of adenoacanthomas of the endometrium. Similarly, some tumors have foci resembling serous or mucinous carcinomas. The survival data cited earlier are modified by the level of differentiation of the epithelial component. The overall five-year survival rate is 40 to 50%.

Clear Cell Adenocarcinoma

This uncommon pattern of surface epithelial tumor of the ovary is characterized by large epithelial cells with abundant clear cytoplasm. Because these tumors sometimes occur in association with endometriosis or endometrioid carcinoma of the ovary, and resemble clear cell carcinoma of the endometrium, they are now thought to be of müllerian duct origin and, indeed, variants of endometrioid adenocarcinoma.[121]

The clear cell tumors of the ovary can be predominantly solid or cystic. In the solid neoplasm, the clear cells are arranged in sheets or tubules. In the cystic variety, the neoplastic cells line the spaces. The five-

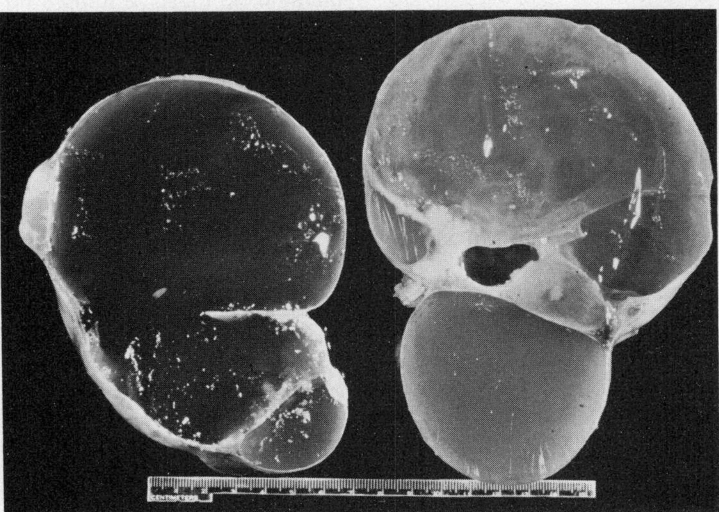

Fig. 24–45

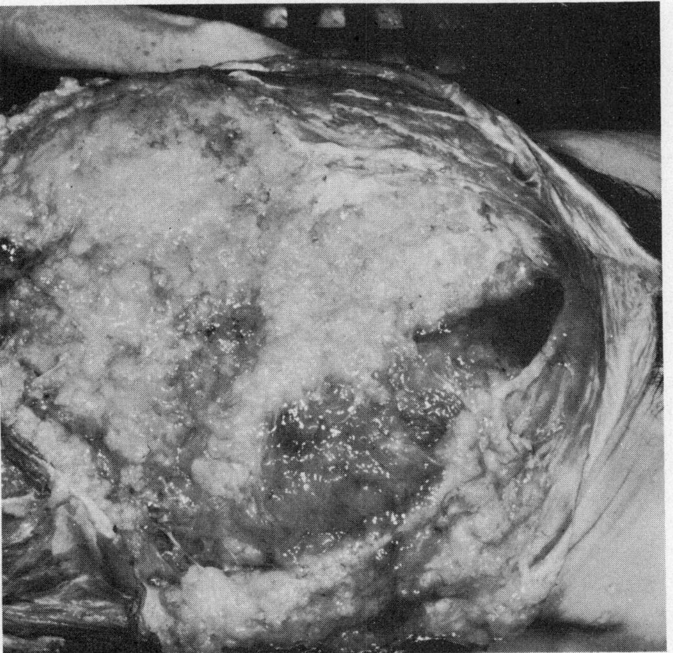

Fig. 24–46

Figure 24–45. Bilateral mucinous cystadenomas of ovary. Tumors were fixed before sectioning to demonstrate gelatinous nature of cystic contents. Note 15-cm rule.

Figure 24–46. Pseudomyxoma peritonei (ovarian), viewed at autopsy with abdominal wall laid back to expose massive overgrowth of gelatinous metastatic tumor.

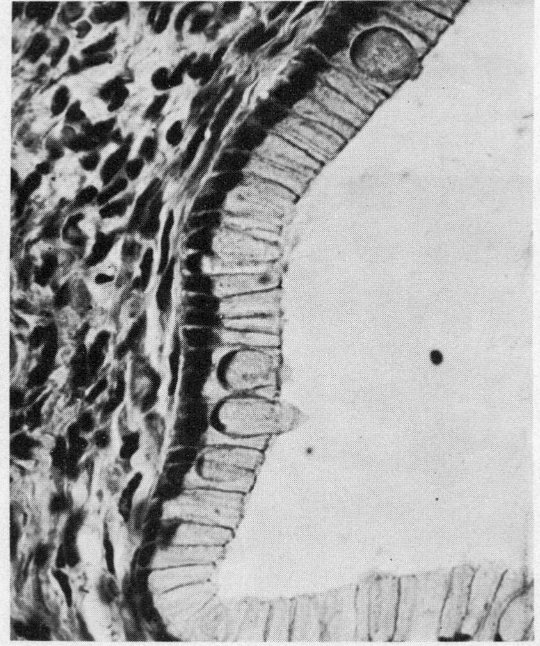

Figure 24–47. Histologic detail of classic nonciliated, mucin-secreting, columnar lining epithelium of a mucinous cystadenoma of ovary. (Courtesy of Dr. Arthur Hertig.)

year survival rate is approximately 50% when the tumors are confined to the ovaries.[121] Some patients with more well-differentiated tumors may have no recurrence. With spread beyond the ovary, five-year survival is exceptional.

Cystadenofibroma

The cystadenofibroma is essentially a variant of the serous cystadenoma in which there is more pronounced proliferation of the fibrous stroma that underlies the columnar lining epithelium. These tumors are usually small and multilocular and have rather simple papillary processes that do not become so complicated and branching as those found in the ordinary cystadenoma. The epithelial lining is usually quite regular. Carcinomatous transformation is rare. Borderline lesions with cellular atypia also occur, but their malignant potential is much less than that of borderline serous tumors.[122]

Brenner Tumor

This usually solid ovarian neoplasm is characterized by a dense fibrous stroma punctuated by nests of transitional cells resembling those lining the urinary bladder. Less frequently, the nests contain microcysts or glandular spaces lined by columnar, mucin-secreting cells. Brenner tumors are uncommon and account for no more than 2% of ovarian neoplasms. They are encountered at all ages, from childhood to the advanced years of life, with a peak incidence between the ages of 40 and 70. As cited earlier, Brenner tumors are occasionally encountered in mucinous cystadenomas. This and other evidence suggest that these tumors arise from coelomic epithelial inclusion cysts through metaplasia of the cyst lining to transitional epithelium.[123]

These neoplasms are usually unilateral (approximately 90%) and vary in size from small lesions less than 1 cm in diameter to massive tumors up to 20 and 30 cm. Although generally solid, they occasionally are cystic. The fibrous stroma, resembling that of the normal ovary, is marked by sharply demarcated nests of epithelial cells (Fig. 24–48). The epithelial cells consist of solid nests resembling the epithelium of the urinary tract, often with mucinous glands in their center. Infrequently, the stroma is composed of somewhat plump fibroblasts resembling theca cells. Such neoplasms may have hormonal activity, and in support of such a notion are the reported instances of the concurrence of Brenner tumors and endometrial carcinoma. The vast majority of Brenner tumors are benign, but borderline and malignant counterparts have been reported.[124]

Clinical Course of Surface Epithelial Tumors

All these tumors of the ovary tend to produce the same clinical manifestations. The two most prominent complaints are low abdominal pain and abdominal enlargement. Gastrointestinal complaints, urinary frequency, dysuria, pelvic pressure, and many other symptoms may appear. When benign, the lesions are easily

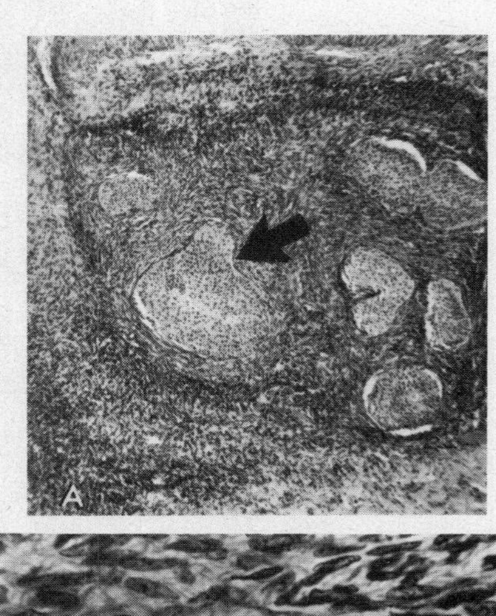

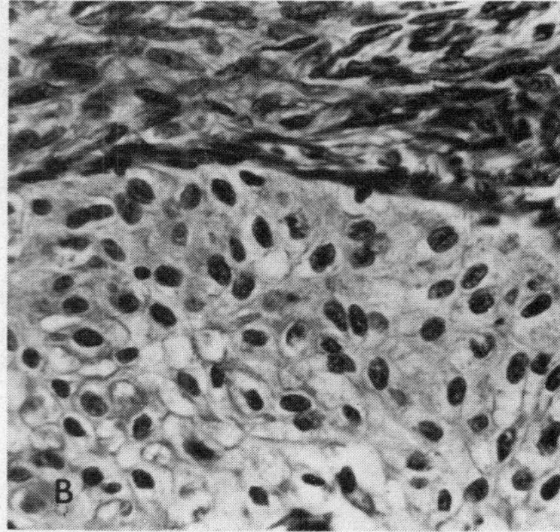

Figure 24–48. Brenner tumor. *A,* Low-power micrograph showing spindle cell component and nests of epithelial cells *(arrow)*. *B,* High-power detail of characteristic epithelial nests.

resected with cure. However, the malignant forms tend to cause the progressive weakness, weight loss, and cachexia characteristic of all malignancies.

The carcinomas extend through the capsule of the tumor to seed the peritoneal cavity. Massive ascites is common with such dissemination to the abdominal cavity. Characteristically, this fluid is filled with diagnostic exfoliated tumor cells. The peritoneal seeding that these malignancies produce is quite distinctive: they tend to seed all serosal surfaces diffusely with 0.1- to 0.5-cm nodules of tumor. These surface implants rarely invade the underlying parenchyma of the organ. The regional nodes are often involved and intraparenchymal visceral mestatases may be found in the liver, bones, and lungs and elsewhere. Metastasis across the midline to the opposite ovary is discovered in about half the cases by the time of laparotomy, and from this point the patients usually run a progressive downhill course to death within one to two years.

Several complications may punctuate the course of these neoplasms. The large, bulky ovarian masses may become twisted on their pedicles (torsion) and undergo hemorrhagic infarction, and thus evoke symptoms of an acute abdomen. The cystic lesions may rupture spontaneously or during palpation, to produce acute abdominal symptoms.

These tumors grow slowly and often remain undiagnosed until very large; thus, many patients with ovarian carcinoma are first seen with lesions that are no longer confined to the ovary. This is perhaps the primary reason for the relatively poor five- and ten-year survival rates for these patients, compared with rates in cervical and endometrial carcinoma. Similarly, follow-up of such patients after surgical therapy, radiotherapy, or chemotherapy can be difficult, since recurrences and spread cannot easily be detected. For these reasons, specific biochemical markers for tumor antigens or tumor products in the plasma of these patients are being sought vigorously.[125] Relative success has been achieved with the measurement of alpha-fetoprotein levels in germ cell tumors (p. 1097), but a radioimmunoassay using monoclonal antibody for ovarian tumor–associated antigen has recently been described and is under evaluation.

GERM CELL TUMORS

Germ cell tumors represent 15 to 20% of all ovarian tumors.[126, 127] The vast majority (95%) are benign cystic teratomas, but the remainder, which are found principally in children and young adults, have a higher incidence of malignant behavior and pose problems in histologic diagnosis and in therapy.

Teratomas

Teratomas are divided into three categories: (1) mature (benign), (2) immature (malignant), and (3) monodermal or highly specialized.

MATURE (BENIGN) TERATOMAS. The vast majority of benign teratomas are cystic and are better known in clinical parlance as *dermoid cysts*. This designation alludes to the fact that they are lined by apparent skin with all of its associated adnexal structures and are typically filled with a sebaceous cheesy secretion in which is found matted hair. These neoplasms are invariably benign and are presumably derived from the ectodermal differentiation of totipotential cells, although mesodermal and endodermal elements are often encountered within the wall of the cyst. Cystic teratomas are usually found in young women during the active reproductive years.

The tumors are unilateral in about 80% of cases and are relatively small compared with other ovarian neoplasms; three-quarters are less than 10 cm in diameter. Characteristically, they are unilocular cysts that on section have a thin wall lined by an opaque, gray-white, wrinkled, apparent epidermis. From this epidermis, hair shafts frequently protrude. Within the wall, it is common to find tooth structures and areas of calcification that prove to be bony spicules. The lumen of the cyst is filled with a sebaceous secretion that is more or less heavily admixed with matted strands of hair (Fig. 24–49).

Histologically, the cyst wall is composed of stratified squamous epithelium with underlying sebaceous glands, hair shafts, and other skin adnexal structures (Fig. 24–50). In most cases, structures from other germ layers can be identified, such as cartilage, bone, thyroid tissue, or other organoid formations (Fig. 24–51). Dermoid cysts are sometimes incorporated within the wall of a pseudomucinous cystadenoma. In less than 1% of the dermoids, malignant transformation of the epithelium is found.

The clinical symptoms are those of all ovarian neoplasms, i.e., abdominal pain, mass, and, occasionally, gastrointestinal complaints or disturbances in the menstrual cycle. There is apparently some unknown influence of these tumors upon the uterus and contralateral ovary, since these patients have a higher than

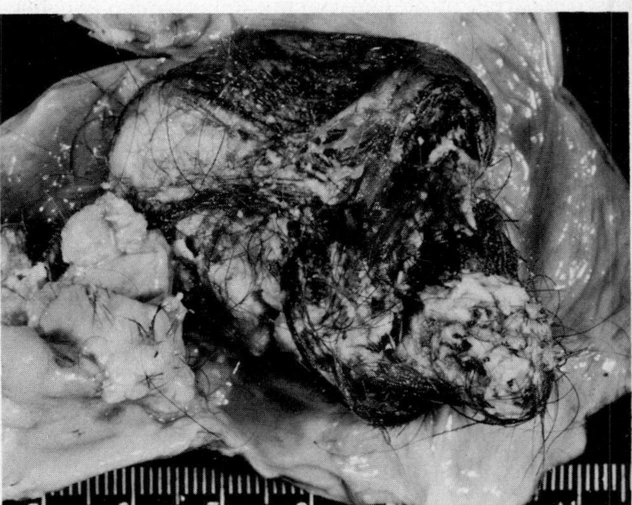

Figure 24–49. Opened dermoid cyst of ovary. Abundant hair and sebaceous material is evident.

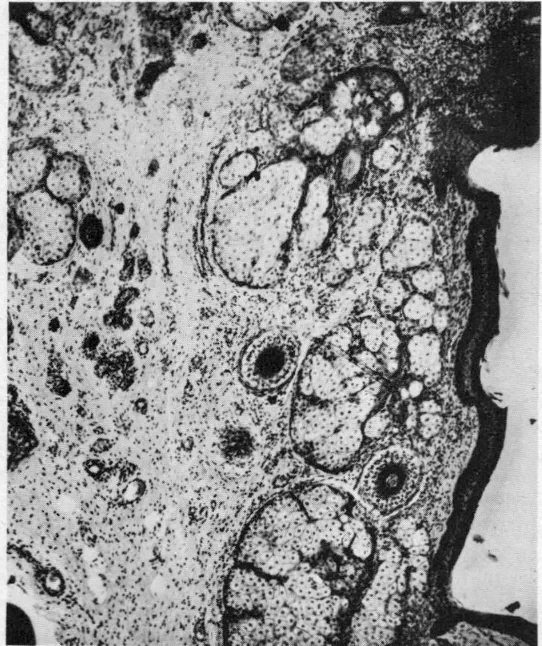

Figure 24–50. Dermoid cyst. Low-power view of lining epithelium, illustrating almost complete resemblance to skin. (Courtesy of Dr. Arthur Hertig.)

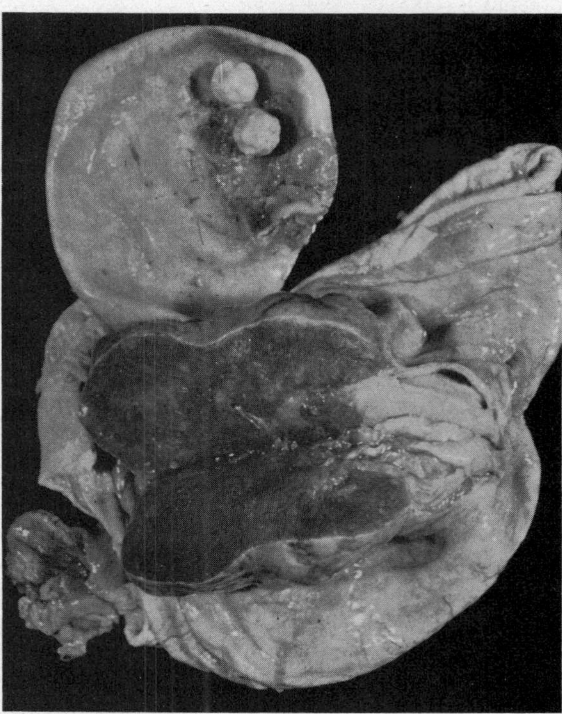

Figure 24–51. Dermoid cyst of ovary, opened to illustrate several abortive tooth structures *(above)* and a darker area of thyroid substance *(below)*.

usual rate of sterility. Torsion of a dermoid tumor on its pedicle is a not uncommon complication that produces signs and symptoms of an acute abdominal emergency. Occasionally, the diagnosis of a dermoid can be made radiographically by the shadows caused by teeth, bones, or areas of calcification, or even the markedly thickened epidermal lining of the cyst. Except in the rare instance of malignant transformation (1% or less), these tumors are resectable and curable. The malignant component may take the form of a squamous cell carcinoma, a thyroid carcinoma, malignant melanoma, or sarcoma.

In rare instances, a teratoma is solid but is composed entirely of benign-looking heterogeneous collections of tissues and organized structures derived from all three germ layers. These tumors presumably have the same histogenetic origin as dermoid cysts, but there is no preponderant differentiation into ectodermal derivatives. These tumors behave in a benign fashion and can be adequately treated by simple surgical extirpation. They should be differentiated from the malignant, immature teratomas, which almost always are largely solid.

The origin of teratomas has been a matter of fascination for centuries. Some common beliefs blamed witches, nightmares, or adultery with the devil. The parthenogenetic theory suggests origin from a primordial germ cell. The karyotypes of all benign ovarian teratomas are 46,XX. From the results of chromosome-banding techniques and the distribution of electrophoretic variants of enzymes in the normal and teratoma cells, Linder and his group suggested that these tumors arise from an ovum after the first meiotic division.[128]

IMMATURE (MALIGNANT) TERATOMAS. These are rare tumors composed of a wide variety of tissue elements in varying stages of differentiation, but they differ from benign teratomas in that *embryonic* (rather than adult) *elements* derived from more than one of the three germ layers are usually present (Fig. 24–52). The tumor is found chiefly in prepubertal adolescents and young women, the mean age being 18.[129]

The tumors are bulky and have a smooth external surface. On section they have a solid or predominantly solid structure containing small locules or cystic spaces. Rarely, the cysts may be quite large. There are areas of necrosis and hemorrhage. Hair, grumous material, cartilage, bone, or calcification may be present. Microscopically, there are varying amounts of immature tissue differentiating toward cartilage, glands, bone, muscle, nerve, and others. The main determinant of extraovarian spread and life expectancy in immature teratomas is the histologic grade of tumor (I–III), which depends primarily on **(1) the degree of immaturity of the various tissue elements and (2) the presence of neuroepithelium.** Grade I tumors contain abundant mature cartilage and a few neuroepithelial elements, whereas higher grades contain fewer mature elements and more neuroepithelial structures that frequently merge with sarcomatous tissue.

Immature teratoma is a malignant tumor that usually grows rapidly and penetrates its capsule early. Spread and metastases are common. With Grade I histology and tumors confined to the ovary, the five-year survival rate is excellent, but unfortunately most patients seen are more far advanced with a poor overall five-year survival rate.

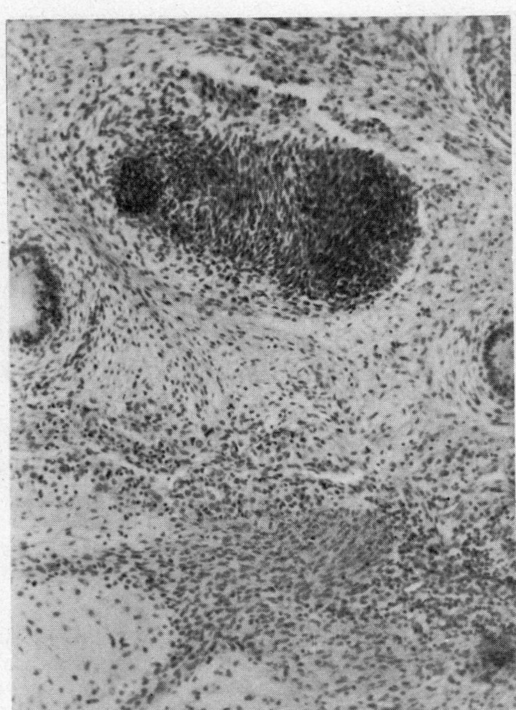

Figure 24–52. Immature teratoma of ovary, illustrating heterogeneity of embryonal organoid structures.

In some cases there is coexistence of immature teratoma with other germ cell tumor elements (choriocarcinoma, endodermal sinus tumor, and embryonal carcinoma) within the same tumor mass.

MONODERMAL OR SPECIALIZED TERATOMAS. These specialized teratomas are a remarkable group of tumors, the most common of which are *struma ovarii* and *carcinoid.*[130] Struma ovarii is entirely composed of mature thyroid tissue. Interestingly, these thyroidal neoplasms may hyperfunction, producing hyperthyroidism. The ovarian carcinoid, which presumably arises from intestinal epithelium in a teratoma, might in fact be functioning, producing 5-hydroxytryptamine and the carcinoid syndrome. Primary ovarian carcinoid must be distinguished from ovarian metastasis of an intestinal carcinoid. Most fascinating is the *strumal carcinoid,* a combination of struma ovarii and carcinoid in the same ovary.

Dysgerminoma

The dysgerminoma[131] is best remembered as the ovarian counterpart of the seminoma of the testis. Like the latter, it is composed of large vesicular cells having a cleared cytoplasm, well-defined cell boundaries, and centrally placed regular nuclei. These cells are derived from primordial germ cells and recapitulate the state of the sexually undifferentiated embryonic gonad. Relatively uncommon tumors, the dysgerminomas account for about 2% of all ovarian cancers, yet form about half of malignant germ cell tumors. They may occur in childhood, but 75% occur in the second and third decades. Some, but by no means all, occur in patients with gonadal dysgenesis of varying degrees, including pseudohermaphroditism. Most of these tumors have no endocrine function but are associated with menstrual bleeding. A few produce elevated levels of chorionic gonadotropin and may have syncytiotrophoblastic giant cells histologically.

Usually unilateral (80 to 90%), they most frequently are solid tumors, ranging in size from barely visible nodules to masses that virtually fill the entire abdomen. On cut surface, they have a yellow-white to gray-pink appearance and are often soft and fleshy. Histologically, the dysgerminoma cells are dispersed in sheets or cords separated by scant fibrous stroma. As in the seminoma, the fibrous stroma is infiltrated with mature lymphocytes and occasionally has focal granulomatous foci reminiscent of tuberculosis or sarcoidosis. Occasionally, small nodules of dysgerminoma are encountered in the wall of an otherwise benign cystic teratoma; conversely, predominantly dysgerminomatous tumor may contain a small cystic teratoma. Dysgerminoma may also be a component of mixed germ cell tumors containing teratoma, choriocarcinoma, embryonal carcinoma, and endodermal sinus tumor.

All dysgerminomas are malignant, but the degree of histologic atypia is variable and only about one-third are aggressive. Thus, a unilateral tumor that has not broken through the capsule and has not spread has an excellent prognosis (up to 96% cure rate) by simple salpingo-oophorectomy. These neoplasms are radiosensitive, and even those that have extended beyond the ovary can generally be controlled or eradicated by such therapy, yielding an overall five-year survival rate between 70 and 90%.

Endodermal Sinus (Yolk Sac) Tumor

This tumor is rare but is the second most frequent malignant tumor of germ cell origin. Its derivation from the extraembryonic yolk sac is now well accepted.[120] Like the yolk sac, the tumor is rich in alpha-fetoprotein and alpha-1-antitrypsin. Its characteristic histologic feature, papillary projections composed of a central blood vessel enveloped by immature epithelium, is a recapitulation of the yolk sac endodermal sinus of Duval.[132] Conspicuous intracellular and extracellular hyaline droplets are present in all tumors and some of these can be stained for alpha-fetoprotein by immunoperoxidase techniques.

Most patients are children or young women presenting with abdominal pain and a pelvic mass. The tumors grow rapidly and aggressively, and once were almost uniformly fatal within two years of diagnosis, but recent combination chemotherapy has measurably improved their outcome.

Choriocarcinoma

More commonly of placental origin, the choriocarcinoma may arise in the ovary from the teratogenous development of germ cells. It is generally held that such an origin can only be certified in the prepubertal girl, since after this age the neoplasm may well have arisen in an ovarian ectopic pregnancy.

Most ovarian choriocarcinomas exist in combination with other germ cell tumors, and pure choriocarcinomas are extremely rare. Histologically, they are identical with the more common placental lesions (p. 1160). These ovarian primaries are ugly tumors that generally have metastasized widely through the bloodstream to the lungs, liver, bone, and other viscera by the time of diagnosis.

As with all choriocarcinomas, they elaborate high levels of chorionic gonadotropins that are sometimes helpful in establishing the diagnosis or in highlighting recurrences. In contrast to choriocarcinomas arising in placental tissue, those arising in the ovary are highly fatal cancers.

Other Germ Cell Tumors

These include (1) *embryonal carcinoma,* another highly malignant tumor of primitive embryonal elements, histologically similar to tumors arising in the testes (p. 1094); (2) *polyembryoma,* a malignant tumor containing so-called "embryoid bodies" (p. 1094); and (3) *mixed germ cell tumors* containing various combinations of dysgerminoma, teratoma, endodermal sinus tumor, and choriocarcinoma.

SEX CORD–STROMAL TUMORS

Included within this category are all ovarian neoplasms originating either from the sex cords of the embryonic gonad (which precede the differentiation of gonadal mesenchyme into male or female) or from the stroma of the ovary.[133] Thus, granulosa cell, theca cell, and luteal cell neoplasms having such histogenetic origins fall within this category. Moreover, since theca cells are the source of ovarian steroids, many of these neoplasms are functional and have feminizing effects.[133] The embryonic sex cords may differentiate along masculine lines to give rise to Sertoli-Leydig cell tumors, also known as androblastomas or arrhenoblastomas. However, some of these Sertoli-Leydig cell tumors either have no function or have estrogenic effects.

Granulosa-Theca Cell Tumors

This designation embraces ovarian neoplasms composed of varying proportions of granulosa cells and theca cells, which may be luteinized. At one end of the spectrum are tumors composed almost entirely of granulosa cells, and at the other are pure *thecomas.* Collectively, these neoplasms account for about 5% of all ovarian tumors. Although they may be discovered at any age, approximately two-thirds occur in postmenopausal women.

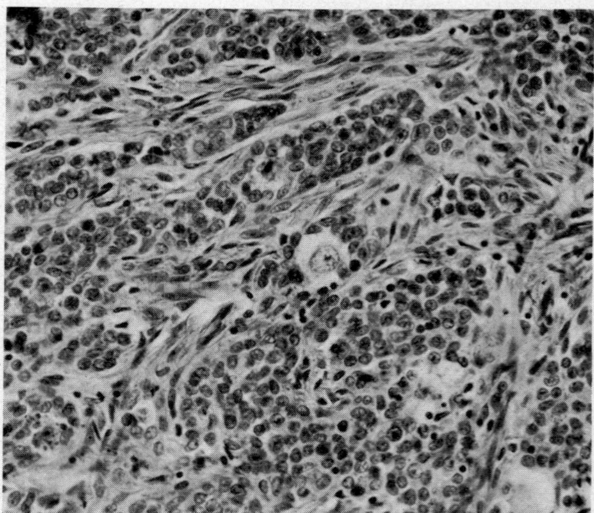

Figure 24–53. Granulosa cell tumor with cuboidal epithelial cells.

Granulosa cell tumors are usually unilateral and vary from microscopic foci to large, solid, and cystic encapsulated masses up to 20 to 30 cm in diameter. Generally, they range from about 5 to 10 cm in diameter. Tumors that are endocrinologically active have a yellow coloration to their cut surfaces, produced by contained lipids, and in the most active tumors, such as the relatively pure thecomas, the coloration may be a bright orange-yellow. The pure thecomas are solid-firm tumors.

The granulosa-cell component of these tumors takes one of many histologic patterns. The small, cuboidal-to-polygonal, epithelial-appearing follicle cells may grow in anastomosing cords, sheets, or strands. In occasional cases, small, distinctive, glandlike structures are produced that are filled with an acidophilic material (Call-Exner bodies) (Fig. 24–53). When these structures are evident, the diagnosis is rendered considerably more simple. In the thecoma component, the cells may be disposed in large sheets of cuboidal-to-polygonal cells that gradually change into plump spindle cells resembling the theca lutein cells. The theca cells, in turn, blend rather deceptively with the surrounding stroma of the ovary.

The variation in architectural pattern of these tumors makes it quite difficult, in certain instances, to determine whether the cells are granulosal in nature or are more like theca cells. Pure thecomas are composed of large sheets or poorly defined areas of plump spindle cells that closely resemble those of the fibroma (Fig. 24–54). The distinction between the theca cell and the fibrocyte cannot be made with certainty. Characteristically, theca cells contain sudanophilic droplets, many of which can be proved by special procedures to give the staining reaction of lipid steroids. Ultrastructurally, thecoma cells resemble fibroblasts but have larger numbers of lipid droplets. However, only clinical or biochemical evidence of hormone production by the tumor distinguishes functional theca cells from fibroblasts.

Most predominantly granulosa cell patterns contain only a scant amount of lipid substance, and most of these tumors are relatively inactive endocrinologically. The finding is consonant with the well-established belief that the granulosa cell of the ovarian follicle does not produce the estrogens, but rather that the endocrinologic activity of the follicle resides in the theca cells.

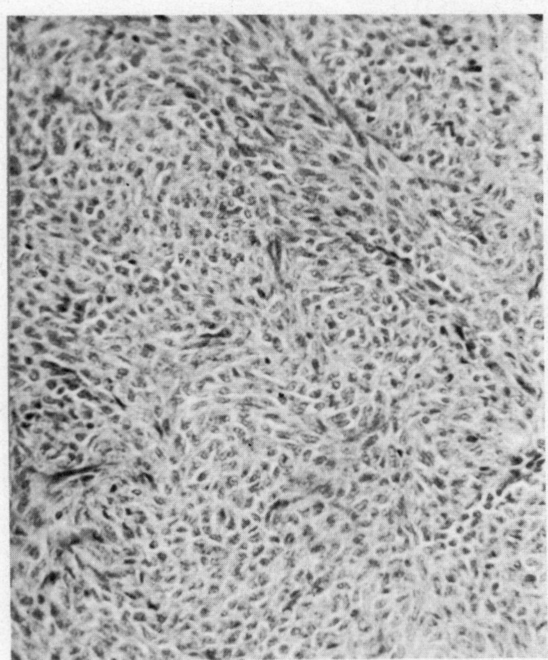

Figure 24–54. Theca luteoma composed of plump, differentiated stromal cells. Note resemblance to a fibroma. (Courtesy of Dr. Arthur Hertig and Armed Forces Institute of Pathology.)

These mesenchymal tumors have clinical importance for two reasons: (1) their potential elaboration of large amounts of estrogen and (2) the definite hazard of malignancy in the granulosa cell forms. Functionally active tumors (usually those having a large thecal component) may produce precocious sexual development in prepubertal girls. In adult women, the elaboration of estrogens leads to a variety of important consequences, including endometrial hyperplasia, cystic disease of the breast, breast carcinoma, and endometrial carcinoma.[134] About 10 to 15% of patients with steroid-producing tumors eventually develop an endometrial carcinoma. In the postmenopausal woman with a functionally active tumor, the incidence of endometrial carcinoma may be as high as 25%. Occasional granulosa cell tumors produce androgens, virilizing the patient.

The additional clinical significance of these tumors lies in the fact that all are potentially malignant. It is not implied that a benign tumor becomes malignant but, rather, that granulosa cell neoplasms range de novo from those that are benign to those that are overtly cancerous. It is difficult, from the histologic evaluation of granulosa cell tumors, to predict their biologic behavior.[135] The estimates of clinical malignancy (recurrence, extension) range from 5 to 25%, but recurrences are amenable to surgical therapy. Recurrences are within the pelvis and abdomen and may appear many years (10 to 20) after removal of the original tumor. The ten-year survival rate is approximately 85%. Tumors composed predominantly of theca cells are almost never malignant.

Fibroma

Fibromas arising in the ovarian stroma are a relatively common form of ovarian neoplasm and account for about 5% of all types. Some are pure fibromas, but others contain theca elements and are termed fibrothecomas. Pure fibromas are nonfunctioning.

The fibromas of the ovary are unilateral in about 90% of cases and usually are solid, spherical, or slightly lobulated, encapsulated, hard, gray-white masses covered by glistening, intact ovarian serosa (Fig. 24–55). Commonly, they have a diameter of 5 to 10 cm when excised, but larger masses have been described. Histologically, they are composed of well-differentiated fibroblasts having a more or less scant collagenous connective tissue interspersed between the cells. The cells are uniform and mature, and mitotic figures are, on the whole, uncommon. Rare mitoses may be found in completely benign lesions.

In addition to the characteristic nonspecific findings of pain, pelvic mass, and possibly intestinal disturbances due to pressure, ascites is found in about 40% of cases in which the tumors measure more than 6 cm in diameter. The genesis of the ascites in these cases is obscure. Uncommonly, these patients with ascites also have hydrothorax, usually only of the right side. This combination of findings, i.e., *ovarian tumor, hydrothorax, and ascites,* is designated *"Meigs' syndrome."* This curious association of ovarian neoplasm with abdominal and pleural fluid has also been reported in other forms of ovarian neoplasms, but not in the same high incidence as with fibromas. An awareness of Meigs' syndrome is of clinical importance, because all too frequently the findings of ovarian tumor, ascites, and pleural fluid are interpreted as indicative of a malignancy with peritoneal and pleural metastases. Rare fibrous tumors with few or more mitotic figures per ten high-power fields have a malignant course and are regarded as fibrosarcomas.[136]

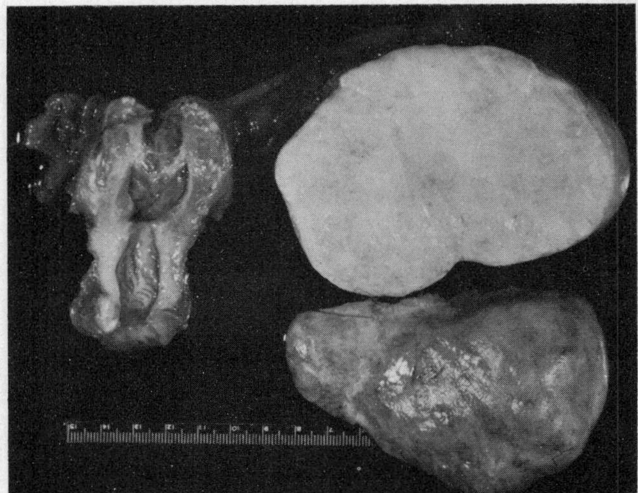

Figure 24–55. Large bisected fibroma of ovary apparent as a white, firm mass.

Sertoli-Leydig Cell Tumors (Androblastoma, Arrhenoblastoma)

These tumors recapitulate, to a certain extent, the cells of the testis at various stages of development.[137] They commonly produce masculinization or at least defeminization, but a few have estrogenic effects. They occur in women of all ages and have been recorded as early as the first decade of life, although the peak incidence is in the second and third. When masculinizing, they inhibit ovulation and are responsible for sterility. Virilization is usually associated with increased urinary excretion of 17-ketosteroids but in some patients the levels are not unusually high or may even be normal, and the elaboration of small amounts of more potent testosterone is postulated. The embryogenesis of such male-directed stromal cells remains a puzzle, and it can be only theorized that it represents masculine differentiation of the mesenchyme derived from the embryonic "ambisextrous" primitive gonads.

These tumors are unilateral and resemble granulosa-theca cell neoplasms. The cut surface is usually gray-white and solid. Larger tumors may have areas of hemorrhage and necrosis and sometimes small cysts.

Histologically, they present a great variation in cytologic detail, so much so that it is difficult at times to establish the identity of this neoplasm unless clear clinical evidence of masculinization is present. The well-differentiated tumors exhibit tubules composed of Sertoli cells or Leydig cells interspersed with stroma. The intermediate forms show only outlines of immature tubules and large eosinophilic Leydig cells. The poorly differentiated tumors have a sarcomatous pattern with a disorderly disposition of epithelial cell cords (Fig. 24–56). Leydig cells may be absent. Heterologous elements, such as mucinous glands, bone, and cartilage, may be present in some tumors.[137]

The incidence of recurrence or metastasis by Sertoli-Leydig cell tumors is less than 5%. These neoplasms may cause defeminization of adult females manifested by atrophy of the breasts, amenorrhea, and loss of hair. This syndrome may progress to striking virilization, i.e., hirsutism, male distribution of hair, hypertrophy of the clitoris, and lowering of the voice. In the prepubertal child, the tumors block normal female sexual development and eventually lead to virilization.

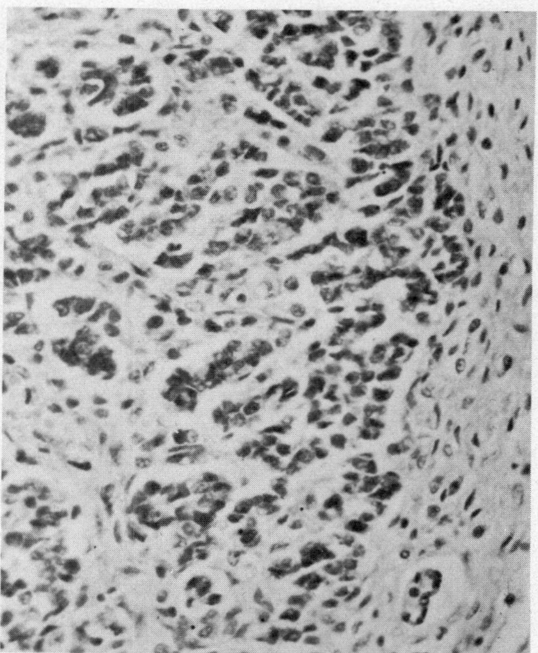

Figure 24–56. Sertoli-Leydig cell tumor growing in poorly developed cords that are not distinctive or pathognomonic. (Courtesy of Dr. Arthur Hertig and Armed Forces Institute of Pathology.)

Other Sex Cord–Stromal Tumors

Hilus cell tumor (pure Leydig cell tumor) is rare and is characterized histologically by large, lipid-laden cells with distinct borders and a granular cytoplasm, and clinically by evidence of masculinization, with hirsutism, voice changes, and clitoral enlargement. Because the cells contain lipochrome pigment as well as Reinke crystals resembling those of the testicular interstitial cells, it is thought that the tumor is derived from the hilus cells of the ovary. The tumors are unilateral. The most consistent laboratory finding is an elevated 17-ketosteroid excretion level unresponsive to cortisone suppression. Treatment is surgical excision. True hilus cell tumors are almost always benign. Occasionally such pure Leydig cell tumors occur in the stroma, not in the hilus (nonhilar Leydig cell tumor).

Lipid cell tumor is an imprecise term used for ovarian tumors with large, vacuolated cells that cannot be clearly categorized as Leydig cell tumors (hilar or stromal), stromal luteoma, or pregnancy luteoma. Malignancy is found in 25% of such tumors, but no histologic criteria have proved useful in predicting their metastatic potential. They are frequently virilizing.

Stromal luteoma is a small, benign tumor rarely over 3 cm in diameter composed of pure lutein cells. The tumor may produce the clinical effects of androgen, estrogen, or progestogen stimulation.

Pregnancy luteoma is a specific lesion, almost certainly not a neoplasm, occurring in women in the last trimester of pregnancy or immediately post partum. The cells resemble those of the corpus luteum of pregnancy, being large and eosinophilic but with little fat. They have been associated with virilization in patients and in female infants born to some of the patients.

Gonadoblastoma is an uncommon tumor thought to be composed of germ cells and sex cord–stroma derivatives.[138] It occurs in individuals with abnormal sexual development and in gonads of indeterminate nature. Patients usually present with amenorrhea, virilization, and abnormal genitalia. Eighty per cent are phenotypic females and 20% are phenotypic males with undescended testicles and female internal secondary organs. This neoplasm has also been observed in hermaphrodites and among phenotypic females with normal menstrual cycles. All patients are under 30 years of age. The tumor is solid and often shows calcifications that may be detected radiologically. Microscopically, it consists of nests of a mixture of germ cells and sex cord

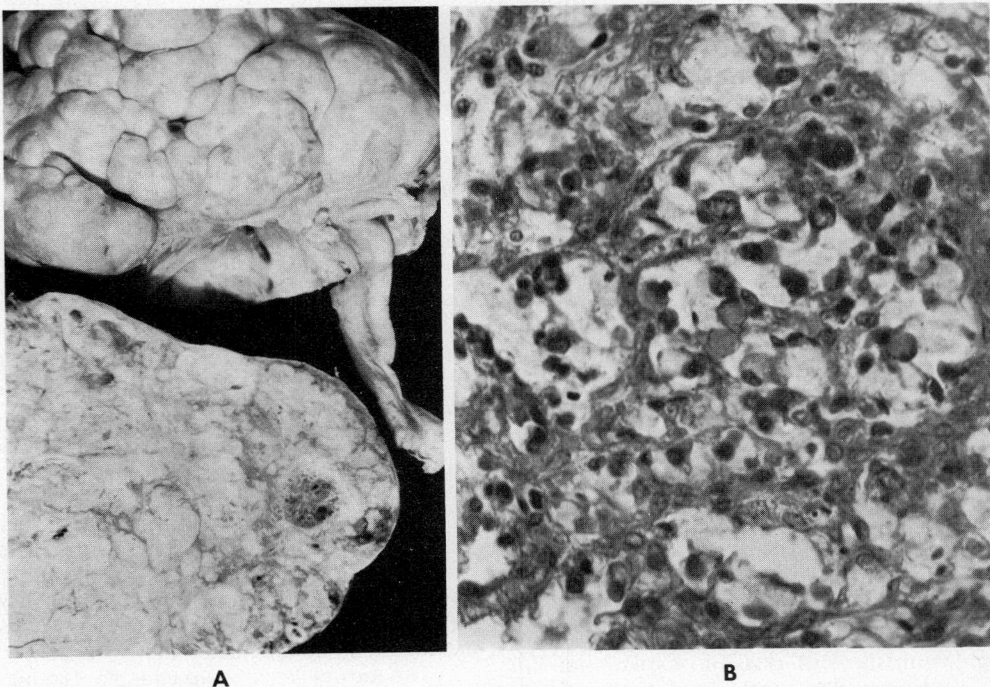

Figure 24–57. *A,* Bilateral Krukenberg tumors of ovary metastatic from stomach. *B,* Krukenberg tumor of ovary, illustrating signet-ring forms dispersed through fibrous stroma.

derivatives resembling immature Sertoli and granulosa cells. A coexistent dysgerminoma occurs in 50% of the cases. The prognosis is excellent if the tumor is completely excised.

METASTATIC TUMORS

The ovary is more often involved by metastatic processes than any of the other pelvic genital organs.[139] Three groups of malignancies contribute to high incidence: carcinomas arising within the other pelvic organs; carcinomas arising in the upper gastrointestinal tract, i.e., stomach, biliary tract, and pancreas; and carcinoma of the breast. The term Krukenberg tumor is sometimes applied to bilateral metastatic ovarian tumors composed of mucin-producing, signet-ring cancer cells, and the vast majority of such metastases are of gastric origin and cause massive enlargement of the ovaries (Fig. 24–57).

Placental Diseases

Toxemia of Pregnancy (Preeclampsia and Eclampsia)
Inflammations
Spontaneous Abortion
Ectopic Pregnancy
Gestational Trophoblastic Neoplasms (GTN)
Hydatidiform mole
Invasive mole (chorioadenoma destruens)
Choriocarcinoma
Placental site trophoblastic tumor

This discussion concerns itself only with disorders of the placenta in which a knowledge of the morphologic lesions contributes to an understanding of the clinical problem.

TOXEMIA OF PREGNANCY (PREECLAMPSIA AND ECLAMPSIA)

Toxemia of pregnancy refers to a symptom complex characterized by hypertension, proteinuria, and edema (preeclampsia). It occurs in about 6% of pregnant women, usually in the last trimester, and more commonly in primiparas than in multiparas. Certain of these patients become more seriously ill, developing frank coma, and some have episodes of convulsions. To this more severe form, the term *eclampsia* is applied. Patients with eclampsia develop *disseminated intravascular coagulation* (DIC) with lesions in the liver, kidneys, heart, placenta, and sometimes the brain. This is not true of all cases. Moreover, there is no absolute correlation between the severity of eclampsia and the magnitude of the anatomic changes.

PATHOGENESIS. The many theories on the nature of toxemia of pregnancy[140] are beyond our scope, and only brief comments will be made on the two events that seem to be of prime importance in this disorder: *hypertension and DIC*.

The mechanism of toxemic hypertension appears to involve the renin-angiotensin mechanism and prostaglandins. Normal pregnant women develop a resistance to the vasoconstrictive and hypertensive effects of angiotensin, but women with toxemia lose such resistance, developing a tendency to hypertension. Prostaglandin E, produced in the uteroplacental vascular bed during pregnancy, is thought to mediate the normal resistance of pregnant women to angiotensin, and prostaglandin production is indeed decreased in the placenta of toxemic women. Thus, the increase in angiotensin hypersensitivity, characteristic of toxemia, may be due to decreased synthesis of prostaglandin. There is also evidence that renin production by the toxemic placenta is increased, another potentially vasoconstrictive event.

The initial cause of the hormonal disturbances (decreased prostaglandins, increased renin) by the placenta is unclear, but clinical and experimental data suggest that reduced *ureteroplacental blood flow* and consequent placental ischemia are early events that mark the critical point for the development of symptoms and lesions of eclampsia.[141] A possible explanation for such reduced flow may lie in the vascular changes occurring in the uterine spiral arteries, consisting of fibrinoid necrosis and accumulation of foamy macrophages in the necrotic vessel wall, a condition called *acute atherosis* (Fig. 24–58). Because these vascular changes are similar to those that occur in immunologic reactions (such as allograft rejection), an immunologic basis for the initial vascular lesion in uteroplacental vessels has been suggested. A speculative sequence of events would then be as follows: immunologic injury to uterine vessels → placental ischemia → increased renin and decreased prostaglandin production → increased sensitivity of arterioles to angiotensin → hypertension. The hypertension itself may then lead to further vascular changes and a vicious cycle.

As to the pathogenesis of DIC in toxemia, it is thought that the coagulation system in pregnancy is under constant activation by slow release of thromboplastic material from the placenta. During toxemia the ischemic placenta leads to a higher output of thromboplastic substances and overt intravascular coagulation. The characteristic lesions in eclampsia are in large part due to thrombosis of arterioles and capillaries throughout the body, particularly in the liver, kidneys, brain, pituitary, and placenta.

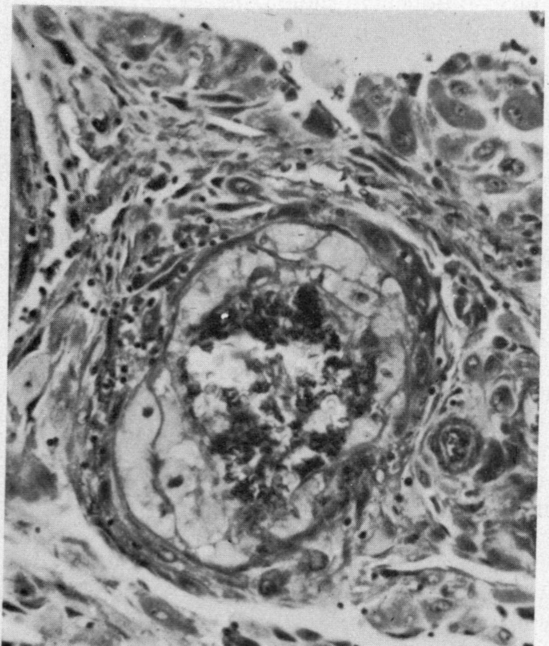

Figure 24–58. Acute atherosis of vessels in an eclamptic placenta. Note foamy subendothelial macrophages.

MORPHOLOGY. The **liver** lesions, when present, take the form of irregular, focal, subcapsular, and intraparenchymal hemorrhages. On histologic examination, there are fibrin thrombi in the portal capillaries with foci of characteristic peripheral hemorrhagic necrosis. These foci of necrosis are accompanied by an inflammatory reaction.[142]

The **kidney** lesions are variable. Glomerular lesions are diffuse, at least when assessed by electron microscopy. These consist of striking swelling of endothelial cells, the deposition of fibrinogen-derived amorphous dense deposits on the endothelial side of the basement membrane, and mesangial cell hyperplasia. Immunofluorescent studies confirm the abundance of fibrin in glomeruli. In the more well-defined cases, fibrin thrombi are present in the glomeruli and capillaries of the cortex. These lead to microinfarcts throughout the cortex. When the lesion is far advanced, it may produce complete destruction of the cortex in the pattern referred to as bilateral renal cortical necrosis (p. 1050).

The **brain** may have gross or microscopic foci of hemorrhage along with small-vessel thromboses. Similar changes are often found in the **heart** and the **anterior pituitary**. It is entirely possible that this type of vascular lesion may account for significant degrees of **pituitary** infarction to reproduce the entity known as Sheehan's postpartum pituitary necrosis (p. 1198).

The **placenta** is the site of variable changes.[143, 144] The principal alterations may be interpreted as **premature aging.** Occasionally, this overall pattern is accompanied by large, pale, retracted areas of infarction that affect whole cotyledons or only a part of one. The aging changes consist principally of an accentuated atrophy of the syncytial trophoblast during the last trimester. Normally in the first two trimesters of pregnancy, the villi are covered by fairly evenly distributed cytotrophoblast and syncytiotrophoblast. In the last trimester, the syncytiotrophoblast undergoes atrophy so that it is disposed unevenly about the villi to create areas devoid of syncytium punctuated by small, piled-up masses of trophoblast—the so-called syncytial knots. In the normal process of maturation and aging of the placenta during the last trimester, about one-third of the villi pass through this phase of epithelial atrophy. However, in eclampsia, this alteration may affect as many as 90 to 100% of the villi. These alterations are often accompanied by capillary thromboses and, once in a while, by florid alterations in the walls of the small vessels characterized by fibrinoid necrosis and intramural lipid deposition (acute atherosis) (Fig. 24–58).

Clinical Course. Preeclampsia usually starts after the 32nd week of pregnancy, but begins earlier in patients with hydatidiform mole, or when there is preexisting kidney disease or hypertension. The onset is usually insidious, characterized by hypertension and edema, with proteinuria following within several days. Headaches, visual disturbances, abdominal distress, and a sense of apprehension are common. Eclampsia is heralded by central nervous system involvement, including convulsions and eventual coma. Mild and moderate forms of eclampsia can be controlled by bed rest, a balanced diet, and antihypertensive agents, but termination of pregnancy is the only definitive treatment of established preeclampsia and eclampsia. Preeclampsia remains one of the leading causes of death among obstetric patients, but mortality can be dramatically reduced by proper prenatal care and management of preeclampsia and its complications. Proteinuria and hypertension usually disappear within one or two weeks after delivery, except in patients whose proteinuria and hypertension predated the pregnancy.[145]

INFLAMMATIONS

Bacterial infections may occur in the placenta *(placentitis)* and in the fetal membranes *(chorioamnionitis)*.[146] In most instances these bacterial invasions arise as ascending infections through the birth canal, and in almost all such instances premature rupture of the membranes provides the portal of entry for the organisms. The hazard of infection is much increased by prolapse of the umbilical cord or one of the extremities. However, bacterial infections may also be introduced in the course of an induced abortion. Very uncommonly, bacterial infections of the placenta and fetal membranes may arise by the hematogenous spread of bacteria, and under these circumstances the fetal membranes may be intact. The amniotic fluid is cloudy and contains purulent exudate. The chorioamnion, when involved, is thickened and opalescent, and histologically is the site of a leukocytic polymorphonuclear infiltration with accompanying edema and congestion of the vessels. When the infection extends beyond the membranes, it may involve the placental villi with similar inflammatory changes. The vessels often have acute vasculitis. In general, in the usual form of chorioamnionitis encountered in induced abortions, the infection is limited to the fetal membranes.

Syphilis at one time was not uncommon in the placenta. It is very rare at present. It is characterized by enlargement of the placenta caused by bulbous swelling and fibrosis of the villi. Histologically, there is plasma cell and lymphocytic infiltration, but the lesions are not specific for syphilis.

Tuberculous infections of the placenta are almost invariably initiated by hematogenous miliary tuberculosis. Although such placental seeding is an infrequent localization of miliary tuberculosis, it provides the possible genesis for the development of congenital tuberculosis in the offspring. *Listeriosis, toxoplasmosis, candidiasis, and various viral (rubella, cytomegalovirus, herpes simplex) and mycoplasma infections* can also affect the placenta.

Villous inflammation may occur without obvious cause, but infections or environmental factors are suspected.[147]

SPONTANEOUS ABORTION

Approximately 15% of pregnancies terminate in spontaneous abortion, most often in the 10th to 13th weeks of gestation. The term abortion implies miscarriage of a pregnancy of less than six months' gestation. Spontaneous abortion represents the natural processes of selection whereby defective ova and fetuses that are either nonviable or have reduced viability are shed. Thus, fetuses that are less defective may survive longer, only to die in the last trimester of pregnancy or immediately following delivery.

The causes of spontaneous abortion are both fetal and maternal. Defective implantation, inadequate to support fetal development, or death of the ovum or fetus in utero because of some genetic or acquired abnormality constitute the major origins of spontaneous abortion. Numerous studies have indicated bizarre chromosomal abnormalities in over one-half of spontaneous abortuses.[148] Induced abortions are now commonplace; in most of these instances, the abortus is normal.

Maternal influences are less well understood and include vaguely postulated inflammatory diseases, both localized to the placenta and systemic, uterine abnormalities, and possibly trauma. The role of trauma is generally overemphasized and it must be considered a rare-to-exceptional cause of spontaneous abortion. Toxoplasmosis as well as Mycoplasma and viral infections have been implicated as causes of abortion, but the evidence is equivocal.

The morphologic changes depend, of course, on the time interval between fetal death and passage of the products of conception.[149–151] Generally, there are focal areas of decidual necrosis with intense neutrophilic infiltrations, thromboses within decidual blood vessels, and considerable amounts of hemorrhage, both recent and old, within the necrotic decidua. The changes encountered in the ovum or fetus are highly variable. In many spontaneous abortions, no fetal products can be identified. In others, the fetus has undergone almost total autolysis. Placental villi may be markedly distended with fluid and devoid of blood vessels (hydropic degeneration of placenta). Such changes are interpreted as a *blighted ovum*, with failure of development of fetal circulation within the villus leading to the progressive accumulation of hydropic fluid.

As indicated earlier, chromosomal studies often yield striking abnormalities in many of the defective fetuses. Such studies are recommended in three circumstances: (1) habitual or recurrent abortion; (2) after prenatal diagnosis of karyotypic abnormality; and (3) when there is a malformed fetus.

ECTOPIC PREGNANCY

Ectopic pregnancy is the nonspecific term applied to implantation of the fetus in any site other than normal uterine location. The most common abnormal location is within the tubes (approximately 90%). The other, far less frequently involved sites are the ovary, the abdominal cavity, and the intrauterine portion of the fallopian tube (interstitial pregnancy). Ectopic pregnancies are by no means uncommon and occur about once in every 150 pregnancies. The most important pathologic condition predisposing to ectopic pregnancy is chronic salpingitis, commonly of gonococcal origin. Other predisposing factors include peritubal adhesions due to appendicitis or endometriosis, leiomyomas, previous surgery, and benign tubular tumors and cysts. Fifty per cent, however, occur in tubes that are apparently normal. These have been ascribed to functional disturbances of tubal physiology, delayed ovulation, and other factors. In women with intrauterine contraceptive devices, almost 5% of all pregnancies (contraceptive failures) are ectopic.

Ovarian pregnancy is presumed to result from the rare fertilization and trapping of the ovum within the follicle just at the time of its rupture. Abdominal pregnancies may develop when the fertilized ovum drops out of the fimbriated end of the tube. In all these abnormal locations, the fertilized ovum undergoes its usual development with the formation of placental tissue, amniotic sac, and fetus, and the host implantation site develops decidual changes.

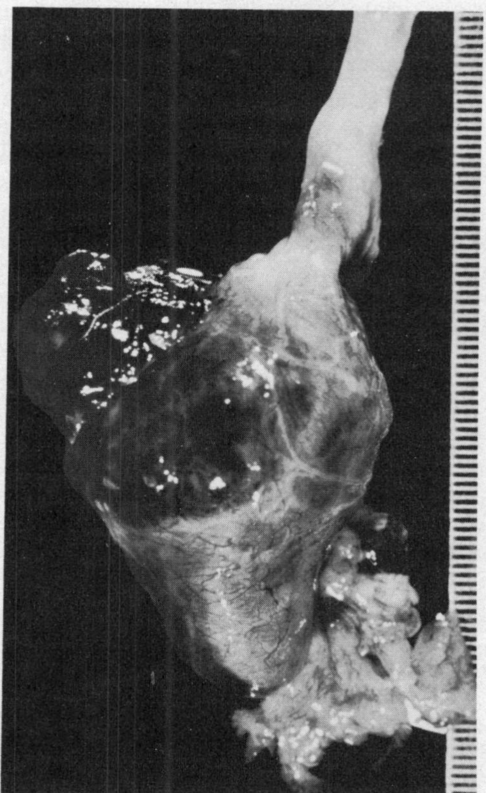

Figure 24–59. Tubal pregnancy with marked dilatation and rupture of distal end of tube by the contained pregnancy and subsequent hemorrhage.

In tubal pregnancy the placenta is poorly attached to the wall of the tube. *Intratubal hemorrhage* may thus occur from partial placental separation without tubal rupture (Fig. 24–59). Tubal pregnancy is the most common cause of hematosalpinx, and when such intratubal hemorrhage is found, this underlying cause should always be suspected. More often the burrowing, invasive placental tissue invades the wall, weakens the tubal wall, and causes *tubal rupture and intraperitoneal hemorrhage.* This is the usual fate of tubal pregnancies, commonly occurring two to six weeks after onset of pregnancy. Less commonly, the tubal pregnancy may undergo *spontaneous regression* due to the poor placental attachment, leading to necrosis of the products of conception, followed by proteolytic digestion, and resorption of the entire gestation.

Still less commonly, the tubal pregnancy is extruded through the fimbriated end into the abdominal cavity *(tubal abortion).* Under these circumstances, the placenta may retain its original site of attachment within the tube or may follow the fetus and become implanted on adjacent intrapelvic or intra-abdominal structures. The capacious abdominal cavity may then permit the full-term development of the fetus, but fetal mortality is 90%.

The clinical course of the usual form of ectopic pregnancy is punctuated by the onset of severe abdominal pain when rupture of the tube leads to a pelvic hemorrhage. Very often, with tubal rupture, the patients rapidly pass into a shocklike state, accompanied by all the classic signs of an acute abdomen. Early diagnosis becomes critical. Physical examination may disclose the tenderness in the tubal regions as well as an apparent tubal mass. In only about half the cases, pregnancy tests are positive. The diagnosis sometimes can also be supported by aspiration of fresh blood from the pouch of Douglas through the posterior vaginal fornix. The most effective diagnostic approach is to carry out laparoscopy or culdoscopy almost immediately on patients suspected of having ectopic pregnancy.

Endometrial biopsy may be helpful. Decidual changes develop here in less than half the cases and, in the absence of chorionic villi, are consistent with ectopic pregnancy. It must be remembered that rupture of a tubal pregnancy constitutes a major medical emergency, since about one in 400 of these patients dies before the hemorrhage can be controlled.

GESTATIONAL TROPHOBLASTIC NEOPLASMS (GTN)

These conditions constitute a spectrum of tumors characterized by proliferation of pregnancy-associated trophoblastic tissue of progressive malignant potential. The lesions include the *benign hydatidiform mole*, the *invasive mole* (chorioadenoma destruens), and the frankly malignant *choriocarcinoma.*[152] GTN are important for the following reasons: (1) the benign mole is a common complication of gestation, occurring about once in every 2000 pregnancies; (2) it has become possible, by monitoring the circulating levels of human chorionic gonadotropin (HCG), to determine the early development of the more malignant forms; and (3) choriocarcinoma, once a dreaded and uniformly fatal complication, is now highly responsive to chemotherapy in most cases.

HYDATIDIFORM MOLE

Hydatidiform mole is a cystic, hydropic swelling of the chorionic villi, accompanied by variable hyperplastic and anaplastic changes in the chorionic epithelium. An embryo or fetus is only exceptionally present. *The most important reason for the correct recognition of true moles is that they are the most common precursors of choriocarcinoma.*[153–155] Most patients present at the fourth or fifth month of pregnancy with vaginal bleeding and with a uterus that is usually, but not always, larger than expected for the duration of pregnancy.

INCIDENCE. These moles can occur at any age during active reproductive life, but the risk is increased in pregnant women between the ages of 40 and 50. For poorly explained reasons, the incidence varies considerably in different regions of the world: one in 2000 pregnancies in the U.S. but as many as one in 120 to 200 in Taiwan, the Philippines, and India.

PATHOGENESIS. Many factors have been implicated in the causation of moles and gestational trophoblastic disease. The geographic distribution alluded to above has suggested both dietary and genetic components. An early theory of Hertig and Mansell[154] postulated that a mole represented an accentuation of the hydropic swelling encountered in a blighted ovum, possibly because the mole is not delivered until the fourth or fifth month of gestation. Cytogenetic studies of moles show that over 90% have 46XX diploid patterns.[156] Chromosome banding patterns of cells from molar tissues and both parents strongly suggest that the entire chromosome complement of the mole comes from the sperm, a phenomenon termed *androgenesis.*[157] The possible mechanism of androgenesis and how it may lead to mole formation are now being explored. Whatever the pathogenesis, the favorite concept today is that *the mole is a true neoplasm and that the trophoblastic lesions are a spectrum of tumors with increasing malignant potential.*[153] In support of the theory of the neoplastic nature of moles are cytogenetic studies showing that aneuploidy in these tumors is associated with aggressive behavior.[158]

MORPHOLOGY. In most instances, hydatid moles develop within the uterus, but they may occur in any ectopic site of pregnancy. When discovered, usually in the fourth or fifth month of gestation, the uterus is usually larger (but may be normal, or even smaller) than anticipated for the duration of the pregnancy. The uterine cavity is filled with a delicate, friable mass of thin-walled, translucent, cystic, grapelike structures (Fig. 24–60). Careful dissection may disclose a small, usually collapsed amniotic sac. Even when the sac is intact and filled with fluid, no ovum or, at best, only a small blighted nubbin representing the ovum can be demonstrated. Theca lutein cysts are found in the ovaries bilaterally in about one-fifth of these cases.

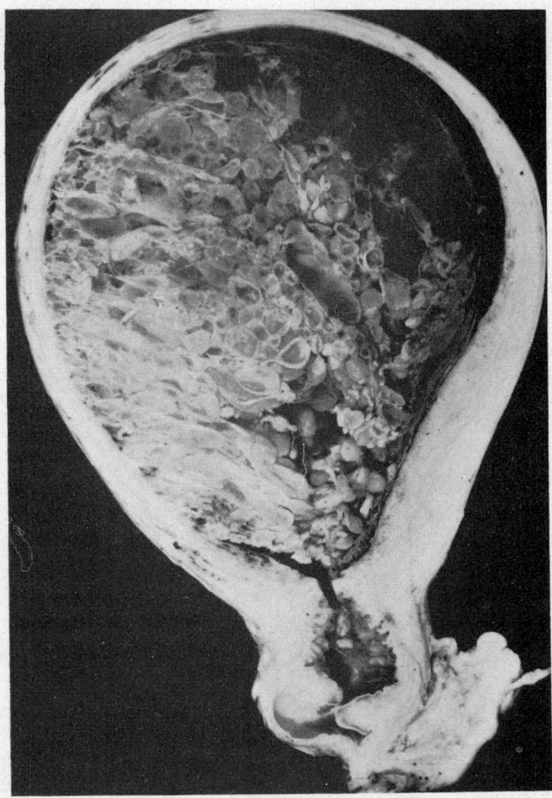

Figure 24–60. Hydatidiform mole. Uterus is filled with the classic mass of grapelike clusters. (Courtesy of Dr. Arthur Hertig. From Anderson, W.A.D.: Textbook of Pathology. St. Louis, C. V. Mosby Co., 1971.)

Microscopically, the mole shows hydropic swelling of chorionic villi, virtual absence or inadequate development of vascularization of villi, and variable degrees of hyperplasia and anaplasia of the chorionic epithelium. The central substance of the villi is a loose, myxomatous, edematous stroma, and they may be covered by a thin layer of chorionic epithelium, both cytotrophoblast and syncytial trophoblast (Fig. 24–61).

At the opposite end of the spectrum are moles having similar cystic dilation of villi, accompanied, however, by striking proliferation of the chorionic epithelium to produce sheets and masses of both cuboidal and syncytial cells. The degree of hyperplasia and anaplasia of epithelium varies considerably and may be difficult to grade, since even normal epithelium is characterized by marked variability in cell morphology. Nevertheless, according to Driscoll,[153] moles can be subdivided into three grades of increasing atypia, decreasing differentiation, and generally worsening prognosis. This grading can be correlated with gonadotropin secretion and is generally predictive of responsiveness to chemotherapy.[159]

The term **incomplete or partial mole** deserves some comment. This refers to the presence of diffuse and massive villous edema **without trophoblastic proliferation** occurring in the presence of a fetus or amnion in specimens from

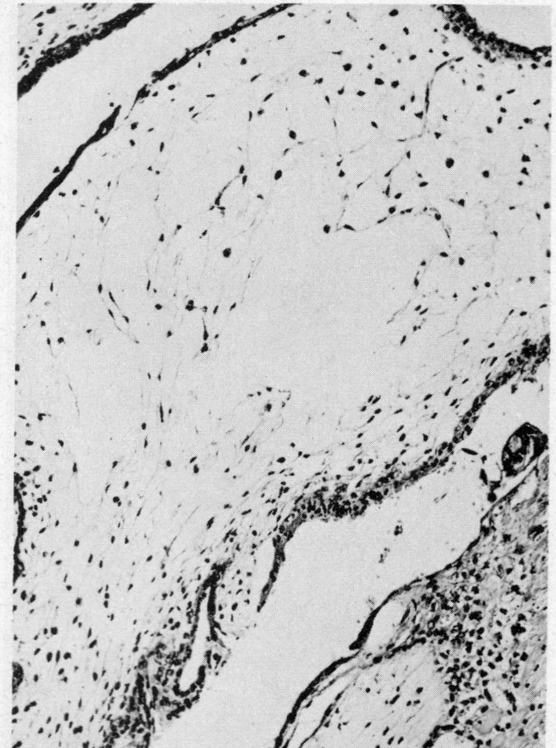

Figure 24–61. Hydatidiform mole. Histologic appearance of cystically edematous villi.

spontaneous abortions. In contrast to true moles, partial moles have a triploid karyotype and are rarely followed by choriocarcinoma.[154]

CLINICAL COURSE. Most patients have abnormal uterine bleeding that usually begins early in the course of the pregnancy and is frequently accompanied by the passage of a thin, watery fluid and bits of tissue seen as small, grapelike masses. The uterine enlargement is more rapid than anticipated. No fetus can be palpated or visualized radiographically, but ultrasound examination permits a definite diagnosis in most cases.

In the classic case, quantitative analysis of HCG shows levels of hormone in both blood and urine greatly exceeding those produced by a normal pregnancy of similar age. Serial hormone determinations will indicate a rapidly mounting level that climbs faster than the usual normal single or even multiple pregnancies.

Once the diagnosis is made, the mole must be removed by thorough curettage. In patients over 35 not desirous of further childbearing, hysterectomy is advocated by most gynecologists. The course following curettage alone depends on the malignant potential of the removed uterine contents. From many studies, it is clear that at least 80% of these moles remain benign and give no further difficulty. The remaining 20%, including those falling into the category of invasive mole, may cause further complications. The incidence of the development of choriocarcinoma in hydatidiform moles is not greater than 2 to 3%. Prophylactic chemotherapy probably diminishes this incidence further but is not widely advocated, since a proper follow-up program should promptly detect malignant transformations in their early curable phase. *The most critical factor in such follow-up is periodic determination of HCG levels.* A rise in such levels for the β subunit of the hormone heralds complications such as persistence of molar fragments or, more ominously, the development of invasive mole or choriocarcinoma.

INVASIVE MOLE (CHORIOADENOMA DESTRUENS)

This is defined as a cellular invasive mole that penetrates and may even perforate the uterine wall. There is invasion of the myometrium by well-developed embryonic villi, accompanied by proliferation of both cuboidal and syncytial chorionic epithelial components. The tumor is locally destructive and may invade parametrial tissues. Hydropic villi may embolize to distant sites such as lungs and brain but do not grow in these organs as true metastases, and even before the advent of chemotherapy they eventually regressed. Clinically, the tumor is manifested by vaginal bleeding and irregular uterine enlargement. It is *always* associated with a persistently elevated chorionic gonadotropin level and varying degrees of luteinization of the ovaries. The tumor responds very well to chemotherapy. Although it is biologically benign, rupture of the uterus may lead to hemorrhage, sepsis, and even death.

CHORIOCARCINOMA

Gestational choriocarcinoma is an epithelial malignancy of trophoblastic cells derived from any form of previous normal or abnormal pregnancy. Although most cases arise in the uterus, ectopic pregnancies provide extrauterine sites of origin. Choriocarcinoma should be differentiated from the locally invasive but nonmetastasizing forms of trophoblastic disease such as invasive mole and placental site trophoblastic tumor (p. 1162), because the choriocarcinoma is one of the most rapidly invasive, widely metastasizing malignancies.

INCIDENCE. This is, fortunately, an uncommon condition that arises in probably not more than one in 20,000 to 30,000 pregnancies in the U.S. It is much more frequent in some Asian and African countries, e.g., one in 2500 pregnancies in Ibadan. It is preceded by the following conditions: 50% arise in hydatidiform moles, 25% in previous abortions, approximately 22% in normal pregnancies, and the rest in ectopic pregnancies and genital and extragenital teratomas. (It should be realized that choriocarcinomas may also occur in males.) It can be further computed that about one in 40 hydatidiform moles may be expected to give rise to a choriocarcinoma, in contrast to one in approximately 150,000 normal pregnancies. It is evident, then, that the more abnormal the pregnancy, the greater is the hazard of the development of this tumor.

MORPHOLOGY.[160] Choriocarcinoma is a purely epithelial cellular malignancy that does not produce chorionic villi and grows, as do other cancers, by the abnormal proliferation of both the cuboidal and syncytial cells of the placental epithelium. It is sometimes possible to identify anaplasia within such abnormal proliferation replete with abnormal mitoses. The tumor invades the underlying myometrium, frequently penetrates blood vessels and lymphatics, and in some cases extends out onto the uterine serosa and adjacent structures (Figs. 24–62 and 24–63). In its rapid growth, it is subject to hemorrhage, ischemic necrosis, and secondary inflammatory infiltration. From this histologic pattern, the characteristic macroscopic features can be deduced.

Classically, the choriocarcinoma is a soft, fleshy, yellow-white tumor with a marked tendency to form large pale areas of ischemic necrosis, foci of cystic softening, and extensive hemorrhage. This pattern of friable hemorrhagic tissue may be encountered as a small area within a previous mole, as a small mural mass recurring after previous evacuations of the uterus, or less frequently as a large tumor that fills the uterine cavity.

Not uncommonly metastatic, unmistakable choriocarcinoma is found in the lungs, bone marrow, liver, and other favored sites of spread in the complete absence of a primary lesion in the uterus or any extrauterine site. This paradoxical situation is encountered not only in the female but also in the male when the tumor may be primary in the testis or some teratoid tumor. (Immunoperoxidase staining of tumor tissue for HCG aids in the histologic diagnosis of such aberrant tumors.) Under such circumstances, it is postulated that the primary focus undergoes total necrosis and resorption after it has metastasized.

CLINICAL COURSE. Classically, the uterine choriocarcinoma does not produce a large, bulky mass. It becomes manifest only by irregular spotting of a bloody, brown, sometimes foul-smelling fluid. This discharge may appear in the course of an apparently normal pregnancy, may begin after a miscarriage, or may become manifest following a curettage for retained products of conception. Sometimes the tumor does not appear until months later. Usually, by the time the tumor is discovered locally, x-ray films of the chest and bones already disclose the presence of metastatic lesions. The HCG titers are markedly elevated by choriocarcinoma to levels above those encountered in hydatidiform moles. When such extreme elevations are found, the diagnosis of choriocarcinoma is virtually established. However, occasional tumors have been recorded as not having produced any hormone, and many tumors have become so necrotic as to become functionally inactive. The final diagnosis must rest on the histologic demonstration of unmistakable cancerous invasiveness in the curettings or other tissue biopsies.

Widespread metastases are characteristic of these tumors. Favored sites of involvement are the lungs (50%) and vagina (30 to 40%), followed in descending order of frequency by the brain, liver, and kidney. However, in the dissemination of this tumor through the vascular system, any organ or tissue may be involved.

The *treatment* of trophoblastic neoplasms depends on the type and stage of tumor, and includes evacuation of the contents of the uterus, surgery, and chemotherapy with methotrexate and actinomycin. Elaborate schemes for the "therapeutic" classification of trophoblastic disease based on levels of HCG, histology, and clinical staging have been devised. One such classification[150] divides trophoblastic disease into:

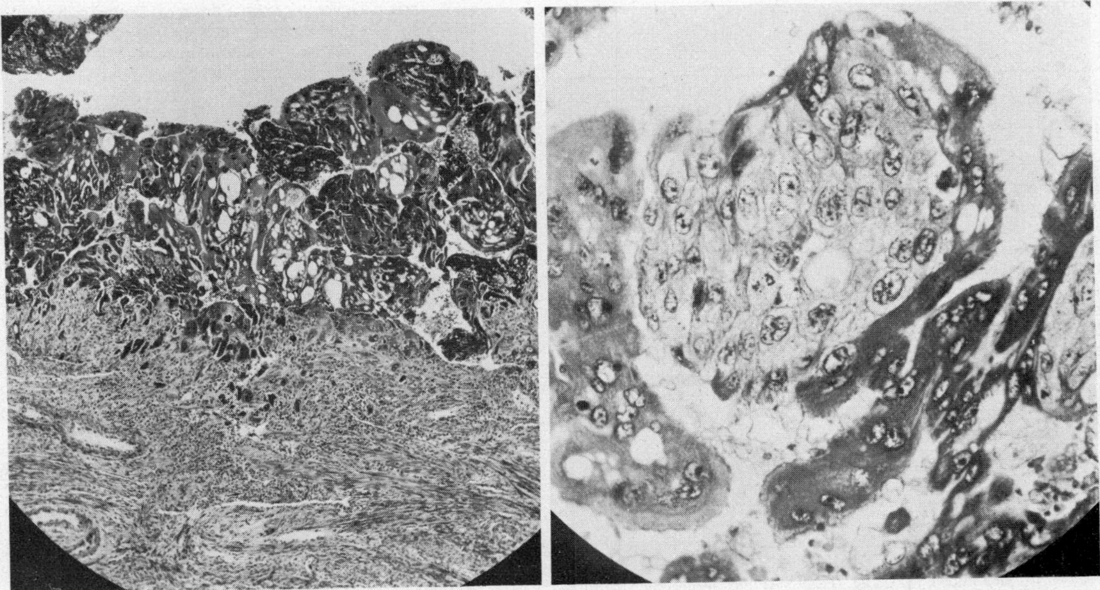

Fig. 24–62 Fig. 24–63

Figure 24–62. Low-power view of choriocarcinoma of uterine wall showing invasion of underlying myometrium.

Figure 24–63. High-power detail of choriocarcinoma illustrating the two types of epithelial cells–cytotrophoblast and syncytiotrophoblast.

Stage 0. Molar pregnancy (usually benign mole).

Stage 1. Trophoblastic neoplasm limited to the uterine corpus with persistent HCG elevation.

Stage 2. Trophoblastic neoplasm outside the uterus but confined to the vagina and pelvic structures.

Stage 3. Trophoblastic neoplasm with metastasis to the lung.

Stage 4. Metastasis to the brain, liver, and other organs.

The results of chemotherapy for gestational choriocarcinoma are indeed spectacular: the protocol used in the New England Trophoblastic Disease Center[152, 161] has resulted in up to 100% cure or remission in all patients except some who had high-risk metastatic trophoblastic disease. Many of the cured patients have had normal subsequent pregnancies and deliveries. These very gratifying results cannot be matched in nongestational choriocarcinomas arising in the ovaries and testes (p. 1151).

PLACENTAL SITE TROPHOBLASTIC TUMOR

This relatively new term has been suggested to encompass conditions previously known as trophoblastic pseudotumor, chorioepithelioma, syncytioma and others.[162] It refers to the presence of proliferating syncytiotrophoblastic tissue deeply invading the myometrium. It differs from choriocarcinoma by the absence of cytotrophoblastic elements and by the low level of HCG production. Despite their locally invasive histologic pattern, most of these lesions are benign and subject to cure by curettage. However, a rare malignant variant has been reported, identified by a high mitotic index, extreme cellularity, extensive necrosis, local spread, or even widespread metastases.[163]

---

1. Noyes, R. W.: Normal phases of endometrium. *In* Norris, H., et al. (eds.): The Uterus. Baltimore, Williams & Wilkins Co., 1973, pp. 110–135.
2. Blaustein, A.: Pathology of the Female Genital Tract. 2nd ed. New York, Springer-Verlag, 1982.
3. Gompel, E., and Silverberg, S.: Pathology in Gynecology and Obstetrics. 2nd ed. Philadelphia, J. B. Lippincott Co., 1977.
4. Haines, M., and Taylor, C. W.: Gynaecologic Pathology. 3rd ed. Edinburgh, Churchill Livingstone, 1984.
5. Jones, H. W., Jr., and Jones, G. S.: Novak's Textbook of Gynecology. 10th ed. Baltimore, Williams & Wilkins Co., 1981.
6. Danforth, D. N. (ed.): Obstetrics and Gynecology. 4th ed. Philadelphia, Harper & Row, 1982.
7. Rosai, J.: Ackerman's Surgical Pathology. 6th ed. St. Louis, C. V. Mosby Co., 1981.
8. Silverberg, S. G. (ed.): Principles and Practice of Surgical Pathology. New York, John Wiley & Sons, 1983.
9. Editorial: The bacteriology of acute pelvic inflammatory disease, Lancet *1*:430, 1982.
10. Josey, W. E.: Viral infections of the vulva. Clin. Obstet. Gynecol. *21*:1053, 1978.
11. Corey, L., et al.: A trial of topical acyclovir in genital herpes simplex virus infections. N. Eng. J. Med. *306*:1313, 1982.
12. Sanchez, N. P., and Mihm, M. C., Jr.: Reactive and neoplastic epithelial alterations of the vulva. J. Am. Acad. Dermatol. *6*:378, 1982.
13. Gardner, H. L., et al.: The vulvar dystrophies, atypias and carcinoma in situ. An invitational symposium. J. Reprod. Med., *17*:131, 1976.
14. Kaufman, R. H., and Gardner, H. L.: Vulvular dystrophies. Clin. Obstet. Gynecol. *21*:1081, 1978.
15. Hart, W. R., et al.: Relation of lichen sclerosus et atrophicus of the vulva to the development of carcinoma. Obstet. Gynecol., *45*:369, 1975.
16. Kryzek, R. A., et al.: Anogenital warts contain several distinct pieces of human papilloma virus. J. Virol. *36*:236, 1980.
17. Kurman, R. J., et al.: Immunoperoxidase localization of papilloma virus antigens in cervical dysplasias and vulvar condylomas. Am. J. Obstet. Gynecol. *140*:931, 1981.
18. Shevchuk, M. M., and Richart, R. M.: DNA content of condyloma acuminatum. Cancer. *49*:489, 1982.
19. Crum, C.: Vulvar intraepithelial oncoplasia: The concept and its application. Hum. Pathol. *13*:127, 1982.
20. Morley, J. W.: Cancer of the vulva: A review, Cancer, *48*:597, 1981.
21. Buscema, J., et al.: Carcinoma in situ of the vulva. Obstet. Gynecol. *55*:225, 1980.
22. Kaufman, R. H.: Intraepithelial carcinoma of the vulva. Obstet. Gynecol. Annu. *6*:317, 1977.
23. Friedrich, E. J., et al.: Carcinoma in situ of the vulva: A continuing challenge. Am. J. Obstet. Gynecol. *136*:830, 1980.
24. Kaufman, R. H., et al.: Herpesvirus-induced antigens in squamous cell carcinoma in situ of the vulva. N. Engl. J. Med. *305*:483, 1981.
25. Schwartz, P. E., and Naftolin, F.: Type 2 herpes simplex virus and vulvar carcinoma. N. Engl. J. Med. *305*:517, 1981.
26. Isaac, J. H.: Verrucous carcinoma of the female genital tract. Gynecol. Oncol. *4*:259, 1976.
27. Jones, R. E., et al.: Extramammary Paget's disease. A critical reexamination. Am. J. Dermatopathol. *1*:101, 1979.
28. Woodruff, D. J.: Lesions of the vulva and vagina. *In* Danforth, D. N. (ed.): Obstetrics and Gynecology. 4th ed. Philadelphia, Harper & Row, 1982, pp. 1023–1040.
29. Mazoujian, G., et al.: Extramammary Paget's disease—evidence for an apocrine origin: An immunoperoxidase study of gross cystic disease fluid protein-15, carcinoembryonic antigen, and keratin proteins. Am. J. Surg. Pathol., *8*:43, 1984.
30. Hart, W. R., and Millman, J. B.: Progression of intraepithelial Paget's disease of the vulva to invasive carcinoma. Cancer *42*:333, 1977.
31. Silvers, D. N., and Halpern, J. A.: Cutaneous and vulvar melanomas. An update. Clin. Obstet. Gynecol. *21*:1117, 1978.
32. Chung, A. F., et al.: Malignant melanomas of the vulva. Obstet. Gynecol. *45*:638, 1975.

32A. Pride, G. L., et al.: Primary invasive squamous carcinoma of the vagina. Obstet. Gynecol. *53*:218, 1979.

33. Herbst, A. L., et al.: Adenocarcinoma of the vagina. Association of maternal stilbestrol therapy with tumor appearance in young women. N. Engl. J. Med. *284*:878, 1971.
34. Herbst, A. L.: Clear cell adenocarcinoma and the current status of DES exposed females. Cancer *48*:484, 1981.
35. Scully, R. E., and Welch, W. R.: Pathology of the female genital tract after prenatal exposure to diethylstilbestrol. *In* Herbst, A. L., and Bern, H. A. (eds.): Developmental Effects of Diethylstilbestrol in Pregnancy. New York, Thieme-Stratton, 1981, pp. 26–45.
36. Robboy, S. J., et al.: Topographic relation of cervical ectropion and vaginal adenosis to clear cell adenocarcinoma. Obstet. Gynecol. *60*:546, 1982.
37. Hilgers, R. D., et al.: Embryonal rhabdomyosarcoma of the vagina. Am. J. Obstet. Gynecol. *107*:484, 1970.
38. Davos, L., and Abell, M. R.: Sarcomas of the vagina. Obstet. Gynecol. *47*:342, 1976.
39. Silverberg, S. G.: Cancer statistics, 1984. CA *34*:7, 1984.
40. Pollack, E. S., and Horm, J. W.: Trends in cancer incidence and mortality in the United States. J. Natl. Cancer Inst. *64*:1091, 1980.
41. Abell, M. A.: Invasive carcinoma of the uterine cervix. *In* Norris, H., et al. (eds.): The Uterus. Baltimore, Williams & Wilkins Co., 1973, pp. 413–456.
42. Ferenczy, A.: Anatomy and histology of the cervix; benign lesions of the cervix; cervical intraepithelial neoplasia; carcinoma and other malignant tumors of the cervix. *In* Blaustein, A. (ed.): Pathology of the Female Genital Tract. 2nd ed. New York, Springer-Verlag, 1982, pp. 119–135.
43. Berg, J., and Lampe, J.: High risk factors in gynecological cancer. Cancer *48*:429, 1981.
44. Devesa, S. S., and Diamond, E. L.: Association of breast cancer and cervical cancer incidence with income and education among whites and blacks. J. Natl. Cancer Inst. *65*:515, 1980.
45. Creagan, E. T., and Fraumeni, J. F., Jr.: Cancer mortality among American Indians. J. Natl. Cancer Inst. *49*:959, 1982.
46. Kessler, I. I.: Venereal factors in human cervical cancer: evidence from marital clusters. Cancer *39*:1912, 1977.
47. Lambert, B., et al.: An etiological survey of clinical factors in cervical intraepithelial neoplasia: A transverse retrospective study, J. Reprod. Med. *24*:26, 1980.
48. Persuad, U. V.: Geographical pathology of cancer of uterine cervix. Trop. Geogr. Med. *29*:235, 1977.
49. Editorial. Oral contraceptives and neoplasia. Lancet *2*:947, 1983.

50. Swan, S. H., and Brown, W. L.: Vasectomy and cancer of the cervix. N. Engl. J. Med. *301*:46, 1979.
51. Stellman, S. D., et al.: Cervix cancer and cigarette smoking: A case control study. Am. J. Epidemiol. *111*:383, 1980.
52. Zur Hansen, H.: Human genital cancer: Synergism between two virus infections or synergism and initiation? Lancet *2*:1370, 1982.
53. Rawls, W. E., and Adams, E.: Herpes simplex viruses and human malignancies. *In* Hyatt, R. et al. (eds.): Origins of Human Cancer, Book B, Mechanisms of Carcinogenesis. Cold Spring Harbor Conferences on Cell Proliferation *4*:1133, 1979.
54. Nahmias, A. J., and Roizman, B.: Infection with herpes simplex virus I and II. N. Engl. J. Med. *289*:667, 719, 781, 1973.
55. Aurelian, L. et al: Viruses and gynecological cancers. Herpes virus protein (ICP10) stroke AG-4, a cervical tumor antigen that fulfills the criteria for a marker of carcinogenicity. Cancer *48*:455, 1981.
56. McDougal, J. K., et al.: Cervical carcinoma: Detection of herpes simplex virus RNA in cells undergoing neoplastic change. Int. J. Cancer *225*:1, 1980.
57. Kurman, R. J., et al.: Papilloma virus infection of the cervix. II. Relationship to intraepithelial neoplasia based on the presence of specific viral structural proteins. Am. J. Surg. Pathol. *7*:39, 1983.
58. Kaufman, R., et al.: Statement of caution in the interpretation of papilloma virus–associated lesions of the epithelium of the uterine cervix. Acta Cytol. *27*:107, 1983.
59. Zoler, M. L.: Human papilloma virus limited to cervical (and other) cancers. J.A.M.A. *249*:2997, 1983.
60. Scully, R. E.: Definitions of precursors in gynecologic cancer. Cancer *48*:531, 1981.
61. Richart, R. M.: Cervical intraepithelial neoplasia. Pathol. Annu., *8*:301, 1973.
62. Christopherson, W. M.: Dysplasia, carcinoma-in-situ and microinvasive carcinoma of the uterine cervix. Hum. Pathol. *8*:481, 1977.
62A. Koss, L. G.: Dysplasia—a real concept or a misnomer. Obstet. Gynecol. *51*:374, 1978.
63. Buckley, C. H., et al.: Cervical intraepithelial neoplasia. J. Clin. Pathol. *35*:1, 1982.
64. Burghardt, E.: Premalignant conditions of the cervix. Clin. Obstet. Gynecol. *3*:257, 1976.
65. Poulsen, H. E., et al.: International Histologic Typing of Female Genital Tract Tumors. Geneva, W.H.O., 1975.
66. Hall, J. E., and Walton, L.: Dysplasia of the cervix: A prospective study of 206 cases. Am. J. Obstet. Gynecol. *105*:386, 1969.
67. Richart, R. M., and Barron, B. B.: A follow-up study of patients with cervical dysplasia. Am. J. Obstet. Gynecol. *105*:386, 1969.
68. Christopherson, W. M., et al.: Cervical cancer control. Cancer *38*:1357, 1976.
69. Lohe, K. J., et al.: Early squamous cell carcinoma of the uterine cervix. Gynecol. Oncol. *6*:10, 1978.
70. Creasman, W. T., et al.: The abnormal Pap smear—what to do next. Cancer *48*:515, 1981.
71. Rotman, M., et al.: Prognostic factors in cervical carcinoma: Implications in staging and management. Cancer *48*:560, 1981.
72. Disaia, A. J.: Surgical aspects of cervical carcinoma. Cancer *48*:548, 1981.
73. Richart, R. M., et al.: An analysis of long-term follow-up results in patients with cervical intraepithelial neoplasia treated by cryotherapy. Am. J. Obstet. Gynecol. *137*:823, 1980.
74. Taylor, H. B., et al.: Atypical endocervical hyperplasia in women taking oral contraceptives. J.A.M.A. *202*:637, 1967.
75. Wilkinson, E., and Dufour, D. R.: Pathogenesis of microglandular hyperplasia. Obstet. Gynecol. *47*:189, 1976.
76. Rotterdam, H.: Chronic endometritis. A clinicopathologic study. Pathol. Annu. *13*(Part 2):209, 1978.
77. Owolabi, T. O., and Stickler, R. C.: Adenomyosis. A neglected diagnosis. Obstet. Gynecol. *50*:424, 1970.
78. Ranney, B.: Endometriosis. Obstet. Gynecol. Annu. *7*:219, 1978.
79. Kistner, R. W.: Infertility with endometriosis. Fertil. Steril. *13*:237, 1962.
80. Askell, S., and Jones, G. S.: Etiology and treatment of dysfunctional uterine bleeding. Obstet. Gynecol. *44*:1, 1970.
81. Jones, G. E.: Luteal phase insufficiency. Clin. Obstet. Gynecol. *16*:255, 1973.
82. Hertig, A. T., and Sommers, S. C.: Genesis of endometrial carcinoma. I. Study of prior biopsies. Cancer *2*:964, 1949.
83. Velios, F.: Endometrial hyperplasias. Precursors of endometrial carcinoma. *In* Sommers, S. C. (ed.): Genital and Mammary Pathology Decennial. New York, Appleton-Century-Crofts, 1975, pp. 55–84.
84. Welch, W. R., and Scully, R. E.: Precancerous lesions of the endometrium. Hum. Pathol. *8*:503, 1977.
85. Gusberg, S. B.: The individual at high risk for endometrial carcinoma. Am. J. Obstet. Gynecol. *126*:535, 1976.
86. Sherman, A. J., and Brown, S.: The precursors of endometrial carcinoma. Am. J. Obstet. Gynecol. *135*:947, 1979.
87. Henderickson, M. R., and Kempson, R. L.: The differential diagnosis of endometrial adenocarcinoma. Some viewpoints concerning a common diagnostic problem. Pathology *12*:35, 1980.
88. Ferenczy, A.: Cytodynamics of endometrial hyperplasia and neoplasia. Part II. *In vitro* DNA histoautoradiography. Hum. Pathol. *14*:77, 1983.
88A. Norris, H. J., et al.: Endometrial hyperplasia and carcinoma: Diagnostic considerations. Am. J. Surg. Pathol. *7*:839, 1983.
89. Kurman, R. J., and Norris, H. J.: Endometrial neoplasia: Hyperplasia and carcinoma. *In* Blaustein, A. (ed.): Pathology of the Female Genital Tract. 2nd ed. New York, Springer-Verlag, 1982, pp. 311–351.
90. Shanklin, D. R.: Endometrial carcinoma. Diagnostic criteria, pathogenesis, natural history and associations. Pathol. Annu. *13*(Part 2):233, 1978.
91. Ober, W. B.: Effects of oral and intrauterine administration of contraceptives on the uterus. Hum. Pathol. *8*:513, 1977.
92. Weiss, N. S., and Sayvetz, T. A.: Incidence of endometrial cancer in relation to the use of oral contraceptives. N. Engl. J. Med. *302*:551, 1980.
93. Hendrickson, M. R., and Kempson, R. L.: Surgical Pathology of the Uterine Corpus. Philadelphia. W. B. Saunders Co., 1980.
94. Merrill, J.: Benign lesions of the corpus uteri. *In* Danforth, D. (ed.): Obstetrics and Gynecology. 4th Ed. Philadelphia, Harper & Row, 1982, p. 1076.
95 Jick, H., et al.: The epidemic of endometrial cancer. Am. J. Public Health *70*:264, 1980.
96. Davies, J. C., et al.: A review of risk factors for endometrial carcinoma. Obstet. Gynecol. Surv. *36*:107, 1981.
97. Henderson, B. E., et al.: The epidemiology of endometrial cancer in young women. Br. J. Cancer *47*:749, 1983.
98. Hammond, C.B., et al.: Effect of long-term estrogen replacement therapy. II. Neoplasia. Am. J. Obstet. Gynecol. *133*:537, 1979.
98A. Antunes, C. M., et al.: Endometrial cancer and estrogen use. N. Engl. J. Med. *300*:9, 1979.
99. Scully, R. E.: Estrogen and endometrial carcinoma. Hum. Pathol. *8*:481, 1977.
100. Siiteri, P. K., and McDonald, P. C.: The role of extraglandular estrogen in human endocrinology. *In* Greep, R. D., and Astwood, A. B. (eds.): Handbook of Physiology. Section VII. Vol. 2. Part I. Washington, D.C., American Physiological Society, 1975, pp. 615–629.
101. Christopherson, W. M., et al.: Carcinoma of the endometrium. I. A clinical and pathological study of clear cell carcinoma and secretory carcinoma. Cancer *49*:1511, 1982.
102. Hendrickson, M., et al.: Uterine papillary serous carcinoma: A highly malignant form of endometrial adenocarcinoma. Am. J. Surg. Pathol. *6*:93, 1982.
103. Glassburn, J. R.: Carcinoma of the endometrium. Cancer *48*:575, 1981.
104. Salazar, H., et al.: Uterine sarcomas. Natural history, treatment and prognosis. Cancer *42*:1152, 1978.
105. Zalondek, C. J., and Norris, H. J.: Sarcomas of the uterus. *In* Fenoglio, C. M., and Wolff, M. (eds.): Progress in Surgical Pathology III. New York, Masson, 1981, pp. 1–35.
106. Bard, D. S., and Zuna, R. E.: Sarcomas and related neoplasms of the uterine corpus. A brief review of the natural history, prognostic factors and management. Obstet. Gynecol. Annu. *10*:237, 1981.
107. Christopherson, W. M., and Richardson, M.: Uterine mesenchymal tumors. Pathol. Annu. *16*:215, 1981.
108. Zalondek, C. J., and Norris, H. J.: Adenofibroma and adenosarcoma. A study of 35 benign and low grade variants of mixed mesodermal tumors. Cancer *48*:354, 1981.
109. Serov, S. F., et al.: International histological classifications of tumors No. 9. Histological Typing of Ovarian Tumors. Geneva, World Health Organization, 1973.
110. Scully, R. E.: Ovarian tumors. A review. Am. J. Pathol. *87*:686, 1977.
111. Fox, H., and Langley, F. A.: Tumors of the Ovary. London, William Heinemann Medical Books, Ltd., 1976.
112. McGowan, L., et al.: The woman at risk for developing ovarian cancer. Gynecol. Oncol. *73*:25, 1979.
113. Cramer, D. W., et al.: Factors affecting the association of oral contraceptives and ovarian cancer. N. Engl. J. Med. *307*:1047, 1982.
114. Blaustein, A.: Surface (germinal) epithelium and related ovarian neoplasms. Pathol. Annu. *16*:247, 1981.
115. Hart, W. R.: Ovarian epithelial tumors of borderline malignancy (carcinomas of low malignant potential). Hum. Pathol. *8*:541, 1977.
116. Katzenstein, A. L.: Proliferative serous tumors of the ovary. Am. J. Surg. Pathol. *2*:339, 1978.
117. Hart, W. R., and Norris, H. J.: Borderline and malignant mucinous tumors of the ovary. Histologic criteria and clinical behavior. Cancer *3*:1031, 1973.
118. Czernobilsky, B., et al.: Endometrioid carcinoma of the ovary. Cancer *26*:1141, 1970.
119. Scully, R. E., et al.: The development of malignancy and endometriosis. Clin. Obstet. Gynecol. *9*:384, 1966.

120. Teilum, G.: Special Tumors of Ovary and Testis and Related Extragonadal Lesions. Philadelphia, J. B. Lippincott Co., 1976.
121. Shevchuk, M. M., et al.: Clear cell carcinoma of the ovary: A clinicopathologic study and review of the literature. Cancer *47*:1344, 1981.
122. Kao, G., and Norris, H. J.: Cystadenofibroma of the ovary with atypia. Am. J. Surg. Pathol. *2*:357, 1978.
123. Shevchuk, M. M., et al.: Histogenesis of Brenner tumors. I. Histology and ultrastructure. II. Histochemistry and CEA. Cancer *46*:2607, 2617, 1980.
124. Balasa, R. W., et al.: The Brenner tumor: A review. Obstet. Gynecol. *50*:120, 1977.
125. Van Nagell, J.R., et al.: Biochemical markers in the plasma and tumors of patients with gynecologic malignancies. Cancer *48*:495, 1981.
126. Kurman, R., and Norris, H. J.: Germ cell tumors of the ovary. Pathol. Annu. *13*:291, 1978.
127. Talerman, A.: Germ cell tumors of the ovary. *In* Blaustein, A. (ed.): Pathology of the Female Genital Tract. New York, Springer-Verlag, 1982, pp. 602–664.
128. Linder, D., et al.: Pathogenetic origin of benign ovarian teratomas. N. Engl. J. Med. *292*:63, 1975.
129. Norris, H. J., et al.: Immature (malignant) teratoma of the ovary. A clinical and pathological study of 58 cases. Cancer *37*:2359, 1976.
130. Robboy, S. J., et al.: Insular carcinoid primary in the ovary. A clinicopathologic study of 48 cases. Cancer *36*:404, 1975.
131. Gordon, T., et al.: Dysgerminoma, a review of 158 cases from the Emil Novak ovarian tumor registry. Obstet. Gynecol. *58*:497, 1981.
132. Kurman, R., and Norris, H.: Endodermal sinus tumor of the ovary: A clinical and pathological analysis of 71 cases. Cancer *38*:2404, 1976.
133. Young, R. H., and Scully, R.: Ovarian sex cord–stromal tumors. Recent progress. Int. J. Gynecol. Pathol. *1*:101, 1982.
134. Mansell, H., and Hertig, A. T.: Granulosa theca cell tumors and endometrial carcinoma: A study of their relationship in a survey of 80 cases. Obstet. Gynecol. *6*:385, 1955.
135. Norris, H. J., and Taylor, H. B.: Prognosis of granulosa–theca cell tumors of the ovary. Cancer *21*:255, 1968.
136. Prat, J., and Scully, R. E.: Cellular fibromas and fibrosarcomas of the ovary. Cancer *47*:2663, 1981.
137. Roth, L. M., et al.: Sertoli-Leydig cell tumors: A clinicopathologic study of 34 cases. Cancer *48*:187, 1981.
138. Scully, R. E.: Gonadoblastoma. Cancer *25*:1314, 1970.
139. Blaustein, A.: Metastatic carcinoma of the ovary. *In* Blaustein, A. (ed.): Pathology of the Female Genital Tract. 2nd ed. New York, Springer-Verlag, pp. 705–716.
140. Ober, W. B.: Experimental toxemia of pregnancy. Review and speculation. Pathol. Annu. *12*:383, 1977.
141. Gant, N. F., et al.: Control of vascular responsiveness during human pregnancy. Kidney Int. *18*:253, 1980.
142. Sheehan, H. L., and Lynch, J. B.: Pathology of Toxemia of Pregnancy. London, Churchill Livingstone, 1973.
143. Benirschke, R., and Driscoll, S.: The Pathology of the Human Placenta. New York, Springer-Verlag, 1967.
144. Fox, H.: Pathology of the Placenta. Philadelphia, W. B. Saunders Co., 1978.
145. Chesley, L. C., et al.: Long term follow up study of eclamptic women: Sixth periodic report. Am. J. Obstet. Gynecol. *124*:446, 1976.
146. Altschuler, G.: Placentitis, with a new light on an old torch. Obstet. Gynecol. Annu. *6*:197, 1977.
147. Russell, P.: Histopathology of placental villitis of unknown etiology. Placenta *1*:227, 1980.
148. Boné, J., and Boné, A.: Chromosomal anomalies in early spontaneous abortion. *In* Gropp, A. (ed.): Current Topics in Pathology 62. Developmental Biology and Pathology. Berlin, Springer-Verlag, 1977.
149. Arnoy, A., et al.: Placental findings in spontaneous abortions and still births. Teratology *24*:243, 1981.
150. Porter, I. H., and Hook, E. G. (eds.): Human Embryonic and Fetal Death. New York, Academic Press, 1980.
151. Rushton, D. I.: Examination of products of conception from previable human pregnancies. J. Clin. Pathol. *34*:819, 1981.
152. Goldstein, D. P., and Berkowitz, R. S.: Gestational Trophoblastic Neoplasms: Clinical Principles of Diagnosis and Management. Vol. 14. Philadelphia, W. B. Saunders Co., 1982.
153. Driscoll, S.G.: Gestational trophoblastic neoplasms: Morphologic considerations. Hum. Pathol. *8*:529, 1977.
154. Hertig, A. T., and Mansell, H.: Tumors of the female sex organs. Part 1; Hydatidiform mole and choriocarcinoma. Washington, D.C., A.F.I.P. Fascicle, 1956.
155. Elston, C. W.: Gestational tumors of trophoblast. *In* Anthony, P. P., and MacSween, R. (eds.): Recent Advances in Histopathology. New York, Churchill Livingstone, 1981, pp. 149–161.
156. Szulman, E., and Surti, U.: Syndromes of a hydatidiform mole. I. Cytogenetic and morphological correlations. Am. J. Obstet. Gynecol. *131*:665, 1978.
157. Wake, N., et al.: Androgenesis as a cause of highly deformed mole. J. Natl. Cancer Inst. *60*:51, 1978.
158. Vassilakos, P., et al.: Hydatidiform mole: Two entities. A morphologic and cytogenetic study with some clinical consideration. Am. J. Obstet. Gynecol. *127*:167, 1977.
159. Deligdisch, L., et al.: Gestational trophoblastic neoplasms: Morphologic correlates of therapeutic response. Am. J. Obstet. Gynecol. *130*:81, 1978.
160. Bigelow, D.: Gestational trophoblastic disease. *In* Blaustein, A.: Pathology of The Female Genital Tract. New York, Springer-Verlag, 1982, pp. 791–803.
161. Goldstein, D., et al.: The current management of molar pregnancy. Curr. Probl. Obstetr. Gynecol. *3*:6, 1979.
162. Kurman, R. J., et al.: Trophoblastic pseudotumor of the uterus. An exaggerated form of "syncytial endometritis" simulating a malignant tumor. Cancer *38*:1214, 1976.
163. Scully, R. E., and Young, R. H.: Trophoblastic pseudotumor—a reappraisal: Editorial comment. Am. J. Surg. Pathol. *5*:75, 1981.

THE BREAST 25

NORMAL

EMBRYOLOGY. The breast is a modified skin sweat gland that develops into a complex functional structure in the female, but remains as a rudimentary organ in the male. It arises from an epidermal thickening on the ventral surface of the body at approximately the sixth week of fetal development. Bilateral ridges (the milk line) develop between the upper and lower limb buds. These ridges totally atrophy except for several persistent thickenings, which later give rise to the nipples. During the second trimester of fetal life, cords of cells grow downward from the basal layer of the epidermis and later give rise to the primary mammary ducts. At first solid, the cords eventually develop lumina so that, at the time of birth, rudimentary branching ducts are present, which fan out in a small area about the region of the nipple and the areola. Development of the breast is by no means complete at the time of birth. Progressive growth and branching of the mammary ducts occur at a very slow pace during prepubertal life. Mammary development ceases at about this stage in the male. In the female, before the onset of menstruation, the growth rate increases with branching of ducts and proliferation of the interductal stroma. During adolescence, stromal growth is responsible for most of the increases in the mass of the breast, but at the same time the terminal small ducts give rise to many small, blind, saccular outpouchings—rudimentary gland buds. Under the influence of the ovarian hormones and the hormones of pregnancy, further changes occur, to be described.

ANATOMY AND HISTOLOGY. Only a few features of the gross anatomy, of special interest to pathology, bear repetition at this time. It is common to consider each breast as a large, single, secretory gland, but in reality each is composed of five to nine separate branching glands, each of which is totally autonomous and has no anastomotic communications with its neighbors. These individual glands are wedge-shaped segments. Each drains through a separate main excretory or *lactiferous duct* into the nipple. The orifices of these mammary ducts are readily identified about the outer margin of the nipple. There are up to 20 such orifices in each nipple but many are pits ending blindly. The resting mammary gland consists of about 20 lobes, each of which is subdivided into *lobules*, the functional units of the mammary parenchyma.

Commonly a long, tonguelike process of breast tissue, the *axillary appendage*, extends from the main mass up into the anterior axillary line toward and even into the axilla. This minor deviation is sometimes of considerable significance, since it may give rise to tumors or to other abnormalities that are mistaken for involvements of the axillary lymph nodes. The various parts of the microanatomy of the breast and the diseases that affect each are shown in Figure 25–1.

The histology of the female breast is constantly changing under the influence of the ovarian hormones and is markedly modified by the hormones of pregnancy. At the time of puberty, the breast consists only of a complex system of branching ducts that drain into the nipple; each duct terminates at the other end in a number of small saccular gland buds that compose an individual duct lobule. These terminal buddings are enclosed in a loose, delicate, myxomatous stroma that contains a scattering of lymphocytes (*intralobular or intrinsic connective tissue*), and the individual lobules are enclosed within a more dense, collagenous, fibrous, *interlobular or extrinsic stroma*.

Just as the endometrium rises and ebbs with each menstrual cycle, so does the breast. Following the menstrual period, with the progressive rise in estrogen, the ductal epithelium and the epithelium of the gland buds proliferate and continue to develop throughout the menstrual cycle. ^{3}H thymidine labeling studies confirm that proliferative activity is related to estrogen levels.[1] During this time, the ducts and gland buds become slightly dilated and hypertrophied. During the last half of the menstrual cycle, under the influence of progesterone, stromal growth and edema begin. This combined stimulatory effect of estrogen and progesterone on the intralobular breast elements accounts for the sense of fullness commonly experienced by women during the premenstrual phase of the cycle. At this same time in the cycle, abortive secretory activity appears in the gland buds and further accentuates the ductal dilatation. At the time of the menstrual period, the fall in estrogen and progesterone levels is followed by desquamation of epithelial cells, atrophy of the intralobular connective tissue, disappearance of the increased interstitial edema fluid, and overall shrinkage in the size of the ducts and gland buds.

Understanding these cyclic changes, we can now present the basic histology of the breast. The stratified squamous epithelium that covers the areola and nipple

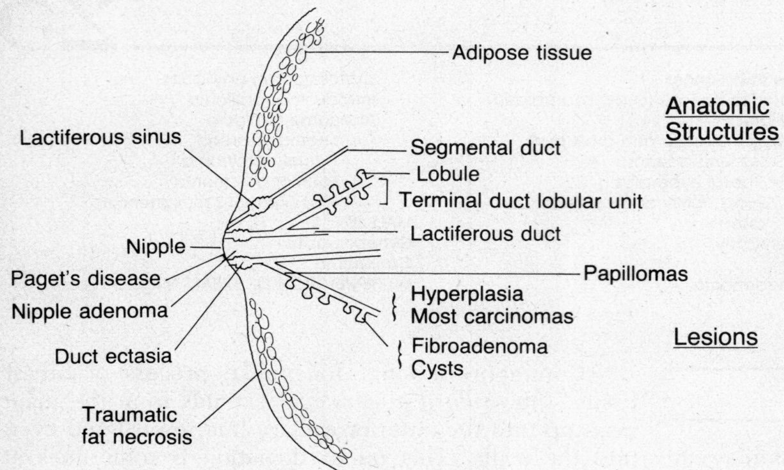

Figure 25–1. Diagram of main anatomic structures *(top)* and major lesions affecting different structures. (Modified from Azzopardi, J. G.: Problems in Breast Pathology. London, W. B. Saunders Co., 1979, pp. 9–10.)

extends only superficially into the mouths of the main lactiferous ducts. It soon becomes transformed into a pseudostratified columnar and then double-layered cuboidal epithelium that lines the major breast ducts. As the ducts branch and become smaller, the epithelium tends to become a single layer of cells but, in the smaller ducts and sometimes even in the gland buds, a low flattened layer of cells (myoepithelial cells) can be identified beneath the more prominent lining epithelium. Myoepithelial cells contain myofilaments oriented parallel to the long axis of the duct. A basement membrane follows faithfully the contour of ducts and ductules.[2] The intralobular and periductal connective tissue has a loose, myxomatous appearance, and therefore is readily distinguished from the surrounding interlobular denser stroma. During the late phases of each menstrual cycle, considerable numbers of lymphocytes accumulate in the periductal tissue.

It is only with the onset of pregnancy that the breast assumes its complete morphologic maturation and functional activity. From each gland bud, numerous true secretory glands pouch out to form grapelike clusters. As a consequence, there is a reversal of the usual stromal-glandular relationship so that, by the end of pregnancy, the breast is composed almost entirely of glands separated by a relatively scant amount of stroma. The secretory glands are lined by a single layer of cuboidal cells, which, in the third trimester, begin to assume secretory activity. Vacuoles of lipid material are found within the cells, and immediately following birth the secretion of milk begins. The lipid material formed before birth accounts for the secretion of colostrum.

Following lactation, the glands once again regress and atrophy, the ducts shrink, and the total breast size diminishes remarkably. However, complete regression to the stage of the normal virginal breast usually does not occur, and some increase of glandular parenchyma remains as a permanent residual.

With the menopause, the ducts and gland buds further atrophy with more shrinkage of the intra- and interlobular stroma. The gland buds may almost totally disappear in the very aged, leaving only ducts to create a morphologic pattern that comes close to that of the male. However, in most women there is sufficient persistent estrogenic stimulation, possibly of adrenal origin, to maintain the vestigial remnants of gland buds that differentiate even the very aged female breast from the male breast.

Before closing the consideration of the normal breast, mention should be made of the influence of maternal hormones on the neonatal breast. These may cause considerable proliferation of the ductal epithelium and periductal connective tissue in the newborn. Accordingly, it is not uncommon to find hypertrophy and swelling of the breasts in the postnatal infant. Sometimes the maternal hormones of pregnancy cause abortive secretory activity with the actual appearance of secretion at the nipple. These changes are entirely normal and should not be confused with inflammation or tumor formation.

PATHOLOGY

Female Breast

Lesions of the breast are preponderantly confined to the female. In the male, the breast is a rudimentary structure relatively insensitive to endocrine influences and apparently resistive to neoplastic growth. In the female, on the other hand, the more complex breast structure, the greater breast volume, and the extreme sensitivity to endocrine influences all predispose this organ to a number of pathologic conditions.

The breast is the most common site of development of cancer in the female and alone accounts for about one-fifth of all malignancies in this sex. Notwithstanding this high incidence, benign tumors and tumor-like conditions are more frequent than these malignant neoplasms.

It is obvious, then, that diseases of the female

breast have great importance in clinical medicine. Therefore, the major portion of this chapter is devoted to exclusive consideration of the female breast. The two disorders of the female breast that assume preponderant importance are fibrocystic disease and carcinomas. Since both these entities give rise to masses or lumps in the breast, the entire consideration of the pathology of this organ should be oriented within the framework of: What lesions produce masses? May it be confused clinically with a carcinoma? Does the lesion have a tendency to become malignant?

CONGENITAL ANOMALIES

These anomalies run the gamut from congenital absence to abnormal numbers of breasts, but as a group these entities are of limited clinical significance.

Supernumerary Nipples or Breasts. These result from the persistence of epidermal thickenings along the line of the ventral ridges, referred to in the embryogenesis of this organ as the milk line. Development of these aberrant foci gives rise to the formation of nipples, or even rudimentary breast structures, along the milk line, both below the adult breast and above it in the anterior axillary fold. Rarely, the disorders that affect the normally situated breast may arise in these heterotopic foci, and occasionally the cyclic changes of the menstrual cycle cause painful premenstrual enlargements of these supernumerary structures.

Accessory Breast Tissue. Extension of breast tissue into the anterior axillary fold or axilla has already been described as being so common that it hardly merits designation as an anomaly. However, these minor aberrations may be the site for the development of tumors or abnormal proliferative or cystic changes. The chief importance of such lesions lies in the fact that they may create masses that appear to be outside the breast, and therefore are commonly misidentified as lesions of the axillary lymph nodes or even as metastases from an occult breast cancer.

Congenital Inversion of Nipples. This occurs in many women, particularly those who have large or pendulous breasts. Commonly, this inversion is corrected during the growth activity of pregnancy, or it may sometimes be corrected by simple traction upon the nipples. Nipple inversion is of clinical significance, since it may frustrate attempts at nursing and may also be confused with acquired retraction of the nipple, sometimes observed in mammary cancer and in inflammations of the breasts.

INFLAMMATIONS

Inflammations of the breast are, on the whole, uncommon and consist of only a relatively few forms of acute and chronic disease. Of these, the most important is nonspecific acute mastitis, virtually confined to the lactating period. Breast abscesses are included under the heading of acute mastitis. The other forms of mastitis consist of posttraumatic lesions and plasma cell mastitis or mammary duct ectasia (an entity of obscure etiology).

ACUTE MASTITIS AND BREAST ABSCESS

During the early weeks of nursing, the breast is rendered vulnerable to bacterial infection by the development of cracks and fissures in the nipples. The disease is not confined to the postpartum state, however, and may be predisposed to by eczema and other dermatologic conditions of the nipples. From this portal of entry, *Staphylococcus aureus* usually, or streptococci less commonly, invade the breast substance.

Usually the disease is unilateral. The staphylococcus tends to produce a localized area of inflammation that may progress to the formation of single or multiple abscesses. The streptococcus tends to cause, as it does in all tissues, a diffuse spreading infection that eventually involves the entire organ. Both agents produce characteristic reddening, swelling, pain, and increased consistency in the affected breast substance, commonly with considerable edema and thickening of the overlying skin. During this early stage, the inflammatory changes may consist largely of the collection of pus within the affected ducts accompanied by periductal neutrophilic infiltration with involvement of the gland buds and surrounding stroma. However, in the course of time, the suppurative necrosis may destroy large, but usually only focal, areas of the breast substance. Surgical drainage and antibiotic therapy may limit the spread of the infection, but when extensive necrosis occurs, the destroyed breast substance is replaced by fibrous scar as a permanent residual of the inflammatory process. Such scarring may create a localized area of increased consistency sometimes accompanied by retraction of the skin or the nipple, changes that may later be mistaken for a neoplasm. The skin and nipple retraction usually regresses in time as the fibrous scar stretches.

MAMMARY DUCT ECTASIA (PLASMA CELL MASTITIS; PERIDUCTAL MASTITIS)

This condition is characterized chiefly by dilatation of ducts, inspissation of breast secretions, and marked periductal and interstitial chronic granulomatous inflammatory reaction, sometimes associated with large numbers of plasma cells. This disorder tends to occur in the fifth decade of life and is much more common in women who have borne children. Its genesis is obscure, but it is thought that it may possibly be due to inspissation of lipid debris and weakening and rupture of ducts. Supporting this theory, about half of the patients have inverted or cracked nipples or difficulties in nursing their young.

Anatomically, the condition usually affects a single area of breast substance drained through one of the major excretory ducts. A poorly defined area of induration, thickening, or ropiness results. Rarely, however, the entire breast is affected when all the ducts are involved, or the disease may even be bilateral. Dilated, firm, ropy ducts are frequently palpable through the skin and become more readily apparent on section. Thick, cheesy material can be extruded from these cut ducts by slight pressure.

On histologic examination, the characteristically dilated ducts are filled by granular, necrotic, acidophilic debris (secretion), which sometimes contains mixed white cells, principally lipid-laden macrophages (Fig. 25–2). The lining epithelial cells of the ducts may persist in small foci, but for the most part are necrotic and atrophic. The periductal and interductal inflammation in the full-blown disease, caused by inflammatory erosion of the duct walls, is manifested by heavy infiltrates of inflammatory cells, i.e., neutrophils, lymphocytes, and histiocytes, with a striking predominance of plasma cells. Occasionally, foci of inflammation about lipid debris create small, granulomatous, inflammatory reactions, composed of central masses of foamy macrophages and precipitated spicules of cholesterol and fatty acids, surrounded by a fibroblastic proliferation and scattered foreign body giant cells. The axillary lymph nodes that drain the focus may also be the site of chronic lymphadenitis and secondary enlargement.

The dilated ducts should not be confused with cysts of fibrocystic disease. The latter form in lobules, not ducts, and thus have no elastic tissue in their walls as do the dilated ducts in plasma cell mastitis.[5]

This lesion is of clinical significance because it produces a focal or ill-defined diffuse area of pain, tenderness, induration, and ropiness in the peri- or subareolar region. Fixation to the skin, with retraction of the skin or nipple, or the presence of nipple discharge may easily cause the lesion to be mistaken for a neoplasm. The concurrence of axillary node enlargement further heightens the similarity by raising the possibility of metastatic spread.

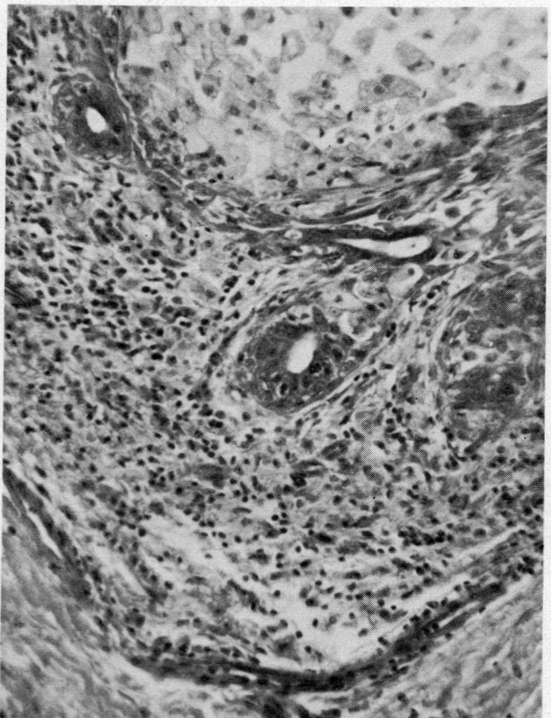

Figure 25–2. Plasma cell mastitis. Duct at top is partially filled with lipid-laden macrophages. Ductal epithelium is destroyed, and periductal tissues are infiltrated with leukocytes, mostly plasma cells.

TRAUMATIC FAT NECROSIS

Focal necrosis of fat tissues in the breast, followed by an inflammatory reaction, is an uncommon lesion that tends to occur as an isolated, sharply localized process in one breast. The subsequent inflammatory scarring may give rise to a focus of increased consistency that is potentially capable of confusion with a new growth, hence the clinical importance of this otherwise innocuous condition. If strict criteria are used to differentiate this entity from mammary duct ectasia, almost all patients give a history of an easily remembered trauma.[5]

The morphologic changes depend on the duration of the lesion and the stage of the inflammatory reaction. In the early stages, the focus may consist of hemorrhage and, later, central liquefactive necrosis of fat surrounded by a zone of increased consistency. Still later, it may be a more or less well-defined nodule of gray-white, increased consistency, containing small foci of chalky white or hemorrhagic debris. In the course of time, the area is converted to a dense fibrous scar, or the central focus of necrosis may become encysted, pigmented, and sometimes calcified. Usually such focal areas are extremely small and are rarely over 2 cm in diameter.[6]

Histologically, the central focus of necrotic fat cells is surrounded by lipid-filled macrophages and an intense neutrophilic infiltration. Then, over the next few days, progressive fibroblastic proliferation, increased vascularization, and lymphocytic and histiocytic infiltration wall off the focus. By this time, the central necrotic fat cells have disappeared and may be represented only by foamy, lipid-laden macrophages and spicules of crystalline lipids (Fig. 25–3). Still later, foreign body giant cells, calcium salts, and blood pigments make their appearance, and eventually the focus is replaced by scar tissue or is encysted and walled off by collagenous tissue.

This condition is without clinical significance save for its possible confusion with a tumor, when fibrosis has created a clinically palpable mass. The tendency for the focus of fibrosis to be attached to the skin, sometimes causing dimpling or retraction, and the focal calcifications seen on mammography further heighten the resemblance to cancer.

GALACTOCELE

A galactocele represents a cystic dilatation of a duct occurring during lactation. It implies some cause for ductal obstruction, such as inflammation, fibrocystic disease, or neoplasia. Occasionally, a single duct is

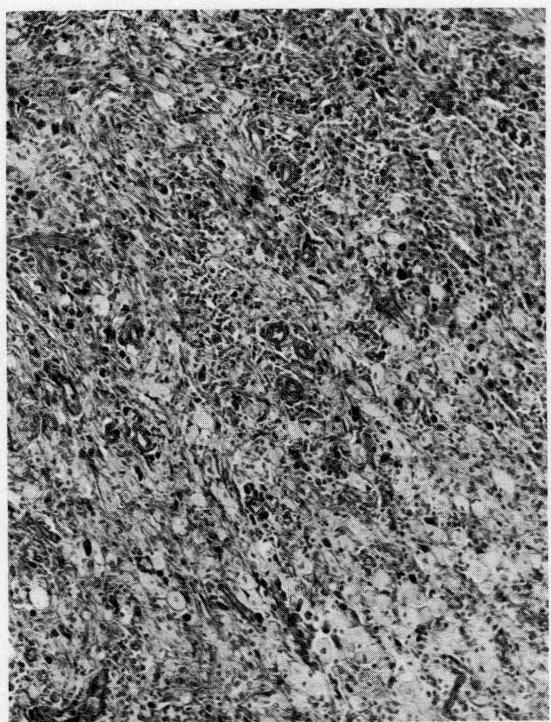

Figure 25–3. Fat necrosis. Lesion is well advanced and now represents a focus of lipophages interspersed with fibroblasts and leukocytes.

affected to produce an isolated cyst, but more often multiple ducts are involved. During the acute phase, the palpable nodules are tender and, when exposed, contain a milky fluid enclosed within thin, dilated ductal walls. In the course of time, the tenderness abates and the cystic dilatations become more firm. At this time, transection may disclose an inspissated cheesy content. Secondary infection may convert these areas to foci of acute mastitis or abscess formation. Occasionally, even in the absence of bacterial contamination, rupture of ducts produces changes similar to those described in mammary duct ectasia.

GRANULOMAS CAUSED BY COSMETIC MAMMARY INJECTIONS

These are uncommon complications of intramammary injection of paraffin or silicone performed for cosmetic reasons.[7] Clinically they present as firm, tender, multiple nodules, and histologically they consist of foreign body granulomatous inflammation surrounding spaces that contain the colorless foreign material.

ENDOCRINE IMBALANCES

FIBROCYSTIC DISEASE (CYSTIC HYPERPLASIA)

This most common involvement of the female breast is included under the heading of endocrine imbalance because it is now almost universally accepted that it results from *an exaggeration and distortion of the cyclic breast changes that normally occur in the menstrual cycle*. The terminology of this condition is unfortunately one of its most confusing aspects, and a complete citation of all the terms that have been used in the past would be nonproductive. Chronic cystic mastitis, mammary dysplasia, mazoplasia, and cystic mastopathy are no longer popular. Cystic hyperplasia is an appropriate term since it at least denotes two of the principal characteristics of this condition. The term fibrocystic disease is currently in vogue as satisfactorily descriptive.

Fibrocystic disease encompasses a wide variety of morphologic changes and resultant clinical manifestations. These run the gamut from lesions that consist principally of an overgrowth of the fibrous stroma to lesions in which both stromal and epithelial proliferation participate, to other types in which epithelial proliferation predominates.[5, 8, 9] It is a notoriously pleomorphic disorder in which variable morphologic patterns are encountered in different patients, in different areas of the same lesion, or even in different microscopic fields of one slide. Despite this marked variability, it is possible to distinguish four dominant patterns of morphologic change: (1) *fibrosis*, (2) *cyst formation*, (3) *sclerosing adenosis*, and (4) *duct epithelial hyperplasia*. The last two are sometimes lumped together under the term "epithelial hyperplasia," but are distinct histologic patterns with different connotations: sclerosing adenosis is characterized by intralobular fibrosis and lobular epithelial proliferation, and has *no* premalignant connotation, whereas duct epithelial hyperplasia is the histologic variant of fibrocystic disease, which *may* predispose to carcinoma.[10–13] Since some of these patterns conform fairly well to specific age distributions, have somewhat distinctive clinical manifestations, and are of differing significance with respect to malignant transformation, they will be presented separately. It should be emphasized, however, that there is much overlap and considerable concurrence in these patterns. It is difficult, therefore, to categorize every case.

INCIDENCE. Together these variants compose the single most common disorder of the breast and account for over one-half of all surgical operations on the female breast. It is difficult to express an incidence of this condition in the general adult female population because of the variable criteria used for its diagnosis and because of the selective nature of the material studied.[14] Indeed, irregular lumps in the breast as well as the histologic spectrum of fibrocystic disease are such common manifestations that some have questioned the usefulness of the term.[15] In a study of the so-called "normal breast," i.e., unselected postmortem cases, significant disease was found in 29% by Frantz et al.[16] Minimal disease was found in an additional 24%. These cases, however, were weighted with older age groups and therefore do not represent a true sample of the general population. It is clear, however, that fibrocystic disease is a commonplace clinical problem. Haagensen estimates that at least 10% of women develop clinically apparent cystic disease.[17] The condition is unusual before adolescence and rarely, if ever, develops after the menopause. However, premenopausal lesions may persist into more advanced life.

PATHOGENESIS. Hormonal imbalances, particularly hyperestrinism, are considered to be basic to the development of this multipatterned disorder.[18] The excess of estrogens may represent an absolute increase, as in the rarely associated functioning ovarian tumors, or may be related to a deficiency of progesterone, as seen in anovulatory women. Experimentally, estrogen injections induce mammary cysts and hyperplastic lesions, particularly in mice.[19] There is also some evidence of abnormal end-organ metabolism of hormones in the pathogenesis of cystic disease.[20] Oral contraceptive use decreases the risk of fibrocystic disease,[21] presumably because it supplies a balanced source of progesterone and estrogen.

Fibrosis

In its pure form, this relatively infrequent variant is characterized principally *by stromal fibrous tissue overgrowth unaccompanied by prominent epithelial hyperplasia.*[13, 17, 22] It is not usually associated with the formation of grossly demonstrable cysts. This pattern tends to occur in women from 35 to 49 years of age and is more usually unilateral, but may affect both breasts. It should be noted that some fibrosis is also a component of all variants of fibrocystic disease, and here we are describing the isolated fibrous lesion only.

Classically, the upper outer quadrant is most often involved and the increase in fibrous tissue results in a poorly defined area of rubbery consistency. On section, the affected area has a dense, rubbery consistency that yields readily to pressure, but resists cutting.

In milder cases, the increase in stromal connective tissue may be so minimal as to appear inadequate as an explanation for the formation of a clinical mass. However, in the more classic examples, the overgrowth of collagenous stroma engulfs the epithelial structures and obliterates the loose periductal and lobular myxomatous stroma. Sometimes it compresses the ducts and buds to the point at which they become markedly flattened or even atrophic (Fig. 25–4). Occasionally, small cysts are also present. However, in the better defined examples, the lesion is principally one of fibrosis, and epithelial changes are insignificant.

The lesion is usually palpable as a reasonably well-delimited, but not sharply circumscribed, area of induration. Sometimes the focus has a sufficiently sharp lateral margin to be described as "saucer-like." It is frequently painful and tender to palpation, particularly in the days preceding menstruation. In the classic case, the tenderness may regress following the menstrual period, with recurrence of pain and tenderness at the next cycle. The significance of this variant and its management will be considered later, along with the other patterns. There is no evidence that it predisposes to carcinoma.

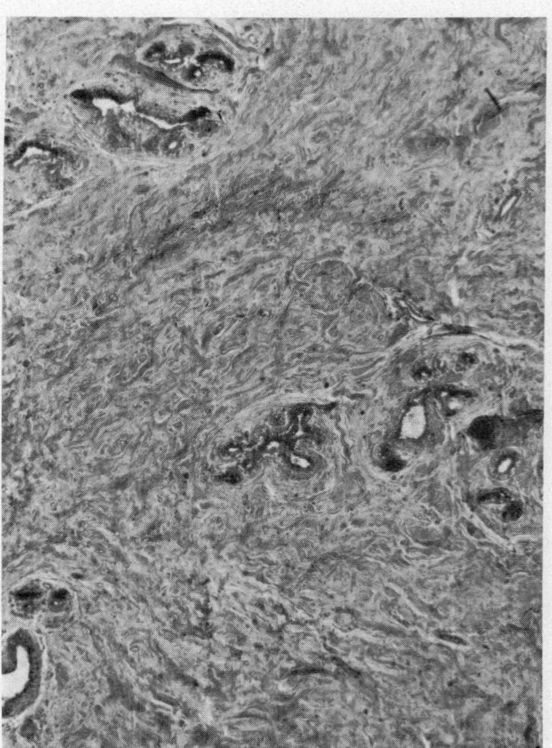

Figure 25–4. Fibrosis of breast. The entire interductal breast substance is replaced by hyaline connective tissue. Ducts and glands are compressed and atrophic.

Cystic Disease and Gross Cysts

This variant, also designated as *Bloodgood's disease, Schimmelbusch's disease,* and *blue dome cyst,* is the form of fibrocystic disease characterized by the *formation of cysts, sometimes accompanied by stromal and epithelial hyperplasia.* Haagensen pleads for differentiating *gross cysts,* over 3 mm in diameter, from *microcysts.*[13, 17] He points out that microcysts are found so commonly in all women in the middle years of life that they cannot be construed as disease nor as justification for surgery. Gross cystic disease usually occurs in women near or at the age of menopause, i.e., between the ages of 45 and 55. Gross cysts occur in about 7% of women.

Rarely, an isolated cyst may be formed within one breast, but the disorder is usually multifocal and often bilateral (Fig. 25–5). As a result of the stromal overgrowth and cystic dilatation of the ducts, the involved areas have an ill-defined diffuse increase in consistency and discrete nodularities. Closely aggregated, small cysts produce a shotty texture. Larger, particularly solitary, cysts evoke the greatest alarm as isolated firm masses that are deceptively unyielding. Occasionally, multiple cysts aggregate to produce a large, irregular, multilobular mass. On section, the cysts vary up to 4 or 5 cm in diameter (some are larger). Unopened, these cysts are brown to blue owing to the contained semitranslucent, turbid fluid (Fig. 25–6). Usually the cysts are filled with serous, turbid fluid that flows out readily to disclose a smooth, glistening, membranous lining devoid of areas of thickening or papillary projection. However, intracystic hemorrhage, inspissation of secretions, or

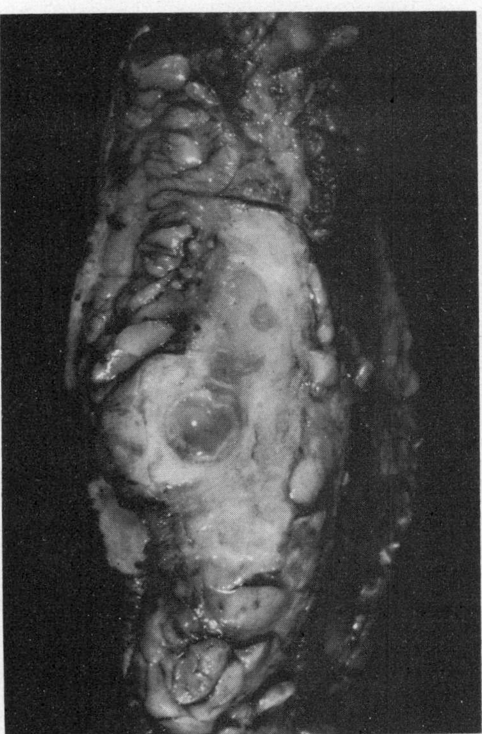

Figure 25–5. Cystic disease of breast. Cross section reveals one large *(center)* and several smaller cysts.

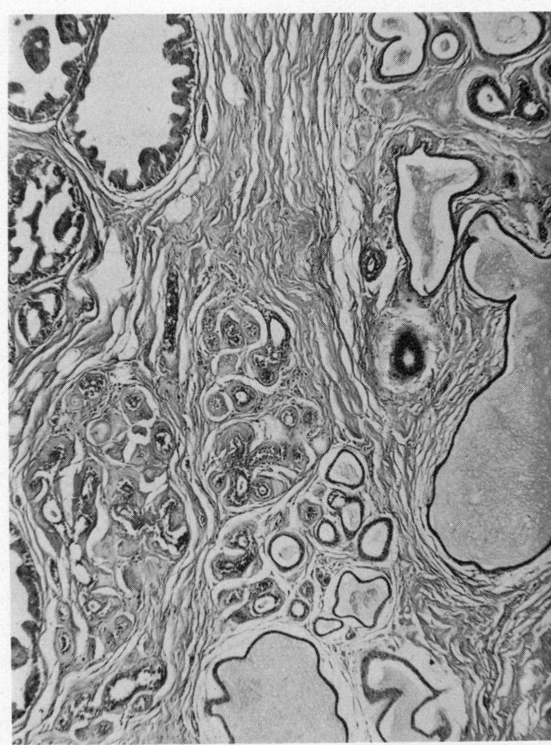

Figure 25–7. Cystic disease of breast. Multiple cystic spaces, some filled with precipitated fluid. Others have a somewhat high epithelium, thrown up into papillary projections.

inflammation may modify the contents. Sometimes the cystic walls are thickened or calcified by complicating hemorrhages and infections.

The histologic hallmark of this variant is formation of cysts. In smaller cysts, the epithelium is more cuboidal to columnar and is sometimes multilayered in focal areas (Figs. 25–7 and 25–8). In larger cysts, the lining epithelium may be flattened or may even be totally atrophic, so that the surface is composed only of compressed collagenous fibrous tissue (Fig. 25–9). Occasionally, epithelial proliferation leads to piled-up masses or small papillary excrescences. In most instances, a clearly defined, intact basal membrane is present, and only rarely are epithelial extensions found outside

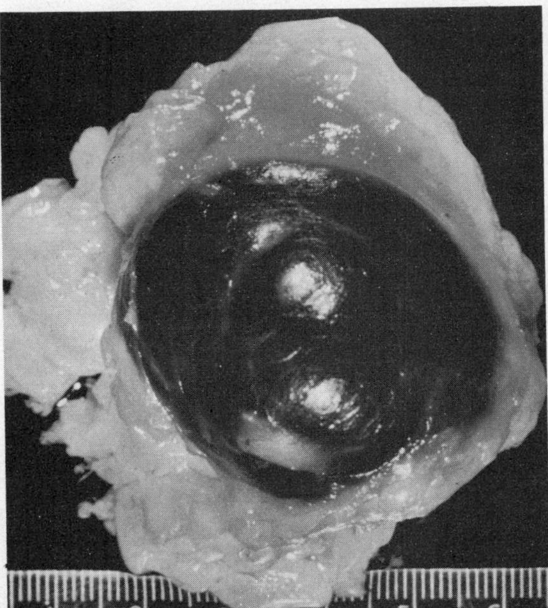

Figure 25–6. Cystic disease of breast. A characteristic excised, unopened, blue dome cyst.

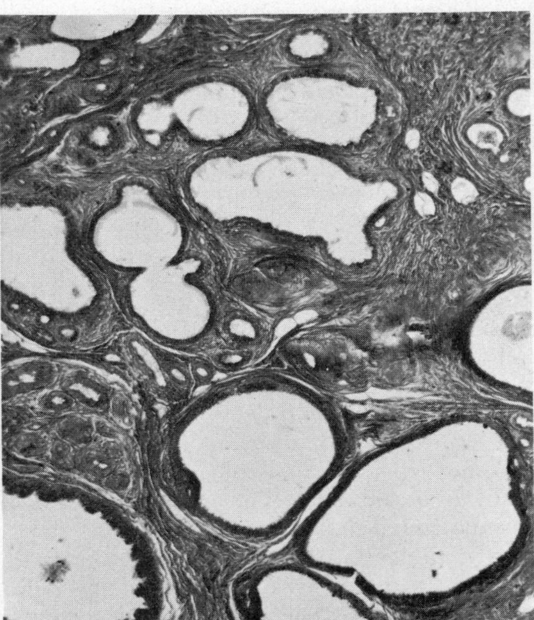

Figure 25–8. Cystic disease of breast. The smaller cysts have preserved cuboidal-to-columnar cell lining epithelium.

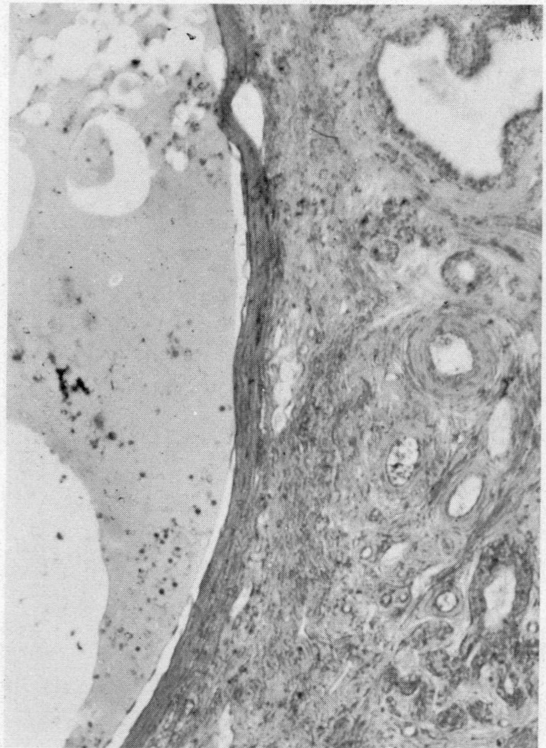

Figure 25–9. Cystic disease of breast. Detail of wall of a large cystic space lined by compressed collagenous connective tissue.

the basement membrane, changes interpreted as "spillage" of the epithelium rather than true invasion. Occasionally, cysts are lined by large polygonal cells having an abundant granular, eosinophilic cytoplasm, with small, round, deeply chromatic nuclei, so-called **apocrine metaplasia**; such apocrine epithelium is found not uncommonly in the normal breast, and is presumed to represent a specialized differentiation of breast parenchyma along the line of sebaceous gland cells. Epithelial overgrowth and papillary projections are common in cysts lined by apocrine epithelium (Fig. 25–10). **Apocrine metaplasia is virtually always benign.**

The stroma about all forms of cysts is usually compressed fibrous tissue, having lost its normal, delicate, myxomatous appearance. Stromal lymphocytic infiltrate is common in this and all other variants of fibrocystic disease, explaining the origin of the older term "chronic cystic mastitis."

The clinical characteristics of this variant of fibrocystic disease have been presented in the morphologic description. When cysts are macroscopic in size, *they are readily palpable as discrete nodules, and since they usually occur multiply and are commonly bilateral, the existence of this diffuse, irregular nodularity is readily distinguished from the characteristic discrete, solitary focus of carcinoma.* However, solitary cysts may be difficult to distinguish from a cancer on gross palpation. Commonly, the cysts produce pain, are tender to palpation, and are more distressing during the period of premenstrual tension. Haagensen holds that gross cystic disease predisposes to carcinoma, with a risk two to three times greater than that for the normal breast.[13]

Sclerosing Adenosis

This variant is characterized histologically by *intralobular fibrosis and proliferation of small ductules or acini.* The lesion may be accompanied by fibrosis and cystic disease, and is most commonly found in women between the ages of 35 and 45. Adenosis is more apt to be unilateral than is cystic disease, and is often focal, affecting the upper outer quadrant of the breast. However, other localizations and bilateral involvement are by no means uncommon.

Depending on the extensiveness of the morphologic changes, the area may have a **hard cartilaginous consistency that begins to approximate that found in breast cancer, or may be only an ill-defined area of firmness.** Cystic nodules are more commonly present in this variant than in the pattern described as fibrosis. On section, the involved area is not well localized, is gray-pink and firm, and on close inspection has small, elevated, pink-gray foci that can be identified later as glandular epithelial structures. Characteristically, however, the chalky yellow-white foci and streaks of necrosis that identify breast carcinoma are absent, an important gross differential feature.

Proliferation of small ducts, canaliculi, and gland buds may yield masses of small gland patterns, or nests and cords of cells within a fibrous stroma. Usually, in such an area, many or at least some well-defined glands can be identified, but frequently they are closely aggregated so that glands lined by single or multiple layers of cells are backed up to each other (**adenosis**). At other times, the stromal overgrowth distorts and compresses the glands;

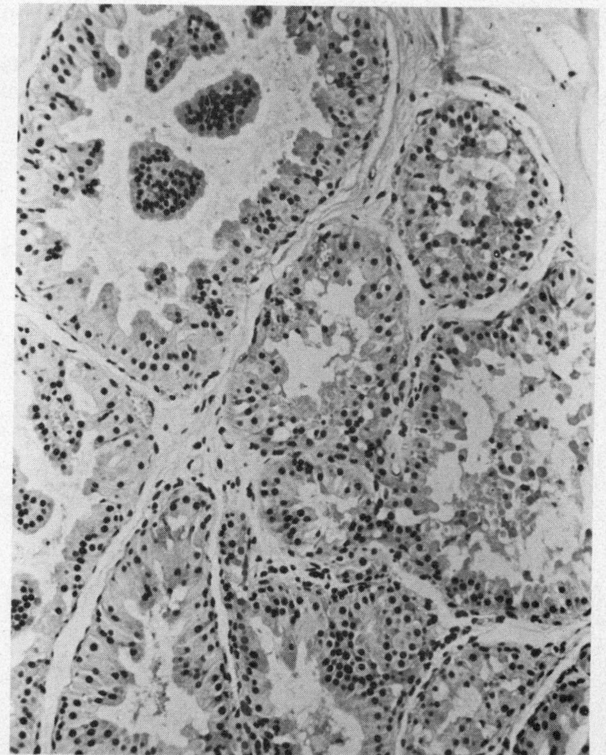

Figure 25–10. Apocrine metaplasia. Lining epithelium is high columnar and faintly staining (eosinophilic with H and E stain).

however, usually the cell aggregates preserve some vestige of a central lumen and some resemblance, therefore, to normal gland patterns. Occasionally, however, the fibrous growth may totally compress the lumina to create the appearance of solid cords or strands of cells lying within the dense stroma, a histologic pattern that at times verges on the appearance of carcinoma.

To the inexperienced, the histologic differentiation of a florid case of sclerosing adenosis from frank cancer is difficult (Figs. 25–11 and 25–12). When clearly defined cysts and apocrine elements are present, or when the epithelial structures preserve their glandular regularity, the distinction is made more readily.

Just as the morphologic differentiation of adenosis from cancer may be difficult, the clinical distinction is equally vague. This lesion characteristically produces a hard localized mass on palpation, reasonably well delimited, but not sharply defined from the surrounding breast substance. It has, therefore, many of the clinical characteristics of malignancy. When the disorder is bilateral, or when cysts are present, the clinical diagnosis is more apparent, but unfortunately such accompanying changes are not invariably present. The pain and tenderness of florid adenosis may also serve to differentiate this lesion from neoplasia. Despite its ominous histologic appearance, sclerosing adenosis does not appear to predispose to carcinoma.[13]

Epithelial Hyperplasia

True epithelial hyperplasia most commonly affects the ducts and ductules, and, as mentioned earlier, *is the histologic variant of fibrocystic disease that is considered by most investigators to increase the risk of the subsequent development of carcinoma.*[3, 5, 10–3, 19, 23] This is not to say that all foci of epithelial hyperplasia (termed *epitheliosis* by British pathologists) are premalignant, leading inevitably to carcinoma; indeed, only a small proportion apparently do. But it is this pattern of alteration that should concern the pathologist, who is called to differentiate among benign hyperplasia, atypical but still noncancerous hyperplasia, and carcinoma. The more severe and atypical the hyperplasia, the greater the risk of developing cancer.[11] These hyperplasias may sometimes coexist with other histologic variants of fibrocystic disease but on occasion they form the predominant pattern. They appear as ill-defined masses in the breasts of women of all ages over 30, but most commonly in those between 35 and 45.

The gross appearance is variable and may be overshadowed by the accompanying fibrosis, cysts, or adenosis. However, many times the ducts have an increased ropy consistency and on pressure exude a pulpy white debris. Microscopically, proliferation causes multilayering of the duct lining epithelium. Sometimes the proliferating epithelium

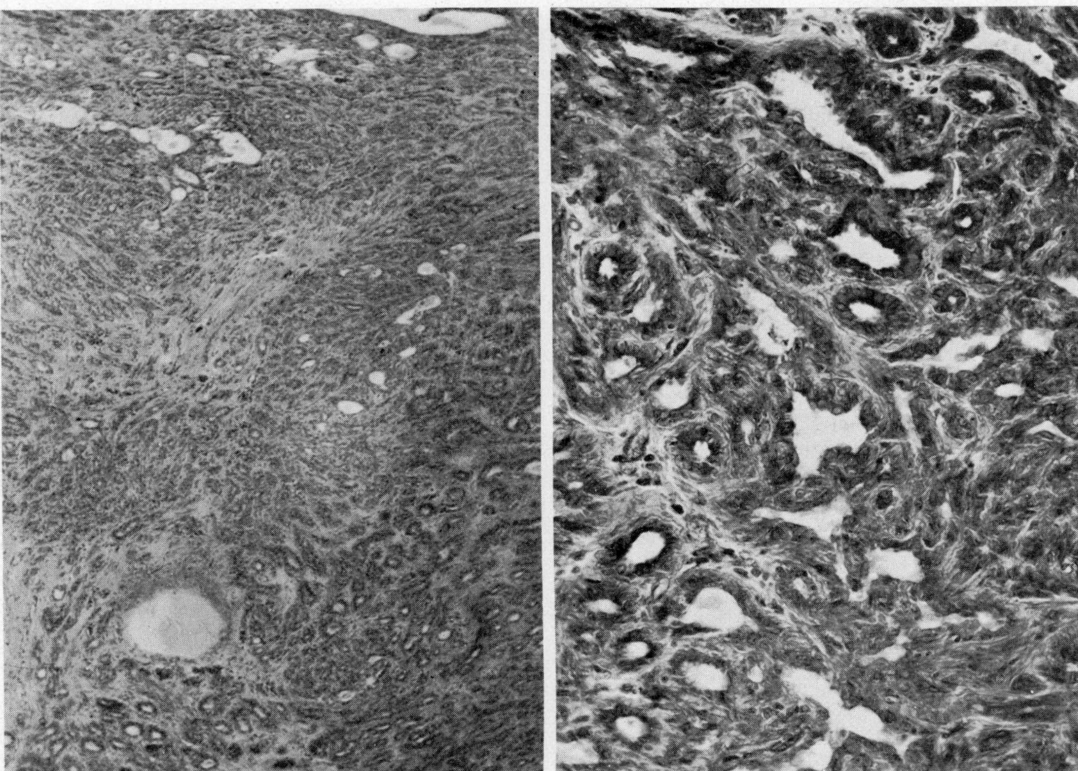

Fig. 25–11 Fig. 25–12

Figure 25–11. Adenosis. Low-power view of a florid case of benign epithelial proliferation, readily mistaken on casual inspection for carcinoma.

Figure 25–12. Adenosis. High-power view of same lesion as in Figure 25–11. Epithelial overgrowth forms many gland patterns that are lined by somewhat distorted but not anaplastic cells.

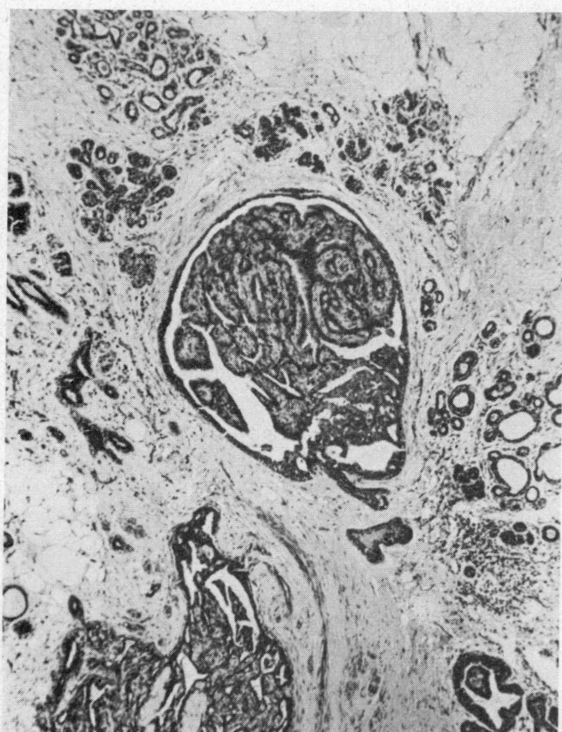

Figure 25–13. Papillary epithelial hyperplasia in fibrocystic disease. Two ducts show hyperplastic epithelium thrown into papillary projections. Note also fibrosis and small cysts.

takes the form of solid masses extending and encroaching into the duct lumen, partially obliterating it, but usually small gland patterns can be discerned within the cellular masses (**cribriform pattern**). Alternatively, papillary epithelial projections may grow into the lumen (**ductal papillomatosis**) (Fig. 25–13). If extensive, this is termed **florid papillomatosis.** Both papillary and solid proliferations may sometimes show various degrees of cellular atypia as well as numerous mitotic figures (**atypical hyperplasia**). The differentiation from intraductal carcinoma (p. 1180) may be difficult in individual cases, especially if the tissue samples examined are inadequate. In general, crowding and loss of polarity of cells, lack of preservation of the duct basement membrane, absence of gland formation, presence of central necrosis, and marked cellular atypicality indicate atypical or malignant transformation. The different patterns of duct hyperplasia are present schematically in Figure 25–14.

Clinically, florid papillomatosis may be associated with a serous or serosanguineous nipple discharge, but most commonly patients with epithelial hyperplasia present with ill-defined breast masses, which may be tender.

Another type of hyperplasia is so-called *atypical lobular hyperplasia.* This is most often an incidental histologic finding, occurring with other variants of fibrocystic disease. Because it may be related to lobular carcinoma in situ, it will be discussed later under this heading (p. 1184).

Clinical Significance of Fibrocystic Disease

The many patterns of breast pathology included under the designation fibrocystic disease have clinical importance for two reasons: (1) they produce masses in the breast that require differentiation from carcinoma and (2) some may predispose to the subsequent development of carcinoma.

Any mass or lump in the breast must be viewed as a possible carcinoma. Certain clinical features of fibrocystic disease tend to differentiate it from cancer, but the only certain way of making this distinction is biopsy and pathologic examination. The following features favor the diagnosis of fibrocystic disease. Bilateral involvement and multiple nodules are more characteristic of fibrocystic disease than of carcinoma. Fibrocystic disease tends to be painful prior to the menstrual period as breast engorgement occurs. These benign lesions occur in a somewhat younger age group but, unless the patient is in the first two decades of life (when carcinoma of the breast is rarely encountered), the age of the patient is a slender thread. Frequently, fibrocystic disease regresses and even disappears during pregnancy. Despite these clinical features, it is an unwise clinician who relies solely on clinical examination of the breast to rule out carcinoma, the more so because carcinoma may supervene on preexisting fibrocystic disease.

What is the relationship between fibrocystic disease and carcinoma? Two viewpoints have long been held equally vehemently: that fibrocystic disease predisposes

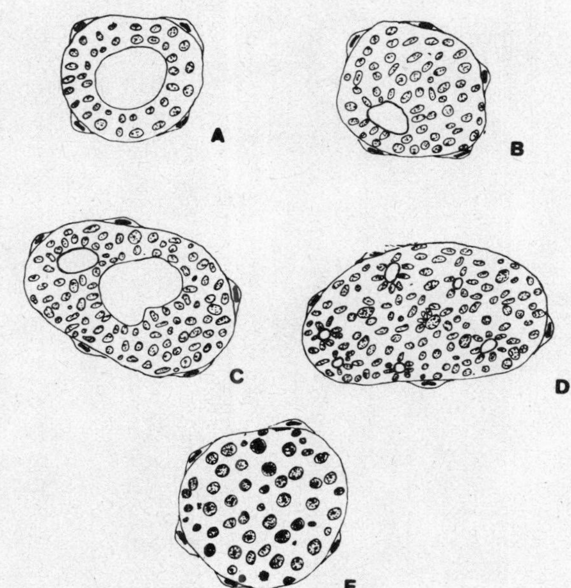

Figure 25–14. Schema of various degrees of epithelial hyperplasia. *A,* Normal lactiferous duct. *B,* Moderate proliferation of cellular layers. *C,* Proliferation with cribriform pattern. *D,* Proliferation with obliteration of lumen and cellular atypia. *E,* Carcinoma in situ. (From Gompel, C., and Van Kerkem, C.: The breast. *In* Silverberg, S. G. (ed.): Principles and Practice of Surgical Pathology. Vol. 1. New York, John Wiley & Sons, 1983. Copyright © 1983. Reprinted by permission of John Wiley & Sons, Inc.)

to cancer and that there is no causal relationship between the two disorders. Although fibrocystic disease shares certain epidemiologic[24] and biochemical[25] characteristics with breast cancer, prospective studies have yielded conflicting results relative to the risk of development of cancer in patients with fibrocystic disease.[15] It is likely that the divergent findings are related to the lack of distinction among the histologic variants of fibrocystic disease and to the lack of a proper control population. *However, the balance of the evidence suggests that patients with some morphologic variants of fibrocystic disease, especially those with epithelial hyperplasia, have a higher than expected attack rate of cancer of the breast.* Warren, in a five-year follow-up of 1200 cases of this disease, cites a cancer rate 4.5 times greater than that in patients with normal breasts.[9] In the patterns that have florid epithelial overgrowth within the ducts, he cites a 12-fold increased attack rate. Others have found a three- to tenfold greater risk of mammary cancer development in patients with previous biopsy-proved fibrocystic disease.[5, 11, 13] *It should be noted, however, that in about half the instances in some series the cancer occurred in the contralateral breast, not in the one with fibrocystic disease.*

Obviously, any meaninful epidemiologic studies must employ precise histologic terminology to describe the findings in benign breast biopsies.[26] If this is done, *the association between fibrocystic disease and cancer is proportional to the degree of epithelial hyperplasia and atypia seen in fibrocystic disease.*[19] In a study of 301 patients in whom a histologic diagnosis of *atypical hyperplasia* was made on biopsy but the breast was not removed, the cumulative risk of breast cancer (both in situ and infiltrating) was 10% at 55 months.[28] As noted, Haagensen also finds an increased risk of cancer in patients with *gross* cysts.[13]

HYPERTROPHY

Abnormal hypertrophy of one or both breasts may occur at any age, presumably when the breast tissue either is excessively sensitive to normal amounts of hormone or is abnormally stimulated by high levels of ovarian hormones. When hypertrophy is unilateral, it is postulated that there is a differential sensitivity of the breasts. Neonatal hypertrophy has already been described. Prepubertal hypertrophy is commonly bilateral and almost invariably suggests abnormal levels of ovarian hormone. This condition is, therefore, encountered in functioning ovarian tumors, choriocarcinomas, adrenal cortical tumors, and pituitary tumors. Control or lowering of hormone production permits regression of breast size. However, in other instances the condition is more obscure and arises without known cause. Sometimes, in the adolescent or preadolescent girl, the hypertrophy of one or both breasts is irreversible. The increase in size may be quite exaggerated, and one or both breasts may assume a bulk three or four times normal. This form of overgrowth is sometimes referred to as virginal hypertrophy. Histologically, there are no distinguishing features, and sections disclose only an abnormal increase of fibrous stroma, accompanied by some proliferation of the ducts and canaliculi.

TUMORS

Neoplasms constitute the most important, albeit not the most common, lesions of the female breast. A great variety of tumors may occur in the female breast, made up as it is of a covering integument, adult fat, mesenchymal connective tissue, and epithelial structures. These tumors run the gamut of virtually all the neoplasms that may arise from stratified squamous epithelium, glandular structures, and mesenchymal connective tissue. Some may be listed as skin papillomas, squamous cell carcinomas of the skin, adenomas, papillomas of ducts, carcinomas of glandular or duct origin, and virtually every variety of benign and malignant mesenchymal tumor, such as fibroma and fibrosarcoma, granular cell myoblastoma, chondroma and chondrosarcoma, lipoma and liposarcoma, osteoma and osteogenic sarcoma, and angioma and angiosarcoma. Only the more common tumors specialized to the breast, however, will be discussed. Most of those listed exactly resemble the analogous neoplasms that occur elsewhere in the body, and do not have any special properties when they arise in the breast.

FIBROADENOMA

The most common benign tumor of the female breast is the fibroadenoma. As the name implies, it is *a new growth composed of both fibrous and glandular tissue*. Occurring at any age within the reproductive period of life, it is somewhat more common before age 30. This tumor is said to develop as the result of increased sensitivity of a focal area of the breast to estrogen. Areas closely resembling a fibroadenoma are found in many cases of cystic disease. Sometimes these areas are poorly defined and merge with the cystic hyperplasia; the term *fibroadenomatosis* is applied to these diffuse lesions to distinguish them from the discrete nodules, fibroadenomas.

The fibroadenoma grows as **a centrifugal, small nodule that is usually sharply circumscribed and freely movable from the surrounding breast substance.** These tumors frequently occur in the upper outer quadrant of the breast. They vary in size up to giant forms 6 to 10 cm in diameter, but most are surgically removed when 2 to 4 cm in diameter (Fig. 25–15). As benign lesions, they are encapsulated and tend to be spherical, but on occasion they may be multilobular and somewhat irregular. On section they are composed of uniform, gray-white tissue punctuated by elevated, minute, yellow-to-pink, softer areas (the glandular structures). Occasionally, soft, somewhat gelatinous areas are present.

The histologic pattern is essentially one of **delicate,**

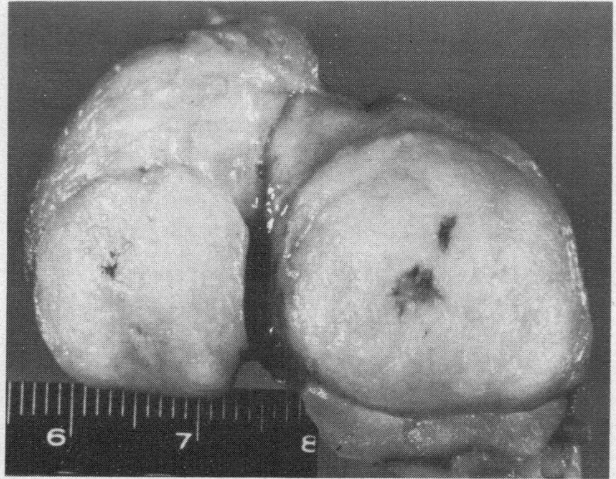

Figure 25–15. Fibroadenoma. Discrete mass bulges above level of surrounding breast tissue.

cellular, fibroblastic stroma enclosing glandular and cystic spaces lined by epithelium. The connective tissue tends to have a loose, reticulated appearance and is sometimes myoxomatous in nature. The glands show variation in form in different tumors, and in different areas within the same tumor. **Intact, round-to-oval gland spaces may be present, lined by single or multiple layers of cells (pericanalicular fibroadenoma)** (Fig. 25–16). The cells are regular and cuboidal to polygonal in shape. The basement membranes of these glands are intact and usually well defined. The connective tissue immediately surrounding these gland spaces tends to be somewhat compressed and denser than the intervening stroma. In other areas, the connective tissue stroma appears to have undergone more active proliferation with compression of the gland spaces. In consequence, **glandular lumina are collapsed or compressed into slitlike, irregular clefts, and the epithelial elements then appear as narrow strands or cords of epithelium lying within the fibrous stroma (intracanalicular fibroadenoma).** Both pericanalicular and intracanalicular patterns often coexist in the same tumor (Fig. 25–17).

Quite rarely, **the connective tissue element is scant in amount, and the entire tumor may be composed of fairly densely packed glandular or acinar spaces lined by a single or double layer of cells.** This pattern is most often encountered in the lactating breast, and frequently the tumor epithelium shows secretory activity similar to that in the surrounding breast substance **(lactating adenoma).**

The clinical characteristics of the fibroadenoma are apparent from the description given. It usually appears as a solitary, discrete, freely movable nodule within the breast. There is no attachment to the overlying skin or underlying fascia. Differentiation from a solitary cyst may at times be difficult. Slight increase in size may occur during the late phases of each menstrual cycle, and pregnancy may stimulate growth. Postmenopausally, regression or calcification may result. Although this lesion presents fairly distinctive clinical characteristics, it nonetheless requires surgical excision for ab-

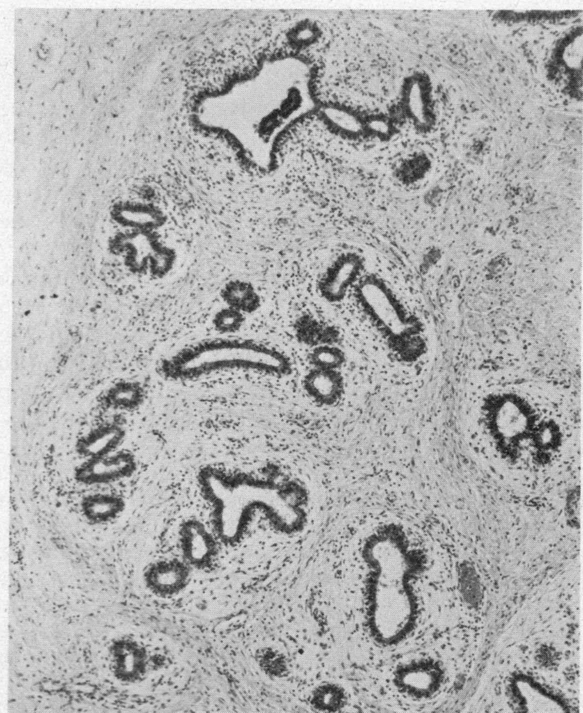

Fig. 25–16

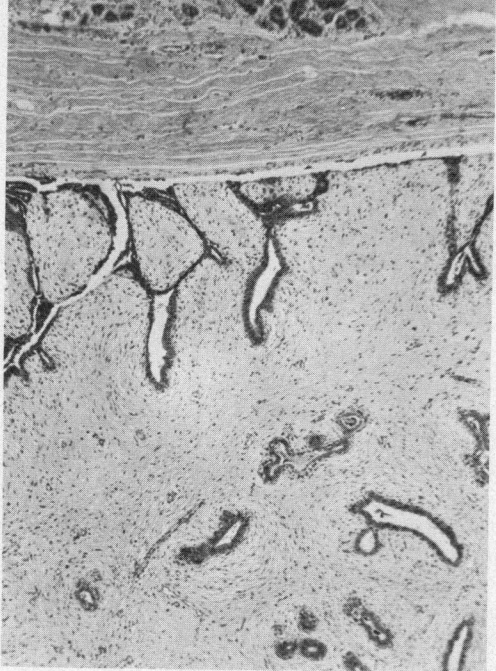

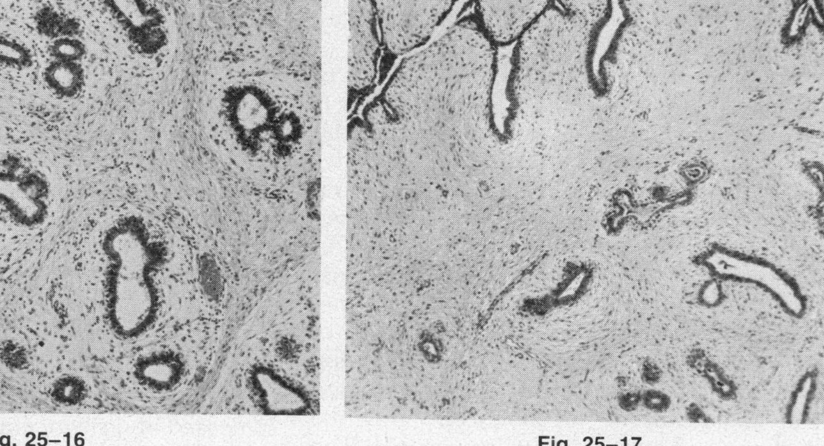

Fig. 25–17

Figure 25–16. Fibroadenoma showing morphology referred to as pericanalicular variant.

Figure 25–17. Fibroadenoma. Margin of nodule, with capsule and separation from compressed breast substance above. Growth is in part intracanalicular, particularly near capsule, with compression of gland spaces. Toward bottom, pattern is pericanalicular.

solute verification of its benign nature, a diagnostic procedure that at the same time effects a cure.

CYSTOSARCOMA PHYLLODES

Infrequently, fibroadenomas may grow to very massive proportions, reaching diameters of 10 to 15 cm, the so-called *giant fibroadenomas.* Some of these large, bulky tumors become lobulated and cystic and hence have been designated *cystosarcoma phyllodes,* an unfortunate term since such lesions can be either benign or malignant. They may distort the breast, produce bulges in the contour of the skin, and even cause pressure necrosis of the overlying skin (Fig. 25–18). In these ulcerated lesions, the capsule of the tumor may rupture, and the growth may fungate through the skin to appear as an irregular mass. However, even this bizarre clinical behavior does not of necessity imply malignancy. Histologically, these lesions tend to have a more cellular myxoid stroma than do the usual fibroadenomas. Lymphomatous, chondromatous, or osteoid foci may appear in the stroma, but the most ominous change is the appearance of increased cellularity, cytologic anaplasia, and high mitotic activity (Fig. 25–18).[29, 20] *Malignant transformation is invariably accompanied by rapid increase in size.* Malignant lesions may recur, but tend to remain as localized lesions for some time. However, in time, metastases to axillary lymph nodes and distant sites occur in about 15% of cases.[31] These tumors, even those that are malignant, can be successfully excised to produce a cure in most cases. Most writers caution that, in many instances, anaplastic changes may be found in masses that nonetheless are innocent clinically, and therefore overdiagnosis and overtreatment must be guarded against. When the term cystosarcoma phyllodes is used for these lesions, the degree of histologic benignity or malignancy should be noted.[3]

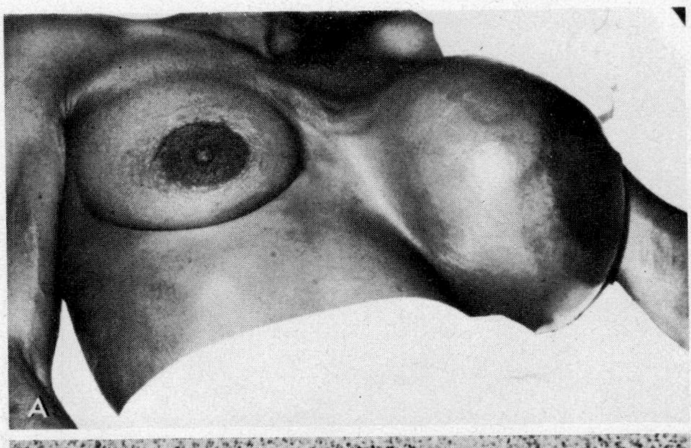

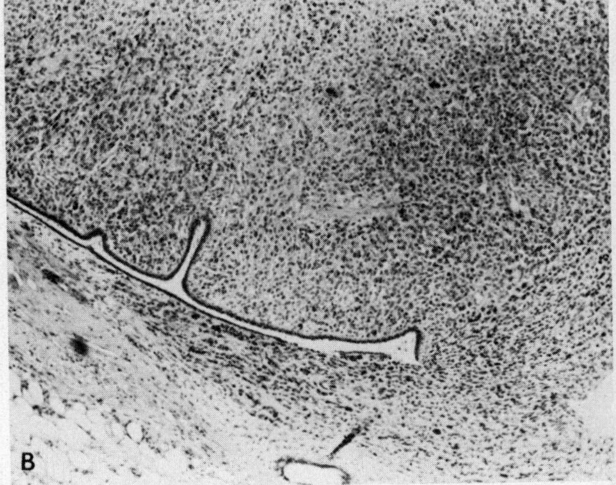

Figure 25–18. Malignant cystosarcoma phyllodes. *A,* Enlargement and distortion of breast. *B,* Pleomorphic hypercellular stromal cells and a compressed ductal structure *(left lower corner).*

INTRADUCTAL PAPILLOMA

It was pointed out that diffuse papillary hyperplasia, called *papillomatosis,* may be a component of fibrocystic disease. In some patients, a neoplastic papillary growth may develop within a duct or a cyst as a *solitary lesion* that is then designated *intraductal papilloma.* Papillomas are most frequently found within the principal lactiferous ducts. They occur at any age but primarily between 30 and 50 years, and present clinically as a result of: (1) the appearance of serous or bloody nipple discharge; (2) the presence of a small subareolar tumor, a few millimeters in diameter; and (3) rarely, nipple retraction.

The tumors are usually very small, rarely more than 1 cm in diameter, and are therefore difficult to locate both clinically and anatomically. As mentioned, they are usually located in the major ducts, close to the nipple. They consist of friable, delicate, villous, branching growths within a dilated duct or cyst. The lesions may be sessile or delicately pedunculated. Histologically, the tumor is composed of multiple papillae, each having a connective tissue axis covered by cuboidal or cylindrical epithelial cells (Fig. 25–19). In areas, there is ramification of these structures so as to form pseudoglandular cavities of diverse size and shape, but solid nests may also be seen. In the truly benign papilloma, two cell types are seen in the centrally situated luminal mass—epithelial and myoepithelial.[5] Apocrine metaplasia may be found and small foci of sclerosis and hyalinization are frequent. Although most of these single papillary lesions are benign, some show significant atypia of epithelium, which should be differentiated from intraductal papillary carcinoma.[5, 13, 32] The distinction between a benign but atypical intraductal papilloma and an intraductal papillary carcinoma may be difficult. In general, severe cytologic atypia, the presence of one rather than two cell types, abnormal mitotic figures, the absence of a vascular connective tissue core, the presence of cell strands bridging the duct lumen (forming a so-called **cribriform pattern**), and the absence of hyalinization and apocrine metaplasia favor a malignant rather than benign papillary tumor. Ultimately, true stromal invasion is the best indication of malignancy.

Complete excision of the duct system should be performed in order to avoid local recurrences. It must be stressed that clearly benign and malignant lesions

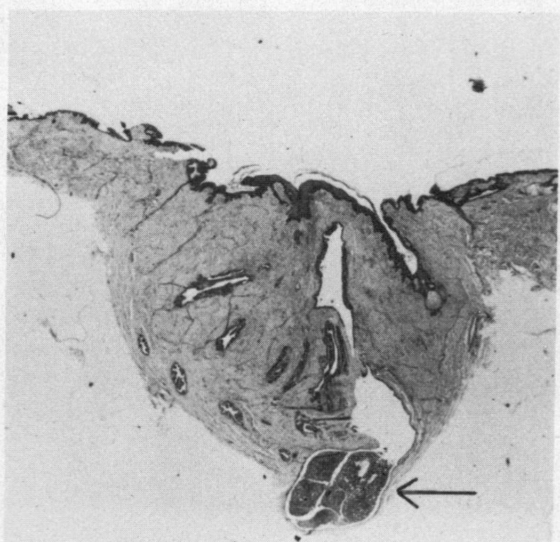

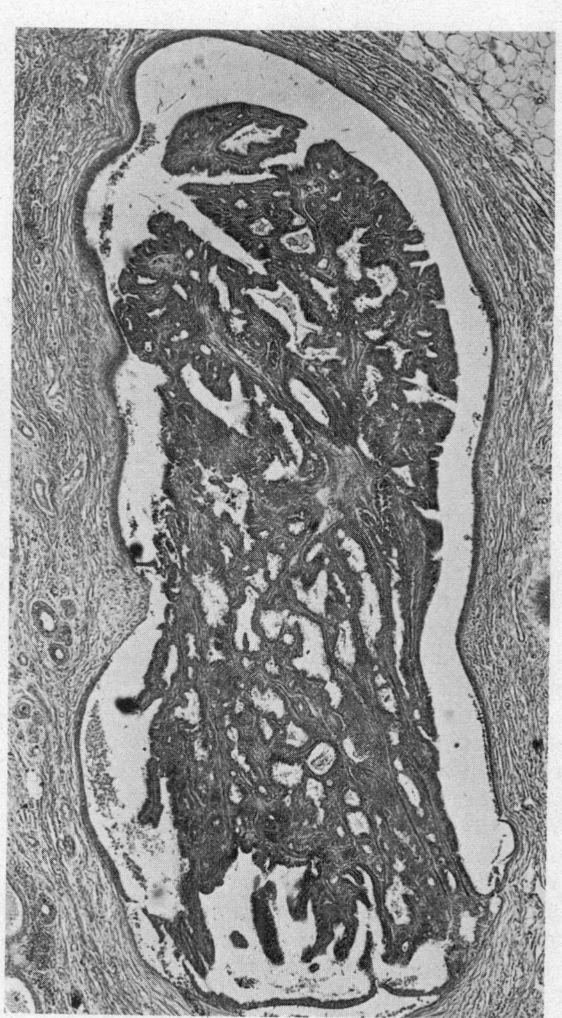

Figure 25–19. Intraductal papilloma. *A,* Low-power view of nipple showing tumor in lactiferous duct *(arrow). B,* High-power view showing well-differentiated papillary tumor.

should be readily differentiated histologically,[5] but some appear to be borderline, producing considerable difficulty in anatomic diagnosis. Fortunately, experience teaches that in these borderline cases, most of the lesions behave in a benign fashion and are effectively cured by local excision. In other words, when the biologic behavior of the growth is that of frank cancer, there is usually little doubt about the anaplastic characteristics of the histologic details.

The present consensus is that solitary intraductal papillomas are benign and are *not* the precursors of papillary carcinoma.[15] However, Haagensen distinguishes *multiple intraductal papillomas* from the group, since he believes they are associated with about a fourfold increased risk of development of papillary carcinoma. These form poorly delineated, palpable tumors in which multiple papillary lesions in ducts occupy peripheral sectors of the breast; these lesions are distinct from the diffuse microscopic papillomatosis seen in fibrocystic disease. Histologically, they resemble the solitary intraductal papilloma.

ADENOMA OF NIPPLE

This is a rare lesion that occurs mostly in elderly women and presents as a nodule immediately beneath the nipple, often with crusting or ulceration of the nipple. Histologically, the appearance is that of a *hidradenoma papilliferum, a type of sweat gland adenoma* (p. 1117). The ducts are lined by papillary projections, which have a central connective tissue axis and a double layer of covering cells: cuboidal, epithelial, and flattened myoepithelial cells. Adenoma of the nipple is a benign tumor cured by local excision.[33]

CARCINOMA OF BREAST

The unqualified term breast cancer implies a carcinoma arising in the glandular and ductal structures of the breast. *Breast carcinoma is the number one cause of cancer deaths among females* and has been called "the foremost cancer" in women. An eloquent justification of this designation was given by H. Marvin Pollard, President of the American Cancer Society: "It is the most feared of cancers, the most frequently self-discovered and the most controversially treated of all cancers. It ranks first among cancers in number of surgical procedures, in radiation therapy treatments, in the number of hormone and chemotherapy administrations. In cancer diagnosis it is first in the number of biopsies. It is the foremost of all cancers, too, from the standpoint of cost in physicians' fees and hospital bills. One cannot compute its ranking to heartache and suffering."[34]

Understandably, then, breast cancer has been the focus of intensive study relative to its origins, diagnostic methods, and treatment. Despite all the efforts, little ground has been gained and the age-adjusted death rate from breast cancer in females in the United States has virtually remained stable over the past 30 years, now being about 22 to 23 per 100,000.[35] In highly personal terms, it has been calculated that six to seven women in every 100 will develop breast cancer.[36] Every 15 minutes about three new cases of breast cancer are diagnosed in the U.S. and one woman is dying of breast cancer. The small gains made in the early diagnosis and treatment of this disease cannot keep pace with its rising incidence in the female. In contrast, cancer of the breast in males is quite rare, the ratio being 100:1. It is both ironic and tragic that a neoplasm arising in an exposed organ, readily accessible to self-examination and clinical diagnosis, continues to exact such a heavy toll.

INCIDENCE. Cancer of the female breast is rarely found before the age of 25. It may occur at any age thereafter, with a peak incidence shortly before, during, or after the menopause. For 1984 the estimated number of new cases of invasive breast cancer in the U.S. was 115,000, and the estimated number of deaths from breast cancer, 37,000.[35]

Few cancers have been subjected to more intensive epidemiologic study. A host of observations has emerged. For example, there are striking geographic differences in its prevalence. The incidence and death rate of breast cancer in Japan and Taiwan is approximately one-fifth that of the U.S. Observations bearing on the incidence of this disease can be summarized as follows:[37–39] breast cancer is more common in:

1. Jews than in Gentiles, by about twofold.
2. Women with increasing age, the incidence curve rising steeply to age 50, then becoming flat for five years, then increasing again but at a much slower place.
3. Women who have had their first child at a late age (over 30).
4. Nulliparous than in multiparous women.
5. Women with late (after age 50) menopause.
6. Women with age of menarche before 13.
7. Obese women.
8. Women with a previous history of breast, ovarian, or endometrial cancer (but breast cancer is less common in women with a history of cervical cancer).
9. Women with fibrocystic disease, particularly epithelial hyperplasia (see earlier discussion).
10. Women with a history of breast cancer in their family, especially if the cancer occurred in young members of the family. A woman whose premenopausal mother and sister have had cancer of the breast has 50 times the control incidence of breast cancer.

Most of the influences productive of a higher attack rate appear to reflect increased exposure to steroid (estrogen) hormones and to familial and genetic influences. Oophorectomy and pregnancy in early fetal life and prolonged lactation in some geographic groups[13, 40] reduce the risk of breast cancer. Some studies show an increased incidence of breast cancer in women taking combination-type oral contraceptives with high progestogen content.[41]

ETIOLOGY AND PATHOGENESIS. The search for the origins of breast cancer has been aided by animal studies but, as with the causation of all cancer, we are still far from an answer. In particular, mammary tumors in mice have been studied extensively. In these animals, it is well documented that four sets of influences are important: (1) genetic factors, (2) hormones, (3) environmental factors, and (4) a virus or viruses. All of these may be directly applicable to women, but it is impossible in humans to establish the rigorous controlled studies of environmental factors achieved with mice. Since a review of breast cancer etiology is beyond our scope, only a few general remarks will be made.[13, 36]

The *role of genetic factors* in the development of cancer, although strongly suggested by family studies, is poorly understood. The risk of breast cancer in women with a familial history of similar disease, particularly premenopausal, is several times greater than that in control groups, but this could be due to either genetic or common environmental influences. A gene transmitted as an autosomal dominant with low penetrance has been described in rare families. Increased prevalence of some cancer-prone haplotypes (HLA-B13) has been claimed.

The *role of hormones* can be summarized thus: unopposed estrogen activity over a long reproductive life span is considered to be highly significant in the genesis of breast cancer. Estrogenic agents readily induce mammary adenocarcinomas in mice and rats. Estrogens are known to induce proliferative changes in the ducts during the normal ebb and flow of hormones in the menstrual cycle. Most breast carcinomas arise in ducts, and it would be reasonable to expect that excessive estrogenic effects might lead to accentuated hyperplasia.

The proliferative effect of steroid hormones is reasonably well characterized. Steroids regulate gene activity, and normal cells, in such target organs as the breast and endometrium, possess specific receptors for estrogens and progesterone. Similar receptors have been identified in breast cancer cells (p. 1188) and these cells may possess enzyme systems not present in normal mammary tissue, rendering them capable of converting androgens to estrogens. The steroid hormone receptor complex serves as a key, which turns on DNA synthesis and replicative activity in target cells through cAMP. In this sense, hormones serve as promoters in the carcinogenic process. Estrogens may also bind covalently to nuclear DNA, and in this way probably act also as initiators. Prolactin, one of the somatotrophins secreted by the anterior pituitary and placenta, has a certain role in maintaining the growth of breast tumors in rats and mice, but its role in human mammary cancer is unsettled.[42]

Much of the epidemiologic data cited earlier supports a role for hyperestrinism in the genesis of breast cancer. The prototype of the unmarried female with no pregnancies and early menarche exemplifies a long reproductive life span, with unremitting exposure to the estrogen peaks of every menstrual cycle. Pregnancies, and a late menarche, shorten such exposure to estrogens. Functioning ovarian tumors and ovarian cortical hyperplasia that elaborate estrogens are associated with breast cancer in postmenopausal women. This neoplasm rarely occurs in the prepubertally castrated. These same hormonal influences are thought to be operative in the genesis of epithelial hyperplasias and probably account for the increased incidence of breast cancer in women with preexisting fibrocystic disease. Recent studies have confirmed associations among excess urinary estrogens, frequency of ovulations, age of menarche, and increased breast cancer risk.[43]

Of the various *environmental factors* implicated (diet, reserpine, caffeine, hair sprays, and so forth), irradiation is the most well established, as shown by increased risk in survivors of atomic bomb exposure and women undergoing radiation therapy.

The most controversial advances have centered on the question of *viral etiology*. The question was raised as early as 1936 by Bittner's discovery that a filterable agent, transmitted through the mother's milk, caused breast cancer in suckling mice.[44] This virus, called mouse mammary tumor virus (MMTV), was subsequently found to be an oncornavirus characterized by type B particles (p. 243). MMTV can produce tumors in vivo and has been shown to be transmitted *horizontally* in the mother's milk and *vertically* through its incorporation in the mother's genome. Genetic strains of mice with a very high incidence of mammary cancer can thus be raised. In recent years, electron microscopic studies of human milk and breast tissue for type B particles have produced conflicting results and, indeed, many of the particles reported had the morphologic appearance of type C viruses, which are not known to be associated with tumor viruses in lower animals. Particularly dramatic were the reports of the presence of reverse transcriptase, an enzyme peculiar to oncogenic RNA viruses, in the same human milk samples containing virus-like particles, as well as nucleic acid hybridization experiments showing similar nucleic-acid sequences in human breast carcinoma and MMTV.[45] More recent studies, however, have cast doubt on these initial reports, and clear documentation of a viral etiology for breast cancer in humans remains as elusive today as it was in 1936.[46]

MORPHOLOGY. Curiously, carcinoma is more common in the left breast than in the right, in a ratio of 110:100. The cancers are bilateral or sequential in the same breast in 4% or more of cases.

Among breast carcinomas small enough for their general areas of origin to be identified, approximately 50% arise in the upper, outer quadrant; 10% in each of the remaining quadrants; and about 20% in the central or subareolar region. As will be seen, the site of origin influences the pattern of nodal metastasis to a considerable degree. Over 90% of breast cancers arise in the ductal epithelium and 10% in the mammary lobules. An overview of the range in tumors types is provided by the following classification.[5,47,48]

- I. Carcinoma arising in mammary ducts
  - A. Noninfiltrating (intraductal) carcinoma
    - 1. Comedo carcinoma
    - 2. Intraductal papillary carcinoma
  - B. Infiltrating duct carcinoma
    - 1. Simple or usual type (also called "not otherwise specified"—NOS)
    - 2. Special types
      - a. Medullary carcinoma with lymphoid infiltration
      - b. Colloid carcinoma (mucinous carcinoma)
      - c. Paget's disease (ductal carcinoma with extension to skin)
      - d. Tubular carcinoma
      - e. Adenoid cystic carcinoma
      - f. Infiltrating comedocarcinoma
      - g. Apocrine carcinoma
      - h. Infiltrating papillary carcinoma
- II. Carcinoma arising in mammary lobules
  - A. Noninfiltrating, in situ lobular carcinoma
  - B. Infiltrating, lobular carcinoma

Only the more common types will be discussed. The incidence of the various types of infiltrating carcinomas collected from a national study is shown in Table 25–1.

Ductal Carcinoma. The noninfiltrating intraductal carcinoma will be discussed first, followed by a presentation of some of the variants of infiltrating tumors arising within the ducts.

INTRADUCTAL CARCINOMA (NONINFILTRATING). As previously stated, over 90% of breast carcinomas arise within the ducts. As long as the tumor remains within the confines of the ductal basement membranes, it constitutes a noninfiltrating intraductal carcinoma. These begin as **atypical proliferations of ductal epithelium that eventually completely fill and plug the ducts with neoplastic cells.** The tumor exists as a poorly defined focus of slightly increased

Table 25–1. INCIDENCE OF HISTOLOGIC TYPES OF INVASIVE BREAST CANCER

	%
Infiltrating duct carcinoma	
Simple or usual type	
Pure	52.6
Combined with other types	22.0
Medullary carcinoma	6.2
Colloid carcinoma	2.4
Paget's disease	2.3
Other pure types	2.0
Other combined types	1.6
Infiltrating lobular carcinoma	4.9
Combined lobular and ductal	6.0

Modified from Fisher, E., et al.: The pathology of invasive breast cancer: A syllabus derived from the findings of the National Surgical Adjuvant Breast Project. Cancer *36*:1, 1975.

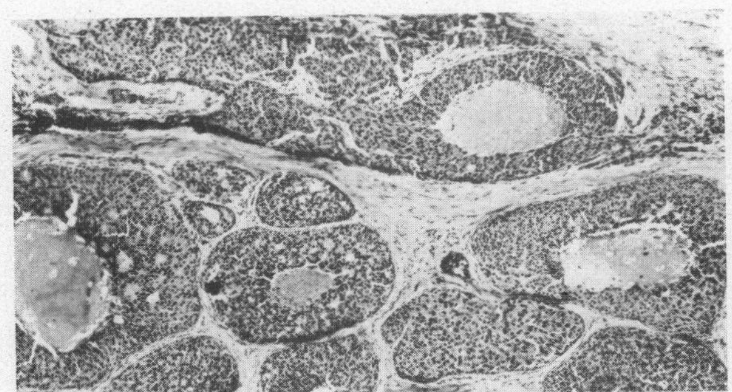

Figure 25–20. Comedocarcinoma. Intraductal proliferation of malignant cells. Note central necrosis.

consistency caused by the marked dilatation and solidification of the ducts. Occasionally, the ductal carcinomas create no change in the consistency of breast substance. It is only when the breast is sectioned that cordlike ducts are found filled with necrotic and cheesy tumorous tissue. This substance can be readily extruded upon slight pressure; hence, the designation **comedocarcinoma**. Histologically, the ducts are dilated and filled with neoplastic epithelial cells that completely plug the lumina. At times, some small glandular pattern or papillary growth may be distinguished, but eventually the proliferation obliterates all architectural detail and only solid cords of anaplastic cells remain, sometimes with central necrosis (Fig. 25–20). As the lesion advances, the intraductal neoplasia eventually extends through the basement membrane, and the tumor becomes an infiltrative ductal carcinoma, to be described. Rarely, these intraductal carcinomas have a predominantly papillary pattern and are called **intraductal papillary carcinomas.**

INFILTRATING DUCT CARCINOMA. As mentioned, this is the most common type of breast cancer. In about 75% of these invasive duct carcinomas, there are no distinguishing histologic features, save for increased dense fibrous tissue stroma, giving the tumor a hard consistency on gross examination. The term **scirrhous carcinoma** was popular for such cancers, denoting their stony-hard consistency. It is now thought that some carcinomas with scirrhous gross features are, in fact, invasive lobular carcinomas, and the term is therefore being discarded. Thus, ductal lesions are now called **infiltrating duct carcinoma, not otherwise specified (NOS) simple or usual types.** These growths occur as fairly sharply delimited nodules of **stony-hard** consistency that average 2 cm in diameter and rarely exceed 4 to 5 cm. On palpation, they may appear deceptively discrete, but in many cases the focus of malignancy is ill defined and obviously has an infiltrative attachment to the surrounding structures with fixation to the underlying chest wall, dimpling of the skin, and retraction of the nipple (Fig. 25–21). Only rarely is there ulceration through the skin. The mass is quite characteristic on cut section. **It is retracted below the cut surface, has a hard cartilaginous consistency, and produces a grating sound when scraped.** Within the central focus, there are small pinpoint foci or streaks of chalky-white, necrotic tumor (Fig. 25–22) and small foci of calcification. Sometimes, obvious long prolongations of fibrous tissue or tumor extend into the surrounding fibrofatty stroma of the breast, with no sharply defined outer limit or encapsulation.

Histologically, the **tumor consists of anaplastic duct lining cells disposed in cords, solid cell nests, tubes, glands, anastomosing masses, and mixtures of all these.** In some, clear-cut intraductal components can also be seen (Fig. 25–23). The cells are disseminated in a fibrous stroma, which varies in amount from one tumor to another, but also from one region to another of a single tumor. The cytologic detail of tumor cells varies from small cells with moderately hyperchromatic regular nuclei to huge cells with large irregular and hyperchromatic nuclei. In many instances, the nuclei are surprisingly uniform in size and shape and display only a small number of mitotic figures. At the margins of the tumor mass, the neoplastic cells infiltrate into the stroma and fibrofatty tissue, and frequently invasion of perivascular and perineural spaces as well as blood and lymphatic vessels is readily evident (Fig. 25–24).

MEDULLARY CARCINOMA WITH LYMPHOID INFILTRATION. This variant accounts for about 5% of all mammary carcinomas and tends to produce large fleshy tumor masses up to 5 to 10 cm in diameter.[49] These tumors do not have the striking desmoplasia (formation of fibrous tissue) of the usual carcinoma, and therefore are distinctly more yielding on external palpation and on cut section. On section, the tumor may bulge above the level of the native tissue and has a soft, fleshy, almost brainlike consistency. These masses grow centrifugally along a broad front and are often deceptively sharply delimited from the surrounding substance (Fig. 25–25). Foci of necrosis and hemorrhage are large and numerous. Histologically, the carcinoma is characterized by (1) solid sheets of large cells with vesicular, often pleomorphic nuclei, containing prominent nucleoli and frequent mitoses; and (2) a moderate-to-marked lymphocytic infiltrate between these sheets, with a scant fibrous component (Fig. 25–26). It is the lymphoid infiltrate that gives these tumors their special significance, since such tumors have a distinctly better prognosis than the usual infiltrating duct carcinomas, even in the presence of axillary lymph node metastases. The ten-year survival rate for these tumors is 84%.[50]

COLLOID OR MUCINOUS CARCINOMA. This unusual variant tends to occur in older women and grows slowly over the course of many years, producing large, gelatinous masses. The tumor is extremely soft and has the consistency and appearance of pale gray-blue gelatin. It may occur in pure form or in association with other types.

Histologically, this tumor usually takes on one of two patterns of growth, which may coexist in a single lesion. There may be large lakes of lightly staining, amorphous mucin that dissect and extend into contiguous tissue spaces and planes of cleavage. Floating within this mucin are small islands and isolated neoplastic cells, sometimes forming glands (Fig. 25–27). Vacuolation of at least some of the cells is characteristic. In other colloid tumors, the histologic appearance may be essentially that of an adenocarcinoma, with well-defined glands, the lumina of which contain mucinous secretions. The cells lining the glands usually contain obvious vacuoles of similar substance. Basic to these variants is the production of abundant mucin, either intra- or extracellularly.

The survival rate is appreciably greater in pure colloid carcinoma than in the usual infiltrating duct carcinoma, and lymph node metastases are infrequent.[51]

PAGET'S DISEASE. Paget's disease of the breast is a specialized form of ductal carcinoma that arises in the main excretory ducts of the breast and extends to involve the skin of the nipple and areola.[52,53] As a consequence of this malignant invasion of the skin, eczematoid changes occur in the nipple and areola. Careful morphologic study of these lesions has demonstrated beyond doubt that **infiltrating ductal carcinoma or, less commonly, intraductal carcinoma invariably antedates the skin change.** This disease

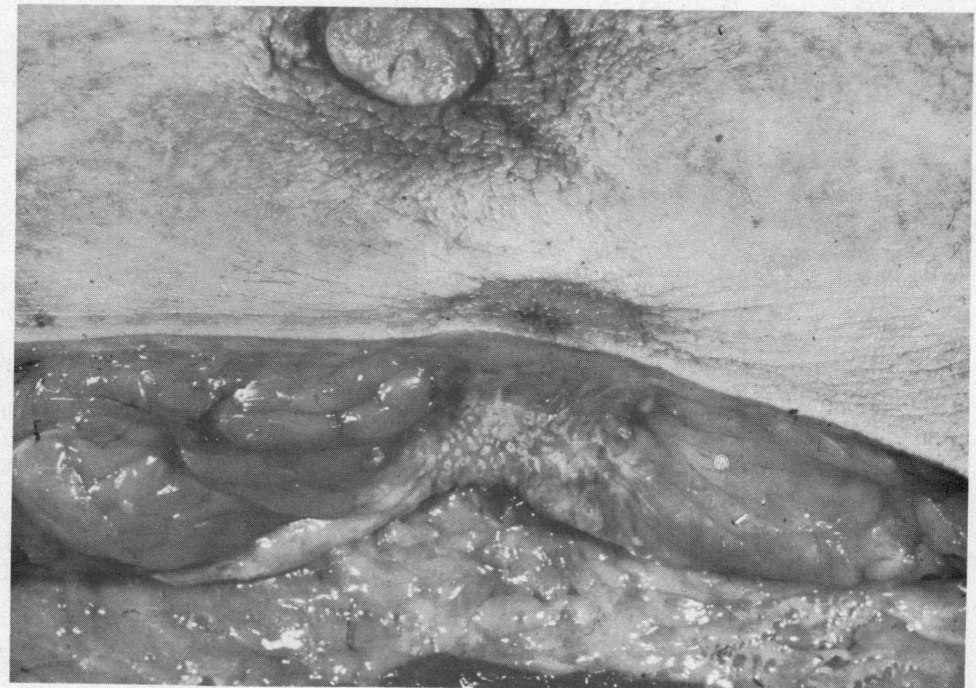

Fig. 25–21

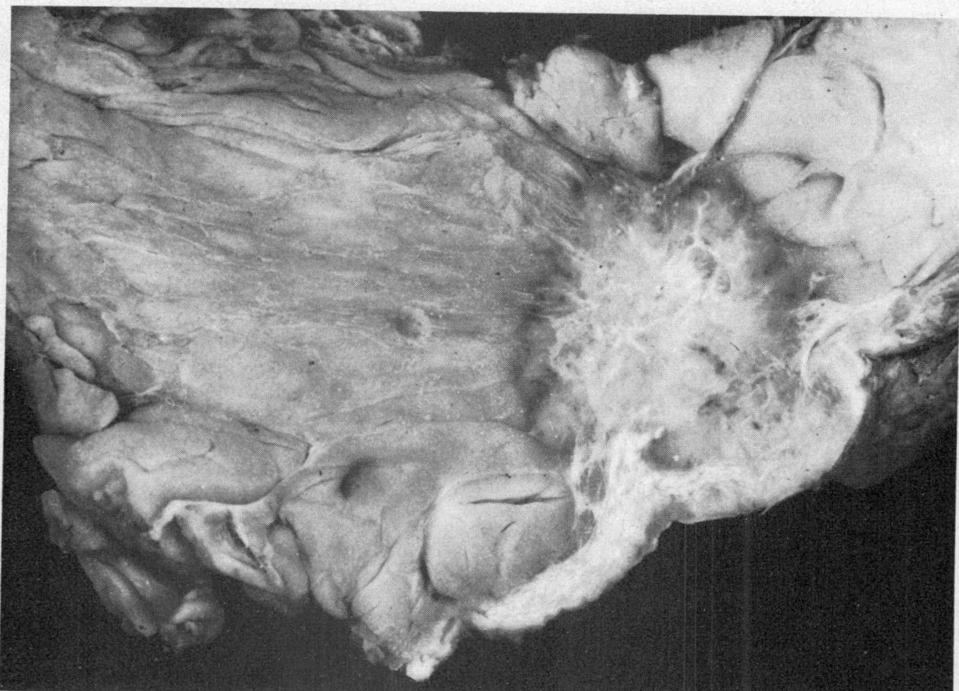

Fig. 25–22

Figure 25–21. Carcinoma of breast, infiltrating. Tumor is transected through middle, and breast is viewed obliquely to illustrate retracted mass and fixation to and dimpling of attached skin.

Figure 25–22. Carcinoma of breast, infiltrating. Cut surface illustrates lack of demarcation, fixation to skin, and chalky foci of necrosis within mass.

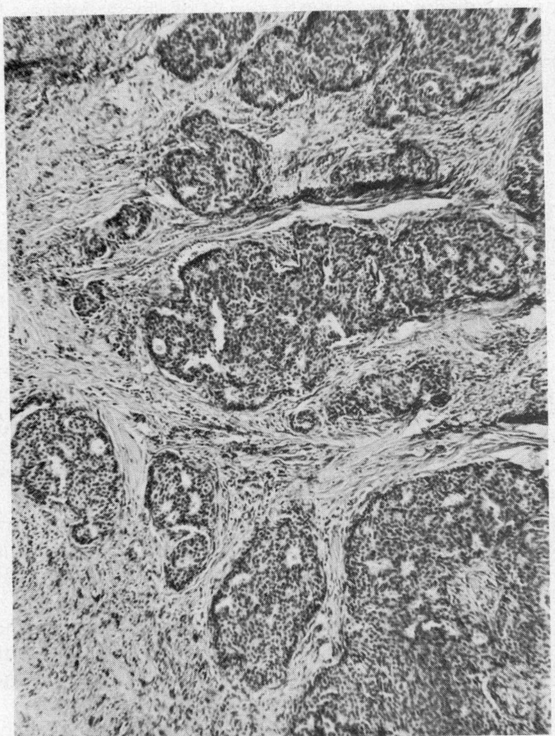

Figure 25–23. Ductal carcinoma. Tumor cells fill ducts and have invaded stroma.

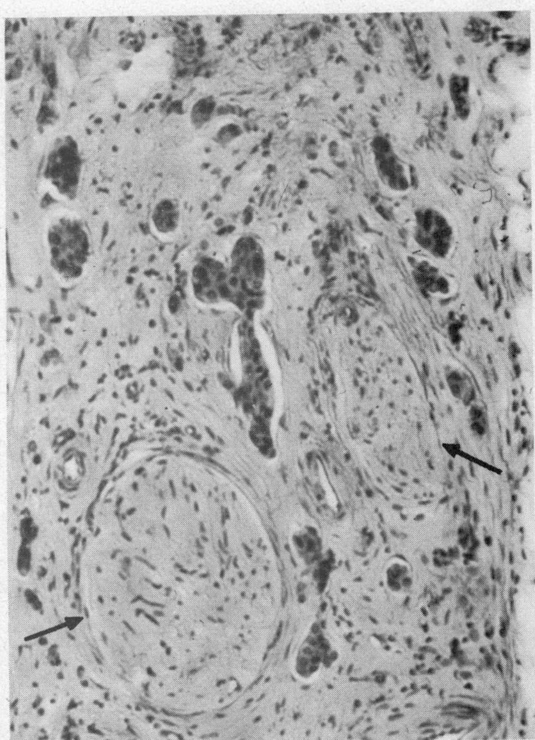

Figure 25–24. Invasive carcinoma of breast. Tumor has surrounded nerve fibers *(arrows)* and is lying within a lymphatic space.

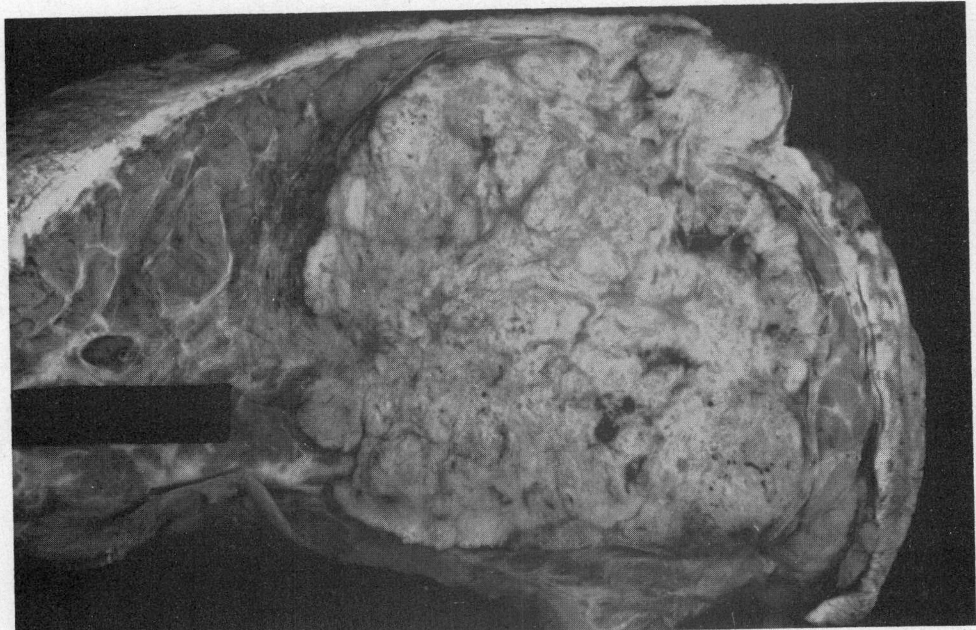

Figure 25–25. Carcinoma of breast, medullary type. The large bulky mass appears deceptively discrete.

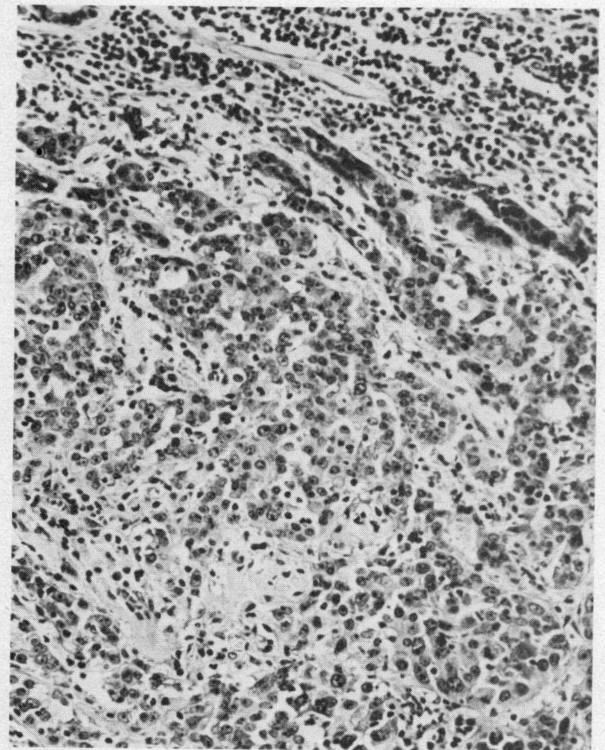

Figure 25–26. Medullary carcinoma with lymphoid infiltrate. Note lymphocytes infiltrating epithelial tumor.

tends to occur in an age group slightly older than that with the common forms of breast carcinoma. Since Paget's disease of the nipple implies extension to the skin, the prognosis is somewhat less favorable than in the simple noninvasive ductal carcinoma. About 30 to 40% of these women have metastases at the time of surgery.

The most striking gross characteristics of this lesion involve the skin. The skin of the nipple and areola is frequently fissured, ulcerated, and oozing. There is surrounding inflammatory hyperemia and edema. In far-advanced cases, total ulceration of the nipple and areola may occur (Fig. 25–28). Superimposed bacterial infection may cause a localized suppurative necrosis, which masks the eczema-like changes. An underlying lump or mass is only rarely present.

Section through the lesion invariably reveals marked proliferation within ducts similar to the other forms of ductal carcinoma. In far-advanced lesions, the tumor extends through the duct basement membrane, at which time the other characteristics of the carcinoma may be present.

The histologic hallmark of this entity is the invasion of the epidermis by malignant cells, referred to as Paget cells. These cells are large, anaplastic, and hyperchromatic and are usually surrounded by a clear zone or halo (Fig. 25–29). The halo, once thought to represent "ballooning degeneration," can be stained with such mucopolysaccharide stains as Alcian blue. In addition to the Paget cells, the other histologic criteria of ductal carcinoma are present. (See also Paget's disease of vulva, p. 1118.)

Lobular Carcinoma. Lobular carcinoma is a relatively distinct morphologic form of mammary cancer[54, 55] that probably arises from the terminal ductules of the breast lobule.[47] Although making up only 5 to 10% of breast carcinomas, **invasive lobular carcinomas** are of particular interest for a number of reasons: (1) they tend to be bilateral far more frequently than those arising in ducts (the likelihood of cancer in the contralateral breast being on the order of 20%); (2) they tend to be multicentric within the same breast; and (3) they have a higher incidence of estrogen receptor positivity (p. 1188).

Grossly, the tumor is rubbery and poorly circumscribed, but sometimes appears as a typical scirrhous type. Histologically, it consists of strands of infiltrating tumor cells, often only one cell in width (in the form of an "Indian file"), loosely dispersed throughout the fibrous matrix (Fig. 25–30). The cells are small and uniform-staining with relatively little cytologic pleomorphism. Irregularly shaped solid nests and sheets may also occur in continuity with the single-file pattern. The tumor cells are frequently arranged in concentric rings about normal ducts, this pattern being virtually diagnostic of invasive lobular carcinoma. However, differentiation between ductal and lobular infiltrating carcinoma may very often be quite difficult, and in some tumors mixed ductal and lobular patterns exist (Table 25–1). When these tumors metastasize to lymph nodes, they rarely form sheets or nests of epithelial cells, and may therefore resemble undifferentiated carcinomas or histiocytic lymphomas.

Lobular carcinoma in situ is a histologically unique lesion manifested by proliferation, in one or more terminal ductules and/or acini, of cells that are loosely cohesive, somewhat larger than normal, and have rare mitoses and oval or round nuclei with small nucleoli (Fig. 25–31). These lesions were initially described as incidental findings in breasts removed for fibrocystic disease or the resection of invasive carcinoma.[57] The frequency with which such change

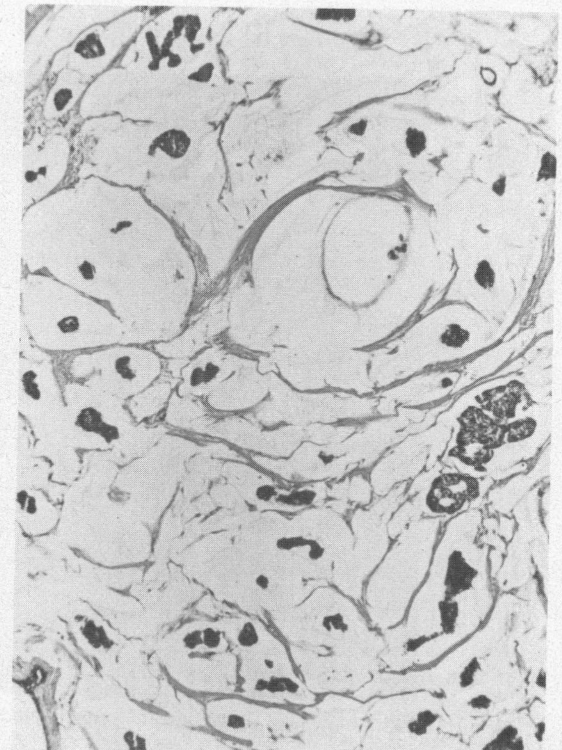

Figure 25–27. Colloid carcinoma. Note lakes of lightly staining mucin with small islands of tumor cells.

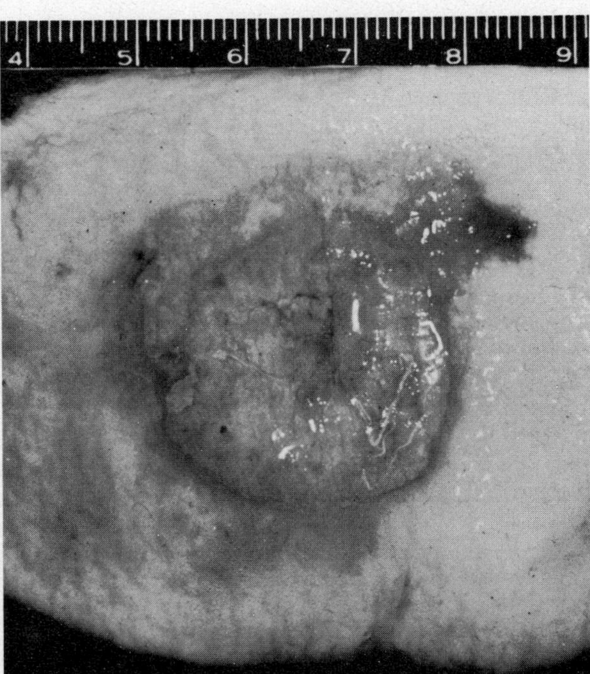

Figure 25–28. Paget's disease of breast. Lesion is far advanced and has destroyed nipple.

may develop into invasive carcinoma in the same breast[58] varies considerably, ranging from 4 to 25%, these differences probably being due to problems of sampling and variable criteria for diagnosis. In particular, differentiation of lobular carcinoma in situ from so-called **atypical lobular hyperplasia** may be difficult, the latter being a somewhat more common accompaniment of fibrocystic disease. In a survey of 99 patients **not** treated with mastectomy and followed for

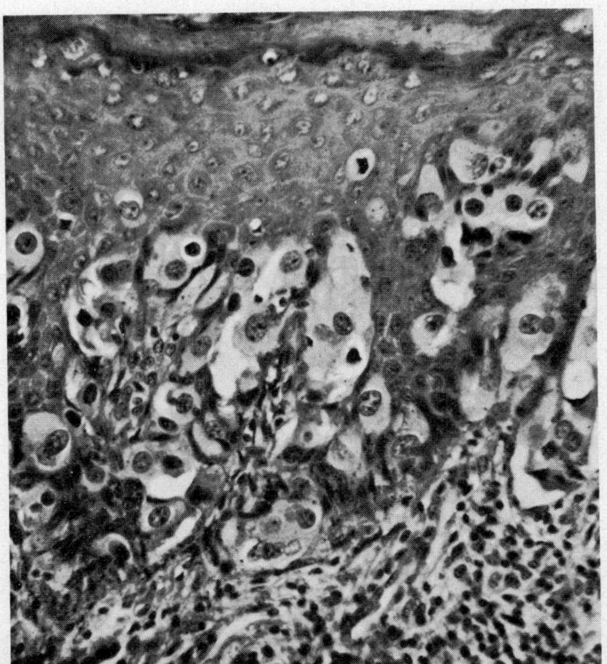

Figure 25–29. Paget's disease of breast. Classic Paget cells dot the epithelium.

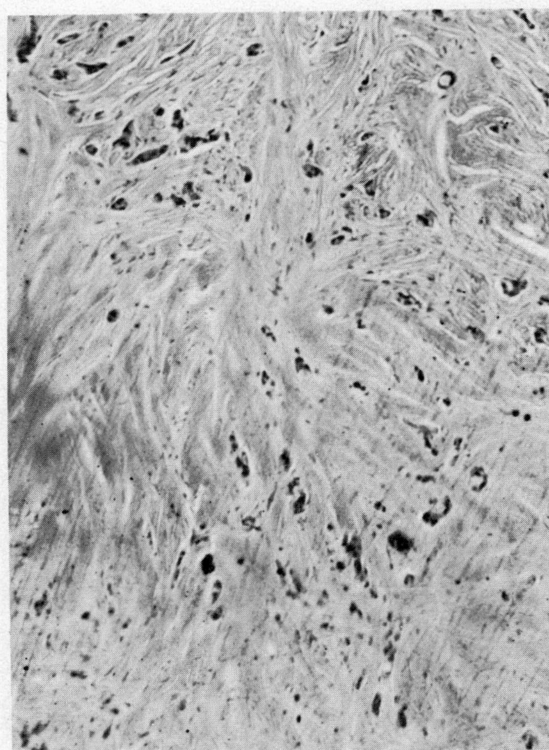

Figure 25–30. Carcinoma of breast, infiltrating lobular type. Small nests of tumor cells are embedded within a dense fibrous stoma.

24 years,[59] the frequency of subsequent carcinoma developing in the same or **contralateral** breast was 36.9%, nine times greater than expected for the general population. In Haagensen's series of 263 patients,[13, 61] the increased risk was 6.9 times greater. The infiltrating carcinomas that subsequently developed in both studies were either ductal or lobular.

There are additional morphologic features common to all infiltrative breast carcinomas, whatever the histologic types. As focal lesions, they extend progressively in all directions. In the course of time, they may become adherent to the deep fascia of the chest wall and thus become **fixed in position.** Extension to the skin may cause not only fixation but **retraction and dimpling of the skin,** an important characteristic of malignant growth. At the same time, the lymphatics may become so involved as to block the local area of skin drainage and cause lymphedema and thickening of the skin, a change that has for years been referred to as **orange peeling.** When the tumor involves the main excretory ducts, particularly in the intraduct variety, **retraction of the nipple** may develop. Certain carcinomas tend to infiltrate widely through the breast substance, involve the majority of the lymphatics, and produce acute swelling, redness, and tenderness of the breast, referred to clinically as **inflammatory carcinoma.** This is not a special morphologic pattern but merely implies widespread dissemination. It tends to develop with pregnancy. Very late lesions may cause ulceration of the skin or extension within the skin to produce the form that was at one time illustrated in medical texts as **carcinoma en cuirasse** (Fig. 25–32).

The ultilization of **mammography** has directed attention to the calcium content of mammary cancers, since the appearance of radiodense deposits has been regarded as an important radiologic feature of carcinoma. Foci of calcifi-

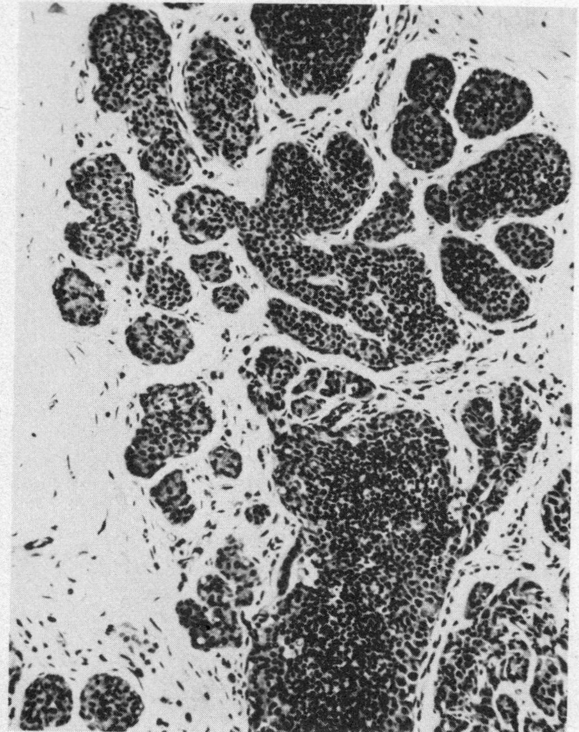

Figure 25–31. Lobular carcinoma in situ. Note proliferation of well-differentiated tumor cells in terminal ducts and acini.

cation are indeed present in 60% of cancers if special stains for calcium are done, although routine H and E sections may miss many of these. However, the incidence of calcific opacifications in benign lesions approaches that in malignant tumors, and furthermore over 40% of cancers are not substantially calcified.

Spread of the tumor eventually occurs through the lymphohematogenous routes. The pathways of lymphatic dissection are in all possible directions: **lateral** to the axilla, **superior** to the nodes above the clavicle and the neck, **medial** to the other breast, **inferior** to the abdominal viscera and lymph nodes, and **deep** to the nodes within the chest, particularly along the internal mammary arteries. The two most favored directions of drainage are the axillary nodes and the nodes along the internal mammary artery.

Overall, about two-thirds of all patients have metastases to lymph nodes at the time of initial diagnosis of breast cancer. **The pattern of nodal spread is heavily influenced by the location of the cancer in the breast.** Tumors arising in the outer quadrants involve the axillary nodes alone in about 50% of cases, and have both internal mammary and axillary involvement in an additional 15% of cases. In contrast, cancers arising in the inner quadrants and center of the breast affect the axilla alone in about 25% of cases. In an additional 40%, internal mammary nodes are affected, often with axillary involvement.[59] The supraclavicular nodes are the third most favored site of nodal spread. As will be seen, nodal involvement seriously prejudices the prognosis. Distant metastases via the bloodstream may affect virtually any organ of the body and, on occasion, extremely widespread dissemination is encountered. Favored sites for dissemination are the lungs, bones, liver, and adrenals. Some of the most bizarre metastatic involvements, such as spread to the pituitary gland, eyes, and skin, are seen in this form of cancer.

GRADING AND STAGING OF BREAST CANCER. The many histologic grades and stages of breast cancer have been subdivided into smaller homogeneous groups to standardize comparisons of results of various therapeutic modalities among clinics.[60] A plethora of classifications has led to mass confusion, but at present three are widely used: one based on histologic details and the other two on the extent of spread of cancer. From the histologic classification described earlier, cancers may be roughly divided as follows:

Nonmetastasizing: intraductal or comedocarcinoma without stromal invasion; in situ lobular carcinoma.

Uncommonly metastasizing: pure extracellular mucinous or colloid cancer; medullary cancer with lymphocytic infiltration; tubular adenocarcinoma, infiltrating papillary.

Moderately to highly metastasizing: all other types.

The American Joint Committee on Cancer Staging more or less follows the recommendations of the TNM terminology of the UICC (p. 229) and divides the clinical stages as follows:

Stage I. A tumor less than 5 cm in diameter without nodal involvement and no metastases.

Stage II. A tumor less than 5 cm in diameter with involved but movable axillary nodes and no distant metastases.

Stage III. All breast cancers of any size with possible skin involvement, pectoral and chest wall fixation, and nodal involvement including axillary nodes, fixed but without disseminated metastases.

Stage IV. Any form of breast cancer with or without nodal involvement, pectoral fixation, skin ulceration, or chest wall fixation, but having disseminated metastases.

The clinical classification more frequently utilized today in the U.S. is the Columbia Clinical Classification, which was proposed more than 20 years ago by Haagensen and colleagues:[13]

Stage A. No skin edema, ulceration, or solid fixation of tumor to chest wall. Axillary nodes not clinically involved.

Stage B. Same as Stage A, but with clinically involved nodes. The latter should be less than 2.5 cm in transverse diameter and not fixed to the skin or deeper tissues of axilla.

Stage C. Any one of five grave signs of breast carcinoma: (1) edema of skin, (2) skin ulceration, (3) fixation of tumor to chest wall, (4) massive involvement of axillary lymph nodes, and (5) fixation of nodes to skin or deeper structures of axilla.

Stage D. All other patients with more advanced cancer including two or more of the signs listed in Stage C.

CLINICAL COURSE. Cancers of the breast are usually first discovered by the patient or physician as a solitary, painless mass in the breast. The older the patient with a single breast mass, the more likely is it to be cancer. When first discovered, these cancers are deceptively

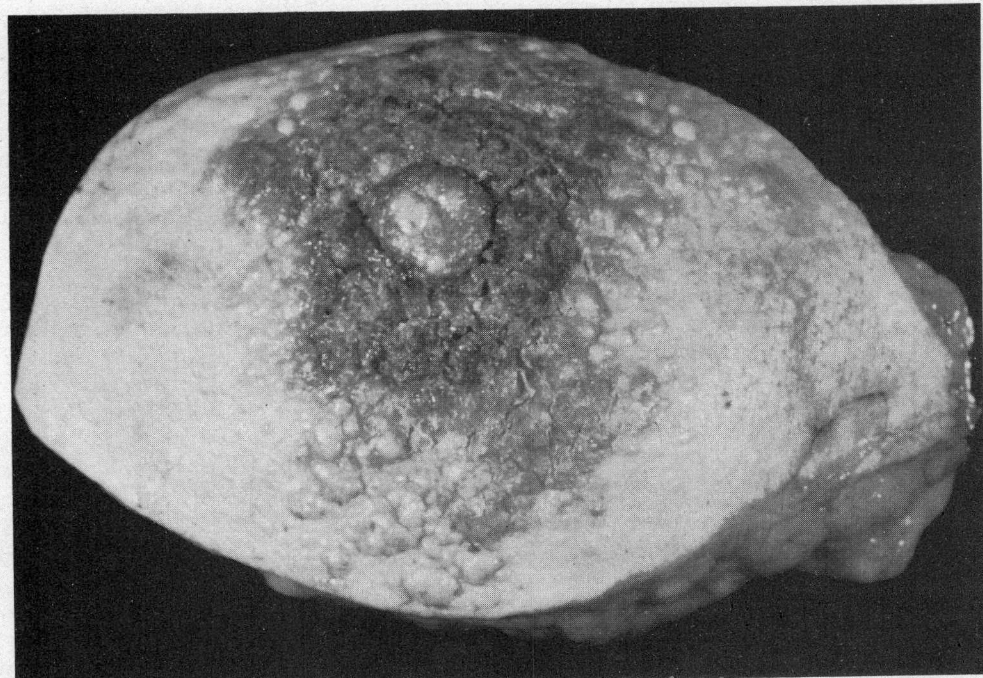

Figure 25–32. Carcinoma of breast. Tumor has extensively invaded skin in pattern referred to as "carcinoma en cuirasse."

freely movable and delimited. Accordingly, the differential diagnosis extends to virtually every disorder in this chapter, including the variants of fibrocystic disease, fat necrosis, scarring of an abscess, and benign tumors. Many cancers are first detected by the patient during self-examination. On the average, these lesions are 4 cm in diameter when first found, and approximately two-thirds have already spread to axillary or other nodes. Intraductal cancers, which rarely produce palpable masses, more often come to attention by the appearance of a discharge (sometimes hemorrhagic) from the nipple.

Because early treatment of localized disease is the best hope of total eradication, an enormous effort is being made to identify breast cancers while they are still in Stages I to II. Health education and frequent self-examination may help but may not accomplish this goal.[62] A number of factors influence the validity of the self-examination technique, principally breast size. Currently, emphasis is being placed on more frequent, regular medical examinations and mammography, xeroradiography, thermography, and ultrasonic studies as screening techniques in high-risk women. With such procedures, it is always necessary to weigh false-negative and false-positive results and risks from the procedures themselves against benefits of early diagnosis.[63] The role of mass screening by mammography is controversial, and the National Cancer Institute Committee report recommended that since no mortality benefit was evident in women under 50 whose carcinoma was detected by mammography, screening should be stopped in such women.[64] A more recent analysis of a screening program, however, strongly supported the efficiency of mammography in detecting early cancers in women 35 to 49 years of age and the low risk of radiation with currently used mammography techniques.[65] At present, the following guidelines are recommended:[64, 66] (1) women 40 to 49 years of age should have a physical examination of the breast annually, and mammography every one to two years;[66] (2) for those with a previous breast cancer or a strong family history, periodic screening should begin at age 35; (3) in women over 50, whether symptomatic or asymptomatic, periodic screening programs are recommended.

At present, it is impossible to present a concise consensus of the most effective methods of treating the varying stages of breast cancer. In particular, contention continues over the effectiveness of the following approaches in the treatment of *early* breast cancer, i.e. cancer localized at presentation:[66] (1) *radical mastectomy* (which includes removal of axillary nodes and pectoral muscles); (2) *supraradical mastectomy* (usually following biopsy of the supraclavicular and internal mammary nodes), which includes, in addition to radical mastectomy, removal of internal mammary nodes and supraclavicular nodes on the same side; (3) *simple mastectomy with axillary lymph node dissection;* (4) *simple mastectomy* or local excision of the lesion along *with intensive irradiation* (McWhirter technique); (5) *modified radical mastectomy with prophylactic, postoperative irradiation;* (6) *radiation alone;* and (7) *radical or simple mastectomy with adjuvant chemotherapy.*

It should be emphasized that even patients with histologically negative axillary nodes cannot be assumed to have localized disease. With radical mastectomy alone there is at least a 24% treatment failure after ten years, suggesting that breast cancer is frequently a systemic disease at the time of operation. For these reasons, prophylactic postoperative therapy with cytotoxic chemotherapeutic agents (adjuvant therapy) has been advocated, and several long-term cooperative studies have suggested a significant benefit in survival over surgery alone.[67]

In addition to surgery, radiation, and chemotherapy, a host of other interventions are employed, either to support the primary treatment or as secondary measures in those who fail to respond or suffer recurrences and metastases. Ovariectomy may be performed in premenopausal women in an effort to reduce levels of circulating estrogens. Adrenalectomy and hypophysectomy are additional measures employed in patients with progressive disease and pain (usually arising in bone metastases), in hope of prolonging life.

Currently, the presence or absence of cytoplasmic *estrogen receptors* (p. 1179) in human breast tumors is being used to predict and monitor their "hormonal dependency," and hence the response of metastatic breast carcinoma to procedures that reduce the level of such hormones. About two-thirds of primary breast cancers are receptor positive with a higher frequency of positivity in premenopausal women. Fifty to 70% of tumors containing estrogen receptors regress after oophorectomy, adrenalectomy, or hypophysectomy, whereas only 5% of estrogen receptor–negative tumors respond to these procedures. Progesterone receptors are also present in breast tumors, and the highest response rates to endocrine ablation are in patients with tumors containing both receptors.[68, 69]

The *prognosis* in breast cancer is modified by the histologic grade and type of lesion, the clinical stage at time of discovery, and such other variables as concomitant pregnancy (the disease appears to be more virulent during pregnancy) and the adequacy of primary treatment. Unfavorable prognostic signs include the following:

1. Extensive edema of the skin over the breast.
2. Edema of the arm.
3. Satellite nodules in the skin over the breast.
4. Extensive skin ulcerations.
5. Fixation to the chest wall.
6. More than three positive axillary nodes, or fixed or enlarged (over 2.5 cm) nodes.
7. Spread to internal mammary nodes.
8. Supraclavicular metastases.
9. Inflammatory carcinoma (redness, swelling, and increased heat in the affected breast due to diffuse permeation of the cancer into the regional lymphatics and blood vessels).
10. Distant metastases.

As to the *histologic type* of tumor, 30-year follow-up of 1458 consecutive operable infiltrating cancers treated by radical mastectomy gives the following results: comedocarcinoma, 74% survival; papillary, 65%; medullary, 58%; colloid, 58%; infiltrating lobular, 34%; simple (scirrhous) infiltrating ductal, 29%.[70]

In the overall view of breast cancers, the five-year survival is about 50%. This rate is heavily weighted by the fact that approximately 25% of breast cancers are found to be inoperable at the time of discovery. The five-year survival rate for all patients treated by radical mastectomy is 50 to 55%. In women with histologically negative lymph nodes, there is an 84% five-year survival rate and a 62% ten-year survival, without evidence of residual disease. The presence of one to three positive axillary lymph nodes only slightly worsens the prognosis. It should be noted that recurrence may appear late, even after ten years, but with each passing year free of disease the prognosis improves. Thus, five years after surgery, those free of disease have an 80% additional five-year survival. With fixed large (over 2.5 cm) nodes, or over three positive nodes in the axilla, five-year survival drops to 30% and ten-year survival to 20%. As stated earlier, there is still much uncertainty as to the best method of treatment of early breast cancer, and more data need to be gathered on carefully controlled and matched series.

Thus, this discussion of breast cancer ends virtually where it began. The clinical problem is monumental; despite great efforts to solve it, there is much yet to be learned.

Miscellaneous Malignancies. Malignant neoplasia may arise from the skin of the breast, sweat glands, sebaceous glands, and hair shafts, or from the connective tissues and fatty stroma. These tumors are identical to their counterparts found in other sites of the body. Those arising from skin grow as basal or squamous cell carcinoma. Cancers arising in the skin adnexa grow as carcinomas of sweat gland or sebaceous gland origin. Malignancies of the stroma are, of course, sarcomas[71, 72] and include fibrosarcomas, myxosarcomas, liposarcomas, angiosarcomas, chondrosarcomas, and osteogenic sarcomas, the last-named primarily derived from metaplastic differentiation of the fibroblasts. Of the same origin are the extremely rare primary malignant lymphomas. As a general rule, sarcomas occur in the same age range as carcinomas and differ chiefly in their rate of growth. They tend to produce large, bulky, fleshy masses that cause rapid increase in breast size with considerable distortion of breast contour. Attachment to the skin surface and ulceration are, perhaps, more common with this rapid growth than with carcinomas. Sarcomas as a group spread via the lymphatics to the axillary nodes, but also frequently metastasize via the blood to distant organs, particularly the lungs. The clinical outlook in these cases is poor. Angiosarcomas, in particular, are the most rapidly fatal of breast tumors.

Male Breast

The rudimentary male breast is relatively free from pathologic involvement. Only two processes occur with sufficient frequency to merit consideration.

GYNECOMASTIA

The embryogenesis and development of the male breast parallel those of the female breast up to the age of puberty. At this point, only the major breast ducts are formed, with a scant amount of secondary duct branching. *Gland lobules are not found in the normal male breast.* As in the female, the male breast is subject to hormonal influences, but is considerably less sensitive than the female. Nonetheless, enlargement of the male breast (gynecomastia) may occur in response to excesses of estrogen. It is encountered under a variety of normal and abnormal circumstances.[73] It may be found at the time of puberty or in the very aged, in the latter presumably owing to a relative increase in adrenal estrogens as the androgenic function of the testis fails. It is one of the manifestations of Klinefelter's syndrome (p. 129) and may occur in those with functioning testicular neoplasms such as Leydig cell and, rarely, Sertoli cell tumors. It may occur at any time during adult life when there is cause for hyperestrinism. The most important cause of hyperestrinism in the male is cirrhosis of the liver, since the liver is responsible for metabolizing estrogen.

Grossly, the lesion may be unilateral or bilateral. Unilateral disease is explained as an increased sensitivity of the tissues in one breast. A button-like, subareolar enlargement develops. In farther advanced cases, the swelling may simulate the adolescent female breast. On section, the breast tissue is white and rubbery and has minute, elevated, pinkish spots dispersed throughout it. This architectural pattern is reminiscent of that found in certain forms of cystic hyperplasia.

Microscopically, there is proliferation of a dense, periductal hyaline, collagenous connective tissue, but more striking are the changes in the epithelium of the ducts.[74] There is marked hyperplasia of the ductal linings with the piling up of multilayered epithelium (Fig. 25–33). The individual cells are fairly regular, columnar to cuboidal with regular nuclei. Occasionally there may be some variation in cell size and considerable disorientation of the heaped-up lining cells. Anaplasia is absent. The basal membranes are intact and the lumina of the ducts are rarely filled. There is minimal periductal lymphocytic and plasma cell infiltration. The microscopic changes, then, are similar to the ductal hyperplasia found in cystic hyperplasia in the female.

The lesion is readily apparent on clinical examination, and must be differentiated only from the seldom-occurring carcinoma of the male breast. Gynecomastia is chiefly of importance as an indicator of hyperestrinism, suggesting the possible existence of a functioning testicular tumor, or the possible presence of cirrhosis of the liver. Gynecomastia may also be seen in chronic marijuana smokers and heroin addicts, and may sometimes occur without apparent cause.

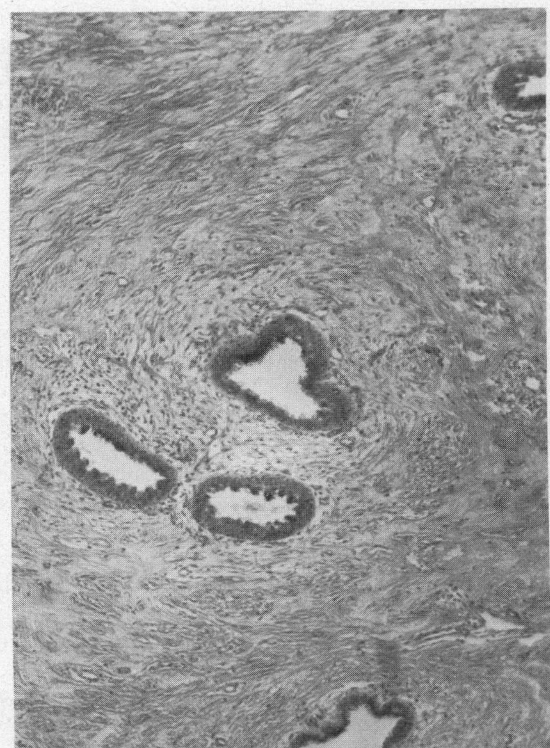

Figure 25–33. Gynecomastia. There is diffuse interductal fibrosis and hyperplasia of lining epithelium.

CARCINOMA

Carcinoma arising in the male breast is a very rare occurrence with a frequency ratio to breast cancer in the female of 1:100. It occurs in advanced age. Because of the scant amount of breast substance in the male, the malignancy rapidly infiltrates to become attached to the overlying skin and underlying thoracic wall. Ulceration through the skin is perhaps more common than in the female. These tumors behave exactly as do the invasive ductal carcinomas in the female, but on the whole tend to have less striking desmoplasia and, hence, less of the hard, scirrhous quality.[75, 76] Some resemble infiltrating lobular carcinoma.[77] Dissemination follows the same pattern as in women, and axillary lymph node involvement is present in about one-half of cases at the time of discovery of the lesion. Distant metastases to the lungs, brain, bone, and liver are common.

Interpretation of Breast Masses

The differential diagnosis of a mass in the female breast is the most important clinical problem that arises in relation to this organ. It is a common clinical problem. The general principle to which most physicians adhere is that *all suspicious areas in the breast must be considered as possible cancer until proved otherwise.* On this basis, the consensus would favor immediate biopsy investigation of all such lesions. This alarmist attitude may result in a certain number of "unnecessary" surgical procedures, but in the long run the greatest good will be done for most patients. Admitting the difficulties in clinical differential diagnosis of breast masses, it is nonetheless desirable to consider the various lesions that may be present according to the age group of the patient. Such a consideration provides a foundation for the clinical approach to the problem and helps to make possible a correct *preoperative* diagnosis.

BREAST MASSES IN WOMEN UNDER 35

FIBROCYSTIC DISEASE. Fibrocystic disease is, without question, the most important cause of breast abnormalities in this age group. These lesions occasionally produce single, unilateral masses but, as has been indicated, many cause multifocal and bilateral involvement that aids in the appropriate diagnosis. Needle aspiration of a solitary cyst may preclude the necessity of "open" biopsy.

FIBROADENOMA. This solitary, circumscribed, well-delimited benign tumor is the most common neoplasm in this age group.

MASTITIS. These focal or diffuse infections develop particularly during pregnancy and nursing. They are usually accompanied by local and systemic signs of inflammation, rendering the diagnosis reasonably apparent. In the presence of these inflammatory reactions, it may be justifiable to observe the process for a reasonable time to determine whether or not it may totally disappear. Persistence of the mass, however, requires biopsy.

TRAUMATIC FAT NECROSIS. This is a rare disorder that can be diagnosed only in the presence of a well-defined clinical history of injury. In the absence of such a history, this diagnosis can be established only by histologic examination.

CARCINOMA OF BREAST. Although malignancy is uncommon in this age group, it cannot be excluded on this basis. In clinical practice, it is distinctly more common than traumatic fat necrosis.

BREAST MASSES IN WOMEN BETWEEN 35 AND 50

This age range is most subject to the development of breast masses.

FIBROCYSTIC DISEASE. This is the most common cause of abnormal lesions in the breast in this age group also. All variants of this disorder may be encountered, but the variants that show epithelial hyperplasia are perhaps more frequent. Since this lesion is associated with a higher-than-usual attack rate of cancer, surgical exploration is strongly indicated. The presence of a diffuse or bilateral involvement cannot be accepted as an indication for nonoperative observation.

CARCINOMA. Mammary cancer is frequent in this age range, and ranks second only to cystic disease as a cause of masses. Any one of the many forms of carcinoma may be present, but the invasive, duct-derived variety is unquestionably the most prevalent.

FIBROADENOMA. This benign tumor is distinctly less common in this age group than in younger women.

TRAUMATIC FAT NECROSIS. Since no age is immune to this lesion, it also occurs in this age group.

MASTITIS. Acute inflammations are less common in this somewhat older age group, presumably because of the lower pregnancy rate.

PAPILLOMA. Papillomas of the breast must be included in the differential diagnosis of lumps, although it is recognized that these lesions are frequently so small as to be entirely occult. The abnormal discharge from the nipple is the most common presenting feature, but occasionally this secretion may be accompanied by alterations in breast consistency.

BREAST MASSES IN WOMEN OVER 50

CARCINOMA. This is the most common cause of abnormal masses in this age group.

FIBROCYSTIC DISEASE. Cystic disease occurs at or just after the menopause, and therefore must also be considered as an important cause of breast pathology in this group.

FAT NECROSIS. In the postmenopausal group, the atrophy of the breast parenchyma causes a relative increase in the amount of fat in the stroma. Accordingly, the breast in this age group is perhaps more subject to injury than in younger women.

PAGET'S DISEASE OF BREAST. This is given a separate heading, because clinically it is often confused with dermatitis. In this age group, involutional atrophy of the skin predisposes to inflammatory conditions, and hence the eczematoid nature of the nipple lesions may deceive the patient into considering the process as a simple dermatitis.

ACUTE MASTITIS. Inflammations in this age group are quite rare.

PAPILLOMA. These benign tumors may occur and produce abnormal discharge.

The chief value of any such differential diagnosis lies merely in the collection of a list of entities that require consideration in the attempt to establish a correct preoperative diagnosis. Under no circumstances is it to be implied that the differential features permit a definite diagnosis without further investigative procedures.

1. Meyer, J. S.: Cell proliferation in normal human breast ducts, fibroadenomas and other ductal hyperplasias measured by nuclear labeling with tritium-labelled thymidine. Hum. Pathol. *8*:67, 1977.
2. Ozzello, L.: Ultrastructure of the human mammary gland. *In* Somers, C. S. (ed.): Pathology Decennial, Genital and Mammary. New York, Appleton-Century-Crofts, 1975, p. 311.
3. Rosai, J.: Ackerman's Surgical Pathology. 6th ed. St. Louis, C. V. Mosby Co., 1981, p. 1087.
4. Rees, B. J., et al.: Nipple retraction in duct ectasia. Br. J. Surg. *64*:577, 1977.
5. Azzopardi, J. G. (ed.): Problems in Breast Pathology. London, W. B. Saunders Co., 1979.
6. Adair, F. E., and Munzer, J. T.: Fat necrosis of the female breast: A report of 110 cases. Am. J. Surg. *74*:117, 1947.

7. Winer, L.H., et al.: Tissue reactions to injected silicone liquids. Arch. Dermatol. *90*:588, 1964.
8. Foote, F. W., and Stewart, H. E.: Comparative study of cancerous vs. noncancerous breasts. Ann. Surg. *121*:6, 197, 1945.
9. Warren, S.: The prognosis of benign lesions of the female breast. Surg. *19*:32, 1946.
10. Fisher, E., et al.: The pathology of invasive breast cancer: A syllabus derived from the findings of the National Surgical Adjuvant Breast Project. Cancer *36*:1, 1975.
11. McDivitt, R. W.: Breast Carcinoma. Hum. Pathol. *9*:3, 1978.
12. Gompel, C., and Van Kerkem, C.: The Breast. *In* Silverberg, S. G. (ed.): Principles and Practice of Surgical Pathology. New York, John Wiley and Sons, 1983, pp. 245–295.
13. Haagensen, C. D., et al. (eds.): Breast Carcinoma: Risk and Detection. Philadelphia, W. B. Saunders Co., 1981.
14. Bartow, S A., et al.: Fibrocystic disease: A continuing enigma. Pathol. Annu. *17*:93, 1982.
15. Love, S. M., et al.: Fibrocystic disease of the breast—a non-disease? N. Engl. J. Med. *307*:1010, 1982.
16. Frantz, V. K., et al.: Incidence of chronic cystic disease in so-called "normal breast." A study based on 225 postmortem examinations. Cancer *4*:762, 1951.
17. Haagensen, C. D.: Diseases of the Breast. Philadelphia, W. B. Saunders Co., 1971.
18. Golinger, R. C.: Hormones and the pathophysiology of cystic mastopathy. Surg. Gynecol. Obstet. *146*:273, 1978.
19. Wellings, S. R.: Development of human breast cancer. Adv. Cancer Res. *31*:287, 1980.
20. Bradlow, H. L., et al.: Steroid hormone accumulation in human breast cyst fluid. Cancer Res. *41*:105, 1981.
21. LiVolsi, V. L., et al.: Fibrocystic disease in oral contraceptive use. A histopathologic evaluation of epithelial atypia. N. Engl. J. Med. *299*:381, 1978.
22. Rivera-Pomar, J. M., et al.: Focal fibrous disease of the breast. Virchow Arch. [Pathol. Anatl.] *386*:59, 1980.
23. Jensen, H. M., et al.: Preneoplastic lesions in human breast. Science *191*:295, 1976.
24. Nomura, A., et al.: Epidemiologic characteristics of benign breast disease. Am. J. Epidemiol. *105*:505, 1977.
25. Haagensen, D. E., Jr.: Biochemical relationship between gross cystic disease and breast carcinoma. *In* Haagensen, C. D., et al. (eds.): Breast Carcinoma: Risk and Detection. Philadelphia, W. B. Saunders Co., 1981, pp. 300–338.
26. Ackerman, L. V., and Katzenstein, A. L.: The concept of minimal breast cancer and the pathologist's role in the diagnosis of carcinoma. Cancer *39*:2755, 1977.
27. Kodlin, D., et al.: Chronic mastopathy and breast cancer: A follow-up study. Cancer *39*:2603, 1977.
28. Ashikari, R., et al.: A clinicopathologic study of atypical lesions of the breast. Cancer *33*:310, 1974.
29. Hart, W. R., et al.: Cystosarcoma phyllodes: A clinicopathologic study of 26 hypercellular periductal stromal tumors of the breast. Am. J. Clin. Pathol. *70*:211, 1978.
30. Blichert-Toft, M., et al.: Clinical course of cystosarcoma phyllodes related to histologic appearance. Surg.Gynecol. Obstet. *140*:929, 1975.
31. Norris, H. J., and Taylor, H.B.: Relationship of the histologic features to behavior of cystosarcoma phyllodes. Cancer *20*:2090, 1967.
32. Kraus, F. T., and Neubecker, R. D.: The differential diagnosis of papillary tumors of the breast. Cancer *15*:444, 1962.
33. Perzin, K. H., and Lattes, R.: Papillary adenoma of the nipple: A clinical pathologic study. Cancer *29*:996, 1972.
34. Pollard, H. M.: Welcoming remarks in a breast cancer symposium. Cancer *28*:1368, 1971.
35. Silverberg, E.: Cancer statistics. Cancer *34*:7, 1984.
36. Leidman, H.: Cancer of the breast. Statistical and epidemiological data. American Cancer Society Professional Education Publication, 1976.
37. Kalache, A., and Vessey, M.: Risk factors for breast cancer. Clin. Oncol. *1*:661, 1982.
38. Wynder, E. L., et al.: The epidemiology of breast cancer in 785 United States Caucasian women. Cancer *41*:2341, 1978.
39. Miller, A., et al.: The epidemiology and etiology of breast cancer. N. Engl. J. Med. *313*:1240, 1981.
40. Ing, R., et al.: Unilateral breast feeding and breast cancer. Lancet *2*:242, 1977.
41. Pike, M. C., et al.: Breast cancer in young women and use of oral contraceptives: Possible modifying effect of formulation and age at use. Lancet *2*:926, 1983.
42. Holdaway, I. M., and Friesen, H.G.: Hormone binding by human mammary carcinomas. Cancer Res. *37*:1946, 1977.
43. McMahon, B., et al.: Urine estrogens, frequency of ovulation and breast cancer risk. J. Natl. Cancer Inst., in press.
44. Bittner, J. J.: Some possible effects of nursing on mammary gland tumor incidence in mice. Science *84*:162, 1936.
45. Speigelman, S.: Viruses and human cancer. Prog. Hematol. *9*:305, 1975.
46. Wyke, J. A.: Oncogenic viruses. J. Pathol. *135*:39, 1981.
47. McDivitt, R. W., et al.: Tumors of the breast. Atlas of Tumor Pathology. Washington, D.C., Armed Forces Institute of Pathology, 1968.
48. Gallager, H. S.: Classification of breast neoplasms. *In* Gallager, H.S., et al. (eds.): The Breast. St. Louis, C. V. Mosby Co., 1978, pp. 61–74.
49. Bloom, H. J., et al.: Host resistance in survival of carcinoma of the breast. Study of 104 cases of medullary carcinoma in a series of 1,411 cases of breast cancer followed for 20 years. Br. Med. J. *3*:181, 1970.
50. Ridolfi, R. L., et al.: Medullary carcinoma of the breast. A clinicopathologic study with a 10-year follow-up. Cancer *40*:1305, 1977.
51. Silverberg, S. G., et al.: Colloid carcinoma of the breast. Am. J. Clin. Pathol. *55*:355, 1971.
52. Toker, C.: Further observations of Paget's disease of the nipple. J. Natl. Cancer Inst. *38*:79, 1967.
53. Ashikari, R., et al.: Paget's disease of the breast. Cancer *26*:680, 1970.
54. Wheeler, J. E., and Enterline, H. T.: Lobular carcinoma of the breast: *in situ* and infiltrating. Pathol. Annu. *11*:61, 1976.
55. Ashikari, R., et al.: Infiltrating lobular carcinoma of the breast. Cancer *31*:110, 1973.
56. Ensebi, V., et al.: Morphofunctional differentiation in lobular carcinoma of the breast. Histopathology *1*:301, 1977.
57. Foote, S. W., and Stewart, S. W.: Lobular carcinoma *in situ:* A rare form of mammary cancer. Am. J. Pathol. *17*:491, 1941.
58. Andersen, J. A.: Lobular carcinoma *in situ:* An approach to rational treatment. Cancer *39*:2597, 1977.
59. Rosen, P. P.: Lobular carcinoma *in situ* of the breast. Am. J. Surg. Pathol. *2*:225, 1978.
60. Silverberg, S.: Staging in the therapy of cancer of the breast. Am. J. Clin. Pathol. *64*:756, 1975.
61. Haagensen, C. D., et al.: Metastasis of carcinoma of the breast to the periphery of the regional lymph node filter. Ann. Surg. *169*:174, 1969.
62. Foster, R. S., Jr., et al.: Breast self-examination practices and breast-cancer stage. N. Engl. J. Med. *299*:265, 1978.
63. Montague, A. C., et al. (eds.): Breast Cancer. New York, Alan R. Liss, 1977, pp. 165, 177, 189, 203, 247.
64. Culliton, B. J.: Mammography controversy. Science *198*:171, 1977.
65. Bland, K. I.: Analysis of breast cancer screening in women younger than 50 years. J.A.M.A. *245*:1037, 1981.
66. Mammography Guidelines 1983: Background statement and update of cancer-related check-up guidelines for breast cancer detection in asymptomatic women age 40–49. Cancer *33*:255, 1983.
67. Bennadonna, G., et al.: Combination chemotherapy as an adjuvant treatment in operable breast cancer. N. Engl. J. Med. *294*:408, 1976.
68. Godolphin, W., et al.: Estrogen receptor quantitation and staging as complementary prognostic indicators in breast cancer. Int. J. Cancer *28*:677, 1981.
69. Lippmann, M. E., and Allegra, J. C.: Current concepts: Receptors in breast cancer. N. Engl. J. Med. *299*:930, 1978.
70. Adair, F. E., et al.: Long-term followup of breast cancer patients: The 30-year report. Cancer *33*:1145, 1974.
71. Oberman, H. A.: Sarcomas of the breast. Cancer *18*:1233, 1965.
72. Barnes, L., and Pietraszkas, M.: Sarcomas of the breast. A clinicopathologic analysis of ten cases. Cancer *40*:1577, 1977.
73. Wilson, J. D., et al.: The pathogenesis of gynecomastia. Adv. Intern. Med. *25*:1, 1980.
74. Bannayan, G. A., and Hadju, S. I.: Gynecomastia: Clinicopathologic study of 351 cases. Am. J. Clin. Pathol. *57*:431, 1972.
75. Norris, H. J., and Taylor, H. B.: Carcinoma of the male breast. Cancer *23*:1428, 1969.
76. Satiani, B., et al.: Cancer of the male breast: A 30-year experience. Ann. Surg. *44*:86, 1978.
77. Giffler, R. F., and Kay, S.: Small cell carcinoma of the male mammary gland. A tumor resembling infiltrating lobular carcinoma. Am. J. Clin. Pathol. *66*:715, 1976.

26 THE ENDOCRINE SYSTEM

In the following sections, each of the endocrine glands is discussed individually. It must not be forgotten, however, that multiple endocrine glands occasionally are affected concomitantly in the individual patient in the complex and intriguing endocrinopathies known as the multiple endocrine neoplasia (MEN) syndromes (p. 988). Also not to be forgotten is the possibility that endocrinopathies may be caused by nonendocrine neoplasms that elaborate hormones or hormone-like products. These so-called "paraneoplastic syndromes" (p. 255) may closely simulate disorders having origin in the endocrine glands.

Pituitary Gland

NORMAL

No organ packs so much critical function into so little space as the pituitary. In the adult it weighs about 0.5 gm and its greatest diameter is in the range of 10 to 15 mm. During pregnancy it enlarges twofold. It is composed of two functionally separate components—the anterior lobe (adenohypophysis) made up of a melange of secretory epithelial cells, and a posterior lobe (neurohypophysis) representing an extension of the brain. The anterior lobe is derived from an evagination of the roof of the primitive oral canal called Rathke's pouch, which extends superiorly toward the base of the brain to come to lie anteriorly to an outpouching of the floor of the third ventricle, constituting the anlage of the posterior lobe. Growth of the sphenoid bone creates the enclosing sella turcica, the floor of which detaches Rathke's pouch from its origins. Occasionally, rests of epithelial cells persist within or below the sphenoid as accessory, sometimes functional, pharyngeal pituitary tissue. In contrast, the connection to the base of the brain persists as the pituitary stalk, providing direct anatomic continuity between the neurohypophysis and hypothalamus. A thick extension of the dura called the diaphragma sellae roofs over the sella; it has a central orifice through which the stalk passes. When this aperture is too large for the stalk or there are other diaphragmatic defects, the arachnoid mater may herniate through when there is a prolonged increase in cerebrospinal fluid (CSF) pressure to compress the pituitary. The blood supply to the pituitary has many similarities to that of the liver.[1] Some is derived from branches of the internal carotid arteries, but most is furnished by a portal system derived from capillaries in the floor of the third ventricle. By coalescence these capillaries form long parallel vessels that course along the surface of the pituitary stalk, eventually to connect with vascular sinusoids in the anterior lobe. There are also portal interconnections between stalk and anterior and posterior lobes. Thus, factors or hormones elaborated in the hypothalamus are readily delivered to the anterior and posterior lobes.

Histologically the posterior and anterior lobes are totally dissimilar. The posterior lobe is composed of tangled nerve fibers through which are scattered occasional glial-like pituicytes. Electron microscopy reveals that the unmyelinated nerve fibers contain numerous membrane-bound, secretory granules of stored posterior pituitary hormones. There is no pars intermedia in the human but its location is sometimes marked by small, colloid-filled cysts or clefts. The anterior lobe, making up about 75 to 80% of the pituitary, is composed of round-to-polygonal epithelial cells disposed in cords and nests (sometimes forming pseudoglandular lumina) separated by a rich fibrovascular network. At one time the cells of the anterior lobe were classified as eosinophils, basophils, or chromophobes on the basis of their uptake of acidic and basic dyes, but the distinctions were at best unsatisfactory. Immunoelectron microscopy and immunocytochemical methods using specific hormonal antibodies now reliably distinguish the various cells responsible for secretion of each of the anterior pituitary hormones. Each tropic hormone is produced by one type of cell and stored in secretory granules of somewhat distinctive size and nature. The gonadotropins, however, are both elaborated by one cell type.[2] By immunocytochemical methods, about 25% of the anterior pituitary cells do not apparently contain any of the known hormones and so conform to the "chromophobes" of the past. Electron microscopy of these cells, however, usually reveals a sparsity of secretory granules, and so they are thought to be degranulated rather than nonfunctional. The salient features of the cells of the anterior pituitary are presented in Table 26–1.

The hypothalamus is a major regulator of both anterior and posterior pituitary secretory activity.[3] The neurohypophyseal hormones, vasopressin (antidiuretic

Table 26–1. CYTOLOGIC DETAILS OF ANTERIOR PITUITARY CELLS

Cell Type/ Relative Frequency	Hormone	H and E	Mallory's Trichrome/ PAS	Granules	Immunocyto-chemistry
Lactotroph (15–20%)	Prolactin (PRL) (polypeptide)	Acidophilic to chromophobic	Acidophilic, PAS negative	Abundant to sparse 200–900 nm	Strong to PRL, may cross-react with GH
Somatotroph (40–50%)	Growth hormone (GH) somatotropin (polypeptide)	Acidophilic rarely chromophobic	Acidophilic, PAS negative	Abundant to sparse 350–450 nm	Strong to GH, may cross-react with PRL
Corticotroph (15–20%)	Corticotropin (ACTH) (polypeptide)	Basophilic	Basophilic, PAS positive	Abundant 300–350 nm	Strong to ACTH
Thyrotroph (5%)	Thyrotropin (TSH) (glycoprotein)	Basophilic	Basophilic, PAS positive	Numerous 90–150 nm	Strong to TSH
Gonadotroph (5%)	Follicle-stimulating (FSH) Luteinizing (LH) (glycoproteins)	Basophilic to chromophobic	Often basophilic, PAS ±	Numerous 250–350 nm	Same cell reacts to FSH and LH
Nonsecretory undifferentiated cell (15–20%)	None	Chromophobic	Chromophobic	None to scant small granules	No reaction to any antibody
Nonsecretory oncocyte (rare)	None	Chromophobic to acidophilic	Acidophilic to chromophobic	More numerous mitochondria	No reaction to any antibody

hormone—ADH) and oxytocin, are produced in neurosecretory cells in the hypothalamus and are then transported within vesicles along the axons that end in the posterior lobe, in which they are stored awaiting secretion. In contrast, adenohypophyseal function is regulated by "releasing" and "inhibiting" factors synthesized in the hypothalamus and carried to the anterior pituitary through the portal system. Without delving into all the details, releasing factors have been well characterized for thyrotropin (TSH), luteinizing hormone (LH), follicle-stimulating hormone (FSH), and corticotropin (ACTH), and less assuredly for growth hormone (GH) and prolactin (PRL). Two release-inhibiting factors of hypothalamic origin have been identified. One is well established, namely, somatostatin, which regulates GH production; the other is prolactin-inhibiting factor (PIF). Somatostatin production is not limited to the hypothalamus and its effects extend beyond the inhibition of GH release. There are some uncertainties about PIF. Dopamine, of neurogenic origin, inhibits PRL secretion, and it is not clear whether dopamine itself serves as the inhibitory factor or instead stimulates the secretion of PIF. Other influences also contribute to the regulation of anterior secretory function. Hormones elaborated by target endocrine glands in negative feedback loops inhibit anterior lobe cells. For example, thyroid hormones inhibit thyrotroph activity and glucocorticoids do the same with corticotrophs.

PATHOLOGY

Disorders of the pituitary must be divided into those involving primarily the anterior lobe and those involving primarily the posterior lobe. However, certain lesions—tumors, for example—may damage both.

Diseases affecting mainly the adenohypophysis come to attention either as the consequence of increased or decreased production of tropic hormones or because of local space-occupying effects. Obviously, small lesions may remain entirely occult whatever their nature and may be discovered only at autopsy. The term *hyperpituitarism* is used to mean increased secretion of one of the tropic hormones of the anterior lobe, generally by a functioning tumor or tumors of the anterior lobe. Rarely it is hypothalamic in origin or related to loss of feedback inhibition by target organ hormones. For example, with destruction of the adrenals, say, by metastatic cancer, the loss of corticosteroids will initiate hyperfunction of the corticotrophs. *Hypopituitarism* has more varied origins and appears whenever there is destruction of at least 75% of the anterior lobe. Infrequently, it is hypothalamic in origin.

The local consequences of anterior pituitary disease can be divided into three patterns.[4] (1) *Enlargement of the sella turcica*, on x-ray or CT scan, is a major marker of pituitary disease and is caused by any expansile lesion such as a neoplasm (primary or secondary) or chronic edematous enlargement of the gland. (2) *Visual disorders* may bring the pituitary pathology to the patient's attention. Classically it takes the form of bilateral homonymous hemianopsia, but other field defects are sometimes encountered. They result from encroachment of an expanding pituitary lesion on the immediately adjacent optic chiasm and/or optic nerves. (3) Infrequently, large pituitary tumors bulge upward into the floor of the brain and *raise intracranial pressure* sufficiently to produce headache, nausea, vomiting, and other manifestations reminiscent of a brain tumor (Fig. 26–1). Frequently the individual patient has more than one of these findings. A functioning pituitary adenoma not only may cause hyperpituitarism but also, with sufficient increase in size, may expand the sella turcica and produce visual disturbances as well as manifestations of a space-occupying lesion. On occasion the hyperpituitarism is suddenly converted to hypopituitarism when a neoplasm undergoes spontaneous infarction as it out-

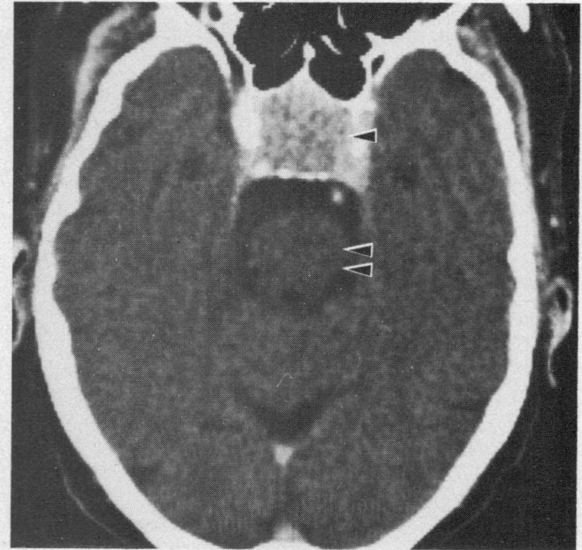

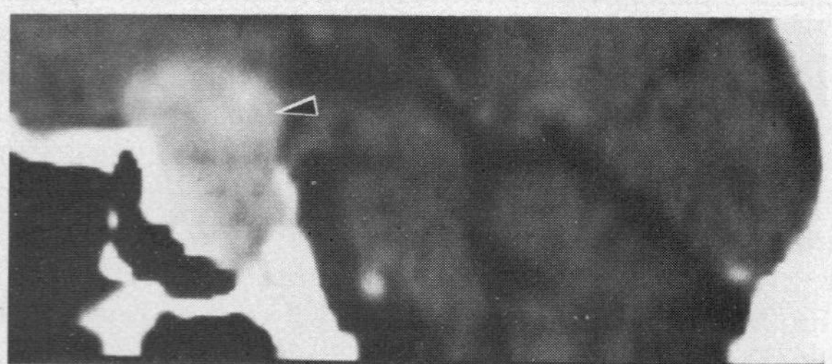

Figure 26–1. *Above,* CT scan of transverse plane of skull at level of pituitary fossa, revealing enlargement of sella caused by an expansile pituitary adenoma *(arrow).* Compare its size with transverse dimension of brain stem *(double arrow). Below,* Computer reconstruction of the same tumor in sagittal plane *(arrow).* It has bulged out of sella turcica, producing a moderately enlarged suprasellar mass. (Courtesy of Dr. Calvin Rumbaugh, Department of Radiology, Brigham and Women's Hospital, Harvard Medical School.)

grows its blood supply. The major anterior pituitary diseases can be encompassed within two categories: (1) hyperpituitarism—anterior lobe tumors and (2) disorders associated with hypopituitarism.

HYPERPITUITARISM—ANTERIOR LOBE TUMORS

For all practical purposes, *hyperfunction of the anterior pituitary means an adenoma;* carcinomas of the anterior lobe are exceedingly rare. The great majority of adenomas are monoclonal and so elaborate a single tropic hormone. *For unknown reasons, PRL-secreting, GH-secreting, and ACTH-secreting adenomas make up 90 to 95% of functional tumors collectively.* Neoplasms producing TSH, LH, and FSH (strangely, the glycoprotein hormones of the anterior lobe) are very uncommon. In one collection of 564 pituitary adenomas, only four elaborated TSH.[5] On occasion an adenoma is associated with the production of two hormones, most often GH and PRL, but, as pointed out in Table 26–1, both of these hormones can sometimes be identified in one cell type. In some other instances the immunoperoxidase method reveals only a single hormone in the tumor cells, and the excess production of the other hormone must be attributed to a secondary effect of the neoplasm on the hypophyseothalamic regulatory apparatus. There are also rare instances of so-called mixed adenomas producing two hormones arising in two distinct populations of cells. On the other extreme are the nonfunctional adenomas (formerly called chromophobe adenomas) that, by virtue of their expansile growth, destroy the surrounding normal parenchyma and so lead to hypopituitarism (discussed on p. 1196). In an analysis of a large series of adenomas, about 25 to 35% were nonfunctional, and the remainder secreted, in order of frequency, PRL (25 to 30%), GH (20 to 25%), ACTH (10 to 15%), and mixed hormones (5%). All the rare types collectively account for only 5%.[6]

MORPHOLOGY. It is impossible on gross examination and light microscopy with routine tissue stains to differentiate one type of adenoma from another reliably. Nonetheless, certain somewhat distinctive features can be identified and highlighted by the trichrome and PAS stains (as detailed in Table 26–1). Ultimate confirmation requires the use of immunocytochemical methods.[7] Adenomas, whatever the cell type, range from microscopic foci (referred to, when less than 10 mm in diameter, as **microadenomas**) to large masses sometimes approaching 10 cm in diameter. Among the functional adenomas, those producing GH generally tend to be the largest, possibly because the endocrinopathy they produce develops insidiously, perhaps over the span of decades, and they achieve large size before being discovered (Fig. 26–2). PRL- and ACTH-secreting lesions range widely in size from microadenomas to expansile masses. Microadenomas are surprisingly common and were found in 27% of an unselected series of autopsies, of which half were PRL secreting.[8] Are such lesions truly minute neoplasms that would, in time, enlarge or are they foci of insignificant hyperplasia? Contributing to the dilemma is the fact that many of these small lesions are poorly encapsulated, an atypical feature for benign neoplasms. However, even large adenomas sometimes have only a delicate capsule that may well be incomplete. Bulkier lesions enlarge the sella turcica, erode the clinoid processes, and sometimes, because of the poor encapsulation, rupture through the diaphragma to injure the optic chiasm or optic nerves. **Large lesions penetrate into surrounding structures.** Thus, adenomas may give the deceptive appearance of invasion into the cavernous sinuses, the nasal sinuses, the base of the brain, or other contiguous structures. Such aggressive local behavior does not imply malignancy. On transection the neoplasms are usually soft, red-brown, and discrete despite the lack of a capsule and despite extension along broad fronts into contiguous structures. Larger lesions may develop foci of ischemic necrosis, cystic softening, and hemorrhages (sometimes called **pituitary apoplexy**). Occasionally, very large adenomas undergo virtual total infarction as the expansile pressure compresses their blood supply. In this connection, you may recall that much of the blood supply is derived from the low-pressure portal system vulnerable to compressive occlusion. The non-neoplastic anterior lobe may be relatively preserved, may be markedly attenuated, or may have disappeared, depending on the size of the neoplasm.

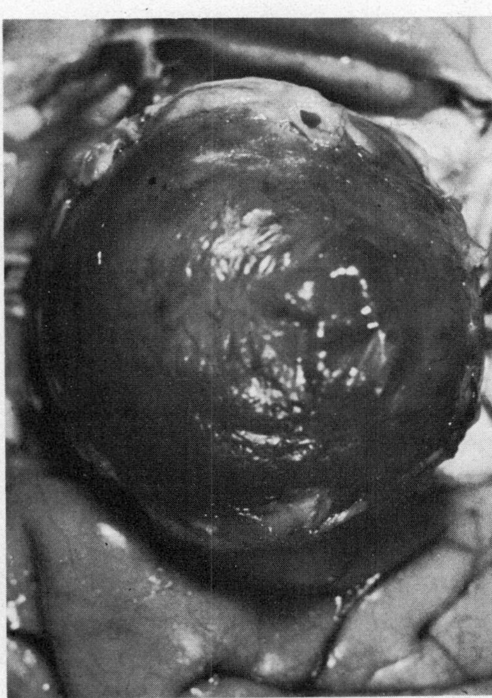

Figure 26–2. Close-up detail of a pituitary adenoma still attached to brain. Compressed vessels and nerves are apparent above periphery.

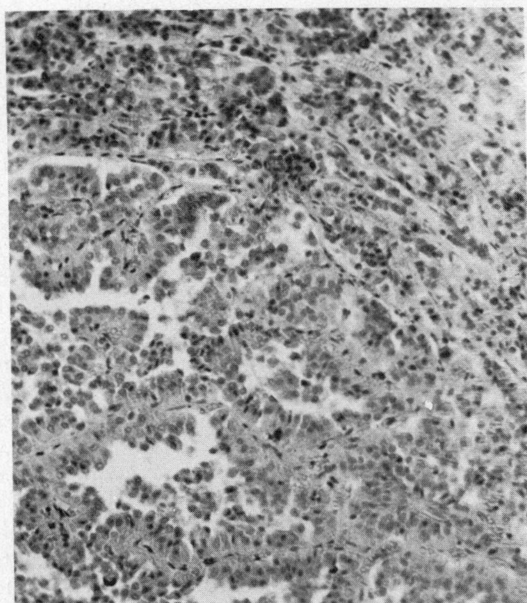

Figure 26–3. A pituitary adenoma illustrating a tendency to papillary growth and poor demarcation from surrounding pituitary substance. Tumor cells are uniform in size and compress adjacent normal gland *(above)*.

Microscopically, all adenomas have a fairly uniform appearance. The cells are disposed in sheets, cords, or nests having only a delicate, vascularized stroma. Sometimes, pseudoglandular or papillary formations are produced (Fig. 26–3). Small or large foci of coagulative necrosis may be present; indeed, in some larger lesions virtually all the cells may have become shadowy carcasses. Cytologically the cells usually are remarkably uniform and closely resemble their normal counterparts. On the other hand, in some neoplasms there is considerable cellular and nuclear pleomorphism bordering on anaplasia. When such cytologic changes are found in neoplasms that have extended beyond the sella, the question arises—is it a cancer? To avoid overdiagnosis, **most experts require evidence of metastatic dissemination for the diagnosis of carcinoma of the anterior pituitary.** As might be expected, the more differentiated the cells, the more abundant are the cytoplasmic granules, but lesions composed almost entirely of sparsely granulated cells may have marked secretory activity, accounting for the past dilemma of so-called "functioning chromophobe adenomas."

Certain correlations can be drawn between the cytologic features mentioned in Table 26–1 and functional activity. Adenomas associated with the production of GH (somatotroph adenomas) and/or PRL are usually composed of richly or sparsely granulated cells. The former reveal brightly eosinophilic, orange-to-red cytoplasmic granules with conventional stains **(eosinophilic adenomas).** Sparsely granulated cells suggest **chromophobe adenomas.** In contrast, neoplasms associated with ACTH secretion (corticotroph adenomas) usually have abundant granules, stain darkly, and react strongly with the PAS stain, and so are called **"basophilic adenomas."** A distinctive alteration, referred to as Crooke's hyaline change and sometimes seen in the corticotrophs, will be discussed in the consideration of Cushing's syndrome (p. 1239).

Primary carcinomas of the anterior lobe should be mentioned. They are rare, are usually sufficiently undifferentiated so that the cell type of origin cannot be identified, and only rarely elaborate hormones. There may be some cytologic anaplasia, but it is rarely enough to differentiate reliably the carcinoma from an adenoma. As already pointed out, local invasion is also unreliable; thus, evidence of metastatic spread is the only valid criterion of malignancy.

CLINICAL COURSE. Pituitary adenomas occur in both sexes at any age but are somewhat more common in men, particularly between the ages of 20 and 50. Rarely, the pituitary tumor is accompanied by lesions in other endocrine glands in MEN I (p. 988). Adenomas may come to clinical attention because of their hormonal function. Alternatively, the local effects of the expanding lesions may constitute the presenting complaints, particularly with the 25% that are nonsecretory and are discussed later as potential causes of hypopituitarism. Many remain occult, however, particularly microadenomas, and are discovered only at autopsy. We need not delve deeply into the endocrinologic manifestations of all functioning adenomas; remarks will be confined largely to brief characterizations of the syndromes associated with the three common types.

Hyperprolactinemia is now recognized to be the most common endocrinopathy caused by pituitary tumors. Classically (but not always) it is marked by the amenorrhea-galactorrhea syndrome in women.[9] Since these manifestations are so overt, PRL-secreting adenomas are usually discovered while very small, i.e., microadenomas. There are, however, many other causes of hyperprolactinemia and/or amenorrhea and galactorrhea; for example, lesions in the hypothalamus, drugs that impair dopaminergic transmission (methyldopa, reserpine), and estrogen therapy. Thus, the clinical diagnosis of a prolactinoma requires not only the confirmation of elevated plasma levels of PRL but also evidence of an anterior lobe neoplasm such as visual field defects or enlargement of the sella. When these neoplasms arise in males they usually come to attention because of local effects, and so the adenomas generally are much larger. Rarely, they cause decreased libido or infertility. Although surgical excision (or sometimes irradiation) is the standard form of treatment for all pituitary adenomas, promising results have been obtained from the administration of bromocriptine. This agent acts as a dopamine agonist and, by stimulating hypothalamic function, increases the output of prolactin-inhibiting factor. Unfortunately, this form of therapy may not reduce the size of the tumor and has other limitations.[10]

Excess secretion of GH by somatotroph adenomas induces gigantism in the prepubertal child and acromegaly in adults. *Gigantism* appears when the epiphyses have not fused and the high plasma levels of somatotropin, perhaps mediated by somatomedins, stimulate extraordinary skeletal growth to produce the pathetic circus giants of the past, sometimes 8 to 9 feet tall. Despite the size of these individuals, myopathies, neuropathies, and arthropathies appear early in life, reducing these giants to tottering hulks. Fortunately, this condition has virtually disappeared because of early recognition and removal of the adenoma. *Acromegaly*, on the other hand, is the second most common hyperpituitary state. The disordered growth is far more insidious than gigantism, and although it may begin in early adult life, the physical changes are usually not recognized until years to decades later. The insidiously appearing somatic changes are often not detectable without earlier photographs for comparison. Most striking is the enlargement and coarsening of the facial features, hands, and feet, namely, "megaly" of the acral parts. When fully expressed, the protruding jaw, thick lips, overly large tongue, and accentuated orbital and frontal ridges can be recognized at a distance (Fig. 26–4). A host of metabolic changes may also be present, among which are glucose intolerance (and sometimes overt diabetes mellitus), osteoporosis, and hypertension. Also, these patients frequently have visual field defects and enlargement of the sella because somatotropic adenomas often become large by the time they are discovered. Surgical excision is the treatment of choice, but some success has been achieved with bromocriptine.

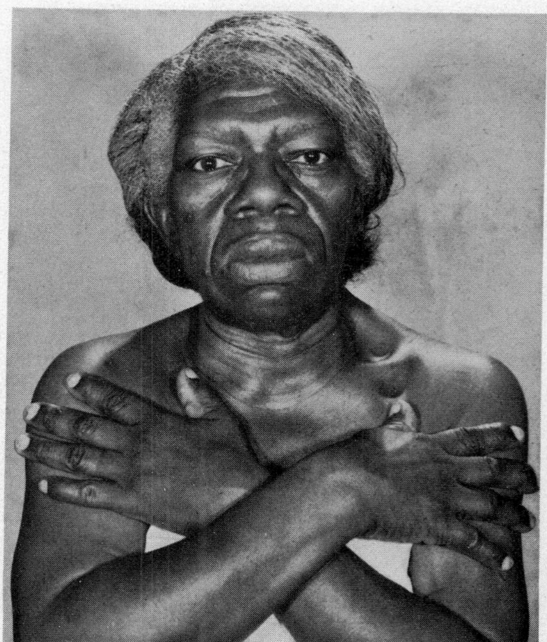

Figure 26–4. Acromegaly in a 60-year-old woman.

Corticotropin-secreting adenomas produce secondary adrenal cortical hyperfunction, known as pituitary *Cushing's syndrome*. An analogous hyperadrenal state (described on p. 1237) may also be caused by adrenal functioning tumors, ectopic production of ACTH by nonendocrine cancers (such as those of the lung), and exogenous adrenal steroids. It is sufficient to note here that the pituitary adenomas giving rise to Cushing's syndrome are usually small, often conform to microadenomas, and (rarely) cause signs and symptoms related to tumorous enlargement of the pituitary.

Secretory pituitary adenomas less regularly induce other syndromes. Most common among these relative rarities are mixed complexes resulting from the simultaneous production of two hormones such as GH and PRL (as noted earlier). Other rarities are TSH-secreting adenomas that induce hyperthyroid syndromes (p. 1203) and the even more exotic gonadotropin-secreting adenomas.

Still other complexities are introduced by the possible effects of the secretory adenoma on the surrounding non-neoplastic pituitary gland. Thus, pressure on the posterior pituitary may impair ADH secretion and add an element of diabetes insipidus to the endocrinopathy. Analogously, an ACTH-secreting adenoma may sometimes lead to hypothyroidism by destruction of the non-neoplastic thyrotrophs. The variable clinical patterns produced by secretory adenomas are almost endless, but it should not be forgotten that they could have their origin in a nonendocrine cancer: for example, the ectopic production of hormones by an undifferentiated bronchogenic carcinoma.

DISORDERS ASSOCIATED WITH HYPOPITUITARISM

Hypofunction of the adenohypophysis may result from lesions in the hypothalamus or in the anterior lobe of the pituitary. Hypothalamic lesions are on the whole extremely rare; only the suprasellar craniopharyngioma, the glioma, and germ cell tumors occur with sufficient frequency to merit description later. Such tumors may produce a variety of clinical syndromes including diabetes insipidus, growth acceleration, stunting of growth, and/or delayed puberty.[11] *More commonly, hypopituitarism arises from destructive processes directly involving the adenohypophysis, the three most common being nonsecretory adenomas, Sheehan's pituitary necrosis, and the empty sella syndrome.* Together they account for over 90% of instances of panhypopituitarism. The remaining causes of pituitary insufficiency include metastatic neoplasms; invasion by a meningioma; disruption of blood supply by systemic arteritis or thrombosis of cavernous venous sinuses; inflammatory destruction of the anterior lobe by sarcoidosis, tuberculosis, or other infections (such as extension of a meningitis); surgical or radiation ablation of the pituitary; and such miscellaneous conditions as Hand-Schüller-Christian disease, Tay-Sachs disease, and hemochromatosis (Fig. 26–5). Whatever the underlying disorder, *pituitary hypofunction is unlikely to be manifest until at least 75% of the anterior lobe is destroyed.* With panlobar destruction, the impairment in tropic hormone production most often becomes evident in the following temporal sequence: gonadotropins, GH (particularly in children), TSH, ACTH, and lastly PRL. Rarely, the pituitary insufficiency manifests itself as an isolated hormone deficiency, most often a lack of GH, less often a gonadotropic insufficiency, and still more infrequently a deficiency of ACTH or TSH. No satisfactory explanation has been offered to explain these unihormonal lacks, but without proof they are attributed to lesions primary in the hypothalamus.[12]

The clinical manifestations of destructive lesions of the adenohypophysis are extremely variable, and many will be mentioned along with the various causative conditions. Only a few comments are necessary here.

Lack of GH per se in the adult is virtually undetectable except by radioimmunoassay. In the prepubertal child it causes retardation of growth, so-called *pituitary dwarfism.* There is symmetric retardation in growth but the legs are often longer in relation to the trunk than in the normal child. Frequently, sexual development is also retarded. This form of dwarfism must be differentiated from that of hypothyroidism (cretinism). The latter is typified by characteristic "mongoloid" facies and, most notably, striking mental retardation that contrast with the normal facial features and mentality of pituitary dwarfs. In female adults the consequences of hypogonadotropism are amenorrhea, loss of axillary and pubic hair, sterility, and atrophy of the ovaries and external genitalia. In the male, hypogonadotropism is manifested by testicular atrophy, sterility, and loss of axillary and pubic hair. Often there is a notable absence of hair or recession of the hairline. All these manifestations in both females and males are directly related to loss of gonadal function followed by atrophy. Other deficits may induce hypothyroidism related to a lack of TSH, or hypoadrenalism related to a deficiency of ACTH, followed in time by atrophy of the thyroid and adrenals. Thus, thyroid, adrenal, or gonadal insufficiency related to deficits of pituitary tropic hormones must be differentiated from primary disorders of these organs. More is said about these difficult differential diagnoses in the consideration of the various endocrine glands, but it suffices here to note that most important are radioimmunoassays for serum levels of tropic hormones. The destructive process, whatever its nature, may also affect the posterior pituitary and add to the symptom complex. It should be noted that panhypopituitarism rarely, if ever, induces weight loss,

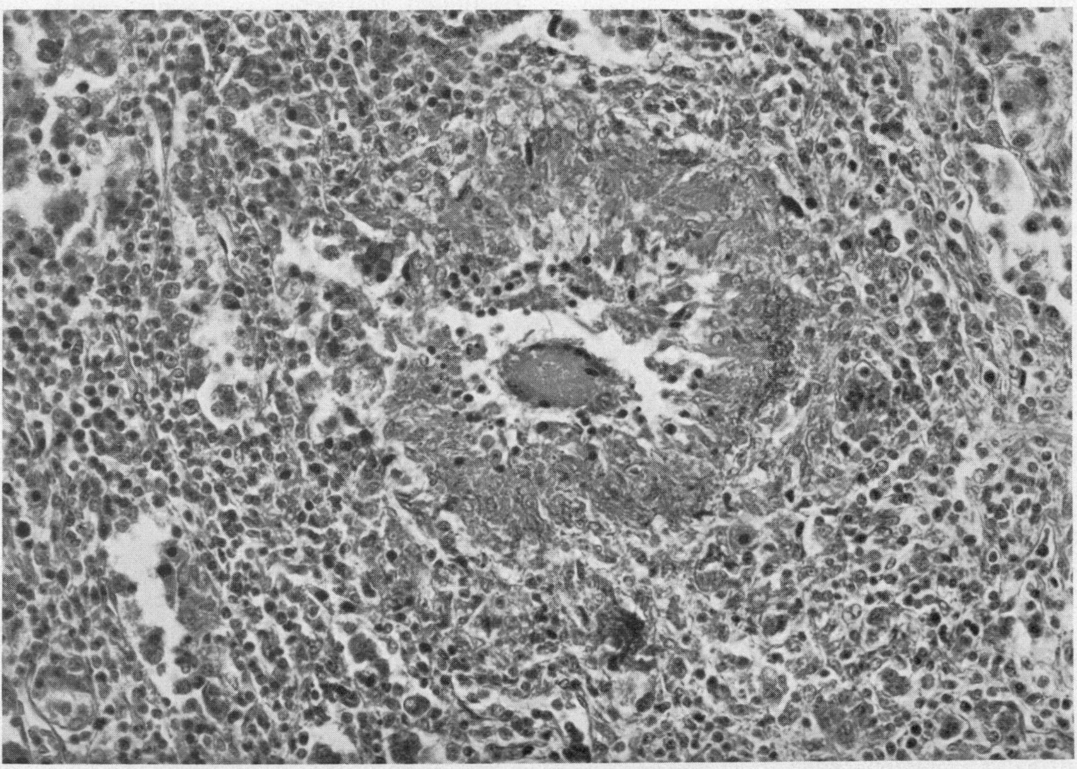

Figure 26–5. Granuloma in anterior lobe of pituitary in a case of generalized sarcoidosis.

and so the older designation of "Simmonds' cachexia" is clearly inappropriate.

Most of the destructive lesions (e.g., tuberculosis, sarcoidosis, and metastatic cancers) that cause hypopituitarism have already been described elsewhere, and remarks will be confined to the four most common causes.

NONSECRETORY (CHROMOPHOBE) PITUITARY ADENOMAS

These tumors may present as space-occupying lesions (discussed on p. 1193) or as tropic hormone insufficiencies. With nonfunctional pituitary adenomas, the hormonal deficits develop slowly over the span of years, and so these nonfunctional tumors often achieve quite large size before they are discovered. On gross inspection they cannot be differentiated from secretory adenomas, but histologically with conventional stains they are apparently composed of chromophobes. The cells may be small and undifferentiated and have only a scant, cleared cytoplasm or an abundant eosinophilic granular cytoplasm that, under the electron microscope, is literally packed with mitochondria. Such cells are called oncocytes, and so the neoplasm is designated an oncocytoma.[6] Immunoelectron microscopy often discloses, in both the chromophobic and oncocytic patterns, small secretory granules about 100 nm in diameter, not sufficient in number to react with any of the antisera to known pituitary tropic hormones.[13] The nonfunction of these cells may, then, be merely a quantitative phenomenon.

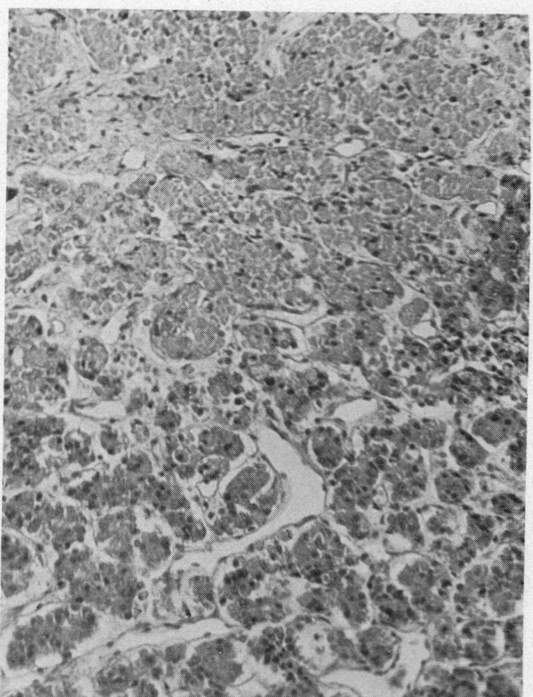

Figure 26–6. Sheehan's syndrome. A recent infarct of pituitary evident as pale-staining shadowy outlines of cells, which contrast with normal nucleated cells immediately below.

SHEEHAN'S SYNDROME

Also known as *postpartum pituitary necrosis, this syndrome results from sudden infarction of the anterior lobe precipitated by obstetric hemorrhage or shock.*[14] It is hypothesized that during pregnancy the anterior pituitary gland enlarges to almost twice its normal size, compressing the vascular sinusoids supplied largely by the portal network at venous pressure. Thus, sudden systemic hypotension precipitates ischemic necrosis of much or all of the anterior lobe, sparing the posterior lobe, which is less vulnerable to anoxia (Fig. 26–6). However, other pathogenetic mechanisms may be involved, such as DIC or (more rarely) sickle cell anemia, cavernous sinus thrombosis, temporal arteritis, or traumatic injury of vessels. With these varied origins, Sheehan's syndrome may be encountered in nonpregnant females as well as in males.[15] In most instances there is destruction of 95 to 99% of the anterior lobe, most evident as a gonadotropic deficiency having the features already described, but possibly accompanied by failure of lactation in the puerperium. Concomitantly the deficiency of TSH and ACTH may induce hypothyroidism and adrenocortical insufficiency.[16] Less extensive destruction of the anterior lobe may be asymptomatic or may present as loss of only one of the tropic hormones. Strangely, the loss of pituitary function may not become evident for years after the initiating event attributed to continued destruction of marginal viable cells as they become trapped in the postinfarction scarring. With substitution therapy or with incomplete destruction of the pituitary, long survival is possible, as indeed is childbearing.

Whatever the pathogenesis, the infarcted adenohypophysis at the outset appears soft, pale, and ischemic or hemorrhagic. Over time the ischemic area is resorbed and replaced by fibrous tissue. In some long-standing cases, the gland scars down to a fibrous nubbin weighing less than 0.1 gm attached to the wall of an empty sella.

EMPTY SELLA SYNDROME

This uncommon condition has a number of origins. Most often it is related to herniation of the arachnoid through some deficit in the diaphragma sellae—either an abnormally large aperture through which the hypophyseal stalk passes or a defect elsewhere. The CSF pressure eventually causes atrophy of the pituitary, creating the appearance of an empty sella (Fig. 26–7). Sometimes, leakage of CSF produces persistent rhinorrhea. Other possible causes are Sheehan's syndrome, total infarction of an adenoma followed by fibrous scarring, and ablation of the gland either by surgery or radiation.[17] In most individuals with this condition, sufficient parenchyma is preserved to prevent pituitary

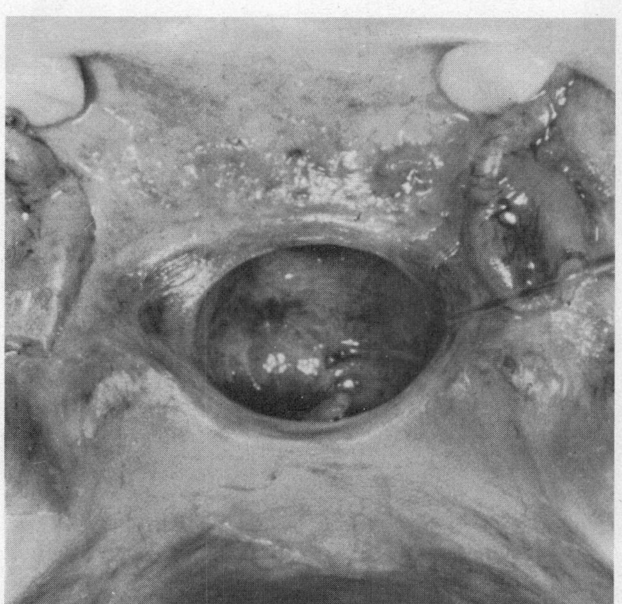
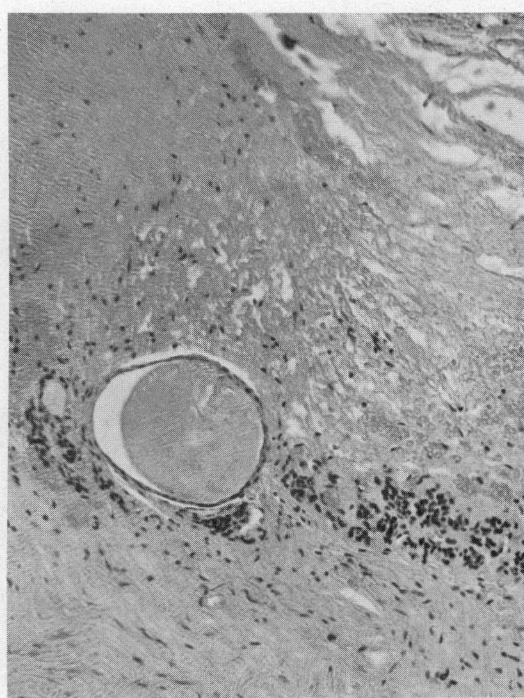

Figure 26–7. *A,* In situ view of sella turcica in a patient dying of far-advanced pituitary insufficiency. Residual gland substance remains in situ and can be seen as a minute nubbin of tissue protruding from midline of posterior wall of sella *(below). B,* Microscopic view of anterior lobe of pituitary illustrated in *A.* Complete fibrous atrophy of anterior lobe is evident above pars intermedia, indicated in photograph by cystic space. Posterior lobe is below and appears normal.

insufficiency, but occasionally there is either panhypopituitarism or inadequate secretion of one or more of the tropic hormones.[18] In some cases the sella is not only empty but also enlarged, and so on radiography or CT scan is readily mistaken for an expansile pituitary neoplasm.

HYPOTHALAMIC SUPRASELLAR TUMORS

Neoplasms in this location are extremely uncommon but may induce hypofunction or hyperfunction of the anterior pituitary, diabetes insipidus, or combinations of these manifestations.[19] The most commonly implicated lesions are gliomas (sometimes arising in the chiasm) and craniopharyngiomas; germ cell tumors and lipomas may also appear as extreme rarities. Only the craniopharyngioma among these tumors is not considered elsewhere. Derived from vestigial remnants of Rathke's pouch, some arise within the sella but most are suprasellar. Most commonly seen in children and young adults, they are usually benign but occasionally cancerous.

Up to 8 to 10 cm in diameter, they may be encapsulated and solid, but more commonly are cystic and sometimes multiloculated.[19] The cysts contain dark-brown, oily fluid in which can be found granular debris as well as glittering cholesterol crystals. Over three-fourths of these tumors contain sufficient calcification to be visualized radiographically, providing an important clinical diagnostic aid. In their strategic location, they often encroach on the optic chiasm or nerves and not infrequently bulge into the floor of the third ventricle and base of the brain.

The histologic pattern is quite variable and recapitulates the enamel organ of the tooth (Fig. 26–8). Thus, these tumors are also known as **adamantinomas** or **ameloblastomas.** Nests or cords of stratified squamous or columnar epithelium are embedded in a loose fibrous stroma. Often the nests of squamous cells gradually merge into a peripheral layer of columnar cells. In the cystic variants the lining stratified squamous or columnar epithelium may be flat and regular, or thrown up into papillary projections. Calcification and metaplastic bone formation occur in the necrotic centers of the solid tumors as well as in the cystic variety. Infrequently, anaplastic changes are encountered in the epithelial cells, but cancerous behavior is rare.

POSTERIOR PITUITARY SYNDROMES

Disorders arising out of posterior pituitary dysfunction are exceedingly rare. Most relate to primary suprasellar hypothalamic lesions that will be detailed below. The consequences of dysfunction of the posterior pituitary take the forms of ADH deficiency or inappropriate release. The only known functions of oxytocin are potentiation of uterine contraction during labor, and stimulation of contraction of lactating glands in the breast to force milk into the excretory ducts during suckling. No well-defined syndrome associated with excessive or inappropriate release has been described.

ADH deficiency induces diabetes insipidus, char-

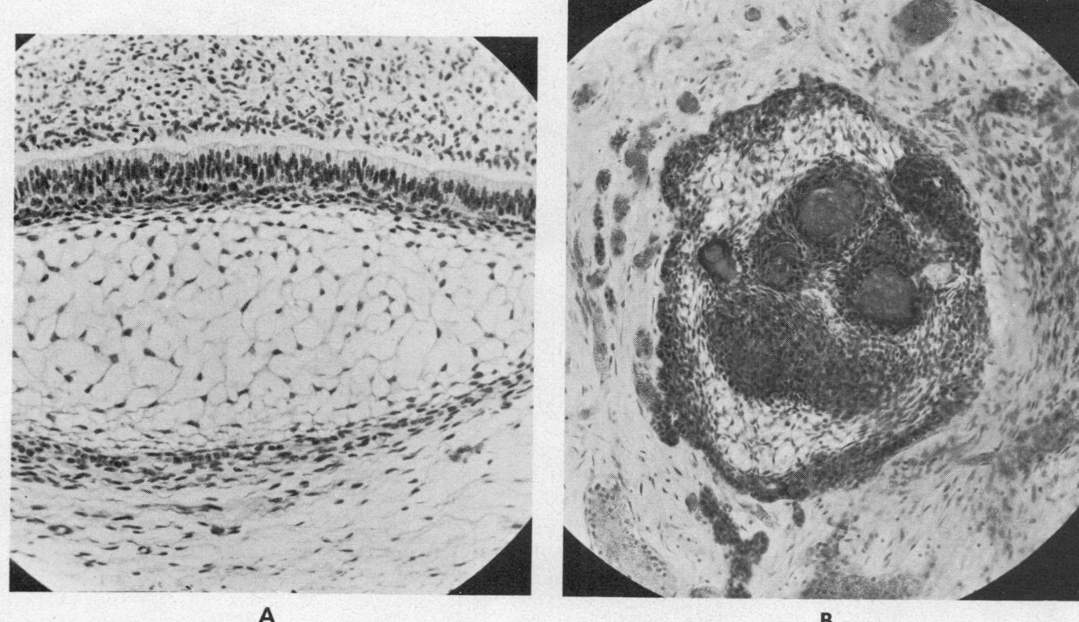

Figure 26–8. *A,* Embryonic tooth bud to illustrate similarity of cytology to cells of adamantinoma. *B,* Craniopharyngioma (adamantinoma). A nest of cells illustrating central squamous elements embedded in a loose cellular structure.

acterized by polyuria and excessive thirst (polydipsia). The origins of this syndrome include (1) neoplastic or inflammatory involvement of the hypothalamo-hypophyseal axis (such as pituitary adenomas, metastatic cancer, abscesses, meningitis, tuberculosis, and sarcoidosis); (2) surgical or radiation injury to the hypothalamo-hypophyseal axis (such as surgical or irradiation hypophysectomy); and (3) severe head injuries; or (4) may be idiopathic. Occasionally, patients with idiopathic diabetes insipidus have regressive alterations of ganglion cells in the hypothalamus of obscure etiology. Rarely, the idiopathic form of this syndrome is familial and apparently inherited as a mendelian dominant.

Inappropriate ADH secretion implies persistent release of ADH unrelated to the plasma osmolarity. Thus, there is excessive reabsorption of water from the glomerular filtrate, abnormal retention of water with expansion of the extracellular fluid volume, consequent hyponatremia and hemodilution, and the inability to excrete a dilute urine. The most common cause of inappropriate ADH secretion is paraneoplastic elaboration of ADH by nonendocrine tumors, particularly oat cell bronchogenic carcinoma, accounting for more than four-fifths of all cases. Other neoplasms associated with ectopic production of ADH include thymoma, carcinoma of the pancreas, and lymphoma. Infrequently, disorders of the central nervous system underlie this syndrome, such as intracerebral hemorrhages or thromboses, subarachnoid hemorrhage, subdural hematoma, and infections in and about the CNS.

Thyroid Gland

NORMAL

The thyroid gland develops as a tubular evagination from the root of the tongue, called the foramen cecum. It grows downward in front of the trachea and thyroid cartilage to reach the position it will occupy as the adult gland. The distal end of this structure proliferates to form the adult gland, while the remainder degenerates and disappears, usually by the fifth to sixth week of fetal development. Persistence of the vestigial tubular structure provides a source for the later development of thyroglossal cysts or ducts. Incomplete descent may lead to the formation of the thyroid at loci abnormally high in the neck, producing, for example, a lingual thyroid or aberrant subhyoid thyroid tissue. Excessive descent leads to substernal thyroid glands. Infrequently, lateral aberrant thyroid nodules develop, but these developmental anomalies are largely confined to the anterior triangle of the neck medial to the sternocleidomastoid muscle. Any of these aberrantly located thyroid glands may be the site of origin of tumors, identical with those arising in the definitive thyroid. Malformations of branchial pouch differentiation may result in intrathyroidal sites for the thymus or parathyroid glands. The implication of these deviations from the norm may become all too evident in the patient who has a total thyroidectomy and subsequently develops hypoparathyroidism.

In the adult, the thyroid gland weighs between 20 and 25 gm. Two large lateral lobes are connected in the midline by a broad isthmus from which, on occasion, a pyramidal lobe may protrude superiorly. Occasionally, in a very thin person, this normal pyramidal structure may be mistaken for a thyroid nodule. The close relationship of the recurrent laryngeal nerve and the parathyroid glands makes them extremely vulnerable to injury during thyroid surgery, and also to involvement by spreading malignancy or inflammation.

Histologically, the thyroid is composed of follicles or acini of variable size that, in three dimensions, comprise spheroidal sacs. These are lined by regular cuboidal cells. Ultrastructural studies disclose, in addition to the usual organization of organelles, numerous fine microvilli extending from the apical surface of the cell into the follicular colloid, within which is stored the thyroglobulin.[20] The microvilli participate in the mobilization of thyroid hormone from the thyroglobulin. In the normal thyroid, the follicles are separated by a delicate fibrous tissue stroma, which is compacted in some places into fibrous septa that traverse the gland. Small collections of lymphocytes are occasionally found in the stroma. Dispersed within the interstitial tissue or the follicles are the parafollicular calcitonin-secreting C cells, the histogenetic source of the medullary thyroid carcinoma.

In the normal state of functional activity, the follicles are filled with the glycoprotein thyroglobulin synthesized by thyroid epithelial cells. In the usual tissue stain, it has a pink, refractile appearance and is termed colloid. Release of active thyroid hormones involves proteolysis of the colloid (thyroglobulin) and splitting the polypeptide thyroid hormones out of the larger thyroglobulin molecule.

The active, circulating hormones of the thyroid are triiodothyronine (T_3) and thyroxine (T_4). The synthesis of these hormones has been described in detail.[21, 22] The following steps are involved:

1. Iodide trapping, an active process requiring energy. Normally the thyroid–serum iodide ratio in humans is about 50:1.
2. Oxidation of iodide within the thyroid cell to some form capable of iodinating tyrosine residues in the thyroglobulin. The oxidation is effected by an iodide peroxidase.
3. Iodination occurring at the microvillous interface between colloid and thyroid cell to form mono- and diiodotyrosine (MIT and DIT).
4. Coupling of MIT and DIT to form T_3 or coupling of two DITs to form T_4, again involving the peroxidase.

The release of T_3 and T_4 from the thyroglobulin involves the endocytosis of thyroglobulin and the proteolysis of the thyroglobulin. The villi apparently reach out and close over small fragments of the colloid to form membrane-bound vesicles that fuse with lysosomes to produce phagolysosomes.[23, 24] The phagolysosome migrates to the basal portion of the epithelial cells and, during this passage, lysosomal proteases and peptidases split out T_3 and T_4, which are discharged at the base of the cell into the perifollicular capillaries. During this process some MITs and DITs are simultaneously released and deiodinated for salvage of the iodides.

Once released into the blood, T_4 is almost totally (99.95%) bound mainly to an alpha globulin—thyroxine or thyronine-binding globulin (TBG). Other plasma proteins, including a prealbumin and albumin, participate to a lesser extent in this binding. T_3 is bound less firmly by TBG and very little by the other plasma proteins. Because the metabolic state of cells is regulated by the unbound fraction, unbound or free T_3 is more available to the cells of the body than is the small fraction of free T_4. Alterations in the plasma levels of TBG may modify the metabolic state. With increased levels of TBG, more thyroid hormone is bound, leaving a lower concentration of free hormones. This in turn reduces the inhibition of the anterior pituitary and leads to increased amounts of TSH, with resultant thyroid stimulation. The increased thyroid activity raises the concentration of thyroid hormones in the serum until the level of free hormone is restored to normal. The converse ensues when the concentration of TBG declines. Situations associated with increased TBG levels are pregnancy, ingestion of oral contraceptives and other forms of estrogen, diffuse liver disease, and possibly some genetic derangements. Decreased levels of TBG are seen with advanced liver disease, protein-losing nephropathies, adrenogenic steroid therapy, and possibly genetically conditioned syndromes.

Control of thyroid function and hormone output is exerted by two mechanisms: (1) hypothalamic and hypophyseal (as noted on p. 1193) and (2) feedback inhibition of TSH secretion by thyroid hormones. Release of TSH is dependent on a hypothalamic TSH-releasing hormone. TSH stimulates synthesis of thyroidal hormones through two separate pathways: by activating membrane-bound adenylate cyclase and by inducing synthesis of nucleic acids and proteins, leading to cellular hypertrophy and hyperplasia. In turn, through a feedback loop, thyroid hormones act upon the anterior pituitary and possibly the hypothalamus to suppress TSH release. There is also some evidence for yet another level of regulation of thyroid function. It also takes the form of a feedback loop in which the thyroid iodine content modifies the metabolic activity of the thyroid cell, perhaps by altering the adenylate cyclase response to TSH. This autoregulation becomes important when, for example, the diet is low in iodine and the follicular cell becomes more efficient in extracting and concentrating the meager amounts.

The metabolic function of the thyroid hormones is a large and complex subject, well reviewed elsewhere.[25, 26] It can be grossly oversimplifed by stating that at the cellular level thyroid hormone appears to interact with the nucleus, probably through nuclear hormone-binding receptors, and also with mitochondria to stimulate oxidative phosphorylation with the formation of ATP. Thyroidal hormones also enhance transmembrane transport and enzyme activity. With all these actions the hormones, more specifically the unbound or free fractions, stimulate virtually all metabolic processes, both synthetic and catabolic. In effect, then, the hormones provide the spark that keeps the metabolic machine running. As will be seen, a deficiency of the hormones significantly slows the machine, whereas an excess speeds it to the point at which it begins to consume itself.

From the physiologic standpoint, the thyroid gland is one of the most sensitive organs in the body. It responds to many stimuli and is in a constant state of adaptation. During puberty, pregnancy, and physiologic stress from any source, the gland increases in size and becomes more active functionally. Changes in activity and size may even be noted during a normal menstrual period. This extreme functional lability is reflected in transient hyperplasia of the thyroidal epithelium. At this time, thyroglobulin is resorbed and the follicular cells become tall and columnar, sometimes forming small infolded buds. When the stress abates, involution occurs, i.e., the height of the epithelium falls, colloid accumulates, and the follicular cells resume their normal size and architecture. Failure of this normal balance between hyperplasia and involution may produce major or minor deviations from the usual histologic pattern.

The function of the thyroid gland can be inhibited by a variety of chemical agents, collectively referred to as *goitrogens*. Because they suppress T_3 and T_4 synthesis, increased levels of TSH and subsequent hyperplastic enlargement of the gland (*goiter*) follow. Most important among these compounds are certain drugs used in the treatment of hyperthyroidism. The antithyroid agents thiourea and mercaptoimidazole inhibit the oxidation of iodide and block coupling of the iodotyrosines into T_3 and T_4. Thus, thyroid hormones cannot be produced; there is diminished negative feedback on the pituitary, and the result is increased levels of TSH with futile stimulation of the gland, resulting in thyroid hyperplasia and enlargement. Iodide, when given to patients with thyroid hyperfunction, also blocks the release of thyroid hormones, but through different mechanisms. Iodides in large doses inhibit proteolysis of thyroglobulin. Thus, thyroid hormone is synthesized and incorporated within increasing amounts of colloid, but it is not released into the blood. *The gland following thiourea therapy lacks thyroglobulin-colloid and is extremely cellular, but with iodine treatment the follicles become distended with thyroglobulin-colloid*, creating the appearance of an inactive gland.

Some of the numerous tests currently available to assay normal thyroid gland function include measurement of serum TSH by radioimmunoassay. The serum levels of total T_3 and T_4 and the precise levels of free T_3 and T_4 can be determined. Less precise but nonetheless widely used is the protein-bound iodine (PBI) determination, which estimates the level of thyroid hormones by quantitating the concentration of iodine in the serum precipitable by protein-denaturing agents. Another measure of thyroid activity is its ability to take up an administered dose of radioactive iodine (RAI uptake). A functional evaluation of the gross anatomy of the thyroid is provided by a scintiscan, after administration of a radionuclide of iodide or technetium pertechnetate. The scan will disclose focal lesions such as tumors that are nonfunctioning ("cold nodules") or hyperactive masses ("hot nodules"), and aberrant thyroid tissue and functioning metastases of thyroid cancer, wherever they are located.

Other procedures are also available, but it suffices to note that it is now possible to detect very precisely aberrations in the function of the thyroid and to study noninvasively the anatomy of the gland.

PATHOLOGY

Diseases of the thyroid, although not common in clinical practice, are nonetheless of great importance because most are amenable to medical or surgical management. They present principally as *hyperthyroidism, hypothyroidism,* or *enlargement of the thyroid gland* known as goiter. The enlargement may be diffuse and symmetric or irregular and focal (nodular). Some concept of the relative frequency of the more common forms of thyroid disease can be gained from a screening survey of individuals in a small northeastern town in the United States.[27] A total of 5.8% of the population was found to have thyroid abnormalities. In order of frequency, the following conditions were identified: simple (nonfunctional) symmetric enlargement, hyperthyroidism, multinodular goiter, thyroiditis, and a solitary nodular goiter (presumably an adenoma). No cases of cancer were identified. An essentially similar distribution of the various thyroid disorders was reported from a British community.[28] Thus, goitrous thyroid enlargement without manifestations of thyroid hyperfunction is the most common disease in these two surveys, followed in frequency by hyperthyroidism.

There is no simple correspondence between morphologic lesions of the thyroid and resultant clinical manifestations. For example, a multinodular goiter in one instance may be associated with normal thyroid function, in another with hyperfunction, and in yet another with hypofunction. It is best, therefore, at the outset to present the clinical syndromes of hyperthyroidism and hypothyroidism and then discuss the various thyroid lesions in some rational morphologic sequence, relating each to its possible clinical significance.

CLINICAL SYNDROMES ASSOCIATED WITH THYROID DISEASE

HYPERTHYROIDISM

Hyperthyroidism, also known as thyrotoxicosis, is a hypermetabolic state encountered much more often in females, caused by an increased output of thyroid hormones, namely, T_4 *and* T_3. It is manifested by nervousness, palpitation, rapid pulse, fatigability, muscular weakness, weight loss with good appetite, diarrhea, heat intolerance, warm skin, excessive perspiration, emotional lability, menstrual changes, a fine tremor of the hand (particularly when outstretched), eye changes, and sometimes prominence of the thyroid gland. The changes in the skin, eyes, and cardiovascular system are particularly significant.

Typically, the skin is warm, moist, and flushed, related both to peripheral vasodilatation to increase the heat loss, and to the general hyperdynamic circulatory state. **The eye changes often call attention to the thyrotoxicosis.** Typically, patients have a wide-eyed stare produced by retraction of the upper eyelid and upper lid lag as it falls behind the globe on slow downward gaze. In the thyrotoxicosis of Graves' disease there is also protrusion of the globe (proptosis) secondary to immunoinflammatory (infiltrative) changes in the retro-orbital tissues (Fig. 26–9). **Cardiac manifestations are among the earliest and most consistent features of hyperthyroidism.** Tachycardia, palpitations, and cardiomegaly are common. Cardiac arrhythmias occasionally appear, often supraventricular. The basis for these arrhythmias is not clear. Morphologic myocardial changes, such as foci of lymphocytic and eosinophilic infiltration, mild fibrosis in the interstitium, fatty change in myofibers, and an increase in size and number of mitochondria, have been described.[29] These changes are not frequent and other possible concomitant pathogeneses have not been rigorously ruled out, so that debate continues about so-called **thyrotoxic cardiomyopathy.** The cardiomegaly is equally obscure and is vaguely attributed to a cardiac hyperdynamic state induced by increased formation of or response to catecholamines. An alternative explanation involves the recent observation in thyroid hormone–treated rabbits of a new myosin in the myofibers having a higher level of ATPase activity, permitting increased contractility and thereby possibly leading to hypertrophy.[30] Other explanations have been offered, but it suffices that much is uncertain; only uncommonly does cardiac failure occur in these patients, usually in the elderly when other cardiac diseases are often present.

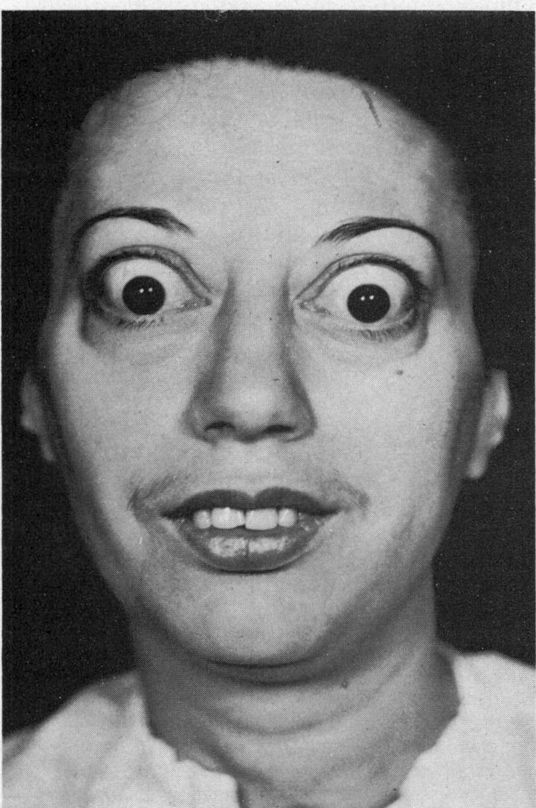

Figure 26–9. Hyperthyroidism in a 27-year-old woman.

Other findings throughout the body are variable and generally not significant, including atrophy and fatty infiltration of skeletal muscle, sometimes with focal interstitial lymphocytic infiltrates; minimal fatty changes in the liver, sometimes accompanied by mild, periportal fibrosis and a mild lymphocytic infiltrate; and osteoporosis.

Hyperthyroidism or thyrotoxicosis may be caused by a variety of disorders (Table 26–2). The three common causes collectively account for virtually 99% of cases. Among these, Graves' disease is the most frequent, particularly in patients under 40 years of age. This disease is also known as diffuse toxic goiter to differentiate it from the thyrotoxicosis related to toxic nodular goiter, whether it is a solitary nodule (presumably an adenoma) or multinodular.[31] Only a few brief comments are merited on the rare causes of hyperthyroidism. Metastatic, well-differentiated thyroid carcinoma may sometimes elaborate sufficient thyroid hormones to cause thyrotoxicosis. Similarly, acute or subacute thyroiditis during the stage of active cell injury may be associated with sufficient release of stored hormones to induce transient manifestations. Incongruously, choriocarcinomas and hydatidiform moles not only produce chorionic gonadotropin, but sometimes also a TSH-like material.[32] Increased levels of thyroid hormones are rarely caused by TSH-secreting pituitary tumors or pituitary stimulation by excessive hypothalamic release of TRH.[33] Thyroid hyperfunction can be also induced by excess iodine ingestion in patients with various thyroid disorders. This pattern of the disease is sometimes referred to as *jodbasedow disease.* It is unclear at present how the iodine ingestion precipitates the thyrotoxicosis.[34] Equally rarely, patients receiving thyroid hormone medication for hypothyroidism or for other reasons (misguided attempts at weight control) may develop iatrogenic or factitious hyperthyroidism. In all the above situations, the same hypermetabolic syndrome results.

The diagnosis of thyrotoxicosis may be readily apparent from the clinical manifestations, or the signs and symptoms may be so subtle that resort must be made to laboratory evidence. Characteristically, there is an increase in the basal metabolic rate (BMR) and serum concentrations of T_4 and T_3, particularly the latter.

Table 26–2. DISORDERS ASSOCIATED WITH HYPERTHYROIDISM

Common
Diffuse toxic hyperplasia (Graves' disease)
Toxic multinodular goiter
Toxic adenoma
Uncommon
Acute or subacute thyroiditis
Hyperfunctioning thyroid carcinoma
Choriocarcinoma or hydatidiform mole
TSH-secreting pituitary or pituitary tumor
Neonatal thyrotoxicosis (mother with Graves' disease)
Struma ovarii (teratomatous thyroid tissue within ovary)
Iodide-induced hyperthyroidism (jodbasedow disease)
Iatrogenic (exogenous) hyperthyroidism

Sometimes a decrease of thyroxine-binding globulin increases both the proportion and the amount of free T_4 and T_3. Also present are an increased protein-bound iodine (PBI) and radioactive iodine uptake (RAIU). With Graves' disease, there are additional immunologic findings, and with thyrotoxicosis secondary to neoplastic or nodular goitrous involvement of the gland, there may be abnormalities in the scintiscan.

Finally, brief mention should be made of *thyrotoxic crisis* or *storm.* Although poorly understood, this clinical emergency usually occurs in patients with unrecognized or inadequately treated thyrotoxicosis. It is precipitated by subtotal thyroidectomy before adequate control of the thyrotoxic state has been established, but may also arise with severe infection, trauma, or any other form of acute stress. Severe hypermetabolism erupts marked by fever, tachycardia, and often cardiac irregularities and failure, leading soon to progressive mental obtundation and coma. Emergency measures are necessary to control the desperate situation, but it is nonetheless fatal in 20 to 25% of patients.

HYPOTHYROIDISM

Any structural or functional derangement of the thyroid that significantly impairs its output of hormone will lead to the hypometabolic state of hypothyroidism. The clinical manifestations of the hormone lack depend on the age when it first appears. When present during development and infancy it results in *cretinism* with its associated physical and mental retardation. The term "cretin" was once derived from the French "chrétien," meaning "Christian" or "Christ-like," and was applied to these unfortunates because they were considered to be so mentally retarded as to be incapable of sinning! When hypothyroidism first appears in older children or adults, it is termed *myxedema.* This designation calls attention to the accumulation of hydrophilic mucopolysaccharides in connective tissue throughout the body, leading to a distinctive, edematous, doughy thickening of the skin that is resistant to pitting.

The causes of hypothyroidism in both infants and adults can be divided into several categories, as in Table 26–3. Among these various disorders, the most frequent cause in the United States today is ablation of the gland by either surgery or radiation. Sometimes an overly generous subtotal thyroidectomy for the treatment of hyperthyroidism is followed by insufficient thyroid function. On occasion it is necessary to remove the thyroid to excise a primary neoplasm adequately. The gland may also be ablated by radiation, whether in the form of radioiodine administered for the treatment of hyperthyroidism or in the form of exogenous irradiation employed in the treatment of some nearby neoplasm, e.g., lymphoma. The next most common cause of hypothyroidism is so-called *primary idiopathic myxedema.* There is now substantial evidence that this condition is autoimmune in origin.[35] Autoimmunity is also believed to underlie several forms of thyroid disease, notably

Table 26–3. CAUSES OF HYPOTHYROIDISM

Deficiency Thyroid Parenchyma (Thyroprivic)
Surgical or radiation ablation
Primary idiopathic myxedema (? autoimmune)
Agenesis, hypoplasia, or dysplasia of thyroid
Goitrous Hypothyroidism
Hashimoto's thyroiditis
Endemic iodine deficiency
Exogenous goitrogenic agents (para-aminosalicylic acid, cruciferous plants, phenylbutazone, lithium, cassava)
Congenital, often heritable biosynthetic defects
Iodide-induced
Suprathyroidal Disorders (Trophoprivic)
Hypopituitarism
Hypothalamic lesions
Peripheral Resistance to Thyroid Hormone

Hashimoto's thyroiditis and Graves' disease, and this subject is discussed later (p. 1210). It suffices for now to note that autoantibodies that block the TSH receptors have been identified and proposed as the cause of primary hypothyroidism.[36] Together, these two forms of thyroidal inadequacy account for 80 to 90% of all cases of hypothyroidism. Infrequently, hypothyroidism stems from a developmental failure, synthetic defect, or forms of thyroid disease that produce, among other things, a goiter (enlargement of the thyroid gland). Even more infrequently, hypothyroidism arises because of some hypophyseothalamic disorder that reduces serum TSH levels, or because of some peripheral resistance to thyroid hormone.

Cretinism

This usually preventable, and therefore all the more tragic, condition is marked by retardation of both physical and intellectual growth. It is seldom apparent at birth but, depending on the severity of hormone lack, becomes evident over ensuing weeks to months. By the time the changes become unmistakably evident they are largely irreversible, and so a strong case can be made for routine screening of neonates for possible thyroid hormone lack. The first and most sensitive laboratory abnormality to appear is an increase in serum TSH level related to loss of feedback inhibition. In time, serum T_4 and then T_3 concentrations falls. Other laboratory findings include decreased BMR and elevated serum cholesterol, but these are rarely necessary to establish the diagnosis. The initial clinical manifestations are feeding problems; constipation; a hoarse, husky cry; somnolence; and failure to thrive. With time, the abdomen becomes protuberant, the skin grows dry, and there is delay in the appearance of the deciduous teeth, accompanied by impaired skeletal growth leading to dwarfism. The fully developed syndrome is characterized by dry, rough skin; widely set eyes; periorbital puffiness, a flattened, broad nose; and an overly large protuberant tongue. There is delay in closure of the fontanelles and, later in life, delay in closure of the epiphyses along with other epiphyseal abnormalities. The radiographic findings are so distinctive as to be virtually diagnostic. Most important is the neurologic deficit, which varies somewhat depending on the time of onset of the thyroid hormone lack. Two somewhat distinctive syndromes can be distinguished. When the thyroid deficit is present during early fetal development, as may occur with severe iodine lack, agenesis of the thyroid, or a congenital biosynthetic defect, there is retarded development of the brain and the child manifests deaf-mutism, spasticity, and severe mental deficiency, giving rise to the term *neurologic cretinism.*[37] If the hormone lack is less severe or appears later in development, there is milder impairment but still some degree of mental deficiency, called *hypothyroid cretinism.*

The sometimes used terms *endemic cretinism* and *sporadic cretinism* should be clarified here. Endemic cretinism occurs wherever endemic goiter is prevalent, generally related to a dietary lack of iodine. Often, both parents of the affected infant are goitrous. Sporadic cretinism, in contrast, is usually caused by some congenital developmental failure in thyroid gland formation (sporadic athyreotic cretinism) or by some biosynthetic defect in thyroid hormone formation.[38] In most instances, the hormonal lack in the neonate is not so severe as in endemic cretinism, and so the mental retardation is more subtle at birth and difficult to detect. However, it also provides a greater opportunity, if recognized relatively early, to institute appropriate therapy and prevent fully developed cretinism.

Myxedema

The term myxedema is applied to hypothyroidism in the older child or adult. The clinical manifestations vary with the age of onset of the deficiency. The older child shows signs and symptoms intermediate between those of the cretin and the adult with hypothyroidism. In the adult the condition appears very insidiously and may take years to reach the level of clinical suspicion. Basically it is characterized by slowing of physical and mental activity. The initial symptoms are tiredness, lethargy, cold intolerance, and general listlessness and apathy. Speech and intellectual functions become slowed. With the passage of time, periorbital edema develops along with a thickened, dry, coarse skin. Eventually the facial features become thickened and the tongue enlarged, and the distinctive peripheral edema described earlier worsens. At this time there is extreme physical and mental torpor. Other systems share in the general lethargy with decreased sweating, constipation, and slowness of motor function. The cardiac output is also decreased because of a reduction in both stroke volume and heart rate. An increase in peripheral vascular resistance and a decrease in blood volume result in narrowing of the pulse pressure, prolongation of the circulation time, and decreased flow to the peripheral tissues. It is the reduced circulation in the skin that accounts for the sensitivity to the cold. In well-advanced myxedema the heart is flabby and enlarged with dilated chambers. Histologically, there is sometimes swelling of the myofibers with some loss of striations, accompanied by an increase of interstitial mucopolysaccharide-rich edema fluid. A similar fluid sometimes accumulates within the pericardial sac. To these changes, the term *myxedema heart* or *hypothyroid cardiomyopathy* has been applied. The skeletal muscles may also reveal changes similar to those found in the myocardium. Pleural effusions are common. The general retardation of growth and activity leads to decreased production of erythropoietin and often a mild, normocytic, normochromic anemia. Defective absorption of vitamin B_{12} may in some cases induce a macrocytic anemia. There may also be some retardation in skeletal growth and in CNS development; however, the latter is more characteristic of cretinism.

Although the diagnosis of myxedema can often be made on the basis of the clinical findings, it usually requires laboratory confirmation. As in the infant and child with cretinism, the BMR is depressed and the serum levels (total and free) of T_4 and T_3 are subnormal. The TSH level is of particular importance. In primary hypothyroidism, such as occurs with thyroid disease, the TSH level is elevated owing to loss of feedback inhibition of the pituitary. However, in the uncommon instance when the hypothyroidism is related to some hypophyseothalamic disorder and loss of tropic stimulation of the thyroid gland, the TSH levels are abnormally low. Recognition of this form of so-called *trophoprivic hypothyroidism* is of great importance because it is often accompanied by depressed ACTH levels and adrenocortical insufficiency. In such circumstances, treatment of the hypothyroid state with thyroid hormone and stimulation of the general metabolic activity of the body may precipitate a crisis of adrenal insufficiency. With this overview of the clinical consequences of disturbed thyroid function, we can turn to the disorders causing it.

THYROIDITIS

A variety of ill-defined forms of thyroiditis may be produced by microbial seeding of the thyroid. Almost always the infection is primary elsewhere and the agents blood-borne; rarely, there is direct traumatic seeding of the gland. Sometimes, immunologic incompetence potentiates these infective forms of thyroiditis. The most frequent causes are *Staphylococcus aureus*, streptococci, Salmonella, Enterobacter, tuberculosis, and fungi (Candida, aspergilli, Mucormycetes). Viral thyroiditis is a special case, discussed later. The thyroid may also be involved in systemic sarcoidosis. Whatever the cause, the inflammatory involvement may cause painful enlargement of the gland, but almost always the condition is transient and self-limited or controllable with appropriate therapy. Thyroid function usually is not significantly affected and there are few residuals except for possible small foci of scarring. Much more common and clinically significant are the following more or less well-defined forms of thyroiditis: (1) Hashimoto's thyroiditis, (2) subacute granulomatous thyroiditis, (3) subacute lymphocytic thyroiditis, and (4) Riedel's thyroiditis (struma).[39, 40, 41]

HASHIMOTO'S THYROIDITIS

Marked by an intense infiltrate of lymphocytes admixed with plasma cells that virtually replaces the thyroid parenchyma (Fig. 26–10), this chronic form of thyroiditis is of importance on several scores: (1) it is the most common cause of goitrous hypothyroidism in regions having a sufficiency of iodine; (2) it is a major cause of nonendemic goiter in children; and (3) it is the first-described and archetype of organ-specific autoimmune diseases. The thyroid enlargement is generally painless; although diffuse, it may be asymmetric and may sometimes appear lobulated (possibly mimicking tumorous involvement). Most patients with long-standing Hashimoto's disease become hypothyroid, but a few in mid-course develop typical hyperthyroidism, sometimes called "hashitoxicosis." This concurrence is more than fortuitous: there are many similarities in the autoimmune reactions in Hashimoto's thyroiditis and Graves' thyrotoxicosis. Because of all the immunologic abnormalities, Hashimoto's thyroiditis is also sometimes called *autoimmune thyroiditis*. Another synonym is

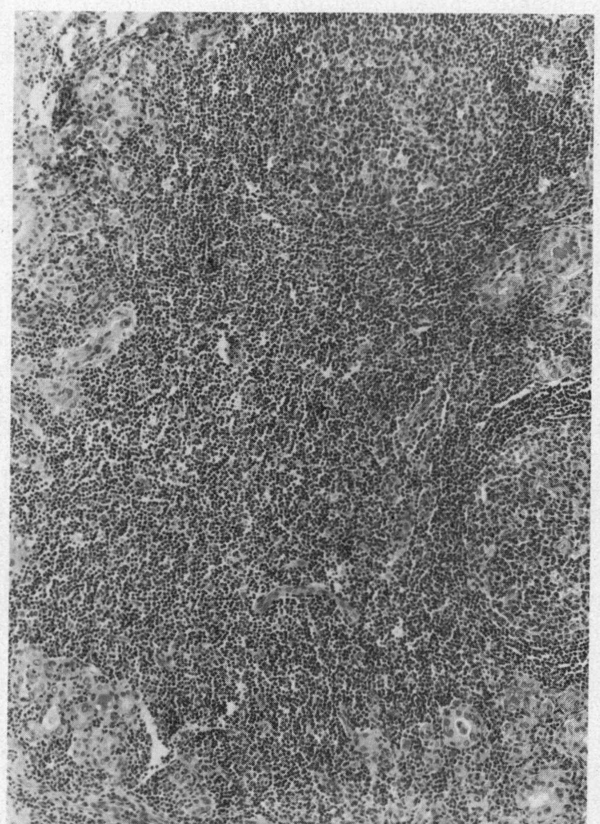

Figure 26–10. Hashimoto's thyroiditis. The thyroid parenchyma is largely replaced by a heavy lymphocytic infiltrate containing two evident lymphoid follicles. Only some marginal thyroid follicles are present in the field.

struma lymphomatosa, denoting the striking replacement of the thyroid parenchyma with lymphoid cells.

Hashimoto's thyroiditis is predominantly a disease of women, with a female:male ratio of 10:1. Most cases occur between the ages of 30 and 50, but some are noted in children. The possibility of some genetic predisposition is suspected because of the familial occurrence of the disease and because of a well-defined association with HLA-DR5. There is also a greater-than-chance association with other diseases of presumed autoimmune origin, including systemic lupus erythematosus, Sjögren's syndrome, rheumatoid arthritis, pernicious anemia, adult-onset diabetes and (as mentioned before) Graves' disease. However, it should be noted that the last-named condition tends to be associated with HLA-DR3 in whites.

ETIOLOGY AND PATHOGENESIS. A large body of evidence supports the theory of an autoimmune origin of this form of chronic thyroiditis.[42] *The basic defect is thought to be a genetically conditioned deficiency in antigen-specific suppressor T cells. As a consequence, there is uncontrolled attack on the follicular cells by cytotoxic T cells, and simultaneously unregulated T-helper cell participation in the B-cell formation of autoantibodies.* The supporting evidence is as follows. A variety of autoantibodies against thyroid-cell antigens can be identified in virtually all patients with this condition, most consistently thyrotropin-receptor (TSH) antibodies and thyroid microsomal antibodies.[43] About half of the patients also have antibodies to thyroglobulin and, less constantly, to follicular cell membranes, thyroid hormones themselves, and a colloid component other than thyroglobulin. *The TSH-receptor autoantibodies* are of particular interest; by binding to receptors, *they mimic the action of TSH*, but studies indicate that these receptor autoantibodies can be separated into those that stimulate hormone synthesis (thyroid-stimulating immunoglobulins—TSI) and those that initiate thyroid growth (thyroid-growth immunoglobulins—TGI).[44] To complicate matters further, "blocking" antibodies for each of these subsets can be identified, i.e., "TSI-block" and "TGI-block."[36] Two scenarios can therefore be proposed in the pathogenesis of Hashimoto's disease: (1) the TSH-receptor autoantibodies may be largely TGI, i.e., those that stimulate growth with a relative paucity of TSI, which stimulate hormone synthesis; or (2) both TSI and TGI autoantibodies are present, but also TSI-blocking antibodies. These issues are now under investigation, but in either instance *goitrous enlargement occurs without hyperfunction.*[45] It is speculated, therefore, that HLA-DR5 individuals are in some way genetically predisposed to the production of the pathogenetic antibodies. Interestingly, patients with Graves' hyperthyroidism have virtually an identical complement of thyroidal autoantibodies but, with the HLA-DR3 genotype, express more of the TSI.

Hashimoto's thyroiditis is characterized by extensive loss of thyroid parenchyma, but despite all the immunologic alterations, the precise mechanism(s) of follicular cell destruction is/are uncertain. Cytotoxic T cells, antibody-dependent cellular cytotoxicity, or complement activation, singly or in concert, could account for the attack on the follicle cells.

MORPHOLOGY. There are two major morphologic variants of Hashimoto's thyroiditis. The **classic form** is characterized by rubbery, firm, usually symmetric, moderate enlargement of the gland. The capsule is intact and only rarely adherent to surrounding structures. Transection discloses a pale-gray, fleshy cut surface with accentuation of normal lobulations. Although the macroscopic changes could be mistaken for neoplastic replacement, the symmetry of the involvement and the integrity of the capsule argue against a neoplasm. The differentiation can be more difficult when there is asymmetric enlargement.

Microscopically, **there is extensive replacement of the native architecture by lymphoid cells, including plasma cells, immunoblasts, transformed lymphocytes, and macrophages with the formation of lymphoid germinal centers.**[40] Here and there, isolated follicles or clusters of follicles persist, but they are often atrophic and contain sparse, deeply-staining colloid. The persistent follicular epithelium is transformed into so-called **Hürthle cells or oncocytes** having an abundant brightly eosinophilic granular cytoplasm packed with mitochondria and lysosomes. Despite the mitochondria with their oxidative enzymes, Hürthle cells are functionally inactive and do not produce T_4, T_3, or thyroglobulin. They are thought to represent a degenerated state of the follicular epithelium, are not specific for Hashimoto's thyroiditis, and are found in many other forms of thyroid injury.[46] Such fibrosis as is present is usually delicate and largely confined to the interlobular septa.

The other, much less common morphologic pattern is called **fibrosing** Hashimoto's thyroiditis[47] and is characterized by modest thyroid enlargement, a more intense fibrosis, and a less prominent lymphoid infiltrate. The follicular atrophy is often more severe with conversion of persistent follicular epithelium into either Hürthle cells or squamous cells. The fibrosing reaction does not extend beyond the capsule, differentiating this pattern of Hashimoto's disease from Riedel's struma, to be described.

CLINICAL COURSE. *The cardinal clinical features of Hashimoto's thyroiditis are goitrous enlargement of the thyroid gland associated with hypothyroidism in a middle-aged woman.* At the outset only a goiter may be present, but in those with the fibrosing variant the enlargement may be subtle and the major feature is hypothyroidism. Only infrequently does the thyroid enlarge rapidly enough to cause pain and tenderness. In time, hypothyroidism becomes evident in most patients, but it worsens only very slowly over the course of years and is sometimes virtually static. Thus, early in the disease the patient is metabolically normal but the serum TSH levels may be mildly elevated. At this time the RAI uptake (RAIU) and PBI may be mildly increased because of deranged thyroidal function with the secretion of hormonally inactive iodoproteins. Notably, the serum T_4 and T_3 levels are normal. As the hypothyroidism becomes more established, the RAIU, PBI, and T_4 and T_3 levels decline. Radioimmunoassays or hemagglutination tests almost always reveal one or more of the circulating autoantibodies previously described. Despite all the clinical evidence, needle biopsy is often required to confirm the diagnosis histologically. Treatment with replacement doses of thyroid hormone is all that is required and is sometimes accompanied by regression of the goiter. There is no increased prevalence of thyroid carcinoma in these glands, but possibly some predisposition to lymphoma (p. 1224).

SUBACUTE GRANULOMATOUS (DE QUERVAIN'S) THYROIDITIS

The term subacute thyroiditis might include the various forms of bacterial or fungal infection, but by common practice it is restricted to a distinctive form of self-limited inflammation of the thyroid gland of probable viral etiology.[49] This entity is also referred to as *giant cell* or *pseudogranulomatous thyroiditis.* The peak incidence is in the second to fifth decades of life, with a female:male ratio of 3–6:1.[50]

Although the cause is still uncertain, considerable circumstantial evidence suggests a viral etiology:[51]

1. There is a more-than-chance association between onset of the thyroiditis and some form of viral infection, e.g., mumps, upper respiratory infection, pneumonitis, or infectious mononucleosis.
2. Antibodies to the causative agents of these infections can be identified in about half the cases.
3. The condition is reminiscent of an infection with fever, painful tender enlargement of the thyroid gland, and a self-limited course measured in months.[52]

A possible role for autoimmunity has also been raised but has been largely excluded. In theory, a viral infection might either alter thyroid antigens or, by damaging the thyroid gland, release large amounts of antigens to initiate an autoimmune reaction. However, significant levels of thyroid autoantibodies are present in only a minority of patients, do not correlate with the course of the disease, and are transitory. The same can be said about cell-mediated immunity. "Thyroid-stimulating immunoglobulins" (p. 1207) have been identified by a few investigators during the early phase of this condition, but are found in only a few patients and are not correlated with the clinical course. Moreover, they disappear soon after the onset, suggesting that they are secondary events and not pathogenetic.[53]

MORPHOLOGY. The gland may be subtly or markedly enlarged (threefold). Sometimes, the enlargement appears asymmetric or focal on palpation of the neck, but more often the whole gland is involved, although irregularly. It may be slightly adherent to surrounding structures. On cut section the involved areas are firm and yellow-white and stand out from the more rubbery, yielding, normal brown thyroid substance. Histologically, the changes are patchy and depend on the stage of the disease. Early in the active inflammatory phase, scattered follicles may be entirely disrupted and replaced by neutrophils forming microabscesses. **Later, the more characteristic features appear in the form of aggregations of macrophages about damaged follicles, admixed with multinucleate giant cells enclosing naked pools or fragments of colloid** (Fig. 26–11).[40] The inflammatory foci more or less resemble granulomas, hence the designation "granulomatous thyroiditis." In the later stages of the disease, a chronic inflammatory infiltrate and fibrosis may replace the foci of injury. Different histologic stages are sometimes found in the same gland, suggesting waves of destruction over a period of time. Despite all the pathogenetic evidence cited earlier, electron microscopy has failed to disclose viral inclusion bodies.

CLINICAL COURSE. The presentation of this condition is extremely variable. Basically, three patterns can be identified: (1) an acute systemic febrile reaction; (2) sudden painful enlargement of the gland, sometimes mimicking "sore throat"; or (3) less painful enlargement accompanied by transient manifestations of hyperthyroidism. Obviously, more than one may coexist in the same patient. Whatever form the condition takes at onset, the condition is self-limited, and over the span of weeks to months the tenderness usually abates along with the fever and manifestations of hyperthyroidism. Indeed, with extensive destruction of the gland, transient hypothyroidism may supervene. Laboratory tests of thyroid function can be anticipated to a considerable extent. During the stage of follicular damage, there is leakage of a variety of iodinated products into the blood with an increase in PBI. There may also be an elevation

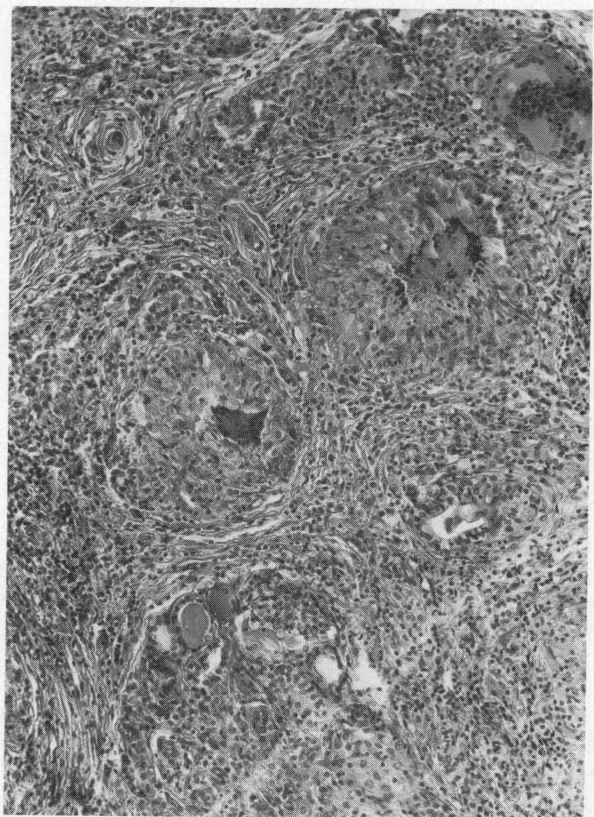

Figure 26–11. Subacute thyroiditis. Two granulomatous foci enclosing remnants of colloid are evident in midfield. Note large giant cell *(above right).* (Courtesy of Dr. Merle Legg, New England Deaconess Hospital.)

of serum T_4 and T_3 levels, indicating cleavage of thyrogobulin with the release of thyroid hormones. Extensive damage to the gland may induce a transient phase of hypothyroidism with a fall in plasma hormone levels. Following recovery, generally within five to six months, normal thyroid function resumes and the various laboratory test results return to normal. At this time the goiter disappears and the only residual may be scattered foci of fibrous scarring, rarely sufficient to cause asymmetry of the gland or to masquerade as tumorous involvement.

SUBACUTE LYMPHOCYTIC (PAINLESS) THYROIDITIS

This poorly understood condition constitutes, in essence, a *painless* variant of subacute granulomatous thyroiditis. It is also distinctive anatomically inasmuch as the only changes in the gland are foci of lymphocytic infiltration, sometimes accompanied by an increase in interstitial fibrous tissue. There is no tendency to formation of lymphoid germinal centers and few, if any, plasma cells such as are found in Hashimoto's thyroiditis. The acute follicular destruction or granulomatous reaction characteristic of de Quervain's disease are not noted. Subacute painless thyroiditis usually comes to attention because of either goitrous enlargement of the gland or hyperthyroidism, or both. One survey indicated that subacute lymphocytic thyroiditis was responsible for about 15% of all hyperthyroidism in North America.[54] In the absence of hyperthyroidism and with only modest goitrous enlargement, the condition may well pass unrecognized, particularly since it is self-limited and without sequelae.

The origin of this form of thyroiditis and its place in the spectrum of thyroiditis are obscure. There is no association with previous viral infections and the autoimmune reactions are inconstant and evanescent. There is no evidence that it constitutes a precursor of Hashimoto's disease or that it leads to so-called primary idiopathic myxedema and permanent hypothyroidism.

RIEDEL'S THYROIDITIS (STRUMA)

This rare form of chronic thyroiditis is characterized pathologically by a fibrosing reaction that destroys more or less all the thyroid gland while simultaneously extending beyond the thyroid capsule into surrounding structures in the neck. Because of the woody hardness of the thyroid, it is sometimes called *ligneous thyroiditis.* The female:male ratio is approximately 3:1, and most affected individuals are in the fourth to seventh decades of life. The disease, although rare, assumes importance because it is easily confused with a thyroid malignancy. Patients may have manifestations of an obstructive, invasive process, including stridor, dysphagia, recurrent laryngeal nerve paralysis, dyspnea, or even suffocation. More often, however, the chief complaint is merely a painless lump in the neck.

The etiology of this condition is unknown.[55] All the available evidence argues against its being an end stage of any other form of thyroiditis, despite many morphologic overlaps with the fibrosing variant of Hashimoto's disease. Riedel's thyroiditis is not accompanied by thyroid autoantibodies, or at most they are present in very low titer. The fibrosing reaction, as mentioned, extends beyond the gland, and there is none of the exuberant lymphoid infiltration seen in Hashimoto's disease. Similar fibrosing reactions sometimes are also present elsewhere, suggesting some systemic, possibly familial, fibrosclerosing derangement.[56]

MORPHOLOGY. The entire thyroid may be normal in size or slightly enlarged but is usually markedly contracted. **It is stony hard, pale gray, and asymmetric, having apparent nodularity on clinical palpation.** Sometimes, only a lobe or portion of a lobe is involved. The capsule is involved in the inflammatory process, producing dense adherence to surrounding structures such as the carotid sheath, trachea, and neck muscles—hence, the simulation of cancer. On section, the tissue is hard and woody.

From the histologic standpoint, there is no specific diagnostic feature of this disorder. In advanced cases, the parenchyma is markedly atrophic and is replaced by masses of dense collagenous fibrous tissue (Fig. 26–12). Scattered throughout this scarring, there is a delicate-to-moderate lymphocytic infiltration. Such epithelial elements or acini as remain show varying stages of pressure atrophy and atypi-

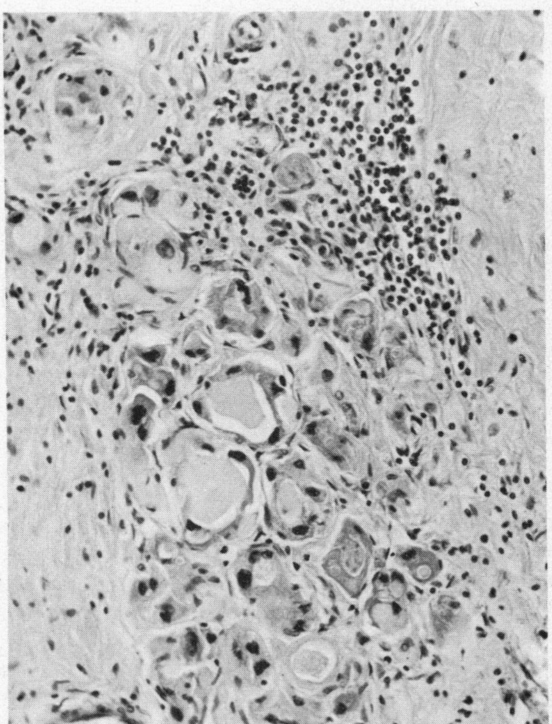

Figure 26–12. High-power view of a Riedel's struma illustrating extensive fibrosis, scant lymphocytic infiltration, and a few residual distorted thyroid follicles.

cality of cells. Often the trapped epithelial cells are transformed into Hürthle cells (p. 1207).

Clinical Course. The prominent clinical features of this condition have already been cited. About 25 to 50% of patients are hypothyroid; the remainder are euthyroid. The major clinical significance of this condition is its differentiation from thyroid cancer. Because needle biopsy of the woody thyroid is difficult, surgical exploration may be necessary. Moreover, splitting the isthmus surgically may be required to relieve pressure on the trachea. Overall, the prognosis is good and the fibrosing reaction rarely progresses to the extent that surgical excision is necessary.

GRAVES' DISEASE

The term Graves' disease is restricted to a syndrome marked by thyrotoxicosis caused by a hyperfunctioning diffuse hyperplastic goiter, accompanied by ophthalmopathy and sometimes dermopathy. Thyrotoxicosis may also be produced by other disorders such as subacute thyroiditis, toxic multinodular goiter, and a functioning (toxic) adenoma, but these syndromes are differentiated from Graves' disease because the eye and skin changes are less prominent. As intimated previously, the hyperplastic goiter is thought to be autoimmune in origin. The most striking features of the ophthalmopathy, when present, are lid lag, upper lid retraction, stare, weakness of eye muscles, diplopia, periorbital edema, and notably proptosis to the point at which the lids cannot close. More consistent is an increase in intraocular pressure, only evident on special testing.[57] All these ocular abnormalities are believed to arise from chronic edematous inflammation of the extraocular muscles and retro-orbital tissues caused by autoimmune reactions. The dermopathy takes the form of localized areas of edematous skin thickening (orange-peeling) over the dorsum of the legs or feet. The lesions are quite discrete and may have a plaquelike or nodular conformation. Little is known about the origins of these changes. Despite the fact that the dermopathy is typical of Graves' disease, it is present in only 10 to 15% of cases. Perplexingly, it has been referred to as localized myxedema. Thus, *although Graves' disease is said to consist of a triad of major abnormalities, the dermopathy may be lacking and the ophthalmopathy may not be readily evident, so that diagnosis rests largely on the documentation of thyrotoxicosis related to diffuse toxic goiter.* As will become evident, there are reasons for believing that all three components are independent, albeit related, disorders that often do not pursue parallel courses.

Graves' disease is relatively common and may arise at any age, with a peak incidence in the third and fourth decades. The female:male ratio is 5:1. There is a well-defined association with HLA-DR3, and familial predisposition has been frequently noted.[58] There is also a well-defined association between Graves' disease and other autoimmune thyroid disorders, notably Hashimoto's thyroiditis and, less strikingly, primary (? autoimmune) myxedema. You may recall that hyperthyroidism sometimes supervenes on preexisting Hashimoto's thyroiditis, and conversely the morphologic changes in the thyroid gland in Graves' disease have some similarities to those of Hashimoto's thyroiditis. As might be expected, other autoimmune diseases such as pernicious anemia occur with greater-than-chance frequency in patients with Graves' disease.

Etiology and Pathogenesis. The evidence is quite compelling that the goitrous, hyperfunctioning, diffuse hyperplasia of the thyroid gland is autoimmune in origin and initiated by IgG autoantibodies that stimulate both thyroid growth and function.[42] The essential nature of the autoimmune reaction is almost identical to that described in Hashimoto's thyroiditis (p. 1207), arising because of a deficiency of antigen-specific suppressor T cells. Thus, the stage is set for an abnormal humoral reaction with the formation of autoantibodies to TSH-receptor antigens. It is theorized that immune response genes of the HLA-DR3 genotype account for the defect in antigen-specific suppressor T cells. TSH autoantibodies, which subsume the function of TSH by binding to the follicular cell receptors, can be identified in nearly all patients with Graves' disease.[59] As indicated in the discussion of Hashimoto's disease (p. 1206), the TSH autoantibodies are of two categories: thyroid-stimulating immunoglobulins (TSI) that induce hyperfunction, and thyroid-growth immunoglobulins (TGI) that initiate growth.[44] As mentioned earlier, blocking antibodies for each of these immunoglobulins have been identified. Thus, *in Graves' disease both the TSI and the TGI fractions account for the increased output of thyroid hormones and the glandular hyperplasia.* By contrast, in Hashimoto's thyroiditis associated with the HLA-DR5 genotype, there is expression mainly of TGI with either a failure in production of TSI or the elaboration of TSI-blocking antibody.[35]

The question must be raised—if genetic predisposition underlies the development of Graves' disease, why does it appear only in the third and fourth decades of life? One hypothesis invokes the concept that the disease only appears when chance mutation gives rise to autoreactive B cells that cannot be held in check because of the genetic defect in suppressor-cell function. Alternatively, progressive decline in suppressor-cell function may occur with the passing years, leading eventually to a critical threshold. Yet again, cumulative stress, either physical or emotional, may impair lymphocyte function in genetically predisposed individuals to potentiate the development of Graves' disease.[60] Whatever the initiating mechanism, the thyroid hyperfunction, once begun, may be self-perpetuating. Thyrotoxicosis in animals depresses suppressor T-cell function, and in humans control of the hyperfunction with therapy tends to restore suppressor function to normal.[61]

Evidence is accumulating that the ophthalmopathy of Graves' disease is also autoimmune in origin. A fairly intense lymphocytic infiltrate is present in the intra- and extraocular eye muscles as well as in the retro-orbital fibrofatty tissues, and a circulating autoantibody against a soluble eye-muscle antigen can be identified in most patients.[62] The association of this ocular autoimmune reaction with past, present, or future thyroid dysfunction in 80 to 90% of cases may be explicable by more recent findings that monoclonal antibodies to eye-muscle antigens cross-react with thyroid microsomes.[63] So it is that the thyroid and orbital autoimmune reactions are separate but related.

MORPHOLOGY. In most cases of diffuse hyperplasia, the gland is usually uniformly but not markedly enlarged. It is **uncommon** to observe **more than threefold** increases in weight up to 80 to 90 gm. The capsule is intact and not adherent. On cut section, the parenchyma has a soft, yielding, red-brown, meaty appearance closely resembling the cross section of normal muscle. Preoperative iodine administration causes the accumulation of colloid and alters this gross appearance.

The dominant histologic feature is that of excessive cellularity of the parenchyma. This is imparted by two alterations: an increase in height of the lining epithelial cells to form tall columnar cells, and an increase in the number of cells, causing them to pile up in papillary buds and encroach on the colloid (Figs. 26–13 and 26–14). For the most part, these papillae represent **simple, nonbranching** projections, which are usually slightly elevated above the level of the surrounding epithelium. Occasionally, the papillae are sufficiently large to mushroom out and virtually fill the follicles. The cells may show slight variation in size and shape, but no striking atypicality is present. The Golgi apparatus is hypertrophied, the mitochondria increased in number, and the microvilli more abundant. Colloid is markedly diminished in amount and, when present, has a thin, pale pink, watery appearance. The interfollicular stroma shows a striking increase in the amount of lymphoid tissue and, in some areas, large lymphoid follicles are produced. The accumulation of lymphoid tissue in the thyroid is only one aspect of the generalized lymphoid hypertrophy found throughout the body with enlargement of lymph nodes and thymus and hyperplasia of the lymphoid tissue of the spleen. There is inevitably a markedly increased vascularization of the thyroid gland.

This classic histologic pattern may be significantly altered by preoperative medication. Iodine promotes colloid storage, devascularization, and involution of the gland, whereas thiouracil tends to produce marked hyperplasia. Thus, it is impossible to evaluate correctly, from histologic examination, the amount of functional activity of pretreated surgical specimens.

When present, the exophthalmos is related to an increase in the volume of the extraocular muscles and orbital tissues secondary to edema, increased deposits of hydrophilic mucopolysaccharides, fibrosis, and lymphocytic infiltrates (infiltrative ophthalmopathy). The compressive forces account for the increased intraocular pressure. Later, there is fibrosis and contractures of the extraocular muscles, accounting for the incoordination of eye movements, diplopia, and sometimes ophthalmoplegia.[64]

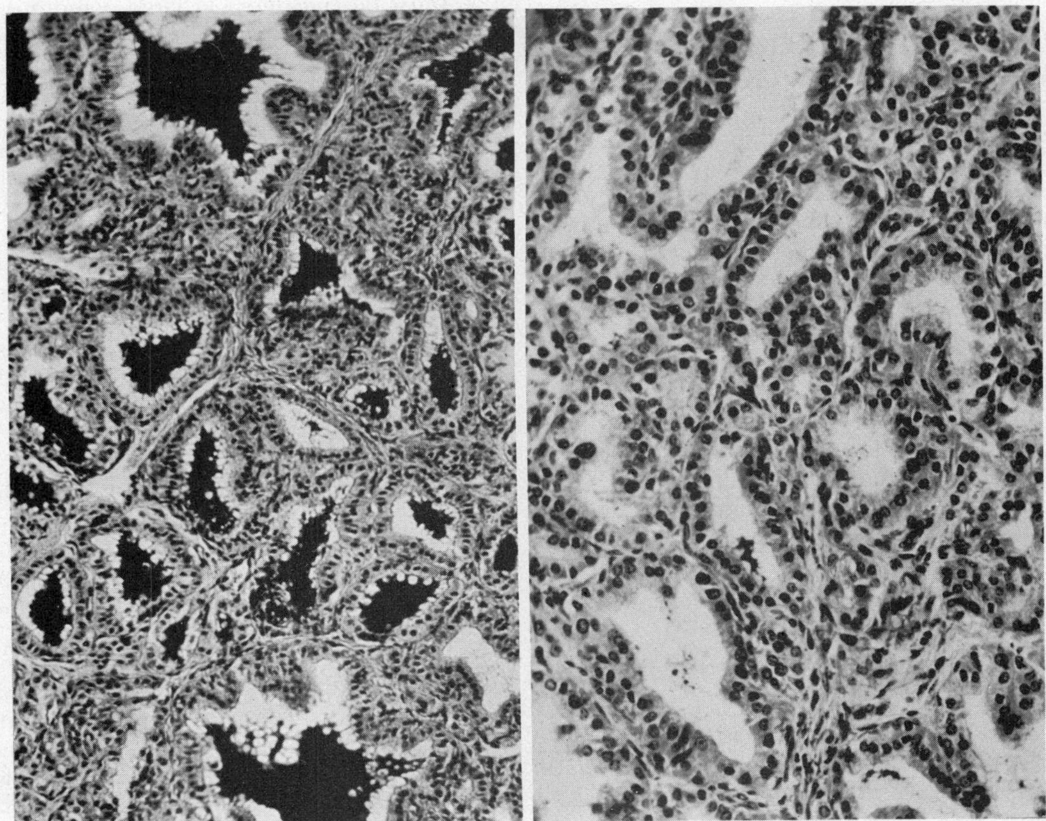

Fig. 26–13 Fig. 26–14

Figure 26–13. Microscopic view of diffuse thyroid hyperplasia. Cellularity of follicles and resorption of colloid are evident. High columnar epithelium and small projections into follicular spaces are visible.

Figure 26–14. High-power view of diffuse thyroid hyperplasia, illustrating total absence of colloid, increase in height of epithelium, and buckling of lining cells into follicular spaces.

Clinical Course. Graves' disease presents, principally in young women, as thyrotoxicosis (p. 1203) associated with modest symmetric enlargement of the thyroid gland. When the ophthalmopathy and the dermopathy already described are also present, the diagnosis is almost certain. Confirmation usually requires one or more of the following findings: an elevated BMR, increased radioactive iodine uptake, and above-normal serum levels of T_4, T_3, and free T_4 and T_3.

In most cases of Graves' disease the thyrotoxicosis is persistent, but it may wax and wane in severity over time. There are, however, many ways of controlling it, including antithyroid drugs such as thiourea derivatives, iodides, a therapeutic dose of radioiodine, and subtotal thyroidectomy, each of which has its indications and contraindications. However, control of the thyrotoxicosis is without effect on the ophthalmopathy. In most cases the eye changes run a benign course and spontaneously remit. The condition can, however, become progressively worse when the proptosis precludes closure of the lids with corneal injuries and ulcerations and, ultimately, loss of the eye(s). Anti-immune therapy such as steroids may stem the tide, but in some instances orbital decompression is necessary to preserve vision. On a happier note, there is no evidence of an increased frequency of thyroidal cancer in patients with Graves' disease.

DIFFUSE NONTOXIC GOITER AND MULTINODULAR GOITER

Diffuse nontoxic goiter and multinodular goiter are the consequences of compensatory hypertrophy and hyperplasia of follicular epithelium secondary to some derangement that hampers thyroid hormone output. The degree of thyroid enlargement is proportional to the level and duration of thyroid hormone lack, but optimally, in most cases, the increased thyroid mass eventually achieves a euthyroid state, although hypo- or hyperthyroidism may result. At the outset the goitrous enlargement is diffuse, but for poorly understood reasons and in the course of time it is likely to become nodular, as described below. This progression is not inevitable and indeed, during the diffuse stage, the gland may revert to normal if, for example, the impediment to thyroid hormone output abates.

DIFFUSE NONTOXIC (SIMPLE) GOITER

This designation specifies a form of goiter that: (1) diffusely involves the entire gland without producing nodularity and (2) is not associated with either hyper- or hypofunction. Because the enlarged follicles are filled with colloid, the term *colloid goiter* has also been applied to this condition. It occurs in both an endemic and sporadic distribution.

The term *endemic goiter* simply refers to the high incidence of simple goiter in particular geographic locales, namely, in over 10% of the population. It is extremely common throughout the world and is thought to affect over 200 million individuals. It is most prevalent in mountainous areas such as the Alps, Andes, and Himalayas, but may also occur in nonmountainous regions remote from the sea. With this distribution a deficient intake of iodine is the dominant cause of the disease.[65] Simple goiter was at one time moderately prevalent in the Great Lakes region of North America but the incidence has markedly decreased with the use of iodized salt. The lack of iodine leads to decreased synthesis of thyroid hormone and a compensatory increase in TSH, causing follicular cell hypertrophy and hyperplasia with the generation of new follicles and goitrous enlargement. The enlarged mass of follicular cells increases hormone output and eventually achieves a euthyroid state.

Variations in the prevalence of endemic goiter in locales with similar levels of iodine deficiency point to the existence of other causative influences, particularly dietary substances referred to as *goitrogens.*[66] Calcium and fluorides in the water supply promote goiter formation. A number of foods, including cabbage, cassava, cauliflower, Brussels sprouts, turnip, and others belonging to the Brassica and Cruciferae plants, have been documented to be goitrogenic in animals and associated with goiter in humans. To be clinically significant the food must be consumed in large quantity or represent the major portion of the diet, as noted in native populations subsisting largely on cassava root.[67] Cassava contains a thiocyanate that inhibits iodide transport within the thyroid, worsening any possible concurrent iodine deficiency. Pollution of water supplies may also in some way be goitrogenic. Depending on the severity of iodine lack and goitrogenic influences, the thyroid enlargement may appear in early childhood, but usually it peaks at about puberty or soon thereafter, affecting females more often than males. Severe iodine deficiency during fetal development may produce cretinism.

Nonendemic or sporadic simple goiter is much less common than the endemic variety. There is a striking female preponderance in the ratio of 8:1, with a peak incidence at puberty or in young adult life. The cause of this condition is rarely evident. Although it is natural to assume that increased levels of TSH stimulate the glandular enlargement, it has not been possible to document elevated levels of the pituitary hormone in all patients, perhaps because the elevations are slight or are intermittent and missed. Alternatively, an intrathyroidal mechanism has been invoked. Earlier (p. 1202) it was pointed out that a reduction in the intrathyroidal level of iodine, whatever the basis, enhances the adenyl cyclase response to TSH, initiating growth, but there is as yet no proof of this mechanism in sporadic goiter. Conceivably, a number of influences act in concert. For example, a minimal iodine lack, when coupled with increased demand for thyroid hormones, might lead to goiter formation. Sporadic goiters, especially in girls, are prone to appear first at puberty, a time of increased physiologic demand. During pregnancy, increased levels of the thyroid-binding globulins (TBG), perhaps estrogen induced, and raised iodide clearance by the kidney may lower the levels of free T_4 and T_3 and reduce feedback inhibition of TSH. Dietary goitrogens may be superimposed on these causal influences. Other very uncommon causes of sporadic goiter are a hereditary defect in hormone transport and synthesis of excess amounts of TBG, reducing the proportion of free thyroid hormones.[68, 69] Finally, there are the inborn biosynthetic errors in iodine metabolism.

The four major *hereditary biosynthetic defects* in thyroid hormone synthesis, all transmitted as autosomal recessive conditions, can be characterized as (1) iodide transport defect, (2) organification defect, (3) dehalogenase defect, and (4) iodotyrosine coupling defect.[70] In the *transport defect*, the thyroid and salivary glands and stomach are unable to trap or concentrate iodide or other anions such as perchlorate; the precise basis of the transport defect remains unclear. In the *organification defect*, an apparent lack of peroxidase limits the redox reaction, in which an electron is split off iodide before it combines with tyrosine. A subset of this group has concomitant deafness, referred to as *Pendred's syndrome*. The *dehalogenase defect* is characterized by an inability to recapture the iodide in MIT and DIT released from colloid along with T_4 and T_3. The fourth syndrome constitutes an *inability to couple iodotyrosyl residues to form T_4 and T_3*, and may actually embrace a number of defects, all leading to impaired hormone synthesis. Depending on the severity of the biosynthetic defect, the development of a goiter may permit the output of sufficient thyroid hormone to maintain the euthyroid state. Obviously, with more severe biosynthetic defects, there is hypothyroidism along with the goitrous enlargement. Indeed, such errors in hormone synthesis may be responsible for cretinism.

MORPHOLOGY. **Two stages can be identified in the evolution of the diffuse nontoxic goiter, whether endemic or sporadic, the first being the hyperplastic stage and the second the colloid involution.** In the stage of hyperplasia, the gland is modestly enlarged and rarely exceeds 100 to 150 gm. It is diffusely, symmetrically involved and markedly hyperemic. Histologically, the follicular epithelium is tall and columnar and the newly generated follicles small with only scanty colloid. The duration of the hyperplastic stage is extremely variable. With the increased mass of cells a euthyroid state is achieved, and follicular cell growth ceases and is followed by colloid accumulation.[71] Now the follicles enlarge as they become filled with colloid and the epithelium undergoes progressive flattening (Fig. 26–15). Indeed, it may be reduced to a thin layer of pavemented attenuated cells. For reasons that are unclear, **the accumulation of colloid is not uniform throughout the gland, and some follicles are hugely distended, while others remain small and may even retain small papillary infoldings of hyperplastic cells.** Now the thyroid becomes markedly enlarged, sometimes to 500 gm or more. The accumulated colloid produces a marked increase in consistency and a gelatinous, glistening cut surface. It is this phase of nontoxic diffuse enlargement that is referred to as **colloid goiter.** The pathogenetic mechanism underlying such colloid involution is obscure but presumably reflects the synthesis of thyroid hormone–poor glycoprotein.

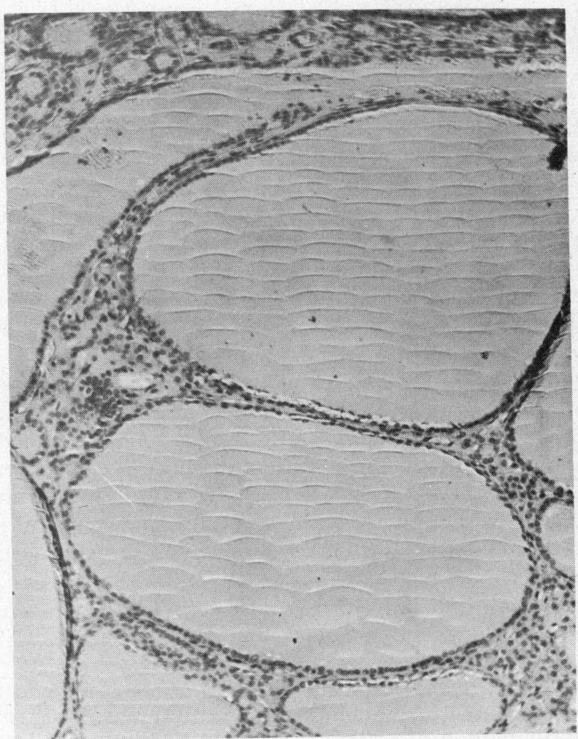

Figure 26–15. Diffuse, nontoxic goiter. Follicles are distended with colloid, and epithelial lining is flattened.

CLINICAL COURSE. The clinical significance of nontoxic diffuse goiter depends largely on its ability to achieve a state of euthyroidism, which is generally the rule. Rare patients are hypothyroid and in these the TSH level is almost invariably elevated, as it may be to a lesser extent in those marginally euthyroid. The goitrous enlargement may be nonvisible, even with the head raised, or plainly evident to the casual observer on the street. By definition, the increase in size is symmetric and sometimes accompanied by a prominent pyramidal lobe. During the early stages, administration of iodine brings about regression of the goiter, but later it is without effect. *Perhaps the major significance of the diffuse goiter is that it is a forerunner of a nodular goiter.*

MULTINODULAR GOITER

Nearly all long-standing simple goiters become transformed in time into multinodular goiters. They may be nontoxic or sometimes induce thyrotoxicosis (*toxic multinodular goiter*), which differs from Graves' disease inasmuch as there is no associated ophthalmopathy or dermopathy and the hypermetabolism is usually less severe. Rarely, multinodular goiters are associated with hypothyroidism. Whatever their functional state, *multinodular goiters produce the most extreme thyroid enlargements and are more frequently mistaken for neoplastic involvement than any other form of thyroid disease.* Since they derive from simple goiter, they occur in both sporadic and endemic forms, having the same female-to-male distribution and presumably the same origins, but affect older individuals because they are late complications. However, there is no clear understanding of the basis for the transformation into the nodular pattern. It is speculated that, with follicular hyperplasia, generation of new follicles, and uneven accumulation of colloid throughout the follicles, tensions and stresses are produced within the thyroid gland that lead to rupture of follicles and vessels followed by hemorrhages, scarring, and sometimes calcifications. The scarring adds to the tensions, and in this cyclical manner nodularity appears. Moreover, the preexistent stromal framework of the gland may more or less enclose areas of expanded parenchyma contributing to the nodularity.[72] Although individual nodules may closely resemble neoplastic adenomas, it has been shown that the contained follicles are polyclonal and thus appear to represent expansions of preexisting polyclonal normal follicles.[71]

MORPHOLOGY. The multinodular goiter is marked by its heterogeneity. **Typical features are (1) nodularity created by islands of colloid-filled acini or islands of small hyperplastic acini, (2) random irregular scarring, (3) focal hemorrhages and hemosiderin pigmentation, (4) focal calcifications in areas of scarring, and (5) microcyst formations.** The goitrous enlargement may be monstrous and achieve weights of over 2000 gm. The pattern of enlargement is quite unpredictable and may involve one lobe far more than the other, producing lateral pressure on midline structures such as the trachea and esophagus (Fig. 26–16). In other instances, the goiter grows behind the sternum and clavicles to produce the so-called **intrathoracic or plunging goiter.** Occasionally, most of it is hidden behind the trachea and esophagus, yet in other instances one nodule may so stand out as to impart the clinical appearance of a solitary nodule. On cut section there is an overall heterogeneous multinodularity; some of the nodules are poorly circumscribed, but others appear to accumulate scarring and condensation of the thyroid stroma about themselves to create the appearance of complete encapsulation similar to that found in the true adenoma. Thus have arisen the terms **adenomatous goiter** or **multiple colloid adenomatous goiter** as synonyms for this condition.

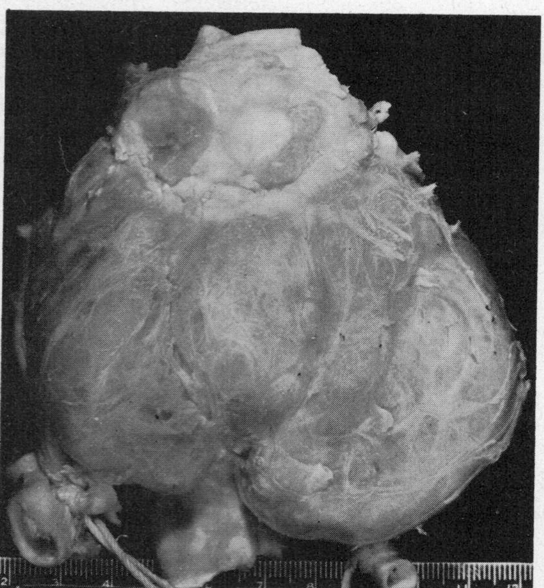

Figure 26–16. Multinodular goiter removed with trachea attached. Asymmetry and enlargement of gland are apparent.

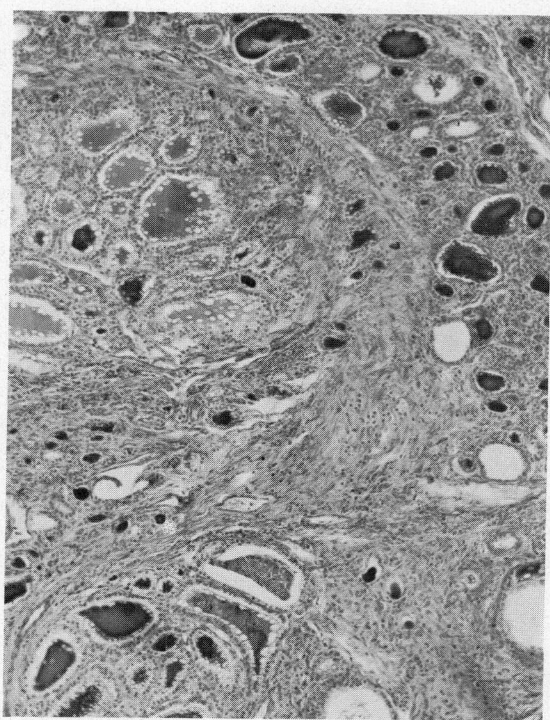

Figure 26–17. Multinodular goiter illustrating scarring and variation in size of follicles.

The histology of the multinodular lesion is characterized above (Fig. 26–17). The differentiation of a nodule in this condition from a true adenoma is at best treacherous and is discussed in some detail on page 1216.

CLINICAL COURSE. From the clinical standpoint, multinodular goiters are of importance because of (1) size and location of the goitrous mass; (2) possible abnormal function, usually thyrotoxicosis; and (3) their differentiation from neoplasms. When sufficiently enlarged, the goiter may cause not only cosmetic disfigurement but also dysphagia, a choking sensation, and (with compression of the trachea) an inspiratory stridor. These manifestations are particularly prominent when the goiter enlarges into the thoracic inlet behind the sternum. Such lesions may induce a superior vena caval syndrome, i.e., distention of the veins of the neck and upper extremities, edema of the eyelids and conjunctiva, and syncope on coughing. Hemorrhages into the goiter may induce sudden painful enlargement, worsening the obstructive symptoms.

In less than half of the cases, hyperfunction appears—toxic multinodular goiter. Although it basically resembles the thyrotoxicosis of Graves' disease, there are several significant differences. Ophthalmopathy and dermopathy do not appear and, when present, probably represent the super-imposition of Graves' disease; the thyrotoxicosis is in general mild to moderate; and cardiovascular manifestations tend to predominate, possibly because toxic multinodular goiter usually appears in older patients likely to have underlying heart disease. Thus, atrial fibrillation, tachycardia, and sometimes heart failure may be encountered. The radioactive iodine uptake and serum levels of T_3 and T_4 may be only slightly elevated. Scintiscans of the gland reveal one of two patterns: the radioiodine may accumulate in patchy foci throughout the gland or, less commonly, in only one or a few nodules. What accounts for this variation is not known, but the latter pattern suggests suppression of much of the parenchymal function by hyperfunction of one or a few foci.

The differentiation of a multinodular goiter, toxic or nontoxic, from a neoplasm may be simple or difficult, both clinically and anatomically. When the multinodularity involves the entire gland, it is highly likely to represent a goiter rather than a neoplasm. Thyroid cancer sometimes spreads throughout the gland, but in such circumstances the nodular enlargement is usually of relatively short duration and not present for decades, as is generally the case with multinodular goiter. The major difficulty arises when the enlargement of a single focus outpaces the rest of the gland. It is beyond our scope to dig deeply into this clinical dilemma, which taxes all diagnostic methods and often ultimately requires needle biopsy or surgical excision. Ultrasonography and CT scan may be helpful in ruling out neoplasia by revealing widespread diffuse multinodularity. Suppression of TSH by the administration of thyroid hormone is more likely to induce regression of a non-neoplastic nodule than of an autonomous tumor, but functioning adenomas also sometimes respond, and the converse is true about nodules within a goiter. A vast amount of literature has accumulated on the differential diagnosis, as discussed below.[73, 74]

TUMORS

Nodules in the thyroid have always commanded a great deal of attention because they are sometimes visible, are often palpated by the patient, and raise the question of cancer.[75] According to most authorities, clinically palpable thyroid nodules are present in 4 to 7% of adults in the United States, but cancers of the thyroid are rare.[76] Postmortem studies reveal one or more nodules much more often, but in most instances they are small anatomic lesions of no clinical significance. The annual incidence of thyroid cancer in the U.S. is approximately 25 to 35 cases per million population, accounting for about 0.4% of cancer deaths.[77] It follows, therefore, that only a few clinically palpable nodules of the order of one to two per 1000 are cancers. Reports from surgical clinics, however, point to a much higher incidence of cancer in nodular glands, with estimates ranging up to 20 to 30%. Such data can only reflect selection bias with surgical exploration of only the most ominous lesions. *It can reasonably be concluded that thyroid nodules are very common, but thyroid cancer is very uncommon.*

Despite all the epidemiologic data, the patient is not a statistic, and so every nodule demands careful appraisal. Short of anatomic study, there are no certain methods of differentiating nontumorous nodules from neoplasms and the benign from the malignant. One study of thyroid nodules that were considered to be sufficiently obscure to merit needle biopsy revealed the data set out in Table 26–4. It is evident from these findings that many lesions of the thyroid may present as nodules and, indeed, in 10% of the cases no thyroid abnormality is present.

A discussion of current diagnostic approaches is far beyond our scope, but a few deserve mention because of their anatomic relevance. For years the cornerstone of clinical appraisal of a nodular thyroid has been the scintiscan, following the administration of radioiodine. Most thyroid cancers, and many adenomas, cannot accumulate significant quantities of radioiodine and so appear as nonfunctioning *"cold" nodules.* Although most adenomas and carcinomas are "cold" lesions, so are nonfunctioning nodules in multinodular goiter and focal enlargements in Hashimoto's thyroiditis. It is estimated that only about 20% of "cold" nodules prove to be malignant. Moreover, some adenomas and a rare cancer may be "hot," i.e., may take up radioiodine. Thus, although scintiscans suggest probabilities, they are not definitive. Another approach has been the search for serum tumor markers. Only one has proved to be of great worth, namely, elevated serum titers of calcitonin with medullary carcinomas of the thyroid. Modest increases of the serum carcinoembryonic antigen level have been identified in a small fraction of patients with other forms of thyroid cancer, but this marker has not proved to be of significant diagnostic value. As reliable as any are the following simple observations. A solitary nodule is more suspect of being neoplastic than multiple nodules, for reasons that must now be obvious. The younger the patient (under the age of 40), the greater is the likelihood of neoplasia, because non-neoplastic nodularity, such as may be produced by Hashimoto's

Table 26–4. NEEDLE BIOPSIES OF SUSPICIOUS NODULES*

		Percentage
Hashimoto's thyroiditis	291	32.1%
Adenoma	275	30.3
Colloid nodule or nodular goiter	78	8.6
Nonspecific thyroiditis	61	6.7
Cancer	40	4.4
Subacute thyroiditis	36	4.0
Hyperplasia	24	2.7
Fibrosis	10	1.1
No abnormality	91	10.0

*Adapted from Yao, Y.: Thyroid nodules—benign or malignant? Postgrad. Med. *61*:65, 1977.

thyroiditis or multinodular goiter, tends to appear in older individuals. Both of these non-neoplastic disorders are significantly more common in women than in men, and thus a nodule in a male is more ominous than one in a female. With this cursory look at the diagnostic problem, we can turn to consider the major forms of neoplasia.

Adenomas

Virtually all adenomas of the thyroid gland present as solitary, discrete, small (under 4 cm) nodules (Figs. 28–18 and 28–19). As noted above, many thyroid lesions and even normal glands may at times give the clinical impression of a nodule. In general, only 30 to 50% of seemingly solitary nodules prove to be adenomas of one type or another. The classification of adenomas continues to be unsettled. On histologic grounds, a variety of patterns can be identified that recapitulate stages in the embryogenesis of the normal thyroid, and hence are sometimes specified as *fetal*, *embryonal*, *simple*, and *colloid adenomas*. However, all adenomas contain follicles of varying size and in variable proportions. Hence, all might well be called *follicular adenomas*. A somewhat less common variant has branching papillary excrescences protruding into microcystic spaces; such lesions have been referred to as *papillary cystadenomas*. However, although most of these lesions pursue an innocent course, some that are histologically innocent invade locally and even spread to regional nodes. Conversely, some anaplastic variants are very indolent and almost never kill. It seems best, therefore, to consider all as papillary carcinomas having a range of histologic atypicality and clinical behavior. One additional rare lesion is the so-called *Hürthle cell adenoma*.

MORPHOLOGY. All adenomas will be described as a more or less cohesive group, indicating such distinctive patterns as can be discerned. As stated, they are generally solitary lesions rarely exceeding 3 cm in diameter, readily defined from the surrounding thyroid substance. Infrequently, two or even more adenomas are present. On cross section they range from pale-tan to gray, are soft and fleshy, and sometimes have foci of softening, hemorrhage, or central fibrosis with calcification.

The histologic differentiation of a nodule within a multinodular goiter from an adenoma is difficult not only clinically but also anatomically. **The morphologic criteria used to identify an adenoma are (1) complete fibrous encapsulation, (2) a clear distinction between the architecture inside and outside the capsule, (3) compression of the thyroidal parenchyma about the adenoma, and (4) the lack of multinodularity in the remaining gland** (Fig. 26–20). None of these features alone is sufficient, but collectively they are quite reliable. All adenomas are characterized by considerable variation in the size and number of follicles as well as in the abundance of interfollicular stroma. At one extreme is the lesion composed of closely packed cells forming cords or trabeculae, with only here and there a small abortive follicle. This architecture is reminiscent of embryonic thyroid parenchyma before the development of well-formed follicles, accounting for the sometimes-used designations **embryonal** or **trabecular adenomas.** Another pattern is

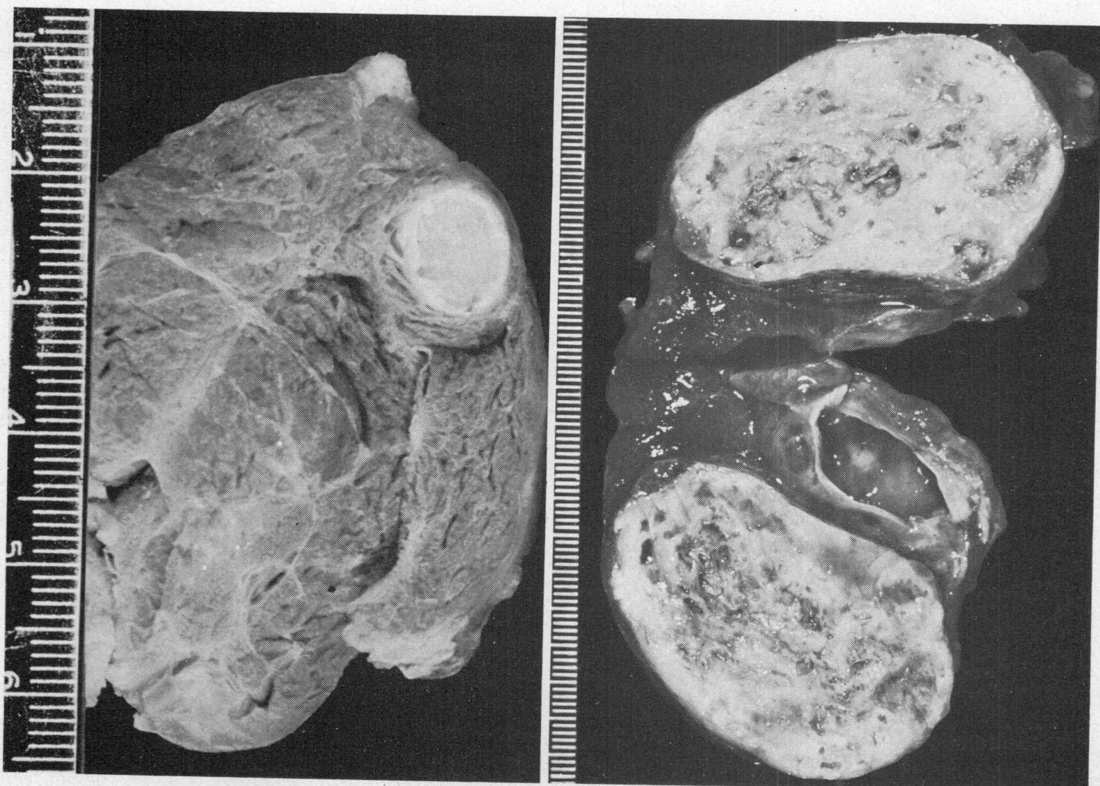

Fig. 26–18

Fig. 26–19

Figures 26–18 and 26–19. Adenomas of thyroid. View of cross section of nodules against background of darker normal thyroid tissue.

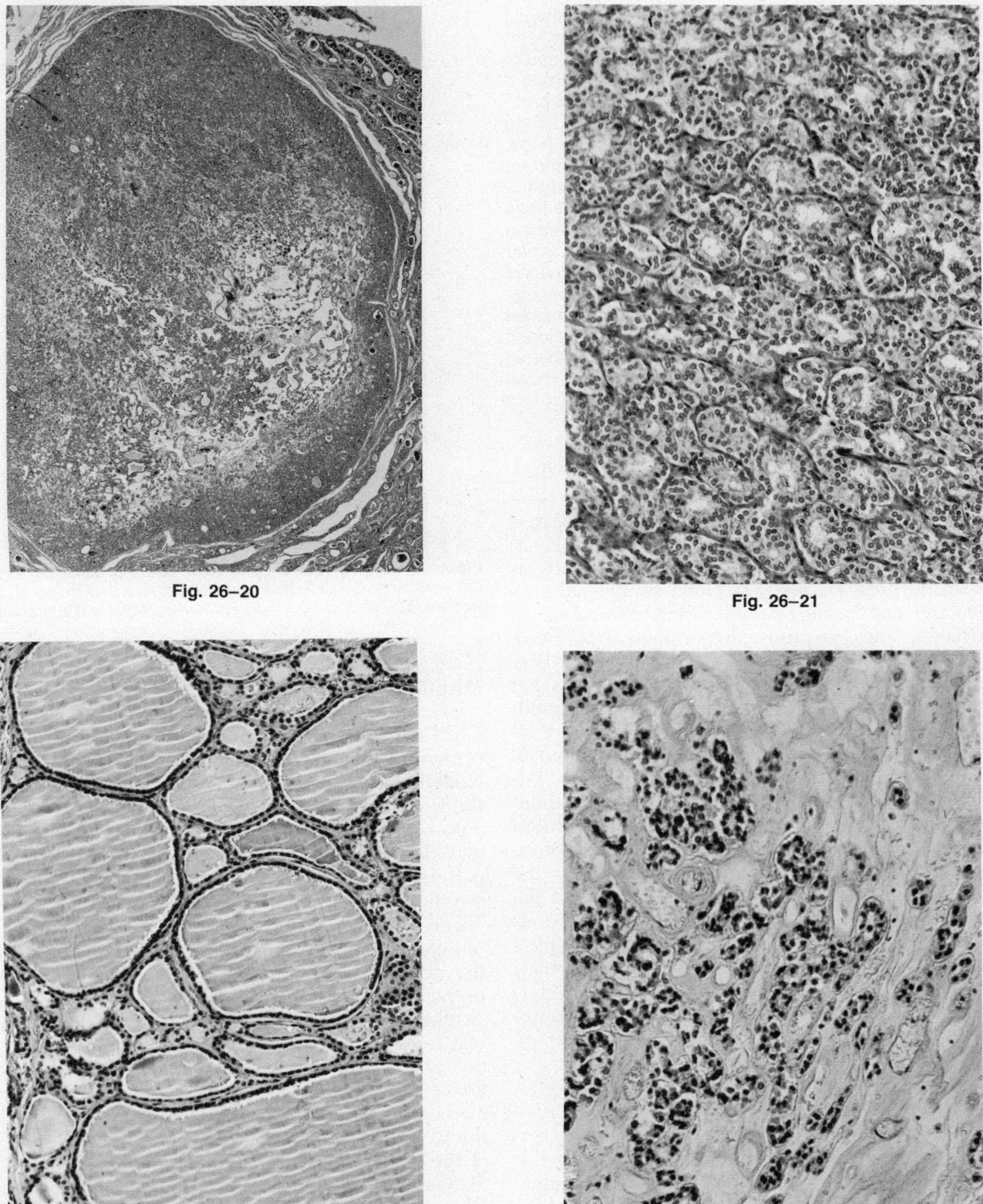

Figure 26–20. Low-power view of follicular adenoma of thyroid, illustrating discrete encapsulation and demarcation from surrounding thyroid substance.

Figures 26–21 to 26–23. Three types of follicular adenoma, illustrating variability in acinar size, colloid content, and amount of interstitial connective tissue. Figure 26–23 represents the type formerly referred to as a fetal adenoma.

composed of small follicles containing little or no colloid separated by an abundant, loose connective tissue. Here the architecture mimics the embryogenesis of the thyroid gland one step after the embryonal stage; hence, the term **fetal adenoma.** The next identifiable variant is composed of closely packed follicles of normal size, sometimes termed a **simple adenoma.** Proceeding along this inexact and probably futile hair-splitting is the **colloid adenoma,** having large follicles filled with colloid and lined by flat epithelium (Figs. 26–21, 26–22, and 26–23). A reasonable argument can be made to merely divide all these adenomas into **microfollicular** and **macrofollicular** patterns, recognizing that all have the same clinical significance. Only the Hürthle cell adenoma is histologically distinctive, being composed of large granular cells identical to those encountered in various non-neoplastic thyroidal lesions (p. 1207), usually arranged in a trabecular pattern (Fig. 26–24). Infrequently, follicular adenomas exhibit some variability in cell morphology or have poorly developed capsules, and so seem to extend into the surrounding thyroid parenchyma. To express such changes, the term **atypical adenomas** has been applied, but it should not be construed as implying a drift toward cancer.

The principal importance of adenomas is their clinical differentiation from cancers, as has already been emphasized. In addition, they may (1) slowly increase in size to cause pressure symptoms in the neck; (2) achieve a certain size and then plateau, apparently as the expansile pressure restricts blood supply; (3) suddenly enlarge and become painful owing to intralesional hemorrhages; and (4) rarely, hyperfunction to cause thyrotoxicosis. The resultant hyperthyroidism differs from Graves' disease inasmuch as it is not associated with ophthalmopathy and is usually relatively mild. Most adenomas are "cold" nodules, but some, particularly those associated with hyperfunction, accumulate sufficient radioiodine to appear as "hot" nodules. Although theoretically autonomous, an adenoma occasionally has some dependence on TSH and so can be induced to regress by the administration of thyroid hormones, which suppress TSH secretion. Finally, there is the issue of malignant transformation of an adenoma. At one time these benign lesions were thought to be a serious risk, but there currently is doubt that even the "atypical adenomas" ever become cancerous. Past impressions probably reflect biopsy sampling errors of well-differentiated follicular carcinomas at one time inappropriately labeled "angioinvasive adenomas" (p. 1221).

Other Benign Tumors

As many as 10 to 25% of solitary nodules of the thyroid gland prove to be cysts.[78] The great preponderance of these represent cystic degeneration of a follicular adenoma; the remainder probably arise in multinodular goiters. They are often filled with a brown, turbid fluid containing changed blood, hemosiderin pigment, and cell debris. Additional benign rarities include dermoid cysts, lipomas, hemangiomas, and teratomas (seen mainly in infants).

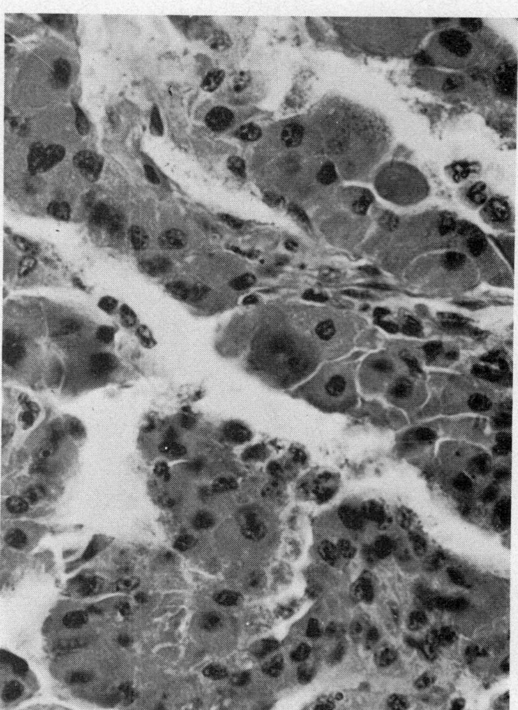

Figure 26–24. High-power detail of the cells that constitute a Hürthle cell adenoma. Considerable variability in size and shape of cells is evident. The abundant cytoplasm demonstrates a fine granularity.

MALIGNANT

Comment has already been made about the rarity of thyroid cancers in the general population (p. 1215). Nonetheless, they cause about 7000 deaths annually in the United States, with a 2–3:1 female:male ratio. There are a number of anatomic subtypes of thyroid carcinoma, as indicated in Table 26–5.[79] Each of these anatomic patterns has its own distinctive biology and clinical significance. At one end of the spectrum are the often "benign" papillary carcinomas; at the other end are the undifferentiated carcinomas that must be rated among the ugliest cancers of humans. Fortunately, the great preponderance of carcinomas fall into the so-called "well-differentiated" category, i.e., papillary and follicular lesions.

Since 1935 the overall incidence of thyroid carcinoma has tripled, but it is not certain whether this increase is real or artifactual. Favoring a real increase is the well-documented contribution of external radiation of the thyroid gland to the induction of cancer.[80] Irradiation during childhood has incurred the greatest risk.[81] From 4 to 9% of individuals irradiated during infancy for such trivial conditions as tonsillar or thymic enlargement, acne, and other skin disorders have developed thyroid carcinoma after a mean latent period of 20 years. From a different vantage point, 80% of children who develop thyroid carcinoma have received therapeutic radiation. Among the Japanese, 6.7% of individuals

Table 26–5. MORPHOLOGIC CLASSIFICATION OF CANCER OF THYROID

	Carcinoma
Well-differentiated	Papillary adenocarcinoma (60–70%)
	Pure papillary adenocarcinoma
	Mixed papillary and follicular carcinoma
	Follicular carcinoma (20–25%
	Pure follicular carcinoma
	Clear cell carcinoma
	Oxyphil cell carcinoma
Poorly differentiated	Medullary carcinoma (5–10%)
	Undifferentiated carcinoma (10–15%)
	Small cell carcinoma
	Giant cell carcinoma
	Epidermoid carcinoma
	Other Malignant Tumors
	Lymphoma
	Sarcoma
	Secondary tumor

exposed to the atomic bomb have developed thyroid cancers.[82] Small wonder that there is present concern in the U.S. about the disposal of nuclear wastes. The nuclear accident at Three Mile Island in 1979 also gives pause for thought despite reassurances that the risk is less than one case per 10 million exposed.[83] The only dubious comfort regarding the relationship of thyroid cancer to irradiation derives from the fact that the great preponderance of associated thyroid cancers are either papillary or follicular, and only very rarely one of the "uglies." There is no current evidence of an increased incidence of thyroid cancer in patients receiving either the relatively small doses of radiant energy involved in scintiscans or the larger doses inherent in the treatment of hyperthyroidism with radioiodine.[84] Moreover, it is no longer believed that preexistent thyroid disease such as multinodular goiter, Graves' disease, Hashimoto's thyroiditis, and adenomas predispose to thyroid cancer.

Before turning to the various anatomic patterns, the clinical staging of thyroid cancers should be presented. The following is most widely used:

Stage I. Intrathyroidal lesions.

Stage II. Cancers lacking fixation to surrounding structures but with movable cervical metastases.

Stage III. Cancers with local fixation or fixed cervical nodes.

Stage IV. Cancers with distant metastases.

The staging of thyroid cancers is obviously of importance in estimating the prognosis, but the histologic type is of much greater significance.

Papillary Carcinoma

Under this designation are included the benign-appearing lesions, formerly termed papillary adenoma, as well as the overt carcinomas, because experience has taught that all papillary neoplasms have the potential for spread and cancerous behavior. As Table 26–5 indicates, papillary carcinomas may be "pure," but over half contain an admixture of follicular carcinoma, just as follicular lesions are also frequently mixed with papillary growths. Even Solomon would have difficulty in appropriately subclassifying the infinite range of mixtures encountered. Long-term follow-up of patients with these mixed lesions, however, indicates that, *regardless of the precise proportions, all neoplasms containing some papillary growth have identical biologic behavior;* the great majority of all papillary lesions are indolent with an excellent prognosis. About 10 to 20% first come to attention by spread to regional nodes with the production of cervical lymphadenopathy. As noted earlier, many are associated with previous exposure to ionizing radiation.[85]

Whether pure or mixed, papillary adenocarcinomas are the most common form of thyroid cancer (60 to 70%).[86] They tend to occur rather evenly through the third to seventh decades, but these neoplasms account for at least 80% of thyroid cancers in individuals under 40 years of age, largely because the less well-differentiated neoplasms tend to occur in older persons. Females are affected two to three times as often as males. The tumors usually present as an incidental, nonpainful lump in the neck, but occasionally may be sufficiently large to produce obvious masses. *Not infrequently, the primary lesion remains occult and the first sign of the disease is metastatic enlargement of a cervical lymph node.*

Papillary adenocarcinomas range from microscopic foci found incidentally in thyroids or lymph nodes removed for other reasons to nodules up to 10 cm in diameter (Fig. 26–25). The microscopic foci are often found within scarred areas and sometimes crop up in numerous foci within the gland. Indeed, about 20 to 75% of these cancers are multifocal in the gland, and this is now proved by cell marker studies to be due to intraglandular spread. Larger nodules are generally unencapsulated and invasive locally but may have apparent, poorly developed encapsulation. Penetration of the capsule of the thyroid gland occurs in about 20% of cases and is somewhat more common in the more anaplastic lesions and those having a follicular component. Such extension worsens the prognosis. Sometimes there are cystic spaces into which papillary fronds project, giving rise to the term papillary cystadenocarcinoma. The cut surface of these neoplasms may be furry, owing to the myriads of tiny papillae. Occasional tumors show dense fibrous sclerosis throughout the neoplasm, sometimes punctuated by focal calcification. **The pathognomonic histologic feature of the lesions is a complicated, branching, treelike pattern most sharply outlined by the papilliform axial fibrovascular stroma.** In the benign-appearing so-called adenomas, this framework is covered by a single layer of well-oriented regular cuboidal epithelium (Fig. 26–26). Some papillae are cut in cross section to produce apparent isolated islands; elsewhere follicles may be formed, sometimes filled with colloid. All degrees of atypicality and disorientation of cells, piling up of epithelium, invasion of the stalk and capsule, and formation of glands or sheets of cells may be encountered in the more obviously malignant lesions. Moreover, a wide range of histologic changes is often found from one

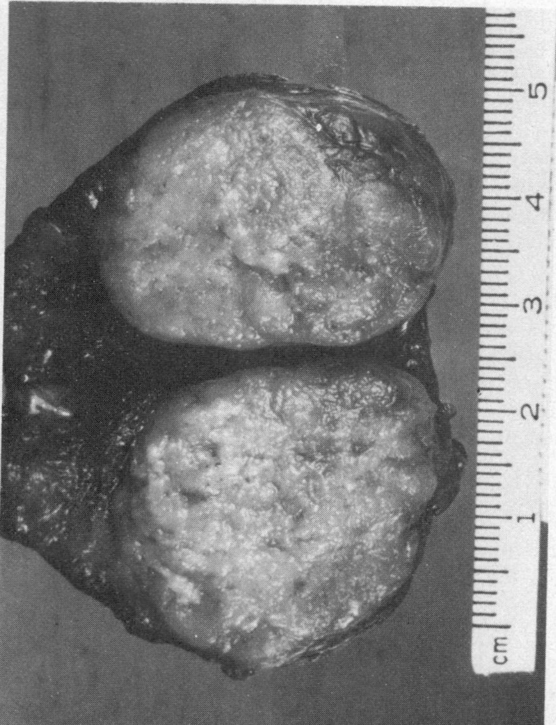

Figure 26–25. A papillary carcinoma showing deceptive apparent encapsulation. (Courtesy of Dr. Merle Legg, New England Deaconess Hospital.)

microscopic field to another within the same lesion, underscoring the difficulty of trying to differentiate so-called adenomas from carcinomas.

In more than half of these neoplasms the nuclei assume a distinctive "ground-glass" appearance.[87] The nuclear membranes are distinct, but the nucleoli and nuclear chromatin are barely discernible. Ground-glass nuclei have been used as the sole criterion for classifying a tumor as papillary, even in the absence of papillae.[88] Almost half of all papillary lesions contain laminated calcific spherules known as **psammoma bodies.** They range in size up to 0.1 nm and often are located in the fibrous axial stroma of the tip of a papilla (Fig. 26–27). Psammoma bodies are rarely encountered in other forms of thyroid neoplasia, and so when present point strongly to the diagnosis of a papillary adenocarcinoma. In the great majority of papillary lesions there is a smaller or greater follicular component (described in the next section). Ultrastructural studies reveal numerous mitochondria; an abundant, rough endoplasmic reticulum; and apical microvilli, similar to those seen in normal follicular cells.[20]

Papillary adenocarcinomas are notorious for their extremely indolent growth and their propensity to metastasize to lymph nodes, particularly in the neck, while not spreading through blood vessels. Many appear as an incidental asymptomatic nodule that has been present for months to years before being brought to clinical attention. In one study, patients reported that the

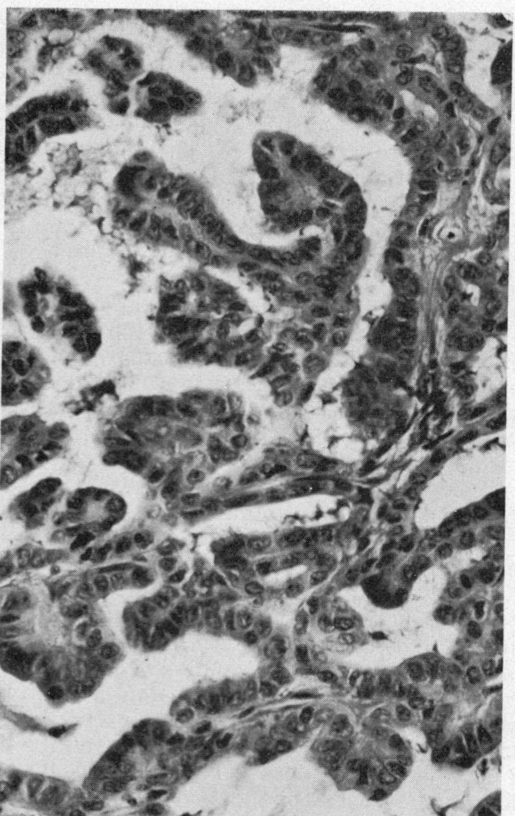

Figure 26–26. High-power detail of a well-differentiated papillary carcinoma illustrating papillary growth pattern and regular alignment of covering epithelium, producing a unicellular layer.

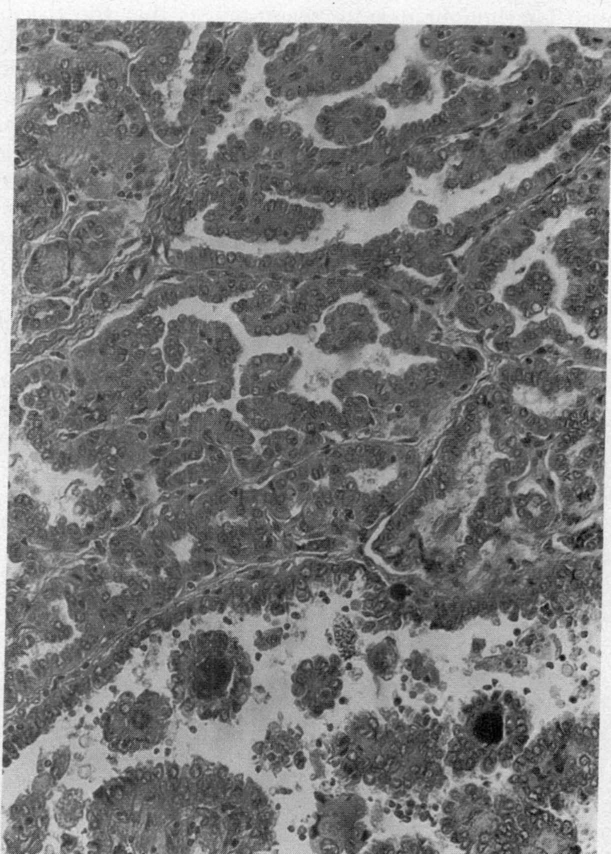

Figure 26–27. Papillary carcinoma of thyroid, showing obvious piling up and anaplasia of cells with some gland formations. Compare with better differentiated lesion of Figure 26–26. Note psammoma bodies within papillae in lower field. (Courtesy of Dr. Merle Legg, New England Deaconess Hospital.)

nodule had been present for an average of six years before they sought medical attention.[77] Others slowly but progressively enlarge and rarely induce disfiguring masses, dysphagia, dysphonia, or dyspnea. Whatever the presentation, all slowly increase in size and sometimes spread beyond the confines of the gland. In one analysis of a large series of cases, about 40% of the lesions had spread beyond the thyroid capsule at the time of initial diagnosis; a similar proportion had metastasized to regional lymph nodes; and 10% had metastasized more widely, e.g., to lungs, bones, and other areas.[89] Overall, 70 to 80% of patients with this form of neoplasia survive at least ten years. Despite an innocuous facade, however, some of these lesions behave as usual cancers. Bearing on the outlook are the following factors: (1) the prognosis is significantly worse with extrathyroidal extension; (2) prognosis and cure are correlated with the level of anaplasia, although this factor is less important than local spread; (3) there is a tendency to greater malignancy with advancing age of the patient; and (4) the duration of the tumor is significant—there is a suggestion that highly malignant neoplasms emerge over time from preexisting low-grade lesions.[89] The patient's age appears to be the most important factor; only rarely does papillary carcinoma cause death in young adults.

Follicular Carcinoma

This pattern accounts for about one-quarter of all thyroid cancers; it is a more aggressive form than papillary carcinomas. As mentioned earlier, mixtures of follicular and papillary growth are frequent and behave as papillary carcinomas. The categorization of a cancer as "follicular" has great clinical significance, since it implies up to a 70% mortality rate at five years.[90] *Critical to the segregation of follicular from papillary carcinomas is the absence of (1) ground-glass nuclei, (2) well-formed papillae, and (3) psammoma bodies.* The presence of these morphologic features, even in neoplasms composed largely of follicular elements, seems to portend the biologic course of papillary carcinoma. Follicular carcinoma occurs more often in females than males and at any age, with a peak incidence in the fifth and sixth decades.

Anatomically, these tumors take one of two gross forms: (1) a small nodule, seemingly encapsulated, closely resembling a follicular adenoma; and (2) an obvious invasive mass, perhaps occupying an entire lobe.[91] The adenoma-like lesion has been described earlier as an **angioinvasive adenoma,** more properly called an **angioinvasive encapsulated carcinoma.** The more common pattern is that of an obvious cancerous mass causing irregular enlargement of the gland. The tumorous gray-white tissue overgrows the thyroid, replaces large parts of it, and extends through the capsule to become adherent to or invade the trachea, muscles, skin, and great vessels of the neck (Fig. 26–28). In this infiltrative progression, the recurrent laryngeal nerves are often trapped. Both the localized and invasive forms often have an abundant fibrous stroma, particularly in the central regions, that is sometimes calcified. Hemorrhages, cyst formations, and areas of necrosis are frequently present.

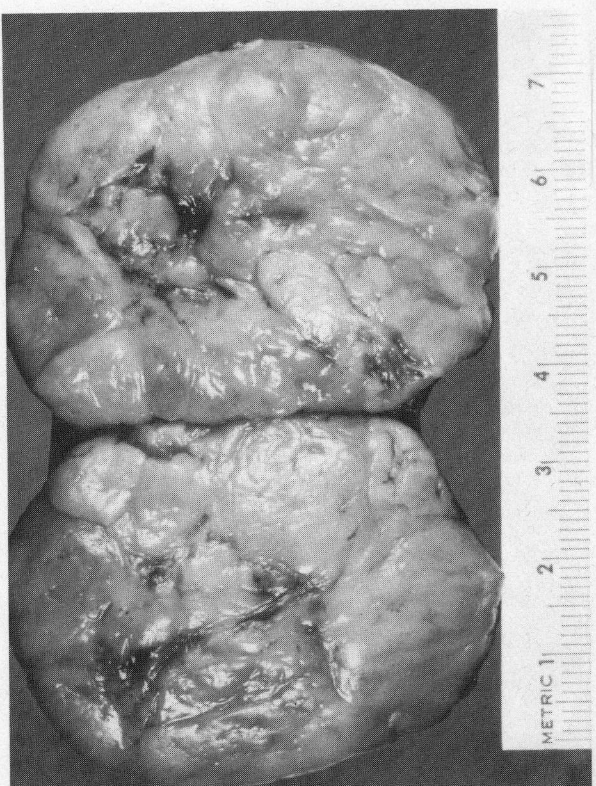

Figure 26–28. Cut surface of a follicular carcinoma with complete replacement of thyroid lobe. (Courtesy of Dr. Merle Legg, New England Deaconess Hospital.)

Microscopically, the pattern is that of an adenocarcinoma with considerable range in the size and differentiation of the gland (follicle) formations. This range conforms to that encountered in the several variations of the adenoma. Thus, some carcinomas have a basically trabecular pattern with only small abortive gland formations, resembling the embryonal pattern of follicular adenoma, whereas others produce well-defined glands or follicles containing colloid (Fig. 26–29). In such lesions, the differentiation from normal thyroid architecture is difficult. These extremely well-differentiated, colloid-producing adenocarcinomas, when found in metastatic sites, have in former years been referred to as **benign, metastasizing struma** (Fig. 26–30). The invasiveness of these lesions is also quite variable. As pointed out, in the localized, adenoma-like pattern there may be only penetration of the apparent capsule, and in the more overt, aggressive, lesions there is frequently extension beyond the gland capsule and vascular invasion, both features serving to differentiate these lesions from adenomas. In contrast to the papillary adenocarcinoma, follicular carcinomas have a strong tendency to invade blood vessels and metastasize, but lymphatic and lymph node dissemination is much less common (Fig. 26–31).

There are two rare variant histologic patterns of the follicular adenocarcinoma. In one the cells have a very clear cytoplasm and closely resemble the clear cell renal carcinoma (hypernephroma) (p. 1054). In the other variant the cells are large and have an abundant acidophilic cytoplasm with small pyknotic central nuclei, closely simulating Hürthle (oxyphil) cells. Neither of these histologic variations alters the biologic course of these neoplasms.

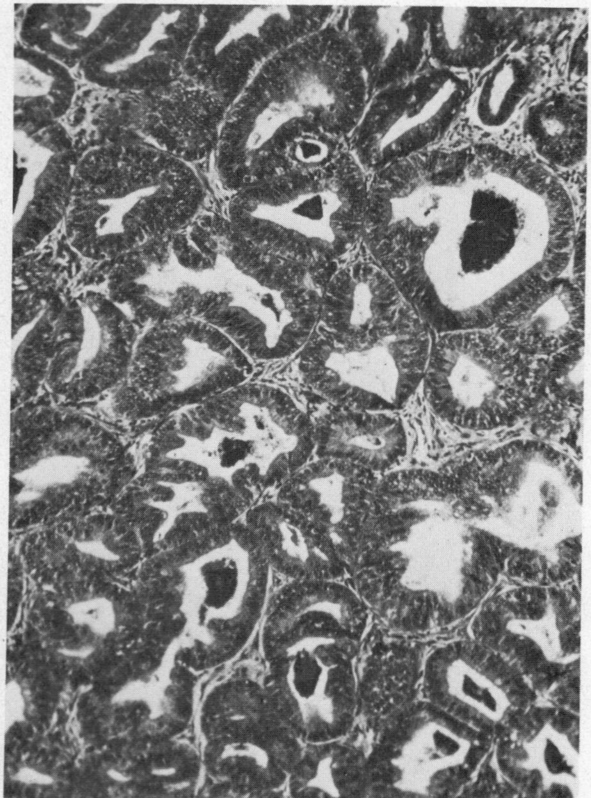

Figure 26–29. Follicular carcinoma of thyroid. A few of the glandular lumina contain recognizable colloid.

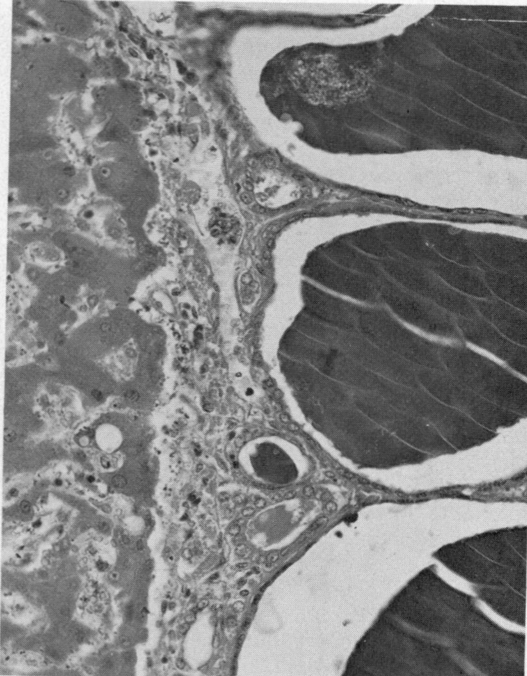

Figure 26–30. High-power detail of follicular cancer of thyroid that has metastasized to liver. Normal liver cells *(on left)* can be seen in approximation to extremely well-differentiated thyroid tissue, demonstrating abundant colloid and deceptively benign-appearing follicular epithelium.

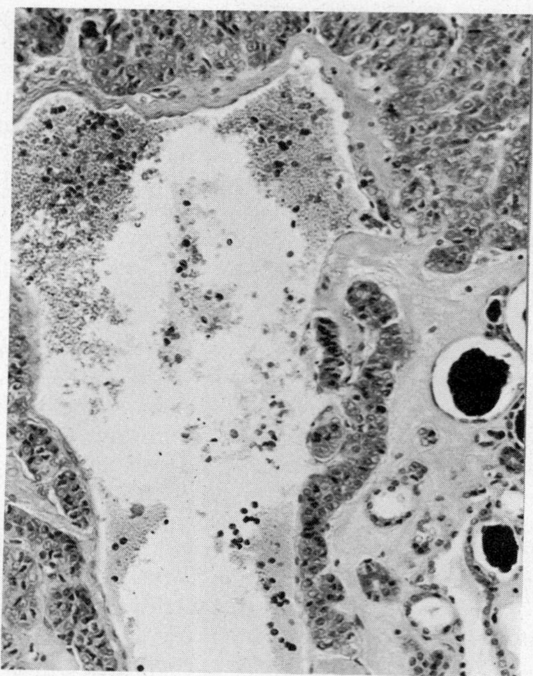

Figure 26–31. High-power detail of cancer of thyroid, illustrating extension of neoplasm through wall of a vessel. Several small nests of cells are seen lying within lumen.

The clinical presentation of this form of thyroid cancer is either that of a solitary enlarging nodule or (more often) irregular, firm, nodular thyroid enlargement. In both presentations the mass slowly expands over the years but at a somewhat more rapid pace than that of the papillary adenocarcinoma. Metastases may not become evident for some time, but eventually most lesions, when left untreated, disseminate through the bloodstream to the lungs, bones, and other distant sites. As mentioned, lymph node spread within the neck may appear, but is not common.

The prognosis is heavily dependent on the stage of the neoplasm at the time diagnosed and on its response to therapy. Stages I and II cancers are generally curable by surgery. Because many of the well-differentiated lesions elaborate thyroglobulin and colloid, these neoplasms, even in Stages III and IV, can sometimes be remarkably controlled by the administration of TSH, followed by radioiodine.

Medullary Carcinoma

This form of cancer, although one of the less frequent patterns (approximately 5 to 10%), is the most versatile of the thyroid carcinomas. Derived from parafollicular (C) cells of neurosecretory origin within and between thyroid acini, *the medullary carcinoma belongs to the family of APUD tumors. It has three distinctive features: (1) its amyloid stroma, (2) its genetic associations, and (3) its elaboration of a variety of polypeptide products.*[92] Amyloid deposits are present in the stroma of most, but not all medullary carcinomas. The amyloid stains in the usual manner and appears to be produced by the parenchymal cells of the neoplasm. With respect to genetic associations, perhaps 80 to 90% of these neoplasms occur sporadically, usually in adults, but 10 to 15% are encountered in children and teenagers in well-defined genetic syndromes, all transmitted by autosomal dominant inheritance.[93] The *Sipple syndrome* constitutes the association of pheochromocytoma with medullary carcinoma of the thyroid, sometimes coupled with either an adenoma or hyperplasia of the parathyroid gland. Thus, the Sipple syndrome is one of the multiple endocrine neoplasia (MEN) syndromes, classified as type IIa (p. 988). In MEN IIb, medullary carcinoma of the thyroid and pheochromocytomas are associated with mucosal neuromas without parathyroid involvement. Much less well characterized are the familial clusterings of medullary thyroid carcinoma unassociated with pheochromocytoma. Clinicoanatomic differences in the presentation of the sporadic and genetic forms of this cancer are mentioned later.[94] Approximately 80 to 90% of medullary cancers secrete calcitonin, providing the opportunity to screen for this neoplasm by radioimmunoassay.[95] Less frequently, these tumors elaborate histaminase, prostaglandins, and (more rarely), ACTH and serotonin. Calcitonin and/or prostaglandins induce diarrhea in about 30% of patients. The ACTH may be responsible for Cushing's syndrome, and the serotonin has in rare instances led to the carcinoid syndrome. It is evident that medullary carcinoma is associated with a variety of clinical presentations.

Grossly, two patterns can be discerned—discrete tumors in one lobe, or numerous nodules that usually infiltrate both lobes. The sporadic neoplasms tend to be localized to one lobe and are often quite large because of late diagnosis, whereas the genetic familial lesions are often multinodular and bilobar, but generally are small lesions confined within the capsule because the associated endocrinopathies call attention to them early. In both, the tumor tissue is firm and gritty and ranges from gray-white to yellow-brown. There may be foci of hemorrhage and necrosis in larger lesions, and some may have spread outside the thyroid capsule. About half of the sporadic larger tumors have metastasized at time of diagnosis. Histologically, these neoplasms have a range of cytologic patterns from round-to-polygonal cells mimicking the histology of endocrine cell tumors (argentaffinomas) (p. 843) to spindled cells having a sarcomatoid appearance. Either cellular pattern may be disposed in organoid nests separated by a fibrovascular, amyloid-containing stroma; sometimes the nests acquire a pseudopapillary appearance (Fig. 26–32). Alternatively, the cells, usually the spindled pattern, may be disposed in sheets. Ultrastructural studies usually disclose in all cytologic patterns both argentaffin- and argyrophil-positive neurosecretory granules characteristic of carcinoids. With immunoperoxidase techniques, calcitonin can also be localized within the cells.[96] The amyloid is stained by Congo red and yields an apple-green fluorescence by polarized light. Multiple foci of C-cell hyperplasia occasionally accompany the neoplasm in familial cases, but are rarely if ever found in the sporadic pattern.[97]

As mentioned earlier, there are significant differences in the clinical presentation of the sporadic and familial lesions.[98] The mean age of diagnosis of the sporadic disease is the fifth to sixth decade; of the familial, the second decade. The familial disease may also be marked by the clinical manifestations emanating from an associated pheochromocytoma or parathyroid lesion (p. 1244). However, diarrhea related to calcitonin secretion is a common manifestation in both forms. The diagnosis of medullary carcinoma can often be made by stimulating calcitonin secretion with pentagastrin and/or calcium infusions. With early diagnosis often possible in the familial form, a 60 to 70% ten-year survival can be anticipated following resection of the tumor. However, with the larger, more advanced sporadic neoplasms, the mean survival approaches five years. Death is usually related to recurrence, extension beyond the capsule, and metastasis, commonly to regional nodes, lung, liver, and bone.

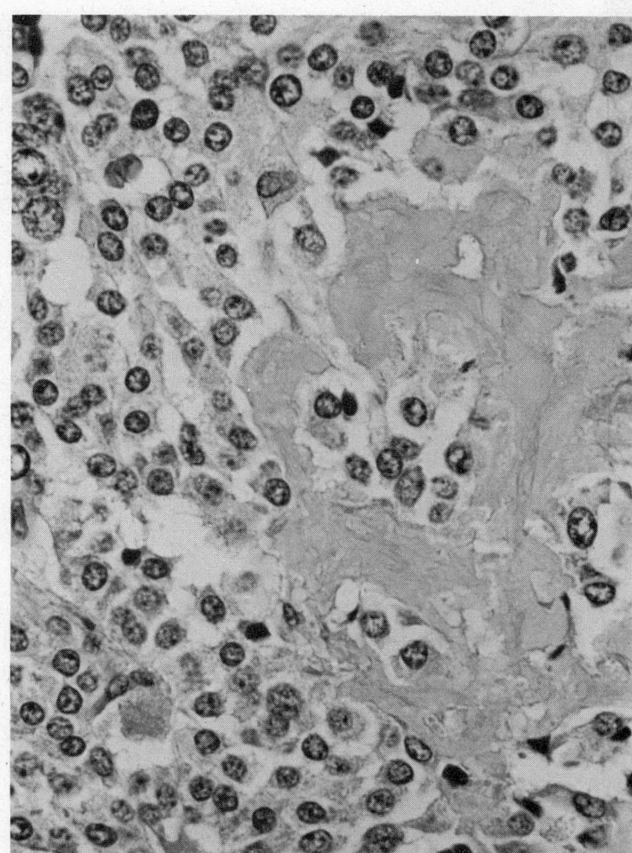

Figure 26–32. Medullary carcinoma with amyloid stroma. High-power detail revealing round-to-polygonal, neurosecretory-like tumor cells with an abundant intercellular amyloidic stroma. (Courtesy of Drs. M. Warhol and L. Weiss, Department of Pathology, Brigham and Women's Hospital, Harvard Medical School.)

Undifferentiated Carcinoma

About 10 to 15% of all thyroid carcinomas belong to this group. These tumors usually occur in the seventh and eighth decades of life and include some of the most malignant neoplasms encountered in man.

By the time these patients are seen clinically, most neoplasms have usually involved large areas of the thyroid gland and, indeed, have extended beyond its confines to produce bulky masses, readily apparent on clinical inspection. Several histologic variants can be identified. **Small cell carcinomas** are made up of compact, closely packed, cuboidal-to-polygonal cells, growing in cords or clusters, separated by a fibrous but non–amyloid-containing stroma. Numerous mitoses are present but giant cells are infrequent. In another variant of small cell carcinoma, there are sheets of extremely small cells, having round, dark nuclei that indeed closely resemble atypical lymphocytes. Such neoplasms are readily mistaken for a lymphoma.

The **giant cell carcinoma** is one of the most bizarre human neoplasms and is composed of highly anaplastic cells, some of which are extremely large and pleomorphic, having multiple or multilobate nuclei; other cells may assume a spindle shape; still others may appear as elongated cytoplasmic ribbons. Numerous mitoses, bizarre mitoses, and giant nuclei are characteristic. Infrequently there are admixtures of papillary and gland formations. Invasion beyond the capsule, blood vessel involvement, and foci of infarct necrosis highlight the aggressive rapid growth of these forms of neoplasia (Fig. 26–33).

The clinical course of these anaplastic cancers is somewhat variable but always grim. Progressive local invasion and widespread metastases account for about a 20% one-year survival with an average duration from the time of diagnosis to death of less than six months.

Other Malignant Tumors

Both Hodgkin's disease and non-Hodgkin's lymphoma may involve the thyroid in the course of their systemic dissemination, but both types of disease may also *arise* in the *thyroid* in the absence of systemic dissemination of a lymphoma primary elsewhere. Although most non-Hodgkin's lymphomas have been classified as histiocytic, cell marker studies now suggest that they are transformed B cells and, in the terminology of Lukes and Collins, would be referred to as immunoblastic lymphomas (p. 664).[99] The mean age at the time of diagnosis is 60 to 70 years, and females are involved three or four times more commonly than males. In one small series of cases, Hashimoto's thyroiditis was frequently present as a preexisting lesion.[100] However, the pathogenetic role of this benign condition in the initiation of the lymphoma is still uncertain.

Sarcomas of the thyroid gland—fibrosarcoma, hemangiosarcoma, osteogenic sarcoma—are extremely rare primary cancers of the thyroid. The diagnosis of such lesions must be made with due consideration for the fact that undifferentiated carcinomas may assume a sarcomatoid appearance.

MISCELLANEOUS LESIONS

This noncommittal heading is adopted to cover some congenital anomalies of the thyroid gland and sundry other involvements, some encountered in systemic diseases.

CONGENITAL ANOMALIES

Thyroglossal duct or cyst is the most common clinically significant congenital anomaly. A persistent sinus tract may remain as a vestigial remnant of the tubular development of the thyroid gland. Parts of this tube may be obliterated, leaving small segments to form

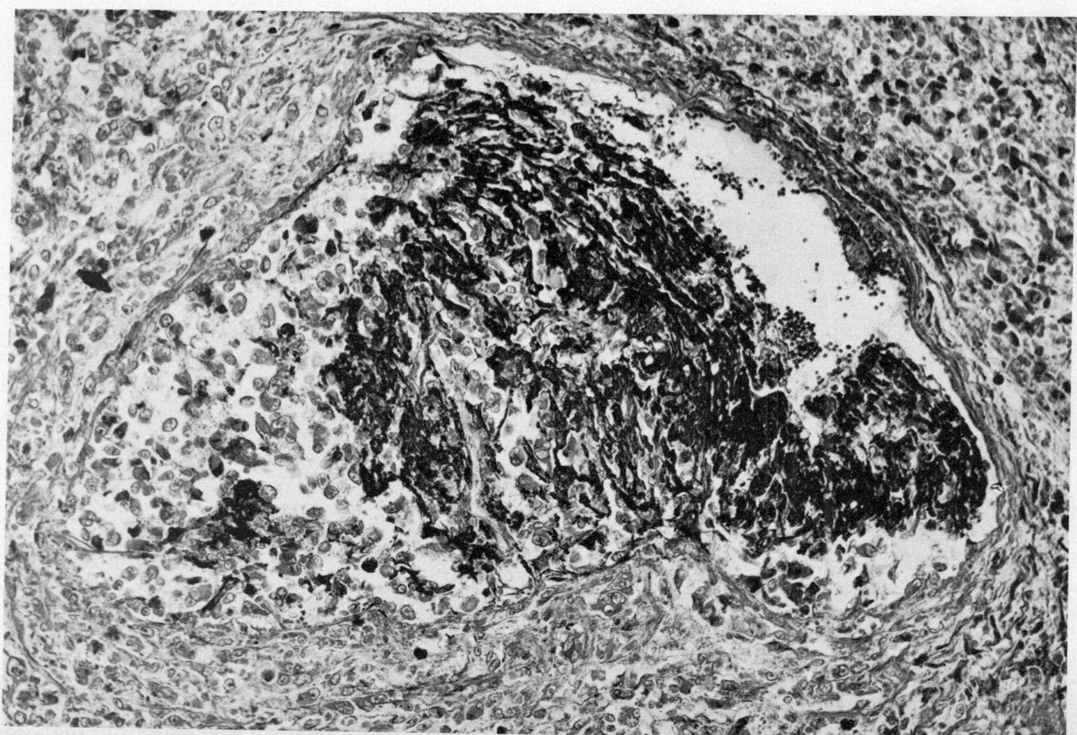

Figure 26–33. A highly undifferentiated anaplastic cancer of thyroid showing vascular invasion and thrombosis of the involved vessel.

cysts. These occur at any age and may not become evident until adult life. Mucinous, clear secretion may collect within these cysts to form either spherical masses or fusiform swellings, rarely over 2 to 3 cm in diameter. These are present in the midline of the neck anterior to the trachea. Segments of the duct and cysts that occur high in the neck are lined by stratified squamous epithelium, which is essentially identical with that covering the posterior portion of the tongue in the region of the foramen cecum. Those anomalies that occur in the lower neck more proximal to the thyroid gland are lined by epithelium resembling the thyroidal acinar epithelium. Characteristically, subjacent to the lining epithelium there is an intense lymphocytic infiltrate. Superimposed infection may convert these lesions into abscess cavities.

The main significance of these lesions is that (1) they create masses in the neck requiring differentiation from more serious neoplasms; (2) they may communicate with the skin to produce persistent draining sinuses; (3) sometimes the persistent duct drains into the base of the tongue; and (4) these anomalous structures are rare sources for the development of malignancy.[101]

Agenesis and dysgenesis of the thyroid gland are uncommon congenital anomalies. In many instances there appears to be total failure of development of the normally situated thyroid gland. Aberrant rests of *ectopic thyroid* are rare congenital anomalies. They are located most often at the base of the tongue but sometimes along the course of the thyroglossal duct. As mentioned at the outset, the ectopic rests are almost always located within the anterior triangle of the neck, and so may be mistaken for an enlarged lymph node or sometimes for a metastasis from a very well-differentiated carcinoma of the thyroid. In most cases, these remnants are supernumerary to the definitive thyroid gland. Only infrequently do they represent the only thyroid tissue in the individual. When the definitive thyroid is lacking and there is little or no aberrant tissue to replace it, athyreotic cretinism may result.

ATROPHY OF THYROID

Atrophy of the thyroid gland is a nonclinical term applied by morphologists to total or near-total replacement of the thyroidal substance by fibrous tissue when the cause is uncertain. Often, only scattered rests of thyroid parenchyma persist along with foci of lymphocytic infiltration in the fibrous atrophy. Such follicular cells as persist may have undergone squamous metaplasia or transformation into Hürthle cells having abundant, finely granular eosinophilic cytoplasm. It is impossible from the morphologic examination to determine the cause of the atrophic process, but the possibilities include (1) panhypopituitarism, (2) acute or subacute thyroiditis (bacterial, viral), (3) irradiation, and (4) primary, idiopathic (autoimmune) hypothyroidism.

SYSTEMIC THYROIDAL CHANGES

Notable in this category are systemic amyloidosis, with deposits in the stromal connective tissue chiefly about vessels, and hemochromatosis, with the accumulation of hemosiderin pigment within thyroidal epithelium and within fibroblasts in the stroma. These involvements rarely produce functional abnormalities. The thyroid may be seeded by any blood-borne infection or disseminated disease, as pointed out in the consideration of thyroiditis (p. 1206). It is sometimes seeded by metastatic cancers, including lymphomas and leukemias. Necropsy studies have identified thyroid involvement in 4 to 24% of patients dying of disseminated cancer.[102] Almost any solid tissue cancer may involve the thyroid, but the usual primary lesions are carcinomas of the breast, lung, and kidney and malignant melanoma of the skin. In most instances the seedings or leukemic infiltrates are small and of no significance; on occasion, however, they are sufficiently extensive to cause thyroidal enlargement and sometimes functional insufficiency, but usually in a patient already terminally ill.

Parathyroid Glands

NORMAL

The parathyroid glands are derived from the pharyngeal pouches—the upper glands from the endoderm of the fourth pouch, and the lower pair from the third pouch. About 90% of individuals have four parathyroid glands, but there may be as many as six or as few as two. There is, therefore, hazard in unnecessarily removing even a single gland in a patient who might have only one gland left. In the adult, the parathyroid is a yellow-brown, ovoid, encapsulated nodule weighing approximately 35 to 40 mg. It measures between 4 to 6 mm in length, 2 to 4 mm in width, and 0.5 to 2 mm in thickness. The superior glands are almost always located close to the upper posterior aspect of the thyroid, but the inferior glands are much more footloose and found anywhere from the lower pole of the thyroid down to the deepest recesses of the thymus.

In early infancy and in the child, the parathyroids are composed almost entirely of solid sheets of chief cells. With increasing age, oxyphil and water-clear cells appear as well as fat, but a recent study indicates that most normal parathyroids accumulate on average only about 15 to 20% of fat and almost never more than 50% at any age.[103]

Chief cells vary from light to dark pink with H and E stain in the light microscope, depending on their glycogen content: the more glycogen, the lighter the cell. They are polygonal, 12 to 20 μ in diameter with slightly acidophilic cytoplasm and central, round, uniform nuclei. In addition to having the usual cellular organelles, they have a large Golgi complex, a moderate number of mitochondria, lipofuscin pigment granules, and numerous secretory granules. The *water-clear* cell is a variant of the chief cell, having few secretory and lipofuscin granules and large lakes of glycogen. *Oxyphil cells*, found throughout the normal parathyroid in adults, either singly or in small clusters, are slightly larger than chief cells, have a brightly acidophilic cytoplasm, and under the electron microscope are classically tightly packed with mitochondria. Glycogen granules are also present in these cells, but there are no secretory granules. The chief cell is the progenitor of the other forms and is the major source of parathyroid hormone. Transitional oxyphils are indeed more numerous than oxyphils.

Parathyroid hormone (PTH) is a peptide containing 84 amino acids derived from a longer "pre-pro" form by sequential cleavage within chief cells. The steps involved in these cleavages are available in standard texts. Following secretion, PTH is rapidly split (within a half-life of minutes) into an amino-terminal (N) fragment of 34 amino acids having an even shorter half-life and a carboxy-terminal (C) fragment with a half-life of several hours. Most radioimmunoassays measure the serum level of the C fragments, which are more readily titered because of their longer half-life, but the biologic activity of PTH resides in the N fragments. The C fragment, so far as is known, has no biologic activity. Thus, it is possible for nonendocrine tumors to elaborate biologically active fragments of PTH that will not be detectable by radioimmunoassays or for elevated immunoassays to not be associated with hyperfunction.[104]

As is well-known, the function of PTH is the maintenance of normal levels of calcium (more accurately, ionized calcium) in the extracellular fluid. At the cell level, the hormone binds to membrane receptors on target cells to stimulate adenylate cyclase, leading to an increase in intracellular cAMP. At the same time it facilitates the flow of calcium out of blood into cells. It thus appears that both cAMP and calcium cooperate in serving as the ultimate mediators of the physiologic actions of PTH, but the precise steps involved are unknown. Maintenance of normocalcemia is mediated by direct effects on kidney and bone and indirect effects on the intestines. Absorption of calcium from the gut is enhanced largely by the vitamin D metabolite $1\alpha,25\text{-}(OH)_2D_3$ whose synthesis in the kidney is regulated by PTH, as detailed on page 406. At the same time it directly reduces renal excretion of calcium by enhancing its reabsorption from the glomerular filtrate and increases the rate of dissolution of bone mineral, involving two separable sequences. First, there is an immediate efflux of calcium from bone into blood within minutes. This is followed by a more prolonged release of bone calcium as a consequence of increased resorption of bone. Whether this action is related to increased osteoclastic activity or reduced osteoblastic activity, leading to a net catabolic effect, is not clear.[105] All actions of PTH serve to increase serum calcium. In turn, PTH secretion is regulated by the serum calcium level in a classic feedback loop. The complex relationships among phosphate, vitamin D, and PTH in the maintenance of normocalcemia were discussed earlier (p. 406).

PATHOLOGY

The anatomic disorders of the parathyroid gland are best considered in relation to their effects on function, i.e., hyperparathyroidism and hypoparathyroidism. The former can further be divided into primary hyperparathyroidism, which results from disorders intrinsic to the glands that produce hypersecretion of PTH with hypercalcemia and hypophosphatemia, and *secondary hyperparathyroidism*, also associated with excessive production of PTH, but basically characterized by some apparent resistance in the target tissues to the action of the hormone. Thus, in secondary hyperparathyroidism the physiologic actions of PTH are more or less blocked, with resultant hypocalcemia and hyperphosphatemia. The low serum calcium levels stimulate parathyroid function and, in time, induce hyperplastic changes. The following discussion, therefore, covers primary hyperparathyroidism, secondary hyperparathyroidism, and hypoparathyroidism.

PRIMARY HYPERPARATHYROIDISM

The major biochemical features that characterize primary hyperparathyroidism and are found in almost all patients are (1) elevated serum levels of PTH by radioimmunoassay, (2) hypercalcemia, (3) hypophosphatemia, and (4) excessive urinary excretion of calcium. A number of clinical consequences follow, some early, others only after some long period of hyperfunction, and thus the clinical presentation depends on the duration of the metabolic derangement.[106] Neuromuscular weakness and fatigability appear early and insidiously in most patients. Less regularly, neuropsychiatric disturbances develop ranging from depression, anxiety, and psychoses to mental obtundation and even coma. More specific is the appearance of renal stones or nephrocalcinosis (p. 1053) incident to the hypercalciuria. These abnormalities were once found in 50 to 70% of patients, but with earlier diagnosis of the condition, for reasons given later, they are now present in less than 25%. Increased mobilization of skeletal calcium followed by bone resorption and remodeling may in time give rise to so-called "osteitis fibrosa cystica" (p. 1329), diagnostic of hyperparathyroidism. These bony changes appear only after some long period (years) of parathyroid hyperfunction. They were once present in 80 to 90% of cases, but now are found in only 10 to 15%.[107] A number of other changes may also be present but they are less constant and it is less certain that they are directly caused by hyperparathyroidism. Hypertension and its associated cardiovascular consequences is a common finding in over half of the patients. However, the hypertension may not be alleviated by surgical removal of the causal parathyroid lesion, calling into question cause and effect. However, it is possible that perpetuation of the hypertension may be due to the development of renovascular changes incident to the prolonged hypertension. Pancreatitis is sometimes associated with hyperparathyroidism, as noted on page 963, but for reasons that are not entirely clear. Peptic ulcers are also more prevalent, and this is attributed to increased secretion of gastrin secondary to elevated serum levels of calcium or PTH. However, a direct causal association between primary hyperparathyroidism and peptic ulcer has been challenged. Cholelithiasis has been reported in 25 to 35% of patients, presumably owing to increased calcium levels in the bile with the formation of insoluble calcium bilirubinates. Finally, the hypercalcemia may give rise to metastatic calcifications in soft tissues, vessels, and joints, as described on page 35. The deposit of calcium pyrophosphate in the joints causes disabling chondrocalcinosis in about 15 to 20% of cases (p. 1362).[108]

As indicated, the clinical picture of primary hyperparathyroidism has undergone change over the past years. At one time the condition passed unrecognized until "stone and bone" disease brought it to attention. Today, the diagnosis is often made fortuitously by a routine determination of serum calcium as one of the multiphasic laboratory tests routinely employed in clinical practice. Thus, most patients are asymptomatic or only in retrospect have vague complaints.[109] However, it must be cautioned that the mere identification of hypercalcemia by the laboratory cannot be equated with hyperparathyroidism. It may have many causes, as indicated in Table 26–6.

Hypercalcemia is at least as frequently caused by nonparathyroid cancers as it is by hyperparathyroidism. In some of these cases the elevated serum calcium is related to direct resorption of bone by the cancer (multiple myeloma) or by its osteolytic metastases (from cancers of the breast, lung, and other areas). Sometimes, however, the hypercalcemia occurs in the absence of skeletal metastases related to the elaboration of some calcium-mobilizing humoral agent such as prostaglandin E_2, osteoclast-activating factor, PTH, or PTH-like substances.[110] There is a regrettable tendency to refer to these syndromes as "pseudohyperparathyroidism" when in reality they represent paraneoplastic syndromes.

Table 26–6. CLINICAL CAUSES OF HYPERCALCEMIA*

Diagnosis	Percentage of Cases
Malignancy	34.4
Hyperparathyroidism	34.2
Vitamin D excess	12.1
Hyperthyroidism	3.9
Milk-alkali syndrome	3.9
Immobilization	2.3
Idiopathic	0.9
Sarcoidosis	0.9
Dysproteinemias	0.6
Addison's disease	0.6
Laboratory error	13.4

*Taken from Schmidt, N.: Hyperparathyroidism, a review. Am. J. Surg. *139*:657, 1980.

Analyses of large series of cases of primary hyperparathyroidism reveal the following distribution of glandular abnormalities.[111]

Lesion	*Percentage*
Single adenoma	80
Double adenoma (? hyperplasia)	2–3
Primary hyperplasia	15
Carcinoma	2–3

Specifically excluded are the nonparathyroid cancers producing hypercalcemia, since paraneoplastic syndromes do not constitute primary hyperparathyroidism. However, included in this compilation are instances in which the parathyroid pathology is a component of familial polyendocrine syndromes such as multiple endocrine neoplasia (MEN) I, MEN IIa, and other more rare familial hypercalcemic hyperparathyroid constellations.[106] The MEN syndromes are discussed on page 988 and it suffices to note here that they may be associated with either adenomas or hyperplasia of the parathyroids.

ADENOMAS

These benign tumors are generally extremely small and difficult to locate even at surgical exploration. They may occur in either sex at any age, with a peak incidence in the middle decades of life. As the above listing indicates, they usually occur singly, although occasionally two adenomas are found dispersed among the four glands. The interpretation of double adenomas is uncertain. Are they merely coincidental neoplasms, or is the enlargement of two glands an incomplete form of hyperplasia that usually involves all four glands, but sometimes asymmetrically, giving the false impression of multiple adenomas? Relevant to this issue is the finding that at least some parathyroid adenomas are polyclonal in origin.[112] If adenomas were true neoplasms, is it likely that they, like most neoplasms, would be monoclonal? Thus, a slender thread of evidence suggests that adenomas may arise as hyperplastic lesions that are converted into autonomous neoplasms. What the stimulus to such hyperplasia may be is a mystery. Nonetheless, it is evident that, in the surgical excision of an adenoma, all four glands must be visualized to discover possible double or polyglandular enlargements.

Adenomas are generally small, averaging 0.5 to 5.0 gm in weight. Occasionally, however, they are as large as 10 to 20 gm, and extreme weights of over 100 gm have been reported. For obscure reasons, the neoplasm is most often located in the inferior parathyroid glands.[113] However, they may be found in such ectopic sites as the thymus, thyroid, or pericardium or behind the esophagus, sometimes creating the proverbial surgical problem of "the needle in the haystack." They are well encapsulated, soft, yielding, yellow-to-tan-to-red lesions. **Some are composed of pure cell types, but others display mixed cell populations** (Fig. 26–34). The most common variant is composed principally of chief cells, but many transitional and oxyphil cells are often also present. The chief cells are frequently slightly larger than normal, with variations in cell and nuclear size. Sometimes, hyperchromatic pleomorphic nuclei are present in these benign lesions, with occasional binucleate forms—features that are of some importance since they help to distinguish primary adenomas from hyperplasia. In the latter, the cell types are much more uniform. Infrequently, the adenoma is composed largely of water-clear cells; however, here again chief cells and oxyphils may be found (Fig. 26–35). A functioning adenoma composed largely of oxyphil cells is extremely rare. Whatever the cell type, they are disposed in solid sheets or masses, but occasionally the tumor is separated into apparent lobules by traversing bands of fibrous tissue. At other times, a well-vascularized stroma produces cords of cells, and occasionally glandlike patterns are seen. **Sometimes a rim of normal parathyroid tissue can be seen external to the capsule, serving to differentiate the adenomatous lesion from diffuse hyperplasia.**

Electron microscopy of these adenomas has not revealed many differences between these neoplastic cells and their normal counterparts.[114] Distinctive in many cells is a concentric laminated pattern of smooth-faced cisternae, termed annulate lamellae, in the region of the Golgi complex.[115] This structure has been identified in many experimental tumors, and there is the suggestion that it is involved in protein synthesis or some other synthetic activity and perhaps accounts for the growth potential of these cells.

No correlation has been noted between the cell type predominating in the adenoma and the level of resultant hyperfunction.

CARCINOMA

Carcinoma of the parathyroid glands is a rare cause of primary hyperfunction. The manifestations are similar to those of "benign" hyperparathyroidism but tend to be exaggerated, with more marked and earlier bone changes and a greater tendency to renal stones—"bone and stone disease."[116] All agree that there are undoubted cases of nonfunctioning carcinomas of the parathyroid glands, but the close anatomic similarity between such lesions and carcinomas arising in the thyroid has led to the commonly accepted criterion that the diagnosis of a carcinoma arising in the parathyroid requires the dem-

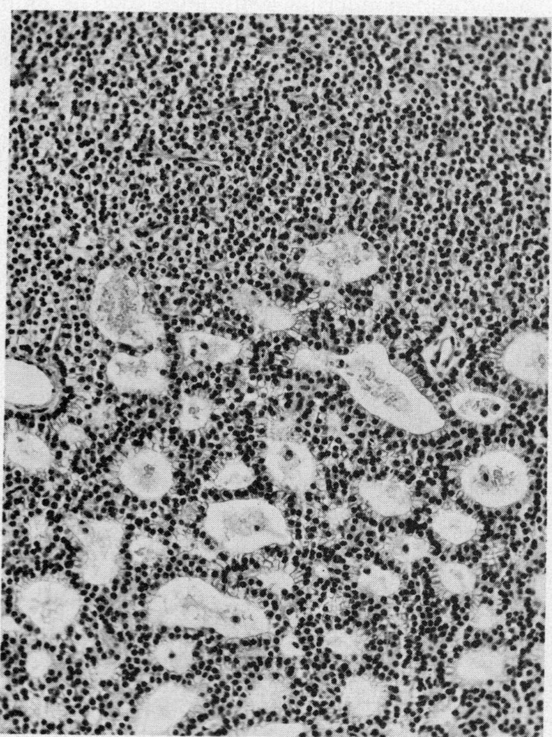

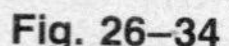

Fig. 26–34

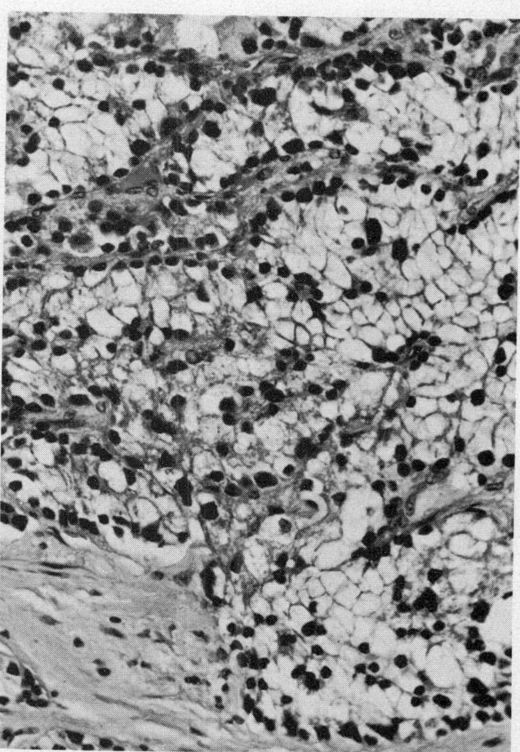

Fig. 26–35

Figure 26–34. Parathyroid adenoma containing chief cells, oxyphils, and a few water-clear ("wasserhelle") cells growing in sheets and glandular patterns.

Figure 26–35. Parathyroid adenoma, chiefly of "wasserhelle" cell type. Note the slight variability in cell and nuclear size.

onstration of hyperfunction. There is great difficulty in distinguishing between the pleomorphism of adenomas and the mild anaplasia of some carcinomas. As a consequence, it has also been proposed that, for a diagnosis of malignancy, one of the three following features must be present: (1) metastases, either to regional nodes or to distant organs; (2) capsular invasion; or (3) local recurrence following resection.

Most of the carcinomas described have been small and, in fact, some have been less than 1 gm in weight. They are often irregular in shape and show lobulation and pseudopod formation and sometimes adherence to surrounding structures. They are usually considerably more firm than adenomas. The major histologic features that may help to distinguish a carcinoma from an adenoma are (1) a trabecular pattern, (2) mitotic figures, (3) thick fibrous bands, (4) capsular invasion, and (5) blood vessel invasion.[117]

When these lesions metastasize, they usually affect the regional nodes alone. Rarely, they spread to distant organs such as the lungs, as well as below the diaphragm. Survival for many years is the rule, and death results more often from the complications of hyperparathyroidism than from the spread of the lesion.

PRIMARY HYPERPLASIA

This designation is applied to diffuse hyperplastic enlargement, usually of all four parathyroid glands. However, as pointed out earlier, the hyperplasia may be asymmetric and leave one or two glands deceptively unenlarged, accounting for the controversy relative to multiple adenomas versus asymmetric hyperplasia. The dispute is heightened by a lack of understanding of the basis of the hyperplasia. Many highly hypothetical explanations have been offered invoking excessive urinary excretion of calcium leading to a mild hypocalcemia, subtle end-organ resistance to PTH calling for increased parathyroid gland function, and previous neck irradiation stimulating cell replication. In the last analysis, however, the cause of the primary hyperplasia is unknown. Whatever its origins, primary hyperplasia accounts for 15% of cases of primary hyperparathyroidism, and is caused most often by chief cell hyperplasia (12%) and less commonly by clear cell hyperplasia (3%).

Chief cell hyperplasia must be described separately from clear cell hyperplasia since there are both gross and microscopic differences. In **chief cell hyperplasia,** the total weight of all glands may be less than 1 gm, although an upper range on the order of 10 gm has been recorded. Often, one or two glands are significantly larger than the remainder.[118] It would be easy to interpret such a presentation as that of an adenoma or double adenomas. The glands vary in color from yellow to tan to red-brown and often contain small cysts.

The histologic pattern of the hyperplastic glands is quite variable. The chief cells are laid down in cords, sheets, and occasionally glandular patterns, sometimes with dispersed stromal fat cells. However, **usually there are areas of solid parathyroid cells devoid of fat cells, a microscopic feature of great importance in distinguishing hyperplasia from normal glands.** Rarely, in chief cell hyperplasia, the glands are composed almost completely of oxyphil cells, or a mixture of groups of chief cells, oxyphils, and transitional cells.[118] Ultrastructurally, many of the chief cells and oxyphils contain numerous secretory vacuoles.

In contrast, **clear cell hyperplasias** are usually marked by greater enlargement of the glands than in chief cell hyperplasia. Aggregate weights of over 10 gm are not uncommon. In clear cell hyperplasias the glands are most often characterized by a uniform distribution of variably enlarged cells (8 to 40 μm) with pale, amphophilic cytoplasm. Usually, all four parathyroid glands are completely replaced by the clear cells and there are few residual fat cells or oxyphil cells (Fig. 26–36). The cytoplasm is not actually cleared, but can be resolved under the electron microscope as being filled by small, seemingly empty vacuoles of uncertain origin—either derived from the Golgi apparatus or from the granular endoplasmic reticulum.[119]

SECONDARY HYPERPARATHYROIDISM

Secondary hyperparathyroidism is characterized by compensatory hypersecretion of PTH in response to end-organ resistance to PTH, leading to an inability to maintain blood calcium levels. *Primary hyperparathyroidism is usually marked by hypercalcemia, whereas secondary is characterized by hypocalcemia,* albeit sometimes mild. The most important cause of secondary hyperparathyroidism is chronic renal insufficiency. Chronic hypocalcemia and secondary hyperparathyroid-

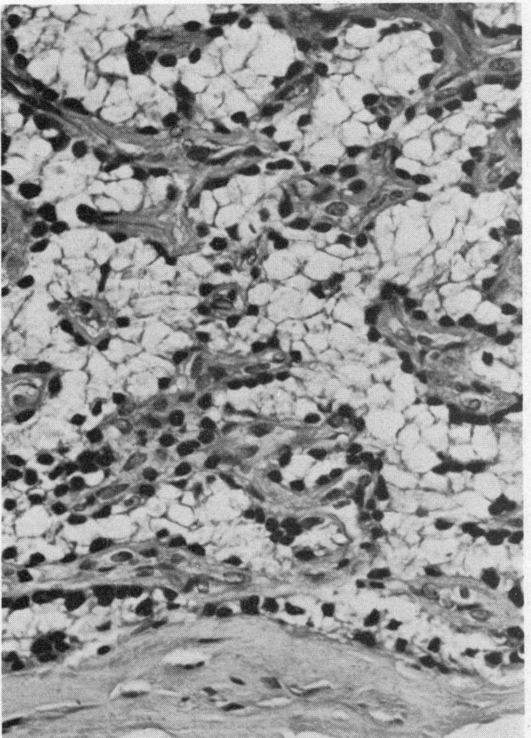

Figure 26–36. A detail of marked primary parathyroid hyperplasia showing characteristic clear cell pattern.

ism may also be encountered in vitamin D deficiency, intestinal malabsorption syndromes with inadequate absorption of vitamin D and calcium, and pseudohypoparathyroidism (p. 1131). Rarely, medullary thyroid carcinomas producing an excess of calcitonin may be accompanied by secondary hyperplasia of the parathyroid glands.

The sequence of events leading to the parathyroid compensatory hyperfunction in the various clinical circumstances mentioned is poorly understood. Although resistance to PTH and hypocalcemia are postulated, they are difficult to establish in many instances. Moreover, many more complexities are probably involved. For example, in chronic renal failure the initial stimulus is probably reduction of ionized calcium in the extracellular fluid secondary to renal retention of phosphate. The hyperphosphatemia and damaged renal parenchyma (underlying the renal failure) combine to reduce the renal production of $1\alpha,25\text{-}(OH)_2D_3$. Decreased intestinal absorption of calcium follows. There is also impaired mobilization of calcium from the skeleton, attributed to resistance to PTH. Compensatory hyperfunction of the parathyroids ensues. Generally, however, the manifestations of such hyperfunction are less prominent than those associated with primary hyperparathyroidism.

The anatomic changes in the parathyroid glands consist principally of hyperplasia of the chief cells. This usually affects all glands but, not infrequently, one, two, or even three may be spared. The basis for such asymmetric involvement is obscure. Islands of oxyphils are often present, and the fat is usually largely replaced by hyperplastic cells (Figs. 26–37 and 26–38). In general, more fat remains than in cases of primary hyperplasia.

In many instances the glands revert to normal if the basic clinical derangement is brought under control by, for example, renal transplantation or vitamin D supplementation. With long-standing secondary hyperplasia and greater glandular enlargement, however, reversion to normal may not occur, contributing to the possibility that *secondary hyperplasia may in time convert into autonomous primary hyperplasia, which in turn may induce adenoma formation.*

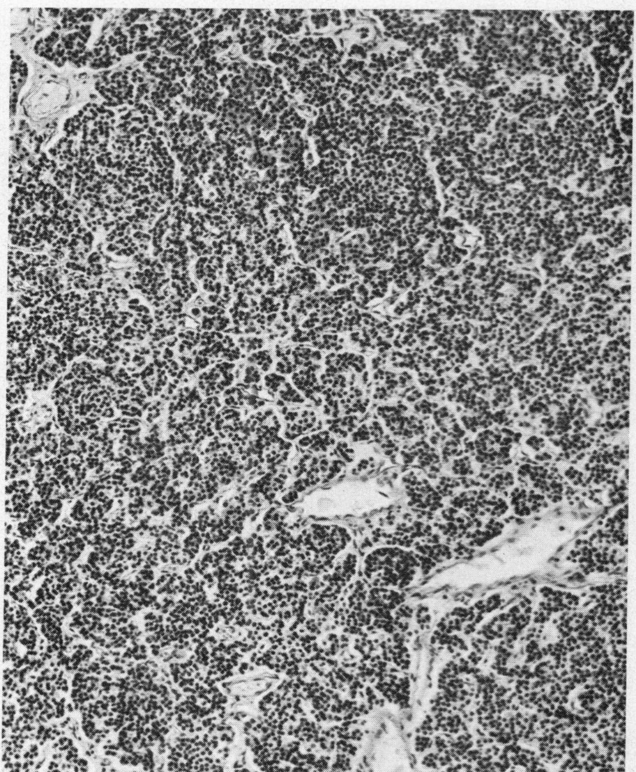

Figure 26–37. Diffuse secondary hyperplasia of parathyroid, illustrating extensive replacement of the normally contained fat.

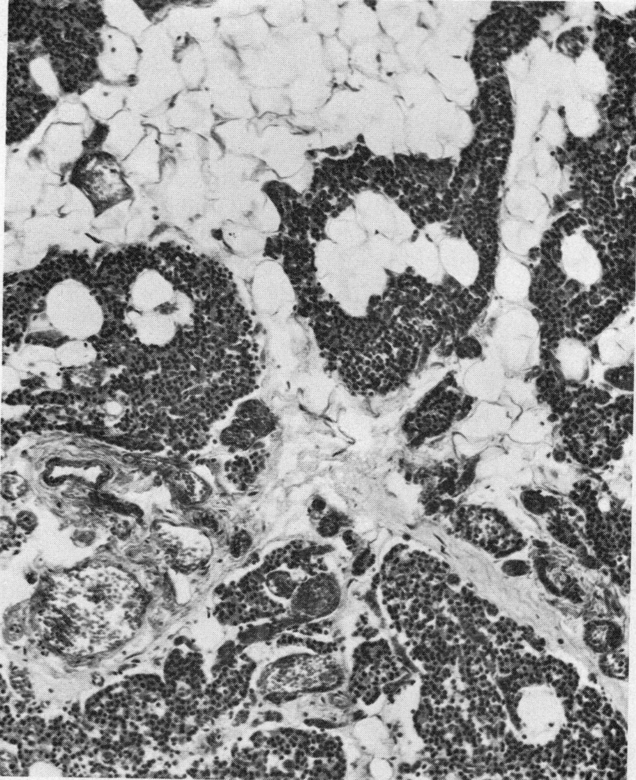

Figure 26–38. Normal parathyroid for comparison with Figure 26–37 to illustrate usual content of fat and abundant connective tissue stroma.

HYPOPARATHYROIDISM

Hypoparathyroidism may arise whenever there is inadequate secretion of PTH or the hormone is biologically ineffective. Under these circumstances the diminished physiologic action of PTH on the kidney and bone leads to hypocalcemia and hyperphosphatemia. On occasion, reduced end-organ sensitivity to PTH may induce *hypo*parathyroidism that in time may convert to secondary *hyper*parathyroidism. A constellation of clinical changes are associated with hypoparathyroidism, but since the resultant syndrome is largely metabolic and clinical with scant anatomic changes, it will be discussed only briefly. With milder expressions of the syndrome, the clinical manifestations are exceedingly subtle and almost undecipherable without the documentation of hypocalcemia. On the other extreme are the more overt expressions marked by the following:

1. *Increased neuromuscular excitability* may be noted, related to the decreased serum ionized calcium concentration. Classically, this is elicited by tapping along the course of the facial nerve, which induces contractions of the muscles of the eye, mouth, or nose (*Chvostek's sign*). More dramatic is the development of tetany with muscle cramps, carpopedal spasms, laryngeal stridor, and convulsions.

2. *Mental changes* ranging from irritability to depression and frank psychosis may appear.

3. *Neurologic signs suggesting an intracranial tumor* may appear with elevated CSF pressure and papilledema.

4. *Intracranial calcifications* can be visualized by skull x-rays in approximately 20% of patients with chronic hypoparathyroidism, sometimes leading to a parkinsonian-like syndrome.

5. *The lens may become calcified, leading to cataract formation.*

6. The lowered serum calcium causes *abnormalities in cardiac conduction* (mainly prolongation of the Q-T interval and T-wave changes).

7. *Abnormalities in dentition* are common in children, taking the forms of defective enamel, dental hypoplasia, and delayed eruption of teeth.

A number of other changes may be present, depending on the particular cause of the hypoparathyroidism.

Many disorders may induce hypoparathyroidism. Their relative frequency differs in adults and children, as indicated in the following listing, cited in order of frequency:[120]

In Adults

Postsurgical removal of glands
Idiopathic isolated hypoparathyroidism
Familial (? autoimmune) hypoparathyroidism
DiGeorge's syndrome

In Neonates and Children

Idiopathic isolated hypoparathyroidism
Familial (? autoimmune) hypoparathyroidism
DiGeorge's syndrome
Postsurgical removal of glands

Postsurgical hypoparathyroidism has been reported following thyroidectomy, surgery for hyperparathyroidism, and radical neck dissections for cancer; its reported frequency ranges from 0.2 to 10%. The familial syndrome of uncertain mode of transmission is thought to represent some form of autoimmune disease, but apparent autoimmune disease may also appear without an obvious hereditary background. In both instances the hypoparathyroidism is often accompanied by hypoadrenalism, autoimmune thyroid disease, insulin-dependent diabetes mellitus, and pernicious anemia, all suspected of also being autoimmune.[121] There is frequently an associated mucocutaneous candidiasis, and studies point to deranged T-suppressor cell function as the basis of the autoimmune reactions and vulnerability to fungal infections.[122] DiGeorge's syndrome, as discussed on page 207, is a form of congenital immunodeficiency state characterized by a T-cell deficiency secondary to thymic hypoplasia, but, for our interest, also accompanied by parathyroid hypoplasia. There are still other causes of hypoparathyroidism such as postradiation, metastases to the parathyroid glands, and suppression of PTH secretion by prolonged hypercalcemia, but all are exceedingly uncommon.

PSEUDO- AND PSEUDOPSEUDOHYPOPARATHYROIDISM

Pseudohypoparathyroidism and *pseudopseudohypoparathyroidism* are rare and merit only brief characterizations of their intriguing qualities. *Pseudohypoparathyroidism is a hereditary disorder, perhaps transmitted as an X-linked dominant, characterized by signs and symptoms of hypoparathyroidism, with hypocalcemia and hyperphosphatemia, associated, however, with normal or even elevated levels of circulating PTH.* End-organ unresponsiveness mainly in the kidney is postulated because the circulating hormone can be proved to be biologically active. Rare reports suggest restoration of normal sensitivity to PTH following the administration of large doses of $1\alpha,25\text{-}(OH)_2D_3$. The distinctive features of pseudohypoparathyroidism are short stature, round face, short neck, abnormally short metacarpal and metatarsal bones, and particularly an abnormally short fourth and fifth metacarpal and metatarsal. Many patients are mentally deficient. Soft tissue calcifications and bony changes similar to those in hyperparathyroidism sometimes appear. You may recall that end-organ resistance to PTH may lead to secondary hyperparathyroidism, and it is likely that some patients with pseudohypoparathyroidism develop some of the stigmata of secondary hyperparathyroidism.

Pseudopseudohypoparathyroidism is characterized by a clinical picture identical to that of pseudohypoparathyroidism except that these patients have no hypocalcemia or hyperphosphatemia and apparently have a normal renal response to PTH. It, too, may be an X-linked hereditary disorder, but the rarity of the condition has not permitted mendelian analysis.

Adrenal Cortex

NORMAL

The adrenals, although small and tucked away as seeming appendages to the kidneys, are remarkably crucial to homeostasis and adaptation to stress. We do not know why the cortex and medulla are in such close relationship, for they have little in common. The medulla is of neural crest ectodermal origin and thus is essentially a neurosecretory organ. The cortex is mesodermal in origin, derived from the urogenital ridge. Before birth the adrenal cortex is composed largely of a wide juxtamedullary fetal zone, but after birth the fetal zone begins to atrophy. In a few months the three definitive cortical zones appear: the subcapsular zona glomerulosa, the intermediate zone fasciculata, and the inner zona reticularis.

The normal adrenal in the adult weighs 4 to 5 gm. Significant increases above this weight may be the chief evidence of hyperplasia, just as reductions would point to atrophy. The normal adrenal cortex is yellow-brown owing largely to its content of lipochrome pigment and in some part to stored steroid precursors—free and esterified cholesterol, triglycerides, and phospholipids. The *zona glomerulosa* makes up approximately 10 to 15% of the cortex. It consists of closely packed groups and clusters of cuboidal-to-columnar cells with darkly staining nuclei and scanty cytoplasm containing only a few lipid droplets. Under the electron microscope the most prominent feature is an abundant anastomosing network of smooth endoplasmic reticulum. The mitochondria are filamentous and have lamellar cristae like those in most other organs. Differences in mitochondrial morphology in the cells of the three cortical layers may help in identifying the precise cells of origin of cortical neoplasms.

The *zona fasciculata* constitutes 80% of the cortex. It is organized into long cords or columns of polyhedral cells somewhat larger than those of the glomerulosa that have a central darkly-staining nucleus and a cytoplasm stuffed with fine vacuoles. The lipids within these vacuoles are mostly cholesterol and cholesteryl esters, which are dissolved out in the usual paraffin sections submitted to organic solvents. Such cells are variously referred to as "clear" or "light" cells. With electron microscopy, an elaborate smooth endoplasmic reticulum is seen, as well as a Golgi apparatus somewhat larger than that present in the zona glomerulosa. However, mitochondria are less numerous, more variable in size and shape, and the cristae are tubulovesicular invaginations of the inner membrane. Histochemical stains disclose scant amounts of oxidases and dehydrogenases in the mitochondria. The abundant storage of cholesterol is interpreted as reserve substrate for the biogenesis of the corticosteroids and is taken to mean that fasciculata cells in the normal state of health are inactive in terms of synthetic function.

In the *zona reticularis,* the parallel cords give way to irregularly arranged clusters that abut on the adrenal medulla and in the aggregate make up about 5 to 10% of the total cortex. The cells basically resemble those of the fasciculata, but the cytoplasm is nonvacuolated and darkly acidophilic and contains large accumulations of lipochrome pigment. Thus, these cells are called "dark" or "compact" cells. They possess an abundant smooth endoplasmic reticulum, numerous mitochondria having cristae intermediate between those in the other two zones, and are rich in oxidative enzymes, alkaline, and acid phosphatases and ribonucleic acid. It is proposed that reticularis cells are the major source of glucocorticoids and adrenal androgens under normal conditions of health. With prolonged stress, as during a chronic illness or after exogeneous ACTH stimulation, the fasciculata cells are converted from within outward into nonvacuolated "dark" cells as the stored precursors are used up in the synthesis of corticosteroids (Fig. 26–39). Thus, the zonae fasciculata and reticularis represent a single functional zone, with the fasciculata constituting a ready reserve, capable of being activated into steroidogenesis.

A few comments on the biosynthesis of the cortical steroids are in order to facilitate an understanding of the clinical significance of cortical diseases. As you may know, all the steroids are synthesized from acetate and cholesterol precursors.[123] A simplified flow diagram of steroid synthesis is presented in Figure 26–40. Pregnenolone is derived from cholesterol and it in turn may be converted by a 3-β-hydroxysteroid dehydrogenase into progesterone or by a 17-hydroxylase into a 17-α-hydroxypregnenolone. Progesterone is a key intermediate; from it flows all aldosterone secretion. Cortisol and testosterone may also be derived from it, although other pathways exist for these steroids. Critical enzymes involved in biosynthesis are 3-β-hydroxysteroid dehydrogenase, and 11-, 17-, and 21-hydroxylases. A hereditary deficiency of one of these enzymes not only blocks the synthesis of specific steroids but also channels the precursors into alternative pathways.

There are associations between cortical zones and specific corticosteroids. The *mineralocorticoids,* the most important of which is *aldosterone,* are synthesized in the zona glomerulosa, although certain glucocorti-

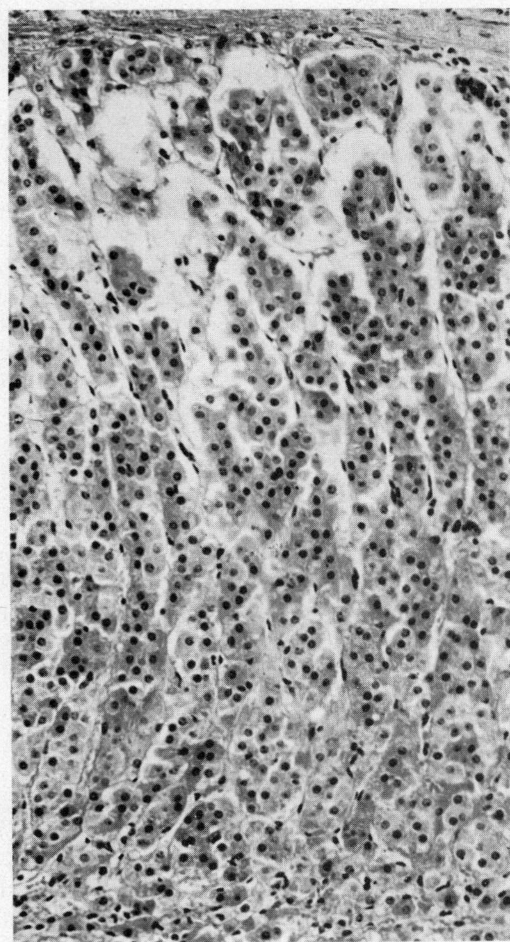

Figure 26–39. Human adrenal cortex in stress—complete lipid depletion. Cells of cortex are exclusively "dark" (compact) in type.

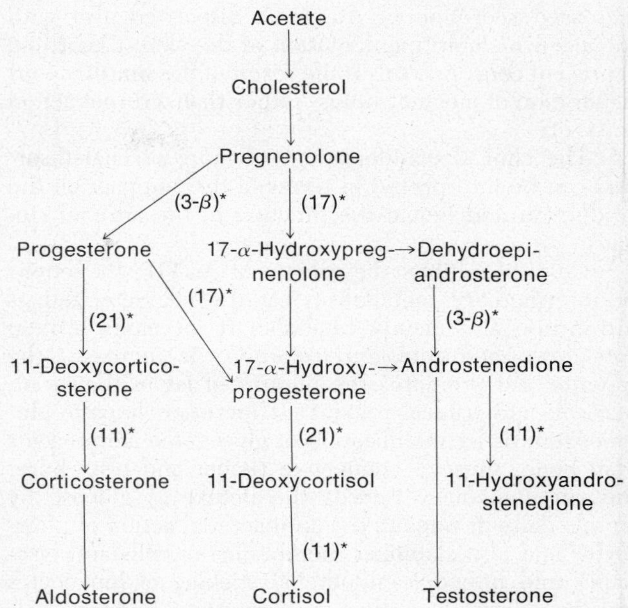

Figure 26–40. Pathways of steroid synthesis.

coids, e.g., cortisol, have similar but weaker effects. The *glucocorticoids*, of which the most active is cortisol, are synthesized in the zonae reticularis and fasciculata. Analogously, testosterone, the major adrenal *androgen*, is also synthesized in the inner two zones. Estrogens probably are not synthesized by the normal adrenal gland. The feminization associated with certain disorders is most likely the consequence of the action of liver enzymes on androgenic precursors secreted by the cortex. Although synthesis of the glucocorticoids and adrenal androgens is under hypothalamic-anterior pituitary ACTH control, aldosterone secretion is largely independent of ACTH and is regulated by the serum levels of potassium and renin-angiotensin. However, physiologic levels of ACTH may be necessary to potentiate aldosterone secretion. Thus, increased levels of ACTH, whether of exogenous or endogenous origin, induce hyperplasia of the inner two zones, not affecting the zona glomerulosa and, conversely, loss of anterior pituitary function leaves the zona glomerulosa relatively unaffected, while causing atrophy of the remainder of the cortex. Indeed, it has been said that the cortex functions as two separate glands, the zona glomerulosa being quite apart from the zonae fasciculata and reticularis.

As pointed out earlier (p. 1193), ACTH is stored in and released from corticotrophs in the anterior pituitary. It is an unbranched polypeptide composed of 39 amino acids and derived from a much longer peptide, which is cleaved first into a carboxy-terminal fragment containing not only ACTH but also beta lipotropin, beta endorphin, and beta melanotropin (a melanocyte-stimulating factor). The amino-terminal fragment has no steroidogenic effect but contains a gamma melanotropin.[124] Thereafter, ACTH is cleaved from the carboxy-terminal fragment. Hence, ACTH production is accompanied by the formation of melanotropins. Certain extrapituitary neoplasms such as bronchogenic carcinomas and others (p. 255) may also elaborate ACTH or ACTH-like substances (presumably carboxy-terminal fragments). Release of ACTH in the anterior pituitary is effected by corticotropin-releasing factor (CRF) secreted into the pituitary stalk–portal vascular system by the hypothalamus. Three influences regulate CRF and therefore ACTH release: (1) plasma free-cortisol levels, (2) stress, and (3) the diurnal cycle. Thus, there is a feedback loop in which ACTH stimulates cortisol secretion, which in turn inhibits the corticotrophs and possibly the hypothalamus to suppress ACTH secretion. ACTH in time induces morphologic changes in the adrenal gland, principally depletion of lipid and cortical hyperplasia, accounting for an increase in adrenal weight and transformation of fasciculata "light" cells into "dark" cells actively engaged in steroid synthesis (Fig. 26–39).

Increased secretion of ACTH is associated also with enhanced melanin pigmentation of the skin. According to present concepts, this is the result of the simultaneous elaboration of melanotropins, rather than a direct action of ACTH.

The clinical manifestations of most adrenal disorders can be interpreted in terms of their impact on the production and hence the function of the adrenal steroids.

Cortisol inhibits the release of ACTH. Its actions on intermediary metabolism can be characterized as anti-insulin and mainly catabolic. It increases protein breakdown and nitrogen excretion. It increases the appetite and promotes the deposit of fat in the facial, cervical, and truncal regions. It increases hepatic gluconeogenesis by mobilization of glycogenic amino acids from bone, muscle, connective tissue, and elsewhere, and simultaneously retards the uptake of glucose by muscle cells. It impairs the antibacterial action of phagocytes and also stabilizes membranes of cells and lysosomes and impedes endothelial sticking of leukocytes and diapedesis. By unknown pathways it induces lysis of lymphoid tissues, particularly T cells. It is evident that this steroid blocks inflammatory and immunologic responses and may predispose to serious infections. By its membrane actions, cortisol inhibits the migration of water into cells and tends to expand the extracellular fluid (ECF) volume. Derangements in these functions are readily observed in patients with disorders that increase or decrease the synthetic activity of the inner two zones of the adrenal cortex.

Aldosterone has two principal actions: (1) it is a major regulator of ECF volume and (2) it is the major regulator of potassium metabolism. An excess of aldosterone leads to sodium retention, loss of potassium, expansion of ECF volume, and hypertension. A deficiency induces the converse.

Testosterone and the androgenic steroids accentuate male characteristics (cause masculinization) and inhibit female characteristics (cause defeminization). Thus, excesses of androgens lead to virilization in the female, manifested principally by hirsutism, amenorrhea, clitoral enlargement, atrophy of the breasts and uterus, deepening of the voice, acne, and receding hairline. Masculinization is difficult to detect in the adult male but can lead to precocity in the prepubertal boy.

PATHOLOGY

The pathology of the adrenal cortex can be divided essentially into three categories: (1) disorders that reduce the output of adrenal steroids, (2) disorders characterized by excess steroid production, and (3) lesions that have no functional effect.

Inflammatory and regressive processes and, rarely, some tumors may destroy sufficient functioning cortical tissue to lead to adrenocortical hypofunction. The adrenal cortex has an enormous reserve of functional activity. The destructive processes, then, must wipe out most of the functioning cortical tissue before insufficiency develops.

On the other hand, hyperplastic or neoplastic processes, by the production of increased amounts of steroids, lead to adrenocortical hyperfunction. To understand these syndromes, the biosynthesis of the steroids and the enzyme systems that play a role in this synthetic process must be known. In this area of pathology, as in so many others, function cannot be separated from structure. In the sections that follow, the major disorders of the adrenals will be discussed under the headings of hypo- and hyperadrenalism. Developmental anomalies and nonfunctioning tumors are dealt with separately.

DEVELOPMENTAL ANOMALIES

Adrenocortical hyperplasias are the most important of the congenital disorders. Because all cause striking alterations and increases in steroid synthesis resulting in adrenogenital syndromes, they will be discussed in the section on hyperadrenalism. Several rare anomalies remain to be considered here.

CONGENITAL ADRENAL HYPOPLASIA

Two distinct adrenal lesions occur in the newborn or young child. In one, the small adrenals are seen in the anencephalic, usually stillborn fetus, and the term *anencephalic type* is applied. The gland consists only of a provisional or adult cortex and no fetal zone. The cause is either cerebral, hypothalamic, or pituitary in origin.

In the second, the *cytomegalic type*, an equally small adrenal (combined weight less than 1 gm) and a distinctive histologic pattern are found. The cortex consists uniformly of large, compact eosinophilic cells several times the size of normal adrenal cells, referred to as cytomegaly. They extend in irregular columns up to the capsule of the gland. They resemble the large cells seen occasionally in the fetal zone. This cytomegalic type of adrenal hypoplasia should not be confused with cytomegalic inclusion disease, which is a very different condition. The cause of cytomegalic adrenal hypoplasia is still unknown, but is possibly familial. When it is recognized promptly and replacement steroid therapy is instituted, long survival is possible.[125]

ECTOPIC ADRENALS

Accessory adrenal tissue may be found retroperitoneally anywhere from the diaphragm to the pelvis. Surprisingly, some of these aberrant adrenals contain both cortex and medulla. Rests of adrenal cortex are also found in the subcapsular regions of the kidney, testis, and ovarian cortex. These curious ectopias may assume importance, as in the patient with advanced breast cancer who is ovariectomized and adrenalectomized to ablate all sources of estrogen.

HYPOFUNCTION OF ADRENAL CORTEX (HYPOADRENALISM)

Adrenocortical hypofunction may be caused by any anatomic or metabolic lesion of the cortex that impairs the output of cortical steroids, or it may be secondary to a deficiency of ACTH. These varied origins of adrenocortical insufficiency are classified in Table 26–7.

The distinctive clinicoanatomic patterns of adrenocortical insufficiency consist of (1) primary chronic adrenocortical insufficiency (Addison's disease), (2) primary acute adrenocortical insufficiency (adrenal crisis), and (3) secondary adrenocortical insufficiency.

PRIMARY CHRONIC ADRENOCORTICAL INSUFFICIENCY (ADDISON'S DISEASE)

Addison's disease is a rare condition caused by any chronic destructive process in the adrenal cortex. Clinical manifestations appear insidiously at any age, but not until at least 90% of the functioning cells have been destroyed.

ETIOLOGY AND PATHOGENESIS. Among the many possible origins of primary chronic adrenal insufficiency listed below only two—idiopathic adrenalitis/atrophy and tuberculosis—account for most cases. All the remaining potential causes, such as amyloidosis, metastatic cancer, sarcoidosis, and hemochromatosis, are extremely rare, and moreover when present may not destroy over 90% of the functional reserve. Tuberculosis, usually secondary to pulmonary disease, was once the dominant cause of Addison's disease, but it now accounts for less than 20 to 25% of cases, having been supplanted by so-called idiopathic adrenalitis/atrophy. In some cases of Addison's disease, small atrophic adrenal glands are found. There may be a cortical infiltrate of lymphocytes, or merely marked cortical atrophy. Presumably the noninflammatory glands represent the end stage of a previously more active destructive process. There are many hints that this condition is autoimmune in origin. Adrenal autoantibodies can be identified in 60 to 75% of patients, and their absence in tuberculous involvement suggests that they are not merely secondary phenomena but instead play a causal role.[126] So-called *autoimmune Addison's disease* has been described in association with pernicious anemia, insulin-dependent diabetes mellitus, chronic mucocutaneous candidiasis, hypoparathyroidism, hypogonadism, and autoimmune thyroid disorders. This polyglandular autoimmune syndrome has been broken down into two distinctive subsets, both of which occur as sporadic and familial diseases.[121] Type I is characterized by at least two of the triad of Addison's disease, hypoparathyroidism and mucocutaneous candidiasis. Other autoimmune disorders may or may not be present. The other, Type II, also known as *Schmidt's syndrome*, is characterized by Addison's disease with autoimmune thyroid disease and/or insulin-dependent diabetes mellitus, but hypoparathyroidism or candidiasis is not present. This subset is clearly associated with HLA-A1 and B8 haplotypes, which is not true of the other subgroup. The autoimmune reactions in Type I have been related to a defect in T-suppressor cell function.[122] However, in the Type II subset, genetic predisposition is postulated. In any event, although adrenocortical insufficiency may be the sole disorder in a patient, it is more often accompanied by some other form of endocrinopathy or systemic disease.[127]

Table 26–7.

Primary Adrenocortical Insufficiency
Anatomic loss of cortex
Idiopathic (? autoimmune) adrenalitis/atrophy
Infection (tuberculous, fungal, others)
Hemorrhage (neonatal, bacteremic, traumatic)
Metastatic cancer
Amyloidosis
Bilateral adrenalectomy for metastatic breast cancer
Others (sarcoidosis, hemochromatosis)
Metabolic failure in hormone production
Congenital adrenal hyperplasia
Drug-induced inhibition of cortical cell function
Secondary Adrenocortical Insufficiency (Lack of ACTH)
Hypothalamic-pituitary disease
Hypothalamic-pituitary suppression
Chronic administration of steroids
Steroid-producing neoplasms

MORPHOLOGY. A variety of anatomic changes may be present in the cortex, depending on the cause of the cortical destruction. When associated with a systemic disease (e.g., tuberculosis) or primary cancer elsewhere, specific histologic changes are present. With so-called idiopathic atrophy, the anatomic changes are less specific. The glands are small and irregularly contracted, and may have a combined weight of as little as 2 to 3 gm (Fig. 26–41). Indeed, it may be difficult to identify such glands in the periadrenal fat. The medulla is unaltered, but the cortex appears to have collapsed about it. There is focal or general absence of cortical epithelium, and such intervening cells as are present are usually large with an abundant eosinophilic cytoplasm and atypical nuclei. A loose fibrous tissue, heavily infiltrated with lymphocytes, may occupy the areas between and about the

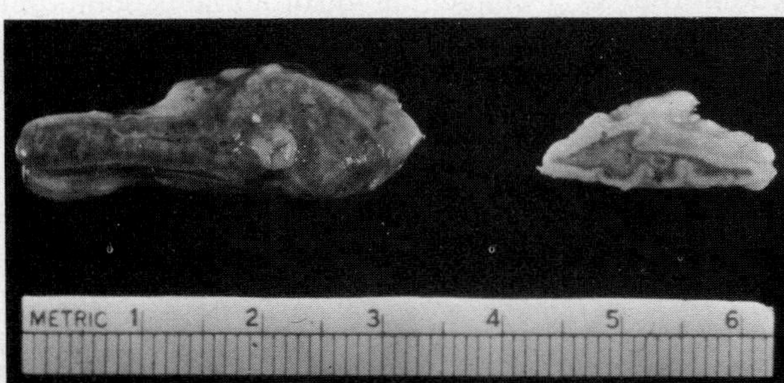

Figure 26–41. Cross section of an atrophic adrenal *(right)*. Compare with normal adrenal cross section *(left)*.

islands of residual epithelial cells, or the cortical cells may be merely atrophic with little or no lymphocytic infiltrate.

Clinical Course. Nearly all patients with primary chronic adrenocortical insufficiency insidiously and progressively develop weakness, fatigability, anorexia, nausea and vomiting, weight loss, hypotension, and hyperpigmentation of the skin and sometimes of the mucous membranes. Less consistently present are diarrhea, constipation, salt craving, and ill-defined abdominal pain that sometimes becomes sufficiently severe to mimic an "acute abdomen." The weakness may become so profound as to confine the individual to bed and even impair speech. Blood pressure may fall below 80/50 and induce syncope on sudden standing. The pigmentation appears as an accentuated sun tan on both exposed and unexposed skin, apparently as a consequence of loss of feedback inhibition of pituitary function and increased synthesis of both ACTH and melanotropin. Sometimes the mucous membranes develop brown-black patches. All the laboratory values may be within the normal range in mild expressions of Addison's disease. However, as the adrenocortical insufficiency becomes more marked, the serum levels of sodium, chloride, bicarbonate, and glucose fall, as well as the plasma cortisol and urinary steroid excretory products such as 17-ketosteroids and 17-hydroxycorticoids. The serum potassium is elevated largely because of aldosterone deficiency, contributing to the salt wasting, lowered circulating blood volume, and hypotension.

When the diagnosis of adrenocortical insufficiency has been established, it is necessary to determine whether it is primary, related to adrenal dysfunction, or secondary, having its origins in the anterior pituitary or hypothalamus. The skin pigmentation may be of value in the differential diagnosis since it is not seen in secondary adrenocortical insufficiency. More direct and definitive is measurement of the plasma ACTH level or testing of the adrenocortical functional reserve by ACTH administration. Although Addison's disease is readily managed by steroids, death may occur when the disease is unrecognized because of acute adrenal insufficiency superimposed on the chronic condition, hyperkalemic cardiac arrhythmias, or a hypoglycemic cerebral crisis. Any of these complications may be precipitated by any form of stress, including intercurrent illness in an already fragile metabolic state.

Brief mention should be made of an uncommon form of *selective aldosterone insufficiency*, which is encountered as a congenital disorder and sometimes following removal of an aldosterone-secreting adenoma. It usually presents as a hyperkalemic salt-wasting syndrome.

PRIMARY ACUTE ADRENOCORTICAL INSUFFICIENCY

Acute adrenocortical insufficiency may appear in three settings: (1) it can occur as a "crisis" in patients with chronic Addison's disease, precipitated by any form of stress such as infection, trauma, surgery, or significant hemorrhage, all of which require an immediate increase in steroid output from glands incapable of responding; (2) it most frequently results from too rapid withdrawal of steroids from patients whose adrenal glands have been suppressed by chronic steroid administration,or from failure to increase the level of administered steroids during stress in a bilaterally adrenalectomized patient; (3) it can occur in otherwise healthy individuals as the result of massive hemorrhagic destruction of the adrenals (adrenal apoplexy). In neonates, extensive adrenal hemorrhages may follow prolonged and difficult delivery associated with considerable trauma and hypoxia. The neonatal adrenal is particularly predisposed since it is large for the body size, it has little periadrenal fat, and its large medullary venous sinuses are fragile and have poorly developed muscular walls. Moreover, newborn infants are often deficient in prothrombin for at least several days after birth. In adults, the hemorrhagic destruction of the adrenals is most often related to a bacteremic infection, and in this setting is called the Waterhouse-Friderichsen syndrome.

Waterhouse-Friderichsen Syndrome

This catastrophic cause of acute adrenocortical insufficiency is most often caused by meningococcemia.[128] Sometimes these patients have a preceding overt meningitis, but in other instances the first manifestations of the meningococcal infection relate to the meningococcemia. Less commonly, the Waterhouse-Friderichsen syndrome is seen with bacteremic infections due to pneumococci, staphylococci, or *Hemophilus influenzae*. Whatever the causative organism, the disease may be literally explosive. Soon after the onset of the infectious febrile reaction, systemic hemorrhagic manifestations appear. Showers of cutaneous petechiae and purpura can be seen in the skin. Presumably at the same time there are hemorrhages into the adrenals and other internal organs and surfaces. The patient may go into circulatory collapse and die within 24 hours. Blood cultures invariably disclose the causative organism. It can also sometimes be cultured from the hemorrhagic skin lesions that may become focally necrotic if the patient survives long enough. However, more often the skin lesions are related to the development of disseminated intravascular coagulation (DIC) and therefore may not reveal organisms.

Anatomically, widespread petechiae, purpura, and hemorrhages are found throughout the body, particularly in the skin, mucous membranes and serosal surfaces. The adrenals are likewise hemorrhagic and partially necrotic. In some children, the adrenals appear as virtual sacs of clotted blood (Fig. 26–42). The bleeding begins in the zona reticularis or the medulla and may be confined to these regions. More often, it extends throughout the medulla and cortex, at first penetrating between the cords of cortical cells toward the capsule and eventually engulfing these cells. Classically, even in those cases in which the entire adrenal appears to

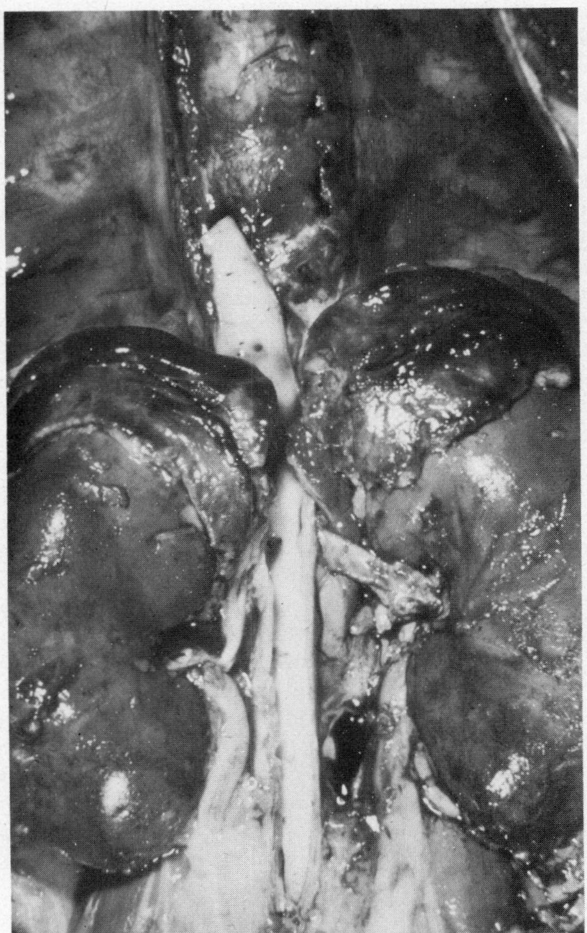

Figure 26–42. Waterhouse-Friderichsen syndrome in a child. The dark, hemorrhagic adrenal glands are distended with blood.

be replaced by blood clot, microscopic examination discloses nests and strands of preserved cortical cells. In essence, the morphologic changes are those of a bleeding diathesis, probably related to the development of DIC. Sometimes the endotoxemia causes an acute interstitial myocarditis.

The cause of the circulatory collapse appears to be predominantly the overwhelming bacteremia and toxemia; however, cardiac failure, arrhythmias, and the acute adrenocortical insufficiency may play significant contributory roles. When this condition is recognized promptly (within hours) and appropriately treated with massive doses of antibiotics and steroids, survival and complete recovery are possible.

Uncommonly, the meningococcemia pursues a chronic or recurrent course and produces a vasculitis indistinguishable from hypersensitivity leukocytoclastic vasculitis (p. 522).

SECONDARY ADRENOCORTICAL INSUFFICIENCY

Any disorder of the hypophyseal-thalamic axis such as metastatic cancer, infection, infarction, or irradiation that reduces the output of ACTH will lead to a syndrome of hypoadrenalism having many similarities to Addison's disease. Analogously, prolonged administration of exogenous glucocorticoids will suppress the output of ACTH to induce a similar syndrome. *With secondary disease the hyperpigmentation of primary Addison's disease is lacking, since tropic hormones are low.* The manifestations also differ inasmuch as secondary hypoadrenalism is characterized by deficient cortisol and androgen output but normal or near-normal aldosterone synthesis. Thus, in adrenal insufficiency secondary to pituitary malfunction there is no marked hyponatremia and hyperkalemia, although a liberal intake of water may induce dilutional lowering of the serum sodium level.

ACTH deficiency may be selective, but in some instances it is only one part of panhypopituitarism, associated with multiple primary tropic hormone deficiencies. For example, in Sheehan's anterior pituitary necrosis (p. 1198), infarction of the anterior lobe leads to depressed function of multiple end-organ targets, including not only the adrenals but also the thyroid and gonads. The differentiation of secondary disease from Addison's disease can be confirmed with demonstration by radioimmunoassay of low levels of plasma ACTH in the former. Because of the technical difficulties inherent in this assay, a further differential test is the administration of ACTH. In patients with primary disease, the destruction of the adrenal cortex does not permit a response in the form of increased plasma levels of cortisol, whereas in those with secondary hypofunction, there is a prompt rise in plasma cortisol levels.

Depending on the extent of ACTH lack, the adrenals may be moderately-to-markedly reduced in size. They may come to have a leaflike appearance and, indeed, be difficult to find in the periadrenal fat. The cortex may be reduced to a thin ribbon having an unusually heavy fibrous capsule and scattered subcapsular cortical cells composed largely of zona glomerulosa. The medulla is unaffected.

HYPERFUNCTION OF ADRENAL CORTEX (HYPERADRENALISM)

Just as there are three basic types of corticosteroids elaborated by the adrenal cortex—glucocorticoids, mineralocorticoids, and androgens—so there are three distinctive hyperadrenal clinical syndromes: (1) Cushing's syndrome, characterized by an excess of cortisol; (2) aldosteronism, with excess production of aldosterone; and (3) congenital adrenal hyperplasia, with an excess of adrenal androgens. As might be anticipated, however, there is sometimes overlap among these conditions.

CUSHING'S SYNDROME

Cushing's syndrome is a distinctive constellation of clinical features associated with prolonged overproduction of cortisol. The most characteristic findings are summarized in Table 26–8.[129] Other changes may also be present, including impaired glucose tolerance, overt diabetes (in approximately 20%), "moon facies," "buffalo hump," abdominal striae, and (in men) loss of libido, impotence, and oligospermia. Some of these abnormalities, such as the obesity, deranged glucose metabolism, and mental disorders (ranging from emotional lability to psychoses), are directly attributable to the increase of cortisol or other glucocorticoids, but many have more complex origins. Excess production of testosterone probably contributes to the appearance of the hirsutism and acne in women. The testosterone and the cortisol inhibition of pituitary release of gonadotropins accounts for the menstrual irregularities. The bruisability and osteoporosis are poorly understood, but it is speculated that steroid suppression of collagen synthesis deprives subcutaneous vessels of their connective tissue support, and similar suppression of osteoid matrix formation underlies the osteoporosis. It suffices to note that, although Cushing's syndrome is characterized by overproduction of cortisol, other secondary derangements contribute to its full expression.

PATHOGENESIS. The term "Cushing's syndrome" encompasses four distinct pathogenetic syndromes all marked by hypercortisolism.[130]

1. *About 60 to 70% of cases can best be identified as "pituitary Cushing's syndrome,"* which was the first type to be described by Harvey Cushing.[131] Perhaps because he was a neurosurgeon, most of his patients had well-defined pituitary basophilic adenomas, presumably composed of corticotropin-secreting cells. On this account, Cushing's *syndrome* related to an adenoma (some would include all forms of the pituitary subgroup) is sometimes referred to as Cushing's *disease* or Cushing's *basophilism.* This practice is regrettable since it is unnecessarily confusing. More recently, it has become evident that many patients with pituitary Cushing's syndrome do not have a discrete solitary adenoma, but instead have multiple corticotroph microadenomas. Moreover, a significant minority have no apparent pituitary tumor(s), giving rise to the concept of "hypothalamic Cushing's syndrome."[132] Not rigorously ruled out in some of the cases attributed to hypothalamic origins are undetected microadenomas. In any event, *pituitary Cushing's syndrome is characterized by bilateral adrenal hyperplasia and, in most cases, readily measurable elevated plasma levels of ACTH.* Sometimes, however, the elevations are very modest or indeed undetectable. No satisfactory explanation has been offered for the failure to find elevated levels of ACTH, but the possibilities have been raised of abnormal sensitivity of adrenal cortical cells to even normal levels of ACTH, or loss of the normal circadian rhythm of ACTH secretion inducing unremitting stimulation of the adrenals by low levels of ACTH.[133] *Whatever the nature of the pituitary dysfunction, the hypercortisolism can be suppressed by large doses of administered glucocorticoids such as dexamethasone, inducing a fall in levels of serum cortisol and its urinary excretory products (e.g., 17-hydroxycorticosteroid). This response serves as a clinical diagnostic test of the pituitary variant of Cushing's syndrome.*

2. *About 20 to 25% of cases are best termed "adrenal Cushing's syndrome."* The source of the excess cortisol is a functioning neoplasm of the adrenal cortex, more often an adenoma than a carcinoma. Rarely, there is no well-defined neoplasm but only apparently autonomous nodular hyperplasia. The origin of bilateral nodular hyperplasia is not evident but it is not clearly neoplastic in origin. The adrenocortical carcinomas tend to produce the most marked hypercortisolism. In those instances due to a unilateral neoplasm, the uninvolved adrenal cortex and that in the opposite gland undergo atrophy because of suppression of ACTH secretion. *Adrenal Cushing's syndrome is marked by low serum levels of ACTH and failure of administered large doses of glucocorticoid to suppress the levels of serum cortisol and its urinary excretory products.*

3. *About 10 to 15% of cases are "ectopic Cushing's syndrome"* in which nonendocrine cancers elaborate ACTH or some biologically active fragment as a paraneoplastic syndrome.[134] Most commonly implicated are bronchogenic carcinoma (60%), malignant thymoma (15%), and pancreatic neoplasms—usually islet cell (10%), but a variety of other tumors have also been implicated. An elevated plasma level of ACTH is almost uniformly present. In passing, sensitive radioimmunoassays have documented that the great majority of bronchogenic carcinomas contain ACTH-like material, but in most instances it represents a nonbiologically active fragment of the large precursor peptide from which ACTH is cleaved.[135] Very rarely, a visceral cancer produces corticotropin-releasing factor or a closely related product as the basis for the ectopic Cushing's syndrome. *As in the pituitary variant, the adrenal glands undergo bilateral cortical hyperplasia, but with ectopic disease the ACTH secretion cannot be suppressed by large doses of glucocorticoid, and so there is no fall in levels of serum cortisol or its excretory products.*

4. *Iatrogenic Cushing's syndrome* is uncommon but may arise from the long-term use of glucocorticoids, for example, as an immunosuppressant in transplant recipients or those having an autoimmune disorder. Prolonged use of ACTH would have similar effect. Little need be said about this category save that it is uncom-

Table 26–8. CUSHING'S SYNDROME

Symptoms	Percentage
Truncal obesity	59–100
Plethoric face	50–100
Hypertension	50–90
Hirsutism	28–93
Muscle weakness	18–96
Menstrual disorders	40–85
Acne	26–82
Bruising	23–62
Mental disorders	31–70
Osteoporosis (backache, fractures)	22–70

mon, because incipient manifestations are usually recognized and therapy discontinued. Should a patient receiving long-term steroids die, bilateral cortical atrophy may be present related to suppression of ACTH secretion.

MORPHOLOGY. The basic lesions of Cushing's syndrome are found in the pituitary and adrenal glands.

In the **pituitary**, irrespective of the cause of Cushing's syndrome, the increased levels of cortisol produce apparent feedback effects on the nontumorous corticotrophs, referred to as **Crooke's hyaline degeneration of the basophils.** Infrequently, the corticotrophs in adenomas display the same changes.[136] The perinuclear or patchy foci of cytoplasm take on a basophilic hyalinization that obscures underlying details. Electron microscopy indicates that the hyaline is made up of aggregates of microfilaments in which secretory granules are scattered.[137] The basis for this change is not known. In most cases of the pituitary variant of Cushing's syndrome, adenomas or microadenomas composed of densely granulated or sparsely granulated corticotrophs also are present. These lesions have already been described in the consideration of the pituitary (p. 1194), and so it suffices to note that they are distinctive by virtue of their content of ACTH, demonstrable by immunocytochemical methods. There are no adequate data on how often the anterior pituitary lacks any evidence of neoplasia (suggesting only a hypothalamic dysfunction) in cases that otherwise satisfy the criteria of the "pituitary" syndrome, but this is rare.[138]

The changes in the **adrenals** are varied, as may be anticipated from the preceding discussion. **They may take the form of (1) bilateral cortical hyperplasia, which is sometimes nodular in response to ACTH of either pituitary or ectopic origin** (Fig. 26–43); **(2) an adrenal cortical neoplasm, benign or malignant; (3) nodular hyperplasia morphologically indistinguishable from that encountered in ACTH-driven glands; or (4) adrenocortical atrophy, either iatrogenic in origin or secondary to an autonomous cortical neoplasm.** The hyperplasia induced by ACTH is usually diffuse and bilateral, but sometimes a nodularity appears. The extent of the hyperplasia is obviously a function of the duration and level of the ACTH excess. It may be subtle, with an aggregate weight of the glands in the range of 10 to 12 gm. It is therefore said that Cushing's syndrome sometimes may be associated with "normal adrenal glands." However, the term "normal" only depicts the subtlety of the hyperplasia compatible with excess elaboration of cortisol. With more marked ACTH production, as is encountered in some nonendocrine cancers, the adrenals are markedly enlarged, sometimes to a collective weight of 25 gm. There is almost always an increase in width of the cortex. Histologically, the enlargement is caused primarily by marked widening of the zona reticularis that occupies the inner half of the cortex, accompanied by some widening of the zona fasciculata. Most prominent in such glands are large, so-called "clear cells" that, under the electron microscope, exhibit dilation and hyperplasia of the hyperfunctioning smooth endoplasmic reticulum.[139] The adenomas or carcinomas of the adrenal cortex, as the source of the cortisol secretion, are not macroscopically distinctive from nonfunctioning adrenal neoplasms (to be described) or from those encountered in the adrenogenital syndrome. Histologically, the adenomas present varying admixtures of "clear" and "compact" cells similar to those of the normal zona fasciculata, but compact cells usually predominate. Electron microscopy indicates a rich endowment of smooth endoplasmic reticulum and mitochondria of variable size and shape.[140] Similarly, the adrenal cancers in Cushing's syndrome display the same range in cellular pleomorphism encountered in nonfunctioning cancers (p. 1243). Ultrastructurally, the anaplastic cells possess less smooth endoplasmic reticulum and more mitochondria.[141] The atrophic adrenal is a small, shrunken organ having a barely visible rim of cortex surrounding the medulla. The glands may be reduced in size to a collective weight of 3 to 6 gm. Histologically, it is evident that the atrophy affects primarily the inner two zones of the cortex, sparing to an extent the aldosterone-secreting zona glomerulosa, which is nondependent on ACTH. The severity of these atrophic changes is, of course, a function of the level of suppression of ACTH secretion and its duration.

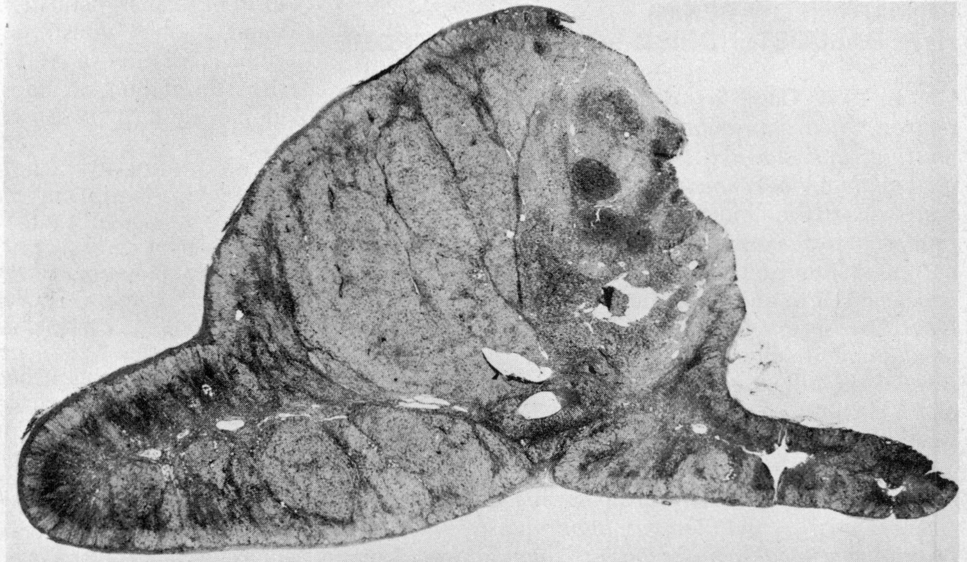

Figure 26–43. Irregular, nodular adenomatous hyperplasia of adrenal from a patient with Cushing's syndrome.

Clinical Course. Cushing's syndrome generally appears in middle adult life, and three times more often in women than in men. When it occurs in childhood it is most often related to an adrenal carcinoma. The presenting features mentioned at the outset are more or less the same irrespective of the underlying cause of the hypercortisolism. However, when related to ectopic production of ACTH by a nonadrenal cancer, the shortened clinical course may truncate the full development of the complete syndrome. Most commonly observed under these circumstances are weakness, muscle wasting, hypokalemia, hyperglycemia, and (sometimes) hyperpigmentation related to the elaboration of melanotonins. Truncal obesity, hirsutism, bruisability, and osteoporosis may not have time to develop.

It is beyond our scope to go into the diagnosis of Cushing's syndrome and the differential diagnosis of the various patterns. It is enough to note that the diagnosis rests mainly on the documentation of hypercortisolism, and the differential diagnosis on the cortisol-secretory response to an administered large dose of corticosteroid (dexamethasone), the measurement of the plasma ACTH level, and evidence of a pituitary lesion based largely on radiography and CT scan. For example, a drop in serum cortisol and urinary excretory products points to "pituitary Cushing's syndrome." Lack of response implies either an "ectopic" or "adrenal" syndrome. Differentiation between these two possibilities rests largely on the plasma ACTH level.

Brief mention should be made of *Nelson's syndrome*, encountered in patients with pituitary corticotroph adenomas who are bilaterally adrenalectomized because the primary pituitary tumor cannot be eradicated. Under these circumstances, progressive enlargement of the pituitary adenoma may follow as the feedback inhibition of cortisol is removed, often accompanied by intense pigmentation, presumably related to excess production of ACTH and melanotonin.

PRIMARY (LOW-RENIN) HYPERALDOSTERONISM—CONN'S SYNDROME

In 1955, Conn first described a patient with *hypertension, neuromuscular symptoms, renal potassium wasting, and elevated levels of aldosterone, all associated with an adrenocortical adenoma.* These features were all attributable to the "autonomous" hypersecretion of aldosterone, which promotes sodium retention and potassium excretion. The sodium retention leads to expansion of extracellular fluid volume and elevation of blood pressure, with concomitant suppression of renin production. In the absence of circulatory insufficiency, physiologic adjustments prevent progressive expansion of ECF volume and overt edema. The renal potassium wasting induces hypokalemia, hypokalemic alkalosis, and muscular weakness, as well as other neuromuscular abnormalities and electrocardiographic changes.

Primary or autonomous hyperaldosteronism must be differentiated from secondary hyperaldosteronism. The latter is not a disease process, but rather the appropriate secretion of aldosterone in response to increased levels of renin-angiotensin. Overproduction of renin by the kidneys occurs mainly with (1) any cause of renal ischemia, (2) any edematous state, and (3) a renin-producing neoplasm. Decreased renal blood flow and/or perfusion pressure occurs, for example, in renal artery stenosis and malignant nephrosclerosis with its hyperplastic arteriolosclerosis. Secondary aldosteronism is also encountered in situations with developing edema as sodium is retained, e.g., in the nephrotic syndrome. Rarely, a renin-producing tumor or oral contraceptives induce elevated levels of aldosterone. A special form of secondary disease is known as *Bartter's syndrome*, characterized by renal juxtaglomerular cell hyperplasia, hyperreninemia, hyperaldosteronism, hypokalemia, and failure to thrive. Inappropriately, blood pressure is often low, raising the issue of blood pressure refractoriness to the actions of renin-angiotensin.[142] Whatever its origins, *secondary aldosteronism is associated with sodium retention and potassium wasting, but notably with high renin output, in contrast to the low renin levels of primary aldosteronism.*

Pathogenesis. *There are three distinctive clinicoanatomic forms of primary aldosteronism.*[143] *The most common form in adults is caused by an aldosterone-producing adenoma, accounting for 50 to 90% of cases.* Very rarely, an adrenal carcinoma induces this pattern of the condition. Second, particularly common in children but sometimes encountered in adults, is *idiopathic hyperaldosteronism*, sometimes called *congenital hyperaldosteronism*, when the onset is in childhood owing to bilateral adrenal hyperplasia. This pattern has also been called pseudoprimary aldosteronism. Third and much more rare is a subset called *glucocorticoid-suppressible hyperaldosteronism.*[144] Little is known about the adrenal histologic findings in this third pattern, but adrenal hyperplasia was observed in several surgical patients. Parenthetically, the glucocorticoid suppressibility of this form of primary aldosteronism has aroused great excitement among "aldosteronists" since it suggests the possible mediation of ACTH or some fragment thereof in the stimulation of aldosterone secretion by the zona glomerulosa (p. 1232).

Morphology. Aldosterone-secreting adenomas are usually less than 2 cm in diameter but may be larger. For obscure reasons, in most reported series the left adrenal gland is involved in slightly more than 60% of cases. Macroscopically, they are not distinctive from nonfunctioning adenomas.[145] Large tumors may show areas of necrosis and hemorrhage or cystic change. Cytologically they show a mixture of cell types, including lipid-laden "clear" cells, compact cells, and hybrid forms (Fig. 26–44). Electron microscopic studies indicate that cells of the adenoma sometimes possess lamellar mitochondrial cristae identical to those in glomerulosa cells, whereas others interestingly possess tubulovesicular cristae identical to those in the cells of the zona fasciculata. When cells of such adenomas are cultured in vitro, they produce, as would be expected of such a mixture of cell types, aldosterone and cortisol.[146]

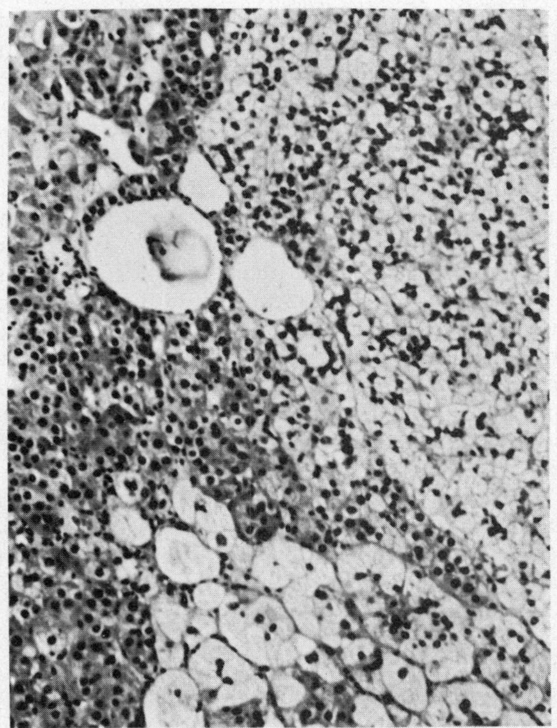

Figure 26–44. Conn's syndrome with a mixture of cell types within adenoma. To left are dark "compact" cells. Below and to right is a nest of light "clear" cells, and in upper right are some hybrid forms.

In cases in which there is no adrenal neoplasm, most patients have bilateral hyperplasia of the cortex, sometimes nodular. Very rarely, the hyperplasia is unilateral as judged by measurement of the aldosterone levels in the venous efflux of each gland. Supporting this surprising finding is the fact that unilateral adrenalectomy is curative in these cases. The cells making up the diffuse and nodular hyperplasia are largely lipid-laden, with occasional masses of compact cells (Fig. 26–45). The hyperplastic foci may extend into the inner cortex in tonguelike fashion. It is of interest that functional studies in vitro indicate that the hyperplastic cortical cells, as exemplified by those in the macronodules, synthesize not only aldosterone but also cortisol. Thus, the micronodular and the diffuse adrenal hyperplasia may reflect some unknown proliferative stimulus that induces simultaneously hyperfunction and hyperplasia of zona glomerulosa cells and glucocorticoid-secreting cells.

The adrenal carcinomas associated with hyperaldosteronism are not morphologically different from nonfunctioning neoplasms.[147]

CLINICAL COURSE. Primary aldosteronism is generally an insidious disease that can only be diagnosed with a high index of suspicion. *Moderate hypertension (diastolic pressure 100 to 125 mm Hg) is the predominant manifestation*, sometimes associated with mild frontal headaches, chronic fatigue, and weakness, but obviously these are quite nonspecific. It must be appreciated, however, that less than 1% of hypertensives have primary aldosteronism. Rarely, there are more distinctive neuromuscular findings in the form of paralyses or tetany secondary to hypokalemia. *Only the laboratory evidence is diagnostic—hypernatremia, hypokalemia, alkalosis, excessive potassium excretion, low plasma-renin activity, and (with adenomas) elevated nonsuppressible aldosterone levels.*[148]

Even more difficult than establishing the diagnosis of primary aldosteronism is determining its cause. The identification of an adenoma is both difficult and critical: difficult because the lesions are frequently small, and critical because the decision must be made about which side to operate on. Radioscans and CT scans may suffice, but in most instances adrenal vein catheterization (a difficult procedure with many limitations) is necessary to measure the levels of aldosterone in the venous efflux from each gland. When it is equally elevated in the effluent of both adrenal veins, bilateral hyperplasia is most likely, but rarely it is also unilateral. A number of other clinical approaches can be used and have been briefly characterized by Ganguly and colleagues.[149] It need only be emphasized in closing that recognition of an aldosterone-producing adenoma offers the satisfying opportunity of curing a form of hypertension.

ADRENAL VIRILISM AND CONGENITAL ADRENAL HYPERPLASIA (CAH)

Adrenal virilism, most readily recognized in females although males may also be affected, can appear at any age with an androgen-secreting adenoma or carcinoma. *More often it arises as a congenital metabolic disorder*

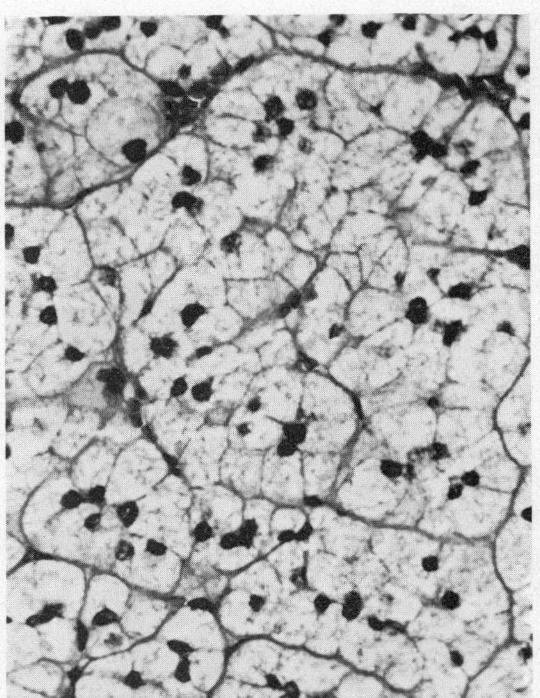

Figure 26–45. Conn's syndrome caused by diffuse hyperplasia composed of lipid-laden cells.

related to some enzymatic defect in the biosynthesis of cortical steroids leading to cortisol deficiency. The resultant increased levels of ACTH stimulate unaffected pathways of steroidogenesis, notably those involved in the production of adrenal androgens. Depending on the specific enzymatic defect and its effects on steroid biosynthesis, these inborn errors of metabolism may present as "pure" virilization or as a "mixed" syndrome characterized by both virilization and some of the features of Cushing's syndrome (when there is concomitant increased production of a glucocorticoid). As might be anticipated, the elevated levels of ACTH induce congenital adrenal hyperplasia (Fig. 26–46).

At least eight distinctive clinical syndromes are encompassed under the term "congenital adrenal hyperplasia." All are characterized by a congenital deficiency of a specific biosynthetic enzyme. All variants are autosomal recessive, and within a particular family all members inherit the same enzyme deficiency.[150] *The clinical manifestations of each syndrome are determined largely by the functional properties of the steroid intermediates that build up because of the enzyme lack, and by the completeness of the enzyme block and resultant cortisol deficiency.* Three clinical patterns account for 95 to 98% of cases of CAH; all are characterized by virilism—hence, the term *adrenogenital syndromes.*

1. *Simple virilizing CAH* alone accounts for about 90% of all cases. It is the consequence of a 21-hydroxylase deficiency. From the biosynthetic pathways depicted in Figure 26–40, this enzymatic deficiency impairs the synthesis of cortisol and shunts steroidogenesis into androgen production. There is no lack of aldosterone in this pattern.

2. *A salt-losing form of virilizing CAH* is also associated with a 21-hydroxylase deficiency, accompanied, however, by deficient production of aldosterone. The basis of the defective synthesis of aldosterone is not understood. Infants with this condition have hyponatremia, hyperkalemia, dehydration, and vomiting and are at great risk of dying unless replacement steroid, fluid, and electrolyte therapy is instituted at birth.

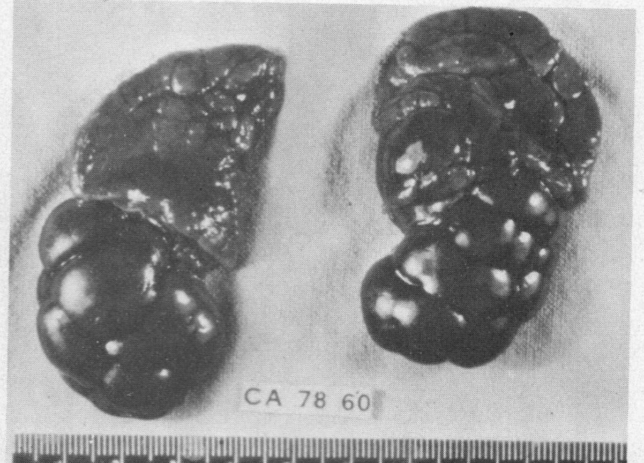

Figure 26–46. Adrenogenital syndrome in an infant with massive nodular enlargement of adrenals to the point at which they approximate size of kidneys.

3. *An 11-hydroxylase deficiency* is best characterized as the *hypertensive form of CAH.* There is not only excessive secretion of androgens but also impaired conversion of 11-deoxycorticosterone to corticosterone. Like aldosterone, 11-deoxycorticosterone is a potent mineralocorticoid, causing the hypertension.

The remaining forms of CAH are all too uncommon to merit consideration, but they are not associated with virilization. For example, a lack of 17-hydroxylase results in diminished secretion of glucocorticoids and sex steroids, and shunts steroidogenesis into the mineralocorticoid pathway. As a consequence, hypertension and hypokalemia develop, analogous to that in primary aldosteronism. The deficiency of androgens in males suppresses male differentiation and results in pseudohermaphroditism. Untreated females have sexual infantilism.

The adrenal hyperplasia in CAH may be either diffuse or nodular and resembles that found in Cushing's syndrome related to excess ACTH secretion. Biochemical analysis of the adrenal glands revealing a specific enzyme deficiency is the only laboratory method to differentiate the various forms of CAH. On clinical grounds, differentiation depends on the specific manifestations, serum levels of the various steroids, and the urinary levels of their excretory products. When one of the virilizing syndromes is diagnosed early in life, the daily administration of glucocorticoids to suppress pituitary ACTH will stop the virilization, but reconstructive surgery may be necessary to correct abnormalities in the genitals.[151]

CORTICAL NEOPLASMS

It is evident from preceding sections that the proliferative lesions of the adrenal cortex range from diffuse hyperplasia to nodular hyperplasia to benign and malignant tumors, and that all these proliferative processes may be associated with steroidogenesis. In addition, there are nonfunctional benign and malignant tumors of the adrenal cortex, as well as rare neoplasms, that synthesize specific steroids. Occasionally, as mentioned, virilization is related to the autonomous elaboration of androgens by a neoplasm. Even more uncommon is the adrenal tumor that elaborates either estrogens or precursors that are converted into estrogenic compounds. It is extremely difficult, if not impossible, from morphologic examination alone to determine whether a neoplasm is functional or not. The only reliable criteria are biochemical and hormonal assay of fresh tissue.

Adrenal adenomas are found in about 2% of adult autopsies, and most are non–steroid-producing. For years, however, the controversy has persisted as to whether some apparently nonfunctional adenomas may produce hypertension in the nature of a "forme fruste" of Conn's syndrome.[152] It is also important to remember that adrenal adenomas may be one part of the multiple endocrine neoplasia syndrome (p. 988). Usually, adenomas are poorly encapsulated masses of yellow-orange adrenocortical tissue ranging from

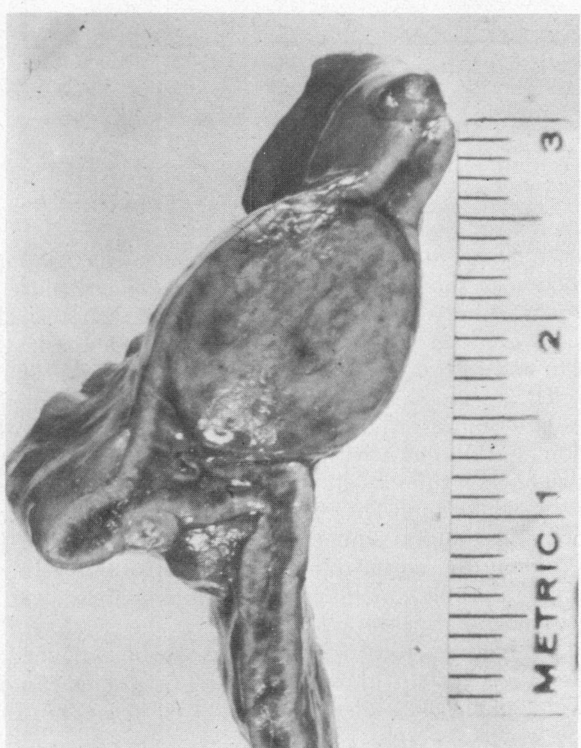

Figure 26–47. A small adrenal adenoma productive of Cushing's syndrome.

1 to 5 cm in diameter. Some nestle within the adrenal cortex, others appear to be within the medulla, and still others protrude under the capsule (Fig. 26–47). They may achieve much larger size and exhibit areas of hemorrhage, cystic degeneration, and calcification. The encapsulation may be poorly defined and may appear at places to be deficient. The non–steroid-producing adenomas differ from their functioning relatives principally because they are composed of lipid-filled cells that reflect their secretory inactivity. **The cells may show some variation in size and nuclear characteristics that, indeed, verges on anaplasia.** Thus, many lesions fall into an intermediate category and are neither clearly benign nor clearly malignant.

Even more difficult is the differentiation of a true adenoma from a focus of nodular hyperplasia. Adenomas, as you recall, are not necessarily well encapsulated and so may be easily mistaken for a focus of hyperplasia. In general, nodules larger than 1 cm in diameter are likely to be adenomas. If nodules are multiple, bilateral, or located in the capsule or outside of it, they are more likely to be expressions of nodular hyperplasia.

Cortical carcinomas usually produce steroids (90%) and are associated with one of the hyperadrenal syndromes; however, some are nonfunctional. They are rare, and most are highly malignant. Usually large when discovered, many exceed 20 cm in diameter. On cut surface, they are predominantly yellow but frequently have hemorrhagic, cystic, and necrotic areas (Fig. 26–48). Many appear to be more or less encapsulated. Histologically, they range from lesions showing mild degrees of atypia, not dissimilar from that seen in some large adenomas, to wildly anaplastic neoplasms composed of monstrous giant cells (Fig. 26–49). Between these extremes are found cancers with moderate degrees of anaplasia, some predominantly composed of spindle cells.

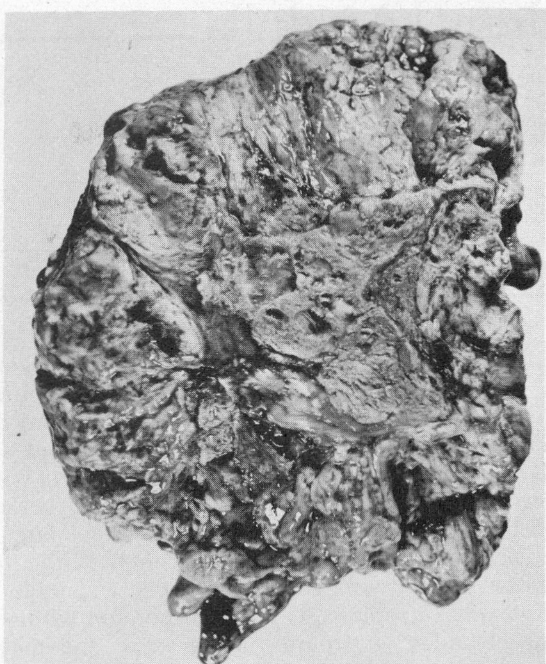

Figure 26–48. Adrenal carcinoma. Tumor is large, hemorrhagic, and necrotic. Very little viable tissue is present.

Adrenal cancers have a strong tendency to invade the adrenal vein, vena cava, and lymphatics. Metastases to regional and periaortic nodes are common, as well as distant hematogenous spread to the lungs and other viscera. Bone metastases are unusual.[153]

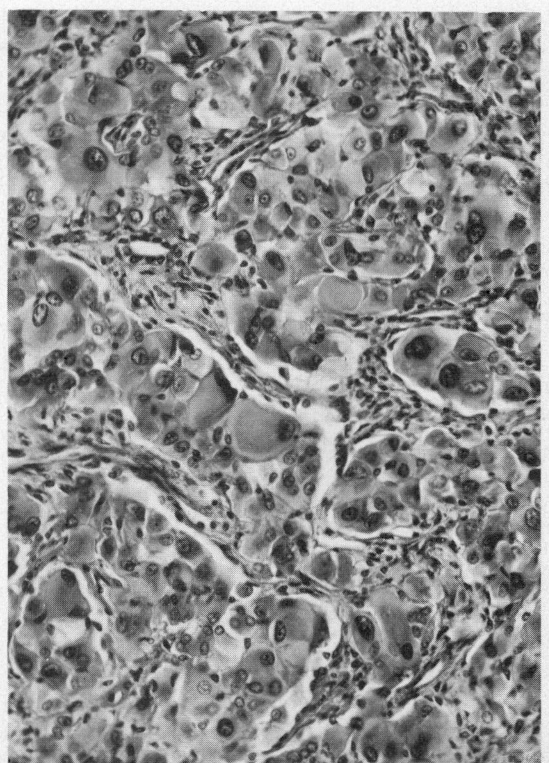

Figure 26–49. Adrenal carcinoma. There is marked anaplasia and pleomorphism of neoplastic cells.

Adrenal Medulla

NORMAL

The adrenal medulla, like other components of the APUD system, is a neurosecretory organ. Embryologically, it is derived from cells of the primitive neuroectoderm (neural crest) that differentiate along two lines to form chromaffin cells (pheochromocytes) and autonomic ganglion cells. Neural crest cells are found widely dispersed through the body in the organs of Zuckerkandl (paired structures lying just anterior to the bifurcation of the aorta) and in the sympathetic ganglia of the neck, posterior mediastinum, retroperitoneum, and abdomen. Occasionally, ectopic rests are incorporated within the urinary bladder, gastrointestinal system, and gonads. These ectopic islands are usually replaced by lymphatic tissue shortly after birth, but may persist and lead to extra-adrenal medullary neoplasms.

The chromaffin cell is characterized by intracytoplasmic granules that appear brown after fixation in dichromates (e.g., Zenker's) as the result of oxidation and polymerization of the catecholamines stored in the granules. The granules are sharply delineated and electron dense. Epinephrine is the major catecholamine, but also present is norepinephrine, the ratio of these two in the normal state being 9:1. The principal metabolites of these catecholamines are metanephrine, normetanephrine, vanillylmandelic acid (VMA), and 3-methoxy-4-hydroxyphenoglycol. Involved in these conversions are hepatic catechol-O-methyltransferase and monamine oxidase.

PATHOLOGY

The only significant disorders arising in the medulla are neoplasms. As can be surmised from the cell types indigenous to the medulla, these are pheochromocytomas, neuroblastomas, and ganglioneuromas.

PHEOCHROMOCYTOMA

This neoplasm is uncommon but of great interest because it usually induces hypertension related to the production of catecholamines. Most of these neoplasms secrete a combination of norepinephrine and epinephrine, predominantly the former. Occasionally a tumor elaborates only one or the other, and a rare tumor produces only dopamine and is not associated with hypertension.[154] Although *only about 0.1 to 0.2% of hypertensives have an underlying pheochromocytoma*, resection of the neoplasm produces a dramatic cure of what is otherwise a potentially lethal disease. The tumors occur at any age, with a peak incidence in the fourth and fifth decades.

These neoplasms may arise wherever chromaffin cells are found. About 97% are situated within the abdomen, 70 to 90% within the adrenals, more often on the right than the left. In about 10 to 20% of cases there are bilateral neoplasms. The small remainder of intra-abdominal tumors, sometimes several tumors, are located along the aorta, often at the bifurcation.[155] Infrequently, a solitary neoplasm or multiple neoplasms arise in thoracic paravertebral ganglia, in the wall of the urinary bladder, or in other sites harboring ectopic neural crest rests. Although 5 to 10% of adrenal tumors are malignant, 30% of extra-adrenal neoplasms in one study were cancerous.[156]

Approximately 80 to 90% of pheochromocytomas occur sporadically, and most often these are solitary neoplasms. The remaining 10 to 20% are associated with four, possibly more, familial syndromes, some of which are characterized by multiple endocrine neoplasms (MEN) and other lesions. You recall that the adrenal medullary cells belong to the category of endocrine or APUD cells. Thus, pheochromocytomas represent endocrine cell tumors (APUDomas), and the associated neoplasms in the familial syndromes are sometimes also APUDomas. The concurrence of multiple endocrine tumors raises the possibility of some widespread stimulus to neoplasia in this family of cells. In the familial syndromes, the pheochromocytomas more often arise outside of the adrenals.

One hereditary pattern is simply familial predisposition to pheochromocytomas transmitted as an autosomal dominant trait with incomplete penetrance. The tumors tend to arise in childhood and are multiple or bilateral in more than half of the cases. *A second familial syndrome is MEN, Type IIa, also known as Sipple's syndrome* (described in more detail on p. 1223). Briefly, it constitutes the concurrence of pheochromocytoma, medullary carcinoma of the thyroid, and parathyroid hyperplasia or adenoma. This condition is thought to be transmitted by autosomal dominant inheritance with a high degree of penetrance. It is distinguished from the simple familial syndrome by a later onset (fourth decade of life), a greater tendency to intermittent or paroxysmal hypertension, fewer pheochromocytomas outside of the adrenals, a strong tendency (60 to 100%) to bilaterality, and an increased frequency of malignant pheochromocytomas. *A third familial subgroup, designated MEN, Type IIb* (or sometimes MEN III) is characterized by pheochromocytoma, medullary carcinoma of the thyroid, and mucosal neuromas, but rarely parathyroid lesions; there may be an associated marfanoid habitus. This subset is also transmitted as an autosomal dominant trait, but the two MEN syndromes are distinct within families. *A fourth familial syndrome is the association of pheochromocytoma with von Recklinghausen's neurofibromatosis.* Conversely, about 1% of patients with neurofibromatosis have a pheochromocytoma. A less well-defined subset is marked by the association of pheochromocytoma with von Hippel-Lindau disease. It is evident that the pheochromocytoma is a "social animal" that may live a solitary life, but often consorts with a number of interesting conditions.

MORPHOLOGY. It should be noted at the outset that, in the MEN syndromes, the adrenal medullary involvement may take the form of diffuse or nodular hyperplasia, sometimes accompanied by one or more discrete neoplasms. There is the suggestion, then, that the pheochromocytoma may arise through a sequence of diffuse hyperplasia, nodular hyperplasia, and, finally, an overt neoplasm. Significantly, occasional intramedullary tumors are associated with hyperplasia in the opposite medulla and/or in the extra-adrenal chromaffin tissue.

The average weight of a pheochromocytoma is 100 gm, but variations from just over 1 to almost 4000 gm have been recorded. The tumors are well demarcated by either connective tissue or compressed adrenocortical tissue. Fibrous trabeculae, richly vascularized, pass into the tumor and produce a lobular pattern. In many tumors, remnants of the adrenal gland can be seen, stretched over the surface or attached at one pole. On section, the cut surface has a pale gray or light brown color, and areas of hemorrhage or necrosis can be observed, particularly in the larger lesions (Fig. 26–50). When a suitable dichromate fixative (Zenker's or Helly's solution) is used, the tumor turns brown-black owing to oxidation of stored catecholamines—hence, the term chromaffin.

The cytologic patterns in pheochromocytomas are quite variable.[157] The tumors are composed of mature pheochromocytes, which possess an abundant basophilic cytoplasm in which secretory granules about 1 micron in size[158] can be seen in dichromate-fixed tissue or with the electron microscope. The functional activity of a neoplasm cannot be judged by the abundance of granules since the preservation and fixation of the tissue may deplete the stored catecholamines. The cells are arranged in either large trabeculae, punctuated by thin-walled sinusoids often lined by the tumor cells themselves (Fig. 26–51), or in small alveoli, each surrounded by fibrovascular stroma derived from the tumor capsule (Fig. 26–52). Various patterns may be found in any one tumor. Cellular and nuclear pleomorphism are often noted, especially in the alveolar group of lesions, and giant and bizarre cells are commonly seen. Mitotic figures usually are not present in these lesions, but they can occur in tumors that subsequently behave in a benign fashion. Occasionally, tumor cells can be found lying in the capillaries or sinusoids. This is not indicative of malignancy, as it has been observed in tumors that are benign in their behavior.

Since malignant and benign pheochromocytomas may have a similar histologic appearance, the diagnosis of malignancy cannot be made by histologic examination of the tumor alone. The general histologic criteria of malignancy when applied to pheochromocytomas only lead to misdiagnosis. The only absolute criterion upon which a diagnosis of malignancy can be made is the presence of distant metastases. Overall, about 10% of pheochromocytomas are malignant, with higher frequencies in the familial syndromes. Metastases occur most frequently in the related lymph nodes, liver, lungs, and bones, and survival after diagnosis rarely exceeds three years.

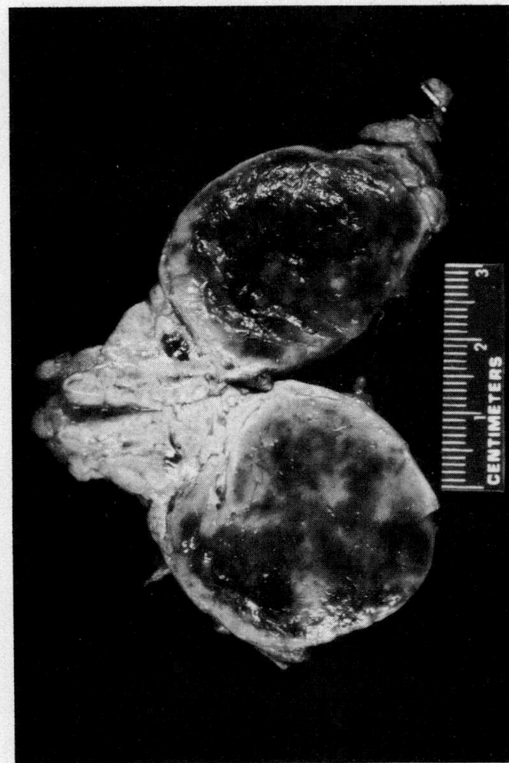

Figure 26–50. Pheochromocytoma of adrenal. Tumor is well encapsulated and exhibits hemorrhagic dark mottling.

An important part of the evaluation of these neoplasms is the demonstration of increased levels of catecholamines in fresh tissue samples of the neoplasms.

CLINICAL COURSE. *The dominant clinical feature in patients with pheochromocytoma is hypertension.*[159] About one-third of patients have sustained hypertension rendered distinctive by attacks or paroxysms of more severe elevation of blood pressure. In another third, the hypertension is intermittent; in the remaining third, it is sustained without paroxysms. The paroxysms may be precipitated by emotional stress, exercise, changes in posture, and (to be noted) palpation in the region of the tumor. The elevations of pressure are induced by the sudden release of catecholamines that may acutely precipitate congestive heart failure, pulmonary edema, myocardial infarction, ventricular fibrillation, cerebral hemorrhage, and even death. The cardiac complications are attributable, at least in some instances, to what has been called *catecholamine cardiomyopathy* or *catecholamine heart muscle disease.* The myocardial changes have been attributed to ischemic damage secondary to the catecholamine-induced vasomotor constriction of the myocardial circulation. Histologically, there are focal

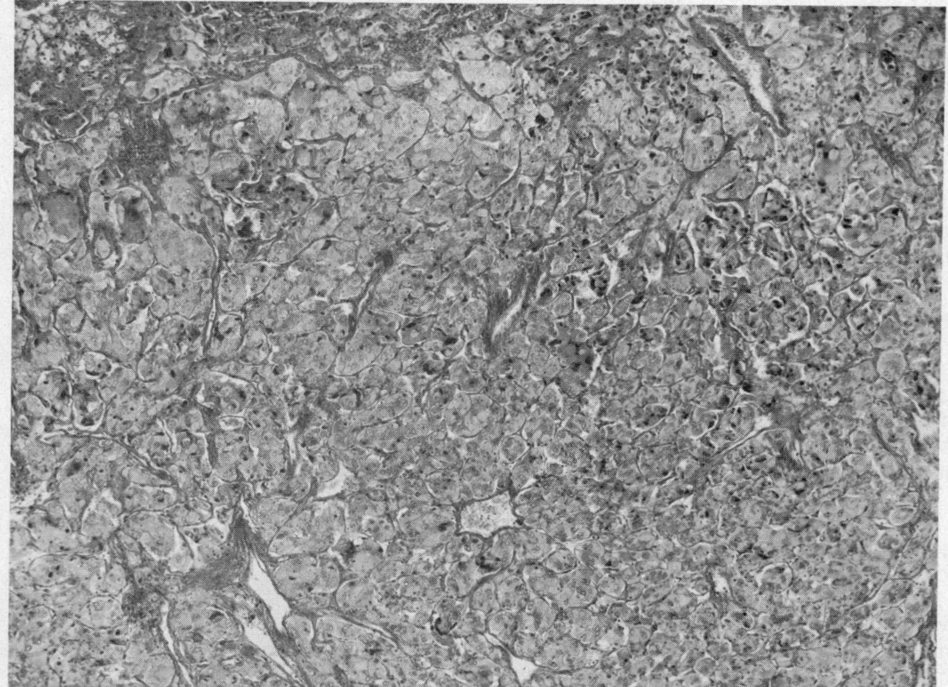

Fig. 26–51

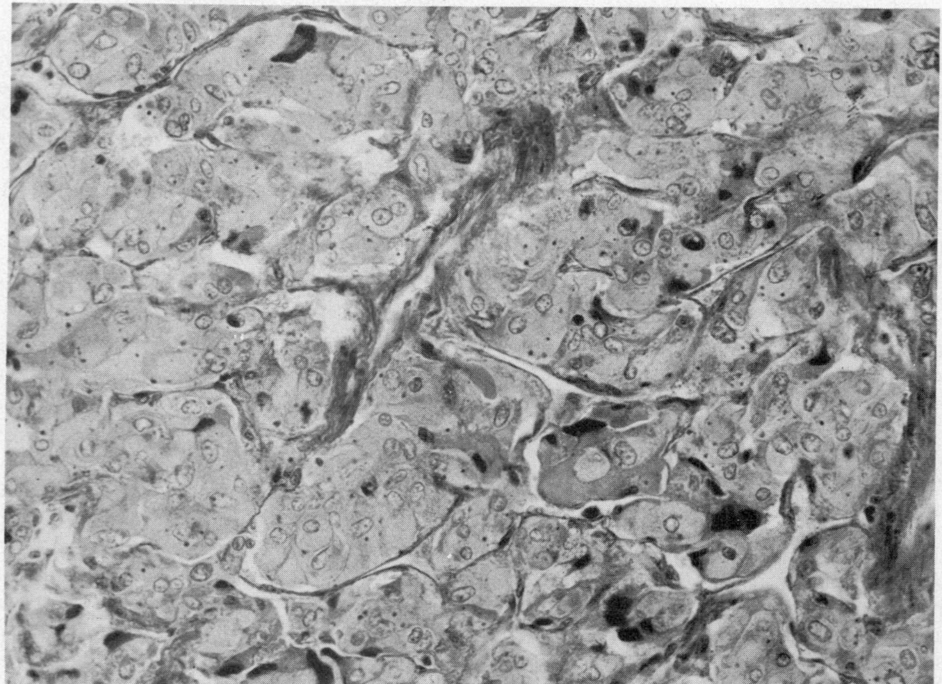

Fig. 26–52

Figure 26–51. Low-power microscopic view of a pheochromocytoma, showing nests of cells resembling those normally found in the medulla.

Figure 26–52. High-power detail of a field from Figure 26–51, illustrating cellular detail consisting of fairly regular nuclei and abundant granular cytoplasm. The chromaffin pigment is not visible in the photograph.

areas of myocytolysis, occasionally myofiber necrosis and interstitial fibrosis, sometimes with mononuclear inflammatory infiltrates.[160] These cardiac lesions are often superimposed upon hypertensive changes and/or alterations incident to coronary artery disease, and so, not surprisingly, patients may have anginal chest pain.

The sudden release of catecholamines may provoke a number of other symptoms during or following the paroxysm, including headache, sweating, anxiety or fear of impending death, tremor, fatigue, nausea and vomiting, abdominal pain, and visual disturbances. These findings in combination with the hypertension, particularly if paroxysmal, point strongly to the appropriate diagnosis. Measurement of urinary catecholamines and their metabolites, principally metanephrine and VMA, are necessary to confirm it. Other diagnostic approaches are also available, such as a hypertensive response to provocative agents, a hypotensive response to adrenergic blockade, plasma assays of catecholamines, and others. Even when excess production of catecholamines has been established, the questions arise, is it caused by a neoplasm and where is it located? You recall that multiple neoplasms may be present or uncommonly there may be no neoplasm, only hyperplastic lesions in chromaffin tissues. Most tumors are larger than 2 cm and can be detected reliably in the CT scan. In some instances, however, resort must be made to intra-abdominal exploration. Finally, it should be recalled that, in 10 to 20% of cases, these neoplasms occur in familial syndromes and so may be accompanied by a variety of other endocrinopathies and systemic disorders.

NEUROBLASTOMA AND GANGLIONEUROMA

Neuroblastoma is one of the most common tumors of childhood and ranks along with Wilms' tumor, glioma, and leukemia as a principal form of cancer in the young. Approximately 80% of these neoplasms are found in children under the age of 5, 35% are found in those under 2, and only infrequently are they encountered in those over the age of 15. There is a striking correlation between the age of the patient and the prognosis.

Although the neuroblastoma may occur sporadically, there is evidence that at least some cases have a heredofamilial basis. In such cases the neoplasms may involve both adrenals or have multiple primary sites of origin. Transmission by an autosomal dominant gene has been proposed, with reports of several pairs of twins being affected and another family in which each of four siblings had a neuroblastoma.

MORPHOLOGY. Arising in neural crest cells, neuroblastomas are found in a variety of locations. The adrenal medulla or cells in the adjacent retroperitoneal tissues on the posterior abdominal wall account for 50 to 80% of neoplasms in most reported series. The second most common location is within the posterior mediastinum, usually in paravertebral sites. The remaining neoplasms occur in derivatives of the neural crest within the pelvis, in the cervical region, in the lower abdominal sympathetic chain, rarely within the posterior cranial fossa, or in other locations. **A closely related tumor in the retina is called a retinoblastoma.**

Macroscopically, the growths are lobular and soft in consistency and weigh between 80 and 150 gm. The cut surface is red-gray in color, and areas of hemorrhage and necrosis may be obvious as the tumor increases in size. Calcification is not infrequent, and this can help in radiologic localization.

Histologically, the cells are small and dark like lymphocytes and frequently are arranged in masses without any true pattern. In characteristic lesions, rosettes are formed where the tumor cells occupy the periphery and young nerve fibrils grow into the center of each rosette (Fig. 26–53). Careful search of any tumor will almost always reveal this type of structure.

Metastases develop rapidly and widely. In addition to local infiltration and lymph node metastases, there is a pronounced tendency to spread by the blood to liver, lungs, and bones. Profuse bony metastases, particularly to the skull and orbit, with exophthalmos is referred to clinically as **Hutchinson-type neuroblastoma.** Widespread dissemination throughout the bone marrow is another distinctive pattern of spread. Many putative cases of Ewing's tumor of

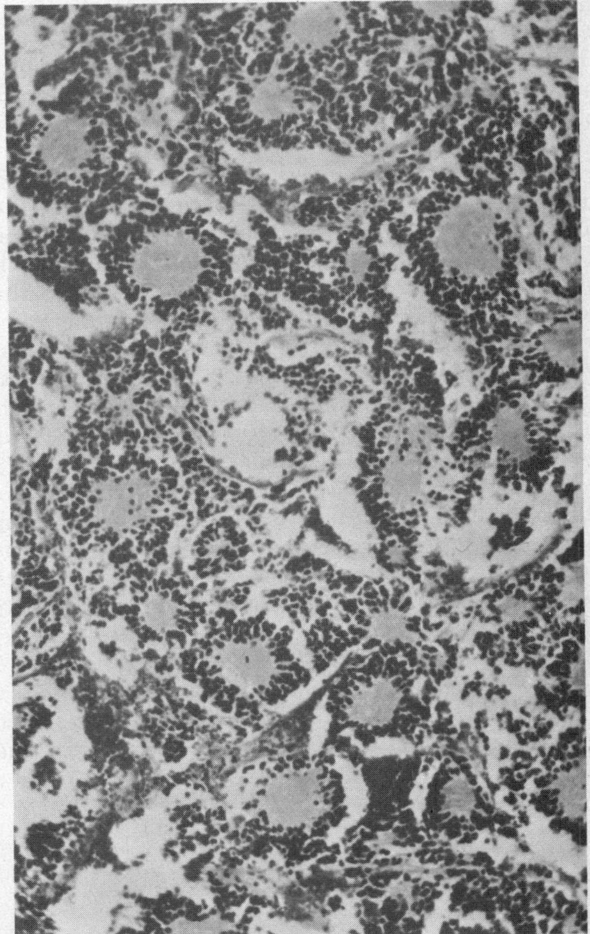

Figure 26–53. Neuroblastoma of adrenal, clearly demonstrating numerous rosettes.

bone represent metastases from an occult primary neuroblastoma. Massive metastasis to the liver is designated the **Pepper-type syndrome.**

Differentiation to varying levels is found in most neuroblastomas. The tumor may completely differentiate to a **ganglioneuroma** composed of a fibrous stromal background through which ganglion cells are scattered. All intermediate levels of differentiation between the pure neuroblastoma and the pure ganglioneuroma may be encountered, referred to as **ganglioneuroblastomas** (p. 1406).

CLINICAL COURSE. The manifestations of neuroblastomas are extremely varied and relate to two essential features, the rapid growth of the malignant neoplasm and its secretory products. Loss of energy and weight, pallor, abdominal protrusion, irregular fever, and generalized malaise are all probably related to rapid tumor growth and resorption of necrotic tumor products. Also, more than 90% of neuroblastomas elaborate catecholamines, principally norepinephrine. There is additional evidence that some tumors elaborate prostaglandins.[161] Thus, assays of catecholamine and prostaglandins' metabolites provide diagnostic screening technics as well as supportive diagnostic evidence. Metastases may be located in bizarre locations, such as in the orbit or scalp, subcutaneously, and elsewhere. Sometimes the appearance of these metastases precedes the identification of the primary neoplasm. Indeed, except for patients in whom the neoplasm is present at or before birth, metastatic dissemination is already present in approximately three-fourths of cases by the time diagnosis is made.[162]

The most intriguing features of these neoplasms are the well-documented instances of spontaneous regression. This occurs mostly in infants (with a median age of 3 months) having small primary tumors and possibly metastases to soft tissues, *but not to bones*. This pattern is categorized as Stage IV-S (special)[163] to differentiate it from instances also having bone metastases—Stage IV. Conceivably, immunologic influences induce the spontaneous regression.[165] One study points out that with Stage IV disease, but not with Stage IV-S, there are high serum ferritin levels and inhibition of T-cell E-rosette formation in vitro, indicating possibly impaired cell-mediated immunity in these individuals.[164] Sometimes the regression takes the form of disappearance of the primary and its metastases. In other instances the highly malignant neuroblastoma undergoes differentiation into a benign ganglioneuroma. In children above 1 year of age, spontaneous regression is rare.

When the neoplasm does not regress, the course of the disease is modified by the location of the lesion and its differentiation. Extra-adrenal neuroblastomas have a better outlook than adrenal neoplasms. The prognosis is also improved when ganglion cells are present in the lesion. Surgery, coupled with radiotherapy or chemotherapy, has yielded somewhat improved survival rates, but generally few children over the age of 1 with metastatic pure neuroblastomas live longer than a year.[166]

TUMORS OF CHEMORECEPTOR SYSTEM

The chemoreceptor system is represented principally by the carotid, vagal and, jugulotympanic bodies, although similar collections of cells have been demonstrated in other sites such as the paranasal or laryngeal regions. These collections of cells respond to variations in the blood oxygen and carbon dioxide tensions and may be concerned with the regulation of respiration. Tumors that arise from them are called chemodectomas or paragangliomas;[167] they resemble pheochromocytomas, described earlier (p. 1244).

Paragangliomas are rare, occur in both males and females, and are found mostly in persons between the ages of 30 and 60 years. They most often occur singly and sporadically, but may be familial and, in some cases, multiple. They can be of great clinical importance, because 10 to 50% of these tumors recur following resection and overall about 10% metastasize widely to cause death.[167]

Typically, these tumors range from 1 to 6 cm in diameter and are firm and tan-red. Despite encapsulation, well developed or scant, they are often densely adherent to adjacent vessels and difficult to excise. Histologically, most are composed of well-differentiated epithelioid cells disposed in small clusters (zellballen) or cords separated by prominent fibrovascular stroma. Distinctive within the cells in most tumors are dark neurosecretory granules when stained with silver impregnations (Grimelius). This feature casts these neoplasms into the category of APUDomas and, indeed, some have been shown to elaborate catecholamines. Sometimes the epithelioid cells are spindle shaped, producing a close resemblance to a glomus tumor. Mitoses are usually infrequent, but occasional tumors are overtly anaplastic and pleomorphic and contain numerous mitoses. Although most are benign, about 10% of those in the carotid body and as many as 50 to 60% of paragangliomas arising elsewhere recur following resection. The more obviously anaplastic lesions may disseminate widely and cause death.[168]

Thymus

NORMAL

Once an organ buried in obscurity within the mediastinum, the thymus has risen to a star role in cell-mediated immunity, as detailed in Chapter 5. Here our interest centers on the disorders of the gland itself.

The thymus is embryologically derived from the third and, inconstantly, the fourth pair of pharyngeal pouches, along with the lower pair of parathyroid glands. Not surprisingly, one or two parathyroids occasionally become enclosed within the thymic capsule, an aberrance that may plague the parathyroid surgeon. At birth it weighs 10 to 35 gm and continues to grow in size until puberty, when it achieves a maximum weight of 20 to 50 gm. Thereafter it undergoes progressive atrophy to little more than 5 to 15 gm in the elderly. This age involution is accompanied by replacement of the thymic parenchyma by fibrofatty tissue. The rate of thymic growth in the child and involution in the adult is extremely variable, and so it is difficult to determine weight appropriate for age, unless there is a marked discrepancy.

The fully-developed thymus is pyramidal shaped, encapsulated, and composed of two fused lobes. Fibrous extensions of the capsule divide each lobe into numerous lobules. The thymus basically consists of epithelial cells. These are admixed with a large number of T lymphocytes having OKT-6 markers of thymocytes, and occasional B cells and macrophages. Scattered so-called "myoid" cells are also present having many ultrastructural and antigenic similarities to skeletal muscle, which may bear on the pathogenesis of myasthenia gravis. In addition, other cell types are present in scant numbers, as pointed out in the discussion of tumors. The epithelial cells, which often have long extended reticular processes (not readily seen in usual sections), form a loose meshwork within the lobule. Ultrastructural studies of these cells reveal unmistakable evidence of their epithelial nature, such as desmosomes, cytoplasmic tonofilaments, and the many other organelles found in epithelial cells. The large spaces between the epithelial cells are filled with lymphocytes. The division of each lobule into a dark cortex and a lighter medulla is the consequence of a greater concentration of lymphocytes in the cortex as compared with the medulla.

Here and there within the medulla, *the epithelial cells are aggregated into concentric onionskin layers of keratinized cells, creating Hassall's corpuscles* (Fig. 26–54) Two special histologic features should be emphasized. Well-developed B-cell lymphoid follicles with germinal centers are on the whole rare in the normal thymus. When numerous and prominent, they must be construed as pathologic and, as will be seen, are associated with a number of extrathymic disorders, notably myasthenia gravis. Similarly, plasma cells are usually absent in the normal thymus and, when present, imply some inflammatory change.

There is no longer doubt that the thymus in its role as a central lymphoid organ in cell-mediated immunity is a secretory organ. Several factors have been described, each by an independent group of investigators, and variously named thymic humoral factor, thymosin, thymin, and thymopoietin. Whether these are truly distinctive is presently unclear, but without doubt one or more is necessary to maintain immunologic compe-

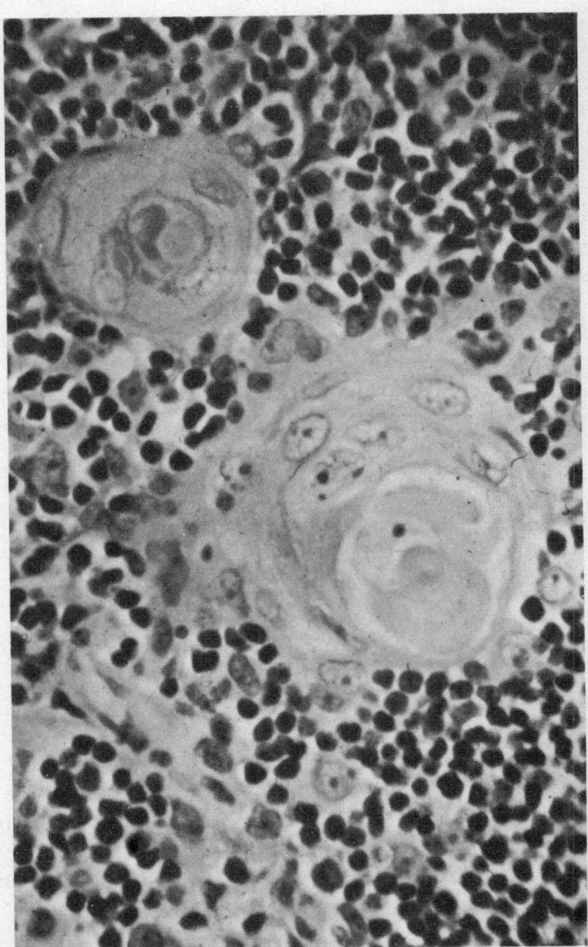

Figure 26–54. Hassall's corpuscles within normal thymus.

tence of peripheral T cells. Also, the thymus plays some role in the maintenance of tolerance and immune surveillance.

PATHOLOGY

Morphologic lesions in the thymus are associated with a diversity of conditions ranging from immunologic to hematologic to neoplastic. Fortunately, thymic lesions are limited in type and can be adequately encompassed within the following categories: (1) thymic agenesis and hypoplasia, (2) thymic hyperplasia, and (3) thymic neoplasia. The thymic changes associated with myasthenia gravis are dealt with on page 1310.

THYMIC AGENESIS AND HYPOPLASIA

Despite the difficulty in estimating thymic size normal for age, there can be no doubt that under certain clinical circumstances the thymus is abnormally small, either as a congenital defect or an acquired disorder. Congenital thymic agenesis or hypoplasia is encountered in neonates and infants having one of the following immunodeficiency states—reticular dysgenesis, combined immunodeficiency disease, ataxia telangiectasia, or the DiGeorge or Nezelof syndromes. In the DiGeorge syndrome there is concomitant agenesis of the parathyroid glands. The thymus in these conditions may be completely absent and represented by a fibrous pad, or sometimes is composed of scattered lymphocytes embedded within fibrous tissue. All these immunodeficiencies are marked by severe T-cell and variable B-cell defects.

Acquired hypoplasia is a normal consequence of aging but it may appear suddenly in the young as a result of severe stress, malnutrition, or irradiation or following the use of cytotoxic drugs or glucocorticoids. The histologic changes depend on the time elapsed since the insult. Early there are focal areas of cytolysis that may later be replaced by fibrosis. Undoubtedly, previous episodes of cytolysis are masked by subsequent regeneration, but some foci of fibrosis may persist.

THYMIC HYPERPLASIA

Thymic hyperplasia is exceedingly difficult to evaluate by the weight of the gland, because of the wide range of normal variation at every age level. *The most reliable criterion of hyperplasia is the appearance of lymphoid follicles within the thymus,* creating what is referred to as *thymic follicular hyperplasia.* Although true hyperplasia has been said to develop in the absence of follicle formation, the onus is on those who make such a diagnosis.

In follicular hyperplasia, the gland may be normal in weight but is more often slightly enlarged. Germinal centers are located principally in the medulla, resulting in compression and atrophy of the cortex. The lymphoid follicles are not different from those encountered in lymph nodes and contain both dendritic reticular cells and, not surprisingly, B lymphocytes.[169] Immunofluorescence generally discloses large amounts of immunoglobulins within the germinal centers.

Although follicular hyperplasia may occur in chronic inflammatory and immunologic states, it is most frequently encountered in myasthenia gravis. In this condition, autoantibodies to acetylcholine receptors at neuromuscular junctions impair transmission of motor impulses, and it is thought that in some cases thymic hyperplasia with the formation of activated lymphoid follicles of B cells participates in the formation of the autoantibodies. More is said on this subject on page 1311. Follicular thymic hyperplasia is not exclusive to myasthenia gravis, and is also found in Graves' disease, Addison's disease, systemic lupus erythematosus, scleroderma, and rheumatoid arthritis, all having autoimmune origins, and in a variety of liver diseases less clearly immunologic in origin. The relationship between the thymic changes and these disorders is unclear. Uncommonly, germinal centers are found in the thymic glands of patients who have died of apparently unrelated disease.

TUMORS

In the past, there has been a practice of referring to all tumors primary in the thymus as thymomas. As pointed out, the basic cell type in the thymus is the epithelial cell; the rich component of lymphocytes is viewed as a migratory population coming and going. Thus, *the term thymoma is now restricted to neoplasms of thymic epithelial cells, regardless of the abundance or scarcity of the lymphoid component.* Both non-Hodgkin's lymphomas and Hodgkin's disease may also arise in the thymus. The latter was once called a granulomatous thymoma, but now is recognized as Hodgkin's disease arising in the thymus. Similarly, there are many other cell types scattered through the thymus, e.g., argentaffin cells, fibroblasts, myoid cells, vascular elements, and sometimes sequestered rests of germ cells. A tumor composed of argentaffin cells is thus termed a thymic carcinoid or argentaffinoma. Germ cell tumors such as teratoma, choriocarcinoma, or germinoma may also be located within the thymus. Despite the diversity of neoplasms that may arise in the thymus, only those having a component of thymic epithelial cells are called thymomas.

THYMOMAS

True thymomas are rare but nonetheless are one of the most common mediastinal neoplasms, particularly those in the anterosuperior mediastinum. They are intriguing tumors because of poorly understood but well-defined associations with a number of systemic disorders, notably myasthenia gravis, hematologic cytopenias, hypogammaglobulinemia, various collagen-vascular diseases, and nonthymic cancers, to mention only the more frequent. Most thymomas (about 90%) are benign and are composed of epithelial cells having a rich or scant lymphocytic infiltration. The lymphocytes are not neoplastic and possess markers of normal thymocytes (OKT-6 antigens); some observations suggest that the more of these that are present, the more likely it is that the tumor will follow a benign course.[170] About 10% of thymomas are malignant. Most of these cancers have little or no cytologic atypia, and so the determination of malignancy rests entirely on demonstration of invasion beyond the capsule or, more certainly, on the presence of lymphatic or hematogenous spread, admittedly uncommon.[169] *Rarities are cytologically malignant tumors segregated from malignant thymomas by being called thymic carcinomas. These display a variety of epithelial differentiations.* It is thus possible to divide all primary thymic neoplasms as shown in Table 26–9.

Thymic carcinomas, like all cancers, have the potential of aggressive local spread and metastasis. They have been well reviewed recently and will not be further discussed because of their great rarity.[171] The following comments, therefore, are largely directed to benign thymomas and the features that suggest aggressive behavior.

MORPHOLOGY. Whatever their histology, all thymomas are gray, yellow, or tan, lobulated, apparently encapsulated masses ranging in size from 1 to 20 cm in greatest diameter. They vary from soft to firm and frequently have focal areas of hemorrhage. Cysts are often present in the larger lesions, sometimes many centimeters in diameter. As pointed out, most are encapsulated, but uncommonly there is invasion beyond the capsule and, even more uncommonly, extension to regional lymph nodes and more widely to lungs, liver, bone, or other sites.

The parenchymatous epithelial component of benign thymomas displays a range of patterns. In most neoplasms the epithelial cells resemble those of the normal cortex, having poorly defined cytoplasmic outlines and visible mostly as large, pale, vesicular nuclei. Their epithelial nature can be documented by the identification of desmosomes and tonofilaments with the electron microscope. The next most frequent variant has oval- to spindle-shaped epithelial cells. Uncommonly, the cells assume a sarcomatoid appearance, readily mistaken for some form of mesenchymal neoplasm. The term "spindle-cell thymoma" is sometimes applied to this morphologic pattern; it tends to be associated with hypogammaglobulinemia and red cell aplasia but not with myasthenia gravis.[172] Other epithelial patterns include reticular and squamoid differentiation. In the latter, there may be formation of Hassall's corpuscles, but they are not frequent.

All epithelial variants have a rich or scant lymphocytic infiltrate of T cells (Figs. 26–55 and 26–56). The lymphocytes appear to be activated and are therefore larger than T cells in the peripheral circulation, have vesicular large nuclei, prominent nucleoli, and sometimes pyroninophilic cytoplasm, meriting the designation "immunoblasts." The abundance of mitotic figures in these cells suggests some form of mitogenic stimulus. Neoplasms having a great many lymphocytes are readily mistaken histologically for non-Hodgkin's lymphoma. Careful scrutiny, however, will disclose epithelial cells or, in a few cases, Hassall's corpuscles indicative of a thymomatous origin.

As noted, malignant thymomas, as distinct from benign thymomas and thymic carcinomas, can be differentiated only by penetration and extension beyond the fibrous capsule or more distant spread.

Table 26–9. CLASSIFICATION OF THYMOMAS

I Benign thymoma (with abundant or scant lymphocytic infiltration)

II Malignant thymoma (with little or no cytologic atypia)
  a. Locally invasive (majority)
  b. With dissemination (rare)

III Thymic carcinoma (with overt cytologic atypia)
  a. Mixed undifferentiated–squamous cell
  b. Basaloid
  c. Mucoepidermoid
  d. Clear cell
  e. Sarcomatoid
  f. Others

CLINICAL COURSE. The mean age of patients with thymomas is 50 years; in children they are rare but have a poor prognosis. Males and females are affected equally often, as are whites and blacks.[173] The clinical presentation is extremely varied, but can be categorized into three basic patterns: (1) neoplasms that are entirely asymptomatic and are discovered incidentally on chest

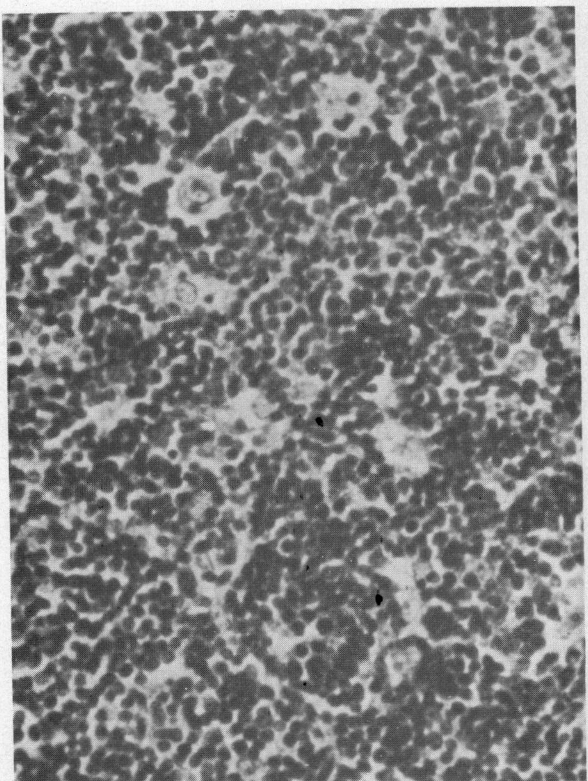

Figure 26–55. Low-power view of a predominantly lymphocytic thymoma.

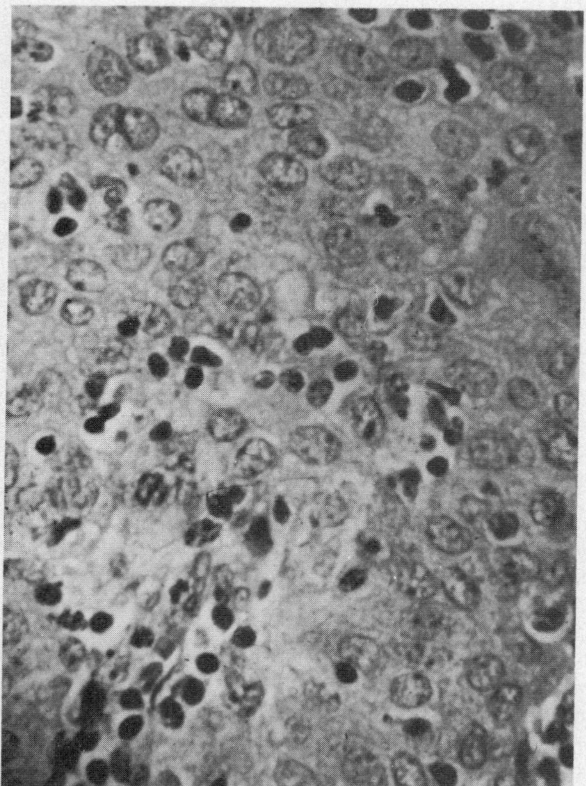

Figure 26–56. Microscopic detail of a predominantly epithelial thymoma.

radiography or at autopsy; (2) neoplasms that cause local pressure effects such as cough, dyspnea, difficulty in swallowing, or signs of vena caval compression; and (3) neoplasms associated with systemic disorders. There is no consensus in the literature on the frequency of each of these three presentations, but the following ranges can be offered. About 10 to 50% of patients are asymptomatic, 10 to 30% have local signs and symptoms, and 30 to 40% have an associated disease. The broad range of associated systemic diseases reported raises the questions how many are coincidental and how many are causally related to the thymic lesion? Only the major associations are presented in Table 26–10.[174]

Most of these associated systemic diseases are probably of autoimmune origin. Intriguing speculations can be made as to why thymic tumors should predispose to such conditions. Tumorous destruction of the thymus might lead to a loss of some T-cell function responsible for immunologic surveillance or maintenance of self-tolerance. Loss of surveillance could also explain the increased incidence of cancer in these individuals. In many instances, however, all normal thymic tissue is not destroyed by the neoplasm. More attractive is the notion of the development, in either the tumors or the nontumorous thymic tissue, of self-reactive or "forbidden" clones. Indeed, thymic follicular hyperplasia is sometimes present in the residual thymic tissue, calling into question the role of the neoplasm. Much is uncertain, underscored by the frequent lack of improvement in the associated disorder following removal of the neoplasm.

Table 26–10. THYMOMAS AND ASSOCIATED DISEASES

Disease	% of Patients with Thymoma
Myasthenia gravis	44
Cytopenias (pure red cell aplasia, thrombocytopenia, neutropenia, pancytopenia)	21
Cancer (nonthymic)	17
Hypogammaglobulinemia	6
Polymyositis	5
Systemic lupus erythematosus	2
Others: thyroiditis, rheumatoid arthritis, chronic ulcerative colitis, regional enteritis, dermatomyositis, scleroderma, pernicious anemia, various endocrine disorders, etc.	Rare

The prognosis in patients with thymic neoplasms is directly related to the aggressiveness of the lesion and to the presence and nature of an associated systemic disease. The following generalizations can be made. Benign thymomas are slow-growing neoplasms. When well encapsulated and noninvasive, they can be completely excised and cured, but recurrence (still benign) rarely follows. In the small minority of malignant thymomas or thymic carcinomas with spread to the pleura or elsewhere, despite surgical resection and postoperative irradiation, over half may be expected to die of their neoplasm within five to ten years. A concomitant systemic disease has a strong adverse effect; about two-thirds of such individuals followed for three to five years died, most often of an uncontrolled infection, sometimes of another complication related to the associated disease.[175]

Pineal Gland

NORMAL

The rarity of clinically significant lesions (only tumors) justifies considerable brevity in the consideration of the pineal gland. It is a minute, pinecone-shaped organ—hence its name—weighing 100 to 180 mg, lying between the superior colliculi at the base of the brain. It is composed of a loose, neuroglial stroma enclosing nests of large, epithelial-appearing pineocytes. Silver impregnations reveal that these cells have long, slender processes reminiscent of primitive neuronal precursors. Although a large number of neurotransmitter substances such as dopamine, octopamine, serotonin, and others can be extracted from the pineal, the only abundant biologically active substance secreted by it is melatonin. The functions of melatonin in humans are poorly understood, but it can be found in the blood, cerebrospinal fluid, and urine. The levels of this hormone have a diurnal rhythm significantly higher during the night than in the day. Administration of melatonin to humans induces sleepiness, and so this secretory product may play some role in maintaining the awake-asleep rhythm. Despite anecdotal observations to the contrary, large pathology texts do not stimulate melatonin secretion! In addition, melatonin is believed to suppress, at least in animals, the release of gonadotropic hormones, and so it may be more than coincidental that pineal tumors that destroy the gland cause precocious puberty almost exclusively in males. However, injury to the immediately adjacent hypothalamus may simultaneously destroy structures normally involved in pubertal development.

Calcification of the pineal occurs with age. It often first becomes visible at the time of puberty, but calcification has also been seen in infants. There appears to be no correlation between the level of calcification and pineal function.[176]

PATHOLOGY

The only lesions of importance in this gland are tumors, accounting for less than 1% of brain neoplasms. Most (50 to 70%) arise from embryonic germ cells sequestered in the midline pineal. As with testicular tumors arising in germ cells, they most commonly take the form of so-called *germinomas* replicating the testicular seminoma (p. 1092). Other lines of germ-cell differentiation include embryonal carcinomas; choriocarcinomas; mixtures of germinoma, embryonal carcinoma and choriocarcinoma; and, uncommonly, typical teratomas (usually benign).[177] Whether to characterize these germ-cell neoplasms as pinealomas is still a subject of debate. Thought today favors the restriction of the term to neoplasms arising from the parenchymal and stromal elements of the pineal gland itself.

PINEALOMAS

These neoplasms are divided into two categories, pineoblastomas and pineocytomas, based on their level of differentiation, which in turn correlates with their neoplastic aggressiveness.

Pineoblastomas are encountered mostly in young people and appear as soft, friable, gray masses punctuated with areas of hemorrhage and necrosis. They typically invade surrounding structures, i.e., hypothalamus, midbrain, and lumen of the third ventricle. Histologically, they are composed of masses of pleomorphic cells two to four times the diameter of an erythrocyte. Large hyperchromatic nuclei appear to occupy almost the entire cell, and mitoses are frequent. The cytology is that of the medulloblastoma-neuroblastoma (p. 1406) of the brain. Large, poorly formed rosettes are sometimes present in the pineoblastoma, reminiscent of these "first cousins" in the brain. A further similarity is the tendency of pineoblastomas to spread via the cerebrospinal fluid. As might be expected the enlarging mass may compress the aqueduct of Sylvius, giving rise to internal hydrocephalus and all its consequences. Survival beyond one to two years is rare.

In contrast, *pineocytomas* occur mostly in adults and are much slower growing than the pineoblastomas. They tend to be well-circumscribed, gray, or hemorrhagic masses that compress but do not infiltrate surrounding structures. *Histologically, these neoplasms exhibit divergent glial and neuronal differentiation.* On the one hand, the neoplasm may be largely astrocytomatous (p. 1401). On the other hand, it may be composed largely of neuronal precursor cells, which are uniform round cells having darkly staining, round-to-oval, fairly regular nuclei. Particularly distinctive of the pineocytoma is the creation of large rosettes rimmed by rows of pineocytes. The centers of these rosettes are filled with eosinophilic cytoplasmic material representing tumor-cell processes. These cells are set against a background of thin, fibrovascular, anastomosing septa that divide the tumor into lobular masses. Occasional mitotic figures and giant cells are present.[178]

In addition to the monomorphic pineocytomas composed largely of one line of differentiation, there are many instances in which mixed patterns are encountered, in part astrocytic, in part pineocytomatous sometimes having neuronal-type cells. Such neoplasms are highly reminiscent of the ganglioglioma (p. 1406).

The clinical course of patients with pineocytomas is prolonged, averaging seven years. The manifestations are the consequence of its compressive effects and consist of visual disturbances, headache, mental deterioration, and sometimes dementia-like behavior. Located where they are, it is understandable that successful excision is at best very difficult.

---

1. Besser, G. M.: The hypothalamus and pituitary. Clin. Endocrinol. *6*:1, 1977.
2. Pelletier, G., et al.: Identification of human anterior pituitary cells by immunoelectron microscopy. J. Clin. Endocrinol. Metab. *46*:534, 1978.
3. Daughaday, W. H.: The adenohypophysis. *In* Williams, R. H. (ed.): Textbook of Endocrinology. 6th ed. Philadelphia, W. B. Saunders Co., 1981, pp. 73–116.
4. Cook, D. M.: Pituitary tumors—current concepts of diagnosis and therapy. West J. Med. *133*:189, 1980.
5. Saeger, W., and Ludecke, D. K.: Pituitary adenomas with hyperfunction of TSH. Virchows. Arch. [Pathol. Anat.] *394*:255, 1982.
6. Kovacs, K., et al.: Pituitary adenomas. Pathol. Annu. *12*:341, 1977.
7. Adelman, L. S.: The pathology of pituitary adenomas. *In* Post, K. D., et al. (eds.): The Pituitary Adenoma. New York, Plenum Medical Book Co., 1980, p. 47.
8. Burrow, G. N., et al.: Microadenomas of the pituitary and abnormal sellar tomograms in an unselected autopsy series. N. Engl. J. Med. *304*:156, 1981.
9. McCarty, K. S., Jr., et al.: Pituitary pathology associated with abnormalities of prolactin secretion. Clin. Obstet. Gynecol. *23*:367, 1980.
10. Editorial: Prolactinomas: Bromocriptine rules OK? Lancet *1*:430, 1982.
11. Sung, D. I.: Suprasellar tumors in children. A review of clinical manifestations and managements. Cancer *50*:1420, 1982.
12. Jialal, I., et al.: Hypopituitarism. A 3-year study. S. Afr. Med. J. *59*:590, 1981.
13. Landolt, A. M., and Oswald, U. W.: Histology and ultrastructure of an oncocytic adenoma of the human pituitary. Cancer *31*:1099, 1973.
14. Sheehan, H. L.: Post partum necrosis of the anterior pituitary. J. Pathol. Bacteriol. *45*:189, 1937.
15. McKay, D. G., et al.: The pathologic anatomy of eclampsia, bilateral cortical necrosis, pituitary necrosis, and other fatal complications of pregnancy and its possible relationship to the generalized Shwartzman phenomenon. Am. J. Obstet. Gynecol. *66*:507, 1953.
16. Grimes, H. G., and Brooks, M. H.: Pregnancy in Sheehan's syndrome. Report of a case and review. Obstet. Gynecol. Surv. *35*:481, 1980.
17. Sachdev, Y., et al.: The empty sella syndrome. Postgrad. Med. J. *52*:703, 1976.
18. Spaziante, R.: The empty sella. Surg. Neurol. *16*:418, 1981.
19. Russell, D. S., and Rubinstein, L. J.: Pathology of Tumors of the Nervous System. 3rd ed. Baltimore, Williams and Wilkins. 1971, p. 233.
20. Johannesen, J. V., et al.: The fine structure of human thyroid cancer. Hum. Pathol. *9*:385, 1978.
21. Rapoport, B., and DeGroot, L. J.: Current concepts of thyroid physiology. Semin. Nucl. Med. *1*:265, 1971.
22. Davies, A. G.: Thyroid physiology. Br. Med. J. *2*:206, 1972.
23. Stein, O., and Gross, J.: Metabolismn of 125-I in the thyroid gland studied with electron microscopic radioautography. Endocrinology *75*:787, 1964.
24. Seljelid, R.: Endocytosis of thyroglobulin and the release of thyroid hormone. Scand. J. Clin. Lab. Invest. (Suppl.) *22*:106, 1968.
25. Sterling, K.: Thyroid hormone action at the cell. N. Engl. J. Med. *300*:117, 173, 1979.
26. Oppenheimer, J. H.: Thyroid hormone action at the cellular level. Science *203*:971, 1979.
27. Baldwin, D. B., and Rowett, D.: Incidence of thyroid disorders in Connecticut. J.A.M.A. *239*:742, 1978.
28. Tunbridge, W. M. G., et al.: The spectrum of thyroid disease in a community: the Whickham survey. Clin. Endocrinol. *7*:481, 1977.
29. Skelton, C. L.: The heart and hyperthyroidism. N. Engl. J. Med. *307*:1206, 1982.
30. Chizzonite, R. A., et al.: Isolation and characterization of two molecular variants of myosin heavy chain from rabbit ventricle: Change in their content during normal growth and after treatment with thyroid hormone. J. Biol. Chem. *257*:2056, 1982.
31. Werner, S. C.: Toxic goiter. *In* Werner, S. C., and Ingbar, S. H. (eds.): The Thyroid. 4th ed. Hagerstown, MD, Harper & Row, 1978, p. 591.
32. Amir, S. M., et al.: In vitro responses to crude and purified hCG in human thyroid membranes. J. Clin. Endocrinol. Metab. *51*:51, 1980.
33. Emerson, C. H., and Utiger, R. D.: Hyperthyroidism and excessive thyrotropin secretion. N. Engl. J. Med. *287*:328, 1972.
34. Dorfman, S. G.: Hyperthyroidism, usual and unusual causes. Arch. Intern. Med. *137*:995, 1977.
35. Doniach, D.: Hashimoto's thyroiditis and primary myxoedema viewed as separate entities. Eur. J. Clin. Invest. *11*:245, 1981.
36. Drexhage, H. A., et al.: Thyroid growth–blocking antibodies in primary myxedema. Nature *289*:594, 1981.
37. Hamilton, W.: Endemic cretinism. Dev. Med. Child. Neurol. *18*:386, 1976.
38. Hamilton, W.: Sporadic cretinism. Dev. Med. Child. Neurol. *18*:384, 1976.
39. Hurley, J. R.: Thyroiditis. DM *24*:3, 1977.
40. Volpe, R.: The pathology of thyroiditis. Hum. Pathol. *9*:429, 1978.
41. LiVolsi, V. A.: Chronic thyroiditis. Pathologic Aspects. *In* LiVolsi, V. A., and LoGerfo, P. (eds.): Thyroiditis. Boca Raton, CRC Press, 1981.
42. Strakosch, C. R., et al.: Immunology of autoimmune thyroid disease. N. Engl. J. Med. *307*:1499, 1982.
43. Volpe, R.: Autoimmunity in the endocrine system. Monogr. Endocrinol. *20*:19, 1981.
44. Drexhage, H. A., et al.: Evidence for thyroid-growth–stimulating immunoglobulins in some goitrous thyroid diseases. Lancet *2*:287, 1980.
45. Rose, N. R., et al.: T-cell regulation in autoimmune thyroiditis. Immunol. Rev. *55*:299, 1981.
46. Friedman, N. B.: Cellular involution in the thyroid gland: Significance of the Hürthle cells in myxedema, exhaustion atrophy, Hashimoto's disease and the reactions to irradiation, thiouracil therapy and subtotal resection. J. Clin. Endocrinol. Metabl. *9*:874, 1949.
47. Katz, S. M., and Vickery, A. L.: The fibrosing variant of Hashimoto's thyroiditis. Hum. Pathol. *5*:161, 1974.
48. Crile, G., Jr.: Struma lymphomatosa and carcinoma of the thyroid. Surg. Gynecol. Obstet. *147*:350, 1978.
49. De Pauw, B. E., and De Rooy, H. A. M.: De Quervain's subacute thyroiditis. Neth. J. Med. *18*:70, 1975.
50. Greene, J. N.: Subacute thyroiditis. Am. J. Med. *51*:97, 1971.
51. Volpe, R.: Subacute thyroiditis. *In* Soto, R. J., et al. (eds.): Progress in Clinical and Biological Research. New York, Alan R. Liss, 1981, p. 115.
52. Volpe, R.: Subacute (de Quervain's) thyroiditis. Clin. Endocrinol. Metab. *8*:81, 1979.
53. Strakosch, C. R., et al.: Thyroid-stimulating antibodies in patients with subacute thyroiditis. J. Clin. Endocrinol. Metab. *46*:345, 1978.
54. Dorfman, S. G., et al.: Painless thyroiditis and transient hyperthyroidism without goiter. Ann. Intern. Med. *86*:24, 1977.
55. Katsikas, D., et al.: Riedel's thyroiditis. Br. J. Surg. *63*:929, 1976.
56. Meyer, S., and Hausman, R.: Occlusive phlebitis in multifocal fibrosclerosis. Am. J. Clin. Pathol. *65*:274, 1976.
57. Gamblin, G. T., et al.: Prevalence of increased intraocular pressure in Grave's disease—evidence of frequent subclinical ophthalmopathy. N. Engl. J. Med. *308*:420, 1983.
58. Farid, N. R., and Bear, J. C.: The human major histocompatibility complex and endocrine disease. Endocrine Rev. *2*:50, 1981.
59. Smyth, P. P. A., et al.: The prevalence of thyroid-stimulating antibodies in goitrous disease assessed by cytochemical section bioassay. J. Clin. Endocrinol. Metab. *54*:357, 1982.
60. Monjan, A. A., and Collector, M. I.: Stress-induced modulation of the immune response. Science *196*:307, 1977.
61. Aoki, N., et al.: Studies on suppressor cell function in thyroid diseases. J. Clin. Endocrinol. Metab. *48*:803, 1979.
62. Kodama, K., et al.: Demonstration of a circulating autoantibody against a soluble I-muscle antigen in Graves' ophthalmopathy. Lancet *2*:1353, 1982.
63. Editorial: Autoimmune endocrine exophthalmos. Lancet *2*:1378, 1982.
64. Gorman, C.: Ophthalmopathy of Graves' disease. N. Engl. J. Med. *308*:453, 1983.
65. Clements, F. W.: Endemic goitre. W.H.O. Mongr. Ser. *62*:83, 1976.
66. Editorial: Dietary goitrogens. Lancet *1*:394, 1982.
67. Delange, F., et al.: Nutritional factors involved in the goitrogenic action of cassava. Ottawa Int. Develop. Res. Ctr., 1982.
68. Refetoff, S., and Selenkow, H. A.: Familial thyroxine-binding globulin deficiency in a patient with Turner's syndrome (XO). N. Engl. J. Med. *278*:1081, 1968.
69. Beierwaltes, W. H., et al.: Hereditary increase in the thyroxin-binding sites in the serum alpha globulin. Trans. Assoc. Am. Physicians *74*:170, 1961.
70. Zonana, J., and Rimoin, D. L.: Genetic disorders of the thyroid gland. Med. Clin. North Am. *59*:1263, 1975.
71. Studer, H., and Ramelli, F.: Simple goiter and its variants: Euthyroid and hyperthyroid multinodular goiters. Endocrine Rev. *3*:40, 1982.
72. Ramelli, F., et al.: Pathogenesis of thyroid nodules in multinodular goiter. Am. J. Pathol. *109*:215, 1982.

73. Taylor, S.: Sporadic nontoxic goiter. *In* Werner, S. C., and Ingbar, S. H. (eds.): The Thyroid. A Fundamental and Clinical Text. 4th ed. Hagerstown, MD, Harper & Row, 1978, p. 505.
74. Van Herle, A. J., and Uller, R. P.: Thyroid cancer classification. Clinical features, diagnosis and therapy. Pharmacol. Ther. 2:215, 1977.
75. Klonoff, D. C., and Greenspan, F. S.: The thyroid nodule. Adv. Intern. Med. *27*:101, 1982.
76. Vander, J. B., et al.: The significance of nontoxic thyroid nodules. Final report of a 15-year study of the incidence of thyroid malignancy. Ann. Intern. Med. *69*:537, 1968.
77. DeGroot, L. J.: Thyroid carcinoma. Med. Clin. North Am. *59*:1233, 1975.
78. Wang, C. A., et al.: The role of needle biopsy in evaluating solitary cold thyroid nodules. Proc. 7th Intl. Thyroid Conf. Thyroid Research. Excerpta Med. Int. Serv. *378*:568, 1975.
79. Meissner, W. A.: Diseases of the thyroid. *In* Werner, S. C., and Ingbar, S. H. (eds.): The Thyroid. A Fundamental and Clinical Text. 4th ed. Hagerstown, MD, Harper & Row, 1978, p. 444.
80. Roudebush, C. P., et al.: Natural history of radiation-associated thyroid cancer. Arch. Intern. Med. *138*:1631, 1978.
81. Refetoff, S., et al.: Continuing occurrence of thyroid carcinoma after irradiation to the neck in infancy and childhood. N. Engl. J. Med. *292*:171, 1975.
82. Sampson, R. J., et al.: Thyroid carcinoma in Hiroshima and Nagasaki. J.A.M.A. *209*:65, 1969.
83. Editorial: The worst nuclear power plant accident yet. Lancet *1*:909, 1979.
84. Rall, J. E.: The effects of radiation on the thyroid gland. A quantitative analysis. *In* Soto, R. J., et al. (eds.): Physiopathology of Endocrine Diseases and Mechanisms of Hormone Action. New York, Allen R. Liss, 1981, p. 29.
85. LiVolsi, V. A., and Merino, M. J.: Histopathologic differential diagnosis of the thyroid. Pathol. Annu. *2*:357, 1981.
86. Frauenhoffer, C. M., et al.: Thyroid carcinoma. A clinical and pathologic study of 125 cases. Cancer *43*:2414, 1979.
87. Selzer, G., et al.: Primary malignant tumors of the thyroid gland. Cancer *40*:1501, 1977.
88. Chen, K. T. K., and Rosai, J.: Follicular variant of thyroid papillary carcinoma. A clinicopathologic study of six cases. Am. J. Surg. Pathol. *1*:123, 1977.
89. Tscholl-Ducommun, J., and Hedinger, C. E.: Papillary thyroid carcinomas: Morphology and prognosis. Virchows Arch. [Pathol. Anat.] *396*:19, 1982.
90. Franssila, K.: Is the differentiation between papillary and follicular carcinoma valid? Cancer *32*:853, 1973.
91. Meissner, W. A.: Follicular carcinoma of the thyroid. Am. J. Surg. Pathol. *1*:171, 1977.
92. Hazard, J. B.: The C cells (parafollicular cells) of the thyroid gland and medullary thyroid carcinoma. Am. J. Pathol. *88*:213, 1977.
93. Editorial: Sipple families. Lancet *1*:939, 1977.
94. Brown, J. S., and Steiner, A. L.: Medullary thyroid carcinoma and the syndromes of multiple endocrine adenomas. DM *28*:1, 1982.
95. Deftos, L. F.: Radioimmunoassay for calcitonin in medullary thyroid carcinoma. J.A.M.A. *227*:403, 1974.
96. DeLellis, R. A., and Balogh, K.: Histochemical characteristics of parafollicular cells in medullary carcinoma. Am. J. Pathol. *72*:119, 1973.
97. DeLellis, R. A., et al.: Adrenal medullary hyperplasia. Am. J. Pathol. *83*:177, 1976.
98. Block, M. A., et al.: Clinical characteristics distinguishing hereditary from sporadic medullary thyroid carcinoma. Treatment implications. Arch. Surg. *115*:142, 1980.
99. Burke, J. S., et al.: Malignant lymphomas of the thyroid, a clinicopathologic study of 35 patients including ultrastructural observations. Cancer *39*:1587, 1977.
100. Kapadia, S. B., et al.: Malignant lymphoma of the thyroid gland: A clinicopathologic study. Head Neck Surg. *4*:270, 1982.
101. Saharia, P. C.: Carcinoma arising in thyroglossal duct remnant: Case reports and review of the literature. Br. J. Cancer *62*:689, 1975.
102. Woolner, L. B., et al.: Classification and prognosis of thyroid carcinoma. Am. J. Surg. *102*:354, 1961.
103. Dufour, D. R., et al.: The normal parathyroid revisited. Hum. Pathol. *13*:717, 1982.
104. Martin, K. J.: The peripheral metabolism of parathyroid hormone. N. Engl. J. Med. *301*:1092, 1979.
105. Raisz, L. G., and Kream, B. E.: Regulation of bone formation. N. Engl. J. Med. *309*:29, 83, 1983.
106. Wells, S. A., Jr., et al.: Primary hyperparathyroidism. Curr. Probl. Surg. *17*:398, 1980.
107. Mallette, L. E., et al.: Primary hyperparathyroidism: Clinical and biochemical features. Medicine *53*:127, 1974.
108. Heath, H., III, et al.: Primary hyperparathyroidism. Incidence, morbidity, and potential economic impact in a community. N. Engl. J. Med. *302*:189, 1980.
109. Coffey, R. J., et al.: The surgical treatment of primary hyperparathyroidism: A 20-year experience. Ann. Surg. *185*:518, 1977.
110. Sharp, C. F., Jr., et al.: Abnormal bone and parathyroid histology in carcinoma patients with pseudohyperparathyroidism. Cancer *49*:1449, 1982.
111. Thompson, N. W., et al.: The anatomy of primary hyperparathyroidism. Surgery *92*:814, 1982.
112. Fialkow, P. J., et al.: Multicellular origin of parathyroid "adenomas." N. Engl. J. Med. *297*:696, 1977.
113. Kay, S.: The abnormal parathyroid. Hum. Pathol. *7*:127, 1976.
114. Nilsson, O.: Studies on the ultrastructure of the human parathyroid glands in various pathological conditions. Acta Pathol. Microbiol. Scand. [A] *263*(Suppl.):5, 1977.
115. Elliott, R. L., and Arhelger, R. B.: Fine structure of parathyroid adenomas. Arch. Pathol. *81*:200, 1966.
116. Shane, E., and Bilezikian, J. P.: Parathyroid carcinoma: A review of 62 patients. Endocrine Rev. *3*:218, 1982.
117. Schantz, A., and Castleman, B.: Parathyroid cancer, a study of 70 cases. Cancer *31*:600, 1973.
118. Castleman, B., et al.: Parathyroid hyperplasia in primary hyperparathyroidism. A review of 85 cases. Cancer *38*:1668, 1976.
119. Roth, S. I.: The ultrastructure of primary water cell hyperplasia of the parathyroid gland. Am. J. Pathol. *61*:233, 1970.
120. Daneman, D., et al.: Hypoparathyroidism and pseudohypoparathyroidism in childhood. Clin. Endocrinol. Metab. *11*:211, 1982.
121. Neufeld, M., et al.: Two types of autoimmune Addison's disease associated with polyglandular autoimmune (PGA) syndromes. Medicine *60*:335, 1981.
122. Arulanantham, K., et al.: Evidence for defective immunoregulation in the syndrome of familial candidiasis endocrinopathy. N. Engl. J. Med. *300*:164, 1979.
123. Neelon, F. A.: Adrenal physiology and pharmacology. Urol. Clin. North Am. *4*:179, 1977.
124. Eipper, B. A., and Mains, R. E.: Structure and biosynthesis of proadenocorticotropin/endorphin and related peptides. Endocrine Rev. *1*:1, 1980.
125. Lindgren, S.: Congenital primary adrenal hypoplasia. Acta Pathol. Microbiol. Scand. *70*:541, 1967.
126. Maisey, M. N., and Lessof, M. H.: Addison's disease: A clinical study. Guy's Hosp. Rep. *118*:363, 1969.
127. Williams, G. H.: The adrenal manifestations of systemic diseases. Clin. Endocrinol. Metab. *8*:527, 1979.
128. Bohm, N.: Adrenal cutaneous and myocardial lesions in fulminating endotoxinemia. Pathol. Res. Pract. *174*:92, 1982.
129. Ross, E. J., et al.: Cushing's syndrome: Diagnostic criteria. Q. J. Med. *35*:149, 1966.
130. Gold, E. M.: The Cushing's syndromes: Changing view of diagnosis and treatment. Ann. Intern. Med. *90*:829, 1979.
131. Cushing, H.: The basophil adenomas of the pituitary body and their clinical manifestations (pituitary basophilism). Bull. Johns Hopkins Hosp. *50*:137, 1932.
132. Krieger, D. T.: The central nervous system and Cushing's disease. Med. Clin. North Am. *62*:261, 1978.
133. Fehm, H. L., and Voigt, K. H.: Pathophysiology of Cushing's disease. Pathobiol. Annu. *9*:225, 1979.
134. Imura, H., et al.: Studies on ectopic ACTH-producing tumors. II. Clinical and biochemical features of 30 cases. Cancer *35*:1430, 1975.
135. Gewirtz, G., and Yalow, R. S.: Ectopic ACTH production in carcinoma of the lung. J. Clin. Invest. *53*:1022, 1974.
136. Felix, I. A., et al.: Massive Crooke's hyalinization in corticotroph cell adenomas of the human pituitary. A histological, immunocytological, and electron microscopic study of three cases. Acta Neurochirurg *58*:235, 1981.
137. DeCicco, F. A., et al.: Fine structure of Crooke's hyaline change in the human pituitary gland. Arch. Pathol. *94*:65, 1972.
138. Tyrrell, J. B., et al.: Cushing's disease. Selective trans-sphenoidal resection of pituitary microadenomas. N. Engl. J. Med. *298*:753, 1978.
139. Hashida, Y., et al.: Ultrastructure of the adrenal cortex in Cushing's disease in children. Hum. Pathol. *1*:595, 1970.
140. Kano, K., and Sato, S.: Fine structure of adrenal adenomata causing Cushing's syndrome. Virchows Arch. [Pathol. Anat.] *374*:157, 1977.
141. Mitschke, H., and Saeger, W.: Ultrastructural pathology of the adrenal glands in Cushing's syndrome. Curr. Top. Pathol. *60*:113, 1975.
142. Editorial: Bartter's syndrome. Lancet *2*:721, 1976.
143. Ferriss, J. B., et al.: Primary hyperaldosteronism. Clin. Endocrinol. Metab. *10*:419, 1981.
144. Ganguly, A., et al.: Anomalous postural aldosterone response in glucocorticoid-suppressible hyperaldosteronism. N. Engl. J. Med. *305*:991, 1981.
145. Neville, A. M., and Symington, T.: Pathology of primary aldosteronism. Cancer *19*:1854, 1966.
146. Hornsby, P. J., et al.: Functional and morphological observations on rat

adrenal zona glomerulosa cells in monolayer culture. Endocrinology *95*:1240, 1974.
147. Neville, A. M., and MacKay, A. M.: The structure of the human adrenal cortex in health and disease. Clin. Endocrinol. Metab. *2*:361, 1972.
148. McGuffin, W. L., Jr., and Gunnells, J. C., Jr.: Primary aldosteronism. Urol. Clin. North Am. *4*:227, 1977.
149. Ganguly, A., et al.: Primary aldosteronism. The etiologic spectrum of disorders and their clinical differentiation. Arch. Intern. Med. *142*:813, 1982.
150. New, M. I., et al.: An update of congenital adrenal hyperplasia. Recent Prog. Horm. Res. *37*:105, 1981.
151. Ross, G., Jr., et al.: Our experience with the adrenogenital syndrome. A review of 16 cases. J. Urol. *115*:462, 1976.
152. Russell, R. P., et al.: Adrenal cortical adenomas and hypertension. A clinical pathologic analysis of 690 cases with matched controls and a review of the literature. Medicine *51*:211, 1972.
153. Hutter, A. M., and Kayhoe, D. E.: Adrenal cortical carcinoma. Am. J. Med. *41*:572, 1966.
154. Falterman, C. J., and Kreisberg, R.: Pheochromocytoma: Clinical diagnosis and management. South. Med. J. *75*:321, 1982.
155. Atuk, N. O.: Pheochromocytoma: Diagnosis, localization and treatment. Hosp. Pract. *18*:187, 1983.
156. Melicow, M. M.: One hundred cases of pheochromocytoma (107 tumors) at the Columbia Presbyterian Medical Center 1926–1976. Cancer *40*:1987, 1977.
157. Symington, T., and Goodall, A. L.: Studies in phaeochromocytoma. Pathological aspects. Glasgow Med. J. *34*:75, 1953.
158. Wilson, R. A., and Ibanez, M. L.: A comparative study of 14 cases of familial and nonfamilial pheochromocytomas. Hum. Pathol. *9*:181, 1978.
159. Goldfien, A.: Phaeochromocytoma. Clin. Endocrinol. Metab. *10*:607, 1981.
160. Garcia, R., and Jennings, J.: Pheochromocytoma masquerading as a cardiomyopathy. Am. J. Cardiol. *29*:568, 1972.
161. Sandler, M., et al.: Prostaglandins in amine-peptide–secreting tumours. Lancet *2*:1053, 1968.
162. Koop, C. E., and Schnaufer, L.: The management of abdominal neuroblastoma. Cancer *35*:905, 1975.
163. Evans, A. E.: Staging and treatment of neuroblastoma. Cancer *45*:1799, 1980.
164. Hann, H. L., et al.: Biologic differences between neuroblastoma stages IV-S and IV: Measurement of serum ferritin and E rosette inhibition in 30 children. N. Engl. J. Med. *305*:423, 1981.
165. Hellstrom, K. E., and Hellstrom, I.: Some aspects of the immune defense against cancer. J. Cancer *28*:1266, 1971.
166. Report of the Subcommittee on Childhood Solid Tumor Task Force, National Cancer Institute: Comparison of survival curves 1956 vs. 1962 in children with Wilms' tumor and neuroblastoma. Pediatrics *45*:800, 1970.
167. Lack, E. E., et al.: Paragangliomas of the head and neck region. A pathobiologic study of tumors from 71 patients. Hum. Pathol. *10*:191, 1979.
168. Someren, A., and Karcoiglu, Z.: Malignant vagal paraganglioma. Report of a case and review of the literature. Am. J. Clin. Pathol. *68*:400, 1977.
169. Levine, G. D., and Rosai, J.: Thymic hyperplasia and neoplasia. A review of current concepts. Hum. Pathol. *9*:495, 1978.
170. Masaoka, A., et al.: Study of the ratio of lymphocytes to epithelial cells in thymoma. Cancer *40*:1222, 1977.
171. Snover, D. C., et al.: Thymic carcinoma. Five distinctive histological variants. Am. J. Surg. Pathol. *6*:451, 1982.
172. Robins-Browne, R. M., et al.: Thymoma, pure red cell aplasia, pernicious anaemia and candidiasis: A defect in immunohomeostasis. Br. J. Haematol. *36*:5, 1977.
173. Salyer, W. R., and Eggleston, J. C.: Thymoma, a clinical and pathological study of 65 cases. Cancer *37*:229, 1976.
174. Souadjian, J. V., et al.: The spectrum of diseases associated with thymoma. Coincidence or syndrome? Arch. Intern. Med. *134*:374, 1974.
175. LeGolvan, D. P., and Abell, M. R.: Thymomas. Cancer *39*:2142, 1977.
176. De Martino, C., et al.: Electron microscopic study of impuberal and adult rats pineal body. Experientia *20*:556, 1964.
177. Rubinstein, L. J.: Cytogenesis and differentiation of pineal neoplasms. Hum. Pathol. *12*:441, 1981.
178. Borit, A., et al.: The separation of pineocytoma from pineoblastoma. Cancer *45*:1408, 1980.

THE SKIN 27

GEORGE F. MURPHY, M.D.,*
THEODORE H. KWAN, M.D.,†
and MARTIN C. MIHM, JR., M.D.‡

NORMAL

To the casual observer, the skin is a passive, somewhat dull body covering. It does not do anything as vivid as pumping blood or thinking, running, or jumping. Yet one needs only to think of a seriously burned patient to realize the problems generated by lack of skin.

The skin is an organ of sharp contrasts. It is our most visible and accessible organ, and yet perhaps the most overlooked clinically. Skin is passive and relatively immobile, but it is composed of numerous highly specialized cells actively engaged in protective functions and reception of at times eloquent tactile messages. Celebrated for its softness, flexibility, and elastic qualities, the skin is surprisingly resistant to blunt trauma, corrosive liquids and the effects of light and other irradiation. On continuous rubbing, the skin hardens and is even capable of forming horns!

Perhaps the most important function of the skin is protection. As our major interface with the environment, the skin produces a scaling surface impermeable to many substances. Pigment produced by specialized cells in the skin filter out harmful rays of ultraviolet light from the sun. An elaborate network of immunocompetent cells in the skin constantly monitors for antigens potentially harmful to us.

Temperature regulation and metabolic functions such as irradiation of vitamin D precursors, excretion of urea, and storage of carbohydrate and fat occur in the skin. As a visual expression of individual phenotype, the skin historically has figured in social interactions. However, despite the differences in pigmentation among the races, the skin from all peoples is remarkably similar histologically and reacts to a variety of stimulants in an identical manner. As our most accessible organ for study, the skin represents a window into mechanisms of many basic biologic processes.

Embryologically, ectoderm, neuroectoderm, and mesoderm all contribute to the varied components of skin. The ectoderm gives rise to epidermis, hair and sebaceous glands (pilosebaceous units), sweat glands (eccrine units), and nails. Neuroectodermal derivatives include melanocytes, nerves, and special neuroreceptors. From the mesenchyme arise collagen, reticulin and elastic fibers, blood vessels, muscle, and fat.

The basic structure of the skin consists of epidermis and a basement membrane zone overlying dermis and subcutaneous fat. Appendageal structures including pilosebaceous units and eccrine and apocrine glands are located in the dermis, but maintain connections with the epidermis from which they arise during embryonic life.

The major components of *epidermis* include *keratinocytes, melanocytes,* and *Langerhans cells.* Nerve processes extend from the dermis a short distance into the epidermis where they associate with the infrequently encountered *Merkel cell,* a slowly adapting cutaneous mechanoreceptor. Blood and lymphatic channels are absent. The epidermis normally may contain immigrant lymphocytes and histiocytes in low numbers, which along with similar cells in the dermis and epider-

*Assistant Professor of Pathology, Brigham and Women's Hospital and Harvard Medical School.
†Instructor in Pathology, Beth Israel Hospital and Harvard Medical School.
‡Professor of Pathology, Massachusetts General Hospital and Harvard Medical School.

mal Langerhans cells constitute the immunologically important *skin-associated lymphoid tissue* (SALT).[1]

Keratinocytes are classified by their location and degree of differentiation. Nucleated keratinocytes make up the *malpighian* layer and include *basal, spinous,* and *granular cells. Cornified cells* are anucleate and are superficial to the malpighian layer.

Basal or *germinative cells* (stratum basale) are located closest to the dermis, and consist of a monolayer of ribosome- and organelle-rich basophilic cuboidal cells. Basal keratinocytes contain melanin, which is synthesized in nearby melanocytes. *Spinous cells* (stratum spinosum) are located above the basal cells, and have more abundant and more eosinophilic cytoplasm than basal cells because of their higher keratin content. Spinous cells are named for their intercellular connections, which resemble spines. These spinous processes, as seen by electron microscopy, contain *desmosomes* at sites of cell-to-cell contact (Fig. 27–1). The cytoplasm of spinous cells contains numerous tonofilaments. *Granular cells* (stratum granulosum), flattened cells located above the spinous layer, contain numerous cytoplasmic keratohyaline granules that appear basophilic in H and E–stained tissue. These granules are osmiophilic and are without apparent internal structure as viewed by electron microscopy. Also visualized ultrastructurally are cytoplasmic structures called *keratinosomes,* which are apparently discharged into the intercellular space where they probably contribute to the relatively impermeable barrier of the stratum corneum. *Cornified cells* (stratum corneum), are located most superficially and consist of very flat, anucleate, orange, eosinophilic cells, each cornified cell covering approximately 25 basal cells. The transition from granular to cornified cells is abrupt. Ultrastructurally, anucleate cornified cell cytoplasm is diffusely filamentous and lacks organelles except for melanosomes. The stratum corneum seems to play an important role in the conservation of moisture and is thickened in areas subject to a lot of friction, such as the palms and soles.

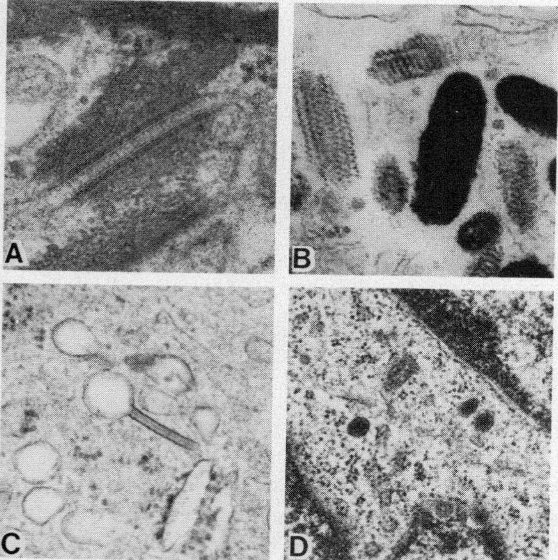

Figure 27–1. Characteristic ultrastructural features of various types of epidermal cells. *A*, Desmosomes are present at sites of cell-to-cell contact between keratinocytes. *B*, Melanosomes, at various stages of melanization, are produced in melanocytes. *C*, Birbeck granules, resembling tennis racquets, are found in Langerhans cells. *D*, Dense-core granules are characteristic of the rarely encountered Merkel cell.

In summary, the following events occur during differentiation of keratinocytes: (1) ribosomes and other cellular organelles decrease; (2) tonofilament content and number of desmosomes increase; (3) shape of cells changes from cuboidal to polygonal to very flattened cells; and (4) nucleus disappears. These changes correlate with progressive synthesis of keratin protein, which constitutes the protective superficial layer of the skin.

As the upper layers of the epidermis are shed, the lower layers regenerate. Normal turnover time for the epidermis has been estimated to be 28 days. It seems likely that, at any given time, only certain groups of basal cells are in a proliferative phase, while others are in a resting phase.[2] *Mitoses are normally present no higher than one cell above the basal layer.*

Melanocytes are usually located in the basal layer of the epidermis where they appear as cells with clear cytoplasm and small dark nuclei pushed to one side of the cell. They also may be found in the hair bulb, uveal tract, retina, inner ear, and leptomeninges, and rarely in the ovary, adrenal medulla, bladder, and substantia nigra of the brain. Melanocytes are dendritic cells *derived from the neural crest* that are capable of production of melanin pigment. Unless filled with melanin, dendritic processes are not apparent on routinely prepared sections. *Melanin* (derived from the Greek word *melas,* meaning black) is an endogenous, non–hemoglobin-derived, brown-black pigment formed when the enzyme tyrosinase catalyzes the oxidation of tyrosine to dihydroxyphenylalanine (DOPA) in melanocytes. Ultrastructurally, melanocytes contain organelles called *melanosomes,* which consist of membrane-bound round or ellipsoidal structures having internal concentric lamellae of constant periodicity (10 nm) (Fig. 27–1). It is in these melanosomes that tyrosinase-dependent melanization occurs, causing these structures to become darker and electron dense by electron microscopy. The process of melanin formation is governed by numerous factors, including genetic, metabolic, and hormonal influences. Hyperpigmentation, for example, may result from excessive production of substances producing effects akin to melanocyte-stimulating hormone (MSH), such as melatonins and ACTH in primary adrenocortical insufficiency (Addison's disease, p. 1235). Hypopigmentation, on the other hand, may be the result of contact with substances that interfere with melanin synthesis, such as hydroquinones.

Each melanocyte supplies numerous basal and spinous cells with melanin. Transfer of melanin occurs as keratinocytes engulf melanin-filled tips of melanocytic dendrites. If one observes a sheet of epidermis en face, melanocytes visualized histochemically are arranged in an orderly, evenly spaced fashion (Fig. 27–2), to ensure effective transfer and distribution of melanin pigment to nearby keratinocytes. It is this melanocyte-keratino-

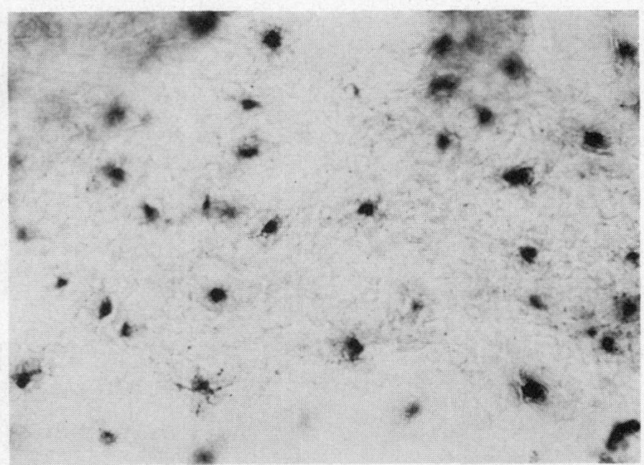

Figure 27–2. Melanocytes visualized histochemically by DOPA technique and viewed en face in an isolated sheet of epidermis are numerous and evenly distributed among keratinocytes, to which they donate melanin pigment.

cyte interaction that provides an internal protective screen against the deleterious effects of ultraviolet radiation. The density of melanocytes is greatest in genital and intertriginous areas, intermediate on the face, and lowest on the trunk.

Langerhans cells cannot be reliably detected on routine sections. Like melanocytes, Langerhans cells are also dendritic, but they stain with gold chloride, and ultrastructurally they contain distinctive cytoplasmic organelles *(Birbeck granules)* whose configuration has been likened to that of tennis racquets (Fig. 27–1). These cells belong to the mononuclear phagocyte system and have many immunologic surface markers characteristic of monocytes and macrophages (Table 15–3, p. 666). Interestingly, Langerhans cells have also been shown to have a thymocyte differentiation antigen (T6)

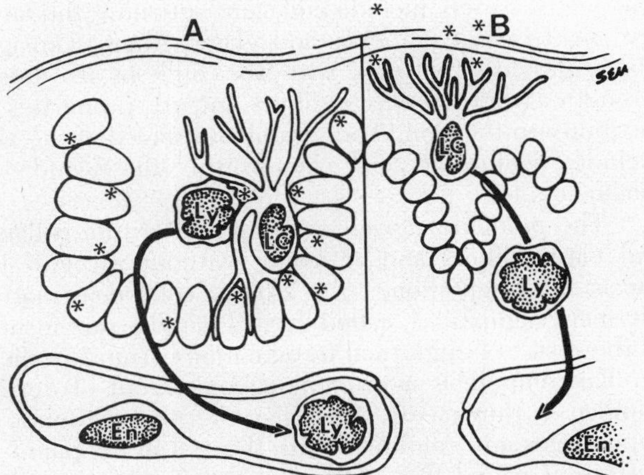

Figure 27–3. Skin-associated lymphoid tissue consists of antigen-presenting dendritic cells, or Langerhans cells and T lymphocytes. Antigens (*) theoretically *(A)* present on certain tumor cells or *(B)* present in the external environment may be taken up by Langerhans cells and presented to T cells locally or in regional lymph nodes after entrance into dermal lymphatics *(arrows)*. Sensitized T cells may then produce an antigen-directed local tissue reaction.

on their surface.[3] Recent evidence indicates that Langerhans cells are capable of antigen processing and presentation to T lymphocytes, and therefore represent important initiators of the afferent limb of the cutaneous immune response (Fig. 27–3).

Merkel cells, like Langerhans cells, cannot be identified in routine sections, and of all types of epidermal cells they are the least numerous. They contain neurosecretory-type "dense-core" granules ultrastructurally (Fig. 27–1) and probably represent in humans a vestige of a mechanoreceptor important in lower animals.

In summary, the epidermis is composed of specialized cells that function to protect us against potentially injurious agents in the external environment. Because physical and chemical agents, ultraviolet radiation, and antigenic substances are ubiquitous in our environment, it is not surprising that the three major component cells of the epidermis deal with each of these factors in a highly specific fashion.

Specialized extensions of the epidermis into the dermis constitute the appendages. *Hair* arises from hair follicles, and is colored by melanin pigment and composed of proteins akin to epidermal keratin. Despite the striking variability in size, color, and shape of hair, the basic structure of all hair follicles is similar. The hair follicle consists of a specialized epidermal invagination associated at its base with a specialized fibrovascular structure, the dermal hair papilla. This latter structure is largely responsible for the growth and maintenance of the hair follicle. For example, plucking hair can damage the follicle, but the hair regenerates as long as the dermal hair papilla is unaffected.

Associated with the hair are melanocytes, sensory nerves, a smooth muscle bundle called arrector pili, sebaceous glands, and sometimes apocrine glands. Cycles of growth, involution, and rest characterize the generation of hair. *Anagen* refers to the growth phase; *catagen*, to the phase of involution; and *telogen*, to the resting phase.

Sebaceous glands and the hair follicle form the pilosebaceous unit; almost all sebaceous glands occur in association with hair follicles. Exceptions include sebaceous glands on the lip, prepuce, labia minora, and eyelids (meibomian glands). Sebaceous glands have a sacular or lobular structure composed of secretory cells. The cytoplasm of cells near the lumen has a bubbly appearance, whereas cells near the periphery of the lobule have a basaloid appearance. The former cells, rich in triglycerides and lipids, are shed into the lumen, so-called holocrine secretion. The short duct, lined by squamous epithelium, opens into the hair follicle at a point roughly one-third the length of the follicle from the skin surface. The secretory product of sebaceous glands is lipid rich and probably functions as a lubricant for hairs and the skin. It is believed to be of importance in the pathogenesis of acne. The control of sebaceous gland secretion is probably mediated by hormonal factors.

Apocrine glands may originate from pilosebaceous units or communicate directly with the epidermis. Apocrine glands are characteristically present in the axillae, genital and perianal areas, areolae, periumbilical areas, external ear canal (ceruminous glands), and eyelids (Moll's glands). The apocrine gland consists of a coiled tubuloglandular structure located in the deep dermis or subcutis. A relatively straight duct leads to a hair follicle or directly to the skin surface. The luminal surface of the gland is lined by large pink cells with apical protrusions in which secretory products consist of budded-off portions of cytoplasm. Apocrine gland secretion is regulated by adrenergic nerves in response to rubbing or pharmacologic or emotional factors, and consists of odiferous fluid that, in certain lower mammals is milky, and serves to regulate olfactory-mediated behavior (pheromone-like substance).

Eccrine sweat glands, numbering 2 to 3 million in each person and widely distributed over the skin, are most numerous in palms, soles, and axillae. Only the lips and certain parts of the genitalia are free of eccrine glands. Each gland consists of a coiled tubuloglandular structure located at or near the junction of dermis and subcutis. A relatively straight duct extends from the gland through the dermis into the epidermis. The intraepidermal portion of the duct assumes a spiral course to the surface. The gland is lined by two types of cells on the luminal surface. Dark cuboidal cells rich in neutral mucopolysaccharides and cells with clear cytoplasm rich in glycogen line the lumen, and in turn are enclosed by myoepithelial cells. Eccrine secretions consist of thin watery fluid. Secretion is merocrine, i.e., it occurs without destruction of part or all of the cell. Cholinergic fibers of the autonomic nervous system control secretion in response to thermal stimulation and psychogenic factors, with lowering of body temperature. Secretion is easily blocked at the duct orifice, especially in infants and children, resulting in the familiar prickly heat rash called miliaria.[4] Electrolytes are present in normal eccrine sweat; in disorders affecting the formation of these secretions such as cystic fibrosis (p. 493), they may be detected in significantly increased quantities. In some patients with cystic fibrosis, loss of excessive amounts of sodium and chloride in eccrine sweat has resulted in acute salt depletion and even death.

A *basement membrane zone* seen particularly well in PAS-stained tissue as a fine violet line is present at the dermoepidermal junction. As seen with the electron microscope, the basement membrane zone consists of: (1) *the plasma membrane and hemidesmosomes of the basal cell;* (2) *the lamina lucida*—an electron-lucent band located below the basal layer; (3) *the basal lamina*—an electron-dense band of finely granular material below the lamina lucida; and (4) *the subbasal lamina fibrous elements* (anchoring fibrils, dermal microfibrillar bundles, and collagen fibers), which merge with the papillary dermis (Fig. 27–4). The first three components of the basement membrane zone are produced by the epidermis, and the subbasal fibrous elements are produced by connective tissue cells in the dermis. The basement membrane zone is of interest in the study of the blistering diseases (p. 1293). For example, in bullous pemphigoid, IgG and complement are deposited in the lamina lucida, whereas in dermatitis herpetiformis, IgA is deposited below the basal lamina.

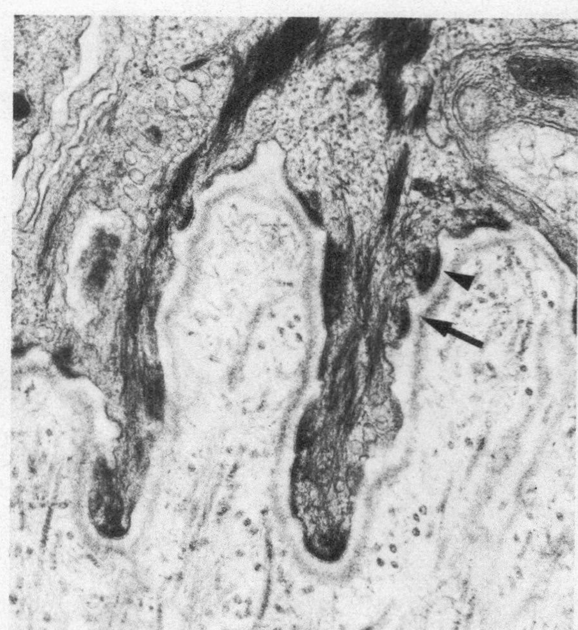

Figure 27–4. Electron micrograph of basement membrane zone at dermoepidermal junction: (1) basal cell plasma membrane and hemidesmosome *(arrowhead)*, (2) lamina lucida, (3) basal lamina *(arrow)*, and (4) subbasal lamina fibrous elements and papillary dermis.

The *dermis* is divided into a thin superficial area called the *papillary dermis* and a thicker deep area, rich in thick collagen bundles, called the *reticular dermis*. Both the papillary dermis and reticular dermis are composed of cellular, fibrous, and ground substance components; the last-named two undergo constant synthesis and degradation. The cellular elements include fibroblasts, histiocytes, endothelial cells, pericytes, and mast cells. Fibers include collagen, reticulin (the latter are small collagen fibers), and elastic fibers. Collagen fibers provide the skin with the bulk of its tensile strength, whereas elastic fibers impart properties of flexibility to the skin. The ground substance of the skin includes hyaluronic acid, chondroitin sulfate, and dermatan sulfate.

The *papillary dermis* is composed of thin collagen and elastic fibers and reticulin, without recognizably consistent orientation, in a ground substance matrix. Dermal evaginations, called dermal papillae, are formed as the result of epidermal invaginations. The superficial capillary venule is a prominent component of dermal papillae. A thin sheath of papillary dermis surrounds all appendages and combined with the rest of the papillary dermis, is called the *adventitial dermis*. The papillary dermis together with the epidermis can apparently act as a functional unit. In some inflammatory disorders such as psoriasis, epidermal and papillary dermal alterations occur in concert, whereas the reticular dermis is relatively uninvolved.

The *reticular dermis* is composed of thick collagen bundles interspersed with elastic and reticulin fibers in a ground substance matrix. The collagen bundles have an interlacing crisscrossed pattern that is predominantly oriented parallel to the surface of the skin. Vessels, nerves, and adnexae are present in the reticular dermis.

Subcutaneous fat. The basic structure of the subcutis consists of *lobules* of fat cells (or lipocytes) separated by *fibrous septa* (or trabecula). Within these septa run nerves and blood and lymphatic channels that supply the overlying skin. Eccrine and apocrine glands, all rimmed by lipocytes, are located near the junction of reticular dermis and subcutis.

Vascular supply of the skin. Arteries and veins form deep and superficial plexuses, with communicating vessels running between them. The *superficial vascular plexus* is located in the high reticular dermis near the junction of the reticular and papillary dermis and is oriented parallel to the surface of the skin. The *superficial capillary venule* arises from the superficial plexus; it is called a capillary venule, because the flow of blood can be arterial to venous or vice versa. Blood flow in the skin results in transport of nutrients and waste products. Control of temperature is affected by vascular regulatory shunts and is mediated by the hypothalamus and sympathetic nervous system. Specialized groups of smooth muscle cells called *glomus bodies* control some of these vascular shunts.

Lymphatics are numerous throughout the dermis but are inconspicuous in histologic sections of normal skin. They arise in the papillary dermis and form plexuses that parallel the other vascular plexuses of the skin.

Innervation of the skin. Nerve fibers in the skin occur free and encapsulated, myelinated and unmyelinated. Many nerves end in microscopically distinctive receptors, e.g., pacinian and Meissner corpuscles. The motor fibers of the skin are all autonomic. Adrenergic fibers mediate the contraction of arrector pili and smooth muscle of arteriolar walls, the glomus body, and apocrine gland myoepithelial cells. Cholinergic fibers supply eccrine glands. Sensory fibers of the skin mediate touch, pressure, temperature, pain, itching, and other sensations. In the past, it was hypothesized that each particular sensation was mediated by a particular anatomically distinct end organ; present hypotheses propose that specific sensations are the result of central summation of patterns of impulses generated by different types of receptors.

PATHOLOGY

The eyes may be the mirror of the soul, but the skin often reflects the state of the internal milieu. Skin disorders are frequently encountered in medical practice, and the astute clinician is able to judge the significance of cutaneous eruptions. In some cases the eruption is a sign of covert or incipient internal disease. In other cases the disorder is limited to the skin.

Definition of Terms

Before describing the clinical features and characteristic histology of skin disorders, we will define some descriptive terms used in dermatopathology.

Macroscopic Terms

Macule: Circumscribed area of any size characterized by its flatness and usually distinguished from surrounding skin by its coloration.

Papule: Elevated solid area 5 mm or less across.

Nodule: Elevated solid area greater than 5 mm across.

Plaque: Elevated flat-topped area, usually greater than 5 mm across.

Vesicle: Fluid-filled raised area 5 mm or less across.

Bulla: Fluid-filled raised area greater than 5 mm across; a large blister.

Blister: Common term used for vesicle or bulla.

Pustule: Discrete, pus-filled, raised area.

Wheal: Itchy, transient, elevated area with variable blanching and erythema formed as the result of dermal edema.

Scale: Dry, horny, platelike excrescence; usually the result of imperfect cornification.

Lichenification: Thickened and rough skin characterized by prominent skin markings; usually the result of repeated rubbing in susceptible persons.

Excoriation: A traumatic lesion characterized by breakage of the epidermis causing a raw linear area, i.e., a deep scratch. Such lesions are often self-induced.

Onycholysis: Loss of integrity of the nail substance.

Microscopic Terms

Hyperkeratosis: Hyperplasia of the stratum corneum often associated with a qualitative abnormality of the keratin.

Parakeratosis: Mode(s) of keratinization characterized by the retention of nuclei in the stratum corneum. On mucous membranes, parakeratosis is normal.

Acanthosis: Epidermal hyperplasia.

Dyskeratosis: Abnormal keratinization occurring prematurely within individual cells or groups of cells below the stratum granulosum.

Acantholysis: Loss of intercellular connections resulting in loss of cohesion between keratinocytes.

Papillomatosis: Hyperplasia of the papillary dermis with elongation and/or widening of the dermal papillae.

Spongiosis: Intercellular edema of the epidermis.

Exocytosis: Infiltration of the epidermis by inflammatory or circulating blood cells.

Erosion: Discontinuity of the skin, exhibiting incomplete loss of the epidermis.

Ulceration: Discontinuity, often excavative, of skin exhibiting complete loss of the epidermis and portions of the dermis and even subcutaneous fat.

Vacuolization: Formation of vacuoles within or adjacent to cells; often refers to basal cell–basement membrane zone area.

The most common tumors encountered in day-to-day medical practice are tumors of the skin. In the following sections they are classified by their anatomic location (e.g., epidermis or dermis) and by their biologic behavior (benign or malignant).

BENIGN EPIDERMAL TUMORS

Benign keratinocytic tumors are the most common types of benign epidermal tumor and are primarily a cosmetic problem. Clinically, they may sometimes be mistaken for malignant tumors. For example, malignant melanoma, a tumor of pigment cells or melanocytes, is frequently confused clinically with pigmented seborrheic keratosis, a benign tumor of keratinocytes. The benign keratoacanthoma is often misdiagnosed as squamous cell carcinoma. In all cases in which the clinical diagnosis is in doubt, biopsy for histopathologic examination should be performed.

SEBORRHEIC KERATOSIS

This is a common benign tumor of basaloid (basal cell–like) cells, occurring most frequently after middle age. Tumors arise spontaneously, sometimes rapidly and in crops (Fig. 27–5). The sudden enlargement or shower-like appearance of numerous seborrheic keratoses may follow hormonal therapy or inflammatory dermatoses. Rarely, crops of these lesions are associated with an internal malignancy. If the malignancy is of gastrointestinal origin, this sudden appearance of seborrheic keratoses is called the sign of *Leser-Trélat.*

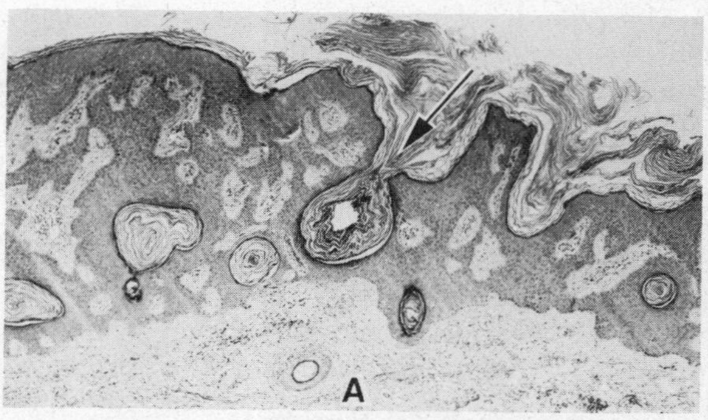

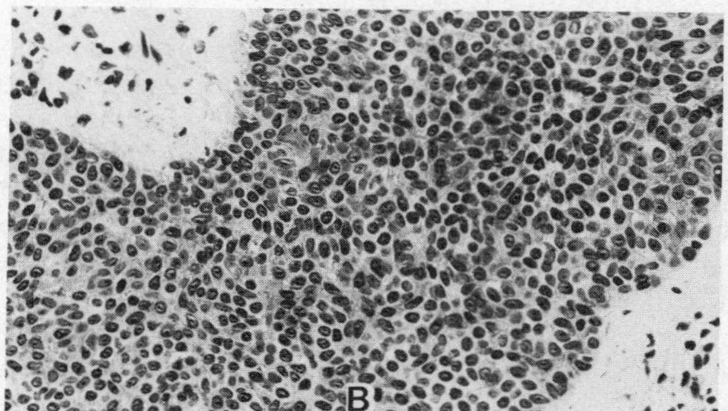

Figure 27–6. *A*, Seborrheic keratosis architecturally is abruptly demarcated and shows hyperkeratosis and epidermal and papillary dermal hyperplasia, and contains horn cysts and "pseudohorn cysts" (keratotic cysts that communicate with the epidermal surface, *arrow*). *B*, Cytologically, these lesions are composed of uniform basaloid cells.

Seborrheic keratoses are usually bilateral, occurring most frequently on the trunk, face, and extremities. Individual lesions vary in size from millimeters to centimeters and present as a variety of plaques, some with greasy surfaces, others with surfaces that can be velvety, granular, or verrucous. The lesions are usually soft and friable and show slight-to-marked pigmentation. In blacks, seborrheic keratosis is called **dermatosis papulosa nigra.** These pigmented lesions are characteristically smaller and smoother than the corresponding lesions in whites.

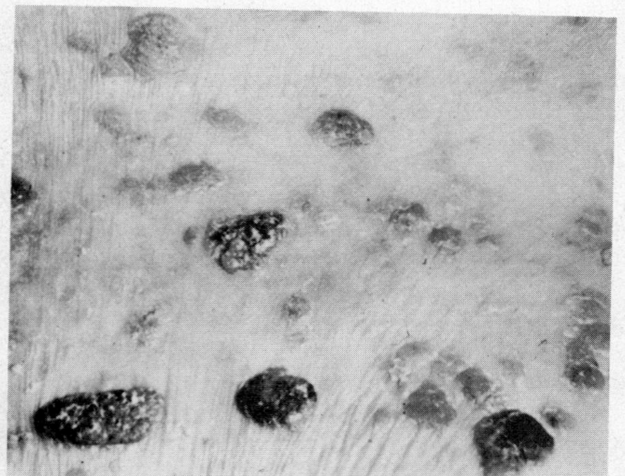

Figure 27–5. Seborrheic keratoses are often multiple and consist of tan-to-brown, well-demarcated plaques exhibiting variable degrees of hyperkeratosis and containing keratotic plugs.

Histologically, seborrheic keratoses may assume widely varying patterns (Fig. 27–6). As a general rule, all are exophytic and composed of basaloid cells. The exophytic nature of the lesion is evident on low-power examination; **the base of the seborrheic keratosis is flat and level with the base of the adjacent normal epidermis**. The basal cells form cords and sheets in the middle of which are epidermal cysts filled with keratin, so-called "horn cysts." These cysts may communicate with the surface of the lesion, resulting in multiple small keratin plugs, a feature visible with a hand lens and not usually present in tumors of melanocytes. Interwoven with the basaloid aggregates are tracts of hyperplastic papillary dermis associated with a variable chronic inflammatory infiltrate. Hyperpigmentation of the basaloid cells may be present. The **irritated seborrheic keratosis**[5] is a special type, which, although fundamentally a basaloid tumor, shows numerous squamous cells arranged in solid sheets, with some cells in a "whorling" pattern. Numerous lymphocytes are present in the dermis. **Inverted follicular keratosis** is an endophytic growth usually associated with a pilosebaceous follicle, and otherwise exhibiting features of an irritated seborrheic keratosis.

Seborrheic keratoses are usually left untreated unless they are removed for itching or pain associated with inflammation, or for cosmetic reasons. They do not recur unless they have been incompletely treated. At times, pigmented seborrheic keratoses resemble melanoma or pigmented basal cell carcinoma. Whenever the clinical diagnosis is uncertain, biopsy for histopathologic evaluation is indicated.

FIBROEPITHELIAL POLYP

Also called skin tag or acrochordon, this very common tumor often is seen as an incidental finding in middle-aged persons.

Skin tags occur most often on the neck and intertrigines and appear as soft papules or soft, pedunculated, baglike tumors. Histologically, they consist of benign squamous epithelium surrounding a fibrovascular core.

Multiple skin tags sometimes develop during pregnancy and are also associated with other disorders such as diabetes and intestinal polyposis. Unless they are extremely numerous, however, skin tags do not seem to be a significant marker of internal disease.

EPIDERMAL CYST (WEN)

Epidermal cysts[6] are derived from the epidermis or the epithelium of the hair follicle. These tumors are formed by cystic enclosures of epithelium within the dermis that become filled with keratin admixed with variable amounts of lipid-rich debris.

There are two major types of epidermal cysts. The *pilar cyst* usually occurs as a firm, well-circumscribed, subepidermal nodule on the scalp and is formed by an outer wall of keratinizing squamous epithelium *without* a granular layer, similar to the normal epithelium of the hair follicle at and distal to the sebaceous duct. The *epidermal inclusion cyst* occurs as a well-circumscribed, subepidermal mobile nodule on the head, neck, and trunk and is formed by keratinizing squamous epithelium *with* a granular layer, similar to the normal epithelium of the follicular infundibulum. Both these cysts contain keratin, although the contents of the pilar cyst are usually more homogenous and lipidized than those of the epidermal inclusion cyst. Less common variants of epidermal cysts include the *dermoid cyst*, which is similar to the epidermal inclusion cyst but has cutaneous appendages originating from its wall, and the *steatocystoma multiplex*, an epithelial cyst without a granular layer and with compressed sebaceous lobules adjacent to its wall. Cutaneous dermoid cysts, unlike benign cystic teratomas or dermoid cysts of the ovary, are not derived from germ cells and are composed only of mature ectodermal elements.

Although all epidermal cysts are benign, they are frequently removed for cosmetic reasons, for histologic identification, or after they rupture. Ruptured cysts elicit considerable inflammation replete with foreign body–type giant cells when keratin escapes into the adjacent dermis. Rarely, large pilar cysts may erode the calvarium, and some may proliferate and grow to become ulcerated tumors that mimic squamous cell carcinomas *(pilar tumor of the scalp)*.

KERATOACANTHOMA

This benign but rapidly growing tumor appears most commonly on the central face, but can arise anywhere on the head or upper extremities. Generally occurring at or after middle age, it begins as a firm, round, flesh-colored or red papule. Within a few weeks this papule can grow remarkably to 1 to 2 cm in diameter or larger, characteristically forming a central crater filled with keratin. Following this phase of rapid growth there may be a static period, but involution with scarring eventually ensues. Keratoacanthomas are generally considered to be neoplasms of the follicular infundibulum. Theories of possible viral etiology exist, but have not been substantiated. In general, keratoacanthomas are biopsied or excised to exclude the possibility of a squamous cell carcinoma, which they may resemble both clinically and histologically.[7]

Histologically, an important feature of the keratoacanthoma is its exophytic cup-shaped architecture. The tumor cells are arranged in lobules and tongues. More centrally, large squamoid cells have a characteristic homogeneous and pale-pink ("glassy") cytoplasm; at the periphery of the lobules the cells are basaloid (Fig. 27–7). Although these lobules may penetrate deeply into the dermis and even surround dermal nerve twigs, they retain a well-defined smooth contour and basaloid differentiation at their periphery. In addition, keratoacanthomas generally show only slight cellular pleomorphism, although mitotic figures may be numerous in the rapid-growth phase. These features aid in excluding squamous cell carcinoma, which generally has a less well-defined pattern of infiltration, squamatization and dyskeratosis at the periphery of invasive tongues, and considerable cellular pleomorphism and anaplasia.

Clinically, squamous cell carcinomas are less symmetric and occur in older individuals as slow-growing tumors. However, no histologic or clinical criterion exists to permit differentiation of all keratoacanthomas from squamous cell carcinomas, and careful evaluation of multiple criteria and clinicopathologic correlation are frequently required to assign the correct diagnosis.

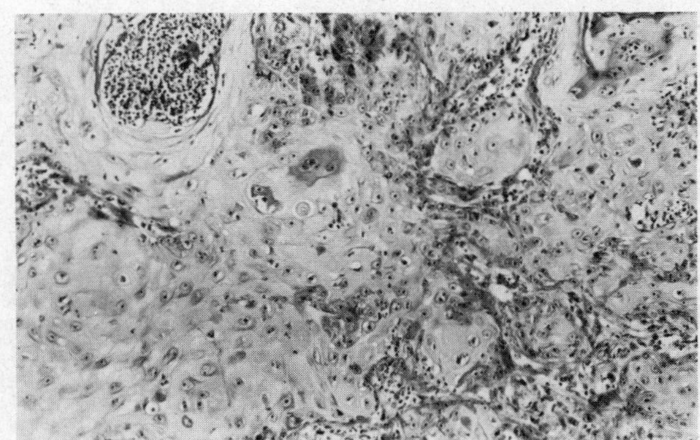

Figure 27–7. Keratoacanthomas are composed centrally of pale, glassy squamous cells and peripherally of a single layer of darker, more basaloid cells. These and other features help to differentiate the dermal component of this tumor from invasive squamous cell carcinoma.

ADNEXAL (APPENDAGE) TUMORS

Adnexal tumors are usually benign neoplasms arising from or differentiating toward cutaneous appendages. It is likely that they originate from pluripotential epithelial cells capable of pilosebaceous, eccrine, or apocrine differentiation. Because these tumors exhibit a wide range of differentiation, their histologic appearance may bear little resemblance to their mature appendageal counterparts. However, electron microscopy and enzyme histochemistry of these tumors often reveals similarities suggesting directions of histodifferentiation in these tumors.[8] For example, *trichoepithelioma* shows hair formation and *cylindroma* contains enzymes considered to be most characteristic of apocrine glands.

The common adnexal tumors include nevus sebaceus, trichoepithelioma, pilomatrixoma, cylindroma, syringocystadenoma papilliferum, syringoma, and eccrine spiradenoma. *Nevus sebaceus* is a congenital hamartoma probably derived from basal cells. Occurring on the face or scalp of children, it usually consists of a slightly raised, flesh-colored plaque, but in adults it consists of a verrucous nodular lesion several centimeters across. The histologic appearance after puberty is characterized by many sebaceous glands, some of which open directly to the surface; papillary epidermal hyperplasia; and the presence of ectopic apocrine glands in the deep dermis (Fig. 27–8*A*). In 10% of cases, basal cell carcinoma develops in these lesions.

Trichoepithelioma refers to benign, usually multiple tumors that recapitulate hair follicles. Lesions first appear in adolescence on the face and scalp, and less commonly on the neck and trunk, as flesh-colored papules and small nodules. The histologic appearance is characterized by aggregates of basal cells similar to those of the hair bulb as well as numerous horn cysts, both surrounded by an inflammatory fibrous stroma.

Pilomatrixoma (calcifying epithelioma of Malherbe) is a benign tumor of hair follicle origin. It usually arises before age 20 and appears clinically as a hard deep nodule usually located on the face or upper extremity. Histologically, pilomatrixoma exhibits a fibrous stroma surrounding nests of basophilic cells and shadow or ghost cells. The latter are keratinized cells that have an unstained central area where their nuclei were formerly located. When special stains are performed, calcium deposits are found in all tumors.

Cylindroma (turban tumor) refers to a usually benign tumor of either apocrine or eccrine origin. It generally arises in early adulthood as single or multiple nodules located on the scalp and less often on the face or extremities. Dominant inheritance is usually associated with multiple lesions. Turban tumor describes the classic appearance of multiple large nodules covering the scalp. Histologically, the tumor consists of nests of small basophilic cells surrounded by pink hyaline sheaths.

Syringocystadenoma papilliferum refers to a benign tumor of eccrine or apocrine origin. It arises at puberty as a papillomatous hyperkeratotic plaque or nodule located on the scalp or face, usually associated with nevus sebaceus. Histologically, the tumor exhibits papillary epidermal hyperplasia communicating with invaginations into the dermis. The invaginations form papillae and are lined by two rows of cells. The stroma of these papillae characteristically is densely infiltrated with

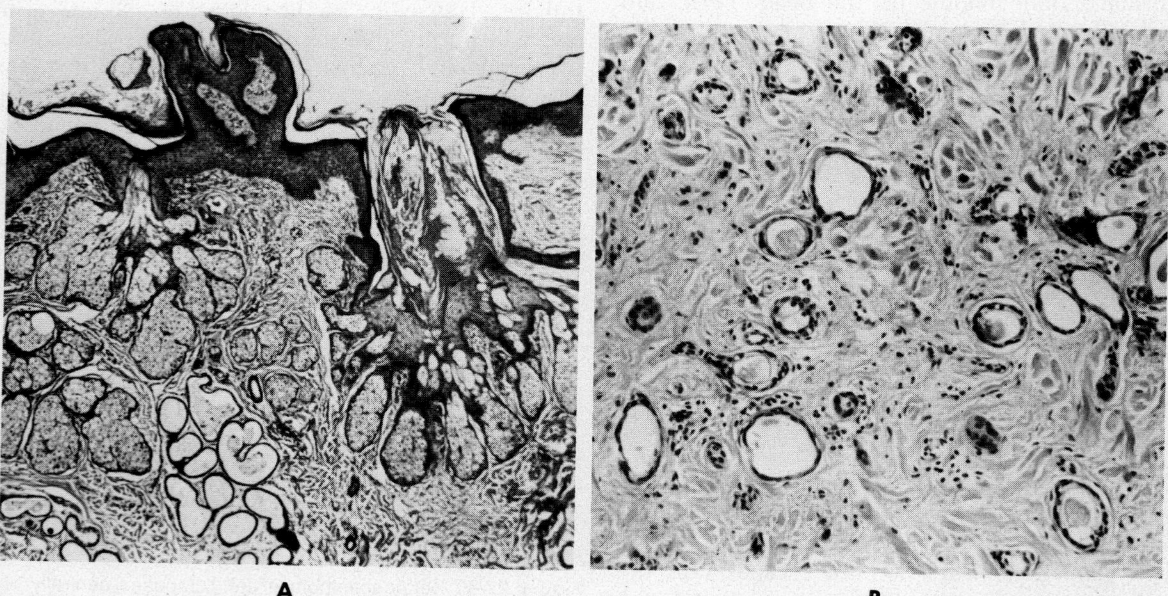

Figure 27–8. *A*, Adnexal tumor–nevus sebaceus. This hamartomatous lesion exhibits numerous sebaceous glands (some opening directly to surface), papillary epidermal hyperplasia, and ectopic apocrine glands. *B*, Adnexal tumor—syringoma. Numerous ductal structures are present embedded in a fibrous stroma. Characteristic tadpole-like shapes result from extreme tortuosity of ductal structures.

plasma cells. Syringocystadenoma papilliferum, like basal cell carcinoma, may also arise within a preexisting nevus sebaceus.

Syringoma is a benign tumor located in the dermis that probably arises from the intraepidermal portion of the eccrine duct. The lesions arise at puberty or later, usually as multiple, 1- to 2-mm, faintly yellow or skin-colored papules located on the face and especially the lower eyelids, abdomen, or vulva. The histologic appearance consists of numerous ductal structures and keratin-filled cysts in a fibrous stroma (Fig. 27–8*B*). The ductal structures have two layers of cells and assume odd shapes, e.g., comma-like tails resembling tadpoles.

Eccrine spiradenoma refers to a benign tumor probably of eccrine origin arising in young adults, and the usually solitary nodule is tender or even painful. It has no characteristic location. The histologic appearance is of one or several well-demarcated lobules composed of small basophilic cells. The latter are organized into clusters, intertwining cords, and ductal structures alternating with thin fibrous stroma.

Although most adnexal tumors are benign, malignant variants do exist. *Sebaceous carcinoma* arising from the meibomian gland of the eyelid, for example, is an aggressive neoplasm that frequently metastasizes. Benign appendage tumors may be markers for internal malignancy. Some patients with multiple *sebaceous adenomas*, a benign tumor of sebaceous glands, have been found to have gastrointestinal adenocarcinomas, and others with multiple *trichilemmomas*, benign plate-like proliferations of follicular epithelium, may have breast carcinoma (Cowden's syndrome).[9]

PREMALIGNANT AND MALIGNANT EPIDERMAL TUMORS

ACTINIC KERATOSIS (SOLAR KERATOSIS)

Actinic keratosis is a premalignant skin lesion characterized by focal areas of epidermal atypia and usually induced by chronic exposure to sunlight. It is very common among fair-complexioned middle-aged persons who have a history of chronic sun exposure. There is a particularly high incidence in the southern United States, South Africa, and Australia. Exposure to ionizing radiation and hydrocarbons and ingestion of arsenicals may induce similar lesions.

Clinically, actinic keratoses are small (less than 1 cm across), erythematous, scaling papules or plaques. They often have a rough or "sandpaper" texture, and may even produce a firm conical excrescence of keratin called a "cutaneous horn."[10] Biopsy is often performed in these latter lesions because squamous cell carcinomas may also produce cutaneous horns. When atypical proliferations of cells occur in the oral cavity, the clinical appearance of leukoplakia may be present (p. 780). When they are premalignant, the cause of these white plaques is less clear than that of actinic keratoses. Most lesions producing leukoplakia, however, are not atypical but show the common histologic features of hyperkeratosis and chronic inflammation.

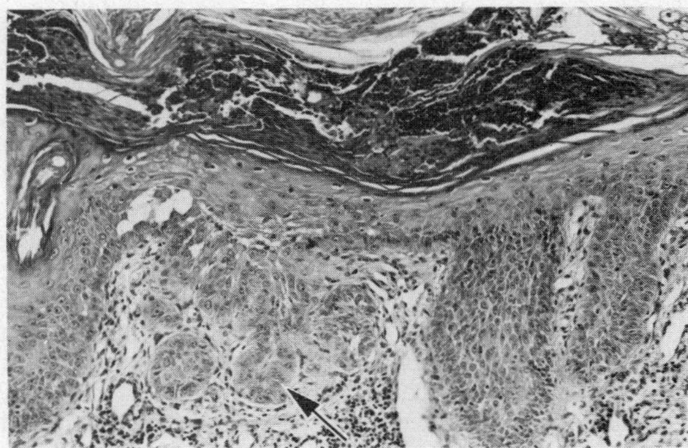

Figure 27–9. Actinic keratoses often show buds of atypical cells *(arrow)* from lower portion of epidermis that protrude into an inflamed and sun-damaged papillary dermis. These lesions are usually covered by parakeratotic scale.

The essential microscopic feature of actinic keratosis is focal atypism of the keratinocytes of the **lower layers** of an atrophic or hyperplastic epidermis. Atypical cells may proliferate in the form of buds into the dermis (Fig. 27–9) but do not invade beyond the basement membrane. Hyperkeratosis and parakeratosis are generally present and are responsible for the texture of these lesions clinically. The papillary dermis frequently contains pale, gray-blue amorphous material, so-called "solar elastosis." These deposits of abnormal connective tissue with properties of elastic tissue are also the result of chronic exposure to ultraviolet light.

BASAL CELL CARCINOMA

This is a common, locally aggressive, rarely metastasizing epidermal tumor, so designated because its cells resemble basal cells of the epidermis. Light-skinned races are most susceptible; the tumor rarely arises before age 40; blacks and Orientals are rarely affected.

Basal cell carcinoma usually presents on the face and hair-bearing areas as a pearly-gray, semitranslucent papule with marked telangiectasis. Non–hair-bearing epithelia (e.g. mucosal surfaces) are generally not affected. Tumors may also appear as brown or black nodules, plaques, or indurated areas with ulceration.

Interestingly, basal cell carcinoma is uncommon on the backs of the hands and forearms, areas of considerable sun exposure. It is common on eyelids and the inner canthus, areas more protected from sunlight but dense with pilosebaceous follicles. Arsenicals, formerly widely available in patent medicines, increase the risk of basal cell carcinoma and squamous cell carcinoma. The rare *basal cell nevus syndrome*[11] is a dominantly inherited disorder associated with the development in early life of numerous basal cell carcinomas and abnormalities of bone, skin, nervous system, eyes, and reproductive system. Patients with *xeroderma pigmentosum* (p. 241) (a group of dominantly inherited disorders characterized by defective DNA replication–repair mechanisms) are also at increased risk of developing basal cell carcinomas. Finally, immunocompromised patients, such as renal transplant recipients, are prone to develop basal and squamous cell carcinomas of the skin.

Histologically, the tumor cells form dermal nests, cords, and islands that, in a given plane or section, may or may not communicate with the overlying epidermis. The cells forming these nests are small and round and resemble basal keratinocytes. At the periphery of the nests, these cells elongate in parallel array, forming a palisading pattern (Fig. 27–10). The tumor cells have little pleomorphism, and mitoses are infrequent. Deposition of melanin pigment in some lesions explains their occasional brown coloration clinically, and cystic spaces in tumor nests may result from central necrosis or appendageal (eccrine) differentiation. A variety of histologic variants exist, including multiple superficial tumors, keratinizing types, and tumors associated with marked dermal sclerosis or with the formation of glandlike (adenoidal) structures. Tumors showing keratinization may form "horn cysts" filled with keratin, and may mimic both benign and malignant squamous cell neoplasms. However, foci of typical basal cell carcinoma can usually be identified in these lesions. The variation in histologic apperance has no effect on the rare metastatic potential of these lesions.[12] However, the presence of a characteristic loose fibrous stroma of the basal cell carcinoma appears necessary for growth of tumor cells in rare instances when metastases occur. Recent data suggest that local cellular immunity may in part relate to the indolent course of these neoplasms.[13]

When completely excised, most basal cell carcinomas are cured. *Superficial basal cell carcinomas,* which consist of nests of tumor budding from multiple epidermal sites, and sclerosing or *morphea-like basal cell carcinomas,* which are associated with marked dermal fibrosis, have ill-defined borders clinically and may recur locally after attempted removal. Long-standing tumors or more aggressive ones may produce deep ulcerations ("rodent ulcers"). Such lesions may involve underlying bone, cartilage, the orbit, and perineural spaces and may require extensive radical surgery.

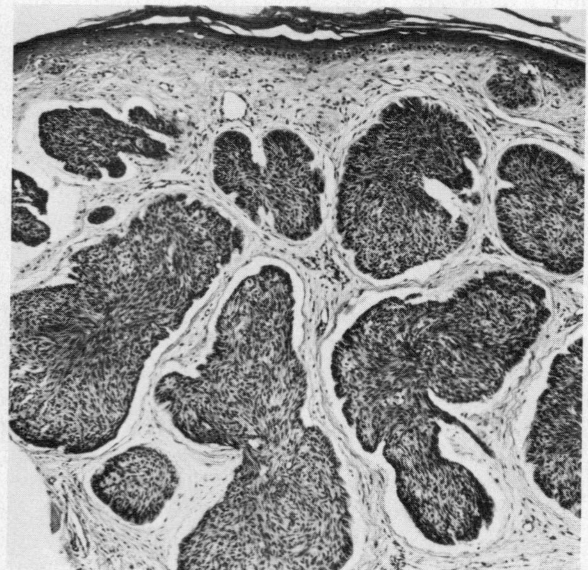

Figure 27–10. Basal cell carcinoma, exhibiting nests of basaloid cells, palisading of cells at periphery of nests, and dense stroma that surrounds tumor nests. Origin of tumor from epidermis can also be seen.

SQUAMOUS CELL CARCINOMA

Squamous cell carcinomas have a low but *significant potential for metastasis.* These tumors have a peak incidence at 60 years and affect women more frequently than men. The most common predisposing factor is chronic sun exposure. Other less common factors include ingestion of arsenicals; chronic ulcers or sinus tracts (such as those draining osteomyelitis); prolonged contact with organic hydrocarbons, tobacco, and betel nuts; radiation or thermal injury; xeroderma pigmentosum (p. 241); and immunosuppression. Most squamous cell carcinomas occur on sun-exposed skin but, in contrast to basal cell carcinomas, any area of skin and mucous membrane may be affected.

In situ (noninvasive) squamous cell carcinomas appear as sharply defined, red-brown plaques with slightly elevated borders. Early invasion is heralded by the development of a painless, firm, red papule or nodule with scaling or cutaneous horn formation. More advanced deeply invasive lesions frequently ulcerate and have wide, raised, indurated borders. On skin not exposed to sunlight, both in situ (Bowen's disease) and early invasive squamous cell carcinomas appear as red oozing patches. Paramucosal and mucosal lesions frequently show whitish discoloration, and this appearance produced by a variety of malignant and benign proliferative and inflammatory conditions is sometimes called **leukoplakia** (see also p. 780).

In situ squamous cell carcinoma is composed of atypical squamous cells, which, unlike actinic keratoses, **entirely replace** the normal epidermis (Fig. 27–11). The superficial dermis contains a lymphocytic infiltrate, but invasion through the basement membrane is not present. **Invasive squamous cell carcinoma** occurs when atypical keratinocytes break through the basement membrane and proliferate downward into the dermis (Fig. 27–12). Tumor cells of both in situ and invasive lesions are pleomorphic, have numerous and atypical mitoses, and show dyskeratosis

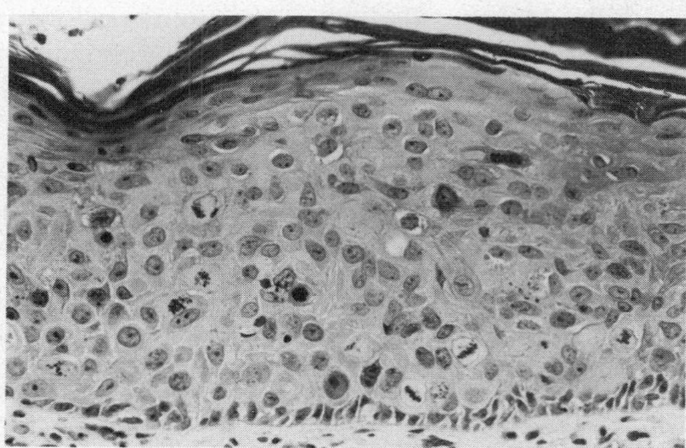

Figure 27–11. Squamous cell carcinoma in situ. Note highly pleomorphic cells at all levels of epidermis and the numerous mitotic figures.

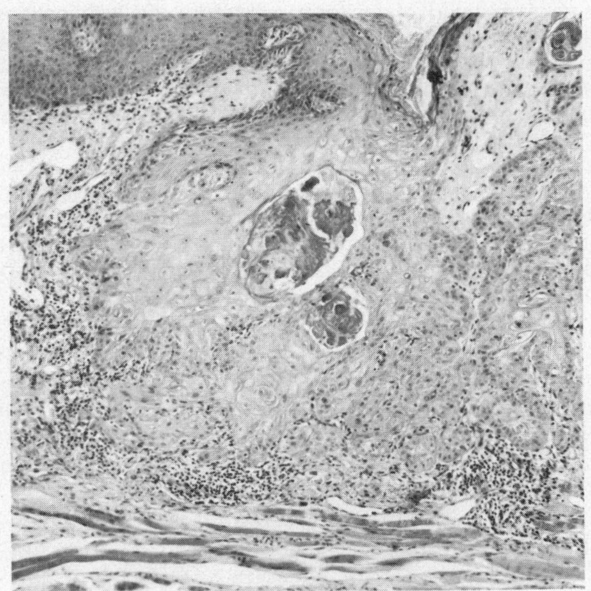

Figure 27–12. Well-differentiated squamous cell carcinoma. Tumor shows squamous differentiation and invades to level of skeletal muscle.

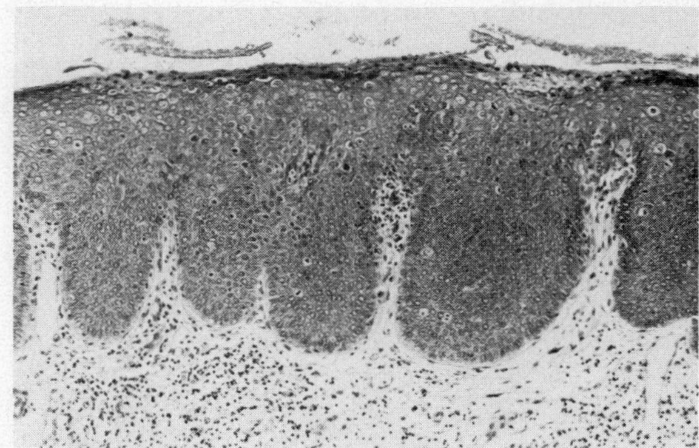

Figure 27–13. Bowenoid papulosis involving vulva. Epidermis is replaced by atypical cells, and lesion resembles squamous cell carcinoma in situ.

and "horn pearl" formation (concentric layers of squamous cells with increasing keratinization centrally). Rare histologic variants of squamous cell carcinomas include pseudoglandular[14] types, the result of acantholysis within tumor nests, and spindle cell[15] types. **Verrucous carcinomas** are an uncommon variety of squamous cell carcinoma. They have a fungating appearance and slow growth, and often are deeply invasive without metastases. Histologically, these tumors are extremely well differentiated and form endophytic, club-shaped projections of epithelium into the underlying dermis.

When squamous cell carcinoma occurs on sun-exposed skin, less than 2% of patients develop metastases. Cure may be expected with complete excision if invasion is not deep and metastases have not occurred.[16] Twenty to 50% of patients develop metastases when squamous cell carcinoma arises on mucosal surfaces, on genitalia, in burn scars, on areas of radiodermatitis, and in chronic ulcers.

Pseudocarcinomatous (pseudoepitheliomatous) hyperplasia, a disorder that must be differentiated from invasive squamous cell carcinoma, refers to benign proliferation of squamous epithelium in the form of tongues growing downward into the dermis. The changes usually occur at the edge of healing wounds and chronic ulcers. This picture is also regularly observed in granuloma inguinale, bromoderma (epithelial hyperplasia associated with ingestion of bromides), cutaneous blastomycosis, and other inflammatory disorders. In addition, it commonly occurs in epithelium overlying granular cell tumors, where it may be mistaken for squamous cell carcinoma in superficial biopsies that do not include the underlying primary tumor. Histologic examination of multiple biopsies is necessary in these cases to distinguish benign hyperplasia from malignant tumor. Pseudocarcinomatous hyperplasia lacks anaplasia and other cytologic features of malignancy, but in certain cases differentiation from squamous cell carcinoma is difficult.

Bowenoid papulosis[17] (Fig. 27–13) is a recently recognized lesion that histologically bears a close resemblance to squamous cell carcinoma in situ. It is a disorder quite distinct from the latter and from Bowen's disease, and usually occurs on the shaft of the penis or vulva as multiple small (less than 0.5-cm) flat papules. Younger patients are affected, and lesions may spontaneously regress. Clinically unlike squamous cell carcinoma in situ at these sites, which presents as a larger (greater than 1-cm) solitary lesion on the glans or vulva of older patients, bowenoid papulosis is now thought to be associated with cutaneous infection by an undefined virus. Although histologic parameters alone do not permit a diagnosis in all instances, some keratinocytes in bowenoid papulosis may appear more uniform and less atypical than in squamous cell carcinoma in situ.

TUMORS OF DERMIS

FIBROUS HISTIOCYTOMA

Fibrous histiocytoma *(dermatofibroma, sclerosing hemangioma, fibrous xanthoma, and nodular subepidermal fibrosis)* refers to a benign dermal proliferation of fibroblasts and histiocytes. The synonyms underlie the heterogeneity of the microscopic appearance and the uncertainty as to precise histogenesis. This group of common lesions usually occurs in adults, frequently on the legs of young to middle-aged women. A history of antecedent trauma in 20% of cases suggests that some of these tumors represent a proliferative response to trauma.

In most tumors the predominant morphologic picture is a dermal proliferation of benign fibroblasts and histiocytes (Fig. 27–14*A*). From a mid-dermal location the proliferation extends upward, downward, or laterally and the borders are usually poorly demarcated. In most cases, fibrocytes are

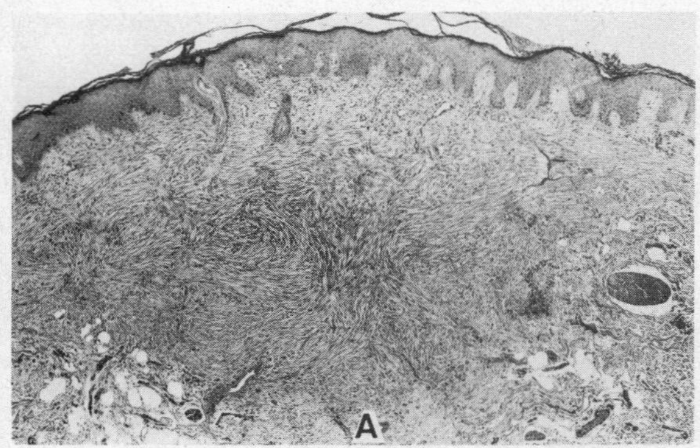

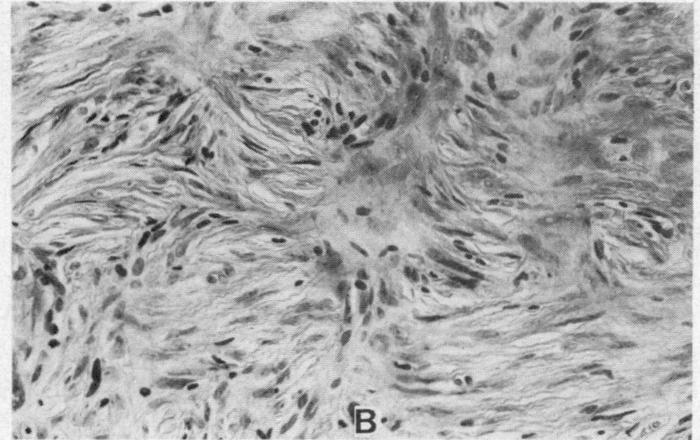

Figure 27–14. Fibrous histiocytoma (dermatofibroma) showing *A*, proliferation of fibroblasts and histiocytes beneath an area of epidermal hyperplasia and *B*, formation of cartwheel or storiform patterns by these proliferating cells.

more numerous than histiocytes, and collagen and reticulin are present in large amounts. Intertwining and anastomosing bands of collagen and tumor cells radiate from a central hub, forming a cartwheel or **storiform** pattern (Fig. 27–14B). In many lesions, scattered or nested histiocytes have a foamy, lipid-laden cytoplasm, giving the tumor the appearance of a "fibrous xanthoma." Because small vascular channels may form a prominent component of the tumor, these lesions have also been called "sclerosing hemangiomas." Extravasation of erythrocytes and deposits of hemosiderin may be present in all types.

In addition to these dermal changes, epidermal hyperplasia with elongation of rete ridges and basal hyperpigmentation are often present (Fig. 27–14*A*). Rarely, epidermal hyperplasia overlying dermatofibroma may resemble basal cell carcinoma.[18]

DERMATOFIBROSARCOMA PROTUBERANS

Dermatofibrosarcoma protuberans is an uncommon, slow-growing, and locally aggressive tumor of the dermis.[19] Clinically, lesions consist of solitary or multiple nodules often arising within an indurated plaque. These tumors arise most frequently on the trunk, but the extremities, neck, scalp, and face may be affected. Although locally invasive, only a few of these neoplasms have been documented to metastasize.[20]

The histologic appearance of dermatofibrosarcoma protuberans is that of a nonencapsulated, cellular dermal neoplasm composed of fusiform cells admixed with collagen and frequently having a storiform pattern. This has been likened to that of a low-grade fibrosarcoma. In general, dermatofibrosarcoma protuberans differs from dermatofibroma in that the former is more cellular, contains more pleomorphic and atypical cells, and has some degree of mitotic activity. In addition, the overlying epidermis is often thinned or ulcerated in dermatofibrosarcoma protuberans, whereas it is frequently hyperplastic in dermatofibroma. Both tumors may infiltrate dermal and subcutaneous tissue, although deep extension into fat and fascial planes is more typical of dermatofibrosarcoma protuberans.

Both dermatofibromas and dermatofibrosarcoma protuberans are believed to be primarily derived from fibroblasts, and the presence of variable proliferations of histiocytes in these lesions is regarded as a secondary event. Local recurrences after presumed adequate excision of dermatofibrosarcoma protuberans is likely to be the result of its insidious and infiltrative growth deep within the skin.

HEMANGIOMA

Benign and malignant tumors of blood and lymphatic vessels are discussed in Chapter 12. Here we shall discuss only the cutaneous hemangiomas, as they are extremely common disorders in dermatologic practice.

Capillary hemangioma (strawberry mark) refers to a common benign vascular tumor that usually regresses by childhood. It is unclear whether this disorder represents a malformation, benign neoplasia, or reactive process (see also p. 538).

Capillary hemangioma presents anywhere on the skin as a hypopigmented area with red stippling. This lesion arises at 3 to 5 weeks of age and evolves into a soft, bright red, lobulated exophytic mass up to 6 cm in diameter. The lesion is usually solitary; when multiple it may be rarely associated with visceral hemangiomas. Spontaneous resolution begins usually at 1 to 3 years of age and is complete within five years in 80% of cases. The resolved lesion appears as normal or slightly wrinkled erythematous skin. Ulceration and infection of a hemangioma may cause scarring.

Histologically, growing capillary hemangiomas exhibit dense dermal proliferation of thin-walled small vessels admixed with zones of dense pericytic proliferation (Fig. 27–15). In mature lesions, capillaries and vessels are present, but areas of pericytic proliferation are no longer identifiable. Involuting hemangiomas exhibit fewer vessels entrapped by dermal fibrosis.

Tumors are left to resolve spontaneously unless they are very large, ulcerated, or in critical locations (e.g., near the eye), in which case they are excised. Biopsy can be helpful in determining treatment; lesions composed of mature vessels are less likely to resolve, whereas lesions of less mature angioblastic tissue can be expected to involute spontaneously.

Pyogenic granuloma of the skin refers to a benign, common, solitary proliferation of capillaries occurring at

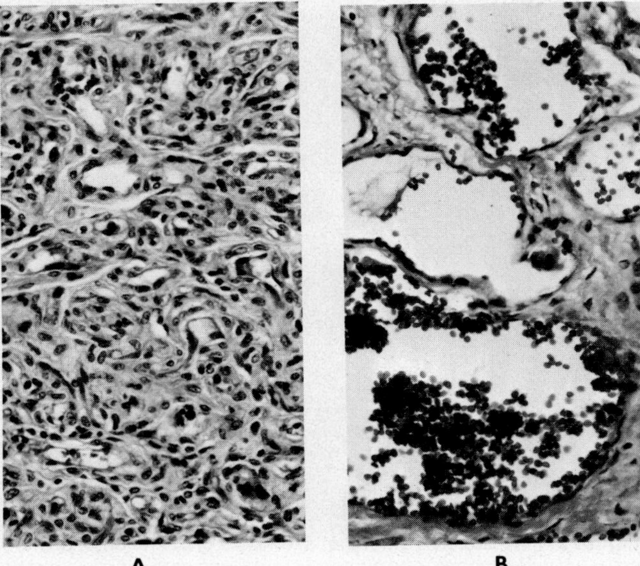

Figure 27–15. Comparison of capillary *(A)* and cavernous *(B)* hemangiomas. Both photomicrographs were taken at same magnification. Note differences in size of lumina and vessel walls, and pericytic proliferation in *A*.

any age of life. The lesion is often associated with a history of trauma and begins as a small erythematous papule that enlarges rapidly and ulcerates. It rarely exceeds 1 cm in diameter and is usually treated by excision. Histologically, there is proliferation of capillaries with endothelial swelling associated with stromal edema and numerous inflammatory cells.

Senile hemangioma (cherry hemangioma) refers to a common, benign, tiny capillary hemangioma that occurs in adult life. Senile hemangiomas are usually multiple and appear as 1- to 3-mm bright red or purple papules that sometimes persist. The histologic appearance is that of a small capillary hemangioma.

Cavernous hemangioma refers to a dermal or subcutaneous vascular tumor characterized by the relatively large size of its vessels. Less common than other types of hemangioma, it affects males more often than females. Superficial lesions usually cause irregularity of the skin surface and exhibit bright-to–dark red coloration. Deep lesions have a smooth surface and appear blue in color. Histologically, this tumor exhibits vessels with large vascular lumens and thick walls (Fig. 27–15).

Cavernous hemangiomas of the skin usually arise independently of systemic disorders; however, the following rare associations are of note. The *Kasabach-Merritt syndrome*[21] refers to an extensive cavernous hemangioma associated with thrombocytopenia. The platelets are apparently trapped in thrombi within the cavernous spaces, resulting in purpura. *Maffucci's syndrome* consists of cavernous hemangiomas with dyschondroplasia and ossification; patients with this congenital but not hereditary syndrome are at high risk for development of chondrosarcoma. *Blue rubber bleb nevus syndrome* refers to large, soft, compressible, cutaneous cavernous hemangiomas associated with gastrointestinal hemangiomas that tend to bleed slowly and chronically.

NEVUS FLAMMEUS

Nevus flammeus is a common benign malformation of telangiectatic vessels. Present in over one-third of infants, it clinically is a large, irregularly shaped, flat pink or orange patch. Most lesions slowly involute during childhood; those that persist are called port-wine stains (or nevi).[22] As the name indicates, these lesions develop dark red–purple or even blue coloration and may be raised. Port-wine nevus usually occurs on the face or neck; when located laterally, it may be associated with other vascular malformations, such as the Sturge-Weber and Klippel-Trenaunay syndromes. The *Sturge-Weber syndrome* (oculomeningeal nevus flammeus) refers to unilateral nevus flammeus located in the trigeminal nerve distribution of the face. Ipsilateral angiomatosis of the retina and meninges may be associated with hemiparesis, epilepsy, or calcifications outlining cerebral sulci and gyri in this condition. The *Klippel-Trenaunay syndrome* (osteohypertrophic nevus flammeus) refers to nevus flammeus involving one or more of the extremities associated with vascular malformation and hypertrophy of underlying soft tissues and bones. It is generally believed that the osteohypertrophy is a consequence of venous hypertension caused by these arteriovenous fistulas.

Histologically, clinically apparent nevus flammeus is indistinguishable from normal skin at birth (Fig. 27–16). Within several years, dilated thin-walled vessels are present

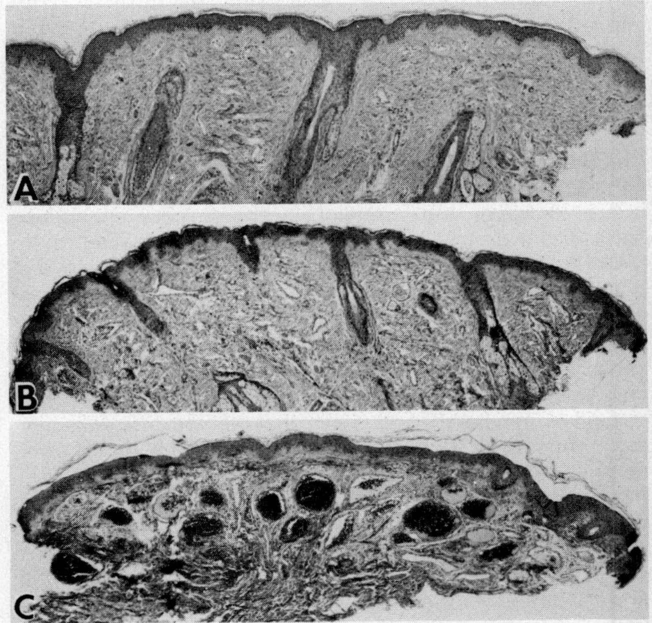

Figure 27–16. Nevus flammeus (port-wine stain). *A*, Lesion in infancy with normal-appearing vessels. *B*, Lesion in childhood with dilatation of some vessels. *C*, Lesion in adulthood with numerous dilated vessels filled with blood. (Courtesy of Seymour Rosen, M.D.)

within the upper dermis, and by adulthood, these vessels become increasingly dilated and filled with blood. Congeries of such vessels are responsible for the marked surface irregularities that characterize the older port-wine stain. Occasionally, polypoid masses develop showing the histologic features of arteriovenous malformations. These vessel changes correlate with the color changes (pink to purple) observed clinically. Nevus flammeus probably arises because of congenital weakness of capillary walls within the dermis or weakness in the supporting connective tissue, and therefore does not represent a true vascular neoplasm of the skin. It is important to recognize, however, that a small number of port-wine stains have an associated cavernous hemangioma. Argon laser therapy in carefully selected patients has provided good-to-excellent cosmetic results.[23]

KAPOSI'S SARCOMA

In its most characteristic form in the United States, this disease is a slowly progressive but malignant mesenchymal neoplasm that most commonly occurs on the lower extremities of men (male:female ratio is 10:1) aged 40 to 70 years.[24, 25] Clinically, lesions consist of red-to-purple plaques containing multiple small papules and nodules on the legs, although lesions may occur anywhere on the skin. Eventually, lesions enlarge and become coalescent to form purple-red spongy tumors that may be 7 cm or more in diameter. As hemosiderin becomes progressively deposited, these tumors acquire a brown color on clinical examination. In disseminated disease, cervical lymph nodes, salivary glands, and ocular glands are usually first involved, and hemorrhage from intestinal lesions is a common complication. This type of disseminated disease is characteristic in African children, in whom lymph node involvement often precedes cutaneous and visceral lesions. Recently, a more aggressive form of Kaposi's sarcoma has been recognized predominantly in young adult male homosexuals with the acquired immunodeficiency syndrome (AIDS) (see p. 208).

Histologically, early lesions of Kaposi's sarcoma may be extremely difficult to diagnose, resembling granulation tissue. However, the formation in anatomically anomalous parts of the dermis of angulated vessels containing endothelial cells with hyperchromatic nuclei and associated with a scant infiltrate of lymphocytes and plasma cells all suggest the possibility of an early lesion of Kaposi's sarcoma. More advanced tumoral nodules of Kaposi's sarcoma generally show (1) proliferation of small vessels lined with endothelial cells having large hyperchromatic nuclei; (2) proliferation of groups of spindle-shaped, somewhat pleomorphic cells having prominent dark nuclei; and (3) the presence of red blood cells in slitlike spaces **not** lined by endothelial cells (Fig. 27–17). Hemosiderin-laden macrophages and spindle cells are frequently interspersed with proliferating vascular and slitlike spaces. At times, Kaposi's sarcoma may resemble stasis dermatitis, other neoplasms of vessels and pericytes, fibrosarcoma, and certain neural tumors. It is generally believed that the cell of origin in Kaposi's sarcoma is a multipotential mesenchymal cell that gives rise to both the vascular and the spindle-cell components of the tumor (see p. 543).

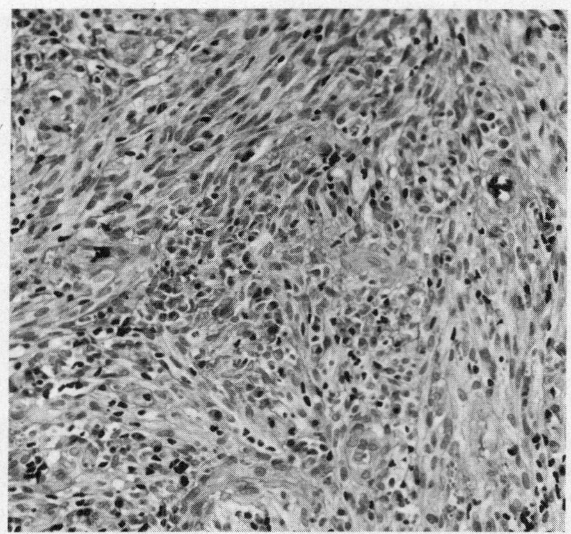

Figure 27–17. Kaposi's sarcoma, showing a proliferation of spindle cells, vascular spaces, and numerous red blood cells (darkly staining cells). The latter are present both in vascular lumina and within slitlike spaces unlined by endothelial cells.

In the U.S., Kaposi's sarcoma is an uncommon disorder, representing only 0.02% of all malignant tumors. In certain parts of Africa, however, it accounts for up to 12% of all malignancies of both children and adults. Unlike the U.S. form in which 10 to 20% of affected individuals die of the disease, the African variety frequently disseminates and has a fulminant course. In patients with AIDS, however, dissemination of the disease is more common, with a clinical course more akin to the African variety.

XANTHOMAS

Xanthomas are tumors characterized by collections of foamy histiocytes. They occur in all races and both sexes, in many cases in association with familial (p. 515) or acquired disorders leading to hyperlipidemia (e.g., biliary cirrhosis, pancreatitis, and diabetes mellitus). Xanthomas also occur in association with malignancies,[26] especially lympho- and myeloproliferative types. In many individuals, however, xanthomas arise without an underlying disorder. On the basis of their clinical appearance and location, xanthomas are classified into five principal types; eruptive, tuberous, and tendon xanthomas; plane xanthoma; and xanthelasma. To some extent, metabolic abnormalities can be correlated with the type of xanthoma.

Eruptive xanthomas usually occur as sudden showers of numerous small, soft, yellow papules that come and go as plasma triglycerides and lipids wax and wane. They occur on the buttocks, posterior thighs, knees, and elbows. **Tuberous and tendinous xanthomas** occur as yellow nodules; the latter frequently are found on the Achilles tendon and the extensor tendons of fingers. **Plane xanthomas** occur in the skin folds, especially palmar creases. **Xanthelasma** refers to soft yellow plaques on the eyelids.

All xanthomas are characterized by the presence of histiocytes with foamy or granular pink cytoplasm. Cholesterol (free and esterified), phospholipids, and triglycerides are found in these cells. The histologic picture varies from case to case depending on the number of foamy histiocytes, the presence or absence of inflammatory cells, and the degree of fibrosis. Xanthelasma, for example, characteristically exhibits foam cells with no accompanying inflammation or fibrosis.

MASTOCYTOSIS (INCLUDING URTICARIA PIGMENTOSA)

The term *mastocytosis* refers to a group of uncommon but fascinating disorders characterized by increased numbers of mast cells in the skin and other organs. The condition is manifested clinically by skin lesions, usually small brown papules and plaques; urticarial lesions may develop after trauma to these sites. It is believed that release of chemical mediators from mast cell granules in these lesions is responsible for urticaria and flushing (two common symptoms of the disease) in patients with mastocytosis.

Over 50% of patients with mastocytosis are children and infants who develop a localized cutaneous form of the disease called *urticaria pigmentosa*. In adults, the disease may be localized to the skin or may also involve other organs, e.g., liver, spleen, lymph nodes, and most frequently bone, where both localized and generalized osteoclastic and osteoblastic lesions are present *(systemic mastocytosis)*. There is evidence that in a small number of patients the disease is inherited.[27]

Many of the signs and symptoms of mastocytosis are due to the effects of histamine, heparin, and other substances released by mast cells. Although approximately 50% of patients with cutaneous lesions are asymptomatic, others experience some of the following classical signs and symptoms: (1) Darier's sign, an erythematous wheal that occurs on firm rubbing of lesions; (2) *dermatographism*, an urticaria that occurs on firm rubbing of apparently normal skin in patients with mastocytosis; (3) *pruritus and flushing*, triggered by hot baths, rubbing, spicy foods, cheese, alcohol, and drugs, including morphine, codeine, and aspirin; (4) *rhinorrhea*, excessive nasal discharge; (5) formation of vesicles and bullae following rubbing or minor trauma of infantile skin; (6) *melena* and *epistaxis*, uncommon symptoms probably due to the anticoagulant effect of heparin; and (7) *bone pain*, due to osteoclastic and osteoblastic lesions in systemic disease.

Clinically, there are five variants of mastocytosis: urticaria pigmentosa, solitary mastocytoma, systemic mastocytosis, telangiectasia macularis eruptiva perstans (TMEP), and diffuse cutaneous mastocytosis. The last two variants are rare and will not be discussed in this section. *Urticaria pigmentosa* is the most common type and usually occurs in infancy, throughout childhood, and in young adulthood. Skin lesions are multiple and widely distributed, and consist of oval-to-round, red-brown macules and papules. The prognosis for these patients is generally good. *Solitary mastocytoma* represents approximately 10% of cases of mastocytosis and occurs at birth or within a few weeks thereafter. Consisting of one to several grouped skin nodules, these lesions are often pruritic and blistering, or flushing may be observed. Like urticaria pigmentosa, the prognosis is generally favorable. Another 10% of patients with mastocytosis have *systemic mastocytosis;* this type affects patients of all ages and is characterized by mast cell infiltrates of bone, liver, spleen, and lymph nodes, as well as skin. The course is progressive, with attacks of syncope, hypotension, tachycardia, and sometimes shock, and the prognosis is poor.

In all types of mastocytosis, the common denominator is the increased number of mast cells in the skin. In **macular** and **papular lesions,** there are increased numbers of spindle- to stellate-shaped mast cells loosely distributed in the papillary dermis. **Nodules** or **erythematous plaques** may have large numbers of tightly packed, round-to-oval mast cells within the upper to mid dermis. Melanin incontinence (loss of melanin pigment into the papillary dermis and phagocytosis by dermal macrophages) frequently occurs in lesions and is responsible for their brown coloration on clinical examination. Exudation of fluid, presumably due to excessive release of histamine, may lead to subepidermal vesicles and bullae in some lesions.

Mast cell granules are best visualized by metachromatic stains such as Giemsa and toluidine blue. Lesions in which mast cells have partially or completely degranulated (e.g., traumatized lesions) may be difficult or impossible to diagnose histologically.

OTHER TUMORS

The cutaneous tumors discussed above arise from either the epidermis or the dermis. In contrast, some tumors arise at distant sites or involve cells of other organ systems (e.g., hematopoietic system, lymphoid organs, or other viscera) and either begin in or show a tropism for the skin, so that their initial clinical presentation may be that of a cutaneous lesion. Three disorders with these characteristics are mycosis fungoides, histiocytosix X, and metastatic carcinoma to the skin.

MYCOSIS FUNGOIDES

This T-cell lymphoproliferative disorder of the skin in some cases evolves into generalized lymphoma.[28] Males are more often involved than females, in a ratio of 2:1. Mycosis fungoides may occur at any age but usually affects persons aged 40 to 60 years. The clinical course can vary from chronic (lasting up to 20 years) to rapidly progressive. One-third of patients die from causes unrelated to their disease. A minority follow a rapid downhill course after the first presentation of disease. Lymph node, hematogenous, and visceral involvement foreshadow a rapid decline.

Lesions characteristic of mycosis fungoides include **eczema-like, plaquelike, and tumor-type or nodular lesions.** Eczema-like lesions are usually seen in early phases of mycosis fungoides and consist of pruritic red, purple, or brown patches with irregular but well-defined borders. They resemble those of eczematous dermatitis not related to mycosis fungoides, but tend to be refractory to conventional therapy. Visceral involvement by mycosis fungoides is not associated with the eczema-like phase.

Plaquelike lesions develop as the disease progresses and consist of irregularly outlined, slightly indurated, rubbery plaques and nodules. The face and scalp are often involved. In the plaque stage, lymph node and visceral involvement may become evident. Despite persistent treatment, clearing of plaques is often only temporary.

Tumor-type lesions are seen in the late stages of mycosis fungoides and consist of multiple large (up to 10 cm and more across), round or irregularly shaped, red-brown tumors that are frequently ulcerated. The name mycosis fungoides refers to the mushroom-like appearance of tumor-type lesions. There is usually evidence of involvement of lymph nodes and other viscera (spleen, lungs, liver, kidney, and gastrointestinal tract) in the tumor stage.

Histologically, the eczema-like phase exhibits epidermal hyperplasia and prominent exocytosis. A loose polymorphous infiltrate of lymphocytes, histiocytes, eosinophils, plasma cells, and mast cells is present in the upper dermis around and between vessels. Findings that permit the diagnosis of mycosis fungoides include the presence of numerous **mycosis cells** in the dermal infiltrate and **Pautrier's microabscesses**. Mycosis cells are atypical lymphoid cells with hyperchromatic, markedly convoluted nuclei. Cell marker studies indicate that these cells are derived from T cells predominantly of the helper/inducer phenotype.[29, 30]

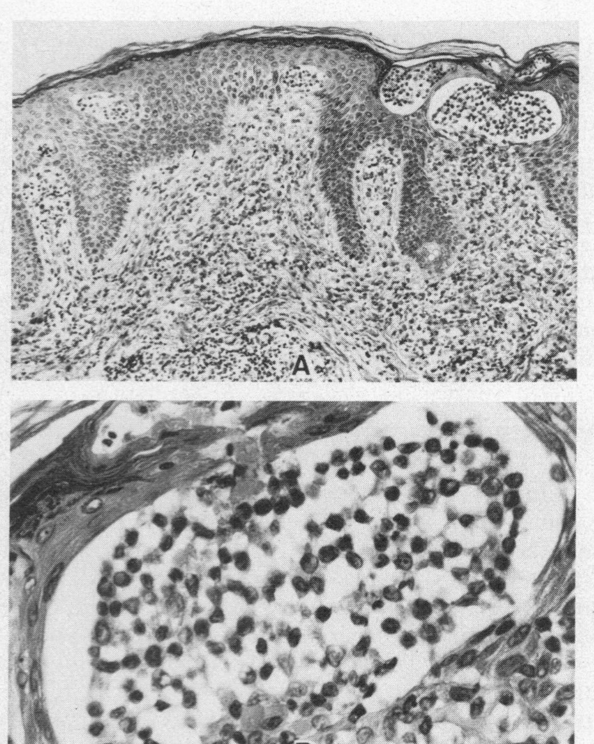

Figure 27–18. Mycosis fungoides, plaque stage. *A*, Dense polymorphous infiltrate including many hyperchromatic lymphoid cells fills dermis and extends into epidermis, forming *B*, Pautrier's microabscesses.

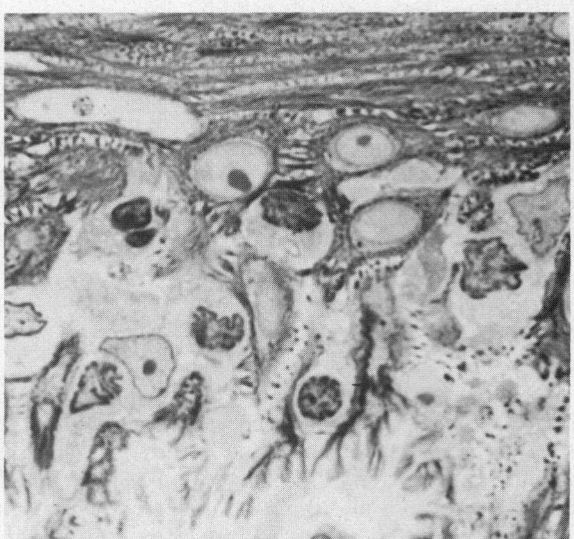

Figure 27–19. Mycosis fungoides, early (eczema-like) stage. In 1-micron thick, plastic-embedded sections, characteristic mycosis cells with convoluted nuclear contours are evident within epidermis.

Pautrier's microabscesses consist of mycosis cells located within nonspongiotic intraepidermal vesicles. Interestingly, recent immunologic studies have demonstrated that these microabscesses consist of malignant T lymphocytes clustered about epidermal Langerhans cells,[30] a relationship reminiscent of interactions occurring during antigen presentation in allergic contact dermatitis!

Plaquelike lesions (Fig. 27–18) exhibit epidermal hyperplasia and exocytosis, with the formation of well-defined Pautrier's microabscesses. A dense, bandlike, polymorphous infiltrate of the upper dermis and a perivascular infiltrate of the mid and lower dermis are typical. The number of mycosis cells is increased over that seen in eczema-like lesions and can compose 20% or more of infiltrating cells.

Tumor-type lesions may be associated with epidermal hyperplasia as in the preceding phases, but a thin or even ulcerated epidermis can be present overlying the tumor. The tumor-type lesions are characterized by extensive dense polymorphous infiltrates involving the dermis and sometimes the subcutis. Mycosis cells may make up 40 to 100% of the infiltrate.

In early lesions of mycosis fungoides, the histologic changes may mimic eczematous dermatitis (p. 1282). However, **spongiosis** is generally **not** associated with exocytosis in mycosis fungoides,[31] as is the case in exocytosis seen in eczematous dermatitis. In difficult cases, thin, plastic-embedded sections of tissue (1-micron sections) aid in revealing characteristic mycosis cells in the epidermis (Fig. 27–19). A premalignant forerunner of mycosis fungoides, parapsoriasis en plaques (p. 1293), shows some but not all of the histologic features described above, and serial biopsies over time are required to assess the evolution of this disorder.

HISTIOCYTOSIS X

Histiocytosis X has been described in detail in a previous chapter (p. 694). However, because this condition appears to represent an abnormal proliferation of Langerhans cells, its histology in the skin will be briefly discussed here. Like neoplastic T cells in mycosis fungoides, the cells in histiocytosis X are not derived primarily from the skin. Langerhans cells are believed to originate in the bone marrow, and histiocytosis X cells, like Langerhans cells, contain *Birbeck granules*. Interestingly, histiocytosis X cells also express thymocyte differentiation antigens (T6 and T4),[32, 33] antigens common to Langerhans and T cells.[3] Thus, it appears that these cells are indeed abnormal Langerhans cells. Because T cells show a propensity for migration into the epidermis, the expression of T-cell antigens by histiocytosis X cells may relate to their tendency to be found in the epidermis (epidermotropism).

Histologically, histiocytosis X involving the skin may have several patterns, all of which may show marked epidermal involvement. The first takes the form of a dermal infiltrate of large, round-to-ovoid cells with pale pink cytoplasm containing reniform and indented nuclei admixed with variable numbers of eosinophils. A second pattern is of similar cells but grouped in aggregates resembling granulomas. A third is characterized by cells with abundant, foamy (xanthomatous) cytoplasm. Variations in histology, including nuclear atypia, do not appear to correlate with biologic behavior.[34] When lesions are poorly differentiated, electron microscopy to document Birbeck granules[35] may aid in assigning a correct diagnosis.

METASTATIC CARCINOMA

Metastatic carcinoma to the skin occurs in 3 to 4% of all visceral malignancies.[36] The primary tumor can also be located in the skin itself. The breast is the most common primary site in women (63%); in men, the most common sites are the lung (28%) and colon (25%).

Clinically, metastatic tumors to the skin present as dermal or subcutaneous nodules that are firm and sometimes ulcerated. Metastases may also appear as papules or plaques and, in the case of inflammatory carcinoma of the breast, as swollen, warm, deeply erythematous areas of the skin. Sclerotic patches of alopecia resembling scleroderma are sometimes associated with metastatic breast carcinoma. Carcinoma *en cuirasse* (French, breastplate), also associated with breast carcinoma, consists of diffuse infiltration of chest skin and soft tissue by cancer cells, whereas *inflammatory carcinoma* refers to brawny induration resulting from lymphatic obstruction by tumor cells in superficial dermal lymphatic vessels (p. 1185).

Histologically, most cases of metastatic carcinoma usually involve primarily the dermis; subsequent spread upward into the epidermis and downward into the subcutis may be seen. Breast carcinoma may infiltrate the dermis in cords (Fig. 27–20) and resemble dermal nevus cells, or may elicit a marked fibrotic response resembling scar tissue. Certain tumors, however, characteristically involve the epidermis, e.g., Paget's disease associated with breast carcinoma (p. 1181). Alternatively, some forms of Paget's disease appear to arise primarily from totipotential cells of the epidermis and adnexae. In these cases the malignant cells within the epidermis often show features of apocrine differentiation, although they may at times be confused with melanoma cells, and malignant squamous cells. Paget's disease arising independent of an underlying dermal or visceral malignancy is more common in apocrine-rich, extramammary sites, such as the perineum, genital skin, and axilla.

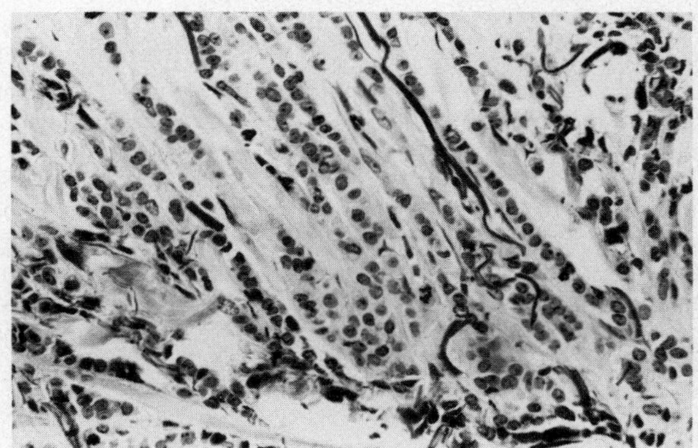

Figure 27–20. Metastatic breast carcinoma. Cords of malignant cells infiltrate among bundles of reticular dermal collagen.

COMMON DISORDERS OF PIGMENTATION

The biology of skin pigmentation is a vast and colorful subject. Description of the common disorders that follow only begins to touch upon the large number of complex pigmentary disorders that have been studied.

FRECKLES

The freckle (ephelis) is the most common pigmented lesion of childhood in light-skinned Caucasians.

Freckles are tan-to–light brown macules, varying in size from 1 to 10 mm and having slightly irregular borders. Freckles first appear in early childhood after exposure to the summer sun. They characteristically fade in winter and reappear after sun exposure in summer. Histologically, there is increased melanin deposition in the basal cell layer. Melanocytes in a freckle are larger than normal and number the same as or slightly less than those in adjacent normal skin.

MELASMA

Melasma is a masklike hyperpigmentation, commonly occurring in pregnant women; hence, its name "the mask of pregnancy."

Melasma affects the face as a large flat area of blotchy light and dark brown pigmentation involving portions of the cheeks, temples, and forehead; often the hyperpigmentation is bilateral. Apart from its association with pregnancy, melasma may occur following administration of progestational agents or hydantoins or may be of idiopathic origin in both sexes. Sunlight accentuates the areas of hyperpigmentation. Melasma associated with pregnancy often resolves spontaneously.

Histologically, two patterns have been recognized;[37] an **epidermal type** in which there is increased melanin deposition in the basal and suprabasal layers, and a **dermal type** characterized by melanin-laden macrophages in the papillary dermis. These two types may be histologically distinguished by examination with a Wood's light. This is important because melasma of the epidermal type may respond to topically applied hydroquinone.

The pathogenesis of melasma appears to relate to functional alterations in melanocytes leading to increased melanin production and transfer. These alterations may be induced in certain individuals by a variety of factors, including persistent exposure to sunlight, circulating hormones, and genetic predisposition.

VITILIGO

Vitiligo[38] is a common disorder of unknown etiology characterized by skin depigmentation. All races are affected, but vitiligo is more noticeable in dark-skinned persons and may be the cause of severe emotional stresses and (in some countries) of social and economic discrimination. It is marked clinically by completely depigmented flat patches of bizarre and irregular configuration (Fig. 27–21). The size of depigmented areas varies considerably, from inches to feet. Vitiligo primarily involves the wrists, axillae, and perioral, periorbital, and anogenital skin, although any part of the body may be involved.

Histologically, there is complete absence of melanocytes; this change can be documented by electron microscopy or sections stained for DOPA (dihydroxyphenylalanine, a melanin precursor). This is in contrast to **albinism**, in which melanocytes are present but no melanin is produced because of a lack of or defect in tyrosinase.

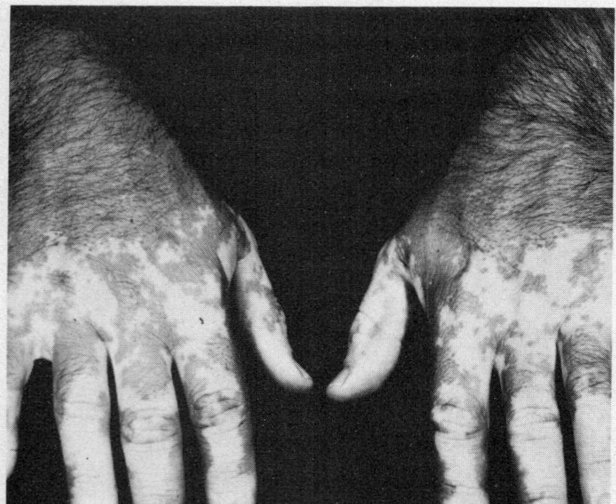

Figure 27–21. Vitiligo. The highly irregular pattern of depigmentation is associated with loss of melanocytes. The small round areas of pigmentation may represent repigmentation and repopulation by melanocytes associated with hair follicles.

Although the etiology and pathogenesis of vitiligo are unclear, there is often a family history of the condition. Theories of pathogenesis include (1) autoimmune causation, (2) neurohumoral factors, and (3) self-destruction of melanocytes by toxic intermediates of melanin synthesis. Most evidence supports autoimmune causation and focuses on the presence of circulating antibody against melanocytes and other melanin-producing cells,[39] and the association of vitiligo with disorders possibly involving autoimmune mechanisms such as pernicious anemia, Addison's disease, and thyroid disease.

ACANTHOSIS NIGRICANS

This term describes a clinical lesion characterized by thickened, pigmented skin most commonly involving flexural areas including the axillae, back and sides of the neck, groin, and anogenital areas. Any area of the skin may be involved, however, including the palms, soles, and mucous membranes, especially the oral cavity. Although this condition may at times resemble *postinflammatory hyperpigmentation*, it has distinctive clinical and histologic features.

Acanthosis nigricans may be associated with underlying benign or malignant conditions,[40] and is accordingly divided into two types.[41] The *benign type* develops gradually and is not extensive, sparing the distal extremities. It is more common in childhood and puberty and constitutes about 80% of all cases. It can occur (1) as an autosomal dominant trait of variable penetrance; (2) in association with obesity or endocrine abnormalities, especially pituitary and pineal tumors and diabetes; and (3) as part of a variety of congenital syndromes (e.g., Lawrence's, Rud's). The *malignant type* affects middle-aged and older individuals and is associated with adenocarcinoma, especially of gastric origin. Lymphoreticular malignancies and squamous cell carcinoma are less frequent associations. In more than 50% of cases, skin changes and tumor present simultaneously, but either feature alone may precede the other.

Histologically, all types of acanthosis nigricans show hyperkeratosis and papillomatosis of the epidermis, but not true thickening (acanthosis). Slight basal layer hyperpigmentation may also be present, although both the texture and color of this lesion clinically appear to result from the epidermal changes and not the increased melanin pigment.

MELANOCYTIC PROLIFERATIVE LESIONS

These include a number of commonly occurring pigmented lesions such as lentigines and nevi as well as malignant melanoma, an awesome tumor of melanocytes that is the most common fatal malignant tumor of the skin.

LENTIGO

Lentigo (nevus spilus,[42] lentigo simplex) refers to a common benign pigmented proliferation of epidermal melanocytes occurring at all ages but often in infancy and childhood. It has no sex or racial predilection, and its etiology and pathogenesis are unknown. These lesions may involve mucous membranes as well as skin, and appear as small (5- to 10-mm), oval, tan-brown macules.

The essential histologic features of lentigo (Fig. 27–22) are hyperplasia of melanocytes and hyperpigmentation of the basal layer of the epidermis. The melanocytes are disposed singly along the dermoepidermal junction. Elongation of rete ridges is also commonly noted in lentigo. In contrast, *freckles* exhibit hyperpigmentation of the basal layer but only normal or decreased numbers of melanocytes. In addition, freckles darken on exposure to ultraviolet light, whereas lentigines do not.

NEVOCELLULAR NEVUS (PIGMENTED NEVUS, MOLE)

The term "nevus" denotes any congenital lesion of the skin (e.g., nevus flammeus, p. 1269). *Nevocellular nevus*, however, specifically refers to a benign *acquired or congenital* tumor of neural crest-derived cells that include modified melanocytes of variable shapes (*nevus cells*). Clinically, nevocellular nevi generally are tan-to-deep brown, uniformly pigmented, small papules with well-defined, rounded borders (Fig. 27–23). There are numerous clinical and histologic types of nevocellular nevi, and the clinical appearance may be quite variable. For example, true *congenital nevocellular nevi* may be large and contain numerous hairs; *blue nevi*, which may be congenital or acquired, have a blue-black color that may be confused with certain malignancies of melanocytes; and the usually acquired *spindle* and *epitheloid nevi* in children are rapidly growing lesions with a characteristic pink-to-red color. The more common nevocellular nevi are the acquired type (noncongenital) that appear during childhood and early adulthood. Congenital nevocellular nevi are less common than acquired nevocellular nevi and are usually noted at birth.

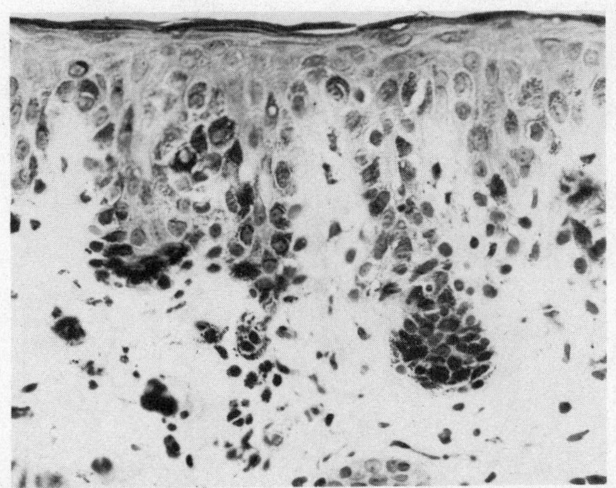

Figure 27–22. Lentigo, showing elongation of rete ridges and basal layer hyperpigmentation. Dark cells in dermis are melanin-laden macrophages.

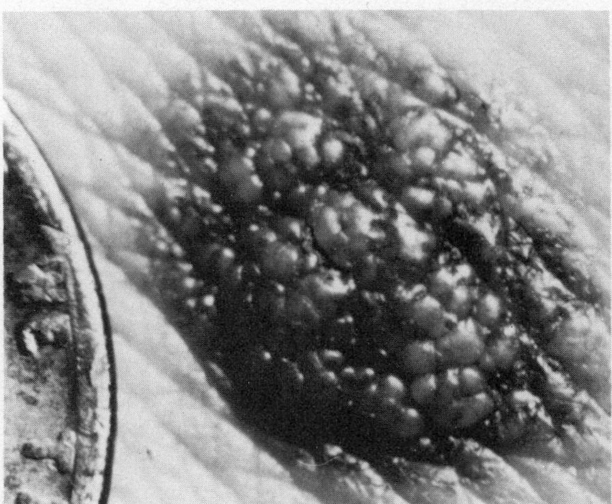

Figure 27–23. Nevocellular nevus. Lesion consists of a small, uniformly pigmented papule with regular, well-defined borders.

Histologically, all nevocellular nevi, both acquired and congenital, are composed of aggregates of nevus cells. These cells are more rounded than normal melanocytes and contain ovoid, uniform nuclei without prominent nucleoli. However, this morphologic appearance may vary considerably according to the various types of nevi, and cells may appear cuboidal, epithelioid, fusiform, dendritic, multinucleated, or ballooned. Although certain histologic variations may be more typical of acquired versus congenital nevocellular nevi, no single cell type is absolutely characteristic for either. Thus, all nevocellular nevi, regardless of their time of origin, may show considerable variability in histologic appearance.

Most nevi begin as well-defined rounded aggregates of nevus cells **(nests)** within the **lower epidermis** at the dermoepidermal junction (Fig. 27–24). Lesions with this histologic appearance are called **junctional nevi** and generally are small and flat or only slightly raised clinically. Pigmented moles on the central surface of the hands and feet and on the genitalia tend to be of the junctional type at time of biopsy.

Eventually, nevus cells begin to grow into the dermis, and when the junctional (intraepidermal) and dermal components are present together, the lesion is called a **compound nevus** (Fig. 27–25). Eventually, the junctional component is lost and the nevus cells lie exclusively within the dermis **(dermal nevus).** Both compound and dermal nevi tend to be more elevated than junctional nevi. When nevus cells grow into the dermis, they begin to differentiate into a variety of patterns. Large pigmented nevus cells in nests within the superficial dermis (type A cells) may elongate into cords of less heavily pigmented cells (type B cells) as they

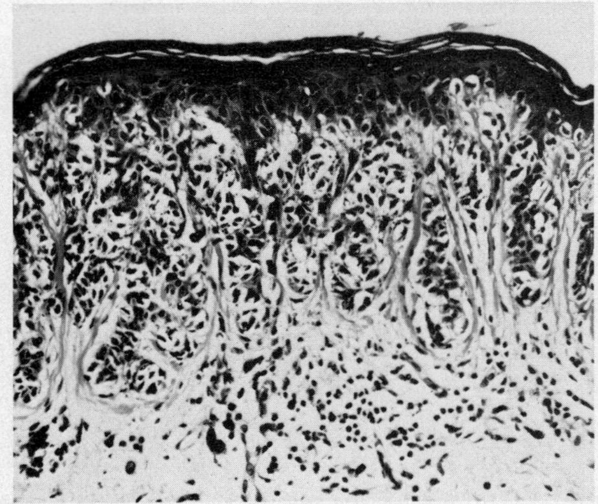

Figure 27–24. Junctional nevus. Nests of nevus cells are located in lower epidermis and at tips of rete ridges.

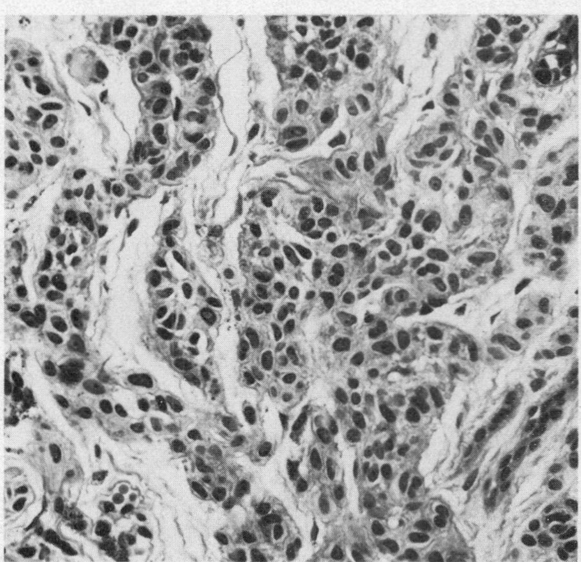

Figure 27–26. Dermal nevus, showing cordlike growth of small, uniform, round-to-ovoid nevus cells (type B cells) within papillary dermis.

extend more deeply into the dermis (Fig. 27–26). Within the deepest portion of the dermis, and particularly in older lesions, nevus cells become smaller and more elongate, and begin to resemble cells comprising neural structures (type C cells). This process, termed **neurotization,** may be dramatic, and nevus cells may be organized in such a way as to tend to recapitulate normal neural structures, such as Meissner corpuscles (Fig. 27–27). These sequential changes of nevus cells in the dermis indicate normal "maturation" of the lesion with age and constitute an important histologic indication of their benign nature.

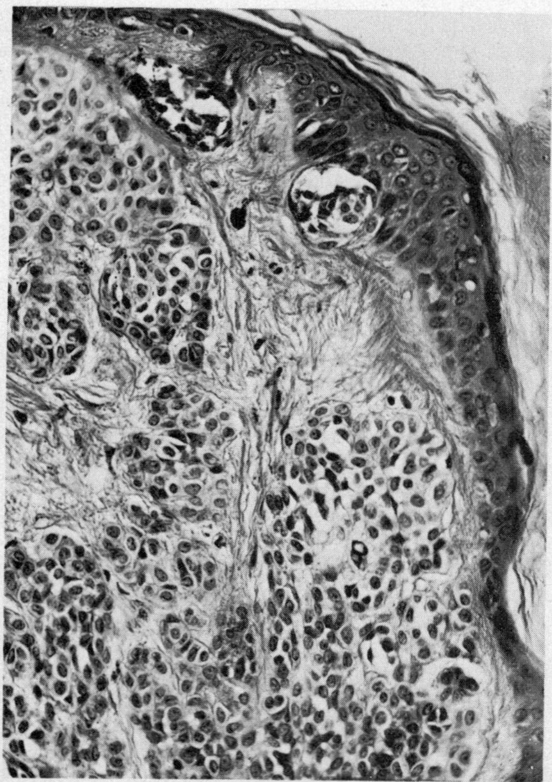

Figure 27–25. Compound nevus. Nests of nevus cells are present both at dermoepidermal junction and within dermis.

Congenital pigmented nevocellular nevi[43] vary widely in size. Some involve large areas of the body surface in a garment-like distribution (giant hairy nevi and bathing trunk nevi), whereas others range in diameter from 1 mm to several centimeters (Fig. 27–28). Unlike acquired nevi, congenital nevi have nests in the external root sheath of hair follicles, along ductular epithelium, and even in sebaceous glands and hair bulbs, in addition to within the epidermis. The nevus cells are indistinguishable from those of acquired nevi and, as lesions age, pass from intraepidermal nests into the dermis, or may be present in the dermis at birth.

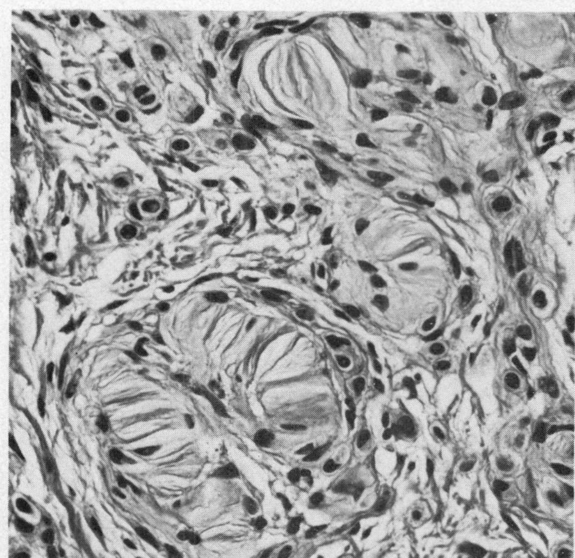

Figure 27–27. Dermal nevus cells with marked neural differentiation at deepest portion of lesion. Structures resembling Meissner corpuscles are formed by the nevus cells.

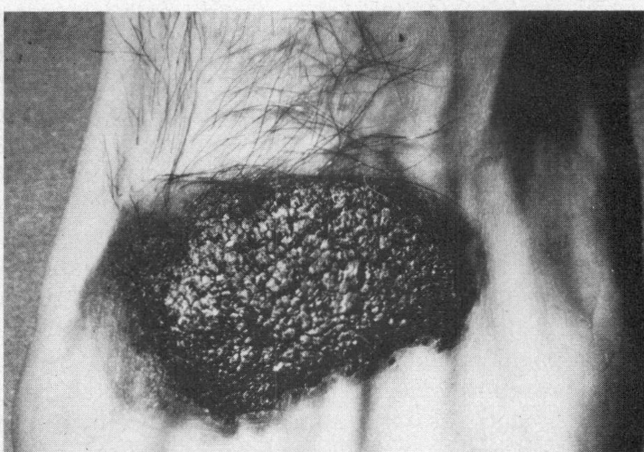

Figure 27–28. Congenital nevus of foot. The large size and animal skin–like quality of this pigmented lesion are characteristic of large congenital nevi.

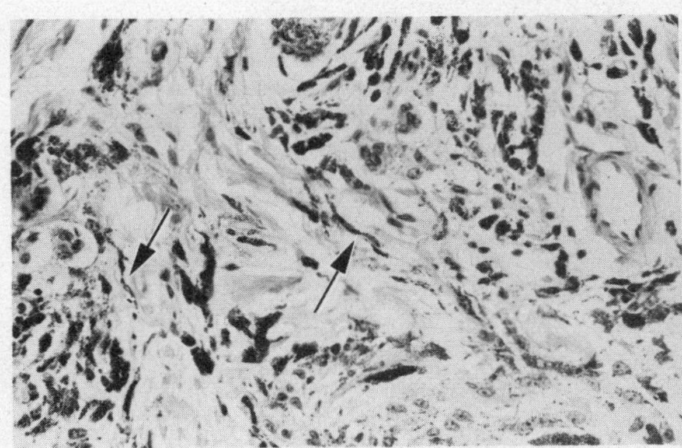

Figure 27–30. Blue nevus in deep dermis. Elongate nevus cells are characteristically heavily pigmented, and dendritic processes may be easily observed *(arrows)*.

Abnormalities and deformities of follicular epithelium, sweat ducts, and arrectores pilorum muscles are frequently associated with congenital nevocellular nevi. Nevus cells are commonly found in intimate association with neurovascular bundles within the dermis. Furthermore, nevus cells commonly extend deeply into the dermis (Fig. 27–29), may involve subcutaneous fat, and (when present on the scalp) may infiltrate the galea aponeurotica. Thus, the disposition of the nevus cells and associated structural abnormalities suggests a diffuse hamartomatous process. This characteristic of diffuse permeation of abnormal dermis and subcutis by nevus cells frequently results in difficulty in adequate surgical removal of congenital nevocellular nevi.

Specific morphologic variants of nevocellular nevi include the blue nevus, the cellular blue nevus, the halo nevus, and the Spitz nevus. In general, these specific variants are acquired lesions.

The **blue nevus** is composed of dendritic, spindle-shaped melanoctyes localized in the dermis. These dendritic melanocytes (blue nevus cells) have slender cytoplasmic processes and contain fine melanin granules. They are often associated with melanin-laden macrophages in a sclerotic dermis (Fig. 27–30).

The **cellular blue nevus** shows a biphasic cell population of melanin-laden dendritic blue nevus cells alternating with whorled bundles of spindle cells occurring in the dermis and subcutaneous fat. Macrophages are usually numerous. Clinically, the cellular blue nevus is a dark plaque or nodule that usually occurs on the buttock or sacrococcygeal area.

The **halo nevus** appears clinically as a central pigmented mole with a peripheral halo of depigmented (and sometimes erythematous) skin (Fig. 27–31). Histologically, the central mole shows nevus cells with abundant eosinophilic cytoplasm and large nuclei intimately admixed with lymphocytes, histiocytes, and melanophages (Fig. 27–32). The halo is characterized by absence of pigmentation and of melanocytes.

The **Spitz nevus** (spindle and epithelioid cell nevus) is composed of spindle and epithelioid cells located predominantly in the dermis (Fig. 27–33). These cells are often highly infiltrative, but unlike melanoma, are arranged in discrete fascicles in which nevus cells appear to "rain down" into the dermis. Mitoses are sometimes present in the Spitz nevus, whereas they are extremely rare in the dermal components of other nevi. Large atypical cells and multinucleate cells may be prominent.

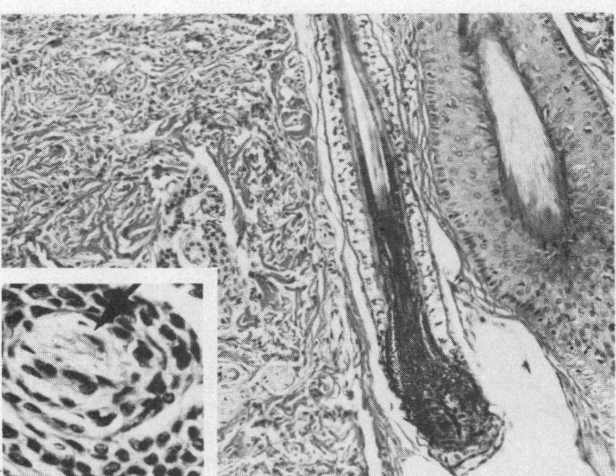

Figure 27–29. Congenital nevocellular nevus. Reticular dermis is permeated by small nevus cells that surround appendages and small nerve twigs *(inset)*.

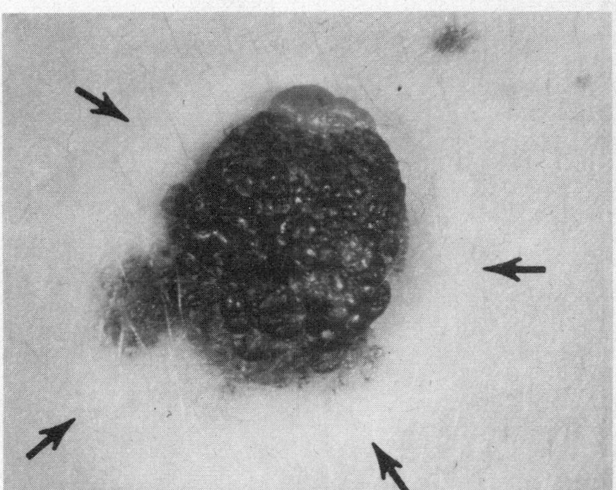

Figure 27–31. Halo nevus. Central pigmented mole is surrounded by a hypopigmented rim *(arrows)*. Because of hypopigmentation, the borders of these benign lesions may become irregular in contour.

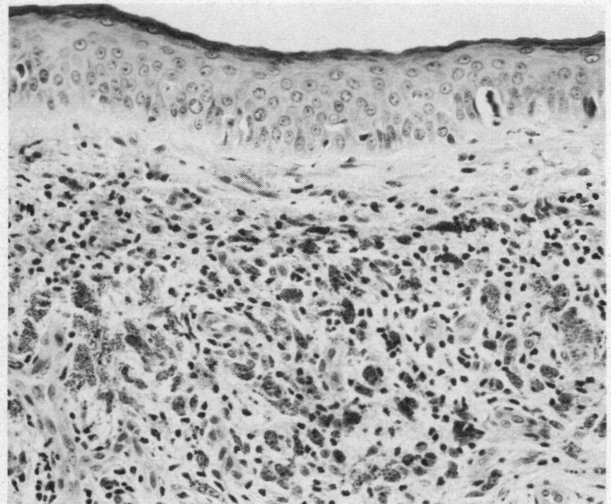

Figure 27–32. Halo nevus. Superficial dermis contains numerous lymphocytes, melanin-laden macrophages, and rare residual nevus cells.

The presence of dermal mitoses and nuclear atypism may invoke the possibility of melanoma, but the Spitz nevus (once termed "juvenile melanoma") is clearly benign. Clinically, the Spitz nevus appears as a pink-tan papule or nodule, most often present on the face or extremities. It occurs more often in children than in adults.[44]

Relationship Between Moles and Melanomas. Having discussed the histologic range of various nevi, we can now address the question of the relationship between nevi and malignant melanoma. Moles are very frequent; malignant melanoma is uncommon so that, at worst, malignant transformation of common moles must be very rare. However, some relationship is suggested by the fact that between 20 and 40% of patients with malignant melanoma have evidence histologically of an associated nevus. It would, therefore, be of interest to determine which of the histologic types of nevi are more likely to undergo malignant transformation.[45] It is not clear whether junctional or compound nevi are more likely to undergo malignant change. Two exceptions to this, however, are certain large congenital nevocellular nevi and the dysplastic nevus (see below).

Although the risk of malignant transformation in small congenital nevi is as yet undefined, 9% to 10% of giant congenital nevocellular nevi at some point evolve into malignant melanoma. Estimates of frequency vary widely, however, and may be misleadingly high, since only those patients with congenital nevocellular nevi who develop melanoma tend to be reported. Malignant change often occurs at an early age (generally by age 10). Why congenital nevi give rise to malignant melanoma is not currently understood. It is possible that nevus cells that proliferate during fetal development may prove to be immunologically or biochemically different populations from those that evolve after birth.

One recognized pigmented nevus with a clear association with malignant transformation is the *large atypical (or B-K) mole*, also known as the *dysplastic nevus.*[45A] Clinically, large atypical moles are slightly elevated, pink-brown lesions with irregular borders and almost invariably a flat (macular) component with a diameter often greater than 1 cm (Fig. 27–34). Patients may have hundreds of these lesions; unlike ordinary acquired moles, they frequently are present on skin not exposed to sun, as well as on sun-exposed sites. Such nevi have been reported to occur as multiple lesions in families exhibiting a tendency to develop malignant melanoma (*heritable melanoma syndrome*).[46] Histologically, large atypical moles or dysplastic nevi are compound nevi with lentigo-like (lentiginous) melanocytic hyperplasia, variable atypism of intraepidermal melan-

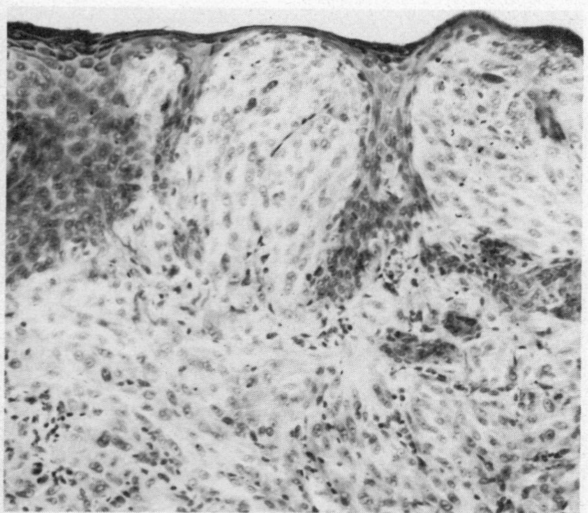

Figure 27–33. Spitz (spindle and epithelioid cell) nevus. The nevus cells are large, pale, and spindle shaped. Nevus cells tend to be arranged in fascicles and often appear to be "raining down" from epidermis into dermis.

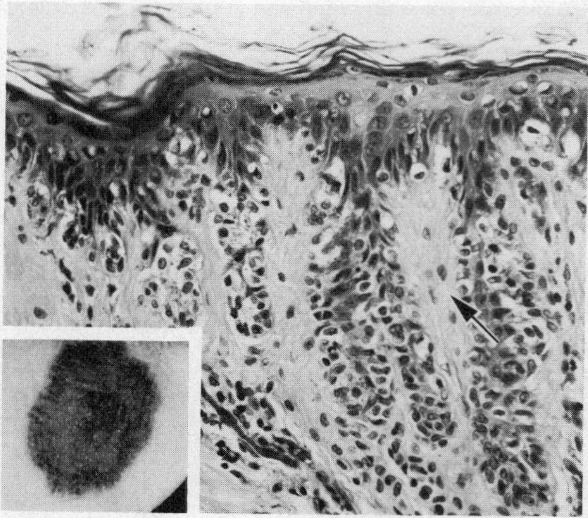

Figure 27–34. Large atypical (B-K) mole or the so-called dysplastic nevus. The lesion histologically is a lentiginous compound nevus with cytologic dysplasia of nevus cells and characteristic sclerosis of papillary dermal collagen *(arrow)*. Clinically *(inset)*, lesions are unevenly pigmented and have irregular borders.

ocytes and nevus cells, and distinctive fibrosis of the superficial papillary dermis (Fig. 27–34). Lymphocytic infiltration, vascular proliferation, and melanin pigment incontinence are frequently present in the papillary dermis. When melanoma arises in these lesions, it appears to originate from lentiginous dysplastic melanocytes. The characteristic clinical and histologic appearances of many of these lesions allow for the identification of individuals and kindreds statistically at risk of developing malignant melanoma, and careful observation of these patients should lead to the detection of melanoma at surgically curable stages.

MALIGNANT MELANOMA

Malignant melanoma[47, 48] refers to a malignant neoplasm of melanocytes and accounts for 1 to 3% of all cancers. Although the peak incidence of melanoma is between the ages of 40 and 60 years, it has been observed in every age group. This tumor occurs most often in the skin but also in the oral cavity, esophagus, anal canal, vagina, leptomeninges, on conjunctivae or within the eye. Malignant melanoma is classified into four types: (1) *superficial spreading melanoma*, (2) *lentigo maligna melanoma*, (3) *acral-lentiginous melanoma*, and (4) *nodular melanoma*.[49, 50] Each type exhibits distinct histologic features, but the following clinical observations pertain to all types.

Most melanomas apparently arise de novo, but some (20% or more, depending on the series reviewed) appear to arise in association with a preexisting benign nevus. The large atypical mole (p. 1278) and some congenital nevocytic nevi are regarded as definite precursor lesions of malignant melanoma. A small number of melanomas arise in association with xeroderma pigmentosum (p. 241) or as cases of familial melanoma. Melanoma has also been reported following trauma, as at the site of a vaccination scar.

Clinical differentiation between benign moles and melanoma is important and is possible with our current knowledge of the clinical manifestations of melanoma. The informed observer can today diagnose melanoma with a clinical accuracy approaching 90%, whereas results in a 1952 study[51] indicate accurate clinical diagnosis in only 30% of cases. Two distinct features of these lesions[52] help in the clinical differentiation–*color* and *border*. Nevi usually exhibit only shades of tan to dark brown, whereas melanomas show areas of red, white, or blue in addition to brown and black. Melanomas typically show irregular borders with notching and striking protrusions (Fig. 27–35), whereas nevi have regular, well-circumscribed borders.

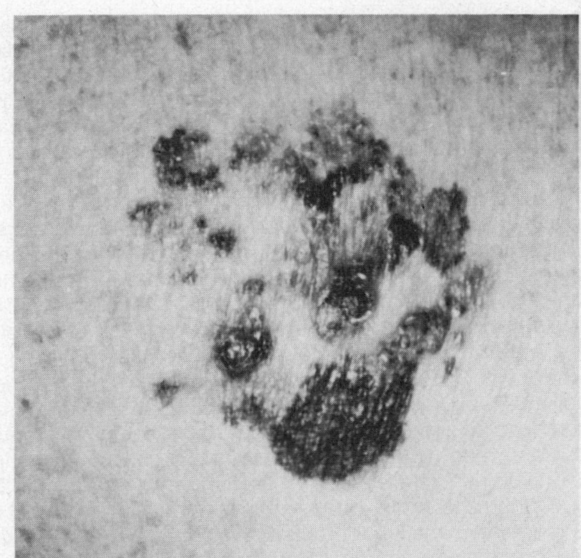

Figure 27–35. Malignant melanoma, superficial spreading type. Raised and flat areas, marked variability of pigmentation, and extremely irregular borders with notching and protrusions are present.

Fundamental to the biology of malignant melanoma are two distinct patterns of growth, **monophasic** and **biphasic** (Fig. 27–36).[53, 54] The monophasic pattern characterizes a melanocytic neoplasm that probably originates within the epidermis, but infiltrates into the papillary and reticular dermis before significant intraepidermal growth occurs. The biphasic pattern consists of an initial **radial** or predominantly intraepidermal growth phase, characterized by proliferation of malignant melanocytes within the epidermis, often accompanied by single-cell invasion of the papillary dermis; and a **vertical** growth phase, typified by formation of an expansile nodule that widens the papillary dermis and invasion of the reticular dermis and subcutaneous fat by malignant cells. Melanomas with biphasic growth patterns may exist in the radial phase for many months to years, and usually do not acquire metastatic potential until vertical growth develops. The development of a vertical growth phase is heralded clinically by elevation or nodularity in a lesion that previously was relatively flat. The level and depth of vertical growth is of prognostic significance and will be discussed in detail

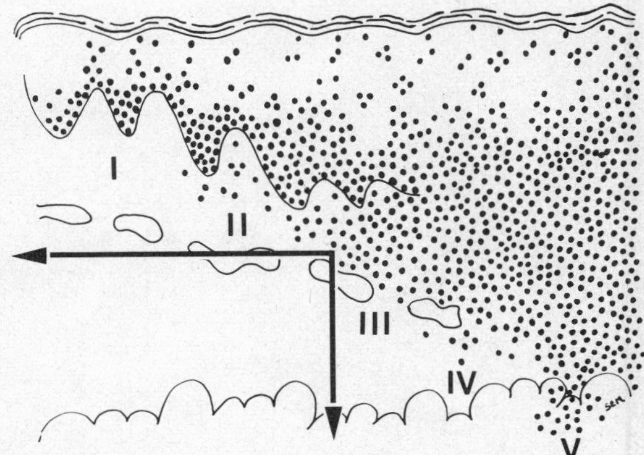

Figure 27–36. Schematic representation of growth patterns in malignant melanoma. Radial growth *(horizontal arrow)* is growth confined to epidermis with or without single cell invasion of papillary dermis; vertical growth *(vertical arrow)* is signified by filling and expansion of papillary dermis and invasion of reticular dermis and subcutaneous fat. Anatomic levels of invasion are I, malignant cells confined to epidermis; II, single cell invasion of papillary dermis: III, filling and expansion of papillary dermis; IV, invasion of reticular dermis; and V, infiltration of subcutaneous fat.

later in this section. Nodular melanoma exhibits only a monophasic (vertical) pattern of growth, whereas superficial spreading melanoma, lentigo maligna melanoma, and acral-lentiginous/mucosal melanoma demonstrate a biphasic pattern of growth. Recognition of the monophasic and biphasic growth patterns facilitates understanding of the clinical behavior and histologic evolution of malignant melanoma.

Superficial spreading melanoma occurs anywhere on the skin or mucosa, but common sites are the lower legs of women and the chest and back of men. The mean age of patients is 56 years. This type of melanoma is rarely more than 2 to 3 cm across and appears as a slightly raised nodule or plaque with bizarre coloration. Brown, black, pink, rose, gray,white, and blue colors may be observed. Irregular borders with indentations and protrusions are characteristic (Fig. 27–35). Unlike nevus cells, superficial spreading melanoma cells are large, and have abundant pink granular cytoplasm and highly pleomorphic nuclei containing peripherally clumped chromatin and prominent nucleoli (Fig. 27–37). During the radial phase of growth, which may last for many months, malignant cells grow primarily in the epidermis, forming aggregates as well as single cells at various levels of the epidermis. This single-cell invasion of the epidermis may superficially resemble Paget's disease in breast skin and is called **pagetoid spread.** Eventually, tumor cells begin to invade the dermis, filling and expanding the papillary dermis, and then extending into the reticular dermis and subcutaneous fat (Fig. 27–38). At this point, unlike tumors growing principally within the epidermis, the melanoma has acquired the potential for metastatic spread.

Lentigo maligna melanoma is a type of melanoma in the vertical phase of growth that arises in a radial growth phase called **lentigo maligna** (melanotic freckle of Hutchinson). Characteristically, lentigo maligna arises on sun-damaged facial skin in middle-aged to elderly patients. Clinically, lentigo maligna is a large (up to 6 cm or more), solitary, brown-black macule with irregular borders, and has been likened to an "ink stain" (Fig. 27–39). Lentigo maligna may grow slowly for years before it invades the dermis and becomes lentigo maligna melanoma. Histologically, lentigo maligna is characterized by linear growth of atypical melanocytes along the basal portion of an atrophic epidermis (Fig. 27–40). Unlike the situation in superficial spreading melanoma, these atypical cells extend down the external root sheaths of hair follicles, and in both radial and vertical growth phases are variable and fusiform in shape and contain pleomorphic, hyperchromatic nuclei (Fig. 27–41). Pagetoid spread into the epidermis is unusual. The vertical growth phase of lentigo maligna melanoma often shows a spindle-cell composition and may mimic malignant tumors of fibroblasts, smooth muscle, or neural elements.

Acral-lentiginous melanoma describes a variant of malignant melanoma that shows some histologic similarities to lentigo maligna melanoma, but arises in association with epidermal hyperplasia (Fig. 27–42) and often contains malignant cells with prominent dendrites. This type of melanoma also commonly involves mucosal surfaces. Acral-lentiginous melanomas usually present on the distal extremities, partic-

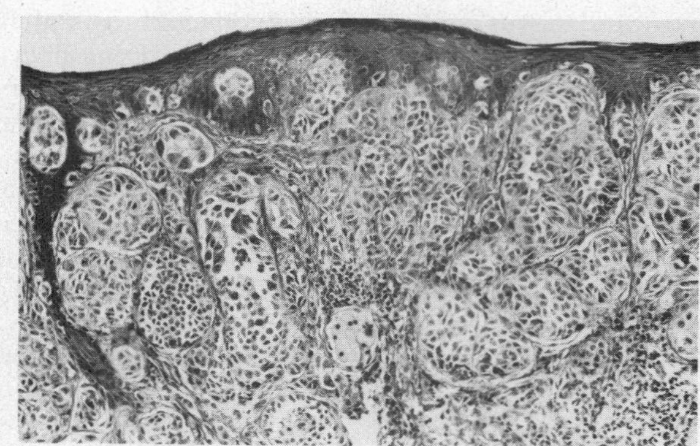

Figure 27–38. Superficial spreading melanoma, vertical growth phase. Coalescent nests of malignant cells are filling and expanding papillary dermis and invading into reticular dermis.

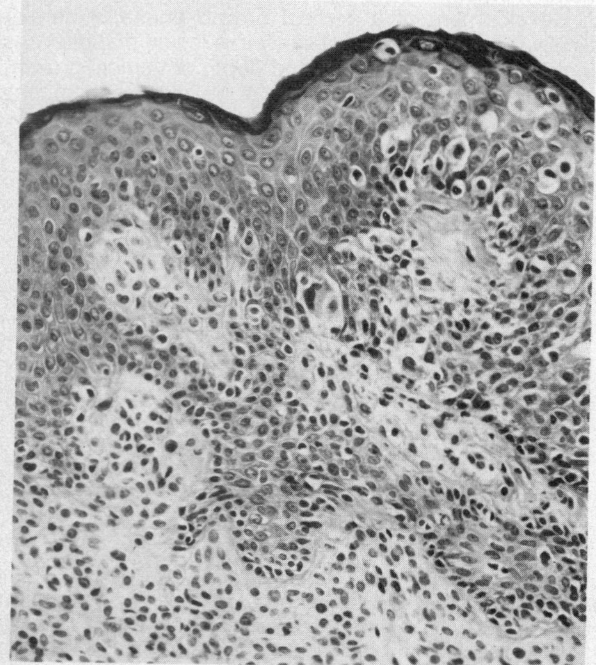

Figure 27–37. Superficial spreading melanoma, radial growth phase. The highly pleomorphic malignant cells show prominent pagetoid invasion of epidermis *(right side of picture)*. The lesion is arising in association with nevocellular nevus *(left side of picture)*.

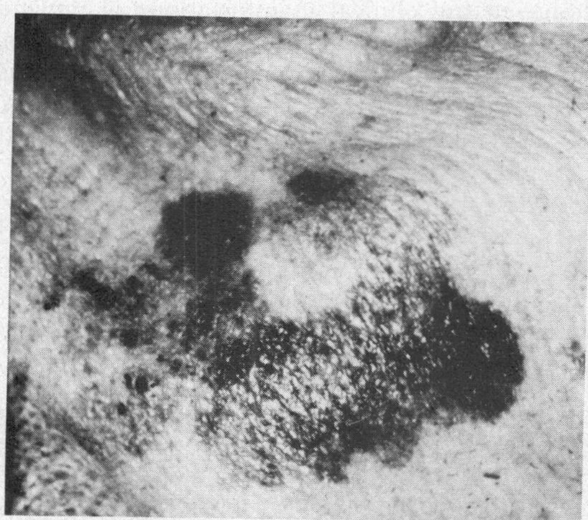

Figure 27–39. Lentigo maligna. This large macule on sun-damaged skin of cheek exhibits irregular borders and irregularities in coloration.

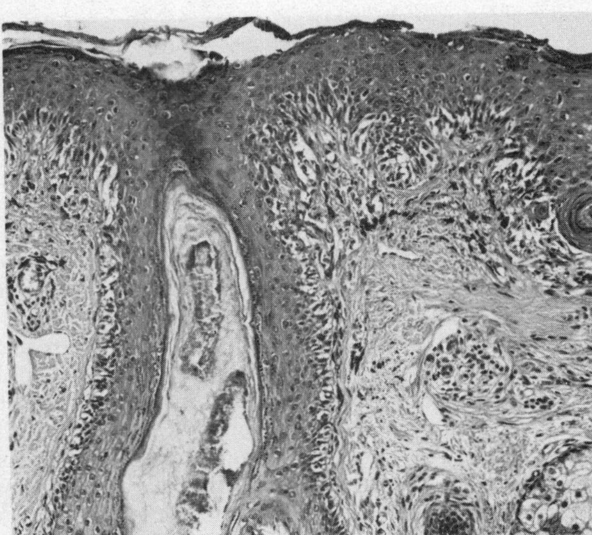

Figure 27–40. Lentigo maligna, showing pleomorphic and atypical melanocytes at dermoepidermal junction extending down along external root sheaths of hair follicles. Dermal invasion is absent.

ularly in Orientals. These lesions may go undiscovered for long periods, particularly when they occur in the web space. Unlike the other types of malignant melanoma with biphasic growth, acral-lentiginous melanomas often develop extensive vertical growth phases without becoming raised or nodular clinically. Mucosal melanomas most commonly arise on the vulva or vaginal mucosa, and account for 3% to 7% of all melanomas in women and for 8% to 11% of all vulvar malignancies.[55] The vertical growth phase of mucosal melanoma may resemble that of any type of melanoma but often shows a spindle-cell composition. Multifocal vertical growth phases may exist in one lesion.

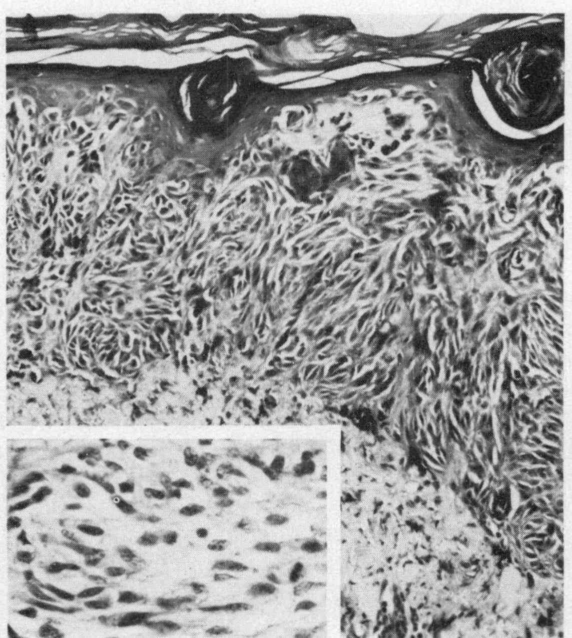

Figure 27–41. Lentigo maligna melanoma. Spindle-shaped malignant melanocytes containing ovoid, hyperchromatic nuclei *(inset)* are invading papillary and reticular dermis beneath an atrophic epidermis.

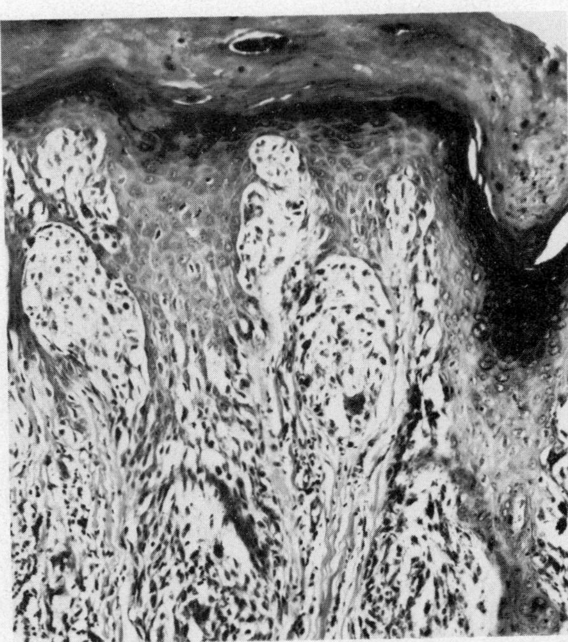

Figure 27–42. Acral-lentiginous melanoma. Spindle-shaped malignant melanocytes infiltrate from a hyperplastic epidermis into underlying papillary dermal collagen. There is relative absence of pagetoid spread into epidermis.

Nodular melanoma clinically is dark brown to black without a perceptible radial growth phase (macular hyperpigmentation at the periphery of the lesion) (Fig. 27–43). The histologic appearance most resembles that of superficial spreading melanoma, but radial or intraepidermal growth, arbitrarily defined as tumor cells exclusively confined to the epidermis for three or more rete ridges at the edge of the vertical growth phase, is absent (Fig. 27–44).

In addition to classifying melanoma by type, it is important to determine the level and depth of invasion as follows:

Level I. Tumor is confined to the epidermis. Also called "severely atypical melanocytic hyperplasia" because of its lack of potential for metastasis.

Level II. Tumor invades but does not fill the papillary dermis.

Level III. Tumor invades through the papillary dermis to the border of the reticular dermis, "filling" and widening the papillary dermis.

Level IV. Tumor invades into the reticular dermis.

Level V. Tumor invades into subcutaneous fat.

Although histologic type and level of invasion have been regarded as important in determining the prognosis in malignant melanoma, pathologists have now begun to quantify the thickness of the tumor in millimeters (measured from the stratum granulosum to the deepest extent of the tumor cells in the dermis, excluding extension down periappendageal adventitial collagen).[56] This has become regarded as another important indicator of prognosis. In general, tumors that have acquired a vertical growth phase acquire the potential for metastatic spread; this potential is related to the level and measured depth of invasion of the tumor cells within the dermis: the greater the level and depth of invasion, the greater the risk. Recent data suggest that combinations of

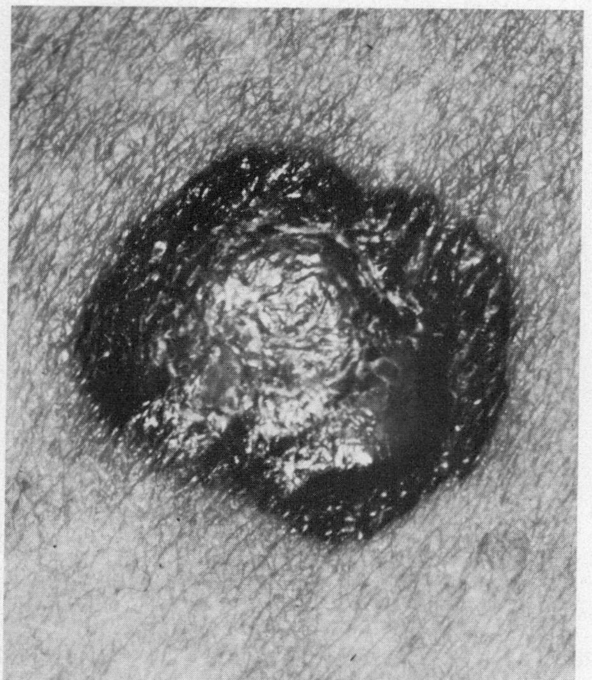

Figure 27–43. Malignant melanoma, nodular type. This nodule exhibits highly variable pigmentation with intense coloration. Irregular erythema of adjacent skin is also present, but macular pigmentation corresponding to a radial growth phase is absent.

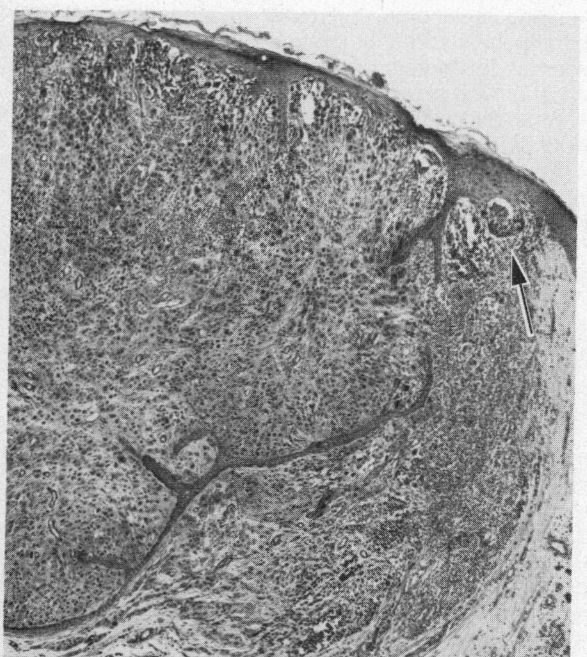

Figure 27–44. Nodular malignant melanoma. Monophasic growth pattern is evidenced by absence of significant intraepidermal spread at edge of vertical growth phase *(arrow)*.

other variables may also be of significance.[57] These variables include anatomic site of the primary tumor, mitotic rate of tumor cells, presence of epidermal ulceration, separate nodules of tumor within the dermis ("microscopic satellites"), lymphocytic response to the tumor, and morphology of the melanoma cells in the vertical phase of growth.

Management of malignant melanoma includes complete surgical excision and microscopic assessment of type, level, depth, and other pertinent prognostic variables. Early recognition is essential to successful treatment because melanoma in its early phase is virtually curable by complete excision. When metastases occur, they first involve the regional and then distal lymph nodes, but hematogenous metastases also occur, resulting in spread to virtually every internal organ.

Extensive regional disease and metastases can be treated by systemic chemotherapy, regional perfusion with cytotoxic drugs, and/or immunotherapy.

INFLAMMATORY DERMATOSES OF PROBABLE HYPERSENSITIVITY ORIGIN

Individual disorders in this important category of dermatologic diseases are classified by a combination of clinical features and gross and microscopic morphology. It should be noted that each entity is less a specific disease than a characteristic pattern of inflammation in the skin, probably immunologically mediated, and associated with diverse etiologic agents. A causative agent is often difficult to identify. Nevertheless, the diagnosis of a disorder of this group is a signal that an underlying etiologic agent should be sought.

ECZEMATOUS DERMATITIS

Eczematous dermatitis refers to a very common and large category of skin lesions characterized by severe pruritus and distinctive gross and microscopic features. One-third of all patients coming to dermatology clinics are seeking relief from the persistent discomfort of eczematous dermatitis.

Because so many types of eczematous dermatitis exist, clinical classification is based on etiology. The most common types include (1) contact dermatitis; (2) atopic dermatitis;[58–61] (3) lichen simplex chronicus; (4) drug-related eczematous dermatitis; (5) photoeczematous dermatitis; and (6) one form of erythroderma. For a summary of the clinicopathologic features of these conditions, see Table 27–1.

When the etiology is unknown, lesions are classified according to distribution, clinical appearance, and history of associated diseases. Histologically, there are only three categories: acute, subacute, and chronic. Microscopic evaluation can suggest causative agents or processes but may not reveal etiology.

The term "eczema," derived from the Greek word meaning "to boil over," vividly describes the clinical appearance

Table 27–1. CLASSIFICATION OF ECZEMATOUS DERMATITIS

Type	Etiology and/or Pathogenesis	Histology	Clinical Features
Contact dermatitis	Topically applied chemicals. Two types of pathogenesis: primary irritant and delayed hypersensitivity	Acute, subacute, and chronic	Marked itching and/or burning. Primary irritant damages without antecedent exposure. Allergic contact usually requires antecedent exposure
Atopic dermatitis	Unknown, may be heritable	Acute in infancy; subacute and chronic in children and adults	Erythematous plaques in flexural areas. Family history of eczema, hay fever, or asthma
Lichen simplex chronicus	Hereditary predisposition, seems induced by repeated rubbing or picking	Chronic; perineural fibrosis and hyperplasia of nerves observed in fibrotic dermis	Lichenified plaques; dry, scaly papules
Drug-related eczematous dermatitis	Systemically administered drug (e.g., penicillin)	Subacute; eosinophils often present in infiltrate	Eruption occurs with administration of drug; remits when drug is discontinued
Photoeczematous eruption	Ultraviolet light	Usually subacute; may be acute	Occurs on sun-exposed skin; photo testing may help in diagnosis
Erythroderma or exfoliative dermatitis	Large number of dermatoses, systemic diseases, and drugs	Subacute or chronic	Erythema of entire skin; scaling and sometimes oozing

of **acute eczematous dermatitis.** The most obvious example of such dermatitis is contact dermatitis, caused by poison ivy and characterized by pruritic, edematous, oozing erythematous plaques, often showing outright blister formation. The histologic alterations in the epidermis include intra- and intercellular edema with the formation of spongiotic vesicles and parakeratosis with coagulated serum. Within the dermis, edema and perivenular infiltrate of lymphocytes, monocytes, and eosinophils can be seen. Inflammatory cells often infiltrate the epidermis (Fig. 27–45).

Subacute eczematous dermatitis, exemplified by childhood atopic eczema, consists of pruritic, moist, erythematous, rather well-defined papules and plaques. Well-developed acanthosis and parakeratosis are present within the epidermis; vesicles are absent but focal areas of edema can be seen. Dermal changes include infiltration of lymphocytes, mononuclear cells, and sometimes eosinophils. Edema is present to a lesser degree than in acute dermatitis.

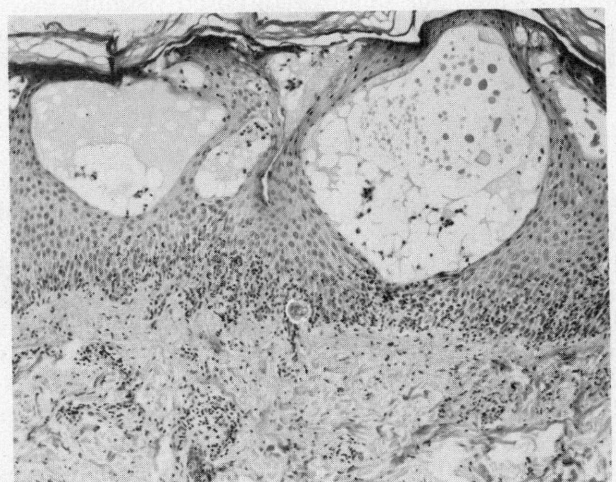

Figure 27–45. Acute eczematous dermatitis showing perivascular infiltrate that extends to lower epidermis, spongiosis (intercellular edema), and spongiotic vesicles.

Chronic eczematous dermatitis consists of markedly pruritic, dry, scaly, well-defined plaques with thickening of the skin and accentuation of skin lines (lichenification). A good clinical example of this form is lichen simplex chronicus. Epidermal alterations include acanthosis with elongation and thickening of rete ridges. Hyperkeratosis and parakeratosis are common; edema is mild or absent. There is a dermal infiltrate of lymphocytes and mononuclear cells.

Although the histologic classification of eczema implies that all types begin with the acute phase and progress to the subacute and chronic, this implication is not valid for every type. Most examples of eczema vary between the acute and subacute or between the subacute and chronic. The precise pathogenesis of each type of eczematous dermatitis is not known (Table 27–1). Although it is almost certain that contact dermatitis is partly due to a Type IV delayed hypersensitivity reaction (p. 169), the sequence of events leading to the more chronic forms of eczema is unclear. It appears, however, that the *scratch-itch phenomenon* is important in the pathogenesis of chronic changes. This vicious cycle consists of itching leading to scratching, scratching leading to lichenification, and lichenification in turn lowering the threshold for itching, and so on.

Immunologic events potentially responsible for eczematous dermatitis resulting from contact antigens include the local uptake, processing, and presentation of these antigens by Langerhans cells to T lymphocytes. Indeed, most lymphocytes so characteristic of the infiltrates of contact dermatitis are T cells. The clinical effects of therapeutic agents such as topical steroids in these lesions may in part relate to their ability to impair the function of antigen-presenting cells and lymphocytes locally in the skin.

URTICARIA

Urticaria (hives) refers to a *common disorder of the skin characterized histologically by dermal edema and clinically by itchy pink or white wheals.* More than 20% of all people experience urticaria at some time during their lives. Clinically, urticaria is classified into acute and chronic types. It can also be classified according to etiology or pathogenesis, but many cases are idiopathic. *Angioedema* is closely related to urticaria and is characterized by edema of both dermis and subcutaneous fat.

It seems likely that the final common pathway in the pathogenesis of urticaria involves localized increases in vascular permeability, with resulting dermal edema. It is now clear that Types I and III hypersensitivity reactions (p. 163) as well as nonimmunologic reactions can all lead to such increases in permeability. Table 27–2 lists the causes of urticaria according to the most probable initiating mechanism. Only a few comments on these will be made here.

In Type I immediate reactions, mast cell degranulation occurs, and histamine is presumed to be an important chemical mediator in the pathogenesis of urticaria. Antihistamines, however, fail to control urticaria, probably because other vasoactive agents, such as the kinins, leukotrienes C4, D4, and E4, prostaglandins, and acetylcholine, are also involved.

Table 27–2. CLASSIFICATION OF URTICARIA BY PROBABLE PATHOGENIC MECHANISMS*

I. Immunologic Urticaria
- A. Type I reaction, IgE-mediated
  1. Atopy
  2. Specific antigen sensitivity: Pollens, foods (nuts, fish), drugs, Hymenoptera venom, and helminths
  3. Physical agents: Dermatographism, cold, light, heat and exercise
- B. Type III reaction, complement-mediated
  1. Hereditary angioedema
  2. Acquired angioedema with lymphoma
  3. Necrotizing vasculitis
  4. Serum sickness
  5. Reactions to serum products

II. Nonimmunologic Urticaria
- A. Direct mast cell releasing agents
  1. Opiates
  2. Antibiotics
  3. Curare, *d*-tubocurarine
  4. Radiocontrast media
- B. Agents that probably alter arachidonic acid metabolism
  1. Aspirin and nonsteroid inflammatory agents
  2. Azo dyes and benzoates

III. Idiopathic Urticaria

*From Soter, N. A., and Wasserman, S. I.: IgE-dependent urticaria, angioedema and anaphylaxis. *In* Fitzpatrick, T. B., et al. (eds.): Dermatology in General Medicine. 2nd ed. New York. McGraw-Hill Book Co., 1979. Copyright © 1979 by McGraw-Hill, Inc. Used by permission of McGraw-Hill Book Company.

You will recall that *hereditary angioneurotic edema* refers to recurrent attacks of angioedema involving the skin, gastrointestinal tract, and larynx, caused by an inherited deficiency of C1 activator (C1 esterase inhibitor) that results in uncontrolled activation of the early components of the complement system (p. 210).

Nonimmunologic urticaria may be caused by substances that themselves cause degranulation of mast cells; examples are included in Table 27–2. Another postulated cause of nonimmunologic urticaria includes suppression of prostaglandin synthesis by chemicals that affect the metabolism of arachidonic acid, such as aspirin and indomethacin.

All types of urticaria exhibit dermal edema, which is manifested histologically by separation of dermal collagen bundles. A perivenular infiltrate of lymphocytes is usually present, sometimes accompanied by neutrophils and eosinophils. Usually, this infiltrate is confined to the superficial dermis where lymphatic and venular ectasia is also sometimes present. Occasionally, as in drug- or insect bite–related urticaria, deep dermal infiltrates with nuclear debris can be observed. A minority of cases show necrotizing venulitis with neutrophils, nuclear debris, hemorrhage, and fibrinoid necrosis of vessel walls.

Lesions of urticaria may occur anywhere on the body, either localized or in a widely distributed, multifocal pattern. The individual lesion is a very itchy wheal varying in size from millimeters to centimeters with a blanched center and an erythematous border. **The transient quality of individual lesions (which characteristically last no longer than 36 hours) distinguishes urticaria from other dermatoses.**

An episode of urticaria lasting less than three weeks is considered acute; one lasting longer than three weeks is chronic. Chronic urticaria indicates the need for a thorough work-up to rule out obscure etiologic agents or related disease. Urticaria does not itself constitute a threat to life, but some predisposed patients may be faced with sudden life-threatening systemic anaphylaxis (p. 165).

ERYTHEMA MULTIFORME

Erythema multiforme is an uncommon, self-limited dermatosis that appears to be a hypersensitivity response to infections and drugs; it may also be of idiopathic origin. In the average dermatologic practice, only about one of 500 patients has erythema multiforme. Persons of any age may be affected. Although the pathogenesis of erythema multiforme is unclear, association with the following conditions is well established: infections (especially herpes virus and mycoplasma infections, but also histoplasmosis, coccidioidomycosis, typhoid, leprosy, and others); the administration of certain drugs (sulfonamides, penicillins, barbiturates, salicylates, hydantoins, and antimalarials); malignancy (carcinomas and lymphomas); and collagen-vascular diseases (lupus erythematosus, dermatomyositis, and periarteritis nodosa).

The lesions are multiform, appearing as macules, papules, vesicles, bullae, or so-called *target lesions*, the most characteristic lesions of erythema multiforme (Fig. 27–46). The latter begin as red macules or papules that develop a pale, bullous, or eroded center. The lesions may be distributed anywhere on the body, although there is a predilection for symmetric involvement of the extremities.

Clinically, it is useful to classify erythema multiforme into minor (simplex) or major (multiplex) forms. In the minor form, patients have few or moderate numbers of skin lesions and minor mucous membrane involvement. More important, these patients do not have systemic symptoms and they feel well. The disease is self-limited, lasting two to six weeks. The major form (also called the *Stevens-Johnson syndrome*), more common in children, is characterized by extensive skin and mucous membrane involvement, fever, prostration, and respiratory symptoms. Typically, erosions and hemorrhagic crusts involve the mouth and lips,[62] but the conjunctivae, urethra, and genital and perianal areas may also be affected. Often, involved areas become infected, leading to life-threatening sepsis.

Histologically, erythema multiforme shows a wide range of changes that reflect the stage of clinical evolution of a given lesion or the site of biopsy within an established lesion.[63] Early lesions or the edges of well-developed lesions show a superficial perivascular lymphocytic infiltrate, dermal edema, alignment or "tagging" of lymphocytes along the basement membrane zone, vacuolization of basal cells, and rare dyskeratotic cells within the epidermis (Fig. 27–47).

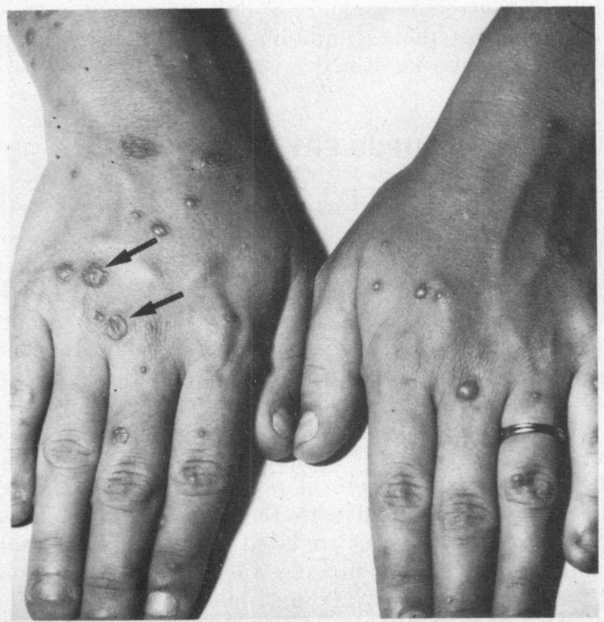

Figure 27–46. Erythema multiforme. Macules, papules, bullae, and target lesions *(arrows)* are present.

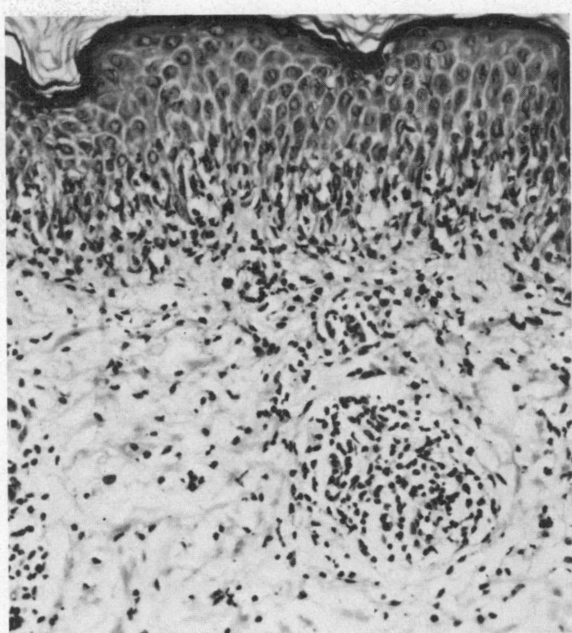

Figure 27–47. Erythema multiforme, early phase, showing epidermal dyskeratosis, basal cell vacuolization, and a lymphohistiocytic infiltrate disposed about vessels and along dermoepidermal junction.

Fully developed lesions or biopsies from the centers of early target lesions show a more prominent perivascular lymphocytic infiltrate with endothelial swelling and degeneration, striking destruction of the basal layer of the epidermis with occasional bulla formation, and exocytosis of lymphocytes into the epidermis, which frequently shows clusters of necrotic keratinocytes (zonal necrosis). In lesions associated with certain drugs, eosinophils may be present in the dermal infiltrate.

Because erythema multiforme is a self-limited dermatosis, usually lasting no more than six weeks, treatment is symptomatic and supportive.

CUTANEOUS NECROTIZING VASCULITIS

This term refers to a group of disorders characterized clinically by palpable purpura and histologically by inflammatory damage to vessel walls. As in other necrotizing vasculitides (p. 519), an immunologic pathogenesis, notably of the Type III antigen-antibody complex–mediated variety, is suspected in most cases (Fig. 27–48).

Histologically, cutaneous necrotizing vasculitis appears as partial or nearly complete fibrinoid necrosis of vessel walls with extravasation of erythrocytes and fluid (Fig. 27–49). Neutrophils and nuclear debris ("dust") are usually present in and about the walls of damaged vessels, creating the picture of leukocytoclastic vasculitis (p. 522), and fibrin thrombi may be observed. Lymphocytes and occasionally eosinophils and other inflammatory cells can be identified in the infiltrate. When vascular changes are severe, epidermal and dermal necrosis can result.

In the skin, superficial venules are involved almost exclusively so that in most cases the term cutaneous nec-

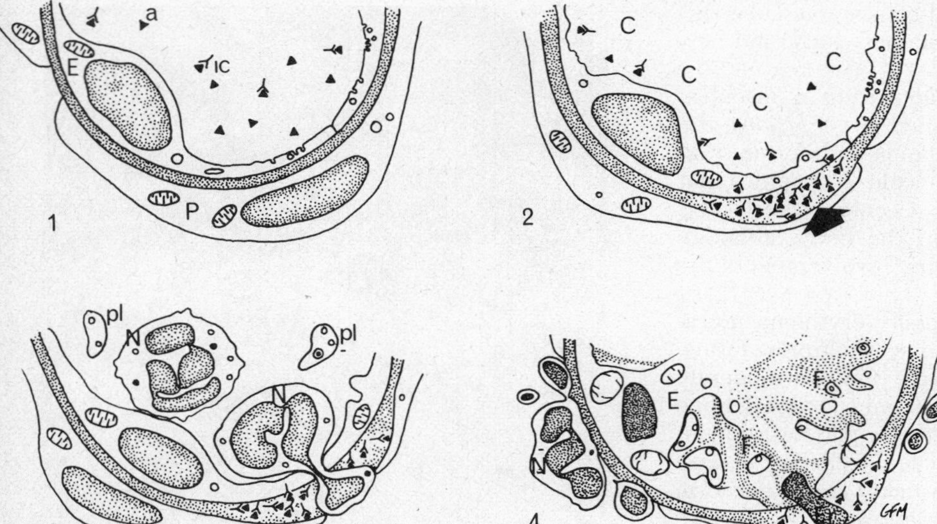

Figure 27–48. Probable pathogenesis of cutaneous necrotizing vasculitis is that (1), immune complexes (IC) form in instances of antigen (a) excess and (2), become deposited in vicinity of basement membranes of small cutaneous venules. As complement (C) becomes activated, (3), neutrophils (N) are recruited to these sites where release of lysosomal enzymes leads to (4), endothelial cell (E) damage, platelet (pl) and fibrin (F) thrombi, hemorrhage and transudation through damaged vessel walls, and fragmentation of neutrophil nuclei ("nuclear dust"). (P = pericyte.)

rotizing **venulitis** is more accurate. Arterioles are involved in rare cases. Larger and deeper vessels in the deep dermis and subcutis can also be affected, often in association with systemic vessel involvement.

Ultrastructural studies disclose the presence of partially degranulated mast cells and debris-laden macrophages, endothelial cell swelling and necrosis, as well as vascular basement membrane reduplication. Interendothelial cell gaps have been described. Immunofluorescence studies in a large number of patients show immunoglobulin and complement in and about vessels of early lesions. In Henoch-Schönlein purpura, IgA may be present in affected cutaneous vessels. Biopsies taken 24 or more hours after the clinical onset of a lesion of cutaneous vasculitis may show negative immunofluorescence, the presumed result of rapid local clearance of immune complexes.[64]

The clinical hallmark of vasculitis is palpable nonblanchable purpura, occurring in crops. They are usually present on dependent areas of bedridden patients or on the lower extremities of those who are ambulatory.

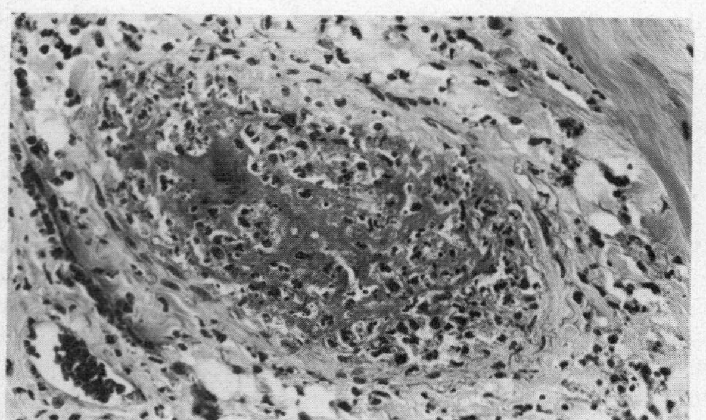

Figure 27–49. Cutaneous necrotizing vasculitis. Wall of this vessel exhibits fibrinoid necrosis and is extensively infiltrated by neutrophils and lymphoid cells. Lumen is occluded by a fibrin thrombus containing fragmented nuclei.

Lesions may affect persons of all ages. A single episode of cutaneous vasculitis usually lasts two to four weeks but may recur. Vasculitis may also present as chronic urticaria without purpura.[65] Fever, malaise, and arthralgia are not uncommon and may indicate the presence of vasculitis in visceral organs; the kidneys, lungs, joints, gastrointestinal tract, central nervous system, and other organs may be involved.

Numerous conditions are associated with cutaneous vasculitis: allergy to drugs, sensitivity to foreign protein (serum sickness), bacterial infections, viral infections (notably hepatitis B), collagen-vascular diseases (lupus erythematosus, rheumatoid arthritis, dermatomyositis), Henoch-Schönlein purpura, malignancies (lymphoma, leukemia, carcinoma), and C2 deficiency. Often, however, none of these conditions exist and an etiologic agent cannot be identified.

CUTANEOUS LUPUS ERYTHEMATOSUS

Lupus erythematosus has been described in detail in a previous chapter (p. 180). Cutaneous lesions consist of facial (malar) erythema and discoid plaques anywhere on the body surface. When the latter lesions are the only manifestation, the condition is referred to as cutaneous lupus erythematosus; such lesions may also occur in association with involvement of other organs (systemic lupus erythematosus, SLE).

Although the histology of the malar erythema of lupus erythematosus is usually nonspecific, the lesions of *discoid lupus erythematosus* have characteristic changes that correlate with their clinical appearance. Plaques of discoid lupus are large and well defined, with scaling, erythematous surfaces. Centripetal compression of such lesions may produce multiple fine wrinkles, suggesting epidermal atrophy. Zones of hyper- and hypopigmentation may be observed, and dilated tortuous vessels, or telangiectasia, are often visible beneath the epidermis.

Histologically, lesions of discoid lupus show hyperkeratosis, epidermal atrophy with loss of the rete ridges, dyskeratosis and vacuolization of the basal layer, a variable infiltrate of lymphocytes disposed in bandlike array along the dermoepidermal junction, and incontinence of melanin pigment into the papillary dermis (Fig. 27–50). Superficial vessels are often widely dilated and there is a variable degree of dermal edema and mucopolysaccharide deposition. Hair follicles may be widened and filled with keratin, and the lymphocytic infiltrate will commonly surround adnexal structures and deep dermal vessels. Infiltration of the subcuticular fat by lymphocytes, histiocytes, and plasma cells, often without significant epidermal change, is seen in a rare cutaneous manifestation of lupus called **lupus profundus**.

PAS stains frequently reveal thickening of the epidermal basement membrane in discoid lupus, although similar change may occur with aging or in chronically sun-damaged skin. Immunofluorescence of lesional skin reveals IgG, IgM, at times IgA, and complement in granular array along the epidermal and follicular basement membrane zone in most cases **(lupus band test).**[66] This granular band of immunoglobulins and complement may also be present in clinically normal, non–sun-exposed skin in patients with SLE and represents one of many criteria for establishing that diagnosis.[67] The pathogenesis of cutaneous lupus erythematosus is unclear, but many investigators believe that both humoral and cell-mediated mechanisms are involved, resulting in the immunologic destruction of pigment-containing basal cells.[68] Recent evidence suggests that the pathogenesis of lesions is related to deposition of both immune complexes and C5b–C9 ("membrane attack" complex).[68A] Whether the initial event is humoral or cell mediated is presently not known.

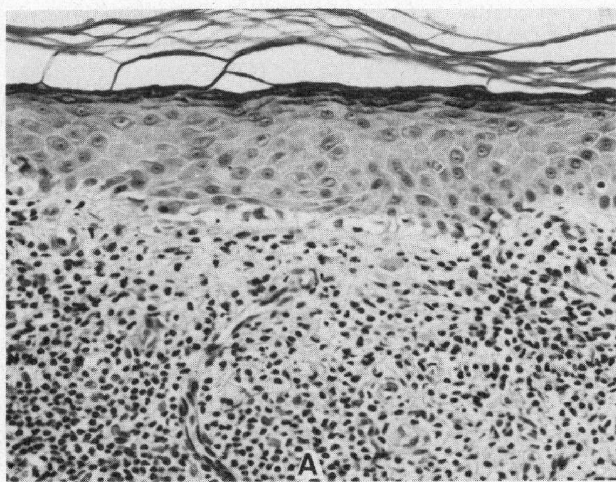

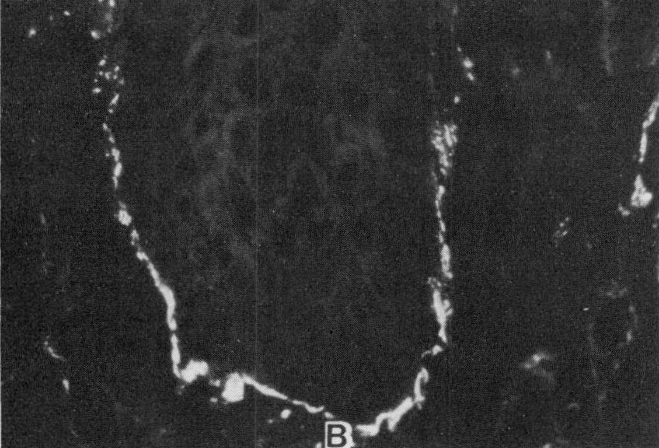

Figure 27–50. Discoid lupus erythematosus. *A*, Epidermis shows hyperkeratosis, atrophy, and vacuolization of basal cell layer; upper dermis is infiltrated by a bandlike aggregate of lymphocytes. B, Direct immunofluorescence shows an intense granular band for IgG, IgM, and complement along dermoepidermal junction.

GRAFT-VERSUS-HOST DISEASE

This disorder most commonly follows transplantation of tissue containing immunocompetent allogeneic lymphocytes to immunosuppressed individuals. These lymphocytes react against a variety of sites including skin, liver, and the gastrointestinal tract. An *acute phase* (several weeks after transplantation) and a *chronic phase* (several months to one year after transplantation) have been recognized. Although either phase may occur without the other, many patients show manifestations of both at some time during their course after transplantation. Approximately 70% of patients receiving bone marrow transplants for leukemia or immunodeficiency states develop some form of graft-versus-host disease.[69] Clinically, an extensive erythematous macular eruption is seen acutely, at times with scaling or bulla formation. Chronic lesions may resemble lichen planus (p. 1290) or show areas of dermal sclerosis and epidermal atrophy.

The histology of acute graft-versus-host disease is subtle and must be distinguished from other causes of similar cutaneous lesions in this patient population (e.g., drug reactions, viral exanthems). The epidermis generally shows disarray of keratinocytes as they progress from vertically oriented basal cells to horizontally oriented, more superficial cells. There may be foci of dyskeratosis and exocytosis of lymphocytes, which often surround necrotic cells **(satellite necrosis).** Vacuolization of the basal cell layer, focal melanin pigment incontinence, and a sparse superficial lymphocytic infiltrate are usually present (Fig. 27–51). Chronic lesions generally show more melanin pigment incontinence and either epidermal hyperplasia or atrophy. Epidermal hyperplasia is associated with a bandlike infiltrate of lymphocytes and thus resembles lichen planus. Atrophic lesions are associated with marked dermal sclerosis and entrapment of adnexal structures by sclerotic collagen, which may extend into the subcutaneous tissue. These changes resemble scleroderma.

The pathogenesis of graft-versus-host disease is the subject of intensive investigations. One possibility is that donor T lymphocytes react against histocompatibility antigens on recipient cells (e.g., endothelium and possibly Langerhans' cells and keratinocytes, in the case of skin). Other workers speculate that humoral immunity may play a role because of the finding by immunofluorescence studies of immunoglobulins and complement at the basement membrane zone and in dermal vessels in more chronic skin lesions.[70]

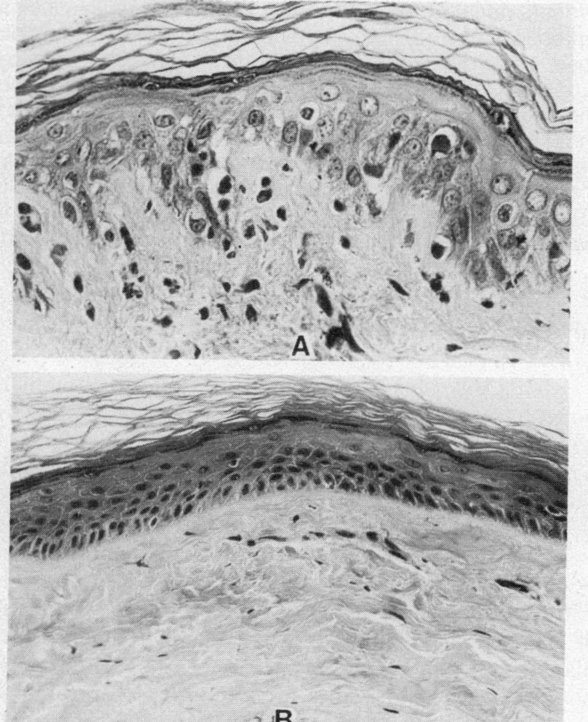

Figure 27–51. Graft-versus-host disease. *A*, Acute lesion shows abnormal epidermal maturation, dyskeratosis and vacuolization of basal cells, and a sparse superficial lymphocytic infiltrate with melanin pigment incontinence. *B*, One type of chronic lesion shows epidermal atrophy and marked dermal sclerosis (sclerodermoid variant).

PANNICULITIS (ERYTHEMA NODOSUM, ERYTHEMA INDURATUM, AND WEBER-CHRISTIAN DISEASE)

The term *panniculitis* describes an inflammatory reaction of the subcutaneous fat that may affect (1) the connective tissue septa separating fat lobules, as in erythema nodosum; (2) the septa, lobules, and vessels, as in erythema induratum; or (3) the fat lobules, as in Weber-Christian disease.

Erythema nodosum is the most common type of panniculitis and is sometimes associated with infections and drugs, but often is of idiopathic origin. The lesions are exquisitely tender, brawny, erythematous plaques and nodules, 1 to 5 cm across, that most often occur on the lower legs of women aged 20 to 30 years. Involution occurs in three to six weeks, leaving a bruiselike lesion; scarring does not result. Although pathogenetic mechanisms are unclear, erythema nodosum is commonly associated with beta-hemolytic streptococcal infections, tuberculosis, and the administration of certain drugs, especially sulfonamides. Less common associations include coccidioidomycosis, histoplasmosis, leprosy, use of oral contraceptives, sarcoidosis, inflammatory bowel disease, and malignancy.

Early histologic alterations include widening of connective tissue **septa** due to edema, fibrin exudation, and neutrophilic infiltration. Later, there is infiltration by lymphocytes, histiocytes, multinucleate giant cells, and occasionally eosinophils; focal necrosis of venules and small veins is often present. Subsequently, septal fibrosis occurs. True granulomas and large vessel vasculitis are not characteristic of erythema nodosum.

Erythema induratum refers to a type of panniculitis characterized histologically by the presence of granulomas, vasculitis, and caseation necrosis. Formerly considered a manifestation of tuberculosis, erythema induratum is today an uncommon disorder of uncertain etiology that most frequently affects adolescent and menopausal women. Cold weather initiates or exacerbates the disease. Tuberculin reactions are sometimes positive, and because of an occasional response to antituberculous therapy, the hypothesis has been advanced that erythema induratum represents a *tuberculid*, i.e., a hypersensitivity response to mycobacterial antigens.

The most frequent clinical presentation is that of either single or multiple dark red, dusky (erythrocyanotic) nodules or plaques located on the calves. Ulcerations are frequent. Recurrences are common, especially in cold weather.

Early lesions occur in the subcutis, involving both **lobular** and septal areas of fat. More advanced lesions can also involve the dermis and epidermis. Three features characterize erythema induratum: granulomas, vasculitis, and caseation necrosis. True granulomas composed of epithelioid and multinucleate histiocytes are found in multiple foci. The walls of small and medium-sized arteries and veins, as well as smaller vessels, are extensively infiltrated by inflammatory cells. Some vessels exhibit necrosis associated with neutrophils; others show infiltration by lymphocytes and histiocytes. In well-developed lesions, caseation necrosis is present in multiple foci. Mycobacteria have been identified on very rare occasions in these lesions in persons with systemic tuberculosis.

Weber-Christian disease (relapsing febrile nodular panniculitis) refers to a rare type of panniculitis characterized by distinctive histologic changes.[71] It usually occurs in women aged 30 to 60 years but can arise in both sexes and at any age. The etiology and pathogenesis are uncertain, but a hypersensitivity reaction is suggested by the histologic alterations. The disorder is usually limited to subcutaneous fat but has been described in internal fat depots such as omentum, liver and spleen, and bone marrow.

Crops of tender, slightly erythematous, sometimes fluctuant boggy nodules and plaques, often several inches wide, appear predominantly on the lower extremities and are associated with mild fever. The trunk, arms, and rarely the face may be involved. Involution of nodules is usually associated with a slight saucer-like depression.

In adults the disease is limited to the subcutis and the prognosis is usually good. The disorder subsides after several months but can last up to five years before spontaneous remission. In children the disease is frequently accompanied by high fevers and can be associated with systemic life-threatening involvement.[72]

Histologically, lobular involvement with relative sparing of septa is seen. Three stages are recognized. The **early stage** consists of marked neutrophilic infiltration of fat and focal fat necrosis. Lymphocytes and histiocytes may also be observed. This stage is relatively transient. The **intermediate stage** is characterized by the presence of numerous foamy histiocytes within and largely replacing fat lobules. In addition, foreign body giant cells, lymphocytes and plasma cells are present. This stage is believed to be the one most characteristic of Weber-Christian disease histologically. In the **late stage,** fibrous tissue replaces the fat lobule. Lymphocytes and plasma cells are often observed but foamy histiocytes are absent. Epidermal and dermal changes are usually absent in all stages of this disorder.

OTHER INFLAMMATORY DERMATOSES NOT USUALLY ASSOCIATED WITH SYSTEMIC DISEASE

The disorders discussed under this heading are usually localized to the skin and are rarely associated with a specific internal disease. These disorders, which include among others acne vulgaris and psoriasis, represent some of the most common cutaneous disorders. Although rarely a threat to life, they can measurably alter its quality. Occasionally, these disorders may be accompanied by systemic signs and symptoms. For example, most patients with generalized pustular psoriasis exhibit fever and electrolyte disturbances.

ACNE VULGARIS

Acne vulgaris is a chronic inflammatory disorder that is virtually universal in the mid to late teenage years. It is characterized clinically by comedones, papules, nodules, and cysts. Both males and females are affected, but males tend to have more severe lesions. Although seen in all races, acne is said to be milder in Orientals.

Adolescent acne is regarded as a *physiologic state.* In addition, acne may be induced or exacerbated by *drugs, occupational contactants* (cutting oils, chlorinated hydrocarbons, and coal tars), and *occlusive conditions* such as heavy clothing in tropical climates. Drugs that promote acne in susceptible persons include ACTH, corticosteroids, testosterone, gonadotropins, contraceptives, trimethadone, iodides, and bromides. Sometimes families seem particularly affected by acne, which suggests a heritable factor. Dietary factors have been overemphasized in the past.

The pathogenesis of acne[73, 74] is poorly understood. Endocrine factors have been implicated (especially androgens), because castrates never develop acne. However, simple androgen excess does not cause acne.[75] Fatty acids are also known to be highly irritating in the dermis, and it has been postulated that bacterial lipases (of the bacterium *Propionibacterium acnes*) break down sebum, liberating fatty acids, which then cause development of the inflammatory lesions of acne.[76] Inhibition of lipase production is a rationale for administration of antibiotics to patients with inflammatory acne.[77]

The lesions of acne are divided into noninflammatory and inflammatory types, characteristically distributed on the oily skin of the face (with sparing of periorbital areas), back, chest, and shoulders. Noninflammatory lesions include open and closed comedones ("blackheads" and "whiteheads"). An open comedo consists of a small flat or raised area with a central pore filled with impacted keratin and lipid; the comedo is actually a pilosebaceous follicle filled with a keratin plug. The tip of the plug is dark owing to oxidation and melanin pigment deposition into the plug (not dirt). A closed comedo pore is largely covered by epithelium; hence, it is manifested as a papule unless the skin overlying it is stretched apart. Because the impacted keratin is trapped, a closed comedo is believed to be a potential source of inflammatory lesions, which consist of erythematous papules, nodules and cysts. Cystic lesions are abscesses admixed with keratin and sebaceous material.

Histologically, comedo formation begins at midfollicle level as an expanding mass of lipid-impregnated keratin and sometimes hair. As the keratin mass expands, the follicular wall becomes thin, and sebaceous glands atrophy. The open comedo has a large patulous orifice; the closed comedo, a tiny orifice. Inflammatory lesions all show marked lymphocytic infiltration in and about follicles in the dermis; extensive acute and chronic inflammation accompanies rupture of follicles, and dermal abscesses form. Scarring follows the marked inflammation usually associated with cysts.

ROSACEA

Rosacea (formerly called acne rosacea) is a relatively common inflammatory dermatosis. The disorder is most frequent between the ages of 30 and 50 years. Women are more often affected than men in a ratio of 3:1; however, the disorder is usually more severe in men than in women.

Rosacea usually involves the central face and, in contrast to acne vulgaris, generally does not affect the back or chest. The lesions fall into three categories: vascular, acneiform, and hyperplastic (rhinophyma). **Vascular** lesions begin insidiously and consist of intermittent flushing and erythema of the face. This erythema later becomes permanent, and telangiectasia develops. **Acneiform** lesions such as papules, pustules, and cystic nodules arise upon erythematous skin. The characteristic lesion of rosacea is an erythematous papule surmounted by a pustule. **Rhinophyma** consists of telangiectasia and hyperplasia of the soft tissues of the nose (the W. C. Fields nose) and can occur independent of vascular and acneiform lesions. However, it is usually seen on a background of flushing exacerbated by alcohol abuse. Rhinophyma occurs almost exclusively in males and the affected skin is predisposed to the development of basal cell carcinoma.

Histologically,[78] the vascular lesions show a dermal lymphohistiocytic infiltrate loosely disposed about vessels of the superficial plexus. Ectasia of capillaries and venules is present. The acneiform lesion is associated with follicular pustules and perifollicular abscesses with acute and chronic inflammation and foreign body giant cell reaction. Other lesions commonly show only a lymphocytic and histiocytic infiltrate about dilated and plugged hair follicles; in some lesions, the infiltrate may be frankly granulomatous. Areas of rhinophyma exhibit hyperplasia of sebaceous glands, connective tissue, and vessels.

LICHEN PLANUS

This term refers to a relatively common disorder of skin and mucous membranes having a particularly distinctive gross and microscopic appearance. Clinically, the cutaneous lesions consist of itchy, violaceous, flat-topped papules highlighted by white dots or lines called *Wickham's striae*. The disease may present with a single lesion, but in time multiple lesions arise, varying from few to hundreds in number. They are distributed most commonly on the extremities, particularly around wrists and elbows, and occasionally on the glans penis. In 70% of cases, oral lesions accompany cutaneous lesions and appear as white reticulate or plaquelike areas.

The fully developed lesion of lichen planus (Fig. 27–52) shows three basic histologic features: (1) wedgelike hyperplasia of the stratum granulosum; (2) vacuolization and dyskeratosis of the basal cell layer, leaving residual squamous cells interfacing in a "sawtooth" pattern with the dermis ("squamatization of the basal layer"); and (3) a bandlike infiltrate of lymphocytes in the papillary dermis, closely applied to the epidermis. Small dyskeratotic and necrotic basal cells may become incorporated into the inflamed papillary dermis, where they are seen as small pink bodies **(Civatte or colloid bodies).** At times, the destruction of the basal cell layer is so severe that cleftlike spaces develop (so-called **Max Joseph spaces**) and bullous and ulcerative lesions exist clinically. Lichen planus involving the hair follicle is referred to as **lichen planopilaris**.

The etiology and pathogenesis are unknown. Immunologic studies show the dermal infiltrate to be composed almost exclusively of helper/inducer T lymphocytes, and there is hyperplasia of Langerhans' cells within the epidermis,[79] suggesting the possibility of a delayed hypersensitivity-type response, possibly to an epidermal-associated antigen.

Lichen planus usually resolves spontaneously one or two years after onset but leaves residual postinflammatory hyperpigmentation and atrophy. Oral lesions tend to last longer, and malignant change has been described but is controversial.[80] Some centers are presently employing ultraviolet light therapy in an effort to expedite resolution of lesions.

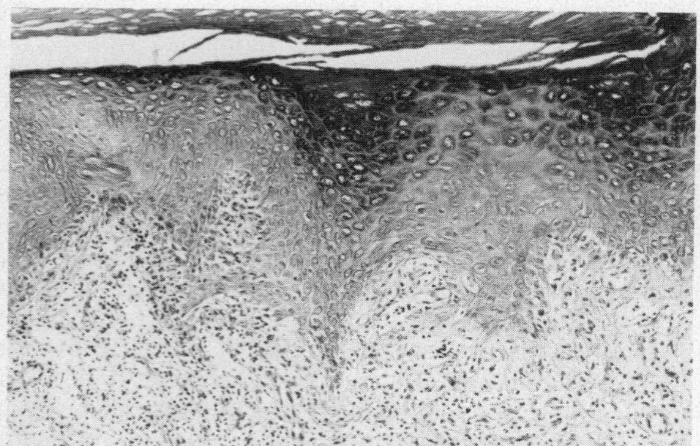

Figure 27–52. Lichen planus, showing wedge-shaped hypergranulosis, squamatized basal layer with "sawtooth" pattern of rete ridges, and a dense dermal lymphocytic infiltrate "hugging" dermoepidermal junction.

LICHEN SCLEROSUS ET ATROPHICUS

Lichen sclerosus et atrophicus[81] is a rare disorder that most commonly involves the genital area of women 45 to 60 years of age (p. 1115). In men it occurs on the foreskin and glans penis, where it is called *balanitis xerotica obliterans*. Extragenital skin in both sexes may also be involved.

Clinically, lichen sclerosus et atrophicus is first recognized as multiple, small, white macules or slightly raised, flat-topped white papules with angulated borders. Centrally there is often a depression or so-called dell. In the early stages individual lesions measure no more than several millimeters across, but with time the papules coalesce to form white plaques that show atrophy, hyperkeratosis, and plugged hair follicles.

Histologically, there is edema and homogenization of the upper dermis (Fig. 27–53). Below the altered dermis

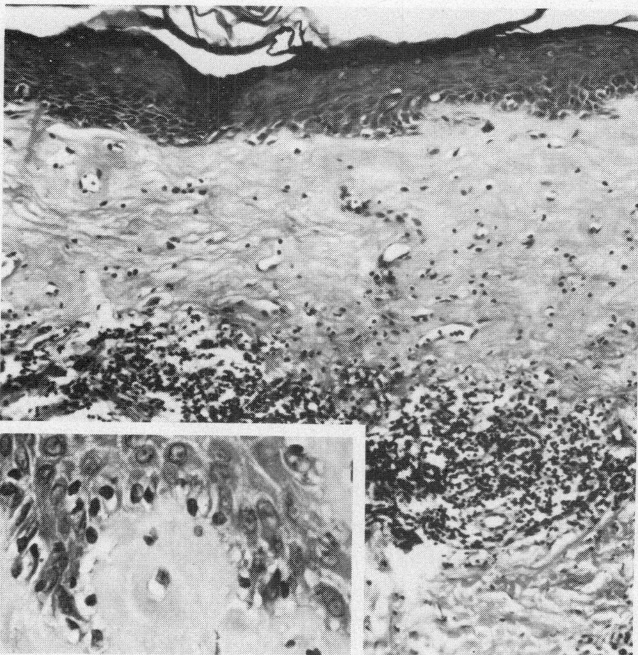

Figure 27–53. Lichen sclerosus et atrophicus. "Homogenization" of papillary dermis with an underlying lymphocytic infiltrate is evident. *Inset:* Vacuolization at dermoepidermal junction is seen in another field of the same biopsy specimen.

there is a dense lymphocytic infiltrate, which is sparse or absent in very long-standing lesions. Epithelial atrophy, hyperkeratosis, and follicular plugging also are often present.

In the vulva, labial atrophy and a narrowed introitus may develop over the course of years. In men, involvement of the foreskin and glans may impinge on the urethral meatus, causing stenosis.

PITYRIASIS ROSEA

This is a relatively common self-limited dermatosis characterized by salmon-colored oval patches with a peripheral thin scale. These are classically distributed over the trunk in a "Christmas-tree" pattern. Persons aged 10 to 35 years are most frequently affected. A viral etiology has been suspected but never substantiated.

Eighty per cent of cases begin with a "herald patch," which consists of a single, sharply defined, scaling red plaque, usually 2 to 6 cm across. Days or weeks later a generalized eruption occurs, usually on the trunk or extremities, along the lines of flexural cleavage. Individual lesions appear as round or oval, salmon-colored patches less than 2 cm across with a collarette of fine cigarette paper–like scale. The long axis of the oval lesion is oriented along lines of cleavage so that the lesions on the trunk may appear to fall in a fir-tree pattern. Successive crops of lesions develop until spontaneous resolution occurs in two to 14 weeks. Hands, feet, and face are rarely affected except in children.

The histologic features are relatively characteristic and include strikingly focal parakeratosis, mild acanthosis, focal mild spongiosis, and focal exocytosis. Dermal changes include a loose, focal, superficial, perivascular infiltrate predominantly composed of lymphocytes.

Often there is slight hemorrhage in the superficial papillary dermis. The focality of the tightly compacted parakeratotic scale suggests the diagnosis, although other disorders (e.g., parapsoriasis and PLEVA—see below) may show a similar scale pattern.

The "herald patch" is often mistaken for tinea corporis (fungus infection of the skin, p. 1300) and is usually not recognized until the generalized eruption blossoms forth. Eruptions that must be considered in the differential diagnosis of pityriasis rosea include drug reaction and secondary syphilis. A pityriasis rosea–like rash has been seen in patients receiving gold therapy, persisting as long as gold is administered, in contrast to the self-limited nature of non–drug-induced pityriasis rosea. Finally, because the cutaneous lesions of secondary syphilis can masquerade as pityriasis rosea, serologic tests to rule out lues must be performed.

PITYRIASIS LICHENOIDES ET VARIOLIFORMIS ACUTA

Usually abbreviated PLEVA, this term refers to an uncommon acute or subacute papulovesicular disorder of unknown etiology. It most commonly affects young adults, but sometimes children and the elderly also. PLEVA can last weeks, months, or even years and then remit spontaneously.

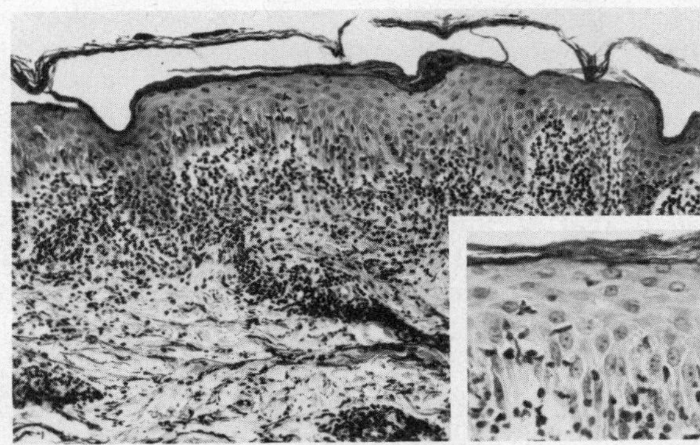

Figure 27–54. Pityriasis lichenoides et varioliformis acuta (PLEVA). Focal parakeratosis, dyskeratosis, and basal cell layer vacuolization overlie a dense lymphocytic infiltrate at dermoepidermal junction and around superficial and deep vessels. Exocytosis of lymphocytes and erythrocytes *(inset)* is a prominent feature of PLEVA.

Lesions usually involve the trunk and extremities and arise in successive crops. They begin as erythematous edematous papules 2 to 5 mm across that are later surmounted by vesicles. Vesicles can be hemorrhagic or pustular. When vesicles rupture, punched-out ulcers and necrotic areas result. Papules can also become scaly and hyperpigmented. An outstanding feature of PLEVA is that lesions in all stages (papules, vesicles, ulcers, necrotic areas, small scars) are typically present together once the disease has developed.

Histologic changes in PLEVA involve both epidermis and dermis. There is focal, tightly compacted parakeratotic scale often containing neutrophils, exocytosis of lymphocytes and erythrocytes into the epidermis, and vacuolization of the basal cell layer (Fig. 27–54). There is a superficial and deep perivascular lymphocytic infiltrate in the dermis, as well as a bandlike infiltrate in the papillary dermis. Venules may exhibit marked endothelial cell swelling and luminal obliteration. **Lymphomatoid papulosis** is a variant of PLEVA in which atypical, hyperchromatic lymphoid cells are present in the dermal infiltrate.[82]

PSORIASIS

Psoriasis refers to a group of chronic disorders characterized clinically by scaly erythematous plaques and histologically by epidermal proliferation. In the U.S., 1 to 2 % of the population is affected by psoriasis. The most common type is *psoriasis vulgaris*, whereas *pustular psoriasis* is rare. The mean age of onset of psoriasis is 27 years, but persons of all age groups from infancy to old age can be affected.

The etiology and pathogenesis are unclear. A polygenic inheritance pattern is suggested by familial clustering of cases and by higher concordance rates in monozygotic than in dizygotic twins. Known precipitating factors include trauma, infection (hemolytic streptococcal infection), and endocrine changes. In women the first onset of psoriasis sometimes occurs after parturition. However, most cases of psoriasis occur without any identifiable precipitating factor. Related to pathogenesis is the extremely rapid turnover time of psoriatic skin, three to four days compared with 28 days in control skin. Indeed, the mitotic rate of psoriatic skin exceeds that of squamous cell carcinoma. Decreased levels of cyclic AMP are also noted in psoriatic skin.[83] Cyclic AMP is normally associated with differentiation of cells.

Psoriasis is sometimes associated with disease in other organ systems. *Psoriatic arthritis*[84] occurs in 7% of patients with psoriasis. Various patterns of involvement can be seen in psoriatic arthritis, including some that resemble rheumatoid arthritis. Besides arthritis, myopathy, enteropathy, and spondylitic heart disease are sometimes associated with psoriasis.

The clinical features of **psoriasis vulgaris** are highly variable but characteristic (Fig. 27–55). Lesions may occur anywhere on the skin; frequently affected sites include elbows, knees, scalp, lumbosacral areas, intergluteal cleft, and glans penis. Nails are involved in 30% of cases. Mucosal lesions are unusual. The most common lesion of psoriasis is the plaquelike lesion, characterized by well-demarcated pink or salmon-colored plaques surmounted by a loosely adherent silver-white scale. The **Auspitz sign,** positive in psoriasis, consists of pinpoint bleeding sites revealed when the scale is removed. This sign correlates with the microscopic findings of thinning of the suprapapillary epidermis and dilation of superficial capillaries.

Plaque-type lesions may be large or very small, numerous or few. They may occur in annular, linear, gyrate, or serpiginous configurations. Bacterial flora is altered in psoriatic skin so that higher numbers of staphylococci are present. Nail changes[85] include pitting, dimpling, onycholysis, thickening, and crumbling. Characteristic of psoriasis is a yellow-brown discoloration of the nailplate that has been likened to the appearance of an oil slick. Diseased nails are often infected with Candida or Pseudomonas species.

Histologically,[86] the fully developed lesion (Fig. 27–56) shows the following characteristic features: parakeratosis, hyperkeratosis, hypogranulosis, epidermal hyperplasia with elongation and thickening of rete ridges, and marked thinning of the epidermis above dermal papillae. **The most distinctive findings in well-developed psoriasis are the spongiform pustule of Kogoj and Munro's microabscess.** The spongiform pustule refers to a focal **subcorneal** area of epidermal spongiosis where neutrophils are present in the intercellular spaces. Monro's microabscess refers to an **intracorneal** collection of four or more neutrophils. It is to be stressed that the spongiform pustule and Munro's microabscess are not pathognomonic of psoriasis, since they occur in other dermatologic conditions not discussed in this chapter (e.g., seborrheic dermatitis and Reiter's disease). Mitoses are frequent in cells as high as two layers above the basal cells. About the superficial plexus is a mononuclear and neutrophilic infiltrate. The capillary loops located in the dermal papillae show marked dilation and abnormal tortuosity; by electron microscopy, capillary walls appear attenuated and intercellular gaps are present.

The earliest changes in psoriasis have recently been described to be the exocytosis of neutrophils into the epidermis, an event that appears to precede abnormal epidermal proliferation.[87] This suggests that chemoattractants for neutrophils, either immunologic (immune complexes) or nonimmunologic (prostaglandins, activation of complement by proteolytic enzymes), may be present in psoriatic epidermis, and that the epidermal proliferation so characteristic of this disorder is a secondary repair mechanism resulting from the persistence of neutrophils in the epidermis.

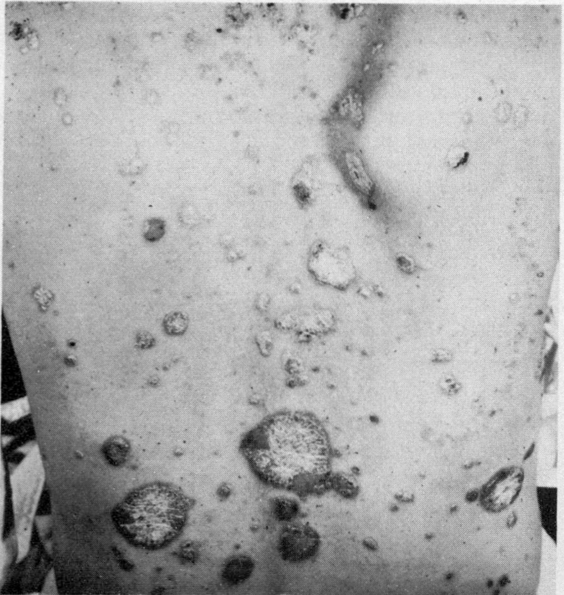

A

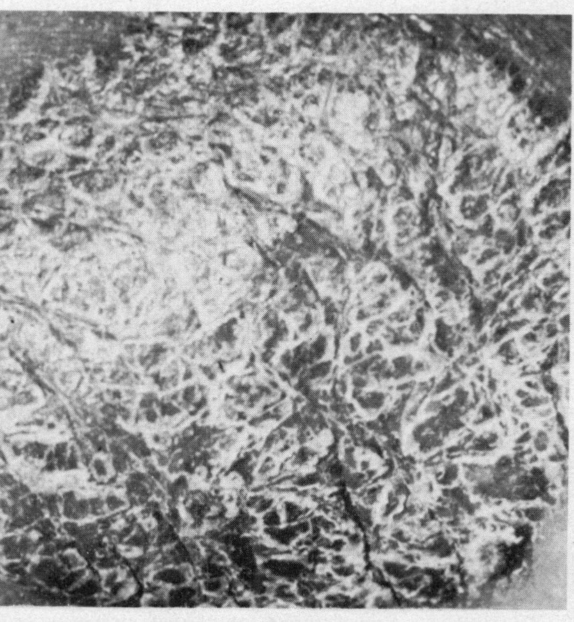

B

Figure 27–55. Psoriasis. *A*, The extensive distribution and variable size of lesions is common in psoriasis. *B*, Close-up view of a large plaque covered with characteristically "silvery" scales.

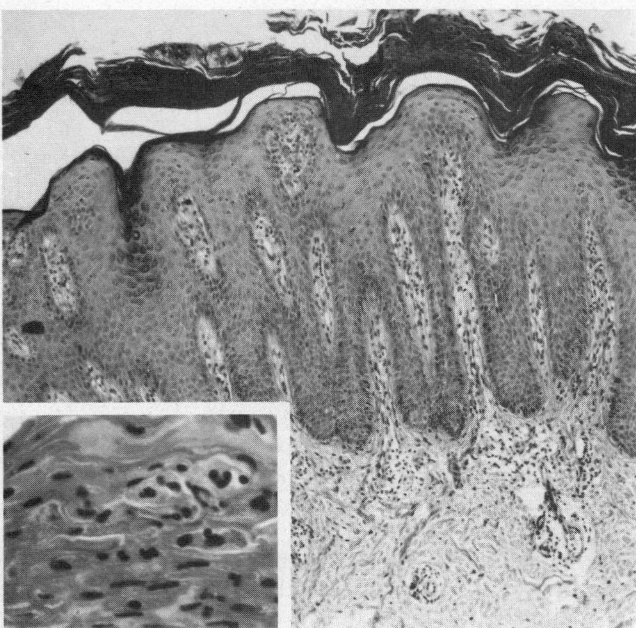

Figure 27–56. Psoriasis. Note thickening and elongation of rete ridges, hyperkeratosis, parakeratosis, and focal diminution of granular layer (hypogranulosis). *Inset:* Munro's microabscess (neutrophils in stratum corneum) characteristic of psoriasis.

Pustular psoriasis is subdivided into *localized* (primarily on hands and feet) and *generalized* variants. Morphologic changes are similar for both, although the generalized form may be a life-threatening disorder, with fever, leukocytosis, arthralgias, diffuse cutaneous and mucosal pustules around plaque-type lesions, and secondary infection and electrolyte disturbances.[88] An intraepidermal or subcorneal abscess or pustule filled with neutrophils and nuclear debris is the central feature of pustular psoriasis. At the edge of the abscess, spongiotic foci filled with neutrophils (spongiform pustules) may be observed. Epidermal hyperplasia is variable. Dermal changes are similar to those of psoriasis vulgaris.

PARAPSORIASIS

This uncommon group of chronic dermatoses is confusing for the following reasons: (1) these disorders have *no relation to psoriasis*, (2) the group consists of several biologically unrelated disorders, and (3) the clinical and histologic appearances of lesions are frequently nonspecific.[89] Nonetheless, this term has persisted so that we frequently consider benign and malignant forms of this disorder as if they were a part of a common entity.

Guttate parapsoriasis usually affects the trunk and proximal extremities of male adolescents and young adults. It is characterized by red-brown infiltrated plaques and papules, 1 to 10 mm across, with a thin adherent scale. The histologic features include focal or diffuse parakeratosis, mild-to-moderate epidermal hyperplasia, and spongiosis. There is usually prominent perivascular lymphohistiocytic infiltration with variable endothelial cell activation. The chronic clinical course (five to ten years) is characterized by periods of remission and exacerbation. Eventual permanent resolution can be expected.

Parapsoriasis en plaques of the benign type is uncommon and usually affects middle-aged men and women. The trunk and proximal extremities show round-oval, poorly-defined flat patches without infiltration. On close inspection, shades of yellow, pink, and brown may be observed. The histologic features of the benign form include focal parakeratosis, slight thinning of the epidermis, and minimal spongiosis. A slight dermal lymphocytic infiltrate is usually limited to the upper dermis. This type follows a chronic and unremitting course.

The premalignant type of parapsoriasis en plaques[90, 91] is a rare dermatosis that affects middle-aged persons of either sex. Common areas of involvement include flexural creases, buttocks, and breasts. The distribution of premalignant lesions tends to be more localized than the distribution of lesions of the benign type. Premalignant plaques appear as large lesions with thin, shiny, telangiectatic skin covered by fine scales, and exhibit patchy hyperpigmentation. Later changes that portend the development of lymphoma include a retiform or netlike grouping of red and brown, flat-topped shiny papules. A striped or variegate pattern of hyperpigmentation associated with markedly erythematous plaques and violaceous papules is also seen in late lesions of the premalignant type.

Some authors have stressed that parapsoriasis occurring primarily as small plaques generally shows a benign course, whereas larger lesions more often become malignant.

The histologic features of the premalignant type include marked epidermal thinning, focal exocytosis, and Pautrier-like microabscesses. Vacuolization of basal cells overlies a dermal bandlike infiltrate of lymphoid cells with vascular ectasia, erythrocyte extravasation, and melanin-laden macrophages. As malignancy supervenes, increasing numbers of atypical lymphocytes with hyperchromatic convoluted nuclei are recognized in the epidermis and dermis, and the picture resembles that described for mycosis fungoides.

The transition period between premalignant forms of parapsoriasis and mycosis fungoides may involve years, and serial biopsies may be necessary to assess the progression of this disorder accurately.

BLISTERING (BULLOUS) DISEASES

Vesicles and bullae (blisters) occur to a variable extent in many skin conditions such as viral infections (smallpox), impetigo, eczematous dermatitis, erythema multiforme, and lesions induced by mechanical, thermal, or chemical agents. However, blisters are the distinctive primary features of a group of diseases of

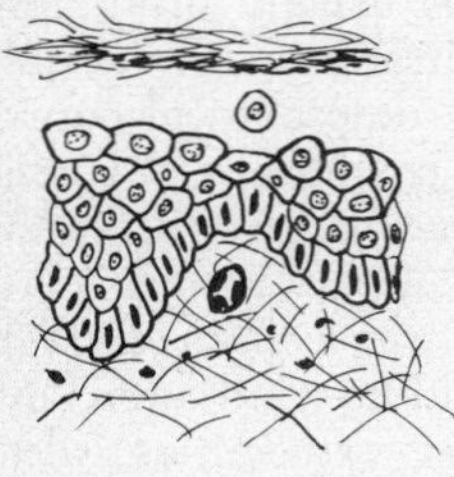

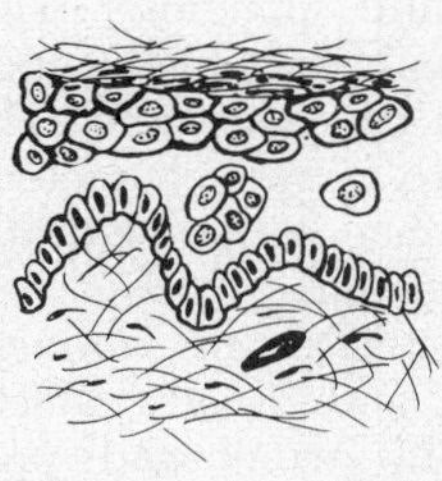

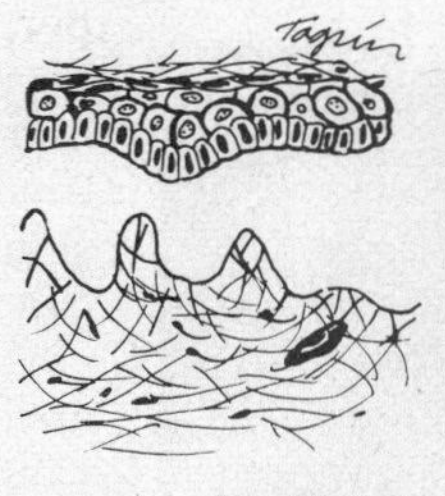

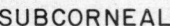

Figure 27–57. Schematic representation of sites of blister formation. In *subcorneal blister*, stratum corneum forms roof of bulla (as in impetigo or pemphigus foliaceus). In a *suprabasal blister*, a portion of epidermis including stratum corneum forms the roof (as in pemphigus vulgaris). In *subepidermal blister*, entire epidermis separates from dermis (as in bullous pemphigoid and dermatitis herpetiformis).

unknown cause referred to as blistering or bullous diseases. Among these are *pemphigus, bullous pemphigoid,* and *dermatitis herpetiformis.* Although these three diseases have distinctive clinical features, they share a number of histologic alterations and, perhaps, overlapping pathogenetic mechanisms.

The blistering disorders are the most visually dramatic of the skin diseases. The sight of vesicles, bullae, ulcerations, and peeling epidermis may be shocking to both seasoned and inexperienced observers. Pemphigus vulgaris, the most dreaded of these diseases, is uniformly fatal if untreated. The other two, though less serious, cause considerable pain and systemic manifestations. In this section we will also briefly discuss *porphyria*, a metabolic disorder occasionally associated with vesicles and bullae. Figure 27–57 is a schematic representation of the three common sites of blister formation within the skin.

PEMPHIGUS

Pemphigus[92] refers to a group of uncommon diseases of the skin characterized clinically by vesicles and bullae and histologically by acantholysis. These disorders are associated with serum autoantibodies directed against antigens in the intercellular zones of the epidermis. There are four types of pemphigus: *pemphigus vulgaris, pemphigus vegetans, pemphigus foliaceus,*[93] and *pemphigus erythematosus*, but by far the most common and the most important for the physician to recognize is pemphigus vulgaris.

PATHOGENESIS. *Acantholysis* is central to all types of pemphigus (Fig. 27–58). Very simply, this refers to a loss of intercellular connections of keratinocytes. As the cells become acantholytic, they lose their polygonal configuration and become round. It must be stressed that, although acantholysis is typical of pemphigus, it occurs in other disorders such as impetigo, herpes simplex, and zoster, but these conditions are usually easy to distinguish from pemphigus by their clinical and histologic features.

There is strong evidence that autoantibodies directed against antigens in the intercellular spaces of the keratinocytes are the cause of acantholysis in pemphigus. Immunofluorescence studies show both immunoglobulin and complement intercellularly in the skin of all patients with active disease (Fig. 27–59). Further, patient's serum contains antibodies that react with intercellular junctions when tested against the patient's own unaffected skin or against normal skin. In addition, there is a direct correlation between serum antibody titers and the severity of the disease in some, but not all, patients. Evidence of activation of the complement system in the blister fluid has also been found. Finally, steroids as well as immunosuppressive drugs not only reverse the skin lesions but also cause reduction in the titer of autoantibodies. What triggers this autoimmune reaction to the patient's own intercellular proteins, however, is completely unknown.

Pemphigus vulgaris most frequently affects those between ages 40 and 60 and usually begins as a small vesiculobullous eruption focally on the skin and often also on the oral mucosa. The lesions then spread in an unpredictable fashion to the other parts of the body, although normally rubbed or traumatized skin and mucous membranes are most likely to be affected. The bullae of pemphigus are characteristically flaccid with a tendency to enlarge. *Nikolsky's sign* refers to bulla formation induced by firm sliding pressure on the skin

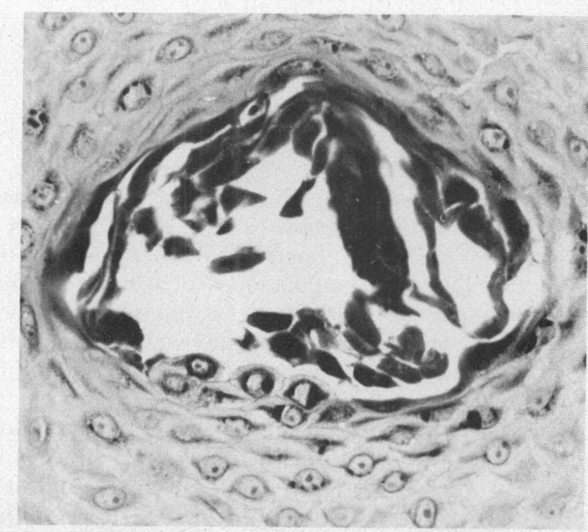

Figure 27–58. Pemphigus foliaceus. In this rare form, a blister results from acantholysis at level of granular cell layer.

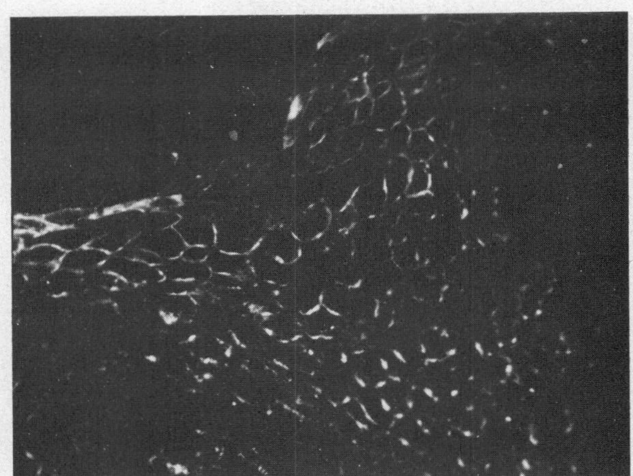

Figure 27–59. Pemphigus vulgaris. Direct immunofluorescence study utilizing patient's skin as substrate, and fluorescein-tagged antibody against IgG demonstrates intercellular staining. The uneven staining of intercellular areas is frequently observed in pemphigus.

by a finger. The bullae are transient, presumably because they are superficial (intraepidermal rather than subepidermal), fragile, and easily rubbed away. Thus, the clinical picture of pemphigus vulgaris is dominated by extensive erosions of skin and mucous membranes. The frequently tender erosions ooze, bleed, and are susceptible to infection. Occasionally, extensive skin surfaces may be denuded, resulting in serious problems in electrolyte balance similar to those occurring in extensively burned patients (p. 462).

Histologically, the earliest change consists of intercellular edema in the lower epidermis. Loss of intercellular bridges follows, leading to loss of cohesion between the epidermal cells (acantholysis) and to the formation of mid-epidermal or suprabasal clefts filled with fluid and round acantholytic cells. Basal cells are separate from one another but remain attached to the dermis, much like a row of tombstones. The roof of the vesicle may be absent if special care has not been taken at the time of biopsy, as it is easily sheared from the epidermis by the trauma associated with biopsy. Dermal inflammation is slight in early lesions and prominent in well-developed ones. Lymphocytes, histiocytes, and eosinophils may be seen in the dermal inflammatory infiltrate, and rarely eosinophils may be present in the epidermis before the development of acantholysis, a finding referred to as "eosinophilic spongiosis."

Before the availability of corticosteroid therapy, patients usually died within 14 months from secondary infection or electrolyte disturbances. With corticosteroid therapy, pemphigus still remains a serious disease, but its course has become more chronic and its mortality has been reduced to 40%.

Pemphigus foliaceus, a variant of pemphigus with a more benign course, presents as blisters that rapidly become crusted plaques. It differs histologically from pemphigus vulgaris by the presence of acantholysis that is predominantly subcorneal.

BULLOUS PEMPHIGOID

This form of blistering disease is characterized by subepidermal bullae and a chronic, relatively self-limited course.[94] Although quite rare, bullous pemphigoid is more common than the other two major blistering disorders, dermatitis herpetiformis and pemphigus. Bullous pemphigoid usually occurs after the age of 60 and is very infrequent before the age of 40.

Lesions of bullous pemphigoid can occur anywhere on the skin, but there is a predilection for the lower abdomen, groin, inner aspects of the thighs, and flexor surfaces of the forearms. In one-third of patients the mouth is involved, but these lesions are small, heal quickly, and are much less significant than those of pemphigus. The development of typical lesions of bullous pemphigoid may be heralded by one or more years of generalized pruritus in certain individuals.[95]

Histologically, early changes consist of vacuolization at the dermoepidermal junction and small collections of eosinophils and mast cells in the dermal papillae. The vacuoles coalesce to form a subepidermal bulla; within and below the bulla there is an infiltrate of eosinophils, mast cells, lymphocytes, histiocytes, and neutrophils. Epidermal regeneration begins within two days of bulla formation at the edges of the bulla and extends toward the bulla center. Acantholysis is **not** a feature of bullous pemphigoid. In urticarial lesions, which may antecede the development of bullae in some individuals, the dermal infiltrate may predominate, with the epidermis showing only subtle basal layer vacuolization.

Immunofluorescence microscopy discloses deposition of complement usually with IgG at the dermoepidermal junction in a linear pattern (Fig. 27–60) at the level of the lamina lucida of the basement membrane. Circulating antibody directed against the dermoepidermal junction is exhibited in 70% of patients.[96] It appears, then, that bullous pemphigoid may be caused by autoantibodies, but, in contrast to pemphigus, these are directed against some component of the lamina lucida of the basement membrane of the epidermis rather than against intercellular antigens.[97] A proposed sequence of events in the development of bullous pemphigoid is the deposition of immunoglobulin and complement at the dermoepidermal junction followed by degranulation of mast cells, resulting in the release of eosinophil chemotactic factors.[98] Release of proteolytic enzymes by degranulating eosinophils may then result in damage to the lamina lucida of the basement membrane zone and the formation of blisters.

DERMATITIS HERPETIFORMIS

This rare disorder of the skin is characterized by itchy papulovesicular lesions and the presence of IgA at the dermoepidermal junction.[99] Adults 25 to 50 years old are the most commonly affected group, although children may occasionally present with this disorder. In the overwhelming majority of cases of dermatitis herpetiformis, IgA and C3 are present at the dermoepider-

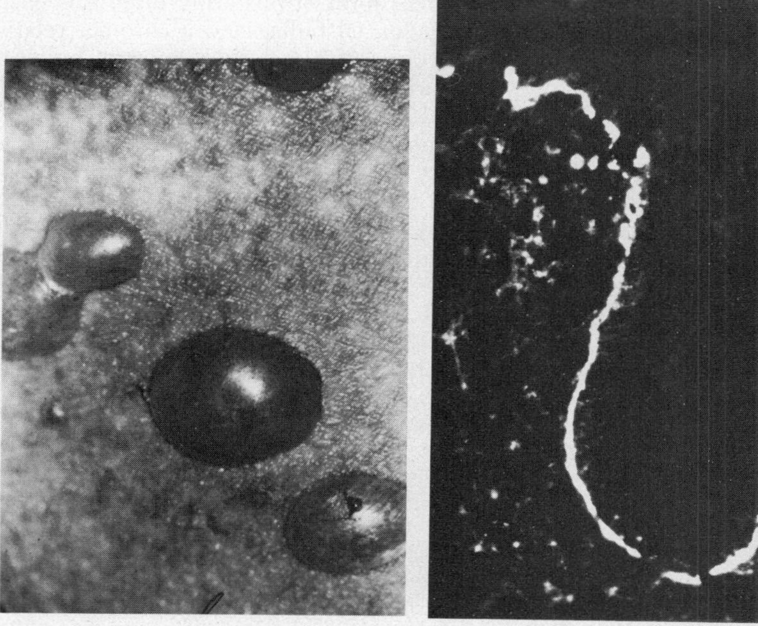

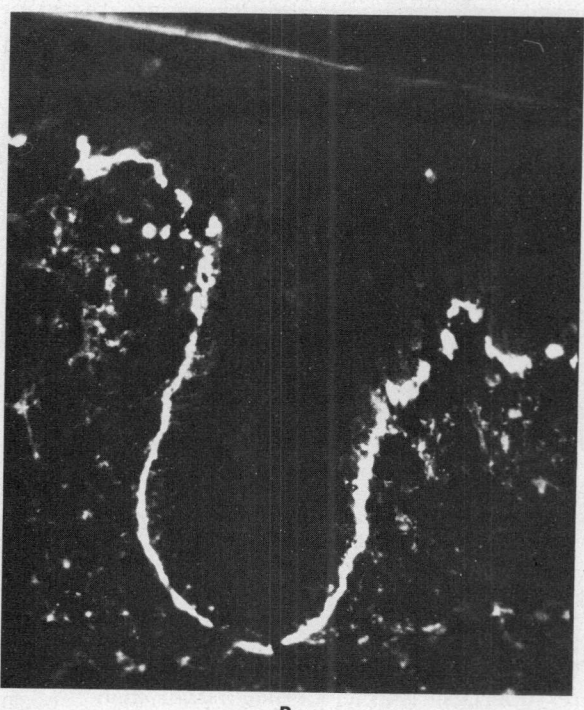

Figure 27–60. Bullous pemphigoid. *A*, Skin surface showing typical tense bullae on an erythematous base. *B*, Direct immunofluorescence study using patient's skin as substrate and fluorescein-tagged antibody against C3. Epidermis is on top. Linear staining of dermoepidermal junction for C3, and in many cases for IgG, is characteristic of bullous pemphigoid.

mal junction of perilesional skin. In addition, there is evidence for activation of the alternate complement pathway. It is plausible, then, that release of chemotactic agents and the influx of inflammatory cells are responsible for damage leading to vesicle formation. There is also a strong association between dermatitis herpetiformis and a usually mild or asymptomatic gluten-sensitive enteropathy (p. 847). A relationship between these two diseases is also suggested by the association of both diseases with the HLA antigens B8 and DW3.

Histologically, early changes include fibrin deposition in tips of the dermal papillae. The fully developed lesion consists of a subepidermal vesicle with predominantly neutrophils and lymphocytes present within and below the vesicle (Fig. 27–61). Adjacent to the vesicle are characteristic microabscesses in dermal papillae, together with neutrophils and nuclear debris scattered along the dermoepidermal junction. The site of cleavage, as seen by electron microscopy, is usually below the basal lamina. Immunofluorescence microscopy shows IgA and C3 in a granular pattern at the dermoepidermal junction, with accentuation in the dermal papillae in perilesional and clinically normal skin. Immunoelectron microscopic studies have localized these IgA deposits to dermal microfibrillar bundles below the basal lamina.[100, 101] In some children and adults, IgA deposits are not granular but linear in character. These individuals do not have gluten-sensitive enteropathy, and this special subset of dermatitis herpetiformis has been termed **linear IgA bullous dermatosis**.

Clinically, dermatitis herpetiformis is characterized by symmetric distribution of grouped (hence, herpetiform) vesicles. The earliest sign of incipient eruption is marked pruritus and burning, followed 24 to 48 hours later by erythematous urticarial lesions. Close inspection with a hand lens allows one to see clusters of minute vesicles surmounting the erythematous urticarial areas.

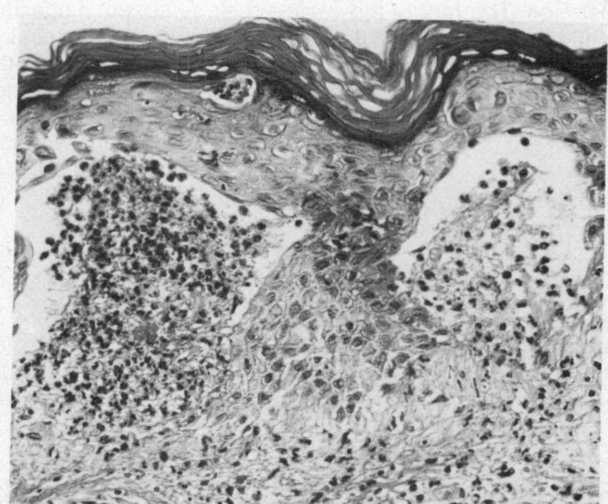

Figure 27–61. Dermatitis herpetiformis. Separation just below dermoepidermal junction is associated with microabcesses of neutrophils in dermal papillae.

Table 27–3. COMPARISON OF PEMPHIGUS, BULLOUS PEMPHIGOID, AND DERMATITIS HERPETIFORMIS

	Level of Blister	Acantholysis	Immunofluorescence
Pemphigus	Intraepidermal	Yes	Intercellular staining for IgG and C3
Bullous pemphigoid	Subepidermal	No	Linear staining at the dermo-epidermal junction for IgG and C3
Dermatitis herpetiformis	Subepidermal	No	Granular staining at the dermoepidermal junction for IgA and usually C3

Fully developed lesions are characterized by bilateral, symmetric, markedly pruritic, grouped vesicles involving shoulders, buttocks, and extensor surfaces of extremities.

The pathogenesis of dermatitis herpetiformis is intriguing. Studies have shown that IgG and IgA antibodies that cross-react with gluten proteins are present in many patients with this condition.[102] These antibodies react with reticulin fibrils directly beneath the basement membrane of the skin or may be deposited there as circulating immune complexes. Genetic factors may play a role in prolonged circulation of immune complexes in these patients.[103] Skin lesions usually respond to oral administration of sulfonamides. Therapy with a gluten-free diet[104] is indicated in persons with gastrointestinal lesions and may, in fact, cause remission of skin lesions. Table 27–3 compares the main features of the three blistering diseases: pemphigus, bullous pemphigoid, and dermatitis herpetiformis.

PORPHYRIA

Porphyria refers to a group of uncommon inborn or acquired metabolic disturbances of porphyrin metabolism.[105] Porphyrins are pigments normally present in hemoglobin, myoglobin, and cytochromes.

The classification of porphyrias is based on clinical and biochemical features. The five major types include *congenital erythropoietic porphyria, erythrohepatic protoporphyria, acute intermittent porphyria, porphyria cutanea tarda,* and *mixed porphyria.* The most commonly observed is the acquired type, porphyria cutanea tarda. Another acquired form occurs after ingestion of specific hepatotoxins such as hexachlorobenzene. Epidemics of acquired porphyria have been described in persons who ingested wheat treated with this hepatotoxic fungicide.

The pathogenesis of these skin manifestations is not completely understood. However, it is clear that cutaneous photosensitivity occurs at wavelengths of maximal absorption of ultraviolet light by the porphyrin molecule.

Cutaneous manifestations of hypersensitivity to light usually occur in both inherited and acquired types of porphyria, and consist of urticarial lesions and vesicles that heal with scarring and thickening of the skin.

Histopathologic changes in porphyria include edema of the papillary body, vesicle formation, and scarring around vessels.[106] The subepidermal vesicle of porphyria cutanea tarda characteristically exhibits deformed dermal pegs jutting into the blister cavity, a picture described as "festooning." Sun-exposed skin exhibits deposition of eosinophilic material in the dermis, particularly about vessels (Fig. 27–62); this material is PAS positive and diastase resistant. The substance is filamentous when viewed under the electron microscope and is apparently produced by fibroblasts.

INFECTION AND INFESTATION

The skin is subject to attack by a variety of microorganisms, parasites, and insects. In most instances there is successful resistance of the skin to invading organisms. Depending on the virulence of the infecting agent, however, and the competence of the host's response, infections and infestations may result.

Many disorders such as herpes simplex and zoster, the viral exanthems, and the deep mycoses are discussed in Chapter 8. Here, we shall cover a small number of rather common infections and infestations whose primary clinical manifestations are in the skin.

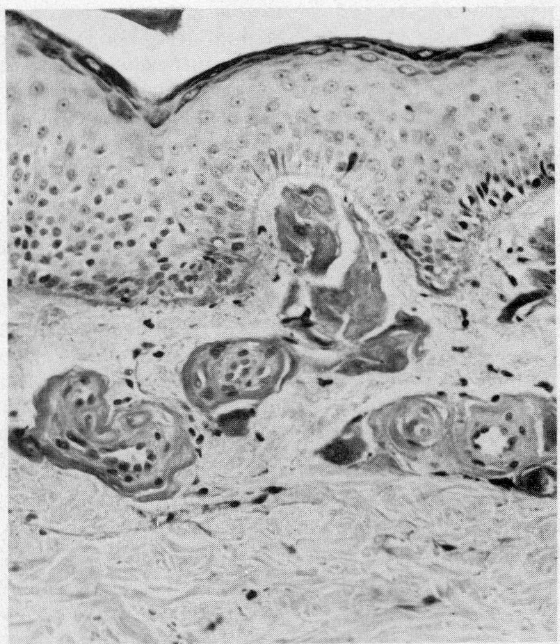

Figure 27–62. Porphyria (erythrohepatic protoporphyria). PAS-positive material is present at dermoepidermal junction and about dermal vessels.

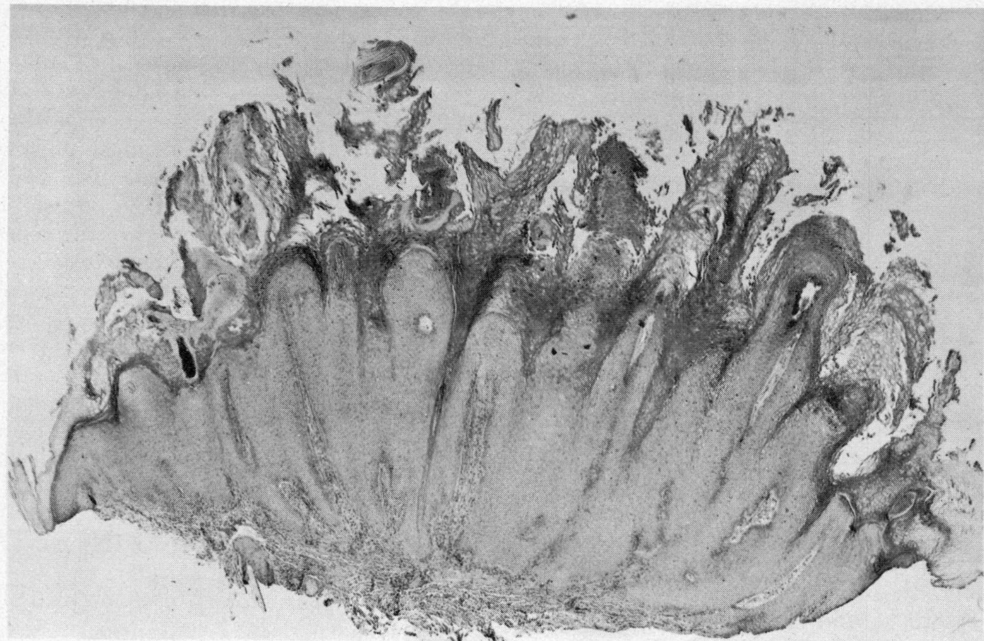

Figure 27–63. Verruca vulgaris, low power, showing hyperkeratosis, hypergranulosis, and papillary epidermal hyperplasia.

VERRUCAE (WARTS)

Verrucae are very common hyperplastic epidermal lesions prevalent in children and adolescents and caused by papovaviruses.[107] The presumed mode of transmission of virus includes contact and autoinoculation.

The classification of verrucae is based largely on gross morphology and location. **Verruca vulgaris** is the most frequent type of wart and may occur anywhere on the skin or oral mucosa; common areas of involvement are the hands, particularly the dorsal surfaces and periungual areas (Fig. 27–63). In these areas, verrucae appear as gray-white or brown and are covered with a rough, horny surface; their sizes vary from 1 to 10 mm. **Verruca plana** or flat wart is common on the face and dorsal surfaces of hands. These verrucae are slightly elevated, flat, smooth, tan papules, measuring 2 to 5 mm across.

Verruca plantaris or **palmaris** occurs on the soles or palms, respectively. These hyperkeratotic lesions measure 3 to 15 mm across. When the keratin is removed, soft white-tan granular tissue is seen. Further curettage reveals pin-point bleeding points. **Condyloma acuminatum** or **venereal wart** occurs on the penis, female genitalia, urethra, perianal areas, and rectum. These lesions appear as soft, tan, raspberry- or cauliflower-like masses (p. 1082).

Histologic features characteristic of all verrucae include epidermal hyperplasia, vacuolization of the cytoplasm of keratinocytes, and the presence of eosinophilic cytoplasmic inclusions and deeply basophilic nuclei (Fig. 27–64). Clumped keratohyaline granules are also common in all types of verrucae, except condyloma acuminatum. Numerous intranuclear viral particles are seen by electron microscopy, and viral antigens may be demonstrated immunologically in tissue showing the cytopathic alterations described.

The viruses causing the different types of verrucae are called papilloma viruses and belong to the DNA-containing papovavirus group. Serologically different types of these viruses have been shown to cause the different clinical and histologic types of verrucae.

MOLLUSCUM CONTAGIOSUM

Molluscum contagiosum is a common viral disease of the skin that gives rise to characteristically umbilicated papules.[108] The etiologic agent is a poxvirus that is characteristically brick shaped, measuring 300 × 240

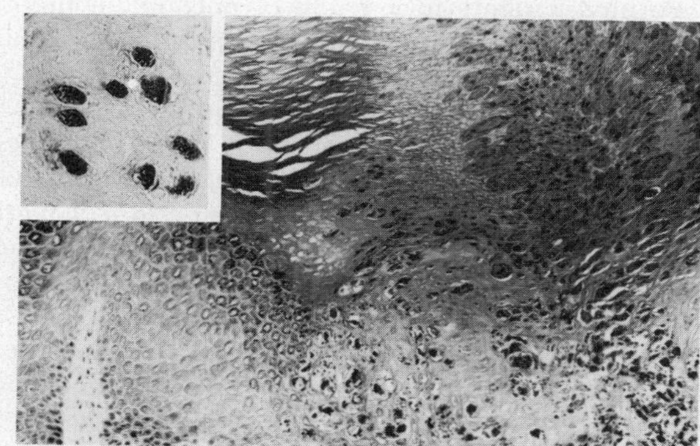

Figure 27–64. Verruca vulgaris, early lesion. Normal epidermis *(left)* is adjacent to epidermis showing cytopathic effects of virus infection (ballooning cells, nuclear inclusions). Antibodies to papilloma virus antigens show reactivity in these morphologically altered cells by the immunoperoxidase technique *(inset)*.

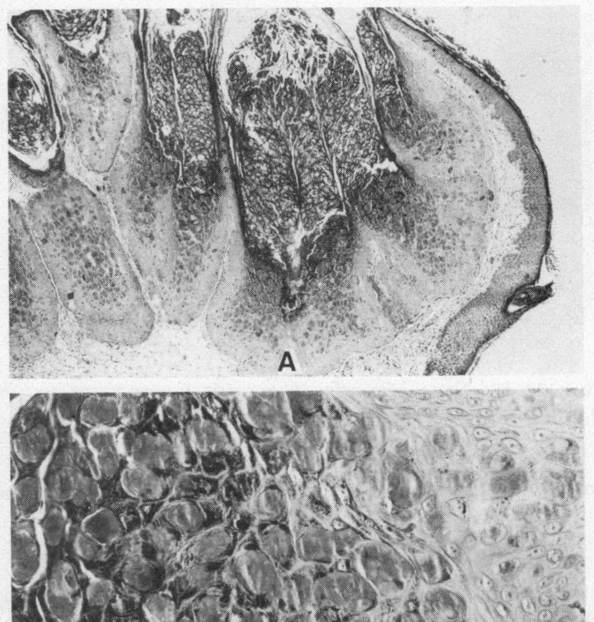

Figure 27–65. Molluscum contagiosum. *A*, Architecturally lesions are cup shaped with distinct edges. B, Numerous epidermal cells contain "molluscum bodies," cytoplasmic aggregates of virions in an altered cytoplasmic material.

× 230 nm with a dumbbell-shaped DNA core. Spread of infection occurs by direct contact and autoinoculation, but fomites may also be a means of transmission.

Molluscum contagiosum is most common in children and young adults, especially males. Multiple lesions, between 3 and 30, occur on skin and mucous membranes, especially the trunk and anogenital areas. Individual lesions appear as waxy pink or skin-colored, firm, pruritic papules with umbilicated centers. These papules measure 2 to 4 mm in diameter but can attain a size of 6 to 10 mm across. A curdlike material can be expressed from the central umbilication. With Giemsa stain this material shows characteristic **molluscum bodies**.

Histologically, there is epithelial hyperplasia with epidermal growth downward in lobules (Fig. 27–65). The pathognomonic structure is the "molluscum body," which occurs as a large (up to 35-micron) homogeneous cytoplasmic inclusion in the stratum granulosum and stratum corneum. These inclusions contain replicating virions.

Spontaneous involution of these lesions usually occurs within two months, but occasionally some persist as new lesions develop.

IMPETIGO

This common superficial staphylococcal or streptococcal infection of the skin is characterized by erosive lesions covered with honey-colored crusts. Impetigo tends to affect children and adults in poor health. Among infants, impetigo is highly infectious.

Impetigo usually involves exposed skin, particularly that of the face and hands. It begins as a group of small red macules that become pustular. The pustules break, leading to the appearance of erosions, usually less than 2 cm across. Over the erosions, drying serum forms a **honey-colored crust**, the clinical hallmark of impetigo. If the crust is not removed, the process tends to expand laterally, forming satellite lesions. Neglected cases show deep extension with destruction of the full thickness of the epidermis. **Ecthyma** refers to ulcerated impetigo. Fever, adenopathy, and other systemic signs often accompany the more severe patterns of involvement.

The characteristic microscopic feature is a subcorneal blister filled with neutrophils and acantholytic keratinocytes (Fig. 27–66). Special stains may reveal the presence of organisms within the blister. Below the blister the epidermis shows spongiosis, and neutrophils can be observed extending from the dermis into the epidermis. In the dermis, a perivascular infiltrate of lymphocytes and neutrophils is apparent. The pustule is short-lived and it ruptures, resulting in an erosion covered by a crust composed of serum, neutrophils, and nuclear and keratinaceous debris.

The etiologic agents are usually coagulase-positive staphylococci and/or group A beta-hemolytic streptococci. Nephritogenic strains of streptococcus cause impetigo, particularly in tropical areas and the southern United States.[109] In some epidemics, 4% of patients with impetigo have had associated glomerulonephritis.

FUNGAL INFECTIONS OF SKIN

Fungal infections of the skin are classified into superficial and deep types. The superficial fungal infections are also referred to as *ringworm* or *dermatophytosis*.[110] The infecting organisms are limited to the cornified layer (or sometimes the granular layer) of the epidermis and hair. Exceptionally, there is erosion of a hair follicle and release of organisms into the dermis (Majocchi's granuloma). Organisms often responsible for superficial fungal infections include *Trichophyton ru-*

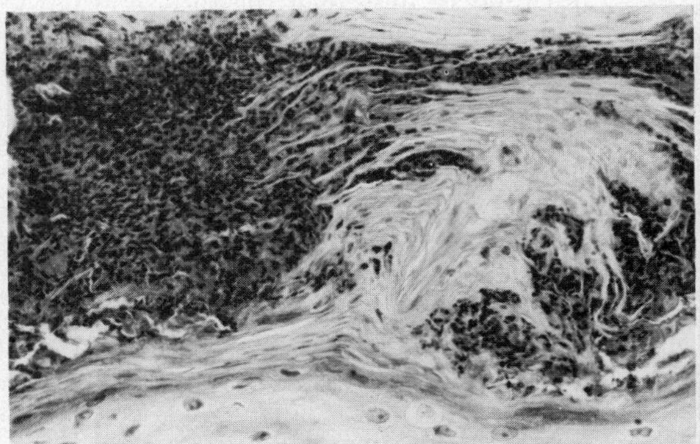

Figure 27–66. Impetigo. Aggregates of neutrophils associated with bacteria are within stratum corneum; subcorneal blisters containing neutrophils and acantholytic keratinocytes also occur.

brum, *Microsporum canis*, and *Malassezia furfur*. Deep fungal infections (p. 352) involve the epidermis, dermis, and subcutis; visceral involvement is common, especially in immunosuppressed patients. Although infections by most Candida species are superficial, deep and visceral involvement can be observed in patients with decreased immunity.

Superficial Fungal Infections

Dermatophytes grow in soil, on animals, and on human beings. *Tinea capitis* refers to dermatophytosis of the scalp; *tinea barbae*, of the beard; *tinea corporis*, of the trunk and extremities; *tinea cruris*, of the anogenital region (jock itch); *tinea manus and pedis*, of the hands and feet (athlete's foot); and *onychomycosis*, of the nails.

Tinea capitis usually occurs in children, rarely in infants or adults. Mild tinea capitis is characterized by symptomless, apparently hairless patches on the scalp associated with mild erythema, crust, and scale. The markedly inflammatory types of tinea capitis, called *kerion*, exhibit painful, boggy, inflamed nodules associated with pustular folliculitis.

Tinea barbae affects adult men and is a relatively uncommon disorder. It may exhibit lesions of the mildly or markedly inflammatory types described above.

Tinea corporis affects all ages, but children seem to be the most susceptible. Conditions that predispose to infection include excessive heat and humidity, exposure to infected animals, and chronic tinea pedis or onychomycosis. The most common type of tinea corporis begins as a papule that expands centrifugally with a leading red circinate border, which is elevated and scaling and may show papulovesicles. Other clinical manifestations of tinea corporis include large scaling plaques, mounds of vesicles, kerion-like lesions (see above), and scaling patches associated with red nodules. The latter, usually on the legs of women, represents an uncommon variant of tinea corporis called *Majocchi's granuloma*, or granulomatous folliculitis and perifolliculitis.[111]

Tinea cruris ("jock itch") occurs most frequently in obese men during warm weather. Conditions that predispose to infection include heat, friction, and maceration. This infection usually first appears on the upper inner thighs with gradual extension of well-demarcated moist red patches with raised scaling borders.

Tinea pedis affects 30 to 40% of the population. Clinical manifestations of tinea of the hands or feet include (1) persistent diffuse erythema and scaling, (2) vesiculobullous lesions, and (3) macerated tissue between the toes associated with malodor, pruritus, and sometimes erythema.

In *onychomycosis*, peripheral discoloration of the nailplate, which gradually extends proximally, is associated with thickening and deformity of the nail and subungual disintegration.[112]

Tinea versicolor usually occurs on the upper trunk and is highly distinctive in its appearance. Caused by *Malassezia furfur*, the lesions consist of groups of macules of all sizes, lighter or darker than surrounding skin, with a fine peripheral scale.

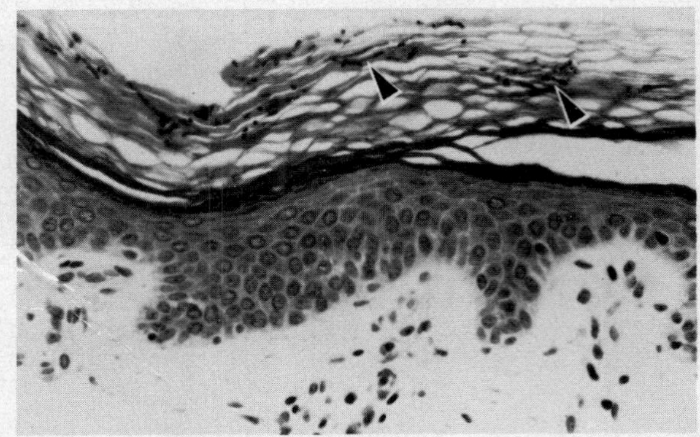

Figure 27–67. Tinea versicolor. Numerous fungal forms *(arrowheads)* are present in the stratum corneum.

The histology of all dermatophytoses varies according to host response to infecting organisms. Fungal cell walls, rich in mucopolysaccharides, stain bright pink to red with the PAS stain. They are present in the anucleate cornified layer of the skin, hair, or nails, since dermatophytes live on and digest keratin (Fig. 27–67). A dermal lymphohistiocytic infiltrate loosely disposed about vessels is usually present. Eosinophils are sometimes seen. Epidermal spongiosis, acanthosis, hyperkeratosis, and parakeratosis are variable features and can be expected to correlate with the clinical appearance of the lesions, e.g., the degree of exudation, thickening, and scaling of the skin.

ARTHROPOD BITES AND STINGS

Arthropods are virtually ubiquitous, and most human beings are prone to their bites and stings and the other discomforts they cause. The arthropods include *Arachnida:* spiders, scorpions, ticks, mites; *Insecta*: lice, bedbugs, bees, wasps, fleas, flies, mosquitoes; and *Chilopoda* (centipedes). All can cause skin lesions, but there is wide variability in the reaction patterns of individuals. Some persons suffer minimal symptoms, others considerable discomfort, and some may die as a consequence of a bite or sting. Arthropods can produce lesions in several ways: (1) the lesions may be caused by a direct irritant effect of arthropod parts or of substances excreted by the arthropod; (2) some venoms may cause specific effects—e.g., that of the black widow spider causes severe cramping and excruciating pain; (3) in some cases, immediate or delayed hypersensitivity to body parts or secretions occurs; (4) arthropods can serve as vectors for bacteria, rickettsia, or parasites.

Insect bites usually manifest themselves at the site of the bite by a firm papule or nodule, sometimes with ulceration, which may last several weeks. Histologically, there is a relatively dense cellular infiltrate in the dermis and underlying subcutaneous tissue. It is composed chiefly of eosinophils, lymphocytes, and monocytes.

Occasionally, parts of the insect may actually be seen in the dermis surrounded by a foreign body reaction. Lymphoid hyperplasia in the skin may also be seen in some patients.

Scabies is a contagious pruritic dermatosis caused by the itch mite *Sarcoptes scabiei.*[113] The female mite produces burrows (linear, poorly defined streaks, 2 to 6 mm in length) on the interdigital skin, palms, fingers, and wrists, the periareolar region in women, and the genital area in men. Excoriations are commonly seen. Histologically, the burrow traverses the keratin layer, and the female mite may be seen in the blind end of the burrow. Usually there is edema of the epidermis in the regions affected. The underlying dermis shows a nonspecific, chronic inflammatory infiltrate composed chiefly of lymphocytes.

Pediculosis is caused by the head louse, crab louse, and body louse. The disease is pruritic, and the louse or its eggs attached to the hair shafts can usually be seen with the unaided eye. In pediculosis of the scalp, impetigo and enlarged cervical lymph nodes may be frequent complications, especially in children. The pubic louse may be transmitted through sexual contact. Infection with the body louse ("vagabond's disease") is usually characterized by areas of hyperpigmentation and scratch marks. Occasionally, a peculiar bluish pigmentation occurs in spots. The pigmentation is thought to be due to small hemorrhages induced by the bite of the insect. The histologic picture is nonspecific.

ACKNOWLEDGMENTS

Dr. Seymour Rosen provided valuable review comments and illustrative material for the section on nevus flammeus. The authors gratefully acknowledge the expert technical assistance of Ms. Ellie Manseau and Mr. Richard Shepard. Mrs. Sharon E. Murphy provided the excellent medical illustrations (Figs. 27–3 and 27–36).

GENERAL REFERENCES

Ackerman, A. B.: Histologic Diagnosis of Inflammatory Skin Disease. Philadelphia, Lea & Febiger, 1978.
Beutner, E. H., et al. (eds.): Immunopathology of the Skin: Labelled Antibody Studies. Stroudsburg, PA, Dowden, Hutchinson & Ross, 1973.
Braverman, I. M.: Skin Signs of Systemic Disease. 2nd ed. Philadelphia, W. B. Saunders Co., 1981.
Breathnach, A. S.: An Atlas of the Ultrastructure of Human Skin. London, J. & A. Churchill, 1971.
Emmons, C. W., et al.: Medical Mycology. 3rd ed. Philadelphia, Lea & Febiger, 1977.
Fitzpatrick, T. B., et al. (eds.): Dermatology in General Medicine. 2nd ed. New York, McGraw-Hill Book Co., 1979.
Fitzpatrick, T. B., et al. (eds.): Sunlight and Man. Tokyo, University of Tokyo Press, 1974.
Gibbs, R. C.: Skin Diseases of the Feet. St. Louis, Warren H. Green, 1974.
Goldsmith, L. A. (ed.): Biochemistry and Physiology of the Skin. Oxford, Oxford University Press, 1983.
Helwig, E. B., and Mostofi, F. K. (eds.): The Skin. Baltimore, Williams & Wilkins Co., 1971.
Jarrett, A., et al. (eds.): The Physiology and Pathophysiology of the Skin. New York, Academic Press, 1973.
Lever, W. F., and Schaumberg-Lever, G.: Histopathology of the Skin. 6th ed. Philadelphia, J. B. Lippincott Co., 1983.
Moschella, S. L., et al. (eds.): Dermatology. Philadelphia, W. B. Saunders Co., 1975.
Pinkus, H., and Mehregan, A. H.: A Guide to Dermatohistopathology. 2nd ed. New York, Appleton-Century-Crofts, 1976.
Reed, R. J.: New Concepts in Surgical Pathology of the Skin. New York, John Wiley & Sons, 1976.
Rook, A., et al.: Textbook of Dermatology. Oxford, Blackwell Scientific Publications, 1972.
Zelickson, A. S.: Ultrastructure of Normal and Abnormal Skin. Philadelphia, Lea & Febiger, 1967.

REFERENCES

1. Toews, G. B., et al.: Langerhans cells: Sentinels of skin-associated lymphoid tissue. J. Invest. Dermatol. *75*:78, 1980.
2. Gelfant, S.: A New Concept of Tissue and Tumor Cell Proliferation. Cancer Res. *37*:3845, 1977.
3. Murphy, G. F., et al.: Characterization of Langerhans cells by the use of monoclonal antibodies. Lab. Invest. *45*:465, 1981.
4. Shelley, W. B., and Harvarth, P. N.: Experimental miliaria in man. J. Invest. Dermatol. *14*:193, 1950.
5. Mevorah, B., and Mishima, Y.: Cellular response of seborrheic keratoses following croton oil irritation and surgical trauma. Dermatologica *113*:452, 1965.
6. McGavran, M. H., and Binnington, B.: Keratinous cysts of the skin. Arch. Dermatol. *94*:499, 1966.
7. Fisher, E. R., et al.: Analysis of histopathologic and electron microscopic determinants of keratoacanthoma and squamous cell carcinoma. Cancer *29*:1387, 1972.
8. Hashimoto, K., and Lever, W. F.: Appendage Tumors of the Skin. Springfield, IL, Charles C Thomas, 1968.
9. Brownstein, M. H., et al.: The dermatopathology of Cowden's syndrome. Br. J. Dermatol. *100*:667, 1979.
10. Bart, R. S., et al.: Cutaneous horn. Acta Derm. Venereol. (Stockh.) *48*:507, 1968.
11. Gorlin, R. J., et al.: The multiple basal cell nevi syndrome. Cancer *18*:89, 1965.
12. Cotran, R. S.: Metastasizing basal cell carcinomas. Cancer *14*:1036, 1961.
13. Murphy, G. F., et al.: Local immune response in basal cell carcinoma: Characterization by transmission electron microscopy and monoclonal anti-T6 antibody. J. Am. Acad. Dermatol. *8*:477, 1983.
14. Miller, S. A., et al.: Adenoid squamous cell carcinoma. Arch. Dermatol. *89*:589, 1964.
15. Underwood, L. J., et al.: Squamous cell epithelioma that simulates sarcoma. Arch. Dermatol. Syphilol. *64*:149, 1951.
16. Epstein, E., et al.: Metastases from squamous cell carcinoma of the skin. Arch. Dermatol. *97*:245, 1968.
17. Wade, T. R., et al.: Bowenoid papulosis of the genitalia. Arch. Dermatol. *115*:306, 1979.
18. Caron, G. A., and Chink, H. M.: Clinical association of basal cell epithelioma with histiocytoma. Arch. Dermatol *90*:271, 1964.
19. Hashimoto, K., et al.: Dermatofibrosarcoma protuberans. Arch. Dermatol. *110*:874, 1974.
20. Brenner, V., et al.: Dermatofibrosarcoma protuberans metastatic to regional lymph nodes. Cancer *36*:1897, 1975.
21. Straub, P. W., et al.: Chronic intravascular coagulation in Kasabach-Merritt syndrome. Arch. Intern. Med. *129*:475, 1972.
22. Barsky, S. H., et al.: The nature and evolution of port wine stains: A computer-assisted study. J. Invest. Dermatol. *74*:154, 1980.
23. Noe, J. M., et al.: Port wine stains and the response to argon laser therapy: Successful treatment and the predictive role of color, age, and biopsy. Plast. Reconstr. Surg. *65*:130, 1980.
24. Cox, F. H., and Helwig, E. B.: Kaposi's sarcoma. Cancer *12*:289, 1959.
25. Templeton, A. C.: Studies in Kaposi's sarcoma. Cancer *30*:854, 1972.
26. Maize, J. C., et al.: Xanthoma disseminatum and multiple myeloma. Arch. Dermatol. *110*:758, 1974.
27. Shaw, V. M.: Genetic aspects of urticaria pigmentosa. Arch. Dermatol. *97*:137, 1968.
28. Rappaport, H., and Thomas, L.: Mycosis fungoides. Cancer *34*:634, 1974.
29. Van Leeowen, A. W., et al.: T-cell membrane characteristics of mycosis cells in the skin and lymph node. J. Invest. Dermatol. *65*:367, 1975.
30. Thomas, J. A., et al.: The relationship between T lymphocyte subsets and Ia-like antigen positive nonlymphoid cells in early stages of cutaneous T cell lymphoma. J. Invest. Dermatol. *78*:169, 1982.
31. Sanchez, J. L., and Ackerman, A. B.: The patch stage of mycosis fungoides. Am. J. Dermatopathol. *1*:5, 1979.
32. Murphy, G. F., et al.: Distribution of T cell antigens in histiocytosis X cells: Quantitative immunoelectron microscopy using monoclonal antibodies. Lab. Invest. *48*:90, 1983.
33. Harrist, T. J., et al.: Histiocytosis X: In situ characterization of cutaneous infiltrates using monoclonal antibodies and heteroantibodies. Am. J. Clin. Pathol. *79*:294, 1983.
34. Risdall, R. J., et al.: Histiocytosis X (Langerhans cell histiocytosis). Arch. Pathol. Lab. Med. *107*:59, 1983.

35. Murphy, G. F., et al.: The role of diagnostic electron microscopy in dermatology. *In* Moschella, S. (ed.): Dermatology Update. New York, Elsevier North-Holland, 1982, p. 355.
36. Brownstein, M. H., and Helwig, E. B.: Metastatic tumors of the skin. Cancer *29*:1298, 1972.
37. Sanchez, N. P., et al.: Melasma: A clinical, light microscopic, ultrastructural, and immunofluorescence study. J. Am. Acad. Dermatol. *4*:698, 1981.
38. Ortonne, J. P., et al.: Vitiligo and Other Hypomelanoses of Skin and Hair. New York, Plenum Press, 1982.
39. Hertz, K. C., et al.: Autoimmune vitiligo, detection of antibodies to melanin-producing cells. N. Engl. J. Med. *297*:634, 1977.
40. Brown, J., and Winklemann, K. K.: Acanthosis nigricans—a study of 90 cases. Medicine *47*:33, 1968.
41. Curth, H. O.: Classification of acanthosis nigricans. Int. J. Dermatol *15*:592, 1976.
42. Cohn, H. J., et al.: Nevus spilus. Arch. Dermatol. *102*:433, 1970.
43. Murphy, G. F., and Mihm, M. C.: Origin and fate of pigmented nevi. *In* Williams, H. B. (ed.): Symposium on Vascular Malformations and Melanocytic Lesions. St. Louis, MO, C.V. Mosby Co., 1983, p. 268.
44. Weedon, D., and Little, J. H.: Spindle and epithelioid cell nevi in children and adults. Cancer *40*:217, 1977.
45. Allen, A. C., and Spitz, S.: Histogenesis and clinicopathologic correlation of nevi and malignant melanomas. Arch. Dermatol. Syphilol. *69*:150, 1954.
45A. Elder, D. E., et al.: Dysplastic nevus syndrome. Cancer *46*:1787, 1980.
46. Clark, W. H., et al.: Origin of familial malignant melanomas from heritable melanocytic lesions. Arch. Dermatol. *114*:732, 1978.
47. Clark, W. H., et al.: Current concepts of the biology of human cutaneous malignant melanoma. Adv. Cancer Res. *24*:267, 1977.
48. Kopf, A. W., et al.: Malignant melanoma: A review. J. Dermatol. Surg. Oncol. *3*:1, 1977.
49. Clark, W. H., et al.: The histogenesis and biologic behavior of primary human malignant melanomas of the skin. Cancer Res. *29*:705, 1969.
50. Clark, W. H., et al.: The developmental biology of malignant melanomas. Semin. Oncol. *2*:83, 1975.
51. Swerdlow, M.: Nevi: A problem of misdiagnosis. Am. J. Clin. Pathol. *22*:1054, 1952.
52. Mihm, M. C., et al.: Early detection of primary cutaneous melanoma—a color atlas. N. Engl. J. Med. *289*:989, 1973.
53. Mihm, M. C., et al.: The clinical diagnosis, classification, and histogenetic concepts of the early stages of cutaneous malignant melanomas. N. Engl. J. Med. *284*:1078, 1971.
54. Mihm, M. C., and Murphy, G. F.: Classification of malignant melanoma. *In* Williams, H. B. (ed.): Symposium on Vascular Malformations and Melanocytic Lesions. St. Louis, MO, C.V. Mosby Co., 1983, p. 339.
55. Mihm, M. C., and Lopansri, S.: A review of the classification of malignant melanoma. J. Dermatol. *6*:131, 1979.
56. Wanebo, H. J., et al.: Malignant melanoma of the extremities: A clinicopathological study using levels of invasion (microstage). Cancer *35*:666, 1975.
57. Day, C. L., et al.: Cutaneous malignant melanoma: Prognostic guidelines for physicians and patients. CA *32*:113, 1982.
58. Blaylock, W. K.: Atopic dermatitis: Diagnosis and pathobiology. J. Allergy Clin. Immunol. *57*:62, 1976.
59. Hanifin, J. M., and Cobitz, W. C.: Newer concepts of atopic dermatitis. Arch. Dermatol. *113*:663, 1977.
60. Norins, A. L.: Atopic dermatitis. Pediatr. Clin. North Am. *18*:801, 1971.
61. Mihm, M. C., Jr., et al.: The structure of normal skin and the morphology of atopic eczema. J. Invest. Dermatol. *67*:305, 1976.
62. Wooten, J. W., et al.: Development of oral lesions in erythema multiforme exudativum. Oral Surg. *24*:808, 1967.
63. Bedi, T. R., and Pinkus, H.: Histopathological spectrum of erythema multiforme. Br. J. Dermatol. *95*:243, 1976.
64. Cochrane, C. G., et al.: The role of polymorphonuclear leukocytes in the initiation and cessation of the arthus vasculitis. J. Exp. Med. *110*:481, 1959.
65. Soter, N. A.: Chronic urticaria as a manifestation of necrotizing venulitis. N. Engl. J. Med. *296*:1440, 1977.
66. Harrist, T. J., and Mihm, M. C.: Cutaneous immunopathology. The use of direct and indirect immunofluorescence techniques in dermatologic disease. Hum. Pathol. *10*:625, 1979.
67. Harrist, T. J., and Mihm, M. C.: The specificity and usefulness of the lupus band test. Arthritis Rheum. *23*:479, 1980.
68. Rubenstein, M. H., et al.: Lichen planus and lupus erythematosus: Two disorders with pigment incontinence of possible immunologically-mediated origin. *In* Fitzpatrick, T. B., et al. (eds.): Biology and Diseases of Dermal Pigmentation. Tokyo, University of Tokyo Press, 1981, p. 151.
68A. Biesecker, G., et al.: Cutaneous localization of the membrane attack complex in discoid and systemic lupus erythematosus. N. Engl. J. Med. *306*:264, 1982.
69. Glucksberg, H., et al.: Clinical manifestations of graft-versus-host disease in human recipients of marrow from HLA-matched sibling donors. Transplantation *18*:295, 1975.
70. Ullman, S.: Immunoglobulins and complement in skin in graft-versus-host disease. Ann. Intern. Med. *85*:205, 1976.
71. Hoyos, N., et al.: Liquefying nodular panniculitis. Dermatologica *101*:332, 1958.
72. Hendricks, W. M., et al.: Weber-Christian syndrome in infancy. Br. J. Dermatol. *98*:175, 1978.
73. Freinkel, R. K.: Pathogenesis of acne vulgaris. N. Engl. J. Med. *280*:1161, 1969.
74. Leyden, J. J.: Pathogenesis of acne vulgaris. Int. J. Dermatol. *15*:490, 1976.
75. Strauss, J. S., and Pochi, P. E.: Recent advances in androgen metabolism and their relation to the skin. Arch. Dermatol. *100*:621, 1969.
76. Voss, J. G.: Acne vulgaris and free fatty acids. Arch. Dermatol. *109*:849, 1974.
77. Webster, G. F., et al.: Inhibition of lipase production in Propionibacterium acnes by sub-minimal-inhibitory concentrations of tetracycline and erythromycin. Br. J. Dermatol. *104*:453, 1981.
78. Marks, R., and Harcourt-Webster, J. N.: Histopathology of rosacea. Arch. Dermatol. *100*:623, 1969.
79. Bhan, A. K., et al.: T cell subset populations in lichen planus: In situ characterization using monoclonal anti-T cell antibodies. Br. J. Dermatol. *105*:617, 1981.
80. Kronenberg, K., et al.: Malignant degeneration of lichen planus. Arch. Dermatol. *104*:304, 1971.
81. Bergfeld, W. F., and Lesowitz, S. A.: Lichen sclerosus et atrophicus. Arch. Dermatol. *101*:247, 1970.
82. Harrist, T. J., et al.: Lymphomatoid vasculitis: A subset of lymphocytic vasculitis. *In* Moschella, S. L. (ed.): Dermatology Update. New York, Elsevier North-Holland, 1982, p. 115.
83. Voorhees, J. J., et al.: Cyclic AMP, cyclic GMP, and glucocorticoids as potential metabolic regulators of epidermal proliferation and differentiation. J. Invest. Dermatol. *65*:179, 1975.
84. Moll, J. M. H., and Wright, V.: Psoriatic arthritis. Semin. Arthritis Rheum. *3*:55, 1973.
85. Zaias, N.: Psoriasis of the nail. A clinical-pathologic study. Arch. Dermatol. *99*:567, 1969.
86. Cox, A. J., and Watson, W.: Histologic variations in lesions of psoriasis. Arch. Dermatol. *106*:503, 1972.
87. Chowaniec, O., et al.: Earliest clinical and histologic changes in psoriasis. Dermatologica *163*:42, 1981.
88. Baker, H., and Ryan, T. J.: Generalized pustular psoriasis. Br. J. Dermatol. *80*:771, 1968.
89. Marks, R., et al.: Pityriasis lichenoides: A reappraisal. Br. J. Dermatol. *86*:215, 1972.
90. Samman, P. D.: Survey of reticuloses and premycotic eruptions. Br. J. Dermatol. *76*:1, 1964.
91. Kawala, A., et al.: A case of parapsoriasis en plaques of 18 year duration terminating in reticulum cell sarcoma. Dermatologica *138*:19, 1969.
92. Lever, W. F. (ed.): Pemphigus and Pemphigoid. Springfield, IL, Charles C Thomas, 1965.
93. Bystryn, J. C., et al.: Pemphigus foliaceus, subcorneal intercellular antibodies of unique specificity. Arch. Dermatol. *110*:857, 1974.
94. Person, J. R., and Rogers, R. S. III: Bullous and cicatricial pemphigoid. Mayo Clin. Proc. *52*:54, 1977.
95. Barriere, H., et al.: Prurit 'sine materia' et pemphigoïde bulleuse. Ann. Dermatol. Venereal. *108*:445, 1981.
96. Jordon, R. E., et al.: The complement system in bullous pemphigoid. II. Immunofluorescent evidence for both classic and alternate pathway activation. Clin. Immunol. Immunopathol. *3*:307, 1975.
97. Schaumberg-Lever, G., et al.: Ultrastructural localization of *in vivo* bound immunoglobulins in bullous pemphigoid—preliminary report. J. Invest. Dermatol. *64*:47, 1975.
98. Dvorak, A. M., et al.: Bullous pemphigoid, an ultrastructural study of the inflammatory response: Eosinophil, basophil, and mast cell granule changes in multiple biopsies from one patient. J. Invest. Dermatol. *78*:91, 1982.
99. Katz, S. I., and Strober, W.: The pathogenesis of dermatitis herpetiformis. J. Invest. Dermatol. *70*:63, 1978.
100. Yaoita, H., and Katz, S. I.: Immunoelectronmicroscopic localization of IgA in skin of patients with dermatitis herpetiformis. J. Invest. Dermatol. *67*:502, 1976.
101. Yaoita, H.: Identification of IgA binding structures in skin of patients with dermatitis herpetiformis. J. Invest. Dermatol. *71*:213, 1978.

102. Ljunghall, K., et al.: Circulating reticulin autoantibodies of IgA class in dermatitis herpetiformis. Br. J. Dermatol. *100*:173, 1979.
103. Lawley, T. J., et al.: Defective Fc-receptor functions associated with the HLA-B8/DRw3 haplotype. Studies in patients with dermatitis herpetiformis and normal subjects. N. Engl. J. Med. *304*:185, 1981.
104. Reunala, T., et al.: Gluten-free diet in dermatitis herpetiformis. Br. J. Dermatol. *97*:473, 1977.
105. Harber, L. C., and Bickers, D. R.: The porphyrias: Basic science aspects, clinical diagnosis and management. *In* Malkinson, F. D., and Pearson, R. W. (eds.): Year Book of Dermatology, Chicago, Year Book Medical Publishers, 1975.
106. Epstein, J. H., et al.: Cutaneous changes in porphyrias. A microscopic study. Arch. Dermatol. *107*:689, 1973.
107. Almeida, J. D., et al.: Electron microscopic study of human warts; sites of production and nature of the inclusion bodies. J. Invest. Dermatol. *38*:337, 1962.
108. Lutzner, M. A.: Molluscum contagiosum, verruca and zoster viruses. Arch. Dermatol. *87*:436, 1963.
109. Dillion, H. C.: Streptococcal skin infection and glomerulonephritis. *In* Hoeprick, P. D. (ed.): Infectious Diseases, 2nd ed. New York, Harper & Row, 1977.
110. Rebell, G., and Iaplin, D.: Dermatophytes: Their Recognition and Identification. Revised ed. Coral Gables, FL, University of Miami Press, 1970.
111. Wilson, J. W., et al.: Nodular granulomatous perifolliculitis of the legs caused by *Trichophyton rubrum*. Arch. Dermatol. *69*:258, 1954.
112. Zaias, N.: Onychomycosis. Arch. Dermatol. *105*:256, 1972.
113. Fernandez, N., et al.: Pathologic findings in human scabies. Arch. Dermatol. *113*:320, 1977.

28 THE MUSCULOSKELETAL SYSTEM

The consideration of the musculoskeletal system will be divided into the following subdivisions: (1) muscles, (2) bones, (3) joints, and (4) tendons, fasciae, and supporting structures.

Skeletal Muscle

NORMAL

The muscle cell is a marvelous example of adaptation of structure to function. A wealth of literature is available pertaining to its structural organization.[1–5] Remarks here will be limited to those essentials necessary for an understanding of the subsequent discussions. The striated muscle cell (myofiber) has a diameter ranging from 10 to 100μ and is of considerable length. Indeed, in short muscles, the cell may extend from one tendinous insertion to the other. It is enclosed within a plasma membrane itself surrounded by an extracellular structureless layer of polysaccharides, resembling the glycocalyx of epithelial cells. A thin connective tissue investment—the endomysium—encloses each fiber and separates adjacent fibers. A similar investment—the perimysium—encloses groups or fascicles of fibers.

The nuclei are dispersed along the length of the myofiber closely approximated to the plasma membrane. The sarcoplasm contains mitochondria, Golgi apparatus, ribosomes, sarcoplasmic reticulum, other tubules, and an abundance of myofibrils. The number of mitochondria varies with the specific functional activity of the cell. Thus, cardiac muscle cells contain many more mitochondria than the cells of skeletal muscle, which have lower oxidative requirements.

Most of the myofiber mass is made up of a parallel array of delicately spindled thick and thin myofilaments that lie in register across the width of the myofiber. It is the transverse registration of the thick, myosin-containing filaments that creates the dark A band (anisotropic), which is bisected in its midregion by a pale H zone having a central dark M band (Fig. 28–1). Analogously, the thin actin myofilaments lie in register attached at one end to a thin dense Z line and interdigitating at the other end with the thick filaments. The zone adjacent to the Z line made up of only actin filaments creates the light-appearing I (isotropic) band. The alternation of A and I bands produces the well-known cross striations of skeletal and cardiac muscle. The segment of myofiber demarcated by adjacent Z bands comprises a functional contractile unit, the sarcomere. It was Huxley who first proposed that muscle shortening occurs by sliding of the thin filaments between the thick filaments toward the center of the sarcomere. The summation of shortening of all sarcomeres accounts for contraction of the entire myofiber and muscle. Overcontraction causes approximation of A bands obscuring the lighter I bands to create darkly staining *contraction bands*. Although the entire myofiber constitutes a single muscle cell, disease may involve only one or more sarcomeres leaving the remainder to degenerate or regenerate.

Certain ultrastructural specializations of the myofiber are intrinsic to its contractile function. One is a system of cross bridges linking the thick and thin filaments. These are small, regularly spaced lateral projections of the thick myofilaments that are thought to play a role in the integration of their function across the width of the myofiber. A second specialization is a transverse tubular (T) system quite separate from the endoplasmic reticulum, also called "sarcoplasmic reticulum." The T tubules arise at the periphery of the myofibers as deep invaginations of the plasma membrane. Thus, their lumina are extensions of the interstitial space and so provide a pathway for the transmission of ionic shifts during contraction to the myofilaments within the sarcomere. The numerous close approximations of the sarcoplasmic reticulum to the T system provide a structural network for the delivery of calcium ions to myofilaments, initiating contraction. Another highly important specialization of each muscle fiber is the *neuromuscular junction* also referred to as *motor endplate*. The junction is marked by a shallow depression in the myofiber surface from which synaptic troughs invaginate the plasma membrane. An unmyelinated terminal nerve branch of a motor nerve lies within each

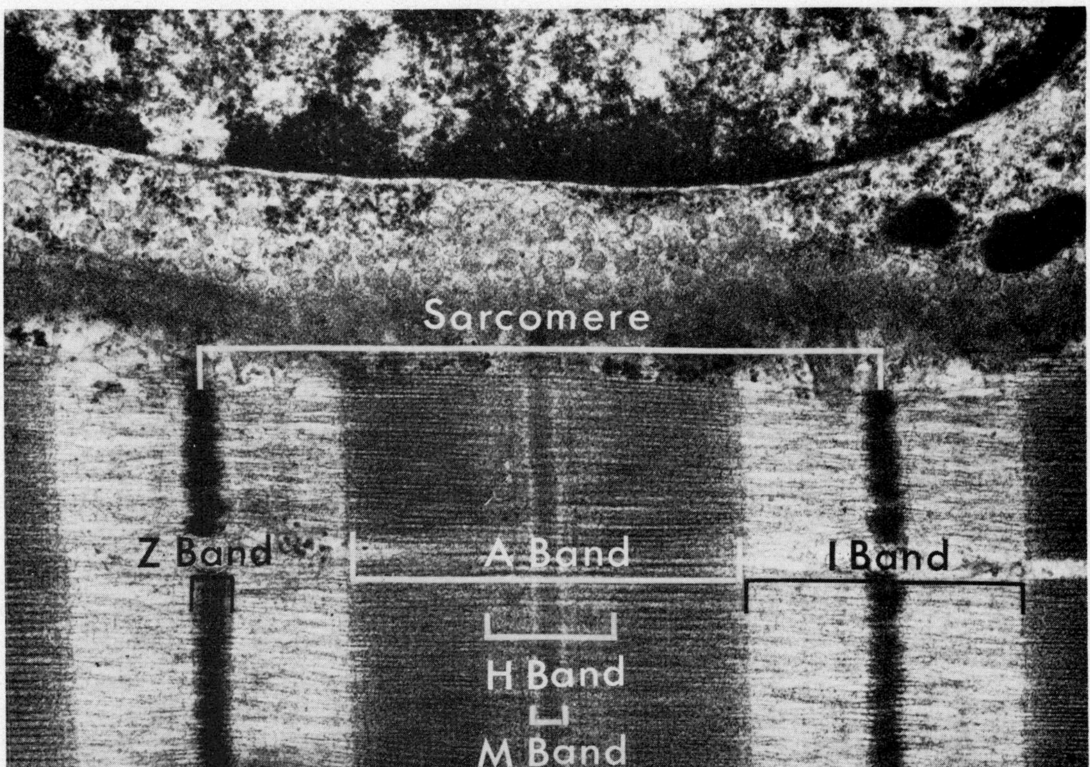

Figure 28–1. Electron micrograph of parts of two muscle fibers with the nucleus of one *(above)* and the most superficial myofibrils of the other *(below)*. Principal features of pattern of cross striations are identified on figure. (×34,000.) (Courtesy of Bloom, W., and Fawcett, D. W.: A Textbook of Histology. 9th ed. Philadelphia, W. B. Saunders Co., 1968, p. 277.)

synaptic trough, separated from the myofiber membrane by a thin extension of a Schwann cell and a scant amount of basement membrane–like material. The terminal axons have numerous small, synaptic vesicles containing acetylcholine. It is the release of this neurotransmitter and its contact with the myofiber membrane that invokes the calcium shift and so induces myofiber contraction. Groups of myofibers, not necessarily contiguous, innervated by a single anterior horn cell constitute a *motor unit*.

The muscles of the body can be divided into two classes, although there are additional subsets. One is designated "slow-twitch" and is involved predominantly in tonic contraction in the maintenance of posture. The myofibers in these muscles (type I) stain darkly and are rich in myoglobin and oxidative enzymes. The other class comprises the "fast-twitch" muscles involved mainly in phasic movement. These muscles are made of light-staining fibers rich in glycolytic enzymes. All the myofibers within a motor unit are of the same type. The difference between type I and type II fibers presumably reflects functional activity since reversal of their innervation is followed by reversal of fiber type.[6] In some of the disorders of muscle, in particular the congenital myopathies, certain fiber types tend to show the most marked morphologic changes.

Regeneration of muscle cells is a poorly understood but important feature of many forms of muscular disease. If only some of the sarcomeres degenerate, the remainder of the muscle cell may die, or it may break and regenerate by "budding" of the severed ends. Sarcolemmal nuclei by migration create a terminal bud that fuses with primitive myoblasts found between myofibers. Myoblasts are normally present between muscle cells as small, spindle-shaped "satellite cells" capable of becoming activated and myogenic in response to injury.[7] The elaboration of sarcoplasm and its ultrastructural components by the myoblasts may thus regenerate a muscle fiber in continuity with the preserved fragment. Often, however, the regeneration produces a misshapen, multinucleated, sarcoplasmic mass seen as a *muscle giant cell* in tissue sections. With death of an entire fiber, mononuclear myoblasts align in a single row and fuse. There follows a process recapitulating the fetal development of muscle cells. The spindled myoblasts acquire more cytoplasm, and myofilaments and cross striations appear. The myofilaments are at first confined to the periphery of the cells, leaving a central, clear, cytoplasmic zone that gives the appearance of a hollow tube. Increased synthesis of myofibrils eventually fills the cytoplasm and pushes the nuclei to their peripheral characteristic sarcolemmal location. These processes account for the varying cytologic patterns seen in sarcomas of muscle cell origin (rhabdomyosarcomas), as will be evident later. Against this background we can turn to the disorders of skeletal muscle.

PATHOLOGY

Disorders of skeletal muscle (myopathies) occur in a variety of systemic diseases as well as in certain primary muscular disorders. In general, these myopathies comprise a relatively small and peripheral area of pathologic practice. To recount all the conditions in which the skeletal muscles may be affected would entail listing many of the disorders that have already been presented. For example, staphylococcic infections may secondarily involve muscle fibers. Muscular involvement is a prominent feature of scleroderma and dermatomyositis. Muscle cell injury is encountered in chronic alcoholism, trichinosis, and typhoid fever, to cite only a few examples. Immobilization of an extremity either by an injury or by paralysis (e.g., stroke, poliomyelitis) is followed by muscular atrophy. Thus, the skeletal muscles are the seat of numerous morphologic changes in many different states.

The present consideration will be largely confined to a description of the basic reactions of muscle to various forms of injury. The number of these morphologic reactions is limited because the same basic reaction may have different causes. To interpret the meaning of these reaction patterns, and thus establish a pathogenetic mechanism and a clinical diagnosis of muscular disease, it is necessary to: (1) identify the basic pattern of muscle injury, (2) determine the distribution of muscle involvement, and (3) ascertain the coexistence of other organ involvements and possible etiologic mechanisms.

After a review of some basic reactions of muscle to injury, a few specific categories of disease will be discussed.

BASIC REACTIONS OF SKELETAL MUSCLE TO INJURY

The basic morphologic reflections of injury in muscle cells can be encompassed within the following categories: (1) muscle atrophy, (2) segmental necrosis, (3) myofiber disfigurative changes, and (4) myofiber volumetric changes.

MUSCULAR ATROPHY

Atrophic changes may result from very diverse derangements. Atrophy of muscle occurs with aging, perhaps related to gradual reduction of blood supply, and with immobilization, malnutrition, and chronic illness and particularly in denervation. Whatever the setting, the anatomic changes are more or less uniform and have been best studied in denervated muscles.

The first observable change involves the sarcolemmal nuclei, which become rounded, plump, somewhat hyperchromatic, and sometimes internalized within the myofiber to assume central or eccentric intrasarcoplasmic locations. There follows over the span of weeks slow, imperceptible diminution in myofiber size, which is responsible for some loss of the total muscle mass. Despite this contraction, cross striations persist, although longitudinal striations may be somewhat obscured. Lipofuscin pigmentation now becomes evident. Accompanying such loss of myofiber mass, there may be some apparent increase in the endomysial and perimysial connective tissue, which may now accumulate scattered fat cells. As the atrophic process continues, myofiber degenerative changes make their appearance. Scattered fibers become more opaque, with progressive disappearance of cross striations and clumping of the cytoplasm. Such fibers are of uneven diameter and in places are narrowed to slender tubes of collapsed sarcolemmal membrane. Phagocytic macrophages and scattered lymphocytes accumulate about such disintegrating myofibers. The sarcolemmal tube may appear to fragment and the macrophages proceed to engulf the cellular debris. Condensation of the sarcolemmal sheaths and endomysium contributes to the accumulation of apparent fibrous tissue.

Electron microscopic and biochemical studies confirm that with loss of fiber size there is progressive disappearance of myofilaments, beginning in the periphery of the myofiber. These changes are accompanied by a decrease in size and number of mitochondria, progressive loss of glycogen granules, an increase in lysosomes and lipofuscin granules, and progressive depletion of oxidative and glycolytic enzymes.[8, 9]

These microscopic changes, when sufficiently marked, cause shrinkage and flabbiness of the entire muscle mass. The muscle loses its normal red-brown color and becomes yellow to brown, depending on the amount of deposition of fat and lipochrome pigment. In far-advanced cases, the replacement fibrosis imparts a pale-gray, fibrous quality to the shrunken muscle.

Although the causes of muscular atrophy are legion, the most extreme examples are found in disorders that deprive motor units of their innervation—denervation atrophy. The neural lesion may be located within either the *spinal cord or peripheral nerves*. The atrophy that occurs then in poliomyelitis, in peripheral neuritis such as is caused by thiamine chloride deficiency and diabetic neuritis, and in injuries to peripheral nerves follows the pattern of morphologic changes described. The distribution of the atrophy depends on the pattern of innervation of affected motor nerves. Denervation atrophy may differ slightly from the other forms of atrophy in that, in the plane of section, one may find affected muscle fibers that have lost their innervation adjacent to normal-appearing muscle fibers having an independent nerve supply. The diagnosis of denervation atrophy can frequently be supported by the demonstration of degenerated nerve filaments within the muscle section. This type of apparent denervation atrophy is also encountered in certain specific neuromuscular diseases, e.g., infantile muscular atrophy, amyotonia congenita, progressive muscular atrophy of Aran-Duchenne, and amyotrophic lateral sclerosis of Charcot.

SEGMENTAL NECROSIS

In different forms of injury, the myofibrillar-sarcoplasmic content of the myofiber is damaged without apparently the endomysial or perimysial connective tissue being affected. Indeed, a few or many, but not all, of the sarcomeres in a myofiber are often affected, but not the entire myofiber. Such changes can be produced by sudden ischemia, physical trauma, extremes of temperatures, and microbiologic invasion.

The process of necrosis begins with acidophilic hyalinization of affected sarcomeres. This morphologic alteration has in the past been called "Zenker's hyaline degeneration." A variety of events may then ensue. The myofiber may sustain transverse fractures, often through the Z lines. Multiple fracture lines may induce so-called "shredding" of the fiber. The muscle nuclei become pyknotic, the cross striations disappear, and, in the course of a few days, neutrophils and macrophages invade the necrotic fiber and begin the process of removal of the amorphous sarcoplasmic debris both by enzymatic digestion and by engulfment. Sometimes the sarcoplasm is evacuated, leaving collapsed, hollow, sarcolemmal tubes and endomysial cords. In the course of time, muscle regeneration can usually be seen from adjacent preserved sarcolemmal nuclei or sarcomeres, as described earlier.

MYOFIBER DISFIGURATIVE CHANGES

The term muscle cell disfiguration has been invoked for a diversity of ultrastructural changes associated with a range of congenital and hereditary diseases.

Some of these disfigurations can be identified under the light microscope, but most require electron microscopic studies of appropriately preserved and processed tissue. It should be cautioned that inappropriate fixation and processing of muscle fibers can lead to a variety of artifacts readily misinterpreted as disfigurative. In many instances, the disfigurations are diagnostic of specific forms of congenital myopathies, discussed later (p. 1310). For example, dense cores of sarcoplasm devoid of myofilaments are found in the center of myofibers in central core myopathy. Electron-dense rods are typical of nemaline (rod-body) myopathy. Abnormalities in mitochondrial size, shape, and number are seen in the so-called mitochondrial myopathies. Accumulation of glycogen granules with disarray of the myofilaments and sarcoplasmic reticulum are encountered in certain glycogen storage diseases.

These disfigurative changes are encountered much less frequently than such basic reactions as myofiber atrophy and necrosis.

MYOFIBER VOLUMETRIC CHANGES

Abnormalities in fiber size may take the form of shrinkage of fibers—as in atrophy—or hypertrophy of fibers, for example, in the adaptation to increased workloads. Both forms of volumetric change may occur together. Denervation of a motor unit may lead to decrease in the size of a group of fibers, which in turn imposes an increased workload on adjacent fibers having normal neural connections, which then undergo "work" hypertrophy. Thus, abnormally large fibers are frequently encountered in diseases when there have been focal, atrophic, or degenerative changes in muscles. *Volumetric abnormalities are particularly prominent in Duchenne muscular dystrophy.* Enlargement of certain muscles, particularly in the leg but sometimes in the upper extremities, is encountered in this hereditary syndrome, accounting for the synonym pseudohypertrophic muscular dystrophy. Whether the myofiber hypertrophy is an early stage of the dystrophy that will in time lead to progressive shrinkage of the dystrophic fibers is uncertain. It should be cautioned that true myofiber hypertrophy, which may produce abnormal enlargement of the entire muscle mass, must be differentiated clinically from the spurious increase in muscle mass produced by the accumulation of fat cells accompanying myofiber atrophy.

MICROBIOLOGIC INJURIES TO MUSCLE

Damage to muscle cells may occur from direct invasion by bacteria, viruses, parasites, or fungi. Also, many bacterial toxic products, such as those produced by *Clostridium perfringens*, injure muscle cells.

Any of these forms of myopathy, better called myositis, may involve one or many muscles and, in the affected muscles, may present as sharply focalized or diffuse lesions. The pattern of reaction has already been described as segmental necrosis (p. 1306). In the foci of damage, there is usually a fairly prominent inflammatory cell infiltration accompanying the cytologic changes within the muscle cells. Depending on the underlying cause, injured muscle cells or totally necrotic muscle cells that have undergone fatty changes or coagulative necrosis are found, along with inflammatory white cell infiltration. The leukocytic response comprises neutrophils if the process is acute, or lymphocytes, histiocytes, and monocytes if the process is chronic. In later stages, there is more or less fibrous replacement of damaged cells and compensatory hypertrophy of marginal preserved cells. When the muscle is actually invaded by the causative agent (as occurs in abscess formation caused by staphylococci or streptococci, infection by trichinae or the spreading infections of **Clostridium perfringens,** toxoplasmosis, cysticercosis, or trypanosomiasis), serial sections, special stains, and cultural techniques sometimes permit identification of the underlying etiologic agent at the site of injury.

In the forms of myopathy encountered in typhoid fever, influenza, pneumonia, and smallpox, the muscle cell injury is usually confined to the sarcoplasmic substance of the muscle cell. Generally, the sarcolemmal sheath, the interstitial connective tissue, and the perimysium are little affected and the inflammatory infiltrate is correspondingly less prominent.

These inflammatory diseases of muscle differ histologically from the muscular dystrophies. In the latter, the leukocytic reaction is more scant and regenerative activity is minimal, whereas in the inflammatory conditions, considerable regrowth of injured or partially damaged muscle cells may occur and compensatory hypertrophy of unaffected cells fills in the gap produced by the loss of muscle cells.

In addition to the various diseases already mentioned, inflammatory myositis may be encountered in any of the so-called *connective tissue diseases*, but in these instances the nature of the muscle involvement can be identified only by the characteristic alterations in blood vessels and organs that accompany the muscle changes (Chapter 5). Myositis is one of the most prominent features of *Weil's disease.* An obscure form of primary myositis involving many muscles simultaneously is termed polymyositis. In all forms of myositis, the inflammatory changes are similar and may only be termed myositis. Differentiation of one condition from the other requires a knowledge of associated anatomic changes and the clinical findings.

MUSCULAR DYSTROPHIES

Muscle weakness, atrophy, and loss of tendon reflexes may have their origins in (1) primary disorders of muscle fibers, (2) spinal cord damage, or (3) peripheral nerve lesions. Here we are concerned with a group of genetic disorders, usually familial, that lead to weakness of muscle—the *muscular dystrophies.* Although there are many overlaps, differentiation among these syndromes depends on (1) age of onset, (2) mode of genetic transmission, (3) the clinical pattern and sequence of the appearance of muscle weaknesses, and (4) the rate of progression and ultimate gravity. These differences are cited in Table 28–1. Although all the dystrophies are considered to be inherited disorders, involvement of family members cannot be identified in many cases. A latent recessive trait in forebears or sporadic spontaneous mutation may account for the remaining cases. Despite clinical differences, *the myofiber changes in the various dystrophic syndromes are basically the same.* In contrast, a number of muscular disorders that closely *simulate the dystrophies clinically but are marked by fairly specific morphologic changes in the myofibers,* as pointed out later, are referred to as *congenital myopathies.*

MORPHOLOGY. The anatomic changes in all dystrophic muscles have been characterized as "living, dying, dead and regenerating muscle fibers in varying proportions according to the stage of the disease."[10] Moreover, each cell is affected individually, leading to juxtaposition of healthy cells with those dead, dying, or regenerating. Macroscopically, involved muscles may appear normal in size; may be shrunken, flabby, and pale, as myofibers are replaced by fibrous tissue and fat; or may even be deceptively enlarged by the accumulation of fat and fibrous tissue. Long before such gross alterations become apparent, individual cells become necrotic. The dying process involves a sequence of changes, often beginning with acidophilic "contraction bands," described earlier (p. 1304). This is followed by disorganization of the parallel myofilaments, creating sarcoplasmic masses. Thereafter, clumping and fragmentation of the sarcoplasm occurs, sometimes accompanied by internalization of sarcolemmal nuclei. An increase of autophagic vacuoles, residual bodies (lipofuscin), and intrafiber fat vacuoles accompanies this process. Less frequently, death of myofibers is first marked by loss of the A or I bands.

Table 28–1. MUSCULAR DYSTROPHIES

	Inheritance	Age at Onset	Major Clinical Features	Course
Duchenne type	X-linked recessive	Early childhood	Symmetric weakness; initially pelvifemoral; later weakness in leg, shoulder girdle, and then trunk muscles; "pseudohypertrophy" of calves; reduced intelligence; cardiac involvement	Progressive; inability to walk by puberty; death by age 20
Becker type	X-linked recessive	Second decade	Milder variant of Duchenne type	"Benign"; ability to walk into adult life
Facioscapulohumeral	Autosomal dominant	Childhood to late adult life	Usually facial weakness first; scapular weakness; humeral weakness	"Benign" course not progressive
Limb-girdle	Autosomal recessive	Variable onset first to sixth decade	Two variants: (1) pelvifemoral weakness; (2) shoulder girdle weakness	Variable progression; disability within 20 years
Myotonic dystrophy	Autosomal dominant	Infancy to middle adult life	Weakness and myotonia (difficulty in relaxation) of distal muscles, e.g., hands and feet; frontal baldness; cataracts; testicular atrophy; cardiac involvement	"Benign"; does not shorten life
Ocular myopathy	?Autosomal dominant	Variable	Group of syndromes all having weakness in extraocular muscles initially; sometimes involvement of face, neck, limbs	Rarely progressive

Accompanying the regressive alterations is a loss of histochemical differentiation between type I and type II fibers, but neither fiber type is spared. Inconstant and variable abnormalities of the plasma membrane have been described and accorded pathogenetic significance. Thereafter, macrophages move in to remove the cellular carcasses. Uninvolved, immediately contiguous myofibers may undergo hypertrophic enlargement. Fully developed disease is characterized then by a random pattern of preserved and unaffected myofibers, enlarged fibers, shrunken fibers and collapsed sheaths bearing recognizable sarcolemmal nuclei, and a variable interstitial accumulation of fat and fibrous tissue (Fig. 28–2). Continued active cell necrosis may or may not be present at this late stage. It is this distinctive, irregular pattern of clustered myofiber involvement that principally differentiates the dystrophies from the "motor unit atrophies" of spinal and neural denervations.

ETIOLOGY AND PATHOGENESIS. The origins of the muscular dystrophies remain unknown. Theories involving myoneural abnormalities or vascular insufficiency related to vasoconstrictive influences have largely been discarded.[11] Their occurrence, in many instances, as familial disorders would logically point to some inborn metabolic or biochemical abnormality (e.g., a missing enzyme or some abnormality in structural protein), but none that can be considered a fundamental defect have been identified. In current favor, but without substantial proof, is the possibility of some membrane defect.[12] Abnormalities in muscle plasma membranes have been visualized with scanning and electron microscopes, especially in Duchenne muscular dystrophy. Similar membrane alterations in erythrocytes and impaired capping of membrane receptors on lymphocytes derived from these patients in response to antigenic or mitogenic challenge have been described, pointing to a generalized membrane defect.[13] However, some of the parents in familial cases also had similar capping abnormalities without evidence of muscular disease. In the last analysis, it is not certain whether these putative membrane abnormalities are primary or secondary, but in either event all of the dystrophies are characterized by increased serum levels of a variety of muscle enzymes, particularly creatine kinase (CK), and are also marked by creatinuria, pointing to abnormally leaky cell membranes.

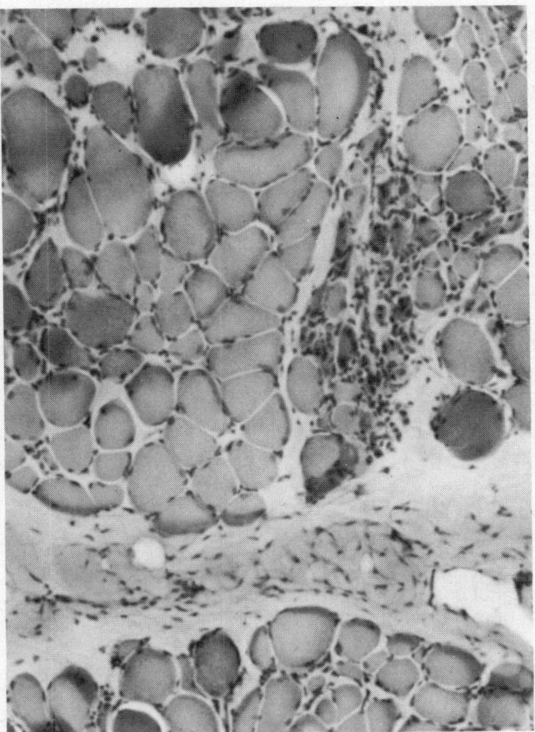

Figure 28–2. Duchenne's muscular dystrophy. Biopsy of calf muscle. There is an obvious focus of active necrosis containing occasional mononuclears, reduplicated sarcolemmal nuclei, and some necrotic and necrotizing muscle fibers with internalization of sarcolemmal nuclei. The surrounding, better-preserved fibers reveal marked inequality of cross-sectional diameter with a slight interstitial fibrosis. (Courtesy of Dr. William Schoene, Department of Pathology, Brigham and Women's Hospital, Boston, and Harvard Medical School.)

CLINICAL SYNDROMES. All the dystrophies are rare and have a prevalence of about 5 to 40 per million population. Only the more common Duchenne type and myotonic dystrophy will be briefly characterized.[14]

The *Duchenne (pseudohypertrophic) muscular dystrophy* is the most disastrous; it appears early in life, is rapidly progressive in most cases, and usually causes death by 20 years of age. As a sex-linked recessive condition it is limited to males, who generally have unaffected mothers unless those mothers are concurrently suffering from Turner's syndrome. Occasionally, female carriers have mild symptoms. The fully expressed condition typically begins in infancy with pelvifemoral muscle weakness that appears insidiously. As a consequence there is a delay in walking, a waddling gait, frequent falls, and difficulty in rising from the floor or climbing stairs. Progressively the muscles of the lower leg are affected and then those of the shoulder girdle, arms, neck, and trunk. Enlargement of the calf muscles, because of the excessive accumulation of fat and fibrous tissue, is particularly distinctive of this dystrophy and accounts for the term "pseudohypertrophic." Usually by age 10 to 12 years the child is reduced to a wheelchair with all manner of grotesque, fixed-flexion deformities. For uncertain reasons, about one-third of these individuals also have significant reduction of intelligence that is apparent from the outset.

The morphologic alterations in Duchenne's dystrophy are basically those common to all of these syndromes, as already detailed. However, because of the rapid progression of the condition, the myofiber necrosis and the interstitial accumulation of fat and fibrous tissue tend to be more florid than in the other forms of dystrophy. Similar changes may appear within the myocardium and lead to abnormalities in the ECG, but cardiac failure is uncommon, perhaps because physical activity is restricted. Ultimately, the progressive involvement of the muscles of the trunk, leading to serious respiratory difficulties and pulmonary infection, is the most common cause of death, although occasionally it is caused by a cardiac arrhythmia.

A milder form of sex-linked dystrophy having many similarities to Duchenne dystrophy is referred to as *Becker dystrophy*. Linkage studies make clear that it is a distinct entity because the two conditions are not encountered in the same family.

Myotonic dystrophy is the most prevalent of the dystrophies. It usually appears in early adult life, although it may begin in infancy and childhood with weakness of the distal muscles of the hands and feet, particularly the adductors of the forearms and thumbs. The weakness is accompanied by myotonia (tonic contraction, e.g., inability to let go after shaking hands). Soon thereafter, ptosis, facial weakness, and dysarthria appear, and are not seen with other forms of dystrophy. Next, more proximal muscle groups in the arms and legs become involved, but generally the motor involvement progresses slowly, is not totally incapacitating, and is compatible with long survival (except in the most extreme instances).

Although this condition is conventionally called "myotonic dystrophy," there are many differences between it and the other dystrophies, notably involvement of many extramuscular systems, as indicated in Table 28–1. Also, there is often mental retardation or dementia and cardiac involvement, sometimes leading to arrhythmias and occasionally to cardiac failure in older patients. The morphologic changes in the muscles, although basically similar to those in the other slowly progressive dystrophies, include two distinctive features. Sometimes seen are "sarcoplasmic masses" constituting accumulations of sarcoplasm free of myofilaments and "ring fibers," where one myofiber transversely encircles the other fibers in the same bundle. When present, they provide the opportunity to identify morphologically a particular form of dystrophy. For the remaining syndromes, as already emphasized, the differential diagnosis rests on clinical grounds.

CONGENITAL MYOPATHIES

In contrast to the muscular dystrophies in which each syndrome is characterized by a fairly specific skeletal distribution of muscle involvement, but with no morphologic changes to permit differentiation among the various syndromes, *the congenital myopathies are not distinctive clinically, but are highly distinctive morphologically*. From a clinical standpoint, all the myopathies tend to present in a similar manner, characterized as "floppy infant syndrome"—muscle weakness appearing in early infancy or later. Sometimes the weakness assumes girdle or proximal limb distributions reminiscent of the muscular dystrophies. In the congenital myopathies, however, the muscle weakness is generally not progressive (although there are exceptions), so these conditions are compatible with long survival.

Because these muscular involvements are extremely rare, the major forms are briefly characterized in Table 28–2.[15]

MYASTHENIA GRAVIS (MG)

Myasthenia gravis is an autoimmune disorder characterized by muscle weakness caused by antibodies that localize in the neuromuscular junctions and impair transmission of neural impulses. *The trigger initiating the development of the antibodies is unknown but the antigenic target is the acetylcholine receptors of the postsynaptic membrane at the motor endplate.* The following features distinguish MG from other muscular disorders:

1. The first and most consistently affected muscles are those in most active use, more or less in descending order of frequency: oculomotor, facial, laryngeal, pharyngeal, and respiratory. With advance of the disease in severity and time, girdle and then proximal muscles are affected and, in the most severe cases nearly all muscles of the body.

2. Particularly distinctive is the progression of the muscular weakness with persistent use, and recovery of strength following a period of rest.

3. Thymic abnormalities are present in 70 to 80% of patients (thymic follicular hyperplasia, "thymitis," in 60 to 65%; thymoma in 10 to 15%).

Table 28–2. CONGENITAL MYOPATHIES

Disease	Inheritance	Histologic Features
Central core disease	Autosomal dominant	Amorphous central core in fibers (principally type I) with partial or complete lack of myofilaments and oxidative and glycolytic enzymes
Nemaline (rod body) myopathy	Sporadic Autosomal dominant Autosomal recessive	Dark-staining ovoid or elongated rods within types I and II fibers composed of filamentous structures with periodic lines perpendicular and parallel to long axis
Centronuclear (myotubular) myopathy	Variable	Nuclei occupy center of fiber, often absence of myofibrils about nuclei, numerous mitochondria and glycogen vacuoles
Congenital fiber–type disproportion	?Autosomal recessive ?Autosomal dominant	Type I fiber predominance; abnormally small type I fibers, normal or enlarged type II, various ultrastructural alterations
Mitochondrial myopathies	?	Variety of myofiber abnormalities in different patients—mitochondria are abnormally large, increased in number, abnormal shapes, abnormalities of cristae

4. The disease may appear at any age, but the peak incidence for females is in the third decade and for males in later adult life.

5. Overall, females are affected twice as often as males, the disproportion being about 4 to 5:1 in the first decade, with some reversal of this ratio in the later years.

6. There are well-defined correlations between age at onset and the thymic abnormalities. Thymic follicular hyperplasia is associated with an early age of onset, i.e., the second to third decades. In contrast, the peak incidence of disease associated with thymoma is in the fifth decade, males being involved more often than females.

7. Also characteristic of myasthenia is the marked improvement in muscle strength in response to anticholinesterase drugs, until the disease becomes advanced.

Still unsettled is the issue of genetic and familial predisposition.[16] Although the classic disease is not clearly familial, an association particularly with HLA-B8, and less strongly with A1 and DW3, has been repeatedly noted, but the association is not invariable and may relate to predisposition to autoimmune disease. In this connection, patients and their families have an increased incidence of autoimmune thyroid diseases, pernicious anemia, and NIDDM diabetes. An early onset form (which may represent a special subset) is thought to be an autosomal recessive condition.

Etiology and Pathogenesis. The evidence linking causation of MG to autoantibodies to acetylcholine receptors is strong despite a few persisting and perplexing incongruities. Electron microscopy discloses morphologic abnormalities in the neuromuscular junctions of affected muscles. Both IgG and C3 can be identified here by the immunoperoxidase method.[17] Circulating antireceptor antibodies can be identified in most patients with active disease.[18] It was always assumed that these antibodies led to the destruction of the receptors, perhaps by activating lytic fractions of complement. Recent studies, however, indicate that in addition to accelerated degradation they may also impair transmission of impulses by blockade of the acetylcholine receptors. Indeed, 98% of a series of myasthenic patients were shown to have antibodies producing either accelerated degradation or blockade of receptors.[19]

The relationship of the thymic abnormalities to the autoimmune reaction is still poorly understood but a number of relevant observations have been made. There is wide, but not universal, agreement that the normal thymus has myoid cells bearing acetylcholine receptors or receptor-like antigens.[20] The follicular hyperplasia encountered in most young patients is characterized by the formation of germinal centers containing B lymphocytes, and receptor antibodies can be shown to be present in these lymphoid follicles. However, the thymus is not a major site of antibody production because serum levels of receptor antibody do not usually fall immediately after thymectomy. Instead, they decline slowly over the span of many months in association with clinical improvement.[21] Relevant to this observation is the ability of cells derived from the thymic glands to selectively enhance production of receptor antibody by autologous circulating lymphocytes.[22] Conceivably some of the thymocytes are specifically sensitized T-helper cells that only slowly disappear from the circulation, accounting for the slow decline in the level of antireceptor antibodies.

The role of the thymoma in the causation of MG is even more obscure. Generally, these patients have higher antibody titers, more progressive disease, and a worse outlook whether the tumor is excised or not. Scattered reports suggest that cultured thymoma cells are able to transform into myoid cells and that there is a higher incidence of lymphoid follicles in the non-neoplastic thymus than in nonthymoma cases.[23] These findings suggest that the thymoma in some way initiates "thymitis," but this proposal awaits further confirmation.

Despite all the cited evidence, pieces are still missing from the puzzle. What initiates the autoimmune reaction? Without proof, viral involvement of the thymus in individuals genetically predisposed by their complement of immune response genes is questioned. How to account for the infrequent cases of MG that appear many years after thymectomy? Why are the benefits of thymectomy largely limited to early or mild disease, and of limited value late in the course? Other questions remain.

Morphology. Anatomic study of the skeletal muscles in MG has been surprisingly unrewarding, since no consistent abnormalities have been noted. In some patients there are focal collections of lymphocytes within the muscles and, occasionally, myofiber atrophy or myofiber necrosis. In most patients the muscles are not obviously atrophic, nor are there myofiber changes by usual histologic techniques. However, with chronic paralysis, disuse atrophy of motor units develops, accompanied by ingrowth of fat and fibrous tissue. As pointed out earlier, electron microscopy in some patients has disclosed abnormalities in the postsynaptic membrane and immune complex deposits at the myoneural junctions, which can be shown by immunoperoxidase techniques to contain IgG and C3. Nonetheless, the terminal motor nerves and anterior horn cells remain unaffected.

The thymus may be normal or show follicular hyperplasia or, in a few patients, a thymoma. These thymic abnormalities were reviewed earlier (p. 1250) (Fig. 28–3).

Rarely, lymphocytic infiltrates have been observed in the liver, thyroid glands, adrenals, and other organs.

Clinical Course. The onset of this condition may be extremely insidious or relatively sudden. The first manifestation is usually weakening of the eye muscles leading to diplopia, often accompanied by drooping of the eyelids. The other muscle groups mentioned earlier may then be affected, with immobility of the face, impaired motion of the tongue, aspiration of food and choking, and alterations in voice quality. The subsequent course is extremely variable. In the fortunate patient, the course is extremely benign and is almost limited to involvement of the eye muscles. In such instances, it may spontaneously disappear. In others

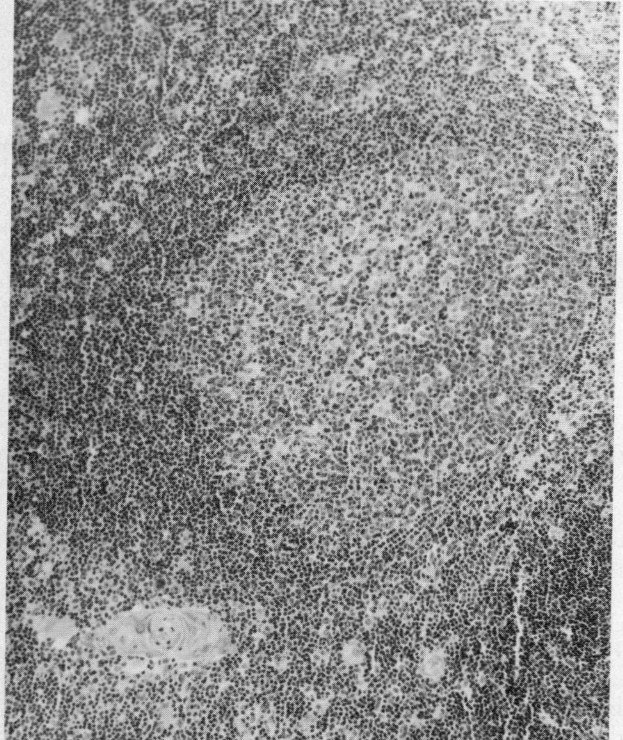

Figure 28–3. Thymus in myasthenia gravis, with follicular hyperplasia. A Hassall's corpuscle may be noted at lower left.

only slightly less fortunate, the muscle weakness does not progress into the trunk or extremities, or the disease may remit partially or completely for months to a few years. At the other end of the spectrum, the motor weakness relentlessly extends over a period to involve the trunk and extremities, or there may be repeated remissions and relapses with progression of the disease with each relapse. Fatigue, infections, alcohol intake, and all forms of stress are thought to precipitate relapses. In such progressive disease, the muscles of respiration and movement are eventually involved, creating a breathless invalid.

During the early so-called "active stage," the weakness is dramatically improved by such anticholinesterase drugs as neostigmine, but with progressive disease thymectomy, corticosteroids, or other immunosuppressive methods may be required. Regrettably, even these therapies may not stem the tide. The major threats to life are respiratory infections secondary to the ventilatory deficit. It is ironic that persons with mild or restricted disease respond best to drugs and thymectomy, whereas those with severe progressive involvement whose lives hang in the balance respond poorly. Most deaths occur within the first year when the probable prognosis is established by the speed and spread of the motor weakness.

The role of thymic surgery in the control of this disorder remains controversial. About two-thirds of patients with no thymic tumor are improved with thymectomy, especially when this is performed early in the course. Those with a thymoma do worse whether the neoplasm is excised or not.

Infants born of myasthenic mothers may manifest so-called congenital myasthenia caused by transplacental passage of maternal IgG antireceptor antibodies. The motor weakness lasts only a few weeks and spontaneous recovery is the rule, but severe impairment of muscle function may threaten life.

TUMORS AND TUMOR-LIKE LESIONS OF MUSCLES

Under this heading are included not only true neoplasms arising in the skeletal muscle cells but also several non-neoplastic conditions—traumatic myositis ossificans and fibromatoses that may simulate neoplasms both morphologically and clinically.

TRAUMATIC MYOSITIS OSSIFICANS

Traumatic injury to muscle, usually accompanied by considerable hemorrhage, is followed by the deposit of fibrous tissue and bone in the site of injury. The fibrous and osseous reaction can readily be mistaken both clinically and morphologically for a neoplasm. This type of muscle injury is most likely to occur in young males following an overt blow or more subtle injury in the course of their work, athletics, or military service. Most often affected are the quadriceps femoris and the brachialis anticus. Following the muscle tear or damage, *the hemorrhage is organized by the characteristic formation of granulation tissue and progressive fibrous scarring*. Regenerating muscle giant cells may be trapped within the scar. In the course of this process, *cartilage may form and be followed by endochondral ossification. Alternatively, calcification may occur en masse and be followed by ossification.* The origin of the osteoblasts that lay down the bone is uncertain, but they either arise in situ from mesenchymal cells or are derived from adjacent periosteum that is involved in the muscular injury. Aside from the attendant pain, swelling, and tenderness, the major significance of myositis ossificans lies in its possible confusion with a bone tumor. The hard, localized, bony mass; the roentgenographic demonstration of bone density outside the normal bone; and the histologic pattern of proliferating fibroblasts associated with bone formation may all be confused by the unwary with an osteogenic sarcoma. Rare instances of transformation to osteogenic sarcoma have been reported.

DESMOID TUMOR (AGGRESSIVE FIBROMATOSIS)

Despite the designation "desmoid tumor" these curious, stubbornly infiltrative fibroblastic lesions are not considered to be neoplasms, do not metastasize, and may even undergo "spontaneous" cure.[24] Instead, they lie in the interface between an exuberant proliferation and a low-grade fibrosarcoma. They arise in the supporting connective tissue and aponeuroses of skeletal muscle; hence, the synonym *musculoaponeurotic fibromatosis*.

Desmoids may occur at any age but the peak incidence is in the third decade. There is a strong female preponderance of 5:1. In females most lesions arise in the anterior abdominal wall, but in males and sometimes in females there is a wide scatter in relation to almost every other muscle in the body.[25] The nature of these fibromatoses is mysterious. One study calls attention to multiple bone malformations, often minor, in patients with desmoid tumors, raising the possibility of some systemic (? genetic) defect in connective tissue formation.[26] Two other major associations are previous trauma at the site of the lesion and multiple pregnancies. These correlates support roles for trauma and estrogen stimulation in their causation. Estrogen receptors can frequently be identified in these growths. Desmoid-like tumors have been produced in guinea pigs by the injection of estrogens, but they did not appear when progesterone or testosterone was administered simultaneously. Conceivably, then, there is an underlying systemic connective tissue derangement that accounts for the bone malformations and becomes expressed when acted on by trauma or estrogens. Slender evidence that the underlying derangement is genetic in origin derives from the occurrence of desmoids with intestinal polyposis in the familial Gardner's syndrome.

MORPHOLOGY. Morphologically, these lesions occur as unicentric, gray-white, firm, unencapsulated, poorly demarcated masses varying from 1 to 15 cm in greatest diameter. They are rubbery and tough and infiltrate between muscles, muscle bundles, and individual muscle cells. Histologically, the more central regions, presumably the oldest part of the growth, are largely densely collagenous, whereas the periphery is made up of plump, typical fibroblasts having moderate variation in cell and nuclear size, resembling a "low-grade" fibrosarcoma.[27] Mitoses are infrequent and, when present, are regular. Muscle cells or groups trapped within the growth are destroyed or atrophic. Sometimes, regenerative activity creates muscle giant cells having many sarcolemmal nuclei and abundant sarcoplasm.

The obvious importance of desmoids is their differentiation from sarcomas. In addition to their possible cosmetic disadvantages, they are occasionally painful. Although curable by adequate excision, they stubbornly recur in the local site when incompletely removed. The rare reports of metastatic dissemination of a desmoid must be interpreted as misidentification of a low-grade fibrosarcoma.

PALMAR FIBROMATOSIS

In addition to desmoids within the musculoaponeuroses, fibromatoses may arise in other connective tissue sites, e.g., in relation to neck muscles (fibromatosis colli), in the penis (Peyronie's disease), in the feet (plantar fibromatosis), and in the fascia of the palms (palmar fibromatosis) giving rise to *Dupuytren's contracture*. When the palmar fascia becomes heavily laden with connective tissue and collagen, the process may trap tendons and extend to the overlying skin. Progressive shrinkage of the collagen leads to flexion contractions of the fingers and hands and, in time, deformity and limitation of motion of the affected parts. Typically, the contractures first become evident in the fifth finger and then sequentially in contiguous fingers. The dense, white fibromatous tissue is easily mistaken for a tumor grossly, and can be misinterpreted as a low-grade fibrosarcoma histologically. These lesions are not neoplastic, but are difficult to manage clinically because of the technical problems involved in total excision of the lesion.

NODULAR (PSEUDOSARCOMATOUS) FASCIITIS

This non-neoplastic lesion is considered here not because it arises in skeletal muscle but because it is basically a fibromatosis, sometimes called *pseudosarcomatous fibromatosis*. Typically, these fibroblastic proliferations arise in subcutaneous locations anywhere in the body with a predilection for the forearm, leg, arm, and face, in that order. Despite the designation "fasciitis," these fibromatoses, unlike desmoid tumors, do not arise primarily in fascia but may in their growth become attached to it.

Grossly, nodular fasciitis is typically a small (less than 2 cm), gray-white, firm-to-myxoid mass that, although well circumscribed, is not encapsulated. The periphery often exhibits streaming extensions into the surrounding fat, fascia, and sometimes muscle, and is readily interpreted as sarcomatous. Four histologic subtypes have been described but all are variations on a common theme. The basic histologic pattern is that of an exuberant overgrowth of "active-looking" fibroblasts intermediate between an inflammatory reparative reaction and a sarcoma (Fig. 28–4). The lesion is mainly composed of thick-to-thin spindle-shaped fibroblasts varying in size. The larger cells have abundant cytoplasm with large nuclei and prominent nucleoli. These spindled cells may be disposed randomly, may suggest a storiform (whorled) pattern, or may be laid down in interconnecting bundles. Scattered, usually normal-appearing mitoses are present as well as larger, multinucleated giant cells. In some instances the giant cells represent regenerating skeletal muscle fibers trapped in the infiltrating lesions, but in other instances they may be of fibroblastic or histiocytic origin.[28] It is apparent that the microscopic changes can readily be mistaken for a sarcoma, but the following features are helpful in the differential diagnosis: **(1) often the center of the nodular fasciitis is myxoid with increasing cellularity toward the periphery, but some lesions are cellular throughout; (2) characteristically, histiocytic cells are scattered throughout the lesion as well as occasional lymphocytes, particularly at the periphery (neutrophils or plasma cells are seldom present); (3) newly formed capillary channels are often radially arrayed at the advancing front of the nodule; (4) in some cases there are foci of osteoid and chondroid metaplasia; and (5) tumor**

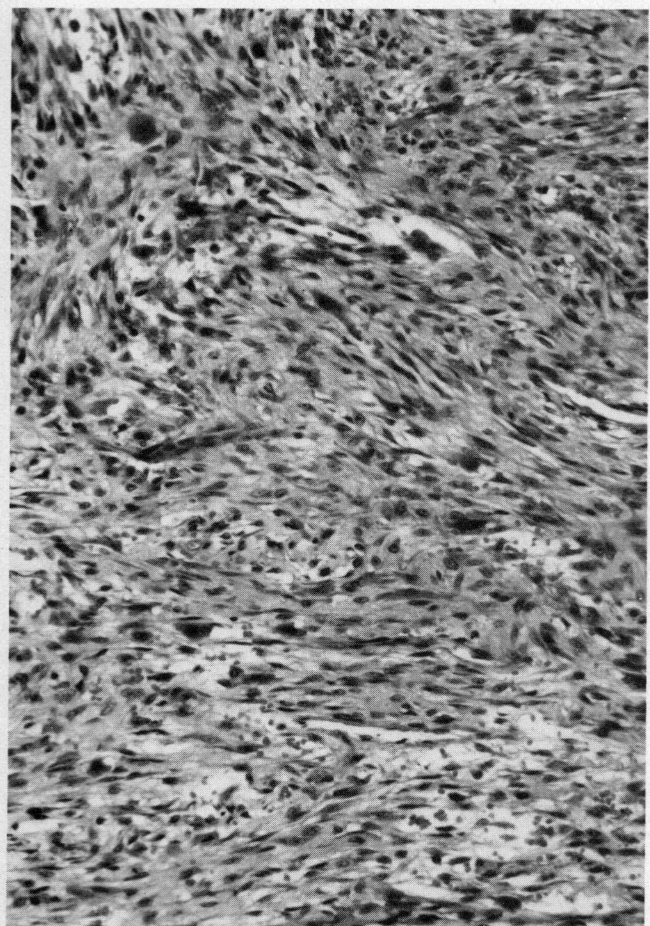

Figure 28–4. Nodular fasciitis. Cellular active margin of a lesion. There is considerable variation in nuclear size of "active-looking" fibroblasts with occasional cells approaching giant cells. Basis for term "pseudosarcomatous fibromatosis" is evident.

giant cells with "ugly" hyperchromatic nuclei are not found.

Nodular fasciitis may present clinically as a subcutaneous tumor and, although most are small, they uncommonly produce firm masses many centimeters in diameter that become attached to the deeper fascial planes and muscles. Most often, they rapidly increase in size over the span of a few weeks after discovery, a growth rate that is unusual for even very aggressive neoplasms. On surgical exposure the lack of encapsulation and pseudoinvasiveness are deceptive. Moreover, the unwary microscopist may misinterpret the lesion and classify it as a cancer, most often a malignant fibrous histiocytoma, fibrosarcoma, or other mesenchymal neoplasm. Correct identification assumes great importance because even incompletely resected lesions do not recur.[29]

RHABDOMYOMA

Cardiac rhabdomyomas were described on page 606. Extracardiac rhabdomyomas are so rare that they fall into the category of "exotic" and thus receive brief comment. The skeletal rhabdomyomas have been subdivided into two types, adult and fetal, based on their histogenesis. The *adult form* occurs almost exclusively in adults in the head and neck region, particularly in the larynx and pharynx, at sites where there is skeletal muscle. They are well-encapsulated, lobulated tumors composed of large, round-to-oval cells with a pale, granular eosinophilic cytoplasm and round-to-ovoid eccentrically located nuclei. Often, large cytoplasmic vacuoles containing glycogen produce so-called "spider cells." Some of the cells almost always reveal cross striations typical of skeletal muscle; ultrastructurally, myofilaments as well as A and I bands and Z lines can be seen.[30]

The *fetal rhabdomyoma* is mainly a tumor of infants that usually is located subcutaneously in the head and neck region with a predilection for the posterior auricular area. However, it may arise in adults, particularly females, in the vulvovaginal region. It is composed of spindled fetal myoblasts having variable degrees of skeletal muscle differentiation. Although circumscribed, it is not encapsulated, and its lack of recurrence following local excision has raised the suggestion that it may be a hamartoma, just as the cardiac rhabdomyoma is thought to be a hamartoma.

Both adult and fetal variants are cured by local excision, and recurrence or aggressive behavior is exceptional.

RHABDOMYOSARCOMA

Although uncommon, rhabdomyosarcomas are one of the most frequent forms of cancer of soft parts (muscle, fibrous tissue, fatty tissue), particularly in children under the age of 15. Four distinctive morphologic variants are recognized: (1) embryonal, (2) alveolar, (3) pleomorphic, and (4) botryoid.[31] The first three are differentiated on cytologic grounds, but the fourth on its gross morphology. The botryoid sarcoma is in reality an embryonal rhabdomyosarcoma rendered distinctive by its outgrowth into an open space (e.g., the vagina, bladder, or nasopharynx), permitting the formation of multiple bulbous projections having some resemblance to a cluster of grapes—hence, botryoid. Although all patterns are presumed to arise in primitive myoblasts that undergo variable levels of myogenic differentiation, in some instances (e.g., the embryonal pattern) the myogenic differentiation is minimal and the neoplastic cells closely resemble those of undifferentiated mesenchymal origin. Significantly, the botryoid pattern arises in locations remote from skeletal muscle. However, studies with immunocytochemical methods document that all four anatomic variants usually contain myoglobin as a tumor marker for striated muscle differentiation.[32] Although myosin or actin can also be identified by similar methods in many of these neoplasms, these markers are less specific because they are not limited to skeletal muscle cells.[33]

Rhabdomyosarcomas may occur at any age from birth to the advanced years of life; however, in children they are the most common form of soft tissue sarcoma.[34] Although the correlations are imperfect, embryonal rhabdomyosarcomas generally arise within the first two decades of life; indeed, they may be present at birth. Most patients with alveolar tumors are adolescent; in contrast, pleomorphic rhabdomyosarcomas usually affect elderly individuals. Thus, the older the patient, the more likely is it that the rhabdomyosarcoma represents the pleomorphic variant.

Before the various morphologic patterns are described, a few words are in order relative to the staging and prognosis of all rhabdomyosarcomas. As cancers, all histologic variants are locally invasive and spread to regional nodes and more widely to almost any site in the body, including the heart and central nervous system. Overall, distant metastases are already present in 20 to 40% of patients at the time of diagnosis. Histologic type exerts little influence.[35] Site of origin is, however, material. Spread of the cancer is most likely with those arising in the trunk, followed in descending order by the genitourinary tract, extremities, and head and neck region. Several staging systems are in use to express the extent of the neoplasia in the patient. Although there are differences among them, the following criteria generally apply:

Stage I— Localized disease; tumor resectable; no nodal or distant spread.
Stage II— Regional disease; tumor questionably resectable; no nodal or distant spread.
Stage III—Regional disease; incomplete gross resection with regional node involvement.
Stage IV—Distant metastasis.

More specific details are available in the report of Green and Jaffe.[36] The prognosis for these neoplasms is difficult to express because it is modified by type and location of lesion, stage of disease, and resectability. Overall, including all patterns of tumors in all locations, a 10 to 30% five-year survival rate has been achieved by surgery alone.[37] The combination of surgery and chemotherapy has greatly improved the outlook, yielding about an 85% disease-free interval for at least two years in persons grossly free of tumor following surgery.[38] Two subsets fared less well than the group as a whole: those with the alveolar histologic pattern and those with neoplasms in the head in parameningeal locations and in the neck region.

Pleomorphic Rhabdomyosarcoma

About three-quarters of pleomorphic rhabdomyosarcomas arise in the soft tissues of the extremities and trunk in adults. Generally, they are deeply situated within muscles, but some appear to arise within the subcutaneous tissues and even fungate through the skin. It is likely, however, that these subcutaneous lesions arise in the superficial layers of the skeletal muscles and then expand toward the skin. They are extremely malignant lesions and metastasize early.

These cancers vary in size from small to large bulky masses, sometimes over 15 cm in diameter. They are often dark-red, lobulated masses that may even give the appearance of multicentricity. Hemorrhages and necroses may produce mottled red-white foci within the center of the mass. Their histology is extremely variable. Basically, four types of cells may be present: (1) large round cells of uncertain characterization, with abundant acidophilic cytoplasm and one or two central nuclei; (2) more distinctive strap-shaped or ribbon-shaped cells with one or several nuclei in which longitudinal fibrils and cross striations may be discernible; (3) racket-shaped cells with a single nucleus in the expanded end and a tapering, acidophilic body; and (4) tumor giant cells, rounded or ovoid, with peripherally arranged vacuoles separated by thin strands of cytoplasm, referred to as "spider cells" (Fig. 28–5).[27] The vacuoles are PAS positive and contain glycogen. These four cell types may be scattered randomly or be arranged in whorls, clusters, or even fascicles. Tumors composed of very undifferentiated cells are difficult to distinguish from other forms of connective tissue sarcoma. **The diagnosis rests on identification of longitudinal myofibrils, cross striations within the myoblastic cells, and/or the identification of myoglobin** (as pointed out above).

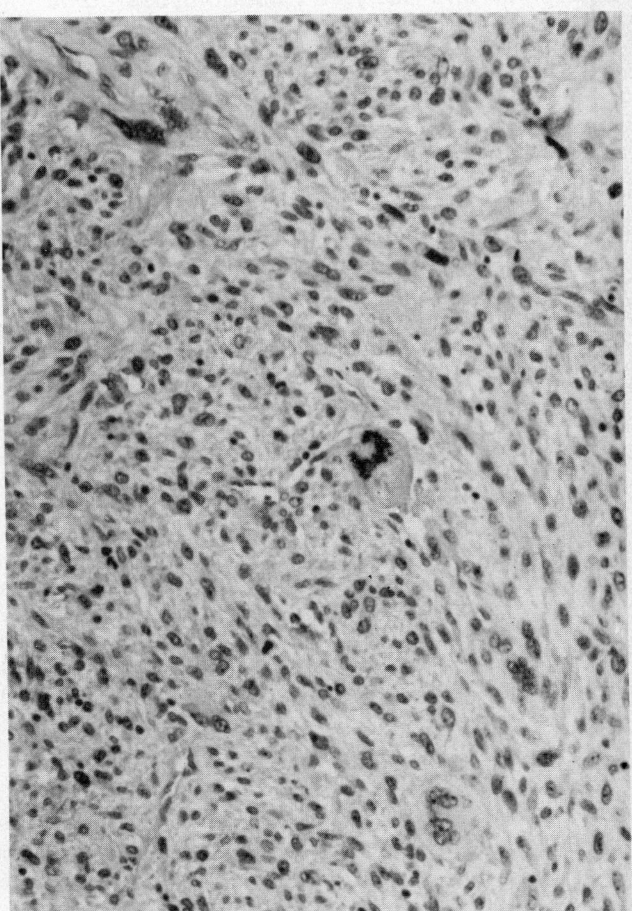

Figure 28–5. Pleomorphic rhabdomyosarcoma. There is marked variability in cell and nuclear size and shape with several obvious tumor giant cells. The central giant cell reveals an atypical mitotic figure and abundant cytoplasm, partially vacuolated.

Alveolar Rhabdomyosarcoma

The alveolar rhabdomyosarcoma most often arises in the muscles of the upper and lower extremities, most often in children and young adults. However, about one-fifth occur in the trunk and an equal number in the head and neck region. Aggressive lesions, they tend to metastasize early and widely.

Grossly, the presentation of these tumors is similar to that of pleomorphic rhabdomyosarcomas. Histologically, they are distinctive by virtue of the tendency for the tumor cells to form islands (alveoli) or broad cords, separated by fibrovascular stroma.[39] The cells more or less represent the hollow tube stage of fetal development. The preponderant cell type is round or oval with scant cytoplasm, easily confused with undifferentiated carcinoma, lymphoma, or Ewing's sarcoma. Scattered within this background are fetal-appearing myocytes and more characteristic strap cells, racquet-shaped cells, or giant cells, having more abundant cytoplasm and myofibrils, as well as cross striations. Myoglobin can usually be demonstrated by immunoperoxidase methods.

Embryonal and Botryoid Rhabdomyosarcoma

As mentioned earlier, sarcoma botryoides is basically an embryonal rhabdomyosarcoma having a distinctive gross morphologic appearance (p. 1314). Both the embryonal and botryoid patterns occur in the young, often in infancy and sometimes at birth. The embryonal variant may arise anywhere in the body including the trunk, extremities, and head and neck region, where it is the predominant type encountered. The botryoid variant has already been described elsewhere (p. 1121). Although embryonal lesions infiltrate and metastasize they are less aggressive than the pleomorphic and alveolar forms.

Embryonal rhabdomyosarcomas may appear grossly as solid, gray-white, infiltrative cancers, or more frequently as loose, myxoid, gelatinous masses. They contain both round and spindled neoplastic cells that have scant-to-moderate amounts of eosinophilic material. Very undifferentiated cells with little cytoplasm may closely resemble malignant lymphoid cells, and indeed some tumors defy light microscopic categorization. The spindle cells may be indistinguishable from fibroblasts except that occasional cells may show greater differentiation with more abundant cytoplasm that can be shown to contain myoglobin as a marker. Nuclear pleomorphism is usually evident, as are scattered-to-abundant mitoses. These cells are disposed in undifferentiated sheets and masses separated by an abundant myxomatous ground substance.

It is important to emphasize that many neoplasms do not fit neatly into a single niche. The range of histologic patterns makes the morphologic diagnosis difficult, and the highly undifferentiated lesions are diagnostic challenges that may well require proof of myoglobin in the neoplastic cells to identify them as rhabdomyosarcomas.[40]

GRANULAR CELL TUMOR

These histologically distinctive, almost always benign neoplasms have many points of interest. Debate about their histogenesis has persisted for years. Early observations attributed these tumors to myoblastic cells, and so they were called *granular cell myoblastomas.* Succeeding reports have variously suggested mesenchymal, fibroblastic, or histiocytic derivations. Favored today is neural derivation from the precursors of Schwann cells, thus making the granular cell tumor and schwannoma first cousins. In support of this concept is the presence of neuron-specific enolase in many of these neoplasms.[41] The two most common locations are the tongue and the subepidermal (and subcutaneous) tissues, particularly in the trunk and upper extremities.[42] However, they have occurred in almost every other site in the body including the breast; oral mucous membranes; gastrointestinal, respiratory, and biliary tracts; urinary bladder; and genitalia. Although rarely malignant they are often poorly encapsulated, with tonguelike

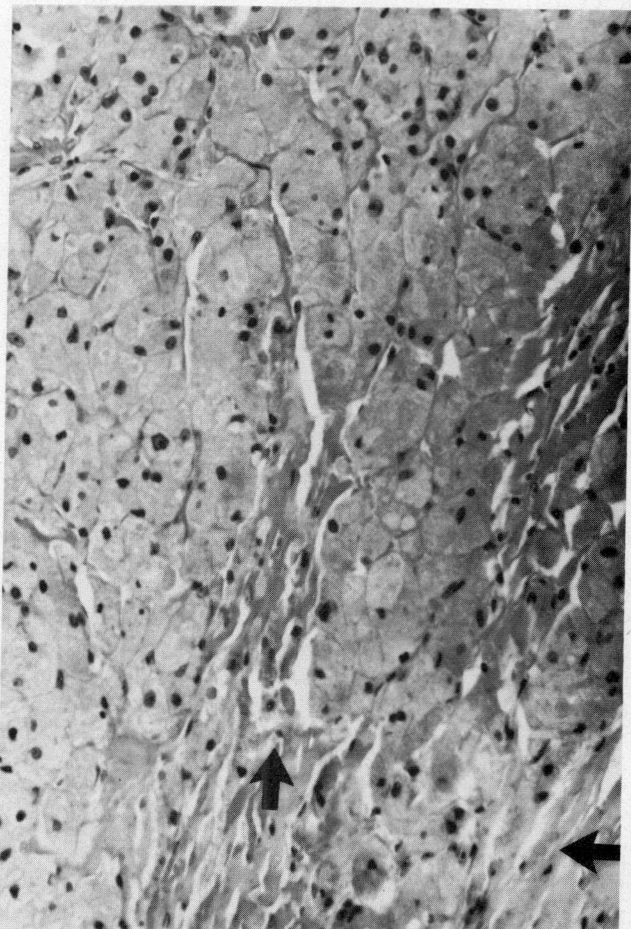

Figure 28–6. Granular cell tumor, the poorly demarcated border penetrating into subcutaneous collagenous fibrous tissue *(arrows)*. The rounded tumor cells have abundant granular cytoplasm, extremely small dark nuclei, and, for the most part, distinct cell borders.

projections simulating local invasiveness. *When located close to the skin, they induce pseudoepitheliomatous hyperplasia of the overlying epithelium that can easily be mistaken for a squamous cell carcinoma.*

Granular cell tumors are generally small (less than 2 cm), firm, discrete, gray-white–to–yellow nodules on cross section. Almost invariably they are composed of nests and sheets of round-to-polygonal cells with distinct borders enclosing an abundant eosinophilic granular cytoplasm evenly distributed about small, usually centrally located, uniform nuclei (Fig. 28–6). Multinucleation, nuclear pleomorphism, and mitotic activity may be present, but only rarely. Myelinated nerve bundles, frequently surrounded by granular cells arranged in concentric whorls, are seen in about half. The histologic hallmark of these lesions is the prominent cytoplasmic granules that are PAS positive and diastase resistant. Under the electron microscope the granules are membrane-limited, autophagic vacuoles or phagolysosomes containing electron-dense amorphous material that can sometimes be resolved as disintegrating cellular organelles. Smaller vesicular bodies may also be present, contributing to the granularity.

Malignant granular cell tumors are rarities. Generally they are of larger size (over 8 to 10 cm), grow more rapidly, and are more obviously infiltrative at their margins. Nuclear hyperchromasia, pleomorphism, and mitoses are more prominent than in benign lesions, but the line of differentiation is at best tenuous.

There are no distinguishing clinical features of granular cell tumors apart from their propensity for unusual locations, such as the tongue. Excision with a comfortable margin is curative. However, infiltrative projections left behind lead to a recurrence rate of 5 to 10%.[42] Secondary and tertiary reexcisions may still be curative. Perplexingly, in some instances, the benign granular cell tumor has failed to recur despite apparent incomplete removal. This repeated observation has raised the possibility that some of these lesions are not neoplastic but, instead, reactive or degenerative processes.[43] Whatever their nature, they are almost always innocent lesions except for their induction of pseudoepitheliomatous hyperplasia of the epidermis, which invites a serious overdiagnosis.

Bones

NORMAL

Despite its seemingly static appearance, bone is a remarkably labile tissue throughout life. Remodeling—formation and resorption—occurs continuously, even after the skeleton has been fully formed. Almost one-fifth of the total skeletal calcium is turned over yearly in the adult. A brief survey of bone as a tissue and of its renewal will facilitate an understanding of the diseases of bone.

BONE AS A TISSUE

No material devised by man can match bone in its durability, adaptability, and capacity to absorb stress over the decades. It consists of a solid mineral phase, an organic matrix of osteoid, and bone cells—osteocytes, osteoblasts, and osteoclasts. *Osteocytes* are merely osteoblasts that become incorporated within the matrix. Both the osteocytes and osteoblasts are uninucleate cells derived from primitive mesenchymal precursors. *Osteoblasts* are found along bone-forming surfaces. Subperiosteally and endosteally, they may form a tight layer or sheet of cells interconnected by tight junctions, but along the surfaces of the trabeculae they are more widely scattered.[44] They contain an abundance of ribosomes involved in the synthesis of mainly collagen polypeptides and are rich in *alkaline* phosphatase. *Osteoclasts* are multinucleated cells disposed mainly along the endosteal surface of the cortex and, here and there, about trabeculae. They have a different histogenetic origin from osteoblasts and may be of the monocyte-macrophage line. Involved in bone resorption, they are generally found within "eaten-out" scalloped bays in the adjacent bone surface *(Howship's lacunae)* (Fig. 28–7). The surface of the osteoclast actively resorbing bone is ruffled, which can be resolved under the electron microscope as villous-like projections that close over crystals or

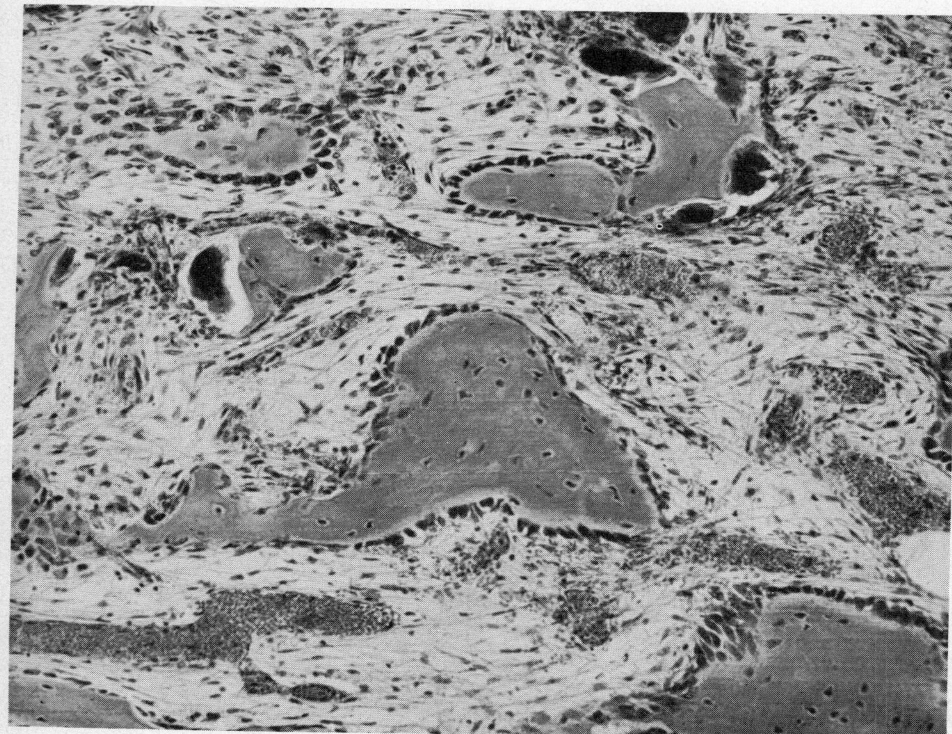

Figure 28–7. Normal bone with active osteoblastic and osteoclastic activity. There is slight fibrosis of marrow spaces.

fragments of bone to form intracytoplasmic vesicles or vacuoles in which the osteolysis is completed. These cells contain *acid* phosphatase, collagenase, dehydrogenases, proteases, and carbonic anhydrase, which undoubtedly play roles in the resorption of bone, as discussed later.

The organic matrix of bone, synthesized by osteoblasts, is called osteoid before it is mineralized. It is 90 to 95% type I collagen embedded within a ground substance of glycosaminoglycans linked to some noncollagenous proteins, principally osteocalcin and osteonectin, both of which are involved in the deposition of calcium (see below). Understandably, hereditary disorders in the metabolism of glycoproteins, e.g., Hurler's or Hunter's syndromes (p. 150), result in skeletal abnormalities. Collagen provides the structural strength of the osteoid, which is buttressed in fully formed bone by the deposition of minerals. Particularly important in collagen are proline and lysine; after hydroxylation they provide the intra- and intermolecular links and bonding, conferring stability on the collagen fibers. Molecular defects in procollagen molecules impair its secretion by osteoblasts into the extracellular ground substance as occurs in osteogenesis imperfecta (p. 1320). When disorders cause increased bone turnover, there is a commensurate increase in urinary excretion of both free and peptide-bound hydroxyproline.

When active neo-osteogenesis is occurring the collagen is first laid down in feltlike sheets producing lamellae along the endosteal and periosteal surfaces, as well as in and about trabeculae. At the outset the collagen fibers are haphazardly arranged and when this osteoid is mineralized it is referred to as *woven bone.* With remodeling the collagen fibers are deposited largely in the long axis of the bone, contributing to the structural strength. Mineralization of this mature osteoid produces lamellar bone (the lamellae being about 10 microns thick). Much of the remodeling, involving coupled osteoclastic resorption and osteoblastic formation, is centered about vessel-bearing haversian canals, creating concentric layers of lamellar bone that constitute an *osteon.* Slender cytoplasmic processes extend out from osteoblasts and osteocytes to create canaliculi through the lamellae to interconnect eventually with the haversian canals. Thus, an elaborate system is provided for the sustenance and coordination of the so-called "bone-lining cells" and for the transfer of minerals into and out of bone.

There is a 12- to 15-day delay between the formation of osteoid and its mineralization, leaving unmineralized osteoid seams up to 15 microns in thickness at bone-forming fronts. *A deficiency in the width and extent of the osteoid seams implies impaired osteoblastic function and reduced bone formation and, conversely, an increase in their width signifies unusually active bone formation and/or a delay in mineralization* (p. 409). Osteoid is recognized histologically by its eosinophilic appearance, in contrast to the basophilia of mineralized osteoid, namely bone.

The mineral phase of bone is largely crystals of hydroxyapatite–empiric formula $Ca_{10}(PO_4)_6\ (OH)_2$. The mineralization initially is in an amorphous form, but with maturation is converted into the crystalline hydroxyapatite. The process of mineralization is poorly understood, as pointed out later. Trace amounts of other minerals such as magnesium, sodium, potassium, and fluorides are also present in bone, particularly in the interface with extracellular fluid. Fluoride ions favor the formation of crystals from the amorphous deposits and thus harden bones (and teeth).

BONE MODELING AND REMODELING

The two pathways by which the bones of the skeleton are formed in the fetus and growing child—intramembranous and endochondral—have already been presented (p. 408). Throughout life there is continuous resorption closely coupled with formation—the two processes constituting remodeling.[45] Obviously, during development of the skeleton, formation far outpaces resorption, but beginning in the fourth or fifth decade the balance reverses. Thus, the skeletal mass declines with advancing age at the impressive rate of about 0.7% of the total mass annually. Bone formation and resorption are complex processes involving (a) calcium and phosphorus metabolism, (2) local influences and (3) humoral endocrine regulators.[46]

Adequate concentrations of calcium and phosphorus in the plasma and in the interstitial fluid that bathes the osteoblast are requisite for mineralization of the osteoid laid down by osteoblasts. Maintenance of the normal levels of calcium and phosphorus within the plasma depends mostly on the parathyroid glands (p. 1226), the vitamin D hormone (p. 406), and calcitonin. It is customary to speak of a "solubility product" for calcium and phosphorus below which mineralization will not occur, but the precise threshold level is not known. One widely held theory is that serum is supersaturated with respect to bone mineral, and so once a crystal is formed it provides a nidus for further accretion of bone salts. Electron microscopic studies reveal within the membranes of osteoblasts minute vesicles less than 1 micron in diameter at sites of mineralization.[47] Needlelike inclusions have been seen within these vesicles and appear later to break out of the vesicles, possibly to start the process of mineralization. Other local influences also play roles. Osteoblasts synthesize osteocalcin, which is a vitamin K–dependent α-carboxyglutamic acid protein that binds calcium. Another product of osteoblasts is osteonectin (analogous to fibronectin) that binds to both calcium and collagen. Bone is known also to remodel in response to stress, which creates so-called piezoelectric currents. How these electrical fields are translated into directed osteoblastic activity is a mystery. Inorganic pyrophosphate, which is present in bone, is a potent inhibitor of mineralization. The alkaline phosphatase of osteoblasts may hydrolyze the pyrophosphate in the local area to permit mineralization. Significantly, elevated plasma levels of "bone" alkaline phosphatase (heat labile compared with the isoenzymes of placental or hepatic origin) are seen whenever there is active bone formation as in childhood and various bone disorders. Local production of prostaglandins E_2 has been observed in bone that has been shown to modulate osteoblast function and may indeed mediate stress-induced bone formation or, under other circumstances, bone resorption.[48]

Bone resorption involves solubilization of the mineral phase first and then the organic phase. Although osteoclasts and macrophages are most important, osteocytes also contribute. The latter possess alkaline phosphatase, proteases and lysosomal acid hydrolases, which could play roles in bone resorption. It is thought that osteocytic activity accounts for the rapid mobilization of calcium in such conditions as hyperparathyroidism, osteomalacia, and thyrotoxicosis, whereas osteoclasts and macrophages act in the slower remodeling involved in the normal turnover of bone during life and the maintenance of normocalcemia. In this connection, activated lymphocytes release an "osteoclast-activating factor" that may turn on "resorbing cells" in some bone disorders.[49] The mobilization of bone mineral is another poorly understood area of bone metabolism. Although osteoclasts contain acid phosphatase, this enzyme is not known to affect the mineral phase. More likely, the carbonic anhydrase and dehydrogenases in these cells catalyze the formation of hydrogen ions and organic acids that could serve to solubilize the bone salts. The proteolytic enzymes are obvious candidates for degradation of the organic phase.

Many hormones affect bone growth and bone loss. Parathyroid hormone (PTH) and the vitamin D–derived calcitriol stimulate bone resorption and have a direct inhibitory effect on osteoblasts. PTH, after binding to membrane receptors, increases adenylate cyclase activity and intracellular levels of cAMP, which leads to a reduction in collagen synthesis and a fall in alkaline phosphatase activity. The actions of the vitamin D hormone were reviewed on page 406, but for our purposes here it involves mobilization of calcium from bone leading to resorption. Calcitonin inhibits resorption and so may favor bone formation. Growth hormone, as is well-known, stimulates skeletal growth, both in children and adults. The effect is probably mediated through increased production of somatomedins by the liver. Sex hormones inhibit bone resorption, albeit indirectly perhaps, by increasing intestinal calcium absorption and calcitonin secretion. A decrease in sex hormone levels may then lead to accelerated bone resorption, accounting possibly for the bone loss in senile and postmenopausal osteoporosis (p. 1327). Adrenal corticoids inhibit the development of osteoblasts from precursors, stimulate osteoclasts, and decrease intestinal absorption of calcium. Thyroid hormones stimulate osteoclastic bone resorption, accounting for the bone loss in hyperthyroidism. Insulin stimulates collagen synthesis by osteoblasts. Thus, it is apparent that many influences are involved in bone formation and resorption.

Bone constitutes an enormous reservoir of calcium and phosphorus. Up to 1 gm of calcium is mobilized from and returned to the skeleton each day. Most of this exchangeable calcium, which forms the largest part of the miscible calcium pool, is derived from the surfaces of bone, i.e., the mineralizing front where bone is constantly being resorbed by osteoclasts before it is reformed. Large demands for calcium bring into play monocytes-macrophages, capable of mobilizing it from the vast surface represented by the bone lacunae and canaliculi. It is apparent that bone, far from being static, is a restless, vital tissue.

PATHOLOGY

The skeletal system is subject to vascular, inflammatory, neoplastic, and endocrine diseases, as are the soft tissues of the body. Besides the minerals, matrix, and associated specialized cells, bone contains within its marrow spaces the wide variety of differentiated and primitive cells of the hematopoietic system. Skeletal tumors may arise from any of the component cellular elements of the bone as well as from the lymphoreticular and myeloid cells contained within the marrow spaces. Many hormones affect bone maintenance, and so hormonal disorders such as Cushing's disease and thyrotoxicosis impact on bone. The bones are also the reluctant hosts to a number of disorders of primary origin elsewhere, such as metastatic tumors. It is no surprise, therefore, that the primary and secondary diseases of bone are varied and numerous.

As if the number of bone diseases were not sufficient, the confusion has been compounded by the zeal that has been displayed in attempting to segregate every involvement of each bone into a distinctive entity and then attaching to these entities an eponymic name. The basic disorder might be the same in all sites, but when aseptic necrosis affects the tibial tubercle, it is called Osgood-Schlatter disease; when this same necrosis affects the navicular bone, it is called Köhler's disease; and when it affects the head of the femur, it is called Legg-Calvé-Perthes disease. In all, ten such eponymic diseases have been created out of a single anatomic derangement. In the face of this complexity, an attempt will be made to select only the more common disorders that represent distinctive morphologic derangements.

CONGENITAL AND HEREDITARY DISORDERS

Congenital and hereditary disorders of bone include a variety of relatively innocuous abnormalities that are confined to one or several bones, and a number of systemic diseases that result in striking skeletal changes and some times great morbidity and mortality. Some of the more simple and less serious anomalies consist of failure of development of a bone so that there is congenital absence of a phalanx, rib, clavicle, or, more important, the femur or other long bone. Occasionally, extra bones are formed, such as supernumerary ribs. Other anomalies take the form of the fusion of two adjacent digits (syndactylism), the duplication of digits resulting in extra fingers or toes (polydactylism), or the development of long spider-like digits (arachnodactylism). The association of the last anomaly with Marfan's syndrome was discussed on p. 137. Other anomalies affect the skull and vertebral column and are frequently of great clinical importance, such as craniorachischisis (failure of closure of the spinal column and skull). This anomaly produces a persistent defect through which the meninges and central nervous system may herniate to produce a meningomyelocele or meningoencephalocele. In addition to these localized developmental defects, there are the more important systemic disorders described below.

OSTEOGENESIS IMPERFECTA (FRAGILITAS OSSIUM, BRITTLE BONES)

Osteogenesis imperfecta, better known as *"brittle bone disease,"* constitutes in reality a constellation of hereditary disorders of connective tissue resulting in abnormalities mainly in the skeleton, eyes, ears, joints, and teeth. The basic defect is thought to be some abnormality in collagen synthesis or resorption, although its precise nature is unknown. Tentative observations suggest that it is either a structural abnormality in the procollagen molecule or some alteration of a pre- or postpeptide segment that impairs secretory formation of type I collagen. Subsets of this condition, differentiated by (1) age of onset, (2) mode of transmission, and (3) severity, can be divided into two categories: *osteogenesis imperfecta congenita* and *osteogenesis imperfecta tarda.* There is also further phenotypic heterogeneity within each of these categories. The highly lethal "congenita" category is marked by clinical manifestations from birth, fractures at or before birth, and skeletal deformities with shortness of stature. The inheritance of this phenotype is uncertain. In some patients it appears to be an autosomal recessive trait; in others, autosomal dominant; and even more frequently, sporadic without a familial background. Most often the bones are soft and very delicate and, although survival is possible, it is complicated by multiple fractures and skeletal deformities. Another phenotypic variant of the "congenita" disease is referred to as "thick bone disease." Inheritance is autosomal recessive and death usually occurs in utero or soon after birth.[50]

The most common variety of osteogenesis imperfecta is the "tarda" subset in which fractures are rare at birth but appear generally in early childhood. In most instances inheritance is autosomal dominant, but occasional cases conform to an autosomal recessive mode of transmission.

The following morphologic features are variably present in most patients with this condition:

The **bones** in the more severe expressions of "congenita" disease may be malformed, thick, and often "crumpled" at time of birth, because they are largely formed of bone salts lacking well-formed osteoid matrix. The skull too may be malformed. With milder "tarda" disease compatible with postnatal survival, they are usually extremely thin and delicate and are often deformed by recent, old, and unhealed fractures. Both cortical and trabecular bone is abnormally thin with increased bone resorption and abnormal disarray of collagen fibers. Although fractures may reunite, the bone callus is weak and susceptible to recurrent fracture.

Eye changes, particularly distinctive, may be present in the more severe involvements. The sclerae are thin, translucent and appear blue because of visualization of the underlying vitreous. The unusual scleral color often calls attention to this skeletal disorder.

The **ear** abnormalities take the form of various levels of hearing impairment to the point of complete deafness resulting from fractures of the ossicle in the middle ear.

The **joints** are abnormally lax, as are the supporting ligaments and tendons of the skeleton, predisposing to joint dislocations, kyphoscoliosis and flat feet.

The **teeth** are characteristically small, misshapen, and blue-yellow owing to hypoplasia of dentine and pulp.

Other features include a predisposition to hernias; cardiovascular abnormalities, particularly mitral valve prolapse; and thin, fragile skin deficient in collagen 1.

Clinical recognition of osteogenesis imperfecta may pose no problem when fully expressed but in these instances is not compatible with long survival. However, there is a wide range in phenotypic expression, and in the milder forms it may go unrecognized for many years unless the blue sclerae or predisposition to fracture bring it to attention. The bone fragility may diminish at puberty only to be reexacerbated in females during pregnancy or after the menopause when bone loss normally occurs. Mild involvements permit normal longevity and so must be considered in the differential diagnosis of all forms of osteopenia (reduced bone mass), particularly osteoporosis.

ACHONDROPLASIA

This autosomal dominant hereditary disease is characterized by impaired proliferation of cartilage cells, and hence decreased epiphyseal bone growth. The bones of the head and vertebral column are unaffected, and thus arises the characteristic dwarf with head and body too large for shortened arms and legs.

Anatomically, the deranged cartilaginous growth produces thick, knobby epiphyses that calcify early and irregularly. Sometimes, exuberant cartilaginous tissue protrudes beyond the contour of the bony cortex. The long bones are abnormally short, but since appositional bone growth is undisturbed, they are relatively thick for their length. Histologically, there is complete disarray of the epiphyseal cartilaginous plates.

Although death may occur in utero or soon after birth, most individuals live to an advanced age in otherwise good health.

OSTEOPETROSIS (OSTEOSCLEROSIS)

Osteopetrosis is also known as *Albers-Schönberg disease* or, more graphically, as *"marble bones" to denote the principal characteristics of overgrowth and sclerosis of bone with resultant marked thickening of the bony cortex and narrowing or even filling of the marrow cavity.* Despite the "too much" bone, the skeleton is abnormally brittle and fractures readily.

This is an uncommon hereditary disorder having two modes of transmission. The autosomal recessive disease is called malignant because, with homozygosity, bony changes appear in utero or in infancy and often result in early death. In contrast, the pattern with an autosomal dominant mode of transmission is relatively benign.[51] Although present from birth, this form often is not recognized until childhood or adult life. Both sexes are affected equally.

The vertebral column, pelvic bones, and ribs are most often involved, but any bone in the body may be affected. Membranous bones such as the skull are usually spared. The characteristic morphologic changes consist of extreme density and overgrowth of solid cortical bone. Depending on the severity and duration of the disease, **the marrow cavity may be narrowed down to a slender central core or, in far-advanced cases, the marrow cavity may be obliterated.** However, the bones are not unusually shortened or deformed so that the individuals are of normal stature. Usually the marked overgrowth of bone is manifested by the wideness of the spicules of cancellous bone and the monotonous solidity of the cortical bone. Sometimes, within the centers of these solid plates of bone and within the cores of the bone spicules, there is preserved cartilage, suggesting that the normal process of resorption of cartilage at the time of provisional calcification did not occur. Such marrow space as may be present is extremely fibrotic, and almost no hematopoietic elements are found.

Many different clinical manifestations are produced by the morphologic changes described. Although the bones are extremely hard and brittle, they have been likened to a stick of peppermint candy that fractures with relatively slight stress. Anemia reflects the replacement of the marrow and is often accompanied by extramedullary hematopoiesis and resultant hepatosplenomegaly. Visual disturbances and blindness follow the progressive constriction of the foramina of the optic nerves. Deafness reflects the overgrowth of bone within the middle ear and inner ear. Cranial nerve palsies and hydrocephalus are further possible clinical manifestations. The diagnosis of this condition is usually obvious from the roentgenograms showing the markedly increased density of bone, along with narrowing of the medullary cavity. In the malignant form of the disease, severe encroachment on the marrow spaces may cause death in utero or in infancy, owing to profound anemia. The milder, dominant pattern is compatible with a near-normal life span, although fractures occur with even mild trauma. Infections, particularly osteomyelitis, are a constant threat to life (possibly related to neutropenia).

OSTEOCHONDROMATOSIS (HEREDITARY MULTIPLE EXOSTOSES)

An osteochondroma is also known as an *exostosis. In essence, these lesions are the result of misdirected epiphyseal bone growth producing cartilage-capped bony projections from the lateral contours of endochondral bones.* It is likely that they are hamartomatous rather than neoplastic, but rarely they are the site of origin of a sarcoma, usually chondrosarcoma. *Exostoses may occur as solitary sporadic lesions and may be called osteochondromas,* but in osteochondromatosis some hereditary defect leads to the formation of multiple exostoses, usually bilateral and often symmetric. The mode of transmission of the hereditary condition is uncertain, but familial pedigrees suggest autosomal dominant with involvement of both male and female offspring of an affected parent. For reasons that are not clear, males are afflicted three times more often than females.

Exostoses most frequently appear on the long bones of the extremities in the metaphyses close to the epiphyseal region. Occasionally the pelvis, scapula, and ribs are involved, but only rarely the small bones of the hands and feet (Fig. 28–8). Although they arise from the epiphyseal cartilage, with growth of the long bones they are left behind, progressively extending the distance from their points of origin. Sometimes there is concomitant derangement in the development of the long bones of the extremities, causing bowing and shortening. Analogously, the pelvic and pectoral girdles may be deformed. Exostoses assume many shapes: some are conical with broad bases attached to the underlying bone; others are mushroom-shaped with slender pedicles and bulbous heads; and still others are platelike. They usually project out 3 to 5 cm from the normal contour of the bone. All have at their outermost extent a layer of mature cartilage resembling an articular surface, but also serving as an epiphyseal site of growth. The body of the lesion is composed of well-formed bone having an outer cortex enclosing trabecular bone (Fig. 28–9). Microscopically, the cartilage is usually mature and resembles that in the normal epiphysis, but foci of cartilage may persist within the cancellous centers of these lesions. The histologic details of the bone structure are otherwise normal.

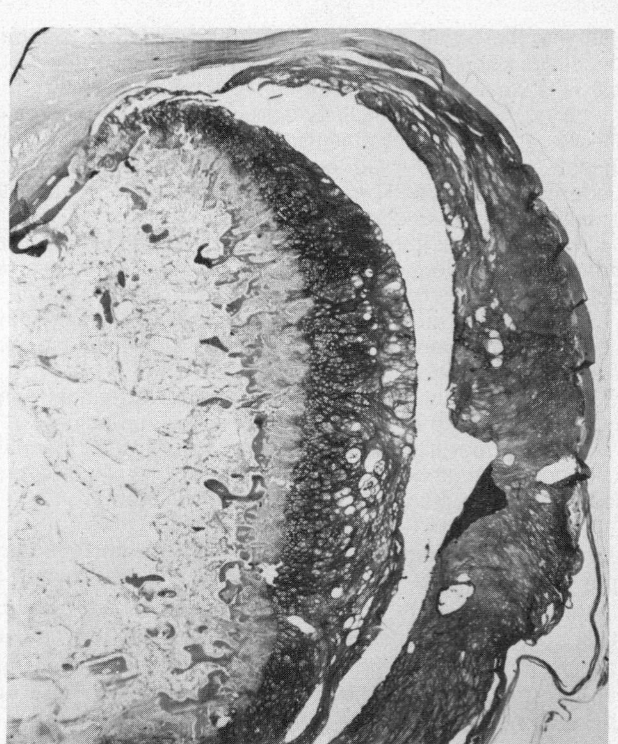

Figure 28–9. Cartilaginous exostosis at low power. The cartilaginous cap has been artifactually partially lifted off.

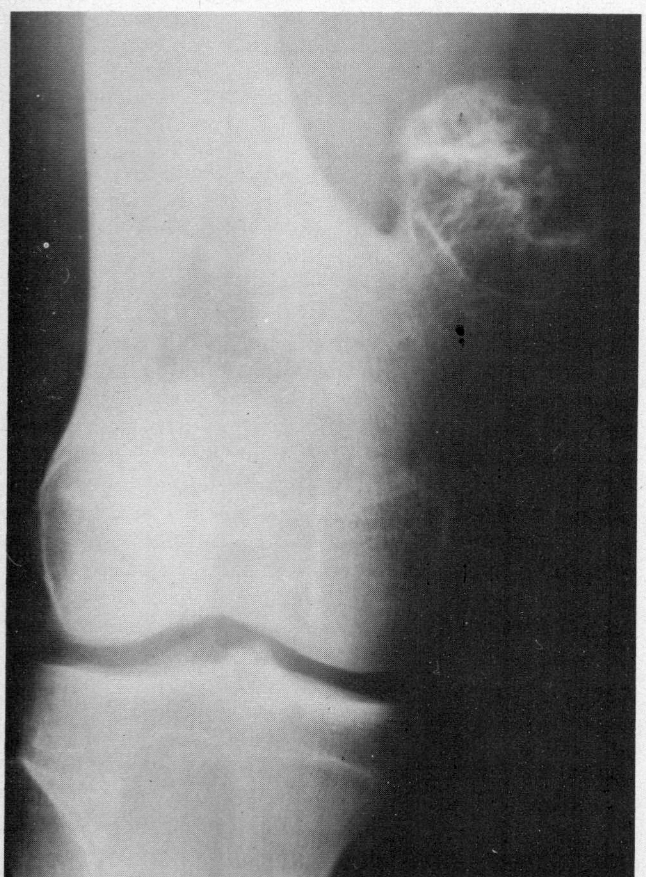

Figure 28–8. Mushroom-shaped osteochondroma (exostosis) of lower end of femur with its long axis pointing away from region of adjacent epiphysis. (Courtesy of Dr. Ashley Davidoff, Department of Radiology, Brigham and Women's Hospital, Boston.)

Solitary exostoses have no apparent hereditary background. Whether solitary or multiple in the hereditary syndrome, they are rarely discovered before late childhood or adolescence, perhaps reflecting the time required for their development. Growth of the lesion usually stops at the time of epiphyseal closure but occasionally continues into adult life. Usually symptomless, they come to attention as a chance radiographic finding. However, they can produce obvious external deformities or uncommonly impinge on a blood vessel or nerve. More important, in 3 to 5% of hereditary cases one of the exostoses gives rise to a fibrosarcoma, osteosarcoma, or (more usually) a chondrosarcoma. The risk for the individual is substantially less with a solitary lesion, presumably because there are fewer lesions. In a rare instance, osteochondromatosis appears in the hereditary Gardner's syndrome (p. 868), characterized also by desmoid tumors, sebaceous cysts, and, most significantly, polyps (papillary adenomas) of the colon that sometimes become carcinomatous.

ENCHONDROMATOSIS (OLLIER'S DISEASE)

An enchondroma is a benign, cartilaginous mass located within the medullary cavity of a bone. As discussed later, solitary enchondromas may appear as sporadic lesions; here we are concerned with the multiple enchondromas in Ollier's disease. Most frequently affected are the bones of the hands and feet, and less often the long tubular bones. Because these are all endochondral bones, it is speculated that in Ollier's disease there is some disturbance in epiphyseal bone growth leaving behind rests of cartilage within the metaphyses that later enlarge to produce the enchondromas. According to this view, the cartilaginous masses are hamartomatous rather than neoplastic.

The condition is usually discovered in early childhood as the proliferation of cartilage causes thinning and expansion of the surrounding cortex leading to pain and eventual skeletal distortions or fractures. With this early age of onset it is natural to assume some congenital derangement, but clear evidence of hereditary and familial influences are lacking. On occasion, enchondromatosis is associated with multiple cavernous hemangiomas, usually of the skin: this particular subset is called *Maffucci's syndrome.*

Since the morphologic appearance of the lesions is identical to that of sporadic enchondromas, they are described on page 1341. Sometimes they rupture through the cortex to produce disfiguring, soft tissue masses, and (most important) they may give rise to chondrosarcomas. The incidence of malignant transformation has been reported variously as 5 to 50%; this range may merely reflect the number of enchondromas within the individual patient, the risk being proportional to the number of lesions. Whatever the level, nearly 50% of chondrosarcomas arise from enchondromas, so that the patient with Ollier's disease is at particular risk.

OTHER HEREDITARY SKELETAL DISORDERS

In this context, mention might be made of three conditions considered elsewhere in this text: Marfan's syndrome (p. 137), Ehlers-Danlos syndrome (p. 155), and the mucopolysaccharidoses (p. 150). Marfan's syndrome is characterized by striking elongation of the skeleton, particularly prominent in the long, spider-like fingers (arachnodactyly). Ehlers-Danlos syndrome is marked by disorders of the supporting tissues of the skeleton, leading to striking hypermobility of the joints. Several variants of the mucopolysaccharidoses are characterized by massive accumulations of mucopolysaccharides within marrow phagocytic cells, sometimes leading to sufficient distortion of the skeleton, and in particular the bones of the face and skull, to have given rise to the term gargoylism.

INFECTIONS

Bacterial infections of bone occur under different circumstances. In any blood-borne systemic disease, such as brucellosis, typhoid fever, the mycoses, tuberculosis, and bacterial endocarditis, the bone marrow may be seeded with organisms to produce small foci of infection. Usually these inflammatory lesions are of microscopic size, do not contribute materially to the clinical disease, and are of significance only as anatomic findings that aid in establishing the nature of the primary systemic disease. However, in addition to these insignificant lesions, more serious bacterial infections occur in bone. Both the bone marrow and bone are often affected concomitantly to produce an *osteomyelitis*. The three most serious infections of bone are (1) pyogenic osteomyelitis, (2) tuberculosis, and (3) syphilis.

PYOGENIC OSTEOMYELITIS

Osteomyelitis represents a pyogenic infection of the bone and bone marrow. Characteristically, it begins as an acute infection. Acute hematogenesis osteomyelitis is almost limited to those under the age of 21, and affects, in descending order of frequency, the femur, tibia, humerus, and radius. The rare cases in adults tend to localize in the spine.[52] Many of these infections spontaneously resolve or are aborted by appropriate treatment. Indeed, in the present era of effective antibacterial therapy, most are brought under prompt control, accounting for a decrease in the incidence of this disease today. If unrecognized or inadequately treated, however, the infection may persist to become chronic, as still occurs in 20% of cases.[53]

ETIOLOGY AND PATHOGENESIS. Osteomyelitis may complicate an overt systemic or distant extraosseous infection, when organisms are blood-borne, but more often it arises as an apparent primary infection in previously healthy individuals. Bacteremias, sometimes extremely fleeting, are known to occur frequently from such trivial sources as insignificant injury to the intestinal mucosa; the mere vigorous chewing of hard foods, with or without apparent dental infection; and commonplace cuts and bruises of the skin. Local trauma may influence the location of the bone infection, but often it appears to be purely chance. Not unexpectedly, these infections are common and more severe in persons suffering from debilitation or some immunodeficiency.

Almost any pathogen may cause osteomyelitis, but most often it is S. *aureus* followed in order of importance by streptococci, pneumococci, gonococci, and influenzal and coliform organisms. In the neonatal period, group B streptococci are frequent offenders. Osteomyelitis is a particular hazard in patients with sickle cell disease; for unknown reasons, with this condition it is often caused by the salmonellae. In drug addicts, Pseudomonas is the most common offender.[54]

Blood-borne infections usually begin in the marrow space of the metaphysis where capillary flow is slowest, favoring lodgement of organisms. The evolution of these infections differs somewhat from those in soft tissues because inflammatory edema in the bony encasement rapidly constricts the blood supply. There is a tendency then for bone fragments to become devitalized and produce *sequestra* (see below). In infants the periosteum is loosely attached and the epiphyseal cartilage traversed by capillaries, favoring subperiosteal spread and extension into the joint space, with resultant suppurative arthritis. In contrast, after the first year or two of life, septic arthritis is uncommon. Rarely, osteomyelitis follows trauma to soft tissues and bone or contiguous soft tissue infection, e.g., direct contamination of an open fracture, direct extension of a periapical tooth abscess, or gangrenous necrosis of the foot or toes.

MORPHOLOGY. During the phase of acute osteomyelitis, a characteristic suppurative reaction occurs, which tends to develop considerable exudative pressure and thus extends in both directions within the marrow cavity. The vascular supply is often compromised as the inflammatory pressure builds up. The inflammation **penetrates the endosteum** and enters the haversian and lacunar systems of the bone to reach the subperiosteum. Sometimes it ruptures through this membrane into the surrounding soft tissues. This pattern of penetration of the cortex may occur at one or several points to eventually cause multiple **sinus tracts** through the cortical bone. When spread to the subperiosteum occurs, the infection dissects in this plane to further impair the blood supply in the affected region. The suppurative and ischemic injury may then cause necrosis of a small or large fragment of bone known as a **sequestrum.** This devitalized sequestrum, in the course of time, may be resorbed or is sometimes sloughed to form a free foreign body that on occasion dissects through to the skin. In this fashion, or by the direct penetration of the spreading infection, inflammatory **skin sinuses** may develop.

Except in infants in the first year of life, the epiphyseal cartilaginous plate resists bacterial invasion, and therefore the osteomyelitis rarely extends into the head of the bone, the epiphysis, or the joint cavity. However, when the infection is sufficiently severe, spread into the soft tissue and then along the outer or inner surface of the periosteum provides a pathway to the head of the bone and the joint cavity. Such a complicating **suppurative arthritis** may result in extensive destruction of the joint and permanent disability (p. 1348).

Not all instances of acute hematogenous osteomyelitis follow such a spreading destructive pattern as described. In certain instances, the initial infection is localized to a small area and becomes walled off by inflammatory fibrous tissue to create a localized abscess that may undergo spontaneous sterilization or become a chronic nidus of infection **(Brodie's abscess).** In other instances, the infection, after having spread through a localized region of the bone, is contained by the natural resistive forces of the host or is controlled by therapy.

In the course of time, all these infections are modified by the reactive reparative responses that come into play even while underlying smoldering infection persists. At this stage, the disease is better called **chronic osteomyelitis.** Osteoblastic activity, particularly from the periosteum, forms new bone subperiosteally **(involucrum)** that encloses and envelops the inflammatory focus. Also, a considerable amount of new bone is laid down about the focus of infection within the marrow cavity to produce increased density and bony sclerosis at the periphery of the infection. This reaction further localizes the infection. This neo-osteogenesis, if continued long enough, gives rise to a densely sclerotic pattern of osteomyelitis referred to as **Garré's sclerosing osteomyelitis** (Fig. 28–10).

The histologic changes depend entirely on the stage of the osteomyelitis and its duration. **Basically, two elements can be identified: suppurative and ischemic destructive necrosis** and **fibrous and bony repair.**

CLINICAL COURSE. Hematogenous osteomyelitis usually manifests itself as an acute, febrile, systemic illness accompanied by symptoms referable to the local lesion. These children have malaise, fever, chills, and leukocytosis as well as marked-to-intense local pain that is frequently described as throbbing. Often there is redness, swelling, and tenderness in the overlying soft tissues. However, the presentation may be much more subtle with only unexplained fever, particularly in infants. The diagnosis is confirmed by radiologic evidence of bone destruction. It should be cautioned, however, that in the early stages of osteomyelitis (during the first ten days) the devitalization and necrosis of bone may not be sufficiently advanced to produce radiographic changes. In about 60% of instances, blood cultures are positive, particularly during the stage of development of bone infection.

In most cases, massive antibiotic therapy successfully aborts the infection before much bone necrosis has

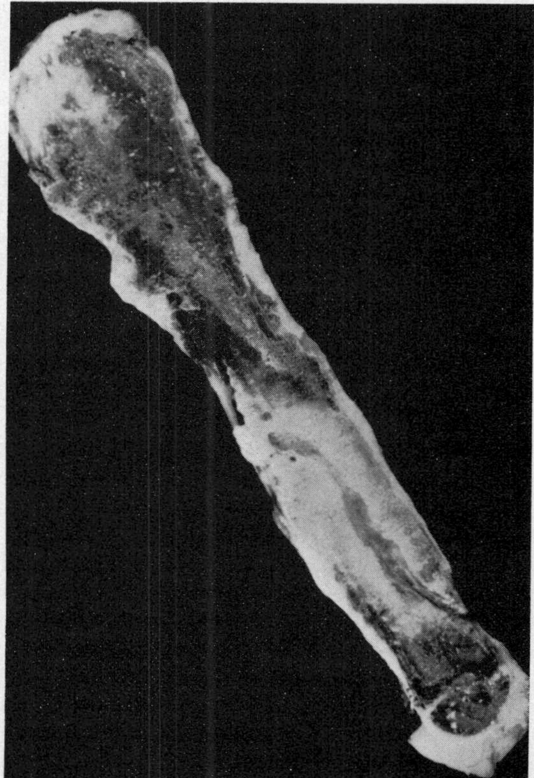

Figure 28–10. Sclerosing osteomyelitis as evidenced by dense, sclerotic, pale-appearing area in shaft.

occurred. Rarely, surgical drainage and débridement of sequestered fragments is necessary. Sometimes the course is complicated by spontaneous fracture of the weakened bone or by the extension of infection into adjacent joints. In addition to the local destruction, osteomyelitis is an important source for the hematogenous dissemination of infection, with the production of pyemic abscesses and focal soft tissue lesions elsewhere in the body, sometimes on the heart valves. The development of osteomyelitis is a feared complication of compound fractures that seriously delays and prejudices the quality of eventual repair. Amyloidosis is a potential complication of persistent chronic infections.

TUBERCULOSIS

Clinically, significant tuberculous infections of bone are now rarities. At present, the usual osseous infection takes the form of miliary seeding of the marrow cavity in the course of hematogenous dissemination of this organism. Such miliary tubercles are generally of little consequence to the patient. However, on bone marrow biopsy they can provide the explanation for a fever of unknown origin (FUO). More serious spreading tuberculous osteomyelitis is now very uncommon and is generally a complication of uncontrolled pulmonary tuberculosis. Usually the organisms originate in cavitary pulmonary lesions, but rarely they spread to the bone from a caseous focus in the lymph nodes in the mediastinum, or from those along the aorta in the abdominal cavity. Children are more frequently affected than adults, but not in the great preponderance encountered in the acute pyogenic osteomyelitis described.

Unlike pyogenic osteomyelitis, *tuberculous osteomyelitis tends to arise as an insidious chronic infection that is characteristically much more destructive and resistant to control.* The long bones of the extremities and the spine are the favored sites of localization. Other less favored sites are the skull, hands, feet, and ribs. Commonly, the infection extends through large areas of the medullary cavity and causes extensive ulcerative inflammatory necrosis of cortical bone, with the production of large and multiple sinuses. The necrosis progresses through the periosteum into the soft tissues and frequently produces skin sinuses. Extension through the epiphyseal cartilage into joint spaces and destruction of intervertebral discs make this disease a most disabling one. When it occurs in the spine *(Pott's disease)*, compression fractures are prone to develop that result in serious deformities (kyphosis and scoliosis) and often lead to permanent damage as new bone formation fixes the spine in this malalignment. The tuberculous exudation may extend from the vertebral bodies into the paravertebral muscles and, in one characteristic pattern, it extends along the sheath of the psoas muscle to produce a *psoas abscess.* Sometimes these infections present as cold fluctuating abscesses in the inguinal regions and inguinal nodes. The morphologic changes are those characteristic of all tuberculous lesions and need not be reiterated. Systemic amyloidosis may develop in protracted cases.

SYPHILIS

Today, in the United States, syphilitic involvement of bone is indeed an uncommon lesion. It may occur in both congenital and acquired syphilis. In the *congenital form,* the involvement affects principally the junction of the metaphysis and the epiphysis and is designated *osteochondritis.* When the periosteum, principally of the long bones, is involved alone, it is referred to as *periostitis.* The osteochondritis causes considerable disarray and destruction of the epiphyseal cartilage by the characteristic fibroproliferative inflammatory reaction of syphilis. This invasive granulation tissue may destroy the lateral margins of the epiphyseal plate or invade the epiphyseal plate, sometimes almost separating the epiphyseal head of the bone from the metaphysis. The inflammatory tissue may extend into the medullary cavity to cause widespread fibrosis.

The characteristic histologic hallmarks of syphilis can be found in this inflammatory response in the form of obliterative endarteritis and striking perivascular mononuclear cell infiltrations, principally of plasma cells. Reactive bone formation occurs from the surrounding vital periosteum. The periostitis produces a similar syphilitic granulation tissue between the cortical bone and the periosteum and is accompanied by the laying down of new bone to produce a characteristic "crew haircut" appearance or sclerosis of the cortex roentgenographically. When this thickening occurs on the tibia, it gives rise to the deformity recognized as *saber shin.*

Acquired syphilis may result in osteochondritis and periostitis, but may also be manifested by the development of a frank syphilitic osteomyelitis, usually by the production of characteristic gummas within the marrow cavity of the bone. In the acquired forms, in addition to the long bones, the skull and vertebral column are affected.

FRACTURES

The speed of healing and perfection of repair of a fracture depend on whether the break has occurred in a previously normal bone or at some site of preexistent disease *(pathologic fracture).* They also depend on the extent and nature of the fracture. Fractures may be *complete* or *incomplete (greenstick), closed (simple)* with intact overlying tissue, *comminuted* when the bone has been splintered, and *compound* when the fracture site communicates with the skin surface. Incomplete closed fractures heal most rapidly with almost complete reconstruction of the preexisting architecture. On the other hand, comminuted and compound fractures heal much more slowly with less satisfactory results. In the former, the devitalized bone splinters constitute impediments to repair; in the latter, possible infection contributes to bone destruction and impairment of blood supply and stimulates fibrosis, which gets in the way of bony healing. On this basis, the morphologic changes that are encountered in the healing of a fracture depend, to a considerable extent, on the nature of the fracture and the collateral problems involved. With this understanding, the basic sequence of events in the repair of a simple closed fracture will be presented, since this pattern is followed in the healing of all fractures and is only slowed and more or less impaired by the complications mentioned.

Healing of a fracture represents a continuous process, but it can be divided for convenience into three distinct stages: (1) **organization** of hematoma at the fracture site, leading to a soft tissue so-called **procallus;** (2) conversion of the procallus to fibrocartilaginous callus, which more effectively immobilizes the bone fragments; and (3) replacement of the fibrocartilaginous callus by osseous callus, which eventually will be remodeled along lines of weight-bearing to complete the repair.

Immediately after a fracture, there is considerable **hemorrhage** into the fracture site from ruptured vessels within the bone as well as from the torn periosteum and surrounding soft tissues. A hematoma is thus formed that fills the fracture cleft and surrounds the area of bone injury. The coagulation of this blood gives rise to a **loose fibrin mesh** that more or less seals off the fracture site and, at the same time, serves as a framework for the ingrowth of fibroblasts and new capillary buds. As occurs with a soft tissue injury, the clot undergoes organization to produce eventually a soft tissue callus that provides some anchorage for the bone fragments, but no structural rigidity (Fig. 28–11).

However, the healing of a bone injury differs from the healing of a soft tissue injury from this point on. After the first few days, **newly formed cartilage and bone matrix** are evident in the fibrovascular response. The origin of this osteoid and cartilaginous tissue is somewhat obscure. Some of the osteoblasts and chondroblasts that form it are undoubtedly derived from periosteum and endosteum of the preserved margins of bone. However, regional fibroblasts may differentiate into osteoblasts and chondroblasts and participate in this activity. By the end of the first week, well-developed new bone and cartilage are dispersed through the soft tissue callus (Fig. 28–12). In the course of succeeding days, these bone spicules become sufficiently numerous and aggregated to create a large, fusiform, temporary bony union of the fracture known as the **provisional** or **procallus.**

This provisional callus is considerably wider than the normal diameter of the bone and extends for some distance up over the fractured ends, thus to create a spindle-shaped, fairly effective splint. In an uncomplicated fracture, the provisional callus usually attains its maximal size at about the end of the second or third week. Over the subsequent course of time, this provisional callus is increasingly strengthened by the widening of the newly formed delicate bone spicules and is at the same time remodeled by osteoblastic and osteoclastic activity.

The remodeling process is directed by the muscle and weight-bearing stresses imposed on the bone. If the fracture has been well aligned and the original weight-bearing strains are restored, nearly perfect reconstruction of the bone is accomplished. In such reconstruction, the internal callus that fills the marrow space is also resorbed and, at some later date, roentgenograms may completely fail to demonstrate the site of previous injury.

Perfect repair may be not only impeded but also blocked by many complications. Malalignment and comminution of

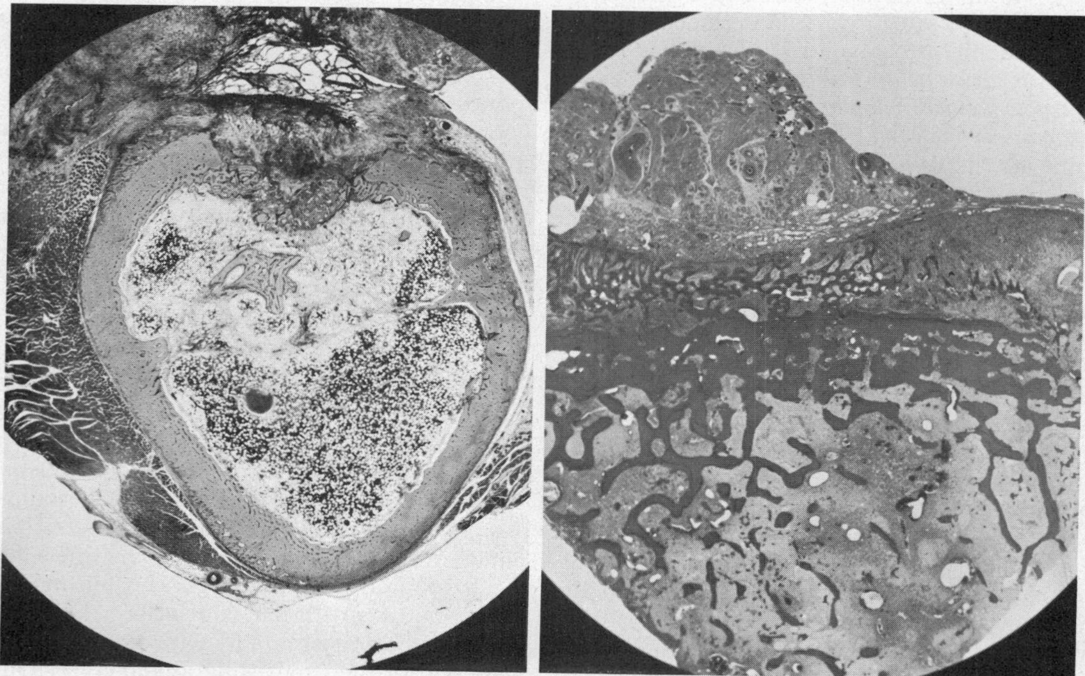

Fig. 28–11

Fig. 28–12

Figure 28–11. Experimental demonstration of bone repair. Hole drilled in femur is filled with hemorrhage and granulation tissue. Fibrous tissue fills adjacent marrow space, and bone spicules are found within this soft tissue callus.

Figure 28–12. New bone formation (slender spicules) outside old cortex in healing of a fracture.

the bone are almost inevitably followed by some permanent deformity. Moreover, the devitalized spicules of comminuted bone must be demineralized and the osteoid material resorbed. These processes delay healing, enlarge the provisional callus, and favor the formation of an overly large, deforming, permanent callus. Permanent obliteration of the marrow cavity may occur. Inadequate immobilization of the bone permits the continuance of twisting, shearing, and bending stresses. Under these circumstances, the laying down of an osteoid and chondromatous matrix is slow and, in fact, in many instances is nearly blocked, so that the callus may be composed of only fibrous tissue and cartilage that perpetuate the abnormal mobility. An osseous callus may not form under these circumstances and a dense fibrous tissue remains as the end stage of the repair process, producing a **false joint (pseudoarthrosis).** Interposition of soft tissues tends to give rise to such fibrous, inadequate bony union. However, in any of these complications, if the interposed soft parts can be removed at a later date, or adequate immobilization eventually effected, ultimate adequate repair can be anticipated except perhaps in advanced age groups suffering from arterial and venous inadequacies. Perhaps the most serious impediment to healing is infection of the fracture site, as feared in comminuted fractures. In this circumstance, the infection must be brought under control before bony union can be effected.

Systemic derangements may further unfavorably affect the end results. Inadequate levels of calcium and phosphorus, avitaminoses, systemic infections, generalized atherosclerosis that renders the area ischemic, and preexistent osteomalacia or osteoporosis (p. 1329) are some of these unfavorable influences. Generally, with children and young adults, in whom most uncomplicated fractures are found, practically perfect reconstruction may be anticipated. In older age groups in whom more of the unfavorable influences are prone to complicate the problem, less favorable union occurs.

OSTEOPOROSIS

Osteoporosis can be defined as an excessive but proportional reduction in the amounts of both the mineral and matrix phases of bone unaccompanied by any abnormality in structure of the residual bone. The reduction in skeletal mass involves both cortical bone, mainly along the endosteal surface, and the trabecular bone. Although the entire skeleton is usually affected, osteoporosis may be restricted under certain circumstances to an extremity, as explained below. The bone loss assumes greatest importance in the vertebrae, femoral necks, pelvis, and ribs where it leads to increased skeletal fragility with predisposition to microfractures, pain, deformities, and overt fractures. Osteoporosis must be viewed in the context that bone loss is almost inevitable, beginning in women at about 45 years of age and in men between 50 and 60 years of age.[55] *Implied, therefore, in the clinical usage of the term "osteoporosis" is a reduction in bone mass sufficient to produce clinical manifestations.* Symptomatic osteoporosis is encountered in three ill-defined and overlapping age groups. The dominant group consists of postmenopausal women, in whom the condition is referred to as *postmenopausal osteoporosis.* Next most common are elderly individuals of both sexes—*senile osteoporosis.* Much less frequently it is encountered in those under the age of 40, and then is referred to as *idiopathic osteoporosis.* When the disorder appears in children or adolescents, it is called *juvenile osteoporosis.* However, the use of these clinical terms should not obscure the fact that, so far as is known, the basic bony disorder is the same in all the clinical subsets.

A major clinical problem in the diagnosis of osteoporosis is its differentiation from other bone-losing disorders, collectively referred to as *osteopenias* (discussed below). Osteomalacia related to a deficiency in adults of vitamin D (or its metabolites), calcium, and/or phosphorus is another skeletal disorder characterized by "too little" bone. Basically, it is marked by impaired mineralization of bone matrix and the accumulation of excess osteoid matrix. In osteoporosis, there is no disturbance in the mineral/organic ratio and no excess of osteoid. Hyperparathyroidism, hyperthyroidism, and widespread malignant infiltrations as in leukemia, multiple myeloma, and disseminated carcinoma also induce increased destruction of bone. Skeletal loss is also seen with glucocorticoid excess, chronic liver disease, alcoholism, and heparin administration.[56] Radiographically, all these disorders produce very similar or identical "osteopenia." To compound the problem further, there is difficulty in determining clinically the severity and indeed the existence of the bone loss in all forms of osteopenia, particularly in osteoporosis. One would assume that it could be established radiographically, but standard x-ray techniques and experienced radiologists cannot detect demineralization until 30 to 50% of bone mineral is lost. Other more specialized procedures (to be cited later) have been developed, but it suffices to note that osteoporosis is difficult to diagnose clinically and difficult to segregate from other forms of osteopenia.[57]

PATHOGENESIS. The origins of osteoporosis in most cases are unknown. Only in a few instances is there a plausible mechanism, as, for example, the skeletal loss in Cushing's syndrome attributed to glucocorticoid excess (p. 1237).[58] Indeed, it is entirely possible that osteoporosis represents a common end point of multiple pathogenetic pathways and, conceivably, several must act in concert to produce significant clinical disease. *Three general, not mutually exclusive, propositions are entertained, any or more of which may be applicable to a particular case: (1) genetic or constitutional predisposition in the form of a delicate skeleton less well able to sustain a negative bone balance, (2) a normal rate of bone loss but slowed bone formation, and (3) a normal rate of bone formation but an accelerated rate of bone loss.*

The *"delicate skeleton" theory* derives support from the following observations. Most cases of osteoporosis become clinically symptomatic after age 50 when progressive, slow attrition of the skeleton is a physiologic phenomenon. With a preexistent slender endowment, the threshold of structural stability is readily passed. Genetic influences may contribute to the skeletal endowment. Osteoporosis is much more common in whites than in blacks, possibly related to a greater bone mass in the latter. A high concordance in both bone mass and age-related loss has been reported in identical twins. However, a poor skeletal endowment cannot readily account for the appearance of osteoporosis at puberty or in young adults when there is normally progressive increase in the bone mass, unless some pathologic process initiates a negative balance.

Slowing of bone formation could account for symptomatic osteoporosis even with a normal rate of bone loss. Immobilization and reduced physical activity are both clearly associated with the appearance of osteoporosis, and both are marked by reduced bone formation.[59] Indeed, immobilization of an extremity, as, for example, following a fracture, is followed by osteoporosis limited to the immobilized portion of the skeleton. In these clinical circumstances, it is theorized that reduction of stress-related piezoelectrical stimuli (mentioned earlier) in some unknown manner reduces bone formation. Theoretically, these influences could contribute to the development of postmenopausal and senile osteoporosis, but there is no documentation that they are related to osteoporosis in younger individuals.

The weight of evidence favors accelerated bone loss, which would, of course, have greatest effect on an already delicate skeleton.[60] With symptomatic osteoporosis, there is increased urinary excretion of both hydroxyproline and calcium, reflecting breakdown of both the organic and mineral phases of bone. Often there is also slightly increased serum alkaline phosphatase, indicative of enhanced osteoblastic activity, and therefore no impairment in bone formation. Indeed, the fact that osteoblastic activity is normal or enhanced is itself suggestive of a compensatory reaction to abnormal bone breakdown. Female and male sex hormones must certainly play a role in the pathogenesis of postmenopausal and senile osteoporosis. As pointed out earlier (p. 1319), these hormones inhibit resorption, and so with a deficiency bone and calcium are lost. Estrogen therapy stems the urinary calcium loss, at least for a time. However, there is no evidence of estrogen receptors in bone that might mediate a direct effect. Instead, it is proposed that sex steroids have indirect effects.[61] Deranged calcium metabolism might also potentiate bone loss. A negative calcium balance is seen in elderly patients with osteoporosis attributed to aging changes in the intestinal mucosa with impaired calcium absorption and to reduced formation of calcitriol from vitamin D. In addition, aged individuals tend to have restricted intakes of calcium, vitamin D, and protein, so that dietary supplementation of each is sometimes beneficial in slowing or preventing the progression of osteoporosis. More speculation might be offered, but it is better to admit ignorance of the origins of this bony disorder and thus permit an unbiased search for new leads.

Save in the rare instances in which only an extremity is immobilized, osteoporosis is a systemic disorder. It is most marked in the axial skeleton (vertebrae, ribs, and pelvis), but other bones, particularly the femoral necks, may also be involved. The loss of bone is generally more marked in the trabeculae than in the cortex. Because the vertebrae are predominantly trabecular bone, they bear the brunt of the disease. In contrast, the ulna, for example, is largely cortical bone, the ratio of cortex to trabeculae being higher in the midshaft than at the ends. A fall is therefore more likely to cause a fracture of the wrist than of the midshaft in individuals with osteoporosis. There is thinning and sometimes complete resorption of bone trabeculae. Cortical thinning due largely to endosteal resorption also occurs; hence, the external surfaces of the bone are smooth and unaffected and their overall diameter is not diminished. Such bone as remains is histologically normal and there is no increase of osteoid matrix or accentuation of the osteoid seams. Compression fractures of the vertebrae and fractures of the femoral necks are the two most common consequences of osteoporosis, the predisposition being proportional to the severity of bone loss.

CLINICAL COURSE. Osteoporosis by itself is asymptomatic. Often it is discovered by noting bone demineralization on x-rays taken for other reasons. However, as indicated, the radiographic demonstration of decreased bone density is nonspecific and is only well defined when the bone loss is already well advanced. Sometimes there are no symptoms but only loss of height due to compression microfractures of the vertebrae accompanied by increased kyphosis of the dorsal spine. Symptomatic osteoporosis presents with: (1) midline back pain in the thoracic or lumbar areas related to vertebral compression microfractures; (2) severe back pain caused by collapse of one or more of the weight-bearing vertebrae (T-7 and lower), causing loss of height and sudden increase in the lumbar lordosis; or (3) sometimes a fracture of the femoral neck, wrist, or other bone. In these patients the rate of hip fractures in women quadruples each decade after the age of 50 and, significantly, up to 20% of elderly patients die within six months after such fractures.

The lack of simple methods for assessing reduction in bone mass complicates clinical diagnosis. The serum calcium and phosphorus levels are characteristically normal or near normal. Although there may be an increase in urinary excretion of hydroxyproline and calcium, the increased levels are often within the range encountered in age-matched controls. Special radiographic studies measuring cortical thickness relative to the overall width or external diameter of the bone are a valuable index of bone loss. Favored sites for these measurements are the iliac crest and metacarpals. More accurate, but not widely available, is dual-beam photon absorptiometry, which provides a remarkably accurate assessment of bone mineral content.[62] Other methods are available, including the CT scan, but often the diagnosis depends largely on the classic clinical findings in the appropriate age setting.

The therapy of osteoporosis is beyond our scope. It suffices to note that, although estrogens in the postmenopausal woman, calcium, fluoride, calcitonin, and vitamin D supplementation, as well as many other agents, singly or in combination, have been reported to be of help in slowing the progression of osteoporosis, such claims have been refuted, and no agent or combination clearly reverses the condition.

OSTEOMALACIA

This systemic bone disorder assumes great importance to the physician because it is the most common *remediable* bone disease of the elderly. Literally, osteomalacia means "softness of bone." *In essence, it represents the adult counterpart of childhood rickets and is characterized by inadequate mineralizaton of bone matrix, resulting in an increase in the relative amount of osteoid tissue.*[63, 64] The excess of osteoid is a consequence of the failure of mineralization to keep pace with new synthesis of bone matrix. Hence, the bone displays an increase of osteoid seams, and an abnormally large fraction of the total bone surface is covered by nonmineralized osteoid *(hyperosteoidogenesis)*. Thus, osteomalacia differs from osteoporosis insofar as the former is characterized by a relative deficiency of mineral and an excess of osteoid, whereas in the latter the proportional composition of the bone is essentially normal. The differential features can indeed be subtle, however, as pointed out on page 1327.

PATHOGENESIS. The pathogenesis of osteomalacia in the adult is the same as that of rickets in the growing child, and was discussed on page 407. The nutritional deficit, whether primary or conditioned, and usually of vitamin D or calcium, induces not only a failure of mineralization but also prolongation of the time interval between osteoid synthesis and mineralization, resulting in abnormally wide osteoid seams. Instead of the normal delay of 12 to 15 days, the time lag for mineralization may be as long as two to three months. Moreover, some areas completely fail to mineralize, leaving residuals of osteoid.

MORPHOLOGY. Osteomalacia is characterized by the inadequate mineralization of newly formed osteoid matrix. With inadequate mineralization, there is some slowing or impairment of the continued formation of matrix so that ultimately the bones are softer and more fragile than normal, as in osteoporosis. Fractures are common as in osteoporosis but, bending and stress deformities also develop because the bones are of decreased brittleness as well as being weaker. Microscopically, there is an excess of osteoid matrix with widening of the seams or external layer of osteoid on surfaces where neo-osteogenesis is occurring. However, these changes are also seen in conditions of active bone formation. More definitive is evidence of inadequate mineralization, such as disappearance of the granular layer of amorphous calcium before it is reorganized into crystalline hydroxyapatite, best brought out by tetracycline labeling (p. 409).[65] The inadequate mineralization makes the matrix a poor substitute for normally calcified bone.

CLINICAL COURSE. Osteomalacia is a disease of economically deprived nations and of the elderly throughout the world. In deprived populations, it is usually the consequence of an inadequate diet worsened by parasitic infections and malabsorption. In the elderly, dietary deficiency is also involved but it is often compounded by avoidance of sunlight, with reduced endogenous synthesis of vitamin D, the use of drugs that alter the metabolism or absorption of the critical nutrients, and renal and intestinal disorders that cause malabsorption or affect the metabolism of vitamin D, calcium, and phosphorus. No better capsule characterization of this disease can be given than that of Habener and Mahaffey: "In its mild form the disease may remain asymptomatic for years. In more advanced forms the disease presents with the typical findings of diffuse bone pain, muscle weakness, hypophosphatemia, hyperphosphatasia, low to low-normal serum calcium, diminished urinary calcium, a roentgenographic appearance of diffuse osteopenia (lack of bone) with or without characteristic pseudofractures and a bone biopsy that reveals the pathognomonic widening of the osteoid seams."[66] The bone pain, like that in osteoporosis, is especially prominent in the back and about the hips, and in some instances may be related to microfractures. The muscular weakness is poorly understood but may be sufficiently severe to limit mobility and mimic that of primary muscle disorders. There is experimental evidence that vitamin D deficiency affects muscle metabolism.[67] Whatever its origin, the myopathy is sometimes alleviated by dietary supplementation with vitamin D and bone minerals. The diagnosis of osteomalacia usually depends on the clinical setting because the radiographic changes are indistinguishable from those of osteoporosis. Particularly helpful are radiolucent bands, known as *Looser's zones*, presumably caused by the erosive pulsation of abutting arteries. They are best seen at the inner aspects of the femur (near the femoral neck), and at the upper fibula, scapula, and pelvis.

Rarely, when the osteomalacia is related to renal tubular disorders or chronic renal failure, there is increased radiographic density of the bones, but they are still subject to fracture with minor trauma.

SKELETAL CHANGES IN HYPERPARATHYROIDISM (OSTEITIS FIBROSA CYSTICA GENERALISATA, VON RECKLINGHAUSEN'S DISEASE OF BONE)

Prolonged or severe hyperparathyroidism, whether primary or secondary, causes progressive resorption and destruction of bone. *Although it has always been classically taught that these changes produce a specific anatomic pattern known as osteitis fibrosa cystica, it is now appreciated that many earlier alterations affecting the bone do not fit into this anatomic pattern.* Osteitis fibrosa cystica is the late lesion that only develops in the advanced stages of hyperparathyroidism. The earlier manifestations consist first of demineralization and then loss of bone that produces changes very similar to those of osteomalacia-osteoporosis. In time, these changes may progress to von Recklinghausen's disease of bone.

PATHOGENESIS. The pathologic physiology of both primary and secondary hyperparathyroidism has already been considered in Chapter 26. For brief review, in the primary disease, an excess of parathormone is produced usually by hyperplasia or neoplasia of the parathyroid gland. Secondary hyperparathyroidism is believed to be caused by end-organ resistance to parathormone leading to compensatory hyperactivity of the parathyroid glands. It is encountered in chronic renal insufficiency, vitamin D deficiency, intestinal malabsorption syndromes, and rarely in other settings described on page 1229. When caused by renal dysfunction, the bony changes have been called *renal osteodystrophy*. In both primary and secondary hyperparathyroidism, there is increased resorption of bone mainly related to inhibition of osteoblastic activity accompanied by increased mobilization of phosphorus and calcium (p. 1319), but the changes are usually much more marked in the primary form.

In the growing child, skeletal changes may appear that are similar to those of rickets (p. 409). In the adult, the osseous lesions can be characterized as **a relative excess of osteoclastic over osteoblastic activity accompanied by fibrous replacement of the marrow that sometimes leaves micro- or macrocysts.** The most characteristic change is an apparent or real increase along the endosteal and trabecular surfaces in the number of osteoclasts lying within scalloped resorption cavities. In this manner the cortex and trabeculae are thinned, and sometimes the latter are completely transected. The bone loss is particularly evident as subperiosteal resorption of the phalanges and loss of the lamina dura (a dense, opaque, radiographic line normally surrounding the tooth socket). Along with the bone resorption, fibrous tissue fills the marrow spaces. It is of a peculiar type, having widely scattered fibroblasts separated by a loose, delicate ground substance. The fibrous tissue may enclose microcysts or, in other areas, large, macroscopically visible cysts. Scattered within this background there may be so-called **"brown tumors,"** a particularly inappropriate designation since the lesions are not neoplastic. They represent foci of hemorrhage, perhaps related to microfractures that undergo organization with the release of hemosiderin and the accumulation of macrophages, fibroblasts, and osteoclastic giant cells. These lesions have more than a passing similarity to true giant cell tumors (described on p. 1345), but are better referred to in osteitis fibrosa cystica as **reparative giant cell granulomas** having none of the neoplastic and malignant potential of true giant cell tumors.

The microscopic alterations may induce gross bony deformities in the form of irregular, abnormal cystic enlargements; fusiform dilatations of the shaft; and, with resorption and softening of the bone, bending and fractures of the more severely affected regions (Fig. 28–13). It is worth reemphasizing that the full-blown changes of osteitis fibrosa cystica are seen only late and in severe cases. The earlier alterations consisting of, in essence, loss of bone may be difficult to differentiate from those of osteomalacia and osteoporosis, both microscopically and radiologically. Soft tissue metastatic calcifications sometimes appear in these individuals.

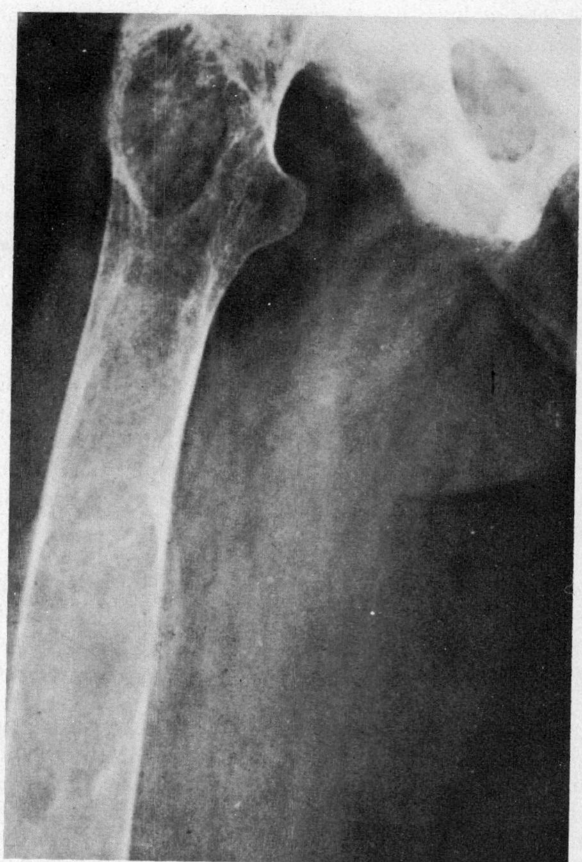

Figure 28–13. Advanced osteitis fibrosa cystica of femur in primary hyperparathyroidism due to a functioning adenoma. Cystic rarefaction is evident throughout shaft.

The skeletal changes of osteitis fibrosa cystica were once clinically detectable in 80 to 90% of cases of primary hyperparathyroidism. Now this endocrine disorder is often first detected by the discovery of hypercalcemia in multiphasic analyses of the blood during a routine check-up or clinical investigation of an illness. Thus, hyperparathyroidism is now being diagnosed much earlier at a time when only 10 to 15% of patients have clinically evident skeletal changes. In all likelihood, early distinctive microscopic changes would be present in most instances. Only rarely is secondary hyperparathyroidism sufficiently severe or prolonged to induce well-defined osteitis fibrosa cystica.

The clinical manifestations relating to the disease of bone are almost invariably overshadowed by the other manifestations of hyperparathyroidism. However, as indicated, there is sometimes a predisposition to fracture, to skeletal deformities under the stress of weight-bearing, and to joint pains and dysfunctions as the lines of normal weight-bearing are disturbed. Morphometry of metacarpal cortical thickness and photon-beam densitometry can confirm bone loss, but not reliably differentiate among the various causes of osteopenia. Sometimes the macroscopic cysts and/or brown tumors produce distinctive localized rarefactions and bony deformity that, in combination with the overall cortical thinning, permit a fairly secure radiographic diagnosis. Depending on their severity, the bony changes may regress or completely disappear following removal of the hyperplastic glands or functioning tumor in primary hyperparathyroidism.

PAGET'S DISEASE OF BONE (OSTEITIS DEFORMANS)

When Sir James Paget noted the increased warmth overlying skeletal deformities (now known to be related to increased vascularity, rather than inflammation), he understandably called the condition "osteitis deformans." *It is a disorder of middle or later life characterized initially by excessive osteoclastic resorption and, later, marked bone formation yielding in affected areas a haphazard arrangement of osteons demarcated by osteoid seams*—a so-called histologic "mosaic." Although it is essentially a focal disorder and may involve only a single bone (monostotic), the involvement in some individuals is more widespread (polyostotic). Most patients are over 40 years of age, with a slight male preponderance. It is an extremely common disorder; the asymptomatic form of the disease has been identified in 1 to 3% of the populations of the United States and United Kingdom.[68] Its cause is best considered in the context of the morphologic changes.

MORPHOLOGY. The microscopic changes can be divided into three progressive phases: (1) the initial so-called osteolytic phase, (2) the active stage of mixed osteolysis and osteogenesis, and (3) the inactive or osteoblastic sclerotic phase of the disease.[69] At the outset, there is irregular, haphazard, osteoclastic bone resorption. The osteoclasts tend to have bizarre shapes and often contain an increased number of nuclei. Even during this osteolytic phase, there is some evidence of an osteoblastic response with the deposition of irregular, woven bone. In an area of active involvement, virtually 100% of the bone surface is covered by osteoclasts and osteoblasts. The bone replacement is not complete, however, and some of the resorbed bone may be replaced by a highly vascularized connective tissue. Concomitantly, there is replacement of the contiguous fatty or hematopoietic marrow by loose, highly vascularized, fibrous connective tissue. In this manner, there is progressive erosion of the cancellous spicules of bone as well as the cortex (beginning at the endosteum) and extensive replacement by fibrous tissue.

With progression, the mixed stage of full pagetic activity becomes apparent. During this active phase, there is prominence of both osteoclasts and osteoblasts. Now the osteoclastic resorption is matched by active bone formation. As the original bony structure with its ordered lamellar pattern is destroyed, it is progressively replaced by a vascular connective tissue in which is laid down, first, woven bone, and later, remodeled lamellar bone. Because the mineralization of the newly laid down matrix lags, osteoid seams persist at the margins of the new osteons to create the so-called **pathognomonic feature of active Paget's disease, a tilelike or mosaic pattern** (Fig. 28–14). The mosaic is evident in both the cortical and cancellous regions, and may completely replace the preexisting bone. Because this new bone is laid down in bits and pieces, it is poorly organized and lacks the structural strength of the original bony tissue. Concomitantly, there may be subperiosteal new bone formation, also of this inadequate, poorly mineralized type. **Therefore, although the thickness of the cortex and trabeculae and the overall size of the bone are increased, the bone is soft, almost rubbery, and porous, composed largely of poorly mineralized matrix and vascular connective tissue.**

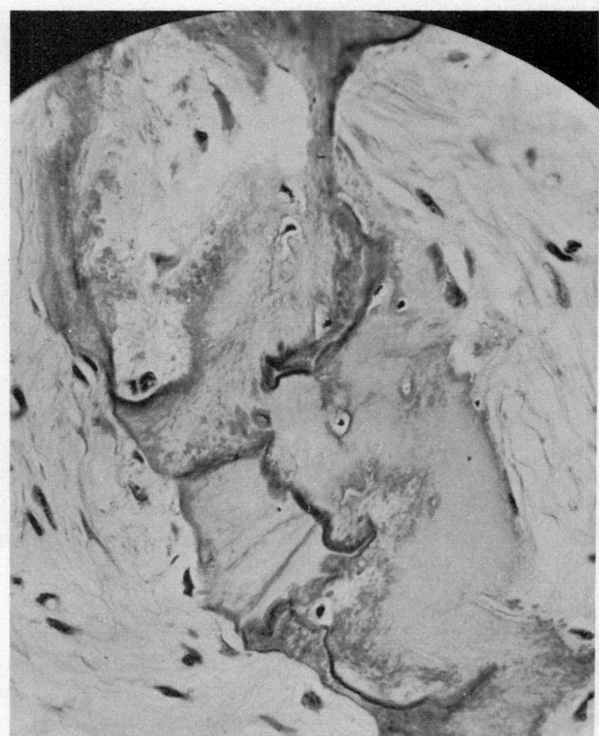

Figure 28–14. Paget's disease of bone. Histologic detail of a single bone spicule to illustrate "mosaic" pattern produced by irregular bone formation.

Eventually, after many years, osteoclastic activity may wane and there is predominantly osteoblastic production of new bone. However, this neo-osteogenesis is still irregular and accompanied by fibroblastic activity in the adjacent marrow space. In this way, the bone volume builds up, but it lacks structural strength.

The bones affected by Paget's disease, in decreasing order of frequency, are the pelvis, skull, femur, spine, tibia, humerus, and scapula and only occasionally other bones including the mandible.[70] Because of their softness, the bones are characteristically deformed by weight-bearing. All manner of distortion of the pelvis occurs. Compression of the vertebral bodies gives rise to kyphosis, scoliosis, and lordosis; the tibias and femurs bend; and the femoral necks may yield under the pressure. Although the bones are increased in size, they are **unusually light, soft, and porous and almost have the consistency of dry bread.** The outer cortical tables are usually thinned or totally replaced. Paget's disease of the skull is particularly striking by virtue of the irregular thickening of the skull (Fig. 28–15), but the bone can be sliced by a knife, and the calvarium, when filled with water, leaks like the proverbial sieve. Similar enlargement, softening, and porosity characterize all the bony involvements wherever they occur. However, during the late, so-called burned-out stage of Paget's disease, the enlarged bones become well mineralized, thoroughly ossified, and densely sclerotic. As mentioned, this process does not necessarily affect the entire skeleton. Sometimes it is monostotic and, even within a single bone, may involve a sharply localized region well demarcated from the adjacent uninvolved bone.

ETIOLOGY. The etiology of Paget's disease is still unknown. Over the years the condition has at one time

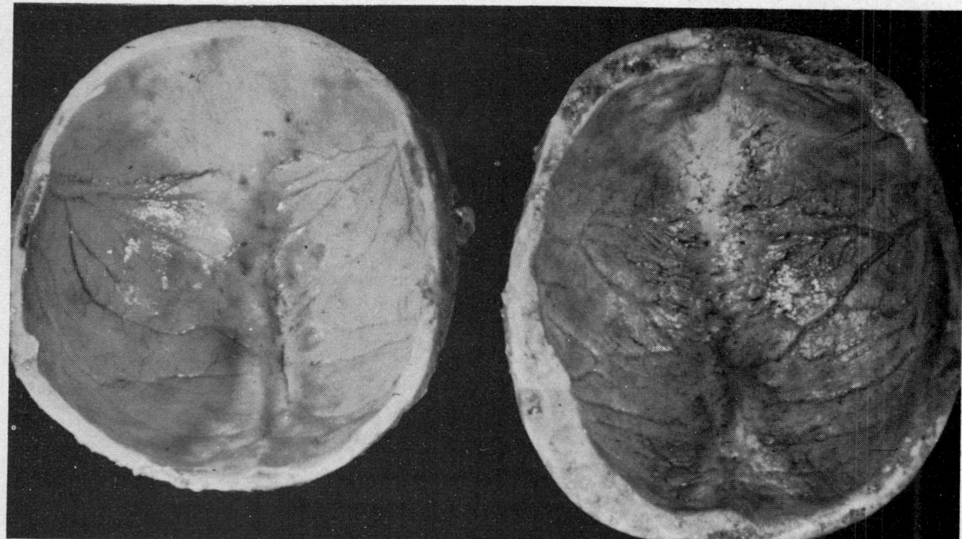

Figure 28–15. Paget's disease of skull. Irregular thickening of right calvarium is well brought out by comparison with normal control on left.

or another been considered to be (1) an inborn error of connective tissue, (2) related to hyperparathyroidism, (3) the consequence of some vascular abnormality mediated by the autonomic nervous system, and (4) an autoimmune derangement. All of these theories cannot be reconciled with the essentially focal nature of the bone involvement. Currently favored is the concept of viral infection, more specifically a slow virus infection such as causes subacute sclerosing panencephalitis (p. 1385).[71] Tubular structures similar to the nucleoprotein subunits of viruses have been visualized within inclusions in the nuclei of the giant osteoclasts.[72] The virus-like tubules closely resemble those found in mumps and measles caused by paramyxoviruses, and antisera to measles react with the cellular inclusions in the immunoperoxidase method.[73] However, it has not been possible to isolate any virus from affected bone either by cell culture or by co-cultivation—the method that was successful in recovering virus from subacute sclerosing panencephalitis. Moreover, there is no consistent evidence of an active antibody response to measles virus in patients with developing or developed bone disease, and there is, in fact, a greater prevalence of antibodies to other viruses in random patients with Paget's disease.[74] It is clear that the viral causation of this skeletal involvement remains to be established.

Clinical Course. Many individuals have monostotic or localized Paget's disease, which is asymptomatic and discovered only incidentally on radiographs or by the chance finding of an elevated serum alkaline phosphatase level. *The alkaline phosphatase level is generally higher in this condition than in any other bone disorder.* Despite the increased bone turnover, the serum concentrations of calcium, phosphorus, and parathyroid hormone remain normal. When symptomatic, the manifestations are extremely variable, depending on the extent of the disease, the particular bones involved, and the development of superimposed complications. The usual initial manifestations consist of either pain or deformity related to underlying skeletal changes. The pain is the result of microfractures, compression of nerves as they pass through bony foramens or secondary osteoarthritis.[75] Pain in the face and headache may be related to enlargement of facial or skull bones, with compression of cranial nerve foramina. A similar mechanism may be involved in hearing loss, with impingement on the eighth cranial nerve, but sometimes it is also caused by direct pagetic changes in the ossicles of the inner ear. Pain in the back and lower extremities may be caused by pressure on nerve roots or by vertebral microfractures, and indeed vertebral fractures with compression of the spinal cord may cause paraplegia. Vertebral column involvement may cause deformities of the trunk, sometimes with grotesque, dwarflike distortions. The skeletal changes may take the form of bowing of the tibias and femurs. Radiologically, affected bones are enlarged, the skull thickened, and the weight-bearing bones bent, but all are characterized by increased radiolucency during the stages of osteolytic and active disease. Later, the deposition of sclerotic bone may cause a patchy, mottled radiographic pattern or, in far-advanced, burned-out cases, an overall increased bone density.

Three additional features may be encountered in Paget's disease: (1) hemodynamic changes, (2) overt pathologic fractures, and (3) the development of a sarcoma in involved bones. Bony hypervascularity, as mentioned, accounts for the warmth of the skin overlying affected areas of the skeleton. When the involvement is polyostotic and widespread, the expansion of the peripheral vascular bed acts as an arteriovenous shunt that sometimes leads to high output failure or exacerbation of any underlying cardiac disease.[76]

The second complication is the appearance of pathologic fractures during the stages of active disease. Fractures are often incomplete but nonetheless may reactivate the disease, causing considerable bone resorption in the area. Occasionally in the late stages of bony sclerosis, complete transverse fractures occur, as though a piece of chalk had been snapped.

The third and most ominous complication is the development of a cancer in an involved bone. *Sarcomas, generally osteogenic sarcomas, but sometimes fibrosarcomas or other forms of sarcoma, arise in pagetic bones in about 1% of patients.*[77] Indeed, when a patient over 40 develops an osteosarcoma, the likelihood of underlying Paget's disease is approximately 20 to 25%.[78] The most frequent locations of the osteosarcomas, in contrast to the usual distribution of de novo tumors (p. 1338), are the pelvis, femur, humerus, tibia, skull, and mandible, in descending order of frequency. The tumors tend to be more aggressive than those in individuals without Paget's disease, and survival for longer than a year is exceptional.

Although a discussion of therapy is beyond our scope, brief mention should be made of the significant benefits that have been reported with the use of calcitonin and diphosphonates. The latter inhibit both bone resorption and formation, and sometimes appear to interrupt the progression of the disease.

HYPERTROPHIC OSTEOARTHROPATHY

This enigmatic disorder is characterized by (1) periosteal inflammation at the ends of bones (long bones of the forearm and lower leg, metacarpals, and metatarsals) with lifting of the periosteum and subjacent new bone formation, accompanied by (2) arthritis of the adjacent joints. The clinical hallmark of osteoarthropathy is painful periarticular or joint swelling over the wrists, elbows, ankles, or knees. It is frequently but not invariably associated with *clubbing of the fingers.* This condition consists of edema with fibrous overgrowth of the tips of the fingers and increased vascularization in the nailbed, with rounding or "watchglass" deformity of nails. The normal inclination of the nail relative to the axis of the bone may be lost. The tips of the digits become enlarged and often are dusky or cyanotic. Occasionally, there is some periosteal reaction of the terminal phalanges known as tufting. *Just as hypertrophic osteoarthropathy may be present without clubbing of the fingers, so clubbing sometimes appears without hypertrophic osteoarthropathy.*

Both these curious conditions may appear in a wide variety of clinical settings. The most frequent clinical accompaniments are primary intrathoracic cancers, notably bronchogenic carcinoma, pleural mesothelioma, and malignant thymoma; intrathoracic sepsis; infective endocarditis; and cyanotic, congenital heart disease.[79] Less frequent clinical associations include ulcerative colitis, regional enteritis, cirrhosis of the liver, cystic fibrosis of the pancreas, metastatic cancer to the lungs, and carcinoma of the thyroid gland. In this roster of underlying disorders, bronchogenic carcinoma stands out as preeminent. Osteoarthropathy and clubbing are said to appear in 10% of these cases, accounting for the sometimes-used designation *hypertrophic pulmonary osteoarthropathy.* Rarely, hypertrophic osteoarthropathy and/or clubbing may appear in patients without an underlying disorder and is also seen within families as an apparently hereditary disorder.

The origins of both hypertrophic osteoarthropathy and clubbing of the fingers are completely obscure, but two theories dominate current thinking, postulating (1) neurovascular abnormalities and (2) hormonal imbalances. It is well documented that both processes can be relieved in patients with bronchogenic carcinoma by dividing the vagus nerves above the hilum without removing the tumor.[80] It is proposed that neurogenic impulses acting through the autonomic nerve centers in some way lead to vasodilatation in the affected areas and that the increased blood flow then induces the anatomic changes previously mentioned. However, high blood flow has not been confirmed by direct plethysmographic measurements. The hormonal theory involving possibly estrogens or human growth hormone is equally poorly established. However, there is a report of increased levels of prostaglandins in cystic fibrosis patients who have digital clubbing.[81] No studies have yet been reported on the prostaglandin levels in the many other conditions associated with osteoarthropathy and finger clubbing, so at present the etiology and pathogenesis of these skeletal changes must be considered unknown.

Both the arthropathy and the digital clubbing are reversible following removal of the primary neoplasm, correction of the congenital heart disease, clearance of the intrathoracic sepsis, or control of the other related conditions. The major significance of these mysterious changes derives from the fact that they sometimes precede and call attention to the more ominous underlying disorder.

FIBROUS DYSPLASIA

This benign disorder of bone is best characterized as slow, progressive replacement of a localized area of bone by an abnormal proliferation of isomorphic fibrous tissue intermixed with poorly formed, haphazardly arranged trabeculae of woven bone. The changes seem to represent a focus of disordered maturation of bone with arrest at an immature stage of woven bone. The lesions appear in three distinctive but sometimes overlapping clinical patterns: (1) involvement of a single bone (monostotic); (2) involvement of several or many, but never all, bones (polyostotic); and (3) a special category of polyostotic fibrous dysplasia associated with skin pigmentations and endocrine dysfunctions, especially precocious sexual development.[82]

Monostotic fibrous dysplasia accounts for about 70 to 75% of all cases. It usually becomes manifest in both sexes in childhood and often comes to an arrest at puberty. The following sites are involved in descending order of frequency—ribs, femur, tibia, maxilla, mandible, calvarium, humerus, and other bones. The condition is often asymptomatic, being discovered incidentally in a radiograph taken for other reasons. However, the lesions may cause tumorous distortion of the bony contours, disfigurement of the face or skull, or sometimes pain related to the expanding bone mass or to pressure on nerves. The monostotic pattern does not appear to be a precursor to the polyostotic form; transition from one to the other has not been recorded.

Polyostotic fibrous dysplasia without endocrine disorders accounts for about 30% of all cases. It tends to appear at a slightly earlier age than the monostotic pattern and may progress into middle adult life. Both sexes are affected equally. The bony sites affected, in descending order of frequency, are the femur, skull, tibia, humerus, ribs, fibula, radius and ulna, mandible, vertebrae, and others. The lesions may be limited to a single limb or one side of the skeleton, but there is sometimes a bilateral distribution. In the polyostotic disease the craniofacial bones are affected in about 50% of persons with moderate dissemination of lesions, but reaches 100% in those with extensive disease. Also distinctive is a tendency to involve the shoulder and pelvic girdles; the development of severe, sometimes crippling deformities (e.g., shepherd-crook deformity of the proximal femur); and a marked predisposition to the development of spontaneous and often recurrent fractures.[83]

Polyostotic fibrous dysplasia in association with endocrinopathies accounts for about 3% of all cases. When accompanied by skin pigmentations and precocious sexual development, the multisystem disorder is referred to as Albright's syndrome. However, many other endocrine disorders may accompany these skeletal lesions, including hyperthyroidism, Cushing's syndrome, hyperparathyroidism, so-called "hypothalamic diabetes mellitus," and pituitary-induced abnormal skeletal growth.[84] In the most common clinical presentation with precocious sexual development, females are affected much more often than males. There is a tendency for the bone lesions to be unilateral and for the skin pigmentations to be confined to the same side of the body. The areas of pigmentation may be large, dark- to light-brown macules having irregular serpiginous borders found primarily on the neck, chest, back, shoulder, and pelvic region. There is no clear understanding of the association of the skeletal, skin, and endocrine derangements, but increased secretion of pituitary trophic hormones, possibly related to hypothalamic influences, is suspected.[85] However, no satisfactory explanation has yet been offered as to how the neurohumoral derangement induces the bony lesions.

MORPHOLOGY. Grossly in all clinical patterns, the bone lesions take the form of localized defects in cortical and cancellous bone, ranging from a few centimeters to massive lesions that distort the normal bony contour. The foci of involvement would appear to arise within the marrow cavities or endosteal region, because frequently a thin shell of subperiosteal cortical bone persists. Rarely, they totally erode the cortex. The gray-red fibrous tissue that fills these lesions may be gritty or sandy to touch. Occasionally, cystic spaces, small hemorrhages, or foci of chondroid or myxomatous tissue are present. Histologically, the lesions are composed of a mature connective tissue that may sometimes be sufficiently cellular to resemble a fibroma in which is laid down trabecular, woven bone. The osseous component is of variable prominence and sometimes is virtually absent. The haphazardly arranged bony trabeculae are thin and appear to be formed through osseous metaplasia of the background fibrous tissue (Fig. 28–16). **The bone is not lamellar in type but is poorly organized, woven bone.** Occasionally, there are calcified spherules or islands of cartilage within the connective tissue, sometimes with ossification of the cartilaginous inclusions. Osteoclastic giant cells are generally sparse and the vascularization varies from scant to abundant. Sequential biopsies have failed to show any evolution of the histologic changes with time. The woven bone trabeculae are not converted into lamellar bone, nor do the lesions become more sclerotic.

CLINICAL COURSE. Fibrous dysplasia pursues an unpredictable course. As mentioned, patients with monostotic lesions remain asymptomatic throughout life. In some instances, however, sufficient destruction of cortical bone leads to fracture. In other instances, particularly in persons with disseminated disease, there is a tendency to skeletal deformity and fracture, and when the facial bones are involved there may be severe distortions of the orbit, nose, and jaw. Generally, the earlier the age of onset, the more progressive is the condition. In about 0.5% of cases, the lesions of fibrous dysplasia undergo sarcomatous change.[86] In some of these instances there has been previous radiation therapy, but malignant transformation has been noted in the absence of such intervention.[87]

FIBROUS CORTICAL DEFECT (NONOSSIFYING FIBROMA)

Fibrous cortical defects are extremely common *non-neoplastic developmental aberrations* seen chiefly in children, almost always in the femur, tibia, and fibula. They create irregular, sharply demarcated, lobular, radiolucent defects in the metaphyseal cortex that usually leave intact a thin, subperiosteal layer of cortical bone. The margins of these lesions are sometimes slightly sclerotic. Multiple and bilateral lesions are found in about half the cases. Often they consist of minute lesions only a few millimeters in diameter, but occasionally larger defects up to 4 to 5 cm are seen. Because the larger lesions may seemingly erode into the marrow cavity, these are sometimes referred to as *nonossifying fibromas*, an unfortunate designation since both the smaller and larger lesions are of developmental origin, rather than being neoplastic.

The major clinical significance of these osseous lesions derives from the following facts: *(1) being non-neoplastic, they do not become transformed into sarcomas; (2) they are generally asymptomatic, but larger lesions may cause pain and predispose to fracture; (3) they are extremely common and have been reported in*

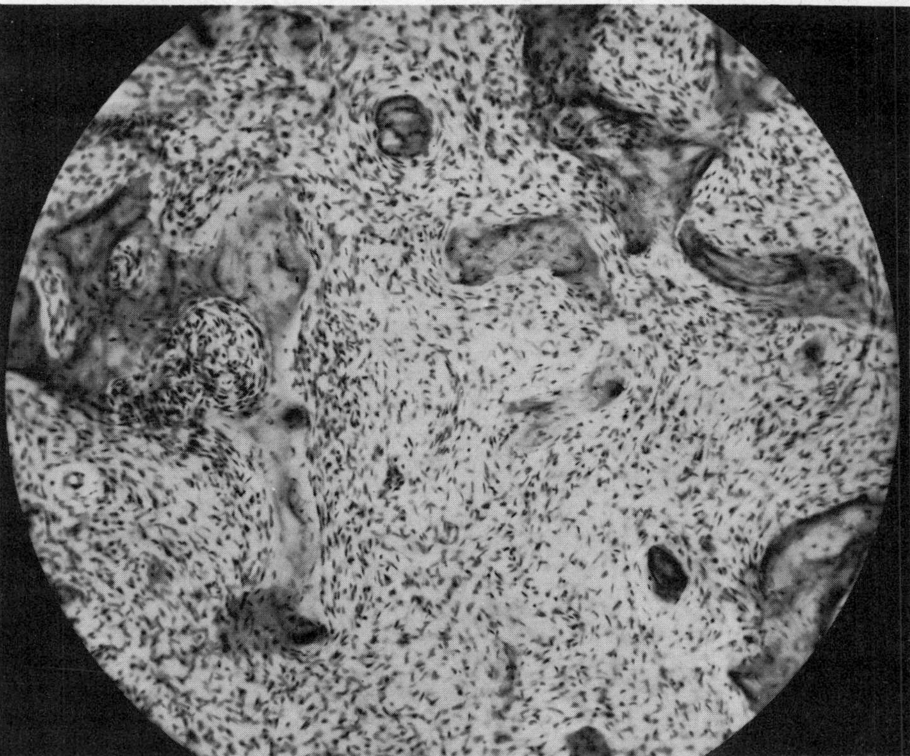

Figure 28–16. Fibrous dysplasia of bone, illustrating characteristic overgrowth of fibrous tissue and haphazardly scattered trabeculae of woven bone.

almost one-third of apparently normal children, both boys and girls; and (4) they usually disappear spontaneously within a few years.

The defects are composed of soft, yellow-gray tissue, usually lying subjacent to a thin shell of overlying intact cortical bone. They are found only in the metaphysis of the bone and have lobulated or scalloped margins. The larger lesions are elongated in the long axis of the bone. Microscopically, they are composed of cellular connective tissue laid down in a whorled, sometimes palisaded arrangement. The cells are usually mature and not anaplastic. Often there are interspersed lipid-laden foam cells and occasional multinucleate osteoclast-like giant cells. Unless fracture has occurred through one of these defects, there is no evidence of new bone formation within the lesion.[88]

As pointed out, awareness of these innocuous lesions is of importance since they are potentially mistaken, both clinically and anatomically, for more ominous bone tumors. In particular, multinucleate giant cells within the fibrous background make possible their misinterpretation as giant cell tumors of bone (p. 1345).

TUMORS

Although tumors of bones are infrequently encountered in clinical practice, they are nonetheless of great clinical significance because of the possibility that any such lesion may be malignant and because certain of these malignancies are among the most lethal, widely metastasizing cancers of humans. The large array of these tumors, their diverse origins from the multiple cell types found in bones, and their extremely variable biologic significance all make of these osseous neoplasms a highly challenging area of clinical and morphologic diagnosis. Before some useful generalizations are made, a few words about the classification of these neoplasms are required.

Primary bone tumors may arise from any of the elements indigenous to bone, including the diverse marrow cells as well as the vascular and neural components. A listing of the more common forms, drawn from the W.H.O. classification, is provided in Table 28–3. Before the number of specific tumors produces a relapse, it should be pointed out that many of these neoplasms, e.g., those derived from marrow, vascular, and neural cells, have been described elsewhere. Remaining for consideration here are the more common and important neoplasms of osseous tissue, cartilage, and uncertain origin.

Certain useful generalizations can be offered about the frequency and clinical presentation of bone tumors. Excluding malignant neoplasms of marrow origin (myeloma and leukemia), *osteosarcoma is the most common cancer of bone*, followed by Ewing's sarcoma, chondrosarcoma, and malignant giant cell tumors. These four neoplasms together constitute the vast bulk of bone cancers. Among the benign tumors the exostoses (osteochondromas) predominate, followed by benign giant cell

Table 28–3. TUMORS OF BONE*†

I Bone-forming Tumors	**IV Marrow Tumors**
Benign	*Malignant*
Osteoma	Ewing's sarcoma
Osteoid osteoma and osteoblastoma	Plasma cell (multiple) myeloma
Indeterminate	Lymphoma
Aggressive osteoblastoma	**V Vascular Tumors**
Malignant	*Benign*
Osteosarcoma, conventional	Hemangioma
Osteosarcoma, variants	Glomangioma
II Cartilage-forming Tumors	*Malignant*
Benign	Angiosarcoma
Osteochondroma (exostosis)	**VI Other Tumors**
Enchondroma (chondroma)	*Benign*
Chondromyxoid fibroma	Neurilemmoma
Chondroblastoma (epiphyseal chondroblastoma)	Neurofibroma
Malignant	*Malignant*
Chondrosarcoma	Malignant fibrous histiocytoma
III Giant Cell Tumors	Liposarcoma
Benign	Undifferentiated sarcoma
Indeterminate	Adamantinoma
Malignant	**VII Tumor-like Lesions**
	Bone cyst
	Fibrous dysplasia
	Reparative giant cell granuloma (e.g., epulis)
	Fibrous cortical defect
	Eosinophilic granuloma

*Partial listing.
†Drawn from the W.H.O. classification as modified by Spjut, H. J., and Ayala, A. G.: Skeletal tumors in children and adolescents. Hum. Pathol. *14*:628, 1983.

tumors. *Age of the patient, skeletal location, and radiographic appearance are important considerations in the differential diagnosis of these neoplasms.*[89] Osteosarcomas tend to occur during childhood and adolescence, a period of active skeletal growth. Indeed, a rough correlation has been drawn between the frequency of such tumors and skeletal height.[90] Chondrosarcoma and giant cell tumors, in contrast, most often arise in the middle years of life. However, it should be cautioned that these age ranges merely express peaks in incidence, and osteosarcoma, for example, may arise in infancy or in the elderly, and chondrosarcoma may arise in the young. Another striking feature is the tendency for each type of tumor to arise in particular skeletal locations. Over half of all osteosarcomas occur about the knee, most often in the distal femoral metaphysis, or less frequently in the proximal tibial metaphysis, the sites of greatest skeletal growth activity. Chondroblastomas and giant cell tumors are almost always located in the epiphyseal ends of long bones. In contrast, Ewing's sarcoma may arise anywhere within a bone, but is frequently diaphyseal in location. The radiographic changes induced by the lesion are also of great differential value. Certain neoplasms often are osteoblastic (e.g., the osteosarcoma), yielding radiodensities within the central region of the tumor and often in the extraskeletal extension of the invasive cancer. On the other hand, radiodensities within a lesion would be strong presumptive evidence against the diagnosis of Ewing's sarcoma. Thus, in the evaluation of a bone neoplasm, the age of the patient, the location of the lesion, its radiographic appearance, and the frequency of the various neoplasms are all important considerations.

BONE-FORMING (OSTEOBLASTIC) TUMORS

Tumors in this category were at one time referred to as osteogenic neoplasms, and the malignant variant was referred to as osteogenic sarcoma. The term "osteogenic" is subject to several interpretations. It could apply to all tumors arising in bone as well as to those producing bone. It is preferable, therefore, to use the designation "bone-forming" or "osteoblastic" tumors, since *the common denominator among all is the synthesis of osteoid matrix that may become mineralized.*

Osteoma

Benign tumors composed of densely sclerotic, well-formed bone, found jutting out from the cortical surface involving most often the skull and facial bones, are osteomas. They often protrude into one of the air sinuses (frontal, ethmoid, and others) and sometimes from the mandible, maxilla, and inner and outer skull tables. These neoplasms may arise at any age, slightly more frequently in men than in women. They can be briefly characterized morphologically as sclerotic lesions composed of mature, irregularly laid down, broad bony trabeculae (Fig. 28–17). The intertrabecular spaces are filled with fibrous tissue that is sometimes highly vascularized and may even contain foci of hematopoiesis. Osteomas are generally of little clinical significance and need not even be excised, unless they cause obstruction to a sinus cavity, impinge on the brain, or are disturbing cosmetically. They do not transform into other lesions but occasionally are associated with Gardner's syndrome.

Osteoid Osteoma and Osteoblastoma

The osteoid osteoma is a small benign neoplasm having no malignant potential. In contrast, the osteoblastoma is best viewed as a larger osteoid osteoma having different clinical significance. Most of the following remarks are directed to the more common osteoid osteoma. It produces a distinctive radiographic pattern and evokes a surprising amount of pain for its small size. Almost 90% of these lesions are encountered in persons between 5 and 25 years of age, slightly more often in males, and most frequently in the diaphyses of the long bones of the lower extremities, particularly the tibia and femur. *Radiographically, they appear as a small radiolucent focus (the nidus), rarely over 1 cm in diameter, surrounded by densely sclerotic bone that may become so radiopaque as to hide the buried nidus.*

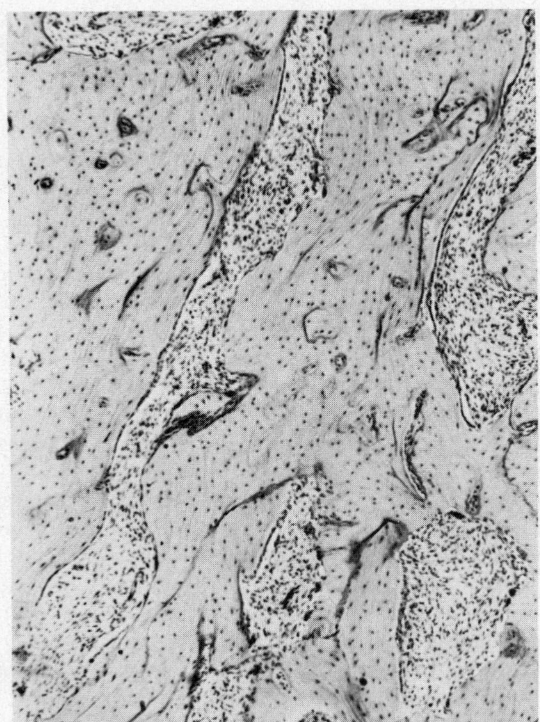

Figure 28–17. Osteoma. Histologic detail to demonstrate broad, well-formed, mature bony spicules.

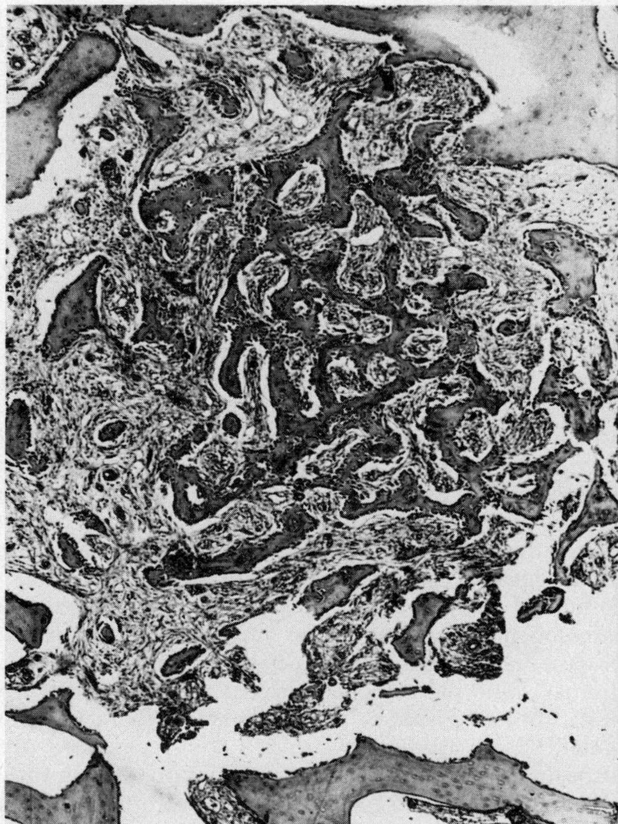

Figure 28–18. Osteoid osteoma. Low-power view of an entire lesion enclosed within sclerotic wide bone spicules. Lesion is composed of fibrous tissue and numerous anastomosing spicules of osteoid.

With lesions located close to the periosteum there may be marked, sclerotic, subperiosteal bone formation sufficient to produce a smooth fusiform thickening of the cortex overlying the nidus.[91] The pain, characteristically more severe at night, may be localized to the site of the lesion, but may radiate widely. When it is located in bones close to the skin, there is often tenderness on palpation.

Most experts believe that this lesion is a neoplasm, but the invariable small size of the lesion, its pain and tenderness, and the striking surrounding reactive bone formation raise the possibility of an inflammatory origin. However, ultrastructural studies indicate that the major cell elements within the nidus are osteoblasts, a finding that would be inconsistent with the notion of an inflammatory reaction.[92]

As pointed out, osteoid osteomas are most commonly located in the diaphyses of the tibia and femur, but nearly every other bone in the body has been involved at one time or another, with the possible exceptions of the skull, sternum, and clavicles. Most lesions are intracortical, but some may arise close to the endosteum or within cancellous bone. The nidus itself is composed of firm, red-gray tissue that is sometimes gritty because of the contained mineralized osteoid trabeculae. The surrounding bone is densely sclerotic. Microscopically, the nidus is composed of a tangled array of branching and anastomosing partially mineralized osteoid trabeculae that are sometimes broad and leave scant, intervening vascularized connective tissue (Fig. 28–18). At other times, the trabeculae are delicate and separated by abundant, richly vascularized intertrabecular tissue. Osteoblasts are often present along the margins of the osteoid trabeculae and blend imperceptibly into the more fibroblastic-looking cells within the soft tissue stroma. In many cases the trabeculae are sharply demarcated from the adjacent stroma, but in some instances the margins are irregular and frayed and merge imperceptibly into the osteoblast-fibroblast stroma. Occasional multinucleate apparent osteoclasts are present, but these are rarely prominent or numerous.

These benign lesions are readily managed by en bloc excision. Removal by curettage may be followed by recurrence, but even with recurrence (which may be years later) malignant transformation does not occur.

The closely related *osteoblastoma,* sometimes called a *giant osteoid osteoma,* has a similar histology but tends to be larger, is frequently located in the vertebrae, does not cause pain, and, although usually benign, may be malignant and an aggressive recurrent lesion.[93]

Osteosarcoma (Osteogenic Sarcoma)

The osteosarcoma is best defined as a malignant tumor of mesenchymal cells, characterized by the direct formation of osteoid or bone by the tumor cells. There is great variability in the histologic appearance of osteosarcomas. Some are composed largely of fibroblastic cells, others have abundant bone formation, some show chondroid differentiation, and still others are highly vascular (telangiectatic), but all have tumor-produced osteoid marked by trapping of anaplastic tumor cells within the lacunae of the osteoid matrix.[94] Osteosarcomas are the second most common form of primary cancer in bones, preceded only by multiple myeloma. They are clearly the most common form in children and young adults.

These neoplasms have been variously subclassified on the basis of (1) the clinical setting in which they appear, (2) their presumed point of origin in relation to a bone, and (3) their dominant histomorphology (discussed later). On the basis of clinical setting, these neoplasms can be divided into two large categories, primary and secondary. *Primary osteosarcomas* arise de novo in the apparent absence of underlying bone disease or recognized carcinogenic influences. Most of these cancers appear in young persons under 20 years of age before the epiphyses have closed. *Secondary osteosarcomas* develop against a background of preexisting bone pathology or previous exposure to some potentially carcinogenic influence. Most important is underlying disease, e.g., Paget's disease of bone, multiple enchondromas, multiple osteochondromas, chronic osteomyelitis, fibrous dysplasia, and infarcts and fractures of bone.[95] Bone irradiation also is a well-recognized predisposing influence and was present in 4% of these neoplasms in one large series.[96] Both external radiation for benign bone disorders and internal radiation derived from bone-seeking radioisotopes such as ^{224}Ra have been implicated.[97] Secondary osteosarcomas rarely arise in childhood or young adult life, but usually the patients are considerably older, particularly when the neoplasms are superimposed on Paget's disease. As pointed out, although the risk of developing a neoplasm with this skeletal disorder is only 1%, the frequency of Paget's disease in older individuals accounts for the fact that about 10 to 15% of all osteosarcomas arise in persons over the age of 30.

On the basis of primary site of origin, osteosarcomas have been divided into the following subsets: (1) conventional (medullary), (2) parosteal (juxtacortical), (3) periosteal, (4) intracortical, and (5) extraskeletal (arising in soft tissues). We need not delve deeply into all the subsets; the following remarks relate mainly to "conventional" neoplasms that usually appear as primary lesions.

Most osteosarcomas (70%) fall into the primary, conventional category. As mentioned, they occur in young individuals, with a 2:1 male:female ratio. Whites and blacks are affected equally. The age and sex distribution has been related to the level of activity of bone growth. Before puberty both sexes are affected equally often, but with the more active bone growth in postpubertal boys a male predisposition becomes apparent. It is of interest that large breeds of dogs such as the St. Bernard and Great Dane have 13 times the frequency of bone sarcoma of smaller breeds. There are also hints of genetic influences. Osteosarcoma is the most common second primary neoplasm in individuals with genetically determined retinoblastoma.[98] Such hereditary conditions as multiple enchondromatosis and multiple osteochondromas are also documented predispositions to this form of bone cancer.[99] Additional evidence of genetic influences is seen in the rare families in which multiple members are affected, often siblings. However, most conventional osteosarcomas occur sporadically without apparent predisposing influences.

PATHOGENESIS. In addition to the radiation and genetic predisposing influences, there are clues pointing to contributory roles for reactive bone formation and viruses. The correlation between active normal bone growth and these neoplasms has already been pointed out. Similarly, Paget's disease is associated with marked new bone formation, as are a number of the various skeletal disorders known to favor the development of osteosarcomas. The evidence implicating viruses is at best tenuous. Bone tumor viruses have been characterized in mice, and a cell-free agent derived from human osteosarcomas, when injected into hamsters, has been reported to produce an increased incidence of a variety of mesenchymal sarcomas, the most common being osteosarcoma.[100] Also relevant is the fragmentary evidence of immunologic reactions to apparent tumor antigens, not only among patients harboring these neoplasms but also within family members.[101] Both humoral antibodies and cell-mediated immune reactions have been reported, but their lack of specificity for "private" tumor antigens, the failure to exclude natural-killer cell reactions, and the fact that healthy persons without exposure to patients with sarcomas have also been found to have low levels of immune reactivity to tumor cells all render the interpretation of these immunologic findings uncertain. At present, it seems wisest to conclude that, with the possible exception of radiation, the origins of these neoplasms are no less mysterious than they are for most cancers.

MORPHOLOGY. Most conventional osteosarcomas arise in the medullary cavity of the metaphyseal end of the long bones of the extremities: in decreasing order of frequency, in the lower end of the femur, upper end of the tibia, upper end of the humerus, and upper end of the femur. Almost 70% of all these tumors arise close to the knee. However, any bone of the body may be involved, and in persons over the age of 25 the incidence in flat bones and long bones is almost equal. By the time of diagnosis, most osteosarcomas are bulky masses that often cause obvious swelling of the extremity. The neoplasms appear as gray-white, aggressive masses that often contain areas of hemorrhage and cystic softening. They vary in consistency depending on the amount of osteoid production. About 50% of osteosarcomas contain sufficiently large amounts of osteoid to merit the designation **osteoblastic or sclerosing osteosarcomas** (Fig. 28–19). The tumor tissue here may be hard and have a gritty feeling. About one-fourth of these neoplasms show predominant **chondroid differentiation**, and in these the neoplastic tissue may appear opalescent and bluish-gray. The remaining one-quarter are largely fibroblastic and have a more typical fish-flesh sarcomatous appearance. Almost invariably the tumor penetrates the cortex and invades the soft tissues; in this process, it lifts

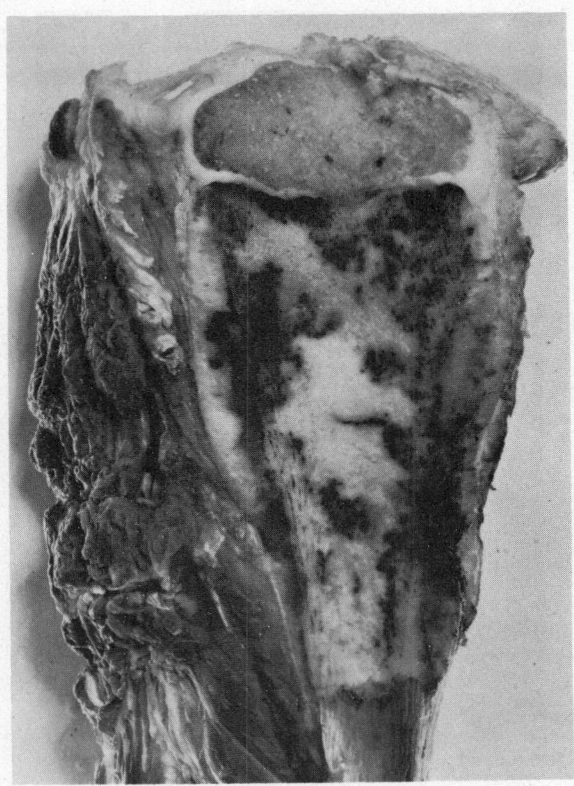

Figure 28–19. Osteogenic sarcoma, sclerosing type, of upper end of tibia. Hard white tumor fills marrow cavity but has not penetrated epiphyseal plate. It has infiltrated through cortex and lifted periosteum on both lateral aspects.

the periosteum and a characteristic so-called Codman's triangle is produced—the angle between the plane of the outer surface of the cortex and the elevated periosteum. This anatomic feature can often be visualized in radiographs, and although it is characteristic of osteogenic sarcoma, it is not pathognomonic. Despite its aggressiveness, osteosarcoma rarely penetrates the epiphyseal plate to involve the joint space; this may, however, occur after epiphyseal closure.

Histologically, these tumors vary in the richness of the osteoid or cartilaginous or vascular components, but **common to all is a basically anaplastic mesenchymal parenchyma that in places is punctuated by the formation of osteoid matrix by tumor cells.** Thus, frankly anaplastic cells are found lying within the lacelike patterns of osteoid matrix (Fig. 28–20). Islands of cartilage formed by tumor cells may or may not be present or may indeed dominate the microscopic fields. The mesenchymal cells between the osteoid and/or cartilaginous matrix are often wildly anaplastic, with numerous tumor giant cells, atypical mitoses, and striking hyperchromasia (Fig. 28–21). Some of the better-differentiated spindled cells appear on electron microscopy to be myofibroblasts.[102] Osteoclastic giant cells may or may not be present and are sometimes numerous (Fig. 28–21). Similarly, the vascularization may be subtle or take the form of large, cavernous telangiectatic channels, distributed throughout the tumor—**telangiectatic osteosarcomas.**

Parosteal sarcomas arise in juxtacortical locations also in the metaphysis. They tend to be well-differentiated lesions with well-formed, irregular bony trabeculae.[103] **Periosteal osteosarcoma,** although arising in the metaphyseal area, usually has a minimal attachment to the cortex or penetrates it only partially. These lesions often contain large areas of chondroid tissue, and some experts consider them to be chondrosarcomas.[103A] The **intracortical osteosarcoma** is a

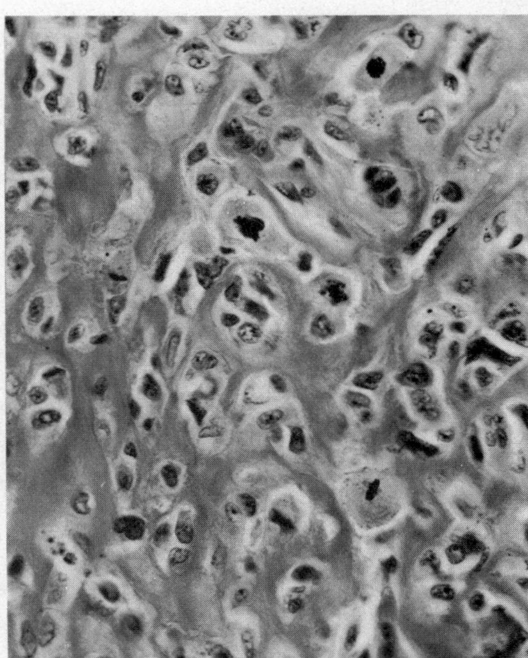

Figure 28–20. Osteoid produced by an osteogenic sarcoma. Note anaplasia and mitotic figures within trapped tumor cells.

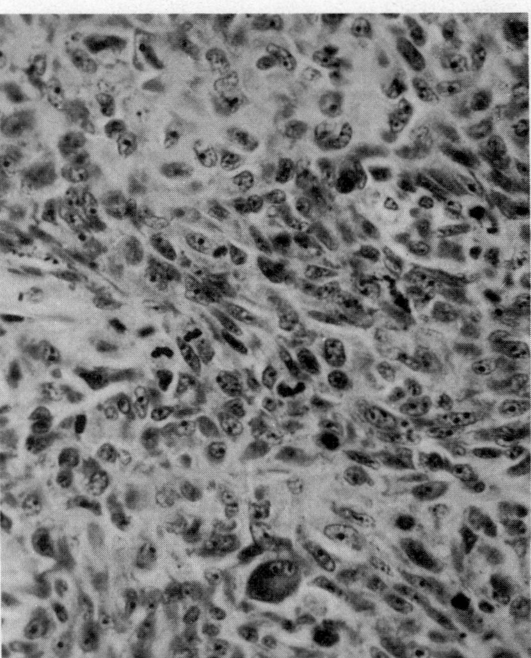

Figure 28–21. Low-power view of anaplastic mesenchymal cells in an osteogenic sarcoma. An osteoclast-like giant cell is present in lower midfield.

rare variant that appears to arise within cortical bone and then penetrate the medullary cavity and the adjacent soft tissue. The major significance of this pattern lies in its differentiation radiographically from a focus of osteomyelitis. **Extraskeletal osteosarcomas** are equally rare. The most common sites of origin are the retroperitoneum, mediastinum, and breast, but sometimes they arise in internal organs such as the uterus or lungs.

Whatever the morphologic variant and site of origin, all osteosarcomas are aggressive lesions that metastasize widely through the bloodstream, usually first to the lungs, but also to other parenchymal organs and other osseous sites. In contrast, lymph node involvement, even in the local region, is unusual. Approximately 20 to 30% of patients have demonstrable metastases when first seen, and more than 90% of those who die of the neoplasm have metastases to the lung.

Numerous efforts have been made to identify microscopic features of prognostic significance. Thus, these neoplasms have been graded I to III based on the degree of anaplasia, but it is generally agreed that there is little correlation between these grades and survival.[104] **More important is the predominant line of differentiation, e.g., osteoblastic, telangiectatic, or chondroblastic** (see below).

CLINICAL COURSE. As with most malignant tumors of bone, the presenting clinical complaints are those of pain, tenderness, and swelling of the affected parts. Occasionally, however, these tumors remain entirely silent and are called to clinical attention by the sudden fracture of the involved bone. Rapid growth is characteristic of many and may actually cause progressive expansion and enlargement of the limb as the neoplasm enlarges. Usually, these tumors follow a rapid clinical course and may be observed to increase in bulk under observation. The serum alkaline phosphatase may be elevated, but is usually of no diagnostic significance. Radiographs are distinctive in many instances. The lifting of the periosteum at Codman's triangle can sometimes be visualized, but may be absent. Another characteristic feature on the x-ray film is produced by the tumorous penetration of the cortical bone with extension into the soft tissue. This subperiosteal and soft tissue tumor with its bony osteoid content produces extraosseous radiodensities (Fig. 28–22). The radiodensity or radiolucency of the tumor varies according to the extent of bone formation, as described previously. However, the early lesion may be difficult to recognize by x-ray examination. In almost all cases, biopsy of the soft tissue extension of these neoplasms is necessary to confirm the diagnosis before such radical surgical procedures as amputation are performed. In the past, with only surgical resection or amputation for conventional osteosarcomas, the three-year survival rate was 50% and the five-year rate less than 25%.[96, 105] Recurrence usually became apparent within one to two years. There is some correlation between the size of the tumor and the prognosis, and it has been rare for a patient to survive even three years with a lesion exceeding 15 cm in greatest dimension. This generally dismal picture has brightened considerably at the present time: the combination of surgery and chemotherapy has yielded an overall survival rate at three years of approximately 65 to 75% in patients with nonmetastatic disease.[106] Recurrences are also delayed with this therapeutic regimen, so that five-year survival does not necessarily indicate a cure. Generally, osteoblastic lesions tend to respond better to chemotherapy than do telangiectatic or chondroblastic tumors.

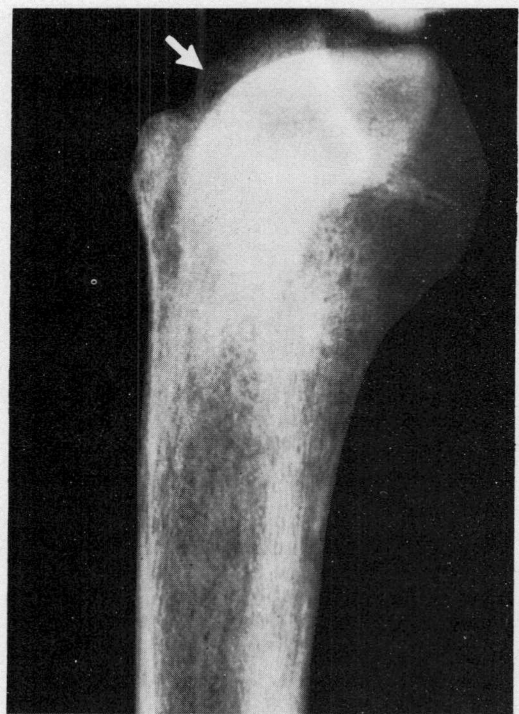

Figure 28–22. Osteogenic sarcoma of humerus. Note bone formation visible external to cortex *(arrow)*.

Secondary Osteosarcoma

As noted at the outset, conventional osteosarcoma generally arises de novo in the young and in the appendicular skeleton. Secondary osteosarcomas may appear at any age, and frequently in the advanced years of life in those with Paget's disease. In this setting the bones most often involved are the pelvis, femur, humerus, tibia, skull, facial bones, and scapula, in descending order of frequency. Although the tumor is morphologically similar to the conventional lesions, it is usually more aggressive, and few cases survive more than two years despite therapy.

Another variant is osteosarcoma of the jawbones, arising generally in middle to later life. These neoplasms tend to have marked chondroid differentiation, and distant metastases are less frequent. Radical resection yields a significantly higher cure rate than is achieved with conventional neoplasms. Other secondary patterns are too rare to merit discussion here, but are well described in the Armed Forces Institute of Pathology Fascicle on Tumors of Bone and Cartilage.[107]

CHONDROMATOUS TUMORS

Osteochondroma (Exostosis Cartilaginea)

These benign neoplasms may occur as solitary, sporadic lesions but are otherwise indistinguishable from their counterparts in the familial disorder osteochondromatosis (p. 1321).

Enchondroma

The term *chondroma* is often used to designate a benign tumor occurring within the interior of a bone composed of mature hyaline cartilage. However, the tumor is best designated as an *enchondroma*. Cartilaginous tumors that occur on the surface of bones and jut out from the bony contour almost invariably fall into the pattern of the exostosis cartilaginea, and therefore are not included within the present category. Solitary enchondromas occur in individuals up to the age of 50 but rarely in those under 10 years old.

Enchondromas may occur in multiple sites, often in childhood in a nonhereditary condition designated *enchondromatosis* or Ollier's disease. When these skeletal lesions are familial and accompanied by hemangiomas of the skin, they have been called *Maffucci's syndrome* (p. 1323). The enchondromas of these systemic patterns tend to be more cellular and more atypical than the isolated lesions, and have a higher incidence of malignant transformation.[108]

Most solitary lesions occur in the small bones of the hands and feet. However, tumors also have been found in the long tubular bones and rarely in the flat bones of the skull and pelvis. These lesions consist of firm, slightly lobulated, rounded, glassy, gray-blue, translucent tissue embedded within the spongiosa of the bone. They abut on and erode the overlying cortical bone. In the small bones of the hand, these lesions may progressively encroach upon the cortex and cause expansion and deformity of the bone. Usually, however, reactive bone formation maintains a thin outer bony shell. External deformity rarely occurs in the long tubular bones of the extremities. These gross characteristics are rarely evident in surgical specimens since the standard form of treatment is curettage of the lesion.

Histologically, the tumor is composed of **small masses or islands of hyaline cartilage, separated by a scant, sometimes richly vascularized fibrous stroma.** The cartilage cells are irregularly dispersed through the matrix and are contained within clearly defined lacunar spaces. Not infrequently, one to three nuclei may be found within a single lacuna. Toward the margins of the islands where they abut on the fibrous tissue, the cells become flattened and gradually assume the appearance of spindled fibroblasts, so that there is no well-defined transition between the cartilage cells and connective soft tissue cells. **Foci of calcification and even ossification are sometimes encountered in the cartilage, but the cells trapped within the bony matrix are not anaplastic,** differentiating such osteoid deposition from that found in osteogenic sarcomas.

Erosion of the adjacent cortex by the expansile lesions may cause pain and swelling, but often the tumors are totally unsuspected until discovered incidentally by roentgenogram or until attention is called to them by a pathologic fracture. Lesions in the small bones of the hands and feet are almost always innocuous and rarely become malignant. Those in the long bones of the extremities have a greater, but still only slight, tendency to undergo malignant transformation. Cartilaginous tumors in the pelvic bones are often malignant, but it is not certain whether these arise as benign chondromas or were chondrosarcomas from the outset.

Chondromyxoid Fibroma (Fibromyxoid Chondroma)

This is a comparatively uncommon lesion, principally of young adults, that is of importance because it is often misinterpreted as malignant. These tumors tend to occur about the knee joint in the lower metaphysis of the femur, the upper metaphysis of the tibia, and the lower end of the fibula.[109] The small bones of the foot may also be affected. As can be seen, this distribution is virtually confined to the lower extremity. Rarely these have been described in the ribs, small bones of the hands and wrist, vertebrae, scapulae, and mastoid. The tumor arises eccentrically within the marrow cavity, and progressively erodes the overlying cortex, causing a focus of radiolucency and sometimes total erosion of the cortical bone. They seldom cause obvious clinical deformity and are usually brought to the patient's attention by pain.

The neoplasm is firm, gray-white, lobulated, and rubbery, and rarely has a sufficient myxoid element to cause sliminess.

On microscopic examination, it is composed of a loose myxomatous tissue containing characteristic spindled fibroblasts, stellate myxoma cells, and, in areas of increased maturity, large amounts of collagenous hyaline fibrous tissue. There may be small-to-large areas of chondroid differentiation. Generally, there is no bone or osteoid formation. The most ominous feature of the tumor is scattered or sometimes aggregated multinucleate giant cells, some of which appear similar to osteoclasts. Other giant cells may have fewer nuclei with considerable hyperchromatism and variation in nuclear size and shape. These cells have the appearance of malignancy and are responsible for the overdiagnosing of these tumors as chondrosarcomas or myxosarcomas.

Experience, to date, indicates that these are entirely benign and do not recur after thorough curettage.

Chondroblastoma

This uncommon benign tumor assumes importance because it can be misinterpreted both clinically and anatomically for more ominous neoplasms such as osteosarcoma, chondrosarcoma, or giant cell tumor. Its clinical and radiographic characteristics are highly distinctive. *It usually arises within the epiphysis of long tubular bones in individuals between 10 and 20 years of age, with a male:female ratio of 2:1.* Radiographically, it appears as a spherical, sometimes lobulated radiolucent defect in the epiphyseal end of the bone. By progressive expansion, it may erode the adjacent cortex and extend through the articular cartilage or epiphyseal plate. Delicate calcifications within the lesion may create so-called cotton-wool opacities within the x-ray of the tumor. Its apparent destructiveness can be mistaken for a malignant neoplasm.

MORPHOLOGY. On gross inspection, chondroblastomas appear as gray-to-yellow-to-brown lesions lying within the epiphyseal end, usually of a long tubular bone. Less frequent locations include the pelvis, scapula, ribs, and calcaneus. The neoplastic tissue is frequently punctuated by foci of hemorrhage, cysts, and gritty calcific deposits. They generally are small neoplasms and rarely exceed 5 cm in diameter. However, they may erode through the articular surface, bony cortex, or (as mentioned) epiphyseal plate.

Microscopic examination of numerous fields of a single tumor may reveal wide variation in patterns. The dominant theme comprises sheets of round-to-oval cells with large, prominent nuclei containing nucleoli. These cells are believed to be chondroblasts. In areas, the cells become more spindled to resemble fibroblasts. Scattered within this richly cellular background are giant cells of two types: (1) small multinucleated giant cells; and (2) larger multinucleated giant cells resembling osteoclasts.[110] Another histologic feature consists of poorly delimited islands of poorly formed chondroid matrix laid down between the osteoblastic cells. This matrix does not recreate the gelatinous appearance of well-developed cartilage, nor are lacunae well formed, such as are seen in the chondrosarcoma. Another feature is spotty calcification within the cellular areas. True bone formation or the deposition of osteoid matrix is infrequent.

The rich cellularity of these neoplasms and the various histologic features cited makes evident why it is possible to interpret this benign neoplasm as an osteosarcoma, chondrosarcoma, or giant cell tumor. Indeed, in the past the chondroblastoma was known as an *epiphyseal giant cell tumor* or *chondromatous giant cell tumor*. Chondroblastomas are usually benign in their behavior and can be adequately treated by local excision or thorough curettage. Incomplete removal will be followed by local recurrence, however, and there are rare instances in which, following several attempts at removal, the recurrence has assumed a more aggressive behavior, such as local invasion or even metastatic dissemination.[111] Regrettably, histologic features are poor prognosticators of behavior.

Chondrosarcoma

Chondrosarcomas are one of the more common forms of cancer of bone, preceded in frequency by multiple myeloma, osteosarcoma, and Ewing's sarcoma. They vary widely in their clinical aggressiveness, depending on their level of anaplasia, but overall are much more amenable to surgical removal and cure than osteosarcomas. A minority arise in preexisting benign lesions —solitary enchondroma, enchondromatosis, multiple exostoses, fibrous dysplasia, and Paget's disease—and these are referred to as secondary osteochondromas. *Most (80 to 90%) arise de novo as primary chondrosarcomas.* Although secondary chondrosarcomas arising in hereditary disorders may affect individuals in the second and third decades of life, the peak incidence of the primary neoplasm is in the sixth and seventh decades.[112] The male:female ratio is approximately 2:1.

MORPHOLOGY. About one-half of these cartilaginous cancers involve the pelvic bones, but additional sites of origin include the humerus, femur, ribs, vertebral bodies, tibia, fibula, and sternum, in approximate descending order of frequency. They may be centrally located within the bones and permeate the marrow space, or may appear to arise in the periphery, to produce masses that extend into the surrounding soft tissues. Central lesions may cause expansion of the cortex, accompanied by peripheral reactive bone formation, but whether peripheral or central in origin, **they tend to be large, bulky, translucent, gray-white lobular growths, having a gelatinous consistence** (Fig. 28–23). Diameters in excess of 25 cm have been recorded. Central necrosis of tumor lobules, spotty calcifications, and ossification are sometimes present. Erosion of bone, destruction of cortex, and extension along broad, lobulated fronts into the surrounding soft tissues are evident in many.

The histologic diagnosis of chondrosarcomas is frequently difficult. The essential feature is the identification of anaplasia within the cells trapped within the cartilaginous lacunae (Fig. 28–24). Typical features of such anaplasia include enlarged hyperchromatic nuclei, multiple nuclei within a single cell, multilobate and grotesque nuclei, and

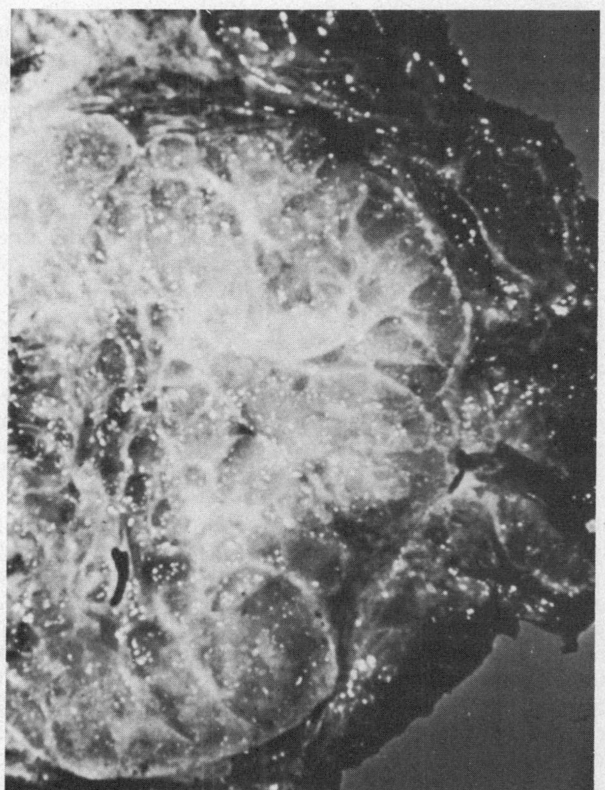

Figure 28–23. Lobulated translucent appearance of transection of a chondrosarcoma.

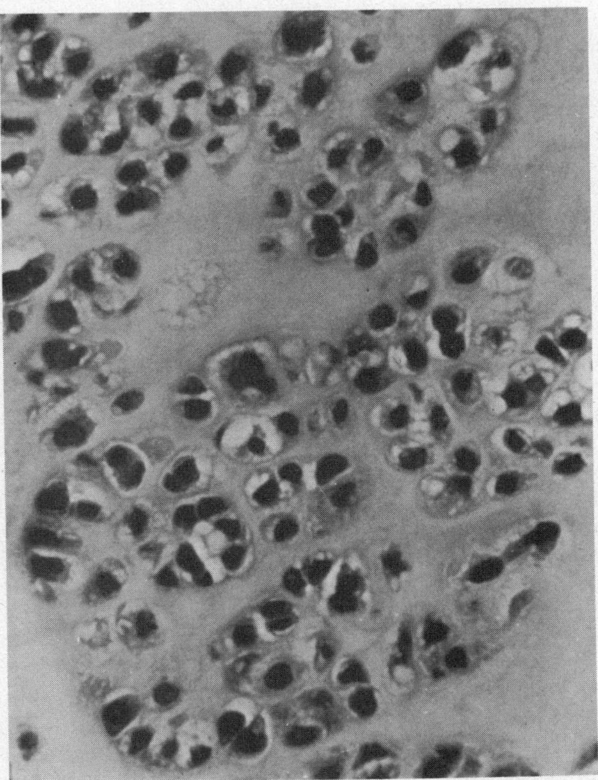

Figure 28–24. Anaplastic chondrocytes within a chondrosarcoma.

sometimes mitotic figures. As mentioned earlier, however, chondrosarcomas display a wide range of anaplasia, and the better-differentiated lesions are readily misinterpreted as benign chondromas. Analogously, tumors displaying foci of calcification and ossification are subject to misidentification as osteosarcomas with chondroid differentiation. **In chondrosarcomas with ossification, the bone formation occurs within cartilage, whereas in osteosarcomas the neo-osteogenesis arises out of the background of anaplastic, osteoblastic-fibroblastic cells.**

With these neoplasms, there is a remarkably clear-cut relationship between histopathology and tumor behavior. On the grounds of nuclear size, cellularity, mitotic rate, and frequency of cartilaginous lacunae containing multiple nuclei, they can be divided into Grades I to III.[112] Fortunately, only about 10% of chondrosarcomas are Grade III.

One particularly aggressive variant is referred to as chondrosarcoma with dedifferentiation.[113] It appears to represent reversion of a focus within a chondrosarcoma to a highly anaplastic spindle-cell neoplasm closely resembling a malignant fibrous histiocytoma of bone (p. 1364).

Usually, chondrosarcomas grow slowly. They come to attention because of pain and swelling in the affected part. Often the symptoms have been present for years. Metastatic dissemination may become evident many years after diagnosis. Metastases are seen most commonly in the lungs and occasionally in the liver, kidney, and brain. By contrast, lymph node metastases are rare. The prognosis is materially affected by the grade of the lesion based on cytologic features and number of mitoses.[112] In one analysis, the five-year survival rates of Grades I, II, and III were 90%, 81%, and 43%, respectively, whereas the corresponding ten-year survival rates were 83%, 64%, and 29%. None of the Grade I lesions metastasized, whereas 70% of the Grade III tumors disseminated. Thus, with chondrosarcomas, more than with most primary bone tumors, histologic analysis is of great prognostic significance. It is particularly important with chondrosarcomas having areas of dedifferentiation since survival with these neoplasms for more than two years is exceptional.

TUMORS OF MARROW ORIGIN

Under this heading are included plasma cell myelomas, so-called reticulum cell sarcoma of bone (closely related if not identical to histiocytic lymphoma), liposarcoma, and Ewing's sarcoma. Since the first three have been considered elsewhere, only Ewing's sarcoma remains to be discussed here.

Ewing's Sarcoma

Ewing's sarcoma is a highly malignant form of primary bone tumor. Although considered here as a neoplasm of marrow origin, its precise histogenesis is uncertain. Over the decades it has been variously considered to take origin from endothelial cells, lymphoreticular cells, or primitive mesenchymal cells. Although uncertainty persists, studies suggest that the neoplastic cells are capable of synthesizing collagen, and so are thought to be of primitive mesenchymal origin having no tendency to differentiation along osteoblastic, fibroblastic, or endothelial lines.[114] These tumors occur predominantly in the 5- to 20-year age group, slightly more often in males than in females and only very rarely in blacks. Local pain is a prominent manifestation as it is with most primary bone tumors, but patients with this form of neoplasm typically also have fever, local swelling, increased local heat, anemia, increased sedimentation rate, and debility, even before the tumor has disseminated.

MORPHOLOGY. These tumors arise within the marrow cavity, usually in unicentric foci within a single bone. In occasional cases, multiple lesions are found in several sites, and it is not certain whether these represent metastases or multicentric foci of origin. The long tubular bones of the body in about half the cases and the innominate bones in about one-fifth constitute the two major loci of origin. The remaining tumors arise in the pubis, ischium, ribs, skull, clavicle, and sternum and in almost any other skeletal part.[115] Most begin in the metaphyses, but a diaphyseal origin is common. They almost never arise in the epiphysis. Characteristically, by the time the specimen is obtained, the tumor involves large areas of the bone or even the entire medullary cavity. It appears as a soft, gray, often cystic lesion that has eroded and frequently expanded the cortex. Hemorrhages and necroses are common within the tumor tissue. Perforation of the cortex with subsequent widespread subperiosteal expansion and penetration into the soft tissues, producing larger extraskeletal than intraosseous masses, is more typical of Ewing's sarcoma than it is of any other form of bone cancer. Characteristically, it is taught that reactive new bone formation creates a **concentric onion-skin layering** about the tumor, but this pattern is not found in more than half the cases. It should be emphasized that these neoplasms are rapidly growing and therefore frequently cause bulky, fleshy masses that are readily palpable in the soft tissues.

Histologically, the tumors are extremely undifferentiated and consist of sheets of small, round, or oval cells having prominent nuclei and scant cytoplasm. **Particularly distinctive of the tumor cells are PAS-positive cytoplasmic granules,** present in nearly all neoplasms. This finding is generally held to distinguish Ewing's sarcoma from other highly undifferentiated cancers.[116] Under the light microscope the nuclei tend to be round to oval and quite uniform in size and shape, but electron microscopy usually reveals slight nuclear indentations. Tumor giant cells and pleomorphism are conspicuously absent in untreated tumors, but are prominent in those receiving previous irradiation. This histologic pattern may be modified by large areas of ischemic infarct necrosis (the rapidly growing tumor tends to outgrow its blood supply) so that, in many tumors, the preserved viable cells are found in cords or masses about blood vessels with necrosis of the more remote areas (Figs. 28–25 and 28–26). It is this totally undifferentiated growth that has provided the difficulty in determining the cell type of origin. Thus, the diagnosis of Ewing's sarcoma should not be made without consideration of the possibility that the lesion may represent a metastasis from an undifferentiated carcinoma, undifferentiated sarcoma, neuroblastoma, or, conceivably, a bone lymphoma. The PAS-positive granules are a helpful pointer to Ewing's sarcoma.

The radiographic appearance of these neoplasms may be quite distinctive or similar to that of other forms of bone tumors. These are generally lytic tumors that erode the cancellous trabeculae and then the cortex from within outward. Generally, extensive soft tissue invasion can be visualized. The continuity of the cortex may be interrupted, but usually it is only mottled in appearance. Elevation of the periosteum is typically present and sometimes is accompanied by so-called Codman's triangle (p. 1339). There may be periosteal bone formation about the tumor to create what has been referred to radiographically as onionskin layering. It should be emphasized that this neo-osteogenesis is reactive and not tumorous. Occasionally, there are spotty radiodensities, apparently within the tumor, but on three-dimensional study it is evident that these represent foci of periosteal new bone formation. Any or all of these radiographic changes can be produced by chronic osteomyelitis or other forms of neoplasms. However, the diagnosis of Ewing's sarcoma is almost certain when the neoplasm is diaphyseal in origin; is associated with local pain, swelling, heat, and fever; and is accompanied by radiographic findings of soft tissue extension of an intramedullary neoplasm.

This form of cancer is one of the most aggressive of the primary bone tumors. At least one-fourth of the patients have metastases at the time of initial diagnosis. Metastases may be widespread and involve any organ or tissue in the body. Particularly distinctive is the tendency to disseminate to other bones, most often the skull, and to the lungs; spread to the brain is also common.[117] In previous years, because of this aggressive

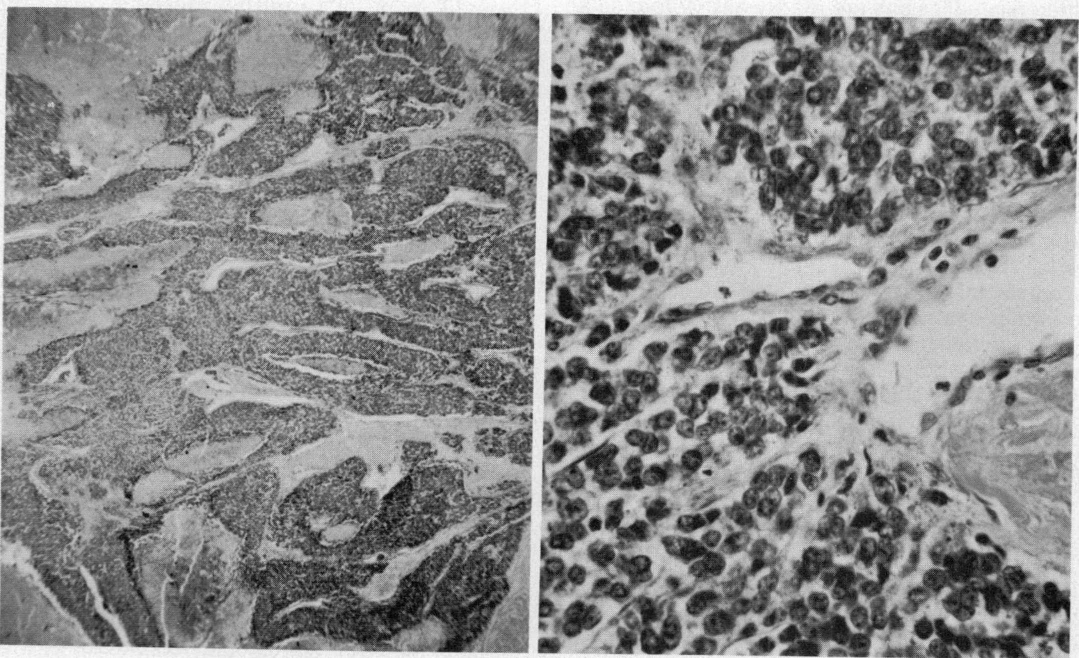

Fig. 28–25

Fig. 28–26

Figure 28–25. Ewing's sarcoma at low power. Broad bands of cells abut on blood vessels and are created by pale ischemic necrosis of intervening areas.

Figure 28–26. Ewing's sarcoma at high power, illustrating characteristic cytology.

behavior, the five-year survival rate based on surgical excision and radiotherapy was approximately 10%. In more recent years, however, chemotherapy has been added to the attack, and with the combined use of surgery, radiation, and chemotherapy a heartening improvement in prognosis has been achieved with a five-year relapse-free survival of approximately 70 to 75%.[118]

GIANT CELL TUMORS

Giant cell tumors are also sometimes referred to as *osteoclastomas* on the basis of the belief that the multinucleated giant cells (such a prominent histologic feature of these neoplasms) are osteoclasts. However, because the precise nature of these giant cells is still unclear, the preferred designation is giant cell tumor. These neoplasms have long been a focus of controversy on three scores: (1) their histogenesis, (2) their differentiation from other giant cell–bearing lesions, and (3) their biologic behavior.

The histogenesis of these neoplasms has long been an enigma.[119] First, it should be emphasized that *the multinucleate giant cells are not the neoplastic element within these tumors, but rather it is the background mononuclear fibroblast-like cells that determine the biologic behavior of these lesions.* Macrophages or histiocytes are numerous in these lesions and the question has been raised as to whether these multipotential mesenchymal cells give origin to both the mononuclear and multinucleate cells.[120] Indeed, some authors believe the giant cell tumor to be a form of fibrohistiocytoma (p. 1364) also having numerous giant cells.[121] Histochemically, however, the giant cells have a high content of acid phosphatase, beta glucuronidase, and succinic dehydrogenase characteristic of osteoclasts. Moreover, electron microscopic studies reveal ultrastructural features nearly identical with those of the osteoclast.[120] Thus, the controversy continues and it seems best to admit the present lack of certainty about the origin of these neoplasms.

Multinucleate giant cells are a feature of many non-neoplastic as well as neoplastic lesions of bone. They are particularly prominent in the so-called "brown tumor" seen in skeletal disease associated with hyperparathyroidism, and in the giant cell granuloma of the gingiva and jawbones (also called epulis). These lesions are better known as *reparative giant cell granulomas* and are not true neoplasms, despite their histologic resemblance to giant cell tumors of bone. Multinucleate giant cells are also encountered in the benign and malignant fibrous histiocytoma, chondromyxoid fibroma, and chondroblastoma, as well as less commonly in other primary bone neoplasms. The chondroblastoma poses a particularly challenging problem because this benign neoplasm usually has many multinucleate giant cells, and moreover the tumor arises in the epiphyseal ends of bone, where giant cell tumors arise. Since the latter are potentially malignant, the importance of the differential diagnosis is obvious.

The biologic behavior of these neoplasms and its predictability from histomorphology are also murky areas. Clearly, about 5 to 15% of these neoplasms classified as Grade III have overt anaplastic changes in the mononuclear cells (the cutting edge of these tumors) associated with aggressive clinical behavior. Most (70 to 75%) are histologically and clinically Grade I lesions. There remains about 10 to 15% of indeterminate lesions in which it is impossible to predict behavior from the microscopic features.[122] More than most neoplasms, the giant cell tumor is an "unreliable critter."

Another vexing issue involves those lesions that at the time of primary excision present a benign histologic appearance, but with incomplete removal and recurrence appear significantly more anaplastic. Does such a sequence represent a primary underdiagnosis or sampling error (with failure to visualize malignant foci) or is there a tendency for benign lesions to become malignant with time, or possibly following surgical or radiation therapy? There are no satisfactory answers to these questions, but the prevailing wisdom holds that the most malignant tumors are such from the outset, although there are undoubted instances in which "benign" lesions subsequently undergo malignant transformation, even in the absence of radiation therapy.[123] The message is clear: the best chance for cure is the first!

MORPHOLOGY. Giant cell tumors nearly always arise within the epiphyses, but may then spread into the metaphyses or even through the articular cartilage into the joint space. A metaphyseal origin is strong evidence against the diagnosis of giant cell tumor. **Over half of these lesions arise about the knee in the distal femur, proximal tibia, or proximal fibula.** Additional primary sites include the distal radius, distal ulna, proximal and distal humerus, sacrum, proximal femur, and vertebrae, as well as other bones.[124] Involvement of the small bones of the hands or feet is rare; giant cell lesions in these locations are more likely to be reparative giant cell granulomas or fibrous histiocytomas. Although most true giant cell tumors occur as solitary neoplasms, multiple or multicentric tumors are encountered rarely.[125]

Characteristically, the tumors begin within the cancellous region of the epiphysis and progressively expand to cause a clublike deformity of the bone (Fig. 28–27). In this expansion the cortex may be thinned or even eroded, but often reactive new bone formation maintains a thin, enclosing bony rim. With progression, they may erode into the joint to involve the neighboring bone. Alternatively, the tumors can penetrate into the surrounding soft tissue. Despite invasive behavior, they tend to grow as cohesive masses along broad lobulated fronts. Characteristically, they are red-brown on cut surface, with prominent areas of hemorrhage, cyst formation, and foci of pale, yellow-white necrosis.

Histologically, these neoplasms are composed mainly of plump, spindled, fibroblast-like cells, or more ovoid, primitive, mesenchymal-appearing cells. Scattered within the background of such mononuclear cells are numerous multinucleate apparent osteoclasts, or foreign body–type giant cells (Figs. 28–28 and 28–29). In areas there may be foci of necrosis, hemorrhage, hemosiderin deposition, and osteoid formation. The interpretation of the osteoid is controversial, and some favor its being reactive, whereas others

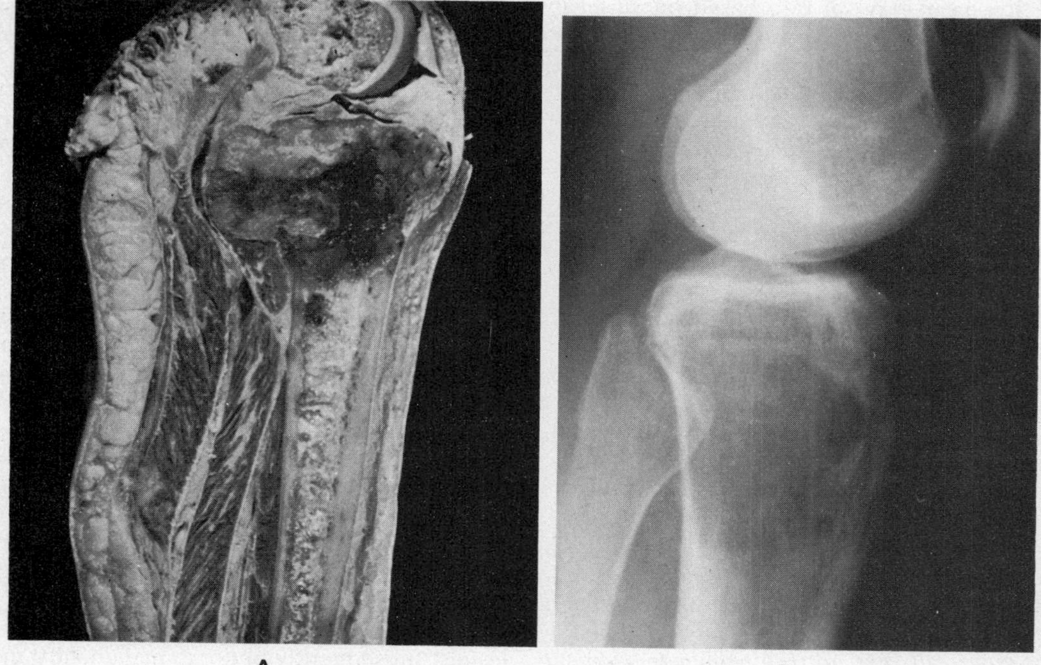

Figure 28–27. *A*, Benign giant cell tumor of upper end of tibia. Tumor has produced an ovoid enlargement, expanding epiphysis. *B*, Radiograph of a similar tumor in upper end of tibia showing lobulated cystic rarefaction of bone extending up to, but not penetrating, the articular surface. (Courtesy of Dr. Ashley Davidoff, Department of Radiology, Brigham and Women's Hospital, Boston.)

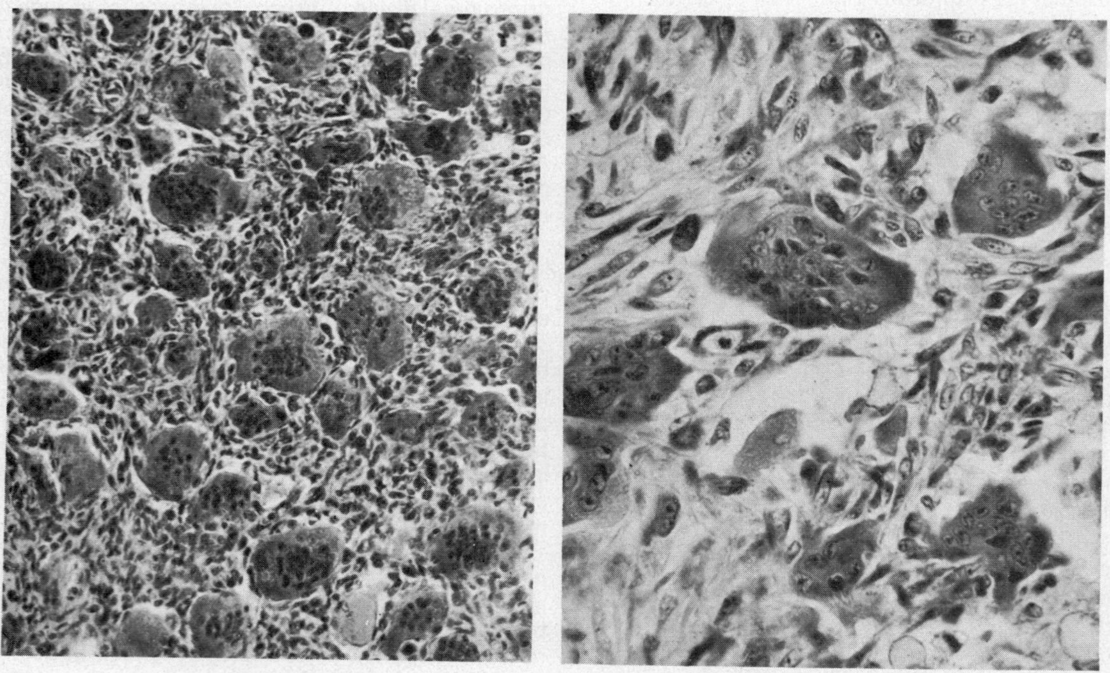

Fig. 28–28 Fig. 28–29

Figure 28–28. Benign giant cell tumor, illustrating abundance of multinucleate giant cells.

Figure 28–29. High-power detail of giant cells and well-differentiated stroma in benign giant cell tumor.

contend that the osteoid matrix is produced by tumor cells themselves. Equally controversial is the issue of cartilage formation within these neoplasms. Some observers deny ever finding cartilage within these tumors, but others point to chondroid areas in as many as one-third of the lesions.[124] **The spindle cell stroma of the giant cell tumors requires the most meticulous attention, for it is upon the regularity or anaplasia in these cells that the clinical behavior of the tumor hinges.** All degrees of cellular atypicality and undifferentiation are encountered, ranging from the Grade I well-differentiated typical tumors having almost mature fibroblastic spindle cells with few, if any, mitoses and no tumor giant cells, to the other extreme of Grade III lesions with cellular pleomorphism, hyperchromasia, abundant mitotic figures, and frank sarcomatous changes (Fig. 28–30).

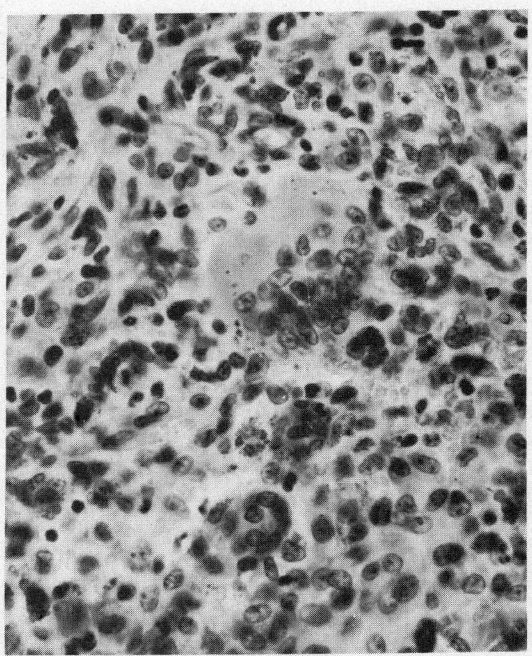

Figure 28–30. Malignant giant cell tumor, illustrating anaplasia within spindle cells that constitute bulk of neoplasm.

Giant cell tumors generally come to diagnosis in persons between the ages of 20 and 55; they are distinctly uncommon in those under 15. Males and females are affected almost equally often, possibly with a slight female preponderance. These patients present the nonspecific complaints of local pain, tenderness, functional disability, and occasionally pathologic fractures. However, in many instances the tumors grow insidiously to massive size to produce externally palpable masses before discovery. Radiographs are distinctive, but not pathognomonic, and show large, roughly spherical cystic areas of bone rarefaction traversed by irregular strands of calcification. Frequently, multiple radiolucent foci create the appearance of a cluster of soap bubbles. A thinned-out but usually preserved cortex surrounds the lesion, although, as pointed out, aggressive neoplasms may destroy the cortex and, indeed, the articular end of the bone. Generally, there is little reactive bone sclerosis in the advancing margins.

The issue of the variable biologic behavior of these neoplasms and its predictability has already been stressed. At the two ends of the morphologic spectrum there is no difficulty. The large center, however, poses a problem because even benign-appearing lesions may recur following therapy; the overall recurrence rate is 25 to 50%, and with each recurrence the horizon darkens.

Joints and Related Structures

NORMAL

The joints are the hinges of the skeleton articulating two or more bones. Where motion is limited the bones are firmly joined by fibrocartilaginous tissue, e.g., the intervertebral discs in the spinal column. The ends of the bone in the diarthrodial joints are capped by articular cartilage, itself covered by a synovial membrane that lines the entire joint space. The membrane consists of a single sheet of cells of two types. The more common, type A synoviocytes, are phagocytic and synthesize degradative enzymes, largely collagenases. Type B synoviocytes, which synthesize mucin, are scattered among the type A cells. The synovial fluid that lubricates diarthrodial joints is composed of a vascular transudate derived from the synovial membrane admixed with mucin derived from the lining cells. Normally the fluid is clear, viscid, and colorless to slightly yellow; contains fewer than 200 white cells per mm^3 (mostly mononuclears); and clots on standing.

The articular cartilage is a unique connective tissue ideally suited to serve as an elastic shock absorber and wear-resistant, weight-bearing surface. Although the ends of apposing bones within a joint are remarkably contoured to fit each other, there is not perfect congruence and so there is uneven load distribution. Articular cartilage, despite its lack of nerves, lymphatics, and blood vessels, is a metabolically active tissue. The relatively few chondrocytes dispersed throughout the fibrocartilaginous matrix are active throughout life in the synthesis of the collagen and the macromolecular proteoglycans of the matrix. These matrix components are in a constant state of turnover. The collagen of cartilage is type II, characterized on page 77. The collagen fibers are largely oriented vertical to the weight-bearing surface, but in the immediate subsynovial region are distributed horizontally and are finer and more dense, constituting a feltlike mesh. This dense layer may serve to contain the proteoglycans and exclude degradative enzymes produced by the synoviocytes or leukocytes in inflammatory states. The vertical orientation of the deeper fibers is maintained by the proteoglycans. These macromolecules have a linear polypeptide backbone to which is attached, at approximately right angles, side chains of glycosaminoglycans (chondroitin-6-sulfate, chondroitin-4-sulfate, and keratan sulfate). Negative surface charges on the side chains repel each other to maintain the proteoglycan molecule stiffly extended in space.[126] The spatial lattice permits the matrix to be hyperhydrated so that articular cartilage is composed of 70 to 80% water, the remainder being about half collagen and half proteoglycans. With each compressive force, water and proteoglycans are displaced to zones bearing less load or possibly in small amounts into the joint space, but normal redistribution follows release of the pressure. Free flow of water out of cartilage is limited by the oncotic pressure of the hydrophilic proteoglycans.

PATHOLOGY

Diseases of joints are commonplace in clinical medicine. Various surveys indicate that about 1.5% of the American population under 45 and 15% of older individuals suffer from complaints probably arising in joint disease. The cost of the loss of productive work exceeds hundreds of millions of dollars annually. Despite this staggering significance, we know little about the precise nature of many of these conditions. Our knowledge is particularly deficient in the most important disorders of the joints, namely, the various types of arthritis. Primary attention is devoted in this section to these forms of disabling arthritis and to the uncommon but clinically significant tumors that arise in the joints and their investing tissues.

ARTHRITIS

Arthritis is a nonspecific term that refers to any inflammatory involvement of a joint. There are a number of classifications based on the acuteness or chronicity of the involvement, the etiology of the inflammation, the specific joints involved, and other considerations. The division employed here is based on distinctive anatomic features.

SUPPURATIVE ARTHRITIS

Suppurative arthritis, almost always acute, refers merely to a suppurative inflammation within a joint space. This type of inflammatory involvement is almost invariably initiated by bacterial invasion. Infrequently, however, physical trauma, bleeding into a joint, or a metabolic disorder such as gout may evoke a leukocytic infiltrate that resembles, but is not, a valid suppurative arthritis. Bacteria usually seed the joint space in the hematogenous dissemination of an infection localized in some other organ of the body. Much less frequently, bacteria may invade the joint either by the direct spread of a neighboring infection or through a perforating injury.

The most common causes of suppurative arthritis are gonococci, staphylococci, streptococci, *Hemophilus influenzae*, and gram-negative bacilli (*Escherichia coli*, Salmonella, Pseudomonas, and others). Most instances of suppurative arthritis occur in adult life, more often in drug addicts and persons with reduced immunocompetence or debilitation (predominantly caused by staphylococci and gram-negative organisms). Gonococcal arthritis is mainly seen in sexually active young adults, more often in females with neglected infections. Acute arthritis may also develop in childhood, when *H. influenzae* is the most common etiologic agent. Suppurative arthritis associated with osteomyelitis is also frequently a childhood disorder. For reasons that are unclear, individuals with sickle cell anemia are particularly prone to Salmonella infections. For many years, oral sepsis and infected tonsils and sinuses were considered important causes of suppurative arthritis. However, repeated studies have deemphasized the significance of these focal infections.

Any joint may be involved, but those most frequently affected are the large joints such as the knee, hip, ankle, elbow, wrist, and shoulder. For obscure reasons, the sternoclavicular joint is an additional favored site. In most instances, the infection is limited to a **monoarticular involvement.** The anatomic changes consist of a **nonspecific, acute suppurative infection virtually identical with similar infections in other regions of the body.** In early and less severe involvements, the synovial membranes are congested, thickened, and edematous, and the joint space contains a thin, cloudy fluid laden with neutrophils. The white cell count may reach 200,000 per mm^3. The fluid is rich in fibrinogen, clots spontaneously, and has poor viscosity. Occasionally, bacteria can be identified in the smear of this fluid, and necrotic microorganisms are often visible within the cytoplasm of the leukocytes. As the process advances, the inflammatory alterations in the synovial membrane become progressively more severe and the fluid is transformed to a thick, characteristic pus. **Depending on the virulence of the causative agent and the chronicity of the infection, the inflammatory synovitis may ulcerate and involve the**

underlying articular cartilage. It is therefore possible for suppurative arthritis to result in extensive destruction of joint surfaces and in fibrous bridging scars that seriously hamper joint function. Calcifications may further limit the mobility, but only infrequently produce permanent ankylosis. In an earlier stage of the disease, the infection may be controlled by appropriate therapy, permitting resolution of the inflammatory changes and restitution of normal structures.

The resultant clinical manifestations are those of any local infection, i.e., redness, swelling, tenderness, and pain. Frequently, a systemic constitutional reaction is also present. Because of the destructive tendencies of chronic, persistent, suppurative infections within joint spaces, these conditions require prompt recognition and effective therapy for the preservation of normal joint function. Overall, however, suppurative arthritis is an uncommon cause of permanent joint damage.

TUBERCULOUS ARTHRITIS

Tuberculous arthritis is almost invariably an insidious chronic disease. It may be encountered in adults but is more common in children, and arises either as a complication of tuberculous osteomyelitis or following hematogenous dissemination of organisms from a pulmonary or other focus of infection. It is usually monoarticular in type. The most common site of localization is the spine *(Pott's disease* or *tuberculous spondylitis).* The second most favored site is the hip joint, but the knee, elbow, wrist, ankle, and sacroiliac joints may also be involved.

As in suppurative arthritis, the tuberculous infection follows the pattern of similar infections elsewhere in the body. The initial involvement consists principally of edema, congestion, and thickening of the synovial membranes. As the infection advances, the lining membrane becomes studded with small foci of inflammatory granulation tissue harboring solitary and confluent tubercles. Because these infections tend to take a chronic course, the inflammatory tissue creates a thick, feltlike covering over the articular surfaces known as a *pannus.* The caseous necrotizing inflammation may extend from the pannus into the underlying articular surface, thus causing considerable ulceration and destruction, and erosion into the head of the bone. Sometimes the tuberculous infection erodes into the bone from the margin of the articular cartilage and, thus undermining it, causes it to fragment and slough. Conversely, tuberculous osteomyelitis may trek into the joint space to cause arthritis.

Tuberculous arthritis tends to be a much more destructive process than suppurative arthritis and frequently results in extensive fibrous bridging and obliteration of the joint space. Late calcification of the inflammatory tissue may lead to ankylosis of the joint. In other instances, the tuberculous infection may erode through the joint capsule to create draining skin sinuses. The precise diagnosis requires the identification of the characteristic morphologic tissue reaction or, more positively, the acid-fast bacilli. When a suppurative arthritis fails to yield a common pyogen by means of usual bacterial cultural methods, tuberculosis should be suspected!

OSTEOARTHRITIS (DEGENERATIVE JOINT DISEASE—DJD)

Osteoarthritis is the most common arthropathy seen principally but not exclusively in elderly individuals.[127] The weight-bearing joints are principally affected by cartilage destruction and erosion followed by subchondral sclerosis and the formation of large calcified osteophytes (spurs) at the joint margins. Pain, deformity, and limitation of motion results.[126] Because the frequency of the condition increases with age, it has long been thought to be a "wear-and-tear" degenerative process and hence is often referred to as *degenerative joint disease (DJD).* However, the growing awareness that the disease may occur in relatively young adults, that in some cases crystals may be found within the joint fluid, and that uncommonly there is joint inflammation all militate toward retention of the time-honored designation osteoarthritis. In most instances when the condition appears in middle adult life or earlier, some previous joint disease or abnormality constitutes a predisposing influence, and hence the osteoarthritis is referred to as secondary. The various predispositions for secondary osteoarthritis can be categorized as follows:[128]

Congenital Aberrations of Joints
- Hypermobility
- Abnormally shaped surfaces

Structural Disorders Arising in Childhood
- Legg-Calvé-Perthes disease
- Slipped femoral epiphysis

Trauma and Mechanical Problems
- Fractures involving the joint surface
- Meniscectomy
- Obesity

Crystal Deposition
- Hydroxyapatite
- Pyrophosphate

Metabolic Abnormality of Cartilage
- Ochronosis

Previous Inflammatory Disease of Joints
- Rheumatoid arthritis
- Gout
- Septic arthritis
- Tuberculous arthritis
- Hemophilia

INCIDENCE. Osteoarthritis has been referred to as the single major cause of disability in the United States.[129] On the basis of radiographic changes, it is estimated that 80% of persons over the age of 70 have this condition, and about half of these have symptoms. Women are affected twice as often as men, and women are prone to develop osteophytic nodules at the base of the terminal phalanges, called *Heberden's nodes;* for unknown reasons, these are rare in men. There are hints of genetic predisposition to osteoarthritis. Siblings, and particularly twins, are likely to develop the arthritic changes at approximately the same age. However, no single pattern of mendelian inheritance has been identified, and both recessive and dominant autosomal transmission have been reported.[130]

PATHOGENESIS. The traditional view of the causation of osteoarthritis invokes biomechanical factors. In the primary form of the disease, it is speculated that the cumulative effects of use ultimately lead to injury to chondrocytes and impaired maintenance of the articular cartilage. As a consequence, there is loss or decreased synthesis of proteoglycans, increased collagen turnover, and possibly molecular or spatial changes in collagen. Central to this theory is the observation that, with decades of weight-bearing, there is remodeling of the conformation of the articular cartilage with redistribution of load stresses. Normal diarthroidal joint surfaces are slightly incongruent with most of the weight load borne by the periphery of the joint. With remodeling the joints become ever more congruent and areas previously not in contact become exposed to weight loads. Chondrocyte integrity depends on normal levels of load, and overloading and underloading induce chondrocyte injury.[131] Moreover, the changed weight-bearing alters the subsynovial weave of collagen fibers, perhaps favoring loss of proteoglycans. Simultaneously the closely approximated articular surfaces are deprived of free flow of synovial fluid. Cartilage injury and erosion ensue, followed by a sequence of changes to be detailed. Many disorders associated with secondary osteoarthritis may reasonably be thought to act by altering joint conformation or weight-bearing loads.

Variations on the biomechanical theory emphasize metabolic and biochemical changes. Chrondrocyte injury may lead to the elaboration or release of degradative enzymes, particularly proteoglycanases and cathepsins.[132] Concomitantly, aging and chondrocyte injury might slow the capacity for proteoglycan synthesis. Different alterations in collagen have also been claimed and disputed, including transition with injury from type II collagen to type I less able to withstand the stress,[133] increased susceptibility of the collagen to protease degradation, and some subtle biochemical or steric change modifying its structural stability. However, the possibility cannot be ruled out that all these changes are responses to cartilage injury rather than primary pathogenetic phenomena.

Yet another dimension has been added to the pathogenesis of osteoarthritis, namely, the observations that well-defined inflammatory changes are sometimes seen in the early stages of the disease and that the joints in a few patients contain crystals of hydroxyapatite and/or pyrophosphate.[134] Whether such individuals represent a special subset of the larger population, or represent a particular stage of the general condition, is not clear at present. Alternatively, the crystals may be seen only in advanced disease secondary to long-standing cartilage injury. It is apparent that we are still groping for an understanding of this common arthropathy.

MORPHOLOGY. The vertebral, hip, knee, and distal interphalangeal joints of the fingers bear the brunt of the disease. The wrists, elbows, and shoulders are seldom involved, as is true of the proximal interphalangeal joints and metacarpophalangeal joints. In contrast, the carpometacarpal joint of the thumb is frequently affected. **The early changes appear to be erosion and flaking of the cartilaginous surface.** This is accompanied by apparent replication of chondrocytes, creating small, clonal clusters of cells within the cartilaginous matrix. Concomitantly, the depletion of proteoglycans leads to a decrease in metachromatic staining, as can be demonstrated by Alcian blue, for example. With advance of the disease, clefts appear within the cartilage at right angles to the surface. These clefts may penetrate to the subchondral bone, producing what is referred to as **cartilage fibrillation.** Sometimes, fragments of cartilage break off to create "joint mice." Perhaps in response to this cartilaginous injury there is ingrowth of blood vessels from the subchondral bone into the articular cartilage. Focal, cystic areas may appear within the subchondral bone, filled with fibrous tissue, presumably a reflection of reactive vascular changes and bone resorption. With further progression, the cartilaginous layer is more deeply eroded or may entirely disappear from focal areas, leaving denuded subchondral bone, which may become dense, smooth, and glistening to resemble ivory (eburnation). The subchondral bone becomes densely sclerotic, and indeed microfractures in this region may occur as an earlier change leading to the bony sclerosis and loss of elasticity of the subchondral cushion. The loss of cartilage accounts for the so-called thinning of the joint space seen radiographically. Concomitantly, osteophytes (bony outgrowths) develop from the margins of the articular cartilage that sometimes extend along ligamentous and capsular attachments to produce the characteristic **bone spurs of osteoarthritis.** These spurs are responsible for the "lipping" found in the vertebral bodies where the spine is affected (Fig. 28–31). When large spurs project from opposing bones, they may come into contact with each other to cause pain and limitation of motion. However, they rarely fuse to produce bony ankylosis as seen in rheumatoid arthritis. It is these bony spurs that account for the nodules referred to previously as Heberden's nodes.

CLINICAL COURSE. Osteoarthritis is an insidious disease that is usually first noticed as transient slight stiffness or decreased mobility, most prominent in the morning on arising. Usually, after resuming motion for a short time, the stiffness, and sometimes the pain, subsides but recurs late in the day with prolonged use or undue activity. These manifestations are most prominent in the hips, knees, and back. With more advanced disease the pain and disability are more protracted. There is usually no evidence of local heat or tenderness, but the joints may have a restricted range of motion, small effusions, and crepitus. The bony outgrowths may impinge on spinal foramina and cause cervical and lumbar nerve root compression, with radicular pain, muscle spasms, muscle atrophy, and neurologic abnor-

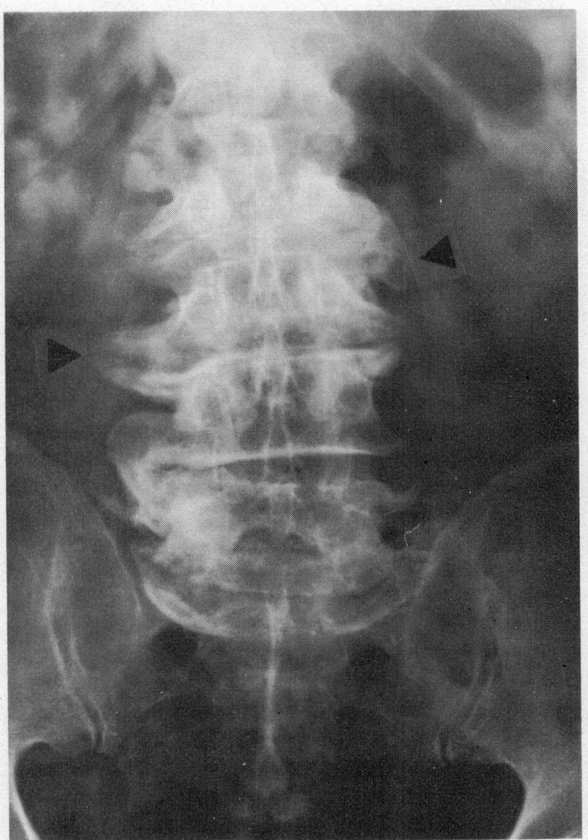

Figure 28–31. Extensive osteoarthritis with marked spur formations *(arrows)* along lateral margins of intervertebral disc spaces. (Courtesy of Dr. John O'Connor, Boston University Medical Center.)

malities. Involvement of the distal interphalangeal joints may cause stiffness and decreased mobility of the fingers.

There is no satisfactory means of preventing this condition nor any method known for its arrest. The disorder usually is slowly progressive over the remaining years of life, and joins atherosclerosis and cancer as a dividend of the "golden years."

RHEUMATOID ARTHRITIS (RA)

Rheumatoid arthritis is a chronic systemic inflammatory disease of unknown etiology. Although the skin, voluntary muscles, bones, eyes, heart, blood vessels, lungs, and possibly other organs may be affected, *the outstanding feature of RA is progressive deforming arthritis.* Classically, multiple joints are affected in a symmetric distribution, notably the small joints of the hands and feet. The disease may take various forms. In most patients it is limited to joint involvement alone, although minor changes in muscle or bone may also be present. In about 20% of patients the arthritis is accompanied by skin rheumatoid nodules. In another group the disease is confined to involvement of the vertebral column (ankylosing spondylitis). In yet another subset the arthritis is accompanied by massive splenomegaly, hypersplenism, and leg ulcers (p. 1355). In hard-coal miners there is prominent involvement of the lungs along with the polyarthritis referred to as Caplan's syndrome (p. 434). In still other instances there is multiorgan and vascular involvement. The question is raised: are these merely variable expressions of a single disorder or are they several closely related disorders, all having in common a similar type of arthritis?

There are other clinical variants of RA. A form of inflammatory synovitis-arthritis closely related to RA is also encountered in juveniles—*juvenile rheumatoid arthritis.* In this age group, however, there are many clinical features that set this disease apart from RA in adults. Psoriasis, ulcerative colitis, regional enteritis, and Whipple's disease also are sometimes accompanied by a closely related form of inflammatory arthritis. In addition, many conditions thought to be immunologic in origin—systemic lupus erythematosus, scleroderma, Sjögren's syndrome, serum sickness, and rheumatic fever—often present joint involvement. However, in these immunologic disorders the arthritis tends to be transitory and does not have the progressive destructive nature of RA. Thus, inflammatory joint involvement of obscure origin is encountered in a diversity of clinical settings. In many cases the disease is not progressive, however, and so differs from classic rheumatoid involvement. Only those with inflammatory disease having the potential of leading to crippling joint destruction are now considered as subsets of RA (cited below) and are referred to as variants of RA.

In RA variants, the anatomic changes within the joints are almost indistinguishable from classic RA, but the clinical course or features of each merit its separation from the parent disease. Thus, the following discussion is restricted to the usual classic form of RA, followed by a brief consideration of the more important variants.

INCIDENCE. RA is a common disorder among adults and is said to affect from 0.5 to 3.8% of women and from 0.15 to 1.3% of men. These ranges reflect varying criteria for establishment of the diagnoses. It may arise at any age, but about 70% of patients are between the third and seventh decades of life. Women are affected three times more often than men. There are hints of genetic predisposition in the form of familial aggregations and a statistically significant association with HLA-D4 or DR4.[135] However, well-defined patterns of inheritance have not been identified.

Before the possible origins of this condition are considered, it is well to review first the morphology.

MORPHOLOGY. Although any joint in the body may be affected, RA tends to begin in the small joints of the hands and feet, particularly the interphalangeal joints. Also commonly affected are the wrists, elbows, ankles, and knees. Occasionally, the cervical spine is involved, but it is uncommon in the lower spine. Sometimes, temporomandibular involvement induces difficulty in chewing. Joint involvement tends to be symmetric, as mentioned earlier. Biopsies reveal that during the early stages there is a nonspecific acute edematous inflammation marked by infiltration of the synovia by neutrophils, lymphocytes, and occasional plasma cells. Similar white cells, predominantly neutrophils, are found within the synovial fluid, which is increased in amount. **With progression, the characteristic changes appear in the form of a diffuse proliferative synovitis** (Fig. 28–32). The synovial lining cells become hypertrophied and multilayered, and the subsynovial connective tissue undergoes similar reactive vascularized hyperplasia. In this manner, **the synovial lining is replaced by a highly vascularized, sometimes polypoid mass of inflammatory tissue, principally infiltrated with lymphocytes, macrophages, and plasma cells to create the pannus.** The mononuclear infiltration may form lymphocytic nodules, particularly prominent about the newly formed vessels. Foci of necrosis and deposits of fibrinoid may appear within this pannus. In time, the pannus and the inflammatory reaction erode into the underlying articular cartilage, beginning at the joint margins where the articular cartilage ends and the joint capsule attaches to bone (Fig. 28–33). The inflammatory process extends to the joint capsule and supporting ligaments, weakening the joint support and contributing to the dysfunction. With erosion of the articular cartilage, the pannus invades the bone, causing rarefaction and foci of cystic softening of the juxta-articular bone. Joint motion may cause erosion of the exuberant pannus, leading to bleeding, fibrin clots, and the formation of granulation tissue that bridges the joint space. Eventually, the total articular surface is eroded and the joint space obliterated. **In the late stages, fibrous adhesions or even bony ankylosis may unite the opposite joint surfaces.**

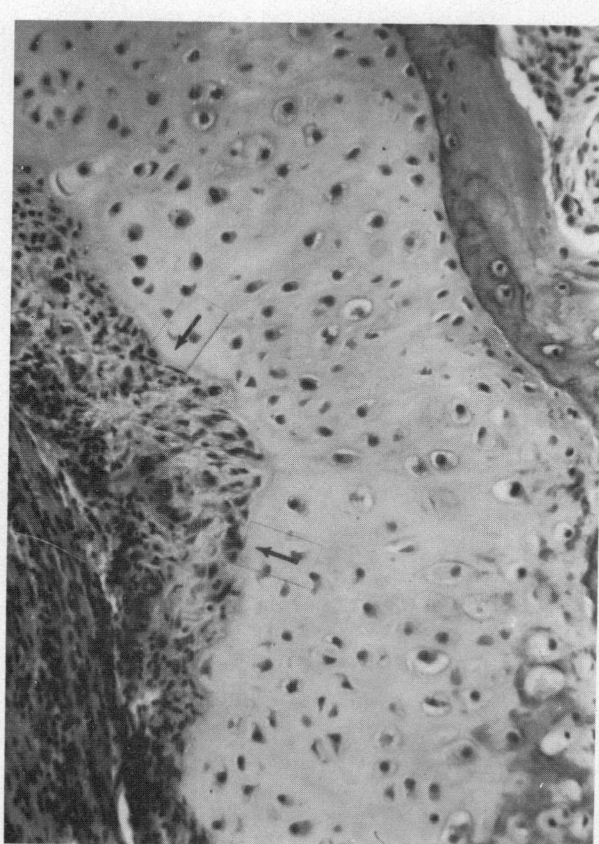

Figure 28–33. Marked chronic rheumatoid arthritis. Joint space to left is filled with inflammatory tissue (pannus) that is simultaneously invading and eroding the articular cartilage *(arrows)*.

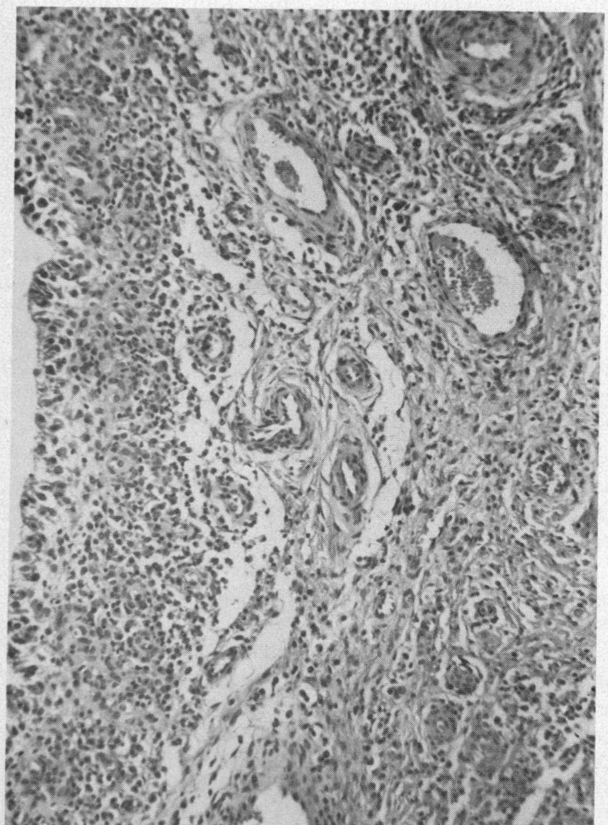

Figure 28–32. Proliferative synovitis of rheumatoid arthritis. Synovial surface seen to left is marked by hypertrophied synoviocytes underlaid by a chronic inflammatory infiltrate. Increased vascularization of subsynovial connective tissue is evident.

As pointed out below, immunofluorescent techniques disclose immune complexes and complement within synovial cells, neutrophils, and macrophages. The fluid aspirated from an involved joint is usually nonviscous and cloudy, and forms a poor mucin clot. Its white cell count is usually moderately elevated, with a predominance of neutrophils. These inflammatory cells too contain immune complexes.

Rheumatoid nodules may appear in the skin, cardiac valves, pericardium, pleura, lung parenchyma, and spleen. They are almost identical to those encountered in some patients with rheumatic fever and are characterized by a focus of central necrosis, surrounded by proliferating connective tissue cells that are usually radially oriented, to thus create a well-defined enclosing palisade (Fig. 28–34). Sometimes the central focus of necrosis contains deposits of fibrinoid. About the palisade, large numbers of lymphocytes and occasional plasma cells accumulate. The skin nodules appear in approximately 20% of patients and are most often found on the extensor surfaces of the arms and elbows; less common sites are the scalp, hands, feet, back, buttocks, and knees. Acute glaucoma may result from involvement of the sclera. The pulmonary involvement may give rise to a diffuse pleuritis or multiple intraparenchymal nodules. The concurrence of rheumatoid pulmonary nodules and pneumoconiosis creates what has been referred to as **Caplan's syndrome.** Sometimes, diffuse interstitial pulmonary fibrosis appears, attributed to immunologically mediated immune complex deposition. Rheumatoid nodules within the heart

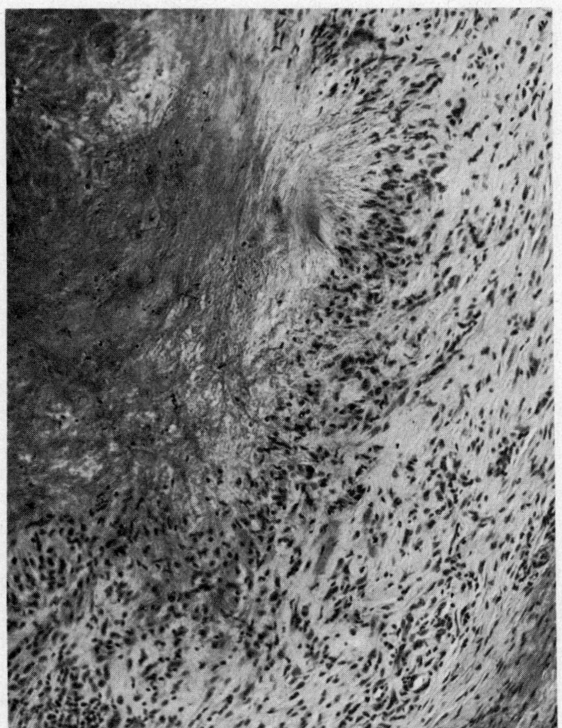

Figure 28–34. Subcutaneous rheumatoid nodule with an area of necrosis *(upper left)* surrounded by a palisade of fibroblasts and white cells.

may induce pericarditis and valvular deformities, particularly in the aortic valve leaflets. Splenomegaly and lymphadenopathy of the nodes about the involved joints may develop. This usually takes the form of nonspecific reactive hyperplasia but rarely is marked by rheumatoid nodules.

Any of the large or small arteries of the body may develop an acute necrotizing vasculitis, characteristic of that seen in other immunologic states. Diffuse involvement of the small arteries of the lungs may lead to pulmonary hypertension. Thromboses of the involved vessels have been responsible for myocardial infarction, cerebrovascular occlusions, mesenteric infarction, and vascular insufficiency in the hands and fingers (Raynaud's phenomenon). Rarely, ulcers of the lower part of the leg or even gangrene develop. The vascular changes are most often encountered in patients receiving steroid therapy, and there is some concern that the therapy may play some role in initiating these lesions.

Muscle changes are quite frequent, but usually take the form of nonspecific atrophy secondary to joint dysfunction. Infrequently, rheumatoid nodules give rise to so-called nodular myositis.

PATHOGENESIS. There is abundant evidence that the synovitis of RA is immune mediated, but the initiating cause of the autoimmune reaction remains unknown. The circulation and joints of nearly all patients with classic RA have antibodies called *rheumatoid factor (RF)* against the Fc fragment of autologous IgG.[136] These autoantibodies are heterogeneous and belong to the IgM, IgG, and IgA classes. Much, but not all, of the RF in the circulation and joints is formed locally in affected joints by the inflammatory infiltrate of activated B cells and plasma cells.[137] The serum titer of RF correlates roughly with the severity of the arthritis.[138] Not only does it form complexes with autologous IgG, but the IgG-RF also preferentially reacts with itself because the self-association permits more stable double bonding. Thus, a whole series of immune complexes are formed of varying size. Complement is bound and activated by the immune complexes, accounting for the characteristic low-complement levels in the rheumatoid synovial effusion. The formation of chemotactic and vasoactive fractions of activated complement undoubtedly participate in the characteristic inflammatory synovitis, particularly in the accumulation of neutrophils in the joint fluid and synovial membranes during the active phase of the arthritis. Phagocytosis of the immune complexes by neutrophils and type A synoviocytes (readily demonstrated by immunofluorescent methods) follows with the release of collagenases and neutral peptidases.[139] By immunofluorescence, collagenase can be identified at the cartilage-pannus junction in inflamed joints.[140] There is abundant evidence that it is capable of degrading articular cartilage. The role of the peptidases in collagen degradation is still uncertain. Prostaglandin E_2 is also present in the synovitis and has been shown to accelerate bone resorption by osteoclasts.[141]

Seductive as this hypothetic sequence may appear, there are still major unanswered questions. What stimulates the autoimmune reaction responsible for the formation of RF? From time to time one or another bacterial or viral agent has been implicated and later dismissed.[142] Theoretically, an exogenous agent might serve as a hapten with autologous proteins or, alternatively, induce immunogens in cells. A favored candidate in this connection is the Epstein-Barr virus (EBV). Lymphocytes transformed by EBV acquire a "rheumatoid arthritis–associated nuclear antigen."[143] There is an additional suggestion that EBV may inhibit T-suppressor cells, leading to abnormal regulation of B-cell formation of antibodies.[144] However, inflammatory synovitis is not a significant feature of infectious mononucleosis, which is known to be caused by EBV. Could genetic predisposition in HLA-D4 and DR4 individuals potentiate the development of joint disease, rather than infectious mononucleosis? Much is speculative and there is no substantial documentation for a role for any microbiologic etiologic agent. IgG itself has been invoked as a possible antigen in rheumatoid synovitis, and scattered reports suggest confirmational alteration of IgG in RA patients.[145] We must accept that, for the present, the trigger for the autoimmune reaction is unknown.

There are other enigmas. If RF is present in the circulation and forms immune complexes by self-association and binding to autologous IgG, why is the major damage in RA localized to the joints? Moreover, is RF central to the pathogenesis of RA? Significantly, RF is also present (albeit in lower concentrations and less consistently) in the sera of patients with many different chronic infections, notably subacute bacterial endocarditis unassociated with chronic arthritis. Similar antibodies can be induced in experimental animals with altered autologous IgG or various bacteria without evoking arthritis. Another question: why are aspirin and other nonsteroidal anti-inflammatory agents usually beneficial in the control of the acute manifestations of rheumatoid synovitis? Does this imply a significant pathogenetic role for the prostaglandins? It is evident that there are more questions than there are answers.

CLINICAL COURSE. RA is a systemic disease of grave nature. Patients generally complain of fatigue, malaise, and low-grade fever even before the onset of actual joint pain or swelling. Eventually, however, the nature of this prodrome becomes evident by the appearance of joint stiffness, most pronounced in the morning immediately on waking. Occasionally, the onset is acute with high fever and prostration.

Affected joints are usually enlarged, tender, and painful on motion and may be red and warm. With chronicity, these acute manifestations are replaced by progressive induration about the joint and increasing stiffness, until eventually ankylosis causes permanent loss of function. *Classically, the enlarged joints have a fusiform tapered appearance with atrophy of the surrounding muscles.* In the hands, clawlike deformities sometimes appear, with characteristic flexion contractures or ulnar deviation of the immobilized fingers (Fig. 28–35). The overlying skin is often shiny, red, and atrophic. It must again be emphasized that such classic joint changes represent the full-blown syndrome; often, at an earlier stage or in other instances, the joint involvement is far more subtle.

As has already been made clear, patients with this disease may develop clinical manifestations of skin nodules, glaucoma, pericarditis, pleuritis; cardiac, pulmonary, and vascular involvement; and the more specific findings relating to the joints. About 15% of patients develop Sjögren's syndrome. Additional findings may include splenomegaly, lymphadenopathy, marked muscular weakness, and Raynaud's phenomenon.

The diagnosis may be readily evident from physical examination or radiography of the involved joint. However, there also are, characteristically, an elevated erythrocyte sedimentation rate, hypergammaglobulinemia, RF in the serum, and, quite typically, a significant anemia. The source of the anemia is still unclear and has been attributed to oozing of blood into joint membranes or to impaired secretion of erythropoietin. Aspiration of the joint fluid with the demonstration of white cells and poor mucin clot formation is an important part of the diagnostic work-up. The major features that differentiate this form of arthritis from the common osteoarthritis are detailed in Table 28–4.

It is impossible to express a prognosis for this unpredictable disorder. Obviously, patients with extraskeletal involvements represent a more grave expression of this disease. With appropriate treatment or sometimes spontaneously, most patients are able to maintain an active life with recurrent exacerbations and varying levels of disability and discomfort. A small fortunate subset remits after the first acute attack, never to have a recurrence. There remain about 10% of patients who suffer progressive joint damage and dysfunction, despite all therapy, leading to crippling disease. RA is now the second commonest antecedent to secondary amyloidosis, seen in about 15 to 25% of patients with long-standing disease.

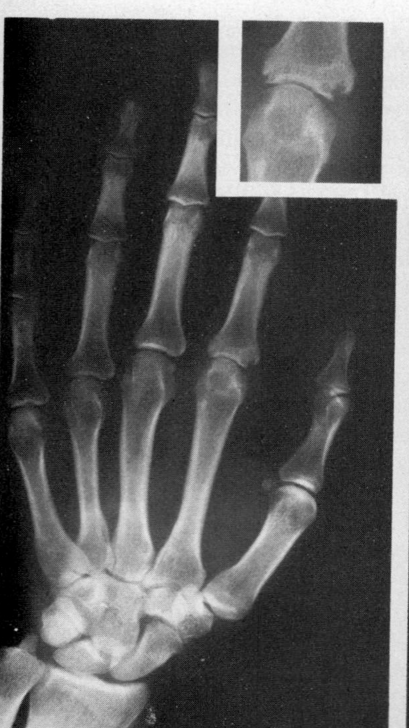

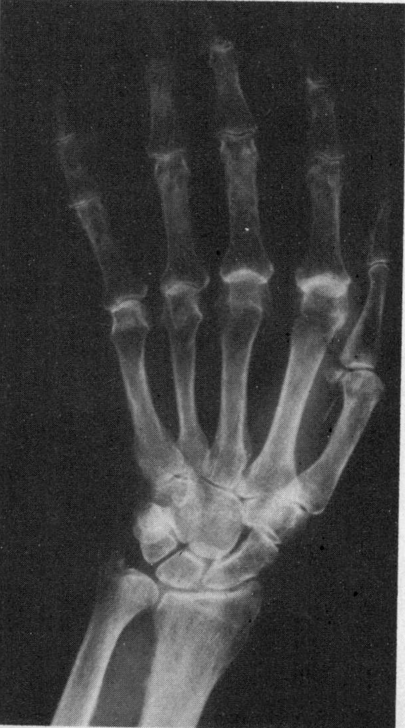

Figure 28–35. Rheumatoid arthritis. *Left*, early disease, most marked in second metacarpophalangeal joint where there is narrowing of joint space and marginal erosions on both radial and ulnar aspects of proximal phalanx *(see inset)*. *Right*, more advanced disease with loss of articular cartilage, narrowing of joint spaces of virtually all the small joints, and ulnar deviation of fingers. There is dislocation of second, third, and fourth proximal phalanges produced by advanced articular disease. (Courtesy of Dr. John O'Connor, Boston University Medical Center.)

Table 28–4. MAJOR DIFFERENCES BETWEEN RHEUMATOID ARTHRITIS AND DEGENERATIVE JOINT DISEASE

	Rheumatoid Arthritis	Degenerative Joint Disease
Age of onset	Third and fourth decades	Fifth and sixth decades
Weight	Normal or underweight	Usually overweight
Constitutional manifestations	Present	Absent
Joints involved	Any joint (classically bilateral symmetric proximal interphalangeal and metacarpophalangeal joints)	Mainly knees, hips, spine, and distal interphalangeal joints
Appearance of joints	Soft tissue swelling	Bony swelling
Special deformities	Fusiform finger joints, ulnar deviation	Heberden's and Bouchard's nodes
Subcutaneous nodules	Present in 20%	Never present
X-ray	Osteoporosis, erosions	Osteosclerosis and osteophytes
Joint fluid	Increased cells, poor mucin	Few cells, good mucin
Rheumatoid factors	Usually present	Usually absent
Blood count	Anemia and leukocytosis	Normal
Erythrocyte sedimentation rate	Markedly elevated	Normal
Course	Often progressive	Slow or stationary
Termination	Ankylosis and deformity; amyloidosis	No ankylosis and no amyloidosis

From Cohen, A. S., et al.: Arthritis and connective tissue disorders. *In* Wilkins, R. W., and Levinsky, N. G. (eds.): Medicine, Essentials of Clinical Practice. 2nd ed. Boston, Little, Brown & Co., 1978, p. 597. Copyright 1978 Little, Brown & Company.

Variants of Rheumatoid Arthritis

Variants of RA include juvenile RA, Felty's syndrome, ankylosing spondylitis, psoriatic arthritis, arthritis associated with ulcerative colitis, arthritis associated with Whipple's disease, and arthritis associated with Sjögren's syndrome. Only the first three are described here; several of the others are discussed on page 1362.

Juvenile rheumatoid arthritis is sometimes referred to as *Still's disease*. Approximately 5% of patients with RA are under 16 years of age and have the juvenile form of the disease. The peak incidence is between 1 and 3 years of age, and in this age group girls are affected more often than boys. The disease differs from that in adults in several respects. It is more often marked by an acute febrile onset, weeks to months before joint manifestations appear. About one-third of patients have involvement of only one or a few joints, most often the knees or ankles. Generalized lymphadenopathy and hepatosplenomegaly are more prominent in this juvenile variant than in the adult disease. RF is present only infrequently. Thus, the possibility must be entertained that the pathogenesis of the joint involvement, which is morphologically similar to that of classic RA, may be distinct from that of the disease that occurs later in life. Moreover, the course of the disease is much more unpredictable. Some patients with involvement of a single or a few joints do not develop persistent, disabling arthritis, and after the acute attack the joint changes remit and do not recur. Those with the acute febrile onset, multiple joint involvement, and RF are more likely to develop crippling deformities.[146]

Felty's syndrome is another variant of RA that comprises the constellation of splenomegaly, manifestations of hypersplenism such as leukopenia, and leg ulcers associated with the characteristic polyarticular RA. In these patients the hematologic derangements (p. 1351) may dominate the clinical course.[147]

Ankylosing spondylitis, also known as *rheumatoid spondylitis* and *Marie-Strümpell disease*, is a distinctive form of inflammatory arthritis, mainly localized to the spine. The sacroiliac joints are always affected, but the hip and shoulder joints only sometimes. The peripheral joints are rarely involved, as in classic RA. It is a disease predominantly of young men and is of unknown etiology. There is, however, a strong association between this condition and HLA-B27, found in approximately 90 to 95% of patients. Hereditary influences appear to play a role, because about one-quarter of close relatives also have symptomatic or asymptomatic spondylitis. There is also a well-defined association of ankylosing spondylitis with ulcerative colitis (p. 859) and regional enteritis (p. 836). All these findings have led to the suspicion that this condition represents an immune response in genetically predisposed individuals to one or more infectious agents or their products. The anatomic changes encountered in the spine, hips, shoulders, and sacroiliac joints are indistinguishable from those of RA and have the same consequences, fibrous and bony ankylosis. As a result, vertebral mobility is impaired, and in severe cases there is fusion of the vertebral bodies and immobilization of affected regions of the spine. A stooped posture, marked dorsal kyphosis, and marked disability may result. These limitations may be worsened by hip and shoulder involvement.

ARTHRITIS ASSOCIATED WITH RHEUMATIC FEVER

It will be remembered that acute rheumatic fever is classically associated with a *migratory polyarthritis*. Although such joint involvement is a principal clinical manifestation of this disease, the arthritic involvement usually spontaneously or with appropriate therapy subsides to leave no permanent residual. It is the heart that bears the brunt of the destructive effects of this systemic inflammation. For further details on the nature of the joint involvement, reference should be made to Chapter 13.

GOUT AND GOUTY ARTHRITIS

Gout may appear in any individual with hyperuricemia. The disease is characterized at the outset by transient but recurrent attacks of acute arthritis, evoked by precipitation into the joint spaces of monosodium urate crystals from supersaturated body fluids. Over the span of years, acute attacks of arthritis lead eventually to chronic disabling arthritis and focal deposits of urates in other tissues, e.g., joint capsules, perichondrial tissues, bursae, heart valves, and kidneys, creating inflammatory foci known as *tophi.* Hypertension is a frequent concomitant, for reasons poorly understood. Although hyperuricemia is fundamental to all these tissue changes, it is not the sole determinant. Therefore, *a clear distinction should be made between hyperuricemia, which is a chemical abnormality, and gout, which is a disease.* A plasma urate level above 7 mg/dl is considered elevated, since it exceeds the saturation value for urate at 37°C and pH 7.4. By this definition, 2 to 18% of the population of the Western world has hyperuricemia, but the incidence of gout ranges from 0.13 to 0.37%. Clearly, factors other than hyperuricemia (some to be discussed later) are also involved in the pathogenesis of gout.

CLASSIFICATION. It is customary to classify gout into primary and secondary groups. *Primary* gout is a genetic disorder in which the underlying biochemical defect causing the hyperuricemia is unknown, or if known, the main manifestation of the defect is gout (Table 28–5). Approximately 90% of all cases of gout are primary, and since the metabolic defect is not known in most of them, they are referred to as *primary idiopathic gout.* Individually rare are those cases of primary gout that are due to well-defined errors of metabolism such as a partial deficiency of hypoxanthine-guanine phosphoribosyltransferase (HGPRT) or increased activity of PP-ribose-P synthetase (Table 28–5). *Secondary gout,* on the other hand, refers to those cases in which hyperuricemia is secondary to some other disorder such as excessive breakdown of cells or some form of renal disease. Also included in this category are certain well-defined genetic diseases such as the Lesch-Nyhan syndrome and Type I glycogen storage disease, in which gout is not the main or the presenting clinical manifestation. Secondary gout accounts for no more than 5 to 10% of all cases, and hence the following remarks will be mostly limited to primary gout, with only scattered references to the less common forms.

INCIDENCE. Primary gout is a familial disease that appears predominantly in adult males (approximately 95% of cases). Affected females are almost always postmenopausal, presumably owing to the normal lower serum urate concentrations during the reproductive period. Gout is rare in children; when encountered in this group, it is usually associated with one of the well-defined errors of metabolism. The mode of transmission of primary gout is poorly understood, and indeed, in view of the large numbers of metabolic errors that can give rise to hyperuricemia (discussed below), many genotypic variants are likely. Multifactorial inheritance,

Table 28–5. CLASSIFICATION OF HYPERURICEMIA AND GOUT

Type	Metabolic Disturbance	Inheritance
Primary (90% of All Cases)		
Molecular defects undefined (idiopathic)		
Normal excretion (85–90% of primary gout)	Overproduction of uric acid or underexcretion of uric acid or both (specific defects undefined)	Multifactorial
Overexcretion (10–15% of primary gout)	Overproduction of uric acid (specific defects undefined)	Multifactorial
Associated with specific enzyme defects		
PRPP variants; increased activity	Overproduction of PRPP and of uric acid	X-linked
Hypoxanthine-guanine phosphoribosyltransferase deficiency (partial)	Overproduction of uric acid; increased purine biosynthesis de novo driven by surplus PRPP	X-linked
Secondary (10% of All Cases)		
Associated with increased nucleic acid turnover	Overproduction of uric acid (chronic hemolysis, polycythemia, leukemia, lymphoma)	
Associated with specific enzyme defects		
Glucose-6-phosphatase deficiency or absence	Overproduction plus reduced renal clearance of uric acid; glycogen storage disease, type I (von Gierke)	Autosomal recessive
Hypoxanthine-guanine phosphoribosyltransferase deficiency "virtually complete"	Overproduction of uric acid; Lesch-Nyhan syndrome	X-linked
Associated with decreased excretion of uric acid	Reduced renal functional mass; inhibited tubular secretion of uric acid or enhanced tubular reabsorption of uric acid, or both	

Adapted from Wyngaarden, J. B., and Kelley, W. N.: Gout. *In* Stanbury, J. B., et al. (eds.): Metabolic Basis of Inherited Disease. 5th ed. New York, McGraw-Hill Book Co., 1982, p. 1043.

with involvement of several genes and environmental factors (e.g., alcohol, diet, and drugs), seems to be the most likely mode of transmission of primary idiopathic gout. As many as 25% of the asymptomatic blood relatives of a patient with familial gout can be shown to be hyperuricemic.

PATHOGENESIS. The pathogenesis of gout is the pathogenesis of hyperuricemia. There are many causes of an increase in the uric acid level in body fluids, and gout therefore has many origins. *It may be more accurate to say that gout is a constellation of hyperuricemic syndromes.* Some result from overproduction of uric acid, others from retention of uric acid because of some renal abnormality, and many from a combination of both.

Metabolic studies indicate that *approximately 70% of patients with primary gout have increased synthesis of uric acid.* Despite overproduction of uric acid, its urinary excretion is normal (580 to 600 mg per day) in 85 to 90% of patients on a purine-free diet.[148] However, normal urinary excretion in the face of hyperuricemia may reflect a state of relative underexcretion of uric acid in these patients. An increased urinary excretion (greater than 600 mg per day) is seen in only 10 to 15% of the overproducers. Approximately *one-third of all patients with primary gout fail to reveal any evidence of increased uric acid synthesis.* In this group, hyperuricemia seems to be a direct result of some primary renal abnormality that selectively impairs the excretion of even normal amounts of uric acid. *Thus, in terms of uric acid synthesis and excretion, patients with primary gout may be divided into three categories: (1) a majority with overproduction and relative underexcretion, (2) a significant minority (approximately 30%) with impaired renal excretion without overproduction, and (3) a small group with overproduction as well as overexcretion of uric acid.* To facilitate further discussion of the pathogenesis of gout, the possible mechanisms of increased uric acid synthesis and reduced renal excretion will be considered separately, although both coexist to some degree in most patients.

Overproduction of uric acid is best considered in the context of normal purine metabolism, presented in skeletal detail in Figure 28–36. For more details, reference may be made to specialized texts.[148] Purine nucleotides (i.e., guanylic acid, inosinic acid, and ad-

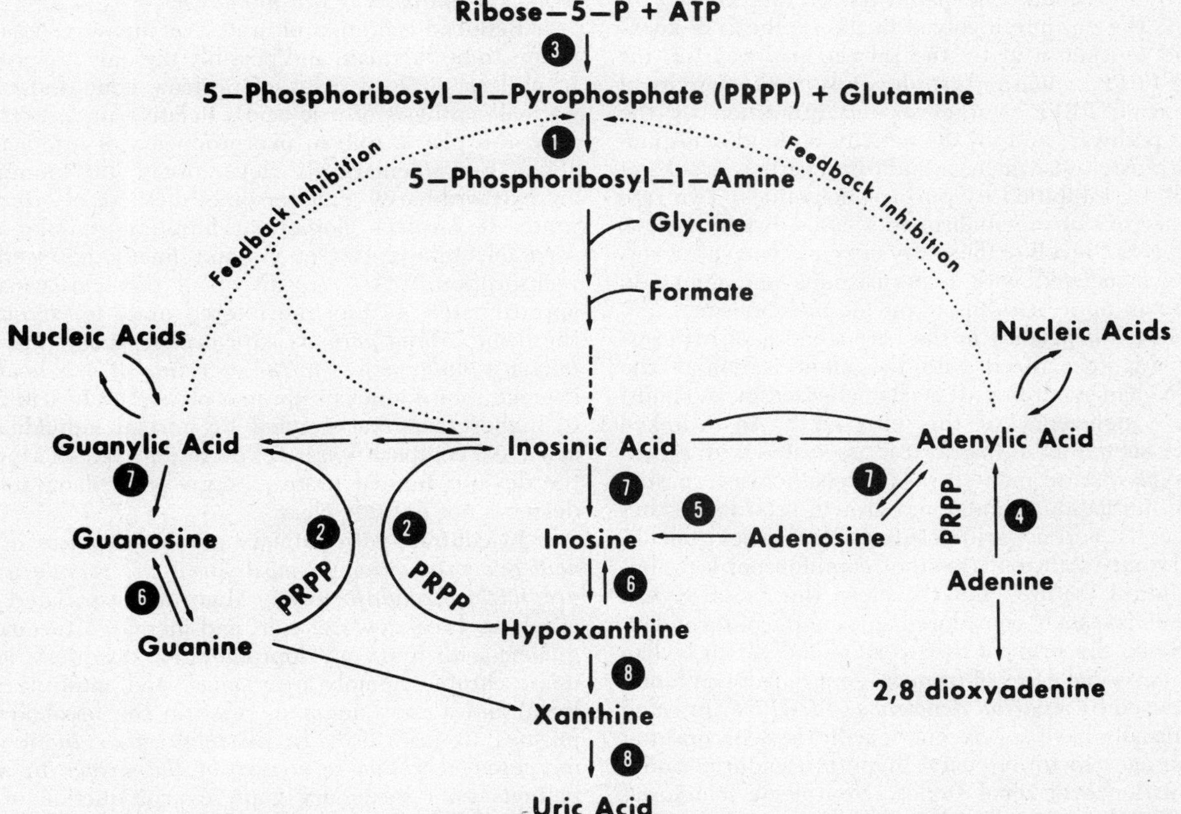

Figure 28–36. Outline of purine metabolism. (1) Amidophoshoribosyltransferase; (2) hypoxanthine-guanine phosphoribosyltransferase; (3) PP-ribose-P synthetase; (4) adenine phosphoribosyltransferase; (5) adenosine deaminase; (6) purine nucleoside phosphorylase; (7) 5′-nucleotidase; (8) xanthine oxidase. (From Kelley, W. N., and Wyngaarden, J. B.: Clinical syndromes associated with hypoxanthine-guanine phosphoribosyl transferase deficiency. *In* Stanbury, J. B., et al. (eds.): Metabolic Basis of Inherited Disease. New York, McGraw-Hill Book Co., 1982, p. 1115. Copyright © 1982 by McGraw-Hill, Inc. Used by permission of McGraw-Hill Book Company.)

enylic acid) can be synthesized by one of two pathways. In the so-called *de novo pathway,* the starting substrate is ribose-5-phosphate, which is converted initially to 5-phosphoribosyl-1-pyrophosphate (PRPP) and then to inosinic acid and other purine nucleotides (Fig. 28–36). The key rate-limiting step in this pathway is the synthesis of 5-phosphoribosyl-1-amine from its precursors glutamine and PRPP. This reaction is catalyzed by amidophosphoribosyltransferase. This enzyme is subject to feedback inhibition by purine nucleotides and is converted to an active form by increased concentration of its substrate PRPP. The other pathway for the synthesis of purine nucleotides involves "salvage" of free purines derived from food or breakdown of nucleic acids. In the so-called *salvage pathway,* hypoxanthine-guanine phosphoribosyltransferase (HGPRT) reconverts hypoxanthine and guanine into inosinic and guanylic acids, respectively, and another enzyme, adenine phosphoribosyltransferase (APRT), catalyzes the formation of adenylic acid from adenosine. In these conversions PRPP, a key substrate in the de novo pathway, is also consumed. Uric acid, the common degradation product of the various purine components, cannot be broken down further because humans lack the enzyme uricase.

Three important control points have been identified in the purine metabolic pathways: (1) *the activity of HGPRT,* the enzyme involved in the synthesis of guanylic and inosinic acid by the salvage pathway; (2) *the level of PRPP,* which in turn depends on the activity of the enzyme PRPP synthetase and utilization by the salvage pathway; and (3) the activity of amidophosphoribosyltransferase, which, as indicated earlier, is subject to feedback inhibition by purine nucleotides. Two rare inborn errors of metabolism (discussed briefly below) that affect the levels of these key enzymes and substrates and are associated with hyperuricemia and gout add much to an understanding of purine metabolism.

HGPRT deficiency in the pathogenesis of hyperuricemia was recognized with the identification of the Lesch-Nyhan syndrome. It is characterized by an almost complete deficiency of this enzyme.[149] An X-linked disorder seen only in males, it is associated with *severe neurologic disease* marked by choreoathetosis, spasticity, self-mutilation, mental and growth retardation, hyperuricemia, and hyperuricosuria with uric acid calculi. Typical gouty arthritis is neither common nor a prominent clinical feature, and therefore the Lesch-Nyhan syndrome is usually considered an example of secondary gout. Since the original discovery of the Lesch-Nyhan syndrome, some cases of primary gout have been found to be caused by a *partial deficiency of HGPRT.* Affected males usually have severe gouty arthritis, with onset at a young age (15 to 30 years), hyperuricaciduria, and a high incidence of renal stones. Neurologic manifestations that dominate the Lesch-Nyhan syndrome are either absent or relatively mild. Two mechanisms may be involved in the overproduction of uric acid in such patients with a partial or complete deficiency of HGPRT and consequent impairment of the salvage pathway. The most important is believed to be an accumulation of PRPP resulting from its underutilization. Second, reduced reconversion of hypoxanthine and guanine to guanylic and inosinic acid dampens the feedback inhibition exerted on amidophosphoribosyltransferase (Fig. 28–36). High levels of PRPP also favor the conversion of amidophosphoribosyltransferase to its active form. All these greatly augment purine biosynthesis by the de novo pathway, resulting eventually in excessive synthesis of the end product, uric acid.

Increased PRPP synthetase activity has been identified in several families with mutant synthetase having increased enzyme activity.[148] As a result, there is an increase in intracellular PRPP, which stimulates purine biosynthesis by the de novo pathway and eventually leads to hyperuricemia. Like HGPRT deficiency, this is an X-linked disorder with the onset of gout in the second or third decade and a high incidence of renal stones.

Still other metabolic errors have been proposed as potential causes of hyperuricemia and primary gout, but these two are the only examples in which the biochemical basis of uric acid overproduction is reasonably well understood. Collectively, however, they account for less than 15% of cases with overproduction of uric acid. *In most patients with primary gout, the cause of increased uric acid synthesis is still unknown.*

Reduced excretion of urates, as mentioned earlier, seems to be the main and possibly the only abnormality in at least 30% of cases of primary gout (those with normal synthesis of uric acid). Relative underexcretion may also play a role in overproducers of uric acid (p. 1357). For a remarkably clever organ, the kidney has an extraordinarily cumbersome method of excreting urate. It involves glomerular filtration, tubular reabsorption, tubular secretion, and finally postsecretory reabsorption.[149] As a result of all this peregrination, approximately 12% of the filtered urate is excreted in the urine. *Many patients with primary idiopathic gout have a tubular defect in the excretion of uric acid.* On average their kidneys require a plasma urate 1 to 2 mg/dl higher than that needed by normal individuals to achieve a comparable rate of excretion. Which aspect of the devious tubular urate pathway is to blame for this defect is not entirely clear.

In contrast with primary gout, *the causes of uric acid overproduction in most forms of secondary gout are fairly straightforward.* Many are associated with excessive breakdown of cells and increased turnover of nucleic acids (e.g., myeloproliferative disorders, leukemias, chronic hemolytic anemias, and multiple myeloma) and a consequent increase in the breakdown of purines to uric acid. *In all these cases there is an increased excretion of urates in the urine.* In a few patients with secondary gout, overproduction of uric acid results from inborn errors of metabolism in which, as mentioned earlier, gout is not the major clinical feature. One such condition is the Lesch-Nyhan syndrome. Another is Type I glycogen storage disease (von Gierke's disease, p. 150), in which the inability to convert glucose-6-phosphate to glucose leads secondarily to excessive production of lactate. Hyperlactic acidemia stimulates purine biosynthesis and impairs the renal clearance of urate by poorly understood mechanisms. As a result, hyperuricemia in these patients is often marked.

Reduced excretion of uric acid in chronic renal diseases such as glomerulonephritis, pyelonephritis, and polycystic kidney disease may also produce secondary gout. Both reduced glomerular filtration and impaired tubular secretion of urate are probably involved. Extrarenal factors may also compromise renal urate clearance. For example, lactic acidosis secondary to uncontrolled diabetes mellitus, alcohol ingestion, or von Gierke's disease can give rise to hyperuricemia, as noted above. The well-known association between diuretic therapy and hyperuricemia may also have renal origins. Still unknown is the basis of the increase in plasma urates associated with endocrinopathies such as hypothyroidism, hyperparathyroidism, and hypoparathyroidism, although reduced renal clearance is suspected. With all these uncommon causes of secondary hyperuricemia, gout is rarely a clinical problem.

MORPHOLOGY. Both morphologically and clinically, the distinctive features of gout are (1) acute arthritis, (2) chronic tophaceous arthritis, and (3) tophi in soft tissues.

Acute arthritis represents an acute inflammatory synovitis accompanied by a rich outpouring of polymorphonuclear leukocytes and macrophages, secondary to the formation of microcrystals of urates in the joint effusion. In order of frequency, joints of the great toe (85% of patients), instep, ankle, heel, and knee are involved, but ultimately any joint in the body may be affected. In most patients, however, involvement is limited to the legs. Typically, one or two joints are affected at one time, but rarely the disease is polyarticular. There is little doubt that the acute attack of arthritis is triggered by the formation of monosodium urate (MSU) crystals within the joint fluid and the synovial membrane. However, the precise sequence of events leading to crystal formation and the relative roles of various inflammatory mediators are still uncertain. Some mechanisms believed to be relevant are (1) crystal-induced activation of Hageman factor, which in turn leads to the generation of a variety of proinflammatory molecules including kallikrein, kinins, and complement fractions (p. 53); (2) direct activation of complement, particularly C5, with the formation of chemotactic split products; and (3) phagocytosis of the MSU crystals by leukocytes. The following sequence is thought to occur: (1) MSU crystals avidly adsorb proteins, particularly albumin and IgG, in the synovial fluid, which facilitates their ingestion by neutrophils;[150] (2) the neutrophils release a chemotactic glycoprotein (molecular weight 8400) derived presumably from lysosomes, and there is some leakage of lysosomal enzymes during phagocytosis; (3) digestion of the protein coat of the crystals in the phagolysosome brings them into direct contact with the inner lysosomal membranes, where their weakly acidic groups damage the phagolysosomal membranes by hydrogen bonding with the phosphate esters of the phospholipids; (4) further leakage of lysosomal enzymes follows, with eventual destruction of the leukocytes; and (5) the released crystals are once again coated by proteins and reingested by incoming leukocytes, thus perpetuating the inflammatory cycle. As discussed in Chapter 2, lysosomal enzymes are powerful promoters of the inflammatory response, and high levels of several inflammatory mediators (kinins, complement fractions), discussed above, are found in the synovial fluid during spontaneous attacks of gout. The most recent addition to this list is leukotriene B_4 (p. 54), a powerful chemotactic agent that also causes aggregation of leukocytes along the venular endothelium.[151] The relative role and specificity of various chemical mediators in the pathogenesis of acute gouty arthritis are still not clear, but the significance of the leukocyte-crystal interaction is well established. Indeed, the therapeutic effect of colchicine in terminating an acute attack of gout is best explained by its ability to block several leukocyte functions (adhesiveness, migration, and movement of lysosomal granules), which depend on the integrity of the cytoskeleton.

Although the mechanisms outlined above provide a reasonable explanation for joint inflammation, unresolved questions persist. What favors the microcrystallization of urates in joint fluids rather than in the normal transudates found within the pericardial and pleural cavities? Why are some joints affected while others are spared? Why is there no good relationship between the level of hyperuricemia and the frequency of attacks of gout? Why are the acute attacks of gout self-limited? Some suggestions have been offered. Since the solubility of urates is significantly reduced at lower temperatures, the tendency for the involvement of peripheral joints may be related to their lower temperature. Cartilage and synovial fluid contain proteoglycans, some of which enhance the solubility of urates. Alterations in the structure or content of proteoglycans brought about by trauma, aging, or perhaps genetic factors may favor local decrease in the solubility with formation of crystals. It is interesting to note that MSU crystals have also been found in the synovial fluid of asymptomatic hyperuricemic subjects, but these differ in shape and size from the crystals seen in inflamed joints. Thus, the structure of the crystals may also be a variable. To explain the self-limited nature of acute gouty arthritis, it has been suggested that elevation of the local temperature brought about by inflammation favors the solubilization of urate crystals, and the increased blood flow tends to wash the dissolved urates out of the joint.

Chronic arthritis evolves from the progressive precipitation of urates into the synovial linings of joints following recurrent attacks of acute arthritis. The urates may heavily encrust the articular surfaces (Fig. 28–37). Synovial proliferation and pannus formation follows and destroys the underlying articular cartilage. With progression, the subarticular bone becomes involved. In time, destruction of subchondral bone, proliferation of marginal bone, and sometimes fibrous or bony ankylosis ensue, ultimately to cause chronic disabling arthritis. Deposits of urates may appear in the periarticular tissues (Fig. 28–38).

The tophus is the pathognomonic lesion of gout—a mass of urates, crystalline or amorphous, surrounded by an intense inflammatory reaction, composed of macrophages, lymphocytes, fibroblasts, and extraordinary foreign body giant cells (Fig. 28–39). The giant cells are distinctive and often appear as extended cytoplasmic masses, partially encircling the central aggregation of urates. Tophi commonly occur in the helix or antihelix of the ear, the olecranon and patellar bursae, and periarticular ligaments and connective tissues. In the kidney, tophi tend to be deposited in the medulla or pyramids and evoke a surrounding typical inflammatory reaction in the tubular interstitium. Less frequently, tophi are found in the skin of the fingertips, palms, or soles; nasal cartilages; aorta; myocardium; and aortic or mitral valves. Very rarely, tophi form in

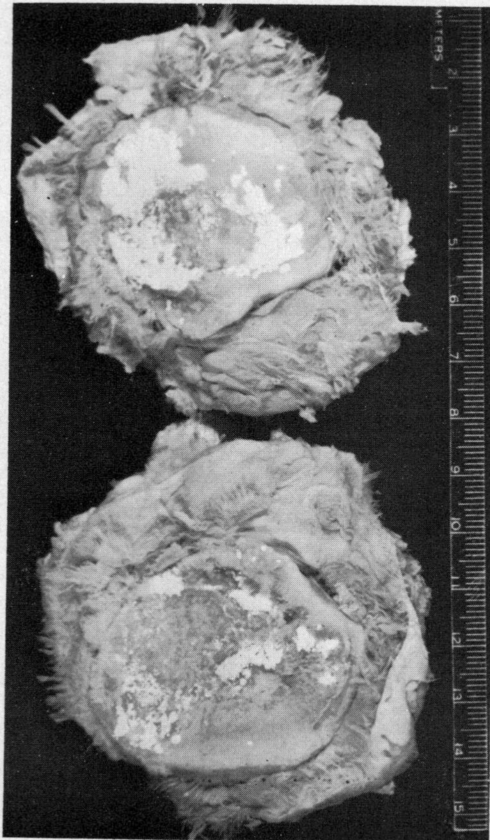

Figure 28–37. Gouty deposits on patella. Articular surfaces of patellas are encrusted with white deposits of urates.

the eyes, tongue, larynx, penis, testis, or marrow cavities of bone, such as in the marrow spaces adjacent to intervertebral discs of the spine.[152] Tophi do not develop in the central nervous system, because of the relative impermeability of the blood-brain barrier to uric acid. The urate crystals are water soluble, and nonaqueous fixatives such as absolute alcohol are necessary to preserve them in histologic section. When preserved, they are brilliantly anisotropic when viewed with polarized light, or are demonstrable as crystalline or amorphous masses with silver staining techniques.

The kidneys are often involved in gout. The most distinctive renal change is the formation of tophi within the pyramids or medulla seen grossly as small white specks or radiating lines. Several other changes may be present, including hyalinization of glomeruli, tubular atrophy or dilatation, interstitial fibrosis, pyelonephritis, and arteriolar nephrosclerosis; these are described in detail in Chapter 21. In the belief that they are somehow caused by hyperuricemia, these lesions collectively have been designated "gouty nephropathy." However, careful studies indicate that chronic hyperuricemia itself does not injure the kidney, and that the incidence of renal dysfunction in patients with gout is no greater than in age-matched groups with a comparable degree of hypertension, diabetes, primary renal disease, and urinary obstruction.[153] It has been suggested that, in some patients at least, concomitant chronic lead toxicity may play a role.

Uric acid stones are found in the urinary tract in 10 to 25% of patients with gout. Their formation is related to both the serum and urinary urate levels. In persons who excrete more than 1100 mg of urate per 24 hours, the incidence of stones reaches 50%. Secondary complications of obstructive uropathy follow in these patients.

There are several other poorly understood associations with gout. Patients with gout seem to have a higher incidence of obesity, hypertriglyceridemia, diabetes mellitus, and hypertension. In none of these instances has a causal relationship with high uric acid levels been established.

CLINICAL CORRELATION. The natural history of gout evolves through three well-defined clinical phases: (1) asymptomatic hyperuricemia, (2) recurrent attacks of acute gouty arthritis interspersed with asymptomatic (intercritical) intervals, and (3) chronic gouty arthritis.

A long period of asymptomatic hyperuricemia almost always precedes the first acute attack of arthritis. As mentioned earlier, most hyperuricemic patients never develop symptomatic gout. The likelihood of developing the disease is correlated with both the duration and level of the hyperuricemia. Long-term studies indicate that patients who develop clinical dis-

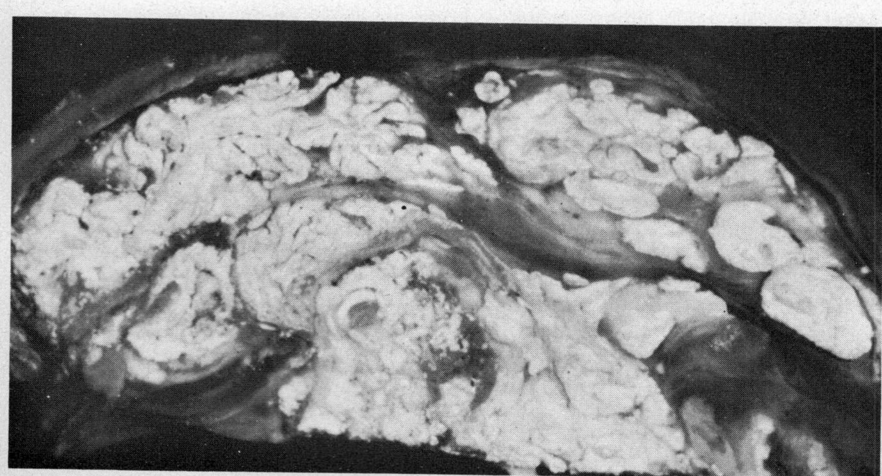

Figure 28–38. Cross section of periarticular tissues of metatarsophalangeal joint with massive white amorphous urate deposition in all layers up to the skin.

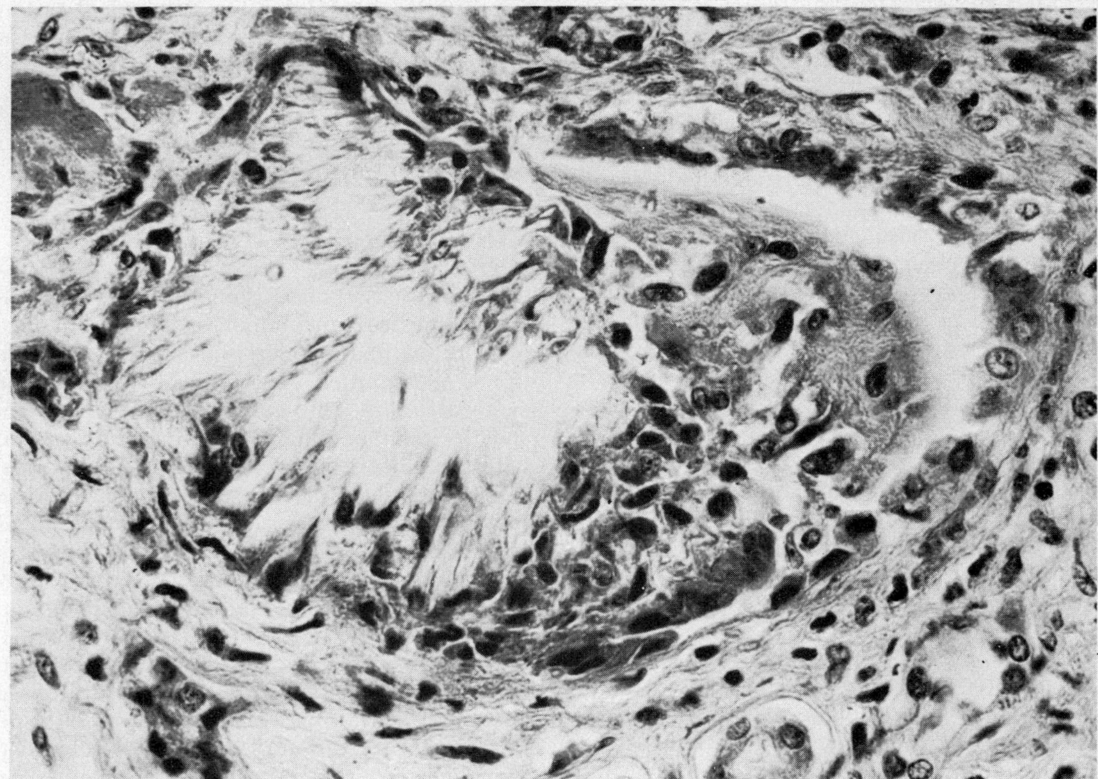

Figure 28–39. A tophus of gout. The group of slender urate crystals is surrounded by a reaction of fibroblasts, occasional lymphocytes, and giant cells.

ease, most often in the fifth or sixth decades of life, usually have had an abnormal level of uric acid in the blood since puberty in the male and the menopause in the female.

Acute gouty arthritis is characterized by the sudden onset of pain, almost always in a peripheral joint, usually in the lower extremity. At least 50% of the initial attacks involve the first metatarsophalangeal joint. The affected joints are swollen and exquisitely tender. Chills and fever may also accompany the acute attack. In some patients a history can be obtained of some unusual form of stress immediately preceding the acute attack, e.g., physical or emotional fatigue, an alcoholic spree, or dietary overindulgence. The initial attack usually subsides with therapy or spontaneously in a few days to a few weeks, and is followed by an asymptomatic phase that may last from a few months to many years, or, in the particularly fortunate patient, for a lifetime. More often, however, a recurrence of the arthritis is experienced within several months to a few years, with increased likelihood of other joint involvement, longer duration of the acute phase, and more severe signs and symptoms.

Chronic gouty arthritis is the most disabling phase of the disease. It generally follows multiple recurrences of acute arthritis over the span of years. The time from the initial attack to chronic gouty arthritis averages about a decade, but may range up to four decades. Obviously, treatment for hyperuricemia and acute arthritis significantly reduces the risk of development of this chronic phase of disease, which appears now in only 15 to 20% of patients under treatment. The appearance of the chronic involvement is insidious and may not become apparent until tophi can be palpated in the soft tissues about the joint, or until it is documented by radiographic evidence of joint damage. Limitation of motion ranges from mild to severe. Surprisingly, the soft tissue tophi are remarkably painless and nontender. With progression, the skin overlying affected joints sometimes becomes tense, shiny, and red, with obvious distortion of the symmetry of the affected part. For unknown reasons, with the development of the chronic phase of the disease, the attacks of acute arthritis tend to subside.

Gouty patients are at increased risk of developing uric acid urinary stones, particularly those who excrete excessive amounts of uric acid. Evidence of renal disease is encountered in 20 to 40% of patients, but its relationship to hyperuricemia is unclear (p. 1052).

The diagnosis of gout should not be missed by clinicians, because it affords them the uncommon and splendid opportunity of "doing good." An extensive armamentarium of drugs is available to inhibit uric acid synthesis, lower serum uric acid levels, abort or prevent acute attacks of arthritis, and mobilize tophaceous deposits. Generally, gout does not materially shorten the span of life, but it certainly may impair its quality.

OTHER FORMS OF ARTHRITIS

Joint disease not conforming to any of the well-defined patterns already described is encountered in association with a number of systemic disorders. The anatomic changes in these diverse arthropathies are not sufficiently well characterized to merit detailed description, and so are included here in capsule form.

Chondrocalcinosis, also called *pseudogout,* is an inflammatory arthritis caused by the deposition of calcium pyrophosphate crystals in the synovial fluid and articular cartilage. The knee and other large joints are most frequently affected. This pattern of articular disease is associated with hemochromatosis, ochronosis, hyperparathyroidism, hypothyroidism, Wilson's disease, diabetes mellitus, and other metabolic disorders. The calcification of the joint cartilage and synovium may lead to an acute edematous arthropathy or, in the later stages, to degeneration and fragmentation of the cartilage. The sudden onset of the arthritis in some individuals accounts for the designation pseudogout. In other instances it is more insidious and chronic in nature and may mimic rheumatoid disease.

Reiter's syndrome is an uncommon disorder characterized by arthritis, urethritis, conjunctivitis, and mucocutaneous lesions. It usually begins with urethritis (after a sexual exposure), followed by the other features of the syndrome in days to a few weeks. Although it is currently thought to represent a chlamydial infection with involvement of multiple sites in the body, no etiologic agent has been firmly implicated. There is, however, a strong association with HLA-B27. The arthritis is a nonspecific, acute inflammatory reaction indistinguishable from other arthropathies of infectious or immunologic origin.

Arthritis is a common complication of ulcerative colitis that appears in 20 to 25% of patients. It may involve peripheral joints or the vertebral column (spondylitis). The arthropathy of the peripheral joints takes the form of a nonspecific, acute inflammatory synovitis analogous to that seen in acute rheumatoid disease, except that it is not progressive, is not accompanied by pannus formation, and usually subsides without residuals within weeks to months. The involvement of the vertebral column takes the form of ankylosing spondylitis indistinguishable from that already described (p. 1351).

Psoriatic arthritis appears in approximately 5% of patients with this common skin disease (p. 1291). A number of clinical subsets can be distinguished, but the three most common patterns of arthropathy are (1) monoarticular or oligoarticular arthritis of the small joints of the hands and feet, (2) a symmetric multijoint involvement simulating rheumatoid arthritis, and (3) ankylosing spondylitis and sacroiliitis. Whatever the clinical pattern and particular joint involved, the changes closely resemble those described in rheumatoid disease, and indeed may lead to joint destruction and limitation of motion. As with the ankylosing spondylitis described earlier, psoriatic spondylitis has a strong association with HLA-B27. Although it is tempting to consider all forms of psoriatic arthritis as rheumatoid disease in patients with the skin condition, rheumatoid factor is almost never present.

TUMORS

SYNOVIOSARCOMA

Synoviosarcomas, sometimes erroneously called synoviomas, are uncommon malignant tumors that occur most often in the deep soft tissues of the lower and upper extremities. They are thought to arise from synovial lining cells more often of bursae and tendon sheaths than of joints, and thus are generally found within or in proximity to skeletal muscle. A significant number of these lesions occur at sites apparently removed from normal synovium, usually in association with fascial sheaths of muscle. In support of a synovial derivation of synoviosarcomas wherever they arise is their usual biphasic histology—one component being epithelial-like cells resembling synoviocytes that often form slitlike clefts or ductal spaces, and the other component taking the form of spindled fibroblastic mesenchymal cells. This concurrence of cell types recapitulates the derivation of cuboidal-to-columnar synovial lining cells from more primitive mesenchymal cells. Not surprisingly, about one-third of these cancers are *monophasic* and composed solely of either fibroblast-like mesenchymal cells or, more rarely, only epithelial-like cells.[154] There is still considerable controversy about the interpretation of monophasic lesions as synoviosarcomas, because obviously there are many other forms of spindle cell sarcomas (e.g., fibrosarcoma, leiomyosarcoma, and neurogenic sarcoma) and the monophasic tumor composed only of epithelial-like cells must be differentiated from carcinoma.

The synoviosarcoma may appear at any age, with a peak incidence in the third and fourth decades of life. Both sexes are affected about equally. Two-thirds arise in the lower extremity from the buttock and groin to the foot; almost all the remainder are located from the shoulder to the forearm. Rarely, they arise in the neck but almost never within the mediastinum and retroperitoneum.[155]

Grossly, the neoplasm appears as a deceptively circumscribed, gray-white mass sometimes having focal areas of pale necrosis and hemorrhage and, of particular importance, areas of gritty calcification that provide diagnostic clues on radiography (Fig. 28–40). Occasional lesions are overtly infiltrative. More readily recognized microscopically are the biphasic lesions. The epithelial-like element may appear as solid nests of polygonal cells sometimes having cleared cytoplasm, or may take the form of cuboidal-to-columnar cells enclosing slitlike spaces or surrounding apparent tubules or ducts (Fig. 28–41). Occasionally, small papillary excrescences project into the enclosed spaces, which often contain mucicarmine-positive and PAS-positive secretion (Fig. 28–42). Enclosing this epithelioid component is a

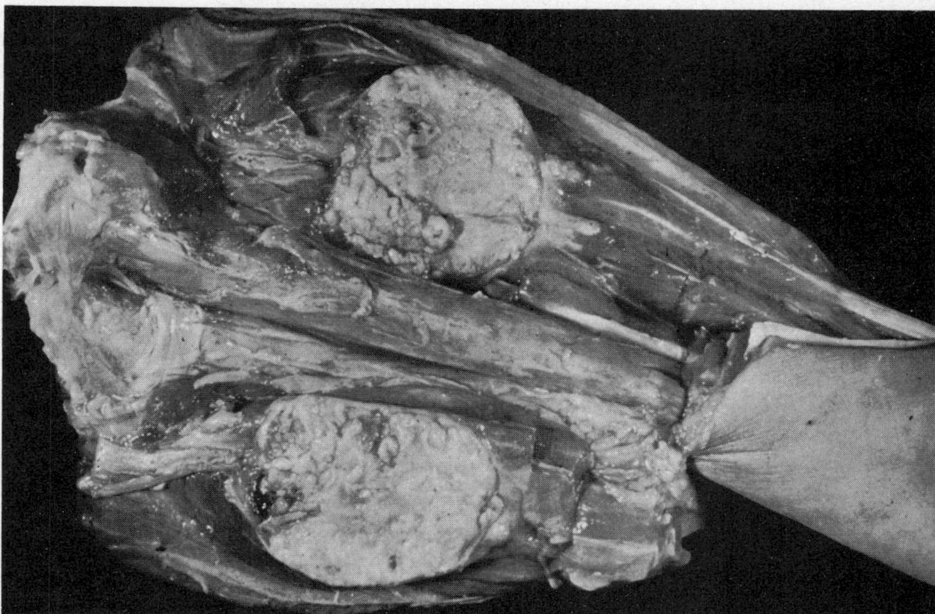

Figure 28–40. Synoviosarcoma. Deceptively discrete mass arising in tendon sheaths.

monotony of spindle cells resembling those in many other types of sarcoma. Transition forms between spindle and epithelioid cells are occasionally seen. Monophasic synoviosarcomas are composed solely of one or the other of the two components described.

Certain features help to identify synoviosarcomas, particularly the monophasic variants. Within the spindle cell areas there may be thick collagen bundles that sometimes appear almost osteoid-like. Focal calcifications are seen in both biphasic and monophasic patterns, and sometimes in the former there are psammoma-like bodies within the tips of papillary excrescences. On electron microscopy, both epithelioid and spindle cells often reveal microfilaments as well as surface microvilli or filopodia. Both types of cells may also have desmosomes and hemidesmosomes.[156] Also helpful is the recent observation that both the spindle-cell and epithelial-like components often contain keratin proteins when stained with the immunoperoxidase method, analogous to the positive reaction encountered with malignant mesotheliomas.[157]

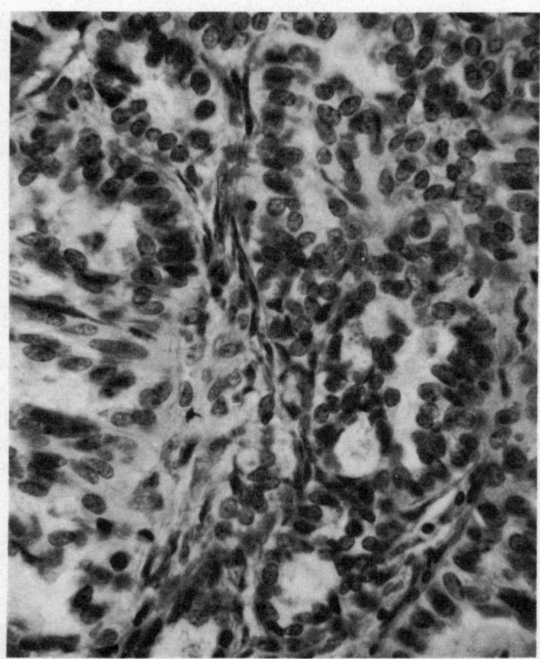

Figure 28–41. High-power detail of biphasic cell morphology.

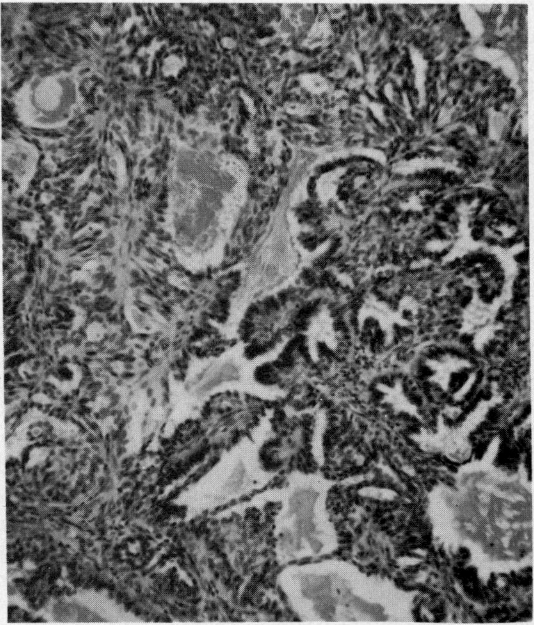

Figure 28–42. Low-power detail of a synoviosarcoma, illustrating cleftlike spaces lined by glandlike epithelium and the formation of papillary projections.

Clinically, these tumors present as slowly enlarging, painless masses either palpable in the deep soft tissues or readily evident as distortions of the contour of the extremity. They are highly aggressive cancers and often have metastasized widely by the time of diagnosis, particularly to the lungs and pleura. Often, cardiopulmonary insufficiency is the cause of death. Even in the absence of metastases, recurrences follow wide surgical excision or amputation in over half of the patients. The recurrence may be delayed for decades. Until recently, the five-year survival with surgery alone averaged about 50%. Factors favorably influencing the prognosis are small size (i.e., less than 5 cm in diameter)—about 70% five-year survival—and peripheral primary location—about 55% five-year survival. Still unsettled is the question whether the biphasic or monophasic tumor carries a better prognosis.[154, 156] Currently, additional modalities of therapy have been added to surgical excision, including radiation, chemotherapy, and regional perfusion, but the five-year results of these varying combinations are not yet available.

MALIGNANT FIBROUS HISTIOCYTOMA

A number of seemingly disparate neoplasms are composed of varying proportions of spindled fibroblastic cells; plump, sometimes lipid-laden histiocytes; and intermediate forms admixed with a variable number of foreign body–type, multinucleate giant cells. The benign variants are also called fibrous xanthomas, xanthofibromas, dermatofibromas, sclerosing hemangiomas, and giant cell tumors of tendon sheath origin. These were described on page 1267. Despite the dominant contributions of apparent fibroblasts and histiocytes to the morphology of these neoplasms, the precise histogenesis of these cell types is still controversial. On the one hand, it is proposed that multipotential mesenchymal cells are the progenitors of all the cell types; on the other, the histiocyte is held to be the progenitor, which then differentiates into the other mesenchymal types. This issue is still under study and need not concern us further.[158] It suffices that, under the electron microscope, cells having the ultrastructural features of fibroblasts and/or histiocytes admixed with occasional myofibroblasts and undifferentiated cells can be identified in all the benign and malignant variants.

Here our attention is directed to the malignant fibrous histiocytoma (MFH) of bones and soft tissues. Basically it is a pleomorphic sarcoma having fibroblast-like and histiocyte-like cells usually accompanied by pleomorphic tumorous giant cells. Occasional neoplasms are largely monomorphic and mimic fibrosarcomas or malignant histiocytosis. In still other instances they have a rich myxoid component simulating rhabdomyosarcoma, or are sufficiently lipid laden to be confused with liposarcoma.[159] The diagnosis of MFH involves, then, the exclusion of many histologically similar neoplasms.

These cancers may arise in soft tissues or bones, most often in adults, with a 2:1 male preponderance. Although it is distinctly uncommon before the fourth decade of life, children and adolescents are sometimes affected. The soft tissue lesions are found in the lower extremity (approximately 50%), upper extremity (approximately 20%), or abdominal cavity including retroperitoneum (approximately 20%). Over half arise in relation to skeletal muscle but some involve the deep fascia or, less often, subcutaneous tissues. The osseous tumors tend to occur as unifocal lesions in the bones around the knee, but more proximal and distal lower extremity locations and origin in the pelvis or upper extremity have also been recorded. Rarely, MFH of bone appears to be multicentric, arising in two or more bones simultaneously.[160]

The soft tissue MFH presents as a multilobulated, gray-white, sarcomatous mass, usually deceptively circumscribed. Some neoplasms, however, are obviously infiltrative, and others are sufficiently hemorrhagic to mimic a hematoma. Bony lesions may arise in any location within the individual bone, usually somewhere within the metaphyseal region. As osteolytic tumors they may erode through the cortex to invade surrounding soft tissues and so mimic osteogenic sarcoma, particularly radiographically. In other instances the neoplasm permeates the bone rather widely to thus resemble a Ewing's sarcoma.

The histology of MFH, as pointed out, is highly variable. Three basic patterns predominate: storiform, pleomorphic, and fascicular.[161] **The storiform pattern** has short fascicles of plump spindled cells arranged in a cartwheel or storiform configuration (Fig. 28–43). Occasional cells are more rounded or plump and contain hemosiderin pigment or fine lipid vacuoles. Mitotic figures, occasional tumor giant cells, and mononuclear inflammatory cells may also be present. **The pleomorphic pattern** is most common and presents a random, haphazard array of cells ranging from spindle forms to rounded, sometimes lipid-laden histiocytes to multinucleate giant cells. The giant cells often have abundant brightly eosinophilic cytoplasm with huge nuclei and sometimes multiple nuclei. Often the giant cells have foamy cytoplasm. As with the storiform pattern, there is sometimes an inflammatory component. The **fascicular pattern** may predominate throughout a specific neoplasm, but more often occurs focally within a storiform or pleomorphic background. The term "fascicular" alludes to the tendency for the plump fibroblast-like cells to be arrayed in broad bands or fascicles. Occasional giant cells, lipid-laden histiocytes, and inflammatory cells are present, helping to differentiate these tumors from fibrosarcomas.

Additional myxoid and lipid-rich elements may be present, but it suffices to note that the diagnosis of MFH is treacherous and often requires ultrastructural or immunohistochemical studies to characterize the critical histiocytic element. Helpful in this connection are the identification by immunoperoxidase techniques of lysozyme or chymotrypsin in the tumor cells, enzymes that are typically present in normal histiocytes.[162]

It is difficult to express a prognosis for these highly variable sarcomas. Overall, for both soft tissue and bony lesions, there is about a 50% survival rate for two to three years. However, the prognosis is materially influenced by site of origin and histologic pattern, and mostly by size of neoplasm and time of discovery. Tumors arising in subcutaneous locations tend to be found

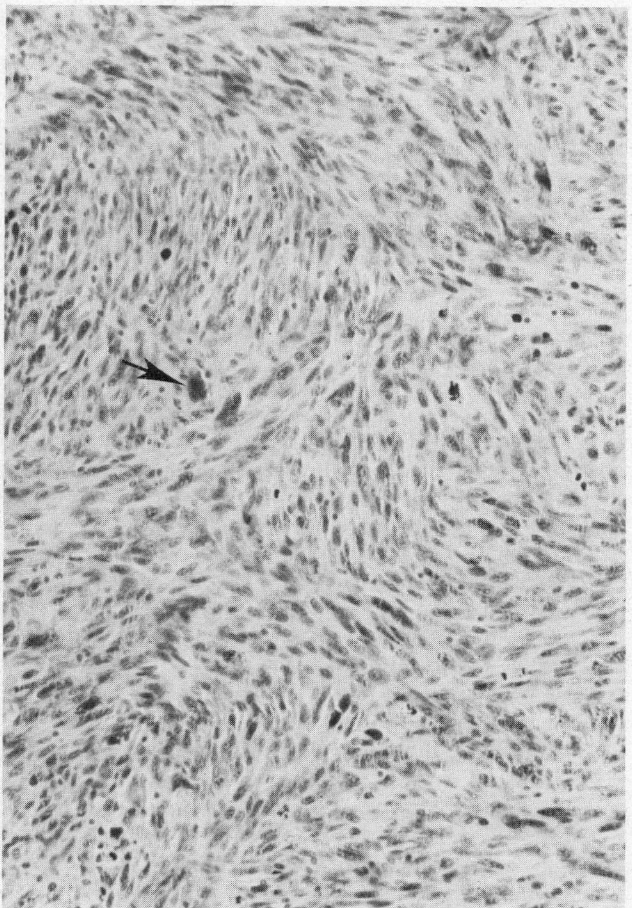

Figure 28–43. Malignant fibrous histiocytoma revealing fascicles of plump spindled cells of varying size arranged in a swirling (storiform) pattern. Giant cells *(arrow)* are present.

earliest, have rarely metastasized, and have the best prognosis. Myxoid histology also improves the outlook and, analogously, the smaller the mass, the better the prognosis. When the primary lesions are small and amenable to radical excision, sometimes coupled with radiotherapy, about one-third of patients have no evidence of recurrence or dissemination over a five- to 12-year follow-up.[163] Death is usually related to metastatic spread to the lungs (approximately 80%) and internal organs. Regional lymph nodes are affected in only 30% of cases, calling into question the value of prophylactic lymph node dissections at the time of excision of the primary mass.

MISCELLANEOUS LESIONS

PIGMENTED VILLONODULAR SYNOVITIS (PIGMENTED VILLONODULAR TENOSYNOVITIS)

This curious condition of uncertain nature can be best characterized as a proliferative lesion of joints and tendon sheaths, marked by hemosiderin deposition within villous overgrowths of the synovium. The synovial overgrowth may be sufficient to induce tumor-like masses that project into the joint or tendon sheath spaces. Indeed, as will be seen, one view is that this lesion is basically neoplastic and a form of fibrous histiocytoma. In this theory the *giant cell tumor of tendon sheaths* is a circumscribed form of nodular tenosynovitis.[164] In joints, however, the entire synovial lining is usually involved, particularly in the knee and less often the hip. The strict limitation of the process to the joint spaces, the lack of cellular atypism, and the benign nature of the multinucleate giant cells, thought to be derived from fusion of synoviocytes or macrophages, all militate against a neoplastic origin for this lesion. Females tend to be affected slightly more often than males. Frequently, there is effusion into the joint space or tendon sheath, accompanied by pain, swelling, and sometimes locking of the joint.

Grossly, the lesion in tendon sheaths takes the form of a small, ovoid swelling, rarely greater than 3 cm in diameter, which on transection is usually golden-yellow to red-brown, depending on the amount of contained lipid and hemosiderin. In joint spaces, more or less of the entire synovial lining is transformed into a tangled mat by numerous brown-to-rusty-colored sessile or villous projections (Fig. 28–44). Sometimes discrete, yellow-brown nodules having the appearance of neoplasms develop either within the thickened synovial membrane or as pedunculated lesions.

The histologic changes are variable and are undoubtedly modified by traumatic injury to the exuberant synovial tissue. Basically, there are two components: a subsynovial accumulation of mononuclear cells thought to be derived from the synovial lining cells, and a florid proliferative response of the surface layer of synoviocytes, creating polypoid projections. The proliferative response creates a population of spindled, cylindrical, or, less often, polyhedral

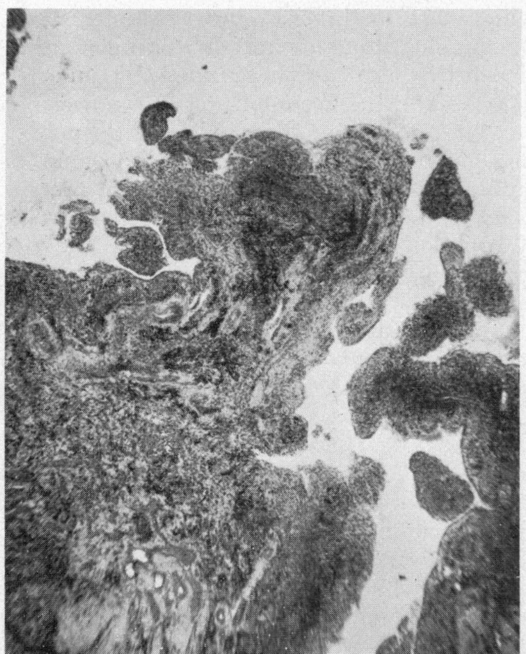

Figure 28–44. Villonodular synovitis, illustrating filamentous strands of inflammatory synovia.

cells, through which are scattered lipid-laden histiocytes, pigment-laden histiocytes, and multinucleate giant cells, sometimes also bearing hemosiderin pigment. Whether the phagocytic cells are of local origin (synoviocytes) or derived from monocytes is not known.[165] This histologic pattern closely resembles that of the fibrous histiocytoma and, as mentioned, this disorder has been interpreted as a fibrous histiocytoma of the tendon sheaths or joint spaces.

The pathogenesis of this lesion is completely obscure. It has been viewed variously as (1) a neoplastic process, as mentioned above; (2) inflammatory in origin, although no specific agents have been isolated; (3) a localized disturbance of lipid metabolism leading to accumulation of lipids within phagocytic cells with secondary traumatic changes; and (4) a reactive response to chronic trauma with repeated hemorrhages. Most observations favor the last hypothesis.[166] The fact that the lesion frequently recurs following incomplete excision has been taken as evidence for a neoplastic origin, but such behavior does not rule out a recurrent stimulus to a reactive process. We must leave it that this disabling but not life-threatening condition is still a complete enigma.

TENOSYNOVITIS

Tenosynovitis denotes an inflammation of the tendon sheaths and contained tendons. This condition is most often encountered in persons who place great stress upon certain tendons in the course of their occupation. Thus, tenosynovitis is most often found in the upper extremities of laborers and artisans, and in the wrists and hands of stenographers. On the basis of this clinical distribution, trauma is believed to play an important role. However, tenosynovitis occasionally may be caused by direct bacterial seeding.

Several anatomic forms of this inflammation are produced by these various causations. *Traumatic synovitis* consists of the accumulation of synovial fluid and fibrin within a tendon sheath. The fibrin may cause a grating sound on motion and may also, in time, become organized to produce fibrous adhesions. Direct bacterial invasion gives rise to a *suppurative tenosynovitis*. The most common offending organisms are the pyogens. Such pyogenic infection may also be initiated by penetrating injuries, as when a surgeon accidentally punctures a tendon sheath in the course of placing sutures. *Tuberculous tenosynovitis* is an uncommon pattern that usually represents a hematogenous focus of seeding, but may occur by direct inoculation of infective material through the skin. These tuberculous infections are characterized by the development of small granulomas on the synovial lining that often protrude and are sloughed off into the fluid of the tendon sheath to produce the characteristic "*rice bodies*." These conditions are extremely painful on motion and cause some disability because of this pain. Adequate rest and other supportive measures usually promote healing. Sometimes, however, residual fibrous adhesions limit, to some extent, the movement of the tendon. In time, these adhesions usually stretch sufficiently to restore function.

As noted in the previous discussion, the giant cell tumor of tendon sheath origin is considered by some to be also a form of tenosynovitis related to pigmented villonodular synovitis. However, it is not associated with pain or other inflammatory manifestations, and so behaves more like a benign tumor.

BURSITIS

Bursitis is an inflammation of the bursa. Although we may so define the lesion, there is considerable dispute as to the exact nature of the bursa. Standard textbooks of anatomy describe numerous cystic spaces between joints and supporting ligaments and tendon sheaths that are presumed to act as gliding surfaces facilitating the mobility of these supporting ligaments over the adjacent bony prominences. Despite these well-ordered descriptions, there is some doubt whether bursae are present in the normal individual. According to this view, they arise as pathologic alterations in connective tissue in response to the constant mobility of the connective tissue at sites of pressure. A bursa, then, may be a pathologic lesion from the outset but, unless further complicated by superimposed inflammation, does not cause symptoms. It is to these additional complications that our present interest is directed.

Bursitis tends to be more common in males than in females, perhaps because of greater physical activity. These lesions are most often encountered in the subdeltoid bursa of the shoulder, the olecranon bursa of the elbow, the prepatellar bursa, and the radiohumeral bursa of the lateral radial head.

The cause of bursitis is unknown. Trauma is believed to play an important role, but whether this acts as an initiating influence or a precipitating factor is still unclear. Bacterial invasion may be responsible for occasional flareups, but in most instances the aspirated fluid is sterile. Most often, no precise initiating influence can be identified except possibly a history of excessive exercise, e.g., tennis elbow.

In the early acute stages of the inflammatory condition, the bursa is distended with a watery or mucoid fluid. As the chronic stage is reached, the stage at which the lesion is usually excised, the bursal space is filled with a granular, brown, inspissated changed blood heavily admixed with gritty calcific precipitations. The wall is thick, tough, and fibrous and is often pigmented by the contained hemorrhage and hardened by calcification. The inner surface is usually shaggy and trabeculated, and often thick, fibrous briding cords traverse the inner space.

Histologically, the walls are composed of dense fibrous tissue focally infiltrated by lymphocytes, plasma cells, and macrophages. The lining of the bursa is usually composed of granulation tissue or precipitated fibrin. Characteristically, there is marked focal vascularization of the wall of the cyst that often produces small, hemangiomatoid collections of capillary channels. Basophilic calcium deposits may be found trapped within the fibrinous lining material and within the wall.

The conditions are more painful than serious and presently are treated by supportive measures, the local instillation of cortisone or similar steroids, and, in the calcific stages, by surgical excision.

GANGLION

A ganglion is a small (1 to 1.5 cm) cystic lesion, almost always found in the collagenous connective tissue of a joint capsule or tendon sheath. A favorite location is the small joints of the wrist, where it is usually palpable as a firm but yielding, pea-sized subcutaneous nodule. Ganglions are thought to arise from a focus of myxoid degeneration and cystic softening of connecting tissue. The central myxoid tissue, perhaps because of motion of the joint, becomes cystic, and condensation of the periphery yields an enclosing collagenous capsule. The lesion may be multilocular and may enlarge through coalescence of adjacent areas of myxoid cystic changes. The older concept that these cysts communicate with the joint space has proved erroneous, and these innocuous lesions are of trivial significance and readily excised. The older "Bible treatment," namely, administering a sound whack to the nodule with a heavy Bible, is far more dramatic, but alas less effective.

---

1. Huxley, H. E.: The double array of filaments in cross-striated muscle. J. Biophys. Biochem. Cytol. *3*:631, 1957.
2. Huxley, H. E.: Electron microscope studies on the structure of natural and synthetic protein filaments from striated muscle. J. Mol. Biol. *7*:281, 1963.
3. Huxley, H. E.: Recent x-ray diffraction and electron microscope studies of striated muscle. *In* The Contractile Process, Proceedings of a Symposium of the New York Heart Association. Boston, Little, Brown & Co. 1967, p. 71.
4. Nelson, D. A., and Benson, E. S.: On the structural continuities of the transverse tubular system of rabbit and human myocardial cells. J. Cell Biol. *16*:297, 1963.
5. Smith, D. S.: Organization and function of the sarcoplasmic reticulum and T-system of muscle cells. Prog. Biophys. *16*:109, 1966.
6. Romanul, F. C. A.: Reversal of energy metabolism and myosin characteristics of white muscles after chronic stimulation. Trans. Am. Neurol. Assoc. *98*:297, 1973.
7. Bischoff, R.: Regeneration of single skeletal muscle fibers in vitro. Anat. Rec. *182*:215, 1975.
8. Stonnington, H. H., and Engel, A. E.: Normal and denervated muscle. Neurology (Minneap.) *23*:714, 1973.
9. Pellegrino, C., and Franzini, C.: An electron microscopic study of denervation atrophy in red and white muscles. J. Cell. Biol. *17*:327, 1963.
10. Cullen, M. J., and Mastaglia, F. L.: Morphological changes in dystrophic muscle. Br. Med. Bull. *36*:145, 1980.
11. Furukawa, T., and Peter, J. B.: The muscular dystrophies and related disorders. I. The muscular dystrophies. J.A.M.A. *239*:1537, 1978.
12. Rowland, L. T.: Biochemistry of muscle membranes of Duchenne muscular dystrophy. Muscle Nerve *3*:3, 1980.
13. Pickard, N. A., et al.: Systemic membrane defect in proximal muscular dystrophies. N. Engl. J. Med. *299*:841, 1978.
14. Gardner-Medwin, D.: Clinical features and classification of the muscular dystrophies. Br. Med. Bull. *36*:109, 1980.
15. Bender, A. N.: Congenital myopathies. Handbook Clin. Neurol. *41*:1, 1979.
16. Simpson, J. A.: Myasthenia gravis and myasthenic syndromes. *In* Walton, Sir J. (ed.): Disorders of Voluntary Muscle. 4th ed. Edinburgh, Churchill Livingstone, 1981, p. 585.
17. Engel, A. G., et al.: Immune complexes (IgGC and C_3) at the motor end-plate in myasthenia gravis. Ultrastructural and light microscopic localization and electrophysiologic correlations. Mayo Clin. Proc. *52*:267, 1977.
18. Vincent, A.: Immunology of acetylcholine receptors in relation to myasthenia gravis. Physiol. Rev. *60*:756, 1980.
19. Drachman, D. B., et al.: Functional activities of autoantibodies to acetylcholine receptors and the clinical severity of myasthenia gravis. N. Engl. J. Med. *307*:769, 1982.
20. Kao, I., and Drachman, D. B.: Thymic muscle cells bear acetylcholine receptors: Possible relation to myasthenia gravis. Science *195*:74, 1977.
21. Editorial: Management of myasthenia gravis. Lancet *2*:135, 1982.
22. Newsom-Davis, J., et al.: Thymus cells in myasthenia gravis selectively enhance production of anti–acetylcholine-receptor antibody by autologous blood lymphocytes. N. Engl. J. Med. *305*:1313, 1981.
23. Tanaoki, N., et al.: Thymus pathology and effects of thymectomy. *In* Satoyoshi, E. (ed.): Myasthenia Gravis. Tokyo, University of Tokyo Press, 1981, p. 269.
24. Caldwell, E. H.: Desmoid tumor: Musculoaponeurotic fibrosis of the abdominal wall. Surgery *79*:104, 1976.
25. Reitamo, J. J., et al.: The desmoid tumor. I. Incidence, sex-, age-, and anatomical distribution in the Finnish population. Am. J. Clin. Pathol. *77*:665, 1982.
26. Häyry, P., et al.: The desmoid tumor. II. Analysis of factors possibly contributing to the etiology and growth behavior. Am. J. Clin. Pathol. *77*:674, 1982.
27. MacKenzie, D. H.: The fibromatoses. A clinicopathological concept. Br. Med. J. *4*:277, 1972.
28. Chung, E. G., and Enzinger, F. M.: Proliferative fasciitis. Cancer *36*:1450, 1975.
29. Bernstein, K. E., and Lattes, R.: Nodular (pseudosarcomatous) fasciitis, a nonrecurrent lesion: Clinicopathologic study of 134 cases. Cancer *49*:1668, 1982.
30. Di Sant'Agnese, P. A., and Knowles, D. M.: Extracardiac rhabdomyoma: A clinicopathologic study and review of the literature. Cancer *46*:780, 1980.
31. Bale, P. M., et al.: Diagnosis and behavior of juvenile rhabdomyosarcoma. Hum. Pathol. *14*:596, 1983.
32. Brooks, J. J.: Immunohistochemistry of soft tissue tumors. Myoglobin as a tumor marker for rhabdomyosarcoma. Cancer *50*:1757, 1982.
33. Mukai, K., et al.: Immunohistochemical localization of actin: Applications in surgical pathology. Am. J. Surg. Pathol. *5*:91, 1981.
34. Feldman, B. A.: Rhabdomyosarcoma of the head and neck. Laryngoscope *92*:424, 1982.
35. Batsakis, J. G.: The pathology of head and neck tumors: Fibroadipose tissue and skeletal muscle. Part 8. Head Neck Surg. *3*:145, 1980.
36. Green, D. M., and Jaffe, N.: Progress and controversy in the treatment of childhood rhabdomyosarcoma. Cancer Treat. Rev. *5*:7, 1978.
37. Ariel, I. M., and Briceno, M.: Rhabdomyosarcoma of the extremities and trunk: Analysis of 150 patients treated by surgical resection. J. Surg. Oncol. *7*:269, 1975.
38. Gaiger, A. M., et al.: Pathology of rhabdomyosarcoma: Experience of the Intergroup Rhabdomyosarcoma Study 1972–78. Natl. Cancer Inst. Monogr. *56*:19, 1981.
39. Enzinger, F. M., and Shiraki, M.: Alveolar rhabdomyosarcoma. An analysis of 110 cases. Cancer *24*:18, 1969.
40. Corson, J., and Pinkus, G.: Intracellular myoglobin: A specific marker for skeletal muscle differentiation in soft tissue sarcomas. Am. J. Pathol. *103*:384, 1981.
41. Rode, J.: Immunohistochemical staining of granular cell tumor for neuron-specific enolase: Evidence in support of a neural origin. Diagnost. Histopathol. *5*:205, 1982.
42. Lack, E. E., et al.: Granular cell tumor: A clinicopathologic study of 110 patients. J. Surg. Oncol. *13*:301, 1980.
43. Cooper, P. H., and Goodman, M. D.: Multilayering of capillary basal laminae in the granular cell tumor, a marker of cellular injury. Hum. Pathol. *5*:327, 1974.
44. Owen, M.: Histogenesis of bone cells. Calcif. Tissue Res. *25*:205, 1978.
45. Parfitt, A. M.: The coupling of bone formation to bone resorption: A critical analysis of the concept and of its relevance to the pathogenesis of osteoporosis. Metab. Bone. Dis. Relat. Res. *4*:1, 1982.
46. Raisz, L. G., and Kream, B. E.: Regulation of bone formation. N. Engl. J. Med. *309*:29, 1983.
47. Anderson, H. C.: Introduction to the Second Conference on Matrix Vesicle Calcification. Metab. Bone Dis. Relat. Res. *1*:83, 1978.
48. Somjen, D., et al.: Bone remodeling induced by physical stress is prostaglandin E_2 mediated. Biochim. Biophys. Acta *627*:91, 1980.
49. Coccia, P. F.: Cells that resorb bone. N. Engl. J. Med. *310*:456, 1984.
50. Ibsen, K. H.: Distinct varieties of osteogenesis imperfecta. Clin. Orthop. *50*:279, 1967.
51. Johnston, C. C., Jr., et al.: Osteopetrosis: A clinical, genetic, metabolic

and morphological study of the dominantly inherited benign form. Medicine *47*:149, 1968.
52. Dich, V. Q., et al.: Osteomyelitis in infants and children. A review of 163 cases. Am. J. Dis. Child. *129*:1273, 1975.
53. McHenry, M. C., et al.: Hematogenous osteomyelitis. Cleve. Clin. Q. *42*:125, 1975.
54. Waldfogel, F. A., and Vasey, H.: Osteomyelitis: The past decade. N. Engl. J. Med. *303*:360, 1980.
55. Courpon, P.: Bone tissue mechanisms underlying osteoporoses. Orthop. Clin. North Am. *12*:513, 1981.
56. Raisz, L. G.: Osteoporosis. J. Am. Geriatr. Soc. *30*:127, 1983.
57. Lukert, B. P.: Osteoporosis. Arch. Phys. Med. Rehabil. *63*:480, 1982.
58. Bressot, C., et al.: Histomorphometric profile, pathophysiology and reversibility of corticosteroid-induced osteoporosis. Metab. Bone Dis. Relat. Res. *1*:303, 1979.
59. Editorial: Osteoporosis and activity. Lancet *1*:1365, 1983.
60. Nordin, B. E. C., et al.: Bone formation and resorption as the determinants of trabecular bone volume in post-menopausal osteoporosis. Lancet *2*:277, 1981.
61. Stevenson, J. C., et al.: Calcitonin and the calcium-regulating hormones in post-menopausal women: Effect of oestrogens. Lancet *1*:693, 1981.
62. Dunn, W. L., et al.: Measurement of bone mineral content in human vertebrae and hip by dual photon absorptiometry. Radiology *136*:485, 1980.
63. Arnstein, A. R., et al.: Recent progress in osteomalacia and rickets. Ann. Intern. Med. *67*:1296, 1967.
64. Winn, E.: Osteoporosis, osteomalacia, and osteitis fibrosa cystica with special reference to the parathyroid and calcium metabolism. Am. Pract. Dig. Treatm. *2*:921, 1951.
65. Felsenfeld, A., and Llach, F.: Vitamin D and metabolic bone disease: A clinicopathologic overview. Pathol. Annu. *17*:383, 1982.
66. Habener, J. F., and Mahaffey, J. E.: Osteomalacia and disorders of vitamin D metabolism. Annu. Rev. Med. *29*:327, 1978.
67. Birge, S. J., and Haddad, J. G.: 25-Hydroxycholecalciferol stimulation of muscle metabolism. J. Clin. Invest. *56*:1100, 1975.
68. Krane, S. M.: Paget's disease of bone. Clin. Orthop. Rel. Res. *127*:24, 1977.
69. Milgram, J. W.: Radiographical and pathological assessment of the activity of Paget's disease of bone. Clin. Orthop. Rel. Res. *127*:43, 1977.
70. Ibbertson, H. K., et al.: Paget's disease of bone: Assessment and management. Drugs *18*:33, 1979.
71. Editorial: Viruses and Paget's disease of bone. Lancet *2*:1198, 1982.
72. Gherardi, G., et al.: Fine structure of nuclei and cytoplasm of osteoclasts in Paget's disease of bone. Histopathology *4*:63, 1980.
73. Redel, A., et al.: Viral antigens in osteoclast from Paget's disease of bone. Lancet *2*:344, 1980.
74. Singer, F. R., et al.: Elevated serum paramyxovirus antibodies in patients with Paget's disease of bone. Clin. Res. *26*:533A, 1978.
75. Ouslander, J. G., and Beck, J. C.: Paget's disease of bone. J. Am. Geriatr. Soc. *30*:410, 1982.
76. Henley, J. W., et al.: The cardiovascular system in Paget's disease of bone and the response to therapy with calcitonin and diphosphonate. Aust. N.Z. J. Med. *9*:390, 1979.
77. Wick, M. R., et al.: Sarcomas of bone complicating osteitis deformans (Paget's disease)—fifty years' experience. Am. J. Surg. Pathol. *5*:74, 1981.
78. McKenna, R. J., et al.: Osteogenic sarcoma arising in Paget's disease. Cancer *17*:42, 1964.
79. Editorial: Finger clubbing and hypertrophic pulmonary osteoarthropathy. Br. Med. J. *2*:785, 1977.
80. Editorial: Finger clubbing. Lancet *1*:1285, 1975.
81. Lemen, R. J., et al.: Relationships among digital clubbing disease severity and serum prostaglandins $F_{2\alpha}$ and E concentrations in cystic fibrosis patients. Am. Rev. Respir. Dis. *117*:639, 1978.
82. Nager, G. T., et al.: Fibrous dysplasia: A review of the disease and its manifestations in the temporal bone. Ann. Otol. Rhinol. Laryngol. (Suppl.) *92*:5, 1982.
83. Harris, W., et al.: The natural history of fibrous dysplasia. J. Bone Joint Surg. *44A*:207, 1962.
84. Danon, M., et al.: Cushing's syndrome. Sexual precocity and polyostotic fibrous dysplasia in infancy. J. Pediatr. *87*:917, 1975.
85. Hall, R., and Warrick, C. H.: Hypersecretion of hypothalamic releasing hormones: A possible explanation of the endocrine manifestations of polyostotic fibrous dysplasia (Albright's syndrome). Lancet *1*:1313, 1972.
86. Schwartz, B. T., and Alpert, M.: The malignant transformation of fibrous dysplasia. Am. J. Med. Sci. *247*:350, 1964.
87. Huvos, A. G., et al.: Bone sarcomas arising in fibrous dysplasia. J. Bone Joint Surg. *54A*:1047, 1972.
88. Cunningham, J. B., and Ackerman, L. V.: Metaphyseal fibrous defects. J. Bone Joint Surg. *38A*:797, 1956.
89. Sweetnam, R.: Primary malignant tumours of bone. Br. Med. J. *2*:1367, 1976.
90. Fraumeni, J. F., Jr.: Stature and malignant tumors of bone in childhood and adolescence. Cancer *20*:967, 1967.
91. Byers, P. D.: Solitary benign osteoblastic lesions of bone: Osteoid, osteoma and osteoblastoma. Cancer *22*:43, 1968.
92. Steiner, G. C.: Ultrastructure of osteoid osteoma. Hum. Pathol. *7*:309, 1976.
93. Jackson, R. P.: Recurrent osteoblastoma. Clin. Orthop. *131*:229, 1978.
94. Dahlin, D. C.: Osteosarcoma of bone and a consideration of prognostic variables. Cancer Treat. Rep. *62*:189, 1978.
95. Dorfman, H. D.: Malignant transformation of benign bone tensions. Proc. Natl. Cancer Conf. *7*:901, 1973.
96. Dahlin, D. C., and Coventry, M. B.: Osteogenic sarcoma, a study of 600 cases. J. Bone Joint Surg. *49A*:101, 1967.
97. Miller, R. W.: Contrasting epidemiology of childhood osteosarcoma, Ewing's tumor and rhabdomyosarcoma. Natl. Cancer Inst. Mongr. *56*:9, 1981.
98. Francois, J.: Retinoblastoma and osteogenic sarcoma. Ophthalmologica *175*:185, 1977.
99. Miller, R. W.: Etiology of childhood bone cancer. Epidemiologic observations. Recent Res. Cancer Res. *54*:50, 1976.
100. Finkel, M. P.: Pathogenesis of radiation and virus-induced bone tumors. Recent Res. Cancer Res. *54*:92, 1976.
101. Sinkovizs, J. G.: Bone sarcomas: Etiology and immunology. Can. J. Surg. *20*:494, 1977.
102. Komiya, S.: Electron microscopy of bone tumors—osteosarcoma, chondrosarcoma, giant cell tumor of bone. J. Jap. Orthop. Assoc. *56*:635, 1982.
103. Bubis, J. J.: Pathology of osteosarcoma. *In* Katznelson, A., and Nerubay, J. (eds.): Osteosarcoma: New Trends in Diagnosis and Treatment. New York, Alan R. Liss, 1982, p. 3.
103A. Schajowicz, F.: Juxtacortical chondrosarcoma. J. Bone Joint Surg. (Br.) *59*:473, 1977.
104. Gravanis, M. B., and Whitesides, T. E., Jr.: The unreliability of prognostic criteria in osteosarcoma. Am. J. Clin. Pathol. *53*:15, 1970.
105. Taylor, W. F., et al.: Trends and variability in survival from osteosarcoma. Mayo Clin. Proc. *53*:695, 1978.
106. Copeland, M. M., and Sutow, W. W.: Osteogenic sarcoma: The past, present, and future. *In* Murphy, G. P. (ed.): International Advances in Surgical Oncology. Vol. 2. New York, Alan R. Liss, 1979, p. 177.
107. Spjut, H. J., et al.: Tumors of Bone and Cartilage. Fascicle V. Washington, D.C., Armed Forces Institute of Pathology, 1971, p. 29.
108. Lewis, R. J., and Ketcham, A. S.: Maffucci's syndrome: Functional and neoplastic significance. J. Bone Joint Surg. *55A*:1465, 1979.
109. Rahimi, A., et al.: Chondromyxoid fibroma. A clinicopathologic study of 76 cases. Cancer *30*:726, 1972.
110. Sundaram, T. K. S.: Benign chondroblastoma. J. Bone Joint Surg. *48B*:92, 1966.
111. Reyes, C. V., et al.: Recurrent and aggressive chondroblastoma of the pelvis with late malignant neoplastic changes. Am. J. Surg. Pathol. *3*:449, 1979.
112. Evans, H. L., et al.: Prognostic factors in chondrosarcoma of bone. A clinicopathologic analysis with emphasis on histologic grading. Cancer *40*:818, 1977.
113. McCarthy, E. G., and Dorfman, H. B.: Chondrosarcoma of bone with dedifferentiation: A study of 18 cases. Hum. Pathol. *13*:36, 1982.
114. Dickman, P. S., et al.: Ewing's sarcoma. Characterization in established cultures and evidence of its histogenesis. Lab. Invest. *47*:375, 1982.
115. Falk, L., and Alpert, M.: The chemical and roentgen aspects of Ewing's sarcoma. Am. J. Med. Sci. *250*:492, 1965.
116. Mahoney, J. P., and Alexander, R. W.: Ewing's sarcoma: A light- and electron-microscopic study of 21 cases. Am. J. Surg. Pathol. *2*:283, 1978.
117. Telles, N. C., et al.: Ewing's sarcoma. An autopsy study. Cancer *41*:2321, 1978.
118. Rosen, G., et al.: Curability of Ewing's sarcoma and considerations for future therapeutic trials. Cancer *41*:888, 1978.
119. Johnston, J.: Giant cell tumor of bone. The role of the giant cell in orthopedic pathology. Orthop. Clin. North Am. *8*:751, 1977.
120. Yoshida, H., et al.: Giant cell tumor of bone. Virchows Arch. [Pathol. Anat.] *395*:319, 1982.
121. Alguacil-Garcia, A., et al.: Malignant giant cell tumor of soft parts. Cancer *40*:244, 1977.
122. Sanerkin, N. G.: Malignancy aggressiveness and recurrence in giant cell tumor of bone. Cancer *46*:1641, 1980.
123. Dahlin, D. C., et al.: Giant cell tumor, a study of 195 cases. Cancer *25*:1061, 1970.
124. Goldenberg, R. R., et al.: Giant cell tumor of bone. An analysis of 218 cases. J. Bone Joint Surg. *52A*:619, 1970.
125. Sim, F. H., et al.: Multicentric giant cell tumor of bone. J. Bone Joint Surg. *59A*:1052, 1977.

126. Mankin, H. J.: The reaction of articular cartilage to injury and osteoarthritis. N. Engl. J. Med. *291*:1285, 1335; 1974.
127. Gardner, D. L.: The nature and causes of osteoarthritis. Br. Med. J. *286*:418, 1983.
128. Huskisson, E. C.: Osteoarthritis: Changing concepts in pathogenesis and treatment. Postgrad. Med. *65*:97, 1979.
129. Roberts, J., and Burch, T. A.: Prevalence of osteoarthritis in adults. United States 1960–1962. United States Public Health Service Publication No. 1000. Series II. No. 15. Washington, D.C., United States Government Printing Office, 1966.
130. Hughes, G. R. V.: Osteoarthritis. Age Aging *8*(Suppl.):1, 1979.
131. Teitelbaum, S. L., and Bullough, P. G.: The pathophysiology of bone and joint disease. Am. J. Pathol. *96*:283, 1979.
132. Howell, D. S., et al.: A view on the pathogenesis of osteoarthritis. Bull. Rheum. Dis. *29*:996, 1978/79.
133. Nimni, M., and Deshmukh, K.: Differences in cartilage metabolism between normal and osteoarthritic human articular cartilage. Science *181*:751, 1973.
134. Editorial: Crystals in joints. Lancet *1*:1006, 1980.
135. Hazelton, R. A., et al.: Immunogenetic insights into rheumatoid arthritis: A family study. Q. J. Med. *51*(New Series):336, 1982.
136. Ziff, M.: Immunopathogenesis of rheumatoid arthritis. Eur. J. Rheumatol. Inflamm. *5*:469, 1982.
137. Hay, F. C., et al.: Intra-articular and circulating immune complexes and antiglobulins (IgG and IgM) in rheumatoid arthritis: Correlation with clinical features. Ann. Rheum. Dis. *38*:1, 1979.
138. Hollingsworth, J. W., and Saykaly, R. J.: Systemic complications of rheumatoid arthritis. Med. Clin. North Am. *61*:217, 1977.
139. Mainardi, C. L., et al.: Rheumatoid synovial collagenase: Proposed mechanisms for its release, activation and protection from inhibition in vivo. Arthr. Rheumatol. *19*:809, 1976.
140. Woolley, D. E., et al.: Collagenase at sites of cartilage erosion in the rheumatoid joint. Arthritis Rheum. *20*:1231, 1977.
141. Dayer, J. M., et al.: Production of collagenase and prostaglandins by isolated adherent rheumatoid synovial cells. Proc. Natl. Acad. Sci. U.S.A. *73*:945, 1976.
142. Williams, R. C.: Immunopathology of rheumatoid arthritis. Hosp. Pract. *13*:53, 1978.
143. Alspaugh, M. A., et al.: Lymphocytes transformed by Epstein-Barr virus. Induction of nuclear antigen reactive with antibody in rheumatoid arthritis. J. Exp. Med. *147*:1018, 1978.
144. Depper, J. M., et al.: Abnormal regulation of Epstein-Barr virus transformation of rheumatoid lymphoid cells. Arthritis Rheum. *22*:605, 1979.
145. Johnson, P. M., et al.: Antiglobulin production to altered IgG in rheumatoid arthritis. Lancet *1*:611, 1975.
146. Schaller, J.: Juvenile rheumatoid arthritis. Postgrad. Med. *61*:177, 1977.
147. Editorial: Felty's syndrome. Lancet *1*:540, 1978.
148. Wyngaarden, J. B., and Kelley, W. N.: Gout. *In* Stanbury, J. B., et al. (eds.): Metabolic Basis of Inherited Disease. 5th ed. New York, McGraw-Hill Book Co., 1982, p. 1043.
149. Boss, G. R., and Seegmiller, J. E.: Hyperuricemia and gout. Classification, complications and management. N. Engl. J. Med. *300*:1459, 1979.
150. Kozin, F., et al.: Polymorphonuclear response to monosodium urate crystals: Modification by absorbed serum proteins. J. Rheumatol. *6*:519, 1979.
151. Rae, S. A., et al.: Leukotriene B_4, an inflammatory mediator in gout. Lancet *2*:1122, 1982.
152. Chung, E. B.: Histologic changes in gout. Georgetown Med. Bull. *15*:269, 1962.
153. Reif, M. C., et al.: Chronic gouty nephropathy: A vanishing syndrome. N. Engl. J. Med. *304*:535, 1981.
154. Evans, H. L.: Synovial sarcoma. A study of 123 biphasic and 17 probable monophasic examples. Pathol. Annu. *15*(Part 2):309, 1980.
155. Hajdu, S. I., et al.: Tendosynovial sarcoma. A clinicopathologic study of 136 cases. Cancer *39*:1201, 1977.
156. Krall, R. A., et al.: Synovial sarcoma. A clinical, pathological and ultrastructural study of 26 cases supporting the recognition of a monophasic variant. Am. J. Surg. Pathol. *5*:137, 1981.
157. Corson, J. M., et al.: Keratin proteins in synovial sarcoma (letter). Am. J. Surg. Pathol. *7*:107, 1983.
158. Harris, M.: The ultrastructure of benign and malignant fibrous histiocytomas. Histopathology *4*:29, 1980.
159. Reddick, R. L., et al.: Malignant soft tissue tumors (malignant fibrous histiocytoma, pleomorphic liposarcoma, and pleomorphic rhabdomyosarcoma): An electron microscopic study. Hum. Pathol. *10*:327, 1979.
160. McCarthy, E. F., et al.: Malignant fibrous histiocytoma of bone. A study of 35 cases. Hum. Pathol. *10*:57, 1979.
161. Weiss, S. W., and Enzinger, F. M.: Malignant fibrous histiocytoma. An analysis of 200 cases. Cancer *41*:2250, 1978.
162. Meister, P., et al.: Malignant fibrous histiocytoma: Histological patterns and cell types. Pathol. Res. Pract. *168*:193, 1980.
163. Ekfors, T. O., and Rantakokko, V.: An analysis of 38 malignant fibrous histiocytomas in the extremities. Acta Pathol. Microbiol. Scand. (A) *86A*:25, 1978.
164. Myers, B. W., et al.: Pigmented villonodular synovitis and tenosynovitis: A clinical epidemiologic study of 166 cases and literature review. Medicine *59*:223, 1980.
165. Schumacher, H. R., et al.: Pigmented villonodular synovitis: Light and electron microscopic studies. Semin. Arthritis Rheum. *12*:32, 1982.
166. Ghadially, F. N., et al.: Ultrastructure of pigmented villonodular synovitis. J. Pathol. *127*:19, 1979.

29 THE NERVOUS SYSTEM

JAMES H. MORRIS, B.M., B.Ch.* and
WILLIAM C. SCHOENE, M.D.†

*Pathologist, Brigham and Women's Hospital, and Assistant Professor, Harvard Medical School, Boston.
†Pathologist, Brigham and Women's Hospital, and Associate Professor, Harvard Medical School, Boston.

NORMAL

On first encounter the nervous system appears to be an impossibly complex assembly of neurons and glia, but on further acquaintance the principles of its organization become clearer. Similarly, neuropathology initially seems to be a forbidding array of obscure, and usually eponymous, diseases with few counterparts in general pathology. Again, a few principles can bring some order to this apparent chaos.

1. Diseases of the nervous system fall into two general categories:
   a. Pathologic processes, such as infections, trauma, and neoplasms, found in both the nervous system and other organs.
   b. Diseases unique to the nervous system. This category includes the diseases of myelin and system degenerations of neurons. They are much rarer than diseases with systemic counterparts.
2. The *localization* or *distribution of function* in the nervous system has important effects on the presentation and progression of diseases involving it:
   a. Localization of function makes the brain *inherently vulnerable to focal lesions* that, in other organs, where function is more uniformly distributed, might go unremarked or produce only trivial symptoms. For example, the destruction of quite small areas of brain can severely impair specific activities such as speech or the ability to move one side of the body. By contrast, two-thirds of the renal mass can be destroyed without fatally compromising renal function. This susceptibility of the brain to focal lesions is compounded by its strictly limited capacity to reconstitute damaged tissue. There has clearly been a serious oversight by the celestial committee in its design of an organ that is so important for biologic survival and is both the most vulnerable to and the least tolerant of focal damage.
   b. The localization of function in the nervous system *causes the same pathologic process to present in a completely different way when it affects a different part of the system.* For example: a meningioma (p. 1407) in the olfactory groove might become manifest only insidiously with unilateral anosmia, but when located in the foramen magnum could cause a rapidly progressive and immediately life-threatening quadriplegia from spinal cord compression.
3. Another type of localizing effect in the brain is the *selective vulnerability* of groups of neurons or specific regions of the brain to particular pathologic processes or etiologic agents. For example, Purkinje cells of the cerebellum and hippocampal neurons are particularly susceptible to ischemia; herpes simplex virus I attacks the temporal lobes; amyotrophic lateral sclerosis (ALS) is a degenerative disease affecting only upper and lower motor neurons. The basis for these differences in susceptibility is largely unknown.
4. Yet another aspect of localization derives from the fact that the histologic reactions of the nervous system are to a degree nonspecific so that different diseases may induce a rather similar histologic appearance. Diagnosis may, therefore, depend as much on the localization, or distribution, of the changes as on their character. For instance, neurofibrillary tangles (described below), when primarily localized in the cerebral cortex suggest Alzheimer's disease, but when found predominantly in the substantia nigra, they are diagnostic of postencephalitic Parkinson's disease, a condition with a completely different clinical presentation and course.
5. A number of anatomic and physiologic features are peculiar to the nervous system and critically affect the nature, growth, spread, presentation, and treatment of disease within it. Prominent among these features are the presence of a blood-brain barrier; the fact that the nervous system is an immunologically privileged site; the presence of the cerebrospinal fluid–filled cerebral ventricles and subarachnoid space; and the limited and fixed volume of the intracranial contents. Some of these factors are interrelated and operate in conjunction, but all are important in the pathophysiology of disease in the nervous system.

It is apparent, therefore, that clinicopathologic correlation is important to the understanding and diagnosis of disease in the nervous system. Because the system is so complex and widespread, it is nearly impossible to examine all its parts in detail, and so it is vital to determine which part is involved clinically before it is examined pathologically. In many cases, a diagnosis can be made only by correlating the clinical and pathologic findings.

NORMAL CELLS AND THEIR BASIC REACTIONS TO INJURY

The principal cells of the nervous system are neurons, glial cells, and microglia. The reactions of the cells of the brain to injury are different from those of the somatic organs, and so it is appropriate to review them before considering specific pathologic processes.

NEURONS

The neuron is the basic communicating unit of the nervous system and possesses the dendrites, axons, and synapses required for this role. Microscopically, the typical neuron is the pyramidal cortical neuron, of triangular shape and with a large pale nucleus containing a prominent nucleolus. Although classically pyramidal, there is an enormous range of neuronal size and shape, well illustrated by the felicitous juxtaposition of the large Purkinje and small granular neurons in the cerebellar cortex. When it can be seen, neuronal cytoplasm is distinguished by the presence of Nissl substance, which the electron microscope shows to be clumps of rough surfaced endoplasmic reticulum and free ribosomal rosettes. Other special features of neuronal cytoplasm are neurofilaments, microtubules, and different types of synaptic vesicles.[1] Neurofilaments are intermediate filaments (p. 28) specific to neurons and are composed of three polypeptide chains with molecular weights of 68K, 150K, and 200K daltons.[2]

In disease a variety of changes occur in neurons that are, to varying degrees, associated with specific etiologic agents or pathologic processes.

1. *Ischemic cell change (red neurons).* Ischemia causes neuronal shrinkage and angulation; the cytoplasm becomes eosinophilic, hence the appellation red, and the nucleus pyknotic and triangular. Once these changes occur, they are irreversible and indicate cell death.

2. *Simple atrophy.* In this process the neuron gradually degenerates and disappears without inciting any inflammatory reaction, but usually with some consequent gliosis (see below). It is the underlying process in the system degenerations such as the spinocerebellar degenerations (p. 1418). Its cause is obscure and is probably different in different diseases.

3. *Transsynaptic degeneration.* Death or injury of one system of neurons may provoke degeneration in another dependent system with which it synapses. Removal of an eye causes degeneration of the optic nerve and tract and, subsequently, "transsynaptic degeneration" of the neurons in the lateral geniculate body with which the axons of the optic tract synapse. The degeneration takes the form of a simple atrophy.

4. *Intraneuronal bodies.* A number of the degenerative diseases have specific intraneuronal cytoplasmic bodies. These include Lewy bodies, Pick bodies, and Hirano bodies; each will be discussed with the appropriate diseases.

5. *Neurofibrillary tangle* formation is a particular type of neuronal degeneration that occurs in a number of diseases. With the light microscope, tangles appear as a skein of basophilic, silver (Bodian) staining filaments in the cytoplasm, which displace or encircle the nucleus (Fig. 29–1). Electron microscopically, they are mostly paired, helically wound filaments with a filament diameter of 7 to 9 nm and a period of 80 nm.[3] In some tangles, especially those seen in progressive supranuclear palsy (p. 1418), the filaments are not always helically wound, but it is not clear that this indicates any fundamental difference.[4] Unsuccessful attempts to analyze tangles probably relate to their being insoluble, as a result of covalent glutamyl-lysine cross-linking of their filaments.[5] Immunologic studies suggest that a major component of these tangles is neurofilaments.[6, 7] Interestingly, positive reactions can be obtained with antibodies to whole neurofilaments but only inconsistently with antibodies to the purified polypeptide chain subunits, a finding that is possibly a reflection of the highly insoluble nature of the tangles, which allows only certain groups to be exposed to immunologic recognition. To date there is no good explanation for the stable cross-linking of the neurofilaments into neurofibrillary tangles.[5]

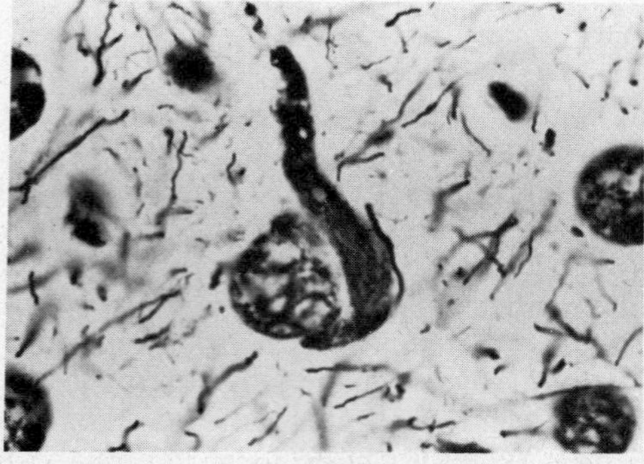

Figure 29–1. Neurofibrillary tangle consisting of a skein of silver-positive material within a neuron (Bodian stain).

At one time neurofibrillary tangles were most notably associated with Alzheimer's disease (p. 1414), but their presence in other diseases suggests that they are the final common pathway of a number of pathophysiologic processes, all of which are currently mysterious. Other conditions in which neurofibrillary tangles are found include postencephalitic Parkinson's disease (p. 1417); progressive supranuclear palsy (p. 1418); Down's syndrome (p. 126); dementia pugilistica;[8] ALS/parkinsonism/dementia complex of Guam.[9]

6. *Storage in neurons.* Neurons may be the depository of various stored substances such as lipids and polysaccharides in the inborn errors of metabolism (e.g., Niemann-Pick disease, p. 145). Microscopically, the neurons are large and round with an eccentrically placed nucleus. The cytoplasm contains the stored material and often has a granular appearance regardless of the composition of the material. Electron microscopy shows details of the ultrastructure of the material, which is sometimes diagnostic. Biochemical evaluation of either brain tissue or some other organ is usually the definitive investigation.[10]

7. *Central chromatolysis* (axonal reaction). If its axon is cut or damaged the cell body swells up, becoming round and pale, and there is loss of stainable Nissl substance. The nucleus is displaced to the periphery of the cell. This change is most dramatically seen in anterior horn cells after there has been damage to a peripheral nerve.

8. *Damage to axons.* Neuronal dysfunction may be manifested by a failure to maintain the axon, which undergoes a process of degeneration starting at its peripheral end—a process called "*dying back.*" This is most frequently seen in the peripheral nervous system (p. 1428), but may also become apparent in the central nervous system, notably at the upper end of the dorsal columns and the lower end of the corticospinal tract.

9. *Spheroids. Spheroids* are local dilatations of axons that often contain many organelles and appear histologically as circular, eosinophilic, granular bodies. They are seen around the edges of infarcts and in axonal dystrophies, and in these circumstances are an indicator of axonal damage, but they may also be seen at the growing tips of regenerating axons.

NEUROGLIA

The neuroglial cells are the proletarians of CNS society, providing shelter and maintenance for the aristocratic neurons. They consist of astrocytes, oligodendrocytes, ependymal cells, and microglial cells.

Astrocytes and Their Reactions. Routine stains demonstrate only astrocyte nuclei that are round or oval and have a fine granular chromatin. With special stains that demonstrate their cytoplasm, they emerge as stellate cells with processes that ramify as an interstitial framework for the parenchymal cells of the brain (Fig. 29–2). They have terminal specializations ending on blood vessels that are called *foot processes* or *end feet.* Astrocytes are divided into *protoplasmic* and *fibrous* forms on the basis of the geometry of their processes; the protoplasmic form occurs mostly in gray matter and has frequently branched processes, whereas the fibrous astrocytes have long thin processes and are found mostly in white matter.

The functions of astrocytes are incompletely understood but probably include the provision of biochemical and physical support, and aid in insulation of the receptive surfaces of neurons. In addition to their activities in normal brain, they also react to CNS injury by glial scar formation. The process is called *gliosis;* it involves the proliferation of fibrillary astrocytes with the formation of many glial fibers that, despite their name, are cellular processes of the astrocytes. Unlike the fibrosis that occurs in the somatic organs, no collagen or equivalent extracellular fibrous protein is formed in gliosis. There are abundant intermediate filaments in these glial fibers, some of which are specific glial fibrillary acidic protein (GFAP), but most are vimentin.[2] The former are well demonstrated by immunoperoxidase preparations for GFAP, but are also stained by phosphotungstic acid–hematoxylin (PTAH) and Holzer. Some astrocytes are further described as *gemistocytic* because of their "stuffed" appearance with abundant eosinophilic homogenous cytoplasm that extends into their processes. This type of astrocyte usually appears in response to a crude tissue injury such as an infarct. If disease damages a specific tract, the resultant gliosis conforms to the pattern of that tract and is called *isomorphic gliosis.* When there is gross tissue destruction, the gliosis is random and is called *anisomorphic gliosis.*

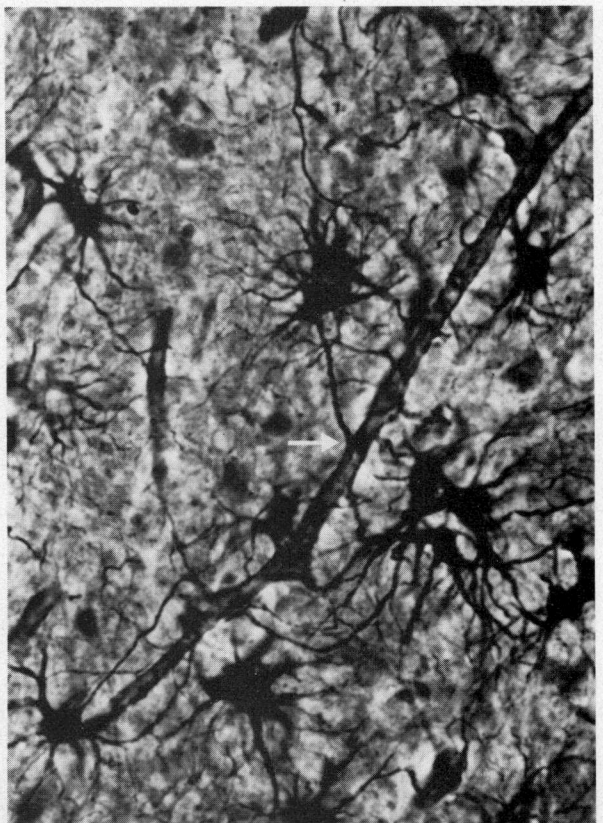

Figure 29–2. Astrocytes and their processes. Some processes are attached to blood vessels (*arrow*) (Cajal gold sublimate).

Rosenthal fibers may be seen in astrocytic processes. They are eosinophilic, opaque, elongated, tapering or globular bodies that are strongly PTAH positive but GFAP negative. With the electron microscope they appear as irregular, amorphous, electron-dense material surrounded by a dense feltwork of intermediate filaments.[11] They are found where there is long-standing progressive gliosis, but are also present in juvenile pilocytic astrocytomas (p. 1403), which are very slowly growing tumors, and in Alexander's disease, an extremely rare leukodystrophy.

Alzheimer II astrocytes have dilated vesicular nuclei with a thickened irregular nuclear membrane and a small eosinophilic intranuclear body containing glycogen, called a *glycogen dot.* Cytoplasmic processes are not prominent and are not seen in routine stains. Alzheimer II astrocytes are seen in conditions in which the blood ammonia level is raised, principally hepatic failure. In certain other metabolic disturbances and toxic states, astrocyte nuclei also become dilated and vesicular but do not develop the glycogen dot.

Polyglucosan bodies[12] are spherical or elongated, basophilic, PAS-positive, sometimes concentrically layered structures with diameters ranging between 1 and 150 μm. Electron microscopically they are seen to be composed of branched filaments approximately 8 nm in diameter, having both granular and amorphous associated material. Biochemical analysis shows their principal component to be glucose polymers (polyglucosans) with a small and variable content of phosphate and sulphate groups and not more than 5% protein. They are seen in different conditions but are not biochemically distinguishable. The most well-known form of polyglucosan bodies are *corpora amylacea.* In astrocyte processes, these accumulate with aging and are found principally in the subpial and subependymal regions, and also around blood vessels. The *Lafora bodies* seen in the perikarya of neurons in myoclonus epilepsy (Lafora's disease) are polyglucosan bodies biochemically indistinguishable from corpora amylacea. In *type IV* glycogenosis (amylopectinosis) (p. 150), in which there is a deficiency of branching enzyme, small polyglucosan bodies are present in astrocytes. Polyglucosan bodies are also found in a number of rare neurologic conditions. Although these bodies develop with branching enzyme deficiency, a lack of this enzyme is not likely to be fundamental to their origin, because it is known to function normally in Lafora's disease.

Oligodendrocytes. These glial cells are so called because, when visualized by special stains, they have fewer and shorter processes than do astrocytes. Routine stains, however, demonstrate only the nucleus, which is round and lymphocyte-sized and has uniformly dense chromatin. Electron microscopically, the nucleus is eccentrically located in a cytoplasm distinguished by many microtubules, which makes it difficult to distinguish between oligodendrocyte processes and dendrites. Oligodendrocytes are found in both white and gray matter. In white matter they are frequently lined up along the myelinated fibers in an interfascicular arrangement, whereas in gray matter they commonly cluster around neurons, where they are called *satellite cells.* Their principal function is the production and maintenance of CNS myelin. Unlike the Schwann cells (p. 1428) of the peripheral nervous system, oligodendrocytes contribute segments of myelin sheath to multiple axons. Because they produce the myelin, diseases of oligodendrocytes manifest themselves as disorders of myelin and myelination. The two principal categories are the *leukodystrophies* (p. 1424), which are generalized, usually hereditary disorders of myelin metabolism, and the acquired *demyelinating diseases* (p. 1410), such as multiple sclerosis with focal myelin loss.

Ependyma. A single layer of cuboidal-to-columnar ependymal cells lines the cerebral ventricles, the aqueduct, and the central canal of the spinal cord. Ependyma reacts to injury mainly by cell loss, and the ensuing gaps are filled with glial fibers produced by the subependymal astrocytes (ependymitis granularis). Inclusion bodies can also be seen in ependymal cells in some viral disorders, such as cytomegalic inclusion disease.

Microglia. These are small cells with elongated nuclei and are scattered throughout the white and gray matter. Routine stains are taken up only by the nucleus, but with special stains they can be seen to have long angular cytoplasmic processes having few organelles but scattered dense bodies. In response to injury or destruction of the brain they become activated and assume the shape of a macrophage *(gitter cells, compound granular corpuscles),* or they proliferate and adopt a rodlike form. Sometimes, swarms of rod cells can be seen surrounding a tiny focus of necrosis or a dead neuron, forming a glial *nodule.* Microglial degradation of dead neurons is called *neuronophagia.*

Historically, there have been two schools of thought about the origin of these cells, one holding that they are ectodermally derived and the other that they are of mesodermal origin like the rest of the mononuclear phagocyte (reticuloendothelial) system (MPS). Recent work shows that, when activated, they yield histochemical reactions similar to macrophages and other members of the MPS but quite different from the reactions of true glial cells.[13] It now seems likely that they are in fact the nervous system representative of the MPS. As such, the name microglia, which tends to link them with the true glial cells, is misleading but probably unchangeable.

Table 29–1. SPECIAL STAINS USED IN NEUROPATHOLOGY

Stains	Demonstrates
Nissl *(cresyl violet)*	Neurons, glial nuclei
Phosphotungstic acid–hematoxylin (PTAH)	(a) Glial fibers, e.g., in *astrocytomas and gliosis* (b) Connective tissue
Holzer	Gliosis
Myelin stain, e.g., *Woelcke, Luxol-fast-blue*	Myelin sheaths
Marchi and Oil-Red-O	Myelin breakdown
Silver, e.g., (a) *Bielschowsky, Cajal, Golgi;*	(a) Neurons and axons
(b) *Hortega carbonate*	(b) Oligodendrocytes, microglia
Cajal gold sublimate	Astrocytes

SPECIAL STAINS IN NEUROPATHOLOGY

Because many diseases of the nervous system affect only certain of its elements, there is a need for equally selective stains. In multiple sclerosis, for example, there is loss of myelin without equivalent loss of axons, best revealed by selective stains for myelin and for axons. Special stains are available for neurons, astrocytes, axons, and myelin. Immunocytochemical techniques are also used. Currently, the most widely available one is an immunoperoxidase method for GFAP that is specific for astrocytes and some ependymal tumors.[14, 15] Many more specific antibodies will undoubtedly be discovered, and early reports suggest that it might become possible to identify subpopulations of neurons.[16] This might be helpful in the elucidation of degenerative diseases in which there is selective loss of neurons, such as Alzheimer's disease where there appears to be a disproportionate loss of cholinergic neurons. Some of the available stains are listed in Table 29–1.

PATHOLOGY

COMMON PATHOPHYSIOLOGIC COMPLICATIONS

Among the unique anatomic and physiologic features of the nervous system, the fixed and restricted volume of the cranial vault is particularly important. It renders the brain susceptible to a group of pathophysiologic complications, particularly *increased intracranial pressure, cerebral edema,* and *hydrocephalus,* which occur in different pathologic processes. *Increased intracranial pressure* occurs with all *space-occupying lesions* that increase the volume of the intracranial contents; it has several seriously detrimental or life-threatening effects. Frequently encountered examples of such space-occupying lesions include hemorrhage, neoplasm, abscess, cerebral edema, and hydrocephalus. Of these, *cerebral edema* and *hydrocephalus* are secondary effects that occur in a number of diseases, and the presence of either or both exacerbates increased intracranial pressure from any other cause. This interaction is one of the most often met, important, dangerous complications occurring in CNS disease.

INCREASED INTRACRANIAL PRESSURE AND HERNIATIONS OF BRAIN

Increased intracranial pressure is defined as elevation of the mean cerebrospinal fluid (CSF) pressure above 200 mm of water (15 mm of mercury) when measured with the patient in the lateral decubitus position.[17] It occurs whenever the volume of intracranial contents increases beyond the slight leeway allowed for expansion. Clinically, it presents with symptoms such as periodic headache, mental slowness, confusion, and papilledema. Because increased intracranial pressure may be caused by many pathologic processes, diagnosis and treatment depend on identifying the underlying cause and understanding the ways in which the brain is thereby affected.

Most cases of increased intracranial pressure are associated with some sort of mass effect that may be either diffuse, as in the case of the generalized edema of the brain in lead encephalopathy, or focal, such as that seen with tumors, abscesses, or hematomas. Regardless of the cause, *it is the compression of or hemorrhage into the brain stem that is most life threatening.*

On gross examination when the increase in pressure is due to some expansile process within the brain, there is either focal or diffuse flattening of the cortical gyri, sometimes associated with compressed or distorted ventricles. The cranial vault is partitioned by relatively rigid dural folds that form the falx cerebri and the tentorium cerebelli. Localized expansion of the brain causes it to be displaced in relation to these partitions, producing **brain herniations.**

Herniations are classified on the basis of the part that is herniated and the structure under which it has been pushed (Fig. 29–3). Expansion of one hemisphere may cause the cingulate gyrus to herniate under the falx, producing **subfalcine herniation.** The same expansion will also cause the medial temporal lobe to be forced into the gap between the cerebral peduncles and the tentorium, producing **uncinate (uncal) or transtentorial herniation.** This may damage the oculomotor nerve, producing the well-known fixed dilated pupil, and also compress the contralateral cerebral peduncle against the free edge of the tentorium, resulting in a paralysis ipsilateral to the lesion, a famous false localizing sign. Downward movement of the posterior fossa contents may produce **herniation of the cerebellar tonsils into the foramen magnum,** a process often called **coning,** which compresses the medulla and its vital respiratory center. This medullary compression causes death in

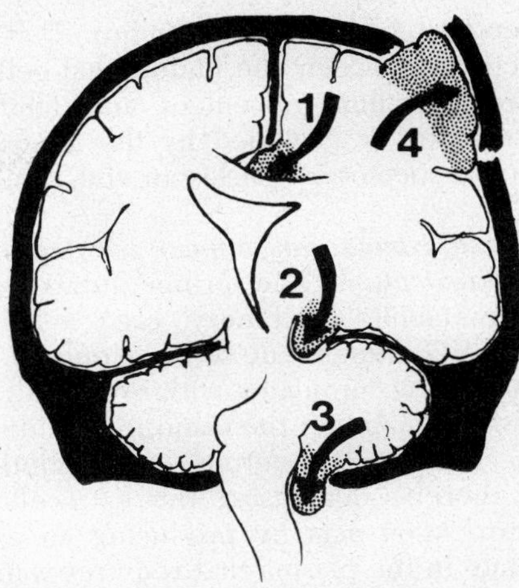

Figure 29–3. Herniations of the brain: (1) cingulate, (2) uncal (hippocampal), (3) cerebellar, and (4) transcalvarial. (From Fishman, R. A.: Brain edema. N. Engl. J. Med. *293*:706, 1975. Reprinted, by permission, from The New England Journal of Medicine.)

patients with tonsillar herniation. Upward herniation of the posterior fossa contents can occur when a mass is located in the posterior fossa. Finally, brain may herniate through skull defects.

Herniations may produce two other effects on the brain. First, they compress surface arteries against the unyielding edge of dural folds, which may occlude the vessels and cause brain infarction. This is seen in the posterior cerebral artery when it is compressed against the free edge of the tentorium in uncinate herniation, and in the callosal marginal branches of the anterior cerebral artery where they pass underneath the falx in subfalcine herniation. Second, in rapidly expanding supratentorial processes, there is compression and downward displacement of the midbrain where it passes through the tentorium. By mechanisms that are not understood, this produces linear hemorrhages in the mesencephalon and upper pons **(Duret hemorrhages).** Brain swelling severe enough to cause this complication is almost invariably fatal.

CEREBRAL EDEMA

Cerebral edema occurs when there is an increase in CNS water content. If the excess water accumulates intracellularly, it is called *cytotoxic edema;* if in the extracellular space, it is termed *vasogenic edema.*[17] The particular susceptibility to and significance of edema in the CNS is conditioned by special anatomic and physiologic features of the brain. In addition to the already discussed restricted volume of the cranial contents, there is (1) the *blood-brain barrier* (BBB), which restricts osmotic movement of particles such as the plasma proteins across the cerebral capillaries; and (2) *the absence in the brain of lymphatics to carry away excess fluid.* The existence of a BBB was first suspected when it was noticed that albumin-bound intravital dyes such as trypan blue do not generally stain the brain.[18] Subsequent ultrastructural and tracer studies using agents such as horseradish peroxidase have located the barrier at the cerebral capillary endothelium.[19, 20] There are tight junctions between the endothelial cells that prevent intercellular fluid movement, and significant intracellular transport is excluded by the almost complete absence of pinocytotic vesicles in the capillary endothelial cells.

Cytotoxic edema may appear with either ischemia or water intoxication. The former induces a defect in the cells' metabolic machinery, e.g., a failure in the membrane ATP-dependent sodium pump. When this occurs, sodium accumulates within the cell and water then follows to maintain the osmotic equilibrium, causing all the brain cells (neurons, glia, endothelial cells) to swell, thereby decreasing the extracellular space. Water intoxication acts by producing an acute hypo-osmolar state in the plasma that requires water to move into the cerebral cells to maintain osmotic equilibrium.

Vasogenic edema is the most common form of cerebral edema. It occurs in association with primary and metastatic tumors, abscesses, hemorrhages, infections, contusions, and lead encephalopathy. The edema fluid leaks into the extracellular space either through damaged capillary endothelial cells that have lost their barrier function or through newly formed capillaries that have not yet established a barrier. Neovascularization is particularly pronounced in tumors, especially metastatic tumors, and in the capsule of abscesses. White matter is conspicuously more affected than gray and the edema may be focal or diffuse. If focal, it is more intense immediately adjacent to the process causing the edema.

Interstitial edema is a third form of cerebral edema seen in obstructive hydrocephalus. In this type of edema, fluid crosses the ventricular lining and accumulates in the periventricular white matter.

Grossly, all forms of cerebral edema produce focal or diffuse brain swelling with gyral flattening. Vasogenic edema causes loosening of the tissue with separation of the myelin sheaths and generally poor staining. Lucent halos are seen around the cell nuclei, particularly oligodendrocytes and astrocytes. In cytotoxic edema there is diffuse swelling of cells without significant enlargement of the extracellular space. Electron microscopic examination of experimental models of vasogenic edema show increased extracellular space with, however, distention of the astrocytic foot processes.[21]

So many conditions secondarily produce cerebral edema that it is a very common clinical problem and major contributor to cerebral herniation and even death. In many cases there is both cytotoxic and vasogenic edema, as, for instance, in arterial occlusion or purulent meningitis when osmotic and metabolic processes combine to damage both cells and blood vessels, resulting in increases in both extracellular and intracellular water.

HYDROCEPHALUS

Hydrocephalus refers to distention of the ventricles with an increase in CSF volume (Figs. 29–4 and 29–5). CSF is produced by the choroid plexus, after which it travels through the ventricles, foramen of Monro, aqueduct of Sylvius, fourth ventricle, and cerebellar foramina to finally reach the subarachnoid space. The CSF is resorbed for the most part by the arachnoid villi.

Hydrocephalus may result from one of two mechanisms: (1) overproduction of CSF or (2) much more commonly, decreased absorption of CSF. Decreased absorption of CSF, may in turn, result from either (a) inability of the arachnoid villi to transfer CSF to the venous system or (b) a block in the CSF pathway to the villi. In the latter situation, CSF backs up behind the

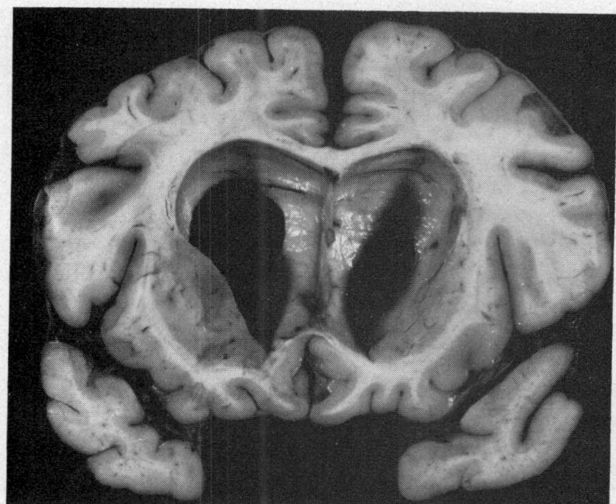

Figure 29–4. Hydrocephalus. Dilated lateral ventricles seen in a coronal section through frontal lobes.

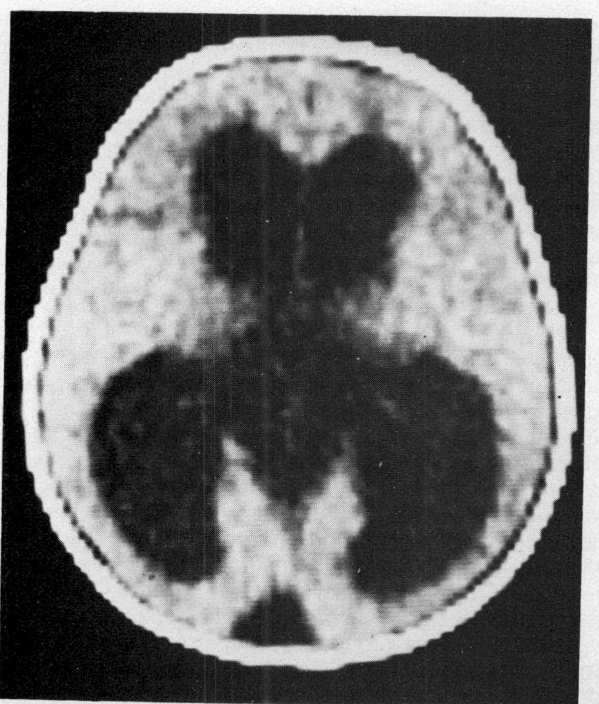

Figure 29–5. CT scan showing massively dilated ventricular system characteristic of hydrocephalus.

block. When the block is in the CSF pathway within the brain, the hydrocephalus is known as *noncommunicating* or *obstructive*. If, on the other hand, CSF is able to pass into the subarachnoid space and is subsequently prevented from being absorbed by the arachnoid villi, the hydrocephalus is known as the *communicating* type. In the latter situation, the blockage either is in the subarachnoid space proper or is the result of damage to or malfunction of the arachnoid villi.

In infants and children, before fusion of the cranial sutures occurs, hydrocephalus may be manifested most dramatically by enlargement of the head. The incidence of such childhood hydrocephalus varies from 0.2 to 5 per 1000 births.[22] Hydrocephalus in children may have many causes including congenital malformations, infections, trauma, subarachnoid hemorrhage, and tumors (Table 29–2). Genetic abnormalities, viruses, irradiation, and vitamin deficiencies have been linked experimentally with congenital abnormalities associated with hydrocephalus.

Hydrocephalus in adults, occurring after the bones of the skull are fused, does not produce enlargement of the head. The onset of adult hydrocephalus may be either acute and rapidly symptomatic, or slow in developing and insidious. Acute hydrocephalus is usually manifested by signs of increased intracranial pressure, and it is frequently associated with trauma, infection, subarachnoid hemorrhage, and brain tumors (Table 29–2). In contrast, slowly developing hydrocephalus is usually productive of progressive dementia, gait disturbance, and incontinence. These patients often have normal CSF pressures and the clinical syndrome is called *normal-pressure hydrocephalus*.[23] Differentiation of normal-pressure hydrocephalus from other causes of dementia is exceedingly important, as patients with the former condition have a dramatic reversal of neurologic disabilities if a ventricular shunt is installed early in the course of the disorder. Examination by CT scan often facilitates the clinical diagnosis of all types of hydrocephalus (Fig. 29–5). Most cases of normal-pressure hydrocephalus are of unknown etiology; some are secondary to subarachnoid hemorrhage.

Table 29–2. CAUSES OF HYDROCEPHALUS*

Obstructive or Noncommunicating Hydrocephalus
- ***Congenital Malformation***
  - Stenosis of aqueduct of Sylvius (a few cases are familial)
  - Forking or atresia of aqueduct of Sylvius
  - Gliosis of aqueduct of Sylvius
  - Occlusion of foramina of Magendie and Luschka (Dandy-Walker syndrome) (with large cystic fourth ventricle)
  - Arnold-Chiari malformation (usually with myelomeningocele)
  - Vascular malformations (e.g., aneurysm of great vein of Galen)
- ***Neoplasms***
- ***Inflammatory Processes***
  - Subarachnoid hemorrhage
  - Meningitis and postmeningitic states
  - Other infections (e.g., toxoplasmosis, cytomegalic inclusion disease)

Communicating Hydrocephalus
- ***Overproduction of Cerebrospinal Fluid***
  - Adenomata of choroid plexus (?)
  - Other causes (?)
- ***Deficient Reabsorption of Cerebrospinal Fluid***
  - Postmeningitic states
  - Posthemorrhagic states
  - Thrombosis of dural sinuses
  - Deficiency of arachnoid villi (?)

*Modified from Paine, R. S.: Hydrocephalus. Pediatr. Clin. North Am. *14*:781, 1967.

On gross examination, both obstructive (or noncommunicating) and communicating types of hydrocephalus show progressive active dilation of the brain's ventricles by CSF (Figs. 29–4 and 29–5). The ependyma and adjacent white matter are secondarily injured as dilation increases. Following injury to the ependyma, fluid passes into the surrounding brain, causing interstitial edema. On microscopic examination, the ependymal lining may be lost and the surrounding white matter is pale and rarefied. The overlying cortex is spared unless the dilation is severe and long-standing.

Hydrocephalus ex vacuo refers to compensatory enlargement of the ventricular system associated with severe brain atrophy, and results from actual loss of CNS tissue. CSF is produced and absorbed normally. The condition occurs most frequently in association with Alzheimer's and Pick's diseases (p. 1414).

IATROGENIC DISEASE

Many modern forms of treatment produce immunosuppression, either as a side effect or, in the case of organ transplantation, as a therapeutic aim. This has resulted in the emergence of a number of opportunistic infections and altered the occurrence and natural history of other infections.[24] With impairment of the usual inflammatory and immune reactions, the clinical presentation of disease and the pathologic appearance of infected tissues is altered. Generally, these infections are more fulminant and less easy to diagnose than in the normal patient. Progressive multifocal leukoencephalopathy (PML) (p. 1386) is a viral disease of oligodendrocytes that is almost unknown outside the immunocompromised population. Toxoplasmosis (p. 373) in the normal adult produces a lymphadenopathy that is

Table 29–3. IATROGENIC DISEASES

Infectious	(1) Bacterial—Meningitides with unusual organisms, e.g., Citrobacter
	(2) Viral—Progressive multifocal leukoencephalopathy (PML)
	(3) Fungal and protozoal—e.g., aspergillosis, candidiasis, toxoplasmosis
Toxic	(1) Radiation necrosis
	(2) Chemotherapy/radiation necrosis
	(3) Peripheral neuropathy—e.g., vinca alkaloids
	(4) Central pontine myelinolysis
Immune	(1) Encephalitis following vaccination
	(2) Acute idiopathic polyneuritis following vaccination

self-limiting, but in the immunosuppressed patient it may produce a fulminant multifocal necrotizing encephalitis that may be rapidly fatal.[25] Anticancer treatment such as radiation and chemotherapeutic agents may also be neurotoxic, and other forms of therapy may produce immune reactions in the nervous system. Individual diseases are discussed in the appropriate sections, but the major types of iatrogenic disease that affect the nervous system are indicated in Table 29–3 (p. 1377).

INFECTIONS

Anatomic and physiologic features of the nervous system influence the pathophysiology of its infections. The most obvious of these is that the brain is bathed in cerebrospinal fluid (CSF), which provides both a congenial culture medium for the infecting organisms and a rapid means of dissemination of the infection throughout the system once the outer defenses have been breached. Further, all the arterial supply and venous drainage of the brain has to pass through this CSF-filled subarachnoid space. This is particularly important in the meningitides, as will be pointed out. Because the nervous system is so well shielded from outside influences, organisms infecting it must first involve other regions of the body and so sometimes evoke prodromal syndromes related to these extracranial involvements.

There are four ways in which infection can enter the nervous system.

1. *Via the bloodstream.* This is the most frequent mode of entry with many bacterial, fungal, and viral infections. Occasionally, as in the case of subacute bacterial endocarditis, a septic embolus combines infarction with infection. Retrograde venous spread may also occur, usually through the veins of the face with anastomotic connections through the orbit to the cerebral circulation.

2. *Direct implantation.* This route of infection is almost invariably traumatic, though it may also be iatrogenic, as by lumbar puncture, infected foreign bodies such as ventricular shunts and rarely by corneal transplant or EEG needles.

3. *Local extension.* Skull fractures may expose the brain or meninges to the bacterially colonized air sinuses. Established infections in an air sinus (most often the mastoid and frontal) may erode through the bone and meninges to the brain. Local extension may also occur in patients, particularly neonates, who have midline fusion defects such as meningomyeloceles, where there is a connection between an external epithelial surface and the nervous system.

4. *From the peripheral nervous system.* Some viral diseases gain entrance to the CNS by ascent up the peripheral nerves to the brain. Rabies is the outstanding example, in which a bite from an infected animal implants the virus into the subcutaneous peripheral nerve twigs. Herpes simplex (p. 1383) also probably gains entrance to the brain by first becoming established in the trigeminal ganglion.

Finally, bacteria that produce exotoxins can seriously affect the nervous system without having to invade it, as in the case of tetanus (p. 324) and diphtheria (p. 317).

Infections of the nervous system are most conveniently discussed by dividing them into the *meningitides* and the *encephalitides*, these being infections of the meninges and brain parenchyma, respectively. It should, however, be realized that infections may extend from the meninges into the brain parenchyma and vice versa, to produce a *meningoencephalitis*. Within the general categories of meningitis and encephalitis, individual infections are classified by the type of syndrome they produce (e.g., acute lymphocytic meningitis) and the etiologic agent (i.e., bacterial, viral, and fungal).

MENINGITIS

A meningitis is an inflammation limited to the leptomeninges (meninges) and the subarachnoid space. Usually the inflammation is caused by an infection, but chemical meningitis (p. 1379) may also occur, and infiltration of the subarachnoid space by tumor cells is called carcinomatous meningitis, in spite of the fact that there is usually no inflammatory response. Infectious meningitis can be broadly classified as *acute pyogenic meningitis* (usually bacterial), *acute lymphocytic meningitis* (generally viral), and *chronic meningitis* (which may be caused by bacteria or fungi).

Acute Pyogenic Meningitis

The most frequently encountered causal organisms are *Escherichia coli* in the neonate and particularly the neonate with a neural tube defect; *Hemophilus influenzae* in infants and children; *Neisseria meningitidis* in adolescents and young adults (also the most frequent cause of epidemic meningitis since it is an oral commensal and can be transmitted through the air);[27] and the *pneumococcus*, particularly in the very young and the old, and in meningitis following trauma.[28] Once the leptomeninges are infected, dissemination of the organisms occurs through the subarachnoid space.

At an early stage the brain and spinal cord are swollen and congested. The subarachnoid space contains exudate that varies in location (Fig. 29–6). In **H. influenzae** meningitis, for example, it is usually basal, but in **pneumococcal** meningitis it is more often located over the cerebral convexities near the longitudinal sinus. From the areas of greatest accumulation, tracts of pus can be followed around the blood vessels. Even in those areas where there is no gross exudate, the leptomeninges are opaque and congested. When the process is fulminant, and especially if it is prolonged, the inflammation will extend to the ependymal surface or even spread downward to the spinal cord.

On microscopic examination, there is a typical neutrophilic exudation in the subarachnoid space with varying amounts of fibrin. In the more severely affected areas, the entire subarachnoid space is replaced by the exudate; in less severely affected areas, only the tissue around the

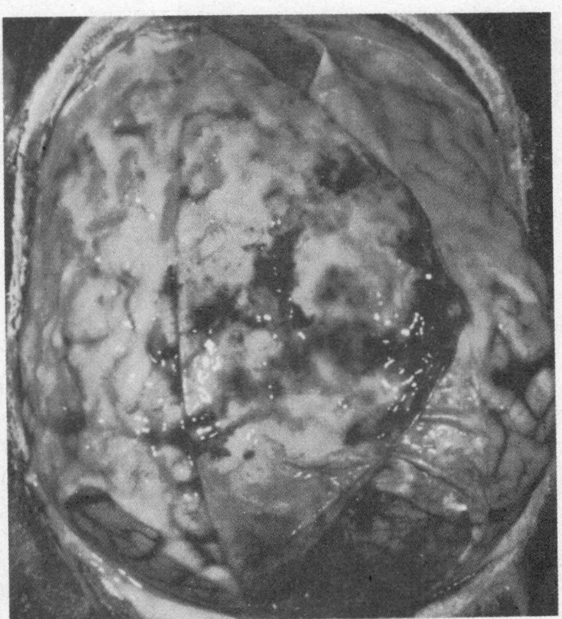

Figure 29–6. Pyogenic meningitis. A thick layer of suppurative exudate is disclosed beneath the folded-back dura.

leptomeningeal blood vessels contains cells. In fulminant infections, the inflammatory cells infiltrate the walls of the leptomeningeal veins, producing vasculitis. Arteritis is not a common complication unless the process is prolonged, because arterial resistance to sepsis is greater than venous resistance. Venous occlusion may produce hemorrhagic infarction of the cortex and underlying white matter, often inducing convulsions that are resistant to therapy.

The prototypic patient with acute pyogenic meningitis has a fever and the general signs of an infection with the symptoms and signs of meningeal irritation: headache, photophobia, irritability, clouding of consciousness, and a stiff neck. *A spinal tap yields cloudy or frankly purulent CSF, under increased pressure, with up to 90,000 polymorphs per mm,^{3} a raised protein, and a strikingly reduced sugar content.*[26] Bacteria can be seen on smear or cultured easily on appropriate media, sometimes hours before the polymorphs appear.

In the past the usual outcome of pyogenic meningitis, if untreated, was death. Recovery, when it did occur, was accompanied by fibroblastic proliferation, producing adhesions between the meninges and the brain. In many cases, a basal adhesive arachnoiditis followed, obliterating the subarachnoid space around the brain stem and occluding the foramina of Magendie and Luschka. The resulting hydrocephalus was often fatal. Even with modern antibiotic treatment, hydrocephalus may still be a sequela, particularly in pneumococcal meningitis in which large quantities of the capsular polysaccharide of the organism produce an especially glutinous exudate that encourages arachnoid fibrosis. A particular current problem is meningitis in the immunosuppressed patient. It is often caused by an unusual agent, pursues a particularly fulminant course, and has atypical CSF findings, all of which render the diagnosis more urgent and more difficult.

An acute so-called *chemical meningitis* can be caused by the release or insertion of irritative substances such as procaine and methotrexate, into the CSF. In such instances there is a CSF polymorph pleocytosis with a raised protein but usually a *normal* sugar content, and of course no organisms can be seen or cultured.[26]

Acute Lymphocytic Meningitis

Viral meningitis presents in much the same way as bacterial meningitis with the clinical signs and symptoms of meningeal irritation, but the course is generally less fulminant and the CSF findings are markedly different. *There is a lymphocytic rather than neutrophilic pleocytosis; protein elevation is only moderate and the sugar content is nearly always normal in sharp contrast to the reduced CSF sugar content in the bacterial meningitides.* The acute viral meningitides are self-limiting and only symptomatic treatment is necessary; there are none of the life-threatening secondary complications that occur in pyogenic meningitis. Many different viruses have been isolated from these cases, including mumps, ECHO viruses, Coxsackie, Epstein-Barr virus, and herpes simplex type II, but viruses can be identified in only two-thirds of the cases at best.

Chronic Meningitis

Several different agents produce a much more slowly evolving type of meningeal infection. The prototypic form of chronic meningitis is that produced by *Mycobacterium tuberculosis*, but all the indolent infections in the meninges may produce similar changes.

With tuberculosis, the meninges are filled with a gelatinous or fibrinous exudate in which focal densities may be visible grossly. These changes are usually most obvious around the base of the brain and extending into the lateral sulcus. Microscopically, the meningeal exudate is composed of varying mixtures of chronic inflammatory cells including lymphocytes, plasma cells, macrophages, and fibroblasts. The focal densities are tubercles, sometimes with caseous centers and giant cells. They are most frequently seen along the course of the cerebral vessels. In late cases there may be a dense fibrous arachnoiditis, most conspicuous around the base of the brain.

Clinically, tuberculous meningitis presents with relatively generalized neurologic complaints of headache and malaise, mental confusion, and vomiting.[29] The CSF has only a moderate pleocytosis of up to about 1000 cells (the usual value is around 100), which are composed of either entirely mononuclear cells or a mixture of polymorphs and mononuclear cells. The protein is elevated, often strikingly so, and the sugar typically is moderately reduced, but may be normal. The most feared, and sometimes devastating, complications of this type of meningitis are consequences of the continuing chronic inflammatory reaction in the subarachnoid space. The arachnoid fibrosis, already alluded to, produces hydrocephalus. The inflammatory reaction around the vessels of the subarachnoid space may cause obliterative endarteritis. Affected vessels may be occluded to produce infarctions in the underlying brain. The clinical consequences depend on which vessel is occluded, but may be catastrophic, as, for instance, with occlusion of the anterior spinal artery. The cranial nerves, which necessarily pass through the subarachnoid space, may also be affected, either directly by the infection, or by the associated inflammatory reaction. A continuing infectious process in the subarachnoid space also increases the likelihood of spread of infection into the parenchyma of the brain, thereby producing a meningoencephalitis.

Other organisms that produce meningitis with similar chronic inflammatory and granulomatous features include bacteria such as *Treponema pallidum* (syphilis) and Brucella sp., and many of the fungi such as Coccidioides and Candida. The complications of obliterative endarteritis and cranial nerve damage may occur with these organisms and also in other conditions that are granulomatous in character but not known to be infective, e.g., sarcoid[30] and granulomatous arteritis.[31] Clinically, all these involvements tend to present with rather nonspecific complaints similar to those of tuberculous meningitis. Likewise, the CSF usually has a moderate pleocytosis, a raised protein, and a variably reduced sugar content. Etiologic diagnosis can sometimes be made serologically, or occasionally by visualization or culture of the causative organism.

CRYPTOCOCCAL MENINGITIS

The meningeal infection caused by the cryptococcus differs from the general run of fungal meningitides, mostly by virtue of its clinical and pathologic variability. Pathologically, this organism sometimes elicits only a trivial inflammatory response, even in the presence of many organisms. Clinically, its course may be fulminant and fatal in as little as two weeks, or indolent over months or even years. The CSF, particularly in indolent cases, may have few cells but a notably high protein (over 500 mg/dl), and often the mucoid encapsulated yeasts seen in the CSF,[26] can be visualized by India ink preparations. The most reliable diagnostic test is, however, identification of cryptococcal antigen in the CSF.[66]

Subdural Empyema

Bacterial, or occasionally, fungal infection of the skull bones or air sinuses can spread, through either the bones themselves or the air sinuses, to the subdural space and produce a subdural empyema. The underlying arachnoid mater and subarachnoid space are usually unaffected, but the pus may form a layer thick enough to compress the underlying brain. Further, a thrombophlebitis may develop in the cerebral veins that cross the affected subdural space and cause venous infarction of the brain with permanent sequelae. Resolution of the empyema occurs from the dural side, and if the patient recovers completely, a thickened dural undersurface may be the only residual.

Most patients with a subdural empyema have an accompanying sinusitis with fever. Subsequently, lethargy, coma, and focal neurologic signs develop. Neck stiffness is almost always present. As with other parameningeal infective foci (e.g., cerebral abscesses), the CSF has an elevated pressure, protein, and white cell count, but a normal glucose content. If diagnosis and treatment are prompt, patients usually recover without neurologic deficits.

ENCEPHALITIS

In principle, it would be correct to call any infection of the brain an encephalitis, since this term implies an inflammatory state in the brain and is not etiologically specific. In practice, however, it is used inconsistently, being most often employed for the more diffuse types of infection typified by the arbovirus encephalitides (p. 1383), but it may also be used for focal disease as in herpes simplex encephalitis (p. 1383). Pathologically, parenchymal infections of the brain are best classified by their causative organisms and divided into bacterial, viral, and fungal infections.

Bacterial Infections

Most CNS bacterial infections manifest as meningitis, but bacteria may invade the brain from a preexisting meningitis to produce a meningoencephalitis. However, parenchymal infection may occur without meningitis, as in the parenchymal forms of tuberculosis and neurosyphilis.

TUBERCULOSIS

As well as a chronic meningitis (p. 1379), tuberculosis may occur in the nervous system as an intraparenchymal tuberculoma. The organisms seed the brain by blood-borne infection and produce tuberculomas that are well-circumscribed masses with a central core of caseous necrosis surrounded by a typically tuberculous cellular reaction. Organisms can often be seen with acid-fast stains. Calcification may occur in inactive lesions.

Although now rare in the United States and Europe, tuberculomas represent up to 25% of intracranial masses in India and South America. In about 25% of patients they are multiple, and only about 50% of patients have a previous history of tuberculosis.[31] Curiously, in children they are usually found in the posterior fossa, whereas in adults they are predominantly supratentorial. They present, like other expanding intracranial masses, with focal brain dysfunction together with the more generalized signs of raised intracranial pressure (p. 1375). By CT scan they appear as focal lesions. Treatment is by antituberculous chemotherapy, followed if necessary by surgery.

Tuberculosis of the spine (Pott's disease) (p. 1325) may, by vertebral collapse, produce spinal cord injury through compression.

Neurosyphilis

It is traditional to devote a large amount of space to a detailed description of neurosyphilis, but in modern practice in the Western world new cases of neurosyphilis are rarely encountered. What follows is a greatly abbreviated account; fuller discussions can be found elsewhere.[33]

Neurosyphilis is the tertiary stage of the disease. All patients have to pass through the primary and secondary stages, during which time the infection may be deliberately or inadvertently treated or may die out of its own accord. Only about 10% of those at risk develop neurosyphilis. The major types of neurosyphilis are:

Meningitic. Meningitic neurosyphilis is a chronic low-grade meningitis (p. 1379) in which the principal damage to the nervous system is produced by endarteritis obliterans.

Paretic. This form is produced by diffuse parenchymal invasion by the treponema. *The persistent infection produces diffuse brain atrophy.* Microscopically, there is loss of cortical neurons with proliferation of the microglia (rod cells) and gliosis, which produces the "windswept" cortical appearance. Appropriate stains demonstrate enormous numbers of spirochetes. As might be surmised from the diffuse pathologic involvement, this variant of neurosyphilis presents as an initially insidious but relentlessly progressive loss of mental and physical functions with mood alterations (including the well-known delusions of grandeur), terminating in a dementia of the most extreme and bizarre variety. Once the disease becomes symptomatic, treatment can only arrest but not reverse the decline in neurologic function.

Tabes Dorsalis (Locomotor Ataxia). In tabes, the spirochete attacks the sensory nerves in the dorsal roots and produces, among other features, impaired joint position sense leading to ataxia (the *locomotor ataxia*); loss of pain sensation leading to skin and joint damage (*Charcot joints*); and other sensory disturbances, particularly the characteristic "lightning pains," and absent deep tendon reflexes. Less well explained, but typically present, are Argyll-Robertson pupils, which react to accommodation but not to light. Microscopically, there is fibrosis and loss of axons and myelin in the dorsal roots, with consequent atrophy in the dorsal columns of the spinal cord.

Although these forms of neurosyphilis are described as separate entities, patients often show incomplete and mixed pictures.

Brain Abscess

Abscesses in the substance of the brain may arise from direct implantation of organisms by trauma, by extension from nearby foci of infection (especially mastoiditis), or by hematogenous spread, particularly from a primary source in lung, heart, or distal bones. Although acute bacterial endocarditis may produce miliary multiple abscesses, it does not usually cause a large solitary abscess. Cyanotic congenital heart disease is associated with a high incidence of cerebral abscesses. This is thought to be due to a right-to-left shunt and loss of pulmonary filtration of organisms. The microflora of intracranial abscesses is varied but includes many anaerobic organisms, of which the anaerobic streptococci and Bacteroides fragilis are the most common. Other common organisms are aerobic streptococci and Staphylococcus species.[34]

An abscess due to mastoiditis is usually preceded by an epidural extension from the infecting site, with spread into either the cerebellar hemisphere or the temporal lobe. During the stage of invasion, the changes are those of an abscess occurring anywhere. There may be a "cellulitis" of brain substance, which then settles down into a nidus of organisms and necrotic tissue. Adhesions of the meninges then usually seal off the point of entry from the rest of the subarachnoid space. Gradually, as elsewhere, an abscess expands, destroying and compressing tissues in the process (Fig. 29–7). As in the somatic organs, brain abscesses are surrounded by a fibrous capsule. This is one of the few instances in which there is fibrosis with collagen production in the brain. The fibroblasts that produce this collagen are derived from the walls of the blood vessels that proliferate around the edge of the necrotic brain. Outside the fibrous capsule is a zone of conventional gliosis. It is probable that this exuberant formation of new vessels is responsible for the pronounced vasogenic edema (p. 1375) so characteristic around brain abscesses. The inflammatory reaction, both acute and chronic, associated with this advancing infection is reflected in the CSF by an increased pressure and raised white cell count and protein, but a normal sugar content. No organisms are present in the CSF unless the abscess has ruptured into a ventricle or the subarachnoid space.

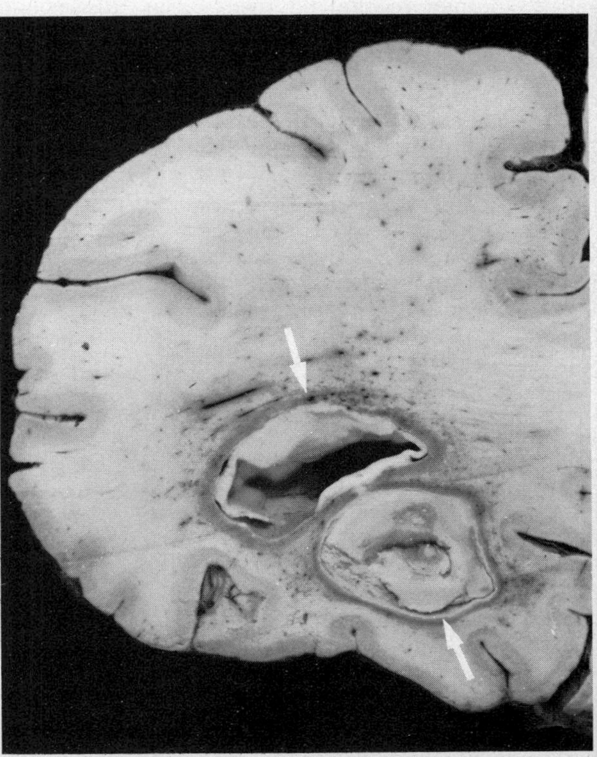

Figure 29–7. Frontal abscesses (*arrows*).

The patient with a brain abscess presents with general complaints relating to the raised intracranial pressure caused by the mass effect, and focal complaints referable to the area of brain involved. Abscesses are so destructive of tissue that a focal deficit is almost always present. Hemiparesis and convulsions in cerebral abscesses, and cerebellar incoordination in cerebellar abscesses[35] are among the more dramatic signs. A systemic or local source of infection is usually detectable, but a small systemic focus may have ceased to be symptomatic by the time the patient presents with evidence of brain involvement. Death may result from increased intracranial pressure and secondary herniation. Rupture of the abscess may lead to ventriculitis, meningitis, and sinus thrombosis. With surgery and antibiotics, the otherwise inevitable mortality can be reduced to less than 20%.

Viral Diseases

Viral diseases in general have been discussed already (p. 277); here, reference will be made only to those aspects not already covered that are particularly germane to disease of the nervous system.

The CNS can be affected by a multitude of viruses that may produce a meningitis or may affect primarily the brain or spinal cord. In these latter types of infection there is almost always some reaction in the leptomeninges, so that in the early stages at least there are inflammatory cells in the CSF. Almost always, viral disease of the nervous system has been preceded by a primary infection, or at least colonization, elsewhere. Sometimes, as with varicella zoster, the primary infection is another recognized disease, in this example chickenpox; however, it is often nonspecific, as in the gastroenteritis of poliomyelitis, or even unknown, as in progressive multifocal leukoencephalopathy (PML) in which there is only serologic evidence of previous infection. Rabies is an exception in that the virus is directly inoculated into the peripheral nerves, through which it ascends to the brain.

The most characteristic histologic change in viral diseases is a mononuclear cell infiltrate (lymphocytes, plasma cells, and macrophages), generally located around blood vessels (Fig. 29–8). The presence of **glial nodules** (p. 1374) and **neuronophagia** (p. 1374) also suggest viral disease. However, too much reliance should not be placed on these histologic features, since both mononuclear infiltrates and glial nodules can be seen in conditions in which viruses are not thought to be involved. A more direct expression of viral involvement is seen in the intranuclear **inclusion bodies** seen in some forms of viral infection. The only diagnostic inclusion is the intracytoplasmic **Negri body** of rabies (p. 1384).

A particularly striking feature of viral infections of the nervous system is the degree of tropism exhibited by some viruses.[36] Herpes zoster and poliomyelitis virus, for example, affect only specific subpopulations of neurons, the dorsal root ganglion cells, and the anterior horn motor neurons, respectively. Other viruses affect whole classes of cells; the virus of PML infects primarily oligodendroglia, and rabies virus attacks only neurons. Herpes simplex, although it infects all types of neural cells, is geographically restricted, affecting principally the temporal lobes. The basis for these different specificities is not clear, but they probably reflect surface receptor interactions between the host cells and the infecting virus.

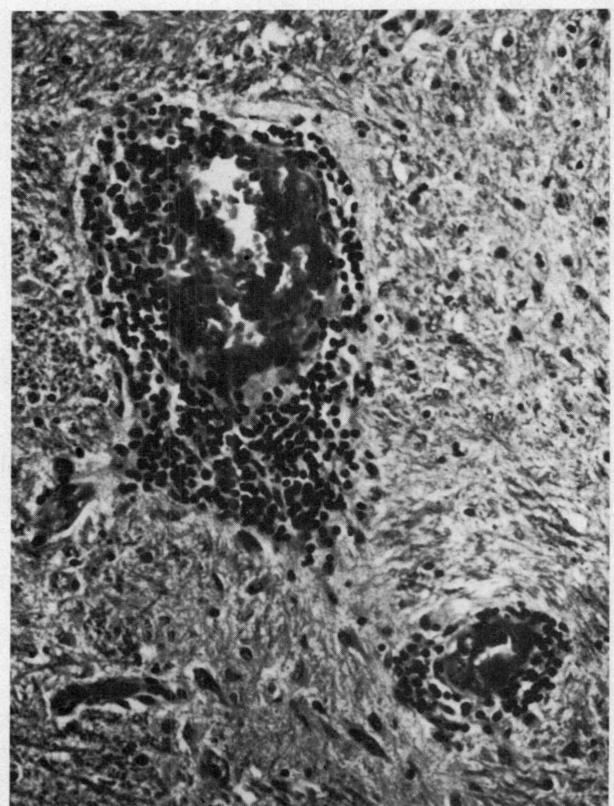

Figure 29–8. Perivascular mononuclear cell infiltrate typical of a viral infection (H and E stain).

The capacity of some viruses for *latency* is important in viral diseases of the nervous system. Herpes simplex (p. 284) and varicella zoster (p. 1384) can remain latent in their host cells in the nervous system, to be reactivated months or years after the initial infection. The *slow virus diseases* (p. 1385) have both a long latent period and an illness that, when it finally becomes manifest, pursues a prolonged clinical course, evolving like a slow motion picture of an acute disease that is quite unlike the usual pattern of infection.

It should not be thought that infections, overt or otherwise, make up the full gamut of viral effects on the nervous system. Systemic viral infections may occasionally be followed by an immune-mediated *perivenous encephalitis* (p. 1412) with no viral penetration of the nervous system. *Reye's syndrome* (p. 941), a condition of unknown but possibly toxic etiology, occurs most frequently after viral infection, usually influenza or chickenpox,[37] and is associated with severe, often fatal, brain edema. *Congenital malformations* can also be attributed to intrauterine viral infection, as occurs with rubella.

A few words are appropriate about the diagnosis of viral disease in the nervous system. At one time, virus identification depended on culture and serologic detection. When no effective treatment was available, these somewhat leisurely methods were quite appropriate. Today, when treatment is possible, speedier recognition is desirable. Brain biopsy permits direct immunofluorescent localization and identification of the virus, giving a specific diagnosis in minutes.[38] This is particularly important in the diagnosis of herpes simplex encephalitis. In other parts of the diagnostic jungle, however, and particularly with the latent and slow viruses, these agents have become so adept at camouflage that they can sometimes be detected only by more arcane methods such as co-cultivation and nucleic acid hybridization. Despite this array of diagnostic sophistication, it must be admitted that a virus is identified in only 30% of cases of presumed "viral encephalitis" and in only about 40% of fatal cases.[39]

Viral Encephalitis

Diffuse viral infection of the brain is usually manifested clinically by global deficits such as seizures, confusion, stupor, coma, or delirium. Often there are also focal nervous system impairments such as reflex asymmetry, involuntary movements, or ocular palsies. *The CSF is usually colorless, but with slightly elevated pressure, and initially a polymorph pleocytosis that rapidly converts to lymphocytes. The CSF protein is usually raised, but glucose and chloride levels are almost invariably normal.* To give an idea of the size of the problem in the U.S., about 1500 cases of presumed viral encephalitis are reported each year to the Centers for Disease Control.[39] Of these, only about 500 actually have a virus identified. Almost all the diagnosed cases fall into five general groups (number of cases for 1978 in parentheses): arboviral (143); enteroviral (40); associated with childhood infections (measles, mumps, chickenpox, rubella) (80); respiratory (70); other known agents (cytomegalovirus, herpes simplex, herpes zoster, Epstein-Barr virus (99), as the major culprits. Because so many types of virus cause encephalitis, it is impractical to consider each separately. Only the most common, and those with specific or illustrative features, will be discussed here.

Arthropod-borne encephalitides are generalized encephalitides characterized by a panencephalitis without conspicuous localizing features, and associated with a perivascular mononuclear reaction and a moderate CSF pleocytosis. Most outbreaks of epidemic encephalitis are due to arthropod-borne viruses (arboviruses). The specific causative agents differ around the world. In the Western hemisphere, the most important ones are eastern and western equine, Venezuelan, St. Louis, and California encephalitis. Types found elsewhere include Japanese B (Far East), tick-borne (U.S.S.R. and eastern Europe), and Murray Valley (Australia and New Guinea). All have vertebrate hosts and mosquito vectors, except for the tick-borne. These viruses have many common properties, so that some investigators wish to group them collectively as *encephaloviruses*.

Eastern equine encephalitis (EEE) may serve as the example for all the arbovirus encephalitides. It was initially described in horses in 1933, and the first human cases were reported in 1939 when an outbreak in children followed an epidemic in horses. Serologic studies indicate that only about 5% of exposed persons develop encephalitis, but the mortality rate is 80%. Some survivors recover completely, but others, especially young children, are left with serious residual disability.

EEE is a meningoencephalitis with perivascular inflammatory cells, many focal areas of necrosis, and selective neuronal necrosis with neuronophagia. In severe cases there may be a vasculitis with vascular necrosis. The location of the most severe damage varies, some cases having a predominantly cortical involvement, whereas in others the basal ganglia bear the brunt. In both eastern and western equine encephalitis, large numbers of polymorphs appear in the brain and CSF early in the disease. However, the CSF sugar is not decreased even when the cell count is exclusively polymorphonuclear.

The other arbovirus encephalitides differ in epidemiology and prognosis, but pathologically their appearance is very similar except for variations in severity and a tendency for there to be fewer polymorphs. There are no consistently reliable morphologic distinguishing features.

In the arbovirus encephalitides, the brain is the principal site of significant infection, but there are other viral diseases in which encephalitis is an occasional and sometimes severe complication, e.g., measles, rubella, and chickenpox. Most of these cases are probably examples of allergic perivenous encephalomyelitis (p. 1412), but in some cases such as EB virus and mumps the fact that virus can be recovered from the CSF is suggestive of direct neurotropic infection.

Herpes simplex (p. 284) in the nervous system illustrates features seen in some infections: i.e., the same agent may produce a number of different diseases, depending on the location of the injury and the state of the patient. HSV I (herpes labialis) has been implicated in at least four conditions:

1. *Herpes labialis,* the common cold sore, from which HSV I can be isolated. The virus can also be isolated from the cells of the geniculate ganglion both during and between crops of skin vesicles.
2. *HSV I encephalitis (adult form)* typically involves the inferior and medial regions of the temporal lobes and the orbital gyri of the frontal lobes. Hemorrhagic necrosis and perivascular infiltrates are usually present, and inclusion bodies (p. 1382) may be found in neurons and glial cells. It may occur in any age group, but is most often seen in children and young adults. Many cases are fatal, but some patients survive with severe dementia and, because of the temporal lobe damage, a striking memory loss. Others may make a complete recovery. Most cases of so-called "acute necrotizing encephalitis" are probably due to herpes simplex. The emergence of effective therapy for HSV I encephalitis (adenine arabinoside A or acyclovir) has generated a requirement for rapid diagnosis, which can be achieved

by the immunofluorescent or electron microscopic demonstration of virus in brain biopsy material. Treatment of this disease has reduced mortality to about 30%, compared with 70% in controls.[40]

3. *HSV I encephalitis (neonatal)* differs from the adult form in that the encephalitis affects the entire brain. The basis for this dissimilarity is not known, but it is speculated that there are differences in surface receptors in neonatal and adult brains.

4. *Benign recurrent (Mollaret) meningitis* is a rare, self-limiting, recurrent meningitis. HSV I has been isolated from at least one case,[41] but it is probable that not all cases of this disease have the same cause.

In addition to these HSV I syndromes, HSV II (genitalis) also affects the nervous system and is responsible for most cases of *herpetic viral meningitis*. More ominously, it causes a generalized and severe *encephalitis* in neonates. With the current prevalence and resistance to treatment of herpes genitalis, obstetric practice is moving toward recommending cesarean section in cases of active herpes genitalis rather than submitting the baby to the risk of encephalitis engendered by delivery through an infected birth canal.

Rabies, usually transmitted by the bite of a rabid dog, produces a characteristic and severe encephalitis that is almost always fatal.

On gross examination, the brain shows intense edema and vascular congestion. Microscopically, there is widespread and severe neuronal degeneration. The severity and extent of the inflammatory reaction is greatest in the basal nuclei, the midbrain, and the floor of the fourth ventricle, particularly in the medulla. **Negri bodies are the diagnostic histologic feature.** These are eosinophilic cytoplasmic inclusions, usually rounded, oval, or bullet shaped, and often multiple. Found only in neurons, they are most frequently seen in the large neurons of Ammon's horn in the temporal lobe, and in the Purkinje cells of the cerebellum. In addition to the brain changes, there may be involvement of the spinal cord and dorsal root ganglia.[42, 43]

The virus enters the CNS by ascending along peripheral nerves from the wound. The incubation period depends on the distance of the wound from the brain and varies between one and three months. Clinically, the onset is nonspecific with general malaise, headache, and moderate fever. The conjunction of these symptoms with local paresthesias around the wound is diagnostic. In the advanced clinical syndrome the patient presents a picture of extraordinary CNS excitability; the slightest touch is painful and minute movements provoke myriad motor responses, progressing to violent convulsions. There are signs of meningeal irritation and, as the disease progresses, flaccid paralysis. Periods of alternating mania and stupor progress to coma and death from respiratory center failure.

Herpes zoster infection, usually of adults (p. 285) in its most common clinical form, is a *vesicular, often painful, skin eruption in the distribution of one or more spinal or cranial sensory nerve roots*. This disease is a recrudescence of varicella infection, with viral persistence in sensory ganglion neurons. Often, it appears in persons with underlying cancer or systemic disease, or who are predisposed owing to chemotherapy or immunodeficiency. The skin lesions are always associated with involvement of the corresponding dorsal root ganglion or gasserian ganglion, with varying degrees of spread both distally and proximally in nervous structures. In a small percentage of cases, segmental motor impairment can accompany the sensory change. Rarely, a widespread encephalomyelitis can occur.[44] Varicella zoster virus is recoverable from the lesions either of skin or of nervous tissue in most cases.

On gross examination, the affected dorsal root ganglion and the nearby root are congested, edematous, and often hemorrhagic. Even when there is no corresponding skin lesion, the adjacent ipsilateral ganglia may participate in the pathologic process. On histologic examination, the affected ganglia show an infiltration by lymphocytes, sometimes accompanied by hemorrhage and necrosis. Ganglion cells can be seen in various stages of disintegration. Inclusion bodies (p. 1382) may be found in satellite cells and in remaining ganglion cells.

Most patients recover, albeit sometimes slowly, from herpes neuritis, ganglionitis, radiculitis, or myelitis. In severe cases, however, the involved structures are destroyed, and secondary degeneration is seen in peripheral nerve and posterior columns of the spinal cord. Such patients have so-called "residual postherpetic neuralgia." Interferon administration seems to have a beneficial effect in the treatment of severe herpes zoster.

Poliomyelitis, at one time a fearsome infection, is an enterovirus disease that extends to the nervous system, specifically the lower motor neurons. The virus exists in at least three variants, known as Brunhilde (type I), Lansing (type II), and Leon (type III). Type I is generally the most virulent. Outbreaks of the disease occur principally in summer, although sporadically at other times. The synonym is "infantile paralysis," but in the last several outbreaks older children and adults were more often affected, and some of the most catastrophic paralyses occurred in adults. In recent years, immunization has greatly reduced the number of cases of crippling acute anterior poliomyelitis, and there is reason to hope that this disease will never again be a serious threat. However, there remains in the population a large number of patients who have suffered the crippling effects of this disease, and for this reason alone it is still worthy of study.

On gross examination of acute cases, the brain and cord are congested and edematous, and small hemorrhages may be seen. These changes are nonspecific and are often seen in patients dying of respiratory failure. Cavitation in the anterior horns is a rare finding. Microscopically, there are often a few lymphocytes in the meninges, and mononuclear cells form perivascular cuffs around meningeal and parenchymal blood vessels. The most important feature is the change in the nerve cells. Experimentally, when virus gains access to the nerve cells it produces cytoplasmic swelling, chromatolysis, and nuclear displacement. Presumably, some cells are affected to the extent that their function is lost, but their capacity for recovery remains. There may be no cellular reaction around such cells. The next step is cell destruction, and all degrees of swollen and shrunken cells can be seen, their nuclear and cytoplasmic envelopes broken down. In early cases, these cells may be surrounded by neutrophils, but sometimes only a microglial and histiocytic reaction is present. The dead cells are eventually replaced by gliosis.

The major target of the injury is the anterior horn cell of the spinal cord. The motor nuclei of the cranial nerves may be involved, but only rarely is there destruction of large numbers of nerve cells. Occasionally, in very fulminant cases, the posterior horns and even the white matter of the cord are affected. In such cases it is not unusual to find some cell loss and inflammatory nodules in the pons, midbrain, and diencephalon. Grossly, long-standing cases show visible atrophy of anterior roots, peripheral nerves, and dependent muscle, and microscopically, gliosis of the affected anterior horns with loss of neurons.

Clinically, the CNS involvement is marked by the development of headache, stiff neck, and stiff back, which occur within a few days of the appearance of the generalized somatic complaints. In most patients, the disease remits at this stage or even earlier, but in a few it goes on to produce focal nervous system destruction that manifests as lower motor neuron paralysis. In the affected spinal segments the paralysis is often permanent, but this is rare in the cranial nerve (bulbar) territories. Although poliovirus may affect the diencephalic nuclei and even the cerebral cortex, a truly encephalitic picture is rare. When death occurs it is usually due to paralysis of the respiratory muscles, which is secondary to infection of the anterior horn cells of the phrenic and intercostal nerves, although the medullary respiratory center may also be directly involved. *The only permanent neurologic residual of poliomyelitis is a lower motor neuron paralysis.* Severe myocarditis occasionally complicates or terminates the clinical course. Rarely, Coxsackie viruses cause diagnostic confusion because they may mimic poliomyelitis, but the paralysis in such infections, although occasionally severe, is usually transitory.

Postencephalitic parkinsonism (von Economo's disease) is a late sequela of a presumed viral epidemic that spread throughout the world around 1915, particularly in eastern Europe, and which in some cases produced an acute encephalitis (encephalitis lethargica). The condition is discussed in more detail in the section on degenerative diseases on page 1414.

Slow Virus Diseases

So far we have been discussing viruses that may be latent but, when they produce disease, cause an acute febrile illness that is recognizably infective in character. The agents that cause *slow virus diseases* not only have a long latent period but also, when they produce disease, cause one that evolves at a much slower pace than normal infection and does not clinically resemble an infection at all. Since 1958, when the concept was first formulated,[45] advances in our understanding of these diseases have made it appropriate to divide them into two groups.[46]

1. *True slow virus infections* have a recognizable or known viral cause, such as subacute sclerosing panencephalitis (SSPE), progressive multifocal leukoencephalopathy (PML), and progressive rubella panencephalitis.[47]

2. The *unconventional agent (spongiform) encephalopathies* (Kuru and Jakob-Creutzfeldt disease in humans) have a distinct histologic appearance and are caused by agents not yet identified, which have some resemblance to conventional viruses but clearly lack many of their characteristics.

Subacute sclerosing panencephalitis (SSPE) is a slow virus infection of relatively recent recognition. In 1933, Dawson described an "inclusion body encephalitis" characterized clinically by involuntary movements and progressive mental retardation. Van Bogaert (1945) reported a clinically similar disease that he called subacute sclerosing leukoencephalitis. It is clear that both authors were describing the same disease, now called subacute sclerosing panencephalitis (SSPE). The disease generally attacks children, although it can sometimes be seen in adolescents and young adults. It has always been preceded by an attack of measles, often unusually early in life, or, occasionally by previous immunization against measles. The onset of the condition is usually heralded by personality changes, followed by the development of involuntary movements. The electroencephalogram exhibits characteristic bursts of high-voltage activity. In most cases the disease progresses relentlessly to death.

On gross examination, the brain may be normal or unusually firm and may contain regions of granularity and focal destruction. Microscopically, there is a perivascular mononuclear cell infiltrate, and inclusion bodies are seen in neurons and oligodendroglia. Neuronophagia and extensive neuronal loss are present in severely involved regions. Dense fibrillary gliosis follows as the process becomes older. Electron microscopy shows that the inclusion bodies contain particles similar to measles virus (p. 282).[48]

The epidemiologic and electron microscopic evidence strongly favors measles virus as the cause of SSPE. Much other recent data are available that throw a light on the course as well as the cause of the disease. Although many inclusion bodies and viral particles are seen in the brain, measles virus can be grown only by co-cultivation with other types of cells. The reason for this requirement has become apparent from studies of the CSF. The CSF in SSPE contains large amounts of oligoclonal immunoglobulins; analysis of these has shown that many of them are directed against components of the measles virus.[49] However, no antibody is present to the nonglycosylated M protein associated with the inner surface of the viral membrane and apparently important in the assembly of the virus particle. It appears that, for reasons currently unknown, the brain cells do not synthesize the M protein and thus are unable to produce fully assembled virus.[50, 51] This probably explains the necessity for co-cultivation for the production of virus particles. It may also help to explain the protracted course of the disease in the presence of what appear to be large quantities of virus.

Progressive multifocal leukoencephalopathy (PML) is a rare viral infection of oligodendrocytes that causes primary demyelination (p. 1410) as its principal pathologic effect. It was first described in 1958 and occurs in association with advanced hematologic malignancies,[52] immunosuppressive therapy, immunodeficiency diseases (including acquired immune deficiency syndrome, AIDS),[53] and chronic debilitating disease (tuberculosis, sarcoidosis, and rheumatoid arthritis). In most cases, the associated illnesses have been present for months or years before PML becomes clinically manifest. Given the nature of the associated conditions, most cases are in middle-aged patients, but the condition does occur in children. It becomes clinically apparent by the development of protean but focal and relentlessly progressive neurologic symptoms and signs. CT scans show extensive, often multifocal areas of lucency in the hemispheric and/or cerebellar white matter. All attempts at treatment, including large doses of interferon, have so far been unavailing.

Grossly, the affected white matter has irregular margins; a sunken, gray, translucent appearance; and a soft texture. Microscopically, there are numerous areas of demyelination, ranging in size from minute foci to huge confluent lesions affecting whole lobes. The cerebrum, brain stem, cerebellum, and (rarely) spinal cord can all be involved. The appearance of the oligodendrocytes is diagnostic; their nuclei are still spherical but grossly enlarged, and contain inclusion bodies that range from violet smudges to discrete homogeneous eosinophilic masses. They are most frequently seen at the edges of the lesions. There are also characteristic bizarre giant astrocytes, with irregular, hyperchromatic, sometimes multiple nuclei. Reactive fibrillary astrocytes are scattered among the bizarre forms, but there is strikingly little inflammatory reaction. Axons transversing the lesions are conspicuously preserved. Electron microscopy shows that the enlarged oligodendrocyte nuclei contain numerous papovavirus-like particles, often in paracrystalline arrays. Isolated virus particles are sometimes seen in astrocyte nuclei.

Two closely related papovaviruses have been implicated in this disorder, one called JC (the initials of a patient and unrelated to Jakob-Creutzfeldt disease) (p. 1387), which accounts for almost all the cases, and SV40, which has been found in at least two patients.[54] About 65% of normal persons show serologic evidence, in the form of specific antibodies, of exposure to JC virus by the age of 12 years.[55] However, it is not known whether the development of PML represents the rekindling of old infection or a new infection in a particularly susceptible host.

UNCONVENTIONAL AGENT (SPONGIFORM) ENCEPHALOPATHIES

A major advance in the understanding of diseases of the nervous system is the recognition of conditions caused by transmissible agents that lack many of the characteristics of conventional viruses and have incubation periods measured in months to years.[56] These unconventional agents are implicated in at least two diseases of humans—kuru and subacute spongiform encephalopathy (Jakob-Creutzfeldt disease)—and in related conditions in animals—scrapie in sheep and goats and transmissible encephalopathy in mink. Microscopically, all these conditions are characterized by a spongiform change in gray matter (Fig. 29–9), and their similarity is emphasized by the fact that scrapie and Jakob-Creutzfeldt tissue when injected into monkeys produce the same disease. Kuru and Jakob-Creutzfeldt disease have both been transmitted from humans to primates[57] by intracerebral, intramuscular, intraperitoneal, and subcutaneous inoculation of infected tissue. After a long latent period (generally about 18 months), the inoculated animals develop CNS changes identical to those seen in humans.

In some ways these agents are similar to conventional viruses: they are filterable, titrate cleanly, and have distinctive host specificities. On the other hand, they differ from conventional viruses in that they are (1) resistant to formalin and to inactivation by other physicochemical agents; (2) have an atypical resistance to ultraviolet and ionizing radiation; (3) are not visible in the electron microscope; and (4) do not invoke either an immune or an inflammatory reaction in the host. They are inactivated by autoclaving, hypochlorite solutions, and alcoholic iodine. Recent work on the scrapie agent may have gone some way toward clarification of the general nature of these unconventional agents.[58, 59] The results suggest that the agent contains a protein of

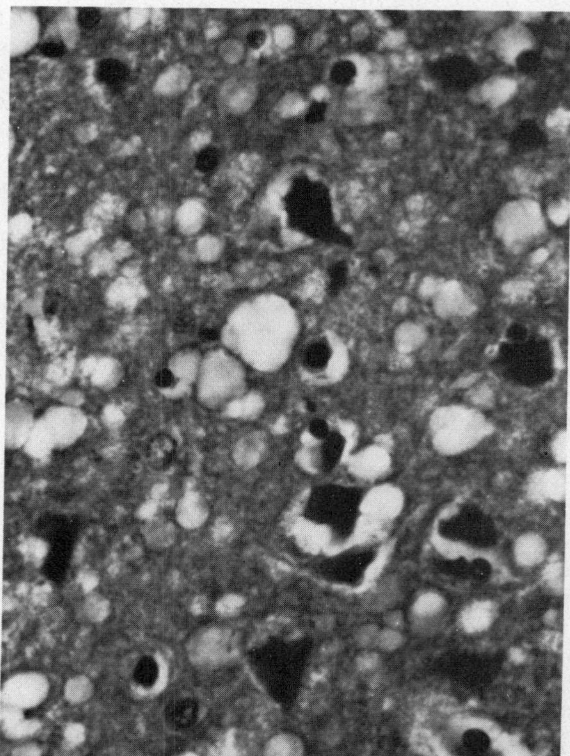

Figure 29–9. Status spongiosus—characteristic of unconventional "slow" virus infections. Vacuoles are located in the neuropil. Note absence of an inflammatory infiltrate. (H and E stain.)

molecular weight between 27K and 30K daltons. The infectious properties of this protein are abolished by procedures that denature proteins, but are unaffected by methods that disrupt nucleic acids, all of which suggests that nucleic acid may not be an essential part of the infectious particle. If this work is confirmed, this agent is unconventional indeed and quite different from all other viruses, viroids, and plasmids. Immediate questions arise about its mechanism of replication and infectivity, to name only the most obvious problems. Much work remains to be done and radical changes may occur in our ideas about these agents. As putative *pro*teinaceous *in*fective particles, they have been tentatively called "prions."

Subacute spongiform encephalopathy (Jakob-Creutzfeldt disease, transmissible agent dementia) are all synonyms for a rare but well-characterized disease that presents clinically as a rapidly progressive dementia. Despite the demonstrated experimental transmissibility of its causative agent, it is sporadic in its occurrence with a worldwide incidence of about one per million, and there is no discernible pattern of exposure in the patient population. The natural mode of transmission in humans is wholly obscure,[62] although in a few cases iatrogenic transmission by medical procedures, such as corneal transplantation, has occurred.[63]

Morphologically, the diagnostic feature is the presence of spongiform change ("bubbles and holes") in the cortex (Fig. 29–9), and sometimes the basal ganglia.[60] In the later stages there is also gross neuronal loss and an accompanying marked fibrillary gliosis. An inflammatory infiltrate is notably absent. By electron microscopy the "holes" appear as intracytoplasmic membrane-bound vacuoles in neuronal and glial processes. They contain curled membranous structures (Fig. 29–10).[61] Kuru plaques (see below) occur in about 10% of cases in the affected cortex. The progress of the disease is usually so rapid that, despite the degree of neuronal loss, there is little if any gross atrophy of the brain.

The clinical picture is quite typical. Abnormalities of personality and visual/spatial coordination are generally the first signs of illness and are rapidly followed by a progressive severe dementia with myoclonus. The CSF is normal except for an occasional mild elevation of protein. The EEG picture is initially normal but later develops a characteristic pattern. The disease is uniformly fatal, with an average duration of seven months, although survival for three years has been recorded. All treatments have so far been unavailing.

Kuru is confined to the Fore tribe of the eastern highlands of Papua–New Guinea, among whom the disease was transmitted by cannibalism. At one time it was the cause of death in 90% of women of the tribe since they mainly come into contact with or ate the brains of the deceased. With the termination of cannibalism in this tribe, the disease has all but disappeared.[56] Clinically, it is characterized by cerebellar ataxia and a "shivering tremor" that progresses to complete motor incapacity and death from intercurrent infection or

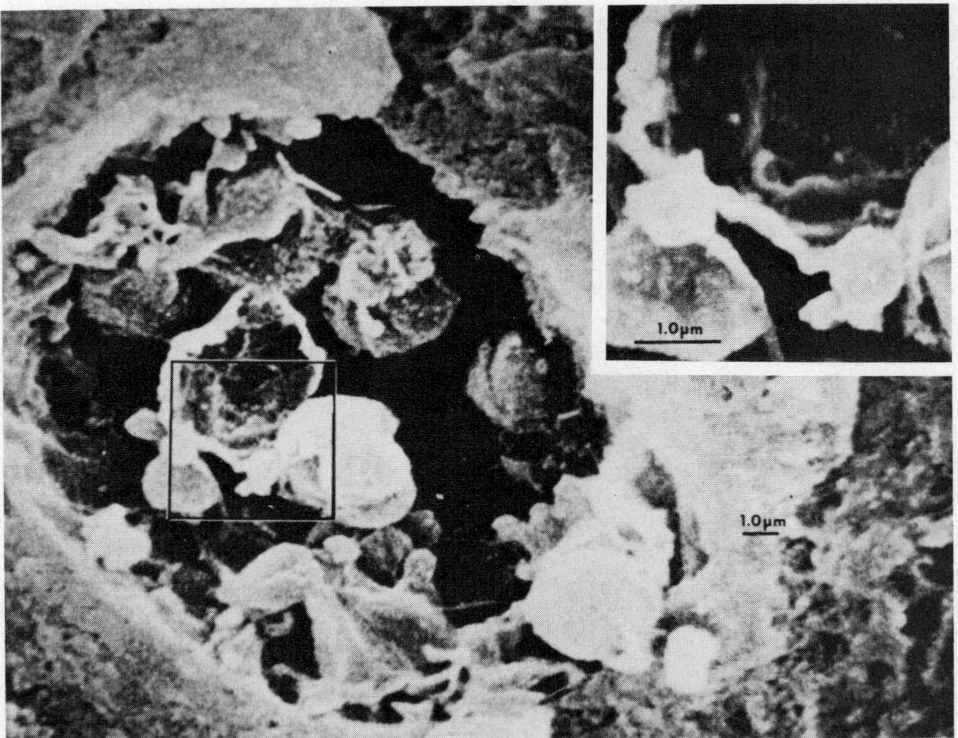

Figure 29–10. Scanning electron micrograph of a large vacuole in a monkey with transmitted Jakob-Creutzfeldt disease. Inset shows an enlargement of the area inside the small square. (From Chou, S. M., et al.: Transmission and scanning electron microscopy of spongiform change in Creutzfeldt-Jakob disease. Brain *103*:885, 1980.)

malnutrition in less than one year after its onset. Dementia is not a prominent feature but may occur in the terminal stage. Qualitatively, the morphologic changes in the CNS are similar to those in Jakob-Creutzfeldt disease. However, in contrast to the latter, they are most prominent in the cerebellum and striatum. Amyloid bodies with radially arranged spicules (kuru plaques) occur in about 60% of cases.

Fungal Infections

As with the systemic deep mycoses (p. 352), fungal disease of the CNS, in modern Western practice, is most frequently encountered in patients with cancer and lymphomas,[64, 65] or in those who are immunocompromised.[24] In these settings the brain usually is involved only late in the disease when there is widespread hematogenous dissemination of the organism, most often *Candida albicans, Phycomycetes, Aspergillus fumigatus,* and *Cryptococcus neoformans (Torula histolytica).* Less frequently seen, and then usually in the endemic areas, are the more traditional agents such as *Histoplasma capsulatum, Coccidioides immitis,* and *Blastomyces dermatitidis.* A broad range of other agents have also been found on rare occasions.

There are three basic patterns of fungal infection in the CNS: *chronic meningitis, fungal vasculitis,* and *parenchymal invasion.*

Chronic meningitis has already been discussed on page 1379, and will not be further considered here.

Fungal vasculitis is most frequently seen with *Phycomycetes* and *Aspergillus* infections, both of which have a marked predilection for invasion of blood vessel walls, but it may also occasionally be found with other organisms, including Candida. This causes thrombosis of the affected vessel, producing a cerebral infarction that is often strikingly hemorrhagic, and subsequently becomes septic from ingrowth of the causative fungus. Clinically, brain involvement is usually indicated by the appearance of a cerebral infarction or infarctions, in patients having systemic infections with these fungi.

Most of the fungi that can affect the nervous system are capable of *parenchymal invasion,* usually in the form of granulomas or abscesses. The two most commonly encountered are *Candida albicans* and *Cryptococcus neoformans.* Candida usually produces multiple microabscesses, with or without giant cell and granuloma formation; these are not generally large enough to produce focal symptoms. In cryptococcosis, parenchymal invasion is seen as cysts, which may be numerous, and measure up to 2 to 3 mm in diameter. Organisms are present within these cysts, but there is strikingly little gliosis or inflammatory reaction around them. With all these fungi, parenchymal invasion may, and often does, coexist with a fungal meningitis.

Although most fungi arrive in the brain by hematogenous dissemination, direct extension may also occur, particularly with the *Phycomycetes,* that have a predilection for growth in air sinuses, and *Actinomyces,* which in its craniofacial form may occasionally invade the brain.

Other Infections

Protozoal diseases such as malaria, toxoplasmosis, amebiasis, and trypanosomiasis; rickettsial infections (typhus, Rocky Mountain spotted fever); and metazoal diseases such as echinococcosis and cysticercosis may also involve the CNS and are discussed in Chapter 8. Of these, *cerebral toxoplasmosis* merits a brief mention because, in its acquired adult form, it occurs only in the immunosuppressed population, is particularly common in AIDS, and is treatable. Pathologically, it is a rapidly progressive, multifocal, necrotizing, and often hemorrhagic encephalitis. The organisms are present in the characteristic pseudocysts and free in the tissue, and usually are most easily seen at the margins of the necrotic areas.

In this brief summary of infections, there has been a considerable bias toward diseases encountered in Western European and North American practice. Outside these privileged areas, however, cerebral malaria, cysticercosis, and tuberculosis are probably the most common infections of the nervous system.

VASCULAR DISEASES

The importance of vascular disease of the brain can hardly be overstated because, notwithstanding a recent and gratifying decrease in its incidence,[67] it has been estimated to account for 50% of the neurologic problems encountered in general hospitals. The major categories to be discussed are (1) *hypoxia, ischemia, and infarction;* (2) *intracranial hemorrhage and vascular malformations;* and (3) *hypertensive encephalopathy.*

HYPOXIA, ISCHEMIA, AND INFARCTION

Although the brain makes up only 2% of body weight, it receives one-sixth of resting cardiac output and accounts for 20% of oxygen consumption. In considering the consequences of oxygen deprivation, it is important to distinguish carefully between hypoxia and ischemia.[68] *Hypoxia is deprivation of oxygen with maintained blood flow,* whereas *ischemia occurs when blood flow is greatly reduced or interrupted.* The cellular pathophysiology of these two situations is quite different,[69] and the brain has a very different sensitivity to them. *Hypoxia* is seen in circumstances such as exposure to reduced atmospheric pressure; patients show euphoria, listlessness, drowsiness, apathy, and defective judgement. If the hypoxia is severe, and especially when it is sudden, unconsciousness and convulsions may occur. Contrary to popular belief, however, neurons are actually quite tolerant of pure hypoxia and capable of substantial anaerobic respiration. In animal experiments in which the circulation is artificially maintained, a Po_2 of 20 torr has been tolerated for as long as 25 minutes. Pure hypoxic brain damage is not often seen pathologically, because most of the more severe hypoxic states rapidly induce a concomitant cardiac arrest, thereby producing an ischemic state.

In contrast to their response to hypoxia, neurons are especially vulnerable to *ischemia,* being able to tolerate it for only three to four minutes without permanent damage. Lesser degrees of ischemia produce individual cell necrosis of neurons, but when the ischemia is sufficiently severe and/or prolonged, parenchymal necrosis occurs, embracing all the cellular elements (i.e., an *infarction*). There is thus a gradation of severity between ischemic damage and infarction, with no absolute dividing line between them. Although there is a pathophysiologic continuum between these two states, the two terms in clinical practice are usually attached to specific types of clinical syndrome. By convention, *ischemic encephalopathy* is used when there has been a *generalized reduction of cerebral perfusion* producing widespread ischemic damage that may even include areas of crude tissue necrosis (such as border zone infarcts, described later). The term *cerebral infarction* is usually reserved for the focal brain necrosis that follows obstruction of blood flow to a *localized area of the brain.*

The cerebral circulation is specially adapted for maintenance of adequate flow in a number of ways. There is autoregulation of cerebral perfusion so that blood flow is constant and independent of systemic blood pressure over a wide range of pressures. This is achieved by control of the cerebrovascular resistance. Also, interconnections between cerebral vessels ameliorate the consequence of single vessel obstruction. Occlusion of an artery such as the internal carotid can be, and often is, compensated for by anastomoses of the circle of Willis. Thus, vascular occlusion, particularly if it occurs gradually in an extracranial vessel, does not necessarily result in an infarction, or even ischemic damage. Although rather less complete, there is also some degree of anastomosis between the major intracerebral arteries. However, it is widely held that infarctions may occasionally occur without a vascular occlusion if there is both a severe stenosis in an artery and a sudden reduction in cerebral perfusion, such as occurs in a brief cardiac arrest, or during surgery if there is a major hemorrhage.

Ischemic Encephalopathy

The mechanisms that operate to protect the brain against ischemia become ineffective in the more extreme degrees of change and in the presence of preexisting cerebrovascular disease. In the normal person, the systolic blood pressure may drop acutely to 70 mm Hg without necessarily producing brain dysfunction. However, a patient with severe cerebral atherosclerosis or established hypertension may suffer ischemic damage with lesser falls in systolic blood pressure.

The changes seen in the brain depend on the duration and intensity of the ischemia and on the length of survival. When the insult has been slight, the nerve cells recover function and no anatomic change occurs. In patients who survive only a few minutes or hours, no changes are seen regardless of the severity of the insult. The first demonstrable change, seen after survival for 12 to 24 hours, is in the nerve cells. The large cells of Sommer's sector of the hippocampus and the Purkinje cells of the cerebellum seem to be the most vulnerable. All forms of ischemia initially result in either swelling or shrinkage of neurons. Shortly thereafter, affected neurons may develop ischemic cell change (p. 1372). In the cortex, the process is usually widespread but not completely uniform; clusters of damaged cells may be found next to unaffected cells, even in the same cortical lamina. Subsequently, the nerve cells die and disappear, to be replaced by fibrillary gliosis. Frank cortical necrosis followed by gliosis occurs in areas of greater destruction, so that laminar necrosis interrupts the normal continuity of the cerebral cortex. In long-term survivors, the degree of cortical atrophy is proportional to the degree of cortical destruction. In generalized reductions of cerebral perfusion, the most severe ischemia is suffered by tissue supplied by the most distal branches of the arteries. This may be severe enough to result in wedge-shaped areas of tissue necrosis in the junctional zones between the major arterial territories, called **border zone** or **watershed** infarcts. In the cerebral hemispheres, the border zone between the anterior and middle cerebral artery territories seems to be most at risk. Damage to this region produces a linear parasagittal infarction, usually with some expansion over the lateral occipital gyri, the precise geometry of the infarct being governed by the degree of ischemia and the extent of the local vessel narrowing in the affected region. Border zone infarcts are invariably seen in the context of generalized severe ischemic encephalopathy.

Ischemic encephalopathy occurs in circumstances of profound systemic hypotension and, probably most often, in cardiac arrest when resuscitation has not been sufficiently expeditious. With lesser degrees of ischemia, there may be only a transient postischemic confusional state. When the ischemia is more severe and/or prolonged, a picture of decortication may emerge, characterized by head retraction, arm flexion, and rigid extension of the legs. When there is sufficient associated brain swelling, herniation may occur, and decorticate posturing may be converted into the more severe decerebrate state. Patients who survive these degrees of ischemic encephalopathy are invariably left with a considerable deficit; they may be demented or have bilateral spasticity, and some become liable to recurrent convulsions.

Cerebral Infarction

Most cerebral infarctions are caused by a local vascular obstruction of some sort and are either *thrombotic* or *embolic*. However, infarction also occurs when cerebral arteries are *compressed against unyielding dural folds* during cerebral herniation, and occasionally it occurs without obstruction when there is a severe reduction in cerebral *perfusion* and marked narrowing of one or more vessels.

Both embolic and compressive arterial occlusions are often only temporary and, either by relief of obstruction or the establishment of collateral flow, reflow of blood may occur into the infarcted area. When this happens, blood enters vessels rendered abnormally permeable by ischemia and, not surprisingly, leaks out, converting a previously anemic (bland) infarct into a hemorrhagic one.

On gross examination, **anemic (bland) infarctions** are not detectable with any certainty until six to 12 hours after their occurrence. The earliest visible change is a slight discoloration and softening of the affected area, so that the gray matter structure becomes blurred and the white matter loses its normal fine-grained appearance (Fig. 29–11). Within 48 to 72 hours, necrosis is well established and there is softening and disintegration of the ischemic area with pronounced circumlesional swelling that may, in lesions of sufficient size, produce brain herniations. As resolution proceeds there is liquefaction, resulting in cyst formation with lesions of sufficient size. These cysts are traversed by trabeculations of blood vessels and surrounded by firm glial tissue (Fig. 29–12). The leptomeninges, when involved, become thickened and opaque and may form the outer wall of the cyst.

The first histologic change, seen after six to 12 hours, is a diffuse reduction in the staining intensity of the tissue. In chromatic stains, the first discrete change is in the nerve cell bodies, with disarrangement and disorganization of the cytoplasm and nuclear chromatin. In addition, but probably following the initial swelling of the cells, there are large numbers of red neurons (p. 1372) suffering from ischemic damage. Special stains reveal fragmentation of axons and early disintegration of myelin sheaths; there is also loss of oligodendrocytes and astrocytes.

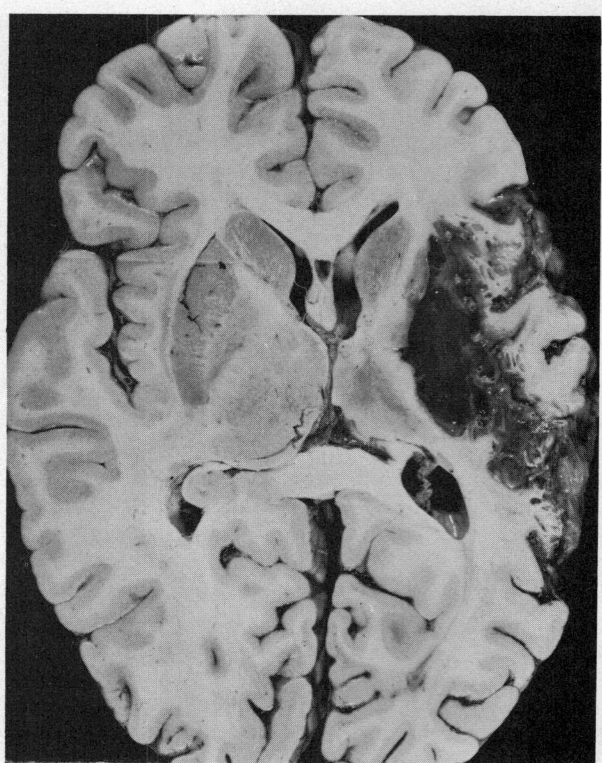

Figure 29–12. Old cystic infarct.

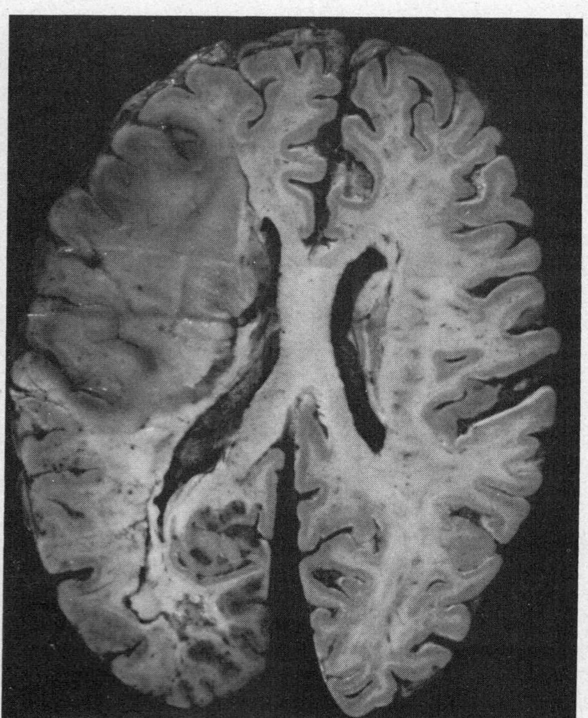

Figure 29–11. Section of brain showing both bland and hemorrhagic infarcts. The bland infarct is the large oval discolored region in the middle of the hemisphere (*upper left*). The hemorrhagic infarct involves the cortex over the posterior-medial region of the same hemisphere.

At about 48 hours, the blood vessels stand out prominently, and some neutrophils begin to pass through the vessel walls and into the tissue. Occasionally, this response is so intense as to simulate a septic infarct, but usually it is replaced at 72 to 96 hours by the aggregation of macrophages around blood vessels. At this stage the macrophages are the dominant reactive cells, attaining their maximal number at about two weeks. After this they gradually disappear, but even years later they may still be found in the interstices of old infarcts. Astrocytosis becomes prominent during the second week and eventually, as the final stage in the resolution of an infarct, results in fibrillary gliosis, which encloses or replaces the necrotic region. The time required for an infarct to resolve ranges from weeks to many months, depending on its size.

Hemorrhagic infarcts, as already indicated, are usually seen in embolic or compressive infarcts. Grossly, the hemorrhage in these infarcts is confined to the cortex (Fig. 29–11); the infarcted white matter does not become hemorrhagic. This difference probably reflects the different caliber of vessel in the cortex and white matter. Hemorrhage does not seem to affect the processes of infarct resolution, except that, histologically, many of the macrophages contain hemosiderin.

Lacunes (little lakes) are small infarcts ranging from a few millimeters to 15 mm in diameter, most commonly found in the deep portions of the brain, especially the putamen, thalamus, internal capsule, basis pontis, and hemispheric white matter.[73] Their occurrence is particularly associated with systemic arterial hypertension and they are thought to result from the occlusion of deep arterioles, either by emboli or by hypertensive hyalinization of these arterioles.[74] Pigmented macrophages can be found in some lacunes, suggesting that a hemorrhagic component may have been present or that they may have been minute hemorrhages.

The symptoms and signs produced by a cerebral infarction depend on the location of the infarcted area and its size. Good descriptions of the many syndromes of infarction can be found in neurology texts, but a few generalizations and some examples are helpful to an understanding of the variety of their pathophysiology.

Stupor and/or *coma* accompanying cerebral infarction is usually a consequence of either extensive bilateral hemispheric injury or damage to the ascending reticular formation in the midbrain and pons. With hemispheric lesions, any depression in the level of consciousness implies a large infarct with associated cerebral swelling. In contrast, damage to the reticular formation can be produced by small infarctions. The distinction between these two situations is made by the other localizing signs and symptoms that accompany the loss of consciousness.

Convulsions at the onset of an infarct are uncommon. When they occur they are most frequently associated with embolic infarcts and cerebral hemorrhages. However, they are relatively common as a late consequence of infarcts and can usually be correlated with scarring of the cortex.

Of all the arterial occlusion syndromes, those associated with obstruction of the *internal carotid artery* produce the most varied symptomatology, ranging from being symptomless to the production of a catastrophic hemiplegia. The reason for this variability lies in the ability of the anastomotic connections of the circle of Willis to compensate for the occlusion. As might be expected, gradual occlusion is more likely to be symptomless than is rapid obstruction. Conversely, a sudden obstruction may produce infarction in the territory of the middle, anterior, and even sometimes posterior cerebral artery on the affected side. Infarcts of this size are particularly likely to produce depression in the level of consciousness secondary to herniation. Atherosclerotic stenosis of the internal carotid artery without complete obstruction may also be symptomatic. The stenosis usually occurs at the bifurcation of the common carotid artery. Most of the symptoms take the form of *transient ischemic attacks (TIAs)* (p. 1394). There is still controversy about the best treatment for symptomatic carotid stenosis, surgical or medical.

Obstructions of the major intracranial arteries produce stereotyped syndromes, specific to each artery. Most of these occlusions are embolic. Involvement of the *middle cerebral artery* and its branches is the most frequent and provides good examples of the type of syndromes to be expected. Total infarction of the territory supplied by the middle cerebral artery will involve much of the caudate, all of the lentiform nucleus, and the intervening internal capsule, all supplied by the lenticulostriate branches. Also, the cortex of the insula and the superior and inferior lips of the sylvian fissure will be infarcted, thereby involving parts of the frontal, parietal, and temporal lobes. Clinically, because of the infarction of the internal capsule, there will be a dense hemiplegia involving both contralateral limbs and the face, a cortical hemisensory deficit, and usually a visual field quadrantanopia. If the left hemisphere is infarcted, there will also be severe aphasia in 95% of cases.

The middle cerebral artery usually has two major branches, a superior division that supplies the frontal and parietal cortex making up the upper lip of the sylvian fissure, and an inferior division that supplies the temporal lobe component of the middle cerebral territory. Obstruction of the left superior division produces a hemiparesis worse in the face and arm (because only the cortical and not the internal capsule motor fibers are affected), a cortical hemisensory deficit, and a nonfluent (Broca) type of aphasia. With a lower division infarction there will be a fluent (Wernicke) type of aphasia and usually a visual field cut, but no hemiparesis or sensory defect since no motor or sensory cortex is infarcted. Infarctions in smaller branches of the artery produce correspondingly smaller deficits. Infarctions in other vascular territories produce equally distinctive clinical syndromes that, when elicited by history and examination, usually permit identification of the affected arterial territory.

Mention must also be made of the infarctions that follow *venous obstruction*. Because of the great collateralization of the cerebral venous drainage, infarction only follows either occlusion of a large sinus or widespread smaller vein obstruction. It is most commonly seen in occlusion of the superior sagittal sinus, which is itself most often the consequence of the predisposition to thrombosis associated with cancer.[72] The infarctions are characteristically bilateral, parasagittal, multiple, and hemorrhagic, with hemorrage in both gray and white matter. Clinically, these infarctions are often distinguished by the occurrence of particularly intractable seizures.

INTRACRANIAL HEMORRHAGE

Intracranial hemorrhage, as in hemorrhage in other organs may be due either to actual physical disruption of vessel walls or to a hemorrhagic diathesis (p. 643). Intracranial hemorrhage is classified according to its location as follows:

1. *Cerebral hemorrhage*, which is hemorrhage into the brain parenchyma and is most commonly due to hypertension.
2. *Subarachnoid* (sometimes with adjacent intracerebral) *hemorrhage* (nontraumatic), caused most commonly by a ruptured berry aneurysm.
3. *Epidural* and *subdural hemorrhage*, seen most frequently in association with trauma and therefore discussed under that heading (p. 1396).
4. *Mixed types* of 1, 2, and 3, often caused by vascular malformations.

Cerebral Hemorrhage

Hemorrhage into the brain substance is most commonly caused by hypertensive vascular disease, but trauma, rupture of aneurysms, angiomas, blood dyscrasias, and bleeding into tumors also cause intracerebral hemorrhage. Atherosclerosis without hypertension is not a cause. In routine autopsies in large general hospitals, hypertension is 10 to 20 times more frequent than all the other causes. Hypertensive hemorrhage into the brain is also the most common cause of death among the cerebral vascular diseases. Although infarcts are more common, they do not cause death unless they are massive or are in critical locations (e.g., brain stem). In contrast, recovery after hypertensive hemorrhage, although possible, is infrequent.

The mechanism of hypertensive cerebral hemorrhage is not understood, although certain facts are generally agreed. It occurs in patients who have had significant systolic-diastolic elevations for at least several years. The occurrence of the hemorrhage is usually related to at least mild exertion; it almost never happens during sleep. Some have theorized that arteriolar necrosis or microaneurysms (Charcot-Bouchard aneurysms) in the small arteries precipitate the hemorrhage. However, there is no good explanation of the pathogenesis. What is known is that a blood vessel may burst within the brain substance in a hypertensive patient.

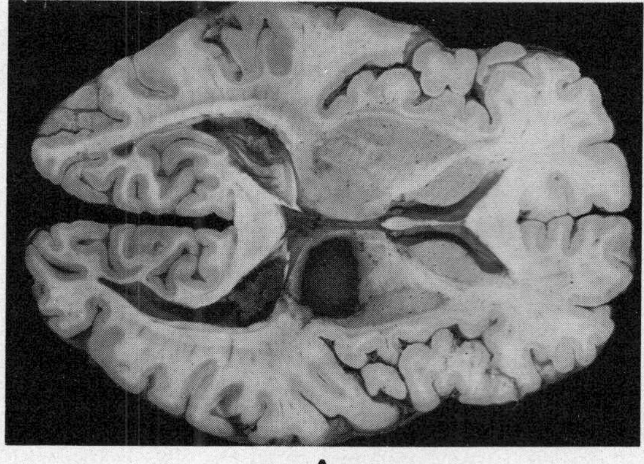

A

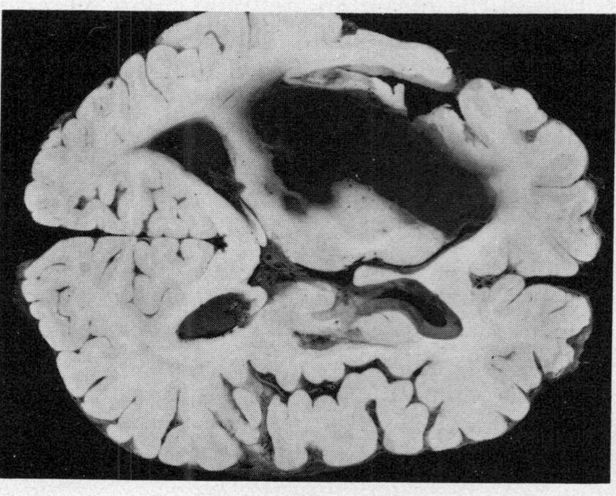

B

Figure 29–13. *A,* Hypertensive hemorrhage, thalamus. *B,* Massive hypertensive hemorrhage, rupturing into lateral ventricle.

Major sites of bleeding in large series are the putamen (55%); cortex and subcortex (15%); thalamus (10%); pons (10%); and cerebellar hemisphere (10%). Whatever their size, shape, or location, these hemorrhages tend to push parenchymal structures aside rather than destroy them. This may account for the improvement in neurologic function in the rare surviving patient. It is important to distinguish between a true hemorrhage and a hemorrhagic infarct. A hemorrhagic infarct corresponds to the supply of a given artery; a hemorrhage often overlaps arterial supplies. In the former, the architecture of the tissue remains, with diapedesis of red blood cells into the tissue surrounding the blood vessels; in the latter, the architecture is displaced and replaced by blood. Under some circumstances, an infarct may be so hemorrhagic that it may be difficult to distinguish from a true hemorrhage.

Most hemorrhages are of large size. Infrequently, one sees a relatively small, slitlike lesion beneath the cortex or in the lateral basal ganglia, or a small rounded lesion in the thalamus (Fig. 29–13*A*) or cerebellum, but for the most part hypertensive hemorrhage is a massive lesion, occupying 25 to 80% of the entire hemisphere (Fig. 29–13*B*). The tissue in the path is displaced by the bleeding, and around the edge the remaining tissue is compressed, distorted, and discolored. Peripheral hemorrhages of small and large size around vessels are common. Edema is massive; the ventricles are displaced, the ipsilateral one compressed. Herniations are the rule: tentorial and subfalcial in cerebral hemorrhage, foraminal in brain stem and cerebellar hemorrhage. Rupture into the ventricle occurs in almost all large intracerebral hemorrhages, and into the subarachnoid space in some.

Resolution of a hemorrhage begins with the appearance of macrophages and reactive fibrillary astrocytes. Macrophages eventually clear the tissue of blood, resulting in a cavity surrounded by dense, fibrillary gliosis and hemosiderin-laden macrophages. An old healed hemorrhage may be difficult to distinguish from a similarly resolved old infarct, although a resolved hemorrhage in most cases contains more hemosiderin-laden macrophages.

Hypertensive cerebral vascular disease is essentially a disorder of smaller arteries and arterioles. Therefore, in hypertensive hemorrhage the vascular changes seen are thickening of the walls of these vessels; increase in cellularity of some; and hyalinization, sometimes with necrosis, of others. Although in many cases of hypertension there is concomitant severe atherosclerosis, this is not a necessary association, and in many cases of hypertensive hemorrhage there is no atherosclerosis of the circle of Willis or of the smaller vessels.

Supratentorial hemorrhages tend to present as hemiplegias, often with an eye-movement disorder. In the posterior fossa, cerebellar hematomas produce symptoms such as intractable vomiting, whereas pontine bleeding may generate bilateral long tract signs from involvement of the corticospinal tracts in the basis pontis and extraocular movement disorders secondary to disruption of the visual apparatus in the floor of the fourth ventricle. If there is substantial bleeding and consequent mass effect, the signs of raised intracranial pressure, coma, and the syndromes of herniation (p. 1375) rapidly begin to dominate the clinical picture.

Subarachnoid Hemorrhage (Berry Aneurysm)

Aneurysms (p. 529) are a common cause of significant subarachnoid hemorrhage. Aneurysms can be developmental (saccular, "congenital," berry), arteriosclerotic (fusiform), inflammatory (mycotic), or traumatic. Here we shall discuss only the developmental berry aneurysm, because 95% of ruptured intracranial aneurysms are of this type. In 20 to 30% of cases, there is more than one aneurysm.

Most berry aneurysms bleed into the subarachnoid space and, to a lesser extent, into the adjacent CNS tissue (Fig. 29–14). Some aneurysms, however, such as those on the anterior communicating artery, may rupture into the CNS with very little bleeding into the subarachnoid space. The location of resultant hemorrhage depends on the site and orientation of the ruptured aneurysm, but the magnitude of the hemorrhage bears no relation to the size of the aneurysm. Often the entire subarachnoid space is filled with blood.

On gross examination, a saccular aneurysm is characterized by ballooning of the vessel wall into a "berry-like" structure that is attached to the vessel by a neck (Figs. 29–15 and 29–16). On microscopic examination, the dome of the aneurysm shows fragmentation of the internal elastica and degeneration or absence of its smooth muscle wall. Only a thin fibrous wall may remain and is the most common site for these aneurysms to rupture. Characteristically, saccular aneurysms occur in the major branches of the circle of Willis. About 94% are located in the internal carotid artery circulation, as contrasted to 6% in the vertebral-basilar artery circulation. The most common sites of rupture are the posterior communicating artery (25%), anterior communicating artery (23%), and middle cerebral bifurcation (16%).

Two theories have been proposed concerning the pathogenesis of aneurysm formation. One postulates a congenital defect in the internal elastic lamina and muscle wall. The other contends that wall degeneration is secondary to such "acquired" processes as atherosclerosis, hypertension, and abnormal hemodynamics. Because of the uncertainty, the terms berry, developmental, or saccular aneurysm are preferred to congenital.

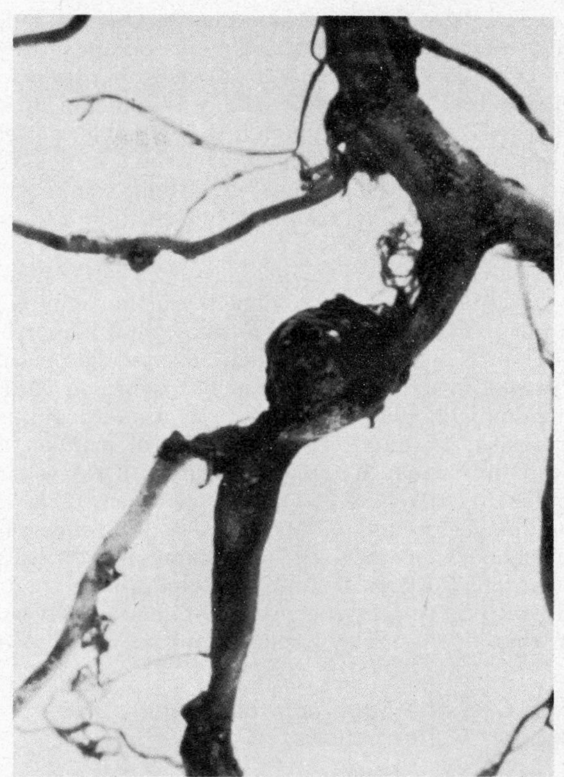

Figure 29–15. Berry aneurysm of middle cerebral artery. The vessels have been dissected away from the brain.

Rupture may occur at any age—rarely in infancy and childhood, most commonly in young and middle-aged adults, and with a greater than usually realized frequency in old age. *Rupture of an aneurysm is not inevitable;* not infrequently, intact berry aneurysms are found at autopsy as incidental findings. The prognosis of rupture appears to be enhanced by significant hypertension. Rupture usually, but not always, follows some exertion. The clinical course of a ruptured aneurysm is quite characteristic. Patients usually complain of a rapidly developing occipital headache and suddenly become unconscious. In most cases, they improve and are awake again within minutes. Arteriography (Fig. 29–16), CT

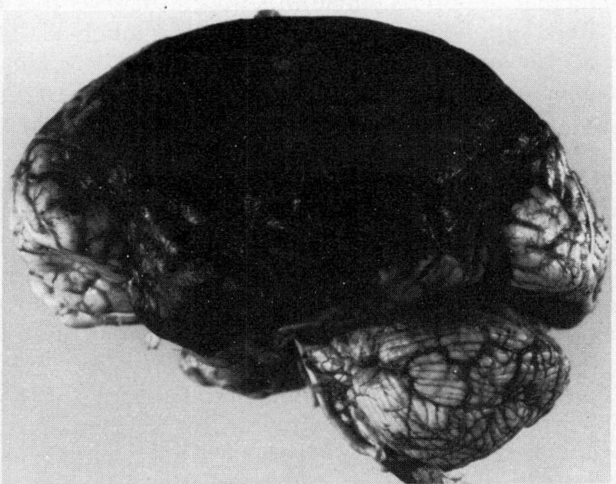

Figure 29–14. Subarachnoid hemorrhage covering the left cerebral hemisphere.

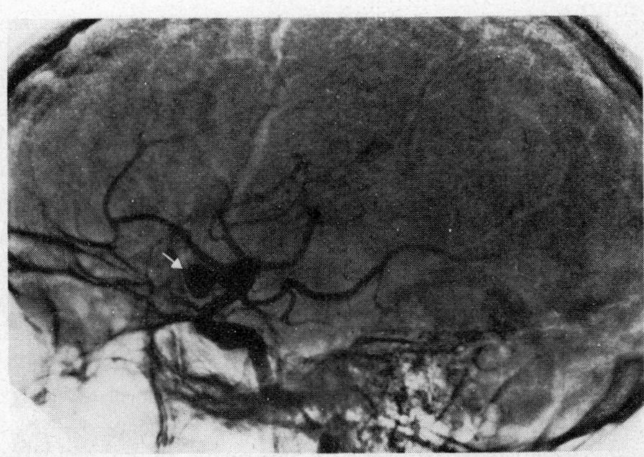

Figure 29–16. Cerebral arteriogram showing berry aneurysm arising from anterior communicating artery.

scan, and the presence of blood in the CSF are helpful in the diagnosis of a ruptured aneurysm and in determining its location. About 25 to 50% of patients die with the first rupture. Rebleeding is common in individuals who survive, although it is impossible to predict in which patient this will occur; when it does, the prognosis is much more grave. Other complications include infarction, hydrocephalus, herniation, and brain stem hemorrhage.

Four to nine days following rupture, some patients show additional neurologic deficits such as hemiplegia, caused by either penetrating intracerebral hemorrhage or ischemic necrosis associated with vascular spasm or narrowing.[76] Arterial spasm can be confirmed with arteriography in about 40% of patients with ruptured aneurysms. Postmortem examination of patients with vasospasm frequently discloses infarcts in the territory supplied by the vessel with the aneurysm or by surrounding vessels without thromboses.[77] The effect of the subarachnoid hemorrhage on surrounding vessels is controversial. Experimentally, platelet products and red cell lysates have caused constriction in cerebral vessels, but whether these play a role in humans is unknown.[78]

Mixed CNS and Subarachnoid Hemorrhage (Vascular Malformations)

Hemorrhage from a vascular malformation occurs within both the CNS and the subarachnoid space in up to 67% of cases. It is confined to the subarachnoid space in about 25% and to the CNS in about 8% of cases. Vascular malformations are traditionally divided into arteriovenous malformations (AVM), capillary telangiectases, and cavernous angiomas.[11]

Arteriovenous malformations consist of tangles of abnormal vessels or channels of various sizes that have characteristics of arteries and veins. Ninety per cent of AVMs are in the cerebral hemispheres; half of these are predominantly located on the surface of the brain and the other half more deeply. The abnormal vessels within brain substance are separated by gliotic tissue in which there is either recent hemorrhage or evidence of old bleeding, in the form of hemosiderin-laden macrophages. Irregular feeding arteries supply the vascular tangle, and veins that drain the malformation can usually be found.

Bleeding from AVMs is clinically most frequent between the ages of 10 and 30; after 60 it is rare. Males are affected twice as often as females. Subarachnoid and intracerebral hemorrhage associated with seizures is the most common clinical presentation. The most frequent site of bleeding is in the region of the middle cerebral artery. Pure venous malformations have also been described.

Capillary telangiectases and *cavernous angiomas* can be briefly discussed together. Capillary telangiectasias are composed of small capillary-like vessels that are separated from each other by brain tissue, as contrasted to cavernous angiomas, which are composed of larger, irregular, thin-walled channels frequently back-to-back without intervening brain tissue. These two types of vascular malformation are sometimes seen together. Capillary telangiectases almost never bleed, although cavernous angiomas sometimes do.

INFARCTION, HEMORRHAGE, AND "STROKE"

"Stroke" or *cerebrovascular accident (CVA)* is the term applied to the acute onset of a focal neurologic deficit, such as a hemiparesis, caused by a vascular event of some sort. As described in the foregoing paragraphs, several different types of vascular event can cause stroke, notably *thrombosis, embolism, lacunar infarction,* and *intracerebral hemorrhage.* Clinically, it is important to distinguish among these processes, and typically each has a characteristic clinical presentation and course that assists etiologic diagnosis.

Thromboses are usually *atherosclerotic* and generally occur in the larger arteries of the brain, notably the internal carotid, vertebral, and lower basilar. Infrequently, but significantly for therapeutic and prognostic reasons, thrombi follow other pathologic processes such as *arteritides* and *hypercoagulable states.* In contrast to atherosclerotic occlusions, these processes may affect arteries of all diameters. *Atherosclerotic thromboses* usually form gradually, producing a "stuttering" clinical course over several days during which time the patients may plateau and then deteriorate further. In most cases only one region, supplied by a single vessel, is affected. About 50% of the patients who eventually develop a thrombotic infarct with permanent neurologic deficits have preceding transient attacks of neurologic impairment. The pathologic basis of these episodes is uncertain, but they are probably caused by either fleeting reductions of flow in the affected vessel or the production of ephemeral emboli, e.g., cholesterol[75] from atherosclerotic plaques. Whatever their etiology, which may be multiple, these episodes are called *transient ischemic attacks (TIAs).* They last from seconds up to 24 hours, most being less than ten minutes long, and their specific neurologic features indicate the territory of the brain or artery involved. For example, transient monocular blindness (amaurosis fugax) suggests that the territory supplied by the carotid artery is involved. TIAs are particularly associated with subsequent thrombosis, but in a large study they have also been shown to occur in 23% of lacunar strokes, 11% of embolic infarcts, and 8% of cerebral hemorrhages.[71]

Emboli usually impact in the smaller cerebral arteries, often at bifurcations. The most frequently affected territory is that of the middle cerebral artery, in which 90% of occlusions are embolic in origin. Despite their frequency, emboli are rarely found at postmortem examination, probably because they fragment, migrate, or lyse. Their origins are extremely diverse and include atherosclerotic debris from ulcerated plaques, vegetations in subacute bacterial endocarditis and nonbacterial thrombotic endocarditis, ventricular and atrial thrombi in myocardial infarction and atrial fibrillation respectively, and bone marrow emboli after trauma. *Embolic strokes* typically have a sudden onset without any premonitory warning. Depending on the source of the emboli, both sides of the brain or regions with different arterial supply may be affected. The clinical pattern is often that of a maximal initial deficit with subsequent recovery. Although most patients survive the first embolus, others may follow. In conformity with the frequently hemorrhagic nature of the infarct in embolic strokes, the CSF often contains red cells.

Lacunar strokes may have an abrupt or gradual onset, but their diagnosis usually rests on the development of one of the recognized lacunar syndromes such as a pure motor hemiparesis or a pure sensory stroke. The volume of brain damaged by this process is so small that unless they strike at a particularly vulnerable spot they are asymptomatic. The most vulnerable areas of the brain in this context are the internal capsule and the basis pontis, where major tracts are compressed into a small volume. *In a large unselected series of cerebral infarcts, 37% of vascular occlusions were considered to be embolic, 41% were large vessel thromboses, and 22% were considered to be lacunar strokes.*[71]

Cerebral hemorrhage typically manifests as the smooth progressive or sudden onset of a stroke syndrome, usually accompanied by generalized signs of acutely raised intracranial pressure (p. 1375). In current practice the CSF is not often sampled, but if it is, the presence of blood corroborates the diagnosis; its absence does not exclude it.

These different pathophysiologic entities can usually be distinguished by a combination of angiography and CT scan. The clinical presentation is not an invariably reliable guide to pathophysiology, so that strokes that would be diagnosed on clinical grounds as infarctions, prove to be hemorrhages, and so forth. One study[71] suggests that clinical diagnoses in all categories have to be changed in between 5 and 10% of cases; this has a measurable impact on treatment. Despite its great utility, CT has certain limitations, most notably with ischemic events, since it takes 24 to 48 hours for the changes in x-ray density to become apparent. More recent developments are positron emission tomography (PET) and nuclear magnetic resonance (NMR) scanning, which provide a more direct look at cerebral metabolic function. This gives a more rapid indication of the location of the damage and also shows areas in which there is ischemia short of infarction. Although currently under development, these techniques are likely to become widely available and have many applications to processes unrelated to ischemia.

HYPERTENSIVE ENCEPHALOPATHY

Hypertensive encephalopathy occurs as an acute clinical condition in which there is a severe and usually abrupt elevation of systolic and diastolic blood pressure, headache, clouding of consciousness, and convulsions, leading to stupor or coma. Also usually present are retinal changes with papilledema, exudates, hemorrhages, and a degree of renal failure. The patient may die or may recover. The pathogenesis is related to acute, severe increases in intravascular pressure. Long-standing hypertension is not necessary for its development, since it can occur in eclampsia and other acute hypertensive episodes, and can be produced acutely in experimental animals. Lowering of blood pressure also can produce the most extraordinary relief of signs and symptoms.

Because this is essentially an acute disturbance in the hemodynamics of smaller arteries and arterioles, it is not surprising that there is no consistent clinicopathologic correlation. A few findings at autopsy are relatively constant. The brain is swollen, even to the development of herniation. On microscopic examination, there are the vascular changes of hypertensive disease in patients with long-standing hypertension, and in some of these individuals there may be fibrinoid necrosis of some vessel walls. Microinfarcts and petechial hemorrhages appear in some cases. There may be perivascular deposits of high-protein fluid, fibrin, or round cells in longer-lasting cases. But this functional disorder may kill the patient before any of these morphologic changes appear.

VASCULAR DISEASES OF SPINAL CORD

The spinal cord has a unique pattern of blood supply with one anterior and two posterior spinal arteries that are reinforced at each vertebral level by tributaries of varying sizes from the intercostal arteries. This arterial arrangement makes the spinal cord vulnerable to ischemic damage from reduced flow to the spinal arteries if there is complete interruption of a sufficient number of the tributaries. The latter is the most common mechanism of vascular injury to the cord, is most frequently seen in dissecting aortic aneurysms, and usually produces damage to the mid and lower thoracic cord. Occlusion of the anterior or other spinal arteries is much more rare but may occur by compression from a herniated disc, obliterative endarteritis (p. 1379), or occasionally embolism. Spinal cord hemorrhage is most commonly associated with trauma (p. 1399), although vascular malformations and tumors can sometimes bleed.

TRAUMA

Injury to the nervous system is a common and often dramatic accompaniment of trauma. In discussing the effect of mechanical injury, we will consider the brain, spinal cord, and peripheral nerves separately, because the mechanisms producing injury and the results incurred differ for each of these structures. The effects of trauma to the skull and brain depend on the shape of the object causing the trauma, the force of impact, and whether the head is in motion at the time of impact. A blow to the head may be penetrating or blunt and may result in either an open or a closed injury. It is important to realize that *severe brain damage can occur in the absence of external injury, and conversely that severe external lacerations and even skull fractures do not necessarily indicate injury to the underlying brain.* A traumatic force may pass through the skull, dura, leptomeninges, and subarachnoid space and finally into the brain. None, some, or all of these structures may be physically disrupted. In the following discussion, injury to specific anatomic structures is considered individually. Figure 29–17 is a diagrammatic summary of the various effects of trauma.

SKULL FRACTURES

Fractures of the skull are common complications of trauma to the head. These fractures may be closed or open, linear or comminuted, and may or may not be depressed. They may be occult, or evident from the presence of blood or CSF draining from the nose or ears. Radiographic examinations are essential to an evaluation of patients with possible skull fractures.

INJURY TO DURA AND LEPTOMENINGES

Injury to the dura may produce lacerations in its blood vessels resulting in *epidural* or *subdural hematoma.*

Epidural Hematoma

An *epidural hematoma* is a localized collection of blood between the skull and dura mater and is usually the result of a tear in the middle meningeal artery or, more rarely, a vein (Fig. 29–18). It occurs in 1 to 3% of all head injuries. An overlying skull fracture is almost always present.[22] Because they are usually a product of

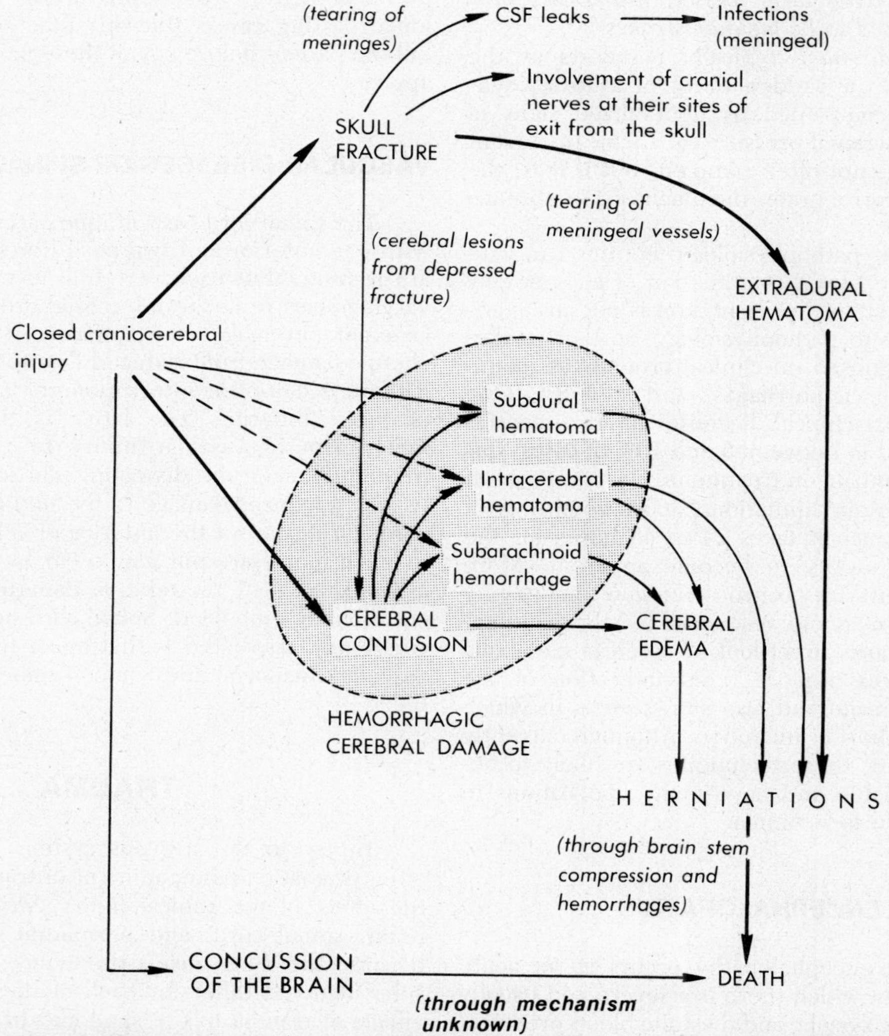

Figure 29–17. Major complications of closed craniocerebral injury. (From Escourolle, R., and Poirier, J.: Manual of Basic Neuropathology. 2nd ed. Philadelphia, W. B. Saunders Co., 1978, p. 65.)

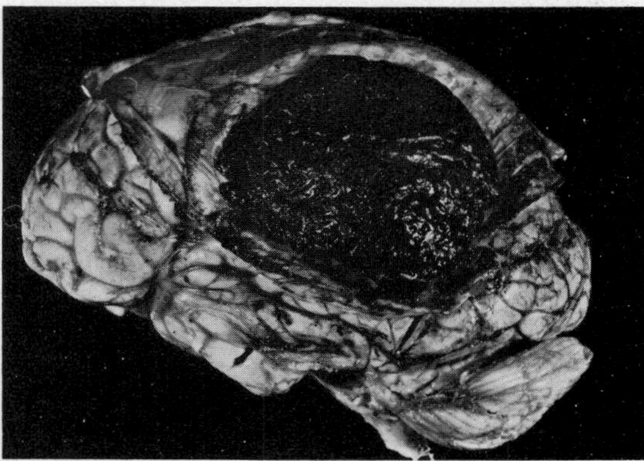

Figure 29–18. Epidural hematoma, the result of laceration of middle meningeal artery caused by fracture of skull.

arterial bleeding, epidural hematomas cause a rapid and progressive rise in intracranial pressure, which usually develops within minutes to a few hours of the trauma. *Typically, patients recover from the initial trauma, the so-called lucid interval, only to slip back into a progressively deepening coma.* Epidural hematomas are surgical emergencies that, if not immediately drained, will produce, in rapid succession, uncinate herniation, tonsillar herniation, medullary compression, respiratory paralysis, and death.

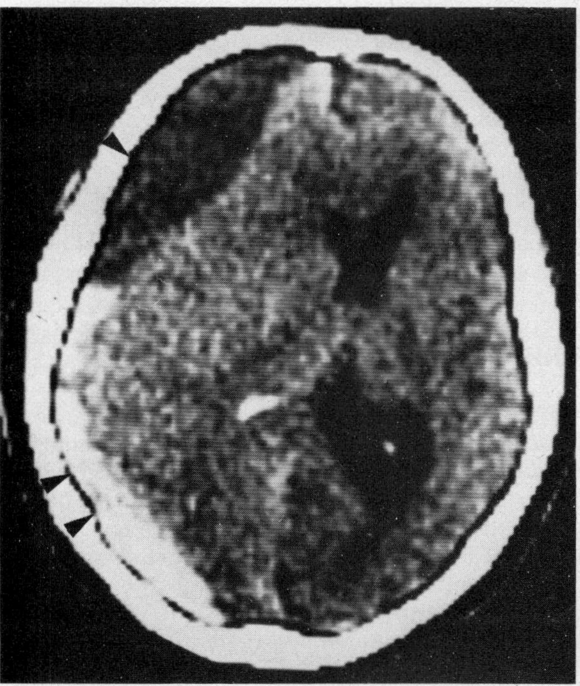

Figure 29–20. CT scan of subdural hematoma overlying and compressing left cerebral hemisphere and distorting ventricular system. Note that less dense blood elements remain in upper zone (*single arrow*) and heavier elements remain in lower dependent zone (*double arrow*).

Subdural Hematoma

A *subdural hematoma* is a collection of blood between the dura and arachnoid (Figs. 29–19 and 29–20). Subdural hematomas often result from blunt trauma without skull fractures, and may be either acute or chronic. They are most frequently located over the convexities of the cerebral hemispheres (bilaterally in 15% of cases), occurring more rarely in the posterior fossa.

Acute subdural hematomas are usually associated with obvious trauma, frequently with a laceration or contusion of the brain. Bleeding occurs from a tear of a bridging vein between the venous sinus and the cortex or from torn vessels in the underlying damaged CNS. *In contrast to epidural hematomas, the onset of symptoms is generally delayed and is manifested clinically by fluctuating levels of consciousness.* The outcome of an acute subdural hematoma depends not only on the effectiveness of surgical treatment but also on whether the adjacent brain is injured.

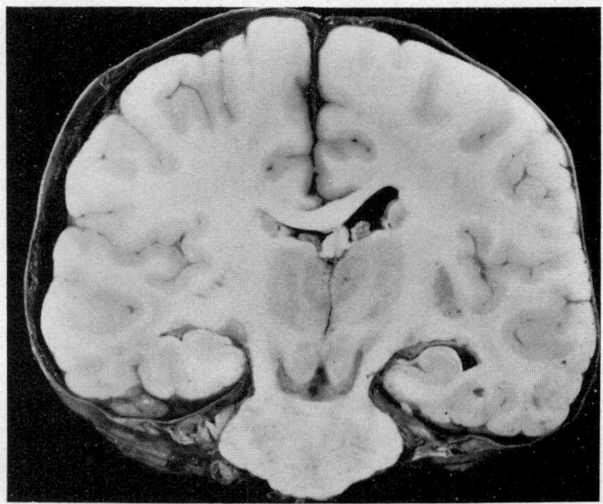

Figure 29–19. Subdural hematoma. The thin inner membrane can be seen between the clot and the leptomeninges (coronal section).

Chronic subdural hematoma is a less dramatic lesion and may be one of the most difficult of all neurologic conditions to diagnose. These hematomas often follow insignificant, sometimes forgotten trauma and are usually of insidious onset. Confusion, inattention, and rarely seizures and coma develop slowly and progressively. Elderly patients and alcoholics are frequent victims. Previous diffuse CNS impairment such as dementia may mask the presence of a subdural hematoma. The symptoms produced are often attributed to other processes, such as neoplasm, brain infarction, and hemorrhage, and for this reason these hematomas are sometimes referred to as "great mimickers."

The sites of bleeding in most chronic subdural hematomas are the bridging veins between the dura and meninges. On histologic examination, these hematomas consist of accumulations of blood encased by an outer membrane underlying the dura and an inner membrane that separates the blood from the adjacent arachnoid. Both membranes are composed of granulation tissue derived from the dura. Electron microscopy shows that the vascular channels within the membranes have incompletely endothelialized walls. This makes them susceptible to rebleeding with only minimal trauma and this may result in a progressive enlargement of the hematoma (Figs. 29–20 and 29–21). The theory of enlargement by oncotic pressure effects has now been discredited. Treatment consists of surgical drainage, but rebleeding from the membranes sometimes leads to reaccumulation, which may necessitate a craniotomy to remove the membranes. A closely related lesion is the subdural hygroma, a subdural collection of CSF, sometimes blood-tinged, which can result from trauma. It is thought to result usually from a tear in the arachnoid membrane.[79]

INJURY TO BRAIN

Traumatic brain injury produces combinations of *contusion*, *laceration*, *intraparenchymal hemorrhage*, and *diffuse axonal injury*. The separate category of birth injury is discussed on page 478. Before the pathologically well-defined entities are discussed, a few words are in order about the poorly defined but common phenomenon of cerebral concussion.

Cerebral concussion is a transient loss of consciousness that occurs immediately following nonpenetrating blunt impact to the head. Generally, this occurs when the head, *while moving*, strikes or is struck by an object. The duration of unconsciousness is usually short—from seconds to minutes—although it may last several hours. Patients normally recover completely without neurologic deficits; on rare occasions, however, they do not regain consciousness, and death is sudden. No satisfactory explanation has been advanced to account for all the observed clinical phenomena. Concussion is probably the result of some type of "physiologic disturbance." On autopsy, brain swelling is apparent in a few patients who die in the acute stage of cerebral concussion, whereas in others who die later of a cause unrelated to the past trauma, old healed contusions are sometimes found.

A *contusion* is an area of hemorrhagic necrosis that occurs when a blunt force crushes or bruises CNS tissue (Fig. 29–22). The most common site of injury is the surface of the brain, especially the crowns of the gyri, frequently in the subfrontal, anterior temporal, and occipital regions. Injury may occur at the site of impact (a *coup lesion*) or at a distance away from the point of impact, usually on the opposite side of the brain (a *contrecoup lesion*). The impacting force may either rotate the brain or pass through it. In either case, the brain—a semisolid structure in a solid box— strikes the supporting structures, such as the tentorium cerebelli and falx cerebri, and slams against the bony projections of the cranial vault, such as the orbital ridge and wing of the sphenoid bone. On histologic examination, acute contusions show foci of hemorrhagic necrosis. Later, macrophages remove dead tissue, and the area gradually resolves into an irregular, yellow-brown, rugose crater with a floor of glial tissue that is often covered by leptomeningeal fibrosis. Because of their color, these old contusions are referred to as "plaques jaunes."

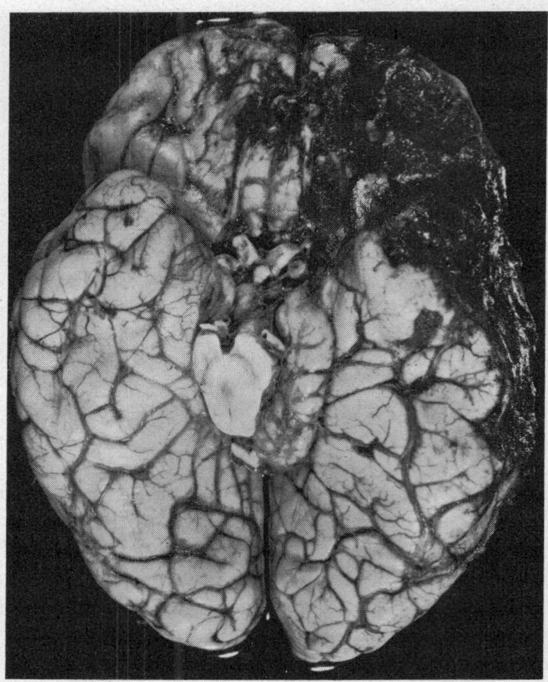

Figure 29–22. Severe contusions of left frontal and temporal lobes. There is also massive left uncal (hippocampal) herniation and compression of right cerebral peduncle.

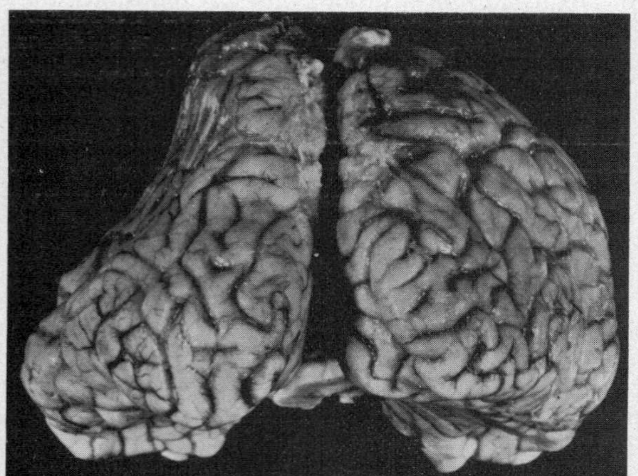

Figure 29–21. Deformed left cerebral hemisphere secondary to massive subdural hematoma.

A *laceration*, in contrast to a contusion, is a tear produced by a crude penetrating injury to CNS tissue, with subsequent hemorrhage and necrosis. A laceration may result from an external penetrating object or from penetration of a sharp fragment of skull. Resolution of a laceration is similar to that of a contusion, except that it leads to an irregular, yellow-brown, frequently linear gliotic scar that involves not only cortex, but also the deep underlying structures, including the white matter and sometimes the basal ganglia.

Traumatic intraparenchymal hemorrhage usually occurs when there has also been contusion and/or laceration of the brain, but very occasionally is seen in their absence. These types of parenchymal trauma also frequently result in sometimes substantial leakage of blood into the subarachnoid space, thereby adding a *traumatic subarachnoid hemorrhage* to the already existing damage.

Diffuse axonal injury occurs in a group of patients who have severe neurologic impairment but do not have massive, grossly visible brain damage. Characteristically, these patients are deeply comatose from the moment of injury and recover only to the point of a persistent vegetative state. Microscopic examination of the brain shows widespread diffuse white matter damage in the form of *ruptured axons* and *spheroids* (p. 1372). Older cases show microglial reaction, myelin degeneration, and sometimes microcavitation.[81, 82] There is some dispute over the pathogenesis of this lesion, but the most likely explanation is that shearing forces during the acceleration/deceleration of the brain cause physical rupture of axons.[83]

COMPLICATIONS OF TRAUMA

Various complications may develop in patients who survive the initial insult (Fig. 29–17). Posttraumatic *brain edema* may occur, especially in children, and *herniation, brain stem compression,* and *Duret hemorrhages* may follow (Fig. 29–22). The pathogenesis of posttraumatic brain swelling is not well understood but seems to be due in part to an increase in the cerebral circulating blood volume, perhaps related to a defect in autoregulation. The cerebral edema accompanying this increased blood volume appears to be attributable to a functional disruption of the blood-brain barrier. Less frequently, skull fracture may provide a conduit for *infection*, especially from the ear or nose; *hydrocephalus* may develop secondary to blood or infection in the ventricular system, aqueduct, or subarachnoid space.

In a few patients, death may follow shortly after trauma when there is no apparent physical disruption of tissue. How and why death occurs in these cases is unknown.

Delayed sequelae of trauma include *posttraumatic epilepsy*, which usually occurs in patients who have sustained a cortical contusion or laceration. Its genesis is poorly understood. *Delayed intracerebral hemorrhage*, the so-called "spät apoplexy," may also follow trauma, for totally obscure reasons.

TRAUMA TO SPINAL CORD

Mechanical injury to the spinal cord occurs by *penetration* and/or *compression* injuries. *Penetrating wounds* are usually secondary to stabbing or shooting, and produce *lacerations* of the cord, sometimes combined with hemorrhage into the cord parenchyma *(hematomyelia). Compression injuries* produce *contusions* of the cord and are most commonly caused by *subluxation, dislocation,* or *fracture* of the vertebrae. These occur most often in the cervical or lumbar regions. Parenthetically, the most frequently encountered cause of cord compression is metastatic tumor in and around the spinal canal. Vertebral dislocation without permanent bone displacement sometimes causes only momentary cord compression, and the resulting "concussion" induces a transient loss of cord function from which there is usually complete recovery. More severe trauma may produce displacement and fracture of the vertebrae, with *contusion, laceration,* or even *transection* of the cord from which there is rarely any significant recovery. If, as in cervical spondylosis, the spinal canal is already narrowed, even small vertebral displacements may severely damage the cord.

Particularly in spinal cord injury, associated vascular damage is often an important contributing factor, adding local ischemia, infarction, edema, and hemorrhage to the direct physical disruption. Epidural bleeding may also exacerbate damage from other causes. Further, because of the arrangement of the spinal arterial supply, ischemia and infarction may occur at some distance from the point of vascular injury. Finally, vascular damage may affect the cord without direct cord injury, because severe thoracic or abdominal trauma can tear the intercostal arteries to the spinal cord and produce an infarction through reduced blood flow (p. 1395).

Pathologically, neurons, axons, and myelin sheaths are variably sheared or crushed, and there is often local necrosis and hemorrhage. Subsequent fibrosis and gliosis may produce a dense collagenous scar or gliotic cavity at the site of the trauma.

There are two different clinical presentations of spinal cord damage. In *traumatic complete transections*, the findings are dramatic: the initial spinal shock produces a hyporeflexic flaccid paralysis, with anesthesia below the level of the lesion, and an atonic bladder. Later, the characteristic spastic picture with hyperreflexia emerges. In *more slowly developing compressions*, such as those caused by metastatic tumor, there is often local pain and tenderness at the site of the compression, and the initial weakness, hyperreflexia, and (often) bowel and bladder dysfunction (typically urinary retention with overflow) progress to spastic paralysis and anesthesia, usually with a sensory level. Confirmation of the compression may be obtained by lumbar puncture and myelography, which, unless it is contraindicated, should rapidly be followed by a decompressive laminectomy if permanent damage is to be minimized. CT scan of the spinal cord is also used to evaluate damage to it.

TUMORS OF NERVOUS SYSTEM

In general usage, the term *brain tumor* is often used to mean any tumor found within the cranial cavity, but properly speaking it should be used only for *neoplasms arising from the constituent cells of the brain,* i.e., *neurons, neuroglia, and cerebral vasculature. Primary intracranial tumors* include various tumors of non–brain tissues such as meninges, cranial nerves, pituitary, as well as the primary brain tumors. Finally, there are *metastatic tumors*.

CLASSIFICATION. Although no current classification is ideal, the one suggested by the World Health Organization (as modified in Table 29–4) is perhaps the best and allows standardization of diagnosis throughout the world. As the table shows, each kind of cell in the nervous system is represented by at least one type of tumor. Tumors arising from nervous system parenchyma may also develop from more than one cell type, e.g., ganglioglioma, or from primitive neuroectodermal cells that can differentiate along neuronal and/or glial lines within the same tumor, e.g., medulloblastoma. A major diagnostic difficulty arises from the wide range of histologic appearances that tumors of the nervous system can exhibit. This can lead to close morphologic similarities between tumors of widely different origin, e.g., a fibrous meningioma and a fibrillary astrocytoma, which may have quite different prognoses. Special stains and, increasingly, specific immunocytochemical markers are helping to resolve these diagnostic problems.

BIOLOGIC PROPERTIES. In considering the prognosis of primary intracranial, and particularly primary brain, tumors, *biologic malignancy* must be distinguished carefully from *histologic malignancy*. There are many intracranial tumors that are histologically benign but cannot be removed, and thus shorten the life of the patient, thereby having biologic malignancy. These tumors may be unresectable for two reasons. First, they may be located in a part of the brain that makes it impossible to remove even a well-circumscribed or trivially invasive neoplasm, as, for example, an ependymoma in the floor of the fourth ventricle. Second, some brain tumors, notably astrocytomas, have a marked propensity for infiltrative growth so that individual tumor cells extend well beyond the margins of the grossly visible tumor. Even allowing for the daunting prognosis of these tumors, an attempt at curative resection requires the sacrifice of so much functioning brain tissue that the subsequent reduction in the quality of life is too great to justify the procedure.

Table 29–4. CLASSIFICATION OF NERVOUS SYSTEM TUMORS

Tumors of Neuroglia
Astrocytes
Astrocytoma—differentiated
—anaplastic
Juvenile pilocytic astrocytoma
Oligodendrocytes
Oligodendroglioma—differentiated
—anaplastic
Ependyma and its homologues
Ependymoma—differentiated
—anaplastic
Ependymoblastoma
Subependymoma
Choroid plexus papilloma
Filum terminale tumor, myxopapillary ependymoma
Undifferentiated neuroglia
Glioblastoma multiforme
Tumors of Neurons
Neuroblastoma
Ganglioneuroma
Tumors of Neurons and Neuroglial Cells
Ganglioglioma
Tumors of Primitive Undifferentiated Cells
Medulloblastoma
Tumors of Pineal Cells
Tumors of Meninges
Meningioma
Meningeal sarcoma
Tumors of Nerve Sheath Cells
Neurofibroma
Schwannoma (neurilemmoma)
Lymphomas—Primary and Secondary
Malformative Tumors
Craniopharyngioma
Epidermoid cyst
Dermoid cyst
Colloid cyst
Metastatic Tumors
Unclassified Tumors

Tumors that break through to the meninges or cerebral ventricles may be spread throughout the nervous system via the CSF, thereby exhibiting a form of *intraneural seeding*, to produce disseminated tumor nodules on the brain, spinal cord, and nerve roots, and which clinically often presents as a *carcinomatous meningitis*. Among the primary brain tumors, medulloblastomas and pineal tumors frequently spread in this manner, but sometimes neuroglial tumors also. Of the metastatic tumors, lung and breast cancers are the principal offenders. *Extraneural metastasis* from primary intracranial tumors is distinctly uncommon, although when encountered is most likely to be from a glioblastoma or medulloblastoma. Its occurrence is encouraged by surgical procedures such as ventriculoperitoneal shunts and other operative procedures that disrupt the integrity of the dura and subarachnoid space.

CLINICAL EFFECTS. The variation in the location, growth rate, and biologic behavior of intracranial tumors makes it impossible to give even the barest outline of the variety of their presenting symptoms, signs, and natural course. However, as with other space-occupying lesions within the cranial cavity, they produce both local and general effects.

Their *local effects* usually are not clinically distinguishable from those of other types of space-occupying lesion, and are determined more by the size and location of the mass than by its nature. Hemiparesis, seizures, ataxia, or weakness are frequent but not diagnostic presentations. CT scans usually show a focal mass lesion of either increased or reduced density, often a midline shift and other effects, e.g., edema (Fig. 29–23). The *general effects* of raised intracranial pressure by any mass lesion have already been described (p. 1375), but the primary intracranial tumors, particularly if located in a so-called silent area such as the frontal lobe, may reach a large size before either local or general symptoms become sufficiently troublesome to bring the patient to medical attention. This insidious onset is more likely to occur with primary intracranial than with metastatic tumors, because the latter are more often surrounded by a zone of edema that renders even small masses rapidly symptomatic.

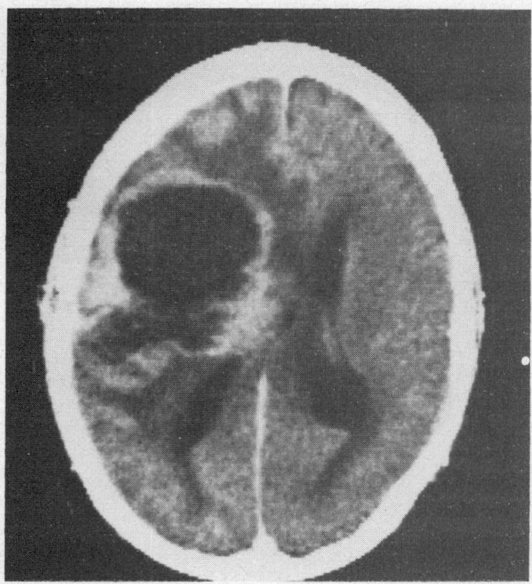

Figure 29–23. Large tumor in cerebral hemisphere showing ring enhancement with contrast material and pronounced peritumor edema.

INCIDENCE. In unselected series, primary *intracranial* tumors are present in about 1.2% of all autopsies and make up approximately 9.2% of all primary neoplasms. They are one of the most common groups of neoplasms in infants and children, become rarer in young adults and then increase again with age, but again become unusual after the age of 70 years. As will be seen, different tumors predominate in different age groups. Medulloblastomas, for example, are principally tumors of children and young adults. In children, 70% of intracranial tumors are infratentorial, whereas in adults the converse is true, 70% being supratentorial. The approximate relative incidence of the more common intracranial tumors in adults is shown in Table 29–5.

NEUROGLIAL TUMORS

Generically called *gliomas*, these are the tumors derived from the neuroectodermal glial cells and comprise *astrocytomas*, *glioblastoma multiforme*, *oligodendrogliomas*, and *ependymomas*.

Astrocytoma

Astrocytic neoplasms range from the histologically well differentiated to the very anaplastic. In well-differentiated lesions, the tumor cells have strong resemblances to the normal reactive forms of astrocytes (p. 1373), and the anaplastic tumors merge into the glioblastomas (p. 1402), into which many of them develop. Collectively, astrocytomas (excluding glioblastomas) account for between 20 and 30% of adult glial tumors; if the glioblastomas are included, the figure is raised to 80 to 90%. The highest incidence is in children and there is a male:female ratio of 2:1. There is a strong correlation between age and both histologic type and

Table 29–5. INCIDENCE OF INTRACRANIAL TUMORS*

100 Intracranial Neoplasms	
Secondary metastases	25–30
Primary neoplasms	70–75
Gliomas	40–50
Glioblastoma	25–30
Astrocytoma	8–12
Ependymoma	2–3
Oligodendroglioma	2–3
Medulloblastoma	2–3
Meningioma	12–15
Acoustic nerve tumor	5–10

*Modified from W.H.O.

topographic location. In children and young adults, pilocytic astrocytomas of the cerebellum, hypothalamus and third ventricle, and chiasm are frequent, as also are pontine gliomas. In adults, most astrocytomas are in the cerebral hemispheres and not infrequently are very anaplastic. With the exception of the pilocytic astrocytomas of the cerebellum and optic nerve, which frequently behave more like hamartomas than tumors and often can successfully be resected, all astrocytomas, whatever their location and level of differentiation, may enter a rapid growth phase.

Grossly, well-differentiated astrocytomas, although occasionally circumscribed, are usually poorly defined, gray-white, fleshy, infiltrative lesions that enlarge and distort the underlying brain (Fig. 29–24). They range from a few centimeters in diameter to enormous masses that can replace the major part of a cerebral hemisphere and even spread into the opposite hemisphere through the corpus callosum. They are generally solid, although they sometimes contain small cysts, and, depending on their fibrillary content, may be firm or soft and gelatinous.

Histologically, differentiated astrocytomas may be composed largely of protoplasmic, pilocytic, or gemistocytic

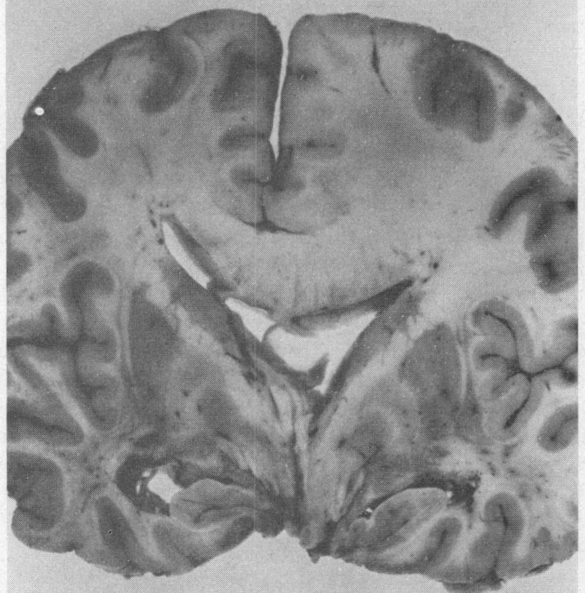

Figure 29–24. Diffuse astrocytoma. Expanded white matter of right cerebral hemisphere and thickened corpus callosum (coronal section).

astrocytes. The **protoplasmic astrocytoma,** the rarest of the differentiated forms, is made up of small, dark, round cells, each consisting of a nucleus surrounded by a scant rim of cytoplasm, from which delicate protoplasmic processes extend. Neuroglial fibers are scant in these tumors. **Pilocytic astrocytomas** are composed of bipolar, spindle-shaped astrocytes with "hairlike" processes and indistinct cytoplasmic borders. **Gemistocytic astrocytomas** are characterized by distended cells with abundant cytoplasm having numerous extended cellular processes. Ultrastructurally, the cytoplasm of these cells is packed with ribosomes and mitochondria. Both the pilocytic and gemistocytic variants have many neuroglial fibers, and if their formation is sufficiently exuberant, the tumor may be called a **fibrillary astrocytoma.** In tissue sections, neuroglial fibers are usually best demonstrated with the PTAH stain, rendering the fibers blue to magenta. Despite this separation of the differentiated astrocytomas into distinctive categories on the basis of the particular line of differentiation of the tumor cells, most tumors are composed of a mixture of these cell types. In all these tumors, mitotic figures are rare, and vascular endothelial hyperplasia either scant or absent.

Another form of astrocytoma usually encountered in the second and third decades of life is called **gliomatosis** or **gliomatosis cerebri,** because a large region of the brain, and sometimes the whole brain, is diffusely infiltrated by a "sprinkling" of neoplastic astrocytes.

Anaplastic astrocytomas verging on glioblastomas multiforme tend to be larger, more obviously infiltrative lesions. Foci of bland necrosis, cystic softening, and hemorrhages are more common than in the better differentiated lesions. However, it is impossible from gross inspection to differentiate unequivocally between anaplastic and well-differentiated astrocytomas. Microscopically, they possess anaplastic features such as increased cellularity, nuclear pleomorphism, hyperchromatism, a variable number of mitotic figures, and vascular endothelial proliferation (Fig. 29–25). Areas of well-differentiated glioma, usually astrocytoma, may also be present. Indeed, well-differentiated astrocytomas exhibit a marked tendency to become more anaplastic with time, so that, for example, a gemistocytic astrocytoma may evolve into an anaplastic astrocytoma or a glioblastoma multiforme.

Clinically, astrocytomas present with general and/or local symptoms and signs, their nature depending largely on the location of the tumor. These symptoms and signs may remain static or progress only slowly for a number of years. Eventually, however, patients usually enter a period of more rapid clinical deterioration, which is generally correlated with the development of anaplasia and rapid growth in the tumor. Once this occurs the prognosis is grave, since rapid tumor growth usually leads to death within months or a few years. The anatomic location of the astrocytoma materially influences the prognosis. For example, a differentiated astrocytoma in the cerebral hemisphere has a much better prognosis than one in the brain stem. Overall, with surgical resection and radiotherapy, supratentorial tumors have a one-year survival rate of about 70%, which falls to between 25 and 35% at five years.

Glioblastoma Multiforme

Glioblastomas multiforme are the most anaplastic of all the gliomas. It may be difficult to determine the origin of the neoplastic cells in these tumors, but careful study of most usually reveals regions characteristic of differentiated or undifferentiated astrocytomas. Indeed, although they may arise de novo, *glioblastomas usually develop in preexisting astrocytomas by progressive loss of differentiation.* They account for more than 50% of all gliomas and may occur at any age, although they are rare under 30 and have a peak incidence between 45 and 55 years. Males are more frequently affected than females. Most glioblastomas arise in the cerebral hemisphere, particularly in the frontal lobes. Rarely, they occur in the spinal cord, but foci of glioblastoma frequently can be found in astrocytomas of the pons and medulla, especially in children. Peculiarly, they almost never arise in the cerebellum.

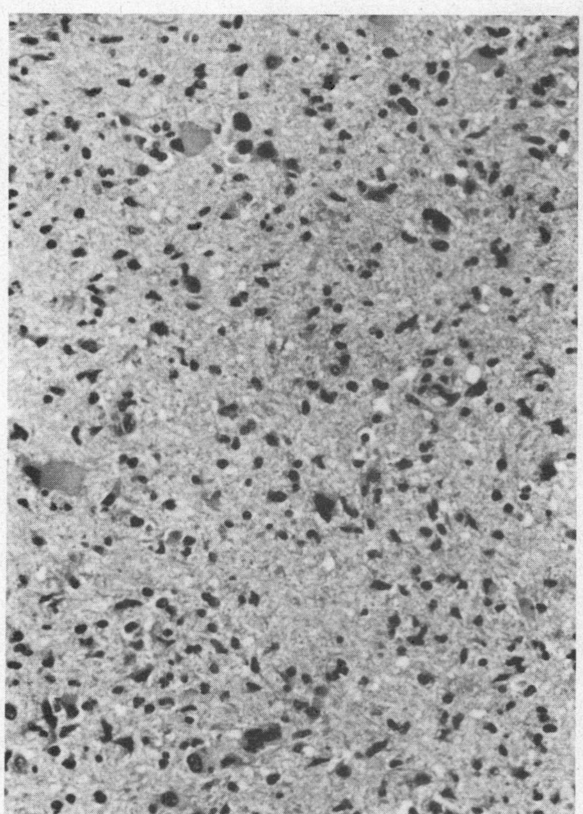

Figure 29–25. Diffuse astrocytoma. Note hypercellularity and pleomorphic astrocytes. (H and E stain.)

Grossly, glioblastomas often appear to be well circumscribed, although they always infiltrate the surrounding brain at their edges. Variation in their gross appearance from region to region is highly characteristic, and gave rise to the appelation "multiforme." Some regions may be white and firm, others yellow and soft. Cystic softenings, foci of necrosis, and hemorrhages are more typical of glioblastomas than of any other brain tumor (Fig. 29–26*A*). In some cases, they spread widely and implant in the meninges or on the spinal cord at some distance from the primary lesion.

Microscopically, they generally are highly anaplastic, with hypercellularity and a striking cellular pleomorphism, ranging from small, elongated, irregular, undifferentiated cells to giant bizarre forms. Necrosis with pseudopalisading of nuclei, abnormal mitoses, and endothelial proliferations

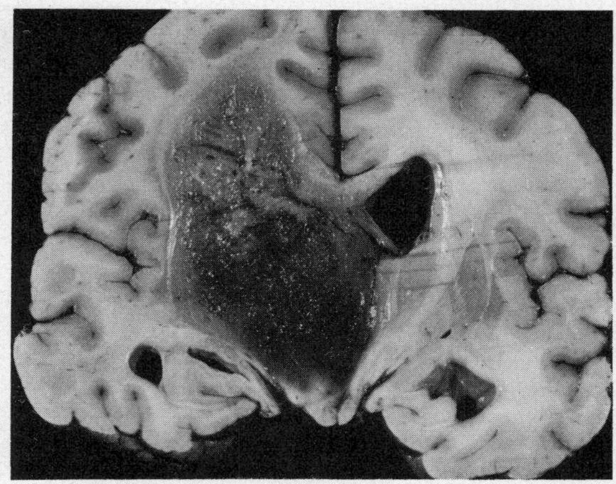

A

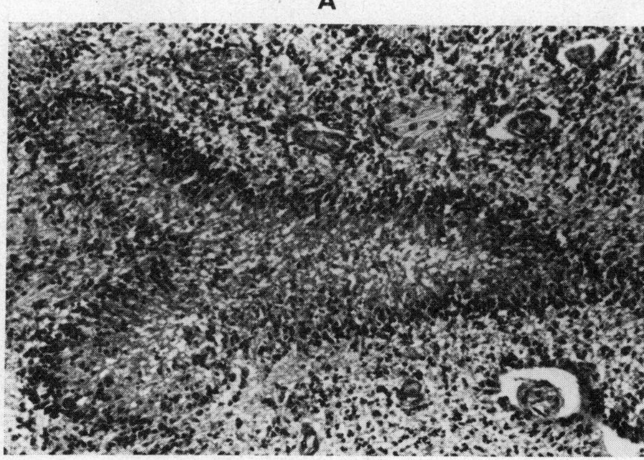

B

Figure 29–26. *A,* Glioblastoma multiforme appearing as a necrotic hemorrhagic infiltrating mass. *B,* Pseudopalisading (neoplastic cells aligned around a region of necrosis), hypercellularity, and pleomorphism in glioblastoma multiforme (H and E stain).

are usually prominent (Fig. 29–26*B*). Almost always, some areas contain recognizable astrocytes.

Clinically, the signs and symptoms evoked by these neoplasms are similar to those produced by astrocytomas, except that they appear more acutely and progress more rapidly. The prognosis is very poor: 90% of patients die within two years of diagnosis. Treatment, consisting of various combinations of surgery, radiotherapy, and chemotherapy, has not been successful to date.

The issue of the pathologic grading of astrocytomas must be addressed briefly. Astrocytomas are often graded on a scale of 1 to 4 with increasing anaplasia; glioblastoma multiforme in this scheme being a grade 4 astrocytoma. However, in the brain, and particularly with astrocytomas, this process is more than usually fraught with difficulty, principally because the degree of anaplasia in a large brain tumor may vary greatly throughout the neoplasm. Thus, the grade as determined by a biopsy, or even several biopsies, may not be representative of the tumor as a whole. Also, judgment of the level of anaplasia is notoriously subjective, and, to compound the problem further, the degree of anaplasia may itself change at any time. Finally, the location of the lesion and its size and accessibility to surgical excision materially affect the outcome, whatever the degree of anaplasia. Thus, the grading of these neoplasms, although often performed, must be interpreted with an understanding of its limitations.

Juvenile Pilocytic Astrocytoma of Cerebellum

This special subtype of astrocytoma has some of the characteristics of a hamartoma, and must be separated from other astrocytomas because of its different biologic behavior and pathologic characteristics.

These astrocytomas are usually located in the cerebellum, though identical-appearing tumors can be found on the floor of the third ventricle, hypothalamus, and optic chiasm and nerve. Grossly, they are well circumscribed, although they may have indistinct borders and cysts of various sizes. Most frequently they occur as a mural nodule in the wall of a large cyst (Fig. 29–27). Microscopically, there are pilocytic astrocytes, which are spindle-shaped cells with thin "hairlike" processes, Rosenthal fibers (p. 1373), and microcysts. Although features of anaplasia are almost never present, there is often vascular endothelial proliferation.

Clinically, these tumors are most common in childhood and present with unsteadiness, headache, and sometimes vomiting. Their *prognosis is excellent* and there are recorded cases of patients living more than 40 years following even incomplete resection.

Oligodendroglioma

About 5% of all intracranial gliomas are oligodendrogliomas. These are among the most unpredictable of the gliomas and, indeed, may be found as incidental lesions at autopsy. However, they are capable of rapid progression and may run a short course to death. The sexes are affected equally, and the peak incidence is in the fourth and fifth decades.

These tumors are usually located in the cerebral hemispheres, but they can occur in the spinal cord and cerebellum. On gross examination, they appear as deceptively well-defined globular gray masses in which cystic foci, spontaneous hemorrhages, and calcifications are frequently found. An occasional tumor extends to the subarachnoid space and disseminates via the cerebrospinal fluid to other sites within the CNS. X-ray examination and CT scan can sometimes suggest an oligodendroglioma because of its tendency to calcify.

On microscopic examination, they consist of monotonous sheets of uniform cells with finely stippled, compact, spherical nuclei surrounded by clear cytoplasm, giving the appearance of a cleared ring or halo (Fig. 29–28). Neuroglial fibers cannot be demonstrated. A delicate-appearing vascular stroma is often present, separating the neoplastic cells into small clusters. Endothelial proliferation and bizarre giant cells can sometimes be found. Calcifications ranging from microscopic foci to massive depositions may occur in these tumors. Electron microscopy has shown concentrically arranged lamellae in some neoplastic oligodendrocytes, suggesting that these cells may be attempting to form sheathlike structures. Mixed oligodendrogliomas and astrocytomas occur with fair frequency. If the astrocytic elements are ana-

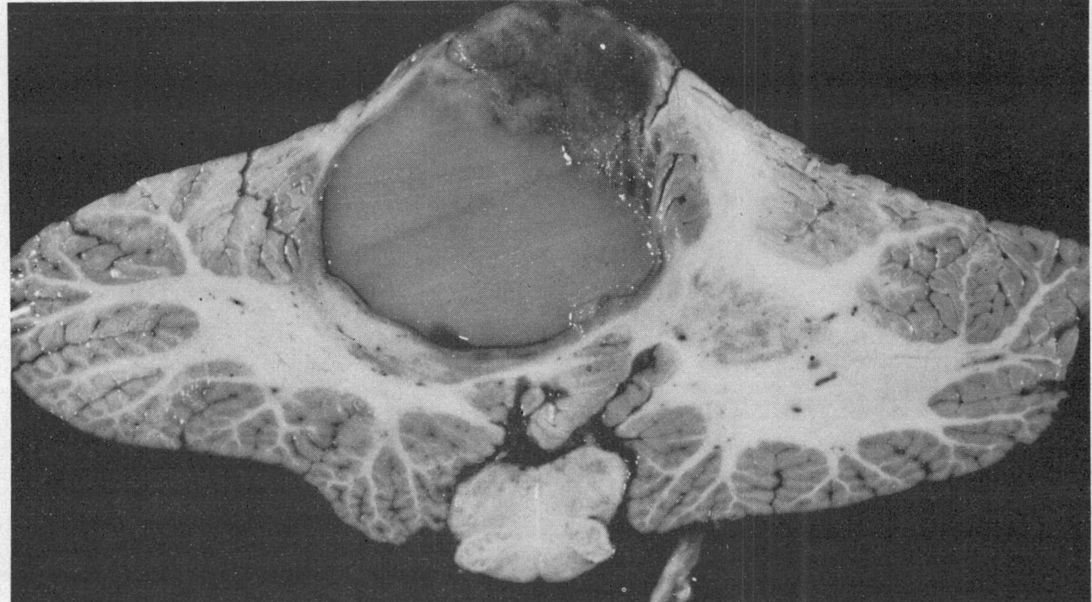

Figure 29–27. Juvenile pilocytic astrocytoma in cerebellum with nodule of tumor and cyst.

plastic, the prognosis is the same as for an anaplastic astrocytoma.

Most oligodendrogliomas grow slowly and produce only focal symptoms such as epileptic seizures. The history of such attacks may go back many years (five to 20). On the other hand, some in their rapid growth mimic glioblastomas. It is important to note that *there is no correlation between the microscopic features of an oligodendroglioma and its biologic behavior*. The treatment is surgical followed by postoperative radiation, yielding an average survival of approximately five years, although, as pointed out, the prognosis in individual cases is difficult to determine. The use of chemotherapy as an adjunct is being explored.

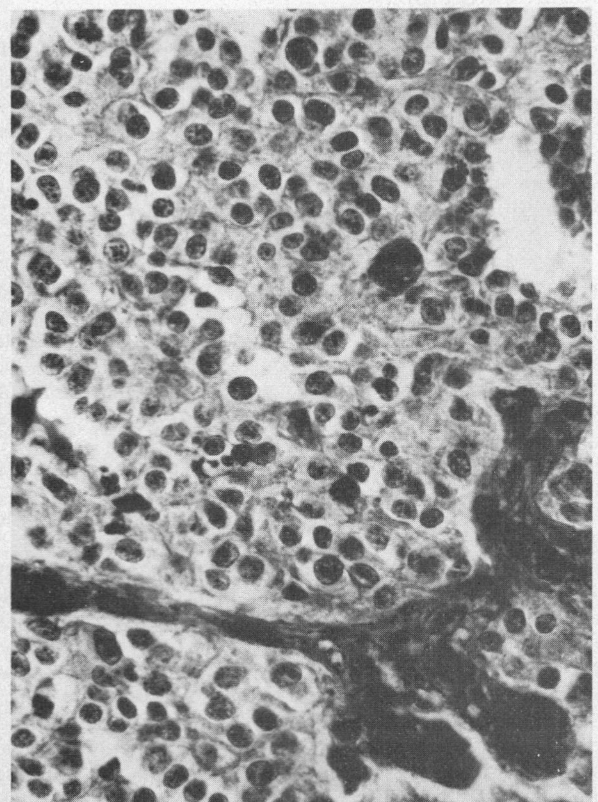

Figure 29–28. Oligodendroglioma. Cells are round and small and have perinuclear halos. (H and E stain.)

Ependymoma and Related Tumors

EPENDYMOMA

The cells of origin for this tumor are the ependymal cells that line the ventricular surfaces and form the central canal in the spinal cord. Ependymomas occur most commonly between childhood and adolescence, although they have been observed at all ages. They represent about 5 to 6% of all intracranial gliomas, but 63% of intraspinal gliomas.[56] Spinal lesions are most prevalent in the lumbosacral and cauda equina regions. One variant, the "myxopapillary ependymoma," tends to occur in the filum terminale.

On gross examination, cranial ependymomas usually appear as fairly well-defined masses that grow by expansion and frequently project into the ventricles. Sometimes these masses assume an extremely papillary form (papillary ependymoma) and must be differentiated from choroid plexus papillomas. Differentiation between these two types of papillary ventricular tumors using the naked eye can be impossible.

On microscopic examination, ependymomas are composed of a uniform population of spindled or carrot-shaped cells with finely basophilic, stippled, uniform nuclei. **Particularly diagnostic are rosette formations in which the tumor cells align themselves in a ring around a canal or space to create a tubule or a likeness to the normal**

ependymal cavity (Fig. 29–29). Neuroglial fibers are seen frequently within these cells. Individual cells may also show so-called blepharoplasts, which appear in the PTAH stain as a cluster of small dark cytoplasmic spots. These structures are associated with cilia formation and, when found, are diagnostic of ependymal cells. Neoplastic cells are arranged frequently around blood vessels in pseudorosette formations (Fig. 29–29). Anaplastic features are rare in these tumors, although they may appear. The name "malignant ependymoma" is applied to these tumors. Rare ependymomas blend in histology into a glioblastoma multiforme. Some pathologists have designated an ependymoma with anaplastic features as an "ependymoblastoma." However, it is preferable to reserve the term ependymoblastoma to distinguish a rarely occurring tumor that is composed only of cells with features of **primitive** ependymal cells.[11]

Clinically, well-differentiated ependymomas grow slowly and cause symptoms by their expansion. Hydrocephalus can be a complication of those arising in the ventricular system. Lesions arising in the spinal cord give rise to symptoms referable to that spinal level. Even though most of these tumors are histologically benign and slow growing, they carry an extremely poor prognosis. Their location often renders them inaccessible to surgical excision. Some spread within the subarachnoid spaces, and rare lesions have given rise to extraneural metastases. Fokes and Earle reported an average survival of 53 months following surgery and radiotherapy in patients with posterior fossa ependymomas.[87]

VARIANTS OF EPENDYMOMA

Subependymomas are well-circumscribed neoplasms that originate from neuroglial tissue just beneath the ependymal lining. These are small, hard, lobulated tumors composed of an admixture of ependymal and astrocytic elements. Often, they protrude as pedunculated nodules into one of the ventricles, and sometimes several totally separate lesions arise concurrently. Generally, they are asymptomatic and are frequently found incidentally at autopsy. On rare occasions, they may grow to a large size and cause hydrocephalus.

Myxopapillary ependymoma is almost exclusively a tumor of the filum terminale. Most occur in the fourth decade of life. This tumor is grouped with the ependymomas because ependymal cells are in most cases the most prominent constituents. However, myxopapillary ependymomas should be thought of as a separate clinicopathologic entity, and the name *"filum terminale tumor"* might be more appropriate.

On gross examination, the myxopapillary ependymoma appears as a mass in the filum terminale, sometimes involving the lower end of the spinal cord. On microscopic examination, its structure is reminiscent of the normal filum terminale. Cuboidal cells, sometimes with clear cytoplasm, are often arranged around papillary cores consisting of connective tissue and blood vessels. These vacuolated cells may also form tubular structures located between the papillary formations. Mucin-positive material may be demonstrated in the connective tissue elements of these tumors. In some cases, this tumor infiltrates surrounding nervous tissue and bone. Very rare examples have metastasized. The prognosis is excellent when the tumor can be completely removed surgically.

Choroid Plexus Papilloma

These rare, usually benign tumors constitute 1 to 2% of all intracranial neoplasms. They may occur at any age, but most often are diagnosed in the first decade of life, principally in males.

Quite distinctive, they appear as well-defined, cauliflower-like papillary masses originating from the choroid

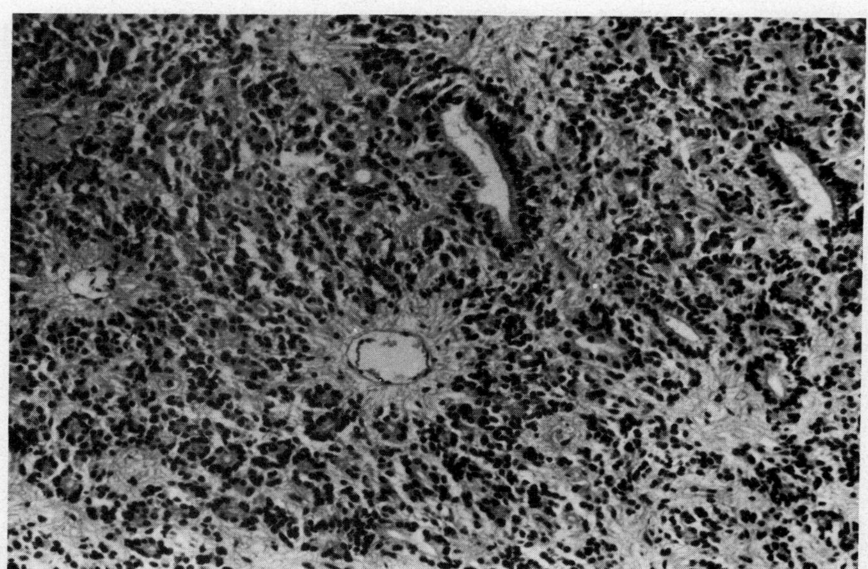

Figure 29–29. Ependymoma. Note tumor cells align themselves around tubular spaces resembling the ependymal cavity and also around blood vessels. (H and E stain.)

plexus and protruding into a ventricular cavity (most often the fourth ventricle). On microscopic examination, the papillary structures are reminiscent of normal choroid plexus characterized by vascular connective tissue stalks covered with cuboidal epithelial cells, which sometimes contain vacuoles of mucin. Choroid plexus papillomas are usually well differentiated. On rare occasions, they can become anaplastic with infiltrative rapid growth, which is designated "choroid plexus carcinoma." Such malignant forms may be difficult to differentiate from metastatic adenocarcinoma.

The papillomas grow by slow expansion and principally cause problems by inducing internal hydrocephalus and/or spontaneous hemorrhages. Treatment consists of surgical removal. In cases of choroid plexus carcinoma, radiation is recommended following surgery.

TUMORS OF NEURONAL ORIGIN

Included under this heading are cerebral neuroblastoma, ganglioneuroma, and ganglioglioma. Neuroblastomas and mature ganglion-cell tumors can occur in the CNS, especially in the cerebral hemispheres; however, they arise more frequently in peripheral nerve ganglia and the adrenal medullae. Very rarely, they are seen in the mediastinum, where they are presumed to be of teratoid origin.

Cerebral Neuroblastoma

Neuroblastomas are rare brain tumors, presumably having origin in precursor cells of neurons. They may arise anywhere in the cerebral hemisphere, perhaps with a slight preference for the frontal lobes. They are most common during the first ten years of life. Occasional tumors mature or show areas of maturation toward ganglion cells.

On gross examination, they are usually located in the cerebral hemispheres, where they appear as well-defined gray granular masses (averaging 6 to 7 cm in diameter) that may contain cysts and regions of necrosis and hemorrhage. Sometimes they have a lobular appearance on cut surface. On microscopic examination, three variants have been described by Horten and Rubinstein: classic, desmoplastic, and transitional types.[88] In the **classic variant**, the tumor is highly cellular and composed of dark, round, sometimes fusiform cells with a scant amount of cytoplasm. The polar extensions of the fusiform cells may be aligned to create rosettes identical to those seen in adrenal neuroblastomas. Similar palisades may be formed around blood vessels. Silver stains sometimes show a transition between undifferentiated cells and mature ganglion cells. Often, there is an abrupt transition between tumor and adjacent brain. This feature is of great aid in surgical enucleation and is helpful in differentiating a cerebral neuroblastoma from other neuroectodermal tumors. The **desmoplastic variant** is characterized by abundant connective tissue stroma. The third variant, **the transitional pattern**, contains both classic and desmoplastic features. In the desmoplastic and transitional variants, the tumor shows less tendency to differentiate into mature ganglion cells.

Clinically, the cerebral neuroblastoma behaves as a malignant neoplasm, with a high recurrence rate following surgery, although some have not recurred for years. Forty per cent of these tumors disseminate by way of the CSF pathway. Rare extraneural metastases occasionally develop. Unlike the neuroblastoma of the adrenal, they rarely elaborate catecholamines. The prognosis of cerebral neuroblastomas is difficult to determine in the individual case, because of their rarity. Whether those lesions showing mature differentiation have a better prognosis than the undifferentiated lesions has not been established. Treatment consists of surgery, total CNS axis radiation, and chemotherapy.

Ganglioglioma and Ganglioneuroma

Tumors composed of mature neurons arise in the peripheral nervous system, the adrenal medulla, or less frequently in the CNS. The stroma in tumors arising in the periphery consists of spindled Schwann cells in which can be found calcospherites. Such tumors are called *ganglioneuromas* or *gangliocytomas*. On the other hand, in tumors within the CNS, when the stroma consists of neuroglial tissue, they are designated *gangliogliomas*. These CNS neoplasms are extremely rare and generally occur in children and young adults.

On gross examination, gangliogliomas are usually well-defined masses with a granular cut surface in which calcifications and small cysts can sometimes be seen. Typically, they occur in the floor of the third ventricle, hypothalamus, and temporal lobe. On microscopic examination, gangliogliomas are characterized by a mixture of well-differentiated neuronal and glial elements that may resemble a hamartoma. On rare occasions, however, either the neuroglial or the neuronal elements may show transition to primitive cells resembling anaplastic astrocytes or neuroblasts. When such features are present, the tumor becomes more indistinct grossly, infiltrates the surrounding brain, undergoes rapid growth, and behaves in a malignant manner.

Overall, the prognosis with these neoplasms is favorable, depending on the anatomic location of the tumor and whether anaplastic features are present. Treatment consists of surgical excision.

TUMORS OF PRIMITIVE OR UNDIFFERENTIATED CELLS

Medulloblastoma

Medulloblastomas are among the more common CNS tumors in children, second in frequency only to astrocytomas. In this age group, they account for 25% of all intracranial tumors. However, they are not restricted to children and have been found in adults up to the sixth decade of life. Males are affected more often than females.

Medulloblastomas arise predominantly in the cerebellum, probably from the fetal external granular layer, although this latter point is controversial.[21] In childhood, they are most common in the vermis of the cerebellum, but are found in the lateral cerebellar hemispheres in adults.

On gross inspection, they usually appear as fairly well-demarcated, gray-white masses with indistinct edges (Fig. 29–30*A*). Histologically some tumors are composed of sheets of small, dark, carrot-shaped cells with poorly defined margins, dense nuclei, and little cytoplasm (Fig. 29–30*B*).

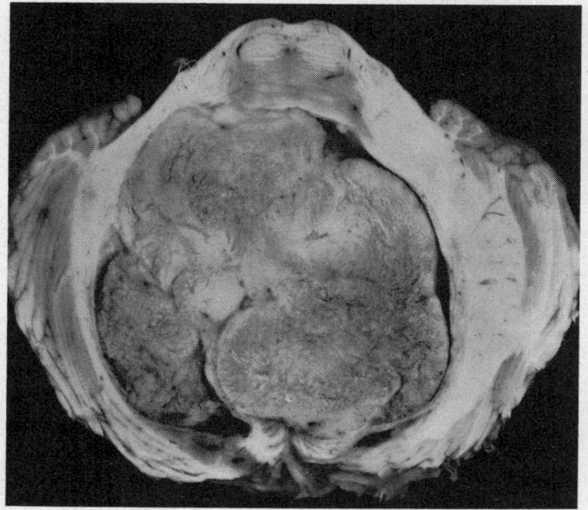

A

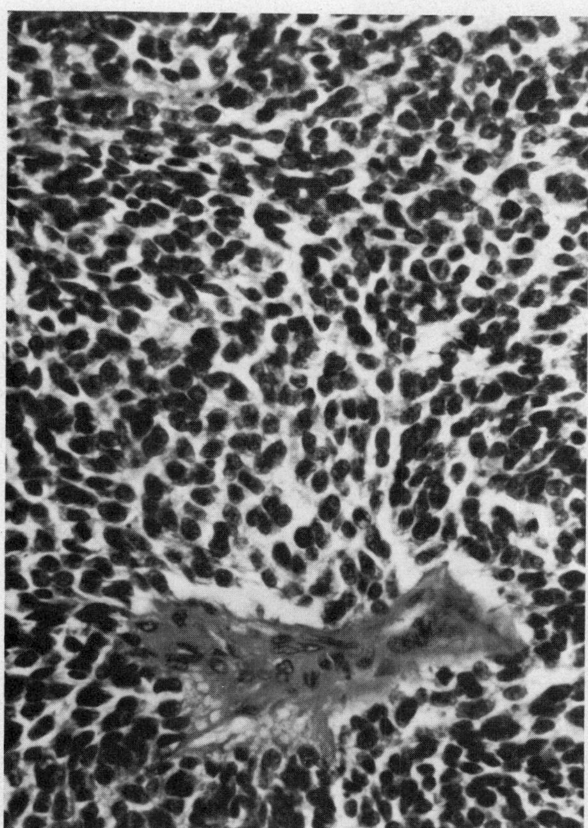

B

Figure 29–30. *A,* Medulloblastoma growing into fourth ventricle, distorting, compressing, and infiltrating surrounding structures. *B,* Medulloblastoma (H and E stain).

Sometimes rosettes are formed, in the center of which silver-positive fibrils can be demonstrated. Occasionally, readily recognized mature ganglion cells are encountered. This pattern of growth is characteristic of neuronal (neuroblastic) differentiation. More commonly, however, these neoplasms have regions of decreased cellularity interspersed with broad bands of undifferentiated cells. These focal, less cellular regions may have a blue fibrillary background with the PTAH stain. Occasionally, neoplastic cells in such regions have cytoplasmic processes and greatly resemble astrocytes. These features are indicative of neuroglial or spongioblastic differentiation. Rare cases simultaneously show both forms of differentiation. **The hallmark, then, of a medulloblastoma that separates it from other neuroectodermal tumors is its origin from primitive cells having the potential to develop along both neuronal and neuroglial lines.**

Medulloblastomas are infiltrative, invasive tumors and commonly spread throughout the CNS axis via the spinal fluid pathway. In some cases, particularly in adults, these tumors infiltrate the overlying meninges and elicit a remarkably desmoplastic reaction. Rare cases have metastasized, most commonly to bone marrow and regional lymph nodes.

Previously, the prognosis for these tumors was bleak. In some recent cases, however, remarkable success has been obtained with the combination of surgical removal, radiation, and chemotherapy.

TUMORS OF MENINGES

Meningioma

A primary tumor of the meninges may originate from any of the meningeal constituents such as arachnoid cells, fibroblasts, or blood vessels. Most arise from arachnoid cells within the arachnoid villi, and so the localization of these neoplasms more or less parallels the sites where villi are most numerous. On the whole, they are slowly growing, benign tumors that may remain silent. At autopsy, especially in patients over 70 years of age, it is quite common to find small asymptomatic meningiomas composed of arachnoid cells. Symptomatic meningiomas nonetheless constitute about 14% of all intracranial tumors. They can occur at any age, but are most frequent in middle-aged adults, especially women.

Meningiomas may occur within the cranial vault or in the spinal canal. The most frequent site of intracranial lesions is the parasagittal region, followed by the lateral cerebral convexity, and then the falx cerebri. Less common locations are the sphenoid ridge, olfactory groove, cerebellar pontine angle, foramen magnum, and spinal canal, especially at the thoracic levels. Intracranial meningiomas are more than twice as common as spinal meningiomas.

On gross examination, the tumors tend to be irregular-to-round, lobulated, tough, white-gray masses that are well circumscribed and indent (from pressure) the adjacent nervous tissue (Fig. 29–31*A*). There is usually a definite cleavage plane between the tumors and the underlying nervous system tissue. Occasionally, they grow en plaque to cover wide areas, e.g., an entire cerebral hemisphere. The cut surface of some tumors is gritty, owing to the presence of numerous psammoma bodies (described below). Two dis-

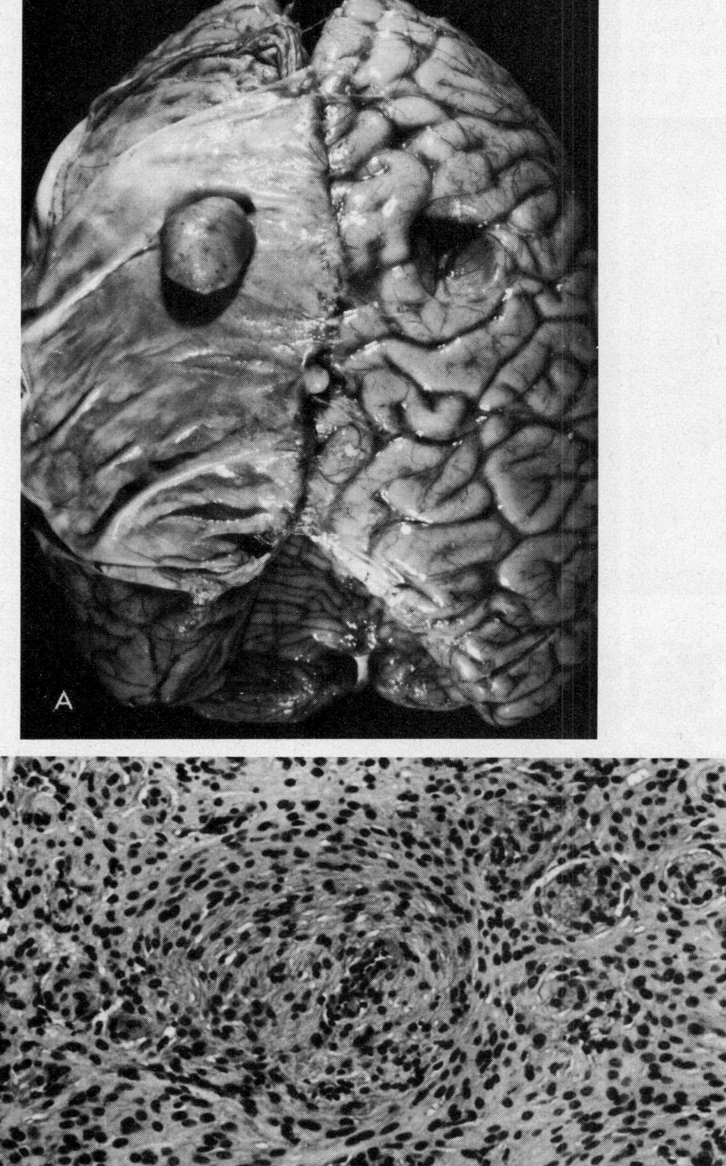

Figure 29–31. *A,* Reflected dura (*on left*) showing one large and one small (*in middle of illustration*) meningioma. Note prominent indentation of right cerebral hemisphere by the larger tumor. *B,* Transitional meningioma with hypercellularity, whorled pattern of cells, and psammoma bodies (H and E stain).

tinctive features are sometimes present: (1) hyperostosis of the contiguous region of the skull and (2) penetration of the tumor into the adjacent bone.

On microscopic examination, meningiomas can be subclassified into meningotheliomatous (syncytial), fibroblastic, transitional, and angioblastic forms. A single tumor may have several patterns, but is classified according to the most prominent one.

Syncytial or meningotheliomatous lesions are composed of epithelial-like cells with abundant cytoplasm, indistinct cytoplasmic borders, and delicate, well-defined oval nuclei. There is no definite cellular arrangement other than lobulated groups of cells reminiscent of the appearance of normal arachnoid granulations.

Fibroblastic tumors are marked by long, tapering spindle cells growing in interlacing bands. There is a tendency toward alignment of the nuclei into palisades. Reticulin and collagen fibers are usually conspicuous between the spindle cells. Psammoma bodies are sometimes present. These comprise concentrically laminated structures formed by the deposition of calcium salts in degenerated tumor cells. This subtype of meningioma is very firm on palpation.

Transitional tumors have features of both syncytial and fibroblastic meningiomas and thus constitute a morphologic bridge between the two preceding patterns. Whorls of neoplastic cells are a conspicuous feature, often enclosing psammoma bodies (Fig. 29–31*B*). The term **psammomatous meningioma** may be applied to any meningioma that contains a large number of psammoma bodies.

Angioblastic meningiomas have evoked considerable nosologic controversy, for which reference may be made to Russell and Rubinstein.[11] Two variants are recognized, the hemangioblastic and hemangiopericytic. Briefly, these tumors are highly cellular and composed of cells with poorly defined cytoplasm and oval nuclei. Such cells usually lie immediately adjacent to capillary-like channels. Larger cells with a foamy appearance can also sometimes be found. Reticulin is usually conspicuous with use of special stains.

Hemorrhages; calcifications; xanthomatous changes within cells, cartilage, bone, and melanin; and myxomatous changes may be present in any of the patterns described. Occasionally, some of these tumors assume a papillary growth pattern, sometimes designated a "papillary meningioma."

Most meningiomas behave in a benign manner. Invasion of the adjacent skull, when present, is not accompanied by widespread dissemination, metastasis, or infiltration of contiguous nervous tissue. Symptoms relating to these tumors usually consist of headaches, visual impairment, and focal seizures. The separation histologically of the syncytial, transitional, and fibroblastic subtypes is of little value in terms of clinical outcome. The prognosis is more dependent on the location of the tumor and its accessibility for surgery. Most are amenable to excision.[23] Overall, the recurrence rate of most meningiomas five years after surgical removal is 15%. The angioblastic pattern, however, should be separated from the other variants because of its more aggressive growth, increased tendency to recur and spread, and consequently less optimistic prognosis.

Rarely, meningiomas show definite anaplastic features, even to the point of being indistinguishable from a spindle cell sarcoma (which can also arise in the meninges and the brain). Such anaplastic variants sometimes metastasize to extraneural sites, principally the lungs and lymph nodes. The papillary pattern is also worrisome, since it is correlated with more rapid growth, recurrence, and occasionally metastasis.

LYMPHOMAS (PRIMARY AND SECONDARY)

The CNS is sometimes seeded by secondary lymphomatous infiltration but, more surprisingly, is also occasionally the site of development of a primary lymphoma. In the past, these primary tumors were called microgliomas, on the assumption that they were derived from microglial cells (p. 1374). However, marker studies show that many of them are of B-lymphocyte origin and could not be derived from a cell of the monocyte-phagocyte series such as the microglial cell.[89] Current practice is to use the same classification as for extracranial lymphomas (p. 658), and older terminology such as microglioma and reticulum cell sarcoma should now be discarded. Statistically, they make up 0.4% of primary brain tumors, and 0.02% of lymphomas. They are met more often in association with mycosis fungoides, dysproteinemias, and renal transplantation.[90] Whatever the setting, they appear most frequently in the fifth and sixth decades of life. Interestingly, even with use of modern diagnostic criteria, no unequivocal case of primary intracranial Hodgkin's disease has yet been described.

On gross examination, a primary CNS lymphoma may take the form of multiple nodules or diffuse infiltration of the nervous tissue. The latter pattern can be extremely widespread without disturbing the underlying architecture of the brain. It may therefore be very difficult to diagnose these tumors by means of x-ray, pneumoencephalogram, arteriogram, or CT scan. The microscopic details of these lesions have been presented earlier under the consideration of systemic lymphoma (p. 658).

Secondary lymphomas of the CNS are much more common than primary lymphomatous involvement. In the secondary disease, the lymphoma usually infiltrates the dura and leptomeninges and, less commonly, the parenchyma of the brain. This is in contrast to the primary lymphomas just described, which infiltrate the brain.

Leukemias, like the secondary lymphomas, may involve the dura and leptomeninges, but rarely show parenchymal infiltration. The peripheral and CNS nerve roots may also be involved in such cases. Focal intracranial hemorrhage may occur secondary to the low platelet count frequently encountered in these disorders. Sometimes, multiple bleeding sites are scattered throughout the brain. Such hemorrhages constitute serious complications that often lead to death.

OTHER INTRACRANIAL TUMORS

Colloid Cyst of Third Ventricle

This entity occurs generally (though not exclusively) in young adults. It constitutes about 2% of all intracranial neoplasms. The nature and origin of these lesions have been the subject of considerable controversy; they may be more of a malformation than a neoplasm and of either ependymal or paraphyseal (choroid plexus) origin.

They are invariably located in the third ventricle anteriorly. They appear as round, soft, white masses ranging from 1 to 4 cm in diameter, attached by their walls or by a short pedicle to the ventricular wall. On cut surface, they consist of a fibrous capsule that surrounds a cystic cavity containing a jelly-like substance. On microscopic examination, the cyst is lined with cuboidal to low columnar, sometimes ciliated, epithelium. Mucous goblet cells are frequently interspersed.

Clinically, patients with these lesions often complain of headache caused by hydrocephalus, which may be aggravated by particular positions of the head. Apparently, these tumors can move about and intermittently obstruct the flow of CSF through the foramen of Monro. Features of anaplasia are not encountered and these lesions behave as slowly growing, noninfiltrating masses. Surgical excision can be curative.

Metastases to CNS

Metastases to the brain account for approximately 20 to 25% of all intracranial tumors. With rare exceptions, e.g., basal cell carcinoma of the skin, all cancers have the potential of disseminating to the brain, but certain primaries have a propensity for such ugly behavior, namely, bronchogenic and breast carcinomas. Following at some distance behind such front runners are carcinomas of the kidney and gastrointestinal tract, and melanocarcinomas. Usually, the intracranial metastases appear in patients who already have far-advanced cancers with widespread dissemination of the tumor throughout the body. However, to the dismay of many a neurosurgeon, an apparent "primary brain tumor" is sometimes found to represent a metastasis. In such cases, the intracranial lesion usually became symptomatic before there were other manifestations of the extracranial neoplasm. Thus, in the morphologic evaluation of a presumed primary CNS tumor, the possibility must always be entertained that it could represent a metastasis from an occult cancer elsewhere in the body.

On gross examination, metastases within the brain are usually discrete, well-circumscribed, firm nodules, 1 cm to several centimeters in diameter, clearly set apart from the surrounding brain substance. Multiple implants are the rule, but occasionally only a single nodule is present. They are frequently located at the junction of gray and white matter. Sometimes the metastases become necrotic or hemorrhagic, or both, thus simulating a malignant glioma. The brain tissue surrounding metastatic deposits can be extensively swollen and edematous. On microscopic examination, these lesions usually recapitulate the architecture and cytology of the primary neoplasm.

The signs and symptoms evoked by metastases to the brain are as varied as the size, number, and location of the implants. Very rarely, the metastases grow diffusely in the meninges and subarachnoid space to masquerade as a form of meningitis. More often, the expanding metastatic deposits and surrounding edema of the brain cause an increase in intracranial pressure that can lead to fatal herniation of the brain stem and cerebellar tonsils. Almost always, patients with brain metastases are close to the end of the road. Rarely, a solitary implant is amenable to surgical excision, permitting some prolongation of life.

DEMYELINATING DISEASES

Primary demyelination is loss of myelin sheaths with relative preservation of the demyelinated axons. It results either from damage to the oligodendroglia, which make the myelin, or from a direct, usually immunologic or toxic attack on the myelin itself. *Secondary demyelination*, in contrast, occurs following axonal degeneration. The *demyelinating diseases* are a group of CNS conditions characterized by *extensive primary demyelination*. They comprise (1) *multiple sclerosis* and its variants and (2) the *perivenous encephalitides*. There are several other diseases in which the principal pathologic change is primary demyelination but which are more conveniently classified in other categories, notably the inborn errors of metabolism (the *leukodystrophies*) (p. 1424); viral disease (progressive multifocal leukoencephalopathy—*PML*) (p. 1386); and several rare disorders of unclear etiology (e.g., *central pontine myelinosis*) (p. 1422).

MULTIPLE SCLEROSIS (MS)

Since Charcot first described the essential characteristics of multiple sclerosis in 1868, it has been the subject of exhaustive but inconclusive study. In about two-thirds of the cases, onset is between 20 and 40 years of age; it is rare in persons over 50. There is a slight female preponderance. The natural history of this disease is as variable as the number and distribution of the brain lesions. Some patients have only a brief episode of slight nervous system disability with rapid recovery, whereas others have a relentless downhill course to death in weeks or months. By far the most common pattern is an episodic course over many years, punctuated by relapses and remissions. Frequent early manifestations are paresthesias, diplopia, central scotomata, mild sensory or motor disorder in a limb, or cerebellar incoordination. Intellectual deterioration is not usually an early feature. As the disease progresses, remissions become less complete. Although not all patients become totally disabled, the end stage is often that of ataxia, incontinence, and paraplegia due to widespread cerebral and spinal cord demyelination. There is no effective treatment, although ACTH is often administered with some benefit during relapses.

MORPHOLOGY. The external appearance of the brain and spinal cord is usually normal. On cut section, multiple, irregularly shaped, sharp-edged lesions called **plaques** are seen. Less frequently, plaques have a diffuse rather than a sharp border and/or may be only faintly visible (shadow plaques). Plaques occur in gray and white matter, vary from 0.1 cm to many centimeters in diameter, and may be sparsely scattered or involve a large fraction of the brain and spinal cord. Although they have a predilection for the angles of the ventricles (Fig. 29–32), they may occur anywhere in the CNS. Their appearance varies with age, being initially slightly pink and swollen, but later becoming gray, retracted, and opalescent.

Microscopically, the earliest loss of myelin is located around small veins and venules (perivenous demyelination). Mononuclear cells and lymphocytes are frequently present around these vessels. As demyelination progresses, the perivenular foci expand to form the macroscopically visible plaques. In actively enlarging plaques, there is an inflammatory mononuclear phalanx at the border between the demyelinated and normal areas. Within the plaque, there is loss of oligodendroglia, but a pronounced reactive astrocytosis and numerous neutral lipid-laden macrophages. The axons traversing the plaque are conspicuously spared. Old inactive plaques have sharply defined edges, profound myelin loss, an almost total absence of oligodendroglia, and scattered fibrillary astrocytes. Although they are relatively preserved, some loss of axons is often detectable. In shadow plaques, the demyelinated area shades gradually into the normal white matter without a sharply defined border, or there may be only partial demyelination throughout the plaque.

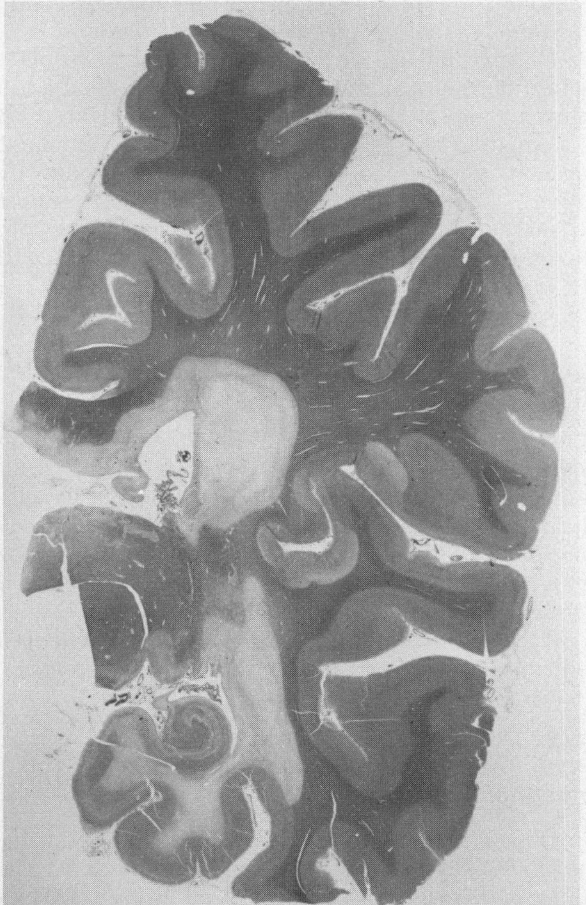

Figure 29–32. Multiple sclerosis. Unstained regions of demyelination (MS plaques) around lateral ventricle and in temporal lobe. (Luxol-fast-blue, PAS stain for myelin.)

PATHOGENESIS. There is much fascinating and provocative evidence about the pathogenesis of MS and many theories have been advanced to account for its epidemiology, clinical course, and pathologic features. Most current work relates to putative viral[91] or autoimmune[92] etiologies, but there is no coherent theory of the pathogenesis of this disease, and it should not be assumed that these must necessarily be the only candidates or that they are mutually exclusive. Data currently regarded as having an important bearing on the pathogenesis of MS are summarized below.

1. The disease is more prevalent in the temperate higher latitudes of both the northern and southern hemispheres.[93, 94] For example, the prevalence is 80 per 100,000 in southern Norway; 41 per 100,000 in Boston, Massachusetts; but only 15 per 100,000 in New Orleans, Louisiana. There are interesting exceptions, however, such as Japan, where the disease is uncommon at any latitude.

2. People who move from a low-risk to a high risk area before adolescence acquire a high risk of developing MS, whereas those who make the same move after adolescence retain their low risk. Thus, it seems that an initial event in the development of the disease occurs in early life.

3. It has been noted that first-degree relatives of MS patients are more likely to develop the disease than the general population. HLA, A3, B7, and DW2 antigens are present in increased frequency in North European and white American patients.[95] Curiously, a similar association is not present in Israeli Jews or Japanese.

4. The suggestion that an infectious agent may be involved in the pathogenesis of MS has been reinforced by the investigation of an outbreak of the disease that occurred in the Faroe Islands during the 1940s and 1950s.[96] The outbreak had the characteristics of a point source epidemic, and present evidence implicates the British occupation of the islands during W.W. II as its source. The agent currently under suspicion is the canine distemper virus (CDV), which was not present on the Faroe Islands before the occupation but is thought to have been introduced by dogs accompanying the occupying force. During and shortly after the occupation, an epidemic of canine distemper occurred in native dogs of the islands. Subsequently, canine distemper has disappeared and, interestingly, new cases of MS also in the resident, native-born Faroese. However, search for evidence of canine distemper infection in MS patients has so far been unfruitful. Some patients have an apparent rise in the antibody titer to CDV, but this is accompanied by a rise in the titer to measles virus (MV) which is antigenically a very similar virus and difficult serologically to distinguish from CDV. Recent results suggest that there are no unique CDV antigens in MS patients,[97] making it unlikely that there is a direct etiologic relationship between MS and CDV.

5. Measurement of the CSF protein in MS shows

an increase in the immunoglobulin content, which, on immunoelectrophoresis, is found to contain oligoclonal bands that are not present in the serum. This implies synthesis of immunoglobulins within the nervous system. The difficulty arises in the interpretation of this finding. Oligoclonal bands found in subacute sclerosing panencephalitis (p. 1385) are immunoglobulins directed against various antigens of the measles virus, but in MS no antigen has yet been discovered against which the antibodies are directed.[98] Further, different bands are found in different patients and it has been shown that, in the same patient, the immunoglobulins eluted from individual MS plaques may be different.[99] These findings tend to suggest that the immunoglobulin production within the blood-brain barrier in MS may be an epiphenomenon, perhaps occurring as a consequence of trapping of activated B cells, rather than being of direct pathophysiologic significance.

6. It has been found that relapses in MS coincide with a reduction in the numbers of circulating suppressor/cytotoxic T5/8 lymphocytes.[100] It has also been shown that the lymphocytes that accumulate in the acute plaques of demyelination are mostly helper T4 cells, so that the decline in the suppressor/cytotoxic T5/8 cells is not a consequence of their sequestration within lesions. Studies of the distribution of lymphocyte subsets within plaques have shown that helper T4 cells are concentrated at the expanding border of the plaque and extend into the surrounding, as yet not demyelinated, white matter, whereas suppressor/cytotoxic T5/8 cells are found mostly within the lesion.[101]

7. Some light has been shed on the process of demyelination in MS by studies of the pattern of disappearance of two of the myelin antigens, myelin basic protein (MBP) and myelin-associated glycoprotein (MAG) from plaques of demyelination. In both MS plaques and the lesions of progressive multifocal leukoencephalopathy, which is a virus disease of oligodendroglia, these two proteins have different time courses of disappearance.[102, 103] Further, in experimental allergic encephalitis (EAE), an experimental autoimmune disease directed against myelin antigens, MAG and MBP are lost simultaneously.[104] The detailed interpretation of these findings is not clear, but they tend to suggest that the pathophysiologic process in MS is not a straightforward immunologic assault on the myelin.

8. Clinical trials of immunosuppression in MS have shown that, in children at least, high levels of immunosuppression can temporarily arrest the progression of the disease.[105]

Present evidence concerning the pathogenesis of MS, therefore, is both confusing and incomplete, but it is suggestive of a role for infective and immune mechanisms, perhaps operating at different times in the lifetime of the patient.[106]

VARIANTS OR CONDITIONS CLOSELY RELATED TO MULTIPLE SCLEROSIS

A problem in the discussion of MS is its highly variable clinical presentation and the differences in the pathologic appearances of the lesions at various stages of the disease. Historically, this led to the emergence of a number of eponyms for what are probably only variants of the basic disease.[107] In addition to the classical *Charcot* type, these include the *Marburg* and *Balo* variants and *neuromyelitis optica* (Devic's disease). In this latter condition there are typical MS-like plaques in the optic nerves together with spinal cord lesions that may either be typical of MS or be a necrotic myelitis and quite unlike MS. Nowhere, however, is the terminology of MS more confusing than in the vexed question of *Schilder's disease*. A major part of the difficulty arises from the fact that Schilder himself, between 1911 and 1924, described what we now recognize to be at least two, and possibly three, morphologically similar but quite different diseases, all of which were called Schilder's disease. One is what we now call adrenoleukodystrophy (p. 1425). The second is probably a variant of MS characterized by giant plaques symmetrically affecting major portions of the cerebral hemispheres. These large lesions often, but not invariably, coexist with other typical plaques of MS elsewhere in the neuraxis. This appearance is usually seen in children but may occur in adults; the clinical course is one of relentless progression, although occasionally a chronic relapsing and remitting pattern is seen. The two entities of adrenoleukodystrophy and the MS variant have a similar morphology in the brain, and it was only the realization that some of these patients also had adrenal failure that led to the discovery of adrenoleukodystrophy as a separate entity. From Schilder's description, it is not now possible to decide which disease his third patient suffered from. In discussing these probable variants of MS, given our current ignorance of its etiology, it should not automatically be assumed that MS is necessarily a single disease.

PERIVENOUS ENCEPHALOMYELITIS

The term perivenous encephalomyelitis is applied to disorders associated with perivenous and perivenular demyelination and a pronounced mononuclear cell infiltration. They usually follow a viral infection, vaccination, or a vague respiratory illness and are characterized by a *monophasic*, rapid, and relentless course that frequently terminates in death. The two major disorders in this category are *acute disseminated encephalomyelitis* and *acute necrotizing hemorrhagic leukoencephalitis*.

Acute Disseminated Encephalomyelitis (Postinfectious and Postvaccinal Encephalomyelitis)

This is a rare condition that may appear during or shortly after a virus infection (measles, mumps, chickenpox, or smallpox) or, rarely, following vaccination against smallpox, rabies, or typhoid. There is compelling evidence that the lesions are induced by an autoimmune reaction to myelin triggered by virus (or vaccination) rather than by viral infection. In the first place, no virus has been consistently isolated from these patients. Second, lymphocytes from these patients exhibit cell-mediated immunity to myelin-basic protein. Third, the disease is strikingly similar to experimental allergic encephalomyelitis (EAE), which can be induced in various experimental animals by injections of brain emulsions in Freund's adjuvant.[108] Injected animals develop typical perivascular infiltrates associated with demyelination. The experimental disease can be transferred by T cells (though not by B cells). It is now established that the antigenic moiety is the basic protein of myelin, and, indeed, the precise amino acid composition of the protein has been mapped for several experimental species.

On gross examination, the brain is usually normal, or it may show slight congestion. Microscopically, perivenular lesions are seen characterized by a region of primary demyelination around veins. A cuff of lymphocytes and mononuclear cells surrounds these veins. Similar cells and macrophages are also scattered in the demyelinated regions (Fig. 29–33). The subpial region of the brain stem and spinal cord may also show demyelination, and the meninges may be infiltrated by mild-to-moderate numbers of inflammatory cells. Axons are preserved, at least in the very early lesions.

The disease has its onset within two to four days of the rash in the spontaneous viral diseases, or 10 to 13 days after vaccination. Neurologic manifestations are heralded by headaches, neck stiffness, and lethargy. Paralysis and coma ensue. Thirty to 50% of patients die in the acute phase. Those who survive the acute episode have severe residual neurologic impairment. Exceptional patients appear to have recovered with no sequelae.

Acute Necrotizing Hemorrhagic Leukoencephalitis

This is a rapidly fatal disorder that fortunately is quite rare. The disease is usually preceded by a nonspecific respiratory infection. Neurologic impairment develops abruptly, heralded by headache and fever, which proceed to paralysis and coma. Death is swift, usually within several days, although rare patients recover.

On gross examination, the brain exhibits asymmetric, soft and sometimes liquefied, gray-red areas flecked with tiny hemorrhages, particularly visible in the white matter of the cerebral hemispheres and brain stem. On histologic examination, there is necrosis and fibrin deposition in and around blood vessel walls, together with a vigorous inflammatory infiltrate. Neutrophils and, later on, lymphocytes and plasma cells infiltrate vessel walls and perivascular spaces. Initially, there appears to be some preservation of axons; however, necrosis quickly ensues. Morphologically, acute necrotizing hemorrhagic leukoencephalitis is distinguished from acute disseminated encephalomyelitis by the presence of more extensive necrosis, a more acute inflammatory infiltrate, the occurrence of perivascular hemorrhages, and its more focal distribution within the cerebral hemispheres or brain stem.

Although the cause of this devastating condition is unknown, an autoimmune basis is suspected, for the same reasons given for acute disseminated encephalomyelitis. In one study, lymphocytes from a patient with acute hemorrhagic leukoencephalitis were sensitized to myelin-basic protein.[109] Some authors regard acute necrotizing hemorrhagic leukoencephalitis as simply a more severe and acute variety of acute disseminated leukoencephalitis.

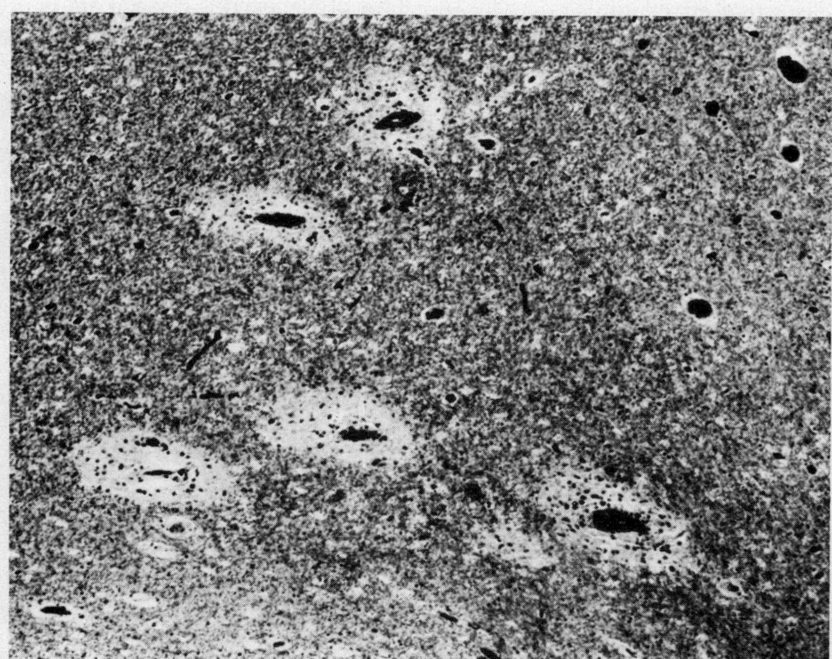

Figure 29–33. Postvaccinal encephalomyelitis. Note demyelination (lack of stain) around venules (stained black) (Woelcke stain).

DEGENERATIVE DISEASES

The application of the label degenerative to the diseases discussed in this section should not be allowed to disguise the fact that it is a confession of ignorance. There is no coherent, or even incoherent, theory for the etiology or pathophysiology of these diseases, and no compelling reason to assume that they all have the same, or even a similar, etiology. Progress in the understanding of these diseases has so far consisted of reassigning them to a more specific etiologic category, as for instance in the case of Jakob-Creutzfeldt disease (p. 1387), which was comfortably ensconced with the degenerative diseases until its transmissibility was demonstrated, thereby causing its removal to the unconventional agent (spongiform) encephalopathies.

Despite these taxonomic strictures, disorders that remain in the category of degenerative diseases do have some general similarities. They are diseases of neurons, and tend to be selective, affecting one or more functional systems of neurons, while leaving others intact; for example, in paralysis agitans there is selective degeneration of the striatonigral dopaminergic system. They are generally symmetric and progressive. There is great variation within syndromes, and clinical and pathologic overlap between ostensibly different syndromes, such as spinocerebellar degenerations.

In other ways, these diseases differ sharply among themselves; some have a clear pattern of heritability, whereas others are sporadic; some have intracellular abnormalities of greater or lesser specificity associated with them (e.g., Lafora bodies, Lewy bodies, neurofibrillary tangles), whereas in others the pathologic process seems to be one of simple atrophy and disappearance of the affected neurons.

Degenerative diseases that affect similar regions of the brain tend to produce clinical syndromes with many similarities, so that, for example, cortical and basal ganglia diseases tend to manifest as dementias and extrapyramidal movement disorders, respectively. With involvement of a particular region, a diagnosis can often be made only by correlation of the clinical and pathologic findings. In this chapter, the diseases are grouped according to the part of the brain most severely affected. Within each group there is usually no reason to suppose a closer etiologic relationship than that of topography.

DEGENERATIVE DISEASES AFFECTING CEREBRAL CORTEX

The major cortical degenerative diseases are *Alzheimer's disease* and *Pick's disease*, and their principal clinical manifestation is *dementia*. They are, of course, not the only causes of dementia; there are many others, including cerebrovascular disease, encephalitis, hydrocephalus, Jakob-Creutzfeldt disease, and metabolic diseases. By convention, dementias are divided into *presenile* and *senile; presenile dementia is defined as progressive mental deterioration leading to dementia, starting before the age of 65.* Despite its widespread employment, this division is not diagnostically or therapeutically helpful, and derives from an old idea that dementia was an age-related condition. Further, there does not seem to be any consistently definable clinical or pathologic difference between these idiopathic dementias that occur before and after the age of 65. Thus, for example, Alzheimer's disease and the so-called "senile dementia of the Alzheimer type" cannot reliably be distinguished from each other, either clinically or pathologically. If there is a difference, it is improbable that it will be on the basis of anything so biologically arbitrary as chronologic age.

Alzheimer's Disease

Alzheimer's disease usually becomes clinically apparent between 50 and 65 years of age (although it may occur earlier), with general impairment of higher intellectual functions or subtle emotional lability in the absence of focal neurologic defects. Characteristically, it progresses steadily over five to ten years to severe dementia and death, usually related to dehydration and respiratory infection. CT scans show marked brain atrophy (Fig. 29–34). There is some tendency to familial occurrence, although most cases are sporadic. Occasionally, localized symptoms of aphasia, agnosia, or apraxia occur, and convulsive disorders may be prominent during the course of some patients.

On gross examination, there is cortical atrophy, usually most pronounced in the frontal, parietal, and temporal regions (Fig. 29–35). Cut sections of the brain show compensatory ventricular enlargement secondary to tissue loss (hydrocephalus ex vacuo). The significant microscopic features of Alzheimer's disease are **neurofibrillary tangles** (p. 1372), **senile plaques, granulovacuolar degeneration,** and **Hirano bodies. Senile plaques** are focal extracellular

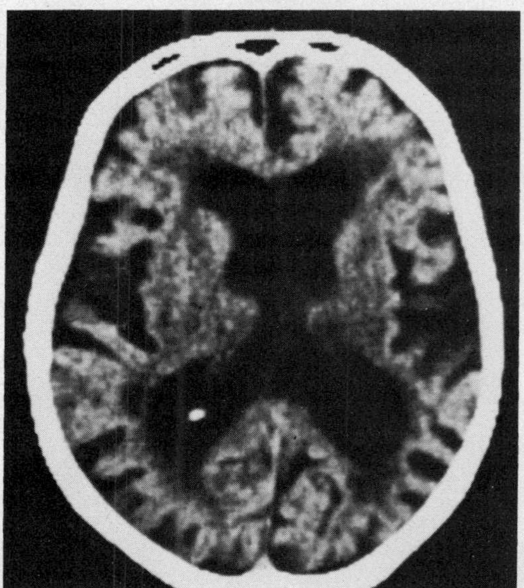

Figure 29–34. CT scan showing severe atrophy with gross dilatation of lateral ventricles and widening of cortical sulci.

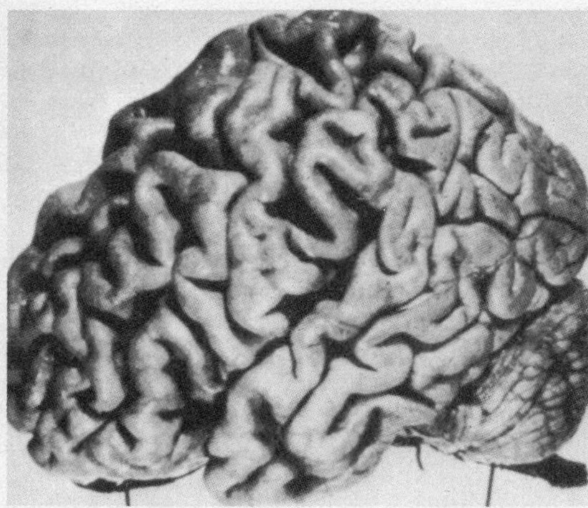

Figure 29–35. Alzheimer's disease. The brain shows diffuse cortical atrophy, particularly marked in frontal, parietal, and temporal lobes, with narrowing of gyri and widening of sulci. (Courtesy of Dr. Robert D. Terry.)

structures (20 to 150 μ in diameter) of dilated, tortuous, presynaptic axon terminals (and probably dendrites) found almost exclusively in the cerebral cortex. Microglial cells are often seen at the periphery of the plaque, and sometimes astrocytosis. Early plaques contain only the enlarged tortuous terminals, but later in their evolution they develop a central extracellular core of amyloid that contains prealbumin, immunoglobulin, and other fractions. Senile plaques are best demonstrated by silver stains and appear as irregular round formations of silver-positive fibers and particulate material that surrounds, but is separated from, the central silver-positive amyloid core by a clear halo (Fig. 29–36). With the electron microscope the axonal terminals contain paired helical filaments similar to those seen in neurofibrillary tangles, together with degenerating lysosomes and mitochondria.[110] **Granulovacuolar degeneration** appears as small (5 μ in diameter), clear, intraneuronal cytoplasmic vacuoles each of which contains an argyrophilic granule. The constituents of this granule are unknown, as is the pathophysiologic significance of this form of degeneration. This latter qualification also applies to **Hirano bodies,** seen in proximal dendrites as glassy eosinophilic inclusions. Ultrastructurally they consist of regular arrays of beaded filaments, which biochemical analyses show to be mostly actin filaments.[111]

All these structures can be seen in patients who do not have any known disease, and it is their numbers and distribution, rather than their mere presence, that allow the diagnosis of Alzheimer's disease to be made. Microscopic examination of the temporal lobe in older persons who are not demented frequently reveals the presence of some granulovacuolar degeneration and occasional Hirano bodies in the hippocampus, and scattered neurofibrillary tangles and senile plaques in the hippocampus, subiculum, and hippocampal gyrus. In Alzheimer's disease, Hirano bodies are numerous, and granulovacuolar degeneration is present in more than 10% of the neurons of the hippocampus. Plaques and tangles are found extensively in the amygdala and in the whole of the cerebral cortex, with the striking exception of the primary motor and sensory cortical areas; the tangles, but not plaques, are also present in the basal forebrain nuclei (basal nucleus of Meynert), and scattered in the raphe nuclei and the locus ceruleus.

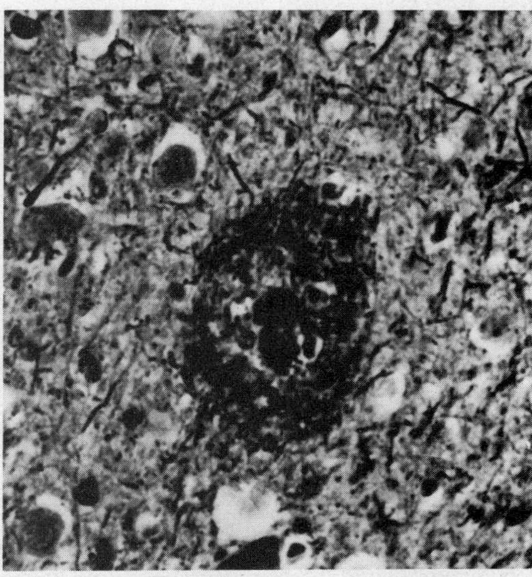

Figure 29–36. A senile (neuritic) plaque composed of a central, silver-positive amyloid core surrounded by a ring of cellular processes (Bielschowsky stain).

Pathogenesis. The basic defect in Alzheimer's disease is unknown. The number of neurofibrillary tangles and senile plaques can be roughly correlated with the degree of dementia, but the mechanisms underlying the formation of these structures are obscure. Recent biochemical findings have spurred a new interest in the distribution of the tangles and plaques. The most consistent biochemical abnormalities in Alzheimer's disease are deficiencies in acetylcholine and associated enzymes choline acetyltransferase and acetylcholinesterase in the cerebral cortex, amygdala, and hippocampus.[112] The cortical muscarinic receptor for acetylcholine remains strikingly intact, suggesting that the defect is in the cholinergic input to the affected areas. These findings not unnaturally provoked examination of the major cortical cholinergic input from the basal nucleus of Meynert. It was found to be severely depleted of cells in Alzheimer's disease,[113] and some of the remaining cells exhibited neurofibrillary tangles and/or granulovacuolar change. Subsequent investigations have shown depletion of other basal forebrain nuclei, i.e., the nucleus of the diagonal band of Broca and the medial septal nuclei, which are major cholinergic inputs to the cortex and hippocampus. In the cortex, the dilated axonal profiles of the senile plaques show large amounts of cholinesterase and a decrease in the amount of this material in the plaques with increasing maturity and the appearance of the central amyloid core. It is not clear, however, that the senile plaque is a direct expression of a disturbance in the terminal axonal arborization of the neurons of the basal nucleus of Meynert. The only other consistent finding in Alzheimer's disease is a decrease in the cortical somatostatin content, a finding that does not yet have an explanation.

As already mentioned, *senile dementia* is the term applied to dementias beginning after age 65. Many patients over this age have pathologic changes identical to those seen in Alzheimer's disease and are conventionally referred to as having *"senile dementia of the Alzheimer type."*[114, 115] Whether this condition and Alzheimer's disease are the same, or have different pathogenetic mechanisms, is controversial.

Pick's Disease

Although far less common than Alzheimer's, Pick's disease is often considered to be its "second cousin" because of its occurrence in the presenium and its frequently indistinguishable clinical symptoms and course. It affects women more often than men and there are occasional familial clusterings. The disease generally begins in middle or late middle life, with symptoms and signs of local cerebral cortical disease, which eventually become submerged in a "sea of mindlessness." Two-thirds of the patients have speech disturbances, manifested by utterance of incomprehensible jargon. The course is progressive, terminating in death within two to ten years.

On gross examination, the brain shows pronounced cortical atrophy in the frontal and temporal regions, with remarkable sparing of the posterior two-thirds of the first temporal gyrus. This is characteristic of this condition and distinguishes it on gross examination from Alzheimer's disease. Atrophy of the gyri can be so extreme as to reduce them to a thin wafer, so-called "knife-blade" atrophy or "walnut brain." Cerebral involvement is symmetric in about one-third of the cases, but there is some left-sided predominance in about half. This has been called lobar atrophy. In contrast to Alzheimer's disease, parietal atrophy is unusual and involvement of the occipital lobe is rare. Microscopically, neuronal loss is most severe in the outer three cortical layers. Remaining neurons frequently contain cytoplasmic, round-to-oval, filamentous inclusions—**Pick bodies.** They are weakly eosinophilic, in H and E preparations, but are strongly argentophilic to silver stains. Electron microscopically, they are probably composed of neurofilaments, paired helical filaments, and vesiculated endoplasmic reticulum. Their neurofilament content has been confirmed by immunochemical methods.[116] The formation of Pick bodies is thought by some investigators to represent retrograde or transsynaptic degeneration, or recent axonal injury near the cell of origin. Neurofibrillary tangles are less frequent than in Alzheimer's disease, and senile plaques are rare, but granulovacuolar change is frequent. Subcortical white matter degeneration is seen in severe cases.

DEGENERATIVE DISEASES OF BASAL GANGLIA AND MESENCEPHALON

Diseases affecting these regions of the brain frequently damage the extrapyramidal motor system and cause various types of movement disorder, such as rigidity, abnormal posturing, and chorea. For this reason, they are sometimes referred to collectively as *extrapyramidal diseases.*

Huntington's Chorea

This disease usually first appears in persons between 20 and 50 years of age, and is characterized clinically by extrapyramidal or choreiform movements combined with a progressive dementia. It is inherited as an autosomal dominant, with the interesting but unexplained property that those who inherit the disease from their fathers tend to manifest it much earlier in life than those who inherit from their mothers. The combination of autosomal dominant inheritance with symptomatic onset, often delayed until middle life, turns this disease into a medical sword of Damocles over the heads of the children of affected persons. For these offspring, an already difficult personal situation is exacerbated by the dilemma whether they themselves should have children and perhaps pass on the disease. The recent discovery that a genetic defect in these patients is located on chromosome 4[117] may lead to the removal of this sword, for although the precise nature of the defect has not yet been identified, its localization to a fragment of a chromosome offers the hope of eventual antenatal diagnosis, and intervention if desired.

On gross examination, the brain is small (less than 1000 gm) and shows striking atrophy of the caudate nucleus and, less dramatically, of the putamen. The globus pallidus may be secondarily atrophied, whereas the lateral and third ventricles are enlarged. Atrophy of the frontal lobes, occasionally of the parietal lobes, and (more rarely) of the entire cortex may be present.

Microscopically, there is preferential loss of the small neurons of the striatum accompanied by fibrillary gliosis. Loss of small neurons and gliosis are also seen in the ventrolateral nucleus of the thalamus and the substantia nigra. By electron microscopy, there are membranous whorls and increased numbers of dense synaptic vesicles in the presynaptic nerve terminals, but the postsynaptic terminals and the synaptic cleft appear normal.

Clinically, delusions, paranoia, neurosis, dementia, and abnormal eye movements are seen, and a hypothalamic component is suggested by abnormalities in glucose metabolism, aberrant growth hormone levels, and altered prolactin release in some patients. The disease is relentlessly progressive, with an average course of 15 years, terminating in death. Biochemically, there is a marked decrease in endogenous γ-amino butyric acid (GABA) and in glutamic acid decarboxylase (GAD). GABA receptors seem to be intact. There is also a decrease in choline-acetyltransferase and in the muscarinic cholinergic receptors. It is thought that these deficiencies lead to a decrease in the "filtering ability" of the striatum, allowing uncontrolled stimulation of the lower centers by the globus pallidus, resulting in the abnormal voluntary movements and chorea.

Hallervorden-Spatz Disease

This rare, and probably autosomal recessive disease affects the globus pallidus and the pars reticulata of the substantia nigra. Clinical features include (1) onset at a young age, generally in early childhood; (2) mainly extrapyramidal signs, with dystonic posturing, choreoathetoid or tremulous movements, and muscular rigidity, but also having spasticity, hyperreflexia, and extensor plantar responses indicative of corticospinal dysfunction; (3) dementia; and (4) a relentlessly progressive course to death in early adult life.

The most striking pathologic feature is the rust-brown gross appearance of the globus pallidus and substantia nigra. Microscopically, the condition is characterized by axonal spheroids (p. 1372), neuronal loss, gliosis, and the deposition of brown-yellow pigment, variably positive for iron. Pigment granules are found either free in the extraneuronal spaces, encrusted on remaining neurons and astrocytes, or in macrophages. Calcifications may also be present. The pathogenesis is unknown.[118]

Lafora's Syndrome (Progressive Familial Myoclonic Epilepsy)

This autosomal recessive disease begins in childhood or early adult life with seizures, myoclonus, a characteristic EEG picture, and eventual mental deterioration and dementia. The course is relentlessly progressive over five to ten years, terminating in death, usually before the age of 30.

The diagnostic feature of this disease is the **Lafora body,** which is one of the types of polyglucosan body (p. 373).[12] Lafora bodies are intracytoplasmic, variable in diameter (1 to 20 μ), and found in neurons or, occasionally, in the extracellular space. They are present throughout the CNS, although most frequent in the basal ganglia and dentate nuclei. In some cases, similar bodies have been seen in the liver and myocardium. By light microscopy, they are round, homogeneous, or concentrically laminated bodies with a dense irregular core, and (frequently) radial striations. Electron microscopy shows them to consist of fibrils, sometimes branched, and associated with endoplasmic reticulum and ribosomal material.

Parkinsonism

Parkinsonism is the name given to a disturbance of motor function characterized by expressionless facies, a stooped posture, slowness of voluntary movement, a festinating gait (progressively shortened, accelerated steps), rigidity, and sometimes a characteristic tremor. It is named after James Parkinson who described idiopathic parkinsonism in 1817, but *this type of motor disturbance is seen in many different disease states that have in common damage to the striatonigral dopaminergic system.* It may also be produced by drugs, particularly dopamine antagonists, that affect this system. The principal diseases that involve the striatonigral system are *idiopathic parkinsonism (paralysis agitans); postencephalitic parkinsonism; striatonigral degeneration; Shy-Drager syndrome;* and *progressive supranuclear palsy.*

IDIOPATHIC PARKINSONISM (PARALYSIS AGITANS)

This is a progressive disorder appearing spontaneously in persons between 50 and 80 years of age. Such biochemical brain abnormalities as have been observed are included below in the discussion of the postencephalitic form of the disease.

Grossly, the substantia nigra and locus ceruleus are depigmented (Fig. 29–37); microscopically, there is loss of the melanin-containing neurons in these regions. **Lewy bodies** may be present in some of the remaining neurons. These are intracytoplasmic, eosinophilic, round-to-elongated inclusions, having a dense core surrounded by a lighter rim. They are composed of filaments that are densely packed in the core but quite loose at the rim.

POSTENCEPHALITIC PARKINSONISM

This is regarded as a sequela of encephalitis that occurred during the great "influenza" epidemics of 1914 to 1918. Brain examinations of patients who died during the acute illness showed perivascular cuffing and meningeal infiltrates of lymphocytes and mononuclear cells, findings suggestive of a viral encephalitis, although a virus was neither isolated nor identified at the time. After months, or more commonly years, some patients who recovered from the encephalitis developed parkinsonism, clinically similar to that seen in paralysis agitans but differing in that it usually occurred at an earlier age and was not a *progressive* disease. The incidence of this disease is decreasing as fewer patients survive who were exposed to the 1914–18 epidemic.

As in idiopathic parkinsonism, there is depigmentation of the substantia nigra and locus ceruleus, with loss of melanin-containing neurons and consequent gliosis. However, instead of Lewy bodies, some of the remaining neurons contain **neurofibrillary tangles** (p. 1372).

Pathologically, both idiopathic and postencephalitic parkinsonism are characterized by degeneration of the

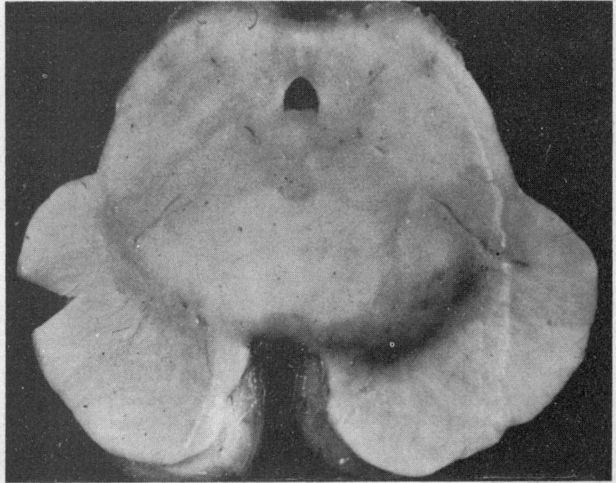

Figure 29–37. Idiopathic Parkinson's disease (paralysis agitans). Unilateral loss of pigment (*left*) in substantia nigra. This is a rare occurrence; most cases show bilateral depigmentation.

dopaminergic nigrostriatal pathway, with loss of cell bodies from the substantia nigra, degeneration of their axons and synapses in the striatum, and consequently a reduction in striatal dopamine content. In idiopathic parkinsonism the reduction is greatest in the putamen, whereas in the postencephalitic form it is marked in both the putamen and the caudate.[119] Neurochemically, the severity of the parkinsonian syndrome is directly proportional to the dopamine deficiency, a deficiency that can, at least in part, be corrected by replacement therapy with levodopa (the immediate precursor of dopamine), which, unlike dopamine, crosses the blood-brain barrier. However, treatment does not reverse the morphologic changes or arrest the progress of the disease.

Striatonigral Degeneration and Shy-Drager Syndrome

Striatonigral degeneration is clinically similar to idiopathic parkinsonism, but pathologically different. There is grossly visible atrophy of the caudate and putamen, both of which, microscopically, show severe neuronal loss, particularly of the small neurons, and a striking gliosis. Loss of pigmented neurons also occurs, particularly in the zona compacta of the substantia nigra, but neither Lewy bodies nor neurofibrillary tangles are seen.

In the *Shy-Drager syndrome*, autonomic system failure is present in addition to parkinsonism. The findings in the brain are variable, some cases being similar to idiopathic parkinsonism with Lewy bodies, whereas others are similar to striatonigral degeneration, with widespread neuronal loss. In the spinal cord, there is loss of neurons in the intermediolateral column, these being the neurons of origin of the sympathetic system. There is great variation in the pathologic findings in these two diseases.

Progressive Supranuclear Palsy

Patients with this disorder usually present with loss of vertical gaze progressing to difficulty with all eye movements, associated with back rigidity, paroxysmal dysequilibrium, expressionless facies, and (often) increasing dementia. Onset is usually between the fifth and seventh decades, and death often occurs within five to seven years.[120]

Morphologically, there is widespread neuronal loss in the globus pallidus, subthalamic nucleus, substantia nigra, tectum, periaqueductal gray matter, and dentate nuclei. The cerebral and cerebellar cortices are usually not involved. Neurofibrillary tangles (p. 1372) are present and are generally, but not invariably, composed of bundles of straight rather than helically wound filaments.[121]

SPINOCEREBELLAR DEGENERATIONS

These are a group of degenerative diseases that affect, in varying degrees, the basal ganglia, brain stem, cerebellum, spinal cord, and peripheral nerves. Clinically, they present with combinations of parkinsonian symptoms and signs, ataxia, spasticity, and motor and sensory deficits reflecting damage to different anatomic areas and/or neuronal systems in the CNS. Pathologically, there is simple neuronal atrophy in the affected regions, together with varying, usually slight degrees of gliosis.

The spinocerebellar degenerations are a confusing area of neuropathology, and there is no satisfactory classification of them. Genetically, they can be dominantly inherited, recessively inherited, or sporadic. Historically, there have been many different, usually eponymous syndromes described. In the inherited degenerations, however, within single affected pedigrees there is great variation in clinical presentation. To compound the problem, even in an individual, the disease may evolve over time from, for example, a predominantly spinal to a predominantly cerebellar symptomatology. The result of this variability is that there are often many similarities among patients suffering from what are nominally different syndromes. Pathologically, patients are often found to have more widespread disease than their symptoms would suggest, so that syndromes that are clinically different may have similar, or overlapping, pathologic findings. The *olivopontocerebellar atrophy* complex provides a good illustration of the types of syndrome and the taxonomic difficulties encountered in these diseases. An alternative approach, which has substantial practical merit, is to classify all these patients as dominant, recessive, or sporadic ataxia and allow each affected individual or pedigree to define the course and prognosis of the disease. Taxonomic nihilism should not, however, be carried too far. Some spinocerebellar degenerations are relatively consistent or have sufficiently characteristic systemic associations to allow them to be reliably defined. An example is *Friedreich's ataxia*, which has a reasonably distinctive neurologic presentation combined with a typical and prognostically significant cardiac lesion.

Olivopontocerebellar Atrophy

Of all the neuronal degenerative diseases, this form has the most inconstant and varied expression, to the extent that the term "heterogeneous system degeneration" is sometimes used. No two cases are exactly alike, even in the same family, and the heredity is no less varied: most cases are autosomal dominant (Menzel type), but others are autosomal recessive and still others are clearly nonfamilial. Neuronal loss is usually concentrated in the olive, pons, and cerebellum, but the basal ganglia and spinal cord can also be involved. Clinically, symptoms and signs include (to varying degrees) ataxia, eye and somatic movement disorders, dysarthria, and rigidity, in varying combinations.

Friedreich's Ataxia

The average age of onset of this usually autosomal recessive condition is 11 years, although a less frequent, dominantly inherited variant comes on at about 20 years of age. There is a male preponderance. Ataxia of gait heralds its onset, followed by clumsiness of hand movements and dysarthria. Deep tendon reflexes are absent, but the Babinski reflex is characteristically present. Joint position and vibratory sense are impaired, and there is sometimes loss of the sensations of pain, temperature, and light touch. The average progression is over a period of about 20 years, and most patients eventually become paralyzed. Some patients show pes cavus and kyphoscoliosis, and there is a high incidence of concomitant diabetes and cardiac disease, the last being manifested as cardiac arrhythmias and congestive heart failure.[122]

The spinal cord is usually small. There is loss of nerve fibers and gliosis in the posterior columns, distal corticospinal tracts, and spinocerebellar tracts. There is neuronal loss in Clark's column; the VIII, X, and XII cranial nerve nuclei; and the dentate nucleus. There is also disappearance of Purkinje cells from the superior vermis and of dorsal root ganglion cells. The ganglion cell loss is the cause of the visible degeneration in the dorsal columns. The heart is frequently enlarged and may have pericardial adhesions. An interstitial myocarditis may be seen with focal and/or diffuse inflammatory infiltrates, myofiber hypertrophy, and, more rarely, myofiber necrosis.

The pathogenesis of this disease is unknown but attention is currently focused on reductions, found in some patients, in the activities of mitochondrial enzymes including pyruvate and oxoglutarate dehydrogenases, and malic enzyme.[123] How these findings relate to the morphologic findings is unclear.

DEGENERATIVE DISEASES AFFECTING MOTOR NEURONS

Motor Neuron Disease (Amyotrophic Lateral Sclerosis [ALS] Complex)

Nowhere is the term "system degeneration" more appropriately applied than with this complex of clinical variants. All are marked by degeneration confined to the pyramidal motor system with its two levels of motor neurons in series. The upper motor neuron is in the motor cortex and its axon traverses the internal capsule, brain stem, and corticospinal tract to synapse on the *lower motor neuron* in the cranial motor nuclei or in the anterior horns of the spinal cord.

Clinically, four variants are recognized. The most frequent is *amyotrophic lateral sclerosis* in which patients show evidence of both lower motor neuron impairment (muscular atrophy and weakness) and upper motor neuron damage (hyperreflexia and a positive Babinski reflex). In *progressive bulbar palsy* there is a predominance of cranial nerve and brain stem involvement; in *progressive muscular atrophy* there is lower motor neuron dysfunction in the absence of clinical evidence of corticospinal tract damage; and in *primary lateral sclerosis* the patients have only upper motor neuron signs and symptoms.

Grossly, lower motor neuron loss is reflected in muscular atrophy and a grey discoloration and atrophy of the anterior (motor) roots of the spinal cord. Degeneration of the upper motor neuron is manifested in the lateral corticospinal tracts, which develop a dense bone-white appearance, and occasionally, in severe or long-standing cases, atrophy of the precentral gyrus. The pathologic findings usually reflect the clinical presentation, so that in primary lateral sclerosis the principal change is fiber loss and gliosis in the lateral corticospinal tract (Fig. 29–38) which may be traceable up to the motor cortex. In progressive muscular atrophy there is a disappearance of the anterior horn neurons with very little consequent gliosis. In amyotrophic lateral sclerosis there is both degeneration in the lateral corticospinal tract and loss of anterior horn cells. Cranial nerve motor nuclei, particularly V, IX, X, XI, and XII, may show neuronal depletion, especially in patients with pronounced bulbar signs. Occasional neuronophagia (p. 1374), indicating continuing neuronal loss, may be seen in affected populations, and the remaining neurons may be shrunken or have a ghostlike appearance.

Most cases of motor neuron disease are sporadic, although a few familial cases have been reported. Males are more often affected than females, and the onset is typically in late middle age with a progressive and inevitably fatal course over two to six years. Progressive bulbar palsy tends to run a shorter course, probably because of earlier involvement of the respiratory and pharyngeal musculature.

The pathogenesis of motor neuron disease is unknown. A high prevalence of HLA-A2, A3, and A28 haplotypes has been described, and interestingly some patients with progressive muscular atrophy have a past history of paralytic poliomyelitis. Many possible causes have been explored, including all varieties of viral, immunologic, and metabolic disease, but as yet no serious etiologic candidates have emerged. A spontaneous lower motor neuron disease in wild mice has been reported, apparently caused by an indigenous C-RNA virus, but it is not clear what relevance this has to human disease. There is also a most curious form of motor neuron disease that occurs in the Chamorro Indians on the island of Guam. In the same population there is also a high incidence of parkinsonism and dementia, and all three conditions are associated with the presence of neurofibrillary tangles.[9] Although this condition, whatever it is, is very interesting, it does not seem to have any relationship to the more conventional type of sporadic motor neuron disease.

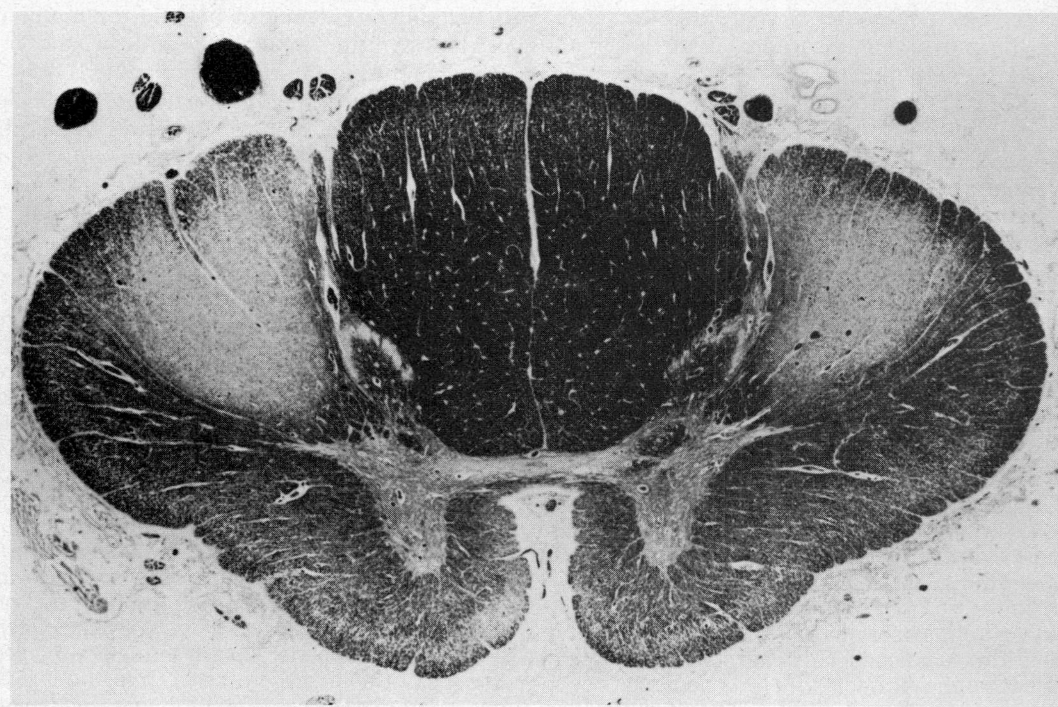

Figure 29–38. Amyotrophic lateral sclerosis. Cross section of spinal cord showing loss of myelinated fibers (lack of stain) in corticospinal tracts. At higher magnification, loss of anterior horn neurons can also be seen (Woelcke stain).

Infantile Progressive Spinal Muscular Atrophy (Werdnig-Hoffmann Disease)

This autosomal recessive condition presents either at birth as a "floppy infant" syndrome or in the first months of life with rapidly progressive muscular weakness. Death usually ensues within a few months from respiratory failure and/or aspiration pneumonia. Morphologically, there is severe loss of anterior horn cells and cranial nerve motor neurons. Necessarily, there is also degeneration of the motor axons in the peripheral nerves and profound neurogenic atrophy in the muscles.

NUTRITIONAL, ENVIRONMENTAL, AND METABOLIC DISORDERS

All the diseases discussed in this section could be considered as metabolic because, although they often subsequently produce gross structural damage, they are characterized initially by a disturbance in nervous system function that is primarily biochemical. More precisely, *nutritional* diseases begin with reductions in or lack of an essential biochemical component; *environmental* illnesses have exposure to a physical or chemical toxin; and conditions labeled as *metabolic* have disordered proportions of normal constituents. Pathologically, the interpretation of these diseases is often complicated by secondary effects such as respiratory failure and cerebral ischemia that are superimposed on the primary metabolic effects.

NUTRITIONAL DEFICIENCY DISORDERS

The major vitamin deficiencies with an effect on the adult nervous system are those of *thiamine, nicotinamide,* and *cobalamin.* As these have already been discussed in Chapter 9, reference will be made here only to those aspects not already covered.

Thiamine Deficiency

In the nervous system, the principal syndromes caused by thiamine deficiency are the *Wernicke-Korsakoff syndrome* and a *peripheral neuropathy.* Clinically, they are most frequently encountered in alcoholics, but are not toxic effects of alcohol, because they are seen in other conditions of thiamine deficiency in which alcohol does not play a part, such as sprue, gastric cancer, and prolonged fasting. Another important cause of a particularly acute thiamine deficiency is prolonged parenteral nutrition, which, if not adequately supplemented with thiamine, can be complicated by fulminant Wernicke's encephalopathy.

Wernicke-Korsakoff Syndrome. The two components of this syndrome may occur separately or together. *Wernicke's encephalopathy* is characterized clinically by the acute onset of mental confusion progressing to coma, nystagmus, extraocular palsies, and prostration. It is a medical emergency and, if left untreated, is frequently fatal. Prompt administration of thiamine can reverse the condition.

Grossly, the most constant and impressive focal lesions are found in the mamillary bodies, but they may also be present in the walls of the third ventricle (Fig. 29–39), around the aqueduct of Sylvius, and in the floor of the fourth ventricle. The vestibular and dorsal motor nuclei of the vagi and the cranial nerve nuclei controlling the extraocular muscles are also commonly involved. In all sites the individual lesions appear congested, have a brown-gray discoloration, and rarely exceed a few millimeters in diameter.

Microscopically, there is vacuolation and degeneration of the affected neuropil, but severe neuronal loss is infrequent. Reactive astrocytosis and macrophage accumulation occur in proportion to the amount of tissue destruction. The most impressive, and probably the most important, change is in the smaller blood vessels, which, although only slightly increased in number, are strikingly conspicuous because they are hypercellular and dilated. In the acute stage, perivascular ring hemorrhages are often seen.

Korsakoff's psychosis is a memory disorder in which the patient cannot form new memories, has difficulty in retrieving old ones, and, classically, fills the resultant gaps by ingenious confabulation. Other aspects of mental function are relatively preserved. The histologic changes are similar to those seen in Wernicke's syndrome, except that the medial dorsal nucleus of the thalamus and, often, the pulvinar are involved.

A *peripheral neuropathy* (p. 1429) is frequently present in alcoholics, but is probably due to thiamine deficiency.

Vitamin B_{12} Deficiency (Subacute Combined Degeneration of Spinal Cord, SACD)

The mechanism by which vitamin B_{12} deficiency (pernicious anemia) affects the nervous system is not understood, but it is clear that it is unrelated to the megaloblastic anemia, since SACD can occur in its absence. Clinically, patients present with a subacute progressive spastic paraparesis, sensory ataxia, and marked paresthesias in the lower limbs. Untreated, this rapidly progresses to a severe ataxic paraplegia or total paralysis, with trunk and lower limb anesthesia. Treatment with vitamin B_{12} can completely reverse the early symptoms and signs, but untreated they rapidly become permanent.

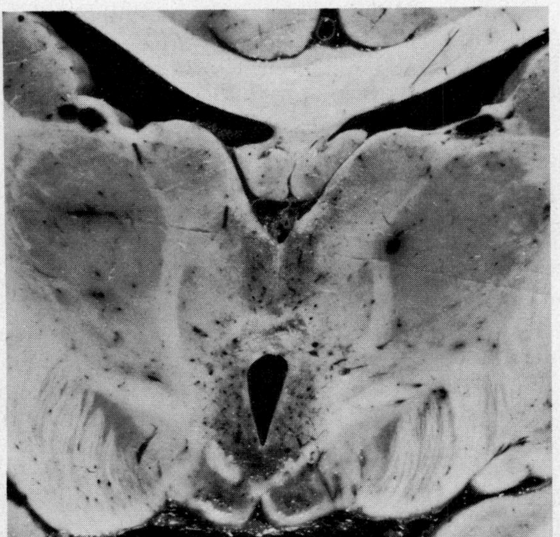

Figure 29–39. Wernicke's encephalopathy. Wall of third ventricle is discolored and there are many small hemorrhages.

Pathologically, there is degeneration in the white matter of the spinal cord, usually confined to the posterior and lateral white columns, and most marked in the midthoracic region. In severe cases the affected areas are grossly atrophic and gray. Characteristically, the earliest lesions are seen in the body of the affected white column and extend outwards from these initial foci. Microscopically, there is early swelling of the myelin sheaths, and their later breakup and degradation by macrophages is followed by secondary degeneration of the axons and a variable amount of gliosis. This disappearance of the axons and their associated myelin gives the tissue a characteristic loose and vacuolated appearance on light microscopy. The gray matter is usually unaffected.

Other lesions encountered in the nervous system in vitamin B_{12} deficiency are optic atrophy, a predominantly axonal peripheral neuropathy, and (rarely) a perivascular demyelination in the hemispheric white matter, similar in histologic character to the lesions in the spinal cord.

ENVIRONMENTAL DISORDERS

The principal environmental disorders are discussed in Chapter 10 and, except for the effects of *alcohol*, will not be further considered here. However, in this era of increasing therapeutic rigor, the iatrogenic causes of brain damage are of increasing importance. A wide and enlarging variety of cerebral toxic effects caused by therapeutic agents have been identified. Three of the best described are *radiation necrosis*, the *radiation/chemotherapy lesion*, and *central pontine myelinolysis*, discussed below.

Alcohol-related Conditions

No medical student needs to be told of the intoxicating properties of ethyl alcohol. Its acute effect is a generalized cerebral depression that, in acute alcohol poisoning, can be severe enough to cause death. In chronic alcohol abuse the incidence of the *Wernicke-Korsakoff syndrome*, *peripheral neuropathy*, *cerebellar degeneration*, and *central pontine myelinolysis* are all greatly increased, but they are not specific to alcoholism and there is no conclusive evidence for any morphologic damage caused by alcohol itself. As already discussed, the first two are caused by thiamine deficiency, and central pontine myelinolysis (see below) probably results from therapeutic manipulation of the serum sodium level. Similarly, *hepatic encephalopathy* and the more severe *hepatocerebral degeneration* (p. 1423) are also seen in alcoholics, but are consequences of liver failure rather than direct toxic effects of alcohol.

Cerebellar degeneration. This disease is characterized by degeneration of cerebellar neurons, particularly Purkinje cells, in the anterior superior vermis. In severe cases, the anterior portion of the anterior lobe can also be involved. Men are more prone to develop this condition than women, in a ratio of 11:1. Clinically, there is truncal ataxia but little limb ataxia, consistent with the predominant involvement of the cerebellar vermis.

In contrast to ethyl alcohol, *methyl alcohol*, through its metabolite formic acid, produces a direct toxic effect on the retina,[133] and there is often widely distributed cerebral damage, which is probably the result of histotoxic anoxia.[134]

Radiation Necrosis

The effects of ionizing radiation have been addressed in Chapter 10. In the brain, radiation-induced vascular damage may result in progressive parenchymal ischemia and even infarction. Because cranial irradiation is given in most cases as part of the treatment for tumor, the neurologic deficits produced by this ischemia or infarction can, by mimicking tumor recurrence, lead to diagnostic confusion.

Radiation/Chemotherapy Lesion

The changes, as in radiation necrosis, are usually delayed in onset and occur in patients given a combination of radiotherapy and various chemotherapeutic agents. Initially, the lesions were thought to be associated with the intrathecal administration of methotrexate, but it has been seen in patients known not to have received this agent[130] and in those to whom no intrathecal medication has been given.

Grossly, the lesions occur as irregularly shaped areas of white matter necrosis, which, in the cerebral hemispheres, are often periventricular. Microscopically, there is a distinctive appearance because the necrotic areas contain many dilated axon profiles that have a tendency to mineralization. There is little or no inflammatory reaction, and although vascular changes similar to those seen in radiation necrosis have been described, they are not consistently present.[127, 128] Although usually seen in the cerebral hemispheres, multiple tiny but histologically similar lesions have also been described in the basis pontis.[129] Although the lesions are well characterized histologically, their pathogenesis is unknown.

Central Pontine Myelinolysis

As implied by the name, this lesion consists of an area of demyelination in the midpart of the pons. The demyelination is symmetrically distributed about the midline, and in severe cases may occupy almost the whole of the basis pontis.[131] Smaller lesions are probably asymptomatic, but in the large lesions a flaccid quadriplegia may develop. Microscopically, despite the profound loss of myelin and oligodendrocytes, there is preservation of the axons and, depending on the stage of its evolution, a reactive astrocytosis and lipid-laden macrophages. When first described, the condition was thought to be particularly associated with alcoholism, but it has now been described in many nonalcoholics. The pathogenesis is not known, but the development is most consistently related to rapid rises, sometimes from a very low level, in serum sodium.[132] These rises are most frequently associated with the intravenous administration of sodium-containing solutions, so that the lesion is arguably iatrogenic in most cases.

METABOLIC ENCEPHALOPATHY

The blood-brain barrier ensures that the CNS neurons are insulated from the normal vagaries of the systemic biochemical milieu, but these defenses can be overcome by large or prolonged changes. Effects can be seen with changes in both electrolytes and nonelectrolytes. The resulting disturbance in cerebral function is referred to as a *metabolic encephalopathy.* Frequently encountered causes include diabetes, in which acute hypoglycemia induces a correspondingly acute confusional state that can be rapidly reversed by the administration of glucose. Hyperglycemic coma is more complicated, with additional changes in pH, electrolytes, and osmotic pressure, all contributing to a cerebral dysequilibrium that can persist for several days after restitution of normality in the serum parameters. This persistence of cerebral dysfunction presumably reflects the time required to reestablish intracellular biochemical normality. Other frequent causes of a more chronic metabolic encephalopathy are uremia, hypercalcemia, and hepatic failure. Despite the sometimes profound disturbance in cerebral function, there is often little or nothing to be seen morphologically, a finding that reflects the predominantly biochemical nature of the cerebral disorder.

Although CNS function is being discussed here, there are also peripheral nervous system effects in some of these conditions, notably diabetes and uremia, both of which produce a peripheral neuropathy.

Hepatic Encephalopathy

Patients with hepatic failure exhibit a characteristic clinical picture, with a peculiar flapping tremor of the extremities called *asterixis*, and a disturbance in consciousness, progressing to coma and even death in severe cases (p. 893). The course of the encephalopathy mimics that of the hepatic failure, with exacerbations of the one producing worsening of the other. A similar encephalopathy can be produced, and marginally compensated patients precipitated into encephalopathy, by portocaval shunting. Although the severity of the encephalopathy is generally correlated with the raised blood ammonia level seen in hepatic failure, it has not been shown that the encephalopathy is a direct toxic effect of the hyperammonemia.

Pathologically, the only consistent change seen in the nervous system is the proliferation of protoplasmic astrocytes with enlarged, watery, deformed nuclei containing a "glycogen dot" (Alzheimer II astrocytes). They are found predominantly in gray matter, being especially prominent in the lenticular nucleus, thalamus, red nucleus, substantia nigra, and deeper layers of the cerebral cortex. Similar nuclei, but without the "glycogen dot," can be seen in many of the other encephalopathies. Tissue well fixed for electron microscopy does not show enlarged watery astrocytic nuclei. This has led some investigators to conclude that the appearance of Alzheimer II astrocytes in formalin-fixed tissue is an artifact.

Severe and long-standing hepatic encephalopathy can lead to a cerebral degeneration morphologically similar to that seen in Wilson's disease (p. 1423).

INBORN ERRORS OF METABOLISM

The variety and range of effects of the inborn errors of metabolism on the nervous system is legion, and only a few of the more important or illustrative will be mentioned in this section. Many of these diseases have effects both inside and outside the nervous system, and in some diseases it is the balance of these effects that determines whether they present clinically as diseases of the nervous system or as systemic diseases. For example, in *Wilson's disease* (p. 932), some patients present with hepatic failure with little nervous system involvement, whereas others present with disease of the brain with choreoathetosis and dementia. In *phenylketonuria* (p. 490), although the inborn error is common to all tissues, the clinical manifestations are overwhelmingly in the nervous system.

To universal regret, there is no easily assimilable classification of these diseases, mostly because disorders affecting a single metabolic system can produce quite different clinical syndromes, and conversely because different disorders produce the same manifestations.[101] Thus, for example, the *sphingolipidoses*, which are a subcategory of the lysosomal storage diseases (p. 142), include *systemic storage diseases*, e.g., Gaucher's disease; *neuronal storage diseases* (Fig. 29–40), exemplified by Tay-Sachs disease (p. 142) and Niemann-Pick disease (p. 145); and *leukodystrophies*, in the form of metachromatic leukodystrophy and globoid cell leukodystrophy (Krabbe's disease). Other general categories of inborn error that may produce effects on the nervous system include the *mucopolysaccharidoses* (p. 150) and the *glycogen storage diseases* (p. 150). This general topic is considered in detail in Chapter 4. In this section we will discuss only *Wilson's disease, Leigh's disease*, and the *leukodystrophies*.

Wilson's Disease

This disorder of copper metabolism is discussed on page 932. Here we shall describe only the neuropathologic changes.

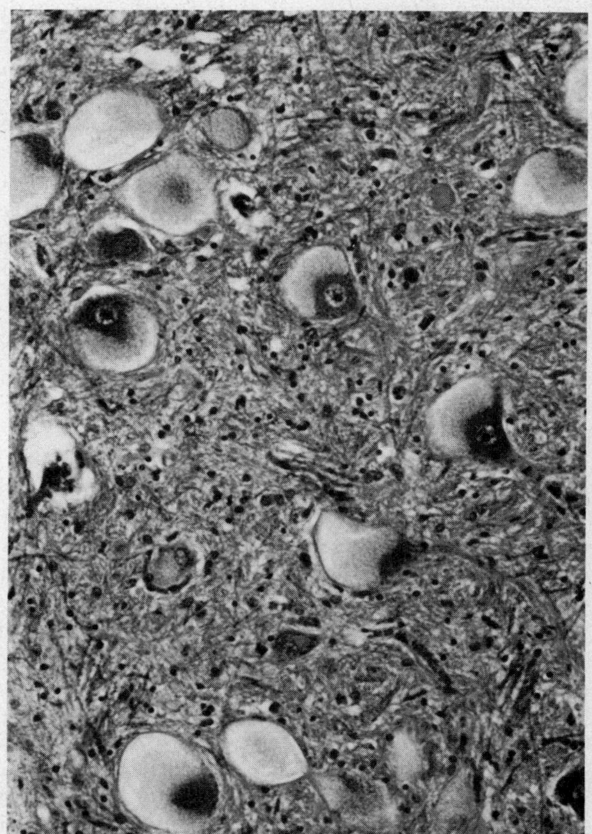

Figure 29–40. Neuronal storage disease. Anterior horn neurons are distended with stored lipid. (H and E stain.)

The changes in the brain are not restricted to the lenticular nucleus but are widespread, justifying the term **hepatocerebral degeneration** used by some authors. In the dystonic (wilsonian) variety, with early onset and rapid evolution, there are always gross changes, the most dramatic being cavitation in the lenticular nucleus. When cavitation is not present, there is a brownish discoloration with some atrophy of the affected nuclear masses. In the Westphal-Strümpell form of late onset and less rapid deterioration, the brain may be grossly normal, or there may be mild atrophy and discoloration of the basal nuclei.

The microscopic changes are widespread, but are maximal in the lenticular nucleus and especially in its putaminal component. The thalamus, red nucleus, and dentate nucleus of the cerebellum also are occasionally affected. The major histologic features are large numbers of Alzheimer II astrocytes, sometimes large multinucleate (Alzheimer I) astrocytes, and neuronal loss. The cavitation appears to be related to the confluence of areas of intense degeneration of nerve cells and astrocytes.

Subacute Necrotizing Encephalomyelopathy (Leigh's Disease)

This disease, inherited as an autosomal recessive trait, is characterized by bilateral symmetric regions of necrosis; cribriform change; vascular proliferation; and gliosis in the thalamus, midbrain, pons, medulla, and spinal cord. In some cases, the peripheral nerves may show regions of demyelination. Although apparently a metabolic disorder, the pathogenesis is not understood. Elevated blood lactate and pyruvate levels and a mild acidosis are usually found, but these appear to be secondary changes. Although some patients have a depression in activity of the mitochondrial pyruvate dehydrogenase complex,[135] this is not always found and the precise biochemical defect is not yet identified. Clinically, onset is in the first year of life, with deterioration of motor skills (e.g., loss of head control and poor sucking), seizures, and myoclonic jerking. The disease is usually fatal within six to 12 months.

LEUKODYSTROPHIES

These are diseases of white matter in which the inborn error is known, or presumed, to be in the pathways of myelin metabolism. In all the leukodystrophies in which the biochemical defect has been identified, it is a deficiency of a lysosomal degradative enzyme. Pathologically, the principal process is primary demyelination (p. 1410), but there may also be some neuronal storage. In view of the nature of the biochemical defect, it is perhaps more helpful to think of them as *dysmyelinating* rather than *demyelinating* diseases. From their biochemical origin it might be expected that all leukodystrophies would become manifest in early childhood as symmetric disorders of myelination, affecting the entire neuraxis. In many cases, such as the childhood form of metachromatic leukodystrophy, they conform quite well to this archetype, but, as exemplified by adrenoleukodystrophy, there can also be a large degree of variation in the clinical expression of these diseases, in spite of the apparently stereotypic nature of the biochemical defect.

Metachromatic Leukodystrophy

This is an autosomal recessive disorder of sphingomyelin metabolism in which there is a deficiency of arylsulfatase A (cerebroside sulfatase), leading to the accumulation of galactosyl sulfatide and other lipids containing a galactosyl-3-sulfatide moiety.[136] Pathologically, the demyelination affects both the central and peripheral nervous systems, and there is also some lipid storage in neurons. There are a few cases of metachromatic leukodystrophy without arylsulfatase A deficiency, and is thought that in these cases there is a deficiency of the sulfatase activator.[10]

The accumulated sulfatide appears as spherical granular masses, 15 to 20 μ in diameter, which stain positively with PAS and metachromatically with acid cresyl violet on frozen sections. In the CNS, these masses may be free in tissue spaces or within macrophages in the perivascular spaces. Subcortical axons and myelin (U fibers) are relatively spared (Fig. 29–41). In the peripheral nervous system (PNS) there is nerve fiber loss and segmental demyelination. Metachromatic material is also found in Schwann cells and macrophages. Accumulation of the material also occurs in renal epithelial cells, in the mucosal cells of the gallbladder, and in the liver, pancreas, pituitary, adrenal cortex, and testis.

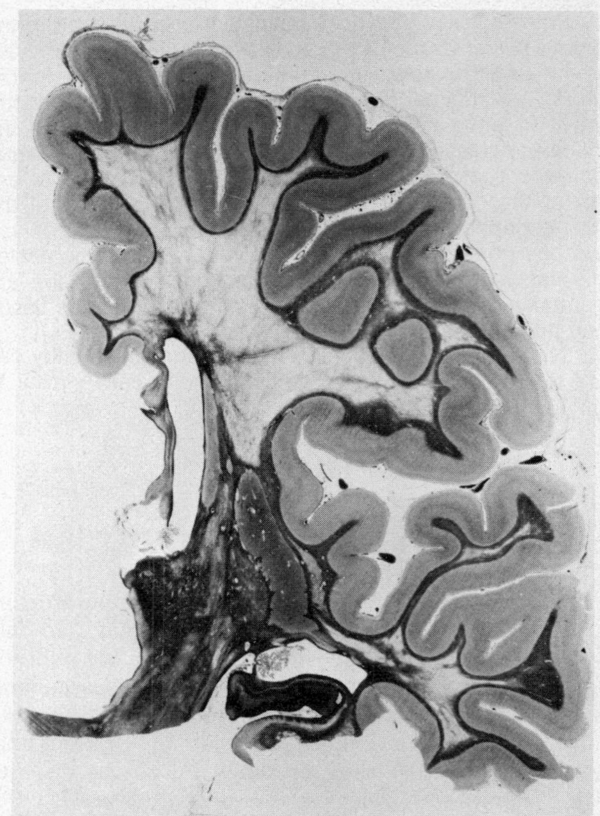

Figure 29–41. Metachromatic leukodystrophy. Demyelination is extensive. Subcortical fibers in cerebral hemisphere are spared. (Luxol-fast-blue, PAS stain.)

The disease usually becomes manifest clinically between the first and fourth year of life, although there are rare adult forms. It presents as progressive motor impairment with mental deterioration and, sometimes, a peripheral neuropathy. Diagnosis is made by measuring urinary arylsulfatase A, which is decreased or absent. Peripheral nerve biopsy can also be helpful by showing myelin breakdown and sulfatide accumulation.

Krabbe's Disease (Globoid Cell Leukodystrophy, Galactocerebroside Lipidosis)

Krabbe's disease is another autosomal recessive leukodystrophy resulting from a deficiency of galactocerebroside β-galactosidase with the accumulation of galactocerebroside.[137] Histologically, in addition to the demyelination, there are characteristic large, sometimes multinucleate, histiocytic cells (globoid cells), usually seen around blood vessels. The PNS may also show degeneration, although it is less common than in metachromatic leukodystrophy. By electron microscopy, the globoid cells have the characteristics of macrophages and contain cytoplasmic inclusions made up of straight or curved hollow tubular profiles, often with longitudinal striations of variable density and approximately 6 nm in width. Cleftlike cytoplasmic inclusions have been found in Schwann cells when there is PNS demyelination.

The onset of Krabbe's disease is in early infancy, generally in the first six months of life, and is marked by rigidity, instability, and decreased alertness. The disease is fatal, usually within six to 12 months of onset, with terminal blindness and deafness.

Adrenoleukodystrophy and Adrenomyeloneuropathy

This interesting disease until recently was classified under *Schilder's disease* (p. 1412), which was originally described as a demyelinating disease characterized by large, often symmetric plaques of demyelination in the hemispheres. Some young male patients thus diagnosed had adrenal failure, and subsequent investigation showed that this group had a distinct familial sex-linked condition, which was then given the name *adrenoleukodystrophy.*[138] Most of these patients were under 10 years of age and pursued a relentless downhill course to death within three to four years of the onset of symptoms. Grossly, and by light microscopy, the brain in these cases has a similar appearance to that of the so-called Schilder variety of multiple sclerosis in children. However, electron microscopy in these patients showed specific diagnostic inclusions in the cerebral macrophages and adrenal cortical cells consisting of dense, long, thin leaflets enclosing an electron-lucent space (Fig. 29–42).[139] Similar inclusions are found in Leydig cells of the testis and Schwann cells. It has been discovered that there is another and quite different form of this disease in adults, also with adrenal insufficiency, but with a much later developing spastic paraparesis and peripheral neuropathy, together with cerebellar ataxia, varying degrees of intellectual deterioration, and hypogonadism. This variant is called *adrenomyeloneuropathy.*[140] Transitional cases occur, and both variants may be seen in the same family.[141] Biochemical studies have not yet definitively identified a defect, but have shown the consistent presence of an excess of long-chain (C24–30) fatty acid esters of cholesterol and an apparent inability to hydrolyze the long-chain fatty acids.[142] Currently, the diagnosis is made by determining the ratio of the C26 to C20 fatty acids in either serum or fibroblast culture.[10] It is now possible to identify most of the female carriers, some of whom are symptomatic, so that they can be given genetic counseling.

These three diseases obviously do not constitute all the leukodystrophies; their catalog is long and includes subtypes ranging from the simple sudanophilic to the eponymous, indeed euphonious, leukodystrophy eternally associated with Messrs. Pelizaeus and Merzbacher.

DEVELOPMENTAL DISEASES AND MALFORMATIONS OF NERVOUS SYSTEM

Developmental malformations of the CNS may be caused by genetic or environmental factors. The trisomies are an example of a genetic cause of CNS malformation (p. 126). Environmental factors known or suspected to result in malformations include (1) fetal anoxia and circulatory insufficiency, (2) maternal and fetal infections (e.g., German measles), (3) physical agents such as ionizing radiation, (4) drugs (e.g., thalidomide), (5) nutritional deficiencies and excesses, and (6) mechanical forces. In most cases of malformation, an etiologic agent cannot be identified.

Genetic and exogenous factors may produce identical-appearing malformations. One of the most critical variables determining the type and severity of malformation is the time of gestation during which particular agents act on the developing nervous system. For example, experimental irradiation of a fetus in animals during the first few days of pregnancy has little effect on CNS development, whereas irradiation given after the first few days results in a series of predictable malformations.[143]

MALFORMATIONS OF CEREBRUM

ANENCEPHALY. In this condition, a fetus develops "without a brain." The cranial vault is absent. The cerebral hemispheres may be completely missing or may be represented by small masses attached to the base of the skull. The condition is at least three times

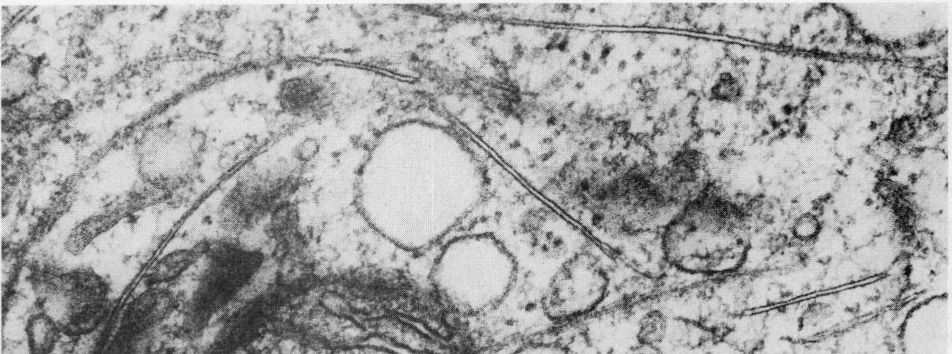

Figure 29–42. Electron micrograph of the characteristic curvilinear profiles seen in adrenoleukodystrophy. (From Schaumberg, H. H., et al.: Adreno-leukodystrophy (sex linked Schilder's disease): ultrastructural demonstration of specific cytoplasmic inclusions in the central nervous system. Arch. Neurol. *31*:210, 1974.)

more common in females than in males and, for unknown reasons, is extremely common in Ireland. It is thought to be due to failure of the neuronal tube at the level of the encephalon to close. Some investigators have suggested that it may be due to destruction of a previously formed brain in the early stages of development.[144] It has also been proposed that anencephaly may be related to lack of vascularization occurring between the third and fifth fetal week of life, at a time when major cerebral arteries are developing.[145]

ARRHINENCEPHALY. In this case, lack of development of the olfactory portion of the brain is usually associated with the lack of development of the nasal portions of the face. *Holoprosencephaly* is a variant of this anomaly in which the forebrain fails to divide so that there is only one massive hemisphere with a single ventricle. Some cases of arrhinencephaly are associated with chromosomal abnormalities such as trisomies 13 and 15.

PORENCEPHALY. This term implies that a "pore" or cavity connects the surface of the brain and subarachnoid space to the lateral ventricles. There are no microscopic changes suggestive of an old destructive process in the walls of the porencephalic cavity. Unfortunately, the term "porencephalic cyst" is often used to designate any old destructive lesion, such as an infarct in the fetal brain. The latter, however, has reactive inflammatory tissue in its wall.

HYDRANENCEPHALY. In this anomaly, the cerebral hemispheres are almost absent, leaving only a thin, saclike structure filled with fluid. The posterior temporal lobes, basal ganglia, brain stem, and cerebellum are usually spared. The skull is absent. It has been suggested that hydranencephaly is caused by obstruction of the carotid artery flow during fetal life.[144]

MENINGOENCEPHALOCELE. In this condition, the brain and the meninges herniate through a defect or opening in the cranial vault, producing a fluctuant, bulging mass under the skin. This condition is discussed later in the section on spinal cord malformation (p. 1427).

MICROCEPHALY VERA. By convention, this term is restricted to an adult brain that weighs less than 900 gm. The term "true microcephaly" should be reserved to mean an abnormally small brain that is the result of an autosomal recessive or sex-linked inherited defect.

Externally, true microcephalic brains have a simplified broad gyral pattern with fewer secondary gyri. On cut surface, the internal structure of the brain is relatively intact and normally arranged, although microscopically the cortical lamination of neurons is abnormal. Microcephalic individuals may have an anthropoid appearance and are usually mentally retarded.

MEGALENCEPHALY. In this condition, the brain weighs more than 1800 gm. Megalencephaly is not necessarily associated with any functional abnormality or mental retardation. Heavy brains are seen in individuals with extraordinary intelligence but also in some with severe mental retardation. Mental retardation is more likely when macroencephaly is associated with an underlying structural abnormality such as abnormal gyral patterns, glial hamartomas, or other associated conditions such as tuberous sclerosis or cerebral lipidoses.

Malformations may be localized to a particular anatomic region of the brain.

AGYRIA, LISSENCEPHALY, AND PACHYGYRIA. These three terms refer to the cortical alterations that result from arrested development before mature gyral formation has been accomplished. The gyral pattern is smooth and has a reduced number of secondary gyri, an appearance characteristic of a brain that has not progressed beyond the seventh fetal month. These gyral malformations may be localized to only one portion of the brain or may be diffuse, involving both cerebral hemispheres.

MICROPOLYGYRIA AND ULEGYRIA. In contrast to agyria, or reduced numbers of gyri, micropolygyria and ulegyria represent the formation of "too many gyri." Micropolygyria implies excessive formation of secondary gyri that are true miniature gyri having a four-layer cortex, sometimes with a festooned second layer. Atrophy, shrinkage, and scarring are not present. Ulegyria, in contrast shows evidence of previous injury resulting in scarring and atrophy. On microscopic study, these gyri do not form true miniature gyri. Anoxic, circulatory, or mechanical factors are blamed for this condition.

ÉTAT MARBRÉ OR STATUS MARMORATUS. These terms are used to designate hypermyelination in the basal ganglia. Usually, the aberrant myelin pattern resembles that of veined marble, hence the term état marbré.

AGENESIS OF CORPUS CALLOSUM. This condition is caused by failure of the corpus callosum and the septum pellucidum to form properly, resulting in a single cerebral ventricle. Agenesis of the corpus callosum is often associated with other malformations. Mental retardation is usually present.

MALFORMATIONS OF CEREBELLUM AND BRAIN STEM

AGENESIS OF CEREBELLUM. Lack of cerebellar development can range from slight hypoplasia to almost complete absence or agenesis. Generally, both hemispheres are involved; however, single-hemisphere agenesis has been reported. These defects are compatible with normal life.

ARNOLD-CHIARI MALFORMATIONS. This group of malformations consists of (1) caudal displacement of the cerebellum and vermis, and elongation of the medulla and fourth ventricle (Fig. 29–43) with herniation into the foramen magnum; (2) platybasia (flattening of the base of the skull; (3) stenosis and forking of the cerebral aqueduct, hydrocephalus, and spina bifida; and (4) meningomyelocele. Not all these defects are present in every patient, and various combinations of Arnold-Chiari malformation may be seen. In all, progressive hydrocephalus is the major clinical complication (p. 1376). The genesis of these malformations is controver-

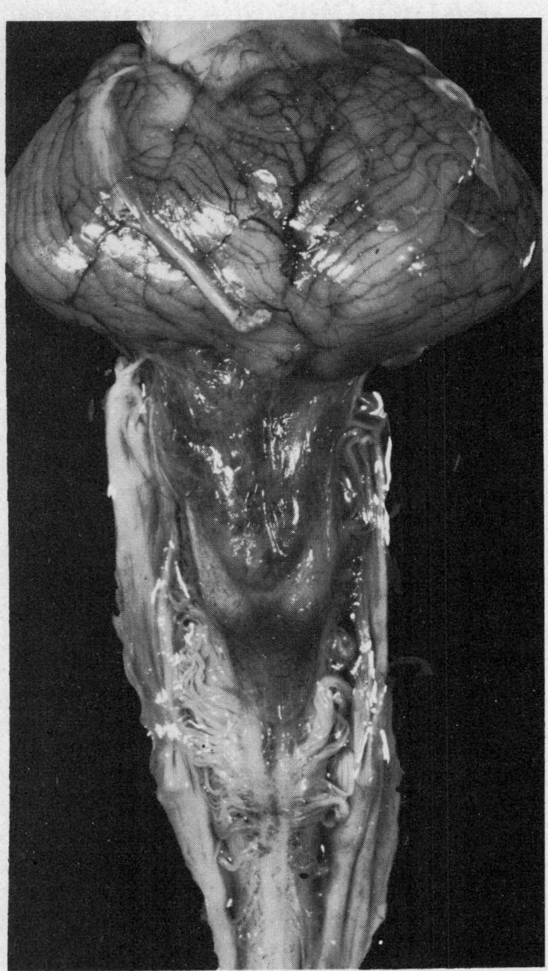

Figure 29–43. Arnold-Chiari malformation. Cerebellar tonsils are displaced into cervical canal.

sial. One view is that the cerebellar malformation leads to hydrocephalus and that increased CSF pressure is translated downward, with "splitting" of the neural tube. Another suggests that traction on the spinal cord, which is fixed to the walls of the meningomyelocele, pulls the posterior fossa contents down into the foramen magnum.

The severity of these malformations varies. Some (such as complete obstruction of the aqueduct) are incompatible with life. Others may not become manifest until adulthood.

DANDY-WALKER SYNDROME. In this condition, the vermis of the cerebellum fails to develop, with resultant occlusion or obliteration of the foramina of Magendie and Luschka. This results in marked dilatation of the fourth ventricle, forming a cyst lined with ependyma covered by meninges. Hydrocephalus is usually present.

MALFORMATIONS OF SPINAL CORD

SPINA BIFIDA. In this abnormality, the bony spinal canal fails to close, thus exposing underlying structures, which may or may not herniate through the bony defect. The meninges alone (meningocele) or meninges and spinal cord (meningomyelocele) may herniate. Spina bifida, meningocele, and meningomyelocele may occur as isolated defects or may be accompanied by other abnormalities, such as the Arnold-Chiari malformation discussed earlier. In some patients, intact skin covers the bony defect, and the region is marked by only a hirsute dimple or a sinus tract. This is called *spina bifida occulta*. Clinically, many of these cases are symptomatic. Involvement of the lower spinal cord is manifested by bladder dysfunction, weakness, and loss of sensation in the lower extremities. Infection (meningitis or meningomyelitis) is a major complication of these conditions.

SYRINGOMYELIA. Derived from the Greek word "syrinx" (a tube), this term refers to a slowly progressive disorder characterized by the development of tubular cavities in the spinal cord. These cavities may be secondary to other lesions, such as a tumor, trauma, infarction, or hemorrhage (secondary syringomyelia),[146] or may be primary, without known cause (idiopathic syringomyelia).

Most commonly, lesions are localized to the cervical region, although they may extend up into the medulla (syringobulbia) or down into the thoracic region. The neurologic deficits are dependent on the location of the cavities, and usually consist of segmental muscle weakness and atrophy accompanied by a *dissociated sensory loss*, i.e., loss of pain and temperature sensation, and preservation of touch sensation. Thoracic kyphoscoliosis also is usually present.

On gross examination, the spinal cord is enlarged and fluctuant over the cavities. Cut section reveals an asymmetric cavity frequently located transversely in the spinal cord, usually involving both gray and white matter. The cavity often crosses the ventral commissure, accounting for the dissociated sensory loss. Syringomyelic cavities may or may not be connected with the central canal. The main cavity is usually lined by a dense collar of glial tissue, whereas the portions involving the central canal are lined with ependyma. Bundles of peripheral nerve can be found in the walls of the cavities, probably owing to ingrowth of regenerating, previously damaged dorsal root nerves.[146] Although the pathogenesis of syringomyelia is unknown, it is considered by most workers to be a developmental anomaly.

HYDROMYELIA. This term denotes dilatation of the central canal by cerebrospinal fluid. The hydromyelic cavity is lined with ependyma. Hydromyelia may be seen alone or in association with spinal cord lesions, including tumors, meningomyelocele, and the Arnold-Chiari syndrome.

PHACOMATOSES

These conditions represent familial, slowly progressive neurocutaneous disorders that "bridge the borderland between neoplasia and malformations." They include *neurofibromatosis* (p. 138), *von Hippel-Lindau disease* (p. 139), *Sturge-Weber disease* (p. 541), and *tuberous sclerosis*. Only the last of these will be described here.

Tuberous Sclerosis (Epiloia, Bourneville's Disease)

Tuberous sclerosis is characterized clinically by a combination of *mental retardation, epileptic fits, and adenoma sebaceum of the skin*. Its pathogenesis is unknown, but it is frequently associated with visceral lesions, e.g., rhabdomyoma of the heart, angiomyolipoma of the kidney, or pancreatic cysts. It is a heredofamilial disorder, inherited as an autosomal dominant trait. It begins in infancy or childhood and may progress intermittently or only up to a given point of disability. The fully developed case is relatively rare, but probably there are many "formes frustes."

In the fully developed form, the cortical surface of the brain presents nodules of firm whitish tissue of pinhead to thumbnail size or even larger. Overgrowth and protrusion of subependymal glia produce an appearance of "candle dripping" on the surface of the ventricles. On microscopic examination, the nodules in the cortex are characterized by loss or distortion of the usual cytoarchitecture, with an excess of glia and many deformed, bizarre, often enlarged neurons. These nerve cells have no definable chromatin, and their processes are poorly developed. Frequently, they are multinucleated. Calcification within the nodules is often sufficiently intense to permit radiographic visualization.

THE PERIPHERAL NERVOUS SYSTEM

The peripheral nervous system (PNS) consists of the motor and sensory components of the cranial and spinal nerves, the autonomic nervous system with its sympathetic and parasympathetic divisions, and the peripheral ganglia. It is the conduit for sensory information to the CNS and effector signals to the peripheral organs such as muscle. Peripheral nerves are composed of groups of intermingling fascicles, each of which consists of a bundle of individual nerve fibers embedded in loose connective tissue containing collagen and fibroblasts *(endoneurium)*, the whole being surrounded by a multilayered membrane of flattened cells *(perineurium)*. The groups of fascicles are bound together by fibrous tissue *(epineurium)*. Nerve axons vary in diameter between 0.5 and 15μ, and if greater than 2μ have a myelin sheath that is produced by *Schwann cells*. The myelin is arranged in segments separated by *nodes of Ranvier*, and, unlike the multiple nodes produced by CNS oligodendroglia, each peripheral nerve myelin internode is produced by a single Schwann cell. Larger diameter axons generally have thicker myelin sheaths.

PATHOLOGIC REACTIONS

In contrast to the brain, which has no ability to regenerate, the pathologic reactions of the PNS include both *degeneration* and *regeneration*. There are three basic processes: *wallerian degeneration, axonal degeneration*, and *segmental demyelination*.

Wallerian degeneration follows peripheral transection of the axon. Proximal to the site of transection, there is degeneration back to the nearest node of Ranvier, and if the transection is sufficiently proximal, there will be chromatolysis (p. 1372) in the cell body of the transected axon. Distal to the transection, there is degeneration of the axon and its myelin sheath, both of which are digested by the Schwann cells that proliferate to accomplish this task (Fig. 29–44).

Regeneration occurs by the outgrowth of multiple sprouts from the distal end of the surviving segment of the axon. If there is no obstruction to their growth, the regenerating axons grow back down the nerve trunk in association with the Schwann cells that remain after digesting the degenerated axon. In optimal conditions, regeneration occurs clinically at a rate of about 1 mm per day. If, as is frequently the case, the cause of the wallerian degeneration is a traumatic injury to the nerve with disruption of its structure, the regenerating sprouts may be prevented from entering the distal part of the nerve by interposed hematoma or fibrous scar. In this circumstance, the obstructed regenerating axons form a tangled, often painful, mass of intertwined nerve fibers called an *amputation*, or *traumatic, neuroma*.

Axonal degeneration also occurs as a manifestation of neuronal dysfunction in which the neuron is unable to maintain its axon, which therefore starts to degenerate. This type of degeneration begins at the distal, or peripheral, end of the axon and proceeds back toward the cell body, a process called "dying back" (Fig. 29–44.)[147] There is often chromatolysis (p. 1372) of the cell body. Schwann cell proliferation occurs in the region of active axonal degeneration, although this is less pronounced than that seen in wallerian degeneration.

If the neuronal dysfunction can be halted or reversed, regeneration and some recovery of nerve function can occur.

Segmental demyelination is analogous to primary demyelination in the brain and is the selective loss of individual myelin internodes with preservation of the underlying axon (Fig. 29–44). Following an episode of demyelination, remyelination can be accomplished by the remaining Schwann cells. which proliferate. An important characteristic of this remyelination is that the reconstituted myelin sheaths are thinner than normal and have shorter internodal lengths. Both these features can be measured and are important in the diagnosis of the demyelinating peripheral neuropathies. Repeated episodes of demyelination and remyelination can occur, generating a concentric arrangement of alternating Schwann cell processes and collagen called "onion bulbs," which are found in the hypertrophic neuropathies (p. 1432) (Fig. 29–45).

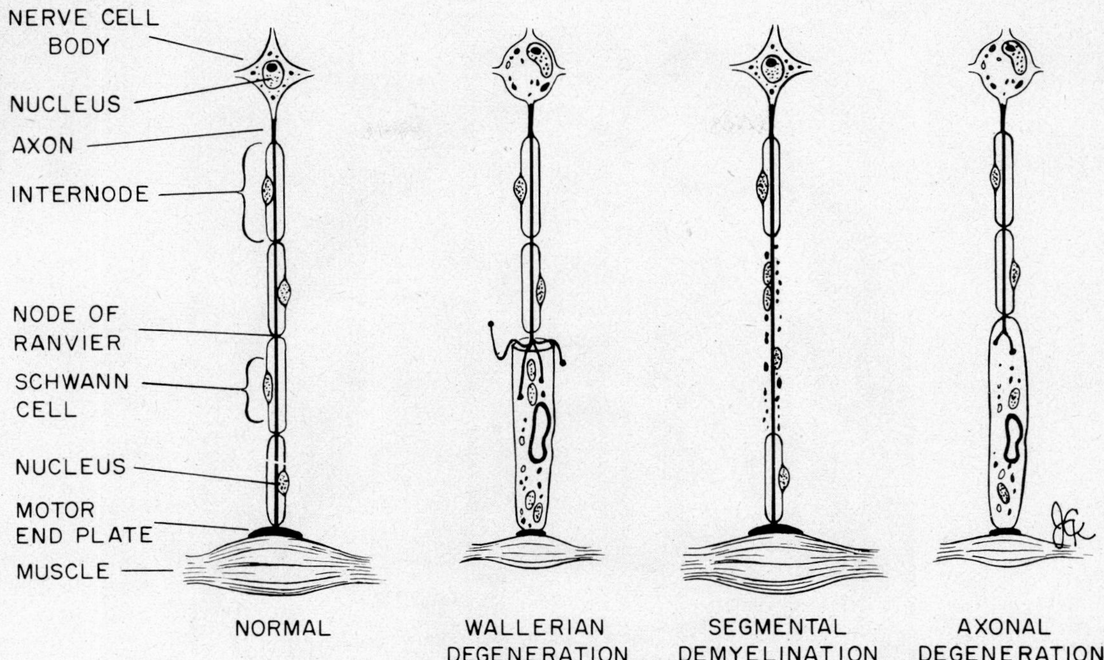

Figure 29–44. Pathologic reactions affecting peripheral nerve. (From Asbury, A. K., and Johnson, P. C.: Pathology of Peripheral Nerve. Philadelphia, W. B. Saunders Co., 1978, p. 51.)

PERIPHERAL NEUROPATHY

In conformity with the restricted range of pathologic changes, peripheral nerve disease has only a limited range of clinical expression, so that a wide range of etiologic agents cause somewhat similar syndromes. This has made the pathogenesis of the peripheral neuropathies difficult to unravel.

Both diffuse demyelination and axonal degeneration tend to affect the longest axons first and produce a syndrome called a *polyneuropathy*. Polyneuropathies are typically symmetric and present with distal signs and symptoms in the limbs, such as motor weakness and loss of deep tendon reflexes, peripheral paresthesias, and/or a "glove and stocking" sensory loss, or if the autonomic system is affected, findings such as postural hypotension, constipation, and impotence. When there is muscle weakness, axonal degeneration can be distinguished clinically from demyelination, because in axonal degeneration there is denervation, which produces muscle fasciculation and wasting. In demyelination, in which there is conduction failure but no denervation, these are not present. Clinically, different etiologic agents preferentially affect axons of different diameters, or sensory, motor, and autonomic axons, to different degrees. The balance of symptoms and signs reflect the axons principally involved. Neuropathies also may be mild or severe; may be acute, subacute, or chronic in time course; and may have relapses and remissions.

Although many etiologic agents produce generalized damage, there are also pathologic processes that are focal (e.g., vasculitis) and that affect only individual nerves, producing a *mononeuritis* or, if more than one nerve is affected, a *mononeuritis multiplex*. If sufficiently widespread, even pathologically focal processes present as a *polyneuropathy*, although often an asymmetric one.

Most clinical classifications of peripheral neuropathies are based on the type of clinical syndrome that develops. A simplified version of a widely used one is given in Table 29–6 with an indication in each clinical category of the predominant pathologic process encountered. Although there is a good general agreement between clinical expression and the type of pathologic process, the concordance is by no means complete. In diabetic neuropathy, for example, there is frequently acute and chronic demyelination, as well as the indicated axonal degeneration.

The classification in Table 29–6 offers an impressively wide choice of possible etiologies, but in most clinical series 30 to 70% of peripheral neuropathies remain undiagnosed in etiologic terms. Intensive evaluation of a series of such cases has shown that no less than 42% were probably hereditary, whereas 20% proved to be inflammatory/demyelinating.[148] However, despite the intensity of this evaluation, one-quarter remained undiagnosed. As can be seen from the number of entries in this by no means exhaustive classification, it would be impossible in this chapter to give even the briefest pathologic account of all the causes of peripheral neuropathy. The following text offers a few examples, selected to illustrate particular points, and has no pretensions to either balance or comprehensiveness.

ACUTE IDIOPATHIC POLYNEURITIS (LANDRY-GUILLAIN-BARRÉ SYNDROME)

This acute demyelinating neuropathy has been associated with a bewildering variety of antecedent events.

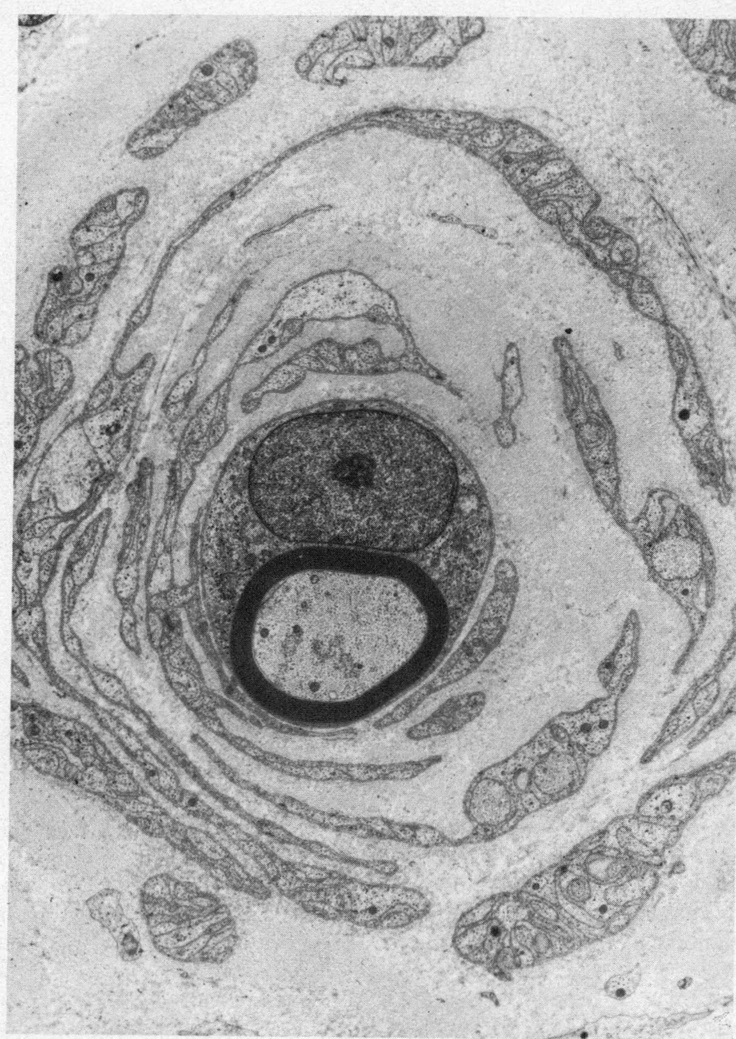

Figure 29–45. Electron micrograph showing onion-bulb formation (hypertrophic neuropathy). Myelinated fiber in center is surrounded by concentrically arranged Schwann cell cytoplasmic processes. Collagen is longitudinally oriented between these processes. (From Asbury, A. K., and Johnson, P. C.: Pathology of Peripheral Nerve. Philadelphia, W. B. Saunders Co., 1978, p. 142.)

About 40% of cases are associated with a "viral prodrome," and studies suggest that in this group cytomegalovirus is the offending agent in about 15%. The Epstein-Barr virus is implicated in 5% of the total number of cases; mycoplasma in about 5%; 10% have had other allergic phenomena; 25% have a wide variety of other associations, including surgery; and the residual 15% have no known antecedent event.[149] The disease presents as a rapidly progressive motor neuropathy with variable sensory features. In severe cases, the muscular weakness may be so profound and proceed so far proximally as to produce potentially fatal respiratory paralysis and facial diplegia. The CSF often, but not invariably, shows the classical "dissociation albuminocytologique," in which there is a strikingly raised protein with a normal or only slightly raised cell count.

Pathologically, there are focal inflammatory lesions scattered throughout the peripheral nerves, although there is some predilection for the proximal nerve trunks.[150] In the lesions, there is demyelination and an accumulation of lymphocytes and macrophages. With the electron microscope, the earliest change that can be seen is splitting of the myelin lamellae. Later, the myelin is apparently stripped off the axon and digested by macrophages, leaving the Schwann cells intact. This demyelination apparently occurs without the direct participation of the lymphocytes.

Although an immunologic component to this disease is widely accepted, its precise nature remains elusive. Lymphocytes accumulate within the nerve, but no B- or T-cell preference is evident and there is no evidence of cytotoxic T-cell activity directed against Schwann cells or myelin.[151] Passive transfer to experi-

Table 29–6. PRINCIPAL NEUROPATHIC SYNDROMES*

Acute Ascending Motor Paralysis with Variable Sensory Disturbance—*Acute demyelinating neuropathies*
- Acute idiopathic polyneuritis (Landry-Guillain-Barré syndrome)
- Infectious mononucleosis with polyneuritis
- Hepatitis and polyneuritis
- Diphtheritic polyneuropathy
- Toxic polyneuropathies, e.g., triorthocresyl phosphate

Subacute Sensorimotor Polyneuropathy
- (1) Symmetric—*Mostly axonal neuropathies*
  - Alcoholic polyneuropathy and beriberi
  - Arsenic polyneuropathy
  - Lead polyneuropathy
  - Vinca alkaloids and other intoxications
- (2) Asymmetric—*Axonal neuropathies with focal and/or diffuse pathology*
  - Diabetic neuropathy
  - Polyarteritis nodosa and other arteritides
  - Sarcoidosis

Chronic Sensorimotor Polyneuropathy
- (1) Acquired—*Axonal neuropathies with focal and/or diffuse pathology*
  - Carcinomatous
  - Paraproteinemias (demyelinating)
  - Uremia
  - Diabetes
  - Connective tissue diseases
  - Amyloidosis
  - Leprosy
- (2) Inherited—*Mostly chronic demyelination with hypertrophic changes*
  - Peroneal muscular atrophy (Charcot-Marie-Tooth disease)
  - Hypertrophic polyneuropathy (Dejerine-Sottas disease)
  - Refsum's disease

Chronic Relapsing Polyneuropathy—*Mixed pathology*
- Idiopathic polyneuritis
- Porphyria
- Beriberi and intoxications.

Mono or Multiple Neuropathy—*Focal axonal or demyelinating pathology*
- Pressure palsies
- Traumatic palsies
- Serum neuritis
- Zoster
- Tumor invasion with neuropathy
- Leprosy

*Adapted from Adams, R. D., and Asbury, A. K.: Diseases of the peripheral nervous system. *In* Petersdorf, R. G., et al. (eds.): Harrison's Principles of Internal Medicine. 10th ed. New York, McGraw-Hill Book Co., 1983, p. 2158.

mental animals with lymphocytes has not been achieved. However, the intraneural injection of sera from patients with Guillain-Barré polyneuritis (GBN) has produced perivenular demyelination.[152] The implication of a humorally mediated effect is reinforced by the finding of C3b and immunoglobulin (mostly IgG or IgM) in the nerves of many patients.[153] There are indications, however, that this may be a passive accumulation, a caveat reinforced by the persistent failure in GBN to find antibodies to the by now well-characterized myelin antigens.[154] Furthermore, plasmapheresis, which removes antibodies from the circulation, does not produce a consistent improvement in patients with GBN.[155] These findings make it difficult to envisage an active role for humoral immunity in a disease in which myelin is the principal target of the pathophysiologic process.

An important experimental model for GBN is experimental allergic neuritis (EAN), which is histologically very similar to GBN[156] but has many pathogenetic dissimilarities.

DIPHTHERITIC PERIPHERAL NEURITIS

The peripheral nerve effects of *Corynebacterium diphtheriae* are produced by the bacterial exotoxin, which causes an acute noninflammatory demyelination. The interesting aspect of this demyelination is its distribution, being almost entirely concentrated in the region of the dorsal root ganglia and the adjacent motor and sensory roots. In this region, there is a naturally occurring defect in the blood peripheral nerve barrier (analogous to the blood-brain barrier) that allows penetration of the toxin at this point but nowhere else in the peripheral nerve. Not surprisingly, the demyelination is confined to areas where the toxin can enter the nerve. Its mechanism of action is poorly understood, but in vitro experiments suggest that it might act in part by inhibiting the synthesis of myelin basic protein and proteolipid.

VINCA ALKALOID TOXICITY

This class of agents includes the chemotherapeutic drugs vinblastine and vincristine, which produce a dose-dependent axonal neuropathy. As antimitotic agents, they inhibit the aggregation of tubulin subunits into microtubules, and hence the formation of the mitotic spindle on which the chromosomes segregate. They have a similar effect on microtubules in axons, which can be seen to possess fewer microtubules than usual and to accumulate neurofilaments.[157, 158] Although these findings are consistent, it is not known how they relate to the axonal degeneration. It is hypothesized that these agents may act by disrupting axonal transport, but this is not proved.

The vinca alkaloids are only one of a large number of classes of neurotoxic agents in the environment. Some are therapeutic agents, but many others are encountered in industrial processes. Although our example produces axonal degeneration, others produce demyelination, and many have effects on both the CNS and PNS.

DIABETIC NEUROPATHY

Peripheral neuropathy frequently develops in diabetics and is often one of its most troublesome complications. One of its outstanding clinical features is its capricious occurrence, sometimes not being present even after 40 years of poorly controlled juvenile-onset diabetes, whereas in other cases it may even antedate measurable hyperglycemia. However, most cases occur late in the course of the disease. Clinically, it is a distal, symmetric, predominantly sensory polyneuropathy; pathologically, it is principally an axonopathy, but with features suggesting the presence of a demyelinating component.

Several possible pathophysiologic mechanisms have been considered and extensively investigated, including ischemic effects, and the metabolic disturbance that occurs in diabetes. Much attention, without conclusive result, has been lavished on the question whether strict diabetic control does or does not alter the likelihood of development of the neuropathy. Current metabolic research is focused on the role of the carbohydrates in the polyol pathway, particularly sorbitol, which increases in diabetes, and myoinositol, which is decreased.[159] In experimental animals, measures that prevent the drop in myoinositol, without altering the other disturbed metabolites such as glucose, sorbitol, and fructose, prevent the occurrence of nerve damage in these animals.[160] Further work is in progress to confirm and possibly extend these early findings.

AMYLOID NEUROPATHY

Amyloid deposition may affect peripheral nerve in three ways:[162] (1) vascular amyloid deposited in epineurial arterioles can produce a generalized ischemic neuropathy; (2) amyloid may be deposited as focal masses within the nerve fascicle, causing local distortion and compression of individual nerve fibers—this may lead to local demyelination and axonal degeneration; and (3) amyloid in ligamentous structures can cause external compression of nerve trunks at sites such as the carpal tunnel.

Many of the hereditary forms of amyloidosis have an associated peripheral neuropathy. In the acquired amyloidoses, primary amyloidosis (immunocyte-derived) more commonly causes neuropathy.

PERIPHERAL NEUROPATHY ASSOCIATED WITH MONOCLONAL GAMMOPATHY

A demyelinating peripheral neuropathy is occasionally seen in association with monoclonal gammopathies, both the benign[163] and the myeloma-associated varieties.[164] Recent work has gone some way toward clarifying the pathogenesis of at least some of these cases. The use of immunochemical techniques has shown the deposition of the monoclonal globulin in the affected nerve, where it usually appears to be associated with the myelin.[165] In one group of patients, all the involved IgM paraproteins were shown to be directed against myelin-associated glycoprotein.[166–168] So far, this has been shown to be the case only with some IgM paraproteins, although similar neuropathies with intraneural deposition of immunoglobulin also occur in patients with IgG and IgA monoclonal gammopathies.

LEPROSY

The neuropathy in leprosy is caused by the growth of the *Mycobacterium leprae* in and around the peripheral nerves.[162] The organisms grow and multiply within Schwann cells, thereby damaging the nerves. The form of neuropathy depends on the type of leprosy. In lepromatous leprosy, in which there is exuberant growth of the organism, the distribution of neuropathy is governed by the localization of the organism and is unique to this disease. Because the mycobacterium grows best in cooler temperatures, the cool parts of the body, notably the extremities, tip of the nose, and ears, are first and most profoundly affected, whereas the axillae and crural areas tend to be spared. Another effect of the temperature sensitivity of the organism is that the affected nerves are superficial and the neuropathy predominantly sensory. There is very little damage to the deeper-lying motor nerves. In tuberculoid leprosy, in which there are few organisms and a pronounced granulomatous reaction, the neuropathy is patchy, but again governed by the location of the reaction to the infection.

PERONEAL MUSCULAR ATROPHY (CHARCOT-MARIE-TOOTH DISEASE)

This is a dominantly inherited, slowly progressive sensorimotor neuropathy. Its major peripheral manifestations are wasting and weakness in the lower leg and foot, giving the characteristic "inverted champagne bottle limb." Pathologically, two forms of this disease are seen, one with thickened hypertrophic nerve and onion bulbs, and the other with a purely axonal neuropathy without the palpable nerves and hypertrophic changes of the more frequent type.[125]

Mention must also be made of two other types of hypertrophic neuropathy.[169] *Dejerine-Sottas disease* is a severe neuropathy occurring in young children.[170] *Refsum's disease* merits mention because of its association with raised levels of *phytanic acid*.

PERIPHERAL NERVE TUMORS

SCHWANNOMAS (NEURILEMMOMAS) AND NEUROFIBROMAS

Despite their usually distinct clinical presentations and histologic features, these tumors are derived from Schwann cells. Previous suggestions of their derivation from fibroblasts or perineurial cells have now been largely discounted by electron microscopic findings and the immunohistochemical demonstration of S-100 protein in these tumors.[171] Parenthetically, the presence of

S-100 protein in *granular cell tumors* (p. 1316)[172] is suggestive of a Schwann cell origin for these tumors also.

Grossly, both types of tumor have a white-to-gray color and a firm texture, but schwannomas are typically solitary, circumscribed, and encapsulated lesions, eccentrically located on proximal nerves or spinal nerve roots (Fig. 29–46). An interesting, although wholly unexplained, observation is that when found on spinal nerve roots they are almost invariably on the sensory root. By contrast, neurofibromas are more often multiple, are usually but not always unencapsulated, and appear as fusiform enlargements on distal nerves. Many are subcutaneous. Microscopically, schwannomas are distinguished by the presence of areas of high and low cellularity, called **Antoni A** and **B** tissue, respectively. In the Antoni A tissue there may be foci of palisaded nuclei called **Verocay bodies.** Blood vessels in schwannomas often have **hyaline thickening** around which there may be pseudopalisading of the tumor nuclei. Neurofibromas have none of these features and usually consist of a loose pattern of interlacing bands of delicate spindle cells with elongated, slender, and sometimes wavy nuclei. In the two types of tumor, there may be quite marked nuclear pleomorphism and irregularity, and occasionally even giant cells, but these are not necessarily ominous findings. Myxoid or xanthomatous degeneration may also be seen. An important point in the distinction between these two tumors is the distribution of nerve fibers in them as visualized by silver (Bodian) stains. In schwannomas, no nerve fibers are present in the body of the tumor, although the residual nerve of origin of the tumor may be seen compressed to one side. In neurofibromas, nerve fibers are found scattered throughout the tumor mass, as though it had arisen by expansion of the entire nerve fascicle. This distinction has practical significance, since the compression to one side of the nerve of origin in a schwannoma raises the possibility of its removal without requiring transection of the nerve, a course of action not possible in neurofibromas in which the entire nerve is involved in the tumor process.

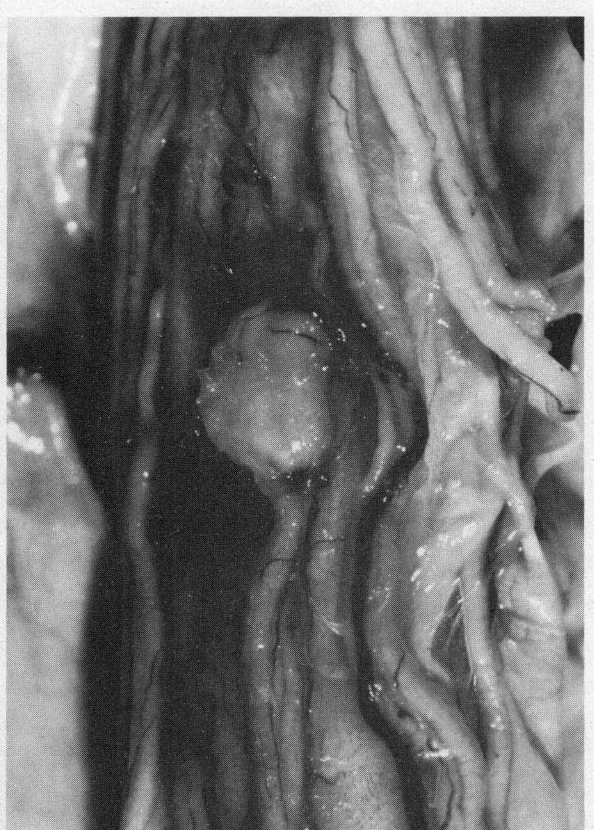

Figure 29–46. Schwannoma in cauda equina region.

Malignant transformation may occur in both types of tumor but is much less frequent in schwannomas.[173, 174] It is characterized by hypercellularity, pleomorphism, mitoses, and blood vessel proliferation, so that the tumor resembles a fibrosarcoma. Most cases of malignant neurofibroma are encountered in patients with von Recklinghausen's neurofibromatosis (p. 138).[175]

Except in von Recklinghausen's disease, these are usually tumors of adults, presenting most frequently in the fifth and sixth decades. The most serious symptoms are those produced by schwannomas on the spinal and cranial nerve roots. Acoustic schwannomas typically present with complaints of deafness and tinnitus associated, if the tumor is large enough, with pressure palsies of the adjacent fifth and seventh cranial nerves, or evidence of brain stem compression and hydrocephalus. Spinal root neurilemmomas may present as slowly progressive cord compression or a cauda equina syndrome. With more distal tumors on nerve trunks, there may be local complaints in the territory of the affected nerve, and finally, there are the ubiquitous subcutaneous "lumps and bumps," which, if of neural origin, usually prove to be neurofibromas.

EPILOGUE

It is evident at the conclusion of this broad overview of the diseases of the nervous system that in number and diversity they rival the wondrous complexities of the nervous system itself. It can be hoped that the capsule descriptions of the less common disorders, if nothing else, provide a glossary of terms and an appreciation of the range of problems that may confront the neurologist and neuropathologist.

1. Peters, A., et al.: The Fine Structure of the Nervous System: The Neurons and Supporting Cells. Philadelphia, W. B. Saunders Co., 1976.
2. Lazarides, E.: Intermediate filaments as mechanical integrators of cellular space. Nature *283*:249, 1980.
3. Wisniewski, H. M., et al.: Neurofibrillary tangles of paired helical filaments. J. Neurol. Sci. *27*:173, 1976.
4. Yagishita, S., et al.: Reappraisal of the fine structure of Alzheimer's neurofibrillary tangles. Acta Neuropathol. (Berl.) *54*:239, 1981.
5. Selkoe, D. J., et al.: Alzheimer's disease: Insolubility of partially purified paired helical filaments in sodium dodecyl sulfate and urea. Science *215*:1243, 1982.
6. Dahl, D., et al.: Immunostaining of neurofibrillary tangles in Alzheimer's senile dementia with a neurofilament antiserum. J. Neurosci. 2:113, 1982.

7. Gambetti, P., et al.: Alzheimer neurofibrillary tangles: An immunohistochemical study. *In* Amaducci, L., et al. (eds.): Aging of the Brain and Dementia. New York, Raven Press, 1980, pp. 55–64.
8. Corsellis, J. A. N., et al.: The aftermath of boxing. Psychol. Med. *3*:270, 1973.
9. Wisniewski, H. M., et al.: Neurofibrillary pathology. J. Neuropathol. Exp. Neurol. *29*:163, 1970.
10. Kolodney, E. H., and Cable, W. J. L.: Inborn errors of metabolism. Ann. Neurol. *11*:221, 1982.
11. Russell, D. S., and Rubinstein, L. J.: Pathology of Tumors of the Nervous System. 4th ed. Baltimore, Williams & Wilkins Co., 1977.
12. Robitaille, Y., et al.: A distinct form of adult polyglucosan body disease with massive involvement of central and peripheral neuronal processes and astrocytes. Brain *103*:315, 1980.
13. Oehneichen, M.: Enzyme-histochemical differentiation of neuroglia and microglia: A contribution to the cytogenesis of microglia and globoid cells. Pathol. Res. Pract. *168*:344, 1980.
14. Bignami, A., and Schoene, W. C.: Glial fibrillary acidic protein in human brain tumors. *In* DeLellis, R. A. (ed.): Diagnostic Immunohistochemistry. New York, Masson Publishing USA. *13*:213, 1981.
15. Velasco, M. E., et al.: Immunohistochemical localization of glial fibrillary acidic protein in human glial neoplasms. Cancer *45*:484, 1980.
16. Zipser, B., and McKay, R.: Monoclonal antibodies distinguish identifiable neurones in the leech. Nature *289*:549, 1981.
17. Fishman, R. A.: Brain edema. N. Engl. J. Med. *293*:706, 1975.
18. Brightman, M. W., et al.: The blood-brain barrier to proteins under normal and pathological conditions. J. Neurol. Sci. *10*:215, 1970.
19. Reese, T. S., and Karnovsky, M. S.: Fine structural localization of a blood-brain barrier to exogenous peroxidase. J. Cell Biol. *34*:207, 1967.
20. Brightman, M. W.: Morphology of blood-brain interface. *In* Bito, L. Z., et al. (eds.): The Ocular and Cerebrospinal Fluids. London, Academic Press, 1977, pp. 1–25.
21. Manz, H. J.: The pathology of cerebral edema. Hum. Pathol. *5*:291, 1974.
22. Katzmann, R., and Pappius, H. M.: Brain electrolytes and fluid metabolism. Baltimore, Williams & Wilkins Co., 1973.
23. Adams, R. S., and Victor, M.: Principles of Neurology. New York, McGraw-Hill Book Co., 1977.
24. Hooper, D. C., et al.: Central nervous system infection in the chronically immunosuppressed. Medicine *61*:166, 1982.
25. Ruskin, J., and Remington, J. S.: Toxoplasmosis in the compromised host. Ann. Intern. Med. *84*:193, 1976.
26. Fishman, R. A.: Cerebrospinal Fluid in Diseases of the Nervous System. Philadelphia, W. B. Saunders Co., 1980.
27. Feigin, R. D., et al.: Epidemic meningococcal disease in an elementary school classroom. N. Engl. J. Med. *307*:1255, 1982.
28. Carpenter, R. R., and Petersdorf, R. G.: The clinical spectrum of bacterial meningitis. Am. J. Med. *33*:262, 1962.
29. Case Records of the Massachusetts General Hospital (Case 2–1982): N. Engl. J. Med. *306*:91, 1982.
30. Delaney, P.: Neurologic manifestations in sarcoidosis: Review of the literature, with a report of 23 cases. Ann. Intern. Med. *87*:336, 1977.
31. Sabharwal, U. K., et al.: Granulomatous angiitis of the nervous system: Case report and review of the literature. Arthritis Rheum. *25*:342, 1982.
32. DeAngelis, L. M.: Intracranial tuberculoma: Case report and review of the literature. Neurology *31*:1133, 1982.
33. Harriman, D. G. F.: Bacterial infections of the central nervous system. *In* Blackwood, W., and Corsellis, J.A.N. (eds.): Greenfield's Neuropathology. 3rd ed. London, Arnold, Ltd., 1976, pp. 238–268.
34. Brewer, N. S., et al.: Brain abscess: A review of recent experience. Ann. Intern. Med. *82*:571, 1975.
35. Shaw, M. D. M., and Russell, J. A.: Cerebellar abscesses: A review of 47 cases. J. Neurol. Neurosurg. Psychiatry *38*:429, 1975.
36. Johnson, R. T.: Selective vulnerability of neural cells to viral infections. Brain *103*:447, 1980.
37. Sullivan-Bolyai, J. Z., et al.: Epidemiology of Reye's syndrome. Epidemiol. Rev. *3*:1, 1981.
38. Tomlinson, A. H., et al.: Immunofluorescence staining for the diagnosis of herpes encephalitis. J. Clin. Pathol. *27*:495, 1974.
39. Centers for Disease Control: Encephalitis surveillance. Annual Summary 1978, issued May, 1981.
40. Whitley, R. J., et al.: Herpes simplex encephalitis: Vidarabine therapy and diagnostic problems. N. Engl. J. Med. *304*:313, 1981.
41. Steel, J. G., et al.: Isolation of herpes simplex virus type I in recurrent (Mollaret) meningitis. Ann. Neurol. *11*:17, 1982.
42. Dupont, J. R., and Earle, K. M.: Human rabies encephalitis. A study of 49 fatal cases with a review of the literature. Neurology *15*:1023, 1965.
43. Sandhyamari, S., et al.: Pathology of rabies: A light and electron-microscopical study with particular reference to the changes with prolonged survival. Acta Neuropathol. (Berl.) *54*:247, 1981.
44. Horten, B., et al.: Multifocal varicella-zoster virus leukoencephalitis temporally remote from herpes zoster. Ann. Neurol. *9*:251, 1981.
45. Sigurdsson, B.: Observations on the slow infections of sheep. Br. Vet. J. *110*:255, 307, 341, 1954.
46. Manz, H. J.: Pathology and pathogenesis of viral infections of the central nervous system. Hum. Pathol. *8*:3, 1977.
47. Townsend, J. J., et al.: Neuropathology of progressive rubella panencephalitis after childhood rubella. Neurology *32*:185, 1982.
48. Oyanagi, S., et al.: Histopathology and electron microscopy of three cases of subacute sclerosing panencephalitis (SSPE). Acta Neuropathol. *18*:58, 1971.
49. Tourtellotte, W. W., et al.: Quantification of *de novo* central nervous system IgG measles antibody synthesis in SSPE. Ann. Neurol. *9*:551, 1981.
50. Hall, W. W., et al.: Measles and SSPE virus proteins: Lack of antibodies to the M protein in patients with subacute sclerosing panencephalitis. Proc. Natl. Acad. Sci. U.S.A. *76*:2047, 1979.
51. Choppin, P. W.: Measles virus and chronic neurological diseases. Ann. Neurol. *9*:17, 1981.
52. Aström, K. E., et al.: Progressive multifocal leukoencephalopathy: A hitherto unrecognised complication of chronic lymphatic leukaemia and Hodgkin's disease. Brain *81*:93, 1958.
53. Miller, J. R., et al.: Progressive multifocal leukoencephalopathy in a male homosexual with T-cell immune deficiency. N. Engl. J. Med. *307*:1436, 1982.
54. Walker, D. L.: Progressive multifocal leukoencephalopathy and opportunistic viral infection of the central nervous system. *In* Vinken, P. J., and Bruyn, G. W. (eds.): Handbook of Clinical Neurology. Vol. 34. Infection of the Nervous System, Part II. Amsterdam, North-Holland Publishing Co., 1978, pp. 307–329.
55. Podgett, B. L., and Walker, D. L.: Prevalence of antibodies in human sera against JC virus, and isolate from a case of progressive multifocal leukoencephalopathy. J. Infect. Dis. *127*:467, 1973.
56. Gajdusek, D. C.: Unconventional viruses and the origin and disappearance of kuru. Science *197*:943, 1977.
57. Gibbs, C. J., Jr., et al.: Creutzfeldt-Jakob disease (spongiform encephalopathy): Transmission to the chimpanzee. Science *161*:388, 1968.
58. Prusiner, S. B.: Novel proteinaceous particles cause scrapie. Science *216*:136, 1982.
59. Bolton, D. C., et al.: Identification of a protein that purifies with the scrapie prion. Science *218*:1309, 1982.
60. Masters, C. L., and Richardson, E. P., Jr.: Subacute spongiform encephalopathy (Creutzfeldt-Jakob disease). Brain *101*:333, 1978.
61. Chou, S. M., et al.: Transmission and scanning electron microscopy of spongiform change in Creutzfeldt-Jakob disease. Brain *103*:885, 1980.
62. Masters, C. L., et al.: Creutzfeldt-Jakob disease: Patterns of worldwide occurrence and the significance of familial and sporadic clustering. Ann. Neurol. *5*:177, 1979.
63. Duffy, P., et al.: Possible person-to-person transmission of Creutzfeldt-Jakob disease. N. Engl. J. Med. *291*:692, 1974.
64. Chernik, N. L., et al.: Central nervous system infections in patients with cancer. Cancer *40*:268, 1977.
65. Parker, J. C., et al.: The emergence of candidosis: The dominant postmortem cerebral mycosis. Am. J. Clin. Pathol. *70*:31, 1978.
66. Snow, R. M., and Dismukes, W. E.: Cryptococcal meningitis: Diagnostic value of cryptococcal antigen in cerebrospinal fluid. Arch. Intern. Med. *135*:1155, 1975.
67. Levy, R. I., and Moskowitz, J.: Cardiovascular research: Decades of progress, a decade of promise. Science *217*:121, 1982.
68. Garcia, J. H., and Conger, K. A.: Ischaemic brain injuries: Structural and biochemical effects. *In* Grenvile, A. K., and Safar, P. (eds.): Brain Failure and Resuscitation. London, Churchill Livingstone, 1981.
69. Plum, F.: What causes infarction in ischemic brain?: The Robert Wartenberg lecture. Neurology (N.Y.) *33*:222, 1983.
70. Meyers, R. E., et al.: Failure of marked hypoxia with maintained blood pressure to produce brain injury in cats. J. Neuropathol. Exp. Neurol. *39*:378, 1980.
71. Mohr, J. P.: The Harvard cooperative stroke registry: A prospective registry. Neurology *28*:754, 1978.
72. Sigsbee, B., et al.: Non-metastatic superior sagittal sinus thrombosis complicating systemic cancer. Neurology (N.Y.) *29*:139, 1979.
73. Fisher, C. M.: Lacunar strokes and infarcts: A review. Neurology (N.Y.) *32*:871, 1982.
74. Fisher, C. M.: The arterial lesions underlying lacunes. Acta Neuropathol. (Berl.) *12*:1, 1969.
75. Beal, M. F., et al.: Cholesterol embolism as a cause of transient ischemic attacks and cerebral infarction. Neurology (N.Y.) *31*:860, 1981.
76. Weir, B., et al.: Time course of vasospasm in man. J. Neurosurg. *48*:173, 1978.
77. Hughes, J. T., and Schianchi, P. M.: Cerebral artery spasm. A histological study at necropsy of the blood vessels in cases of subarachnoid hemorrhage. J. Neurosurg. *48*:515, 1978.
78. Osaka, K.: Cerebral vasospasm—re-evaluation of the factors which have been claimed to be the cause of vasospasm. Arch. Jap. Chir. *46*:380, 1977.
79. Strich, S. J.: Cerebral trauma. *In* Blackwood, W., and Corsellis, J. A. N. (eds.): Greenfield's Neuropathology. 3rd ed. London, Arnold, Ltd., 1976, pp. 327–360.

80. Dawson, S. L., et al.: The contrecoup phenomenon. Hum. Pathol. *11*:155, 1980.
81. Hume-Adams, J.: Diffuse brain damage of immediate impact type. Brain *100*:489, 1977.
82. Hume-Adams, J., et al.: Diffuse axonal injury due to non-missile head injury in humans: An analysis of 45 cases. Ann. Neurol. *12*:557, 1982.
83. Gennarelli, T. A., et al.: Diffuse axonal injury and traumatic coma in the primate. Ann. Neurol. *12*:564, 1982.
84. Rorke, L. B.: The cerebellar medulloblastoma and its relationship to primitive neuroectodermal tumors. J. Neuropathol. Exp. Neurol. *42*:1, 1983.
85. Rubinstein, L. J.: Tumors of the Central Nervous System. Atlas of Tumor Pathology. 2nd series. Washington, D.C., Armed Forces Institute of Pathology, 1972.
86. Slooff, J. L., et al.: Primary Intramedullary Tumors of the Spinal Cord and Filum Terminale. Philadelphia, W. B. Saunders Co., 1964.
87. Fokes, E. C., Jr., and Earle, K. M.: Ependymomas: Clinical and pathological aspects. J. Neurosurg. *30*:585, 1969.
88. Horten, B. C., and Rubinstein, L. J.: Primary cerebral neuroblastoma. A clinicopathological study of 35 cases. Brain *99*:735, 1976.
89. Taylor, C. R., et al.: An immunohistological study of immunoglobulin content of primary central nervous system lymphomas. Cancer *41*:2197, 1978.
90. Hoover, R., and Fraumeni, J. F.: Risk of cancer in renal-transplant recipients. Lancet *2*:55, 1973.
91. Cook, S. D., and Dowling, P. C.: Multiple sclerosis and viruses: An overview. Neurology (N.Y.) *30*:80, 1980.
92. Lisak, R. P.: Multiple sclerosis: Evidence for immunopathogenesis. Neurology (N.Y.) *30*:99, 1980.
93. Kurtzke, J. F.: Epidemiologic contributions to multiple sclerosis: An overview. Neurology (N.Y.) *30*:61, 1980.
94. Fischman, H. R.: Multiple sclerosis: A new perspective on epidemiologic patterns. Neurology (N.Y.) *32*:864, 1982.
95. Visscher, B. R., et al.: HLA types and immunity in multiple sclerosis. Neurology (N.Y.) *29*:1561, 1979.
96. Kurtzke, J. F., and Hyllested, K.: Multiple sclerosis in the Faroe Islands. 1. Clinical and epidemiological features. Ann. Neurol. *5*:6, 1979.
97. Krakowka, S. et al.: Antibody responses to measles virus and canine distemper virus in multiple sclerosis. Ann. Neurol. *14*:533, 1983.
98. Chou, C-H. J., et al.: Failure to detect antibodies to myelin basic protein or peptic fragments of myelin basic protein in CSF of patients with MS. Neurology (N.Y.) *33*:24, 1983.
99. Mehta, P. O., et al.: Oligoclonal IgG bands in plaques from multiple sclerosis brains. Neurology (N.Y.) *32*:372, 1982.
100. Hauser, S. L., et al.: Childhood multiple sclerosis: Clinical features and demonstration of changes in T cell subsets with disease activity. Ann. Neurol. *11*:463, 1982.
101. Traugott, U., et al.: Multiple sclerosis: distribution of T cell subsets within active chronic lesions. Science *219*:308, 1983.
102. Itoyama, Y., et al.: Immunocytochemical observations on the distribution of myelin-associated glycoprotein and myelin basic protein in multiple sclerosis lesions. Ann. Neurol. *7*:167, 1980.
103. Itoyama, Y., et al.: Distribution of papovavirus, myelin-associated glycoprotein, and myelin basic protein in progressive multifocal leucoencephalopathy lesions. Ann. Neurol. *11*:396, 1982.
104. Itoyama, Y., et al.: Immunocytochemical observations on demyelinating lesions in experimental allergic encephalomyelitis (EAE). Soc. Neurosci. (abstr.) *5*:512, 1979.
105. Hauser, S. L., et al.: Intensive immunosuppression in multiple sclerosis. N. Engl. J. Med. *308*:173, 1983.
106. Poskanzer, D. C.: The etiology of multiple sclerosis: Temporal-spatial clustering indicating two environmental exposures before onset. Neurology (N.Y.) *31*:708, 1981.
107. Oppenheimer, D. R.: Demyelinating diseases. *In* Blackwood, W., and Corsellis, J. A. N. (eds.): Greenfield's Neuropathology. 3rd ed. London, Arnold, Ltd., 1976, pp. 470–499.
108. Paterson, P. Y.: Experimental autoimmune (allergic) encephalomyelitis: Induction, pathogenesis and suppression. *In* Miescher, P. A., and Müller-Eberhard, H. J. (eds.): Textbook of Immunopathology. Vol. I, 2nd ed. New York, Grune & Stratton, 1976, pp. 179–213.
109. Behan, P. O., et al.: Delayed hypersensitivity to encephalitogenic protein in disseminated encephalomyelitis. Lancet *2*:1009, 1968.
110. Gonatas, N. K., et al.: The contribution of altered synapses in the senile plaque: An electron microscopic study in Alzheimer's dementia. J. Neuropathol. Exp. Neurol. *26*:25, 1967.
111. Goldman, J. E., and Suzuki, K.: Association of actin with Hirano bodies in human and brindled mouse CNS. J. Neuropathol. Exp. Neurol. (abstr.) *41*:359, 1982.
112. Marchbanks, R. M.: Biochemistry of Alzheimer dementia. J. Neurochem. *39*:9, 1982.
113. Whitehouse, P. J., et al.: Alzheimer's disease and senile dementia: Loss of neurones in the basal forebrain. Science *215*:1237, 1982.
114. Tomlinson, B. E., et al.: Observations on the brains of the demented old people. J. Neurol. Sci. *11*:205, 1970.
115. Terry, R. D.: Aging, senile dementia and Alzheimer's disease. *In* Katzman, R., et al. (eds.): Alzheimer's Disease: Senile Dementia and Related Disorders. New York, Raven Press, 1978, pp. 11–14.
116. Gambetti, P., et al.: Neurofibrillary changes in human brain. An immunocytochemical study with a neurofilament antiserum. J. Neuropathol. Exp. Neurol. *42*:69, 1983.
117. Gusella, J. F., et al.: A polymorphic DNA marker genetically linked to Huntington's disease. Nature *306*:234, 1983.
118. Dooling, E., et al.: Hallervorden-Spatz syndrome. Arch. Neurol. *30*:70, 1974.
119. Calne, D. B., et al.: Advances in the neuropharmacology of parkinsonism. Ann. Intern. Med. *90*:219, 1979.
120. Steele, J. C.: Progressive supranuclear palsy. Brain *95*:693, 1972.
121. Ghatak, N. R., et al.: Neurofibrillary pathology in progressive supranuclear palsy. Acta Neuropathol. (Berl.) *52*:73, 1980.
122. Stumpf, D. A.: Friedreich's ataxia and other hereditary ataxias. *In* Tyler, H. R., and Dawson, D. M. (eds.): Current Neurology. Vol. I. Boston, Houghton-Mifflin Medical Division, 1978, pp. 86–111.
123. Blass, J. P., et al.: Low activities of the pyruvate and oxoglutarate dehydrogenase complexes in five patients with Friedreich's ataxia. N. Engl. J. Med. *295*:62, 1976.
124. Brownell, B., et al.: The central nervous system in motor neurone disease. J. Neurol. Neurosurg. Psychiatry *33*:338, 1970.
125. Dyck, P. J., et al.: The nature of myelinated fiber degeneration in dominantly inherited hypertrophic neuropathy. Mayo Clin. Proc. *49*:34, 1974.
126. Price, R. A., and Jamieson, P. A.: The central nervous system in childhood leukemia. II. Subacute leukoencephalopathy. Cancer *35*:306, 1975.
127. Smith, T. W., et al.: Charcot-Marie-Tooth disease associated with hypertrophic neuropathy. J. Neuropathol. Exp. Neurol. *39*:420, 1980.
128. Rubinstein, L. J., et al.: Disseminated necrotizing leukoencephalopathy: A complication of treated central nervous system leukemia and lymphoma. Cancer *35*:291, 1975.
129. Breuer, A. C., et al.: Multifocal pontine lesions in cancer patients treated with chemotherapy and CNS radiotherapy. Cancer *41*:2112, 1978.
130. Burger, P. C., et al.: Encephalomyelopathy following high-dose B.C.N.U. therapy. Cancer *48*:1318, 1981.
131. Adams, R. D., et al.: Central pontine myelinolysis: A hitherto undescribed disease occurring in alcoholics and malnourished patients. Arch. Neurol. Psychiatry *81*:154, 1959.
132. Norenberg, M. D., et al.: Association between rise in serum sodium and central pontine myelinolysis. Ann. Neurol. *11*:128, 1982.
133. Sharpe, J. A., et al.: Methanol optic neuropathy: A histopathological study. Neurology *32*:1093, 1982.
134. McLean, D. R., et al.: Methanol poisoning: A clinical and pathological study. Ann. Neurol. *8*:161, 1980.
135. Gilbert, E. F., et al.: Leigh's necrotizing encephalopathy with pyruvate carboxylase deficiency. Arch. Pathol. Lab. Med. *107*:162, 1983.
136. Dulaney, J. T., and Moser, H. W.: Sulfatide lipidosis: Metachromatic leukodystrophy. *In* Stanbury, J. B., et al. (eds.): The Metabolic Basis of Inherited Disease. 4th ed. New York, McGraw-Hill Book Co., 1978, pp. 770–809.
137. Suzuki, K., and Suzuki, Y.: Galactosylceramide lipidosis: Globoid cell leukodystrophy (Krabbe's disease). *In* Stanbury, J. B., et al. (eds.): The Metabolic Basis of Inherited Disease. 4th ed. New York, McGraw-Hill Book Co., 1978, pp. 747–769.
138. Schaumberg, H. H., et al.: Adrenoleukodystrophy: A clinical and pathological study of 17 cases. Arch. Neurol. *32*:577, 1975.
139. Schaumburg, H. H., et al.: Adrenoleukodystrophy (sex-linked Schilder disease): Ultrastructural demonstration of specific cytoplasmic inclusions in the central nervous system. Arch. Neurol. *31*:210, 1974.
140. Schaumburg, H. H., et al.: Adrenomyeloneuropathy: A probable variant of adrenoleukodystrophy. II. General pathologic, neuropathologic and biochemical aspects. Neurology (Minneap.) *27*:1114, 1977.
141. O'Neill, B. P., et al.: The adrenoleukomyeloneuropathy complex: Expression in four generations. Neurology (N.Y.) *31*:151, 1981.
142. Singh, I., et al.: Adrenoleukodystrophy: Impaired oxidation of long-chain fatty acids in cultured skin fibroblasts and adrenal cortex. Biochem. Biophys. Res. Commun. *102*:1223, 1981.
143. Hicks, S. P.: Developmental malformations produced by radiation. A timetable of their development. Am. J. Roentgenol. *69*:279, 1953.
144. Urich, H.: Malformations of the nervous system, perinatal damage and related conditions in early life. *In* Blackwood, W., and Corsellis, J. A. N. (eds.): Greenfield's Neuropathology. 3rd ed. London, Arnold, Ltd., 1976, pp. 361–469.
145. Vogel, F. S., and McClenahan, J. L.: Anomalies of major cerebral arteries associated with congenital malformations of the brain with special reference to the pathogenesis of anencephaly. Am. J. Pathol. *28*:701, 1952.
146. Hughes, J. T.: Disease of the spine and spinal cord. *In* Blackwood, W., and Corsellis, J. A. N. (eds.): Greenfield's Neuropathology. 3rd ed. London, Arnold, Ltd., 1976, pp. 652–687.
147. Cavanagh, J. B.: The "dying back" process: A common denominator in

many naturally occurring and toxic neuropathies. Arch. Pathol. Lab. Med. *103*:659, 1979.
148. Dyck, P. J., et al.: Intensive evaluation of referred unclassified neuropathies yields improved diagnosis. Ann. Neurol. *10*:222, 1981.
149. Dowling, P. C., and Cook, S. D.: Role of infection in Guillain-Barré: Laboratory confirmation of herpes viruses in 41 cases. Ann. Neurol. *9*:(Suppl.) 44, 1981.
150. Prineas, J. W.: Pathology of the Guillain-Barré syndrome. Ann. Neurol. *9*:(Suppl.) 6, 1981.
151. Iqbal, A., et al.: Cell-mediated immunity in idiopathic polyneuritis. Ann. Neurol. *9*:(Suppl.) 65, 1981.
152. Feasby, T. E., et al.: Passive transfer studies in Guillain-Barré polyneuropathy. Neurology (N.Y.) *32*:1159, 1982.
153. Nyland, H., et al.: Immunological characterization of sural nerve biopsies from patients with Guillain-Barré syndrome. Ann. Neurol. *9*:(Suppl.) 80, 1981.
154. Whitaker, J. N.: The protein antigens of peripheral nerve myelin. Ann. Neurol. *9*(Suppl.) 56, 1981.
155. Dyck, P. J.: The causes, classification and treatment of peripheral neuropathy. N. Engl. J. Med. *307*:283, 1982.
156. Saida, T., et al.: Experimental allergic neuritis induced by galactocerebroside. Ann. Neurol. *9*(Suppl.): 87, 1981.
157. Bradley, W. G., et al.: The neuropathy of vincristine in man. Clinical electrophysiological and pathological studies. J. Neurol. Sci. *10*:107, 1970.
158. Shelanski, M. L., and Wisniewski, H. M.: Neurofibrillary degeneration induced by vincristine therapy. Arch. Neurol. *20*:199, 1969.
159. Simmons, D. A., et al.: Significance of tissue myoinositol concentrations in metabolic regulation in nerve. Science *217*:848, 1982.
160. Greene, D. A., et al.: Effects of insulin and dietary myoinositol on impaired peripheral motor nerve conduction in acute streptozotocin diabetes. J. Clin. Invest. *55*:1326, 1975.
161. Judzewitsch, R. G., et al.: Aldose reductase improves nerve condition velocity in diabetic patients. N. Engl. J. Med. *308*:119, 1983.
162. Asbury, A. K., and Johnson, P. C.: Pathology of Peripheral Nerve. Philadelphia, W. B. Saunders Co., 1978.
163. Read, D. J., et al.: Peripheral neuropathy and benign IgG paraproteinaemia. J. Neurol. Neurosurg. Psychiatry *41*:215, 1978.
164. Kelly, J. J., et al.: The spectrum of peripheral neuropathy in myeloma. Neurology (N.Y.) *31*:24, 1981.
165. Bosch, E. P., et al.: Peripheral neuropathy associated with monoclonal gammopathy. Studies of intraneural injections of monoclonal immunoglobulin sera. J. Neuropathol. Exp. Neurol. *41*:446, 1982.
166. Latov, N., et al.: Plasma cell dyscrasia and peripheral neuropathy: Identification of the myelin antigens that react with human paraproteins. Proc. Natl. Acad. Sci. U.S.A., *75*:7131, 1981.
167. Braun, P. E., et al.: MAG is the antigen for a monoclonal IgM in polyneuropathy. Trans. Am. Soc. Neurochem. *13*:230, 1982.
168. Steck, A. J., et al.: Demyelinating neuropathy and monoclonal IgM antibody to myelin-associated glycoprotein. Neurology (N.Y.) *33*:19, 1983.
169. Thomas, P. K., and Lascelles, R. G.: Hypertrophic neuropathy. Q. J. Med. *36*:223, 1967.
170. Dyck, P. J., et al.: Severe hypomyelination and marked abnormality of conduction in Dejerine-Sottas hypertrophic neuropathy: Myelin thickness and compound action potential of sural nerve in vitro. Mayo Clin. Proc. *46*:432, 1971.
171. Stefansson, K., et al.: S-100 protein in soft tissue tumors derived from Schwann cells and melanocytes. Am. J. Pathol. *106*:261, 1982.
172. Stefansson, K., and Wollmann, R. L.: S-100 protein in granular cell tumors. Cancer *49*:1834, 1982.
173. Trojanowski, J. Q., et al.: Malignant tumors of nerve sheath origin. Cancer *46*:1202, 1980.
174. Storm, F. K., et al.: Neurofibrosarcoma. Cancer *45*:126, 1980.
175. Riccardi, V. M.: von Recklinghausen's neurofibromatosis. N. Engl. J. Med. *305*:1617, 1981.

INDEX

Page numbers in *italics* denote figures; page numbers followed by *t* indicate tables.